Heart Disease

A TEXTBOOK OF CARDIOVASCULAR MEDICINE

Edited by

EUGENE BRAUNWALD,
M.D., M.D. (hon), Sc.D. (hon), F.R.C.P.

Vice President for Academic Programs, Partners HealthCare System
Distinguished Hersey Professor of Medicine
Faculty Dean for Academic Programs at Brigham and Women's Hospital and
    Massachusetts General Hospital
Harvard Medical School
Boston, Massachusetts

DOUGLAS P. ZIPES, M.D.

Distinguished Professor of Medicine, Pharmacology, and Toxicology
Director, Krannert Institute of Cardiology
Director, Division of Cardiology
Indiana University School of Medicine

Attending Physician
University Hospital, Wishard Memorial Hospital, and Roudebush Veterans
    Affairs Hospital
Indianapolis, Indiana

PETER LIBBY, M.D.

Mallinckrodt Professor of Medicine
Harvard Medical School
Chief, Cardiovascular Medicine
Brigham and Women's Hospital
Boston, Massachusetts

Heart Disease

6TH EDITION

A TEXTBOOK OF CARDIOVASCULAR MEDICINE

Volume 2

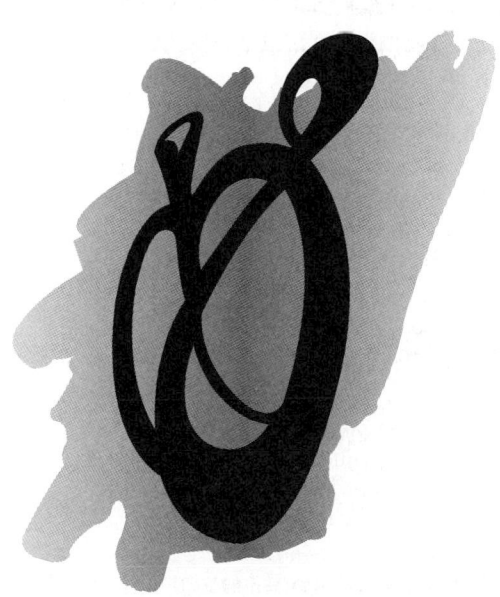

W.B. SAUNDERS COMPANY
A Harcourt Health Sciences Company
Philadelphia   London   New York   St. Louis   Sydney   Toronto

W.B. SAUNDERS COMPANY
A Harcourt Health Sciences Company

The Curtis Center
Independence Square West
Philadelphia, Pennsylvania 19106

Library of Congress Cataloging-in-Publication Data

Heart disease: a textbook of cardiovascular medicine/[edited by] Eugene
Braunwald, Douglas P. Zipes, Peter Libby.—6th ed.

p.   cm.

Includes bibliographical references and index.

ISBN 0–7216–8561–7
1. Heart—Diseases.   2. Cardiovascular system—Diseases.   I. Braunwald,
  Eugene.   II. Zipes, Douglas P.   III. Libby, Peter.   [DNLM: 1. Heart
  Diseases.   2. Cardiovascular Diseases.   WG 210 H43445 2001]

RC681. H36 2001   616.1′2—dc21   00–025391

Editor-in-Chief: Richard Zorab
Developmental Editor: Lynne Gery
Manuscript Editors: Sue Reilly, Anne Ostroff
Production Manager: Frank Polizzano
Illustration Specialist: Rita Martello
Book Designer: Karen O'Keefe Owens

Heart Disease: A Textbook of Cardiovascular Medicine   0–7216–8549–8 (Single Volume)
                                                            0–7216–8561–7 (2-Volume Set)
                                                            0–7216–8562–5 (Volume 1)
                                                            0–7216–8563–3 (Volume 2)
                                                            0–8089–2258–0 (International Edition)

Printed in the United States of America.

Last digit is the print number: 9   8   7   6   5   4   3   2   1

Contents

v

▼ PART III

NORMAL AND ABNORMAL CARDIAC FUNCTION

▼ PART IV

HYPERTENSIVE AND ATHEROSCLEROTIC CARDIOVASCULAR DISEASE

▼ PART V

DISEASES OF THE HEART, PERICARDIUM, AND PULMONARY VASCULAR BED

HYPERTENSIVE AND ATHEROSCLEROTIC CARDIOVASCULAR DISEASE

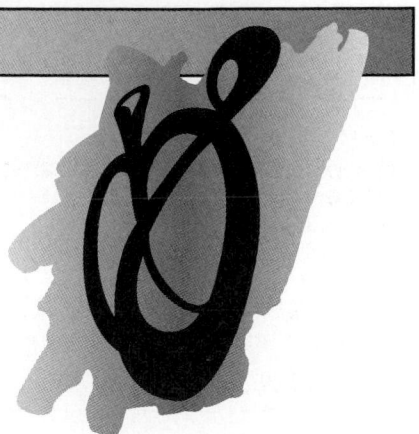

Chapter 34

Coronary Blood Flow and Myocardial Ischemia

PETER GANZ • WILLIAM GANZ

HYPOXIA AND ISCHEMIA

Ischemia is characterized by an imbalance between myocardial oxygen supply and demand (Fig. 34–1). In some situations this imbalance is caused by a reduction of blood flow and oxygen supply secondary to increased coronary vascular tone, intracoronary platelet aggregation, or thrombus formation (see Fig. 36–1); This condition, termed *supply ischemia* or *low-flow ischemia,* is responsible for myocardial infarction and most episodes of unstable angina. In other instances, usually in the presence of chronic coronary obstruction, exercise, tachycardia, or emotion leads to an increase in coronary blood flow that is insufficient to meet the rise in myocardial oxygen demand. This condition is termed *demand ischemia* or *high-flow ischemia.* It is responsible for many episodes of chronic stable angina. Typically, myocardial ischemia results from both an increase in oxygen demand and a reduction in myocardial oxygen supply. For example, although exercise leads to an overall increase in coronary blood flow, most of the additional flow is distributed toward the subepicardium, whereas subendocardial blood flow may even drop below its resting level. The ischemia of the subendocardium is then caused by both an increase in myocardial oxygen demand and a reduction in regional blood flow. *Hypoxia* is the condition in which oxygen supply is reduced despite adequate perfusion. It may be present in asphyxiation, carbon monoxide poisoning, cyanotic congenital heart disease, and cor pulmonale.

Low-flow ischemia, in contrast to *high-flow ischemia or hypoxia,* is characterized not only by oxygen deprivation but also by inadequate removal of metabolites consequent to reduced perfusion and by loss of vascular turgor.[1] Coronary flow and coronary perfusion pressure augment left ventricular systolic performance (Gregg effect) and reduce left ventricular diastolic distensibility (Salisbury effect). Buildup of tissue metabolites, especially inorganic phosphate, reduces calcium sensitivity of myofilaments, thereby diminishing contractility. Accordingly, in patients with low-flow ischemia, left ventricular systolic performance is lower and left ventricular diastolic distensibility greater than when the same patients were exposed to high-flow ischemia or hypoxia[1] (Fig. 34–2). Myocardial ischemia may be manifest as anginal discomfort, breathlessness, deviation of the ST segment on the electrocardiogram, reduced uptake of a tracer substance in myocardial perfusion images, or regional or global impairment of ventricular function.

In this chapter, we consider first the determinants of myocardial oxygen consumption, then the control of coronary blood flow, and, finally, the hemodynamic consequences of ischemia.

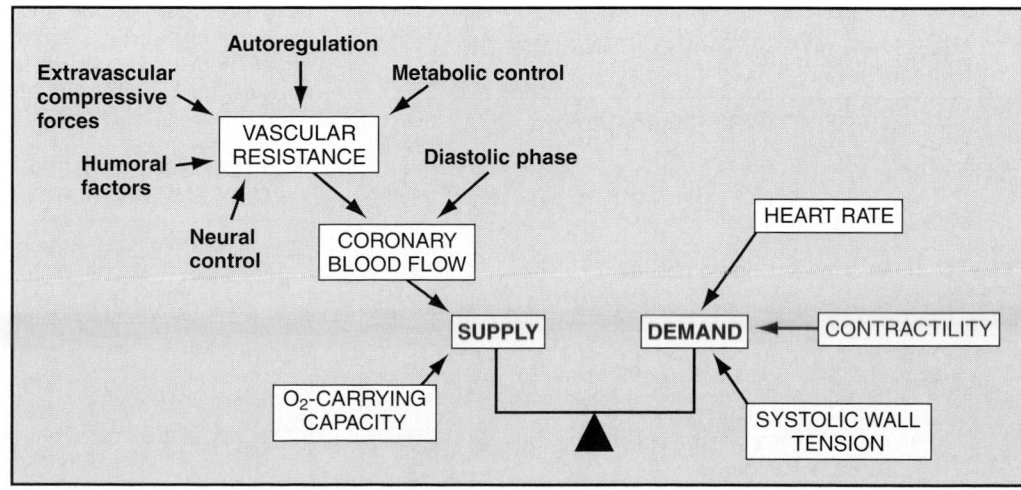

FIGURE 34–1. Factors influencing myocardial oxygen supply and demand. (From Ardehali A, Ports TA: Myocardial oxygen supply and demand. Chest 98: 699, 1990.)

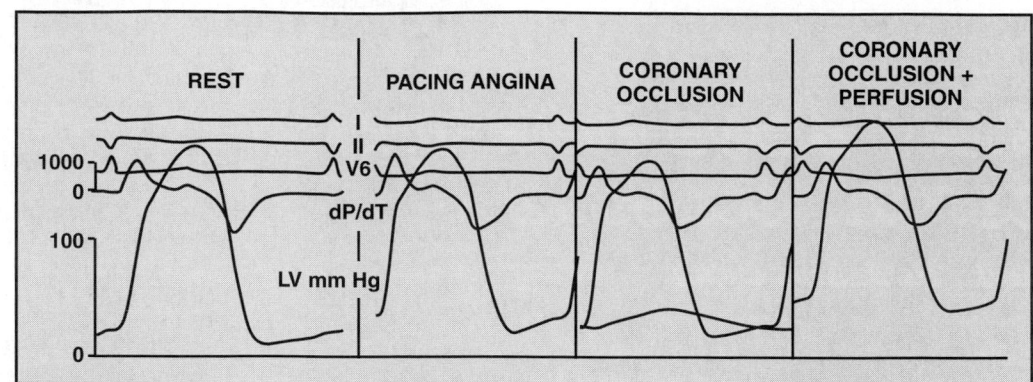

FIGURE 34–2. Differences among the left ventricular hemodynamic responses during low-flow versus high-flow ischemia. Tracings from a patient undergoing cardiac catheterization and balloon coronary angioplasty of two surface leads (I and II) and one precordial lead (V_5) of the electrocardiogram; the left ventricular dP/dt signal; and the left ventricular pressure recording at rest, at cessation of pacing during pacing-induced angina, at the end of a regular angioplasty balloon coronary occlusion, and at the end of an equally long angioplasty balloon coronary occlusion with distal hypoxic perfusion. Left ventricular diastolic pressure was higher (and left ventricular compliance lower) during pacing angina and at the end of balloon coronary occlusion with distal perfusion of hypoxic fluid (examples of high-flow ischemia) than at the end of the regular balloon coronary occlusion (example of low-flow ischemia). (From De Bruyne B, Bronzwaer JG, Heyndrickx GR, Paulus WJ: Comparative effects of ischemia and hypoxemia on left ventricular systolic and diastolic function in humans. Circulation 88:461, 1993. Copyright 1993, American Heart Association.)

DETERMINANTS OF MYOCARDIAL OXYGEN CONSUMPTION

The heart is an aerobic organ; it relies almost exclusively on the oxidation of substrates for the generation of energy, and it can develop only a small oxygen debt. Therefore, in a steady state, myocardial oxygen consumption (MVO_2) provides an accurate measure of its total metabolism.[2] The total metabolism of the arrested, quiescent heart is only a small fraction of that of the working organ. The MVO_2 of the beating canine heart ranges from 8 to 15 ml/min/100 gm, whereas the MVO_2 of the noncontracting heart is approximately 1.5 ml/min/100 gm. The latter is required for those physiological processes not directly associated with contraction. Increases in the frequency of depolarization of the noncontracting heart are accompanied by only small increases of MVO_2[2-4] (Tables 34–1 and 34–2).

MYOCARDIAL TENSION. As early as 1916 Evans and Matsuoka concluded from studies of the Starling heart-lung preparation that "there is a relation between the tension set up on contraction and the metabolism of the contractile tissue."[5] In a systematic investigation of the relative effects of ventricular pressure, stroke volume, and heart rate on MVO_2, it was found that ventricular pressure development is a key determinant of MVO_2. These investigations suggested that MVO_2 per beat correlates well with the area

under the left ventricular pressure curve, termed the *tension-time index*.[5a] Subsequently, it was emphasized that the myocardial wall tension time integral is a more accurate determinant of MVO_2 than is the developed pressure.[6, 7] Later studies demonstrated that frequency of contraction is an important determinant as well. An augmentation of heart rate elevates MVO_2 by increasing the frequency of tension development per unit of time, as well as by increasing contractility.[6, 8]

Rooke and Feigl have provided evidence that MVO_2 is influenced by the degree of myocardial shortening during ejection of stroke volume, although less so than by tension development.[9] They also provided an experimental basis for the use of the systolic pressure-rate product as an estimate of MVO_2 in the clinical setting. This index, frequently referred to as "double product," is used widely to estimate changes in MVO_2 during stimuli such as exercise or pacing tachycardia, although with only limited accuracy.[10] Reexamination of the determinants of MVO_2 has emphasized that they correlate closely with the left ventricular systolic pressure volume area,[11, 12] which consists of the sum of the area within the systolic pressure-volume loop, that is, the external mechanical work and the end-systolic elastic potential energy in the ventricular wall, the area enclosed by the systolic pressure-volume trajectory, and the E_{max} line[12, 13] (Fig. 34–3).

MYOCARDIAL CONTRACTILITY. In addition to the systolic pressure-volume area and heart rate, myocardial contractility is the third major determinant of MVO_2.[13a] The net effect of positive inotropic stimuli (e.g., Ca^{2+} and catecholamines) on MVO_2 is the end result of their influence on two

▼ **TABLE 34–1.** MYOCARDIAL O_2 CONSUMPTION COMPONENTS

TOTAL: 6–8 ml/min/100 gm			
Distribution			
Basal	20%	Volume work	15%
Electrical	1%	Pressure work	64%
Effects on MVO_2 of 50% Increases In			
Wall stress	25%	Heart rate	50%
Contractility	45%	Volume work	4%
Pressure work	50%		

The table demonstrates the dominant contribution to myocardial O_2 consumption (MVO_2) made by pressure work and prominent effects of increasing pressure work and heart rate on MVO_2.

From Gould KL: Coronary Artery Stenosis, New York, Elsevier, 1991, p 8.

▼ **TABLE 34–2.** DETERMINANTS OF MYOCARDIAL OXYGEN CONSUMPTION

Tension development
Contractile state
Heart rate
Shortening against a load (Fenn effect)
Maintenance of cell viability in basal state
Depolarization
Activation
Maintenance of active state
Direct metabolic effect of catecholamines
Fatty acid uptake

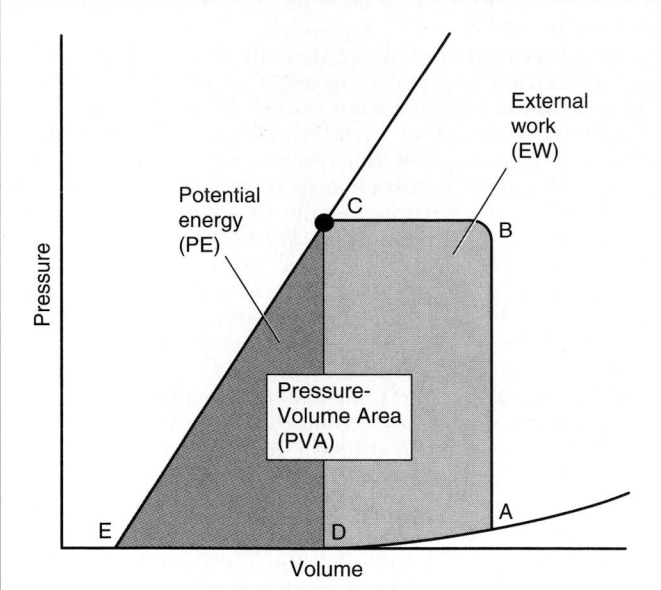

FIGURE 34-3. Myocardial oxygen consumption correlates with the left ventricular pressure-volume area (PVA). PVA is the area in the P-V diagram that is circumscribed by the end-systolic P-V line (E-C), the end-diastolic P-V relation curve (D-A), and the systolic segment of P-V trajectory (E-A-B-C-E). PVA consists of the external work (EW) performed during systole and the end-systolic elastic potential energy (PE) stored in the ventricular wall at end systole. EW is the area within the P-V loop trajectory (A-B-C-D-A), and PE is the area between end-systolic P-V line and end-diastolic P-V relation curve to the left of EW (E-C-D-E). (From Kameyama T, et al: Energy conversion efficiency in human left ventricle. Circulation 85:988, 1992. Copyright 1992, American Heart Association.)

major determinants that change in opposite direction in the intact heart.[2] These are wall tension, which declines as a consequence of reduction in heart size, and myocardial contractility, which, by definition, is augmented by inotropic stimuli. In the failing, dilated ventricle, the increased contractility reduces the left ventricular pressure and volume. On the basis of the Laplace relation, the reduction in ventricular volume leads to a reduction in myocardial tension, which reduces MVO_2. However, the decrease in MVO_2 that might be expected to result from falling ventricular wall tension is opposed by the increase in contractility, which tends to augment MVO_2. Thus, the change in MVO_2 consequent to an inotropic stimulus depends on the extent to which intramyocardial tension is reduced in relation to the extent to which contractility is augmented. In the absence of heart failure, drugs that stimulate myocardial contractility elevate MVO_2 because heart size and therefore wall tension are not reduced substantially and do not offset the effect on metabolism of the stimulation of contractility.

It has been suggested by Suga that almost the entire increase in MVO_2 produced by the administration of positive inotropic agents such as Ca^{2+} and epinephrine results from the energy costs of enhanced excitation-contraction coupling.[11] Specifically, the increased energy costs result from the greater and more rapid Ca^{2+} uptake by the sarcoplasmic reticulum (see Chap. 14) as well as from the increased contractile activity, rather than from a direct stimulating effect of positive inotropic agents on basal myocardial metabolism. In experiments in which the relative effects of changes in tension development and in myocardial contractility on MVO_2 were assessed in the same heart, the quantitative effects of changes of MVO_2 in contractility and tension development were found to be both substantial and of the same order of magnitude.[14]

MVO_2 is also influenced by the substrate used. Specifically, it correlates directly with the fraction of energy derived from the metabolism of fatty acids, which varies directly with the arterial concentration of fatty acids and inversely with that of glucose and insulin.[15]

During diastole, when the aortic valve is closed, aortic diastolic pressure is transmitted without impediment through the dilated sinuses of Valsalva to the coronary ostia. The aortic arch and sinuses then act as a miniature reservoir, facilitating maintenance of relatively uniform coronary inflow through diastole. The major coronary arteries and their principal branches that course across the epicardial surface of the heart serve as conductance (or conduit) vessels. Normal epicardial coronary arteries in humans are typically 0.3 to 5 mm in caliber and do not offer appreciable resistance to blood flow. Even at the highest level of blood flow, there is no detectable pressure drop along the length of human epicardial arteries.[16] Conductance arteries give rise to arterioles, which are resistance vessels 10 to 200 μm in diameter across which a larger pressure drop occurs. The dense network of about 4000 capillaries per square millimeter ensures that each myocyte is adjacent to a capillary. Capillaries are not uniformly patent because precapillary sphincters appear to serve a regulatory function in accordance with the flow needs of the myocardium. This capillary density is reduced in the presence of ventricular hypertrophy.

As in any vascular bed, blood flow in the coronary bed depends on the driving pressure and the resistance offered by this bed. Coronary vascular resistance, in turn, is regulated by several control mechanisms that will be reviewed: myocardial metabolism (metabolic control), endothelial (and other humoral) control, autoregulation, myogenic control, extravascular compressive forces, and neural control. These control mechanisms may be impaired in diseases and thereby contribute to the development of myocardial ischemia.

HETEROGENEITY IN THE CORONARY RESISTANCE VESSELS. Experimental methods to visualize coronary resistance vessels in the beating hearts of animals have become available,[17] and it has been learned that arterioles are specialized according to their size. For example, metabolic vasodilation occurs predominantly in the smallest arterioles less than 30 μm; intermediate arterioles 30 to 60 μm are the principal site of myogenic regulation, whereas the large arterioles 100 to 150 μm appear to be the sites of flow-mediated dilation.[17, 18] The system of multiple valves permits fine control of the coronary circulation. For example, according to a scheme proposed by Chilian,[17] the smallest arterioles dilate during metabolic stress, resulting in reduced microvascular resistance and increased myocardial perfusion. As the upstream arteriolar pressure decreases owing to a fall in distending pressure, myogenic dilation of slightly larger arterioles upstream occurs and causes an additional decrease in resistance. Increased flow in the largest arterioles augments shear stress and triggers flow-mediated dilation, further reducing the resistance of this network. Thus, coronary arterioles appear to have specialized regulatory elements along their length that operate "in series" in an integrated manner.

Metabolic Regulation

RELATIONSHIP BETWEEN CORONARY BLOOD FLOW AND MYOCARDIAL OXYGEN CONSUMPTION. Coronary blood flow is closely coupled to MVO_2 in normal hearts.[7] This linkage is necessary because (1) the myocardium depends almost entirely on aerobic metabolism; (2) the oxygen saturation of coronary venous blood is low (25 to 30 percent at rest), permitting little additional oxygen extraction; and (3) oxygen stores in the heart are meager.

Changes in myocardial oxygen requirement lead to alterations in coronary vascular resistance with great rapidity, generally in less than 1 second. For example, occlusion of a coronary artery for less than 1 second produces an increase in coronary blood flow above baseline after release of the occlusion.[19] This response is called *reactive hyperemia*. The mechanisms that link increases in metabolic activity to reductions in coronary vascular resistance have been investigated extensively, but uncertainty still remains regarding the role of various mediators released from the myocytes and the endothelium.

ADENOSINE. Adenosine has been investigated most extensively.[20] Adenosine is formed by degradation of adenine nucleotides under conditions in which ATP utilization exceeds the capacity of myocardial cells to resynthesize high-energy phosphate compounds (a process dependent on oxidative phosphorylation in mitochondria). This results in the production of adenosine monophosphate (AMP), and the enzyme 5'-nucleotidase is responsible for the formation of adenosine from AMP[21] (Fig. 34–4). Accordingly, adenosine diffuses from myocytes into the interstitial fluid and the coronary venous effluent.[22, 23] Adenosine is a powerful coronary dilator and is considered to be an important, perhaps the critical, mediator of local metabolic regulation.[22, 23] Its production increases at times of an imbalance in the supply-to-demand ratio for oxygen,[20] and the rise in the interstitial concentration of adenosine parallels the increase in coronary blood flow.[24]

Many investigators believe that adenosine fulfills most of the criteria of a metabolic regulator of blood flow.[20] However, inhibition of adenosine, either by its destruction by adenosine deaminase or by administration of adenosine receptor antagonists, does not always reduce the magnitude of the hyperemia in response to metabolic stimuli in animals[25] or humans.[24] Thus, despite its acknowledged importance, adenosine is almost certainly not the *only* vasoactive factor involved in the metabolic regulation of coronary blood flow. Others may include nitric oxide (NO), vasodilator prostaglandins, adenosine triphosphate (ATP)–sensitive K^+ channels (K^+_{ATP} channels; see later), as well as myocardial oxygen and carbon dioxide tensions.[26]

NITRIC OXIDE (NO). This substance increases blood flow during metabolic stimuli. Inhibition of NO reduces the magnitude of metabolic dilation in animals[22, 23, 27] and in the peripheral[28] and coronary circulation in humans.[29] NO production is augmented in response to metabolic stimuli by at least two mechanisms. Hypoxia is a stimulus to release of NO from the endothelium.[30] Furthermore, NO is a principal mediator of flow-mediated dilation. Although hypoxia may initiate hyperemia, flow-mediated dilation sus-

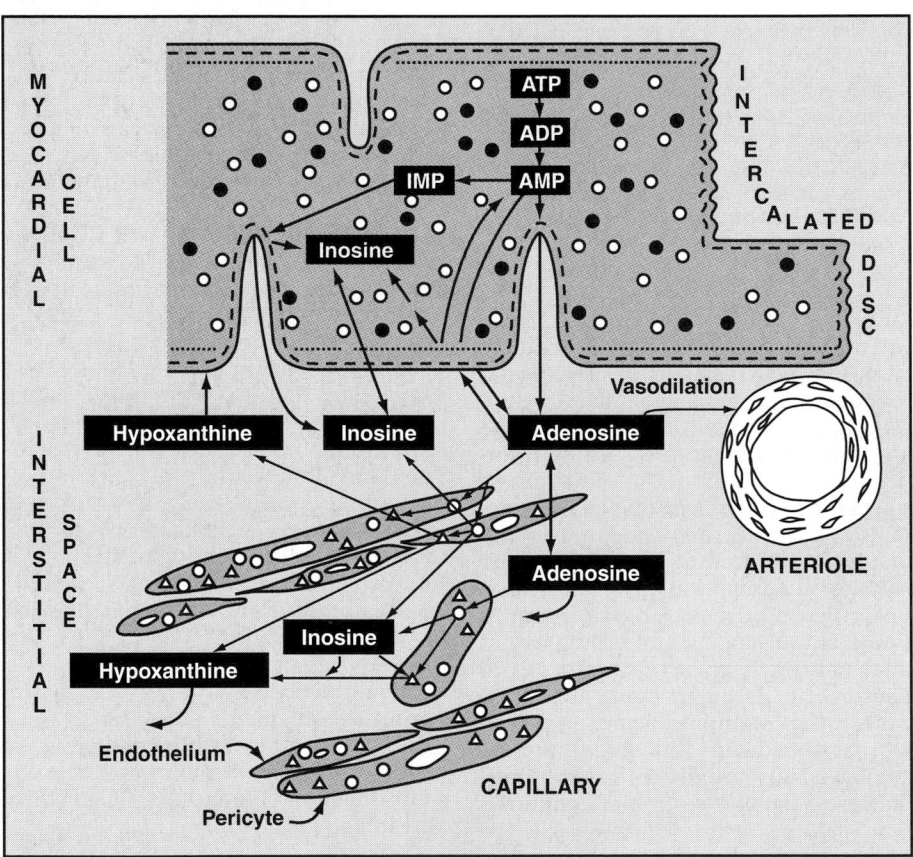

FIGURE 34–4. Schematic depiction of a myocardial interstitial space, an arteriole, and a capillary with the localization of enzymes involved in the formation and fate of adenosine. Adenosine formed by 5'-nucleotidase from adenosine monophosphate (AMP) (which in turn arises from adenosine triphosphate) can enter the interstitial space. There it can induce arteriolar dilation and reenter the myocardial cell, where it is either phosphorylated to AMP by adenosine kinase or deaminated to inosine monophosphate (IMP) by adenosine deaminase, or it can enter the capillaries and leave the tissue. A large fraction of adenosine that crosses the capillary wall is deaminated to inosine, which in turn is split to hypoxanthine and ribose-1-PO₄ by nucleoside phosphorylase located in the endothelial cells, pericytes, and erythrocytes. Most of the adenosine is taken up by the myocardial cells, and that escaping into the circulation is largely in the form of inosine and hypoxanthine. Because adenylic acid deaminase (which deaminates AMP to IMP) is in low concentration in heart muscle, the major degradative pathway from AMP is by means of dephosphorylation to adenosine. Open circles = adenosine deaminase; closed circles = adenylic acid deaminase; triangles = nucleoside phosphorylase; dashed lines = 5'-nucleotidase; dotted lines = adenosine kinase. (From Berne RM, Rubio R: Coronary circulation. *In* Berne RM, Sperelakis N, Geiger SR [eds]: Handbook of Physiology, Section 2. The Cardiovascular System. Bethesda, MD, American Physiological Society, 1979, p 924.)

tains and amplifies it. In support of this, inhibition of nitric oxide attenuates the late phase of reactive hyperemia, when flow-mediated dilation would be expected to occur.[28]

OTHER METABOLIC MEDIATORS. Inhibition of the synthesis of vasodilator prostaglandins[29] and inhibition of K^+_{ATP} channels[31] also reduces metabolic vasodilation. It is likely that vasoactive factors act in concert to regulate coronary flow in response to metabolic needs. A loss or inhibition of one mediator is compensated for by upregulation of others. Although the inhibition of K^+_{ATP} channels, adenosine, and NO individually has at most a modest effect on the increase in coronary blood flow during exercise in dogs, inhibition of all three simultaneously nearly abolishes the flow increase.[32]

Endothelial Control of Coronary Vascular Tone

Vasoactive agents that influence the tone of large and small coronary vessels can be carried in the blood plasma (e.g., epinephrine, vasopressin) or released from circulating blood elements such as platelets (e.g., serotonin, adenosine diphosphate) or from nerve endings in the vascular adventitia (e.g., norepinephrine, vasoactive intestinal peptide). Furthermore, vasoactive factors can be formed locally by the vascular endothelium.

The vascular endothelium performs a wide array of homeostatic functions within normal blood vessels. Located between the vascular lumen and the smooth muscle cells of the vessel wall, the monolayer of endothelial cells is able to transduce blood-borne signals, sense mechanical forces within the lumen, and regulate vascular tone through the production of a variety of factors.[33, 34] Endothelium produces both potent vasodilators, such as endothelium-derived relaxing factor (EDRF, NO), prostacyclin, and endothelium-derived hyperpolarizing factor (EDHF), and vasoconstrictors, such as endothelin-1. Endothelium-derived vasoactive factors are of great interest because endothelium can be damaged by atherosclerosis and by cardiovascular risk factors. Endothelial dysfunction may then lead to disturbances in coronary blood flow, can contribute to the pathogenesis of myocardial ischemia, and is a central feature in the evolution of atherosclerosis and thrombosis[35] (Fig. 34–5) (see also Chap. 30).

ENDOTHELIUM-DERIVED RELAXING FACTOR. Perhaps the most important vasodilator substance produced by endothelial cells is endothelium-derived relaxing factor (EDRF).[36] The discovery of EDRF in 1980 by Furchgott resulted from the observation that intact endothelium is required for acetylcholine-induced vasodilation.[37] In the presence of endothelium, acetylcholine produces dose-dependent vasodilation. When the endothelium is removed, only constriction is induced by acetylcholine. It became apparent that acetylcholine has two distinct and opposite actions on blood vessels: an endothelium-mediated dilation and a smooth muscle–mediated constriction (Fig. 34–6). In any blood vessel, the net response is related to the sum of these two actions. In most healthy arteries, endothelium-dependent vasodilation predominates over direct vasoconstriction.[33]

EDRF has been identified as the nitric oxide (NO) radical.[38, 39] NO is formed in endothelial cells from the substrate L-arginine by the action of NO synthase (Fig. 34–7). In this reaction, the terminal nitrogen from the guanadino group of L-arginine gives rise to NO. This reaction requires molecular oxygen, tetrahydrobiopterin (THB$_4$), NADPH, flavin adenine dinucleotide, and flavin mononucleotide as cofactors and produces L-citrulline as a byproduct that can be recycled to L-arginine. The activity of the enzyme is controlled by calcium and calmodulin.[38, 39] The relaxing effect of NO is mediated by its diffusion to smooth muscle cells,

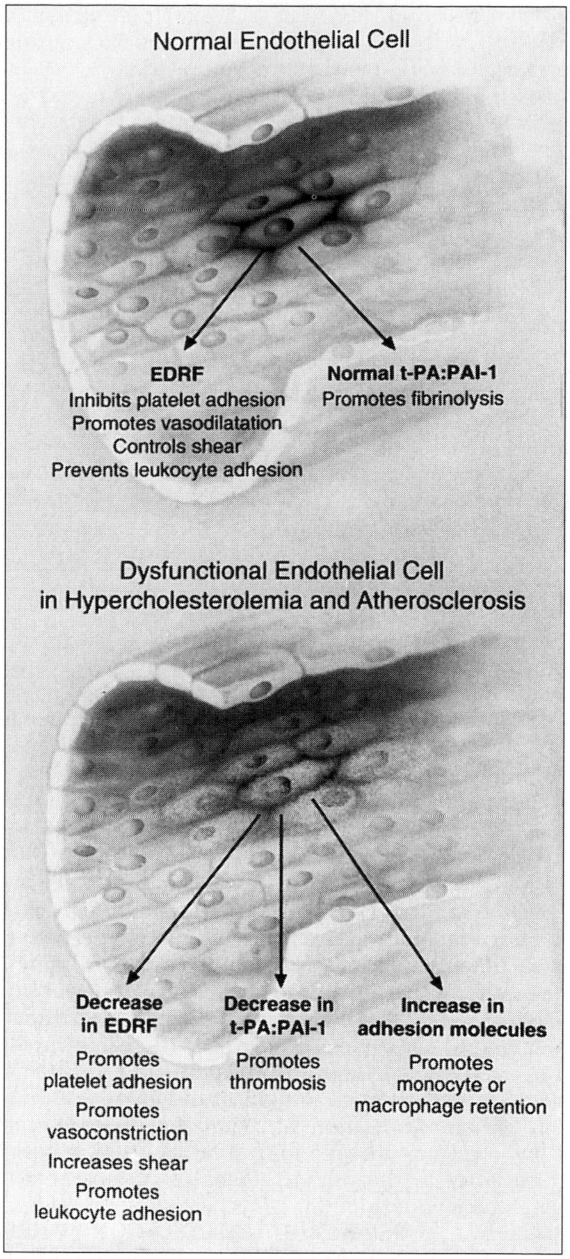

FIGURE 34–5. Normal and dysfunctional endothelial cells, with some of the functions adversely influenced by hypercholesterolemia and atherosclerosis, which may contribute to acute coronary syndromes. t-PA:PAI-1 = the ratio of tissue plasminogen activator to plasminogen-activator inhibitor type 1. EDRF = endothelial derived relaxing factor. (From Levine GN, Keaney JF, Vita JA: Cholesterol reduction in cardiovascular disease. N Engl J Med 332:312, 1995. Copyright 1995, Massachusetts Medical Society.)

where it causes an activation of intracellular guanylate cyclase, a rise in cyclic guanosine monophosphate (GMP), and a consequent fall in intracellular calcium.[40] Once released from endothelial cells NO has a very short half-life, limited by interaction with other free radicals in tissues, principally superoxide, and by entering red blood cells to react with oxyhemoglobin.[41]

In many vascular beds, NO is released continuously, contributing to the maintenance of a vasodilator state. Aside from acetylcholine, the release of NO above this basal level is stimulated by products of thrombosis (thrombin), aggregating platelets (serotonin, ADP), other chemical stimuli (histamine, bradykinin), and increased shear stress resulting from an increase in blood flow; the latter is responsible for so-called flow-mediated vasodilation[33] (Fig.

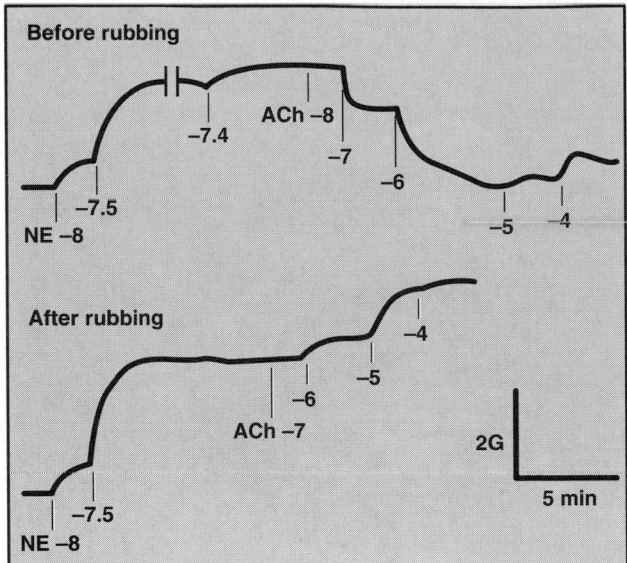

FIGURE 34–6. Relaxation by acetylcholine (ACh) of rings of rabbit thoracic aorta precontracted by norepinephrine (NE). Aortic rings were exposed to increasing concentrations of ACh with endothelium either intact or removed by rubbing with a wooden applicator stick. This representative tracing shows loss of relaxation in response to ACh with removal of endothelium and appearance of mild constriction. (From Furchgott RF: Role of endothelium in responses of vascular smooth muscle. Circ Res 53:557, 1983. Copyright 1983, American Heart Association.)

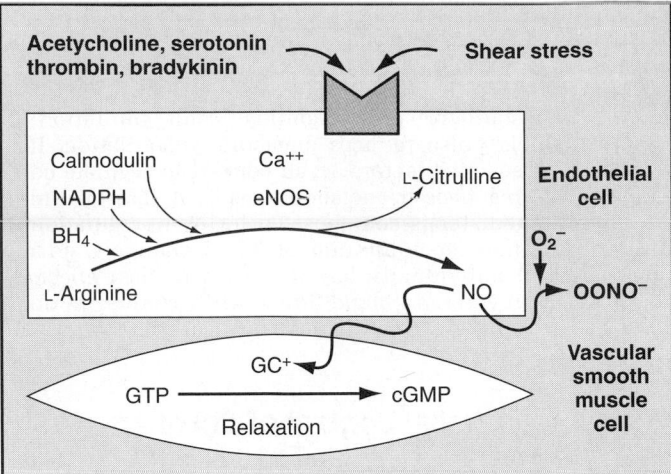

FIGURE 34–7. Endothelial cell production of nitric oxide (NO) by the action of nitric oxide synthase (eNOS) on L-arginine. This reaction requires a number of cofactors such as tetrahydrobiopterin (BH$_4$), calmodulin, and NADPH. eNOS stimulation by vasodilator agonists or shear stress is mediated by rise in intracellular calcium (Ca^{2+}). NO may be broken down by free radicals (O$_2^-$), producing peroxinitrite (OONO$^-$), which is vasoinactive. NO acts on vascular smooth muscle cells to cause relaxation by activating guanylate cyclase (GC), thereby increasing intracellular cyclic guanosine monophosphate (cGMP).

34–8). Vasoconstrictors, such as alpha-adrenergic agonists, may also stimulate the release of NO. Although their net effect on the blood vessel may be vasoconstriction, the presence of an endothelium-dependent vasodilating influence attenuates this constriction. Only a few vasodilators can act independently of the endothelium and directly on vascular smooth muscle. These include the nitrovasodilators (e.g., nitroglycerin, nitroprusside) and prostacyclin.[33] Adenosine elicits both endothelium-independent and endothelium-dependent dilation; at high concentration of adenosine, endothelium-independent dilation dominates while NO contributes to the dilator effects of adenosine at lower adenosine concentration.[42]

ENDOTHELIUM-DEPENDENT VASODILATION IN HEALTHY HUMAN EPICARDIAL ARTERIES. Endothelium-dependent vasodilation as an important mechanism has been documented in many vascular beds throughout animal kingdom, including mammals, birds, and reptiles. The importance of

NO secretion in vasodilation of healthy human epicardial arteries was first demonstrated by intracoronary infusion of acetylcholine at the time of cardiac catheterization.[33] This vasodilation can be inhibited by specifically blocking NO synthesis with N^G-monomethyl-L-arginine (L-NMMA). Likewise, L-NMMA inhibits flow-mediated dilation of human epicardial arteries.[29] Other endothelium-dependent substances that have been shown to dilate healthy human coronary arteries include serotonin, histamine, bradykinin, and substance P.[33]

IMPAIRMENT OF ENDOTHELIUM-DEPENDENT VASODILATION IN HUMAN EPICARDIAL ARTERIES. Evidence has accumulated that the tendency to inappropriate vasoconstriction that characterizes atherosclerosis is related to vasodilator dysfunction of the endothelium, permitting unopposed constriction of vascular smooth muscle. Responses to endothelium-dependent stimuli that dilate healthy human coronary arteries have been found to be markedly impaired in patients with both early and advanced atherosclerosis. Acetylcholine constricts atherosclerotic coronary arteries, reflecting the loss of NO and acetylcholine's unopposed

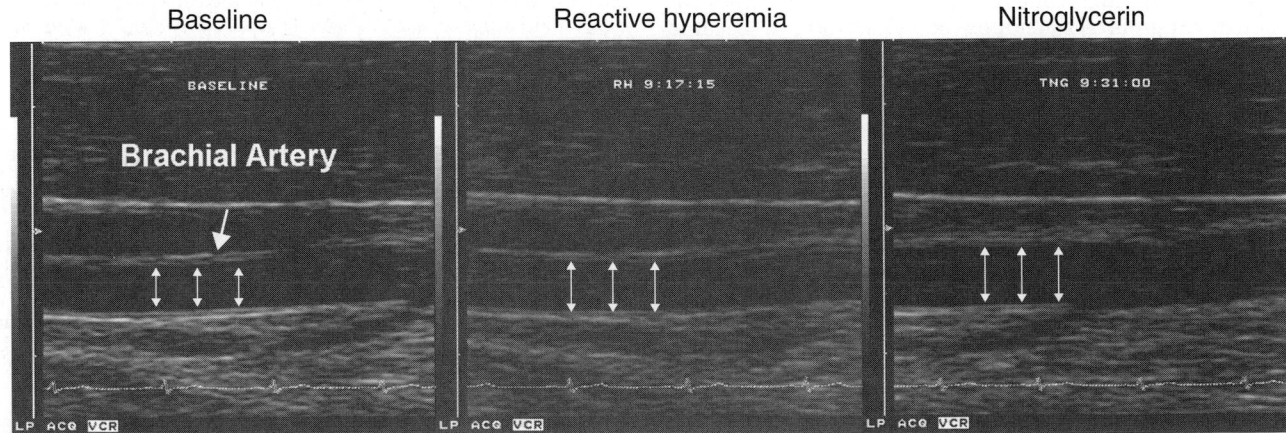

FIGURE 34–8. High-resolution ultrasound images of the human brachial artery at baseline; dilation during reactive hyperemia following the release of a 5-minute occlusion (i.e., flow-mediated dilation); and dilation after the administration of sublingual nitroglycerin (endothelium-independent dilation). This flow-mediated dilation is mediated principally by nitric oxide.

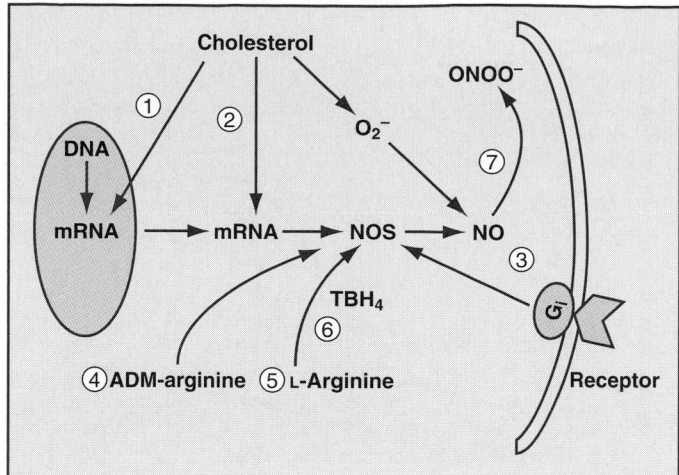

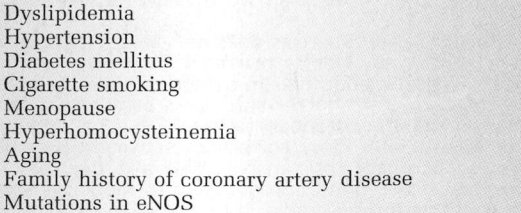

Dyslipidemia
Hypertension
Diabetes mellitus
Cigarette smoking
Menopause
Hyperhomocysteinemia
Aging
Family history of coronary artery disease
Mutations in eNOS

FIGURE 34–9. Mechanisms of endothelial dysfunction with cardiovascular risk factors. Cardiovascular risk factors, including cholesterol, reduce the bioavailability of nitric oxide by reducing the transcription (1) or stability (2) of messenger RNA encoding for nitric oxide synthase; (3) interfering with coupling of endothelial receptors to associated pertussis-sensitive G-proteins; (4 and 5) causing accumulation of asymmetric dimethyl arginine (ADM-arginine), a competitive antagonist to L-arginine, the substrate for nitric oxide synthesis; (6) reducing the availability of tetrahydrobiopterin (TBH$_4$), a cofactor for nitric oxide synthase; and (7) increasing the generation of superoxide (O$_2^-$), which combines with nitric oxide to generate a vasoinactive product ONOO$^-$.

All of the traditional risk factors and several newly described risk factors have been shown to be associated with a loss of endothelium-dependent dilation in human arteries (Table 34–3). One of the first risk factors found to be associated with loss of endothelium-dependent dilation was dyslipidemia.[33] Although native LDL may be involved in this process, there is much evidence that damaging effects on endothelial NO bioavailability are mediated by its most atherogenic forms, including oxidized LDL[49–51] and small, dense LDL particles.[33] Lipoprotein lipases act on triglyceride-rich particles, such as chylomicrons and very low-density lipoprotein, to produce remnant particles. Remnant particles are also highly atherogenic and associated with endothelial dysfunction and reduced NO.[52] Subjects with lipoprotein lipase deficiency, less able to generate remnant particles, have preserved endothelial function despite having a marked elevation in triglycerides.[53] Lipoprotein (a) also leads to a reduction in NO, especially when levels of LDL cholesterol are concomitantly elevated,[54] whereas HDL appears to be protective.[55]

Cause and effect between risk factors and loss of endothelial function was established when risk factors were introduced experimentally (and temporarily) into healthy volunteers. Infusion of high concentration of glucose (to mimic an aspect of diabetes mellitus),[56] methionine loading (to raise homocysteine concentration),[57] or ingestion of fatty meal (to raise the concentration of lipoprotein remnant particles)[58] promptly reduced the availability of NO. Surgical ovariectomy in women free of cardiovascular disease (which produces premature menopause) is also followed by a rapid loss of NO, which can be reversed with estrogen replacement therapy.[59] Mutations in the enzyme NO synthase can be associated with impaired production of NO and are clinically manifested by propensity to coronary vasospasm, hypertension, and myocardial infarction.[60–62] This genetic aberration provides further proof of the importance of the NO system in the clinical setting.

ENDOTHELIUM-DEPENDENT VASODILATION IN HUMAN CORONARY RESISTANCE VESSELS. Endothelium-dependent vasodilation operates not only in large (conductance) arteries, but it is also an important mechanism that controls dilation in small (resistance) vessels (Fig. 34–10). Studies in the human forearm have suggested that *continuous* basal release of NO is an important determinant of resting vascular resistance and blood flow. When a specific inhibitor of NO synthesis, L-NMMA, was infused into the forearm of healthy subjects, resting blood flow was cut in half.[63] Systemic administration of L-NMMA induces hypertension in normal volunteers, suggesting that NO acts to lower systemic vascular resistance.[64] NO release also reduces basal coronary vascular resistance and contributes to dilation in response

constrictor effects on vascular smooth muscle.[33, 43] Although abnormal vasomotor responses to acetylcholine have served as a convenient marker of endothelial dysfunction, the role of acetylcholine in the physiological regulation of vascular tone has not been established. The finding of endothelial vasodilator dysfunction in human coronary atherosclerosis has been confirmed for other more physiological stimuli that release NO, including serotonin, ADP, and increased coronary blood flow (flow-mediated dilation). For example, whereas serotonin, a product released from aggregating platelets, dilates normal human coronary arteries it constricts atherosclerotic arteries.[33, 44, 45]

The loss of endothelium-dependent dilation occurs early in atherosclerosis, even prior to its detection by angiography.[46, 47] This loss of NO bioavailability is related to risk factors for atherosclerosis[48] and is caused by reduced synthesis as well as accelerated breakdown of NO (Fig. 34–9).

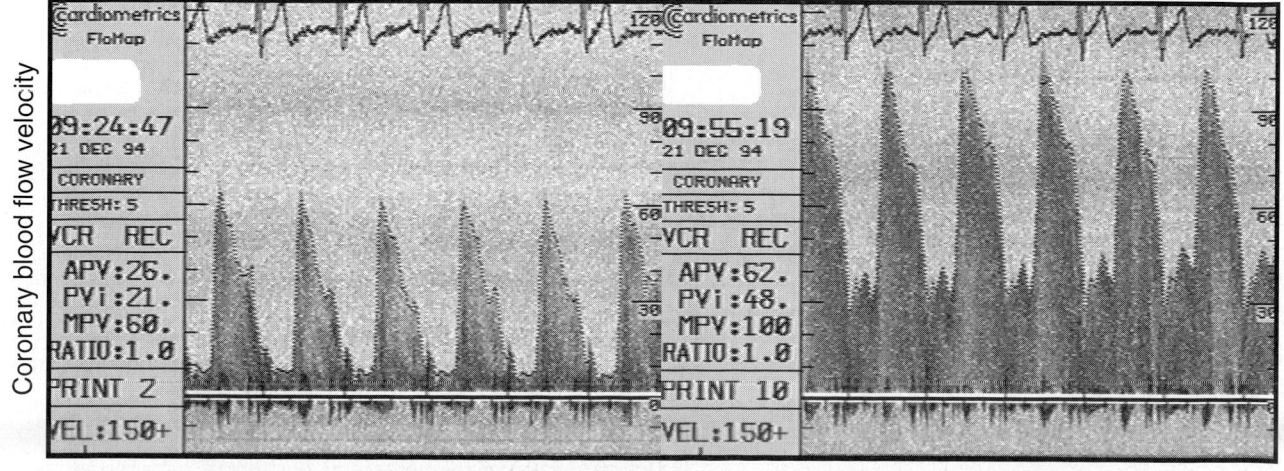

FIGURE 34–10. Increase in coronary blood flow velocity in response to acetylcholine, an endothelium-dependent agonist, in a patient free of coronary atherosclerosis. Coronary blood flow velocity was measured with a Doppler flow wire and increased 2.4-fold during acetylcholine administration; this increase in flow velocity (and blood flow) is indicative of normal endothelial function of resistance arterioles.

to a variety of endothelium-dependent agonists.[43] However, L-NMMA typically inhibits less than half of the vasodilation *stimulated* by various agonists in coronary and most other resistance vessels, suggesting that factors other than NO may play a role in the dilation of arterioles.[43, 65, 66]

Although atherosclerosis does not directly involve resistance vessels, coronary risk factors markedly impair the responses of resistance vessels to endothelium-dependent vasodilator stimuli.[33, 67, 68] This may not be altogether surprising, because risk factors are "systemic" in nature, potentially affecting the endothelial lining of all blood vessels.[69] The close correlation between the extent of NO deficiency in coronary resistance vessels and the failure of coronary blood flow to respond appropriately to metabolic stimuli suggests that endothelial dysfunction in resistance vessels may be an important factor in preventing coronary blood flow from rising during times of increased metabolic stress.[70] An inadequate augmentation of coronary blood flow in the presence of an increased metabolic demand may represent one of the mechanisms by which disturbances in endothelial function can lead to the development of myocardial ischemia in the setting of risk factors and atherosclerosis.

ENDOTHELIAL DYSFUNCTION AS A CAUSE OF MYOCARDIAL ISCHEMIA. Impairment of endothelial function that occurs in atherosclerosis and in the presence of risk factors for atherosclerosis plays an important role in the subsequent development of coronary syndromes. When superimposed on coronary artery stenoses, loss of endothelium-dependent dilation and resultant unopposed coronary constriction predisposes to myocardial ischemia.[71] Several studies have documented the physiological importance of this mechanism in patients with stable angina. With exercise, performed at the time of coronary angiography, epicardial arteries of healthy subjects were noted to dilate. In patients with stable angina, however, paradoxical vasoconstriction typically occurred at the site of coronary stenoses or even mildly irregular arterial segments.[72] Changes during exercise parallel the responses observed in response to the endothelium-dependent agent acetylcholine. Exercise causes dilation of the arteries with normal endothelium (evidenced by a normal response to acetylcholine) but constriction of vessels with evidence of endothelial dysfunction.

A similar pattern of dilation of normal coronary arteries and paradoxical constriction of atherosclerotic coronary arteries with dysfunctional endothelium has been observed with mental stress, the cold pressor test, and increase in heart rate.[68, 71, 73] These stimuli are normally accompanied by activation of the sympathetic nervous system, by an increase in circulating catecholamines, and by increases in coronary blood flow secondary to a rise in myocardial oxygen demand. In patients with dysfunctional endothelium,

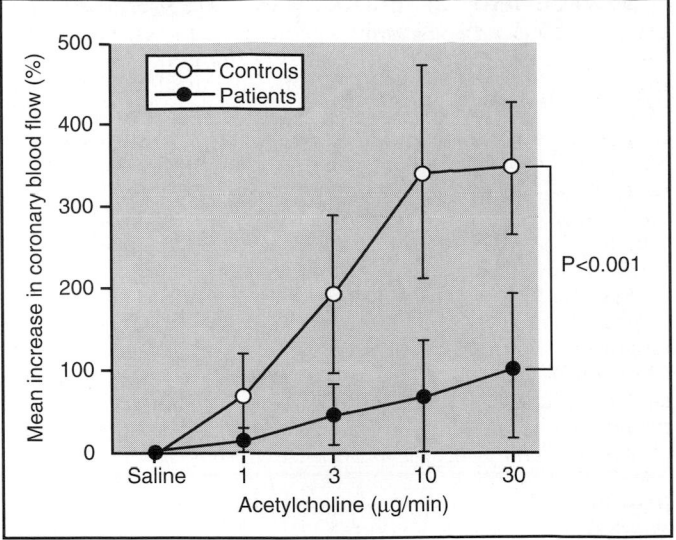

FIGURE 34–12. Increase in coronary blood flow evoked by graded doses of acetylcholine in control subjects and patients with microvascular angina. The dose-dependent increases in coronary blood flow produced by acetylcholine were significantly smaller in patients with microvascular angina than in control subjects ($p < 0.001$ by two-way analysis of variance). Bars indicate the standard deviation. (From Egashira K, et al: Evidence of impaired endothelium-dependent coronary vasodilatation in patients with angina pectoris and normal coronary angiograms. N Engl J Med 328:1659, 1993. Copyright 1993, Massachusetts Medical Society.)

the loss of flow-mediated and catecholamine-stimulated NO release permits unopposed constriction by catecholamines. Thus, the loss of NO may contribute to impaired dilation or exaggerated constriction of epicardial and resistance vessels and thereby to myocardial ischemia. Conversely, improvement in endothelial vasodilator function, achieved by cholesterol lowering therapy, is paralleled by a reduction in myocardial ischemia.[74]

Plaque fissuring or rupture with superimposed platelet aggregation and thrombus is a hallmark of unstable angina and myocardial infarction, but coronary constriction also plays an important role in these conditions.[75] The products of platelet aggregation and thrombosis, although dilating normal arteries, can severely constrict the atherosclerotic arteries of patients with coronary disease. As already noted, intracoronary administration of serotonin, a product released by aggregating platelets, constricts atherosclerotic coronary arteries.[76] The clinical significance of these findings is supported by the observations that patients with unstable coronary syndromes and complex plaques demonstrate augmented release of serotonin into the coronary circulation.[76] Patients with a recent history of myocardial infarction or unstable angina show evidence of endothelial vasodilator dysfunction in the infarct-related artery when tested with acetylcholine that is more pronounced than in arteries with stable stenoses of similar severity.[77]

Reductions in NO are associated not only with enhanced vasoconstriction at sites of disrupted atherosclerotic plaques but also with a predilection toward the destabilization of plaques. Such plaque destabilization is characterized by an infiltration of inflammatory cells, release of enzymes that degrade extracellular matrix, and thinning of the overlying fibrous cap with propensity to rupture.[68, 78] Enhanced production of highly thrombogenic tissue factor by inflammatory cells also plays a central role in this syndromes.[79] NO is a multipotent molecule (see Fig. 34–5) that inhibits the recruitment and differentiation of inflammatory cells by inhibiting the production of chemoattractant cytokines, leukocyte adhesion molecules, and factors that encourage the differentiation of monocytes into macrophages[75] (Fig. 34–11). NO also reduces the production of tissue factor. For these reasons, nitric oxide has become viewed as an important antiatherogenic[80] and plaque stabilizing[68] molecule.

The coronary resistance vessels may be affected by endothelial dysfunction in the *absence* of obstructive epicardial artery disease. Impaired endothelium-dependent dilation of coronary resistance vessels accounts for some of the cases of syndrome X, that is, anginal discomfort, evidence of myocardial ischemia on stress testing, and angiographically normal coronary arteries[81, 82] (Fig. 34–12) (see also Chap. 37).

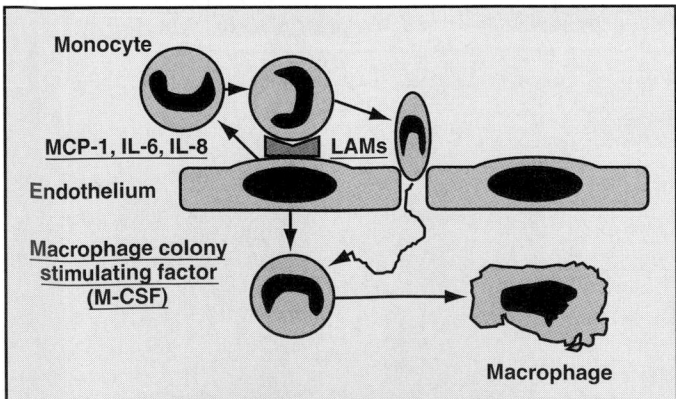

FIGURE 34–11. Nitric oxide, a multipotent molecule, inhibits recruitment of inflammatory cells, including monocytes, into the subendothelial space and their differentiation into macrophages. Specifically, nitric oxide inhibits the production of proinflammatory cytokines and chemokines (e.g., monocyte chemotactic protein-1 [MCP-1], interleukin-6 [IL-6], and interleukin-8 [IL-8]), reduces the expression of leukocyte adhesion molecules (LAMs), and inhibits factors that facilitate differentiation of monocytes into macrophages (e.g., macrophage colony stimulating factor [M-CSF]).

MANAGEMENT OF ENDOTHELIAL DYSFUNCTION. The use of cholesterol-lowering agents (statins or cholestyramine) in patients with hypercholesterolemia has led to a rapid and significant improvement in endothelium-dependent dilation of coronary and peripheral arteries in patients with hypercholesterolemia[33, 68, 83, 84] (Figs. 34–13 and 34–14). Interestingly, such rapid improvement in endothelial function could not be demonstrated in patients with relatively low serum concentrations of cholesterol, a finding that has a clinical counterpart in the results of several recent clinical event trials.

Aggressive reduction in cholesterol is associated with improved myocardial perfusion on positron-emission tomography[85] and a reduction in myocardial ischemia.[74, 86] Cholesterol-lowering markedly reduced evidence of myocardial ischemia on ambulatory electrocardiographic monitoring in patients with stable coronary disease and hypercholesterolemia over a period of 4 to 6 months, a time period that parallels the observed improvement in endothelium-dependent dilation observed in similar patients and duration of treatment[74, 86] (Fig. 34–15).

Other strategies are effective at restoring endothelium-dependent dilation, augmenting myocardial perfusion, and reducing the severity of myocardial ischemia or symptoms of angina. These include the use of angiotensin-converting enzyme inhibitors,[87] antioxidants[88, 89] and the oral administration of L-arginine.[89]

ENDOTHELIUM-DERIVED HYPERPOLARIZING FACTOR. Convincing evidence has accumulated that factors other than NO and prostacyclin (see later) can mediate endothelium-dependent vasodilation by hyperpolarizing the underlying smooth muscle. This hyperpolarization occurs through activation of Ca^{2+}-activated K^+ channels in vascular smooth muscle cells and has been attributed to a diffusible factor termed *endothelium-derived hyperpolarizing factor (EDHF)*.[90] EDHF appears to be far more important in small arterioles than in larger conduit arteries.[91, 92] It is released by many of the same stimuli that stimulate NO, including acetylcholine, bradykinin, substance P, and shear stress.[90, 93–95] Although there may be more than one EDHF molecule, cytochrome P450 (CYP)-dependent metabolites of arachidonic acid (AA), especially the epoxide 11,12-epoxyeicosatrienoic acid, fulfill the essential criteria as mediators of endothelium-dependent hyperpolarization.[96]

EDHF has been demonstrated in human coronary[91] and peripheral arterioles in vitro. NO inhibits the production of EDHF.[97] It has been therefore suggested that when diseases reduce NO bioavailability, release of this intrinsic inhibition may maintain endothelial vasodilator function by up-regulation of EDHF.[90, 97] Nevertheless, aging and long-standing hypercholesterolemia appear to reduce EDHF as well as NO in human peripheral arterioles. Just as NO, EDHF (11,12-epoxyeicosatrienoic acid) is a multipotent molecule with antiinflammatory properties.[96] The full significance of EDHF in normal human coronary physiology and abnormal pathophysiology remains to be established and awaits the availability of specific inhibitors of this pathway.

PROSTACYCLIN. This is a potent vasodilator derived from the endothelium through the actions of cyclooxygenase. The role of prostacyclin in the control of vascular tone in humans has been controversial, at least until recently.[29] Administration of aspirin has little effect on arterial blood pressure in humans, suggesting that inhibition of cyclooxygenase does not cause generalized systemic vasoconstriction. Administration of indomethacin does reduce resting coronary blood flow in humans.[98] It has been suggested, however, that these coronary constrictor effects of indomethacin are not due to inhibition of prostacyclin synthesis.[98]

Although vascular prostacyclin production under physiological conditions appears to be low, patients with atherosclerosis have increased prostacyclin production.[99] In patients with coronary atherosclerosis or risk factors, administration of aspirin to inhibit cyclooxygenase has revealed that prostacyclin contributes importantly to resting vasodilator tone in epicardial arteries and resistance arteri-

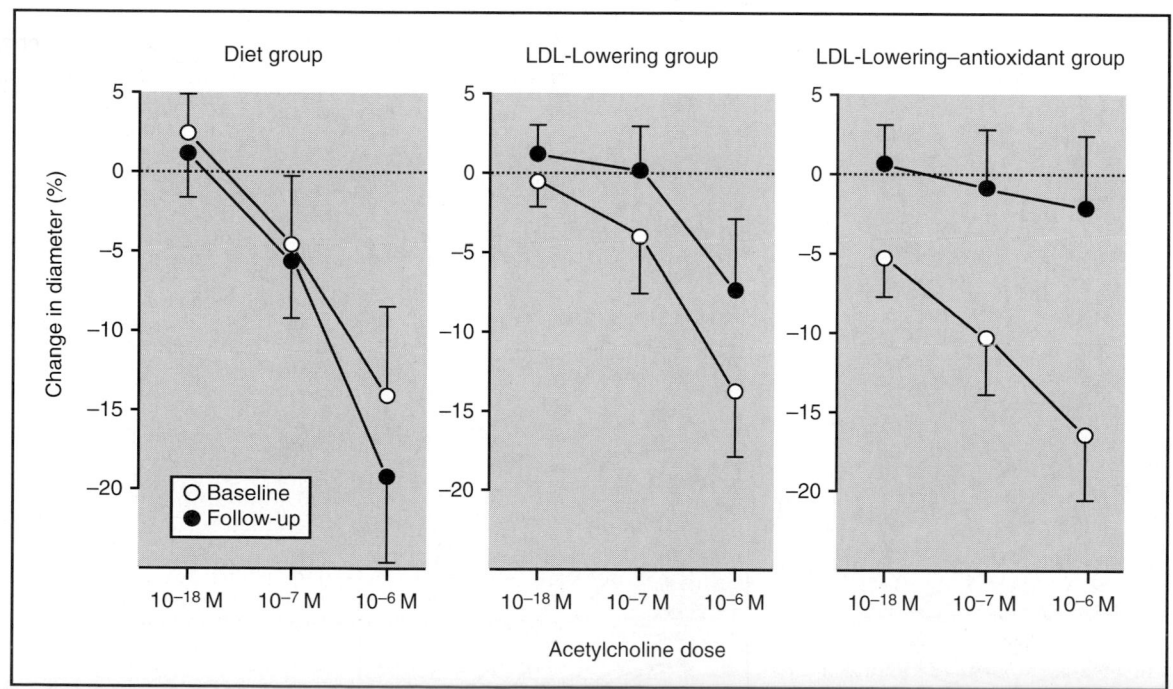

FIGURE 34–13. Mean (+SE) change in coronary artery diameter in response to serial infusions of acetylcholine at baseline and after 1 year of therapy in the three study groups. The improvement in the response from baseline to follow-up in the LDL-lowering-antioxidant group was significantly greater than that in the diet group ($p > 0.05$). Negative numbers indicate vasoconstriction. (From Anderson TJ, Meredith IT, Yeung AC, et al: The effect of cholesterol-lowering and antioxidant therapy on endothelium-dependent coronary vasomotion. N Engl J Med 332:488, 1995. Copyright 1995, Massachusetts Medical Society.)

Initial Study

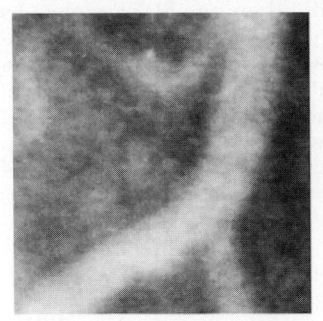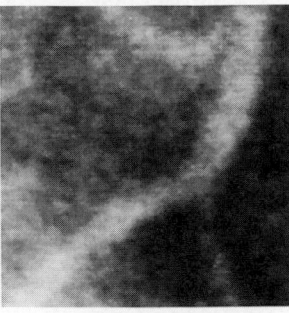

Follow-up Study

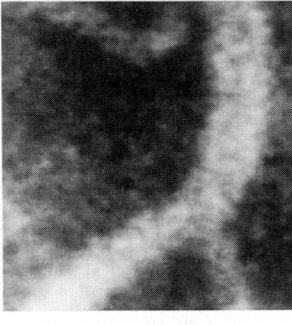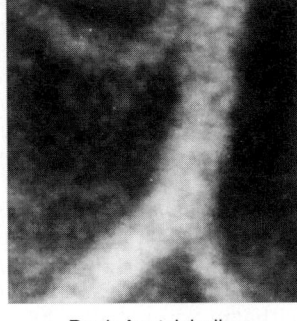

Control   Peak Acetylcholine

FIGURE 34–14. Segment of the circumflex coronary artery at initial and follow-up (5.5 months) studies in a patient with coronary atherosclerosis assigned to lovastatin. Both left panels demonstrate baseline (control) arteriograms; both right panels demonstrate post-acetylcholine arteriograms. Substantial vasoconstriction occurs in response to the peak infusion of acetylcholine in the initial study, with marked improvement (a mild vasodilator response) in the follow-up study. (From Treasure CB, et al: Beneficial effects of cholesterol-lowering therapy on the coronary endothelium in patients with coronary artery disease. N Engl J Med 332:481, 1995. Copyright Massachusetts Medical Society.)

oles and plays a role in flow-mediated coronary dilation and metabolic vasodilation.[29] Thus, the prostacyclin-mediated coronary vasodilation appears to be most important in a setting characterized by a deficiency of nitric oxide and may provide a useful compensatory mechanism.

ENDOTHELIUM-DERIVED CONSTRICTING FACTORS. The endothelium not only mediates vasodilation but it is a source of vasoconstrictor factors as well (Fig. 34–16). The best characterized of these are the endothelins.[100, 101] Endothelin-1 (ET-1) is a 21-amino-acid peptide that has a potent vasoconstrictor activity. Two other isoforms of endothelin have been discovered (ET-2 and ET-3), but endothelium produces only ET-1. Synthesis of ET-1 is complex, starting with a large precursor molecule, preproendothelin, which is processed to "big endothelin" and finally converted by the action of endothelin-converting enzyme to the fully active ET-1.[100]

Unlike NO, which can be released rapidly in response to vasodilator stimuli and then inactivated within seconds, ET-1—mediated constriction is slow in onset and lasts over minutes to hours.[100, 101] Agents that stimulate ET-1, such as thrombin, angiotensin II, epinephrine, or vasopressin, do so by de novo transcription of messenger RNA. On the basis of these considerations, it is likely that ET-1 contributes to the regulation of vascular tone primarily by exerting a tonic vasoconstrictor influence. In addition to its vasoactive properties, ET-1 also stimulates smooth muscle proliferation,[102] vascular remodeling,[103] and leukocyte adhesion and recruitment[104]; it may thereby play a role in inflammation and in atherogenesis.

Plasma concentrations of ET-1 are elevated in a number of cardiovascular disorders,[101, 105] including hypercholesterolemia, hypertension, atherosclerosis, acute myocardial infarction, and congestive heart failure (see also Chap. 16). Aside from the endothelium, macrophages and activated smooth muscle cells are a rich source of ET-1 in the vessel wall. These cells are numerous in vulnerable or ruptured plaques. Consistent with this finding the culprit plaques of patients with acute coronary syndromes express significantly greater ET-1 immunoreactivity than plaques of patients with stable angina.[106] These plaques are also rich in lipid, and oxidized LDL is a potent stimulus to ET-1 synthesis.[107, 108]

ENDOTHELIN RECEPTORS. ET-1 exerts its vascular effects by binding to two specific receptors named ET_A and ET_B. ET_A receptors are present on vascular smooth muscle cells and promote vasoconstriction[109] and smooth muscle proliferation.[102] ET_B receptors are located on endothelial cells where they mediate endothelium-dependent dila-

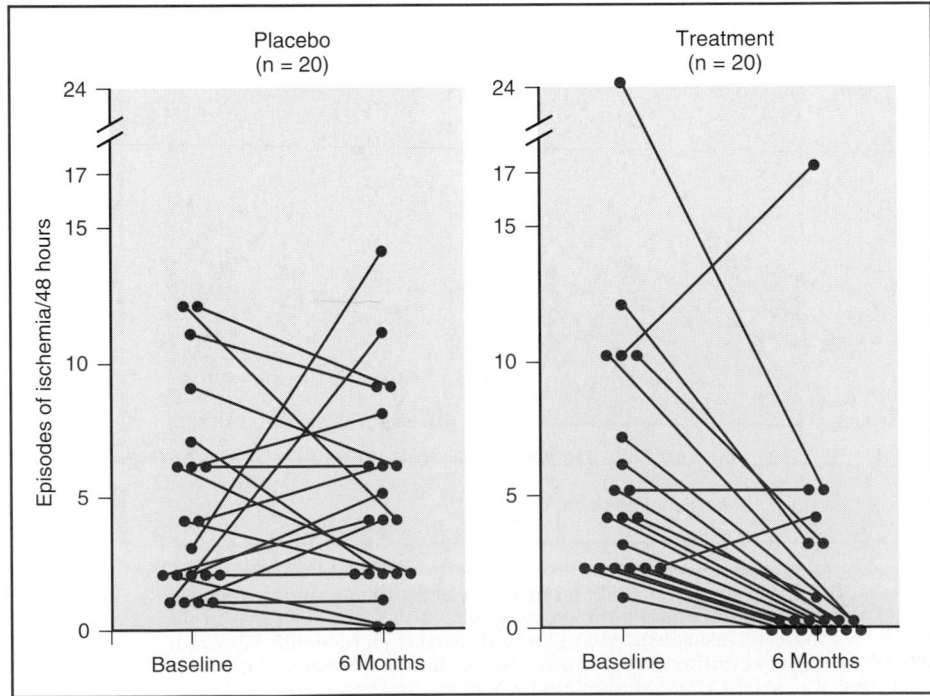

FIGURE 34–15. Effect of cholesterol lowering or placebo over 6 months on the number of episodes of ischemic ST-segment depression in patients with coronary disease. Two of 20 in the placebo group vs. 13 of 20 in the treatment group show resolution of ischemia. (From Andrews TC, Raby K, Barry J, et al: The effect of LDL cholesterol reduction on myocardial ischemia in patients with coronary disease. Circulation 95:324–328, 1997.)

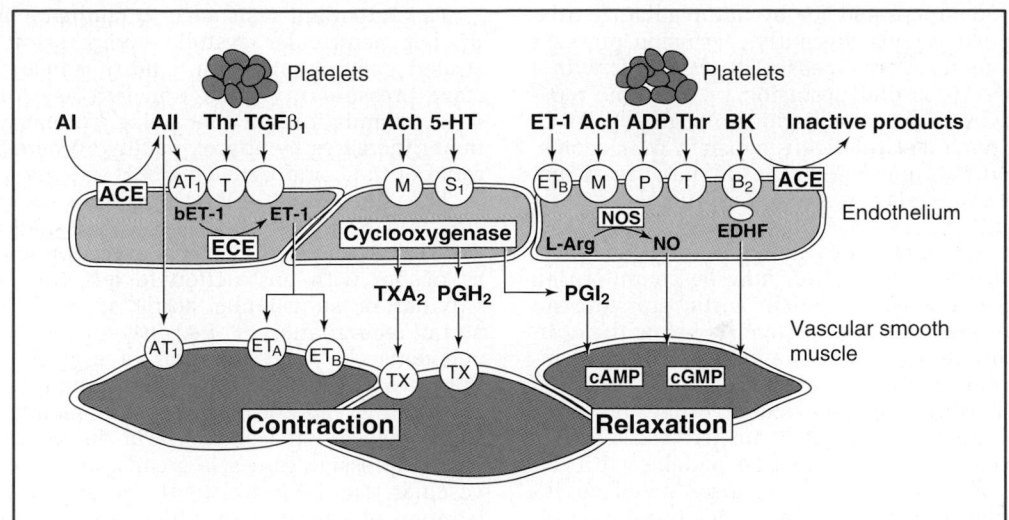

FIGURE 34–16. Endothelium-derived vasoactive substances. The endothelium is a source of relaxins (bottom right) and contracting (bottom left) factors. ACE = angiotensin converting enzyme; Ach = acetylcholine; ADP = adenosine diphosphate; BK = bradykinin; cAMP/cGMP = cyclic adenosine/guanosine monophosphate; ECE = endothelin-converting enzymes; EDHF = endothelium-derived hyperpolarizing factor; ET-1 = endothelin-1; 5HT = 5-hydroxytryptamine (serotonin); L-arg = L-arginine; NO = nitric oxide; PGH_2 = prostaglandin; PGI_2 = prostacyclin; TGF $\beta 1$ = transforming growth factor $\beta 1$; Thr = thrombin; TXA_2 = thromboxane A_2. Circles represent receptors (AT = angiotensinergic; B = bradykinergic; M = muscarinic; P = purinergic; T = thrombin receptor). (From Luscher TF, Noll G: The endothelium in coronary vascular control. *In* Braunwald E [ed]: Heart Disease—Update 3. Philadelphia, WB Saunders Company, 1995, p 2.)

tion by releasing NO and are also located on smooth muscle cells where they mediate constriction.[110] Antagonists of the ET receptors and inhibitors of the endothelin-converting enzyme have become available and are helpful in assessing the role of ET-1 in cardiovascular diseases. Bosentan, a mixed ET_A/ET_B receptor antagonist, was found to lower blood pressure in patients with essential hypertension,[111] which suggests a role for ET-1 in the pathogenesis of hypertension.[112] Inhibition of ET_A receptor by intracoronary infusion of a specific antagonist BQ-123 results in significant dilation of normal human epicardial arteries. This finding suggests that ET-1, through the ET_A receptor, is important to the maintenance of tonic coronary tone in humans. The use of ET inhibitors will be helpful in assessing the role that ET-1 plays in exaggerated constriction in patients with atherosclerotic coronary arteries.

Autoregulation of Coronary Blood Flow

When sudden alterations in perfusion pressure are imposed in many arterial beds (including the coronary), the resulting abrupt changes in blood flow are only transitory, with flow returning promptly to the previous steady-state level[113] (Fig. 34–17). This ability to maintain myocardial perfusion at constant levels in the face of changing driving pressure is termed *autoregulation*. Demonstration of autoregulation in the coronary bed is difficult in intact animals because aortic pressure is not only the perfusion pressure for the coronary circulation, but it is also the afterload for the left ventricle, a major determinant of MVo_2. Coronary autoregulation has therefore been studied under experimental conditions where the coronary circulation is cannulated and perfused separately.[114] Under such controlled conditions perfusion pressure is altered, but ventricular pressure, cardiac contractility and heart rate—the principal determinants of MVo_2 (see p. 1088)—are maintained constant and autoregulation is clearly evident. In dogs the upper limit of autoregulation is 130 mm Hg, whereas the lower limit of autoregulation is 40 mm Hg.[115] That is to say, when mean aortic pressure is within this range, coronary perfusion is relatively constant. When aortic pressure falls below 40 mm Hg, coronary blood flow precipitously declines. When aortic pressure exceeds 130 mm Hg, coronary flow rises sharply.

Although autoregulation cannot be studied in detail in humans, it is perhaps the principal reason why patients with coronary artery disease and epicardial stenoses do not have evidence of resting perfusion deficits or myocardial ischemia at all times! Reductions in perfusion pressure dis-

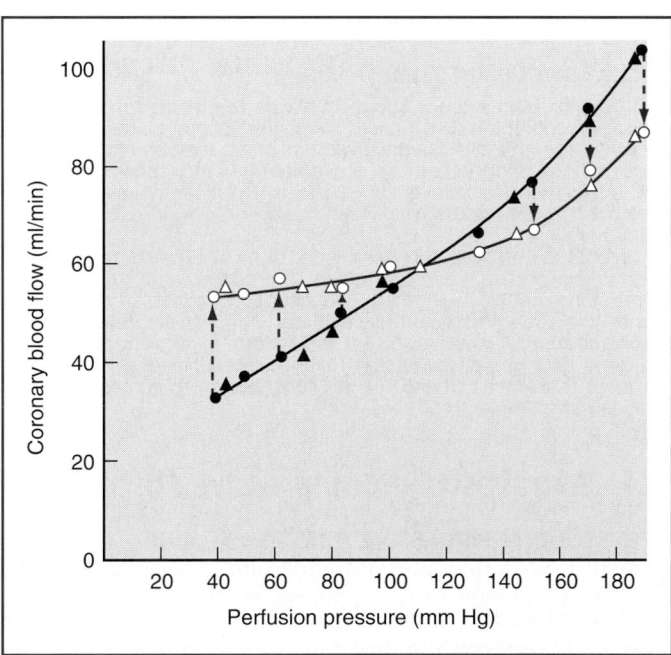

FIGURE 34–17. Autoregulation of coronary blood flow in the beating dog heart. The point where the curves cross represents the control steady-state pressure and flow. A sudden, sustained charge in perfusion pressure caused an abrupt change in flow represented by the filled symbols and black line (transient flow). The open symbols and red line represent the steady-state flows obtained at each perfusion pressure. The points represented by triangles were obtained after blockade of cardiac prostaglandin synthesis with indomethacin. (From Rubio K, Berne KM: Regulation of coronary blood flow. Prog Cardiovasc Dis 18:105, 1975.)

tal to stenoses are compensated for by autoregulatory dilation of the resistance vessels. Recently, perfusion pressure distal to coronary stenoses was measured in patients with a pressure wire and myocardial perfusion in the same territory was assessed by positron emission tomography. Myocardial perfusion remained relatively constant over a pressure range of 45 to 125 mm Hg.[116] These data suggest that the autoregulatory range may be as large in humans as it is in conscious dogs.[115]

The ability of autoregulation to compensate for the effect of a proximal epicardial obstruction may be compromised in several clinical situations. A fall in aortic pressure can lower perfusion pressure distal to a stenosis below the critical levels at which autoregulation is effective, thereby compromising myocardial perfusion, intensifying myocardial ischemia, and increasing left ventricular filling pressure, which reduces the perfusion gradient further. These events may cause a vicious cycle, especially in patients with left main or three-vessel coronary disease. Insertion of an intraaortic balloon pump in this setting raises diastolic perfusion pressure and restores coronary pressure so that autoregulation is reestablished and myocardial ischemia is lessened.

Chronic hypertension and left ventricular hypertrophy narrow the range of autoregulation, especially in the subendocardium, in which autoregulation is ordinarily more limited than in the subepicardium.[117] This amplifies the detrimental effects of coronary stenoses on myocardial perfusion and in patients with severe hypertrophy may lead to subendocardial ischemia even in the absence of coronary stenosis.

Conditions that alter the function of vascular smooth muscle in coronary arterioles attenuate autoregulation. For example, adenosine and dipyridamole abolish autoregulation. In the setting of stenoses, this may cause myocardial ischemia, especially in the subendocardium.[118] In endotoxemic shock, the myocardium produces massive amounts of nitric oxide, a potent vasodilator, which causes autoregulatory dysfunction and potentially predisposes to myocardial ischemia.[119]

MECHANISMS OF AUTOREGULATION

NITRIC OXIDE. Evidence suggests a role for NO in coronary autoregulation. Inhibition of NO raises the lower autoregulatory threshold by about 15 mm Hg.[120] The involvement of NO may be related to the ability of the endothelium to sense changes in perfusion pressure through pressure-sensitive ion channels.[121] Currently, there is little evidence to support the role of adenosine or K^+_{ATP} in coronary autoregulation.[122]

MYOGENIC CONTROL. Arteriolar smooth muscle reacts to increased intraluminal pressure by contracting. The consequent augmentation of resistance tends to return blood flow toward normal despite the higher perfusion pressure. This regulatory mechanism, referred to as *myogenic control*, is an important mechanism in some vascular beds. Although data demonstrate that myogenic responses are present in coronary resistance arteries,[123] their contribution to autoregulation is relatively small.[124]

Extravascular Compressive Forces

SYSTOLIC COMPRESSIVE FORCES. Because systolic ventricular wall compresses intramyocardial vessels, most of the coronary blood flow to the left ventricle occurs during diastole. Thus, the contracting heart obstructs its own blood supply. At peak systole, there is even backflow in the coronary arteries, particularly in the intramural and small epicardial arteries.[125]

The extravascular systolic compressive force has two components. The first is left ventricular systolic intracavitary pressure, which is transmitted fully to the subendocardium but falls off to almost zero at the epicardial surface. The second, and perhaps even more important, is the vascular narrowing caused by compression and bending of vascular arterioles coursing through the ventricular wall as the heart contracts.[126]

The important resistance to coronary blood flow caused by left ventricular systolic compression can be demonstrated experimentally in a beating heart perfused at constant pressure in which transient asystole is induced by vagal stimulation. At that point, coronary blood flow suddenly increases by approximately 50 percent because of the relief of the compressive effect.[127]

The "throttling" effect of systole on myocardial perfusion is particularly important when systolic intraventricular pressure is elevated to levels exceeding coronary perfusion, as occurs with obstruction to left ventricular outflow by valvular or subvalvular aortic stenosis,[128] or with severe aortic regurgitation.[129] Because an increase in heart rate augments the total duration of systolic time per minute during which coronary vascular compression occurs, while augmenting myocardial oxygen demand, tachycardia may cause myocardial ischemia. The importance of extravascular compressive forces is greatly magnified when coronary vascular tone is diminished[130] as may occur during administration of arteriolar vasodilators or during metabolic vasodilation associated with physical activity.

Because compressive forces exerted by the right ventricle are ordinarily far smaller than those of the left ventricle, ventricular perfusion is reduced but not interrupted during systole. When the right ventricular systolic pressure is elevated by disease (e.g., pulmonic stenosis), the phasic blood flow pattern of the arteries perfusing the right ventricle resembles that of the left ventricle.

DIASTOLIC COMPRESSIVE FORCES. The coronary perfusion or effective driving pressure has been assumed to be the pressure gradient between the coronary arteries and the pressure in either the right atrium or the left ventricle in diastole, because coronary flow drains primarily into these two chambers during this phase of the cardiac cycle. When coronary perfusion pressure is lowered, diastolic blood flow ceases when coronary driving pressure reaches 40 to 50 mm Hg, the so-called pressure at zero flow (P_{zf}).[131] This pressure is determined largely by diastolic compressive forces.

Transmural Distribution of Myocardial Blood Flow

Extravascular compressive forces are greater in the subendocardium than in the subepicardial layer (Fig. 34–18). Subendocardial arterioles are particularly susceptible to compression as they arborize from long, transmural vessels.[132] Therefore, *systolic* flow is more reduced in the subendocardium than the subepicardium. Nevertheless, in conscious dogs under resting physiological conditions, the ratio of endocardial to epicardial flow averaged throughout the cardiac cycle is approximately 1.25:1 due to preferential dilatation of the subendocardial arterioles, causing a large increase in diastolic flow in the subendocardium.[133, 134] The greater subendocardial blood flow appears to be secondary to the wall stress (and therefore oxygen consumption per unit weight), which is normally about 20 percent greater than that of subepicardial muscle.[135]

SUBENDOCARDIAL ISCHEMIA. The subendocardium is more vulnerable to ischemic damage than the midmyocardium or subepicardium.[136] Epicardial coronary stenoses are associated with reductions in the subendocardial to subepicardial flow ratio.[134] When coronary arteries were constricted sufficiently to reduce total coronary flow to approximately 40 percent of control, endocardial to epicardial flow ratio fell from 1.16 at baseline to 0.37. This pattern of redistribution of flow away from the endocardium is further exaggerated during exercise, mental stress, and pacing-induced tachycardia.[137] Potent arteriolar vasodilators, such as dipyridamole or adenosine, also cause redistribution of blood flow from the endocardium to the epicardium.

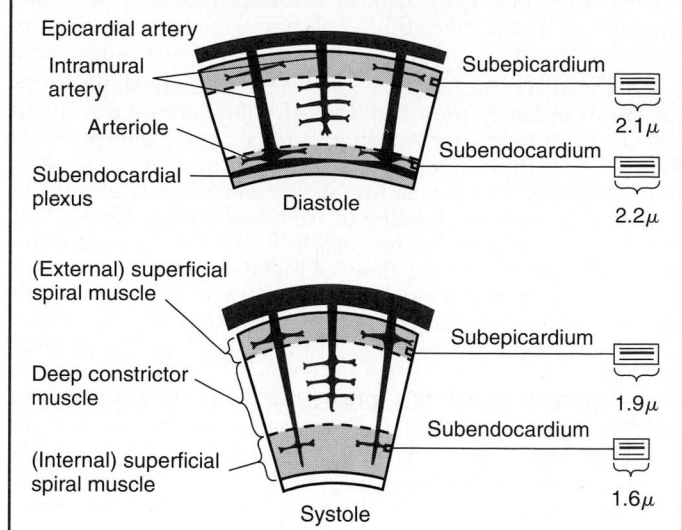

Figure 34–18. Cross-section of the left ventricular wall in diastole and systole. Factors involved in the susceptibility of the subendocardium to the development of ischemia include the greater dependence of this region on diastolic perfusion and the greater degree of shortening, and therefore of energy expenditure, of this region during systole. (From Bell JR, Fox AC: Pathogenesis of subendocardial ischemia. Am J Med Sci 268:2, 1974.)

When the absolute amount of blood flow is restricted, as in the presence of epicardial stenoses, this transmural redistribution leads to a "coronary steal," with the subendocardial flow even falling below resting values. Severe pressure-induced left ventricular hypertrophy,[133] as well as heart failure with elevated left ventricular end-diastolic pressure,[138] may also reduce the endocardial-to-epicardial flow ratio. When the markedly elevated left ventricular end-diastolic pressure in heart failure is corrected, subendocardial coronary flow reserve is restored and the endocardial-to-epicardial flow ratio is normalized.[138] Thus, impairment of endocardial perfusion in heart failure may be a direct consequence of the elevated left ventricular diastolic pressure and the *diastolic* compressive forces exerted on subendocardial perfusion.

A low subendocardial-to-subepicardial flow ratio can be increased by elevation of aortic pressure, which preferentially increases perfusion of the subendocardial region whose arterioles are maximally dilated and in which flow is pressure dependent. Overperfusion of the epicardial region is prevented by autoregulatory arteriolar constriction. Potent vasoconstrictors such as endothelin-1 and alpha-adrenergic agonists[139] or inhibitors of adenosine-induced arteriolar dilation such as theophylline[140] cause arteriolar constriction and redistribution of blood flow to the endocardium. As long as the absolute blood flow is not reduced appreciably, this may result in lessening of myocardial ischemia. Reduction of myocardial oxygen demand, for example by beta blockers, also decreases epicardial blood flow and increases perfusion pressure and thereby flow to the ischemic subendocardial region.[141]

Neural and Neurotransmitter Control

Coronary blood flow is controlled predominantly by local metabolic, autoregulatory and endothelial factors that match coronary blood flow to myocardial oxygen demand and to the driving perfusion pressure. Neural control of the coronary circulation complements these local effects.[142] Epicardial arteries and coronary arterioles are extensively innervated by sympathetic and parasympathetic fibers,[142] and adrenergic and muscarinic receptors are expressed in these locations.[143–145] Investigations of the control of coronary circulation by the autonomic nervous system have been challenging because autonomic activation almost invariably leads to changes in myocardial oxygen demand and, therefore myocardial blood flow, through alterations in heart rate, blood pressure, and contractility. Experiments have been designed to separate the direct from the indirect (metabolic) actions of the sympathetic and the parasympathetic nervous systems. The problems of investigating the sympathetic system are compounded by the opposing actions of vasoconstrictor alpha-adrenergic receptors and vasodilator beta-adrenergic receptors.

Sympathetic Control

ALPHA-ADRENERGIC VASOCONSTRICTION. When its cardiac inotropic and chronotropic actions are blocked by beta-adrenoreceptor antagonists, electrical activation of sympathetic fibers results in coronary vasoconstriction. This constriction is mediated by means of alpha receptors (it is attenuated by alpha-adrenergic antagonists) and competes with metabolic regulation.[142, 142a]

Reflex Alpha-adrenergic Vasoconstriction. The carotid baroreceptor reflex responds to changes in blood pressure. Hypotension leads to activation of sympathetic fibers and inhibition of vagal discharge. The resultant increase in myocardial oxygen demand and blood flow is countered by alpha-adrenergic mediated vasoconstriction.[142, 143] This restraint imposed by the alpha-adrenergic system results in increased myocardial oxygen extraction.[142] In humans, alpha-adrenergic coronary constriction can be demonstrated by activation of another reflex sympathetic pathway by the cold pressor test (immersion of a hand into ice-cold water). In some patients, the cold pressor stimulation results in coronary vasoconstriction that can be blocked by a selective alpha$_1$-adrenergic antagonist.[146]

Alpha-adrenergic coronary vasoconstriction has also been observed during exercise in conscious dogs. During near-maximal exercise in dogs, myocardial oxygen delivery increased markedly but not maximally, because the increase in blood flow was blunted by alpha-adrenergic activation[147] (Fig. 34–19). Feigl has proposed an explanation for the apparent paradox of sympathetic coronary constriction during exercise by its potentially beneficial effects on the transmural distribution of blood in the left ventricular wall.[148] Alpha-adrenergic blockade during exercise results in adverse transmural flow redistribution away from the endocardium.[149] This effect of the alpha-adrenergic activation is not simply due to a reversal of intramural steal but is associated with a reduction in vascular compliance and backward arterial systolic blood flow with each systole.[142]

BETA-ADRENERGIC VASODILATION. Under experimental conditions during which adrenergic activation does not alter myocardial oxygen demand, beta-receptor activation leads to coronary vasodilation. This is mediated predominantly by a beta$_1$ receptor in conduit arteries and by beta$_2$ receptors in resistance arterioles.[142]

PARASYMPATHETIC CONTROL

When myocardial oxygen demand is held constant, stimulation of the parasympathetic nervous system leads to dilation of epicardial arteries and coronary arterioles in dogs[143] and baboons,[150] whereas it leads to constriction in pigs.[151] This species variability can be accounted for by the dual actions of the neurotransmitter acetylcholine, which causes smooth muscle constriction and endothelium-dependent dilation by release of NO and other factors. Although release of acetylcholine from nerve terminals occurs at the medial-adventitial junction, sufficient amount diffuses to stimulate the endothelium. However, in pigs, muscarinic receptors are absent on the endothelium and only smooth muscle constriction is observed. In humans, the coronary response to acetylcholine is vasodilation in healthy subjects. However, vasoconstriction predominates in patients with atherosclerosis or its risk factors.[48]

REFLEX PARASYMPATHETIC VASODILATION. Reflex parasympathetic control has been studied extensively in the canine circulation. Presumably, similar regulation applies to healthy humans with normal

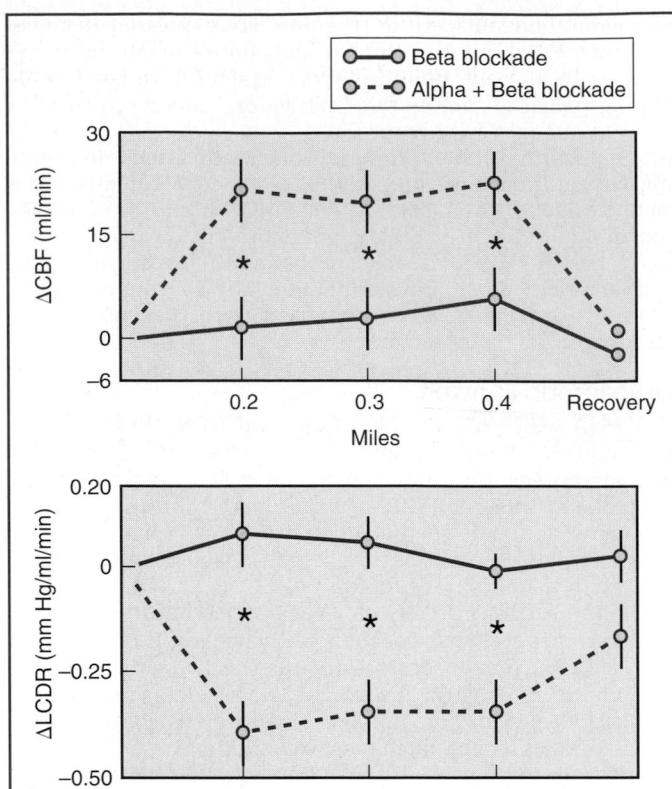

FIGURE 34–19. Comparison of the effects of exercise on changes in mean left circumflex coronary blood flow (CBF, top panel) and late diastolic coronary resistance (LDCR, bottom panel) in the same dogs studied in the presence of beta-adrenergic receptor blockade with propranolol (solid lines) and combined beta- and alpha-adrenergic receptor blockades (broken lines). Increases in coronary blood flow and reductions in coronary resistance were greater after alpha blockade, indicating that sympathetic stimulation increases coronary vascular resistance during exercise by alpha-receptor stimulation. (From Murray PA, Vatner SF: Alpha-adrenoceptor attenuation of the coronary vascular response to severe exercise in conscious dogs. Circ Res 45:654, 1979.)

endothelial function but reflex parasympathetic control has not been characterized in patients with atherosclerosis or its risk factors. In dogs, parasympathetic reflex stimulation leads to coronary vasodilation through several pathways, including (1) carotid baroreceptors that respond to changing blood pressure, (2) carotid bodies that are activated by hypoxia and hypercarbia, and (3) cardiac mechanoreceptors that are stimulated by reduced cardiac filling or small end-systolic volume.[142]

Much remains to be learned about the neural control of the coronary circulation. As was noted previously, coronary arterioles have specialized functions according to their size, a feature that may facilitate finer control of blood flow. It is, therefore, of interest that sympathetic stimulation leads to dilation of the larger arterioles (through the beta-adrenergic system) and constriction of the smaller arterioles.[152] The physiological advantage of this specialized regulation will require further study.

Effects of Coronary Stenoses

Limitation of coronary blood flow imposed by atherosclerosis is related principally to the geometric features of stenoses, including their severity and length, their stiffness or partial distensibility permitting active or passive vasomotion, and the presence of superimposed platelet aggregation and thrombosis.

As blood traverses a stenosis, pressure (energy) is lost. Principles of fluid dynamics have been applied to estimate this pressure loss and validated in animals models as well as in patients. Although the formulas are complex, they can been simplified as follows:

$$\Delta P = \frac{1.8 \cdot Q}{d^4_{sten}} + \frac{6.1 \cdot Q^2}{d^4_{sten}}$$

where ΔP is the pressure drop across a stenosis in millimeters of mercury (mm Hg), Q is the flow across the stenosis in milliliters per second, and d_{sten} is the minimal diameter of the stenosis lumen in millimeters. The first term accounts for viscous friction between layers of fluid in the stenotic segment leading to frictional energy losses. The second term reflects energy losses when the "pressure energy" of normal arterial flow is transferred first to the kinetic energy of high-velocity flow and then, at the exit from the stenosis, to the turbulent energy of distal flow eddies (separation losses due to disturbed laminar flow) (Fig. 34–20).

RELATIONS BETWEEN CORONARY FLOW AND RESISTANCE. At normal levels of coronary arterial flow, both frictional and separation losses contribute to the stenosis resistance and to the presence of a pressure gradient. As flow increases, separation losses, which increase with the square of the flow, become increasingly prominent and viscous losses become negligible. Thus, increases in blood flow and pressure drops across the stenosis are related in an exponential manner (Fig. 34–21). Augmentation of coronary blood flow is associated with elevations in pressure gradient across the stenotic orifice and reductions in poststenotic perfusion pressure (driving pressure for myocardial perfusion).

Brown and colleagues[153] have called attention to several common clinical situations in which reduction in poststenotic pressure contributes to the pathogenesis of myocardial ischemia. First, pharmacological dilators of coronary resistance arterioles, such as adenosine or dipyramidole, increase transstenotic blood flow and reduce poststenotic pressure. When subendocardial resistance vessels become near fully dilated their perfusion becomes pressure dependent (autoregulation fails). Redistribution of flow away from the subendocardium to the subepicardium develops. This is one mechanism of "coronary steal." Second, during physical activity, coronary blood flow rises to meet the increase in myocardial oxygen demand, leading to an increase in transstenotic pressure gradient and a fall in the distal perfusion pressure. This results in a reduction of blood flow from to the subendocardium while the flow to the subepicardium continues to increase, an effect similar to that observed with the administration of pharmacological vasodilators. Furthermore, the fall in intraluminal distending pressure may lead to a passive collapse of the artery at the site of the obstruction, exaggerating the degree of stenosis. Third, the reduced oxygen-carrying capacity of anemia is

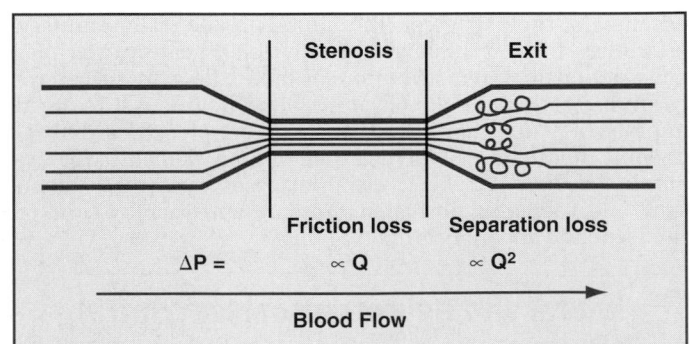

FIGURE 34–20. Energy losses across a stenosis. The pressure gradient due to friction losses within the stenosis (ΔP) is directly proportional to blood flow (Q), whereas separation losses at the exit to the stenosis due to formation of eddies increase with blood flow squared (Q^2). Separation losses predominate at high blood flows.

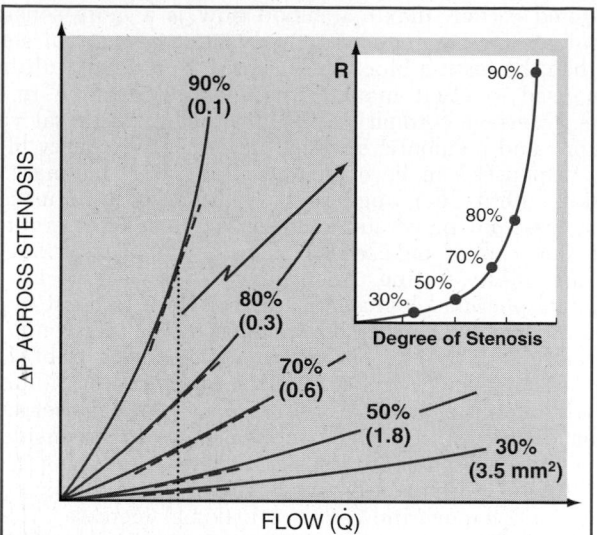

FIGURE 34–21. Relation between pressure reduction across a stenosis (ΔP) and flow through the stenosis (Q). Relations are shown for concentric stenoses of 30, 50, 70, 80, and 90 percent internal diameter. The numbers in parentheses below each percent diameter stenosis represent residual luminal cross-sectional area, calculated on the basis of a normal internal diameter of 3 mm and cross-sectional area of 7.1 mm². The level of flow corresponding to basal metabolic needs is represented by the vertical dotted line; stenosis resistances for this level of flow are shown as the dashed tangent lines to the individual pressure-flow relations. In the inset at right, stenosis resistance (R) is plotted as a function of degree of stenosis. (From Klocke FJ: Measurements of coronary blood flow and degree of stenosis: Current clinical implications and continuing uncertainties. Newsletter of the Council on Clinical Cardiology of the American Heart Association. Vol 7, No. 3, July 1982.)

compensated for by increase in coronary blood flow because the myocardium cannot increase its oxygen extraction significantly. This decreases poststenotic pressure and compromises subendocardial perfusion. Not surprisingly, therefore, anemia is poorly tolerated in patients with coronary artery disease.

SEVERITY OF STENOSIS. At any level of blood flow, the single most important determinant of stenosis resistance is the minimum diameter of the stenosis. The transstenotic pressure drop is inversely proportional to the *fourth* power of the minimum luminal diameter. As a consequence, a relatively small change in luminal diameter (such as caused by active or passive vasomotion) is amplified to produce marked hemodynamic effects in the presence of severe stenoses (see Fig. 34–21). For example, when the diameter stenosis is increased from 80 to 90 percent, the resistance of a stenosis rises nearly threefold.

ENTRANCE AND EXIT EFFECTS. Blood flow velocity (kinetic energy) increases and pressure (static energy) decreases in a narrowed arterial segment. The conversion of static to kinetic energy would occur with little loss of energy if the flow remained laminar, according to the Bernoulli principle. Laminar flow can be preserved if the entrance and the exit of the stenotic segment taper gradually. However, most stenoses have abrupt transitions where energy losses associated with separation of laminar flow into eddy currents (vortices) occurs. The separation energy losses are particularly pronounced at the exits of stenoses.

LENGTH OF STENOSES. For most stenoses, the length of the narrowing has only a modest effect on its physiological significance. However, in very long narrowed segments, significant turbulence occurs along the wall of the stenotic segment and energy is dissipated as heat when eddies impact on the wall; stenosis may become important under these conditions.

DYNAMIC CHANGES IN STENOSIS SEVERITY. Examination of the morphology of pressure-fixed human coronary arteries has revealed eccentricity of atherosclerotic plaques. In many cases, plaques involve only a portion of the arterial wall whereas the remaining arc of the wall is relatively normal and often compliant. This provides a mechanism by which changes in vascular tone may alter luminal caliber and stenosis resistance. For example, most atherosclerotic stenoses in patients can dilate actively in response to nitroglycerin or constrict in response to acetylcholine, ergovine, or alpha-adrenergic stimuli.

Dynamic changes in stenosis severity and resistance can also occur passively due to alterations in intraluminal distending pressure. Such changes can be demonstrated both in experimental models and in patients with coronary artery disease. As blood flow velocity rises in the stenotic segments, distending pressure falls, leading to passive collapse of a pliable segment. Passive collapse of a stenosis associated with the use of vasodilators occurs with agents that selectively dilate distal resistance vessels. The administration of dipyridamole to patients with coronary artery disease can cause narrowing of severely stenotic pliable segments as well as of the normal arterial segments distal to the stenoses. Passive collapse of pliable stenoses may also occur when central aortic pressure is lowered.

EFFECTS OF CORONARY STENOSIS IN THE INTACT CORONARY BED. The physiological effect of a coronary stenosis depends on the degree to which the resistance to flow caused by the stenosis can be compensated for by dilation of arterioles distal to the stenosis. Gould and Lipsomb concluded that in normal dogs, resting coronary flow is not altered until the constriction reaches at least 85 percent of the diameter. Therefore, resting coronary flow is not impeded by mild or moderate stenoses and is an insensitive measure for evaluation of coronary artery disease. *Maximal* coronary blood flow, however, begins to decline when diameter stenosis exceeds 30 to 45 percent (Fig. 34–22). The capacity to increase coronary blood flow in response to

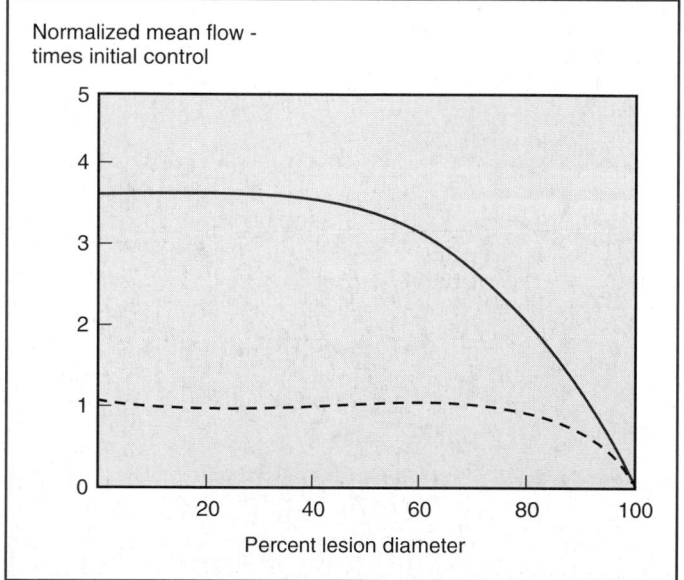

FIGURE 34–22. Relationship between resting (dashed line) and maximal coronary blood flow (solid line) and percentage of diameter stenosis in a dog. Progressive coronary stenosis was achieved by progressively narrowing a short segment of a proximal coronary artery. Resting coronary blood flow did not change until coronary diameter stenosis exceeded 80 percent. (From Marcus ML: The Coronary Circulation in Health and Disease. New York, McGraw-Hill, 1983, and modified from Gould KL, Lipscomb L: Effects of coronary stenoses on coronary flow reserve and resistance. Am J Cardiol 34:50, 1974.)

increased oxygen demand is abolished when diameter stenosis exceeds 90 percent.

Insights derived from such animal studies must be applied cautiously in clinical practice. The simple use of relative percent diameter stenosis determined by coronary arteriography has important limitations, because it does not account for other geometric characteristics of the stenosis such as its absolute diameter, length, entrance and exit angles, or eccentricity. The determination of relative percent diameter narrowing may be misleading in the setting of diffuse disease where segments adjacent to the stenosis are also reduced in caliber. The hemodynamic effects of serial stenoses are also difficult to assess from arteriograms. It is not surprising, then, that the correlation between percent diameter stenosis and the physiological significance of a given obstruction in patients is poor, especially for lesions of moderate severity.[154-158]

Coronary Flow Reserve and Reactive Hyperemia

Severe myocardial ischemia produces maximal coronary dilation.[159] Therefore, when a coronary artery is occluded, release of the occlusion is followed by a marked increase in coronary flow. This response is termed *reactive hyperemia* (Fig. 34-23). Reactive hyperemia follows an occlusion as short at 200 milliseconds. *Maximal reactive hyperemia* follows coronary occlusion of 20 seconds. Longer occlusion increases the duration but not the amplitude of the hyperemic response.

Reactive hyperemia is partly a response driven by a requirement to repay oxygen debt. However, the hyperemic response is less pronounced when coronary arteries are perfused with deoxygenated blood for the same duration.[160] This suggests that factors other than the mere lack of oxygen stimulate the hyperemic response, including the local accumulation of adenosine (see p. 1090), prostacyclin (see p. 1095) and NO (see p. 1090–1094).[28]

After the release of coronary occlusion, the coronary resistance vessels are maximally dilated. Under this condition, autoregulation is abolished and coronary blood flow is directly related to the driving pressure. Therefore, maximal hyperemic coronary blood flow is closely dependent on the coronary arterial (or central aortic) pressure at the time of the measurement.[161]

Assessment of the Physiological Significance of Coronary Stenoses

Because of the limitations inherent in coronary angiography, attention has been directed to using physiological approaches for determining the severity of coronary stenoses.

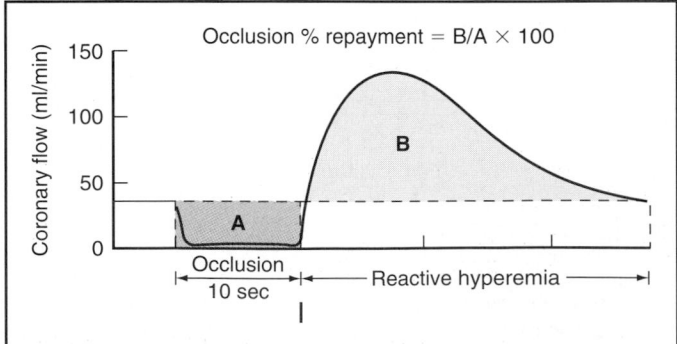

FIGURE 34–23. Mean coronary flow before, during, and after coronary occlusion. Arrow indicates the release of occlusion. Area A represents the flow debt, and area B its repayment. (From Gould KL: Coronary Artery Stenosis. New York, Elsevier, 1991, p 13.)

As noted earlier, maximal blood flow is a more sensitive stimulus for assessing the hemodynamic severity of stenoses than the resting blood flow. Three types of stimuli have been used to elicit maximal coronary blood flow in humans: transient coronary occlusion, pharmacological vasodilators, and metabolic stresses. In humans, coronary blood flow responses can be evaluated after a brief coronary occlusion with balloon angioplasty.[162] A potent stimulus causing a threefold or greater increase in blood flow coronary occlusion cannot be used for diagnostic purposes outside the angioplasty setting. Adenosine and papaverine are the principal pharmacological vasodilators used to elicit hyperemia. Adenosine can be administered by the intravenous or intracoronary route. It has a rapid onset and a brief duration of action and is generally safe. Papaverine is administered by the intracoronary route. It has a slower onset and a longer duration of action. Although it has been considered to be the gold standard for maximally stimulating blood flow, it tends to have more side effects. In appropriate concentrations, papaverine causes a maximal increase in coronary blood flow similar to that obtained with reactive hyperemia after balloon angioplasty.[162] Intense treadmill or bicycle exercise, a potent metabolic stimulus, also yield near maximal flow increases. Exercise is the most physiological stress particularly suited for the noninvasive laboratory, but it is difficult to apply at the time of catheterization. Rapid atrial pacing produces only modest, submaximal increases in coronary blood flow.[163]

INVASIVE MEASUREMENT OF FLOW RESERVE. Several techniques for determining coronary flow reserve have been developed for use during cardiac catheterization. Doppler wires have a miniaturized Doppler crystal placed at the tip of an angioplasty guidewire, permitting measurement of phasic and mean coronary blood flow velocities.[155, 164] Because this technique does not measure absolute coronary blood flow, several indices of flow *velocity* have been used for assessing the physiological significance of coronary stenoses. Coronary flow velocity reserve is the ratio of maximum to baseline flow velocity. Patients with a coronary flow velocity ratio less than 2 typically have other, corroborating evidence of myocardial ischemia[165] and improve symptomatically with revascularization. Conversely, patients with a ratio greater than 2 usually lack other objective evidence of myocardial ischemia and have a favorable outcome with conservative management (Fig. 34–24). Hence, flow velocity measurements can be helpful in the management of patients with coronary lesions of intermediate severity. Diastolic to systolic velocity ratio has also been used to evaluate stenosis severity. While in normal arteries, diastolic flow velocity far exceeds systolic velocity, the two are more equal distal to significant stenoses. A ratio less than 1.7 has been used to define significant coronary lesions.[166]

During coronary interventions, the Doppler guidewire can be used to judge the adequacy with which stenosis severity has been reduced. Patients with higher coronary flow reserve at completion of the procedure have a lower incidence of abrupt reocclusion and restenosis.[167]

Myocardial fractional flow reserve (FFR) is a recently developed index of the functional severity of coronary stenoses that is calculated only from simultaneous pressure measurements proximal and distal to a stenosis obtained with a pressure monitoring guidewire.[168] FFR represents the fraction of the normal maximal coronary flow that can be achieved in an artery in which flow is restricted by a coronary stenosis. The concept of FFR is founded in the observation noted previously, that during maximal hyperemia, myocardial perfusion is entirely pressure dependent. Therefore, maximal blood flow in the presence of a stenosis is determined by the driving pressure distal to the stenosis (P_d) while the theoretical normal maximal blood flow is determined by the pressure proximal to the stenosis (P_p).

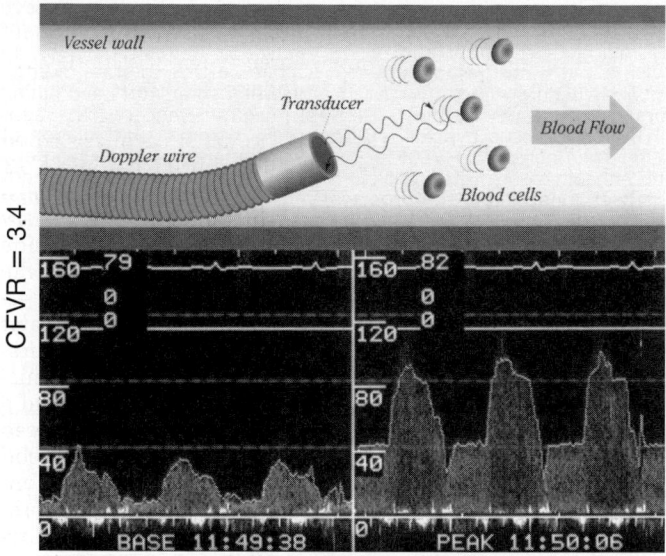

Baseline Adenosine I.C.

FIGURE 34–24. Recording of blood flow velocity using a Doppler wire (schematic illustration in top panel) in the left anterior descending artery of a patient with an "intermediate" stenosis by angiography and exercise testing negative for ischemia. Blood flow velocity increased 3.5-fold after intracoronary (I.C.) adenosine (right lower panel) compared with baseline (left lower panel). Coronary flow velocity ratio (CFVR) = 3.5 indicates that the "intermediate" stenosis is not hemodynamically significant.

FFR is calculated during maximal hyperemia, obtained with adenosine or papaverine as

$$FFR = Pd/Pp.$$

FFR less than 0.75 is typically associated with other objective evidence of myocardial ischemia (Fig. 34–25). Measurement of FFR in patients with coronary stenoses of moderate severity has been shown to be a useful index of the functional severity of the stenoses and the need for coronary revascularization.[158, 169, 170] Measurement of FFR can

also guide the adequacy of reducing coronary stenosis severity with balloon angioplasty[171] or stenting.[172]

NONINVASIVE MEASUREMENT OF FLOW RESERVE. Radionuclide stress myocardial perfusion imaging (thallium-201, sestamibi) is used widely to quantify coronary flow reserve (see Chap. 9). Some laboratories are using positron-emission tomography and nuclear magnetic resonance imaging for the same purpose.[173, 174] Flow reserve is typically assessed by these techniques during exercise or with pharmacological coronary vasodilators. In contrast to invasive techniques that measure an index of *absolute* flow reserve (an index related to the quotient of maximal and basal flow), cardiac imaging techniques assess *relative* coronary flow reserve by comparing the perfusion of ischemic regions of the left ventricle with presumably normally perfused reference regions.

Imaging techniques yield a less quantitative index of flow reserve than do catheter-based techniques. In addition, results can be misleading in the setting of diffuse coronary disease when a normal reference region is not available. However, unlike most measures of absolute flow reserve, relative flow reserve is independent of the loading conditions, because these affect all regions of the left ventricle equally. Taken together, absolute and relative coronary flow reserve provide a more complete description of physiological stenosis severity than does either alone.[175]

STENOSIS SEVERITY AND CLINICAL EVENTS. There is a poor correlation between the severity of stenoses and their propensity to cause myocardial infarction, unstable angina, or sudden coronary death. Pathological studies have revealed that myocardial infarctions and unstable angina are most often caused by rupture of atherosclerotic plaques with formation of a superimposed occlusive thrombus (see Chap. 35). The majority of atherosclerotic lesions responsible for these serious events are mild stenoses of inconsequential hemodynamic significance and are characterized by abundance of lipid, numerous inflammatory cells, and a thin, fragile fibrous cap.[75, 78, 176] These observations suggest that although measurements of coronary flow reserve may be useful in the assessment of the severity of stenoses and in the identification of lesions responsible for effort angina, they are *not* likely to identify the more dangerous plaques responsible for unstable angina, acute myocardial infarction, and ischemic sudden death.

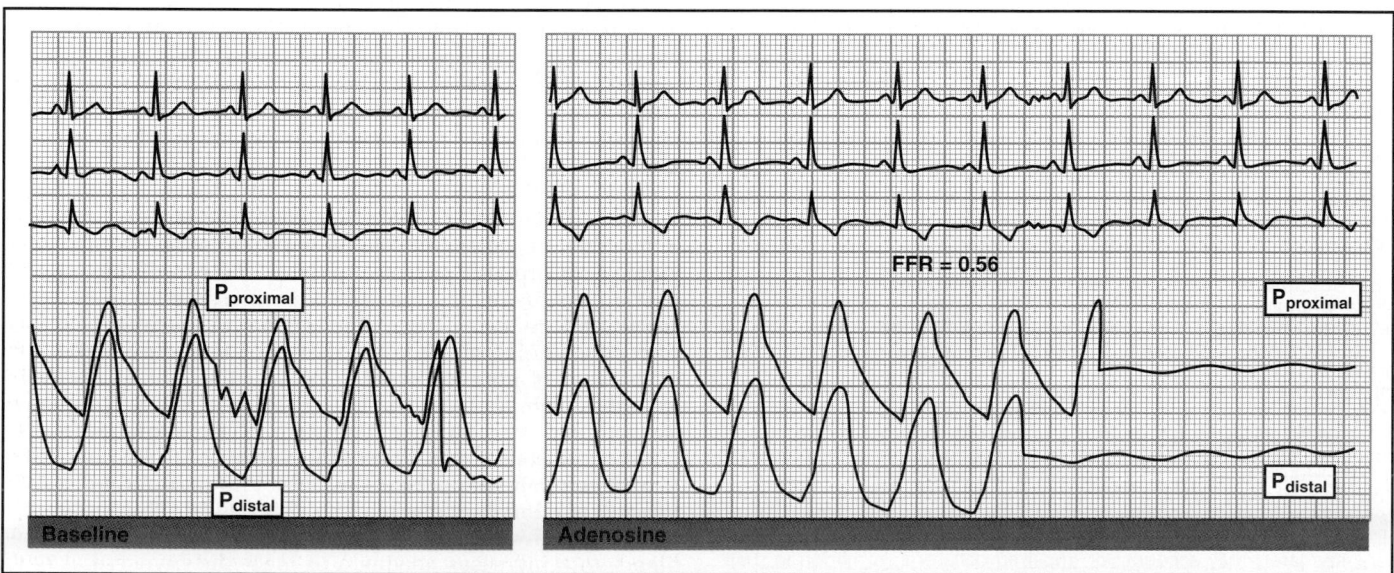

FIGURE 34–25. Recording of arterial pressure (P) proximal to (by means of coronary catheter) and distal to (by means of a pressure wire) an "intermediate" stenosis in the left anterior descending coronary artery of a patient with exercise test positive for ischemia. Fractional flow reserve (FFR, a ratio of distal-to-proximal pressure after adenosine) = 0.56 indicates that the "intermediate" stenosis is hemodynamically significant.

CORONARY COLLATERAL CIRCULATION AND ANGIOGENESIS

Coronary Collateral Vessels

After total or near-total occlusion or a coronary artery, perfusion of ischemic myocardium occurs by way of collaterals—vascular channels that interconnect epicardial arteries.[177] Preexisting collaterals are thin-walled structures ranging in diameter from 20 to 200 μm.[178] The density of preexisting collaterals varies greatly among different species.[179] Acute coronary occlusion produces no infarction at all in guinea pigs because of an exceptionally well developed network of preexisting collaterals. The dog has an intermediate density of preexisting collaterals that can deliver, on average, 5 to 10 percent of preocclusional, basal flow. Pigs, rats, and rabbits have virtually no preexisting collaterals, and infarcts develop rapidly and completely with acute coronary occlusion.[179] The density of preexisting collateral channels in humans appears to be somewhat more modest than in dogs.

COLLATERAL FORMATION (ARTERIOGENESIS)

Preexisting collaterals are normally closed and nonfunctional, because no pressure gradient exists between the arteries they connect. After coronary occlusion, the distal pressure drops precipitously and preexisting collaterals open virtually instantly. The transformation of preexisting collaterals into mature collaterals is called *arteriogenesis* and occurs in three stages. The initial stage (first 24 hours) involves *passive widening* of the preexisting channels facilitating increased flow. Endothelial cells become *activated* by increased blood flow velocity and shear stress and secrete proteolytic enzymes that fragment the basement membrane and dissolve extracellular matrix, an essential process in the upcoming migration of endothelial cells.[180] The second stage (1 day to 3 weeks) is characterized by *inflammation and cellular proliferation*.[177, 178, 181–183]

Monocytes migrate into the vascular wall and secrete cytokines and growth factors. This phase of vascular enlargement is marked by cellular proliferation involving the endothelium, smooth muscle cells, and fibroblasts.[177, 184] Endothelial cells and inflammatory cells also secrete matrix degrading enzymes, which create spaces necessary to accommodate the expanded collateral vessels as well as facilitate cell migration. These enzymes belong to the plasminogen activator/plasmin and matrix metalloproteinase families.[185, 186] Additional space for the larger vessels is created by the process of apoptosis.[177, 187] Over several weeks, endothelial and smooth muscle cells arrange themselves into circular and longitudinal layers. During these first two phases, the luminal diameter of collateral channels increases nearly 10-fold. The third stage of collateral maturation (3 weeks to 6 months) involves thickening of the vessel wall due to *deposition of extracellular matrix* and further cellular proliferation.[177] In its final stage, the mature collateral vessel may reach 1 mm in luminal diameter. Its three-layer structure is nearly indistinguishable from a normal coronary artery of the same size.[177, 178]

MECHANISMS PROMOTING COLLATERAL GROWTH

SHEAR STRESS. Mechanical forces determine the size of collateral channels in the early minutes and hours after coronary occlusion. Pressure gradients across preexisting rudimentary collaterals augment blood flow velocity and shear stress. Shear stress induces widespread functional changes in the endothelium, many of which reflect new gene expression. These include upregulation in leukocyte adhesion molecules[188] and increased production of proinflammatory cytokines (monocyte chemoattractant protein-1, tumor necrosis factor-alpha, granulocyte-macrophage colony-stimulating factor).[184] The end result of this process is an inflammatory environment.

INFLAMMATION. Inflammatory cells are a rich source of matrix degrading enzymes (see earlier) and growth factors.[189] The invasion of inflammatory cells is rapidly followed by mitosis of endothelial and smooth muscle cells.[181]

GROWTH FACTORS. More than 15 growth factors that can stimulate collateral growth (arteriogenesis) or angiogenesis have been identified.[180, 190] Among these, vascular endothelial growth factor (VEGF) and fibroblast growth factor (FGF) are believed to play the most important roles in vivo. Angiogenesis in response to VEGF is mediated by NO, and deficiency of NO (e.g., in the presence of coronary risk factors; see later) may account for impaired collateral formation in that setting.[191]

INHIBITORY FACTORS. Growth factors can be detected in adult tissues in which endothelial cells are quiescent. Absence of angiogenesis in the presence of growth-promoting factors can be partly attributed to the presence of endogenous inhibitors of this process.[180] Potent angiogenesis inhibitors include angiostatin (a fragment of plasminogen),[192] endostatin (a proteolytic fragment of collagen XVIII),[193] and thrombospondin-1.[194] It is believed that the rate of angiogenesis is determined by a balance between stimulators and inhibitors.[194a]

HYPOXIA. Tissue hypoxia is associated with rapid upregulation of VEGF. This increase in VEGF occurs by augmented mRNA synthesis and enhancement of its stability.[184, 195, 196] A hypoxia-sensitive element has been identified in the promoter region of VEGF gene.[197] Furthermore, hypoxia upregulates the number of VEGF receptors.[198] This latter observation may provide an explanation by which intravenous administration of growth factors could induce angiogenesis preferentially and selectively in ischemic tissues.

Nevertheless, hypoxia is not likely an essential requirement for the formation of collaterals. In many cases, the collateral artery originates from a vessel far removed from the site of ischemia.[184]

SEVERITY OF OBSTRUCTION. The severity of coronary obstruction is a critical determinant of the development of coronary collateral channels. In dogs, the growth of collaterals is not stimulated until a coronary stenosis reduces the luminal cross-sectional area by at least 80 percent. In patients, coronary collaterals do not develop until a coronary stenosis of at least 70 percent diameter narrowing is present. Beyond this threshold value, the growth of collateral channels is directly related to the severity of stenosis.[199]

CORONARY RISK FACTORS. Patients with diabetes mellitus have an impaired ability to develop collateral blood vessels in the setting of obstructive coronary artery disease.[200] Similarly, rabbits with experimental hyperlipidemia have a limited collateral growth in response to arterial restriction.[201] Thus, the same risk factors that predispose to atherosclerosis may limit a major compensatory mechanism—formation of collateral pathways.

EXERCISE. This has no effect on the preexisting (rudimentary) collaterals in the absence of coronary occlusions or stenoses. Even in the presence of severe coronary stenoses, the effects of exercise training have been inconsistent and overall neutral in animals.[179] In the clinical studies that used serial angiographic follow-up, increase in collaterals occurred with progression in the severity of coronary artery stenoses, rather than with long-term exercise programs.[202] The reduction of myocardial ischemia associated with exercise is likely the result of improved conditioning.

REGULATION OF COLLATERAL TONE. The mature coronary collaterals can appreciably dilate or constrict in respond to vasoactive stimuli. The release of endogenous vasodilators NO[203] and prostacyclin maintains collaterals in a dilated state. Conditions that reduce endothelium-derived NO, including coronary risk factors, may reduce the dilator reserve of coronary collaterals, a condition correctable by the administration of exogenous nitrates.[203]

Conversely, serotonin[204] and vasopressin[205] constrict collaterals. Serotonin is released into the circulation during episodes of ischemia triggered by platelet aggregation or thrombosis and may exacerbate myocardial ischemia by reducing collateral blood flow.

CORONARY COLLATERALS IN PATIENTS WITH CORONARY ARTERY DISEASE. Because coronary collaterals develop in patients whose symptoms of angina pectoris tend to be severe,[199] controversy arose in the past about their clinical utility.[179] However, it is now clear that coronary collaterals can mitigate the severity of myocardial ischemia[206] and, in acute myocardial infarction, collateral circulation can contribute significant amount of blood flow, decrease infarct size, improve left ventricular function, reduce the likelihood of left ventricular aneurysm formation, and improve survival.[207, 208]

Recently, it has become possible to quantify collateral blood flow in conscious humans undergoing coronary angioplasty. Coronary pressure distal to the site of angioplasty balloon occlusion (coronary wedge pressure) can be measured and reflects recruitable collateral perfusion.[209] Patients in whom recruitable collateral blood flow exceeded 28 percent of normal maximal myocardial blood flow were free of ischemia at the time of coronary occlusion induced by balloon angioplasty. Conversely, ischemia was frequently present at the time of coronary occlusion when recruitable collateral blood flow was less than 28 percent of normal maximal myocardial blood flow.[209] This approach has also shown that collateral circulation rarely provides blood flow increases adequate to meet the myocardial oxygen demand of maximal physical exercise; it is typically limited to less than 50 percent of maximal coronary flow reserve.[209]

Angiogenesis

Arteriogenesis (discussed earlier) refers to formation of mature collaterals by enlargement of *preexisting rudimentary collaterals*. Typically, epicardial collaterals fall into this category. *Angiogenesis* refers to *sprouting of new vessels* from preexisting blood vessels and usually results in formation of smaller, capillary-like structures. Subendocardial collaterals may be formed in this manner. In *therapeutic angiogenesis*, exogenous angiogenic growth factors (or genes encoding these growth factors) are administered to stimulate neovascularization of ischemic issues.[177, 190, 210, 210a]

MECHANISMS OF ANGIOGENESIS. Angiogenic stimuli initiate activation of endothelial cells of capillaries or post-capillary venules. This results in local vasodilation, increased vascular permeability, and degradation of the basement membrane. Migration and proliferation of endothelial cells occurs with formation of capillary sprouts. Furthermore, endothelial proliferation elongates the sprouts and adjacent sprouts connect to form capillary loops that can carry blood flow. Maturation of the sprouts is associated with deposition of basement membrane.[180]

THERAPEUTIC ANGIOGENESIS: PRECLINICAL STUDIES. Preclinical studies in several animal species have established that angiogenic growth factors can promote formation of new collateral channels in models of peripheral and myocardial ischemia.[190, 210] The angiogenic growth factors used in these studies were administered as recombinant protein or by gene transfer and included vascular endothelial growth factor (VEGF), fibroblast growth factor-1 (FGF-1) and FGF-2, hepatocyte growth factor (HGF), and hypoxia inducible factor-1 (HIF-1). Each of these growth factors can stimulate the critical steps in angiogenesis, including endothelial activation and mitogenesis and upregulation of matrix proteins and matrix proteinases.[210]

Much interest has focused on the role of VEGF because it is a potent angiogenic factor and because the receptors for VEGF are relatively specific for endothelial cells.[211] This specificity favors a targeted therapeutic response and limits the potential for pathological angiogenesis.[190] Four forms of VEGF are formed by alternative splicing of the messenger RNA from a single gene. These forms encode for protein molecules of 121, 165, 189, and 206 amino acids that vary in heparin-binding properties and therefore the avidity with which they bind to cell membranes and extracellular matrix. All forms of VEGF are mitogenic for endothelial cells.

FGF comprises a family of growth factors that are potent stimulants of angiogenesis. Unlike VEGF, FGF also stimulates the proliferation of smooth muscle cells and fibroblasts.

Although potentially associated with adverse effects, stimulation of smooth muscle cell growth and its incorporation into the vascular wall might permit formation of a muscular conduits resembling true collaterals rather than capillaries.

The initial demonstration by Isner and colleagues that intraarterial injection of VEGF augmented collateral formation in the ischemic rabbit hind limb has generated great interest in therapeutic angiogenesis[212] (Fig. 34–26). Therapeutic angiogenesis has since been carried out successfully in several animal species for the treatment of peripheral ischemia using intraarterial and intramuscular routes of injection and for the treatment of myocardial ischemia using intracoronary, intravenous, intrapericardial, and intramyocardial routes of administration. In the rabbit hind limb model, morphometric analysis has revealed a significant increase in capillary density, accompanied by an increase in vascular conductance (a reduction in resistance).[181] Premortem angiography has also demonstrated growth of larger collaterals.[210] Whether these formed from preexisting rudimentary collaterals by arteriogenesis or whether they are

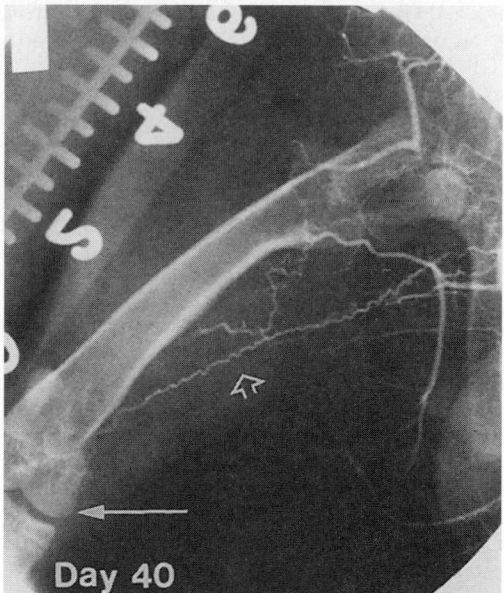

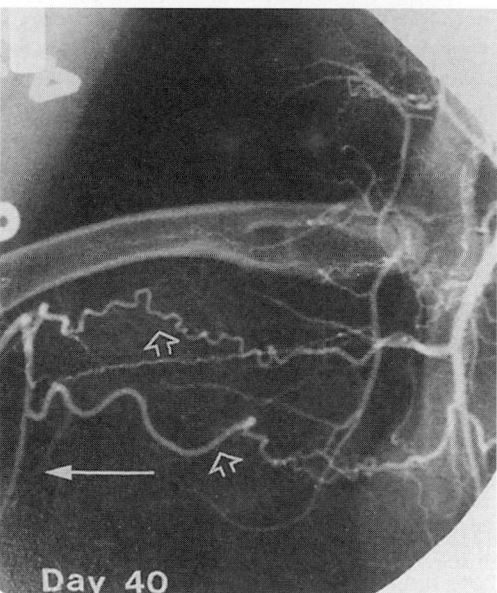

FIGURE 34–26. Selective internal iliac angiography of control rabbit performed at day 40 (control, untreated, top) and of vascular endothelial growth factor (VEGF)-treated rabbit at day 40 (bottom). VEGF was administered as a single intraarterial bolus into the internal iliac artery of rabbits with severe ipsilateral ischemia. The angiogram shown here has yielded angiographic scores of 0.17 and 0.41. Distal reconstitution, barely apparent in the control group (arrows), was evident in the VEGF-treated group (arrows). Direct and linear extension of internal iliac artery to popliteal and/or saphenous arteries was also more evident in the VEGF-treated group (open arrows). (From Takeshita S, et al: Therapeutic angiogenesis. J Clin Invest 93:662, 1994. Copyright, 1994 American Society of Clinical Investigation.)

newly vessels formed by angiogenesis remains to be determined.

THERAPEUTIC ANGIOGENESIS: CLINICAL STUDIES. Demonstration of successful angiogenesis in preclinical studies has led to its application in a number of small-scale trials. In patients with critical limb ischemia, the administration of VEGF by intramuscular injection of plasmid DNA resulted in improved angiographic evidence of collateral blood flow, healing of ulcers, and resolution of rest pain.[213] In another study, administration of FGF improved blood flow to the calf and reduced the symptoms of intermittent claudication.[190] In patients with ischemic heart disease, administration of intramyocardial or intracoronary growth factors (VEGF or FGF) led to an improvement in myocardial perfusion and apparent reduction in symptoms.[214, 215] These early uncontrolled results, while exciting, need to be validated by controlled, randomized trials.

A number of issues will have to be addressed systematically to optimize therapeutic angiogenesis. These involve methodology (e.g., optimal angiogenic factor(s) and synergistic combinations; methods of delivery and dosing schedule) and potential for pathological angiogenesis at undesired sites (e.g., growth of tumors, proliferative retinopathy, progression of atherosclerosis). Furthermore, further advances in the understanding of the biology of angiogenesis are needed to create muscular collaterals with large perfusion capacity rather than a blush of capillaries.

THERAPEUTIC VASCULOGENESIS. *Vasculogenesis* is the formation of new blood vessels that typically occurs during early embryonic development. Endothelial stem cells and circulating endothelial precursors, angioblasts, may persist into adult life.[216] The concept that circulating angioblasts could be harvested and used to create new blood vessels in adults is under investigation.[210]

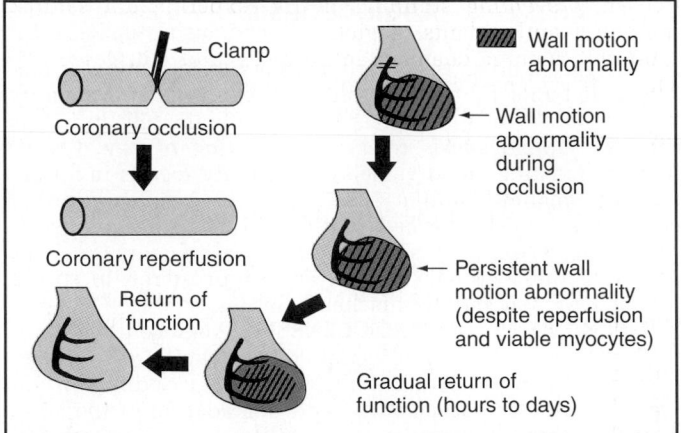

FIGURE 34–27. Schematic diagram of stunned myocardium. During coronary occlusion, a wall motion abnormality of the left ventricle is present in the region supplied by the occluded artery. With relief of ischemia and reestablishment of coronary blood flow, there is a persistent wall motion abnormality despite reperfusion and viable myocytes. There is then gradual improvement in function that requires hours to days for recovery. (From Kloner RA, Przyklenk K, Patel B: Altered myocardial states: The stunned and hibernating myocardium. Am J Med 86[Suppl 1A]:14, 1986.)

CONSEQUENCES OF MYOCARDIAL ISCHEMIA

Myocardial Stunning (See also Chap. 14)

For four decades after Tennant and Wiggers's classic observation on the effects of coronary occlusion on myocardial contraction,[217] it was believed that transient severe ischemia caused either irreversible cardiac injury, that is, infarction, or prompt recovery. However, in the 1970s Heyndrickx and colleagues reported that regional contraction remained depressed for more that 3 hours after a 5-minute coronary occlusion and for more than 6 hours after a 15-minute occlusion in conscious dogs.[218] It became clear that after a brief episode of severe ischemia, prolonged myocardial dysfunction with gradual return of contractile activity occurs, a condition termed *myocardial stunning* (Fig. 34–27). Subsequently, myocardial stunning was observed by other investigators under a variety of additional experimental conditions, including multiple, brief episodes of ischemia; prolonged ischemia resulting in an admixture of myocardial necrosis and stunning of adjacent, viable myocardium; global myocardial ischemia (e.g., cardioplegia arrest); and stunning after exercise-induced ischemia.[219–221]

Myocardial stunning has been observed in patients with coronary artery disease in a variety of clinical conditions. It also has been observed after exercise-induced ischemia.

Persistent wall motion abnormalities can be observed by echocardiography at a time when chest pain, ST segment deviation, and regional perfusion had recovered.[219, 222] It affects both systolic and diastolic function.[223]

Clinically, global myocardial stunning occurs most frequently in patients who have undergone ischemic cardiac arrest during cardiopulmonary bypass, despite modern cardioplegia techniques.[224] Such hearts may not recover for days, and many patients require inotropic support. In patients with a myocardial infarction (both with and without the administration of thrombolytic therapy), stunned myocardium lies adjacent to infarcted myocardium. Improvement in ventricular function occurs gradually over the course of days to weeks.[219, 221] Myocardial stunning is also an important feature of unstable angina.[225]

Coronary angioplasty in patients parallels the observations in animal studies of brief coronary occlusion and reperfusion and provides a useful clinical model of stunning. Occlusions of 1 minute or less induce diastolic dysfunc-

tion, whereas longer occlusions (over 5 minutes) induce systolic dysfunction that persists 24 to 36 hours.[219]

CELLULAR AND MOLECULAR MECHANISMS OF STUNNING. A number of factors converge in the pathogenesis of myocardial stunning (see Fig. 14–35). Probably, the three most important are (1) generation of oxygen derived free radials, (2) calcium overload, and (3) reduced sensitivity of myofilaments to calcium and loss of myofilaments.[219, 220] These mechanisms interact synergistically in the pathophysiological process of stunning.

Transient myocardial ischemia followed by reperfusion results in increased production of superoxide radicals and hydroxyl radicals. Free radicals inactivate enzymes and cause lipid peroxidation. The generation of free radicals in the ischemia-reperfusion setting has been documented by a direct measurement (spin-trapping and aromatic hydroxylation techniques) and by reduction of stunning with administration of antioxidants. The damaging free radicals are generated in the first minute after reperfusion as antioxidant therapy can reduce stunning if administered at the time of reperfusion but not if it is begun 1 minute later. The presumed targets of oxygen derived free radicals include sarcolemmal Na^+,K^+-ATPase and calcium-stimulated ATPase and, in the sarcoplasmic reticulum, calcium-stimulated ATPase. The result is increased influx of calcium through the sarcolemma, diminished calcium reuptake by the sarcoplasmic reticulum resulting in cellular calcium overload, and, ultimately, in impaired excitation-contraction coupling.[219, 220] Calcium overload can also activate enzymes that further damage the sarcolemma and sarcoplasmic reticulum. Ischemia followed by reperfusion also results in decreased calcium sensitivity of myofilaments, at least in part due to oxidation of critical thiol groups and in part due to partial proteolysis of troponin.[219, 220, 226] Recent evidence suggests that calcium overload may activate calpains, resulting in selective proteolysis of myofibrils.[220]

Although antioxidants are effective, they do not prevent stunning completely. It has been postulated that stunning involves two components, one related to ischemia (not responsive to antioxidants) and a larger component related to reperfusion.[219]

TREATMENT OF MYOCARDIAL STUNNING. Myocardial stunning is an important clinical problem because it contributes to heart failure. Various therapies have been effective in *preventing* stunning in the experimental setting, including antioxidants, angiotensin-converting enzyme inhibitors, calcium channel antagonists, and nitrates.[227, 228] Their effectiveness in the clinical setting remains to be established. Once stunning develops, it can be *reversed* with inotropic agents.

Hibernation (See also Chap. 14 and Chap. 37)

The term *hibernating myocardium* refers to the presence of impaired resting left ventricular function, owing to reduced coronary blood flow that can be restored toward normal by revascularization.[229] Hibernation was first noted in patients with coronary artery disease who had no evidence of ongoing ischemia yet whose left ventricular function improved after coronary artery bypass grafting. Even akinetic segments can occasionally regain systolic contraction after revascularization. These observations led to the concept that myocardium can reduce its contractility (and myocardial oxygen demand) to match reduced perfusion, preserving its viability.[219, 230, 231]

Hibernating myocardium is present in approximately one third of patients with coronary artery disease and impaired left ventricular function.[232, 233] The time course of recovery of hibernating myocardium after revascularization is quite variable, ranging from days to months.[219] Slower recovery is typically associated with longer duration of hibernation. Revascularization can be effective whether achieved by coronary bypass grafting as described originally or by coronary angioplasty.[234]

Detection of hibernation (Fig. 37–18) is of great practical significance because it can alleviate symptoms of heart failure and, in the long term, can forestall myocardial necrosis (see later). Detection of hibernating myocardium consists of finding that akinetic or hypokinetic segments of the left ventricular segment are still viable (see Chaps. 9 and 13). This viability can be detected either by the persistence of metabolic activity within the regions of dysfunctional myocardium or by demonstrating improvement in the contraction of the hibernating myocardial segment with appropriate stimulation, such as inotropic stimulation. The improvement in function would not have occurred if the dysfunction had been due to myocardial infarction and scarring.[231] None of the available methods for the detection of myocardial viability is clearly superior to others. Such methods include dobutamine stress echocardiography, thallium-201 redistribution study, imaging with technetium-99m sestamibi, and positron-emission tomography with agents that detect residual metabolic activity such as ^{18}F-fluorodeoxyglucose or ^{11}C-acetate.[219, 231]

Histopathological studies of hibernating myocardium have revealed changes consistent with myocyte dedifferentiation. It has been assumed that these findings are reversible after revascularization. However, areas of hibernating myocardium also show evidence of apoptosis,[194a, 235] necrosis, and fibrosis.[229, 236] Finding of these irreversible changes suggests that revascularization of hibernating myocardium should be performed on an urgent basis.

Unlike stunning, which was described first in the experimental laboratory, hibernation was described initially in the clinical setting, and suitable animal models have been lacking.

Therefore, the cellular and molecular basis of hibernation has not been as extensively investigated. A recent study suggested that in hibernation it is the mitochondria that sense hypoxia. Partial inhibition of cytochrome oxidase during hypoxia allows mitochondria to function as the oxygen sensors, limiting ATP utilization and oxygen consumption.[237]

HIBERNATION VERSUS REPETITIVE STUNNING (see Table 14–6). There is a debate as to whether hibernation is always caused by a chronic reduction in resting myocardial blood flow or whether, at least in some cases, the same syndrome might be caused by repeat episodes of myocardial stunning. Animal models of short-term hibernation have clearly revealed that reductions in blood flow achieved by placement of stenoses are directly correlated with a decrease in contractile function.[238, 239] However, clinical studies have suggested that some patients with coronary artery disease who appear to have hibernating myocardium (poorly contracting but viable myocardium) have normal resting myocardial blood flow but diminished coronary flow reserve. It is likely that these patients suffer episodes of ischemia each time oxygen demand is increased. The final effect of multiple episodes of ischemia is cumulative stunning, mimicking hibernation.[238, 239]

Ultimately, with either scenario, revascularization therapy should improve left ventricular function.

Hemodynamic Consequences of Ischemia

Because the heart has virtually no stores of oxygen and relies almost entirely on aerobic metabolism, within seconds of coronary occlusion its relatively high rate of energy expenditure results in a sudden, striking decline of myocardial oxygen tension and impairment in left ventricular function. For example, sudden coronary occlusion in conscious dogs that produces regional myocardial ischemia is associated with evidence of systolic dysfunction within four beats of occlusion and diastolic dysfunction within nine beats.[240] Impairment of systolic and diastolic function are likely related to alterations in intracellular calcium handling, because calcium is ultimately responsible for regulating both systolic and diastolic function.[241, 242] Because left ventricular dysfunction is so readily induced by ischemia, its detection by echocardiography (see Chap. 7) or radionuclide imaging (see Chap. 9) has become a valuable diagnostic tool in the clinical diagnosis of coronary artery disease.[240]

Clinical evidence of heart failure occurs when regional asynergy is so severe and extensive that the uninvolved myocardium cannot sustain the normal hemodynamic burden (systolic failure). Symptoms of left ventricular failure usually develops when contraction ceases in 20 to 25 percent of the left ventricle. With loss of 40 percent or more of

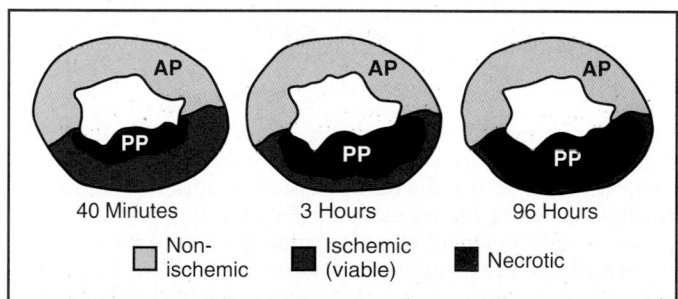

FIGURE 34–28. Progression of cell death versus time after circumflex coronary occlusion in dogs. Necrosis occurs first in the subendocardial myocardium. With longer occlusions, a wavefront of cell death moves from the subendocardial zone across the wall to involve progressively more of the transmural thickness of the ischemic zone. In contrast, the lateral margins in the subendocardial region of the infarct are established as early as 40 minutes after occlusion and are sharply defined by the anatomic boundaries of the ischemic bed. AP = anterior papillary muscle; PP = posterior papillary muscle. (From Reimer KA, Hill ML, Jennings RB: Prolonged depletion of ATP and of the adenine nucleotide pool due to delayed resynthesis of adenine nucleotides following reversible myocardial ischemic injury in dogs. J Mol Cell Cardiol 13:229, 1981.)

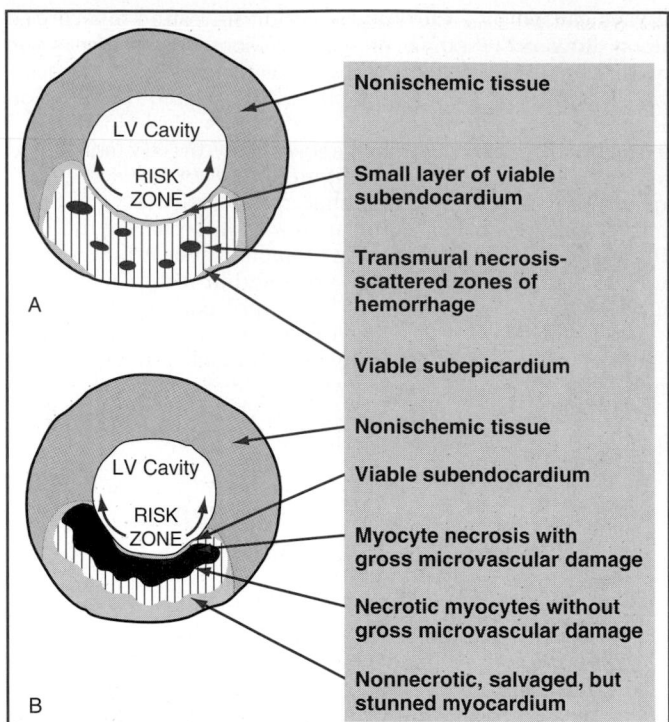

Nonischemic tissue

Small layer of viable subendocardium

Transmural necrosis-scattered zones of hemorrhage

Viable subepicardium

Nonischemic tissue

Viable subendocardium

Myocyte necrosis with gross microvascular damage

Necrotic myocytes without gross microvascular damage

Nonnecrotic, salvaged, but stunned myocardium

FIGURE 34–29. *A,* Schematic diagram showing a transverse section through a canine left ventricle subjected to a permanent coronary occlusion without reperfusion. The white area represents nonischemic myocardium supplied by the nonoccluded vessel. The infarct (hatched area) is transmural or near-transmural. There are scattered zones of hemorrhage (solid black). A small layer of viable subendocardium is present that derives its oxygen directly from the ventricular cavity. Where collateral flow is high, there may be a small rim of surviving subepicardium (shaded areas). *B,* Schematic diagram showing a transverse section through a canine left ventricle subjected to coronary occlusion followed within 1 or 2 hours by coronary reperfusion. The hatched and solid black areas represent the infarct that is confined to the inner half of the myocardium. The solid black areas represent the zone of gross microvascular damage, including zones of no-reflow and hemorrhage. It is smaller than and contained within the total infarct. The remainder of the infarct without severe microvascular damage is represented by the hatched area and is located in the mid myocardium. The epicardial portion of the ischemic zone (stippled area) has been salvaged by coronary reperfusion. It is nonnecrotic but stunned (postischemic ventricular dysfunction) for hours to days after coronary reperfusion. (From Braunwald E, Kloner RA: Myocardial reperfusion: A double-edged sword? J Clin Invest 76:1715, 1985. Copyright 1985, American Society for Clinical Investigation.)

the left ventricular myocardium, severe pump failure ensues, and, if this loss is acute, cardiogenic shock may develop. A shift in the diastolic pressure-volume relationship (diastolic failure) increases the resistance to ventricular filling and leads to elevated ventricular filling pressures, causing symptoms of pulmonary congestion.[243]

The "Wavefront" of Necrosis

As already noted (see p. 1104), within seconds of a coronary occlusion, blood begins to flow through preexisting collateral channels to the occluded segment of the artery. Collateral flow is lowest and myocardial oxygen consumption highest in the subendocardium, and therefore ischemia is most severe in this region. In the normal myocardium, thickening and shortening are greater in the subendocardium, as is wall stress, accounting for the higher subendocardial energy requirements.[244, 245] Consistent with these findings, higher rates of metabolic activity, lower tissue

oxygen tension,[246] and greater oxygen extraction have been found in this region.[247] As a consequence, ischemia becomes most severe and myocardial cells undergo necrosis first in the subendocardium, beginning as early as 15 to 20 minutes after coronary artery occlusion. Necrosis progresses toward the epicardium, gradually involving the less severely ischemic outer layers (Figs. 34–28 and 34–29). The progression of the wavefront of necrosis[248] is slowed by the presence of residual blood flow when the coronary occlusion is incomplete or when mature collaterals are present at the time of occlusion.[248] The progression of the wavefront of necrosis is accelerated when myocardial ischemia is unusually severe, when collateral blood flow is low, in the presence of marked arterial hypotension (e.g., in patients in cardiogenic shock), and in the presence of elevated myocardial oxygen demand, as may be caused by inotropic stimulation, tachycardia, or fever.

In dogs with acute coronary occlusion, the subendocardial lateral boundaries of myocardial infarcts are established early in the first hour, whereas the myocardial infarct enlarges in the transmural direction over 4 to 6 hours.[248] Transmural progression of myocardial infarction has also been observed in humans.[249] The recognition of the time-dependent progression of necrosis is the basis of interventions designed to arrest the progression of necrosis as rapidly as possible by reperfusion of occluded coronary arteries, using thrombolytic therapy or angioplasty (see Chap. 35). Functional recovery that occurs in the subepicardial regions after reperfusion therapy is a mechanism for improvement in regional and global ejection fraction.[249]

Acknowledgment

Dr. E. Braunwald co-wrote this chapter in the fifth edition of this text. Some of the material from the fifth edition has been carried over into this chapter.

REFERENCES

DETERMINANTS OF MYOCARDIAL OXYGEN CONSUMPTION

1. De Bruyne B, Bronzwaer JG, Heyndrickx GR, Paulus WJ: Comparative effects of ischemia and hypoxemia on left ventricular systolic and diastolic function in humans. Circulation 88:461–471, 1993.
2. Braunwald E: Control of myocardial oxygen consumption: Physiologic and clinical considerations. Am J Cardiol 27:416–432, 1971.
3. Klocke FJ, Braunwald E, Ross J Jr: Oxygen cost of electrical activation of the heart. Circ Res 18:357–365, 1966.
4. Loiselle DS: Cardiac basal and activation metabolism. *In* Jacob R, Just HJ, Holubarsch DH (eds): Cardiac Energetics: Basic Mechanisms and Clinical Implications. New York, Springer-Verlag, 1987, pp 37–50.
5. Evans CL, Matsuoka Y: The effect of various mechanical conditions on the gaseous metabolism and efficiency of the mammalian heart. J Physiol 49:378, 1915.
5a. Braunwald E: Myocardial oxygen consumption: The quest for its determinants and some clinical fallout. J Am Coll Cardiol 35:45B, 2000.
6. Sarnoff SJ, Braunwald E, Welch GH Jr, et al: Hemodynamic determinants of oxygen consumption of the heart with special reference to the tension-time index. Am J Physiol 192:148, 1958.
7. Braunwald E, Sarnoff SJ, Case RB, et al: Hemodynamic determinants of coronary flow: Effect of changes in aortic pressure and cardiac output on the relationship between myocardial oxygen consumption and coronary blood flow. Am J Physiol 192:157, 1958.
8. Boerth RC, Covell JW, Pool PE, Ross J Jr: Increased myocardial oxygen consumption and contractile state associated with increased heart rate in dogs. Circ Res 24:725–734, 1969.
9. Rooke GA, Feigl EO: Work as a correlate of canine left ventricular oxygen consumption, and the problem of catecholamine oxygen wasting. Circ Res 50:273–286, 1982.
10. Kal JE, Van Wezel HB, Vergroesen I: A critical appraisal of the rate pressure product as index of myocardial oxygen consumption for the study of metabolic coronary flow regulation. Int J Cardiol 71:141–148, 1999.
11. Suga H: Ventricular energetics. Physiol Rev 70:247–277, 1990.
12. Kameyama T, Asanoi H, Ishizaka S, et al: Energy conversion efficiency in human left ventricle. Circulation 85:988–996, 1992.
13. Takaoka H, Takeuchi M, Odake M, et al: Comparison of hemodynamic determinants for myocardial oxygen consumption under different contractile states in human ventricle. Circulation 87:59-69, 1993.

13a. Braunwald E: Myocardial oxygen consumption: The quest for its determinants and some clinical fallout. J Am Coll Cardiol 34:1365–1369, 1999.

14. Graham TP Jr, Covell JW, Sonnenblick EH, et al: Control of myocardial oxygen consumption: Relative influence of contractile state and tension development. J Clin Invest 47:375–385, 1968.

15. Vik-Mo H, Mjos OD: Influence of free fatty acids on myocardial oxygen consumption and ischemic injury. Am J Cardiol 48:361–365, 1981.

REGULATION OF CORONARY BLOOD FLOW

16. Pijls NH, Van Gelder B, Van der Voort P, et al: Fractional flow reserve: A useful index to evaluate the influence of an epicardial coronary stenosis on myocardial blood flow. Circulation 92:3183–3193, 1995.

17. Chilian WM: Coronary microcirculation in health and disease. Summary of an NHLBI workshop. Circulation 95:522–528, 1997.

18. Stepp DW, Nishikawa Y, Chilian WM: Regulation of shear stress in the canine coronary microcirculation. Circulation 100:1555–1561, 1999.

Metabolic Regulation

19. Dube GP, Bemis KG, Greenfield JC Jr: Distinction between metabolic and myogenic mechanisms of coronary hyperemic response to brief diastolic occlusion. Circ Res 68:1313–1321, 1991.

20. Belardinelli L, Linden J, Berne RM: The cardiac effects of adenosine. Prog Cardiovasc Dis 32:73–97, 1989.

21. Sparks HV Jr, Bardenheuer H: Regulation of adenosine formation by the heart. Circ Res 58:193–201, 1986.

22. Headrick JP, Emerson CS, Berr SS, et al: Interstitial adenosine and cellular metabolism during beta-adrenergic stimulation of the in situ rabbit heart. Cardiovasc Res 31:699–710, 1996.

23. Minamino T, Kitakaze M, Matsumura Y, et al: Impact of coronary risk factors on contribution of nitric oxide and adenosine to metabolic coronary vasodilation in humans. J Am Coll Cardiol 31:1274–1279, 1998.

24. Rossen JD, Oskarsson H, Minor RL Jr, et al: Effect of adenosine antagonism on metabolically mediated coronary vasodilation in humans. J Am Coll Cardiol 23:1421–1426, 1994.

25. Yada T, Richmond KN, Van Bibber R, et al: Role of adenosine in local metabolic coronary vasodilation. Am J Physiol 276:H1425-H1433, 1999.

26. Broten TP, Romson JL, Fullerton DA, et al: Synergistic action of myocardial oxygen and carbon dioxide in controlling coronary blood flow. Circ Res 68:531–542, 1991.

27. Embrey RP, Brooks LA, Dellsperger KC: Mechanism of coronary microvascular responses to metabolic stimulation. Cardiovasc Res 35:148–157, 1997.

28. Meredith IT, Currie KE, Anderson TJ, et al: Postischemic vasodilation in human forearm is dependent on endothelium-derived nitric oxide. Am J Physiol 270:H1435–H1440, 1996.

29. Duffy SJ, Castle SF, Harper RW, Meredith IT: Contribution of vasodilator prostanoids and nitric oxide to resting flow, metabolic vasodilation, and flow-mediated dilation in human coronary circulation. Circulation 100:1951–1957, 1999.

30. Brown IP, Thompson CI, Belloni FL: Role of nitric oxide in hypoxic coronary vasodilatation in isolated perfused guinea pig heart. Am J Physiol 264:H821-H829, 1993.

31. Duncker DJ, van Zon NS, Ishibashi Y, Bache RJ: Role of K+ ATP channels and adenosine in the regulation of coronary blood flow during exercise with normal and restricted coronary blood flow. J Clin Invest 97:996–1009, 1996.

32. Ishibashi Y, Duncker DJ, Zhang J, Bache RJ: ATP-sensitive K+ channels, adenosine, and nitric oxide-mediated mechanisms account for coronary vasodilation during exercise. Circ Res 82:346–359, 1998.

Endothelial Control

33. Kinlay S, Selwyn AP, Delagrange D, et al: Biological mechanisms for the clinical success of lipid-lowering in coronary artery disease and the use of surrogate end-points. Curr Opin Lipidol 7:389–397, 1996.

34. Mombouli JV, Vanhoutte PM: Endothelial dysfunction: From physiology to therapy. J Mol Cell Cardiol 31:61–74, 1999.

35. Ross R: Atherosclerosis—an inflammatory disease. N Engl J Med 340:115–126, 1999.

36. Xu WM, Liu LZ: Nitric oxide: From a mysterious labile factor to the molecule of the Nobel Prize. Recent progress in nitric oxide research. Cell Res 8:251–258, 1998.

37. Furchgott RF: The 1996 Albert Lasker Medical Research Awards. The discovery of endothelium-derived relaxing factor and its importance in the identification of nitric oxide. JAMA 276:1186–1188, 1996.

38. Moncada S: Nitric oxide: Discovery and impact on clinical medicine. J R Soc Med 92:164–169, 1999.

39. Ignarro LJ, Cirino G, Casini A, Napoli C: Nitric oxide as a signaling molecule in the vascular system: An overview. J Cardiovasc Pharmacol 34:879–886, 1999.

40. Murad F: Nitric oxide signaling: Would you believe that a simple free radical could be a second messenger, autacoid, paracrine substance, neurotransmitter, and hormone? Recent Prog Horm Res 53:43–59, 1998.

41. Beckman JS, Koppenol WH: Nitric oxide, superoxide, and peroxynitrite: The good, the bad, and ugly. Am J Physiol 271:C1424–C1437, 1996.

42. Smits P, Williams SB, Lipson DE, et al: Endothelial release of nitric oxide contributes to the vasodilator effect of adenosine in humans. Circulation 92:2135–2141, 1995.

43. Quyyumi AA, Dakak N, Mulcahy D, et al: Nitric oxide activity in the atherosclerotic human coronary circulation. J Am Coll Cardiol 29:308–317, 1997.

44. Britten MB, Zeiher AM, Schachinger V: Clinical importance of coronary endothelial vasodilator dysfunction and therapeutic options. J Intern Med 245:315–327, 1999.

45. Drexler H: Endothelial dysfunction: Clinical implications. Prog Cardiovasc Dis 39:287–324, 1997.

46. Thorne S, Mullen MJ, Clarkson P, et al: Early endothelial dysfunction in adults at risk from atherosclerosis: Different responses to L-arginine. J Am Coll Cardiol 32:110–116, 1998.

47. Celermajer DS: Testing endothelial function using ultrasound. J Cardiovasc Pharmacol 32:S29–S32, 1998.

48. Kinlay S, Ganz P: Role of endothelial dysfunction in coronary artery disease and implications for therapy. Am J Cardiol 80:11I–16I, 1997.

49. Anderson TJ, Meredith IT, Yeung AC, et al: The effect of cholesterol-lowering and antioxidant therapy on endothelium-dependent coronary vasomotion. N Engl J Med 332:488–493, 1995.

50. Anderson TJ, Meredith IT, Charbonneau F, et al: Endothelium-dependent coronary vasomotion relates to the susceptibility of LDL to oxidation in humans. Circulation 93:1647–1650, 1996.

51. Steinberg D: Lewis A. Conner Memorial Lecture: Oxidative modification of LDL and atherogenesis. Circulation 95:1062–1071, 1997.

52. Inoue T, Saniabadi AR, Matsunaga R, et al: Impaired endothelium-dependent acetylcholine-induced coronary artery relaxation in patients with high serum remnant lipoprotein particles. Atherosclerosis 139:363–367, 1998.

53. Chowienczyk PJ, Watts GF, Wierzbicki AS, et al: Preserved endothelial function in patients with severe hypertriglyceridemia and low functional lipoprotein lipase activity. J Am Coll Cardiol 29:964–968, 1997.

54. Raitakari OT, Adams MR, Celermajer DS: Effect of Lp(a) on the early functional and structural changes of atherosclerosis. Arterioscler Thromb Vasc Biol 19:990–995, 1999.

55. Toikka JO, Ahotupa M, Viikari JS, et al: Constantly low HDL-cholesterol concentration relates to endothelial dysfunction and increased in vivo LDL-oxidation in healthy young men. Atherosclerosis 147:133–138, 1999.

56. Williams SB, Goldfine AB, Timimi FK, et al: Acute hyperglycemia attenuates endothelium-dependent vasodilation in humans in vivo. Circulation 97:1695–1701, 1998.

57. Chao CL, Chien KL, Lee YT: Effect of short-term vitamin (folic acid, vitamins B_6 and B_{12}) administration on endothelial dysfunction induced by post-methionine load hyperhomocysteinemia. Am J Cardiol 84:1359–1361, A8, 1999.

58. Plotnick GD, Corretti MC, Vogel RA: Effect of antioxidant vitamins on the transient impairment of endothelium-dependent brachial artery vasoactivity following a single high-fat meal. JAMA 278:1682–1686, 1997.

59. Pinto S, Virdis A, Ghiadoni L, et al: Endogenous estrogen and acetylcholine-induced vasodilation in normotensive women. Hypertension 29:268–273, 1997.

60. Nakayama M, Yasue H, Yoshimura M, et al: T-786→C mutation in the 5′-flanking region of the endothelial nitric oxide synthase gene is associated with coronary spasm. Circulation 99:2864–2870, 1999.

61. Hibi K, Ishigami T, Tamura K, et al: Endothelial nitric oxide synthase gene polymorphism and acute myocardial infarction. Hypertension 32:521–526, 1998.

62. Yoshimura M, Yasue H, Nakayama M, et al: A missense Glu298Asp variant in the endothelial nitric oxide synthase gene is associated with coronary spasm in the Japanese. Hum Genet 103:65–69, 1998.

63. Calver A, Collier J, Vallance P: Forearm blood flow responses to a nitric oxide synthase inhibitor in patients with treated essential hypertension. Cardiovasc Res 28:1720–1725, 1994.

64. Stamler JS, Loh E, Roddy MA, et al: Nitric oxide regulates basal systemic and pulmonary vascular resistance in healthy humans. Circulation 89:2035–2040, 1994.

65. Egashira K, Katsuda Y, Mohri M, et al: Role of endothelium-derived nitric oxide in coronary vasodilatation induced by pacing tachycardia in humans. Circ Res 79:331–335, 1996.

66. Tagawa T, Mohri M, Tagawa H, et al: Role of nitric oxide in substance P–induced vasodilation differs between the coronary and forearm circulation in humans. J Cardiovasc Pharmacol 29:546–553, 1997.

67. Selwyn AP, Kinlay S, Libby P, Ganz P: Atherogenic lipids, vascular dysfunction, and clinical signs of ischemic heart disease. Circulation 95:5–7, 1997.

68. Ganz P, Creager MA, Fang JC, et al: Pathogenic mechanisms of atherosclerosis: Effect of lipid lowering on the biology of atherosclerosis. Am J Med 101:4A10S–4A16S, 1996.

69. Anderson TJ, Gerhard MD, Meredith IT, et al: Systemic nature of endothelial dysfunction in atherosclerosis. Am J Cardiol 75:71B–74B, 1995.

70. Quyyumi AA, Dakak N, Andrews NP, et al: Contribution of nitric oxide to metabolic coronary vasodilation in the human heart. Circulation 92:320–326, 1995.

71. Selwyn AP, Kinlay S, Creager M, et al: Cell dysfunction in atherosclerosis and the ischemic manifestations of coronary artery disease. Am J Cardiol 79:17–23, 1997.

72. Gordon JB, Ganz P, Nabel EG, et al: Atherosclerosis influences the

vasomotor response of epicardial coronary arteries to exercise. J Clin Invest 83:1946–1952, 1989.

73. Yeung AC, Vekshtein VI, Krantz DS, et al: The effect of atherosclerosis on the vasomotor response of coronary arteries to mental stress. N Engl J Med 325:1551–1556, 1991.

74. Andrews TC, Raby K, Barry J, et al: Effect of cholesterol reduction on myocardial ischemia in patients with coronary disease. Circulation 95:324–328, 1997.

75. Kinlay S, Selwyn AP, Libby P, Ganz P: Inflammation, the endothelium, and the acute coronary syndromes. J Cardiovasc Pharmacol 32:S62-S66, 1998.

76. Willerson JT: Conversion from chronic to acute coronary heart disease syndromes: Role of platelets and platelet products. Tex Heart Inst J 22:13–9, 1995.

77. Okumura K, Yasue H, Matsuyama K, et al: Effect of acetylcholine on the highly stenotic coronary artery: Difference between the constrictor response of the infarct-related coronary artery and that of the noninfarct-related artery. J Am Coll Cardiol 19:752–728, 1992.

78. Lee RT, Libby P: The unstable atheroma. Arterioscler Thromb Vasc Biol 17:1859–1867, 1997.

79. Aikawa M, Voglic SJ, Sugiyama S, et al: Dietary lipid lowering reduces tissue factor expression in rabbit atheroma. Circulation 100:1215–1222, 1999.

80. Maxwell AJ, Cooke JP: The role of nitric oxide in atherosclerosis. Coron Artery Dis 10:277–286, 1999.

81. Hasdai D, Lerman A: The assessment of endothelial function in the cardiac catheterization laboratory in patients with risk factors for atherosclerotic coronary artery disease. Herz 24:544–547, 1999.

82. Hasdai D, Gibbons RJ, Holmes DR Jr, et al: Coronary endothelial dysfunction in humans is associated with myocardial perfusion defects. Circulation 96:3390–3395, 1997.

83. Tamai O, Matsuoka H, Itabe H, et al: Single LDL apheresis improves endothelium-dependent vasodilatation in hypercholesterolemic humans. Circulation 95:76–82, 1997.

84. Vogel RA, Corretti MC, Gellman J: Cholesterol, cholesterol lowering, and endothelial function. Prog Cardiovasc Dis 41:117–136, 1998.

85. Huggins GS, Pasternak RC, Alpert NM, et al: Effects of short-term treatment of hyperlipidemia on coronary vasodilator function and myocardial perfusion in regions having substantial impairment of baseline dilator reserve. Circulation 98:1291–1296, 1998.

86. van Boven AJ, Jukema JW, Zwinderman AH, et al: Reduction of transient myocardial ischemia with pravastatin in addition to the conventional treatment in patients with angina pectoris. REGRESS Study Group. Circulation 94:1503–1505, 1996.

87. Mancini GB, Henry GC, Macaya C, et al: Angiotensin-converting enzyme inhibition with quinapril improves endothelial vasomotor dysfunction in patients with coronary artery disease: The TREND (Trial on Reversing ENdothelial Dysfunction) Study. Circulation 94:258–265, 1996.

88. Timimi FK, Ting HH, Haley EA, et al: Vitamin C improves endothelium-dependent vasodilation in patients with insulin-dependent diabetes mellitus. J Am Coll Cardiol 31:552–557, 1998.

89. Diaz MN, Frei B, Vita JA, Keaney JF Jr: Antioxidants and atherosclerotic heart disease. N Engl J Med 337:408–416, 1997.

90. Quilley J, Fulton D, McGiff JC: Hyperpolarizing factors. Biochem Pharmacol 54:1059–1070, 1997.

91. Miura H, Liu Y, Gutterman DD: Human coronary arteriolar dilation to bradykinin depends on membrane hyperpolarization: Contribution of nitric oxide and Ca^{2+}-activated K^+ channels. Circulation 99:3132–3138, 1999.

92. Waldron GJ, Ding H, Lovren F, et al: Acetylcholine-induced relaxation of peripheral arteries isolated from mice lacking endothelial nitric oxide synthase. Br J Pharmacol 128:653–658, 1999.

93. Feletou M, Vanhoutte PM: The alternative: EDHF. J Mol Cell Cardiol 31:15–22, 1999.

94. Campbell WB, Harder DR: Endothelium-derived hyperpolarizing factors and vascular cytochrome P450 metabolites of arachidonic acid in the regulation of tone. Circ Res 84:484–488, 1999.

95. Takamura Y, Shimokawa H, Zhao H, et al: Important role of endothelium-derived hyperpolarizing factor in shear stress–induced endothelium-dependent relaxations in the rat mesenteric artery. J Cardiovasc Pharmacol 34:381–387, 1999.

96. Node K, Huo Y, Ruan X, et al: Anti-inflammatory properties of cytochrome P450 epoxygenase-derived eicosanoids. Science 285:1276–1279, 1999.

97. Bauersachs J, Popp R, Fleming I, Busse R: Nitric oxide and endothelium-derived hyperpolarizing factor: Formation and interactions. Prostaglandins Leukot Essent Fatty Acids 57:439–446, 1997.

98. Edlund A, Berglund B, van Dorne D, et al: Coronary flow regulation in patients with ischemic heart disease: Release of purines and prostacyclin and the effect of inhibitors of prostaglandin formation. Circulation 71:1113–1120, 1985.

99. FitzGerald GA, Smith B, Pedersen AK, Brash AR: Increased prostacyclin biosynthesis in patients with severe atherosclerosis and platelet activation. N Engl J Med 310:1065–1068, 1984.

100. Ortega Mateo A, de Artinano AA: Highlights on endothelins: A review. Pharmacol Res 36:339–351, 1997.

101. Haynes WG, Webb DJ: Endothelin as a regulator of cardiovascular function in health and disease. J Hypertens 16:1081–1098, 1998.

102. Hafizi S, Allen SP, Goodwin AT, et al: Endothelin-1 stimulates proliferation of human coronary smooth muscle cells via the ET(A) receptor and is co-mitogenic with growth factors. Atherosclerosis 146:351–359, 1999.

103. Kirchengast M, Munter K: Endothelin-1 and endothelin receptor antagonists in cardiovascular remodeling. Proc Soc Exp Biol Med 221:312–325, 1999.

104. Zouki C, Baron C, Fournier A, Filep JG: Endothelin-1 enhances neutrophil adhesion to human coronary artery endothelial cells: Role of ET(A) receptors and platelet-activating factor. Br J Pharmacol 127:969–979, 1999.

105. Kelly JJ, Whitworth JA: Endothelin-1 as a mediator in cardiovascular disease. Clin Exp Pharmacol Physiol 26:158–161, 1999.

106. Zeiher AM, Goebel H, Schachinger V, Ihling C: Tissue endothelin-1 immunoreactivity in the active coronary atherosclerotic plaque: A clue to the mechanism of increased vasoreactivity of the culprit lesion in unstable angina. Circulation 91:941–947, 1995.

107. Chen TH, Tseng HP, Yang JY, Mao SJ: Effect of antioxidant in endothelial cells exposed to oxidized low-density lipoproteins. Life Sci 62:L277–L282, 1998.

108. He Y, Kwan WC, Steinbrecher UP: Effects of oxidized low density lipoprotein on endothelin secretion by cultured endothelial cells and macrophages. Atherosclerosis 119:107–118, 1996.

109. Haynes WG, Strachan FE, Webb DJ: Endothelin ETA and ETB receptors cause vasoconstriction of human resistance and capacitance vessels in vivo. Circulation 92:357–363, 1995.

110. Verhaar MC, Strachan FE, Newby DE, et al: Endothelin-A receptor antagonist-mediated vasodilatation is attenuated by inhibition of nitric oxide synthesis and by endothelin-B receptor blockade. Circulation 97:752–756, 1998.

111. Krum H, Viskoper RJ, Lacourciere Y, et al: The effect of an endothelin-receptor antagonist, bosentan, on blood pressure in patients with essential hypertension. Bosentan Hypertension Investigators. N Engl J Med 338:784–790, 1998.

112. Taddei S, Virdis A, Ghiadoni L, et al: Vasoconstriction to endogenous endothelin-1 is increased in the peripheral circulation of patients with essential hypertension. Circulation 100:1680–1683, 1999.

Autoregulation

113. Johnson PC: Autoregulation of blood flow. Circ Res 59:483–495, 1986.

114. Feigl EO: Coronary autoregulation. J Hypertens Suppl 7:S55–S58; discussion S59, 1989.

115. Canty JM Jr: Coronary pressure-function and steady-state pressure-flow relations during autoregulation in the unanesthetized dog. Circ Res 63:821–836, 1988.

116. Pijls NHJ, De Bruyne B: Coronary Pressure. Dodrecht, The Netherlands, Kluwer Academic Publishers, 1997, pp 12–13.

117. Harrison DG, Florentine MS, Brooks LA, et al: The effect of hypertension and left ventricular hypertrophy on the lower range of coronary autoregulation. Circulation 77:1108–1115, 1988.

118. Rouleau J, Boerboom LE, Surjadhana A, Hoffman JI: The role of autoregulation and tissue diastolic pressures in the transmural distribution of left ventricular blood flow in anesthetized dogs. Circ Res 45:804–815, 1979.

119. Avontuur JA, Bruining HA, Ince C: Nitric oxide causes dysfunction of coronary autoregulation in endotoxemic rats. Cardiovasc Res 35:368–376, 1997.

120. Smith TP Jr, Canty JM Jr: Modulation of coronary autoregulatory responses by nitric oxide: Evidence for flow-dependent resistance adjustments in conscious dogs. Circ Res 73:232–240, 1993.

121. Lansman JB, Hallam TJ, Rink TJ: Single stretch-activated ion channels in vascular endothelial cells as mechanotransducers? Nature 325:811–813, 1987.

122. Stepp DW, Kroll K, Feigl EO: K+ATP channels and adenosine are not necessary for coronary autoregulation. Am J Physiol 273:H1299–H1308, 1997.

123. Jones CJ, Kuo L, Davis MJ, Chilian WM: Myogenic and flow-dependent control mechanisms in the coronary microcirculation. Basic Res Cardiol 88:2–10, 1993.

124. Rajagopalan S, Dube S, Canty JM Jr: Regulation of coronary diameter by myogenic mechanisms in arterial microvessels greater than 100 microns in diameter. Am J Physiol 268:H788–H793, 1995.

Extravascular Compression

125. Morita K, Mori H, Tsujioka K, et al: Alpha-adrenergic vasoconstriction reduces systolic retrograde coronary blood flow. Am J Physiol 273:H2746–H2755, 1997.

126. Marcus ML, Harrison DG: Physiologic basis for myocardial perfusion imaging. In Marcus ML, Schelbert HR, Skorton DJ, Wolf GL (eds): Cardiac Imaging, a Companion to Braunwald's Heart Disease. Philadelphia, WB Saunders, 1991.

127. Berne RM, Rubio R: Coronary circulation. In Berne RM, et al (eds): Handbook of Physiology: Section 2, The Cardiovascular System. Bethesda, MD, American Physiological Society, 1979, p 897.

128. Zhang J, Duncker DJ, Ya X, et al: Effect of left ventricular hypertrophy secondary to chronic pressure overload on transmural myocardial 2-deoxyglucose uptake: A ^{31}P NMR spectroscopic study. Circulation 92:1274–1283, 1995.

129. Braunwald E, Ross J Jr, Sonnenblick EH: Regulation of Coronary Blood Flow: Mechanisms of Contraction of the Normal and Failing Heart. Boston, Little, Brown, 1976, p 200.
130. Austin RE Jr, Smedira NG, Squiers TM, Hoffman JI: Influence of cardiac contraction and coronary vasomotor tone on regional myocardial blood flow. Am J Physiol 266:H2542–H2553, 1994.
131. Farhi ER, Klocke FJ, Mates RE, et al: Tone-dependent waterfall behavior during venous pressure elevation in isolated canine hearts. Circ Res 68:392–401, 1991.

Transmural Distribution of Myocardial Blood Flow

132. Chilian WM: Microvascular pressures and resistances in the left ventricular subepicardium and subendocardium. Circ Res 69:561–570, 1991.
133. Duncker DJ, Ishibashi Y, Bache RJ: Effect of treadmill exercise on transmural distribution of blood flow in hypertrophied left ventricle. Am J Physiol 275:H1274–H1282, 1998.
134. Duncker DJ, Traverse JH, Ishibashi Y, Bache RJ: Effect of NO on transmural distribution of blood flow in hypertrophied left ventricle during exercise. Am J Physiol 276:H1305–H1312, 1999.
135. Weiss HR, Neubauer JA, Lipp JA, Sinha AK: Quantitative determination of regional oxygen consumption in the dog heart. Circ Res 42:394–401, 1978.
136. Hoffman JI: Transmural myocardial perfusion. Prog Cardiovasc Dis 29:429–464, 1987.
137. Gallagher KP, Osakada G, Matsuzaki M, et al: Myocardial blood flow and function with critical coronary stenosis in exercising dogs. Am J Physiol 243:H698-H707, 1982.
138. Shannon RP, Komamura K, Shen YT, et al: Impaired regional subendocardial coronary flow reserve in conscious dogs with pacing-induced heart failure. Am J Physiol 265:H801–H809, 1993.
139. Nathan HJ, Feigl EO: Adrenergic vasoconstriction lessens transmural steal during coronary hypoperfusion. Am J Physiol 250:H645–H653, 1986.
140. Heller GV, Barbour MM, Dweik RB, et al: Effects of intravenous theophylline on exercise-induced myocardial ischemia: I. Impact on the ischemic threshold. J Am Coll Cardiol 21:1075–1079, 1993.
141. Kumada T, Gallagher KP, Shirato K, et al: Reduction of exercise-induced regional myocardial dysfunction by propranolol: Studies in a canine model of chronic coronary artery stenosis. Circ Res 46:190–200, 1980.

Neural Control

142. Feigl EO: Neural control of coronary blood flow. J Vasc Res 35:85–92, 1998.
142a. Heusch G; Baumgart D, Camici P, et al: Alpha adrenergic coronary vasoconstriction and myocardial ischemia in humans. Circulation 101:689, 2000.
143. Young MA, Knight DR, Vatner SF: Autonomic control of large coronary arteries and resistance vessels. Prog Cardiovasc Dis 30:211–234, 1987.
144. Trivella MG, Broten TP, Feigl EO: Beta-receptor subtypes in the canine coronary circulation. Am J Physiol 259:H1575–H1585, 1990.
145. Feigl EO, Van Winkle DM, Miyashiro JK: Cholinergic vasodilatation of coronary resistance vessels in dogs, baboons and goats. Blood Vessels 27:94–105, 1990.
146. Kern MJ, Horowitz JD, Ganz P, et al: Attenuation of coronary vascular resistance by selective alpha 1-adrenergic blockade in patients with coronary artery disease. J Am Coll Cardiol 5:840–846, 1985.
147. Murray PA, Vatner SF: Alpha-adrenoceptor attenuation of the coronary vascular response to severe exercise in the conscious dog. Circ Res 45:654–660, 1979.
148. Feigl EO: The paradox of adrenergic coronary vasoconstriction. Circulation 76:737–745, 1987.
149. Huang AH, Feigl EO: Adrenergic coronary vasoconstriction helps maintain uniform transmural blood flow distribution during exercise. Circ Res 62:286–98, 1988.
150. Knight DR, Shen YT, Young MA, Vatner SF: Acetylcholine-induced coronary vasoconstriction and vasodilation in tranquilized baboons. Circ Res 69:706–713, 1991.
151. Kawamura A, Fujiwara H, Onodera T, et al: Response of large and small coronary arteries of pigs to intracoronary injection of acetylcholine: Angiographic and histologic analysis. Int J Cardiol 25:289-302, 1989.
152. Chilian WM, Layne SM, Eastham CL, Marcus ML: Heterogeneous microvascular coronary alpha-adrenergic vasoconstriction. Circ Res 64:376–88, 1989.

Effects of Coronary Stenoses

153. Brown BG, Bolson EL, Dodge HT: Dynamic mechanisms in human coronary stenosis. Circulation 70:917–922, 1984.
154. Ferrari M, Schnell B, Werner GS, Figulla HR: Safety of deferring angioplasty in patients with normal coronary flow velocity reserve. J Am Coll Cardiol 33:82–87, 1999.
155. Bach RG, Kern MJ: Practical coronary physiology: Clinical application of the Doppler flow velocity guide wire. Cardiol Clin 15:77–99, 1997.

156. Kern MJ, de Bruyne B, Pijls NH: From research to clinical practice: Current role of intracoronary physiologically based decision making in the cardiac catheterization laboratory. J Am Coll Cardiol 30:613–620, 1997.
157. Wilson RF: Assessing the severity of coronary-artery stenoses. N Engl J Med 334:1735–1737, 1996.
158. Pijls NH, De Bruyne B, Peels K, et al: Measurement of fractional flow reserve to assess the functional severity of coronary-artery stenoses. N Engl J Med 334:1703–1708, 1996.
159. Canty JM Jr, Smith TP Jr: Adenosine-recruitable flow reserve is absent during myocardial ischemia in unanesthetized dogs studied in the basal state. Circ Res 76:1079–1087, 1995.
160. Kelley KO, Gould KL: Coronary reactive hyperaemia after brief occlusion and after deoxygenated perfusion. Cardiovasc Res 15:615–622, 1981.
161. Dole WP, Montville WJ, Bishop VS: Dependency of myocardial reactive hyperemia on coronary artery pressure in the dog. Am J Physiol 240:H709–H715, 1981.
162. Serruys PW, Di Mario C, Meneveau N, et al: Intracoronary pressure and flow velocity with sensor-tip guidewires: A new methodologic approach for assessment of coronary hemodynamics before and after coronary interventions. Am J Cardiol 71:41D–53D, 1993.
163. Nabel EG, Selwyn AP, Ganz P: Paradoxical narrowing of atherosclerotic coronary arteries induced by increases in heart rate [see comments]. Circulation 81:850–859, 1990.
164. Verberne HJ, Piek JJ, van Liebergen RA, et al: Functional assessment of coronary artery stenosis by Doppler derived absolute and relative coronary blood flow velocity reserve in comparison with (99m)Tc MIBI SPECT. Heart 82:509–514, 1999.
165. Miller DD, Donohue TJ, Younis LT, et al: Correlation of pharmacological ^{99m}Tc-sestamibi myocardial perfusion imaging with poststenotic coronary flow reserve in patients with angiographically intermediate coronary artery stenoses. Circulation 89:2150–2160, 1994.
166. Donohue TJ, Kern MJ, Aguirre FV, et al: Assessing the hemodynamic significance of coronary artery stenoses: Analysis of translesional pressure-flow velocity relations in patients. J Am Coll Cardiol 22:449–458, 1993.
167. Serruys PW, di Mario C, Piek J, et al: Prognostic value of intracoronary flow velocity and diameter stenosis in assessing the short- and long-term outcomes of coronary balloon angioplasty: The DEBATE Study (Doppler Endpoints Balloon Angioplasty Trial Europe). Circulation 96:3369–3377, 1997.
168. Segers P, Fostier G, Neckebroeck J, Verdonck P: Assessing coronary artery stenosis severity: In vitro validation of the concept of fractional flow reserve. Cathet Cardiovasc Interv 46:375–379, 1999.
169. Bech GJ, De Bruyne B, Bonnier HJ, et al: Long-term follow-up after deferral of percutaneous transluminal coronary angioplasty of intermediate stenosis on the basis of coronary pressure measurement. J Am Coll Cardiol 31:841–847, 1998.
170. Pijls NH, De Bruyne B: Coronary pressure measurement and fractional flow reserve. Heart 80:539–542, 1998.
171. Bech GJ, Pijls NH, De Bruyne B, et al: Usefulness of fractional flow reserve to predict clinical outcome after balloon angioplasty. Circulation 99:883–888, 1999.
172. Hanekamp CE, Koolen JJ, Pijls NH, et al: Comparison of quantitative coronary angiography, intravascular ultrasound, and coronary pressure measurement to assess optimum stent deployment. Circulation 99:1015–1021, 1999.
173. Rutishauser W: The Denolin Lecture 1998. Towards measurement of coronary blood flow in patients and its alteration by interventions. Eur Heart J 20:1076–1083, 1999.
174. Baller D, Notohamiprodjo G, Gleichmann U, et al: Improvement in coronary flow reserve determined by positron emission tomography after 6 months of cholesterol-lowering therapy in patients with early stages of coronary atherosclerosis. Circulation 99:2871–2375, 1999.
175. Gould KL, Kirkeeide RL, Buchi M: Coronary flow reserve as a physiologic measure of stenosis severity. J Am Coll Cardiol 15:459–474, 1990.
176. Newby AC, Libby P, van der Wal AC: Plaque instability–the real challenge for atherosclerosis research in the next decade? Cardiovasc Res 41:321–322, 1999.

CORONARY COLLATERALS

177. Schaper W, Ito WD: Molecular mechanisms of coronary collateral vessel growth. Circ Res 79:911–919, 1996.
178. Wolf C, Cai WJ, Vosschulte R, et al: Vascular remodeling and altered protein expression during growth of coronary collateral arteries. J Mol Cell Cardiol 30:2291–2305, 1998.
179. Schaper W, Gorge G, Winkler B, Schaper J: The collateral circulation of the heart. Prog Cardiovasc Dis 31:57–77, 1988.
180. Pepper MS: Manipulating angiogenesis: From basic science to the bedside. Arterioscler Thromb Vasc Biol 17:605–619, 1997.
181. Arras M, Ito WD, Scholz D, et al: Monocyte activation in angiogenesis and collateral growth in the rabbit hindlimb. J Clin Invest 101:40–50, 1998.
182. Majno G: Chronic inflammation: Links with angiogenesis and wound healing. Am J Pathol 153:1035–1039, 1998.
183. McCourt M, Wang JH, Sookhai S, Redmond HP: Proinflammatory medi-

ators stimulate neutrophil-directed angiogenesis. Arch Surg 134:1325–1331; discussion 1331–1332, 1999.

184. Schaper W, Buschmann I: Collateral circulation and diabetes. Circulation 99:2224–2226, 1999.

185. Stetler-Stevenson WG: Matrix metalloproteinases in angiogenesis: A moving target for therapeutic intervention. J Clin Invest 103:1237–1241, 1999.

186. Haas TL, Madri JA: Extracellular matrix-driven matrix metalloproteinase production in endothelial cells: Implications for angiogenesis. Trends Cardiovasc Med 9:70–77, 1999.

187. Majno G, Joris I: Apoptosis, oncosis, and necrosis: An overview of cell death. Am J Pathol 146:3–15, 1995.

188. Chappell DC, Varner SE, Nerem RM, et al: Oscillatory shear stress stimulates adhesion molecule expression in cultured human endothelium. Circ Res 82:532–539, 1998.

189. Cavaillon JM: Cytokines and macrophages. Biomed Pharmacother 48:445–453, 1994.

190. Henry TD: Therapeutic angiogenesis. BMJ 318:1536–1539, 1999.

191. Shizukuda Y, Tang S, Yokota R, Ware JA: Vascular endothelial growth factor–induced endothelial cell migration and proliferation depend on a nitric oxide–mediated decrease in protein kinase C delta activity. Circ Res 85:247–256, 1999.

192. O'Reilly MS, Holmgren L, Shing Y, et al: Angiostatin: A novel angiogenesis inhibitor that mediates the suppression of metastases by a Lewis lung carcinoma. Cell 79:315–328, 1994.

193. Moulton KS, Heller E, Konerding MA, et al: Angiogenesis inhibitors endostatin or TNP-470 reduce intimal neovascularization and plaque growth in apolipoprotein E-deficient mice. Circulation 99:1726–1732, 1999.

194. Chen D, Asahara T, Krasinski K, et al: Antibody blockade of thrombospondin accelerates reendothelialization and reduces neointima formation in balloon-injured rat carotid artery. Circulation 100:849–854, 1999.

194a. Lim H, Fallavollita JA, Hard R, et al: Profound apoptosis-mediated regional myocyte loss and compensatory hypertrophy in pigs with hibernating myocardium. Circulation 100:2380–2386, 1999.

195. Shweiki D, Itin A, Soffer D, Keshet E: Vascular endothelial growth factor induced by hypoxia may mediate hypoxia-initiated angiogenesis. Nature 359:843–845, 1992.

196. Liu Y, Cox SR, Morita T, Kourembanas S: Hypoxia regulates vascular endothelial growth factor gene expression in endothelial cells. Identification of a 5′ enhancer. Circ Res 77:638–643, 1995.

197. Levy AP, Levy NS, Wegner S, Goldberg MA: Transcriptional regulation of the rat vascular endothelial growth factor gene by hypoxia. J Biol Chem 270:13333–13340, 1995.

198. Tuder RM, Flook BE, Voelkel NF: Increased gene expression for VEGF and the VEGF receptors KDR/Flk and Flt in lungs exposed to acute or to chronic hypoxia: Modulation of gene expression by nitric oxide. J Clin Invest 95:1798–1807, 1995.

199. Piek JJ, Koolen JJ, Hoedemaker G, et al: Severity of single-vessel coronary arterial stenosis and duration of angina as determinants of recruitable collateral vessels during balloon angioplasty occlusion. Am J Cardiol 67:13–17, 1991.

200. Abaci A, Oguzhan A, Kahraman S, et al: Effect of diabetes mellitus on formation of coronary collateral vessels. Circulation 99:2239-2242, 1999.

201. Bucay M, Nguy J, Barrios R, et al: Impaired adaptive vascular growth in hypercholesterolemic rabbit. Atherosclerosis 139:243–251, 1998.

202. Ferguson RJ, Petitclerc R, Choquette G, et al: Effect of physical training on treadmill exercise capacity, collateral circulation and progression of coronary disease. Am J Cardiol 34:764–769, 1974.

203. Klassen CL, Traverse JH, Bache RJ: Nitroglycerin dilates coronary collateral vessels during exercise after blockade of endogenous NO production. Am J Physiol 277:H918–H923, 1999.

204. Hollenberg NK, Monteiro K, Sandor T: Endothelial injury provokes collateral arterial vasoconstriction: Response to a serotonin 2 antagonist, thromboxane antagonist or synthetase inhibition. J Pharmacol Exp Ther 244:1164–1168, 1988.

205. Harrison DG, Simonetti I: Neurohumoral regulation of collateral perfusion. Circulation 83:III62–III67, 1991.

206. Vanoverschelde JL, Wijns W, Depre C, et al: Mechanisms of chronic regional postischemic dysfunction in humans: New insights from the study of noninfarcted collateral-dependent myocardium. Circulation 87:1513–1523, 1993.

207. Charney R, Cohen M: The role of the coronary collateral circulation in limiting myocardial ischemia and infarct size. Am Heart J 126:937–945, 1993.

208. Sabia PJ, Powers ER, Ragosta M, et al: An association between collateral blood flow and myocardial viability in patients with recent myocardial infarction. N Engl J Med 327:1825–1831, 1992.

209. Pijls NH, Bech GJ, el Gamal MI, et al: Quantification of recruitable coronary collateral blood flow in conscious humans and its potential to predict future ischemic events. J Am Coll Cardiol 25:1522–1528, 1995.

Angiogenesis

210. Isner JM, Asahara T: Angiogenesis and vasculogenesis as therapeutic strategies for postnatal neovascularization. J Clin Invest 103:1231–1236, 1999.

210a. Lee SH, Wolf PL, Escudero R, et al: Early expression of angiogenesis factors in acute myocardial ischemia and infarction. N Engl J Med 342:626–633, 2000.

211. Engler DA: Use of vascular endothelial growth factor for therapeutic angiogenesis [editorial; comment]. Circulation 94:1496–1498, 1996.

212. Takeshita S, Zheng LP, Brogi E, et al: Therapeutic angiogenesis: A single intraarterial bolus of vascular endothelial growth factor augments revascularization in a rabbit ischemic hind limb model. J Clin Invest 93:662–670, 1994.

213. Baumgartner I, Pieczek A, Manor O, et al: Constitutive expression of phVEGF165 after intramuscular gene transfer promotes collateral vessel development in patients with critical limb ischemia. Circulation 97:1114–1123, 1998.

214. Rosengart TK, Lee LY, Patel SR, et al: Angiogenesis gene therapy: Phase I assessment of direct intramyocardial administration of an adenovirus vector expressing VEGF121 cDNA to individuals with clinically significant severe coronary artery disease. Circulation 100:468–474, 1999.

215. Losordo DW, Vale PR, Symes JF, et al: Gene therapy for myocardial angiogenesis: Initial clinical results with direct myocardial injection of phVEGF165 as sole therapy for myocardial ischemia. Circulation 98:2800–2804, 1998.

216. Shi Q, Rafii S, Wu MH, et al: Evidence for circulating bone marrow-derived endothelial cells. Blood 92:362–367, 1998.

CONSEQUENCES OF MYOCARDIAL ISCHEMIA

217. Tennant R, Wiggers CJ: The effect of coronary occlusion on myocardial contractions. Am J Physiol 112:351, 1935.

218. Heyndrickx GR, Millard RW, McRitchie RJ, et al: Regional myocardial functional and electrophysiological alterations after brief coronary artery occlusion in conscious dogs. J Clin Invest 56:978–985, 1975.

219. Kloner RA, Bolli R, Marban E, et al: Medical and cellular implications of stunning, hibernation, and preconditioning: An NHLBI workshop. Circulation 97:1848–1867, 1998.

220. Bolli R, Marban E: Molecular and cellular mechanisms of myocardial stunning. Physiol Rev 79:609–634, 1999.

221. Bolli R: Basic and clinical aspects of myocardial stunning. Prog Cardiovasc Dis 40:477–516, 1998.

222. Rinaldi CA, Masani ND, Linka AZ, Hall RJ: Effect of repetitive episodes of exercise induced myocardial ischaemia on left ventricular function in patients with chronic stable angina: Evidence for cumulative stunning or ischaemic preconditioning? Heart 81:404–411, 1999.

223. Fragasso G, Benti R, Sciammarella M, et al: Symptom-limited exercise testing causes sustained diastolic dysfunction in patients with coronary disease and low effort tolerance. J Am Coll Cardiol 17:1251–1255, 1991.

224. Kloner RA, Przyklenk K, Kay GL: Clinical evidence for stunned myocardium after coronary artery bypass surgery. J Card Surg 9:397–402, 1994.

225. Gerber BL, Wijns W, Vanoverschelde JL, et al: Myocardial perfusion and oxygen consumption in reperfused noninfarcted dysfunctional myocardium after unstable angina: Direct evidence for myocardial stunning in humans. J Am Coll Cardiol 34:1939–1946, 1999.

226. Perez NG, Marban E, Cingolani HE: Preservation of myofilament calcium responsiveness underlies protection against myocardial stunning by ischemic preconditioning. Cardiovasc Res 42:636–643, 1999.

227. Morales C, Rodriguez M, Scapin O, Gelpi RJ: Comparison of the effects of ACE inhibition with those of angiotensin II receptor antagonism on systolic and diastolic myocardial stunning in isolated rabbit heart. Mol Cell Biochem 186:117–121, 1998.

228. Shinmura K, Tang XL, Takano H, et al: Nitric oxide donors attenuate myocardial stunning in conscious rabbits. Am J Physiol 277:H2495–H2503, 1999.

229. Elsasser A, Schlepper M, Klovekorn WP, et al: Hibernating myocardium: An incomplete adaptation to ischemia. Circulation 96:2920–2931, 1997.

230. Rahimtoola SH: Concept and evaluation of hibernating myocardium. Annu Rev Med 50:75–86, 1999.

231. Wijns W, Vatner SF, Camici PG: Hibernating myocardium. N Engl J Med 339:173–181, 1998.

232. Afridi I, Qureshi U, Kopelen HA, et al: Serial changes in response of hibernating myocardium to inotropic stimulation after revascularization: A dobutamine echocardiographic study. J Am Coll Cardiol 30:1233–1240, 1997.

233. Auerbach MA, Schoder H, Hoh C, et al: Prevalence of myocardial viability as detected by positron emission tomography in patients with ischemic cardiomyopathy. Circulation 99:2921–2926, 1999.

234. Fath-Ordoubadi F, Beatt KJ, Spyrou N, Camici PG: Efficacy of coronary angioplasty for the treatment of hibernating myocardium. Heart 82:210–216, 1999.

235. Chen C, Ma L, Linfert DR, et al: Myocardial cell death and apoptosis in hibernating myocardium. J Am Coll Cardiol 30:1407–1412, 1997.

236. Schwarz ER, Schoendube FA, Kostin S, et al: Prolonged myocardial hibernation exacerbates cardiomyocyte degeneration and impairs recovery of function after revascularization. J Am Coll Cardiol 31:1018–1026, 1998.

237. Budinger GR, Duranteau J, Chandel NS, Schumacker PT: Hibernation during hypoxia in cardiomyocytes: Role of mitochondria as the O_2 sensor. J Biol Chem 273:3320–3326, 1998.

238. Camici PG, Rimoldi O: Myocardial hibernation vs. repetitive stunning in patients. Cardiol Rev 7:39-43, 1999.

239. Camici PG, Wijns W, Borgers M, et al: Pathophysiological mechanisms of chronic reversible left ventricular dysfunction due to coronary artery disease (hibernating myocardium). Circulation 96:3205–3214, 1997.

240. Ihara T, Komamura K, Shen YT, et al: Left ventricular systolic dysfunction precedes diastolic dysfunction during myocardial ischemia in conscious dogs. Am J Physiol 267:H333–H343, 1994.

241. Stoddard MF, Wagner SG, Ikram S, et al: Effects of nifedipine and nitroglycerin on left ventricular systolic dysfunction and impaired diastolic filling after exercise-induced ischemia in humans. J Am Coll Cardiol 28:915–923, 1996.

242. Mochizuki T, Eberli FR, Ngoy S, et al: Effects of brief repetitive ischemia on contractility, relaxation, and coronary flow: Exaggerated postischemic diastolic dysfunction in pressure-overload hypertrophy. Circ Res 73:550–558, 1993.

243. Grossman W: Diastolic dysfunction in congestive heart failure. N Engl J Med 325:1557–1564, 1991.

244. Yin FC: Ventricular wall stress. Circ Res 49:829–842, 1981.

245. Dunn RB, Griggs DM Jr: Transmural gradients in ventricular tissue metabolites produced by stopping coronary blood flow in the dog. Circ Res 37:438–445, 1975.

246. Moss AJ: Intramyocardial oxygen tension. Cardiovasc Res 2:314–318, 1968.

247. Weiss HR, Sinha AK: Regional oxygen saturation of small arteries and veins in the canine myocardium. Circ Res 42:119–126, 1978.

248. Jennings RB, Steenbergen C Jr, Reimer KA: Myocardial ischemia and reperfusion. Monogr Pathol 37:47–80, 1995.

249. Bogaert J, Maes A, Van de Werf F, et al: Functional recovery of subepicardial myocardial tissue in transmural myocardial infarction after successful reperfusion: An important contribution to the improvement of regional and global left ventricular function. Circulation 99:36–43, 1999.

Chapter 35

Acute Myocardial Infarction

ELLIOTT M. ANTMAN · EUGENE BRAUNWALD

CHANGING PATTERNS IN CLINICAL CARE OF PATIENTS WITH ACUTE MYOCARDIAL INFARCTION

Despite impressive strides in diagnosis and management over the past three decades, acute myocardial infarction (AMI) continues to be a major public health problem in the industrialized world and is becoming an increasingly important problem in developing countries.[1] In the United States, nearly 1.0 million patients annually suffer from AMI.[2] More than 1 million patients with suggested AMI are admitted yearly to coronary care units (CCUs) in the United States.[2] Although the death rate from AMI has declined by about 30 percent over the past decade, its development is still a fatal event in approximately one third of patients. About 50 percent of the deaths associated with AMI occur within 1 hour of the event and are attributable to arrhythmias, most often ventricular fibrillation. Because AMI may strike an individual during the most productive years, it can have profoundly deleterious psychosocial and economic ramifications.

Of particular concern from a global perspective are projections from the World Heart Federation that the burden of disease in developing countries will become more closely aligned with that now afflicting developed countries[2, 3] (see Chap. 1). With a decline in infectious disease–related deaths accompanied by accelerated economic development and life style change promoting atherosclerosis, developing countries especially in Eastern Europe, Asia, and parts of Latin America are expected to experience a sharp increase in ischemic heart disease and AMI.[3] Given the wide disparity of available resources to treat AMI in developing countries, major efforts are needed on an international level to strengthen primary prevention programs at the community level.[1]

IMPROVEMENTS IN OUTCOME. A steady decline in the mortality rate from AMI has been observed across several population groups since 1960.[1, 4] This appears to be caused by a fall in the incidence of AMI (replaced in part by an increase in the rate of unstable angina[5]) and a fall in the case-fatality rate once an MI has occurred[6, 7] (Fig. 35–1).

Several phases in the management of patients have contributed to the decline in mortality from AMI.[8, 9] The "clinical observation phase" of coronary care consumed the first half of the 20th century and focused on a detailed recording of physical and laboratory findings; treatment consisted of strict bed rest and sedation. Subsequently, the "coronary care unit phase" beginning in the mid-1960s occurred and was notable for detailed analysis and vigorous management of cardiac arrhythmias. The "high-technology phase" was ushered in by the introduction of the pulmonary artery balloon flotation catheter, setting the stage for bedside hemodynamic monitoring and more precise management of heart failure and cardiogenic shock associated with AMI. The modern "reperfusion era" of coronary care was introduced by intracoronary and then intravenous thrombolysis, increased use of aspirin, and development of primary percutaneous transluminal coronary angioplasty (PTCA) and implantation of coronary stents for AMI. A battery of tests sometimes providing overlapping information was typically ordered during the high-technology phase.

Driven in large part by the need for cost-saving measures, contemporary care of patients with AMI has entered the "evidence-based coronary care phase" and is becoming increasingly influenced by managed care systems and guidelines for clinical practice[10, 11] Although increased responsibility has been placed in the hands of primary care physicians, they have begun to express concern about the potential adverse impact of an excessive increase in the scope of care they are being asked to provide.[12] Coronary care practice is better equipped than other areas of cardiology to face this transition from pathophysiologically based decision-making to evidence-based decision-making, given the rich data base of patients with suspected AMI studied in clinical trials and registries and efforts at summarizing a vast amount of data using metaanalysis.[13–16] New therapies for AMI are being evaluated not only for evidence of safety and efficacy but also for their cost-effectiveness in caring for patients and their impact on quality of life. However, despite an abundance of cost-effectiveness information analyzed from a societal perspective with data from clinical trials, clinicians weighing the risk-benefit ratio at the bedside of an individual patient with AMI may have difficulty applying the findings for several reasons: uncertainty whether the benefits observed in a strictly defined trial population are applicable to a wider selection of patients,[17] limited data on specific subgroups, vari-

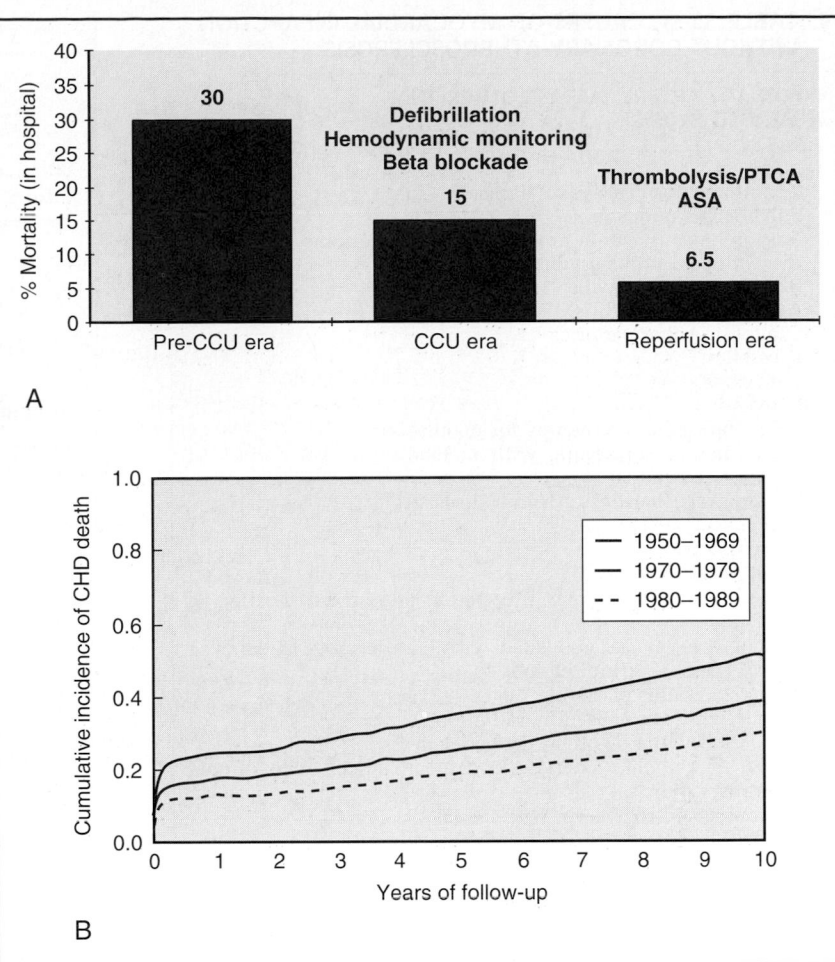

FIGURE 35–1. *A,* The impact of medical therapy for AMI on short-term mortality. In the pre-CCU era AMI short-term mortality (30-day) was estimated to be 30 percent. Implementation of the CCU concept with defibrillation, sophisticated hemodynamic monitoring, and beta blockade reduced this to 15 percent. A further mortality reduction was ushered in by the reperfusion era; combinations of thrombolysis, primary percutaneous transluminal coronary angioplasty, and aspirin are now employed. (Modified from Antman EM: General hospital management. *In* Julian D, Braunwald E (eds): Management of Acute Myocardial Infarction. London, WB Saunders, 1994, p 31.) *B,* Cumulative incidence of CHD death as function of time period of initial Q-wave MI. (Modified from Guidry UC, et al: Temporal trends in event rates after Q-wave myocardial infarction: The Framingham Heart Study. Circulation 100:2054–2059, 1999. Copyright 1999, American Heart Association.)

ations in the absolute level of baseline risk,[18] and variations in patient preferences. The information in this chapter on various treatment strategies should therefore be used as a guide and not a substitute for carefully reasoned clinical decision-making on a case-by-case basis.

LIMITATIONS OF CURRENT THERAPY AND VARIATIONS IN CLINICAL RESPONSE IN KEY SUBGROUPS. Despite the gratifying success of medical therapy for AMI, several observations indicate that considerable room for improvement exists. The short-term mortality of patients with AMI who receive aggressive pharmacological reperfusion therapy as part of a randomized trial is in the range of 6.5 to 7.0 percent,[19-22] whereas observational data bases such as The National Registry of Myocardial Infarction and Cooperative Cardiovascular Project suggest that the mortality rate in AMI patients is about 20 percent.[16] In addition, the mortality rate from AMI in patients enrolled in randomized trials is considerably lower than that observed among patients who are excluded from such trials.

Although the survival of elderly patients (> age 65) after AMI has improved significantly, advanced age consistently emerges as one of the principal determinants of mortality in AMI.[23] Despite reluctance to use potentially life-saving drug therapies in the elderly,[23a, 23b] cardiac catheterization and other invasive procedures are being performed more commonly at some point during hospitalization in elderly AMI patients. Nevertheless, evidence suggests that the greatest reductions in mortality for elderly patients are derived from those strategies employed during the first 24 hours, the time frame in which prompt and appropriate use of life-saving pharmacotherapy is of paramount importance, emphasizing the need to extend advances in drug therapy for AMI to the elderly.[24]

Despite trends toward greater use of mortality-reducing therapies such as thrombolytics, aspirin, and beta-adrenoceptor blockers in patients with AMI, these drugs still appear to be underused.[25-29a] Considerable variation exists in practice patterns for management of patients with AMI. This variation is seen not only on an international level but also regionally within countries[26, 30] and across medical specialties[26, 31, 32]; such variations in practice are correlated with differences in outcome after AMI.[33] Intriguing data have indicated that mortality rates for AMI are lower in hospitals with a high clinical volume, a high rate of invasive procedures, and a top ranking in quality reports.[33-35a]

Variation has also been observed in the treatment patterns of certain population subgroups with AMI, notably women and blacks.[29a, 36] Although the unadjusted rates of thrombolytic use and referral for cardiac catheterization and angioplasty are lower and unadjusted mortality rates are higher in women with AMI, gender differences are less apparent (but may not disappear entirely) once adjustment is made for baseline variables such as comorbidities and age[29a, 37] (see Chap. 58). Of interest, after AMI, younger women but not older women have higher rates of in-hospital mortality than do men of the same age.[38]

Pathology

Almost all MIs result from coronary atherosclerosis, generally with superimposed coronary thrombosis. Nonatherogenic forms of coronary artery disease are discussed on pages 1123 and 1336, and causes of AMI without coronary atherosclerosis are shown in Table 35–1.

Before the thrombolytic era, clinicians typically divided AMI patients into those suffering a Q-wave or non-Q-wave infarct, based on the evolution of the pattern on the electrocardiogram (ECG) over several days after AMI. The term "Q-wave infarction" was frequently considered to be virtu-

▼ TABLE 35–1. CAUSES OF MYOCARDIAL INFARCTION WITHOUT CORONARY ATHEROSCLEROSIS

CORONARY ARTERY DISEASE OTHER THAN ATHEROSCLEROSIS
Arteritis
  Luetic
  Granulomatous (Takayasu disease)
  Polyarteritis nodosa
  Mucocutaneous lymph node (Kawasaki) syndrome
  Disseminated lupus erythematosus
  Rheumatoid spondylitis
  Ankylosing spondylitis
Trauma to coronary arteries
  Laceration
  Thrombosis
  Iatrogenic
  Radiation (radiation therapy for neoplasia)
Coronary mural thickening with metabolic disease or intimal proliferative disease
  Mucopolysaccharidoses (Hurler disease)
  Homocysteinuria
  Fabry disease
  Amyloidosis
  Juvenile intimal sclerosis (idiopathic arterial calcification of infancy)
  Intimal hyperplasia associated with contraceptive steroids or with the postpartum period
  Pseudoxanthoma elasticum
  Coronary fibrosis caused by radiation therapy
Luminal narrowing by other mechanisms
  Spasm of coronary arteries (Prinzmetal angina with normal coronary arteries)
  Spasm after nitroglycerin withdrawal
  Dissection of the aorta
  Dissection of the coronary artery

EMBOLI TO CORONARY ARTERIES
Infective endocarditis
Nonbacterial thrombotic endocarditis
Prolapse of mitral valve
Mural thrombus from left atrium, left ventricle, or pulmonary veins
Prosthetic valve emboli
Cardiac myxoma
Associated with cardiopulmonary bypass surgery and coronary arteriography
Paradoxical emboli
Papillary fibroelastoma of the aortic valve ("fixed embolus")
Thrombi from intracardiac catheters or guidewires

CONGENITAL CORONARY ARTERY ANOMALIES
Anomalous origin of left coronary from pulmonary artery
Left coronary artery from anterior sinus of Valsalva
Coronary arteriovenous and arteriocameral fistulas
Coronary artery aneurysms

MYOCARDIAL OXYGEN DEMAND-SUPPLY DISPROPORTION
Aortic stenosis, all forms
Incomplete differentiation of the aortic valve
Aortic insufficiency
Carbon monoxide poisoning
Thyrotoxicosis
Prolonged hypotension

HEMATOLOGICAL (IN SITU THROMBOSIS)
Polycythemia vera
Thrombocytosis
Disseminated intravascular coagulation
Hypercoagulability, thrombosis, thrombocytopenic purpura

MISCELLANEOUS
Cocaine abuse
Myocardial contusion
Myocardial infarction with normal coronary arteries
Complication of cardic catheterization

Modified from Cheitlin M, et al: Myocardial infarction without atherosclerosis. JAMA 231:951, 1975. Copyright 1975, American Medical Association.

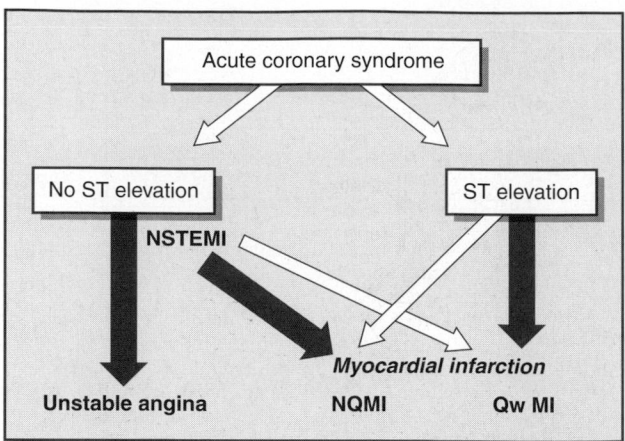

FIGURE 35–2. Nomenclature of acute coronary syndromes. Patients with ischemic discomfort may present with or without ST segment elevation on the ECG. The majority of patients with ST segment elevation (large arrows) ultimately develop a Q-wave acute myocardial infarction (QwMI), whereas a minority (small arrow) develop a non-Q-wave AMI (NQMI). Patients who present without ST segment elevation are either experiencing unstable angina or a non–ST segment elevation MI (NSTEMI). The distinction between these two diagnoses is ultimately made based on the presence or absence of a cardiac marker detected in the blood. Most patients with NSTEMI do not evolve a Q wave on the 12-lead ECG and are subsequently referred to as having sustained a non-Q-wave MI (NQMI); only a minority of NSTEMI patients develop a Q-wave AMI and are later diagnosed as having a Q-wave MI. The spectrum of clinical conditions ranging from unstable angina to non-Q-wave AMI comprise the acute coronary syndromes (ACS). (From Braunwald E, Antman EM, Beasley JW, et al: ACC/AHA guidelines for the management of patients with unstable angina: A report of the American College of Cardiology/American Heart Association Task Force on Practice Guidelines (Committee on the Management of Patients With Unstable Angina). J Am Coll Cardiol 36:970–1062, 2000.)

ally synonymous with "transmural infarction," whereas "non-Q-wave infarction" was often referred to as a "subendocardial infarction." Phibbs and colleagues have summarized the arguments that previous distinctions between Q-wave infarction and non-Q-wave infarction were based on erroneous interpretation of pathological data and should not serve as the basis for designing therapy.[39] A more suitable framework is based on the pathophysiology of AMI, leading to a reorganization of clinical presentations into what is now referred to as the *acute coronary syndromes* (Fig. 35–2) (see p. 1118).

ROLE OF ACUTE PLAQUE CHANGE

Slowly accruing high-grade stenoses of epicardial coronary arteries may progress to complete occlusion but do not usually precipitate AMI, probably because of the development of a rich collateral network (see p. 1123) over time. However, during the natural evolution of atherosclerotic plaques, especially those that are lipid laden, an abrupt and catastrophic transition may occur, characterized by plaque rupture. Evidence exists that some patients have a systemic predisposition to plaque rupture that is independent of traditional risk factors.[40–40a] After plaque rupture there is exposure of substances that promote platelet activation and aggregation, thrombin generation, and, ultimately, thrombus formation[41–42b] (Figs. 35–3 and 35–4). The resultant thrombus that is formed interrupts blood flow and leads to an imbalance between oxygen supply and demand and, if this imbalance is severe and persistent, to myocardial necrosis (Fig. 35–5).

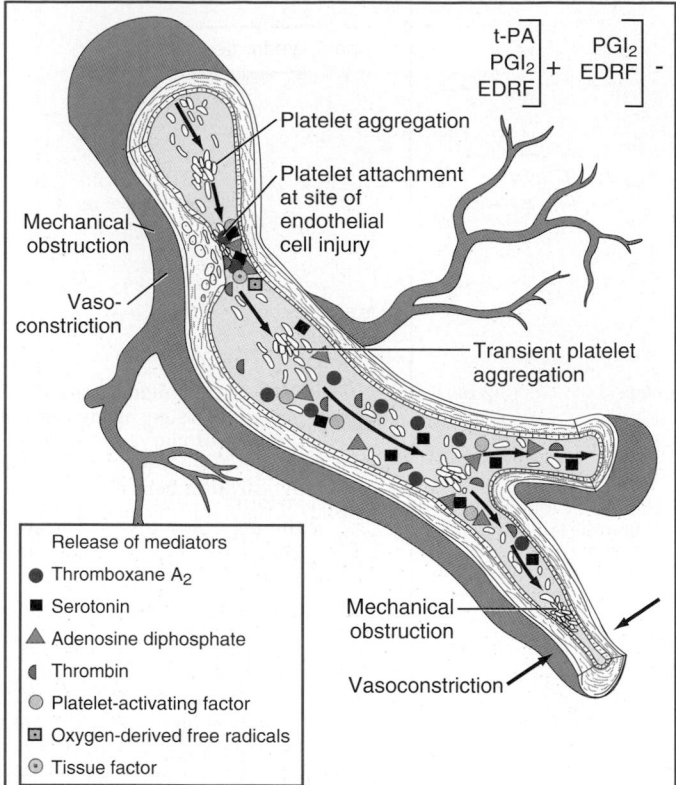

FIGURE 35–3. Schematic diagram suggesting probable mechanisms responsible for the conversion from chronic coronary heart disease to acute coronary artery disease syndromes. In this scheme, endothelial injury, usually at sites of atherosclerotic plaques and usually plaque ulceration or fissuring, is associated with platelet adhesion and aggregation and the release or activation of selected mediators, including thromboxane A_2, serotonin (5HT), adenosine diphosphate (ADP), platelet-activating factor (PAF), thrombin, tissue factor, and oxygen-derived free radicals. The accumulation of these mediators promotes platelet aggregation and mechanical obstruction of the narrowed artery. Thromboxane A_2, 5HT, thrombin, and PAF are vasoconstrictors at sites of endothelial injury. ADP, 5HT, and tissue factor have mitogenic influences and promote the development of neointimal proliferation. Therefore, the conversion from chronic stable to acute unstable coronary heart disease syndromes is most likely associated with endothelial injury, platelet aggregation, accumulation of platelet and other cell-derived mediators, further platelet aggregation, and vasoconstriction, with consequent dynamic narrowing of the coronary artery lumen. The relative absence of prostacyclin (PGI_2), tissue plasminogen activator (t-PA), and endothelium-derived relaxing factor (EDRF; nitrous oxide) at sites of endothelial injury contributes to the development of thrombosis, vasoconstriction, and neointimal proliferation. There are many different reasons for endothelial injury in addition to atherosclerotic plaque fissuring or ulceration, including flow shear stress, hypertension, immune complex deposition with complement activation, and mechanical injury to the endothelium as it occurs with coronary artery angioplasty, atherectomy, and stent placement and after heart transplantation. (From Willerson JT, Cohen LS, Maseri A: Pathophysiology and clinical recognition. *In* Willerson JT, Cohen JN [eds]: Cardiovascular Medicine. New York, Churchill Livingstone, 1995, p 335.)

COMPOSITION OF PLAQUES. At autopsy, the atherosclerotic plaque of patients who died of MI is composed primarily of fibrous tissue of varying density and cellularity with superimposed thrombus. Calcium, lipid-laden foam cells, and extracellular lipid each constitute 5 to 10 percent of the remaining area. The atherosclerotic plaques that are associated with thrombosis and a total occlusion, located in infarct-related vessels, are generally more complex and irregular than those in vessels not associated with MI.[43] Histological studies of these lesions often reveal plaque rup-

ture or erosion.[43] Angiographic morphology suggestive of plaque rupture has been identified in the majority of stenoses associated with AMI or abrupt onset of unstable angina.[44] This finding is rare in the non–infarct-related vessels of AMI patients and in the vessels of patients with chronic, stable angina.

Platelet-rich thrombi are often associated with the surface of the most advanced atherosclerotic lesions, called complicated plaques, which are characterized by fibrocalcific degeneration, deposition of lipid, calcium, fibrous tissue, necrotic debris, extravasated blood, and a fibrous cap (see Fig. 35–3). Impaired endothelial cell function may contribute to atherogenesis through release of growth factors. Luminal narrowing may potentiate platelet activation through augmentation of shear forces.

In patients with MI, coronary thrombi are usually superimposed on or adjacent to atherosclerotic plaques (see Figs. 35–3 and 35–4).[45] These coronary arterial thrombi, which are approximately 1 cm in length in most cases, adhere to the luminal surface of an artery and are composed of platelets, fibrin, erythrocytes, and leukocytes. The composition of the thrombus may vary at different levels: a white thrombus is composed of platelets, fibrin, or both; and a red thrombus is composed of erythrocytes, fibrin, platelets, and leukocytes.[46] Early thrombi are usually small and nonocclusive and are composed predominantly of platelets.[40a, 47]

PLAQUE FISSURING AND RUPTURE. The process of plaque fissuring is an area of intense investigation and is likely to be multifactorial in nature (see Fig. 35–3). In atherosclerotic plaques prone to rupture there is an increased rate of formation of metalloproteinase enzymes such as collagenase, gelatinase, and stromelysin that degrades components of the protective interstitial matrix.[48] These proteinases may be elaborated by activated macrophages and mast cells that have been shown to accumulate in high concentration at the site of atheromatous erosions and plaque rupture in patients who died of AMI.[45] Examination of specimens from atherectomy reveals a much higher content of macrophages and tissue factor in patients with unstable angina or AMI compared with patients with chronic stable angina.[49] In addition to these structural as-

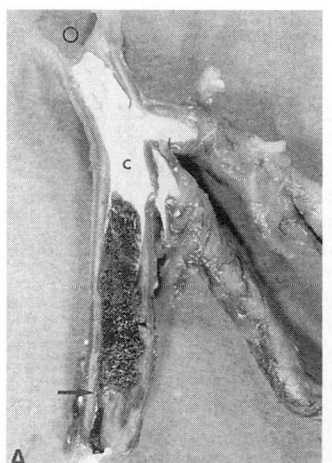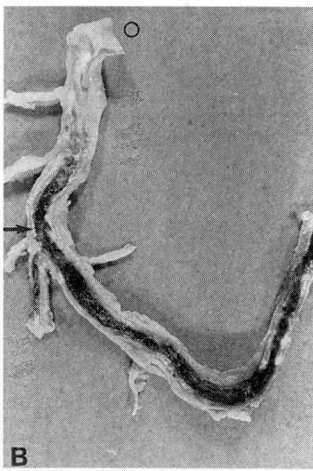

FIGURE 35–4. Thrombus propagation. *A,* Left anterior descending coronary artery cut open longitudinally, showing a dark (red) stagnation thrombosis propagating upstream from the initiating rupture/platelet-rich thrombus at the arrow. In this case, the thrombus has propagated proximally up to the nearest major side branch (the first diagonal branch). *B,* The right coronary artery cut open longitudinally, showing a huge stagnation thrombosis propagating downstream from the initiating rupture/platelet-rich thrombus at the arrow. Unlike upstream thrombus propagation, downstream propagation may, as in this case, occlude major side branches. O = coronary ostium; c = contrast medium injected postmortem. (From Falk E: Coronary thrombosis: Pathogenesis and clinical manifestations. Am J Cardiol 68:28B, 1991.)

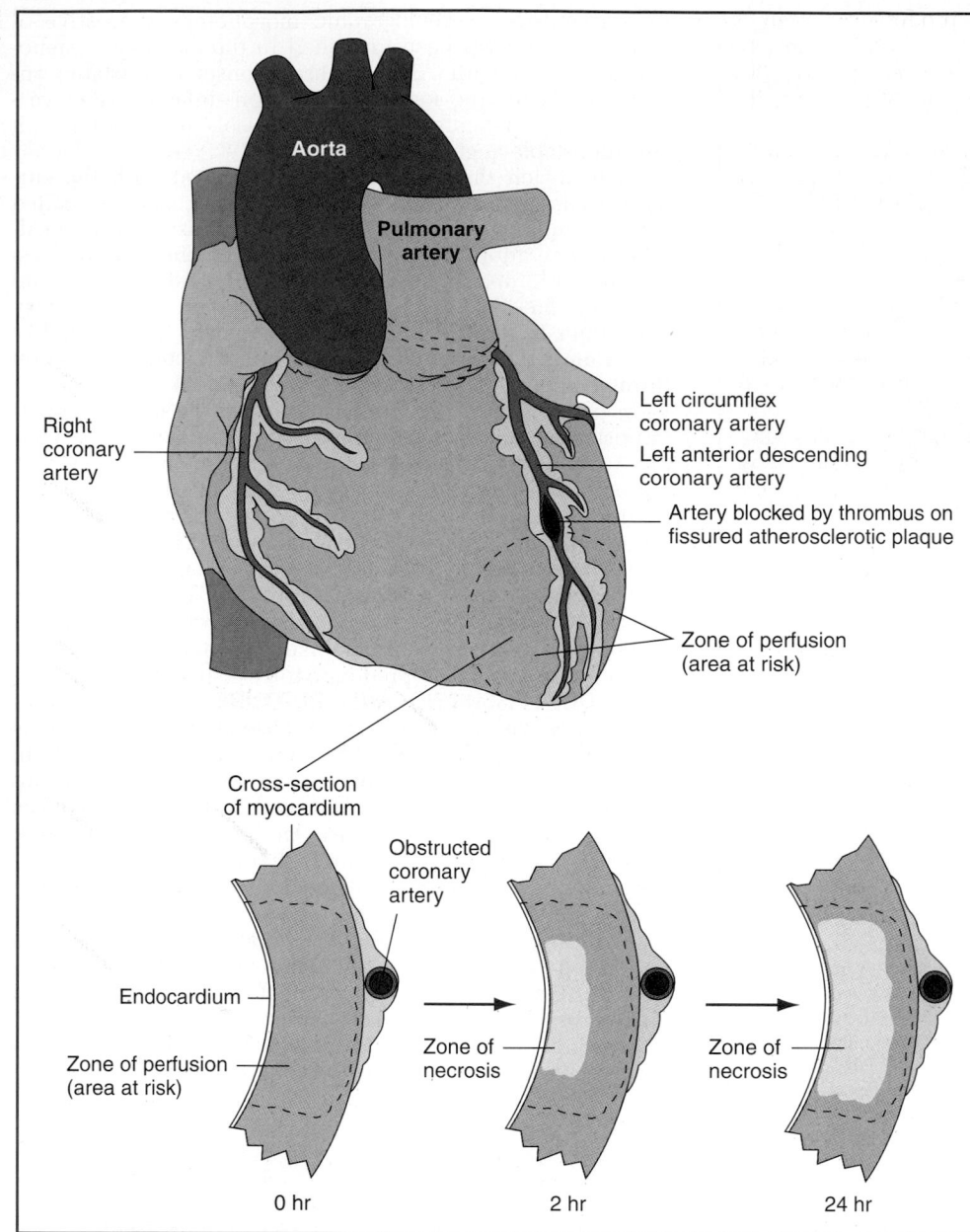

FIGURE 35–5. Schematic representation of the progression of myocardial necrosis after coronary artery occlusion. Necrosis begins in a small zone of the myocardium beneath the endocardial surface in the center of the ischemic zone. This entire region of myocardium (dashed outline) depends on the occluded vessel for perfusion and is the area at risk. Note that a very narrow zone of myocardium immediately beneath the endocardium is spared from necrosis because it can be oxygenated by diffusion from the ventricle. (Redrawn with permission from Schoen FJ: The heart. In Cotran RS, Kumar V, Collins T (eds): Pathologic Basis of Disease. 6th ed. Philadelphia, WB Saunders, 1999, p 557.)

pects of vulnerable plaques, stresses induced by intraluminal pressure, coronary vasomotor tone, tachycardia (cyclic stretching and compression), and disruption of nutrient vessels combine to produce plaque rupture at the margin of the fibrous cap near an adjacent plaque-free segment of the coronary artery wall (shoulder region of plaque).[41, 43] A number of key physiological variables such as systolic blood pressure, heart rate, blood viscosity, endogenous tissue plasminogen activator (t-PA) activity, plasminogen activator inhibitor-1 (PAI-1) levels, plasma cortisol levels, and plasma epinephrine levels that exhibit circadian and seasonal variations and are increased at times of stress act in concert to produce a heightened propensity for plaque rupture and coronary thrombosis, yielding the clustering of AMI in the early morning hours and especially in the winter and after natural disasters.[50, 51]

Acute Coronary Syndromes

If a sufficient quantity of thrombogenic substances is exposed when plaque rupture occurs, the coronary artery lumen may become obstructed by a combination of fibrin, platelet aggregates, and red blood cells (see Figs. 35–3 and 35–4).[51a] An adequate collateral network that prevents necrosis from occurring can result in clinically silent episodes of coronary occlusion. The rupture of plaques is now considered to be the common pathophysiological substrate of the *acute coronary syndromes* (see Fig. 35–2).[5, 42a, 52, 52a] The dynamic process of plaque rupture may evolve to a completely occlusive thrombus, typically producing ST segment elevation on the ECG. Typically, such completely occlusive thrombi lead to a large zone of necrosis involving the full or nearly full thickness of the ventricular wall in the myocardial bed subtended by the affected coronary artery (see Fig. 35–5). The infarction process alters the sequence of depolarization ultimately reflected as changes in the surface of the QRS complex.[39] The most characteristic change in the QRS complex that develops in about 75 percent of patients initially presenting with ST segment elevation is the evolution of Q waves in the leads overlying the infarct zone, leading to the term "Q-wave infarction" (see Fig. 35–2). In about 25 percent of patients presenting with ST segment elevation, no Q waves develop[53] but other abnormalities of the QRS are seen, such as diminution in R wave height and notching or splintering of the QRS complex.

Less obstructive thrombi and/or those that are constituted by less robust fibrin formation and a greater proportion of platelet aggregates typically produce ST segment depression and/or T wave inversion on the ECG (see Fig. 35–2). Relief of transient vasospasm (induced by thromboxane A_2 and serotonin released from activated platelets) (see Fig. 35–3) or spontaneous lysis and restoration of antegrade flow in the culprit coronary vessel in less than 20 minutes usually does not result in histological evidence of necrosis, the release of biochemical markers of necrosis, or persistent changes on the ECG. Episodes of plaque rupture more prolonged and more severe typically result in release of biochemical markers of necrosis but a less extensive pattern of necrosis than found in patients with ST segment elevation MI (STEMI). Patients presenting without ST segment elevation are initially diagnosed as suffering either from a non–ST segment elevation MI (NSTEMI) or unstable angina (see Fig. 35–2). The distinction between NSTEMI and unstable angina is based on whether a cardiac marker indicative of necrosis is detected in the blood, a finding that is now possible in a greater number of patients using sensitive markers such as cardiac-specific troponin T or I (see p. 1133). The majority of patients presenting with NSTEMI do not develop Q waves on the ECG and are ultimately diagnosed as having had a non-Q-wave MI. However, a minority of patients with NSTEMI develop Q waves and are ultimately diagnosed as having had a Q-wave MI (see Fig. 35–2).

The acute coronary syndrome spectrum concept, organized around a common pathophysiological substrate, is a useful framework for developing therapeutic strategies.[52a, 54] Patients presenting with persistent ST segment elevation are candidates for reperfusion therapy (either pharmacological or catheter-based) to restore flow in the occluded epicardial infarct–related artery. Patients presenting without ST segment elevation are not candidates for pharmacological reperfusion but should receive vigorous antiischemic therapy (see Chap. 36). Antithrombin therapy and antiplatelet therapy should be administered to all patients with an acute coronary syndrome regardless of the presence or absence of ST segment elevation. Thus, the 12-lead ECG remains at the center of the decision pathway for management of patients with an acute coronary syndrome to distinguish between presentations with ST segment elevation and those without ST elevation (see Fig. 35–2).[55, 56] The ECG lacks sufficient sensitivity and specificity to permit reliable distinction of transmural from subendocardial infarcts. Categorization of patients into those with Q-wave and non-Q-wave infarction patterns is best conceived of as only a crude guide to the extent of ventricular damage. Prognostic considerations must take into account other important factors, such as whether the ECG abnormality is due to a first infarct versus subsequent infarct, the location of infarction (anterior vs. inferior), infarct size, and demographic factors such as patient age.[39]

Some patients with stenotic atherosclerotic lesions experience AMI without evidence of plaque rupture or superimposed thrombosis. AMI occurs in clinical circumstances that produce a marked reduction in myocardial oxygen supply (e.g., prolonged severe vasospasm, as in Prinzmetal's variant angina [see Chap. 37], or associated with a marked increase in myocardial oxygen demand [see later]). These infarcts are located along the least well-perfused inner one third to one half of the ventricular wall and often extend beyond the target territory perfused by a single coronary vessel.[57] The ECG in such patients may show deep T wave inversions or diffuse ST segment depression.

GROSS PATHOLOGICAL CHANGES

The location and extent of AMI can be assessed on pathological examination (Fig. 35–6). On gross inspection, AMI may be divided into two major types: (1) transmural in-

FIGURE 35–6. See color plate 21.

farcts, in which myocardial necrosis involves the full thickness (or nearly full thickness) of the ventricular wall, and (2) subendocardial (nontransmural) infarcts, in which the necrosis involves the subendocardium, the intramural myocardium, or both without extending all the way through the ventricular wall to the epicardium.[57]

An occlusive coronary thrombus appears to be far more common when the infarction is transmural and localized to the distribution of a single coronary artery (see Fig. 35–4). Nontransmural infarctions, however, frequently occur in the presence of severely narrowed but still patent coronary arteries. Patchy nontransmural infarction may arise from thrombolysis or PTCA of an originally occlusive thrombus with restoration of blood flow *before* the wave front of necrosis has extended from the subendocardium across the full thickness of the ventricular wall (see Fig. 35–5). The histological pattern of necrosis may differ, with contraction band injury (see later) occurring almost twice as often in nontransmural as in transmural infarction. Paradoxically, before their infarction, patients with nontransmural infarcts have, on average, a more severe stenosis in the infarct-related coronary artery than do patients suffering from transmural infarcts. This finding suggests that a more severe obstruction occurring before infarction protects against the development of transmural infarction, perhaps by fostering the development of collateral circulation. It also accords with the concept that less severely stenotic but lipid-laden plaques with a fragile cap are responsible for the abrupt presentation of ST segment elevation that may evolve into transmural infarctions.

THE FIRST HOURS. Gross alterations of the myocardium are difficult to identify until at least 6 to 12 hours have elapsed after the onset of necrosis (Fig. 35–7). However, a variety of histochemical stains can be used to identify zones of necrosis that can be discerned after only 2 to 3 hours. Tissue slices of suspected infarct sites are immersed in a solution of triphenyltetrazolium chloride (TTC), which stains viable myocardium brick red (because of preserved dehydrogenase enzymes that form a red formazan precipitate) and leaves the infarcted region pale as a result of failure of uptake of the vital dye (see Fig. 35–6). The nitroblue tetrazolium (NBT) staining technique can similarly distinguish viable zones of myocardium, which stain dark blue, from necrotic areas of myocardium that therefore remain uncolored and identifiable. Other approaches include autofluorescence staining, immunohistochemical analysis, and, more recently, special DNA staining techniques to identify apoptotic bodies in myocardial sections.[58]

Initially, the myocardium in the affected region may appear pale and slightly swollen. Eighteen to 36 hours after the onset of the infarct, the myocardium is tan or reddish purple (due to trapped erythrocytes), with a serofibrinous exudate evident on the epicardium in transmural infarcts. These changes persist for approximately 48 hours; the infarct then turns gray, and fine yellow lines, secondary to neutrophilic infiltration, appear at its periphery. This zone gradually widens and during the next few days extends throughout the infarct.

THE FIRST DAYS. Eight to 10 days after infarction the thickness of the cardiac wall in the area of the infarct is reduced as necrotic muscle is removed by mononuclear cells. The cut surface of an infarct of this age is yellow, surrounded by a reddish purple band of granulation tissue that extends through the necrotic tissue by 3 to 4 weeks. Commencing at this time and extending over the next 2 to 3 months, the infarcted area gradually acquires a gelatinous, ground-glass, gray appearance, eventually converting into a shrunken, thin, firm scar that whitens and firms

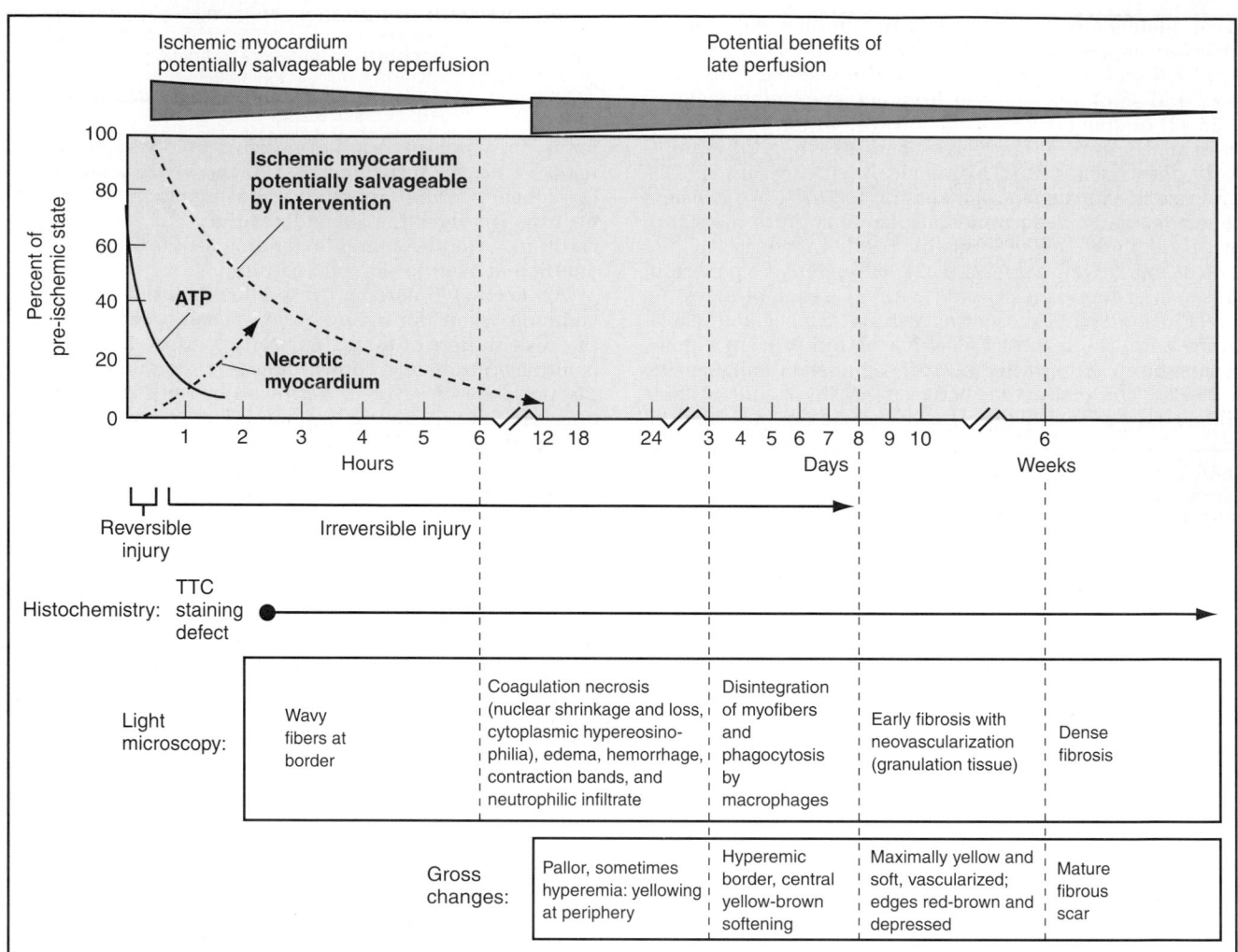

FIGURE 35-7. Temporal sequence of early biochemical, ultrastructural, histochemical, and histological findings after onset of MI. At the top of the figure are schematically shown the time frames for early and late reperfusion of the myocardium supplied by an occluded coronary artery. For approximately one-half hour after the onset of even the most severe ischemia, myocardial injury is potentially reversible; after that there is progressive loss of viability that is complete by 6 to 12 hours. The benefits of reperfusion (both early and late) are greatest when it is achieved early, with progressively smaller benefits occurring as reperfusion is delayed. (From Schoen FJ: Pathologic considerations of the surgery of adult heart disease. *In* Edmunds LH [ed]: Cardiac Surgery in the Adult. New York, McGraw-Hill, 1997, p 85.)

progressively with time[57] (see Fig. 35-6). This process begins at the periphery of the infarct and gradually moves centrally. The endocardium below the infarct increases in thickness and becomes gray and opaque.

Histological and Ultrastructural Changes

ELECTRON MICROSCOPY. In experimental infarction, the earliest ultrastructural changes in cardiac muscle after ligation of a coronary artery, noted within 20 minutes, consist of reduction in the size and number of glycogen granules, intracellular edema, and swelling and distortion of the transverse tubular system, the sarcoplasmic reticulum, and the mitochondria[58] (see Fig. 35-7). These early changes are reversible. Changes after 60 minutes of occlusion include myocardial cell swelling, mitochondrial abnormalities such as swelling and internal disruption, development of amorphous, flocculent aggregation and margination of nuclear chromatin, and relaxation of myofibrils. After 20 minutes to 2 hours of ischemia, changes in some cells become irreversible, and there is progression of these alterations; additional changes include indistinct, tight junctions at the intercalated discs, swollen sacs of the sarcoplasmic reticulum at the level of the A band, greatly enlarged mitochondria with few cristae, thinning and fractionation of myofilaments, disappearance of the heterochromatin, rarefaction of the euchromatin and peripheral aggregation of chromatin in the nucleus, disorientation of myofibrils, and clumping of mitochondria. Cells irreversibly damaged by ischemia are usually swollen, with an enlarged sarcoplasmic space; the sarcolemma may peel

off the cells, defects in the plasma membrane may appear, and the mitochondria are fragmented. The swollen mitochondria obtained from ischemic myocardium contain deposits of calcium phosphate and amorphous matrix densities. Many of these changes become more intense when blood flow is restored.[57]

LIGHT MICROSCOPY. It was previously believed that no light microscopic changes could be seen in infarcted myocardium until 8 hours after interruption of blood flow. However, in some infarcts a pattern of wavy myocardial fibers may be seen 1 to 3 hours after onset, especially at the periphery of the infarct (see Figs. 35-7 and 35-8). It is hypothesized that wavy fibers result from the stretching and buckling of noncontractile fibers as forces are transmitted to them from adjacent viable contractile fibers.[57] After 8 hours, edema of the interstitium becomes evident, as do increased fatty deposits in the muscle fibers, along with infiltration of neutrophilic polymorphonuclear leukocytes and red blood cells. Muscle cell nuclei become pyknotic and then undergo karyolysis, and small blood vessels undergo necrosis.

By 24 hours there is clumping of the cytoplasm and loss of cross striations, with appearance of focal hyalinization and irregular cross bands in the involved myocardial fibers. The nuclei become pyknotic and sometimes even disappear. The myocardial capillaries in the involved region dilate, and polymorphonuclear leukocytes accumulate, first at the periphery and then in the center of the infarct. During the first 3 days, the interstitial tissue becomes edematous and red blood cells may extravasate (see Fig. 35-7). Generally, on about the fourth day after infarction, removal of necrotic fibers by macrophages begins, again commencing at the periphery (see Figs. 35-7 and 35-8). Later, lymphocytes, macrophages, and fibroblasts infiltrate between myocytes, which become fragmented. At 8 days, the necrotic muscle fibers have become dissolved; by about 10 days, the number of poly-

FIGURE 35–8. See color plate 21.

morphonuclear leukocytes is reduced and granulation tissue first appears at the periphery (see Figs. 35–7 and 35–8). Ingrowth of blood vessels and fibroblasts continues, along with removal of necrotic muscle cells, until the fourth to sixth week after infarction, by which time much of the necrotic myocardium has been removed. This process continues along with increasing collagenization of the infarcted area. By the sixth week, the infarcted area has usually been converted into a firm connective tissue scar with interspersed, intact muscle fibers (see Figs. 35–7 and 35–8).

PATTERNS OF MYOCARDIAL NECROSIS

COAGULATION NECROSIS. This results from severe, persistent ischemia and is usually present in the central region of infarcts, which results in the arrest of muscle cells[59] in the relaxed state and the passive stretching of ischemic muscle cells. On light microscopy the myofibrils are stretched, many with nuclear pyknosis, vascular congestion, and healing by phagocytosis of necrotic muscle cells (see Fig. 35–7). There is evidence of mitochondrial damage with prominent amorphous (flocculent) densities but no calcification.

NECROSIS WITH CONTRACTION BANDS. This form of myocardial necrosis, also termed "contraction band necrosis" or "coagulative myocytolysis," results primarily from severe ischemia followed by reflow.[57] It is caused by increased calcium ion (Ca^{2+}) influx into dying cells, resulting in the arrest of cells in the contracted state. It is seen in the periphery of large infarcts and is present to a greater extent in nontransmural than in transmural infarcts. The entire infarct may show this form of necrosis when reperfusion occurs experimentally or by surgery[59] (see Figs. 35–8 and 35–9). Although patches of contraction band necrosis are found after successful reperfusion by thrombolytic therapy, their presence in a large segment of the infarcts of patients who did not receive such therapy suggests that reperfusion through spontaneous thrombolysis or the release of spasm or both have occurred. It is characterized by hypercontracted myofibrils with contraction bands and mitochondrial damage, frequently with calcification, marked vascular congestion, and healing by lysis of muscle cells.

MYOCYTOLYSIS. Ischemia without necrosis generally causes no acute changes that are visible by light microscopy. However, severe prolonged ischemia can cause myocyte vacuolization, often termed "myocytolysis." Prolonged severe ischemia, which is potentially reversible, causes cloudy swelling, as well as hydropic, vascular, and fatty degeneration. Frequently seen at the borders of an infarct as well as in patchy areas of infarction in patients with chronic ischemic heart disease, myocytolysis is characterized by edema and cell swelling, lysis of myofibrils and nuclei, no neutrophilic response, and heal-

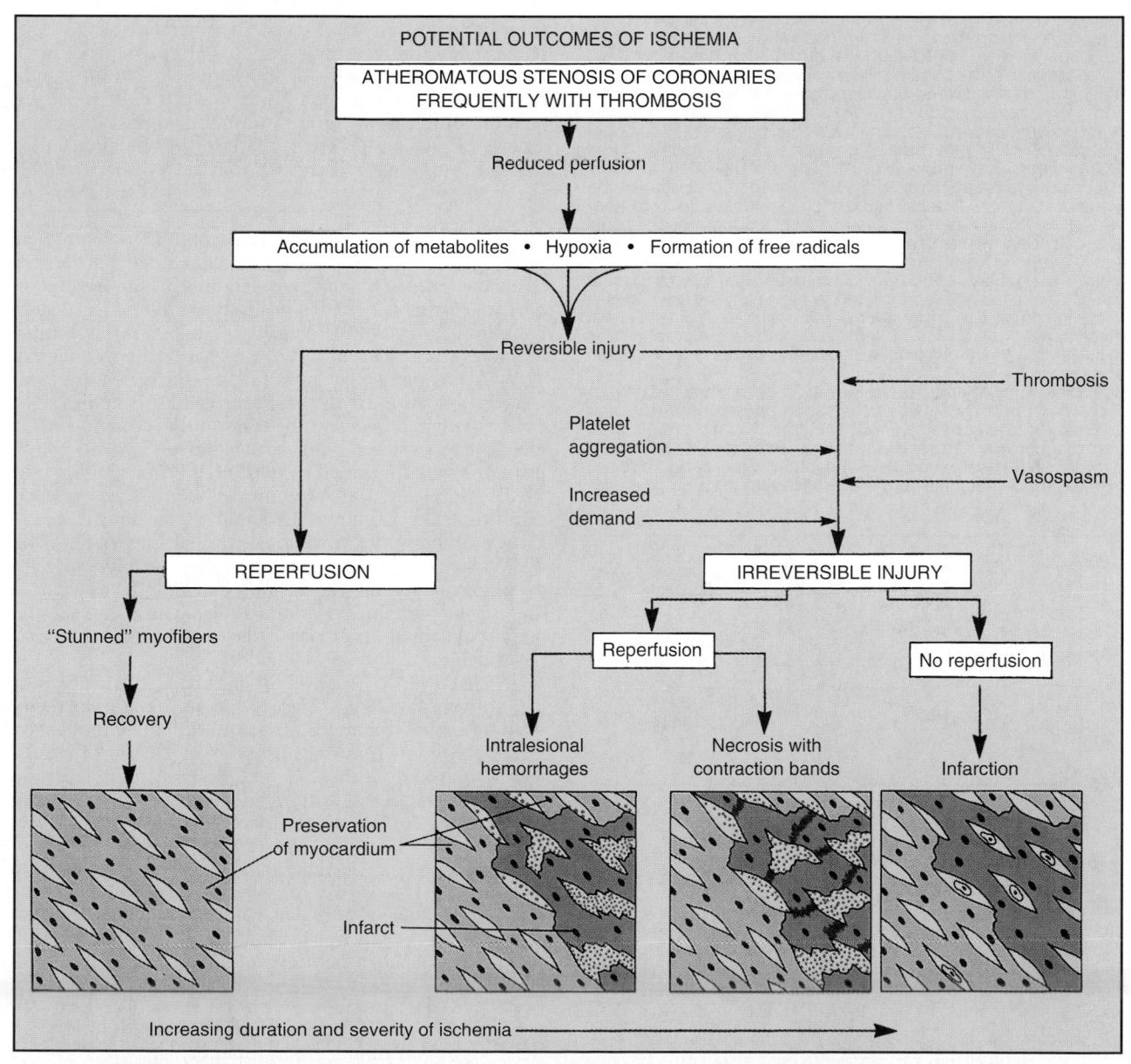

FIGURE 35–9. Several potential outcomes of reversible and irreversible ischemic injury to the myocardium. (From Schoen FJ: The heart. *In* Cotran RS, Kumar V, Robbins SL (eds): Pathologic Basis of Disease. 5th ed. Philadelphia, WB Saunders, 1994, p 538.)

ing by lysis and phagocytosis of necrotic myocytes and ultimately scar formation.

MODIFICATION OF PATHOLOGICAL CHANGES BY REPERFUSION

Early after the onset of ischemia, contractile dysfunction is observed that is believed to be due in part to shortening of the action potential duration, reduced cytosolic free calcium levels, and intracellular acidosis. When reperfusion of myocardium undergoing the evolutionary changes from ischemia to infarction occurs sufficiently early (i.e., within 15 to 20 minutes), it may successfully prevent necrosis from developing. Beyond such a very early stage, the number of salvaged myocytes and therefore the amount of salvaged myocardial tissue (area of necrosis/area at risk) is directly related to the length of time the coronary artery has been totally occluded, the level of myocardial oxygen consumption, and the collateral blood flow (see Fig. 35–9). Typical pathological findings of reperfused infarcts include a histological mixture of necrosis, hemorrhage within zones of irreversibly injured myocytes, coagulative myocytolysis with contraction bands, and distorted architecture of the cells in the reperfused zone[58] (see Fig. 35–9). After reperfusion, mitochondria in nonviable myocytes develop deposits of calcium phosphate and ultimately a large fraction of the cells may calcify. Reperfusion of infarcted myocardium also accelerates the washout of intracellular proteins ("serum cardiac markers"), producing an exaggerated and early peak value of substances such as the MB isoenzyme of creatine kinase (CK-MB) and cardiac-specific troponin T and I[60] (see p. 1134).

CORONARY ANATOMY AND LOCATION OF INFARCTION

In over 75 percent of patients with MI who come to autopsy, more than one coronary artery is severely narrowed. One third to two thirds of patients with AMI have critical obstruction (to less than 25 percent of luminal area) of all three coronary arteries, whereas the remainder are equally divided between those having one-vessel disease and those having two-vessel disease. Coronary arteriographic studies in surviving patients show that a higher percentage have one-vessel disease. Angiographic studies performed in the earliest hours of AMI in patients presenting with ST segment elevation have revealed approximately a 90 percent incidence of total occlusion of the infarct-related vessel.[61] Recanalization from spontaneous thrombolysis[62] as well as attrition due to some mortality among those patients with total occlusion results in a diminishing incidence of angiographically totally occluded vessels in the period after MI (Fig. 35–10). Pharmacological thrombolysis markedly increases the proportion of patients with a patent infarct-related artery early after AMI (see Fig. 35–10). In contrast to patients presenting with ST segment elevation, those patients who present without ST segment elevation have a much lower incidence of complete occlusion of the infarct-related coronary artery.

Thus, transmural infarcts occur distal to an acutely totally occluded coronary artery with thrombus superimposed on a ruptured plaque. However, the converse is not the case, in that chronic total occlusion of a coronary artery is not always associated with myocardial infarction. Collateral blood flow and other factors—such as the level of myocardial metabolism, the presence and location of steno-

ses in other coronary arteries, the rate of development of the obstruction, and the quantity of myocardium supplied by the obstructed vessel—all influence the viability of myocardial cells distal to the occlusion. In many series of patients studied at necropsy or by coronary arteriography, a small number (5 percent) of patients with AMI are found to have normal coronary vessels. In these patients, an embolus that has lysed, a transiently occlusive platelet aggregate, or a prolonged episode of severe coronary spasm may have been responsible for the reduction in coronary flow.

Studies of patients who ultimately develop AMI after having undergone coronary angiography at some time before its occurrence have been helpful in clarifying coronary anatomy before infarction. Although high-grade stenoses, when present, more frequently lead to AMI than do less severe lesions, the majority of occlusions actually occur in vessels with a previously identified stenosis of less than 50 percent on angiograms performed months to years earlier. This finding supports the concept that AMI occurs as a result of sudden thrombotic occlusion at the site of rupture of previously nonobstructive but lipid-rich plaques.

Rather frequently, when an area of the ventricle is perfused by collateral vessels, an infarct occurs at a distance from a coronary occlusion. For example, after the gradual obliteration of the lumen of the right coronary artery, the inferior wall of the left ventricle may be maintained viable by collateral vessels arising from the left anterior descending coronary artery. In this circumstance, an occlusion of the left anterior descending artery may cause an infarct of the diaphragmatic wall.

RIGHT VENTRICULAR INFARCTION. Depending on the criteria used, approximately 50 percent of patients with inferior infarction have some involvement of the right ventricle.[63, 63a] Among these patients, right ventricular infarction occurs exclusively in those with transmural infarction of the inferoposterior wall and the posterior portion of the septum. Right ventricular infarction almost invariably develops in association with infarction of the adjacent septum and left ventricular myocardium, but isolated infarction of the right ventricle is seen in 3 to 5 percent of autopsy-proven cases of MI.

Regardless of whether it is combined with involvement of the left ventricle, right ventricular infarction is generally associated with obstructive lesions of the right coronary artery. However, right ventricular infarction occurs less commonly than would be anticipated from the frequency of atherosclerotic lesions involving the right coronary artery. This discrepancy probably can be explained by the lower oxygen demands of the right ventricle, because right ventricular infarcts occur more commonly in conditions associated with increased right ventricular oxygen needs, such as pulmonary hypertension and right ventricular hypertrophy.[63] Moreover, the intercoronary collateral system of the right ventricle is richer than that of the left, and the thinness of the right ventricular wall allows the chamber to derive some nutrition from the blood within the right ventricular cavity. For the reasons just noted, the right ventricle can sustain long periods of ischemia but still demonstrate excellent recovery of contractile function after reperfusion.[64]

ATRIAL INFARCTION. This may be seen in up to 10 percent of patients with AMI if PR segment displacement is used as the criterion for atrial infarction. Although isolated atrial infarction may be observed in 3.5 percent of autopsies of patients with AMI, it often occurs in conjunction with ventricular infarction and can cause rupture of the atrial wall. This type of infarct is more common on the right than the left side, occurs more frequently in the atrial appendages than in the lateral or posterior walls of the atrium, and can result in thrombus formation. The difference in incidence between right and left atrial infarction might be explained by the considerably higher oxygen content of left atrial blood. Atrial infarction is frequently accompanied by atrial arrhythmias.[65, 66] It has also been reported to be associated with reduced secretion of atrial natriuretic peptide and a low cardiac output syndrome when right ventricular infarction coexists.

CORONARY ARTERY SPASM. In addition to causing AMI in patients with Prinzmetal angina (see p. 1324), coronary artery spasm may also

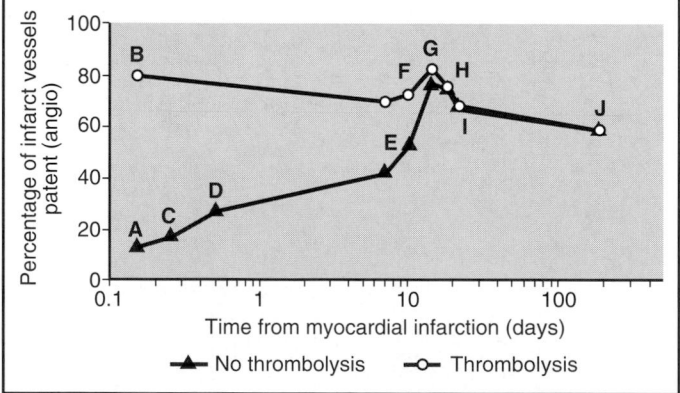

FIGURE 35–10. Comparison of angiographically documented infarct-related coronary artery patency rates in 10 separate clinical studies and time from MI as modulated by early administration of a thrombolytic agent versus nonthrombolytic (conventional) therapy. The x axis is a semilogarithmic scale of time in days from myocardial infarction. Note that the difference in patency rates becomes diminishingly small within the first 2 to 3 weeks after infarction. (From Rumberg JA, Gersh BJ: Coronary artery patency and left ventricular remodeling after myocardial infarction: mechanisms and mechanics. In Califf RM, Mark DB, Wagner GS [eds]: Acute Coronary Care. St. Louis, Mosby–Year Book, 1995, p 122.)

cause intimal damage that can initiate formation of an atherosclerotic plaque. Epicardial coronary artery spasm has been identified in patients with fixed atherosclerotic coronary artery stenosis before, during, and after AMI. An association between coronary artery spasm and coronary artery thrombosis has also been documented clinically.

COLLATERAL CIRCULATION IN ACUTE MYOCARDIAL INFARCTION

The coronary collateral circulation is particularly well developed in patients with (1) coronary occlusive disease, especially when it is severe, with the reduction of the luminal cross-sectional area by more than 75 percent in one or more major vessels; (2) chronic hypoxia, as occurs in severe anemia, chronic obstructive pulmonary disease, and cyanotic congenital heart disease; and (3) left ventricular hypertrophy, which intensifies coronary collateral vessels.

The magnitude of coronary collateral flow is one of the principal determinants of infarct size. Indeed, it is rather common for patients with abundant collateral vessels to have totally occluded coronary arteries without evidence of infarction in the distribution of that artery; thus, the survival of the myocardium distal to such occlusions must depend on collateral blood flow. Even if collateral perfusion existing at the time of coronary occlusion is not successful in improving contractile function, it may still exert a beneficial effect by preventing the formation of a left ventricular aneurysm. Some collaterals are seen in nearly 40 percent of patients with an acute total occlusion, and more begin to appear soon after the total occlusion occurs.[61] It is likely that the presence of a high-grade stenosis (90 percent), possibly with periods of intermittent total occlusion, permits the development of collateral vessels that remain only as potential conduits until a total occlusion occurs or recurs. The latter event then brings these channels into full operation.[67]

The incidence of collateral vessels 1 to 2 weeks after AMI varies considerably and may be as high as 75 to 100 percent in patients with persistent occlusion of the infarct vessel or as low as 17 to 42 percent in patients with subtotal occlusion.

NONATHEROSCLEROTIC CAUSES OF ACUTE MYOCARDIAL INFARCTION

Numerous pathological processes other than atherosclerosis can involve the coronary arteries (see p. 1336) and result in MI (see Table 35–1). For example, coronary arterial occlusions can be the result of embolization of a coronary artery. Emboli most frequently lodge in the distribution of the left anterior descending coronary artery, commonly in the distal epicardial and intramural branches. The causes of coronary embolism are numerous: infective endocarditis and nonbacterial thrombotic endocarditis (see Chap. 47), mural thrombi, prosthetic valves, neoplasms, air that is introduced at the time of cardiac surgery, and calcium deposits from manipulation of calcified valves at operation. In situ thrombosis of coronary arteries can occur secondary to chest wall trauma (see Chap. 51).

VASCULAR INFLAMMATION. A variety of inflammatory processes can be responsible for coronary artery abnormalities, some of which mimic atherosclerotic disease and may predispose to true atherosclerosis. Epidemiological evidence suggests that viral infections, particularly with Coxsackievirus B, may be an uncommon cause of AMI. Viral illnesses precede AMI occasionally in young persons who are later shown to have normal coronary arteries.

Syphilitic aortitis may produce marked narrowing or occlusion of one or both coronary ostia, whereas Takayasu arteritis may result in obstruction of the coronary arteries (see Chap. 40). Necrotizing arteritis, polyarteritis nodosa, mucocutaneous lymph node syndrome (Kawasaki disease) (see Chap. 45), systemic lupus erythematosus (see Chap. 67), and giant cell arteritis (see Chap. 67) can cause coronary

occlusion. Therapeutic levels of mediastinal radiation can cause thickening and hyalinization of the walls of coronary arteries, with subsequent infarction. AMI may also be the result of coronary arterial involvement in amyloidosis (see Chap. 48), Hurler syndrome, pseudoxanthoma elasticum, and homocystinuria.

COCAINE. As cocaine abuse has become more common, reports of AMI after the use of cocaine have appeared with increasing frequency. Cocaine may cause AMI in patients with normal coronary arteries, preexisting MI, documented coronary artery disease, or coronary artery spasm.[52] AMI associated with cocaine has also been reported after its topical use in nasal septoplasty and in neonates whose mothers used the drug. Recurrent MI after further cocaine abuse has been reported as well.

Cocaine may cause AMI by at least three mechanisms: (1) increasing myocardial oxygen demand through increases in heart rate and blood pressure, (2) diminishing coronary artery flow resulting from either coronary vasospasm or thrombosis, and (3) active myocarditis (either hypersensitivity or toxicity). In very high doses, cocaine appears to have a direct toxic effect on heart muscle that may produce cardiac failure and sudden death with extensive myocyte necrosis.

MYOCARDIAL INFARCTION WITH ANGIOGRAPHICALLY NORMAL CORONARY VESSELS

Approximately 6 percent of all patients with AMI and perhaps four times that percentage of patients with this diagnosis younger than the age of 35 years do not have coronary atherosclerosis demonstrated by coronary arteriography or at autopsy.[61] Perhaps half the patients of this group, in turn, have a variety of other lesions involving the coronary vessels or myocardium (see Table 35–1), whereas the others have no detectable coronary obstructive lesions. Patients with AMI and normal coronary arteries tend to be young and to have relatively few coronary risk factors, except that they often have a history of cigarette smoking. Usually, they have no history of angina pectoris before the infarction. The infarction in these patients is usually not preceded by any prodrome, but the clinical, laboratory, and ECG features of AMI are otherwise indistinguishable from those present in the overwhelming majority of patients with AMI who have classic obstructive atherosclerotic coronary artery disease. In patients who recover, areas of localized dyskinesis and hypokinesis can often be demonstrated by left ventricular angiography. Many of these cases are caused by coronary artery spasm and/or thrombosis, perhaps with underlying endothelial dysfunction or small plaques that are not apparent on coronary angiography. Additional suggested causes include (1) coronary emboli (perhaps from a small mural thrombus, a prolapsed mitral valve, or a myxoma); (2) coronary artery disease in vessels too small to be visualized by coronary arteriography or coronary arterial thrombosis with subsequent recanalization (see Table 35–1); (3) a variety of hematological disorders causing in situ thrombosis in the presence of normal coronary arteries (polycythemia vera, cyanotic heart disease with polycythemia, sickle cell anemia, disseminated intravascular coagulation, thrombocytosis, and thrombotic thrombocytopenic purpura); (4) augmented oxygen demand (thyrotoxicosis, amphetamine use); (5) hypotension secondary to sepsis, blood loss, or pharmacological agents; and (6) anatomical variations such as anomalous origin of a coronary artery (see Chap. 44), coronary arteriovenous fistula (see Chap. 44), or a myocardial bridge (see Chap. 12).

PROGNOSIS. The long-term outlook for patients who have survived an AMI with angiographically normal coronary vessels on arteriography appears to be substantially better than that for patients with MI and obstructive coronary artery disease. After recovery from the initial infarct, recurrent infarction, heart failure, and death are unusual in patients with normal coronary arteries. Indeed, most of these patients have normal exercise ECGs and only a minority develop angina pectoris.

▼ Pathophysiology

LEFT VENTRICULAR FUNCTION

Systolic Function

On interruption of antegrade flow in an epicardial coronary artery, the zone of myocardium supplied by that vessel immediately loses its ability to shorten and perform contractile work. Four abnormal contraction patterns develop in sequence: (1) dyssynchrony (i.e., dissociation in the time course of contraction of adjacent segments), (2) hypokinesis (reduction in the extent of shortening), (3) akinesis (cessation of shortening), and (4) dyskinesis (paradoxical expansion, systolic bulging).[68, 69] Accompanying dysfunction of the infarcting segment initially is hyperkinesis of the remaining normal myocardium. The early hyperkinesis of the noninfarcted zones is believed to be the result of acute compensatory mechanisms, including increased activity of the sympathetic nervous system and the Frank-Starling mechanism. A portion of this compensatory hyperkinesis is ineffective work because contraction of the noninfarcted segments of myocardium causes dyskinesis of the infarct zone. Increased motion of the noninfarcted region subsides within 2 weeks of infarction, during which time some degree of recovery can be seen in the infarct region as well, particularly if reperfusion of the infarcted area occurs and myocardial stunning diminishes.

Patients with AMI often also show reduced myocardial contractile function in noninfarcted zones. This may result from previous obstruction of the coronary artery supplying the noninfarcted region of the ventricle and loss of collaterals from the freshly occluded infarct-related vessel, a condition that has been termed "ischemia at a distance."[70] Conversely, the presence of collaterals developing before MI may allow for greater preservation of regional systolic function in an area of distribution of the occluded artery and improvement in left ventricular ejection fraction early after infarction.

If a sufficient quantity of myocardium undergoes ischemic injury, LV pump function becomes depressed; cardiac output, stroke volume, blood pressure, and peak dP/dt are reduced[69]; and end-systolic volume is increased. The degree to which end-systolic volume increases is perhaps the most powerful predictor of mortality after AMI.[71] Paradoxical systolic expansion of an area of ventricular myocardium further decreases LV stroke volume. As necrotic myocytes slip past each other, the infarct zone thins and elongates, especially in patients with large anterior infarcts, leading to infarct expansion. As the ventricle dilates during the first few hours to days after infarction, regional and global wall stress increases according to Laplace's law. In some patients a vicious cycle of dilatation begetting further dilatation is initiated.[72, 73] The degree of ventricular dilatation, which depends closely on infarct size, patency of the infarct-related artery,[74] and activation of the local renin-angiotensin system in the noninfarcted portion of the ventricle, can be favorably modified by angiotensin-converting enzyme (ACE) inhibition therapy even in the absence of symptomatic LV dysfunction.[75]

With the passage of time, edema, cellular infiltration, and ultimately fibrosis, increase the stiffness of the infarcted myocardium back to and beyond control values. Increasing stiffness in the infarcted zone of myocardium improves LV function because it prevents paradoxical systolic wall motion.

A linear relationship exists between specific parameters of LV function and the likelihood of developing clinical symptoms such as dyspnea and ultimately a shocklike state. The earliest abnormality is a reduction in diastolic compliance (see later), which can be observed with infarcts that involve only 8 percent of the total left ventricle on angiographic examination. When the abnormally contracting segment exceeds 15 percent, the ejection fraction may be reduced and elevations of LV end-diastolic pressure and volume occur. The risk of developing physical signs and symptoms of LV failure also increases proportionally to increasing areas of abnormal left ventricular wall motion.[69] Clinical heart failure accompanies areas of abnormal contraction exceeding 25 percent, and cardiogenic shock, often fatal, accompanies loss of more than 40 percent of the left ventricular myocardium.

Unless infarct extension occurs, some improvement in wall motion takes place during the healing phase, as recovery of function occurs in initially reversibly injured (stunned) myocardium (see Fig. 35–9). Regardless of the age of the infarct, patients who continue to demonstrate abnormal wall motion of 20 to 25 percent of the left ventricle are likely to manifest hemodynamic signs of LV failure.

Diastolic Function (See Chap. 15)

Left ventricular diastolic properties are altered in infarcted and ischemic myocardium, leading initially to an increase but later to a reduction in LV compliance. These changes are associated with a decrease in the peak rate of decline in left ventricular pressure (peak [−] dP/dt), an increase in the time constant of the fall in left ventricular pressure, and an initial rise in LV end-diastolic pressure. Over a period of several weeks, end-diastolic volume increases and diastolic

pressure begins to fall toward normal. As with impairment of systolic function, the magnitude of the diastolic abnormality appears to be related to the size of the infarct.

CIRCULATORY REGULATION

The abnormality in circulatory regulation that is present in AMI is diagrammed in Figure 35–11. The process begins with an anatomical or functional obstruction in the coronary vascular bed, which results in regional myocardial ischemia and, if the ischemia persists, in infarction. If the infarct is of sufficient size, it depresses overall left ventricular function so that LV stroke volume falls and filling pressures rise. A marked depression of LV stroke volume ultimately lowers aortic pressure and reduces coronary perfusion pressure; this condition may intensify myocardial ischemia and thereby initiate a vicious cycle (see Fig. 35–11). The inability of the left ventricle to empty also leads to an increased preload, that is, it dilates the well-perfused, normally functioning portion of the left ventricle. This compensatory mechanism tends to restore stroke volume to normal levels but at the expense of a reduced ejection fraction. However, the dilatation of the left ventricle also elevates ventricular afterload, because Laplace's law dictates that at any given arterial pressure the dilated ventricle must develop a higher wall tension. This increased afterload not only depresses left ventricular stroke volume but also elevates myocardial oxygen consumption, which in turn intensifies myocardial ischemia. When regional myocardial dysfunction is limited and the function of the remainder of the left ventricle is normal, compensatory mechanisms sustain overall LV function. If a large portion of the left ventricle becomes necrotic, pump failure occurs; that is, overall left ventricular function becomes so depressed that the circulation cannot be sustained despite the dilatation of the remaining viable portion of the ventricle.

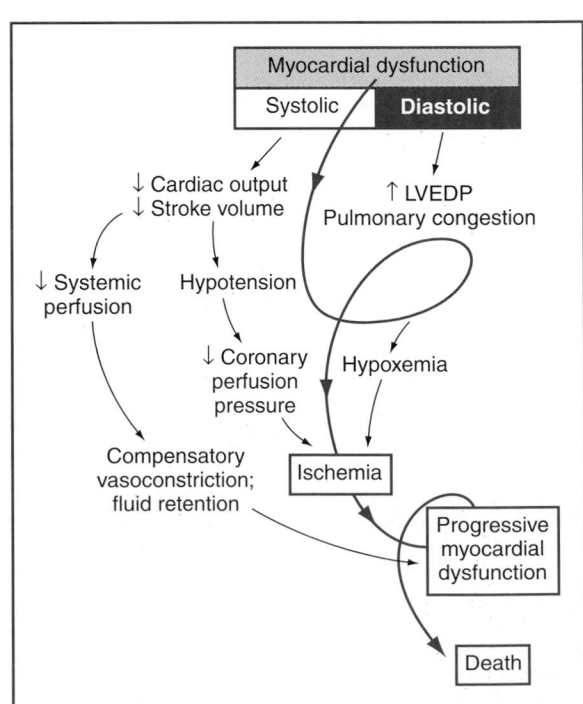

FIGURE 35–11. The vicious circle in cardiogenic shock. LVEDP = left ventricular end-diastolic pressure. (From Hollenberg SM, Kavinsky CJ, Parrillo JE: Cardiogenic shock. Ann Intern Med 131:47–59, 1999.)

As a consequence of MI, the changes in left ventricular size, shape, and thickness involving both the infarcted and the noninfarcted segments of the ventricle just described occur and are collectively referred to as *ventricular remodeling*. This process, in turn, can influence ventricular function and prognosis.[72] A combination of changes in left ventricular dilation and hypertrophy of residual noninfarcted myocardium is responsible for remodeling.[72a] After the size of infarction, the two most important factors driving the process of left ventricular dilatation are ventricular loading conditions and infarct artery patency[72, 74, 76] (Fig. 35–12). Elevated ventricular pressure contributes to increased wall stress and the risk of infarct expansion, and a patent infarct artery accelerates myocardial scar formation and increases tissue turgor in the infarct zone, reducing the risk of infarct expansion and ventricular dilatation.

INFARCT EXPANSION. An increase in the size of the infarcted segment, known as infarct expansion, is defined as "acute dilatation and thinning of the area of infarction not explained by additional myocardial necrosis."[77] Infarct expansion appears to be caused by (1) a combination of slippage between muscle bundles, reducing the number of myocytes across the infarct wall; (2) disruption of the normal myocardial cells; and (3) tissue loss within the necrotic zone.[77] It is characterized by disproportionate thinning and dilation of the infarct zone before formation of a firm, fibrotic scar.[72a] The degree of infarct expansion appears to be related to the preinfarction wall thickness, with existing hypertrophy possibly protecting against infarct thinning. The apex is the thinnest region of the ventricle and an area of the heart that is particularly vulnerable to infarct expansion.[78] Infarction of the apex secondary to occlusion of the left anterior descending coronary artery causes the radius of curvature at the apex to increase, exposing this normally thin region to a marked elevation in wall stress.

When it is present, infarct expansion is associated with both a higher mortality and a higher incidence of nonfatal complications, such as heart failure and ventricular aneurysm.[79] Infarct expansion has been noted in more than three fourths of the hearts of patients succumbing to AMI and in one third to one half of all patients with anterior Q-wave infarctions.[79] Infarct expansion is best recognized echocardiographically as elongation of the noncontractile region of the ventricle. When expansion is severe enough to cause symptoms, the most characteristic clinical finding is deterioration of systolic function associated with new or louder gallop sounds and new or worsening pulmonary congestion. Rupture of the ventricle may be considered to be a consequence of extreme infarct expansion.

VENTRICULAR DILATATION. Although infarct expansion plays an important role in the ventricular remodeling that occurs early after MI, remodeling is also caused by dilatation of the viable portion of the ventricle, commencing immediately after AMI and progressing for months or years thereafter (Fig. 35–12).[72a] As opposed to distention, dilatation may be accompanied by a shift of the pressure-volume curve of the left ventricle to the right, resulting in a larger left ventricular volume at any given diastolic pressure. This global dilatation of the noninfarct zone may be viewed as a compensatory mechanism that maintains stroke volume in the face of a large infarction. However, ventricular dilatation is also associated with nonuniform repolarization of the myocardium that predisposes the patient to life-threatening ventricular arrhythmias.

After AMI, an extra load is placed on the residual functioning myocardium, a load that presumably is responsible for the compensatory hypertrophy of the uninfarcted myocardium. This hypertrophy could help to compensate for

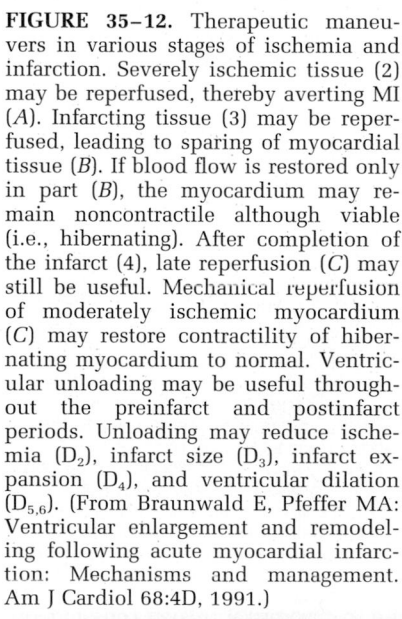

FIGURE 35–12. Therapeutic maneuvers in various stages of ischemia and infarction. Severely ischemic tissue (2) may be reperfused, thereby averting MI (*A*). Infarcting tissue (3) may be reperfused, leading to sparing of myocardial tissue (*B*). If blood flow is restored only in part (*B*), the myocardium may remain noncontractile although viable (i.e., hibernating). After completion of the infarct (4), late reperfusion (*C*) may still be useful. Mechanical reperfusion of moderately ischemic myocardium (*C*) may restore contractility of hibernating myocardium to normal. Ventricular unloading may be useful throughout the preinfarct and postinfarct periods. Unloading may reduce ischemia (D_2), infarct size (D_3), infarct expansion (D_4), and ventricular dilation ($D_{5,6}$). (From Braunwald E, Pfeffer MA: Ventricular enlargement and remodeling following acute myocardial infarction: Mechanisms and management. Am J Cardiol 68:4D, 1991.)

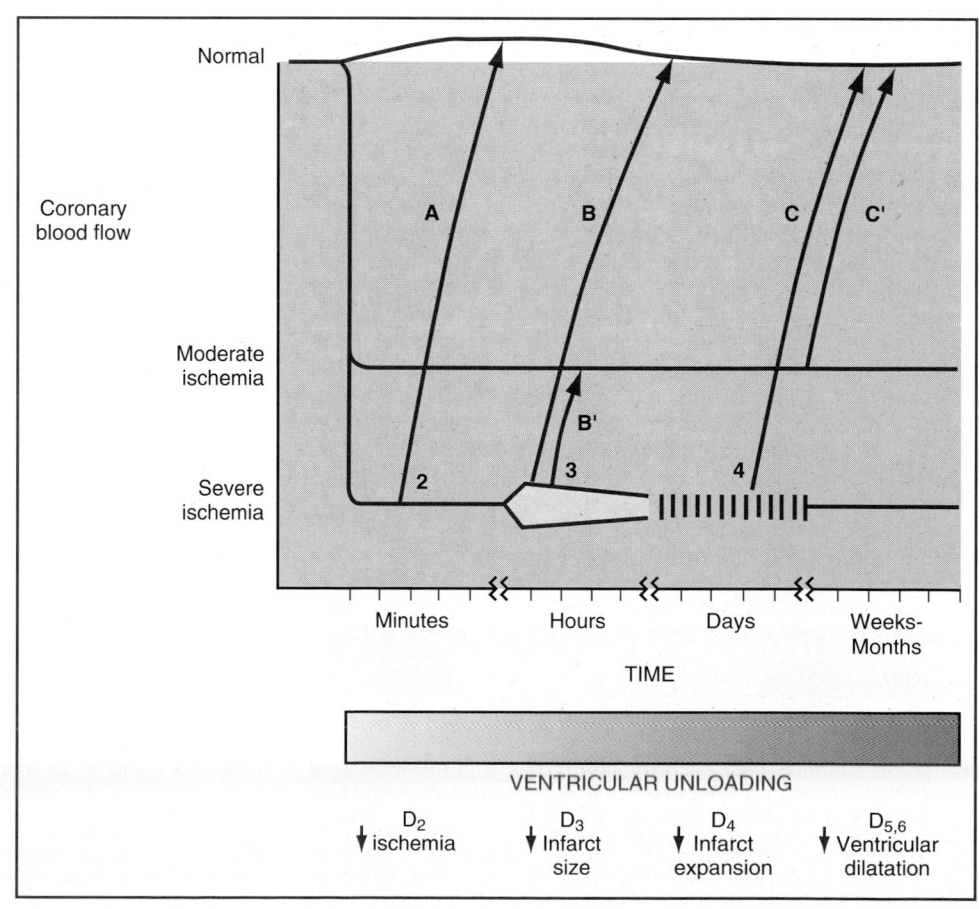

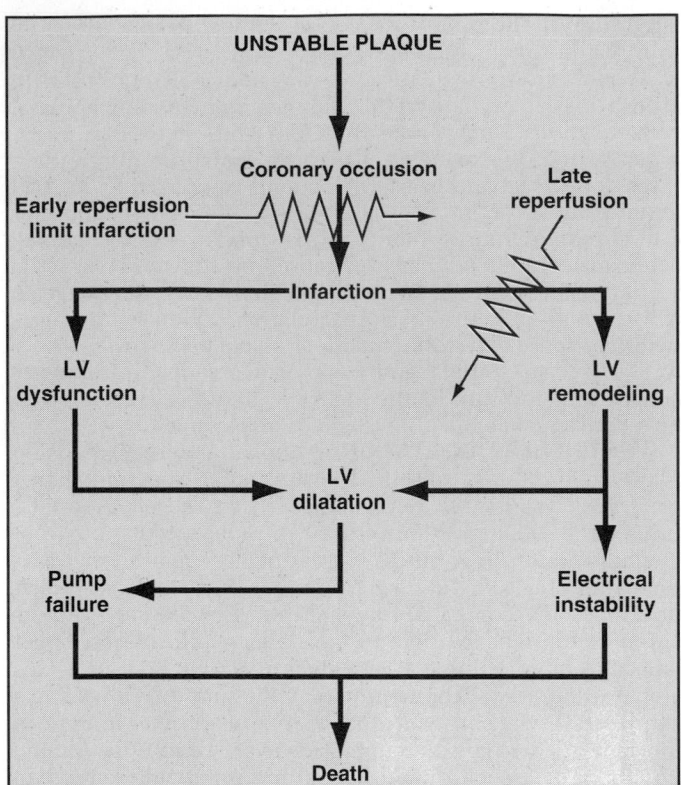

UNSTABLE PLAQUE

Coronary occlusion

Early reperfusion limit infarction

Late reperfusion

Infarction

LV dysfunction

LV remodeling

LV dilatation

Pump failure

Electrical instability

Death

FIGURE 35–13. Flow chart showing postulated sequence of events from an unstable atherosclerotic plaque to death. The original paradigm emphasizing early reperfusion is shown at the left; the expanded paradigm illustrating the benefits of late reperfusion is shown at the right. (From Kim CB, Braunwald E: Potential benefits of late reperfusion of infarcted myocardium: The open artery hypothesis. Circulation 88:2426, 1993. Copyright 1993, American Heart Association.)

the functional impairment caused by the infarct and may be responsible for some of the hemodynamic improvement seen in the months after infarction in some patients.[72a]

EFFECTS OF TREATMENT. Ventricular remodeling after AMI can be affected by several factors, the first of which is infarct size (see Fig. 35–12). Acute reperfusion and other measures to restrict the extent of myocardial necrosis limit the increase in ventricular volume after AMI, and evidence suggests that an open infarct artery per se achieved even late after coronary occlusion also attenuates ventricular enlargement[72a, 74] (Fig. 35–13). The second factor is scar formation in the infarct. Glucocorticosteroids and nonsteroidal anti-inflammatory agents given early after MI can cause scar thinning and greater infarct expansion, whereas ACE inhibitors[72] attenuate ventricular enlargement (see p. 1169 and Figs. 35–12 and 35–13). Additional beneficial consequences of inhibition of angiotensin II that may contribute to myocardial protection include attenuation of endothelial dysfunction and direct antiatherogenic effects.[72a, 80]

PATHOPHYSIOLOGY OF OTHER ORGAN SYSTEMS

PULMONARY FUNCTION

Changes in pulmonary gas exchange, ventilation, and distribution of perfusion all occur with AMI. Hypoxemia is a frequent consequence, with a severity, in general, proportional to that of left ventricular failure. There is an inverse relation between pulmonary artery diastolic pressure and arterial oxygen tension in patients with AMI. This suggests that increased pulmonary capillary hydrostatic pressure leads to interstitial edema, which results in arteriolar and bronchiolar compression that ultimately causes perfusion of poorly ventilated al-

veoli with resultant hypoxemia. In addition to hypoxemia, there is a fall in diffusing capacity. Hyperventilation often occurs in patients with AMI and may cause hypocapnia and respiratory alkalosis, particularly in restless, anxious patients with pain. With reversal of heart failure, hypoxemia and intrapulmonary shunting diminish.

INCREASE IN INTERSTITIAL WATER. A positive correlation has been demonstrated between pulmonary extravascular (interstitial) water content, left ventricular filling pressure, and the clinical signs and symptoms of left ventricular failure. The increase in pulmonary extravascular water may be responsible for the alterations in pulmonary mechanics observed in patients with AMI (i.e., reduction of airway conductance, pulmonary compliance, forced expiratory volume, and midexpiratory flow rate and an increase in closing volume—the last presumably related to the widespread closure of small, dependent airways during the first 3 days after AMI). Ultimately, severe increases in extravascular water may lead to pulmonary edema. Recovery of LV function or diuresis reduces abnormally elevated values for closing volumes (i.e., the lung volume at which airway closure commences) to normal.

The "closing volume" can encroach on and sometimes exceed functional residual volume. This can lead to arterial hypoxemia by the shunting of blood through alveoli that are not well ventilated.

REDUCTION OF VITAL CAPACITY. Virtually all lung volume indices—total lung capacity, functional residual capacity, and residual volume, as well as vital capacity—fall in the presence of AMI.[81] These reductions correlate with the elevations of left-sided filling pressures and are most probably due to increases in pulmonary extravascular water. Lung volumes, oxygenation, and airway resistance all return toward normal by the time of hospital discharge for most patients.[81] Increased pulmonary venous pressure also results in redistribution of pulmonary blood flow from the bases to the apices of the lung in patients with AMI, altering the relationship between ventilation and perfusion. However, at follow-up examination 3 to 25 weeks after MI, the ventilation-perfusion relationship has usually returned to normal or almost so.

REDUCTION OF AFFINITY OF HEMOGLOBIN FOR OXYGEN. In patients with MI, particularly when complicated by LV failure or cardiogenic shock, the affinity of hemoglobin for oxygen is reduced (i.e., the P_{50} is increased). The increase in P_{50} results from increased levels of erythrocyte 2,3-diphosphoglycerate (2,3-DPG), which constitutes an important compensatory mechanism, responsible for an estimated 18 percent increase in oxygen release from oxyhemoglobin in patients with cardiogenic shock.

ENDOCRINE FUNCTION

PANCREAS. Hyperglycemia and impaired glucose tolerance are common in patients with AMI. Although the absolute levels of blood insulin are often in the normal range, they are usually inappropriately low for the level of blood sugar, and there may be relative insulin resistance as well. Stress-induced hyperglycemia in the setting of AMI is associated with an increased risk of mortality even in patients without diabetes mellitus.[81a] Patients with cardiogenic shock often demonstrate marked hyperglycemia and depressed levels of circulating insulin, often with complete suppression of insulin secretion in response to tolbutamide.[82] These abnormalities in insulin secretion and the resultant impaired glucose tolerance appear to be secondary to a reduction in pancreatic blood flow as a consequence of splanchnic vasoconstriction accompanying severe LV failure. In addition, increased activity of the sympathetic nervous system with augmented circulating catecholamines inhibits insulin secretion and augments glycogenolysis, also contributing to the elevation of blood sugar.[83]

Glucose appears to be a more favorable energy source than free fatty acids for the ischemic myocardium by more efficiently replenishing the Krebs cycle and stimulating contractile performance.[84] Because hypoxic heart muscle derives a considerable portion of its energy from the metabolism of glucose (see Chap. 63) and because insulin is essential for the uptake of glucose by the myocardium as well as for myocardial protein synthesis and inhibition of lysosomal activity, the deleterious effects of insulin deficiency are clear. These metabolic considerations, combined with epidemiological observations that diabetic patients have a markedly worse prognosis, have served as the foundation for efforts to more aggressively administer insulin-glucose infusions to diabetics with AMI (see p. 1172).

ADRENAL MEDULLA. Excessive secretion of catecholamines produces many of the characteristic signs and symptoms of AMI. The plasma and urinary catecholamine levels are highest during the first 24 hours after the onset of chest pain,[83] with the greatest rise in plasma catecholamine secretion occurring during the first hour after the onset of MI. These high levels of circulating catecholamines in patients with AMI correlate with the occurrence of serious arrhythmias and result in an increase in myocardial oxygen consumption, both directly and indirectly, as a consequence of catecholamine-induced elevation of circulating free fatty acids. As might be anticipated, the concentration of circulating catecholamines correlates with the extent of myocardial damage and incidence of cardiogenic shock, as well as both early and late mortality rates.

Circulating catecholamines enhance platelet aggregation; when this occurs in the coronary microcirculation, the release of the potent vasoconstrictor thromboxane A_2 may further impair cardiac perfusion. The marked increase in sympathetic activity associated with AMI serves as the foundation for beta-adrenoceptor blocker regimens in the acute phase (see p. 1168).

LOCAL MYOCARDIAL AND SYSTEMIC RENIN-ANGIOTENSIN SYSTEM. Noninfarcted regions of the myocardium appear to exhibit activation of the tissue renin-angiotensin system with increased angiotensin II production. Both locally and systemically generated angiotensin II may stimulate the production of various growth factors, such as platelet-derived growth factor and transforming growth factor, that promote compensatory hypertrophy in the noninfarcted myocardium as well as control the structure and tone of the infarct-related coronary and other myocardial vessels.[72a] Additional potential actions of angiotensin II that have a more negative impact on the infarction process include release of endothelin, PAI-1, and aldosterone, which may cause vasoconstriction, impaired fibrinolysis, and increased sodium retention, respectively. Inhibition of generation of circulating and tissue angiotensin II is one of the proposed mechanisms of benefit from ACE inhibitors in AMI.

NATRIURETIC PEPTIDES. The peptides atrial natriuretic factor (ANF) and N-terminal pro-ANF are released from cardiac atria in response to elevation of atrial pressure. In a case-control study from the Thrombolysis in Myocardial Infarction (TIMI) II trial, Hall and colleagues have shown that elevated N-terminal pro-ANF levels within the first 12 hours of AMI are highly predictive of an increased mortality risk in the year after infarction. A novel protein, brain natriuretic peptide (BNP), originally isolated from porcine brain, has been shown to be secreted by human ventricular myocardium. It appears to be released early after AMI, peaking at about 16 hours. Patients with anterior infarction, lower cardiac index, and more significant congestive heart failure after AMI have higher levels of BNP and also show a second peak of BNP release about 5 days after infarction. These intriguing observations suggest that BNP levels may be a marker of the degree of left ventricular dysfunction in AMI and that markedly elevated levels of BNP correlate with a worse prognosis.

ADRENAL CORTEX. Plasma and urinary 17-hydroxycorticosteroids and ketosteroids, as well as aldosterone, are also markedly elevated in patients with AMI.[83] Their concentrations correlate directly with the peak level of serum creatine kinase, implying that the stress imposed by larger infarcts is associated with greater secretion of adrenal steroids. The magnitude of the elevation of cortisol correlates with infarct size and mortality. Glucocorticosteroids also contribute to the impairment of glucose tolerance.

THYROID GLAND. Although patients with AMI are generally euthyroid, evidence indicates a significant transient decrease in serum triiodothyronine (T_3) levels, a fall that is most marked on about the third day after the infarct. This fall in T_3 is usually accompanied by a rise in reverse T_3, with variable changes or no change in thyroxine (T_4) and thyroid-stimulating hormone (TSH) levels. The alteration in peripheral T_4 metabolism appears to correlate with infarct size and may be mediated by the rise in endogenous levels of cortisol that accompanies AMI.

RENAL FUNCTION

Both prerenal azotemia and acute renal failure can complicate the marked reduction of cardiac output that occurs in cardiogenic shock.

On the other hand, an increase in circulating atrial natriuretic peptide occurs after AMI, an increase that is correlated with the severity of left ventricular failure. An increase in atrial natriuretic peptide is also found when right ventricular infarction accompanies inferior wall infarction, suggesting that this hormone may play a role in the hemodynamic disturbances that accompany right ventricular infarction.

HEMATOLOGICAL FUNCTION

PLATELETS. AMI generally occurs in the presence of extensive coronary and systemic atherosclerotic plaques, which may serve as the site for the formation of platelet aggregates, a sequence that has been suggested as the initial step in the process of coronary thrombosis, coronary occlusion, and subsequent MI. Circulating platelets are hyperaggregable in patients with AMI. The role of platelets in AMI is discussed in Chapter 62. Platelets from AMI patients have an increased propensity for aggregation locally in the area of a disrupted plaque and also release vasoactive substances such as thromboxane A_2 (see Fig. 35–3).

HEMOSTATIC MARKERS. Elevated levels of serum fibrinogen degradation products, an end product of thrombosis—as well as release of distinctive proteins when platelets are activated (i.e., platelet factor 4 and beta-thromboglobulin)—have been reported in some patients with AMI. Fibrinopeptide A, a protein released from fibrin by thrombin, is a marker of ongoing thrombosis and is increased during the early hours of AMI. Marked elevation of hemostatic markers such as FPA, TAT, and F1&2 is associated with an increased risk of mortality in AMI patients[85] (see Chap. 62 and Fig. 35–7). The interpretation of the coagulation tests in patients with AMI may be complicated by elevated blood levels of catecholamines, concomitant shock, and/or pulmonary embolism, conditions that are all capable of altering various tests of platelet and coagulation function. Thus, it is not yet clear whether the aforementioned changes are the causes or consequences of AMI.

LEUKOCYTES. An elevated leukocyte count is an epidemiologic marker for coronary heart disease.[86] AMI is usually accompanied by leukocytosis, which is related to the magnitude of the necrotic process, elevated glucocorticoid levels, and possibly inflammation in the coronary arteries. The magnitude of elevation of the leukocyte count is associated with in-hospital mortality after AMI.[87, 87a] Activation of neutrophils may produce important intermediaries, such as leukotriene B_4 and oxygen free radicals, that have important microcirculatory effects.

BLOOD VISCOSITY. Clinical and epidemiological studies suggest that several hemostatic and hemorheological factors (e.g., fibrinogen, factor VII, plasma viscosity, hematocrit, red blood cell aggregation, total white blood cell count) are involved in the pathophysiology of atherosclerosis and also play an integral role in acute thrombotic events. An increase in blood viscosity also occurs in patients with AMI. During the first few days after infarction, this is mainly attributable to hemoconcentration, but later the increases in plasma viscosity and red cell aggregation correlate with elevated serum concentrations of alpha$_2$-globulin and fibrinogen, which are nonspecific reactions to tissue necrosis and are also responsible for the elevated sedimentation rate characteristic of AMI. The high values of blood viscosity indices are observed most frequently in patients with complications such as left ventricular failure, cardiogenic shock, and thromboembolism.

▼ Clinical Features

PREDISPOSING FACTORS

The risk factors for atherosclerosis and coronary artery disease are discussed in Chapter 31.

In as many as one half of patients with AMI, a precipitating factor or prodromal symptoms can be identified.[88] Evidence suggests that unusually heavy exercise (particularly in fatigued or emotionally stressed, habitually inactive patients) may play a role in precipitating AMI.[89, 90] Such infarctions could be the result of marked increases in myocardial oxygen consumption in the presence of severe coronary arterial narrowing. It has been suggested that unusually heavy exertion or mental stress such as that caused by anger[91] may trigger plaque disruption, leading to AMI. Patients with known coronary artery disease who have been hospitalized for treatment of an acute coronary syndrome–related event and who subsequently report a high level of stress in their life have an increased risk of rehospitalization for cardiovascular reasons and also for "hard" events such as death and MI. Of interest, however, one study has provided evidence that, in a multivariate analysis adjusting for other cardiac risk factors, job strain did not affect the outcome (including nonfatal AMI) in patients with angiographically proven coronary artery disease.[92]

Accelerating angina and rest angina, two patterns of unstable angina (see Chap. 36), may culminate as AMI (see Fig. 35–2).[40a] Noncardiac surgical procedures have also been noted as precursors of AMI (see Chap. 61). Perioperative risk stratification and the use of beta blockers may reduce the likelihood of AMI and cardiac-related mortality.[93, 94] Reduced myocardial perfusion secondary to hypotension (e.g., hemorrhagic or septic shock) and increased myocardial oxygen demands secondary to aortic stenosis, fever, tachycardia, and agitation can also be responsible for myocardial necrosis. Other factors reported as predisposing to AMI include respiratory infections, hypoxemia of any cause, pulmonary embolism, hypoglycemia, administration of ergot preparations, use of cocaine, sympathomimetics, serum sickness, allergy, and on rare occasion wasp stings. In patients with Prinzmetal's angina (see Chap. 37), AMI may develop in the territory of the coronary artery that repeatedly undergoes spasm.[95] Rarely, munitions workers exposed to high concentrations of nitroglycerin may develop MI when they are withdrawn from this exposure, suggesting that it is caused by vasospasm.[96]

Trauma may precipitate an AMI in one of two ways. Myocardial contusion and hemorrhage into the myocardium may actually cause cell necrosis, or the injury may involve a coronary artery, causing occlusion of that vessel with resultant AMI (see Chap. 51). Neurological disturbances (transient ischemic attacks or strokes) may also precipitate AMI. Concern has been raised on the basis of a case-control study that patients with hypertension who are receiving short-acting calcium antagonists, particularly in high doses, are at increased risk of developing AMI. Because of possible selection bias in the patients who received calcium antagonists, these results must be viewed cautiously and clinicians should await the results of ongoing multicenter trials (e.g., ALLHAT) before withdrawing calcium antagonists from patients who might be benefiting from their antihypertensive effect (reduction of stroke).

CIRCADIAN PERIODICITY. An analysis of a large number of patients hospitalized with MI, studied as a part of the Multicenter Investigation of Limitation of Infarct Size (MILIS), revealed a pronounced circadian periodicity for the time of onset of AMI, with peak incidence of events between 6 a.m. and 12 p.m. Circadian rhythms affect many physiological and biochemical parameters; the early morning hours are associated with rises in plasma catecholamines and cortisol and increases in platelet aggregability.[97] Interestingly, the characteristic circadian peak was *absent* in patients receiving beta blocker or aspirin therapy before their presentation with AMI. The concept of "triggering" an AMI is a complex one and likely involves the superimposition of multiple factors such as time of day, season, and the stress of natural disasters.[50, 98]

HISTORY

PRODROMAL SYMPTOMS. Despite recent advances in the laboratory detection of AMI, the history remains of substantial value in establishing a diagnosis. The prodrome is usually characterized by chest discomfort, resembling classic angina pectoris (see Chap. 37), but it occurs at rest or with less activity than usual and can therefore be classified as unstable angina. However, the latter is often not disturbing enough to induce patients to seek medical attention; if they do, they may not be hospitalized. Of the patients with AMI presenting with prodromal symptoms of unstable angina, approximately one third have had symptoms from 1 to 4 weeks before hospitalization; in the remaining two thirds, symptoms predated admission by 1 week or less, with one third of these patients (20 percent of all with prodromes) having had symptoms for 24 hours or less. A feeling of general malaise or frank exhaustion often accompanies other symptoms preceding AMI.

NATURE OF THE PAIN. The pain of AMI is variable in intensity; in most patients it is severe and in some instances intolerable. The pain is prolonged, usually lasting for more than 30 minutes and frequently for a number of hours. The discomfort is described as constricting, crushing, oppressing, or compressing; often the patient complains of a sensation of a heavy weight or a squeezing in the chest. Although the discomfort is typically described as a choking, viselike, or heavy pain, it may also be characterized as a stabbing, knifelike, boring, or burning discomfort. The pain is usually retrosternal in location, spreading frequently to both sides of the anterior chest, with predilection for the left side. Often the pain radiates down the ulnar aspect of the left arm, producing a tingling sensation

in the left wrist, hand, and fingers. Some patients note only a dull ache or numbness of the wrists in association with severe substernal or precordial discomfort. In some instances, the pain of AMI may begin in the epigastrium and simulate a variety of abdominal disorders, a fact that often causes MI to be misdiagnosed as "indigestion." In other patients the discomfort of AMI radiates to the shoulders, upper extremities, neck, jaw, and interscapular region, again usually favoring the left side. In patients with preexisting angina pectoris, the pain of infarction usually resembles that of angina with respect to location. However, it is generally much more severe, lasts longer, and is not relieved by rest and nitroglycerin.

In some patients, particularly the elderly, AMI is manifested clinically not by chest pain but rather by symptoms of acute left ventricular failure and chest tightness or by marked weakness or frank syncope.[98a, 98b] These symptoms may be accompanied by diaphoresis, nausea, and vomiting. The pain of AMI may have disappeared by the time the physician first encounters the patient (or the patient reaches the hospital), or it may persist for many hours. Opiates—in particular morphine—usually relieve the pain. Both angina pectoris and the pain of AMI are thought to arise from nerve endings in ischemic or injured, but not necrotic, myocardium. Thus, in MI, stimulation of nerve fibers in an ischemic zone of myocardium surrounding the necrotic central area of infarction probably gives rise to the pain.

Pain often disappears suddenly and completely when blood flow to the infarct territory is restored. In patients in whom reocclusion occurs after thrombolysis, pain recurs if the initial reperfusion has left viable myocardium. Thus, what has previously been thought of as the "pain of infarction," sometimes lasting for many hours, probably represents pain caused by ongoing ischemia. The recognition that pain implies ischemia and not infarction heightens the importance of seeking ways to relieve the ischemia, for which the pain is a marker. This finding suggests that the clinician should not be complacent about ongoing cardiac pain under any circumstances.

OTHER SYMPTOMS. Nausea and vomiting occur in more than 50 percent of patients with transmural MI and severe chest pain, presumably owing to activation of the vagal reflex or to stimulation of left ventricular receptors as part of the Bezold-Jarisch reflex. These symptoms occur more commonly in patients with inferior MI than in those with anterior MI. Moreover, nausea and vomiting are common side effects of opiates. When the pain of AMI is epigastric in location and is associated with nausea and vomiting, the clinical picture may easily be confused with that of acute cholecystitis, gastritis, or peptic ulcer. Occasionally, a patient complains of diarrhea or a violent urge to evacuate the bowels during the acute phase of MI. Other symptoms include feelings of profound weakness, dizziness, palpitations, cold perspiration, and a sense of impending doom. On occasion, symptoms arising from an episode of cerebral embolism or other systemic arterial embolism are the first signs of AMI. The aforementioned symptoms may or may not be accompanied by chest pain.

Differential Diagnosis

The pain of AMI may stimulate the pain of acute pericarditis (see Chaps. 3 and 50), which is usually associated with some pleuritic features; that is, it is aggravated by respiratory movements and coughing and often involves the shoulder, ridge of the trapezius, and neck. An important feature that distinguishes pericardial pain from ischemic discomfort is that ischemic discomfort never radiates to the trapezius ridge, a characteristic site of radiation of pericardial pain.[99] Pleural pain is usually sharp, knifelike, and aggravated in a cyclical fashion by each breath, which distinguishes it from the deep, dull, steady pain of AMI. Pulmonary embolism (see Chap. 52) generally produces pain laterally in the chest, is often pleuritic, and may be associated with hemoptysis. The pain due to acute dissection of the aorta (see Chap. 40) is usually localized in the center of the chest, is extremely severe and described by the patient as a "ripping" or "tearing" sensation, is at its maximal intensity shortly after onset, persists for many hours, and often radiates to the back or the lower extremities. Often one or more major arterial pulses are absent. Pain arising from the costochondral and chondrosternal articulations may be associated with localized swelling and redness; it is usually sharp and "darting" and is characterized by marked localized tenderness. Episodes of retrosternal discomfort induced by peristalsis in patients with increased esophageal stiffness and also episodes of sustained esophageal contraction can mimic the pain of AMI.[100, 101]

SILENT MI AND ATYPICAL PRESENTATION. Population studies suggest that between 20 and 60 percent of nonfatal MIs are unrecognized by the patient and are discovered only on subsequent routine ECG or postmortem examinations. Of these unrecognized infarctions, approximately half are truly silent, with the patients unable to recall any symptoms whatsoever. The other half of patients with so-called silent infarction can recall an event characterized by symptoms compatible with acute infarction when leading questions are posed after the ECG abnormalities are discovered. Unrecognized or silent infarction occurs more commonly in patients without antecedent angina pectoris and in patients with diabetes[98a] and hypertension.[102] Silent MI is often followed by silent ischemia (see p. 1330). The prognoses of patients with silent and symptomatic presentations of AMI appear similar.

Atypical presentations of AMI include the following: (1) congestive heart failure—beginning de novo or worsening of established failure; (2) classic angina pectoris without a particularly severe or prolonged attack; (3) atypical location of the pain; (4) central nervous system manifestations, resembling those of stroke, secondary to a sharp reduction in cardiac output in a patient with cerebral arteriosclerosis; (5) apprehension and nervousness; (6) sudden mania or psychosis; (7) syncope; (8) overwhelming weakness; (9) acute indigestion; and (10) peripheral embolization.

PHYSICAL EXAMINATION

GENERAL APPEARANCE. Patients suffering an AMI often appear anxious and in considerable distress. An anguished facial expression is common, and—in contrast to patients with severe angina pectoris, who often lie, sit, or stand still, recognizing that all forms of activity increase the discomfort—some patients suffering an AMI may be restless and move about in an effort to find a comfortable position. They often massage or clutch their chests and frequently describe their pain with a clenched fist held against the sternum (the "Levine" sign, named after Dr. Samuel A. Levine). In patients with left ventricular failure and sympathetic stimulation, cold perspiration and skin pallor may be evident; they typically sit or are propped up in bed, gasping for breath. Between breaths, they may complain of chest discomfort or a feeling of suffocation. Cough productive of frothy, pink, or blood-streaked sputum is common.

Patients in cardiogenic shock often lie listlessly, making few if any spontaneous movements. The skin is cool and clammy, with a bluish or mottled color over the extremities, and there is marked facial pallor with severe cyanosis of the lips and nailbeds. Depending on the degree of cerebral perfusion, the patient in shock may converse normally or may evidence confusion and disorientation.

HEART RATE. The heart rate may vary from a marked bradycardia to a rapid regular or irregular tachycardia, depending on the underlying rhythm and the degree of left ventricular failure. Most commonly, the pulse is rapid and regular initially (sinus tachycardia at 100 to 110 beats/min), slowing as the patient's pain and anxiety are relieved; ventricular premature beats (VPBs) are common, occurring in more than 95 percent of patients evaluated within the first 4 hours after the onset of symptoms.

BLOOD PRESSURE. The majority of patients with uncomplicated AMI are normotensive, although the reduced stroke volume accompanying the tachycardia may cause declines in systolic and pulse pressures and elevation of diastolic pressure. Among previously normotensive patients, a hypertensive response occasionally is seen during the first few hours, with the arterial pressure exceeding 160/90 mm Hg, presumably as a consequence of adrenergic discharge secondary to pain and agitation. It is common for previously hypertensive patients to become normotensive without treatment after AMI, although many of these previously hypertensive patients eventually regain their elevated levels of blood pressure, generally 3 to 6 months after infarction. In patients with massive infarction, arterial pressure falls acutely, owing to left ventricular dysfunction and venous pooling secondary to administration of morphine or nitrates or both; as recovery occurs, the arterial pressure tends to return to preinfarction levels.

Patients in cardiogenic shock (see p. 1178), by definition, have systolic pressures below 90 mm Hg and evidence of end-organ hypoperfusion. However, hypotension alone does not necessarily signify cardiogenic shock because some patients with inferior infarction in whom the Bezold-Jarisch reflex is activated may also transiently have systolic blood pressure below 90 mm Hg. Their hypotension eventually resolves spontaneously, although the process can be accelerated by intravenous atropine (0.5 to 1.0 mg) and assumption of the Trendelenburg position. Other patients who are initially only slightly hypotensive may demonstrate gradually falling blood pressures with progressive reduction in cardiac output over several hours or days as they develop cardiogenic shock as a consequence of increasing ischemia and extension of infarction (see Fig. 35-11). Evidence of autonomic hyperactivity is common, varying in type with the location of the infarction. At some time in their initial presentation, more than half of patients with inferior MI have evidence of excess parasympathetic stimulation, with hypotension, bradycardia, or both, whereas about half of patients with anterior MI show signs of sympathetic excess, having hypertension, tachycardia, or both.[103]

TEMPERATURE AND RESPIRATION. Most patients with extensive AMI develop fever, a nonspecific response to tissue necrosis, within 24 to 48 hours of the onset of infarction. Body temperature often begins to rise within 4 to 8 hours after the onset of infarction, and rectal temperature may reach 101° to 102°F. Fever usually resolves by the fourth or fifth day after infarction.

The respiratory rate may be slightly elevated soon after the development of an AMI; in patients without heart failure, it results from anxiety and pain because it returns to normal with treatment of physical and psychological discomfort. In patients with left ventricular failure, the respiratory rate correlates with the severity of failure; patients with pulmonary edema may have respiratory rates exceeding 40 breaths/min. However, the respiratory rate is not necessarily elevated in patients with cardiogenic shock. Cheyne-Stokes (periodic) respiration (see Chap. 17) may occur in elderly individuals with cardiogenic shock and heart failure, particularly after opiate therapy and in the presence of cerebrovascular disease.

JUGULAR VENOUS PULSE. The height and contour of the jugular venous pulse reflect right atrial and right ventricular diastolic pressures (see Chap. 4). Because these pressures are usually normal or only slightly elevated in patients with AMI (even in the presence of mild to moderate LV failure), it is not surprising that usually the jugular venous pulse fails to show any abnormalities. The a wave may be prominent in patients with pulmonary hypertension secondary to LV failure or reduced compliance. In contrast, right ventricular infarction (whether or not it accompanies left ventricular infarction) often results in marked jugular venous distention and, when it is complicated by necrosis or ischemia of right ventricular papillary muscles, tall c-v waves of tricuspid regurgitation are evident. In patients with AMI and cardiogenic shock, the jugular venous pressure is usually elevated. In patients with AMI, hypotension, and hypoperfusion (findings that may resemble those of patients with cardiogenic shock) but who have flat neck veins, it is likely that the depression of left ventricular performance may be related, at least in part, to hypovolemia. The differentiation can be made only by assessing left ventricular performance using echocardiography or by measuring left ventricular filling pressure with a pulmonary artery flotation catheter.

CAROTID PULSE. Palpation of the carotid arterial pulse provides a clue to the left ventricular stroke volume; a small pulse suggests a reduced stroke volume, whereas a sharp, brief upstroke is often observed in patients with mitral regurgitation or ruptured ventricular septum with a left-to-right shunt. Pulsus alternans reflects severe left ventricular dysfunction.

THE CHEST. Moist rales are audible in patients who develop left ventricular failure and/or a reduction of left ventricular compliance with AMI. Diffuse wheezing may be present in patients with severe left ventricular failure. Cough with hemoptysis, suggesting pulmonary embolism with infarction, may also occur. In 1967 Killip and Kimball proposed a prognostic classification scheme based on the presence and severity of rales detected in patients presenting with AMI.[104] Class I patients are free of rales and a third heart sound (S_3). Class II patients have rales but to only a mild-moderate degree (<50 percent of lung fields) and may or may not have an S_3. Patients in Class III have rales in more than half of each lung field and frequently have pulmonary edema. Finally, Class IV patients are in cardiogenic shock. Despite overall improvement in mortality in each class, compared with data observed during the original development of the classification scheme, the latter remains useful today, as evidenced by data from more recently conducted large MI trials.[15, 22]

Cardiac Examination

PALPATION. Despite severe symptoms and extensive myocardial damage, the findings on examination of the heart may be quite unremarkable in patients with AMI. Palpation of the precordium may yield normal findings, but in patients with transmural AMI it more commonly reveals a presystolic pulsation, synchronous with an audible fourth heart sound (S_4), reflecting a vigorous left atrial contraction filling a ventricle with reduced compliance. In the presence of left ventricular systolic dysfunction, an outward movement of the left ventricle may be palpated in early diastole, coincident with an S_3. When the anterior or lateral portion of the ventricle is dyskinetic, an abnormal systolic pulsation is present in the third, fourth, or fifth intercostal space to the left of the sternum. In some patients, this paradoxical precordial impulse is clearly separable from the point of maximal impulse, which is more lateral and to the left. In other patients, the abnormal impulse is a diffuse, rippling, precordial movement, approximately 5 to 10 cm in diameter, not clearly separable from the point of maximal impulse and can be appreciated near the left anterior axillary line. Patients with long-standing hypertension or previous infarction with left ventricular hypertrophy often demonstrate a laterally displaced, sustained apical impulse.

AUSCULTATION. The heart sounds, particularly the first sound (S_1), are frequently muffled and occasionally inaudible immediately after the infarct, and their intensity increases during convalescence. A soft S_1 may also reflect prolongation of the PR interval. Patients with marked ventricular dysfunction and/or left bundle branch block may have paradoxical splitting of the second heart sound (S_2) (see Chap. 4). Patients with postinfarction angina may also develop a transient, paradoxically split S_2 during anginal episodes.

Third and Fourth Heart Sounds. An S_3 in AMI usually reflects severe left ventricular dysfunction with elevated ventricular filling pressure. It is caused by rapid deceleration of transmitral blood flow during protodiastolic filling of the left ventricle with resultant oscillations of the cardiohemic system (i.e., myocardium and stream of blood flowing from left atrium to left ventricle) and is usually heard in patients with large infarctions. This sound is detected best at the apex, with the patient in the left lateral recumbent position, and is more common in patients with transmural anterior infarctions than in those with inferior or nontransmural infarctions. The mortality of patients who manifest an S_3 during the acute phase of MI is higher than that of patients without such a sound. An S_3 may be caused not only by left ventricular failure but also by increased inflow into the left ventricle, as occurs when mitral regurgitation or ventricular septal defect complicates AMI. The S_3 and S_4 emanating from the left ventricle are heard best at the apex; in patients with right ventricular infarcts, these sounds may be heard along the left sternal border and are intensified by inspiration.

An S_4 is almost universally present in patients with AMI in sinus rhythm and is usually best heard between the left sternal border and the apex. This sound reflects the atrial contribution to ventricular filling and is particularly prominent in AMI patients due to a reduction in LV compliance and elevation of LV end-diastolic pressure (LV-EDP), even in the absence of left ventricular systolic dysfunction. This finding is of limited diagnostic value because it is commonly audible in most patients with chronic ischemic heart disease and is recordable, although not often audible, in many normal subjects older than 45 years.

Murmurs. *Systolic murmurs,* transient or persistent, are commonly audible in patients with AMI and generally result from mitral regurgitation secondary to dysfunction of the mitral valve apparatus (papillary muscle dysfunction, left ventricular dilatation). A new, prominent apical holosystolic murmur, accompanied by a thrill, may represent rupture of a head of a papillary muscle (see p. 1184). The findings in rupture of the interventricular septum are similar, although the murmur and thrill are usually most prominent along the left sternal border and may be audible at the right sternal border as well. The systolic murmur of tricuspid regurgitation (caused by right ventricular failure due to pulmonary hypertension and/or right ventricular infarction or by infarction of a right ventricular papillary muscle) is also heard along the left sternal border. It is characteristically intensified by inspiration and is accompanied by a prominent c-v wave in the jugular venous pulse and a right ventricular S_4.

Pericardial Friction Rubs. These may be heard in patients with AMI, especially those sustaining large transmural infarctions.[99] Rubs are notorious for their evanescence and, hence, are probably even more common than reported; frequent auscultation in patients with transmural infarction often results in the discovery of a rub that might otherwise have gone unnoticed. Although friction rubs may be heard within 24 hours or as late as 2 weeks after the onset of infarction, most commonly they are noted on the second or third day.[99] Occasionally, in patients with extensive infarction, a loud rub may be heard for many days. Patients with AMI and a pericardial friction rub may have a pericardial effusion on echocardiographic study, but only rarely are the classic ECG changes of pericarditis (see Chap. 5) seen.[99] Delayed onset of the rub and the associated discomfort of pericarditis (as late as 3 months' postinfarction) are characteristic of the now rare post-MI (Dressler) syndrome (see p. 1196).

Pericardial rubs are most readily audible along the left sternal border or just inside the point of maximal impulse. Loud rubs may be audible over the entire precordium and even over the back. Occasionally, only the systolic portion of a rub is heard; it may be confused with a systolic murmur, and the diagnosis of rupture of the ventricular septum or mitral regurgitation may be incorrectly considered.

OTHER FINDINGS

FUNDI. Hypertension, diabetes, and generalized atherosclerosis commonly accompany AMI, and because these conditions may produce characteristic changes in the fundus, a careful funduscopic examination may provide information concerning the underlying vascular status; this is particularly useful in patients unable to provide a detailed history.

ABDOMEN. As already noted, in patients with AMI, particularly in an inferior location with diaphragmatic irritation, the pain may be localized to the epigastrium or the right upper quadrant. Pain in the abdomen associated with nausea, vomiting, restlessness, and even abdominal distention is often interpreted by patients as a sign of "indigestion," resulting in self-medication with antacids, and it may suggest an acute abdominal process to the physician. Right-sided heart failure, characterized by hepatomegaly and a positive abdominojugular reflux, is unusual in patients with acute left ventricular infarction but does occur in patients with severe and prolonged left ventricular failure or right ventricular infarction.

EXTREMITIES. Coronary atherosclerosis is often associated with systemic atherosclerosis, and it is therefore common for patients with AMI to have a history of intermittent claudication and to demonstrate physical findings of peripheral vascular disease. Thus, diminished peripheral arterial pulses, loss of hair, and atrophic skin in the lower extremities are noted frequently in patients with coronary artery disease. Peripheral edema is a manifestation of right ventricular failure and, like congestive hepatomegaly, is unusual in patients with acute left ventricular infarction. Cyanosis of the nailbeds is common in patients with severe left ventricular failure and is particularly striking in patients with cardiogenic shock.

NEUROPSYCHIATRIC FINDINGS. Except for the altered mental status that occurs in patients with AMI who have a markedly reduced cardiac output and cerebral hypoperfusion, the neurological examination is normal unless the patient has suffered cerebral embolism secondary to a mural thrombus. Indeed, an underlying MI is common in patients with cerebral embolic stroke. The coincidence between these two conditions may be explained by systemic hypotension due to MI precipitating a cerebral infarction and the converse, as well as by mural emboli from the left ventricle causing cerebral emboli.

Patients with AMI often exhibit alterations of the emotional state, including intense anxiety, denial, and depression. Medical staff caring for AMI patients must be sensitive to changes in the patient's emotional state: a calm, professional atmosphere, with thorough explanations of equipment and prognosis, can help alleviate the distress associated with AMI.

LABORATORY EXAMINATIONS

Markers of Cardiac Damage

The classic World Health Organization (WHO) criteria for the diagnosis of AMI require that at least two of the following three elements be present: (1) a history of ischemic-type chest discomfort, (2) evolutionary changes on serially obtained ECG tracings, and (3) a rise and fall in serum cardiac markers.[105] There is considerable variability in the pattern of presentation of AMI with respect to these three elements, as exemplified by the following statistics. ST segment elevation and Q waves on the ECG, two features that are highly indicative of AMI, are seen in only about half of AMI cases on presentation. Approximately one third of patients with AMI do not present with classic chest pain,[98a] and the event would go unrecognized unless an ECG were recorded fortuitously in temporal proximity to the infarction or permanent pathological Q waves were are seen on later tracings. Nondiagnostic ECGs are recorded in approximately half of patients presenting to emergency departments with chest pain suggestive of MI who ultimately are shown to have an AMI. Among patients admitted to the hospital with a chest pain syndrome, fewer than 20 percent are subsequently diagnosed as having had an AMI. Therefore, in the majority of patients, clinicians must obtain serum cardiac marker measurements at periodic intervals to either establish or exclude the diagnosis of AMI; such measurements may also be useful for a rough quantitation of the size of infarction.[106] The availability of new serum cardiac markers with markedly enhanced sensitivity for myocardial damage enables clinicians to diagnose AMI in about an additional one third of patients who would not have fulfilled criteria for AMI in the past.[107] The increased use of more sensitive biomarkers of AMI combined with more precise imaging techniques has necessitated establishment of new criteria for AMI (Table 35–2).

As myocytes become necrotic, the integrity of the sarcolemmal membrane is compromised and intracellular macromolecules (serum cardiac markers) begin to diffuse into the cardiac interstitium and ultimately into the microvasculature and lymphatics in the region of the infarct[60] (Fig. 35–14 and Table 35–3). The rate of appearance of these macromolecules in the peripheral circulation depends on several factors, including intracellular location, molecular weight, local blood and lymphatic flow, and the rate of elimination from the blood.[60, 108, 109]

Given the accelerated pace of decision-making in patients with acute coronary syndromes and emphasis on reduction of length of hospital stay, there is considerable interest in evaluating new serum cardiac markers,[60] shortening assay time in the central chemistry laboratory,[110] and designing rapid whole blood bedside assays.[111] For optimal specificity, a serum marker of MI should be present in high concentration in the myocardium and be absent from nonmyocardial tissue and serum.[60, 108] For optimal sensitivity it should be rapidly released into the blood after myocardial injury, and there should be a stoichiometric relationship between the plasma level of the marker and the extent of myocardial injury. For ease of clinical use, the marker should persist in blood for an appropriate length of time to provide a convenient diagnostic time window (see Table 35–3). Finally, the assay methodology should be inexpensive and easy to perform.

CREATINE KINASE (CK). Serum CK activity exceeds the normal range within 4 to 8 hours after the onset of AMI and declines to normal within 2 to 3 days (see Fig. 35–14).

▼ **TABLE 35–2. CRITERIA FOR THE DIAGNOSIS OF ACUTE MYOCARDIAL INFARCTION (AMI)**

INCREASED BIOMARKERS PLUS ONE OR MORE OF THE FOLLOWING	PATHOLOGICAL FINDINGS OF AMI	TYPICAL SYMPTOMS OF AMI PLUS ONE OF THE FOLLOWING	PROCEDURAL MYOCARDIAL DAMAGE
Typical symptoms of myocardial ischemia Q waves in the ECG ST segment elevation or depression in the ECG	No other findings required	ST segment elevation in the ECG Increased levels of cardiac biomarkers	Increased levels of cardiac biomarkers to prespecified levels; symptoms may be absent; ECG changes may be absent or nonspecific

Modified from Alpert J, Thygesen K, et al: Towards a new definition of myocardial infarction for the 21st century. J Am Coll Cardiol 2000, in press.

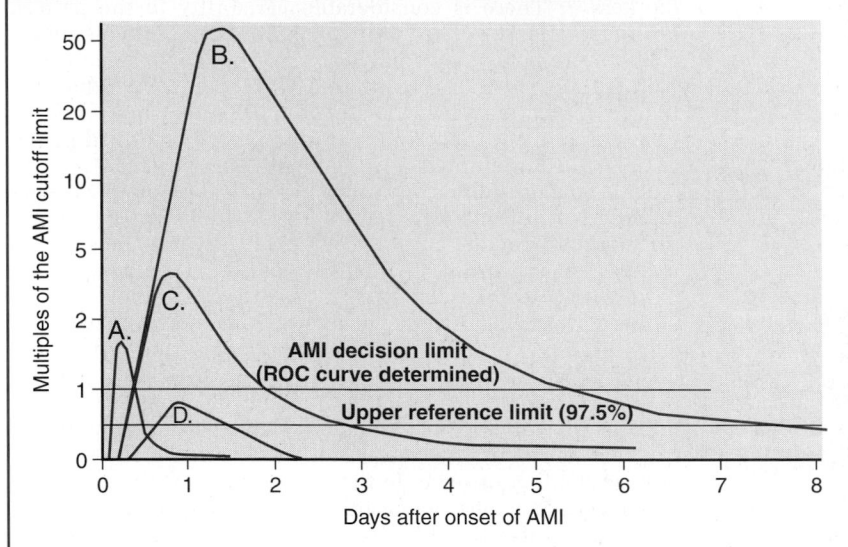

FIGURE 35–14. Plot of the appearance of cardiac markers in blood versus time after onset of symptoms. Peak A, early release of myoglobin or CK-MB isoforms after AMI; peak B, cardiac troponin after AMI; peak C, CK-MB after AMI; peak D, cardiac troponin after unstable angina. Data are plotted on a relative scale, where 1.0 is set at the AMI cutoff concentration. (From Wu AH, Apple FS, Gibler WB, et al: National Academy of Clinical Biochemistry Standards of Laboratory Practice: Recommendations for the use of cardiac markers in coronary artery diseases. Clin Chem 45:1104–1121, 1999.)

Although the peak CK occurs on average at about 24 hours, peak levels occur earlier in patients who have had reperfusion as a result of the administration of thrombolytic therapy or mechanical recanalization (as well as in patients with early spontaneous thrombolysis). Because the time-activity curve of serum CK is influenced by reperfusion, and because reperfusion itself influences infarct size, reperfusion interferes with estimation of infarct size by enzyme analysis.[60, 112]

Although elevation of the serum CK is a sensitive enzymatic detector of AMI that is routinely available in most hospitals,[60] important drawbacks include false-positive results in patients with muscle disease, alcohol intoxication, diabetes mellitus, skeletal muscle trauma, vigorous exercise, convulsions, intramuscular injections, thoracic outlet syndrome, and pulmonary embolism.[60, 109, 113]

CK ISOENZYMES. Three isoenzymes of CK (MM, BB, and MB) have been identified by electrophoresis. Extracts of brain and kidney contain predominantly the BB isoenzyme, skeletal muscle contains principally MM but does contain some MB (1 to 3 percent), and both MM and MB isoenzymes are present in cardiac muscle. The MB isoenzymes

of CK may also be present in minor quantities in the small intestine, tongue, diaphragm, uterus, and prostate. Strenuous exercise, particularly in trained long-distance runners or professional athletes, may cause elevation of both total CK and CK-MB.[114] Because CK-MB can be detected in the blood of healthy subjects, the cutoff value for abnormal elevation of CK-MB is usually set a few units above the end of the reference (normal) range for a given laboratory. Despite the fact that small quantities of CK-MB isoenzyme are found in tissues other than the heart, elevated levels of CK-MB may be considered, for practical purposes, to be the result of AMI (except in the case of trauma or surgery on the aforementioned organs).

Earlier CK-MB assay methods that were in common use included radioimmunoassay and agarose gel electrophoresis techniques; these have now been largely supplanted by highly sensitive and specific enzyme immunoassays that use monoclonal antibodies directed against CK-MB.[115] Mass assays report results in nanograms per milliliter rather than units per milliliter and have been confirmed to be more accurate than CK-MB activity assays, especially in patients presenting within 4 hours of the onset of AMI. It has been

▼ **TABLE 35–3.** MOLECULAR MARKERS USED OR PROPOSED FOR USE IN THE DIAGNOSIS OF ACUTE MYOCARDIAL INFARCTION

MARKER	MW (D)	RANGE OF TIMES TO INITIAL ELEVATION (hr)	MEAN TIME TO PEAK ELEVATIONS (NONTHROMBOLYSIS)	TIME TO RETURN TO NORMAL RANGE	MOST COMMON SAMPLING SCHEDULE
hFABP	14,000–15,000	1.5	5–10 hr	24 hr	On presentation, then 4 hr later
Myoglobin	17,800	1–4	6–7 hr	24 hr	Frequent; 1–2 hr after CP
MLC	19,000–27,000	6–12	2–4 d	6–12 d	Once at least 12 hr after CP
cTnI	23,500	3–12	24 hr	5–10 d	Once at least 12 hr after CP
cTnT	33,000	3–12	12 hr–2 d	5–14 d	Once at least 12 hr after CP
MB-CK	86,000	3–12	24 hr	48–72 hr	Every 12 hr × 3*
MM-CK tissue isoform	86,000	1–6	12 hr	38 hr	60–90 min after CP
MB-CK tissue isoform	86,000	2–6	18 hr	Unknown	60–90 min after CP
Enolase	90,000	6–10	24 hr	48 hr	Every 12 hr × 3
LD	135,000	10	24–48 hr	10–14 d	Once at least 24 hr after CP
MHC	400,000	48	5–6 d	14 d	Once at least > 2 d after CP

*Increased sensitivity can be achieved with sampling every 6 or 8 hours.
hFABP = heart fatty acid binding proteins; MLC = myosin light chain; cTnI = cardiac troponin I; cTnT = cardiac troponin T; MB-CK = MB isoenzyme of creatinine kinase (CK); MM-CK = MM isoenzyme of CK; LD = lactate dehydrogenase; MHC = myosin heavy chain; CP = chest pain.
Modified from Adams J III, Abendschein D, Jaffe A: Biochemical markers of myocardial injury. Is MB creatine kinase the choice for the 1990s? Circulation 88:750, 1993. Copyright 1993, American Heart Association.

PLATE 21

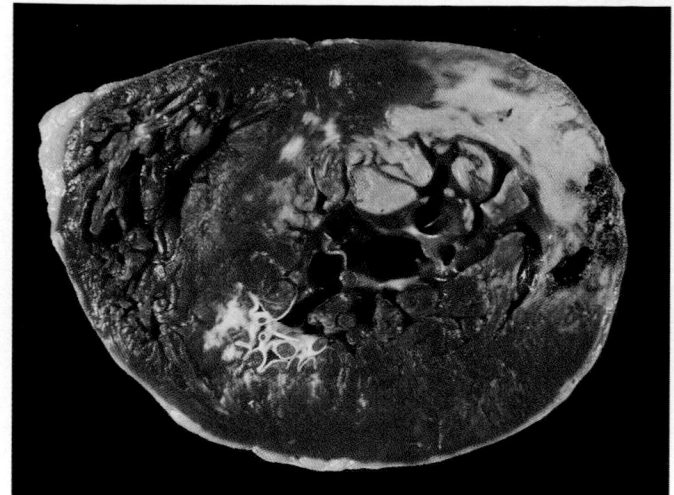

FIGURE 35–6. Acute myocardial infarct, predominantly of the posterolateral left ventricle, demonstrated histochemically by a lack of staining by the triphenyltetrazolium chloride (TTC) stain in areas of necrosis. The staining defect is due to the enzyme leakage that follows cell death. Note the myocardial hemorrhage at one edge of the infarct that was associated with cardiac rupture (at the 3 o'clock position) and the anterior scar (at the 7 o'clock position), indicative of old infarct. (Specimen oriented with posterior wall at top.) (From Schoen FJ: The heart. *In* Cotran RS, Kumar V, Collins T [eds]: Pathologic Basis of Disease. 6th ed. Philadelphia, WB Saunders, 1999, p 559.)

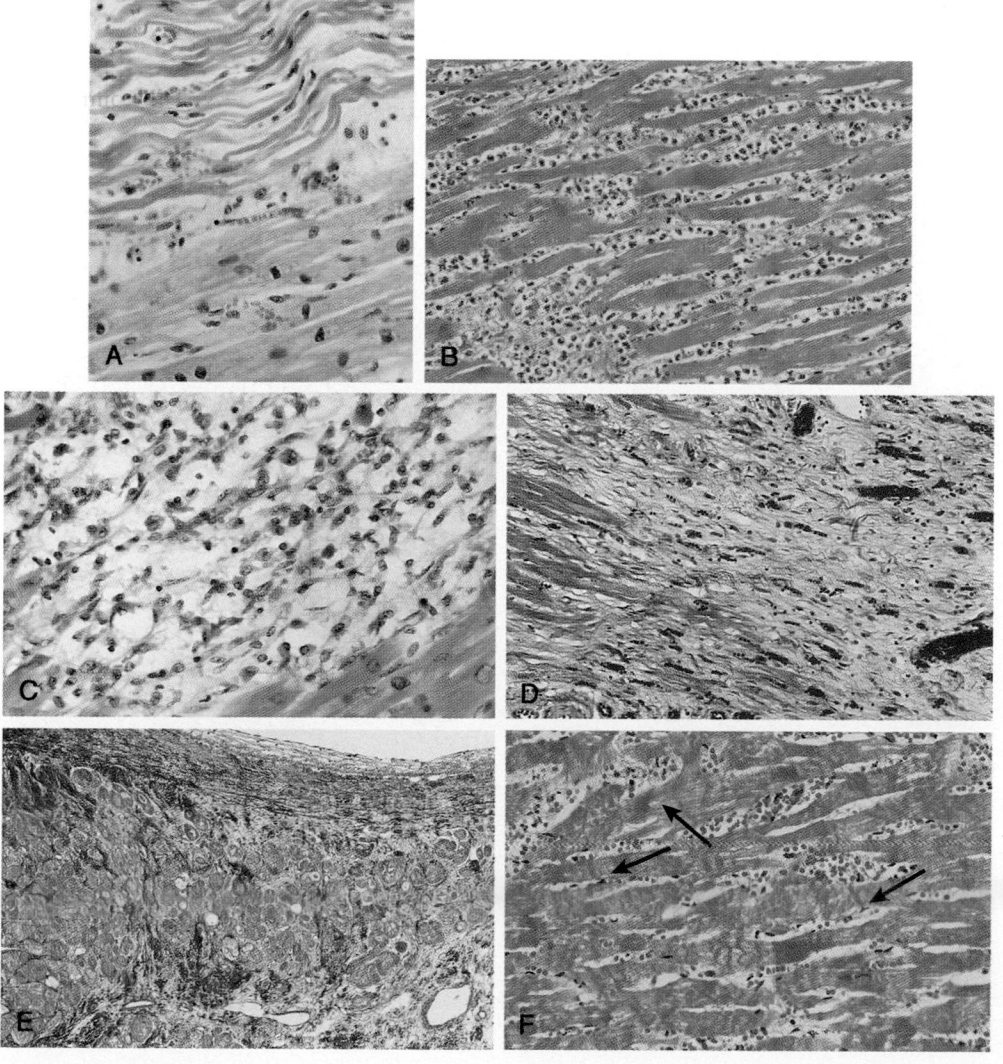

FIGURE 35–8. Microscopic features of myocardial infraction. *A,* One-day-old infarct showing coagulative necrosis, wavy fibers with elongation, and narrowing, compared with adjacent normal fibers (lower right). Widened spaces between the dead fibers contain edema fluid and scattered neutrophils. *B,* Dense polymorphonuclear leukocytic infiltrate in an area of acute myocardial infarction of 3 to 4 days' duration. *C,* Nearly complete removal of necrotic myocytes by phagocytosis (7 to 10 days). *D,* Granulation tissue with a rich vascular network and early collagen deposition, approximately 3 weeks after infarction. *E,* Well-healed myocardial infarct with replacement of the necrotic fibers by dense collagenous scar. A few residual cardiac muscle cells are present. (In *D* and *E,* collagen is highlighted as blue in this Masson trichrome stain). *F,* Myocardial necrosis with hemorrhage and contraction bands, visible as dark bands spanning some myofibers (arrows). This is the characteristic appearance of markedly ischemic myocardium that has been reperfused. (From Schoen FJ: The heart. *In* Cotran RS, Kumar V, Collins T (eds): Pathologic Basis of Disease. 6th ed. Philadelphia, WB Saunders, 1999, pp 560–561.)

PLATE 22

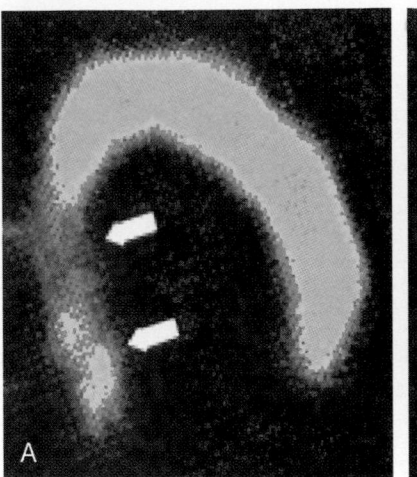 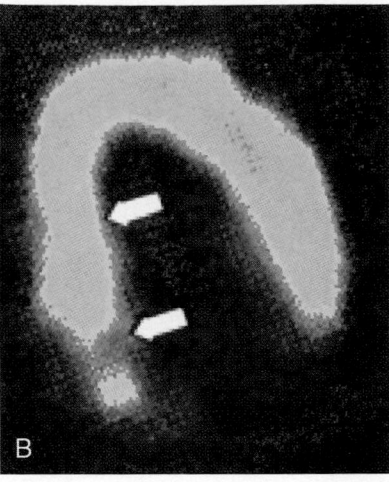

FIGURE 35–23. Myocardial perfusion in AMI. *A,* 99mTc-sestamibi SPECT before reperfusion; vertical long-axis slice; reduced tracer uptake of basal inferior left ventricular myocardium (arrows). *B,* 99mTc-sestamibi SPECT 7 days after stenting of left circumflex coronary artery; nearly normal tracer uptake of basal inferior left ventricular myocardium. (From Horcher J, et al: Myocardial perfusion in acute coronary syndrome. Circulation 99:e15, 1999. Copyright 1999, American Heart Association.)

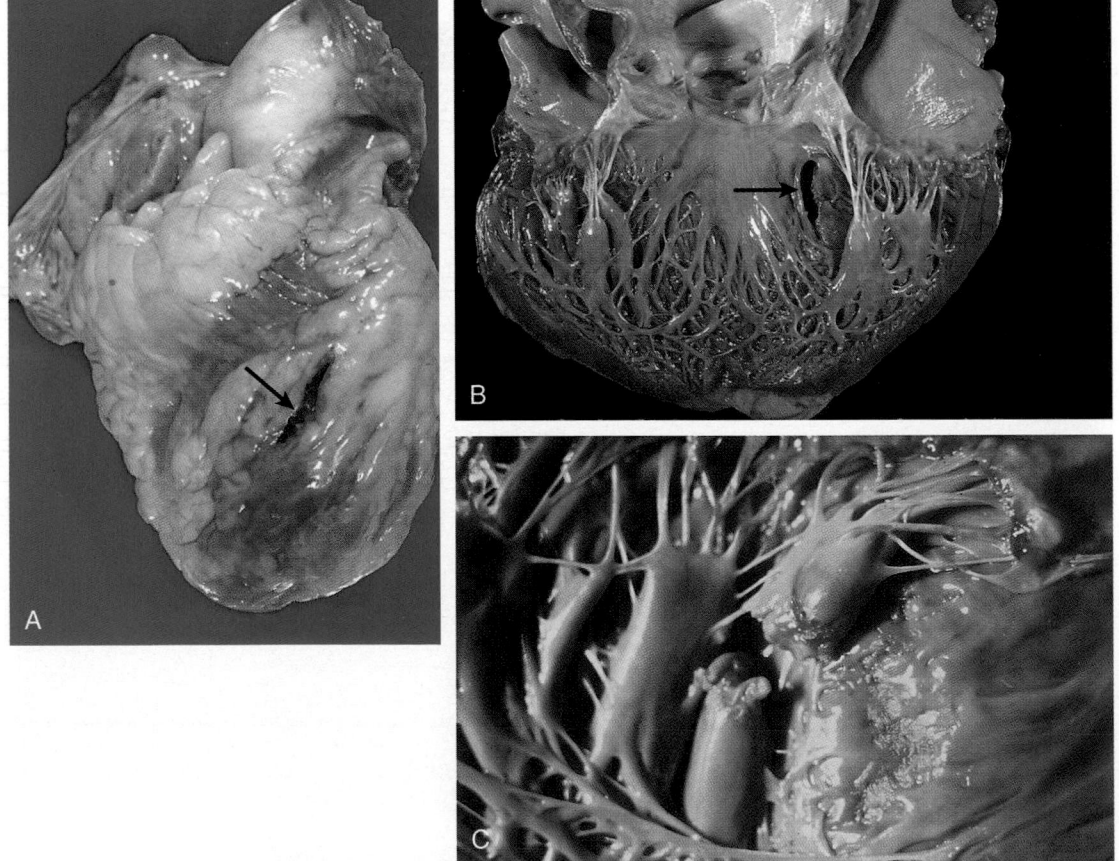

FIGURE 35–45. Cardiac rupture syndromes complicating acute myocardial infarction. *A,* Anterior myocardial rupture in an acute infarct (arrow). *B,* Rupture of the ventricular septum (arrow). *C,* Complete rupture of a necrotic papillary muscle. (From Schoen FJ: The heart. *In* Cotran RS, Kumar V, Collins T [eds]: Pathologic Basis of Disease. 6th ed. Philadelphia, WB Saunders, 1999, p 562.)

proposed that a ratio (relative index) of CK-MB mass/CK activity of about 2.5 is indicative of a myocardial rather than a skeletal source of the CK-MB elevation. Although this ratio may be satisfied by many patients with AMI, it is inaccurate in several circumstances: (1) when high levels of total CK are present because of skeletal muscle injury (a large quantity of CK-MB must be released from the myocardium to satisfy criteria); (2) chronic skeletal muscle injury releases large amounts of CK-MB; and (3) total CK measurements are within the normal reference range for the laboratory and CK-MB is elevated (possibly indicating that a microinfarction has occurred). Patients with minimally elevated CK-MB and normal CK levels have a prognosis that is generally worse than that for patients with suspected MI but no CK-MB elevation. Elevation of CK-MB after percutaneous coronary artery revascularization is associated with increased late (1–3 years) cardiac mortality.[116]

Clinicians should not rely on measurements of CK and CK-MB at a single point in time but instead should evaluate the temporal rise and fall of serially obtained values; skeletal muscle release of CK-MB generally remains elevated for a longer time than myocardial release of CK-MB and produces a "plateau" pattern of CK-MB values over several days, in contrast to the shorter time course of skeletal muscle CK-MB elevation, as depicted in Figure 35–7. Of note, since the cardiac-specific troponin I and T (cTnI and cTnT) (see Fig. 35–14 and Tables 35–2 and 35–3) accurately distinguish skeletal from cardiac muscle damage, the troponins are now considered the preferred biomarkers for diagnosing AMI.[117]

In addition to AMI secondary to coronary obstruction, other forms of injury to cardiac muscle—such as those resulting from myocarditis, trauma, cardiac catheterization, shock, and cardiac surgery—may also produce elevated serum CK-MB levels.[114] These latter causes of elevation of serum CK-MB values can usually be readily distinguished from AMI by the clinical setting.

CK ISOFORMS. Isoforms of the MM and MB isoenzymes have been identified.[118] These are subtypes of the individual isoenzymes and are formed in the circulation when the enzyme carboxypeptidase cleaves lysine residues from the carboxy terminus of the myocardial form of the enzyme (CK-MM3 and CK-MB2), producing isoforms with a different electrophoretic mobility (CK-MM2, CK-MM1, and CK-MB1). Certain isoforms appear to be released into the blood quite rapidly, perhaps as soon as 1 hour, after the onset of infarction. An absolute level of CK-MB2 isoform greater than 1.0 U/liter or a ratio of CK-MB2/CK-MB1 greater than 2.5 has a sensitivity for diagnosing AMI of 46.4 percent at 4 hours and of 91.5 percent at 6 hours.[119] A rapid high-voltage electrophoretic assay for these isoforms is available, and results in experienced research laboratories suggest it may permit early identification of patients with AMI and early detection of successful reperfusion (peak CK-MB2/CK-MB1 > 3.8 at 2 hours).[120]

MYOGLOBIN. This low-molecular-weight heme protein is released into the circulation from injured myocardial cells and can be detected within a few hours after the onset of infarction (see Fig. 35–14 and Table 35–3). Peak levels of serum myoglobin are reached considerably earlier (1 to 4 hours) than peak values of serum CK.[120] Because of its lack of cardiac specificity, an isolated measurement of myoglobin within the first 4 to 8 hours after onset of chest discomfort in patients with a nondiagnostic ECG should not be relied on to make the diagnosis of AMI but should be supplemented by a more cardiac-specific marker such as cTnI or cTnT.[117]

In contrast to CK, myoglobin is readily excreted into the urine. A more rapid rise in serum myoglobin has been observed after reperfusion, and its measurement has been suggested as a useful index of successful reperfusion[120] (Fig. 35–15) and even infarct size. In patients presenting less

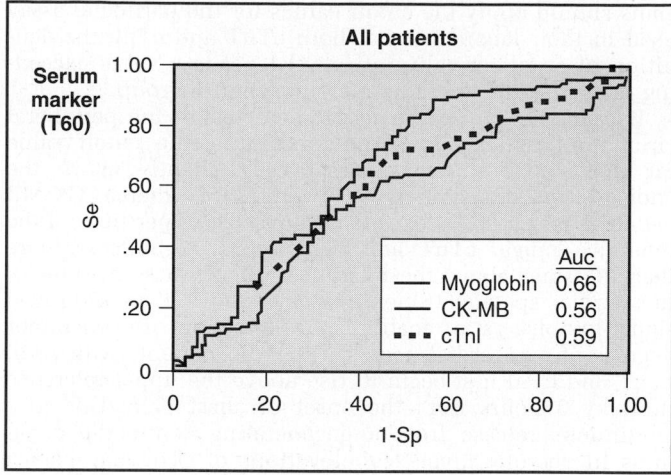

FIGURE 35–15. Receiver operator curves (ROC) of the 60-min value of myoglobin, CK-MB and cardiac troponin-I (cTnI), for noninvasive prediction of occlusion after thrombolysis. Auc = area under curve; Se = sensitivity; Sp = specificity. (Modified from Tanasijevic MJ, Cannon CP, Antman EM, et al: Am Coll Cardiol 1999;34:739–747.)

than 6 hours from symptoms and with ST segment elevation where the diagnosis of AMI is not in doubt, an elevated myoglobin level is associated with an increased risk of mortality.[121] The adverse prognostic significance of an elevated myoglobin level at presentation is probably due to a combination of a large amount of myocardial damage and a delay of at least several hours from onset of symptoms to blood sampling.

CARDIAC-SPECIFIC TROPONINS. The troponin complex consists of three subunits that regulate the calcium-mediated contractile process of striated muscle. These include troponin C, which binds Ca^{2+}; troponin I (TnI), which binds to actin and inhibits actin-myosin interactions; and troponin T (TnT), which binds to tropomyosin, thereby attaching the troponin complex to the thin filament (see Chap. 14). Although the majority of TnT is incorporated in the troponin complex, approximately 6 percent is dissolved in the cytosol; about 2 to 3 percent of TnI is found in a cytosolic pool.

Although both TnT and TnI are present in cardiac and skeletal muscle, they are encoded by different genes and the amino acid sequence differs.[122] This permits the production of antibodies that are specific for the cardiac form (cTnT and cTnI) and has led to the development of quantitative assays for cTnT and cTnI that have been approved by the Food and Drug Administration (FDA) for clinical use[117] (see Fig. 35–14 and Table 35–3). Several studies have confirmed the reliability of these new quantitative assays for detecting myocardial injury, and measurement of cTnT or cTnI is now at the center of a new diagnostic criterion for AMI.[52, 123, 123a] Qualitative, rapid, bedside assays for cTnT and cTnI have also been approved for diagnosing AMI.[124]

When interpreting the results of assays for cTnT or cTnI, clinicians must be cognizant of several analytical issues.[124a] The first-generation assay for cTnT exhibited some nonspecific binding to skeletal muscle troponin, but this was corrected in subsequent generations of assays. The cTnT assays are produced by a single manufacturer, leading to relative uniformity of cutoffs, whereas multiple manufacturers produce cTnI assays. The majority of cTnI released into the bloodstream in AMI is complexed with cardiac troponin C.[125] Variations in the cutoff concentration for abnormal levels of cTnI in the clinically available immunoassays may be due in part to different specificities of the antibodies used for detecting free and complexed cTnI.[125] Thus, when using the measurement of cTnI for diagnosing AMI, clinicians should apply the cutoff values for the particular assay used in their laboratory. For both cTnT and cTnI, the definition of an abnormally increased level is a value exceeding that of 99 percent of a reference control group.[123]

Because cTnT or cTnI is not detected in the peripheral circulation under normal circumstances, the cutoff value for these analytes may be set only slightly above the "noise" level of the assay.[109] Furthermore, whereas CK-MB usually increases 10- to 20-fold above the upper limit of the reference range, cTnT and cTnI typically increase more than 20 times above the reference range. These features of the cardiac-specific troponin assays provide an improved signal-to-noise ratio, enabling the detection of even minor degrees of myocardial necrosis.[52a, 111] In patients with AMI, cTnT and cTnI first begin to rise above the upper reference limit by 3 hours from the onset of chest pain. Due to a continuous release from a degenerating contractile apparatus in necrotic myocytes, elevations of cTnI may persist for 7 to 10 days after AMI; elevations of cTnT may persist for up to 10 to 14 days. The prolonged time course of elevation of cTnT and cTnI is advantageous for the late diagnosis of AMI.

Patients with AMI who undergo successful recanalization of the infarct-related artery have a rapid release of cardiac troponins that may be useful as an indicator of reperfusion, although myoglobin appears slightly more efficient in this regard.[126, 127]

Troponins vs. CK-MB. When comparing the diagnostic efficiency of the cardiac troponins versus CK-MB for AMI, it is important to bear in mind that the troponin assays are probably capable of detecting episodes of myocardial necrosis that are below the detection limit of the current CK-MB assays, leading to a number of "false-positive" cases of troponin elevations if CK-MB is used as the gold standard.[52a] The somewhat vague terms *minor myocardial damage* and *microinfarction* have been used to describe the pathological process in patients who have a chest pain syndrome and elevated cardiac troponin but in whom CK-MB is in the normal range.[128] From a clinical perspective, it is desirable to have diagnostic tests for AMI with increased sensitivity to increase the number of AMI cases identified and increased specificity to reduce the number of cases incorrectly diagnosed and treated for AMI. In addition, cardiac troponin measurements have been shown to have prognostic value for identifying patients with an acute coronary syndrome at risk for adverse clinical outcomes and who also exhibit enhanced responsiveness to new therapies such as glycoprotein (GP) IIb/IIIa inhibitors and low-molecular-weight heparins.[129] The prognostic value of the troponins is independent of other risk factors, such as age and ECG abnormalities, as well as the measurement of classic biomarkers such as CK-MB. The exact mechanism(s) by which troponins convey adverse prognostic potential is not clearly established. They may provide a more accurate reflection of the amount of myocardial necrosis sustained by the patient, but they may also reflect an increased propensity for thromboembolization from an unstable coronary plaque.

Interpretation of Elevated Troponin. Both cTnI and cTnT have been detected in the blood of patient with end-stage heart failure, including those with a nonischemic cardiomyopathy.[130] Observations such as these emphasize that the troponins detect myocyte damage regardless of the cause.

Balanced against the advantages of the troponins for improved detection of AMI and prognostication of risk are the epidemiological, social, and health care delivery implications of assigning a diagnosis of AMI to a larger cohort of patients than was the case in an earlier era (see Table 35–2). Revised criteria for AMI impact on the ability to monitor trends in the incidence of AMI and draw comparisons with previous observations, the psychological status of the patient, ability to obtain driving and pilot licenses, disability applications, and hospital reimbursement.[123] There is no clear solution to the issues just cited. It has been proposed that two decision limits are needed for optimal interpretation of troponin tests: a low abnormal value indicating myocardial damage and a higher value indicating the diagnosis of AMI according to traditional criteria.[128] There is a quantitative relationship between the amount of cardiac troponin released into the blood and the risk for adverse clinical outcomes.[5] We consider patients without elevation of cTnI or cTnT not to have had an AMI, those with elevated troponin but normal CK-MB to have microinfarction and a slight increase in risk compared with patients without troponin elevations, and those with elevation of both troponin and CK-MB to fulfill the "classic" definition of AMI with a larger amount of myocardial infarction and the greatest risk of adverse outcome.

LACTATE DEHYDROGENASE (LDH). The activity of this enzyme exceeds the normal range by 24 to 48 hours after the onset of AMI, reaches a peak 3 to 6 days after the onset of pain, and returns to normal levels 8 to 14 days after the infarction. LDH comprises five isoenzymes, which are numbered in the order of the rapidity of their migration toward the anode of an electrophoretic field. LDH$_1$ moves most rapidly, whereas LDH$_5$ is the slowest. Fractionation of the serum LDH into its five isoenzymes increases diagnostic accuracy because the heart contains principally LDH$_1$. However, LDH isoenzyme analysis for the diagnosis of AMI is no longer recommended because it has been superseded by newer, more cardiac-specific late markers such as cTnT or cTnI (see Table 35–3).[117]

OTHER SERUM CARDIAC MARKERS. Other promising serum cardiac markers that are under development include heart fatty acid binding proteins (hFABP), myosin light chains (MLC), myosin heavy chains (MHC), and glycogen phosphorylase isoenzyme BB (GPBB).[113] These markers offer the potential for earlier diagnosis (hFABP, GPBB) and a longer diagnostic window (MLC, MHC), but their relative roles compared with traditional markers such as CK-MB and newer markers such as CK-MB isoforms, cTnT, or cTnI remain to be defined and we do not recommend their routine use for diagnosing AMI.[117]

RECOMMENDATIONS FOR MEASUREMENT OF SERUM MARKERS. It seems reasonable for clinicians to measure either cTnT or cTnI in patients with suspected AMI. From a cost-effectiveness perspective, it is unnecessary to measure both a cardiac-specific troponin and CK-MB at all time points.[131] Routine diagnosis of AMI can be accomplished within 12 hours using CK-MB, cTnT, or cTnI by obtaining measurements approximately every 8 to 12 hours (see Table 35–2). Retrospective diagnosis or diagnosis of AMI in the presence of skeletal muscle injury is more readily accomplished with cTnT or cTnI. Future directions for research with the cardiac troponins involve evaluating their ability to aid in the diagnosis of AMI that occurs after cardiac and noncardiac surgery[132] and interventional catheterization procedures and in identifying myocardial injury from conditions other than AMI, such as myocarditis.

Although serum cardiac markers have been used successfully to stratify patients for risk of cardiac events when the presenting ECG does not show ST segment elevation, bedside assays for troponin or myoglobin either alone or in combination with the ECG also are useful for stratifying risk in patients with STEMI.[121, 133]

OTHER LABORATORY MEASUREMENTS

Numerous nonspecific manifestations may be recognized in patients with AMI. Although they are not generally employed in establishing the diagnosis, awareness of their coexistence with infarction is important to avoid misinterpretation or erroneous diagnosis of other disorders.

SERUM LIPIDS. These are often determined in patients with AMI. However, the results may be misleading because numerous factors that can alter the values are operating at the time of the patient's admission to the hospital. Serum triglycerides are affected by caloric intake, intravenous glucose, and recumbency.

During the first 24 to 48 hours after admission, total cholesterol and high-density lipoprotein (HDL) cholesterol remain at or near baseline values but generally fall precipitously after that. The fall in HDL cholesterol after AMI is greater than the fall in total cholesterol; thus, the ratio of total cholesterol to HDL cholesterol is no longer useful for risk assessment early after MI. A lipid profile should be obtained on all AMI patients who are admitted within 24 to 48 hours of symptoms. Based on the success of lipid-lowering therapy in primary and secondary prevention studies and evidence that hypolipidemic therapy improves endothelial function and inhibits thrombus formation,[134, 135] it has been argued that early management of serum lipids in patients hospitalized for AMI is advisable.[136] For patients admitted beyond 24 to 48 hours, more accurate determinations of serum lipid levels are obtained about 8 weeks after the infarction has occurred.

HEMATOLOGICAL MANIFESTATIONS. The elevation of the white blood cell count usually develops within 2 hours after the onset of chest pain, reaches a peak 2 to 4 days after infarction, and returns to normal in 1 week; the peak white blood cell count usually ranges between 12 and $15 \times 10^3/mm^3$ but occasionally rises to as high as $20 \times 10^3/mm^3$ in patients with large transmural AMI. Often there is an increase in the percentage of polymorphonuclear leukocytes and a shift of the differential count to band forms.

The erythrocyte sedimentation rate (ESR) is usually normal during the first 1 or 2 days after infarction, even though fever and leukocytosis may be present. It then rises to a peak on the fourth or fifth day and may remain elevated for several weeks. The increase in the ESR is secondary to elevated plasma alpha$_2$-globulin fibrinogen, but the peak does not correlate well with the size of the infarction or with the prognosis. The hematocrit often increases during the first few days after infarction as a consequence of hemoconcentration.

Electrocardiographic Findings

(See also Chap. 5)

In the majority of patients with AMI, some change can be documented when serial ECGs are compared. However, many factors limit the ability of the ECG to diagnose and localize MI: the extent of myocardial injury, the age of the infarct, its location, the presence of conduction defects, the presence of previous infarcts or acute pericarditis, changes in electrolyte concentrations, and the administration of cardioactive drugs. Changes in the ST segment and T wave are quite nonspecific and may occur in a variety of conditions, including stable and unstable angina pectoris, ventricular hypertrophy, acute and chronic pericarditis, myocarditis, early repolarization, electrolyte imbalance, shock, and metabolic disorders and after the administration of digitalis. Serial ECGs may be of considerable aid in differentiating these conditions from AMI. Transient changes favor angina or electrolyte disturbances, whereas persistent changes argue for infarction if other causes, such as shock, administration of digitalis, and persistent metabolic disorders, can be eliminated. Nevertheless, serial standard 12-lead ECGs remain a potent and extremely clinically useful method for the detection and localization of MI.[55, 137, 138] Analysis of the constellation of ECG leads showing ST segment elevation may also be useful for identifying the site of occlusion in the infarct artery.[139, 140] The extent of ST deviation on the ECG, location of infarction, and QRS duration correlate with risk of adverse outcomes.[56, 141] Even when left bundle branch block is present on the ECG, MI can be diagnosed when striking ST segment deviation is present beyond that which can be explained by the conduction defect.[142] In addition to the diagnostic and prognostic information contained within the 12-lead ECG, it also provides valuable noninvasive information about the success of reperfusion for STEMI.

Although general agreement exists on ECG and vectorcardiographic criteria for the recognition of infarction of the anterior and inferior myocardial walls, less agreement is found on criteria for lateral and posterior infarcts[143]; here even the terminology may be confusing. It has been reported that patients with an abnormal R wave in V_1 (0.04 second in duration and/or R/S ratio ≥ 1 in the absence of preexcitation or right ventricular hypertrophy) with inferior or lateral Q waves have an increased incidence of isolated occlusion of a dominant left circumflex coronary artery without collateral circulation; such patients have a lower ejection fraction, increased end-systolic volume, and higher complication rate than patients with inferior infarction due to isolated occlusion of the right coronary artery.

More sophisticated forms of ECG recordings including high-resolution ECG, body surface potential mapping of ST segments, and continuous vectorcardiography have all been reported in small series of patients to augment the 12-lead ECG in diagnosing AMI, but the lack of ready availability of equipment and the special expertise required limit the use of these techniques.

Although most patients continue to demonstrate the ECG changes from an infarction for the rest of their lives, particularly if they evolve Q waves, in a substantial minority the typical changes disappear, Q waves can regress, and the ECG can even return to normal after a number of years. Under many circumstances Q-wave patterns may simulate MI. Conditions that may mimic the ECG features of MI by producing a pattern of "pseudoinfarction" include ventricular hypertrophy, conduction disturbances, preexcitation, primary myocardial disease, pneumothorax, pulmonary embolus, amyloid heart disease, primary and metastatic tumors of the heart, traumatic heart disease, intracranial hemorrhage, hyperkalemia, pericarditis, early repolarization, and cardiac involvement with sarcoidosis. Normalization of negative T waves on serial ECGs is a useful marker of recovery of regional ventricular function after AMI.[143a]

Q-WAVE AND NON-Q-WAVE INFARCTION. As noted earlier (see p. 1116), the presence or absence of Q waves on the surface ECG does not reliably predict the distinction between transmural and nontransmural (subendocardial) AMI.[39] Q waves on the ECG signify abnormal electrical activity but are not synonymous with irreversible myocardial damage. Also, the absence of Q waves may simply reflect the insensitivity of the standard 12-lead ECG, especially in the posterior zones of the left ventricle. True pathological subendocardial AMI, as recognized at autopsy, is seen with ST segment depression and/or T wave changes only about 50 percent of the time.[144] Angiographic studies in AMI patients without ST segment elevation show a higher incidence of subtotal occlusion of the culprit coronary vessel and greater collateral flow to the infarct zone. Observational data suggest that AMI without ST segment elevation is seen more commonly in elderly patients and patients with a prior MI.

ISCHEMIA AT A DISTANCE. Patients with new Q waves and ST segment elevation diagnostic for AMI in one territory often have ST segment depression in other territories. These additional ST segment changes may be caused either by ischemia in a territory other than the area of infarction, termed "ischemia at a distance," or by reciprocal electrical phenomena. A good deal of attention has been directed to associated ST segment depression in the anterior leads when it occurs in patients with acute inferior MI. However, despite the clinical importance of differentiation among causes of anterior ST segment depression in such patients—including anterior ischemia, posterior wall infarction, and true reciprocal changes—such a differentiation cannot be made reliably by ECG or even vectorcardiographic techniques. Although precordial ST segment depression is more commonly associated with extensive infarction of the posterior, lateral, or inferior septal segments—rather than anterior wall subendocardial ischemia—imaging techniques such as two-dimensional echocardiography are necessary to ascertain whether an anterior wall motion abnormality is present.[145, 146] Regardless of whether the anterior ST segment changes reflect anterior wall ischemia or are reciprocal to changes elsewhere, this finding, as with ischemia at a distance, implies a poorer prognosis than if such changes are not present.[147]

RIGHT VENTRICULAR INFARCTION. ST segment elevation in right precordial leads (V_1, V_3R–V_6R) is a relatively sensitive and specific sign of right ventricular infarction.[63a, 148] Occasionally, ST segment elevation in leads V_2 and V_3 may be due to acute right ventricular infarction; this appears to occur only when the injury to the left inferior wall is minimal.[149] Usually, the concurrent inferior wall injury suppresses this anterior ST segment elevation resulting from right ventricular injury. Likewise, right ventricular infarction appears to reduce the anterior ST segment depression often observed with inferior wall MI. A QS or QR pattern in leads V_3R and/or V_4R also suggests right ventricular myocardial necrosis but has less predictive accuracy than ST segment elevation in these leads.[52]

ATRIAL INFARCTION. The most common ECG patterns are depression or elevation of the PR segment, alterations in the contour of the P wave, and abnormal atrial rhythms, including atrial flutter, atrial fibrillation, wandering atrial pacemaker, and atrioventricular (AV) nodal rhythm.

Imaging

ROENTGENOGRAPHY. The initial chest roentgenogram in patients with AMI is almost invariably a portable film obtained in the emergency department or the CCU. When present, prominent pulmonary vascular markings on the roentgenogram reflect elevated left-ventricular end-diastolic pressure, but significant temporal discrepancies may occur because of what have been termed diagnostic lags and posttherapeutic lags. Up to 12 hours may elapse before pulmonary edema accumulates after ventricular filling pressure has become elevated. The posttherapeutic phase lag represents a longer time interval; up to 2 days are required for pulmonary edema to resorb and the radiographic signs of pulmonary congestion to clear after ventricular filling pressure has returned toward normal. The degree of congestion and the size of the left side of the heart on the chest film are useful for defining groups of patients with AMI who are at increased risk of dying after the acute event.[150]

Echocardiography

(See Figs. 7-104, 7-105, and 7-106)

TWO-DIMENSIONAL ECHOCARDIOGRAPHY. The relative portability of echocardiographic equipment makes this technique ideal for the assessment of patients with AMI hospitalized in the CCU or even in the emergency department before admission. In patients with chest pain compatible with AMI but with a nondiagnostic ECG, the finding on echocardiography of a distinct region of disordered contraction can be helpful diagnostically because it supports the diagnosis of myocardial ischemia. Echocardiography is also useful in evaluating patients with chest pain and a nondiagnostic ECG who are suspected of having an aortic dissection. The identification of an intimal flap consistent with an aortic dissection is a crucial observation because it represents a major contraindication to thrombolytic therapy (see Chap. 40).

Areas of abnormal regional wall motion are observed almost universally in patients with AMI, and the degree of wall motion abnormality can be categorized with a semiquantitative wall motion score index. Of note, abnormal wall motion is less often noted echocardiographically when the infarction is small and the age of regional wall motion abnormality cannot always be determined.[52] Left ventricular function estimated from two-dimensional ECGs correlates well with measurements from angiography and is useful in establishing prognosis after AMI.[145] Furthermore, the early use of echocardiography can aid in the early detection of potentially viable but stunned myocardium (contractile reserve), residual provocable ischemia, patients at risk for the development of congestive heart failure after AMI, and mechanical complications of AMI.[145]

Whereas transthoracic imaging is adequate in most patients, occasional patients have poor echo windows, especially if they are undergoing mechanical ventilation. In such patients transesophageal echocardiography can be safely performed and can be useful in evaluating ventricular septal defects and papillary muscle dysfunction.[146]

DOPPLER ECHOCARDIOGRAPHY (see Fig. 7-28). This technique allows for assessment of blood flow in the cardiac chambers and across cardiac valves. Used in conjunction with two-dimensional echocardiography, it is helpful in detecting and assessing the severity of mitral or tricuspid regurgitation after AMI. Identification of the site of acute ventricular septal rupture, as well as quantification of shunt flow across the resulting defect, is also possible.[146]

Other Imaging Modalities

NUCLEAR IMAGING. Radionuclide angiography, perfusion imaging, infarct-avid scintigraphy, and positron-emission tomography have been used to evaluate patients with AMI. Nuclear cardiac imaging techniques (see Figs. 9-15 and 9-16) can be useful for detecting AMI; assessing infarct size, collateral flow, and jeopardized myocardium; determining the effects of the infarct on ventricular function; and establishing prognosis of patients with AMI.[151] However, the necessity of moving a critically ill patient from the CCU to the nuclear medicine department limits their practical application unless a portable gamma camera is available. Cardiac radionuclide imaging for the diagnosis of MI should be restricted to special, limited situations in which the trial of clinical history, ECG findings, and serum marker measurements is unavailable or unreliable.[52]

COMPUTED TOMOGRAPHY (CT) (see Chap. 10). This technique can provide useful cross-sectional information in patients with MI. In addition to the assessment of cavity dimensions and wall thickness, left ventricular aneurysms may be detected and, of particular importance in AMI, intracardiac thrombi can be identified. Although cardiac CT is a less convenient technique, it probably is more sensitive for thrombus detection than is echocardiography.

MAGNETIC RESONANCE IMAGING (MRI) (see Fig. 10-9). In addition to localizing and sizing the area of infarction, MRI techniques are capable of early recognition of MI and of providing an assessment of the severity of the ischemic insult.[152] This modality is attractive because of its ability to assess perfusion of infarcted and noninfarcted tissue as well as of reperfused myocardium; to identify areas of jeopardized but not infarcted myocardium; to identify myocardial edema, fibrosis, wall thinning, and hypertrophy; to assess ventricular chamber size and segmental wall motion; and to identify the temporal transition between ischemia and infarction[153] but has limited practical application because of the need to transport patients with AMI to the MRI facility.

ESTIMATION OF INFARCT SIZE

ELECTROCARDIOGRAPHY. Interest in limiting infarct size, in large part because of the recognition that the quantity of myocardium infarcted has important prognostic implications, has focused attention on the accurate determination of MI size. The sum of ST segment elevations measured from multiple precordial leads correlates with the extent of myocardial injury in patients with anterior MI.[154] QRS scoring systems and planar or vectorcardiographic techniques to estimate infarct size have also been developed. Although they demonstrate good correlations with infarct size at autopsy and with enzymatic estimates, formal sizing of infarcts by ECG technique is not necessary in most patients. Of note, however, there is a relationship between the number of ECG leads showing ST segment elevation and mortality: patients with 8 or 9 of 12 leads with ST segment elevation have three to four times the mortality of those with only 2 or 3 leads with ST segment elevation. The duration of ischemia time as estimated from continuous ST segment monitoring is correlated with infarct size, the ratio of infarct size to area at risk, and the extent of regional wall motion abnormality observed at 7 days and 30 days after AMI.[154]

CARDIAC MARKER METHODS. To estimate infarct size by analysis of serum cardiac marker levels, it is necessary to account for the quantity of the marker lost from the myocardium, its volume of distribution, and its release ratio.[60] Serial measurements of proteins released by necrotic myocardium are helpful in determining AMI size. Clinically, the peak CK or CK-MB provides an approximate estimate of infarct size and is widely used prognostically. In the prethrombotic era, quantification of the cumulative release of CK or CK-MB correlated with other techniques for estimating infarct size in vivo as well as with the area of necrosis at autopsy. However, coronary artery reperfusion dramatically changes the washout kinetics of CK and other markers from myocardium, resulting in early and exaggerated peak levels and limiting the usefulness of such curves as a measure of infarct size.

NONINVASIVE IMAGING TECHNIQUES. Echocardiography (see Chap. 7), radionuclide scintigraphy[52] (see Chap. 9), CT (see Chap. 10), and MRI (see Chap. 10) have all been used for the clinical and experimental

assessment of infarct size. Infarct-avid scintigraphy and myocardial perfusion imaging have been used to quantify infarct size. Estimation of infarct size by quantitative tomographic employing technetium-99m (^{99m}Tc)-sestamibi imaging appears to be less limited by ventricular geometry and can distinguish small infarcts and ischemia from infarcted myocardium more readily than other noninvasive methods.[155] Tomography has improved on planar techniques employing ^{99m}Tc pyrophosphate to image AMI (see Chap. 9).[156] Contrast medium–enhanced MRI has been helpful in demonstrating the regional heterogeneity of infarction patterns in patients with persistently occluded infarct arteries versus those with successfully reperfused vessels.

▼ Management

PREHOSPITAL CARE

The prehospital care of patients with suspected AMI is a crucial element bearing directly on the likelihood of survival. Most deaths associated with AMI occur within the first hour of its onset and are usually due to ventricular fibrillation[157] (see also Chap. 26). Accordingly, the importance of the immediate implementation of definitive resuscitative efforts and of rapidly transporting the patient to a hospital cannot be overemphasized.[52] Major components of the delay from the onset of symptoms consistent with AMI to reperfusion include the following[157]: (1) the time for the patient to recognize the seriousness of the problem and seek medical attention; (2) prehospital evaluation, treatment, and transportation; (3) the time for diagnostic measures and initiation of treatment in the hospital (e.g., "door-to-needle" time for patients receiving a thrombolytic and "door-to-balloon" time for patients undergoing a catheter-

based reperfusion strategy); and (4) the time from initiation of treatment to restoration of flow (Fig. 35–16).

Patients with previously diagnosed coronary heart disease have the same delay times (median of 2.0 hours) as those without prior AMI or coronary heart disease.[158, 159] Therefore, patients must be educated to seek immediate medical attention should they develop manifestations of AMI. Patient-related factors that correlate with longer decision to seek medical attention include older age; female gender; African-American race; low socioeconomic status; low emotional or somatic awareness; history of angina, diabetes, or both; consulting a spouse or other relative; and consulting a physician.[159, 160]

Health care professionals should heighten the level of awareness of patients at risk for AMI (e.g., those with hypertension, diabetes, history of angina pectoris).[158] They should review and reinforce with patients and their families the need for seeking urgent medical attention for a

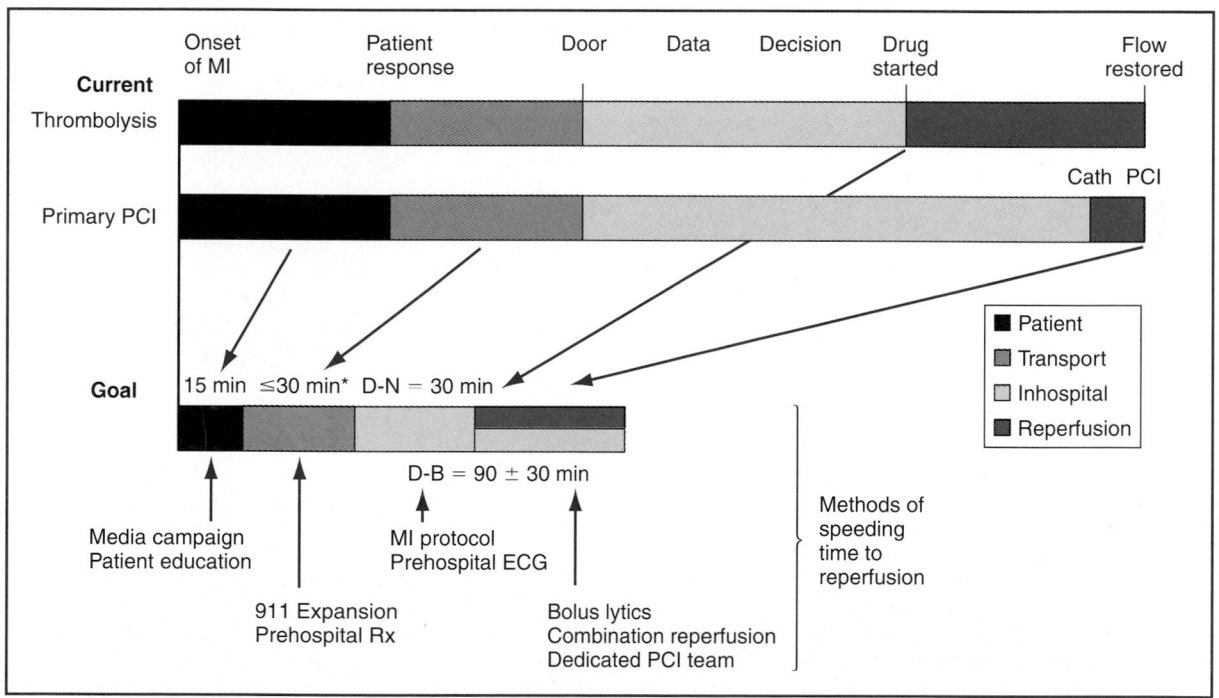

FIGURE 35–16. Major components of time delay between onset of infarction and restoration of flow in the infarct-related artery. Plotted sequentially from left to right are shown the time for patients to recognize symptoms and seek medical attention, transportation to the hospital, in-hospital decision-making and implementation of reperfusion strategy, and time for restoration of flow once the reperfusion strategy has been initiated. The time to initiate thrombolytic therapy is the "door-to-needle" (D-N) time; this is followed by the period of time required for pharmacological restoration of flow. More time is required to move the patient to the catheterization laboratory for a percutaneous coronary interventional (PCI) procedure, referred to as the "door-to-balloon" (D-B) time, but restoration of flow in the epicardial infarct-related artery occurs promptly after PCI. At the bottom are shown a variety of methods for speeding the time to reperfusion along with the goals for the time intervals for the various components of the time delay. (Cannon CP, Antman EM, Walls R, Braunwald E: Time as an adjunctive agent to thrombolytic therapy. J Thromb Thrombol 1:27–34, 1994.)

pattern of symptoms including chest discomfort, extreme fatigue, and dyspnea, especially if accompanied by diaphoresis, lightheadedness, palpitations, or a sense of impending doom[52] (see Fig. 35–16). Although many patients shun such discussions and tend to minimize the likelihood of ever needing emergency cardiac treatment, emphasis should be placed on the prevention and treatment of potentially fatal arrhythmias as well as salvage of the jeopardized myocardium by reperfusion, for which time is crucial.[161] Patients should also be instructed in the proper use of sublingual nitroglycerin, which should be taken as one tablet at the onset of ischemic-type discomfort and repeated at 5-minute intervals for a total of three doses. If the symptoms have not dissipated within 15 minutes, the patient should be rapidly transported to a medical facility that has the capability of recording and interpreting an ECG, providing advanced cardiac life support and cardiac monitoring, and initiating reperfusion therapy with either thrombolysis or angioplasty if indicated. Primary care physicians play an important role in helping implement strategies to facilitate early treatment.[158]

THE NATIONAL HEART ATTACK ALERT PROGRAM. This program has stressed the importance of community-wide planning for strategies allowing rapid recognition and triage of patients potentially suffering from AMI[162] (see Fig. 35–16). Well-equipped ambulances and helicopters staffed by personnel trained in the acute care of the infarction victim (mobile CCUs) allow definitive therapy to commence while the patient is being transported to the hospital[163] (Table 35–4). To be used effectively, they must be placed strategically within a community, and excellent radio communication systems must be available. These units should be equipped with battery-operated monitoring equipment, a direct-current defibrillator, oxygen, endotracheal tubes and suction apparatus, and commonly used cardiovascular drugs. Radiotelemetry systems that allow transmission of the ECG signal to the hospital are highly desirable and are becoming increasingly available in many communities (see Fig. 35–16). The effectiveness of such a prehospital system depends on the competency of paramedics,[160, 164] transmission distances, and the availability of expert consultation on the receiving end.[165] Observations of simple variables such as heart rate and blood pressure permit initial classification of patients into high- or low-risk subgroups[166] because those patients initially presenting with hypotension have a mortality in excess of 30 percent, whereas young patients with isolated sinus bradycardia and a normal or elevated blood pressure appear to have a mortality that is under 5 percent.[15]

In addition to prompt defibrillation, the efficacy of prehospital care appears to depend on several factors, including early relief of pain with its deleterious physiological sequelae, reduction of excessive activity of the autonomic nervous system, and abolition of prelethal arrhythmias, such as ventricular tachycardia. However, these efforts must not inhibit rapid transfer to the hospital.[52]

PREHOSPITAL THROMBOLYSIS. The potential benefits of prehospital thrombolysis have been evaluated in several

▼ **TABLE 35–4. CHEST PAIN CHECKLIST FOR USE BY EMT/PARAMEDIC FOR DIAGNOSIS OF ACUTE MYOCARDIAL INFARCTION AND THROMBOLYTIC THERAPY SCREENING**

Check each finding below. If all [yes] boxes are checked and ECG indicates ST segment elevation or new BBB, reperfusion therapy with thrombolysis or primary PTCA may be indicated. Thrombolysis is generally not indicated unless all [no] boxes are checked and BP ≤180/110 mm Hg.

	Yes	No
Ongoing chest discomfort (≥20 min and <12 hr)	☐	—
Oriented, can cooperate	☐	—
Age > 35 (>40 if female)	☐	—
History of stroke or transient ischemic attack		—
Known bleeding disorder	—	☐
Active internal bleeding in past 2 weeks	—	☐
Surgery or trauma in past 2 weeks	—	☐
Terminal illness	—	☐
Jaundice, hepatitis, kidney failure	—	☐
Use of anticoagulants	—	☐

Systolic/diastolic blood pressure
  Right arm: ____/____
  Left arm: ____/____

	Yes	No
ECG done	☐	—

High-risk profile*	**Yes**	**No**
Heart rate ≥ 100 beats/min	☐	—
BP ≤ 100 mm Hg	☐	—
Pulmonary edema (rales greater than halfway up)	☐	—
Shock	☐	—

*Transport to hospital capable of angiography and revascularization if needed.

Pain began	_____	AM/PM
Arrival time	_____	AM/PM
Begin transport	_____	AM/PM
Hospital arrival	_____	AM/PM

EMT = emergency medical technician; ECG = electrocardiogram; BBB = bundle branch block; PTCA = percutaneous transluminal coronary angioplasty; BP = blood pressure.
Adapted from the Seattle/King County EMS Medical Record. From 1999 Updated ACC/AHA AMI Guideline (Web version), p 16.

randomized trials.[167] Although none of the individual trials showed a significant reduction in mortality with prehospital-initiated thrombolytic therapy, there was a generally consistent observation of benefit from earlier treatment, and meta-analyses of all the available trials demonstrate a significant 17 percent reduction in mortality.[167, 167a]

Several factors must be weighed when communities consider whether their ambulances and emergency transport vehicles should have capabilities of initiating thrombolytic therapy. The greatest reduction in mortality is observed when reperfusion can be initiated within 60 to 90 minutes of the onset of symptoms.[15, 168] It has been suggested that the streamlining of emergency department triage practices so that treatment can be started within 30 minutes, when coupled with the 15- to 30-minute transport time that is common in most urban centers, may be more cost-effective than equipping all ambulances to administer prehospital thrombolytic therapy[52] (see Fig. 35–16). The latter would require extensive training of personnel (see Table 35–4), installation of computer-assisted electrocardiographs or systems for radio transmission of the ECG signal to a central station, and stocking of medicine kits with the necessary drug supplies[165, 169–171] (see Fig. 35–16). However, in selected communities where transport delays may be 60 to 90 minutes or longer and experienced personnel or physicians are available on ambulances, prehospital thrombolytic therapy is probably beneficial.[52, 172, 173]

MANAGEMENT IN THE EMERGENCY DEPARTMENT

Physicians evaluating patients in the emergency department must confront the difficult task of rapidly identifying patients who require urgent reperfusion therapy, triaging lower risk patients to the appropriate facility within the hospital, and not discharging patients home inappropriately while avoiding unnecessary admissions.[157, 168, 174–174b] As emphasized in Figure 35–17, a history of ischemic-type discomfort and the initial 12-lead ECG (Fig. 35–18) are the primary tools for screening patients with acute coronary syndromes in the emergency department. ST segment elevation on the ECG of a patient with a history compatible with AMI is highly suggestive of thrombotic occlusion of an epicardial coronary artery,[61] and its presence should serve as the trigger for a well-rehearsed sequence of rapid assessment of the patient for contraindications to thrombolysis and initiation of a reperfusion strategy[157, 168, 175–177] (see Fig. 35–17).

Because lethal arrhythmias can occur suddenly in patients with an acute coronary syndrome, all patients should have a 12-lead ECG performed immediately while a brief targeted history is taken[157, 168] (see Fig. 35–17). Patients should then be attached to a bedside ECG monitor and intravenous access obtained for infusion of 5 percent dextrose in water. If the initial ECG shows ST segment elevation of 1 mm or more in at least two contiguous leads (see Fig. 35–18) or a new or presumably new bundle branch block, the patient should be screened immediately for any contraindications to thrombolysis (Table 35–5) to help facilitate expeditious initiation of reperfusion therapy.[178] The National Heart Attack Alert Program recommends that emergency departments strive for a goal of treating eligible AMI patients with thrombolytic therapy within 30 minutes[157, 168, 177] (see Figs. 35–16 and 35–17). As door-to-needle times increase beyond 30 minutes, there is a progression in mortality and the likelihood of developing an ejection fraction less than 40 percent.[179] Evidence exists that for patients undergoing primary PTCA for AMI, delays in door-to-balloon times in excess of 2 hours are associated with increased mortality, emphasizing the need for expeditious transfer to the catheterization laboratory if primary PTCA is selected as the reperfusion strategy.[179a]

The available data fail to show a benefit of thrombolysis in AMI patients who do not present with ST segment elevation[15, 180] (see Fig. 35–17). Patients with an initial ECG that reveals new or presumably new ST segment depression and/or T wave inversion, while not considered candidates for thrombolytic therapy, should be treated as though they are suffering from AMI without ST segment elevation or unstable angina (a distinction to be made subsequently after scrutiny of serial ECGs and cardiac marker measurements) (see Figs. 35–2 and 35–14 and Chap. 36).

Management of the AMI patient without ST segment elevation is an important problem because 40 to 50 percent of patients with AMI are not considered candidates for thrombolysis on the basis of an initial ECG that does not show ST segment elevation.[5] Some patients without ST segment elevation on the initial ECG may subsequently experience a worsening of ischemic discomfort, develop ST segment elevation (presumably when a subtotal occlusion of the culprit coronary artery progresses to total occlusion), and become candidates for reperfusion therapy (see Table 35–5). Therefore, patients whose ECG is highly suggestive of myocardial ischemia should be admitted to a hospital unit with facilities for continuous monitoring of the ECG (either the CCU or intermediate care unit) that will alert the staff if arrhythmias or ST segment elevation occurs.[181, 182] Arrangements should be made for 12-lead ECGs to be obtained approximately every 8 hours for the first 24 hours, or more frequently if ischemic discomfort recurs.

Patients with a history suggestive of AMI (see p. 1128) and an initial nondiagnostic ECG (i.e., no obvious ST segment deviation or T wave inversion) should have serial tracings obtained while being evaluated in the emergency department for AMI (see Fig. 35–17). Emergency department staff may be alerted to the sudden development of ST segment elevation by periodic visual inspection of the bedside ECG monitor, by continuous ST segment recording, or by auditory alarms when the ST segment deviation exceeds programmed limits. Decision aids such as computer-based diagnostic algorithms, identification of high-risk clinical indicators, rapid determination of cardiac serum markers,[111] two-dimensional echocardiographic screening for regional wall motion abnormalities, and myocardial perfusion imaging are of greatest clinical utility when the ECG is nondiagnostic. In an effort to improve the cost-effectiveness of care of patients with a chest pain syndrome, nondiagnostic ECG, and low suspicion of AMI but in whom the diagnosis has not been entirely excluded, many medical centers have developed critical pathways that involve a coronary observation unit with a goal of ruling out AMI in less than 12 hours (see Fig. 35–17).[183, 184]

General Treatment Measures

ASPIRIN. This agent is effective across the entire spectrum of acute coronary syndromes (see Fig. 35–2) and now forms part of the initial management strategy of patients with suspected AMI (see Fig. 35–17). The pharmacology of aspirin is presented in Chapter 62. The goal of aspirin treatment is to quickly block formation of thromboxane A_2 in platelets by cyclooxygenase inhibition. Because low doses (40 to 80 mg) take several days to achieve full antiplatelet effect, at least 160 to 325 mg should be administered acutely in the emergency department.[52] To achieve therapeutic blood levels rapidly, the patient should chew the tablet, thus promoting buccal absorption rather than absorption through the gastric mucosa.

CONTROL OF CARDIAC PAIN. Analgesia is an important element of management of AMI patients in the emergency department. Often there is a tendency to underdose the

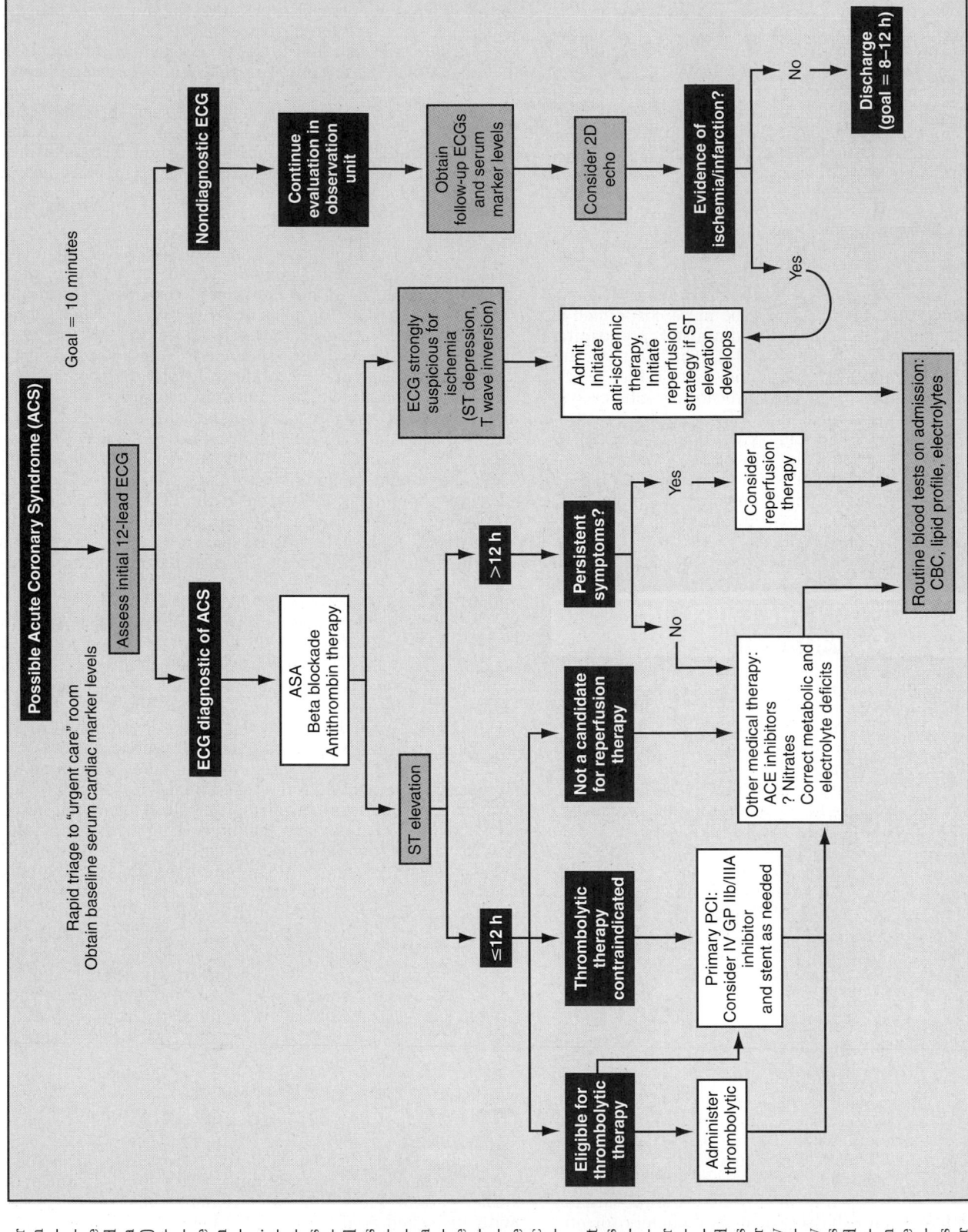

FIGURE 35–17. Algorithm for management of patients with suspected acute coronary syndrome in emergency department. All patients with possible ischemic-type discomfort should be rapidly evaluated and have a 12-lead electrocardiogram (ECG) performed. If the ECG is diagnostic of an acute coronary syndrome, patients should receive aspirin (ASA), beta blockers (in the absence of contraindications), and an antithrombin. Patients with ST segment elevation should be considered candidates for reperfusion, whereas those without ST segment elevation whose ECG and clinical history are strongly suspicious for ischemia should be admitted for initiation of antiischemic therapy. Patients with a nondiagnostic ECG should undergo further evaluation in the emergency department or short-term observation unit with ultimate disposition based on the results of serial serum cardiac marker levels and echocardiographic findings.

Patients with ST segment elevation treated within 12 hours who are eligible for thrombolytics should expeditiously receive thrombolytic therapy or be considered for primary percutaneous coronary intervention (PCI). Primary PCI should be supported by an intravenous glycoprotein IIb/IIIa inhibitor and stent as needed. Primary PCI is also to be considered when thrombolytic therapy is contraindicated. Individuals treated after 12 hours should receive the initial medical therapy noted earlier and on an individual basis and may be candidates for angiotensin-converting enzyme (ACE) inhibitors (particularly if left ventricular function is impaired).

Routine blood tests that should be obtained in all patients admitted by means of the algorithm include a complete blood cell count (CBC), lipid profile, and electrolyte levels. After discharge, all patients should receive aspirin and a beta blocker (in the absence of contraindications). Dietary modifications and, if needed, treatment to reduce low-density lipoprotein cholesterol and elevated high-density lipoprotein cholesterol are strongly encouraged, as is life style modification (including regular physical exercise and cessation of cigarette smoking).

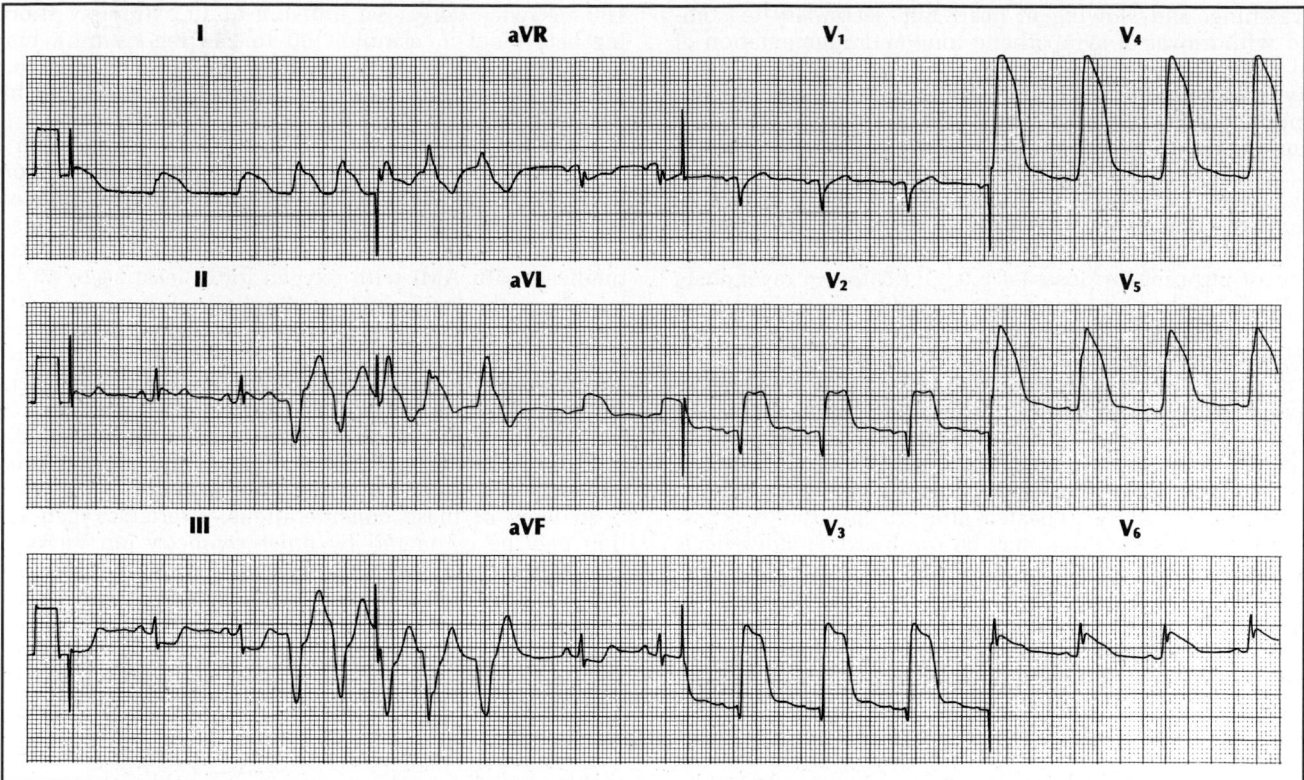

FIGURE 35–18. This 12-lead ECG was obtained from a middle-aged man admitted with an extensive anterior AMI. (Note pathological Q waves in the precordial leads and marked repolarization abnormalities in the anterior and lateral leads.) A five-beat salvo of nonsustained ventricular tachycardia is seen extending over the transition between leads III and aV$_f$. (From Antman EM, Rutherford JD: Coronary Care Medicine. Boston, Martinus Nijhoff Publishing, 1986, p 81.)

▼ **Table 35–5. CONTRAINDICATIONS AND CAUTIONS FOR THROMBOLYTIC USE IN MYOCARDIAL INFARCTION***

CONTRAINDICATIONS
- Previous hemorrhagic stroke at any time; other strokes or cerebrovascular events within 1 year
- Known intracranial neoplasm
- Active internal bleeding (does not include menses)
- Suspected aortic dissection

CAUTIONS/RELATIVE CONTRAINDICATIONS
- Severe uncontrolled hypertension on presentation (blood pressure > 180/110 mm Hg)†
- History of prior cerebrovascular accident or known intracerebral pathology not covered in contraindications
- Current use of anticoagulants in therapeutic doses (INR ≥ 2–3); known bleeding diathesis
- Recent trauma (within 2–4 weeks), including head trauma or traumatic or prolonged (> 10 min) CPR or major surgery (< 3 wk)
- Noncompressible vascular punctures
- Recent (within 2–4 weeks) internal bleeding
- For streptokinase/anistreplase: prior exposure (especially within 5 d–2 yr) or prior allergic reaction
- Pregnancy
- Active peptic ulcer
- History of chronic severe hypertension

*Viewed as advisory for clinical decision making and may not be all-inclusive or definitive.

†Could be an absolute contraindication in low-risk patients with myocardial infarction (see text).

INR = international normalized ratio; CPR = cardiopulmonary resuscitation.

From 1999 Updated ACC/AHA AMI Guideline (Web version), p 38.

patient for fear of obscuring response to antiischemic or reperfusion therapy. This should be avoided because pain contributes to the heightened sympathetic activity that is particularly prominent during the early phase of AMI. Control of cardiac pain is typically accomplished with a combination of nitrates, analgesics (e.g., morphine), oxygen, and beta-adrenoceptor blockers. Similar pharmacological principles apply in the CCU, where many of the therapies discussed in this section are continued after initial dosing in the emergency department. Because the pain associated with MI is related to ongoing ischemia, many interventions that act to improve the oxygen supply-demand relationship (by either increasing supply or decreasing demand) may lessen the pain associated with AMI.

Analgesics. Although a wide variety of analgesic agents has been used to treat the pain associated with AMI, including meperidine, pentazocine, and morphine, the last one remains the drug of choice, except in patients with well-documented morphine hypersensitivity. Four to 8 mg of morphine should be administered intravenously and doses of 2 to 8 mg repeated at intervals of 5 to 15 minutes until the pain is relieved or evident toxicity (i.e., hypotension, depression of respiration, or severe vomiting) precludes further administration of the drug. In some patients, remarkably large cumulative doses of morphine (2 to 3 mg/kg) may be required and are usually tolerated.[185]

The reduction of anxiety resulting from morphine diminishes the patient's restlessness and the activity of the autonomic nervous system, with a consequent reduction of the heart's metabolic demands. The beneficial effect of morphine in patients with pulmonary edema is unequivocal and may relate to several factors, including peripheral arterial and venous dilatation (particularly among patients with excessive sympathoadrenal activity), reduction of the work of breathing, and slowing of heart rate secondary to combined withdrawal of sympathetic tone and augmentation of vagal tone.[185]

Hypotension after the administration of nitroglycerin and morphine can be minimized by maintaining the patient in a supine position and elevating the lower extremities if systolic arterial pressure declines below 100 mm Hg. Obviously, such positioning is undesirable in the presence of pulmonary edema, but morphine rarely produces hypotension under these circumstances. The concomitant administration of atropine in doses of 0.5 to 1.5 mg intravenously may be helpful in reducing the excessive vagomimetic effects of morphine, particularly when hypotension and bradycardia are present before it is administered.[52] Respiratory depression is an unusual complication of morphine in the presence of severe pain or pulmonary edema, but as the patient's cardiovascular status improves, impairment of ventilation may supervene and should be watched for. It can be treated with naloxone, in doses of 0.1 to 0.2 mg intravenously initially, repeated after 15 minutes if necessary. Nausea and vomiting may be troublesome side effects of large doses of morphine and may be treated with a phenothiazine.

NITRATES. By virtue of their ability to enhance coronary blood flow by coronary vasodilation and to decrease ventricular preload by increasing venous capacitance, sublingual nitrates are indicated for most patients with an acute coronary syndrome. At present, the only groups of patients with AMI in whom sublingual nitroglycerin should *not* be given are those with inferior MI and suspected right ventricular infarction[63, 63a] or marked hypotension (systolic pressure < 90 mm Hg), especially if accompanied by bradycardia.

Once it is ascertained that hypotension is not present, a sublingual nitroglycerin tablet should be administered and the patient observed carefully for improvement in symptoms or change in hemodynamics. If an initial dose is well tolerated and appears to be of benefit, further nitrates should be administered, with careful monitoring of the vital signs. Even small doses may produce sudden hypotension and bradycardia, a reaction that can be life threatening but can usually be easily reversed with intravenous atropine if it is recognized quickly. Long-acting oral nitrate preparations should be avoided in the very early course of AMI because of the frequently changing hemodynamic status of the patient. In patients with a prolonged period of waxing and waning chest pain, intravenous nitroglycerin may be of benefit in controlling symptoms and correcting ischemia, but frequent monitoring of blood pressure is required.[185]

BETA-ADRENOCEPTOR BLOCKERS. These drugs relieve pain, reduce the need for analgesics in many patients, and reduce infarct size.[186] Patients most suited for the use of beta blockers early in the course of AMI are those who also have sinus tachycardia and hypertension because beta blockers lower both the heart rate and arterial blood pressure, thereby lowering myocardial oxygen demand. A popular and relatively safe protocol for the use of a beta blocker in this situation is as follows:

1. Patients with heart failure (rales > 10 cm up from diaphragm), hypotension (BP < 90 mm Hg), bradycardia (heart rate < 60 beats/min), or heart block (PR > 0.24 sec) are first excluded.[187]

2. Metoprolol is given in three 5-mg boluses.

3. Patients are observed for 2 to 5 minutes after each bolus, and if the heart rate falls below 60 beats/min or systolic blood pressure falls below 100 mm Hg, no further drug is given; a total of three intravenous doses (15 mg) is administered.

4. If hemodynamic stability continues, 15 minutes after the last intravenous dose, the patient is begun on oral metoprolol, 50 mg every 6 hours for 2 days, then switched to 100 mg twice daily. An infusion of an extremely short-acting beta blocker, esmolol (50 to 250 mg/kg/min), may be useful in patients with relative contraindications to beta blockade in whom heart rate slowing is considered highly desirable.[188]

OXYGEN. Hypoxemia may occur in patients with AMI and is usually secondary to ventilation-perfusion abnormalities that are sequelae of left ventricular failure; pneumonia and intrinsic pulmonary disease are additional causes of hypoxemia. It is common practice to treat all patients hospitalized with AMI with oxygen for at least 24 to 48 hours, based on the empirical assumption of hypoxia and evidence that increased oxygen in the inspired air may protect ischemic myocardium.[189] However, this practice may not be cost-effective. Augmentation of the fraction of oxygen in the inspired air does not elevate oxygen delivery significantly in patients who are not hypoxemic. Furthermore, it may increase systemic vascular resistance and arterial pressure and thereby lower cardiac output slightly.

In view of these considerations, arterial oxygen saturation may be estimated by pulse oximetry (an increasingly available technology), and oxygen therapy may be omitted if it is normal. On the other hand, oxygen should be administered to patients with AMI when arterial hypoxemia is clinically evident or can be documented by measurement (e.g., SaO_2 < 90%).[52] In these patients, serial arterial blood gas measurements may be employed to follow the efficacy of oxygen therapy.

In general, the delivery of 2 to 4 liters/min of 100 percent oxygen by mask or nasal prongs for 6 to 12 hours is satisfactory for most patients with mild hypoxemia. If arterial oxygenation is still depressed on this regimen, the flow rate may have to be increased and other causes for hypoxemia should be sought. In patients with pulmonary edema, endotracheal intubation and positive-pressure controlled ventilation may be necessary.

Limitation of Infarct Size

Infarct size is an important determinant of prognosis in patients with AMI. Patients who succumb from cardiogenic shock generally exhibit either a single massive infarct or a small to moderate-sized infarct superimposed on multiple prior infarctions.[190] Survivors with large infarcts frequently exhibit late impairment of ventricular function, and the long-term mortality rate is higher than that for survivors with small infarcts, who tend not to develop cardiac decompensation.[78, 191]

In view of the prognostic importance of infarct size, the concept that modification of infarct size is possible has attracted a great deal of experimental and clinical attention[192] (see Fig. 35–17). Efforts to limit the size of the infarct have been divided among several different (sometimes overlapping) approaches: (1) early reperfusion,[193] (2) reduction of myocardial energy demands, (3) manipulation of sources of energy production in the myocardium, and (4) prevention of reperfusion injury. Although early reperfusion ("time-dependent effect of reperfusion") has been the major focus of modern management strategies for AMI, it is important to note that in addition to the limitation of infarct size, even late reperfusion of ischemic myocardium conveys several benefits that contribute to mortality reduction ("time-independent effect of reperfusion")[74] (see Fig. 35–17).

THE DYNAMIC NATURE OF INFARCTION. AMI is a dynamic process that does not occur instantaneously but evolves over hours (see Fig. 35–5). The fate of jeopardized, ischemic tissue may be affected favorably by interventions that restore myocardial perfusion, reduce microvascular damage in the infarct zone, reduce myocardial oxygen requirements, inhibit accumulation of or facilitate washout of noxius metabolites, augment the availability of substrate for anaerobic metabolism,[84, 194] or blunt the effects of mediators of injury (e.g., calcium overload or oxygen free radicals)[84, 194-197] that compromise the structure and function of intracellular organelles and constituents of cell membranes. Strong evidence in experimental animals and suggestive evidence in patients indicate that ischemic preconditioning, a form of endogenous protection against AMI, before sustained coronary occlusion decreases infarct size and is associated with a more favorable outcome and with decreased risk of extension of infarction and recurrent ischemic events.[198] Brief episodes of ischemia in one coronary vascular bed may precondition myocardium in a remote zone, attenuating the size of infarction in the latter when sustained coronary occlusion occurs.[199] Intriguing data have been reported that the expression of angiogenesis factors early after the onset of AMI may also contribute to the limitation of infarct size by promoting neovascularization in the infarct zone.[199a]

The perfusion of the myocardium in the infarct zone appears to be reduced maximally immediately after coronary occlusion. Up to one third of patients may develop spontaneous recanalization of an occluded infarct-related artery beginning at 12 to 24 hours. This delayed spontaneous reperfusion has been associated with improvement of left ventricular function because it improves healing of infarcted tissue, prevents ventricular remodeling, and reperfuses hibernating myocardium. However, in order to *maximize* the amount of myocardium salvaged by *accelerating* the process of reperfusion and also implementing it in those patients who would otherwise have an occluded infarct-related artery, the strategies of pharmacologically induced and catheter-based reperfusion of the infarct vessel have been developed (see page 1145).

Additional factors that may contribute to limitation of infarct size in association with reperfusion include relief of coronary spasm, prevention of damage to the microvasculature, improved systemic hemodynamics (augmentation of coronary perfusion pressure and reduced LV-EDP), and development of collateral circulation. The prompt implementation of measures designed to protect ischemic myocardium and support myocardial perfusion may provide sufficient time for the development of anatomical and physiological compensatory mechanisms that limit the ultimate extent of infarction (see Figs. 35-10 and 35-12). It is possible that interventions designed to protect ischemic myocardium during the initial event may also reduce the incidence of extension of infarction or early reinfarction.

ROUTINE MEASURES FOR INFARCT SIZE LIMITATION. Whereas reperfusion of ischemic myocardium is the most important technique for limiting infarct size, several routine measures to accomplish this goal are applicable to all patients with AMI, whether or not reperfusion therapy is prescribed. The treatment strategies discussed in this section may be initiated in the emergency department (see Fig. 35-17) and then continued in the CCU.

It is important to maintain an optimal balance between myocardial oxygen supply and demand so that as much as possible of the jeopardized zone of the myocardium surrounding the most profoundly ischemic zones of the infarct can be salvaged. During the period before irreversible injury has occurred, myocardial oxygen consumption should be minimized by maintaining the patient at rest, physically and emotionally, and by using mild sedation and a quiet atmosphere, which may lower heart rate, a major determinant of myocardial oxygen consumption. If the patient was receiving a beta-adrenoceptor blocking agent at the time the clinical manifestations of the infarction began, the drug should be continued unless a specific contraindication develops, such as left ventricular systolic failure or bradyarrhythmia. Marked sinus bradycardia (heart rate less than approximately 50 beats/min) and the frequently coexisting

hypotension should be treated with postural maneuvers (the Trendelenburg position) to increase central blood volume and atropine and electrical pacing, but not with isoproterenol. On the other hand, the routine administration of atropine, with the resultant increase in heart rate, to patients without serious bradycardia is contraindicated. All forms of tachyarrhythmias require prompt treatment because they increase myocardial oxygen needs.[52]

Congestive heart failure should be treated promptly. Given their multiple beneficial actions in AMI patients, ACE inhibitors are the first line of drugs indicated in the treatment of congestive heart failure associated with AMI unless the patient is hypotensive (see p. 1169).[199b] Drugs such as isoproterenol that increase myocardial oxygen consumption should be avoided.

As discussed earlier, arterial oxygenation should be restored to normal in patients with hypoxemia, such as occurs in patients with chronic pulmonary disease, pneumonia, or left ventricular failure. Oxygen-enriched air should be administered to patients with hypoxemia, and bronchodilators and expectorants should be used when indicated. Severe anemia, which can also extend the area of ischemic injury, should be corrected by the cautious administration of packed red cells, accompanied by a diuretic if there is any evidence of left ventricular failure. Associated conditions, particularly infections and the accompanying tachycardia, fever, and elevated myocardial oxygen needs, require immediate attention.

Systolic arterial pressure should not be allowed to deviate by more than approximately 25 to 30 mm Hg from the patient's usual level unless marked hypertension had been present before the AMI. It is likely that each patient has an optimal range of arterial pressure; as coronary perfusion pressure deviates from this level, the unfavorable balance between oxygen supply (which is related to coronary perfusion pressure) and myocardial oxygen demand (which is related to ventricular wall tension) that ensues increases the extent of ischemic injury.

REPERFUSION OF MYOCARDIAL INFARCTION

GENERAL CONCEPTS. Although reperfusion occurs spontaneously in some patients, persistent thrombotic occlusion is present in the majority of patients with STEMI while the myocardium is undergoing necrosis.[62] Timely reperfusion of jeopardized myocardium represents the most effective way of restoring the balance between myocardial oxygen supply and demand. The extent of protection appears to be related directly to the rapidity with which reperfusion is implemented after the onset of coronary occlusion[166, 193, 200] (see Fig. 35-7). Preliminary data exist suggesting that after thrombolytic therapy more rapid reperfusion (and smaller infarcts) occurs in patients with AMI preceded by unstable angina compared with those without preinfarction angina.[201]

In some patients, particularly those with cardiogenic shock, tissue damage occurs in a "stuttering" manner rather than abruptly, a condition that might more properly be termed subacute infarction. This concept of the nature of the infarction process, as well as the observation that the incidence of complications of AMI in both the early and late postinfarction periods is a function of infarct size, underscores the need for careful history-taking to ascertain whether the patient appears to have had repetitive cycles of spontaneous reperfusion and reocclusion. "Fixing" the time of onset of the infarction process in such patients can be difficult. In such patients with waxing and waning ischemic discomfort, a rigid time interval from the first episode of pain should not be used when determining whether a patient is "outside the window" for benefit from acute reperfusion therapy.

PATHOPHYSIOLOGY OF MYOCARDIAL REPERFUSION.
Prevention of cell death by the restoration of blood flow depends on the severity and duration of preexisting ischemia. Substantial experimental and clinical evidence exists indicating that recovery of left ventricular systolic function, improvement in diastolic function, and reduction in overall mortality are more favorably influenced the earlier that blood flow is restored[15, 193] (see Fig. 35–7). Collateral coronary vessels also appear to play a role in the successful left ventricular function after reperfusion.[67] They provide sufficient perfusion of myocardium to retard cell death and are probably of greater importance in patients having reperfusion later rather than 1 to 2 hours after coronary occlusion.

Even after successful reperfusion and despite the absence of irreversible myocardial damage, a period of postischemic contractile dysfunction can occur—a phenomenon referred to as *myocardial stunning*[202] (see Chap. 34). Animal data suggest that selective proteolysis of troponin I may contribute to myocardial stunning.[202a] Periods of myocardial stunning are well described in experimental animals but have also been confirmed in AMI patients by Gerber and coworkers using positron emission tomography after PTCA to measure myocardial blood flow and oxygen consumption.[203]

Reperfusion Injury

The process of reperfusion, although beneficial in terms of myocardial salvage, may come at a cost owing to a process known as *reperfusion injury*[204–204a] (see Fig. 35–9). Kloner and Przyklonk have summarized the data on the four types of reperfusion injury that have been observed in experimental animals.[205] These consist of (1) lethal reperfusion injury—a term referring to reperfusion-induced death of cells that were still viable at the time of restoration of coronary blood flow; (2) vascular reperfusion injury—progressive damage to the microvasculature such that there is an expanding area of no reflow and loss of coronary vasodilatory reserve[206, 207]; (3) stunned myocardium—salvaged myocytes display a prolonged period of contractile dysfunction after restoration of blood flow owing to abnormalities of intracellular biochemistry leading to reduced energy production[196] (see Chap. 34) (see Fig. 35–9); and (4) reperfusion arrhythmias—bursts of ventricular tachycardia and, on occasion, ventricular fibrillation that occur within seconds of reperfusion. The available evidence suggests that vascular reperfusion injury, stunning, and reperfusion arrhythmias can all occur in patients with AMI. The concept of lethal reperfusion injury of potentially salvageable myocardium remains controversial, both in experimental animals and in patients.[57, 205, 208]

Reperfusion increases the cell swelling that occurs with ischemia. Reperfusion of the myocardium in which the microvasculature is damaged leads to the creation of a hemorrhagic infarct (see Fig. 35–9). Thrombolytic therapy appears more likely to produce hemorrhagic infarction than reperfusion by mechanical means. Although concern has been raised that this hemorrhage may lead to extension of the infarct, this does not appear to be the case. Histological study of patients not surviving in spite of successful reperfusion has revealed hemorrhagic infarcts, but this hemorrhage usually does not extend beyond the area of necrosis.[57]

The loss of magnesium with ischemia, followed during reperfusion by the sudden exposure of severely ischemic cells to both calcium and oxygen on restoration of flow, has been observed to affect the severity of ischemic damage in several animal species.[195, 196, 209] Toxicity from oxygen-derived free radicals mediated at least in part by stimulated leukocytes has attracted considerable attention for its possible role in extending myocardial injury and contributing to calcium overload and inability to regulate cell volume. It has been proposed that necrotic myocytes expose cardiac antigens that lead to T-cell activation and generation of cytokines such as interferon gamma, interleukin-3, and granulocyte-monocyte colony stimulating factor.[210] These cytokines ultimately increase the expression of integrins such as Mac-1 on monocytes promoting adhesion to the endothelium in the ischemic territory and microvascular plugging (i.e., no-reflow phenomenon). Interest has therefore arisen in development of antibodies that interrupt leukocyte-leukocyte and leukocyte-endothelium interactions in patients with AMI.[210] Experimental models of AMI have revealed a consistent message: interventions that attenuate reperfusion injury exert their maximal beneficial effect if blood levels (and presumably myocardial tissue concentrations) are elevated at the time reperfusion occurs.[204a, 211] The effectiveness of agents such as superoxide dismutase and magnesium rapidly declines the later they are administered after reperfusion; eventually no beneficial effect is detectable in animal models after 45 to 60 minutes of reperfusion has elapsed.[208] Drugs such as beta-adrenoceptor blockers, which delay the death of ischemic cells, may, if administered prophylactically to patients at high risk of occlusion (or reocclusion) or in the earliest phases of the development of an AMI, enhance the quantity of myocardium salvaged by early reperfusion.[212, 213]

Ischemic Preconditioning

Brief periods of experimental coronary occlusion and reperfusion before a more sustained period of occlusion result in marked reduction in the amount of necrosis that develops has led to the concept of *ischemic preconditioning*[198, 214] (see Chap. 14). Data suggest that during the period of brief coronary occlusion adenosine receptors are activated that initiate a cascade of intracellular events culminating in phosphorylation of a membrane protein that is responsible for the protective effect. The leading candidate is the mitochondrial adenosine triphosphate (ATP)-dependent potassium channel that, when activated, causes a decrease in calcium influx, a reduction in contractile force generation, and thereby an energy-sparing effect.[215] The implications of ischemic preconditioning, including a possible modification of the severity of MI, are profound and have stimulated interest in ATP-dependent potassium channel openers such as nicorandil, bimakalim, and other "preconditioning mimetic" agents for potential use in patients with AMI.[198, 216] A second window of protection after preconditioning has been described.[198] It may be mediated by such processes as molecular adaptation leading to the production of heat shock protein or antioxidant enzymes, augmentation of inducible NO synthase, and opening of mitochondrial ATP-sensitive potassium channels.[215] Preconditioning appears to be associated with a more oxidized cellular redox state, which may contribute to protection against subsequent bouts of ischemia. In experimental animals the infarct size–limiting effect of ischemic preconditioning is blunted by hypercholesterolemia but is restored by treatment with pravastatin.[217]

Clinical observations consistent with the concept of ischemic preconditioning include the "warm-up phenomenon" reported by many angina patients (i.e., angina early in exercise necessitating a brief rest period followed by a resumption of exercise without angina) and a lower 30-day cardiac event rate (mortality, recurrent MI, congestive heart failure, or shock) in AMI patients who have a history of angina within the 48-hour period that precedes infarction.[218] A history of preinfarction angina in patients with a first Q-wave MI has been reported to be associated with lower peak CK activity, lower in-hospital incidence of sustained ventricular tachycardia (VT) and ventricular fibrillation, and a lower incidence of pump failure and cardiac mortality. Of interest, in patients with a first anterior MI, a history of preinfarction angina was associated with a greater degree of recovery of left ventricular function.[219] The greater protective effect of a longer time interval between angina pectoris and AMI suggests that the beneficial effect of prior angina is due to a delayed response to preconditioning.[219]

Reperfusion Arrhythmias

Transient sinus bradycardia occurs in many patients with inferior infarcts at the time of acute reperfusion; it is most often accompanied by some degree of hypotension. This combination of hypotension and bradycardia with a sudden increase in coronary flow has been ascribed to the activation of the Bezold-Jarisch reflex. Premature ventricular contractions, accelerated idioventricular rhythm, and nonsustained VT are also seen commonly after successful reperfusion. In experimental animals with AMI, ventricular fibrillation occurs shortly after reperfusion, but this arrhythmia is not as frequent in patients as in the experimental setting. Although some investigators have postulated that early afterdepolarizations participate in the genesis of reperfusion ventricular arrhythmias, Vera and colleagues have shown that early afterdepolarizations are present both during ischemia and during reperfusion and are therefore unlikely to be involved in the development of reperfusion VT or ventricular fibrillation.

When present, rhythm disturbances may actually be a marker of successful restoration of coronary flow. However, although reperfusion arrhythmias have a high sensitivity for detecting successful reperfusion, the high incidence of identical rhythm disturbances in patients without successful coronary artery reperfusion limits their specificity for detection of restoration of coronary blood flow. In general, clinical features are poor markers of reperfusion, with no single clinical finding or constellation of findings being reliably predictive of angiographically demonstrated coronary artery patency.[220]

Although reperfusion arrhythmias may show a temporal clustering at the time of restoration of coronary blood flow in patients with successful thrombolysis, the overall incidence of such arrhythmias appears to be similar in patients not receiving a thrombolytic agent who may develop these arrhythmias as a consequence of spontaneous coronary artery reperfusion or the evolution of the infarct process itself. These considerations, as well as the fact that the brief "electrical storm" occurring at the time of reperfusion is generally innocuous, indicate that no prophylactic antiarrhythmic therapy is necessary when thrombolytics are prescribed.[221]

Late Establishment of Patency of the Infarct Vessel

It has been suggested that improved survival and ventricular function after successful reperfusion are not due entirely to limitation of infarct size.[74, 222] Both experimental and clinical evidence indicates that the benefits of a patent artery include a favorable effect on ventricular remodeling (improved healing of infarcted tissue and prevention of infarct expansion),[72, 78, 191, 223] enhancement of collateral flow, improvement in diastolic and systolic function, increased electrical stability, and reduced long-term mortality.[224, 225] Late reperfusion of the artery perfusing an infarction provides a vascular scaffolding in the infarct zone and increases the influx of inflammatory cells that participate in the formation of a mature fibrous scar. The vascular scaffold and firmer myocardial scar prevent infarct segment lengthening and decrease the tendency toward infarct expansion and aneurysm formation.[222] Poorly contracting or noncontracting myocardium in a zone that is supplied by a stenosed infarct-related artery with slow antegrade perfusion may still contain viable myocytes. This situation is referred to as *hibernating* myocardium[204] (see Chap. 37), and its function can be improved by PTCA to augment flow

in the infarct-related artery.[226] Late reperfusion of the infarct-related artery by thrombolysis or late restoration of flow by PTCA enhances the electrical stability of the infarcted zone and is probably related to the reduced incidence of ventricular fibrillation and automatic firing of implantable cardioverter-defibrillator devices.[227, 228] The beneficial effect of late reperfusion of the infarct-related artery is independent of left ventricular function and other mortality-reducing therapies such as ACE inhibitors.[224] Several clinical trials are under way testing the benefits of late reperfusion of an occluded infarct artery in asymptomatic patients (OAT, ACTOR).

Summary of Effects of Myocardial Reperfusion

As illustrated in Figure 35–13, rupture of an unstable plaque in the culprit vessel produces complete occlusion of the infarct-related coronary artery. AMI occurs with the ensuing development of left ventricular dilatation and ultimate death through a combination of pump failure and electrical instability. Early reperfusion (i.e., thrombolysis, primary PTCA) shortens the duration of coronary occlusion, minimizes the degree of ultimate LV dysfunction and dilatation, and reduces the probability that the AMI patient will develop pump failure or malignant ventricular tachyarrhythmias. Late reperfusion may favorably affect the process of infarct healing and minimize LV remodeling and the ultimate development of pump dysfunction and electrical instability.

CORONARY THROMBOLYSIS

Many years elapsed between the first report of intracoronary clot lysis in an experimental animal and the widespread use of thrombolytic agents in AMI. With publication of the first Gruppo Italiano per lo Studio della Streptochinasi nell'Infarto Miocardico (GISSI) trial of over 11,000 patients in 1986,[229] in which intravenous streptokinase was shown to result in a significant reduction in mortality in patients treated within 6 hours of the onset of symptoms, the routine use of thrombolytic therapy in AMI was established. It is now clear that thrombolysis recanalizes thrombotic occlusion associated with AMI (see Fig. 35–10) and that restoration of coronary flow reduces infarct size and improves myocardial function and survival over both the short and the long term.[230, 231] The majority of the mortality benefit seen at 10-year follow-up in the GISSI trial was obtained before hospital discharge because no survival difference was seen in thrombolysed and control patients discharged alive except for those treated within the first hour after symptoms.[230]

INTRACORONARY THROMBOLYSIS. Clinical investigation of pharmacological reperfusion of ischemic myocardium initially focused on intracoronary thrombolysis in the early hours of AMI.[193, 232, 233] The fact that viability could be maintained in a portion of the successfully reperfused myocardium was reflected in studies showing the restoration of contractile activity.[234] Most reported experience with intracoronary thrombolysis has not been in randomized controlled trials, largely because it has been thought difficult to withhold thrombolytic therapy once a thrombotic coronary artery occlusion has been visualized angiographically and because it has not been considered ethical to catheterize patients if randomization to no thrombolytic therapy were possible for a portion of the patients. Because of the delay involved in catheterizing patients with AMI, current consensus is that intracoronary administration of thrombolytic therapy should be reserved for patients who develop coronary thrombosis during the course of an angiographic procedure and in whom either a coronary catheter is already in place or such placement is easily and rapidly achieved.

INTRAVENOUS THROMBOLYSIS. This form of thrombolytic therapy has several important advantages over intracoronary use. Because only the placement of a peripheral intravenous line is required, therapy may be initiated early, in a variety of locations (home, ambulance, helicopter,

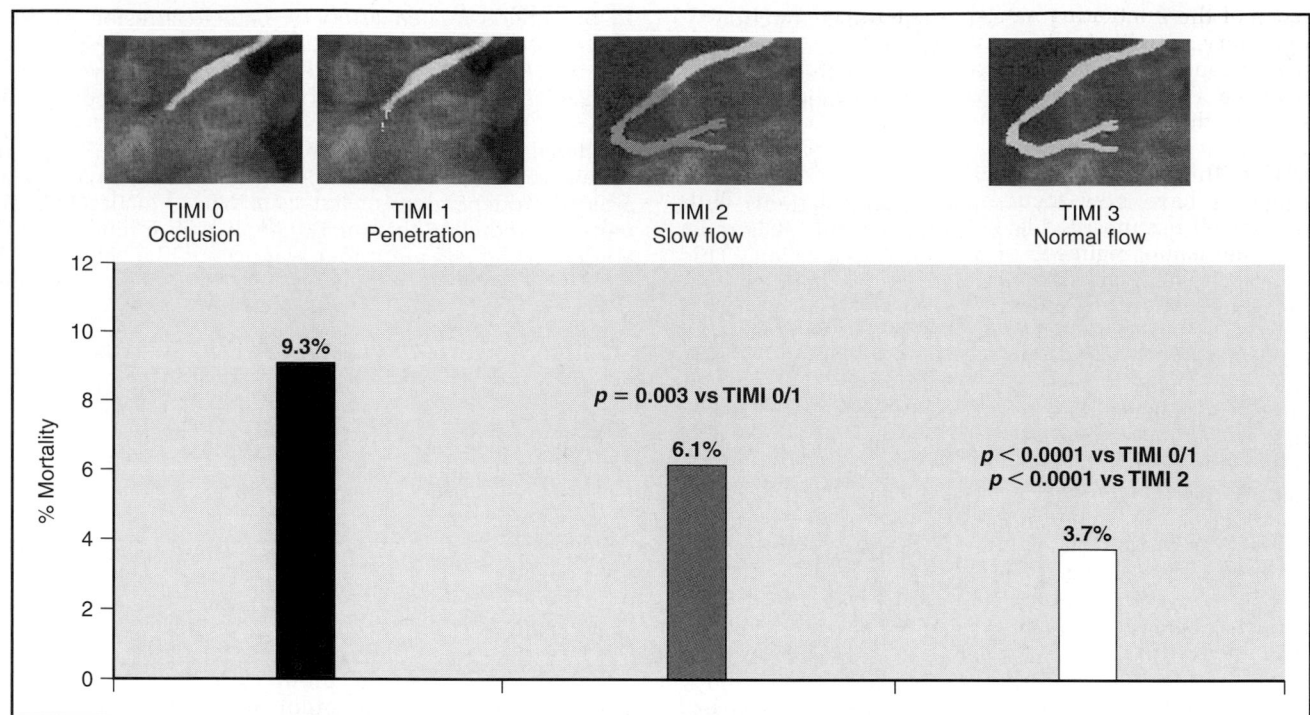

FIGURE 35–19. Correlation of Thrombolysis in Myocardial Infarction (TIMI) flow grade and mortality. A pooled analysis of data from 5498 patients in several angiographic trials of reperfusion for ST segment elevation MI showed a gradient of mortality when the angiographic findings were stratified by TIMI flow grade. Patients with TIMI 0 or TIMI 1 flow had the highest mortality; TIMI 2 flow was associated with an intermediate mortality; lowest mortality was observed in patients with TIMI 3 flow. (Personal communication, Dr. Michael Gibson, 2000.)

emergency department) and at relatively low cost. The subject of intravenous thrombolysis has perhaps been one of the most rapidly evolving areas in the management of patients with AMI, especially over the past decade.

To provide a level of standardization for comparison of the various regimens, most investigators describe the flow in the infarct vessel according to the TIMI grading system:

Grade 0 = complete occlusion of the infarct-related artery.

Grade 1 = some penetration of the contrast material beyond the point of obstruction but without perfusion of the distal coronary bed.

Grade 2 = perfusion of the entire infarct vessel into the distal bed but with delayed flow compared with a normal artery.

Grade 3 = full perfusion of the infarct vessel with normal flow.[235, 236]

When evaluating reports of angiographic studies of thrombolytic agents, it must be kept in mind that only in studies in which a pretreatment coronary arteriogram documents occlusion of the culprit vessel can the term *recanalization* be applied if flow is restored. If the status of the culprit vessel is not known before treatment, the only fact that can be stated with certainty is the *patency rate* of the vessel at the moment contrast medium is injected. This snapshot in time does not reflect the fluctuating status of flow in the infarct vessel that characteristically undergoes repeated cycles of patency and reocclusion, as has been documented angiographically and by continuous ST segment monitoring.

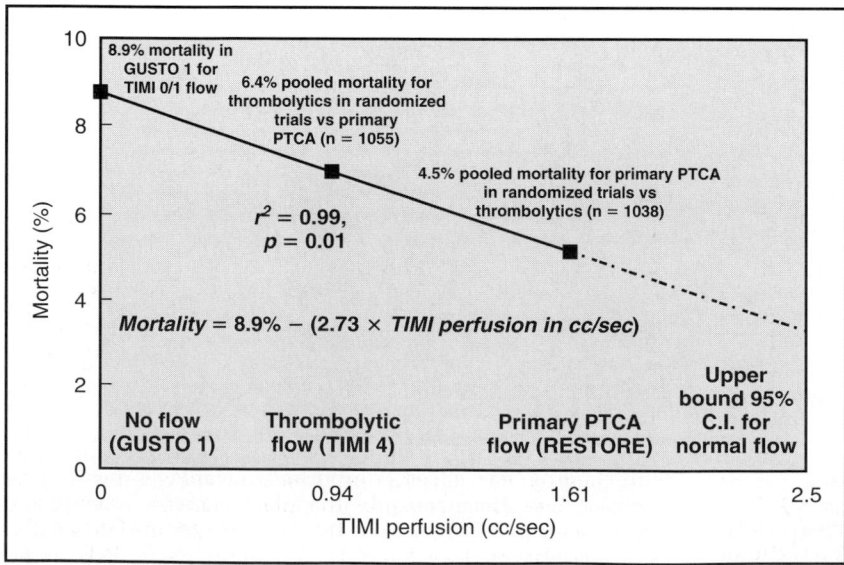

FIGURE 35–20. Relationship between coronary blood flow and mortality in AMI. (From Gibson CM: Primary angioplasty, rescue angioplasty, and new devices. *In* Hennekens CH (ed): Clinical Trials in Cardiovascular Disease: A Companion to Braunwald's Heart Disease. Philadelphia, WB Saunders, 1999, p 194.)

Issues of the fluctuating nature of patency of the infarct-related artery notwithstanding, the majority of angiographic studies of reperfusion regimens for STEMI used an assessment of the TIMI flow grade at 90 minutes as the primary endpoint of the trial. With an increasing number of angiographers being able to perform diagnostic catheterizations in patients with AMI more expeditiously than in the past, investigators have now focused on the TIMI grade flow assessed at 60 minutes. Evidence exists that differences between reperfusion regimens with respect to the rate and extent of thrombolysis can be discriminated better at 60 rather than 90 minutes after initiation of therapy: earlier opening of infarct-related arteries is expected to reduce infarct size further and translate into a reduction in mortality.[237]

Initially, combined TIMI grade 2 and grade 3 flow was lumped into the favorable category of coronary patency that was compared with a combined TIMI grade 0 and grade 1 flow into an unfavorable category of persistent occlusion. However, TIMI grade 2 flow should not be lumped with grade 3 flow because it has been recognized that TIMI grade 3 flow is far superior to grade 2 flow in terms of infarct size reduction and both short-term[238] and long-term[239] mortality benefit. Therefore, TIMI grade 3 flow should be considered to be the goal of reperfusion therapy[240, 241] (Fig. 35–19). In an effort to provide a more quantitative statement of the briskness of coronary blood flow in the infarct artery and also to account for differences in the size and length of vessels (e.g., left anterior descending artery vs. right coronary artery) and interobserver variability, Gibson and co-workers have developed the *TIMI frame count*—a simple count of the number of angiographic frames elapsed until the contrast medium arrives in the distal bed of the vessel of interest. The TIMI frame count, an objective and quantitative index of coronary blood flow, is an independent predictor of in-hospital mortality from AMI and also discriminates patients with TIMI grade 3 flow into low- and high-risk groups.[242, 243] The TIMI frame count can also be used to quantitate coronary blood flow (milliliters per second) calculated at 21/(observed TIMI frame count) $\times$ 1.7 (based on Doppler velocity wire data showing normal flow equals 1.7 cm^3/sec, which is proportional to 21 frames). The relationship between calculated coronary perfusion and mortality for patients treated with thrombolytics and primary PTCA is illustrated in Figure 35–20.

MYOCARDIAL PERFUSION. Despite the intense interest in development of reperfusion regimens that normalize flow in the epicardial infarct-related artery, the real goal of reperfusion in STEMI is to improve myocardial perfusion in the infarct zone. Of course, myocardial perfusion cannot be improved adequately without restoration of flow in the occluded infarct-related artery (Fig. 35–21). However, even patients with TIMI grade 3 flow may not achieve adequate myocardial perfusion.[207, 244] The two major impediments to normalization of myocardial perfusion are microvascular damage[245] (see Fig. 35–21) and reperfusion injury. Obstruction of the distal microvasculature in the downstream bed of the infarct-related artery is caused by platelet microemboli and thrombi. Microembolization of platelet aggregates may actually be exacerbated by thrombolysis by means of the exposure of clot-bound thrombin, an extremely potent platelet agonist. Spasm may also occur in the microvasculature owing to the release of substances from activated platelets such as serotonin and thromboxane A$_2$ (see Fig. 35–3). Reperfusion injury, discussed earlier (see p. 1144), results in cellular edema, free radical formation, and calcium overload. In addition, cytokine activation leads to neutrophil accumulation and inflammatory mediators that contribute to tissue injury.

Several techniques have been used to evaluate the adequacy of myocardial perfusion. ST segment resolution on the ECG is a strong predictor of outcome in AMI patients (Fig. 35–22); its absence is a better predictor of an occluded rather than patent infarct-related artery.[207, 246–250] Absence of early ST segment resolution after angiographically successful primary PTCA identifies patients with a higher risk of left ventricular dysfunction and mortality, presumably because of microvascular damage in the infarct zone.[251, 252] Thus, the 12-lead ECG can serve as a clinically useful marker of the biological integrity of myocytes in the infarct zone and can reflect inadequate myocardial perfusion even in the presence of TIMI 3 flow.[207] Given the dynamic nature of coronary occlusion, it has been proposed that continuous ST segment monitoring is more informative than static 12-lead ECG recordings, but practical limitations have prevented continuous ST segment monitoring from

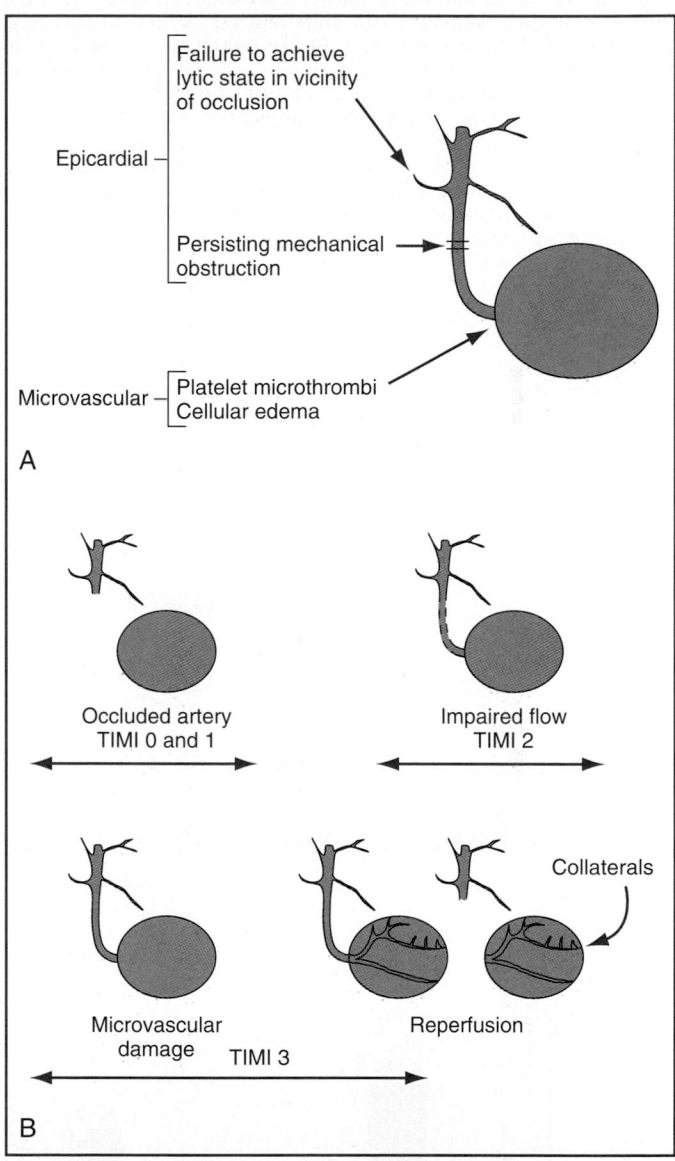

FIGURE 35–21. Patterns of response to thrombolysis. *A,* Failure of epicardial reperfusion can occur owing to failure to induce a lytic state or to mechanical factors at the site of occlusion. Failure of microvascular reperfusion is due to a combination of platelet microthrombi followed by endothelial swelling and myocardial edema ("no reflow"). *B,* Thrombolysis may fail owing to persistent occlusion of the epicardial infarct-related artery (TIMI 0 and 1), patency of an epicardial artery in the presence of impaired (TIMI 2) flow, or microvascular occlusion in the presence of angiographically normal flow (TIMI 3). Successful reperfusion requires a patent artery with an intact microvascular network. Conversely, reperfusion may occur despite an occluded epicardial artery due to the presence of collateral vessels. (From Davies CH, Ormerod OJ: Failed coronary thrombolysis. Lancet 351:1191–1196, 1998.)

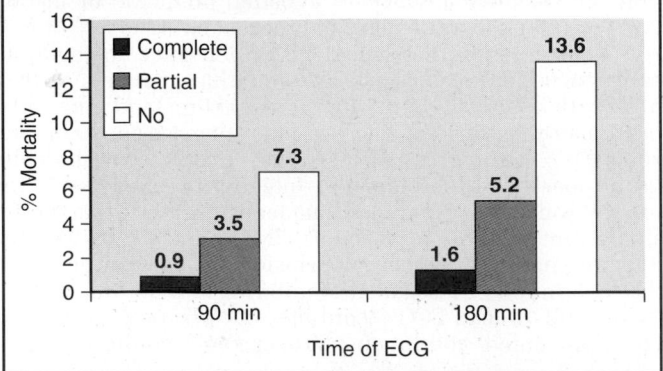

FIGURE 35–22. Relationship between ST segment resolution and 30-day mortality. Patients with complete (> 70 percent) ST segment resolution have the lowest 30-day mortality followed by patients with partial (30–70 percent) and no (< 30 percent) ST segment resolution. The gradient of mortality stratified by ST segment resolution is evident at both 90 minutes and 180 minutes after initiation of thrombolytic therapy. (Adapted from data in Schroder R, et al: Comparison of the predictive value of ST segment elevation resolution at 90 and 180 min after start of streptokinase in acute myocardial infarction: A substudy of the Hirudin for Improvement of Thrombolysis [HIT]-4 study. Eur Heart J 20:1563–1571, 1999.

FIGURE 35–23. See color plate 22.

by the availability of new echo contrast agents that may be injected intravenously.[257, 257a] Doppler flow wire studies, MRI, and nuclear imaging with positron emission tomography (Fig. 35–23) have also been used to define abnormalities of myocardial perfusion.[245, 258–260]

A new angiographic method for assessing myocardial perfusion has also been introduced by Gibson and colleagues—the TIMI myocardial perfusion grade (Fig. 35–24). Abnormalities of increasing myocardial perfusion as assessed by the TIMI myocardial perfusion grade correlate with mortality risk even after adjusting for the presence of TIMI grade 3 flow or a normal TIMI frame count.[261]

A variety of treatments have been tested for increasing myocardial perfusion. A generally consistent theme is that myocardial protective agents should be administered either before or concurrent with efforts at restoration of flow in the epicardial infarct–related artery to minimize damage that may occur as a consequence of reperfusion strategies. Administration of adenosine in the Acute Myocardial Infarction Study of Adenosine (AMISTAD) trial was associated with a reduction in infarct size in patients with an anterior wall MI.[262] Efforts to treat vasospasm with vasodilators such as nicorandil, papavarine, verapamil, and trimetazidine have been associated with improvement in myocardial perfusion in several small series.[216] The most promising intervention to date for treating obstruction of the microvasculature is the administration of an intravenous GPIIb/IIIa inhibitor either in conjunction with a reduced dose of thrombolytic or in association with a catheter-based reperfusion strategy.

widespread clinical application.[253, 254] Defects in perfusion patterns seen with myocardial contrast echocardiography correlate with regional wall motion abnormalities[255] and lack of myocardial viability on dobutamine stress echocardiography.[256] A practical limitation to myocardial contrast echocardiography is the need for intracoronary injection of echo contrast medium, although this may be circumvented

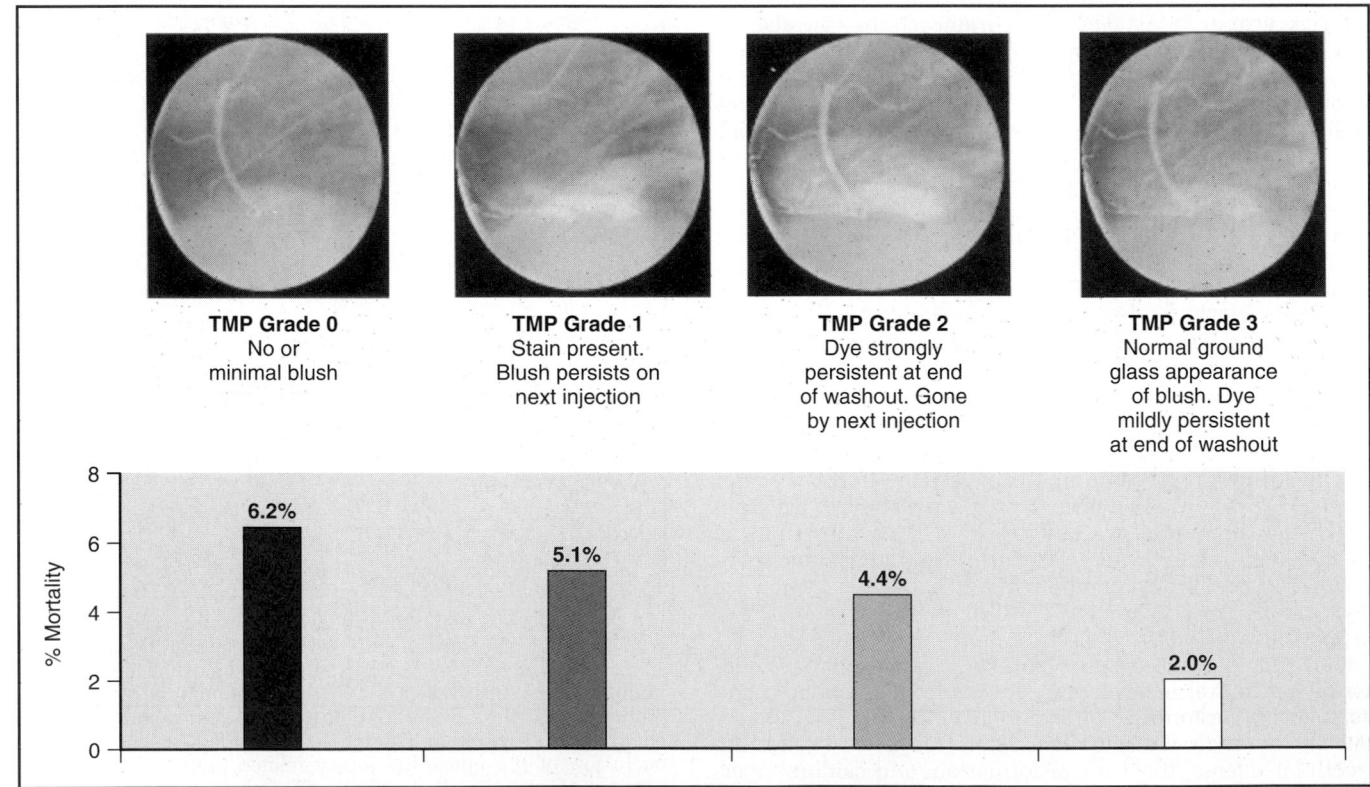

FIGURE 35–24. Relationship between TIMI myocardial perfusion grade and mortality. TIMI myocardial perfusion (TMP) grade 0 or no perfusion of the myocardium is associated with the highest mortality. If the stain of the myocardium is present (grade 1), mortality is also high. A reduction in mortality is seen if the dye enters the microvasculature but is still persistent at the end of the washout phase (grade 2). The lowest mortality is observed in those patients with normal perfusion (grade 3) in whom the dye is minimally persistent at the end of the washout phase. (From Gibson CM, et al: Circulation 101:125–130, 2000. Copyright 2000, American Heart Association.)

With the exception of intravenous GPIIb/IIIa inhibitors, no intervention can be recommended definitively for the specific purposes of improving myocardial perfusion, although this situation may change as more data become available.

Effect on Mortality

There is no doubt that early intravenous therapy and thrombolytic drugs improve survival in patients with AMI[15, 52] (Fig. 35–25). Mortality varies considerably depending on patients included for study and adjunctive therapies employed. The benefit of thrombolytic therapy appears to be greatest when agents are administered as early as possible, with the most dramatic results when the drug is given less than 1 to 2 hours after symptoms begin.[166, 263, 264] The Fibrinolytic Therapy Trialists' (FTT) collaborative group has performed a comprehensive overview of nine trials of thrombolytic therapy, each of which enrolled more than 1000 patients[15] (Fig. 35–26). The data base for the FTT overview consisted of a total of 58,600 patients, including 6,177 (10.5 percent) who died, 564 (1.0 percent) who sustained a stroke, and 436 (0.7 percent) who sustained major noncerebral hemorrhages. The absolute mortality rates for the control and fibrinolytic groups stratified by presenting features are shown in Figure 35–26. The overall results indicated an 18 percent reduction in short-term mortality, but as much as a 25 percent reduction in mortality for the subset of 45,000 patients with ST segment elevation or bundle branch block. Two trials, Late Assessment of Thrombolytic Efficacy (LATE) and Estudio Multi-centrico Estreptquinasa Republicas de America del Sur (EMERAS), viewed together provide evidence that a mortality reduction may still be observed in patients treated with thrombolytics between 6 and 12 hours from the onset of ischemic symptoms.[265, 266] The data from LATE and EMERAS and the FTT overview form the basis for extending the "window" of treatment with thrombolytics up to 12 hours from the onset of symptoms. Boersma and colleagues pooled the trials in the FTT overview, 2 smaller studies with data on time to randomization, and 11 additional trials of more than 100 patients. Patients were divided into six time categories from symptom onset to randomization. A regression analysis revealed there was a nonlinear relationship of treatment benefit to time.

MORTALITY REDUCTIONS IN SUBGROUPS. The mortality effect of thrombolytic therapy in elderly patients is of considerable interest and controversy.[23a, 23b] Whereas patients older than the age of 75 were initially excluded from randomized trials of thrombolytic therapy, they now constitute about 15 percent of the patients studied in recent megatrials of thrombolysis and are being analyzed in registries of AMI patients.[19, 267, 268] Barriers to initiation of therapy in older patients with AMI include a protracted period of delay in seeking medical care, a lower incidence of ischemic discomfort and greater incidence of atypical symptoms and concomitant illnesses, and an increased incidence of nondiagnostic ECGs.[158] Younger patients with AMI achieve a slightly greater relative reduction in mortality compared with elderly patients, but the higher absolute mortality in the elderly results in similar absolute mortality reductions. Thus, as seen in Figure 35–26, there was a 26 percent decrease in mortality in patients who were younger than 55 years of age (11 lives saved per 1000 with thrombolytic therapy) and a 4 percent reduction in mortality in patients older than age 75 (10 lives saved per 1000 treated). Observational data from the Cooperative Cardiovascular Project (CCP) have raised concern about increased mortality in patients over age 75 years.[23a] However, such observations should not be considered definitive given the nonrandomized nature of the dataset.[23b] Nevertheless clinicians should consider the risks of thrombolysis, especially intracranial hemorrhage, when selecting a reperfusion strategy for elderly patients.[23b]

Other important baseline characteristics that have an impact on the mortality effect of thrombolytic therapy include the vital signs at presentation and the presence of diabetes mellitus (see Fig. 35–26). For example, there was an 18 percent decrease in mortality for patients presenting with a systolic pressure less than 100 mm Hg (62 lives saved per 1000 treated), compared with a 12 percent reduction in mortality for patients with a systolic pressure of 175 mm Hg or more (10 lives saved per 1000 treated). Patients with a history of diabetes mellitus experienced a mortality reduction of 21 percent (37 lives saved per 1000 treated), compared with a mortality reduction of 15 percent (15 lives saved per 1000 treated) in patients without a history of diabetes.

A number of models have been developed to integrate the many clinical variables that affect a patient's mortality risk before administration of thrombolytic therapy. In the TIMI II trial, patients were classified as low risk if they *lacked* any of the following: age of 70 years or older, previous infarction, atrial fibrillation, anterior infarction, rales in more than one third of the lung fields, hypotension and sinus tachycardia, female gender, and diabetes mellitus (see Table 35–4). A more comprehensive, convenient, bedside, simple risk-scoring system for predicting 30-day mortality at presentation for fibrinolytic-eligible patients with ST-elevation MI was developed by Morrow et al using the InTIME-2 trial database[268a] (Fig. 35–27). However, modeling of mortality risk cannot cover all clinical scenarios and should not substitute for clinical judgment in individual cases. For

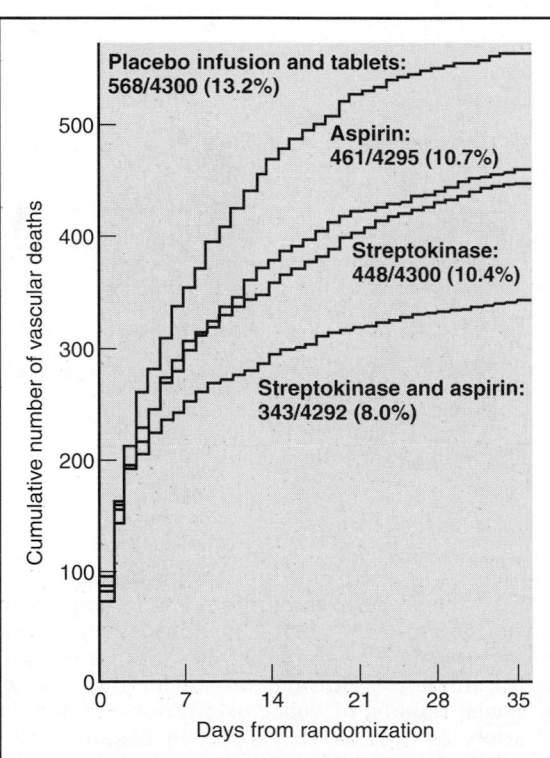

FIGURE 35–25. Cumulative vascular mortality (deaths from cardiac, cerebral, hemorrhagic, or other known vascular disease, or unknown causes) in days 0 to 35 of the Second International Study of Infarct Survival (ISIS-2). The four curves describe mortality for patients allocated (i) active streptokinase only, (ii) active aspirin only, (iii) both active treatments, and (iv) neither. Note that individually aspirin and streptokinase have a favorable effect of similar magnitudes and together the benefits appear additive. (From ISIS-2 [Second International Study of Infarct Survival] Collaborative Group: Randomized trial of intravenous streptokinase, oral aspirin, both, or neither among 17,187 cases of suspected acute myocardial infarction: ISIS-2. Lancet 2:349, 1988.)

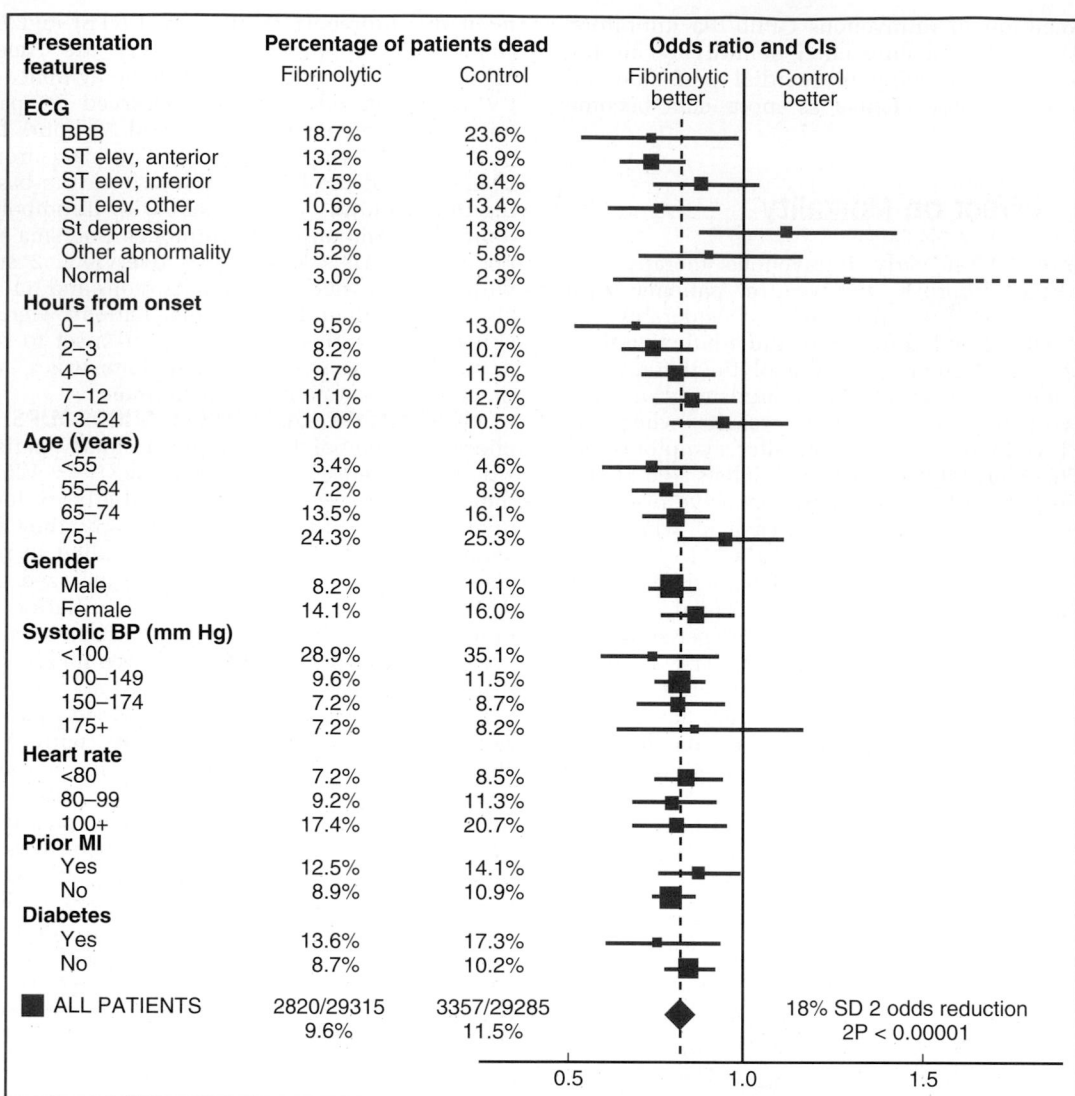

Presentation features	Percentage of patients dead		Odds ratio and CIs	
	Fibrinolytic	Control	Fibrinolytic better	Control better
ECG				
BBB	18.7%	23.6%		
ST elev, anterior	13.2%	16.9%		
ST elev, inferior	7.5%	8.4%		
ST elev, other	10.6%	13.4%		
St depression	15.2%	13.8%		
Other abnormality	5.2%	5.8%		
Normal	3.0%	2.3%		
Hours from onset				
0–1	9.5%	13.0%		
2–3	8.2%	10.7%		
4–6	9.7%	11.5%		
7–12	11.1%	12.7%		
13–24	10.0%	10.5%		
Age (years)				
<55	3.4%	4.6%		
55–64	7.2%	8.9%		
65–74	13.5%	16.1%		
75+	24.3%	25.3%		
Gender				
Male	8.2%	10.1%		
Female	14.1%	16.0%		
Systolic BP (mm Hg)				
<100	28.9%	35.1%		
100–149	9.6%	11.5%		
150–174	7.2%	8.7%		
175+	7.2%	8.2%		
Heart rate				
<80	7.2%	8.5%		
80–99	9.2%	11.3%		
100+	17.4%	20.7%		
Prior MI				
Yes	12.5%	14.1%		
No	8.9%	10.9%		
Diabetes				
Yes	13.6%	17.3%		
No	8.7%	10.2%		
ALL PATIENTS	2820/29315 9.6%	3357/29285 11.5%		18% SD 2 odds reduction 2P < 0.00001

0.5   1.0   1.5

FIGURE 35–26. Mortality differences during days 0 to 35 subdivided by presentation features in a collaborative overview of results from nine trials of thrombolytic therapy. The absolute mortality rates are shown for fibrinolytic and control groups in the center portion of the figure for each of the clinical features at presentation listed on the left side of the figure. The odds ratio for death in the fibrinolytic group to that in the control group is shown for each subdivision (colored square), along with its 99 percent confidence interval (horizontal line). The summary odds ratio at the bottom of the figure corresponds to an 18 percent proportional reduction in 35-day mortality and is highly statistically significant. This translates to a reduction of 18 deaths per 1000 patients treated with thrombolytic agents. (From Fibrinolytic Therapy Trialists' [FTT] Collaborative Group: Indications for fibrinolytic therapy in suspected acute myocardial infarction: Collaborative overview of mortality and major morbidity results from all randomized trials of more than 1000 patients. Lancet 343:311, 1994.)

example, patients with inferior MI who might otherwise be considered to have a low risk of mortality and for whom many physicians have questioned the benefits of thrombolytic therapy might be in a much higher mortality risk subgroup if their inferior infarction is associated with right ventricular infarction, precordial ST segment depression, or ST segment elevation in the lateral precordial leads. The Global Use of Strategies to Open Occluded Coronary Arteries (GUSTO) I investigators developed a regression model to illustrate the relative importance of clinical characteristics on 30-day mortality in contemporary thrombolytic-treated patients.[269] Much greater proportions of the risk of mortality are contributed by the systolic blood pressure and heart rate at presentation than precisely which thrombolytic agent is selected.

CLINICAL BENEFIT. As a result of greater patency of the infarct vessel in patients treated with thrombolytic agents, the clinical benefits that appear to accrue and contribute to the reduction in mortality include reductions in left ven-

tricular failure, malignant arrhythmias,[270] and serious complications of AMI such as septal rupture and cardiogenic shock.[270–272] The short-term survival benefit enjoyed by patients who receive thrombolytic therapy is maintained over the 1- to 10-year follow-up that has been reported in a number of studies.[230] However, room for improvement remains, given reports of reocclusion rates of the infarct-related artery as high as 10 percent in hospital and up to 30 percent by 3 months[273] and reinfarction rates as high as 5 percent in hospital and 7 percent within the first year in thrombolytic-treated patients.

Comparison of Thrombolytic Agents

(See also Chap. 62)

There has been considerable controversy regarding the efficacy of various thrombolytic agents[274] (Table 35–6). In the GUSTO I trial, 41,021 patients were randomized into one of four treatment arms: strepto-

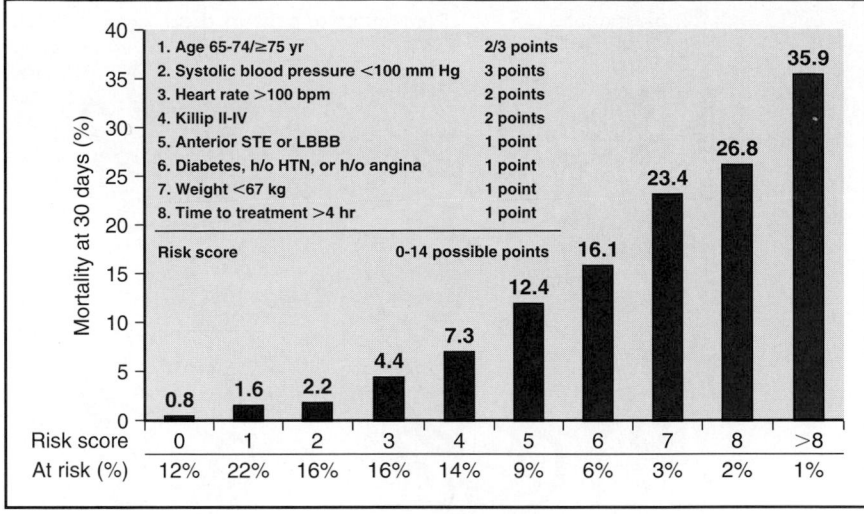

FIGURE 35-27. TIMI Risk Score for STEMI for predicting 30-day mortality. STE = ST elevation; LBBB = left bundle branch block; h/o = history of; HTN = hypertension. (From Morrow DA, Antman EM, Charlesworth A, et al: The TIMI risk score for ST elevation myocardial infarction: A convenient, bedside, clinical score for risk assessment at presentation: An InTIME II substudy. Circulation, in press.)

kinase, 1.5 MU over 60 minutes with immediate intravenous heparin to a target activated partial thromboplastin time of 60 to 85 seconds; accelerated t-PA with immediate intravenous heparin; a combination arm of intravenous t-PA (1 mg/kg over 60 minutes) and streptokinase (1.0 MU over 60 minutes); and streptokinase, 1.5 MU over 60 minutes with subcutaneous heparin. The 30-day mortality for the accelerated t-PA group was 6.3 percent; streptokinase plus subcutaneous heparin, 7.2 percent; streptokinase plus intravenous heparin, 7.4 percent; and streptokinase plus t-PA combination plus intravenous heparin, 7.0 percent.

In the GUSTO angiographic substudy involving 2431 patients, those with TIMI grade 0 or 1 flow had a 30-day mortality of 9.8 percent that was reduced to 7.9 percent in patients with TIMI grade 2 flow and to 4.3 percent in those with TIMI grade 3 flow.[238] The 90-minute patency rates for the infarct-related artery in the four treatment arms were as follows: accelerated t-PA, 81 percent (54 percent grade 3 flow); combination t-PA plus streptokinase, 73 percent (38 percent grade 3 flow); streptokinase plus intravenous heparin, 60 percent (32 percent grade 3 flow); and streptokinase plus subcutaneous heparin, 54 percent (29 percent grade 3 flow). This early gradient in patency rates favoring t-PA was no longer apparent beyond 180 minutes, presumably because of a "catch-up" phenomenon whereby late patency rates with streptokinase approach those of front-loaded t-PA, albeit beyond a time when as much myocardial salvage is possible as with t-PA. A related observation on early arterial patency was made in the TIMI 4 trial that randomized patients with AMI presenting within 6 hours to receive front-loaded t-PA, anistreplase (APSAC, anisoylated plasminogen streptokinase activator complex), or a combination of a reduced dose of both t-PA and anistreplase.[275] The 90-minute patency rate for front-loaded t-PA was 84 percent (60 percent grade 3); anistreplase, 73 percent (43 percent grade 3); and the combination, 68 percent (45 percent grade 3). A mortality trend favoring t-PA com-pared with both of the other treatment regimens was seen at 1 year.[275]

TISSUE PLASMINOGEN ACTIVATOR. The t-PA molecule contains the following five domains: finger, epidermal growth factor, kringle 1 and kringle 2, and serum protease[276] (Fig. 35-28). In the absence of fibrin, t-PA is a weak plasminogen activator; fibrin provides a scaffold on which t-PA and plasminogen are held in such a way that the catalytic efficiency for plasminogen activation of t-PA is increased manyfold. Plasma clearance of t-PA is mediated to a varying degree by residues in each of the domains except the serine protease domain, which is responsible for the enzymatic activity of t-PA. The accelerated dose regimen of t-PA over 90 minutes produces more rapid thrombolysis than the standard 3-hour infusion of t-PA. A double-bolus regimen of t-PA was not shown to be equivalent to the accelerated dose regimen[277-279] and was associated with a slightly higher rate of intracranial hemorrhage; the double-bolus regimen has not been recommended for clinical use.

Modifications of the basic t-PA structure have been made to yield a group of third-generation fibrinolytics (see Fig. 35-28 and Table 35-6). A common feature among the third-generation fibrinolytics is prolonged plasma clearance, allowing them to be administered as a bolus rather than the

▼ TABLE 35-6. KEY PROPERTIES OF NEW FIBRINOLYTIC AGENTS AS COMPARED WITH t-PA AND STREPTOKINASE

PROPERTY	SK	t-PA	r-PA	TNK-tPA	SAK
Molecular weight (daltons)	47,000	70,000	39,000	70,000	16,500
Plasma half-life (min)	23-29	4-8	15	±20	6
Fibrin specificity	—	++	+	+++	++++
Plasminogen activation	Indirect	Direct	Direct	Direct	Indirect
Dose*	1.5 MU/60 min	100 mg/90 min	2 × 10 MU bolus 30 min apart	0.5 mg/kg bolus	20-30 mg/30 min
Antigenic	+	–	–	–	+
Hypotension	+	–	–	–	–
Patency at 90 min	+	+++	++++	+++	+++(+?)
Hemorrhagic stroke	+	++	++	++	?
Mortality reduction	+	++	++	++	?
Cost	+	+++	+++	+++(?)	++(?)
Concomitant heparin†	?	+	+	+	+
Bleeding (noncerebral)	+++	++	++	+	?

*Most frequently used/tested.

†With the exception of SK and t-PA, the need for concomitant heparin has not been formally tested.

Modified from White HD, van de Werf F: Thrombolysis for acute myocardial infarction. Circulation 97:1632-1646, 1998. Copyright 1998, American Heart Association.

SK = streptokinase; t-PA = recombinant tissue-type plasminogen activator (alteplase); SAK = recombinant staphylokinase; TNK-tPA = TNK variant of tissue-type plasminogen activator; r-PA = reteplase.

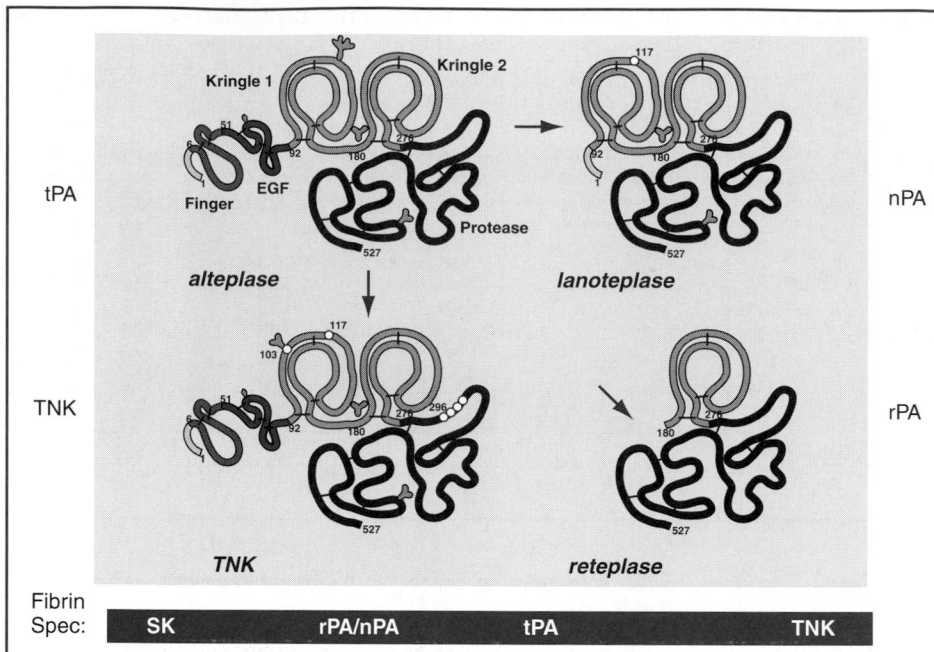

FIGURE 35–28. Molecular structure of alteplase (t-PA), lanoteplase (n-PA), reteplase (r-PA), and tenecteplase. Streptokinase is the least fibrin-specific thrombolytic agent in clinical use; the progressive increase in relative fibrin specificity for the various thrombolytics is shown at the bottom. (Modified from Brener SJ, Topol EJ: Third-generation thrombolytic agents for acute myocardial infarction. *In* Topol EJ [ed]: Acute Coronary Syndromes. New &York, Marcel Dekker, Inc., 1998, p. 169.)

bolus and double infusion technique by which accelerated dose t-PA is administered.[276]

RETEPLASE (rPA). This is a recombinant deletion mutant form of t-PA lacking the finger, epidermal growth factor, and kringle 1 domains as well as the carbohydrate side chains (see Fig. 35–28 and Table 35–6). After a series of four phase II angiographic trials were performed (GRECO,[280] GRECO-DB,[281] Recombinant Plasminogen Activator Angiographic Phase II International Dose Finding Study [RAPID]-1,[282] RAPID-2[283]), it was determined that the optimum dose and administration schedule for reteplase was 10 + 10 units delivered as two separate intravenous boluses separated by 30 minutes. The TIMI 3 flow rate with a 10 + 10-unit regimen of reteplase was 51.2 percent at 60 minutes and 59.5 percent at 90 minutes compared with 37.4 percent and 45.2 percent at 60 and 90 minutes, respectively, for 100 mg of accelerated dose t-PA.[283]

The International Joint Efficacy Comparison of Thrombolytics (INJECT) trial was the first equivalence trial in the field of thrombolytic therapy for STEMI.[284] A total of 6010 patients were randomized to a double bolus 10 + 10-unit reteplase regimen given 30 minutes apart or 1.5 million units of streptokinase over 60 minutes. Mortality at 35 days was 9.02 percent in the reteplase group and 9.53 percent in the streptokinase group. The 95 percent confidence intervals of the differences in mortality range from −1.98 percent to 0.96 percent, satisfying the prespecified definition for equivalence between reteplase and streptokinase. The intracranial hemorrhage rate with reteplase was 0.77 percent compared with 0.37 percent for streptokinase.

The GUSTO III trial compared the 10 + 10-unit regimen of reteplase with accelerated t-PA in 15,059 patients.[20] The 30-day mortality rate was 7.47 percent in the reteplase group and 7.24 percent in the t-PA group, corresponding to an absolute difference of 0.23 percent, with a 95 percent confidence interval of −0.66 percent to +1.1 percent (Fig. 35–29). The results of GUSTO III did not demonstrate superiority of reteplase over t-PA; using a 1 percent absolute difference as a boundary for equivalence, the mortality results also do not formally demonstrate equivalence.[278, 279] The intracranial hemorrhage rate was 0.91 percent with reteplase and 0.87 percent with t-PA. The secondary composite endpoint of net clinical benefit (death or disabling stroke) was 7.89 percent with reteplase and 7.91 percent with accelerated t-PA.

Although GUSTO III did not fulfill formal criteria for equivalence of reteplase and t-PA, many clinicians consider the two agents to be therapeutically similar and consider the double bolus method of administration of reteplase to be an advantage over t-PA.

LANOTEPLASE. Lanoteplase (nPA, novel plasminogen activator) is a mutant of t-PA lacking the finger and epidermal growth factor domains and also containing an amino acid substitution in the kringle 1 domain, leading to deletion of a glycosylation site (see Fig. 35–28 and Table 35–6). The phase II dose-ranging angiographic trial InTIME I suggested that lanoteplase at a dose of 120 kU/kg was superior to accelerated dose t-PA in that the TIMI 3 flow rate at 90 minutes was 57.1

percent with lanoteplase versus 46.4 percent with t-PA.[285] InTIME II was a phase III double-blind equivalence trial in 15,078 patients comparing 120 kU/kg of lanoteplase with 100 mg of accelerated dose t-PA. The 30-day mortality was 6.61 percent in the t-PA group and 6.75 percent in the lanoteplase group[21] (relative risk 1.02; *p* = 0.075 for equivalence) (Fig. 35–29). The intracranial hemorrhage rate was 0.64 percent for t-PA and 1.12 percent for lanoteplase (*p* = 0.004).

TENECTEPLASE. Tenecteplase (TNK–t-PA) is a mutant of t-PA with specific amino acid substitutions in the kringle 1 domain and protease domain introduced to decrease plasma clearance, increase fibrin specificity, and reduce sensitivity to PAI-1[286] (see Fig. 35–28 and Table 35–6). The phase II angiographic dose-ranging studies TIMI 10A and TIMI 10B defined the optimum dose of tenecteplase with respect to efficacy.[287, 288] A single bolus of 40 mg of tenecteplase over 5 to 10 seconds was associated with a 63 percent rate of TIMI 3 flow at 90 minutes; 50 mg of tenecte-

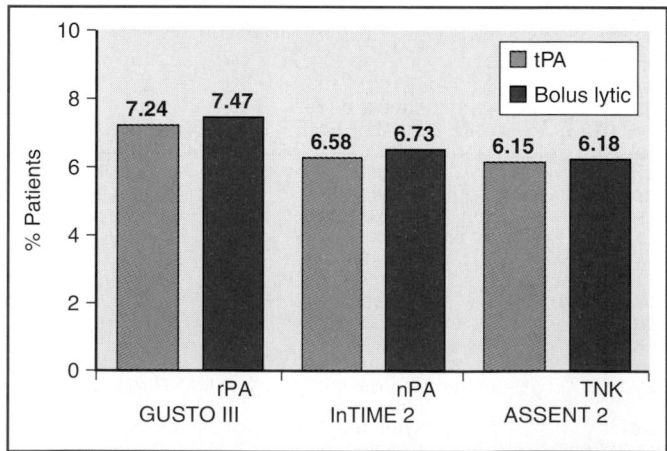

FIGURE 35–29. Mortality rates in trials of bolus thrombolytics. A 30-day mortality rate was similar in patients receiving the bolus thrombolytics in the trials shown compared with patients receiving the accelerated dose regimen of tissue plasminogen activator. (Adapted from data in [1] The Global Use of Strategies to Open Occluded Coronary Arteries [GUSTO III] Investigators. N Engl J Med 337:1118–1123, 1997. [2] Neuhaus KL: InTIME-2 results. Presented at the Scientific Sessions of the American College of Cardiology, New Orleans, March 9, 1999; and [3] Assessment of the Safety and Efficacy of a New Thrombolytic [ASSENT-2] Investigators. Lancet 354:716–722, 1999.)

plase produced a 66 percent TIMI 3 flow rate. An analysis comparing the weight-adjusted dose of tenecteplase compared with TIMI 3 flow indicated that a dose of 0.53 mg/kg was optimal for achieving high rates of TIMI 3 flow.[288]

The safety of tenecteplase was evaluated in both TIMI 10B and another large phase II clinical trial called ASSENT 1.[289] Initially, tenecteplase doses of 30, 40, and 50 mg were tested in ASSENT 1, but the 50-mg dose was discontinued and replaced by the 40-mg dose because of increased bleeding observed in the TIMI 10B study. An overall rate of intracranial hemorrhage of 0.77 percent was observed in the total ASSENT 1 study population. Observations made in the combined data set of TIMI 10B and ASSENT 1 suggested that a reduction in the dose of adjunctive unfractionated heparin was associated with a reduction in the risk of intracranial hemorrhage.

ASSENT 2 was a randomized double-blind phase III equivalence trial comparing single-bolus tenecteplase with accelerated dose t-PA in 16,949 patients.[22] The 30-day mortality rate with tenecteplase was 6.179 percent and with t-PA 6.151 percent ($p = 0.0059$ for equivalence) (see Fig. 35–29). The rate of intracranial hemorrhage was 0.93 percent with tenecteplase and 0.94 percent with t-PA. Major bleeding occurred in 4.66 percent of tenecteplase-treated patients compared with 5.94 percent of t-PA–treated patients (peak was 0.0002). There was no specific subgroup of patients in whom tenecteplase or t-PA was significantly better, with the exception of patients treated after 4 hours from the onset of symptoms in whom the mortality rate was 7.0 percent with tenecteplase and 9.2 percent with t-PA ($p = 0.018$).

OTHER THROMBOLYTIC AGENTS. SPB, a naturally occurring plasminogen activator, has been undergoing evaluation for treatment of AMI for at least three decades. Although it offers the potential advantage of less antigenicity than that with streptokinase, infarct artery patency rates are about the same as those achieved with streptokinase. Although it is prescribed in an intravenous regimen for AMI in some countries, given its high cost and lack of advantage over streptokinase, its use in the United States is almost exclusively for intracoronary infusion (6000 IU/min to an average cumulative dose of 500,000 IU) to lyse intracoronary thrombi that are believed to be responsible for an evolving AMI. Anistreplase, usually administered in a dose of 30 mg over 2 to 5 minutes intravenously, has a side effect profile similar to that of streptokinase, a patency profile similar to that of conventional-dose t-PA, and a mortality benefit similar to that of streptokinase or t-PA (double-chain form, duteplase). The lack of any compelling advantages (other than bolus administration) and costs higher than streptokinase have relegated anistreplase to an extremely infrequently prescribed drug for AMI in the United States.

SPB (scuPA or prourokinase) has been produced both in nonglycosylated (e.g., saruplase) and glycosylated (e.g., Abbott-74187) forms. Angiographic studies of saruplase (PRIMI,[290] Saruplase and Urokinase in the Treatment of Acute Myocardial Infarction [SUTAMI[291], Study in Europe with Saruplase and Alteplase in Myocardial Infarction [SESAMI][292]) have shown it to have thrombolytic efficacy similar to streptokinase, urokinase, and a 3-hour infusion of t-PA; and the Practical Applications of Saruplase Study (PASS) suggested it could be administered safely (intracranial hemorrhage rate of 0.5 percent in 1698 patients).[276,293] In the Comparison Trial of Saruplase and Streptokinase (COMPASS), the 30-day mortality was 5.8 percent for saruplase versus 6.7 percent for streptokinase; intracranial hemorrhage occurred in 0.9 percent of saruplase patients and 0.3 percent of streptokinase patients.[294] In the Bolus versus Infusion in Rescuepase Development (BIRD) trial, single-bolus administration of saruplase, 80 mg, was found to be similar to a 1 hour infusion.[295]

Staphylokinase. This is a highly fibrin-specific plasminogen activator that requires priming on the surface of a clot.[296] (see Table 35–6). Recombinant forms of staphylokinase have shown high degrees of thrombolytic efficiency (STAR trial[297]), and dose-ranging studies are the ongoing Collaborative Angiographic Patency Trial of Recombinant Staphylokinase [CAPTORS].[298] Of concern is the fact that recombinant staphylokinase is highly antigenic, which may limit its use beyond a single administration unless pegilated variants with reduced immunogenicity prove to be clinically safe and effective.

Effect on Left Ventricular Function

Although precise measurements of infarct size would be an ideal endpoint for clinical reperfusion studies, such measures have been found to be impractical. Attempts to use LV ejection fraction as a surrogate for infarct size have not been productive because little difference is seen in ejection fraction between treatment groups that show a significant difference in mortality. Alternative methods of assessing left ventricular function, such as end-systolic volume[299] or quantitative echocardiography,[300] are more revealing because patients with smaller volumes and better-preserved ventricular shape have an improved survival.

As with survival, improvement in global LV function is related to the time of thrombolytic treatment, with greatest improvement occurring with earliest therapy. Greater improvement in left ventricular function has been reported with anterior than with inferior infarcts. Earlier trials failed to demonstrate any difference in global left ventricular function when streptokinase and t-PA were compared.[301] The angiographic substudy in GUSTO I reported detailed regional wall motion analyses stratified by thrombolytic regimen.[238] Patients who received the accelerated t-PA regimen had significantly less depression of regional wall motion in the ischemic zone, as evidenced by fewer abnormal chords when their ventricular silhouettes were subjected to segmental wall motion analysis. In addition, this patient group tended to have a slightly higher global ejection fraction and slightly reduced end-systolic volume index at 90 minutes after initiation of thrombolytic therapy. The totality of the data presented in the GUSTO angiographic substudy[238] is consistent with the hypothesis that more rapid and complete restoration of normal coronary blood flow in the infarct-related artery with t-PA was associated with an improvement in regional and global left ventricular function (presumably through greater myocardial salvage in the ischemic zone) and that this difference in function compared with that obtained with streptokinase may have contributed to the mortality differences observed at 30 days and beyond.

Complications of Thrombolytic Therapy

Recent (< 1 year) exposure to streptococci or streptokinase produces some degree of antibody-mediated resistance to streptokinase (and anistreplase) in most patients. Although this is of clinical consequence only rarely, it is recommended that patients not receive streptokinase for AMI if they have been treated with a streptokinase product within the past year. Bleeding complications are, of course, the most common and potentially the most serious. Most bleeding is relatively minor with all agents, with more serious episodes occurring in patients requiring invasive procedures.[302, 303] Overall, 70 percent of bleeding episodes occur at the site of vascular punctures.[302-304] Intracranial hemorrhage is the most serious complication of thrombolytic therapy[305, 306]; its frequency varies with the clinical characteristics of the patient and the thrombolytic prescribed[306, 307] (Table 35–7).

Collaborators from the European Cooperative Society Group (ECSG) and GISSI, TAMI, TIMI, and ISAM groups pooled their respective data bases on thrombolytic-treated patients with AMI to develop a statistical model for individual risk assessment for intracranial hemorrhage using a case-control format.[307] The following four clinical variables known at hospital admission were shown to predict an increased risk of intracranial hemorrhage: age older than 65 years (odds ratio for intracranial hemorrhage = 2.2), weight less than 70 kg (2.1), hypertension on presentation (2.0), and use of t-PA as opposed to streptokinase (1.6). Assuming an overall incidence of intracranial hemorrhage of 0.75 percent, the expected incidence of intracranial hemorrhage stratified by the number of risk factors would be 0.26 percent for no risk factors, 0.96 percent for one risk factor, 1.32 percent for two risk factors, and 2.17 percent for three risk factors. The incremental incidence of intracranial hemorrhage with thrombolysis appears to be at least partially

▼ TABLE 35-7. INTRACRANIAL HEMORRHAGE IN RECENT THROMBOLYTIC TRIALS WITH TISSUE PLASMINOGEN ACTIVATORS

PATIENT CHARACTERISTICS	GUSTO-I	GUSTO-II	COBALT	GUSTO-III	ASSENT-2	IN TIME-II
Number	41,021	3473	7169	15,059	16,950	15,078
Average age (yr)	62	62.5	62.4	63		
>75 yr (%)	10.5	11.8	13.0	13.6		
Female (%)	25.2	22.4	23.4	27.4		
Intracranial hemorrhage rates						
SK	0.51	0.37	Double bolus 1.12	0.87	0.94	0.64
t-PA	0.70	0.72	Accl infusion 0.81			
t-PA				0.91		
TNK-tPA	0.7	0.72			0.94	
nPA						1.13

Accl = accelerated; nPA = lanoteplase; rPA = reteplase; TNK-tPA = a genetically engineered variant of t-PA; t-PA = recombinant tissue-type plasminogen activator; SK = streptokinase.

Modified from Ryan TJ, Antman EM, Brooks NH, et al: 1999 update: ACC/AHA Guidelines for the Management of Patients With Acute Myocardial Infarction: Executive Summary and Recommendations: A report of the American College of Cardiology/American Heart Association Task Force on Practice Guidelines (Committee on Management of Acute Myocardial Infarction). Circulation 100:1016–1030, 1999. Copyright 1999, American Heart Association.

offset by a lower frequency of thrombotic strokes, so that the overall incidence of stroke is usually not much higher in patients receiving thrombolytic therapy than in control patients.[229, 305, 308] Gurwitz and colleagues analyzed 71,073 patients in the National Registry of Myocardial Infarction 2 who had received t-PA for AMI.[309] Multivariable analysis indicated the following patient characteristics were associated with an increased risk of intracranial hemorrhage: older age, female sex, black ethnicity, systolic blood pressure of 140 mm Hg or more, diastolic blood pressure of 100 mm Hg or more, history of stroke, t-PA dose more than 1.5 mg/kg, and a low body weight (Table 35–8).

There have been reports of an "early hazard" with thrombolytic therapy, that is, an excess of deaths in the first 24 hours in thrombolytic-treated patients compared with controls (especially in elderly patients treated >12 hours).[15] However, this excess early mortality is more than offset by the deaths prevented beyond the first day, culminating in an 18 percent (13 to 23 percent) reduction in mortality by 35 days.[15] The mechanisms responsible for this early hazard are not clear but probably are multiple, including an increased risk of myocardial rupture (particularly in the elderly), fatal intracranial hemorrhage,[305] inadequate myocardial reperfusion resulting in pump failure and cardiogenic shock,[310] and possible reperfusion injury of reperfused myocardium.[205] Reports of more unusual complications such as splenic rupture, aortic dissection, and cholesterol embolization have also appeared.

Recommendations for Thrombolytic Therapy

NET CLINICAL BENEFIT OF THROMBOLYSIS. Perhaps one of the most important messages from all of the available evidence is that thrombolytic therapy is underused in patients with AMI.[311] Hesitancy in prescribing a thrombolytic agent is often the result of uncertainty about the risk of bleeding, and analysis from GUSTO-1 shows that moderate to severe bleeding occurred more often in patients who were older, female, lighter, shorter, and of African ancestry and who underwent an invasive procedure.[312] The specific profile of patients at risk for intracranial hemorrhage was discussed previously. Patients with a higher baseline risk of mortality are more likely to benefit from thrombolytic therapy.

Against the mortality benefit associated with thrombolytic therapy must be weighed the excess risk of stroke. By using the net clinical benefit composite endpoint of 30-day mortality or nonfatal stroke, a small but statistically signifi-

cant benefit is seen for accelerated dose t-PA compared with streptokinase. Given the data from the GUSTO-3 and Assessment of the Safety and Efficacy of a New Thrombolytic (ASSENT)-2 trials, it appears that the net clinical benefit of accelerated dose t-PA is similar to that obtained with reteplase or tenecteplase.[20, 22] Of interest, the rate of noncerebral major bleeding was lower with tenecteplase than t-PA in the ASSENT-2 trial, possibly due to the greater fibrin specificity of tenecteplase.[22]

CHOICE OF AGENT. Analysis of the net clinical benefit and cost-effectiveness of t-PA versus streptokinase does not easily yield recommendations for treatment because clinicians must weigh the risk of mortality and risk of intracranial hemorrhage when confronting a thrombolytic-eligible patient with AMI; additional considerations may be the constraints placed on physicians' therapeutic decision-mak-

▼ TABLE 35-8. ADJUSTED ODDS RATIOS RELATING PATIENT CHARACTERISTICS TO INTRACRANIAL HEMORRHAGE

CHARACTERISTIC	ADJUSTED ODDS RATIO (95% CI)
Age	
< 65 yr	1.00
65–74 yr	2.71
≥ 75 yr	4.34
Sex	
Male	1.00
Female	1.59
Ethnicity	
White	1.00
Black	1.70
History of stroke	
No	1.00
Yes	1.90
Systolic blood pressure	
< 140 mm Hg	1.00
140–159 mm Hg	1.33
≥ 160 mm Hg	1.48
Diastolic blood pressure	
< 80 mm Hg	1.00
80–99 mm Hg	1.09 (p = NS)
≥ 100 mm Hg	1.40
Dose of tissue plasminogen activator	
< 1.5 mg/kg	1.00
≥ 1.5 mg/kg	1.49

Modified from Gurwitz JF, Gore JM, Goldberg RJ, et al: Risk for intracranial hemorrhage after tissue plasminogen activator treatment for acute myocardial infarction. Participants in the National Registry of Myocardial Infarction 2. Ann Intern Med 129:597–604, 1998.

ing by the health care system in which they are practicing.[313] We are in agreement with the general recommendations by Martin and Kennedy[193] and Simoons and Arnold[314] that categorize patients into those that are at high risk of death (advanced age, female gender, depressed left ventricular function, anterior MI, bundle branch block, total magnitude of ST segment elevation, diabetes, heart rate greater than 100 beats/min, systolic pressure less than 100 mm Hg, long delay since onset of ischemic discomfort),[193, 314] and high risk of intracranial hemorrhage. In the subgroup of patients presenting within 4 hours of symptom onset, the speed of reperfusion of the infarct vessel is of paramount importance, and a high-intensity thrombolytic regimen such as accelerated t-PA or tenecteplase is the preferred treatment, except in those individuals in whom the risk of death is low (e.g., a young patient with a small inferior MI) and the risk of intracranial hemorrhage is increased (e.g., acute hypertension), in whom streptokinase and accelerated t-PA are approximately equivalent choices. Of note, for those patients presenting between 4 and 12 hours from symptom onset with a low mortality risk but an increased risk of intracranial hemorrhage (e.g., elderly patients with inferior MI, blood pressure greater than 100 mm Hg, and heart rate less than 100 beats/min), streptokinase is probably preferable to t-PA because of cost considerations if thrombolytic therapy is prescribed at all in such a patient.

In those patients considered appropriate candidates for thrombolysis and in whom t-PA would have been selected as the agent of choice in the past, we believe clinicians should now consider using a bolus thrombolytic such as reteplase or tenecteplase. The rationale for this recommendation is that bolus thrombolysis has the advantage of ease of administration and a lower chance of medication errors (and the associated increase in mortality when such medication errors occur) and also offers the potential for prehospital thrombolysis.

LATE THERAPY. No mortality benefit was demonstrated in the LATE and EMERAS trials when thrombolytics were routinely administered to patients between 12 and 24 hours,[265, 266] although we believe it is still reasonable to consider thrombolytic therapy in appropriately selected patients with persistent symptoms and ST segment elevation on ECG beyond 12 hours (see Fig. 35–17). Persistent chest pain late after the onset of symptoms correlates with a higher incidence of collateral or antegrade flow in the infarct zone and is therefore a marker for patients with viable myocardium that might be salvaged.[315] Because elderly patients treated with thrombolytics more than 12 hours after the onset of symptoms are at increased risk of cardiac rupture, it is our practice to restrict late thrombolytic administration to younger patients (<65 years) with ongoing ischemia, especially those with large anterior infarctions. The elderly patient with ongoing ischemic symptoms but presenting late (>12 hours) is probably better managed with direct (primary) PTCA (discussed subsequently) than with thrombolytic therapy.

Before the institution of thrombolytic therapy, consideration should be given to the patient's need for intravascular catheterization, as would be required for the placement of an arterial pressure monitoring line, a pulmonary artery catheter for hemodynamic monitoring, or a temporary transvenous pacemaker. If any of these are required, ideally they should be placed as expeditiously as possible *before* infusion of the thrombolytic agent. If such procedures require an additional delay of more than 30 minutes, they should be deferred as long as possible after thrombolytic therapy is begun. In the early hours after institution of thrombolytic therapy, such catheterization should be performed only if crucial to survival, and then sites where excessive bleeding can be controlled should be chosen (e.g., subclavian vein catheterization should be avoided).

As noted earlier, all patients with suspected AMI should receive aspirin (160 to 325 mg) regardless of the thrombolytic agent prescribed. Aspirin should be continued indefinitely. The issues surrounding antithrombin therapy as an adjunct to thrombolysis are complex and are discussed in detail in a subsequent section (see p. 1162).

CATHETER-BASED REPERFUSION
(See also Chap. 38)

It is now established that reperfusion can be achieved by emergency percutaneous coronary intervention (PCI). By using a guidewire and balloon catheter, it is technically easier to cross a total occlusion consisting of a fresh thrombus than to cross a long-standing occlusion of a coronary artery. Thus, wire-guided balloon angioplasty can be useful to achieve reperfusion in two quite different circumstances: (1) in lieu of thrombolytic therapy where it is referred to as *direct* or *primary angioplasty*[316] and (2) as adjunctive therapy with thrombolysis or as a management strategy in the subacute phase of AMI (days 2 to 7) in patients who do not receive thrombolysis. Several clinical scenarios have been described that represent different categories of use of PCI when it is not selected as the primary reperfusion strategy. When thrombolysis has failed to reperfuse the infarct vessel or a severe stenosis is present in the infarct vessel, a *rescue PCI* may be performed as soon as possible. Alternatively, strategies of empirical *immediate* (i.e., performed urgently within a few hours) or *deferred* (i.e., performed within the first week) PCI have been proposed for all patients with residual critical stenosis (> 70 percent of lumen diameter) who receive thrombolysis. Finally, a more conservative approach of *elective* PCI may be used to manage AMI patients only when spontaneous or exercise-provoked ischemia occurs whether or not they have received a previous course of thrombolytic therapy.

Catheter-based strategies for reperfusion of the occluded infarct-related artery in patients with AMI is a rapidly evolving field. Coronary artery stenting, originally introduced for elective percutaneous procedures, was originally withheld in patients with AMI because of concerns over acute stent thrombosis. However, with advances in stent deployment (high pressure inflations, intravascular ultrasound guidance), improvements in antiplatelet therapy (GPIIb/IIIa inhibitors) and operator experience have fueled interest in primary coronary artery stenting as a new catheter-based strategy for reperfusion.[316, 317]

Primary Angioplasty

ADVANTAGES. An important advantage of primary PCI in AMI is the ability to achieve reperfusion of the infarct vessel without the risk of bleeding associated with thrombolytic therapy. In addition, primary PCI (performed predominantly in experienced centers) as compared with thrombolytic therapy has been shown in several randomized trials and registries to yield higher patency rates of the infarct vessel both at 90 minutes (85 to 90 percent for PCI vs. 65 percent for thrombolysis).[238, 273, 318] Systematic overviews of trials of primary PTCA versus thrombolysis collectively enrolling 2635 patients revealed lower 30-day and 6-month mortality rates for patients treated with primary PTCA versus thrombolysis[319, 320] (Fig. 35–30). The rate of recurrent infarction was also lower for patients treated with primary PTCA[320] (see Fig. 35–30). Primary PTCA was also associated with significant reductions in total stroke and hemorrhagic stroke. Thus, primary PCI appears to be superior to thrombolytic therapy when it is performed in experi-

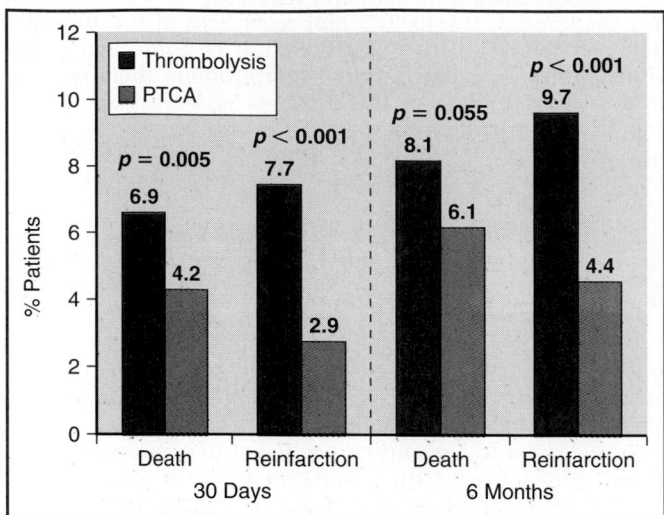

FIGURE 35–30. Comparison of mortality and reinfarction in AMI patients treated with thrombolysis vs. primary percutaneous transluminal coronary angioplasty (PTCA). Pooled data from 11 randomized trials revealed significant reductions in the 30-day and 6-month rates of mortality and reinfarction in patients treated with primary PTCA. (Adapted from Grines CL, Ellis SG, Jones M, et al: Primary coronary angioplasty vs. thrombolytic therapy for acute myocardial infarction (MI): Long term follow-up of ten randomized trials. Circulation [Suppl] I-499, 1999.)

enced centers with a well-staffed invasive angiography team. It is also associated with a shorter length of hospital stay and reduced costs because of fewer patients with recurrent ischemia and recurrent MI when treated with primary PCI.[321, 322]

Primary PCI appears to have a particular advantage over thrombolysis for the management of high-risk AMI patients such as diabetics and the elderly.[323, 324] In an analysis of Medicare patients in the Cooperative Cardiovascular Project data base, primary PCI was associated with improved 30-day survival (hazard ratio 0.74, 95 percent confidence interval 0.63–0.88) and also 1-year survival (hazard radio 0.88, 95 percent confidence intervals 0.73–0.94).[325] The benefits of primary PCI in the elderly persisted after stratification by the volume of AMI patients cared for at individual hospitals and the presence of on-site angiography.

Why have these dramatic differences favoring primary PCI over thrombolytic therapy been observed? In addition to the high level of technical expertise in the dedicated centers that have reported promising results with primary PCI, differences in the adequacy of reperfusion and responses of ischemic myocardium to restoration of flow by thrombolysis and mechanical means should be considered. Early patency of the infarct-related artery is higher with direct PCI, full reperfusion (TIMI grade 3 flow) is higher, the degree of residual stenosis is less, reocclusion rates are lower,[273] and collateral flow to non–infarct-related myocardial zones is probably increased—all features that promote better healing in the infarct zone, less left ventricular dilatation, and reduced morbidity and mortality.[326–328] Mechanical recanalization of the infarct vessel does not produce the interstitial edema, contraction band necrosis, and microvascular hemorrhage seen with thrombolytic therapy (see Figs. 35–8 and 35–9).

OBSTACLES TO IMPLEMENTATION. The clinical trial results and intriguing experimental observations cited earlier must be placed in perspective when one considers implementing primary PCI as a treatment strategy for the majority of patients with AMI. Because PCI is performed only in patients with suitable angiographic anatomy, a bias may have been introduced in the available data bases excluding patients at higher risk of events from being treated by PCI.[329] The MITRA Registry of 54 university and community hospitals in Germany found that in clinical practice patients treated with primary PTCA are more often given beta blockers and ACE inhibitors than patients treated with thrombolytics, drug treatment practices that could contribute to a reduction in mortality that is not a direct result of PTCA.[330] Although reports from individual community hospitals replicating the results in randomized trials can be found in the literature, fewer than 20 percent of hospitals in the United States and less than 10 percent of hospitals in Europe can perform primary PCI, and an even smaller proportion are capable of performing it on an emergency basis 24 hours a day, 7 days a week.[331]

It remains to be determined whether lower-volume PCI centers with less-experienced investigators can replicate the encouraging results reported to date. In addition, it is unclear whether on-site cardiac surgical backup is a necessary component of a primary PCI strategy for AMI.[332] The problem of lack of on-site surgical backup is being evaluated in studies such as Air PAMI in which patients who present to a community hospital that does not perform primary PCI and who are thrombolytically eligible with at least one high-risk criterion are randomized to either immediate intravenous thrombolysis or emergency transfer for PCI.[333] The randomized population in Air PAMI will be compared with a separate registry of Air PAMI–eligible patients who have PCI performed in hospitals with catheterization laboratories but no on-site surgery (No S.O.S. Registry).[333] Preliminary results from the No S.O.S. Registry are encouraging in that the in-hospital death rate was 2.7 percent and the stroke rate was 2.7 percent in 500 patients.[332] The PRAGUE study compared the incidence of death/MI/stroke at 30 days in a randomized trial of aspirin plus streptokinase with management in a community hospital (Group A); aspirin plus streptokinase with transfer to a nearby interventional center (Group B); and aspirin plus heparin (10,000 U) with transfer to a nearby interventional center (Group C). All patients received fraxiparine for 3 days and ticlopidine for 1 month.[334] There were no deaths during or within 30 minutes of transport. The primary composite endpoint occurred in 23 percent of group A, 15 percent of group B, and 8 percent of group C patients, respectively ($p < 0.02$), indicating that interhospital transport for primary PCI is feasible and safe and may be associated with a lower event rate after AMI. The potential cost implications of offering primary PCI to all eligible patients with AMI are staggering and have been the subject of considerable ongoing debate in several countries.[316]

Primary Stenting

Although it has been agreed that primary PTCA has an advantage over thrombolysis in AMI patients with a prior CABG, observations from the National Registry of Myocardial Infarction (NRMI)-2 suggest the outcome is similar to the two reperfusion strategies.[335] Interventionalists have begun to embrace new strategies such as stenting and intravenous GPIIb/IIIa inhibitors (see Chap. 38) to improve on results with PTCA in AMI. Experience gained with elective coronary stenting (see Chap. 38) led to a series of reports of implantation of coronary stents in AMI patients.[336] A high procedural success rate was reported and the subacute thrombosis rate was low (< 3 percent), largely due to aggressive use of antiplatelet therapy with aspirin and ticlopidine. Table 35–9 summarizes major randomized trials of primary stenting versus primary PTCA in AMI. In general, the procedural success rate was high with both stenting and PTCA. Of interest, in the largest of the trials, PAMI-STENT, a slightly lower rate of TIMI grade 3 flow was seen with stenting compared with PTCA, raising the possibility of embolization of platelet aggregates at the time of stent deployment.[337] Mortality rates were generally low, with

▶ TABLE 35–9. RANDOMIZED TRIALS OF PRIMARY STENT PLACEMENT VS. PRIMARY PERCUTANEOUS TRANSLUMINAL CORONARY ANGIOPLASTY (PTCA) IN ACUTE MYOCARDIAL INFARCTION

	ESCOBAR	FRESCO	GRAMI	PASTA	PRISAM	PAMI-STENT
No. of patients						
Stent	112	75	52	67	39	452
PTCA	115	75	52	69	49	448
Enrollment criteria	≥ 6 hr after symptoms onset; 6–24 hr of persistent symptoms	≥ 6 hr after symptoms onset; 6–24 hr of persistent symptoms; ST segment elevation	< 30 min after symptoms onset; ST segment elevation; ≤ 24 hr after symptoms onset; ≤ 75 years old	≤ 12 hr after symptom onset	≤ 24 hr after symptom onset	≤ 12 hr after symptom onset
Randomization criteria	Lesion suitable for stenting	Optimal PTCA result	Lesion suitable for stenting	Lesion suitable for stenting	Lesion suitable for stenting	Lesion suitable for stenting
Length of follow-up	6 mo	6 mo	1 yr	≤1 yr	6 mo	30 d
Crossover (bailout), No. (%)	15 (13)	0 (0)	13 (25)			68 (15.1)
TIMI grade 3 flow, %						
Stent		100	98			88.9
PTCA		99	$p < 0.03$ 83			92.7
Mortality, %*						
Stent	2	1	3.8	4.8	0	3.5
PTCA	3	0	$p = NS$ 7.6	9.1	0	1.8
Target vessel revascularization, %						
Stent	4	7	14	18.6	11	0.9
PTCA	$p = 0.0016$ 17	$p = 0.002$ 25	$p = NS$ 21	$p = 0.009$ 37.6	$p = 0.01$ 36	$p = 0.006$ 3.5

*All differences in mortality are nonsignificant.

From Every NR: Thrombolysis and Interventional Therapy in Acute Myocardial Infarction. Presented at the George Washington University 15th International Workshop on Thrombolysis and Interventional Therapy in Acute Myocardial Infarction, November 6, 1999, Atlanta, GA.

slight nonsignificant trends favoring stenting. The major benefit of stenting was seen in a significant reduction in the incidence of the subsequent target vessel revascularization.[337]

Angioplasty as an Adjunct to Thrombolysis

Ellis and associates have summarized the heterogeneous outcomes reported in observational series of *rescue* PTCA after failed thrombolysis. Although procedural success was obtained in about 80 percent of patients, the average rate of reocclusion was 18 percent and the average mortality was 10.6 percent. The RESCUE trial focused on the subset of AMI patients with an anterior infarction and reported a reduction in the composite endpoint of death or congestive heart failure by 30 days in the PTCA group.[338]

After thrombolytic therapy, the majority of patients are found to have a significant residual stenosis.[338a] Even in patients who clinically appear to have reperfused, PTCA, whether applied immediately or deferred, has the theoretical benefit of further opening of a stenosed coronary artery to increase flow, perhaps enhancing myocardial recovery and diminishing the possibility of reocclusion. Several trials have compared immediate, early (within several hours to a few days), or deferred (delayed for 4 days) PTCA versus no PTCA, whereas others have compared immediate versus deferred PTCA or immediate versus deferred versus no PTCA. A summary of the design features and main findings of 16 trials that collectively enrolled about 6200 patients in these categories has been published along with meta-analysis of the mortality results.[339] Although none of the individual comparisons of strategies achieved conventional statistical significance, a consistent theme was observed—the *routine empirical* use of PTCA (either immediate or delayed) after thrombolysis was associated with a trend toward *increased* mortality.[339] In addition, there were higher rates of abrupt reclosure of the infarct-related coronary artery and complications, including reinfarction and the need for urgent CABG while providing no benefit in terms of recovery of ventricular function.[340, 341] Possible explanations for the increased hazard associated with PTCA soon after thrombolysis include exacerbation of platelet activation and thrombosis at the site of plaque rupture and increased bleeding, including hemorrhagic dissections of the target vessel.[212, 340, 342, 343]

There is also no evidence to support *empirically deferred* PCI in patients without evidence of recurrent or provocable ischemia. The TOPS trial randomized patients with a negative exercise test several days after thrombolysis to either medical therapy or medical therapy plus PCI. There was no benefit in terms of rest or exercise ejection fraction, but there were disturbing trends toward a higher rate of abrupt vessel closure and non-Q-wave MI acutely and a lower rate of infarct-free survival at 1-year follow-up in the PTCA-treated patients.

Because many of the previous trials of PCI early after full-dose thrombolytics were undertaken during the thrombolytic infusion or shortly thereafter, which potentially contributed to a lower success rate of PCI, higher bleeding, and a trend toward higher rates of adverse outcomes, the Plasminogen-activator Angioplasty Compatibility Trial (PACT) was undertaken.[344] After aspirin and heparin, 606 AMI patients were randomized within 6 hours of symptoms to a 50-mg bolus of t-PA over 3 minutes or placebo followed by angiography and rescue PTCA for less than TIMI 3 flow. Patency of the infarct artery was 61 percent (TIMI 3 = 33 percent, TIMI 2 = 28 percent) in the t-PA group versus 34 percent (TIMI 3 = 15 percent, TIMI 2 = 19 percent) in the placebo group ($p = 0.001$) before PCI (median of 98 minutes from pharmacological reperfusion). Rescue PCI was successful in over 90 percent of patients in both groups as was left ventricular ejection fraction at 5 to 7 days. However, left ventricular function was significantly higher in those patients achieving TIMI 3 flow by the time of diagnostic angiography and those patients who had rescue PCI within 1 hour of the bolus of the study drug. The rates of major bleeding and reinfarction were similar in the t-PA and placebo groups. Thus, PACT reaffirmed the time-dependent nature of the open artery hypothesis with greater preservation of left ventricular function in patients with earlier attainment of TIMI 3 flow. This trial also showed that a tailored combination of reduced dose lytic and rescue PCI as needed could be performed safely.[345] However, only 26 percent of patients in PACT underwent stenting, and GPIIb/IIIa inhibitors were used in only 5 percent of patients.[344, 346] Whether the improved equipment available now for PTCA, the use of stents,[347] and modified pharmacological reperfusion regimens such as reduced-dose thrombolytics, intravenous GPIIb/IIIa inhibitors, or the combination of reduced dose thrombolytics and GPIIb/IIIa inhibitors (see p. 1164) would swing the evidence in favor of routine angiography followed by catheter-based reperfusion as needed after MI is an intriguing question that needs to be addressed.

Recommendations for Catheter-Based Reperfusion in AMI

It appears that primary PCI, when carried out by experienced interventional cardiologists in high-volume angiography laboratories, is superior to thrombolytic therapy. It is our practice to refer thrombolytic-ineligible patients to primary PCI and also to select primary PCI as the reperfusion method of choice if the patient is at relatively high risk of intracerebral hemorrhage consequent to thrombolytic therapy (see p. 1153), or if the anticipated time to placement of angioplasty catheters is less than 1 hour from the patient's presentation to the emergency department. In the special circumstances of cardiogenic shock, provided no other life-threatening comorbidities are present, we refer patients for revascularization (see p. 1179).

Patients in whom thrombolytic therapy fails to achieve reperfusion represent candidates for rescue PCI, and in such patients this can usually be safe and effective. The practical issue is the difficulty in reliably identifying patients who fail to reperfuse after thrombolytic therapy using noninvasive indices either alone or in combination.[127, 348–348a] Therefore, until there are better ways to recognize patients who might benefit from "rescue PCI," the question of optimal treatment of thrombolytic failure remains unresolved. However, we consider patients with evolving chest pain and ST segment elevations that persist for 90 minutes after the onset of administration of a thrombolytic agent to be candidates for emergency catheterization and, if the infarct-related vessel is occluded, for rescue PCI. Elective PCI can be considered for most patients receiving thrombolytic therapy in whom ischemia develops at rest, during ambulation in the hospital, or during a prehospital discharge exercise test.[349] We do not consider it necessary to carry out routine coronary arteriography on asymptomatic patients with negative prehospital discharge exercise tests to identify patients who have severe obstruction in whom PCI can be performed.

Although some reports suggested that prophylactic intraaortic balloon counterpulsation may be useful to maintain vessel patency after PCI, subsequent randomized trials in high-risk patients showed that balloon counterpulsation did not decrease the rates of infarct-related artery reocclusion or reinfarction, promote myocardial recovery, or improve overall clinical outcome.[350] We believe that intraaortic balloon pumping should be reserved for hemodynamically unstable patients.[351]

SURGICAL REPERFUSION

There have been extensive improvements in intraoperative myocardial preservation with cardioplegia and hypothermia and in surgical techniques. These have allowed surgical reperfusion in patients with AMI to be carried out at quite low short- and long-term mortality rates—approximately 2 percent in hospital and 25 percent 10-year mortality rates in selected centers. This has kept alive the concept of emergency coronary revascularization as a possible measure to protect jeopardized myocardium in patients suffering AMI.[352] As appears to be the case for all methods designed to limit infarct size, salvage of myocardium is most successful if surgery is performed within the first 4 to 6 hours of the onset of the acute event. In the usual patient who develops an AMI outside the hospital, it is logistically almost impossible to bring the patient to the hospital, carry out a clinical evaluation, outline the coronary anatomy by arteriography, assemble the surgical team, commence operation, and place the patient on cardiopulmonary bypass in less than 4 to 6 hours after the onset of the event. It is therefore unlikely that surgical reperfusion can or will be applied in the *routine* treatment of AMI. Indeed, the operation is contraindicated in patients with uncomplicated transmural infarcts more than 6 hours after the onset of the event. When carried out at this time, surgical reperfusion appears to produce marked hemorrhage into the area of infarction. In some patients with AMI, including some with cardiogenic shock, infarction appears to occur in a stuttering manner over an interval of several days.[353] Revascularization carried out more than 6 hours after the onset of the event might be of benefit in this group, but this has yet to be rigorously established.

Ten to 20 percent of AMI patients are currently referred for CABG for one of the following indications: persistent or recurrent chest pain despite thrombolysis or PCS, high-risk coronary anatomy (e.g., left main artery stenosis) discovered at catheterization, or a complication of AMI such as ventricular septal rupture or severe mitral regurgitation due to papillary muscle dysfunction. Patients with AMI with continued severe ischemic and hemodynamic instability are likely to benefit from emergency revascularization. PCI with stenting as needed is the preferable technique when revascularization is needed in the first 48 to 72 hours after AMI; surgery should be reserved for those in whom PCI has been unsuccessful or whose anatomy dictates the need for CABG, such as patients with left main or extensive multivessel coronary artery disease.

Patients undergoing successful thrombolysis but with important residual stenoses, who on anatomical grounds are more suitable for surgical revascularization than for PCI, have undergone CABG with quite low mortality (about 4 percent) and morbidity *provided* that they are operated on more than 24 hours after AMI; those patients requiring urgent or emergency CABG within 24 to 48 hours of AMI have mortality rates between 15 and 20 percent.[352] When surgery is performed under urgent conditions with active and ongoing ischemia or cardiogenic shock, operative mortality rises steeply. At autopsy, such patients have extensive myocardial necrosis that is often hemorrhagic. Patients who are referred urgently for CABG within 6 to 12 hours of receiving a thrombolytic should receive aprotinin and fresh-frozen plasma to correct their coagulation system deficit and minimize the requirements for blood transfusion (see

Chap. 60). Although postoperative chest tube drainage with relatively minor bleeding occurs more commonly than after elective bypass surgery, this problem is not of major concern.

ANTITHROMBOTIC AND ANTIPLATELET THERAPY
(See also Chap. 62)

Antithrombotic Therapy

Despite more than 30 years of active clinical investigation, the use of antithrombotic agents after AMI remains controversial. The rationale for administering heparin acutely in AMI includes prevention of deep venous thrombosis, pulmonary embolism, ventricular thrombus formation, and cerebral embolization. In addition, establishing and maintaining patency of the infarct-related artery, whether or not a patient receives thrombolytic therapy, is another common rationale for heparin therapy in AMI.

EFFECT ON MORTALITY. Randomized trials in AMI conducted in the prethrombolytic era (between 1969 and 1973) showed that the risks of pulmonary embolism, stroke, and reinfarction were reduced in patients who received intravenous heparin. This formed the basis for the use of heparin in AMI patients not treated with thrombolytic therapy. With the introduction of the thrombolytic era and importantly after the publication of the Second International Study of Infarct Survival (ISIS-2),[308] the situation became more complicated because of strong evidence of a substantial mortality reduction with aspirin alone and confusing and conflicting data regarding the risk-benefit ratio of heparin used as an adjunct to aspirin or in combination with aspirin and a thrombolytic agent (Table 35–10).

In the SCATI trial of streptokinase for AMI, in which patients were randomized to receive either delayed subcutaneous heparin or placebo as the *sole* adjunctive therapy (i.e., no aspirin), there was a trend toward lower mortality in the heparin group. In the combined data set of GISSI-2 and ISIS-3 (totaling over 62,000 patients), the 35-day mortality was 10.0 percent in the patients receiving subcutaneous heparin versus 10.2 percent in the patients not receiving any subcutaneous heparin. In addition, in the GUSTO study, no difference was seen in the 35-day mortality rate in patients receiving streptokinase plus subcutaneous heparin (7.2 percent) or intravenous heparin (7.4 percent).[19] Nonrandomized subgroup analyses from the LATE trial of 2821 patients who received t-PA showed a 35-day mortality of 7.6 percent when intravenous heparin was administered, compared with 10.4 percent when no heparin was given.[265] Thus, the available information suggests that intravenous heparin is probably of no benefit in patients receiving streptokinase but may be helpful in patients receiving t-PA.[274] Heparin was administered as adjunctive therapy in randomized trials of reteplase and tenecteplase under the supposition that those agents were more fibrin specific than streptokinase and required concomitant use of heparin.[289, 354]

EFFECT ON PATENCY OF INFARCT ARTERY

A number of angiographic studies have examined the role of heparin in establishing and maintaining patency of the infarct-related artery in patients with AMI. Comparison of these trials is difficult because of potentially important differences in study design, including whether aspirin was administered along with heparin, the thrombolytic agent that was administered, and variations in the time of diagnostic coronary arteriography. The Bleich and coworkers[355] and HART[356] studies showed a higher infarct-related artery patency rate in AMI patients treated with t-PA plus heparin than t-PA plus placebo (71 to 82 per-

▼ **TABLE 35–10.** EFFECTS OF HEPARIN IN THE ABSENCE AND IN THE PRESENCE OF ASPIRIN: OVERVIEW OF 26 RANDOMIZED TRIALS

	TRIALS WITH ROUTINE ASPIRIN (68,000 PATIENTS: 93% ALSO HAD FIBRINOLYTIC AGENT)		
	Aspirin + Heparin (34,053)	Aspirin Only (34,055)	Effect per 1000 Allocated to Aspirin and Heparin
Death (generally in hospital)	8.6% 2932	9.1% 3092	5 ± 2 less (2p = 0.03)
Reinfarction	3.0% 1009	3.3% 1103	3 ± less (2p = 0.04)
Stroke	1.2% 397	1.1% 375	1 ± 1 more (NS)
Pulmonary embolism	0.3% 82	0.4% 117	1 ± 0.4 less (2p = 0.01)
Major bleed	1.0% 342	0.7% 234	3 ± 1 more (2p < 0.00001)

Modified from Baigent C, Collins R: Aspirin and heparin. *In* Hennekens CH [ed]: Clinical Trials in Cardiovascular Disease: Companion to Braunwald's Heart Disease. Philadelphia, WB Saunders, 1999, p 60.

cent vs. 43 to 52 percent infarct-related artery patency at 7 to 72 hours). The European Cooperative Study Group performed angiograms relatively late (i.e., 48 to 120 hours after t-PA) and still showed a somewhat greater patency rate of the infarct-related artery in the heparin-treated patients.[357] The TAMI-3 study suggested that in patients receiving aspirin plus t-PA no patency benefit was achieved by the immediate intravenous administration of heparin and that it could therefore be delayed for at least 60 to 90 minutes after thrombolysis.

Although a slightly better 90-minute infarct-related artery patency rate was observed in the OSIRIS (streptokinase plus aspirin) study in patients who received heparin versus placebo (82 percent patency vs. 72 percent), the GUSTO angiographic substudy[238] showed no benefit of intravenous heparin versus subcutaneous heparin in patients who received streptokinase plus aspirin with respect to 90-minute infarct-related artery patency (60 percent vs. 54 percent). Although preliminary observations suggested that extremely high doses of intravenous unfractionated heparin (300 U/kg) alone were associated with an increase in patency rates of the infarct-related artery, this was not confirmed on follow-up in a larger trial.[358, 359]

EFFECT ON LEFT VENTRICULAR THROMBUS. Anticoagulant therapy significantly reduces the incidence of echocardiographically documented left ventricular thrombi.[360] These benefits are observed most prominently in patients with anterior MI, particularly those with a large area of wall motion abnormality. In the thrombolytic era, the incidence of left ventricular thrombi is reduced.[361] Although co-administration of heparin does not appear to affect the incidence of left ventricular thrombus formation in patients who receive thrombolytic therapy, the thrombi protrude less into the ventricular cavity when heparin is administered.

COMPLICATIONS OF ANTITHROMBOTIC THERAPY

Although heparin may induce thrombocytopenia through an immunological mechanism, this is seen only rarely, probably occurring in only 2 to 3 percent of patients.[362] The most serious complication of antithrombotic therapy is bleeding (especially intracranial hemorrhage) when thrombolytic agents are prescribed. Major hemorrhagic events occur more frequently in patients of low body weight, advanced age, female gender, marked prolongation of the activated partial thromboplastin time (> 90 to 100 seconds), and the performance of invasive procedures.[302, 303, 312, 363] Frequent monitoring of the activated partial thromboplastin time (facilitated by use of a bedside testing device) reduces the risk of major hemorrhagic complications in patients treated with heparin. However, during the first 12 hours after thrombolytic therapy, the activated partial thromboplastin time may be elevated from the thrombolytic agent alone (particularly if streptokinase is administered), making it difficult to accurately interpret the effects of a heparin infusion on the patient's coagulation status.

The optimal dose of unfractionated heparin as an adjunct to thrombolysis and its potential causative role in intracranial hemorrhage is unclear. Giugliano and associates examined the data from four sets of trials: (1) TIMI trials studying accelerated t-PA and intravenous heparin, (2) studies with t-PA and intravenous unfractionated

heparin in which the heparin regimen was changed during the course of the trial, (3) phase III trials with accelerated dose t-PA and intravenous unfractionated heparin, and (4) trials of new single-bolus thrombolytics.[364] The intracranial hemorrhage rate in the angiographic TIMI trials was nearly double that in the nonangiographic TIMI trials (1.42 percent vs. 0.76 percent). Lower rates of intracranial hemorrhage were observed among studies of t-PA that reduced the dose of unfractionated heparin midtrial (TIMI 9A–9B, 1.87 percent–1.07 percent; GUSTO IIA-IIb, 0.92 percent–0.7 percent; TIMI 10B, 2.80 percent–1.16 percent). The rates of intracranial hemorrhage with accelerated-dose t-PA gradually increased from GUSTO I (0.72 percent) conducted in 1990–1993 to ASSENT 2 (0.94 percent) conducted in 1997–1998. Potential explanations for the increase in intracranial hemorrhage rates over time include enrollment of higher-risk patients and greater ascertainment of intracranial hemorrhage due to increased availability of imaging modalities such as CT and MRI. This trend in intracranial hemorrhage with t-PA was reversed in the InTIME-II trial, which used the lowest dose of heparin and most aggressive activated partial thromboplastin time monitoring and observed an intracranial hemorrhage rate of 0.64 percent. Observations regarding the benefit of a reduction in the dose of intravenous unfractionated heparin with t-PA also were extended to tenecteplase and lanoteplase.

NEW ANTITHROMBOTIC AGENTS

Potential disadvantages of unfractionated heparin include dependency on antithrombin III for inhibition of thrombin activity, sensitivity to platelet factor 4, inability to inhibit clot-bound thrombin, marked interpatient variability in therapeutic response, and the need for frequent activated partial thromboplastin time monitoring.[365] In an effort to circumvent these disadvantages of unfractionated heparin, there has been interest in the development of novel antithrombotic compounds.

HIRUDIN. The prototypical direct antithrombin hirudin was compared with heparin in several phase III trials: TIMI 9A, GUSTO IIA, and r-Hirudin for Improvement of Thrombolysis (HIT) III.[302, 303, 366] A feature common to all three trials was that they were stopped prematurely because of unacceptable rates of serious bleeding, particularly intracranial hemorrhage. This excessive rate of bleeding appeared to be attributable to high levels of anticoagulation in both the heparin and hirudin groups. Possible explanations for the unexpectedly high rates of bleeding were low estimates of the hemorrhagic risk of the doses of hirudin infused owing to the relatively small number of patients previously evaluated in phase II studies and attempts to push the heparin dose to achieve activated partial thromboplastin time levels in an effort to prevent reocclusion of successfully reperfused vessels.[302] After downward modification of the dose of antithrombins, the TIMI 9B and GUSTO IIb trials were initiated.[354, 367] The results of a prospectively planned meta-analysis of the TIMI 9B and GUSTO IIB data are shown in Table 35–11.[368] Mortality rates were similar at 30 days in both trials. A generally consistent reduction in the rate of reinfarction was seen in the two trials, but this was of borderline statistical significance in the pooled data set: no statistically significant reduction

| GROUP | NO. | MORTALITY | | |
		Heparin (%)	Hirudin (%)	OR (95% CI)
TIMI 9	3002	5.1	6.1	1.21 (0.88–1.65)
GUSTO II Lytic	3052	6.5	6.0	0.91 (0.68–1.23)
Combined	6054			1.04 (0.84–1.29)

| GROUP | NO. | REINFARCTION | | |
		Heparin (%)	Hirudin (%)	OR (95% CI)
TIMI 9	3002	5.2	4.5	0.85 (0.61–1.18)
GUSTO II Lytic	3052	6.8	5.3	0.77 (0.58–1.04)
Combined	6054			0.81 (0.65–1.00)

| GROUP | NO. | DEATH + REINFARCTION | | |
		Heparin (%)	Hirudin (%)	OR (95% CI)
TIMI 9	3002	9.5	9.7	1.02 (0.80–1.31)
GUSTO II Lytic	3052	12.1	10.2	0.84 (0.66–1.03)
Combined	6054			0.91 (0.77–1.08)

Modified from Antman EM, Bittl JA: Direct thrombin inhibitors. *In* Hennekens CH [ed]: Clinical Trials in Cardiovascular Disease: A Companion to Braunwald's Heart Disease. Philadelphia, WB Saunders, 1999, p 155.

was seen in the composite endpoint of death and nonfatal reinfarction.

By inhibiting the coagulation cascade upstream from thrombin, heparin has an advantage over the direct antithrombins because of its additional ability to decrease thrombin generation along with its ability to inhibit thrombin activity. Hirudin has a greater ability than heparin to decrease thrombin activity, but once the thrombin inhibitory capacity is exceeded (by virtue of the local concentration of hirudin), free thrombin may be generated in an explosive fashion. The net result of this balance of actions is that use of heparin or the direct antithrombins in a dose that is safe results in an equivalent decrement in thrombus formation in the infarct-related artery.

EFEGATRAN. Efegatran, another direct antithrombin, was compared with unfractionated heparin as an adjunct to streptokinase in the ESCALAT study.[369] Efegatran was not superior to heparin in achieving coronary patency and was associated with high rates of bleeding.

HIRULOG. It has been argued by the Hirulog Early Reperfusion/ Occlusion (HERO) trial investigators that in order to truly expose the benefits of a direct antithrombin, it must be administered before a thrombolytic.[370] The ongoing HERO II trial is comparing hirulog with unfractionated heparin for reduction in mortality in patients receiving streptokinase.[371]

LOW-MOLECULAR-WEIGHT HEPARINS. These are formed by controlled enzymatic or chemical depolymerization producing chains of glycosaminoglycans of varying length but with a mean molecular weight of approximately 5000 daltons.[365] Advantages of low-molecular-weight heparins include a stable, reliable anticoagulant effect, high bioavailability permitting administration by means of the subcutaneous route, and a high anti-factor Xa:anti-factor IIa ratio producing blockade of the coagulation cascade in an upstream location resulting in a marked decrement in thrombin generation. Preliminary observations suggest that low-molecular-weight heparins facilitate thrombolysis and prevent recurrent ischemic events.[372–374] Low-molecular-weight heparin preparations are now being examined in AMI patients both in the presence (AMISK, HART-2, ENTIRE-TIMI 23) and absence (TETAMI) of thrombolytic therapy.

Recommendations for Antithrombin Therapy

Given the pivotal role played by thrombin in the pathogenesis of AMI, antithrombotic therapy remains an important therapeutic intervention. All patients with an acute coronary syndrome should receive antiplatelet therapy (aspirin remains the recommended agent at this time). For patients who do *not* receive thrombolytic therapy, overviews of the available data indicate that heparin reduces mortality and morbidity from serious complications such as reinfarction and thromboembolism.[52] Therefore, in the absence of contraindications to anticoagulation we routinely use antithrombin therapy in *all* AMI patients presenting with ST segment elevation who are not candidates for thrombolysis and also prescribe it for AMI patients presenting without ST segment elevation. Although intravenous unfractionated heparin for 48 to 72 hours is an acceptable choice, given the greater ease of use we prefer subcutaneous injections of a low-molecular-weight heparin instead of either subcutaneous or intravenous unfractionated heparin for such patients.[375] In view of its superiority over unfractionated heparin[376] in patients with an acute coronary syndrome presenting without ST segment elevation, we prefer to prescribe enoxaparin, 1 mg/kg twice daily, for the duration of the hospitalization.[376] In patients at high risk for systemic emboli (large or anterior MI, atrial fibrillation, previous embolus, known left ventricular thrombus), intravenous unfractionated heparin is the preferred form of anticoagulation because of insufficient data to formulate recommendations for treatment with a low-molecular-weight heparin.

For patients receiving thrombolytic therapy with either streptokinase or anistreplase, there is no apparent mortality benefit of immediate intravenous heparin, and we do not recommend its use if those thrombolytics are prescribed. The only exception to this are patients who have another compelling indication for anticoagulation, such as a large anterior MI with a significant wall motion abnormality[360] or atrial fibrillation; in this case we generally use intravenous heparin administered to a target activated partial thromboplastin time of 50 to 70 seconds. The relative benefits of routine use of delayed (4 to 12 hours), high-dose (12,500 IU twice daily) subcutaneous heparin in patients receiving streptokinase remain unresolved.[377]

On the basis of the principle that t-PA is a more fibrin-specific lytic agent and the evidence that infarct-related artery patency rates are higher in patients receiving intravenous heparin adjunctively with t-PA, it is commonly recommended that with t-PA, intravenous heparin should be administered.[360] A similar line of reasoning can be applied to reteplase and tenecteplase. Nevertheless, the dose of heparin in thrombolytic-treated patients remains controversial. Lessons learned from clinical trials over the past 5 to 10 years suggest that the target activated partial thromboplastin time values should be lower than was previous practice; the current recommendation is an activated partial thromboplastin time of 50 to 70 seconds.[312] In addition, unfractionated heparin should be administered using a weight-based regimen with lower total maximum doses than was previous practice. An initial 60-unit/kg bolus (maximum 4000 units) should be followed by a maintenance infusion of 12 units/kg/hr (maximum 1000 units/hr).[52] It is important to emphasize that it is difficult to provide a heparin adjustment nomogram that is universally applicable because of varying responsiveness of the thromboplastin reagent used in local laboratories for measuring the activated partial thromboplastin time. The appropriate therapeutic range must be established for each local laboratory reagent, with nomograms developed corresponding to the defined therapeutic range. Whereas for patients with venous thrombosis or pulmonary embolism, the target activated partial thromboplastin time should be equivalent to a heparin level of 0.3 to 0.7 unit/ml by anti-factor Xa heparin levels, the therapeutic range should be lower in patients receiving thrombolytics and/or GPIIb/IIIa inhibitors. Although no large-scale studies are available, we are in agreement with the recommendation of Hochman and coworkers, who proposed a therapeutic range corresponding to anti-factor Xa levels of 0.14 to 0.34 unit/ml.[378]

Because of concern about the possibility of a rebound increase in thrombin generation and recurrent ischemia after cessation of heparin therapy, some clinicians have suggested a tapering of heparin infusions rather than abrupt discontinuation together with continued aspirin.[379]

Antiplatelet Therapy

As discussed earlier (see p. 1116), platelets play a major role in the thrombotic response to rupture of a coronary artery plaque[380] (see Fig. 35-3). Platelets are activated in response to thrombolysis and platelet-rich thrombi are also more resistant to thrombolysis than are fibrin and erythrocyte-rich thrombi[381] (Fig. 35-31). Thus, there is a sound scientific basis for inhibiting platelet aggregation in *all* AMI patients, regardless of whether a thrombolytic agent is prescribed. Comprehensive overviews of randomized trials of antiplatelet therapy have summarized the overwhelming evidence of the benefit of antiplatelet therapy for a wide range of vascular disorders.[14, 382-384] In patients at risk for AMI, patients with a documented prior AMI, and patients in the acute phase of an AMI, dramatic reductions (between 25 to 50 percent in relative risk) in mortality, nonfatal reduction of recurrent infarction, and nonfatal stroke are achieved by antiplatelet therapy[14] (Fig. 35-32). Not unexpectedly, the *absolute* benefits are greatest in those patients at highest baseline risk.[14] Although several antiplatelet regimens have been evaluated, the agent most extensively tested has been aspirin, and this also is the drug for which the most compelling evidence of benefit exists.[274]

The ISIS-2 study was the largest trial of aspirin in AMI and provides the single strongest piece of evidence that aspirin reduces mortality in AMI[308] (see Fig. 35-25). Of interest, in contrast to the observations of a time-dependent mortality effect of thrombolytic therapy, the mortality reduction with aspirin was similar in patients treated within 4 hours (25 percent reduction in mortality), between 5 and 12 hours (21 percent reduction), and between 13 and 24 hours (21 percent reduction). There was an overall 23 percent reduction in mortality from aspirin in ISIS-2 that was largely additive to the 25 percent reduction in mortality from streptokinase, so that patients receiving both therapies experienced a 42 percent reduction in mortality.[308] The mortality reduction was as high as 53 percent in those patients who received both aspirin and streptokinase within 6 hours of symptoms. Of particular interest was the finding that the combination of streptokinase and aspirin reduced mortality from 23.8 to 15.8 percent (34 percent reduction) *without* increasing the risk of stroke or hemorrhage. Fibrinogen bound to the GPIIb/IIIa receptor on platelets interacts with leukocytes by means of the CD116/CD18 (Mac-1) receptor, providing a link between platelet activation and inflammatory processes in AMI.[385, 386]

Obstructive arterial thrombi that are platelet rich are resistant to thrombolysis and have an increased tendency to produce reocclusion after initial successful reperfusion in patients with ST segment elevation AMI.[47, 51a, 387] Despite the inhibition of cyclooxygenase by aspirin, platelet activation continues to occur through thromboxane A2-independent pathways, leading to platelet aggregation and increased thrombin formation. Activation of platelets by a variety of agonists results in the expression of functional receptors for fibrinogen and other ligands on the platelet surface—the GPIIb/IIIa receptor.[388] GPIIb/IIIa inhibition accelerates thrombolysis and prevents reocclusion in several animal species with experimentally induced platelet-rich coronary thromboses.[237, 389] Potential mechanistic explanations for the beneficial effects of GPIIb/IIIa inhibition when combined with thrombolytics center around important interactions between thrombolytics and platelets (see Fig. 35-31). Platelets can be stimulated by thrombolytics (e.g., by the exposure of clot-bound thrombin). A narrowed lumen and a highly stenosed infarct-related artery generate high shear forces, a potent stimulus to platelet activation. Activated platelets may inhibit thrombolysis through the release of substances such as PAI-1, alpha2-plasminogen inhibitor, and factor XIII, which stabilize the clot and also enhance clot retraction, all features that make the clot more resistant to thrombolysis. Observations such as those just noted served as the foundation for testing the hypothesis that GPIIb/IIIa inhibition is a potent and safe addition to thrombolytic regimens and introduced the concept of *combination reperfusion* for STEMI.[390]

GPIIb/IIIa INHIBITION. Reperfusion in AMI represents a potent stimulus for platelet activation and aggregation as well as activation of the coagulation cascade. Thus, GPIIb/IIIa inhibition has also been used to support PCI and stenting in AMI patients with the hopes of decreasing the risk of acute thrombotic occlusion of the infarct artery and also reducing the risk of death and cardiac ischemic events.[390]

Aspirin only partially inhibits platelet aggregation by inhibiting the thromboxane A_2 pathway. Thienopyridines such as ticlopidine and clopidogrel inhibit binding to the adenosine diphosphate receptor and also block adenosine diphosphate–dependent pathways for platelet activation. Platelet inhibition by aspirin and the thienopyridines blocks only a limited number of the pathways of platelet activation. Irrespective of the stimulus for platelet activation, the final common pathway is expression of the GPIIb/IIIa receptor on the platelet surface.[47] Therefore, direct inhibition of the GPIIb/IIIa receptor with intravenous agents such as abciximab, tirofiban, and eptifibatide has been studied in patients with AMI[391] (see Fig. 35-31).

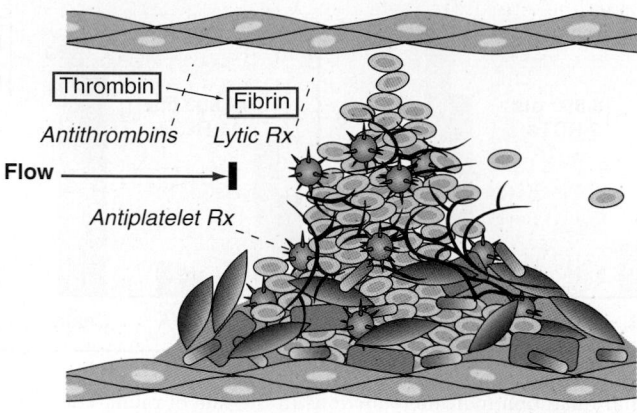

Thrombosis of epicardial coronary artery...

Thrombin → Fibrin

Antithrombins   *Lytic Rx*

Flow →

Antiplatelet Rx

...the cause of ST ↑ MI

A

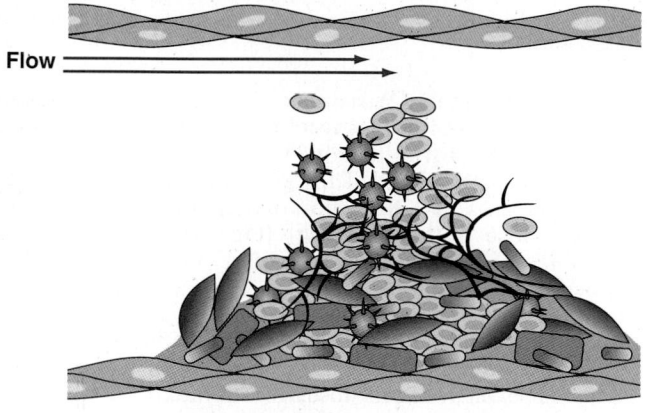

Persistent platelet aggregates and fibrin mesh...

Flow

...incomplete reperfusion with full dose lytic.

B

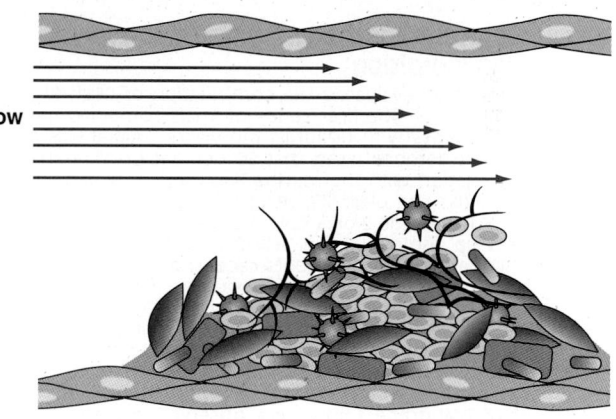

Weakened clot structure...greater penetration by lytic...

Flow

...enhanced reperfusion.

C

FIGURE 35–31. Pharmacological dissolution of thrombus in infarct-related artery. The three panels shown in this figure are schematic views of a longitudinal section of an infarct-related artery at the level of the obstructive thrombus. *A,* After rupture of a vulnerable plaque (bottom center), the coagulation cascade is activated, ultimately leading to the deposition of fibrin strands (black curvilinear arcs); platelets are activated and begin to aggregate (transition from flat discs representing inactive platelets to spiked ball elements representing activated and aggregating platelets). The mesh of fibrin strands and platelet aggregates obstructs flow (normally moving from left to right) in the infarct-related artery; this would correspond to TIMI grade 0 on angiography. Pharmacological reperfusion is a multipronged approach consisting of thrombolytics that digest fibrin, antithrombins that prevent the formation of thrombin and inhibit the activity of thrombin that is formed, and antiplatelet therapy. *B,* Full-dose thrombolysis results in incomplete reperfusion in about 50 percent of patients because of persistent platelet aggregates and fibrin strands. On angiography, this would correspond to TIMI flow grade 2. *C,* Combination reperfusion therapy with an intravenous glycoprotein IIb/IIIa inhibitor and reduced dose thrombolytic facilitates the rate and extent of thrombolysis. Prevention of platelet aggregates allows deeper penetration of the thrombolytic into the weakened clot structure, and full reperfusion (TIMI flow grade 3) is achieved. (Courtesy of Luke Welles, The Exeter Group.)

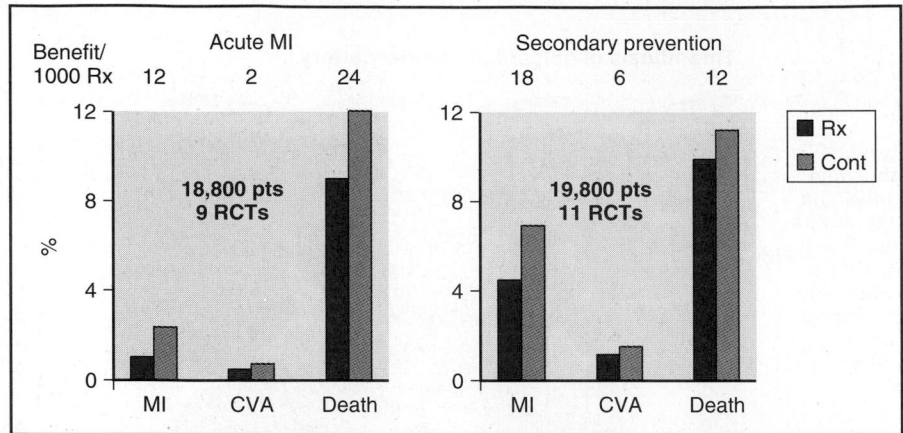

FIGURE 35–32. Antiplatelet therapy in myocardial infarction. Pooled data from randomized control trials (RCTs) of acute myocardial infarction indicate reductions in the rate of reinfarction, stroke (cerebrovascular accident [CVA]), and death in patients receiving antiplatelet therapy compared with control. Similarly, reductions in reinfarction, CVA, and death are seen in the pooled data from trials of secondary prevention with antiplatelet therapy after AMI. Based on the absolute event rates and the treatment effect for each endpoint, the benefit per 1000 patients treated with an antiplatelet agent can be calculated. (Adapted from data in Antiplatelet Trialists' Collaboration: Collaborative overview of randomised trials of antiplatelet therapy: I. Prevention of death by myocardial infarction and stroke by prolonged antiplatelet therapy in various categories of patients. BMJ 308:81–106, 1994.)

Pharmacological Reperfusion with Thrombolytic and GPIIb/IIIa Inhibition

Several clinical studies evaluated the combination of GPIIb/IIIa inhibitors and thrombolytics. The first series of trials combined full doses of thrombolytic agents with GPIIb/IIIa inhibitors. TAMI-8 was a dose-ranging study that demonstrated that 80 percent or more inhibition of platelet aggregation with the murine Fab fragments of a monoclonal antibody against the GPIIb/IIIa receptor (m7E3) could be accomplished safely.[392] TIMI grade 2 or 3 flow was seen in the infarct-related artery at follow-up angiography at day 5 in 56 percent of 9 control patients and 92 percent of 37 patients receiving m7E3 (*p* = 0.02). The IMPACT AMI trial demonstrated that patients receiving doses of eptifibatide achieving 50 to 60 percent of platelet aggregation in combination with full-dose t-PA showed an increased rate of TIMI grade 3 flow at 90 minutes (66 percent compared with 39 percent in the placebo group).[393] The streptokinase-eptifibatide trial combined full-dose streptokinase with ascending doses of eptifibatide. Although increased rates of TIMI grade 3 flow were observed in the combination arms, unacceptably high rates of major hemorrhage were also observed, leaving the investigators to conclude that eptifibatide could not be safely combined with full doses of streptokinase.[394] The Platelet Aggregation Receptor Antagonist Dose Investigation and Reperfusion Gain in Myocardial Infarction (PARADIGM) investigators compared different doses of lamifiban with either t-PA or streptokinase at standard doses.[395] Lamifiban was associated with improved ST segment resolution on continuous ECG monitoring, suggesting improved myocardial perfusion.

The combination of a reduced dose thrombolytic agent and GPIIb/IIIa inhibitor was tested in a subsequent series of trials. The TIMI 14 trial demonstrated that abciximab facilitated the rate and extent of thrombolysis, producing early, marked increases in TIMI 3 flow when combined with half the usual dose of t-PA (50 mg) (Fig. 35–33).[237] The improvement in epicardial reperfusion with reduced-dose t-PA occurred without an increase in major bleeding. Although modest improvements in TIMI 3 flow were seen when abciximab was combined with reduced doses of streptokinase, there was an increased risk of bleeding suggesting that even reduced doses of streptokinase could not be safely combined with a GPIIb/IIIa inhibitor.[237] In multivariate logistic regression analyses, after adjusting for infarct location and time from symptom onset to administration of the reperfusion regimen when compared with a full-dose thrombolytic, use of abciximab with a reduced-dose thrombolytic was associated with a significant in-

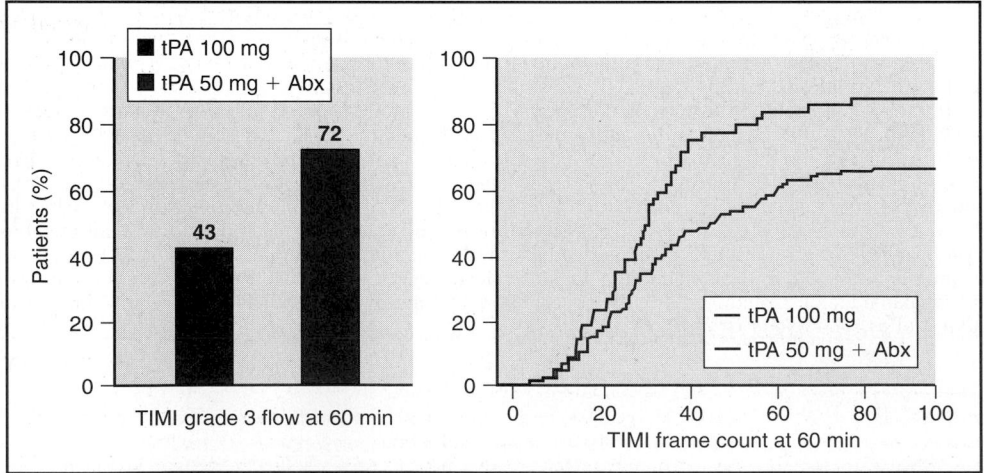

FIGURE 35–33. Abciximab (Abx) facilitates the rate and extent of thrombolysis. Compared with patients receiving full-dose t-PA (100 mg), patients receiving abciximab and reduced-dose t-PA (50 mg) had a significantly higher rate of TIMI grade 3 flow at 60 minutes after initiation of reperfusion therapy. A significantly greater proportion of patients treated with the combination reperfusion regimen had lower frame counts (i.e., faster flow).

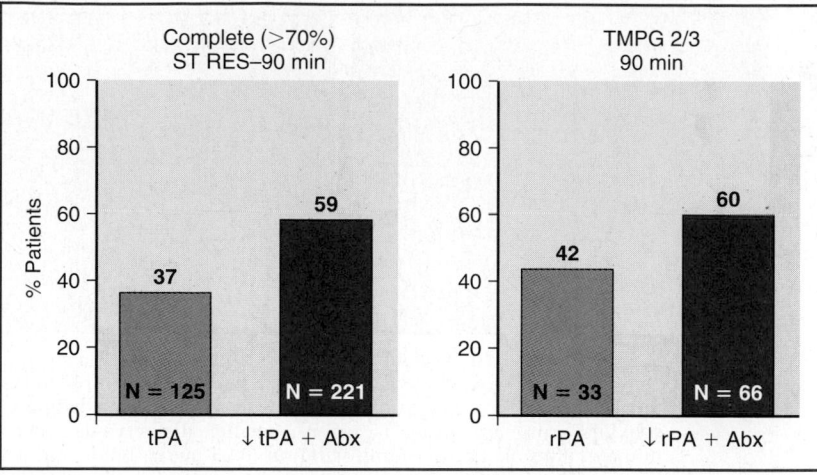

FIGURE 35–34. Improved myocardial perfusion with combination therapy. Abciximab in combination with reduced-dose thrombolytics increased the proportion of patients achieving complete ST segment resolution at 90 minutes and TIMI myocardial perfusion grade 2 or 3 at 90 minutes. TMPG = TIMI myocardial perfusion grade. (Modified from data in de Lemos JA, Antman EM, Gibson CM, et al: Circulation. 2000;101:239–43 and Antman EM, Gibson CM, de Lemos JA, et al: Combination reperfusion therapy with abciximab and reduced dose reteplase: Results from TIMI 14. Eur Heart J, 2000, in press.)

crease in the probability of achieving TIMI 3 flow and complete ST segment resolution at 90 minutes.[396] Improvement in ST segment resolution and TIMI myocardial perfusion grade was observed even among patients with normal epicardial flow, indicating that abciximab improves not only epicardial flow but also myocardial perfusion (Fig. 35–34).[396a] Combination reperfusion therapy for STEMI is being studied in GUSTO IV, a large phase III trial that will provide data on the impact of abciximab with reduced doses of reteplase on clinical outcome.

The Strategies for Patency Enhancement in the Emergency Department (SPEED) and INTRO-AMI trials evaluated abciximab with low-dose reteplase and eptifibatide with low-dose t-PA, respectively.[397, 398] Both studies showed that combination therapy with intravenous GPIIb/IIIa inhibitors and reduced doses of lytics increased the proportion of patients achieving TIMI 3 flow by 60 to 90 minutes and also facilitated rescue PTCA procedures.

GPIIb/IIIa Inhibition to Support Catheter-Based Reperfusion

Interest in the use of intravenous GPIIb/IIIa inhibitors to support primary PTCA for AMI began with a small series of patients studied by Gold and colleagues and a subset of patients in the EPIC trial.[399, 400] Promising observations included improvements in TIMI 3 flow and a

reduction in the primary composite endpoint of death, MI, or urgent revascularization in patients treated with abciximab and primary PTCA. Neumann and colleagues reported that improvement in papaverine-induced peak flow velocities and wall motion indices was seen in patients undergoing stenting for AMI when the procedure was supported by abciximab[260] (Fig. 35–35). Schömig and associates reported that in patients with AMI, coronary stenting plus abciximab led to a greater degree of myocardial salvage and a better clinical outcome than did fibrinolysis with t-PA.[260a]

Abciximab given in the emergency department in patients awaiting primary angioplasty increases the probability of achieving TIMI grade 3 flow before the procedure. Compared with an 8 percent incidence of TIMI 3 flow in the GUSTO IIB trial in patients receiving heparin and aspirin, a time-dependent increase in the proportion of patients with TIMI 3 flow was seen with 18 percent in the Glycoprotein Receptor Antagonist Patency Evaluation (GRAPE) trial (45 minutes), 23 percent in the SPEED trial (60 minutes), and 32 percent in TIMI 14 (90 minutes).[401] The ReoPro and Primary PTCA Organization and Randomized Trial (RAPPORT) was a double-blind comparison of abciximab versus placebo.[402] The composite endpoint of death, MI, or urgent target vessel revascularization was reduced from 17.8 percent in the placebo group to 11.6 percent in the abciximab group, the benefit being driven almost entirely by a 64 percent reduction in the odds of requiring urgent target vessel revascularization when abciximab was used. Major bleeding occurred significantly more frequently in the abciximab group (16.6 percent vs. 9.5 percent, $p = 0.02$) mostly at the arterial access site. The Abciximab before Direct angioplasty and stenting in Myocardial Infarction Regarding Acute and Long-term follow-up (ADMIRAL) investigators randomized AMI patients with 12 hours of symptoms to either abciximab or placebo, which was administered in the ambulance, emergency department, or catheterization

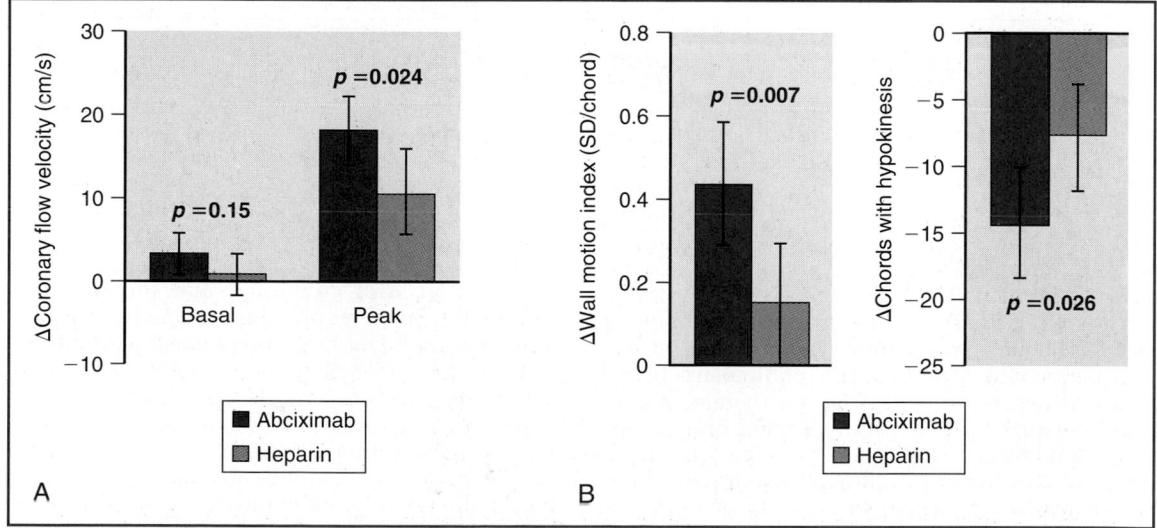

FIGURE 35–35. Effect of abciximab on myocardial flow and contractile function. *A*, Plot of differences between 14-day follow-up and initial postinterventional study in basal flow velocity and papaverine-induced flow velocity in patients treated with primary percutaneous intervention for acute MI. The columns represent mean differences. *B*, Plot of differences between 14-day follow-up and initial postinterventional study in wall motion index and in number of cords with an infarct region. (From Neumann FJ, Blasini R, Schmitt C, et al: Effect of glycoprotein IIb/IIIa receptor blockade on recovery of coronary flow and left ventricular function after the placement of coronary-artery stents in acute myocardial infarction. Circulation 98:2695–2701, 1998. Copyright 1998, American Heart Association.)

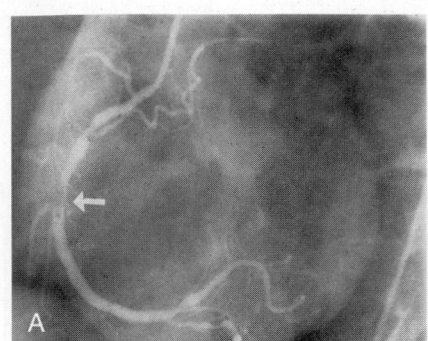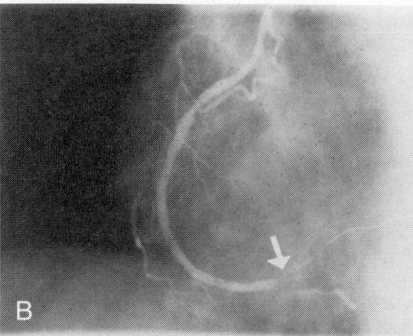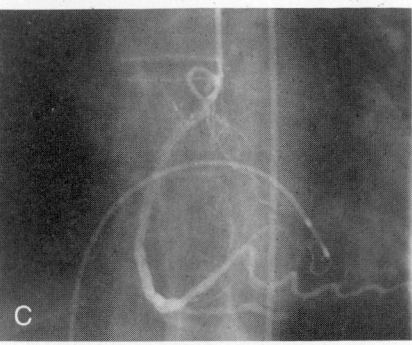

FIGURE 35–36. Glycoprotein IIb/IIIa receptor antagonists for failed rescue angioplasty. *A,* Before balloon angioplasty there is acute inferior MI with hampered flow and cardiogenic shock. A thrombus is seen in the middle of the right coronary artery (arrow). *B,* After balloon angioplasty, there is no reflow. Although proximal coronary artery is patent, smaller distal vessels are occluded (arrow). *C,* Approximately 10 minutes after abciximab administration (0.25-mg/kg bolus and a 10-μg/min infusion), coronary artery flow is restored to TIMI 3 flow. (Reproduced from Ronner E, et al: IIb/IIIa receptor antagonists for failed rescue angioplasty. Circulation 101:214–215, 2000. Copyright 2000, American Heart Association.)

laboratory as soon as AMI was diagnosed and before sheath insertion. The incidence of death/recurrent MI/urgent target vessel revascularization at 30 days was reduced by 46.5 percent with abciximab from 20.0 percent in the placebo group to 10.7 percent in the abciximab group (*p* < 0.03).[403] As was observed in the RAPPORT trial, the major benefit of abciximab was in reducing urgent target vessel revascularization.

The CADILLAC trial was designed to compare in a 2 × 2 factorial fashion the effects of balloon angioplasty (with or without abciximab) and stenting (with or without abciximab) in AMI patients presenting within 12 hours of symptoms. TIMI 3 flow was obtained after PTCA in about 95 percent of patients both with and without abciximab treatment. There was a slight reduction in the rate of TIMI 3 flow to 92.1 percent in the stent group without abciximab, which rose to 96.7 percent in patients receiving a stent in combination with abciximab. Use of abciximab was associated with reductions in target vessel revascularization and recurrent ischemia both in patients undergoing primary PTCA without stenting and those patients undergoing primary stenting.[404]

Recommendations for Antiplatelet Therapy

Some uncertainty about the optimal dose of aspirin for acute treatment of AMI remains. In general, high doses of aspirin are not more effective than lower doses but are more likely to provoke gastrointestinal side effects. However, adequate cyclooxygenase inhibition (and reduction in thromboxane A_2 production) takes several days to accomplish with less than 75 mg of aspirin, and loading doses of 160 to 325 mg (preferably chewed) are therefore recommended for all AMI patients without a history of aspirin allergy whether they present with ST segment elevation or not and whether they undergo reperfusion with thrombolytics or PTCA or are treated with a more conservative medical regimen (see Fig. 35–17). Active peptic ulcer disease is a relative contraindication to antiplatelet therapy. For patients with severe nausea and vomiting, aspirin suppositories (325 mg) can be used. Aspirin should be continued indefinitely in patients with AMI.

In patients with AMI who cannot tolerate aspirin, clopidogrel, 75 mg orally, is an acceptable alternative. Administration of intravenous GPIIb/IIIa inhibitors cannot be recommended as a routine measure after full-dose thrombolytic therapy has been given. However, as reviewed earlier they are useful to support primary PCI (Fig. 35–36).[405–407]

 ## Hospital Management

CORONARY CARE UNITS

Deaths from primary ventricular fibrillation in AMI have been prevented because the CCU allows continuous monitoring of cardiac rhythm by highly trained nurses with the authority to initiate immediate treatment of arrhythmias in the absence of physicians and because of the specialized equipment (defibrillators, pacemakers) and drugs available. Although all of these benefits can be achieved for patients scattered throughout the hospital, the clustering of patients with AMI in the CCU has greatly improved the efficient use of the trained personnel, facilities, and equipment. In recent years, with increasing emphasis on hemodynamic monitoring and treatment of the serious complications of AMI with such modalities as thrombolytic therapy, afterload reduction, and intraaortic balloon counterpulsation, the CCU has assumed even greater importance.[185] Improvements in the 30-day survival of elderly patients with AMI can be traced to advances in therapy delivered in CCUs.[408] As interventional strategies including thrombolytic therapy and acute coronary angioplasty are used more routinely in AMI patients, facilities in which patients may undergo diagnostic and therapeutic angiographic procedures are being integrated into the CCU structure.

At the same time, the value of CCUs for patients with uncomplicated AMI has been questioned and restudied.[185] With increasing attention directed to the limitation of resources and to the economic impact of intensive care, there have been efforts to select patients for whom hospitalization in a CCU would likely be of benefit. The ECG, on presentation, particularly in conjunction with previous tracings[409] and an immediate general clinical assessment, can be useful both for predicting which patients will have the diagnosis of AMI confirmed and identifying low-risk patients who may require less intensive care.[55] Among patients with a history of typical chest pain but with a normal ECG in the emergency department, less than 20 percent ultimately have an AMI on that admission, and less than 1 percent develop any significant complication. Thus, a patient with a normal ECG may not require admission to a full-fledged CCU. Careful analysis of the quality of pain may help identify such low-risk patients as well. Patients without a history of angina pectoris or MI presenting with pain that is sharp or stabbing and pleuritic, positional, or reproduced by palpation of the chest wall are extremely unlikely to have an AMI. Computer-guided decision protocols are being developed to aid clinicians in identifying those AMI patients who require admission to the CCU as opposed to a less intensive hospital ward.[174]

Contemporary CCUs typically have equipment available

for noninvasive monitoring of single or multiple ECG leads, cardiac rhythm, ST segment deviation, arterial pressure, and arterial oxygen saturation. Computer algorithms for detection and analysis of arrhythmias are superior to visual surveillance by skilled CCU staff. However, even the most sophisticated ECG monitoring systems are susceptible to artifacts due to patient movement or noise on the signal from poor skin preparation when monitoring electrodes are applied.[185] Noninvasive monitoring of arterial blood pressure using a sphygmomanometric cuff that undergoes cycles of inflation and deflation at programmed intervals is suitable for the majority of patients admitted to a CCU. Invasive arterial monitoring is preferred in patients with a low output syndrome under circumstances in which inotropic therapy is initiated for severe left ventricular failure.[185]

The CCU remains the appropriate hospital unit for patients with complicated infarctions (e.g., hemodynamic instability, recurrent arrhythmias) and those patients requiring intensive nursing care for devices such as an intraaortic balloon pump.[44] For patients with a low risk of mortality from AMI (Fig. 35–27), the clinician should consider admission to an intermediate care facility (see later) equipped with simple ECG monitoring and resuscitation equipment.[52] This strategy has been shown to be cost-effective and may reduce CCU utilization by one third, shorten hospital stays, and have no deleterious effect on patients' recovery. Intermediate-care units for low-risk AMI patients may also be appealing to patients who stand to gain little benefit from the high staffing, intense activity, and elaborate technology available in current CCUs (with their attendant high costs) and who may be disturbed by that activity and equipment.[410, 411]

RECOMMENDATIONS FOR ADMISSION TO THE CCU. The following should be considered:

1. Patients with clear-cut AMI, presenting within 12 to 24 hours of symptoms, should, in general, be admitted to a CCU. A possible exception are patients who are taken directly from the emergency department to the catheterization laboratory where they undergo a successful and uncomplicated revascularization procedure. Such patients may be considered for admission to an intermediate-care unit rather than the CCU.

2. Patients with severe unstable angina should also be admitted to the CCU, particularly if episodes of chest pain occur at rest, high doses of intravenous nitroglycerin (e.g., ≥300 mg/min) are required to relieve chest pain, or frequent adjustments of intravenous nitroglycerin infusions are required because of fluctuating symptoms and hemodynamic status (see Chap. 36).

3. Once an AMI is ruled out (ideally by 12 hours) and symptoms are controlled with oral or topical pharmacological agents, discharge from the CCU should be considered.

4. AMI patients with an uncomplicated status, such as those without a history of previous infarction, persistent ischemic-type discomfort, congestive heart failure, hypotension, heart block, or hemodynamically compromising ventricular arrhythmias, may be safely transferred out of the CCU within 24 to 36 hours.

5. In patients with a complicated AMI, the duration of the CCU stay should be dictated by the need for "intensive" care, that is, hemodynamic monitoring, close nursing supervision, intravenous vasoactive drugs, and frequent changes in the medical regimen.

General Measures for Management of AMI

The CCU staff must be sensitive to patient concerns about mortality, prognosis, and future productivity. A calm, quiet atmosphere and the "laying on of hands" with a gentle but confident touch help allay anxiety and reduce sympathetic tone, ultimately leading to a reduction in hypertension, tachycardia, and arrhythmias.[185] To reduce the risk of nausea and vomiting early after infarction and to reduce the risk of aspiration, during the first 4 to 12 hours after admission patients should receive either nothing by mouth or a clear liquid diet (Table 35–12). Subsequently, a diet with 50 to 55 percent of calories from complex carbohydrates and up to 30 percent from mono- and unsaturated fats should be given. The diet should be enriched in foods that are high in potassium, magnesium, and fiber but low in sodium (see Table 35–12).

The results of laboratory tests obtained in the CCU should be scrutinized for any derangements potentially contributing to arrhythmias, such as hypoxemia, hypovolemia, disturbances of acid-based balance or of electrolytes, and drug toxicity. Oxazepam, 15 to 30 mg orally four times a day, is useful to allay the anxiety that is common in the first 24 to 48 hours (see Table 35–12). Delirium may be provoked by medications frequently used in the CCU, including antiarrhythmic drugs, histamine-2 blockers, narcotics, and beta blockers. Potentially offending agents should be discontinued in patients with an abnormal mental status. Haloperidol, a butyrophenone, may be used safely in patients with AMI beginning with a dose of 2 mg intravenously for mildly agitated patients and 5 to 10 mg for progressively more agitated patients. Hypnotics, such as temazepam, 15 to 30 mg, or an equivalent, should be provided as needed for sleep. Dioctyl sodium sulfosuccinate, 200 mg daily, or another stool softener should be used to prevent constipation and straining (see Table 35–12).

"Coronary precautions" that do not appear to be supported by evidence from clinical research include the avoidance of iced fluids,[412] hot beverages, caffeinated beverages, rectal examinations, back rubs, and assistance with eating.[185]

PHYSICAL ACTIVITY. In the absence of complications, patients with AMI need not be confined to bed for more than 12 hours and, unless they are hemodynamically compromised, they may use a bedside commode shortly after admission (see Table 35–12). Progression of activity should be individualized depending on the patient's clinical status, age, and physical capacity.

In patients without hemodynamic compromise, early ambulation (including dangling feet on the side of the bed,

▼ **TABLE 35–12. SAMPLE ADMITTING ORDERS**

Condition:	Serious
IV:	NS or D$_5$W to keep vein open
Vital signs:	q 1/2 hr until stable, then q 4 h and prn. Notify if HR < 60 or > 110; BP < 90 or > 150; RR < 8 or > 22. Pulse oximetry × 24 hr.
Activity:	Bed rest with bedside commode and progress as tolerated after approximately 12 hr
Diet:	NPO until pain free, then clear liquids. Progress to a heart-healthy diet (complex carbohydrates = 50–55% of kilocalories), monounsaturated and unsaturated fats (≤ 30% of kilocarlories), including foods high in potassium (e.g., fruits, vegetables, whole grains, dairy products), magnesium (e.g., green leafy vegetables, whole grains, beans, seafood), and fiber (e.g., fresh fruits and vegetables, whole-grain breads, cereals).
Medications:	• Nasal O$_2$ L/min × 3 hr • Enteric-coated ASA daily (165 mg) • Stool softener daily • Beta-adrenoceptor blockers? • Consider need for analgesics, nitroglycerin, anxiolytics

NS = normal saline; D$_5$W = dextrose 5% in water; HR = heart rate; BP = blood pressure; RR = respiratory rate; NPO = nothing by mouth; ASA = acetylsalicylic acid.
From 1999 Updated ACC/AHA AMI Guidelines (Web version), p 54.

sitting in a chair, standing, and walking around the bed) does not cause important changes in heart rate, blood pressure, or pulmonary wedge pressure. Although heart rate increases slightly (usually by less than 10 percent), pulmonary wedge pressures fall slightly as the patient assumes the upright posture for activities. Early ambulatory activities are rarely associated with any symptoms; when symptoms do occur, they generally are related to hypotension. Thus, when Levine and Lown proposed the "armchair" treatment of AMI in 1952, they were undoubtedly correct that stress to the myocardium is less in the upright position.[413] As long as blood pressure and heart rate are monitored carefully, early ambulation offers considerable psychological and physical benefit without any clear medical risk.

The Intermediate Coronary Care Unit

AMI patients are at risk for late in-hospital mortality from recurrent ischemia or infarction, hemodynamically significant ventricular arrhythmias, and severe congestive heart failure after discharge from the CCU. Therefore, continued surveillance in intermediate CCUs (also called step-down units) is justifiable. Risk factors for mortality in the hospital after discharge from the CCU include significant congestive heart failure, evidenced by persistent sinus tachycardia for more than 2 days and rales greater than one third of the lung fields; recurrent VT and ventricular fibrillation; atrial fibrillation or flutter while in the CCU; intraventricular conduction delays or heart block; anterior location of infarction; and recurrent episodes of angina with marked ST segment abnormalities at low activity levels. Although it has not been shown rigorously, it is likely that a reduction in late hospital mortality can be achieved with the use of intermediate CCUs, which permits prolonged continuous monitoring of the ECG and prompt, effective treatment of ventricular fibrillation and other serious arrhythmias.

The availability of intermediate care units may also be helpful in identifying those patients who remain free of complications and are suitable candidates for early discharge from the hospital. Aggressive reperfusion protocols with angioplasty or thrombolytics can reduce length of hospital stay.[322] In patients who are believed to have undergone successful reperfusion, the *absence* of early sustained ventricular tachyarrhythmias, hypotension, or heart failure, coupled with a well-preserved LV ejection fraction, predicts a low risk of late in-hospital complications.[414] Such patients are suitable candidates for discharge from the hospital in less than 5 days from the onset of symptoms,[410] although decisions regarding the length of stay must also factor in the need to optimize medication dosages and the patient's psychological state and support systems at home.[411]

After AMI, patients are often eager for information, in need of reassurance, confused by misinformation and prior impressions, capable of counterproductive denial, and simply frightened.[185] Intermediate care facilities provide ideal settings and ample opportunities to begin the rehabilitation process.[52, 414b] The capacity for the early detection of problems after AMI and the social and educational benefits of grouping such patients together strongly argue for continued utilization of intermediate CCUs. Furthermore, the economic advantage of grouping such patients together for sharing of skilled personnel and resources outweighs any questions raised by the lack of a clear consensus regarding reduced mortality. An additional potential advantage is the facilitation of patient education in a group setting with lectures and audiovisual programs.

PHARMACOLOGICAL THERAPY

The rationale and recommendations for initiation of several pharmacological measures to treat AMI in the emergency department have been reviewed previously (see p. 1139; see Fig. 35–18). The early use of beta blockers, ACE inhibitors, calcium antagonists, nitrates, and other therapies such as magnesium and glucose-insulin-potassium is discussed in this section. Secondary prevention with some of these agents is discussed subsequently (see p. 1203).

Beta Blockers

The effects of beta blockers on AMI can be divided into those that are immediate, when the drug is given very early in the course of infarction, and long term (secondary prevention), when the drug is initiated sometime after infarction. The intravenous administration of beta-adrenoceptor blockers reduces cardiac index, heart rate, and blood pressure.[186] The net effect is a reduction in myocardial oxygen consumption per minute and per beat. Favorable effects of acute intravenous administration of beta-adrenoceptor blockers on the balance of myocardial oxygen supply and demand are reflected in reductions in chest pain, in the proportion of patients with threatened infarction who actually evolve AMI, and in the development of ventricular arrhythmias.[415] Because beta-adrenoceptor blockade diminishes circulating levels of free fatty acids by antagonizing the lipolytic effects of catecholamines and because elevated levels of fatty acids augment myocardial oxygen consumption and probably increase the incidence of arrhythmias, these metabolic actions of beta-blocking agents may also be beneficial to the ischemic heart.

Objective evidence of beneficial effects of beta blockers in AMI has been reported using the precordial ST segment mapping technique. Acute beta blockade probably reduces infarct size in AMI. Reduction in release of cardiac enzymes with beta blockade[416] is suggestive of a smaller infarct, as is the preservation of R waves and reduction in the development of Q waves.

At least 29 randomized beta blocker trials involving more than 28,970 patients have been undertaken. Intravenous, followed by oral, beta-blocker therapy is associated with about a 13 percent relative reduction in the risk of mortality[417] (Fig. 35–37). Although antagonism of sympathetic stimulation to the heart might be expected to exacerbate pulmonary edema in patients with occult heart failure, usually only small changes in pulmonary capillary wedge pressure occur when the drug is used in patients with AMI. Thus, in appropriately selected patients (Table 35–13) the

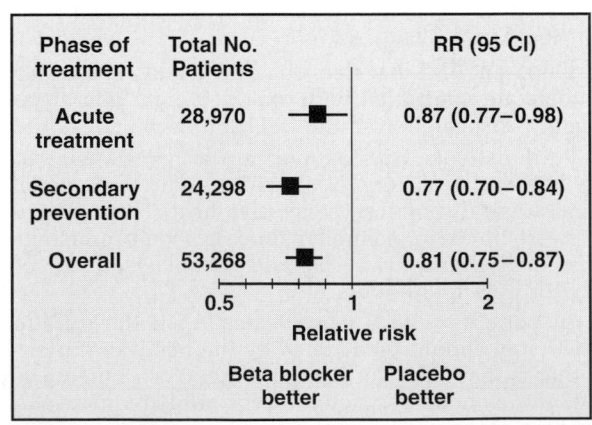

Phase of treatment	Total No. Patients	RR (95 CI)
Acute treatment	28,970	0.87 (0.77–0.98)
Secondary prevention	24,298	0.77 (0.70–0.84)
Overall	53,268	0.81 (0.75–0.87)

FIGURE 35–37. Effect of beta blockers on mortality in myocardial infarction. The relative risk of mortality is reduced with beta blockers both during the acute phase of treatment and when prescribed as secondary prevention after acute myocardial infarction. (Adapted from data in Chae CU, Hennekens CH: Beta blockers. In Hennekens CH [ed]: Clinical Trials in Cardiovascular Disease: A Companion to Braunwald's Heart Disease. Philadelphia, WB Saunders, 1999, p 84.)

▼ **TABLE 35–13. CONTRAINDICATIONS TO BETA-ADRENOCEPTOR BLOCKER THERAPY IN ACUTE MYOCARDIAL INFARCTION**

Heart rate < 60 beats/min
Systolic arterial pressure < 100 mm Hg
Moderate or severe left ventricular failure
Signs of peripheral hypoperfusion
PR interval > 0.24 second
Second- or third-degree atrioventricular block
Severe chronic obstructive pulmonary disease
History of asthma
Severe peripheral vascular disease
Insulin-dependent diabetes mellitus

From 1999 Updated ACC/AHA AMI Guidelines (Web version), p 109.

benefits just noted occur at a cost of about a 3 percent incidence of provocation of congestive heart failure or complete heart block and a 2 percent incidence of the development of cardiogenic shock.

Because reduction of infarct size in AMI patients treated with beta blockers is likely to occur only with early treatment (4 hours from the onset of pain), investigators have sought other explanations for the reduction in the mortality in the acute phase that has been observed. Intriguing observations from the ISIS-1 trial raise the possibility that a reduction in the development of cardiac rupture or electromechanical dissociation during the first day is achieved with early beta blockade.[418]

In the TIMI-II trial the addition of a beta blocker (metoprolol) to thrombolytic therapy was studied.[349] Although recurrent ischemia and reinfarction were reduced by immediate intravenous versus delayed use of metoprolol, mortality was not reduced nor was ventricular function improved. Thus, immediate intravenous beta blockade, although clinically beneficial, may not enhance salvage of myocardium in the setting of early reperfusion but may confer clinical benefit by means of its antiischemic effect.[213]

Substantial proportions of elderly patients who are hospitalized with AMI and are ideal candidates for early beta blocker therapy do not receive this treatment.[419] Compared with elderly patients who receive early beta blockade in AMI, those who do not receive beta blockade are older, more likely to be women, and less likely to be white. Elderly patients who receive early beta-blocker therapy have significantly lower in-hospital mortality rates than those who do not receive beta blockers (5.1 percent compared with 8.1 percent; $p \leq 0.001$).

RECOMMENDATIONS. Given the overwhelming evidence of benefits of early blockade in AMI, patients without a contraindication who can be treated within 12 hours of the onset of infarction, irrespective of administration of concomitant thrombolytic therapy or performance of primary angioplasty, should receive beta blockers. We do not draw a distinction between AMI patients presenting with ST segment elevation and those presenting without ST segment elevation and therefore consider early beta blockade applicable across the entire spectrum of acute coronary syndromes. For patients presenting within 12 hours of the onset of symptoms or for those presenting with overactivity of the sympathetic nervous system, we prefer to begin beta-blocker therapy intravenously. For patients presenting after 12 hours, especially if there is little sympathetic overactivity, it is our practice to begin beta-blocker therapy orally. Beta blockers are especially helpful in patients in whom infarction is complicated by persistent or recurrent ischemic pain, by progressive or repetitive serum enzyme elevations suggestive of infarct extension, or by tachyarrhythmias early after the onset of infarction. If adverse effects of beta blockers develop or if patients present with complica-

tions of infarction that are contraindications to beta blockade such as heart failure or heart block, the beta blocker should be withheld. Unless there are contraindications (see p. 1243), beta blockade probably should be continued in patients who develop AMI.

Selection of Beta Blocker. Favorable effects have been reported with atenolol, timolol, and alprenolol; these benefits probably occur with propranolol and with esmolol, an ultra–short-acting agent, as well. In the absence of any favorable evidence supporting the benefit of agents with intrinsic sympathomimetic activity, such as pindolol and oxprenolol, and with some unfavorable evidence for these agents in secondary prevention,[420] beta blockers with intrinsic sympathomimetic activity probably should not be chosen for treatment of AMI. Occasionally, the clinician may wish to proceed with beta-blocker therapy even in the presence of relative contraindications, such as a history of mild asthma, mild bradycardia, mild heart failure, or first-degree heart block. In this situation, a trial of esmolol may help determine whether the patient can tolerate beta blockade.[188, 420] Because the hemodynamic effects of this drug, with a half-life of 9 minutes, disappear in less than 30 minutes, it offers considerable advantage over longer-acting agents when the risk of a beta blocker complication is relatively high.

ACE Inhibitors

In 1992, with the publication of the Survival and Ventricular Enlargement (SAVE) trial,[421] ACE inhibitors were established as an important addition to the list of treatments for AMI. The rationale for their use includes experimental and clinical evidence of a favorable impact on ventricular remodeling, improvement in hemodynamics, and reductions in congestive heart failure.[78, 191] There is now unequivocal evidence from randomized, placebo-controlled mortality trials that ACE inhibitors reduce death from AMI.[199b] These trials may be grouped into two categories. The first *selected* AMI patients for randomization, based on features indicative of increased mortality such as left ventricular ejection fraction less than 40 percent,[421] clinical signs and symptoms of congestive heart failure,[422] anterior location of infarction,[423] and abnormal wall motion score index[424] (Fig. 35–38). The second group were *unselective* trials that randomized all patients with AMI provided they had a minimum systolic pressure of approximately 100 mm Hg (ISIS-4,[425] GISSI-3,[426] Cooperative North Scandinavian Enalapril Survival Study [CONSENSUS] II,[427] and Chinese Captopril Study[428]) (Fig. 35–39). With the exception of the Survival

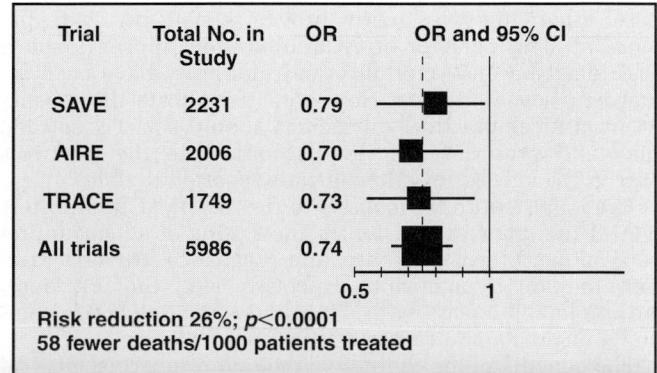

FIGURE 35–38. Effect of angiotensin-converting enzyme inhibitors on mortality after myocardial infarction: Results from the long-term trials. (From Flather MD, Pfeffer MA: Angiotensin-converting enzyme inhibitors. *In* Hennekens CH [ed]: Clinical Trials in Cardiovascular Disease: A Companion to Braunwald's Heart Disease. Philadelphia, WB Saunders, 1999, p 97.)

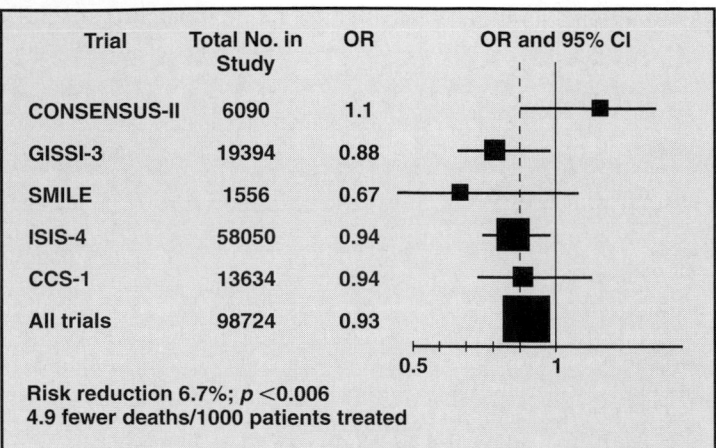

Trial	Total No. in Study	OR	OR and 95% CI
CONSENSUS-II	6090	1.1	
GISSI-3	19394	0.88	
SMILE	1556	0.67	
ISIS-4	58050	0.94	
CCS-1	13634	0.94	
All trials	98724	0.93	

Risk reduction 6.7%; $p < 0.006$
4.9 fewer deaths/1000 patients treated

FIGURE 35–39. Effects of angiotensin-converting enzyme inhibitors on mortality after myocardial infarction: results from the short-term trials. (From Flather MD, Pfeffer MA: Angiotensin-converting enzyme inhibitors. *In* Hennekens CH [ed]: Clinical Trials in Cardiovascular Disease: A Companion to Braunwald's Heart Disease. Philadelphia, WB Saunders, 1999, p 101.)

of Myocardial Infarction Long-term Evaluation (SMILE) trial,[423] all of the selective trials initiated ACE inhibitor therapy between 3 and 16 days after AMI and maintained it for 1 to 4 years, whereas the unselective trials all initiated treatment within the first 24 to 36 hours and maintained it for only 4 to 6 weeks.

A consistent survival benefit was observed in all of the trials already noted, except for CONSENSUS II, the only study that used an intravenous preparation early in the course of AMI.[427] Estimates of the mortality benefit of ACE inhibitors in the unselective, short duration of therapy trials was 5 per 1000 patients treated.[429, 430] Analysis of these unselective short-term trials indicates that approximately one third of the lives saved occurred within the first 1 to 2 days. Certain subgroups such as those with anterior infarction showed proportionately greater benefit from early administration (11 lives saved/1000) of ACE inhibitors. Not unexpectedly, greater survival benefits of 42 to 76 lives saved per 1000 patients treated were obtained in the *selective, long* duration of therapy trials. Of note, there was generally a 20 percent reduction in the risk of death attributable to ACE inhibitor treatment in the selective trials. The mortality reduction with ACE inhibitors is accompanied by significant reductions in the development of congestive heart failure, supporting the underlying pathophysiological rationale for administering this class of drugs in AMI.[421, 422, 424, 426] In addition, some data suggest that ischemic events, including recurrent infarction and the need for coronary revascularization, can also be reduced by chronic administration of ACE inhibitors after an AMI.[431]

The mortality benefits of ACE inhibitors are additive to those achieved with aspirin and beta blockers.[421, 426] Thus, ACE inhibitors should not be considered a substitute for these other therapies with proven benefit in AMI patients.[199b] The benefits of ACE inhibition appear to be a class effect because mortality and morbidity have been reduced by several agents. However, to replicate these benefits in clinical practice, physicians should select a specific agent and prescribe the drug according to the protocols used in the successful clinical trials reported to date.

The major *contraindications* to the use of ACE inhibitors in AMI include hypotension in the setting of adequate preload, known hypersensitivity, and pregnancy. Adverse reactions include hypotension, especially after the first dose, and intolerable cough with chronic dosing; much less commonly angioedema can occur (see Chap. 18).

The benefits of an alternative method of pharmacological inhibition of the renin-angiotensin system by angiotensin-II receptor antagonists is being evaluated in the VALIANT[431a] and Optimal Therapy in Myocardial Infarction with the Angiotensin II Antagonist Losartan, (OPTIMAAL) trials.[432]

RECOMMENDATIONS. After administration of aspirin and initiating reperfusion strategies and, where appropriate, beta blockade, *all* AMI patients should be considered for ACE inhibition therapy. Although there is little disagreement that high-risk AMI patients (elderly, anterior infarction, prior infarction, Killip class II or greater, and asymptomatic patients with evidence of depressed global ventricular function on an imaging study) should receive life-long treatment with ACE inhibitors,[191, 433] therapy to a broader group of patients has also been proposed based on the pooled results of the unselective mortality trials.[425] Considering all the available data, we favor a strategy of an initial trial of oral ACE inhibitors in all AMI patients with congestive heart failure as well as in hemodynamically stable patients with ST segment elevation or left bundle branch block, commencing within the first 24 hours.[430, 434] Recommendations for chronic use of ACE inhibitors are discussed on p. 1203.

Nitrates

Sublingual nitroglycerin very rarely opens occluded coronary arteries. However, in patients with AMI the potential for reductions in ventricular filling pressures, wall tension, and cardiac work coupled with improvement in coronary blood flow, especially in ischemic zones, and antiplatelet effects make nitrates a logical and attractive pharmacological intervention in AMI.[435, 436]

In patients with AMI, the administration of nitrates reduces pulmonary capillary wedge pressure and systemic arterial pressure, left ventricular chamber volume, infarct size, and the incidence of mechanical complications. As with other interventions to spare ischemic myocardium in AMI, intravenous nitroglycerin appears to be of greatest benefit in patients treated earliest after the onset of symptoms.

CLINICAL TRIAL RESULTS. In the prethrombolytic era, 10 randomized trials of acute administration of intravenous nitroglycerin (or nitroprusside, another nitric oxide donor) collectively enrolled 2042 patients. A meta-analysis of these trial results showed a reduction in mortality of 35 percent associated with nitrate therapy.

In the thrombolytic era two megatrials of nitrate therapy have been conducted—GISSI-3[426] and ISIS-4.[425] In GISSI-3, there was no independent effect of nitrates on short-term mortality.[426] Similarly, in ISIS-4, no effect of a mononitrate on 35-day mortality was observed. A pooled analysis of over 80,000 patients treated with nitrate-like preparations intravenously or orally in 22 trials revealed a mortality rate of 7.7 percent in the control group, which was reduced to 7.4 percent in the nitrate group. These data are consistent with a small treatment effect of nitrates on mortality such that three to four fewer deaths would occur for every 1000 patients treated.[425]

**NITRATE PREPARATIONS AND MODE OF ADMINISTRA-
TION.** Intravenous nitroglycerin can be administered safely to patients with evolving MI as long as the dose is titrated carefully to avoid induction of reflex tachycardia or systemic arterial hypotension. Patients with inferior wall infarction are particularly sensitive to an excessive fall in preload, particularly if concurrent right ventricular infarction is present.[52] In such cases nitrate-induced venodilatation could impair cardiac output and reduce coronary block flow, thus worsening myocardial oxygenation rather than improving it.

A useful regimen employs an initial infusion rate of 5 to 10 μg/min with increases of 5 to 20 μg/min until the mean arterial blood pressure is reduced by 10 percent of its baseline level in normotensive patients and by 30 percent for hypertensive patients, but in no case below a systolic pressure of 90 mm Hg. Alternatively, nitroglycerin may be administered as a sustained-release oral preparation (30 to 60 mg/d) or as an ointment (1 to 3 inches every 6 to 8 hours for patients with a systolic pressure greater than 120 mm Hg). Nitroglycerin can also be given sublingually at doses of 0.3 to 0.6 mg. This route may be more hazardous because the rate of absorption is difficult to control and arterial pressure may decline precipitously.

ADVERSE EFFECTS. Clinically significant methemoglobinemia has been reported to occur during administration of intravenous nitroglycerin. Although uncommon, this problem is seen when unusually large doses of nitrates are administered. It is important not only for its potential to cause symptoms of lethargy and headache but also because elevated methemoglobin levels can impair the oxygen-carrying capacity of blood, potentially exacerbating ischemia. Dilatation of the pulmonary vasculature supplying poorly ventilated lung segments may produce a ventilation-perfusion mismatch.

Tolerance to intravenous nitroglycerin (as manifested by increasing nitrate requirements) develops in many patients, often as soon as 12 hours after the infusion is started. Despite the theoretical and demonstrated benefit of sulfhydryl agents in diminishing tolerance, their use has not become widespread.

RECOMMENDATIONS. Nitroglycerin is indicated for the relief of persistent pain and as a vasodilator in patients with infarction associated with left ventricular failure. In the absence of recurrent angina or congestive heart failure, we do not routinely prescribe them in AMI patients. Higher-risk patients such as those with large transmural infarctions, especially of the anterior wall, have the most to gain from nitrates in terms of reduction of ventricular remodeling, and we therefore routinely use intravenous nitrates for 24 to 48 hours in such patients. There is no clear benefit to empirical long-term cutaneous or oral nitrates in the asymptomatic patient, and we therefore do not prescribe nitrates beyond the first 48 hours unless angina or ventricular failure is present.

Calcium Antagonists

Despite sound experimental and clinical evidence of an antiischemic effect, calcium antagonists have *not* been found to be helpful in the acute phase of AMI; concern has been raised in several systematic overviews about an increased risk of mortality when they are prescribed on a routine basis to AMI patients.[186, 437, 438] Perhaps in response to the lack of compelling data showing a beneficial effect and concerns about the risk of excess mortality coupled with more convincing evidence of benefit from aspirin and beta blockers, many clinicians have decreased their use of calcium antagonists in the setting of AMI.[26, 439] A distinction should be made between the dihydropyridine type of calcium antagonists (e.g., nifedipine) and the nondihydro-

pyridine calcium antagonists (e.g., verapamil and diltiazem).[437]

NIFEDIPINE. In multiple trials involving a total of over 5000 patients, the immediate-release preparation of nifedipine has not shown any reduction in infarct size, prevention of progression to infarction, control of recurrent ischemia, or lowering of mortality. When trials of the immediate-release form of nifedipine are pooled in a meta-analysis, evidence suggests a dose-related increased risk of in-hospital mortality (especially above 80 mg of nifedipine),[438, 440] although post-hospital mortality does not appear to be increased in nifedipine-treated patients.[441] Nifedipine does not appear to be helpful in conjunction with either thrombolytic therapy or beta blockade.[442] A potential mechanism by which the immediate-release form of nifedipine may be harmful in AMI is coronary hypoperfusion due to an abrupt fall in systolic pressure from peripheral vasodilatation. The abrupt fall in arterial pressure may also provoke a reflex action of the renin-angiotensin system and sympathetic discharge that produces tachycardia. Thus, we do not recommend use of immediate-release nifedipine early in the treatment of AMI. No trials of the sustained-release preparations of nifedipine in AMI have been reported to date.

VERAPAMIL AND DILTIAZEM. When administered during the acute phase of AMI, these drugs have not had any demonstrated favorable effect on infarct size or other important endpoints in patients with AMI, with the exception of control of supraventricular arrhythmias.[443] Although the possibility has been raised that verapamil and diltiazem in the first few days after AMI may be helpful in preventing reinfarction in patients with non-Q-wave infarction,[443-445] the data supporting this contention are not statistically robust and require further evaluation in future studies. Subgroup analyses of the Multicenter Diltiazem Postinfarction Trial (MDPIT) and the Danish Verapamil Infarction Trial (DAVIT)-II with both diltiazem and verapamil have suggested that mortality is reduced in patients free of heart failure in the CCU.[446, 447] These subgroup analyses must be interpreted with caution because in the MDPIT study about 50 percent of patients in the placebo and diltiazem groups were also receiving beta blockers that may have contributed to the observed mortality reduction[446]; in the DAVIT-II study patients with an indication for beta blockers were excluded from the trial.[447] Furthermore, both the MDPIT and DAVIT-II studies were conducted in an era when aspirin, ACE inhibitors, and early use of coronary angiography for recurrent ischemia were not as common as they are now. The Incomplete Infarction Trial of European Research Collaborators Evaluating Prognosis Post-Thrombolysis (INTERCEPT) trial is testing the hypothesis that sustained-release diltiazem will decrease death and cardiac ischemic events in patients receiving thrombolytic therapy for a first AMI.[448]

RECOMMENDATIONS. Based on the available data, we do *not* recommend the routine use of either verapamil or diltiazem in AMI regardless of whether it is believed that the patient is suffering from a Q-wave or non-Q-wave infarction.[449] Verapamil and diltiazem may be given for relief of ongoing ischemia or slowing of a rapid ventricular response in atrial fibrillation in patients for whom beta blockers are ineffective or contraindicated.[52] Their use should be avoided in patients with Killip class II or greater hemodynamic findings.

MAGNESIUM

Patients with AMI may have a total body deficit of magnesium because of a low dietary intake, advanced age, or prior diuretic use. They may also acquire a functional deficit of available magnesium due to trapping of free magnesium in adipocytes, because soaps are formed when free fatty acids are released by catecholamine-induced lipolysis with the onset of infarction. Myocardial and urinary losses of magnesium that occur during AMI may increase a patient's magnesium requirement. The magnesium cation serves as a critical cofactor in over 300 intracellular enzymatic processes, including several that are integrally involved in mitochondrial function, energy production, maintenance of trans-sarcolemmal ionic gradients, cell volume control, and resting membrane potential.[450] Experimental models of AMI in at least four different animal species have shown that supplemental administration of magnesium before coronary occlusion, during occlusion, coincident with reperfusion, or for a short time interval (15 to 45 minutes) after reperfusion reduces infarct size and prevents myocardial stunning due to reperfusion injury.[208] However, delayed administration of magnesium beyond a very short interval (15 to 60 minutes) after reperfusion is no longer effective in reducing myocardial damage.[208]

Since 1984, several trials of routine supplemental administration of intravenous magnesium in patients with suspected AMI have been conducted. Synthesis of all the trials published before ISIS-4 suggests that the treatment effect of magnesium is greatest in patients at highest risk of mortality and decreases progressively as the mortality risk in the control population decreases.[208] Despite its large sample size, the negative results for magnesium in ISIS-4 do not conclusively exclude benefits of magnesium in AMI. The control group mortality was 7.2 percent in ISIS-4 compared with 7.6 percent in the magnesium group.[425] Given the low control group mortality rate in ISIS-4, the lack of a beneficial effect of magnesium was not unexpected. In addition, ISIS-4 required that acute phase treatment for MI, including lytic therapy, be administered before randomization and that study drugs such as magnesium be administered beyond the "early" lytic phase (e.g., first hour). Because the time for randomization to actual administration of magnesium was not recorded in ISIS-4, the actual relationship between reperfusion and timing of administration of magnesium cannot be determined with certainty but the available information suggests that magnesium was administered relatively late in ISIS-4—a second feature that may have biased ISIS-4 toward a null effect of magnesium. In contrast, Shechter and associates reported a reduction in mortality with magnesium in a high-risk population of patients who were considered unsuitable for thrombolysis.[451] Because of the trivial cost of magnesium, its ease of administration, widespread availability, and the fact that it has the potential to reduce mortality in high-risk AMI patients, another large-scale randomized multicenter trial (Magnesium in Coronaries [MAGIC]) is underway to define more explicitly the role of magnesium in AMI.[452]

RECOMMENDATIONS. Because of the risk of cardiac arrhythmias when electrolyte deficits are present in the early phase of infarction, all patients with AMI should have a serum magnesium measurement on admission. We advocate repleting magnesium deficits to maintain a serum magnesium level of 2.0 mEq/liter or more. In the presence of hypokalemia (< 4.0 mEq/liter) during the course of treatment of AMI, the serum magnesium level should be rechecked and repleted if necessary because it is often difficult to correct a potassium deficit in the presence of a concurrent magnesium deficit. Episodes of torsades de pointes should be treated with 1 to 2 gm of magnesium delivered as a bolus over about 5 minutes. Although routine early (ideally < 6 hours from the onset of chest pain) supplemental magnesium administration may be helpful in certain high-risk patients such as the elderly or those for whom reperfusion therapy is contraindicated,[52] additional data are needed before definite recommendations regarding patient selection and dosing can be made. There does not appear to be any benefit to routine late (> 6 hours) administration of magnesium to patients with uncomplicated AMI who do not have electrolyte deficits.

Because it may cause vasodilation and hypotension, magnesium infusions should not be administered in patients with a systolic pressure less than 80 to 90 mm Hg. Patients with renal failure may not excrete magnesium normally and should not be considered candidates for supplemental magnesium infusions.

Other Approaches

GLUCOSE-INSULIN-POTASSIUM. Administration of a solution of glucose-insulin-potassium (300 gm of glucose, 50 units of insulin, and 80 mEq of KCl in 1000 ml of water administered at a rate of 1.5 ml/kg/hr) lowers the concentration of plasma free fatty acids and improves ventricular performance, as reflected in systolic arterial pressure, cardiac output, and stroke work at any level of left ventricular filling pressure; also the frequency of VPBs decreases.[453] Fath-Ordoubadi and Beatt reported in a meta-analysis of nine studies conducted be-

tween 1965 and 1987 enrolling a cumulative total of 1932 patients that the mortality rate was reduced from 21 percent in the placebo group to 16.1 percent in the glucose-insulin-potassium group (OR 0.72, 95 percent CI 0.57–0.90; p = 0.004).[454] Subsequently, the Estudios Cardiologicos Latinoamerica (ECLA) group performed a randomized trial of AMI patients treated within 24 hours of onset of symptoms.[455] Mortality was reduced from 15.2 percent in the control group to 5.2 percent in the glucose-insulin-potassium group for the subset of patients who received thrombolysis (OR 0.34; 95 percent CI 0.15–0.77; p = 0.01). The findings from the ECLA study raise the possibility that therapeutic metabolic manipulation in AMI patients may be a fruitful avenue of investigation, particularly in specific patient subgroups such as those with left ventricular hypertrophy and those for whom there is a delay until the performance of a primary catheter-based reperfusion procedure.[456, 457]

The Diabetes Mellitus Insulin–Glucose Infusion in Acute Myocardial Infarction (DIGAMI) study reported a significant 30 percent relative decrease in mortality at 1 year in diabetics with AMI who received a strict regimen of an insulin-glucose infusion for 24 hours, followed by 3 months of subcutaneous injections of insulin four times daily as compared with standard therapy[458] (Fig. 35–40). Thus, "infusions of glucose-insulin-potassium (GIK) may provide necessary metabolic support for the ischemic myocardium; this may be particularly important in patients with large anterior infarcts and cardiogenic shock."[84]

INTRAAORTIC BALLOON COUNTERPULSATION. (See also Chap. 19.) From a theoretical standpoint, intraaortic balloon counterpulsation might be expected to limit infarct size for several reasons. In experimental animals, intraaortic balloon counterpulsation decreases preload, increases coronary blood flow, and improves cardiac performance. No definitive information is available, indicating that intraaortic balloon counterpulsation alters the prognosis in patients with relatively uncomplicated infarction. The Second Primary Angioplasty in Myocardial Infarction (PAMI-II) investigators randomized high-risk patients undergoing primary PTCA to 36 to 48 hours of intraaortic balloon counterpulsation treatment versus traditional care. There was no significant difference in the predefined composite endpoint of death, reinfarction, infarct-related artery reocclusion, stroke, or new-onset heart failure/hypotension in patients treated with an intraaortic balloon counterpulsation versus those treated conservatively.[350] Intraaortic balloon counterpulsation also did not result in enhanced myocardial recovery after PTCA.

Given the relatively frequent rate of complications after intraaortic balloon insertion and the absence of convincing data for infarct size reduction, intraaortic balloon pumping should be reserved for hemodynamically compromised patients and for those with refractory ischemia. Although noninvasive external forms of counterpulsation have been developed, these approaches have not been rigorously studied in patients with AMI.

OTHER AGENTS. Oxygen-derived free radicals are abundant in ischemic tissue and may contribute to myocardial injury, particularly after

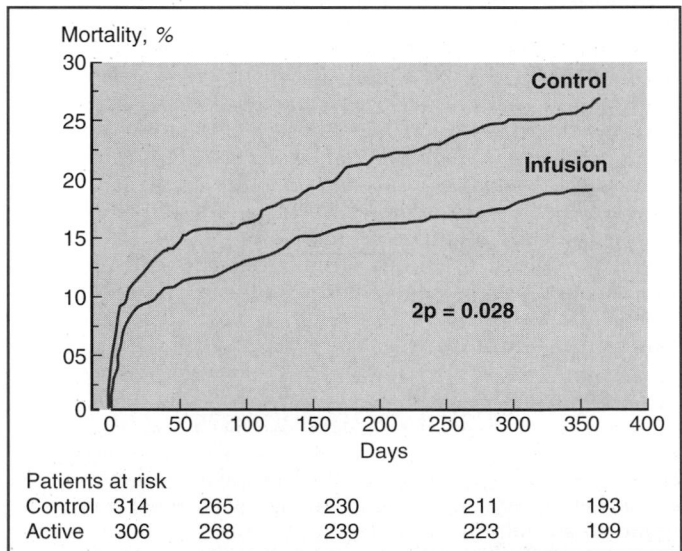

FIGURE 35–40. Actuarial mortality curves in patients receiving insulin-glucose infusion and in control subjects of the Diabetes Mellitus Insulin-Glucose Infusion in Acute Myocardial Infarction (DIGAMI) study during 1 year of follow-up. Numbers below graph indicate the number of patients at different times of observation. Active = patients receiving infusion. (From Malmberg K, Ryden L, Efendic S, et al: Randomized trial of insulin glucose infusion followed by subcutaneous insulin treatment in diabetic patients with acute myocardial infarction (DIGAMI Study): Effects on mortality at 1 year. J Am Coll Cardiol 26:57, 1995.)

reperfusion (see Chap. 34). Although evidence from studies in animals suggested that the extent of myocardial necrosis and postischemic dysfunction can be affected favorably by treatment with oxygen free radical scavengers such as superoxide dismutase,[195] initial results in patients have not been encouraging. Given the important role that nitric oxide (NO) plays in regulating platelet activation, interest has arisen in developing techniques for increasing NO production or providing exogenous NO donors in the setting of AMI other than the nitrates discussed earlier. Adenosine, a widely used pharmacological stress agent for detection of coronary artery disease, has been shown in animal models of reperfusion injury to decrease infarct size. The AMISTAD trial tested the hypothesis that a 3-hour infusion of adenosine as an adjunct to thrombolysis would reduce myocardial infarct size.[262] Although there was a reduction in infarct size as determined by single-photon emission computed tomographic cardiac im-

aging, this observation was restricted to patients with an anterior infarction. Despite the reduction in left ventricular infarct size in the adenosine group, in-hospital clinical outcomes were similar between the two treatment groups.

Previous studies suggested that poloxamer 188 (RheothRx) reduces infarct size and improves left ventricular function. However, the Collaborative Organization for RheothRx Evaluation (CORE) trial showed no effect on the composite endpoint of mortality, reinfarction, or cardiogenic shock but did increase the risk of renal failure in patients with AMI.[459] The HALT-AMI trial tested whether a humanized IgG4 monoclonal antibody that binds to CD11b/CD18 receptors on leukocytes, would reduce MI size in patients treated with primary angioplasty.[460] Although the study drug was well tolerated when given just before angioplasty, no significant reduction in infarct size or major cardiac adverse events was seen.

▼ Hemodynamic Disturbances

HEMODYNAMIC ASSESSMENT

In patients with clinically uncomplicated AMI, invasive hemodynamic monitoring is *not* necessary because the status of the circulation can be assessed by careful clinical evaluation. This ordinarily consists of monitoring of heart rate and rhythm, repeated measurement of systemic arterial pressure by cuff, obtaining chest roentgenograms to detect heart failure, careful and repeated auscultation of the lung fields for pulmonary congestion, measurement of urine flow, examination of the skin and mucous membranes for evidence of the adequacy of perfusion, and arterial sampling for PO_2, PCO_2, and pH when hypoxemia or metabolic acidosis is suspected.

In contrast, in patients with AMI whose ventricular contractile performance is not normal, it is important to assess the degree of hemodynamic compromise to initiate therapy with drugs such as vasodilators and diuretics. In the past, central venous or right atrial pressure was used to gauge the degree of left ventricular failure in patients with AMI. However, this technique is fraught with error because central venous pressure actually reflects right rather than left ventricular function. Right ventricular function and therefore systemic venous pressure may be normal or nearly so in patients with significant left ventricular failure. Conversely, patients with right ventricular failure due to right ventricular infarction or pulmonary embolism may exhibit elevated right atrial and central venous pressures despite normal left ventricular function. Low values for right atrial and central venous pressures imply hypovolemia, whereas elevated right atrial pressures usually result from right ventricular failure secondary to left ventricular failure, pulmonary hypertension, or right ventricular infarction or less commonly from tricuspid regurgitation or pericardial tamponade.

Major advances in the management of AMI have resulted from the hemodynamic monitoring that has become widespread in CCUs[461, 462] (Table 35–14). This often consists of both an intraarterial catheter and a pulmonary artery catheter for measurement of pulmonary artery, pulmonary artery occlusive (equivalent to pulmonary wedge) and right atrial pressures, and cardiac output by thermodilution. In patients with hypotension, a Foley catheter provides accurate and continuous measurement of urine output.

NEED FOR INVASIVE MONITORING. The use of invasive hemodynamic monitoring is based on the following principal factors:

1. Difficulty of interpreting clinical and radiographic findings of pulmonary congestion because of phase lags, such as those occurring after diuretic therapy. Severe depression of cardiac index and/or elevation of left ventricular filling pressure may be unsuspected in as many as 15 percent of patients when estimates are based exclusively on clinical criteria.

2. Need for identifying noncardiac causes of arterial hypotension, particularly hypovolemia.

3. Possible contribution of reduced ventricular compliance to impaired hemodynamics, requiring judicious adjustment of intravascular volume to optimize left ventricular filling pressure.

4. Difficulty in assessing the severity and sometimes even determining the presence of lesions such as mitral regurgitation and ventricular septal defect when the cardiac output or the systemic pressures are depressed.

5. Establishing a baseline of hemodynamic measurements and guiding therapy in patients with clinically apparent pulmonary edema or cardiogenic shock.

6. Underestimation of systemic arterial pressure by the cuff method in patients with intense vasoconstriction.

The prognosis and the clinical status are related to both the cardiac output and the pulmonary artery wedge pressure. Patients with normal cardiac output after AMI have an extremely low expected mortality; prognosis worsens as cardiac output declines. Patients with intraventricular conduction defects, AV block, or both after anterior infarction have lower cardiac indices and higher pulmonary capillary wedge pressures than do patients without these conduction disturbances. On the other hand, patients with these conduction defects and inferior MI usually do not demonstrate such hemodynamic abnormalities.

PULMONARY ARTERY PRESSURE MONITORING. Patients most likely to benefit from pulmonary artery catheter moni-

▼ TABLE 35–14. INDICATIONS FOR HEMODYNAMIC MONITORING OF ACUTE MYOCARDIAL INFARCTION

Management of complicated AMI
  Hypovolemia vs. cardiogenic shock
  Ventricular septal rupture vs. acute mitral regurgitation
  Severe left ventricular failure
  Right ventricular failure
Refractory ventricular tachycardia
Differentiating severe pulmonary disease from left ventricular
  failure
Assessment of cardiac tamponade
Assessment of therapy in *selected* individuals
  Afterload reduction in patients with severe left ventricular
    failure
  Inotropic agent therapy
  Beta blocker therapy
  Temporary pacing (ventricular vs. atrioventricular)
  Intraaortic balloon counterpulsation
  Mechanical ventilation

From Gore JM, Zwernet PL: Hemodynamic monitoring of acute myocardial infarction. *In* Francis GS, Alpert JS (eds): Modern Coronary Care. Boston, Little, Brown & Co, 1990, p 138.

toring include those whose AMI is complicated by (1) hypotension that is not easily corrected by fluid administration; (2) hypotension in the presence of congestive heart failure; (3) hemodynamic compromise severe enough to require intravenous vasopressors or vasodilators or intraaortic balloon counterpulsation; (4) mechanical lesions (or suspected ones) such as cardiac tamponade, severe mitral regurgitation, and a ruptured ventricular septum; and (5) right ventricular infarction.[63] Other indications for hemodynamic monitoring include assessment of the effects of mechanical ventilation, differentiating pulmonary disease from left ventricular failure as the cause of hypoxemia, and management of septic shock[185] (see Table 35–14).

Before inserting a pulmonary artery catheter into a patient with an AMI, the physician must decide that the potential benefit of the information to be obtained outweighs any potential risks. Major complications from pulmonary artery catheters are relatively rare (3 to 5 percent of cases), but severe problems can occur, including sepsis, pulmonary infarction, and pulmonary artery rupture. By minimizing the duration of catheterization and by strict adherence to aseptic techniques, risk can be diminished.[462a] Catheter-related bloodstream infections can also be reduced by using antiseptic-impregnated catheters.[463]

Accurate determination of hemodynamics by clinical assessment is difficult in critically ill patients. The use of a pulmonary artery catheter often leads to important changes in therapy that would not have occurred if the hemodynamic information had not been available. Of note, reports exist that complications and mortality may be higher in patients who undergo pulmonary artery catheterization, although such patients are often at higher risk initially. These observations emphasize the importance of patient selection, meticulous technique, and correct interpretation of the data obtained.

Hemodynamic Abnormalities

In 1976, Swan, Forrester, and their associates measured the cardiac output and wedge pressure simultaneously in a large series of patients with AMI and identified four major hemodynamic subsets of patients (Table 35–15): (1) patients with normal perfusion and without pulmonary congestion (normal cardiac output and normal wedge pressure), (2) patients with normal perfusion and pulmonary congestion (normal cardiac output and elevated wedge pressure), (3) patients with decreased perfusion but without pulmonary congestion (reduced cardiac output and normal wedge pressure), and (4) patients with decreased perfusion and pulmonary congestion (reduced cardiac output and elevated wedge pressure). This classification, which overlaps with a crude clinical classification proposed earlier by Killip and Kimball (see Table 35–15), has proved to be quite useful, but it should be noted that patients frequently pass from one category to another with therapy and sometimes apparently even spontaneously.

HEMODYNAMIC SUBSETS. These are usually reflected in the patient's clinical status. Hypoperfusion usually becomes evident clinically when the cardiac index falls below approximately 2.2 liters/min/m², whereas pulmonary congestion is noted when the wedge pressure exceeds approximately 20 mm Hg. However, approximately 25 percent of patients with cardiac indices less than 2.2 liters/min/m² and 15 percent of patients with elevated pulmonary capillary wedge pressures are not recognized clinically. Discrepancies in hemodynamic and clinical classification of patients with AMI arise for a variety of reasons. Patients may exhibit "phase lags" as clinical pulmonary congestion develops or resolves, symptoms secondary to chronic obstructive pulmonary disease may be confused with those resulting from pulmonary congestion, or longstanding left ventricular dysfunction may mask signs of hypoperfusion secondary to compensatory vasoconstriction.[69]

The hemodynamic findings shown in Tables 35–15 and 35–16 allow for rational approaches to therapy. The goals of hemodynamic therapy are to maintain ventricular performance, support blood pressure, and protect jeopardized myocardium. Because these goals occasionally may be at cross-purposes, recognition of the hemodynamic profile, as assessed clinically or as available from hemodynamic monitoring, is required before optimal therapeutic interventions can be designed along the lines discussed here.

Hypotension in the Prehospital Phase

During the prehospital phase of AMI, invasive hemodynamic monitoring is not feasible; during this period, therapy should be guided by frequent clinical assessment and measurement of arterial pressure by cuff, with the recognition that intense vasoconstriction can provide a falsely low pressure measured by this method. Hypotension associated with bradycardia often reflects excessive vagotonia. Relative or absolute hypovolemia is often present when hypotension occurs with a normal or rapid heart rate, particularly among patients receiving diuretics just before the occurrence of infarction. Marked diaphoresis, reduction of fluid intake, or vomiting during the period preceding and accompanying the onset of AMI may all contribute to the development of hypovolemia. Even if the effective vascular volume is normal, relative hypovolemia may be present because ventricular compliance is reduced in AMI and a left ventricular filling pressure as high as 20 mm Hg may be needed to provide an optimal preload.

MANAGEMENT. In the absence of rales involving more than one third of the lung fields, the patient should be put in the reverse Trendelenburg position, and in those with

▼ **TABLE 35–15.** HEMODYNAMIC CLASSIFICATIONS OF PATIENTS WITH ACUTE MYOCARDIAL INFARCTION

A. BASED ON CLINICAL EXAMINATION[a]		B. BASED ON INVASIVE MONITORING[b]	
Class	**Definition**	**Subset**	**Definition**
I	Rales and S₃ absent	I	Normal hemodynamics PCWP < 18, CI > 2.2
II	Rales over < 50% of lung	II	Pulmonary congestion PCWP > 18, CI < 2.2
III	Rales over > 50% of lung fields (pulmonary edema)	III	Peripheral hypoperfusion PCWP < 18, CI > 2.2
IV	Shock	IV	Pulmonary congestion and peripheral hypoperfusion PCWP > 18, CI < 2.2

PCWP = pulmonary capillary wedge pressure; CI = cardiac index.
Modified from Killip T, Kimball J: Treatment of myocardial infarction in a coronary care unit: A two year experience with 250 patients. Am J Cardiol 20:457, 1967; and Forrester J, Diamond G, Chatterjee K, et al: Medical therapy of acute myocardial infarction by the application of hemodynamic subsets. N Engl J Med 295:1356, 1976.

CARDIAC CONDITION	CHAMBER PRESSURE (mm Hg)				
	RA	RV	PA	PCW	CI
Normal	0–6	25/0–6	25/0–12	6–12	≥ 2.5
AMI without LVF	0–6	25/0–6	30/12–18	≤ 18	≥ 2.5
AMI with LVF	0–6	30–40/0–6	30–40/18–25	> 18	> 2.0
Biventricular failure	> 6	50–60/>6	50–60/25	18–25	> 2.0
RVMI	12–20	30/12–20	30/12	≤ 12	< 2.0
Cardiac tamponade	12–16	25/12–16	25/12–16	12–16	< 2.0
Pulmonary embolism	12–20	50–60/12–20	50–60/12	< 12	< 2.0

AMI = acute myocardial infarction; CI = cardiac index; LVF = left ventricular failure; PA = pulmonary artery; PCW = pulmonary capillary wedge; RA = right atrium; RV = right ventricle; RVMI = right ventricular myocardial infarction.

From Gore JM, Zwerner PL: Hemodynamic monitoring of acute myocardial infarction. In Francis GS, Alpert JS (eds): Modern Coronary Care, pp 139–164, 1990.

sinus bradycardia and hypotension, atropine should be administered (0.3 to 0.6 mg intravenously repeated at 3- to 10-minute intervals up to 2.0 mg). If these measures do not correct the hypotension, normal saline should be administered intravenously, beginning with a bolus of 100 ml followed by 50-ml increments every 5 minutes. The patient should be carefully observed and the infusion stopped when the systolic pressure returns to approximately 100 mm Hg, if the patient becomes dyspneic, or if pulmonary rales develop or increase. Because of the poor correlation between LV filling pressure and mean right atrial pressure, assessment of systemic (even central) venous pressure is of limited value as a guide to fluid therapy.

Administration of cardiotonic agents is indicated during the prehospital phase if systemic hypotension persists despite correction of hypovolemia and excessive vagotonia. In the absence of invasive hemodynamic monitoring, assessment of peripheral vascular resistance must be based on clinical observations. If cutaneous vasoconstriction is present, therapy with dobutamine, which stimulates cardiac contractility without unduly accelerating heart rate and which does not increase the impedance to ventricular outflow, may be helpful (see Chap. 18). In hypotensive patients with AMI with clinical evidence of vasodilatation, an uncommon circumstance, phenylephrine hydrochloride, is preferable, although this agent, which increases coronary as well as peripheral vascular tone, should be used with caution.

Hypovolemic Hypotension

Recognition of hypovolemia is of particular importance in hypotensive patients with AMI because of the hazard it poses and because of the improvement in circulatory dynamics that can be achieved so readily and safely by augmentation of vascular volume. Because hypovolemia is often occult, it is frequently overlooked in the absence of invasive hemodynamic monitoring. Hypovolemia may be absolute, with low LV filling pressure (8 mm Hg) or relative, with normal (8 to 12 mm Hg) or even modestly increased (13 to 18 mm Hg) left ventricular filling pressures. Because of the reduction of left ventricular compliance that occurs with acute ischemia and infarction (see Chap. 34), LV filling pressures between 13 and 18 mm Hg, although above the upper limits of normal, may actually be suboptimal.

Exclusion of hypovolemia as the cause of hypotension requires the documentation of a reduced cardiac output despite left ventricular filling pressure exceeding 18 mm Hg. If, in a hypotensive patient, the pulmonary capillary wedge pressure (ordinarily measured as the pulmonary artery occlusive pressure) is below this level, fluid challenge should be carried out as described previously. If hypovolemia is documented or suspected, the fluid replaced should resemble the fluid lost. Thus, when a low hematocrit complicates AMI, infusion of packed red blood cells or whole blood is the treatment of choice. On the other hand, crystalloid or colloid solutions should be administered when the hematocrit is normal or elevated.

Hypotension caused by right ventricular infarction may be confused with that caused by hypovolemia because both are associated with a low, normal, or minimally elevated LV filling pressure. The findings and management of right ventricular infarction are discussed on page 1180.

The Hyperdynamic State

When infarction is not complicated by hemodynamic impairment, no therapy other than general supportive measures and treatment of arrhythmias is necessary. However, if the hemodynamic profile is of the hyperdynamic state (i.e., elevation of sinus rate, arterial pressure, and cardiac index, occurring singly or together in the presence of a normal or low LV filling pressure) and if other causes of tachycardia such as fever, infection, and pericarditis can be excluded, treatment with beta-adrenoceptor blockers is indicated. Presumably, the increased heart rate and blood pressure are the result of inappropriate activation of the sympathetic nervous system, possibly secondary to augmented release of catecholamines, pain and anxiety, or some combination of these.

LEFT VENTRICULAR FAILURE

Even in the thrombolytic era, left ventricular dysfunction remains the single most important predictor of mortality after AMI (Fig. 35–41).[20, 22] In patients with AMI, heart failure is characterized either by systolic dysfunction alone or by both systolic and diastolic dysfunction. Left ventricular diastolic dysfunction leads to pulmonary venous hypertension and pulmonary congestion, whereas systolic dysfunction is principally responsible for a depression of cardiac output and of the ejection fraction. Clinical manifestations of left ventricular failure become more common as the extent of the injury to the left ventricle increases. In addition to infarct size, other important predictors of the development of symptomatic left ventricular dysfunction include advanced age and diabetes.[464] Mortality increases in association with the severity of the hemodynamic deficit.[69]

THERAPEUTIC IMPLICATIONS. Classification of patients with AMI by hemodynamic subsets has therapeutic relevance. As already noted, patients with normal wedge pressures and hypoperfusion often benefit from infusion of fluids, because the peak value of stroke volume is usually not attained until LV filling pressure reaches 18 to 24 mm Hg. However, a low level of left ventricular filling pressure

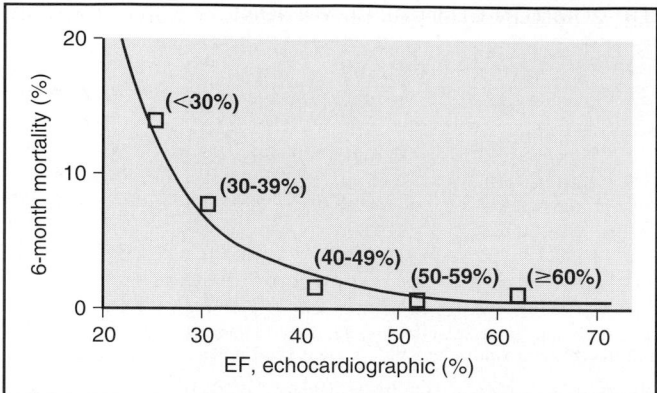

FIGURE 35–41. Impact of left ventricular function on survival after myocardial infarction. The curvilinear relationship between left ventricular ejection fraction (LVEF) for patients treated in the thrombolytic era is shown. Among patients with an LVEF below 40 percent, mortality is markedly increased at 6 months. Thus, interventions such as thrombolysis, aspirin, and angiotensin-converting enzyme (ACE) inhibitors should be of considerable benefit in patients with acute myocardial infarction to minimize the amount of left ventricular damage and interrupt the neurohumoral activation seen with congestive heart failure. (Adapted from Volpi A, De VC, Franzosi MG, et al: Determinants of 6-month mortality in survivors of myocardial infarction after thrombolysis: Results of the GISSI-2 data base. The Ad Hoc Working Group of the Gruppo Italiano per lo Studio della Sopravvivenza nell'Infarto Miocardico (GISSI)-2 Data Base. Circulation 88:416–429, 1993. Copyright 1993, American Heart Association.)

does not imply that left ventricular damage is necessarily slight. Such patients may be relatively hypovolemic and/or may have suffered a right ventricular infarct with or without severe left ventricular damage.

The relation between ventricular filling pressure and cardiac index when preload is increased by an infusion of saline or dextran can provide valuable hemodynamic information, in addition to that obtained from baseline measurements. For example, the ventricular function curve rises steeply (marked increase in cardiac index, small increase in filling pressure) in patients with normal left ventricular function and hypovolemia, whereas the curve rises gradually or remains flat in those patients with a combination of hypovolemia and depressed cardiac function.

Invasive hemodynamic monitoring is essential to guide therapy for patients with severe left ventricular failure (pulmonary capillary wedge pressure > 18 mm Hg *and* cardiac index < 2.5 liters/min/m²).

AVOIDANCE OF HYPOXEMIA. Patients whose AMI is complicated by congestive heart failure characteristically develop hypoxemia due to a combination of pulmonary vascular engorgement (and in some cases pulmonary interstitial edema), diminished vital capacity, and respiratory depression from narcotic analgesics. Hypoxemia can impair the function of ischemic tissue at the margin of the infarct and thereby contribute to establishing or perpetuating the vicious circle (see Fig. 35–11). The ventilation-perfusion mismatch that results in hypoxemia requires careful attention to ventilatory support. Increasing fractions of inspired oxygen (FIO₂) via face mask should be used initially, but if the oxygen saturation of the patient's blood cannot be maintained above 85 to 90 percent on 100 percent FIO₂, strong consideration should be given to endotracheal intubation with positive-pressure ventilation. The improvement of arterial oxygenation and hence myocardial oxygen supply may help to restore ventricular performance. Positive end-expiratory pressure (PEEP) may diminish systemic venous return and reduce effective left ventricular filling pressure. This may require reduction in the amount of PEEP, normal saline infusions to maintain LV filling pressure, ad-

justment of the rate of infusion of vasodilators such as nitroglycerin, or some combination. Because myocardial ischemia frequently occurs during the return to unsupported spontaneous breathing, the weaning process should be accompanied by observation for signs of ischemia and is potentially facilitated by a period of intermittent mandatory ventilation or pressure support ventilation before extubation. Continuous ST segment monitoring has been recommended for these patients.

When wheezing complicates pulmonary congestion, bronchodilators that act primarily on beta₂-adrenoceptors, such as metaproterenol, given as an aerosol, or terbutaline, are more desirable than conventional bronchodilators such as isoproterenol or epinephrine. The latter act primarily on beta₁-receptors, which, by increasing myocardial oxygen consumption, can increase ischemia. Racemic beta₂ agonists are composed of a 50:50 mixture of R and S isomers. The R isomers exhibit virtually all the bronchodilation, whereas the S isomers enhance bronchial reactivity to methacholine, eosinophil activation, and histamine-induced influx of fluid, proteins, and neutrophils into the airspaces. As suggested by Handley, use of pure R isomers of beta₂-adrenoceptor agonists may permit bronchodilation with few beta-adrenoceptor–mediated side effects.[465]

Although positive inotropic agents may be useful, they do not represent the initial therapy of choice in patients with AMI. Instead, heart failure is managed most effectively first by reduction of ventricular preload and then, if possible, by lowering afterload. Arrhythmias may contribute to hemodynamic compromise and should be treated promptly in patients with left ventricular failure.

DIURETICS. (See also Chap. 18.) Mild heart failure in patients with AMI frequently responds well to diuretics such as furosemide, administered intravenously in doses of 10 to 40 mg, repeated at 3- to 4-hour intervals if necessary. The resultant reduction of pulmonary capillary pressure reduces dyspnea, and the lowering of LV wall tension that accompanies the reduction of LV diastolic volume diminishes myocardial oxygen requirements and may lead to improvement of contractility and augmentation of the ejection fraction, stroke volume, and cardiac output. The reduction of elevated LV filling pressure may also enhance myocardial oxygen delivery by diminishing the impedance to coronary perfusion attributable to elevated ventricular wall tension. It may also improve arterial oxygenation by reducing pulmonary vascular congestion.

The intravenous administration of furosemide reduces pulmonary vascular congestion and pulmonary venous pressure within 15 minutes, before renal excretion of sodium and water has occurred; presumably this action results from a direct dilating effect of this drug on the systemic arterial bed. It is important not to reduce left ventricular filling pressure much below 18 mm Hg, the lower range associated with optimal left ventricular performance in AMI, because this may reduce cardiac output further and cause arterial hypotension. Excessive diuresis may also result in hypokalemia, with its attendant risk of digitalis intoxication.

AFTERLOAD REDUCTION. (See also Chap. 18.) Myocardial oxygen requirements depend on LV wall stress, which in turn is proportional to the product of peak developed left ventricular pressure, volume, and wall thickness. Vasodilator therapy is recommended in patients with AMI complicated by (1) heart failure unresponsive to treatment with diuretics, (2) hypertension, (3) mitral regurgitation, or (4) ventricular septal defect. In these patients, treatment with vasodilator agents increases stroke volume and may reduce myocardial oxygen requirements and thereby lessen ischemia. Hemodynamic monitoring of systemic arterial and, in many cases, pulmonary capillary wedge (or at least pulmonary artery) pressure and cardiac output in patients treated with these agents is important. Improvement of cardiac performance and energetics requires three simultaneous effects: (1) reduction of LV afterload, (2) avoidance of excessive systemic arterial hypotension in order to maintain effective coronary perfusion pressure, and (3) avoidance of excessive reduction of ventricular filling pressure with consequent diminution of cardiac output. In general, pulmonary capillary wedge pressure should be maintained at approximately 20 mm Hg and arterial pressure above 90/60 mm Hg in patients who were normotensive before developing the AMI.

Vasodilator therapy is particularly useful when AMI is complicated by mitral regurgitation or rupture of the ventricular septum. In such patients, vasodilators alone or in combination with intraaortic balloon counterpulsation can sometimes serve as a "holding maneuver" and provide hemodynamic stabilization to permit definitive catheterization and angiographic studies to be carried out and to prepare the patient for early surgical intervention. Because of the precarious state of patients with complicated infarction and the need for meticulous adjustment of dosage, therapy is best initiated with agents that can be administered intravenously and that have a short duration of action, such as nitroprusside, nitroglycerin, or isosorbide dinitrate. After initial stabilization, the medication of choice is generally an ACE inhibitor, but long-acting nitrates given by mouth, sublingually, or by ointment may also be useful.

Nitroglycerin. (See also Chap. 36.) This drug has been shown in animal experiments to be less likely than nitroprusside to produce a "coronary steal" (i.e., to divert blood flow from the ischemic to the nonischemic zone). Therefore, apart from consideration of its routine use in AMI patients discussed earlier (see p. 1170), it may be a particularly useful vasodilator in patients with AMI complicated by left ventricular failure. Ten to 15 μg/min is infused, and the dose is increased by 10 μg/min every 5 minutes until (1) the desired effect (improvement of hemodynamics or relief of ischemic chest pain) is achieved or (2) a decline in systolic arterial pressure to 90 mm Hg, or by more than 15 mm Hg, has occurred. Although both nitroglycerin and nitroprusside lower systemic arterial pressure, systemic vascular resistance, and the heart rate/systolic blood pressure product, the reduction of LV filling pressure is more prominent with nitroglycerin because of its relatively greater effect than nitroprusside on venous capacitance vessels. Nevertheless, in patients with severe left ventricular failure, cardiac output often increases despite the reduction in LV filling pressure produced by nitroglycerin.

Oral Vasodilators. The use of oral vasodilators in the treatment of chronic congestive heart failure is discussed in Chapter 21. In patients with AMI and persistent heart failure, long-term treatment with a converting enzyme inhibitor should be carried out. This reduced ventricular load decreases the remodeling of the left ventricle that occurs commonly in the period after MI and thereby reduces the development of heart failure and risk of death.[72]

DIGITALIS. (See also Chap. 18.) Although digitalis increases the contractility and the oxygen consumption of normal hearts, when heart failure is present the diminution of heart size and wall tension frequently results in a net reduction of myocardial oxygen requirements. In animal experiments it fails to improve ventricular performance immediately after experimental coronary occlusion, but salutary effects are elicited when it is administered several days later. The absence of early beneficial effects may be due to the inability of ischemic tissue to respond to digitalis or the already maximal stimulation of contractility of the normal heart by circulating and neuronally released catecholamines.

Although the issue is still controversial, arrhythmias may be increased by digitalis glycosides when they are given to patients in the first few hours after the onset of MI, particularly in the absence of hypokalemia. Also, undesirable peripheral systemic and coronary vasoconstriction may

result from the rapid intravenous administration of rapidly acting glycosides such as ouabain.

Administration of digitalis to patients with AMI in the hospital phase should generally be reserved for the management of supraventricular tachyarrhythmias such as atrial flutter and fibrillation and of heart failure that persists despite treatment with diuretics, vasodilators, and beta-adrenoceptor agonists. There is no indication for its use as an inotropic agent in patients without clinical evidence of left ventricular dysfunction, and it is too weak an inotropic agent to be relied on as the principal cardiac stimulant in patients with overt pulmonary edema or cardiogenic shock. It may, however, be useful as a supplement to vasodilator agents and in the maintenance phase of treatment for persistent or recurrent left ventricular failure.[466]

Cardiac glycosides appear to become progressively more effective in the treatment of heart failure as the interval from onset of infarction lengthens; that is, they are more effective in the treatment of chronic than of acute heart failure secondary to ischemic heart disease. Of note, in a direct comparison of captopril versus digoxin for prevention of left ventricular remodeling and dysfunction after AMI, patients in whom captopril therapy was initiated 7 to 10 days after onset of infarction had less left ventricular remodeling and better preserved global left ventricular function than patients receiving digitalis. In addition, the possibility that continued administration of digitalis might contribute to late mortality in the 2 years after AMI has been raised[467–469] and debated.[470, 471] Although it is clear that mortality is greater in patients treated with digoxin after AMI, it is not clear that this increase in mortality is due to digoxin itself or to confounding variables that correlate with use of digoxin.[471] At this time, digoxin appears to be indicated in AMI patients only if they exhibit supraventricular tachyarrhythmias or overt heart failure that is not adequately controlled by ACE inhibitors and diuretics.

BETA-ADRENOCEPTOR AGONISTS. When left ventricular failure is severe, as manifested by marked reduction of cardiac index (< 2 liters/min/m²), and pulmonary capillary wedge pressure is at optimal (18 to 24 mm Hg) or excessive (> 24 mm Hg) levels despite therapy with diuretics, beta-adrenoceptor agonists are indicated. Although isoproterenol is a potent cardiac stimulant and improves ventricular performance, it should be avoided in AMI patients. It also causes tachycardia and augments myocardial oxygen consumption and lactate production; in addition, it reduces coronary perfusion pressure by causing systemic vasodilation and in animal experiments it increases the extent of experimentally induced infarction. Norepinephrine also increases myocardial oxygen consumption because of its peripheral vasoconstrictor as well as positive inotropic actions.

Dopamine and dobutamine (see Chap. 18) may be particularly useful in patients with AMI and reduced cardiac output, increased left ventricular filling pressure, pulmonary vascular congestion, and hypotension. Fortunately, the potentially deleterious alpha-adrenergic vasoconstrictor effects exerted by dopamine occur only at higher doses than those required to increase contractility. Its vasodilating actions on renal and splanchnic vessels and its positive inotropic effects generally improve hemodynamics and renal function. In patients with AMI and severe left ventricular failure, this drug should be administered at a dose of 3 μg/kg/min while monitoring pulmonary capillary wedge and systemic arterial pressures as well as cardiac output. The dose may be increased stepwise to 20 μg/kg/min, to reduce pulmonary capillary wedge pressure to approximately 20 mm Hg and elevate cardiac index to exceed 2 liters/min/m². However, it must be recognized that doses exceeding 5 μg/kg/min activate peripheral alpha receptors and cause vasoconstriction.

Dobutamine has a positive inotropic action comparable to that of dopamine but a slightly less positive chronotropic effect and less vasoconstrictor activity. In patients with AMI, dobutamine improves left ventricular performance without augmenting enzymatically estimated infarct size.[472] It may be administered in a starting dose of 2.5 μg/kg/min and increased stepwise to a maximum of 30 μg/kg/min. Both dopamine and dobutamine must be given carefully and with constant monitoring of the ECG, systemic arterial pressure, and pulmonary artery or pulmonary artery occlusive pressure and, if possible, with frequent measurements of cardiac output. The dose must be reduced if the heart rate exceeds 100 to 110 beats/min, if supraventricular or ventricular tachyarrhythmias are precipitated, or if ST segment changes increase.

OTHER POSITIVE INOTROPIC AGENTS. Milrinone is a noncatecholamine, nonglycoside, phosphodiesterase inhibitor with inotropic and vasodilating action (see Chap. 18). It is useful in selected patients whose heart failure persists despite treatment with diuretics, who are not hypotensive, and who are likely to benefit from both an enhancement in contractility and afterload reduction. Milrinone should be given as a loading dose of 50 μg/kg over 10 minutes, followed by a maintenance infusion of 0.375 to 0.75 μg/kg/min.

CARDIOGENIC SHOCK

This severest clinical expression of left ventricular failure is associated with extensive damage to the left ventricular myocardium (about 40 percent) in more than 80 percent of AMI patients in whom it occurs; the remainder have a mechanical defect such as ventricular septal or papillary muscle rupture or predominant right ventricular infarction.[473, 473a] In the past, cardiogenic shock has been reported to occur in up to 20 percent of patients with AMI,[474] but estimates from recent large randomized trials of thrombolytic therapy and observational data bases report an incidence rate in the range of 7 percent.[192, 475] About 10 percent of patients with cardiogenic shock present with this condition at the time of admission, whereas 90 percent develop it during hospitalization. This low-output state is characterized by elevated ventricular filling pressures, low cardiac output, systemic hypotension, and evidence of vital organ hypoperfusion (e.g., clouded sensorium, cool extremities, oliguria, acidosis).[190] Patients with cardiogenic shock due to AMI are more likely to be older, to have a history of a prior MI or congestive heart failure, and to have sustained an anterior infarction at the time of development of shock.[190, 475a] Of note, although the incidence of cardiogenic shock in AMI has been relatively stable since the mid 1970s, the short-term mortality decreased from 70 to 80 percent in the 1970s to 50 to 60 percent in the 1990s.[475] Cardiogenic shock is the cause of mortality in about 60 percent of patients dying after thrombolysis for AMI.[476]

PATHOLOGICAL FINDINGS. At autopsy, more than two thirds of patients with cardiogenic shock demonstrate stenosis of 75 percent or more of the luminal diameter of all three major coronary vessels, usually including the left anterior descending coronary artery. Almost all patients with cardiogenic shock are found to have thrombotic occlusion of the artery supplying the major region of recent infarction with loss of about 40 percent of the left ventricular mass.[473] Other causes of cardiogenic shock in AMI include mechanical defects such as rupture of the ventricular septum, a papillary muscle, or a free wall with tamponade; right ventricular infarction[473]; or marked reduction of preload due to conditions such as hypovolemia.[477]

Patients who die as a consequence of cardiogenic shock often have "piecemeal" necrosis, that is, progressive myocardial necrosis from marginal extension of their infarct into an ischemic zone bordering on the infarction. This is generally associated with persistent elevation of CK-MB. Early deterioration in left ventricular function secondary to apparent extension of infarction may, in some cases, result from expansion of the necrotic zone of myocardium without actual extension of the necrotic process (Fig. 35-42). Shear forces that develop during ventricular systole can disrupt necrotic myocardial muscle bundles, with resultant expansion and thinning of the akinetic zone of myocardium, which in turn results in deterioration of overall left ventricular function.

At autopsy, patients with cardiogenic shock consistently demonstrate marginal extension of recent areas of infarction. Additionally, focal areas of necrosis are frequently found in regions of the left and right ventricles that are not adjacent to the major area of recent infarction. Such extensions and focal lesions are probably in part the result of the shock state itself, because they can also be found in the hearts of patients dying of noncardiogenic shock. Infarction of the ischemic periinfarction zone can be precipitated by a number of factors that adversely affect the supply of oxygen or the metabolic demand in this zone of myocardium. These include a reduction of coronary perfusion pressure that causes impaired myocardial perfusion in the presence of atherosclerotic obstructions of the nonculprit artery. An augmentation of myocardial oxygen demand resulting from the local release of catecholamines from ischemic adrenergic nerve endings in the heart as well as from circulating

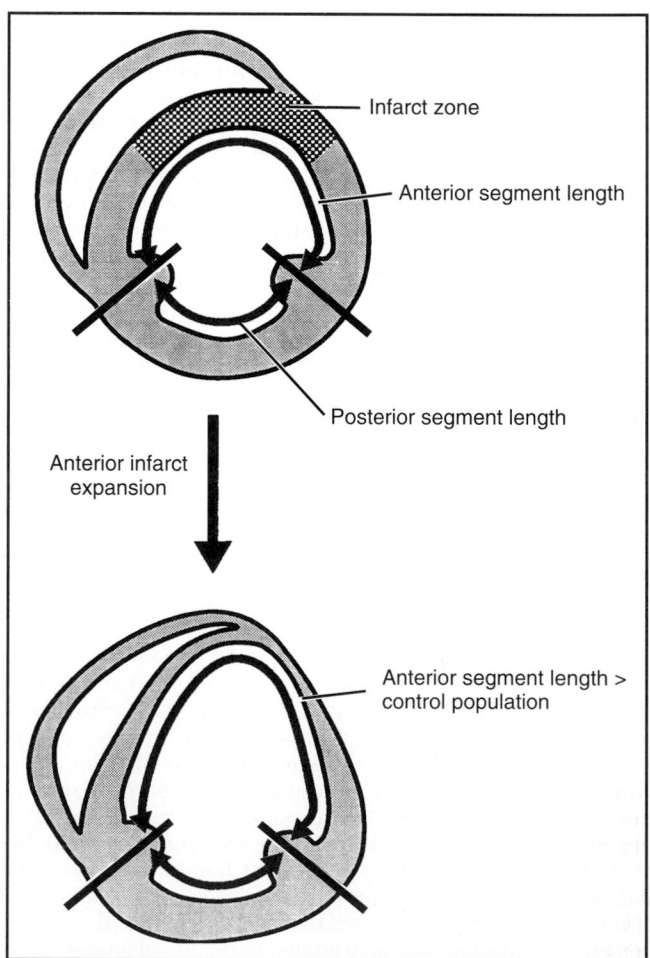

FIGURE 35-42. Infarct expansion after transmural anterior myocardial infarction. (From Tice FD, Kisslo J: Echocardiographic assessment and monitoring of the patient with AMI: Prospects for the thrombolytic era. *In* Califf RM, Mark DB, Wagner GS (eds): Acute Coronary Care. St. Louis, Mosby–Year Book, 1995, p 496.)

endogenous or infused catecholamines may also play a role. Patients with shock due to a mechanical defect often have smaller infarcts than do those with cardiogenic shock secondary to ventricular failure without a mechanical lesion. The prognosis is better in such patients because the smaller infarct allows their left ventricle to support the circulation if the mechanical defect has been corrected surgically.

PATHOPHYSIOLOGY. The shock state in patients with AMI appears to be the result of a vicious circle, demonstrated in Figure 35–11 (see p. 1124).[190] According to this formulation, coronary obstruction leads to myocardial ischemia, which impairs myocardial contractility and ventricular performance. This, in turn, reduces arterial pressure and therefore coronary perfusion pressure, leading to further ischemia and extension of necrosis until the left ventricle has insufficient contracting myocardium to sustain life. The progressive nature of the myocardial insult in this syndrome is reflected in the stuttering and progressive evolution of elevations in the plasma enzyme–time activity curves of markers specific for myocardial injury. Consideration of the vicious circle also points to the hazard of hypovolemic hypotension in patients with AMI but without cardiogenic shock. Hypotension, whatever its cause, reduces coronary perfusion, especially of myocardium in the territory of obstructive arteries, and thereby may enhance necrosis.

DIAGNOSIS. Cardiogenic shock is characterized by marked and persistent (> 30 min) hypotension with systolic arterial pressure less than 80 mm Hg and a marked reduction of cardiac index (generally < 1.8 liters/mm/m²) in the face of elevated LV filling pressure (pulmonary capillary wedge pressure > 18 mm Hg). Spurious estimates of LV filling pressure based on measurements of the pulmonary artery wedge pressure can occur in the presence of marked mitral regurgitation, in which the tall v wave in the left atrial (and pulmonary artery wedge) pressure tracing elevates the mean pressure above LV end-diastolic pressure. Accordingly, mitral regurgitation and other mechanical lesions, such as ventricular septal defect, ventricular aneurysm, and pseudoaneurysm, must be excluded before the diagnosis of cardiogenic shock due to impairment of left ventricular function can be established. Mechanical complications should be suspected in any patient with AMI in whom circulatory collapse occurs.[190] Immediate hemodynamic, angiographic, and echocardiographic evaluations are necessary in patients with cardiogenic shock. It is important to exclude mechanical complications because primary therapy of such lesions usually requires immediate operative treatment with intervening support of the circulation by intraaortic balloon counterpulsation.

Medical Management

When the aforementioned mechanical complications are not present, cardiogenic shock is due to impairment of left ventricular function. Although dopamine or dobutamine usually improves the hemodynamics in these patients, unfortunately neither appears to improve hospital survival significantly. Similarly, vasodilators have been used in an effort to elevate cardiac output and to reduce left ventricular filling pressure. However, by lowering the already markedly reduced coronary perfusion pressure, myocardial perfusion can be compromised further, accelerating the vicious circle illustrated in Figure 35–11. Vasodilators may nonetheless be used in conjunction with intraaortic balloon counterpulsation and inotropic agents in an effort to increase cardiac output while sustaining or elevating coronary perfusion pressure.[190]

The systemic vascular resistance is usually elevated in patients with cardiogenic shock, but occasionally resistance is normal and in a few cases vasodilation actually predominates. When systemic vascular resistance is not elevated (i.e., < 1800 dyne-sec/cm⁵) in patients with cardiogenic

shock, norepinephrine, which has both alpha- and beta-adrenoceptor agonist properties (in doses ranging from 2 to 10 g/min), may be employed to increase diastolic arterial pressure, maintain coronary perfusion, and improve contractility. Norepinephrine should be used only when other means, including balloon counterpulsation, fail to maintain arterial diastolic pressure above 50 to 60 mm Hg in a previously normotensive patient. The use of alpha-adrenoceptor agents such as phenylephrine and methoxamine is contraindicated in patients with cardiogenic shock (unless systemic vascular resistance is inordinately low).

Intraaortic Balloon Counterpulsation
(See also Chap. 19)

INDICATIONS. Intraaortic balloon counterpulsation is used in the treatment of AMI in three groups of patients[478]: (1) those whose conditions are hemodynamically unstable and in whom support of the circulation is required for the performance of cardiac catheterization and angiography carried out to assess lesions that are potentially correctable surgically or by angioplasty; (2) those with cardiogenic shock that is unresponsive to medical management; and (3) rarely, those with persistent ischemic pain that is unresponsive to treatment with inhalation of 100 percent oxygen, beta-adrenoceptor blockade, and nitrates. Unfortunately, among patients with cardiogenic shock, improvement is often only temporary and "balloon dependence" commonly develops. Patients with cardiogenic shock treated with this modality can be successfully weaned from the supporting system only occasionally. Counterpulsation alone does not improve overall survival in patients either with or without a surgically remediable mechanical lesion.

COMPLICATIONS. These occur infrequently but include damage to or perforation of the aortic wall, ischemia distal to the site of insertion of the balloon in the femoral artery, thrombocytopenia, hemolysis, renal emboli, and mechanical failure such as rupture of the balloon. Those at highest risk include patients with peripheral vascular disease, the elderly, and women, particularly if they are small. These factors should be taken into consideration before an attempt is made to institute intraaortic balloon counterpulsation. Because of the potential for vascular bleeding complications, there has been reluctance to use intraaortic pumps in patients who have undergone thrombolytic therapy. However, despite the increased bleeding risk, because of the poor outcome among patients with shock after thrombolysis (usually ineffective thrombolysis), this modality should be considered in selected patients who are candidates for an aggressive approach to revascularization.

Revascularization

Reversal of cardiogenic shock by acute reperfusion has been reported, usually with thrombolytic therapy, emergency PTCA, or a combination of these measures.[190] In uncontrolled reports, the mortality of patients with cardiogenic shock appears to have been reduced by about 30 percent by early angioplasty or coronary artery bypass surgery.[479] Encouraging evidence favoring early angiography and revascularization has been reported in a cardiogenic shock registry. Another small retrospective series reported that patients with cardiogenic shock who underwent a successful angioplasty had a better 1-year survival than either those who did not undergo a successful angioplasty or those who received only medical therapy. These promising results must be interpreted cautiously because selection bias due to exclusion of elderly and moribund patients may have inflated the estimate of the beneficial effect of angioplasty.

Of the five therapies frequently used to treat patients with cardiogenic shock (vasopressors, intraaortic balloon counterpulsation, thrombolysis, angioplasty, and CABG), the first two are useful temporizing maneuvers. Surgical

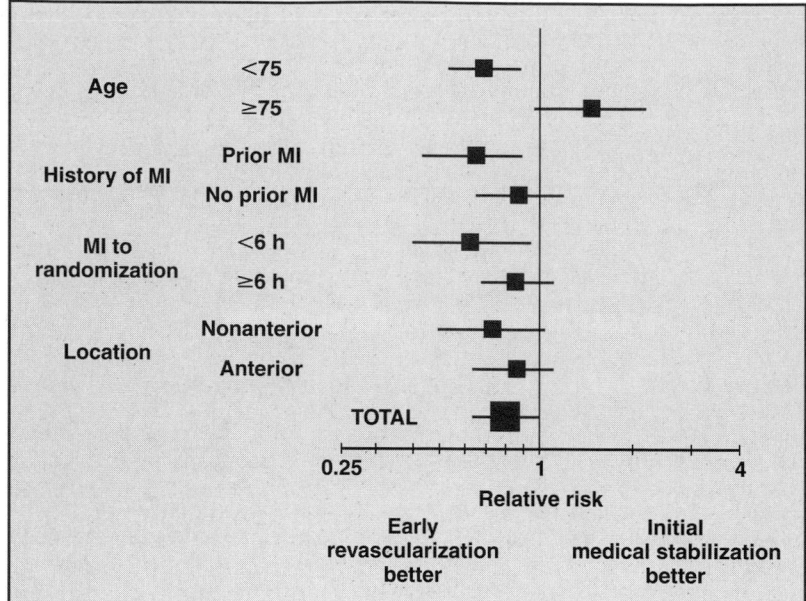

FIGURE 35-43. Effect of early revascularization in cardiogenic shock. The 6-month mortality is lower in patients with cardiogenic shock from myocardial infarction who were randomized to early revascularization in the SHOCK trial. Subgroups of patients that showed a particular benefit from early revascularization include those patients younger than age 75, a history of prior myocardial infarction, and randomization in less than 6 hours from the onset of symptoms. (Adapted from data in Hochman JS, Sleeper LA, Webb JG, et al: Early revascularization in acute myocardial infarction complicated by cardiogenic shock. SHOCK Investigators. Should We Emergently Revascularize Occluded Coronaries for Cardiogenic Shock. N Engl J Med 341:625-634, 1999.)

treatment in cardiogenic shock (aside from correcting mechanical abnormalities) may involve bypassing occluded as well as severely obstructed nonoccluded vessels. Occlusion of one major vessel may cause left ventricular dysfunction and hypotension, which can then lead to hypoperfusion and ischemia of myocardium subserved by the other diseased vessels. Left ventricular function may be improved by relief of this ischemia with revascularization.

The SHOCK study evaluated early revascularization for the treatment of patients with AMI complicated by cardiogenic shock. Patients with shock due to left ventricular failure complicating MI were randomized to emergency revascularization (n = 152), accomplished by either CABG or angioplasty, or initial medical stabilization (n = 150). In 86 percent of patients in both groups, intraaortic balloon counterpulsation was performed. The primary endpoint was all-cause mortality at 30 days; a secondary endpoint was mortality at 6 months. At 30 days, overall mortality was 46.7 percent in the revascularization group, not significantly different from the 56.0 percent mortality rate observed in the medical-therapy group ($p = 0.11$). However, 6-month mortality was significantly lower in the revascularization group than in the medical-therapy group, with rates of 50.3 percent versus 63.1 percent, respectively ($p = 0.027$).[480] Subgroups of patients in the SHOCK trial that showed particular benefit from the early revascularization strategy (i.e., reduced 6-month mortality) were those who were younger than 75 years of age, had a prior AMI, and were randomized in less than 6 hours from onset of infarction (see Fig. 35-43).

RECOMMENDATIONS. We recommend assessment of patients on an individualized basis to determine their desire for aggressive care and overall candidacy for further treatment (e.g., age, mental status, comorbidities). Patients who are potential candidates for revascularization should then rapidly receive intraaortic balloon counterpulsation and be referred for coronary arteriography. Those with suitable anatomy should be revascularized with angioplasty or CABG. In appropriately selected patients, emergency cardiac transplantation has also been used successfully to manage cardiogenic shock.

RIGHT VENTRICULAR INFARCTION

A characteristic hemodynamic pattern (Table 35-17) has been observed in patients with right ventricular infarction,

which frequently accompanies inferior left ventricular infarction or rarely occurs in isolated form. Right-sided heart filling pressures (central venous, right atrial, and right ventricular end-diastolic pressures) are elevated, whereas left ventricular filling pressure is normal or only slightly raised; right ventricular systolic and pulse pressures are decreased, and cardiac output is often markedly depressed. Rarely,

▼ **TABLE 35-17. FEATURES OF RIGHT VENTRICULAR MYOCARDIAL INFARCTION**

Clinical Findings
Normal or depressed right ventricular function
Shock
Tricuspid regurgitation
Ruptured ventricular septum

Hemodynamic Measurements
Abnormally elevated right atrial pressure
Normal right ventricular and pulmonary artery systolic pressures
Increased ratio of right ventricular to left ventricular filling presure
Depressed right ventricular function curve

Scintigraphy
Uptake in right ventricular free wall
Increased right ventricular dimensions and decreased wall motion

Echocardiography
Increased right ventricular dimension
Absence of pericardial effusion

Cardiac Enzymes
Increased magnitude of enzyme values relative to degree of left ventricular dysfunction

Cardiac Catheterization
Involvement of right (usually) or left (rarely) circumflex coronary arteries
Right ventricular akinesis

Differential Diagnosis
Hypotension with acute myocardial infarction
Pericardial tamponade
Constrictive pericarditis
Pulmonary embolus

Modified from Rackley CE, Russell RO Jr, Mantle JA, et al: Right ventricular infarction and function. Am Heart J 101:215, 1981.

this disproportionate elevation of right-sided filling pressure causes right-to-left shunting through a patent foramen ovale. This possibility should be considered in patients with right ventricular infarction who have unexplained systemic hypoxemia. The finding of an elevation in atrial natriuretic factor in this condition has led to the suggestion that abnormally high levels of this peptide might be in part responsible for the hypotension seen in right ventricular infarction. Of note, the same protective effect of ischemic preconditioning that has been described in infarction of the left ventricle has also been reported in patients with infarction of the right ventricle.[481, 482]

Diagnosis

Right ventricular infarction is common among patients with inferior left ventricular infarction. Therefore, otherwise unexplained systemic arterial hypotension or diminished cardiac output or marked hypotension in response to small doses of nitroglycerin in patients with inferior infarction should lead to the prompt consideration of this diagnosis.

Many patients with the combination of normal left ventricular filling pressure and depressed cardiac index have right ventricular infarcts (with accompanying inferior left ventricular infarcts). The hemodynamic picture may superficially resemble that seen in patients with acute pericarditis (see Chap. 50). It includes elevated right ventricular filling pressure; steep, right atrial *y* descent; and an early diastolic drop and plateau (square root sign) in the right ventricular pressure tracing. Moreover, Kussmaul's sign (an increase in jugular venous pressure with inspiration, see Chap. 4) and pulsus paradoxus (a fall in systolic pressure of greater than 10 mm Hg with inspiration, see Chap. 4) may be present in patients with right ventricular infarction.[52] In fact, Kussmaul's sign in the setting of inferior wall AMI is highly predictive of right ventricular involvement.

ELECTROCARDIOGRAPHY. The ECG may provide the first clue that right ventricular involvement is present in the patient with inferior wall MI (see Chap. 5). Most patients with right ventricular infarction have ST segment elevation in lead V_4R (right precordial lead in V_4 position).[63a, 482] Transient elevation of the ST segment in any of the right precordial leads may occur with right ventricular MI, and the presence of ST segment elevation of 0.1 mV or more in any one or combination of leads V_4R, V_5R, and V_6R in patients with the clinical picture of acute MI is highly sensitive and specific for the diagnosis of right ventricular MI.[483] Wellens has emphasized that, in addition, noting the presence or absence of convex upward ST segment elevation in V_4R, clinicians should determine if the T wave is positive or negative; such distinctions help distinguish proximal versus distal occlusion of the right coronary artery versus occlusion of the left circumflex artery[140] (Fig. 35–44). Elevation of the ST segments in leads V_1 through V_4 due to right ventricular infarction can be confused with that due to anteroseptal infarction. Although the elevated ST segments are oriented anteriorly in both cases, it is the frontal plane that provides important clues—the ST segments are oriented to the right in right ventricular infarction (e.g. +120 degrees) whereas they are oriented to the left in anteroseptal infarction (e.g. −30 degrees).[484]

ECHOCARDIOGRAPHY AND RADIONUCLIDE ANGIOGRAPHY. Echocardiography is helpful in the differential diagnosis because in right ventricular infarction, in contrast to pericardial tamponade, no significant quantities of pericardial fluid are seen. On two-dimensional echocardiography, abnormal wall motion of the right ventricle as well as right ventricular dilatation and depression of right ventricular ejection fraction are noted.[52] Gated equilibrium radionuclide angiography is also useful for recognizing right ventricular MI. Serial studies have shown that some degree of recovery of an initially depressed right ventricular ejection fraction is the rule with right ventricular MI,[424] whereas this is less apparent in left ventricular ejection fraction.

HEMODYNAMICS. Loss of atrial transport in patients with right ventricular infarction can result in marked reductions in stroke volume and arterial blood pressure. As already noted, disproportionate elevation of the right-sided filling pressure is the hemodynamic hallmark of right ventricular infarction. Therefore, ventricular pacing may fail to increase cardiac output, and atrioventricular sequential pacing may be required.

Management

Because of their ability to reduce preload, medications routinely prescribed for left ventricular infarction may produce profound hypotension in patients with right ventricular in-

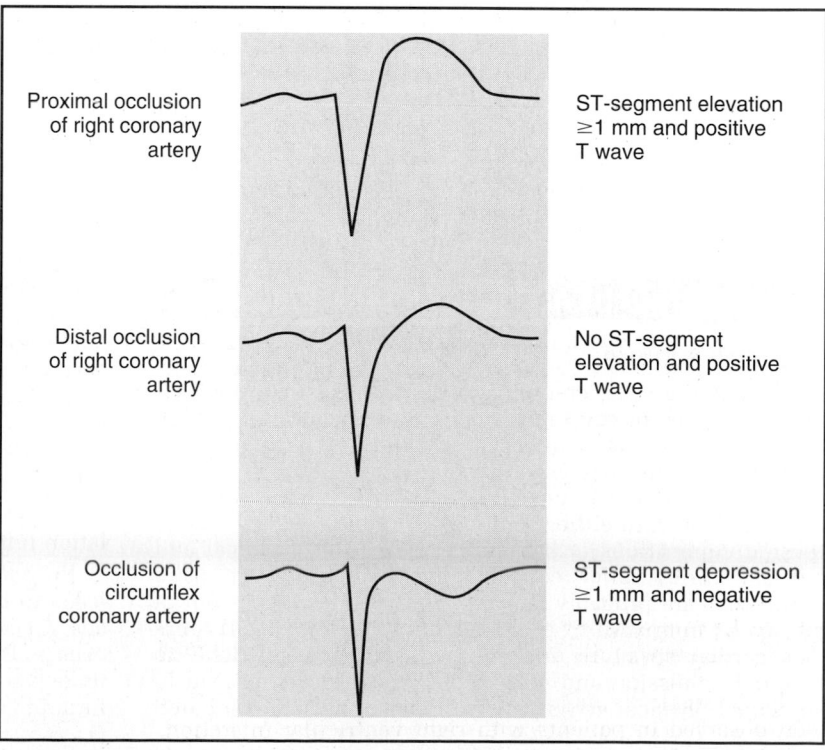

FIGURE 35–44. ST segment and T wave configurations in lead V_4R in inferoposterior myocardial infarction. Proximal occlusion of the right coronary artery is characterized by ST segment elevation of at least 1 mm and a positive T wave. Distal occlusion of the right coronary artery is characterized by a positive T wave but no ST segment elevation. Occlusion of the circumflex coronary artery is characterized by a negative T wave and ST segment depression of at least 1 mm. (Reproduced with permission from Wellens HJ: The value of the right precordial leads of the electrocardiogram. N Engl J Med 340: 381–383, 1999.)

Proximal occlusion of right coronary artery — ST-segment elevation ≥1 mm and positive T wave

Distal occlusion of right coronary artery — No ST-segment elevation and positive T wave

Occlusion of circumflex coronary artery — ST-segment depression ≥1 mm and negative T wave

▼ **TABLE 35–18.** TREATMENT STRATEGY FOR RIGHT VENTRICULAR ISCHEMIA/INFARCTION

Maintain Right Ventricular Preload
  Volume loading (IV normal saline)
  Avoid use of nitrates and diuretic
  Maintain AV synchrony
    AV sequential pacing for symptomatic high-degree heart block unresponsive to atropine
  Prompt cardioversion for hemodynamically significant SVT
Inotropic Support
  Dobutamine (if cardiac output fails to increase after volume loading)
Reduce Right Ventricular Afterload with Left Ventricular Dysfunction
  Intraaortic balloon pump
  Arterial vasodilators (sodium nitroprusside, hydralazine)
  ACE inhibitors
Reperfusion
  Thrombolytic agents
  Primary PTCA
  CABG (in selected patients with multivessel disease)

IV = intravenous; AV = atrioventricular; SVT = supraventricular tachycardia; ACE = angiotension-converting enzyme; PTCA = percutaneous transluminal coronary angioplasty; CABG = coronary artery bypass graft.
From 1999 Updated ACC/AHA AMI Guidelines (Web version), p 66.

FIGURE 35–45. See color plate 22.

farction.[52] In patients with hypotension due to right ventricular MI, hemodynamics may be improved by a combination of expanding plasma volume to augment right ventricular preload and cardiac output and, when left ventricular failure is present, arterial vasodilators[63] (Table 35–18). The initial therapy for hypotension in patients with right ventricular infarction should almost always be volume expansion. However, if hypotension has not been corrected after one or more liters of fluid has been administered briskly, consideration should be given to hemodynamic monitoring with a pulmonary artery catheter, because further volume infusion may be of little use and may produce pulmonary congestion.[485] Vasodilators reduce the impedance to left ventricular outflow and, in turn, left ventricular diastolic, left atrial, and pulmonary (arterial) pressures, thereby lowering the impedance to right ventricular outflow and enhancing right ventricular output (see Table 35–18).

In view of the importance of atrial transport, patients requiring pacing should have atrial or AV sequential pacing. Successful reperfusion of the right coronary artery significantly improves right ventricular mechanical function and lowers in-hospital mortality in patients with right ventricular infarction.[64] Replacement of the tricuspid valve and repair of the valve with annuloplasty rings have been carried out in the treatment of severe tricuspid regurgitation secondary to right ventricular infarction.

MECHANICAL CAUSES OF HEART FAILURE

Free Wall Rupture

The most dramatic complications of AMI are those that involve tearing or rupture of acutely infarcted tissue[486] (Fig. 35–45). The clinical characteristics of these lesions vary considerably and depend on the site of rupture, which may involve the papillary muscles, the interventricular septum, or the free wall of either ventricle. The overall incidence of these complications is hard to assess because clinical and autopsy series differ considerably.[487, 488] However, as a group they are probably responsible for about 15 percent of all deaths from AMI.[486, 489] In general, patients with rupture of a cardiac structure during AMI have a greater delay to hospital admission and are more likely to have engaged in sustained physical activity after the onset of AMI compared

with those AMI patients who do not experience cardiac rupture.[490] The comparative clinical profile of these complications, as gathered from different studies, is shown in Table 35–19. The incidence of myocardial rupture has increased since the late 1960s.[487] The prior use of corticosteroids or nonsteroidal antiinflammatory agents has been implicated as predisposing to rupture as a result of impaired healing. Controversy remains about the actual relationship between the use of such agents and the frequency of rupture, with several series suggesting a correlation of rupture with their use[491] and others not.[488] Conversely, the early use of thrombolytic therapy appears to reduce the incidence of cardiac rupture, an effect that is responsible in part for improved survival with effective thrombolysis. Late thrombolytic therapy may actually *increase* the risk of cardiac rupture despite improving overall survival.

Rupture of the free wall of the infarcted ventricle (see Fig. 35–45) occurs in up to 10 percent of patients dying in the hospital of AMI.[486] Thinness of the apical wall, marked intensity of necrosis at the terminal end of the blood supply, poor collateral flow, the shearing effect of muscular contraction against an inert and stiffened necrotic area, and aging of the myocardium with laceration of the myocardial microstructure have all been proposed as the local factors that lead to rupture.

CLINICAL FEATURES. The following are some features that characterize this serious complication of AMI:

1. It occurs more frequently in the elderly and possibly more frequently in women than in men with infarction.[492]

2. It appears to be more common in hypertensive than in normotensive patients.

3. It occurs more frequently in the left than the right ventricle and seldom occurs in the atria.

4. It usually involves the anterior or lateral walls[486] of the ventricle in the area of the terminal distribution of the left anterior descending coronary artery.

5. It is usually associated with a relatively large transmural infarction involving at least 20 percent of the left ventricle.

6. It occurs between 1 day and 3 weeks, but most commonly 1 to 4 days, after infarction.

7. It is usually preceded by infarct expansion (i.e., thinning and a disproportionate dilatation within the softened necrotic zone).

8. Most commonly it results from a distinct tear in the myocardial wall or a dissecting hematoma that perforates a necrotic area of myocardium (see Fig. 35–45).

9. It usually occurs near the junction of the infarct and the normal muscle.

10. It occurs less frequently in the center of the infarct, but when rupture occurs here, it is usually during the second rather than the first week following the infarct.

11. It rarely occurs in a greatly thickened ventricle or in an area of extensive collateral vessels.

12. It most often occurs in patients *without* previous infarction.[488]

13. There is no evidence that the intensity of anticoagulation influences the occurrence of rupture.[492]

Rupture of the free wall of the left ventricle usually leads to hemopericardium and death from cardiac tamponade. Occasionally, rupture of the free wall of the ventricle occurs as the first clinical manifestation in patients with undetected or silent MI, and then it may be considered a form of "sudden cardiac death."

VARIABLE	VENTRICULAR SEPTAL DEFECT	FREE WALL RUPTURE	PAPILLARY MUSCLE RUPTURE
Age (mean, years)	63	69	65
Days post-MI	3–5	3–6	3–5
Anterior MI	66%	50%	25%
New murmur	90%	25%	50%
Palpable thrill	Yes	No	Rare
Previous MI	25%	25%	30%
Echocardiographic findings			
Two-dimensional	Visualize defect	May have pericardial effusion	Flail or prolapsing leaflet
Doppler	Detect shunt		Regurgitant jet in LA
PA catheterization	Oxygen step-up in RV	Equalization of diastolic pressure	Prominent c-v wave in PCW tracing
Mortality			
Medical	90%	90%	90%
Surgical	50%	Case reports	40–90%

MI = myocardial infarction; LA = left atrium; PA = pulmonary artery; RV = right ventricle; PCW = pulmonary capillary wedge.
Modified from Labovitz AJ, et al: Mechanical complications of acute myocardial infarction. Cardiovasc Rev Rep 5:948, 1984.

The course of rupture varies from catastrophic, with an acute tear leading to immediate death, to subacute, with nausea, hypotension, and pericardial type of discomfort being the major clinical clues to its presence.[486] Survival depends on the recognition of this complication, on hemodynamic stabilization of the patient (usually with inotropic agents and/or intraaortic balloon pump), and, most importantly, on prompt surgical repair.

PSEUDOANEURYSM. Incomplete rupture of the heart may occur when organizing thrombus and hematoma, together with pericardium, seal a rupture of the left ventricle and thus prevent the development of hemopericardium (Fig. 35–46). With time, this area of organized thrombus and pericardium can become a pseudoaneurysm (false aneurysm) that maintains communication with the cavity of the left ventricle. In contrast to true aneurysms, which always contain some myocardial elements in their walls, the walls of pseudoaneurysms are composed of organized hematoma and pericardium and lack any elements of the original myocardial wall. Pseudoaneurysms can become quite large, even equaling the true ventricular cavity in size, and they communicate with the left ventricular cavity through a narrow neck. Frequently, pseudoaneurysms contain significant quantities of old and recent thrombus, superficial portions of which can cause arterial emboli. Pseudoaneurysms can drain off a portion of each ventricular stroke volume exactly as do true aneurysms. The diagnosis of pseudoaneurysm can usually be made by two-dimensional echocardiography (see Chap. 7) and contrast angiography, although at times differentiation between true aneurysm and pseudoaneurysm may be difficult by any imaging technique.

DIAGNOSIS. The rupture usually is first suggested by the development of sudden profound shock, often rapidly leading to electromechanical dissociation due to pericardial tamponade. Immediate pericardiocentesis confirms the diagnosis and relieves the pericardial tamponade, at least momentarily. If the patient's condition is relatively stable, echocardiography may help in establishing the diagnosis of tamponade.[52] Under the most favorable conditions, cardiac catheterization can be carried out, not necessarily to confirm the diagnosis of rupture but to delineate the coronary anatomy. This is helpful so that, in addition to ventricular repair, CABG can be performed in patients in whom high-grade obstructive lesions are present. In patients in whom hemodynamics are critically compromised, establishment of the diagnosis should be followed immediately by surgical resection of the necrotic and ruptured myocardium with primary reconstruction (Fig. 35–47). When rupture is subacute and a pseudoaneurysm is suspected or present, prompt elective surgery is indicated because rupture of the pseudoaneurysm occurs relatively frequently.

Rupture of the Interventricular Septum

Although rupture of the interventricular septum previously was reported in up to 11 percent of autopsied cases and 2 percent of AMI patients in the prethrombolytic era, it occurs in 0.2 percent of patients in recent thrombolytic trials.[486, 493, 494] Clinical features associated with an increased risk of rupture of the interventricular septum include lack of development of a collateral network, advanced age, hypertension, anterior location of infarction, and possibly thrombolysis.[493, 494] Patients who develop a rupture of the

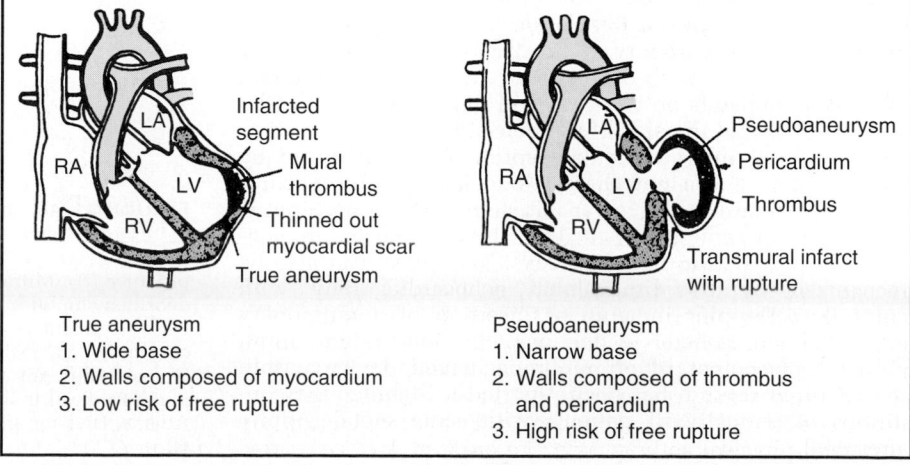

FIGURE 35–46. Differences between a pseudoaneurysm and a true aneurysm. (From Shah PK: Complications of acute myocardial infarction. *In* Parmley W, Chatterjee K [eds]: Cardiology. Philadelphia, JB Lippincott, 1987.)

True aneurysm
1. Wide base
2. Walls composed of myocardium
3. Low risk of free rupture

Pseudoaneurysm
1. Narrow base
2. Walls composed of thrombus and pericardium
3. High risk of free rupture

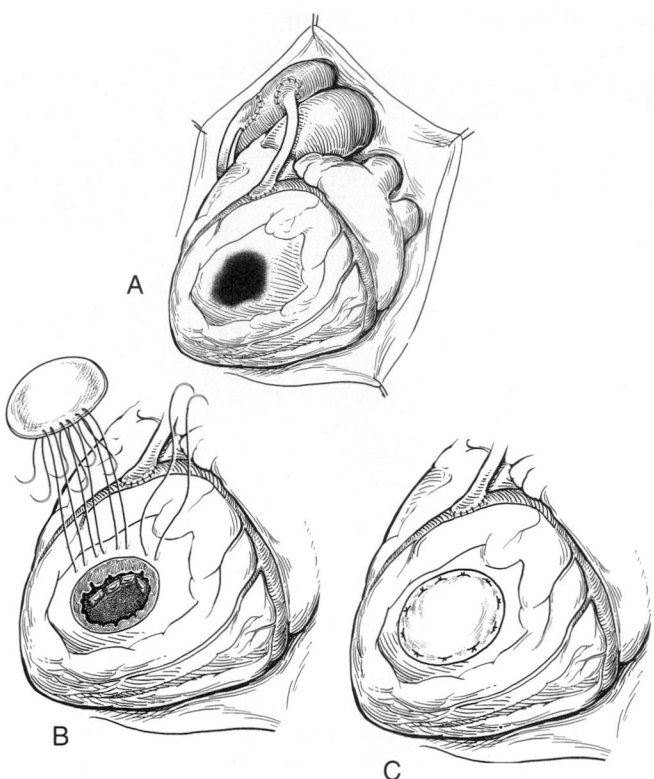

FIGURE 35–47. Management of free wall rupture. Typically, the rupture site is within a larger area of necrotic muscle *(A)*. After débridement, pledgeted sutures are placed inside the ventricle and through a tailored prosthetic patch *(B)*. The patch is then secured to the free wall *(C)*. (Courtesy of Dr. David Adams, Division of Cardiac Surgery, Brigham and Women's Hospital.)

interventricular septum after AMI have a higher 30-day mortality (74 percent) compared with those patients who do not develop this complication (7 percent).[493]

The perforation may range in length from one to several centimeters (see Fig. 35–45). It may be a direct through-and-through opening, or it may be more irregular and ser-piginous. The size of the defect determines the magnitude of the left-to-right shunt and the extent of hemodynamic deterioration, which in turn affects the likelihood of sur-vival.[486] As in rupture of the free wall of the ventricle, transmural infarction underlies rupture of the ventricular septum. Rupture of the septum with an anterior infarction tends to be apical in location, whereas inferior infarctions are associated with perforation of the basal septum and with a worse prognosis than those in an anterior location. In contrast to rupture of the free wall, rupture of the ven-tricular septum is more likely (20 to 30 percent of cases) to be associated with complete heart block, right bundle branch block, and atrial fibrillation.[495] Virtually all patients have multivessel coronary artery disease, with the majority exhibiting lesions in all of the major vessels. The likelihood of survival depends on the degree of impairment of ventric-ular function and the size of the defect.[496]

A ruptured interventricular septum is characterized by the appearance of a new harsh, loud holosystolic murmur that is heard best at the lower left sternal border and that is usually accompanied by a thrill.[52] Biventricular failure gen-erally ensues within hours to days. The defect can also be recognized by two-dimensional echocardiography with color flow Doppler imaging or insertion of a pulmonary artery balloon catheter to document the left-to-right shunt. Catheter placement of an umbrella-shaped device within the ruptured septum has been reported to stabilize the con-ditions of critically ill patients with acute septal rupture after AMI.

Papillary Muscle Rupture

Partial or total rupture of a papillary muscle is a rare but often fatal complication of transmural MI[486] (see Fig. 35–45). Inferior wall infarction can lead to rupture of the pos-teromedial papillary muscle,[497] which occurs more com-monly than rupture of the anterolateral muscle, a conse-quence of anterolateral MI. Rupture of a right ventricular papillary muscle is rare but can cause massive tricuspid regurgitation and right ventricular failure. Complete tran-section of a left ventricular papillary muscle is incompati-ble with life because the sudden massive mitral regurgita-tion that develops cannot be tolerated. Rupture of a portion of a papillary muscle, usually the tip or head of the muscle, resulting in severe, although not necessarily overwhelming, mitral regurgitation, is much more frequent and is not im-mediately fatal. Unlike rupture of the ventricular septum, which occurs with large infarcts, papillary muscle rupture occurs with a relatively small infarction in approximately one half of the cases seen. The extent of coronary artery disease in these patients sometimes is modest as well.

In a small number of patients, rupture of more than one cardiac structure is noted clinically or at postmortem exam-ination; all possible combinations of rupture of the free left ventricular wall, the interventricular septum, and the papil-lary muscles have been described.[495]

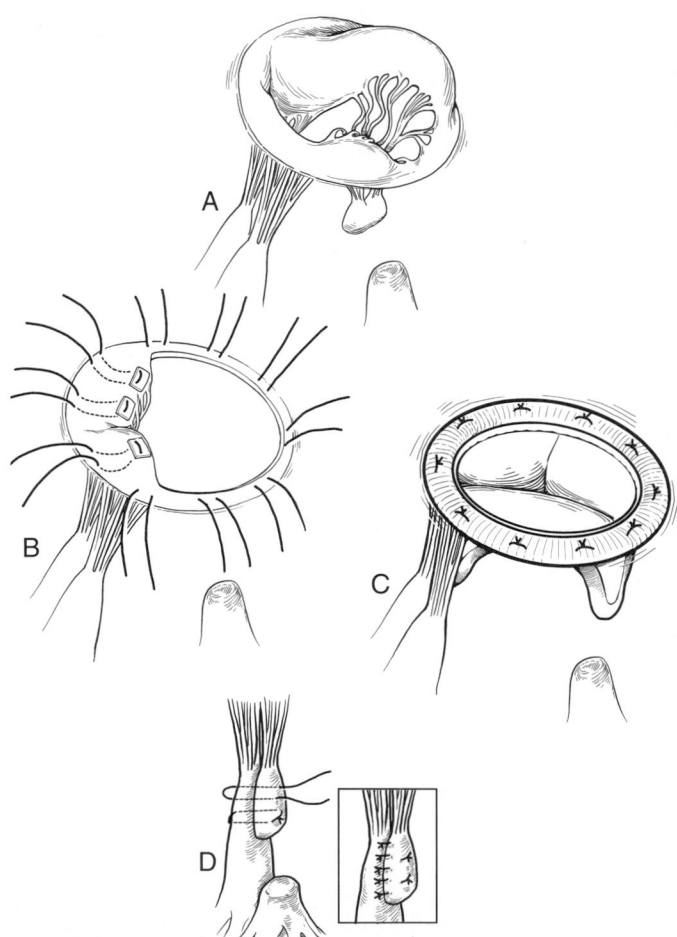

FIGURE 35–48. Surgical management of mitral regurgitation due to ruptured papillary muscle. Acute papillary muscle rupture re-sults in severe mitral regurgitation due to leaflet and commissural prolapse *(A)*. Mitral valve replacement is usually necessary. Mitral débridement with retention of the unruptured commissural and leaflet segment is performed to preserve partial annular papillary continuity *(B)*. Mitral valve replacement is then performed *(C)*. Occasionally, mitral valve repair can be performed by transfer of a papillary head to a nonrupture segment *(D)*. (Courtesy of Dr. David Adams, Division of Cardiac Surgery, Brigham and Women's Hospi-tal.)

As with patients who have a ruptured ventricular septal defect, those with papillary muscle rupture manifest a new holosystolic murmur and develop increasingly severe heart failure. In both conditions the murmur may become softer or disappear as arterial pressure falls. Mitral regurgitation due to partial or complete rupture of a papillary muscle may be promptly recognized echocardiographically.[498] Color flow Doppler imaging is particularly helpful in distinguishing acute mitral regurgitation from a ventricular septal defect in the setting of AMI (Table 35–19).[499] Therefore, an echocardiogram should be obtained immediately on any patient in whom the diagnosis is suspected, because hemodynamic deterioration can ensue rapidly. Echocardiography also often permits differentiation of papillary muscle rupture from other, generally less severe forms of mitral regurgitation that occur with AMI.

Differentiation Between Ventricular Septal Rupture and Mitral Regurgitation

It may be difficult, on clinical grounds, to distinguish between acute mitral regurgitation and rupture of the ventricular septum in patients with AMI who suddenly develop a loud systolic murmur. This differentiation can be made most readily by color flow Doppler echocardiography. In addition, a right-heart catheterization with a balloon-tipped catheter can readily distinguish between these two complications. As already noted, patients with ventricular septal rupture demonstrate a "step-up" in oxygen saturation in blood samples from the right ventricle and pulmonary artery compared with those from the right atrium. Patients with acute mitral regurgitation lack this step-up; they may demonstrate tall c-v waves in both the pulmonary capillary wedge and pulmonary arterial pressure tracings.

Invasive monitoring, which is essential in these patients, also allows for the critically important assessment of ventricular function.[52] Right and left ventricular filling pressures (right atrial pressure and pulmonary capillary wedge pressure) dictate fluid administration or the use of diuretics, whereas measurements of cardiac output and mean arterial pressure are obtained for calculation of systemic vascular resistance as a guide for vasodilator therapy. Unless systolic pressure is below 90 mm Hg, this therapy, generally using nitroglycerin or nitroprusside, should be instituted as soon as possible once hemodynamic monitoring is available. This may be critically important for stabilizing the patient's condition in preparation for further diagnostic studies and surgical repair. If vasodilator therapy is not tolerated or if it fails to achieve hemodynamic stability, intraaortic balloon counterpulsation should be rapidly instituted.

Surgical Treatment

Operative intervention is most successful in patients with AMI and circulatory collapse when a surgically correctable mechanical lesion such as ventricular septal defect or mitral regurgitation can be identified and repaired.[493] In such

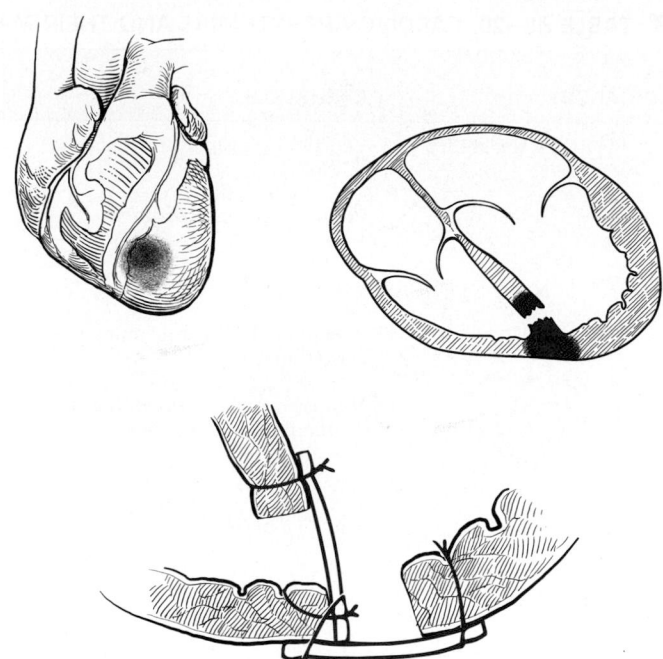

FIGURE 35–49. Repair of ischemic ventricular septal defect. The infarct typically involves a free wall and septum (*A* and *B*). Repair of the defect is performed through an incision in the ventricular wall infarct. The septal defect is closed with a prosthetic patch, and a second patch is used to close the incision in the free wall (*C*). (Courtesy of Dr. David Adams, Division of Cardiac Surgery, Brigham and Women's Hospital.)

patients the circulation should at first be supported by intraaortic balloon pulsation and a positive inotropic agent such as dopamine or dobutamine in combination with a vasodilator, unless the patient is hypotensive. Operation should not be delayed in patients with a correctable lesion who agree to an aggressive management strategy and require pharmacological and/or mechanical (counterpulsation) support.[494] Such patients frequently develop a serious complication (infection, adult respiratory distress syndrome, extension of the infarct, or renal failure) if operation is delayed. Surgical survival is predicted by early operation, short duration of shock, and mild degrees of right and left ventricular impairment.[494] When the hemodynamic status of a patient with one of these mechanical lesions complicating an AMI remains stable after the patient has been weaned from pharmacological and/or mechanical support, it may be possible to postpone operation for 2 to 4 weeks to allow some healing of the infarct to occur. Surgical repair may involve correction of mitral regurgitation, insertion of a prosthetic mitral valve repair, or closure of a ventricular septal defect, usually accompanied by coronary revascularization (Figs. 35–48 and 35–49).[52]

▼ Arrhythmias

The genesis, diagnosis, and treatment of cardiac arrhythmias are presented in Chapters 22 to 26. The role of arrhythmias in complicating the course of patients with AMI and the prevention and treatment of these arrhythmias in this setting are discussed here and summarized in Table 35–20.

The incidence of arrhythmias is higher in those patients seen earlier after the onset of symptoms. Many serious arrhythmias develop before hospitalization, even before the patient is monitored.[500] Some abnormality of cardiac rhythm also occurs in the majority of patients with AMI treated in CCUs.[501] When patients are seen very early during the course of MI, they almost invariably exhibit evidence of increased activity of the autonomic nervous system. Thus, sinus bradycardia, sometimes associated with AV block, and hypotension reflect augmented vagal activity.

MECHANISM OF ARRHYTHMIAS IN MYOCARDIAL INFARCTION. Owing to the difficulty of studying cardiac ar-

CATEGORY	ARRHYTHMIA	OBJECTIVE OF TREATMENT	THERAPEUTIC OPTIONS
1. Electrical instability	Ventricular premature beats	Correction of electrolyte deficits and increased sympathetic tone	Potassium and magnesium solutions, beta blocker
	Ventricular tachycardia	Prophylaxis against ventricular fibrillation, restoration of hemodynamic stability	Antiarrhythmic agents; cardioversion/defibrillation
	Ventricular fibrillation	Urgent reversion to sinus rhythm	Defibrillation; bretylium tosylate
	Accelerated idioventricular rhythm	Observation unless hemodynamic function is compromised	Increase sinus rate (atropine, atrial pacing); antiarrhythmic agents
	Nonparoxysmal atrioventricular junctional tachycardia	Search for precipitating causes (e.g., digitalis intoxication); suppress arrhythmia only if hemodynamic function is compromised	Atrial overdrive pacing; antiarrhythmic agents; cardioversion relatively contraindicated if digitalis intoxication present
2. Pump failure/ excessive sympathetic stimulation	Sinus tachycardia	Reduce heart rate to diminish myocardial oxygen demands	Antipyretics; analgesics; consider beta blocker unless congestive heart failure present; treat latter if present with anticongestive measures (diuretics, afterload reduction)
	Atrial fibrillation and/or atrial flutter	Reduce ventricular rate; restore sinus rhythm	Verapamil, digitalis glycosides; anticongestive measures (diuretics, afterload reduction); cardioversion; rapid atrial pacing (for atrial flutter)
	Paroxysmal supraventricular tachycardia	Reduce ventricular rate; restore sinus rhythm	Vagal maneuvers; verapamil; cardiac glycosides; beta-adrenergic blockers; cardioversion; rapid atrial pacing
3. Bradyarrhythmias and conduction disturbances	Sinus bradycardia	Acceleration of heart rate only if hemodynamic function is compromised	Atropine; atrial pacing
	Junctional escape rhythm	Acceleration of sinus rate only if loss of atrial "kick" causes hemodynamic compromise	Atropine; atrial pacing
	Atrioventricular block and intraventricular block		Insertion of pacemaker

Modified from Antman EM, Rutherford JD (eds): Coronary Care Medicine: A Practical Approach. Boston, Martinus Nijhoff Publishing, 1986, p 78.

rhythmias in patients with acute myocardial ischemia and infarction, investigators have resorted to animal models of coronary occlusion and release in an attempt to elucidate the causes of arrhythmias in the clinical setting and identify potential therapeutic targets.[502, 503] Animal models have generally been divided into arrhythmias occurring during the early phase of MI (first 30 minutes after coronary occlusion) and arrhythmias occurring during later phases in the infarction process (occurring hours to days and even weeks after infarction).[504] When interpreting animal models to draw correlations to clinical arrhythmias, several factors must be considered: the mode of coronary artery occlusion (thrombotic occlusion versus coronary ligation), number of successive coronary occlusions (e.g., preconditioning), the size of the myocardial ischemic zone, the level of activity of the autonomic nervous system, and the presence or absence of collateral vessels.[505] Electrophysiological disturbances during the acute phase of coronary occlusion in experimental animals that are probably relevant in patients with AMI include a loss of transmembrane resting potential, alterations in refractoriness and excitability, slowing of conduction, and the emergence of abnormal mechanisms of automatic impulse formation. A leading hypothesis for a major mechanism of arrhythmias in the acute phase of coronary occlusion is micro-reentry due to inhomogeneity of the electrical characteristics of ischemic myocardium. Cells at the center of the ischemic zone have a relatively uniform increase in extracellular potassium concentration, whereas

cells in the border zone between the ischemic region and normal myocardium are only partially depolarized and therefore have action potentials with a larger amplitude. Slowing of impulse conduction and block occurs in markedly depressed areas leading to arrhythmias such as polymorphic VT and ventricular fibrillation.[506]

The cellular electrophysiological mechanisms for reperfusion arrhythmias appear to include washout of various ions such as lactate and potassium and toxic metabolic substances that have accumulated in the ischemic zone. Cells in reperfused myocardial zones can exhibit action potentials of the slow response type.[504] In animal models in which reperfusion does not take place and a permanent occlusion of the infarct artery occurs, delayed afterdepolarizations and triggered automaticity have been demonstrated. It is unclear whether such phenomena also occur in patients with AMI.

The treatment of tachyarrhythmias involves not only the use of antiarrhythmic drugs but also correction of abnormalities of plasma electrolyte concentrations, acid-base balance disturbances, hypoxemia, anemia, and digitalis intoxication. In addition, it is essential to treat pericarditis, pulmonary emboli, and pneumonia or other infections, which may give rise to sinus tachycardia or other supraventricular tachyarrhythmias.

Arrhythmias occurring in patients with AMI require aggressive treatment when they (1) impair hemodynamics, (2) compromise myocardial viability by augmenting myocardial oxygen requirements, or (3) predispose to malignant ventricular arrhythmias (i.e., VT, ventricular fibrillation, or asystole). Evidence indicates that both the diminished threshold to ventricular fibrillation[507] and the incidence of malignant ventricular arrhythmias associated with infarction are affected by the extent of the underlying infarction.[508]

HEMODYNAMIC CONSEQUENCES. Patients with significant left ventricular dysfunction have a relatively fixed stroke volume and depend on changes in heart rate to alter cardiac output. However, there is a narrow range of heart rate over which the cardiac output is maximal, with significant reductions occurring at both faster and slower rates. Thus, all forms of bradycardia and tachycardia may depress the cardiac output in patients with AMI. Although the optimal rate insofar as cardiac output is concerned may exceed 100 beats/min, it is important to consider that heart rate is one of the major determinants of myocardial oxygen consumption and that at more rapid heart rates myocardial energy needs can be elevated to levels that adversely affect ischemic myocardium. Therefore, in patients with AMI, the optimal rate is usually lower, in the range of 60 to 80 beats/min.

A second factor to consider in assessing the hemodynamic consequences of a particular arrhythmia is the loss of the atrial contribution to ventricular preload. Studies in patients without AMI have demonstrated that loss of atrial transport decreases left ventricular output by 15 to 20 percent.[509] However, in patients with reduced diastolic left ventricular compliance of any cause (including AMI), atrial systole is of greater importance for left ventricular filling. In patients with AMI, atrial systole boosts end-diastolic volume by 15 percent, end-diastolic pressure by 29 percent, and stroke volume by 35 percent.

VENTRICULAR ARRHYTHMIAS
(See also Chap. 25)

Ventricular Premature Beats

Before the widespread use of reperfusion therapy, aspirin, beta blockers, and intravenous nitrates in the management of AMI, it was believed that frequent VPB (more than five per minute), VPBs with multiform configuration, early coupling (the "R-on-T" phenomenon), and repetitive patterns in the form of couples or salvos presaged ventricular fibrillation. However, it is now clear that such "warning arrhythmias" are present in as many patients who do not develop fibrillation as those who do. Several reports have shown that primary ventricular fibrillation (see later) occurs without antecedent warning arrhythmias and may even develop in spite of suppression of warning arrhythmias.[510] On the other hand, frequent and complex VPBs and R-on-T beats are commonly observed in patients with AMI who never develop ventricular fibrillation.[510] Both primary ventricular fibrillation and VPBs, especially R-on-T beats, occur during the early phase of AMI when considerable heterogeneity of electrical activity is present. Although R-on-T beats expose this heterogeneity and can precipitate ventricular fibrillation in a small minority of patients, the ubiquitous nature of VPBs in AMI and the extremely infrequent nature of ventricular fibrillation in the current era of AMI management produce unacceptably low sensitivity and specificity of ECG patterns observed on monitoring systems for identifying patients at risk of ventricular fibrillation.

MANAGEMENT. Because the incidence of ventricular fibrillation in AMI seen in CCUs over the past three decades appears to be declining, the prior practice of prophylactic suppression of VPBs with antiarrhythmic drugs is no longer necessary and there is the possibility that its use may actually be associated with an increased risk of fatal bradycardic and asystolic events.[511-515] Therefore, we pursue a conservative course when VPBs are observed in AMI and do not routinely prescribe antiarrhythmic drugs but instead determine whether recurrent ischemia or electrolyte (Fig. 35-50) or metabolic disturbances are present.[510]

When, at the very inception of an infarction, VPBs are encountered in the presence of sinus tachycardia, augmented sympathoadrenal stimulation is often a contributing factor and may be treated by beta-adrenoceptor blockade. In fact, early administration of an intravenous beta blocker is effective in reducing the incidence of ventricular fibrillation in evolving MI.[516, 517]

Accelerated Idioventricular Rhythm

Commonly defined as a ventricular rhythm with a rate of 60 to 125 beats/min, and frequently called "slow ventricular tachycardia," this arrhythmia is seen in up to 20 percent of patients with AMI. It occurs frequently during the first 2 days, with about equal frequency in anterior and inferior infarctions, and probably results from enhanced automaticity of Purkinje fibers. Most episodes are of short duration, and the arrhythmia may terminate abruptly, slow gradually before termination, or be overdriven by acceleration of the basic cardiac rhythm. Variation of the rate is common.

Accelerated idioventricular rhythm is often observed shortly after successful reperfusion has been established.[518] However, the frequent occurrence of these rhythms in patients without reperfusion limits their reliability as markers of restoration of patency of the infarct-related coronary artery.[519] In contrast to rapid ventricular tachycardia, accelerated idioventricular rhythms are thought not to affect prognosis. There is no definitive evidence that this arrhythmia, when left untreated, increases the incidence of either ventricular fibrillation or death. Therefore, we do not routinely treat accelerated idioventricular rhythms. In the rare patient with clear-cut hemodynamic compromise or recurrent angina related to accelerated idioventricular rhythms, we attempt to accelerate the sinus rate with atropine or atrial pacing; suppressive antiarrhythmic therapy with lidocaine or procainamide is usually not used unless there is unequivocal precipitation of more serious ventricular tachyarrhythmias.

Ventricular Tachycardia

Nonsustained ventricular tachycardia (VT) is usually defined as three or more consecutive ventricular ectopic beats (at a rate > 100 beats/min and lasting < 30 seconds; see Fig. 35-18); sustained VT refers to similar rhythms that last longer than 30 seconds or cause hemodynamic compromise *that requires intervention.* (Although most brief runs of VT

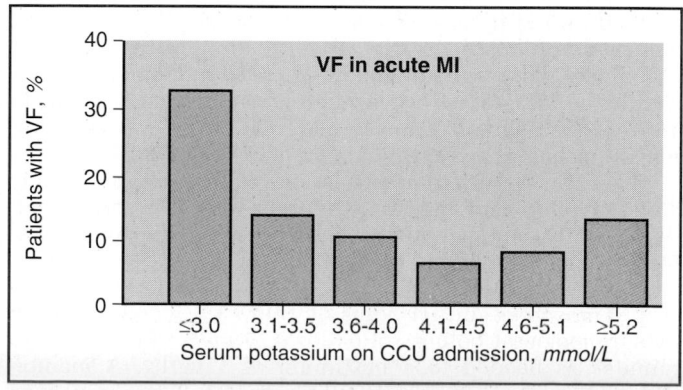

FIGURE 35–50. Importance of electrolyte deficits, as shown in this study in which the risk for ventricular fibrillation was strikingly increased in patients who presented to the critical care unit (CCU) with hypokalemia. (From Nordrehaug JE, van der Lippe G: Hypokalemia and ventricular fibrillation in acute myocardial infarction. Br Heart J 50:525, 1983.)

cause some reduction in blood pressure that is observed on arterial line pressure tracings, the majority of such episodes are not recognized by the patient). Additional descriptive features of note for sustained VT are whether the ECG appearance is monomorphic or polymorphic.[520] This may be of importance because the former is more likely to be due to a myocardial scar and require aggressive strategies to prevent its recurrence and the latter may be more responsive to measures directed against ischemia. When continuous ECG recordings during the first 12 hours of AMI are analyzed, nonsustained paroxysms of monomorphic or polymorphic VT may be seen in up to 67 percent of patients.[521] These *nonsustained* runs of ventricular tachycardia do not appear to be associated with an increased mortality risk, either during hospitalization or over the first year. Data from the GUSTO-I trial indicate that in the thrombolytic era, sustained VT occurs in 3.5 percent of patients, ventricular fibrillation in 4.1 percent of patients, and a combination of sustained VT and ventricular fibrillation in 2.7 percent of patients.[522] Patients who experience sustained VT either in isolation or in combination with ventricular fibrillation have larger infarcts than patients who do not experience sustained VT or ventricular fibrillation. Not unexpectedly, the larger infarcts in patients with sustained VT are associated with a significantly higher risk of congestive heart failure, cardiogenic shock, and atrial fibrillation. The in-hospital mortality rate for patients experiencing only sustained VT is 18.6 percent, whereas those experiencing both sustained VT and ventricular fibrillation have a 44 percent in-hospital mortality.[522] Patients with sustained VT or both VT and ventricular fibrillation who survive to 30 days have a higher 1-year mortality rate (approximately 7 percent) compared with patients who do not experience either arrhythmia (approximately 3 percent).[522]

VT occurring late in the course of AMI is more common in patients with transmural infarction and left ventricular dysfunction, is likely to be sustained, usually induces marked hemodynamic deterioration, and is associated with both an increased hospital mortality and long-term mortality.

MANAGEMENT. Because hypokalemia may increase the risk of developing VT,[523] low serum potassium levels should be identified quickly after a patient's admission for AMI and should be treated promptly. The serum potassium level should be maintained above 4.5 mEq/liter, and the serum magnesium level should be above 2 mEq/liter.[185]

Rapid abolition of sustained VT in patients with AMI is mandatory because of its deleterious effect on pump function and because it frequently deteriorates into ventricular fibrillation. When the ventricular rate is rapid (150 beats/min) and/or there is a decline in arterial pressure, a single attempt at "thumpversion" (i.e., striking a sharp blow to the precordium) is indicated. Rapid polymorphic VT should be managed similar to ventricular fibrillation, with an unsynchronized discharge of 200 J, whereas monomorphic VT should be treated with a synchronized discharge of 50 to 100 J.[52] Occasionally, lower-energy (10 to 20 J) synchronized discharges can terminate monomorphic VT.

When the ventricular rate is slower than approximately 150 beats/min and the arrhythmia is well tolerated hemodynamically, antiarrhythmic therapy with one of the following regimens should be attempted[52]:

1. *Lidocaine*—initial bolus of 1.0 to 1.5 mg/kg followed by supplemental boluses of 0.5 to 0.75 mg/kg every 5 to 10 minutes as needed to a maximum of 3 mg/kg. A maintenance infusion of 20 to 50 μg/kg/min (1 to 4 mg/min) may then be started. The metabolism of lidocaine is slowed not only in patients with heart failure or hypotension but also in those with diminution of hepatic blood flow due to effects of pharmacological agents such as propranolol. The rate of infusion should be lower in patients with renal

failure. Therefore, careful titration is needed to avoid toxicity, manifested primarily by central nervous system hyperactivity, as well as by depression of intraventricular and atrioventricular conduction and cardiac contractility. Saturation of an extravascular pool normally occurs after a continuous infusion of approximately 3 hours, at which time blood levels increase despite maintenance of a constant infusion rate. At this time, it may be desirable to reduce the rate of administration by about 25 percent.

2. *Procainamide*—loading infusion of 12 to 17 mg/kg over about 20 to 30 minutes, followed by a maintenance infusion of 1 to 4 mg/min (see also Chap. 23).

3. *Amiodarone*—loading infusion of 150 mg, followed by a constant infusion of 1.0 mg/min for up to 6 hours and then a maintenance infusion at 0.5 mg/min (see also Chap. 23).

After reversion to sinus rhythm, every effort should be made to correct underlying abnormalities such as hypoxia, hypotension, acid-base or electrolyte disturbances, and digitalis excess. Although no definitive data are available, it is a common clinical practice to continue maintenance infusions of antiarrhythmic drugs for several days after an index episode of VT and to discontinue the drug and either observe the patient for recurrence or perform a diagnostic electrophysiology study. Patients with recurrent or refractory VT should be considered for specialized procedures such as implantation of antitachycardia devices or surgery (see Chap. 24). Occasionally, urgent attempts at revascularization with angioplasty or CABG may help control refractory VT.[520]

Ventricular Fibrillation

This arrhythmia may occur in three settings in hospitalized patients with AMI. (Its occurrence as a mechanism of sudden death is discussed in Chapter 26.) *Primary* ventricular fibrillation occurs suddenly and unexpectedly in patients with no or few signs or symptoms of left ventricular failure.[520a] Although primary ventricular fibrillation occurred in up to 10 percent of patients hospitalized with AMI several decades ago, analyses suggest that its incidence has declined.[511, 524] Approximately 60 percent of episodes occur within 4 hours and 80 percent within 12 hours of the onset of symptoms.[521] *Secondary* ventricular fibrillation, on the other hand, is often the final event of a progressive downhill course with left ventricular failure and cardiogenic shock. So-called *late* ventricular fibrillation develops more than 48 hours after AMI and frequently but not exclusively occurs in patients with large infarcts and ventricular dysfunction. Patients with intraventricular conduction defects and anterior wall infarction, patients with persistent sinus tachycardia, atrial flutter, or fibrillation early in the clinical course, and those with right ventricular infarction who require ventricular pacing are at higher risk for suffering late in-hospital ventricular fibrillation than are patients without these features.

PROGNOSIS. The effect of primary ventricular fibrillation on prognosis continues to be debated.[515] The MILIS study, conducted in the prethrombolytic era, suggested that it does not have an adverse effect on hospital mortality, whereas the GISSI investigators, reporting observations in large cohorts of thrombolytic-treated patients, suggest that there is an excess mortality due to primary ventricular fibrillation during the hospital phase but not thereafter.[525] Observations from the GUSTO I trial indicate that the in-hospital mortality of patients with early (within the first 48 hours) ventricular fibrillation is 19.8 percent but survivors to 30 days have a 1-year mortality of 2.7 percent, similar to the 1-year mortality of 30-day survivors who do not experience ventricular fibrillation or VT during the initial hospitalization for AMI.[522] On the other hand, secondary ventricular fibrillation occurring in association with marked left ventricular failure or cardiogenic shock, an arrhythmia that typically occurs late (> 48 hours) after presentation with AMI, entails a poor prognosis, with an in-hospital mortality rate of 40 to 60 percent.[521, 526] With the availability of amiodarone and new antitachycardia devices, the prognosis of late ventricular fibrillation is improving and is probably driven more by residual ventricular function and recurrent ischemia than the arrhythmic risk per se.[510]

PROPHYLAXIS. In the early years of MI care in CCUs, concern about the risk of primary ventricular fibrillation led to aggressive monitoring for "warning" ventricular arrhythmias and the initiation of antiarrhythmic therapy when they appeared. Later, when it was shown that warning arrhythmias could not be relied on to predict the risk of ventricular fibrillation, arrhythmia prophylaxis became routine.[527, 528] Lidocaine has been studied most extensively in this regard and has been shown to reduce the incidence of ventricular fibrillation,[529] leading to its widespread routine use in CCUs in patients with known or suspected AMI. However, we no longer endorse that CCU practice for the following reasons:

1. As already noted, the incidence of ventricular fibrillation in patients hospitalized for AMI is decreasing so that the risk for the arrhythmia is now much lower than it was several decades ago (probably under 5 percent). The reasons for this reduction in ventricular fibrillation are not clear but probably include general improvements in the care of AMI patients, greater use of beta blockers, aggressive repletion of electrolytes, prompt treatment of ischemia and congestive heart failure, and reduction in infarct size from reperfusion strategies.[511]

2. There is no evidence that prophylaxis with lidocaine actually reduces mortality in hospitalized patients with AMI because they can almost always be promptly defibrillated.[515] Furthermore, there appear to be trends to excess mortality risk when lidocaine is used on a routine prophylactic basis.[512-514, 529]

3. Beta-adrenoceptor blockers, which should be administered promptly to the majority of patients with AMI (see p. 1168), have been shown to reduce not only ventricular fibrillation[517] but also mortality from AMI.[510, 530]

4. There is an association between hypokalemia and the risk of ventricular fibrillation in the CCU.[531, 532] (see Fig. 35-50)

Although it has not been conclusively shown that correction of hypokalemia to a level of 4.5 mEq/liter actually reduces the incidence of ventricular fibrillation, our experience suggests that this probably is protective and of little risk. The data on magnesium and the risk of ventricular fibrillation are incomplete at present. Despite the fact that no consistent relationship between hypomagnesemia and ventricular fibrillation has been observed,[532] magnesium deficits may still be involved in the risk of ventricular fibrillation because intracellular magnesium levels are reduced in AMI and are not adequately reflected by serum measurements. For these reasons, plus the fact that it is often difficult to repair a potassium deficit without administering supplemental magnesium, we routinely replete magnesium to a level of 2 mEq/liter.

The only situation in which we might consider prophylactic lidocaine (bolus of 1.5 mg/kg followed by 20 to 50 μg/kg/min) would be the unusual circumstance in which a patient within the first 12 hours of an AMI must be managed in a facility where cardiac monitoring is not available and equipment for prompt defibrillation is not readily accessible.

MANAGEMENT. (See also Chap. 25.) The likelihood of successful restoration of an effective cardiac rhythm declines rapidly with time after the onset of uncorrected ventricular fibrillation. Irreversible brain damage may occur within 1 to 2 minutes, particularly in elderly patients. The

treatment of ventricular fibrillation is an unsynchronized electrical countershock with at least 200 to 300 J, implemented as rapidly as possible.[52] This interrupts fibrillation and restores an effective cardiac rhythm in patients under direct medical observation in the CCU. When ventricular fibrillation occurs outside an intensive care unit, resuscitative efforts are much less likely to be successful, primarily because the time interval between the onset of the episode and the institution of definitive therapy tends to be prolonged. Because closed-chest cardiopulmonary resuscitation with external cardiac compression provides only a marginal cardiac output even under optimal circumstances, countershock could be implemented as soon as possible after the detection of ventricular fibrillation rather than deferred under the mistaken impression that adequate circulatory and respiratory support can be maintained in the interim. Failure of electrical countershock to restore an effective cardiac rhythm is due almost always to rapidly recurrent VT or ventricular fibrillation, to electromechanical dissociation, or, very rarely, to electrical asystole.

Ventricular fibrillation often recurs rapidly and repeatedly when the metabolic milieu of the heart has been compromised by severe or prolonged hypoxemia, acidosis, electrolyte abnormalities, or digitalis intoxication. Under these conditions, continued cardiopulmonary resuscitation, prompt implementation of pharmacological and ventilatory maneuvers designed to correct these abnormalities, and rapidly repeated attempts with electrical countershock may be effective. Even though repeated shocks with excessive energy may damage the myocardium and elicit arrhythmias, speed is essential and prompt efforts with high-intensity shocks (generally 300 to 400 watt-seconds) are justified. When ventricular fibrillation persists without documented interruption by electrical countershock, administration of epinephrine either by the intracardiac route (up to 10 ml of a 1:10,000 concentration) or intravenous route (1 mg initially) may facilitate a subsequent defibrillation attempt.

Successful interruption of ventricular fibrillation or prevention of refractory recurrent episodes may also be facilitated by administration of bretylium tosylate, 5 mg/kg intravenously, repeated 5 to 20 minutes later if necessary, or amiodarone (75 to 150 mg bolus). When synchronous cardiac electrical activity is restored by countershock but contraction is ineffective (i.e., during electromechanical dissociation), the usual underlying cause is very extensive myocardial ischemia or necrosis or rupture of the ventricular free wall or septum. If rupture has not occurred, intracardiac administration of calcium gluconate or epinephrine may promote restoration of an effective heartbeat. We do *not* usually administer bicarbonate injections to correct acidosis because of the high osmotic load they impose and the fact that hyperventilation of the patient is probably a more suitable means of clearing the acidosis.

BRADYARRHYTHMIAS

Sinus Bradycardia

Sinus bradycardia is a common arrhythmia occurring during the early phases of AMI, and it is particularly frequent in patients with inferior and posterior infarction.[52] Observations in mobile CCUs indicate that 25 to 40 percent of patients with AMI have ECG evidence of sinus bradycardia within the first hour after the onset of symptoms; however, 4 hours after infarction commences the incidence of sinus bradycardia has declined to 15 to 20 percent.[500] Stimulation of cardiac vagal afferent receptors (which are more common in the inferoposterior than the anterior or lateral portions of the left ventricle), with resulting efferent cholinergic stimulation of the heart, produces vagotonia with resultant bradycardia and hypotension. This is a manifestation of the

Bezold-Jarisch reflex[533] that is mediated by the vagus nerves and occurs during reperfusion, particularly of the right coronary artery.[277, 308, 534] Often sinus bradycardia is a component of vasovagal or vasodepressor response, which may be intensified by severe pain as well as by morphine, and may be related to vasovagal syncope (see Chap. 27).[535]

On the basis of data obtained in experimental infarction and from some clinical observations, it appears that the increased vagal tone that produces sinus bradycardia during the early phase of AMI may actually be protective, perhaps because it reduces myocardial oxygen demands.[536] Thus, the acute mortality rate appears to be as low in patients with sinus bradycardia as in patients without this arrhythmia.

MANAGEMENT. Isolated sinus bradycardia, unaccompanied by hypotension or ventricular ectopy, should be observed rather than treated initially. In the first 4 to 6 hours after infarction, if the sinus rate is extremely slow (under 40 to 50 beats/min), administration of intravenous atropine in aliquots of 0.3 to 0.6 mg every 3 to 10 minutes (with a total dose not exceeding 2 mg) to bring heart rate up to approximately 60 beats/min often abolishes the VPBs commonly associated with this degree of sinus bradycardia.[537] Atropine often contributes to restoration of arterial pressure and hence coronary perfusion and should be employed if hypotension accompanying any degree of sinus bradycardia is present. The favorable effects of atropine may be accompanied by regression of ST segment elevation. Elevation of the lower extremities also often elevates arterial pressure by redistributing blood from the systemic venous bed to the thorax, thereby augmenting ventricular preload, cardiac output, and arterial pressure.

Sinus bradycardia occurring more than 6 hours after the onset of the AMI is often transitory, is caused by sinus node dysfunction or atrial ischemia rather than vagal hyperactivity, is usually not accompanied by hypotension, and does not usually predispose to ventricular arrhythmias. Treatment is not required unless ventricular performance is compromised or the administration of a beta-adrenoceptor blocker or high doses of antiarrhythmic drugs (which may slow the sinus rate further) is planned. When atropine is ineffective and the patient is symptomatic and/or hypotensive, electrical pacing is indicated.[52] In patients with depressed ventricular performance, who require the atrial contribution to ventricular filling, atrial pacing or atrioventricular sequential pacing is superior to simple ventricular pacing.

Atrioventricular and Intraventricular Block

Ischemic injury can produce conduction block at any level of the AV or intraventricular conduction system. Such blocks may occur in the AV node and the bundle of His, producing various grades of AV block; in either main bundle branch, producing right or left bundle branch block; and in the anterior and posterior divisions of the left bundle branch, producing left anterior or left posterior (fascicular) divisional blocks.[538] Disturbances of conduction can, of course, occur in various combinations. The mechanisms and recognition of intraventricular and AV conduction disturbances are discussed in Chapter 22.

First-Degree AV Block

First-degree AV block occurs in less than 15 percent of patients with AMI admitted to CCUs. His bundle ECG studies have shown that almost all patients with first-degree AV block have disturbances in conduction above the bundle of His (i.e., intranodal). The localization of the site of block is important because development of complete heart block and ventricular asystole is restricted almost exclusively to

those patients with first-degree block in whom the conduction disturbance is *below* the bundle of His; this occurs more commonly in patients with anterior infarction and those with associated bifascicular block.

First-degree AV block generally does not require specific treatment. However, if digitalis intoxication is suspected as the cause, this drug should be discontinued. Beta blockers and calcium antagonists (other than nifedipine) prolong AV conduction and may be responsible for first-degree AV block as well. However, discontinuation of these drugs in the setting of AMI has the potential to increase ischemia and ischemic injury. Therefore, it is our practice not to decrease the dosage of these drugs unless the PR interval is greater than 0.24 second. Only if higher-degree block or hemodynamic impairment occurs should these agents be stopped. If the block is a manifestation of excessive vagotonia and is associated with sinus bradycardia and hypotension, administration of atropine, as already outlined, may be helpful. Continued ECG monitoring is important in such patients in view of the possibility of progression to higher degrees of block.

Second-Degree AV Block

MOBITZ TYPE I OR WENCKEBACH AV BLOCK. Mobitz type I block occurs in up to 10 percent of patients with AMI admitted to CCUs and accounts for about 90 percent of all patients with AMI and second-degree AV block. This type of block (1) generally occurs within the AV node, (2) is usually associated with narrow QRS complexes, (3) is presumably secondary to ischemic injury, (4) occurs more commonly in patients with inferior than anterior MI, (5) is usually transient and does not persist for more than 72 hours after infarction, (6) may be intermittent, and (7) rarely progresses to complete AV block (Table 35–21). First-degree and type I second-degree AV blocks do not appear to affect survival, are most commonly associated with occlusion of the right coronary artery, and are caused by ischemia of the AV node.

Specific therapy is not required in patients with second-degree AV block of the Mobitz type I variety when the ventricular rate exceeds 50 beats/min and ventricular irritability, heart failure, and bundle branch block are absent. However, if these complications develop or if the heart rate falls below approximately 50 beats/min and the patient is symptomatic, immediate treatment with atropine (0.3 to 0.6 mg) is indicated; temporary pacing systems are almost never needed in the management of this arrhythmia.

MOBITZ TYPE II AV BLOCK. This is a rare conduction defect after AMI, occurring in only 10 percent of all cases of second-degree block. Thus, the overall incidence of Mobitz type II block after infarction is less than 1 percent. In contrast to Mobitz type I block, type II second-degree block (1) usually originates from a lesion in the conduction system below the bundle of His, (2) is associated with a wide QRS complex, (3) often but not invariably reflects trifascicular block with impaired conduction distal to the bundle of His, (4) often progresses suddenly to complete AV block, and (5) is almost always associated with anterior rather than inferior infarction (see Table 35–21).

Because of its potential for progression to complete heart block, Mobitz type II second-degree AV block should be treated with a temporary external or transvenous demand pacemaker with the rate set at approximately 60 beats/min.[52]

Complete (Third-Degree) AV Block

The AV conduction system has a dual blood supply: the AV branch of the right coronary artery and the septal perforating branch from the left anterior descending coronary artery. Therefore, complete AV block can occur in patients

	LOCATION OF AV CONDUCTION DISTURBANCE	
	Proximal	Distal
Site of block	Intranodal	Infranodal
Site of infarction	Inferoposterior	Anteroseptal
Compromised arterial supply	RCA (90%), LCX (10%)	Septal perforators of LAD
Pathogenesis	Ischemia, necrosis, hydropic cell swelling, excess parasympathetic activity	Ischemia, necrosis, hydropic cell swelling
Predominant type of AV nodal block	First-degree (PR > 200 msec) Mobitz type I second-degree	Mobitz type II second-degree Third-degree
Common premonitory features of third-degree AV block	(a) First–second-degree AV block (b) Mobitz I pattern	(a) Intraventricular conduction block (b) Mobitz II pattern
Features of escape rhythm following third-degree block		
(a) Location	(a) Proximal conduction system (His bundle)	(a) Distal conduction system (bundle branches)
(b) QRS width	(b) < 0.12/sec*	(b) > 0.12/sec
(c) Rate	(c) 45–60/min but may be as low as 30/min	(c) Often < 30/min
(d) Stability of escape rhythm	(d) Rate usually stable; asystole uncommon	(d) Rate often unstable with moderate to high risk of ventricular asystole
Duration of high-grade AV block	Usually transient (2–3 days)	Usually transient but some form of AV conduction disturbance and/or intraventricular defect may persist
Associated mortality rate	Low unless associated with hypotension and/or congestive heart failure	High because of extensive infarction associated with power failure or ventricular arrhythmias
Pacemaker therapy		
(a) Temporary	(a) Rarely required; may be considered for bradycardia associated with left ventricular power failure, syncope, or angina	(a) Should be considered in patients with anteroseptal infarction and acute bifascicular block
(b) Permanent	(b) Almost never indicated because conduction defect is usually transient	(b) Indicated for patients with high-grade AV block with block in His-Purkinje system and those with transient advanced AV block and associated bundle branch block

*Some studies suggest that a wide QRS escape rhythm (> 0.12 sec) following high-grade AV block in inferior infarction is associated with a worse prognosis.

RCA = right coronary artery; LCX = left circumflex coronary artery; LAD = left anterior descending coronary artery.

Modified from Antman EM, Rutherford JD: Coronary Care Medicine: A Practical Approach. Boston, Martinus Nijhoff, 1986; Dreifus LS, et al: Guidelines for implantation of cardiac pacemakers and antiarrhythmia devices. J Am Coll Cardiol 18:1, 1991. Reprinted with permission from the American College of Cardiology.

with either anterior or inferior infarction. Complete AV block occurs in about 5 percent of patients in the thrombolytic era, although the incidence may be higher in patients with right ventricular infarction.[63, 539, 540] As with other forms of AV block, the prognosis depends on the anatomical location of the block in the conduction system and the size of the infarction.[541]

Complete heart block in patients with inferior infarction usually results from an intranodal or supranodal lesion[542] and develops gradually, often progressing from first-degree or type I second-degree block (see Table 35–21). The escape rhythm is usually stable without asystole and often junctional, with a rate exceeding 40 beats/min and a narrow QRS complex in 70 percent of cases and a slower rate and wide QRS in the others. This form of complete AV block is often transient, may be responsive to pharmacological antagonism of adenosine with methylxanthines,[543, 544] and resolves in the majority of patients within a few days. The mortality may approach 15 percent unless right ventricular infarction is present, in which case the mortality associated with complete AV block may be more than doubled.

In patients with anterior infarction, third-degree AV block often occurs suddenly, 12 to 24 hours after the onset of infarction, although it is usually preceded by intraventricular block and often Mobitz type II (not first-degree or Mobitz type I) AV block (see Table 35–20). Such patients have unstable escape rhythms with wide QRS complexes and rates less than 40 beats/min; ventricular systole may occur quite suddenly. The mortality in this group of patients is extremely high, 70 to 80 percent.

PROGNOSIS. This depends on the extent and secondarily on the anatomical site of the myocardial injury.[539, 545] Patients with inferior infarction often have concomitant ischemia or infarction of the AV node secondary to hypoperfusion of the AV nodal artery. However, the His-Purkinje system usually escapes injury in such individuals. Patients with inferior MI who develop AV block usually have lesions in both the right and left anterior descending coronary arteries. Likewise, patients with inferior MI and AV block have larger infarcts and more depressed right ventricular and left ventricular function than do patients with inferior infarct and no AV block. As already noted, junctional escape rhythms with narrow QRS complexes occur commonly in this setting. In patients with anterior infarction, AV block usually develops as a result of extensive septal necrosis that involves the bundle branches. The high mortality in this group of patients with slow idioventricular rhythm and wide QRS complexes is the consequence of extensive myocardial necrosis resulting in severe left ventricular failure and often shock.

Although data suggest that complete AV block is *not* an independent risk factor for mortality, whether temporary transvenous pacing per se improves survival of patients with anterior AMI remains controversial. Some investigators contend that ventricular pacing is useless when employed to correct complete AV block in patients with anterior infarction in view of the poor prognosis in this group regardless of therapy. However, pacing may protect against transient hypotension with its attendant risks of extending infarction and precipitating malignant ventricular tachyarrhythmias. Also, pacing protects against asystole, a particular hazard in patients with anterior infarction and infranodal block. Improved survival with pacing probably occurs in only a small fraction of patients with complete AV block and anterior wall infarcts because the extensive destruction of the myocardium that almost invariably accompanies this condition results in a very high mortality rate, even in paced patients. Given these considerations, an extremely large series of patients would be required to demonstrate the small reduction of mortality that might be achieved by pacing. The absence of data supporting such an effect, however, by no means excludes the possibility that it may be present.

Pacing is not usually needed in patients with inferior wall infarction and complete AV block that is often transient in nature, but it is indicated if the ventricular rate is very slow (< 40 to 50 beats/min), if ventricular irritability or hypotension is present, or if pump failure develops; atropine is only rarely of value in these patients. Only when complete heart block develops in less than 6 hours after the onset of symptoms is atropine likely to abolish the AV block or cause acceleration of the escape rhythm. In such cases the AV block is more likely to be transient and related to increases in vagal tone than the more persistent block seen later in the course of MI, which generally requires cardiac pacing.

Intraventricular Block

In the prethrombolytic era, studies of intraventricular conduction disturbances, such as a block within one or more of the three subdivisions (fascicles) of the His-Purkinje system (the anterior and posterior divisions of the left bundle and the right bundle), had been reported to occur in 5 to 10 percent of patients with AMI.[532, 546, 547] Several series in the thrombolytic era suggest that intraventricular blocks occur in 2 to 5 percent of patients with AMI.[540, 548] The right bundle branch and the left posterior division have a dual blood supply from the left anterior descending and right coronary arteries, whereas the left anterior division is supplied by septal perforators originating from the left anterior descending coronary artery. Not all conduction blocks observed in patients with AMI can be considered to be complications of infarcts because almost half are already present at the time the first ECG is recorded, and they may represent antecedent disease of the conduction system.[547, 549] Compared with patients without conduction defects, AMI patients with bundle branch blocks have more comorbid conditions; are less likely to receive therapies such as thrombolytics, aspirin, and beta blockers; and have an increased in-hospital mortality rate.[550]

ISOLATED FASCICULAR BLOCKS. Isolated left anterior divisional block is unlikely to progress to complete AV block.[546, 551, 552] Mortality is increased in these patients, although not as much as in patients with other forms of conduction block. The posterior fascicle is larger than the anterior fascicle, and, in general, a larger infarct is required to block it. As a consequence, mortality is markedly increased. Complete AV block is not a frequent complication of either form of isolated divisional block.[546, 551, 552]

RIGHT BUNDLE BRANCH BLOCK. This defect alone occurs in approximately 2 percent of patients with AMI and may lead to AV block because it is often a new lesion, associated with anteroseptal infarction.[547] Isolated right bundle branch block is associated with an increased mortality risk in patients with anterior MI even if complete AV block does not occur, but this appears to be the case only if it is accompanied by congestive heart failure.[547, 551, 553]

BIFASCICULAR BLOCK. The combination of right bundle branch block with either left anterior or posterior divisional block or the combination of left anterior and posterior divisional blocks (i.e., left bundle branch block) is known as bidivisional or bifascicular block. If a new block occurs in two of the three divisions of the conduction system, the risk of developing complete AV block is quite high. Mortality is also high because of the occurrence of severe pump failure secondary to the extensive myocardial necrosis required to produce such an extensive intraventricular block.[548, 552] Left bundle branch block occurs in 2 to 5 percent of patients with AMI. Although the latter defect progresses to complete AV block only half as frequently as does right bundle branch block, it is associated with as high a mortality as right bundle branch block and the other two forms of bifascicular block[551] and with a high late mortality. Patients with intraventricular conduction defects, particularly right bundle branch block, account for the majority of patients who develop ventricular fibrillation late in their hospital stay. However, the high mortality in these patients occurs even in the absence of high-grade AV block and appears to be related to cardiac failure and massive infarction rather than to the conduction disturbance.[550]

Preexisting bundle branch block or divisional block is less often associated with the development of complete heart block in patients with AMI than are conduction defects acquired during the course of the infarct.[551] Bidivisional block in the presence of prolongation of the PR interval (first-degree AV block) may indicate disease of the third subdivision rather than of the AV node. In such cases, termed "trifascicular block," nearly 40 percent progress to complete heart block, a risk that is considerably greater than the risk of complete heart block without first-degree AV block.[546]

Complete bundle branch block (either left or right), the combination of right bundle branch block and left anterior divisional (fascicular) block, and any of the various forms of trifascicular block are all more often associated with anterior than inferoposterior infarction. All these forms are more frequent with large infarcts and in older patients and have a higher incidence of other accompanying arrhythmias than is seen in patients without bundle branch block.

Asystole

This arrhythmia has been reported to occur in 1 to 14 percent of patients with AMI admitted to CCUs. This wide variation in incidence reflects differences in the definition of this event. The lower incidence rates include only patients who develop asystole either as a primary event or after abnormalities of AV or intraventricular conduction, whereas the higher rates include patients who develop asystole as a terminal complication. In either event, the mortality is very high.

The presence of apparent ventricular asystole on monitor displays of continuously recorded ECGs may be misleading, because the mechanism may in fact be fine ventricular fibrillation. Because of the predominance of ventricular fibrillation as the cause of cardiac arrest in this setting, initial therapy should include electrical countershock, even if definitive ECG documentation of this arrhythmia is not available. In the rare instance in which asystole can be documented to be the responsible electrophysiological disturbance, immediate transcutaneous pacing (or stimulation with a transvenous pacemaker if one is already in place) is indicated.[52]

Use of Pacemakers in AMI

(See also Chap. 24)

TEMPORARY PACING. Just as is the case for complete AV block, transvenous ventricular pacing has not resulted in statistically demonstrable improvement in prognosis among patients with AMI who develop intraventricular conduction defects. However, temporary pacing is advisable in some of these patients because of the high risk of developing complete AV block. This includes patients with new bilateral (bifascicular) bundle branch block (i.e., right bundle branch block with left anterior or posterior divisional block and alternating right and left bundle branch block); first-degree AV block adds to this risk. Isolated new block in only one of the three fascicles even with PR interval prolongation and preexisting bifascicular block and normal PR interval poses somewhat less risk; these patients should be monitored closely, with insertion of a temporary pacemaker deferred unless higher-degree AV block occurs.

It has been proposed on the basis of results of an analysis of several large series of well-characterized patients that the risk of developing complete heart block after AMI can be predicted.[552] The presence (new or preexisting) of any of the following conduction disturbances is considered a risk factor: first-degree AV block, Mobitz type I second-degree AV block, Mobitz type II second-degree AV block, left anterior hemiblock, left posterior hemiblock, right bundle branch block, and left bundle branch block. Each risk factor was assigned a score of 1, and the risk score was calculated as the sum of these ECG risk factors. The incidence of complete heart block occurred as follows: risk score 0, 1.2 to 6.8 percent incidence; risk score 1, 7.8 to 10.4 percent incidence; risk score 2, 25.0 to 30.1 percent incidence; and risk score 3, 36 percent or greater incidence.[552] Some authorities have pointed out deficiencies in this scoring system in that Mobitz type II AV block is assigned a score of only 1 point but appears to carry more significance; also there is no differentiation between preexisting and newly appearing bundle branch block.

We believe that failure to demonstrate improved prognosis statistically does not belie the potential value of pacemaker therapy; it probably reflects the overriding impact on mortality of the extensive infarction responsible for the development of the conduction abnormality and the large number of patients required to permit statistical documentation of reduction of mortality.

In assessing the need for temporary pacing (see Table 35–21), the clinician must keep in mind that between 10 and 20 percent of patients develop pacemaker-related complications. A pericardial friction rub develops in approximately 5 percent of patients but does not necessarily indicate cardiac perforation, nor is such a finding an indication for withdrawal of the pacemaker electrode. Arrhythmias requiring cardioversion, right ventricular perforation, and local infectious complications occur in 1 to 3 percent of cases. Pacemaker malfunction also occurs rather frequently and is, in part, related to the experience of the clinical team in managing the device and its insertion.

Although external temporary cardiac pacing was introduced in 1952, its widespread clinical use did not occur until relatively recently owing to technical refinements making the technique safe, quickly applicable, and relatively well tolerated. Noninvasive external temporary cardiac pacing is now possible routinely in conscious patients and is acceptable to many but not all patients because of the discomfort.[554] Used in a standby mode, it is virtually free of complications and contraindications and provides an important alternative to transvenous endocardial pacing.[52] Once it is clinically evident that continuous pacing is required, external pacing, which is generally not well tolerated for more than minutes to hours, should be replaced by a temporary transvenous pacemaker.

PERMANENT PACING. The question of permanent pacing in survivors of AMI associated with conduction defects is still controversial (see Table 35–21). Patients with inferior infarction with transient type II second-degree block or complete AV block without an associated intraventricular conduction defect do not appear to require permanent pacing. Some contend that prophylactic pacing makes little

difference in the long-term survival of patients with AMI and bundle branch block complicated by transient high-degree block. On the other hand, in a retrospective multicenter study, survivors of AMI and bundle branch block who experienced transient high-degree (Mobitz type II second-degree or third-degree) block had a high incidence of recurrent high-degree AV block and sudden death, and this incidence was reduced by insertion of a permanent demand pacemaker.[546, 551] Thus, these findings suggest a role for prophylactic permanent pacing in patients with AMI and bundle branch block with transient high-degree AV block.

The question of the advisability of permanent pacemaker insertion is complicated by the fact that not all sudden deaths in this population are due to recurrent high-degree block. A high incidence of late in-hospital ventricular fibrillation occurs in CCU survivors with anteroseptal MI complicated by either right or left bundle branch block. If the propensity for this arrhythmia continued, ventricular fibrillation rather than asystole due to failure of AV conduction and of the infranodal pacemaker could be responsible for late sudden death.

Long-term pacing is often helpful when complete heart block persists throughout the hospital phase in a patient with AMI, when sinus node function is markedly impaired, or when Mobitz II second- or third-degree block occurs intermittently.[52] When high-grade AV block is associated with newly acquired bundle branch block or other criteria of impairment of conduction system function, prophylactic long-term pacing may be justified as well. Thus, despite the difficulty of proving that long-term pacing improves survival after MI because of the high mortality associated with extensive infarction frequently responsible for high degrees of heart block, prophylactic long-term pacing is prudent.

SUPRAVENTRICULAR TACHYARRHYTHMIAS
(See also Chap. 25)

SINUS TACHYCARDIA. This arrhythmia is typically associated with augmented sympathetic activity and may provoke transient hypertension or hypotension. Common causes are anxiety, persistent pain, left ventricular failure, fever, pericarditis, hypovolemia, pulmonary embolism, and the administration of cardioaccelerator drugs such as atropine, epinephrine, or dopamine; rarely it occurs in patients with atrial infarction. Sinus tachycardia is particularly common in patients with anterior infarction, especially if there is significant accompanying left ventricular dysfunction. It is an undesirable rhythm in patients with AMI because it results in an augmentation of myocardial oxygen consumption, as well as a reduction in the time available for coronary perfusion, thereby intensifying myocardial ischemia and/or external myocardial necrosis. Persistent sinus tachycardia may signify persistent heart failure and under these circumstances is a poor prognostic sign associated with an excess mortality.[52] An underlying cause should be sought and appropriate treatment instituted (e.g., analgesics for pain, diuretics for heart failure, oxygen, beta blockers and nitroglycerin for ischemia, and aspirin for fever or pericarditis).

Administration of beta-adrenoceptor blocking agents, may be helpful in the treatment of sinus tachycardia, particularly when this arrhythmia is a manifestation of hyperdynamic circulation, which is seen particularly in young patients with an initial MI without extensive cardiac damage. However, beta blockade is contraindicated in patients in whom the sinus tachycardia is a manifestation of hypovolemia or of pump failure, the latter reflected by a systolic arterial pressure below 100 mm Hg, rales involving more than one third of the lung fields, a pulmonary capillary wedge pressure exceeding 20 to 25 mm Hg, or a cardiac index below approximately 2.2 liters/min/m². A possible exception to this is a patient in whom persistent ischemia is believed to be the cause or the result of tachycardia: cautious administration of an ultrashort-acting beta-adrenoceptor blocker such as esmolol (25 to 200 μg/kg/min) may be tried to ascertain the patient's response to slowing of the heart rate.[188]

ATRIAL PREMATURE CONTRACTIONS. Atrial premature contractions, and the atrial tachyarrhythmias (paroxysmal supraventricular tachycardia, atrial flutter, and atrial fibrillation) that they often herald, may be caused by atrial distention secondary to increases in left ventricular diastolic pressure, by pericarditis with its associated atrial epicarditis, or, less commonly, by ischemic injury to the atria and sinus node. Atrial premature beats per se are not associated with an increase in mortality, and cardiac output is unaffected. No specific therapy is needed, but it should be kept in mind that these beats may indicate excessive autonomic stimulation or the presence of overt or occult heart failure—conditions that may be assessed by physical examination, chest roentgenography, and echocardiography.

PAROXYSMAL SUPRAVENTRICULAR TACHYCARDIA. This arrhythmia occurs in less than 10 percent of patients with AMI but requires aggressive management because of the rapid ventricular rate.[462] Augmentation of vagal tone by manual carotid sinus stimulation may restore sinus rhythm. The drug of choice for paroxysmal supraventricular tachycardia in the non-AMI patient is adenosine (6 to 12 mg).[462] Few data exist to guide therapy with adenosine in the AMI patient, but we believe that it can be used safely provided that hypotension (systolic pressure 100 mm Hg) is not present before its administration. Intravenous verapamil (5 to 10 mg), diltiazem (15 to 20 mg), and metoprolol (5 to 15 mg) are suitable alternatives in patients without significant left ventricular dysfunction. In the presence of congestive heart failure or hypotension, direct-current countershock or rapid atrial stimulation via a transvenous intraatrial electrode should be used. Although digitalis glycosides may be useful in augmenting vagal tone, thereby terminating the arrhythmia, their effect is often delayed.

ATRIAL FLUTTER AND FIBRILLATION. Atrial flutter is the least common major atrial arrhythmia associated with AMI. Atrial flutter is usually transient, and in AMI it is typically a consequence of augmented sympathetic stimulation of the atria, often occurring in patients with left ventricular failure or pulmonary emboli in whom the arrhythmia intensifies hemodynamic deterioration.[500, 555]

Atrial fibrillation is far more common than flutter, occurring in 10 to 20 percent of patients with AMI.[556, 557] As with atrial premature contractions and atrial flutter, fibrillation is usually transient and tends to occur in patients with left ventricular failure but is also observed in patients with pericarditis and ischemic injury to the atria and right ventricular infarction.[63, 558] The increased ventricular rate and the loss of the atrial contribution to left ventricular filling result in a significant reduction in cardiac output. Atrial fibrillation during AMI is associated with increased mortality and stroke, particularly in patients with anterior wall infarction.[557, 559] However, because it is more common in patients with clinical and hemodynamic manifestations of extensive infarction and a poor prognosis, atrial fibrillation is probably a marker of poor prognosis, with only a small independent contribution to increased mortality.

Management. Atrial flutter and fibrillation in patients with AMI are treated in a manner similar to these conditions in other settings (see Chap. 23). Because of the possibility that the rapid ventricular rate and hypotension associated with these arrhythmias can increase infarct size and because of the important role played by atrial contraction in the support of cardiac output in patients with AMI, treatment must be prompt, especially when the ventricular rate exceeds 100 beats/min. When hemodynamic decompensation is prominent, electrical cardioversion is indicated, beginning with 25 to 50 J for atrial flutter and 50 to 100 J for atrial fibrillation, with gradual increase if the initial shock is not successful. For patients without hemodynamic compromise, the first maneuver should be to slow the ventricular rate. Ideally, a beta-adrenoceptor blocker (e.g., metoprolol in 5-mg intravenous boluses every 5 to 10 minutes to a total dose of 15 to 20 mg, followed by 25 to 50 mg orally every 6 hours) should be used because of the combined effects of ischemia and sympathetic tone that are usually present in patients with atrial fibrillation. If there is concern about the patient's ability to tolerate beta blockade, esmolol may be used. Intravenous doses of verapamil or diltiazem are attractive alternatives because of their ability to slow the ventricular rate promptly, but they should be used with caution if at all in patients with pulmonary congestion. In patients with congestive heart failure, digitalis is

the principal agent used to slow the ventricular response, although the onset of its effect may be delayed for several hours. Digitalis may be supplemented by small intravenous doses of a beta blocker, which also prolongs the AV nodal refractory period: 1 to 4 mg of propranolol in divided doses is often quite effective in reducing the ventricular rate and is well tolerated, even in patients with mild heart failure and a rapid ventricular rate. An additional important option for the treatment of atrial flutter is the use of rapid atrial stimulation through a transvenous intraatrial electrode. Because of the increased risk of embolism in atrial fibrillation, intravenous anticoagulation with heparin should be instituted in the absence of any contraindications.

Attention should be directed to the management of the underlying cause (usually heart failure), and then a decision must be made about the advisability of antiarrhythmic therapy to restore and maintain sinus rhythm. In patients who have acute atrial flutter or fibrillation without a history of atrial fibrillation and in whom congestive symptoms are either absent or easily controlled, we usually administer intravenous procainamide (2 to 4 mg/min) for 24 to 48 hours. The goal is to achieve pharmacological cardioversion or secondarily to establish a therapeutic concentration of the drug in preparation for direct-current cardioversion.

In view of the mounting evidence of an increased risk of proarrhythmia from antiarrhythmic drugs prescribed for atrial fibrillation, as well as an adverse interaction between recurrent ischemia and antiarrhythmic drugs, we are reluctant to prescribe type I antiarrhythmic agents over the intermediate or long term in patients with AMI.[510, 560] Amiodarone appears to be an increasingly attractive antiarrhythmic drug for suppression of recurrences of atrial fibrillation. This drug is also useful for prevention of ventricular arrhythmias and can block the AV node should atrial fibrillation recur, both desirable features after AMI. It may be prescribed in a low dose (200 mg/d), thereby reducing the risk of toxicity. Although experience is limited, we believe that amiodarone is a logical choice for suppression of atrial fibrillation after AMI; often only a short course of treatment (6 weeks) is needed because the risk of atrial fibrillation decreases as time passes after infarction.

Patients with recurrent episodes of atrial fibrillation should be treated with oral anticoagulants (to reduce the risk of stroke), even if sinus rhythm is present at the time of hospital discharge, because no antiarrhythmic regimen can be relied on to be completely effective in suppressing atrial fibrillation. In the absence of contraindications, the majority of patients should receive a beta blocker after AMI; in addition to their several other beneficial effects in MI and post-MI patients, these agents are helpful in slowing the ventricular rate should atrial fibrillation recur.

JUNCTIONAL RHYTHMS. These arrhythmias are often transient, occur during the first 48 hours of the infarction, typically develop and terminate gradually, and are characterized by QRS complexes that resemble those of normally conducted beats. Retrograde P waves may be evident, or AV dissociation may occur, with the junctional rate slightly in excess of the underlying sinus rate. Junctional rhythms fall into two categories:

1. AV junctional rhythm at a rate of 35 to 60 beats/min in which the AV junctional tissue simply assumes the role of the dominant pacemaker when the sinus node is depressed. This arrhythmia is generally a benign protective escape rhythm that is commonly seen among patients with a slow sinus rate in the presence of inferior MI. When there is hemodynamic impairment, transvenous sequential AV pacing may be required to facilitate ventricular performance and maintain adequate peripheral perfusion.

2. Accelerated junctional rhythm (nonparoxysmal junctional tachycardia) is less common and occurs when there is increased automaticity of the junctional tissue, which

usurps the role of pacemaker, usually appearing at a rate of 70 to 130 beats/min. This arrhythmia is seen more commonly with inferior than anterior AMI and may also appear in patients with digitalis intoxication. In studies conducted during the prethrombolytic era, the appearance of accelerated junctional rhythm in the setting of anterior infarction was associated with a poor prognosis, but this was not observed when it occurred in patients with inferior infarction.

OTHER COMPLICATIONS

Recurrent Chest Discomfort

Evaluation of postinfarction chest discomfort may be complicated by previous abnormalities on the ECG and a vague description of the discomfort by the patient who either may be exquisitely sensitive to fleeting discomfort or may deny a potential recrudescence of symptoms. The critical task for clinicians is to distinguish recurrent angina or infarction from nonischemic causes of discomfort that might be caused by infarct expansion, pericarditis, pulmonary embolism, and noncardiac conditions. Important diagnostic maneuvers include a repeat physical examination, repeat ECG, and assessment of the response to sublingual nitroglycerin, 0.4 mg. (The use of noninvasive diagnostic evaluation for recurrent ischemia in patients whose symptoms only appear with moderate levels of exertion is discussed on page 1199.)

RECURRENT ISCHEMIA AND INFARCTION. The incidence of postinfarction angina without reinfarction is between 20 and 30 percent.[349] It does not appear to be reduced by the use of thrombolytic therapy as the management strategy during the acute phase[19] but has been reported to be lower in patients who undergo primary PTCA for AMI, especially if stents are used.[337] When accompanied by ST segment and T wave changes in the same leads where Q waves have appeared, it may be due to occlusion of an initially patent vessel, reocclusion of an initially recanalized vessel, or coronary spasm.

Extension of the original zone of necrosis or *reinfarction* in a separate myocardial zone can be a difficult diagnosis, especially within the first 24 hours after the index event.[79] It is more convenient to refer to both extension and reinfarction collectively under the more general term *recurrent infarction.* Circulating cardiac markers may still be elevated from the initial infarction, and it may not be possible to distinguish the ECG changes that are part of the normal evolution after the index infarction from those due to recurrent infarction. Because the cardiac-specific troponins (see p. 1134) remain elevated for more than 1 week after the index event, they are of less value for diagnosing recurrent infarction than are more rapidly rising and falling markers such as CK-MB. Within the first 18 to 24 hours after the initial infarction, when serum cardiac markers may not have returned to the normal range, recurrent infarction should be strongly considered when there is repeat ST segment elevation on the ECG. Although pericarditis remains a possibility in such patients, the two can usually be distinguished by the presence of a rub and the lack of responsiveness to nitroglycerin in patients with pericardial discomfort.

Beyond the first 24 hours, cardiac markers such as CK-MB have usually returned to the normal range; thus, recurrent infarction may be diagnosed either by reelevation of the CK-MB above the upper limit of normal and increased by at least 50 percent of the previous value or by the appearance of new Q waves on the ECG.[52] Because of variations in patient populations and definitions of recurrent infarction, estimates of the incidence of this complication vary; recent large thrombolytic trials report reinfarction rates of 5 to 6 percent.[20, 22] Reinfarction is more common in patients with diabetes mellitus and those with a previous

MI, but it cannot be predicted reliably from the angiographic appearance of the coronary artery early after infarction, at least when thrombolytic therapy has been given.

Regardless of whether postinfarction angina is persistent or limited, its presence is important because short-term morbidity is higher among such patients; mortality may be increased if the recurrent ischemia is accompanied by ECG changes and hemodynamic compromise.[52, 561] Recurrent infarction (due in many cases to reocclusion of the infarct-related coronary artery) carries serious adverse prognostic information because it is associated with a twofold to fourfold higher rate of in-hospital complications (congestive heart failure, heart block) and mortality. The mortality rate at 1 to 3 years after the initial infarction is higher in those patients who suffered from recurrent infarction during their index hospitalization.[562] Presumably, the higher mortality is related to the larger mass of myocardium whose function becomes compromised.

Of the standard therapies that are routinely prescribed during the acute phase of AMI, aspirin and beta blockers have been associated with a reduction in the incidence of recurrent infarction.[52, 349, 563] The data on heparin are less convincing.

Management. As with the acute phase of treatment of AMI, algorithms for management of patients with recurrent ischemic discomfort at rest center on the 12-lead ECG (Fig. 35–51). Those patients with ST segment reelevation should either receive repeat thrombolysis[52, 564] or be referred for urgent catheterization and PTCA. Insertion of an intraaortic balloon pump may help stabilize the patient while other procedures are being arranged. For patients believed to have recurrent ischemia who do not have evidence of hemodynamic compromise, an attempt should be made to control symptoms with sublingual or intravenous nitroglycerin and intravenous beta blockade to slow the heart rate to 60 beats/min. When hypotension, congestive heart failure, or ventricular arrhythmias develop during recurrent ischemia, urgent catheterization and revascularization are indicated.

Pericardial Effusion and Pericarditis
(See also Chap. 50.)

PERICARDIAL EFFUSION. Effusions are generally detected echocardiographically, and their incidence varies with technique, criteria, and laboratory expertise. Effusions are more common in patients with anterior MI and with larger infarcts and when congestive heart failure is present.[565] The majority of pericardial effusions that are

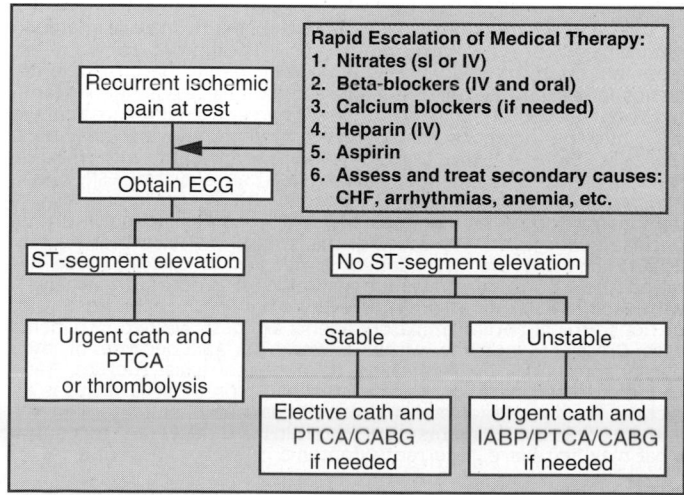

FIGURE 35–51. Treatment of recurrent ischemic events. (From Cannon CP, Ganz LI, Stone PH: Complicated myocardial infarction. *In* Rippe JM, Irwin RS, Fink MP, Cerra FB [eds]: Intensive Care Medicine. 3rd ed. Boston, Little, Brown & Co, 1995.)

seen after AMI do not cause hemodynamic compromise; when tamponade occurs, it is usually due to ventricular rupture or hemorrhagic pericarditis.[99]

The reabsorption rate of a postinfarction pericardial effusion is slow, with resolution often taking several months. The presence of an effusion does not indicate that pericarditis is present; although they may occur together, the majority of effusions occur without other evidence of pericarditis.

PERICARDITIS. When secondary to transmural AMI, pericarditis may produce pain as early as the first day and as late as 6 weeks after MI. The pain of pericarditis may be confused with that resulting from postinfarction angina, recurrent infarction, or both. An important distinguishing feature is the radiation of the pain to either trapezius ridge, a finding that is nearly pathognomonic of pericarditis and rarely seen with ischemic discomfort.[99] Transmural MI, by definition, extends to the epicardial surface and is responsible for local pericardial inflammation. An acute fibrinous pericarditis (pericarditis epistenocardica) occurs commonly after transmural infarction, but the majority of patients do not report any symptoms from this process.[99] Although transient pericardial friction rubs are relatively common among patients with transmural infarction within the first 48 hours, pain or ECG changes occur much less often. However, the development of a pericardial rub appears to be correlated with a larger infarct and greater hemodynamic compromise. The discomfort of pericarditis usually becomes worse during a deep inspiration, but it may be relieved or diminished when the patient sits up and leans forward.

Although anticoagulation clearly increases the risk for hemorrhagic pericarditis early after MI, this complication has not been reported with sufficient frequency during heparinization or after thrombolytic therapy to warrant absolute prohibition of such agents when a rub is present, but the detection of a pericardial effusion on an echocardiogram is usually an indication for discontinuation of anticoagulation.[99] In patients in whom continuation or initiation of anticoagulant therapy is strongly indicated (such as during cardiac catheterization or after coronary angioplasty), heightened monitoring of clotting parameters and observation for clinical signs of possible tamponade are needed. Late pericardial constriction due to anticoagulant-induced hemopericardium has been reported.

Treatment of pericardial discomfort consists of aspirin, but usually in higher doses than prescribed routinely after infarction: doses of 650 mg orally every 4 to 6 hours may be needed. Nonsteroidal antiinflammatory agents and corticosteroids should be avoided because they may interfere with myocardial scar formation.[566]

DRESSLER SYNDROME. Also known as the postmyocardial infarction syndrome,[567] Dressler syndrome usually occurs 1 to 8 weeks after infarction. Its incidence is difficult to define because it often blends imperceptibly with the more common early post-MI pericarditis. Dressler cited an incidence of 3 to 4 percent of all AMI patients in 1957, but the incidence has decreased dramatically since that time. Clinically, patients with Dressler syndrome present with malaise, fever, pericardial discomfort, leukocytosis, an elevated ESR, and a pericardial effusion. At autopsy, patients with this syndrome usually demonstrate localized fibrinous pericarditis containing polymorphonuclear leukocytes.[567] The cause of this syndrome is not clearly established, although the detection of antibodies to cardiac tissue has raised the notion of an immunopathological process. Treatment is with aspirin, 650 mg, as often as every 4 hours. Glucocorticosteroids or nonsteroidal antiinflammatory agents are best avoided in patients with Dressler syndrome within 4 weeks of AMI because of their potential to impair infarct healing, to cause ventricular rupture,[568] and to increase coronary vascular resistance. Aspirin in large doses is effective. Four weeks after AMI, nonsteroidal antiinflammatory agents and in occasional patients corticosteroids are necessary to control what may be severe, recurrent symptoms.

Venous Thrombosis and Pulmonary Embolism

Almost all pulmonary emboli originate from thrombi in the veins of the lower extremities (see Chap. 52); much less commonly, they originate from mural thrombi overlying an area of right ventricular infarction. Bed rest and heart failure predispose to venous thrombosis and subsequent pulmonary embolism, and both of these factors occur commonly in patients with AMI, particularly those with large infarcts. Several decades ago, at a time when patients with AMI were routinely subjected to prolonged periods of bed rest, significant pulmonary embolism was found in more than 20 percent of patients with MI coming to autopsy, and massive pulmonary embolism accounted for 10 percent of deaths from AMI.[569] In recent years, with early mobilization and the widespread use of low-dose anticoagulant prophylaxis, especially using low-molecular-weight heparins, pulmonary embolism has become an uncommon cause of death in this condition. When pulmonary embolism does occur in patients with AMI, management is generally along the lines described for noninfarction patients.

Left Ventricular Aneurysm

The term *left ventricular aneurysm* (often termed *true aneurysm*) is generally reserved for a discrete, dyskinetic area of the left ventricular wall with a broad neck (to differentiate it from pseudoaneurysm due to a contained myocardial rupture). True left ventricular aneurysms probably develop in less than 5 to 10 percent of all patients with AMI and perhaps somewhat more frequently in patients with transmural infarction (especially anterior).[57] The wall of the true aneurysm is thinner than the rest of the left ventricle (Fig. 35–46), and it is usually composed of fibrous tissue as well as necrotic muscle, occasionally mixed with viable myocardium. Aneurysm formation presumably occurs when intraventricular tension stretches the noncontracting infarcted heart muscle, thus producing infarct expansion; a relatively weak, thin layer of necrotic muscle; and fibrous tissue that bulges with each cardiac contraction. With the passage of time, the wall of the aneurysm becomes more densely fibrotic, but it continues to bulge with systole, causing some of the left ventricular stroke volume during each systole to be ineffective.

When an aneurysm is present after anterior MI, there is generally a total occlusion of a poorly collateralized left anterior descending coronary artery. An aneurysm is rarely seen with multivessel disease when there are either extensive collaterals or a nonoccluded left anterior descending artery. Aneurysms usually range from 1 to 8 cm in diameter. They occur approximately four times more often at the apex and in the anterior wall than in the inferoposterior wall. The overlying pericardium is usually densely adherent to the wall of the aneurysm, which may even become partially calcified after several years. True left ventricular aneurysms (in contrast to pseudoaneurysms) rarely rupture soon after development. Late rupture, when the true aneurysm has become stabilized by the formation of dense fibrous tissue in its wall, almost never occurs.

Mortality in patients with a left ventricular aneurysm is up to six times higher than in patients without aneurysms, even when compared with that in patients with comparable left ventricular ejection fraction.[570] Death in these patients is often sudden and presumably related to the high incidence of ventricular tachyarrhythmias that occur with aneurysms.[510]

The presence of persistent ST segment elevation in an ECG area of infarction, classically thought to suggest aneurysm formation, actually indicates a large infarct but does not necessarily imply an aneurysm. The diagnosis of aneurysm is best made noninvasively by an echocardiographic study by radionuclide ventriculography or at the time of cardiac catheterization by left ventriculography. With the loss of shortening from the area of the aneurysm, the remainder of the ventricle must be hyperkinetic in order to compensate. With relatively large aneurysms, complete compensation is impossible. The stroke volume falls or, if maintained, it is at the expense of an increase in end-diastolic volume, which in turn leads to increased wall tension and myocardial oxygen demand. Heart failure may ensue, and angina may appear or worsen.

TREATMENT. Aggressive management of AMI, including coronary thrombolysis, may diminish the incidence of ventricular aneurysms. Surgical aneurysmectomy (Fig. 35–52) generally is successful only if there is relative preservation of contractile performance in the nonaneurysmal portion of the left ventricle. In such circumstances, when the operation is performed for worsening heart failure or angina, operative mortality is relatively low and clinical improvement can be expected.[571]

Left Ventricular Thrombus and Arterial Embolism

Mural thrombi occur in approximately 20 percent of patients with AMI who do not receive anticoagulant therapy; the incidence rises to 40 percent with anterior infarction and to as high as 60 percent in patients with large anterior infarcts that involve the apex of the left ventricle.[346] The most convenient and accurate method for diagnosing left ventricular thrombosis is two-dimensional echocardiography (see Chap. 7). It is hypothesized that endocardial inflammation during the acute phase of infarction provides a thrombogenic surface for clots to form in the left ventricle. With extensive transmural infarction of the septum, however, mural thrombi may overlie infarcted myocardium in both ventricles. Prospective studies have suggested that patients who develop a mural thrombus early (within 48 to 72 hours of infarction) have an extremely poor early prognosis,[494] with a high mortality from the complications of a large infarction (shock, reinfarction, rupture, and ventricular tachyarrhythmia), rather than emboli from the left ventricular thrombus.

Although a mural thrombus adheres to the endocardium overlying the infarcted myocardium, superficial portions of it can become detached and produce systemic arterial emboli. Although estimates vary based on patient selection, about 10 percent of mural thrombi result in systemic embolization.[346] Echocardiographically detectable features that suggest a given thrombus is more likely to embolize include increased mobility and protrusion into the ventricular chamber, visualization in multiple views, and contiguous zones of akinesis and hyperkinesis.

MANAGEMENT. Over the past decade six randomized trials involving only 560 patients tested whether anticoagulant therapy reduced the incidence of *left ventricular thrombus formation*.[572, 573] Collectively, these smaller trials showed that anticoagulation (intravenous heparin or high-dose subcutaneous heparin) reduced the development of *thrombi* by 50 percent, but, because of the low event rate, it was not possible to demonstrate a reduction in the incidence of *systemic embolism*. Additional data from thrombolytic trials suggest that thrombolysis reduces the rate of thrombus formation and the character of the thrombi so that they are less protuberant. Of note, however, the data from thrombolytic trials are difficult to interpret because of the confounding effect of antithrombotic therapy with heparin.[573] Recommendations for anticoagulation vary considera-

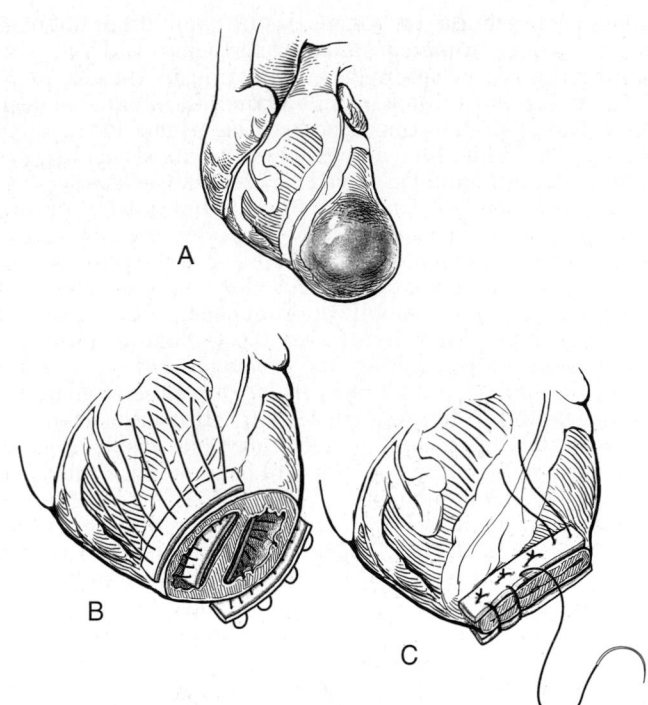

FIGURE 35–52. Surgical repair of ventricular aneurysm. In this case the aneurysm is located at the apex (*A*). The aneurysmal segment is resected, and felt pledget strips are used to reinforce interrupted suture closure of the apex (*B*). Completed repair partially restores apical geometry (*C*). (Courtesy of Dr. David Adams, Division of Cardiac Surgery, Brigham and Women's Hospital.)

bly,[574, 575] and thrombolysis has precipitated fatal embolization. Nevertheless, anticoagulation for 3 to 6 months with warfarin is advocated for many patients with demonstrable mural thrombi.

Based on the available data, it is our practice to recommend anticoagulation (intravenous heparin to elevate the activated partial thromboplastin time one and one-half to two times control, followed by a minimum of 3 to 6 months of warfarin) in the following clinical situations: (1) an embolic event has already occurred or (2) the patient has a large anterior infarction whether or not a thrombus is visualized echocardiographically. We are also inclined to follow the same anticoagulation practice in patients with infarctions other than those in the anterior distribution if a thrombus or large wall motion abnormality is detected.

Aspirin, although probably not capable of affecting thrombus size in most patients, may prevent further platelet deposition on existing thrombi and also is protective against recurrent ischemic events. It should be prescribed in conjunction with warfarin to patients who are candidates for long-term anticoagulation therapy based on the indications discussed earlier.

Convalescence, Discharge, and Post–Myocardial Infarction Care

Prolonged hospitalization and enforced bed rest for any illness may lead to complications (particularly in elderly patients) such as constipation, decubitus ulcers, excessive resorption of bone with formation of renal calculi, atelectasis, thrombophlebitis, pulmonary emboli, urinary retention, mild anemia due to repetitive blood sampling for diagnostic tests, impaired oral intake of fluids, bleeding from the gastrointestinal tract due to stress ulcers, and deconditioning of cardiovascular reflex responses to postural changes. Because of the precarious status of the heart recovering from AMI, avoidance of such complications is of primary importance. For example, constipation may lead to straining, transitory reduction of venous return and diminution of cardiac output, impaired coronary perfusion, and ventricular arrhythmias, occasionally culminating in ventricular fibrillation. Early use of a bedside commode, stool softeners, and a bed-chair regimen appear to be useful in avoiding many of the difficulties encountered previously among patients with AMI confined to bed for several weeks.

Although concern has been raised from studies in animals that early physical activity might unfavorably influence ventricular remodeling, perhaps by causing infarct extension, no evidence indicates that this concern is relevant to patients, and early mobilization appears to be warranted in most stable AMI patients. For the patient with an uncomplicated AMI, washing and personal care may begin within the first 12 to 24 hours. If the convalescence continues uneventfully, limited ambulation within the room can be begun on the second or third day (see Table 35–12). Once early ambulatory activities are begun, advancement in the activity should depend on the patient's condition. A shower may be allowed some time after the third day.

TIMING OF HOSPITAL DISCHARGE. The time of discharge from the hospital is variable. Patients who have undergone aggressive reperfusion protocols and have no significant ventricular arrhythmias, recurrent ischemia, or congestive heart failure have been safely discharged in less than 5 days. More commonly, discharge occurs 5 or 6 days after admission for patients who experience no complications, who can be followed readily at home, and whose family setting is conducive to convalescence. Most complications that would preclude early discharge occur within the first day or two of admission; therefore, patients suitable for early discharge can be identified early during the hospitalization.[410, 576] However, as noted previously, even if no complications have occurred by hospital day 3, many clinicians find it useful to keep the patient hospitalized for another 1 to 2 days to finalize the discharge prescriptions, provide additional patient education, and confirm the adequacy of the patient's support systems at home.[411]

For patients who have experienced a complication, discharge is deferred until their condition has been stable for several days and it is clear that they are responding appropriately to necessary medications such as antiarrhythmic agents, vasodilators, or positive inotropic agents or that they have undergone the appropriate work-up for recurrent ischemia.

COUNSELING. Before discharge from the hospital, all patients should receive detailed instruction concerning physical activity. Initially, this should consist of ambulation at home but avoidance of isometric exercise such as lifting; several rest periods should be taken daily. In addition, the patient should be given fresh nitroglycerin tablets and instructed in their use and should receive careful instructions about the use of any other medications prescribed. As convalescence progresses, graded resumption of activity should be encouraged. Many approaches have been used, ranging from formal rigid guidelines to general advice advocating moderation and avoidance of any activity that evokes symptoms. Sexual counseling is often overlooked during recovery from MI and should also be included as part of the educational process. Such counseling should begin early after AMI and should include the recommendation that sexual activity be resumed after successful completion of either early submaximal or later symptom-limited exercise stress testing.[52]

Some evidence indicates that behavioral alteration is possible after recovery from MI and that this may improve prognosis. A cardiac rehabilitation program with supervised physical exercise and an educational component has been recommended for most MI patients after discharge. Although the overall clinical benefit of such programs continues to be debated, there is little question that most people derive considerable knowledge and psychological security from such interventions and they continue to be endorsed by experienced clinicians.[52] Meta-analyses of randomized trials of medically supervised rehabilitation programs versus usual care that were conducted in an era before the widespread use of beta-adrenoceptor blockers and thrombolytics have shown a reduction in cardiovascular death but no change in the incidence of nonfatal reinfarction.[577] Given the relationship between a history of depression and risk for AMI,[578] interest has arisen in psychosocial intervention programs in the convalescent phase of AMI.[579, 580] Psychosocial intervention programs alone have not been proven to be helpful, but they are a useful adjunct to standard cardiac rehabilitation programs after AMI.[581, 581a] More detailed information on physical and psychological aspects of rehabilitation of patients convalescing from AMI is discussed in Chapter 38.

RISK STRATIFICATION

The process of risk stratification after AMI occurs in several stages: initial presentation, in-hospital course (CCU, intermediate care unit), and at the time of hospital discharge. The tools used to form an integrated assessment of the patient consist of baseline demographic information,[268a] serial ECGs and serum cardiac marker measurements, hemodynamic monitoring data, a variety of noninvasive tests, and, if performed, the findings at cardiac catheterization.[414, 582]

INITIAL PRESENTATION. Certain demographic and historical factors are associated with a poor prognosis in patients with AMI, including female gender, age older than 70 years, a history of diabetes mellitus, prior angina pectoris, and previous MI.[414] Diabetes mellitus, in particular, appears to confer a threefold to fourfold increase in risk. Whether this is due to accelerated atherosclerosis or some other characteristic induced by the diabetic state (such as a larger infarct size) is unclear. (Surviving diabetic patients also experience a more complicated post-MI course, including a greater incidence of postinfarction angina, infarct extension, and heart failure.)[52]

In addition to playing a central role in the decision pathway for management of patients with AMI based on the presence or absence of ST segment elevation, the 12-lead ECG carries important prognostic information. Mortality is greater in patients experiencing anterior wall MI than after inferior MI, even when corrected for infarct size.[52] Patients with right ventricular infarction complicating inferior infarction, as suggested by ST segment elevation in V_4R, have a greater mortality rate than patients sustaining an inferior infarction without right ventricular involvement.[63] Patients with multiple leads showing ST segment elevation and those with a high sum of ST segment elevation have an increased mortality, especially if their infarct is anterior.[582] Patients whose ECG demonstrates persistent advanced heart block (e.g., Mobitz type II, second-degree, or third-degree AV block) or new intraventricular conduction abnormalities (bifascicular or trifascicular) in the course of an AMI have a worse prognosis than do patients without these abnormalities. The influence of high degrees of heart block is particularly important in patients with right ventricular infarction, for such patients have a markedly increased mortality. Other ECG findings that augur poorly are persistent horizontal or downsloping ST segment depression, Q waves in multiple leads, evidence of right ventricular infarction accompanying inferior infarction,[63] ST segment depressions in anterior leads in patients with inferior infarction,[583] and atrial arrhythmias (especially atrial fibrillation).

Data from the thrombolytic era have confirmed that important determinants of short- and long-term prognosis appear to be similar in patients who have received thrombolytic therapy compared with those who have not.[414] A constellation of clinical factors can be detected at the time of presentation to help select patients at particularly high risk of death in the first 4 to 6 weeks after AMI (see Fig. 35–27, p. 1151).

HOSPITAL COURSE. Soon after CCUs were instituted, it became apparent that left ventricular function is an important early determinant of survival. Hospital mortality from AMI depends directly on the severity of left ventricular dysfunction.[414] Risk stratification by means of clinical findings, estimation of infarct size, and, in appropriate patients, invasive hemodynamic monitoring in the CCU (see p. 1174) provides an assessment of the likelihood of a complicated hospital course[584] and may also identify important abnormalities such as hemodynamically significant mitral regurgitation that convey an adverse long-term prognosis.

Recurrent ischemia and infarction after AMI, either in the same location as the index infarction or "at a distance," influence prognosis adversely. Poor prognosis comes from the loss of viable myocardium, with the resulting larger area of infarction creating a greater compromise in ventricular function. Postinfarction angina generally connotes a less favorable prognosis because it indicates the presence of jeopardized myocardium.[582] In the current era of aggressive revascularization, early postinfarction angina often leads to early interventions that tend to improve outcome, diminishing the long-term impact and significance of angina early after AMI.[585]

Assessment at Hospital Discharge

Both short-term and long-term survival after AMI depend on three factors: (1) resting left ventricular function, (2) residual potentially ischemic myocardium, and (3) susceptibility to serious ventricular arrhythmias. The most important of these factors is the state of left ventricular function[586] (see Fig. 35–41). The second most important factor is how the severity and extent of the obstructive lesions in the coronary vascular bed perfusing residual viable myocardium impacts the risk of recurrent infarction, additional myocardial damage, and serious ventricular arrhythmias.[582] Thus, survival relates to the quantity of myocardium that has become necrotic and the quantity at risk of becoming necrotic. At one extreme, the prognosis is best for the patient with normal intrinsic coronary vessels whose completed infarction constitutes a small fraction (5 percent) of the left ventricle as a consequence of a coronary embolus and who has no jeopardized myocardium. At the other extreme is the patient with a massive infarct with left ventricular failure whose residual viable myocardium is perfused by markedly obstructed vessels. Obviously, progression of atherosclerosis or lowering of perfusion pressure in these vessels impairs the function and viability of the residual myocardium on which left ventricular function depends. The situation may not be hopeless even in such a patient, however, because revascularization may reduce the threat to the jeopardized myocardium. The third risk factor, the susceptibility to serious arrhythmias, is reflected in ventricular ectopic activity and other indicators of electrical instability such as reduced heart rate variability or baroreflex sensitivity and an abnormal signal-averaged ECG. All of these identify patients at increased risk of death.

In addition, as noted earlier, patients with an occluded infarct-related artery late (e.g., 1 to 2 weeks) after AMI have a higher long-term mortality.[74] Persistent occlusion of the culprit artery is associated with an increased incidence of abnormal late potentials on the ECG[587] and appears to have an adverse prognostic effect independent of the level of ventricular function (Fig. 35–53).[224]

ASSESSMENT OF LEFT VENTRICULAR FUNCTION. Left ventricular ejection fraction may be the most easily as-

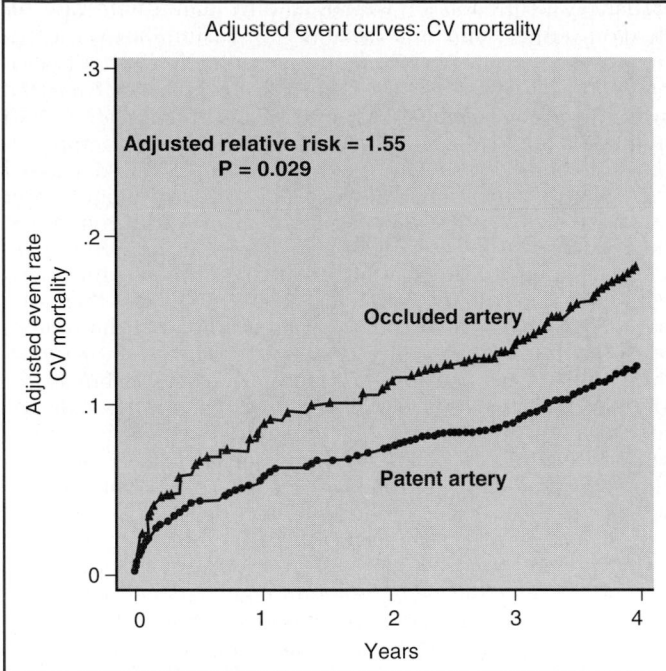

FIGURE 35–53. Impact of patency of the infarct-related artery on long-term mortality. In patients with a patent infarct-related coronary artery at 2 weeks after infarction, the long-term mortality is significantly reduced compared with that of patients with an occluded infarct-related vessel. The beneficial effect of infarct-related artery patency was independent of the number of obstructed coronary arteries or of left ventricular function. (From Lamas GA, Flaker GC, Mitchell G, et al: Effect of infarct artery patency on prognosis after acute myocardial infarction. Circulation 92:1101, 1995. Copyright 1995, American Heart Association.)

sessed measurement of left ventricular function, and this measurement is extremely useful for risk stratification (see Fig. 35–41). However, imaging of the left ventricle at rest may not distinguish adequately between infarcted, irreversibly damaged myocardium and stunned or hibernating myocardium. To circumvent this difficulty, a variety of techniques has been investigated to assess the extent of residual viable myocardium, including exercise and pharmacological stress echocardiography, stress radionuclide ventricular angiography, perfusion imaging in conjunction with pharmacological stress, and positron emission tomography (see Chap. 13). All of these techniques can be performed safely in postinfarction patients. Because no study has clearly shown one imaging modality to be superior to others, clinicians should be guided in their selection of ventricular imaging technique by the availability and level of expertise with a given modality at their local institution.[414]

In patients with low left ventricular ejection fraction, the measurement of exercise capacity is useful for further identifying those patients at particularly high risk and also for establishing safe exercise limits after discharge.[588] Patients with a good exercise capacity despite a reduced ejection fraction have a better long-term outcome than those who cannot perform more than modest exercise.

ASSESSMENT OF MYOCARDIAL ISCHEMIA. Because of the potent adverse consequences of recurrent MI after AMI,[562] it is important to assess a patient's risk for future ischemia and infarction. Given the increasing array of pharmacological, interventional catheterization, and surgical options available to modify the likelihood of developing recurrent episodes of myocardial ischemia, most clinicians find it helpful to identify patients at risk for provocable myocardial ischemia before discharge. A predischarge evaluation for ischemia allows clinicians to select patients who might benefit from catheterization and revascularization after AMI and to assess the adequacy of medical therapy for those patients who are suitable for a more conservative management strategy. Although it may be argued that coronary arteriography for risk stratification after AMI has the advantage of permitting simultaneous identification and treatment (angioplasty) of coronary obstructions, important limitations of this strategy should be noted.[589] As discussed previously (see p. 1116), the coronary artery plaques that are most likely to rupture (and produce future events) are those that are lipid laden and have a thin fibrous cap. These plaques cannot be adequately identified with arteriography because they may be associated with less than a 75 percent stenosis of the coronary artery lumen at the time of angiography after an index AMI. Furthermore, coronary arteriography does not provide information on the functional significance of coronary lesions. Previous studies comparing routine use of coronary angiography versus selected use only in patients with spontaneous or provoked ischemia showed no advantage to the routine catheterization strategy with respect to 6-week mortality and reinfarction.[52, 589]

An exercise test also offers the clinician an opportunity to formulate a more precise exercise prescription and is helpful in boosting patients' confidence in their ability to conduct their daily activities after discharge. Patients who are unable to exercise may be evaluated using a pharmacological stress protocol such as an infusion of dobutamine or dipyridamole with echocardiography or perfusion imaging.

Treadmill exercise testing after AMI has traditionally used a submaximal protocol that requires the patient to exercise until symptoms of angina appear, ECG evidence of ischemia is seen, or a target workload (approximately 5 METS) has been reached (see Chap. 6). It has been proposed that symptom-limited exercise tests may be safely performed before discharge in patients with an uncomplicated postinfarction course in hospital.[590] Variables derived from exercise tests after AMI that have been evaluated for their ability to predict the occurrence of death or recurrent nonfatal infarction include the development and magnitude of ST segment depression, the development of angina, exercise capacity, and the systolic blood pressure response during exercise.[586]

Myocardial perfusion with ^{99m}Tc sestamibi during exercise or pharmacological (e.g., dipyridamole, adenosine, or dobutamine) stress increases the sensitivity for detection of patients at risk for death or recurrent infarction (see Chap. 9). Similar results have been reported for dipyridamole stress echocardiography. Although perfusion imaging may be helpful for risk stratification in patients with uninterpretable ECGs or the inability to exercise, the regular use of these more expensive procedures in patients with interpretable ECGs and the ability to exercise has been questioned.[414, 591] An increasing number of patients are treated with thrombolysis, angioplasty, or surgery and have a more favorable natural history than that reported in patients who have not undergone aggressive reperfusion and revascularization for AMI.[591] Until clinical trials relating the findings of a postinfarction perfusion imaging test to long-term outcome in cohorts of patients receiving contemporary therapy for AMI are available, we do not advocate the *routine* use of perfusion imaging for risk stratification after AMI. At present its use should be restricted to patients who are candidates for further revascularization procedures and have physical limitations preventing them from exercising to an adequate workload or those with conduction abnormalities, significant resting ST segment and T wave abnormalities, or repolarization abnormalities on the ECG due to ventricular hypertrophy or digitalis therapy.[592] We have also used perfusion imaging studies when a conventional exercise ECG is mildly abnormal and there is uncertainty about the significance of the finding or uncertainty about the potential culprit vessel or vessels. In such cases perfusion imaging may help guide decisions after catheterization if multiple coronary vessels have important stenoses.

The Danish Trial in Acute MI (DANAMI) investigators reported that when patients with provokable ischemia after infarction were randomized to catheterization and revascularization versus conservative medical therapy, they experienced a lower requirement for antianginal medications, less unstable angina, and fewer nonfatal infarctions.[585]

ASSESSMENT FOR ELECTRICAL INSTABILITY. After AMI, patients are at greatest risk for the development of sudden cardiac death due to malignant ventricular arrhythmias over the course of the first 1 to 2 years.[593, 594] Several techniques have been devised to stratify patients into those who are at increased risk of sudden death after AMI: measurement of QT interval dispersion (variability of QT intervals between ECG leads), ambulatory ECG recordings for detection of ventricular arrhythmias (Holter monitoring; see Chap. 22), invasive electrophysiological testing, recording a signal-averaged ECG (a measure of delayed, fragmented conduction in the infarct zone), and measuring heart rate variability (beat-to-beat variability in RR intervals) or baroreflex sensitivity (slope of a line relating beat-to-beat change in sinus rate in response to alteration of blood pressure).[510]

Given the risks associated with routine use of type I antiarrhythmics prescribed to suppress VPBs that are detected on ambulatory ECG recordings, we do not recommend routine Holter monitoring to determine which patients should receive antiarrhythmic therapy after AMI. The value of empirical administration of the type III antiarrhythmic drug amiodarone after infarction is discussed on p. 1204.

A variety of noninvasive tests have been used to assess patients for electrical instability after AMI.[510] The presence of a filtered QRS complex duration greater than 120 milliseconds and abnormal late potentials recorded on a signal-averaged ECG after AMI have a positive predictive value between 8 and 27 percent and a negative predictive value of over 95 percent for serious arrhythmic events. When viewed in isolation, the signal-averaged ECG suffers from a high false-positive rate, which may be improved by combining it with other variables, such as left ventricular ejection fraction. Electrophysiological testing also appears to suffer from a high false-positive rate and has the additional disadvantage of being invasive. The ability of electrophysiological testing to identify patients at risk for arrhythmic events after AMI appears to be improved if it is performed in patients who also have an ejection fraction less than 40 percent, an abnormal signal-averaged ECG, and VPBs. Depressed heart rate variability (HRV) is an independent predictor of mortality and arrhythmic complications after AMI, especially if cutoffs of standard deviation of the average interval between normal beats below 50 milliseconds and HRV triangular index (a geometric method for integrating the distribution of intervals between normal beats) less than 15 are used. A depressed baroreflex sensitivity value (3.0 msec/mm Hg) is associated with about a threefold increase in the risk of mortality.[595]

Despite the increased risk of arrhythmic events after AMI in patients who are found to have abnormal results on one or more of the noninvasive tests described earlier, several points should be emphasized. The low positive predictive value (< 30 percent) for the noninvasive screening tests limits their usefulness when viewed in isolation. Although the predictive value of screening tests can be improved by combining several of them together, the therapeutic implications of an increased risk profile for arrhythmic events have not been established. The mortality reductions achievable with the general use of beta blockers, ACE inhibitors, aspirin, and revascularization when appropriate after infarction, coupled with concerns about efficacy and safety of antiarrhythmic drugs and cost of implanted defibrillators, leave considerable uncertainty about the therapeutic implications of an abnormal noninvasive test for electrical instability in an asymptomatic patient. Additional data on patient outcomes when clinicians act on the results of an abnormal finding are required before definitive recommendations can be made for asymptomatic patients.[52] The management of patients with sustained, hemodynamically compromising arrhythmias is discussed in Chapter 23.

Recommendations for Predischarge Management

An algorithm for predischarge management of patients at varying levels of risk after infarction is outlined in Figure 35–54. Initially, a judgment is made as to the presence of clinical variables indicative of high risk for future cardiac events. Patients with spontaneous episodes of ischemia or depressed left ventricular function who are considered suitable candidates for revascularization based on their overall medical condition should be referred for cardiac catheterization (Fig. 35–54). The former group of patients is at increased risk of recurrent infarction (and subsequent increased mortality risk[562]), whereas the latter group may benefit from revascularization surgery if multivessel coronary artery disease is identified at catheterization (see Chap. 37).[562a] Patients with sustained VT or ventricular fibrillation that occurs more than 48 hours after the acute event (see Fig. 35–54) are at increased risk of sudden cardiac death and should be considered for diagnostic electrophysiology study and treatment as outlined in Chapter 25.

In the absence of high-risk clinical indicators, two management strategies are possible; the choice between them may be influenced by patient and physician preferences and the availability of resources in the patient's local community for the necessary follow-up procedures (see Fig. 35–54). Initial exercise testing can use conventional ECG with supplementation by a perfusion imaging study for patients with uninterpretable resting ECGs or an equivocal (i.e., mildly abnormal) initial ECG result. Submaximal exercise testing can be performed before discharge to triage patients to an early catheterization strategy or medical therapy strategy. Plans for a follow-up symptom-limited exercise test in patients without clear indications for catheterization are formulated based on the patient's life style and occupation. Patients who undergo aggressive reperfusion therapy and have an uncomplicated course in the CCU may be suitable candidates for early hospital discharge with plans for a symptom-limited exercise test 2 to 3 weeks later. Subsequent decisions about continued medical therapy or referral for cardiac catheterization can then be made as outlined in Figure 35–54.

SECONDARY PREVENTION OF RECURRENT ACUTE MYOCARDIAL INFARCTION

The concept of secondary prevention of reinfarction and death after recovery from an AMI has been investigated actively for several decades. Problems in proving the efficacy of various interventions have been related both to the ineffectiveness of certain strategies and to the difficulty in proving a benefit as mortality and morbidity have improved after AMI. Nevertheless, patients who survive the initial course of AMI are at increased risk because of coronary artery disease and its complications; therefore, it is imperative that efforts be made to reduce this risk. Although secondary prevention drug trials generally have tested one form of therapy against placebo in an attempt to demonstrate a benefit of that therapy, the physician must remember that disciplined clinical care of the individual patient is far more important than rote use of an agent found beneficial in the latest drug trial.[17, 596]

LIFE STYLE MODIFICATION. Efforts to improve survival and the quality of life after MI that relate to life style modi-

fication of known risk factors are considered in Chapter 36. Of these, cessation of smoking and control of hypertension are probably most important. It has been shown that within 2 years of quitting smoking, the risk of a nonfatal MI in these former smokers falls to a level similar to that in patients who never smoked. Being hospitalized for an AMI is a powerful motivation for patients to cease cigarette smoking, and this is an ideal time to encourage that clearly beneficial and highly cost-effective life style change.[597] It is also an ideal time to begin to treat hypertension, to counsel patients to achieve optimal body weight, and to consider various strategies to improve the patient's lipid profile (see later).

Physicians caring for patients after an AMI need to be sensitive to the fact that some patients experience major depression after infarction, and the development of this problem is an independent risk factor for mortality.[598] In addition, lack of an emotionally supportive network in the patient's environment after discharge is associated with an increased risk of mortality and recurrent cardiac events.[599] The precise mechanisms relating depression and lack of social support to worse prognosis after AMI are not clear, but one possibility is lack of adherence to prescribed treatments, a behavior that has been shown to be associated with increased risk of mortality after infarction.[600] Evidence exists that a comprehensive rehabilitation program using primary health care personnel who counsel patients and make home visits favorably impacts the clinical course of patients after infarction and reduces the rate of rehospitalization for recurrent ischemia and infarction. A supportive physician attitude can also have a positive impact on the rate of return to work after AMI.

MODIFICATION OF LIPID PROFILE. Compelling evidence now exists that an increased cholesterol level, and most importantly an increased low-density lipoprotein (LDL) cholesterol level, is associated with an increased risk of coronary heart disease (see Chap. 33). Based on this observation and the finding that lowering cholesterol reduces the risk of coronary heart disease,[601, 602] a target LDL cholesterol level of less than 100 mg/dl has been recommended in patients with clinically evident coronary heart disease.[603] This recommendation clearly applies to patients with AMI, and it is therefore important to obtain a lipid profile on admission in all patients admitted with acute infarction. (It should be recalled that cholesterol levels may fall 24 to 48 hours after infarction.) In addition to lowering LDL cholesterol, therapy with statins reduces levels of C-reactive protein, suggesting an antiinflammatory effect.[604]

Surveys of physician practice in the past have revealed a disappointingly low rate of treatment of hypercholesterolemia in patients with proven coronary artery disease, indicating considerable room for improvement in this aspect of secondary prevention after AMI.[603]

Recommendations. All patients recovering from AMI should be considered potential candidates for modification of their lipid profile. Initial therapy should consist of an AHA Step II diet (< 7 percent of total calories as saturated fat and cholesterol < 200 mg/d). Patients with an LDL cholesterol level greater than 125 mg/dl despite the AHA Step II diet should be placed on drug therapy to reduce the LDL cholesterol level to less than 100 mg/dl.[52] Our preference at present is to prescribe an HMG-CoA reductase inhibitor before hospital discharge in patients with an LDL cholesterol level greater than 130 mg/dl on admission.[605] For many patients recovering from AMI, a low HDL cholesterol level is their primary lipid abnormality. Gemfibrozil (1200 mg/d) reduces the risk of death, reinfarction, and stroke in such patients.[606]

ANTIPLATELET AGENTS. On the basis of 11 randomized trials in 20,000 patients with a prior infarction, the Antiplatelet Trialists' Collaboration reported a 25 percent reduction in the risk of recurrent infarction, stroke, or vascular

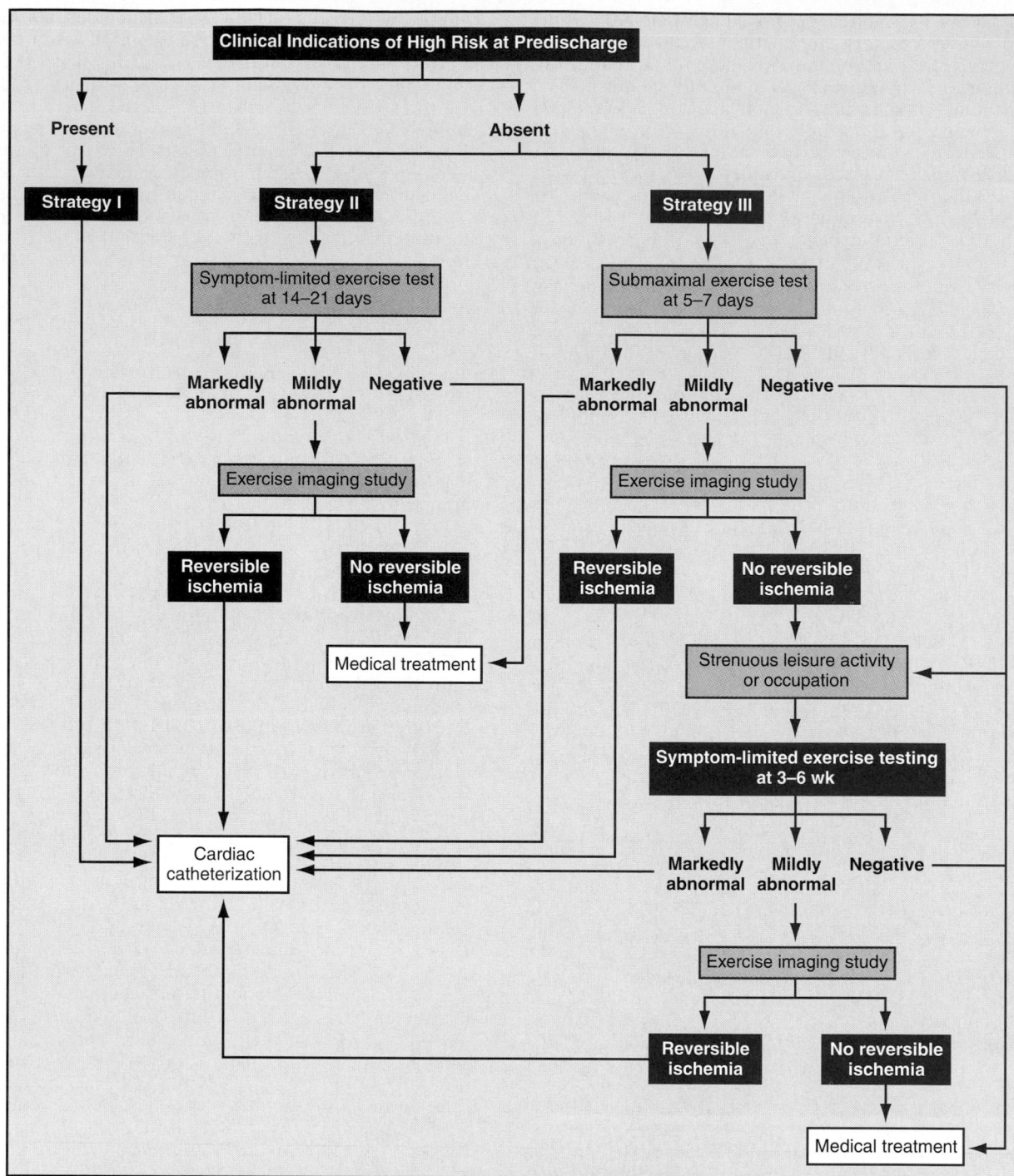

FIGURE 35–54. Management algorithm for risk stratification after acute myocardial infarction. Patients with clinical indicators of high risk at hospital discharge such as recurrent ischemia at rest or depressed left ventricular function should be considered candidates for revascularization and referral to cardiac catheterization for ultimate triage to either angioplasty/coronary artery bypass surgery or medical therapy and risk factor reduction (strategy I). Patients with life-threatening arrhythmias such as sustained ventricular tachycardia or ventricular fibrillation should be considered for diagnostic cardiac catheterization, electrophysiology study, and management with implantation of a cardioverter-defibrillator either alone or in conjunction with Amiodarone (strategy I). Patients without indicators of high risk at hospital discharge can be evaluated with either a symptom-limited exercise test at 14 to 21 days (strategy II) or a submaximal exercise test before discharge (strategy III). Patients with either a markedly abnormal exercise test or evidence of reversible ischemia on an exercise imaging study in strategy II or III should be referred for cardiac catheterization. Patients with a negative exercise test or no evidence of reversible ischemia on an exercise imaging study can be managed with medical therapy and risk factor reduction. (From Ryan TJ, Antman EM, Brooks NH, et al: 1999 update: ACC/AHA Guidelines for the Management of Patients With Acute Myocardial Infarction: Executive Summary and Recommendations: A report of the American College of Cardiology/American Heart Association Task Force on Practice Guidelines [Committee on Management of Acute Myocardial Infarction]. Circulation 100:1016–1030, 1999.)

death in patients receiving prolonged antiplatelet therapy (36 fewer events for every 1000 patients treated).[14] No antiplatelet therapy proved superior to aspirin, and daily doses of aspirin between 80 and 325 mg appear to be effective.[607] Data from the Worcester Heart Attack Study suggest that when an AMI occurs in chronic users of aspirin, it is likely to be smaller and non-Q wave in nature.[608] Experimental data on late reperfusion in a rat model of coronary occlusion suggest that aspirin treatment after AMI increases the patency of the microvasculature in the infarcted area, resulting in less infarct expansion and thicker myocardial walls in the infarct zone.[609] The compelling arguments cited earlier serve as the basis for the recommendation that all patients recovering from AMI should, in the absence of contraindications, remain on aspirin for an indefinite period.[596, 610] Patients with true aspirin allergy may be treated with sulfinpyrazone (400 mg twice daily), ticlopidine (250 mg twice daily),[14] or clopidogrel (75 mg once daily),[611] although the data indicating that these agents reduce mortality after AMI are not nearly as robust as those for aspirin.

ACE INHIBITORS. The rationale for the acute use of ACE inhibitors after AMI has been discussed earlier (see p. 1169). To prevent late remodeling of the left ventricle and also to decrease the likelihood of recurrent ischemic events,[421, 431] we advocate indefinite therapy with an ACE inhibitor to all patients with clinically evident congestive heart failure, a moderate decrease in global ejection fraction, or a large regional wall motion abnormality, even in the face of a normal global ejection fraction.[52] A decision-analytic model that tested strategy of prescription of ACE inhibitors to hypothetical 50- to 80-year-old patients with an ejection fraction of 40 percent or less after AMI reported incremental cost-effectiveness ratios of $4,000 to $10,000 per quality-adjusted life-year (QALY). These calculations compare quite favorably with the costs of other commonly accepted medical procedures such as angioplasty for one- or two-vessel coronary artery disease ($8,000 to $111,000 per QALY).

The optimum duration of therapy with ACE inhibitors after AMI is an intriguing question. Evidence exists that long-term (at least 3 to 5 years) treatment with ACE inhibitors in patients with severely reduced left ventricular function after AMI prolongs survival,[612, 613] especially in diabetic patients.[614] Although the benefit of ACE inhibitors in patients with symptomatic congestive heart failure is greater with higher doses, some protection against death and hospitalization for heart failure is obtained even if lower doses of ACE inhibitors are used.[615] Finally, ACE inhibitors are associated with a reduction in sudden death after AMI,[616] profession of renal failure in insulin-dependent diabetics,[617] and prevention of death, AMI, and stroke when used for primary prevention in patients at high risk for cardiovascular events but without left ventricular dysfunction or heart failure.[618] The observations cited earlier along with data suggesting that ACE inhibitors have direct antiatherosclerotic effects and favorably influence remodeling of vascular walls pose a persuasive argument for a more widespread use of ACE inhibitors for all patients after AMI.

BETA-ADRENOCEPTOR BLOCKERS. Meta-analyses of trials from the prethrombolytic era involving over 24,000 patients who received beta-adrenoceptor blockers in the convalescent phase of AMI have shown a 23 percent reduction in long-term mortality[417] (see Fig. 35–37). When beta blockade is initiated early (6 hours) in the acute phase of infarction and continued in the chronic phase of treatment, some of the benefit may result from a reduction in infarct size. However, in the majority of patients who have beta blockade initiated during the convalescent phase of AMI, reduction in long-term mortality is probably due to a combination of an antiarrhythmic effect (prevention of sudden death) and prevention of reinfarction.[417]

Overviews of the results of trials of beta-adrenoceptor blockers with agonist activity have not shown a beneficial effect on mortality compared with more convincing evidence of a beneficial effect and little evidence of harm for trials of beta blockers without agonist activity (odds ratio 0.69 [0.61–0.79]).[186] No differences are seen when cardioselective and noncardioselective agents are compared. The greatest mortality benefit from chronic beta blockade after AMI is seen in patients with the greatest baseline risk—those with compromised ventricular function and ventricular arrhythmias. The results of the Beta-Blocker Pooling Project, in which data were examined from nine separate studies involving more than 10,000 patients, suggest a highly significant reduction in overall mortality among treated patients with pump failure.[619] Treatment with beta blockers after AMI is particularly helpful for reducing mortality in patients who do not undergo revascularization.[620] Mortality is reduced even in patients who receive less than 50 percent of the dosage found to be effective in preventing cardiac death in large randomized trials.[621]

Recommendations. Given the well-documented benefits of beta-adrenoceptor blockade, it is disturbing that this form of therapy continues to be underused, especially in high-risk groups such as the elderly.[622] We are in agreement with the "Quality Care Alert" issued jointly by several authoritative bodies that beta-adrenoceptor blockers be prescribed to all high-risk patients regardless of whether the event was a Q-wave or non-Q-wave AMI, as long as no contraindications are present.[623] Patients with a relative contraindication to beta blockade (moderate heart failure, bradyarrhythmias) should undergo a monitored trial of therapy in the hospital. The dosage should be sufficient to blunt the heart rate response to stress or exercise. Much of the impact of beta blockers in preventing mortality occurs in the first weeks; treatment should commence as soon as possible. Evidence exists that programs providing physician feedback improve adherence to guidelines such as those noted earlier for prescription of beta-adrenoceptor blockers after AMI.[624]

Some controversy exists as to how long patients should be treated.[625] The collective data from five trials providing information on long-term follow-up of beta-adrenoceptor blockers after infarction suggest that therapy should be continued for at least 2 to 3 years.[626, 627] At that time, if the beta blocker is well tolerated and if there is no reason to discontinue therapy, such therapy probably should be continued in most patients.[628]

Not all patients derive the same benefit from beta-blocker therapy. The cost-effectiveness of treatment in medium- or high-risk persons compares very favorably with that of many other accepted interventions such as coronary bypass surgery, angioplasty, and lipid-lowering therapy.[625] In patients with an extremely good prognosis (first AMI, good ventricular function, no angina, negative stress test, and no complex ventricular ectopy) in whom a mortality rate of approximately 1 percent per year can be anticipated, beta blockers would have a smaller impact on survival. However, it is our preference to prescribe beta blockers to such patients for whatever postinfarction benefit is achieved and also to have them as part of the patient's usual regimen should AMI recur at an unpredictable time in the future.

NITRATES. Although these agents are suitable for management of specific conditions after AMI such as recurrent angina or as part of a treatment regimen for congestive heart failure, little evidence indicates that they reduce mortality over the long term when prescribed on a routine basis to all patients with infarction.[425, 426]

ANTICOAGULANTS. (See also Chap. 62.) At least three theoretical reasons exist for anticipating that anticoagulants might be beneficial in the long-term management of patients after AMI.

1. Because the coronary occlusion responsible for the AMI is often due to a thrombus, anticoagulants might be expected to halt, slow progression, or prevent the development of new thrombi elsewhere in the coronary arterial tree.

2. Anticoagulants might be expected to diminish the formation of mural thrombi and resultant systemic embolization.

3. Anticoagulants might be expected to reduce the incidence of venous thrombosis and pulmonary embolization.

After several decades of evaluation, the weight of evidence now suggests that anticoagulants have a favorable effect on late mortality, stroke, and reinfarction among patients hospitalized with AMI.[13, 629] Long-term anticoagulant therapy has also been shown to be a cost-effective intervention after AMI, with the major cost savings coming from reductions in the rate of recurrent infarction and related interventions.[630]

Previous small trials of aspirin versus oral anticoagulation have led to conflicting results, with no clear consensus regarding superiority of either antithrombotic strategy. The APRICOT investigators reported that after initially successful thrombolysis, aspirin-treated patients had lower rates of reinfarction, need for revascularization, and mortality than did warfarin-treated patients.[273] As expected, cost-effectiveness calculations show that aspirin is associated with a very favorable economic profile, but its true efficacy compared with or combined with oral anticoagulation remains unknown. The Coumadin Aspirin Reinfarction Study (CARS) was discontinued prematurely owing to lack of evidence of benefit of reduced-dose aspirin (80 mg/d) with either 1 or 3 mg of warfarin daily compared with aspirin 160 mg alone daily.[631] The Combination Hemotherapy and Mortality Prevention (CHAMP) study found no benefit of using warfarin (to an international normalized ratio of 1.5–2.5) plus aspirin 81 mg/d versus aspirin 162 mg/d with respect to total mortality, cardiovascular mortality, stroke, and nonfatal MI (mean follow-up 2.7 years) after an index AMI.[632]

Therefore, at present we recommend routine use of aspirin in all AMI patients without contraindications and add warfarin only to patients with clear indications for anticoagulation such as deep vein thrombosis, pulmonary embolism, mural thrombus seen at echocardiography, a large regional wall motion abnormality (especially anterior) seen at echocardiography even in the absence of a visualized thrombus, atrial fibrillation, and a history of embolic cerebrovascular accident.

CALCIUM ANTAGONISTS. At present we do *not* recommend the routine use of calcium antagonists for secondary prevention of infarction. A possible exception is a patient who cannot tolerate a beta-adrenoceptor blocker because of adverse effects on bronchospastic lung disease but who has well-preserved left ventricular function; such patients may be candidates for a rate-slowing calcium antagonist such as diltiazem or verapamil.

ANTIARRHYTHMICS. Although it has been recognized for decades that antiarrhythmic therapy can control atrial and ventricular arrhythmias effectively in many patients, careful reviews of clinical trials after AMI have reported an increased risk of mortality with type I drugs[633, 634] (Table 35–22). The most notable postinfarction trial in this area was the Cardiac Arrhythmia Suppression Trial (CAST), which tested whether encainide, flecainide, or moricizine for suppression of ventricular arrhythmias detected on ambulatory ECG monitoring would reduce the risk of cardiac arrest and death over the long term. Both the first phase of the trial (encainide or flecainide vs. placebo) and the second phase of the trial (moricizine vs. placebo) were stopped prematurely because of increased mortality in the active treatment groups.[634–636] The mechanism of the increased risk after

AMI remains a subject of investigation, but one hypothesis that has been put forth is an adverse interaction between recurrent ischemia and the presence of an antiarrhythmic drug because the risk of death or cardiac arrest was greater in patients with non-Q-wave AMI than with Q-wave AMI.[637] Sodium channel blockade by antiarrhythmics may exacerbate electrophysiological differences between subepicardial and subendocardial zones of myocardium, rendering the latter more susceptible to ischemic injury.[638]

Subsequent to CAST, another postinfarction prophylactic antiarrhythmic drug trial was undertaken with oral d-sotalol (Survival With ORal D-sotalol = SWORD). This trial was designed to test the hypothesis that prophylactic administration of d-sotalol to patients with depressed left ventricular function (ejection fraction = 40 percent) and either a recent (6 to 42 days) or remote (42 days) AMI would reduce total mortality. SWORD also was stopped prematurely after enrollment of only 3121 of a planned 6400 patients because statistical evidence of increased mortality emerged in the active treatment group[639] (Fig. 35–55).

The Canadian Amiodarone Myocardial Infarction Trial (CAMIAT) showed that amiodarone reduced ventricular premature depolarization frequency in patients with recent MI; this correlated with a reduction in arrhythmic death or resuscitation from ventricular fibrillation[640] (see Fig. 35–55). However, 42 percent of patients discontinued amiodarone during maintenance therapy in CAMIAT because of intolerable side effects. The European Amiodarone Myocardial Infarction Trial (EMIAT) showed a reduction in arrhythmic death after MI in patients with depressed left ventricular function, but there was no reduction in total mortality or other cardiovascular-related mortality[641] (see Fig. 35–55).

At the present time, the *routine* use of antiarrhythmic agents (including amiodarone) cannot be recommended.[641a] Given the data cited earlier on the protective effects of beta-adrenoceptor blockers against sudden death (see p. 1203) and the ability of aspirin to reduce the risk of reinfarction (see p. 1201), it is unclear whether additional mortality reductions would be achieved by the empirical addition of amiodarone in the patient who is convalescing from an AMI and is free of symptomatic sustained ventricular arrhythmias. Although several trials that included postinfarction patients in the study population have shown mortality reductions in patients randomized to implantable cardioverter-defibrillator implantation versus antiarrhythmic therapy, the profound financial and societal implications have prevented adoption of widespread implantable cardioverter-defibrillator implantation to asymptomatic patients recovering from AMI but with an abnormal noninvasive test (e.g., ejection fraction < 40 percent, frequent ventricular premature depolarizations).[570, 642–644] Whether subgroups of patients with indicators of high risk of sudden death, such as abnormal heart rate variability or reduced baroreflex sensitivity, should be treated and, if so, by what strategy remains to be determined.

HORMONE REPLACEMENT THERAPY. (See also Chap. 58.) Estrogen replacement therapy has been reported to possibly be helpful in the primary prevention of coronary heart disease, improves the coronary artery disease risk factor profile in postmenopausal women,[645] and appears to reduce mortality in women with moderate coronary heart disease. However, the decision to prescribe hormone replacement therapy is often a complex one that involves weighing risks of breast and endometrial cancer versus modification of a coronary artery disease risk factor profile.[646] Of note, despite improvement in lipid profiles, hormone replacement therapy with estrogen plus progestin to postmenopausal women with established coronary heart disease in the Heart and Estrogen/Progestin Replacement Study (HERS) did not prevent recurrent coronary events and was associated with significantly increased risk of venous thromboembolic

▶ TABLE 35–22. IMPORTANT ARRHYTHMIA TRIALS IN PATIENTS AFTER ACUTE MYOCARDIAL INFARCTION

TRIAL	OBJECTIVE	NO. OF PATIENTS	ENTRY CRITERIA	TREATMENT ARMS	MAIN RESULTS	CLINICAL IMPORTANCE
CAST	To test whether PVC suppression (asymptomatic or mildly symptomatic) reduced arrhythmia-related mortality.	2309	6 d to 2 yr post-MI ≥ 6 PVCs/hr LVEF ≤ 40% if MI 90 d to 2 yr	1) Open-label titration during which three drugs (encainide, flecainide, and moricizine) at two doses were tested 2) Titration phase terminated when PVCs suppressed 3) Patients excluded if intolerant or arrhythmia worsened 4) Patients assigned to active drug that suppressed arrhythmia, or placebo	1) 7.7% mortality in encainide/flecainide group vs. 3% in placebo group (p = 0.0004). 2) Arrhythmic death was more common in the encainide/flecainide group vs. placebo (4.5% vs. 1.2%, p = 0.0004).	Both encainide and flecainide were associated with increased mortality even though PVC suppression was demonstrated.
CAST II	To test whether PVC suppression (asymptomatic or mildly symptomatic) by moricizine reduced mortality.	1325	6–90 days post-MI ≥ 6 PVCs/hr LVEF ≤ 55% if MI within 90 d LVEF ≤ 40% if MI 90 d to 2 yr	Two blinded randomized phases: 1) Early phase to assess risk of starting moricizine post-MI (200 mg tid × 14 d vs. placebo) 2) Long-term phase evaluated the effect of moricizine on survival in patients whose PVCs were suppressed	CAST II was stopped early because of increased mortality in the early 14-d phase.	Similar to CAST, moricizine effectively suppressed PVCs, but it was associated with increased mortality.
SWORD	To test whether a pure potassium channel blocker without beta blocking activity reduced mortality	3121	LVEF ≤ 40% and either recent (6–42 days) MI or symptomatic heart failure with a remote (242 days) MI	d-sotalol vs. placebo	SWORD was stopped prematurely due to higher mortality in d-sotalol (5% vs. 3.1%; p = 0.006).	Subgroup analysis showing higher mortality with d-sotalol in patients with better LVEF (31–40%) compared with patients with lower LVEF (≤ 30%) lends support to concept of proarrhythmia.
CAMIAT	To evaluate the efficacy of amiodarone in reducing arrhythmic death.	1202	6–45 days post-MI > 10 PVCs/hr or any run ≥ 3 beats VT > 100 beats/min	Amiodarone vs. placebo	1) Amiodarone did not affect total cardiac mortality but reduced SD or recurrent VF (p < 0.05) 2) There was concordance between PVC suppression and reduced SD and recurrent VF. 3) Early discontinuation of amiodarone for side effects was common (42.3%).	Amiodarone did not improve overall mortality, but reduced SD or recurrent VF. Improvement was concordant with PVC suppression.
EMIAT	To assess the efficacy of prophylactic antiarrhythmic therapy in patients with asymptomatic complex ventricular ectopy.	1486	5–21 d post-MI LVEF ≤ 40% 18–75 yr 24-hr ambulatory monitoring before entry but not used as part of inclusion criteria	Amiodarone vs. placebo	1) No difference in overall mortality. 2) Reduction in arrhythmic death in the amiodarone group (p = 0.052). 3) Drug discontinuation due to side effects or intolerance was high in the amiodarone group (45% by 2 yr).	Amiodarone did not decrease overall mortality but reduced SD.

PVC = premature ventricular contraction; LVEF = left ventricular ejection fraction; VT = ventricular tachycardia; VF = ventricular fibrillation; SD = sudden death.
Modified from Tracy GM: Current review of arrhythmia trials. Cardiology Special Edition 5(1):17–23, 1999.

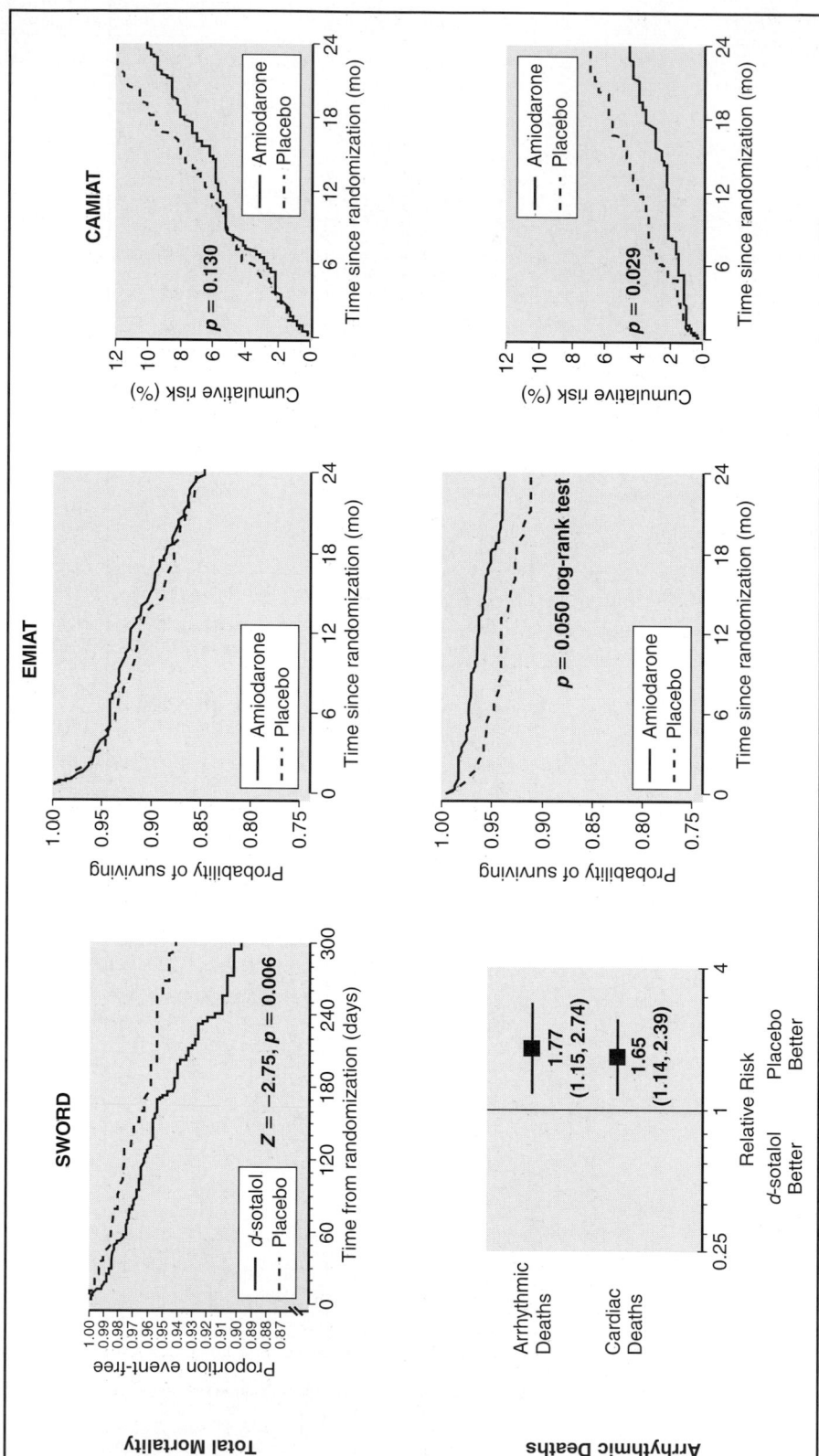

FIGURE 35–55. Effect of type III antiarrhythmic drugs after acute myocardial infarction. The results of the SWORD, EMIAT, and CAMIAT trials are shown with total mortality plotted in the top panels and arrhythmic deaths plotted in the bottom panels. The SWORD trial was stopped prematurely owing to increased total mortality in patients receiving *d*-sotalol compared with placebo; arrhythmic mortality was also significantly increased. Both the EMIAT and CAMIAT trials showed no signifcant reduction in total mortality with amiodarone, but there was a reduction in arrhythmic deaths in patients receiving amiodarone. However, the rate of discontinuation due to intolerable side effects was high with amiodarone in both the EMIAT and CAMIAT trials. (Adapted from Waldo AL, Camm AJ, deRuyter H, et al: Effect of *d*-sotalol on mortality in patients with left ventricular dysfunction after recent and remote myocardial infarction. The SWORD Investigators. Survival With Oral *d*-Sotalol. Lancet 348:7–12, 1996; Julian DG, Camm AJ, Frangin G, et al: Randomised trial of effect of amiodarone on mortality in patients with left-ventricular dysfunction after recent myocardial infarction: EMIAT. European Myocardial Infarct Amiodarone Trial Investigators. Lancet 349:667–674, 1997; and Cairns JA, Connolly SJ, Roberts R, Gent M: Randomised trial of outcome after myocardial infarction in patients with frequent or repetitive ventricular premature depolarisations: CAMIAT. Canadian Amiodarone Myocardial Infarction Arrhythmia Trial Investigators. Lancet 349:675–682, 1997.)

events and a trend toward an early (year 1) increase in coronary events.[647] At present, we recommend continuing hormone replacement therapy in postmenopausal women after AMI but not starting it in women who have not been on hormone replacement previously until more data are available and longer-term follow-up in HERS has been reported.

REFERENCES

CHANGING PATTERNS OF CARE

1. Chockalingam A, Balaguer-Vintro I: Impending Global Pandemic of Cardiovascular Diseases; Challenges and Opportunities for the Prevention and Control of Cardiovascular Diseases in Developing Countries and Economies in Transition. Barcelona, Prous Science, 1999.
2. American Heart Association: 1999 Heart and Stroke Statistical Update. Dallas, American Heart Association, 1998.
3. Bayes de Luna A: International cooperation in world cardiology: The role of the World Heart Federation. Circulation 99:986–989, 1999.
4. Tunstall-Pedoe H, Mahonen M, Tolonen H, et al, for the WHO MONICA (monitoring trends and determinants in cardiovascular disease) Project: Contribution of trends in survival and coronary-event rates to changes in coronary heart disease mortality: 10-year results from 37 WHO MONICA Project populations. Lancet 353:1547–1557, 1999.
5. Braunwald E, Antman EM, Beasley JW, et al: ACC/AHA guidelines for the management of patients with unstable angina. A report of the American College of Cardiology/American Heart Association Task Force on Practice Guidelines (Committee on the Management of Patients With Unstable Angina). J Am Coll Cardiol 36:970–1062, 2000.
6. Guidry UC, Evans JC, Larson MG, et al: Temporal trends in event rates after Q-wave myocardial infarction: The Framingham Heart Study. Circulation 100:2054–2059, 1999.
7. Goldberg RJ, Yarzebski J, Lessard D, Gore JM: A two-decades (1975 to 1995) long experience in the incidence, in-hospital and long-term case-fatality rates of acute myocardial infarction: A community-wide perspective. J Am Coll Cardiol 33:1533–1539, 1999.
8. Braunwald E: Evolution of the management of acute myocardial infarction: A 20th century saga. Lancet 352:1771–1774, 1998.
9. Braunwald E, Antman EM: Evidence-based coronary care. Ann Intern Med 126:551–553, 1997.
10. Iezzoni LI: How much are we willing to pay for information about quality of care? Ann Intern Med 126:391–393, 1997.
11. Pine M, Norusis M, Jones B, Rosenthal GE: Predictions of hospital mortality rates: A comparison of data sources. Ann Intern Med 126:347–354, 1997.
12. St Peter RF, Reed MC, Kemper P, Blumenthal D: Changes in the scope of care provided by primary care physicians. N Engl J Med 341:1980–1985, 1999.
13. Antman E, Lau J, Kupelnick B, et al: A comparison of results of meta-analyses of randomized control trials and recommendations of clinical experts. JAMA 268:240–248, 1992.
14. Antiplatelet Trialists' Collaboration: Collaborative overview of randomised trials of antiplatelet therapy: I. Prevention of death myocardial infarction and stroke by prolonged antiplatelet therapy in various categories of patients. BMJ 308:81–106, 1994.
15. Fibrinolytic Therapy Trialists (FTT) Collaborative Group: Indications for fibrinolytic therapy in suspected acute myocardial infarction: Collaborative overview of early mortality and major morbidity results from all randomised trials of more than 1000 patients. Lancet 343:311–322, 1994.
16. Every NR, Frederick PD, Robinson M, et al: A comparison of the National Registry of Myocardial Infarction 2 with the Cooperative Cardiovascular Project. J Am Coll Cardiol 33:1886–1894, 1999.
17. Hampton JR: The limits of evidence-based cardiovascular therapy. Cardiovasc Drugs Ther 12:487–491, 1998.
18. Schmid CH, Lau J, McIntosh MW, Cappelleri JC: An empirical study of the effect of the control rate as a predictor of treatment efficacy in meta-analysis of clinical trials. Stat Med 17:1923–1942, 1998.
19. The GUSTO Investigators. An international randomized trial comparing four thrombolytic strategies for acute myocardial infarction. N Engl J Med 329:673–682, 1993.
20. The Global Use of Strategies to Open Occluded Coronary Arteries (GUSTO III) Investigators: A comparison of reteplase with alteplase for acute myocardial infarction. N Engl J Med 337:1118–1123, 1997.
21. Neuhaus KL: InTime-2 results. Presented at the Scientific Sessions of the American College of Cardiology, New Orleans, March 9, 1999.
22. Assessment of the Safety and Efficacy of a New Thrombolytic (ASSENT-2) Investigators: Single-bolus tenecteplase compared with front-loaded alteplase in acute myocardial infarction: The ASSENT-2 double-blind randomised trial: Assessment of the Safety and Efficacy of a New Thrombolytic Investigators. Lancet 354:716–722, 1999.
23. Barakat K, Wilkinson P, Deaner A, et al: How should age affect management of acute myocardial infarction? A prospective cohort study. Lancet 353:955–959, 1999.
23a. Thiemann DR, Coresh J, Schulman SP, et al: Lack of benefit for intravenous thrombolysis in patients with myocardial infarction who are older than 75 years. Circulation 101:2239–46, 2000.
23b. Ayanian JZ, Braunwald E: Thrombolytic therapy for patients with myocardial infarction who are older than 75 years. Do the risks outweigh the benefits? Circulation 101:2224–6, 2000.
24. Chen J, Marciniak TA, Radford MJ, et al: Beta-blocker therapy for secondary prevention of myocardial infarction in elderly diabetic patients. Results from the National Cooperative Cardiovascular Project. J Am Coll Cardiol 34:1388–1394, 1999.
25. European Secondary Prevention Study Group. Translation of clinical trials into practice: A European population-based study of the use of thrombolysis for acute myocardial infarction. Lancet 347:1203–1207, 1996.
26. Kizer JR, Cannon CP, McCabe CH, et al: Trends in the use of pharmacotherapies for acute myocardial infarction among physicians who design and/or implement randomized trials versus physicians in routine clinical practice: The MILIS-TIMI experience. Multicenter Investigation on Limitation of Infarct Size. Thrombolysis in Myocardial Infarction. Am Heart J 137:79–92, 1999.
27. McCormick D, Gurwitz JH, Lessard D, et al: Use of aspirin, beta-blockers, and lipid-lowering medications before recurrent acute myocardial infarction: Missed opportunities for prevention? Arch Intern Med 159:561–567, 1999.
28. Saketkhou BB, Conte FJ, Noris M, et al: Emergency department use of aspirin in patients with possible acute myocardial infarction. Ann Intern Med 127:126–129, 1997.
29. Goldberg RJ, Gurwitz JH: Disseminating the results of clinical trials to community-based practitioners: Is anyone listening? Am Heart J 137:4–7, 1999.
29a. Gan SC, Beaver SK, Houck PM, et al: Treatment of acute myocardial infarction and 30-day mortality among women and men. N Engl J Med 343:8–15, 2000.
30. O'Connor GT, Quinton HB, Traven ND, et al: Geographic variation in the treatment of acute myocardial infarction: The Cooperative Cardiovascular Project. JAMA 281:627–633, 1999.
31. Jollis JG, DeLong ER, Peterson ED, et al: Outcome of acute myocardial infarction according to the specialty of the admitting physician. N Engl J Med 335:1880–1887, 1996.
32. Frances CD, Go AS, Dauterman KW, et al: Outcome following acute myocardial infarction: Are differences among physician specialties the result of quality of care or case mix? Arch Intern Med 159:1429–1436, 1999.
33. Chen J, Radford MJ, Wang Y, et al: Do "America's Best Hospitals" perform better for acute myocardial infarction? N Engl J Med 340:286–292, 1999.
34. Thiemann DR, Coresh J, Oetgen WJ, Powe NR: The association between hospital volume and survival after acute myocardial infarction in elderly patients. N Engl J Med 340:1640–1648, 1999.
35. Selby JV, Fireman BH, Lundstrom RJ, et al: Variation among hospitals in coronary-angiography practices and outcomes after myocardial infarction in a large health maintenance organization. N Engl J Med 335:1888–1896, 1996.
35a. Canto JG, Shlipak MG, Rogers WJ, et al: Prevalence, clinical characteristics, and mortality among patients with myocardial infarction presenting without chest pain. JAMA 283:3223–3229, 2000.
36. Kravitz RL: Ethnic differences in use of cardiovascular procedures: New insights and new challenges. Ann Intern Med 130:231–233, 1999.
37. Malacrida R, Genoni M, Maggioni AP, et al: A comparison of the early outcome of acute myocardial infarction in women and men. The Third International Study of Infarct Survival Collaborative Group. N Engl J Med 338:8–14, 1998.
38. Vaccarino V, Parsons L, Every NR, et al: Sex-based differences in early mortality after myocardial infarction. National Registry of Myocardial Infarction 2 Participants. N Engl J Med 341:217–225, 1999.

PATHOLOGY

39. Phibbs B, Marcus F, Marriott HJC, et al: Q-wave versus non-Q-wave myocardial infarction: A meaningless distinction. J Am Coll Cardiol 33:576–582, 1999.
40. Rothwell PM, Villagra R, Gibson R, et al: Evidence of a chronic systemic cause of instability of atherosclerotic plaques. Lancet 355:19–24, 2000.
40a. Maseri A: From syndromes to specific disease mechanisms. The search for the causes of myocardial infarction. Ital Heart J 1:253–257, 2000.
41. Malek AM, Alper SL, Izumo S: Hemodynamic shear stress and its role in atherosclerosis. JAMA 282:2035–2042, 1999.
42. Rosenberg RD, Aird WC: Vascular-bed–specific hemostasis and hypercoagulable states. N Engl J Med 340:1555–1564, 1999.
42a. Davies MJ: The pathophysiology of acute coronary syndromes. Heart 83:361–6, 2000.
42b. Dahlback B: Blood coagulation. Lancet 355:1627–32, 2000.
43. Lee RT, Libby P: The unstable atheroma. Arterioscler Thromb Vasc Biol 17:1859–1867, 1997.
44. Fuster V: 50th anniversary historical article: Acute coronary syndromes: The degree and morphology of coronary stenoses. J Am Coll Cardiol 34:1854–1856, 1999.

45. Davies MJ: Stability and instability: Two faces of coronary atherosclerosis. Circulation 94:2013–2020, 1996.

46. Fuster V: Mechanisms of arterial thrombosis: Foundation for therapy. Am Heart J 135:S361–S366, 1998.

47. Gawaz M, Neumann FJ, Schomig A: Evaluation of platelet membrane glycoproteins in coronary artery disease: Consequences for diagnosis and therapy. Circulation 99:E1–E11, 1999.

48. Ross R: Atherosclerosis—an inflammatory disease. N Engl J Med 340:115–126, 1999.

49. Ardissino D, Merlini PA, Ariens R, et al: Tissue-factor antigen and activity in human coronary atherosclerotic plaques. Lancet 349:769–771, 1997.

50. Kloner RA, Leor J: Natural disaster plus wake-up time: A deadly combination of triggers. Am Heart J 137:779–781, 1999.

51. Feng DL, Tofler GH: Diurnal physiologic processes and circadian variation of acute myocardial infarction. J Cardiovasc Risk 2:494–498, 1995.

51a. Rentrop KP: Thrombi in acute coronary syndromes: Revisited and revised. Circulation 101:1619–26, 2000.

52. Ryan TJ, Antman EM, Brooks NH, et al: 1999 update: ACC/AHA Guidelines for the Management of Patients With Acute Myocardial Infarction: Executive Summary and Recommendations: A report of the American College of Cardiology/American Heart Association Task Force on Practice Guidelines (Committee on Management of Acute Myocardial Infarction). Circulation 100:1016–1030, 1999.

52a. Fox KA: Acute coronary syndromes: Presentation-clinical spectrum and management. Heart 84:93, 2000.

53. Goodman SG, Langer A, Ross AM, et al: Non-Q-wave versus Q-wave myocardial infarction after thrombolytic therapy: Angiographic and prognostic insights from the global utilization of streptokinase and tissue plasminogen activator for occluded coronary arteries: I. Angiographic substudy. GUSTO-I Angiographic Investigators. Circulation 97:444–450, 1998.

54. Zaacks SM, Liebson PR, Calvin JE, et al: Unstable angina and non-Q-wave myocardial infarction: Does the clinical diagnosis have therapeutic implications? J Am Coll Cardiol 33:107–118, 1999.

55. Savonitto S, Ardissino D, Granger CB, et al: Prognostic value of the admission electrocardiogram in acute coronary syndromes. JAMA 281:707–713, 1999.

56. Hathaway WR, Peterson ED, Wagner GS, et al: Prognostic significance of the initial electrocardiogram in patients with acute myocardial infarction. GUSTO-I Investigators. Global Utilization of Streptokinase and t-PA for Occluded Coronary Arteries. JAMA 279:387–391, 1998.

57. Schoen FJ: The heart. In Cotran FS, Kumar V, Collins T (eds): Pathologic Basis of Disease. 6th ed. Philadelphia, WB Saunders, 1999, pp 543–599.

58. Vargas SO, Sampson BA, Schoen FJ: Pathologic detection of early myocardial infarction: A critical review of the evolution and usefulness of modern techniques. Mod Pathol 12:635–645, 1999.

59. Kloner RA, Ellis SG, Lange R, et al: Studies of experimental coronary artery reperfusion: Effects on infarct size, myocardial function, biochemistry, ultrastructure and microvascular damage. Circulation 68:15–18, 1983.

60. Adams J III, Abendschein D, Jaffe A: Biochemical markers of myocardial injury. Is MB creatine kinase the choice for the 1990s? Circulation 88:750–763, 1993.

61. DeWood MA, Spores J, Notske RN, et al: Prevalence of total coronary artery occlusion during the early hours of transmural myocardial infarction. N Engl J Med. 303:897–902, 1980.

62. DeWood MA, Notske RN, Simpson CS, et al: Prevalence and significance of spontaneous thrombolysis in transmural myocardial infarction. Eur Heart J 6:33, 1985.

63. Kinch JW, Ryan TJ. Right ventricular infarction. N Engl J Med 330:1211–1217, 1994.

63a. Haji SA, Movahed A: Right ventricular infarction-diagnosis and treatment. Clin Cardiol 23:473–482, 2000.

64. Bowers TR, O'Neill WW, Grines C, et al: Effect of reperfusion on biventricular function and survival after right ventricular infarction. N Engl J Med 338:933–940, 1998.

65. Hod H, Lew AS, Keltai M, et al: Early atrial fibrillation during evolving myocardial infarction: A consequence of impaired left atrial perfusion. Circulation 75:146–150, 1987.

66. Kyriakidis M, Barbetseas J, Antonopoulos A, et al: Early atrial arrhythmias in acute myocardial infarction: Role of the sinus node artery. Chest 101:944–947, 1992.

67. Fujita M, Nakae I, Kihara Y, et al: Determinants of collateral development in patients with acute myocardial infarction. Clin Cardiol 22:595–599, 1999.

PATHOPHYSIOLOGY

68. Swan HJC, Forrester JS, Diamond G, et al: Hemodynamic spectrum of myocardial infarction and cardiogenic shock. Circulation 45:1097, 1972.

69. Forrester JS, Wyatt HL, Daluz PL, et al: Functional significance of regional ischemic contraction abnormalities. Circulation 54:64, 1976.

70. Schuster EH, Bulkley BH: Ischemia at a distance after acute myocardial infarction: A cause of early postinfarction angina. Circulation 62:509–515, 1980.

71. White HD, Norris RM, Brown MA, et al: Left ventricular end-systolic volume as the major determinant of survival after recovery from myocardial infarction. Circulation 76:44–51, 1987.

72. Pfeffer MA, Braunwald E: Ventricular remodeling after myocardial infarction: Experimental observations and clinical implications. Circulation 81:1161–1172, 1990.

72a. Sutton MG, Sharpe N: Left ventricular remodeling after myocardial infarction: Pathophysiology and therapy. Circulation 101:2981–2988, 2000.

73. Braunwald E, Pfeffer MA: Ventricular enlargement and remodeling following acute myocardial infarction: Mechanisms and management. Am J Cardiol 68:1D–6D, 1991.

74. Braunwald E, Kim CB: Late establishment of patency of the infarct-related artery. In Julian D, Braunwald E (eds): Acute Myocardial Infarction. London, WB Saunders, 1994, pp 147–162.

75. Pfeffer MA, Lamas GA, Vaughan DE, et al: Effect of captopril on progressive ventricular dilatation after anterior myocardial infarction. N Engl J Med 319:80–86, 1988.

76. Pfeffer JM, Pfeffer MA, Fletcher PJ, Braunwald E: Progressive ventricular remodeling in rat with myocardial infarction. Am J Physiol 260:H1406–H1414, 1991.

77. Weisman HF, Bush DE, Mannisi JA, et al: Cellular mechanisms of myocardial infarct expansion. Circulation 78:186–201, 1988.

78. Pfeffer MA: Left ventricular remodeling after acute myocardial infarction. Ann Rev Med 46:455–466, 1995.

79. Weisman HF, Healy B: Myocardial infarct expansion, infarct extension, and reinfarction: pathophysiologic concepts. Prog Cardiovasc Dis 30:73–110, 1987.

80. Schmermund A, Lerman LO, Ritman EL, Rumberger JA: Cardiac production of angiotensin II and its pharmacologic inhibition: Effects on the coronary circulation. Mayo Clin Proc 74:503–513, 1999.

81. Gray BA, Hyde RW, Hodges M, Yu PN: Alterations in lung volume and pulmonary function in relation to hemodynamic changes in acute myocardial infarction. Circulation 59:551, 1979.

81a. Capes SE, Hunt D, Malmberg K, Gerstein HC: Stress hyperglycaemia and increased risk of death after myocardial infarction in patients with and without diabetes: A systemic overview. Lancet 355:773–8, 2000.

82. Vetter NJ, Adams W, Strange RC, Oliver MF: Initial metabolic and hormonal response to acute myocardial infarction. Lancet 1:284, 1974.

83. Ceremuzynski L: Hormonal and metabolic reactions evoked by acute myocardial infarction. Circ Res 48:767, 1981.

84. Taegtmeyer H: Metabolic support of the postischaemic heart. Lancet 345:1552–1555, 1995.

85. Li YH, Teng JK, Tsai WC, et al: Prognostic significance of elevated hemostatic markers in patients with acute myocardial infarction. J Am Coll Cardiol 33:1543–1548, 1999.

86. Danesh J, Collins R, Appleby P, Peto R: Association of fibrinogen, C-reactive protein, albumin, or leukocyte count with coronary heart disease: Meta-analyses of prospective studies. JAMA 279:1477–1482, 1998.

87. Furman MI, Becker RC, Yarzebski J, et al: Effect of elevated leukocyte count on in-hospital mortality following acute myocardial infarction. Am J Cardiol 78:945–948, 1996.

87a. Kyne L, Hausdorff JM, Knight E, et al: Neutrophilia and congestive heart failure after acute myocardial infarction. Am Heart J 139:94–100, 2000.

88. Braunwald E: Acute myocardial infarction—the value of being prepared. N Engl J Med 334:51–52, 1996.

CLINICAL FEATURES

89. Stewart RA, Robertson MC, Wilkins GT, et al: Association between activity at onset of symptoms and outcome of acute myocardial infarction. J Am Coll Cardiol 29:250–253, 1997.

90. Giri S, Thompson PD, Kiernan FJ, et al: Clinical and angiographic characteristics of exertion-related acute myocardial infarction. JAMA 282:1731–1736, 1999.

91. Gullette EC, Blumenthal JA, Babyak M, et al: Effects of mental stress on myocardial ischemia during daily life. JAMA 277:1521–1526, 1997.

92. Hlatkly MA, Lam LC, Lee KL, et al: Job strain and the prevalence and outcome of coronary artery disease. Circulation 92:327–333, 1995.

93. Lee TH, Marcantonio ER, Mangione CM, et al: Derivation and prospective validation of a simple index for prediction of cardiac risk of major noncardiac surgery. Circulation 100:1043–1049, 1999.

94. Poldermans D, Boersma E, Bax JJ, et al: The effect of bisoprolol on perioperative mortality and myocardial infarction in high-risk patients undergoing vascular surgery. N Engl J Med 341:1789–1794, 1999.

95. Maseri A, L'Abbate A, Baroldi G, et al: Coronary vasospasm as a possible cause of myocardial infarction. N Engl J Med 299:1271, 1978.

96. Lange RL, Reid MS, Tresch DD, et al: Nonatheromatous ischemic heart disease following withdrawal from chronic industrial nitroglycerin exposure. Circulation 46:666, 1972.

97. Muller JE, Abela GS, Nesto RW, Tofler GH: Triggers, acute risk factors and vulnerable plaques: The lexicon of a new frontier. J Am Coll Cardiol 23:809–813, 1994.

98. Spencer FA, Goldberg RJ, Becker RC, Gore JM: Seasonal distribution of acute myocardial infarction in the second National Registry of Myocardial Infarction. J Am Coll Cardiol 31:1226–1233, 1998.

98a. Canto JG, Every NR, Magid DJ, et al: The volume of primary angioplasty procedures and survival after acute myocardial infarction. National Registry of Myocardial Infarction 2 Investigators. N Engl J Med 342:1573–80, 2000.

98b. Sheifer SE, Gersh BJ, Yanez ND 3rd, et al: Prevalence, predisposing factors, and prognosis of clinically unrecognized myocardial infarction in the elderly. J Am Coll Cardiol 35:119–26, 2000.

99. Spodick DH: Pericardial complications of myocardial infarction. *In* Francis GS, Alpert JS (eds): Coronary Care. Boston, Little, Brown & Co, 1995, pp 333–341.

100. Goyal RK. Changing focus on unexplained esophageal chest pain. Ann Intern Med 124:1008–1011, 1996.

101. Balaban DH, Yamamoto Y, Liu J, et al: Sustained esophageal contraction: A marker of esophageal chest pain identified by intraluminal ultrasonography. Gastroenterology 116:29–37, 1999.

102. McGuire DK, Granger CB: Diabetes and ischemic heart disease. Am Heart J 138:366–375, 1999.

103. Webb SW, Adgey AA, Pantridge JF: Autonomic disturbance at onset of acute myocardial infarction. BMJ 818:89, 1982.

104. Killip T, Kimball JT: Treatment of myocardial infarction in a coronary care unit: A two year experience with 250 patients. Am J Cardiol 20:457–464, 1967.

105. Pedoe-Tunstall H, Kuulasmaa K, Amouyel P, et al: Myocardial infarction and coronary deaths in the World Health Organization MONICA Project. Circulation 90:583–612, 1994.

106. Fox AC, Levin RI: Ruptured plaques and leaking cells: Cost-effectiveness in the diagnosis of acute coronary syndromes. Ann Intern Med 131:968–970, 1999.

107. Ravkilde J, Horder M, Gerhardt W, et al: Diagnostic performance and prognostic value of serum troponin T in suspected acute myocardial infarction. Scand J Clin Lab Invest 53:677–685, 1993.

108. Ellis AK: Serum protein measurements and the diagnosis of acute myocardial infarction. Circulation 83:1107–1109, 1991.

109. Mair J, Dienstl F, Puschendorf B: Cardiac troponin T in the diagnosis of myocardial injury. Crit Rev Clin Lab Sci 29:31–57, 1992.

110. Puleo PR, Meyer D, Wathen C, et al: Use of a rapid assay of subforms of creatine kinase MB to diagnose or rule out acute myocardial infarction. N Engl J Med 331:561–566, 1994.

111. Antman EM, Grudzien C, Sacks DB: Evaluation of a rapid bedside assay for detection of serum cardiac troponin T. JAMA 273:1279–1282, 1995.

112. Roberts R: Enzymatic estimation of infarct size: Thrombolysis induced its demise: Will it now rekindle its renaissance? Circulation 81:707–710, 1990.

113. Adams JE, Bodor GS, Davila-Roman VG, et al: Cardiac troponin I: A marker with high specificity for cardiac injury. Circulation 88:101–106, 1993.

114. Apple FS: Tissue specificity of cardiac troponin I, cardiac troponin T and creatine kinase-MB. Clin Chim Acta 284:151–159, 1999.

115. Christenson RH, Vaidya H, Landt Y, et al: Standardization of creatine kinase-MB (CK-MB) mass assays: The use of recombinant CK-MB as a reference material. Clin Chem 45:1414–1423, 1999.

116. Ohman EM, Tardiff BE: Periprocedural cardiac marker elevation after percutaneous coronary artery revascularization: Importance and implications. JAMA 277:495–497, 1997.

117. Wu AH, Apple FS, Gibler WB, et al: National Academy of Clinical Biochemistry Standards of Laboratory Practice: Recommendations for the use of cardiac markers in coronary artery diseases. Clin Chem 45:1104–1121, 1999.

118. Roberts R, Kleiman N: Earlier diagnosis and treatment of acute myocardial infarction necessitates the need for a "new diagnostic mind-set." Circulation 89:872–881, 1994.

119. Zimmerman J, Fromm R, Meyer D, et al: Diagnostic marker cooperative study for the diagnosis of myocardial infarction. Circulation 99:1671–1677, 1999.

120. Apple FS: Creatine kinase isoforms and myoglobin: Early detection of myocardial infarction and reperfusion. Coron Artery Dis 10:75–79, 1999.

121. de Lemos JA, Antman EM, Schroder R, et al: Very early risk stratification after thrombolytic therapy using a bedside myoglobin assay and the 12-lead ECG. Am Heart J, in press.

122. Hamm CW: New serum markers for acute myocardial infarction. N Engl J Med 331:607–608, 1994.

123. The Joint European Society of Cardiology/American College of Cardiology Committee: Myocardial infarction redefined—A consensus document of The Joint European Society of Cardiology/American College of Cardiology Committee for the Redefinition of Myocardial Infarction. J Am Coll Cardiol 36:959–969, 2000.

123a. Jaffe AS, Ravkilde J, Roberts R, et al: It's time for a change to a troponin standard. Circulation 102:1216–1220, 2000.

124. Hamm CW, Goldmann BU, Heeschen C, et al: Emergency room triage of patients with acute chest pain by means of rapid testing for cardiac troponin T or troponin I. N Engl J Med 337:1648–1653, 1997.

124a. Hamm CW, Braunwald E: A classification of unstable angina revisited. Circulation 102:118–122, 2000.

125. Katrukha AG, Bereznikova AV, Esakova TV, et al: Troponin I is released in bloodstream of patients with acute myocardial infarction not in free form but as complex. Clin Chem 43:1379–1385, 1997.

126. Tanasijevic MJ, Cannon CP, Antman EM, et al: Myoglobin, creatine-kinase-MB and cardiac troponin-I 60-minute ratios predict infarct-related artery patency after thrombolysis for acute myocardial infarction: Results from the Thrombolysis in Myocardial Infarction study (TIMI) 10B. J Am Coll Cardiol 34:739–747, 1999.

127. Stewart JT, French JK, Theroux P, et al: Early noninvasive identification of failed reperfusion after intravenous thrombolytic therapy in acute myocardial infarction. J Am Coll Cardiol 31:1499–1505, 1998.

128. Panteghini M, Apple FS, Christenson RH, et al: Use of biochemical markers in acute coronary syndromes. IFCC Scientific Division, Committee on Standardization of Markers of Cardiac Damage. International Federation of Clinical Chemistry. Clin Chem Lab Med 37:687–693, 1999.

129. Heeschen C, Hamm CW, Goldmann B, et al: Troponin concentrations for stratification of patients with acute coronary syndromes in relation to therapeutic efficacy of tirofiban. PRISM Study Investigators. Platelet Receptor Inhibition in Ischemic Syndrome Management. Lancet 354:1757–1762, 1999.

130. Del Carlo CH, O'Connor CM: Cardiac troponins in congestive heart failure. Am Heart J 138:646–653, 1999.

131. Polanczyk CA, Kuntz KM, Sacks DB, et al: Emergency department triage strategies for acute chest pain using creatine kinase-MB and troponin I assays: A cost-effectiveness analysis. Ann Intern Med 131:909–918, 1999.

132. Adams JE, Sicard GA, Allen BT, et al: Diagnosis of perioperative myocardial infarction with measurement of cardiac troponin I. N Engl J Med 330:670–674, 1994.

133. Ohman EM, Armstrong PW, White HD, et al: Risk stratification with a point-of-care cardiac troponin T test in acute myocardial infarction. Am J Cardiol 84:1281–1286, 1999.

134. Szczeklik A, Musial J, Undas A, et al: Inhibition of thrombin generation by simvastatin and lack of additive effects of aspirin in patients with marked hypercholesterolemia. J Am Coll Cardiol 33:1286–1293, 1999.

135. Dangas G, Badimon JJ, Smith DA, et al: Pravastatin therapy in hyperlipidemia: Effects on thrombus formation and the systemic hemostatic profile. J Am Coll Cardiol 33:1294–1304, 1999.

136. Amsterdam EA: The rationale for early initiation of cholesterol lowering therapy after myocardial infarction. Prev Cardiol 2:38–41, 1999.

137. Bayes de Luna A: Clinical Electrocardiography: A Textbook. Armonk, NY, Futura Publishing, 1998.

138. Panju AA, Hemmelgarn BR, Guyatt GH, Simel DL: Is this patient having a myocardial infarction? JAMA 280:1256–1263, 1998.

139. Engelen DJ, Gorgels AP, Cheriex EC, et al: Value of the electrocardiogram in localizing the occlusion site in the left anterior descending coronary artery in acute anterior myocardial infarction. J Am Coll Cardiol 34:389–395, 1999.

140. Wellens HJ: The value of the right precordial leads of the electrocardiogram. N Engl J Med 340:381–383, 1999.

141. Holmvang L, Clemmensen P, Wagner G, Grande P: Admission standard electrocardiogram for early risk stratification in patients with unstable coronary artery disease not eligible for acute revascularization therapy: A TRIM substudy. ThRombin Inhibition in Myocardial Infarction. Am Heart J 137:24–33, 1999.

142. Sgarbossa EB, Pinski SL, Barbagelata A, et al: Electrocardiographic diagnosis of evolving acute myocardial infarction in the presence of left bundle-branch block. N Engl J Med 334:481–487, 1996.

143. Cooksey JD, Dunn M, Massie E: Clinical Vectorcardiography and Electrocardiography. Chicago, Year Book Medical Publishers, 1977.

143a. Bosimini E, Giannuzzi P, Temporelli PL, et al: Electrocardiographic evolutionary changes and left ventricular remodeling after acute myocardial infarction: Results of the GISSI-3 Echo substudy. J Am Coll Cardiol 35:127–35, 2000.

144. Levine HD: Subendocardial infarction in retrospect: Pathologic, cardiographic, and ancillary features. Circulation 72:790, 1985.

145. Cheitlin MD, Alpert JS, Armstrong WF, et al: ACC/AHA guidelines for the clinical application of echocardiography: Executive summary. A report of the American College of Cardiology/American Heart Association Task Force on practice guidelines (Committee on Clinical Application of Echocardiography): Developed in collaboration with the American Society of Echocardiography. J Am Coll Cardiol 29:862–879, 1997.

146. Reimold SC, Antman EM: Noninvasive cardiac imaging in chest pain syndromes. J Thromb Thrombol 6:239–252, 1998.

147. Mirvis DM: Physiologic bases for anterior ST segment depression in patients with acute inferior wall myocardial infarction. Am Heart J 116:1308, 1988.

148. Lopez-Sendon J, Coma-Canella I, Alcasena S, et al: Electrocardiographic findings in acute right ventricular infarction: Sensitivity and specificity of electrocardiographic alterations in right precordial leads V4R, V3R, V1, V2, and V3. J Am Coll Cardiol 6:1273–1279, 1985.

149. Geft IL, Shah PK, Rodriguez L, et al: ST elevations in leads V1 to V5 may be caused by right coronary artery occlusion and acute right ventricular infarction. Am J Cardiol 53:991, 1984.

150. Brattler A, Karliner JS, Higgins CB, et al: The initial chest x-ray in acute myocardial infarction: Prediction of early and late mortality and survival. Circulation 61:1004, 1980.

151. Schwaiger M, Melin J: Cardiological applications of nuclear medicine. Lancet 354:661–666, 1999.

152. Gotte MJ, van Rossum AC, Marcus JT, et al: Recognition of infarct localization by specific changes in intramural myocardial mechanics. Am Heart J 138:1038–1045, 1999.

153. Konermann M, Sanner BM, Horstmann E, et al: Changes of the left ventricle after myocardial infarction—estimation with cine magnetic resonance imaging during the first six months. Clin Cardiol 20:201–212, 1997.

154. Hasche ET, Fernandes C, Freedman SB, Jeremy RW: Relation between ischemia time, infarct size, and left ventricular function in humans. Circulation 92:710–719, 1995.

155. Gibbons RJ, Miller TD, Christian TF: Infarct size measured by single photon emission computed tomographic imaging with (99m)Tc-sestamibi: A measure of the efficacy of therapy in acute myocardial infarction. Circulation 101:101–108, 2000.

156. Miller TD, Christian TF, Hopfenspirger MR, et al: Infarct size after acute myocardial infarction measured by quantitative tomographic 99mTc sestamibi imaging predicts subsequent mortality. Circulation 92: 334–341, 1995.

MANAGEMENT

157. National Heart Attack Alert Program Coordinating Committee—60 Minutes to Treatment Working Group. Emergency department: Rapid identification and treatment of patients with acute myocardial infarction. Ann Emerg Med 23:311–329, 1994.

158. National Heart Attack Alert Program Coordinating Committee Working Group on Educational Strategies to Prevent Prehospital Delay in Patients at High Risk for Acute Myocardial Infarction. Educational strategies to prevent prehospital delay in patients at high risk for acute myocardial: A report by the National Heart Attack Alert Program. J Thromb Thromol 6:000–000, 1998.

159. Goff DC Jr, Feldman HA, McGovern PG, et al: Prehospital delay in patients hospitalized with heart attack symptoms in the United States: The REACT trial. Am Heart J 138:1046–1057, 1999.

160. Cannon CP, Sayah AJ, Walls RM: Prehospital thrombolysis: An idea whose time has come. Clin Cardiol 22:IV10–IV19, 1999.

161. Hand M, Brown C, Horan M, Simons-Morton D: The National Heart Attack Alert Program: Progress at 5 years in educating providers, patients and the public, and future directions. J Thromb Thromol 6:9–17, 1998.

162. National Heart Attack Alert Program Coordinating Committee: Access to timely and optimal care of patients with acute coronary syndromes—community planning considerations: A report by the National Heart Attack Alert Program. J Thromb Thromol 6:19–46, 1998.

163. Lombardi G, Gallagher J, Gennis P: Outcome of out-of-hospital cardiac arrest in New York City. The Pre-Hospital Arrest Survival Evaluation (PHASE) Study. JAMA 271:678–683, 1994.

164. Sandler DA: Paramedic direct admission of heart-attack patients to a coronary-care unit. Lancet 352:1198, 1998.

165. National Heart Attack Alert Program: 9-1-1: Rapid Identification and Treatment of Acute Myocardial Infarction (NIH publication 94-3302). Department of Health and Human Services Public Health Service, National Institutes of Health. Bethesda, MD, National Heart, Lung, and Blood Institute, 1994, pp 1–6.

166. Weaver WD, Cerqueira M, Hallstrom AP, et al: Prehospital-initiated vs. hospital-initiated thrombolytic therapy. The Myocardial Infarction Triage and Intervention Trial. JAMA 270:1211–1216, 1993.

167. The European Myocardial Infarction Project Group: Prehospital thrombolytic therapy in patients with suspected acute myocardial infarction. N Engl J Med 329:383–389, 1993.

167a. Morrison LJ, Verbeek PR, McDonald AC, et al: Mortality and prehospital thrombolysis for acute myocardial infarction: A meta-analysis. JAMA 283:2686–92, 2000.

168. National Heart Attack Alert Program: Emergency Department: Rapid Identification and Treatment of Patients with Acute Myocardial Infarction (NIH publication 93-3278). Bethesda, MD, National Heart, Lung, and Blood Institute, 1993.

169. National Heart Attack Alert Program: Emergency Medical Dispatching: Rapid Identification and Treatment of Acute Myocardial Infarction (NIH publication 94-3287). Bethesda, MD, National Heart, Lung, and Blood Institute, 1994, pp 1–14.

170. National Heart Attack Alert Program: Staffing and Equipping Emergency Medical Services Systems: Rapid Identification and Treatment of Acute Myocardial Infarction (NIH publication 93-3304). Bethesda, MD, National Heart, Lung, and Blood Institute, 1994, pp 1–20.

171. Canto JG, Rogers WJ, Bowlby LJ, et al: The prehospital electrocardiogram in acute myocardial infarction: Is its full potential being realized? National Registry of Myocardial Infarction 2 Investigators. J Am Coll Cardiol 29:498–505, 1997.

172. Rawles JM: Quantification of the benefit of earlier thrombolytic therapy: Five-year results of the Grampian Region Early Anistreplase Trial (GREAT). J Am Coll Cardiol 30:1181–1186, 1997.

173. The pre-hospital management of acute heart attacks. Recommendations of a Task Force of The European Society of Cardiology and The European Resuscitation Council. Eur Heart J 19:1140–1164, 1998.

174. Selker HP, Zalenski RJ, Antman EM, et al: An evaluation of technologies for identifying acute cardiac ischemia in the emergency department: Executive summary of a National Heart Attack Alert Program Working Group Report. Ann Emerg Med 29:1–12, 1997.

174a. Lee TH, Goldman L: Evaluation of the patient with acute chest pain. N Engl J Med 342:1187, 2000.

174b. Pope JH, Aufderheide TP, Ruthazer R, et al: Missed diagnoses of acute cardiac ischemia in the emergency department. N Engl J Med 342: 1163–70, 2000.

175. Selker HP, Griffith JL, Beshansky JR, et al: Patient-specific predictions

176. of outcomes in myocardial infarction for real-time emergency use: A thrombolytic predictive instrument. Ann Intern Med 127:538–556, 1997.

176. Lambrew CT, Bowlby LJ, Rogers WJ, et al: Factors influencing the time to thrombolysis in acute myocardial infarction. Time to Thrombolysis Substudy of the National Registry of Myocardial Infarction-1. Arch Intern Med 157:2577–2582, 1997.

177. Zalenski RJ, Selker HP, Cannon CP, et al: National Heart Attack Alert Program position paper: Chest pain centers and programs for the evaluation of acute cardiac ischemia. Ann Emerg Med 35:462–471, 2000.

178. Shlipak MG, Lyons WL, Go AS, et al: Should the electrocardiogram be used to guide therapy for patients with left bundle-branch block and suspected myocardial infarction? JAMA 281:714–719, 1999.

179. Cannon CP, Gibson CM, Lambrew CT, et al: Longer thrombolysis door-to-needle times are associated with increased mortality in acute myocardial infarction: An analysis of 85,589 patients in the National Registry of Myocardial Infarction 2 & 3. J Am Coll Cardiol 35(Suppl. A): 376A, 2000.

179a. Cannon CP, Gibson CM, Lambrew CT, et al: Relationship of symptom-onset-to-balloon time and door-to-balloon time with mortality in patients undergoing angioplasty for acute myocardial infarction. JAMA 283:2941–7, 2000.

180. The TIMI IIIB Investigators: Effects of tissue plasminogen activator and a comparison of early invasive and conservative strategies in unstable angina and non-Q-wave myocardial infarction: Results of the TIMI IIIB Trial. Circulation 89:1545–1556, 1994.

181. Ornato JP: Chest pain emergency centers: Improving acute myocardial infarction care. Clin Cardiol 22:IV3–IV9, 1999.

182. Farkouh ME, Smars PA, Reeder GS, et al: A clinical trial of a chest-pain observation unit for patients with unstable angina. Chest Pain Evaluation in the Emergency Room (CHEER) Investigators. N Engl J Med 339: 1882–1888, 1998.

183. Nichol G, Walls R, Goldman L, et al: A critical pathway for management of patients with acute chest pain who are at low risk for myocardial ischemia: Recommendations and potential impact. Ann Intern Med 127:996–1005, 1997.

184. Roberts RR, Zalenski RJ, Mensah EK, et al: Costs of an emergency department–based accelerated diagnostic protocol vs hospitalization in patients with chest pain: A randomized controlled trial. JAMA 278: 1670–1676, 1997.

185. Antman EM: General hospital management. In Julian DG, Braunwald E (eds): Management of Acute Myocardial Infarction. London, WB Saunders, 1994, pp 29–70.

186. Chamberlain D: E-blockers and calcium antagonists. In Julian D, Braunwald E (eds): Management of Acute Myocardial Infarction. London, WB Saunders, 1994, pp 193–221.

187. Hjalmarson A, Elmfeldt D, Herlitz J, et al: Effect on mortality of metoprolol in acute myocardial infarction, a double-blind randomized trial. Lancet 2:823–827, 1981.

188. Kirshenbaum JM, Kloner RA, Antman EM, Braunwald E: Use of an ultra short-acting beta-blocker in patients with acute myocardial ischemia. Circulation 72:873–880, 1985.

189. Maroko P, Radvany P, Braunwald E, Hale S: Reduction of infarct size by oxygen inhalation following acute coronary occlusion. Circulation 52:360, 1975.

190. Califf RM, Bengtson JR: Cardiogenic shock. N Engl J Med 330:1724–1730, 1994.

191. Pfeffer M: ACE inhibition in acute myocardial infarction. N Engl J Med 332:118–120, 1995.

192. Maroko PR, Braunwald E: Modification of myocardial infarct size after coronary occlusion. Ann Intern Med 79:720–733, 1973.

193. Martin GV, Kennedy JW: Choice of thrombolytic agent. In Julian D, Braunwald E (eds): Management of Acute Myocardial Infarction. London, WB Saunders, 1994, pp 71–105.

194. Taegtmeyer H: Energy metabolism of the heart: From basic concepts to clinical applications. Curr Probl Cardiol 19:57–116, 1994.

195. Bolli R: Oxygen-derived free radicals and postischemic myocardial dysfunction ("stunned myocardium"). J Am Coll Cardiol 12:239–249, 1988.

196. Bolli R: Myocardial "stunning" in man. Circulation 86:1671–1691, 1992.

197. Przyklenk K, Kloner RA: Oxygen radical scavenging agents as adjuvant therapy with tissue plasminogen activator in a canine model of coronary thrombolysis. Cardiovasc Res 27:925–934, 1993.

198. Tomai F, Crea F, Chiariello L, Gioffre PA: Ischemic preconditioning in humans: Models, mediators, and clinical relevance. Circulation 100: 559–563, 1999.

199. Przyklenk K, Bauer B, Ovize M, et al: Regional ischemic "preconditioning" protects remote virgin myocardium from subsequent sustained coronary occlusion. Circulation 87:893–899, 1993.

199a. Lee SH, Wolf PL, Escudero R, et al: Early expression of angiogenesis factors in acute myocardial ischemia and infarction. N Engl J Med 342: 626–33, 2000.

199b. Latini R, Tognoni G, Maggioni AP, et al: Clinical effects of early angiotensin-converting enzyme inhibitor treatment for acute myocardial infarction are similar in the presence and absence of aspirin: Systematic overview of individual data from 96,712 randomized patients. Angiotensin-converting Enzyme Inhibitor Myocardial Infarction Collaborative Group. J Am Coll Cardiol 35:1801–7, 2000.

200. Gersh BJ, Anderson JL: Thrombolysis and myocardial salvage: Results of clinical trials and the animal paradigm—paradoxic or predictable? Circulation 88:296–306, 1993.

201. Ottani F, Galvani M, Ferrini D, Nicolini FA: Clinical relevance of pro-

dromal angina before acute myocardial infarction. Int J Cardiol 68(Suppl 1):S103–S108, 1999.

202. Bolli R, Marban E: Molecular and cellular mechanisms of myocardial stunning. Physiol Rev 79:609–634, 1999.

202a. Murphy AM, Kogler H, Georgakopoulos D, et al: Transgenic mouse model of stunned myocardium. Science 287:488–91, 2000.

203. Gerber BL, Wijns W, Vanoverschelde JL, et al: Myocardial perfusion and oxygen consumption in reperfused noninfarcted dysfunctional myocardium after unstable angina: Direct evidence for myocardial stunning in humans. J Am Coll Cardiol 34:1939–1946, 1999.

204. Kloner RA, Przyklenk K: Understanding the jargon: A glossary of terms used (and misused) in the study of ischaemia and reperfusion. Cardiovasc Res 27:162–166, 1993.

204a. Theroux P: Myocardial cell protection: A challenging time for action and a challenging time for clinical research. Circulation 101:2874–2876, 2000.

205. Kloner RA: Does reperfusion injury exist in humans? J Am Coll Cardiol 21:537–545, 1993.

206. Ito H, Tomooka T, Sakai N, et al: Lack of myocardial perfusion immediately after successful thrombolysis: A predictor of poor recovery of left ventricular function in anterior myocardial infarction. Circulation 85:1699–1705, 1992.

207. Davies CH, Ormerod OJ: Failed coronary thrombolysis. Lancet 351:1191–1196, 1998.

208. Antman E: Magnesium in acute myocardial infarction: Overview of available evidence. Am Heart J 132:487–494, 1996.

209. Kloner RA, Yellon D: Does ischemic preconditioning occur in patients? J Am Coll Cardiol 24:1133–1142, 1994.

210. Meisel SR, Shapiro H, Radnay J, et al: Increased expression of neutrophil and monocyte adhesion molecules LFA-1 and Mac-1 and their ligand ICAM-1 and VLA-4 throughout the acute phase of myocardial infarction: Possible implications for leukocyte aggregation and microvascular plugging. J Am Coll Cardiol 31:120–125, 1998.

211. Horwitz LD, Kong Y, Robertson AD: Timing of treatment for myocardial reperfusion injury. J Cardiovasc Pharmacol 33:19–29, 1999.

212. TIMI Study Group: Comparison of invasive and conservative strategies after treatment with intravenous tissue plasminogen activator in acute myocardial infarction. Results of the Thrombolysis in Myocardial Infarction (TIMI) Phase II Trial. N Engl J Med 320:618–627, 1989.

213. Roberts R, Rogers WJ, Meuller HS, for the TIMI Investigators: Immediate versus deferred β-blockade following thrombolytic therapy in patients with acute myocardial infarction: Results of the Thrombolysis in Myocardial Infarction (TIMI) II-B Study. Circulation 83:422–437, 1991.

214. Murry CE, Jennings RB, Reimer KA: Preconditioning with ischemia: A delay of lethal cell injury in ischemic myocardium. Circulation 74:1124–1136, 1986.

215. Sato T: Signaling in late preconditioning: Involvement of mitochondrial K(ATP) channels. Circ Res 85:1113–1114, 1999.

216. Ito H, Taniyama Y, Iwakura K, et al: Intravenous nicorandil can preserve microvascular integrity and myocardial viability in patients with reperfused anterior wall myocardial infarction. J Am Coll Cardiol 33:654–660, 1999.

217. Ueda Y, Kitakaze M, Komamura K, et al: Pravastatin restored the infarct size-limiting effect of ischemic preconditioning blunted by hypercholesterolemia in the rabbit model of myocardial infarction. J Am Coll Cardiol 34:2120–2125, 1999.

218. Kloner RA, Shook T, Antman EM, et al: Prospective temporal analysis of the onset of preinfarction angina versus outcome: An ancillary study in TIMI-9B. Circulation 97:1042–1045, 1998.

219. Noda T, Minatoguchi S, Fujii K, et al: Evidence for the delayed effect in human ischemic preconditioning: Prospective multicenter study for preconditioning in acute myocardial infarction. J Am Coll Cardiol 34:1966–1974, 1999.

220. Califf RM, O'Neill W, Stack RS, et al: Failure of simple clinical characteristics to predict perfusion status after intravenous thrombolysis. Ann Intern Med 108:658–662, 1988.

221. Solomon SD, Ridker PM, Antman EM: Ventricular arrhythmias in trials of thrombolytic therapy for acute myocardial infarction: A meta-analysis. Circulation 88:2575–2581, 1993.

222. Kim C, Braunwald E: Potential benefits of late reperfusion of infarcted myocardium: The open artery hypothesis. Circulation 88:2426–2436, 1993.

223. Hochman JS, Choo H: Limitation of myocardial infarct expansion by reperfusion independent of myocardial salvage. Circulation 75:299–306, 1987.

224. Lamas GV, Flaker GC, Mitchell G, et al: Effect of infarct artery patency on prognosis after acute myocardial infarction. Circulation 92:1101–1109, 1995.

225. White HD, Cross DB, Elliott JM, et al: Long-term prognostic importance of patency of the infarct-related coronary artery after thrombolytic therapy for acute myocardial infarction. Circulation 89:61–67, 1994.

226. Wilson JM: Reversible congestive heart failure caused by myocardial hibernation. Tex Heart Inst J 26:19–27, 1999.

227. Gang ES, Lew AS, Hong M, et al: Decreased incidence of ventricular late potentials after successful thrombolytic therapy for acute myocardial infarction. N Engl J Med 321:712–716, 1989.

228. Horvitz LL, Pietrolungo JF, Suri RS, et al: An open infarct-related artery is associated with a lower risk of lethal ventricular arrhythmias in patients with a left ventricular aneurysm. Circulation 86:I-315, 1992.

229. Gruppo Italiano per lo Studio della Streptochinasi nell'Infarto Miocardico (GISSI): Effectiveness of intravenous thrombolytic treatment in acute myocardial infarction. Lancet 1:397–401, 1986.

230. Franzosi MG, Santoro E, De Vita C, et al: Ten-year follow-up of the first megatrial testing thrombolytic therapy in patients with acute myocardial infarction: Results of the Gruppo Italiano per lo Studio della Sopravvivenza nell'Infarto-1 study. The GISSI Investigators. Circulation 98:2659–2665, 1998.

231. Califf RM: Ten years of benefit from a one-hour intervention. Circulation 98:2649–2651, 1998.

232. Van de Werf F, Ludbrook PA, Bergmann SR, et al: Coronary thrombolysis with tissue-type plasminogen activator in patients with evolving myocardial infarction. N Engl J Med 310:609–613, 1984.

233. Kennedy J, Ritchie J, Davis K, et al: The Western Washington randomized trial of intracoronary streptokinase in acute myocardial infarction: A 12-month follow-up report. N Engl J Med 312:1073–1078, 1985.

234. Tiefenbrunn AJ, Sobel BE: Thrombolysis and myocardial infarction. Fibrinolysis 5:1–15, 1991.

235. TIMI Study Group: The Thrombolysis in Myocardial Infarction (TIMI) Trial: Phase I findings. N Engl J Med 312:932–936, 1985.

236. Chesebro JH, Knatterud G, Roberts R, et al: Thrombolysis in Myocardial Infarction (TIMI) Trial, phase 1: A comparison between intravenous tissue plasminogen activator and intravenous streptokinase. Circulation 76:142–154, 1987.

237. Antman EM, Giugliano RP, Gibson CM, et al: Abciximab facilitates the rate and extent of thrombolysis: Results of the thrombolysis in myocardial infarction (TIMI) 14 trial. The TIMI 14 Investigators. Circulation 99:2720–2732, 1999.

238. The GUSTO Angiographic Investigators: The comparative effects of tissue plasminogen activator, streptokinase, or both on coronary artery patency, ventricular function and survival after acute myocardial infarction. N Engl J Med 329:1615–1622, 1993.

239. Lenderink T, Simoons ML, Van Es G-A, et al: Benefit of thrombolytic therapy is sustained throughout five years and is related to TIMI perfusion grade 3 but not grade 2 flow at discharge. Circulation 92:1110–1116, 1995.

240. Gibson CM: Primary angioplasty, rescue angioplasty, and new devices. In Hennekens CH (ed): Clinical Trials in Cardiovascular Disease: A Companion to Braunwald's Heart Disease. Philadelphia, WB Saunders, 1999, pp 185–197.

241. Fath-Ordoubadi F, Huehns TY, Al-Mohammad A, Beatt KJ: Significance of the Thrombolysis in Myocardial Infarction scoring system in assessing infarct-related artery reperfusion and mortality rates after acute myocardial infarction. Am Heart J 134:62–68, 1997.

242. Gibson CM, Murphy SA, Rizzo JM, et al: Relationship between TIMI frame count and clinical outcomes after thrombolytic administration. Thrombolysis In Myocardial Infarction (TIMI) Study Group. Circulation 99:1945–1950, 1999.

243. Gibson CM, Murphy S, Menown IB, et al: Determinants of coronary blood flow after thrombolytic administration. TIMI Study Group. Thrombolysis in Myocardial Infarction. J Am Coll Cardiol 34:1403–1412, 1999.

244. Ito H, Okamura A, Iwakura K, et al: Myocardial perfusion patterns related to thrombolysis in myocardial infarction perfusion grades after coronary angioplasty in patients with acute anterior wall myocardial infarction. Circulation 93:1993–1999, 1996.

245. Wu KC, Zerhouni EA, Judd RM, et al: Prognostic significance of microvascular obstruction by magnetic resonance imaging in patients with acute myocardial infarction. Circulation 97:765–772, 1998.

246. Schroder R, Wegscheider K, Schroder K, et al: Extent of early ST segment elevation resolution: A strong predictor of outcome in patients with acute myocardial infarction and a sensitive measure to compare thrombolytic regimens. A substudy of the International Joint Efficacy Comparison of Thrombolytics (INJECT) trial. J Am Coll Cardiol 26:1657–1664, 1995.

247. Schroder K, Wegscheider K, Neuhaus KL, et al: Significance of initial ST segment changes for thrombolytic treatment in first inferior myocardial infarction. Heart 77:506–511, 1997.

248. Wegscheider K, Neuhaus KL, Dissmann R, et al: Prognostic significance of ST segment change in acute myocardial infarct. Herz 24:378–388, 1999.

249. Schroder R, Zeymer U, Wegscheider K, Neuhaus KL: Comparison of the predictive value of ST segment elevation resolution at 90 and 180 min after start of streptokinase in acute myocardial infarction: A substudy of the hirudin for improvement of thrombolysis (HIT)-4 study. Eur Heart J 20:1563–1571, 1999.

250. van't Hof AW, Liem A, de Boer MJ, Zijlstra F: Clinical value of 12-lead electrocardiogram after successful reperfusion therapy for acute myocardial infarction. Zwolle Myocardial Infarction Study Group. Lancet 350:615–619, 1997.

251. Matetzky S, Freimark D, Chouraqui P, et al: The distinction between coronary and myocardial reperfusion after thrombolytic therapy by clinical markers of reperfusion. J Am Coll Cardiol 32:1326–1330, 1998.

252. Matetzky S, Novikov M, Gruberg L, et al: The significance of persistent ST elevation versus early resolution of ST segment elevation after primary PTCA. J Am Coll Cardiol 34:1932–1938, 1999.

253. Langer A, Krucoff MW, Klootwijk P, et al: Prognostic significance of ST segment shift early after resolution of ST elevation in patients with

myocardial infarction treated with thrombolytic therapy: The GUSTO-I ST Segment Monitoring Substudy. J Am Coll Cardiol 31:783–789, 1998.

254. Drew BJ, Krucoff MW: Multilead ST-segment monitoring in patients with acute coronary syndromes: A consensus statement for healthcare professionals. ST-Segment Monitoring Practice Guideline International Working Group. Am J Crit Care 8:372–386, 1999.

255. Agati L, Voci P, Hickle P, et al: Tissue-type plasminogen activator therapy versus primary coronary angioplasty: Impact on myocardial tissue perfusion and regional function 1 month after uncomplicated myocardial infarction. J Am Coll Cardiol 31:338–343, 1998.

256. Gassler JP, Topol EJ: Reperfusion revisited: Beyond TIMI 3 flow. Clin Cardiol 22:IV20–IV29, 1999.

257. Horcher J, Blasini R, Martinoff S, et al: Myocardial perfusion in acute coronary syndrome. Circulation 99:E15, 1999.

257a. Lepper W, Hoffmann R, Kamp O, et al: Assessment of myocardial reperfusion by intravenous myocardial contrast echocardiography and coronary flow reserve after primary percutaneous transluminal coronary angiography in patients with acute myocardial infarction. Circulation 101:2368–74, 2000.

258. Stewart RE, Miller DD, Bowers TR, et al: PET perfusion and vasodilator function after angioplasty for acute myocardial infarction. J Nucl Med 38:770–777, 1997.

259. Iwakura K, Ito H, Nishikawa N, et al: Early temporal changes in coronary flow velocity patterns in patients with acute myocardial infarction demonstrating the "no-reflow" phenomenon. Am J Cardiol 84:415–419, 1999.

260. Neumann FJ, Blasini R, Schmitt C, et al: Effect of glycoprotein IIb/IIIa receptor blockade on recovery of coronary flow and left ventricular function after the placement of coronary-artery stents in acute myocardial infarction. Circulation 98:2695–2701, 1998.

260a. Schömig A, Kastrati A, Dirschinger J, et al: Coronary stenting plus platelet glycoprotein IIb/IIIa blockade compared with tissue plasminogen activator in acute myocardial infarction. N Engl J Med 343:385–391, 2000.

261. Gibson CM, Cannon CP, Murphy SA, et al: Relationship of TIMI myocardial perfusion grade to mortality after administration of thrombolytic drugs. Circulation 101:124–130, 2000.

262. Mahaffey KW, Puma JA, Barbagelata NA, et al: Adenosine as an adjunct to thrombolytic therapy for acute myocardial infarction: Results of a multicenter, randomized, placebo-controlled trial: The Acute Myocardial Infarction STudy of ADenosine (AMISTAD) trial. J Am Coll Cardiol 34:1711–1720, 1999.

263. Weaver WD: Time to thrombolytic treatment: Factors affecting delay and their influence on outcome. J Am Coll Cardiol 25:3S–9S, 1995.

264. Boersma E, Maas AC, Deckers JW, Simoons ML: Early thrombolytic treatment in acute myocardial infarction: Reappraisal of the golden hour. Lancet 348:771–775, 1996.

265. LATE (Late Assessment of Thrombolytic Efficacy) Study Group: Late Assessment of Thrombolytic Efficacy (LATE) Study with alteplase 6–24 hours after onset of acute myocardial infarction. Lancet 342:759–766, 1993.

266. EMERAS (Estudio Multicentrico Estreptoquinasa Republicas de America del Sur) Collaborative Group: Randomized trial of late thrombolysis in acute myocardial infarction. Lancet 342:767–772, 1993.

267. ISIS-3 (Third International Study of Infarct Survival) Collaborative Group: ISIS-3: A randomized trial of streptokinase vs tissue plasminogen activator vs anistreplase and of aspirin plus heparin vs aspirin alone among 41,299 cases of suspected acute myocardial infarction. Lancet 339:753–770, 1992.

268. Chandra NC, Ziegelstein RC, Rogers WJ, et al: Observations of the treatment of women in the United States with myocardial infarction: A report from the National Registry of Myocardial Infarction-I. Arch Intern Med 158:981–988, 1998.

268a. Morrow DA, Antman EM, Charlesworth A, et al: The TIMI risk score for ST elevation myocardial infarction: A convenient, bedside, clinical score for risk assessment at presentation: An InTIME II substudy. Circulation, in press.

269. Lee KL, Woodlief LH, Topol EJ, et al: Predictors of 30-day mortality in the era of reperfusion for acute myocardial infarction: Results from an international trial of 41,021 patients. GUSTO-I Investigators. Circulation 91:1659–1668, 1995.

270. Wilcox RG, von der Lippe G, Olsson CG, et al: Trial of tissue plasminogen activator for mortality reduction in acute myocardial infarction. Anglo-Scandinavian Study of Early Thrombolysis (ASSET). Lancet 1:525–530, 1988.

271. ISAM (Intravenous Streptokinase in Acute Myocardial Infarction) Study Group: A prospective trial of intravenous streptokinase in acute myocardial infarction (ISAM). N Engl J Med 314:1465–1471, 1986.

272. Becker RC, Gore JM, Lambrew C, et al: A composite view of cardiac rupture in the United States National Registry of Myocardial Infarction. J Am Coll Cardiol 27:1321–1326, 1996.

273. Meijer A, Verheugt FWA, Werter CJPJ, et al: Aspirin versus coumadin in the prevention of reocclusion and recurrent ischemia after successful thrombolysis: A prospective placebo-controlled angiographic study: Results of the APRICOT Study. Circulation 87:1524–1530, 1993.

274. Collins R, Peto R, Baigent C, Sleight P: Aspirin, heparin, and fibrinolytic therapy in suspected acute myocardial infarction. N Engl J Med 336:847–860, 1997.

275. Cannon CP, McCabe CH, Diver DJ, et al: Comparison of front-loaded recombinant tissue-type plasminogen activator, anistreplase and combi-

nation thrombolytic therapy for acute myocardial infarction: Results of the Thrombolysis in Myocardial Infarction (TIMI) 4 trial. J Am Coll Cardiol 24:1602–1610, 1994.

276. Van de Werf FJ: The ideal fibrinolytic: Can drug design improve clinical results? Eur Heart J 20:1452–1458, 1999.

277. The Continuous Infusion versus Double-Bolus Administration of Alteplase (COBALT) Investigators: A comparison of continuous infusion of alteplase with double-bolus administration for acute myocardial infarction. The Continuous Infusion versus Double-Bolus Administration of Alteplase (COBALT) Investigators. N Engl J Med 337:1124–1130, 1997.

278. Ware JH, Antman EM: Equivalence trials. N Engl J Med 337:1159–1161, 1997.

279. White HD: Thrombolytic therapy and equivalence trials. J Am Coll Cardiol 31:494–496, 1998.

280. Neuhaus KL, von Essen R, Vogt A, et al: Dose finding with a novel recombinant plasminogen activator (BM 06.022) in patients with acute myocardial infarction: Results of the German Recombinant Plasminogen Activator Study. A study of the Arbeitsgemeinschaft Leitender Kardiologischer Krankenhausarzte (ALKK). J Am Coll Cardiol 24:55–60, 1994.

281. Tebbe U, von Essen R, Smolarz S, et al: Open, noncontrolled dose-finding study with a novel recombinant plasminogen activator (BM 06.022) given as a double bolus in patients with acute myocardial infarction. Am J Cardiol 72:518–524, 1993.

282. Smalling RW, Bode C, Kalbfleisch J, et al: More rapid, complete, and stable coronary thrombolysis with bolus administration of reteplase compared with alteplase infusion in acute myocardial infarction. RAPID Investigators. Circulation 91:2725–2732, 1995.

283. Bode C, Smalling RW, Berg G, et al: Randomized comparison of coronary thrombolysis achieved with double-bolus reteplase (recombinant plasminogen activator) and front-loaded, accelerated alteplase (recombinant tissue plasminogen activator) in patients with acute myocardial infarction. The RAPID II Investigators. Circulation 94:891–898, 1996.

284. International Joint Efficacy Comparison of Thrombolytics: Randomised, double-blind comparison of reteplase double-bolus administration with streptokinase in acute myocardial infarction (INJECT): Trial to investigate equivalence. Lancet 346:329–336, 1995.

285. den Heijer P, Vermeer F, Ambrosioni E, et al: Evaluation of a weight-adjusted single-bolus plasminogen activator in patients with myocardial infarction: A double-blind, randomized angiographic trial of lanoteplase versus alteplase. Circulation 98:2117–2125, 1998.

286. Keyt BA, Paoni NF, Refino CJ, et al: A faster-acting and more potent form of tissue plasminogen activator. Proc Natl Acad Sci U S A 91:3670–3674, 1994.

287. Cannon CP, McCabe CH, Gibson CM, et al: TNK-tissue plasminogen activator in acute myocardial infarction: Results of the Thrombolysis in Myocardial Infarction (TIMI) 10A dose-ranging trial. Circulation 95:351–356, 1997.

288. Cannon CP, Gibson CM, McCabe CH, et al: TNK-tissue plasminogen activator compared with front-loaded alteplase in acute myocardial infarction: Results of the TIMI 10B trial. Thrombolysis in Myocardial Infarction (TIMI) 10B Investigators. Circulation 98:2805–2814, 1998.

289. Van de Werf F, Cannon CP, Luyten A, et al: Safety assessment of single-bolus administration of TNK tissue-plasminogen activator in acute myocardial infarction: The ASSENT-1 trial. The ASSENT-1 Investigators. Am Heart J 137:786–791, 1999.

290. PRIMI Trial Study Group: Randomised double-blind trial of recombinant pro-urokinase against streptokinase in acute myocardial infarction. Lancet 1:863–868, 1989.

291. Michels R, Hoffmann H, Windeler J, et al: A double-blind multicenter comparison of the efficacy and safety of saruplase and urokinase in the treatment of acute myocardial infarction: Report of the SUTAMI study group. J Thromb Thrombol 2:117–124, 1995.

292. Bar FW, Meyer J, Vermeer F, et al: Comparison of saruplase and alteplase in acute myocardial infarction: SESAM Study Group. The Study in Europe with Saruplase and Alteplase in Myocardial Infarction. Am J Cardiol 79:727–732, 1997.

293. Vermeer F, Bosl I, Meyer J, et al: Saruplase is a safe and effective thrombolytic agent; Observations in 1,698 patients: Results of the PASS study. Practical Applications of Saruplase Study. J Thromb Thrombol 8:143–150, 1999.

294. Tebbe U, Michels R, Adgey J, et al: Randomized, double-blind study comparing saruplase with streptokinase therapy in acute myocardial infarction: The COMPASS Equivalence Trial. Comparison Trial of Saruplase and Streptokinase (COMPASS) Investigators. J Am Coll Cardiol 31:487–493, 1998.

295. Bar WF, Hopkins G, Dickhoet S: The Bolus versus Infusion in Rescueplase (saruplase) Development (BIRD) Study in 2410 patients with myocardial infarction. Circulation 98:I-505, 1998.

296. Collen D. Staphylokinase: A potent, uniquely fibrin-selective thrombolytic agent. Nat Med 4:279–284, 1998.

297. Vanderschueren S, Barrios L, Kerdsinchai P, et al: A randomized trial of recombinant staphylokinase versus alteplase for coronary artery patency in acute myocardial infarction. The STAR Trial Group. Circulation 92:2044–2049, 1995.

298. Armstrong PW, Burton JR, Palisaitis D, et al: Collaborative Angiographic Patency Trial of Recombinant Staphylokinase (CAPTORS). Circulation 100:I-650, 1999.

299. White HD, Norris RM, Brown MA, et al: Effect of intravenous streptokinase on left ventricular function and early survival after acute myocardial infarction. N Engl J Med 317:850–855, 1987.

300. St. John Sutton M, Pfeffer MA, Plappert T, et al: Quantitative two-dimensional echocardiographic measurements are major predictors of adverse cardiovascular events after acute myocardial infarction: The protective effects of captopril. Circulation 89:68–75, 1994.

301. Gruppo Italiano per lo Studio della Sopravvivenza nell'Infarto Miocardico: GISSI-2: A factorial randomised trial of alteplase versus streptokinase and heparin versus no heparin among 12,490 patients with acute myocardial infarction. Lancet 336:65–71, 1990.

302. Antman EM, for the TIMI 9A Investigators: Hirudin in acute myocardial infarction: Safety report from the Thrombolysis and Thrombin Inhibition in Myocardial Infarction (TIMI) 9A trial. Circulation 90:1624–1630, 1994.

303. The Global Use of Strategies to Open Occluded Coronary Arteries (GUSTO) IIa Investigators: A randomized trial of intravenous heparin versus recombinant hirudin for acute coronary syndromes. Circulation 90:1631–1637, 1994.

304. Sane DC, Califf RM, Topol EJ, et al: Bleeding during thrombolytic therapy for acute myocardial infarction: Mechanisms and management. Ann Intern Med 111:1010, 1989.

305. Gore JM, Granger CB, Simoons ML, et al: Stroke after thrombolysis: Mortality and functional outcomes in the GUSTO-I Trial. Circulation 92:2811–2818, 1995.

306. Maggioni AP, Franzosi MG, Santoro E, et al: The risk of stroke in patients with acute myocardial infarction after thrombolytic and antithrombotic treatment. N Engl J Med 327:1–6, 1992.

307. Simoons ML, Maggioni AP, Knatterud G, et al: Individual risk assessment for intracranial haemorrhage during thrombolytic therapy. Lancet 342:1523–1528, 1993.

308. ISIS-2 (Second International Study of Infarct Survival) Collaborative Group: Randomised trial of intravenous streptokinase, oral aspirin, both, or neither among 17,187 cases of suspected acute myocardial infarction: ISIS-2. Lancet 2:349–360, 1988.

309. Gurwitz JH, Gore JM, Goldberg RJ, et al: Risk for intracranial hemorrhage after tissue plasminogen activator treatment for acute myocardial infarction: Participants in the National Registry of Myocardial Infarction 2. Ann Intern Med 129:597–604, 1998.

310. Kleiman NS, Terrin M, Mueller H, et al: Mechanisms of early death despite thrombolytic therapy: Experience from the Thrombolysis in Myocardial Infarction Investigation Phase II (TIMI II) Study. J Am Coll Cardiol 19:1129–1135, 1992.

311. Hennekens C: The need for wider utilization of thrombolytic therapy. Clin Cardiol 20:III26–III31, 1997.

312. Berkowitz SD, Granger CB, Pieper KS, et al: Incidence and predictors of bleeding after contemporary thrombolytic therapy for myocardial infarction: The Global Utilization of Streptokinase and Tissue plasminogen activator for Occluded coronary arteries (GUSTO) I Investigators. Circulation 95:2508–2516, 1997.

313. Lee TH: Cost effectiveness of tissue plasminogen activator. N Engl J Med 332:1443–1444, 1995.

314. Simoons ML, Arnold AE: Tailored thrombolytic therapy: A perspective. Circulation 88:2556–2564, 1993.

315. Brodie BR, Stuckey TD, Hansen C, et al: Benefit of late coronary reperfusion in patients with acute myocardial infarction and persistent ischemic chest pain. Am J Cardiol 74:538–543, 1994.

CATHETER-BASED REPERFUSION

316. Dangas G, Stone GW: Primary mechanical reperfusion in acute myocardial infarction: The United States experience. Semin Intervent Cardiol 4:21–33, 1999.

317. Antoniucci D, Valenti R, Trapani M, Moschi G: Current role of stenting in acute myocardial infarction. Am Heart J 138:147–152, 1999.

318. Grines CL: Should thrombolysis or primary angioplasty be the treatment of choice for acute myocardial infarction? Primary angioplasty—the strategy of choice. N Engl J Med 335:1313–1316, 1996.

319. Weaver WD, Simes RJ, Betriu A, et al: Comparison of primary coronary angioplasty and intravenous thrombolytic therapy for acute myocardial infarction: A quantitative review. JAMA 278:2093–2098, 1997.

320. Grines CL, Ellis SG, Jones M, et al: Primary coronary angioplasty vs. thrombolytic therapy for acute myocardial infarction (MI): Long term follow-up of ten randomized trials. Circulation 100:I-499, 1999.

321. Stone GW, Grines CL, Rothbaum D, et al: Analysis of the relative costs and effectiveness of primary angioplasty versus tissue-type plasminogen activator: The Primary Angioplasty in Myocardial Infarction (PAMI) trial. The PAMI Trial Investigators. J Am Coll Cardiol 29:901–907, 1997.

322. Grines CL, Marsalese DL, Brodie B, et al: Safety and cost-effectiveness of early discharge after primary angioplasty in low risk patients with acute myocardial infarction. PAMI-II Investigators. Primary Angioplasty in Myocardial Infarction. J Am Coll Cardiol 31:967–972, 1998.

323. Antoniucci D, Valenti R, Santoro GM, et al: Systematic primary angioplasty in octogenarian and older patients. Am Heart J 138:670–674, 1999.

324. Grines CL, Ellis S, Jones M, et al: Primary coronary angioplasty vs. thrombolytic therapy for treatment of acute myocardial infarction (MI): Findings from the PCAT collaboration. Eur Heart J 20:170, 1999.

325. Berger AK, Schulman KA, Gersh BJ, et al: Primary coronary angioplasty vs thrombolysis for the management of acute myocardial infarction in elderly patients. JAMA 282:341–348, 1999.

326. Nunn CM, O'Neill WW, Rothbaum D, et al: Long-term outcome after primary angioplasty: Report from the primary angioplasty in myocardial infarction (PAMI-I) trial. J Am Coll Cardiol 33:640–646, 1999.

327. Zijlstra F, Hoorntje JC, de Boer MJ, et al: Long-term benefit of primary angioplasty as compared with thrombolytic therapy for acute myocardial infarction. N Engl J Med 341:1413–1419, 1999.

328. The Global Use of Strategies to Open Occluded Coronary Arteries in Acute Coronary Syndromes (GUSTO IIb) Angioplasty Substudy Investigators: A clinical trial comparing primary coronary angioplasty with tissue plasminogen activator for acute myocardial infarction. N Engl J Med 336:1621–1628, 1997.

329. Yusuf S, Pogue J: Primary angioplasty compared with thrombolytic therapy for acute myocardial infarction. JAMA 278:2110–2111, 1997.

330. Zahn R, Schuster S, Schiele R, et al: Differences in patients with acute myocardial infarction treated with primary angioplasty or thrombolytic therapy. Maximal Individual Therapy in Acute Myocardial Infarction (MITRA) Study Group. Clin Cardiol 22:191–199, 1999.

331. Ashmore RC, Luckasen GJ, Larson DG, et al: Immediate angioplasty for acute myocardial infarction: A community hospital's experience. J Invas Cardiol 11:61–65, 1999.

332. Wharton TP Jr, McNamara NS, Fedele FA, et al: Primary angioplasty for the treatment of acute myocardial infarction: Experience at two community hospitals without cardiac surgery. J Am Coll Cardiol 33:1257–1265, 1999.

333. Grines CL: Transfer of high-risk myocardial infarction patients for primary PTCA. J Invas Cardiol 9:13B–19B, 1997.

334. Ferguson JJ. Meeting Highlights: Highlights of the 21st Congress of the European Society of Cardiology. Circulation 100:e126–e131, 1999.

335. Peterson LR, Chandra NC, French WJ, et al: Reperfusion therapy in patients with acute myocardial infarction and prior coronary artery bypass graft surgery (National Registry of Myocardial Infarction-2). Am J Cardiol 84:1287–1291, 1999.

336. Jacobs AK: Coronary stents—have they fulfilled their promise? N Engl J Med 341:2005–2006, 1999.

337. Grines CL, Cox DA, Stone GW, et al: Coronary angioplasty with or without stent implantation for acute myocardial infarction. N Engl J Med 341:1949–1956, 1999.

338. Ellis SG, da Silva ER, Heyndrickx G, et al: Randomized comparison of rescue angioplasty with conservative management of patients with early failure of thrombolysis for acute anterior myocardial infarction. Circulation 90:2280–2284, 1994.

338a. Llevadot J, Giugliano RP, McCabe CH, et al: Degree of residual stenosis in the culprit coronary artery after thrombolytic administration (Thrombolysis In Myocardial Infarction [TIMI] trials). Am J Cardiol 85:1409–1413, 2000.

339. Michels KB, Yusuf S: Does PTCA in acute myocardial infarction affect mortality and reinfarction rates? A quantitative overview (meta-analysis) of the randomized clinical trials. Circulation 91:476–485, 1995.

340. Topol EJ, Califf RM, George BS, et al: A randomized trial of immediate versus delayed elective angioplasty after intravenous tissue plasminogen activator in acute myocardial infarction. N Engl J Med 317:581–588, 1987.

341. Rogers WJ, Baim DS, Gore JM, et al: Comparison of immediate invasive, delayed invasive, and conservative strategies after tissue-type plasminogen activator: Results of the Thrombolysis in Myocardial Infarction (TIMI) Phase II-A Trial. Circulation 81:1457–1476, 1990.

342. The TIMI Research Group: Immediate vs delayed catheterization and angioplasty following thrombolytic therapy for acute myocardial infarction: TIMI II A results. JAMA 260:2849–2858, 1988.

343. SWIFT (Should We Intervene Following Thrombolysis) Trial Study Group: SWIFT trial of delayed elective intervention v. conservative treatment after thrombolysis with anistreplase in acute myocardial infarction. BMJ 302:555–560, 1991.

344. Ross AM, Coyne KS, Reiner JS, et al: A randomized trial comparing primary angioplasty with a strategy of short-acting thrombolysis and immediate planned rescue angioplasty in acute myocardial infarction: The PACT trial. PACT investigators. Plasminogen-activator Angioplasty Compatibility Trial. J Am Coll Cardiol 34:1954–1962, 1999.

345. Keeley EC, Weaver WD: Combination therapy for acute myocardial infarction. J Am Coll Cardiol 34:1963–1965, 1999.

346. Keeley EC, Hillis LD: Left ventricular mural thrombus after acute myocardial infarction. Clin Cardiol 19:83, 1996.

347. Rankin JM, Spinelli JJ, Carere RG, et al: Improved clinical outcome after widespread use of coronary-artery stenting in Canada. N Engl J Med 341:1957–1965, 1999.

348. Pomes Iparraguirre H, Conti C, Grancelli H, et al: Prognostic value of clinical markers of reperfusion in patients with acute myocardial infarction treated by thrombolytic therapy. Am Heart J 134:631–638, 1997.

348a. Goldman LE, Eisenberg MJ: Identification and management of patients with failed thrombolysis after acute myocardial infarction. Ann Intern Med 132:556–65, 2000.

349. The TIMI Study Group: Comparison of invasive and conservative strategies after treatment with intravenous tissue plasminogen activator in acute myocardial infarction: Results of the Thrombolysis in Myocardial Infarction (TIMI) phase II trial. N Engl J Med 320:618–627, 1989.

350. Stone GW, Marsalese D, Brodie BR, et al: A prospective, randomized evaluation of prophylactic intraaortic balloon counterpulsation in high risk patients with acute myocardial infarction treated with primary

angioplasty. Second Primary Angioplasty in Myocardial Infarction (PAMI-II) Trial Investigators. J Am Coll Cardiol 29:1459–1467, 1997.

351. van't Hof AW, Liem AL, DeBoer MJ, et al: A randomized comparison of intra-aortic balloon pumping after primary coronary angioplasty in high-risk patients with acute myocardial infarction. Eur Heart J 20:659–665, 1999.

352. Kereiakes DJ, Topol EJ, George BS, et al: Favorable early and long-term prognosis following coronary bypass surgery therapy for myocardial infarction: Results of a multicenter trial. TAMI Study Group. Am Heart J 118:199–207, 1989.

ANTITHROMBOTIC AND ANTIPLATELET THERAPY

353. Kagen L, Scheidt S, Butt A: Serum myoglobin in myocardial infarction: The "staccato phenomenon": Is acute myocardial infarction in man an intermittent event? Am J Med 62:86, 1977.

354. The Global Use of Strategies to Open Occluded Coronary Arteries (GUSTO) IIb investigators: A comparison of recombinant hirudin with heparin for the treatment of acute coronary syndromes. N Engl J Med 335:775–782, 1996.

355. Bleich SD, Nichols T, Schumacher RR, et al: Effect of heparin on coronary patency after thrombolysis with tissue plasminogen activator in acute myocardial infarction. Am J Cardiol 66:1412–1417, 1990.

356. Hsia J, Hamilton WP, Kleiman N, et al: A comparison between heparin and low-dose aspirin as adjunctive therapy with tissue plasminogen activator for acute myocardial infarction. N Engl J Med 323:1433–1437, 1990.

357. de Bono DP, Simoons MI, Tijssen J, et al: Effect of early intravenous heparin on coronary patency, infarct size, and bleeding complications after alteplase thrombolysis: Results of a randomized double blind European Cooperative Study Group trial. Br Heart J 67:122–128, 1992.

358. Verheugt FW, Liem A, Zijlstra F, et al: High dose bolus heparin as initial therapy before primary angioplasty for acute myocardial infarction: Results of the Heparin in Early Patency (HEAP) pilot study. J Am Coll Cardiol 31:289–293, 1998.

359. Liem A, Zijlstra F, Ottervanger JP, et al: High dose heparin as pretreatment for primary angioplasty in acute myocardial infarction: The Heparin in EArly Patency (HEAP) randomized trial. J Am Coll Cardiol 35:600–604, 2000.

360. Cairns JA, Theroux P, Lewis HD Jr, et al: Antithrombotic agents in coronary artery disease. Chest 114:611S–633S, 1998.

361. Vaitkus P, Barnathan E: Embolic potential, prevention and management of mural thrombus complicating anterior myocardial infarction: A meta-analysis. J Am Coll Cardiol 22:1004–1009, 1993.

362. Warkentin TE, Levine MN, Hirsh J, et al: Heparin-induced thrombocytopenia in patients treated with low-molecular-weight heparin or unfractionated heparin. N Engl J Med 332:1374–1376, 1995.

363. Krumholz HM, Hennen J, Ridker PM, et al: Use and effectiveness of intravenous heparin therapy for treatment of acute myocardial infarction in the elderly. J Am Coll Cardiol 31:973–979, 1998.

364. Giugliano RP, Cutler SS, Llevadot J: Risk of intracranial hemorrhage with accelerated tPA: Importance of the heparin dose. Circulation 100 (Suppl 1):I–1650, 1999.

365. Weitz JI: Low-molecular-weight heparins. N Engl J Med 337:688–698, 1997.

366. Neuhaus KL, von Essen R, Tebbe U, et al: Safety observations from the pilot phase of the randomized r-Hirudin for Improvement of Thrombolysis (HIT-III) study: A study of the Arbeitsgemeinschaft Leitender Kardiologischer Krankenhausarzte (ALKK). Circulation 90:1638–1642, 1994.

367. Antman EM: Hirudin in acute myocardial infarction. Thrombolysis and Thrombin Inhibition in Myocardial Infarction (TIMI) 9B trial. Circulation 94:911–921, 1996.

368. Antman EM, Bittl JA: Direct thrombin inhibitors. In Hennekens CH (ed): Clinical Trials in Cardiovascular Disease: A Companion to Braunwald's Heart Disease. Philadelphia, WB Saunders, 1999, pp 145–165.

369. Fung AY, Lorch G, Cambier PA, et al: Efegatran sulfate as an adjunct to streptokinase versus heparin as an adjunct to tissue plasminogen activator in patients with acute myocardial infarction. ESCALAT Investigators. Am Heart J 138:696–704, 1999.

370. White HD, Aylward PE, Frey MJ, et al: Randomized, double-blind comparison of hirulog versus heparin in patients receiving streptokinase and aspirin for acute myocardial infarction (HERO). Hirulog Early Reperfusion/Occlusion (HERO) Trial Investigators. Circulation 96:2155–2161, 1997.

371. French JK, White HD: Antithrombin agents as adjuncts to thrombolytic therapy. J Thromb Thrombol 8:159–166, 1999.

372. Leadley RJ Jr, Kasiewski CJ, Bostwick JS, et al: Comparison of enoxaparin, hirulog, and heparin as adjunctive antithrombotic therapy during thrombolysis with rtPA in the stenosed canine coronary artery. Thromb Haemost 78:1278–1285, 1997.

373. Glick A, Kornowski R, Michowich Y, et al: Reduction of reinfarction and angina with use of low-molecular-weight heparin therapy after streptokinase (and heparin) in acute myocardial infarction. Am J Cardiol 77:1145–1148, 1996.

374. Frostfeldt G, Ahlberg G, Gustafsson G, et al: Low molecular weight heparin (dalteparin) as adjuvant treatment of thrombolysis in acute myocardial infarction—a pilot study: Biochemical markers in acute coronary syndromes (BIOMACS II). J Am Coll Cardiol 33:627–633, 1999.

375. Zed PJ: Low-molecular-weight heparin should replace unfractionated

376. Antman EM, Cohen M, Radley D, et al: Assessment of the treatment effect of enoxaparin for unstable angina/non-Q-wave myocardial infarction. TIMI 11B-ESSENCE meta-analysis. Circulation 100:1602–1608, 1999.

377. White HD, Yusuf S: Issues regarding the use of heparin following streptokinase therapy. J Thromb Thrombol 2:5–10, 1995.

378. Hochman JS, Wali AU, Gavrila D, et al: A new regimen for heparin use in acute coronary syndromes. Am Heart J 138:313–318, 1999.

379. Becker RC, Spencer FA, Li Y, et al: Thrombin generation after the abrupt cessation of intravenous unfractionated heparin among patients with acute coronary syndromes: Potential mechanisms for heightened prothrombotic potential. J Am Coll Cardiol 34:1020–1027, 1999.

380. Falk E, Shah PK, Fuster V: Coronary plaque disruption. Circulation 92:657–671, 1995.

381. Shimomura H, Ogawa H, Arai H, et al: Serial changes in plasma levels of soluble P-selectin in patients with acute myocardial infarction. Am J Cardiol 81:397–400, 1998.

382. Antiplatelet Trialists' Collaboration: Collaborative overview of randomised trials of antiplatelet therapy: II. Maintenance of vascular graft or arterial patency by antiplatelet therapy. BMJ 308:159–168, 1994.

383. Antiplatelet Trialists' Collaboration: Collaborative overview of randomised trials of antiplatelet therapy: III. Reduction in venous thrombosis and pulmonary embolism by antiplatelet prophylaxis among surgical and medical patients. BMJ 308:235–246, 1994.

384. Zusman RM, Chesebro JH, Comerota A, et al: Antiplatelet therapy in the prevention of ischemic vascular events: Literature review and evidence-based guidelines for drug selection. Clin Cardiol 22:559–573, 1999.

385. Weber C, Springer TA: Neutrophil accumulation on activated, surface-adherent platelets in flow is mediated by interaction of Mac-1 with fibrinogen bound to alphaIIb/beta3 and stimulated by platelet-activating factor. J Clin Invest 100:2085–2093, 1997.

386. Mickelson JK, Ali MN, Kleiman NS, et al: Chimeric 7E3 Fab (ReoPro) decreases detectable CD11b on neutrophils from patients undergoing coronary angioplasty. J Am Coll Cardiol 33:97–106, 1999.

387. Nordt TK, Moser M, Kohler B, et al: Augmented platelet aggregation as predictor of reocclusion after thrombolysis in acute myocardial infarction. Thromb Haemost 80:881–886, 1998.

388. Topol EJ, Byzova TV, Plow EF: Platelet GPIIb-IIIa blockers. Lancet 353:227–231, 1999.

389. Gurbel PA, Serebruany VL, Shustov AR, et al: Effects of reteplase and alteplase on platelet aggregation and major receptor expression during the first 24 hours of acute myocardial infarction treatment. GUSTO-III Investigators. Global Use of Strategies to Open Occluded Coronary Arteries. J Am Coll Cardiol 31:1466–1473, 1998.

390. Vorchheimer DA, Badimon JJ, Fuster V: Platelet glycoprotein IIb/IIIa receptor antagonists in cardiovascular disease. JAMA 281:1407–1414, 1999.

391. Harrington RA: Overview of clinical trials of glycoprotein IIb-IIIa inhibitors in acute coronary syndromes. Am Heart J 138:S276–S286, 1999.

392. Kleiman N, Ohman EM, Califf RM, et al: Profound inhibition of platelet aggregation with monoclonal antibody 7E3 Fab after thrombolytic therapy: Results of the Thrombolysis and Angioplasty in Myocardial Infarction (TAMI) 8 pilot study. J Am Coll Cardiol 22:381–389, 1993.

393. Ohman EM, Kleiman NS, Gacioch G, et al: Combined accelerated tissue-plasminogen activator and platelet glycoprotein IIb/IIIa integrin receptor blockade with Integrilin in acute myocardial infarction. Results of a randomized, placebo-controlled, dose-ranging trial. IMPACT-AMI Investigators. Circulation 95:846–854, 1997.

394. SK Eptifibatide Trial. Eur Heart J 2000.

395. The PARADIGM Investigators: Combining thrombolysis with the platelet glycoprotein IIb/IIIa inhibitor lamifiban: Results of the Platelet Aggregation Receptor Antagonist Dose Investigation and Reperfusion Gain in Myocardial Infarction (PARADIGM) trial. J Am Coll Cardiol 32:2003–2010, 1998.

396. Antman EM, Gibson CM, de Lemos JA, et al: For the Thrombolysis in Myocardial Infarction (TIMI) 14 Investigators. Combination reperfusion therapy with abciximab and reduced dose reteplase: Results from TIMI 14. Eur Heart J 2000, in press.

396a. de Lemos JA, Antman EM, ibson CM, et al: Abciximab improves both epicardial flow and myocardial reperfusion in ST-elevation myocardial infarction. Observations from the TIMI 14 trial. Circulation 101:239–43, 2000.

397. Brener SJ, Lopez JF, Vrobel TR, et al: Eptifibatide markedly enhances arterial patency after low-dose tissue plasminogen activator in acute myocardial infarction. J Am Coll Cardiol, submitted for publication.

398. Strategies for Patency Enhancement in the Emergency Department (SPEED) Group: Trial of abciximab with and without low-dose reteplase for acute myocardial infarction. Circulation 101:2788–2794, 2000.

399. Gold HK, Garabedian HD, Dinsmore RE, et al: Restoration of coronary flow in myocardial infarction by intravenous chimeric 7E3 antibody without exogenous plasminogen activators: Observations in animals and humans. Circulation 95:1755–1759, 1997.

400. Lefkovits J, Ivanhoe RJ, Califf RM, et al: Effects of platelet glycoprotein IIb/IIIa receptor blockade by a chimeric monoclonal antibody (abciximab) on acute and six-month outcomes after percutaneous transluminal coronary angioplasty for acute myocardial infarction. EPIC investigators. Am J Cardiol 77:1045–1051, 1996.

heparin in the management of acute coronary syndromes. J Thromb Thrombol 8:79–87, 1999.

401. van den Merkhof LF, Zijlstra F, Olsson H, et al: Abciximab in the treatment of acute myocardial infarction eligible for primary percutaneous transluminal coronary angioplasty. Results of the Glycoprotein Receptor Antagonist Patency Evaluation (GRAPE) pilot study. J Am Coll Cardiol 33:1528–1532, 1999.

402. Brener SJ, Barr LA, Burchenal JE, et al: Randomized, placebo-controlled trial of platelet glycoprotein IIb/IIIa blockade with primary angioplasty for acute myocardial infarction. ReoPro and Primary PTCA Organization and Randomized Trial (RAPPORT) Investigators. Circulation 98:734–741, 1998.

403. Montalescot G, Barragan P, Wittenberg O, et al: Abciximab associated with angioplasty and stenting in acute myocardial infarction: The ADMIRAL study, 30-day final results. Circulation 18:I-87, 1999.

404. CADILLAC Study Presented at 72nd Scientific Sessions of AHA, Atlanta, GA, 1999.

405. White HD: Future of reperfusion therapy for acute myocardial infarction. Lancet 354:695–697, 1999.

406. Kennedy JW, Stadius ML: Combined thrombolytic and platelet glycoprotein IIb/IIIa inhibitor therapy for acute myocardial infarction: Will pharmacological therapy ever equal primary angioplasty? Circulation 99:2714–2716, 1999.

407. Harrington RA, Kleiman NS, Granger CB, et al: Relation between inhibition of platelet aggregation and clinical outcomes. Am Heart J 136:S43–S50, 1998.

HOSPITAL MANAGEMENT

408. Daida H, Kottke TE, Backes RJ, et al: Are coronary-care unit changes in therapy associated with improved survival of elderly patients with acute myocardial infarction? Mayo Clin Proc 72:1014–1021, 1997.

409. Lee TH, Cook EF, Weisberg MC, et al: Impact of the availability of a prior electrocardiogram on the triage of the patient with acute chest pain. J Gen Intern Med 5:381–388, 1990.

410. Newby KL, Eisenstein EL, Califf RM, et al: Cost-effectiveness of early discharge after acute myocardial infarction after uncomplicated myocardial infarction. N Engl J Med 342:749–785, 2000.

411. Antman EM, Kuntz KM: The length of the hospital stay after myocardial infarction. N Engl J Med 342:808–810, 2000.

412. Kirchhoff KT, Holm K, Foreman MD, Rebenson-Piano M: Electrocardiographic response to ice water ingestion. Heart Lung 19:41–48, 1990.

413. Levine SA, Lown B: "Armchair" treatment of acute coronary thrombosis. JAMA 148:1365, 1952.

414. Peterson ED, Shaw LJ, Califf RM: Risk stratification after myocardial infarction. Ann Intern Med 126:561–582, 1997.

415. The MIAMI Trial Research Group: Metoprolol in acute myocardial infarction: Arrhythmias. Am J Cardiol 56:35G–38G, 1985.

416. The MIAMI Trial Research Group: Metoprolol in acute myocardial infarction: Enzymatic estimation of infarct size. Am J Cardiol 56:27G–29G, 1985.

417. Chae CU, Hennekens CH: Beta blockers. In Hennekens CH (ed): Clinical Trials in Cardiovascular Disease: A Companion to Braunwald's Heart Disease. Philadelphia, WB Saunders, 1999, pp 76–94.

418. ISIS-1 (First International Study of Infarct Survival) Collaborative Group: Mechanisms for the early mortality reduction produced by beta-blockade started early in acute myocardial infarction: ISIS-1. Lancet 1:921–923, 1988.

419. Krumholz HM, Radford MJ, Wang Y, et al: Early beta-blocker therapy for acute myocardial infarction in elderly patients. Ann Intern Med 131:648–654, 1999.

420. Yusuf S, Peto R, Lewis J, et al: Beta blockade during and after myocardial infarction: An overview of the randomized trials. Prog Cardiovasc Dis 27:335–371, 1985.

421. Pfeiffer MA, Braunwald E, Moye LA, et al: Effect of captopril on mortality and morbidity in patients with left ventricular dysfunction after myocardial infarction. N Engl J Med 327:669–677, 1992.

422. The Acute Infarction Ramipril Efficacy (AIRE) Study Investigators: Effect of ramipril on mortality and morbidity of survivors of acute myocardial infarction with clinical evidence of heart failure. Lancet 342:821–828, 1993.

423. Ambrosioni E, Borghi C, Magnani B, on behalf of the SMILE Study Investigators: Effects of the early administration of zofenopril on mortality and morbidity in patients with anterior myocardial infarction. Results of the Survival of Myocardial Infarction Long-Term Evaluation Trial. N Engl J Med 332:280–285, 1995.

424. Kobler L, Torp-Pedersen C, Carlsen JE, et al: A clinical trial of the angiotensin-converting-enzyme inhibitor trandolapril in patients with left ventricular dysfunction after myocardial infarction. N Engl J Med 333:1670–1676, 1995.

425. ISIS-4 Collaborative Group: ISIS-4: A randomized factorial trial assessing early oral captopril, oral mononitrate, and intravenous magnesium sulphate in 58,050 patients with suspected acute myocardial infarction. Lancet 345:669–685, 1995.

426. Gruppo Italiano per lo Studio della Sopravvivenza nell'Infarto Miocardico: GISSI-3: Effects of lisinopril and transdermal glyceryl trinitrate singly and together on 6-week mortality and ventricular function after acute myocardial infarction. Lancet 343:1115–1122, 1994.

427. Swedberg K, Held P, Kjekshus J, et al, on behalf of the CONSENSUS II Study Group: Effects of early administration of enalapril on mortality in patients with acute myocardial infarction. Results of the Cooperative North Scandinavian Enalapril Survival Study II (CONSENSUS II). N Engl J Med 327:678–684, 1992.

428. Chinese Cardiac Study Collaborative Group: Oral captopril versus placebo among 13,634 patients with suspected myocardial infarction: Interim report from the Chinese Cardiac Study (CCS-1). Lancet 345:686–687, 1995.

429. ACE Inhibitor Myocardial Infarction Collaborative Group: Indications for ACE inhibitors in the early treatment of acute myocardial infarction: Systematic overview of individual data from 100,000 patients in randomized trials. Circulation 97:2202–2212, 1998.

430. Pfeffer MA: ACE inhibitors in acute myocardial infarction: Patient selection and timing. Circulation 97:2192–2194, 1998.

431. Rutherford JD, Pfeffer MA, Moye LA, et al: Effects of captopril on ischemic events after myocardial infarction: Results of the Survival and Ventricular Enlargement Trial. Circulation 90:1731–1738, 1994.

431a. Pfeffer MA: Enhancing cardiac protection after myocardial infarction: Rationale for newer clinical trials of angiotensin receptor blockers. Am Heart J 139:S23–S28, 2000.

432. Dickstein K, Kjekshus J: Comparison of the effects of losartan and captopril on mortality in patients after acute myocardial infarction: The OPTIMAAL trial design. Optimal Therapy in Myocardial Infarction with the Angiotensin II Antagonist Losartan. Am J Cardiol 83:477–481, 1999.

433. Lindsay HSJ, Zaman AG, Cowan JC: ACE inhibitors after myocardial infarction: Patient selection or treatment for all? Br Heart J 73:397–400, 1995.

434. Pfeffer MA, Greaves SC, Arnold JM, et al: Early versus delayed angiotensin-converting enzyme inhibition therapy in acute myocardial infarction: The healing and early afterload reducing therapy trial. Circulation 95:2643–2651, 1997.

435. Jugdutt BI: Nitrates in myocardial infarction. Cardiovasc Drugs Ther 8:635–646, 1994.

436. Abrams J: The role of nitrates in coronary heart disease. Arch Intern Med 155:357–364, 1995.

437. Yusuf S, Held P, Furberg C: Update of effects of calcium antagonists in myocardial infarction or angina in light of the second Danish Verapamil Infarction Trial (DAVIT-II) and other recent studies. Am J Cardiol 67:1295–1297, 1991.

438. Furberg CD, Psaty BM, Meyer JV: Nifedipine: Dose-related increase in mortality in patients with coronary heart disease. Circulation 92:1326–1331, 1995.

439. Rogers W, Bowlby L, Chandra N, et al: Treatment of myocardial infarction in the United States (1990 to 1993). Observations from the National Registry of Myocardial Infarction. Circulation 90:2103–2114, 1994.

440. Yusuf S: Calcium antagonists in coronary artery disease and hypertension: Time for reevaluation? Circulation 92:1079–1082, 1995.

441. Opie LH, Messerli FH: Nifedipine and mortality: Grave defects in the dossier. Circulation 92:1068–1073, 1995.

442. Report of the Holland Interuniversity Nifedipine/Metoprolol Trial Research Group: Early treatment of unstable angina in the coronary care unit: A randomised, double-blind, placebo-controlled comparison of recurrent ischaemia and thrombolytic therapy in patients treated with nifedipine or metoprolol or both. Br Heart J 56:400, 1986.

443. The Danish Study Group on Verapamil in Myocardial Infarction: Verapamil in acute myocardial infarction. Eur Heart J 54:516–528, 1984.

444. Gibson RS, Boden WE, Theroux P, et al: Diltiazem and reinfarction in patients with non-Q wave myocardial infarction: Results of a double-blind, randomized, multicenter trial. N Engl J Med 315:423–429, 1986.

445. Hansen JF: Treatment with verapamil after an acute myocardial infarction: Review of the Danish studies on verapamil in myocardial infarction (DAVIT I and II). Drugs 2:43–53, 1991.

446. The Multicenter Diltiazem Postinfarction Trial Research Group: The effect of diltiazem on mortality and reinfarction after myocardial infarction. N Engl J Med 319:385–392, 1988.

447. The Danish Study Group on Verapamil in Myocardial Infarction: Effect of verapamil on mortality and major events after acute infarction (the Danish Verapamil Infarction Trial II-DAVIT II). Am J Cardiol 66:779, 1990.

448. Boden WE, van Gilst WH, Scheldewaert RG: Diltiazem in acute myocardial infarction treated with thrombolytic agents: A randomised placebo-controlled trial. Incomplete Infarction Trial of European Research Collaborators Evaluating Prognosis post-Thrombolysis (INTERCEPT). Lancet 355:1751–6, 2000.

449. Leitch JW, McElduff P, Dobson A, Heller R: Outcome with calcium channel antagonists after myocardial infarction: A community-based study. J Am Coll Cardiol 31:111–117, 1998.

450. Shechter M, Kaplinsky E, Rabinowitz B: The rationale of magnesium supplementation in acute myocardial infarction: A review of the literature. Arch Intern Med 152:2189–2196, 1992.

451. Shechter M, Hod H, Kaplinsky E, et al: Magnesium therapy in acute myocardial infarction when patients are not candidates for thrombolytic therapy. Am J Cardiol 75:321–323, 1995.

452. MAGIC Steering Committee: Rationale and design of the Magnesium in Coronaries (MAGIC) study: A clinical trial to reevaluate the efficacy of early administration of magnesium in acute myocardial infarction. Am Heart J 139: 10–14, 2000.

453. Rogers WJ, Segall PH, McDaniel HG, et al: Prospective randomized trial of glucose-insulin-potassium in acute myocardial infarction. Am J Cardiol 43:801, 1979.

454. Fath-Ordoubadi F, Beatt KJ: Glucose-insulin-potassium therapy for treatment of acute myocardial infarction: An overview of randomized placebo-controlled trials. Circulation 96:1152–1156, 1997.

455. Diaz R, Paolasso EA, Piegas LS, et al: Metabolic modulation of acute myocardial infarction. The ECLA (Estudios Cardiologicos Latinoamerica) Collaborative Group. Circulation 98:2227–2234, 1998.

456. Apstein CS: Glucose-insulin-potassium for acute myocardial infarction: Remarkable results from a new prospective, randomized trial. Circulation 98:2223–2226, 1998.

457. Opie LH: Proof that glucose-insulin-potassium provides metabolic protection of ischaemic myocardium? Lancet 353:768–769, 1999.

458. Malmberg K, Ryden L, Efendic S, et al: Randomized trial of insulin-glucose infusion followed by subcutaneous insulin treatment in diabetic patients with acute myocardial infarction (DIGAMI Study): Effects on mortality at 1 year. J Am Coll Cardiol 26:57–65, 1995.

459. Collaborative Organization for RheothRx Evaluation (CORE). Effects of RheothRx on mortality, morbidity, left ventricular function, and infarct size in patients with acute myocardial infarction. Circulation 96:192–201, 1997.

460. HALT-AMI Trial Presented at 72nd Scientific Sessions of the American Heart Association, Atlanta, GA, Nov. 1999.

HEMODYNAMIC DISTURBANCES

461. Swan HJC, Ganz W, Forrester JS, et al: Catheterization of the heart in man with use of a flow-directed balloon-tipped catheter. N Engl J Med 283:447, 1970.

462. Ganz LI, Friedman PL: Supraventricular tachycardia. N Engl J Med 332:162–173, 1995.

462a. Mermel LA: Prevention of intravascular catheter-related infections. Ann Intern Med 132:391–402, 2000.

463. Veenstra DL, Saint S, Saha S, et al: Efficacy of antiseptic-impregnated central venous catheters in preventing catheter-related bloodstream infection: A meta-analysis. JAMA 281:261–267, 1999.

464. Ali AS, Rybicki BA, Alam M, et al: Clinical predictors of heart failure in patients with first acute myocardial infarction. Am Heart J 138:1133–1139, 1999.

465. Handley DA, Anderson AJ, Koester J, Snider ME: New millennium bronchodilators for asthma: Single-isomer beta agonists. Curr Opin Pulm Med 6:43–49, 2000.

466. Marchionni N, Pini R, Vanucci A, et al: Hemodynamic effects of digoxin in acute myocardial infarction in man: A randomized controlled trial. Am Heart J 109:63–68, 1985.

467. Moss AJ, Davis HT, Conard DL, et al: Digitalis-associated cardiac mortality after myocardial infarction. Circulation 64:1150–1156, 1981.

468. Ryan TJ, Bailey KR, McCabe CH, et al: The effects of digitalis on survival in high-risk patients with coronary artery disease. Circulation 67:735–742, 1983.

469. Digitalis Subcommittee of the Multicenter Post-Infarction Research Group. The mortality risk associated with digitalis treatment after myocardial infarction. Cardiovasc Drugs Ther 1:125–132, 1987.

470. Bigger JT, Fleiss JL, Rolnitzky LM et al: Effect of digitalis treatment on survival after acute myocardial infarction. Am J Cardiol 55:623–630, 1985.

471. Muller JE, Turi ZG, Stone PH, et al: Digoxin therapy and mortality after myocardial infarction. N Engl J Med 314:265–271, 1986.

472. Maekawa K, Liang CS, Hood WBJ. Comparison of dobutamine and dopamine in acute myocardial infarction: Effects of systemic hemodynamics, plasma catecholamines, blood flows and infarct size. Circulation 67:750, 1983.

473. Barry WL, Sarembock IJ: Cardiogenic shock: Therapy and prevention. Clin Cardiol 21:72–80, 1998.

473a. Hochman JS, Buller CE, Sleeper LA, et al, for the SHOCK Investigators: Cardiogenic shock complicating acute myocardial infarction—Etiologies, management and outcome: A report from the SHOCK Trial Registry. J Am Coll Cardiol 36(3, suppl 1):1063–1070, 2000.

474. Scheidt S, Ascheim R, Killip T: Shock after acute myocardial infarction: A clinical and hemodynamic profile. Am J Cardiol 26:556–564, 1970.

475. Goldberg RJ, Samad NA, Yarzebski J, et al: Temporal trends in cardiogenic shock complicating acute myocardial infarction. N Engl J Med 340:1162–1168, 1999.

475a. Hasdai D, Califf RM, Thompson TD, et al: Predictors of cardiogenic shock after thrombolytic therapy for acute myocardial infarction. J Am Coll Cardiol 35:136–43, 2000.

476. Holmes DR Jr, Bates ER, Kleiman NS, et al: Contemporary reperfusion therapy for cardiogenic shock: The GUSTO-I trial experience. The GUSTO-I Investigators. Global Utilization of Streptokinase and Tissue Plasminogen Activator for Occluded Coronary Arteries. J Am Coll Cardiol 26:668–674, 1995.

477. Zeymer U, Neuhaus KL, Wegscheider K, et al: Effects of thrombolytic therapy in acute inferior myocardial infarction with or without right ventricular involvement. HIT-4 Trial Group. Hirudin for Improvement of Thrombolysis. J Am Coll Cardiol 32:876–881, 1998.

478. Mueller H, Ayres SM, Conklin EF, et al: The effects of intra-aortic counter pulsation on cardiac performance and metabolism in shock associated with acute myocardial infarction. J Clin Invest 50:1885, 1971.

479. Holmes DR Jr, Califf RM, Van de Werf F, et al: Difference in countries' use of resources and clinical outcome for patients with cardiogenic

480. Hochman JS, Sleeper LA, Webb JG, et al: Early revascularization in acute myocardial infarction complicated by cardiogenic shock. SHOCK Investigators. Should We Emergently Revascularize Occluded Coronaries for Cardiogenic Shock. N Engl J Med 341:625–634, 1999.

481. Shiraki H, Yoshikawa T, Anzai T, et al: Association between preinfarction angina and a lower risk of right ventricular infarction. N Engl J Med 338:941–947, 1998.

482. Inoue K, Ito H, Kitakaze M, et al: Antecedent angina pectoris as a predictor of better functional and clinical outcomes in patients with an inferior wall acute myocardial infarction. Am J Cardiol 83:159–163, 1999.

483. Robalino BD, Whitlow PL, Underwood DA, Salcedo EE: Electrocardiographic manifestations of right ventricular infarction. Am Heart J 118:138, 1989.

484. Hurst JW: Comments about the electrocardiographic signs of right ventricular infarction. Clin Cardiol 21:289–291, 1998.

485. Gewirtz H, Gold HK, Fallon JT, et al: Role of right ventricular infarction in cardiogenic shock associated with inferior myocardial infarction. Br Heart J 42:719, 1979.

486. Reeder GS: Identification and treatment of complications of myocardial infarction. Lancet 70:880–884, 1995.

487. Reddy SG, Roberts WC: Frequency of rupture of the left ventricular free wall or ventricular septum among necropsy cases of fatal acute myocardial infarction since introduction of coronary care units. Am J Cardiol 63:906, 1989.

488. Pohjola-Sintonen S, Muller JE, Stone PH, et al: Ventricular septal and free wall rupture complicating acute myocardial infarction: Experience in the Multicenter Limitation of Infarct Size. Am Heart J 117:809, 1989.

489. Pappas PJ, Cernaianu AC, Baldino WA, et al: Ventricular free-wall rupture after myocardial infarction. Chest 99:892, 1991.

490. Figueras J, Cortadellas J, Calvo F, Soler-Soler J: Relevance of delayed hospital admission on development of cardiac rupture during acute myocardial infarction: Study in 225 patients with free wall, septal or papillary muscle rupture. J Am Coll Cardiol 32:135–139, 1998.

491. Bulkley BH, Roberts WC: Steroid therapy during acute myocardial infarction: A cause of delayed healing and of ventricular aneurysm. Am J Med 56:244, 1974.

492. Becker RC, Hochman JS, Cannon CP, et al: Fatal cardiac rupture among patients treated with thrombolytic agents and adjunctive thrombin antagonists: Observations from the Thrombolysis and Thrombin Inhibition in Myocardial Infarction 9 Study. J Am Coll Cardiol 33:479–487, 1999.

493. Crenshaw BS, Granger CB, Birnbaum Y, et al: Risk factors, angiographic patterns, and outcomes in patients with ventricular septal defect complicating acute myocardial infarction. Circulation 101:27–32, 2000.

494. Held AC, Cole PL, Lipton B, et al: Rupture of the interventricular septum complicating acute myocardial infarction: A multicenter analysis of clinical findings and outcome. Am Heart J 116:1330, 1988.

495. Figueras J, Cortadellas J, Soler-Soler J: Comparison of ventricular septal and left ventricular free wall rupture in acute myocardial infarction. Am J Cardiol 81:495–497, 1998.

496. Radford MJ, Johnson RA, Daggett WM, et al: Ventricular septal rupture: A review of clinical and physiologic features and an analysis of survival. Circulation 64:545, 1981.

497. Manning WJ, Waksmonski CA, Boyle NG: Papillary muscle rupture complicating inferior myocardial infarction: Identification with transesophageal echocardiography. Am Heart J 129:191–193, 1995.

498. Come PC, Riley MF, Weintraub R, et al: Echocardiographic detection of complete and partial papillary muscle rupture during acute myocardial infarction. Am J Cardiol 56:787, 1985.

499. Verma R, Freeman I: Images in clinical medicine: Rupture of papillary muscle during acute myocardial infarction. N Engl J Med 341:247, 1999.

ARRHYTHMIAS

500. Pantridge JF, Adgey AAJ: Pre-hospital coronary care: The mobile coronary care unit. Am J Cardiol 24:666, 1969.

501. Aufderheide TP: Arrhythmias associated with acute myocardial infarction and thrombolysis. Emerg Med Clin North Am 16:583–600, 1998.

502. Coronel R, Wilms-Schopman FJ, Janse MJ: Profibrillatory effects of intracoronary thrombus in acute regional ischemia of the in situ porcine heart. Circulation 96:3985–3991, 1997.

503. Greenspon AJ, Hsu SS, Borge R, et al: Insights into the mechanism of sustained ventricular tachycardia after myocardial infarction in a closed chest porcine model using a multielectrode "basket" catheter. J Cardiovasc Electrophysiol 10:1501–1516, 1999.

504. Karagueuzian HS, Mandel WJ: Electrophysiologic mechanisms of ischemic ventricular arrhythmias: Experimental and clinical correlations. In Mandel WJ (ed): Cardiac arrhythmias: Their mechanisms, diagnosis, and management. Philadelphia, JB Lippincott, 1995, pp 563–603.

505. Janse MJ: Ischemia as a trigger for arrhythmias. ACC Curr J Rev 8:15–17, 1999.

506. Carmeliet E: Cardiac ionic currents and acute ischemia: From channels to arrhythmias. Physiol Rev 79:917–1017, 1999.

507. Bloor CM, Ehsani A, White FC, Sobel BE: Ventricular fibrillation threshold in acute myocardial infarction and its relation to myocardial infarct size. Cardiovasc Res 9:468, 1975.

508. Roque F, Amuchastegui LM, Lopez Morillos MA, et al: Beneficial effects of timolol on infarct size and late ventricular tachycardia in patients with myocardial infarction. Circulation 76:610, 1987.

509. Ruskin J, McHale PA, Harley A, Greenfield JC Jr: Pressure-flow studies in man; Effects of atrial systole on left ventricular function. J Clin Invest 49:472, 1970.

510. Cannom DS, Prystowsky EN: Management of ventricular arrhythmias: Detection, drugs, and devices. JAMA 281:172–179, 1999.

511. Antman EM, Berlin JA: Declining incidence of ventricular fibrillation in myocardial infarction: Implications for prophylactic use of lidocaine. Circulation 86:764–773, 1992.

512. Hine LK, Laird N, Hewitt P, Chalmers TC: Meta-analytic evidence against prophylactic use of lidocaine in acute myocardial infarction. Arch Intern Med 149:2694–2698, 1989.

513. Sadowski ZP, Alexander JH, Skrabucha B, et al: Multicenter randomized trial and a systematic overview of lidocaine in acute myocardial infarction. Am Heart J 137:792–798, 1999.

514. Alexander JH, Granger CB, Sadowski Z, et al: Prophylactic lidocaine use in acute myocardial infarction: Incidence and outcomes from two international trials. The GUSTO-I and GUSTO-IIb Investigators. Am Heart J 137:799–805, 1999.

515. Tan HL, Lie KI: Prophylactic lidocaine use in acute myocardial infarction revisited in the thrombolytic era. Am Heart J 137:770–773, 1999.

516. Yusuf S, Sleight P, Rossi P, et al: Reduction in infarct size, arrhythmias and chest pain by early intravenous beta blockade in suspected acute myocardial infarction. Circulation 67:12, 1983.

517. Norris RM, Brown MA, Clark ED, et al: Prevention of ventricular fibrillation during acute myocardial infarction by intravenous propranolol. Lancet 2:833–836, 1984.

518. Gressin V, Gorgels A, Louvard Y, et al: ST-segment normalization time and ventricular arrhythmias as electrocardiographic markers of reperfusion during intravenous thrombolysis for acute myocardial infarction. Am J Cardiol 71:1436–1439, 1993.

519. Maggioni AP, Zuanetti G, Franzosi MG, et al: Prevalence and prognostic significance of ventricular arrhythmias after acute myocardial infarction in the fibrinolytic era: GISSI-2 results. Circulation 87:312–322, 1993.

520. Wolfe CL, Nibley C, Bhandari A, et al: Polymorphous ventricular tachycardia associated with acute myocardial infarction. Circulation 84:1543–1551, 1991.

520a. Gheeraert PJ, Henriques JP, De Buyzere ML, et al: Out-of-hospital ventricular fibrillation in patients with acute myocardial infarction: Coronary angiographic determinants. J Am Coll Cardiol 35:144–50, 2000.

521. Campbell RWF, Murray A, Julian DG: Ventricular arrhythmias in first 12 hours of acute myocardial infarction: Natural history study. Br Heart J 46:351–357, 1981.

522. Newby KH, Thompson T, Stebbins A, et al: Sustained ventricular arrhythmias in patients receiving thrombolytic therapy: Incidence and outcomes. The GUSTO Investigators. Circulation 98:2567–2573, 1998.

523. Nordehaug JE, Johannessen KA, von der Lippe G: Serum potassium concentration as a risk factor of ventricular arrhythmias early in acute myocardial infarction. Circulation 71:645, 1985.

524. Volpi A, Maggioni A, Franzosi MG, et al: In-hospital prognosis of patients with acute myocardial infarction complicated by primary ventricular fibrillation. N Engl J Med 317:257–261, 1987.

525. Volpi A, Cavalli A, Santoro L, Negri E: Incidence and prognosis of early primary ventricular fibrillation in acute myocardial infarction—results of the Gruppo Italiano per lo Studio della Sopravvivenza nell'Infarto Miocardico (GISSI-2) database. Am J Cardiol 82:265–271, 1998.

526. Behar S, Reicher Ress H, Schechter M, et al: Frequency and prognostic significance of secondary ventricular fibrillation complicating acute myocardial infarction. Am J Cardiol 71:152–156, 1993.

527. Lown B, Fakhro AM, Hood WB, Thorn GW: The coronary care unit: New perspectives and directions. JAMA 199:188–198, 1967.

528. Harrison DC: Should lidocaine be administered routinely to all patients after acute myocardial infarction? Circulation 58:581–584, 1978.

529. MacMahon S, Collins R, Peto R, et al: Effects of prophylactic lidocaine in suspected acute myocardial infarction: An overview of results from the randomized, controlled trials. JAMA 260:1910–1916, 1988.

530. ISIS-1 (First International Study of Infarct Survival) Collaborative Group: Randomized trial of intravenous atenolol among 16,027 cases of suspected acute myocardial infarction. Lancet 2:57–66, 1986.

531. Nordehaug JE, Lippe GVD: Hypokalemia and ventricular fibrillation in acute myocardial infarction. Br Heart J 50:525–529, 1983.

532. Higham PD, Adams PC, Murray A, Campbell RWF: Plasma potassium, serum magnesium and ventricular fibrillation: A prospective study. Q J Med 86:609–617, 1993.

533. Mark AL: The Bezold-Jarisch reflex revisited: Clinical implications of inhibitory reflexes originating in the heart. J Am Coll Cardiol 1:90, 1983.

534. Koren G, Weiss AT, Ben-David J, et al: Bradycardia and hypotension following reperfusion with streptokinase (Bezold-Jarish reflex): A sign of coronary thrombolysis and myocardial salvage. Am Heart J 112:468–471, 1986.

535. Come PC, Pitt B: Nitroglycerin-induced severe hypotension and bradycardia in patients with acute myocardial infarction. Circulation 54:624–628, 1976.

536. Zuanetti G, Mantini L, Hernandez-Bernal F, et al: Relevance of heart rate as a prognostic factor in patients with acute myocardial infarction: Insights from the GISSI-2 study. Eur Heart J 19(Suppl F):F19–F26, 1998.

537. Swart G, Brady WJ Jr, DeBehnke DJ, et al: Acute myocardial infarction complicated by hemodynamically unstable bradyarrhythmia: Prehospital and ED treatment with atropine. Am J Emerg Med 17:647–652, 1999.

538. Simons GR, Sgarbossa E, Wagner G, et al: Atrioventricular and intraventricular conduction disorders in acute myocardial infarction: A reappraisal in the thrombolytic era. Pacing Clin Electrophysiol 21:2651–2663, 1998.

539. Harpaz D, Behar S, Gottlieb S, et al: Complete atrioventricular block complicating acute myocardial infarction in the thrombolytic era. SPRINT Study Group and the Israeli Thrombolytic Survey Group. Secondary Prevention Reinfarction Israeli Nifedipine Trial. J Am Coll Cardiol 34:1721–1728, 1999.

540. Archbold RA, Sayer JW, Ray S, et al: Frequency and prognostic implications of conduction defects in acute myocardial infarction since the introduction of thrombolytic therapy. Eur Heart J 19:893–898, 1998.

541. Goldberg RJ, Zevallos JC, Yarzebski J, et al: Prognosis of acute myocardial infarction complicated by complete heart block (the Worcester Heart Attack Study). Am J Cardiol 69:1135–1141, 1992.

542. Bilbao FJ, Zabalza IE, Vilanova JR, Froupe J: Atrioventricular block in posterior acute myocardial infarction: A clinicopathologic correlation. Circulation 75:733, 1987.

543. Bertolet BD, McMurtrie EB, Hill JA, Bellardinelli L: Theophylline for the treatment of atrioventricular block after myocardial infarction. Ann Int Med 123:509–511, 1995.

544. Altun A, Kirdar C, Ozbay G: Effect of aminophylline in patients with atropine-resistant late advanced atrioventricular block during acute inferior myocardial infarction. Clin Cardiol 21:759–762, 1998.

545. Lilavie CJ, Gersh PJ: Mechanical and electrical complication of acute myocardial infarction. Mayo Clin Proc 65:709–730, 1990.

546. Hindman MC, Wagner GS, JaRo M, et al: The clinical significance of bundle branch block complicating acute myocardial infarction: 2. Indications for temporary and permanent pacemaker insertion. Circulation 58:689–699, 1978.

547. Klein RC, Vera Z, Mason DT: Intraventricular conduction defects in acute myocardial infarction: Incidence, prognosis and therapy. Am Heart J 108:1007–1013, 1984.

548. Sgarbossa EB, Pinski SL, Topol EJ, et al: Acute myocardial infarction and complete bundle branch block at hospital admission: Clinical characteristics and outcome in the thrombolytic era. GUSTO-I Investigators. Global Utilization of Streptokinase and t-PA [tissue-type plasminogen activator] for Occluded Coronary Arteries. J Am Coll Cardiol 31:105–110, 1998.

549. Herlitz J, Karlson BW, Bang A, Sjolin M: Mortality and risk indicators for death during five years after acute myocardial infarction among patients with and without ST elevation on admission electrocardiogram. Cardiology 89:33–39, 1998.

550. Go AS, Barron HV, Rundle AC, et al: Bundle-branch block and in-hospital mortality in acute myocardial infarction. National Registry of Myocardial Infarction 2 Investigators. Ann Intern Med 129:690–697, 1998.

551. Hindman MC, Wagner GS, JaRo M, et al: The clinical significance of bundle branch block complicating acute myocardial infarction: I. Clinical characteristics, hospital mortality, and one-year follow-up. Circulation 58:679–688, 1978.

552. Lamas GA, Mueller JE, Turi AG, et al: A simplified method to predict occurrence of complete heart block during acute myocardial infarction. Am J Cardiol 57:1213, 1986.

553. Scheinman MM, Gonzalez RP: Fascicular block and acute myocardial infarction. JAMA 244:2646–2649, 1980.

554. Zoll PM, Zoll RH, Falk RH, et al: External non-invasive temporary cardiac pacing: Clinical trials. Circulation 71:937, 1985.

555. DeSanctis RW, Block P, Hutter AM: Tachyarrhythmias in myocardial infarction. Circulation 45:681, 1972.

556. Eldar M, Canetti M, Rotstein Z, et al: Significance of paroxysmal atrial fibrillation complicating acute myocardial infarction in the thrombolytic era. SPRINT and Thrombolytic Survey Groups. Circulation 97:965–970, 1998.

557. Pedersen OD, Bagger H, Kober L, Torp-Pedersen C: The occurrence and prognostic significance of atrial fibrillation/flutter following acute myocardial infarction. TRACE Study group. TRAndolapril Cardiac Evaluation. Eur Heart J 20:748–754, 1999.

558. Waldecker B: Atrial fibrillation in myocardial infarction complicated by heart failure: Cause or consequence? Eur Heart J 20:710–712, 1999.

559. Mahaffey KW, Granger CB, Sloan MA, et al: Risk factors for in-hospital nonhemorrhagic stroke in patients with acute myocardial infarction treated with thrombolysis: Results from GUSTO-I. Circulation 97:757–764, 1998.

560. Singh BN: Current antiarrhythmic drugs: An overview of mechanisms of action and potential clinical utility. J Cardiovasc Electrophysiol 10:283–301, 1999.

561. Betriu A, Califf RM, Bosch X, et al: Recurrent ischemia after thrombolysis: Importance of associated clinical findings. GUSTO-I Investigators. Global Utilization of Streptokinase and t-PA [tissue-plasminogen activator] for Occluded Coronary Arteries. J Am Coll Cardiol 31:94–102, 1998.

562. Mueller HS, Forman SA, Manegus MA, et al: Prognostic significance of nonfatal reinfarction during 3-year follow-up: Results of the Thrombolysis in Myocardial Infarction (TIMI) Phase II Clinical Trial. J Am Coll Cardiol 26:900–907, 1995.

562a. Detre KM, Lombardero MS, Brooks MM, et al: The effect of previous coronary-artery bypass surgery on the prognosis of patients with diabetes who have acute myocardial infarction. Bypass Angioplasty Revascularization Investigation Investigators. N Engl J Med 342:989–97, 2000.

563. Roux S, Christeller S, Ludin E: Effects of aspirin on coronary reocclusion and recurrent ischemia after thrombolysis: A meta-analysis. J Am Coll Cardiol 19:671–677, 1992.

564. Simoons ML, Arnout J, van den Brand M, et al: Re-treatment with alteplase for early signs of reocclusion after thrombolysis. The European Cooperative Study Group. Am J Cardiol 71:524–528, 1993.

565. Correale E, Maggioni AP, Romano S, et al: Pericardial involvement in acute myocardial infarction in the post-thrombolytic era: Clinical meaning and value. Clin Cardiol 20:327–331, 1997.

566. Kloner R, Fishbein M, Lew H, et al: Mummification of the infarcted myocardium by high dose corticosteroids. Circulation 57:56, 1978.

567. Dressler W: The post-myocardial infarction syndrome: A report of forty-four cases. Arch Intern Med 103:28, 1959.

568. Reinecke H, Wichter T, Weyand M: Left ventricular pseudoaneurysm in a patient with Dressler's syndrome after myocardial infarction. Heart 80:98–100, 1998.

569. Hellerstein HK, Martin JW: Incidence of thromboembolic lesions accompanying myocardial infarction. Am Heart J 33:443, 1947.

570. Meizlish JL, Berger HJ, Plankey M, et al: Functional left ventricular aneurysm formation after acute anterior transmural myocardial infarction: Incidence, natural history, and prognostic implications. N Engl J Med 311:1001, 1984.

571. Ha JW, Cho SY, Lee JD, Kang MS: Left ventricular aneurysm after myocardial infarction. Clin Cardiol 21:917, 1998.

572. Davis MJE, Ireland MA: Effect of early anticoagulation on the frequency of left ventricular thrombi after anterior wall acute myocardial infarction. Am J Cardiol 57:1244–1247, 1986.

573. Turpie AGG, Robinson JG, Doyle DJ, et al: Comparison of high-dose with low-dose subcutaneous heparin to prevent left ventricular mural thrombosis in patients with acute transmural anterior myocardial infarction. N Engl J Med 320:352–357, 1989.

574. Halperin JL, Fuster V: Left ventricular thrombus and stroke after myocardial infarction: Toward prevention or perplexity? J Am Coll Cardiol 14:912, 1989.

575. Stein B, Fuster V, Halperin JL, Chesebro JH: Antithrombotic therapy in cardiac disease: An emerging approach based on pathogenesis and risk. Circulation 80:1501–1513, 1989.

576. Newby LK, Califf RM, Guerci A, et al: Early discharge in the thrombolytic era: An analysis of criteria for uncomplicated infarction from the Global Utilization of Streptokinase and t-PA for Occluded Coronary Arteries (GUSTO) trial. J Am Coll Cardiol 27:625–632, 1996.

CONVALESCENCE AND POST–MYOCARDIAL INFARCTION CARE

577. O'Connor GT, Buring JE, Yusuf S, et al: An overview of randomized trials of rehabilitation with exercise after myocardial infarction. Circulation 80:234, 1989.

578. Barefoot JC, Schroll M: Symptoms of depression, acute myocardial infarction, and total mortality in a community sample. Circulation 93:1976–1980, 1996.

579. Petrie KJ, Weinman J, Sharpe N, Buckley J: Role of patients' view of their illness in predicting return to work and functioning after myocardial infarction: Longitudinal study. BMJ 312:1191–1194, 1996.

580. Frasure-Smith N, Lesperance F, Prince RH, et al: Randomised trial of home-based psychosocial nursing intervention for patients recovering from myocardial infarction. Lancet 350:473–479, 1997.

581. Linden W, Stossel C, Maurice J: Psychosocial interventions for patients with coronary artery disease: A meta-analysis. Arch Intern Med 156:745–752, 1996.

581a. Thompson DR, Lewin RJ: Management of the post-myocardial infarction patient: Rehabilitation and cardiac neurosis. Heart 84:101–105, 2000.

582. American College of Physicians: Guidelines for risk stratification after myocardial infarction. Ann Intern Med 126:556–560, 1997.

583. Mukharji J, Murray S, Lewis SE, et al: Is anterior ST depression with acute transmural inferior infarction due to posterior infarction? J Am Coll Cardiol 4:28, 1984.

584. Fresco C, Carinci F, Maggioni AP, et al: Very early assessment of risk for in-hospital death among 11,483 patients with acute myocardial infarction. Am Heart J 138:1058–1064, 1999.

585. Madsen JK, Grande P, Saunamaki K, et al: Danish multicenter randomized study of invasive versus conservative treatment in patients with inducible ischemia after thrombolysis in acute myocardial infarction (DANAMI). DANish trial in Acute Myocardial Infarction. Circulation 96:748–755, 1997.

586. Volpi A, De VC, Franzosi MG, et al: Determinants of 6-month mortality in survivors of myocardial infarction after thrombolysis: Results of the GISSI-2 data base. The Ad hoc Working Group of the Gruppo Italiano per lo Studio della Sopravvivenza nell'Infarto Miocardico (GISSI)-2 Data Base. Circulation 88:416–429, 1993.

587. Aguirre FV, Kern MJ, Hsia J, et al: Importance of myocardial infarct artery patency on the prevalence of ventricular arrhythmia and late potentials after thrombolysis in acute myocardial infarction. Am J Cardiol 68:1410–1416, 1991.

588. Fletcher GF, Balady G, Froelicher VF, et al: Exercise standards: A statement for healthcare professionals from the American Heart Association. Circulation 91:580–615, 1995.

589. Bates DW, Miller E, Bernstein SJ, et al: Coronary angiography and angioplasty after acute myocardial infarction. Ann Intern Med 126:539–550, 1997.

590. Jain A, Myers GH, Sapin PM, O'Rourke RA: Comparison of symptom-limited and low level exercise tolerance tests early after myocardial infarction. J Am Coll Cardiol 22:1816–1820, 1993.

591. Committee on Radionuclide Imaging: ACC/AHA Task Force Report: Guidelines for clinical use of cardiac radionuclide imaging. J Am Coll Cardiol 25:521–547, 1995.

592. Kuntz KM, Tsevat J, Weinstein MC, Goldman I: Expert panel vs decision-analysis recommendations for postdischarge coronary angiography after myocardial infarction. JAMA 282:2246–2251, 1999.

593. Moss AJ, Davis HT, DeCamilla J, Bayer LW: Ventricular ectopic beats and their relation to sudden and nonsudden cardiac death after myocardial infarction. Circulation 60:998–1003, 1979.

594. Morganroth J, Bigger JT Jr. Pharmacologic management of ventricular arrhythmias after the Cardiac Arrhythmia Suppression Trial. Am J Cardiol 65:1497–1503, 1990.

595. La Rovere MT, Bigger JT Jr, Marcus FI, et al: Baroreflex sensitivity and heart-rate variability in prediction of total cardiac mortality after myocardial infarction. ATRAMI (Autonomic Tone and Reflexes After Myocardial Infarction) Investigators. Lancet 351:478–484, 1998.

596. Julian D: The practical implications of clinical trials: Putting it all together. In Julian D, Braunwald E (eds): Management of Acute Myocardial Infarction. London, WB Saunders, 1994, pp 407–415.

597. Krumholz HM, Cohen BJ, Tsevat J, et al: Cost-effectiveness of a smoking cessation program after myocardial infarction. J Am Coll Cardiol 22:1697–1702, 1993.

598. Frasure-Smith N, Lesperance F, Talajic M: Depression following myocardial infarction: Impact on 6-month survival. JAMA 270:1819–1825, 1993.

599. Bucher HC: Social support and prognosis following first myocardial infarction. J Gen Intern Med 9:409–417, 1994.

600. Gallagher EJ, Viscoli CM, Horwitz RI: The relationship of treatment adherence to the risk of death after myocardial infarction in women. JAMA 270:742–744, 1993.

601. Knopp RH: Drug treatment of lipid disorders. N Engl J Med 341:498–511, 1999.

602. LaRosa JC, He J, Vupputuri S: Effect of statins on risk of coronary disease: A meta-analysis of randomized controlled trials. JAMA 282:2340–2346, 1999.

603. Ansell BJ, Watson KE, Fogelman AM: An evidence-based assessment of the NCEP Adult Treatment Panel II guidelines. National Cholesterol Education Program. JAMA 282:2051–2057, 1999.

604. Ridker PM, Rifai N, Pfeffer MA, et al: Long-term effects of pravastatin on plasma concentration of C-reactive protein. The Cholesterol and Recurrent Events (CARE) Investigators. Circulation 100:230–235, 1999.

605. Lee TH, Cleeman JI, Grundy SM, et al: Clinical goals and performance measures for cholesterol management in secondary prevention of coronary heart disease. JAMA 283:94–98, 2000.

606. Rubins HB, Robins SJ, Collins D, et al: Gemfibrozil for the secondary prevention of coronary heart disease in men with low levels of high-density lipoprotein cholesterol. Veterans Affairs High-Density Lipoprotein Cholesterol Intervention Trial Study Group. N Engl J Med 341:410–418, 1999.

607. Gutstein DE, Fuster V: Pathophysiologic bases for adjunctive therapies in the treatment and secondary prevention of acute myocardial infarction. Clin Cardiol 21:161–168, 1998.

608. Col NF, Yarzebski J, Gore JM, et al: Does aspirin consumption affect the presentation or severity of acute myocardial infarction? Arch Intern Med 155:1386–1389, 1995.

609. Alhaddad IA, Tkaczevski L, Siddiqui F, et al: Aspirin enhances the benefits of late reperfusion on infarct shape: A possible mechanism of the beneficial effects of aspirin on survival after acute myocardial infarction. Circulation 91:2819–2823, 1995.

610. Hennekens CH, Dyken ML, Fuster V: Aspirin as a therapeutic agent in cardiovascular disease: A statement for healthcare professionals from the American Heart Association. Circulation 96:2751–2753, 1997.

611. CAPRIE Steering Committee: A randomised, blinded, trial of clopidogrel versus aspirin in patients at risk of ischaemic events (CAPRIE). Lancet 348:1329–1339, 1996.

612. Hall AS, Murray GD, Ball SG: Follow-up study of patients randomly allocated ramipril or placebo for heart failure after acute myocardial infarction: AIRE Extension (AIREX) Study. Acute Infarction Ramipril Efficacy. Lancet 349:1493–1497, 1997.

613. Torp-Pedersen C, Kober L: Effect of ACE inhibitor trandolapril on life expectancy of patients with reduced left-ventricular function after acute myocardial infarction. TRACE Study Group. Trandolapril Cardiac Evaluation. Lancet 354:9–12, 1999.

614. Gustafsson I, Torp-Pedersen C, Kober L, et al: Effect of the angiotensin-converting enzyme inhibitor trandolapril on mortality and morbidity in diabetic patients with left ventricular dysfunction after acute myocardial infarction. Trace Study Group. J Am Coll Cardiol 34:83–89, 1999.

615. Packer M, Poole-Wilson PA, Armstrong PW, et al: Comparative effects of low and high doses of the angiotensin-converting enzyme inhibitor, lisinopril, on morbidity and mortality in chronic heart failure. Circulation 100:rt1–rt7, 1999.

616. Domanski MJ, Exner DV, Borkowf CB, et al: Effect of angiotensin con-

verting enzyme inhibition on sudden cardiac death in patients following acute myocardial infarction. A meta-analysis of randomized clinical trials. J Am Coll Cardiol 33:598–604, 1999.

617. The EUCLID Study Group: Randomised placebo-controlled trial of lisinopril in normotensive patients with insulin-dependent diabetes and normoalbuminuria or microalbuminuria. Lancet 349:1787–1792, 1997.

618. The Heart Outcomes Prevention Evaluation and Study Investigators: Effects of an angiotensin-converting-enzyme inhibitor, ramipril, on cardiovascular events in high-risk patients. N Engl J Med 342:145–153, 2000.

619. Beta-Blocker Pooling Project Research Group: The Beta-Blocker Pooling Project (BBPP): Subgroup findings from randomized trials in post-infarction patients. Eur Heart J 9:8, 1988.

620. Barron HV, Viskin S, Lundstrom RJ, et al: Effect of beta-adrenergic blocking agents on mortality rate in patients not revascularized after myocardial infarction: Data from a large HMO. Am Heart J 134:608–613, 1997.

621. Barron HV, Viskin S, Lundstrom RJ, et al: Beta-blocker dosages and mortality after myocardial infarction: Data from a large health maintenance organization. Arch Intern Med 158:449–453, 1998.

622. Krumholz HM, Radford MJ, Wang Y, et al: National use and effectiveness of beta-blockers for the treatment of elderly patients after acute myocardial infarction: National Cooperative Cardiovascular Project. JAMA 280:623–629, 1998.

623. Crockett SE, Davis D, Golden WE, et al: Quality Care Alert: Beta Blocker Prophylaxis after Myocardial Infarction. Chicago, American Medical Association, 1998.

624. Marciniak TA, Ellerbeck EF, Radford MJ, et al: Improving the quality of care for Medicare patients with acute myocardial infarction: Results from the Cooperative Cardiovascular Project. JAMA 279:1351–1357, 1998.

625. Goldman L, Sia STB, Cook EF, et al: Costs and effectiveness of routine therapy with long-term beta-adrenergic antagonists after acute myocardial infarction. N Engl J Med 319:152, 1988.

626. Yusuf S, Wittes J, Friedman L: Overview of results of randomized clinical trials in heart disease: I. Treatments following myocardial infarction. JAMA 260:2088–2093, 1988.

627. Brand DA, Newcomer LN, Freiburger A, et al: Cardiologists' practices compared with practice guidelines: Use of beta-blockade after myocardial infarction. J Am Coll Cardiol 26:1432, 1995.

628. Freemantle N, Cleland J, Young P, et al: β Blockade after myocardial infarction: Systematic review and meta regression analysis. BMJ 318:730–737, 1999.

629. Anticoagulants in the Secondary Prevention of Events in Coronary Thrombosis (ASPECT) Research Group: Effect of long-term oral anticoagulant treatment on mortality and cardiovascular morbidity after myocardial infarction. Lancet 343:499–503, 1994.

630. van Bergen PFMM, Jonker JJC, van Hout BA, et al: Costs and effects of long-term oral anticoagulant treatment after myocardial infarction. JAMA 273:925–928, 1995.

631. Coumadin Aspirin Reinfarction Study (CARS) Investigators: Randomised double-blind trial of fixed low-dose warfarin with aspirin after myocardial infarction. Lancet 350:389–396, 1997.

632. CHAMP Trial Presented at 72nd Scientific Sessions of AHA, Atlanta, GA, 1999.

633. Teo KK, Yusuf S, Furberg CD: Effects of prophylactic antiarrhythmic drug therapy in acute myocardial infarction. JAMA 270:1589–1595, 1993.

634. Epstein AE, Hallstrom AP, Rogers WJ, et al: Mortality following ventricular arrhythmia suppression by encainide, flecainide, and moricizine after myocardial infarction: The original design concept of the Cardiac Arrhythmia Suppression Trial (CAST). JAMA 270:2451–2455, 1993.

635. Echt DS, Liebson PR, Mitchell LB, et al: Mortality and morbidity in patients receiving encainide, flecainide, or placebo. The Cardiac Arrhythmia Suppression Trial. N Engl J Med 324:781–788, 1991.

636. The Cardiac Arrhythmia Suppression Trial II Investigators: Effect of the antiarrhythmic agent moricizine on survival after myocardial infarction. N Engl J Med 327:227–233, 1992.

637. Akiyama T, Pawitan Y, Greenberg H, et al: Increased risk of death and cardiac arrest from encainide and flecainide in patients after non-Q-wave acute myocardial infarction in the Cardiac Arrhythmia Suppression Trial. CAST Investigators. Am J Cardiol 68:1551–1555, 1991.

638. Krishnan SC, Shivkumar K, Garan H, Ruskin JN: Increased vulnerability of the subendocardium to ischaemic injury: An electrophysiological explanation. Lancet 346:1612–1614, 1995.

639. Waldo AL, Camm AJ, deRuyter H, et al: Effect of d-sotalol on mortality in patients with left ventricular dysfunction after recent and remote myocardial infarction. The SWORD Investigators. Survival With Oral d-Sotalol. Lancet 348:7–12, 1996.

640. Cairns JA, Connolly SJ, Roberts R, Gent M: Randomised trial of outcome after myocardial infarction in patients with frequent or repetitive ventricular premature depolarisations: CAMIAT. Canadian Amiodarone Myocardial Infarction Arrhythmia Trial Investigators. Lancet 349:675–682, 1997.

641. Julian DG, Camm AJ, Frangin G, et al: Randomised trial of effect of amiodarone on mortality in patients with left-ventricular dysfunction after recent myocardial infarction: EMIAT. European Myocardial Infarct Amiodarone Trial Investigators. Lancet 349:667–674, 1997.

641a. Elizari MV, Martinez JM, Belziti C, et al: Morbidity and mortality following early administration of amiodarone in acute myocardial infarction. GEMICA study investigators. GEMICA Group, Buenos Aires, Argentina. Grupo de Estudios Multicentricos en Argentina. Eur Heart J 21:198–205, 2000.

642. The Antiarrhythmics versus Implantable Defibrillators (AVID) Investigators: A comparison of antiarrhythmic-drug therapy with implantable defibrillators in patients resuscitated from near-fatal ventricular arrhythmias. N Engl J Med 337:1576–1583, 1997.

643. Buxton AE, Lee KL, Fisher JD, et al: A randomized study of the prevention of sudden death in patients with coronary artery disease. Multicenter Unsustained Tachycardia Trial Investigators. N Engl J Med 341:1882–1890, 1999.

644. Moss AJ, Hall WJ, Cannom DS, et al: Improved survival with an implanted defibrillator in patients with coronary disease at high risk for ventricular arrhythmia. Multicenter Automatic Defibrillator Implantation Trial Investigators. N Engl J Med 335:1933–1940, 1996.

645. Mendelsohn ME, Karas RH: The protective effects of estrogen on the cardiovascular system. N Engl J Med 340:1801–1811, 1999.

646. Sourander L, Rajala T, Raiha I, et al: Cardiovascular and cancer morbidity and mortality and sudden cardiac death in postmenopausal women on oestrogen replacement therapy (ERT). Lancet 352:1965–1969, 1998.

647. Hulley S, Grady D, Bush T, et al: Randomized trial of estrogen plus progestin for secondary prevention of coronary heart disease in postmenopausal women. Heart and Estrogen/progestin Replacement Study (HERS) Research Group. JAMA 280:605–613, 1998.

GUIDELINES

DIAGNOSIS AND MANAGEMENT OF ACUTE MYOCARDIAL INFARCTION

Thomas H. Lee

Key guidelines for the diagnosis and management of acute myocardial infarction (AMI) have been published by the American College of Emergency Physicians (ACEP)[1] and by an ACC/AHA Committee.[2] Additional influential guidelines on management of patients with acute ischemic heart disease syndromes have been published by the National Heart Attack Alert Program (NHAAP),[3] the Agency for Health Care Policy and Research (AHCPR),[4] and an ACC/AHA task force on unstable angina.[5]

Evaluation of Patients with Acute Chest Pain
(Table 35–G–1)

In all of these guidelines, the recommended actions in response to the data that are collected during this evaluation are intended to lead to timely care for patients with AMI, unstable angina, aortic dissection, and pulmonary embolus. The ACC/AHA guidelines on unstable angina and non–ST segment elevation MI emphasize that patients with possible acute coronary syndromes should be evaluated at a facility at which a 12-lead electrocardiogram (ECG) can be performed (as op-

posed to over the telephone).[5] According to these guidelines, patients with suspected acute coronary syndromes of symptom duration of more than 20 minutes, hemodynamic instability, or recent syncope or presyncope are most appropriately seen in an emergency department or specialized chest pain unit. Emergency transport services should be used when available for such patients; private vehicles are acceptable alternatives only if waiting for an emergency vehicle would impose a long delay.

The ACEP statement on the initial evaluation of patients with acute chest pain[1] include "rules" and "guidelines" about the data that should be recorded and the actions that should follow from certain findings. In these guidelines, "rules" are actions that are general principles of good practice; deviation from a "rule" should generally be justified in the record. "Guidelines" are actions that should be considered, but failure to follow a "guideline" does not necessarily imply that care was improper. The ACEP policy statement includes in its appendix forms that can be used to assess compliance with their "rules" and to remind clinicians of their content.

The ACEP statement indicates that the routine evaluation of non-traumatic chest pain should include a history that obtains data on the

TABLE 35–G–1. EVALUATION OF ACUTE CHEST PAIN: EXCERPTS FROM THE CLINICAL POLICY OF THE AMERICAN COLLEGE OF EMERGENCY PHYSICIANS (ACEP) (1995)

Variable	Finding	Rule*	Guideline†
Pain	Ongoing and severe and crushing and substernal or same as previous pain diagnosed as MI	Intravenous access Supplemental oxygen Cardiac monitor ECG Aspirin Nitrates Management of ongoing pain Admit	Serum cardiac markers CXR Anticoagulation
	Severe or pressure or substernal or exertional or radiating to jaw, neck, shoulder, or arm	ECG	Intravenous access Supplemental oxygen Cardiac monitor Serum cardiac markers CXR Nitrates Management of ongoing pain Admit
	Tearing, severe, and radiating to back	Large-bore intravenous access Supplemental oxygen Cardiac monitor CXR, ECG	Differential upper extremity blood pressures Aortic imaging Management of ongoing pain Admit
	Similar to that of previous pulmonary embolus	Intravenous access Supplemental O_2 Cardiac monitor ABG/oximetry Anticoagulation/pulmonary vascular imaging ECG	CXR Admit
	Indigestion or burning epigastric	None	ECG
	Pleuritic	None	CXR ECG
Associated symptoms	Syncope or near-syncope	ECG	Cardiac monitor Hematocrit
	Shortness of breath, dyspnea on exertion, paroxysmal nocturnal dyspnea, or orthopnea	ECG	ABG/oximetry CXR
Past medical history	Previous MI, coronary artery bypass graft, angioplasty, cocaine use within past 96 hours, previous positive cardiac diagnostic studies	ECG	
	Major risk factors for coronary artery disease		ECG

*Rule: An action reflecting principles of good practice in most situations. There may be circumstances when a rule need not or cannot be followed; in these situations, it is advisable that deviation from the rule be justified in writing. Inability to comply with rules should be incorporated in institutional policies.

†Guideline: An action that may be considered, depending on the patient, the circumstances, or other factors. Thus, guidelines are not always followed, and there is no implication that failure to follow a guideline is improper.

CXR = chest radiograph; ECG = electrocardiogram; ABG = arterial blood gas analysis.

From American College of Emergency Physicians: Clinical policy for the initial approach to adults presenting with a chief complaint of chest pain, with no history of trauma. Ann Emerg Med 25:274–299, 1995.

character of pain, age, associated symptoms, and past history. The physical examination should include vital signs, a cardiovascular examination, and a pulmonary examination. The performance of an ECG is a "rule" in all but atypical chest pain syndromes. The ACEP statement emphasizes that the decision to admit the patient must be based primarily on clinical judgment.

The NHAAP report also includes guidelines for specific functions related to evaluation and treatment of patients with chest pain aimed at improving the speed with which patients with AMI are identified and treated,[3] including recommendations for which patient subsets should be placed on the AMI protocol. For registration staff, the NHAAP guidelines recommend that patients older than age 30 with the following chief complaints receive immediate assessment by the triage nurse and be referred for further evaluation:

• Chest pain, pressure, tightness, or heaviness; radiating pain in neck, jaw, shoulders, back, or one or both arms
• Indigestion or "heartburn"/nausea and/or vomiting
• Persistent shortness of breath
• Weakness/dizziness/lightheadedness/loss of consciousness

The triage nurse should immediately assess patients for initiation of the AMI protocol and obtain an ECG if they have any of the following:

• Chest pain
• Associated dyspnea
• Associated nausea/vomiting
• Associated diaphoresis

For physicians, the NHAAP guidelines offer several clinical recommendations and explicitly note that the use of a so-called GI cocktail (usually including an antacid) as a diagnostic test to differentiate between gastrointestinal and cardiac causes of the patient's symptoms is inappropriate because it frequently leads to erroneous conclusions.

ECG and aspirin are strongly recommended for patients with new-onset angina that is exertional, but admission is not considered mandatory in the ACEP policy statement. The AHCPR guidelines also indicate that not all patients with unstable angina require admission but recommend that patients with unstable angina be monitored electrocardiographically during their initial evaluation and that those with ongoing rest pain should be placed at bed rest during the initial phase of stabilization.[4]

EARLY RISK STRATIFICATION. The ACC/AHA guidelines for management of unstable angina emphasize the importance of a search for noncoronary causes that might explain the patient's symptoms but recommend that biochemical cardiac markers be performed for all patients with suspected acute coronary syndromes.[5] This recommendation does not mandate the performance of markers in patients with a very low probability of acute coronary syndromes, for whom discharge without such testing is appropriate.[6] The ACC/AHA task force supports the use of cardiac troponins as a preferred marker for acute ischemic injury (Table 36–G–2).

Specific recommendations for the care of patients with unstable angina are included in the guidelines in Chapter 36.

Urgent Care of AMI (Table 35–G–2)

The 1999 ACC/AHA update of guidelines on AMI[2] seek to ensure timely revascularization of patients who present early in the course of

their infarction by setting a goal for timely evaluations of patients with acute chest pain, including performance of an ECG within 10 minutes and administration of thrombolytic therapy for appropriate patients within 30 minutes. To achieve this goal, the NHAAP guidelines[3] recommend measuring the time at which four specific events occur for patients with AMI:

1. Presentation to the emergency department
2. Performance of the ECG
3. Decision of whether to administer thrombolytic therapy
4. Actual infusion of the thrombolytic agent

Specific time goals can be set for the interval between these events (e.g., 10 minutes). Another critical issue is who gives the order to administer thrombolytic therapy. ACEP guidelines recommend that emergency department physicians be given the authority to administer thrombolytic therapy.[1]

In the ACC/AHA guidelines,[2] thrombolytic therapy is considered appropriate (Class I) for up to 12 hours after the onset of symptoms for patients younger than age 75 years and presenting with ST segment elevation or bundle branch block. The ACC/AHA task force considered the weight of evidence in favor of extending the same approach to patients older than 75. Primary intervention with percutaneous transluminal coronary angioplasty (PTCA) was considered an appropriate (Class I) alternative to thrombolytic therapy within the first 12 hours of infarction and beyond for patients with persisting ischemic symptoms. The ACC/AHA guidelines also define goals for speed and volume for operators and institutions performing primary PTCA. Primary PTCA is also endorsed as a strategy for patients with cardiogenic shock due to MI.

The ACC/AHA guidelines do *not* support routine use of angiogra-

TABLE 35–G–2. ACC/AHA GUIDELINES FOR INITIAL MANAGEMENT OF ACUTE MYOCARDIAL INFARCTION (AMI) AND ISCHEMIC COMPLICATIONS

Indication	Class I	Class IIa	Class IIb	Class III
Telephone triage[5]	Patients with symptoms suggesting possible ACS should be evaluated by a medical practitioner in a facility equipped to record a 12-lead ECG and not over the telephone.			
Emergency department or outpatient facility presentation[5]	Patients with suspected ACS with symptom duration > 20 minutes, hemodynamic instability, or recent syncope or presyncope should be referred to an emergency department or specialized chest pain unit. Other patients with suspected ACS may be seen initially either in an emergency department, chest pain unit, or an outpatient facility.			
Early risk stratification[5]	Patients presenting with chest pain should undergo early risk stratification focusing on anginal symptoms, the presence or absence of traditional risk factors for coronary artery disease, physical findings, and ECG. A 12-lead ECG should be obtained immediately in patients with ongoing chest pain and within 10 minutes of presentation in patients with a history of chest pain consistent with ACS but has resolved by the time of evaluation.	An acceptable but less preferable marker is CK-MB. Mass assays for CK-MB are preferred over activity assays for CK-MB.		Total CK activity, AST, and/or LDH as the serum markers for detecting MI in patients with chest pain suggestive of ACS.

Table continued on following page

1222 **TABLE 35–G–2.** ACC/AHA GUIDELINES FOR INITIAL MANAGEMENT OF ACUTE MYOCARDIAL INFARCTION (AMI) AND ISCHEMIC COMPLICATIONS *Continued*

Ch 35

Indication	Class I	Class IIa	Class IIb	Class III
	Serum cardiac markers should be measured in all patients presenting with chest pain consistent with ACS. A cardiac-specific troponin is the preferred marker and if available should be measured in all patients. For patients presenting within 6 hours of the onset of symptoms, an early marker, myoglobin, should be measured in addition to a cardiac troponin. In patients with negative serum markers within 6 hours of the onset of pain, another determination should be made at 9 hours.			
Oxygen	Overt pulmonary congestion Arterial oxygen desaturation (SaO$_2$ < 90%)	Routine administration to all patients with uncomplicated MI during the first 2 to 3 hours	Routine administration of supplemental O$_2$ to patients with uncomplicated MI beyond 3 to 6 hours	
Intravenous nitroglycerin	For the first 24 to 48 hours in patients with AMI and CHF, large anterior infarction, persistent ischemia, or hypertension Continued use (beyond 48 hours) in patients with recurrent angina or persistent pulmonary congestion		For the first 24 to 48 hours in all patients with AMI who do not have hypotension, bradycardia, or tachycardia. Continued use (beyond 48 hours) in patients with a large or complicated infarction. (Oral or topical preparations may be substituted.)	Patients with systolic blood pressure < 90 mm Hg or severe bradycardia (< 50/min)
Aspirin	160 to 325 mg on day 1 of AMI and continued indefinitely on a daily basis.		Other antiplatelet agents, such as dipyridamole, ticlopidine, or clopidogrel, may be substituted if true aspirin allergy is present or if the patient is unresponsive to aspirin.	
Atropine	Sinus bradycardia with evidence of low cardiac output and peripheral hypoperfusion or frequent PVCs at onset of symptoms of AMI Acute inferior infarction with type I second- or third-degree AV block associated with symptoms of hypotension, ischemic discomfort, or ventricular arrhythmias Sustained bradycardia and hypotension after administration of nitroglycerin For nausea and vomiting associated with administration of morphine Ventricular asystole	Symptomatic patients with inferior infarction and type I second- or third-degree heart block at the level of the AV node	Administration concomitant with administration of morphine in the presence of sinus bradycardia Asymptomatic patients with inferior infarction and type I second-degree heart block or third-degree heart block at the level of the AV node. Second- or third-degree AV block of uncertain mechanism when pacing is not available.	Sinus bradycardia > 40 beats/min without signs or symptoms of hypoperfusion or frequent PVCs. Type II AV block and third-degree AV block and third-degree AV block with new wide QRS complex presumed due to AMI.

TABLE 35–G–2. ACC/AHA GUIDELINES FOR INITIAL MANAGEMENT OF ACUTE MYOCARDIAL INFARCTION (AMI) AND ISCHEMIC COMPLICATIONS *Continued*

1223

Ch 35

Indication	Class I	Class IIa	Class IIb	Class III
Thrombolysis	ST segment elevation (> 0.1 mV, two or more contiguous leads), time to therapy ≤ 12 hr, age < 75 yr BBB (obscuring ST segment analysis) and history suggesting AMI	ST segment elevation, age ≥ 75 yr	ST segment elevation, time to therapy > 12 to 24 hr Blood pressure on presentation > 180 mm Hg systolic and/or > 110 mm Hg diastolic associated with high-risk MI.	ST segment elevation, time to therapy greater than 24 hours, ischemic pain resolved ST segment depression only
Primary percutaneous transluminal coronary angioplasty	As an alternative to thrombolytic therapy in patients with AMI and ST segment elevation or new or presumed new left BBB (LBBB) who can undergo angioplasty of the infarct-related artery within 12 hours of onset of symptoms or beyond 12 hours if ischemic symptoms persist, and performed in a timely fashion* by persons skilled in the procedure† and supported by experienced personnel in an appropriate laboratory environment.‡ In patients who are within 36 hours of an acute ST segment elevation/Q wave or new LBBB MI who develop cardiogenic shock, are < 75 years old, and in whom revascularization can be performed within 18 hours of onset of shock.	As a reperfusion strategy in candidates for reperfusion who have a contraindication to thrombolytic therapy	In patients with AMI who do not present with ST segment elevation but who have reduced (< TIMI grade 2) flow in the infarct-related artery and when PTCA can be performed within 12 hours of onset of symptoms.	Patients with AMI who: 1. Undergo elective PTCA of a non–infarct-related artery at the time of AMI 2. Are beyond 12 hours after onset of symptoms and have no evidence of myocardial ischemia 3. Have received thrombolytic therapy and have no symptoms of myocardial ischemia 4. Are eligible for thrombolysis and are undergoing primary angioplasty performed by a low-volume operator in a laboratory without surgical backup
Early coronary angiography in the ST segment elevation or BBB cohort not undergoing primary PTCA		Patients with cardiogenic shock or persistent hemodynamic instability	Patients with evolving large or anterior infarcts treated with thrombolytic agents in whom it is believed that the artery is not patent and adjuvant PTCA is planned	Routine use of angiography and subsequent PTCA within 24 hours of administration of thrombolytic agents
Emergency or urgent coronary artery bypass graft surgery	Failed PTCA with persistent pain or hemodynamic instability in patients with coronary anatomy suitable for surgery AMI with persistent or recurrent ischemia refractory to medical therapy in patients with coronary anatomy suitable for surgery who are not candidates for PCI. At the time of surgical repair of postinfarction ventricular septal defect or mitral regurgitation	Cardiogenic shock with coronary anatomy suitable for surgery	Failed PTCA and small area of myocardium at risk; hemodynamically stable	When the expected surgical mortality rate equals or exceeds the mortality rate associated with appropriate medical therapy

Table continued on following page

TABLE 35–G–2. ACC/AHA GUIDELINES FOR INITIAL MANAGEMENT OF ACUTE MYOCARDIAL INFARCTION (AMI) AND ISCHEMIC COMPLICATIONS *Continued*

Indication	Class I	Class IIa	Class IIb	Class III
Early coronary angiography and/or interventional therapy in non–ST segment elevation MI	Patients with persistent or recurrent (stuttering) episodes of symptomatic ischemia, spontaneous or induced, with or without associated ECG changes Presence of shock, severe pulmonary congestion, or continuing hypotension			
Glycoprotein IIb/IIIa inhibitors		Patients experiencing an MI without ST segment elevation who have some high-risk features and/or refractory ischemia, provided they do not have a major contraindication due to a bleeding risk		

*Performance standard: balloon inflation within 90 (±30) minutes of admission.
†Individuals who perform > 75 PTCA procedures per year.
‡Centers that perform > 200 PTCA procedures per year and have cardiac surgical capability.
For definition of classes see p. 1353.
ACS = acute coronary syndrome; ECG = electrocardiogram; CK = creatine kinase; CK-MB = MB isoenzyme of creatine kinase; AST = aspartate transaminase; LDH = lactate dehydrogenase; CHF = congestive heart failure; BBB = bundle branch block; PVCs = premature ventricular contractions; AV = atrioventricular; PTCA = percutaneous transluminal coronary angioplasty; PCI = percutaneous coronary intervention
Unless otherwise specified, data from Ryan TJ, Antman EM, Brooks NH, et al: 1999 Update: ACC/AHA guidelines for the management of patients with acute myocardial infarction: Executive summary and recommendations: A report of the American College of Cardiology/American Heart Association Task Force on Practice Guidelines (Committee on Management of Acute Myocardial Infarction). Circulation 100:1016–1030, 1999. Copyright 1999, American Heart Association.

TABLE 35–G–3. ACC/AHA GUIDELINES FOR HEMODYNAMIC MONITORING IN ACUTE MYOCARDIAL INFARCTION (AMI)

Indication	Class I	Class IIa	Class IIb	Class III
Balloon flotation right-sided heart catheter monitoring	Severe or progressive CHF or pulmonary edema Cardiogenic shock or progressive hypotension Suspected mechanical complications of AMI (i.e., VSD, papillary muscle rupture, or pericardial tamponade)	Hypotension that does not respond promptly to fluid administration in a patient without pulmonary congestion		Patients with AMI without cardiac or pulmonary complications
Intraarterial pressure monitoring	Patients with severe hypotension (systolic arterial pressure < 80 mm Hg and/or cardiogenic shock Patients receiving vasopressor agents	Patients receiving intravenous sodium nitroprusside or other potent vasodilators	Hemodynamically stable patients receiving intravenous nitroglycerin for myocardial ischemia Patients receiving intravenous inotropic agents	Patients with acute infarction who are hemodynamically stable
Intraaortic balloon counterpulsation	Cardiogenic shock not quickly reversed with pharmacological therapy as a stabilizing measure for angiography and prompt revascularization Acute MR or VSD complicating MI as a stabilizing therapy for angiography and repair/revascularization Recurrent intractable ventricular arrhythmias with hemodynamic instability Refractory post-MI angina as a bridge to angiography and revascularization	Signs of hemodynamic instability, poor left ventricular function, or persistent ischemia in patients with large areas of myocardium at risk.	In patients with successful PTCA after failed thrombolysis or those with three-vessel coronary disease to prevent reocclusion In patients known to have large areas of myocardium at risk with or without active ischemia	

CHF = congestive heart failure; VSD = ventricular septal defect; MR = mitral regurgitation; PTCA = percutaneous transluminal coronary angioplasty.
For definition of classes see p. 1353.

phy and subsequent PTCA within 24 hours after administration of a thrombolytic agent. Emergency or urgent coronary artery bypass graft (CABG) is endorsed only when patients have severe, persistent ischemia that cannot be addressed by medical therapy and/or PTCA or as part of an effort to correct mechanical complications of MI. Such surgery along with correction of the latter is considered appropriate when these complications cause severe hemodynamic compromise.

For patients with AMI without ST segment elevation, the ACC/AHA guidelines consider early coronary angiography appropriate if they have recurrent ischemia, spontaneous or induced, with or without associated ECG changes. In these patients, glycoprotein IIb/IIIa inhibitors are usually appropriate (Class IIa), assuming that patients do not have major contraindications to these agents. (See guidelines in Chapter 36 for more detail.)

Oxygen therapy is recommended for patients even in the absence of complications in the first 2 to 3 hours, but the evidence was considered weak for this intervention after 3 to 6 hours. Similarly, routine use of intravenous nitroglycerin in patients with uncomplicated courses is not generally advised (Class IIb).

HEMODYNAMIC MONITORING (Table 35–G–3) *Routine* use of right-sided heart catheterization or intraarterial pressure monitoring in the absence of cardiac or pulmonary complications is considered inappropriate by the ACC/AHA guidelines. These interventions are considered clearly appropriate (Class I) in patients who have severe hemodynamic derangements or who require vasopressor agents. Intraaortic balloon counterpulsation is endorsed for patients with cardiogenic shock or other major hemodynamic instability and as a bridge to angiography and revascularization in patients with refractory post-MI angina.

Management of Arrhythmias (Table 35–G–4)

The ACC/AHA guidelines recommend a rapid response to the development of atrial fibrillation, including prompt electrical cardioversion for

TABLE 35–G–4. ACC/AHA GUIDELINES FOR MANAGEMENT OF ARRHYTHMIAS IN ACUTE MYOCARDIAL INFARCTION (AMI)

Indication	Class I	Class IIa	Class IIb	Class III
Atrial fibrillation	Electrical cardioversion for patients with severe hemodynamic compromise or intractable ischemia Rapid digitalization to slow a rapid ventricular response and improve LV function Intravenous beta adrenoceptor blockers to slow a rapid ventricular response in patients without clinical LV dysfunction, bronchospastic disease, or AV block	Either diltiazem or verapamil intravenously to slow a rapid ventricular response if beta-adrenoceptor blocking agents are contraindicated or ineffective		
Ventricular tachycardia (VT)/ ventricular fibrillation (VF)	VF should be treated with an electric shock with an initial energy of 200 J; if unsuccessful, a second shock of 200 to 300 J should be given, and, if necessary, a third shock of 360 J Sustained (> 30 seconds or causing hemodynamic collapse) polymorphic VT should be treated with an unsynchronized electric shock using an initial energy of 200 J; if unsuccessful, a second shock of 200 to 300 J should be given, and, if necessary, a third shock of 360 J. Episodes of sustained monomorphic VT associated with angina, pulmonary edema, or hypotension (systolic pressure < 90 mm Hg) should be treated with a synchronized electric shock of 100 J initial energy. Increasing energies may be used if not initially successful. Sustained monomorphic VT not associated with angina, pulmonary edema, or hypotension (systolic pressure < 90 mm Hg) should be treated with one of the following regimens:	nfusions of antiarrhythmic drugs may be used after an episode of VT/VF but should be discontinued after 6 to 24 hours and the need for further arrhythmia management assessed Electrolyte and acid-base disturbances should be corrected to prevent recurrent episodes of VF when an initial episode of VF has been treated.	Drug-refractory polymorphic VT should be managed by aggressive attempts to reduce myocardial ischemia, including therapies such as beta-adrenoceptor blockade, intraaortic balloon pumping, and emergency PTCA/CABG surgery. Amiodarone, 150 mg infused over 10 minutes followed by a constant infusion of 1.0 mg/min for up to 6 hours and then a maintenance infusion of 0.5 mg/min.	Treatment of isolated VPBs, couplets, runs of accelerated idioventricular rhythm, and nonsustained VT Prophylactic administration of antiarrhythmic therapy when using thrombolytic agents.

Table continued on following page

TABLE 35–G–4. ACC/AHA GUIDELINES FOR MANAGEMENT OF ARRHYTHMIAS IN ACUTE MYOCARDIAL INFARCTION (AMI) *Continued*

Indication	Class I	Class IIa	Class IIb	Class III
	1. Lidocaine: bolus 1.0 to 1.5 mg/kg. Supplemental boluses of 0.5 to 0.75 mg/kg every 5 to 10 minutes to a maximum of 3 mg/kg total loading dose may be given as needed. Loading is followed by infusion of 2 to 4 mg/min (30 to 50 μg/kg/min). 2. Procainamide: 20 to 30 mg/min loading infusion, up to 12 to 17 mg/kg. This may be followed by an infusion of 1 to 4 mg/min. 3. Amiodarone: 150 mg infused over 10 minutes followed by a constant infusion of 1.0 mg/min for 6 hours and then a maintenance infusion of 0.5 mg/min. 4. Synchronized electrical cardioversion starting at 50 J (brief anesthesia is necessary).			
Atropine	Symptomatic sinus bradycardia (generally, heart rate < 50 beats/min associated with hypotension, ischemia, or escape ventricular arrhythmia). Ventricular asystole Symptomatic AV block occurring at the AV nodal level (second-degree type I or third-degree with a narrow-complex escape rhythm)			AV block occurring at an infranodal level (usually associated with anterior MI with a wide-complex escape rhythm). Asymptomatic sinus bradycardia
Temporary pacing: placement of transcutaneous patches and active (demand) transcutaneous pacing	Sinus bradycardia (rate less than 50 beats/min) with hypotension (systolic pressure < 80 mm Hg) unresponsive to drug therapy. Mobitz type II second-degree AV block Third-degree heart block Bilateral BBB (alternating BBB, or RBBB) and alternating LAFB, LPFB (irrespective of time of onset) Newly acquired or age-indeterminate LBBB, LBBB and LAFB, RBBB, and LPFB RBBB or LBBB and first-degree AV block	Stable bradycardia (systolic pressure > 90 mm Hg, no hemodynamic compromise, or compromise responsive to initial drug therapy) Newly acquired or age-indeterminate RBBB	Newly acquired or age-indeterminate first-degree AV block	Uncomplicated AMI without evidence of conduction system disease

TABLE 35–G–4. ACC/AHA GUIDELINES FOR MANAGEMENT OF ARRHYTHMIAS IN ACUTE MYOCARDIAL INFARCTION (AMI) *Continued*

Indication	Class I	Class IIa	Class IIb	Class III
Temporary transvenous pacing	Asystole Symptomatic bradycardia (includes sinus bradycardia with hypotension and type I second-degree AV block with hypotension not responsive to atropine) Bilateral BBB (alternating BBB or RBBB with alternating LAFB/LPFB) (any age) New or indeterminate-age bifascicular block (RBBB with LAFB or LPFB, or LBBB) with first-degree AV block Mobitz type II second-degree AV block	RBBB and LAFB or LPFB (new or indeterminate) RBBB with first-degree AV block LBBB, new or indeterminate Incessant VT, for atrial or ventricular overdrive pacing Recurrent sinus pauses (greater than 3 seconds) not responsive to atropine	Bifascicular block of indeterminate age New or age-indeterminate isolated RBBB	First-degree AV block Type I second-degree AV block with normal hemodynamics Accelerated idioventricular rhythm BBB or fascicular block known to exist before AMI
Permanent pacing after AMI	Persistent second-degree AV block in the His-Purkinje system with bilateral BBB or complete AV block after AMI Transient advanced (second- or third-degree) AV block and associated BBB Symptomatic AV block at any level		Persistent advanced (second- or third-degree) block at the AV node level	Transient AV conduction disturbances in the absence of intraventricular conduction defects Transient AV block in the presence of isolated LAFB Acquired LAFB in the absence of AV block Persistent first-degree AV block in the presence of BBB that is old or age indeterminate

LV = left ventricular; AV = atrioventricular; PTCA = percutaneous transluminal coronary angioplasty; CABG = coronary artery bypass graft; BBB = bundle branch block; RBBB and LBBB = right and left bundle branch block; LAFB and LPFB = left anterior and posterior fascicular block. For definition of classes see p. 1253.

patients who develop hemodynamic compromise or intractable ischemia with this arrhythmia. Intravenous beta blockers are considered appropriate agents to slow a rapid ventricular response in the absence of contraindications.

The guidelines do *not* recommend routine administration of antiarrhythmic therapy for nonsustained ventricular tachycardia or less severe ventricular arrhythmias, nor do they support prophylactic antiarrhythmic therapy for patients receiving thrombolytic agents. Intravenous amiodarone is considered an appropriate agent in patients with sustained monomorphic ventricular tachycardia.

The ACC/AHA guidelines consider temporary pacemaker placement appropriate in patients with second-degree Mobitz type II or third-degree atrioventricular block, as well as various configurations of bifascicular and potentially trifascicular block. Permanent pacemaker placement is supported for symptomatic atrioventricular block at any level but not for uncomplicated unifascicular block.

Pharmacotherapy (Table 35–G–5)

Intravenous heparin therapy is considered clearly appropriate (Class I) for patients undergoing revascularization and probably appropriate (Class IIa) for patients receiving intravenous alteplase therapy or with non–ST segment elevation MI (Table 35G–5). Intravenous heparin is also recommended for patients at high risk for embolic events, such as those with large or anterior MIs.

The ACC/AHA guidelines support a low threshold for initiation of beta-adrenoceptor blocker therapy within 12 hours of the onset of MI in patients without contraindications. Early administration of angiotensin-converting enzyme inhibitors is recommended for patients with ST segment elevation in anterior leads. Initiation of this therapy is consid-

ered clearly (Class I) or probably indicated (Class IIa) in broad classes of patients without contraindications.

In contrast, the use of calcium channel blockers is discouraged. Exceptions include the use of verapamil or diltiazem for patients in whom beta blockers cannot be used or are ineffective for management of arrhythmia or ischemia. The ACC/AHA task force considered diltiazem only marginally appropriate (Class IIb) in the first 24 hours for patients with non–ST segment elevation infarction without left ventricular dysfunction, pulmonary congestion, or congestive heart failure.

The role of intravenous magnesium therapy was considered unestablished, although evidence supported its use in patients with documented magnesium deficits or episodes of *torsades de pointes type* ventricular tachycardia.

Discharge from Hospital (Table 35–G–6)

The ACC/AHA guidelines strongly support performance of noninvasive risk stratification using exercise or pharmacological stress testing. The guidelines indicate that the lowest cost alternative—exercise electrocardiography—is an appropriate first-line test. Imaging and pharmacological stress testing are recommended when clinical or electrocardiographic findings compromise the reliability of exercise electrocardiography. The ACC/AHA task force concluded that there was not strong evidence to support *routine* use of ambulatory (Holter) monitoring or analyses of heart rate variability (Class IIb).

Routine use of coronary angiography and revascularization in patients without evidence of ongoing ischemia was also considered inappropriate (Class III) or weakly supported by evidence (Class IIb). However, invasive evaluation and treatment was recommended (Class I or IIa) when patients had spontaneous or induced evidence

TABLE 35–G–5. ACC/AHA GUIDELINES FOR PHARMACOTHERAPY IN ACUTE MYOCARDIAL INFARCTION (AMI)

Indication	Class I	Class IIa	Class IIb	Class III
Heparin	Patients undergoing percutaneous or surgical revascularization	Intravenously in patients undergoing reperfusion therapy with alteplase Intravenous UFH or LMWH subcutaneously for patients with non–ST segment elevation MI. Subcutaneous UFH (e.g., 7500 U b.i.d.) or LMWH (e.g., enoxaparin 1 mg/kg b.i.d.) in all patients not treated with thrombolytic therapy who do not have a contraindication to heparin. In patients who are at high risk for systemic emboli (large or anterior MI, AF, previous embolus, or known LV thrombus), intravenous heparin is preferred. Intravenously in patients treated with nonselective thrombolytic agents (streptokinase, anistreplase, urokinase) who are at high risk for systemic emboli (large or anterior MI, AF, previous embolus, or known LV thrombus)	Patients treated with non-selective thrombolytic agents, not at high risk, subcutaneous heparin, 7500 U to 12,500 U twice a day until completely ambulatory	Routine intravenous heparin within 6 hours to patients receiving a nonselective fibrinolytic agent (streptokinase, anistreplase, urokinase) who are not at high risk for systemic embolism
Beta-adrenoceptor blocking agents: early therapy	Patients without a contraindication to beta-adrenoceptor blocker therapy who can be treated < 12 hours of onset of AMI, irrespective of administration of concomitant thrombolytic therapy or performance of primary angioplasty Patients with continuing or recurrent ischemic pain Patients with tachyarrhythmias, such as AF with a rapid ventricular response Non–ST segment elevation MI		Patients with moderate LV failure (the presence of bibasilar rales without evidence of low cardiac output) or other relative contraindications to beta-adrenoceptor blocker therapy, provided patients can be monitored closely	Patients with severe LV failure
Angiotensin-converting enzyme (ACE) inhibitors	Patients within the first 24 hours of a suspected AMI with ST segment elevation in > 2 anterior precordial leads or with clinical heart failure in the absence of hypotension (systolic BP < 100 mm Hg) or known contraindications to use of ACE inhibitors Patients with MI and LV ejection fraction < 40% or patients with clinical heart failure on the basis of systolic pump dysfunction during and after convalescence from AMI	All other patients within the first 24 hours of a suspected or established AMI, provided significant hypotension or other clear-cut contraindications are absent Asymptomatic patients with mildly impaired LV function (ejection fraction 40% to 50%) and a history of old MI	Patients who have recently recovered from MI but have normal or mildly abnormal global LV function	

TABLE 35–G–5. ACC/AHA GUIDELINES FOR PHARMACOTHERAPY IN ACUTE MYOCARDIAL INFARCTION (AMI) *Continued*

Indication	Class I	Class IIa	Class IIb	Class III
Calcium channel blockers		Verapamil or diltiazem in patients in whom beta-adrenoceptor blockers are ineffective or contra-indicated (i.e., broncho-spastic disease) for relief of ongoing ischemia or control of a rapid ven-tricular response with AF after AMI in the absence of CHF, LV dysfunction, or AV block	In non–ST segment ele-vation infarction, dilti-azem may be given to patients without LV dys-function, pulmonary congestion, or CHF. It may be added to stan-dard therapy after the first 24 hours and con-tinued for 1 year.	Nifedipine (short acting) is generally contraindicated in routine treatment of AMI because of its nega-tive inotropic effects and the reflex sympathetic activation, tachycardia, and hypotension associ-ated with its use. Diltiazem and verapamil are contraindicated in pa-tients with AMI and asso-ciated LV dysfunction or CHF.
Magnesium		Correction of documented magnesium (and/or po-tassium) deficits, espe-cially in patients receiv-ing diuretics before onset of infarction Episodes of torsades de pointes-type VT associ-ated with a prolonged QT interval should be treated with 1 to 2 gm of magnesium administered as a bolus over 5 min-utes.	Magnesium bolus and in-fusion in high-risk pa-tients such as the el-derly and/or those for whom reperfusion ther-apy is not suitable	

UFH = unfractionated heparin; LMWH = low molecular weight heparin; AF = atrial fibrillation; LV = left ventricular; BP = blood pressure; VT = ventricular tachycardia; AV = atrioventricular; CHF = congestive heart failure.
For definition of classes see p. 1253.

TABLE 35–G–6. ACC/AHA GUIDELINES FOR PREPARATION FOR DISCHARGE FROM HOSPITAL AFTER ACUTE MYOCARDIAL INFARCTION (AMI)

Indication	Class I	Class IIa	Class IIb	Class III
Noninvasive evaluation of low-risk patients	Stress ECG Before discharge for prognostic assessment or functional capacity (submaximal at 4 to 6 days or symptom lim-ited at 10 to 14 days) Early after discharge for prognostic assessment and functional capacity (14 to 21 days) Late after discharge (3 to 6 weeks) for func-tional capacity and prognosis if early stress was submaximal Exercise, vasodilator stress nuclear scintigraphy, or exercise stress echocar-diography when baseline abnormalities of the ECG compromise interpretation	Dipyridamole or adenosine stress perfusion nuclear scintigraphy or dobuta-mine echocardiography before discharge for prognostic assessment in patients judged to be unable to exercise Exercise two-dimensional echocardiography or nu-clear scintigraphy (be-fore or early after dis-charge for prognostic assessment)	Stress testing within 2 to 3 days of AMI Either exercise or pharma-cological stress testing at any time to evaluate patients with unstable postinfarction angina pectoris At any time to evaluate patients with AMI who have uncompensated CHF, cardiac arrhyth-mia, or noncardiac con-ditions that severely limit their ability to exer-cise. Before discharge to evalu-ate patients who have already been selected for cardiac catheteriza-tion	
Assessment of ventric-ular arrhythmia—routine testing			Ambulatory (Holter) moni-toring, signal-averaged ECG, heart rate variabil-ity, baroreflex sensitivity monitoring, alone or in combination for risk as-sessment after MI, es-pecially in patients at higher perceived risk, when findings might in-fluence management is-sues, or for clinical re-search purposes	

Table continued on following page

TABLE 35–G–6. ACC/AHA GUIDELINES FOR PREPARATION FOR DISCHARGE FROM HOSPITAL AFTER ACUTE MYOCARDIAL INFARCTION (AMI) *Continued*

Indication	Class I	Class IIa	Class IIb	Class III
Coronary angiography and possible PTCA	Patients with spontaneous episodes of myocardial ischemia or episodes of myocardial ischemia provoked by minimal exertion during recovery from AMI Before definitive therapy of a mechanical complication of infarction such as acute MR, VSD, pseudoaneurysm, or LV aneurysm Patients with persistent hemodynamic instability	When MI is suspected to have occurred by a mechanism other than thrombotic occlusion at an atherosclerotic plaque. This would include coronary embolism, certain metabolic or hematological diseases, or coronary artery spasm Survivors of AMI with depressed LV systolic function (LV ejection fraction less than or equal to 40%), CHF, prior revascularization, or malignant ventricular arrhythmias Survivors of AMI who had clinical heart failure during the acute episode but subsequently demonstrated well-preserved LV function	Coronary angiography performed in all patients after infarction to find persistently occluded infarct-related arteries in an attempt to revascularize the artery or to identify patients with three-vessel disease All patients after a non-Q-wave MI Recurrent VT or VF or both, despite antiarrhythmic therapy in patients without evidence of ongoing myocardial ischemia	Routine use of coronary angiography and subsequent PTCA of the infarct-related artery within days after receiving thrombolytic therapy Survivors of MI who are thought not to be candidates for coronary revascularization
Routine coronary angiography and PTCA after successful thrombolytic therapy				Routine PTCA of the stenotic infarct-related artery immediately after thrombolytic therapy PTCA of the stenotic infarct-related artery within 48 hours of receiving a thrombolytic agent in asymptomatic patients without evidence of ischemia

ECG = electrocardiogram; CHF = congestive heart failure; MR = mitral regurgitation; VSD = ventricular septal defect; LV = left ventricular; VT = ventricular tachycardia; VF = ventricular fibrillation; PTCA = percutaneous transluminal coronary angioplasty.
For definition of classes see p. 1253.

TABLE 35–G–7. SECONDARY PREVENTION

Indication	Class I	Class IIa	Class IIb	Class III
Management of lipids	The AHA step II diet, which is low in saturated fat and cholesterol in all patients after recovery from AMI Patients with LDLC > 125 mg/dl despite the AHA step II diet should be placed on drug therapy, with the goal of reducing LDLC to < 100 mg/dl Patients with normal plasma cholesterol levels with HDLC < 35 mg/dl should receive nonpharmacological therapy (e.g., exercise) designed to raise it	Drug therapy added to diet in patients with LDLC levels < 130 mg/dl but > 100 mg/dl after an appropriate trial of the AHA step II diet Patients with normal total cholesterol levels but HDLC < 35 mg/dl despite diet and other nonpharmacological therapy may be started on drugs such as niacin to raise HDL levels.	Drug therapy with either niacin or gemfibrozil added to diet regardless of LDLC and HDLC when triglyceride levels are > 200 mg/dl.	
Long-term beta-adrenoceptor blocker therapy in survivors of myocardial infarction	All but low-risk patients without a clear contraindication to beta-adrenoceptor blocker therapy. Treatment should begin within a few days of the event (if not initiated acutely) and continue indefinitely.	Low-risk patients without a clear contraindication to beta-adrenoceptor blocker therapy. Survivors of non–ST segment elevation MI.	Patients with moderate or severe LV failure or other relative contraindications to beta-adrenoceptor blocker therapy, provided patients can be monitored closely	

TABLE 35–G–7. SECONDARY PREVENTION *Continued*

1231

Ch 35

Indication	Class I	Class IIa	Class IIb	Class III
Long-term anticoagulation	Post-MI patients unable to take daily aspirin Post-MI patients in persistent AF Patients with LV thrombus	Post-MI patients with extensive wall motion abnormalities Patients with paroxysmal AF.	Post-MI patients with severe LV systolic dysfunction with or without CHF	
Estrogen replacement therapy and myocardial infarction		HRT with estrogen plus progestin for secondary prevention of coronary events should not be given de novo to postmenopausal women after AMI. Postmenopausal women who are already taking HRT with estrogen plus progestin at the time of AMI can continue this therapy.		

LDLC and HDLC = low- and high-density lipoprotein cholesterol; LV = left ventricular; CHF = congestive heart failure; AF = atrial fibrillation. For definition of classes see p. 1253.

of myocardial ischemia or other complications of ischemic heart disease.

Secondary Prevention (Table 35–G–7)

The ACC/AHA guidelines strongly endorse pharmacological and aggressive dietary interventions to reduce low-density lipoprotein (LDL) cholesterol after acute myocardial infarction. An AHA Step II diet is considered appropriate for all patients after recovery from AMI, and initiation for drug therapy is considered clearly appropriate (Class I) if LDL cholesterol is greater than 125 mg/dl despite this diet. The use of a lower LDL cholesterol threshold (100–125 mg/dl) for initiation of drug therapy was considered to be less clearly established (Class IIa). Exercise and other efforts to raise high-density lipoprotein cholesterol are also recommended.

The guidelines reflect enthusiasm for the benefits of beta blockers for all but low-risk patients if there are no contraindications to these agents. Anticoagulation with warfarin is considered appropriate for patients unable to take daily aspirin or for patients who have atrial fibrillation or left ventricular thrombus. The guidelines are somewhat supportive (Class IIa) of anticoagulation in patients with extensive wall motion abnormalities or paroxysmal atrial fibrillation but not for all patients with severe left ventricular dysfunction.

The guidelines do not support initiation of hormone replacement therapy in postmenopausal patients with the goal of preventing coronary events after AMI but did not oppose their continuation.

References

1. American College of Emergency Physicians: Clinical policy for the initial approach to adults presenting with a chief complaint of chest pain, with no history of trauma. Ann Emerg Med 25:274–299, 1995.
2. Ryan TJ, Antman EM, Brooks NH, et al: 1999 update: ACC/AHA guidelines for the management of patients with acute myocardial infarction: Executive summary and recommendations: A report of the American College of Cardiology/American Heart Association Task Force on Practice Guidelines (Committee on Management of Acute Myocardial Infarction). J Am Coll Cardiol 34: 890–911, 1999.
3. National Heart Attack Alert Program Coordinating Committee 60 Minutes to Treatment Working Group: Emergency Department: Rapid Identification and Treatment of Patients with Acute Myocardial Infarction. NIH publication No. 93-3278. National Heart, Lung, and Blood Institute, Public Health Service, US Department of Health and Human Services, September 1993.
4. Braunwald E, Mark DB, Jones RH, et al: Unstable Angina: Diagnosis and Management. Clinical Practice Guideline Number 10 (amended). AHCPR publication No. 94-0602. Rockville, MD, Agency for Health Care Policy and Research and the National Heart, Lung, and Blood Institute, Public Health Service, US Department of Health and Human Services, May 1994.
5. Braunwald E, Antman EM, Beasley JW, et al: ACC/AHA guidelines for the management of patients with unstable angina: A report of the American College of Cardiology/American Heart Association Task Force on Practice Guidelines (Committee on the Management of Patients with Unstable Angina). J Am Coll Cardiol 36:970–1062, 2000.
6. Nichol G, Walls R, Goldman L, et al: A critical pathway for management of patients with acute chest pain at low risk for myocardial ischemia: Recommendations and potential impact. Ann Intern Med 127:996–1005, 1997.

Chapter 36

Unstable Angina

CHRISTOPHER P. CANNON · EUGENE BRAUNWALD

Unstable angina lies in the center of the spectrum of clinical conditions caused by myocardial ischemia. These range from chronic stable angina pectoris (see Chap. 37) to the acute coronary syndromes. The latter, in turn, consist of acute myocardial infarction (MI) associated with electrocardiographic ST segment elevation (STEMI) (see Chap. 35) and unstable angina/non-ST segment elevation MI (UA/NSTEMI). The former is most commonly caused by acute total coronary occlusion,[1, 2] and urgent reperfusion is the mainstay of therapy, whereas UA/NSTEMI is usually associated with severe coronary obstruction but not total occlusion of the culprit coronary artery.[3, 4] If the myocardial ischemia that results from the coronary obstruction is long in duration and/or great in severity, myocardial necrosis occurs,[5] and the patient is classified as having a non-Q-wave MI or, now more aptly termed, NSTEMI (see Fig. 35–2).

Although, with the advent of thrombolysis and other emergency reperfusion therapies, a great deal of attention has focused on acute MI with ST segment elevation, UA/NSTEMI (the focus of this chapter) occurs with much greater frequency. Every year in the United States, approximately 1.3 million patients are admitted to the hospital with unstable angina or NSTEMI compared with approximately 350,000 patients with acute STEMI.[6]

DEFINITION AND CLASSIFICATION

DEFINITION. This is largely based on the clinical presentation[7] (see p. 1235). *Stable* angina pectoris is characterized by a deep, poorly localized chest or arm discomfort (rarely described as pain) that is reproducibly associated with physical exertion or emotional stress and relieved within 5 to 15 minutes by rest and/or sublingual nitroglycerin. *Unstable* angina is defined as angina pectoris (or equivalent type of ischemic discomfort) with at least one of three features: (1) it occurs at rest (or with minimal exertion) usually lasting more than 20 minutes (if not interrupted by nitroglycerin); (2) it is severe and described as frank pain and of new onset (i.e., within 1 month); and (3) it occurs with a crescendo pattern (i.e., more severe, prolonged, or frequent than previously). Some patients with this pattern of ischemic discomfort, especially those with prolonged rest pain,[5] develop evidence of myocardial necrosis on the basis of the release of cardiac markers and thus have a diagnosis of NSTEMI. Traditionally, this diagnosis has been

based on elevation of serum creatine kinase (CK)-MB, but recently troponin T and I assays have been used to define ischemic myocardial damage based on their higher sensitivity for myocardial necrosis and powerful prognostic ability (see pp. 1236, 1237, and 1240).

CLASSIFICATION. Because unstable angina comprises such a heterogeneous group of patients, classification schemes based on clinical features have been proposed.[7–10] A clinical classification of unstable angina, presented by one of the authors (Table 36–1),[8] has been found to be a useful means of stratifying risk.[11–15] Patients are divided into three groups according to the clinical circumstances of the acute ischemic episode: primary unstable angina, secondary unstable angina (i.e., with unstable angina related to obvious precipitating noncoronary factors such as anemia, infection, or cardiac arrhythmias), and post-MI angina. Patients are also classified according to the severity of the ischemia (acute rest pain, subacute rest pain, or new-onset severe angina)[8] (see Table 36–1). This classification has been shown to be predictive of plaques with thrombus at angiography[11, 16, 17] or in atherectomy specimens[18] and in risk stratification (see p. 1234).[12–14]

Because unstable angina is a clinical syndrome rather than a specific disease (much like hypertension rather than pneumococcal pneumonia), and because it has many potential causes, an etiological approach has been proposed.[10] Five pathophysiological processes that may contribute to the development of unstable angina have been identified (Fig. 36–1):

1. Plaque rupture with superimposed nonocclusive thrombus

2. Dynamic obstruction (i.e., coronary spasm of an epicardial artery, as in Prinzmetal angina [see Chap. 37] or constriction of the small muscular coronary arteries)

3. Progressive mechanical obstruction

4. Inflammation and/or infection

5. Secondary unstable angina, precipitated by increased myocardial oxygen demand or decreased supply (e.g., thyrotoxicosis or anemia)

Individual patients may have several of these processes coexisting as the cause of their episode of unstable angina. Use of this etiological approach will refine the diagnostic approach and help target therapeutic strategies to treat the underlying disease that precipitated the episode of unstable angina.

CLASS	DEFINITION	DEATH OR MYOCARDIAL INFARCTION TO 1 YEAR*
Severity		
Class I	New onset of severe angina or accelerated angina; no rest pain	7.3%
Class II	Angina at rest within past month but not within preceding 48 hr (angina at rest, subacute)	10.3%
Class III	Angina at rest within 48 hr (angina at rest, subacute)	10.8%†
Clinical Circumstances		
A (secondary angina)	Develops in the presence of extracardiac condition that intensifies myocardial ischemia	14.1%
B (primary angina)	Develops in the absence of extracardiac condition	8.5%
C (postinfarction angina)	Develops within 2 weeks after acute myocardial infarction	18.5%‡
Intensity of treatment	Patients with unstable angina may also be divided into three groups depending on whether unstable angina occurs (1) in the absence of treatment for chronic stable angina, (2) during treatment for chronic stable angina, or (3) despite maximal antiischemic drug therapy. The three groups may be designated subscripts 1, 2, or 3, respectively.	
Electrocardiographic changes	Patients with unstable angina may be further divided into those with or without transient ST-T wave changes during pain.	

* Data from TIMI III Registry: Cannon CP, McCabe CH, Stone PH, et al: Prospective validation of the Braunwald classification of unstable angina: Results from the Thrombolysis in Myocardial Ischemia (TIMI) III Registry (abstract). Circulation 92(Suppl I):1–19, 1995. Copyright 1995, American Heart Association.

† $p = 0.057$.

‡ $p < 0.001$.

From Braunwald E. Unstable angina: A classification. Circulation 80:410–414, 1989. Copyright 1989, American Heart Association.

PATHOPHYSIOLOGY

The majority of patients with unstable angina have significant obstructive coronary atherosclerosis (see Chap. 30). Episodes of ischemia can be provoked by an increase in myocardial oxygen demand (e.g., precipitated by tachycardia or hypertension) and/or by a reduction in supply (e.g., due to reduction in coronary lumen diameter by platelet-rich thrombi or vasospasm). Rapid progression of the underlying coronary artery disease has been documented.[19, 20] A sequence of events can be documented in unstable angina in which there is first a reduction in coronary sinus oxygen saturation (signifying a reduction in coronary blood flow), then ST segment depression, followed by chest discomfort.[21] Elevations in blood pressure and/or heart rate sometimes ensue.[21] A patient might have both a small increase in myocardial oxygen demand, in conjunction with a reduction in coronary blood flow, leading to the episode of ischemia. The five major causes of these two broad precipitants of unstable angina are reviewed next.

PLAQUE RUPTURE, FISSURE, OR EROSION. Rupture or erosion of an atherosclerotic plaque with superimposed nonocclusive thrombus is by far the most common cause of UA/NSTEMI. The type of plaque that ruptures, the so-called vulnerable plaques, are usually lesions with less than 50 percent stenosis.[22–24] Plaque rupture can be precipitated by multiple factors, including high plaque lipid content,[25] local inflammation causing breakdown of the thin shoulder of the plaque,[26] coronary artery constriction at the site of the plaque, local shear stress forces, platelet activa-

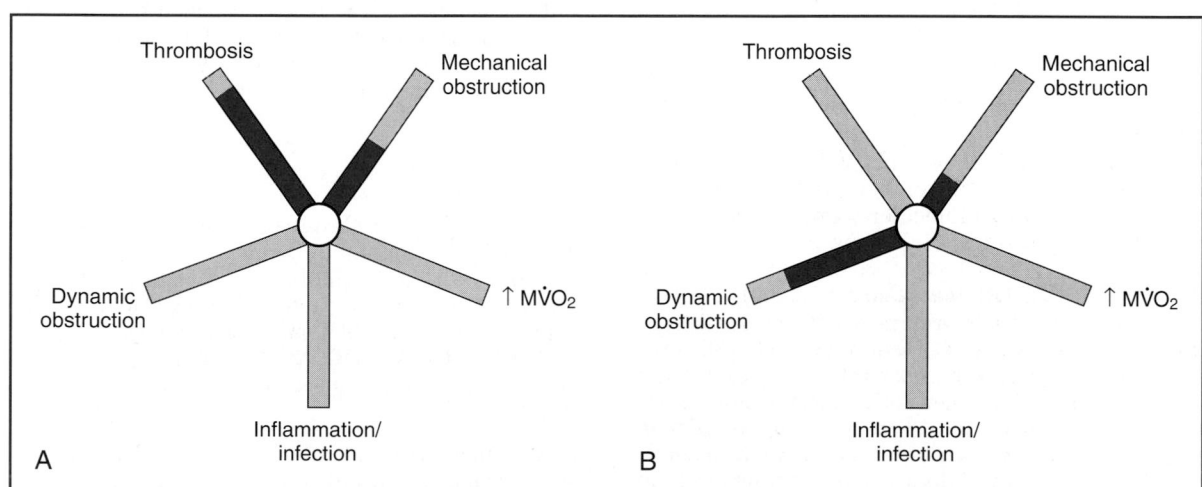

FIGURE 36–1. Schematic representation of the causes of unstable angina. Each of the five bars represents one of the etiologic mechanisms, and the red portion of the bar represents the extent to which the mechanism is operative. *A,* Most common form of unstable angina in which atherosclerotic plaque causes moderate (60 percent diameter) obstruction and acute thrombus overlying plaque causes very severe (90 percent diameter) narrowing. *B,* Mild coronary obstruction, adjacent to which there is intense (90 percent diameter) vasoconstriction. (From Braunwald E: Unstable angina: An etiologic approach to management [editorial]. Circulation 98:2219–2222, 1998. Copyright 1998, American Heart Association.)

tion,[27, 28] and the status of the coagulation system (i.e., a potentially prothrombotic state),[29, 30] all of which culminate in the formation of platelet-rich thrombi at the site of the plaque rupture or erosion and the resultant acute coronary syndrome (see also Chaps. 30 and 35).[31-33] Circadian variation with a morning increase in the onset of UA/NSTEMI has been reported[34] and likely relates to similar factors as in MI, including morning elevations in platelet aggregability[35, 36] and in myocardial oxygen demand with increases in blood pressure, heart rate, emotional stress, and physical exertion.[37]

INFLAMMATION AND/OR INFECTION. Recent evidence has also pointed to a role for inflammation, which appears to play a key role in the development of atherosclerosis (see Chaps. 30 and 31),[38, 39] and in the development and recurrence of unstable angina.[40-43] Infectious agents, notably *Chlamydia pneumoniae,* appear to be one of the underlying causes of diffuse inflammation in the pathogenesis of coronary artery disease.[44-46] Others for which there is some, albeit less strong, evidence include *Helicobacter pylori* and cytomegalovirus.[44] An etiological relationship between these infectious agents to the development of unstable angina (or MI) has not been definitively established.[46-48] On the other hand, evidence from several animal models,[49-51] and pilot treatment trials in patients,[52-54] suggests that *Chlamydia pneumoniae* may be an important and *potentially treatable* cause of unstable angina or MI, and larger trials are ongoing.

THROMBOSIS (see also Chap. 62). The central role of coronary artery thrombosis in the pathogenesis of unstable angina is supported by a substantial body of evidence.[4, 31, 32, 55-57] Six sets of observations contribute to this concept:

1. At autopsy, thrombi can usually be identified at the site of a ruptured plaque[31, 32, 58] or a coronary erosion.[59]

2. Coronary atherectomy specimens obtained from patients with unstable angina demonstrate a high incidence of thrombotic lesions, as compared with those obtained from stable angina patients.[18, 57, 60, 61]

3. Coronary angioscopic observations in unstable angina indicate that thrombus is frequently present.[55, 56, 62-64]

4. Coronary angiography has demonstrated ulceration or irregularities suggesting a ruptured plaque[22, 65] and/or thrombus in many patients (Fig. 36-2). In the Thrombosis in Myocardial Infarction (TIMI) IIIA trial of patients with UA/NSTEMI, 35 percent of patients had definite thrombus and an additional 40 percent had possible thrombus at angiography.[4]

5. Evidence of ongoing thrombosis has been noted with elevation of several markers of platelet activity and fibrin formation.[66-70]

6. The clinical outcome of patients with acute coronary syndromes improves with antithrombotic therapy with aspirin,[71-74] heparin,[73-77] low-molecular-weight heparin,[78-80] and platelet glycoprotein IIb/IIIa inhibitors.[81-83]

PLATELET AGGREGATION (see also Chap. 62). Platelets play a key role in the transformation of a stable atherosclerotic plaque to an unstable lesion (Fig. 36-3). With rupture or ulceration of an atherosclerotic plaque, the subendothelial matrix (e.g., collagen and tissue factor) is exposed to the circulating blood. The first step is *platelet adhesion* by means of the platelet glycoprotein Ib receptor through its interaction with endothelial von Willebrand factor. This is followed by *platelet activation,* which leads to (1) a shape change in the platelet (from a smooth discoid shape to a spiculated form, which increases the surface area upon which thrombin generation can occur); (2) degranulation of the alpha and dense granules, thereby releasing thromboxane A_2, serotonin, and other platelet aggregatory and chemoattractant agents; and (3) expression of

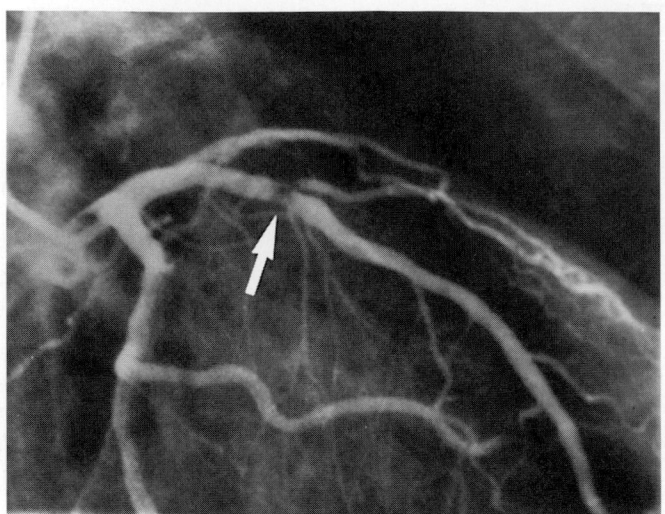

FIGURE 36-2. Coronary artery thrombus in a patient with unstable angina. A 60-year-old man presented with prolonged rest pain and transient anterior ST segment elevations. Coronary angiography shows an irregular hazy filling defect in the left anterior descending artery at the level of the second diagonal branch (arrow). Contrast medium surrounds the globular thrombus, which extends into the diagonal branch.

glycoprotein IIb/IIIa receptors on the platelet surface with activation of the receptor so that it can bind fibrinogen. The final step is *platelet aggregation,* that is, the formation of the platelet plug. Fibrinogen (or von Willebrand factor) binds to the activated glycoprotein IIb/IIIa receptors of two platelets, thereby creating a growing platelet aggregate. Antiplatelet therapy is one of the cornerstones of therapy in unstable angina (see p. 1243) and is directed at decreasing the formation of thromboxane A_2 (aspirin), inhibiting the adenosine diphosphate (ADP) pathway of platelet activation (ticlopidine and clopidogrel), and directly inhibiting platelet aggregation (glycoprotein IIb/IIIa inhibitors) (see Fig. 36-3).

SECONDARY HEMOSTASIS. Simultaneously with formation of the platelet plug, the plasma coagulation system is activated. Release of tissue factor appears to be the predominant mechanism of initiating hemostasis during plaque rupture and coronary thrombosis (see Chap. 62).[84-86] Ultimately, factor X is activated (to factor Xa), leading to the generation of thrombin, which plays a central role in arterial thrombosis. Thrombin has several actions: (1) it converts fibrinogen to fibrin in the final common pathway for clot formation; (2) it is a powerful stimulus for platelet aggregation; and (3) it activates factor XIII, which leads to cross-linking and stabilization of the fibrin clot. Thrombin molecules are incorporated into coronary thrombi and can form the nidus of rethrombosis (i.e., reocclusion or reinfarction) as the thrombus undergoes spontaneous or pharmacologically induced fibrinolysis. Accordingly, effective inhibition of thrombin and factor Xa plays an important part of the therapy of unstable angina (see later).

CORONARY VASOCONSTRICTION. There are three settings in which the process of dynamic coronary obstruction is identified:

1. Prinzmetal variant angina, with intense *focal* spasm of a segment of an epicardial coronary artery, is the prototypical example (see also Chap. 37).[87] This can occur in patients without coronary atherosclerosis or in patients with a nonobstructive atheromatous plaque. The vasospastic angina appears to be due to hypercontractility of vascular smooth muscle and endothelial dysfunction occurring in the region of spasm.[88] Such patients typically present with rest pain accompanied by transient ST segment elevation.

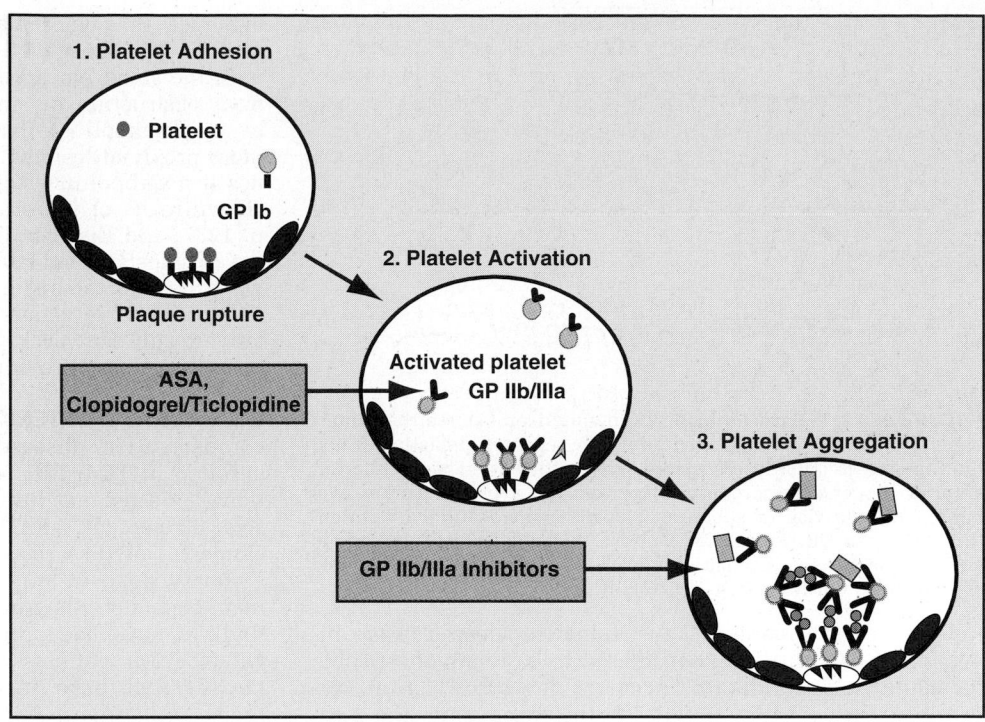

FIGURE 36–3. Primary hemostasis: process of platelet adhesion (a), activation (b), and aggregation (c). Platelets initiate thrombosis at the site of a ruptured plaque: the first step is *platelet adhesion* (1) via the glycoprotein Ib receptor in conjunction with von Willebrand factor. This is followed by *platelet activation* (2), which leads to a shape change in the platelet, degranulation of the alpha and dense granules, and expression of glycoprotein IIb/IIIa receptors on the platelet surface with activation of the receptor, such that it can bind fibrinogen. The final step is *platelet aggregation* (3), in which fibrinogen (or von Willebrand factor) binds to the activated glycoprotein IIb/IIIa receptors of two platelets. Aspirin (ASA) and clopidogrel act to decrease platelet activation (see text for details), whereas the glycoprotein IIb/IIIa inhibitors inhibit the final step of platelet aggregation.

2. Coronary vasoconstriction causing "microcirculatory angina" results from constriction of the small intramural coronary resistance vessels.[89] Although there are no epicardial coronary artery stenoses, coronary flow is usually slowed (see Chap. 37).

3. Probably the most common setting in which vasoconstriction occurs is in the presence of coronary atherosclerotic plaques.

Vasoconstriction can occur as the result of local vasoconstrictors released from platelets, such as serotonin and thromboxane A_2,[66, 69] as well as those present within the thrombus, such as thrombin.[90] A dysfunctional coronary endothelium, with reduced production of nitric oxide and increased release of endothelin (see Chap. 34), can also lead to vasoconstriction. Adrenergic stimuli, cold immersion,[91] cocaine,[92, 93] or mental stress[94] can also cause coronary vasoconstriction.

PROGRESSIVE MECHANICAL OBSTRUCTION. The fourth etiology of unstable angina results from progressive luminal narrowing. This is most commonly seen in the setting of restenosis after percutaneous coronary intervention (PCI) (see Chap. 38). However, angiographic[20] and atherectomy studies[60, 95] have demonstrated that many patients without previous intracoronary procedures have shown progressive luminal narrowing of the culprit vessel that is related to rapid cellular proliferation in the period preceding the onset of unstable angina.

SECONDARY UNSTABLE ANGINA. This form of unstable angina is precipitated by an imbalance in myocardial oxygen supply and demand caused by conditions extrinsic to the coronary arteries in patients with prior coronary stenosis and chronic stable angina.[8] This could occur by either an increased myocardial oxygen demand, a reduction in coronary blood flow, or both. Conditions that increase oxygen demand include tachycardia (e.g., supraventricular tachycardia or new-onset atrial fibrillation with rapid ventricular response), fever, thyrotoxicosis, hyperadrenergic states, and elevations of left ventricular afterload such as hypertension or aortic stenosis. Secondary unstable angina can also occur due to impaired oxygen delivery, as occurs in anemia, hypoxemia (e.g., due to pneumonia or congestive heart failure), and hyperviscosity states or hypotension.

Secondary angina appears to have a worse prognosis than primary unstable angina (see Table 36–1).[14]

CLINICAL PRESENTATION

The clinical profile of patients presenting with unstable angina differs from that of acute ST elevation MI. Unstable angina occurs more frequently in women, who comprise 30 to 45 percent of patients in studies of unstable angina,[96–98] compared with 25 to 30 percent of patients with NSTEMI and 20 percent of patients with STEMI.[96, 97, 99] In comparison to the latter, patients with unstable angina also have higher rates of prior MI, angina, previous coronary revascularization, and extracardiac vascular disease.[97, 99] Indeed, approximately 80 percent of patients with unstable angina have a prior history of coronary artery disease.

HISTORY AND PHYSICAL EXAMINATION. A description of "ischemic pain" is the hallmark of unstable angina (see Chap. 3). Chronic stable angina is usually described as a discomfort or pressure but rarely as a pain; it is usually located in the substernal region, but sometimes is near the epigastrium, and it frequently radiates to the anterior neck, left shoulder and left arm (see Chap. 37). In unstable angina, the discomfort, occurring either on exertion or at rest, is usually severe enough to be considered painful. The physical examination may be unremarkable or may support the diagnosis of cardiac ischemia (see Chap. 4) Signs that suggest unstable angina (or MI) with ischemia involving a larger fraction of the left ventricle are transient diaphoresis, pale cool skin, sinus tachycardia, a third or fourth heart sound, and basilar rales on lung examination. Rarely, the severity of left ventricular dysfunction causes hypotension.

ELECTROCARDIOGRAM (ECG). In unstable angina, ST segment depression (or transient ST segment elevation) and T wave changes occur in up to 50 percent of patients.[83, 100, 101] Three analyses have shown that in patients with the clinical presentation of unstable angina, *new* ST segment deviation, even of only 0.05 mV, is a specific and important measure of ischemia and prognosis.[100, 102, 103] T wave changes are sensitive but nonspecific of acute ischemia,

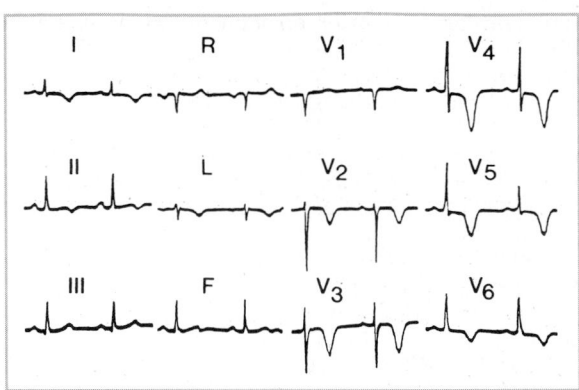

FIGURE 36–4. Electrocardiogram showing deep symmetrical anterolateral T wave inversion without ST segment deviation. Such findings are frequently associated with critical stenosis of the left anterior descending coronary artery and are a useful marker of a patient at high risk of subsequent death or myocardial infarction. (From Haines DE, Raabe DS, Gundel WD, Wackers FJ: Anatomic and prognostic significance of new T-wave inversion in unstable angina. Am J Cardiol 52:14–18, 1983.)

unless they are marked. Thus, transient, deep T wave inversions (≥ 0.3 mV) are considered to be relatively specific for acute ischemia, like ST segment deviations, and to signify high risk[7, 83] (Fig. 36–4). On the other hand, the presence of T wave inversions of 0.1 mV in patients with unstable angina may add little to the clinical history.[100, 103]

CONTINUOUS ECG MONITORING. Continuous ECG monitoring can be used for two purposes in unstable angina: (1) to detect arrhythmias in association with the acute episode and (2) to monitor the ST segments for evidence of recurrent ischemia.[7] Although life-threatening arrhythmias are rare in unstable angina, they may be more common among NSTEMI patients. Guidelines generally recommend continuous monitoring for at least 24 hours in patients hospitalized for UA/NSTEMI.[104, 105] When screening for ischemia, ST segment monitoring appears to be more sensitive than patient's symptoms, and it is a strong marker of adverse short- and long-term outcome.[21, 106–110] Evidence has shown that continuous 12-lead ST segment monitoring provides independent prognostic information even when it is used in conjunction with troponins and clinical variables.[110] Silent ischemia was more frequent and prolonged in patients with NSTEMI compared with those with unstable angina.[111]

CARDIAC MARKERS. Among patients presenting with symptoms consistent with unstable angina, the diagnosis of NSTEMI is made if there is biochemical evidence of myocardial necrosis, that is, positive CK-MB, troponin T or I, or potentially other markers of injury[7, 112] (see also Chap. 35).

The issue of what "cut point" to use for a positive troponin assay is currently being debated. One group has proposed two cut points: one "diagnostic" cut point to define myocardial infarction (derived from a comparison with CK-MB-defined MI) and a second, lower, "prognostic" cut point, generally the upper detectable limit of the assay or more specifically the 97.5th percentile of a normal population of subjects.[113] Each assay may have different cut points. As an example, at Brigham and Women's Hospital for the Dimension R $\times$ L assay for troponin I (Dade-Behring), the cut points are more than 1.5 ng/dl for the diagnosis of MI and 0.1 ng/dl or more for prognosis. Cut points are different for troponin T, and, to date, a cut point of 0.1 ng/dl or more has been used for both diagnosis and prognosis[114, 115]; however, a cut point for prognosis of as low as 0.01 ng/dl or more is being explored as the prognostic cut point with the third-generation assay.[116]

In patients with UA/NSTEMI, values greater than the upper (diagnostic) cut point indicate evidence of NSTEMI. Smaller elevations in troponin are believed also to signify

evidence of myocardial damage, although the extent of myocardial damage has not been documented in patients with the small elevations. The damage is believed to result from obstruction of small, distal coronary vessels, caused by microemboli of thrombus or of plaque debris from a more proximal lesion.[117] Smaller elevations in troponin values (e.g., troponin I between 0.1 and 1.5 ng/dl) have been shown to be of important prognostic value (see Diagnosis, p. 1237, and Risk Stratification, p. 1239) and may assist in the diagnosis of unstable angina when used in conjunction with the clinical history and ECG. Bedside tests can have either a positive versus negative result or provide a quantitative result. However, because each assay is different, each hospital needs to review the specific cut points defined by that assay.

CORONARY ARTERIOGRAPHIC FINDINGS. The extent of coronary artery disease among patients with UA/NSTEMI enrolled in TIMI IIIB was 15 percent with critical obstruction (> 60 percent luminal diameter stenosis) of three vessels, 30 percent with two-vessel disease, 40 percent with single-vessel disease, and 20 percent with no significant coronary stenosis.[101] Five to 10 percent of patients had left main stem stenosis greater than 50 percent.[100, 101, 118] Similar findings have been reported from registries of unselected UA/NSTEMI patients.[100, 118] Women and nonwhites with UA/NSTEMI have less extensive coronary disease than their counterparts,[96–98, 118, 119] whereas patients with NSTEMI have more extensive disease than those who present with unstable angina.[97]

Fifteen to 30 percent of patients who present with symptoms of unstable angina will have no significant coronary stenosis on coronary angiography.[96, 97, 100, 101, 118–120] Women and nonwhites comprise a larger proportion of such patients without epicardial coronary disease,[96, 97, 118–120] suggesting a difficulty in making a firm diagnosis of unstable angina in these groups and/or a different pathophysiological mechanism for their clinical presentation. Approximately one third of patients with unstable angina without a critical epicardial obstruction will have impaired coronary flow, suggesting a pathophysiological role for coronary microvascular dysfunction.[120] The short-term prognosis is excellent in this group of patients.

The culprit lesion in unstable angina typically exhibits an eccentric stenosis with scalloped or overhanging edges and a narrow neck.[4, 22, 65] These angiographic findings may represent disrupted atherosclerotic plaque, thrombus, or a combination.[121] Features suggesting thrombus include globular intraluminal masses with a rounded or polypoid shape[4] (see Fig. 36–2). "Haziness" of a lesion has been used as an angiographic marker of possible thrombus, but this finding is less specific. Patients with angiographically visualized thrombus have impaired coronary flow and worse clinical outcomes, compared with those without thrombus.[122, 123] Of interest, however, is that angiographically documented thrombus is present in only 20 to 40 percent of patients using a rigorous definition.[4, 123, 124] It is likely that the frequency is much greater and that angiography simply is not sensitive enough to detect all but the largest thrombi.

ANGIOSCOPY AND INTRAVASCULAR ULTRASOUND. Greater definition of the culprit lesion has been possible using angioscopy, where "white" (platelet-rich) thrombi are frequently observed as opposed to "red" thrombi, which are more often seen in patients with acute STEMI.[55, 56, 62, 64] Intravascular ultrasound examination identified more soft "echolucent" plaques and fewer calcified lesions among patients with unstable versus stable angina.[17]

OTHER LABORATORY TESTS. A chest roentgenogram may be useful in identifying pulmonary congestion or edema, which would be more likely in patients with NSTEMI involving a significant proportion of the left ventricle or in those with prior known left ventricular dysfunction.[7] The presence of congestion has been shown to confer an adverse prognosis.[125, 126]

Obtaining a serum cholesterol level is useful in identifying an important, treatable cause of coronary atherosclerosis. Because serum cholesterol levels begin to fall 24 hours after acute MI or unstable angina, it should be measured at the time of hospital admission. If only a later sample is obtained, but the value falls into a range that warrants long-term treatment (see Chap. 39) appropriate therapy can be initiated,[127–129] although the optimal timing of initiation of cholesterol-lowering therapy is being studied. Other circulating markers of increased risk are discussed later (see p. 1240). Evaluation for other secondary causes of unstable angina[8] may also be appropriate in selected patients (e.g., checking thyroid function in a patient who presents with unstable angina and a persistent tachycardia).

DIAGNOSIS OF UA/NSTEMI

The diagnosis of unstable angina is a clinical one, based on the patient's description of symptoms, as described earlier. A diagnosis of NSTEMI is made on the basis of a clinical history consistent with UA/NSTEMI and positive circulating cardiac markers[7] (see p. 1240 and Chap. 35). However, in the United States 6 to 7 million persons per year present to an emergency department (ED) with a complaint of chest pain or other symptoms suggestive of possible acute coronary syndrome, of whom only 20 to 25 percent have a final diagnosis of unstable angina or MI.[130, 131]

ASSESSING LIKELIHOOD OF CORONARY ARTERY DISEASE. Thus, the key first step in evaluation of patients with possible UA/NSTEMI is to determine the *likelihood* that coronary artery disease is the cause of the presenting symptoms.[7] From several large studies of patients presenting with chest pain to an ED,[100, 112, 130, 132–145] certain features portend a higher likelihood that the patient actually has unstable angina (Table 36–2). High likelihood exists among patients with prior coronary disease and/or with symptoms

▼ **TABLE 36–2. FEATURES ASSOCIATED WITH HIGHER LIKELIHOOD OF CORONARY ARTERY DISEASE AMONG PATIENTS PRESENTING WITH SYMPTOMS SUGGESTIVE OF UNSTABLE ANGINA**

History
Chest pain as chief complaint similar to prior ACS symptoms
Known history of coronary artery disease, myocardial infarction, percutaneous coronary intervention, coronary artery bypass graft
History of angina
Age > 60
Male gender
More than two major cardiac risk factors
Diabetes
Extracardiac vascular disease (carotid or peripheral)

Physical Examination
Pulmonary rales, hypotension
Transient mitral regurgitation
Diaphoresis

Electrocardiogram
New/presumably new ST deviation >0.05 mV
T wave inversion ≥0.1 mV
Q waves, left bundle branch block

Cardiac Markers
Elevated CK-MB, troponin I or T

Data supporting these factors come from references 100, 130, 132–145, and 412.

that are similar to a prior episode of MI or unstable angina.[130, 132–134, 136, 137] Elevation of cardiac markers or evidence of congestive heart failure or hemodynamic compromise also increase the likelihood of UA/NSTEMI.

CLINICAL AND ECG PREDICTOR RULES. Several groups have developed predictor rules to enhance clinical assessment of patients presenting with chest pain to the ED.[132–139] These "predictor rules" use clinical variables as well as ECG findings to define either MI,[132, 133, 135] any acute coronary syndrome (UA, NSTEMI, or STEMI),[134, 137–139] or subsequent cardiac complications regardless of initial diagnosis.[136] In general, all of these prediction rules can assist the clinician in assessing the likelihood of unstable angina or MI, but because of the numerous questions that are part of the assessment they are not often used in clinical practice. One algorithm, the Acute Cardiac Ischemia—Time Insensitive Prediction Instrument (ACI-TIPI) has been integrated into ECG devices and provides a likelihood of the patient having unstable angina or MI.[137, 139] This device evaluates the ECG for the presence of ST segment deviation, Q waves, and T wave inversion; and the operator enters into the computer the patient's age and gender and whether the patient's primary symptom was chest/left arm pain. The ACI-TIPI algorithm then computes a probability that the patient has an acute coronary syndrome, which is printed with the computer's standard interpretation of the ECG. This device was shown in a randomized trial to reduce unnecessary hospital and coronary care unit admissions and thus provide more cost-effective triage of patients.[139]

CARDIAC-SPECIFIC TROPONINS. The troponins can be used in two ways in the ED to evaluate patients with possible UA/NSTEMI: (1) to diagnose NSTEMI and (2) to define prognosis (i.e., the risk of developing recurrent cardiac ischemic events, including death, recurrent infarction, and recurrent severe ischemia requiring rehospitalization or urgent revascularization). In numerous studies, in patients admitted to the hospital with unstable angina[115, 141–155] (see p. 1240) as well as in the broad group of patients presenting to the ED with chest pain,[141, 143, 144] elevations of either troponin T or I have been shown to be very strong predictors of subsequent cardiac events.

However, "false-positive" troponin tests have been noted among series of patients presenting to the ED with chest pain.[156–158] In patients presenting to the ED with a complaint of chest pain, the clinical suspicion (and prevalence) of coronary artery disease is lower than it is in patients who are admitted to the hospital with unstable angina.[141, 143] Thus, the use of cardiac markers in the ED setting should be integrated with the clinical history and the ECG to arrive at an overall assessment of the likelihood of the patient having unstable angina.[141, 143, 159]

The timing of when blood samples should be obtained during initial evaluation of UA/NSTEMI has been examined in several studies. Most have included a "baseline" sample,[115, 146, 148, 149] which in studies conducted within clinical trials of unstable angina was at the time of randomization (i.e., at least several hours after the patient had presented to the ED). Recent large studies, in which the first blood sample is taken at the time of the patient's initial evaluation in the ED, have shown elevations of troponin T or I to be strongly predictive of subsequent cardiac complications.[141, 144] However, several recent studies have found incremental benefit by adding an additional one or two samples (generally 4, 8, or 16 hours later), with the second or third sample identifying a progressively greater number of patients who are positive and who are found to be high risk.[141, 143, 146, 151, 153]

Serial measurements are definitely needed among patients who present to the hospital within 6 hours from the onset of pain (which comprise the majority of patients[133, 141]) because of the release kinetics of troponins and CK-MB (see Chap. 35). In this early time window, myoglobin or CK-MB isoforms may be useful markers.[112, 160, 161] However, owing to low specificity of myoglobin for myocardial tissue, it should not be used in isolation but rather confirmed with a later sample analyzed for a more cardiac-specific marker (e.g., troponin or CK-MB).[7]

Emergency Department Chest Pain Pathways

The current approach to evaluating patients with chest pain (or related symptoms suggestive of UA/NSTEMI) incorporates four major diagnostic tools—clinical history, ECG, cardiac markers and provocative stress testing. They have three major objectives: (1) to diagnose infarction (using cardiac markers), (2) to evaluate for evidence of ischemia at rest (using symptoms, ECG, and/or continuous ECG monitoring), and (3) to evaluate for significant coronary artery disease (provocative stress testing).

Most pathways, including that shown in Figure 36–5, begin with a clinical assessment of the likelihood of the presenting symptoms being angina.[7] Patients with intermediate or high likelihood of ischemia (i.e., those with any feature shown in Table 36–2) are admitted to the hospital and treated with appropriate therapy for UA/NSTEMI (see p. 1241). On the other hand, patients, with atypical pain, not suggestive of ischemia, are discharged home with follow-up to their primary physicians. The remaining patients with a low likelihood of ischemia (i.e., without any of the factors shown in Table 36–2) are observed in the ED (or chest pain unit or related facility)[162, 163] with a standardized protocol.[164, 165]

These patients are monitored for recurrent rest pain and have a panel of markers (currently CK-MB, troponin I, and myoglobin) at arrival and 6 hours later. If the onset of pain was more than 6 hours before arrival, the baseline sample is frequently considered sufficient to "rule out" MI. If cardiac markers are positive or if the patient develops recur-

rent pain with ECG changes, the patient is admitted to the hospital and treated for UA/NSTEMI. If the patient remains pain free and the markers are negative, the patient goes on to exercise stress testing. For most patients, ECG stress testing is used, but for patients with fixed ECG abnormalities (e.g., left bundle branch block [LBBB]) perfusion imaging is employed and for those who cannot walk, pharmacological stress testing is used. If the clinical history suggests a very low likelihood of acute ischemia, patients are discharged home with subsequent outpatient stress testing. The goal is to carry out the testing and discharge (or admit) patients within 6 to 9 hours from ED arrival with follow-up to their primary physicians.

The safety of early exercise stress testing in patients presenting to the ED with chest pain was initially questioned, but several recent studies have demonstrated no adverse outcomes when applied to appropriately selected patients (as described earlier).[166–168]

CARDIAC IMAGING: SESTAMIBI PERFUSION IMAGING AND ECHOCARDIOGRAPHY. The use of additional imaging techniques is taking on increasing importance in the early diagnosis of patients presenting with suspected unstable angina and MI, especially when the ECG findings are obscured by LBBB or a paced rhythm. Sestamibi (see Chap. 9) has been useful for patients presenting with chest pain in the ED without diagnostic ECG, to discriminate patients with coronary artery disease (in whom perfusion defects are observed) from those with noncardiac chest pain (with normal perfusion scans).[169, 170] Sestamibi scanning (and echocardiography) also can provide information about left ventricular ejection fraction and wall motion that may be useful in triage decisions of the patients.

Some centers have utilized stress echocardiography in evaluating chest pain patients.[171–173] However, in two studies, little additional information was obtained in the *routine* use of echocardiography in all chest pain patients.[162, 174] Echocardiography performed while the patient is at rest in the ED has been used to evaluate whether a wall motion

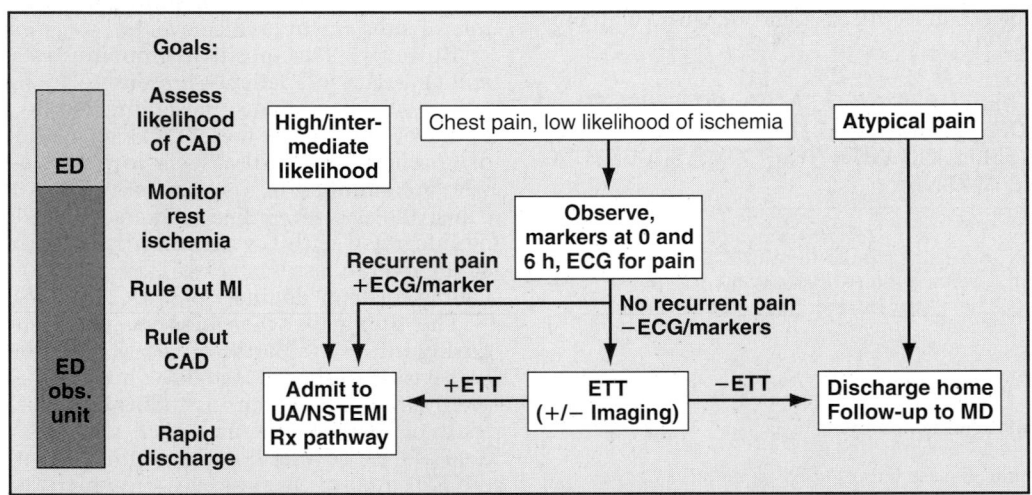

FIGURE 36–5. Brigham and Women's Hospital Emergency Department "Rule Out Myocardial Infarction (MI)" critical pathway. The approach to patients presenting with acute chest pain or other symptoms suggestive of possible UA/NSTEMI is first to assess the likelihood of coronary artery disease (CAD). Patients with high or intermediate likelihood are admitted to the hospital and treated according to the UA/NSTEMI pathway. Those with clearly atypical chest pain are discharged home. Patients with a low likelihood enter the pathway and are observed in a monitored bed in the emergency department (ED) observation unit over a period of 6 hours, and 12-lead electrocardiograms (ECGs) are performed if the patient has recurrent chest discomfort. A panel of cardiac markers (e.g., troponin I, CK-MB, and myoglobin) are drawn at baseline and 6 hours later. If the patient develops recurrent pain, has ST segment or T wave changes, or has positive cardiac markers, he or she is admitted to the hospital and treated for UA/NSTEMI. If the patient has negative markers and no recurrence of pain, he or she is sent for exercise treadmill testing (ETT), with imaging reserved for patients with abnormal baseline ECGs (e.g., left bundle branch block or left ventricular hypertrophy with ST-T wave abnormalities). If the test is positive in a patient presenting with acute chest pain, the patient is admitted; if the test is negative, the patient is discharged home with follow-up to his or her primary physician.

abnormality is present, to help in establishing (or excluding) the diagnosis of ischemic heart disease,[175] and in determining prognosis.[176] However, cost issues have precluded widespread *routine* use of echocardiography, but most centers use echocardiography selectively (i.e., in patients with LBBB or paced rhythms or in patients with suspected valvular disease and/or aortic dissection, especially transesophageal echocardiography for the latter).[177–179]

One study found improved sensitivity of perfusion imaging compared with stress echocardiography or ECG stress testing,[180] whereas another study found similar overall diagnostic capabilities of the two imaging modalities[181] (see also Chap. 13). Both of these modalities can assess global left ventricular function, a powerful determinant of subsequent prognosis after MI[182, 183] (and presumably after unstable angina as well), and this may be important in triaging medical therapy among patients with confirmed MI or unstable angina (e.g., angiotensin-converting enzyme [ACE] inhibitors).[184] However, because most patients presenting to EDs do not have coronary artery disease,[130, 131] such widespread assessment of left ventricular function would likely not be cost effective.

CHEST PAIN CENTERS. Many hospitals have developed "chest pain centers" within or closely related to the ED in which patients with suspected acute coronary syndromes can be triaged. Standardized protocols for acute STEMI can be implemented, thereby reducing door-to-needle time[185] (see Chap. 35), and rapid "rule out MI" protocols for low-risk patients with chest pain can be carried out.[165, 186] Use of such chest pain centers or specialized ED units can reduce by 20 to 30 percent the number of patients who require admission to the hospitals[162, 163, 170, 174, 187] and randomized trials.[163, 174] One multicenter study found that the implementation of a chest pain unit significantly decreased the rate of hospital admission and overall costs, despite an overall increase in the number of patients who underwent "rule-out MI" evaluation instead of being discharged home directly.[187] Thus, there is emerging evidence that chest pain centers or specific protocols/critical pathways in the ED can improve the efficiency of health care for this large population of patients.

Natural History

The outcome of patients with UA/NSTEMI is generally favorable when compared with acute STEMI,[96, 97, 99] although there are several subgroups of patients who can have *higher* mortality (see later). In the TIMI III Registry of patients with UA/NSTEMI, 21 percent "ruled in" for an NSTEMI at the time of admission; 62 percent underwent cardiac catheterization, 22 percent angioplasty, and 13 percent coronary bypass surgery. By 42 days, mortality was 2.4 percent and a new or recurrent MI occurred in 2.9 percent of patients. Within clinical trials, in which inclusion criteria select higher risk patients (see later), rates of death by 30 days ranged from 3.5 to 4.5 percent and rates of new or recurrent MI ranged from 6 to 12 percent.[80, 81, 83]

RISK STRATIFICATION

As already noted, unstable angina is a heterogeneous condition that ranges from one with an excellent outcome with modest adjustments in therapeutic regimen to one in which the risk of death or MI is high and intensive (and expensive) treatment is needed. Evidence is available from recent large clinical trials for important subgroups of patients who are at higher risk of adverse outcomes (Table 36–3).[7] Furthermore, these groups appear to derive greater benefit from more aggressive antithrombotic therapy (see p. 1246). Clinical predictors can be also used to assist in triage of unstable angina patients to the coronary care unit versus a moni-

History
Advanced age (> 65 years)
Diabetes mellitus
Post-myocardial infarction angina
Prior peripheral vascular disease
Prior cerebrovascular disease

Clinical Presentation
Braunwald Class II or III (acute or subacute rest pain)
Braunwald Class B (secondary unstable angina)
Heart failure/hypotension

Electrocardiogram
New/ST segment deviation ≥ 0.05 mV
New T wave inversion ≥ 0.3 mV
Left bundle branch block

Cardiac Markers
Increased troponin T or I or CK-MB
Increased C-reactive protein (CRP)

Angiogram
Thrombus

tored bed.[5, 7, 104] Patients determined to be at high risk should be admitted to the coronary care unit, whereas those with intermediate or lower risk could be admitted to a monitored bed on a cardiac step-down unit.

CLINICAL VARIABLES. The Braunwald classification of unstable angina[8] (see Table 36–1) has been shown in several studies to be useful in identifying high-risk patients.[12–14] In the multicenter TIMI III Registry, which included 3318 consecutive patients with UA/NSTEMI, this classification was an important predictor of rate of death or MI to 1 year—both by the severity of the unstable angina and by the clinical circumstances in which it occurred (see Table 36–1). High-risk groups of patients with unstable angina are those with acute rest pain, those with post-MI unstable angina, and those with secondary unstable angina.[14]

HIGH-RISK SUBGROUPS. Increasing age has been shown to be associated with a significant increase in adverse outcomes in patients with UA/NSTEMI.[100, 188] Diabetic patients with UA/NSTEMI are at approximately 50 percent higher risk than nondiabetics (see Chap. 63).[189, 190] Patients with extracardiac vascular disease (i.e., those with either cerebrovascular disease or peripheral arterial vascular disease) also appear to have approximately 50 percent higher rates of death or recurrent ischemic events compared with patients without previous peripheral or cerebrovascular disease, even after controlling for other differences in baseline characteristics.[191] Patients who present with evidence of congestive heart failure (Killip Class > II) have increased risk of death in the setting of unstable angina.[126, 192] In addition, patients who develop recurrent ischemia after initial presentation have also been found to be at increased risk.[83, 193]

PRIOR ASPIRIN THERAPY. Another group of patients with UA/NSTEMI that has been identified as high risk are those who present with acute ischemia despite chronic aspirin therapy. These patients are sometimes termed "aspirin failures," and a subset of these patients may actually represent "aspirin resistance"[194]; however, the pathophysiology of this observation is not fully defined and is actively being studied.[195] This group represents an increasing proportion of patients (from 60 to 80 percent of patients in recent trials) and, among patients not randomized to a glycoprotein IIb/IIIa inhibitor, their subsequent rate of death or MI was 50 percent higher than those not previously taking aspirin.[196, 197] Treatment with a glycoprotein IIb/IIIa inhibitor appeared to decrease this risk (see p. 1246). In the OPUS-TIMI 16 trial, higher event rates were again observed in prior aspirin users, but this was not an independent predictor of mortality or recurrent cardiac events.[198] Thus, the development of UA/NSTEMI despite aspirin therapy is a useful clinical marker of high risk.

RISK ASSESSMENT BY ECG. The admission ECG is very useful in predicting long-term adverse outcomes. In the TIMI III Registry of patients with UA/NSTEMI, independent predictors of 1-year death or MI included LBBB (risk ratio 2.8) and ST segment deviation of 0.05 mV or greater (risk ratio 2.45) (both $p < 0.001$).[100] The presence of 0.05 mV or more ST segment depression on the admission ECG has also been reported to be an independent determinant of 4-year mortality, with a gradient of increasing risk with increasing ST segment depression.[103] In contrast, the presence of T wave changes of 0.1 mV or more was associated with a modest[103] or no increase in subsequent death or MI compared with patients without ST or T wave changes.[100] Similar findings were observed in predicting 30-day and 6-month outcomes in the Global Use of Strategies to Open Occluded Coronary Arteries (GUSTO) IIb study, in which the presence of ST segment deviation greater than 0.5 mm confers a worse prognosis than T wave changes.[102]

CK-MB AND THE TROPONINS. Patients with NSTEMI have a worse long-term prognosis than those with unstable angina.[73, 101, 199–204] However, the high-risk population extends beyond those who have positive CK-MB fractions, the traditional definition of MI. Studies have found that patients with "microinfarction"[205] or "minor myocardial damage"[206, 207] (i.e., those not meeting usual criteria for MI of elevated CK and CK-MB but with elevated troponin T,[115, 144, 146, 147, 149, 151, 154, 155, 208] troponin I,[148, 150, 152, 155, 209] myosin light chains,[147] or mildly elevated CK-MB[210, 211]) are a high-risk population.

Patients with elevated troponin values are at much higher risk of subsequent cardiac complications, including mortality[115, 144, 146–155, 208] (Fig. 36–6). This has been observed even in patients without CK-MB elevation.[146, 148, 153, 212] Beyond just a positive versus negative test result, there is a linear relationship between the level of troponin T or I in the blood and subsequent risk of death—the higher the troponin, the higher the mortality risk (see Fig. 36–6B). Similar results have been obtained using a bedside rapid assay for troponin T, in which time to positivity is a semi-quantitative measure of serum troponin T and related to increased mortality.[144, 212] Thus, troponin T and I are very useful not only in diagnosing infarction[205] (see p. 1237 and Chap. 35) but also in risk assessment in patients presenting with acute UA/NSTEMI and in "targeting" therapies to high-risk patients (see p. 1241).

C-REACTIVE PROTEIN. Additional markers also appear to be useful in assessing patients with UA/NSTEMI, among which C-reactive protein (CRP) is very promising. Elevated CRP has been related to increased risk of death, MI, and/or need for urgent revascularization.[40–43, 213–216] In TIMI 11A, 14-day mortality for patients with an elevated CRP ($\geq$ 1.55 mg/dl, the 99th percentile of normal subjects) was 5.6 percent compared with 0.3 percent for patients without an elevated CRP (Fig. 36–7A).[43] Even among patients with negative troponin T at baseline, who had a 14-day mortality of 1.5 percent overall, CRP was able to discriminate a high- and low-risk group: mortality for patients with an elevated CRP was 5.8 percent versus 0.4 percent for patients without elevated CRP (see Fig. 36–7A).[43] When using both CRP and troponin T, mortality could be stratified from 0.4 percent for patients with both markers negative, to 4.7 percent if either CRP or troponin were positive, to 9.1 percent if both were positive (see Fig. 36–7B).[43] Thus, the combination of a necrosis marker (troponin T or I) and an inflammatory marker (CRP) provides independent and powerful prognostic information in patients with acute coronary syn-

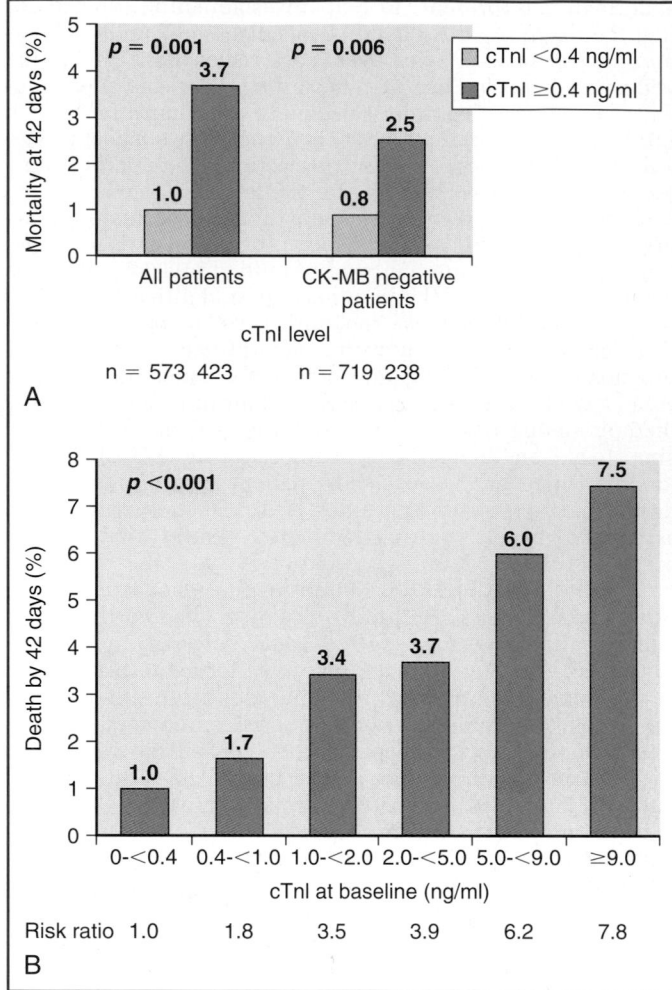

FIGURE 36–6. TIMI IIIB. *A,* The relationship of a positive versus negative troponin I versus 42-day mortality in the total group (left) and those with negative creatine kinase (CK)-MB (right). *B,* A direct relationship was observed between increasing levels of troponin I and a higher 42-day mortality. cTnI = cardiac specific troponin I; Neg = negative. (Adapted from Antman EM, Tanasijevic MJ, Thompson B, et al: Cardiac-specific troponin I levels to predict the risk of mortality in patients with acute coronary syndromes. N Engl J Med 335:1342–1349, 1996, with permission of the New England Journal of Medicine.)

dromes.[43, 214, 216] In another recent study, CRP was not predictive of in-hospital events but was a powerful predictor of 30-day and 6-month events.[215]

CRP measured at the time of hospital discharge has been found to be a very strong predictor of outcome to 3 to 12 months.[217, 218] Other inflammatory markers have offered consistent evidence of an association between systemic inflammation and recurrent adverse events, including serum amyloid A,[219] interleukin-6,[220] CD40 ligand,[221] CD4+ CD28null.[222] These studies indicate that inflammation is related to the instability of patients and an increased risk of recurrent cardiac events.

COMBINED RISK ASSESSMENT SCORES. An emerging approach to unstable angina is to use a comprehensive approach to risk assessment. As illustrated in Figure 36–8, patients with symptoms of unstable angina fall on a spectrum. ST segment deviation or deep T wave inversion defines high-risk patients. CK-MB can be used to define NSTEMI. Troponins are more sensitive markers of necrosis and extend the population that is identified as high risk. Finally, even among patients who are troponin negative, CRP can further identify high-risk patients.

By integrating this approach, comprehensive risk scores

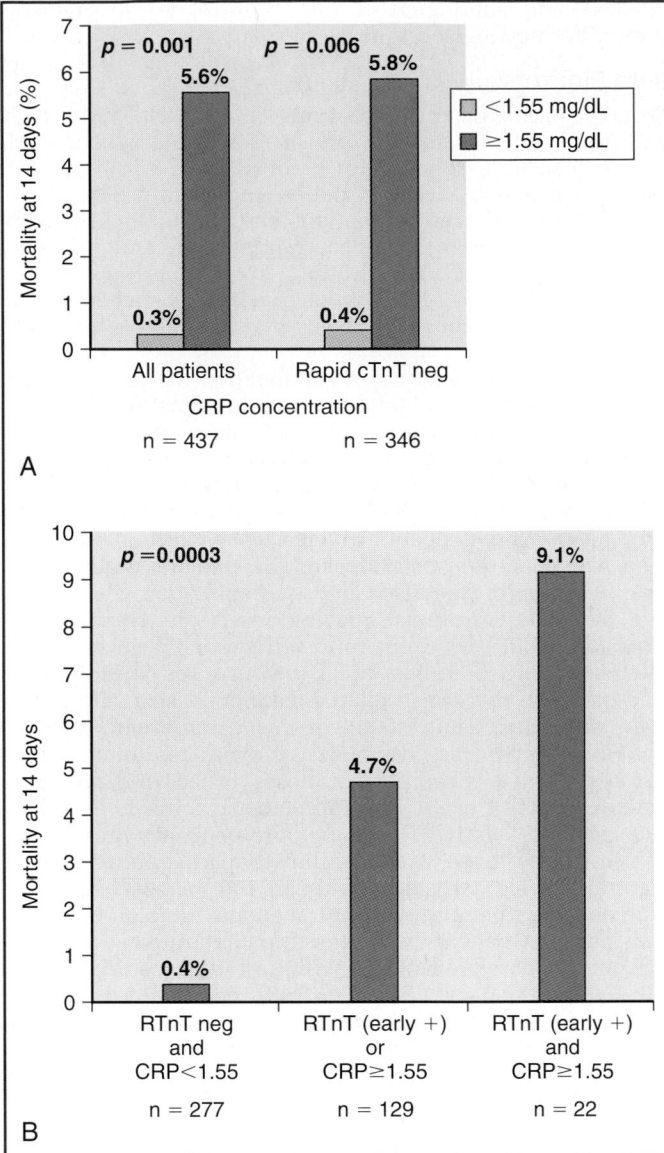

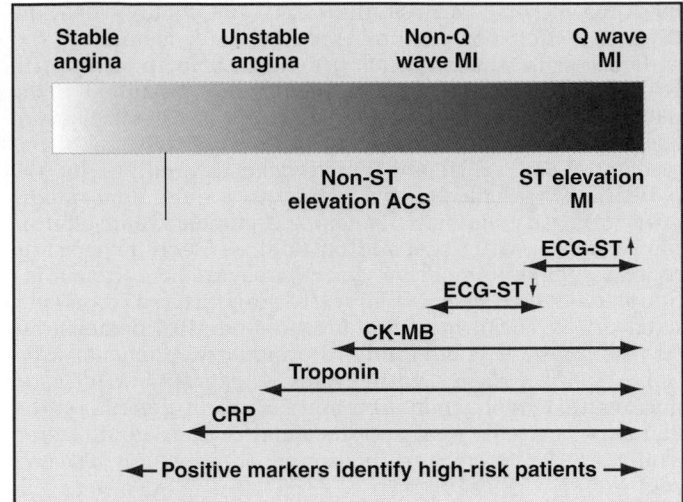

FIGURE 36–8. Risk stratification across the spectrum of acute coronary syndromes (ACS). Positive tests identify higher risk patients. This summary of the risk stratification tools currently available shows that among the broad spectrum of patients with ischemic heart disease, the electrocardiogram (ECG), cardiac markers creatine kinase (CK-MB) and troponin, and C-reactive protein (CRP) can identify increasing proportions of the overall group as being at high risk of recurrent cardiac events or death. For the ECG, markers of high risk include ST depression of 0.05 mV or more. The newer markers troponins and CRP identify a higher percentage of patients than did CK-MB, the only marker used in the mid 1990s.

FIGURE 36–7. TIMI 11A. *A,* Relationship of C-reactive protein (CRP) vs. 14-day mortality in all patients with UA/NSTEMI (left) and those with negative baseline troponin T (right). *B,* Use of both troponin T and CRP to predict mortality. (An "early positive" rapid bedside troponin T assay [RTnT] was defined as positive ≤ 10 minutes.) These data demonstrate that an elevated CRP (the high-sensitivity assay was used in this study) is a potent predictor of increased mortality and extends beyond the prognostic information that troponin provides. CRP is a marker of inflammation, whereas the troponins are markers of myocardial necrosis, and these data demonstrate the complementary information provided by these two markers in patients with UA/NSTEMI. Early + = early positive; neg = negative. (From Morrow DA, Rifai N, Antman EM, et al: C-reactive protein is a potent predictor of mortality independently and in combination with troponin T in acute coronary syndromes: A TIMI 11A substudy. J Am Coll Cardiol 31:1460–1465, 1998.)

can be developed using both clinical variables, as well as variables from the ECG and initial serum cardiac markers. One such analysis used three simple markers: age 65 years or older, ST segment deviation of 0.5 mm or more, and positive serum cardiac markers (either CK-MB or troponin). When these three parameters were used, the risk of death, MI, or urgent revascularization at 43 days rose from 14.5 percent for none or one of these risks to 19.3 percent and 27.3 percent for patients with one, two or all three factors ($p < 0.0001$).[223] The more detailed TIMI risk score was developed using multivariate analysis, which identified seven independent risk factors: age 65 years or older; more than three risk factors for coronary artery disease; documented coronary artery disease at catheterization; ST segment deviation of 0.5 mm or more, more than two episodes of angina in the last 24 hours, aspirin within prior week, and elevated cardiac markers. Use of this scoring system was able to risk-stratify patients across a 10-fold gradient of risk, from 4.7 to 40.9 percent ($p < 0.001$).[224]

MEDICAL THERAPY

TREATMENT GOALS. The treatment objectives for patients with UA/NSTEMI are focused on stabilizing and "passivating" the acute coronary lesion, treatment of residual ischemia, and long-term secondary prevention. Antithrombotic therapy (e.g., aspirin, low or unfractionated molecular weight heparin, glycoprotein IIb/IIIa inhibitors, and clopidogrel) is used to prevent further thrombosis and allow endogenous fibrinolysis to dissolve the thrombus and reduce the degree of coronary stenosis. Antithrombotic therapy is continued long term to reduce the risk of developing future events and/or to prevent progression to complete occlusion of the coronary artery. Antiischemic therapies (e.g., beta blockers, nitrates, and/or calcium antagonists) are used primarily to reduce myocardial oxygen demand. Coronary revascularization is frequently needed to treat recurrent or residual ischemia that occurs despite the medical therapy. After the acute event is stabilized, the many factors that led up to the event need to be reversed (i.e., treatment of atherosclerotic risk factors such as hypercholesterolemia, hypertension, and cessation of smoking, each of which contributes to stabilization of the cholesterol-laden plaque and healing of the endothelium).

General Measures

The approach to the patient with UA/NSTEMI generally includes admission to a monitored bed. In these settings, continuous ECG monitoring (i.e., telemetry) is used to evaluate for cardiac arrhythmias and potentially for new asymptomatic ST deviations as markers of ischemia.[7]

Bed rest is usually prescribed initially for patients with UA/NSTEMI.[7] Ambulation as tolerated is permitted if the patient has been stable hemodynamically without recurrent chest discomfort for at least 12 to 24 hours. Means of improving the physical and emotional surroundings for the patient, such as placing the patient in a quiet atmosphere, away from any emotionally taxing arguments, and offering physician's reassurance and/or mild sedation may act to reduce sympathetic drive and thereby reduce ischemia.[7] Supplemental oxygen is frequently administered to patients with UA/NSTEMI, but there are no studies to demonstrate its usefulness. It is advisable to provide supplemental oxygen only to patients with cyanosis, extensive rales, and documented hypoxemia. Oxygen saturation determined by oximetry is useful with supplemental oxygen administered if the arterial oxygen saturation declines below 92 percent.[7]

Relief of chest pain is an initial goal of treatment. In patients with persistent pain despite therapy with nitrates and beta blockers (see later), morphine sulfate, 1 to 5 mg intravenously, is recommended. Contraindications include hypotension or prior allergy (meperidine can be substituted for the patients who are allergic to morphine). With careful blood pressure monitoring, repeat doses can be administered every 5 to 30 minutes. Morphine may act both as an analgesic and anxiolytic, but its venodilatory effects may produce beneficial hemodynamic effects by reducing preload. The latter is especially useful in the setting of acute pulmonary edema. If hypotension develops after administration of morphine, supine positioning or intravenous saline should restore blood pressure and pressors are rarely needed. If respiratory depression develops, naloxone (0.4 to 2.0 mg) may be given.

Nitrates (see also Chap. 37)

Nitrates are endothelium-independent vasodilators that both increase myocardial blood flow by coronary vasodilatation and reduce myocardial oxygen demand. The latter effect is produced by venodilation leading to reduced myocardial preload and reduction in ventricular wall stress, thereby reducing myocardial oxygen demand. Nitrates should initially be given sublingually or by buccal spray (0.3 to 0.6 mg) if the patient is experiencing ischemic pain. If pain persists after three sublingual tablets (or buccal sprays) each 5 minutes apart and initiation of beta blockade, intravenous nitroglycerin (5 to 10 μg/min using nonabsorbing tubing) is recommended.[7] The rate of the infusion may be increased by 10 μg/min every 3 to 5 minutes until symptoms are relieved or systolic blood pressure falls by more than 30 mm Hg or to below 100 mm Hg. Although there is no absolute maximum dose, a dose of 200 μg/min is generally used as a ceiling. Contraindications to use of nitrates are hypotension or the use of sildenafil (Viagra) within the previous 24 hours.[225]

Topical or oral nitrates can be used if the episode of pain has resolved, or they may replace intravenous nitroglycerin if the patient has been pain free for 12 to 24 hours.[7] Dosing of nitrates depends on the formulation (see Table 37-4), but dosing should attempt to have an 8- to 10-hour nitrate-free interval to avoid the development of tolerance.

The effect of nitrates on mortality was evaluated in the Gruppo Italiano per lo Studio della Sopravvivenza nell'Infarto Miocardico (GISSI)-3 and International Study of Infarct Survival (ISIS)-4 trials for patients with suspected MI (both STEMI and NSTEMI).[226, 227] No benefit on mortality was observed in the overall population or in the subgroup of patients with NSTEMI. Consequently, the goal of nitrate therapy is relief of pain; chronic nitrate therapy can frequently be tapered off in the long-term management of patients, with primary therapy being aspirin and beta

blockers and sublingual or buccal nitroglycerin given as needed for new episodes of pain.

Beta Blockers (see also Chap. 37)

Several placebo-controlled trials in UA/NSTEMI have shown benefit of beta blockers in reducing subsequent MI and/or recurrent ischemia.[228-233] In patients with acute MI (in studies which included patients with both STEMI and NSTEMI in the prethrombolytic era), beta blockers were shown to reduce infarct size, reinfarction, and mortality (see Chap. 35).[234-237] In addition, in subgroup analyses of patients with NSTEMI in three trials, the benefits of beta blockers (intravenous followed by oral) have been observed.[237-240]

Thus, beta blockers are recommended for patients with UA/NSTEMI who do not have contraindications to these agents (e.g., bradycardia, advanced atrioventricular block, persistent hypotension, pulmonary edema, history of bronchospasm).[104, 105] A reduced ejection fraction is no longer a contradiction to beta blockade, and, indeed, such patients may derive added benefit given the benefits on mortality seen with long-term beta blockade in patients with congestive heart failure (see also Chaps. 18 and 21).[241-243] If ischemia and chest pain is ongoing, early intravenous beta blockade should be used, followed by oral beta blockade. The choice of which beta blocker to use can be individualized based on the drug's pharmacokinetics, cost, and physician familiarity (Table 37-6). However, those with intrinsic sympathomimetic activity (ISA), such as pindolol, should not be selected. Examples of doses tested in large trials include atenolol (5–10 mg intravenous bolus followed by 100 mg orally daily)[237] and metoprolol (5 mg intravenous boluses, three given 2 to 5 minutes apart, followed by 50 mg orally twice daily titrated up to 100 mg twice daily).[244] Commencing therapy with intravenous esmolol could be considered in patients with possible contraindications (e.g., a history of possible asthma) with an initial loading dose of 0.5 mg/kg/min over 1 minute, followed by a 0.05 mg/kg/min infusion, with repeat loading doses and increases in the infusion of 0.05 mg/kg/min to achieve the desired heart rate.[245]

Calcium Channel Blockers (see also Chap. 37)

These drugs have vasodilatory effects and lower blood pressure, and some also slow heart rate (Table 37-8). They may be used in patients who have persistent or recurrent symptoms but are currently recommended only in patients who have persistent ischemia after treatment with full-dose nitrates and beta blockers have been used or in patients with contraindications to beta blockade.[7] Such patients should be treated with heart rate–slowing calcium channel blockers (e.g., diltiazem or verapamil).[104, 105] Oral doses of diltiazem and verapamil range from 30 to 90 mg four times daily to 360 mg once daily of the long-acting preparations.

In the Diltiazem Reinfarction Study, involving 576 patients with non-Q-wave MI, diltiazem reduced recurrent MI from 9.3 percent on placebo to 5.2 percent on diltiazem.[201] A more recent pilot study using intravenous diltiazem[246] and a larger clinical trial using long-acting diltiazam[247, 248] in patients after thrombolytic therapy found trends toward benefit of diltiazem versus placebo. In the Danish Study Group on Verapamil in Myocardial Infarction (DAVIT) II trial of patients with suspected MI or unstable angina, of whom nearly half did not have confirmed MI, verapamil tended to reduce recurrent MI or death.[249] However, meta-analyses have found no beneficial effect of the calcium antagonist drugs as a class in reducing mortality or subsequent infarction.[229, 250, 251] One overview did suggest benefit of verapamil alone.[252]

Importantly, in patients with acute MI with left ventricular dysfunction or congestive heart failure, a harmful effect of diltiazem has been observed.[253] Nifedipine, which does not lower heart rate, has been shown to increase the incidence of adverse events in patients with acute MI when not coadministered with a beta blocker.[254, 255] In contrast, no harm was observed in one study with verapamil in patients with congestive heart failure, all of whom were treated with ACE inhibitors.[256] Similarly, no harm with long-term treatment with amlodipine[257] or felodipine[258] was observed in patients with documented left ventricular dysfunction and coronary artery disease, indicating that these vasoselective calcium antagonists may be safely used in patients with unstable angina with left ventricular dysfunction.

In summary, calcium antagonists should be used in patients with UA/NSTEMI if needed for recurrent ischemia despite beta blockade or in patients in whom beta blockade is contraindicated (e.g., bronchospasm);[7] diltiazem should be avoided in patients with left ventricular dysfunction and/or congestive heart failure.

Angiotensin-Converting Enzyme Inhibitors (see also Chap. 29)

ACE inhibitors have been shown to be beneficial in many settings, including patients *post* MI who have demonstrated either impaired left ventricular function (ejection fraction < 40 percent)[184] or congestive heart failure.[259] The GISSI-3, ISIS-4, and Chinese Captopril trials showed a 0.5 percent absolute mortality benefit of early (initiated within 24 hours) ACE inhibition in patients with acute MI.[226, 227, 260] However, in the ISIS-4 study, no benefit was observed in patients without ST segment elevation. Thus, *short-term* ACE inhibition does not appear to confer any benefit for patients with unstable angina or NSTEMI without impaired left ventricular function.

On the other hand, *long-term* use of ACE inhibition is applicable to several groups of patients: those with (1) left ventricular dysfunction,[184] (2) congestive heart failure,[259] and (3) based on recent evidence from the Heart Outcomes Prevention Evaluation (HOPE) trial, it may apply to most patients with all forms of ischemic heart disease, including UA/NSTEMI.[261] Recurrent MI and the need for revascularization were reduced with ACE inhibitors in the Survival and Ventricular Enlargement (SAVE) and Studies of Left Ventricular Dysfunction (SOLVD) trials, suggesting an antiischemic effect of this class of agents,[262, 263] which was confirmed in the HOPE trial (see also Chap. 39).

Lipid-Lowering Therapy (see also Chap. 33)

Long-term treatment with lipid-lowering therapy, especially with statins, has been shown to be beneficial in patients after acute MI and unstable angina[127-129] (see also Chap. 39). In the Scandinavian Simvastatin Survival Study (4S), carried out in hypercholesterolemic patients with a history of MI *or* unstable angina, mortality was reduced by 30 percent ($p = 0.0003$) and coronary deaths were significantly reduced by 42 percent.[128] In addition, recurrent MI was significantly reduced by 37 percent ($p < 0.001$), coronary revascularization by 37 percent ($p < 0.0001$), and rehospitalization for acute cardiovascular disease by 26 percent ($p < 0.001$).[128, 264] The cost savings of these reductions offset nearly all the cost of the simvastatin therapy. Thus, the cost-effectiveness is very favorable: cost per year of life saved ranged from $3,800 for 70-year-old men with a cholesterol level of 309 mg/dl to $27,400 for 35-year-old women with a cholesterol level of 213 mg/dl.[265]

The Cholesterol and Recurrent Events (CARE) and Long-Term Intervention with Pravastatin in Ischaemic Disease (LIPID) studies extended these benefits to patients with average cholesterol levels (i.e., <240 mg/dl), which constitute the majority of patients with acute coronary syndromes. In CARE, treatment with pravastatin for an average of 5 years led to a 24 percent reduction in cardiovascular death or MI ($p = 0.003$), with similar reductions in need for revascularization and stroke.[127] Interestingly, no benefit was observed in the subgroup of patients with a baseline low-density lipoprotein (LDL) of less than 125 mg/dl. The LIPID trial enrolled more than 9000 patients with a history (at least 3 months prior) of MI or unstable angina. In the prespecified subgroup of more than 3200 patients with unstable angina, pravastatin therapy led to a significant 26 percent reduction in total mortality ($p = 0.004$).[129]

Thus, long-term cholesterol lowering has been shown to have dramatic benefits in secondary prevention after infarction[266-268] and is very cost effective. For patients with UA/NSTEMI, testing the cholesterol level is critical. To ensure that all patients would benefit from cholesterol lowering, as demonstrated in these three trials, the total cholesterol and LDL cholesterol levels (calculated or direct measurement) should be obtained and treatment initiated with a statin drug if the LDL is more than 125 mg/dl (as suggested by the CARE and LIPID results). The National Cholesterol Education Panel recommends diet therapy if the LDL is higher than 100 mg/dl and drug therapy if the LDL is 130 mg/dl or more, with a target of reducing LDL to 100 mg/dl or less.[267] The timing of the blood sample is ideally in the first 24 hours after admission, because cholesterol levels fall with acute illness. However, cholesterol should be measured at some time during admission, because if it is high, therapy is warranted. Because treatment with statin drugs was associated with the previously mentioned benefits on mortality and cardiovascular morbidity, these are the current first-line lipid-lowering drugs. Additional or alternate therapy is also warranted according to the National Cholesterol Education Program (see also Chap. 39).[267]

Antithrombotic Therapy in UA/NSTEMI

Aspirin (see also Chap. 62)

Several trials have demonstrated clear beneficial effects of aspirin in patients with UA/NSTEMI, with a more than 50 percent reduction in the risk of death or MI[71-74] (Fig. 36-9). Thus, aspirin has a dramatic effect in reducing adverse clinical events both early and late in the course of treatment of UA/NSTEMI and is primary therapy for these patients (see Chap. 64).

The dose of aspirin in the four randomized trials (Fig. 36-9) ranged from 75 mg to 1300 mg/d, and each trial showed a roughly 50 percent reduction in death or MI.[71-74] Thus, there does not appear to be a dose response in efficacy of aspirin. In the International Study of Infarct Survival (ISIS)-2, a dose of 160 mg/d was shown to be associated with a mortality benefit, so this dose is the minimum initial dose recommended.[269] For safety (e.g., gastrointestinal bleeding), the rate of bleeding appears to be slightly higher with higher doses, and thus a dose of 75 to 81 mg/d could be an appropriate dose for long-term therapy, although major bleeding is relatively rare (<1 percent) even at a dose of 325 mg/d.[270]

Absolute contraindications for aspirin therapy are few but include documented aspirin allergy (e.g., asthma), active bleeding, or a known platelet disorder. In patients who had reported dyspepsia or other gastrointestinal symptoms with long-term aspirin therapy (i.e., intolerance), this would not be expected to be an acute problem of in-hospital treatment, and aspirin therapy is recommended, at least for the short term.

Clopidogrel and Ticlopidine (see also Chap. 62)

Clopidogrel, like its sister drug ticlopidine, is a thienopyridine derivative that inhibits platelet aggregation, increases bleeding time, and reduces blood viscosity by inhibiting ADP action on platelet receptors. *Ticlopidine* was studied in a randomized trial of patients with unstable angina involving 652 patients. The control group did not receive aspirin because at the time of protocol design it was not routinely used to treat unstable angina. At 6-month follow-

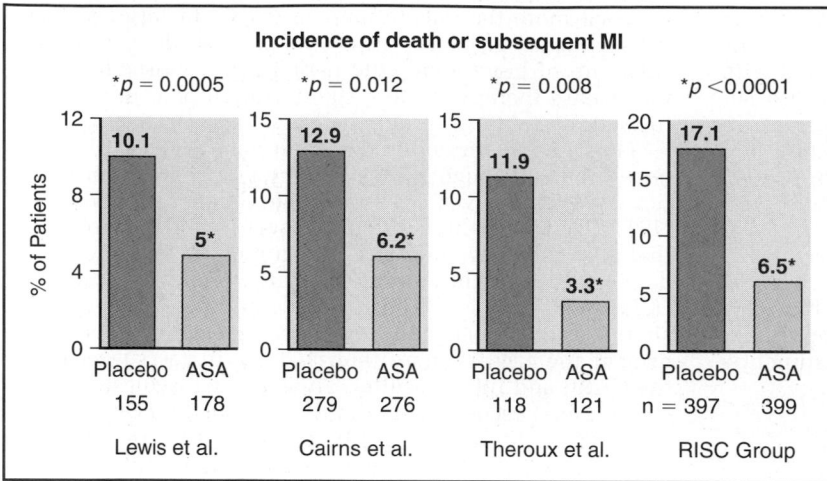

Incidence of death or subsequent MI

FIGURE 36-9. Four randomized trials showing the benefit of aspirin (ASA) in UA/NSTEMI. In UA/NSTEMI, the incidence of death or myocardial infarction was reduced by over 50 percent in each of the four trials. The doses of aspirin in the four trials were 325 mg, 1300 mg, 650 mg, and 75 daily, respectively, indicating no difference in efficacy for aspirin across these doses. (Data from Lewis HD, Davis JW, Archibald DG, et al: Protective effects of aspirin against acute myocardial infarction and death in men with unstable angina. N Engl J Med 309:396–403, 1983; Cairns JA, Gent M, Singer J, et al: Aspirin, sulfinpyrazone, or both in unstable angina. N Engl J Med 313:1369–1375, 1985; Theroux P, Ouimet H, McCans J, et al: Aspirin, heparin or both to treat unstable angina. N Engl J Med 319:1105–1111, 1988; and The RISC Group: Risk of myocardial infarction and death during treatment with low dose aspirin and intravenous heparin in men with unstable coronary artery disease. Lancet 336:827–830, 1990.)

up, ticlopidine led to a significant 46 percent reduction in vascular death or nonfatal MI.[271] Of note, there was no difference in the number of events over the first 10 days, consistent with the delayed onset of the antiplatelet effect of ticlopidine. Thus, ticlopidine appears to be comparable to aspirin for secondary prevention of events post UA/NSTEMI. Ticlopidine has also been demonstrated to be effective in combination with aspirin for prevention of thrombosis and recurrent ischemic events in patients undergoing coronary stent implantation, a portion of whom have recently suffered UA/NSTEMI (see also Chap. 38).[272-274] However, ticlopidine is associated with neutropenia and thrombocytopenia in approximately 1 percent of patients, and quite rarely with thrombotic thrombocytopenic purpura, which can be fatal in 25 to 40 percent of cases.[275, 276] Thus, if ticlopidine is used, short courses (2–3 weeks) and biweekly monitoring of complete blood cell count are generally recommended.

Clopidogrel has been tested for secondary prevention in a broad population of patients with atherosclerosis in the Clopidogrel versus Aspirin in Patients at Risk for Ischemic Events (CAPRIE) trial. An 8.7 percent reduction relative to aspirin in the combined endpoint of ischemic stroke, MI, or vascular death during long-term follow-up was reported (see also Chap. 37).[270] When added to aspirin, clopidogrel also appears to be as effective as ticlopidine in preventing stent thrombosis,[277-280] especially when using a loading dose of 300 mg, which achieves effective platelet inhibition within 2 to 5 hours.[281] Clopidogrel is not associated with neutropenia and an extremely low rate of (approximately four cases per million) thrombotic thrombocytopenic purpura. It was associated with a lower rate of gastrointestinal bleeding compared with aspirin.[270] These data support the use of clopidogrel in patients with unstable angina who cannot take aspirin (e.g., a true aspirin allergy). Trials are in progress for patients with UA/NSTEMI testing the combination of clopidogrel plus aspirin versus aspirin alone.

Heparin (see also Chap. 62)

Heparin also appears to be beneficial in UA/NSTEMI: Several randomized trials suggest that unfractionated heparin (UFH) can improve clinical outcome compared with aspirin alone (see Chap. 62).[73-76] The greatest benefit was observed during the period of intravenous therapy, with "rebound" in recurrent events after stopping UFH observed in one study.[282] A meta-analysis showed a 33 percent reduction in death or MI at 2 to 12 weeks follow-up when comparing UFH plus aspirin versus aspirin alone, although this reduction was of borderline statistical significance (Fig. 36–10).[77]

HEPARIN RESISTANCE. Variability in the anticoagulant

effects of UFH, so-called heparin resistance,[283, 284] is thought to be due to the heterogeneity of heparin and to the neutralization of heparin by circulating plasma factors and by proteins released by activated platelets.[285, 286] Clinically, frequent monitoring of the anticoagulant response using activated partial thromboplastin time (APTT) is recommended, with titrations made according to a standardized nomogram (Table 36–4).[104] The latter minimizes the variability in the dosing adjustments given by various physicians and has been shown to improve the achievement of a target APTT.[287, 288]

THERAPEUTIC RANGE. The exact level of anticoagulation that constitutes the "therapeutic range" is not yet firmly established. Small studies in unstable angina[289] and acute MI[290-293] have suggested that lower APTT values may be related to recurrent ischemic events, suggesting that the lower limit of the target range of APTT is at least 1.5 times control. On the upper boundary of the target range, higher APTT values are associated with an increased risk of hemorrhage.[294] The lowest rate of bleeding (and mortality) in

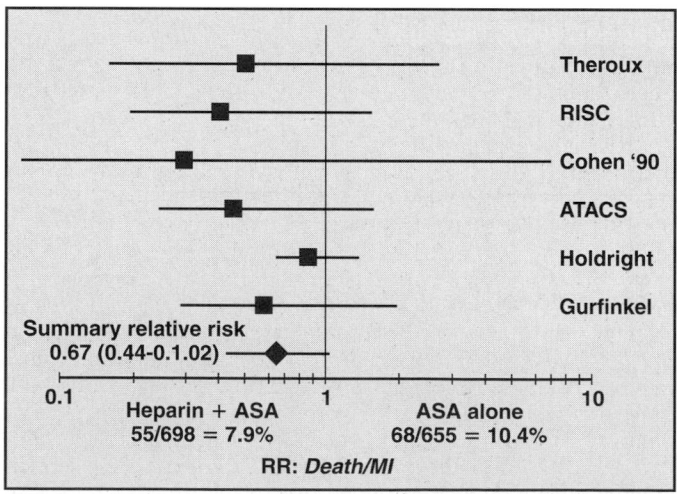

FIGURE 36-10. Meta-analysis of six randomized trials comparing unfractionated heparin plus aspirin (ASA) vs. ASA alone, showing benefit of the combination therapy. The rate of death or myocardial infarction during follow-up (2–12 weeks in these trials) tended to be reduced in patients randomized to aspirin plus heparin. (Adapted from Oler A, Whooley MA, Oler J, Grady D: Adding heparin to aspirin reduces the incidence of myocardial infarction and death in patients with unstable angina: A meta-analysis. JAMA 276:811–815, 1996. Copyright 1996, American Medical Association.)

▼ TABLE 36–4. STANDARDIZED NOMOGRAM FOR TITRATION OF HEPARIN

Initial Dose: 60 U/kg bolus and 12 U/kg/hr infusion
Activated partial thromboplastin time (APTT) should be checked and infusion adjusted at 6, 12, and 24 hours after initiation of heparin, daily thereafter, and 4 to 6 hours after any adjustment in dose.

APTT (secs)	CHANGE	IV INFUSION (U/kg/hr)
<35	70 U/kg bolus	+3
35–49	35 U/kg bolus	+2
50–70	0	0
71–90	0	−2
>100	Hold infusion for 30 min	−3

From Becker RC, Ball SP, Eisenberg P, et al: A randomized, multicenter trial of weight-adjusted intravenous heparin dose titration and point-of-care coagulation monitoring in hospitalized patients with active thromboembolic disease. Am Heart J 137:59–71, 1999.

patients with STEMI treated with thrombolytic therapy was when the 12-hour APTT was between 50 and 70 seconds.[293] Furthermore, in TIMI IIIB, there appeared to be no advantage of higher levels of anticoagulation in reducing ischemic events.[295]

DOSING. Dosing of UFH has traditionally used a 5000-U bolus followed by a 1000-U/hr infusion, which is then titrated according to the APTT.[285] The use of weight-adjusted UFH has been suggested as a means of improving APTT control and safety.[296] Three randomized trials of weight-adjusted UFH in unstable angina have been conducted. In one trial, there was a high percentage of patients who "overshot" in the initial APTT at 6 hours (median 150 seconds).[297] A more recent study examined a 60-U/kg bolus and 12-U/kg/hr infusion and found a higher percentage of patients within range without a large number of APTTs above range at 6 hours.[297a] The third trial tested standard dosing versus weight-adjusted dosing (70-U/kg bolus and 15-U/kg/hr initial infusion), and found no significant difference in control of APTT with weight-adjusted dosing.[298] Another approach uses "on-line" feedback of APTT data to a computer algorithm using a pharmacodynamic model of heparin response in the individual patient, with promising results in an initial pilot trial.[299]

CURRENT RECOMMENDATIONS. Based on available data, the current optimal regimen appears to be a weight-adjusted dose of UFH (60 U/kg bolus and 12 U/kg/hr infusion), frequent monitoring of APTT (every 6 hours until in the target range and every 12 to 24 hours thereafter), and titration of UFH using a standardized nomogram (see Table 36–4) with a target range of APTT between one and one-half to two times control or approximately 50 and 70 seconds.[7]

Low-Molecular-Weight Heparins (see also Chap. 62)

A major advance in the use of heparin has been in the development of low-molecular-weight heparins (LMWH), which *combine* factor IIa and factor Xa inhibition. Thus, they inhibit both the action (anti-IIa action) and generation (anti-Xa action) of thrombin. LMWH are obtained by depolymerization of standard UFH and selecting those with lower molecular weight.[285, 300] As compared with UFH that has nearly equal anti-IIa (thrombin) and anti-Xa activity, LMWH have increased ratios of anti-Xa to anti-IIa activity of either 2:1 (e.g., dalteparin) or 3.8:1 (e.g., enoxaparin) (see Chap. 62).

LMWH have several potential advantages over UFH. First, their greater anti–factor Xa activity inhibits thrombin generation more effectively.[300] LMWH also induce a greater release of tissue factor pathway inhibitor than does UFH, and they are not neutralized by platelet factor 4.[285] LMWH

have been found to have a lower rate of thrombocytopenia compared with UFH.[301] Their high bioavailability allows for subcutaneous administration, which provides a long duration of systemic anticoagulation, so that dosing can be administered twice daily. Finally, LMWH have less binding to plasma proteins (e.g., acute phase reactant proteins) and thus have a more consistent anticoagulant effect in relation to the dose administered. Accordingly, monitoring of the level of anticoagulation (as is necessary using APTT for UFH) is not necessary. These final two differences make LMWH a much simpler anticoagulant to administer than UFH. However, LMWH are more affected by renal dysfunction than UFH, and a reduced dose should be considered in patients with creatinine clearance less than 30 mL/min.

CLINICAL TRIALS. Five trials have compared LMWH with aspirin,[78] or with UFH plus aspirin.[79, 80, 302, 303] In the Fragmin during Instablity in Coronary Artery Disease (FRISC) study, dalteparin plus aspirin was found to reduce death or MI over the first 6 days compared with aspirin alone (1.8 percent vs. 4.8 percent, $p = 0.001$).[78] However, in the Fragmin in Unstable Coronary Artery Disease (FRIC) trial, no difference was observed between intravenous UFH and dalteparin.[302] Similarly, no benefit was seen when nadroparin was compared with UFH in the Fraxiparine in Ischaemic Syndrome (FRAXIS) trial.[303]

On the other hand, in two trials, Evaluation of the Safety and Efficacy of Enoxaparin in Non-ST Elevation Coronary Events (ESSENCE) and TIMI 11B, enoxaparin was found to confer a significant benefit in reducing death, MI, or recurrent ischemia compared with UFH. In ESSENCE, death, MI, or recurrent ischemia at 14 days was significantly lower (16.6 percent vs. 19.8 percent for UFH, $p = 0.019$).[79] The rates of this endpoint at 30 days were 19.8 percent vs. 23.3 percent ($p = 0.016$). Death or MI at 30 days also favored enoxaparin (6.2 percent vs. 7.7 percent).[79] The rates of catheterization (43 percent vs. 46 percent for enoxaparin vs. UFH) and PCI (13 percent vs. 17 percent, respectively) were lower in patients treated with enoxaparin than UFH.[79] A subsequent cost-effectiveness analysis found that there was a minimal increase in the cost for the drug (enoxaparin vs. UFH with APTT measurements) ($75); but with lower rates of catheterization and revascularization, treatment with enoxaparin led to a savings of $1172 per patient treated.[304] Thus, both improved outcomes and lower costs were observed with enoxaparin versus UFH.

The TIMI 11B trial studied high-risk patients with UA/NSTEMI. Death, MI, or severe recurrent ischemia requiring urgent revascularization through day 8 occurred in 12.4 percent of patients treated with enoxaparin versus 14.5 percent of patients treated with UFH ($p = 0.048$), a 15 percent relative risk reduction.[80] Parallel reductions in death and MI were also observed. No additional benefit of continuing enoxaparin beyond hospital discharge was observed.

A meta-analysis of the TIMI 11B and ESSENCE trials showed a consistent 20 percent reduction in both the composite endpoint of death, MI, or urgent revascularization and of death or MI that occurred at 8, 14, and 43 days (Fig. 36–11).[305] Enoxaparin reduced the rate of death, MI, or urgent revascularization from 18.7 to 15.6 percent ($p = 0.0006$).[305] Death or MI at 43 days was reduced from 8.6 to 7.1 percent ($p = 0.02$) (see Fig. 36–11). Thus, in two large randomized trials enoxaparin has been shown to be superior to UFH for the treatment of UA/NSTEMI, a benefit that has not been demonstrated yet for the other LMWH. It is not clear whether these differences in clinical results are related to the patients enrolled in the trials, the trial design, or the specific characteristics of the LMWH.

The effects of prolonged administration of LMWH after hospital discharge have been examined in several of the trials with mixed results. No benefit of 6 weeks of therapy was observed with dalteparin therapy in the FRIC trial,[302] of enoxaparin in the TIMI 11B trial,[80] or of 14 days of

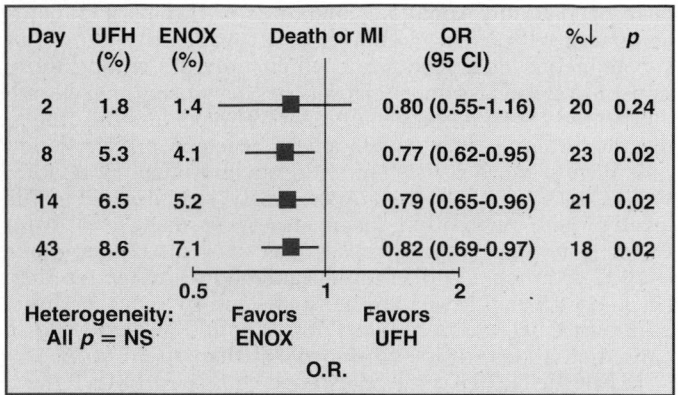

Day	UFH (%)	ENOX (%)	Death or MI	OR (95 CI)	%↓	p
2	1.8	1.4		0.80 (0.55-1.16)	20	0.24
8	5.3	4.1		0.77 (0.62-0.95)	23	0.02
14	6.5	5.2		0.79 (0.65-0.96)	21	0.02
43	8.6	7.1		0.82 (0.69-0.97)	18	0.02

Heterogeneity: All *p* = NS — Favors ENOX / Favors UFH — O.R.

FIGURE 36–11. TIMI 11B/ESSENCE meta-analysis: Data from over 7000 patients randomized in these two trials show a consistent and significant 20 percent reduction in the rate of death or myocardial infarction at each of the four time points in patients treated with enoxaparin (ENOX) vs. unfractionated heparin (UFH). (Adapted from Antman EM, Cohen M, Radley D, et al: Assessment of the treatment effect of enoxaparin for unstable angina/non-Q-wave my-ocardial infarction: TIMI 11B-ESSENCE meta-analysis. Circulation 100:1602–1608, 1999. Copyright 1999, American Heart Association.)

therapy with nadroparin in the FRAXIS trial.[303] On the other hand, in FRISC II, there was a lower rate of death or MI at 1 month but not at 3 or 6 months in patients treated with a 90-day course of dalteparin.[306] This early benefit was present only in patients randomized to the conservative strategy arm.[307] Thus, the FRISC II Investigators proposed a potential role for continued LMWH therapy after hospital discharge in selected higher-risk patients who are managed conservatively or in patients awaiting angiography and re-vascularization.[306] All four trials found higher rates of bleeding in patients receiving LMWH after hospital dis-charge. Thus, the *routine* use of prolonged LWMH therapy is not indicated, but it may be applicable to selected, con-servatively managed patients.

Direct Thrombin Inhibitors

Direct thrombin inhibitors have also undergone extensive evaluation. The prototypic agent is hirudin, a naturally oc-curring anticoagulant from the medicinal leech. Hirudin, which is made by recombinant DNA technology, is a 65 amino acid polypeptide that binds directly to thrombin, independent of antithrombin. The hirudin desirudin was tested in the GUSTO IIb trial involving 12,142 patients with UA/NSTEMI and STEMI. In the entire cohort, the 30-day rate of death or MI tended to be lower, 8.9 percent versus 9.8 percent (*p* = 0.06),[99] with no difference in mortality and a modest reduction in reinfarction (5.4 percent vs. 6.3 percent for heparin, *p* = 0.04). In the 8011 patients with UA/NSTEMI, 30-day death or MI was not significantly re-duced (8.3 percent vs. 9.1 percent, *p* = 0.22).[99]

The Organisation to Assess Strategies for Ischemic Syn-dromes (OASIS-2) trial[308] compared lepirudin to UFH: car-diovascular death or MI at 7 days tended to be lower (3.6 percent vs. 4.2 percent, respectively, *p* = 0.08). Major bleeding requiring transfusion was rare but more frequent with lepirudin (1.2 percent vs. 0.7 percent for heparin, *p* = 0.01). A meta-analysis of all hirudin trials showed a modest 10 percent benefit favoring hirudin, which was not statisti-cally significant for patients with UA/NSTEMI. Other syn-thetic direct thrombin inhibitors have also been tested (e.g., argatroban and bivalirudin [Hirulog]), and, again, only mod-est or no improvements were observed compared with hep-arin,[309–311] although lower rates of bleeding have been ob-served with bivalirudin.[311] The direct thrombin inhibitors have been shown to provide a very stable level of anticoag-ulation, as measured by APTT,[99, 312, 313] and no episodes of

thrombocytopenia were reported for the hirudin class. Of note, lepirudin is approved by the U.S. Food and Drug Administration for use as an anticoagulant in patients with heparin-induced thrombocytopenia and associated thrombo-embolic disease. Additional trials with this class of drugs are ongoing.

Oral Anticoagulation (see also Chap. 62)

Oral anticoagulation with warfarin has been examined in several recent trials, with the rationale that prolonged treat-ment might extend the benefit of early anticoagulation with an antithrombin agent (e.g., UFH, LMWH). Although pilot trials suggested benefit of a strategy of initial UFH followed by warfarin,[76, 314–316] two larger trials have failed to show a significant benefit of long-term warfarin plus aspirin versus aspirin alone. In the OASIS-2 trial of patients with UA/NSTEMI, the rate of cardiovascular death, MI, or stroke at 5 months was 7.4 percent for those receiving warfarin plus aspirin versus 8.2 percent for those receiving aspirin alone (*p* = NS). Similarly, in the Combination Hemotherapy and Mortality Prevention (CHAMP) trial of survivors of MI, there was no difference in the rate of all-cause mortality over an average 2.7-year follow-up between the combina-tion of warfarin plus aspirin versus aspirin alone but there was a higher rate of major bleeding.[317] In addition, fixed-dose warfarin plus aspirin was not better than aspirin alone in the Coumadin Aspirin Reinfarction Study (CARS) trial.[318] Of note, however, a post-hoc analysis of OASIS-2 suggested that if compliance is excellent, a benefit might be observed with the combination of aspirin plus warfarin.[319]

One primary prevention trial in high-risk patients was a 2 × 2 factorial design of aspirin versus placebo and warfa-rin adjusted to an international normalized ratio of 1.5 and placebo found a significant reduction in coronary death or MI of the combination of warfarin plus aspirin (8.7 percent vs. 13.3 percent for placebo) but not significantly better than aspirin alone (10.2 percent) or warfarin alone (10.3 percent).[320] In this trial, however, there was an increase in hemorrhagic strokes among patients treated with the combi-nation: 0.9 percent vs. 0.1 percent for warfarin alone, 0.2 percent for aspirin alone, and 0 percent for placebo (*p* = 0.009).[320] Thus, the *routine* use of the combination of war-farin plus aspirin cannot be recommended.

Warfarin therapy (without aspirin) has been shown to be superior to placebo after MI (both STEMI and NSTEMI)[321–323] and could be considered a suitable *alterna-tive* to aspirin. Furthermore, warfarin is indicated in pa-tients with atrial fibrillation[324, 325] or severe left ventricular dysfunction who are at high risk of systemic embolization (see Chap. 62).[326]

Glycoprotein IIb/IIIa Inhibitors

(See also Chap. 62)

Because plaque rupture in a coronary artery is followed by platelet aggregation and thrombosis and given the dramatic clinical benefits of the relatively weak antiplatelet agent aspirin,[327] attention has focused on the new class of drugs that inhibit platelet aggregation by binding to the platelet glycoprotein IIb/IIIa receptor. By preventing the final com-mon pathway of platelet aggregation (i.e., fibrinogen medi-ated cross-linkage of platelets by means of the glycoprotein IIb/IIIa receptor) (see Fig. 36–3), these agents are potent inhibitors of platelet aggregation from all types of stimuli (e.g., thrombin, ADP, collagen, serotonin). Three agents are now available for use in UA/NSTEMI—abciximab, tirofi-ban, and eptifibatide—with the former currently approved only in patients undergoing PCI. Abciximab is a Fab frag-ment of a monoclonal antibody directed at the glycoprotein IIb/IIIa receptor. Eptifibatide, a synthetic heptapeptide, and tirofiban, a nonpeptide molecule, are antagonists of the gly-coprotein IIb/IIIa receptor whose structure mimics the arginine-glycine-aspartic acid (abbreviated RGD) amino acid sequence by which fibrinogen binds to the glycoprotein IIb/IIIa receptor (see Chap. 62).

Several trials have shown benefit of glycoprotein IIb/IIIa inhibition in UA/NSTEMI either in patients managed predominantly with medical management,[82] with early interventional management,[328] or with both.[81, 83, 329-331] In the Platelet Receptor Inhibition for Ischemic Syndrome Management in Patients Limited by Unstable Signs and Symptoms (PRISM-PLUS) study, tirofiban plus heparin and aspirin significantly reduced the rate of death, MI, or refractory ischemia at 7 days compared with heparin plus aspirin.[83] Death or MI at 30 days was also significantly reduced by 30 percent, from 11.9 percent to 8.7 percent, with improvements generally consistent across all subgroups and management strategies (i.e., medical therapy [25 percent reduction], percutaneous transluminal coronary angioplasty [PTCA, 35 percent reduction], and coronary artery bypass grafting [CABG, 30 percent reduction].[332] In the Platelet Glycoprotein IIb/IIIa in Unstable Angina: Receptor Suppression Using Integrilin Therapy (PURSUIT) trial, involving 10,948 patients, eptifibatide also significantly reduced the rate of death or MI at 30 days.[81] In this trial, a greater benefit of eptifibatide was observed in patients undergoing early angioplasty compared with other treatment strategies.[81] Meta-analyses involving over 30,000 patients found that treatment with a glycoprotein IIb/IIIa inhibitor led to a 21 percent reduction in death or MI at 30 days.[330, 331]

The relative benefits of IIb/IIIa inhibition relative to medical versus interventional treatment have been examined more closely. The PRISM trial, involving patients managed medically for the first 48 hours, found a significant 32 percent reduction in death, MI, or refractory ischemia at 48 hours, suggesting a significant clinical benefit during medical treatment alone.[82] In a recent pooling of data from PRISM-PLUS, PURSUIT, and the Chimeric 7E3 Antiplatelet in Unstable Angina Refractory to Standard Treatment (CAPTURE) trials involving 12,296 patients, there was a 34 percent relative reduction in death or MI during a period of 24 to 72 hours of medical management only (3.8 percent vs. 2.5 percent, $p = 0.001$) (Fig. 36–12).[333] These findings support the use of glycoprotein IIb/IIIa inhibition in the medical management of patients with UA/NSTEMI.[7] However, in the recently reported GUSTO-IV ACS trial, conducted in a relatively low-risk unstable angina population in whom the use of early PCI was discouraged, no clinical benefit was demonstrated when abciximab was added to aspirin and heparin.[333a]

On the other hand, among patients with unstable angina who undergo PCI (i.e., those managed with an early invasive strategy), glycoprotein IIb/IIIa inhibition appears to be beneficial both *before* intervention and especially *during* the intervention. This was first demonstrated in CAPTURE, in which abciximab was shown to reduce death, MI, or the need for urgent revascularization significantly.[328] In the meta-analysis, a significant benefit was seen when the agents are continued during angioplasty (death or MI was reduced from 8.0 to 4.9 percent (see Fig. 36–12). A broader overview of patients with UA/NSTEMI who underwent PCI can be obtained by including patients enrolled in PCI trials (Fig. 36–13).[7] In this overview, the benefit of IIb/IIIa inhibition is quite dramatic, with reductions of death or MI seen ranging from 30 to 70 percent. Thus, glycoprotein IIb/IIIa inhibition appears to have an additional benefit in patients in whom the drug is continued through PCI.[7]

NEED FOR INTRAVENOUS HEPARIN. The long-term effects of glycoprotein IIb/IIIa inhibition appear to be greater when used in conjunction with heparin, as was done in the majority of patients in the PRISM-PLUS and PURSUIT trials.[82, 83, 334] It is not clear whether even greater benefits can be safely achieved when combining glycoprotein IIb/IIIa inhibitors with LMWH. This question is being addressed in several ongoing clinical trials.

SAFETY. The rate of major hemorrhage was slightly higher for patients treated with glycoprotein IIb/IIIa inhibitors than for those receiving aspirin and heparin alone. For example, in the PRISM-PLUS trial, major bleeding occurred in 4.0 percent of patients treated with tirofiban plus heparin plus aspirin versus 3.0 percent for heparin plus aspirin ($p = $ NS).[83] For eptifibatide, the rates of severe or moderate bleeding versus placebo were 12.8 percent versus 9.9 percent ($p < 0.001$).[81]

Thrombocytopenia is an uncommon but important complication of glycoprotein IIb/IIIa inhibitors: For tirofiban in PRISM-PLUS, the rate of severe thrombocytopenia (<50,000 cells/mm³) was 0.5 percent versus 0.3 percent for heparin ($p = $ NS)[83]; in the PURSUIT trial, thrombocytopenia (<20,000 cells/mm³) occurred in 0.2 percent versus less than 0.1 percent for heparin.[81] Thrombocytopenia is associated with increased bleeding and, in a smaller proportion of patients, with recurrent thrombotic events.[335, 336] This syndrome bears resemblance to heparin-induced thrombocytopenia and indicates a need to monitor platelet count daily during the glycoprotein IIb/IIIa infusion.

ORAL GLYCOPROTEIN IIb/IIIa INHIBITION. Because the benefit of the small molecule intravenous glycoprotein IIb/IIIa inhibitors (tirofiban and eptifibatide) occurs only during the infusion, whereas abciximab's action dissipates 12 to 48 hours after cessation of the infusion, it has been hoped that prolonged glycoprotein IIb/IIIa inhibition using oral agents might lead to further, and continued, reduction in recurrent events. Unfortunately, four large trials, one in patients with acute coronary syndromes, OPUS-TIMI 16,[337] two in stabilized patients after an acute coronary syndrome, SYMPHONY,[338, 338a] and one in patients undergoing PCI, EXCITE,[339] all failed to show any benefit of the oral glycoprotein IIb/IIIa inhibitors orbofiban, sibrafiban, and xemilofiban, respectively. A higher degree of variability in the drug level and of the degree of platelet inhibition achieved with oral as compared with intravenous drugs is one potential explanation of the difference in outcomes between the two types of IIb/IIIa inhibitors.[340] It also appears that some of the agents may have intrinsic proaggregatory effects.[341] Trials are continuing to evaluate "second generation" oral glycoprotein IIb/IIIa inhibitors, which have longer half-lives and tighter binding to the glycoprotein IIb/IIIa receptor similar to that of abciximab.[342]

MECHANISM OF BENEFIT. Three new concepts are emerging on the benefit of glycoprotein IIb/IIIa inhibitors in

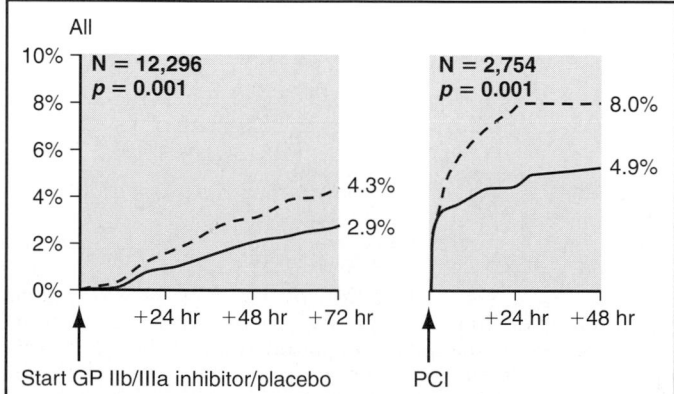

FIGURE 36–12. Pooled data from CAPTURE, PRISM-PLUS, and PURSUIT trials of unstable angina, showing benefit of glycoprotein IIb/IIIa inhibition during medical therapy only (left panel), during, and immediately after percutaneous coronary intervention (PCI, right panel). (From Boersma E, Akkerhuis KM, Theroux P, et al: Platelet glycoprotein IIb/IIIa receptor inhibition in non-ST-elevation acute coronary syndromes: Early benefit during medical treatment only, with additional protection during percutaneous coronary intervention. Circulation 100:2045–2048, 1999. Copyright 1999, American Heart Association.)

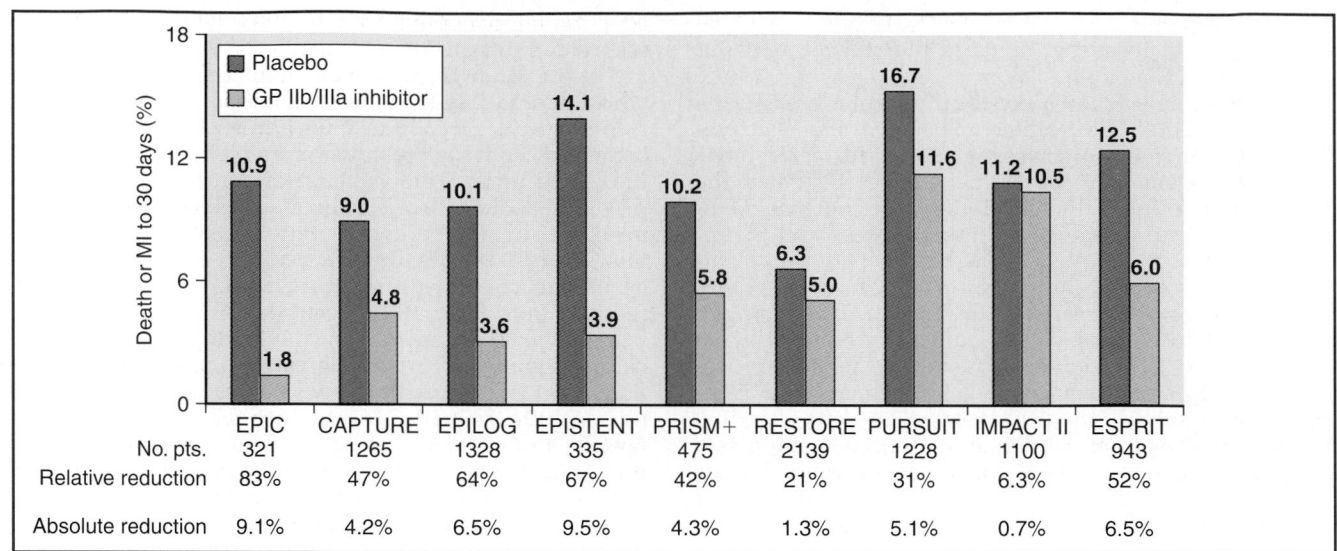

FIGURE 36–13. Benefit of glycoprotein IIb/IIIa inhibition among patients with UA/NSTEMI treated with percutaneous coronary intervention across all large trials. As shown, both the relative benefit and the absolute benefit are quite substantial, ranging from 50 to 100 deaths or myocardial infarctions prevented for every 1000 patients treated. (Adapted from Braunwald E, Antman EM, et al: ACC/AHA guidelines for the management of patients with unstable angina/non-ST segment elevation myocardial infarction: A report of the American College of Cardiology/American Heart Association Task Force on Practice Guidelines [Committee on the Management of Unstable Angina and Non-ST Segment Elevation Myocardial Infarction]. J Am Coll Cardiol 36:970–1062, 2000, with data for ESPRIT provided by Tcheng JE.)

UA/NSTEMI. First, angiographic data from two trials have shown that the IIb/IIIa inhibitors lead to greater resolution of thrombus and improved coronary flow compared with aspirin and heparin alone.[123, 343] In PRISM-PLUS, for example, tirofiban led to a 35 percent overall improvement in TIMI flow grade ($p = 0.002$).[123] Together these data establish the pathophysiological link between the potent platelet inhibition achieved by glycoprotein IIb/IIIa inhibition, a reduction in thrombus, improvement in coronary blood flow, and consequent improvement in clinical outcome.[344]

A second new concept based on evidence from two trials is that glycoprotein IIb/IIIa inhibitors can reduce the size of an evolving NSTEMI (Fig. 36–14).[345, 346] It was observed in the PURSUIT trial that the size of the MI, either index or recurrent, measured by peak CK-MB was significantly smaller in patients treated with eptifibatide. Similarly, in the PRISM-PLUS troponin substudy, those randomized to tirofiban plus heparin had a significantly lower peak troponin (see Fig. 36–14).[346]

The third new concept is that there appears to be a greater benefit of treatment when administered earlier relative to the onset of pain. In an analysis from PURSUIT, the absolute reduction in death or MI with eptifibatide was 2.8 percent for patients treated within 6 hours from the onset of pain and was less for those treated between 6 and 12 and 12 and 24 hours after onset of pain. No benefit was observed in patients treated 24 hours after the onset of pain (Fig. 36–15). Similar data have been observed in PRISM-PLUS (unpublished data).

COST BENEFIT OF GLYCOPROTEIN IIb/IIIa INHIBITION. Thus, intravenous glycoprotein IIb/IIIa inhibition has been shown to be beneficial in patients at intermediate to high risk, on the basis of rest pain and either ECG changes or positive cardiac markers.[81–83] Although these agents add to the expense of therapy, this cost is balanced by a reduction in recurrent cardiac events. A cost-effectiveness analysis from PURSUIT found that the cost per year of life saved was approximately $16,000, well within the generally acceptable range for medical interventions.[346a] As noted later (see p. 1253), benefit of glycoprotein IIb/IIIa inhibition appears to be greatest in patients at higher risk, as evidence by those who have a positive troponin at baseline,[154, 155] those with diabetes,[189] those with recurrent angina,[83, 193] or those with prior aspirin use.[196] In these high-risk subgroups of patients, the absolute benefit is greater and the therapy is even more cost effective.

In conclusion, it appears reasonable to use an intravenous glycoprotein IIb/IIIa inhibitor with aspirin and UFH as antithrombotic therapy in patients who have UA/NSTEMI with high-risk features (see Table 36–3), especially those with a positive troponin value.

Thrombolytic Therapy

Because thrombolytic therapy is beneficial in the treatment of patients with acute STEMI, it was thought that it might also be effective in the other acute coronary syndromes in which thrombosis plays a role. In TIMI IIIB, 1473 patients

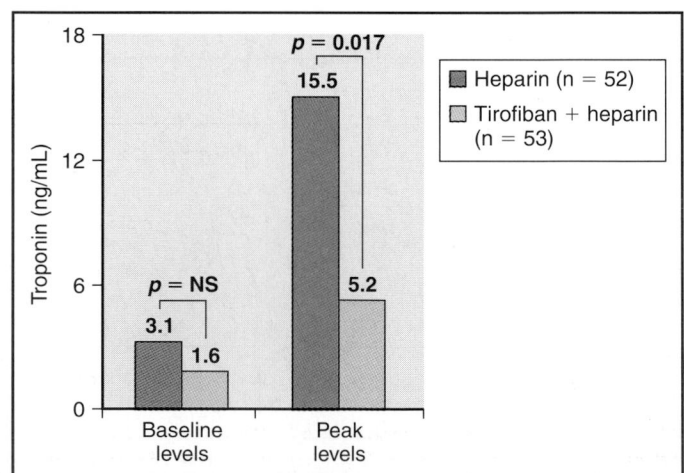

FIGURE 36–14. PRISM-PLUS troponin substudy: Peak levels of troponin I (TnI) were reduced in patients treated with the glycoprotein IIb/IIIa inhibitor tirofiban compared with aspirin and heparin in the trial. These data demonstrate that early treatment (within 12 hours from the onset of chest pain in this study) led to a reduced infarct size among patients with UA/NSTEMI. (Data from Januzzi JL, Hahn SS, et al: Reduction of troponin I levels in patients with acute coronary syndromes by glycoprotein IIb/IIIa inhibition with tirofiban. Am J Cardiol [in press].)

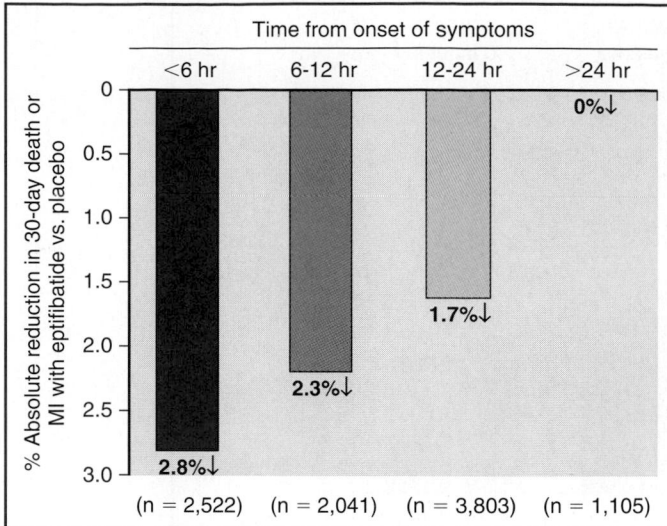

Time from onset of symptoms

FIGURE 36–15. PURSUIT: Evidence showing greater benefit of glycoprotein IIb/IIIa inhibition with more rapid time to treatment. The absolute reduction in death or myocardial infarction to 30 days in patients treated with eptifibatide versus placebo was greatest for patients treated within 6 hours from the onset of chest pain, with lower benefit as time from onset of pain increased. These data underscore the importance of treating patients with UA/NSTEMI rapidly, preferably in the emergency department, with IIb/IIIa inhibitors. (Data from Bhatt, et al: Circulation 98[Suppl. I]:I–561, 1998. Copyright 1998, American Heart Association.)

with UA/NSTEMI were treated with aspirin, UFH, and antiischemic therapy and were randomized to receive either tissue plasminogen activator (t-PA) or placebo. No differences were observed in the incidence of death, postrandomization MI, or recurrent, objectively documented ischemia through 6 weeks.[101] Fatal and nonfatal MI after randomization actually occurred *more frequently* in t-PA–treated patients (7.4 percent) than in placebo-treated patients (4.9 percent) ($p = 0.04$). In addition, t-PA was associated with a 0.6 percent rate of intracranial hemorrhage compared with 0 percent for UFH alone ($p = 0.06$).

The TIMI IIIB results are corroborated by a meta-analysis of all previous smaller trials of thrombolytic therapy in UA/NSTEMI, in which no benefit of thrombolytic therapy was observed.[104] In both ISIS-2 and the Fibrinolytic Therapy Trialists' overview, patients with suspected MI and ST segment depression had a *higher* mortality with thrombolytic therapy compared with placebo.[269, 347] Accordingly, routine thrombolytic therapy *is not indicated* in UA/NSTEMI.[7]

The proposed mechanism for adverse effect of thrombolysis in UA/NSTEMI is a prothrombotic effect of thrombolysis. Thrombolysis is known to activate platelets[348] and increase fibrinopeptide A,[349] and the dissolution of the fibrin clot exposes clot-bound thrombin, which is enzymatically active and can lead to clot formation.[350] Because most patients with UA/NSTEMI have a patent culprit artery, these prothrombotic forces can lead to progression of the thrombus to total occlusion, thereby causing an MI (as was observed in TIMI IIIB).[101] In STEMI, in contrast, the culprit vessel is occluded at baseline and can only improve with successful thrombolysis.

Registry Experience with Compliance

A major problem recently identified in current practice is that a large proportion of patients do not receive guideline-recommended therapies.[98, 100, 118, 351, 352] For example, in the first National Registry of Myocardial Infarction (NRMI) conducted in 1990 to 1993, only 63 percent of patients with NSTEMI received aspirin.[353] In the TIMI III Registry of UA/NSTEMI conducted in 1992 to 1993, 80 percent of patients received aspirin,[98, 100] and in the Global Unstable Angina Registry and Treatment Evaluation (GUARANTEE) registry conducted in 1996, 83 percent of patients received aspirin.[118, 354, 355] This slight improvement suggests a possible benefit of the widespread dissemination and education after the publication of the Unstable Angina Guideline in 1994.[104] However, despite the overwhelming benefits of aspirin (arguably the best studied and most beneficial medication in cardiovascular medicine),[327] significant proportions of patients do not receive this drug. The American Heart Association published a scientific statement strongly urging physicians to use aspirin in appropriate patients,[356] which includes all UA/NSTEMI patients without contraindications. Similar findings have been observed for beta blockers and UFH,[98, 100, 118, 352, 355] with the latter used in only 57 percent of patients in the TIMI III Registry and in 67 percent of patients in the GUARANTEE Registry.[100, 118, 355] Importantly, recent evidence has suggested that if patients are treated according to the Unstable Angina Guideline recommendations, their adjusted 1-year mortality is lower compared with patients who do not receive all guideline-recommended therapies.[357] Thus, a major focus for physicians, hospitals, and health care systems is to improve the use of aspirin, and other important medications, using critical pathways and other methods (see p. 1254).

TREATMENT STRATEGIES AND INTERVENTIONS

Two general approaches to the use of cardiac catheterization and revascularization in UA/NSTEMI exist: (1) an "early invasive" strategy, involving routine early cardiac catheterization and revascularization with PCI or bypass surgery depending on the coronary anatomy, and (2) a more "conservative" approach with initial medical management, with catheterization and revascularization only for recurrent ischemia either at rest or on a noninvasive stress test. The latter has also been termed an "ischemia-guided" strategy.

Four randomized trials have assessed these two general strategies (Fig. 36–16). In the TIMI IIIB trial, 1473 patients were randomized in a 2 × 2 factorial design to receive either t-PA or its placebo and follow either an early invasive strategy with routine angiography 18 to 48 hours after randomization with revascularization as appropriate or an early conservative strategy with angiography and revascularization performed only for recurrent ischemia. All patients received intravenous heparin, aspirin, beta blockers, nitrates, and calcium antagonists as clinically indicated.

There was no difference between the early invasive and conservative strategies in the rate of death, postrandomization MI, or a strongly positive exercise test at 6 weeks (16.2 percent vs. 18.1 percent, $p = NS$).[101] Similarly, there was no difference in the incidence of death or MI at 6 weeks or 1 year (10.8 percent vs. 12.2 percent, $p = NS$)[199] (see Fig. 36–16). It is worth noting that the conservative strategy was truly an "ischemia-guided" strategy, with the indications for catheterization based on very careful assessment for recurrent ischemia (i.e., ischemia at rest with ECG changes, ST segment depression on a Holter monitor, a "high risk" exercise thallium stress test). However, despite this requirement for objective evidence of recurrent ischemia, 49 percent of patients in the conservative arm subsequently required revascularization, evenly split between PTCA and CABG.[101] The results of TIMI IIIB were nearly duplicated in the smaller Medicine versus Angiography in Thrombolytic Exclusion (MATE) trial[358] (see Fig. 36–16).

The Veterans Administration Non-Q-Wave Infarction Strategies in-Hospital (VANQWISH) trial compared invasive

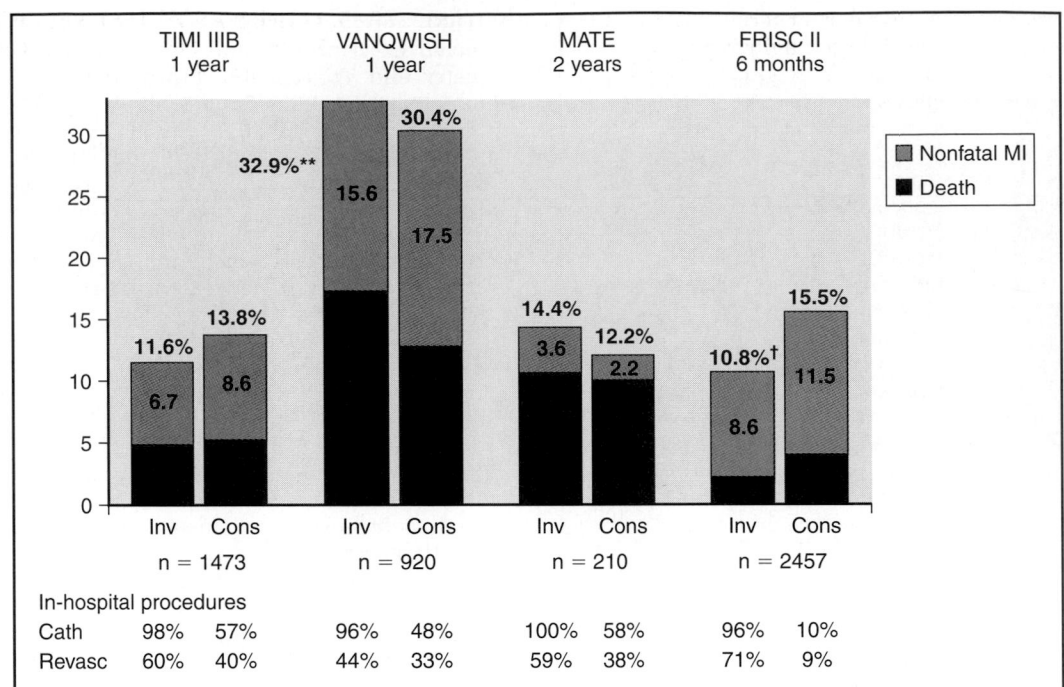

FIGURE 36–16. Results from the four randomized trials of invasive (Inv) vs. conservative (Cons) strategies in UA/NSTEMI. The duration of follow-up is shown for each trial at the top, and the number of patients is shown at the bottom. In addition, the rate of cardiac catheterization (Cath) during the initial hospitalization, as well as the rates of revascularization (revasc) with PCI or CABG are shown. *p = 0.05, **p = 0.025, +p = 0.031. (Data from Anderson, et al.[199]; Boden, et al.[359]; McCollough, et al.[358]; and the Fragmin and Fast Revascularisation during InStability in Coronary artery disease Investigators.[307])

and conservative strategies in 920 patients with non-Q-wave MI (not unstable angina, and including 15 percent STEMI). There was no significant difference in the primary endpoint of death or nonfatal MI during follow-up (approximately 2 years): 26.9 percent in the invasive arm versus 29.9 percent in the conservative arm.[359] However, there were significantly more deaths in patients assigned to the invasive compared with the conservative strategy at hospital discharge (4.5 percent vs. 1.3 percent), a difference that remained significant at 1 year. Of the 21 in-hospital deaths in the invasive group, 11 followed within 30 days of coronary bypass surgery, indicating a 11.6 percent perioperative mortality in the invasive group, which explains some of the early hazard of the early invasive group. Of note, the peri-CABG mortality in patients in the conservative arm was only 3.4 percent, with a more delayed CABG (median 24 days, versus 8 days in the invasive group).

Most recently, the FRISC II trial of 2457 patients with UA/NSTEMI found a significant *benefit* of a delayed invasive strategy.[307] Patients with chest pain within 48 hours with either ST-T wave changes or positive serum markers were enrolled and received subcutaneous dalteparin in hospital. They were then randomized to an invasive versus conservative strategy. In the invasive arm, cardiac catheterization and revascularization were carried out within 3 and 7 days of randomization, respectively, and thus this invasive strategy could be considered a "delayed" invasive strategy. Criteria for catheterization in the conservative strategy were strict and required refractory angina despite maximal medical treatment or a positive ECG exercise test with 0.3 mV or more ST segment depression. Thallium imaging was not performed with the stress testing. With this conservative strategy, only 9 percent of patients underwent revascularization during the first 7 days.[307]

The primary endpoint, death or MI at 6 months, was significantly lower in the invasive versus conservative group (9.4 percent vs. 12.1 percent, p = 0.031).[307] Preliminary 1-year results show a significant reduction in *mortality*

in the invasive versus conservative groups (2.2 percent vs. 4.0 percent, respectively, p = 0.018) and of death or MI (10.5 percent vs. 14.2 percent, respectively, p = 0.007).[360] Additional analyses showed greater benefit of the invasive strategy in higher risk groups identified by age >65 years, ST segment depression on the admission ECG or troponin T of 0.01 ng/dl or more.[116, 361] Of note, the 30-day mortality following CABG was less than 2 percent in this study.[307]

A recent meta-analysis of these four studies has shown that there is an early hazard with an invasive strategy, but that this is balanced by later benefit in the invasive group making overall odds ratio of death or MI 0.94 (95% CI 0.78–1.13).[362] This early hazard was also observed in the Kaplan-Meier event rate curves from the TIMI IIIB and FRISC II trials.[199, 307] One randomized trial of CABG versus medical therapy in patients with unstable angina conducted in the 1980s found no overall difference in mortality at 2 years but a survival benefit in patients with left ventricular dysfunction.[204, 363]

Indications for Invasive Versus Conservative Management Strategies

Thus, balancing the current evidence, either an early conservative or early invasive strategy appears to be appropriate for patients with UA/NSTEMI.[7] However, it may be possible to individualize the approach based on the patient population and the success rates of the coronary interventions. For patients managed in a conservative fashion, indications for coronary angiography are (1) recurrent ischemia at rest or with low-level activity accompanied by ECG changes, (2) congestive heart failure, (3) evidence of ischemia on stress testing,[364] (4) when hemodynamic instability is present,[365] and (5) evidence of sustained ventricular arrhythmias.[7] With regard to the exact criteria for "significant" ischemia on stress testing, the relatively worse outcome of the conservative strategy (with strict criteria) in FRISC II as compared with the invasive group, in contrast to the equal outcomes between invasive versus conservative strategies (with moderately stringent criteria in TIMI IIIB), suggest that criteria for proceeding to angiography in a conservative strategy should not be *too* stringent.

An early invasive strategy can be considered appropriate and more expeditious than an early conservative strategy, and it appears to be *beneficial* in higher risk patients (see Table 36–3). As noted earlier, a significant benefit of an early invasive strategy was observed in FRISC II in patients with ST segment depression on the admission ECG[307, 361] in patients older than 65 years of age.[199, 307] An early invasive approach appears warranted in those with hemodynamic instability, based on studies in acute MI.[365, 366] In addition, an early invasive strategy in those who present with UA/NSTEMI within 6 months of a prior PCI, in whom restenosis may be frequent, may be a more expeditious strategy.

On the other hand, for the very high-risk patients with NSTEMI and multivessel disease requiring bypass surgery (similar to patients in the VANQWISH trial), and/or at hospitals where intervention complication rates are higher, an *initial* more conservative approach may be most appropriate.[7] For such patients, one might pursue a delayed invasive strategy, based on the lower perioperative mortality in the VANQWISH trial comparing patients who underwent delayed versus early CABG.[359] Results from additional trials such as Treat Angina with Aggrastat and Determine Cost of Therapy with Invasive or Conservative Strategy (TACTICS)-TIMI 18, conducted in the current era of glycoprotein IIb/IIIa inhibition and coronary stenting, should provide additional perspective on the issue of invasive versus conservative strategies in UA/NSTEMI, including a cost-benefit analysis.[367, 368]

Noninvasive Testing

In the management of unstable angina, noninvasive testing is used (1) at presentation, usually in the ED to diagnose the presence or absence of coronary artery disease (in patients with low likelihood of coronary disease) (see p. 1234); (2) after hospitalization and medical therapy has been carried out, to evaluate the extent of residual ischemia to guide further therapy, especially an "ischemia-guided" strategy; (3) to evaluate left ventricular function; and (4) to estimate prognosis (i.e., risk stratification).

The results from noninvasive tests that portend high risk of future cardiac events are shown in Table 36–5 (see also Chaps. 7, 9, and 37). These results are derived from studies involving patients with UA, MI, and stable coronary artery disease. The markers of high risk are either evidence of ischemia on stress testing or left ventricular dysfunction (either at rest or stress induced).[369–373]

The need for angiography and revascularization for patients who had a positive stress test (i.e., evidence of ischemia) has long been assumed and has been used in the "conservative" arms of most randomized trials.[101, 244, 307, 359] This benefit of revascularization for provokable ischemia has been documented in patients with a positive ECG stress test following thrombolytic therapy of STEMI.[364]

The safety of early stress testing in patients with UA/NSTEMI has been debated, but evidence from several trials has suggested that pharmacological,[374] or symptom-limited stress testing,[375] is safe after at least 24 to 48 hours of stabilization without recurrent ischemia in patients with UA/NSTEMI. Contraindications to stress testing are a recent recurrence of rest pain, especially if associated with ECG changes or other signs of instability (hemodynamic or significant arrhythmias).

The merits of various modalities of stress testing have been compared in relatively small series of patients (see also Chaps. 6, 7, and 9). Stress myocardial perfusion imaging with sestamibi and stress echocardiographic imaging are slightly more sensitive than ECG stress testing alone and have shown greater prognostic value.[180, 376–378] An overview has suggested that the perfusion imaging tests are

EXERCISE ECG TESTING
Abnormal horizontal or downsloping ST segment depression with
  Onset at heart rate <120 beats/min or ≤6.5 METS
  Magnitude ≥2.0 mm
  Postexercise duration of ≥6 minutes
  Depression in multiple leads
Abnormal systolic blood pressure response
  With sustained decrease of >10 mm Hg or flat blood pressure response ≤130 mm Hg, associated with abnormal electrocardiogram
Other
  Exercise-induced ST segment elevation
  Ventricular tachycardia

RADIONUCLIDE MYOCARDIAL PERFUSION IMAGING
Abnormal myocardial tracer distribution in more than one coronary artery region at rest or with stress or an anterior defect that reperfuses
Abnormal myocardial distribution with increased lung uptake
Cardiac enlargement

LEFT VENTRICULAR IMAGING

Stress Radionuclide Ventriculography
Exercise EF of ≤50%
Rest EF ≤35%
Fall in EF of ≥10% with exercise

Stress Echocardiography
Rest EF ≤35%
Wall motion score index >1

EF = ejection fraction; METS = metabolic equivalents
Data from Schlant RC, Blomqvist CG, Brandenburg RO et al: Guidelines for exercise testing: A report of the Joint American College of Cardiology/American Heart Association Task Force on Assessment of Cardiovascular Procedures (Subcommittee on Exercise Testing). Circulation 1986;74:653A–667A, 1986; O'Rourke RA, Challerjee K, Dodge HT et al. Guidelines for clinical use of cardiac radionuclide imaging, December 1986: A report of the American College of Cardiology/American Heart Association Task Force on Assessment of Cardiovascular Procedures (Subcommittee on Nuclear Imaging). J Am Coll Cardiol 8:1471–1483, 1986; and Cheitlin MD, Alpert JS, Armstrong WF et al. ACC/AHA Guidelines for the Clinical Application of Echocardiography: A report of the American College of Cardiology/American Heart Association Task Force on Practice Guidelines. Circulation 1997;95:1686–1744, 1997.

more sensitive for ischemia than ECG-only stress testing and that such testing is generally cost effective in higher risk patients.[379] A recommended approach is to individualize the choice based on patient characteristics, local availability, and expertise in interpretation.[7] For most patients, ECG stress testing is recommended if the ECG is without significant ST segment abnormalities.[7] If ST segment abnormalities exist, then perfusion or echocardiographic imaging is recommended. Exercise testing is generally recommended unless the patient cannot walk sufficiently to achieve a significant workload, in which case pharmacological stress testing is recommended.[7]

Intraaortic Balloon Counterpulsation

Intraaortic balloon counterpulsation (IABP) is a very effective means of increasing diastolic coronary blood flow and reducing left ventricular afterload, which act in concert to reduce ischemia (see Chap. 19). IABP is usually reserved for patients with UA/NSTEMI who are refractory to maximal medical therapy and those with hemodynamic compromise who are awaiting cardiac catheterization or for those identified to have very high risk coronary anatomy (e.g., left main stenosis) as a bridge to coronary angioplasty or bypass surgery.[7] In the TIMI III Registry, only 1 percent of patients required IABP during hospitalization.[98, 100] No randomized trials are available to document its benefit, but this method is very effective in stabilizing patients with refractory ischemia. However, vascular access site complications are relatively common in the elderly, women, and diabetics.[380, 381]

Revascularization (see also Chap. 38)

PERCUTANEOUS CORONARY INTERVENTION. PCI is an effective means of reducing coronary obstruction, improving acute ischemia, and improving regional and global left ventricular function in patients with UA/NSTEMI.[382] Current angiographic success rates are high, generally more than 95 percent[383] (see also Chap. 38), although the presence of unstable angina or visualized thrombus has been associated with increased risk of acute complications such as abrupt closure or MI (as compared with patients with stable angina or those without visualized thrombus).[123, 384] Thus, use of glycoprotein IIb/IIIa inhibitors in such patients is associated with improved PCI outcomes (Fig. 36–13, p. 1248).

The TIMI III investigators reported a favorable experience with balloon angioplasty in patients with a UA/NSTEMI with a periprocedural MI rate of 2.7 percent, an emergency bypass surgery rate of 1.4 percent, and a mortality of 0.5 percent. Since that time, the advent of coronary stenting has reduced the rate of emergency bypass surgery and the increasing use of glycoprotein IIb/IIIa inhibitors has reduced the rates of death and MI.[81, 328, 385–391] When CK-MB is measured serially during the 24 hours after a procedure, the rates of MI are higher: 5 to 8 percent among patients treated with aspirin and heparin. These rates are markedly reduced when IIb/IIIa inhibitors are used during the PCI.[81, 328, 387–391] (see Fig. 36–13) (see also Chap. 38).

PCI VERSUS CABG. When revascularization is required in patients with UA/NSTEMI, the choice is between PCI and CABG. Five trials have compared PTCA and CABG in patients with ischemic heart disease, many of whom had unstable angina.[392–396] The results of these trials are reviewed in Chapters 37 and 38. Based on the results of these trials, and those of previous trials of CABG versus medical therapy,[397–400] and more recent observational data,[401] CABG is recommended for patients with disease of the left main coronary artery, multivessel disease involving the proximal left anterior descending artery, or multivessel disease and impaired left ventricular function or diabetes.[402] For other patients, either PCI or CABG may be suitable: PCI is associated with a slightly lower initial morbidity and mortality than CABG but a higher rate of repeat procedures, whereas CABG is associated with more effective relief from angina.

TARGETING OF NEW THERAPIES TO SPECIFIC SUBGROUPS

With the large array of new therapies and interventions now available for the treatment of patients with UA/NSTEMI, and in light of the limited resources available for health care, there has been a desire to apply the newer (and generally more expensive) therapies to those who will benefit most. Although it had long been assumed that patients at highest risk would benefit most from more aggressive therapy,[7, 104] there is now a growing body of evidence from large randomized trials to support this hypothesis. Early risk assessment (especially using troponins, but also clinical variables) has been useful in predicting which patients will derive the greatest benefit from newer and more potent antithrombotic therapies such as LMWH and glycoprotein IIb/IIIa inhibitors[153–155, 224, 403, 404] and from an early invasive strategy.[116, 199, 307, 361] Because the high-risk subgroups have a

higher event rate, even a similar *relative* benefit translates into a *greater absolute* number of cardiac events prevented. In addition, there appears to be an *increasing relative* benefit of some of the therapies[80, 405] that would extend further the incremental value of these drugs.

ELDERLY PATIENTS. Outcomes in elderly patients are worse than in younger patients; and, disappointingly, some therapies, notably thrombolysis for STEMI, appear to have *less* relative benefit than in younger patients.[347] In contrast, in UA/NSTEMI, the elderly appear to derive *greater* relative and absolute benefit from the newer more potent antithrombotic therapies. In both the ESSENCE and TIMI 11B trials, the LMWH enoxaparin, compared with UFH, appeared to exert a greater relative and absolute benefit in patients older than 65 years as compared with younger patients.[80, 405] For the glycoprotein IIb/IIIa inhibitors, an equivalent relative benefit has been observed that translated into a greater *absolute* benefit in older versus younger patients.[81–83]

With regard to an invasive versus conservative management strategy, in the FRISC II trial, the benefit of an early invasive strategy was confined to patients older than age 65 years with no difference in outcome by strategy in younger patients.[307] A similar trend was observed in the TIMI IIIB trial.[199] Thus, in unstable angina, elderly patients are at higher risk and appear to derive particular *benefit* from more aggressive antithrombotic or interventional therapy.

CLINICAL SUBGROUPS. Diabetics are known to be at high risk, and there is now evidence of a greater *relative* benefit of intravenous glycoprotein IIb/IIIa inhibition in diabetic patients with UA/NSTEMI, with a dramatic 72 percent risk reduction in 30-day death or MI (15.5 percent for heparin alone vs. 4.7 percent for tirofiban plus heparin), as compared with 13 percent reduction in nondiabetics.[189] Similarly, for patients presenting with unstable angina while already taking aspirin, there was a trend for greater benefit from eptifibatide or enoxaparin in the PURSUIT and TIMI 11B trials, respectively, compared with non–prior-aspirin users.[196, 197] In addition, patients who develop recurrent angina after initial presentation to the hospital are at high risk and derive greater benefit from glycoprotein IIb/IIIa inhibitors.[83, 193]

ELECTROCARDIOGRAPHY. In both the ESSENCE and TIMI 11B trials, patients with ST segment deviation exhibited a significant reduction in cardiac events from enoxaparin compared with UFH, whereas those without ST segment deviation did not.[80, 405] For glycoprotein IIb/IIIa inhibitors, the greatest benefit has been observed in patients with transient ST segment elevation, followed by ST segment depression, with an absolute benefit two to three times greater than for patients without ST segment changes.[83] Evidence from the FRISC II trial of invasive versus conservative strategies found particular benefit of an invasive strategy in patients with ST segment depression at presentation.[361] Thus, ST segment deviation is a marker of increased risk but also of greater benefit from aggressive antithrombotic and interventional therapy.

CARDIAC MARKERS. Elevated circulating cardiac markers have been shown to correlate with a higher rate of thrombus at angiography. This has been demonstrated with both CK-MB[4, 123] and troponin T and I.[124, 154] It has been proposed that minor myocardial damaged as assessed by troponin is a marker of microemboli from coronary thrombi.[117] A greater antithrombotic effect has been observed in patients with positive markers: for example, the degree of resolution of thrombus after 24 hours of therapy with abciximab in the CAPTURE trial was greater in patients who were troponin T positive versus troponin T negative.[154]

Clinical benefits have followed the same pattern: When treating with the IIb/IIIa inhibitor abciximab there was a 68

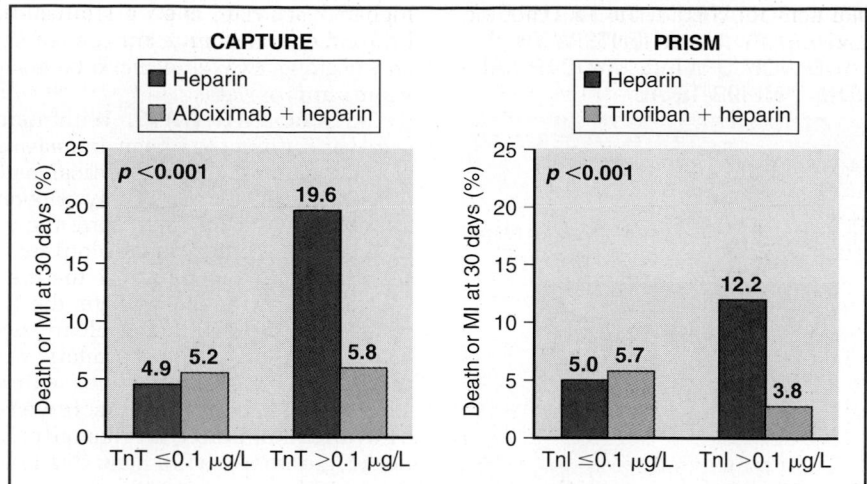

FIGURE 36–17. *Left,* Benefit of abciximab in the CAPTURE trial of patients with refractory unstable angina treated with angioplasty in those with positive versus negative troponin T values at study entry. *Right,* Greater benefit of tirofiban versus heparin in patients with UA/NSTEMI was also seen in those with positive troponin I values in the PRISM trial, with a nearly 70 percent reduction in death or myocardial infarction at 30 days with the IIb/IIIa inhibitor. (Data from Hamm CW, Heeschen C, Goldmann B, et al: Benefit of abciximab in patients with refractory unstable angina in relation to serum troponin T levels. c7E3 Fab Antiplatelet Therapy in Unstable Refractory Angina (CAPTURE) Study Investigators. N Engl J Med 340:1623–1629, 1999; and Heeschen C, Hamm CW, Goldmann B, et al: Troponin concentrations for stratification of patients with acute coronary syndromes in relation to therapeutic efficacy of tirofiban. PRISM Study Investigators. Platelet Receptor Inhibition in Ischemic Syndrome Management. Lancet 354: 1757–1762, 1999.)

percent reduction in death or MI at 6 months in the CAPTURE trial in those who were troponin T positive versus no significant benefit for those who were troponin T negative ($p < 0.001$)[154] (Fig. 36–17). These findings have recently been essentially duplicated with tirofiban versus heparin in the PRISM trial (see Fig. 36–17).[155] However, a benefit of abciximab was not observed in GUSTO IV ACS in troponin-positive patients.[333a] In the TIMI 11B trial, even among patients who were CK-MB negative, those with elevations of troponin I derived a significantly greater benefit from the LMWH enoxaparin versus UFH compared with those with negative troponins.[153] Similar findings may also be emerging for selecting patients for an invasive versus conservative strategy: In the FRISC II study, the majority of the benefit of invasive therapy at 1 year was obtained in

patients with an elevated troponin T level, using an ultra low threshold of 0.01 ng/dl or more, whereas no benefit was observed in patients with troponin T of less than 0.01 ng/dl.[116]

Thus, there is now evidence from several trials that use of troponins can assist in both risk stratification and in determining which patients should be treated with the newer antithrombotic agents, such as LMWH or glycoprotein IIb/IIIa inhibitors, and potentially with an invasive management strategy.[7]

C-REACTIVE PROTEIN. One small study of patients with unstable angina found that a glycoprotein IIb/IIIa inhibitor attenuated the increase in CRP levels as compared with placebo.[406] During long-term treatment of patients after MI, pravastatin has been shown to reduce CRP,[407] and a greater

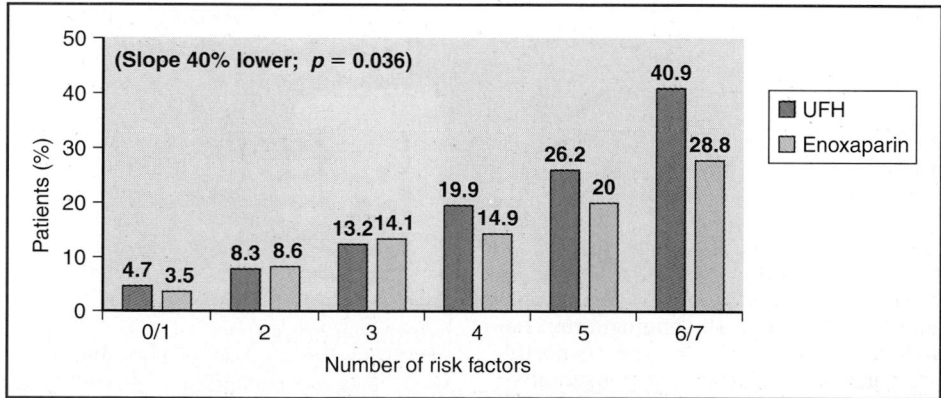

FIGURE 36–18. TIMI 11B: Use of a simple, but comprehensive clinical risk stratification score to identify (1) increasing risk of death, myocardial infarction, or urgent revascularization to day 14, and (2) increasing benefit of enoxaparin versus unfractionated heparin (UFH). The risk factors are age 65 years or older, more than three risk factors for coronary artery disease, documented coronary artery disease at catheterization, ST segment deviation of 0.5 mm or more, more than two episodes of angina in last 24 hours, aspirin within prior week, and elevated cardiac markers. (Adapted from Antman EM, Cohen M, Bernink PJLM, et al: The TIMI Risk Score for unstable angina/non-ST elevation MI: A method for prognostication and therapeutic decision making. JAMA 284:835–842, 2000.)

▼ **TABLE 36–6. FACTORS ASSOCIATED WITH FAILURE OF INITIAL MEDICAL THERAPY IN PATIENTS WITH UNSTABLE ANGINA AND NON-Q-WAVE MYOCARDIAL INFARCTION FROM THE TIMI IIIB TRIAL**

FACTOR	DEATH, MYOCARDIAL INFARCTION, RECURRENT ISCHEMIA (ODDS RATIO)	DEATH, MYOCARDIAL INFARCTION, RECURRENT ISCHEMIA, MARKEDLY POSITIVE TEST (ODDS RATIO)
ST segment depression	2.6*	3.2†
History of angina	1.8	1.9*
Heparin use	1.7*	1.3
Aspirin use	1.4*	1.3
Age (per 10 years)	1.3*	1.2
Family history of coronary artery disease	1.2	1.2

* $p < 0.01$.
† $p < 0.0001$.

Markedly positive test was defined as: 20 minutes of ST depression ≥0.1 mV on a Holter monitor, a "high risk" exercise test (ischemic discomfort before end of stage II, ST depression ≥0.2 mV, or fall in systolic blood pressure >10 mm Hg on two determinations), a "high risk" thallium perfusion imaging with ≥2 regions of reversible hypoperfusion or increased lung uptake and one region of reversible hypoperfusion. From Stone PH, et al. Factors associated with failure of medical therapy in patients with unstable angina and non-Q wave myocardial infarction: A TIMI-IIIB database study. Eur Heart J 20:1084–1093, 1999.

relative benefit of this therapy was observed in patients with elevated baseline levels of CRP compared with patients with normal baseline levels of CRP.[38, 408] Additional studies are ongoing to examine the usefulness of CRP in targeting acute therapies for unstable angina.

COMBINED RISK ASSESSMENT SCORES. Risk scores combining clinical factors have been used to identify patients who derived the greatest benefit from enoxaparin versus UFH (Fig. 36–18)[223, 224] or GP IIb/IIIa inhibitors (Reference Sabative 2000).[224a] Another use of clinical risk stratification score is to predict not just mortality or recurrent MI, but also failure of medical therapy (i.e., recurrent ischemia—either spontaneous or on a provocative test despite therapy). Such an analysis was carried out in the patients randomized to the conservative treatment strategy of the TIMI IIIB trial to identify patients with a high likelihood of failing medical therapy in whom an early invasive strategy might be advisable. Several predictors emerged, including ST segment deviation, history of prior angina, family history of coronary disease, prior use of heparin or aspirin, and advanced age (Table 36–6). By combining these baseline risk characteristics, the likelihood of developing death, MI, recurrent rest ischemia, or a strongly positive test for ischemia ranged from 8 percent if none was present to 63 percent if all six were present.[409] It seems reasonable that if three or more of these risk factors are present, patients could be referred for early coronary angiography, because it will ultimately be required in the majority, whereas if fewer than three were present, a conservative approach is more likely to be successful, without recurrent ischemia. Such a "risk-based" triage approach could be useful in selecting an appropriate management strategy (see Table 36–6).

A proposed treatment algorithm integrating the risk assessment and the targeting of therapy is illustrated in Figure 36–19. Risk assessment based on the clinical history, ECG, and serum markers identifies patients with medium to high risk who are appropriate candidates for aggressive antithrombotic therapy. For patients with uncertain history and negative ECG and markers, a rapid "rule-out MI" pathway is appropriate.

CRITICAL PATHWAYS. With rising restraints on health care costs, there has been increasing focus on the creation and implementation of "critical pathways," with an initial goal to reduce length of stay. However, several other goals are appropriate: (1) improving the use of appropriate medications (e.g., aspirin, beta blockers), (2) improving triage of the patient to the appropriate level of care,[164, 410] and (3) reducing the number of unnecessary tests that are performed (e.g., laboratory blood tests, echocardiography). With regard to triage, coronary care unit admission was standard practice for patients with all forms of acute coronary syndromes in the past. However, at present, coronary care unit admission is generally reserved for STEMI patients and those with hemodynamic compromise or other complications.

The pathway for management of UA/NSTEMI at Brigham and Women's Hospital[411] emphasizes (1) early relief of ischemic pain, which has been found to be a determinant of development of NSTEMI among patients presenting with symptoms of acute ischemia[5]; (2) administration of antithrombotic and antiischemic therapy as outlined earlier; (3) reminders of eligibility criteria of ongoing clinical trials; (4) detailed list of suggested blood and laboratory tests in an effort to reduce unnecessary tests; and (5) choice of either an early conservative strategy or an early invasive strategy, as used in TIMI IIIB.[164] Initial experience with this pathway has shown a reduction in hospital length of stay from a median of 5 days before the pathway to 2 days, as well as an improvement in the use of appropriate medications. As institutions gain experience with implementation of critical pathways, their impact on coronary care will be able to be assessed more clearly.

"CARDIAC CHECKLIST". One simple method of ensuring better compliance with recommended therapies is to use a checklist of the medications when first treating patients with UA/NSTEMI.[411] Indeed, checklists currently are used for preadmission testing and procedures, and thus this notion can be extended to treatments. Table 36–7 shows a proposed "cardiac checklist" for patients with UA/NSTEMI, which includes aspirin, heparin or LMWH, glycoprotein IIb/IIIa inhibition, beta blockers, heart-rate–lowering calcium antagonists (in the absence of congestive heart failure

▼ **TABLE 36–7. CARDIAC CHECKLIST FOR UNSTABLE ANGINA/NON–ST ELEVATION MYOCARDIAL INFARCTION**

MEDICATIONS
- ☐ Aspirin
- ☐ Heparin (or low-molecular-weight heparin)
- ☐ Glycoprotein IIb/IIIa inhibitor
- ☐ Beta blocker
- ☐ Nitrate
- ☐ Heart-rate lowering Ca^{2+} blocker
- ☐ Angiotensin-converting enzyme inhibitor

INTERVENTIONS
- ☐ Catheterization/revascularization for recurrent ischemia or in high-risk patients

SECONDARY PREVENTION
- ☐ Cholesterol: check + treat as needed
- ☐ Treat other risk factors (smoking)

See text for details of specific indications and contraindications for medications. Adapted from Cannon CP: Optimizing the medical management of acute coronary syndromes. J Thromb Thrombolysis 7:171–189, 1999.

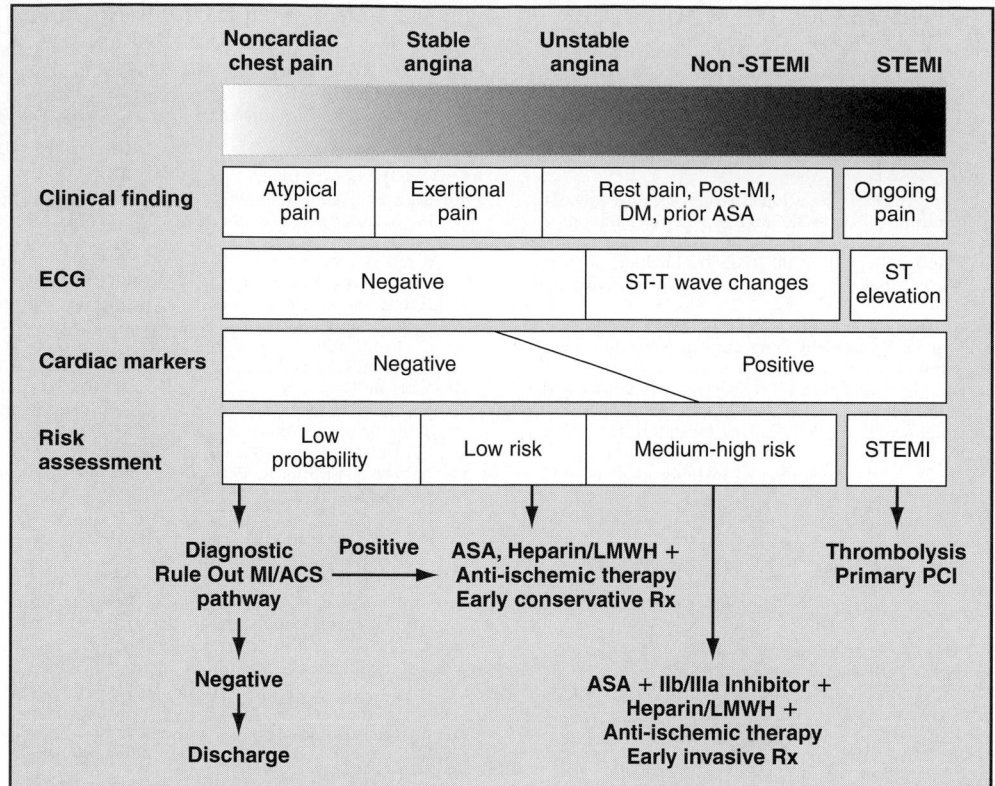

FIGURE 36-19. Algorithm for risk stratification and treatment of patients with UA/NSTEMI. Using the clinical history of the type of pain and prior medical history, the electrocardiogram (ECG), and cardiac markers, one can identify patients who have a low likelihood of UA/NSTEMI, for whom a diagnostic "rule-out" myocardial infarction (MI) or acute coronary syndrome (ACS) is warranted. If this is negative the patient is discharged home; and if it is positive, the patient is admitted and treated for UA/NSTEMI. On the other end of the spectrum patients with acute ongoing pain and ST segment elevation are treated with thrombolysis or percutaneous coronary intervention (PCI) (see Chap. 35). For those with UA/NSTEMI, all patients are given standard treatment with aspirin (ASA), unfractionated or low-molecular-weight heparin [LMWH], and antiischemic therapy with beta blockers and nitrates. Risk stratification is used to identify patients at medium to high risk, for whom aggressive treatment with glycoprotein IIb/IIIa inhibition and an early invasive strategy is warranted. (Data on the safety and efficacy of the combination of LMWH and glycoprotein IIb/IIIa inhibition are still emerging at the time of this writing.) For patients at low risk, standard treatment is likely sufficient, and a more conservative approach could be expected to be equivalent in outcomes to a more invasive one. DM = diabetes mellitus; Rx = treatment; STEMI = ST elevation myocardial infarction.

or left ventricular dysfunction), cholesterol lowering, and other risk factor modifications. This "cardiac checklist" could be used in two ways: (1) physicians who encounter these patients frequently could keep a copy on a small index card in their pocket and run down the list when writing admission orders for patients or (2) it could be used in developing standard orders for unstable angina (either printed order sheets or computerized orders).

Therapy at Hospital Discharge

After the acute treatment of patients with acute coronary syndromes, the focus turns to preventing recurrent ischemic events (i.e., secondary prevention). The drugs that have been proven to be of benefit in long-term treatment are aspirin or clopidogrel as antiplatelet therapy, beta blockers, ACE inhibitors, and statin therapy. Efforts should be undertaken to ensure that patients receive such therapies to ensure optimal outcomes during long-term treatment (see Chap. 39). In patients who have managed on a conservative strategy, a maximal exercise stress test 2 to 6 weeks after discharge is indicated to identify high-risk patients who may benefit from coronary revascularization and who should therefore undergo coronary angiography.

REFERENCES

DEFINITION AND CLASSIFICATION

1. DeWood MA, Spores J, Notske R, et al: Prevalence of total coronary occlusion during the early hours of transmural myocardial infarction. N Engl J Med 303:897–902, 1980.
2. TIMI Study Group: The Thrombolysis in Myocardial Infarction (TIMI) Trial: Phase I findings. N Engl J Med 312:932–936, 1985.
3. DeWood MA, Stifter WF, Simpson CS, et al: Coronary arteriographic findings soon after non–Q wave myocardial infarction. N Engl J Med 315:417–423, 1986.
4. The TIMI IIIA Investigators: Early effects of tissue-type plasminogen activator added to conventional therapy on the culprit lesion in patients presenting with ischemic cardiac pain at rest: Results of the Thrombolysis in Myocardial Ischemia (TIMI IIIA) Trial. Circulation 87:38–52, 1993.
5. Cannon CP, Thompson B, McCabe CH, et al: Predictors of non-Q-wave acute myocardial infarction in patients with acute ischemic syndromes: An analysis from the Thrombolysis in Myocardial Ischemia (TIMI) III Trials. Am J Cardiol 75:977–981, 1995.
6. American Heart Association: 1999 Heart and Stroke Statistical Update. *In* American Heart Association, 1999.
7. Braunwald E, Antman EM, Beasley JW, et al: ACC/AHA guidelines for the management of patients with unstable angina/non-ST segment elevation myocardial infarction: A report of the American College of Cardiology/American Heart Association Task Force on Practice Guidelines (Committee on the Management of Unstable Angina and Non-ST Seg-

ment Elevation Myocardial Infarction). J Am Coll Cardiol 36:970–1062, 2000.

8. Braunwald E: Unstable angina: A classification. Circulation 80:410–414, 1989.

9. Betriu A, Heras M, Cohen M, Fuster V: Unstable angina: Outcome according to clinical presentation. J Am Coll Cardiol 19:1659–1663, 1992.

10. Braunwald E: Unstable angina: An etiologic approach to management (editorial). Circulation 98:2219–2222, 1998.

11. Ahmed WH, Bittl JA, Braunwald E: Relation between clinical presentation and angiographic findings in unstable angina pectoris, and comparison with that in stable angina. Am J Cardiol 72:544–550, 1993.

12. Calvin JE, Klein LW, VandenBerg BJ, et al: Risk stratification in unstable angina: Prospective validation of the Braunwald classification. JAMA 273:136–144, 1995.

13. van Miltenburg-van Sijl AJM, Simoons ML, Veerhoek RJ, Bossuyt PMM: Incidence and follow-up of Braunwald subgroups in unstable angina pectoris. J Am Coll Cardiol 25:1286–1292, 1995.

14. Cannon CP, McCabe CH, Stone PH, et al: Prospective validation of the Braunwald classification of unstable angina: Results from the Thrombolysis in Myocardial Ischemia (TIMI) III Registry (abstract). Circulation 92(Suppl. I):I-19, 1995.

15. Hamm CW, Braunwald E. A classification of unstable angina—revisited. Circulation, 102:118–122, 2000.

16. Rupprecht HJ, Sohn HY, Kearney P, et al: Clinical predictors of unstable coronary lesion morphology. Eur Heart J 16:1526–1534, 1995.

17. De Servi S, Arbustini E, Marsico F, et al: Correlation between clinical and morphologic findings in unstable angina. Am J Cardiol 77:128–132, 1996.

18. Depre C, Wijns W, Robert AM, et al: Pathology of unstable plaque: correlation with the clinical severity of acute coronary syndromes. J Am Coll Cardiol 30:694–702, 1997.

PATHOPHYSIOLOGY

19. Moise A, Theroux P, Taeymans Y, et al: Unstable angina and progression of coronary atherosclerosis. N Engl J Med 309:685–689, 1983.

20. Kaski JC, Chester MR, Chen L, Katritsis D: Rapid angiographic progression of coronary artery disease in patients with angina pectoris. The role of complex stenosis morphology. Circulation 92:2058–2065, 1995.

21. Chierchia S, Brunelli C, Simonetti I, et al: Sequence of events in angina at rest: Primary reduction in coronary flow. Circulation 61:759–768, 1980.

22. Ambrose JA, Winters SL, Arora RR, et al: Angiographic evolution of coronary artery morphology in unstable angina. J Am Coll Cardiol 7: 472–478, 1986.

23. Little WC, Constantinescu M, Applegate RJ, et al: Can coronary angiography predict the site of a subsequent myocardial infarction in patients with mild-to-moderate coronary artery disease? Circulation 78:1157–1166, 1988.

24. Mann JM, Davies MJ: Vulnerable plaque. Relation of characteristics to degree of stenosis in human coronary arteries. Circulation 94:928–931, 1996.

25. Lee RT, Libby P: The unstable atheroma. Arterioscler Thromb Vasc Biol 17:1859–1867, 1997.

26. Moreno PR, Bernardi VH, Lopez-Cuellar J, et al: Macrophages, smooth muscle cells, and tissue factor in unstable angina: Implications for cell-mediated thrombogenicity in acute coronary syndromes. Circulation 94: 3090–3097, 1996.

27. Weiss EJ, Bray PF, Tayback M, et al: A polymorphism of a platelet glycoprotein receptor as an inherited risk factor for coronary thrombosis. N Engl J Med 334:1090–1094, 1996.

28. Ault K, Cannon CP, Mitchell J, et al: Platelet activation in patients after an acute coronary: Results from the TIMI 12 trial. J Am Coll Cardiol 33: 634–639, 1999.

29. Merlini PA, Bauer KA, Oltrona L, et al: Persistent activation of coagulation mechanism in unstable angina and myocardial infarction. Circulation 90:61–68, 1994.

30. Rosenberg RD, Aird WC: Vascular-bed–specific hemostasis and hypercoagulable states. N Engl J Med 340:1555–1564, 1999.

31. Falk E: Unstable angina with fatal outcome: Dynamic coronary thrombosis leading to infarction and/or sudden death. Circulation 71:699–708, 1985.

32. Davies MJ, Thomas A: Plaque fissuring—the cause of acute myocardial infarction, sudden ischemic death, and crescendo angina. Br Heart J 53: 363–373, 1985.

33. Shah PK, Falk E, Badimon JJ, et al: Human monocyte-derived macrophages induce collagen breakdown in fibrous caps of atherosclerotic plaques: Potential role of matrix-degrading metalloproteinases and implications for plaque rupture. Circulation 92:1565–1569, 1998.

34. Cannon CP, McCabe CH, Stone PH, et al: Circadian variation in the onset of unstable angina and non-Q-wave acute myocardial infarction (The TIMI III Registry and TIMI IIIB). Am J Cardiol 79:253–258, 1997.

35. Tofler GH, Brezinski D, Schafer AI, et al: Concurrent morning increase in platelet aggregability and the risk of myocardial infarction and sudden cardiac death. N Engl J Med 316:1514–1518, 1987.

36. Brezinski DA, Tofler GH, Muller JE, et al: Morning increase in platelet aggregability: Association with assumption of the upright posture. Circulation 78:35–40, 1988.

37. Muller JE, Tofler GH, Stone PH: Circadian variation and triggers of onset of acute cardiovascular disease. Circulation 79:733–743, 1989.

38. Ridker PM, Cushman M, Stampfer MJ, et al: Inflammation, aspirin, and the risk of cardiovascular disease in apparently healthy men. N Engl J Med 336:973–979, 1997.

39. Anderson JL, Carlquist JF, Muhlestein JB, et al: Evaluation of C-reactive protein, an inflammatory marker, and infectious serology as risk factors for coronary artery disease and myocardial infarction. J Am Coll Cardiol 32:35–41, 1998.

40. Berk BC, Weintraub WS, Alexander RW: Elevation of C-reative protein in "active" coronary artery disease. Am J Cardiol 65:168–172, 1990.

41. Liuzzo G, Biasucci LM, Gallimore JR, et al: The prognostic value of C-reactive protein and serum amyloid A protein in severe unstable angina. N Engl J Med 331:417–424, 1994.

42. Haverkate F, Thompson SG, Pyke SDM, et al, for the European Concerted Action on Thrombosis and Disabilities Angina Pectoris Study Group: Production of C-reactive protein and risk of coronary events in stable and unstable angina. Lancet 349:462–466, 1997.

43. Morrow DA, Rifai N, Antman EM, et al: C-reactive protein is a potent predictor of mortality independently and in combination with troponin T in acute coronary syndromes: A TIMI 11A substudy. J Am Coll Cardiol 31:1460–1465, 1998.

44. Danesh J, Collins R, Peto R: Chronic infection and coronary heart disease: Is there a link? Lancet 350:430–436, 1997.

45. Libby P, Egan D, Skarlatos S: Roles of infectious agents in atherosclerosis and restenosis: An assessment of the evidence and need for future research. Circulation 96:4095–4103, 1997.

46. Toss H, Gnarpe J, Gnarpe H, et al: Increased fibrinogen levels are associated with persistent Chlamydia pneumoniae infection in unstable coronary artery disease. Eur Heart J 19:570–577, 1998.

47. Nobel M, De Torrente A, Peter O, Genne D: No serological evidence of association between Chlamydia pneumonia infection and acute coronary heart disease. Scand J Infect Dis 31:261–264, 1999.

48. Ridker PM, Kundsin RB, Stampfer MJ, et al: Prospective study of Chlamydia pneumoniae IgG seropositivity and risks of future myocardial infarction. Circulation 99:1161–1164, 1999.

49. Fong IW, Chiu B, Viira E, et al: Rabbit model for Chlamydia pneumoniae infection. J Clin Microbiol 35:48–52, 1997.

50. Muhlestein JB, Anderson JL, Hammond EH, et al: Infection with Chlamydia pneumoniae accelerates the development of atherosclerosis and treatment with azithromycin prevents it in a rabbit model. Circulation 97:633–636, 1998.

51. Moazed TC, Campbell LA, Rosenfeld ME, et al: Chlamydia pneumoniae infection accelerates the progression of atherosclerosis in apolipoprotein E-deficient mice. J Infect Dis 180:238–241, 1999.

52. Gurfinkel E, Bozovich G, Daroca A, et al, for the ROXIS Study Group: Randomised trial of roxithromycin in non-Q wave coronary syndromes: ROXIS pilot study. Lancet 350:404–407, 1997.

53. Gupta S, Leathan EW, Carrington D, et al: Elevated Chlamydia pneumoniae antibodies, cardiovascular events, and azithromycin in male survivors of myocardial infarction. Circulation 96:404–407, 1997.

54. Anderson JL, Muhlestein JB, Carlquist J, et al: Randomized secondary prevention trial of azithromycin in patients with coronary artery disease and serological evidence for Chlamydia pneumoniae infection: The Azithromycin in Coronary Artery Disease: Elimination of Myocardial Infection with Chlamydia (ACADEMIC) study. Circulation 99: 1540–1547, 1999.

55. Sherman CT, Litvack F, Grundfest W, et al: Coronary angioscopy in patients with unstable angina pectoris. N Engl J Med 315:913–919, 1986.

56. Mizuno K, Satumo K, Miyamoto A, et al: Angioscopic evaluation of coronary artery thrombi in acute coronary syndromes. N Engl J Med 326:287–291, 1992.

57. Sullivan E, Kearney M, Isner JM, et al: Pathology of unstable angina: Analysis of biopsies obtained by directional coronary atherectomy. J Thromb Thrombolysis 1:63–71, 1994.

58. Falk E, Shah PK, Fuster V: Coronary plaque disruption. Circulation 92: 657–671, 1995.

59. Farb A, Burke AP, Tang AL, et al: Coronary plaque erosion without rupture into a lipid core: A frequent cause of coronary thrombosis in sudden coronary death. Circulation 93:1354–1363, 1996.

60. Arbustini E, De Servi S, Bramucci E, et al: Comparison of coronary lesions obtained by directional coronary atherectomy in unstable angina, stable angina, and restenosis after either atherectomy or angioplasty. Am J Cardiol 75:675–682, 1995.

61. Harrington RA, Califf RM, Holmes DR Jr, et al: Is all unstable angina the same? Insights from the Coronary Angioplasty Versus Excisional Atherectomy Trial (CAVEAT-I). Am Heart J 137:227–233, 1999.

62. de Feyter PJ, Ozaki Y, Baptista J, et al: Ischemia-related lesion characteristics in patients with stable or unstable angina: A study with intracoronary angioscopy and ultrasound. Circulation 92:1408–1413, 1995.

63. Silva JA, White CJ, Collins TJ, Ramee SR: Morphologic comparison of atherosclerotic lesions in native coronary arteries and saphenous vein grafts with intracoronary angioscopy in patients with unstable angina. Am Heart J 136:156–163, 1998.

64. Nesto RW, Waxman S, Mittleman MA, et al: Angioscopy of culprit coronary lesions in unstable angina pectoris and correlation of clinical presentation with plaque morphology. Am J Cardiol 81:225–228, 1998.

65. Ambrose JA, Hjemdahl-Monsen CE, Borrico S, et al: Angiographic dem-

onstration of a common link between unstable angina and non-Q-wave myocardial infarction. Am J Cardiol 61:244–247, 1988.

66. Hirsch PD, Hillis LD, Campbell WB, et al: Release of prostaglandins and thromboxane into the coronary circulation in patients with ischemic heart disease. N Engl J Med 304:685–691, 1981.

67. Fitzgerald DJ, Roy L, Catella F, Fitzgerald GA: Platelet activation in unstable coronary disease. N Engl J Med 315:983–989, 1986.

68. Theroux P, Latour JG, Leger-Gautier C, Delaria J: Fibrinopeptide A and platelet factor four levels in unstable angina. Circulation 75:156–162, 1987.

69. Willerson JT, Golino P, Eidt J, et al: Specific platelet mediators and unstable coronary artery lesions: Experimental evidence and potential clinical implications. Circulation 80:198–205, 1989.

70. Becker RC, Tracy RP, Bovill EG, et al, for the TIMI-III Thrombosis and Anticoagulation Study Group: The clinical use of flow cytometry for assessing platelet activation in acute coronary syndromes. Coron Artery Dis 5:339–345, 1994.

71. Lewis HD, Davis JW, Archibald DG, et al: Protective effects of aspirin against acute myocardial infarction and death in men with unstable angina. N Engl J Med 309:396–403, 1983.

72. Cairns JA, Gent M, Singer J, et al: Aspirin, sulfinpyrazone, or both in unstable angina. N Engl J Med 313:1369–1375, 1985.

73. Theroux P, Ouimet H, McCans J, et al: Aspirin, heparin or both to treat unstable angina. N Engl J Med 319:1105–1111, 1988.

74. The RISC Group: Risk of myocardial infarction and death during treatment with low dose aspirin and intravenous heparin in men with unstable coronary artery disease. Lancet 336:827–830, 1990.

75. Theroux P, Waters D, Qiu S, et al: Aspirin versus heparin to prevent myocardial infarction during the acute phase of unstable angina. Circulation 88:2045–2048, 1993.

76. Cohen M, Adams PC, Parry G, et al: Combination antithrombotic therapy in unstable rest angina and non-Q-wave infarction in nonprior aspirin users: Primary end points analysis from the ATACS trial. Circulation 89:81–88, 1994.

77. Oler A, Whooley MA, Oler J, Grady D: Adding heparin to aspirin reduces the incidence of myocardial infarction and death in patients with unstable angina: A meta-analysis. JAMA 276:811–815, 1996.

78. Fragmin during Instability in Coronary Artery Disease (FRISC) Study Group. Low-molecular-weight heparin during instability in coronary artery disease. Lancet 347:561–568, 1996.

79. Cohen M, Demers C, Gurfinkel EP, et al: A comparison of low-molecular-weight heparin with unfractionated heparin for unstable coronary artery disease. N Engl J Med 337:447–452, 1997.

80. Antman EM, McCabe CH, Gurfinkel EP, et al: Enoxaparin prevents death and cardiac ischemic events in unstable angina/non-Q-wave myocardial infarction: Results of the Thrombolysis In Myocardial Infarction (TIMI) 11B trial. Circulation 100:1593–601, 1999.

81. The PURSUIT Trial Investigators: Inhibition of Platelet Glycoprotein IIb/IIIa with eptifibatide in patient with acute coronary syndromes. N Engl J Med 339:436–443, 1998.

82. The Platelet Receptor Inhibition for Ischemic Syndrome Management (PRISM) Study Investigators: A comparison of aspirin plus tirofiban with aspirin plus heparin for unstable angina. N Engl J Med 338:1498–1505, 1998.

83. The Platelet Receptor Inhibition for Ischemic Syndrome Management in Patients Limited by Unstable Signs and Symptoms (PRISM-PLUS) Trial Investigators: Inhibition of the Platelet Glycoprotein IIb/IIIa Receptor With Tirofiban in Unstable Angina and Non-Q-Wave Myocardial Infarction. N Engl J Med 338:1488–1497, 1998.

84. Broze GJ Jr: The role of tissue factor pathway inhibitor in a revised coagulation cascade. Semin Hematol 29:159–169, 1992.

85. Furie B, Furie BC: Molecular and cellular biology of blood coagulation. N Engl J Med 326:800–806, 1992.

86. Badimon JJ, Lettino M, Toschi V, et al: Local inhibition of tissue factor reduces the thrombogenicity of disrupted human atherosclerotic plaques: Effects of tissue factor pathway inhibitor on plaque thrombogenicity under flow conditions. Circulation 99:1780–1787, 1999.

87. Prinzmetal M, Kennamer R, Merliss R, et al: A variant form of angina pectoris. Am J Med 1959;27:375, 1959.

88. McFadden EP, Clarke JG, Davies GJ, et al: Effect of intracoronary serotonin on coronary vessels in patients with stable angina and patients with variant angina. N Engl J Med 324:648–654, 1991.

89. Epstein SE, Cannon RO: Site of increased resistance to coronary flow in patients with angina pectoris and normal epicardial coronary arteries. J Am Coll Cardiol 8:459–461, 1986.

90. Eisenberg PR, Kenzora JL, Sobel BE, et al: Relation between ST segment shifts during ischemia and thrombin activity in patients with unstable angina. J Am Coll Cardiol 18:898–903, 1991.

91. Nabel EG, Ganz P, Gordon JB, et al: Dilation of normal and constriction of atherosclerotic coronary arteries caused by the cold pressor test. Circulation 77:43–52, 1988.

92. Daniel WC, Lange RA, Landau C, et al: Effects of the intracoronary infusion of cocaine on coronary arterial dimensions and blood flow in humans. Am J Cardiol 78:288–291, 1996.

93. Pitts WR, Lange RA, Cigarroa JE, Hillis LD: Cocaine-induced myocardial ischemia and infarction: Pathophysiology, recognition, and management. Prog Cardiovasc Dis 40:65–76, 1997.

94. Yeung AC, Vekshtein VI, Krantz DS, et al: The effect of atherosclerosis on the vasomotor response of coronary arteries to mental stress. N Engl J Med 325:1551–1556, 1991.

95. Flugelman MY, Virmani R, Correa R, et al: Smooth muscle cell abundance and fibroblast growth factors in coronary lesions of patients with nonfatal unstable angina: A clue to the mechanism of transformation from the stable to the unstable clinical state. Circulation 88:2493–2500, 1993.

CLINICAL PRESENTATION

96. Hochman JS, McCabe CH, Stone PH, et al: Outcome and profile of women and men presenting with acute coronary syndromes: A report from TIMI IIIB. J Am Coll Cardiol 30:141–148, 1997.

97. Hochman JS, Tamis JE, Thompson TD, et al: Sex, clinical presentation, and outcome in patients with acute coronary syndromes. Global Use of Strategies to Open Occluded Coronary Arteries in Acute Coronary Syndromes IIb Investigators. N Engl J Med 341:226–232, 1999.

98. Stone PH, Thompson B, Anderson HV, et al: Influence of race, sex, and age on management of unstable angina and non-Q-wave myocardial infarction: The TIMI III Registry. JAMA 275:1104–1112, 1996.

99. The Global Use of Strategies to Open Occluded Coronary Arteries (GUSTO) IIb Investigators: A comparison of recombinant hirudin with heparin for the treatment of acute coronary syndromes. N Engl J Med 335:775–782, 1996.

100. Cannon CP, McCabe CH, Stone PH, et al: The electrocardiogram predicts one-year outcome of patients with unstable angina and non-Q wave myocardial infarction: Results of the TIMI III Registry ECG Ancillary Study. J Am Coll Cardiol 30:133–140, 1997.

101. The TIMI IIIB Investigators: Effects of tissue plasminogen activator and a comparison of early invasive and conservative strategies in unstable angina and non-Q-wave myocardial infarction: Results of the TIMI IIIB Trial. Circulation 89:1545–1556, 1994.

102. Savonitto S, Ardissino D, Granger CB, et al: Prognostic value of the admission electrocardiogram in acute coronary syndromes. JAMA 281:707–713, 1999.

103. Hyde TA, French JK, Wong CK, et al: Four-year survival of patients with acute coronary syndromes without ST-segment elevation and prognostic significance of 0.5-mm ST-segment depression. Am J Cardiol 84:379–385, 1999.

104. Braunwald E, Mark DB, Jones RH, et al: Unstable Angina: Diagnosis and Management. Clinical Practice Guideline Number 10. Rockville, MD, Agency for Health Care Policy and Research and the National Heart, Lung, and Blood Institute, Public Health Service, U.S. Department of Health and Human Services, 1994, p 154.

105. Ryan TJ, Anderson JL, Antman EM, et al: ACC/AHA guidelines for the management of patients with acute myocardial infarction: A report of the American College of Cardiology/American Heart Association Task Force on Practice Guidelines (Committee on Management of Acute Myocardial Infarction). J Am Coll Cardiol 28:1328–1428, 1996.

106. Gottlieb SO, Weisfeldt ML, Ouyang P, et al: Silent ischemia predicts infarction and death during 2 year follow-up of unstable angina. J Am Coll Cardiol 10:756–760, 1987.

107. Nadamanee K, Intarachot V, Josephson MA, et al: Prognostic significance of silent myocardial ischemia in patients with unstable angina. J Am Coll Cardiol 10:1–9, 1987.

108. Holdright D, Patel D, Cunningham D, et al: Comparison of the effect of heparin and aspirin versus aspirin alone on transient myocardial ischemia and in-hospital prognosis in patients with unstable angina. J Am Coll Cardiol 24:39–45, 1994.

109. Patel DJ, Knight CJ, Holdright DR, et al: Long-term prognosis in unstable angina: The importance of early risk stratification using continuous ST segment monitoring [see comments]. Eur Heart J 19:240–249, 1998.

110. Jernberg T, Lindahl B, Wallentin L: ST-segment monitoring with continuous 12-lead ECG improves early risk stratification in patients with chest pain and ECG nondiagnostic of acute myocardial infarction. J Am Coll Cardiol 34:1413–1419, 1999.

111. Patel DJ, Knight CJ, Holdright DR, et al: Pathophysiology of transient myocardial ischemia in acute coronary syndromes: Characterization by continuous ST-segment monitoring. Circulation 95:1185–1192, 1997.

112. Zimmerman J, Fromm R, Meyer D, et al: Diagnostic marker cooperative study for the diagnosis of myocardial infarction. Circulation 99:1671–1677, 1999.

113. Panteghini M, Apple FS, Christenson RH, et al: Use of biochemical markers in acute coronary syndromes. IFCC Scientific Division, Committee on Standardization of Markers of Cardiac Damage. International Federation of Clinical Chemistry. Clin Chem Lab Med 37:687–693, 1999.

114. Wu AH, Valdes R Jr, Apple FS, et al: Cardiac troponin-T immunoassay for diagnosis of acute myocardial infarction. Clin Chem 40:900–907, 1994.

115. Ohman EM, Armstrong P, Christenson RH, et al: Cardiac troponin T levels for risk stratification in unstable myocardial ischemia. N Engl J Med 335:1333–1341, 1996.

116. Laqerqvist B, Diderholm E, Lindahl B, et al: An early invasive treatment strategy reduces cardiac events regardless of troponin levels in unstable coronary artery (UCAD) with and without troponin-elevation: A FRISC II substudy (abstract). Circulation 100(Suppl I):I-497, 1999.

117. Hamm CW: Unstable angina: The breakthrough. Eur Heart J 20:1517–1519, 1999.

118. Scirica BM, Moliterno DJ, Every NR, et al: Differences between men and women in the management of unstable angina pectoris (The

GUARANTEE Registry). The GUARANTEE Investigators. Am J Cardiol 84:1145–1150, 1999.

119. Scirica BM, Moliterno DJ, Every NR, et al: Racial differences in the management of unstable angina: Results from the GUARANTEE Registry. Am Heart J 138:1065–1072, 1999.

120. Diver DJ, Bier JD, Ferreira PE, et al: Clinical and arteriographic characterization of patients with unstable angina without critical coronary arterial narrowing (from the TIMI-IIIA trial). Am J Cardiol 74:531–537, 1994.

121. Roberts WC: Qualitative and quantitative comparison of amounts of narrowing by atherosclerotic plaques in the major epicardial coronary arteries at necropsy in sudden coronary death, transmural acute myocardial infarction, transmural healed myocardial infarction and unstable angina pectoris. Am J Cardiol 64:324–328, 1989.

122. Freeman MR, Williams AE, Chisholm RJ, Armstrong PW: Intracoronary thrombus and complex morphology in unstable angina: Relation to timing of angiography and in-hospital cardiac events. Circulation 80:17–23, 1989.

123. Zhao X-Q, Theroux P, Snapinn SM, Sax FL, for the PRISM-PLUS Investigators. Intracoronary thrombus and platelet glycoprotein IIb/IIIa receptor blockade with tirofiban in unstable angina or non-Q-wave myocardial infarction: Angiographic results from the PRISM-PLUS trial (Platelet Receptor Inhibition for Ischemic Syndrome Management in Patients Limited by Unstable Signs and Symptoms). Circulation 100:1609–1615, 1999.

124. Heeschen C, van Den Brand MJ, Hamm CW, Simoons ML: Angiographic findings in patients with refractory unstable angina according to troponin T status. Circulation 100:1509–1514, 1999.

125. Clark LT, Garfein OB, Dwyer EM Jr: Acute pulmonary edema due to ischemic heart disease without accompanying myocardial infarction: Natural history and clinical profile. Am J Med 75:332–336, 1983.

126. Jaber WA, Prior DL, Marso SP, et al: CHF on presentation is associated with markedly worse outcomes among patients with acute coronary syndromes: PURSUIT trial findings (abstract). Circulation 100(Suppl. I): I-433, 1999.

127. Sacks RM, Pfeffer MA, Moye LA, et al: The effect of pravastatin on coronary events after myocardial infarction in patients with average cholesterol levels. N Engl J Med 335:1001–1009, 1996.

128. Scandinavian Simvastatin Survival Study Group: Randomised trial of cholesterol lowering in 4444 patients with coronary heart disease: The Scandinavian Simvastatin Survival Study (4S). Lancet 344:1383–1389, 1994.

129. The Long-Term Intervention with Pravastatin in Ischaemic Disease (LIPID) Study Group. Prevention of cardiovascular events and death with pravastatin in patients with coronary heart disease and a broad range of initial cholesterol levels. N Engl J Med 339:1349–1357, 1998.

DIAGNOSIS

130. Pope JH, Ruthazer R, Beshansky JR, et al: Clinical features of emergency department patients presenting with symptoms suggestive of acute cardiac ischemia: A multicenter study. J Thromb Thrombolysis 6: 63–74, 1998.

131. Kontos MC, Ornato JP, Tatum, JL, et al: How many patients are eligible for treatment with GP IIb/IIIa inhibitors? Results from a clinical database (abstract). Circulation 100(Suppl. I):I-775, 1999.

132. Goldman L, Cook EF, Brand DA, et al: A computer protocol to predict myocardial infarction in emergency department patients with chest pain. N Engl J Med 318:797–803, 1988.

133. Lee TH, Juarez G, Cook EF, et al: Ruling out acute myocardial infarction: A prospective multicenter validation of a 12-hour strategy for patients at low risk. N Engl J Med 324:1239–1246, 1991.

134. Pozen MW, D'Agostino RB, Selker HP, et al: A predictive instrument to improve coronary-care-unit admission practices in acute ischemic heart disease: A prospective multicenter clinical trial. N Engl J Med 310: 1273–1278, 1984.

135. Tierney WM, Roth BJ, Psaty B, et al: Predictors of myocardial infarction in emergency room patients. Crit Care Med 13:526–531, 1985.

136. Goldman L, Cook EF, Johnson PA, et al: Prediction of the need for intensive care in patients who come to emergency departments with acute chest pain. N Engl J Med 334:1498–1504, 1996.

137. Sarasin FP, Reymond J-M, Griffith JL, et al: Impact of the acute cardiac ischemia time-insensitive predictive instrument (ACI-TIPI) on speed of triage decision making for emergency department patients presenting with chest pain: A controlled clinical trial. J Gen Intern Med 9:187–194, 1994.

138. Selker HP, Griffith JL, D'Agostino RB: A time-insensitive predictive instrument for acute myocardial infarction mortality: A multicenter study. Med Care 29:1196–1211, 1991.

139. Selker HP, Beshansky JR, Griffith JL, et al: Use of the acute cardiac ischemia time-insensitive predictive instrument (ACI-TIPI) to assist with triage of patients with chest pain or other symptoms suggestive of acute cardiac ischemia: A multicenter, controlled clinical trial. Ann Intern Med 129:845–855, 1998.

140. Hertzer NR, Beven EG, Young JR, et al: Coronary artery disease in peripheral vascular patients: A classification of 1000 coronary angiograms and results of surgical management. Ann Surg 199:223–233, 1984.

141. Polanczyk CA, Lee TH, Cook EF, et al: Cardiac troponin I as a predictor of major cardiac events in emergency department patients with acute chest pain. J Am Coll Cardiol 32:8–14, 1998.

142. Polanczyk CA, Johnson PA, Cook EF, Lee TH: A proposed strategy for utilization of creatine kinase-MB and troponin I in the evaluation of acute chest pain. Am J Cardiol 83:1175–1179, 1999.

143. Johnson PA, Goldman L, Sacks DB, et al: Cardiac troponin T as a marker for myocardial ischemia in patients seen at the emergency department for acute chest pain. Am Heart J 137:1137–1144, 1999.

144. Hamm CW, Goldmann BU, Heeschen C, et al: Emergency room triage of patients with acute chest pain by means of rapid testing for cardiac troponin T or troponin I [see comments]. N Engl J Med 337:1648–1653, 1997.

145. Rapid Evaluation by Assay of Cardiac Troponin T (REACTT) Investigators Study Group: Evaluation of a bedside whole-blood rapid troponin T assay in the emergency department. Acad Emerg Med 4:1018–1024, 1997.

146. Hamm CW, Ravkilde J, Gerhardt W, et al: The prognostic value of troponin T in unstable angina. N Engl J Med 327:146–150, 1992.

147. Ravkilde J, Nissen H, Horder M, Thygesen K: Independent prognostic value of serum creatine kinase isoenzyme MB mass, cardiac troponin T and myosin light chain levels in suspected acute myocardial infarction: Analysis of 28 months of follow-up in 196 patients. J Am Coll Cardiol 25:574–581, 1995.

148. Antman EM, Tanasijevic MJ, Thompson B, et al: Cardiac-specific troponin I levels to predict the risk of mortality in patients with acute coronary syndromes. N Engl J Med 335:1342–1349, 1996.

149. Lindahl B, Venge P, Wallentin L, for the FRISC Study Group. Relation between troponin T and the risk of subsequent cardiac events in unstable coronary artery disease. Circulation 93:1651–1657, 1996.

150. Galvani M, Ottani F, Ferrini D, et al: Prognostic influence of elevated values of cardiac troponin I in patients with unstable angina. Circulation 95:2053–2059, 1997.

151. Newby LK, Christenson RH, Ohman EM, et al: Value of serial troponin T measures for early and late risk stratification in patients with acute coronary syndromes. The GUSTO-IIa Investigators. Circulation 98: 1853–1859, 1998.

152. Olatidoye AG, Wu AH, Feng YJ, Waters D: Prognostic role of troponin T versus troponin I in unstable angina pectoris for cardiac events with meta-analysis comparing published studies. Am J Cardiol 81:1405–1410, 1998.

153. Morrow DA, de Lemos JA, Rifai N: Troponin I predicts early need for revascularization in acute coronary syndromes: A TIMI 11B substudy (abstract). Circulation 100(Suppl I):I-775, 1999.

154. Hamm CW, Heeschen C, Goldmann B, et al: Benefit of abciximab in patients with refractory unstable angina in relation to serum troponin T levels. c7E3 Fab Antiplatelet Therapy in Unstable Refractory Angina (CAPTURE) Study Investigators. N Engl J Med 340:1623–1629, 1999.

155. Heeschen C, Hamm CW, Goldmann B, et al: Troponin concentrations for stratification of patients with acute coronary syndromes in relation to therapeutic efficacy of tirofiban. PRISM Study Investigators. Platelet Receptor Inhibition in Ischemic Syndrome Management. Lancet 354: 1757–1762, 1999.

156. Wright SA, Sawyer DB, Sacks DB, et al: Elevation of troponin I levels in patients without evidence of myocardial injury. JAMA 278:2144, 1997.

157. deFilippi CR, Parmar RJ, Potter MA, Tocchi M: Diagnostic accuracy, angiographic correlates and long-term risk stratification with the troponin T ultra sensitive Rapid Assay in chest pain patients at low risk for acute myocardial infarction. Eur Heart J 19(Suppl N):N42–N47, 1998.

158. Khan IA, Tun A, Wattanasauwan N, et al: Elevation of serum cardiac troponin I in noncardiac and cardiac diseases other than acute coronary syndromes. Am J Emerg Med 17:225–229, 1999.

159. Lee TH: Chest pain algorithms in the troponin era: Time to integrate expertise (editorial). Am Heart J 138:606–608, 1999.

160. de Lemos JA, Rifai N, Morrow DA, et al: Elevated baseline myoglobin is associated with increased mortality in acute coronary syndromes, even among patients with normal baseline troponin I: a TIMI 11B substudy (abstract). Circulation 100(Suppl I):I-372–I-373, 1999.

161. Puleo PR, Guadagno PA, Roberts R, et al: Early diagnosis of acute myocardial infarction based on assay for subforms of creatine kinase-MB. Circulation 82:759–764, 1990.

162. Gibler WB, Runyon JP, Levy RC, et al: A rapid diagnostic and treatment center for patients with acute chest pain in the emergency department. Ann Emerg Med 25:1–8, 1995.

163. Farkouh ME, Smars PA, Reeder GS, et al: A clinical trial of a chest-pain observation unit for patients with unstable angina. Chest Pain Evaluation in the Emergency Room (CHEER) Investigators. N Engl J Med 339: 1882–1888, 1998.

164. Cannon CP: Optimizing the treatment of unstable angina. J Thromb Thrombolysis 2:205–218, 1995.

165. Nichol G, Walls R, Goldman L, et al: A critical pathway for management of patient with acute chest pain at low risk for myocardial ischemia: Recommendations and potential impact. Ann Intern Med 127:996–1005, 1997.

166. Kerns JR, Shaub TF, Fontanarosa PB: Emergency cardiac stress testing in the evaluation of emergency department patients with atypical chest pain. Ann Emerg Med 22:794–798, 1993.

167. Mikhail MG, Smith FA, Gray M, et al: Cost-effectiveness of mandatory stress testing in chest pain center patients. Ann Emerg Med 29:88–98, 1997.

168. Krasuski RA, Hartley LH, Lee TH, et al: Weekend and holiday exercise testing in patients with chest pain. J Gen Intern Med 14:10–14, 1999.

169. Veretto T, Cantalupi D, Altieri A, Orlandi C: Emergency room technetium-99m sestamibi imaging to rule out acute myocardial ischemic events in patients with nondiagnostic electrocardiograms. J Am Coll Cardiol 22:1804–1808, 1993.

170. Tatum JL, Jesse RL, Kontos MC, et al: Comprehensive strategy for the evaluation and triage of the chest pain patient. Ann Emerg Med 29:116–125, 1997.

171. Colon PJ III, Guarisco JS, Murgo J, Cheirif J: Utility of stress echocardiography in the triage of patients with atypical chest pain from the emergency department. Am J Cardiol 82:1282–1284, A10, 1998.

172. Colon PJ III, Mobarek SK, Milani RV, et al: Prognostic value of stress echocardiography in the evaluation of atypical chest pain patients without known coronary artery disease. Am J Cardiol 81:545–551, 1998.

173. Pellikka PA: Stress echocardiography in the evaluation of chest pain and accuracy in the diagnosis of coronary artery disease. Prog Cardiovasc Dis 39:523–532, 1997.

174. Gomez MA, Anderson JL, Karagounis LA, et al, for the ROMIO Study Group: An emergency department-based protocol for rapidly ruling out myocardial ischemia reduces hospital time and expense: results of a randomized study (ROMIO). J Am Coll Cardiol 28:25–33, 1996.

175. Berning J, Launbjerg J, Appleyard M: Echocardiographic algorithms for admission and predischarge prediction of mortality in acute myocardial infarction. Am J Cardiol 69:1538–1544, 1992.

176. Fleischmann KE, Goldman L, Robiolio PA, et al: Echocardiographic correlates of survival in patients with chest pain. J Am Coll Cardiol 23:1390–1396, 1994.

177. Sommer T, Fehske W, Holzknecht N, et al: Aortic dissection: A comparative study of diagnosis with spiral CT, multiplanar transesophageal echocardiography, and MR imaging. Radiology 199:347–352, 1996.

178. Evangelista A, Garcia-del-Castillo H, Gonzalez-Alujas T, et al: Diagnosis of ascending aortic dissection by transesophageal echocardiography: Utility of M-mode in recognizing artifacts. J Am Coll Cardiol 27:102–107, 1996.

179. Banning AP, Masani ND, Ikram S, et al: Transoesophageal echocardiography as the sole diagnostic investigation in patients with suspected thoracic aortic dissection. Br Heart J 72:461–465, 1994.

180. Santoro GM, Sciagra R, Buonamici P, et al: Head-to-head comparison of exercise stress testing, pharmacologic stress echocardiography, and perfusion tomography as first-line examination for chest pain in patients without history of coronary artery disease. J Nucl Cardiol 5:19–27, 1998.

181. Geleijnse ML, Elhendy A, van Domburg RT, et al: Cardiac imaging for risk stratification with dobutamine-atropine stress testing in patients with chest pain. Echocardiography, perfusion scintigraphy, or both? Circulation 96:137–147, 1997.

182. Multicenter Postinfarction Research Group. Risk Stratification and survival after myocardial infarction. N Engl J Med 309:331–336, 1983.

183. Zaret BL, Wackers FJT, Terrin ML, et al: Value of radionuclide rest and exercise left ventricular ejection fraction is assessing survival of patients after thrombolytic therapy for acute myocardial infarction: Results of the Thrombolysis in Myocardial Infarction (TIMI) Phase II study. J Am Coll Cardiol 26:73–79, 1995.

184. Pfeffer MA, Braunwald E, Moye LA, et al: Effect of captopril on mortality and morbidity in patients with left ventricular dysfunction after myocardial infarction. N Engl J Med 327:669–677, 1992.

185. Cannon CP, Johnson EB, Cermignani M, et al: Emergency department thrombolysis critical pathway reduces door-to-drug times in acute myocardial infarction. Clin Cardiol 22:17–22, 1999.

186. Zalenski RJ, Rydman RJ, Ting S, et al: A national survey of emergency department chest pain centers in the United States. Am J Cardiol 81:1305–1309, 1998.

187. Graff LG, Dallara J, Ross MA, et al: Impact on the care of the emergency department chest pain patient from the Chest Pain Evaluation Registry (CHEPER) Study. Am J Cardiol 80:563–568, 1997.

RISK STRATIFICATION

188. Boersma E, Pieper KS, Steyerberg EW, et al: Predictors of outcome in patients with acute coronary syndromes without persistent ST-segment elevation: Results from an international trial of 9,461 patients. Circulation 2000; 101:2557–2567, 2000.

189. Theroux P, Ghannam A, Nasmith J, et al: Improved cardiac outcomes in diabetic unstable angina/non-Q-wave myocardial infarction patients treated with tirofiban and heparin (abstract). Circulation 98(Suppl I):I-359, 1998.

190. McGuire DK, Emanuelsson H, Charnwood A, et al: Diabetes mellitus is associated with worse clinical outcomes across the spectrum of acute coronary syndromes: Results from GUSTO-IIb (abstract). Circulation 100(Suppl I):I-432, 1999.

191. Cotter G, Cannon CP, McCabe CH, et al: Prior peripheral vascular disease and cerebrovascular disease are independent predictors of increased 1 year mortality in patients with acute coronary syndromes: Results from OPUS-TIMI 16. J Am Coll Cardiol, 35(Suppl A):392a, 2000.

192. Taniguchi H, Iwasaka T, Sugiura T, et al: Acute pulmonary edema in patients with unstable angina: Clinical profile and natural history. Coron Artery Dis 2:529–532, 1992.

193. Klootwijk P, Meij S, Melkert R, et al: Reduction of recurrent ischemia with abciximab during continuous ECG-ischemia monitoring in patients with unstable angina refractory to standard treatment (CAPTURE). Circulation 98:1358–1364, 1998.

194. Helgason CM, Bolin KM, Hoff JA, et al: Development of aspirin resistance in persons with previous ischemic stroke. Stroke 25:2331–2336, 1994.

195. Weber AA, Zimmermann KC, Meyer-Kirchrath J, Schror K: Cyclooxygenase-2 in human platelets as a possible factor in aspirin resistance. Lancet 353:900, 1999.

196. Alexander JH, Harrington RA, Tuttle RH, et al: Prior aspirin use predicts worse outcomes in patients with non-ST-elevation acute coronary syndromes. PURSUIT Investigators. Platelet IIb/IIIa in Unstable angina: Receptor Suppression Using Integrilin Therapy. Am J Cardiol 83:1147–1151, 1999.

197. Santopinto J, Blanca B, Tajer C, et al: Prior aspirin users are at increased risk of cardiac events and should be treated with enoxaparin (abstract). Circulation 100(Suppl. I):I-620, 1999.

198. Sharis PJ, Cannon CP, McCabe CH, et al: Prior aspirin use is a univariate, but not a multivariate predictor of 1 year mortality in 10,302 patients with acute coronary syndromes: Results from OPUS-TIMI 16. J Am Coll Cardiol, 35(Suppl A):392a, 2000.

199. Anderson HV, Cannon CP, Stone PH, et al: One-year results of the Thrombolysis In Myocardial Infarction (TIMI) IIIB clinical trial: A randomized comparison of tissue-type plasminogen activator versus placebo and early invasive versus early conservative strategies in unstable angina and non-Q-wave myocardial infarction. J Am Coll Cardiol 26:1643–1650, 1995.

200. Cohen M, Xiong J, Parry G, et al: Prospective comparison of unstable angina versus non-Q wave myocardial infarction during antithrombotic therapy. J Am Coll Cardiol 22:1338–1343, 1993.

201. Gibson RS, Boden WE, Theroux P, et al: Diltiazem and reinfarction in patients with non-Q wave myocardial infarction. Results of a double-blind, randomized, multicenter trial. N Engl J Med 315:423–429, 1986.

202. Gheorghiade M, Schultz L, Tilley B, et al: Natural history of the first non-Q wave myocardial infarction in the placebo arm of the Beta-Blocker Heart Attack Trial. Am Heart J 122:1548–1553, 1991.

203. Gibson RS: Non-Q wave myocardial infarction: Prognosis, changing incidence, and management. In Gersh BJ, Rahimtoola SH (eds): Acute Myocardial Infarction. New York, Elsevier Science Publishing, 1991, pp 284–307.

204. Luchi RJ, Scott SM, Dupree RH, and the Principal Investigators and their Associates of Veterans Administration Cooperative Study No. 28: Comparison of medical and surgical treatment for unstable angina pectoris. N Engl J Med 316:977–984, 1987.

205. Antman EM, Grudzien C, Mitchell RN, Sacks DB: Detection of unsuspected myocardial necrosis by rapid bedside assay for cardiac troponin T. Am Heart J 133:596–598, 1997.

206. Rottbauer W, Greten T, Muller-Bardorff M, et al: Troponin T: A diagnostic marker for myocardial infarction and minor cardiac cell damage. Eur Heart J 17(Suppl F):3–8, 1996.

207. Simoons ML, van den Brand M, Lincoff M, et al: Minimal myocardial damage during coronary intervention is associated with impaired outcome. Eur Heart J 20:1112–1119, 1999.

208. Stubbs P, Collinson P, Moseley D, et al: Prospective study of the role of cardiac troponin T in patients admitted with unstable angina. BMJ 313:262–264, 1996.

209. Adams JE, Bodor GS, Davila-Roman VG, et al: Cardiac troponin I: A marker with high specificity for cardiac injury. Circulation 88:101–106, 1993.

210. Fung AY, Jue J, Thompson CR, et al: Diagnosis of microinfarction in acute ischemic syndromes is of prognostic value (abstract). J Am Coll Cardiol Special Issue:316A, 1994.

211. Lloyd-Jones DM, Camargo CA Jr, Giugliano RP, et al:. Characteristics and prognosis of patients with suspected acute myocardial infarction and elevated MB relative index but normal total creatine kinase. Am J Cardiol 84:957–962, 1999.

212. Antman EM, Sacks DB, Rifai N, et al: Time to positivity of a rapid bedside assay for cardiac-specific troponin T predicts prognosis in acute coronary syndromes: A Thrombolysis in Myocardial Infarctin (TIMI) 11A Substudy. J Am Coll Cardiol 31:326–330, 1998.

213. Toss H, Lindahl B, Siegbahn A, Wallentin L, for the FRISC Study Group: Prognostic influence of increased fibrinogen and C-reactive protein levels in unstable coronary artery disease. Circulation 96:4204–4210, 1997.

214. Rebuzzi AG, Quaranta G, Liuzzo G, et al: Incremental prognostic value of serum levels of troponin T and C-reactive protein on admission in patients with unstable angina pectoris. Am J Cardiol 82:715–719, 1998.

215. Heeschen C, Hamm CW, Jens B: Predictive value of C-reactive protein and troponin T in patients with unstable angina: A comparative analysis (abstract). Circulation 100(Suppl I):I-371, 1999.

216. de Winter RJ, Bholasingh R, Lijmer JG, et al: Independent prognostic value of C-reactive protein and troponin I in patients with unstable angina or non-Q-wave myocardial infarction. Cardiovasc Res 42:240–245, 1999.

217. Ferreiros ER, Boissonnet CP, Pizarro R, et al: Independent prognostic value of elevated C-reactive protein in unstable angina. Circulation 100:1958–1963, 1999.

218. Biasucci LM, Liuzzo G, Grillo RL, et al: Elevated levels of C-reactive protein at discharge in patients with unstable angina predict recurrent instability. Circulation 99:855–860, 1999.

219. Morrow DA, Antman EM, Rifai N, et al: Serum amyloid A and rapid troponin independently predict mortality in acute coronary syndromes. J Am Coll Cardiol, 35:358–362, 2000.

220. Biasucci LM, Liuzzo G, Fantuzzi G, et al: Increasing levels of interleukin (IL)-1Ra and IL-6 during the first 2 days of hospitalization in unstable angina are associated with increased risk of in-hospital coronary events. Circulation 99:2079–2084, 1999.

221. Aukrust P, Muller F, Ueland T, et al. Enhanced levels of soluble and membrane-bound CD40 ligand in patients with unstable angina: Possible reflection of T lymphocyte and platelet involvement in the pathogenesis of acute coronary syndromes. Circulation 100:614–620, 1999.

222. Liuzzo G, Kopecky SL, Frye RL, et al: Perturbation of the T-cell repertoire in patients with unstable angina. Circulation 100:2135–2139, 1999.

223. Holper EM, Antman EM, McCabe CH, et al: A simple, readily available method for risk stratification of patients with unstable angina or non-Q myocardial infarction: a TIMI 11B substudy (abstract). Circulation 98(Suppl I):I-493, 1998.

224. Antman EM, Cohen M, Bernink PJLM, et al: The TIMI risk score for unstable angina/non-ST elevation MI: A method for prognostication and therapeutic decision making. JAMA 284:835–842, 2000.

224a. Sabatine MS, Snapinn S, Theroux P, et al: Factors influencing outcome and degree of benefit with GP IIb/IIIa inhibition in patients with non-ST-elevation acute coronary syndromes. J Am Coll Cardiol 35 (Suppl A):392A, 2000.

MEDICAL THERAPY

225. Cheitlin MD, Hutter AM Jr, Brindis RG, et al: ACC/AHA expert consensus document: Use of sildenafil (Viagra) in patients with cardiovascular disease. American College of Cardiology/American Heart Association. J Am Coll Cardiol 33:273–282, 1999.

226. Gruppo Italiano per lo Studio della Sopravvivenza nell'Infarto Miocardico. GISSI-3: Effects of lisinopril and transdermal glyceryl trinitrate singly and together on 6-week mortality and ventricular function after acute myocardial infarction. Lancet 343:1115–1122, 1994.

227. ISIS-4 Collaborative Group: ISIS-4: Randomized factorial trial assessing early oral captopril, oral mononitrate, and intravenous magnesium sulphate in 58,050 patients with suspected acute myocardial infarction. Lancet 345:669–685, 1995.

228. Gottlieb SO, Weisfeldt ML, Ouyang P, et al: Effect of the addition of propranolol to therapy with nifedepine for unstable angina: A randomized, double-blind, placebo-controlled trial. Circulation 73:331–337, 1986.

229. Yusuf S, Wittes J, Friedman L: Overview of results of randomized clinical trials in heart disease: II. Unstable angina, heart failure, primary prevention with aspirin and risk factor reduction. JAMA 260:2259–2263, 1988.

230. Muller JE, Turi ZG, Pearle DL, et al: Nifedipine and conventional therapy for unstable angina pectoris: A randomized, double-blind comparison. Circulation 69:728–739, 1984.

231. The Holland Interuniversity Nifedipine/Metoprolol Trial (HINT) Research Group: Early treatment of unstable angina in the coronary care unit: A randomised, double blind, placebo controlled comparison of recurrent ischaemia in patients treated with nifedipine or metoprolol or both. Br Heart J 56:400–413, 1986.

232. Theroux P, Taeymans Y, Morissette D, et al: A randomized study comparing propranolol and diltiazem in the treatment of unstable angina. J Am Coll Cardiol 5:717–722, 1985.

233. Rizik D, Timmis GC, Grines CL, et al: Immediate use of beta blockers, but not calcium blockers, improves prognosis in unstable angina (abstract). Circulation 84(Suppl II):II–345, 1991.

234. The Norwegian Multicenter Study Group: Timolol-induced reduction in mortality and reinfarction in patients surviving acute myocardial infarction. N Engl J Med 304:801–807, 1981.

235. Hjalmarson A, Elmfeldt D, Herlitz J, et al: Effect on mortality of metoprolol in acute myocardial infarction, a double-blind randomized trial. Lancet 2:823–827, 1981.

236. Beta-Blocker Heart Attack Trial Research Group: A randomized trial of propranolol in patients with acute myocardial infarction: I. Mortality results. JAMA 247:1707–1714, 1982.

237. ISIS-1 (First International Study of Infarct Survival) Collaborative Group: Randomised trial of intravenous atenolol among 16,027 cases of suspected acute myocardial infarction. Lancet 2:57–66, 1986.

238. Hjalmarson A, Herlitz J, Holmberg S, et al: The Gotenborg metoprolol trial: Effects on mortality and morbidity in acute myocardial infarction. Circulation 67(Suppl I):I-26–I-32, 1983.

239. Yusuf S, Sleight P, Rossi P, et al: Reduction in infarct size, arrhythmias and chest pain by early intravenous beta blockade in suspected myocardial infarction. Circulation 67(Suppl I):I-32–I-41, 1983.

240. Shivkumar K, Schultz L, Goldstein S, Gheorghiade M: Effects of propranolol in patients entered in the Beta-Blocker Heart Attack Trial with their first myocardial infarction and persistent electrocardiographic ST-segment depression. Am Heart J 135(2 Pt 1):261–267, 1998.

241. Packer M, Bristow MR, Cohn JN, et al: The effect of carvedilol on morbidity and mortality in patients with chronic heart failure. N Engl J Med 334:1349–1355, 1996.

242. The MERIT-HF Investigators: Effect of metoprolol CR/XL in chronic heart failure: Metoprolol CR/XL Randomised Intervention Trial in Congestive Heart Failure (MERIT-HF). Lancet 353:2001–2007, 1999.

243. The CIBIS-II Investigators: The Cardiac Insufficiency Bisoprolol Study II (CIBIS-II): A randomised trial. Lancet 353:9–13, 1999.

244. TIMI Study Group: Comparison of invasive and conservative strategies after treatment with intravenous tissue plasminogen activator in acute myocardial infarction: Results of the Thrombolysis in Myocardial Infarction (TIMI) Phase II Trial. N Engl J Med 320:618–627, 1989.

245. Kirshenbaum JM, Kloner RA, Antman E, Braunwald E: Use of an ultrashort acting β blocker in patients with acute myocardial ischemia. Circulation 72:873, 1985.

246. Theroux P, Gregoire J, Chin C, et al: Intravenous diltiazem in acute myocardial infarction: Diltiazem as adjunctive therapy to activase (DATA) trial. J Am Coll Cardiol 32:620–628, 1998.

247. Boden WE, Scheldewaert R, Walters EG, et al: Design of a placebo-controlled clinical trial of long-acting diltiazem and aspirin versus aspirin alone in patients receiving thrombolysis with a first acute myocardial infarction. Am J Cardiol 75:1120–1123, 1995.

248. Boden WE: Incomplete Infarction Trial of European Research Collaborators Evaluating Prognosis Post-Thrombolysis (INTERCEPT). Presented at the American Heart Association Scientific Sessions, Dallas, November 1998.

249. The Danish Study Group on Verapamil in Myocardial Infarction: Effect of verapamil on mortality and major events after acute infarction (The Danish Verapamil Infarction Trial II—DAVIT II). Am J Cardiol 66:779, 1990.

250. Teo KT, Yusuf S, Furberg CD: Effects of prophylactic antiarrhythmic drug therapy in acute myocardial infarction: An overview of results from randomized controlled trails. JAMA 270:1589–1595, 1993.

251. Hennekens CH, Albert CM, Godfried SL, et al: Adjunctive drug therapy of acute myocardial infarction—evidence from clinical trials. N Engl J Med 335:1660–1667, 1996.

252. Pepine CJ, Faich G, Makuch R: Verapamil use in patients with cardiovascular disease: An overview of randomized trials. Clin Cardiol 21:633–641, 1998.

253. The Multicenter Diltiazem Postinfarction Trial Research Group. The effect of diltiazem on mortality and reinfarction after myocardial infarction. N Engl J Med 319:385–392, 1988.

254. Wilcox RG, Hampton JR, Banks DC, et al: Trial of Early Nifedepine in Acute Myocardial Infarction: The TRENT study. BMJ 293:1204–1208, 1986.

255. The Israeli SPRINT Study Group: Secondary Prevention Reinfarction Israeli Nifedipine Trial (SPRINT): A randomized intervention trial of nifedipine in patients with acute myocardial infarction. Eur Heart J 9:354–364, 1988.

256. Hansen JF, Hagerup L, Sigurd B, et al: Cardiac event rates after acute myocardial infarction in patients treated with verapamil and trandolapril versus trandolapril alone. Am J Cardiol 79:738–741, 1997.

257. Packer M, O'Connor CM, Ghali JK, et al: Effect of amlodipine on morbidity and mortality in severe chronic heart failure. N Engl J Med 335:1107–1114, 1996.

258. Cohn JN, Ziesche S, Smith R, et al: Effect of the calcium antagonist felodipine as supplementary vasodilator therapy in patients with chronic heart failure treated with enalapril: V-HeFT III. Vasodilator-Heart Failure Trial (V-HeFT) Study Group. Circulation 96:856–863, 1997.

259. The Acute Infarction Ramipril Efficacy (AIRE) Study Investigators. Effect of ramipril on mortality and morbidity of survivors of acute myocardial infarction with clinical evidence of heart failure. Lancet 342:821–828, 1993.

260. Chinese Cardiac Study Collaborative Group. Oral captopril versus placebo among 13,634 patients with suspected myocardial infarction: Interim report from the Chinese Cardiac Study (CCS-1). Lancet 345:686–687, 1995.

261. Yusuf S, Sleight P, Pogue J, et al: Effects of an angiotensin-converting-enzyme inhibitor, ramipril, on cardiovascular events in high-risk patients. N Engl J Med 342:145–53, 2000 [published erratum appears in N Engl J Med 2000 Mar 9; 342:748].

262. Rutherford JD, Pfeffer MA, Moye LA, et al: Effects of captopril on ischemic events after myocardial infarction: Results of the Survival and Ventricular Enlargement Trial. Circulation 90:1731–1738, 1994.

263. The SOLVD Investigators. Effect of enalapril on survival in patients with reduced left ventricular ejection fractions and congestive heart failure. N Engl J Med 325:293–302, 1991.

264. Pedersen TR, Kjekshus J, Berg K, et al: Cholesterol lowering and the use of healthcare resources. Results of the Scandinavian Simvastatin Survival Study. Circulation 93:1796–1802, 1996.

265. Johannesson M, Jonsson B, Kjekshus J, et al: Cost effectiveness of simvastatin treatment to lower cholesterol levels in patients with coronary heart disease. N Engl J Med 336:332–336, 1997.

266. LaRosa JC, He J, Vupputuri S: Effect of statins on risk of coronary disease: A meta-analysis of randomized controlled trials. JAMA 282:2340–2346, 1999.

267. Expert Panel on Detection, Evaluation and Treatment of High Blood Cholesterol in Adults: Summary of the second report of the National Cholesterol Education Program (NCEP) Expert Panel on Detection, Evaluation, and Treatment of High Blood Cholesterol in Adults (Adult Treatment Panel II). JAMA 269:3015–3023, 1993.

268. Knopp RH: Drug treatment of lipid disorders. N Engl J Med 341:498–511, 1999.

269. ISIS-2 (Second International Study of Infarct Survival) Collaborative Group: Randomised trial of intravenous streptokinase, oral aspirin, both, or neither among 17,187 cases of suspected acute myocardial infarction: ISIS-2. Lancet 2:349–360, 1988.

270. CAPRIE Steering Committee: A randomised, blinded, trial of clopidogrel versus aspirin in patients at risk of ischaemic events (CAPRIE). Lancet 348:1329–1339, 1996.

271. Balsano F, Rizzon P, Violi F, et al: Antiplatelet treatment with ticlopidine in unstable angina: A controlled multicenter clinical trial. Circulation 82:17–26, 1990.

272. Schömig A, Neumann F-J, Kastrati A, et al: A randomized comparison of antiplatelet and anticoagulant therapy after the placement of coronary-artery stents. N Engl J Med 334:1084–1089, 1996.

273. Leon MB, Baim DS, Popma JJ, et al: A clinical trial comparing three antithrombotic-drug regimens after coronary-artery stenting. Stent Anticoagulation Restenosis Study Investigators. N Engl J Med 339 :1665–1671, 1998.

274. Sharis PJ, Cannon CP, Loscalzo J: The antiplatelet effects of ticlopidine and clopidogrel. Ann Intern Med 129:394–405, 1998.

275. Bennett CL, Weinberg PD, Rozenberg-Ben-Dror K, et al: Thrombotic thrombocytopenic purpura associated with ticlopidine: A review of 60 cases. Ann Intern Med 128:541–544, 1998.

276. Steinhubl SR, Tan WA, Foody JM, Topol EJ: Incidence and clinical course of thrombotic thrombocytopenic purpura due to ticlopidine following coronary stenting. EPISTENT Investigators: Evaluation of Platelet IIb/IIIa Inhibitor for Stenting. JAMA 281:806–810, 1999.

277. Bertrand M: The CLASSICS trial. Presented at the American College of Cardiology Scientific Sessions, Orlando, FL, 1999.

278. Moussa I, Oetgen M, Roubin G, et al: Effectiveness of clopidogrel and aspirin versus ticlopidine and aspirin in preventing stent thrombosis after coronary stent implantation. Circulation 99:2364–2366, 1999.

279. Mishkel GJ, Aguirre FV, Ligon RW, et al: Clopidogrel as adjunctive antiplatelet therapy during coronary stenting. J Am Coll Cardiol 34:1884–1890, 1999.

280. Berger PB, Bell MR, Rihal CS, et al: Clopidogrel versus ticlopidine after intracoronary stent placement. J Am Coll Cardiol 34:1891–1894, 1999.

281. Savcic M, Hauert J, Bachmann F, et al: Clopidogrel loading dose regimens: Kinetic profile of pharmacodynamic response in healthy subjects. Semin Thromb Hemost 25(Suppl 2):15–19, 1999.

282. Theroux P, Waters D, Lam J, et al: Reactivation of unstable angina after the discontinuation of heparin. N Engl J Med 327:141–145, 1992.

283. Maraganore JM, Bourdon P, Adelman B, et al: Heparin variability and resistance: Comparisons with a direct thrombin inhibitor (abstract). Circulation 86(Suppl I):I-386, 1992.

284. Young E, Prins M, Levine MN, Hirsh J: Heparin binding to plasma proteins, an important mechanism for heparin resistance. Thromb Haemostas 67:639–643, 1992.

285. Hirsh J, Fuster V: Guide to anticoagulation therapy: I. Heparin. Circulation 89:1449–1468, 1994.

286. Preissner KT, Muller-Berghaus G: Neutralization and binding of heparin by S-protein/vitronectin in the inhibition of factor Xa by antithrombin III. J Biol Chem 262:12247–12253, 1987.

287. Cruikshank MK, Levine MN, Hirsh J, et al: A standard nomogram for the management of heparin therapy. Arch Intern Med 151:333–337, 1991.

288. Flaker GC, Bartolozzi J, Davis V, et al: Use of a standardized nomogram to achieve therapeutic anticoagulation after thrombolytic therapy in myocardial infarction. Arch Intern Med 154:1492–1496, 1994.

289. Melandri G, Branzi A, Traini AM, et al: On the value of the activated clotting time for monitoring heparin therapy in acute coronary syndromes. Am J Cardiol 71:469–471, 1993.

290. Kaplan K, Davison R, Parker M, et al: Role of heparin after intravenous thrombolytic therapy for acute myocardial infarction. Am J Cardiol 59:241–244, 1987.

291. Camilleri JF, Bonnet JL, Bouvicr JL, et al: Thrombolyse intraveineuse dans l'infarctus du myocarde: Influence de la qualité de l'anticoagulation sur le taux de récidivés précoces danger ou d'infarctus. Arch Mal Coeur 81:1037–1041, 1988.

292. Tracy RP, Kleiman NS, Thompson B, et al: Relation of coagulation parameters to patency and recurrent ischemia in the Thrombolysis In Myocardial Infarction (TIMI) Phase II Trial. Am Heart J 135:29–37, 1998.

293. Granger CB, Hirsh J, Califf RM, et al: Activated partial thromboplastin time and outcome after thrombolytic therapy for acute myocardial infarction: Results from the GUSTO-I Trial. Circulation 93:870–878, 1996.

294. Landefeld CS, Cook EF, Flateley M, et al: Identification and preliminary validation of predictors of major bleeding in hospitalized patients starting anticoagulant therapy. Am J Med 82:703–713, 1987.

295. Becker RC, Cannon CP, Tracy RP, et al: Relationship between systemic anticoagulation as determined by activated partial thromboplastin time and heparin measurements and in-hospital clinical events in unstable angina and non-Q wave myocardial infarction. Am Heart J 131:421–433, 1996.

296. Raschke RA, Reilly BM, Guidry JR, et al: The weight-based heparin dosing nomogram compared with a "standard care" nomogram. Ann Intern Med 119:874–881, 1993.

297. Hassan WM, Flaker GC, Feutz C, et al: Improved anticoagulation with a weight adjusted heparin nomogram in patients with acute coronary syndromes: A randomized trial. J Thromb Thrombolysis 2:245–249, 1996.

298. Becker RC, Ball SP, Eisenberg P, et al: A randomized, multicenter trial of weight-adjusted intravenous heparin dose titration and point-of-care coagulation monitoring in hospitalized patients with active thromboembolic disease. Am Heart J 137:59–71, 1999.

299. Cannon CP, Dingemanse J, Kleinbloesem CH, et al: An automated heparin titration device to control activated partial thromboplastin time: Evaluation in normal volunteers. Circulation 99:751–756, 1999.

300. Hirsh J, Levine M: Low molecular weight heparin. Blood 79:1–17, 1993.

301. Warkentin TE, Levine MN, Hirsh J, et al: Heparin-induced thrombocytopenia in patients treated with low-molecular-weight heparin or unfractionated heparin. N Engl J Med 332:1330–1335, 1995.

302. Klein W, Buchwald A, Hillis SE, et al: Comparison of low-molecular-weight hepairn with unfractionated heparin acutely and with placebo for 6 weeks in the management of unstable coronary artery disease. Fragmin in Unstable Coronary Artery Disease Study (FRIC). Circulation 96:61–68, 1997.

303. The FRAX.I.S. Study Group: Comparison of two treatment durations (6 days and 14 days) of a low molecular weight heparin with a 6-day treatment of unfractionated heparin in the initial management of unstable angina or non-Q wave myocardial infarction: FRAX.I.S. (FRAxiparine in Ischaemic Syndrome). Eur Heart J 20:1553–1562, 1999.

304. Mark DB, Cowper PA, Berkowitz SD, et al: Economic assessment of low-molecular-weight heparin (enoxaparin) versus unfractionated heparin in acute coronary syndrome patients: Results from the ESSENCE randomized trial. Circulation 97:1702–1707, 1998.

305. Antman EM, Cohen M, Radley D, et al: Assessment of the treatment effect of enoxaparin for unstable Angina/Non-Q-wave myocardial infarction: TIMI 11B-ESSENCE meta-analysis. Circulation 100:1602–1608, 1999.

306. FRagmin and Fast Revascularisation during InStability in Coronary artery disease Investigators: Long-term low-molecular-mass heparin in unstable coronary-artery disease: FRISC II prospective randomised multicentre study. Lancet 354:701–707, 1999.

307. FRagmin and Fast Revascularisation during InStability in Coronary artery disease Investigators: Invasive compared with non-invasive treatment in unstable coronary-artery disease: FRISC II prospective randomised multicentre study. Lancet 354:708–715, 1999.

308. Organisation to Assess Strategies for Ischemic Syndromes (OASIS-2) Investigators: Effects of recombinant hirudin (lepirudin) compared with heparin on death, myocardial infarction, refractory angina, and revascularisation procedures in patients with acute myocardial ischaemia without ST elevation: A randomised trial. Lancet 353:429–438, 1999.

309. Gold HK, Torres FW, Garabedian HD, et al: Evidence of a rebound coagulation phenomenon after cessation of a 4-hour infusion of a specific thrombin inhibitor in patients with unstable angina pectoris. J Am Coll Cardiol 21:1039–1047, 1993.

310. Neuhaus KL, Molhoek GP, Zeymer U, et al: Recombinant hirudin (lepirudin) for the improvement of thrombolysis with streptokinase in patients with acute myocardial infarction: Results of the HIT-4 trial. J Am Coll Cardiol 34:966–73, 1999.

311. Kong DF, Topol EJ, Bittl JA, et al: Clinical outcomes of bivalirudin for ischemic heart disease. Circulation 100:2049–2053, 1999.

312. Cannon CP, Braunwald E: Hirudin: Initial results in acute myocardial infarction, unstable angina, and angioplasty. J Am Coll Cardiol 25:30s–37s, 1995.

313. Fuchs J, Cannon CP, and the TIMI 7 Investigators. Hirulog in the treatment of unstable angina: Results of the Thrombin Inhibition in Myocardial Ischemia (TIMI) 7 trial. Circulation 92:727–733, 1995.

314. Williams DO, Kirby MG, McPhearson K, Phear DN: Anticoagulant treatment in unstable angina. Br J Clin Pract 40:114–116, 1986.

315. Williams MJ, Morison IM, Parker JH, Stewart RA: Progression of the culprit lesion in unstable coronary artery disease with warfarin and aspirin versus aspirin alone: Preliminary study. J Am Coll Cardiol 30:364–369, 1997.

316. Anand SS, Yusuf S, Pogue J, et al: Long-term oral anticoagulant therapy in patients with unstable angina or suspected non-Q-wave myocardial infarction: Organization to assess strategies for ischemic syndromes (OASIS) pilot study results. Circulation 98:1064–1070, 1998.

317. Fiore L: CHAMPS trial. Presented at the American Heart Association Scientific Sessions. Atlanta, Georgia, November 1999.

318. Coumadin Aspirin Reinfarction Study (CARS) Investigators: Randomised double-blind trial of fixed low-dose warfarin with aspirin after myocardial infarction. Lancet 350:389–396, 1997.

319. Anand SS, Yusuf S, for the OASIS Investigators: Randomized trial of oral anticoagulation therapy in patient with acute ischemic syndromes without ST elevation: importance of good compliance (abstract). J Am Coll Cardiol 33(Suppl A):396A, 1999.

320. The Medical Research Council's General Practice Research Framework. Thrombosis prevention trial: Randomised trial of low-intensity oral anticoagulation with warfarin and low-dose aspirin in the primary prevention of ischaemic heart disease in men at increased risk. Lancet 351:233–241, 1998.

321. Smith P, Arnesen H, Holme I: The effect of warfarin on mortality and reinfarction after myocardial infarction. N Engl J Med 323:147–152, 1990.

322. The Sixty-Plus Reinfarction Study Research Group: A double-blind trial

to assess long-term oral anticoagulant therapy in elderly patients after myocardial infarction. Lancet 2:989–994, 1980.

323. Anticoagulants in the Secondary Prevention of Events in Coronary Thrombosis (ASPECT) Research Group: Effect of long-term oral anticoagulant treatment on mortality and cardiovascular morbidity after myocardial infarction. Lancet 343:499–503, 1994.

324. Hirsh J, Fuster V: Guide to anticoagulation therapy. II. Oral anticoagulants. Circulation 89:1469–1480, 1994.

325. The Stroke Prevention in Atrial Fibrillation Investigators. Preliminary report of the Stroke Prevention in Atrial Fibrillation Study. N Engl J Med 322:863–868, 1990.

326. Loh E, Sutton MS, Wun CC, et al: Ventricular dysfunction and the risk of stroke after myocardial infarction. N Engl J Med 336:251–257, 1997.

327. Antiplatelet Trialist' Collaboration. Collaborative overview of randomised trials of antiplatelet therapy: I. Prevention of death myocardial infarction and stroke by prolonged antiplatelet therapy in various categories of patients. BMJ 308:81–106, 1994.

328. The CAPTURE Investigators: Randomised placebo-controlled trial of abciximab before and during coronary intervention in refractory unstable angina: The CAPTURE study. Lancet 349:1429–1435, 1997.

329. The PARAGON Investigators: International, randomized, controlled trial of lamifiban (a platelet glycoprotein IIb/IIIa inhibitor), heparin or both in unstable angina. Circulation 97:2386–2395, 1998.

330. Topol EJ, Byzova TV, Plow ER: Platelet GPIIb–IIIa blockers. Lancet 353:227–231, 1999.

331. Kong DF, Califf RM, Miller DP, et al: Clinical outcomes of therapeutic agents that block the platelet glycoprotein IIb/IIIa integrin in ischemic heart disease. Circulation 98:2829–2835, 1998.

332. Barr E, Thornton AR, Sax FL, et al: Benefit of tirofiban + heparin therapy in unstable angina/non-Q wave myocardial infarction patients is observed regardless of interventional treatment (abstract). Circulation 98(Suppl I):I-504, 1998.

333. Boersma E, Akkerhuis KM, Theroux P, et al: Platelet glycoprotein IIb/IIIa receptor inhibition in non-ST-elevation acute coronary syndromes: Early benefit during medical treatment only, with additional protection during percutaneous coronary intervention. Circulation 100:2045–2048, 1999.

333a. Simoons ML: GUSTO IV ACS: Outcomes of 7600 patients with acute coronary syndromes randomised to placebo or abciximab for 1 or 2 days. Presented at XXIIth Congress of the European Society of Cardiology, Amsterdam, August 28, 2000.

334. Peterson JG, Lauer MA, Sapp SK, Topol EJ: Heparin use is required for clinical benefit of GP IIb/IIIa inhibitor eptifibatide in acute coronary syndromes: Insights from the PURSUIT trial (abstract). Circulation 98(Suppl I):I-360, 1998.

335. Berkowitz SD, Sane DC, Sigmon KN, et al: Occurrence and clinical significance of thrombocytopenia in a population undergoing high-risk percutaneous coronary revascularization. Evaluation of c7E3 for the Prevention of Ischemic Complications (EPIC) Study Group. J Am Coll Cardiol 32:311–319, 1998.

336. Mahaffey KW, Harrington RA, Simoons ML, et al: Stroke in patients with acute coronary syndromes: Incidence and outcomes in the platelet glycoprotein IIb/IIIa in unstable angina. Receptor suppression using integrilin therapy (PURSUIT) trial. The PURSUIT Investigators. Circulation 99:2371–2377, 1999.

337. Cannon CP: Orbofiban in Patients with Unstable Coronary Syndromes (OPUS)—TIMI 16 trial. Presented at the American College of Cardiology Scientific Session, New Orleans, March 1999.

338. The SYMPHONY Investigators. Comparison of sibrafiban with aspirin for prevention of cardiovascular events after acute coronary syndromes: A randomised trial. Lancet 355:337–45, 2000.

338a. Newby LK: A Randomized Comparison of Sibrafiban, an Oral Glycoprotein IIb/IIIa Receptor Antagonist, With and Without Aspirin Versus Aspirin after Acute Coronary Syndromes: Results of the 2nd SYMPHONY Trial, American College of Cardiology Scientific Sessions, Anaheim, March 2000.

339. O'Neill WW, Serruys P, Knudtson M, et al: Long-term treatment with a platelet glycoprotein-receptor antagonist after pecutaneous coronary revascularization. N Engl J Med 342:1316–1324, 2000.

340. Cannon CP, McCabe CH, Borzak S, et al: A randomized trial of an oral platelet glycoprotein IIb/IIIa antagonist, sibrafiban, in patients after an acute coronary syndrome: Results of the TIMI 12 trial. Circulation 97:340–349, 1998.

341. Holmes MB, Sobel BE, Cannon CP, Schneider DJ: Increased platelet reactivity in patients given orbofiban after an acute coronary syndrome: An OPUS-TIMI 16 substudy. Am J Cardiol, in press.

341a. Holmes MB, Sobel BE, Schneider DJ: Variable responses to inhibition of fibrinogen binding induced by tirofiban and eptifibatide in blood from healthy subjects. Am J Cardiol 84:203–7, 1999.

342. Mousa SA, Bozarth JM, Lorelli W, et al: Antiplatelet efficacy of XV459, a novel nonpeptide platelet GPIIb/IIIa antagonist: Comparative platelet binding profiles with c7E3. J Pharmacol Exp Ther 286:1277–1284, 1998.

343. van den Brand M, de Scheerder I, Heyndrickx G, et al: Assessment of coronary angiograms prior and after treatment with abciximab, in patients with refractory unstable angina (abstract). Eur Heart J 18(Suppl): 243, 1997.

344. Cannon CP: Overcoming thrombolytic resistance: Rationale and initial clinical experience combining thrombolytic therapy and glycoprotein IIb/IIIa receptor inhibition for acute myocardial infarction. J Am Coll Cardiol 34:1395–1402, 1999.

345. Alexander JH, Sparapani RA, Mahaffey KW, et al: Eptifibatide reduces the size and incidence of myocardial infarction in patients with non-ST-elevation acute coronary syndromes (abstract). J Am Coll Cardiol 33(Suppl. A):331A, 1999.

346. Januzzi JL, Hahn SS, Chae CU, et al: Reduction of troponin I levels in patients with acute coronary syndromes by glycoprotein IIb/IIIa inhibition with tirofiban. Am J Cardiol (in press).

346a. Mark DB, Harrington RA, Lincoff AM, et al: Cost-effectiveness of platelet glycoprotein IIb/IIIa inhibition with eptifibatide in patients with non-ST-elevation acute coronary syndromes. Circulation 101:366–71, 2000.

347. Fibrinolytic Therapy Trialists' (FTT) Collaborative Group. Indications for fibrinolytic therapy in suspected acute myocardial infarction: Collaborative overview of early mortality and major morbidity results from all randomised trials of more than 1000 patients. Lancet 343:311–322, 1994.

348. Coller BS: Platelets and thrombolytic therapy. N Engl J Med 322:33–42, 1990.

349. Owen J, Friedman KD, Grossmann BA, et al: Thrombolytic therapy with tissue-plasminogen activator or streptokinase induces transient thrombin activity. Blood 72:616-620, 1988.

350. Weitz JI, Hudoba M, Massel D, et al: Clot-bound thrombin is protected from inhibition by heparin-antithrombin III but is susceptible to inactivation by antithrombin III-independent inhibitors. J Clin Invest 86:385–391, 1990.

351. Giugliano RP, Camargo CA Jr, Lloyd-Jones DM, et al: Elderly patients receive less aggressive medical and invasive management of unstable angina. Arch Intern Med 158:1113–1120, 1998.

352. Alexander KP, Peterson ED, Granger CB, et al: Potential impact of evidence-based medicine in acute coronary syndromes: Insights from GUSTO-IIb. J Am Coll Cardiol 32:2023–2030, 1998.

353. Rogers WJ, Bowlby LJ, Chandra NC, et al: Treatment of myocardial infarction in the United States (1990 to 1993). Observations from the National Registry of Myocardial Infarction. Circulation 90:2103–2114, 1994.

354. Moliterno DJ, Aguirre FV, Cannon CP, et al: The Global Unstable Angina Registry and Treatment Evaluation (GUARANTEE) Study (abstract). Circulation 94[Suppl I]:I-195, 1996.

355. Cannon CP, Moliterno DJ, Every N, et al: Implementation of AHCPR guidelines for unstable angina in 1996: Unfortunate differences between men & women: Results from the multicenter GUARANTEE registry. (abstract). J Am Coll Cardiol 29(Suppl. A):217A, 1997.

356. Hennekens CH, Dyken ML, Fuster V: Aspirin as a therapeutic agent in cardiovascular disease: A statement for healthcare professionals from the American Heart Association. Circulation 96:2751–2753, 1997.

357. Giugliano RP, Lloyd-Jones DM, Camargo CA Jr, et al: Association of unstable angina guideline care with improved survival. Arch Intern Med 160:1775–1780, 2000.

TREATMENT STRATEGIES AND INTERVENTIONS

358. McCullough PA, O'Neill WW, Graham M, et al: A prospective randomized trial of triage angiography in acute coronary syndromes ineligible for thrombolytic therapy: Results of the medicine versus angiography in thrombolytic exclusion (MATE) trial. J Am Coll Cardiol 32:596–605, 1998.

359. Boden WE, O'Rourke RA, Crawford MH, et al: Outcomes in patients with acute non-Q-wave myocardial infarction randomly assigned to an invasive as compared with a conservative strategy. N Engl J Med 338:1785–1792, 1998.

360. Fragmin and fast revascularisation during instability in coronary artery disease investigators: Invasive compared with non-invasive treatment in unstable coronary-artery disease: FRISC II prospective randomised multicentre study. Lancet 354:708–715, 1999.

361. Diderholm E, Andren B, Frostfeldt G, et al: ST depression in ECG at entry identifies patients who benefit most from early revascularization in unstable coronary artery disease: A FRISC II substudy (abstract). Circulation 100(Suppl I):I-497–I-498, 1999.

362. Mehta S, Yusuf S, Hunt D, Natarajan M: Invasive versus conservative management of unstable angina and non-Q-wave infarction: A meta-analysis (abstract). Circulation 100(Suppl I):I-775, 1999.

363. Sharma GVRK, Deupree RH, Luchi RJ, Scott SM, and the participants of the Veterans Administration Cooperative Study: Identification of unstable angina patients who have favorable outcome with medical or surgical therapy (eight-year follow-up of the Veterans Administration Cooperative Study). Am J Cardiol 74:454–458, 1994.

364. Madsen JK, Grande P, Saunamaki K, et al: Danish multicenter randomized study of invasive versus conservative treatment in patients with inducible ischemia after thrombolysis in acute myocardial infarction (DANAMI). Circulation 96:748–755, 1997.

365. Hochman JS, Sleeper LA, Webb JG, et al: Early revascularization in acute myocardial infarction complicated by cardiogenic shock. N Engl J Med 341:625–634, 1999.

366. Berger PB, Holmes DR Jr, Stebbins AL, et al: Impact of an aggressive invasive catheterization and revascularization strategy on mortality in patients with cardiogenic shock in the Global Utilization of Streptokinase and Tissue Plasminogen Activator for Occluded Coronary Arteries (GUSTO-I) trial: An observational study. Circulation 96:122–127, 1997.

367. Cannon CP, Weintraub WS, Demopoulos LA, et al: Invasive versus conservative strategies in unstable angina and non-Q wave myocardial infarction following treatment with *tirofiban*: Rationale and study design of the international TACTICS-TIMI 18 trial. Am J Cardiol 82:731–736, 1998.

368. Weintraub WS, Culler SD, Kosinski A, et al: Economics, health-related quality of life, and cost effectiveness methods for the TACTICS (Treat Angina with Aggrastat [tirofiban] and Determine Cost of Therapy with Invasive or Conservative Strategy)—TIMI 18 Trial. Am J Cardiol 83:317–322, 1999.

369. O'Rourke RA, Chatterjee K, Dodge HT, et al: Guidelines for Clinical Use of Cardiac Radionuclide Imaging, December 1986. A report of the American College of Cardiology/American Heart Association Task Force on Assessment of Cardiovascular Procedures (Subcommittee on Nuclear Imaging). J Am Coll Cardiol 8:1471–1483, 1986.

370. Gibbons RJ, Balady GJ, Beasley JW, et al: ACC/AHA guidelines for exercise testing: Executive summary. A report of the American College of Cardiology/American Heart Association Task Force on Practice Guidelines (Committee on Exercise Testing). Circulation 96:345–354, 1997.

371. Cheitlin MD, Alpert JS, Armstrong WF, et al: ACC/AHA Guidelines for the Clinical Application of Echocardiography A report of the American College of Cardiology/American Heart Association Task Force on Practice Guidelines (Committee on Clinical Application of Echocardiography). Developed in colloboration with the American Society of Echocardiography. Circulation 95:1686–1744, 1997.

372. Ritchie JL, Bateman TM, Bonow RO, et al: Guidelines for clinical use of cardiac radionuclide imaging: A report of the American College of Cardiology/American Heart Association Task Force on assessment of diagnostic and therapeutic cardiovascular procedures (Committee on Radionuclide Imaging): Developed in collaboration with the American Society of Nuclear Cardiology. J Nucl Cardiol 2(2 Pt 1):172–192, 1995.

373. Severi S, Orsini E, Marraccini P, et al: The basal electrocardiogram and the exercise stress test in assessing prognosis in patients with unstable angina. Eur Heart J 9:441–446, 1988.

374. Heller GV, Brown KA, Landin RJ, Haber SB: Safety of early intravenous dipyridamole technetium 99m sestamibi SPECT myocardial perfusion imaging after uncomplicated first myocardial infarction. Early Post MI IV Dipyridamole Study (EPIDS). Am Heart J 134:105–111, 1997.

375. Larsson H, Areskog M, Areskog NH, et al: Should the exercise test (ET) be performed at discharge or one month later after an episode of unstable angina or non-Q-wave myocardial infarction? Int J Card Imaging 7:7–14, 1991.

376. Amanullah AM, Lindvall K: Prevalence and significance of transient—predominantly asymptomatic—myocardial ischemia on Holter monitoring in unstable angina pectoris, and correlation with exercise test and thallium-201 myocardial perfusion imaging. Am J Cardiol 72:144–148, 1993.

377. Amanullah AM, Lindvall K, Bevegard S: Prognostic significance of exercise thallium-201 myocardial perfusion imaging compared to stress echocardiography and clinical variables in patients with unstable angina who respond to medical treatment. Int J Cardiol 39:71–78, 1993.

378. Brown KA: Prognostic value of thallium-201 myocardial perfusion imaging in patients with unstable angina who respond to medical treatment. J Am Coll Cardiol 17:1053–1057, 1991.

379. Bateman TM, O'Keefe JH Jr, Williams ME: Incremental value of myocardial perfusion scintigraphy in prognosis and outcomes of patients with coronary artery disease. Curr Opin Cardiol 11:613–620, 1996.

380. Arafa OE, Pedersen TH, Svennevig JL, et al: Vascular complications of the intraaortic balloon pump in patients undergoing open heart operations: 15-year experience. Ann Thorac Surg 67:645–651, 1999.

381. Patel JJ, Kopisyansky C, Boston B, et al: Prospective evaluation of complications associated with percutaneous intraaortic balloon counterpulsation. Am J Cardiol 76:1205–1207, 1995.

382. de Feyter PJ, Suryapranata H, Serruys PW, et al: Effects of successful percutaneous transluminal coronary angioplasty on global and regional left ventricular function in unstable angina pectoris. Am J Cardiol 60:993–997, 1987.

383. Williams DO, Braunwald E, Thompson B, et al: Results of percutaneous transluminal coronary angioplasty in unstable angina and non-Q-wave myocardial infarction: Observations from the TIMI IIIB Trial. Circulation 94:2749–2755, 1996.

384. Kamp O, Beatt KJ, De Feyter PJ, et al: Short-, medium-, and long-term follow-up after percutaneous transluminal coronary angioplasty for stable and unstable angina pectoris. Am Heart J 117:991–996, 1989.

385. Fischman DL, Leon MB, Baim DS, et al: A randomized comparison of coronary-stent placement and balloon angioplasty in the treatment of coronary artery disease. N Engl J Med 331:496–501, 1994.

386. Serruys PW, de Jaegere P, Kiemeneij F, et al: A comparison of balloon-expandable-stent implantation with balloon angioplasty in patients with coronary artery disease. N Engl J Med 331:489–495, 1994.

387. The EPIC Investigators: Use of a monoclonal antibody directed against the platelet glycoprotein IIb/IIIa receptor in high risk angioplasty. N Engl J Med 330:956–961, 1994.

388. The EPILOG Investigators: Platelet glycoprotein IIb/IIIa receptor blockade and low-dose heparin during percutaneous coronary revascularization. N Engl J Med 336:1689–1696, 1997.

389. The EPISTENT Investigators: Randomised placebo-controlled and balloon-angioplasty-controlled trail to assess the safety of coronary stenting with use of platelet glycoprotein-IIb/IIIa blockade. Lancet 352:87–92, 1998.

390. The IMPACT-II Investigators: Randomised placebo-controlled trial of effect of eptifibatide on complications of percutaneous coronary intervention: IMPACT-II. Lancet 349:1422–1428, 1997.

390a. Tcheng JE: ESPRIT, American College of Cardiology Scientific Sessions, Anaheim, CA, 2000.

391. The RESTORE Investigators: The effects of platelet glycoprotein IIb/IIIa blockade with tirofiban on adverse cardiac events in patients with unstable angina or acute myocardial infarction undergoing coronary angioplasty. Circulation 96:1445–1453, 1997.

392. RITA Trial Participants: Coronary angioplasty versus coronary artery bypass surgery: The Randomized Intervention Treatment of Angina (RITA) trial. Lancet 341:573–580, 1993.

393. Rodriquez A, Boullon F, Perez-Balino N, et al: Argentine Randomized Trial of Percutaneous Transluminal Coronary Angioplasty versus Coronary Artery Bypass Surgery in Multivessel Disease (ERACI): In-hospital results and 1-year follow-up. J Am Coll Cardiol 22:1060–1067, 1993.

394. Hamm CW, Reimers J, Ischinger T, et al: A randomized study of coronary angioplasty compared with bypass surgery in patients with symptomatic multivessel coronary disease. N Engl J Med 331:1037–1043, 1994.

395. King SB III, Lembo NJ, Weintraub WS, et al: A randomized trial comparing coronary angioplasty with coronary bypass surgery. N Engl J Med 331:1044–1050, 1994.

396. The Bypass Angioplasty Revascularization Investigation (BARI) Investigators: Comparison of coronary bypass surgery with angioplasty in patients with multivessel disease. N Engl J Med 335:217–225, 1996.

397. European Coronary Surgery Study Group: Long-term results of prospective randomized study of coronary artery bypass surgery in stable angina pectoris. Lancet 2:1173–1180, 1982.

398. CASS Principal Investigators and their Associates: Coronary Artery Surgery Study (CASS): A randomized trial of coronary artery bypass surgery: Survival data. Circulation 68:939–950, 1983.

399. The Veterans Administration Coronary Artery Bypass Surgery Collaborative Study Group: Eleven-year survival in the Veterans Administration randomized trial of coronary bypass surgery for stable angina. N Engl J Med 311:1333–1339, 1984.

400. Chaitman BR, Fisher LD, Bourassa MD: Effect of coronary bypass surgery on survival patterns in subsets of patients with left main coronary artery disease: Report of the Collaborative Study in Coronary Artery Surgery (SASS). Am J Cardiol 48:765–777, 1981.

401. Mark DB, Nelson CL, Califf RM, et al: Continuing evolution of therapy for coronary artery disease: Initial results from the era of coronary angioplasty. Circulation 89:2015–2025, 1994.

402. Hillis LD, Rutherford JD: Coronary angioplasty compared with bypass grafting. N Engl J Med 331:1086–1087, 1994.

TARGETING NEW THERAPIES

403. Lindahl B, Venge P, Wallentin L, and the FRISC study group: Troponin T identifies patients with unstable coronary artery disease who benefit from long-term antithrombotic protection. J Am Coll Cardiol 29:43–48, 1997.

404. Antman EM, McCabe CH, Gurfinkel EP, et al: Treatment benefit of enoxaparin in unstable angina/non-Q wave myocardial infarction is maintained at one year in TIMI 11B (abstract). Circulation 100(Suppl I):I-497, 1999.

405. Cohen M, Stinnett S, Fromell G: Effect of low molecular weight heparin on prespecified patient subgroups with rest unstable angina or non-Q-wave myocardial infarction (abstract). Circulation 98(Suppl I):I-559, 1998.

406. Theroux P, Barr E, Snappin S, Sax FL: Rise in C-reactive protein is suppressed with tirofiban + heparin but not with heparin alone in patients with unstable angina/non-Q-wave myocardial infarction (abstract). J Am Coll Cardiol 33(Suppl. A):333A, 1999.

407. Ridker PM, Rifai N, Pfeffer MA, et al: Long-term effects of pravastatin on plasma concentration of C-reactive protein. Circulation 100:230–235, 1999.

408. Ridker PM, Rifai N, Pfeffer MA, et al: Inflammation, pravastatin, and the risk of coronary events after myocardial infarction in patients with average cholesterol levels. Circulation 98:839–844, 1998.

409. Stone PH, Thompson B, Zaret BL, et al: Factors associated with failure of medical therapy in patients with unstable angina and non-Q myocardial infarction: A TIMI-IIIB database study. Eur Heart J 20:1084–1093, 1999.

410. Cannon CP, Antman EM, Walls R, Braunwald E: Time as an adjunctive agent to thrombolytic therapy. J Thromb Thrombolysis 1:27–33, 1994.

411. Cannon CP, O'Gara PT: Critical pathways in acute coronary syndromes. *In* Cannon CP (ed): Management of Acute Coronary Syndromes. Totowa, NJ, Humana Press, 1999, pp 611–627.

412. Haines DE, Raabe DS, Gundel WD, Wackers FJ: Anatomic and prognostic significance of new T-wave inversion in unstable angina. Am J Cardiol 52:14–18, 1983.

GUIDELINES

MANAGEMENT OF UNSTABLE ANGINA/NON–ST SEGMENT ELEVATION MYOCARDIAL INFARCTION

Thomas H. Lee

Key guidelines for management of unstable angina and non–ST segment elevation myocardial infarction (UA/NSTEMI) were issued by an American College of Cardiology/American Heart Association (ACC/AHA) task force in 2000.[1] These guidelines updated and extended recommendations published in 1994 by the Agency for Health Care Policy and Research (AHCPR) and the National Heart, Lung and Blood Institute.[2] Other guidelines relevant to the diagnosis and management of this population have been issued by the American College of Emergency Physicians and other ACC/AHA task forces and are described in the Guidelines to Chapter 35.

The ACC/AHA guidelines on UA/NSTEMI used the customary ACC/AHA classification system to provide recommendations for the appropriateness of indications, described in Chapter 37.

In addition, these ACC/AHA guidelines adapted the AHCPR approach of grading the strength of evidence used to develop these recommendations. The weight of evidence was ranked highest (A) if the data were derived from multiple randomized trials involving large numbers of patients. An intermediate rank (B) was assigned if the data were derived from a limited number of randomized trials with small numbers of patients or from careful analysis of nonrandomized studies or observational data bases. A lower rank of "C" was assigned when the basis of the recommendation was expert consensus.

These guidelines focus on the care of patients with *acute coronary syndrome* (ACS), which includes acute myocardial infarction and UA. UA and NSTEMI are considered closely related conditions that differ primarily in severity. Excluded is the care of patients with acute myocardial infarction and ST segment elevation, who would be eligible for acute reperfusion (see Chap. 35).

Initial Evaluation and Management (Fig. 36–G–1)

The guidelines emphasize the importance of prompt evaluation of patients with acute chest pain in settings in which a 12-lead electrocardiogram (ECG) can be performed, as opposed to over the telephone. Patients with prolonged (>20 minutes) chest pain or symptoms suggesting hemodynamic instability or arrhythmia should be triaged to an emergency department or chest pain unit; transport should ideally occur by emergency medical vehicles. Patients with *possible ACS* should have a 12-lead ECG and undergo observation with serial measurement of cardiac markers. Cardiac-specific troponins are identified as preferred markers, while creatine kinase MB isoenzyme (CK-MB) is considered a less preferable but acceptable marker.

Immediate Management (Table 36–G–1)

After identifying and appropriately treating patients with reperfusion-eligible acute myocardial infarction (see Chap. 35), as well as others with cardiac conditions that are not due to ACS, the clinical findings should be used to assign the remaining patients with chest pain to one of four categories (see Table 36–G–1):

1. A noncardiac diagnosis
2. Chronic stable angina
3. Possible ACS
4. Definite ACS

Management of patients with chronic stable angina is expected to be according to ACC/AHA guidelines on this topic, as summarized in the Guidelines to Chapter 37.

For patients with possible ACS who have no recurrent chest discomfort over a 4- to 8-hour period and have normal results of follow-up 12-lead ECGs and biochemical cardiac markers, stress testing is considered appropriate (Table 36–G–1). Patients with negative stress tests can be discharged for further management as outpatients. Patients with strongly positive stress tests are considered to be at high risk (Table 36–G–2) and should be admitted to the hospital. Management of patients with intermediate test results must be determined by clinical judgment. The ACC/AHA guidelines indicate that exercise ECG is an appropriate first-line test for risk stratification.

Hospital Care (Table 36–G–2, Fig. 36–G–2)

The guidelines recommend that patients with recurrent symptoms, ECG ST segment deviations, positive cardiac markers (CK-MB or troponin), or hemodynamic instability be admitted to an inpatient unit with continuous rhythm monitoring. For this population, observation in such facilities for at least 24 hours without any recurrence of ischemia or major complications is recommended before considering transfer to a lower level of care. Factors that suggest triage to a coronary care unit (as opposed to a unit with a lower nurse/patient ratio) are elevated serum markers or hemodynamic instability.

TABLE 36–G–1. INITIAL EVALUATION AND MANAGEMENT

Issue	Class	Recommendation	Level of Evidence
Immediate management	I	The history, physical examination, 12-lead ECG, and initial serum marker tests should be integrated to assign patients with chest pain to 1 of 4 categories: a noncardiac diagnosis, chronic stable angina, possible ACS, and definite ACS	C
		Patients whose symptoms are suggestive of ACS or are believed to be consistent with definite ACS but whose initial 12-lead ECG and serum cardiac marker levels are normal should be observed in a facility with cardiac monitoring (e.g., chest pain unit), and a repeat ECG and serum marker measurement should be obtained 4–8 hr later	C
			C
		If the follow-up 12-lead ECG and cardiac marker measurements are normal, a stress test to provoke ischemia may be performed. Patients with a negative stress test can be managed as outpatients. Patients with a strongly positive stress test are considered to have myocardial ischemia and, in the presence of a clinical picture of acute ischemia, should be admitted to the hospital for further management. The stress test can be conducted on an outpatient basis in low-risk patients with unstable angina/non–ST segment elevation myocardial infarction	C
			C
		Patients who are unable to exercise or who have an abnormal resting ECG should have stress myocardial perfusion imaging	
		Patients believed to have an ACS with an abnormal initial 12-lead ECG should be managed according to the findings of the 12-lead ECG. Patients with ST elevation should be evaluated for immediate reperfusion therapy. Patients with new ST depression and/or T wave abnormalities should be admitted to the hospital for further management	C
			C

ACS = acute coronary syndrome; ECG = electrocardiogram.

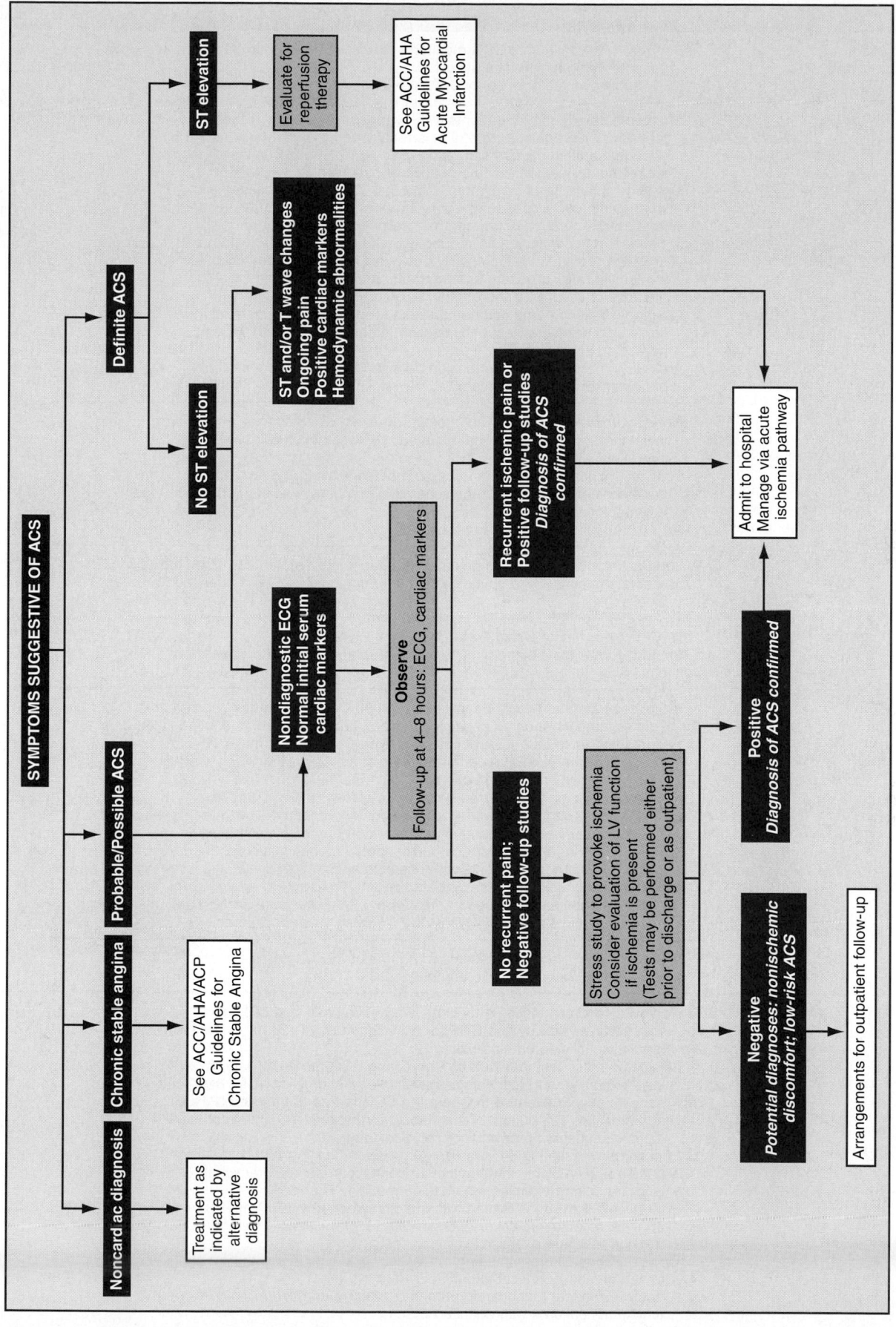

FIGURE 36–G–1. Algorithm for evaluation and management of patients suspected of having acute coronary syndrome (ACS). ACP = American College of Physicians; ECG = electrocardiogram; LV = left ventricular. (From Braunwald E, Antman EM, Beasley JW, et al: ACC/AHA guidelines for the management of patients with unstable angina: A report of the American College of Cardiology/American Heart Association Task Force on Practice Guidelines (Committee on the Management of Patients with Unstable Angina). J Am Coll Cardiol, 36:970–1062, 2000.)

Issue	Class	Recommendation	Level of Evidence
Antiischemic therapy	I	Bed rest with continuous ECG monitoring for ischemia and arrhythmia detection in patients with ongoing pain at rest	C
		NTG, sublingual tablet or spray or IV, for immediate relief of ischemia and associated symptoms	C
		Supplemental oxygen for patients with cyanosis, respiratory distress, or high-risk features. Finger pulse oximetry or arterial blood gas determination to confirm adequate arterial oxygen saturation (SaO$_2$ >92%) and continued need for supplemental oxygen in the presence of hypoxemia	C
		Morphine sulfate IV when symptoms are not immediately relieved with NTG or when acute pulmonary congestion and/or severe agitation is present	C
		A beta blocker, oral or IV, in the absence of contraindications	B
		In patients with continuing or frequently recurring ischemia in whom beta blockers are either contraindicated or fully deployed, a nondihydropyridine calcium antagonist (e.g., diltiazem or verapamil), oral and/or IV, as initial therapy in the absence of severe LV dysfunction or other contraindications	B
		Intraaortic balloon pump counterpulsation for patients with either ischemia that is continuing or recurs frequently despite intensive medical therapy or hemodynamic instability	C
		An ACE inhibitor when hypertension persists despite treatment with NTG and a beta blocker and in patients with LV systolic dysfunction	B
	IIa	Nondihydropyridine calcium antagonist (diltiazem or verapamil), oral and/or IV, as initial therapy in the absence of severe LV dysfunction or other contraindications	B
		Oral long-acting dihydropyridine calcium antagonists in the absence of contraindications for recurrent ischemia when beta blockers and nitrates are fully deployed	C
		An ACE inhibitor for diabetic patients	B
	IIb	Long-acting nondihydropyridine calcium antagonists instead of a beta blocker	B
		Immediate-release dihydropyridine calcium antagonists in the presence of a beta blocker	B
	III	NTG or other nitrate within 24 hr of sildenafil (Viagra) use	C
		Immediate-release dihydropyridine calcium antagonists in the absence of a beta blocker	B
Antiplatelet and anticoagulation therapy	I	Antiplatelet therapy should be initiated promptly. ASA is the first choice and is administered as soon as possible after arrival and then continued indefinitely	A
		Patients unable to take ASA because of hypersensitivity or major GI intolerance should receive an ADP receptor antagonist as a substitute	
		Ticlopidine has been found effective	B
		Clopidogrel may be preferred because of safety	B
		Parenteral anticoagulation with IV unfractionated heparin or with subcutaneous low-molecular-weight heparin should be added to antiplatelet therapy	A
		A platelet GP IIb-IIIa receptor antagonist should be administered, in addition to ASA and heparin, to patients with unstable angina with continuing ischemia or with other high-risk features. Eptifibatide and tirofiban are approved for this use. Abciximab can also be used for 12–24 hr in patients with UA/NSTEMI in whom an interventional procedure within the following 24 hr is planned	A
	III	IV thrombolytic therapy in patients without acute ST segment elevation of a presumably new left bundle branch block	A
Risk stratification	I	Noninvasive stress testing in patients who have been free of angina at rest or with low-level activity and CHF for a minimum of 24–28 hr and who are not otherwise considered high risk	C
		Choice of stress test is based on the resting ECG, ability to perform exercise, local expertise, and technologies available. Treadmill exercise is suitable in patients able to exercise in whom the ECG is free of baseline ST segment abnormalities, left bundle branch block, LV hypertrophy, intraventricular conduction defect, preexcitation, or digoxin effect	C
		In patients with resting ST segment depression (≥1 mm), LV hypertrophy, left bundle branch block, intraventricular conduction defect, preexcitation, or digoxin who are able to exercise, an imaging modality is added	C
		Pharmacological stress testing with imaging when physical limitations (e.g., arthritis, amputation, severe peripheral vascular disease, severe COPD, general debility) preclude exercise	B
		Choice among different imaging modalities used with stress testing should be based primarily on local expertise	C
		A noninvasive test (echocardiogram, radionuclide angiogram) to evaluate LV function in patients with definite ACS	C
		Prompt angiography without noninvasive risk stratification for failure of stabilization with medical treatment	B

TABLE 36-G-2. HOSPITAL CARE—*Continued*

1267

Ch 36

Issue	Class	Recommendation	Level of Evidence
	III	Noninvasive stress testing or coronary angiography in patients with extensive comorbidity in whom revascularization is contraindicated	C
Early conservative vs. invasive strategies	I	An early invasive strategy involving prompt coronary angiography to evaluate for revascularization in patients with any of the following high-risk indicators: Patients receiving intensive antiischemic therapy with recurrent angina/ischemia at rest or with low-level activities or accompanied by CHF symptoms, and S_3 gallop, or new or worsening MR High-risk findings on noninvasive stress testing (see Table 36-G-3) Depressed LV systolic function (EF <0.4) by noninvasive study) Hemodynamic instability Sustained ventricular tachycardia Prior revascularization (PCI or CABG)	C
	IIa	In the absence of findings in Class I, either an early conservative or early invasive strategy may be performed in hospitalized patients without contraindications for revascularization	C
		An early invasive strategy in patients who prefer and have no contraindications to revascularization Repeated attacks of ACS without evidence for ischemia or high risk	C
	III	Coronary angiography in patients with extensive comorbidities (e.g., liver or pulmonary failure, cancer) in whom the risks of revascularization are not likely to outweigh the benefits	
Coronary revascularization using PCI and CABG in patients with UA/NSTEMI	I	CABG for patients with significant left main CAD, as well as in patients with severe multivessel CAD or two-vessel disease involving the proximal LAD and depressed LV systolic function PCI or CABG for nondiabetic patients with multivessel CAD. PCI for patients with coronary anatomy suitable for catheter-based therapy and preserved LV function. Platelet GP IIb-IIIa receptor inhibitor in UA/NSTEMI patients undergoing percutaneous revascularization	A A A A
	IIa	CABG for patients with multivessel disease and diabetes mellitus PCI or CABG for patients with 2-vessel disease not involving the proximal LAD PCI or CABG for patients with single-vessel, proximal LAD disease	B B B
	IIb	PCI for patients with multivessel disease and diabetes of LV dysfunction PCI for patients with significant left main disease in whom CABG cannot be carried out	B C

ACE = angiotensin-converting enzyme; ACS = acute coronary syndrome; ADP = adenosine diphosphate; ASA = acetylsalicylic acid; CABG = coronary artery bypass grafting; CAD = coronary artery disease; CHF = congestive heart failure; COPD = chronic obstructive pulmonary disease; ECG = electrocardiogram; EF = ejection fraction; GI = gastrointestinal; GP = glycoprotein; LAD = left anterior descending artery; LV = left ventricular; MR = mitral regurgitation; NTG = nitroglycerin; PCI = percutaneous coronary intervention; UA/NSTEMI = unstable angina/non—ST segment elevation myocardial infarction.

ANTIISCHEMIC THERAPY. Early initiation of beta blocker therapy in the absence of contraindications is recommended. Calcium antagonists are considered useful primarily for symptom control and appropriate for second or third choices following initiation of nitrates and beta blockers. For agents that slow the heart rate (verapamil and diltiazem), early use is more appropriate because of the lack of controlled trial evidence of harm, and some trends suggest potential benefit. The guidelines consider the use of immediate-release dihydropyridine calcium antagonists in the absence of a beta blocker to be *inappropriate* (Class III).

ANTIPLATELET AND ANTICOAGULATION THERAPY. The guidelines encourage prompt initiation of an array of agents to impede thrombus formation. Antiplatelet therapy should begin immediately, ideally with acetylsalicylic acid (ASA), but with newer agents (clopidogrel or ticlopidine) if the use of ASA is contraindicated. The guidelines also support a low threshold for anticoagulation with intravenous heparin or with subcutaneous low-molecular-weight heparin for patients with ACS. High-risk patients should also be considered for therapy with a platelet glycoprotein (GP) IIb-IIIa receptor antagonist.

Intravenous thrombolytic therapy in the absence of acute ST segment elevation or a presumably new left bundle branch block is considered inappropriate (Class III).

RISK STRATIFICATION (see Table 36-G-2). Early use of noninvasive tests for risk stratification after patients have been free of angina at rest or during low-level activity, heart failure, or other major complications for 24 to 48 hours is recommended. As noted above, an exercise ECG is considered the most appropriate first-line test for patients with adequate functional capacity and appropriate rest ECGs. This recommendation is based on its "simplicity, lower cost, and widespread familiarity with performance and interpretation." For other patients, choices among different imaging modalities should be based on local expertise. Findings on noninvasive testing that predict a high risk for adverse outcomes are shown in Table 36-G-3.

For patients with definite ACS, left ventricular function should be assessed to help guide long-term management strategies. If medical treatment is not able to control symptoms of ischemia, patients should undergo prompt coronary angiography, as long as other considerations (e.g., extensive comorbidity) would not preclude coronary revascularization.

Early Conservative Versus Invasive Strategies
(see Table 36-G-2)

Two strategies for coronary angiography were discussed. In the *early conservative strategy*, patients routinely undergo noninvasive risk stratification, and coronary angiography is reserved for patients identified as being at high risk for adverse outcomes based on their clinical courses or noninvasive test results. In the *early invasive strategy*, patients without obvious contraindications to coronary revascularization are routinely recommended for coronary angiography followed by revascularization, if possible.

A clearly appropriate (Class I) assessment was given to the use of an early invasive strategy for patients with high-risk indicators, includ-

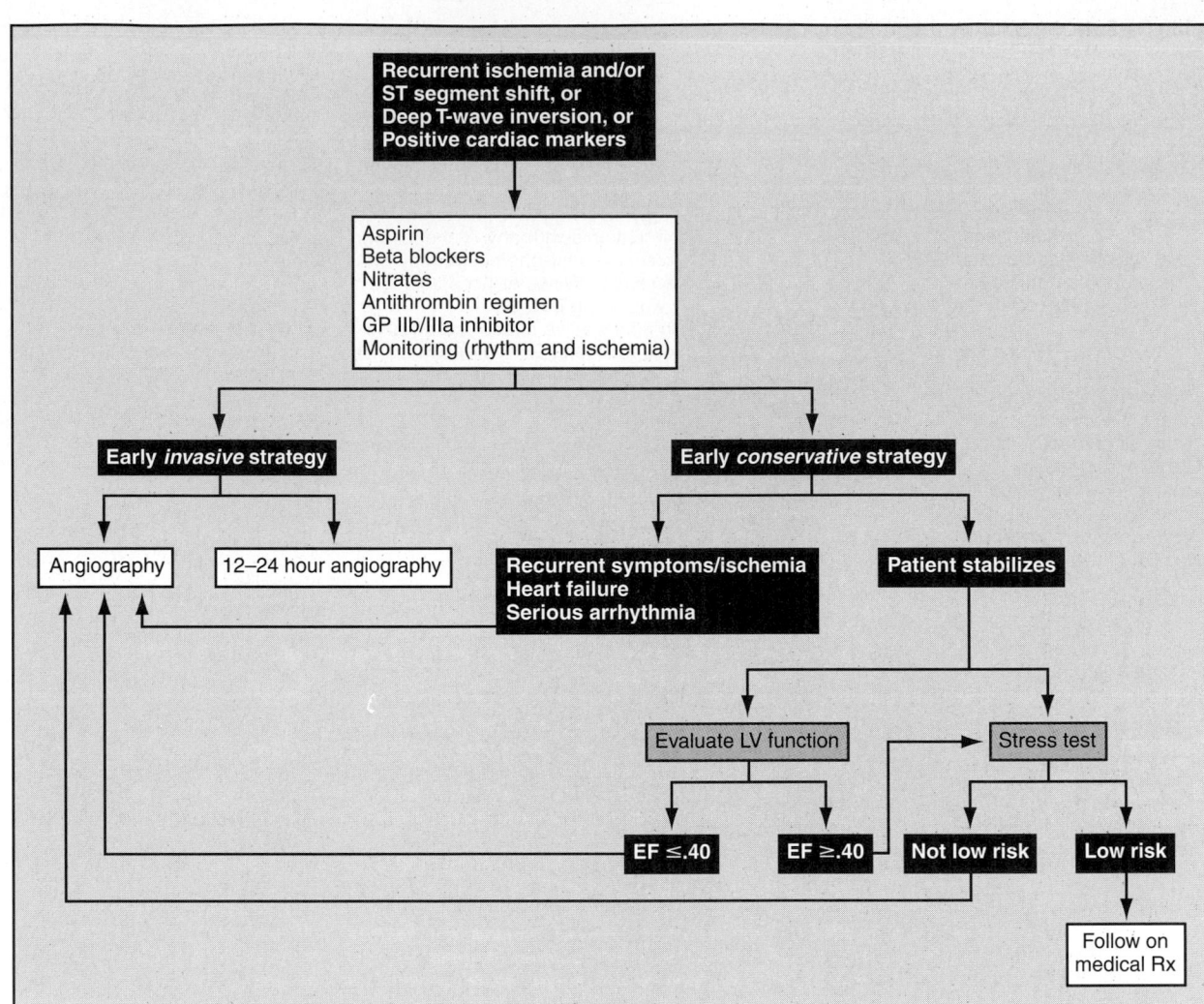

FIGURE 36–G–2. Acute ischemia pathway. EF = ejection fraction; GP = glycoprotein; LV = left ventricular. (From Braunwald E, Antman EM, Beasley JW, et al: ACC/AHA guidelines for the management of patients with unstable angina: A report of the American College of Cardiology/American Heart Association Task Force on Practice Guidelines [Committee on the Management of Patients with Unstable Angina]. J Am Coll Cardiol, 36:970–1062, 2000.)

ing recurrent ischemia, markedly abnormal noninvasive test results (see Table 36–G–2), a history of prior revascularization, depressed left ventricular function, hemodynamic instability, or sustained ventricular tachycardia. In other patients, either strategy is acceptable (Class I). The early invasive approach was considered reasonably appropriate (Class IIa) for patients who prefer revascularization to medical therapy and for patients who have repeated attacks of suspected ACS without evidence of ischemia or increased risk.

CORONARY REVASCULARIZATION. The indications for revascularization in patients with UA/NSTEMI are similar to those for patients with chronic stable angina (see Guidelines to Chap. 37). These guidelines reflect the growing experience with percutaneous coronary interventions (PCIs) and the benefit of platelet GP IIb-IIIa receptor inhibitors in high-risk patients. Coronary artery bypass graft (CABG) surgery remains the appropriate intervention for patients with left main disease, for patients with severe multivessel disease and depressed left ventricular function, and for patients with two-vessel disease that includes the proximal left anterior descending coronary artery (LAD) with depressed left ventricular function (see Table 36–G–2). In addition, the guidelines consider CABG surgery most appropriate for patients with multivessel disease and diabetes (Class IIa). Either CABG or PCI may be used in patients with one- or two-vessel disease without significant proximal LAD obstruction. However, PCI is considered appropriate (Class I) for nondiabetic patients with single or multivessel disease if the coronary anatomy is suitable for such procedures. Use of platelet GP IIb-IIIa receptor inhibitors for patients with UA/NSTEMI who are undergoing PCI is also endorsed by these guidelines.

Hospital Discharge And Post–Hospital Discharge Care (Table 36–G–4)

Long-term medical treatment of patients who have been stabilized with medical therapy or revascularization should include, in the absence of contraindications, ASA and beta blockers. Dietary interventions should be used if low-density lipoprotein (LDL) cholesterol is greater than 100 mg/dl; 3-hydroxy-3-methylglutaryl coenzyme A (HMG-CoA) reductase inhibitors should be started if LDL cholesterol is 125 mg/dl or higher. Angiotensin-converting enzyme inhibitors should be considered, especially in patients with evidence of left ventricular dysfunction.

The ACC/AHA guidelines emphasize the importance of careful follow-up within a few weeks after discharge. Recurrent unstable angina should lead to consideration of coronary revascularization. Explicit recommendations on appropriate educational messages for patients and families are provided (see Table 36–G–4). These discussions should include information about resumption of sexual activity. The guidelines also recommend control of other risk factors besides elevated LDL cholesterol, including consideration of referral of patients who are smokers to a smoking cessation program.

Special Patient Populations (Table 36–G–5)

The guidelines conclude that women with ACS should be managed in a manner similar to men—that is, no evidence supports the use of different management strategies or indications for procedures. They also recommend similar management strategies for patients with dia-

TABLE 36–G–3. NONINVASIVE TEST RESULTS PREDICTING HIGH RISK FOR AN ADVERSE OUTCOME

Exercise ECG Testing
Abnormal horizontal or down-sloping ST segment depression with
    Onset at heart rate <120/min or ≤6.5 METS
    Magnitude ≥2.0 mm
    Postexercise duration ≥6 min
    Depression in multiple leads
Abnormal systolic blood pressure response—with a sustained decrease of >10 mm Hg or a flat blood pressure response (≤130 mm Hg), associated with abnormal ECG findings
Other
    Exercise-induced ST segment elevation
    Ventricular tachycardia
Stress Radionuclide Myocardial Perfusion Imaging
Abnormal myocardial tracer distribution in more than one coronary artery region at rest or with stress or a large anterior defect that reperfuses
Abnormal myocardial distribution with increased lung uptake
Cardiac enlargement
Stress Radionuclide Ventriculography
Exercise EF of ≤0.50
Rest EF ≤0.35
Fall in EF of ≥0.10
Stress Echocardiography
Rest EF ≤0.35
Wall motion score index >1

ECG = electrocardiogram; EF = ejection fraction.

Adapted from Braunwald E, Antman EM, Beasley JW, et al: ACC/AHA guidelines for the management of patients with unstable angina: A report of the American College of Cardiology/American Heart Association Task Force on Practice Guidelines (Committee on the Management of Patients with Unstable Angina). J Am Coll Cardiol, 36:970–1062, 2000. Reprinted with permission from the American College of Cardiology.)

betes mellitus, while emphasizing the importance of diabetes as a risk factor for cardiovascular complications and the importance of glucose control as an approach to minimizing the effects of this condition. If revascularization is needed for patients with diabetes mellitus and multivessel disease, CABG (with particular attention to the use of internal mammary grafts) is preferred over PCI.

In patients who have previously undergone CABG, decisions about medical treatment or the use of revascularization should be similar to those used in other patients with UA/NSTEMI. The ACC/AHA guidelines considered the use of imaging technologies with stress testing appropriate (Class IIa) in this population. The task force also thought that a lower threshold for angiography may be appropriate in post-CABG patients because of the multiple potential causes of ischemia.

The ACC/AHA guidelines do not suggest qualitatively different strategies for the management of elderly patients with UA/NSTEMI but encourage greater attention to the impact of comorbidities, life expectancy, and the pharmacokinetics and side effects of drugs. Since the survival benefit of interventions may not be similar to those demonstrated in randomized trials involving younger patients, clinicians should give particular emphasis to the impact of interventions on quality of life.

For patients with chest pain after cocaine use, the guidelines support the use of nitroglycerin and calcium channel blockers if they have ST segment deviations. Coronary arteriography or thrombolytic therapy should be used for patients with ST segment elevation that persists despite these interventions.

Coronary arteriography, nitrates, and calcium channel blockers are also considered appropriate for patients with demonstrated coronary spasm (Prinzmetal's angina). The guidelines discourage provocative testing for spasm without coronary arteriography.

For patients with syndrome X (angina or angina-like discomfort with exercise, ST segment depression on treadmill testing, and normal or nonobstructed coronary arteries by arteriography), the guidelines recommend reassurance in view of the excellent long-term prognosis for these patients. To help relieve symptoms, the task force recommends medical therapy with antianginal agents, as well as risk factor reduction to help prevent the development of atherosclerotic coronary artery disease.

TABLE 36–G–4. HOSPITAL DISCHARGE AND POSTDISCHARGE CARE

Issue	Class	Recommendation	Level of Evidence
Hospital discharge and postdischarge care	I	Patients who do not undergo coronary revascularization, patients with unsuccessful revascularization, or patients with recurrent symptoms following revascularization should continue taking the regimen required in the hospital to control ischemia after hospital discharge	C
		Postdischarge antianginal therapy is not required for patients with successful revascularization and recurrent ischemia	C
		All patients should be given sublingual NTG and instructed in its use	C
Long-term medical therapy	I	ASA 75–160 mg/d in the absence of contraindications	A
		Beta blockers in the absence of contraindications in patients with prior MI	A
		Beta blockers in the absence of contraindications in patients without prior MI	B
		Lipid-lowering agents and diet in patients with LDL cholesterol >125 mg/dl, including after revascularization	A
		Diet for LDL >100 mg/dl	C
		Angiotensin-converting enzyme inhibitors, especially if LV dysfunction, <40% EF, or CHF is present	A
		HMG-CoA reductase inhibitors for LDL >125 mg/dl	A
Postdischarge follow-up	I	Discharge instructions should include a follow-up appointment. Low-risk medically treated patients and revascularized patients should return in 2–6 wk and higher-risk patients in 1–2 wk	C
		Patients managed initially with a conservative strategy who experience recurrent UA or severe (Canadian class III) chronic stable angina despite medical management should be considered for coronary arteriography if they are suitable for revascularization	B
		Patients who have tolerable stable angina or no anginal symptoms at follow-up visits should be managed with long-term medical therapy for stable CAD	C

Table continued on following page

TABLE 36–G–4. HOSPITAL DISCHARGE AND POSTDISCHARGE CARE *Continued*

Issue	Class	Recommendation	Level of Evidence
Use of medication	I	Prior to hospital discharge, patients and/or designated responsible caregivers should be provided with instruction with respect to medication type, purpose, dose, frequency, and pertinent side effects that are well understood	All C
		Anginal discomfort lasting more than 2 or 3 min should prompt the patient to discontinue the activity or remove himself/herself from the stressful event. If pain does not subside immediately, the patient should be instructed to take NTG. If the first tablet or spray does not provide relief within 5 min, a second and third dose, at 5-min intervals, should be taken. Pain lasting longer than 15–20 min and persistent pain despite 3 NTG doses should prompt the patient to seek immediate medical attention by going to the nearest hospital ED, preferably by ambulance or the quickest available alternative	
		If the pattern of anginal symptoms changes (e.g., pain more frequent or severe, precipitated by less effort, or now occurring at rest), the patient should contact his/her physician to determine the need for additional treatment or testing	
Risk factor modification	I	Specific instructions should be given on	
		Smoking cessation, achievement or maintenance of optimal weight, daily exercise, and diet	B
		Cholesterol-lowering medications for LDL >125 mg/dl	A
		Diet for LDL >100 mg/dl	C
		Hypertension control	B
		Tight control of hyperglycemia in diabetics	B
		Consider referral of patients who are smokers to a smoking cessation program or clinic and/or an outpatient cardiac rehabilitation program	B
Life style issues	I	Health care providers should discuss the safety and timing of resumption of sexual activity (e.g., 1–2 wk for low-risk patients, 4 wk for post–CABG surgery patients)	C
		Beyond the instructions for daily exercise, patients require specific instructions on activities (e.g., heavy lifting, climbing stairs, yard work, household activities) that are permissible and those that should be avoided. Specific mention should be made about when they can resume driving and return to work	C

ASA = acetylsalicylic acid; CAD = coronary artery disease; CHF = congestive heart failure; ED = emergency department; EF = ejection fraction; HMG-CoA = 3-hydroxy-3-methylglutaryl coenzyme A; LDL = low-density lipoprotein; LV = left ventricular; MI = myocardial infarction; NTG = nitroglycerin; UA = unstable angina.

TABLE 36–G–5. MANAGEMENT OF SPECIAL POPULATIONS

Issue	Class	Recommendation	Level of Evidence
Patients with chest pain after cocaine use	I	NTG and calcium channel blockers for patients with ST segment elevation or depression	B
		Immediate coronary arteriography, if possible, in patients whose ST segments remain elevated after NTG and calcium channel blockers. Thrombolysis (with or without PCI) if thrombus is detected	C
	IIa	IV calcium channel blockers for patients with ST segment elevation or depression	B
		Beta blockers for hypertensive patients (systolic B: >150 mm Hg) or those with sinus tachycardia (pulse >100/min)	C
		Thrombolytic therapy if ST segments remain elevated despite NTG and calcium blockers and if coronary angiography is not possible	C
		Coronary arteriography, if available, for patients with ST depression or isolated T wave changes not known to be old and who are unresponsive to NTG and calcium channel blockers	C
	III	Coronary arteriography in patients with chest pain without ST-T wave changes	C
Variant (Prinzmetal) angina	I	Coronary arteriography in patients with episodic chest pain and ST segment elevation that resolves with NTG and/or calcium channel blockers	B

TABLE 36–G–5. MANAGEMENT OF SPECIAL POPULATIONS *Continued*

1271

Ch 36

Issue	Class	Recommendation	Level of Evidence
		Treatment with nitrates and calcium channel blockers in patients whose coronary arteriogram is normal or shows only nonobstructive lesions	B
	IIa	In the absence of significant CAD on coronary arteriography, provocative testing with methylergonovine, acetylcholine, or methacholine when coronary spasm is suspected but there is no ECG evidence of transient ST segment elevation	B
	IIb	Provocative testing in patients with a nonobstructive lesion on coronary arteriography, a clinical picture of coronary spasm, and evidence of transient ST segment elevation	B
		Provocative testing in patients with nonobstructive lesions on coronary arteriography and a clinical picture of coronary spasm and transient ST segment depression	B
	III	Provocative testing carried out without coronary arteriography	C
		Provocative testing in patients with high-grade obstructive lesions on coronary arteriography	B
Syndrome X	I	Reassurance and medical therapy with nitrates, beta blockers, and calcium channel blockers alone or in combination	B
		Risk factor reduction	C
	IIb	Intracoronary ultrasound to rule out missed obstructive lesions	B
		If no ECGs are available during chest pain and coronary spasm cannot be ruled out, coronary arteriography and provocative testing using methylergonovine, acetylcholine, or methacholine should be carried out	C
		Hormone replacement in postmenopausal women unless contraindicated	C
		Imipramine for continued pain despite Class I measures	C

BP = blood pressure; CAD = coronary artery disease; ECG = electrocardiogram; NTG = nitroglycerin; PCI = percutaneous coronary intervention.

References

1. Braunwald E, Antman EM, Beasley JW, et al: ACC/AHA guidelines for the management of patients with unstable angina: A report of the American College of Cardiology/American Heart Association Task Force on Practice Guidelines (Committee on the Management of Patients with Unstable Angina). J Am Coll Cardiol 2000, 36:970–1062, 2000.
2. Braunwald E, Mark DB, Jones RH, et al: Unstable Angina: Diagnosis and Management. Clinical Practice Guideline Number 10 (amended). AHCPR Publication No 94-0602. Rockville, MD, Agency for Health Care Policy and Research and the National Heart, Lung and Blood Institute, Public Health Service, US Department of Health and Human Services, May 1994.
3. Gibbons RJ, Chatterjee K, Daley J, et al: ACC/AHA/ACP guidelines for the management of patients with chronic stable angina. J Am Coll Cardiol 33: 2092–2197, 1999.

Chapter 37

Chronic Coronary Artery Disease

BERNARD J. GERSH · EUGENE BRAUNWALD
ROBERT O. BONOW

Chronic coronary artery disease (CAD) is most commonly due to obstruction of the coronary arteries by atheromatous plaque[1] (the pathogenesis of atherosclerosis is described in Chapter 30). Factors that predispose to this condition are discussed in Chapter 31, the control of coronary blood flow in Chapter 34, acute myocardial infarction in Chapter 35, and unstable angina in Chapter 36; sudden cardiac death, another significant consequence of CAD, is presented in Chapter 26.

No uniform syndrome of signs and symptoms is initially seen in patients with CAD. Chest discomfort is usually the predominant symptom in chronic (stable) angina (see p. 1273), unstable angina (see Chap. 36), Prinzmetal (variant) angina (p. 1324), microvascular angina (p. 1329), and acute myocardial infarction (Chap. 35). However, syndromes of CAD also occur in which ischemic chest discomfort is absent or not prominent, such as asymptomatic (silent) myocardial ischemia (see p. 1330), congestive heart failure, cardiac arrhythmias, and sudden death (Chap. 26). Obstructive CAD also has many nonatherosclerotic causes, including congenital abnormalities of the coronary arteries, myocardial bridging, coronary arteritis in association with the systemic vasculitides, and radiation-induced coronary disease.[2, 3] Whether coronary ectasia is a cause of angina pectoris in the absence of coronary artery obstruction remains to be clarified.[4] Myocardial ischemia and angina pectoris may also occur in the *absence* of obstructive CAD, as in the case of aortic valve disease (see Chap. 46), hypertrophic cardiomyopathy (Chap. 48), and idiopathic dilated cardiomyopathy (Chap. 48). Moreover, CAD may coexist with these other forms of heart disease.

THE MAGNITUDE OF THE PROBLEM

The importance of CAD in contemporary society is attested to by the almost epidemic number of persons afflicted—especially when this number is compared with the anecdotal reports of its occurrence in the medical literature before this century. Moreover, as the challenges posed by infectious, parasitic, and nutritional disorders and perinatal mortality are overcome, particularly in the developing world, a global epidemic of CAD looms large on the horizon (see Chap. 1). It is estimated that 12,200,000 Americans have CAD, 6,300,000 of whom have angina pectoris and 7,200,000 have had myocardial infarction.[5, 6] The economic cost of CAD and stroke in the United States in 2000 is estimated at $326.6 billion ($118.2 billion for CAD).[5] Given the current magnitude of the problem and the increasing prevalence of CAD that is anticipated because of aging of the population, recognition, management, and prevention of CAD are of major public health importance.[5, 6]

CAD mortality rates vary widely among countries and even within a country. Recent 10-year data from the World Health Organization Monitoring of Trials and Determinants in Cardiovascular Disease (MONICA) Project in 37 different populations demonstrated a reduction in CAD events and mortality rates in most countries, but with contradictory results for a few countries, mostly in central and eastern Europe and Asia.[7] Within the United States, death rates from cardiovascular disease among black males and females are substantially higher than those among whites.[5] Among American Indians, not only do rates of CAD exceed those reported for other U.S. populations, but the disease is more often fatal.[8] However, there is encouraging evidence that in the last three decades the age-adjusted death rate from CAD, which had reached pandemic proportions in industrial countries during the middle years of the 20th century, has decreased.[9] For example, between 1961 and 1991, the age-adjusted death rate for CAD declined by 52 percent, more so in men than in women.[5] Similar trends have been observed in many industrialized nations with different health care systems. Multiple causes may have contributed to this favorable trend, including a reduction in risk factors (see Chap. 31), improvements in socioeconomic circumstances such as enhanced access to care, and new methods of diagnosis and treatment. In the United States, it has been estimated that approximately 50 percent of the decrease in CAD mortality during the last decade has resulted from reductions in primary and secondary risk factors, but the contributions from new methods of treatment are also considered substantial.[10]

CLINICAL MANIFESTATIONS

CHARACTERISTICS OF ANGINA (see also Chap. 3). Angina pectoris is a discomfort in the chest or adjacent areas caused by myocardial ischemia. It is usually brought on by exertion and associated with a disturbance in myocardial function, but without myocardial necrosis.[11] Heberden's initial description of the chest discomfort as conveying a sense of "strangling and anxiety" is still remarkably pertinent, although adjectives frequently used to describe this distress include "viselike," "constricting," "suffocating," "crushing," "heavy," and "squeezing." In other patients, the quality of the sensation is more vague and described as a mild pressure-like discomfort, an uncomfortable numb sensation, or a burning sensation. The site of the discomfort is usually retrosternal, but radiation is common and usually occurs down the ulnar surface of the left arm; the right arm and the outer surfaces of both arms may also be involved[11] (see Fig. 3-2). Epigastric discomfort alone or in association with chest pressure is not uncommon. Anginal discomfort above the mandible, below the epigastrium, or confined to the ear is rare. Anginal "equivalents" (i.e., symptoms of myocardial ischemia other than angina), such as dyspnea, faintness, fatigue, and eructations, are common, particularly in the elderly. A history of abnormal exertional dyspnea may be an early indicator of CAD even when angina is absent or no electrocardiographic (ECG) evidence of ischemic heart disease can be found.[12] Dyspnea at rest or with exertion may be a manifestation of severe ischemia and lead to increases in left ventricular filling pressure. Nocturnal angina should raise the suspicion of sleep apnea.[13]

A careful clinical history is key to making the correct diagnosis and is particularly important in this era of cost-conscious practice of medicine because it may obviate more expensive testing. If the quality of the pain and its duration, precipitating factors, and associated symptoms are taken into consideration, it is usually possible to arrive at a correct diagnosis (see Table 3-4). The typical episode of angina pectoris usually begins gradually and reaches its maximum intensity over a period of minutes before dissipating. It is unusual for angina pectoris to reach its maximum severity within seconds, and it is characteristic that patients with angina usually prefer to rest, sit, or stop walking during episodes.[11] Chest discomfort while walking in the cold, uphill, or after a meal is suggestive of angina. Features suggesting the *absence* of angina pectoris include pleuritic pain, pain localized to the tip of one finger, pain reproduced by movement or palpation of the chest wall or arms, and constant pain lasting many hours or, alternatively, very brief episodes of pain lasting seconds. Pain radiating into the lower extremities is also a highly unusual manifestation of angina pectoris.

Typical angina pectoris is relieved within minutes by rest or by the use of nitroglycerin. The response to the latter is often a useful diagnostic tool, although it should be remembered that esophageal pain and other syndromes may also respond to nitroglycerin. A delay of more than 5 to 10 minutes before relief is obtained by rest and nitroglycerin suggests that the symptoms are either not due to ischemia or, alternatively, are due to severe ischemia, i.e., acute myocardial infarction or unstable angina. The phenomenon of "first effort" or "warm-up" angina is used to describe the ability of some patients in whom angina develops with exertion to subsequently continue at the same level of exertion without symptoms after an intervening period of rest. This attenuation of myocardial ischemia observed with repeated exertion has been postulated to be due to ischemic preconditioning.[14]

An important component of the history is to assess the degree of cardiovascular disability caused by angina pectoris. Such assessment is a crucial part of the evaluation for coronary revascularization. Although several classifications for assessing cardiovascular disability are available,[15] the Canadian Cardiovascular Society Functional Classification System (see Table 3-11) is most widely used.[16]

MECHANISMS. The mechanisms of cardiac pain and the neural pathways involved are poorly understood.[1] It is presumed that angina pectoris results from ischemic episodes that excite chemosensitive and mechanoreceptive receptors in the heart. Stimulation of these receptors results in the release of adenosine, bradykinin, and other substances that excite the sensory ends of the sympathetic and vagal afferent fibers. The afferent fibers traverse the nerves that connect to the upper five thoracic sympathetic ganglia and upper five distal thoracic roots of the spinal cord. Impulses are transmitted by the spinal cord to the thalamus and hence to the neocortex. Within the spinal cord, cardiac sympathetic afferent impulses may converge with impulses from somatic thoracic structures, which may be the basis for referred cardiac pain, for example, to the chest. In comparison, cardiac vagal afferent fibers synapse in the nucleus tractus solitarius of the medulla and then descend to excite the upper cervical spinothalamic tract cells, which may contribute to the anginal pain experienced in the neck and jaw.[17] On the basis of positron-emission tomographic (PET) findings on changes in regional cerebral blood flow associated with angina pectoris, it has been proposed that cortical activation is necessary for pain sensation and the thalamus acts as a gate for afferent pain signals.[18]

Differential Diagnosis of Chest Pain
(see Fig. 3-3 and Table 3-4)

Differentiation of various disorders from CAD is challenging because the severity of the chest pain and the seriousness of the underlying disorder are not necessarily related. Compounding the difficulty in differential diagnosis is the common myth that pain in the left arm or left side of the chest is an ominous sign signifying the presence of CAD. However, a host of other disorders can also cause discomfort in these locations.

ESOPHAGEAL DISORDERS. The common esophageal disorders that may simulate or coexist with angina pectoris are gastroesophageal reflux and disorders of esophageal motility, including diffuse spasm as well as "nutcracker" esophagus, which is characterized by high-amplitude peristaltic contractions and vigorous achalasia.[19] Symptomatic esophageal reflux is common and estimated to occur in 7 to 14 percent of an otherwise "healthy" U.S. population. In a comparative study of patients with chest pain and normal coronary angiograms and controls with confirmed CAD, esophageal function testing (including manometry, provocation tests, and 24-hour ambulatory pH monitoring) commonly implicated the esophagus as a cause of pain in patients with normal coronary angiograms. Nonetheless, a similar high frequency of esophageal abnormalities among patients with angina pectoris suggests that the esophagus may be an unrecognized source of pain in both groups of patients.[19] Further evidence of a relationship between esophageal abnormalities and angina pectoris was provided by a prospective study demonstrating that esophageal acid stimulation can cause anginal attacks in association with a significant reduction in coronary blood flow in patients with CAD.[20] A lack of any significant effect in this study in heart transplant recipients with cardiac denervation suggests a neural origin.

The classic manifestation of esophageal pain is "heartburn," particularly in connection with changes in posture and meals and in association with dysphagia. Esophageal spasm may also cause constant retrosternal discomfort of uniform intensity or severe spasmodic pain during or after swallowing. To further compound the difficulty in distinguishing between angina and esophageal pain, both may be relieved by nitroglycerin. However, esophageal pain is often relieved by milk, antacids, foods, or, occasionally, warm liquids.

GASTROESOPHAGEAL REFLUX. The esophageal acid perfusion, or Bernstein, test may be helpful in its use of alternate infusions of dilute acid and normal saline by a nasal gastric catheter with the tip placed at the level of the midesophagus.[19] Infusion of acid produces pain in over 90 percent of patients with subjective and objective evidence of gastroesophageal acid reflux, but it is particularly useful if the patient's symptoms are reproduced. Acid reflux into the esophagus can also be recognized by recording the pH from an electrode at the tip of a catheter inserted into the distal portion of the esophagus.

ESOPHAGEAL MOTILITY DISORDERS. Esophageal motility disorders are not uncommon in patients with retrosternal chest pain of unclear cause and should be specifically excluded or confirmed, if possible.[21] In addition to chest pain, the majority of such patients have dysphagia. Although barium studies may reveal motility problems, esophageal manometry may show diffuse esophageal spasm, increased pressure at the lower esophageal sphincter, and other motility disorders. Provocative pharmacological agents such as methacholine may provoke esophageal pain and manometric signs of spasm.

A more complex problem is determining whether part or all of the symptoms in patients with *known* CAD are due to esophageal disease. Both CAD and esophageal disease are common clinical entities that may coexist. Diagnostic evaluation for an esophageal disorder may be indicated in patients with CAD who have a poor symptomatic response to antianginal therapy in the absence of documentation of severe ischemia or in patients with persistent symptoms despite adequate coronary revascularization.

BILIARY COLIC. Although visceral symptoms are a common association of myocardial ischemia (particularly acute inferior myocardial infarction [see Chap. 35]), cholecystitis and related hepatobiliary disorders may also mimic ischemia and should always be considered in patients with atypical chest discomfort, particularly those with diabetes.[22] The pain is steady, usually lasts 2 to 4 hours, and subsides spontaneously without any symptoms between attacks. It is generally most intense in the right upper abdominal area but may also be felt in the epigastrium or precordium. This discomfort is often referred to the scapula, may radiate around the costal margin to the back, or may in rare cases be felt in the shoulder and suggest diaphragmatic irritation. Ultrasonography is accurate in diagnosing gallstones and allows determination of gallbladder size and thickness and whether the bile ducts are dilated.

COSTOSTERNAL SYNDROME. In 1921, Tietze first described a syndrome of local pain and tenderness, usually limited to the anterior chest wall and associated with swelling of costal cartilage. This condition causes pain that can resemble angina pectoris. The full-blown Tietze syndrome, i.e., pain associated with tender *swelling* of the costochondral junctions, is uncommon, whereas costochondritis causing tenderness of the costochondral junctions (without swelling) is relatively common.[23] Pain on palpation of these joints is a useful clinical sign. Local pressure should be applied routinely to the anterior chest wall during examination of a patient with suspected angina pectoris. In addition, costochondritis is usually well localized. Although palpation of the chest wall often reproduces pain in patients with various musculoskeletal conditions, it should be appreciated that chest wall tenderness may also be associated with and does not exclude symptomatic CAD.[24]

OTHER MUSCULOSKELETAL DISORDERS. Cervical radiculitis may be confused with angina. This condition may occur as a constant ache, sometimes resulting in a sensory deficit. The pain may be related to motion of the neck, just as motion of the shoulder triggers attacks of pain from bursitis. A hyperalgesic area noted by running the finger down the back and exerting pressure may lead to a suspicion of thoracic root pain. Occasionally, pain mimicking angina can be due to compression of the brachial plexus by the cervical ribs, and tendinitis or bursitis involving the left shoulder may also cause angina-like pain. Physical examination may also detect pain brought about by movement of an arthritic shoulder or a calcified shoulder tendon.

OTHER CAUSES OF ANGINA-LIKE PAIN. *Acute myocardial infarction* is usually associated with prolonged (>30 minutes), severe pain occurring at rest that apart from duration and intensity, may be similar to angina pectoris. It is associated with characteristic ECG changes and the release of cardiac markers (see Chap. 35). Unstable angina is a severe form of angina that may also occur at rest and may not be relieved by nitroglycerin (see Chap. 36).

The classic symptom of *dissecting aortic aneurysm* is a severe, often sharp pain that radiates to the back (see Chap. 40). Although aortic dissection is generally part of the differential diagnosis of acute myocardial infarction, the syndrome may be chronic in some patients. The pain is often described as sharp, but its pleuropericarditic quality is usually helpful in the differential diagnosis.

Severe pulmonary hypertension may be associated with exertional chest pain with the characteristics of angina pectoris, and indeed, this pain is thought to be due to right ventricular ischemia that develops during exertion (see Chap. 53). Other associated symptoms include exertional dyspnea, dizziness, and syncope. Associated findings on physical examination, such as parasternal lift, a palpable and loud pulmonary component of the second sound, and right ventricular hypertrophy on the ECG, are usually readily recognized.

Pulmonary embolism is initially characterized by dyspnea as the cardinal symptom, but chest pain may also be present (see Chap. 52). Pleuritic pain suggests pulmonary infarction, and a history of exacerbation of the pain with inspiration, along with a pleural friction rub, usually helps distinguish it from angina pectoris.

The pain of *acute pericarditis* (see Chap. 50) may at times be difficult to distinguish from angina pectoris. However, pericarditis tends to occur in younger patients than does angina, and the diagnosis depends on the combination of chest pain not relieved by rest or nitroglycerin, a pericardial friction rub, and ECG changes.

Chronic CAD can and frequently does coexist with any of the other disorders mentioned above, and noncardiac disease can trigger a true angina attack in a patient with CAD. An additional component of the history is an evaluation of risk factors for CAD because such risk factors in turn have an effect on both the probability of significant obstructive CAD and the overall prognosis.[25]

Physical Examination

GENERAL EXAMINATION. Inspection of the eyes may reveal a *corneal arcus*, and examination of the skin may show xanthomas (see Fig. 4–2). Among patients with heterozygous familial hypercholesterolemia (in whom CAD is common), the presence of a corneal arcus increases with age and, in some studies, correlates positively with levels of cholesterol and low-density lipoprotein (LDL) and also with the prognosis.[26, 27] *Xanthelasma*, in which lipid deposits are intracellular, appears to be promoted by increased levels of triglycerides and a relative deficiency of high-density lipoprotein (HDL). The presence of xanthelasma is a strong marker of dyslipidemia and, often, a family history of cardiovascular disease, and should provide a strong impetus for performing a comprehensive lipid profile.[28] Retinal arteriolar changes are common in patients with CAD and diabetes mellitus or hypertension. Moreover, diabetes-associated visual impairments, including retinopathy, are independent predictors of increased mortality from all causes, including CAD.[29]

Some correlation has been noted between CAD and a *diagonal earlobe crease* (except in American Indians and Asians). A unilateral diagonal earlobe crease is often present in younger persons with CAD and becomes bilateral with advancing age.[30] A hospital-based, case-control study of men admitted with a first nonfatal myocardial infarction demonstrated that the presence of a diagonal earlobe crease was associated with a relative risk of 1.37 for myocardial infarction; the risk is similarly increased in the presence of baldness and thoracic hairiness.[31]

Blood pressure may be chronically elevated or may rise acutely (along with the heart rate) during an angina attack. Changes in blood pressure may precede (and precipitate) or follow (and be caused by) angina.

Other important features of the general physical examination are abnormalities in arterial pulses and the venous system. A rapid pulse may be a clue to cardiac decompensation or to a systemic condition such as thyrotoxicosis or anemia, which can exacerbate angina pectoris. The association between peripheral vascular disease and CAD is strong and well documented.[32, 33] This association is not confined to patients with symptomatic or clinically overt peripheral vascular disease or CAD but is also seen in asymptomatic subjects with a reduced ankle-brachial blood pressure index or evidence of early carotid disease on ultrasonography.[34] The presence of carotid and peripheral arterial disease on palpation and auscultation increases the likelihood that chest discomfort of unclear origin is caused by CAD. Evaluation of the patient's venous system, particularly in the legs, may have an important bearing on the type of grafting procedure used in subsequent coronary bypass surgery.

CARDIAC EXAMINATION. The physical findings of hypertrophic cardiomyopathy (see Chap. 48) or aortic valve disease (Chap. 46) suggest that angina may be due to conditions other than (or in addition to) CAD. It is often helpful to examine the heart *during* an episode of pain because ischemia may produce transient left ventricular dysfunction with a third heart sound and pulmonary rales detectable on physical examination.[35] If massage of the carotid sinus produces pain relief in a patient without a carotid bruit, the pain is probably anginal. Softening of the mitral component of the first heart sound as a result of ischemic left ventricular dysfunction may also be demonstrated during angina. Paradoxical splitting of the second heart sound (see Chap. 4) may occur transiently during angina and appears to be related to asynergy and prolongation of left ventricular contraction, which results in delayed closure of the aortic valve. If other obvious cardiac diseases are absent, a third or loud fourth heart sound suggests ischemia as the basis for the chest pain. These sounds are common in patients with angina at rest, and their frequency is increased during handgrip exercise,[36] even if the latter does not precipitate angina pectoris. A sustained apical cardiac impulse is common in patients with moderate or severe left ventricular dysfunction. A displaced ventricular impulse, particularly if dyskinetic, is a sign of significant left ventricular systolic dysfunction, especially in a patient who previously had a myocardial infarction.

Transient apical systolic murmurs are quite common in CAD and have been attributed to reversible papillary mus-cle dysfunction secondary to transient myocardial ischemia. When persistent, such murmurs may be due to papillary muscle fibrosis, which is often a manifestation of subendocardial infarction or a regional wall motion abnormality altering the alignment of the papillary muscles in relation to other components of the mitral valve apparatus. These murmurs are more prevalent in patients with extensive CAD, especially those with prior myocardial infarction and left ventricular dysfunction, and may indicate an adverse prognosis.[37] Systolic murmurs may assume a variety of configurations (early, late, or holosystolic) and may be accentuated by exertion or during angina. A midsystolic click, often followed by a late systolic murmur produced by mitral valve prolapse (see Chap. 46), also occurs in patients with CAD. A diastolic murmur or a continuous murmur is a rare finding in CAD and has been attributed to turbulent flow across a proximal coronary artery stenosis.[38]

PATHOPHYSIOLOGY

Angina pectoris results from myocardial ischemia, which is caused by an imbalance between myocardial O_2 requirements and myocardial O_2 supply.[1] The former may be elevated by increases in heart rate, left ventricular wall stress, and contractility (see Chap. 34); the latter is determined by coronary blood flow and coronary arterial O_2 content (Fig. 37–1).

ANGINA CAUSED BY INCREASED MYOCARDIAL O_2 REQUIREMENTS. In this condition, sometimes termed "demand angina," the myocardial O_2 requirement increases in the face of a constant and usually restricted O_2 supply. The increased requirement commonly stems from norepinephrine release by adrenergic nerve endings in the heart and vascular bed, a physiological response to exertion, emotion, or mental stress. Of great importance to the myocardial O_2 requirement is the *rate* at which any task is carried out. Hurrying is particularly likely to precipitate angina, as are efforts involving motion of the hands over the head. Mental stress may also precipitate angina, presumably by increased hemodynamic and catecholamine responses to stress, increased adrenergic tone, and reduced vagal activity.[39, 40]

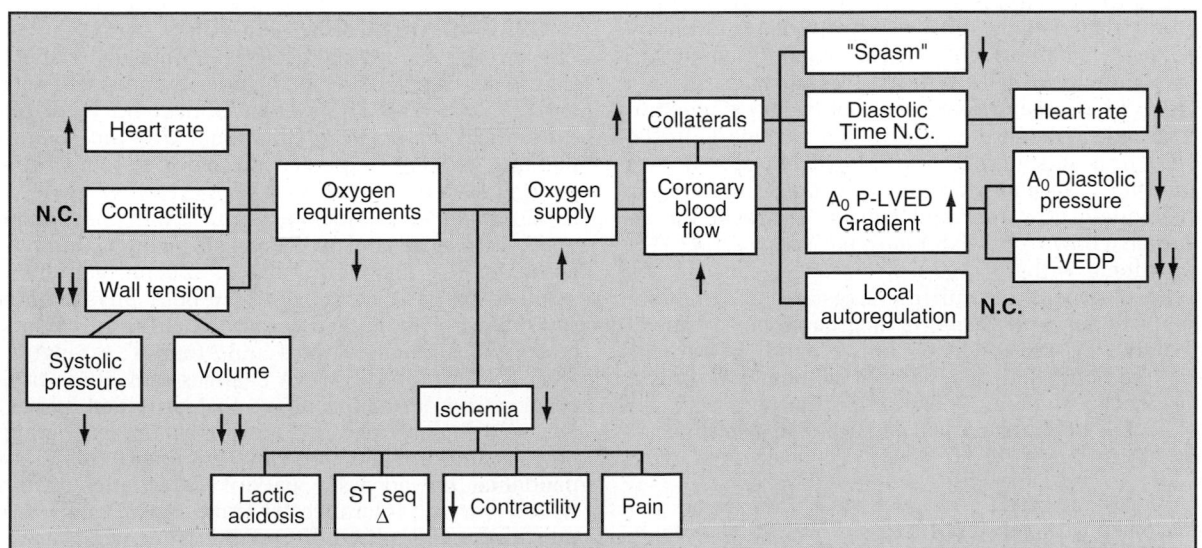

FIGURE 37–1. Factors influencing the balance between myocardial O_2 requirements *(left)* and supply *(right)*. Arrows indicate effects of nitrates. In relieving angina pectoris, nitrates exert favorable effects by reducing O_2 requirements and increasing supply. Although a reflex increase in heart rate would tend to reduce the time for coronary flow, dilation of collaterals and enhancement of the pressure gradient for flow to occur as the left ventricular end-diastolic pressure (LVEDP) falls tend to increase coronary flow. A_oP = aortic pressure; NC = no change. (From Frishman WH: Pharmacology of the nitrates in angina pectoris. Am J Cardiol 56:8I, 1985. By permission of Excerpta Medica.)

The combination of physical exertion and emotion in association with sexual activity commonly precipitates angina pectoris, but sexual activity seldom triggers myocardial infarction.[41] Anger may produce constriction of coronary arteries with preexisting narrowing without necessarily affecting O_2 demand. Other factors causing angina secondary to an increase in myocardial O_2 requirement in patients with obstructive CAD include physical exertion after a heavy meal and the excessive metabolic demands imposed by chills, fever, thyrotoxicosis, tachycardia from any cause, and hypoglycemia. Among patients with stable, fixed obstructive CAD, several studies using ambulatory ECG monitoring have documented the importance of increases in myocardial O_2 requirement and, in particular, tachycardia as a precipitant of ischemia.[42]

In all these conditions, underlying coronary artery obstruction is usually present, and the other factors (e.g., exertion, emotion, or fever) precipitate ischemia and chest discomfort by stimulating myocardial O_2 need in the presence of a relatively fixed and limited myocardial O_2 supply.

ANGINA CAUSED BY TRANSIENTLY DECREASED O_2 SUPPLY. Increasing evidence suggests that not only unstable angina but also chronic stable angina may be caused by transient reductions in O_2 supply as a consequence of coronary vasoconstriction,[1, 43] a condition that is sometimes termed "supply angina" and due to the entity of "dynamic stenosis."[44] The coronary arterial bed is well innervated, and a variety of stimuli alter coronary tone (see Chap. 34). Two main explanations have been offered for the association between coronary vasoconstriction and spasm in the presence of organic stenoses. First, platelet thrombi and leukocytes may elaborate vasoconstrictor substances such as serotonin and thromboxane A_2. Second, endothelial damage in atherosclerotic coronary arteries may result in decreased production of vasodilator substances and an abnormal vasoconstrictor response to exercise and other stimuli. A variable threshold of myocardial ischemia in patients with chronic stable angina may be due to dynamic changes in peristenotic smooth muscle tone and also to constriction of arteries distal to the stenosis.[45] In this setting, calcium antagonists and nitrates are less effective than in patients with variant angina, perhaps because of the nature of the constricting stimuli and the site of constriction.[45]

Patients with angina precipitated by a transient reduction in myocardial O_2 supply may have a spectrum of signs and symptoms that depend on the severity of the underlying fixed defect and the degree of the dynamic change in coronary arterial tone. In a typical patient with chronic stable angina, the degree of fixed obstruction is sufficient to result in an inadequate coronary flow rate to cope with the increased O_2 demands of exercise. However, episodes of transient coronary vasoconstriction may be superimposed on this inadequate flow rate and cause additional limitations to coronary flow reserve in many patients.

In rare patients without organic obstructing lesions, severe dynamic obstruction occurring at rest alone can cause myocardial ischemia and result in angina (see Prinzmetal [Variant] Angina, p. 1324). On the other hand, in patients with severe fixed obstruction to coronary blood flow, only a minor increase in dynamic obstruction is necessary for blood flow to fall below a critical level and cause myocardial ischemia.

FIXED COMPARED WITH VARIABLE-THRESHOLD ANGINA. The threshold for angina differs widely among patients with chronic angina. In patients with fixed-threshold angina precipitated by increased O_2 demands with few if any dynamic (vasoconstrictor) components, the level of physical activity required to precipitate angina is relatively constant. Characteristically, these patients can predict the amount of physical activity that will precipitate angina, e.g., walking up exactly two flights of stairs at a customary pace. When these patients are tested on a treadmill or bicycle, the pressure-rate product (the so-called double product, a correlate of the myocardial O_2 requirement) that elicits angina and/or ECG evidence of ischemia is relatively constant.

In patients with fixed-threshold, demand angina, the specific threshold at which ischemia develops (as reflected in angina and/or ST segment depression) is a function of the myocardial O_2 requirement. As the activity of the left ventricle (and therefore its O_2 requirement) increases, a point is reached at which perfusion distal to a critical coronary arterial obstruction cannot supply sufficient O_2 to myocardium perfused by the obstructed artery; ischemia and angina ensue. This relationship is, however, modified by the effects of coronary vasomotor tone on myocardial O_2 supply.[46] Coronary vascular reserve (or coronary vasodilator or flow reserve) is impaired in patients with significant obstructive CAD and also in those with microvascular disease or endothelial damage from conditions such as hypertension.[47]

The majority of patients with variable-threshold angina have atherosclerotic coronary arterial narrowing, but dynamic obstruction caused by vasoconstriction plays an important role in causing myocardial ischemia. These patients typically have "good days," when they are capable of substantial physical activity, as well as "bad days," when even minimal activity can cause clinical and/or ECG evidence of myocardial ischemia or angina at rest. Often, even in the course of a single day, they may be capable of substantial physical activity at one time while minimal activity results in angina at another. Patients with variable-threshold angina often complain of a circadian variation in angina that is more common in the morning. Angina on exertion and sometimes even at rest may be precipitated by cold temperature,[48] emotion, and mental stress.[49] A cold environment has been shown to increase peripheral resistance, both at rest and during exercise.[50] The rise in arterial pressure, by augmenting myocardial O_2 requirements, lowers the threshold for the development of angina. An alternative or additional explanation is the development of cold-induced coronary vasoconstriction via activation of peripheral and reflex mechanisms.[50]

The entity of postprandial angina has been recognized for about two centuries and may be a marker of severe multivessel CAD.[51] The mechanism has not been explained, but it may be due to redistribution of coronary blood flow away from the territory supplied by severely stenosed vessels.[52] Some evidence indicates that this phenomenon is more prominent after high-carbohydrate than high-fat meals.[51]

MIXED ANGINA. The term *mixed angina* has been proposed by Maseri and colleagues to describe the many patients who fall between the two extremes of fixed-threshold and variable-threshold angina.[53] The pathophysiological and clinical correlations of ischemia in patients with stable CAD may have important implications for the selection of antiischemic agents, as well as for their timing. The greater the contribution from increased myocardial O_2 requirements to the imbalance between supply and demand, the greater the likelihood that beta-blocking agents will be effective, whereas nitrates and calcium channel blocking agents, at least on theoretical grounds, are likely to be especially effective in episodes caused primarily by coronary vasoconstriction. The finding that in most patients with chronic stable angina an increase in myocardial O_2 requirement precedes episodes of ischemia, i.e., that they have demand angina, argues in favor of beta blockers as essential therapeutic agents.[54]

GRADING OF ANGINA PECTORIS. A system of grading the severity of angina pectoris proposed by the Canadian Cardiovascular Society has gained widespread acceptance[16] (see Table 3–11). The system is a modification of the New York Heart Association functional classification but allows patients to be categorized in more specific terms. Other grading systems include a specific activity scale developed by Goldman and associates[15] and an anginal "score" developed by Califf and colleagues.[55] The Goldman scale is based on the metabolic cost of specific activities and appears to be valid when used by both physicians and nonphysicians. The anginal score of Califf and coworkers integrates the clinical features and "tempo" of angina together with ECG ST and T wave changes and offers independent prognostic information above that provided by age, gender, left ventricular function, and coronary angiographic anatomy. A limitation of all these grading systems is their dependence on accurate patient observation and patients' widely varying tolerance for symptoms. Prospective evaluation of the reproducibility of the New York Heart Association estimates of functional class made by two physicians demonstrated a reproducibility of only 56 percent, and only 51 percent of the estimates agreed with treadmill exercise performance. Functional estimates based on the Canadian Cardiovascular Society criteria were more reproducible (73 percent) but still did not correlate well with objective measures of exercise performance.[15]

AGE (yr)	NONANGINAL CHEST PAIN		ATYPICAL ANGINA		TYPICAL ANGINA	
	Men	Women	Men	Women	Men	Women
30–39	4	2	34	12	76	26
40–49	13	3	51	22	87	55
50–59	20	7	65	31	93	73
60–69	27	14	72	51	94	86

*Each value represents the percentage with significant coronary artery disease on catheterization (combined data from Diamond and Forrester[56] and Chaitman et al.[59]).

From Gibbons RJ, Chatterjee K, Daley J, et al: ACC/AHA/ACP-ASIM guidelines for the management of patients with chronic stable angina: A report of the American College of Cardiology/ American Heart Association Task Force on Practice Guidelines (Committee on Management of Patients with Chronic Stable Angina). J Am Coll Cardiol 33:2092, 1999. By permission of The American College of Cardiology and The American Heart Association.

CORRELATION BETWEEN HISTORICAL FEATURES AND CORONARY ANGIOGRAPHY. An important objective of the history and physical examination is to acquire information that can be used to estimate the probability of the presence of obstructive CAD. The importance of this point is emphasized by the impact of the pretest likelihood of CAD on the performance of a standard exercise test.[35] The ability to predict the probability of CAD with reasonable accuracy from the history and physical examination was demonstrated originally by Diamond and Forrester and expanded on by other studies in both men and women referred for cardiac catheterization or stress testing.[56, 58] The inclusion of such risk factors as cigarette smoking, hyperlipidemia, and diabetes mellitus strengthens the predictability of these models, as do certain changes on the ECG.[57] Subsequently, the Diamond and Forrester model was shown to be in strong agreement with the findings of the Coronary Artery Surgery Study (CASS).[59] The joint American College of Cardiology and American Heart Association (ACC/AHA) Guidelines Committee[35] combined data from both studies to illustrate the pretest likelihood of CAD in men and women stratified by age and nature of the chest pain (Table 37-1).

Although the clinical manifestations of CAD, including rest angina and nocturnal and postprandial angina, tend to be more severe in patients with multivessel than single-vessel disease, neither the severity, duration, or nature of the pain nor its precipitating factors correlate with the extent of disease at angiography. Perhaps the most striking example of the lack of historical-arteriographic correlation is in two subgroups of patients—those with advanced obstructive CAD who are asymptomatic with "silent ischemia" (see p. 1330) and those with Prinzmetal, or variant, angina, who may have episodes of very severe anginal discomfort, yet have minimal or no underlying coronary atherosclerosis (see p. 1324).

NONINVASIVE TESTING

Biochemical Tests

In patients with chronic stable angina, metabolic abnormalities that are risk factors for the development of CAD are frequently detected. These abnormalities include hypercholesterolemia and other dyslipidemias (see Chap. 31), carbohydrate intolerance, and insulin resistance.[60, 61] All patients with established or suspected CAD warrant biochemical evaluation of total cholesterol, LDL cholesterol, HDL cholesterol, triglycerides, and fasting blood glucose.[62] New biochemical markers, such as C-reactive protein, lipoprotein Lp(a), and homocysteine, have been shown to increase the likelihood of future cardiovascular events,[63–65] especially in patients with hypercholesterolemia, but no consensus has been reached regarding routine measurement of these markers, and measuring them is not generally recommended.[66]

Serum levels of cardiac markers are normal in patients with chronic stable angina, which serves to differentiate them from patients with acute myocardial infarction.

Resting Electrocardiogram (see also Chap. 5)

The resting ECG is normal in approximately half of patients with chronic stable angina pectoris, and even patients with severe CAD may have a normal tracing at rest. A normal resting ECG suggests the presence of normal resting left ventricular function[67] and is an unusual finding in a patient with an extensive previous infarction. The most common ECG abnormalities in patients with chronic CAD are nonspecific ST-T wave changes with or without abnormal Q waves. Numerous pitfalls must be avoided when using the *resting* ECG for the diagnosis of myocardial ischemia. In addition to myocardial ischemia, other conditions that can produce ST-T wave abnormalities include left ventricular hypertrophy and dilatation, electrolyte abnormalities, neurogenic effects, and antiarrhythmic drugs.[68] In patients with known CAD, however, the occurrence of ST-T wave abnormalities on the resting ECG may correlate with the severity of the underlying heart disease, including the number of vessels involved and the presence of left ventricular dysfunction.[69] This association may explain the adverse impact of ST-T wave changes on prognosis in these patients. In contrast, a normal resting ECG is a more favorable long-term prognostic sign in patients with suspected or definite CAD.[35, 70]

Interval ECGs may reveal the development of Q wave infarctions that have gone unrecognized clinically. Various conduction disturbances, most frequently left bundle branch block and left anterior fascicular block, may occur in patients with chronic stable angina, and they are often associated with impairment of left ventricular function[71] and reflect multivessel disease and previous myocardial damage. Hence, such conduction disturbances are an indicator of a relatively poor prognosis.[35] In patients with chronic stable angina, abnormal Q waves are relatively specific, but insensitive indicators of previous myocardial infarction. Various arrhythmias, especially ventricular premature beats, may be present on the ECG, but they too have low sensitivity and specificity for CAD.

Ambulatory ECG monitoring has shown that many patients with symptomatic myocardial ischemia also have episodes of silent ischemia that would otherwise go unrecognized during normal daily activities (see p. 1330). Although this form of ECG testing provides a quantitative estimate of the frequency and duration of ischemic episodes during routine activities, its sensitivity for detecting CAD is less than that of exercise ECG.

Left ventricular hypertrophy on the ECG is a poor prognostic factor in patients with chronic stable angina. This finding should suggest the presence of underlying hypertension, aortic stenosis, or hypertrophic cardiomyopathy and warrants further evaluation, such as echocardiography to assess left ventricular size, wall thickness, and function.

During an episode of angina pectoris, the ECG becomes abnormal in 50 percent or more of patients with normal resting ECGs. The most common finding is ST segment depression, although ST segment elevation and normalization of previous resting ST-T wave depression or inversion ("pseudonormalization") may develop.

Noninvasive Stress Testing

(see also Chap. 13)

Noninvasive stress testing can provide useful and often indispensable information to establish the diagnosis and estimate the prognosis in patients with chronic stable angina.[35, 72] However, several studies have emphasized that the indiscriminate use of such tests may provide limited *incremental* information over and above that provided by the physician's detailed and thoughtful clinical assessment.[35, 57, 73–76] Appropriate application of noninvasive tests requires consideration of Bayesian principles (see Chap. 6). These principles state that the reliability and predictive accuracy of any test is defined not only by its sensitivity and specificity but also by the prevalence of disease (or pretest probability) in the population under study.

In an era of emphasis on cost-effectiveness, optimal utilization of testing requires an assessment of the *incremental* amount of information provided by a test, over and above what can be obtained from standard clinical variables alone. Noninvasive testing should be performed only if the test result will alter the planned management strategy. The value of noninvasive stress testing is greatest when the pretest likelihood is intermediate because the test result will have the greatest effect on the posttest probability of CAD and, hence, on clinical decision-making in this group of patients.

Exercise Electrocardiography (see also Chap. 6)

DIAGNOSIS OF CORONARY ARTERY DISEASE. As a screening test for CAD, the exercise ECG is useful in that it is relatively simple and inexpensive. It is particularly helpful in patients with chest pain syndromes who are considered to have a moderate probability of CAD and in whom the resting ECG is normal, provided that they are capable of achieving an adequate workload.[77] Although the incremental diagnostic value of exercise testing is limited in patients in whom the estimated prevalence of CAD is either high or low, the test provides useful, additional information about the degree of functional limitation in both groups of patients and about the severity of ischemia and prognosis in patients with a high pretest probability of CAD.[35, 78, 79]

The exercise ECG variable most useful for the detection of CAD and, in particular, multivessel disease is the ST segment shift during exercise and recovery.[78, 80] The sensitivity of the ST segment response increases with age, with the severity of CAD, and with the magnitude of the ST segment change itself (see Fig. 6–7).[35] The predictive value for the detection of CAD is 90 percent if typical chest discomfort occurs during exercise along with horizontal or downward-sloping ST segment depression of 1 mm or more. ST segment depression of 2 mm or more accompanied by typical chest discomfort is virtually diagnostic of significant CAD.[80] In the absence of typical angina pectoris, downsloping or horizontal ST segment depression of 1 mm or more has a predictive value of 70 percent for the detection of significant coronary stenosis, but the predictive value increases to 90 percent with ST segment depression of 2 mm or more. The early onset of ST segment depression during exercise, its long persistence following discontinuation of exercise, a downsloping or horizontal depression, and a low work capacity or exercise duration are all strongly associated with multivessel disease. Exercise-induced QRS prolongation also appears to be a function of exercise-induced ischemia[81] and is related to the extent of exercise-induced segmental contraction abnormalities.

A meta-analysis of 147 published studies involving more than 24,000 patients was performed in the process of establishing the ACC/AHA Guidelines on Exercise Testing.[78] Wide variability in sensitivity and specificity was reported, with a mean sensitivity of 68 percent and mean specificity of 77. The results of stress testing often influence the subsequent decision for angiography and create a posttest referral bias that tends to inflate sensitivity and decrease specificity.[82] When meta-analyses are restricted to studies designed to avoid such work-up bias, the sensitivity is only 45 to 50 percent but the specificity is 85 to 90 percent.[78]

A major factor contributing to the low sensitivity of exercise ECG is that many patients are incapable of reaching the level of exercise required for near-maximal effort (85 percent or more of the maximal predicted heart rate), particularly those receiving beta-adrenergic blockers, those in whom fatigue, leg cramps, or dyspnea develops, and those with musculoskeletal symptoms. ST segment changes have low specificity in patients taking digitalis and those with left ventricular hypertrophy and repolarization abnormalities. ST segment changes cannot be interpreted when patients have left bundle branch block, Wolff-Parkinson-White syndrome, or an artificial pacemaker. In these subsets of patients, noninvasive *imaging* with exercise or pharmacological stress testing or diagnostic coronary angiography may be indicated.

INFLUENCE OF ANTIANGINAL THERAPY. Antianginal pharmacological therapy reduces the sensitivity of exercise testing as a screening tool. Beta blockade increases the exercise duration and suppresses, diminishes, or delays the appearance of ST segment depression and thus obscures the diagnostic interpretation of exercise testing.[78, 83] Because beta blockade reduces the sensitivity of the test, a negative exercise test in patients receiving antianginal drugs does not exclude significant and possibly life-threatening myocardial ischemia.

Therefore, if the purpose of the exercise test is to diagnose ischemia, it should be performed, if possible, in the absence of antianginal medications. However, the advisability of withholding medications in an individual patient before exercise testing is a matter of judgment. Two or 3 days are required for patients receiving long-acting beta blockers. Unless the patient has severe angina, sublingual nitroglycerin for 1 or 2 days is likely to be sufficient to control symptoms if other therapy is withdrawn. For long-acting nitrates, calcium antagonists, and short-acting beta blockers, discontinuing use of the medications the day before testing usually suffices. If the purpose of the exercise test is to identify safe levels of daily activity or the extent of functional disability, the test should be performed while the patient is taking the usual medications.

Nuclear Cardiology Techniques (see Chap. 9)

STRESS MYOCARDIAL PERFUSION IMAGING. Exercise perfusion imaging incorporates all the components of the exercise ECG with images of myocardial blood flow by using either thallium-201 or a technetium-99m (^{99m}Tc)-based perfusion tracer.[84] The radionuclide is injected intravenously at peak exercise or at a symptom-limited endpoint, such as angina pectoris or dyspnea; the patient is encouraged to exercise for another 30 to 45 seconds to ensure that initial myocardial uptake of the tracer reflects the perfusion pattern at peak stress. Acquisition of the stress images is performed several minutes later when the patient is at rest. A separate image acquisition is obtained at rest to compare the stress images with images of resting perfusion. Reversible perfusion defects between stress and rest indicate exercise-induced ischemia, whereas irreversible defects usually represent regions of myocardial fibrosis (see Fig. 9–12). In the case of thallium-201, a stress-redistribution protocol is usually followed, in which rest images are obtained 3 to 4 hours after the stress test without a second injection of tracer. More rapid washout rates of thallium from normal versus ischemic myocardium produce apparent filling in of perfusion defects caused by reversible ischemia, a process termed "redistribution." With ^{99m}Tc perfusion tracers, which do not redistribute appreciably, two separate injections are required, one during stress and the other at rest. This technique can be accomplished by using either 1-day or 2-day imaging protocols.[84, 85]

A hybrid dual-isotope protocol has evolved in which both thallium and a ^{99m}Tc tracer are used.[86, 87] The lower-energy thallium is injected at rest and imaged, followed immediately by stress imaging with the higher-energy, ^{99m}Tc-labeled compound. This latter procedure can be accomplished within 90 minutes and has the advantage of requiring a much shorter time for completing the study than with standard thallium stress-redistribution or ^{99m}Tc stress-rest imaging protocols.

Exercise perfusion imaging with simultaneous ECG is

superior to exercise ECG alone in detecting CAD, in identifying multivessel disease, in localizing diseased vessels, and in determining the magnitude of ischemic and infarcted myocardium (see also Chap. 13). The published results of exercise single-proton emission computed tomographic (SPECT) imaging involving more than 5200 patients with angiographic documentation of the presence or absence of CAD yield an average sensitivity and specificity of 89 and 76 percent, respectively (range, 71 to 98 percent and 43 to 92 percent, respectively).[35] Referral bias may account, in part, for the low specificity of many studies, and the few studies that adjusted for referral bias report a specificity higher than 90 percent.[35] The results with thallium-201 are comparable to those obtained with ^{99m}Tc-sestamibi or ^{99m}Tc-tetrofosmin, so these agents can in general be used interchangeably for the diagnosis of CAD.

Perfusion imaging is valuable for detecting myocardial viability in patients with regional or global left ventricular dysfunction, with or without Q waves[88, 89] (see Chap. 13). Stress perfusion imaging also provides important information in regard to prognosis.[74, 75, 90, 91]

Stress myocardial scintigraphy is particularly helpful in the diagnosis of CAD in patients with abnormal resting ECGs and those in whom ST segment responses cannot be interpreted accurately, such as patients with left ventricular hypertrophy and repolarization abnormalities, those with left bundle branch block, and those receiving digitalis. Because stress myocardial perfusion imaging is a relatively expensive test (three to four times the cost of an exercise ECG), certain issues should be considered: (1) a regular exercise ECG should always be considered first in patients with chest pain and a normal resting ECG for screening and detection of CAD[35, 78]; (2) stress myocardial perfusion scintigraphy should *not* be used as a screening test in patients in whom the prevalence of CAD is low because the majority of abnormal tests will be false-positive results; (3) stress perfusion imaging is more sensitive in detecting CAD, especially in patients with single-vessel CAD, than exercise ECG[35, 84]; (4) perfusion imaging is more accurate in patients with resting ECG abnormalities and those receiving digitalis; and (5) perfusion imaging is more accurate in localizing and quantifying regions of myocardial ischemia, which is of particular importance in patients who previously had revascularization, and in determining the extent of viable myocardium in patients with left ventricular dysfunction.

PHARMACOLOGICAL NUCLEAR STRESS TESTING. For patients unable to exercise adequately, especially the elderly and patients with peripheral vascular disease, pulmonary disease, arthritis, or a previous stroke, pharmacological vasodilator stress with dipyridamole or adenosine may be used.[84, 92, 93] In most nuclear cardiology laboratories, such patients account for approximately 40 percent of those referred for perfusion imaging. A comparison of 2000 patients undergoing adenosine and dipyridamole pharmacological stress testing demonstrated that adverse effects occurred less often with dipyridamole than with adenosine.[94] However, the effects of adenosine are very brief, whereas those associated with dipyridamole are more difficult to manage and necessitate longer monitoring time, as well as fairly frequent intravenous administration of aminophylline for reversal. In patients with asthma, dobutamine stress perfusion imaging is a useful and safe alternative to vasodilator stress imaging,[95] but adenosine and dipyridamole are more sensitive for detecting CAD because they produce a greater increase in coronary blood flow.[96] Although the diagnostic accuracy of pharmacological vasodilator stress perfusion imaging is comparable to that achieved with exercise perfusion imaging,[97] treadmill testing is preferred for patients who are capable of exercising because the exercise component of the test provides additional diagnostic information about ST segment changes, effort tolerance and symptomatic response, and heart rate and blood pressure response.

EXERCISE RADIONUCLIDE ANGIOGRAPHY. The use of radionuclide angiography for detecting and estimating prognosis in CAD has been supplanted largely by exercise echocardiography. Although radionuclide angiography is more accurate than echocardiography in measuring the ejection fraction, failure to augment the ejection fraction with exercise is a nonspecific finding that is influenced by age, gender, and the presence of hypertension. The addition of radionuclide ventriculography in patients with a normal ECG at rest adds little to the diagnostic information provided by clinical and other exercise variables.[84] Echocardiography provides a more accurate assessment of exercise-induced changes in regional wall motion and systolic wall thickening, which are more specific markers of reversible ischemia than are changes in ejection fraction.

Stress Echocardiography (see also Chap. 7)

EXERCISE ECHOCARDIOGRAPHY. Two-dimensional echocardiography is useful in the evaluation of patients with chronic CAD because it can assess global and regional left ventricular function in the absence and presence of ischemia, as well as detect left ventricular hypertrophy and associated valve disease. Echocardiography is relatively inexpensive and safe. Stress echocardiography, in which imaging is performed at rest and immediately after exercise, allows the detection of regional ischemia by identifying new areas of wall motion disorders. Adequate images can be obtained in more than 85 percent of patients, and the test is highly reproducible. The inability to image at peak exercise is only a minor disadvantage because most wall motion abnormalities do not normalize immediately upon cessation of exercise.

Detection of ischemic myocardium has been enhanced with the development of systems that allow simultaneous side-by-side display of rest and postexercise images. Numerous studies have shown that exercise echocardiography can detect the presence of CAD with an accuracy that is similar to that of stress myocardial perfusion imaging and superior to exercise ECG alone.[35, 98, 99] Stress echocardiography is also valuable in localizing and quantifying ischemic myocardium. Published results in more than 3200 patients with angiographic confirmation of the presence or absence of CAD yield an average sensitivity of 85 percent and specificity of 86 percent.[35] As with perfusion imaging, stress echocardiography also provides important prognostic information in patients with known or suspected CAD.[35]

Indications for stress echocardiography are similar to those discussed above for stress myocardial perfusion imaging. Stress echocardiography is an excellent alternative to nuclear cardiology procedures. Although less expensive than nuclear perfusion imaging, stress echocardiography is more expensive and less available than exercise ECG, and a regular exercise ECG should always be considered first for screening and detection of CAD in patients with a normal resting ECG who are capable of performing treadmill exercise.[35, 78]

PHARMACOLOGICAL STRESS ECHOCARDIOGRAPHY. In patients unable to exercise, those unable to achieve adequate heart rates with exercise, and those in whom the quality of the echocardiographic images during or immediately after exercise is poor, alternative approaches are available. The most well studied and clinically available method is dobutamine stress echocardiography,[35, 100, 101] in which constant echocardiographic imaging is performed during the infusion of dobutamine beginning at 5 to 10 μg/kg/min with graded increases to a maximum of 40 to 45 μg/kg/min. Dobutamine increases both the heart rate and contractility and produces diagnostic changes in regional wall motion and systolic wall thickening as ischemia develops. Low-dose dobutamine infusion (5 to 10 μg/kg/min) is also valuable for assessing contractile reserve in regions with hypokinetic or akinetic wall motion at rest, as a means of identifying viable myocardium that may improve in function after revascularization[89, 102, 103] (see Chap. 13). Atropine increases the accuracy of dobutamine stress echocardiography in patients with inadequate heart rate responses,[104] especially those taking beta blockers and those in whom second-degree heart block develops at higher atrial rates. Dobutamine stress imaging achieves diagnostic accuracy comparable to that of exercise echocardiography,[35, 100, 101] but as with myocardial perfusion imaging, exercise stress imaging is preferable in patients capable of performing adequate exercise. An exception to this general policy is a patient with left ventricular dysfunction who is undergoing dobutamine echocardiography to assess myocardial viability. Dobutamine stimulation is safe, especially if the test is terminated at the onset of the first ischemic regional wall motion abnormalities.

An alternative form of pharmacological stress echocardiography is the use of high-dose dipyridamole infusion[105] or adenosine infusion, but exercise and dobutamine stress appear to have greater sensitivity than vasodilator stress in detecting CAD[100, 101] and are superior in assessing the extent of CAD.[100] All forms of stress echocardiography have similar high specificity because a new wall motion abnormality in a patient with normal resting left ventricular function is a highly specific finding for reversible ischemia.

Transesophageal dobutamine stress echocardiography has been shown to be feasible, safe, and accurate for the detection of myocardial ischemia. Although not a readily available technique for large numbers of patients, it may allow extension of dobutamine stress testing to patients with inadequate transthoracic echocardiographic imaging.[106]

STRESS ECHOCARDIOGRAPHY VERSUS STRESS NUCLEAR PERFUSION IMAGING (see also Chap. 13). The two stress imaging methods in general provide similar accuracy in detecting CAD. In studies in which the same patients were studied with both techniques and with coronary angiography, nuclear myocardial perfusion imaging had slightly greater sensitivity and stress echocardiography had greater specificity.[107] The potential advantage of stress echocardiography in terms of enhanced specificity has also been demonstrated in meta-analyses (which did not account for possible posttest referral bias).[99] Stress echocardiography is also associated with lower cost and easier implementation in the physician's office. The choice of diagnostic test to perform, however, depends on several additional factors, including local expertise and available facilities.

CONTRAST ECHOCARDIOGRAPHY (see also Chap. 7). Contrast echocardiography is a rapidly evolving field in noninvasive testing for the diagnosis and assessment of CAD.[108] A major objective is the development of intravenous ultrasonic contrast agents for noninvasive myocardial perfusion imaging. With greater spatial resolution than nuclear perfusion imaging, echocardiography has the potential for evaluating transmural distribution of flow heterogeneity and detecting changes in subendocardial perfusion. Although this goal has not been fully realized with the intravenous administration of ultrasonic contrast agents, early work is promising.[109] An outgrowth of this research is two developments that have improved wall motion assessment during standard stress echocardiography. The first is blood pool opacification with intravenous injection of a contrast agent, which has improved delineation of the left ventricular endocardial surface.[110] The second is the use of harmonic imaging, which can be used even without administration of a contrast agent and, in addition, enhances definition of the endocardial border.[111] Poor visualization of endocardial borders in a sizable subset of patients has been a limitation of stress echocardiography for many years, and these two new developments have significantly improved endocardial border definition, with the potential for enhanced detection of ischemic myocardium.

Clinical Application of Noninvasive Testing

GENDER DIFFERENCES IN THE DIAGNOSIS OF CAD (see also Chap. 58). On the basis of earlier studies that indicated a much higher frequency of false-positive stress test results in women than in men, it is generally accepted that ECG stress testing is not as reliable in women. However, the prevalence of CAD among women in the patient populations under study was low, and the lower positive predictive value of exercise ECG in women can be accounted for, in large part, on the basis of Bayesian principles (Table 37-1).[112] Once men and women are stratified appropriately according to the pretest prevalence of disease, the results of stress testing are similar.[78, 113]

Exercise imaging modalities have greater diagnostic accuracy than exercise ECG in both men and women.[35, 78] Although soft tissue attenuation artifacts, especially those

caused by breast tissue, may reduce the specificity of myocardial perfusion imaging in women, these artifacts can usually be identified by experienced observers without a substantial reduction in diagnostic accuracy, and risk assessment by nuclear perfusion imaging is not diminished in women compared with men.[114] In addition, the use of gated SPECT imaging has greatly improved identification of these artifacts by demonstrating that regions with apparently irreversible perfusion defects have normal wall motion, thereby enhancing diagnostic accuracy.[115] Among women without a history of myocardial infarction, exercise echocardiography was superior to exercise ECG in the detection of CAD.[116, 117]

IDENTIFICATION OF PATIENTS AT HIGH RISK. When applying noninvasive tests to the diagnosis and management of CAD, it is useful to grade the results as "negative"; "indeterminate"; "positive, not high risk"; and "positive, high risk." The criteria for high-risk findings on stress ECG, myocardial perfusion imaging, and stress echocardiography are listed in Table 37-2.

Regardless of the severity of symptoms, patients with high-risk noninvasive test results have a very high likelihood of CAD and, if they have no obvious contraindications to revascularization, should undergo coronary arteriography. Such patients, even if asymptomatic, are at risk for left main or three-vessel CAD, and many will have impaired left ventricular function. Hence, they are at high risk for experiencing coronary events. The prognosis in these patients may often be improved by coronary bypass surgery. In contrast, patients with clearly negative exercise tests, regardless of symptoms, have an excellent prognosis that cannot usually be improved by revascularization. If they do not have serious symptoms, they generally do not require coronary arteriography.

ASYMPTOMATIC PERSONS. In asymptomatic persons or in those with chest pain not likely to be angina, the pretest likelihood of CAD is low (<15 percent). In such patients, a negative exercise ECG, for practical purposes, excludes ischemic heart disease. However, if such a patient has an abnormal exercise ST segment response, several alternatives exist. If the ST segment is abnormal but not high risk (<2-mm depression) and the patient demonstrates excellent exercise capacity (i.e., to stage IV of a Bruce protocol or the

▼ **TABLE 37-2. HIGH-RISK FINDINGS ON NONINVASIVE STRESS TESTING**

EXERCISE ELECTROCARDIOGRAPHY
2.0-mm or greater ST segment depression
1.0-mm or greater ST segment depression in stage I
ST segment depression for longer than 5 min during the recovery period
Achievement of a workload of less than 4 METs or a low exercise maximal heart rate
Abnormal blood pressure response
Ventricular tachyarrhythmias
MYOCARDIAL PERFUSION IMAGING
Multiple perfusion defects (total plus reversible defects) in more than one vascular supply region (e.g., defects in coronary supply regions of the left anterior descending and left circumflex vessels)
Large and severe perfusion defects (high semiquantitative defect score)
Increased lung thallium-201 uptake reflecting exercise-induced left ventricular dysfunction
Postexercise transient left ventricular cavity dilatation
Left ventricular dysfunction on gated single-photon emission computed tomography
STRESS ECHOCARDIOGRAPHY
Multiple reversible wall motion abnormalities
Severity and extent of these abnormalities (high global wall motion score)
Severe reversible cavity dilation
Left ventricular systolic dysfunction at rest

equivalent), the likelihood of left main CAD or multivessel CAD is low, the prognosis is favorable, and the patient may usually be observed without further testing. If, however, such a patient has a high-risk positive exercise ECG, coronary angiography is usually indicated to determine whether left main CAD or severe multivessel disease with left ventricular dysfunction is present. If the patient falls into an intermediate category (a positive but not high-risk exercise test result), a stress imaging study (echocardiography or perfusion scintigraphy) may provide further information. If both studies are abnormal but not high risk, the likelihood of CAD approaches 90 percent.

PATIENTS WITH ATYPICAL ANGINA. In these patients, the pretest probability of CAD is approximately 50 percent. If two noninvasive tests are abnormal, the likelihood of CAD exceeds 95 percent; if both tests are normal, it falls below 5 percent. When test results are discordant, they should be evaluated in light of the exercise level achieved, the presence of accompanying symptoms, and whether one of the tests is positive with high risk. Thus, for example, a patient who has atypical angina and a normal exercise ECG with multiple large perfusion defects on a stress thallium-201 scintigram at a heart rate of 130 beats/min has a much greater likelihood of having CAD than one who has a normal exercise ECG and a single small perfusion defect without chest pain at a heart rate of 185 beats/min. Although the indications for performing a stress imaging test directly in such a patient without an initial exercise ECG are controversial, such an approach is reasonable if the patient with atypical angina also has multiple cardiovascular risk factors, such as smoking, hypercholesterolemia, or a positive family history of premature CAD.

PATIENTS WITH TYPICAL ANGINA. In patients with a high pretest likelihood of disease of approximately 90 percent, noninvasive testing is most valuable for estimating the extent and severity of CAD and thereby the prognosis. The development of a high-risk positive stress test points to multivessel disease and a high risk of subsequent coronary events, and unless the patient has contraindications to revascularization, coronary angiography is indicated.

Chest Roentgenogram

The chest roentgenogram is usually within normal limits in patients with chronic stable angina, particularly if they have a normal resting ECG and have not experienced a myocardial infarction. If cardiomegaly is present, it is indicative of severe CAD with previous myocardial infarction, preexisting hypertension, concomitant valvular heart disease, or an associated nonischemic condition such as cardiomyopathy.

ELECTRON BEAM COMPUTED TOMOGRAPHY
(see also Figs. 10–40, 10–41, and 10–42)

Noninvasive detection of coronary artery calcification has long been possible with fluoroscopy. Such calcific deposits are diagnostic of coronary atherosclerosis.[118] Electron beam cardiac computed tomography (CT) has emerged as a highly sensitive method for detecting coronary calcification and is being used at several centers as a screening technique for CAD. The calcium score is a quantitative index of total coronary artery calcium detected by CT, and this score has been shown to be a good marker of the total coronary atherosclerotic burden.[119] However, the relationship of the coronary calcium score to subsequent cardiac events in asymptomatic persons has not been fully established.[97, 120] Several other uncertainties persist as well, including (1) the value of coronary calcium screening in comparison to multiple risk factor assessment, (2) whether coronary calcium scores add incremental value beyond the standard risk factors, and (3) whether coronary calcium screening is more accurate and cost-effective in asymptomatic persons than are other new methods that assess atherosclerotic burden, such as the ankle-brachial index and ultrasonic carotid intimal-medial thickening.[121, 122]

The *absence* of calcium on CT imaging is predictive of the absence of significant atherosclerotic disease in older persons,[119] but it is possible for young people (men younger than 45 years, women younger than 55) to have obstructive CAD and, hence, a risk for future cardiac events in the absence of detectable calcification or with a low calcium score.[123] Although coronary calcification is a highly sensitive

finding in patients who have CAD and the presence of coronary calcification is an accurate marker of coronary atherosclerosis, the specificity of this finding for identifying patients with obstructive CAD is very low.[124] Thus, in patients with known or suspected CAD, exercise testing is preferable to electron beam CT imaging for determining the extent of CAD and the indications for coronary angiography.[124] An analysis by a committee of the AHA on the potential value of electron beam CT and more recent consensus statements of the ACC and AHA[66, 124] concluded that whereas the technique is highly predictive for the presence of atherosclerosis, the degree of atherosclerosis cannot be predicted and the prognostic importance has not been established. Although this modality was considered to have great potential, it was not recommended for routine screening of patients.[66, 124] The results of several ongoing studies will probably provide important information in regard to defining the role of this promising technique in the future.

MAGNETIC RESONANCE IMAGING (see Chap. 10)

Magnetic resonance imaging is emerging as a versatile noninvasive imaging modality with high spatial resolution that will have many applications for patients with CAD. The potential of this technique for detecting regional myocardial ischemia with dobutamine stress[125] and for identifying viable myocardium in patients with left ventricular dysfunction has been demonstrated.[126] Exciting new developments on the horizon include contrast agents for myocardial perfusion imaging and, ultimately, noninvasive magnetic resonance coronary angiography.[127]

CATHETERIZATION, ANGIOGRAPHY, AND CORONARY ARTERIOGRAPHY

The clinical examination and noninvasive techniques described above are extremely valuable in establishing the diagnosis of CAD and are indispensable to an overall assessment of patients with this condition. However, definitive diagnosis of CAD and precise assessment of its anatomical severity and its effects on cardiac performance still require cardiac catheterization, coronary arteriography, and left ventricular angiography[128] (see Chaps. 11 and 12). Among patients with chronic stable angina pectoris referred for coronary arteriography, approximately 25 percent each have one-, two-, or three-vessel disease (i.e., >70 percent luminal diameter narrowing). Five to 10 percent have obstruction of the left main coronary artery, and in approximately 15 percent no critical obstruction is detectable. Coronary angiographic findings differ between patients with an initial attack of acute myocardial infarction and those with chronic stable angina. Patients with unheralded myocardial infarction have fewer diseased vessels, fewer stenoses and chronic occlusions, and less diffuse disease than do chronic stable angina patients, thus suggesting that the pathophysiological substrate and the propensity for thrombosis differ between these two groups of patients.[129] In patients with chronic angina who have a history of prior infarction, total occlusion of at least one major coronary artery is more common than in those without such a history.

CORONARY ARTERY ECTASIA AND ANEURYSMS. Patulous, aneurysmal dilatation involving most of the length of a major epicardial coronary artery is present in approximately 1 to 3 percent of patients with obstructive CAD at autopsy or angiography. This angiographic lesion does not appear to affect symptoms, survival, or the incidence of myocardial infarction.[130, 131] Most coronary artery ectasia and/or aneurysms are due to coronary atherosclerosis (50 percent), and the rest are due to congenital anomalies and inflammatory diseases such as Kawasaki disease. Despite the absence of overt obstruction, 70 percent of patients with multivessel fusiform coronary artery ectasia/aneurysms demonstrated evidence of cardiac ischemia based on cardiac lactate levels during ergometry and atrial pacing. Moreover, nitroglycerin was of no benefit.[132]

Coronary ectasia should be distinguished from discrete *coronary artery aneurysms*, which are almost never found in arteries without severe stenosis, are most common in the left anterior descending coronary artery, and are usually associated with extensive CAD.[133] These discrete atherosclerotic coronary artery aneurysms do not appear to rupture, and resection of them is not warranted.

CORONARY COLLATERAL VESSELS (see Fig. 12–29). Provided that they are of adequate size, collaterals may protect against myocardial infarction when total occlusion occurs.[134] In patients with abundant collateral vessels, myocardial infarct size is smaller than in patients without collaterals, and total occlusion of a major epicardial artery may not lead to left ventricular dysfunction.[135] In patients with chronic occlusion of a major coronary artery but without infarction, collateral-dependent myocardial segments show nearly normal baseline blood flow and O_2 consumption but severely limited flow reserve. This finding provides an explanation for the ability of collaterals to protect against resting ischemia but not exercise-induced angina.[136]

MYOCARDIAL BRIDGING. Bridging of coronary arteries (see Chap. 12) is observed in angiographically normal coronary arteries and ordinarily does not constitute a hazard. Occasionally, compression of a portion of a coronary artery by a myocardial bridge can be associated with clinical manifestations of myocardial ischemia during strenuous physical activity and may even initiate malignant ventricular arrhythmias.[137]

LEFT VENTRICULAR FUNCTION. *Ventricular relaxation,* as reflected in the early diastolic ventricular filling rate, may be impaired at rest in patients with chronic CAD. Diastolic filling becomes even more abnormal (slowed) during exercise, when ischemia intensifies. In patients with chronic stable angina, the frequency of elevated left ventricular end-diastolic pressure and reduced cardiac output at rest, generally attributed to abnormal left ventricular dynamics, increases with the number of vessels exhibiting critical narrowing and with the number of prior infarctions.[138] However, a great deal of overlap is seen in individual patients, so the severity of coronary arterial disease cannot be predicted from these measurements. Left ventricular end-diastolic pressure may be elevated secondary to reduced ventricular compliance, left ventricular systolic failure, or a combination of these two processes.[139] Both impaired systolic and impaired diastolic function may occur as a consequence of acute, reversible ischemia and/or chronic scar formation. In many patients with normal hemodynamics in the resting state, abnormalities of left ventricular function can be elicited by dynamic or isometric exercise. Elevations of left ventricular end-diastolic pressure usually occur *before* angina develops and before ECG ST segment depression occurs.

Left ventricular function can be assessed by means of biplane contrast ventriculography (see Chap. 15). Global abnormalities of left ventricular function are reflected by elevations in left ventricular end-diastolic and end-systolic volume and depression of the ejection fraction. These changes are, however, quite nonspecific and can occur in many forms of heart disease. Abnormalities of *regional* wall motion (hypokinesis, akinesia, or dyskinesia) are more characteristic of CAD because the latter is usually regional in distribution. Also, hyperkinetic contraction of nonischemic myocardium, detected by left ventriculography, may compensate for hypokinetic or akinetic ischemic or necrotic myocardium, thereby maintaining normal or nearly normal global left ventricular function despite marked depression of function in one region of the ventricle.

Left ventricular function (global or regional) may be normal at rest in patients with chronic CAD without previous myocardial infarction but may become abnormal during or after stress. Abnormalities of left ventricular function detected angiographically may signify irreversible damage, i.e., prior infarction, or they may indicate acute ischemia or chronic hypoperfusion sufficient to maintain viability, but not contractility of the myocardium, i.e., "myocardial hibernation"[140–142] (see Chaps. 13, 14, and 34 and also Chap. 37, p. 1316). Reversibility of this form of left ventricular dysfunction in patients with CAD and chronic stable angina is reflected by improved contraction assessed angiographically after an inotropic stimulus (postextrasystolic potentiation or the infusion of a sympathomimetic amine[102, 103, 143]) or by long-term improvement after myocardial revascularization.

In addition to demonstrating areas of asynergy, left ventriculography may also show mitral valve prolapse, which occurs in approximately 20 percent of patients with obstructive CAD[144] and probably results from impaired contractility of the ventricular myocardium and papillary muscles. Mitral regurgitation secondary to left ventricular

dilatation may be observed in patients with chronic stable angina and ischemic cardiomyopathy.

CORONARY BLOOD FLOW AND MYOCARDIAL METABOLISM. Cardiac catheterization can also document abnormal myocardial metabolism in patients with chronic stable angina. With a catheter in the coronary sinus, arterial and coronary venous lactate measurements are obtained at rest and after suitable stress, such as the infusion of isoproterenol[145] or pacing-induced tachycardia.[146] Because lactate is a byproduct of anaerobic glycolysis, its production by the heart and subsequent appearance in coronary sinus blood is a reliable sign of myocardial ischemia. When combined with coronary arteriography, this technique may be helpful in localizing significant coronary obstructive lesions and myocardial ischemia.[147]

Studies of coronary flow reserve (maximum flow divided by resting flow) and endothelial function are frequently abnormal in patients with CAD and chronic stable angina. They are discussed in Chapter 34.

MEDICAL MANAGEMENT

Comprehensive management of chronic stable angina has five aspects: (1) identification and treatment of associated diseases that can precipitate or worsen angina; (2) reduction of coronary risk factors; (3) application of general and nonpharmacological methods, with particular attention toward adjustments in life style; (4) pharmacological management; and (5) revascularization by percutaneous catheter-based techniques or by coronary bypass surgery. Although discussed individually, all five of these approaches must be considered, often simultaneously, in each patient. Among the medical therapies, only two (aspirin and effective lipid lowering) have been convincingly shown to reduce mortality and morbidity in patients with chronic stable angina and preserved left ventricular function. A single large multicenter randomized trial has provided strong evidence that angiotensin-converting enzyme (ACE) inhibitors may also reduce mortality and ischemic events in such patients. Other therapies such as nitrates, beta blockers, and calcium antagonists have been shown to improve symptomatology and exercise performance, but their effect, if any, on survival has not been demonstrated.

In stable patients with left ventricular dysfunction following myocardial infarction, data consistently indicate that ACE inhibitors and beta blockers reduce both mortality and the risk of repeat infarction, and these agents are recommended in such patients, along with aspirin and lipid-lowering drugs.

TREATMENT OF ASSOCIATED DISEASES. Several common medical conditions that can increase myocardial O_2 demand or reduce O_2 delivery may contribute to the onset of new angina pectoris or the exacerbation of previously stable angina. These conditions include anemia, marked weight gain, occult thyrotoxicosis, fever, infections, and tachycardia. Drugs such as amphetamines and isoproterenol all increase myocardial O_2 demand, as do other agents that stimulate the sympathetic nervous system. Cocaine, which can cause acute coronary spasm and myocardial infarction, is discussed in Chapter 48. Congestive heart failure, by causing cardiac dilatation, mitral regurgitation, or tachyarrhythmias, including sinus tachycardia, can increase myocardial O_2 need, along with an increase in the frequency and severity of angina. Identification and treatment of these conditions are critical to the management of chronic stable angina.

Reduction of Coronary Risk Factors

HYPERTENSION (see also Chaps. 28 and 29). Epidemiological links between increased blood pressure and CAD severity and mortality are well established.[62, 148, 149] Hypertension predisposes to vascular injury, accelerates the development of atherosclerosis, increases myocardial O_2 demand, and intensifies ischemia in patients with preexisting obstructive coronary vascular disease. Although the relationship between hypertension and CAD is linear,[150] left ventricular hypertrophy is a stronger predictor of myocardial infarction and CAD death than is the actual degree of increase in blood pressure.[151] A meta-analysis of clinical trials of treatment of mild to moderate hypertension showed a statistically significant 16 percent reduction in CAD events and mortality in patients receiving antihypertensive therapy.[152] This treatment effect is nearly twice as great in older than younger persons.[153] It is logical to extend these observations on the benefits of antihypertensive therapy on mortality and ischemic events to patients with established CAD. Therefore, blood pressure control is an essential aspect of the management of patients with chronic stable angina.

Dietary and Life Style Modification. Alterations in life style and dietary treatment should be initiated in conjunction with antihypertensive therapy. Attainment of ideal body weight is particularly important in obese patients, in whom weight reduction, in addition to assisting in blood pressure control, greatly aids in control of lipid abnormalities, diabetes, and hyperinsulinemia, which otherwise increase the risk of ischemic events.[62, 154] More directly, weight loss increases the threshold for and may even abolish angina pectoris.

CIGARETTE SMOKING. Smoking remains one of the most powerful risk factors for the development of CAD in all age groups (see Chap. 31), and cardiac events occur at a younger age in smokers, especially among women.[61, 150, 155] Postmortem data suggest that smoking predisposes to atherosclerotic plaque erosion and acute thrombosis,[156] which is consistent with the known effects of smoking on fibrinogen and platelet adhesion.[157] Smoking also aggravates other CAD risk factors. Among patients with angiographically documented CAD, cigarette smokers have a higher 5-year mortality and relative risk of infarction or sudden death than do those who have stopped smoking,[158] and smoking cessation lessens the risk of adverse coronary events in patients with established CAD.[159] In patients who have undergone coronary bypass surgery, cessation of cigarette smoking has been shown to decrease both morbidity and mortality substantially.[160, 161]

Cigarette smoking may be responsible for aggravating angina pectoris other than through the progression of atherosclerosis. It may increase myocardial O_2 demand and reduce coronary blood flow by means of an alpha-adrenergically mediated increase in coronary artery tone and thereby cause acute ischemia.[162] Cigarette smoking also appears to reduce the efficacy of antianginal drugs.[163] Smoking cessation is one of the most effective and certainly the least expensive approach to the prevention of disease progression in native vessels and bypass grafts. Techniques for smoking cessation are discussed in Chapter 39.

Passive cigarette smoking, air pollution, and ascent to high altitude all lower the threshold for angina, and their avoidance represents an important aspect of therapy.

MANAGEMENT OF DYSLIPIDEMIA (see also Chap. 33). The beneficial effect of reducing serum cholesterol in patients with hypercholesterolemia is incontrovertible. Cholesterol lowering by diet and drugs has been shown to reduce the incidence of clinical CAD events in primary prevention trials. Among men with moderate hypercholesterolemia in the West of Scotland trial, treatment with pravastatin significantly reduced the incidence of myocardial infarction and death without adversely affecting the risk of death from noncardiovascular causes.[164] Similarly, lovastatin reduced fatal and nonfatal coronary events in the Air Force/Texas Coronary Atherosclerosis Prevention Study (AFCAPS/TexCAPS), which enrolled both men and women with average levels of total cholesterol and LDL cholesterol for age and gender and low levels of HDL cholesterol.[165] In view of the low-risk characteristics of the population, no significant effect of therapy on mortality alone was observed.

In patients with established CAD, clinical trials have

demonstrated a significant reduction in disease progression and subsequent cardiovascular events in patients with a wide range of serum cholesterol and LDL cholesterol levels who are treated with 3-hydroxy-3-methylglutaryl coenzyme A (HMG-CoA) reductase inhibitors (statins).[166-171] Angiographic trials of cholesterol lowering in patients with chronic CAD, many of whom had chronic stable angina, have shown that the effects on coronary obstruction are modest whereas the reduction in cardiovascular events is quite impressive. Several studies have shown that statins significantly improve endothelium-mediated responses in the coronary and systemic arteries of patients with hypercholesterolemia or known atherosclerosis.[172-174] In addition, pravastatin has been shown to reduce circulating levels of C-reactive protein[175] and decrease thrombogenicity[176]; these effects do not appear to correlate well with the change in serum LDL cholesterol and suggest antiatherothrombotic properties of this and possibly other statin agents.[175-177] These findings may explain the improvement in blood flow,[47, 178] the reduction in inducible myocardial ischemia,[179] and the disproportionate reduction in coronary events in patients treated with statins despite very small degrees of anatomical regression of atherosclerotic stenoses.

Results from the three secondary prevention trials of patients with a history of angina, unstable angina, or previous myocardial infarction provide convincing evidence that effective lipid-lowering therapy significantly improves overall survival and reduces cardiovascular mortality in patients with coronary heart disease[168, 170, 171] (see Chap. 33). These effects have been demonstrated in both men and women and in the elderly[180-182] and provide a cost-effective approach to the management of large numbers of patients with chronic CAD.[183, 184]

The National Cholesterol Education Program Guidelines advocate cholesterol-lowering therapy for all patients with coronary heart disease or extracardiac atherosclerosis to LDL levels below 100 mg/dl, and these guidelines have been adopted by the AHA and ACC.[35]

Low HDL Cholesterol. Patients with low levels of HDL cholesterol represent a subgroup with considerable risk for future coronary events.[61, 185] Low HDL levels are often associated with obesity, hypertriglyceridemia, and insulin resistance[61, 186, 187] and often signify the presence of small lipoprotein remnants and small dense LDL particles that are thought to be particularly atherogenic.[188] Therapy has focused on diet and exercise, as well as LDL cholesterol reduction in patients with a concomitant increase in LDL cholesterol.[61, 189] The Veterans Affairs High-Density Lipoprotein Cholesterol Intervention Trial (VA-HIT) Study Group has demonstrated the efficacy of gemfibrozil treatment in patients with low HDL cholesterol (≤40 mg/dl) without elevations in LDL cholesterol (≤140 mg/dl) or triglycerides (mean, 160 mg/dl).[190] Gemfibrozil resulted in a 6 percent increase in HDL cholesterol and a 31 percent decrease in triglycerides, and these changes were associated with a 24 percent reduction in death, nonfatal myocardial infarction, and stroke ($p = 0.006$). The 22 percent reduction in cardiac death achieved only borderline statistical significance ($p = 0.07$).

DYSLIPIDEMIA AFTER MYOCARDIAL REVASCULARIZATION. In patients who have undergone coronary artery bypass surgery (CABG), elevation of LDL cholesterol is a risk factor for the development of saphenous vein graft occlusive disease, as well as progression of atherosclerosis in the native coronary arteries.[191, 192] In the Post Coronary Artery Bypass Graft Clinical Trial, patients randomly assigned to receive treatment with lovastatin and the addition of cholestyramine as necessary to achieve an LDL cholesterol level less than 100 mg/dl had a 31% reduction in saphenous vein occlusive disease at a mean of 4.3 years in comparison to patients randomly assigned to receive placebo.[191] This effect was observed in both men and women and in both young and old patients.[193] In patients with low HDL cholesterol after bypass surgery, similar benefits have been obtained with gemfibrozil.[194] Lipid-lowering therapy reduces mortality and acute coronary events in patients who have undergone either surgical or percutaneous revascularization,[195] and therapy for dyslipidemia should be given to these patients, as to all patients with chronic CAD. However, lipid-lowering strategies do not have an effect on restenosis at the site of angioplasty.[196]

ESTROGEN REPLACEMENT (see also Chaps. 32 and 58). Male gender and, in women, the postmenopausal state are risk factors for the development and progression of CAD. Epidemiological studies have shown that the favorable cardiovascular risk profile in premenopausal women changes after menopause—the levels of total cholesterol, LDL cholesterol, apolipoprotein B, and triglycerides all increase and HDL cholesterol levels decrease slightly or are unchanged.[197] Several long-term studies have identified reduced HDL cholesterol and increased triglyceride levels as powerful predictors of CAD risk among postmenopausal women,[198] and several large cross-sectional studies[199] and a randomized trial[200] have indicated that hormone replacement therapy with estrogens, alone or in combination with medroxyprogesterone acetate, has a favorable effect on the cardiovascular risk factor lipid profile. These changes are similar to, but less pronounced than, those achieved with therapy with statin agents.[201]

The potential beneficial effect of estrogen replacement therapy is probably not limited to altering the lipid profile favorably. Estrogens have multiple complex and interrelated beneficial effects on vascular structure and function,[202, 203] including immediate, short-term, and long-term effects. The principal short-term pharmacological effect is vasodilatation mediated directly via stimulation of estrogen receptors and indirectly through elaboration of nitric oxide (NO). The long-term effects, mediated via genetic signaling, include a reduction in vascular inflammation and injury, delay in lipid accumulation and LDL oxidation, enhanced function of the vascular endothelium to promote vasodilatation and reduce thrombosis, and reduction in vascular smooth muscle proliferation.

A large data base derived from observational studies suggests an important protective effect of hormone replacement therapy for postmenopausal women, with a 30 to 50 percent reduction in overall mortality from cardiovascular disease.[204, 205] Most of these studies evaluated the effects of estrogen alone, primarily in healthy women. Several randomized primary and secondary prevention trials investigating hormone replacement therapy are under way. The only completed randomized trial to date is the Heart and Estrogen/Progestin Replacement Study (HERS),[206] which randomly assigned postmenopausal women (mean age, 68 years) with established CAD to receive conjugated estrogen plus medroxyprogesterone or placebo, with a follow-up period of 4 years. No difference was seen in cumulative cardiac mortality or total cardiovascular events between the two groups despite a greater decrease in LDL cholesterol and increase in HDL cholesterol in the treatment group. This result has generated considerable discussion and controversy about the efficacy or lack of efficacy as well as the safety of hormone replacement therapy. Most endpoints took place in the first year, when more events occurred in the group randomly assigned to receive hormone therapy. This finding raises the possibility that the potential long-term beneficial antiatherogenic efficacy of therapy is offset by a short-term risk, perhaps related to increased thrombogenicity. This limitation is supported by the finding of greater venous thrombosis in the first year in the treatment group in HERS[206] and other patients who have received hormone replacement therapy.[207] Because of the specific progestin used in HERS, the question has also been raised about a less favorable reduction in lipids than might have occurred with estrogen alone.

In light of the HERS results, the case for estrogen replacement therapy as secondary prevention of CAD is now less strong. The other ongoing secondary prevention trials will help clarify this issue. The HERS findings may not be representative of the effects of estrogen or estrogen-progestin replacement when used as primary prevention in younger women, and this point will also be clarified by current and future trials. While awaiting these results and in view of the increased risk of estrogen alone and estrogen-progesterone combinations on the development of breast cancer and the increased risk of "unopposed estrogen" on uterine cancer, it is *not* advised that hormone replacement therapy be *commenced* in women with CAD. However, such therapy may be *continued* in women who are already receiving it, once CAD is discovered.

ANTIOXIDANTS (see also Chap. 32)

Oxidized LDL particles are strongly linked to the pathophysiology of atherogenesis, and descriptive, prospective cohort, and case-control studies suggest that a high dietary intake of antioxidant vitamins (A, C, and beta-carotene) and flavonoids (polyphenolic antioxidants), naturally present in vegetables, fruits, tea, and wine, is associated with a decrease in coronary heart disease events.[208]

RANDOMIZED TRIALS. All three primary prevention trials, each involving between 18,000 and 29,000 subjects monitored from 4 to 12 years, failed to demonstrate a positive effect of beta-carotene on major cardiac events.[209-211] The single trial that also studied vitamin E showed no cardiovascular benefit but rather an increased risk of death from hemorrhagic stroke in subjects receiving vitamin E.[209] The Cambridge Heart Antioxidant Study (CHAOS) investigators studied 2002 patients with angiographic evidence of CAD who were randomly assigned to receive alpha-tocopherol, 400 and 800 mg daily, versus placebo.[212] During the brief follow-up period (mean, 510 days), patients receiving alpha-tocopherol had a 77 percent reduction in myocardial infarction and a 47 percent reduction in all cardiovascular events. No effect on cardiac mortality was demonstrated. Similar, but less impressive results were obtained in a secondary analysis of 1862 patients with previous myocardial infarction in the Alpha-Tocopherol and Beta-Carotene (ATBC) study, in which vitamin E treatment was associated with a 38 percent reduction in recurrent myocardial infarction.[213] In a third nonrandomized study, analysis of patients who had undergone previous coronary bypass surgery indicated less angiographic progression of CAD in subjects with a supplementary vitamin E intake of 100 IU/d or more than in those with lower intake.[213a] However, the largest trial to date with the longest duration of study has shown no benefit of vitamin E supplementation. The Heart Outcomes Prevention Evaluation (HOPE) investigators randomly assigned more than 9200 patients with known atherosclerotic vascular disease or diabetes and another CAD risk factor to receive vitamin E or placebo and demonstrated no effect of vitamin E supplementation on cardiovascular death, myocardial infarction, or stroke over the course of 5 years.[214]

Taken together, current data bases indicate that beta-carotene, vitamin C, and vitamin E have little cardiovascular benefit and do not support the case for antioxidant vitamin supplementation to reduce cardiovascular events. The use of vitamin E supplementation must be balanced against the potential for increased risk of bleeding, especially in patients who are taking aspirin. Unless new clinical trials in this area provide more positive information, *there is no basis for recommending antioxidant vitamins to patients with chronic CAD.*[215, 216]

However, another possible role for antioxidant therapy is in prevention of restenosis after percutaneous coronary intervention. Two studies have demonstrated that probucol (a lipid-lowering agent with potent additional antioxidant properties) significantly reduces restenosis when administered 1 month before and continued for 6 months after the procedure.[217, 218]

EXERCISE (see also Chap. 39)

The conditioning effect of exercise on skeletal muscles allows a greater workload at any level of total-body O_2 consumption. By decreasing the heart rate at any level of exertion, a higher cardiac output can be achieved at any level of myocardial O_2 consumption. The combination of these two effects of exercise conditioning permits patients with chronic stable angina to increase physical performance substantially following institution of a continuing exercise program.[219]

Most of the information about the physiological effects of exercise and their effect on prognosis in patients with CAD comes from studies on patients entered into cardiac rehabilitation programs,[219, 220] many of whom previously sustained a myocardial infarction. Less information is available on the benefits of exercise in patients with chronic stable CAD, but nine small randomized studies with a total of 980 patients have consistently demonstrated improved effort tolerance, O_2 consumption, and quality of life in patients undergoing exercise training.[35] Six studies have shown a consistent reduction in indexes of myocardial ischemia during the course of conditioning,[35, 221, 222] and a seventh study has demonstrated a striking and direct relationship between the intensity of exercise and favorable changes in the morphology of obstructive lesions on angiography.[223] The question of whether exercise accelerates the development of collateral vessels in patients with chronic CAD remains unsettled.

Exercise is safe if begun under supervision,[219] and if survivors of myocardial infarction can be used as a yardstick, it is probably cost-effective.[224] The psychological benefits of exercise are difficult to evaluate. However, a single nonrandomized study demonstrated significant improvement in well-being scores and positive effect scores, as well as a reduction in disability scores, in patients in a structured exercise program.[225] In addition, exercise conditioning programs may be quite helpful in increasing the self-confidence of patients with chronic CAD (as they are in patients recovering from acute myocardial infarction). Patients who are involved in exercise programs are also more likely to be health conscious, to pay attention to diet and weight, and to discontinue cigarette smoking. Thus, in addition to a conditioning effect on skeletal and cardiac muscle, regular dynamic exercise provides the patient with a feeling of well-being, an important consideration in the management of any chronic disease.

For all the aforementioned reasons, patients should be urged to participate in regular exercise programs—usually walking (see below)—in conjunction with their drug therapy.[35]

ASPIRIN (see also Chaps. 32 and 62). A meta-analysis of 140,000 patients in 300 studies confirmed the prophylactic benefit of aspirin in both men and women with angina pectoris, previous myocardial infarction or stroke, and after bypass surgery.[226] In a Swedish trial of both men and women with chronic stable angina, 75 mg daily of aspirin in conjunction with the beta blocker sotalol caused a 34 percent reduction in acute myocardial infarction and sudden death.[227] In a smaller study confined to men with chronic stable angina but without a history of myocardial infarction, 325 mg of aspirin on alternate days reduced the risk of myocardial infarction during 5 years of follow-up by 87 percent.[228] Therefore, 75 to 325 mg of aspirin daily is advisable in patients with chronic stable angina but without contraindications to this drug.[229]

Two other orally acting drugs that block platelet aggregation are the thienopyridine derivatives ticlopidine and clopidogrel,[230] and they may be substituted for aspirin in patients with aspirin hypersensitivity or those who cannot tolerate this drug (see Chap. 36).

In addition to its antithrombotic effects, aspirin may be beneficial in reducing cardiovascular events in patients with chronic CAD via its antiinflammatory effects, properties not shared by ticlopidine or clopidogrel. Aspirin reduces the risk of subsequent myocardial infarction in healthy men with increased levels of C-reactive protein,[63] and in patients with established CAD and inducible myocardial ischemia, aspirin reduces circulating levels of C-reactive protein, macrophage colony-stimulating factor, and interleukin-6.[231] Aspirin also improves endothelial function in patients with atherosclerosis through a mechanism that may involve blockade of cyclooxygenase-dependent release of endothelium-derived constricting factors.[232]

Although warfarin has proved beneficial in postinfarct patients, no data support the use of chronic anticoagulation in patients with stable angina. However, a single large randomized trial in patients with risk factors for atherosclerosis but without symptoms of angina has shown that low doses of warfarin (achieving a mean international normalized ratio [INR] of 1.47) combined with aspirin decrease the risk of coronary death and myocardial infarction when used for primary prevention in high-risk groups.[233] Any benefit of this combination must be balanced against the potential for increased bleeding, which was also noted in this study.

INTERACTION WITH ACE INHIBITORS. With the increasing use of ACE inhibitors in patients with cardiovascular disease, concern has arisen about a possible adverse interaction between aspirin and these drugs. Aspirin has the potential to inhibit prostaglandin-mediated pathways of ACE inhibition, and evidence of such antagonism has been demonstrated in patients with hypertension and heart failure.[234, 235] In the Second Cooperative New Scandinavian Enalapril Survival Study (CONSENSUS II) of survival after myocardial infarction, evidence for such an interaction was observed.[234] Patients taking aspirin had less benefit of enalapril on survival than did those not taking aspirin, and the enalapril-aspirin interaction term was a significant predictor of mortality ($p = 0.047$). Such an effect has not been reported in patients with chronic stable CAD, and evidence demonstrating no such effect

was reported by the Bezafibrate Infarction Prevention Trial investigators.[236] Among 1247 patients with established CAD treated with ACE inhibitors, 618 (50 percent) were also treated with aspirin. Five-year mortality was significantly lower among patients taking ACE inhibitors and aspirin than those taking ACE inhibitors alone (19 vs. 27 percent, $p < 0.001$). The beneficial effect of aspirin was even more marked in patients with symptomatic heart failure. These data are supported by findings of the HOPE Study investigators, who reported no difference in the cardiovascular benefits of ramipril in patients with or without concomitant aspirin therapy (Fig. 37–2).[214] Thus, current evidence supports aspirin therapy for all patients with CAD, including those taking ACE inhibitors. Ongoing clinical trials in this area will provide additional information.

BETA BLOCKERS. The value of beta blockers in reducing death and recurrent myocardial infarction in patients who have experienced a myocardial infarction is well established[237, 238] (see Chap. 35), as is their usefulness in the treatment of angina (see p. 1290). Whether these drugs are also of value in preventing infarction and sudden death in patients with chronic stable angina is uncertain. However, there is no reason to assume that the favorable effects of beta blockers on ischemia and perhaps on arrhythmias should not apply to patients with chronic stable angina pectoris. Therefore, it is sensible to use these drugs when angina, hypertension, or both are present in patients with chronic CAD and when these drugs are well tolerated.

ANGIOTENSIN CONVERTING-ENZYME (ACE) INHIBITORS. Studies of the effect of ACE inhibitors on the severity of angina pectoris and ischemia are limited by small sample size and brief duration of therapy. ACE inhibitors are not indicated for the treatment of angina. However, ACE inhibitors appear to have important benefits in reducing the risk of future ischemic events.

An unexpected and far-reaching finding from recent randomized trials of ACE inhibitors in postinfarct and other patients with ischemic and nonischemic causes of left ventricular dysfunction is the striking reduction in incidence of subsequent ischemic events such as myocardial infarction, unstable angina, and the need for coronary revascularization procedures.[239-243] Data from four trials including approximately 11,000 patients demonstrated a statistically significant risk reduction in myocardial infarction of 21 percent and in subsequent unstable angina of 15 percent.[243] The potentially beneficial effects of ACE inhibitors include a reduction in left ventricular hypertrophy, vascular hypertrophy, progression of atherosclerosis, plaque rupture, and thrombosis, in addition to a potentially favorable influence on myocardial O_2 supply/demand relationships and cardiac hemodynamics and a reduction in sympathetic activity.[243] Recent evidence also indicates that ACE inhibitors enhance coronary endothelial vasomotor function in patients with CAD,[244] which may contribute to enhanced myocardial blood flow during increases in myocardial demand.[245]

These beneficial effects of ACE inhibitors on vascular structure and function should in theory extend beyond patients with left ventricular dysfunction to a much wider range of patients with CAD, including those with normal left ventricular function. This is the subject of several ongoing randomized multicenter trials. The first of these trials to be completed has provided strong evidence supporting the therapeutic benefit of ACE inhibitors. The HOPE Study enrolled 9297 patients with atherosclerotic vascular disease or diabetes and at least one other CAD risk factor and randomly assigned them to receive ramipril (10 mg daily) or placebo; the mean follow-up was 5 years (Fig. 37–2).[214] Eighty percent of patients had CAD, only 12 percent of whom had a myocardial infarction within 1 year after enrollment. No patient had heart failure symptoms on study entry, and echocardiograms (available for 5183 patients) demonstrated preserved left ventricular function (ejection fraction ≥40%) in 92 percent of patients. Ramipril significantly decreased the risk of the primary composite endpoint of cardiovascular death, myocardial infarction, and stroke from 17.7 to 14.1 percent (relative risk reduction of

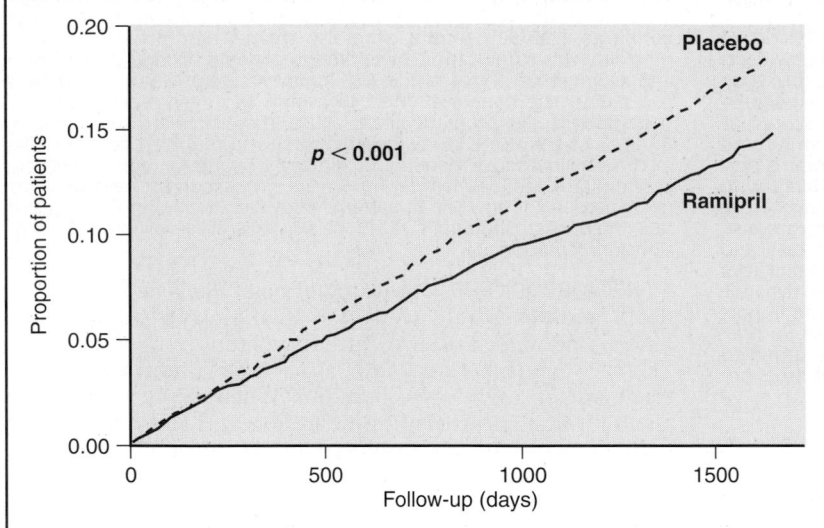

FIGURE 37–2. Kaplan-Meier estimates of the composite outcome of myocardial infarction, stroke, or death from cardiovascular causes in the ramipril group and the placebo group (Heart Outcomes Prevention Evaluation [HOPE] Study). The relative risk of the composite outcome in the ramipril group versus the placebo group was 0.78 (95 percent confidence interval, 0.70 to 0.86). (From Yusuf S, Dagenais G, Pogue J, et al: Vitamin E supplementation and cardiovascular events in high-risk patients. The Heart Outcomes Prevention Evaluation Study Investigators. N Engl J Med 342:154, 2000. By permission of the Massachusetts Medical Society.)

22 percent, $p < 0.001$). The relative decreases in cardiovascular death, myocardial infarction, and stroke were 25, 20, and 31 percent, respectively. Ramipril also reduced secondary endpoints such as myocardial revascularization and all-cause mortality. The results were similar when examined in patient subsets defined by age, sex, known CAD, hypertension, diabetes, left ventricular function, or previous myocardial infarction. Beneficial effects were also similar in patients who were or were not taking aspirin.

The results of the HOPE Study have wide-reaching implications and suggest that all patients with stable CAD should be receiving ACE inhibitor therapy. Although these results were obtained from a large and well-designed and well-executed clinical trial, they represent the results of only a single trial. Definite recommendations should await the findings of two other ongoing randomized trials: Prevention of Events with Angiotensin-Converting Enzyme Inhibition (PEACE) and the European trial on reduction of cardiac events with perindopril in stable coronary artery disease (EUROPA) in patients with stable CAD, which will also clarify whether the benefits in patients with preserved left ventricular function are unique to ramipril (Fig. 37–2).

Counseling and Changes in Life Style

The psychosocial issues faced by a patient with chronic stable angina for the first time are similar to, although usually less intense than, those experienced by a patient with an acute myocardial infarction. Many patients have an unrealistically gloomy perception of their prognosis; they should be offered a realistic appraisal, together with an understandable explanation of the pertinent clinical features of the disease.

An important aspect of the physician's role is to counsel patients in the kinds of work they can do and in their leisure activities, eating habits, vacation plans, and the like.[246] Certain changes in life style may be helpful, such as modifying strenuous activities if they constantly and repeatedly produce angina. These changes may be minor in many instances. For example, golfing could be modified to include the use of a golf cart instead of walking. A history of CAD and stable angina is not inconsistent with the ability to continue to perform vigorous exertion, which is important not only in regard to recreational activities and life style but also for patients in whom some physical exertion is required in their employment. However, isometric activities such as weight lifting[247] and other activities such as snow shoveling, which involves an energy expenditure be-

tween 60 and 65 percent of peak oxygen consumption,[248] and cross-country or downhill skiing[249] are undesirable. In addition, some activities expose the individual to the detrimental effects of cold on the O_2 demand/supply relationship,[50, 250] and these activities should also be avoided if possible.

Thoughtful counseling, which may include supervised exercise sessions simulating the particular activity in question, can play a vital role in maintaining a productive and enjoyable life style in patients with chronic stable angina. Many activities, such as shopping or climbing stairs, need not be discontinued by patients with chronic angina; often, it is necessary merely to perform them more slowly or pause intermittently for brief periods of rest. Patients with chronic stable angina should avoid excessive fatigue and exhaustion. Although it is desirable to minimize the number of bouts of angina, an occasional episode is not to be feared. Indeed, unless patients occasionally reach their angina threshold, they may not appreciate the extent of their exercise capacity. Most patients with chronic stable angina should not be treated as invalids. Often, the propensity for angina actually declines with time, perhaps as a result of the development of collaterals and/or because of training effects.

Eliminating or reducing the factors that precipitate anginal episodes is of obvious importance. Patients learn their usual threshold by trial and error. Because many anginal episodes are precipitated by increases in mechanical activity of the heart (because of increases in myocardial O_2 requirements), patients should avoid *sudden* bursts of activity, particularly after long periods of rest or after meals and in cold weather. Both chronic angina and unstable angina exhibit a circadian rhythm characterized by a lower angina threshold shortly after arising.[251] Therefore, morning activities such as showering, shaving, and dressing should be done at a slower pace and, if necessary, with the use of prophylactic nitroglycerin. The stress of sexual intercourse is approximately equal to that of climbing one flight of stairs at a normal pace or any activity that induces a heart rate of approximately 120 beats/min. With proper precautions, i.e., commencing more than 2 hours postprandially and taking an additional dose of a short-acting beta blocker 1 hour before and nitroglycerin 15 minutes before, the majority of patients with chronic stable angina are able to continue satisfactory sexual activity.

Just as exercise has a role in the management of CAD, so too rest has a role, especially when angina has become frequent or severe. Marked restriction in activity or even complete bed rest, in addition to drug therapy, may occasionally be necessary to control symptoms. In less critical situations, merely reducing the amount of time spent working or increasing the rest periods has a beneficial effect. For example, a long lunch break that includes a short nap may be beneficial. It may be helpful for the patient to use a face mask or scarf to cover the mouth or nose in cold weather. A hot, humid environment may also precipitate angina, and air conditioning may be a necessity rather than a luxury for patients with chronic angina. Large meals can have a similar effect if they are followed by exertion. An effort should be made to minimize emotional outbursts because they too increase myocardial O_2 requirements and sometimes induce coronary vasoconstriction. Occasionally, antianxiety drugs and sedatives or relaxation techniques using biofeedback mechanisms may be helpful. Hostility is an adverse risk factor in CAD.

PHARMACOLOGICAL MANAGEMENT

Nitrates

MECHANISM OF ACTION. Even though the clinical effectiveness of amyl nitrite in angina pectoris was first described in 1867 by Brunton, organic nitrates are still the drugs most commonly used in the treatment of patients with this condition. The action of these agents is to relax vascular smooth muscle.[252] The vasodilator effects of nitrates are evident in both systemic (including coronary) arteries and veins in normal subjects and in patients with ischemic heart disease, but they appear to be predominant in the venous circulation. The venodilator effect reduces ventricular preload,[253] which in turn reduces myocardial wall tension and O_2 requirements. The action of nitrates in reducing both preload and afterload makes them useful in the treatment of heart failure (see Fig. 37–1), as well as angina pectoris.

Posture is important in evaluating the hemodynamic effects of nitrates. In a supine patient, venous return is normally greater and exercise tolerance and the angina threshold are lower than in the upright position. The hemodynamic and angina-relieving effects of nitrates are most marked when patients are sitting or standing, i.e., when the preload-reducing effects of these drugs are most prominent. By reducing the heart's mechanical activity, volume, and O_2 consumption, nitrates increase exercise capacity in patients with ischemic heart disease, thereby allowing a greater total-body workload to be achieved before the angina threshold is reached.

EFFECTS ON THE CORONARY CIRCULATION

Conductance Vessels (see Table 37–3). Quantitative, computer-assisted measurements of coronary arterial diameter have been used to show that nitroglycerin causes dilatation of epicardial stenoses. These stenoses are often eccentric lesions, and nitroglycerin causes relaxation of the smooth muscle in the wall of the coronary artery that is not encompassed by plaque. Even a small increase in a narrowed arterial lumen can produce a significant reduction in resistance to blood flow across obstructed regions[254] (see Fig. 34–21). Nitrates may also exert a beneficial effect in patients with impaired coronary flow reserve by alleviating the vasoconstriction caused by endothelial dysfunction.[255]

REDISTRIBUTION OF MYOCARDIAL BLOOD FLOW. Studies in experimental animals with coronary obstruction have shown that nitroglycerin causes redistribution of blood flow from normally perfused to ischemic areas, particularly in the subendocardium.[256] This redistribution may be mediated in part by an increase in collateral blood flow and in part by lowering of ventricular diastolic pressure, thereby reducing subendocardial compression. In patients with chronic stable angina responsive to nitroglycerin, topical nitroglycerin under resting conditions alters myocardial perfusion by preferentially increasing flow to areas of reduced perfusion with little or no change in global myocardial perfusion.[257]

The results of studies of nitroglycerin on coronary blood flow in patients have been conflicting. Some studies have reported increased blood flow after sublingual or intravenous nitroglycerin,[257] but most report no change or reduced flow.[258] However, because myocardial O_2 demand fell, the net effect on O_2 balance became favorable in the latter studies. Intracoronary injection of xenon-133 (as well as retrograde perfusion during coronary bypass surgery) has been used to demonstrate that blood flow in regions of myocardium perfused by stenotic coronary arteries rises after the administration of nitroglycerin when well-developed collaterals supplying those regions are present. In patients with chronic stable angina, topical nitroglycerin alters myocardial perfusion by preferentially increasing flow to areas of reduced perfusion with little or no change in global myocardial perfusion.[257]

The presence of well-developed collaterals may be an important determinant of a good therapeutic response to nitrates.[259] After systemic nitroglycerin, the heart can be paced to higher rates before

▼ **TABLE 37–3.** EFFECTS OF ANTIANGINAL AGENTS ON INDICES OF MYOCARDIAL OXYGEN SUPPLY AND DEMAND*

| INDEX | NITRATES | BETA-ADRENOCEPTOR BLOCKERS | | | | CALCIUM ANTAGONISTS | | |
| | | ISA | | Cardioselective | | | | |
		No	Yes	No	Yes	Nifedipine	Verapamil	Diltiazem
SUPPLY								
Coronary resistance								
Vascular tone	↓↓	↑	0	↑	0↑	↓↓↓	↓↓↓	↓↓↓
Intramyocardial diastolic tension	↓↓↓	↑	0	↑	↑	↓↓	0↑	0
Coronary collateral circulation	↑	0	0	0	0	↑	0	↑
Duration of diastole	0(↓)	↑↑↑	0↓	↑↑↑	↑↑↑	0↑(↓↓)	↑↑↑(↓)	↑↑(↓)
DEMAND								
Intramyocardial systolic tension								
Preload	↓↓↓	↑	0	↑	↑	↓0	↑0↓	0↓
Afterload (peripheral vascular resistance)	↓	↑	↑	↑↑	↑	↓↓	↓	↓
Contractility	0(↑)	↓↓↓	↓	↓↓↓	↓↓↓	↓(↑↑)†	↓↓(↑)†	↓(↑)†
Heart rate	0(↑)	↓↓↓	0↓	↓↓↓	↓↓↓	0(↑↑)	↓↓(↑)	↓↓(↑)

* ↑ = Increase; ↓ = decrease; 0 = little or no definite effect. The number of arrows represents the relative intensity of effect. Symbols in parentheses indicate reflex-mediated effects.

†Effect of calcium entry on left ventricular *contractility*, as assessed in the intact animal model. The net effect on *left ventricular performance* is variable since it is influenced by alterations in afterload, reflex cardiac stimulation, and the underlying state of the myocardium.

ISA = intrinsic sympathomimetic activity.

From Shub C, Vlietstra RE, McGoon MD: Selection of optimal drug therapy for the patient with angina pectoris. Mayo Clin Proc 60:539, 1985. By permission of the Mayo Foundation.

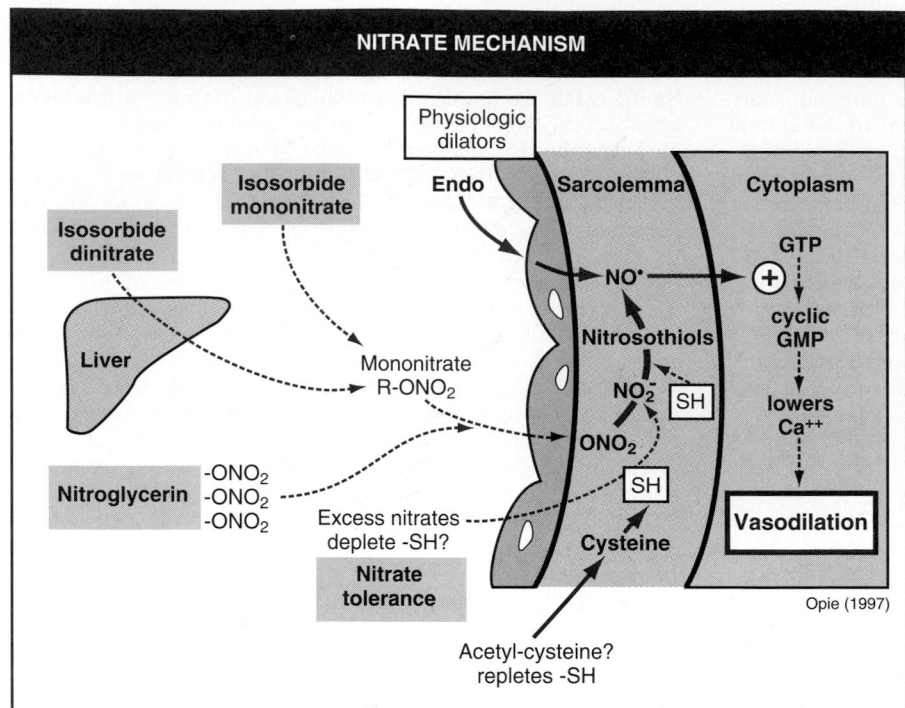

FIGURE 37–3. Mechanisms of the effects of nitrates in the generation of nitric oxide (NO) and stimulation of guanylate cyclase cyclic guanosine monophosphate (GMP), which mediates vasodilation. Sulfhydryl (SH) groups are required for the formation of NO and stimulation of guanylate cyclase. Isosorbide dinitrate is metabolized by the liver, whereas the liver is bypassed by mononitrates. GTP = guanosine triphosphate. (Redrawn from Opie LH: Drugs for the Heart. 4th ed. Philadelphia, WB Saunders, 1995, p 33. By permission.)

angina occurs. However, such is not the case after intracoronary administration, which implies that the systemic effects of nitrates may predominate in patients with pure effort angina.[258] Nitrates have also been shown to improve ventricular wall motion in patients with CAD, as demonstrated by contrast ventriculography, echocardiography, and radionuclide ventriculography, both at rest and during exercise. They also reduce the extent of myocardial ischemia, as reflected in exercise-thallium tomographic perfusion defect severity.[260]

ANTITHROMBOTIC EFFECTS. Stimulation of guanylate cyclase by NO results in inhibitory action on platelets in addition to vasodilation. Although the antithrombotic effects of intravenous nitroglycerin have been demonstrated both in patients with unstable angina and in those with chronic stable angina,[261] the clinical significance of these actions is not clear.

CELLULAR MECHANISM OF ACTION. Nitrates have the ability to cause vasodilation regardless of whether the endothelium is intact. After entering the vascular smooth muscle cell, nitrates are converted to reactive oxygen species, such as nitric oxide (NO) or *S*-nitrosothiols, which activate intracellular guanylate cyclase to produce cyclic guanosine monophosphate,[262] which in turn triggers smooth muscle relaxation and antiplatelet aggregatory effects (Fig. 37–3). Sulfhydryl (SH) groups are required for both formation of NO and stimulation of guanylate cyclase, and nitroglycerin-induced vasodilation can be enhanced by prior administration of *N*-acetylcysteine, an agent that increases the availability of SH groups.[263] This action of *N*-acetylcysteine potentiates peripheral hemodynamic responses[263] and the coronary vasodilator effect of nitroglycerin[264] and reverses the partial tolerance to the coronary vasodilator effect of nitroglycerin.

Types of Preparations and Routes of Administration (see Table 37–4)

Nitroglycerin administered sublingually remains the drug of choice for the treatment of acute angina episodes and for the prevention of angina. Because sublingual administration avoids first-pass hepatic metabolism, a transient but effective concentration of the drug rapidly appears in the circulation. The half-life of nitroglycerin itself is brief, and it is rapidly converted to two inactive metabolites, both of which are found in the urine. The liver possesses large amounts of hepatic glutathione organic nitrate reductase, the enzyme that breaks down nitroglycerin, but there is also evidence that blood vessels (veins and arteries) may metabolize nitrates directly. Within 30 to 60 minutes, hepatic breakdown has abolished the hemodynamic and clinical effects.

The usual sublingual dose is 0.3 to 0.6 mg, and most patients respond within 5 minutes to one or two 0.3-mg tablets. If symptoms are not relieved by a single dose, additional doses of 0.3 mg may be taken at 5-minute intervals, but no more than 1.2 mg should be used within a 15-minute period. The development of tolerance (see below) is rarely a problem with intermittent use. Sublingual nitro-

▼ **TABLE 37–4.** RECOMMENDED DOSING REGIMENS FOR LONG-TERM NITRATE THERAPY

PREPARATION OF AGENT	DOSE	SCHEDULE
NITROGLYCERIN*		
Ointment	0.5–2 inches	2–3 times daily
Buccal or transmucosal	1–3 mg	3 times daily
Transdermal patch	0.2–0.8 mg/hr	q24hr; remove at bedtime for 12–14 hr
Sublingual tablet	0.3–0.6 mg	As needed up to 3 doses 5 min apart
Spray	1–2 sprays	As needed up to 3 doses 5 min apart
Oral sustained release	2.5–6.5 mg	2–3 times daily†
ISOSORBIDE DINITRATE*		
Oral	10–40 mg	2–3 times daily
Oral sustained release	80–120 mg	1–2 times daily (eccentric schedule)
ISOSORBIDE 5-MONONITRATE		
Oral	20 mg	2 times daily (given 7–8 hr apart)
Oral sustained release	30–240 mg	Once daily

*A 10- to 12-hour nitrate-free interval is recommended.
†Very limited data available on efficacy.

glycerin is especially useful when it is taken prophylactically shortly before undertaking physical activities that are likely to cause angina. When used for this purpose, it may prevent angina for up to 40 minutes.

ADVERSE REACTIONS. Adverse reactions are common and include headache, flushing, and hypotension. The latter is rarely severe, but in some patients with volume depletion and in an upright posture, nitrate-induced hypotension is accompanied by a paradoxical bradycardia, consistent with a vasovagal or vasodepressor response. This reaction is more common in the elderly, who are less able to tolerate hypovolemia. Administration of nitrates before a meal, particularly in patients with a tendency toward postprandial hypotension, may enhance venous pooling, preload reduction, and the extent of the fall in blood pressure after the meal.[265] In addition, the partial pressure of O_2 in arterial blood may fall after large doses of nitroglycerin because of a ventilation-perfusion imbalance caused by inability of the pulmonary vascular bed to constrict in areas of alveolar hypoxia, thereby leading to perfusion of less hypoxic tissues.[266] Methemoglobinemia is a rare complication of very large doses of nitrates; commonly used doses of nitrates cause small elevations of methemoglobin that are probably not of clinical significance.

PREPARATIONS (see Table 37–4)

Nitroglycerin Tablets. Nitroglycerin tablets tend to lose their potency, especially if exposed to light, and should thus be kept in dark containers. Other nitrate preparations are available in sublingual, buccal, oral, spray, and ointment forms. An oral nitroglycerin spray that dispenses metered, aerosolized doses of 0.4 mg may be better absorbed than the sublingual form in patients with dry mucosal membranes.[267] It can also be quickly sprayed onto or under the tongue. For prophylaxis, the spray should be used 5 to 10 minutes before angina-provoking activities.

Isosorbide Dinitrate. This drug is an effective antianginal agent but has low bioavailability after oral administration. It undergoes hepatic metabolism rapidly, and marked variation in plasma concentrations may be seen after oral administration. It has two metabolites (one has potent vasodilator action) that are cleared less rapidly than the parent drug and excreted unchanged in the urine. It is available in tablets for sublingual use, in chewable form, in tablets for oral use, and in sustained-release capsules.

Partial or complete nitrate tolerance (see below) develops with regimens of isosorbide dinitrate when it is administered as 30 mg three or four times daily.[268] A dosage schedule should be adopted that allows a 10- to 12-hour nitrate-free interval. If the drug is administered on a three-times-daily schedule (e.g., at 8 A.M., 1 P.M., and 6 P.M.), the antianginal benefit lasts for approximately 6 hours, and the magnitude of the antianginal benefit decreases with each successive dose.[268]

Isosorbide 5-Mononitrate. This active metabolite of the dinitrate is completely bioavailable with oral administration because it does not undergo first-pass hepatic metabolism,[269] and it is efficacious in the treatment of chronic stable angina.[270] Plasma levels of isosorbide 5-mononitrate reach their peak between 30 minutes and 2 hours after ingestion, and the drug has a plasma half-life of 4 to 6 hours. A single 20-mg tablet still exhibits activity 8 hours after administration. Tolerance has not been demonstrated with once-a-day or eccentric dosing intervals but does occur with a twice-daily dosing regimen at 12-hour intervals. The only sustained-release preparation of isosorbide 5-mononitrate is Imdur, which is given once daily in a dose of 30 to 240 mg. Presumably, this preparation avoids tolerance by either providing a sufficiently low nitrate level or a duration of activity of 12 hours or less.

Topical Nitroglycerin

Ointment. Nitroglycerin ointment (15 mg/inch) is efficacious when applied (most commonly to the chest) in strips of 0.5 to 2.0 inches. The delay in onset of action is approximately 30 minutes. Because this form of the drug is effective for 4 to 6 hours, it is particularly useful in patients with severe angina or unstable angina who are confined to bed and chair. Nitroglycerin ointment may also be used prophylactically after retiring by patients with nocturnal angina. Skin permeability increases with increased hydration, and absorption is also enhanced if the paste is covered with plastic whose edges are taped to the skin.

Transdermal Patches. Application of silicone gel or polymer matrix impregnated with nitroglycerin results in absorption for 24 to 48 hours at a rate determined by various methods of preparation of the patch, including a semipermeable membrane placed between the drug reservoir and the skin (usually 7.5 to 10 mg/12 hr patch, to remove after 12 hrs, and 15 mg for the phasic nitroglycerin patch). The release rate of the patches varies from 2.5 to 15 mg per 24 hours. Relatively low doses (2.5 to 5 mg per 24 hours) may not produce sufficient plasma and tissue concentrations to sustain consistent, effective antianginal effects. Transdermal nitroglycerin therapy has been shown to increase exercise duration and maintain antiischemic effects for 12 hours after patch application throughout 30 days of therapy without significant evidence of nitrate tolerance or rebound phenomena,[271] provided that the patch is not applied for more than 12 out of 24 hours.

NITRATE TOLERANCE

A major problem with the use of nitrates is the development of nitrate tolerance, which has been demonstrated with all forms of nitrate administration delivering continuous, relatively stable blood levels of the drug.[253, 268, 271, 272] Although nitrate tolerance is rapid in onset, renewed responsiveness is easily established after a short nitrate-free interval. The problem of tolerance applies to all nitrate preparations and is particularly important in patients with chronic stable angina pectoris, as opposed to those receiving short-acting courses of nitrates (e.g., unstable angina and myocardial infarction). Nitrate tolerance appears to be limited to the capacitance and resistance vessels and has not been noted in the large conductance vessels, including the epicardial coronary arteries and radial arteries, despite continuous administration of nitroglycerin for 48 hours.[273]

A meta-analysis of randomized clinical trials of nitroglycerin patches suggested that in doses of 5 to 10 mg, exercise duration was improved early after administration but, by 24 hours, the effect of nitroglycerin on exercise performance was attenuated by the development of nitrate tolerance. However, a regimen in which transdermal nitroglycerin was applied for 12 hours and removed for 12 hours improved exercise performance for 8 to 12 hours after application of the patch. After 1 month of such therapy, responsiveness to transdermal nitroglycerin remained virtually unchanged. Therefore, after application of a transdermal nitroglycerin patch, one can expect therapeutic efficacy (improved exercise performance) for 8 to 12 hours. Provided that patients have a substantial nitrate-free interval (10 to 12 hours) every 24-hour period, sustained improvement in exercise performance may be maintained. If a state of tolerance is induced, a nitrate-free interval restores responsiveness. If large intermittent doses of transdermal or oral nitrates are used (equivalent to 20 mg per 24 hours of a transdermal patch), rebound angina may occur during the nitrate-free period.

MECHANISMS (Fig. 37–3). Several mechanisms of nitrate tolerance have been proposed,[253] but their relative importance has not been defined.

Depletion of Sulfhydryl Groups. The most widely accepted and most extensively studied explanation of nitrate tolerance is that intracellular SH co-factors are depleted and that they are a crucial component of the metabolic conversion of nitroglycerin to NO or S-nitrosothiols, a conversion necessary for activation of guanylate cyclase.[274]

Neurohormonal Activation. Nonspecific activation of neurohormonal mechanisms may occur in response to the hypotensive effects of nitrates, with a resultant increase in plasma catecholamines, plasma renin activity, and arginine vasopressin causing sodium retention and weight gain.[275, 276] It has been suggested that ACE inhibitors modify nitrate tolerance by blunting the neurohormonal response to nitrate therapy.[277]

Plasma Volume Expansion. Plasma volume expansion occurs during continuous nitrate administration,[275] even in the absence of neurohormonally mediated sodium retention. It may be the result of a fluid shift from the extravascular to the intravascular space in response to the vasodilating or hemodynamic actions of nitrates. However, diuretic therapy appears to have no effect on nitrate tolerance in patients with chronic CAD.[278]

Downregulation of Nitrate Receptors. It has been proposed that high-affinity receptors, which respond to low concentrations of nitrates, are downregulated during the development of tolerance. The activity of low-affinity receptors is maintained, and these continue to respond but require increasing concentrations of nitrate.[279]

Free Radical Generation. A novel mechanism that may contribute to nitrate tolerance is the production of superoxide anions and other free radicals by the endothelium.[280] This mechanism is supported by two small clinical studies reporting positive results of antioxidant vitamin supplements in reducing tolerance in patients with chronic CAD.[281, 282] The mechanism of nitrate-induced free radical generation is uncertain but may involve endothelin and angiotensin II.[283]

MANAGEMENT. The only practical strategy to manage nitrate tolerance is to prevent it by providing a "nitrate-free" interval. The optimal interval is unknown, but with patches or ointment of nitroglycerin or preparations of isosorbide dinitrate or isosorbide 5-mononitrate, a 12-hour off period is recommended.[269] The timing of administration should be adapted to the pattern of symptoms, e.g., whether angina is predominantly exercise related during the day or nocturnal. Moreover, nitroglycerin administered by the sublingual route does not result in tolerance, and even after 2 weeks of therapy, efficacy is not reduced when sublingual nitroglycerin is administered two or three times daily.[284] The use of supplemental antioxidant vitamins to attenuate nitrate tolerance is attractive, but larger-scale studies are needed to confirm the current preliminary findings.

NITRATE WITHDRAWAL. A common form of nitrate withdrawal (rebound) is observed in patients whose angina is intensified after discontinuation of large doses of long-acting nitrates.[285] In this situation, patients may also have heightened sensitivity to constrictor stimuli.[276, 277] The potential for rebound can be modified by adjusting the dose and timing of administration in addition to the use of other antianginal drugs.

Because of the possibility of nitrate dependence, nitrate therapy should be withdrawn carefully. In persons exposed to industrial doses of nitroglycerin, nitrate tolerance, nitrate dependence, and withdrawal symptoms may cause serious problems. During the manufacture of dynamite, substantial levels of nitrates are often present in the atmosphere and can be absorbed through the skin and lungs. After an acute response of headache, hypotension, palpitations, and gastrointestinal disturbances, adaptation occurs.[286] Withdrawal from this environment may result in angina unrelated to exertion or emotion. In fact, spontaneous coronary vasospasm and acute myocardial infarction have been documented during a period of withdrawal.

INTERACTION WITH SILDENAFIL. The combination of nitrates and sildenafil may cause serious, prolonged, and potentially life-threatening hypotension.[287] Nitrate therapy is an absolute contraindication to the use of sildenafil and vice versa. Patients who wish to take sildenafil should be aware of the serious nature of this adverse drug interaction and be warned about taking sildenafil within 24 hours of any nitrate preparation, including short-acting sublingual nitroglycerin tablets.

Beta-Adrenoceptor Blocking Agents

Beta-adrenoceptor blocking drugs (beta blockers) constitute a cornerstone of therapy for angina pectoris. In addition to their antiischemic properties, beta blockers are effective antihypertensives (see Chap. 29) and antiarrhythmics (Chap.

23). They have also been shown to reduce mortality and reinfarction in patients after myocardial infarction (see Chap. 35) and reduce mortality in patients with heart failure (Chap. 18). This combination of actions makes them extremely useful in the management of chronic stable angina. A number of studies have shown that beta blockers, in doses that are generally well tolerated, reduce the frequency of anginal episodes and raise the anginal threshold, both when given alone and when added to other antianginal agents.

The salutary action of these drugs (which have a chemical structure resembling that of beta-adrenoceptor agonists) depends on their ability to cause competitive inhibition of the effects of neuronally released and circulating catecholamines on beta adrenoceptors[288] (Table 37–5). Beta blockade reduces myocardial O_2 requirements, primarily by slowing the heart rate; the slower heart rate in turn increases the fraction of the cardiac cycle occupied by diastole, with a corresponding increase in the time available for coronary perfusion (Fig. 37–4 and Table 37–6; see also Table 37–3). These drugs also reduce exercise-induced increases in blood pressure and limit exercise-induced increases in contractility. Thus, beta blockers reduce myocardial O_2 demand primarily during activity or excitement, when surges of increased sympathetic activity occur.[54] Thus, in the face of impaired myocardial perfusion, the effects of beta blockers on myocardial O_2 demand may critically and favorably alter the imbalance between supply and demand, thereby resulting in the elimination of ischemia.

Beta blockers may reduce blood flow to most organs by means of the combination of unopposed alpha-adrenergic vasoconstriction and beta$_2$ receptor blockade. Complications are relatively minor, but in patients with peripheral vascular disease, the reduction in blood flow to skeletal muscles with the use of nonselective beta blockers may reduce maximal exercise capacity. In patients with preexisting left ventricular dysfunction, beta blockade may increase ventricular volume and thereby enhance O_2 demand.

Characteristics of Different Beta Blockers
(see Table 37–6)

SELECTIVITY. Two major subtypes of beta receptors, designated beta$_1$ and beta$_2$, are present in different proportions in different tissues. Beta$_1$ receptors predominate in the heart, and stimulation of these receptors leads to an increase in heart rate, atrioventricular (AV) conduction, and contractility; release of renin from juxtaglomerular cells in the kidneys; and lipolysis in adipocytes. Beta$_2$ stimulation causes bronchodilation, vasodilation, and glycogenolysis. Nonselective beta-blocking drugs (propranolol, nadolol,

▼ **TABLE 37–5. PHYSIOLOGICAL ACTIONS OF BETA-ADRENERGIC RECEPTORS**

ORGAN	RECEPTOR TYPE	RESPONSE TO STIMULUS
HEART		
SA node	Beta$_1$	Increased heart rate
Atria	Beta$_1$	Increased contractility and conduction velocity
AV node	Beta$_1$	Increased automaticity and conduction velocity
His-Purkinje system	Beta$_1$	Increased automaticity and conduction velocity
Ventricles	Beta$_1$	Decreased automaticity, contractility, and conduction velocity
ARTERIES		
Peripheral	Beta$_2$	Dilatation
Coronary	Beta$_2$	Dilatation
Carotid	Beta$_2$	Dilatation
OTHER	Beta$_1$	Increased insulin release
		Increased liver and muscle glycogenolysis
LUNGS	Beta$_2$	Dilatation of bronchi
UTERUS	Beta$_2$	Smooth muscle relaxation

AV = atrioventricular; SA = sinoatrial.
From Abrams J: Medical therapy of stable angina pectoris. *In* Beller G, Braunwald E (eds): Chronic Ischemic Heart Disease. Atlas of Heart Disease. Vol 5. Philadelphia, Mosby, 1995, p 7.19. By permission of Current Medicine.

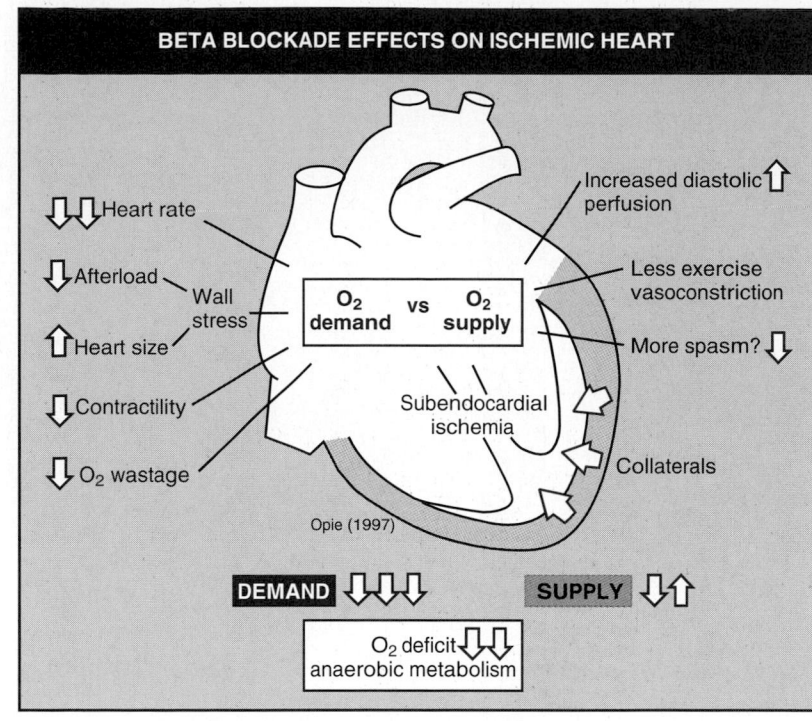

BETA BLOCKADE EFFECTS ON ISCHEMIC HEART

FIGURE 37–4. Effects of beta blockade on the ischemic heart. Beta blockade has a beneficial effect on ischemic myocardium unless (1) the preload rises substantially as in left-sided heart failure or (2) vasospastic angina is present, in which case spasm may be promoted in some patients. Note the recent proposal that beta blockade diminishes exercise-induced vasoconstriction. (Redrawn from Opie LH: Drugs for the Heart. 4th ed. Philadelphia, WB Saunders, 1995. Figure copyright L.H. Opie.)

penbutolol, pindolol, sotalol, timolol, carteolol) block both beta$_1$ and beta$_2$ receptors, whereas cardioselective beta blockers (acebutolol, atenolol, betaxolol, bisoprolol, esmolol, and metoprolol) block beta$_1$ receptors while having less effect on beta$_2$ receptors. Thus, cardioselective beta blockers reduce myocardial O$_2$ requirements while tending to not block bronchodilation, vasodilation, or glycogenolysis. However, as the doses of these drugs are increased, this cardioselectivity diminishes. Because cardioselectivity is only relative, the use of cardioselective beta blockers in doses sufficient to control angina may still cause bronchoconstriction in some susceptible patients.

Some beta blockers also cause vasodilatation. Such drugs include labetalol (an alpha-adrenergic blocking agent and beta$_2$ agonist, see Chap. 29), carvedilol (with alpha- and beta$_1$-blocking activity), and bucindolol (a nonselective beta blocker that causes direct [non–alpha-adrenergic–mediated] vasodilation).[289]

ANTIARRHYTHMIC ACTIONS (see also Chap. 23). Beta blockers have antiarrhythmic properties as a direct effect of their ability to block sympathoadrenal myocardial stimulation, which in certain situations may be arrhythmogenic.[290] Sotalol has combined class II (beta blocking) and class III antiarrhythmic activities; it is an attractive drug when it is desired to treat angina and suppress ventricular tachyarrhythmias.[291]

MEMBRANE-STABILIZING ACTIVITY. This property refers to the "quinidine-like" effect of certain beta blockers in reducing the rate of rise in cardiac action potential. The clinical relevance of this effect is negligible (except perhaps in cases of overdose) because it is observed only at concentrations far exceeding therapeutic levels.[292]

INTRINSIC SYMPATHOMIMETIC ACTIVITY. Beta blockers with intrinsic sympathomimetic activity (ISA), such as acebutolol, carteolol, celiprolol, penbutolol, and pindolol, are partial beta agonists that also produce blockade by shielding beta receptors from more potent beta agonists. Pindolol and acebutolol produce low-grade beta stimulation when sympathetic activity is low (at rest), whereas these partial agonists behave more like conventional beta blockers when sympathetic activity is high. Agents with ISA may not be as effective as those without this property in reducing the heart rate or the frequency, duration, and magnitude of ambulatory ST segment changes or in increasing the duration of exercise in patients with severe angina.[293]

POTENCY. Potency can be measured by the ability of beta blockers to inhibit the tachycardia produced by isoproterenol. All drugs are considered in reference to propranolol, which is given a value of 1.0 (see Table 37–6). Timolol and pindolol are the most potent agents, and acebutolol and labetalol are the least potent.

LIPID SOLUBILITY. The hydrophilicity or lipid solubility of beta blockers is a major determinant of their absorption and metabolism. The lipid-soluble (lipophilic) beta blockers propranolol, metoprolol, and pindolol are readily absorbed from the gastrointestinal tract, are metabolized predominantly by the liver, have a relatively short half-life, and usually require administration twice or more daily to achieve continuing pharmacological effects. The water-soluble (hydrophilic) beta blockers (atenolol, sotalol, and nadolol) are not as readily absorbed from the gastrointestinal tract, are not as extensively metabolized, have relatively long plasma half-lives, and can be administered once daily. If either metoprolol or propranolol is administered intravenously, a much higher concentration reaches the bloodstream, and therefore intravenous dosing has much greater potency than oral dosing.

ALPHA ADRENOCEPTOR BLOCKING ACTIVITY. The alpha-blocking potency of labetalol is approximately 20 percent of its beta-blocking potency, and it is also one of the weaker beta blockers in comparison with propranolol,[294] although it possesses significant ISA (see Table 37–6). Labetalol's combined alpha- and beta-blocking effects make it a particularly useful antihypertensive agent (see Chap. 29), and it is especially so in patients with hypertension and angina. The major side effects of labetalol are postural hypotension and retrograde ejaculation.

OXIDATION PHENOTYPE. Metoprolol and propranolol are lipid-soluble beta blockers noted for the variability of their pharmacokinetics, drug metabolism, and pharmacodynamics. The oxidative metabolism of metoprolol exhibits the debrisoquin type of genetic polymorphism; poor hydroxylators or metabolizers (up to 10 percent of whites) have significant prolongation of the elimination half-life of the drug in comparison to extensive hydroxylators or metabolizers. Thus, angina might be controlled by a single daily dose of metoprolol in poor metabolizers, whereas extensive metabolizers require the same dose two or three times a day.[295] If a patient exhibits an exaggerated clinical response (e.g., extreme bradycardia) following the administration of metoprolol, propranolol, or other lipid-soluble beta blockers, it may be the result of prolongation of the elimination half-life because of slow oxidative metabolism.

EFFECTS ON SERUM LIPIDS. Beta blocker therapy (with agents lacking ISA) usually causes no significant changes in total or LDL cholesterol but increases triglycerides and reduces HDL cholesterol.[296] The most commonly studied drug has been propranolol, which can increase plasma triglyceride concentrations by up to 50 percent and reduce HDL cholesterol by approximately 15 percent. Adverse effects on the lipid profile may be more frequent with nonselective than with beta$_1$-selective blockers. Two drugs possessing ISA—acebutolol and pindolol—do not significantly change total cholesterol, triglycerides, or LDL cholesterol, and pindolol increases serum HDL cholesterol. The effects of these changes in serum lipids by long-term administration of beta blockers must be considered when this therapy is begun or maintained for either hypertension or angina.[296]

DOSAGE. For optimal results, the dosage of a beta blocker should be carefully adjusted. In the case of propranolol, it is usual to start with a dose of 80 mg daily (20 mg four times a day); other beta blockers should be started

▼ TABLE 37-6. PHARMACOKINETICS AND PHARMACOLOGY OF SOME BETA-ADRENOCEPTOR BLOCKERS

CHARACTERISTIC	ATENOLOL	METOPROLOL/XL	NADOLOL	PINDOLOL	PROPRANOLOL/LA	TIMOLOL	ACEBUTOLOL	LABETALOL	BISOPROLOL	BETAXOLOL	CARTEOLOL	PENBUTOLOL	CARVEDILOL	ESMOLOL (IV)	SOTALOL
Extent of absorption (%)	≅50	>95	≅30	>90	>90	>90	≅70	>90	>90	>90	>90	100	ND	ND	ND
Extent of bioavailability (% of dose)	≅40	≅50/77	≅30	≅90	≅30/20	75	≅50	≅25	80	90	85	100	≅30	100	>90
Beta-blocking plasma concentration	0.2–0.5 µg/ml	50–100 ng/ml	50–100 ng/ml	50–100 ng/ml	50–100 ng/ml	50–100 ng/ml	0.2–2.0 µg/ml	0.7–3.0 µg/ml	16–70	20–50 ng/ml	40–160 ng/ml	ND	ND	0.15–2.0 µg/ml	ND
Protein binding (%)	<5	12	≅30	57	93	≅10	30–40	≅50	30	50–60	23–30	80–98	95–98	55	0
Lipophilicity*	Low	Moderate	Low	Moderate	High	Low	Low	Low	Moderate	Moderate	Low	High	High	Low	Low
Elimination half-life (hr)	6–9	3–7	14–25	3–4	3.5 to 6/8–11	3–4	3–4†	≅6	7–15	12–22	5–7	17–26	6–10	4.5 min	12
Drug accumulation in renal disease	Yes	No	Yes		No	No	Yes‡	No	Yes	Yes	Yes	Yes	No	No	Yes
Route of elimination	RE (mostly unchanged)	HM	RE	RE (≅40 unchanged and HM)	HM	RE (≅20% unchanged and HM)	HM‡	HM	HM 50% RE 50%	HM	RE	HM	HM	§	RE
Beta-blocker potency ratio (propranolol = 1)	1.0	1	1.0	6.0	1	6.0	0.3	0.3	10	4	10	1	10	.02	0.3
Adrenergic receptor blocking activity	β₁¶	β₁¶	β₁/β₂	β₁/β₂	β₁/β₂	β₁/β₂	β₁¶	β₁/β₂/α₁	β₁¶	β₁¶	β₁/β₂	β₁/β₂	β₁/β₂/α₁	β₁¶	β₁/β₂
Intrinsic sympathetic activity	0	0	0	+	0	0	+	0	0	0	+	+	0	0	0
Membrane-stabilizing activity	0	0	0	+	++	0	+	0	0	0	0	0	+	0	0
Usual maintenance dose	50–100 mg/d	50–100 mg b.i.d.–q.i.d./ 50–400 mg/d — XL	40–80 mg/d	10–40 mg/d (b.i.d.–t.i.d.)	80–320 mg/d (b.i.d.–t.i.d.)/ 80–160 mg/d — LA	10–30 mg b.i.d.	200–600 mg b.i.d.	100–400 mg b.i.d.	5–20 mg/d	5–20 mg/d	2.5–10 mg/d	10–40 mg/d	3.125–50 mg/b.i.d.	Bolus of 500 µg/kg; infusion at 50–200 µg/kg/min	80–160 mg b.i.d.
FDA-approved indications															
Hypertension	Yes	Yes Yes	Yes	Yes	Yes Yes	Yes	Yes	Yes	Yes	Yes	Yes	Yes	Yes	Yes	No
Angina	Yes	Yes Yes	Yes	No	Yes Yes	No	No	No	No	No	No	No	No	Yes	No
Postmyocardial infarction	Yes	Yes No	No	No	Yes No	Yes	No	No	No	No	No	No	No	No	No

*Determined by the distribution ratio between octanol and water.
†Half-life of the active metabolite, diacetolol, is 12 to 15 hours.
‡Acebutolol is mainly eliminated by the liver, but its major metabolite, diacetolol, is excreted by the kidney.
§Rapid metabolism by esterases in the cytosol of red blood cells.
¶Beta₁ selectivity is maintained at lower doses, but beta₂ receptors are inhibited at higher doses.
FDA = Food and Drug Administration; HM = hepatic metabolism; ND = no data; RE = renal excretion.

at comparable doses. Twenty-four to 48 hours is required for the drug to achieve an antianginal effect. Efficacy is determined by its effect on the heart rate and symptoms, and when these are unclear, its effect on exercise performance can be evaluated by treadmill exercise testing. The resting heart rate should be reduced to between 50 and 60 beats/min, and an increase of less than 20 beats/min should occur with modest exercise[297] (e.g., climbing one flight of stairs). The usual dosage of propranolol ranges from 80 to 320 mg/day, but some patients require (and tolerate) much higher doses. Therapy needs to be individualized and requires repeated clinical evaluation during the initial period of drug administration.

ADVERSE EFFECTS AND CONTRAINDICATIONS. Most of the adverse effects of beta blockers occur as a consequence of the known properties of these drugs and include cardiac effects (severe sinus bradycardia, sinus arrest, AV block, reduced left ventricular contractility), bronchoconstriction, fatigue, mental depression, nightmares, gastrointestinal upset, sexual dysfunction, intensification of insulin-induced hypoglycemia, and cutaneous reactions (Table 37–7). Lethargy, weakness, and fatigue may be caused by reduced cardiac output or may arise from a direct effect on the central nervous system. Bronchoconstriction results from blockade of beta$_2$ receptors in the tracheobronchial tree. As a consequence, asthma and chronic obstructive lung disease are contraindications to beta blockers, even to beta$_1$-selective agents.[298]

In patients who already have impaired left ventricular function, congestive heart failure may be intensified, an effect that can be counteracted in part by the use of digitalis or diuretics. Beginning therapy with a very low dose (e.g., metoprolol, 12.5 mg daily, for the first week) and then gradually increasing the dose over the course of several weeks has been shown to be beneficial in patients with idiopathic dilated cardiomyopathy and those with heart failure caused by ischemic heart disease (see Chap. 18).

Beta blockers should be prescribed with great caution in patients with cardiac conduction disease involving either the sinus node or the AV conduction system. In patients with symptomatic conduction disease, beta blockers are contraindicated unless a pacemaker is in place. In patients with asymptomatic sinus node dysfunction or first-degree AV block, beta blockers may be tolerated, but their administration requires careful observation. Pindolol, because of its ISA activity, may be preferable in this situation. Blockade of noncardiac beta$_2$ receptors inhibits catecholamine-induced glycogenolysis, so noncardioselective beta blockers can impair the defense to insulin-induced hypoglycemia. Blockade of beta$_2$ receptors also inhibits the vasodilating effects of catecholamines in peripheral blood vessels and leaves the constrictor (alpha-adrenergic) receptors unopposed, thereby enhancing vasoconstriction. Noncardioselective beta blockers may precipitate episodes of Raynaud's phenomenon in patients with this condition and may cause uncomfortable coldness in the distal extremities. Reduced flow to the limbs may occur in patients with peripheral vascular disease.[299]

Abrupt withdrawal of beta-adrenoceptor blocking agents after prolonged administration can result in increased total ischemic activity in patients with chronic stable angina. This increased ischemia may be caused by a return to the previously high levels of myocardial O$_2$ demand while the underlying atherosclerotic process has progressed.[300] Occasionally, such withdrawal can precipitate unstable angina and may in rare cases even provoke myocardial infarction. Chronic beta blocker therapy can be safely discontinued by slowly withdrawing the drug in a stepwise manner over the course of 2 to 3 weeks. If abrupt withdrawal of beta blockers is required, patients should be instructed to reduce exertion and manage angina episodes with sublingual nitroglycerin and/or substitute a calcium antagonist.

Calcium Antagonists (see also Chap. 29)

The critical role of calcium ions in the normal contraction of cardiac and vascular smooth muscle is discussed in Chapter 14. Calcium antagonists are a heterogeneous group of compounds that inhibit calcium ion movement through slow channels in cardiac and smooth muscle membranes by noncompetitive blockade of voltage-sensitive L-type calcium channels[301–303a] (see Fig. 14–14). The three major classes of calcium antagonists are the dihydropyridines (nifedipine is the prototype), the phenylalkylamines (verapamil is the prototype), and the modified benzothiazepines (diltiazem is the prototype). The two predominant effects of calcium antagonists result from blocking the entry of calcium ions and slowing recovery of the channel.[303a] Phenylalkylamines have a marked effect on recovery of the channel and thereby exert depressant effects on cardiac pacemakers and conduction, whereas dihydropyridines, which do not impair channel recovery, have little effect on the conduction system.

MECHANISM OF ACTION. The efficacy of calcium antagonists in patients with angina pectoris is related to the reduction in myocardial O$_2$ demand and the increase in O$_2$ supply that they induce[303a] (see Table 37–3). The latter effect is particularly important in patients with conditions in which a prominent vasospastic or vasoconstrictor component may be present, such as Prinzmetal (variant) angina (see p. 1324), variable-threshold angina (p. 1276), and angina related to impaired vasodilator reserve of small coronary arteries.[304] Calcium antagonists may be effective on their own or in combination with beta-adrenoceptor blockers and nitrates in patients with chronic stable angina.[301, 305, 306]

Several calcium antagonists are effective for the treatment of angina pectoris (Table 37–8). Each of these agents is effective in causing relaxation of vascular smooth muscle in both the systemic arterial and coronary arterial beds. In addition, blockade of the entry of calcium into myocytes results in a negative inotropic effect, which is counteracted to some extent by peripheral vascular dilation and by activation of the sympathetic nervous system in response to drug-induced hypotension.[302] However, the negative inotropic effect must be taken into consideration in patients with significant left ventricular dysfunction.

▼ **TABLE 37–7. CANDIDATES FOR USE OF BETA-BLOCKING AGENTS FOR ANGINA**

IDEAL CANDIDATES
Prominent relationship of physical activity to attacks of angina
Coexistent hypertension
History of supraventricular or ventricular arrhythmias
Previous myocardial infarction
Left ventricular systolic dysfunction
Mild to moderate heart failure symptoms (NYHA functional Class II–III)
Prominent anxiety state

POOR CANDIDATES
Asthma or reversible airway component in chronic lung disease patients
Severe left ventricular dysfunction with severe heart failure symptoms (NYHA functional Class IV)
History of severe depression
Raynaud's phenomenon
Symptomatic peripheral vascular disease
Severe bradycardia or heart block
Brittle diabetes

NYHA = New York Heart Association.
Modified from Abrams JA: Medical therapy of stable angina pectoris. *In* Beller G: Chronic Ischemic Heart Disease. *In* Braunwald E (ed): Atlas of Heart Disease. Vol 5. Philadelphia, Mosby, 1995, p 7.22. By permission of Current Medicine.

▼ TABLE 37–8. PHARMACOKINETICS OF CALCIUM ANTAGONISTS USED COMMONLY FOR ANGINA PECTORIS

CHARACTERISTIC	DILTIAZEM/SR	NICARDIPINE	NIFEDIPINE/SR	VERAPAMIL/SR	AMLODIPINE	FELODIPINE	ISRADIPINE	BEPRIDIL	NISOLDIPINE
Usual adult dose	IV: 0.25-mg/kg bolus, then 5–15 mg/hr; Oral: 30–90 mg t.i.d.–q.i.d.; SR: 60–180 mg b.i.d.; CD: 120–480 mg/d	IV: 3–15 mg/hr; Oral: 20–40 mg t.i.d.; SR: 30–60 mg b.i.d.	Oral: 10–30 mg t.i.d.; SR: 90 mg/d	IV: 0.075–0.15 mg/kg; Oral: 80–120 mg t.i.d.–q.i.d.; SR: 180–480 mg/d	Oral 2.5–10 mg/d	Oral SR: 2.5–10 mg/d	Oral CR: 2.5–10 mg b.i.d.	Oral: 200–400 mg/d	Oral SR: 10–40 mg/d
Extent of absorption (%)	80–90	100	90	90	>90	>90	>90	>90	ND
Extent of bioavailability (%)	40–70	30	65–75/86	20–35	60–90	20	25	60	5
Onset of action	IV: 3 min; Oral: 30–60 min	IV: 1 min; Oral: 20 min	20 min	IV: 2–5 min; Oral: 30 min	0.5–1.0 hr	2 hr	20 min	1 hr	1–3 hr
Time to peak serum concentration (hr)	2–3/6–11	0.5–2.0	0.5/6	IV: 3–5 min; Oral: 1–2; SR: 7–9	6–12	2–5	1.5	2–3	6–12
Therapeutic serum levels (ng/ml)	50–200	30–50	25–100	80–300	5–20	1–5	2–10	500–2000	ND
Elimination half-life (hr)	3.5/5–7	2.0–4.0	2.0–5.0	3.0–7.0*	30–50	11–16	8	24	7–12
Elimination	60% metabolized by liver; remainder excreted by kidneys	High first-pass hepatic metabolism	High first-pass hepatic metabolism	85% eliminated by first-pass hepatic metabolism	Hepatic	High first-pass hepatic metabolism	High first-pass hepatic metabolism	Hepatic	Hepatic
Heart rate	↓	↔	↑↔	↓	0	↑↔	0	↓	0
Peripheral vascular resistance	↓	↓	↓↓	↓	↓	↓	↓		↓
FDA-approved indications	IR / SR		IR / SR	IR / SR					
Hypertension	No / Yes	Yes†	No / Yes	Yes / Yes	Yes	Yes	Yes	No	Yes
Angina	Yes / Yes	Yes	Yes / Yes	Yes / No	Yes	No	No	Yes	Yes
Coronary spasm	Yes / No	No	Yes / Yes	Yes / No	Yes	No	No	No	No

*Half-life of 4.5 to 12 hours with multiple dosing; may be prolonged in the elderly.
†The sustained-release formulation may be preferred for hypertension.
CD = combination drug; CR = controlled release; FDA = Food and Drug Administration; IR = immediate release; ND = no data; SR = sustained release.

With a rapid onset of action and metabolism by the liver, calcium antagonists have a limited bioavailability of between 13 and 52 percent and a half-life of between 3 and 12 hours. Amlodipine and bepridil are exceptions in that both drugs have long half-lives and may be administered once daily. In the case of some of the other calcium antagonists, sustained-release preparations have been shown to be effective.

ANTIATHEROGENIC ACTION. Studies in experimental animals, both primates and nonprimates, have suggested that calcium antagonists might have an antiatherogenic effect, and human studies support this conclusion.[307, 308] In multicenter randomized trials using quantitative coronary arteriography, significantly fewer new lesions developed in patients showing mild CAD and taking nifedipine than in patients taking placebo. However, preexisting lesions did not appear to be affected. Prolonged follow-up is necessary to determine whether these angiographic observations are accompanied by clinical benefit. In patients undergoing cardiac transplantation, diltiazem has been reported to be beneficial in reducing the frequency and severity of coronary arteriopathy in the transplanted heart.[309]

First-Generation Calcium Antagonists

NIFEDIPINE. This dihydropyridine is a particularly effective dilator of vascular smooth muscle and is a more potent vasodilator than either diltiazem or verapamil. Although its in vitro actions on myocardium and specialized cardiac tissue are similar to those of other agents, the concentration required to reproduce effects on these tissues is not reached in vivo because of the early appearance of its powerful vasodilating effects. Thus, in clinical practice, the potential negative chronotropic, inotropic, and dromotropic (on AV conduction) effects of nifedipine are seldom a problem, although even nifedipine can worsen heart failure in patients with preexisting chronic congestive heart failure.[310]

In contrast to beta blockers, which decrease the heart rate and the rate-pressure product at rest and during exercise, nifedipine reduces only systolic pressure.[311] Thus, the beneficial effects of nifedipine in the treatment of angina result from its capacity to reduce myocardial O_2 requirements because of its afterload-reducing effect and to increase myocardial O_2 delivery as a result of its dilating action on the coronary vascular bed (see Table 37–3). In patients without heart failure, nifedipine causes modest reflex increases in the ejection fraction, velocity of circumferential fiber shortening, heart rate, and cardiac index; these increases can be blocked by beta-adrenoceptor blockade.

The initial dose is 10 mg orally every 8 hours, increased stepwise to 20 mg every 6 hours guided by the blood pressure response, to a maximal daily dose of 160 mg. An extended-release formulation using the gastrointestinal therapeutic system (GITS) of drug delivery (see Table 37–8) is designed to deliver 30, 60, or 90 mg of nifedipine in a single daily dose at a relatively constant rate over a 24-hour period and is useful for the treatment of chronic stable angina, Prinzmetal angina, and hypertension.[312] The efficacy of the extended-release preparation, either alone or in conjunction with beta blockers, in reducing episodes of angina and ischemia on ambulatory monitoring has been documented.[313]

Adverse Effects. Adverse effects occur in 15 to 20 percent of patients and require discontinuation of medication in about 5 percent. Most adverse effects are related to systemic vasodilation and include headache, dizziness, palpitations, flushing, hypotension, and leg edema (unrelated to heart failure). Gastrointestinal side effects, including nausea, epigastric pressure, and vomiting, are noted in approximately 5 percent of patients. In rare instances, in patients with extremely severe, fixed coronary obstructions, nifedipine aggravates angina, presumably by lowering arterial pressure excessively, with subsequent reflex tachycardia. For this reason, combined treatment of angina with nifedipine and a beta blocker is particularly effective and superior to nifedipine alone.[306, 311] Most of the adverse effects are reduced by the use of extended-release preparations.

Several clinical case-control studies of hypertension and associated reviews have suggested that *short-acting nifedipine* may cause an increase in mortality.[314–317] These findings have not been confirmed by other case-control studies,[318, 319] and these conclusions have not been accepted universally. No firm data indicate that this risk applies to extended-release nifedipine or to other calcium antagonists.[320, 321] Although insufficient data are available to assess the long-term risks (if any) of calcium antagonists in chronic CAD, *long-acting nifedipine* should be considered an effective and safe antianginal drug for the treatment of symptomatic patients with chronic CAD who are already receiving beta blockers, with or without nitrates. Short-acting nifedipine should ordinarily be avoided.

Because of its potent vasodilator effects, nifedipine is contraindicated in patients who are hypotensive or have severe aortic valve stenosis and in patients with unstable angina who are not simultaneously receiving a beta blocker and in whom reflex-mediated increases in the heart rate may be harmful. Nifedipine (or one of the second-generation dihydropyridines) is the calcium antagonist of choice in patients with mild left ventricular dysfunction, sinus bradycardia, sick sinus syndrome, or AV block (particularly if a beta-adrenoceptor blocking agent is administered concurrently and additional drug therapy for angina is indicated).[306] This recommendation is based on nifedipine having fewer negative effects on myocardial contractility, heart rate, and AV conduction than seen with verapamil or diltiazem in doses used clinically. Nonetheless, in patients with more serious left ventricular dysfunction, all calcium antagonists—even nifedipine—can precipitate heart failure.[310]

Nifedipine interacts significantly with prazosin (resulting in excessive hypotension), cimetidine, and phenytoin (resulting in increased bioavailability of nifedipine and increased quinidine clearance). Nifedipine increases blood levels of propranolol, and use of the two drugs together poses the risk of an added negative inotropic and hypotensive effect.[311] In patients with Prinzmetal angina, abrupt cessation of nifedipine therapy may result in a rebound increase in the frequency and duration of attacks.

VERAPAMIL (see also Chap. 23). Verapamil dilates systemic and coronary resistance vessels and large coronary conductance vessels. It slows the heart rate and reduces myocardial contractility. This combination of actions results in a reduction in myocardial O_2 requirement, which is the basis for the drug's efficacy in the management of chronic stable angina. Thrombus formation and thrombin-mediated platelet aggregation are decreased by verapamil,[322] effects also observed with transdermal nitroglycerin. To what extent the clinical benefits of verapamil and nitrates are related to their effects on platelet aggregation and thrombus formation is uncertain.

Verapamil reduces the frequency of angina and prolongs exercise tolerance in patients with symptomatic chronic CAD, and the combination of verapamil and a beta blocker provides clinical benefit that is additive.[323] Despite the marked negative inotropic effects of verapamil in isolated cardiac muscle preparations, changes in contractility are modest in patients with normal cardiac function. However, in patients with cardiac dysfunction, verapamil, like beta blockers, may reduce cardiac output, increase left ventricular filling pressure, and cause clinical heart failure. In clinically useful doses, verapamil inhibits calcium influx into specialized cardiac cells, sometimes causing slowing of the heart rate and AV conduction. Therefore, it is contraindicated in patients with preexisting AV nodal disease or sick sinus syndrome, congestive heart failure, and suspected digitalis or quinidine toxicity.

The usual starting dose of verapamil for oral administration is 40 to 80 mg three times daily to a maximal dose of 480 mg/d (see Table 37–8). Sustained-release capsules of verapamil are available (60, 90, and 120 mg), and starting doses are 60 to 120 mg twice daily with a usual optimal dose range of 240 to 360 mg/d.

Verapamil interacts significantly with several other drugs. Intravenous verapamil should not be used together with a beta blocker (given intravenously or orally), nor should a beta blocker be administered intravenously in patients receiving oral verapamil. The bioavailability of verapamil is increased by cimetidine and carbamazepine, whereas verapamil may increase plasma levels of cyclosporine and digoxin and may be associated with excessive hypotension in patients receiving quinidine or prazosin. Hepatic enzyme inducers such as phenobarbital may reduce the effects of verapamil.

Adverse effects of verapamil are noted in approximately 10 percent of patients and relate to systemic dilation (hypotension and facial flushing), gastrointestinal symptoms (constipation and nausea), and central nervous system reactions such as headache and dizziness. A rare side effect is gingival hyperplasia, which appears after 1 to 9 months of therapy.

DILTIAZEM. Diltiazem's actions are intermediate between those of nifedipine and verapamil. In clinically useful doses, its vasodilator effects are less profound than nifedipine's, and its cardiac depressant action (on the sinoatrial and AV nodes and myocardium) is less than that of verapamil. This profile may explain the remarkably low incidence of adverse effects of diltiazem. This drug is a systemic vasodilator that lowers arterial pressure at rest and during exertion and increases the workload required to produce myocardial ischemia, but it may also increase myocardial O_2 delivery. Although diltiazem causes little vasodilation of epicardial coronary arteries under basal conditions, it may enhance perfusion of the subendocardium distal to a flow-limiting coronary stenosis[324]; it also blocks exercise-induced coronary vasoconstriction. In patients with chronic stable angina receiving maximally tolerated doses of diltiazem, the heart rate is significantly reduced at rest, but no effect on peak blood pressure is achieved during exercise, and the duration of symptom-limited treadmill exercise is prolonged.

The dose of diltiazem is 30 to 60 mg four times daily, although higher doses are sometimes needed. Several sustained-release formulations have been approved and are available for once-daily treatment of systemic hypertension and angina pectoris.[325]

Diltiazem is a highly effective antianginal agent. Atenolol and diltiazem have similar efficacy in increasing nonischemic exercise duration in patients with variable-threshold angina and act primarily by slowing the resting heart rate.[326] High doses (mean dose, 340 mg) have been shown to be a relatively safe addition to maximally tolerated doses of isosorbide dinitrate and a beta blocker and cause increases in exercise tolerance and resting and exercise left ventricular ejection fraction.[325] Major side effects are similar to those of the other calcium channel blockers and are related to vasodilation, but they are relatively infrequent, particularly if the dose does not exceed 240 mg/d. As is the case with verapamil, diltiazem should be prescribed with caution for patients with sick sinus syndrome or AV block. In patients with preexisting left ventricular dysfunction, diltiazem may exacerbate or precipitate heart failure.

Diltiazem interacts with other drugs, including beta-adrenergic blocking agents (causing enhanced negative inotropic, chronotropic, and dromotropic effects), flecainide, and cimetidine (which increases the bioavailability of diltiazem), and diltiazem has been associated with increased plasma levels of cyclosporine, carbamazepine, and lithium carbonate. Diltiazem may cause excessive sinus node depression if administered with disopyramide and may reduce digoxin clearance, especially in patients with renal failure.[327]

Second-Generation Calcium Antagonists

The second-generation calcium antagonists (nicardipine, isradipine, amlodipine, and felodipine) are mainly dihydropyridine derivatives, with nifedipine being the prototypical agent. Considerable experience has also accumulated with nimodipine, nisoldipine, and nitrendipine. These agents differ in potency, tissue specificity, and pharmacokinetics and, in general, are potent vasodilators because of greater vascular selectivity than seen with the first-generation antagonists, i.e., verapamil, nifedipine, and diltiazem.

AMLODIPINE. This agent, which is less lipid soluble than nifedipine, has a slow, smooth onset and ultra-long duration of action (plasma half-life of 36 hours). It causes marked coronary and peripheral dilatation and may be useful in the treatment of patients with angina accompanied by hypertension. It may be used as a once-daily hypotensive or antianginal agent.[328] In a series of randomized placebo-controlled studies in patients with stable exercise-induced angina pectoris, amlodipine was shown to be effective and well tolerated.[329] It has little, if any, negative inotropic action and may be especially useful in patients with chronic angina and left ventricular dysfunction. The Prospective Randomized Amlodipine Survival Evaluation (PRAISE) investigators enrolled 1153 patients with New York Heart Association Class III to IV failure and a mean ejection fraction of 21 percent.[330] When amlodipine versus placebo was added to a full regimen of digoxin, diuretic, and ACE inhibitor therapy, no significant difference in survival was observed in patients with ischemic cardiomyopathy. Although amlodipine did not have a beneficial effect on mortality, these data suggest that in patients with congestive heart failure caused by severe CAD, amlodipine may be safely added for control of hypertension or angina, without an adverse effect on survival.[330]

NICARDIPINE. This drug has a similar half-life to that of nifedipine (2 to 4 hours), but it appears to have greater vascular selectivity. Nicardipine may be used as an antianginal and antihypertensive agent and requires three-times-daily administration, although a sustained-release formulation is available for twice-daily dosing in hypertension. For chronic stable angina pectoris, it appears to be as effective as verapamil or diltiazem, and its efficacy is enhanced when combined with a beta blocker.

FELODIPINE AND ISRADIPINE. In the United States, both drugs are approved by the Food and Drug Administration (FDA) for the treatment of hypertension but not for angina pectoris. A recent study documented similar efficacy between felodipine and nifedipine in patients with chronic stable angina.[331] Felodipine has also been reported to be more vascular selective than nifedipine and to have a mild positive inotropic effect as a result of calcium channel agonist properties. Isradipine has a longer half-life than nifedipine and demonstrates greater vascular sensitivity.

BEPRIDIL. This calcium antagonist interacts with dihydropyridine-binding sites and also has a sodium channel blocking effect. It markedly prolongs the atrial refractory period and may be useful in the treatment of patients with angina and arrhythmias. However, it is also arrhythmogenic and causes QT prolongation and torsades de pointes.[332] Although chemically unrelated to the other calcium channel blockers, bepridil has been shown to be an effective antianginal agent. Nonetheless, because of its potential to prolong the QT interval and to cause torsades de pointes, the drug should be reserved only for patients in whom other antianginal drugs have failed. Interactions with antiarrhythmic agents, tricyclic antidepressants, and cardiac glycosides are potentially hazardous.

Medical Management of Angina Pectoris

RELATIVE ADVANTAGES OF BETA BLOCKERS AND CALCIUM ANTAGONISTS (see Table 37–9). The choice between a beta blocker and a calcium channel antagonist as initial therapy in patients with chronic stable angina is controversial because both classes of agents are effective in relieving symptoms and reducing ischemia.[333] Trials comparing beta blockers and calcium antagonists have not shown any dif-

▼ TABLE 37-9. RECOMMENDED DRUG THERAPY (CALCIUM ANTAGONIST VS. BETA BLOCKER) IN PATIENTS WHO HAVE ANGINA IN CONJUNCTION WITH OTHER MEDICAL CONDITIONS

CLINICAL CONDITION	RECOMMENDED DRUG
CARDIAC ARRHYTHMIA OR CONDUCTION DISTURBANCE	
Sinus bradycardia	Nifedipine or amlodipine
Sinus tachycardia (not caused by cardiac failure)	Beta blocker
Supraventricular tachycardia	Beta blocker (verapamil)
Atrioventricular block	Nifedipine or amlodipine
Rapid atrial fibrillation (with digitalis)	Verapamil or beta blocker
Ventricular arrhythmia	Beta blocker
LEFT VENTRICULAR DYSFUNCTION	
Heart failure	Beta blocker
MISCELLANEOUS MEDICAL CONDITIONS	
Systemic hypertension	Beta blocker (calcium antagonist)
Severe preexisting headaches	Beta blocker (verapamil or diltiazem)
COPD with bronchospasm or asthma	Nifedipine, amlodipine, verapamil, or diltiazem
Hyperthyroidism	Beta blocker
Raynaud's syndrome	Nifedipine or amlodipine
Claudication	Calcium antagonist
Severe depression	Calcium antagonist

COPD = chronic obstructive pulmonary disease.
(alternatives in parentheses)

ference in the rate of death or myocardial infarction,[334-337] although in some studies beta blockers appeared to have greater clinical efficacy.[334, 336, 337] Because long-term administration of beta blockers has been demonstrated to prolong life in patients after acute myocardial infarction and in the treatment of hypertension, it is reasonable to consider beta blockers over calcium antagonists as the agents of choice in treating patients with chronic stable angina. However, it must be recognized that beta blockers (without ISA) increase serum triglycerides and decrease HDL cholesterol with uncertain long-term consequences.[296] In addition, these drugs may produce fatigue, depression, and sexual dysfunction. In contrast, long-term administration of calcium antagonists has not been shown to improve long-term survival after acute myocardial infarction,[338] although diltiazem is apparently effective in preventing severe angina and early reinfarction after non–Q-wave infarction[339] and verapamil reduces reinfarction rates,[340] whereas nifedipine has been associated with the development of fewer new coronary artery lesions[307] in patients with established CAD.

The choice of drug with which to initiate therapy is influenced by a number of clinical factors (see Table 37–9).

1. Calcium antagonists are the preferred agents in patients with a history of asthma, chronic obstructive lung disease, and/or wheezing on clinical examination, in whom beta blockers, even relatively selective agents, are contraindicated.

2. Nifedipine (long acting), amlodipine, and nicardipine are the calcium antagonists of choice in patients with chronic stable angina and sick sinus syndrome, sinus bradycardia, or significant AV conduction disturbances, whereas beta blockers and verapamil should be used only with great caution in such patients. In patients with symptomatic conduction disease, neither a beta blocker nor a calcium channel blocker should be used unless a pacemaker is in place. If a beta blocker is required in patients with asymptomatic evidence of conduction disease, pindolol, which has the greatest ISA, is useful. In the case of calcium channel blockers, nifedipine or nicardipine is preferable to verapamil and diltiazem, but careful observation for deterioration of conduction is mandatory.

3. Calcium antagonists are clearly preferred in patients with suspected Prinzmetal (variant) angina; beta blockers may even aggravate angina under these circumstances.

4. Calcium antagonists may be preferred over beta blockers in patients with significant symptomatic peripheral arterial disease because the latter may cause peripheral vasoconstriction.

5. Beta blockers should usually be avoided in patients with a history of significant depressive illness and should be prescribed cautiously for patients with sexual dysfunction, sleep disturbance, nightmares, fatigue, or lethargy.

6. The presence of moderate to severe left ventricular dysfunction in patients with angina limits the therapeutic options. The beneficial effects of beta blockers on survival in patients with left ventricular dysfunction after myocardial infarction,[237, 238] coupled with their beneficial effects on survival and left ventricular performance in patients with heart failure,[341, 342] has established beta blockers as the drug class of choice for the treatment of angina in patients with left ventricular dysfunction, with or without symptoms of heart failure, together with ACE inhibitors, digitalis, and diuretics. If angina persists despite beta blockade and nitrates, amlodipine can be administered.[330] Verapamil, nifedipine, and diltiazem should be avoided.

7. Short-acting nifedipine should not be used as the initial and only agent in patients with unstable angina (see Chap. 36) because the reflex-mediated tachycardia may aggravate unstable angina.[343] However, long-acting nifedipine may be helpful if symptoms persist despite therapy with a beta blocker, aspirin, nitrates, and antithrombotic agents.

8. Hypertensive patients with angina pectoris do well with either beta blockers or calcium antagonists because both agents have antihypertensive effects. However, beta blockers are the preferred initial agent for treating angina in such patients, as noted above, and an ACE inhibitor should be strongly considered for all patients with CAD who have hypertension.[214]

COMBINATION THERAPY. The combination of a beta blocker, calcium antagonist, and long-acting nitrate is widely used in the management of chronic stable angina.[337] When adrenergic blockers and calcium antagonists are used together in the treatment of angina pectoris, several issues should be considered:

1. The addition of a beta blocker enhances the clinical effect of nifedipine and other dihydropyridines.

2. In patients with moderate or severe left ventricular dysfunction, sinus bradycardia, or AV conduction disturbances, combination therapy with calcium antagonists and beta blockers either should be avoided or should be initiated with caution. In patients with AV conduction system

disease, the preferred combination is long-acting nifedipine or another dihydropyridine and a beta blocker. The negative inotropic effects of calcium antagonists are not usually a problem in combined therapy with low doses of beta blockers but can become significant with higher doses. With such doses, amlodipine is the calcium antagonist of choice, but it should be used cautiously.

3. The combination of a dihydropyridine and a long-acting nitrate (without a beta blocker) is not an optimal combination because both are vasodilators.

Approach to Patients with Chronic Stable Angina

1. Identify and treat precipitating factors, such as anemia, uncontrolled hypertension, thyrotoxicosis, tachyarrhythmias, uncontrolled congestive heart failure, and concomitant valvular heart disease.

2. Initiate risk factor modification, physical exercise, diet, and life style counseling. Initiate therapy with an HMG-CoA reductase inhibitor, as needed, to reduce LDL cholesterol below 100 mg/dl.

3. Initiate pharmacotherapy with aspirin and a beta blocker. Strongly consider an ACE inhibitor as first-line therapy in all patients with chronic CAD.

4. Use sublingual nitroglycerin for alleviation of symptoms and prophylactically.

5. If episodes occur more than two or three times per week, the next step is addition of a calcium antagonist or a long-acting nitrate via eccentric dosing schedules to prevent nitrate tolerance. The decision to add a calcium antagonist or a long-acting nitrate is not based entirely on the frequency and severity of symptoms. The need to treat concomitant hypertension or the presence of left ventricular dysfunction and symptoms of heart failure may be an indi-

cation for the use of one of these agents, even in patients in whom episodes of symptomatic angina are infrequent.

6. If angina persists despite two antianginal agents (a beta blocker with either a long-acting nitrate preparation or a calcium antagonist), add the third antianginal agent.

7. Coronary angiography, with a view to considering coronary revascularization, is indicated in patients with refractory symptoms or ischemia despite optimal medical therapy; it should also be carried out in patients with "high-risk" noninvasive test results (see Table 37-2) and in those with occupations or life styles that require a more aggressive approach.

OTHER THERAPIES

An option for patients with refractory angina who are not candidates for coronary revascularization is spinal cord stimulation using a specially designed electrode inserted into the epidural space. The beneficial effects of neuromodulation via this technique on pain are based on the gate theory, in which stimulation of axons in the spinal cord that do not transmit pain to the brain will reduce input to the brain from axons that do so. Irrespective of the mechanism, several observation studies have reported success rates of up to 80 percent in terms of the frequency and severity of angina.[344] What is less easily explained is the apparent antiischemic effect of this technique. Randomized placebo-controlled trials are impossible to perform, and this approach should be reserved for patients in whom all other treatment options have been exhausted.[345]

The use of enhanced external counterpulsation (EECP) is another promising alternative to treatment of refractory angina. The mechanisms underlying the effects of EECP are currently under evaluation and include (1) hemodynamic changes that reduce myocardial O_2 demand in addition to the potential for increased transmyocardial pressure to open collaterals and (2) the possibility that exposure of the arterial bed to the augmented blood flow produced by EECP could lead to the elaboration of various substances that improve endothelial function and vascular remodeling.[346] Irrespective of the mechanism, in a recent multicenter prospective trial in which active counterpulsation was compared with "inactive counterpulsation," the former reduced angina and extended the time to exercise-induced ischemia over a 4- to 7-week period in patients with symptomatic CAD. Moreover, the treatment was relatively well tolerated, so this modality warrants further investigation.[347]

Translaser myocardial revascularization techniques are addressed on p. 1305.

Percutaneous Coronary Interventions

(see also Chap. 38)

Percutaneous coronary interventions (PCIs), which include percutaneous transluminal coronary angioplasty (PTCA), stenting, and related techniques, represent a major therapeutic advance in the management of chronic stable angina.[348] Their importance to the management of CAD in the United States is reflected by the performance of approximately 447,000 procedures in 1997 (52 percent of which were performed on persons younger than 65 years). This figure represents an increase of 190 percent from 1987 to 1997. The dramatic growth in the use of PCI has not eliminated growth in the use of coronary bypass surgery, and in 1997, the latter procedures were performed on 366,000 patients, which reflects an increase of 227 percent in the number of patients treated from 1979 to 1997. The practice of interventional cardiology has changed radically during the last 5 years following the widespread use of stents, the introduction of new platelet inhibitors, and the development of other devices that have a niche in the context of specific technical issues, e.g., rotablator and atherectomy.[349]

PATIENT SELECTION. Improved technology and increasing operator experience have continued to expand the pool of patients with both single-vessel and multivessel disease who are candidates for PCI (and other catheter-based techniques for revascularization). Factors that need to be considered in patient selection include the following:

1. The need for revascularization (surgical or catheter based) as opposed to medical therapy, including stringent risk factor modification.

2. The likelihood of successful catheter-based revascularization based on the angiographic characteristics of the lesion—type A, B, or C lesions,[350] which characterize complexity as mild, moderate, or severe, respectively (see Chap. 38). Equally important are factors such as vessel size, extent of calcification, tortuosity, and relationships to side-branches.

3. The risk and potential consequences of acute failure of PCI, which are a function, in part, of the coronary artery anatomy and underlying left ventricular function.

4. The likelihood of restenosis.

5. The need for complete revascularization based on the extent of CAD, the severity of ischemia, and the presence or absence of left ventricular dysfunction.

6. The presence of comorbid conditions and the suitability of the patient for surgery.

7. Patient preference.

The patient with chronic stable angina who is ideal for PCI, i.e., who is at low risk for complications and in whom the likelihood of technical success is high, is a male with chronic stable angina who is younger than 70 years and has single-vessel and single-lesion CAD, the anatomical characteristics of a type A lesion with less than 90 percent stenosis, no history of congestive heart failure, and an ejection fraction greater than 40 percent. Although these characteristics define the ideal candidate, excellent technical and clinical results can still be obtained in many patients who do not fulfill these ideal criteria.

Features associated with an increased risk for PCI failure include advanced age, female gender, unstable angina, congestive heart failure, left main coronary artery-equivalent disease, multivessel multi-lesion CAD, and probably recent thrombolytic therapy.[351] Diabetes mellitus in patients with multivessel disease has been associated with increased periprocedural ischemic complications and late mortality in comparison with patients without diabetes. Patients with impaired renal function, particularly those with diabetes, are also at increased risk for periprocedural morbidity and, in particular, contrast agent nephropathy.[351, 352]

The original ACC/AHA criteria for PTCA success based on lesion morphology suggested that the outcome was poorer with type B or C lesions. These data, validated in the early 1990s,[353] were examined more recently in the setting of better guidewires, new devices, and perfusion balloons.[354] In this large study of patients treated between 1994 and 1996, success rates were not shown to differ among patients with A, B1, or B2 lesions, but each was accompanied by higher success rates than seen with type C lesions. Independent predictors of procedural failure were the presence of total occlusion and vessel tortuosity. Predictors of complications were bifurcation lesions, the presence of thrombus, the inability to protect a sidebranch, and degenerative vein graft lesions. The presence of the aforementioned features does not necessarily contraindicate PCI but should certainly raise the threshold for performing the procedure. However, it would appear that in the current era, lesion morphology may be a less powerful predictor of complications than was previously the case.

EARLY OUTCOME. Continued improvement in the technical aspects of PCI, as well as increasing operator experience, has had a favorable impact on the rate of primary success (usually defined as an increase in diameter of >20 percent and a final diameter obstruction <50 percent) and the rate of reductions in complications, i.e., death, myocardial infarction, and emergency coronary bypass surgery.[355] These improvements have occurred despite broadening of the selection criteria for PCI to include older and sicker patients with more complex anatomy.[349, 351] Current expectations for PCI, particularly with the widespread use of coronary stents, are an overall procedural success rate of at least 90 percent with a mortality of less than 1 percent, rate of Q wave myocardial infarction of less than 1.5 percent, and rate of emergency bypass surgery of 1 to 2 percent.

ABRUPT CLOSURE. This complication after initially successful PCI has been defined as total or subtotal occlusion of the target lesion, and it is usually recognized before the patient leaves the laboratory. The entity of "threatened" vessel closure is defined by recurrent stenosis of less than 50 percent and Thrombosis in Myocardial Infarction (TIMI) flow less than grade 3.[356]

The treatment objectives of abrupt closure are to establish adequate coronary perfusion as a bridge to coronary bypass surgery or, in some patients, as a definitive strategy.

LONG-TERM OUTCOME. For the majority of patients undergoing PCI, the intermediate and late outcomes can be characterized by a low mortality or nonfatal myocardial infarction rate.[357] Several recent studies provide reassuring data on the long-term results of PTCA. The 10-year follow-up of the first series of patients undergoing PTCA performed by Gruentzig demonstrated a survival rate of 95 percent in patients with single-vessel disease and 81 per-

cent in those with multivessel disease.[358] In the National Heart, Lung, and Blood Institute (NHLBI) Registry, 5-year survival rates were 93.2, 88.8, and 86 percent in patients with single-, double-, and triple-vessel disease, respectively.[357] Five-year survival rates from 1980 to 1990 in the Emory University data base of over 10,000 patients were 88 and 93 percent, respectively, for patients with and those without diabetes mellitus.[359] Independent correlates of late survival were younger age, preserved left ventricular ejection fraction, and absence of congestive heart failure, multivessel disease, and diabetes.

Restenosis, the Achilles heel of angioplasty, continues to have a major impact on long-term outcome. Also, angina frequently recurs.[349, 357, 360–363] Restenosis and, to a lesser extent, progression of disease are the major reasons for repeat revascularization procedures, which in the randomized trials were performed in 30 to 40 percent of patients at 1 to 2 years and, in the Bypass Angioplasty Revascularization Investigation (BARI), in 60 percent of patients at 5 years.[352] Approximately 50 percent of all repeat revascularization procedures are repeat PCIs, with the rest being coronary artery bypass procedures.[352, 364, 365] What is reassuring is that the need for repeat revascularization tapers off rapidly after the second year.

STENTS. Since their entry into clinical practice in the early 1990s, stents have had an effect on both the early and late results of PCI. In regard to the former, stents have produced a marked reduction in the need for emergency bypass surgery, and in comparison with PTCA, stents have been associated with a significant reduction in the incidence of major cardiac events after discharge.[366] However, these results are not due to any reduction in death or myocardial infarction, but almost entirely to a reduction in the need for and performance of target vessel repeat revascularization, which in turn reflects a reduction in clinical restenosis. The development of newer techniques such as intravascular brachytherapy,[367] techniques for local drug delivery, and new stent coatings may result in a further improvement in long-term results.

COMPARISONS BETWEEN PTCA AND MEDICAL THERAPY. Only four trials have compared PTCA with medical therapy.[183, 368–370] The first major randomized trial involving PTCA was the Veterans Administration Comparison of Angioplasty with Medical Therapy in the treatment of single-vessel CAD, reported in 1992.[371] PTCA was distinctly superior to medical therapy in the relief of angina and in improvement in exercise tolerance, although repeat PTCA or CABG surgery was required in 15 percent of patients by 6 months. A conclusion that can be drawn from this study is that a trial of medical therapy followed by PCI in the event of treatment failure is a reasonable initial strategy for patients with stable angina and single-vessel disease. Nonetheless, indices of quality of life, including functional capacity and the patient's perception of well-being, were significantly better among patients treated with PTCA.[372] At 2 to 3 years, although some of the early benefits of PTCA on exercise tolerance and symptoms were sustained, the subsequent use of CABG and PTCA in the two groups was no different.

Another small randomized trial from Brazil, the Medicine Angioplasty or Surgery Study (MASS), compared PTCA with medical therapy and CABG for patients with proximal stenosis of the left anterior descending coronary artery. After 3 years, no difference was seen between medical therapy and PTCA in the combined endpoints of cardiac death, myocardial infarction, and refractory angina requiring revascularization, but the surgical arm was superior to the two other modalities (3 percent incidence in the surgical arm vs. 24 percent after PTCA and 17 percent with medical therapy). Nonetheless, both revascularization arms were superior to medical therapy for the relief of symptoms and reduction in exercise-induced ischemia. At 5 years of follow-up, surgery using the internal mammary artery (IMA) in all patients was superior to PTCA and medical therapy for the combined endpoints of death, myocardial infarction, unstable angina, and treatment failure requiring revascularization, and the only significant difference between PTCA and medical therapy was in the severity of angina, which was significantly less in the PTCA arm.[369]

The most recent trial of PTCA versus medical therapy and the most relevant to contemporary clinical practice is the Atorvastatin Versus Revascularization Treatment Trial (AVERT).[183] Patients with one- or two-vessel disease who were asymptomatic or had chronic mild to moderate stable angina were randomly assigned to atorvastatin (80 mg/d) or PTCA, followed by usual care, including lipid-lowering therapy in some patients, but this therapy was protocol mandated. The serum LDL cholesterol in the atorvastatin arm exhibited a 46 percent decrease versus an 18 percent decrease in the angioplasty arm. At 18 months, the incidence of ischemic events was 21 percent in the PTCA group in comparison with 13 percent in the atorvastatin group ($p = 0.024$), and among patients with exercise-induced ST segment depression at baseline, the rate of ischemic events was 19 percent versus 8.6 percent in the atorvastatin arm.[183]

The U.K. trial Randomized Intervention Treatment of Angina-2 (RITA-2) enrolled 1018 patients who were generally at low risk in that 80 percent of them had Class 0 to 2 stable angina (patients with unstable angina were excluded), 60 percent had single-vessel disease, 33 percent had double-vessel disease, and only 6 percent had significant left ventricular dysfunction.[370] The rate of death and nonfatal myocardial infarction was 6.3 percent in the PTCA group and 3.3 percent in the medical therapy group ($p = NS$). The difference was attributable primarily to an excess of periprocedural myocardial infarctions in the PTCA group. The benefits of PTCA over medical therapy in the relief of symptoms occurred primarily in patients who at baseline had much more severe symptoms. The results of this trial are consistent with those of other trials comparing PTCA with medical therapy, which have demonstrated that PTCA is more effective in the relief of symptoms but does not produce any apparent reduction in mortality or late myocardial infarction.

The Duke University data base provides important information on the relative benefits of CABG, PTCA, and medical therapy on survival in 9263 patients referred for cardiac catheterization between 1984 and 1990. Adjusted 5-year survival rates for patients with single-vessel disease were similar—95 percent with PTCA and 94 percent with medical therapy; in patients with two-vessel disease, the rates were 91 and 86 percent, respectively, and in patients with three-vessel disease, they were 81 and 72 percent. These trends suggest that PTCA is superior to medical management in patients with multivessel disease (Fig. 37–5).

PCI IN PATIENTS WITH LEFT VENTRICULAR DYSFUNCTION.

Several studies of PCI in patients with left ventricular dysfunction have documented a high initial procedural success rate with successful dilatation of at least one lesion in 88 percent and all lesions in 76 percent. Nonetheless, successful dilatation of all lesions is less than the rate in patients with well-preserved ventricular function, probably a reflection of more extensive CAD and total occlusion,[360] and the long-term results are less favorable. Two-year survival rate among patients with an ejection fraction of 0.40 or less and multivessel disease was only approximately 75 percent.[373] In another series, 23 percent of patients with an ejection fraction less than 0.35 died during mean follow-up period of 21 months.[374] In a 1985–1986 report from the NHLBI Registry, the 4-year survival rate for patients with very poor left ventricular function (ejection fraction <25 percent) was only 45 percent.[360] Nonetheless, 87 percent of patients with a mean ejection fraction of 39.6 percent were alive at the latest follow-up, and 77 percent were alive and free of recurrent myocardial infarction or the necessity for bypass surgery.[360] Another study demonstrated similar results with 3-year survival rates of 83 and 92 percent in patients with ejection fractions of 0.31 to 0.35 and 0.36 to 0.40, respectively, but only 69 percent in patients with an ejection fraction of 0.30 or less.[375] To achieve a good outcome in patients with multivessel disease and left ventricular dysfunction, particularly if angina or ischemia is severe, revascularization should be complete. Complete revascularization, however, is often difficult to achieve with PCI, particularly in the presence of chronic total occlusions, which are not infrequent in these patients. This limitation of PCI in the achievement of complete revascularization is an important factor contributing to its relatively disappointing results in patients with significant left ventricular dysfunction and multivessel disease. It is likely that stents and other devices that have the potential to restore and maintain the patency of vessels with chronic total occlusion will expand the pool of patients with multivessel disease which is amenable to complete revascularization, with the potential for better long-term results.

RESTENOSIS (see also Chap. 38)

Although striking improvement has occurred in the initial results of PTCA during the last 20 years, restenosis continues to dominate late events. The most frequently used definition is greater than 50 percent diameter stenosis and/or greater than 50 percent late loss of the acute luminal gain, but no clear consensus has been reached regarding the optimal angiographic definition.[361] From a clinical perspective, restenosis is considered a recurrent ischemic event, usually angina, but restenosis may be clinically silent in approximately 30 percent of patients.[361] Before the introduction of stents, the incidence was 30 to 50 percent.

MECHANISMS OF AND RISK FACTORS FOR RESTENOSIS. The pathogenesis of restenosis in response to mechanical injury is incompletely understood and multifactorial. Traditionally, restenosis has been considered to be due to the development of neointimal thickening as a result of migration and stimulation of smooth muscle by growth factors. The elastic properties of the vessel undergoing PTCA and its recoil in the development of restenosis have also received attention (Fig. 37–6). Recent concepts of restenosis suggest that intimal proliferation may account for only about 30 percent of the late loss in lumen diameter 6 months after PTCA. The major mechanism appears

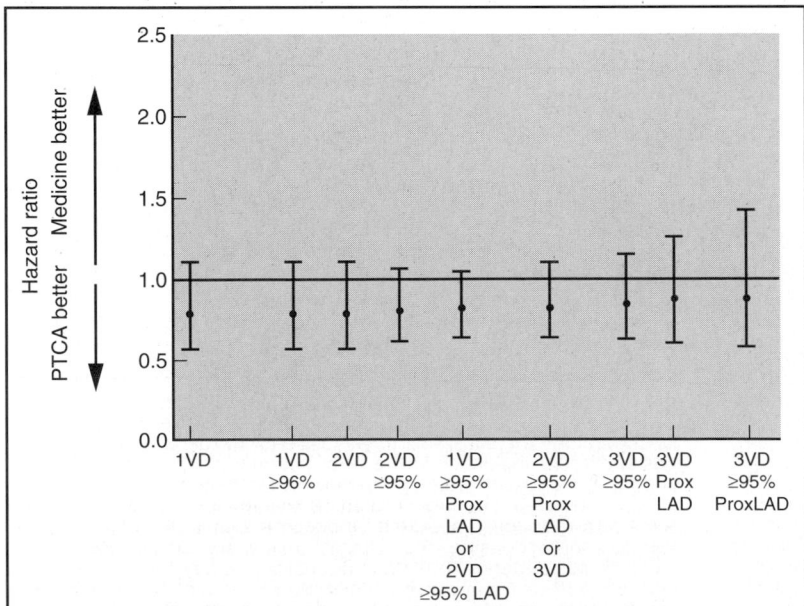

FIGURE 37–5. Hazard ratios for percutaneous transluminal coronary angioplasty (PTCA) versus medicine calculated from the Cox regression model to evaluate relative survival differences. Points indicate hazard ratios for each level of the coronary artery disease index; bars indicate 99 percent confidence intervals. The horizontal line at ratio 1.0 indicates the point of prognostic equivalence between treatments. Hazard ratios below the line favor PTCA; those above the line favor medicine. Prox LAD = proximal left anterior descending coronary artery; VD = vessel disease. (From Mark DB, Nelson CL, Califf RM, et al: Continuing evolution of therapy for coronary artery disease: Initial results from the era of coronary angioplasty. Circulation 89:2015, 1994. By permission of the American Heart Association, Inc.)

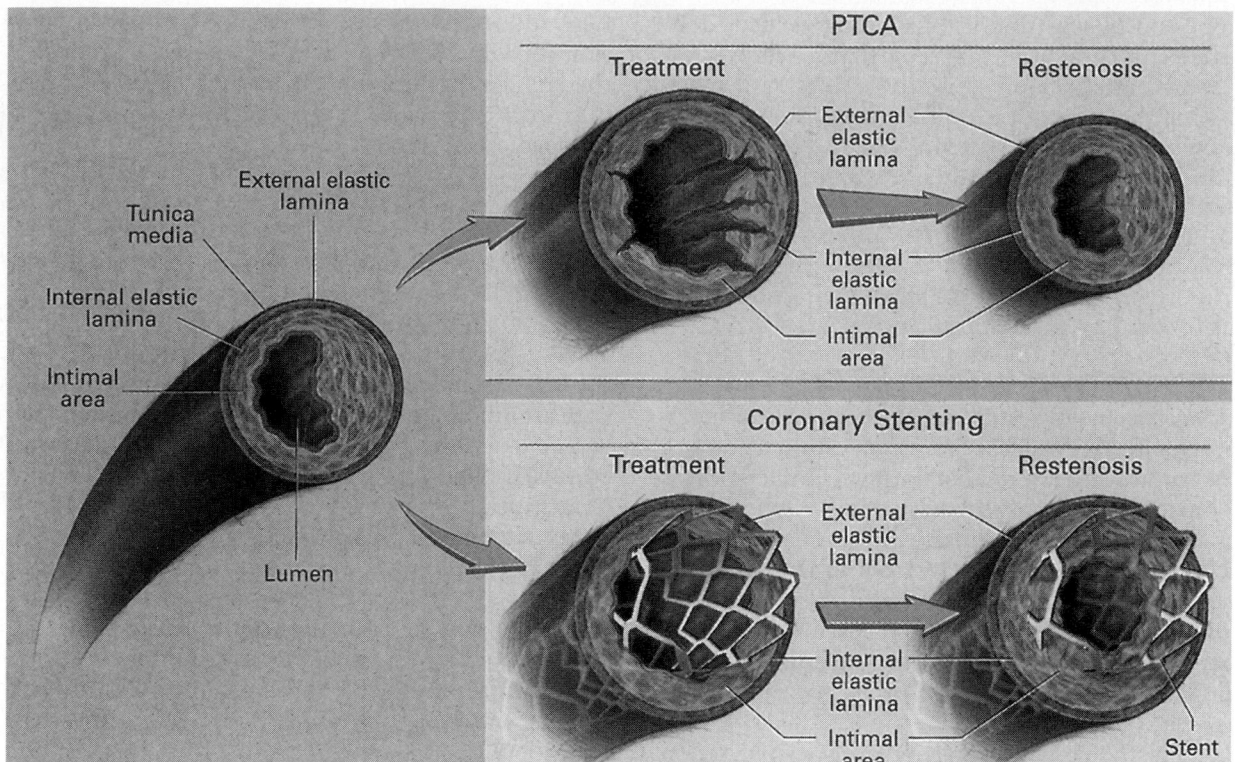

FIGURE 37–6. Possible mechanisms of restenosis after percutaneous transluminal coronary angioplasty (PTCA) and coronary stenting. Serial intravascular ultrasonographic studies suggest that PTCA almost always disrupts plaque without reducing the total intimal area, frequently causes dissections that penetrate into the tunica media through the internal elastic lamina, and transiently enlarges the vessel, measured as the cross-sectional area subtended by the external elastic lamina. Restenosis is caused by pathological arterial remodeling characterized by shrinkage of the area circumscribed by the external elastic lamina and, to a lesser extent, by neointimal thickening. Coronary stenting also enlarges the cross-sectional area of the vessel. The radial force of the stent prevents vessel shrinkage, but neointimal proliferation can be excessive. (From Bittl JA: Advances in coronary angioplasty. N Engl J Med 335:1290, 1996. By permission of the Massachusetts Medical Society.)

to be shrinkage of the dilated segment—a maladaptive form of arterial remodeling.[349, 362] This mechanism would explain why stenting, which produces a larger luminal area, is so effective in decreasing the incidence of restenosis. In contrast to the mechanisms of restenosis in native vessels, stent restenosis is accounted for primarily by neointimal proliferation through the stent.[349] Clinical variables that appear to be associated with increased rates of restenosis include diabetes, severe angina, male sex, smoking, and older age. *Anatomical* factors include total occlusion, left anterior descending coronary artery location, saphenous vein graft lesions, long lesions, and multivessel or multilesion PTCA. *Procedural* variables include greater residual stenosis following PTCA, severe dissection, the absence of an intimal tear, the use of inappropriately sized balloons, and the presence of thrombus.

PREVENTION OF RESTENOSIS. The single major advance in the reduction of restenosis has been the development of stents. In the Belgium Netherlands Stent (BENESTENT) Trial, restenosis rates were 22 percent in the stent group versus 32 percent in the group receiving PTCA alone. This improvement was accompanied by a reduction in clinical events.[376] In the Stent Restenosis Study (STRESS), restenosis rates were 32 and 42 percent in the stent and PTCA groups, respectively. Intracoronary radiation therapy using beta and gamma emitters shows promise in preventing restenosis.[377, 378] Many issues need to be resolved, including cost and logistics, long-term safety, and the potential incidence of "late" restenosis or subacute reocclusion.

MANAGEMENT OF RESTENOSIS. The incidence of restenosis peaks between 3 and 6 months, and this interval is the period of maximal vigilance for detecting restenosis in asymptomatic patients. The role of "routine" cardiac stress testing, particularly in asymptomatic patients, has not been clarified. Angiography after PTCA should be confined to patients with symptoms or abnormal functional studies because angiographic as opposed to clinical follow-up is associated with a marked increase in repeat revascularization procedures.[379]

Restenosis is amenable to repeat PCI, but it is not entirely clear whether lesions in which restenosis has developed are more prone to the development of restenosis after a subsequent percutaneous intervention.[380] Among patients with stable or unstable angina and restenosis, a 93 percent anatomical success rate after repeat angioplasty has been reported, and most patients experienced significant long-term clinical improvement. However, the likelihood of recurrent angina requiring subsequent bypass surgery was greater than in patients undergoing PTCA for the first time.[381] In patients undergoing a third PTCA for restenosis at the same site, an interval of less than 3 months between the second and third procedures was strongly associated with further restenosis, thus suggesting that such patients should be considered for CABG.[382]

CHRONIC TOTAL OCCLUSION. Chronic total occlusions are present in 20 to 40 percent of patients with angiographic documentation of CAD[383] and are particularly frequent in patients with multivessel disease and left ventricular dysfunction, in whom a total occlusion is a formidable obstacle to PCI success and the completeness of revascularization. This problem is particularly relevant in the presence of bridging collaterals, an estimated duration of occlusion of more than 3 months, and vessel diameter less than 3 mm.[384] After initially successful elective coronary angioplasty of total occlusions, the restenosis rate was 45 percent in vessels with total occlusion in comparison with 34 percent in those with subtotal obstruction ($p < 0.001$), primarily because of an increased number of total occlusions at follow-up angiography[385] (19.2 vs. 5.0 percent for stenoses, $p < 0.001$).

Several studies have documented the feasibility of stenting in patients with chronic total occlusions,[386] and the apparent superiority of stenting over PTCA was suggested by the results of small randomized trials in highly selected patients.[387, 388]

PCI IN WOMEN. The in-hospital mortality among women is slightly higher than among men; however, after a successful procedure, the long-term survival for women is excellent and similar to that for men. Still, women are more likely to experience a recurrence of angina.[389] However, in the BARI Trial, after multivariable adjustments, female gender was shown to be an independent predictor of improved 5-year survival after either form of revascularization.[390]

PCI IN THE ELDERLY. Catheter-based revascularization is particularly attractive in the elderly because of age-related changes in cognitive function and cerebrovascular events after CABG surgery and because of the adverse effect of coexisting disease (which is frequent in the elderly) on perioperative outcome.[391] Nonetheless, the increased prevalence of multivessel and diffuse disease and left ventricular dysfunction in the elderly diminishes the proportion of patients likely to have significant long-term benefits in comparison to CABG.[392] The more unfavorable coronary artery anatomy in the elderly population together with left ventricular dysfunction is reflected by the high mortality and periprocedural complication rates in the elderly undergoing PTCA, in addition to greater recurrence of angina in hospital survivors. Still, periprocedural outcomes are improving. Between 1990 and 1992 at the Mayo Clinic, 768 patients 65 years or older had PTCA and were compared with 982 patients who had the procedure between 1980 and 1989.[393] Despite the increased complexity and comorbidity of the latter group, procedural success rates were higher and periprocedural complications lower in the more recent group. However, event-free survival after discharge did not improve and was essentially the same in the two groups, with an overall rate of death from myocardial infarction during the initial hospitalization and 6-month follow-up of approximately 10 percent.[393]

PCI IN CORONARY BYPASS GRAFTS. CABG and PCI are often considered competitive procedures, but it is more appropriate to view them as complementary. An increasing number of patients who have had CABG and later have recurrent ischemia undergo revascularization with a percutaneous interventional technique. At the Mayo Clinic, approximately 20 percent of all PCIs are in patients who have had previous CABG.[394]

The initial and subsequent success rates of PCI in venous bypass grafts are lower than in native vessels. Success rates are approximately 90 percent, with restenosis rates ranging from 40 to 70 percent. The results are better with dilatation of distal graft lesions.

Innovative approaches to the management of vein graft atherosclerosis include catheter-based aspiration systems, in which the techniques of aspiration and filters are combined to prevent distal emboli,[395] glycoprotein IIb/IIIa platelet receptor inhibitors,[396] and the use of coronary ultrasonography to lyse thrombi.[397] The most encouraging development in patients with vein graft stenoses has been the use of elective stent replacement, which in several initial studies appears to have decreased the long-term incidence of restenosis from 40 to 70 percent after PTCA to 17 to 30 percent with stenting.[398] Long-term results from stenting of saphenous vein grafts are not available but appear to be superior to those after PTCA. An ACC Expert Consensus Document stated that in selected patients with saphenous vein graft disease, stents have resulted in improved initial success rates and larger acute angiographic gain, but restenosis rates and longer-term morbidity are still increased in comparison with stenting in large native coronary arteries.[398] Elective stent placement will probably become the treatment of choice in the management of vein graft stenosis. Whether these results will improve with the adjunctive use of other devices such as transluminal extraction cardiac atherectomy remains to be determined.

COMPARISON OF PCI AND CORONARY ARTERY BYPASS SURGERY. See p. 1319.

OTHER CATHETER-BASED TECHNIQUES. Lasers, rotablators, and atherectomy are discussed in Chapter 38.

CONCLUSIONS. PCI represents a major advance in the management of CAD, and new developments in interventional cardiology over the last 5 years have had a substantial effect on outcomes and on expanding the pool of patients eligible for these procedures. The practice of interventional cardiology has been revolutionized by coronary stenting, and further advances in coated stents and antithrombotic agents are likely. However, it must be appreciated that restenosis remains a problem, and management of a patient with chronic total occlusion by PCI is suboptimal. The latter is probably the major reason why patients are deemed unsuitable for PCI and referred for CABG. Also, it must be appreciated that a dilatable lesion represents an isolated target whereas atherosclerosis is a diffuse process. Thus, PCI is but one aspect of a comprehensive therapeutic strategy that should vigorously address the risk factors for CAD.

▼ Coronary Artery Bypass Surgery

In 1964, Garrett, Dennis, and DeBakey first used CABG as a "bailout" procedure.[399] Widespread use of the technique by Favoloro and Johnson and their respective collaborators followed in the late 1960s.[400, 401] Use of the IMA graft was pioneered by Kolessov in 1967 and by Green and colleagues in 1970.[402, 403]

The number of coronary bypass operators in the United States increased by 227 percent from 1979 to 1997, and in 1997, approximately 366,000 patients underwent coronary bypass surgery.[5] The advent of PCI may have blunted the growth of CABG. Nevertheless, CABG remains one of the most frequently performed operations in the United States; approximately 1 in every 1000 persons undergoes CABG on an annual basis, and this procedure results in the expenditure of almost $50 billion annually.

The appropriate use of invasive cardiovascular procedures is undergoing increasing scrutiny. It is therefore reassuring to note that in studies of coronary angiography and bypass surgery in New York State and Canada, only 6 and 4 percent of bypass procedures, respectively, were considered inappropriate.[404] In a study from The Netherlands, 84 percent of decisions to perform CABG were rated appropriate, 12 percent uncertain, and 4 percent inappropriate.[405] A recent review of surgical indications from a consortium of academic medical centers demonstrated that only 1.6 percent of operations were considered inappropriate and 7 percent were uncertain.[406]

Technical Considerations

When a decision has been reached to proceed with CABG, administration of beta blockers, nitrates, and calcium antagonists is continued until surgery. It is crucial to minimize perioperative damage and protect the myocardium. The most commonly used method involves a single period of aortic cross-clamping with intermittent infusion of cold cardioplegia solution. A 1994 trial of cold crystalloid versus warm blood cardioplegia in elective bypass surgery in patients with well-preserved preoperative ventricular function demonstrated low mortality and morbidity with both techniques.[407] Cardioplegic solutions may be sanguineous and have high concentrations of potassium with or without added substances, such as O_2, buffers, and free radical scavengers.[408] Retrograde cardioplegia through the coronary sinus facilitates more uniform distribution of cardioplegic solution. Many surgeons now use a combination of antegrade and retrograde perfusion,[409] as well as topical hypothermia with cold saline or ice slush as an adjunct.

Among patients with satisfactory preoperative cardiac function, a wide range of techniques have produced excellent results. This success is probably a reflection of the extent of myocardial functional reserve in those with well-preserved systolic function. In contrast, among patients with depressed left ventricular function (both acutely and chronically), it is easier to demonstrate a benefit with more

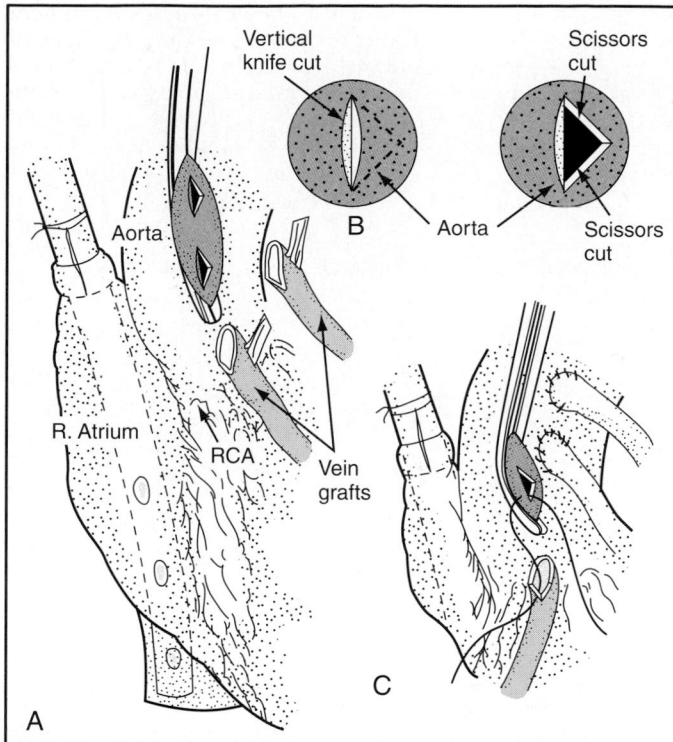

FIGURE 37–7. Aorticovenous anastomosis in a coronary artery–saphenous vein bypass graft. *A,* Direction of the anastomotic site for left-sided grafts. *B,* Details of aortic orifices. *C,* Direction of right coronary artery (RCA) grafts. (From Cohn LH: Surgical techniques of emergency coronary revascularization. *In* Cohn LH [ed]: The Treatment of Acute Myocardial Ischemia: An Integrated Medical-Surgical Approach. Mt Kisco, NY, Futura, 1979, p 87. By permission.)

specialized protocols, including the use of sanguineous cardioplegic techniques, with or without substrate enhancement,[408] and blood cardioplegia.[410] The theoretical advantages of blood cardioplegic solutions, which may be helpful in patients with severe chronic left ventricular dysfunction, include superior buffering capacity, enhanced flow rates at a capillary level, and a reduction in free radicals.[410]

Renewed interest in coronary bypass surgery without cardiopulmonary bypass has been stimulated by the desire to avoid blood transfusions, by economic issues, and by the wish to avoid the damaging neurological effects of bypass, particularly in the elderly and in patients with heavily calcified aortas.[411] An alternative approach to revascularization using the beating heart is off-pump coronary bypass, which frequently entails a conventional median sternotomy and mechanical suction stabilizing systems. This combination enhances surgical exposure and is particularly useful if multivessel bypass grafting is contemplated. This technique is particularly attractive in patients with diffuse aortic atherosclerosis, and preliminary results are encouraging.[412–415]

MINIMALLY INVASIVE CABG. Other approaches are termed "less invasive" or "minimally invasive" and include the use of alternative incisions such as a left thoracotomy with or without cardiopulmonary bypass or fluoroscopic techniques. The ultimate success of these "nontraditional" approaches to CABG will depend on long-term graft patency and the development of new techniques that will increase exposure to allow for more complete revascularization. Initial reports are encouraging in regard to decreasing the number of days spent in the intensive care unit and hospital and reducing neurological complications, but additional large studies are needed.

An innovative approach to coronary revascularization is the "port access" method, which uses small thoracotomy ports for cardiac manipulation; cardiopulmonary bypass is established by groin cannulation. Experience with this technique is limited, although the two largest single-center series and the first report of the Port-Access International Registry, which documented the results of 555 bypass procedures, were encouraging. Nonetheless, follow-up has been short, and the results do not reflect the "learning curve." Limitations to the use of this technique include atherosclerotic involvement of the aortic arch, high cost, long operating times, and the risk of aortic dissection.[415–417]

A novel approach to coronary revascularization integrates coronary artery bypass with PTCA by combining a minimally invasive coronary bypass surgical procedure on the left anterior descending coronary artery with PTCA on the remaining vessels. Further experience is needed to clarify the selection criteria and long-term strategy and whether it offers any advantages over multivessel bypass surgery alone.[101, 418]

"The learning curve" of minimally invasive coronary bypass surgery has led to numerous reports of early graft failure.[419] In many centers, intraoperative or early postoperative angiography is performed to assess the quality of the anastomosis. It should be emphasized that with conventional surgical techniques, the *early* patency rates of an IMA graft are excellent (98.7 percent in one large series), and less than 50 percent stenosis was noted in 91 percent of grafts. The future of minimally invasive and other techniques will depend on their ability to equal these excellent patency rates.[420]

VENOUS CONDUITS. The saphenous vein is used mainly for distal branches of the right and circumflex coronary arteries and for sequential grafts to these vessels and diagonal branches (Figs. 37–7 and 37–8). In emergency situations, many surgeons prefer the saphenous vein, which can be harvested and grafted more rapidly, to the IMA. Arm vein grafts are not as effective as either IMA or saphenous vein grafts.

Eight to 12 percent of saphenous vein grafts become occluded during the early perioperative period. Trauma to the vein during surgical preparation can denude the endothelium, impair the intrinsic fibrinolytic activity of the saphenous vein, and damage the vessel wall, thereby predisposing to early thrombosis.[421] Careful harvesting of the

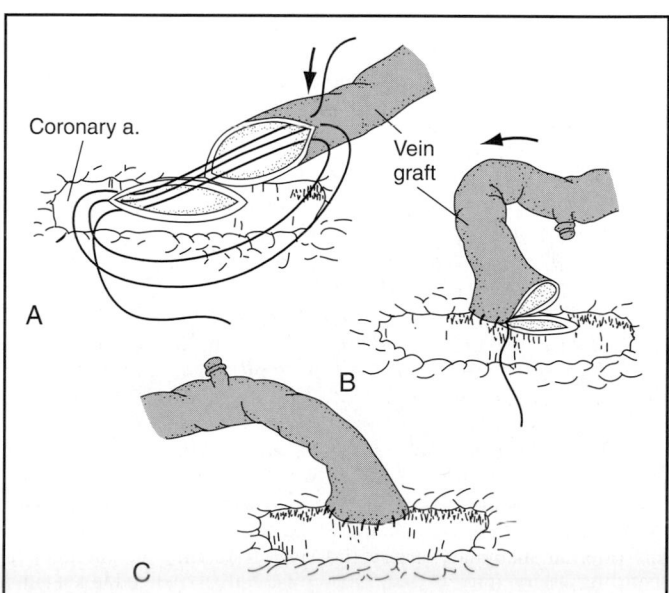

FIGURE 37–8. Venocoronary anastomosis to the proximal portion of the arteriotomy. (From Cohn LH: Surgical techniques of emergency coronary revascularization. *In* Cohn LH [ed]: The Treatment of Acute Myocardial Ischemia: An Integrated Medical-Surgical Approach. Mt Kisco, NY, Futura, 1979, p 87. By permission.)

graft, with particular attention to avoidance of overdistention and the use of modified storage solutions, has been shown to improve patency and preserve the integrity of the graft in both animal models and the clinical setting.

INTERNAL MAMMARY ARTERY BYPASS GRAFTS. The IMA, also known as the internal thoracic artery, is usually remarkably free of atheroma, especially in patients younger than 65 years. When it is grafted to a coronary artery (Figs. 37–9 and 37–10), it appears to be virtually immune to the development of intimal hyperplasia, which is almost universally seen in aortocoronary vein grafts.[422] Atherosclerotic changes in the IMA develop in only a small percentage of patients after coronary bypass surgery. The IMA is delicate, so great care has to be taken to mobilize the vessel without traumatizing it.[423] The procedure is time consuming, and thus, the IMA is not often used for emergency surgery.

Comparative morphological and angiographic studies of IMA and saphenous vein bypass grafts that have been implanted long-term show that accelerated atherosclerosis occurs commonly in saphenous vein grafts but is extremely rare in IMA grafts. Several potential explanations may be offered for the superiority of the IMA graft.[423] The media of the artery may derive nourishment from the lumen as well as from the vasa vasorum, and the internal elastic lamina of the IMA is uniform. Moreover, the finding that the endothelium of the IMA produces significantly more prostacyclin than that of the saphenous vein may explain why endothelium-dependent relaxation is more pronounced, which may allow flow-dependent autoregulation to occur.[424] The diameter of the IMA graft is usually a closer match to that of the recipient coronary artery than is the diameter of a saphenous vein. The increasing popularity of the IMA as a conduit is reflected in the Society of Thoracic Surgeons data base. Among the patients in the United States who had first operations in 1990, the IMA was used in 48.5 percent, but this figure steadily increased to 79.77 percent by 1997.[425]

In one series, IMA grafts and saphenous vein grafts had patency rates of 95 and 93 percent, respectively, at 1 year,

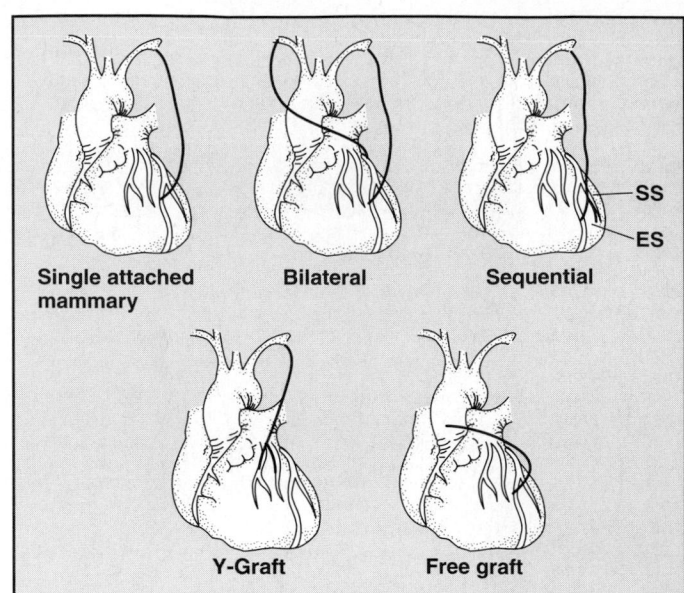

FIGURE 37–10. Different types of internal mammary artery grafts. A single attached internal mammary artery graft (either the right or left) remains attached proximally to the subclavian artery and is connected to the coronary arteries. Bilateral internal mammary artery grafts (right and left) are joined end to side to coronary arteries. Sequential internal mammary artery grafts consist of an attached or free internal mammary artery with one or more side-to-side anastomoses and one end-to-side anastomosis. The internal mammary artery Y graft has two terminal branches of either the attached or free internal mammary artery sutured to two coronary arteries. A free internal mammary graft is placed by transecting the right or left internal mammary artery near its origin in the subclavian artery and anastomosing the proximal portion of the artery to the aorta and the distal end to the coronary artery. (From Tector AJ, Schmahl TM, Canino VR: Expanding the use of the internal mammary artery to improve patency in coronary artery bypass grafting. J Thorac Cardiovasc Surg 91:9, 1986. By permission of Mosby.)

but at 5 and 10 years, the patency rates of the IMA grafts were 88 and 83 percent, superior to the 74 and 41 percent rates for saphenous vein grafts.[426] Excellent long-term results have also been achieved with use of the right IMA as a free or sequential graft.[427] However, fibrointimal proliferation occasionally develops in IMA grafts, and the resultant narrowing may be a factor in late graft closure.[423]

Patients receiving an IMA graft have a decreased risk of late death, myocardial infarction, cardiac events, and reoperations, and this clinical advantage persists for up to 20 years.[428] The contemporary standard for bypass grafting advocates routine use of the left IMA for grafting the left anterior descending coronary artery, with supplemental saphenous vein grafts to other vessels.

Although the benefits of a single IMA graft over a saphenous vein graft alone are not in dispute, the superiority of bilateral IMA grafts over a single IMA graft and one saphenous vein graft is less well accepted.[429] Initial enthusiasm for the use of bilateral IMA grafts was tempered by the higher rate of postoperative complications, including bleeding, wound infection, and prolonged ventilatory support. Subsequent series have shown that bilateral versus single IMA grafting is associated with lower rates of recurrent angina pectoris, reoperation, and myocardial infarction and a trend toward improved survival,[430] but at the cost of a higher rate of sternal wound infections, particularly among patients who are obese or diabetic or require prolonged ventilatory support.

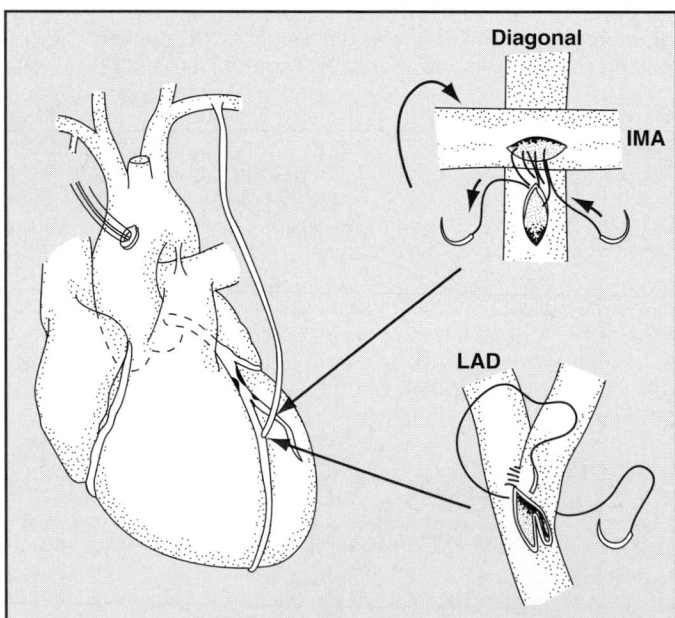

FIGURE 37–9. Internal mammary grafting consisting of an in situ left internal mammary artery (IMA) graft to the left anterior descending artery (end to side) and diagonal branch (side to side), with the diamond anastomotic technique used for the latter. The details show the IMA pedicle rolled up over the diagonal coronary artery to facilitate exposure and the use of continuous suture. (From Jones EL: Extended use of the internal mammary–coronary artery bypass. J Card Surg 1:13, 1986. By permission of Futura Publishing Co.)

COMPLICATIONS OF ARTERIAL CONDUITS. Inadequate flow rates with evidence of myocardial ischemia in the perioperative period are rare after IMA grafts to the left anterior descending coronary artery or its diagonal branches.[423] Perioperative spasm is the presumed cause and can be managed by the administration of sodium nitroprusside or a combination of glyceryl trinitrate and verapamil.[431] Other complications include an increased incidence of sternal wound infections, which is more frequent in obese patients and diabetics and after bilateral IMA implants.

OTHER ARTERIAL CONDUITS. The success of IMA grafts has stimulated interest in the use of other arterial conduits, particularly in patients who are younger, diabetic, or hyperlipidemic or in whom the saphenous veins are unsuitable or unavailable.[423] Initial enthusiasm for use of the radial artery was blunted by reports of high reocclusion rates. More recent experience, in which attention has been paid to avoiding spasm by minimizing manipulation and the use of calcium channel blockers, has been favorable. Brodman and colleagues reported a 95 percent 12-week patency rate in a large series of patients receiving radial artery grafts.[432] Another recent series reported an 84 percent 5-year patency rate in 100 consecutive recipients of radial grafts versus a 90 percent patency rate for the IMA.[433]

The right gastroepiploic artery can be harvested by extending the median sternotomy incision toward the umbilicus. It is frequently placed as a graft to the right coronary artery, but both the circumflex and the left anterior descending coronary arteries can be grafted with this conduit.[434] Early results demonstrated excellent patency rates, but there is a paucity of data on long-term results. Similarly, the inferior epigastric artery has been used as a free graft for coronary revascularization, with good short-term patency rates but without long-term data.[435] Cryopreserved homologous saphenous vein grafts and glutaraldehyde-treated umbilical veins have been used, but the patency rates are not optimal. These grafts should be used only as a last resort, and this restriction also applies to the use of bovine IMA, Dacron, and polytetrafluoroethylene (PTFE) grafts.[436]

THE DISTAL VASCULATURE. The state of the distal coronary vasculature is important for the fate of bypass grafts. Late patency of grafts is related to coronary arterial runoff as determined by the diameter of the coronary artery into which the graft is inserted, the size of the distal vascular bed, and the severity of coronary atherosclerosis distal to the site of insertion of the graft. The highest graft patency rates are found when the lumina of the vessels distal to the graft insertion are greater than 1.5 mm in diameter, perfuse a large vascular bed, and are free of atheroma obstructing more than 25 percent of the vessel lumen. For saphenous veins, optimal patency rates are achieved with a lumen of 2.0 mm or greater.

FLOW RATES. When measured at the time of surgery, flow rates through saphenous vein grafts average nearly 70 ml/min. Flow rates less than 45 ml/min—and especially less than 25 ml/min—are more frequently associated with graft closure than are flow rates exceeding 45 ml/min.[437] The utility of measuring flow rates is enhanced by taking into account the type of conduit used and the size of the distal vasculature. If flow rates are lower than expected, reassessment of the anastomosis with a probe may be helpful. Possible causes of reduced flow include (1) subcritical obstruction of the coronary artery, (2) a technically poor anastomosis with narrowing of the lumen from kinking of the vessel or pinching at the site of anastomosis, (3) a small myocardial mass perfused by the graft, and (4) a diseased distal vascular bed.[438]

Other Surgical Procedures for Ischemic Heart Disease

Coronary bypass surgery may be combined with surgical procedures aimed at correction of atherosclerotic disease elsewhere in the cardiovascular system, such as correction of mechanical complications of myocardial infarction (mitral regurgitation or ventricular septal defect), left ventricular aneurysms, and concomitant valvular heart disease. Not unexpectedly, morbidity and mortality are correspondingly increased because of the added complexity of the procedure and, in many patients who require these other procedures, the presence of underlying left ventricular dysfunction (see below).

TRANSLASER MYOCARDIAL REVASCULARIZATION. Translaser myocardial revascularization, an innovative approach to the treatment of ischemic heart disease, is currently under evaluation.[439, 440] The initial assumption was that laser-mediated channels would provide a network of functional connections between the left ventricular cavity and the ischemic myocardium. Subsequent observations demonstrating closure of the channels within hours or days despite apparent relief of symptoms have led to alternative explanations for the apparent clinical success of the procedure. These explanations include improved perfusion by stimulation of angiogenesis, a potential placebo effect, and an anesthetic effect mediated by the destruction of sympathetic

nerves carrying pain-sensitive afferent fibers[441, 442] or periprocedural infarction. A recent study evaluated sympathetic innervation with [¹¹C]hydroxyephedrine and demonstrated decreased myocardial uptake of this substance in most patients, without significant change in resting or stress myocardial perfusion, which suggests that the improvement in angina after the procedure may be partly due to sympathetic denervation.[442]

Initial clinical studies in patients with severe CAD often amenable to a bypass procedure have been promising in that the majority have demonstrated a clear reduction in anginal severity and improved exercise tolerance. Several small randomized trials of translaser myocardial revascularization have resulted in improvement in comparison with maximal medical therapy.[443-445] The results of one trial suggested improvement in perfusion as assessed by PET, but such improvement was not shown with thallium scintigraphy in another trial.[444, 445] In contrast to the positive studies, Schofield and associates reported no significant improvement in exercise time and 12-minute walking distance up to 1 year after translaser myocardial revascularization with a carbon dioxide laser,[446] although the laser-treated patients had a modest reduction in the frequency of angina. The subjective improvement in the severity of angina found in this study, in the absence of any measurable effect on myocardial perfusion or exercise tolerance, argues for a placebo effect or denervation. Two other randomized trials from the United States confirmed the improvement in angina in patients receiving surgical translaser myocardial revascularization, but no study has demonstrated a reduction in myocardial ischemia as measured objectively, and laser revascularization was not associated in any of the three randomized trials with long-term improvement in left ventricular systolic function.[447, 448] On the basis of data from the randomized trials, it would appear that the widespread use of translaser myocardial revascularization as a "stand-alone" method cannot be justified, but it may still have a role as an adjunctive procedure during CABG in patients who have some vessels suitable for bypass but others that are unsuitable.

After the FDA approved carbon dioxide laser translaser myocardial revascularization for the sole treatment of Class III or IV angina in August 1998, interest has developed in other sources of laser energy, such as percutaneous myocardial revascularization (PCMR) in association with various techniques of left ventricular mapping (Fig. 37–11). Initial results have been promising,[449, 450] and the randomized Potential Angina Class Improvement from Intramyocardial Channels (PACIFIC) Trial of 231 patients with Class III or IV angina suggested that the procedure was safe. Moreover, at 6 months the PCMR group had symptomatic improvement in comparison with the maximal medical therapy group (Osterle S, personal communication). Nonetheless, the placebo effect has not been eliminated, and randomized trials in which both patients and investigators are blinded are currently in progress. Because the mechanisms underlying the observed clinical benefits are not well defined, the future of this technique depends on well-designed randomized trials, but it is possible that translaser myocardial revascularization or PCMR may eventually be combined with other interventions such as incomplete bypass surgery or used as an adjunct to PCI. Whether this technique will fulfill its potential as a vehicle for the delivery of angiogenic factors and other forms of gene therapy remains to be determined.[451]

Surgical Outcomes

OPERATIVE MORTALITY. Risk factors for death following coronary artery surgery may be separated into five categories: (1) preoperative factors related to CAD, including recent acute myocardial infarction, hemodynamic instability, left ventricular dysfunction, extensive CAD, the presence of left main CAD, and severe or unstable angina; (2) preoperative factors related to the aggressiveness of the arteriosclerotic process, as reflected in associated carotid or peripheral vascular disease; (3) preoperative biological factors (older age at surgery, diabetes mellitus, and perhaps female gender); (4) intraoperative factors (intraoperative ischemic damage and failure to use IMA grafts)[452]; and (5) environ-

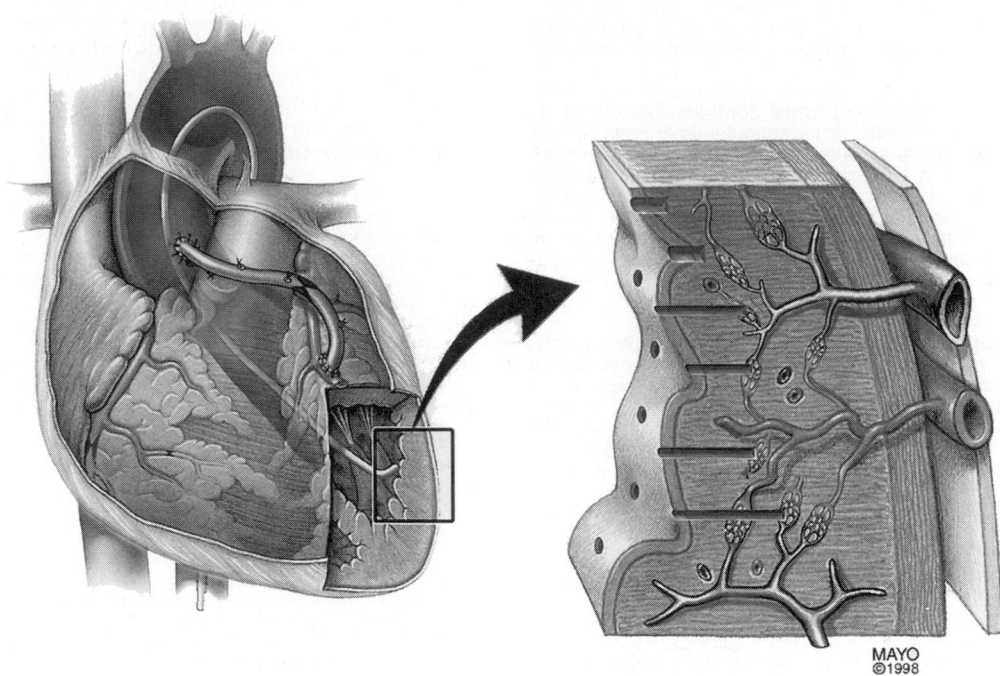

FIGURE 37–11. Schematic demonstrating the mechanism of percutaneous myocardial laser revascularization (PCMR). Left, A ventriculogram and coronary angiogram performed at the beginning of the procedure demonstrate that the left ventricular anatomy is suitable for treatment. A steerable catheter is delivered retrogradely across the aortic valve, and the catheter for energy delivery is advanced through a guiding catheter and placed in the left ventricular chamber. The steerable catheter allows access to the endocardial surface. Right, When the energy delivery catheter is in contact with the endocardium, intramyocardial channels are made by tissue ablation. The channels cause intramyocardial hemorrhage by transecting the microvasculature (bold arrow). A = epicardial artery; v = epicardial vein. (From Kantor B, McKenna CJ, Caccitolo JA, et al: Transmyocardial and percutaneous myocardial revascularization: Current and future role in the treatment of coronary artery disease. Mayo Clin Proc 74:585, 1999. By permission of Mayo Foundation for Medical Education and Research.)

mental or institutional factors, including the specific surgeon and treatment protocols used.[453]

The patient population undergoing CABG has been changing over time, particularly with the wider use of PCI. In comparison with the 1970s, patients undergoing CABG today are older, include a higher percentage of women, and are "sicker" in that a greater proportion have unstable angina, three-vessel disease, previous coronary revascularization with either CABG or PCI, left ventricular dysfunction, and comorbid conditions, including hypertension, diabetes, and peripheral vascular disease.

In-hospital mortality after isolated coronary bypass surgery was characterized by a steady decline from 1967 to the 1980s. Recently, a plateau and perhaps even a slight increase has been noted in morbidity and mortality, findings reflective of the changing demographics toward an older and sicker population of patients undergoing initial surgery and a higher proportion undergoing reoperation.[454] In 1997, perioperative mortality among 174,806 patients undergoing coronary bypass surgery entered into the Society of Thoracic Surgeons data base was 2.8 percent. In patients undergoing an elective first isolated coronary bypass operation, the mortality in 1997 was 1.7 percent.[425]

With increasingly wide scrutiny of procedural results, it has become recognized that absolute rates of morbidity and mortality might not provide a fair basis for comparing institutions and individuals, unless the characteristics of the patients are considered. Several models have been developed and refined with the objective of predicting perioperative mortality.[455] Major determinants are advancing age, poor left ventricular function, and the urgency of surgery, but additional factors such as comorbid conditions and coronary anatomy have added independent predictive value.

A useful perspective of long-term survival after coronary bypass surgery is provided by the most recent follow-up data (mean, 15 years) from the CASS Registry. Ninety percent of patients were alive at 5 years, 74 percent at 10 years, and 56 percent at 15 years. The hazard function for death decreases rapidly after surgery to its nadir at 9 to 12 months, followed by a steady increase with a doubling of the hazard ratio at 15 years in comparison to that at 5 years.

PERIOPERATIVE COMPLICATIONS

Perioperative morbidity (also see Chap. 60) has also increased because of a larger fraction of higher-risk patients.

PERIOPERATIVE MYOCARDIAL INFARCTION. Perioperative myocardial infarction, particularly if it is associated with hemodynamic or arrhythmic complications or preexisting left ventricular dysfunction, has a major adverse effect on early and late prognosis.[456] The cardiac troponins and myocardial creatine phosphokinase-MB (CK-MB) may be useful as markers of perioperative infarction.[457] Predictors of perioperative myocardial infarction in the CASS Trial were female gender, severe perioperative angina pectoris, severe stenosis of the left main coronary artery, and three-vessel disease.[456] Preconditioning the myocardium with short periods of ischemic stress interspersed with reperfusion increases the resistance to infarction and appears to reduce myocardial damage during cardiac surgery, but the appropriateness of this technique as a routine clinical tool has not been determined.

RESPIRATORY COMPLICATIONS. Postoperative changes in pulmonary function after CABG are frequent and troublesome, but rarely serious, except in patients with preexisting chronic lung disease or the elderly. A potentially serious complication is phrenic nerve injury, which may be related to cold-induced damage during myocardial protection strategies or possibly to mechanical injury while harvesting the IMA. The pulmonary consequences vary and range from an asymptomatic radiographic abnormality to severe pulmonary dysfunction requiring prolonged ventilation.[458]

BLEEDING. Impaired hemostasis and bleeding complications are an inherent risk of CABG. Reoperation for bleeding is required in 2 to 5 percent of patients. Cardiopulmonary bypass causes derangement of the intrinsic coagulation and fibrinolytic systems in addition to platelet function. The risk of bleeding is increased with age, a smaller body surface area, reoperation, bilateral internal thoracic artery grafts, and the preoperative use of heparin, aspirin, and thrombolytic agents. Bleeding is less common in obese patients,[459] but this complication may be reduced with aprotinin and lysine analogs such as aminocaproic acid and tranexamic acid.[460]

WOUND INFECTIONS. Major perioperative wound complications, especially mediastinitis and/or wound dehiscence, occur in approximately 1 percent of patients.[458] This risk is substantially increased by the use of double IMA grafts, particularly in diabetic patients,[461] and it is markedly increased in obese patients.[459] Preventive measures include careful skin preparation, increased attention to sterility in the perioperative environment, and preoperative use of antimicrobial agents.[458] Other factors that may decrease perioperative infection include the avoidance of unnecessary blood transfusion in view of the immunosuppressive effect of the latter.

PULMONARY INSUFFICIENCY. In the Society of Thoracic Surgeons data base,[425] postoperative pulmonary insufficiency requiring ventilation for more than 1 day was noted in 5.5 and 10.7 percent of patients undergoing a first operation and reoperation, respectively. The etiology is multifactorial and includes the presence of preexisting pulmonary disease and numerous perioperative factors related directly to anesthesia, cardiopulmonary bypass, incisional pain, chest tube placement, and occasionally, phrenic nerve damage.[458]

Severe chronic obstructive pulmonary disease, as defined by a forced expiratory volume in 1 second (FEV_1) of greater than 50 percent or an FEV_1/forced vital capacity (FVC) ratio less than 0.70, is associated with a high incidence of postoperative pulmonary complications (29 percent).[462] The left ventricular ejection fraction is also an important determinant of prolonged ventilation.[463]

POSTOPERATIVE HYPERTENSION. Hypertension can occur in up to one-third of patients postoperatively. The mechanisms are unclear but may be related to increased levels of circulating catecholamines and other humoral factors in addition to vasoconstriction secondary to activation of the renin-angiotensin system. Control of postoperative hypertension is important to prevent myocardial ischemia, cardiac failure, perioperative bleeding, and diminished tissue perfusion.[464] Regardless of the cause, sodium nitroprusside is an effective approach to afterload reduction, and other drugs such as calcium antagonists, nitrates, and beta blockers, including short-acting esmolol, are helpful.[458]

CEREBROVASCULAR COMPLICATIONS. Neurological abnormalities following cardiac surgery are dreaded complications. Postulated mechanisms include emboli from an atherosclerotic aorta or other vessels, emboli possibly from the cardiopulmonary bypass machine circuit and its tubing, and intraoperative hypotension, particularly in patients with preexisting hypertension.[458, 465, 466] Type I injury is associated with major neurological deficits, stupor, and coma, and type II is characterized by a deterioration in intellectual function and memory.[467] In a recent large multicenter series, the incidence of neurological abnormalities was 6.1 percent, and these abnormalities were almost evenly distributed between type I and type II deficits, with mortality rates of 21 and 10 percent, respectively.[467] Intellectual dysfunction in the early postoperative period, as expressed by a battery of neurocognitive defects, was noted in 75 percent of patients. However, major sequelae were unusual.[468] In regard to the neurological sequelae of cardiopulmonary bypass (including stroke, delirium, and neurocognitive dysfunction), older age in addition to other comorbid conditions associated with atherosclerosis is one of the more powerful predictors.[466] In most studies, atherosclerosis of the proximal aorta has also been a strong predictor of stroke.[465]

Intraoperative manipulation of the aorta is a major cause of atheroemboli and neurological complications. Preoperative or intraoperative screening with transesophageal echocardiography or epiaortic echocardiography to detect mobile aortic atheromas is increasingly being used, although the sensitivity and specificity need to be better defined.[469] An aggressive approach to the management of severe aortic atherosclerosis includes changing the cannulation sites based on echocardiographic findings, no-clamp fibrillatory arrest, and replacement of the ascending aorta.

Bypass surgery performed on the beating heart without the use of cardiopulmonary bypass has less potential for generating cerebral emboli,[411] and it appears to produce a lower incidence of cognitive dysfunction in both short- and intermediate-term postoperative follow-up than does conventional coronary bypass surgery with cardiopulmonary bypass.

ATRIAL FIBRILLATION. Atrial fibrillation is one of the most frequent complications of coronary bypass surgery. It occurs in up to 40 percent of patients, primarily within 2 to 3 days.[470] In the early postoperative period, rapid ventricular rates and loss of atrial transport may compromise systemic hemodynamics, increase the risk of embolization, and lead to a significant increase in duration of the hospital stay and charge and a twofold to threefold increase in postoperative stroke[471] (see also Chap. 60).

CONDUCTION DISTURBANCES AND BRADYARRHYTHMIAS. The incidence of postoperative bradyarrhythmias requiring permanent pacemaker implantation was 0.8 percent in a series of 1614 consecutive patients discharged from the hospital after coronary bypass surgery. Predictive factors were preoperative left bundle branch block, concomitant left ventricular aneurysmectomy, and older age. The majority of patients continued to require permanent pacemaker support during follow-up.

SYMPTOMATIC RESULTS. Coronary bypass surgery is highly effective in the relief of angina and results in improved quality of life. Approximately 80 percent of patients are free of angina at 5 years and 63 percent at 10 years, but by 15 years only about 15 percent are alive and free of an ischemic event.[472, 473] The acceleration in adverse events after 5 to 15 years is due to gradual occlusion of vein grafts in addition to progressive disease in the native coronary vessels. Independent predictors of recurrence of angina are female gender, obesity, preoperative hypertension, and lack of use of the IMA as a conduit.[474] In patients with triple-vessel disease undergoing coronary bypass surgery, the completeness of revascularization was a significant determinant of the relief of symptoms over a 5-year period.[475]

In the bypass surgery arms of recent randomized trials of PTCA and CABG, recurrent angina pectoris was reported in 21.5 to 34 percent of patients at a follow-up ranging from 2 to 3 years, but (Canadian classification) grade III or IV angina was present in only 6 percent at 2.5 years in the RITA Trial[364, 476] (Fig. 37-12).

RETURN TO EMPLOYMENT. Return to full employment has been variable. Among participants in the surgical arm of the Emory Angioplasty Versus Surgery Trial (EAST), whose mean age was 61 years at entry, only 38.5 percent were gainfully employed at 3 years.[364] In contrast, in a study of patients younger than 65 years who were employed at the time of revascularization, 79 percent who had CABG were working at 1 year, and after adjustment for baseline characteristics, 1-year employment rates were the same among patients treated with surgery, PTCA, or medi-

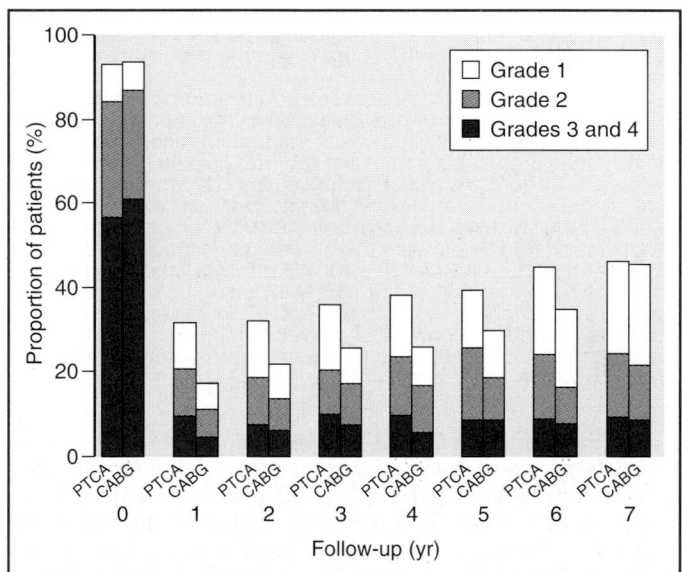

FIGURE 37-12. Prevalence and severity of angina by treatment group for each annual visit up to 7 years in the RITA-1 Trial. The prevalence of severe angina declines markedly from baseline (0-year follow-up) to the first year of follow-up. During the first few years, angina prevalence and severity are greater after percutaneous transluminal coronary angioplasty (PTCA), but no difference is seen at 7 years. CABG = coronary artery bypass graft. (From Henderson RA, Pocock SJ, Sharp SJ, et al: Long-term results of RITA-1 trial: Clinical and cost comparisons of coronary angioplasty and coronary-artery bypass grafting. Randomised Intervention Treatment of Angina. Lancet 352:1419, 1998. © by The Lancet Ltd., 1998.)

cal therapy.[477] Factors that adversely affect the prospects of patients for returning to work include advanced age, postoperative angina, and a period of either unemployment or disability before surgery. Forty-seven percent of patients undergoing bypass surgery in the EAST Trial were able to engage in moderate or strenuous activity 3 years after the procedure.[364]

GRAFT PATENCY. Experimental studies and observations in patients suggest that the development of disease in venous aortocoronary artery bypass grafts occurs in several phases. The occlusion rate, which is high in the first year, decreases substantially between the first and sixth years. Between 6 and 10 years after surgery, the attrition rate for grafts increases again. Early occlusion (before hospital discharge) occurs in 8 to 12 percent of venous grafts, and by 1 year, 15 to 30 percent of vein grafts have become occluded.[478] After the first year, the annual occlusion rate is 2 percent and rises to approximately 4 percent annually between years 6 and 10. At 10 years, approximately 50 percent of vein grafts have become occluded, and significant atherosclerosis is present in the substantial proportion of grafts remaining patent, with significant stenoses in 20 to 40 percent.[423, 473, 478] Patency rates with IMA grafts are superior.

EARLY PHASE (FIRST MONTH). Technical factors that may cause thrombotic closure at the proximal or distal anastomoses include kinking because of excessive length, tension from insufficient length, poor graft flow, and inadequate distal runoff. Surgical manipulation of the saphenous vein during harvesting and preparation prior to grafting play key roles in initiating the sequence of endothelial damage with subsequent platelet and fibrin deposition leading to thrombosis.[421]

INTERMEDIATE PHASE (1 MONTH TO 1 YEAR). Vein grafts that have been implanted in the arterial circulation for 1 month to 1 year are subject to substantial endothelial denudation and proliferation and to migration of medial cells to the intima. Migration of vascular smooth muscle cells through the internal elastic lamina into the intima may also occur.[421] This initial phase of rapid proliferation is followed after several months by a marked increase in the connective tissue matrix, which further increases intimal and medial thickness. This accelerated process of intimal hyperplasia and thickening is an early stage of atherosclerotic plaque formation and is believed to occur because of interaction between platelets and macrophages and endothelial damage. If the proliferation is severe and localized, as may occur at the site of anastomosis between the grafts and the recipient artery, total occlusion can occur within 1 year.

LATE PHASE (BEYOND 1 YEAR). Some investigators believe that the development of atherosclerosis in vein grafts, as in native arteries, is a continuum starting from platelet deposition and advancing to smooth muscle cell proliferation and finally to lipid incorporation into the plaque. By 10 years, nearly half of venous grafts patent at 5 years have become occluded.[479] Beyond the first year, particularly after 3 to 5 years, the histological appearance of occluded or obstructed coronary bypass grafts is consistent with atherosclerosis. There is clear evidence of mature lipid-laden plaque, foam cells, cholesterol clefts, ulceration, and areas of calcification with disruption of the medial layer.[480] Late coronary atherosclerosis is often characterized by an extensive thrombotic burden and marked friability of the lesions; the resultant intermittent distal embolization in turn complicates repeat revascularization procedures either by percutaneous coronary reintervention or reoperation.[397, 481, 482]

DETERMINATION OF GRAFT PATENCY. Although angiography is the most frequently used method for the determination of vein graft patency, the diffuseness of the atherosclerotic process, which in many patients decreases the luminal diameter of the entire vessel, may lead to an underestimation of the severity of a more focal lesion. Alternative approaches to the evaluation of vein graft patency that are being investigated include contrast-enhanced CT, phase-contrast magnetic resonance angiography,[483] and transcutaneous[484] and magnetic resonance measurements of angiographic flow (see Chap. 10).[485]

PROGRESSION OF DISEASE IN NONGRAFTED ARTERIES. Disease progression, defined as worsening of a preexisting lesion or the appearance of a new diameter narrowing of 50 percent or greater, can occur at a rate of 20 to 40 percent over 5 to 10 years in nongrafted native vessels.[486] The rate of disease progression appears highest in arterial segments already showing evidence of disease,[487] and it is between three and six times higher in grafted native coronary arteries than in ungrafted native vessels. Disease progression is also greater in arteries with patent grafts than in arteries with occluded grafts[488] and usually occurs proximal to the site of graft insertion.[486, 487] These data suggest that bypassing an artery with minimal disease, even if initially successful, may ultimately be harmful to patients, who incur both the risk of graft closure and the increased risk of accelerated obstruction of native vessels.

EFFECTS OF THERAPY ON VEIN GRAFT OCCLUSION AND NATIVE VESSEL PROGRESSION

Measures aimed at enhancing long-term patency are generally directed at delaying the overall process of atherosclerosis, and as such, they may have several additional benefits.[482]

ANTIPLATELET THERAPY. A meta-analysis of clinical trials conducted before 1990 suggests that antiplatelet or anticoagulant therapy after coronary artery bypass surgery may prevent graft occlusion.[489] Several trials have demonstrated the efficacy of aspirin therapy when started 1, 7, or 24 hours preoperatively, but the benefit is lost when aspirin is started more than 48 hours postoperatively.[490] Aspirin, 100 to 325 mg/d should be continued indefinitely.[491] The addition of dipyridamole or warfarin in conventional doses has not been shown to provide added benefit.[492] Ticlopidine is effective but not superior to aspirin, and its use should be confined to patients who are intolerant of aspirin. Although the effects of clopidogrel on graft patency have not been studied specifically,[493] it is likely to be at least as effective as aspirin.

LIPID-LOWERING THERAPY. The rationale for lowering lipid levels in patients with CAD was extended to postoperative patients with at least one patent vein graft and LDL cholesterol concentrations between 130 and 175 mg/dl in the Post-Coronary Artery Bypass Graft Trial.[191] Patients who received aggressive treatment with lovastatin and, if needed, cholestyramine to decrease LDL cholesterol to less than 100 mg/dl, in comparison with "moderate" therapy resulting in an LDL cholesterol level of 134 mg/dl, had a lower rate of progressive atherosclerosis in grafts (27 vs. 39 percent, $p < 0.001$) and a lower rate of repeat revascularization procedures over a 4-year period. A similar benefit in both native vessels and grafts was noted in the Cholesterol-Lowering Atherosclerosis Study (CLAS), which used combined colestipol and niacin therapy.[494] The Lipid Coronary Angiography Trial (LOCAT) compared gemfibrozil and placebo in patients with LDL cholesterol concentrations of 175 mg/dl or lower and an HDL cholesterol of less than 42 mg/dl. The treated group had a lower rate of progression of native coronary atherosclerosis and a lower incidence of new lesions in the vein graft (2 vs. 14 percent) after an average 32-month follow-up.[194]

SMOKING CESSATION. Strong evidence from the CASS randomized trial and other series indicates that continued smoking after bypass surgery increases mortality, the recurrence rate of angina, the need for repeat hospitalization, and repeat revascularization procedures.[160, 161] Not unexpectedly, continued smoking has been associated with angiographic progression of graft disease.

Patient Selection

Indications for coronary bypass surgery consist of the need for improvement in the quality and/or the duration of life. Patients whose angina is not controlled by medical management or who have unacceptable side effects with such management should be considered for coronary revascularization. The decision to perform PCI or CABG is based partly on coronary anatomy, left ventricular function, and patient preference. Recent technological developments have enlarged the pool of patients with single-vessel or multivessel disease amenable to PCI. For patients who are suitable for PCI and who do not fulfill the criteria of anatomy requiring surgery (e.g., left main CAD or severe three-vessel disease and left ventricular dysfunction), PCI is generally the procedure of choice. However, if medical therapy has failed, i.e., the symptoms are severe or sufficient to impair quality of life, and the patient is not a good candidate for PCI, CABG should be strongly considered. This procedure is also indicated for patients with CAD, regardless of symptoms, in whom survival is likely to be prolonged,[495] and for patients in whom noninvasive testing suggests "high risk," independent of symptoms.[496]

In making the decision about revascularization, it is important to assess the patient's prognosis (Table 37–10) and

▼ TABLE 37–10. DETERMINANTS OF ADVERSE PROGNOSIS IN PATIENTS WITH CORONARY ARTERY DISEASE

CARDIAC DETERMINANTS
  Left ventricular dysfunction
  Extent of myocardial jeopardy—extent of ischemia at rest and with exercise and the number of large vessels diseased
  Extent of myocardium in jeopardy
  Abnormal arrhythmic substrate
CLINICAL AND ELECTROCARDIOGRAPHIC MODIFYING FACTORS
  Advanced age
  History of congestive heart failure
  Diabetes
  Rapidly accelerating angina
  Resting electrocardiographic abnormalities
  Left ventricular hypertrophy and hypertension
  Peripheral vascular disease
  Hyperlipidemia

how it may be affected by surgery. The key initial step is to stratify patients into categories of risk with continued medical therapy based on an analysis of clinical, noninvasive, and, in some patients, angiographic variables. This process defines the *indications* for revascularization over medical therapy and, by implication, the indications for coronary angiography in patients with chronic stable angina. More recent randomized trial data are helpful in finding which *modality* of revascularization (PCI or surgery) is preferable.[496]

The four major determinants of risk in CAD are the extent of ischemia, the number of vessels diseased, left ventricular function, and the electrical substrate (Fig. 37–13). The major effect of coronary revascularization is on ische-

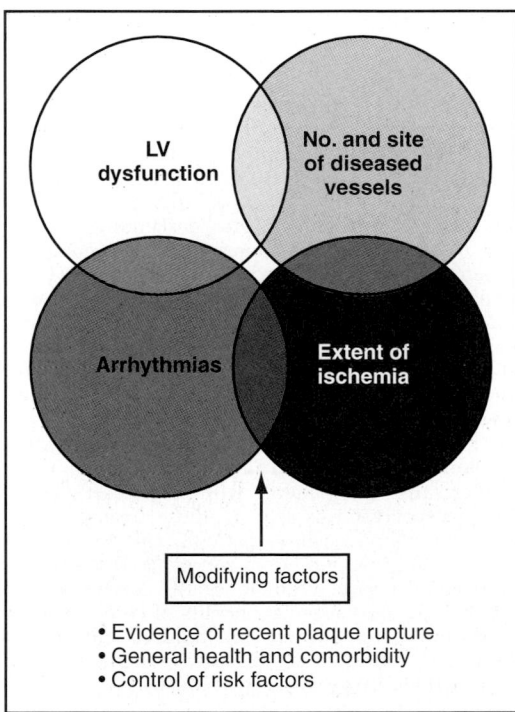

FIGURE 37–13. Risk stratification in coronary artery disease (CAD). A Venn diagram illustrates factors affecting the prognosis of chronic CAD. Major determinants are the severity of symptoms and/or ischemia, presence of multivessel disease and in particular three-vessel disease, extent of myocardial jeopardy as defined by clinical stenoses in the left main coronary artery and proximal left anterior descending coronary artery, and left ventricular dysfunction. Interactions between an abnormal arrhythmic substrate, evidence of recent plaque rupture (acute coronary syndromes), and general health and coexisting conditions are important.

mia, and the magnitude of the benefit compared with that of medical therapy is enhanced with left ventricular dysfunction, particularly in the presence of reversibly ischemic jeopardized myocardium. In this context, patients can be risk-stratified according to the expected benefit of revascularization versus medical therapy. Patients with more extensive and severe CAD have an increasing magnitude of benefit from CABG over medical therapy (Fig. 37–14A and Table 37–11). Selection of patients for surgery is based on clinical, angiographic, and noninvasive testing characteristics that may be considered markers or, in some cases, surrogates of the three major predictors—ischemia, left ventricular function, and, to a lesser extent, arrhythmia. Other factors that must always be considered in the decision are general health and noncoronary comorbid conditions.

Natural History of Angina Pectoris

CLINICAL AND ELECTROCARDIOGRAPHIC CRITERIA. Data from the Framingham Study, obtained before the widespread use of aspirin, beta blockers, and aggressive modification of risk factors, showed that the average annual mortality rate of patients with chronic stable angina was 4 percent.[497] The combination of these treatments has improved prognosis. Nonetheless, a recent study from the United Kingdom of patients evaluated for the first time with typical angina has suggested that the prognosis should be guarded because over a 15-month period, 4 percent mortality and a 7 percent rate of nonfatal myocardial infarction were noted, and only 11 percent had spontaneous remission of angina.[498] Several studies have shown that a composite risk score based on multiple clinical variables (e.g., age, sex, diabetes, previous myocardial infarction, and the nature of the chest pain) may be quite strongly predictive of the presence of severe CAD (triple-vessel or left main CAD) and thus provide a strong indication for angiography[35, 499] (see Fig. 37–14 and Table 37–11). Numerous studies attest to the adverse prognostic effect of congestive heart failure (based on a clinical history of cardiomegaly on chest radiography), previous myocardial infarction, hypertension, and advanced age in patients with stable angina pectoris.[79, 497, 498] A third heart sound is a useful clinical predictor of an abnormal left ventricular ejection fraction and an adverse prognosis in patients with CAD. The severity of angina, especially the tempo of intensification, is also an important predictor of outcome.

On the other hand, a normal resting ECG in patients with stable angina pectoris speaks in favor of well-preserved left ventricular function and a favorable long-term prognosis[364] (see p. 1277). Among 14,507 patients with chest pain enrolled in the CASS Registry, 91.8 percent of those with a normal ECG had an ejection fraction greater than 50 percent and only 0.6 percent had an ejection frac-

▼ TABLE 37–11. IMPACT OF CORONARY BYPASS SURGERY ON SURVIVAL IN SUBSETS OF PATIENTS STUDIED IN THE CORONARY ARTERY SURGERY STUDY (CASS) RANDOMIZED TRIAL AND REGISTRY STUDIES

CATEGORY OF RISK	NUMBER OF VESSELS DISEASED	SEVERITY OF ISCHEMIA	EJECTION FRACTION	RESULTS OF SURGERY ON SURVIVAL
Mild	2	Mild	>0.50	Unchanged*
	3			Unchanged*
Moderate	2	Moderate to severe	>0.50	Unchanged*
	3			Improved†
	2	Mild	<0.50	Unchanged*
	3			Improved†
Severe	2	Moderate to severe	<0.50	Improved†
	3			Improved†

*Randomized trial.
†Survival improved with surgery versus medicine. In the European Coronary Surgery Trial, patients with double-vessel disease and involvement of the paroxysmal left anterior descending coronary artery had improved survival with surgery irrespective of left ventricular function.

tion less than 35 percent.[500] Left ventricular hypertrophy, as determined on the ECG or echocardiogram, is associated with increased mortality.[501] Although the presence of calcium in the coronary arteries on chest radiography, fluoroscopy, or electron beam CT is associated with an adverse prognosis and correlates to some extent with the severity of CAD, the presence and extent of calcification cannot be used at this stage as an indication for angiography or coronary revascularization.[35]

In summary, a comprehensive clinical evaluation pro-

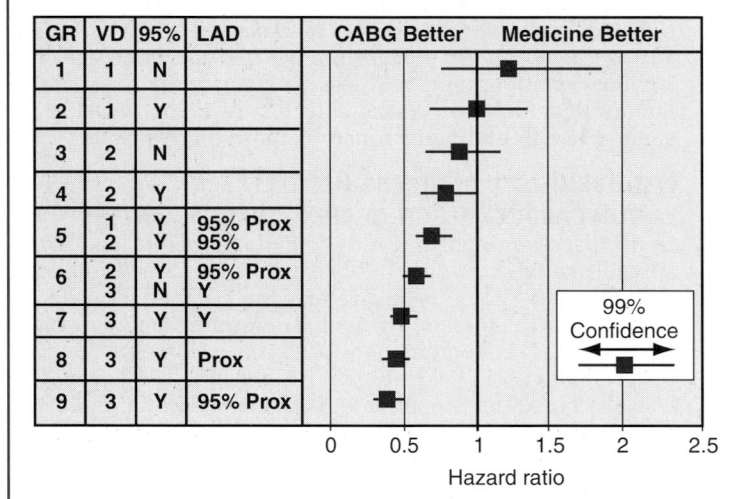

FIGURE 37–14. A, Adjusted hazard (mortality) ratios comparing coronary artery bypass grafting (CABG) and medical therapy for nine coronary anatomy severity groups (GR) according to the number of vessels diseased (VD), the presence or absence of a 95 percent proximal stenosis (95 percent), and involvement of the left anterior descending coronary artery (LAD). B, Adjusted hazard (mortality) ratios comparing CABG and percutaneous transluminal angioplasty (PTCA) for nine coronary anatomy groups according to the number of vessels diseased, the presence or absence of a 95 percent proximal stenosis, and LAD involvement. Among patients with the least severe categories of disease, 5-year survival appears to be better with PTCA (single-vessel disease without proximal stenosis and without LAD involvement), whereas for patients with three-vessel disease and higher-grade, more complex two-vessel disease, a survival benefit is noted with surgery. For other subsets of patients with two-vessel disease, no difference in survival was seen in those treated with CABG or PTCA, and many of these patients are probably similar to those included in the randomized trials. (Data from the Duke University data base. From Jones RH, Kesler K, Phillips HR III, et al: Long-term survival benefits of coronary artery bypass grafting and percutaneous transluminal angioplasty in patients with coronary artery disease. J Thorac Cardiovasc Surg 111:1013, 1996. By permission of Mosby.)

vides useful prognostic information in addition to being an indispensable basis for assessing the risk of a procedure and the likelihood of sustained benefits.

NONINVASIVE STRESS TESTING (see p. 1278). One of the most valuable aspects of noninvasive imaging is the echocardiographic assessment of left ventricular function. Such testing is not necessary for all patients, and among patients with a normal ECG and no previous history of myocardial infarction, the likelihood of preserved left ventricular systolic function is high. In contrast, among patients with a history of myocardial infarction, ST-T wave changes, or conduction defects or Q waves on the ECG, left ventricular function should be measured with echocardiography or an equivalent technique.[35] In patients in whom left ventricular function and coronary anatomy have already been defined, stress testing may provide additional prognostic information about the functional significance of specific angiographic lesions.

The prognostic importance of the treadmill exercise test was determined by several observational studies in the 1980s and early 1990s, and these studies have had a major influence on current indications for coronary revascularization.[35] One of the most important and consistent predictors is the maximal exercise capacity, regardless of whether it is measured by exercise duration or workload achieved or whether the test was terminated because of dyspnea, fatigue, or angina.[35, 502, 503] Other factors with a poor prognosis identified in individual series of patients with chronic stable angina are described in Table 37–2 (see p. 1280).

Prognostic Scores. The impact of the magnitude of exercise-induced ischemia on prognosis as defined by symptoms or ST segment deviation has led to the development of various prognostic scores that appear to work well in both the inpatient and outpatient settings. Mark and colleagues developed a prognostic score that incorporates exercise duration, the magnitude of ST segment deviation, and exercise-induced angina.[502] Patients were stratified into three groups with an average annual mortality of 0.25, 1.25, and 5.0 percent. Moreover, the score contained incremental information beyond that provided by clinical and catheterization data.[502]

Stress Thallium-201 Myocardial Perfusion Imaging (see also Chaps. 9 and 13 and p. 1278). A normal stress thallium study is highly predictive of a favorable prognosis in patients with and without documented CAD.[35, 75, 504] In an analysis of 16 studies involving more than 3500 patients, the rate of cardiac death and myocardial infarction over a mean follow-up period of 29 months was only 0.9 percent. In patients with documented CAD, the single most powerful prognostic factor was the magnitude of the perfusion abnormality on SPECT thallium-201 scintigraphy.[505] Pharmacological stress perfusion imaging techniques with dipyridamole, adenosine, or dobutamine have an established place as an alternative to exercise perfusion imaging in establishing the prognosis in patients with stable CAD.[74, 506]

Stress Echocardiography (see also Chap. 7 and p. 1279). Evidence is increasingly demonstrating that echocardiography with exercise or pharmacological stress (dobutamine, arbutamine, or dipyridamole) is both sensitive and specific for the identification of myocardial ischemia and for risk stratification in patients with chronic stable angina.[98, 507, 508] The presence or absence of inducible regional wall motion abnormalities and the response of the ejection fraction to exercise appear to provide incremental prognostic information in addition to the assessment of cardiac structure and function provided by the resting echocardiogram. Moreover, a negative stress test portends a very low risk for future events.[509] Although most studies demonstrated enhanced diagnostic accuracy for dobutamine stress echocardiography, the prognostic value of dipyridamole and dobutamine may be similar.[510]

The choice of a particular stress testing modality in a

patient with chronic stable angina undergoing assessment for coronary revascularization depends on several clinical issues that may limit the technical quality of the echocardiographic images, such as the presence of obesity or chronic obstructive pulmonary disease. Nonetheless, the most vital factor to be considered is probably the level of expertise that an institution has with each technique.

ANGIOGRAPHIC CRITERIA. The independent impact of multivessel disease and left ventricular dysfunction and their interaction on the prognosis of patients with CAD has been well documented[511, 512] and provides a logical framework for coronary angiography in the assessment of prognosis (Fig. 37–15). These two risk factors are synergistic in that the adverse effects of impaired ventricular function on prognosis are more pronounced as the number of stenotic vessels increases.[511]

Although several indices have been used to quantify the extent of severity of CAD, the simple classification of disease into one-vessel, two-vessel, three-vessel, or left main CAD is the most widely used and is effective.[511, 513] Addi-

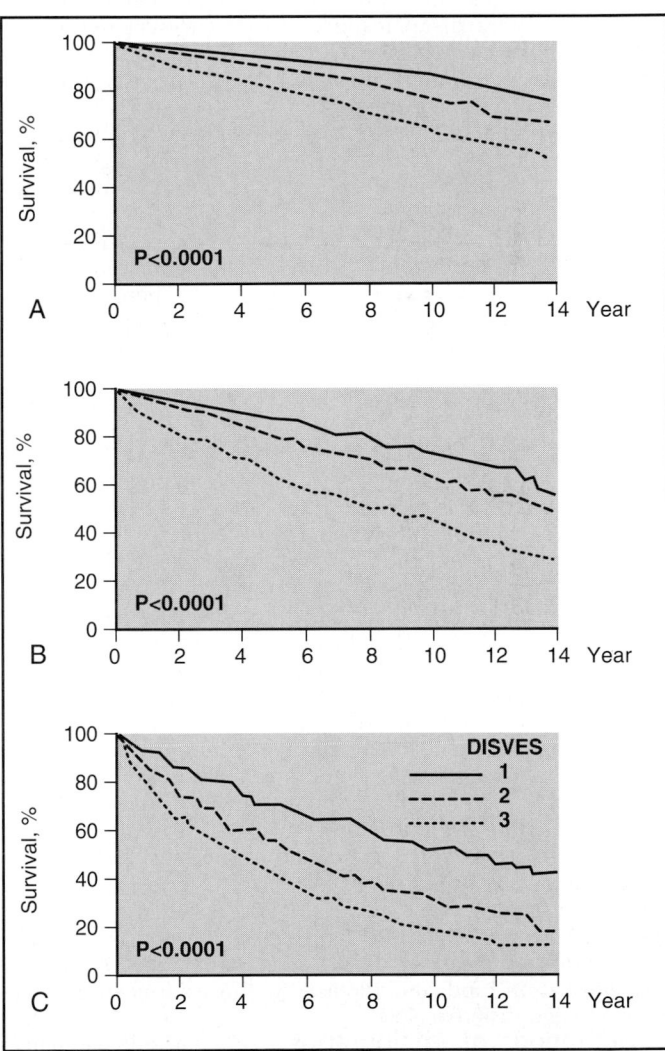

FIGURE 37–15. Graphs showing survival for medically treated CASS patients. *A,* Patients with one-, two-, or three-vessel disease and an ejection fraction of 50 to 100 percent stratified by the number of diseased vessels (DISVES). *B,* Patients with one-, two-, or three-vessel disease and an ejection fraction of 35 to 49 percent stratified by the number of diseased vessels. *C,* Patients with one-, two-, or three-vessel disease and an ejection fraction of 0 to 34 percent stratified by the number of diseased vessels. (From Emond M, Mock MB, Davis KB, et al: Long-term survival of medically treated patients in the Coronary Artery Surgery Study (CASS) Registry. Circulation 90:2645, 1994. By permission of the American Heart Association, Inc.)

tional prognostic information is provided by the severity of obstruction and the location, whether proximal or distal.[35, 514] The concept of the gradient of risk is illustrated in Figure 37–14, which was derived from the Duke University data base of patients treated medically. Among medically treated patients in CASS, the 12-year survival rate was 91 percent among those with chronic angina and angiographically normal vessels. In the presence of single-vessel disease, it was 86 percent for patients with at least one obstruction of 30 to 50 percent, 79 percent for patients with at least one stenosis of 50 to 70 percent, and 74 percent for patients with single-vessel disease and stenosis of 70 percent or more.[511]

Studies of treated symptomatic patients have revealed that if only one of the three major coronary arteries has more than 50 percent stenosis, the annual mortality rate is approximately 2 percent.[515] The importance to survival of the quantity of myocardium that is jeopardized is reflected in the observation that an obstructive lesion proximal to the first septal perforating branch of the left anterior descending coronary artery was associated with a 5-year survival rate of 90 percent in comparison with 98 percent for patients with more distal lesions.[515] The survival rate of patients with isolated right CAD at 5 years appeared to be higher (96 percent) than for patients with disease of the left anterior descending coronary artery (92 percent). The overall survival of medically treated patients with left anterior descending and left circumflex CAD was not significantly different, but both were less than the survival of patients with isolated right CAD.[515]

The impact of left ventricular dysfunction is illustrated by the 12-year survival rates of unoperated patients in the CASS Registry, which were 73, 54, and 21 percent among patients with ejection fractions of 50 percent or higher, 35 to 49 percent, and less than 35 percent, respectively[511] (Fig. 37–15).

In the example used in the ACC/AHA guidelines,[35] a 65-year-old man with three-vessel disease and stable angina has a 5-year survival rate ranging from 93 to 58 percent, according to the presence or absence of congestive heart failure and a decreased ejection fraction.

High-grade lesions of the left main coronary artery or its "equivalents," as defined by severe proximal left anterior descending and proximal left circumflex CAD, are particularly life threatening.[516] Mortality among medically treated patients has been reported to be 29 percent at 18 months, 39 percent at 2 years, and 43 percent at 5 years.[516] Survival is better for patients with 50 to 70 percent stenosis (1- and 3-year survival rates of 91 and 66 percent, respectively) than for patients with a left main coronary artery stenosis greater than 70 percent (1- and 3-year survival rates of 72 and 41 percent).[517] Furthermore, a number of characteristics found at catheterization or on noninvasive examination are predictors of an adverse prognosis in patients with 70 percent or greater left main coronary artery stenosis, including chest pain at rest, ST-T wave changes on resting ECG, cardiomegaly on chest radiography, a history of congestive heart failure, findings of left ventricular dysfunction at catheterization, and an increase in the arterial–mixed venous oxygen difference.[517]

Limitations of Angiography. The pathophysiological significance of coronary stenoses lies in their impact on resting and exercise-induced blood flow, in addition to their potential for plaque rupture with superimposed thrombotic occlusion. It is generally accepted that a stenosis of greater than 60 percent of the luminal diameter is hemodynamically significant in that it may be responsible for a reduction in exercise-induced myocardial blood flow and cause angina and ischemia[518] (see Chap. 34). The functional significance of obstruction of "intermediate" severity (approximately 50 percent diameter stenosis) is less well established. Coronary angiography is not a reliable indica-

tor of the functional significance of stenosis, nor is it sensitive to the presence of thrombus.[519] Moreover, the coronary angiographic determinants of the severity of stenosis are based on a decrease in the caliber of the lumen at the site of the lesion *relative* to adjacent reference segments, which are considered, often erroneously, to be relatively free of disease. This approach may lead to significant underestimation of the severity and extent of atherosclerosis.[520] Furthermore, assessment of left main stem disease, particularly in vessels with lesser degrees of obstruction, is not optimal.[521]

Another limitation to the routine use of coronary angiography for prognosis in patients with chronic stable angina is its inability to identify which coronary lesions can be considered to be at high risk for future events, such as myocardial infarction or sudden death. Although it is widely accepted that myocardial infarction is the result of thrombotic occlusion at the site of plaque rupture (see Chap. 35), a growing body of evidence indicates that it is not necessarily the plaque causing the most severe stenosis that subsequently ruptures.[522] Several studies of patients undergoing serial coronary angiography indicate that myocardial infarction often arises from rupture of the plaque that did *not* cause critical obstruction. Lesions causing mild obstructions can rupture, thrombose, and occlude, thereby leading to myocardial infarction and sudden death.[523–525] In contrast, arteries with severe preexisting stenoses may proceed to clinically silent complete occlusion, often without infarction, presumably because of the formation of collaterals as ischemia gradually becomes more severe.

In summary, angiographic documentation of the extent of CAD is an indispensable step in the selection of patients for coronary revascularization, particularly if the interaction between the anatomical extent of disease, left ventricular function, and the severity of ischemia is taken into account. However, angiography is not helpful in predicting the site of subsequent occlusions that could cause myocardial infarction or sudden cardiac death, particularly in an individual patient.

In the characterization of lesion morphology and severity, intravascular ultrasonography (see Chap. 12) may be helpful, particularly in patients undergoing PCI.[526] Assessment of coronary flow reserve with Doppler techniques and assessment of transstenotic gradients at baseline and during maximal hyperemia (see Chap. 34) are tools that, in an experienced laboratory, may also be helpful in deciding on the flow-limiting significance of a specific lesion and the need for coronary revascularization.[527]

Results

In 1972, a committee of the AHA indicated that the most widely accepted indication for surgical revascularization was "significant disability from moderate to severe angina pectoris, unresponsive to optimal medical care." Three decades later, the realization that CABG prolongs survival in subgroups of patients with either minimal or mild to moderate symptoms has shifted the emphasis toward *ischemia* instead of *symptoms alone* as the target for coronary revascularization. Consequently and appropriately, CABG is currently performed in an increasing number of patients with multivessel disease and/or left ventricular dysfunction (particularly in the face of viable jeopardized dysfunctioning myocardium) and in patients with poor exercise tolerance in the presence of stress-induced ischemia. Severe ischemia and/or reversible left ventricular dysfunction provides a window of opportunity for improving survival (in comparison to medical therapy) that has resulted in an increase in the frequency of CABG in patients with unstable angina and in survivors of acute myocardial infarction. Left ventricular dysfunction, initially a relative contraindication for surgery, has become a major indication. Nonetheless, severe symptoms or even moderate symptoms that interfere with the quality of life despite adequate medical therapy are still as firm an indication for coronary revascularization (PCI or CABG) as they were for CABG almost three decades ago.

Relief of Angina

CABG is highly effective in providing complete relief from angina in some patients and improvement in the severity of symptoms in most of the rest (Fig. 37–12). In a series of patients who received saphenous vein grafts alone, approximately 90 percent were free of angina at 1 year. In the following 4 years, the recurrence rate was approximately 3 percent per year and 5 percent per year thereafter. Approximate rates of freedom from angina were 78 percent at 5 years, which decreased to 52 and 23 percent at 10 and 15 years, respectively.[528] The major randomized trials have all demonstrated greater relief of angina, better exercise performance, and a lower requirement for antianginal medications for surgically versus medically treated patients 5 years postoperatively.[495, 529–531] Beyond 5 years, differences in symptoms between patients initially treated medically and surgically are diminished, in part because of the high "crossover" rate from medical to surgical therapy in patients with continued symptoms and progression of disease in vein grafts and nonbypassed vessels in the surgical group.[529, 530] The 22-year follow-up of the Veterans Administration (VA) Trial demonstrated no difference in the severity of angina between medically and surgically treated groups after 10 years.[532] These results must be tempered by the low rate of initial complete revascularization, absence of the use of an IMA graft, and lack of platelet inhibitor therapy and risk factor reduction in this trial, which reflected the very early part of the "learning curve" of coronary bypass surgery.[533] The reoperation rate for recurrence of symptoms has been reported to be in the range of 6 to 8 percent per year.[534]

For patients with persistent angina despite adequate medical therapy or for patients who do not tolerate medications or who are not suitable candidates for PCI, coronary bypass grafting provides excellent symptomatic relief.[35] With increasing use of IMA grafts, long-term relief from angina and freedom from subsequent cardiac events are improved in comparison to previous patient populations who received vein grafts alone.

In summary, after 5 years, approximately three-fourths of surgically treated patients can be predicted to be free of an ischemic event, sudden death, occurrence of myocardial infarction, or the recurrence of angina; about half remain free for approximately 10 years and about 15 percent for 15 or more years. Symptomatic improvement is best maintained in patients with the most complete revascularization.[453, 528]

Effects on Survival

Current clinical practice has been shaped by three major randomized trials that enrolled patients between 1972 and 1979: the VA Trial, the European Cardiac Society Study (ECSS), and the National Institutes of Health–supported CASS (Fig. 37–16 and Table 37–12).[531, 535–539] These trials antedated widespread use of the IMA for revascularization, as well as the use of aspirin and coronary angioplasty. The extent of the completeness of coronary revascularization, graft patency rates, and perioperative mortality in the VA Trial fall far short of current expectations and reflect, in part, the initial learning experience of coronary bypass surgery.

In the VA Study, no significant difference was found in overall survival between the groups initially assigned to medical or surgical treatment after 11 years of follow-up. However, higher-risk subsets, including patients with left main coronary disease and patients who had three-vessel disease with impaired left ventricular function, initially had a significant survival advantage with surgery, although the magnitude of the difference decreased between 7 and 11 years. On retrospective analysis, a higher-risk subset, those with two or more of the following risk factors—New York Heart Association Class III or IV angina, a history of hypertension, a history of prior myocardial infarction, and ST segment depression on the resting ECG—experienced a survival benefit from surgery.[537]

Patients randomly assigned to an initial surgical approach also experienced an overall survival advantage in the ECSS.[531] Again, the benefits of surgery were greater in patients at higher risk, including those with multivessel disease that included the proximal left anterior descending coronary artery, older patients, those with evidence of ischemia or infarction on the resting ECG, patients with peripheral vascular disease, and those with a markedly positive stress test. No significant difference in survival was seen between medical and surgical treatment in patients with one-vessel disease and those with two-vessel disease without critical stenosis of the proximal left anterior descending coronary artery. In the CASS randomized trial, no difference in overall survival was found between the medically and surgically treated groups.[535, 539] However, survival of patients at higher risk, e.g., those with a left ventricular ejection fraction between 35 and 50 percent, was improved by surgery.[535]

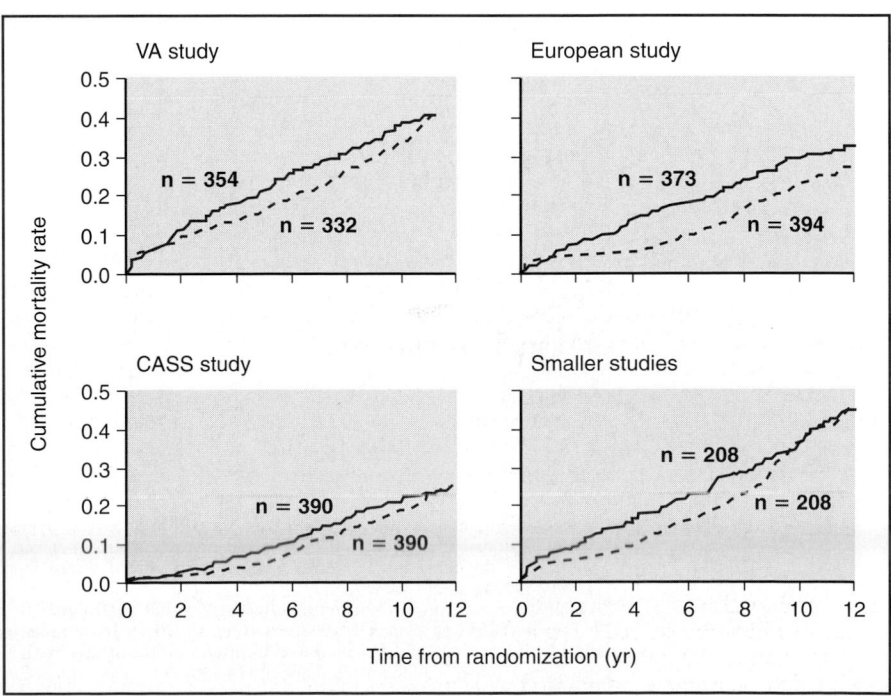

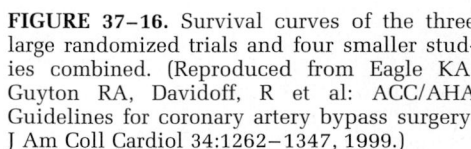

FIGURE 37–16. Survival curves of the three large randomized trials and four smaller studies combined. (Reproduced from Eagle KA, Guyton RA, Davidoff, R et al: ACC/AHA Guidelines for coronary artery bypass surgery. J Am Coll Cardiol 34:1262–1347, 1999.)

LEFT MAIN CORONARY ARTERY STENOSIS. It is widely agreed that surgical treatment improves survival in patients with left main coronary artery obstruction[540] or its "equivalent." The CASS Registry demonstrated that the superiority of revascularization was equivalent in both symptomatic and asymptomatic patients with disease affecting the left main coronary artery.[516, 541]

Whether a "left main equivalent" anatomy exists that has a natural history similar to that of left main CAD is uncertain. The condition in question may consist of disease in the proximal portions of both the left anterior descending and left circumflex coronary arteries. It is likely that significant left main coronary disease has an ominous nature, because a single event (rupture of a single plaque) can cause infarction of a very large quantity of myocardium. Consequently, although combined disease of the proximal left anterior descending and circumflex coronary arteries does identify a subgroup of high-risk patients, the prognosis is not as poor as it is for patients with left main CAD.[542] Nevertheless, patients with combined stenoses of 70 percent or greater in the left anterior descending coronary artery, before the first septal perforating branch, and in the proximal circumflex coronary artery, before the first obtuse marginal branch, who have impaired ventricular function also have improved survival and less angina following surgical revascularization than if they are treated medically, particularly in the face of left ventricular dysfunction. The median survival of surgically treated patients with left main–equivalent disease is 13.1 years versus 6.2 years for those medically treated.[541]

OVERVIEW OF THE RANDOMIZED TRIALS. A systematic overview of the seven randomized trials (the three aforementioned large trials and four smaller trials) that compared coronary bypass surgery with medical therapy between 1972 and 1984 yielded 2649 patients (see Fig. 37–16 and Table 37–12). In interpreting this overview, it must be appreciated that surgical treatment has improved significantly in the past 25 years and that outcomes have been improved, in particular with the widespread use of one or two IMAs. Patients undergoing CABG had a significantly lower mortality at 5, 7, and 10 years, but by 10 years, 41 percent of the patients initially randomly assigned to medical treatment had undergone CABG (so-called crossovers). The advantage for surgery was greatest in patients with left main CAD. An improvement in survival was also noted with surgical treatment in patients with one- or two-vessel disease and stenosis of the proximal left anterior descending coronary artery. Among patients without obstruction of the proximal left anterior descending coronary artery, the reduction in mortality was confined to those with left main coronary artery or three-vessel disease.

To place the relevant and absolute benefits of coronary bypass surgery into perspective, patients were further stratified into high-, moderate- and low-risk subgroups by using criteria developed by the VA Cooperative Study.[537] These criteria were based on clinical findings and included the severity of angina, history of hypertension, prior myocardial infarction, and ST segment depression at rest. Low-risk patients had none of the four risk factors aside from ST segment depression, whereas those with two or three risk factors were considered to be at high risk. In patients at high risk, the mortality reduction was 29 percent at 10 years versus 10 percent for patients at moderate risk. In low-risk patients, a nonsignificant trend was seen toward greater mortality with bypass surgery.

The results of all the trials and registries[538] taken to-

▼ **TABLE 37–12. EFFECTS OF CORONARY ARTERY BYPASS GRAFT SURGERY ON SURVIVAL***

SUBGROUP	MEDICAL TREATMENT MORTALITY RATE (%)	p VALUE FOR CABG SURGERY VS. MEDICAL TREATMENT
VESSEL DISEASE		
One vessel	9.9	0.18
Two vessels	11.7	0.45
Three vessels	17.6	<0.001
Left main artery	36.5	0.004
NO LAD DISEASE		
One or two vessels	8.3	0.88
Three vessels	14.5	0.02
Left main artery	45.8	0.03
Overall	12.3	0.05
LAD DISEASE PRESENT		
One or two vessels	14.6	0.05
Three vessels	19.1	0.009
Left main artery	32.7	0.02
Overall	18.3	0.001
LV FUNCTION		
Normal	13.3	<0.001
Abnormal	25.2	0.02
EXERCISE TEST STATUS		
Missing	17.4	0.10
Normal	11.6	0.38
Abnormal	16.8	<0.001
SEVERITY OF ANGINA		
Class 0, I, II	12.5	0.005
Class III, IV	22.4	0.001

*Systematic overview of the effect of coronary artery bypass graft (CABG) surgery versus medical therapy on survival based on data from the seven randomized trials comparing a strategy of initial CABG surgery with one of initial medical therapy. Subgroup results at 5 years are shown.

LAD = left anterior descending artery; LV = left ventricular.

From Yusuf S, Zucker D, Peduzzi P, et al: Effect of coronary artery bypass surgery on survival: Overview of 10-year results from randomized trials by the Coronary Artery Bypass Surgery Trialists Collaboration. Lancet 344:563, © by The Lancet Ltd., 1994.

gether indicate that the "sicker" the patient (based on the severity of symptoms or ischemia, age, the number of vessels diseased, and the presence of left ventricular dysfunction), the greater the benefit of surgical over medical therapy on survival (see Table 37–12).[348, 514] Among low-risk patients and patients with single-vessel disease, no trial has demonstrated any benefit on survival.

Thus, CABG prolongs survival in patients with significant left main CAD irrespective of symptoms, in patients with multivessel disease and impaired left ventricular function, and in patients with three-vessel disease that includes the proximal left anterior descending coronary artery (irrespective of left ventricular function).[495, 543] Surgical therapy has also been demonstrated to prolong life in patients with *two-vessel disease* and left ventricular dysfunction, particularly those with proximal narrowing of one or more coronary arteries and in the presence of severe angina.[544] Although no study has documented a survival benefit with surgical treatment in patients with *single-vessel disease*, some evidence indicates that such patients who have impaired left ventricular function have a poor long-term survival.[511] Such patients with angina or evidence of ischemia at a low or moderate level of exercise, especially those with obstruction of the proximal left anterior descending coronary artery, may benefit from coronary revascularization by either PCI or bypass surgery.

The only randomized data comparing CABG with medical therapy in the current era are from the Asymptomatic Cardiac Ischemia Pilot (ACIP) Study of 558 patients[545] (Fig. 37–17). This trial of angina-guided versus angina plus ischemia–guided medical therapy (using ambulatory monitoring) in comparison to revascularization by either PTCA (92 patients) or CABG (79 patients) enrolled relatively low-risk patients. After 2 years of follow-up, mortality was significantly lower among the patients assigned to routine revascularization (1.1 vs. 6.6 and 4.4 percent for the two medical groups [*p* < 0.02]), and rates of death or myocardial infarction were 12.1 (angina-guided medical therapy), 8.9 (ischemia-guided medical therapy), and 4.7 percent following coronary revascularization (*p* < 0.04). Although this trial was designed as a pilot study and the number of patients was relatively small, the observed risk reductions were statistically significant and suggest that the benefits of revascularization in the context of current revascularization technique may be greater than previously appreciated. The trial was not designed to assess differences between PTCA and bypass surgery but does point to the need for larger, more definitive randomized trials testing contemporary strategies of revascularization with optimal medical therapy and risk factor reduction.

The major randomized trials of patients with mild to moderate angina suggested that the likelihood of occurrence of myocardial infarction after 5 to 10 years of follow-up was similar in medically and surgically treated patients.[531, 537, 538, 546, 547] In both the VA Study and the CASS, the major benefit of surgery on myocardial infarction does not appear to be mediated by a decrease in the frequency of myocardial infarction but by a decrease in the case fatality rate of patients who subsequently have infarction.[548] Potential explanations are that previous bypass surgery results in smaller infarcts caused by distal occlusions and that the bypass may enhance myocardial perfusion distal to the obstructing lesion.[549]

Patients with Depressed Left Ventricular Function

Depressed *left ventricular function* is one of the most powerful predictors of perioperative and late mortality.[550–553] In the Society of Thoracic Surgeons data base[425] (www.ctsnenet.org), the mean ejection fraction among approximately 161,000 patients undergoing initial coronary bypass in 1997 was approximately 51 percent, and approximately 25 percent had an ejection fraction less than 45 percent. Moreover, as the population ages and the proportion undergoing reoperation increases, the number of patients with preoperative left ventricular dysfunction and clinical heart failure will increase. In the CABG Patch Trial confined to patients with an ejection fraction of 35 percent of less, perioperative mortality was 3.5 percent for patients without clinical signs of heart failure versus 7.7 percent for those with New York Heart Association Class I to IV heart failure.[554] The latter was a powerful independent predictor of increased operative mortality in patients with ventricular dysfunction and a positive signal-averaged ECG[554] (odds ratio, 2.4; *p* = 0.01).

Although the effect of a reduced ejection fraction on operative mortality cannot be eliminated, careful attention to intraoperative metabolic, inotropic, and mechanical support, including preoperative intraaortic balloon counterpulsation in some patients, may decrease perioperative mortality in comparison with the mortality rates expected from prediction models.[555]

The powerful effect of the preoperative ejection fraction on late survival emphasizes that in the current era, the presence of left ventricular dysfunction has changed from a relative contraindication to coronary bypass to a very strong indication.[552] This shift in focus has been due to the realization that viable dysfunctioning myocardium may improve after coronary revascularization.[550, 556] Indeed, the

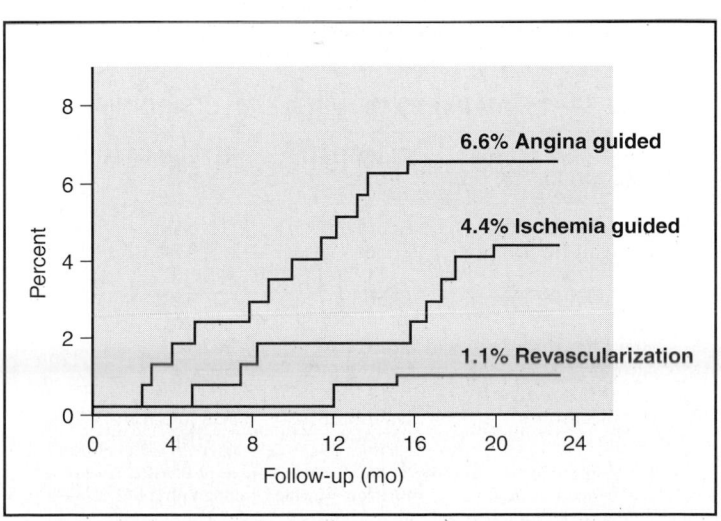

FIGURE 37–17. Two-year cumulative mortality rates for the three treatment strategies in the Asymptomatic Cardiac Ischemia Pilot (ACIP) study. Significant differences were seen between revascularization and angina-guided strategies (*p* ≤ 0.005) and between revascularization and ischemia-guided strategies (*p* ≤ 0.05). Angina-guided and ischemia-guided strategies were not significantly different from each other (*p* = 0.34). Similar results were noted for the endpoints of cumulative rates of death, myocardial infarction, or cardiac hospitalization. (From Davies RF, Goldberg AD, Forman S, et al: Asymptomatic Cardiac Ischemia Pilot [ACIP] study two-year follow-up: Outcomes of patients randomized to initial strategies of medical therapy versus revascularization. Circulation 95:2037, 1997. By permission of the American Heart Association, Inc.)

most striking survival benefits of CABG, as well as symptomatic and functional improvement, are shown by patients with seriously impaired left ventricular function in whom the prognosis of medical therapy is poor.[88, 555-558] In patients with a history of congestive heart failure and multivessel (particularly three-vessel) disease, coronary bypass surgery may also reduce the incidence of sudden cardiac death.[559] Although preoperative left ventricular dysfunction creates the potential for significant benefit, the perioperative risk should not be underestimated, particularly in the setting of clinical congestive heart failure.[550] In the CASS Registry, operative mortality was 1.97 percent and the 5-year survival rate was 92 percent for patients with normal or nearly normal left ventricular function; operative mortality was 4.2 percent and the 5-year survival rate was 80 percent for those with an ejection fraction of 0.35 to 0.49, and for those with an ejection fraction less than 0.35, operative mortality was 6.2 percent and the 5-year survival rate was 65 percent.[560] A more recent series demonstrated an in-hospital operative mortality of 8.4 percent for patients with an ejection fraction of 0.30 or less.[550]

MYOCARDIAL HIBERNATION. Improvement in survival and left ventricular function following CABG depends on successful reperfusion of viable, but noncontractile or poorly contracting myocardium (see Chaps. 13, 14, and 34). Two related pathophysiological conditions have been described to explain reversible ischemic contractile dysfunction[561]: myocardial stunning (prolonged but temporary postischemic ventricular dysfunction without myocardial necrosis) and myocardial hibernation (persistent left ventricular dysfunction when myocardial perfusion is chronically reduced but sufficient to maintain the viability of tissue). The reduction in myocardial contractility in hibernating myocardium conserves metabolic demands and may be protective, but more prolonged and severe hibernation may lead to severe ultrastructural abnormalities, irreversible loss of contractile units, and apoptosis.[562]

Hibernating myocardium can cause abnormal systolic or diastolic ventricular function or both. The predominant clinical feature of myocardial ischemia in these patients may not be angina, but dyspnea secondary to increased left ventricular diastolic pressure. Symptoms of heart failure resulting from chronic left ventricular dysfunction may be inappropriately ascribed to myocardial necrosis and scarring when the symptoms may, in fact, be reversed after the chronic ischemia is relieved by coronary revascularization.[103, 563]

Detection Of Hibernating Myocardium. Several clinical markers may be used to determine the likelihood that a dysfunctional myocardial segment is viable or nonviable (Table 37-13). A severe reduction in the diastolic wall thickness of dysfunctional left ventricular segments is indicative of scarring. On the other hand, akinetic or dyskinetic segments with preserved diastolic wall thickness may

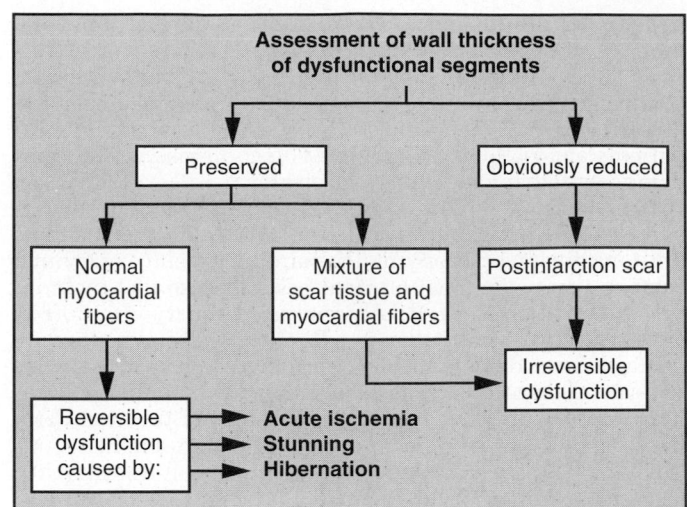

FIGURE 37-18. Flow diagram for the practical assessment of noncontractile segments of myocardial wall potentially recoverable by revascularization procedures. An obviously reduced wall thickness is indicative of a postinfarction scar. Absence of contractile function in segments of the ventricular wall with preserved wall thickness may be caused by different mechanisms. An acute ischemic cause can be excluded by the administration of sublingual nitrates. Stunning can be excluded by repeating the ventricular wall motion study several days after the last ischemic episode. Hibernating myocardium should be distinguished from a mixture of scar tissue and viable myocardial cells. (From Maseri A: Ischemic Heart Disease: A Rational Basis for Clinical Practice and Clinical Research. New York, Churchill Livingstone, 1995. By permission.)

represent a mixture of scarred and viable myocardium. A useful strategy for the assessment of dysfunctional segments has been developed by Maseri (Fig. 37-18). Although a number of imaging tools may be used for this assessment (see Chaps. 7, 9, 10, and 13), the most readily available in most settings is low-dose dobutamine echocardiography.

The term *contractile reserve* describes the ability of hibernating myocardium to exhibit augmented contractility to a suitable temporary stimulus, often causing transient improvement in the global ejection fraction. Contractile reserve underscores the fact that many hypokinetic (and even akinetic) areas of the ventricular wall are composed entirely or in part of viable, hibernating myocardium or a mixture of the latter and fibrous scar. Viable muscle is capable of responding to a sympathomimetic agent. In contrast, necrotic tissue obviously cannot be stimulated to contract by any pharmacological or hemodynamic intervention or by improved perfusion. The most common method of identifying contractile reserve is echocardiographic imaging during infusion of a low dose of dobutamine.[561] Numerous studies have demonstrated that the finding of contractile reserve by low-dose dobutamine echocardiography identifies dysfunctional, but viable myocardium with the potential to improve in function after myocardial revascularization.[89, 102, 103, 561, 564]

PET (see Chap. 9) has emerged as an excellent method for demonstrating viable myocardium in patients with impaired left ventricular function.[89, 561, 563-566] In comparative studies, PET has yielded the highest predictive accuracy of all imaging modalities in detecting dysfunctional myocardium that will improve after revascularization.[89, 564] However, the high cost, technical difficulty, and need for a cyclotron continue to limit this technique's widespread applicability.

Important advances in the assessment of myocardial viability with thallium-201 include rest-redistribution imaging to determine whether regions with hypoperfusion at rest manifest filling in of the resting defect with time and stress-redistribution-reinjection imaging, in which a second injection of thallium is administered to determine whether defects that do not redistribute after exercise represent fi-

▼ **TABLE 37-13. MARKERS OF VIABLE MYOCARDIUM**

CLINICAL INDICATOR	DIAGNOSTIC TEST	ALTERNATIVE TEST
Diastolic wall thickness	Echo	CT, MRI
Systolic wall thickening	Echo	CT, MRI, gated SPECT
Regional wall motion	Echo	CT, MRI, gated SPECT
Regional blood flow	SPECT	PET
Myocardial metabolism	PET	SPECT
Cell membrane integrity	SPECT	PET
Contractile reserve	Dobutamine, Echo	Angiography, CT, MRI

CT = computed tomography; Echo = echocardiography; MRI = magnetic resonance imaging; PET = positron-emission tomography; SPECT = single-photon emission computed tomography.

brotic myocardium or myocardium that is severely ische-mic[88, 89, 102, 561, 567] (see Chap. 9).

Prognostic Implications of Identifying Viable Myocardium. A growing body of evidence indicates that the detection of viable myocardium in patients with CAD and left ventricular dysfunction not only identifies those in whom improvement in cardiac function is likely after revascularization but also identifies a group of high-risk patients in whom revascularization improves survival (Fig. 37–19). Studies with PET, thallium-201, and dobutamine echocardiography have uniformly demonstrated that patients with left ventricular dysfunction and evidence of hibernating myocardium have a high mortality rate during medical therapy and appear to have a better outcome with revascularization.[103, 568–571] All these studies have limitations, including a small number of patients, the retrospective nature of the analysis, and lack of a randomized control group. However, the consistency of the findings has been striking. Recent data point out that viability assessment is also helpful in the selection of patients for revascularization because patients selected for revascularization on the basis of an imaging study demonstrating myocardial viability have lower operative mortality and a higher long-term survival rate than do those who have no evidence of important myocardial viability or those in whom a viability assessment is not performed.[88, 103, 572] Perioperative mortality in the latter patients approaches 10 percent.[88, 103, 572]

The mechanisms for improved survival after revascularization in patients with hibernating myocardium may be related to improvement in left ventricular function, but it is likely that other important factors are also operative. Revascularization of viable myocardium may also reduce left ventricular remodeling, the propensity for serious arrhythmias, and the likelihood of a future fatal acute ischemic event.[89] In this manner, patients with left ventricular dysfunction and hibernating myocardium may be viewed as other high-risk patients with left ventricular dysfunction, multivessel CAD, and jeopardized myocardium, in whom outcome is improved by revascularization. In this regard, survival may be enhanced by revascularization in such patients, even if left ventricular function does not improve after the procedure.

Surgical Treatment in Special Groups

WOMEN (see also Chap. 58). It is clear that CABG use is much lower in women than in men.[573, 574] However, what has not been established is whether these differences represent underutilization in women, overutilization in men, or

both.[458, 575] In comparison with men, women who undergo coronary bypass surgery are "sicker," as defined by age, comorbid conditions, the severity of angina, and history of congestive heart failure.[574, 576] Many series have demonstrated higher morbidity and mortality in coronary surgery in women. The 1997 Society of Thoracic Surgeons data base showed that approximately 30 percent of isolated CABG procedures in the United States were performed in women, with a perioperative mortality of 3.9 percent versus 2.3 percent for men.[425]

Among patients 70 years or older in the Toronto Hospital experience, operative mortality in men in comparison with women was 5.4% vs 11.8% from 1982–1986, 3.8% vs 5.8% from 1987–1991 and 3.8% vs 6.3% from 1992–1996.[577] Perioperative morbidity, including myocardial infarction, respiratory failure, and stroke, was also significantly higher in women. A higher incidence of sternal wound infections may be related to obesity.[458] Most of the differences between men and women are the consequence of age, the "sicker" preoperative status of women, a higher rate of nonelective procedures, and the presence of more diffuse disease and left ventricular dysfunction in women reaching surgery,[578] but the presence of smaller distal vessels (as a function of a smaller body surface area) and lower use of IMA grafts may also be contributing factors.[390, 579] However, a small independent detrimental effect of female gender persists in most multivariate analyses. Despite the increased perioperative mortality and morbidity in women, late survival is similar in men and women,[580] but the relief of anginal symptoms appears to be less in women.[577, 580, 581]

Independent risk factors for long-term prognosis in women are similar to those in men, including older age, previous coronary bypass surgery, previous myocardial infarction, and diabetes.[580] In the BARI Trial, in-hospital mortality was similar for men and women, as were the unadjusted 5.4-year mortality rates of 12.8 percent in women and 12 percent in men (p = NS). After adjustment for the higher risk profiles in women, including age, symptom severity, and comorbid conditions, the relative risk of death in women versus men was actually lower, 0.60 (95 percent confidence intervals, 0.43 to 0.84; p = 0.003). However, these data may not be generalizable outside the confines of a randomized trial.

YOUNGER PATIENTS. Patients 35 years or younger who undergo CABG usually have hyperlipidemia and other major risk factors for CAD.[582] Despite the severity of the underlying disease and the rapidity of the atherosclerotic process, CABG is associated with excellent actuarial survival rates of 94 percent at 5 years and 85 percent at 10 years.[582] Nonetheless, in the CASS Registry, patients younger than 35 years had markedly impaired survival over a 15-year period in comparison with an age- and sex-matched U.S. population.[581] This impaired survival is probably the result of progression of premature atherosclerotic disease, the presence of multiple risk factors, and the development of progressive vein graft disease. The latter underlies the current trend for the use of bilateral IMA grafts and other arterial conduits in younger patients.

THE ELDERLY (see also Chap. 57). A demographic tide in combination with marked improvement in perioperative care and in the outcomes of CABG has resulted in a

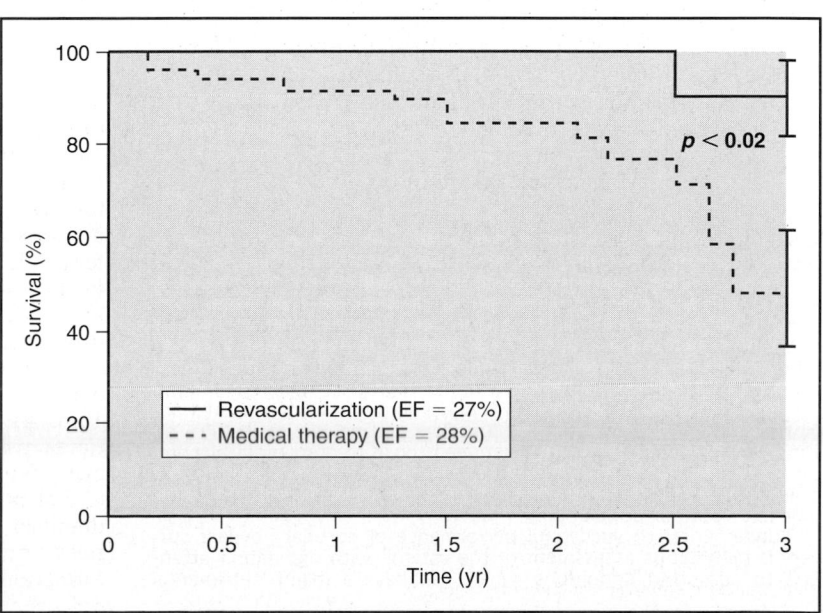

FIGURE 37–19. Survival among 58 patients with coronary artery disease, left ventricular dysfunction, and contractile reserve detected by low-dose dobutamine echocardiography. Patients treated with revascularization have a significantly higher survival rate than those treated medically. EF = ejection fraction. (From Chaudhry FA, Tauke JT, Alessandrini RS, et al: Prognostic implications of myocardial contractile reserve in patients with coronary artery disease and left ventricular dysfunction. J Am Coll Cardiol 34: 730, 1999. Reprinted with permission from the American College of Cardiology.)

burgeoning population of elderly patients with extensive disease undergoing such surgery. In 1997, the median age of patients undergoing an initial coronary bypass procedure was approximately 65 years in the United States and 64 years in Canada.[425] In 1997 in the United States, among 17,806 patients undergoing isolated CABG, 34 percent of patients were older than 70 years, 8872 operations were performed on octogenarians, and 106 new patients were in their 90s.[425] Between 1987 and 1990 in the Medicare population, the number of patients older than 80 years undergoing coronary bypass surgery increased by 67 percent.[583]

Older patients are "sicker" than their younger counterparts in that they have a greater frequency of comorbid conditions, including peripheral vascular and cerebrovascular disease, more extensive triple-vessel and left main CAD, and a higher frequency of left ventricular dysfunction and history of congestive heart failure.[392] Not unexpectedly, these differences are translated into higher perioperative mortality and complication rates, with a sharp increase in the slope of the curve relating mortality to age seen in patients older than 70 years.[425, 458, 577, 581, 584] More encouraging data were recently presented from the Toronto Hospital: Over a 15-year period, despite an increase in the prevalence and severity of risk factors, operative mortality in patients 70 years or older declined from 7.2 percent to less than 5 percent overall, with a mortality of 3 percent for patients defined as "low" or "medium risk."[577]

Perioperative morbidity is also increased in the elderly, with high rates of low-output syndrome, stroke, gastrointestinal complications, wound infection, and postoperative atrial fibrillation.[458, 471] The major predictors of perioperative mortality in the elderly are similar to those in younger patients, but with an increasing emphasis on the number of associated comorbid conditions, including the presence of peripheral and cerebrovascular disease. Although chronological age is not the most powerful independent predictor for perioperative mortality, it is an *independent* predictor, which suggests that other less tangible factors associated with older age increase operative risk.[392] In addition, from an examination of Medicare data from 1987 to 1990, patients older than 70 years, in comparison with those 65 to 70 years old, had longer postoperative hospital stays (mean of 14.3 vs. 10.4 days), higher charges, and greater costs.[583]

Despite the difficulties and expense of performing coronary bypass surgery in the elderly, excellent *long-term* survival rates can be achieved in addition to having the elderly return to an active functional status.[581, 585–587] In the CASS Registry, among patients 65 and 75 years old at the time of surgery, 74 and 59 percent, respectively, were alive 10 years after surgery and 54 and 33 percent 15 years after surgery (now 90 years old).[581] The survival of these patients exceeded that of the average age- and sex-matched U.S. population, which probably reflects in part the benefit of coronary revascularization in addition to selection bias. Similarly, octogenarians who survived the perioperative period had a long-term survival rate similar to that of the general octogenarian population of the United States.[583]

Predictors of late outcome in the elderly are similar to those in younger patients, including left ventricular dysfunction, but the number of associated comorbid conditions in addition to chronological age has a major effect.[588] Although no randomized trials have compared surgical and medical therapy in patients older than 65 years, a nonrandomized analysis of the CASS Registry demonstrated a significant benefit from surgery over medical therapy in the majority of patients who were considered to be at "high risk," whereas among the approximately 15 percent of low-risk patients who had mild angina, relatively good ventricular function, and no left main CAD, no survival differences were seen between those treated medically and those treated surgically. Therefore, the results in this registry are consistent with the randomized trials conducted during the same time in a younger population.[538]

Fundamental to successful performance of coronary bypass surgery is meticulous assessment of the patient, with mandatory attention to comorbid conditions, which can have a major detrimental effect on both perioperative morbidity and mortality and long-term survival. Evaluation of the elderly for coronary bypass surgery should take into account other less tangible factors related to quality of life and the potential ability to benefit from the operation. These factors include not only the chronological age of the patient but also the estimated physiological age, the patient's attitude, including understanding of the risks and expectations of the procedure, and an assessment of the patient's level of activity and current life style.

END-STAGE RENAL DISEASE. Cardiovascular disease is the major predictor of mortality in patients with end-stage renal disease (ESRD) and accounts for 54 percent of deaths[589] (see Chap. 72). Patients with ESRD have numerous risk factors that not only accelerate the development of CAD but also complicate its medical management. These risk factors include diabetes, hypertension with left ventricular hypertrophy, both systolic and diastolic dysfunction, abnormal lipid metabolism, anemia, and increased homocysteine levels.[458] Coronary revascularization with PCI or CABG is feasible and well documented in patients with ESRD, but the mortality and complication rates are increased.[458, 590] It has been suggested that for chronic dialysis patients, CABG is preferred for revascularization over PCI.[590] In one series, the 30-day mortality was 9 percent, but CABG produced a substantial improvement in the quality of life.[591] Another series reported a 68 percent cumulative survival rate over a 5-year period in patients with New York Heart Association Class II to III symptoms, which supports a policy of operating on symptomatic patients receiving dialysis but before the onset of severe congestive heart failure.[592] In the only randomized trial of surgical and medical therapy for insulin-dependent diabetic candidates for renal transplantation, 10 of 13 medically managed patients and 2 of 13 surgically treated ones had a major cardiovascular event during approximately 8 months of follow-up ($p < 0.01$).[593]

In summary, coronary bypass surgery can be performed with an acceptable risk and a reasonable expectation of long-term benefit in carefully selected patients with ESRD. As for all high-risk situations, careful attention to patient selection is essential.

PATIENTS REQUIRING REOPERATION. Currently, approximately 10 percent of coronary artery procedures are reoperations, and in some centers, particularly tertiary care centers, the proportion is increasing rapidly and accounts for 15 to 18 percent of all CABG operations.[458] The major indication for reoperation is late disease of saphenous vein grafts. Moreover, the patient population is elderly, and an added factor underlying recurrent symptoms is progression of disease in native vessels between the first and second operations. Several series have emphasized the "sicker" preoperative status of patients undergoing reoperation, including older age, more extensive comorbidity, associated valvular heart disease, and a greater prevalence of left ventricular dysfunction and greater extent of ischemic jeopardized myocardium.[594] Not unexpectedly, the mortality associated with reoperation is significantly higher than that of initial bypass procedures. In the 1997 data base of the Society of Thoracic Surgeons, the mortality among 99,810 patients undergoing an elective first CABG procedure was 1.7 percent versus 5.2 percent for elective reoperations. For patients undergoing first operations, mortality was 2.6 percent for urgent and 6 percent for emergency procedures in comparison with 7.4 and 13.5 percent, respectively, among patients undergoing repeat bypass surgery. Virtually every large series has demonstrated higher morbidity and twofold to threefold greater mortality for reoperation.[594, 595] The determinants of perioperative mortality are similar to those for a first operation, although a short time interval between the first operation and the repeat procedure is an added major predictor of increased mortality. Third- and even fourth-time coronary reoperations are increasing in frequency and are associated with substantial increases in perioperative complications, including bleeding and myocardial infarction.[595]

More encouraging are the late survival rates of approximately 77 to 90 percent at 5 years and 48 to 83 percent at 10 years.[594, 596] Although in one series 73 percent of patients were free of angina at 5 years, relief of angina is generally less complete than after an initial operation.

Indications for reoperation have not been defined by randomized trials, but in general, the same principles that apply to patients with initial disease should be followed. Information about the effect of graft stenosis on late survival was recently provided by a large retrospective study of patients who had postoperative coronary angiography and in whom a stenosis of 20 percent or more was present in at least one graft (Fig. 37–20). Stenoses in a vein graft to the left anterior descending coronary artery were associated with a reduction in survival, and the major improvement in survival after reoperation was particularly evident for patients in this category. Among these patients, survival rates were 84 and 74 percent for the reoperation group 2 and 4 years after catheterization versus 76 and 53 percent for the medically treated group ($p = 0.004$).[597] Nonetheless, the greater risk and the less favorable outcome after reoperation than after the initial procedure need to be considered, and the indications should probably be more stringent than for patients with native vessel disease alone.

OTHER HIGH-RISK SUBGROUPS. Patients with *familial hyperlipidemia* have long been considered to be at particular risk for an adverse late outcome after CABG. More encouraging results have been reported with the use of an IMA or other arterial conduit in conjunction with aggressive lipid-lowering therapy.[598] In comparison with age-matched nondiabetic patients, elderly *diabetic* patients with angiographically proven CAD are more likely to be female with evidence of peripheral vascular disease and a higher number of coronary occlusions.[599] In a cohort of CASS Registry patients, diabetes was an independent predictor of mortality. However, the relative survival benefit of CABG versus medical therapy was comparable in diabetic and nondiabetic patients, with a significant (44 percent) reduction in mortality provided by surgery over medical therapy in diabetics.[599] Other large studies have emphasized the independent adverse effect of diabetes on mortality after CABG. In the Duke data base, the 5-year unadjusted survival rate was 74 percent among diabetic patients and 86 percent among nondiabetic patients treated surgically.[363] In a diabetic population undergoing coronary revascularization, insulin dependence is an added adverse predictor of 5- and 10-year survival rates.[600]

Summary of Indications for Coronary Revascularization

1. Certain anatomical subsets of patients are candidates for CABG, regardless of the severity of symptoms or left ventricular dysfunction. Such patients include those with significant left main CAD and most patients with three-vessel disease that includes the proximal left anterior descending coronary artery, especially those with left ventricular dysfunction.

2. The benefits of coronary bypass surgery are well documented in patients with left ventricular dysfunction and multivessel disease, regardless of symptoms. In patients whose dominant symptom is heart failure without severe angina, the benefits of coronary revascularization are less well defined, but this approach should be considered in patients who also have evidence of severe ischemia (regardless of angina symptoms), particularly in the presence of a

significant extent of potentially viable dysfunctioning (hibernating) myocardium.

3. The primary objective of coronary revascularization in patients with single-vessel disease is relief of significant symptoms or objective evidence of severe ischemia. For the majority of these patients, PCI is the revascularization modality of choice.

4. In patients with angina who are *not* considered to be at high risk, survival is similar for surgically and medically treated groups.

5. All the indications discussed above relate to the potential benefits of surgery over medical therapy on *survival*. Coronary revascularization with PCI or CABG is highly efficacious in relieving symptoms and may be considered for patients with moderate to severe ischemic symptoms who are dissatisfied with medical therapy, even if they are not in a high-risk subset. For such patients, the optimal method of revascularization is selected on the basis of left ventricular function and arteriographic findings and the likelihood of technical success.

Comparisons Between PTCA and CABG

OBSERVATIONAL STUDIES. Since the catheter-based revascularizations in these comparative studies were limited largely to PTCA, this term instead of PCI is used in this section. Among the many comparative studies of PTCA and CABG in patients with multivessel disease, several included patients with single-vessel disease,[514, 601, 602] but in only five studies were the groups matched for differences in baseline characteristics.[514, 601, 603–605] Regardless of the limitations of these series and the differences in baseline characteristics, the results are quite consistent. Over a period of 1 to 5 years, the rates of mortality and nonfatal infarction were not significantly different between the two groups but recurrent events, including angina pectoris and the need for repeat revascularization procedures, were significantly more frequent in the PTCA than the CABG group. Among patients with left ventricular dysfunction, survival after CABG appears to be better than after PTCA, probably because of the ability to achieve more complete revascularization with the former.[606] Indeed, complete revascularization is achieved by PTCA in only 25 to 50 percent of patients with two-vessel disease and in 10 to 25 percent of those with three-vessel disease.[607] In the future, improvements in transcatheter techniques, particularly in the ability to treat chronic total occlusions, may improve the results of this approach in patients with left ventricular dysfunction.

Outcome data 1 year after PTCA in patients (most of

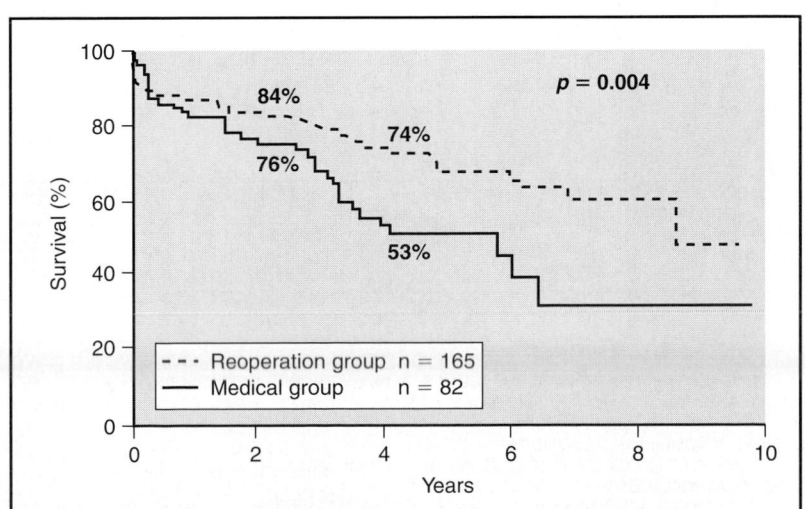

FIGURE 37–20. Survival of patients with late stenoses in saphenous grafts to the left anterior descending coronary artery. In this subgroup, patients undergoing reoperation had improved survival when compared with those receiving medical therapy. (Data obtained from the Cleveland Clinic Series. From Lytle BW, Loop FD, Taylor PC, et al: The effect of coronary reoperation on the survival of patients with stenoses in saphenous vein bypass grafts to coronary arteries. J Thorac Cardiovasc Surg 105:605, 1993. By permission of Mosby.)

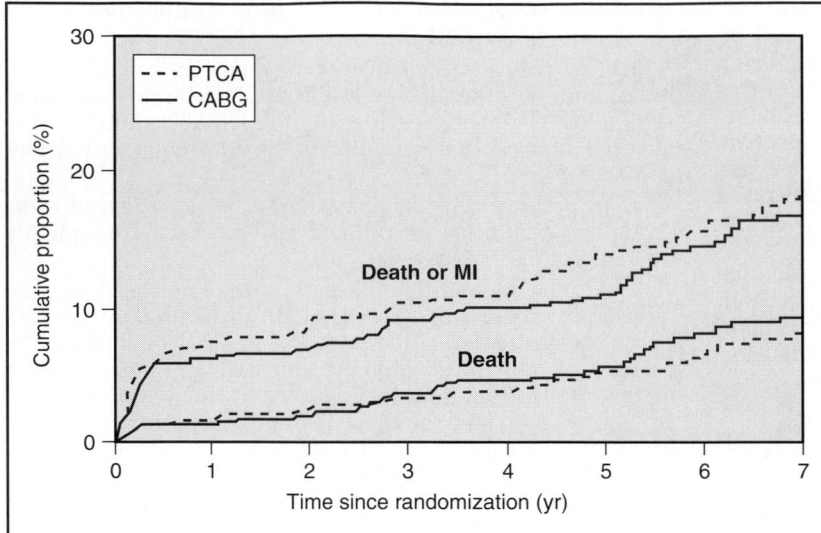

FIGURE 37–21. Hazard ratios for coronary artery bypass graft surgery (CABG) versus percutaneous transluminal coronary angioplasty (PTCA). Points below 1.0 favor CABG. Prox LAD = proximal left anterior descending coronary artery; VD = vessel disease. (From Mark DB, Nelson CL, Califf RM, et al: Continuing evolution of therapy for coronary artery disease: Initial results from the era of coronary angioplasty. Circulation 89:2015, 1994. By permission of the American Heart Association, Inc.)

whom had single-vessel disease) indicate that recurrence of symptoms and/or the need for repeat revascularization procedures is high (approximately 40 percent) and that approximately 20 percent actually undergo CABG. In one report, after approximately 2 years, 49 percent of patients had had one repeat cardiac catheterization and approximately 25 percent had undergone multiple cardiac catheterizations.[603] These results need to be modified by a reduction in the rate of repeat revascularization procedures and recurrent angina in patients currently treated with stents instead of PTCA alone.[366, 608] CABG provided a clear survival benefit over PTCA in the Duke University data base in patients with two-vessel disease that included 95 percent or greater obstruction of the proximal left anterior descending coronary artery and in all forms of three-vessel disease (Fig. 37–14B, p. 1310; and Fig. 37–21). However, the effect of the method of revascularization on survival was equal in patients with two-vessel disease who did not have obstruction of the proximal left anterior descending coronary artery. The New York State procedure registries of PTCA and CABG from 1993 to 1995 demonstrate an approximately 37 percent rate of repeat revascularization after PTCA over a 3-year period in comparison with 3.3 percent after surgery.[608] Hazard ratios for mortality are shown in Figure 37–22, which illus-

trates that the anatomical extent and specific site of the disease influence the results of the treatment chosen, whether PTCA or CABG.

RANDOMIZED TRIALS

PTCA Versus CABG in Patients with Single-Vessel Disease. In the RITA Trial, 45 percent of patients had single-vessel disease, and both the Lausanne Trial and the MASS Trial from Brazil, which included a medical arm, were limited to patients with isolated disease of the proximal left anterior descending coronary artery.[369, 476, 609] The results of these small trials were consistent in that over 2 to 3 years the rates of mortality and myocardial infarction were similar in the two strategies, as was improvement in symptoms, but at the cost of more frequent reintervention in patients treated with PTCA. At 5 years in the Lausanne Trial, mortality rates and functional status were similar for the two groups; however, an excess incidence of non-Q-wave myocardial infarction was noted in patients treated with PTCA, but this complication did not affect vital status or symptomatic outcome.[610]

In summary, the results suggest that PTCA and CABG are highly effective in preventing symptoms in patients with single-vessel disease. Moreover, no difference in mortality is seen between these two methods of revascularization.

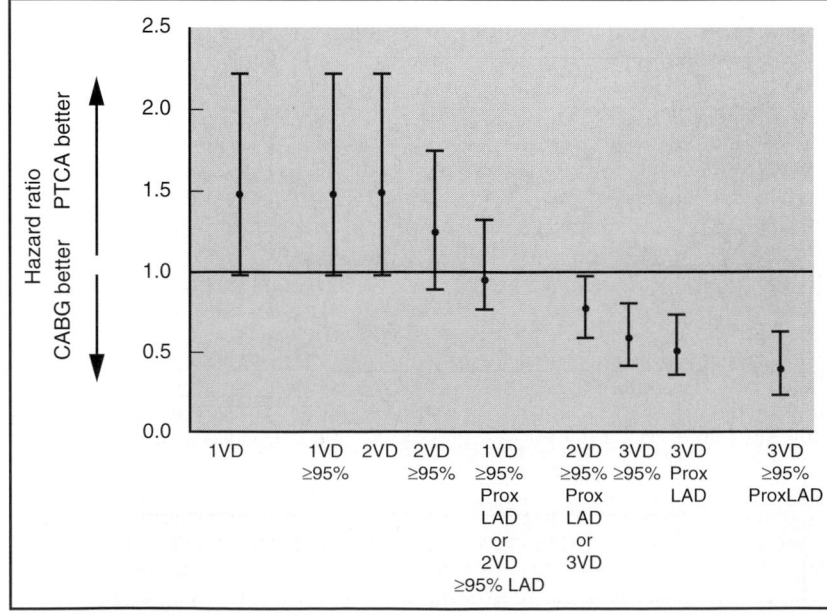

FIGURE 37–22. Differences in adjusted percent survival at 3 years with percutaneous transluminal coronary angioplasty (PTCA) and coronary artery bypass graft surgery (CABG) in the New York State data base (1993 to 1995). Data are stratified according to the number of vessels diseased and whether the left anterior descending (LAD) coronary arteries are involved and according to whether the stenoses are proximal. Note the better survival with CABG among patients with three- or two-vessel disease in combination with proximal LAD involvement. (From Hannan EL, Racz MJ, McCallister BD, et al: A comparison of three-year survival after coronary artery bypass graft surgery and percutaneous transluminal coronary angioplasty. J Am Coll Cardiol 33:63, 1999. Reprinted with permission from the American College of Cardiology.)

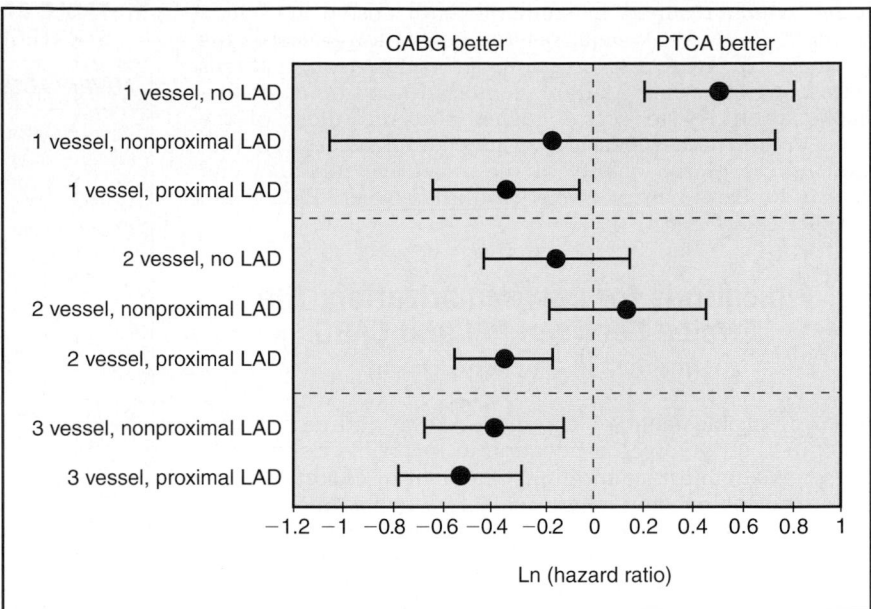

FIGURE 37–23. Cumulative risk of death or myocardial infarction after percutaneous transluminal coronary angioplasty (PTCA) and bypass surgery in the RITA-1 trials (-----, PTCA; ———, CABG). No significant difference was found in either death or the combined endpoint of death or myocardial infarction. (From Henderson RA, Pocock SJ, Sharp SJ, et al: Long-term results of RITA-1 trial: Clinical and cost comparisons of coronary angioplasty and coronary-artery bypass grafting. Randomised Intervention Treatment of Angina. Lancet 352:1419, 1998. © by The Lancet Ltd., 1998.)

Multivessel Disease. Seven published studies have compared PTCA with CABG in patients with multivessel disease. Another study, the Arterial Revascularization Therapy Study (ARTS), has recently been presented.[611] One of these trials (RITA) included patients with single-vessel disease.[352, 364, 476, 612–614a] Despite the heterogeneity of the trials in regard to design, methods, and the patient population enrolled, the results are generally comparable and provide a consistent perspective of CABG and PTCA in selected patients with multivessel disease. A major limitation is that these trials, except for ARTS and ERACI-II,[620] were conducted before the widespread use of stents and other advances in PCI technology and adjunctive therapy, such as ticlopidine and glycoprotein IIb/IIIa platelet inhibition. Also, these trials lacked an aggressive approach to lipid lowering in both groups of patients. In the RITA, the ERACI-I, ARTS, and the French Monocentric trials, the ability to achieve "equivalent" degrees of revascularization in the two groups was an inclusion criterion.[364, 476] Moreover, the majority of patients entered into the trials had well-preserved left ventricular function and a mean ejection fraction exceeding 50 percent. In the main, patients enrolled in these trials were at relatively low risk, with predominantly two-vessel disease and well-preserved left ventricular function, i.e., a high proportion of patients in whom CABG surgery had *not* been previously shown to be superior to medical therapy in regard to survival. Thus, one would not expect a significant mortality difference between PTCA and CABG, particularly with the relatively small sample size of the trials (Fig. 37–23).[365, 615]

The BARI Trial, initiated by the NHLBI, enrolled 1829 patients with multivessel disease in the United States and Canada. This trial is the largest of the randomized trials of PTCA and bypass surgery and the only trial with sufficient statistical power to detect a substantial mortality difference. At 5 years, overall survival rates were not different between the two groups (89.3 percent with CABG and 86.3 percent with PTCA [*p* = 0.19]), nor was any difference noted in the incidence of Q wave myocardial infarction.[352, 616] An initially unexpected finding—but one that is also evident as a trend in the Coronary Angioplasty Versus Bypass Revascularisation Investigation (CABRI) and EAST trials (Rickards A, personal communication; King SB III, personal communication)—was that patients with previously treated diabetes who underwent PTCA had a mortality of 34.5 percent versus 19.4 percent for those who underwent CABG (*p* = 0.003) (see also Chap. 63).

Because of the heterogeneity among the trials, it is reassuring that the results are highly consistent within the trials and with observational studies. In these highly selected patients, neither procedure has demonstrated, after 1 to 5 years of follow-up, a clear superiority over the other for primary outcomes of mortality and Q wave myocardial infarction (Fig. 37–23).[617] Although a meta-analysis by Pocock and colleagues demonstrated a trend in favor of bypass surgery, this trend did not reach statistical significance.[618]

CABG is initially associated with greater improvement in angina, which appears to be proportional to the more complete revascularization in patients with multivessel disease (Fig. 37–12).[619] Moreover, as anticipated from the observational data, repeat revascularization procedures are more frequent after PTCA, although it is likely that more widespread use of stents will reduce the magnitude of the difference in repeat revascularization rates. In the RITA Trial, for example, after 5 years, repeat PTCA was performed in 27 percent of patients in the angioplasty group and CABG was performed in 26 percent; in comparison, among the patients treated initially with surgery only, 3 percent underwent reoperation and 9 percent subsequently required PTCA. What is encouraging among patients assigned to PTCA is the striking decrease in the need for reinterventions after the first 2 years, with a repeat revascularization rate of only 3 percent per year during years 3 to 5 of follow-up. In patients assigned to CABG, the reintervention rate remains steady at 2 percent per year, but it might be expected to increase after approximately 7 to 8 years of follow-up.[617] In the ARTS Trial, which compared multivessel stenting with CABG, repeat revascularization was performed in only 16.9 percent of patients in the stented group. This figure is lower than the repeat procedural rates noted in trials of angioplasty alone. Preliminary results from this study also suggested that 1-year costs were lower in the stented than in the bypass surgery group.[611] In the ERACI-II Study, preliminary results were similar to those in the ARTS Trial, with only 16 percent of patients who had PCI with stenting requiring repeat revascularization in follow-up versus 4.4 percent of bypass surgical patients (mean follow-up, 14.7 ± 6.4 months).[620]

Another consistent, but not unexpected finding was the lower in-hospital cost for patients undergoing PTCA.[364] However, the need for recurrent hospitalization and repeat revascularization procedures over the long term contributed to an increase in postdischarge cost in the PTCA arms, which resulted in similar overall cost over 3 to 5 years.[364, 373, 374, 621] A major determinant of lower cost is the presence of two-vessel disease; in comparison, patients with congestive heart failure, comorbid conditions, or diabetes are likely to accrue higher cost regardless of the procedure.[621] Other measures of procedural success, including indices of the quality of life, cognitive function, and return to employment, were similar between PTCA and CABG.[621, 622]

Indications for Revascularization: The Choice Between PCI and CABG

(Fig. 37–24 and Table 37–14)

Medical management of chronic CAD as outlined on pp. 1282 to 1298 involves a reduction in reversible risk factors, life style alteration counseling, treatment of conditions that intensify angina, and pharmacological management of ischemia. When an unacceptable level of angina persists or the patient has troubling side effects from the antiischemic drugs, the coronary anatomy should be defined to allow selection of the appropriate technique for revascularization. In patients in whom the angina is controlled, noninvasive testing is carried out and coronary arteriography performed in those with a "high-risk" result[365] (see p. 1280). After elucidation of the coronary anatomy, selection of the technique of revascularization is made as follows:

SINGLE-VESSEL DISEASE. Among patients with single-vessel disease in whom revascularization is deemed necessary and the lesion is anatomically suitable, PCI is generally preferred over bypass surgery.

MULTIVESSEL DISEASE. The first step is to decide whether a patient falls into the category of those who were included in randomized trials comparing PTCA and CABG. The majority of patients included in these trials were at lower risk, as defined by two-vessel disease and well-preserved ventricular function. Moreover, three trials required that equivalent degrees of revascularization be achievable

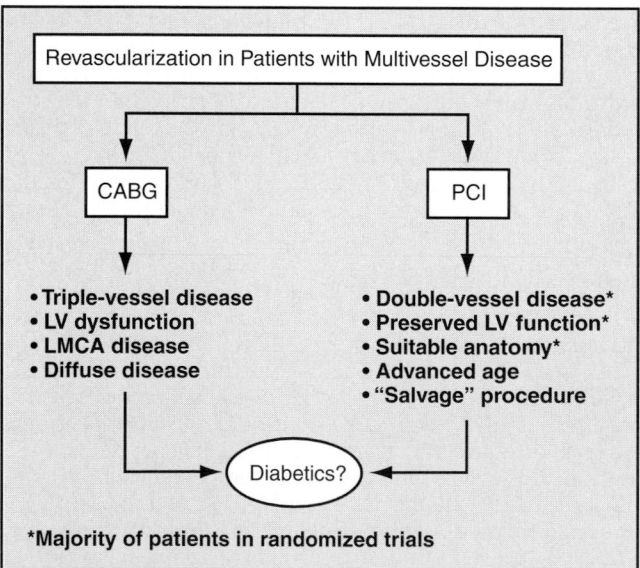

FIGURE 37–24. Indications for coronary revascularization with bypass surgery (CABG) or percutaneous coronary intervention (PCI) in patients with multivessel disease. The combination of triple-vessel disease and left ventricular (LV) dysfunction and/or left main coronary artery (LMCA) disease is primarily surgical, whereas the majority of the patients entered into the randomized trials were suitable for angioplasty on the basis of double-vessel disease, preserved left ventricular dysfunction, and suitable anatomy. Diabetics should be treated individually.

▼ **TABLE 37–14. COMPARISON OF REVASCULARIZATION STRATEGIES IN MULTIVESSEL DISEASE**

ADVANTAGES	DISADVANTAGES
PERCUTANEOUS CORONARY INTERVENTION	
Less invasive	Restenosis
Shorter hospital stay	High incidence of incomplete revascularization
Lower initial cost	
Easily repeated	Relative inefficacy in patients with severe left ventricular dysfunction
Effective in relieving symptoms	
	Uncertain long-term outcome (>10 yr)
	Limited to specific anatomical subsets
CORONARY ARTERY BYPASS GRAFT SURGERY	
Effective in relieving symptoms	Cost
Improved survival in certain subsets	Increased risk of a repeat procedure because of late graft closure
Ability to achieve complete revascularization	Morbidity
Wider applicability	

Modified from Faxon DP: Coronary angioplasty for stable angina pectoris. In Beller G (ed): Chronic Ischemic Heart Disease. In Braunwald E (ed): Atlas of Heart Disease. Vol 5. Philadelphia, Current Medicine, 1995.

by both techniques. Most patients with chronically occluded coronary arteries were excluded, and of those who were clinically eligible, approximately two-thirds were excluded for angiographic reasons. The lack of any difference in late mortality and myocardial infarction between the two groups in such patients indicates that PCI is a reasonable *initial* strategy, provided that the patient accepts the distinct possibility of symptom recurrence and need for repeat revascularization. Patients with a single localized lesion in each affected vessel and preserved left ventricular function fare best with PCI.

NEED FOR COMPLETE REVASCULARIZATION. Complete revascularization is an important goal in patients with left ventricular dysfunction and/or multivessel disease. The major advantage of CABG surgery over PCI is its greater ability to achieve complete revascularization, particularly in patients with three-vessel disease. In the majority of such patients, particularly those with chronic total coronary occlusion, left ventricular dysfunction, or left main CAD, CABG is the procedure of choice.[348, 475] Among patients with borderline left ventricular function (ejection fraction between 40 and 50 percent) and milder degrees of ischemia, PCI may provide adequate revascularization, even if it is not complete anatomically.

In many patients, either method of revascularization is suitable. Other factors that come into consideration include (1) access to a high-quality team and operator with an excellent record of success; (2) patient preference—some patients are made anxious by the idea that after PCI they remain at risk for symptom recurrence and may require reintervention (such patients are better candidates for surgical treatment); (3) advanced patient age and comorbidity—frail, very elderly patients and those with comorbid conditions, such as cancer or serious liver disease with a limited life expectancy, but who have disabling angina—are often better candidates for PCI; and (4) younger patient age—PCI is also often preferable in younger patients (<50 years) with the expectation that they may require CABG at some time in the future and that PCI will postpone the need for surgery; this sequence may be preferable to two operations. Patient preference is a pivotal aspect of the decision to perform PCI or CABG in these patient groups.

PTCA AND CORONARY BYPASS SURGERY IN DIABETIC PATIENTS (see also Chap. 63). The poorer outcomes after PTCA than after CABG in treated diabetic patients in the BARI Trial, together with similar trends in the EAST and CABRI trials, have raised concern about whether all diabetic patients with multivessel disease should be treated surgically. This important issue has significant economic implications, but further analysis suggests that treatment of diabetic patients can be individualized, as in nondiabetic patients. Despite the use of stents for multivessel PCI in the ARTS Trial, preliminary data suggest that the 1-year mortality in diabetic patients who received PCI and stenting was double that of those undergoing bypass surgery (6.3 vs. 3.1 percent).[623]

One explanation for the difference in outcomes may be an altered vascular biological response in diabetic patients to balloon injury and progression of disease in nondilated segments. The diabetic atherosclerotic milieu is characterized by a procoagulant state, decreased fibrinolytic activity, increased proliferation, and inflammation.[624]
Restenosis is more frequent in diabetic patients, as is disease progression. In a study of patients referred for diagnostic angiography 1 month or more after successful PTCA, the number of new narrowings in the arteries of diabetic patients increased by 22 percent, particularly at other sites in the artery that initially underwent PTCA.[625] Thus, CABG, which bypasses the majority of the vessel instead of a specific lesion, may offer a better long-term outcome.[626]
Another explanation for the results of PTCA and CABG is related to the patient selection criteria for enrollment into the trials. In the BARI Registry, in which patients were treated according to the preference of the individual physician, and in two large data base studies, poorer outcomes were noted for both CABG and PTCA in diabetics versus nondiabetics, but among diabetics, no survival difference was noted between PTCA and CABG.[627] Similar trends were noted in two large community studies.[363, 600] Diabetic patients as a group in BARI had a greater prevalence of three-vessel disease, left ventricular dysfunction, and a history of congestive heart failure. It is noteworthy that in the Emory University Study of diabetic patients, approximately 85 percent of those with three-vessel disease underwent bypass surgery, whereas the use of PTCA and CABG was similar among those with two-vessel disease.[600] A plausible explanation for the differences in results in the registry and data base studies and the randomized trials is that in the latter, sicker diabetic patients with three-vessel disease and left ventricular dysfunction, by design, were treated equally with bypass surgery and PTCA, whereas in clinical practice, such patients are referred appropriately for surgery, and earlier data base studies suggest that 3- to 5-year survival after CABG in the higher-risk subgroups is superior to that obtained with PCI.

The therapeutic implications of these observations are evident. The revascularization strategy in diabetic patients should be based on the number of vessels diseased, lesion-related technical factors, the caliber of the distal vessels, and the presence or absence of left ventricular dysfunction.

Coronary Bypass Surgery in Patients with Associated Vascular Disease

Management of patients with combined CAD and peripheral vascular disease involving the carotid arteries, the abdominal aorta, or the vessels of the lower extremities presents many challenges.[32] Combined disease is becoming increasingly frequent as the population of patients under consideration for CABG ages and as technical improvements allow the application of coronary revascularization to ever more complex cases.

IMPACT OF CAD IN PATIENTS WITH PERIPHERAL VASCULAR DISEASE. Clinically apparent CAD occurs frequently in patients with peripheral vascular disease.[32] The prevalence of clinically unrecognized CAD, as documented by angiographic studies, is even higher.[628] Among patients undergoing peripheral vascular surgery, late outcomes are dominated by cardiac causes of morbidity and mortality.[628, 629] Conversely, in patients with CAD, the presence of peripheral vascular disease, even if asymptomatic, is associated with an adverse prognosis, presumably because of the greater total atherosclerotic burden borne by these patients.[33, 630]

If coronary revascularization is performed before vascular surgery in patients with combined peripheral vascular disease and CAD, the perioperative mortality of the vascular procedure is reduced.[32] In seven series totaling 1237 patients undergoing vascular surgical procedures, the mean operative mortality was 1.5 percent among patients with prior CABG surgery, similar to the 1.3 percent mortality rate in patients without clinically apparent CAD and substantially lower than the 6.8 percent mortality rate in patients with clinically suspected but uncorrected CAD.[32] Late mortality in patients with peripheral vascular disease is also reduced among those who have undergone prior CABG.[631] However, because patients with CAD and peripheral atherosclerosis tend to be older and have more widespread vascular disease and end-organ damage than do patients without peripheral atherosclerosis, the perioperative mortality and morbidity consequent to CABG are high and the late outcome not as favorable.[32, 628, 632] In the Northern New England Cardiovascular data base, in-hospital mortality after bypass surgery was 2.4-fold greater in patients with peripheral vascular disease than in those without it, particularly for patients with lower extremity disease.[633] In the BARI Trial, approximately one-third of patients had peripheral vascular disease, among whom the risk of major complications after both bypass surgery and PTCA was markedly increased in comparison to those without peripheral vascular disease, even after controlling for baseline differences.[634] *Diffuse atheroembolism* is a particularly serious complication of coronary bypass surgery in patients with peripheral vascular disease and aortic atherosclerosis. It is a major cause of perioperative death, stroke, neurocognitive dysfunction, and multiple organ dysfunction after CABG.

Not only is perioperative morbidity and mortality increased in patients with peripheral vascular disease, but the latter is also a strong marker of an adverse long-term outcome. At any point during a 10-year period, patients in either the medical or surgical group in the CASS Registry who had peripheral vascular disease had a 25 percent greater likelihood of mortality than did those without this condition.[33] Similarly, in the Northern New England Cardiovascular data base, the 5-year mortality remained approximately twofold greater in patients with peripheral vascular disease than in those without it, even after adjusting for comorbid conditions, which are more frequent in patients with peripheral vascular disease.[633, 635] In the BARI Trial, patients with asymptomatic lower extremity disease, as defined by the ankle-arm index, had an almost fivefold greater mortality than did those without lower extremity arterial disease. Indeed, mortality was similar for patients with symptomatic and patients with asymptomatic lower extremity disease.

It is important to identify CAD and to estimate its severity in patients who are candidates for peripheral vascular surgery. The diagnostic problem is intensified because these patients often have limited walking capacity and may not develop effort angina. Pharmacological stress myocardial perfusion scintigraphy or echocardiography can be used. Identification of "high-risk" patients by these techniques (Table 37–2, p. 1280) should lead to coronary angiography in these patients even if they have no or only mild angina and, depending on the anatomical findings, should lead to coronary revascularization, often before peripheral vascular surgery.

Thus, the presence of peripheral vascular disease suggests that the patient may also have high-risk CAD, with potential benefit from CABG in the long term. In the ECSS, patients with CAD and peripheral vascular disease receiving CABG had a much better survival rate than did those who were treated medically.[531] In the CASS Registry, patients with peripheral vascular disease and three-vessel CAD who received surgical treatment also exhibited a major reduction in late mortality and morbidity in comparison with those who were managed medically.[32] Observations such as these argue for *consideration* of CABG in patients with peripheral vascular disease who have significant CAD. The major indication for coronary revascularization before vascular surgery in patients with known chronic CAD is the intention of improving the *long-term* prognosis. A randomized trial of prophylactic coronary artery revascularization in patients undergoing elective vascular surgery is in progress.[636]

CAROTID ARTERY DISEASE. In patients with stable CAD and *carotid artery disease* in whom coronary endarterectomy is planned, exercise stress testing and consideration of coronary revascularization can ordinarily be performed after the carotid surgery.[32] CAD is significantly associated with an increased risk of stroke after bypass surgery, and this association is also strongly correlated with age.[467, 637] However, many strokes are not ipsilateral to the site of stenosis, and the association most likely reflects the presence of diffuse aortic atherosclerosis.[638] The prevalence of significant carotid disease in an increasingly elderly population coming to CABG is high—approximately 17 to 22 percent have a stenosis of 50 percent or greater, 6 to 12 percent have a stenosis of 80 percent or greater, and the percentage is higher in patients with left main CAD.[458, 639]

In patients for whom surgical treatment is considered for both carotid artery disease and CAD, the merits of a combined versus a staged approach are debated.[640, 641] Neither strategy has been demonstrated to be unequivocally superior to the other, and an individualized approach, depending on the patient's initial condition, the severity of symptoms, the anatomy of the coronary and carotid vessels, and individual institutional experience, is most appropriate.[458, 642]

MANAGEMENT. Patients with severe or unstable coronary disease requiring revascularization can be categorized into two groups according to the severity and instability of the accompanying vascular disease.[32] When the noncoronary vascular procedures are elective, they can generally be postponed until the cardiac symptoms have stabilized, either by intensive medical therapy or by revascularization. A combined procedure is necessary in patients with both unstable CAD and an unstable vascular condition, e.g., frequent recurrent transient ischemic attacks or a rapidly expanding abdominal aortic aneurysm.[640, 643] In some patients in this category, PCI offers the potential for stabilizing the patient's cardiac condition before proceeding with a definitive vascular repair.[644]

Other Manifestations of Coronary Artery Disease

PRINZMETAL (VARIANT) ANGINA

In 1959, Prinzmetal and associates described an unusual syndrome of cardiac pain secondary to myocardial ischemia that occurs almost exclusively at rest, is not usually precipitated by physical exertion or emotional stress, and is associated with ECG ST segment elevations[645] (Fig. 37–25). This syndrome, now known as *Prinzmetal*, or *variant*, *angina*, may be associated with acute myocardial infarction and severe cardiac arrhythmias, including ventricular tachycardia and fibrillation, as well as sudden death. A prevailing clinical impression, at least in North America, is that Prinzmetal angina has become less frequent for reasons that are unclear, perhaps because of the more widespread use of calcium antagonists, better nitrate regimens, or alterations in pathophysiology of the coronary disease process.[646] It appears to remain more common in Japan.

Mechanisms

The original hypothesis of Prinzmetal and colleagues, that variant angina was the result of transient increases in coronary vasomotor tone or vasospasm, was convincingly demonstrated by coronary angiography.[647] Vasospasm causes a transient, abrupt, marked decrease in the diameter of an epicardial (or large septal) coronary artery that results in myocardial ischemia. This event occurs in the absence of any preceding increases in myocardial O_2 demand, as reflected in an increased heart rate or blood pressure. The decrease in diameter can usually be reversed by nitroglycerin, sometimes requiring large doses, and can occur in either normal or diseased coronary arteries. Although the sites of vasospasm may correspond to areas of severe focal stenosis, in some patients with apparently normal vessels at angiography, the vasospastic segments appear to occur at sites of at least minimal atherosclerotic change, as detected

by intravascular ultrasonography.[648] Measurements of great cardiac vein flow and left anterior descending coronary artery diameter in patients with vasospastic angina suggest that not only epicardial but also the coronary resistance arteries are affected by the coronary vasomotion disorder.[649] This focal severe vasospasm should not be confused with vasoconstriction of both the large and small coronary vessels, a *normal* response to stimuli such as cold exposure. The latter response is much less intense and occurs diffusely throughout the coronary vascular bed.

In patients with Prinzmetal angina, basal coronary artery tone may be increased. Although responses to various vasoconstrictor substances, including catecholamines, thromboxane A_2, serotonin, endothelin, and arginine vasopressin, are greater in spastic segments of the coronary arteries, hypersensitivity to vasoconstrictor stimuli also occurs throughout the entire coronary tree,[650] perhaps as a manifestation of a more generalized response to vasoactive stimuli.[651] The precise mechanisms have not been established, but a systemic alteration in NO production or an imbalance between endothelium-derived relaxing and contracting factors has been suggested.[650, 652]

In other patients, the sites of spasm in Prinzmetal angina may be adjacent to atheromatous plaque. It has been suggested that in this subgroup of patients, the basic abnormality may be hypercontractility of the arterial wall associated with the atherosclerotic process itself. Other suggested mechanisms include endothelial injury (which reverses the dilator response to a variety of stimuli, e.g., acetylcholine [see Chap. 34]) and hypercontractility of vascular smooth muscle as a result of vasoconstrictor mitogens, leukotrienes, serotonin, endothelin, angiotensin II, histamine,[653, 654] and higher local concentrations of blood-borne vasoconstrictors in areas adjacent to neovascularized atherosclerotic plaque.

The sequelae of coronary spasm may, but do not consistently, accelerate atherosclerosis and predispose to further spasm. One mechanism may involve the release of potent

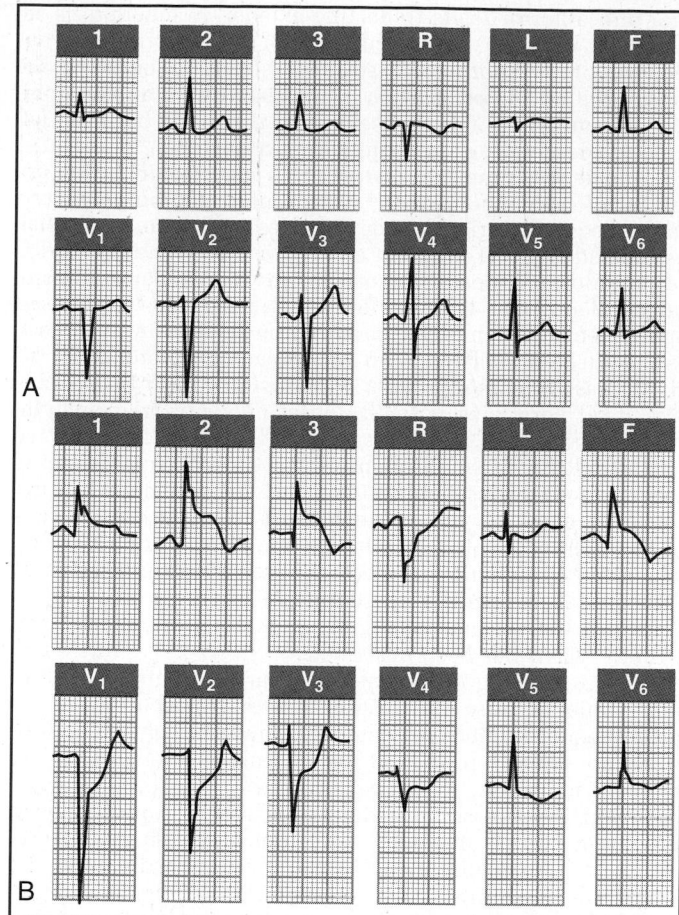

FIGURE 37–25. Electrocardiogram (ECG) before an episode of Prinzmetal angina *(A)* and during an episode of Prinzmetal angina *(B)*. ST segments are now markedly elevated in the inferior leads, with reciprocal depression in the anterior leads. After nitroglycerin was given, the ECG returned to baseline. (From Berman ND, McLaughlin PR, Huckell VF, et al: Prinzmetal's angina with coronary artery spasm. Angiographic, pharmacologic, metabolic and radionuclide perfusion studies. Am J Med 60:727, 1976. By permission of Excerpta Medica.)

concentration, with peak levels occurring from midnight to early morning, in parallel with the frequency of ischemic attacks in these patients.[662] In patients with variant angina, a significant variation in fibrinolytic activity (lowest in the early morning) corresponds with the occurrence of anginal episodes, which are most frequent in the early morning. The possibility that vasospasm may induce leukocyte adhesion in the coronary circulation at an early stage in the initiation of an inflammatory process has been suggested.[663]

Cigarette smoking is an important risk factor for Prinzmetal angina.[664] It has been reported that hypomagnesemia predisposes to variant angina,[665] and magnesium sulfate has been shown to terminate cold pressor–induced anginal attacks and the induction of future attacks[666] and to suppress attacks induced by hyperventilation[667] and exercise in these patients.[668]

Clinical Manifestations

Patients with variant angina tend to be younger than patients with chronic stable angina or unstable angina secondary to coronary atherosclerosis, and many do not exhibit classic coronary risk factors except that they are often heavy cigarette smokers. The anginal discomfort is often extremely severe, is generally referred to as "pain," and may be accompanied by syncope. Associated features in patients with syncope include inferior ST segment elevation and serious arrhythmias, either AV block and asystole or ventricular tachyarrhythmias[669–672] (Fig. 37–26).

Attacks of Prinzmetal angina tend to be clustered between midnight and 8 A.M.[662] Attacks sometimes occur in clusters of two or three within 30 to 60 minutes.[45] Patients studied by means of ambulatory ECG, even those without clinically apparent angina pectoris, show more frequent abnormalities in the morning. In contrast to patients with unstable angina, the pain at rest in patients with Prinzmetal angina has not usually progressed from a period of chronic stable angina. Although exercise capacity is generally well preserved in patients with Prinzmetal angina, some patients experience typical pain and ST segment elevations not only at rest but during or after exertion as well. Acute myocardial infarction in patients with spasm and angiographically normal coronary arteries has been well documented.[673, 674]

Clinical features do not reliably differentiate patients with Prinzmetal angina and normal or mildly abnormal coronary arteriograms from those with this syndrome and severe coronary obstruction.[669] However, the latter may have a combination of fixed-threshold, exertion-induced angina with ST segment depression, as well as episodes of angina at rest with ST segment elevation. In rare cases, Prinzmetal angina develops after coronary artery bypass surgery,[675] and occasionally it appears to be a manifestation of a generalized vasospastic disorder associated with attacks of migraine and Raynaud's phenomenon; it has also been reported in association with aspirin-induced asthma.[676] Coronary spasm with ventricular fibrillation has been observed in thyrotoxicosis.[677] Some patients appear to demonstrate a distinct relationship between emotional distress and episodes of coronary vasospasm, which is consistent with studies suggesting that a sympathovagal imbalance may precipitate spasm in patients with variant angina.[672] Alcohol withdrawal may precipitate variant angina,[678] and conversely, alcohol ingestion may prevent coronary spasm.[679] Variant angina has been reported to be provoked by 5-fluorouracil[680] and by cyclophosphamide[681] (see Chap. 69).

The results of cardiac examination are usually normal in the absence of ischemia (unless the patient has suffered a previous myocardial infarction), but signs of dyskinesia and impaired left ventricular function during episodes of myocardial ischemia are often revealed.

vasoconstrictor substances such as platelet-derived growth factors, in addition to activation of the coagulation system.[655, 656] The combination of a reduction in blood flow and an increase in platelet activation and local thrombosis may accelerate the process of atherosclerosis.[655] Histological findings in patients undergoing coronary atherectomy suggest that repetitive coronary vasospasm may provoke vascular injury and lead to the formation of neointimal hyperplasia at the initial site of spasm. In this respect, coronary spasm may have a key role in the rapid progression of coronary stenosis in some patients.[657] Ergonovine stimulation has been demonstrated to provoke platelet aggregation and an increase in beta-thromboglobulin levels before ECG changes and chest pain in patients with coronary vasospasm.[658]

Imaging with iodine-123–labeled metaiodobenzylguanidine (^{123}I-MIBG) has demonstrated regional myocardial sympathetic dysinnervation, which was not observed in patients with significant obstructive CAD and in subjects with normal coronary arteries.[659] The region of myocardial sympathetic dysinnervation is usually in the area of distribution of the vessel in which vasospasm developed.[659, 660]

Coronary spasm in patients with variant angina may induce stasis and result in the conversion of fibrinogen to fibrin in the coronary vessels, with elevated levels of plasma fibrinopeptide A, an index of fibrin formation.[661] The latter displays significant circadian variation in plasma

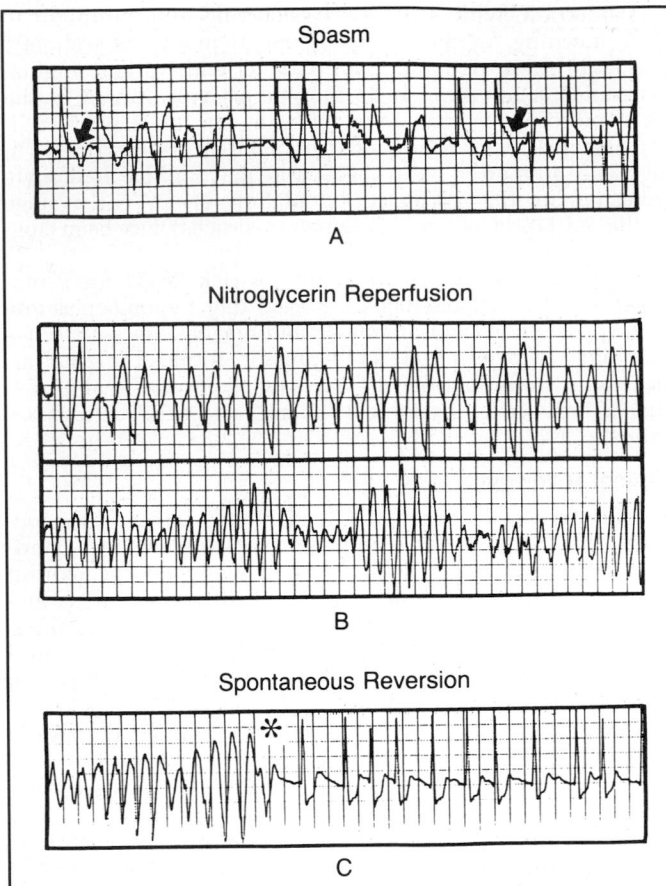

Spasm

A

Nitroglycerin Reperfusion

B

Spontaneous Reversion

C

FIGURE 37-26. Arrhythmia during silent ischemia and reperfusion. Selected strips from a 2.5-minute continuous recording (lead II) in patient during an angiographically documented spasm of the right coronary artery are shown. Tracing A began 24 seconds after the onset of ST segment elevations (arrows) and demonstrates premature ventricular contractions and salvos. The top strip of tracing B was recorded 70 seconds after onset, immediately after the sublingual administration of nitroglycerin (1/150 grain); the bottom strip of tracing B was recorded 36 seconds later. Tracing C was recorded 130 seconds after onset and shows spontaneous reversion (asterisk) and atrial fibrillation. (From Myerburg RJ, Kessler KM, Mallon SM, et al: Life-threatening ventricular arrhythmias in patients with silent myocardial ischemia due to coronary-artery spasm. N Engl J Med 326:1451, 1992. By permission of The Massachusetts Medical Society.)

Electrocardiographic Studies

The key to the diagnosis of variant angina lies in the detection of ST segment elevation with pain (see Fig. 37-25). In a series of patients with variant angina and normal coronary arteries monitored with a computerized 24-hour, 12-lead ECG recording and analysis system, approximately 90 percent of episodes were associated with ST segment elevation, with accompanying arrhythmias in 19 percent, but no arrhythmias were noted in the small proportion of patients with ST segment depression.[669] In some patients, episodes of ST segment depression follow episodes of ST segment elevation and are associated with T wave changes, including peaking of T waves or pseudonormalization of previously depressed segments. ST segment and T wave alternans[682] and increased QT dispersion[683] are the result of ischemic conduction delay and may be associated with potentially lethal ventricular arrhythmias.[684] R wave "growth" may also be associated with the occurrence of ventricular arrhythmias.[685] Many patients exhibit multiple episodes of asymptomatic ST segment elevation (silent ischemia). ST segment deviations may be present in any leads; the concurrent presence of ST segment elevations in both the infe-

rior and anterior leads (reflecting extensive ischemia) is associated with an increased risk of sudden death.[686] A pattern of *alternating* ST segment elevation between the precordial and inferior leads is associated with angiographically documented multivessel spasm involving both the left anterior descending and right coronary systems.[687]

Transient conduction disturbances may occur during episodes of ischemia.[670, 672, 685] Ventricular ectopic activity is more frequent during longer episodes of ischemia, is often associated with ST segment and T wave alternans,[685] and is of ominous prognostic import. In survivors of out-of-hospital cardiac arrest without flow-limiting coronary stenoses, spontaneous or induced focal coronary spasm has been found to be associated with life-threatening ventricular arrhythmias. In some patients, reperfusion rather than ischemia itself correlates with the onset of ventricular arrhythmias[688] (Fig. 37-26). Myocardial cell damage, as reflected by the release of small quantities of CK-MB, may occur in the absence of persistent ECG changes in patients with prolonged attacks of variant angina; transient Q waves have been observed, which may be explained by a transient loss of normal cell membrane electrical activity during spasm.[689] Transmural myocardial infarction caused by coronary artery spasm in the absence of angiographically demonstrable obstructive CAD has been described.[673, 674]

Exercise testing in patients with variant angina is of limited value because the response is so variable. Approximately equal numbers of patients show ST segment depression, no change in ST segments during exercise, or ST segment elevation, which reflects the presence of underlying fixed CAD in some patients, the absence of significant lesions in others, and the provocation of spasm by exercise in the rest. Ambulatory ECG monitoring or the use of a telephone transmitter may be helpful in capturing ST segment elevation during symptomatic episodes.[690]

Hemodynamic and Arteriographic Studies

Spasm of a proximal coronary artery with resultant transmural ischemia and abnormalities in left ventricular function has been convincingly documented arteriographically and is the diagnostic hallmark of Prinzmetal angina.[691]

Significant fixed proximal coronary obstruction of at least one major vessel occurs in the majority of patients, and in these patients spasm usually occurs within 1 cm of the obstruction. The remainder have normal coronary arteries in the absence of ischemia. The process almost always involves large segments of the epicardial vessels at a single site, but at different times other sites may be involved (Fig. 37-27). The right coronary artery is the most frequent site, followed by the left anterior descending coronary artery.[690] Among the 45 percent of patients in one series with multivessel spasm, three different patterns were noted: (1) spasm at a different site on different occasions (migratory spasm), (2) spasm that sequentially affected two different sites, and (3) simultaneous spasm at more than one site. The duration of ST segment elevation was greater in patients with sequential and simultaneous spasm than in those with single-vessel spasm, as was the frequency of arrhythmias.[669] Patients with Prinzmetal angina and normal coronary arteriograms in the absence of pain are more likely to have purely nonexertional angina and ST segment elevations involving the inferior leads during pain. In contrast, patients with Prinzmetal angina who have fixed obstructive lesions with superimposed coronary artery spasm often have associated effort-induced angina and ischemia in the anterolateral leads. Patients with no or mild fixed coronary obstruction tend to experience a more benign course than do patients with associated severe obstructive lesions.[692]

PROVOCATIVE TESTS

THE ERGONOVINE TEST. Several provocative tests for coronary spasm have been developed. Of these, the ergonovine test is the

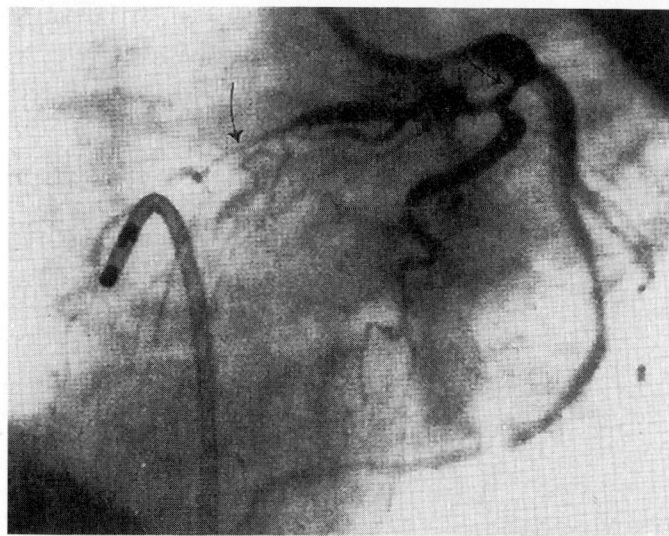

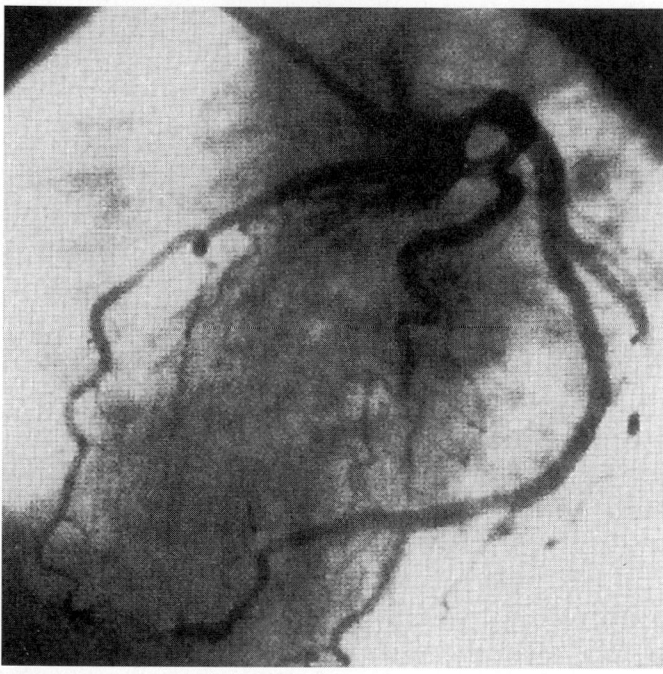

FIGURE 37–27. Angiograms of the left coronary artery in patients with variant angina (left anterior oblique projection). Infusion of 10^{-4} M acetylcholine into the left coronary artery *(top panel)* induced spasm at three focal sites in the left anterior descending artery (arrows). Spasm was reversed after intracoronary nitroglycerin administration *(bottom)*. (From Pepine CJ, el-Tamimi H, Lambert CR: Prinzmetal's angina [variant angina]. Heart Dis Stroke 1: 281, 1992. By permission of The American Heart Association.)

most sensitive. Ergonovine maleate, an ergot alkaloid that stimulates both alpha-adrenergic and serotonergic receptors and therefore exerts a direct constrictive effect on vascular smooth muscle,[693] has been used to induce coronary artery spasm, which results in chest pain and ST segment elevation in patients with Prinzmetal angina. Occasionally, ergonovine may produce a similar response in patients with more typical effort-related anginal symptoms.[690] Coronary arteries that constrict spontaneously appear to be abnormally sensitive to this agent. When administered intravenously in doses ranging from 0.05 to 0.40 mg, ergonovine provides a sensitive and specific test for provoking coronary artery spasm. The majority of patients who have a response to ergonovine do so at a dose of less than 0.2 mg.[690] An inverse correlation is found between the dose of ergonovine required to induce a positive test and the frequency of spontaneous attacks.[694] In low doses and in carefully controlled clinical situations, ergonovine is a relatively safe drug, but prolonged coronary artery spasm precipitated by ergonovine may cause myocardial infarction. Occasionally, conduction disturbances develop (heart block, asystole, or severe tachyarrhythmias).

Because of these hazards, it is recommended that ergonovine be administered only to patients in whom coronary arteriography has demonstrated normal or nearly normal coronary arteries and in gradually increasing doses, beginning with a very low dose. Nitrates and calcium antagonists are usually effective in providing prompt relief from drug-induced spasm, and the intracoronary route is usually the most expeditious in patients already undergoing angiography. To ensure a valid test, nitrates and calcium antagonists must be withdrawn for 48 hours or more before testing. Women are more sensitive than men to ergonovine.[496, 695]

The ergonovine test should be conducted only in a setting where appropriate resuscitative equipment, drugs, and personnel are readily available, usually in the cardiac catheterization laboratory and with a catheter poised to enter the coronary arteries, so that the angiographic diagnosis of spasm can be made and intracoronary nitroglycerin administered to abolish the spasm. Absolute contraindications to ergonovine testing include pregnancy, severe hypertension, severe left ventricular dysfunction, moderate to severe aortic stenosis, and high-grade left main coronary artery stenosis. Relative contraindications include uncontrolled or unstable angina, uncontrolled ventricular arrhythmias, recent myocardial infarction, and advanced CAD.[496]

The response of the *normal* coronary arterial bed to larger doses (≥ 0.40 mg) of ergonovine is a diffuse reduction in arterial caliber.

HYPERVENTILATION. This stimulus has also been demonstrated to provoke some episodes of intense angina,[696] ECG ST segment elevations, angiographic evidence of coronary artery spasm, and ventricular arrhythmias. A recent large series documented the relative specificity of the hyperventilation test in patients with vasospastic angina.[697] Patients with positive tests had a statistically significantly greater frequency of high disease activity (five or more attacks per week), severe arrhythmias during attacks, and multivessel spasm.

ACETYLCHOLINE. Stimulation of acetylcholine receptors produces a uniform endothelium-dependent dilatation of coronary vessels of all sizes that leads to vasoconstriction when endothelial function is impaired.[698] In patients with variant angina, intracoronary injections of acetylcholine have been shown to induce severe coronary spasm and reproduce the clinical syndrome[699] (see Fig. 37–27). This focal spasm should not be confused with the mild diffuse constriction that acetylcholine induces in patients with abnormal coronary endothelium. Because this method allows induction of spasm separately in the left and right coronary arteries, it is useful in patients with known multivessel disease or spasm. Acetylcholine is infused over a 1-minute period into a coronary artery in incremental doses of 10, 25, 50, and 100 μg, and doses should be separated by 5-minute intervals.[496, 695]

Histamine, dopamine, and serotonin can also induce coronary artery spasm.[700, 701] Like ergonovine and acetylcholine, these agents are capable of causing marked coronary artery spasm in patients with variant angina who have severe underlying arteriosclerotic coronary artery narrowing and in those without such fixed stenoses.

Exercise, the cold pressor test, and induced alkalosis can all cause coronary spasm in patients with variant angina, but none of these tests is as sensitive as ergonovine or acetylcholine.

Management

The mainstay of therapy for vasospastic angina is a calcium channel blocker alone or in combination with long-acting nitrates. Nonetheless, several important differences can be seen between the optimal management of Prinzmetal variant angina and classic (stable and unstable) angina.

1. Patients with both variant and classic angina usually respond well to nitrates; sublingual or intravenous nitroglycerin often abolishes attacks of variant angina promptly, and long-acting nitrates are useful in preventing attacks.[702] However, the mechanism of action of the drugs may differ in the two types of angina. As already discussed (see p. 1287), in chronic (effort-induced) stable angina as well as in unstable angina, one important action of nitrates is to reduce myocardial O_2 need and another is to cause coronary vasodilation. In Prinzmetal angina, nitrates abolish or prevent myocardial ischemia *exclusively* by exerting a direct vasodilating effect on the spastic coronary arteries.

2. In patients with classic angina (stable and unstable), beta blockade is usually beneficial, but the response in patients with Prinzmetal angina to these agents is variable.[703] Some, particularly those with associated fixed lesions, exhibit a reduction in the frequency of exertion-induced angina caused primarily by augmentation of myocardial O_2 requirements. In others, however, nonselective beta-adrenoreceptor blockers may actually be detrimental because blockade of beta$_2$ receptors, which subserve coro-

nary dilation, allows unopposed alpha receptor—mediated coronary vasoconstriction to occur; in these patients, the duration of episodes of vasotonic angina may be prolonged by propranolol.[704]

3. In contrast to the variable effectiveness of beta blockers, calcium antagonists are extremely effective in preventing the coronary artery spasm of variant angina,[705, 706] and they should ordinarily be prescribed in maximally tolerated doses. These drugs, along with long- and short-acting nitrates, are the mainstay of therapy. Because calcium antagonists act through a different mechanism than nitrates, the vasodilatory actions of these two classes of drugs may be additive. All first-generation calcium channel antagonists have similar efficacy in producing relief of symptoms: 94 percent for nifedipine, 40 mg/d; 91 percent for diltiazem, 180 mg/d; and 86 percent for verapamil, 240 mg/d.[650, 705–708] In rare instances, a patient responds to only one of these three agents, and even less commonly, the simultaneous administration of two or even three calcium antagonists is required. Some patients need extremely high doses, although side effects are increased.

Slow-release nifedipine has been shown to be highly effective in suppressing not only symptomatic but also asymptomatic myocardial ischemia in patients with variant angina.[707] Second-generation calcium blockers such as the vascular-selective agents felodipine and amlodipine have also been shown to be effective. In addition, once-daily felodipine has been demonstrated to be highly effective in preventing ergonovine-induced myocardial ischemia in patients with variant angina[709] and in patients with spontaneous Prinzmetal angina.[710] In a randomized trial, amlodipine, 5 to 10 mg/d, has also been shown to be effective.[711] Reports have suggested a rebound of symptoms when calcium antagonist therapy is discontinued.[708]

4. *Prazosin*, a selective alpha-adrenoreceptor blocker (see Chap. 29), has also been found to be of value in patients with Prinzmetal angina.[712] *Nicorandil*, a vasodilator that influences coronary arterial tone by acting through potassium channel activation, appears to be effective for the treatment of vasospastic angina, as suggested by studies in Japan and Europe.[713] *Aspirin*, helpful in unstable angina (see Chap. 36), may actually *increase* the severity of ischemic episodes in patients with Prinzmetal angina because it inhibits biosynthesis of the naturally occurring coronary vasodilator prostacyclin.[714] *ACE inhibition* with enalapril was shown to be ineffective in comparison with verapamil in patients with vasospastic angina.[715] Other novel but promising approaches to the management of vasospastic angina include troglitazone, an insulin sensitizer,[716] and denopamine, an adrenergic beta$_1$ agonist,[717] and in a small study of patients in whom vasospastic angina was induced by hyperventilation, the infusion of B-type (brain) natriuretic peptide was highly effective.[718]

5. PCI and occasionally CABG may be helpful in patients with variant angina and discrete, proximal fixed obstructive lesions.[719] Calcium antagonists should be continued for at least 6 months following successful revascularization. PCI and coronary artery bypass surgery are *contraindicated* in patients with isolated coronary artery spasm without accompanying fixed obstructive disease.

Prognosis

Many patients with Prinzmetal angina pass through an acute, active phase, with frequent episodes of angina and cardiac events during the first 6 months after diagnosis. Long-term survival at 5 years is excellent (89 to 97 percent).[686] In a large series of 277 patients with a median follow-up of 7.5 years, recurrent angina was common (39 percent), but cardiac death and myocardial infarction were relatively infrequent and occurred in 3.5 and 6.5 percent of

patients, respectively.[720] However, recurrent myocardial infarction in the setting of normal coronary arteries and angiography has been described.[674] The extent and severity of the underlying CAD and the activity or the tempo of the syndrome have a major effect on the incidence of late mortality and myocardial infarction. Because occlusive coronary spasm may cause stasis with platelet aggregation and thrombosis, the duration of the episodes of spasm is probably a factor in the development of acute infarction.

Patients with variant angina in whom serious arrhythmias (ventricular tachycardia, ventricular fibrillation, high-degree AV block, or asystole) develop during spontaneous episodes of pain have a higher risk of sudden death.[721, 722]

In most patients who survive an infarction or the initial 3- to 6-month period of frequent episodes, the condition stabilizes and symptoms and cardiac events tend to diminish with time. In patients who experience such remissions, cautious tapering of calcium antagonists may be attempted. In one series, 16 percent of patients had spontaneous remission for 3 months after withdrawal of therapy, 44 percent continued to have symptoms despite treatment with calcium antagonists and nitrates, and the other 40 percent were free of angina but receiving treatment. Remission occurred more frequently in patients without significant coronary artery stenoses and in those who stopped smoking.[723]

For reasons that are not clear, some patients, after a relatively quiescent period of months or even years, experience a recrudescence of vasospastic activity with frequent and severe episodes of ischemia.[724] Fortunately, these patients respond to re-treatment with calcium antagonists and nitrates. Most patients in whom symptoms recur after a pain-free period demonstrate, on provocative testing, spasm at the same location as previously demonstrated and respond once more to treatment with nitrates and calcium antagonists.

CHEST PAIN WITH NORMAL CORONARY ARTERIOGRAM

The syndrome of angina or angina-like chest pain with a normal coronary arteriogram, often referred to as *syndrome X* (to be distinguished from the metabolic syndrome X characterized by abdominal obesity, hypertriglyceridemia, low HDL cholesterol, insulin resistance, hyperinsulinemia, and hypertension), is an important clinical entity that should be differentiated from classic ischemic heart disease caused by CAD. In this condition, the prognosis is usually excellent,[725, 726] in contrast to the variable outcome in patients with angina caused by coronary atherosclerosis. Patients with chest pain and normal coronary arteriograms may represent as many as 10 to 20 percent of those undergoing coronary arteriography because of clinical suspicion of angina. The cause(s) of the syndrome is unclear. True myocardial ischemia, reflected in the production of lactate by the myocardium during exercise or pacing, is present in some of these patients.[727] The incidence of coronary calcification on double-helical CT scanning is significantly higher than that of normal controls (63 vs. 22 percent), but lower than that in patients with organic heart disease (96 percent).[728]

It is postulated that the syndrome of angina pectoris with normal coronary arteries reflects a number of conditions. Included in syndrome X are patients with microvascular dysfunction or spasm in whom angina may be the result of ischemia.[729, 730] This condition is frequently referred to as *microvascular angina* (Fig. 37–28). In others, chest discomfort without ischemia may be due to abnormal pain perception or sensitivity. This hypersensitivity may result in an awareness of chest pain in response to stimuli such as arterial stretch or changes in heart rate, rhythm, or contractility. A sympathovagal imbalance with sympathetic

FIGURE 37–28. Proposed pathogenetic mechanisms of microvascular angina. The syndrome results from a variable combination of two components: an increased sensitivity to painful stimuli associated with coronary microvascular dysfunction (indicated by recurring ST segment depression), both of which have a bell-shaped prevalence in the population. Furthermore, within any individual, either component may vary in time (indicated by the horizontal lines). In patients with markedly enhanced sensitivity to pain, even minimal microvascular dysfunction can cause angina. Conversely, some patients with severe microvascular dysfunction (indicated by recurring ST segment depression) may not come to medical attention if they have normal or low sensitivity to pain. (From Maseri A: Ischemic Heart Disease: A Rational Basis for Clinical Practice and Clinical Research. New York, Churchill Livingstone, 1995. By permission.)

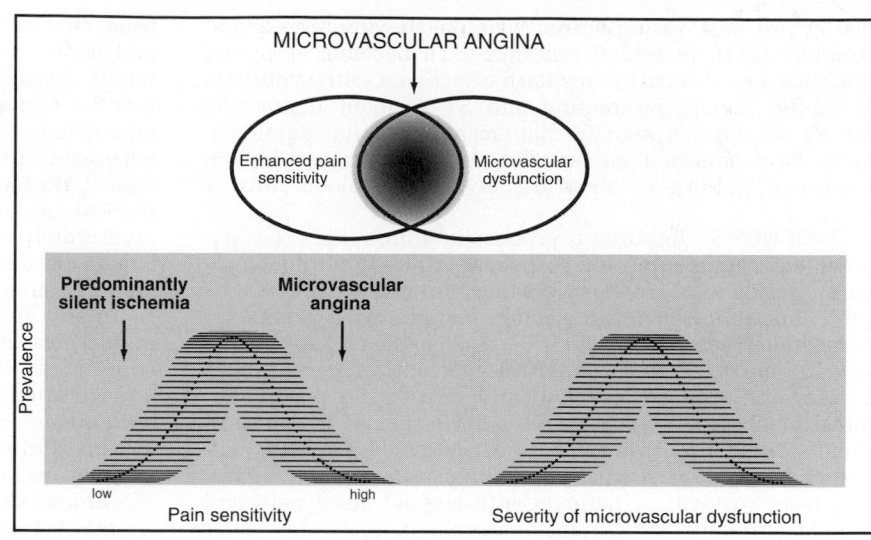

predominance in some of these patients has also been postulated. At the time of cardiac catheterization, some patients with syndrome X are unusually sensitive to intracardiac instrumentation, with typical chest pain being consistently produced by direct right atrial stimulation and saline infusion.[731] Other patients appear to have a combination of microvascular dysfunction and abnormal pain sensitivity. Intravascular ultrasound studies have demonstrated the anatomical and physiological heterogeneity of syndrome X, with a spectrum ranging from normal coronary arteries to vessels with intimal thickening and atheromatous plaque.[732] On the other hand, many patients do not have metabolic evidence of ischemia despite abnormal coronary flow reserve after pacing.[733]

MICROVASCULAR DYSFUNCTION (INADEQUATE VASODILATOR RESERVE) (Fig. 37–28). Patients with chest pain, angiographically normal coronary arteries, and no evidence of large vessel spasm even after an acetylcholine challenge may demonstrate an abnormally reduced capacity to reduce coronary resistance and increase coronary flow in response to stimuli such as exercise, dipyridamole, and atrial pacing. These patients also have an exaggerated response of small coronary vessels to vasoconstrictor stimuli and an impaired response to intracoronary papavarine.[734] Some evidence indicates that increased endothelin concentrations may be associated with reduced coronary flow responses during atrial pacing.[735] This abnormality appears to affect the smaller resistance vessels that are not visible angiographically, whereas the large proximal conductance vessels are normal.[736] The reduced vasodilator reserve in the microcirculation may be associated with exercise-induced regional wall motion abnormalities, as well as abnormalities in diastolic function.[737] The reduced coronary flow reserve may cause abnormalities in myocardial perfusion that are detectable with PET.[738] It has been reported that these patients also have impaired vasodilator reserve in forearm vessels[739] and airway hyperresponsiveness,[740] which suggests that the smooth muscle of systemic arteries and other organs may be affected in addition to that of the coronary circulation.

A link between coronary microvascular dysfunction and ischemia in response to exercise is an attractive concept that could explain abnormal left ventricular function resulting from exercise in some patients with chest pain and normal coronary arteries.[738, 741] Abnormal endothelial function and increased sympathetic drive or responsiveness have been reported.[742, 743]

EVIDENCE FOR ISCHEMIA. Despite general acceptance that microvascular and/or endothelial dysfunction (see Fig. 37–28) is present in many patients with syndrome X, whether ischemia is in fact the putative cause of the symptoms in these patients is not clear.[731, 741] The development

of left ventricular dysfunction and ECG or scintigraphic abnormalities during exercise in some of these patients supports an ischemic cause. However, transesophageal stress echocardiography with dobutamine has failed to demonstrate regional contraction abnormalities consistent with ischemia.[744] The lack of definitive evidence of ischemia in some patients with syndrome X has focused attention on alternative nonischemic causes of cardiac-related pain, including a decreased threshold for pain perception—the so-called sensitive heart syndrome.[731, 745] It is difficult to distinguish patients with syndrome X in whom chest pain is caused by ischemia from patients with noncardiac pain (see p. 1274). Behavioral or psychiatric disorders may be evident.[746, 747] Esophageal dysmotility and reproduction of pain after the infusion of hydrochloric acid into the esophagus (Bernstein test) or intraesophageal balloon distention have been reported in some of these patients.

Clinical Features

The syndrome of angina or angina-like chest pain with normal epicardial arteries occurs more frequently in women,[748] many of whom are premenopausal, whereas obstructive CAD is found more commonly in men and postmenopausal women. Fewer than half of patients with syndrome X have typical angina pectoris; the majority have a variety of forms of atypical chest pain. Although the features are frequently atypical, the chest pain may nonetheless be severe and disabling.[748] The condition may be benign in regard to survival, but it may have markedly adverse effects on the quality of life, employment, and use of health care resources.[749]

In some patients with minimal or no CAD, an exaggerated preoccupation with personal health is associated with the chest pain, and panic disorder may be responsible in a proportion of such patients. Potts and Bass found that two-thirds of patients with chest pain and normal coronary arteries have predominantly psychiatric disorders.[747] Others have reported that the incidence of obstructive CAD is extremely low in patients with atypical chest pain who are anxious and/or depressed.[750] The association between syndrome X and insulin resistance warrants further study.

PHYSICAL AND LABORATORY EXAMINATION. Abnormal physical findings reflecting ischemia, such as a precordial bulge, gallop sound, and the murmur of mitral regurgitation, are uncommon in syndrome X. The resting ECG may be normal, but nonspecific ST-T wave abnormalities are often observed, sometimes occurring in association with the chest pain. Approximately 20 percent of patients with chest pain and normal coronary arteriograms have positive exercise tests. However, many patients with this syndrome do not complete the exercise test because of fatigue or mild chest discomfort. Left ventricular function is usually normal at rest and during stress,[737] unlike the situation in obstructive CAD, in which function often becomes impaired during stress. A small percentage of patients with syndrome X exhibit lactate production and ST segment depression during exercise, a sign of significant ischemia. Some patients have abnormal myocardial perfusion reserve, but no consistent pattern of abnormal myocardial blood flow is seen.

PROGNOSIS. Important prognostic information on patients with angina and either normal or nearly normal coronary arteriograms has been obtained from the CASS Registry.[725] In patients with an ejection fraction of 50 percent or more, the 7-year survival rate was 96 percent for patients with a normal arteriogram and 92 percent for those whose arteriographic study revealed mild disease (50 percent luminal stenosis). In such patients, an ischemic response to exercise was not associated with increased mortality, although a history of smoking or hypertension was. Thus, long-term survival of patients with anginal chest pain and normal coronary angiograms is excellent, markedly better than in patients with obstructive CAD and no different from that in an age-matched general population.[731, 741, 751] Nonetheless, the symptoms are persistent, and most patients continue to experience chest pain that leads to repeated cardiac catheterization and hospital admission.[741, 752]

Management

In patients with angina-like chest pain syndrome and normal epicardial coronary arteries, esophageal abnormalities should be considered (see p. 1273). Such patients may show either motility disorders of the esophagus or abnormal reflux. Exercise ECG and/or myocardial perfusion scintigraphy is often helpful in excluding obstructive CAD. When a noninvasive stress test is positive, or even in patients with serious disability and multiple hospital admissions in whom the test is negative, documentation of normal coronary arteries by coronary angiography provides an objective basis for firm reassurance.

In patients with syndrome X in whom ischemia can be demonstrated by noninvasive stress testing, a trial of antiischemic therapy with nitrates and beta blockers is logical, but the response to this therapy is often poor.[731] In contrast to patients with organic CAD, sublingual nitrates are ineffective in improving exercise tolerance in patients with syndrome X, and in some, exercise tolerance may deteriorate further.[753] Calcium antagonists are effective in reducing the frequency and severity of angina and improving exercise tolerance in some patients. When these conditions are present, treatment of esophageal reflux and dysmotility may be effective.

Estrogen has been shown to attenuate normal coronary vasomotor responses to acetylcholine, increase coronary blood flow, and potentiate endothelium-dependent vasodilation in postmenopausal women.[754] Although estrogen would therefore seem to be a logical treatment for postmenopausal women with syndrome X, only short-term estrogen administration has been studied,[755] and long-term clinical effectiveness of estrogen therapy in these patients has not been documented. Imipramine (50 mg) has been reported to be helpful in some.[746]

Oral aminophylline (an adenosine receptor blocker) may have a favorable effect on the exercise-induced chest pain threshold without any effect on exercise-induced ST segment changes.[756]

SILENT MYOCARDIAL ISCHEMIA

The prognostic importance and the mechanisms of silent ischemia have been the subject of considerable interest for almost 30 years.[757, 758] Patients with silent ischemia have been stratified into three categories by Cohn.[759] The first and least common form, type I silent ischemia, occurs in totally asymptomatic patients with obstructive CAD (which may be severe), and these patients *do not experience angina at any time*; some type I patients do not even experience pain in the course of myocardial infarction. Epidemiological studies of sudden death (see Chap. 26), as well as clinical and postmortem studies of patients with silent myocardial infarction and studies of patients with chronic angina pectoris, suggest that many patients with extensive coronary artery obstruction never experience angina pectoris in any of its recognized forms (stable, unstable, or variant). These patients with type I silent ischemia may be considered to have a *defective anginal warning system*. Type II silent ischemia is the form that occurs in patients with documented previous myocardial infarction.

The third and much more frequent form, designated type III silent ischemia, occurs in patients with the usual forms of chronic stable angina, unstable angina, and Prinzmetal angina. When monitored, patients with this form of silent ischemia exhibit some episodes of ischemia that are associated with chest discomfort and other episodes that are not—i.e., episodes of silent (asymptomatic) ischemia. The "total ischemic burden" in these patients refers to the total period of ischemia, both symptomatic and asymptomatic.

AMBULATORY ELECTROCARDIOGRAPHY. The extensive use of ambulatory ECG monitoring has led to a greater appreciation of the high frequency of type III "silent" ischemia[760] (Fig. 37–29). It has become apparent that anginal pain is a poor indicator and underestimates the frequency of significant cardiac ischemia.[761] Exercise-induced hemodynamic changes indicative of myocardial ischemia (increasing left ventricular end-diastolic pressure and decreasing left ventricular ejection fraction) occur in patients with CAD, regardless of the development of ischemic discomfort.[762]

The role of myocardial O_2 demand in the genesis of myocardial ischemia has been evaluated by measuring the heart rate and blood pressure changes preceding silent ischemic events during ambulatory studies. In one series, 92

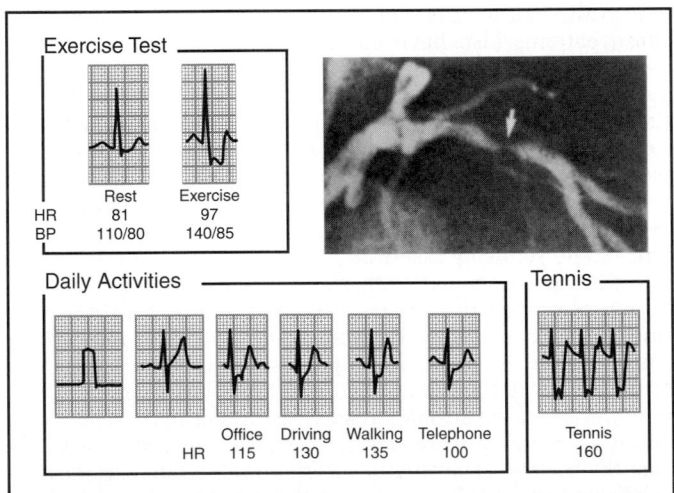

FIGURE 37–29. Ambulatory electrocardiograms and coronary angiogram of a severe left anterior descending stenosis in a patient with fatigue (but not angina) during a tennis match. In stage II of a treadmill exercise test (Bruce protocol), 4 mm of ST segment depression was seen in lead V_5. Ambulatory Holter monitoring of lead V_5 demonstrates ischemic ST segment depression during a number of ordinary activities, e.g., walking, telephoning. During a game of tennis, marked ST segment depression was recorded when the patient was asymptomatic. (From Nabel EG, Rocco MB, Selwyn AB: Characteristics and significance of ischemia detected by ambulatory electrocardiographic monitoring. Circulation 75[Suppl 5]:74, 1987. By permission of the American Heart Association, Inc.)

percent of all episodes were silent, and 60 to 70 percent were preceded by significant increases in heart rate or blood pressure. The circadian variations in heart rate and blood pressure also paralleled the increase in silent ischemic events. This and other studies have suggested that increases in myocardial O_2 demand have a significant role in the genesis of silent ischemia but, in other patients, reductions in myocardial O_2 supply may make an important contribution to the initiation of both symptomatic and asymptomatic episodes.[763] The mechanisms underlying the development of ischemia, as detected by ambulatory ECG and exercise testing, may be different, and in patients in the ACIP Study, concordance between the ambulatory ECG and SPECT was only 50 percent. For identification of silent ischemia, the two techniques probably complement each other.[764]

Transient ST segment depression of 0.1 mV or more that lasts longer than 30 seconds is a very rare finding in normal subjects.[765] Patients with known CAD show a strong correlation between such transient ST segment depression and independent measurements of impaired regional myocardial perfusion and ischemia determined by rubidium-82 uptake as measured by PET.[766] In patients with type III silent ischemia, perfusion defects occur in the same myocardial regions during symptomatic and asymptomatic episodes of ST segment depression. Other methods of detecting "silent" ischemia include measurement of the left ventricular ejection fraction with a "nuclear vest" or the presence of regional wall motion abnormalities and perfusion defects on echocardiography or radionuclide scintigraphy.[764]

Type III silent ischemia is extremely common. Analysis of ambulatory ECG recordings among patients with CAD who had both symptomatic and silent myocardial ischemia found that 85 percent of ambulant ischemic episodes occur without chest pain and 66 percent of angina reports were unaccompanied by ST segment depression.[767] Their frequency is such that it has been suggested that overt angina pectoris is merely the "tip of the ischemic iceberg." Among patients with stable CAD enrolled 1 to 6 months after hospitalization for an acute ischemic event, only 15 percent had angina with exercise, yet 28 percent had ST segment depression and 41 percent had reversible myocardial perfusion defects on thallium scintigraphy.[768] Episodes of silent ischemia have been estimated to be present in approximately half of all patients with angina, although a higher prevalence has been reported in diabetics.[760, 769, 770] Episodes of ST segment depression, both symptomatic and asymptomatic, exhibit a circadian rhythm and are more common in the morning. Asymptomatic nocturnal ST segment changes are almost invariably an indicator of two- or three-vessel CAD or left main coronary artery stenosis.

Pharmacological agents that reduce or abolish episodes of symptomatic ischemia, i.e., nitrates, beta blockers, and calcium antagonists, also reduce or abolish episodes of silent ischemia.[771]

MECHANISMS OF SILENT ISCHEMIA. It is not clear why some patients with unequivocal evidence of ischemia do not experience chest pain whereas others are symptomatic. Maseri has proposed that silent ischemia results from a variable combination of decreased sensitivity to painful stimuli and coronary microvascular dysfunction[1] (Fig. 37-28). Investigation into the causes of silent ischemia has focused primarily on five areas: (1) The association between diabetes and both silent ischemia and "painless infarctions" has been attributed to an autonomic neuropathy.[757, 770, 772, 773] (2) Patients with silent ischemia have been shown to have a high threshold for other forms of pain, such as that resulting from electrical shock, limb ischemia,[774] or cutaneous application of heat[775] or from balloon inflation in the coronary artery.[776] (3) Hypertensive patients who demonstrated a higher incidence of "silent" ischemia

have been shown to have higher pain thresholds and lower reactions to tooth pulp stimulation than normotensive subjects.[776] It has been postulated that these patients produce an excessive quantity of endogenous opioids (and endorphins) that raise the pain threshold, but the existence of such a mechanism is debated.[777] (4) In patients with type III silent ischemia, the asymptomatic episodes may result from a less severe ischemia than the symptomatic episodes. In some of these patients, shorter periods of ischemia on Holter ECG tend to be asymptomatic, whereas longer periods are accompanied by angina.[778, 779] It has been postulated that the pain receptors are not stimulated by the milder episodes of ischemia. (5) A more recent area of investigation suggests that silent ischemia in some patients may not be due to peripheral nerve dysfunction but instead be the result of a defect in the cerebral cortex.[780] Frontal cortical activation appears necessary to experience cardiac pain, and some evidence indicates that in patients with silent ischemia, afferent pain messages from the heart are subject to abnormal neural processing.[764, 780, 781] The role of psychosocial factors in the perception of pain is controversial.[782]

PROGNOSIS. Irrespective of the mechanism(s) responsible, ample evidence supports the view that episodes of myocardial ischemia, regardless of whether they are symptomatic or asymptomatic, are of prognostic importance in patients with CAD. As such, myocardial ischemia, as opposed to symptoms alone, has been identified as a valid therapeutic target. In asymptomatic patients, the presence of exercise-induced ST segment depression has been shown to predict a fourfold to fivefold increase in cardiac mortality in comparison with patients without this finding.[783] In a series of patients in the CASS Registry with ST segment depression on treadmill exercise testing, the risk of subsequent myocardial infarction and sudden cardiac death and the relative benefits of surgery versus medical therapy were determined primarily by angiographic variables of CAD severity and not by the presence or absence of ischemia.[512, 784] A greater benefit was noted with CABG than with medical therapy in those with silent ischemia and three-vessel disease.[784] On the other hand, in some subsets of patients, e.g., stable patients with a previous myocardial infarction, the presence of painless exercise-induced ischemia has not been shown to provide additional prognostic information.[785]

It has been well established that the presence of myocardial ischemia on ambulatory ECG, whether silent or symptomatic, is associated with an adverse cardiac outcome, particularly if the episodes are frequent or accelerating.[334, 771, 786] What previously has been less clear is whether the detection of asymptomatic episodes of ischemia on ambulatory ECG adds *independent* prognostic information over and above that provided by the results of the stress test and the frequency and severity of symptoms.[787, 788] In the ACIP Study, among patients treated medically, myocardial ischemia detected by ambulatory ECG and by an abnormal exercise treadmill test were each *independently* associated with adverse cardiac outcomes.[789] Moreover, ischemia detected by ambulatory ECG monitoring did not correlate with the presence and extent of ischemia as quantified by stress SPECT scintigraphy, which suggests that these techniques detect different pathophysiological manifestations of ischemia.[790] Further support for this concept is provided by angiographic evidence from the ACIP Study data base, in which patients with ischemia and ambulatory ECG were more likely to have multivessel CAD, severe proximal stenoses, and a greater frequency of complex lesion morphology, including intracoronary thrombus, ulceration, and eccentric lesions, than were patients without evidence of ischemia on ambulatory monitoring. The presence of severe and complex CAD may partly explain the apparent independent effect of silent ischemia during ambulatory monitoring on prognosis.[791]

Whether the incremental prognostic information provided by adding an ambulatory ECG to a standard stress test will justify the cost of using this modality as a tool for widespread screening remains to be determined, but it is unlikely. Exercise ECG can identify the majority of patients likely to have significant ischemia during their daily activities and remains the most important screening test for significant CAD. Many patients with type I silent ischemia have been identified because of an asymptomatic positive exercise ECG obtained following myocardial infarction. In such patients with a defective anginal warning system, it is reasonable to assume that asymptomatic ischemia has a significance similar to that of symptomatic ischemia and that their management with respect to coronary angiography and revascularization should be similar.

MANAGEMENT. Drugs that are effective in preventing episodes of symptomatic ischemia (nitrates, calcium antagonists, and beta blockers) are also effective in reducing or eliminating episodes of silent ischemia[757, 792] (Fig. 37-30). In the Atenolol Silent Ischemia Study Trial (ASIST), 4 weeks of atenolol therapy decreased the number of ischemic episodes detected on ambulatory ECG (from 3.6 to 1.7; $p < 0.001$) and also the average duration (from 30 to 16.4 minutes per 48 hours; $p < 0.001$).[334] In another randomized study, long-acting metoprolol taken once daily was as effective as formulations requiring more frequent dosing.[793] In yet another randomized study, metoprolol was shown to be superior to diltiazem in decreasing the mean number of ischemic episodes and the mean duration of ischemia.[794] A combination of a beta blocker and a calcium antagonist is superior to either class of drug alone in suppressing ischemia detected by ambulatory ECG.

Although suppression of ischemia in patients with asymptomatic ischemia is a worthwhile objective, whether treatment should be guided by symptoms or by ischemia as reflected by the ambulatory ECG has not been established. The ACIP Pilot Study showed that the proportion of patients free of ischemia on a 48-hour ambulatory ECG among medically treated patients assigned to an "ischemia-guided" strategy and those assigned to an "angina-guided" strategy was 31 and 36 percent, respectively, at 1 year ($p = $ NS). Among patients treated with coronary revascularization, 57 percent were free of ischemia at 1 year ($p < 0.001$).[795] Similar trends were noted in the results of exercise testing.[796]

Coronary revascularization is superior to medical therapy for the relief of both angina and ambulatory ischemia at 12 weeks.[797] Moreover, the early benefits of revascularization on ischemia are associated with improved clinical outcomes. In this pilot study with over 2 years of follow-up, total mortality was 6.6 percent with the angina-guided strategy, 4.4 percent with the ischemia-guided strategy, and 1.1 percent with the revascularization strategy ($p < 0.02$). The rate of death or myocardial infarction was 12.1 percent in the angina-guided strategy, 8.8 percent in the ischemia-guided strategy (see Fig. 37-17), and 4.7 percent in the revascularization strategy, and a strong reduction was also seen in recurrent hospitalizations and the revascularization strategies. These differences were significant, but no differences were noted between the two strategies of medical therapy.[545]

HEART FAILURE IN ISCHEMIC HEART DISEASE

In the current era, the leading cause of heart failure in developed countries is CAD.[798] In the United States, CAD and its complications account for two-thirds to three-fourths of all cases of heart failure. In many patients, the progressive nature of heart failure reflects the progressive nature of the underlying CAD. The term *ischemic cardiomyopathy* is used for the clinical syndrome in which one or more of the above pathophysiological features result in left ventricular dysfunction and heart failure symptoms. This condition is the predominant form of heart failure related to CAD. Additional complications of CAD that may become superimposed on ischemic cardiomyopathy and precipitate heart failure are the development of left ventricular aneurysm and mitral regurgitation caused by papillary muscle dysfunction.

Ischemic Cardiomyopathy

In 1970, Burch and colleagues first used the term *ischemic cardiomyopathy* to describe the condition in which CAD results in severe myocardial dysfunction, with clinical manifestations often indistinguishable from those of primary dilated cardiomyopathy[799] (see Chap. 48). Symptoms of heart failure caused by ischemic myocardial dysfunction and hibernation, diffuse fibrosis, or multiple infarctions, alone or in combination, may dominate the clinical picture of CAD. In some patients with chronic CAD, angina may be the principal clinical manifestation at one time, but later this symptom diminishes or even disappears as heart failure becomes more prominent. Other patients with ischemic cardiomyopathy have no history of angina or myocardial infarction (type I silent ischemia, see p. 1330), and it is in this subgroup that ischemic cardiomyopathy is most often confused with dilated cardiomyopathy.

It is important to recognize hibernating myocardium in patients with ischemic cardiomyopathy because symptoms resulting from chronic left ventricular dysfunction may be incorrectly thought to result from necrotic and scarred

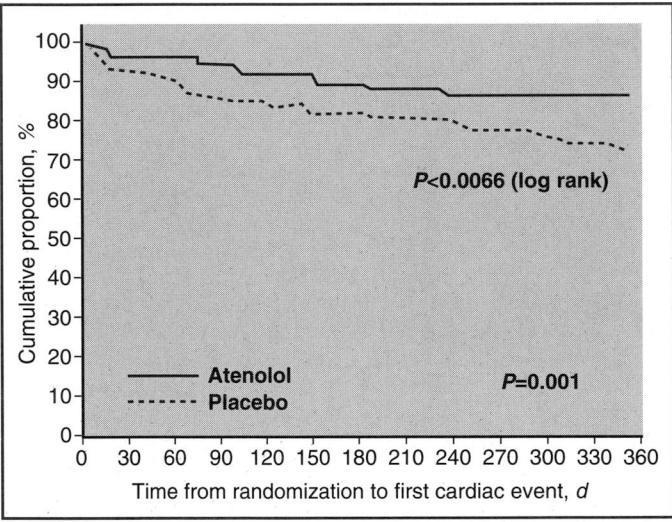

FIGURE 37-30. Atenolol in Silent Ischemia Trial (ASIST). The recently reported ASIST is the first controlled trial to demonstrate modification of cardiac risk through treatment of silent myocardial ischemia (SMI). A total of 306 asymptomatic or minimally symptomatic patients with coronary artery disease, positive exercise tests, and ambulatory electrocardiographic (ECG) episodes of SMI were randomized to receive atenolol or placebo. Ambulatory ECG monitoring was repeated at 4 weeks, and outcome was assessed after 1 year. At 4 weeks, atenolol was associated with a significant reduction in SMI. After 1 year, a significant (56 percent) relative reduction in adverse events (death, resuscitated ventricular tachycardia and fibrillation, nonfatal myocardial infarction, and unstable or worsening angina) was found when patients given atenolol were compared with those given placebo. The presence of ischemia at 4 weeks was the most important independent factor associated with adverse outcomes after 1 year. (From Bertolet BD, Pepine CJ: Silent myocardial ischemia. *In* Beller GA, Braunwald E [eds]: Chronic Ischemic Heart Disease. Atlas of Heart Diseases. Vol 5. Philadelphia, Current Medicine, 1995, p 8.9. By permission of W.B. Saunders Co.)

myocardium rather than from a reversible ischemic process. Hibernating myocardium may be present in patients with known or suspected CAD with a degree of cardiac dysfunction or heart failure not readily accounted for by previous myocardial infarctions (see also p. 1316).

The outlook for patients with ischemic cardiomyopathy treated medically is quite poor, and revascularization or cardiac transplantation may be considered.[800] The prognosis is particularly poor for patients in whom ischemic cardiomyopathy is due to multiple myocardial infarctions, in those with associated ventricular arrhythmias, and in those with extensive amounts of hibernating myocardium. However, this latter group of patients, whose heart failure, even if severe, is due to large segments of reversibly dysfunctional, but viable myocardium, has a significantly better prognosis after revascularization.[564, 568–571] Revascularization in this group also significantly improves heart failure symptoms.[103, 563, 564] Thus, the key to management of patients with ischemic cardiomyopathy is to assess the extent of residual viable myocardium with a view to coronary revascularization of viable myocardium (see Chap. 13 and p. 50–51). Patients with little or no viable myocardium in whom heart failure is secondary to extensive myocardial infarction and/or fibrosis should be managed in a manner similar to those with dilated cardiomyopathy (see Chaps. 21 and 48). Their prognosis is poor.

Left Ventricular Aneurysm

Left ventricular aneurysm is usually defined as a segment of the ventricular wall that exhibits paradoxical (dyskinetic) systolic expansion. Chronic fibrous aneurysms interfere with ventricular performance principally through loss of contractile tissue. Aneurysms made up largely of a mixture of scar tissue and viable myocardium or of thin scar tissue also impair left ventricular function by a combination of paradoxical expansion and loss of effective contraction. *False aneurysms* (pseudoaneurysms) represent localized myocardial rupture in which the hemorrhage is limited by pericardial adhesions, and they have a mouth that is considerably smaller than the maximal diameter (Fig. 37–31). True and false aneurysms may coexist, although the combination is extremely rare.[801]

The frequency of ventricular aneurysms depends on the incidence of transmural myocardial infarction and congestive heart failure in the population studied. Left ventricular aneurysms and the need for aneurysmectomy have declined dramatically during the last 5 to 10 years in concert with the expanded use of acute reperfusion therapy in evolving myocardial infarction. More than 80 percent of left ventricular aneurysms are located anterolaterally near the apex. They are often associated with total occlusion of the left anterior descending coronary artery and a poor collateral blood supply.[802] Approximately 5 to 10 percent of aneurysms are located posteriorly. Three-quarters of patients with aneurysms have multivessel CAD.[803]

Left ventricular aneurysms can develop in patients who sustain a blunt chest injury (see Chap. 51). The condition is attributed to myocardial contusion or to direct vascular damage causing myocardial necrosis; pseudoaneurysms of adjacent vascular structures, including the thoracic aorta, may be present in addition to valvular damage.[804] Death from rupture of a false aneurysm caused by nonpenetrating chest trauma has been described[805] and successfully repaired surgically.[806]

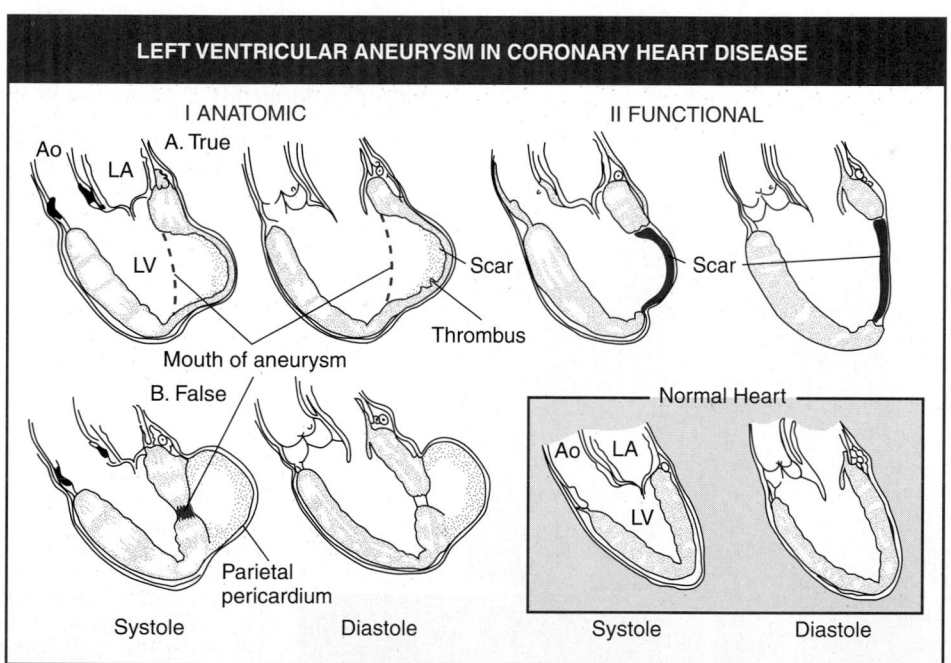

FIGURE 37–31. Hearts in systole and diastole with true and false anatomical and functional left ventricular aneurysms and healed myocardial infarction. A normal heart in systole and diastole is shown for comparison. A true anatomical left ventricular aneurysm protrudes during both systole and diastole, has a mouth that is as wide or wider than the maximal diameter, has a wall that was formerly the wall of the left ventricle, and is composed of fibrous tissue with or without residual myocardial fibers. A true aneurysm may or may not contain thrombus and almost never ruptures once the wall is healed. A false anatomical left ventricular aneurysm protrudes during both systole and diastole, has a mouth that is considerably smaller than the maximal diameter of the aneurysm and represents a myocardial rupture site, has a wall made up of parietal pericardium, virtually always contains thrombus, and often ruptures. A functional left ventricular aneurysm protrudes during ventricular systole but not during diastole and consists of fibrous tissue with or without myocardial fibers. (From Cabin HS, Roberts WC: Left ventricular aneurysm, intraaneurysmal thrombus and systemic embolus in coronary heart disease. Chest 77:586, 1980. By permission of The American College of Chest Physicians.)

Almost 50 percent of patients with moderate or large aneurysms have symptoms of heart failure (with or without associated angina), approximately 33 percent have severe angina alone, and approximately 15 percent have symptomatic ventricular arrhythmias that may be intractable and life threatening.[807] Mural thrombi are found in almost half of patients with chronic left ventricular aneurysms and can be detected by angiography and two-dimensional echocardiography (see Chap. 7). Systemic embolic events in patients with thrombi and left ventricular aneurysm tend to occur early after myocardial infarction. In the Mayo Clinic series of patients with chronic left ventricular aneurysm (documented at least 1 month after infarction), subsequent systemic emboli were extremely uncommon[808] (0.35 per 100 patient-years in patients not receiving anticoagulants).

DETECTION. Clues to the presence of aneurysm include persistent ST segment elevations on the resting ECG (in the absence of chest pain)[809] and a characteristic bulge of the silhouette of the left ventricle on a chest roentgenogram. Marked calcification of the left ventricular silhouette may be present[810] (Fig. 37–32). These findings, when clear-cut, are relatively specific, but they have limited sensitivity. Radionuclide ventriculography and two-dimensional echocardiography can demonstrate ventricular aneurysm more readily; the latter is also helpful in distinguishing between true and false aneurysms based on the demonstration of a narrow neck in relation to cavity size in the latter.[811] Color flow echocardiographic imaging is useful in establishing the diagnosis because flow "in and out" of the aneurysm as well as abnormal flow within the aneurysm can be detected, and subsequent pulsed Doppler imaging can reveal a "to-and-fro" pattern with characteristic respiratory variation in the peak systolic velocity. The use of transesophageal echocardiography and left-heart contrast agents in the assessment of pseudoaneurysms is being evaluated.[812] CT and magnetic resonance imaging are reliable noninvasive techniques for the identification of left ventricular aneurysms (Fig. 37–32; see Fig. 10–8) and screening for resectability.[813]

Tomographic three-dimensional echocardiographic calculation of left ventricular volume and systolic function compares favorably with the accuracy of magnetic resonance imaging and cineangiography and has the advantage of being less time consuming and less invasive; also, patient discomfort may be less.[814] However, biplane left ventriculography is still the most widely used method for outlining a true left ventricular aneurysm and assessing septal motion and the extent of residual functioning myocardium. An assessment of the extent of stunned, hibernating but potentially viable, myocardium within the infarct zone is helpful in many patients, particularly those in whom the left ventricular aneurysm is less discrete.

LEFT VENTRICULAR ANEURYSMECTOMY. True ventricular aneurysms do not rupture, and operative excision is carried out to improve the clinical manifestations, most often heart failure but sometimes also angina, embolization, and life-threatening tachyarrhythmias.[807, 815] Coronary revascularization is frequently performed along with aneurysmectomy, especially in patients in whom angina accompanies heart failure.

A large left ventricular aneurysm in a patient with symptoms of heart failure, particularly if angina pectoris is also present, is an indication for surgery. The operative mortality rate for left ventricular aneurysmectomy is approximately 10 percent (ranging from 0 to 19 percent),[815, 816] with rates of 6 and 7.2 percent reported in more recent series.[816, 817] Among 26 patients undergoing surgery between 1992 and 1994 with the new technique of endoventricular patchplasty, no operative mortality was reported.[817] Risk factors for early death include poor left ventricular function, recent myocardial infarction, the presence of mitral regurgitation, and intractable ventricular arrhythmias.[818] The presence of angina pectoris instead of dyspnea as the dominant preoperative symptom is a determinant of lower operative mortality.[817] Surgery carries a particularly high risk in patients with severe heart failure, a low-output state, and akinesis of the interventricular septum, as assessed echocardiographically.[803] Akinesis or dyskinesis of the pos-

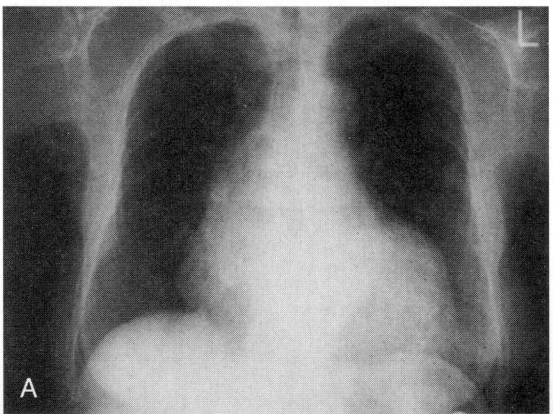
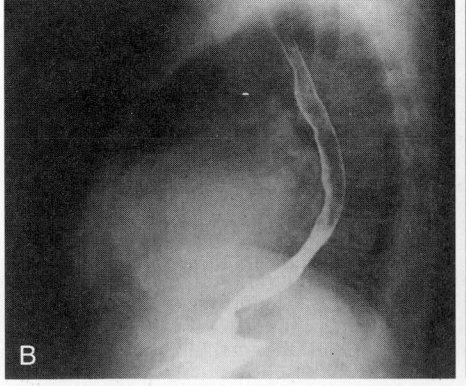
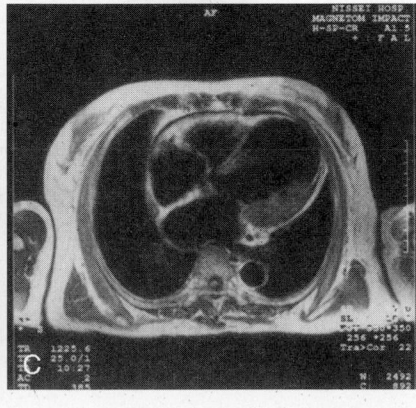

FIGURE 37–32. Evaluation of an 83-year-old woman for chest discomfort. When she was about 50 years old, this woman had been hospitalized because of acute myocardial infarction of the anteroseptal wall. An electrocardiogram showed an abnormal image characteristic of anteroseptal cardiac aneurysm. A plain chest film (A and B) showed marked calcification on the left ventricular silhouette. A magnetic resonance image (C) of the heart showed thinning of the left ventricular wall. The patient's overall condition improved after treatment with isosorbide mononitrate and diuretics. (From Nakajima O, Sano I, Akioka H: Marked calcified left ventricular aneurysm. Circulation 95:1974, 1997. By permission of the American Heart Association, Inc.)

terior basal segment of the left ventricle and significant right coronary artery stenoses are additional risk factors.[803] Pseudoaneurysms rupture frequently and should therefore be resected on an urgent basis as soon as the diagnosis is established.[819]

Risk factors for late mortality following survival from surgery include incomplete revascularization, impaired systolic function of the basal segments of the ventricle and septum not involved by the aneurysm, the presence of a large aneurysm with a small quantity of residual viable myocardium, and the presence of severe cardiac failure as the initial feature.[816, 817, 820]

Improvement in left ventricular function has been reported in survivors of resection of left ventricular aneurysms complicated by cardiac failure.[818, 821] By removing the abnormal mechanical burden, left ventricular aneurysmectomy has been associated with late improvement in overall systolic function and improvement in the performance of regional nonischemic myocardium in zones remote from the left ventricular aneurysm,[822] in addition to improvement in measures of ventricular relaxation and cardiovascular neuroregulatory mechanisms.[821, 823] A concomitant improvement in exercise performance and clinical symptoms may also occur, particularly in patients who have undergone complete revascularization. An early series of carefully selected patients documented a 10-year survival rate of 69 percent among patients undergoing left ventricular aneurysmectomy plus coronary revascularization in comparison with 57 percent after aneurysmectomy alone.

New surgical approaches to the repair of left ventricular aneurysms are designed to restore normal left ventricular geometry by using an alternative method of epicardial closure and/or an endocardial patch to divide the area of the aneurysm from the remainder of the ventricular cavity[824, 825] (Fig. 37–33). Favorable clinical and hemodynamic results following the use of these newer techniques have been reported, with 5-year survival rates ranging from 73 to 87.5 percent[816, 820] and a corresponding improvement in hemodynamics and clinical symptoms. In one series, 88 percent of patients treated with the endoaneurysmorrhaphy technique were in New York Heart Association Class I or II after a mean follow-up of approximately 3.5 years.[826]

Mitral Regurgitation Secondary to Coronary Artery Disease (see also Chap. 46)

Mitral regurgitation is an important cause of heart failure in some patients with CAD. Rupture of a papillary muscle or the head of a papillary muscle usually causes severe acute mitral regurgitation in the course of acute myocardial infarction. The cause of chronic mitral regurgitation in patients with CAD is multifactorial, and the geometrical determinants are complex and include papillary muscle dysfunction from ischemia and fibrosis in conjunction with a wall motion abnormality and changes in ventricular shape in the region of the papillary muscle and/or dilatation of the mitral annulus.[827, 828] Enlargement of the mitral annulus at end systole is asymmetrical, with lengthening primarily involving the posterior annular segments and leading to prolapse of leaflet tissue tethered by the posterior papillary muscle and restriction of leaflet tissue attached to the anterior leaflet.[829] Most patients with chronic CAD and mitral regurgitation have suffered a previous myocardial infarction.

Clinical features that help identify mitral regurgitation secondary to papillary muscle dysfunction as the cause of acute pulmonary edema or the cause of milder symptoms of left-sided failure include a loud systolic murmur and demonstration of a flail mitral valve leaflet on echocardiography. In some patients with severe mitral regurgitation into a small "unprepared" left atrium, the murmur may be unimpressive or inaudible. Doppler echocardiography is helpful in assessing the severity of the regurgitation (see Chap. 7).

As in mitral regurgitation of other causes, the left atrium is not usually greatly enlarged unless mitral regurgitation has been present for more than 6 months. The ECG is nonspecific, and most patients have angiographic evidence of multivessel CAD.

In patients with posterior papillary muscle dysfunction resulting from acute myocardial infarction, reperfusion therapy with thrombolysis or PCI may be attempted initially because urgent surgery is often accompanied by high mortality. In patients with rupture of a papillary muscle or, more frequently, rupture of one or more heads of a papillary muscle, immediate surgery is required because the natural history after apparent stabilization with medical therapy is labile and unpredictable and sudden unexpected deterioration is frequent.[830]

In patients with severe mitral regurgitation, the indications for surgical correction, usually in association with coronary artery bypass, are fairly clear-cut. Mitral valve repair, as opposed to mitral replacement, is the procedure of choice, but the decision is based on the anatomical characteristics of the structures forming the mitral valve apparatus, the urgency of the need for surgery, and the severity of left ventricular dysfunction.[831] A more complex and fre-

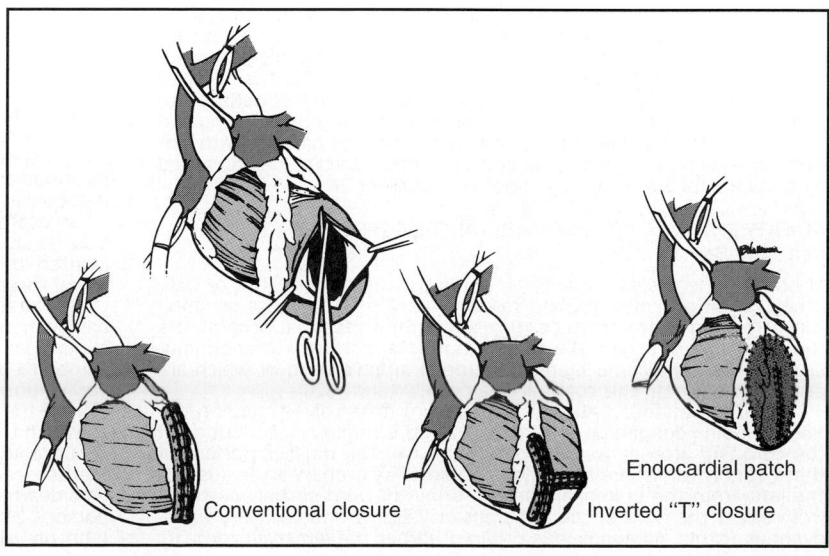

FIGURE 37–33. Operative techniques used in left ventricular aneurysm repair. The figure depicts resection of the ventricular aneurysm enclosure by one of three methods. The conventional closure is illustrated on the left. The "T" closure and the endocardial patch techniques were developed in an attempt to restore normal left ventricular geometry. (From Komeda M, David TE, Malik A, et al: Operative risks and long-term results of operation for left ventricular aneurysm. Ann Thorac Surg 53:22, 1992. By permission of The Society of Thoracic Surgeons.)

Conventional closure   Inverted "T" closure   Endocardial patch

quently encountered problem involves the indications for mitral valve surgery in patients undergoing coronary bypass surgery in whom the severity of mitral regurgitation is moderate. The decision is based partly on the presence or absence of structural abnormalities of the mitral apparatus and the amenability of the valve to repair. Intraoperative transesophageal echocardiography is invaluable in assessing the severity of regurgitation, the reparability of the valve, and the success of the integrity of the repair after discontinuation of cardiopulmonary bypass.[458]

The mortality associated with combined coronary bypass surgery and mitral valve placement in the 1997 Society of Thoracic Surgeons data base was 12.7 percent overall and 8.3 percent for patients undergoing an elective first procedure. For bypass surgery and mitral valve repair, mortality rates were 7.6 percent overall and 4.8 percent for patients undergoing an elective first procedure.[425] Predictors of early mortality include the need for replacement versus repair (in some but not all series) but, in addition, may include other variables such as age, comorbid conditions, the urgency of surgery, and left ventricular function.[831, 832] Late results are strongly influenced by the pathophysiological mechanisms underlying mitral regurgitation and are poorer in patients with regurgitation resulting from annular dilatation or restrictive leaflet motion than in patients with chordal or papillary muscle rupture.[832, 833] It is encouraging that despite the relatively high operative mortality, late survival of hospital survivors is excellent. In patients with very poor left ventricular function and dilatation of the mitral annulus, mitral regurgitation can intensify the severity of left ventricular failure. In such patients, the risk of surgery is high and the benefits less obvious, and a trial of intensive medical therapy, including offload reduction to reduce left ventricular volume and the diameter of the annulus, may be worthwhile.

CARDIAC ARRHYTHMIAS (see also Chap. 25)

In some patients with CAD, cardiac arrhythmias are the dominant clinical manifestation of the disease. Various degrees and forms of ventricular ectopic activity are the most common arrhythmias in patients with CAD, but serious ventricular arrhythmias may be a major component of the clinical findings in other subgroups. Malignant ventricular arrhythmias in CAD may be dynamic, e.g., plaque rupture that causes acute ischemia, which results in polymorphic ventricular tachycardia or ventricular fibrillation.[834] A more frequent manifestation of ventricular arrhythmias in CAD occurs as a consequence of reentrant arrhythmias arising from fixed substrate composed of scar and residual viable myocardium.[835] In this situation, it is presumed that initially stable, sustained monomorphic ventricular tachycardia degenerates into ventricular fibrillation. The former situation is theoretically preventable by coronary revascularization alone, although for patients who have survived an out-of-hospital cardiac arrest, coronary revascularization alone is usually ineffective in preventing occurrences.[559, 836]

Surgical strategies for patients with CAD and ventricular tachycardia, in association with left ventricular aneurysms and/or myocardial scar, were directed primarily at removal of the extensive area of subendocardial scar tissue, with or without electrophysiological mapping.[837, 838] Surgical treatment of ventricular arrhythmias has declined markedly with the advent of the implantable cardioverter-defibrillator and, to a lesser extent, advances in electrophysiological mapping and catheter ablation. Recognition and management of patients with malignant ventricular arrhythmias and/or sudden cardiac death caused by chronic CAD are discussed in detail in Chapter 26.

NONATHEROMATOUS CORONARY ARTERY DISEASE
(see Table 35–1)

Although atherosclerosis is by far the most important cause of CAD, other conditions may also be responsible.[839, 840] The most common causes of nonatheromatous CAD resulting in myocardial ischemia are the syndrome of angina-like pain with normal coronary arteriograms, i.e., so-called syndrome X and Prinzmetal angina, both of which are discussed earlier in this chapter (see pp. 1324 and 1328).

Nonatheromatous CAD may result from other diverse abnormalities, including congenital abnormalities in the origin or distribution of the coronary arteries (see Chaps. 43 and 44). The most important of these abnormalities are anomalous origin of a coronary artery (usually the left) from the pulmonary artery, origin of both coronary arteries from either the right or the left sinus of Valsalva, and coronary arteriovenous fistula. An anomalous origin of either the left main coronary artery or right coronary artery from the aorta with subsequent coursing between the aorta and pulmonary trunk is a rare and sometimes fatal coronary arterial anomaly.[841]

In an autopsy study of 150 cases of sudden death in persons 35 years or younger, death was attributed to CAD in 48. In 16 of these cases, the disease was not atherosclerosis but attributable to abnormalities in the origin and course of the coronary arteries, including a deep intramyocardial course, ostial obstruction, an abnormal origin of the right or left coronary artery, or spontaneous dissection of a coronary artery. In one patient, effort-induced acute myocardial infarction was noted in the presence of an intramural coronary arterial trunk.[842]

Myocardial bridging causing systolic compression of the left anterior descending coronary artery is a well-recognized angiographic phenomenon of questionable clinical significance.

Several inherited connective tissue disorders are associated with myocardial ischemia (see Chap. 56), including the Marfan syndrome (causing aortic and coronary artery dissection), Hurler syndrome (causing coronary obstruction), homocysteinuria (causing coronary artery thrombosis), Ehlers-Danlos syndrome (causing coronary artery dissection), and pseudoxanthoma elasticum (causing accelerated CAD). Kawasaki disease (the mucocutaneous lymph node syndrome) may cause coronary artery aneurysms and ischemic heart disease in children (see Chap. 45).

Spontaneous coronary dissection is a rare cause of myocardial infarction and sudden cardiac death.[843] Chronic dissection manifested as congestive heart failure has been described. In one series, approximately 75 percent of cases were diagnosed at autopsy, and 75 percent occurred in women, half of which were associated with a postpartum state.[844] Some cases are associated with atherosclerosis. Hypertension has been postulated as a cause of multivessel spontaneous coronary dissection in some patients, and in others, no obvious cause has been identified. In the acute phase, thrombolytic therapy may be dangerous, but early angiography may identify patients who could benefit from stenting or bypass surgery.[845] In survivors of spontaneous coronary artery dissection, the subsequent 3-year mortality was 20 percent, but complete healing as defined angiographically may lead to a favorable outcome without intervention.[846]

Coronary vasculitis resulting from connective tissue diseases or autoimmune forms of vasculitis, including polyarteritis nodosa,[847] giant cell (temporal) arteritis,[848] and scleroderma,[849] is well described (see Chap. 67). Coronary arteritis is seen at autopsy in about 20 percent of patients with rheumatoid arthritis but is rarely associated with clinical manifestations.[850] The incidence of CAD is increased in women with systemic lupus erythematosus.[851] In patients with systemic lupus erythematosus, CAD has been attributed to a vasculitis, immune complex–mediated endothelial damage, and coronary thrombosis from antiphospholipid antibodies,[851, 852] as well as accelerated atherosclerosis. Giant coronary artery aneurysm associated with systemic lupus erythematosus is an unusual manifestation that has been associated with the development of acute myocardial infarction despite therapy.[852] The antiphospholipid syndrome, which is characterized by arterial and venous thrombosis and is associated with the presence of antiphospholipid antibodies, may be associated with myocardial infarction, angina, and diffuse left ventricular dysfunction.[853]

In rare cases, *Takayasu arteritis* (see Chap. 67) is associated with angina, myocardial infarction, and cardiac failure in patients younger than 40 years.[854] Coronary blood flow may be decreased by involvement of the ostia or proximal segments of the coronary arteries, but disease in distal coronary segments is rare.[855] The average age at the onset of symptoms is 24 years, and the event-free survival rate 10 years after diagnosis is approximately 60 percent.[854] Luetic aortitis may also produce myocardial ischemia by causing coronary ostial obstruction.

The occurrence of CAD and morbid cardiac events in young persons after mediastinal irradiation is highly suggestive of a cause-and-effect relationship.[856, 857] Pathological changes include adventitial scarring and medial hypertrophy with severe intimal atherosclerotic disease.[858] Radiation injury may be latent and may not be manifested clinically for many years after therapy. Contributory factors include higher doses than currently administered and the presence of cardiac risk factors.[859] Among patients without risk factors who receive an intermediate total dose of 30 and 40 Gy, the risk of cardiac death and myocardial infarction is low.[857]

Myocardial ischemia not caused by coronary atherosclerosis can also result from embolism, infective endocarditis (see Chap. 47), implanted prosthetic cardiac valves (Chap. 46), calcified aortic valves, mural thrombi, and primary cardiac tumors (Chap. 49).

An interesting nonatherosclerotic myocardial ischemic syndrome has been described in workers in the nitrate industry, who apparently experience nitrate withdrawal symptoms on weekends. It is presumed to be secondary to coronary spasm in the absence of counterstimulation to the vasoconstriction that they undergo as an adaptation to the vasodilating actions of the high concentrations of nitrates to which they have been exposed.[860]

Cocaine, because of its widespread use, has become a well-documented cause of chest pain, myocardial infarction, and sudden cardiac death.[861, 862] In a population-based study of sudden death among persons 20 to 40 years old in Olmsted County over a 30-year period, a high prevalence of cocaine abuse was observed in the more recent cohort of young adults who died suddenly.[863] The principal effects of cocaine are mediated by alpha-adrenergic stimulation, which causes an increase in myocardial O_2 demand and a reduction in O_2 supply because of coronary vasoconstriction.[862]

CARDIAC TRANSPLANT–ASSOCIATED CORONARY ARTERIOPATHY (see also Chap. 20).

Worldwide, approximately 4500 patients undergo cardiac transplantation annually (2340 in the United States in 1998), and their survival has been extended by improved immunosuppression. Accelerated coronary atherosclerosis has become the principal cause of late death.[864] The link between chronic immune injury to the coronary endothelium of the donor heart and transplant CAD is unclear, but it is believed to be initiated by immunologically mediated damage, followed by intimal smooth muscle proliferation, accumulation of lipids in the vascular wall, and eventually, diffuse luminal narrowing.[865] Other suggested etiological factors include opportunistic infections (cytomegalovirus infection), immunosuppressive therapy, cyclosporine-induced endothelial injury, and dyslipidemia.[866]

By the time that the disease is diagnosed, it is well advanced, but its progression to myocardial infarction, sudden cardiac death, and diffuse left ventricular dysfunction may not be accompanied by chest pain or typical ECG changes. The diagnosis is usually made at coronary angiography, but this visualization technique may underestimate the severity or the extent of the disease.[867] Noninvasive approaches, including dobutamine stress echocardiography and stress thallium imaging, are promising tools that are being investigated.[868]

MANAGEMENT. Management of cardiac transplant–associated arteriopathy includes retransplantation, PCI in selected patients with focal stenoses (although the incidence of subsequent restenosis is increased), and coronary bypass surgery; however, the latter is confined to a relatively few highly selected patients without distal involvement.[869] A preliminary study suggested that diltiazem may retard the reduction in coronary vessel diameter defined by quantitative angiography, but its clinical impact needs to be determined.[309] In comparison with dietary measures alone, a recent randomized trial demonstrated that the combination of a low-cholesterol diet and simvastatin after heart transplantation led to a significant reduction in cholesterol levels, a significantly higher long-term survival rate, and a lower incidence of accelerated graft vessel disease.[870] Among patients who were not treated with calcium channel blockers, ganciclovir, which is effective in preventing cytomegalovirus illness, appeared to decrease the incidence of CAD in the donor heart in comparison to placebo.

REFERENCES

1. Maseri A: Ischemic Heart Disease: A Rational Basis for Clinical Practice and Clinical Research. New York, Churchill Livingstone, 1995.
2. Virmani R, Forman MB: Nonatherosclerotic Ischemic Heart Disease. New York, Raven, 1989.
3. Manzi S, Meilahn EN, Rairie JE, et al: Age-specific incidence rates of myocardial infarction and angina in women with systemic lupus erythematosus: Comparison with the Framingham Study. Am J Epidemiol 145:408, 1997.
4. Sorrell VL, Davis MJ, Bove AA: Current knowledge and significance of coronary artery ectasia: A chronologic review of the literature, recommendations for treatment, possible etiologies, and future considerations. Clin Cardiol 21:157, 1998.
5. American Heart Association: 2000 Heart and Stroke Statistical Update. Dallas, American Heart Association, 1999.
6. National Center for Health Statistics: National Health and Nutrition Examination Survey III, 1988–94. Hyattsville, MD, US Department of Health and Human Services, Centers for Disease Control and Prevention, National Center for Health Statistics, 1998.
7. Tunstall-Pedoe H, Kuulasmaa K, Mahonen M, et al: Contribution of trends in survival and coronary-event rates to changes in coronary heart disease mortality: 10-year results from 37 WHO MONICA project populations. Monitoring trends and determinants in cardiovascular disease. Lancet 353:1547, 1999.
8. Howard BV, Lee ET, Cowan LD, et al: Rising tide of cardiovascular disease in American Indians. The Strong Heart Study. Circulation 99:2389, 1999.
9. Rosamond WD, Chambless LE, Folsom AR, et al: Trends in the incidence of myocardial infarction and in mortality due to coronary heart disease, 1987 to 1994. N Engl J Med 339:861, 1998.
10. Hunink MG, Goldman L, Tosteson AN, et al: The recent decline in mortality from coronary heart disease, 1980–1990. The effect of secular trends in risk factors and treatment. JAMA 277:535, 1997.

STABLE ANGINA PECTORIS

11. Matthews MB, Julian DG: Angina pectoris: Definition and description. *In* Julian DG (ed): Angina Pectoris. 2nd ed. New York, Churchill Livingstone, 1985, pp 1–2.
12. Cook DG, Shaper AG: Breathlessness, angina pectoris and coronary artery disease. Am J Cardiol 63:921, 1989.

13. Peled N, Abinader EG, Pillar G, et al: Nocturnal ischemic events in patients with obstructive sleep apnea syndrome and ischemic heart disease: Effects of continuous positive air pressure treatment. J Am Coll Cardiol 34:1744, 1999.
14. Bogaty P, Kingma JG Jr, Robitaille NM, et al: Attenuation of myocardial ischemia with repeated exercise in subjects with chronic stable angina: Relation to myocardial contractility, intensity of exercise and the adenosine triphosphate-sensitive potassium channel. J Am Coll Cardiol 32:1665, 1998.
15. Goldman L, Hashimoto B, Cook EF, et al: Comparative reproducibility and validity of systems for assessing cardiovascular functional class: Advantages of a new specific activity scale. Circulation 64:1227, 1981.
16. Campeau L: Grading of angina pectoris (letter). Circulation 54:522, 1976.
17. Foreman RD: Mechanisms of cardiac pain. Annu Rev Physiol 61:143, 1999.
18. Rosen SD, Paulesu E, Frith CD, et al: Central nervous pathways mediating angina pectoris. Lancet 344:147, 1994.
19. Cooke RA, Anggiansah A, Chambers JB, et al: A prospective study of oesophageal function in patients with normal coronary angiograms and controls with angina. Gut 42:323, 1998.
20. Chauhan A, Mullins PA, Taylor G, et al: Cardioesophageal reflex: A mechanism for "linked angina" in patients with angiographically proven coronary artery disease. J Am Coll Cardiol 27:1621, 1996.
21. Borjesson M, Albertsson P, Dellborg M, et al: Esophageal dysfunction in syndrome X. Am J Cardiol 82:1187, 1998.
22. Thomas LR, Baden L, Zaleznik DF: Clinical problem-solving. Chest pain with a surprising course. N Engl J Med 341:1134, 1999.
23. Epstein SE, Gerber LH, Borer JS: Chest wall syndrome. A common cause of unexplained cardiac pain. JAMA 241:2793, 1979.
24. Wise CM, Semble EL, Dalton CB: Musculoskeletal chest wall syndromes in patients with noncardiac chest pain: A study of 100 patients. Arch Phys Med Rehabil 73:147, 1992.
25. 27th Bethesda Conference: Matching the Intensity of Risk Factor Management with the Hazard for Coronary Disease Events. September 14–15, 1995. J Am Coll Cardiol 27:957, 1996.
26. Winder AF, Jolleys JC, Day LB, et al: Corneal arcus, case finding and definition of individual clinical risk in heterozygous familial hypercholesterolaemia. Clin Genet 54:497, 1998.
27. Chambless LE, Fuchs FD, Linn S, et al: The association of corneal arcus with coronary heart disease and cardiovascular disease mortality in the Lipid Research Clinics Mortality Follow-up Study. Am J Public Health 80:1200, 1990.
28. Ribera M, Pinto X, Argimon JM, et al: Lipid metabolism and apolipoprotein E phenotypes in patients with xanthelasma. Am J Med 99:485, 1995.
29. Klein R, Klein BE, Moss SE, et al: Association of ocular disease and mortality in a diabetic population. Arch Ophthalmol 117:1487, 1999.
30. Tranchesi JB, Barbosa V, de Albuquerque CP, et al: Diagonal earlobe crease as a marker of the presence and extent of coronary atherosclerosis. Am J Cardiol 70:1417, 1992.
31. Miric D, Fabijanic D, Giunio L, et al: Dermatological indicators of coronary risk: A case-control study. Int J Cardiol 67:251, 1998.
32. Gersh BJ, Rihal CS, Rooke TW, et al: Evaluation and management of patients with both peripheral vascular and coronary artery disease. J Am Coll Cardiol 18:203, 1991.
33. Eagle KA, Rihal CS, Foster ED, et al: Long-term survival in patients with coronary artery disease: Importance of peripheral vascular disease. J Am Coll Cardiol 23:1091, 1994.
34. Ogren M, Hedblad B, Isacsson SO, et al: Non-invasively detected carotid stenosis and ischaemic heart disease in men with leg arteriosclerosis. Lancet 342:1138, 1993.
35. Gibbons RJ, Chatterjee K, Daley J, et al: ACC/AHA/ACP-ASIM guidelines for the management of patients with chronic stable angina: A report of the American College of Cardiology/American Heart Association Task Force on Practice Guidelines. J Am Coll Cardiol 33:2092, 1999.
36. Cohn PF, Thompson P, Strauss W, et al: Diastolic heart sounds during static (handgrip) exercise in patients with chest pain. Circulation 47:1217, 1973.
37. Lamas GA, Mitchell GF, Flaker GC, et al: Clinical significance of mitral regurgitation after acute myocardial infarction. Survival and Ventricular Enlargement Investigators. Circulation 96:827, 1997.
38. Sangster JF, Oakley CM: Diastolic murmur of coronary artery stenosis. Br Heart J 35:840, 1973.
39. Freedman SB, Wong CK: Triggers of daily life ischaemia. Heart 80:489, 1998.
40. Gullette EC, Blumenthal JA, Babyak M, et al: Effects of mental stress on myocardial ischemia during daily life. JAMA 277:1521, 1997.
41. Muller JE, Mittleman A, Maclure M, et al: Triggering myocardial infarction by sexual activity. Low absolute risk and prevention by regular physical exertion. JAMA 275:1405, 1996.
42. Andrews TC, Fenton T, Toyosaki N, et al: Subsets of ambulatory myocardial ischemia based on heart rate activity. Circadian distribution and response to anti-ischemic medication. Circulation 88:92, 1993.
43. Hillis LD, Braunwald E: Coronary-artery spasm. N Engl J Med 299:695, 1978.
44. Opie LH: The Heart: Physiology, From Cell to Circulation. 3rd ed. Philadelphia, Lippincott-Raven, 1998, p 287.
45. Maseri A, Crea F, Lanza GA: Coronary vasoconstriction: Where do we

stand in 1999? An important, multifaceted but elusive role (editorial). Cardiologia 44:115, 1999.

46. Epstein SE, Talbot TL: Dynamic coronary tone in precipitation, exacerbation and relief of angina pectoris. Am J Cardiol 48:797, 1981.

47. Baller D, Notohamiprodjo G, Gleichmann U, et al: Improvement in coronary flow reserve determined by positron emission tomography after 6 months of cholesterol-lowering therapy in patients with early stages of coronary atherosclerosis. Circulation 99:2871, 1999.

48. Benhorin J, Banai S, Moriel M, et al: Circadian variations in ischemic threshold and their relation to the occurrence of ischemic episodes. Circulation 87:808, 1993.

49. Gottdiener JS, Krantz DS, Howell RH, et al: Induction of silent myocardial ischemia with mental stress testing: Relation to the triggers of ischemia during daily life activities and to ischemic functional severity. J Am Coll Cardiol 24:1645, 1994.

50. Marchant B, Donaldson G, Mridha K, et al: Mechanisms of cold intolerance in patients with angina. J Am Coll Cardiol 23:630, 1994.

51. Kearney MT, Charlesworth A, Cowley AJ, et al: William Heberden revisited: Postprandial angina—interval between food and exercise and meal composition are important determinants of time to onset of ischemia and maximal exercise tolerance. J Am Coll Cardiol 29:302, 1997.

52. Baliga RR, Rosen SD, Camici PG, et al: Regional myocardial blood flow redistribution as a cause of postprandial angina pectoris. Circulation 97:1144, 1998.

53. Maseri A, Chierchia S, Kaski JC: Mixed angina pectoris. Am J Cardiol 56:30E, 1985.

54. Parker JD, Testa MA, Jimenez AH, et al: Morning increase in ambulatory ischemia in patients with stable coronary artery disease. Importance of physical activity and increased cardiac demand. Circulation 89:604, 1994.

55. Califf RM, Mark DB, Harrell FE Jr, et al: Importance of clinical measures of ischemia in the prognosis of patients with documented coronary artery disease. J Am Coll Cardiol 11:20, 1988.

56. Diamond GA, Forrester JS: Analysis of probability as an aid in the clinical diagnosis of coronary-artery disease. N Engl J Med 300:1350, 1979.

57. Pryor DB, Shaw L, McCants CB, et al: Value of the history and physical in identifying patients at increased risk for coronary artery disease. Ann Intern Med 118:81, 1993.

58. Sox HC Jr, Hickam DH, Marton KI, et al: Using the patient's history to estimate the probability of coronary artery disease: A comparison of primary care and referral practices. Am J Med 89:7, 1990.

59. Chaitman BR, Bourassa MG, Davis K, et al: Angiographic prevalence of high-risk coronary artery disease in patient subsets (CASS). Circulation 64:360, 1981.

Non-Invasive Testing in Angina

60. French JK, Elliott JM, Williams BF, et al: Association of angiographically detected coronary artery disease with low levels of high-density lipoprotein cholesterol and systemic hypertension. Am J Cardiol 71:505, 1993.

61. Grundy SM, Balady GJ, Criqui MH, et al: Primary prevention of coronary heart disease: Guidance from Framingham: A statement for healthcare professionals from the AHA Task Force on Risk Reduction. Circulation 97:1876, 1998.

62. Fuster V, Gotto AM, Libby P, et al: 27th Bethesda Conference: Matching the intensity of risk factor management with the hazard for coronary disease events. Task Force 1. Pathogenesis of coronary disease: The biologic role of risk factors. J Am Coll Cardiol 27:964, 1996.

63. Ridker PM, Cushman M, Stampfer MJ, et al: Inflammation, aspirin, and the risk of cardiovascular disease in apparently healthy men. N Engl J Med 336:973, 1997.

64. Ridker PM, Buring JE, Shih J, et al: Prospective study of C-reactive protein and the risk of future cardiovascular events among apparently healthy women. Circulation 98:731, 1998.

65. Malinow MR, Bostom AG, Krauss RM: Homocyst(e)ine, diet, and cardiovascular diseases: A statement for healthcare professionals from the Nutrition Committee, American Heart Association. Circulation 99:178, 1999.

66. Smith SC Jr, Greenland P, Grundy SM: AHA Conference Proceedings. Prevention conference V: Beyond secondary prevention: Identifying the high-risk patient for primary prevention: Executive summary. American Heart Association. Circulation 101:111, 2000.

67. Christian TF, Miller TD, Chareonthaitawee P, et al: Prevalence of normal resting left ventricular function with normal rest electrocardiograms. Am J Cardiol 79:1295, 1997.

68. Mirvis DM, el-Zeky F, Vander Zwaag R, et al: Clinical and pathophysiologic correlates of ST-T-wave abnormalities in coronary artery disease. Am J Cardiol 66:699, 1990.

69. Miranda CP, Lehmann KG, Froelicher VF: Correlation between resting ST segment depression, exercise testing, coronary angiography, and long-term prognosis. Am Heart J 122:1617, 1991.

70. Crenshaw JH, Mirvis DM, el-Zeky F, et al: Interactive effects of ST-T wave abnormalities on survival of patients with coronary artery disease. J Am Coll Cardiol 18:413, 1991.

71. Hamby RI, Weissman RH, Prakash MN, et al: Left bundle branch block: A predictor of poor left ventricular function in coronary artery disease. Am Heart J 106:471, 1983.

72. Peterson MC, Holbrook JA, VonHale D, et al: Contributions of the history, physical examination and laboratory investigation in making medical diagnoses. West J Med 156:163, 1992.

73. Marantz PR, Tobin JN, Wassertheil-Smoller S, et al: Prognosis in ischemic heart disease. Can you tell as much at the bedside as in the nuclear laboratory? Arch Intern Med 152:2433, 1992.

74. Berman DS, Hachamovitch R, Kiat H, et al: Incremental value of prognostic testing in patients with known or suspected ischemic heart disease: A basis for optimal utilization of exercise technetium-99m sestamibi myocardial perfusion single-photon emission computed tomography. J Am Coll Cardiol 26:639, 1995.

75. Hachamovitch R, Berman DS, Shaw LJ, et al: Incremental prognostic value of myocardial perfusion single photon emission computed tomography for the prediction of cardiac death: Differential stratification for risk of cardiac death and myocardial infarction. Circulation 97:535, 1998.

76. Shaw LJ, Hachamovitch R, Berman DS, et al: The economic consequences of available diagnostic and prognostic strategies for the evaluation of stable angina patients: An observational assessment of the value of precatheterization ischemia. Economics of Noninvasive Diagnosis (END) Multicenter Study Group. J Am Coll Cardiol 33:661, 1999.

77. Wilson RF, Marcus ML, Christensen BV, et al: Accuracy of exercise electrocardiography in detecting physiologically significant coronary arterial lesions. Circulation 83:412, 1991.

78. Gibbons RJ, Balady GJ, Beasley JW, et al: ACC/AHA Guidelines for Exercise Testing. A report of the American College of Cardiology/American Heart Association Task Force on Practice Guidelines (Committee on Exercise Testing). J Am Coll Cardiol 30:260, 1997.

79. Chang JA, Froelicher VF: Clinical and exercise test markers of prognosis in patients with stable coronary artery disease. Curr Probl Cardiol 19:533, 1994.

80. Ribisl PM, Morris CK, Kawaguchi T, et al: Angiographic patterns and severe coronary artery disease. Exercise test correlates. Arch Intern Med 152:1618, 1992.

81. Michaelides A, Ryan JM, VanFossen D, et al: Exercise-induced QRS prolongation in patients with coronary artery disease: A marker of myocardial ischemia. Am Heart J 126:1320, 1993.

82. Rozanski A, Diamond GA, Berman D, et al: The declining specificity of exercise radionuclide ventriculography. N Engl J Med 309:518, 1983.

83. Ho SW, McComish MJ, Taylor RR: Effect of beta-adrenergic blockade on the results of exercise testing related to the extent of coronary artery disease. Am J Cardiol 55:258, 1985.

84. Ritchie JL, Bateman TM, Bonow RO, et al: Guidelines for clinical use of cardiac radionuclide imaging. Report of the American College of Cardiology/American Heart Association Task Force on Assessment of Diagnostic and Therapeutic Cardiovascular Procedures (Committee on Radionuclide Imaging), developed in collaboration with the American Society of Nuclear Cardiology. J Am Coll Cardiol 25:521, 1995.

85. Berman DS, Kiat HS, Van Train KF, et al: Myocardial perfusion imaging with technetium-99m-sestamibi: Comparative analysis of available imaging protocols. J Nucl Med 35:681, 1994.

86. Berman DS, Kiat H, Friedman JD, et al: Separate acquisition rest thallium-201/stress technetium-99m sestamibi dual-isotope myocardial perfusion single-photon emission computed tomography: A clinical validation study. J Am Coll Cardiol 22:1455, 1993.

87. Berman DS, Amanullah AM, Hayes S, et al: Dual-isotope myocardial perfusion SPECT with rest thallium-201 and stress technetium-99m sestamibi. In Zaret BL, Beller G (eds): Nuclear Cardiology: State of the Art and Future Directions. 2nd ed. St Louis, Mosby, 1999, pp 281–297.

88. Pagley PR, Beller GA, Watson DD, et al: Improved outcome after coronary bypass surgery in patients with ischemic cardiomyopathy and residual myocardial viability. Circulation 96:793, 1997.

89. Bonow RO: Identification of viable myocardium (editorial). Circulation 94:2674, 1996.

90. Lauer MS, Lytle B, Pashkow F, et al: Prediction of death and myocardial infarction by screening with exercise-thallium testing after coronary-artery-bypass grafting. Lancet 351:615, 1998.

91. Gibbons RJ, Hodge DO, Berman DS, et al: Long-term outcome of patients with intermediate-risk exercise electrocardiograms who do not have myocardial perfusion defects on radionuclide imaging. Circulation 100:2140, 1999.

92. Iskandrian AS, Heo J, Lemlek J, et al: Identification of high-risk patients with left main and three-vessel coronary artery disease by adenosine-single photon emission computed tomographic thallium imaging. Am Heart J 125:1130, 1993.

93. Taillefer R, Amyot R, Turpin S, et al: Comparison between dipyridamole and adenosine as pharmacologic coronary vasodilators in detection of coronary artery disease with thallium 201 imaging. J Nucl Cardiol 3:204, 1996.

94. Johnston DL, Daley JR, Hodge DO, et al: Hemodynamic responses and adverse effects associated with adenosine and dipyridamole pharmacologic stress testing: A comparison in 2,000 patients. Mayo Clin Proc 70:331, 1995.

95. Pennell DJ, Underwood SR, Ell PJ: Safety of dobutamine stress for thallium-201 myocardial perfusion tomography in patients with asthma. Am J Cardiol 71:1346, 1993.

96. Calnon DA, Glover DK, Beller GA, et al: Effects of dobutamine stress on myocardial blood flow, 99mTc sestamibi uptake, and systolic wall thickening in the presence of coronary artery stenoses: Implications for dobutamine stress testing. Circulation 96:2353, 1997.

97. Detrano RC, Wong ND, Doherty TM, et al: Coronary calcium does not accurately predict near-term future coronary events in high-risk adults. Circulation 99:2633, 1999.

98. Cheitlin MD, Alpert JS, Armstrong WF, et al: ACC/AHA Guidelines for the Clinical Application of Echocardiography. A report of the American College of Cardiology/American Heart Association Task Force on Practice Guidelines (Committee on Clinical Application of Echocardiography). Developed in collaboration with the American Society of Echocardiography. Circulation 95:1686, 1997.

99. Fleischmann KE, Hunink MG, Kuntz KM, et al: Exercise echocardiography or exercise SPECT imaging? A meta-analysis of diagnostic test performance. JAMA 280:913, 1998.

100. Dagianti A, Penco M, Agati L, et al: Stress echocardiography: Comparison of exercise, dipyridamole and dobutamine in detecting and predicting the extent of coronary artery disease. J Am Coll Cardiol 26:18, 1995.

101. Beleslin BD, Ostojic M, Stepanovic J, et al: Stress echocardiography in the detection of myocardial ischemia. Head-to-head comparison of exercise, dobutamine, and dipyridamole tests. Circulation 90:1168, 1994.

102. Perrone-Filardi P, Pace L, Prastaro M, et al: Assessment of myocardial viability in patients with chronic coronary artery disease. Rest-4-hour-24-hour ^{201}T1 tomography versus dobutamine echocardiography. Circulation 94:2712, 1996.

103. Bax JJ, Poldermans D, Elhendy A, et al: Improvement of left ventricular ejection fraction, heart failure symptoms and prognosis after revascularization in patients with chronic coronary artery disease and viable myocardium detected by dobutamine stress echocardiography. J Am Coll Cardiol 34:163, 1999.

104. Fioretti PM, Poldermans D, Salustri A, et al: Atropine increases the accuracy of dobutamine stress echocardiography in patients taking beta-blockers. Eur Heart J 15:355, 1994.

105. Marangelli V, Iliceto S, Piccinni G, et al: Detection of coronary artery disease by digital stress echocardiography: Comparison of exercise, transesophageal atrial pacing and dipyridamole echocardiography. J Am Coll Cardiol 24:117, 1994.

106. Tauke JA, Allesandrini A, Cusick DS, et al: Enhanced detection of ischemic myocardium by transesophageal dobutamine stress echocardiography. J Am Soc Echocardiogr, in press.

107. O'Keefe JH Jr, Barnhart CS, Bateman TM: Comparison of stress echocardiography and stress myocardial perfusion scintigraphy for diagnosing coronary artery disease and assessing its severity. Am J Cardiol 75:25D, 1995.

108. Kaul S: Myocardial contrast echocardiography: 15 years of research and development. Circulation 96:3745, 1997.

109. Kaul S, Senior R, Dittrich H, et al: Detection of coronary artery disease with myocardial contrast echocardiography: Comparison with ^{99m}Tc-sestamibi single-photon emission computed tomography. Circulation 96:785, 1997.

110. Cohen JL, Cheirif J, Segar DS, et al: Improved left ventricular endocardial border delineation and opacification with OPTISON (FS069), a new echocardiographic contrast agent. Results of a phase III Multicenter Trial. J Am Coll Cardiol 32:746, 1998.

111. Kasprzak JD, Paelinck B, Ten Cate FJ, et al: Comparison of native and contrast-enhanced harmonic echocardiography for visualization of left ventricular endocardial border. Am J Cardiol 83:211, 1999.

112. Wenger NK, Speroff L, Packard B: Cardiovascular Health and Disease in Women: Proceedings of an NHLBI Conference. Greenwich, CT, Le Jacq Communications, 1993, p 74.

113. Shaw LJ, Miller DD, Romeis JC, et al: Gender differences in the noninvasive evaluation and management of patients with suspected coronary artery disease. Ann Intern Med 120:559, 1994.

114. Hachamovitch R, Berman DS, Kiat H, et al: Effective risk stratification using exercise myocardial perfusion SPECT in women: Gender-related differences in prognostic nuclear testing. J Am Coll Cardiol 28:34, 1996.

115. Taillefer R, DePuey EG, Udelson JE, et al: Comparative diagnostic accuracy of T1-201 and Tc-99m sestamibi SPECT imaging (perfusion and ECG-gated SPECT) in detecting coronary artery disease in women. J Am Coll Cardiol 29:69, 1997.

116. Marwick TH, Anderson T, Williams MJ, et al: Exercise echocardiography is an accurate and cost-efficient technique for detection of coronary artery disease in women. J Am Coll Cardiol 26:335, 1995.

117. Roger VL, Pellikka PA, Bell MR, et al: Sex and test verification bias. Impact on the diagnostic value of exercise echocardiography. Circulation 95:405, 1997.

118. Loecker TH, Schwartz RS, Cotta CW, et al: Fluoroscopic coronary artery calcification and associated coronary disease in asymptomatic young men. J Am Coll Cardiol 19:1167, 1992.

119. Rumberger JA, Simons DB, Fitzpatrick LA, et al: Coronary artery calcium area by electron-beam computed tomography and coronary atherosclerotic plaque area. A histopathologic correlative study. Circulation 92:2157, 1995.

120. Secci A, Wong N, Tang W, et al: Electron beam computed tomographic coronary calcium as a predictor of coronary events: Comparison of two protocols. Circulation 96:1122, 1997.

121. Newman AB, Siscovick DS, Manolio TA, et al: Ankle-arm index as a marker of atherosclerosis in the Cardiovascular Health Study. Cardiovascular Heart Study (CHS) Collaborative Research Group. Circulation 88:837, 1993.

122. O'Leary DH, Polak JF, Kronmal RA, et al: Carotid-artery intima and media thickness as a risk factor for myocardial infarction and stroke in older adults. Cardiovascular Health Study Collaborative Research Group. N Engl J Med 340:14, 1999.

123. Budoff MJ, Georgiou D, Brody A, et al: Ultrafast computed tomography as a diagnostic modality in the detection of coronary artery disease: A multicenter study. Circulation 93:898, 1996.

124. O'Rourke RA, Brundage BH, Froelicher VF, et al: American College of Cardiology/American Heart Association Clinical Expert Consensus Document on electron beam computed tomography for the diagnosis and prognosis of coronary artery disease. J Am Coll Cardiol 36:326, 2000.

125. Nagel E, Lehmkuhl HB, Bocksch W, et al: Noninvasive diagnosis of ischemia-induced wall motion abnormalities with the use of high-dose dobutamine stress MRI: Comparison with dobutamine stress echocardiography. Circulation 99:763, 1999.

126. Ramani K, Judd RM, Holly TA, et al: Contrast magnetic resonance imaging in the assessment of myocardial viability in patients with stable coronary artery disease and left ventricular dysfunction. Circulation 98:2687, 1998.

127. Botnar RM, Stuber M, Danias PG, et al: Improved coronary artery definition with T2-weighted, free-breathing, three-dimensional coronary MRA. Circulation 99:3139, 1999.

Coronary Arteriography

128. Ellis SG: The role of coronary angiography. In Fuster V, Ross R, Topol EJ (eds): Atherosclerosis and Coronary Artery Disease. Philadelphia, Lippincott-Raven, 1996, pp 1433–1450.

129. Bogaty P, Brecker SJ, White SE, et al: Comparison of coronary angiographic findings in acute and chronic first presentation of ischemic heart disease. Circulation 87:1938, 1993.

130. Stajduhar KC, Laird JR, Rogan KM, et al: Coronary arterial ectasia: Increased prevalence in patients with abdominal aortic aneurysm as compared to occlusive atherosclerotic peripheral vascular disease. Am Heart J 125:86, 1993.

131. Hartnell GG, Parnell BM, Pridie RB: Coronary artery ectasia. Its prevalence and clinical significance in 4993 patients. Br Heart J 54:392, 1985.

132. Kruger D, Stierle U, Herrmann G, et al: Exercise-induced myocardial ischemia in isolated coronary artery ectasias and aneurysms ("dilated coronopathy"). J Am Coll Cardiol 34:1461, 1999.

133. Tunick PA, Slater J, Kronzon I, et al: Discrete atherosclerotic coronary artery aneurysms: A study of 20 patients. J Am Coll Cardiol 15:279, 1990.

134. Agarwal JB, Helfant RH: Functional importance of coronary collateral circulation. Int J Cardiol 4:94, 1983.

135. Newman PE: The coronary collateral circulation: Determinants and functional significance in ischemic heart disease. Am Heart J 102:431, 1981.

136. Vanoverschelde JL, Wijns W, Depre C, et al: Mechanisms of chronic regional postischemic dysfunction in humans. New insights from the study of noninfarcted collateral-dependent myocardium. Circulation 87:1513, 1993.

137. Bestetti RB, Costa RS, Kazava DK, et al: Can isolated myocardial bridging of the left anterior descending coronary artery be associated with sudden death during exercise? Acta Cardiol 46:27, 1991.

138. Moraski RE, Russell RO Jr, Smith MK, et al: Left ventricular function in patients with and without myocardial infarction and one, two or three vessel coronary artery disease. Am J Cardiol 35:1, 1975.

139. Mann T, Brodie BR, Grossman W, et al: Effect of angina on the left ventricular diastolic pressure-volume relationship. Circulation 55:761, 1977.

140. Rahimtoola SH: The hibernating myocardium. Am Heart J 117:211, 1989.

141. Braunwald E, Rutherford JD: Reversible ischemic left ventricular dysfunction: Evidence for the "hibernating myocardium." J Am Coll Cardiol 8:1467, 1986.

142. Marban E: Myocardial stunning and hibernation. The physiology behind the colloquialisms. Circulation 83:681, 1991.

143. Nesto RW, Cohn LH, Collins JJ Jr, et al: Inotropic contractile reserve: A useful predictor of increased 5 year survival and improved postoperative left ventricular function in patients with coronary artery disease and reduced ejection fraction. Am J Cardiol 50:39, 1982.

144. Verani MS, Carroll RJ, Falsetti HL: Mitral valve prolapse in coronary artery disease. Am J Cardiol 37:1, 1976.

145. Herman MV, Elliott WC, Gorlin R: An electrocardiographic, anatomic, and metabolic study of zonal myocardial ischemia in coronary heart disease. Circulation 35:834, 1967.

146. Gertz EW, Wisneski JA, Neese R, et al: Myocardial lactate metabolism: Evidence of lactate release during net chemical extraction in man. Circulation 63:1273, 1981.

147. Cannon PJ, Weiss MB, Sciacca RR: Myocardial blood flow in coronary artery disease: Studies at rest and during stress with inert gas washout techniques. Prog Cardiovasc Dis 20:95, 1977.

MEDICAL MANAGEMENT OF STABLE ANGINA

148. Stamler J, Stamler R, Neaton JD: Blood pressure, systolic and diastolic, and cardiovascular risks. US population data. Arch Intern Med 153:598, 1993.

149. Jousilahti P, Vartiainen E, Tuomilehto J, et al: Sex, age, cardiovascular risk factors, and coronary heart disease: A prospective follow-up study

of 14,786 middle-aged men and women in Finland. Circulation 99:1165, 1999.

150. de Lorgeril M, Salen P, Martin JL, et al: Mediterranean diet, traditional risk factors, and the rate of cardiovascular complications after myocardial infarction: Final report of the Lyon Diet Heart Study. Circulation 99:779, 1999.

151. Devereux RB, Roman MJ: Inter-relationships between hypertension, left ventricular hypertrophy and coronary heart disease. J Hypertens 11(Suppl):3, 1993.

152. Hebert PR, Moser M, Mayer J, et al: Recent evidence on drug therapy of mild to moderate hypertension and decreased risk of coronary heart disease. Arch Intern Med 153:578, 1993.

153. Cutler JA, Psaty BM, MacMahon S, et al: Public health issues in hypertension control: What has been learned from clinical trials. In Laragh JH, Brenner BM (eds): Hypertension: Pathophysiology, Diagnosis, and Management. 2nd ed. Vol 1. New York, Raven Press, 1995, pp 253–270.

154. Lempiainen P, Mykkanen L, Pyorala K, et al: Insulin resistance syndrome predicts coronary heart disease events in elderly nondiabetic men. Circulation 100:123, 1999.

155. Frost PH, Davis BR, Burlando AJ, et al: Coronary heart disease risk factors in men and women aged 60 years and older: Findings from the Systolic Hypertension in the Elderly Program. Circulation 94:26, 1996.

156. Burke AP, Farb A, Malcom GT, et al: Coronary risk factors and plaque morphology in men with coronary disease who died suddenly. N Engl J Med 336:1276, 1997.

157. Davis JW, Hartman CR, Lewis HD Jr, et al: Cigarette smoking–induced enhancement of platelet function: Lack of prevention by aspirin in men with coronary artery disease. J Lab Clin Med 105:479, 1985.

158. Vlietstra RE, Kronmal RA, Oberman A, et al: Effect of cigarette smoking on survival of patients with angiographically documented coronary artery disease. Report from the CASS registry. JAMA 255:1023, 1986.

159. Hermanson B, Omenn GS, Kronmal RA, et al: Beneficial six-year outcome of smoking cessation in older men and women with coronary artery disease. Results from the CASS registry. N Engl J Med 319:1365, 1988.

160. Cavender JB, Rogers WJ, Fisher LD, et al: Effects of smoking on survival and morbidity in patients randomized to medical or surgical therapy in the Coronary Artery Surgery Study (CASS): 10-year follow-up. J Am Coll Cardiol 20:287, 1992.

161. Voors AA, van Brussel BL, Plokker HW, et al: Smoking and cardiac events after venous coronary bypass surgery. A 15-year follow-up study. Circulation 93:42, 1996.

162. Czernin J, Sun K, Brunken R, et al: Effect of acute and long-term smoking on myocardial blood flow and flow reserve. Circulation 91:2891, 1995.

163. Deanfield J, Wright C, Krikler S, et al: Cigarette smoking and the treatment of angina with propranolol, atenolol, and nifedipine. N Engl J Med 310:951, 1984.

164. Shepherd J, Cobbe SM, Ford I, et al: Prevention of coronary heart disease with pravastatin in men with hypercholesterolemia. West of Scotland Coronary Prevention Study Group. N Engl J Med 333:1301, 1995.

165. Downs JR, Clearfield M, Weis S, et al: Primary prevention of acute coronary events with lovastatin in men and women with average cholesterol levels: Results of AFCAPS/TexCAPS. Air Force/Texas Coronary Atherosclerosis Prevention Study. JAMA 279:1615, 1998.

166. Pitt B, Mancini GB, Ellis SG, et al: Pravastatin limitation of atherosclerosis in the coronary arteries (PLAC I): Reduction in atherosclerosis progression and clinical events. PLAC I investigation. J Am Coll Cardiol 26:1133, 1995.

167. Blankenhorn DH, Azen SP, Kramsch DM, et al: Coronary angiographic changes with lovastatin therapy. The Monitored Atherosclerosis Regression Study (MARS). Ann Intern Med 119:969, 1993.

168. Scandinavian Simvastatin Survival Study Group: Randomised trial of cholesterol lowering in 4444 patients with coronary heart disease: The Scandinavian Simvastatin Survival Study (4S). Lancet 344:1383, 1994.

169. Byington RP, Jukema JW, Salonen JT, et al: Reduction in cardiovascular events during pravastatin therapy. Pooled analysis of clinical events of the Pravastatin Atherosclerosis Intervention Program. Circulation 92:2419, 1995.

170. Sacks FM, Pfeffer MA, Moye LA, et al: The effect of pravastatin on coronary events after myocardial infarction in patients with average cholesterol levels. Cholesterol and Recurrent Events Trial investigators. N Engl J Med 335:1001, 1996.

171. The Long-Term Intervention with Pravastatin in Ischaemic Disease (LIPID) Study Group: Prevention of cardiovascular events and death with pravastatin in patients with coronary heart disease and a broad range of initial cholesterol levels. N Engl J Med 339:1349, 1998.

172. Anderson TJ, Meredith IT, Yeung AC, et al: The effect of cholesterol-lowering and antioxidant therapy on endothelium-dependent coronary vasomotion. N Engl J Med 332:488, 1995.

173. O'Driscoll G, Green D, Taylor RR: Simvastatin, an HMG-coenzyme A reductase inhibitor, improves endothelial function within 1 month. Circulation 95:1126, 1997.

174. Dupuis J, Tardif JC, Cernacek P, et al: Cholesterol reduction rapidly improves endothelial function after acute coronary syndrome. The RECIFE (Reduction of Cholesterol in Ischemia and Function of the Endothelium) trial. Circulation 99:3227, 1999.

175. Ridker PM, Rifai N, Pfeffer MA, et al: Long-term effects of pravastatin on plasma concentration of C-reactive protein. The Cholesterol and Recurrent Events (CARE) Investigators. Circulation 100:230, 1999.

176. Dangas G, Badimon JJ, Smith DA, et al: Pravastatin therapy in hyperlipidemia: Effects on thrombus formation and the systemic hemostatic profile. J Am Coll Cardiol 33:1294, 1999.

177. Rosenson RS, Tangney CC: Antiatherothrombotic properties of statins: Implications for cardiovascular event reduction. JAMA 279:1643, 1998.

178. Aengevaeren WR, Uijen GJ, Jukema JW, et al: Functional evaluation of lipid-lowering therapy by pravastatin in the Regression Growth Evaluation Statin Study (REGRESS). Circulation 96:429, 1997.

179. Andrews TC, Raby K, Barry J, et al: Effect of cholesterol reduction on myocardial ischemia in patients with coronary disease. Circulation 95:324, 1997.

180. Miettinen TA, Pyorala K, Olsson AG, et al: Cholesterol-lowering therapy in women and elderly patients with myocardial infarction or angina pectoris: Findings from the Scandinavian Simvastatin Survival Study (4S). Circulation 96:4211, 1997.

181. Lewis SJ, Sacks FM, Mitchell JS, et al: Effect of pravastatin on cardiovascular events in women after myocardial infarction: The Cholesterol and Recurrent Events (CARE) trial. J Am Coll Cardiol 32:140, 1998.

182. Lewis SJ, Moye LA, Sacks FM, et al: Effect of pravastatin on cardiovascular events in older patients with myocardial infarction and cholesterol levels in the average range. Results of the Cholesterol and Recurrent Events (CARE) trial. Ann Intern Med 129:681, 1998.

183. Pitt B, Waters D, Brown WV, et al: Aggressive lipid-lowering therapy compared with angioplasty in stable coronary artery disease. Atorvastatin versus Revascularization Treatment Investigators. N Engl J Med 341:70, 1999.

184. Johannesson M, Jonsson B, Kjekshus J, et al: Cost effectiveness of simvastatin treatment to lower cholesterol levels in patients with coronary heart disease. Scandinavian Simvastatin Survival Study Group. N Engl J Med 336:332, 1997.

185. Goldbourt U, Yaari S, Medalie JH: Isolated low HDL cholesterol as a risk factor for coronary heart disease mortality. A 21-year follow-up of 8000 men. Arterioscler Thromb Vasc Biol 17:107, 1997.

186. Schaefer EJ, Lamon-Fava S, Ordovas JM, et al: Factors associated with low and elevated plasma high density lipoprotein cholesterol and apolipoprotein A-I levels in the Framingham Offspring Study. J Lipid Res 35:871, 1994.

187. O'Brien T, Nguyen TT, Zimmerman BR: Hyperlipidemia and diabetes mellitus. Mayo Clin Proc 73:969, 1998.

188. Lamarche B, Tchernof A, Moorjani S, et al: Small, dense low-density lipoprotein particles as a predictor of the risk of ischemic heart disease in men. Prospective results from the Quebec Cardiovascular Study. Circulation 95:69, 1997.

189. Stefanick ML, Mackey S, Sheehan M, et al: Effects of diet and exercise in men and postmenopausal women with low levels of HDL cholesterol and high levels of LDL cholesterol. N Engl J Med 339:12, 1998.

190. Rubins HB, Robins SJ, Collins D, et al: Gemfibrozil for the secondary prevention of coronary heart disease in men with low levels of high-density lipoprotein cholesterol. Veterans Affairs High-Density Lipoprotein Cholesterol Intervention Trial Study Group. N Engl J Med 341:410, 1999.

191. The Post Coronary Artery Bypass Graft Trial Investigators: The effect of aggressive lowering of low-density lipoprotein cholesterol levels and low-dose anticoagulation on obstructive changes in saphenous-vein coronary-artery bypass grafts. N Engl J Med 336:153, 1997.

192. Goldman S, Zadina K, Krasnicka B, et al: Predictors of graft patency 3 years after coronary artery bypass graft surgery. Department of Veterans Affairs Cooperative Study Group No. 297. J Am Coll Cardiol 29:1563, 1997.

193. Campeau L, Hunninghake DB, Knatterud GL, et al: Aggressive cholesterol lowering delays saphenous vein graft atherosclerosis in women, the elderly, and patients with associated risk factors. NHLBI Post Coronary Artery Bypass Graft Clinical trial. Post CABG Trial Investigators. Circulation 99:3241, 1999.

194. Frick MH, Syvanne M, Nieminen MS, et al: Prevention of the angiographic progression of coronary and vein-graft atherosclerosis by gemfibrozil after coronary bypass surgery in men with low levels of HDL cholesterol. Circulation 96:2137, 1997.

195. Flaker GC, Warnica JW, Sacks FM, et al: Pravastatin prevents clinical events in revascularized patients with average cholesterol concentrations. Cholesterol and Recurrent Events CARE Investigators. J Am Coll Cardiol 34:106, 1999.

196. Bertrand ME, McFadden EP, Fruchart JC, et al: Effect of pravastatin on angiographic restenosis after coronary balloon angioplasty. The PREDICT Trial Investigators. Prevention of Restenosis by Elisor after Transluminal Coronary Angioplasty. J Am Coll Cardiol 30:863, 1997.

197. van Beresteijn EC, Korevaar JC, Huijbregts PC, et al: Perimenopausal increase in serum cholesterol: A 10-year longitudinal study. Am J Epidemiol 137:383, 1993.

198. Stensvold I, Tverdal A, Urdal P, et al: Non-fasting serum triglyceride concentration and mortality from coronary heart disease and any cause in middle aged Norwegian women. BMJ 307:1318, 1993.

199. Manolio TA, Furberg CD, Shemanski L, et al: Associations of postmenopausal estrogen use with cardiovascular disease and its risk factors in older women. Circulation 88:2163, 1993.

200. Espeland MA, Marcovina SM, Miller V, et al: Effect of postmenopausal hormone therapy on lipoprotein(a) concentration. PEPI Investigators. Postmenopausal Estrogen/Progestin Interventions. Circulation 97:979, 1998.

201. Sbarouni E, Kyriakides ZS, Kremastinos D: The effect of hormone replacement therapy alone and in combination with simvastatin on plasma lipids of hypercholesterolemic postmenopausal women with coronary artery disease. J Am Coll Cardiol 32:1244, 1998.

202. Koh KK, Blum A, Hathaway L, et al: Vascular effects of estrogen and vitamin E therapies in postmenopausal women. Circulation 100:1851, 1999.

203. Mendelsohn ME, Karas RH: The protective effects of estrogen on the cardiovascular system. N Engl J Med 340:1801, 1999.

204. Grodstein F, Stampfer MJ, Colditz GA, et al: Postmenopausal hormone therapy and mortality. N Engl J Med 336:1769, 1997.

205. Sidney S, Petitti DB, Quesenberry CP Jr: Myocardial infarction and the use of estrogen and estrogen-progestogen in postmenopausal women. Ann Intern Med 127:501, 1997.

206. Hulley S, Grady D, Bush T, et al: Randomized trial of estrogen plus progestin for secondary prevention of coronary heart disease in postmenopausal women. Heart and Estrogen/Progestin Replacement Study (HERS) Research Group. JAMA 280:605, 1998.

207. Daly E, Vessey MP, Hawkins MM, et al: Risk of venous thromboembolism in users of hormone replacement therapy. Lancet 348:977, 1996.

208. Kushi LH, Folsom AR, Prineas RJ, et al: Dietary antioxidant vitamins and death from coronary heart disease in postmenopausal women. N Engl J Med 334:1156, 1996.

209. The Alpha-Tocopherol, Beta Carotene Cancer Prevention Study Group: The effect of vitamin E and beta carotene on the incidence of lung cancer and other cancers in male smokers. N Engl J Med 330:1029, 1994.

210. Hennekens CH, Buring JE, Manson JE, et al: Lack of effect of long-term supplementation with beta carotene on the incidence of malignant neoplasms and cardiovascular disease. N Engl J Med 334:1145, 1996.

211. Omenn GS, Goodman GE, Thornquist MD, et al: Effects of a combination of beta carotene and vitamin A on lung cancer and cardiovascular disease. N Engl J Med 334:1150, 1996.

212. Stephens NG, Parsons A, Schofield PM, et al: Randomised controlled trial of vitamin E in patients with coronary disease: Cambridge Heart Antioxidant Study (CHAOS). Lancet 347:781, 1996.

213. Rapola JM, Virtamo J, Ripatti S, et al: Randomised trial of alpha-tocopherol and beta-carotene supplements on incidence of major coronary events in men with previous myocardial infarction. Lancet 349:1715, 1997.

213a. Hadis HN, Mark WJ, LaBree I, et al: Serial coronary angiographic evidence that antioxidant vitamin intake reduces progression of coronary athorosclerosis JAMA 273:1849–1854, 1995.

214. Yusuf S, Dagenais G, Pogue J, et al: Vitamin E supplementation and cardiovascular events in high-risk patients. The Heart Outcomes Prevention Evaluation Study Investigators. N Engl J Med 342:154, 2000.

215. Diaz MN, Frei B, Vita JA, et al: Antioxidants and atherosclerotic heart disease. N Engl J Med 337:408, 1997.

216. Tribble DL: AHA Science Advisory. Antioxidant consumption and risk of coronary heart disease: Emphasis on vitamin C, vitamin E, and beta-carotene: A statement for healthcare professionals from the American Heart Association. Circulation 99:591, 1999.

217. Tardif JC, Cote G, Lesperance J, et al: Probucol and multivitamins in the prevention of restenosis after coronary angioplasty. N Engl J Med 337:365, 1997.

218. Yokoi H, Daida H, Kuwabara Y, et al: Effectiveness of an antioxidant in preventing restenosis after percutaneous transluminal coronary angioplasty: The Probucol Angioplasty Restenosis Trial. J Am Coll Cardiol 30:855, 1997.

219. Fletcher GF: How to implement physical activity in primary and secondary prevention. A statement for healthcare-professionals from the Task Force on Risk-reduction, American Heart Association. Circulation 96:355, 1997.

220. Hedback B, Perk J, Wodlin P: Long-term reduction of cardiac mortality after myocardial infarction: 10-year results of a comprehensive rehabilitation programme. Eur Heart J 14:831, 1993.

221. Schuler G, Hambrecht R, Schlierf G, et al: Myocardial perfusion and regression of coronary artery disease in patients on a regimen of intensive physical exercise and low fat diet. J Am Coll Cardiol 19:34, 1992.

222. Ades PA, Waldmann ML, Poehlman ET, et al: Exercise conditioning in older coronary patients. Submaximal lactate response and endurance capacity. Circulation 88:572, 1993.

223. Hambrecht R, Niebauer J, Marburger C, et al: Various intensities of leisure time physical activity in patients with coronary artery disease: Effects on cardiorespiratory fitness and progression of coronary atherosclerotic lesions. J Am Coll Cardiol 22:468, 1993.

224. Oldridge N, Furlong W, Feeny D, et al: Economic evaluation of cardiac rehabilitation soon after acute myocardial infarction. Am J Cardiol 72:154, 1993.

225. Denollet J: Emotional distress and fatigue in coronary heart disease: The Global Mood Scale (GMS). Psychol Med 23:111, 1993.

226. Antiplatelet Trialists' Collaboration: Collaborative overview of randomised trials of antiplatelet therapy—I: Prevention of death, myocardial infarction, and stroke by prolonged antiplatelet therapy in various categories of patients. BMJ 308:81, 1994.

227. Juul-Möller S, Edvardsson N, Jahnmatz B, et al: Double-blind trial of aspirin in primary prevention of myocardial infarction in patients with stable chronic angina pectoris. Lancet 340:1421, 1992.

228. Ridker PM, Manson JE, Gaziano JM, et al: Low-dose aspirin therapy for chronic stable angina. A randomized, placebo-controlled clinical trial. Ann Intern Med 114:835, 1991.

229. Hennekens CH, Dyken ML, Fuster V: Aspirin as a therapeutic agent in cardiovascular disease: A statement for healthcare professionals from the American Heart Association. Circulation 96:2751, 1997.

230. Quinn MJ, Fitzgerald DJ: Ticlopidine and clopidogrel. Circulation 100:1667, 1999.

231. Ikonomidis I, Andreotii F, Economou E, et al: Increased proinflammatory cytokines in patients with chronic stable angina and their reduction by aspirin. Circulation 100:793, 1999.

232. Husain S, Andrews NP, Mulcahy D, et al: Aspirin improves endothelial dysfunction in atherosclerosis. Circulation 97:716, 1998.

233. The Medical Research Council's General Practice Research Framework: Thrombosis prevention trial: Randomised trial of low-intensity oral anticoagulation with warfarin and low-dose aspirin in the primary prevention of ischaemic heart disease in men at increased risk. Lancet 351:233, 1998.

234. Nguyen KN, Aursnes I, Kjekshus J: Interaction between enalapril and aspirin on mortality after acute myocardial infarction: Subgroup analysis of the Cooperative New Scandinavian Enalapril Survival Study II (CONSENSUS II). Am J Cardiol 79:115, 1997.

235. Spaulding C, Charbonnier B, Cohen-Solal A, et al: Acute hemodynamic interaction of aspirin and ticlopidine with enalapril: Results of a double-blind, randomized comparative trial. Circulation 98:757, 1998.

236. Leor J, Reicher-Reiss H, Goldbourt U, et al: Aspirin and mortality in patients treated with angiotensin-converting enzyme inhibitors: A cohort study of 11,575 patients with coronary artery disease. J Am Coll Cardiol 33:1920, 1999.

237. Gottlieb SS, McCarter RJ, Vogel RA: Effect of beta-blockade on mortality among high-risk and low-risk patients after myocardial infarction. N Engl J Med 339:489, 1998.

238. Chen J, Marciniak TA, Radford MJ, et al: Beta-blocker therapy for secondary prevention of myocardial infarction in elderly diabetic patients. Results from the National Cooperative Cardiovascular Project. J Am Coll Cardiol 34:1388, 1999.

239. Pfeffer MA, Braunwald E, Moye LA, et al: Effect of captopril on mortality and morbidity in patients with left ventricular dysfunction after myocardial infarction. Results of the Survival and Ventricular Enlargement trial. N Engl J Med 327:669, 1992.

240. The SOLVD Investigators: Effect of enalapril on survival in patients with reduced left ventricular ejection fractions and congestive heart failure. N Engl J Med 325:293, 1991.

241. The SOLVD Investigators: Effect of enalapril on mortality and the development of heart failure in asymptomatic patients with reduced left ventricular ejection fractions. N Engl J Med 327:685, 1992.

242. The Acute Infarction Ramipril Efficacy (AIRE) Study Investigators: Effect of ramipril on mortality and morbidity of survivors of acute myocardial infarction with clinical evidence of heart failure. Lancet 342:821, 1993.

243. Lonn EM, Yusuf S, Jha P, et al: Emerging role of angiotensin-converting enzyme inhibitors in cardiac and vascular protection. Circulation 90:2056, 1994.

244. Prasad A, Husain S, Quyyumi AA: Abnormal flow-mediated epicardial vasomotion in human coronary arteries is improved by angiotensin-converting enzyme inhibition: A potential role of bradykinin. J Am Coll Cardiol 33:796, 1999.

245. Schneider CA, Voth E, Moka D, et al: Improvement of myocardial blood flow to ischemic regions by angiotensin-converting enzyme inhibition with quinaprilat IV: A study using [15O] water dobutamine stress positron emission tomography. J Am Coll Cardiol 34:1005, 1999.

246. Larson CO, Nelson EC, Gustafson D, et al: The relationship between meeting patients' information needs and their satisfaction with hospital care and general health status outcomes. Int J Qual Health Care 8:447, 1996.

247. Featherstone JF, Holly RG, Amsterdam EA: Physiologic responses to weight lifting in coronary artery disease. Am J Cardiol 71:287, 1993.

248. Franklin BA, Hogan P, Bonzheim K, et al: Cardiac demands of heavy snow shoveling. JAMA 273:880, 1995.

249. Kahn JF, Jouanin JC, Espirito-Santo J, et al: Cardiovascular responses to leisure alpine skiing in habitually sedentary middle-aged men. J Sports Sci 11:31, 1993.

250. Luurila OJ, Karjalainen J, Viitasalo M, et al: Arrhythmias and ST segment deviation during prolonged exhaustive exercise (ski marathon) in healthy middle-aged men. Eur Heart J 15:507, 1994.

251. Figueras J, Lidon RM: Early morning reduction in ischemic threshold in patients with unstable angina and significant coronary disease. Circulation 92:1737, 1995.

Pharmacological Management of Angina

252. Robertson RM, Robertson D: Drugs used for the treatment of myocardial ischemia. In Goodman LS, Gilman A, Hardman JG, et al (eds): Goodman & Gilman's The Pharmacological Basis of Therapeutics. 9th ed. New York, McGraw-Hill, 1996, pp 759–779.

253. Parker JD, Parker JO: Nitrate therapy for stable angina pectoris. N Engl J Med 338:520, 1998.

254. Brown BG, Bolson E, Petersen RB, et al: The mechanisms of nitroglycerin action: Stenosis vasodilatation as a major component of the drug response. Circulation 64:1089, 1981.

255. Parker JO: Nitrates and angina pectoris. Am J Cardiol 72:3C, 1993.

256. Bache RJ, Ball RM, Cobb FR, et al: Effects of nitroglycerin on trans-

mural myocardial blood flow in the unanesthetized dog. J Clin Invest 55:1219, 1975.

257. Fallen EL, Nahmias C, Scheffel A, et al: Redistribution of myocardial blood flow with topical nitroglycerin in patients with coronary artery disease. Circulation 91:1381, 1995.

258. Ganz W, Marcus HS: Failure of intracoronary nitroglycerin to alleviate pacing-induced angina. Circulation 46:880, 1972.

259. Ohno A, Fujita M, Miwa K, et al: Importance of coronary collateral circulation for increased treadmill exercise capacity by nitrates in patients with stable effort angina pectoris. Cardiology 78:323, 1991.

260. Mahmarian JJ, Fenimore NL, Marks GF, et al: Transdermal nitroglycerin patch therapy reduces the extent of exercise-induced myocardial ischemia: Results of a double-blind, placebo-controlled trial using quantitative thallium-201 tomography. J Am Coll Cardiol 24:25, 1994.

261. Andrews R, May JA, Vickers J, et al: Inhibition of platelet aggregation by transdermal glyceryl trinitrate. Br Heart J 72:575, 1994.

262. Anderson TJ, Meredith IT, Ganz P, et al: Nitric oxide and nitrovasodilators: Similarities, differences and potential interactions. J Am Coll Cardiol 24:555, 1994.

263. Horowitz JD, Antman EM, Lorell BH, et al: Potentiation of the cardiovascular effects of nitroglycerin by N-acetylcysteine. Circulation 68:1247, 1983.

264. Winniford MD, Kennedy PL, Wells PJ, et al: Potentiation of nitroglycerin-induced coronary dilatation by N-acetylcysteine. Circulation 73:138, 1986.

265. Jansen RW, Lipsitz LA: Postprandial hypotension: Epidemiology, pathophysiology, and clinical management. Ann Intern Med 122:286, 1995.

266. Hales CA, Westphal D: Hypoxemia following the administration of sublingual nitroglycerin. Am J Med 65:911, 1978.

267. Parker JO, Vankoughnett KA, Farrell B: Nitroglycerin lingual spray: Clinical efficacy and dose-response relation. Am J Cardiol 57:1, 1986.

268. Bassan MM: The daylong pattern of the antianginal effect of long-term three times daily administered isosorbide dinitrate. J Am Coll Cardiol 16:936, 1990.

269. de Belder MA, Schneeweiss A, Camm AJ: Evaluation of the efficacy and duration of action of isosorbide mononitrate in angina pectoris. Am J Cardiol 65:6J, 1990.

270. Nordlander R, Walter M: Once- versus twice-daily administration of controlled-release isosorbide-5-mononitrate 60 mg in the treatment of stable angina pectoris. A randomized, double-blind, cross-over study. Eur Heart J 15:108, 1994.

271. Parker JO, Amies MH, Hawkinson RW, et al: Intermittent transdermal nitroglycerin therapy in angina pectoris. Clinically effective without tolerance or rebound. Circulation 91:1368, 1995.

272. Mangione NJ, Glasser SP: Phenomenon of nitrate tolerance. Am Heart J 128:137, 1994.

273. Jeserich M, Munzel T, Pape L, et al: Absence of vascular tolerance in conductance vessels after 48 hours of intravenous nitroglycerin in patients with coronary artery disease. J Am Coll Cardiol 26:50, 1995.

274. Packer M: What causes tolerance to nitroglycerin? The 100 year old mystery continues (editorial). J Am Coll Cardiol 16:932, 1990.

275. Parker JD, Farrell B, Fenton T, et al: Counter-regulatory responses to continuous and intermittent therapy with nitroglycerin. Circulation 84:2336, 1991.

276. Caramori PR, Adelman AG, Azevedo ER, et al: Therapy with nitroglycerin increases coronary vasoconstriction in response to acetylcholine. J Am Coll Cardiol 32:1969, 1998.

277. Heitzer T, Just H, Brockhoff C, et al: Long-term nitroglycerin treatment is associated with supersensitivity to vasoconstrictors in men with stable coronary artery disease: Prevention by concomitant treatment with captopril. J Am Coll Cardiol 31:83, 1998.

278. Parker JD, Parker AB, Farrell B, et al: Effects of diuretic therapy on the development of tolerance to nitroglycerin and exercise capacity in patients with chronic stable angina. Circulation 93:691, 1996.

279. Watanabe H, Kakihana M, Ohtsuka S, et al: Platelet cyclic GMP. A potentially useful indicator to evaluate the effects of nitroglycerin and nitrate tolerance. Circulation 88:29, 1993.

280. Munzel T, Sayegh H, Freeman BA, et al: Evidence for enhanced vascular superoxide anion production in nitrate tolerance. A novel mechanism underlying tolerance and cross-tolerance. J Clin Invest 95:187, 1995.

281. Watanabe H, Kakihana M, Ohtsuka S, et al: Randomized, double-blind, placebo-controlled study of supplemental vitamin E on attenuation of the development of nitrate tolerance. Circulation 96:2545, 1997.

282. Watanabe H, Kakihana M, Ohtsuka S, et al: Randomized, double-blind, placebo-controlled study of the preventive effect of supplemental oral vitamin C on attenuation of development of nitrate tolerance. J Am Coll Cardiol 31:1323, 1998.

283. Kurz S, Hink U, Nickenig G, et al: Evidence for a causal role of the renin-angiotensin system in nitrate tolerance. Circulation 99:3181, 1999.

284. May DC, Popma JJ, Black WH, et al: In vivo induction and reversal of nitroglycerin tolerance in human coronary arteries. N Engl J Med 317:805, 1987.

285. Przybojewski JZ, Heyns MH: Acute coronary vasospasm secondary to industrial nitroglycerin withdrawal. A case presentation and review. S Afr Med J 63:158, 1983.

286. Schwartz AM: The cause, relief and prevention of headaches arising from contact with dynamite. N Engl J Med 235:541, 1948.

287. Cheitlin MD, Hutter AM Jr, Brindis RG, et al: ACC/AHA expert consensus document. Use of sildenafil (Viagra) in patients with cardiovascular

disease. American College of Cardiology/American Heart Association. J Am Coll Cardiol 33:273, 1999.

288. Hoffman BB, Lefkowitz RJ: Catecholamines, sympathomimetic drugs, and adrenergic receptor antagonists. In Goodman LS, Gilman A, Hardman JG, et al (eds): Goodman & Gilman's The Pharmacological Basis of Therapeutics. 9th ed. New York, McGraw-Hill, 1996, pp 199–248.

289. Frishman WH: Carvedilol. N Engl J Med 339:1759, 1998.

290. Steinbeck G, Andresen D, Bach P, et al: A comparison of electrophysiologically guided antiarrhythmic drug therapy with beta-blocker therapy in patients with symptomatic, sustained ventricular tachyarrhythmias. N Engl J Med 327:987, 1992.

291. Hohnloser SH, Meinertz T, Stubbs P, et al: Efficacy and safety of d-sotalol, a pure class III antiarrhythmic compound, in patients with symptomatic complex ventricular ectopy. Results of a multicenter, randomized, double-blind, placebo-controlled dose-finding study. The d-Sotalol PVC Study Group. Circulation 92:1517, 1995.

292. Henry JA, Cassidy SL: Membrane stabilising activity: A major cause of fatal poisoning. Lancet 1:1414, 1986.

293. Frishman WH: Drug therapy. Pindolol: A new beta-adrenoceptor antagonist with partial agonist activity. N Engl J Med 308:940, 1983.

294. Frishman W, Halprin S: Clinical pharmacology of the new beta-adrenergic blocking drugs. Part 7. New horizons in beta-adrenoceptor blockade therapy: Labetalol. Am Heart J 98:660, 1979.

295. Lennard MS: The polymorphic oxidation of beta-adrenoceptor antagonists. Pharmacol Ther 41:461, 1989.

296. Northcote RJ, Todd IC, Ballantyne D: Beta blockers and lipoproteins: A review of current knowledge. Scott Med J 31:220, 1986.

297. Borzak S, Fenton T, Glasser SP, et al: Discordance between effects of anti-ischemic therapy on ambulatory ischemia, exercise performance and anginal symptoms in patients with stable angina pectoris. J Am Coll Cardiol 21:1605, 1993.

298. Opie LH, Sonnenblick EH, Kaplan NM: Beta-agents. In Opie LH, Chatterjee K (eds): Drugs for the Heart. 4th ed. Philadelphia, WB Saunders, 1995, pp 20–23.

299. Hiatt WR, Stoll S, Nies AS: Effect of beta-adrenergic blockers on the peripheral circulation in patients with peripheral vascular disease. Circulation 72:1226, 1985.

300. Miller RR, Olson HG, Amsterdam EA, et al: Propranolol-withdrawal rebound phenomenon. Exacerbation of coronary events after abrupt cessation of antianginal therapy. N Engl J Med 293:416, 1975.

301. Braunwald E: Mechanism of action of calcium-channel-blocking agents. N Engl J Med 307:1618, 1982.

302. Freher M, Challapalli S, Pinto JV, et al: Current status of calcium channel blockers in patients with cardiovascular disease. Curr Probl Cardiol 24:236, 1999.

303. Abernethy DR, Schwartz JB: Calcium antagonist drugs. N Engl J Med 341:1447, 1999.

303a. Katz AM: Cardiac ion channels. N Engl J Med 328:1244, 1993.

304. Cannon RO III, Watson RM, Rosing DR, et al: Efficacy of calcium channel blocker therapy for angina pectoris resulting from small-vessel coronary artery disease and abnormal vasodilator reserve. Am J Cardiol 56:242, 1985.

305. Opie LH: Calcium channel antagonists in the treatment of coronary artery disease: Fundamental pharmacological properties relevant to clinical use. Prog Cardiovasc Dis 38:273, 1996.

306. Cohn PF: Concomitant use of nitrates, calcium channel blockers, and beta blockers for optimal antianginal therapy. Clin Cardiol 17:415, 1994.

307. Lichtlen PR, Hugenholtz PG, Rafflenbeul W, et al: Retardation of angiographic progression of coronary artery disease by nifedipine. Results of the International Nifedipine Trial on Antiatherosclerotic Therapy (INTACT). Lancet 335:1109, 1990.

308. Waters D, Lesperance J: Interventions that beneficially influence the evolution of coronary atherosclerosis. The case for calcium channel blockers. Circulation 86(Suppl 3):111, 1992.

309. Schroeder JS, Gao SZ, Alderman EL, et al: A preliminary study of diltiazem in the prevention of coronary artery disease in heart-transplant recipients. N Engl J Med 328:164, 1993.

310. Elkayam U, Amin J, Mehra A, et al: A prospective, randomized, double-blind, crossover study to compare the efficacy and safety of chronic nifedipine therapy with that of isosorbide dinitrate and their combination in the treatment of chronic congestive heart failure. Circulation 82:1954, 1990.

311. Opie LH, Frishman WH, Thadani U: Calcium channel antagonists (calcium entry blockers). In Opie LH, Chatterjee K (eds): Drugs for the Heart. 4th ed. Philadelphia, WB Saunders, 1995, p 53.

312. Wallace WA, Wellington KL, Chess MA, et al: Comparison of nifedipine gastrointestinal therapeutic system and atenolol on antianginal efficacies and exercise hemodynamic responses in stable angina pectoris. Am J Cardiol 73:23, 1994.

313. Parmley WW, Nesto RW, Singh BN, et al: Attenuation of the circadian patterns of myocardial ischemia with nifedipine GITS in patients with chronic stable angina. J Am Coll Cardiol 19:1380, 1992.

314. Psaty BM, Heckbert SR, Koepsell TD, et al: The risk of myocardial infarction associated with antihypertensive drug therapies. JAMA 274:620, 1995.

315. Furberg CD, Psaty BM, Meyer JV: Nifedipine. Dose-related increase in mortality in patients with coronary heart disease. Circulation 92:1326, 1995.

316. Pahor M, Guralnik JM, Corti MC, et al: Long-term survival and use of

antihypertensive medications in older persons. J Am Geriatr Soc 43: 1191, 1995.

317. Alderman M, Cohen H, Rogue R, et al: Long and short acting calcium channel antagonists differ with regard to cardiovascular outcomes in hypertensive patients. Lancet 349:585, 1997.

318. Aursnes I, Litleskare I, Froyland H, et al: Association between various drugs used for hypertension and risk of acute myocardial infarction. Blood Press 4:157, 1995.

319. Jick H, Derby LE, Gurewich V, et al: The risk of myocardial infarction associated with antihypertensive drug treatment in persons with uncomplicated essential hypertension. Pharmacotherapy 16:321, 1996.

320. Opie LH, Messerli FH: Nifedipine and mortality. Grave defects in the dossier (editorial). Circulation 92:1068, 1995.

321. Yusuf S: Calcium antagonists in coronary artery disease and hypertension. Time for reevaluation? (editorial) Circulation 92:1079, 1995.

322. Lacoste L, Lam JY, Hung J, et al: Oral verapamil inhibits platelet thrombus formation in humans. Circulation 89:630, 1994.

323. Leon MB, Rosing DR, Bonow RO, et al: Clinical efficacy of verapamil alone and combined with propranolol in treating patients with chronic stable angina pectoris. Am J Cardiol 48:131, 1981.

324. Bache RJ: Effects of calcium entry blockade on myocardial blood flow. Circulation 80(Suppl 4):40, 1989.

325. Klinke WP, Baird M, Juneau M, et al: Antianginal efficacy and safety of controlled-delivery diltiazem QD versus an equivalent dose of immediate-release diltiazem TID. Cardiovasc Drugs Ther 9:319, 1995.

326. Nadazdin A, Davies GJ: Investigation of therapeutic mechanisms of atenolol and diltiazem in patients with variable-threshold angina. Am Heart J 127:312, 1994.

327. Piepho RW, Culbertson VL, Rhodes RS: Drug interactions with the calcium-entry blockers. Circulation 75(Suppl 5):181, 1987.

328. Abernethy DR: An overview of the pharmacokinetics and pharmacodynamics of amlodipine in elderly persons with systemic hypertension. Am J Cardiol 73:10A, 1994.

329. Ezekowitz MD, Hossack K, Mehta JL, et al: Amlodipine in chronic stable angina: Results of a multicenter double-blind crossover trial. Am Heart J 129:527, 1995.

330. Packer M, O'Connor CM, Ghali JK, et al: Effect of amlodipine on morbidity and mortality in severe chronic heart failure. Prospective Randomized Amlodipine Survival Evaluation Study Group. N Engl J Med 335:1107, 1996.

331. Ekelund LG, Ulvenstam G, Walldius G, et al: Effects of felodipine versus nifedipine on exercise tolerance in stable angina pectoris. Am J Cardiol 73:658, 1994.

332. Frishman WH: Comparative efficacy and concomitant use of bepridil and beta blockers in the management of angina pectoris. Am J Cardiol 69:50D, 1992.

333. Ryden L, Malmberg K: Calcium channel blockers or beta receptor antagonists for patients with ischaemic heart disease. What is the best choice? (editorial) Eur Heart J 17:1, 1996.

334. Pepine CJ, Cohn PF, Deedwania PC, et al: Effects of treatment on outcome in mildly symptomatic patients with ischemia during daily life. The Atenolol Silent Ischemia Study (ASIST). Circulation 90:762, 1994.

335. Rehnqvist N, Hjemdahl P, Billing E, et al: Treatment of stable angina pectoris with calcium antagonists and beta-blockers. The APSIS study. Angina Prognosis Study in Stockholm. Cardiologia 40(Suppl 1):301, 1995.

336. von Arnim T: Medical treatment to reduce total ischemic burden: Total Ischemic Burden Bisoprolol Study (TIBBS), a multicenter trial comparing bisoprolol and nifedipine. The TIBBS Investigators. J Am Coll Cardiol 25:231, 1995.

337. Savonitto S, Ardissino D, Egstrup K, et al: Combination therapy with metoprolol and nifedipine versus monotherapy in patients with stable angina pectoris. Results of the International Multicenter Angina Exercise (IMAGE) Study. J Am Coll Cardiol 27:311, 1996.

338. Ishikawa K, Nakai S, Takenaka T, et al: Short-acting nifedipine and diltiazem do not reduce the incidence of cardiac events in patients with healed myocardial infarction. Secondary Prevention Group. Circulation 95:2368, 1997.

339. The Multicenter Diltiazem Postinfarction Trial Research Group: The effect of diltiazem on mortality and reinfarction after myocardial infarction. N Engl J Med 319:385, 1988.

340. The Danish Study Group on Verapamil in Myocardial Infarction: Effect of verapamil on mortality and major events after acute myocardial infarction (the Danish Verapamil Infarction Trial II—DAVIT II). Am J Cardiol 66:779, 1990.

341. CIBIS-II Investigators and Committees: The Cardiac Insufficiency Bisoprolol Study II (CIBIS-II): A randomised trial. Lancet 353:9, 1999.

342. MERIT-HF Study Group: Effect of metoprolol CR/XL in chronic heart failure: Metoprolol CR/XL Randomised Intervention Trial in Congestive Heart Failure (MERIT-HF). Lancet 353:2001, 1999.

343. The Holland Interuniversity Nifedipine/Metoprolol Trial (HINT) Research Group: Early treatment of unstable angina in the coronary care unit: A randomised, double blind, placebo controlled comparison of recurrent ischaemia in patients treated with nifedipine or metoprolol or both. Report of The Holland Interuniversity Nifedipine/Metoprolol Trial (HINT) Research Group. Br Heart J 56:400, 1986.

344. Mannheimer C, Eliasson T, Augustinsson LE, et al: Electrical stimulation versus coronary artery bypass surgery in severe angina pectoris: The ESBY study. Circulation 97:1157, 1998.

345. Brodison A, Chauhan A: Spinal-cord stimulation in management of angina. Lancet 354:1748, 1999.

346. Niebauer J, Cooke JP: Cardiovascular effects of exercise: Role of endothelial shear stress. J Am Coll Cardiol 28:1652, 1996.

347. Arora RR, Chou TM, Jain D, et al: The Multicenter Study of Enhanced External Counterpulsation (MUST-EECP): Effect of EECP on exercise-induced myocardial ischemia and anginal episodes. J Am Coll Cardiol 33:1833, 1999.

PERCUTANEOUS CORONARY INTERVENTIONS

348. Gersh BJ: Coronary revascularization in the 1990s: A cardiologist's perspective. Can J Cardiol 10:661, 1994.

349. Bittl JA: Advances in coronary angioplasty. N Engl J Med 335:1290, 1996.

350. Ryan TJ, Bauman WB, Kennedy JW, et al: Guidelines for percutaneous transluminal coronary angioplasty. A report of the American College of Cardiology/American Heart Association Task Force on Assessment of Diagnostic and Therapeutic Cardiovascular Procedures (Committee on Percutaneous Transluminal Coronary Angioplasty). J Am Coll Cardiol 22:2033, 1993.

351. Hirshfeld JW Jr, Ellis SG, Faxon DP: Recommendations for the assessment and maintenance of proficiency in coronary interventional procedures: Statement of the American College of Cardiology. J Am Coll Cardiol 31:722, 1998.

352. The Bypass Angioplasty Revascularization Investigation (BARI) Investigators: Comparison of coronary bypass surgery with angioplasty in patients with multivessel disease. N Engl J Med 335:217, 1996.

353. Kimmel SE, Berlin JA, Strom BL, et al: Development and validation of simplified predictive index for major complications in contemporary percutaneous transluminal coronary angioplasty practice. The Registry Committee of the Society for Cardiac Angiography and Interventions. J Am Coll Cardiol 26:931, 1995.

354. Zaacks SM, Allen JE, Calvin JE, et al: Value of the American College of Cardiology/American Heart Association stenosis morphology classification for coronary interventions in the late 1990s. Am J Cardiol 82:43, 1998.

355. O'Connor GT, Malenka DJ, Quinton H, et al: Multivariate prediction of in-hospital mortality after percutaneous coronary interventions in 1994–1996. Northern New England Cardiovascular Disease Study Group. J Am Coll Cardiol 34:681, 1999.

356. Piana RN, Ahmed WH, Chaitman B, et al: Effect of transient abrupt vessel closure during otherwise successful angioplasty for unstable angina on clinical outcome at six months. J Am Coll Cardiol 33:73, 1999.

357. Ellis SG, Cowley MJ, Whitlow PL, et al: Prospective case-control comparison of percutaneous transluminal coronary revascularization in patients with multivessel disease treated in 1986–1987 versus 1991: Improved in-hospital and 12-month results. Multivessel Angioplasty Prognosis Study (MAPS) Group. J Am Coll Cardiol 25:1137, 1995.

358. King SB III, Schlumpf M: Ten-year completed follow-up of percutaneous transluminal coronary angioplasty: The early Zurich experience. J Am Coll Cardiol 22:353, 1993.

359. Stein B, Weintraub WS, Gebhart SP, et al: Influence of diabetes mellitus on early and late outcome after percutaneous transluminal coronary angioplasty. Circulation 91:979, 1995.

360. Holmes DR Jr, Detre KM, Williams DO, et al: Long-term outcome of patients with depressed left ventricular function undergoing percutaneous transluminal coronary angioplasty. The NHLBI PTCA Registry. Circulation 87:21, 1993.

361. Wurdeman RL, Hilleman DE, Mooss AN: Restenosis, the Achilles' heel of coronary angioplasty. Pharmacotherapy 18:1024, 1998.

362. Landzberg BR, Frishman WH, Lerrick K: Pathophysiology and pharmacological approaches for prevention of coronary artery restenosis following coronary artery balloon angioplasty and related procedures. Prog Cardiovasc Dis 39:361, 1997.

363. Barsness GW, Peterson ED, Ohman EM, et al: Relationship between diabetes mellitus and long-term survival after coronary bypass and angioplasty. Circulation 96:2551, 1997.

364. King SB III, Lembo NJ, Weintraub WS, et al: A randomized trial comparing coronary angioplasty with coronary bypass surgery. Emory Angioplasty versus Surgery Trial (EAST). N Engl J Med 331:1044, 1994.

365. Solomon AJ, Gersh BJ: Management of chronic stable angina: Medical therapy, percutaneous transluminal coronary angioplasty, and coronary artery bypass graft surgery. Lessons from the randomized trials. Ann Intern Med 128:216, 1998.

366. Rankin JM, Spinelli JJ, Carere RG, et al: Improved clinical outcome after widespread use of coronary-artery stenting in Canada. N Engl J Med 341:1957, 1999.

367. Teirstein PS, Massullo V, Jani S, et al: Three-year clinical and angiographic follow-up after intracoronary radiation: Results of a randomized clinical trial. Circulation 101:360, 2000.

368. Hueb WA, Bellotti G, de Oliveira SA, et al: The Medicine, Angioplasty or Surgery Study (MASS): A prospective, randomized trial of medical therapy, balloon angioplasty or bypass surgery for single proximal left anterior descending artery stenoses. J Am Coll Cardiol 26:1600, 1995.

369. Hueb W: The Medicine Angioplasty and Surgery Study (MASS): A prospective randomized trial of medical therapy, balloon angioplasty, or bypass surgery for single proximal left anterior artery stenosis: Five years of follow up. American College of Cardiology Annual Scientific Session, Anaheim, Ca., 1999.

370. RITA-2 Trial Participants: Coronary angioplasty versus medical therapy for angina: The second Randomised Intervention Treatment of Angina (RITA-2) trial. Lancet 350:461, 1997.

371. Parisi AF, Folland ED, Hartigan P: A comparison of angioplasty with medical therapy in the treatment of single-vessel coronary artery disease. N Engl J Med 326:10, 1992.

372. Strauss WE, Fortin T, Hartigan P, et al: A comparison of quality of life scores in patients with angina pectoris after angioplasty compared with after medical therapy. Outcomes of a randomized clinical trial. Circulation 92:1710, 1995.

373. Ellis SG, Cowley MJ, DiSciascio G, et al: Determinants of 2-year outcome after coronary angioplasty in patients with multivessel disease on the basis of comprehensive preprocedural evaluation. Implications for patient selection. Circulation 83:1905, 1991.

374. Kohli RS, DiSciascio G, Cowley MJ, et al: Coronary angioplasty in patients with severe left ventricular dysfunction. J Am Coll Cardiol 16:807, 1990.

375. Eltchaninoff H, Franco I, Whitlow PL: Late results of coronary angioplasty in patients with left ventricular ejection fractions < or = 40%. Am J Cardiol 73:1047, 1994.

376. Serruys PW, de Jaegere P, Kiemeneij F, et al: A comparison of balloon-expandable-stent implantation with balloon angioplasty in patients with coronary artery disease. N Engl J Med 331:489, 1994.

377. Teirstein PS, Massullo V, Jani S, et al: Catheter-based radiotherapy to inhibit restenosis after coronary stenting. N Engl J Med 336:1697, 1997.

378. King SB III: Radiation for restenosis: Watchful waiting (editorial). Circulation 99:192, 1999.

379. Ruygrok PN, Melkert R, Morel MA, et al: Does angiography six months after coronary intervention influence management and outcome? Benestent II Investigators. J Am Coll Cardiol 34:1507, 1999.

380. Moscucci M, Piana RN, Kuntz RE, et al: Effect of prior coronary restenosis on the risk of subsequent restenosis after stent placement or directional atherectomy. Am J Cardiol 73:1147, 1994.

381. Piessens JH, Stammen F, Desmet W, et al: Immediate and 6-month follow-up results of coronary angioplasty for restenosis: Analysis of factors predicting recurrent clinical restenosis. Am Heart J 126:565, 1993.

382. Bauters C, McFadden EP, Lablanche JM, et al: Restenosis rate after multiple percutaneous transluminal coronary angioplasty procedures at the same site. A quantitative angiographic study in consecutive patients undergoing a third angioplasty procedure for a second restenosis. Circulation 88:969, 1993.

383. Delacretaz E, Meier B: Therapeutic strategy with total coronary artery occlusions. Am J Cardiol 79:185, 1997.

384. Berger PB, Holmes DR Jr, Ohman EM, et al: Restenosis, reocclusion and adverse cardiovascular events after successful balloon angioplasty of occluded versus nonoccluded coronary arteries. Results from the Multicenter American Research Trial with Cilazapril after Angioplasty to Prevent Transluminal Coronary Obstruction and Restenosis (MARCATOR). J Am Coll Cardiol 27:1, 1996.

385. Violaris AG, Melkert R, Serruys PW: Long-term luminal renarrowing after successful elective coronary angioplasty of total occlusions. A quantitative angiographic analysis. Circulation 91:2140, 1995.

386. Ozaki Y, Violaris AG, Hamburger J, et al: Short- and long-term clinical and quantitative angiographic results with the new, less shortening Wallstent for vessel reconstruction in chronic total occlusion: A quantitative angiographic study. J Am Coll Cardiol 28:354, 1996.

387. Sirnes PA, Golf S, Myreng Y, et al: Sustained benefit of stenting chronic coronary occlusion: Long-term clinical follow-up of the Stenting in Chronic Coronary Occlusion (SICCO) study. J Am Coll Cardiol 32:305, 1998.

388. Buller CE, Dzavik V, Carere RG, et al: Primary stenting versus balloon angioplasty in occluded coronary arteries: The Total Occlusion Study of Canada (TOSCA). Circulation 100:236, 1999.

389. Bell MR, Grill DE, Garratt KN, et al: Long-term outcome of women compared with men after successful coronary angioplasty. Circulation 91:2876, 1995.

390. Jacobs AK, Kelsey SF, Brooks MM, et al: Better outcome for women compared with men undergoing coronary revascularization: A report from the Bypass Angioplasty Revascularization Investigation (BARI). Circulation 98:1279, 1998.

391. Kaul TK, Fields BL, Wyatt DA, et al: Angioplasty versus coronary artery bypass in octogenarians. Ann Thorac Surg 58:1419, 1994.

392. Gersh BJ, Kronmal RA, Frye RL, et al: Coronary arteriography and coronary artery bypass surgery: Morbidity and mortality in patients ages 65 years or older. A report from the Coronary Artery Surgery Study. Circulation 67:483, 1983.

393. Thompson RC, Holmes DR Jr, Grill DE, et al: Changing outcome of angioplasty in the elderly. J Am Coll Cardiol 27:8, 1996.

394. Mathew V, Clavell A, Grill DE, et al: Percutaneous coronary intervention in patients with prior coronary bypass surgery. Am J Med, in press.

395. Moses JW, Moussa I, Popma JJ, et al: Risk of distal embolization and infarction with transluminal extraction atherectomy in saphenous vein grafts and native coronary arteries. NACI Investigators. New Approaches to Coronary Interventions. Cathet Cardiovasc Interv 47:149, 1999.

396. Mak KH, Challapalli R, Eisenberg MJ, et al: Effect of platelet glycoprotein IIb/IIIa receptor inhibition on distal embolization during percutaneous revascularization of aortocoronary saphenous vein grafts. EPIC Investigators. Evaluation of IIb/IIIa platelet receptor antagonist 7E3 in Preventing Ischemic Complications. Am J Cardiol 80:985, 1997.

397. Rosenschein U, Gaul G, Erbel R, et al: Percutaneous transluminal therapy of occluded saphenous vein grafts: Can the challenge be met with ultrasound thrombolysis? Circulation 99:26, 1999.

398. Holmes DR Jr, Hirshfeld J Jr, Faxon D, et al: ACC Expert Consensus document on coronary artery stents. Document of the American College of Cardiology. J Am Coll Cardiol 32:1471, 1998.

CORONARY ARTERY BYPASS SURGERY

399. Garrett HE, Dennis EW, DeBakey ME: Aortocoronary bypass with saphenous vein graft. Seven-year follow-up. JAMA 223:792, 1973.

400. Favoloro RG: Saphenous vein autograft replacement of severe segmental coronary artery occlusion: Operative technique. Ann Thorac Surg 5:334, 1968.

401. Johnson WD, Flemma RJ, Lepley D Jr, et al: Extended treatment of severe coronary artery disease: A total surgical approach. Ann Surg 170:460, 1969.

402. Kolessov VI: Mammary artery–coronary artery anastomosis as method of treatment for angina pectoris. J Thorac Cardiovasc Surg 54:535, 1967.

403. Green GE, Spencer FC, Tice DA, et al: Arterial and venous microsurgical bypass grafts for coronary artery disease. J Thorac Cardiovasc Surg 60:491, 1970.

404. McGlynn EA, Naylor CD, Anderson GM, et al: Comparison of the appropriateness of coronary angiography and coronary artery bypass graft surgery between Canada and New York State. JAMA 272:934, 1994.

405. Meijler AP, Rigter H, Bernstein SJ, et al: The appropriateness of intention to treat decisions for invasive therapy in coronary artery disease in The Netherlands. Heart 77:219, 1997.

406. Leape LL, Hilborne LH, Schwartz JS, et al: The appropriateness of coronary artery bypass graft surgery in academic medical centers. Working Group of the Appropriateness Project of the Academic Medical Center Consortium. Ann Intern Med 125:8, 1996.

407. Martin TD, Craver JM, Gott JP, et al: Prospective, randomized trial of retrograde warm blood cardioplegia: Myocardial benefit and neurologic threat. Ann Thorac Surg 57:298, 1994.

408. Allen BS, Buckberg GD, Fontan FM, et al: Superiority of controlled surgical reperfusion versus percutaneous transluminal coronary angioplasty in acute coronary occlusion. J Thorac Cardiovasc Surg 105:864, 1993.

409. Ikonomidis JS, Yau TM, Weisel RD, et al: Optimal flow rates for retrograde warm cardioplegia. J Thorac Cardiovasc Surg 107:510, 1994.

410. Christakis GT, Lichtenstein SV, Buth KJ, et al: The influence of risk on the results of warm heart surgery: A substudy of a randomized trial. Eur J Cardiothorac Surg 11:515, 1997.

411. Murkin JM, Boyd WD, Ganapathy S, et al: Beating heart surgery: Why expect less central nervous system morbidity? Ann Thorac Surg 68:1498, 1999.

412. Buffolo E, de Andrade CS, Branco JN, et al: Coronary artery bypass grafting without cardiopulmonary bypass. Ann Thorac Surg 61:63, 1996.

413. Calafiore AM, Teodori G, Di Giammarco G, et al: Minimally invasive coronary artery surgery: The last operation. Semin Thorac Cardiovasc Surg 9:305, 1997.

414. Puskas JD, Wright CE, Ronson RS, et al: Off-pump multivessel coronary bypass via sternotomy is safe and effective. Ann Thorac Surg 66:1068, 1998.

415. Goldstein DJ, Oz MC: Current status and future directions of minimally invasive cardiac surgery. Curr Opin Cardiol 14:419, 1999.

416. Galloway AC, Shemin RJ, Glower DD, et al: First report of the Port Access International Registry. Ann Thorac Surg 67:51, 1999.

417. Ribakove GH, Miller JS, Anderson RV, et al: Minimally invasive port-access coronary artery bypass grafting with early angiographic follow-up: Initial clinical experience. J Thorac Cardiovasc Surg 115:1101, 1998.

418. Izzat MB, Yim AP, Mehta D, et al: Staged minimally invasive direct coronary artery bypass and percutaneous angioplasty for multivessel coronary artery disease. Int J Cardiol 62(Suppl 1):105, 1997.

419. Possati G, Gaudino M, Alessandrini F, et al: Systematic clinical and angiographic follow-up of patients undergoing minimally invasive coronary artery bypass. J Thorac Cardiovasc Surg 115:785, 1998.

420. Berger PB, Alderman EL, Nadel A, et al: Frequency of early occlusion and stenosis in a left internal mammary artery to left anterior descending artery bypass graft after surgery through a median sternotomy on conventional bypass: Benchmark for minimally invasive direct coronary artery bypass. Circulation 100:2353, 1999.

421. Bryan AJ, Angelini GD: The biology of saphenous vein graft occlusion: Etiology and strategies for prevention. Curr Opin Cardiol 9:641, 1994.

422. Loop FD: Internal-thoracic-artery grafts. Biologically better coronary arteries (editorial). N Engl J Med 334:263, 1996.

423. Turina M: Coronary artery surgical technique. Curr Opin Cardiol 8:919, 1993.

424. Chaikhouni A, Crawford FA, Kochel PJ, et al: Human internal mammary artery produces more prostacyclin than saphenous vein. J Thorac Cardiovasc Surg 92:88, 1986.

425. www.ctsnet.org. Society of Thoracic Surgeons Database.

426. Barner HB, Standeven JW, Reese J: Twelve-year experience with internal mammary artery for coronary artery bypass. J Thorac Cardiovasc Surg 90:668, 1985.

427. Palatianos GM, Bolooki H, Horowitz MD, et al: Sequential internal mammary artery grafts for coronary artery bypass. Ann Thorac Surg 56:1136, 1993.

428. Cameron A, Davis KB, Green G, et al: Coronary bypass surgery with internal-thoracic-artery grafts—effects on survival over a 15-year period. N Engl J Med 334:216, 1996.

429. Naunheim KS, Barner HB, Fiore AC: 1990: Results of internal thoracic artery grafting over 15 years: Single versus double grafts. 1992 update. Ann Thorac Surg 1992 53:716.

430. Pick AW, Orszulak TA, Anderson BJ, et al: Single versus bilateral internal mammary artery grafts: 10-year outcome analysis. Ann Thorac Surg 64:599, 1997.

431. He GW, Buxton BF, Rosenfeldt FL, et al: Pharmacologic dilatation of the internal mammary artery during coronary bypass grafting. J Thorac Cardiovasc Surg 107:1440, 1994.

432. Brodman RF, Frame R, Camacho M, et al: Routine use of unilateral and bilateral radial arteries for coronary artery bypass graft surgery. J Am Coll Cardiol 28:959, 1996.

433. Acar C, Ramsheyi A, Pagny JY, et al: The radial artery for coronary artery bypass grafting: Clinical and angiographic results at five years. J Thorac Cardiovasc Surg 116:981, 1998.

434. Jegaden O, Eker A, Montagna P, et al: Technical aspects and late functional results of gastroepiploic bypass grafting (400 cases). Eur J Cardiothorac Surg 9:575, 1995.

435. Puig LB: Inferior epigastric artery (letter). Ann Thorac Surg 68:631, 1999.

436. Suma H, Wanibuchi Y, Takeuchi A: Bovine internal thoracic artery graft for myocardial revascularization: Late results. Ann Thorac Surg 57:704, 1994.

437. Grondin CM, Lepage G, Castonguay YR, et al: Aortocoronary bypass graft. Initial blood flow through the graft, and early postoperative patency. Circulation 44:815, 1971.

438. Alderman EL: Angiographic correlates of graft patency and relationship to clinical outcomes. Ann Thorac Surg 62(Suppl):22, 1996.

439. Kantor B, McKenna CJ, Caccitolo JA, et al: Transmyocardial and percutaneous myocardial revascularization: Current and future role in the treatment of coronary artery disease. Mayo Clin Proc 74:585, 1999.

440. Hughes GC, Abdel-aleem S, Biswas SS, et al: Transmyocardial laser revascularization: Experimental and clinical results. Can J Cardiol 15:797, 1999.

441. Mack CA, Magovern CJ, Hahn RT, et al: Channel patency and neovascularization after transmyocardial revascularization using an excimer laser: Results and comparisons to nonlased channels. Circulation 96(Suppl 2):65, 1997.

442. Al-Sheikh T, Allen KB, Straka SP, et al: Cardiac sympathetic denervation after transmyocardial laser revascularization. Circulation 100:135, 1999.

443. Horvath KA, Cohn LH, Cooley DA, et al: Transmyocardial laser revascularization: Results of a multicenter trial with transmyocardial laser revascularization used as sole therapy for end-stage coronary artery disease. J Thorac Cardiovasc Surg 113:645, 1997.

444. Vincent JG, Bardos P, Kruse J, et al: End stage coronary disease treated with the transmyocardial CO_2 laser revascularization: A chance for the "inoperable" patient. Eur J Cardiothorac Surg 11:888, 1997.

445. Allen KB, Fudge TL, Schoettle GP Jr, et al: Prospective randomized multicenter trial of transmyocardial revascularization versus maximal medical management in patients with refractory class IV angina: 12-month results (abstract). Circulation 98(Suppl 1):476, 1998.

446. Schofield PM, Sharples LD, Caine N, et al: Transmyocardial laser revascularisation in patients with refractory angina: A randomised controlled trial. Lancet 353:519, 1999.

447. Frazier OH, March RJ, Horvath KA: Transmyocardial revascularization with a carbon dioxide laser in patients with end-stage coronary artery disease. N Engl J Med 341:1021, 1999.

448. Allen KB, Dowling RD, Fudge TL, et al: Comparison of transmyocardial revascularization with medical therapy in patients with refractory angina. N Engl J Med 341:1029, 1999.

449. Shawl FA, Domanski MJ, Kaul U, et al: Procedural results and early clinical outcome of percutaneous transluminal myocardial revascularization. Am J Cardiol 83:498, 1999.

450. Lauer B, Junghans U, Stahl F, et al: Catheter-based percutaneous myocardial laser revascularization in patients with end-stage coronary artery disease. J Am Coll Cardiol 34:1663, 1999.

451. Fleischer KJ, Goldschmidt-Clermont PJ, Fonger JD, et al: One-month histologic response of transmyocardial laser channels with molecular intervention. Ann Thorac Surg 62:1051, 1996.

452. Edwards FH, Clark RE, Schwartz M: Impact of internal mammary artery conduits on operative mortality in coronary revascularization. Ann Thorac Surg 57:27, 1994.

453. Kirklin JW, Naftel CD, Blackstone EH, et al: Summary of a consensus concerning death and ischemic events after coronary artery bypass grafting. Circulation 79(Suppl 1):81, 1989.

454. Katz NM, Gersh BJ, Cox JL: Changing practice of coronary bypass surgery and its impact on early risk and long-term survival. Curr Opin Cardiol 13:465, 1998.

455. Shroyer AL, Plomondon ME, Grover FL, et al: The 1996 coronary artery bypass risk model: The Society of Thoracic Surgeons Adult Cardiac National Database. Ann Thorac Surg 67:1205, 1999.

456. Schaff HV, Gersh BJ, Fisher LD, et al: Detrimental effect of perioperative myocardial infarction on late survival after coronary artery bypass.

Report from the Coronary Artery Surgery Study—CASS. J Thorac Cardiovasc Surg 88:972, 1984.

457. Kallner G, Lindblom D, Forssell G, et al: Myocardial release of troponin T after coronary bypass surgery. Scand J Thorac Cardiovasc Surg 28:67, 1994.

458. Eagle KA, Guyton RA, Davidoff R, et al: ACC/AHA Guidelines for Coronary Artery Bypass Graft Surgery: A Report of the American College of Cardiology/American Heart Association Task Force on Practice Guidelines (Committee to Revise the 1991 Guidelines for Coronary Artery Bypass Graft Surgery). J Am Coll Cardiol 34:1262, 1999.

459. Birkmeyer NJ, Charlesworth DC, Hernandez F, et al: Obesity and risk of adverse outcomes associated with coronary artery bypass surgery. Northern New England Cardiovascular Disease Study Group. Circulation 97:1689, 1998.

460. Levi M, Cromheecke ME, de Jonge E, et al: Pharmacological strategies to decrease excessive blood loss in cardiac surgery: A meta-analysis of clinically relevant endpoints. Lancet 354:1940, 1999.

461. Loop FD, Lytle BW, Cosgrove DM, et al: J. Maxwell Chamberlain memorial paper. Sternal wound complications after isolated coronary artery bypass grafting: Early and late mortality, morbidity, and cost of care. Ann Thorac Surg 49:179, 1990.

462. Kroenke K, Lawrence VA, Theroux JF, et al: Operative risk in patients with severe obstructive pulmonary disease. Arch Intern Med 152:967, 1992.

463. Spivack SD, Shinozaki T, Albertini JJ, et al: Preoperative prediction of postoperative respiratory outcome. Coronary artery bypass grafting. Chest 109:1222, 1996.

464. Vandersalm T, Stahl F: Early postoperative care. In Edmunds LH (ed): Cardiac Surgery in the Adult. New York, McGraw-Hill, 1997, p 343.

465. Blauth CI, Cosgrove DM, Webb BW, et al: Atheroembolism from the ascending aorta. An emerging problem in cardiac surgery. J Thorac Cardiovasc Surg 103:1104, 1992.

466. Selnes OA, Goldsborough MA, Borowicz LM, et al: Neurobehavioural sequelae of cardiopulmonary bypass. Lancet 353:1601, 1999.

467. Roach GW, Kanchuger M, Mangano CM, et al: Adverse cerebral outcomes after coronary bypass surgery. N Engl J Med 335:1857, 1996.

468. Shaw PJ, Bates D, Cartlidge NE, et al: Early intellectual dysfunction following coronary bypass surgery. Q J Med 58:59, 1986.

469. Sylivris S, Calafiore P, Matalanis G, et al: The intraoperative assessment of ascending aortic atheroma: Epiaortic imaging is superior to both transesophageal echocardiography and direct palpation. J Cardiothorac Vasc Anesth 11:704, 1997.

470. Campbell RW: Postoperative arrhythmias and the role for implantable cardioverter-defibrillators. Curr Opin Cardiol 8:932, 1993.

471. Aranki SF, Shaw DP, Adams DH, et al: Predictors of atrial fibrillation after coronary artery surgery. Current trends and impact on hospital resources. Circulation 94:390, 1996.

472. Cameron AA, Davis KB, Rogers WJ: Recurrence of angina after coronary artery bypass surgery: Predictors and prognosis (CASS Registry). Coronary Artery Surgery Study. J Am Coll Cardiol 26:895, 1995.

473. Kirklin JW, Akins CW, Blackstone EH, et al: Guidelines and indications for coronary artery bypass graft surgery. A report of the American College of Cardiology/American Heart Association Task Force on Assessment of Diagnostic and Therapeutic Cardiovascular Procedures (Subcommittee on Coronary Artery Bypass Graft Surgery). J Am Coll Cardiol 17:543, 1991.

474. Thourani VH, Weintraub WS, Stein B, et al: Influence of diabetes mellitus on early and late outcome after coronary artery bypass grafting. Ann Thorac Surg 67:1045, 1999.

475. Bell MR, Gersh BJ, Schaff HV, et al: Effect of completeness of revascularization on long-term outcome of patients with three-vessel disease undergoing coronary artery bypass surgery. A report from the Coronary Artery Surgery Study (CASS) Registry. Circulation 86:446, 1992.

476. Anonymous: Coronary angioplasty versus coronary artery bypass surgery: The Randomized Intervention Treatment of Angina (RITA) trial. Lancet 341:573, 1993.

477. Mark DB, Lam LC, Lee KL, et al: Effects of coronary angioplasty, coronary bypass surgery, and medical therapy on employment in patients with coronary artery disease. A prospective comparison study. Ann Intern Med 120:111, 1994.

478. Bourassa MG: Long-term vein graft patency. Curr Opin Cardiol 9:685, 1994.

479. FitzGibbon GM, Leach AJ, Kafka HP, et al: Coronary bypass graft fate: Long-term angiographic study. J Am Coll Cardiol 17:1075, 1991.

480. Cox JL, Chiasson DA, Gotlieb AI: Stranger in a strange land: The pathogenesis of saphenous vein graft stenosis with emphasis on structural and functional differences between veins and arteries. Prog Cardiovasc Dis 34:45, 1991.

481. Fitzgibbon GM, Kafka HP, Leach AJ, et al: Coronary bypass graft fate and patient outcome: Angiographic follow-up of 5,065 grafts related to survival and reoperation in 1,388 patients during 25 years. J Am Coll Cardiol 28:616, 1996.

482. Motwani JG, Topol EJ: Aortocoronary saphenous vein graft disease: Pathogenesis, predisposition, and prevention. Circulation 97:916, 1998.

483. Zund G, Hauser M, Vogt P, et al: New approach to patency and flow assessment after left internal thoracic artery hypoperfusion syndrome with additional saphenous vein graft to the left anterior descending artery with phase-contrast magnetic resonance angiography. J Thorac Cardiovasc Surg 114:428, 1997.

484. Gupta S, Murgatroyd F, Widenka K, et al: Role of transcutaneous ultra-

sound in evaluation of graft patency following minimally invasive coronary surgery. Eur J Cardiothorac Surg 14(Suppl 1):88, 1998.

485. Miller S, Scheule AM, Hahn U, et al: MR angiography and flow quantification of the internal mammary artery graft after minimally invasive direct coronary artery bypass. AJR Am J Roentgenol 172:1365, 1999.

486. Hwang MH, Meadows WR, Palac RT, et al: Progression of native coronary artery disease at 10 years: Insights from a randomized study of medical versus surgical therapy for angina. J Am Coll Cardiol 16:1066, 1990.

487. Goldman S, Copeland J, Moritz T, et al: Saphenous vein graft patency 1 year after coronary artery bypass surgery and effects of antiplatelet therapy. Results of a Veterans Administration Cooperative Study. Circulation 80:1190, 1989.

488. Kroncke GM, Kosolcharoen P, Clayman JA, et al: Five-year changes in coronary arteries of medical and surgical patients of the Veterans Administration Randomized Study of Bypass Surgery. Circulation 78(Suppl 1):144, 1988.

489. Henderson WG, Goldman S, Copeland JG, et al: Antiplatelet or anticoagulant therapy after coronary artery bypass surgery. A meta-analysis of clinical trials. Ann Intern Med 111:743, 1989.

490. Chesebro JH, Fuster V, Elveback LR, et al: Effect of dipyridamole and aspirin on late vein-graft patency after coronary bypass operations. N Engl J Med 310:209, 1984.

491. Goldman S, Copeland J, Moritz T, et al: Internal mammary artery and saphenous vein graft patency. Effects of aspirin. Circulation 82(Suppl 4):237, 1990.

492. Sethi GK, Copeland JG, Goldman S, et al: Implications of preoperative administration of aspirin in patients undergoing coronary artery bypass grafting. Department of Veterans Affairs Cooperative Study on Antiplatelet Therapy. J Am Coll Cardiol 15:15, 1990.

493. Rajah SM, Nair U, Rees M, et al: Effects of antiplatelet therapy with indobufen or aspirin-dipyridamole on graft patency one year after coronary artery bypass grafting. J Thorac Cardiovasc Surg 107:1146, 1994.

494. Blankenhorn DH, Nessim SA, Johnson RL, et al: Beneficial effects of combined colestipol-niacin therapy on coronary atherosclerosis and coronary venous bypass grafts. JAMA 257:3233, 1987.

495. Yusuf S, Zucker D, Peduzzi P, et al: Effect of coronary artery bypass graft surgery on survival: Overview of 10-year results from randomised trials by the Coronary Artery Bypass Graft Surgery Trialists Collaboration. Lancet 344:563, 1994.

496. Scanlon PJ, Faxon DP, Audet AM, et al: ACC/AHA guidelines for coronary angiography. A report of the American College of Cardiology/American Heart Association Task Force on practice guidelines (Committee on Coronary Angiography). Developed in collaboration with the Society for Cardiac Angiography and Interventions. J Am Coll Cardiol 33:1756, 1999.

497. Kannel WB, Feinleib M: Natural history of angina pectoris in the Framingham study. Prognosis and survival. Am J Cardiol 29:154, 1972.

498. Gandhi MM, Lampe FC, Wood DA: Incidence, clinical characteristics, and short-term prognosis of angina pectoris. Br Heart J 73:193, 1995.

499. Hubbard B: Prospective evaluation of a clinical exercise test model. Ann Intern Med 118:81, 1993.

500. Rihal CS, Davis KB, Kennedy JW, et al: The utility of clinical, electrocardiographic, and roentgenographic variables in the prediction of left ventricular function. Am J Cardiol 75:220, 1995.

501. Galderisi M, Lauer MS, Levy D: Echocardiographic determinants of clinical outcome in subjects with coronary artery disease (the Framingham Heart Study). Am J Cardiol 70:971, 1992.

502. Mark DB, Shaw L, Harrell FE Jr, et al: Prognostic value of a treadmill exercise score in outpatients with suspected coronary artery disease. N Engl J Med 325:849, 1991.

503. Roger VL, Jacobsen SJ, Pellikka PA, et al: Prognostic value of treadmill exercise testing: A population-based study in Olmsted County, Minnesota. Circulation 98:2836, 1998.

504. Marie PY, Danchin N, Durand JF, et al: Long-term prediction of major ischemic events by exercise thallium-201 single-photon emission computed tomography. Incremental prognostic value compared with clinical, exercise testing, catheterization and radionuclide angiographic data. J Am Coll Cardiol 26:879, 1995.

505. Iskandrian AS, Chae SC, Heo J, et al: Independent and incremental prognostic value of exercise single-photon emission computed tomographic (SPECT) thallium imaging in coronary artery disease. J Am Coll Cardiol 22:665, 1993.

506. Herman SD, LaBresh KA, Santos-Ocampo CD, et al: Comparison of dobutamine and exercise using technetium-99m sestamibi imaging for the evaluation of coronary artery disease. Am J Cardiol 73:164, 1994.

507. Poldermans D, Arnese M, Fioretti PM, et al: Improved cardiac risk stratification in major vascular surgery with dobutamine-atropine stress echocardiography. J Am Coll Cardiol 26:648, 1995.

508. Coletta C, Galati A, Greco G, et al: Prognostic value of high dose dipyridamole echocardiography in patients with chronic coronary artery disease and preserved left ventricular function. J Am Coll Cardiol 26:887, 1995.

509. McCully RB, Roger VL, Mahoney DW, et al: Outcome after normal exercise echocardiography and predictors of subsequent cardiac events: Follow-up of 1,325 patients. J Am Coll Cardiol 31:144, 1998.

510. Pingitore A, Picano E, Varga A, et al: Prognostic value of pharmacological stress echocardiography in patients with known or suspected coronary artery disease: A prospective, large-scale, multicenter, head-to-head comparison between dipyridamole and dobutamine test.

Echo-Persantine International Cooperative (EPIC) and Echo-Dobutamine International Cooperative (EDIC) Study Groups. J Am Coll Cardiol 34:1769, 1999.

511. Emond M, Mock MB, Davis KB, et al: Long-term survival of medically treated patients in the Coronary Artery Surgery Study (CASS) Registry. Circulation 90:2645, 1994.

512. Weiner DA, Ryan TJ, McCabe CH, et al: Comparison of coronary artery bypass surgery and medical therapy in patients with exercise-induced silent myocardial ischemia: A report from the Coronary Artery Surgery Study (CASS) registry. J Am Coll Cardiol 12:595, 1988.

513. Califf RM, Armstrong PW, Carver JR, et al: 27th Bethesda Conference: Matching the intensity of risk factor management with the hazard for coronary disease events. Task Force 5. Stratification of patients into high, medium and low risk subgroups for purposes of risk factor management. J Am Coll Cardiol 27:1007, 1996.

514. Jones RH, Kesler K, Phillips HR III, et al: Long-term survival benefits of coronary artery bypass grafting and percutaneous transluminal angioplasty in patients with coronary artery disease. J Thorac Cardiovasc Surg 111:1013, 1996.

515. Califf RM, Tomabechi Y, Lee KL, et al: Outcome in one-vessel coronary artery disease. Circulation 67:283, 1983.

516. Caracciolo EA, Davis KB, Sopko G, et al: Comparison of surgical and medical group survival in patients with left main coronary artery disease. Long-term CASS experience. Circulation 91:2325, 1995.

517. Conley MJ, Ely RL, Kisslo J, et al: The prognostic spectrum of left main stenosis. Circulation 57:947, 1978.

518. Vogel RA: Coronary stenosis significance: Lessons learned from recent trials. Curr Opin Cardiol 9:705, 1994.

519. Topol EJ, Nissen SE: Our preoccupation with coronary luminology. The dissociation between clinical and angiographic findings in ischemic heart disease. Circulation 92:2333, 1995.

520. Hong MK, Mintz GS, Popma JJ, et al: Limitations of angiography for analyzing coronary atherosclerosis progression or regression. Ann Intern Med 121:348, 1994.

521. Johnston PW, Fort S, Cohen EA: Noncritical disease of the left main coronary artery: Limitations of angiography and the role of intravascular ultrasound. Can J Cardiol 15:297, 1999.

522. Mann JM, Davies MJ: Vulnerable plaque. Relation of characteristics to degree of stenosis in human coronary arteries. Circulation 94:928, 1996.

523. Little WC, Downes TR, Applegate RJ: The underlying coronary lesion in myocardial infarction: Implications for coronary angiography. Clin Cardiol 14:868, 1991.

524. Giroud D, Li JM, Urban P, et al: Relation of the site of acute myocardial infarction to the most severe coronary arterial stenosis at prior angiography. Am J Cardiol 69:729, 1992.

525. Ambrose JA, Winters SL, Arora RR, et al: Coronary angiographic morphology in myocardial infarction: A link between the pathogenesis of unstable angina and myocardial infarction. J Am Coll Cardiol 6:1233, 1985.

526. Mintz GS, Kent KM, Pichard AD, et al: Contribution of inadequate arterial remodeling to the development of focal coronary artery stenoses. An intravascular ultrasound study. Circulation 95:1791, 1997.

527. Pijls NH, De Bruyne B, Peels K, et al: Measurement of fractional flow reserve to assess the functional severity of coronary-artery stenoses. N Engl J Med 334:1703, 1996.

Results of Surgery

528. van Brussel BL, Plokker HW, Ernst SM, et al: Venous coronary artery bypass surgery. A 15-year follow-up study. Circulation 88(Suppl 2):87, 1993.

529. Rogers WJ, Coggin CJ, Gersh BJ, et al: Ten-year follow-up of quality of life in patients randomized to receive medical therapy or coronary artery bypass graft surgery. The Coronary Artery Surgery Study (CASS). Circulation 82:1647, 1990.

530. The VA Coronary Artery Bypass Surgery Cooperative Study Group: Eighteen-year follow-up in the Veterans Affairs Cooperative Study of Coronary Artery Bypass Surgery for Stable Angina. Circulation 86:121, 1992.

531. Varnauskas E: Survival, myocardial infarction, and employment status in a prospective randomized study of coronary bypass surgery. Circulation 72(Suppl 5):90, 1985.

532. Peduzzi P, Kamina A, Detre K: Twenty-two-year follow-up in the VA Cooperative Study of Coronary Artery Bypass Surgery for Stable Angina. Am J Cardiol 81:1393, 1998.

533. Bonchek LI, Peduzzi P, Kamina A, et al: The Veterans Affairs Cooperative Study of Coronary Artery Bypass Surgery for Stable Angina: A continuing debate after 22 years (letter). Am J Cardiol 83:301, 1999.

534. Cameron A, Kemp HG Jr, Green GE: Reoperation for coronary artery disease. 10 years of clinical follow-up. Circulation 78(Suppl 1):158, 1988.

535. Passamani E, Davis KB, Gillespie MJ, et al: A randomized trial of coronary artery bypass surgery. Survival of patients with a low ejection fraction. N Engl J Med 312:1665, 1985.

536. Detre KM, Takaro T, Hultgren H, et al: Long-term mortality and morbidity results of the Veterans Administration randomized trial of coronary artery bypass surgery. Circulation 72(Suppl 5):84, 1985.

537. The Veterans Administration Coronary Artery Bypass Surgery Cooperative Study Group: Eleven-year survival in the Veterans Administration

randomized trial of coronary bypass surgery for stable angina. N Engl J Med 311:1333, 1984.

538. Gersh BJ, Kronmal RA, Schaff HV, et al: Comparison of coronary artery bypass surgery and medical therapy in patients 65 years of age or older. A nonrandomized study from the Coronary Artery Surgery Study (CASS) registry. N Engl J Med 313:217, 1985.

539. Alderman EL, Bourassa MG, Cohen LS, et al: Ten-year follow-up of survival and myocardial infarction in the randomized Coronary Artery Surgery Study. Circulation 82:1629, 1990.

540. Takaro T, Pifarre R, Fish R: Veterans Administration Cooperative Study of medical versus surgical treatment for stable angina—progress report. Section 3. Left main coronary artery disease. Prog Cardiovasc Dis 28:229, 1985.

541. Caracciolo EA, Davis KB, Sopko G, et al: Comparison of surgical and medical group survival in patients with left main equivalent coronary artery disease. Long-term CASS experience. Circulation 91:2335, 1995.

542. Califf RM, Conley MJ, Behar VS, et al: "Left main equivalent" coronary artery disease: Its clinical presentation and prognostic significance with nonsurgical therapy. Am J Cardiol 53:1489, 1984.

543. Subcommittee on Coronary Artery Bypass Graft Surgery: Guidelines and indications for coronary artery bypass graft surgery. A report of the American College of Cardiology/American Heart Association Task Force on Assessment of Diagnostic and Therapeutic Cardiovascular Procedures. J Am Coll Cardiol 17:543, 1991.

544. Mock MB, Fisher LD, Holmes DR Jr, et al: Comparison of effects of medical and surgical therapy on survival in severe angina pectoris and two-vessel coronary artery disease with and without left ventricular dysfunction: A Coronary Artery Surgery Study Registry study. Am J Cardiol 61:1198, 1988.

545. Davies RF, Goldberg AD, Forman S, et al: Asymptomatic Cardiac Ischemia Pilot (ACIP) study two-year follow-up: Outcomes of patients randomized to initial strategies of medical therapy versus revascularization. Circulation 95:2037, 1997.

546. Murphy ML, Meadows WR, Thomsen J, et al: Veterans Administration Cooperative Study on medical versus surgical treatment for stable angina—progress report. Section 11. The effect of coronary artery bypass surgery on the incidence of myocardial infarction and hospitalization. Prog Cardiovasc Dis 28:309, 1986.

547. CASS Principal Investigators and Their Associates: Myocardial infarction and mortality in the Coronary Artery Surgery Study (CASS) randomized trial. N Engl J Med 310:750, 1984.

548. Davis KB, Alderman EL, Kosinski AS, et al: Early mortality of acute myocardial infarction in patients with and without prior coronary revascularization surgery. A Coronary Artery Surgery Study Registry study. Circulation 85:2100, 1992.

549. Alderman EL: Late benefit of coronary surgery on mortality from myocardial infarction (editorial). Circulation 83:1087, 1991.

550. Elefteriades JA, Tolis G Jr, Levi E, et al: Coronary artery bypass grafting in severe left ventricular dysfunction: Excellent survival with improved ejection fraction and functional state. J Am Coll Cardiol 22:1411, 1993.

551. Baker DW, Jones R, Hodges J, et al: Management of heart failure. III. The role of revascularization in the treatment of patients with moderate or severe left ventricular systolic dysfunction. JAMA 272:1528, 1994.

552. Stahle E, Bergstrom R, Edlund B, et al: Influence of left ventricular function on survival after coronary artery bypass grafting. Ann Thorac Surg 64:437, 1997.

553. Trachiotis GD, Weintraub WS, Johnston TS, et al: Coronary artery bypass grafting in patients with advanced left ventricular dysfunction. Ann Thorac Surg 66:1632, 1998.

554. Argenziano M, Spotnitz HM, Whang W, et al: Risk stratification for coronary bypass surgery in patients with left ventricular dysfunction: Analysis of the coronary artery bypass grafting patch trial database. Circulation 100(Suppl 2):119, 1999.

555. Cimochowski GE, Harostock MD, Foldes PJ: Minimal operative mortality in patients undergoing coronary artery bypass with significant left ventricular dysfunction by maximization of metabolic and mechanical support. J Thorac Cardiovasc Surg 113:655, 1997.

556. Jegaden O, Bontemps L, de Gevigney G, et al: Does the extended use of arterial grafts compromise the myocardial recovery after coronary artery bypass grafting in left ventricular dysfunction? Eur J Cardiothorac Surg 14:353, 1998.

557. Bounous EP, Mark DB, Pollock BG, et al: Surgical survival benefits for coronary disease patients with left ventricular dysfunction. Circulation 78(Suppl 1):151, 1988.

558. Di Carli MF, Maddahi J, Rokhsar S, et al: Long-term survival of patients with coronary artery disease and left ventricular dysfunction: Implications for the role of myocardial viability assessment in management decisions. J Thorac Cardiovasc Surg 116:997, 1998.

559. Holmes DR Jr, Davis KB, Mock MB, et al: The effect of medical and surgical treatment on subsequent sudden cardiac death in patients with coronary artery disease: A report from the Coronary Artery Surgery Study. Circulation 73:1254, 1986.

560. Myers WO, Davis K, Foster ED, et al: Surgical survival in the Coronary Artery Surgery Study (CASS) registry. Ann Thorac Surg 40:245, 1985.

561. Hendel RC, Chaudhry FA, Bonow RO: Myocardial viability. Curr Probl Cardiol 21:145, 1996.

562. Elsasser A, Schlepper M, Klovekorn WP, et al: Hibernating myocardium: An incomplete adaptation to ischemia. Circulation 96:2920, 1997.

563. Di Carli MF, Asgarzadie F, Schelbert HR, et al: Quantitative relation

between myocardial viability and improvement in heart failure symptoms after revascularization in patients with ischemic cardiomyopathy. Circulation 92:3436, 1995.

564. Bax JJ, Wijns W, Cornel JH, et al: Accuracy of currently available techniques for prediction of functional recovery after revascularization in patients with left ventricular dysfunction due to chronic coronary artery disease: Comparison of pooled data. J Am Coll Cardiol 30:1451, 1997.

565. Tamaki N, Kawamoto M, Tadamura E, et al: Prediction of reversible ischemia after revascularization. Perfusion and metabolic studies with positron emission tomography. Circulation 91:1697, 1995.

566. Maddahi J, Schelbert H, Brunken R, et al: Role of thallium-201 and PET imaging in evaluation of myocardial viability and management of patients with coronary artery disease and left ventricular dysfunction. J Nucl Med 35:707, 1994.

567. Udelson JE, Coleman PS, Metherall J, et al: Predicting recovery of severe regional ventricular dysfunction. Comparison of resting scintigraphy with ^{201}T1 and ^{99m}Tc-sestamibi. Circulation 89:2552, 1994.

568. Gioia G, Powers J, Heo J, et al: Prognostic value of rest-redistribution tomographic thallium-201 imaging in ischemic cardiomyopathy. Am J Cardiol 75:759, 1995.

569. Afridi I, Grayburn PA, Panza JA, et al: Myocardial viability during dobutamine echocardiography predicts survival in patients with coronary artery disease and severe left ventricular systolic dysfunction. J Am Coll Cardiol 32:921, 1998.

570. Senior R, Kaul S, Lahiri A: Myocardial viability on echocardiography predicts long-term survival after revascularization in patients with ischemic congestive heart failure. J Am Coll Cardiol 33:1848, 1999.

571. Chaudhry FA, Tauke JT, Alessandrini RS, et al: Prognostic implications of myocardial contractile reserve in patients with coronary artery disease and left ventricular dysfunction. J Am Coll Cardiol 34:730, 1999.

572. Haas F, Haehnel CJ, Picker W, et al: Preoperative positron emission tomographic viability assessment and perioperative and postoperative risk in patients with advanced ischemic heart disease. J Am Coll Cardiol 30:1693, 1997.

573. Ayanian JZ, Epstein AM: Differences in the use of procedures between women and men hospitalized for coronary heart disease. N Engl J Med 325:221, 1991.

574. Cosgrove DM: Coronary artery surgery in women. In Wenger NK, Speroff L, Packard B (eds): Cardiovascular Health and Disease in Women: Proceedings of an N.H.L.B.I. Conference. Greenwich, CT, Le Jacq Communications, 1993, p 117.

575. Schulman KA, Berlin JA, Harless W, et al: The effect of race and sex on physicians' recommendations for cardiac catheterization. N Engl J Med 340:618, 1999.

576. Czajkowski SM, Terrin M, Lindquist R, et al: Comparison of preoperative characteristics of men and women undergoing coronary artery bypass grafting (the Post Coronary Artery Bypass Graft [CABG] Biobehavioral Study). Am J Cardiol 79:1017, 1997.

577. Ivanov J, Weisel RD, David TE, et al: Fifteen-year trends in risk severity and operative mortality in elderly patients undergoing coronary artery bypass graft surgery. Circulation 97:673, 1998.

578. Hammar N, Sandberg E, Larsen FF, et al: Comparison of early and late mortality in men and women after isolated coronary artery bypass graft surgery in Stockholm, Sweden, 1980 to 1989. J Am Coll Cardiol 29:659, 1997.

579. O'Connor NJ, Morton JR, Birkmeyer JD, et al: Effect of coronary artery diameter in patients undergoing coronary bypass surgery. Circulation 93:652, 1996.

580. Davis KB, Chaitman B, Ryan T, et al: Comparison of 15-year survival for men and women after initial medical or surgical treatment for coronary artery disease: A CASS registry study. Coronary Artery Surgery Study. J Am Coll Cardiol 25:1000, 1995.

581. Myers WO, Blackstone EH, Davis K, et al: CASS Registry long term surgical survival. Coronary Artery Surgery Study. J Am Coll Cardiol 33:488, 1999.

582. Lytle BW, Kramer JR, Golding LR, et al: Young adults with coronary atherosclerosis: 10 year results of surgical myocardial revascularization. J Am Coll Cardiol 4:445, 1984.

583. Peterson ED, Cowper PA, Jollis JG, et al: Outcomes of coronary artery bypass graft surgery in 24,461 patients aged 80 years or older. Circulation 92(Suppl 2):85, 1995.

584. Katz NM, Hannan RL, Hopkins RA, et al: Cardiac operations in patients aged 70 years and over: Mortality, length of stay, and hospital charge. Ann Thorac Surg 60:96, 1995.

585. Mullany CJ, Darling GE, Pluth JR, et al: Early and late results after isolated coronary artery bypass surgery in 159 patients aged 80 years and older. Circulation 82(Suppl 4):229, 1990.

586. Gersh BJ, Kronmal RA, Schaff HV, et al: Long-term (5 year) results of coronary bypass surgery in patients 65 years old or older: A report from the Coronary Artery Surgery Study. Circulation 68(Suppl 2):190, 1983.

587. Cane ME, Chen C, Bailey BM, et al: CABG in octogenarians: Early and late events and actuarial survival in comparison with a matched population. Ann Thorac Surg 60:1033, 1995.

588. Boucher JM, Dupras A, Jutras N, et al: Long-term survival and functional status in the elderly after cardiac surgery. Can J Cardiol 13:646, 1997.

589. The National Institutes of Health, the National Institute of Diabetes and Digestive and Kidney Diseases, Division of Kidney, Urologic, and Hematologic Diseases (Bethesda, MD April 1997): Excerpts from United

States Renal Data System 1997 Annual Data Report. Am J Kidney Dis 30(Suppl 1):1, 1997.

590. Rinehart AL, Herzog CA, Collins AJ, et al: A comparison of coronary angioplasty and coronary artery bypass grafting outcomes in chronic dialysis patients. Am J Kidney Dis 25:281, 1995.

591. Owen CH, Cummings RG, Sell TL, et al: Coronary artery bypass grafting in patients with dialysis-dependent renal failure. Ann Thorac Surg 58:1729, 1994.

592. Kaul TK, Fields BL, Reddy MA, et al: Cardiac operations in patients with end-stage renal disease. Ann Thorac Surg 57:691, 1994.

593. Manske CL, Wang Y, Rector T, et al: Coronary revascularisation in insulin-dependent diabetic patients with chronic renal failure. Lancet 340:998, 1992.

594. Brener SJ, Loop FD, Lytle BW, et al: A profile of candidates for repeat myocardial revascularization: Implications for selection of treatment. J Thorac Cardiovasc Surg 114:153, 1997.

595. Rosengart TK: Risk analysis of primary versus reoperative coronary artery bypass grafting. Ann Thorac Surg 56(Suppl):74, 1993.

596. Pick AW, Mullany CJ, Orszulak TA, et al: Third and fourth operations for myocardial ischemia: Short-term results and long-term survival. Circulation 96(Suppl 2):26, 1997.

597. Lytle BW, Loop FD, Taylor PC, et al: The effect of coronary reoperation on the survival of patients with stenoses in saphenous vein bypass grafts to coronary arteries. J Thorac Cardiovasc Surg 105:605, 1993.

598. Takahashi T, Nakano S, Shimazaki Y, et al: Long-term appraisal of coronary bypass operations in familial hypercholesterolemia. Ann Thorac Surg 56:499, 1993.

599. Barzilay JI, Kronmal RA, Bittner V, et al: Coronary artery disease and coronary artery bypass grafting in diabetic patients aged > or = 65 years (report from the Coronary Artery Surgery Study [CASS] Registry). Am J Cardiol 74:334, 1994.

600. Weintraub WS, Stein B, Kosinski A, et al: Outcome of coronary bypass surgery versus coronary angioplasty in diabetic patients with multivessel coronary artery disease. J Am Coll Cardiol 31:10, 1998.

Comparisons Between PTCA and CABG

601. Hochberg MS, Gielchinsky I, Parsonnet V, et al: Coronary angioplasty versus coronary bypass. Three-year follow-up of a matched series of 250 patients. J Thorac Cardiovasc Surg 97:496, 1989.

602. Akins CW, Block PC, Palacios IF, et al: Comparison of coronary artery bypass grafting and percutaneous transluminal coronary angioplasty as initial treatment strategies. Ann Thorac Surg 47:507, 1989.

603. Vacek JL, Rosamond TL, Stites HW, et al: Comparison of percutaneous transluminal coronary angioplasty versus coronary artery bypass grafting for multivessel coronary artery disease. Am J Cardiol 69:592, 1992.

604. O'Keefe JH Jr, Allan JJ, McCallister BD, et al: Angioplasty versus bypass surgery for multivessel coronary artery disease with left ventricular ejection fraction < or = 40%. Am J Cardiol 71:897, 1993.

605. Berreklouw E, Hoogsteen J, van Wandelen R, et al: Bilateral mammary artery surgery or percutaneous transluminal coronary angioplasty for multivessel coronary artery disease? An analysis of effects and costs. Eur Heart J 10(Suppl H):61, 1989.

606. O'Keefe JH Jr, Sutton MB, McCallister BD, et al: Coronary angioplasty versus bypass surgery in patients > 70 years old matched for ventricular function. J Am Coll Cardiol 24:425, 1994.

607. Bourassa MG, Holubkov R, Yeh W, et al: Strategy of complete revascularization in patients with multivessel coronary artery disease (a report from the 1985–1986 NHLBI PTCA Registry). Am J Cardiol 70:174, 1992.

608. Hannan EL, Racz MJ, McCallister BD, et al: A comparison of three-year survival after coronary artery bypass graft surgery and percutaneous transluminal coronary angioplasty. J Am Coll Cardiol 33:63, 1999.

609. Goy JJ, Eeckhout E, Burnand B, et al: Coronary angioplasty versus left internal mammary artery grafting for isolated proximal left anterior descending artery stenosis. Lancet 343:1449, 1994.

610. Goy JJ, Eeckhout E, Moret C, et al: Five-year outcome in patients with isolated proximal left anterior descending coronary artery stenosis treated by angioplasty or left internal mammary artery grafting. A prospective trial. Circulation 99:3255, 1999.

611. Serruys PW, Costa MA, Betriu A, et al: The influence of diabetes mellitus on clinical outcome following multivessel stenting in CABG in the ARTS trial (abstract). Circulation 100 (Suppl I) I-364, 1999.

612. Hamm CW, Reimers J, Ischinger T, et al: A randomized study of coronary angioplasty compared with bypass surgery in patients with symptomatic multivessel coronary disease. German Angioplasty Bypass Surgery Investigation (GABI). N Engl J Med 331:1037, 1994.

613. CABRI Trial Participants: First-year results of CABRI (Coronary Angioplasty versus Bypass Revascularisation Investigation). Lancet 346:1179, 1995.

614. Carrie D, Elbaz M, Puel J, et al: Five-year outcome after coronary angioplasty versus bypass surgery in multivessel coronary artery disease: Results from the French Monocentric Study. Circulation 96(Suppl 2):1, 1997.

614a. Rodriguez A, Mele E, Peyregne E: Three-year follow-up of the Argentine Randomized Trial of Percutaneous Transluminal Coronary Angioplasty versus Coronary Artery Bypass Surgery in Multivessel Disease (ERACI). J Am Coll Cardiol 27:1178, 1996.

615. Rihal CS, Gersh BJ, Yusuf S: Chronic coronary artery disease: Coronary artery bypass surgery vs percutaneous transluminal coronary angio-

plasty vs medical therapy. In Yusuf S, Cairns JA, Camm AJ, et al (eds): Evidence Based Cardiology. London, BMJ Books, 1998, pp 368–392.

616. Chaitman BR, Rosen AD, Williams DO, et al: Myocardial infarction and cardiac mortality in the Bypass Angioplasty Revascularization Investigation (BARI) randomized trial. Circulation 96:2162, 1997.

617. Henderson RA, Pocock SJ, Sharp SJ, et al: Long-term results of RITA-1 trial: Clinical and cost comparisons of coronary angioplasty and coronary-artery bypass grafting. Randomised Intervention Treatment of Angina. Lancet 352:1419, 1998.

618. Pocock SJ, Henderson RA, Rickards AF, et al: Meta-analysis of randomised trials comparing coronary angioplasty with bypass surgery. Lancet 346:1184, 1995.

619. Whitlow PL, Dimas AP, Bashore TM, et al: Relationship of extent of revascularization with angina at one year in the Bypass Angioplasty Revascularization Investigation (BARI). J Am Coll Cardiol 34:1750, 1999.

620. Rodriguez A, Palacios IF, Navia J, et al: Argentine Randomized Study: Coronary angioplasty with stenting vs. coronary artery bypass surgery in patients with multiple vessel disease (ERACI II); 30 day and long-term follow-up results (abstract). Circulation 100(Suppl 1):234, 1999.

621. Hlatky MA, Rogers WJ, Johnstone I, et al: Medical care costs and quality of life after randomization to coronary angioplasty or coronary bypass surgery. Bypass Angioplasty Revascularization Investigation (BARI) Investigators. N Engl J Med 336:92, 1997.

622. Pocock SJ, Henderson RA, Seed P, et al: Quality of life, employment status, and anginal symptoms after coronary angioplasty or bypass surgery. 3-year follow-up in the Randomized Intervention Treatment of Angina (RITA) Trial. Circulation 94:135, 1996.

623. Serruys PW, Costa MA, Betriu A, et al: The influence of diabetes mellitus on clinical outcome following multivessel stenting or CABG in the ARTS Trial (abstract). Circulation 100(Suppl 1):364, 1999.

624. Sobel BE, Woodcock-Mitchell J, Schneider DJ, et al: Increased plasminogen activator inhibitor type 1 in coronary artery atherectomy specimens from type 2 diabetic compared with nondiabetic patients: A potential factor predisposing to thrombosis and its persistence. Circulation 97:2213, 1998.

625. Rozenman Y, Sapoznikov D, Mosseri M, et al: Long-term angiographic follow-up of coronary balloon angioplasty in patients with diabetes mellitus: A clue to the explanation of the results of the BARI study. Balloon Angioplasty Revascularization Investigation. J Am Coll Cardiol 30:1420, 1997.

626. Kuntz RE: Importance of considering atherosclerosis progression when choosing a coronary revascularization strategy: The diabetes-percutaneous transluminal coronary angioplasty dilemma. Circulation 99:847, 1999.

627. Detre KM, Guo P, Holubkov R, et al: Coronary revascularization in diabetic patients: A comparison of the randomized and observational components of the Bypass Angioplasty Revascularization Investigation (BARI). Circulation 99:633, 1999.

628. Rihal CS, Eagle KA, Mickel MC, et al: Surgical therapy for coronary artery disease among patients with combined coronary artery and peripheral vascular disease. Circulation 91:46, 1995.

629. Farkouh ME, Rihal CS, Gersh BJ, et al: Influence of coronary heart disease on morbidity and mortality after lower extremity revascularization surgery: A population-based study in Olmsted County, Minnesota (1970–1987). J Am Coll Cardiol 24:1290, 1994.

630. Smith GD, Shipley MJ, Rose G: Intermittent claudication, heart disease risk factors, and mortality. The Whitehall Study. Circulation 82:1925, 1990.

631. Hertzer NR, Young JR, Beven EG, et al: Late results of coronary bypass in patients with peripheral vascular disease. I. Five-year survival according to age and clinical cardiac status. Cleve Clin Q 53:133, 1986.

632. Shaw PJ, Bates D, Cartlidge NE, et al: Neurologic and neuropsychological morbidity following major surgery: Comparison of coronary artery bypass and peripheral vascular surgery. Stroke 18:700, 1987.

633. Birkmeyer JD, Quinton HB, O'Connor NJ, et al: The effect of peripheral vascular disease on long-term mortality after coronary artery bypass surgery. Arch Surg 131:316, 1996.

634. Rihal CS, Sutton-Tyrrell K, Guo P, et al: Increased incidence of periprocedural complications among patients with peripheral vascular disease undergoing myocardial revascularization in the Bypass Angioplasty Revascularization Investigation. Circulation 100:171, 1999.

635. Eagle KA, Brundage BH, Chaitman BR, et al: Guidelines for perioperative cardiovascular evaluation for noncardiac surgery. Report of the American College of Cardiology/American Heart Association Task Force on Practice Guidelines (Committee on Perioperative Cardiovascular Evaluation for Noncardiac Surgery). J Am Coll Cardiol 27:910, 1996.

636. McFalls EO, Ward HB, Krupski WC, et al: Prophylactic coronary artery revascularization for elective vascular surgery: Study design. Veterans Affairs Cooperative Study Group on Coronary Artery Revascularization Prophylaxis for Elective Vascular Surgery. Control Clin Trials 20:297, 1999.

637. Hogue CW Jr, Murphy SF, Schechtman KB, et al: Risk factors for early or delayed stroke after cardiac surgery. Circulation 100:642, 1999.

638. The French Study of Aortic Plaques in Stroke Group: Atherosclerotic disease of the aortic arch as a risk factor for recurrent ischemic stroke. N Engl J Med 334:1216, 1996.

639. Schwartz LB, Bridgman AH, Kieffer RW, et al: Asymptomatic carotid artery stenosis and stroke in patients undergoing cardiopulmonary bypass. J Vasc Surg 21:146, 1995.

640. Akins CW, Moncure AC, Daggett WM, et al: Safety and efficacy of concomitant carotid and coronary artery operations. Ann Thorac Surg 60:311, 1995.

641. Coyle KA, Gray BC, Smith RB III, et al: Morbidity and mortality associated with carotid endarterectomy: Effect of adjunctive coronary revascularization. Ann Vasc Surg 9:21, 1995.

642. Beebe HG, Clagett GP, DeWeese JA, et al: Assessing risk associated with carotid endarterectomy. A statement for health professionals by an Ad Hoc Committee on Carotid Surgery Standards of the Stroke Council, American Heart Association. Circulation 79:472, 1989.

643. Hertzer NR, Loop FD, Beven EG, et al: Surgical staging for simultaneous coronary and carotid disease: A study including prospective randomization. J Vasc Surg 9:455, 1989.

644. Huber KC, Evans MA, Bresnahan JF, et al: Outcome of noncardiac operations in patients with severe coronary artery disease successfully treated preoperatively with coronary angioplasty. Mayo Clin Proc 67:15, 1992.

PRINZMETAL (VARIANT) ANGINA

645. Prinzmetal M, Kennamer R, Merliss R, et al: Angina pectoris. I. A variant form of angina pectoris: Preliminary report. Am J Med 27:375, 1959.

646. Pepine CJ: Ergonovine echocardiography for coronary spasm: Facts and wishful thinking (editorial). J Am Coll Cardiol 27:1162, 1996.

647. Cohen M: Variant angina pectoris. In Fuster V, Ross R, Topol EJ (eds): Atherosclerosis and Coronary Artery Disease. Philadelphia, Lippincott-Raven, 1996, pp 1367–1376.

648. Yamagishi M, Miyatake K, Tamai J, et al: Intravascular ultrasound detection of atherosclerosis at the site of focal vasospasm in angiographically normal or minimally narrowed coronary segments. J Am Coll Cardiol 23:352, 1994.

649. Nakamura Y, Yamaguro T, Inoki I, et al: Vasomotor response to ergonovine of epicardial and resistance coronary arteries in the nonspastic vascular bed in patients with vasospastic angina. Am J Cardiol 74:1006, 1994.

650. Mayer S, Hillis LD: Prinzmetal's variant angina. Clin Cardiol 21:243, 1998.

651. Okumura K, Yasue H, Matsuyama K, et al: Diffuse disorder of coronary artery vasomotility in patients with coronary spastic angina. Hyperreactivity to the constrictor effects of acetylcholine and the dilator effects of nitroglycerin. J Am Coll Cardiol 27:45, 1996.

652. Cox DJ, Kaski JC, Clague JR: Endothelial dysfunction in the absence of coronary atheroma causing Prinzmetal's angina. Heart 77:584, 1997.

653. McFadden EP, Clarke JG, Davies GJ, et al: Effect of intracoronary serotonin on coronary vessels in patients with stable angina and patients with variant angina. N Engl J Med 324:648, 1991.

654. Sakata Y, Komamura K, Hirayama A, et al: Elevation of the plasma histamine concentration in the coronary circulation in patients with variant angina. Am J Cardiol 77:1121, 1996.

655. Vandergoten P, Benit E, Dendale P: Prinzmetal's variant angina: Three case reports and a review of the literature. Acta Cardiol 54:71, 1999.

656. Ogawa H, Yasue H, Okumura K, et al: Platelet-derived growth factor is released into the coronary circulation after coronary spasm. Coron Artery Dis 4:437, 1993.

657. Suzuki H, Kawai S, Aizawa T, et al: Histological evaluation of coronary plaque in patients with variant angina: Relationship between vasospasm and neointimal hyperplasia in primary coronary lesions. J Am Coll Cardiol 33:198, 1999.

658. Gurevich VS, Mikhailova IA, Kuleshova EV, et al: Platelet activation during provocation of coronary artery spasm by ergonovine and cold pressor testing in patients with angina pectoris. Blood Coagul Fibrinolysis 7:181, 1996.

659. Sakata K, Miura F, Sugino H, et al: Assessment of regional sympathetic nerve activity in vasospastic angina: Analysis of iodine 123-labeled metaiodobenzylguanidine scintigraphy. Am Heart J 133:484, 1997.

660. Takano H, Nakamura T, Satou T, et al: Regional myocardial sympathetic dysinnervation in patients with coronary vasospasm. Am J Cardiol 75:324, 1995.

661. Irie T, Imaizumi T, Matuguchi T, et al: Increased fibrinopeptide A during anginal attacks in patients with variant angina. J Am Coll Cardiol 14:589, 1989.

662. Ogawa H, Yasue H, Oshima S, et al: Circadian variation of plasma fibrinopeptide A level in patients with variant angina. Circulation 80:1617, 1989.

663. Kaikita K, Ogawa H, Yasue H, et al: Soluble P-selectin is released into the coronary circulation after coronary spasm. Circulation 92:1726, 1995.

664. Kim HS, Lee MM, Oh BH, et al: Variant angina is not associated with angiotensin I converting enzyme gene polymorphism but rather with smoking. Coron Artery Dis 10:227, 1999.

665. Igawa A, Miwa K, Miyagi Y, et al: Comparison of frequency of magnesium deficiency in patients with vasospastic angina and fixed coronary artery disease. Am J Cardiol 75:728, 1995.

666. Cohen L, Kitzes R: Prompt termination and/or prevention of cold-pressor-stimulus–induced vasoconstriction of different vascular beds by magnesium sulfate in patients with Prinzmetal's angina. Magnesium 5:144, 1986.

667. Miyagi H, Yasue H, Okumura K, et al: Effect of magnesium on anginal attack induced by hyperventilation in patients with variant angina. Circulation 79:597, 1989.

668. Kugiyama K, Yasue H, Okumura K, et al: Suppression of exercise-induced angina by magnesium sulfate in patients with variant angina. J Am Coll Cardiol 12:1177, 1988.

669. Onaka H, Hirota Y, Shimada S, et al: Clinical observation of spontaneous anginal attacks and multivessel spasm in variant angina pectoris with normal coronary arteries: Evaluation by 24-hour 12-lead electrocardiography with computer analysis. J Am Coll Cardiol 27:38, 1996.

670. Unverdorben M, Haag M, Fuerste T, et al: Vasospasm in smooth coronary arteries as a cause of asystole and syncope. Cathet Cardiovasc Diagn 41:430, 1997.

671. Tsurukawa T, Kawabata K, Miyahara K, et al: Sudden death during Holter electrocardiogram monitoring in a patient with variant angina. Intern Med 35:966, 1996.

672. Pozzati A, Pancaldi LG, Di Pasquale G, et al: Transient sympathovagal imbalance triggers "ischemic" sudden death in patients undergoing electrocardiographic Holter monitoring. J Am Coll Cardiol 27:847, 1996.

673. Gersh BJ, Bassendine MF, Forman R, et al: Coronary artery spasm and myocardial infarction in the absence of angiographically demonstrable obstructive coronary disease. Mayo Clin Proc 56:700, 1981.

674. Lip GY, Gupta J, Khan MM, et al: Recurrent myocardial infarction with angina and normal coronary arteries. Int J Cardiol 51:65, 1995.

675. Waters DD, Theroux P, Crittin J, et al: Previously undiagnosed variant angina as a cause of chest pain after coronary artery bypass surgery. Circulation 61:1159, 1980.

676. Habbab MA, Szwed SA, Haft JI: Is coronary arterial spasm part of the aspirin-induced asthma syndrome? Chest 90:141, 1986.

677. Carey D, Hurst JW Jr, Silverman ME: Coronary spasm and cardiac arrest after coronary arteriography in unsuspected thyrotoxicosis. Am J Cardiol 70:833, 1992.

678. Pijls NH, van der Werf T: Prinzmetal's angina associated with alcohol withdrawal. Cardiology 75:226, 1988.

679. Matsuguchi T, Araki H, Nakamura N, et al: Prevention of vasospastic angina by alcohol ingestion: Report of 2 cases. Angiology 39:394, 1988.

680. Kleiman NS, Lehane DE, Geyer CE Jr, et al: Prinzmetal's angina during 5-fluorouracil chemotherapy. Am J Med 82:566, 1987.

681. Stefenelli T, Zielinski CC, Mayr H, et al: Prinzmetal's angina during cyclophosphamide therapy. Eur Heart J 9:1155, 1988.

682. Chockalingam V, Jaganathan V, Chandrasekar PV, et al: A case of ST-segment and T-wave alternans. Arch Intern Med 143:1792, 1983.

683. Suzuki M, Nishizaki M, Arita M, et al: Increased QT dispersion in patients with vasospastic angina. Circulation 98:435, 1998.

684. Salerno JA, Previtali M, Panciroli C, et al: Ventricular arrhythmias during acute myocardial ischaemia in man. The role and significance of R-ST-T alternans and the prevention of ischaemic sudden death by medical treatment. Eur Heart J 7(Suppl A):63, 1986.

685. Bayes de Luna A, Carreras F, Cladellas M, et al: Holter ECG study of the electrocardiographic phenomena in Prinzmetal angina attacks with emphasis on the study of ventricular arrhythmias. J Electrocardiol 18:267, 1985.

686. Yasue H, Takizawa A, Nagao M, et al: Long-term prognosis for patients with variant angina and influential factors. Circulation 78:1, 1988.

687. Miwa K, Fujita M: Alternate coronary artery spasm with ST-segment "seesaw" phenomenon in variant angina. Jpn Circ J 57:167, 1993.

688. Myerburg RJ, Kessler KM, Mallon SM, et al: Life-threatening ventricular arrhythmias in patients with silent myocardial ischemia due to coronary-artery spasm. N Engl J Med 326:1451, 1992.

689. Kerin NZ, Rubenfire M, Naini M, et al: Prinzmetal's variant angina: Electrocardiographic and angiographic correlations. J Electrocardiol 15:365, 1982.

690. Pepine CJ, el-Tamimi H, Lambert CR: Prinzmetal's angina (variant angina). Heart Dis Stroke 1:281, 1992.

691. Matsuda Y, Ozaki M, Ogawa H, et al: Coronary arteriography and left ventriculography during spontaneous and exercise-induced ST segment elevation in patients with variant angina. Am Heart J 106:509, 1983.

692. Crea F: Variant angina in patients without obstructive coronary atherosclerosis: A benign form of spasm (editorial). Eur Heart J 17:980, 1996.

693. Tatineni S, Kern MJ, Deligonul U, et al: The effects of ionic and non-ionic radiographic contrast media on coronary hyperemia in patients during coronary angiography. Am Heart J 123:621, 1992.

694. Harding MB, Leithe ME, Mark DB, et al: Ergonovine maleate testing during cardiac catheterization: A 10-year perspective in 3,447 patients without significant coronary artery disease or Prinzmetal's variant angina. J Am Coll Cardiol 20:107, 1992.

695. Suzuki Y, Tokunaga S, Ikeguchi S, et al: Induction of coronary artery spasm by intracoronary acetylcholine: Comparison with intracoronary ergonovine. Am Heart J 124:39, 1992.

696. Minoda K, Yasue H, Kugiyama K, et al: Comparison of the distribution of myocardial blood flow between exercise-induced and hyperventilation-induced attacks of coronary spasm: A study with thallium-201 myocardial scintigraphy. Am Heart J 127:1474, 1994.

697. Nakao K, Ohgushi M, Yoshimura M, et al: Hyperventilation as a specific test for diagnosis of coronary artery spasm. Am J Cardiol 80:545, 1997.

698. Marcus ML, Chilian WM, Kanatsuka H, et al: Understanding the coronary circulation through studies at the microvascular level. Circulation 82:1, 1990.

699. Kugiyama K, Ohgushi M, Motoyama T, et al: Enhancement of constrictor response of spastic coronary arteries to acetylcholine but not to

phenylephrine in patients with coronary spastic angina. J Cardiovasc Pharmacol 33:414, 1999.

700. Okumura K, Yasue H, Matsuyama K, et al: Effect of H1 receptor stimulation on coronary artery diameter in patients with variant angina: Comparison with effect of acetylcholine. J Am Coll Cardiol 17:338, 1991.

701. Crea F, Chierchia S, Kaski JC, et al: Provocation of coronary spasm by dopamine in patients with active variant angina pectoris. Circulation 74:262, 1986.

702. Lombardi M, Morales MA, Michelassi C, et al: Efficacy of isosorbide-5-mononitrate versus nifedipine in preventing spontaneous and ergonovine-induced myocardial ischaemia. A double-blind, placebo-controlled study. Eur Heart J 14:845, 1993.

703. De Cesare N, Cozzi S, Apostolo A, et al: Facilitation of coronary spasm by propranolol in Prinzmetal's angina: Fact or unproven extrapolation? Coron Artery Dis 5:323, 1994.

704. Robertson RM, Wood AJ, Vaughn WK, et al: Exacerbation of vasotonic angina pectoris by propranolol. Circulation 65:281, 1982.

705. Antman E, Muller J, Goldberg S, et al: Nifedipine therapy for coronary-artery spasm. Experience in 127 patients. N Engl J Med 302:1269, 1980.

706. Ginsburg R, Lamb IH, Schroeder JS, et al: Randomized double-blind comparison of nifedipine and isosorbide dinitrate therapy in variant angina pectoris due to coronary artery spasm. Am Heart J 103:44, 1982.

707. Morikami Y, Yasue H: Efficacy of slow-release nifedipine on myocardial ischemic episodes in variant angina pectoris. Am J Cardiol 68:580, 1991.

708. Winniford MD, Johnson SM, Mauritson DR, et al: Verapamil therapy for Prinzmetal's variant angina: Comparison with placebo and nifedipine. Am J Cardiol 50:913, 1982.

709. Chimienti M, Negroni MS, Pusineri E, et al: Once daily felodipine in preventing ergonovine-induced myocardial ischaemia in Prinzmetal's variant angina. Eur Heart J 15:389, 1994.

710. Gradman AH: The evolving role of calcium channel blockers in the treatment of angina pectoris: Focus on felodipine. Can J Cardiol 11(Suppl B):14, 1995.

711. Opie LH: Calcium channel antagonists in the management of anginal syndromes: Changing concepts in relation to the role of coronary vasospasm. Prog Cardiovasc Dis 38:291, 1996.

712. Tzivoni D, Keren A, Benhorin J, et al: Prazosin therapy for refractory variant angina. Am Heart J 105:262, 1983.

713. Kaski JC: Management of vasospastic angina—role of nicorandil. Cardiovasc Drugs Ther 9(Suppl 2):221, 1995.

714. Miwa K, Kambara H, Kawai C: Effect of aspirin in large doses on attacks of variant angina. Am Heart J 105:351, 1983.

715. Guazzi M, Agostoni P, Loaldi A: Ineffectiveness of angiotensin converting enzyme inhibition (enalapril) on overt and silent myocardial ischemia in vasospastic angina and comparison with verapamil. Clin Pharmacol Ther 59:476, 1996.

716. Murakami T, Mizuno S, Ohsato K, et al: Effects of troglitazone on frequency of coronary vasospastic-induced angina pectoris in patients with diabetes mellitus. Am J Cardiol 84:92, 1999.

717. Shimizu H, Lee JD, Ogawa KB, et al: Refractory variant angina relieved by denopamine—a case report. Jpn Circ J 55:692, 1991.

718. Kato H, Yasue H, Yoshimura M, et al: Suppression of hyperventilation-induced attacks with infusion of B-type (brain) natriuretic peptide in patients with variant angina. Am Heart J 128:1098, 1994.

719. Gaspardone A, Tomai F, Versaci F, et al: Coronary artery stent placement in patients with variant angina refractory to medical treatment. Am J Cardiol 84:96, 1999.

720. Bory M, Pierron F, Panagides D, et al: Coronary artery spasm in patients with normal or near normal coronary arteries. Long-term follow-up of 277 patients. Eur Heart J 17:1015, 1996.

721. Shimokawa H, Nagasawa K, Irie T, et al: Clinical characteristics and long-term prognosis of patients with variant angina. A comparative study between western and Japanese populations. Int J Cardiol 18:331, 1988.

722. Maseri A, Severi S, Marzullo P: Role of coronary arterial spasm in sudden coronary ischemic death. Ann N Y Acad Sci 382:204, 1982.

723. Tashiro H, Shimokawa H, Koyanagi S, et al: Clinical characteristics of patients with spontaneous remission of variant angina. Jpn Circ J 57:117, 1993.

724. Ozaki Y, Takatsu F, Osugi J, et al: Long-term study of recurrent vasospastic angina using coronary angiograms during ergonovine provocation tests. Am Heart J 123:1191, 1992.

CHEST PAIN WITH NORMAL CORONARY ARTERIOGRAM

725. Kemp HG, Kronmal RA, Vlietstra RE, et al: Seven year survival of patients with normal or near normal coronary arteriograms: A CASS registry study. J Am Coll Cardiol 7:479, 1986.

726. Maseri A, Crea F, Kaski JC, et al: Mechanisms of angina pectoris in syndrome X (editorial). J Am Coll Cardiol 17:499, 1991.

727. Camici PG, Marraccini P, Lorenzoni R, et al: Coronary hemodynamics and myocardial metabolism in patients with syndrome X: Response to pacing stress. J Am Coll Cardiol 17:1461, 1991.

728. Shemesh J, Fisman EZ, Tenenbaum A, et al: Coronary artery calcification in women with syndrome X: Usefulness of double-helical CT for detection. Radiology 205:697, 1997.

729. Mohri M, Koyanagi M, Egashira K, et al: Angina pectoris caused by coronary microvascular spasm. Lancet 351:1165, 1998.

730. Murakami H, Urabe K, Nishimura M: Inappropriate microvascular constriction produced transient ST-segment elevation in patients with syndrome X. J Am Coll Cardiol 32:1287, 1998.

731. Cannon RO III: The sensitive heart. A syndrome of abnormal cardiac pain perception. JAMA 273:883, 1995.

732. Wiedermann JG, Schwartz A, Apfelbaum M: Anatomic and physiologic heterogeneity in patients with syndrome X: An intravascular ultrasound study. J Am Coll Cardiol 25:1310, 1995.

733. Rosano GM, Kaski JC, Arie S, et al: Failure to demonstrate myocardial ischaemia in patients with angina and normal coronary arteries. Evaluation by continuous coronary sinus pH monitoring and lactate metabolism. Eur Heart J 17:1175, 1996.

734. Chauhan A, Mullins PA, Petch MC, et al: Is coronary flow reserve in response to papaverine really normal in syndrome X? Circulation 89:1998, 1994.

735. Cox ID, Botker HE, Bagger JP, et al: Elevated endothelin concentrations are associated with reduced coronary vasomotor responses in patients with chest pain and normal coronary arteriograms. J Am Coll Cardiol 34:455, 1999.

736. Cannon RO III: The microcirculation in atherosclerotic coronary artery disease. In Fuster V, Ross R, Topol EJ (eds): Atherosclerosis and Coronary Artery Disease. Philadelphia, Lippincott-Raven, 1996, pp 773–788.

737. Cannon RO III, Bonow RO, Bacharach SL, et al: Left ventricular dysfunction in patients with angina pectoris, normal epicardial coronary arteries, and abnormal vasodilator reserve. Circulation 71:218, 1985.

738. Geltman EM, Henes CG, Senneff MJ, et al: Increased myocardial perfusion at rest and diminished perfusion reserve in patients with angina and angiographically normal coronary arteries. J Am Coll Cardiol 16:586, 1990.

739. Lekakis JP, Papamichael CM, Vemmos CN, et al: Peripheral vascular endothelial dysfunction in patients with angina pectoris and normal coronary arteriograms. J Am Coll Cardiol 31:541, 1998.

740. Cannon RO III, Peden DB, Berkebile C, et al: Airway hyperresponsiveness in patients with microvascular angina. Evidence for a diffuse disorder of smooth muscle responsiveness. Circulation 82:2011, 1990.

741. Cannon RO III: Chest pain with normal coronary angiograms. In Fuster V, Ross R, Topol EJ (eds): Atherosclerosis and Coronary Artery Disease. Philadelphia, Lippincott-Raven, 1996, pp 1577–1588.

742. Vrints CJ, Bult H, Hitter E, et al: Impaired endothelium-dependent cholinergic coronary vasodilation in patients with angina and normal coronary arteriograms. J Am Coll Cardiol 19:21, 1992.

743. Bugiardini R, Pozzati A, Ottani F, et al: Vasotonic angina: A spectrum of ischemic syndromes involving functional abnormalities of the epicardial and microvascular coronary circulation. J Am Coll Cardiol 22:417, 1993.

744. Panza JA, Laurienzo JM, Curiel RV, et al: Investigation of the mechanism of chest pain in patients with angiographically normal coronary arteries using transesophageal dobutamine stress echocardiography. J Am Coll Cardiol 29:293, 1997.

745. Lagerqvist B, Sylven C, Waldenstrom A: Lower threshold for adenosine-induced chest pain in patients with angina and normal coronary angiograms. Br Heart J 68:282, 1992.

746. Cannon RO III, Quyyumi AA, Mincemoyer R, et al: Imipramine in patients with chest pain despite normal coronary angiograms. N Engl J Med 330:1411, 1994.

747. Potts SG, Bass CM: Psychological morbidity in patients with chest pain and normal or near-normal coronary arteries: A long-term follow-up study. Psychol Med 25:339, 1995.

748. Rosen SD, Uren NG, Kaski JC, et al: Coronary vasodilator reserve, pain perception, and sex in patients with syndrome X. Circulation 90:50, 1994.

749. Atienza F, Velasco JA, Brown S, et al: Assessment of quality of life in patients with chest pain and normal coronary arteriogram (syndrome X) using a specific questionnaire. Clin Cardiol 22:283, 1999.

750. Kaski JC, Rosano GM, Collins P, et al: Cardiac syndrome X: Clinical characteristics and left ventricular function. Long-term follow-up study. J Am Coll Cardiol 25:807, 1995.

751. Pupita G, Kaski JC, Galassi AR, et al: Long-term variability of angina pectoris and electrocardiographic signs of ischemia in syndrome X. Am J Cardiol 64:139, 1989.

752. Romeo F, Rosano GM, Martuscelli E, et al: Long-term follow-up of patients initially diagnosed with syndrome X. Am J Cardiol 71:669, 1993.

753. Lanza GA, Manzoli A, Bia E, et al: Acute effects of nitrates on exercise testing in patients with syndrome X. Clinical and pathophysiological implications. Circulation 90:2695, 1994.

754. Gilligan DM, Quyyumi AA, Cannon RO III: Effects of physiological levels of estrogen on coronary vasomotor function in postmenopausal women. Circulation 89:2545, 1994.

755. Roque M, Heras M, Roig E, et al: Short-term effects of transdermal estrogen replacement therapy on coronary vascular reactivity in postmenopausal women with angina pectoris and normal results on coronary angiograms. J Am Coll Cardiol 31:139, 1998.

756. Elliott PM, Krzyzowska-Dickinson K, Calvino R, et al: Effect of oral aminophylline in patients with angina and normal coronary arteriograms (cardiac syndrome X). Heart 77:523, 1997.

SILENT MYOCARDIAL ISCHEMIA

757. Stern S, Cohn PF, Pepine CJ: Silent myocardial ischemia. Curr Probl Cardiol 18:301, 1993.
758. Stern S, Tzivoni D: Early detection of silent ischaemic heart disease by 24-hour electrocardiographic monitoring of active subjects. Br Heart J 36:481, 1974.
759. Cohn PF: Silent myocardial ischemia: Classification, prevalence, and prognosis. Am J Med 79:2, 1985.
760. Kellermann JJ, Braunwald E (eds): Silent Myocardial Ischemia: A Critical Appraisal. Basel, Karger, 1990.
761. Epstein SE, Quyyumi AA, Bonow RO: Myocardial ischemia—silent or symptomatic. N Engl J Med 318:1038, 1988.
762. Hirzel HO, Leutwyler R, Krayenbuehl HP: Silent myocardial ischemia: Hemodynamic changes during dynamic exercise in patients with proven coronary artery disease despite absence of angina pectoris. J Am Coll Cardiol 6:275, 1985.
763. Deedwania PC, Nelson JR: Pathophysiology of silent myocardial ischemia during daily life. Hemodynamic evaluation by simultaneous electrocardiographic and blood pressure monitoring. Circulation 82:1296, 1990.
764. Krone RJ: Diagnosis and prognosis of silent ischemia. Cardiologia 43:1159, 1998.
765. Deanfield JE, Ribiero P, Oakley K, et al: Analysis of ST-segment changes in normal subjects: Implications for ambulatory monitoring in angina pectoris. Am J Cardiol 54:1321, 1984.
766. Quyyumi AA, Mockus L, Wright C, et al: Morphology of ambulatory ST segment changes in patients with varying severity of coronary artery disease. Investigation of the frequency of nocturnal ischaemia and coronary spasm. Br Heart J 53:186, 1985.
767. Krantz DS, Hedges SM, Gabbay FH, et al: Triggers of angina and ST-segment depression in ambulatory patients with coronary artery disease: Evidence for an uncoupling of angina and ischemia. Am Heart J 128:703, 1994.
768. Krone RJ, Gregory JJ, Freedland KE, et al: Limited usefulness of exercise testing and thallium scintigraphy in evaluation of ambulatory patients several months after recovery from an acute coronary event: Implications for management of stable coronary heart disease. J Am Coll Cardiol 24:1274, 1994.
769. Sigurdsson E, Thorgeirsson G, Sigvaldason H, et al: Unrecognized myocardial infarction: Epidemiology, clinical characteristics, and the prognostic role of angina pectoris. The Reykjavik Study. Ann Intern Med 122:96, 1995.
770. Zarich S, Waxman S, Freeman RT, et al: Effect of autonomic nervous system dysfunction on the circadian pattern of myocardial ischemia in diabetes mellitus. J Am Coll Cardiol 24:956, 1994.
771. Cohn PF: Silent Myocardial Ischemia and Infarction. 3rd ed. New York, Marcel Dekker, 1993, p 73.
772. Shakespeare CF, Katritsis D, Crowther A, et al: Differences in autonomic nerve function in patients with silent and symptomatic myocardial ischaemia. Br Heart J 71:22, 1994.
773. Naka M, Hiramatsu K, Aizawa T, et al: Silent myocardial ischemia in patients with non–insulin-dependent diabetes mellitus as judged by treadmill exercise testing and coronary angiography. Am Heart J 123:46, 1992.
774. Glazier JJ, Chierchia S, Brown MJ, et al: Importance of generalized defective perception of painful stimuli as a cause of silent myocardial ischemia in chronic stable angina pectoris. Am J Cardiol 58:667, 1986.
775. Sheps DS, McMahon RP, Light KC, et al: Low hot pain threshold predicts shorter time to exercise-induced angina: Results from the Psychophysiological Investigations of Myocardial Ischemia (PIMI) study. J Am Coll Cardiol 33:1855, 1999.
776. Falcone C, Auguadro C, Sconocchia R, et al: Susceptibility to pain during coronary angioplasty: Usefulness of pulpal test. J Am Coll Cardiol 28:903, 1996.
777. Sheps DS, Ballenger MN, De Gent GE, et al: Psychophysical responses to a speech stressor: Correlation of plasma beta-endorphin levels at rest and after psychological stress with thermally measured pain threshold in patients with coronary artery disease. J Am Coll Cardiol 25:1499, 1995.
778. Nihoyannopoulos P, Marsonis A, Joshi J, et al: Magnitude of myocardial dysfunction is greater in painful than in painless myocardial ischemia: An exercise echocardiographic study. J Am Coll Cardiol 25:1507, 1995.
779. Klein J, Chao SY, Berman DS, et al: Is 'silent' myocardial ischemia really as severe as symptomatic ischemia? The analytical effect of patient selection biases. Circulation 89:1958, 1994.
780. Crea F, Gaspardone A: New look to an old symptom: Angina pectoris. Circulation 96:3766, 1997.
781. Rosen SD, Paulesu E, Nihoyannopoulos P, et al: Silent ischemia as a central problem: Regional brain activation compared in silent and painful myocardial ischemia. Ann Intern Med 124:939, 1996.
782. Freedland KE, Carney RM, Krone RJ, et al: Psychological determinants of anginal pain perception during exercise testing of stable patients after recovery from acute myocardial infarction or unstable angina pectoris. Am J Cardiol 77:1, 1996.
783. Ekelund LG, Suchindran CM, McMahon RP, et al: Coronary heart disease morbidity and mortality in hypercholesterolemic men predicted from an exercise test: The Lipid Research Clinics Coronary Primary Prevention Trial. J Am Coll Cardiol 14:556, 1989.
784. Weiner DA, Ryan TJ, McCabe CH, et al: Significance of silent myocardial ischemia during exercise testing in patients with coronary artery disease. Am J Cardiol 59:725, 1987.
785. Casella G, Pavesi PC, Medda M, et al: Long-term prognosis of painless exercise-induced ischemia in stable patients with previous myocardial infarction. Am Heart J 136:894, 1998.
786. Pepine CJ, Sharaf B, Andrews TC, et al: Relation between clinical, angiographic and ischemic findings at baseline and ischemia-related adverse outcomes at 1 year in the Asymptomatic Cardiac Ischemia Pilot study. J Am Coll Cardiol 29:1483, 1997.
787. Mulcahy D, Purcell H, Patel D, et al: Asymptomatic ischaemia during daily life in stable coronary disease: Relevant or redundant? Br Heart J 72:5, 1994.
788. Conti CR, Geller NL, Knatterud GL, et al: Anginal status and prediction of cardiac events in patients enrolled in the Asymptomatic Cardiac Ischemia Pilot (ACIP) study. Am J Cardiol 79:889, 1997.
789. Stone PH, Chaitman BR, Forman S, et al: Prognostic significance of myocardial ischemia detected by ambulatory electrocardiography, exercise treadmill testing, and electrocardiogram at rest to predict cardiac events by one year (the Asymptomatic Cardiac Ischemia Pilot [ACIP] study). Am J Cardiol 80:1395, 1997.
790. Mahmarian JJ, Steingart RM, Forman S, et al: Relation between ambulatory electrocardiographic monitoring and myocardial perfusion imaging to detect coronary artery disease and myocardial ischemia: An ACIP ancillary study. J Am Coll Cardiol 29:764, 1997.
791. Sharaf BL, Williams DO, Miele NJ, et al: A detailed angiographic analysis of patients with ambulatory electrocardiographic ischemia: Results from the Asymptomatic Cardiac Ischemia Pilot (ACIP) study angiographic core laboratory. J Am Coll Cardiol 29:78, 1997.
792. TIBET Study Group: Total Ischaemic Burden European Trial (TIBET): Effect of treatment on exercise and Holter ECG in angina (abstract). Circulation 86(Suppl 1):513, 1992.
793. Tzivoni D, Medina A, David D, et al: Comparison between metoprolol orally osmotic once daily and metoprolol two or three times daily in suppressing exercise-induced and daily myocardial ischemia. Am J Cardiol 78:1362, 1996.
794. Portegies MC, Sijbring P, Gobel EJ, et al: Efficacy of metoprolol and diltiazem in treating silent myocardial ischemia. Am J Cardiol 74:1095, 1994.
795. Rogers WJ, Bourassa MG, Andrews TC, et al: Asymptomatic Cardiac Ischemia Pilot (ACIP) study: Outcome at 1 year for patients with asymptomatic cardiac ischemia randomized to medical therapy or revascularization. J Am Coll Cardiol 26:594, 1995.
796. Chaitman BR, Stone PH, Knatterud GL, et al: Asymptomatic Cardiac Ischemia Pilot (ACIP) study: Impact of anti-ischemia therapy on 12-week rest electrocardiogram and exercise test outcomes. J Am Coll Cardiol 26:585, 1995.
797. Knatterud GL, Bourassa MG, Pepine CJ, et al: Effects of treatment strategies to suppress ischemia in patients with coronary artery disease: 12-week results of the Asymptomatic Cardiac Ischemia Pilot (ACIP) study. J Am Coll Cardiol 24:11, 1994.

HEART FAILURE IN ISCHEMIC HEART DISEASE

798. Gheorghiade M, Bonow RO: Chronic heart failure in the United States: A manifestation of coronary artery disease. Circulation 97:282, 1998.
799. Burch GE, Giles TD, Colcolough HL: Ischemic cardiomyopathy. Am Heart J 79:291, 1970.
800. Kron IL, Flanagan TL, Blackbourne LH, et al: Coronary revascularization rather than cardiac transplantation for chronic ischemic cardiomyopathy. Ann Surg 210:348, 1989.
801. Das AK, Wilson GM, Furnary AP: Coincidence of true and false left ventricular aneurysm. Ann Thorac Surg 64:831, 1997.
802. Hirai T, Fujita M, Nakajima H, et al: Importance of collateral circulation for prevention of left ventricular aneurysm formation in acute myocardial infarction. Circulation 79:791, 1989.
803. Barratt-Boyes BG, White HD, Agnew TM, et al: The results of surgical treatment of left ventricular aneurysms. An assessment of the risk factors affecting early and late mortality. J Thorac Cardiovasc Surg 87:87, 1984.
804. Adalia R, Sabater L, Azqueta M, et al: Combined left ventricular aneurysm and thoracic aortic pseudoaneurysm caused by blunt chest trauma. J Thorac Cardiovasc Surg 117:1219, 1999.
805. Arcudi G, Marchetti D: Left ventricular aneurysm caused by blunt chest trauma. Am J Forensic Med Pathol 17:194, 1996.
806. Maselli D, Micalizzi E, Pizio R, et al: Posttraumatic left ventricular pseudoaneurysm due to intramyocardial dissecting hematoma. Ann Thorac Surg 64:830, 1997.
807. Stephenson LW, Hargrove WC III, Ratcliffe MB, et al: Surgery for left ventricular aneurysm. Early survival with and without endocardial resection. Circulation 79(Suppl 1):108, 1989.
808. Lapeyre AC III, Steele PM, Kazmier FJ, et al: Systemic embolism in chronic left ventricular aneurysm: Incidence and the role of anticoagulation. J Am Coll Cardiol 6:534, 1985.
809. Candell-Riera J, Santana-Boado C, Armadans-Gil L, et al: Comparison of patients with anterior wall healed myocardial infarction with and without exercise-induced ST-segment elevation. Am J Cardiol 81:12, 1998.
810. Nakajima O, Sano I, Akioka H: Images in cardiovascular medicine. Marked calcified left ventricular aneurysm. Circulation 95:1974, 1997.
811. Yeo TC, Malouf JF, Oh JK, et al: Clinical profile and outcome in 52 patients with cardiac pseudoaneurysm. Ann Intern Med 128:299, 1998.

812. Waggoner AD, Williams GA, Gaffron D, et al: Potential utility of left heart contrast agents in diagnosis of myocardial rupture by 2-dimensional echocardiography. J Am Soc Echocardiogr 12:272, 1999.

813. Marcus ML, Stanford W, Hajduczok ZD, et al: Ultrafast computed tomography in the diagnosis of cardiac disease. Am J Cardiol 64:54E, 1989.

814. Buck T, Hunold P, Wentz KU, et al: Tomographic three-dimensional echocardiographic determination of chamber size and systolic function in patients with left ventricular aneurysm: Comparison to magnetic resonance imaging, cineventriculography, and two-dimensional echocardiography. Circulation 96:4286, 1997.

815. Couper GS, Bunton RW, Birjiniuk V, et al: Relative risks of left ventricular aneurysmectomy in patients with akinetic scars versus true dyskinetic aneurysms. Circulation 82(Suppl 4):248, 1990.

816. Pasini S, Gagliardotto P, Punta G, et al: Early and late results after surgical therapy of postinfarction left ventricular aneurysm. J Cardiovasc Surg (Torino) 39:209, 1998.

817. Vural KM, Sener E, Ozatik MA, et al: Left ventricular aneurysm repair: An assessment of surgical treatment modalities. Eur J Cardiothorac Surg 13:49, 1998.

818. Louagie Y, Alouini T, Lesperance J, et al: Left ventricular aneurysm complicated by congestive heart failure: An analysis of long-term results and risk factors of surgical treatment. J Cardiovasc Surg (Torino) 30:648, 1989.

819. Ivert T, Almdahl SM, Lunde P, et al: Postinfarction left ventricular pseudoaneurysm—echocardiographic diagnosis and surgical repair. Cardiovasc Surg 2:463, 1994.

820. Di Mattia DG, Di Biasi P, Salati M, et al: Surgical treatment of left ventricular post-infarction aneurysm with endoventriculoplasty: Late clinical and functional results. Eur J Cardiothorac Surg 15:413, 1999.

821. Dalla Vecchia L, Mangini A, Di Biasi P, et al: Improvement of left ventricular function and cardiovascular neural control after endoventriculoplasty and myocardial revascularization. Cardiovasc Res 37:101, 1998.

822. Di Donato M, Sabatier M, Toso A, et al: Regional myocardial performance of non-ischaemic zones remote from anterior wall left ventricular aneurysm. Effects of aneurysmectomy. Eur Heart J 16:1285, 1995.

823. Fantini F, Barletta G, Toso A, et al: Effects of reconstructive surgery for left ventricular anterior aneurysm on ventriculoarterial coupling. Heart 81:171, 1999.

824. Dor V, Montiglio F, Sabatier M, et al: Left ventricular shape changes induced by aneurysmectomy with endoventricular circular patch plasty reconstruction. Eur Heart J 15:1063, 1994.

825. Komeda M, David TE, Malik A, et al: Operative risks and long-term results of operation for left ventricular aneurysm. Ann Thorac Surg 53:22, 1992.

826. Shapira OM, Davidoff R, Hilkert RJ, et al: Repair of left ventricular aneurysm: Long-term results of linear repair versus endoaneurysmorrhaphy. Ann Thorac Surg 63:701, 1997.

827. Komeda M, Glasson JR, Bolger AF, et al: Geometric determinants of ischemic mitral regurgitation. Circulation 96(Suppl 2):128, 1997.

828. Gorman RC, McCaughan JS, Ratcliffe MB, et al: Pathogenesis of acute ischemic mitral regurgitation in three dimensions. J Thorac Cardiovasc Surg 109:684, 1995.

829. Gorman JH III, Gorman RC, Jackson BM, et al: Distortions of the mitral valve in acute ischemic mitral regurgitation. Ann Thorac Surg 64:1026, 1997.

830. Nishimura RA, Schaff HV, Gersh BJ, et al: Early repair of mechanical complications after acute myocardial infarction. JAMA 256:47, 1986.

831. Akins CW, Hilgenberg AD, Buckley MJ, et al: Mitral valve reconstruction versus replacement for degenerative or ischemic mitral regurgitation. Ann Thorac Surg 58:668, 1994.

832. Cohn LH, Rizzo RJ, Adams DH, et al: The effect of pathophysiology on the surgical treatment of ischemic mitral regurgitation: Operative and late risks of repair versus replacement. Eur J Cardiothorac Surg 9:568, 1995.

833. Kishon Y, Oh JK, Schaff HV, et al: Mitral valve operation in postinfarction rupture of a papillary muscle: Immediate results and long-term follow-up of 22 patients. Mayo Clin Proc 67:1023, 1992.

834. Burke AP, Farb A, Malcom GT, et al: Plaque rupture and sudden death related to exertion in men with coronary artery disease. JAMA 281:921, 1999.

835. Meissner MD, Akhtar M, Lehmann MH: Nonischemic sudden tachyarrhythmic death in atherosclerotic heart disease. Circulation 84:905, 1991.

836. Daoud EG, Niebauer M, Kou WH, et al: Incidence of implantable defibrillator discharges after coronary revascularization in survivors of ischemic sudden cardiac death. Am Heart J 130:277, 1995.

837. Morris JJ, Rastogi A, Stanton MS, et al: Operation for ventricular tachyarrhythmias: Refining current treatment strategies. Ann Thorac Surg 58:1490, 1994.

838. Mickleborough LL, Mizuno S, Downar E, et al: Late results of operation for ventricular tachycardia. Ann Thorac Surg 54:832, 1992.

839. Drexler H, Schroeder JS: Unusual forms of ischemic heart disease. Curr Opin Cardiol 9:457, 1994.

840. Harrison DC: Nonatherosclerotic coronary artery disease. In Fuster V, Ross R, Topol EJ (eds): Atherosclerosis and Coronary Artery Disease. Philadelphia, Lippincott-Raven, 1996, pp 757–772.

841. Kragel AH, Roberts WC: Anomalous origin of either the right or left main coronary artery from the aorta with subsequent coursing between aorta and pulmonary trunk: Analysis of 32 necropsy cases. Am J Cardiol 62:771, 1988.

842. Corrado D, Thiene G, Cocco P, et al: Non-atherosclerotic coronary artery disease and sudden death in the young. Br Heart J 68:601, 1992.

843. Hobbs RE, Scally AP, Tan WA: Chronic coronary artery dissection presenting as heart failure. Circulation 100:445, 1999.

844. DeMaio SJ Jr, Kinsella SH, Silverman ME: Clinical course and long-term prognosis of spontaneous coronary artery dissection. Am J Cardiol 64:471, 1989.

845. Hanratty CG, McKeown PP, O'Keeffe DB: Coronary stenting in the setting of spontaneous coronary artery dissection. Int J Cardiol 67:197, 1998.

846. Longheval G, Badot V, Cosyns B, et al: Spontaneous coronary artery dissection: Favorable outcome illustrated by angiographic data. Clin Cardiol 22:374, 1999.

847. Gunal N, Kara N, Cakar N, et al: Cardiac involvement in childhood polyarteritis nodosa. Int J Cardiol 60:257, 1997.

848. Saito S, Arai H, Kim K, et al: Acute myocardial infarction in a young adult due to solitary giant cell arteritis of the coronary artery diagnosed antemortemly by primary directional coronary atherectomy. Cathet Cardiovasc Diagn 33:245, 1994.

849. LeRoy EC: The heart in systemic sclerosis (editorial). N Engl J Med 310:188, 1984.

850. Morris PB, Imber MJ, Heinsimer JA, et al: Rheumatoid arthritis and coronary arteritis. Am J Cardiol 57:689, 1986.

851. Moder KG, Miller TD, Tazelaar HD: Cardiac involvement in systemic lupus erythematosus. Mayo Clin Proc 74:275, 1999.

852. Nobrega TP, Klodas E, Breen JF, et al: Giant coronary artery aneurysms and myocardial infarction in a patient with systemic lupus erythematosus. Cathet Cardiovasc Diagn 39:75, 1996.

853. Vaarala O: Antiphospholipid antibodies and myocardial infarction. Lupus 7(Suppl 2):132, 1998.

854. Subramanyan R, Joy J, Balakrishnan KG: Natural history of aortoarteritis (Takayasu's disease). Circulation 80:429, 1989.

855. Kihara M, Kimura K, Yakuwa H, et al: Isolated left coronary ostial stenosis as the sole arterial involvement in Takayasu's disease. J Intern Med 232:353, 1992.

856. Scholz KH, Herrmann C, Tebbe U, et al: Myocardial infarction in young patients with Hodgkin's disease—potential pathogenic role of radiotherapy, chemotherapy, and splenectomy. Clin Invest 71:57, 1993.

857. Glanzmann C, Kaufmann P, Jenni R, et al: Cardiac risk after mediastinal irradiation for Hodgkin's disease. Radiother Oncol 46:51, 1998.

858. Virmani R, Farb A, Carter AJ, et al: Comparative pathology: Radiation-induced coronary artery disease in man and animals. Semin Interv Cardiol 3:163, 1998.

859. King V, Constine LS, Clark D, et al: Symptomatic coronary artery disease after mantle irradiation for Hodgkin's disease. Int J Radiat Oncol Biol Phys 36:881, 1996.

860. Lange RL, Reid MS, Tresch DD, et al: Nonatheromatous ischemic heart disease following withdrawal from chronic industrial nitroglycerin exposure. Circulation 46:666, 1972.

861. Hollander JE: The management of cocaine-associated myocardial ischemia. N Engl J Med 333:1267, 1995.

862. Pitts WR, Lange RA, Cigarroa JE, et al: Cocaine-induced myocardial ischemia and infarction: Pathophysiology, recognition, and management. Prog Cardiovasc Dis 40:65, 1997.

863. Shen WK, Edwards WD, Hammill SC, et al: Sudden unexpected nontraumatic death in 54 young adults: A 30-year population-based study. Am J Cardiol 76:148, 1995.

864. Fraund S, Pethig K, Franke U, et al: Ten year survival after heart transplantation: Palliative procedure or successful long term treatment? Heart 82:47, 1999.

865. Schmid C, Heemann U, Azuma H, et al: Transplant vasculopathy in rat heart transplantation: A morphologic chameleon determined by antigen-dependent and -independent factors. Transplant Proc 27:2077, 1995.

866. Hoang K, Chen YD, Reaven G, et al: Diabetes and dyslipidemia. A new model for transplant coronary artery disease. Circulation 97:2160, 1998.

867. Buszman P, Zembala M, Wojarski J, et al: Comparison of intravascular ultrasound and quantitative angiography for evaluation of coronary artery disease in the transplanted heart. Ann Transplant 1:31, 1996.

868. Spes CH, Klauss V, Mudra H, et al: Diagnostic and prognostic value of serial dobutamine stress echocardiography for noninvasive assessment of cardiac allograft vasculopathy: A comparison with coronary angiography and intravascular ultrasound. Circulation 100:509, 1999.

869. Musci M, Loebe M, Wellnhofer E, et al: Coronary angioplasty, bypass surgery, and retransplantation in cardiac transplant patients with graft coronary disease. Thorac Cardiovasc Surg 46:268, 1998.

870. Wenke K, Meiser B, Thiery J, et al: Simvastatin reduces graft vessel disease and mortality after heart transplantation: A four-year randomized trial. Circulation 96:1398, 1997.

GUIDELINES

MANAGEMENT OF CHRONIC ISCHEMIC HEART DISEASE

Thomas H. Lee

Multiple guidelines are relevant to the care of patients with chronic ischemic heart disease, including the 1999 guidelines developed by an American College of Cardiology/American Heart Association (ACC/AHA) task force.[1] These guidelines will be summarized, as well as the 1993 guidelines for percutaneous transluminal angioplasty[2] (PTCA) and 1999 guidelines for coronary artery bypass graft (CABG) surgery.[3]

According to the usual format of ACC/AHA guidelines, the appropriateness of various tests and procedures in different clinical settings was categorized into the following:

I.   Conditions for which there is evidence and/or general agreement that a given procedure or treatment is useful and effective.
II. Conditions for which there is conflicting evidence and/or a divergence of opinion about the usefulness/efficacy of a procedure.
IIa. Weight of evidence/opinion is in favor of usefulness/efficacy.
IIb. Usefulness/efficacy is less well established by evidence/opinion.
III. Conditions for which there is evidence and/or general agreement that the procedure/treatment is not useful/effective and in some cases may be harmful.

Diagnosis

The ACC/AHA guidelines emphasize the importance of using clinical data to make a qualitative estimate of the patient's probability of coronary artery disease. Routine laboratory data that are considered appropriate (Class I) include hemoglobin, fasting glucose, a lipid profile, and resting electrocardiogram (ECG). Chest x-rays are considered appropriate for patients with signs or symptoms of cardiovascular disease but were considered to have uncertain appropriateness for other patients (Table 37−G−1).

The exercise ECG is an appropriate first-line test for patients with an intermediate probability of coronary artery disease, including patients with complete right bundle branch block or less than 1 mm of ST depression at rest. Other technologies may be appropriate for patients whose ECG has mild ST depression in the setting of digoxin therapy or criteria for left ventricular hypertrophy or patients who had other ECG abnormalities described in Table 37−G−1. The ACC/AHA guidelines indicate that exercise ECG should be the first-line test for women as well as men.

The ACC/AHA task force was not supportive of echocardiography as a routine test for diagnosis of the cause of acute chest pain unless the patient has a systolic murmur suggesting structural heart disease (Table 37−G−1). The guidelines did, however, support the use of echocardiography to assess the extent or severity of ischemia when the study could be obtained during or shortly after chest pain.

Imaging during physical or pharmacological stress was considered to be appropriate (Class I) in patients at intermediate risk for coronary disease for whom exercise ECG was unlikely to be useful because of baseline ECG abnormalities. Exercise myocardial perfusion imaging was also considered an appropriate test for risk stratification of patients who had undergone prior revascularization with either PTCA or CABG. Pharmacological stress with adenosine or dipyridamole is appropriate for patients who are unable to exercise. Because of abnormal patterns of myocardial activation, stress echocardiography is *discouraged* as an imaging modality for patients with left bundle branch block.

Coronary angiography was not considered clearly appropriate for the diagnosis of chronic stable angina in most patients, except for those who had survived sudden cardiac death. Several patient subsets were considered possibly appropriate (Class II) for coronary angiography, such as patients whose diagnosis was still uncertain after noninvasive testing or those with an occupational requirement for a definitive diagnosis. Coronary angiography is, however, an important test in risk stratification (see below).

Risk Stratification

The ACC/AHA guidelines emphasize that most patients with stable angina do not need routine echocardiography either for initial baseline studies or for reassessment (Table 37−G−1). However, the ACC/AHA guidelines support the use of echocardiography or radionuclide angiography in patients with a history or ECG evidence of a prior myocardial infarction or symptoms or signs of congestive heart failure. Assessment of left ventricular function is also endorsed for patients with complex ventricular arrhythmias.

The ACC/AHA guidelines are supportive of exercise ECG as a first-line test for risk stratification or after a significant change in cardiac symptoms. Exceptions are made for patients in whom imaging technologies would provide more accurate information because of a history of CABG or PTCA or ECG abnormalities (see Table 37−G−1). However, the guidelines do not provide strong support (Class IIb) for routine screening of patients 6 months after revascularization procedures.

Coronary angiography is supported as appropriate for patients with disabling angina despite medical therapy, as well as for those with high-risk exercise test results or signs of congestive heart failure and for survivors of sudden cardiac death. The ACC/AHA guidelines considered coronary angiography inappropriate in patients with Canadian Cardiovascular Society Class I or II angina who respond to medical therapy and have no evidence of ischemia on noninvasive testing (Table 37−G−1).

Treatment

The ACC/AHA guidelines support the use of aspirin and beta blocker therapy in the absence of contraindications. Calcium antagonists or long-acting nitrates can be administered when beta blockers are contraindicated or ineffective. Short-acting dihydropyridine calcium antagonists are to be avoided.

Multiple efforts are endorsed to reduce the risk of progression of atherosclerosis. Lipid-lowering therapy is considered clearly appropriate (Class I) when low-density lipoprotein (LDL) cholesterol is greater than 130 mg/dl and possibly appropriate (Class IIa) when LDL is between 100 and 129 mg/dl. Also supported by the guidelines are interventions to treat hypertension according to Joint National Conference VI guidelines, cigarette smoking, diabetes, and obesity.

Guidelines for revascularization with CABG or PTCA are similar to those described for unstable angina (Table 37−G−2). CABG is appropriate for patients with left main coronary artery disease, three-vessel disease, and subsets of patients with two-vessel disease. PTCA is considered appropriate for multivessel disease in patients who have normal left ventricular function and do not have diabetes. (See below for further information on appropriate indications for these procedures.)

FOLLOW-UP. The same principles that define the appropriateness of the initial use of tests for patients with chronic stable angina characterize their use during follow-up in patients who have new or worsening cardiovascular symptoms (see Table 37−G−1). The guidelines are not supportive of annual treadmill exercise tests or other procedures in patients who have had no change in clinical status. For low-risk stable patients, the guidelines suggest that an interval of 3 years or longer between exercise tests may be appropriate.

Percutaneous Transluminal Coronary Angioplasty

The development of guidelines for PTCA is complicated by several trends, including technological innovations (e.g., stents), broadening of the patient population to which this procedure is applied, and lack of data identifying populations in which PTCA confers a survival advantage. As physicians have become more expert in performing this procedure, they have also become more ambitious, and PTCA is now frequently used for patients with acute myocardial infarction and patients with multivessel coronary artery disease. An additional reason for uncertainty over the optimal role for PTCA is that it is an alternative to more than one major strategy—medical therapy or CABG surgery. Hence, trials in which PTCA is directly compared with another strategy (e.g., CABG) do not address the full range of choices for clinicians.

Recent ACC/AHA guidelines for unstable angina[4] and chronic stable angina[1] are beginning to address the question of which patients should preferentially undergo PTCA or CABG. However, for many patients with chronic stable angina, clinical judgment remains the critical mechanism for deciding which procedure should be performed.

TABLE 37–G–1. ACC/AHA GUIDELINES FOR MANAGEMENT OF STABLE ANGINA

Issue	Class	Recommendation	Level of Evidence
History and physical examination	I	In patients with chest pain, a detailed symptom history, focused physical examination, and directed risk factor assessment should be performed. With this information, the clinician should estimate the probability of significant CAD (i.e., low, intermediate, high)	B
Initial laboratory tests for diagnosis	I	Hemoglobin Fasting glucose Fasting lipid panel, including total cholesterol, HDL cholesterol, triglycerides, and calculated LDL cholesterol	C C C
ECG, chest x-ray, or electron beam computed tomography in the diagnosis of chronic stable angina	I	Rest ECG in patients without an obvious noncardiac cause of chest pain Rest ECG during an episode of chest pain Chest x-ray in patients with signs or symptoms of CHF, valvular heart disease, pericardial disease, or aortic dissection/aneurysm	B B B
	IIa	Chest x-ray in patients with signs or symptoms of pulmonary disease	B
	IIb	Chest x-ray in other patients Electron beam computed tomography	C B
Diagnosis of obstructive CAD with exercise ECG testing without an imaging modality	I	Patients with an intermediate pretest probability of CAD based on age, gender, and symptoms, including those with complete right bundle branch block or <1 mm of ST depression at rest (exceptions are listed below in Classes II and III)	B
	IIa	Patients with suspected vasospastic angina	C
	IIb	Patients with a high pretest probability of CAD by age, gender, and symptoms Patients with a low pretest probability of CAD by age, gender, and symptoms Patients taking digoxin whose ECG has <1 mm of baseline ST segment depression Patients with ECG criteria for LV hypertrophy and <1 mm of baseline ST segment depression	B B B B
	III	Patients with the following baseline ECG abnormalities: Preexcitation (Wolff-Parkinson-White) syndrome Electronically paced ventricular rhythm More than 1 mm of ST depression at rest Complete left bundle branch block Patients with an established diagnosis of CAD from prior MI or coronary angiography; however, testing can assess functional capacity and prognosis	 B B B B B
Echocardiography for diagnosis of cause of chest pain in patients with suspected chronic stable angina pectoris	I	Patients with systolic murmur suggestive of aortic stenosis or hypertrophic cardiomyopathy Evaluation of extent (severity) of ischemia (e.g., LV segmental wall motion abnormality) when the echocardiogram can be obtained during pain or within 30 min after its abatement	C C
	IIb	Patients with a click or murmur to diagnose mitral valve prolapse	C
	III	Patients with a normal ECG, no history of MI, and no signs or symptoms suggestive of heart failure, valvular heart disease, or hypertrophic cardiomyopathy	C
Cardiac stress imaging as the initial test for diagnosis in patients with chronic stable angina who are able to exercise	I	Exercise myocardial perfusion imaging or exercise echocardiography in patients with an intermediate pretest probability of CAD who have one of the following baseline ECG abnormalities: Preexcitation (Wolff-Parkinson-White) syndrome More than 1 mm of ST depression at rest Exercise myocardial perfusion imaging or exercise echocardiography in patients with prior revascularization (either PTCA or CABG) Adenosine or dipyridamole myocardial perfusion imaging in patients with an intermediate pretest probability of CAD and one of the following baseline ECG abnormalities: Electronically paced ventricular rhythm Left bundle branch block	 B B B C B

Issue	Class	Recommendation	Level of Evidence
	IIb	Exercise myocardial perfusion imaging and exercise echocardiography in patients with a low or high probability of CAD who have one of the following baseline ECG abnormalities:	
		Preexcitation (Wolff-Parkinson-White) syndrome	B
		More than 1 mm of ST depression	B
		Adenosine or dipyridamole myocardial perfusion imaging in patients with a low or high probability of CAD and one of the following baseline ECG abnormalities:	
		Electronically paced ventricular rhythm	C
		Left bundle branch block	B
		Exercise myocardial perfusion imaging or exercise echocardiography in patients with an intermediate probability of CAD who have one of the following:	
		Digoxin use with <1-mm ST depression on the baseline ECG	B
		LV hypertrophy with <1-mm ST depression on the baseline ECG	B
		Exercise myocardial perfusion imaging, exercise echocardiography, adenosine or dipyridamole myocardial perfusion imaging, or dobutamine echocardiography as the initial stress test in a patient with a normal rest ECG who is not taking digoxin	B
		Exercise or dobutamine echocardiography in patients with left bundle branch block	C
Cardiac stress imaging as the initial test for diagnosis in patients with chronic stable angina who are unable to exercise	I	Adenosine or dipyridamole myocardial perfusion imaging or dobutamine echocardiography in patients with an intermediate pretest probability of CAD	B
		Adenosine or dipyridamole stress myocardial perfusion imaging or dobutamine echocardiography in patients with prior revascularization (either PTCA or CABG)	B
	IIb	Adenosine or dipyridamole stress myocardial perfusion imaging or dobutamine echocardiography in patients with a low or high probability of CAD in the absence of electronically paced ventricular rhythm or left bundle branch block	B
		Adenosine or dipyridamole myocardial perfusion imaging in patients with a low or a high probability of CAD and one of the following baseline ECG abnormalities:	
		Electronically paced ventricular rhythm	C
		Left bundle branch block	B
		Dobutamine echocardiography in patients with left bundle branch block	C
Coronary angiography to establish a diagnosis in patients with suspected angina, including those with known CAD who have a significant change in anginal symptoms	I	Patients with known or possible angina pectoris who have survived sudden cardiac death	B
	IIa	Patients with an uncertain diagnosis after noninvasive testing in whom the benefit of a more certain diagnosis outweighs the risk and cost of coronary angiography	C
		Patients who cannot undergo noninvasive testing because of disability, illness, or morbid obesity	C
		Patients with an occupational requirement for a definitive diagnosis	C
		Patients who by virtue of young age at onset of symptoms, noninvasive imaging, or other clinical parameters are suspected of having a nonatherosclerotic cause of myocardial ischemia (coronary artery anomaly, Kawasaki disease, primary coronary artery dissection, radiation-induced vasculoplasty)	C
		Patients in whom coronary artery spasm is suspected and provocative testing may be necessary	C
		Patients with a high pretest probability of left main or three-vessel CAD	C
	IIb	Patients with recurrent hospitalization for chest pain in whom a definite diagnosis is judged necessary	C
		Patients with an overriding desire for a definitive diagnosis and a greater than low probability of CAD	C
	III	Patients with significant comorbidity in whom the risk of coronary arteriography outweighs the benefit of the procedure	C
		Patients with an overriding personal desire for a definitive diagnosis and a low probability of CAD	C

Table continued on following page

Issue	Class	Recommendation	Level of Evidence
Measurement of rest LV function by echocardiography or radionuclide angiography in patients with chronic stable angina	I	Echocardiography or radionuclide angiography to assess LV function in patients with a history of prior MI, pathological Q waves, or symptoms or signs suggestive of heart failure	B
		Echocardiography in patients with a systolic murmur suggesting mitral regurgitation to assess its severity and etiology	C
		Echocardiography or radionuclide angiography in patients with complex ventricular arrhythmias to assess LV function	B
	III	Routine periodic reassessment of stable patients for whom no new change in therapy is contemplated	C
		Patients with a normal ECG, no history of MI, and no symptoms or signs suggestive of CHF	B
Exercise testing for risk assessment and prognosis in patients with an intermediate or high probability of CAD	I	Patients undergoing initial evaluation (Exceptions are listed below in Classes IIb and III)	B
		Patients after a significant change in cardiac symptoms	
	IIb	Patients with the following ECG abnormalities:	
		Preexcitation (Wolff-Parkinson-White) syndrome	B
		Electronically paced ventricular rhythm	B
		More than 1 mm of ST depression at rest	B
		Complete left bundle branch block	B
		Patients who have undergone cardiac catheterization to identify ischemia in the distribution of a coronary lesion of borderline severity	C
		Postrevascularization patients who have a significant change in anginal pattern suggestive of ischemia	C
	III	Patients with severe comorbidity likely to limit life expectancy or prevent revascularization	C
Cardiac stress imaging as the initial test for risk stratification of patients with chronic stable angina who are able to exercise	I	Exercise myocardial perfusion imaging or exercise echocardiography to identify the extent, severity, and location of ischemia in patients who do not have left bundle branch block or an electronically paced ventricular rhythm and either have an abnormal rest ECG or are using digoxin	B
		Dipyridamole or adenosine myocardial perfusion imaging in patients with left bundle branch block or electronically paced ventricular rhythm	B
		Exercise myocardial perfusion imaging or exercise echocardiography to assess the functional significance of coronary lesions (if not already known) in planning PTCA	B
	IIb	Exercise or dobutamine echocardiography in patients with left bundle branch block	C
		Exercise, dipyridamole, or adenosine myocardial perfusion imaging or exercise or dobutamine echocardiography as the initial test in patients who have a normal rest ECG and who are not taking digoxin	B
	III	Exercise myocardial perfusion imaging in patients with left bundle branch block	C
		Exercise, dipyridamole, or adenosine myocardial perfusion imaging or exercise or dobutamine echocardiography in patients with severe comorbidity likely to limit life expectation or prevent revascularization	C
Cardiac stress imaging as the initial test for risk stratification of patients with chronic stable angina who are unable to exercise	I	Dipyridamole or adenosine myocardial perfusion imaging or dobutamine echocardiography to identify the extent, severity, and location of ischemia in patients who do not have left bundle branch block or electronically paced ventricular rhythm	B
		Dipyridamole or adenosine myocardial perfusion imaging in patients with left bundle branch block or electronically paced ventricular rhythm	B
		Dipyridamole or adenosine myocardial perfusion imaging or dobutamine echocardiography to assess the functional significance of coronary lesions (if not already known) in planning PTCA	B
	IIb	Dobutamine echocardiography in patients with left bundle branch block	C
	III	Dipyridamole or adenosine myocardial perfusion imaging or dobutamine echocardiography in patients with severe comorbidity likely to limit life expectation or prevent revascularization	C

TABLE 37–G–1. ACC/AHA GUIDELINES FOR MANAGEMENT OF STABLE ANGINA *Continued*

Issue	Class	Recommendation	Level of Evidence
Coronary angiography for risk stratification in patients with chronic stable angina	I	Patients with disabling (CCS classes III and IV) chronic stable angina despite medical therapy	B
		Patients with high-risk criteria on noninvasive testing regardless of anginal severity	B
		Patients with angina who have survived sudden cardiac death or serious ventricular arrhythmia	B
		Patients with angina and symptoms and signs of CHF	C
		Patients with clinical characteristics that indicate a high likelihood of severe CAD	C
	IIa	Patients with significant LV dysfunction (ejection fraction <45%), CCS class I or II angina, and demonstrable ischemia but less than high-risk criteria on noninvasive testing	C
		Patients with inadequate prognostic information after noninvasive testing	C
	IIb	Patients with CCS class I or II angina, preserved LV function (ejection fraction >45%), and less than high-risk criteria on noninvasive testing	C
		Patients with CCS class III or IV angina, which with medical therapy improves to class I or II	C
		Patients with CCS class I or II angina but intolerance (unacceptable side effects) to adequate medical therapy	C
	III	Patients with CCS class I or II angina who respond to medical therapy and have no evidence of ischemia on noninvasive testing	C
		Patients who prefer to avoid revascularization	C
Pharmacotherapy to prevent MI and death and reduce symptoms	I	Aspirin in the absence of contraindications	A
		Beta blockers as initial therapy in the absence of contraindications in patients with prior MI	A
		Beta blockers as initial therapy in the absence of contraindications in patients without prior MI	B
		Calcium antagonists* or long-acting nitrates as initial therapy when beta blockers are contraindicated	B
		Calcium antagonists* or long-acting nitrates in combination with beta blockers when initial treatment with beta blockers is not successful	B
		Calcium antagonists* and long-acting nitrates as a substitute for beta blockers if initial treatment with beta blockers leads to unacceptable side effects	C
		Sublingual nitroglycerin or nitroglycerin spray for the immediate relief of angina	C
		Lipid-lowering therapy in patients with documented or suspected CAD and LDL cholesterol >130 mg/dl, with a target LDL of <100 mg/dl	A
	IIa	Clopidogrel when aspirin is absolutely contraindicated	B
		Long-acting nondihydropyridine calcium antagonists* instead of beta blockers as initial therapy	B
		Lipid-lowering therapy in patients with documented or suspected CAD and LDL cholesterol of 100–129 mg/dl, with a target LDL of 100 mg/dl	B
	IIb	Low-intensity anticoagulation with warfarin in addition to aspirin	B
	III	Dipyridamole	B
		Chelation therapy	B
Treatment of risk factors	I	Treatment of hypertension according to Joint National Conference VI guidelines	A
		Smoking cessation therapy	B
		Management of diabetes	C
		Exercise training program	B
		Lipid-lowering therapy in patients with documented or suspected CAD and LDL cholesterol >130 mg/dl, with a target LDL of <100 mg/dl	A
		Weight reduction in obese patients with hypertension, hyperlipidemia, or diabetes mellitus	C
	IIa	Lipid-lowering therapy in patients with documented or suspected CAD and LDL cholesterol of 100–129 mg/dl, with a target LDL <100 mg/dl	B

Table continued on following page

Issue	Class	Recommendation	Level of Evidence
	IIb	Hormone replacement therapy in postmenopausal women in the absence of contraindications	B
		Weight reduction in obese patients in the absence of hypertension, hyperlipidemia, or diabetes mellitus	C
		Folate therapy in patients with elevated homocysteine levels	C
		Vitamin C and E supplementation	B
		Identification and appropriate treatment of clinical depression	C
		Intervention directed at psychosocial stress reduction	C
	III	Chelation therapy	C
		Garlic	C
		Acupuncture	C
Revascularization with PTCA (or other catheter-based techniques) and CABG in patients with stable angina	I	CABG for patients with significant left main coronary disease	A
		CABG for patients with 3-vessel disease. The survival benefit is greater in patients with abnormal LV function (ejection fraction <50%)	A
		CABG for patients with 2-vessel CAD, with significant proximal LAD disease and either abnormal LV function (ejection fraction <50%) or demonstrable ischemia on noninvasive testing	A
		PTCA for patients with 2- or 3-vessel CAD and significant proximal LAD disease who have anatomy suitable for catheter-based therapy, have normal LV function, and do not have treated diabetes	B
		PTCA or CABG for patients with 1- or 2-vessel CAD without significant proximal LAD disease but with a large area of viable myocardium and high-risk criteria on noninvasive testing	B
		CABG for patients with 1- or 2-vessel CAD without significant proximal LAD disease who have survived sudden cardiac death or sustained ventricular tachycardia	C
		In patients with prior PTCA or CABG for recurrent stenosis associated with a large area of viable myocardium or high-risk criteria on noninvasive testing	C
		PTCA or CABG for patients who have not been successfully treated by medical therapy and can undergo revascularization with acceptable risk	B
	IIa	Repeat CABG for patients with multiple saphenous vein graft stenoses, especially with significant stenosis of a graft supplying the LAD. It may be appropriate to use PTCA for focal saphenous vein graft lesions or multiple stenoses in poor candidates for reoperative surgery	C
		Use of PTCA or CABG for patients with 1- or 2-vessel CAD without significant proximal LAD disease but with a moderate area of viable myocardium and demonstrable ischemia on noninvasive testing	B
		Use of PTCA or CABG for patients with 1-vessel CAD and significant proximal LAD disease	B
	IIb	Compared with CABG, PTCA for patients with 2- or 3-vessel CAD and significant proximal LAD disease who have anatomy suitable for catheter-based therapy and who have treated diabetes or abnormal LV function	B
		Use of PTCA for patients with significant left main coronary disease who are not candidates for CABG	C
		PTCA for patients with 1- or 2-vessel CAD without significant proximal LAD disease who have survived sudden cardiac death or sustained ventricular tachycardia	C
	III	Use of PTCA or CABG for patients with 1- or 2-vessel CAD without significant proximal LAD disease who have mild symptoms that are unlikely to be due to myocardial ischemia or who have not received an adequate trial of medical therapy and Have only a small area of viable myocardium or Have no demonstrable ischemia on noninvasive testing	C
		Use of PTCA or CABG for patients with borderline coronary stenoses (50–60% diameter in locations other than the left main coronary artery) and no demonstrable ischemia on noninvasive testing	C
		Use of PTCA or CABG for patients with insignificant coronary stenosis (<50% diameter)	C
		Use of PTCA in patients with significant left main coronary artery disease who are candidates for CABG	B

Issue	Class	Recommendation	Level of Evidence
Echocardiography, treadmill exercise testing, stress imaging studies, and coronary angiography during patient follow-up	I	Chest x-ray for patients with evidence of new or worsening CHF	C
		Assessment of LV ejection fraction and segmental wall motion in patients with new or worsening CHF or evidence of intervening MI by history or ECG	C
		Echocardiography for evidence of new or worsening valvular heart disease	C
		Treadmill exercise test for patients without prior revascularization who have a significant change in clinical status, are able to exercise, and do not have any of the ECG abnormalities listed below	C
		Stress imaging procedures for patients without prior revascularization who have a significant change in clinical status and are unable to exercise or have one of the following ECG abnormalities:	C C C C
		Preexcitation (Wolff-Parkinson-White) syndrome	
		Electronically paced ventricular rhythm	
		More than 1 mm of rest ST depression	
		Complete left bundle branch block	
		Stress imaging procedures for patients who have a significant change in clinical status and required a stress imaging procedure on their initial evaluation because of equivocal or intermediate-risk treadmill results	C
		Stress imaging procedures for patients with prior revascularization who have a significant change in clinical status	C
		Coronary angiography in patients with marked limitation of ordinary activity (CCS class III) despite maximal medical therapy	C
	IIb	Annual treadmill exercise testing in patients who have no change in clinical status, can exercise, have none of the ECG abnormalities listed above, and have an estimated annual mortality rate >1%	C
	III	Echocardiography or radionuclide imaging for assessment of LV ejection fraction and segmental wall motion in patients with a normal ECG, no history of MI, and no evidence of CHF	C
		Repeat treadmill exercise testing in <3 yr in patients who have no change in clinical status and an estimated annual mortality rate <1% on their initial evaluation, as demonstrated by one of the following:	
		Low-risk Duke treadmill score (without imaging)	C
		Low-risk Duke treadmill score with negative imaging	C
		Normal LV function and a normal coronary angiogram	C
		Normal LV function and insignificant CAD	C
		Stress imaging procedures for patients who have no change in clinical status and a normal rest ECG, are not taking digoxin, are able to exercise, and did not require a stress imaging procedure on their initial evaluation because of equivocal or intermediate-risk treadmill results	C
		Repeat coronary angiography in patients with no change in clinical status, no change on repeat exercise testing or stress imaging, and insignificant CAD on initial evaluation	C

Level of evidence: A = highest; B = intermediate; C = lowest
* Short-acting dihydropyridine calcium antagonists should be avoided.
ACC/AHA = American College of Cardiology/American Heart Association; CABG = coronary artery bypass grafting; CAD = coronary artery disease; CHF = congestive heart failure; CCS = Canadian Cardiovascular Society; ECG = electrocardiography; HDL = high-density lipoprotein; LAD = left anterior descending artery; LDL = low-density lipoprotein; LV = left ventricular; MI = myocardial infarction; PTCA = percutaneous transluminal coronary angioplasty.
From Gibbons RJ, Chatterjee K, Daley J, et al: ACC/AHA/ACP-ASIM guidelines for the management of patients with chronic stable angina: A report of the American College of Cardiology/American Heart Association Task Force on Practice Guidelines (Committee on the Management of Patients with Chronic Stable Angina). J Am Coll Cardiol 33:2092–2197, 1999. Reprinted with permission from the American College of Cardiology.

An ACC/AHA task force published guidelines for PTCA in 1993[2] (new guidelines are being developed) that defined contraindications to *elective* angioplasty, including relative contraindications to coronary angiography. These guidelines stress that PTCA may be appropriate even in patients with these contraindications who are severely symptomatic and not candidates for CABG. *Absolute contraindications* included

1. Absence of a lesion that causes a 50 percent or greater reduction in coronary diameter
2. Presence of significant left main coronary disease unless this coronary distribution is protected by at least one nonobstructed bypass graft
3. Absence of a formal cardiac surgical program in the institution

Relative contraindications included

1. Conditions associated with an unacceptable risk of serious bleeding or thrombotic occlusion or a recently dilated vessel
2. Diffusely diseased saphenous vein grafts without a focal dilatable lesion
3. Diffusely diseased native coronary arteries with distal vessels suitable for bypass grafting
4. The vessel in question is the sole remaining vessel in the coronary circulation
5. Chronic total occlusions with clinical features suggesting a very low anticipated success rate
6. Borderline stenotic lesion (usually less than 50 percent stenosis)
7. Procedure proposed for a non–infarct-related artery in patients

with multivessel disease who are undergoing direct angioplasty for acute myocardial infarction

The ACC/AHA guidelines also considered anatomical features that increase the risk for abrupt closure (see Chap. 38) to be relative contraindications to PTCA. Because of the risk of such complications, the guidelines recommended that for all elective PTCA procedures, an experienced cardiovascular surgical team be present within the hospital to perform emergency CABG should the need arise. The AHA/ACC task force did not consider formal surgical consultation mandatory before PTCA.

Under some circumstances, the AHA/ACC task force considered PTCA reasonable even if surgical back-up were not available. For patients with a high risk of acute myocardial infarction in whom thrombolytic therapy was contraindicated, emergency PTCA was "acceptable treatment" if the patient could not be transferred expeditiously to a center with surgical back-up. However, the guidelines noted that patients with unstable angina could and should usually be transferred to an institution with a cardiac surgical program before consideration of PTCA.

The experience of the operator is also a critical factor in determining the outcome of PTCA. Therefore, several task forces have provided recommendations for the minimum number of cases during PTCA training and for the minimum annual volume required to maintain competency.[5-7] The most recent statement from the ACC, published in 1998, concluded that the relationship between individual operator procedural volume and patient outcomes was statistically valid but complex.[7] These guidelines recommended that an institution performing PTCA have an activity level of at least 400 coronary procedures per year and that an institution performing fewer than 200 procedures per year consider discontinuing this service unless it is in a region that is underserved. Institutions offering coronary interventional services should have a physician-director with experience consisting of at least 500 procedures. The ACC statement indicated that individual operators should perform at least 75 procedures per year and that operators who perform 50 to 75 procedures per year should be very cautious in case selection. Ideally, the guidelines said, operators with annual procedural volumes below 75 should work only at institutions with an activity level greater than 600 procedures per year. Recommendations also included a "mentoring" relationship for low-volume operators with a highly experienced operator who has an annual procedural volume greater than 150 procedures per year.

Indications for PTCA

The 1993 AHA/ACC task force developed assessments of the appropriateness of PTCA in various clinical settings according to the same three classes used in other ACC/AHA guidelines.[2] These indications included consideration of the patient's coronary anatomy, symptomatic status, and the clinical syndrome.

SINGLE-VESSEL CORONARY DISEASE. The ACC/AHA task force included different recommendations for patients with and without symptoms of coronary disease. For patients who were *asymptomatic* or only mildly symptomatic, regardless of whether they had received medical therapy, PTCA was considered appropriate (Class I) in those with a lesion resulting in a 50 percent or greater reduction in the diameter of a coronary artery that supplies a large area of viable myocardium if they also had evidence of myocardial ischemia induced by low levels of exercise (Bruce stage 1, or <4.0 METs, or a heart rate less than 100 beats/min) during noninvasive testing (see Table 37-10). Other Class I indications for PTCA included prior cardiac arrest or sustained ventricular tachycardia in the absence of acute myocardial infarction and the need to undergo major vascular surgery (such as aortic aneurysm repair, iliofemoral bypass, or carotid artery surgery) if patients had clinical evidence of ischemic heart disease.

In patients with less myocardium in jeopardy, the appropriateness of single-vessel angioplasty was less clear-cut. Indications for PTCA were considered equivocal (Class II) in patients whose stenotic coronary artery supplied a moderate- or large-sized area of viable myocardium if they had objective evidence of ischemia and had coronary anatomy suggesting that PTCA could be performed with a moderate likelihood of success and low risk of complications. PTCA was considered inappropriate (Class III) for patients with only a small area of viable myocardium at risk, no evidence of ischemia, or a moderate to high risk of complications.

For patients who are *symptomatic* from single-vessel coronary disease despite medical therapy, the ACC/AHA guidelines considered PTCA appropriate (Class I) even if only a moderate amount of myocardium was supplied by the stenosed vessel—if they showed evidence of ischemia despite medical therapy, had angina pectoris that was inadequately responsive to medical treatment, or were intolerant

of medical therapy. "Inadequately responsive" indicates that the patient and physician agree that angina significantly interferes with the patient's occupation or ability to perform usual activities. All these patients should have at least a moderate likelihood of successful dilation and be at low or moderate risk for morbidity and mortality for PTCA to be considered clearly appropriate.

PTCA was considered to be of equivocal appropriateness (Class II) in patients with an increased risk of complications or failure of the procedure. The ACC/AHA guidelines did not support PTCA's appropriateness in patients with no or only a small area of myocardium at risk in the absence of disabling symptoms or in patients with a high risk of procedural failure or complications.

MULTIVESSEL CORONARY DISEASE. For *asymptomatic* patients with multivessel disease, the AHA/ACC guidelines indicate that PTCA is reasonable (Class I) if dilation of one major coronary artery could lead to nearly complete revascularization and the chance of success was moderate or high. For PTCA to be considered appropriate in this population, patients should have the same clinical indications as for Class I in asymptomatic patients with single-vessel disease, including evidence of severe ischemia. The indications were less clear (Class II) if the amount of myocardium at risk was only moderate or if there were other coronary stenoses that affected a moderate amount of myocardium. PTCA was considered inappropriate if patients had only a small amount of viable myocardium at risk, had chronic total occlusions, or had a high risk of complications.

For symptomatic patients with multivessel coronary disease, appropriate (Class I) indications for PTCA were similar to those for symptomatic patients with single-vessel disease, except that these indications included patients who had lesions in two or more major arteries affecting at least moderately sized areas of viable myocardium. If these patients had a moderate risk for complications or did not have objective evidence of myocardial ischemia, the appropriateness of PTCA was regarded as uncertain (Class II).

The ACC/AHA task force was also uncertain about the appropriateness of PTCA for patients with multivessel coronary disease and angina that was disabling despite medical therapy if these patients were poor candidates for surgery and were at moderate risk for complications from PTCA. The concern reflected in these guidelines is that PTCA might lead to abrupt closure of a coronary artery, thereby creating a dilemma in which the physicians must decide whether to send a poor surgical candidate for CABG.

Coronary Artery Bypass Graft Surgery

Guidelines for the use of CABG surgery were updated in 1999 by an ACC/AHA task force.[3] When compared with the 1991 guidelines for CABG from the ACC/AHA,[8] this revision reflects greater consideration of the impact of this procedure on relief of symptoms, as well as overall survival. For example, the authors of these guidelines considered CABG beneficial for younger patients without left ventricular dysfunction, even if no improvement in survival could be predicted, because CABG can be performed with low mortality in such patients and because their potential for resuming an active life style is high.

Indications (Table 37-G-2)

The 1999 update of the ACC/AHA guidelines designates an appropriateness class for patient subsets defined by major variables:

1. Symptomatic status
2. Severity of ischemia on noninvasive testing
3. Number of diseased coronary arteries
4. Involvement of the left main coronary artery
5. Involvement of the proximal left anterior descending coronary artery
6. Left ventricular function

In these guidelines, coronary stenosis is defined as a 50 percent or greater reduction in lumen diameter. Certain subsets of coronary anatomy have been found to have better prognoses with surgical than medical therapy and are therefore considered indications for CABG regardless of the patient's symptomatic status and severity of ischemia on noninvasive testing. In the ACC/AHA guidelines, CABG surgery is considered appropriate (Class I) for all patients with any of the following criteria:

1. Significant stenosis (>50 percent) of the left main coronary artery
2. Left main equivalent: significant (>70 percent) stenosis of the proximal left anterior descending coronary artery and proximal left circumflex artery

TABLE 37–G–2. APPROPRIATENESS OF CABG FOR SPECIFIC PATIENT SUBSETS

Clinical Subset	Class I	Class IIa	Class IIb	Class III
Asymptomatic or mild angina	Significant left main coronary artery stenosis Left main equivalent: significant (≥70%) stenosis of the proximal LAD and proximal left circumflex artery Three-vessel disease	Proximal LAD stenosis with 1- or 2-vessel disease*	One- or 2-vessel disease not involving the proximal LAD†	Other
Stable angina	Same as for patients with asymptomatic or mild angina, plus Two-vessel disease with significant proximal LAD stenosis and either an EF <0.50 or demonstrable ischemia on noninvasive testing One- or 2-vessel coronary artery disease without significant proximal LAD stenosis but with a large area of viable myocardium and high-risk criteria on noninvasive testing Disabling angina despite maximal medical therapy	Proximal LAD stenosis with 1-vessel disease* One- or 2-vessel coronary artery disease without significant proximal LAD stenosis but with a moderate area of viable myocardium and demonstrable ischemia on noninvasive testing	None	One- or 2-vessel disease not involving significant proximal LAD stenosis in patients who have mild symptoms that are unlikely to be due to myocardial ischemia or who have not received an adequate trial of medical therapy and Have only a small area of viable myocardium or Have no demonstrable ischemia on noninvasive testing Borderline coronary stenoses (50–60% diameter in locations other than the left main coronary artery) and no demonstrable ischemia on noninvasive testing Insignificant coronary stenosis (<50% diameter reduction)
Unstable angina/non-Q-wave MI	Significant left main coronary artery stenosis Left main equivalent: significant (≥70%) stenosis of the proximal LAD and proximal left circumflex artery Ongoing ischemia not responsive to maximal nonsurgical therapy	Proximal LAD stenosis with 1- or 2-vessel disease*	One- or 2-vessel disease not involving the proximal LAD	
ST segment elevation (Q wave) MI	None	Ongoing ischemia/infarction not responsive to maximal nonsurgical therapy	Progressive LV pump failure with coronary stenosis compromising viable myocardium outside the initial infarct area Primary reperfusion in the early hours (≤6 to 12 hr) of an evolving MI with ST segment elevation	Primary reperfusion late (≥12 hr) in evolving MI with ST segment elevation without ongoing ischemia
Poor LV function	Significant left main coronary artery stenosis Left main equivalent: significant (≥70%) stenosis of the proximal LAD and proximal left circumflex artery Proximal LAD stenosis with 2- or 3-vessel disease	Poor LV function with significant viable, noncontracting, revascularizable myocardium without any of the aforementioned anatomical patterns		Poor LV function without evidence of intermittent ischemia and without evidence of significant revascularizable, viable myocardium
Life-threatening ventricular arrhythmias	Left main coronary artery stenosis Three-vessel coronary disease	Bypassable 1- or 2-vessel disease causing life-threatening ventricular arrhythmias‡ Proximal LAD disease with 1- or 2-vessel disease‡		Ventricular tachycardia with scar and no evidence of ischemia

Table continued on following page

Clinical Subset	Class I	Class IIa	Class IIb	Class III
After failed PTCA	Ongoing ischemia or threatened occlusion with significant myocardium at risk Hemodynamic compromise	Foreign body in crucial anatomical position Hemodynamic compromise in patients with impairment of coagulation system and without previous sternotomy	Hemodynamic compromise in patients with impairment of coagulation system and previous sternotomy	Absence of ischemia Inability to revascularize because of target anatomy or no-reflow state
With previous CABG	Disabling angina despite maximal noninvasive therapy	Bypassable distal vessel(s) with a larger area of threatened myocardium by noninvasive studies	Ischemia in the non-LAD distribution with a patent IMA graft to the LAD supplying functioning myocardium, without an aggressive attempt at medical management and/or percutaneous revascularization	

* Becomes Class I if extensive ischemia is documented by noninvasive study and/or the left ventricular ejection fraction is less than 50%.
† Becomes Class I if there is a large area of viable myocardium and high-risk criteria on noninvasive testing.
‡ Becomes Class I if the arrhythmia is resuscitated sudden cardiac death or sustained ventricular tachycardia.
CABG = coronary artery bypass grafting; EF = ejection fraction; IMA = internal mammary artery; LAD = left anterior descending artery; LV = left ventricular; MI = myocardial infarction; PTCA = percutaneous transluminal coronary angioplasty.
From Eagle KA, Guyton RA, Davidoff R, et al: ACC/AHA guidelines for coronary artery bypass graft surgery. A report of the American College of Cardiology/American Heart Association Task Force on Practice Guidelines (Committee to Revise the 1991 Guidelines for Coronary Artery Bypass Graft Surgery). J Am Coll Cardiol 34:1262–1347, 1999.

3. Three-vessel disease, especially if left ventricular function is reduced

CABG is considered appropriate in patients with one or more diseased vessels if they have a large area of viable myocardium and high-risk findings on noninvasive testing. The guidelines recommend a lower threshold for surgery in patients with proximal stenoses of the left anterior descending coronary artery than in other patients with one- or two-vessel disease, particularly if they have extensive evidence of ischemia on noninvasive studies or if they have a left ventricular ejection fraction less than 50 percent. The guidelines assume that surgery can be performed with acceptable risk. They also assume that patients' anginal symptoms are typical; if not, objective evidence of ischemia should be obtained.

ASYMPTOMATIC OR MILD ANGINA. The ACC/AHA task force considered CABG appropriate for patients with no or only mild symptoms even if they had only one- or two-vessel disease as long as they also had evidence of large amounts of myocardium in jeopardy on noninvasive testing. Even in the absence of markedly positive noninvasive tests for ischemia, patients with one- or two-vessel disease were considered to have uncertain (Class II) appropriateness for CABG. These guidelines therefore do not explicitly label as inappropriate any indications for CABG in patients with coronary artery disease. Since these patients are, by definition, free of disabling symptoms, the goal of surgery in this population is to prolong life. Class I subsets represent the groups in which survival benefits are most likely to be realized.

STABLE ANGINA. For patients with stable mild angina, indications for surgery are based on the likelihood of improving survival and on the probability of relieving life-threatening symptoms. Therefore, the ACC/AHA task force concluded that clearly appropriate indications for CABG in this population should include the same factors as for asymptomatic patients, as well as disabling angina. For patients with chronic stable angina and only moderate amounts of myocardium in jeopardy from ischemia on noninvasive stress testing, CABG was considered to be of uncertain appropriateness (Class IIa).

UNSTABLE ANGINA/NON-Q WAVE MYOCARDIAL INFARCTION. The indications for CABG in these patients include those for patients with no or stable angina symptoms but reflect uncertainty about the optimal timing of surgery. The guidelines recommend stabilization with aggressive medical therapy if possible before proceeding to CABG.

ST SEGMENT ELEVATION (Q WAVE) MYOCARDIAL INFARCTION. For patients with ST segment (Q wave) acute myocardial infarction, the ACC/AHA guidelines discourage the use of CABG in favor of thrombolytic therapy or coronary angioplasty. The guidelines recognize that CABG is warranted in certain conditions, such as the presence of left main stenosis, severe three-vessel disease, associated valve disease, and anatomy unsuitable for other forms of therapy. Otherwise, surgery is most likely to be appropriate when patients have not responded to maximal nonsurgical therapy (Class IIa). Recommendations on the optimal timing for repair of the mechanical complications of acute myocardial infarction (e.g., ventricular septal defect) were not included in these guidelines.

IMPAIRED LEFT VENTRICULAR FUNCTION. CABG is considered an appropriate or potentially appropriate strategy for the management of patients with impaired left ventricular ejection fractions because of evidence that ventricular dysfunction may be due to viable but hibernating myocardium in patients with severe multivessel disease. The guidelines consider surgery to be especially appropriate if the patient has clinical evidence of intermittent ischemia and minimal or no congestive heart failure. In patients with clinical heart failure, the decision to operate should be based on objective evidence of hibernating myocardium.[9, 10]

LIFE-THREATENING VENTRICULAR ARRHYTHMIAS. CABG can suppress arrhythmia induction in patients with ventricular arrhythmias, particularly when an ischemic etiology for the arrhythmia can be documented. However, because multiple other factors can contribute to the development of life-threatening ventricular arrhythmias, such as reentry pathways in scarred myocardium, concomitant insertion of an implantable cardioverter-defibrillator may be necessary for many patients who are candidates for CABG.

FAILED PTCA. The decision to perform CABG after failed PTCA must consider a variety of factors, including the mechanism of the failed procedure, the potential to improve the situation surgically, the extent of myocardium in jeopardy, and the patient's ability to tolerate CABG. Surgery is clearly *appropriate* when patients have or are in danger of hemodynamic compromise or when a foreign body such as an undeployed stent must be retrieved. However, CABG is *inappropriate* when patients do not have active ischemia or when CABG is unlikely to lead to revascularization of the myocardium in jeopardy.

AFTER PRIOR CABG. Reoperation after prior CABG is associated with increased risk and lower rates of relief of symptoms. Therefore, repeat CABG should be reserved for relief of disabling symptoms or clear evidence of life-threatening amounts of myocardium at risk. In patients with functioning internal mammary artery grafts to the left anterior descending artery, the potential loss of this graft with any repeat CABG is a significant disincentive to pursue this strategy.

Recommended Management Strategies

The ACC/AHA guidelines also offer recommendations on the evaluation and management of several specific issues before, during, and after CABG (Table 37–G–3). Among interventions aimed at reducing neurological damage after CABG is screening for carotid artery stenoses, which are often asymptomatic. Although the guidelines do not

Timing	Class Indication	Intervention	Comments
Preoperative			
Carotid screening	I	Carotid duplex ultrasound in a defined population	Carotid endarterectomy if stenosis ≥80%
Perioperative			
Antimicrobials	I	Prophylactic antimicrobials	
Antifibrinolytics	IIa	Aprotinin in selected groups	Significant reduction in blood transfusion requirements
Antiarrhythmics	I	Beta blockers to prevent postoperative atrial fibrillation	Propafenone or amiodarone are alternatives if beta blockers are contraindicated
Antiinflammatory drugs	IIa	Minimize diffuse inflammatory response to cardiopulmonary bypass	
Postoperative			
Antiplatelets	I	Aspirin to prevent early vein graft attrition	Ticlopidine or clopidogrel are alternatives if aspirin is contraindicated
Lipid-lowering therapy	I	Cholesterol-lowering agent plus low-fat diet if low-density lipoprotein cholesterol >100 mg/dl	3-Hydroxy-3-methylglutaryl/coenzyme A reductase inhibitors preferred if elevated low-density lipoprotein is major aberration
Smoking cessation	I	Smoking cessation education and possibly counseling and pharmacotherapy	

From Gibbons RJ, Chatterjee K, Daley J, et al: ACC/AHA/ACP-ASIM guidelines for the management of patients with chronic stable angina: A report of the American College of Cardiology/American Heart Association Task Force on Practice Guidelines (Committee on the Management of Patients with Chronic Stable Angina). J Am Coll Cardiol 33:2092–2197, 1999. Reprinted with permission from the American College of Cardiology.

explicitly call for all patients to undergo such screening, they note that many centers screen all those 65 years or older. Other patients who should undergo carotid artery ultrasound screening include those with a prior history of cerebrovascular disease.

Aspirin for the first year after CABG is considered the drug of choice for prophylaxis against early saphenous graft closure from thrombus; most patients continue this therapy indefinitely to reduce the risk for myocardial infarction. Patients with LDL cholesterol levels above 100 mg/dl warrant dietary and nondietary interventions to improve their lipid profile. Smoking cessation counseling should also be a routine part of care. The guidelines also indicate that cardiac rehabilitation should be offered to all eligible patients.

ORGANIZATIONAL CONSIDERATIONS. The ACC/AHA guidelines noted studies suggesting that survival after CABG is worse when performed at institutions or by operators performing a low volume of procedures annually. The guidelines commented that data support close monitoring of institutions or individuals performing fewer than 100 cases annually.

References

1. Gibbons RJ, Chatterjee K, Daley J, et al: ACC/AHA/ACP-ASIM guidelines for the management of patients with chronic stable angina: A report of the American College of Cardiology/American Heart Association Task Force on Practice Guidelines (Committee on the Management of Patients With Chronic Stable Angina). J Am Coll Cardiol 33:2092–2197, 1999.
2. Ryan TJ, Bauman WB, Kennedy JW, et al: Guidelines for percutaneous transluminal coronary angioplasty. A report of the American College of Cardiology/American Heart Association Task Force on Assessment of Diagnostic and Therapeutic Cardiovascular Procedures (Subcommittee on Percutaneous Transluminal Coronary Angioplasty). J Am Coll Cardiol 22:2033–2054, 1993.
3. Eagle KA, Guyton RA, Davidoff R, et al: ACC/AHA guidelines for coronary artery bypass graft surgery. A report of the American College of Cardiology/American Heart Association Task Force on Practice Guidelines (Committee to Revise the 1991 Guidelines for Coronary Artery Bypass Graft Surgery). J Am Coll Cardiol 34:1262–1347, 1999.
4. Braunwald E, Antman EM, Beasley JW, et al: ACC/AHA guidelines for the management of patients with unstable angina: A report of the American College of Cardiology/American Heart Association Task Force on Practice Guidelines (Committee on the Management of Patients with Unstable Angina). J Am Coll Cardiol, 36:970–1062, 2000.
5. The Society for Cardiac Angiography: Guidelines for credentialing and facilities for performance of coronary angioplasty. Cathet Cardiovasc Diagn 15:136–138, 1988.
6. Ryan TJ, Klocke FJ, Reynolds WA: Clinical competence in percutaneous transluminal coronary angioplasty: A statement for physicians from the ACP/ACC/AHA Task Force on Clinical Privileges in Cardiology. J Am Coll Cardiol 15:1469–1474, 1990.
7. Hirshfeld JW, Ellis SG, Faxon DP, et al: Recommendations for the assessment and maintenance of proficiency in coronary intervention procedures. Statement of the American College of Cardiology. J Am Coll Cardiol 31:722–743, 1998.
8. Kirklin JW, Akins CW, Blackstone EH, et al: Guidelines and indications for coronary artery bypass graft surgery. A report of the American College of Cardiology/American Heart Association Task Force on Assessment of Diagnostic and Therapeutic Cardiovascular Procedures (Subcommittee on Coronary Artery Bypass Graft Surgery). J Am Coll Cardiol 17:543, 1991.
9. Afridi I, Grayburn PA, Panza JA, et al: Myocardial viability during dobutamine echocardiography predicts survival in patients with coronary artery disease and severe left ventricular dysfunction. J Am Coll Cardiol 32:921, 1998.
10. Meluzin J, Cerny J, Frelich M, et al: Prognostic value of the amount of dysfunctional but viable myocardium in revascularized patients with coronary artery disease and left ventricular dysfunction. J Am Coll Cardiol 32:912, 1998.

Chapter 38

Percutaneous Coronary and Valvular Intervention

JEFFREY J. POPMA • RICHARD E. KUNTZ

The use of percutaneous coronary intervention (PCI) in patients with ischemic coronary artery disease (CAD) has expanded dramatically over the past two decades. More than 650,000 patients underwent PCI in 1999 in the United States, far exceeding the number of patients undergoing coronary artery bypass graft surgery (CABG). Continual technological improvements (e.g., stents, atherectomy and thrombectomy devices), refinements in periprocedural adjunctive pharmacology (e.g., glycoprotein IIb-IIIa [GP IIb-IIIa] inhibitors), and a better understanding of early and late outcomes in patients with comorbidities have fostered the expanded use of PCI as definitive therapy for ischemic CAD.

This chapter will review (1) the current methods used for PCI, including conventional balloon angioplasty and new coronary devices; (2) the procedural outcomes and complication rates obtained with contemporary PCI methods; (3) the periprocedural pharmacological strategies to reduce acute complications and restenosis after PCI; and (4) recommendations for coronary revascularization in patients with ischemic CAD, with consideration of the alternatives of medical therapy, PCI, and CABG. A discussion of the current issues in patient selection, technical performance, and outcomes associated with percutaneous mitral and aortic valvuloplasty is also included.

HISTORICAL PERSPECTIVE

Balloon angioplasty, or percutaneous transluminal coronary angioplasty (PTCA), was first performed by Andreas Gruentzig in 1977 with the use of a prototype, fixed-wire balloon catheter.[1] The procedure was initially limited to patients with symptomatic CAD who had focal lesions in proximal coronary vessels and was used as an alternative to CABG.[1] Because of an objective reduction in stenosis severity and consistent improvement in clinical ischemia with this novel method,[2] the number of patients treated with balloon PTCA expanded dramatically over the next decade.[3] Operator experience and equipment design also evolved rapidly, with a transition from poorly steerable, fixed-wire balloon dilatation catheters to highly steerable, over-the-wire, and rapid-exchange balloon dilatation systems. These catheter designs resulted in more flexible, trackable, and lower-profile balloon dilatation systems and allowed the expansion of PCI to a broader spectrum of patients, such as those with multivessel disease, "high-risk" anatomy, reduced left ventricular function, and other serious comorbid medical conditions.[3]

It soon became apparent that two major issues limited the widespread use of balloon PTCA in patients with symptomatic CAD. Abrupt vessel closure resulting from angioplasty-induced dissection and thrombus formation occurred in 6.8 to 8.3 percent of cases,[4-6] largely unpredictable in individual patients despite the description of several predisposing factors in a number of series.[7-10] Although in-laboratory abrupt vessel closure was reversible in most patients, emergency CABG was occasionally (3 to 5 percent of cases) required to relieve ongoing transmural ischemia resulting from catheter-based complications. In some cases, the urgency of surgical revascularization mandated that saphenous vein grafts (SVGs) be used instead of the preferred arterial conduits. The second major limitation of balloon PTCA was the development of restenosis, either clinically manifested by symptom recurrence or identified as recurrent arterial narrowing by routine repeat angiography. The pathology of restenosis has remained poorly understood, and pharmacological agents have not consistently reduced its occurrence.

A number of new coronary devices were developed in the early 1990s to improve upon the early and late procedural outcomes achieved with balloon PTCA. These novel methods were designed to remove (e.g., directional, rotational, or extraction atherectomy), ablate (e.g., excimer laser angioplasty), or scaffold (e.g., stents) atherosclerotic plaque. Randomized clinical trials have shown that some devices (e.g., stents) resulted in better early and late clinical outcome while others (e.g., excimer laser angioplasty) imparted no incremental clinical benefit and were potentially detrimental in comparison to balloon PTCA.

Given these devices' diverse mechanisms of benefit and their niche application in selected patients, it became apparent that a "lesion-specific" approach to coronary angioplasty was required, with the specific type of revascularization tailored to the precise characteristics of the vessel wall pathology. Coronary angioplasty then encompassed the use of both balloons and new devices, and the generic term *percutaneous coronary intervention* was introduced.

BALLOON PTCA

Balloon PTCA expands the coronary lumen by stretching and tearing the atherosclerotic plaque and vessel wall and, to a lesser extent, by redistributing atherosclerotic plaque along its longitudinal axis.[11, 12] There is no evidence that balloon PTCA compresses atherosclerotic plaque.

TECHNICAL ASPECTS. Balloon PTCA is performed by over-the-wire, rapid-exchange, or fixed-wire balloon dilatation systems. A 1.0 to 1.1:1.0 balloon-to-artery ratio is optimal for balloon size selection; higher ratios are associated with complications, and lower ones predispose to restenosis.[13] Although "stand-alone" balloon PTCA is usually (>80 percent) effective in improving ischemic symptoms, it is limited by substantial early elastic recoil, which results in an average 30 to 35 percent residual stenosis. On occasion, propagation of a coronary dissection and superimposed platelet thrombus formation after balloon PTCA result in early complications, including abrupt vessel closure. An "optimal" angiographic result (<20 percent residual stenosis) is obtained in less than 25 percent of patients after balloon PTCA but is associated with a favorable late clinical outcome. Documentation of an "optimal" anatomical *and* physiological result with balloon PTCA requires the addition of Doppler flow measurements[14] or determination of transstenosis pressure gradients (e.g., fractional flow reserve)[15] (see Chap. 12). In a prospective study of 225 patients with an angiographically successful result after balloon PTCA, postprocedural distal coronary flow reserve and percent diameter stenosis were correlated with symptoms and the need for target lesion revascularization (TLR) 1 and 6 months later.[14] Distal coronary flow reserve of 2.5 or higher and residual percent diameter stenosis of 35 or less after balloon PTCA identified lesions with lower rates of 6-month symptom recurrence (23 vs. 47 percent; $p = 0.005$), need for reintervention (16 vs. 34 percent; $p = 0.024$), and restenosis (16 vs. 41 percent; $p = 0.002$) when compared with patients who did not meet these criteria.[14]

Assessment of Outcome. A number of indices have been used to assess both early and late procedural outcomes. *Anatomical (or angiographic) success* has been defined as achieving smaller than 50 percent residual diameter stenosis with Thrombolysis in Myocardial Infarction (TIMI) 3 flow (see Chap. 12) after balloon PTCA,[16] with or without a 20 percent or greater improvement in diameter stenosis.[3] Visually determined angiographic success rates may overestimate the results provided by more quantitative angiographic measurements by 10 to 20 percent, although visual assessment by investigators has been correlated with clinical outcomes in at least one study.[17] *Procedural success* is generally defined as angiographic success without the occurrence of major complications (death, myocardial infarction, or CABG)[16, 18] either during the index hospitalization or within the 30 days of the procedure.[19] *Periprocedural vessel closure* is defined as *abrupt* (TIMI 0 or 1 flow), *subacute* (abrupt closure occurring after the patient leaves the catheterization laboratory but within 30 days of the procedure), and *threatened* (presence of two or more of the following: angina; ischemic electrocardiographic changes; residual diameter stenosis greater than 50 percent; National Heart, Lung, and Blood Institute [NHLBI] type B or C dissection, with length greater than 8 mm; or NHLBI type D, E, or F dissection or deteriorating angiographic appearance with TIMI flow of 0 to 2). (See Chapter 12 for definitions of TIMI flow grades and NHLBI dissection types.)

Procedure-induced non-Q-wave myocardial infarction, as defined by an elevation in creatine phosphokinase isoenzyme (CPK-MB) of three times normal or higher,[18, 20, 21] occurs in 5 to 10 percent of procedures,[20, 22] but its causal relationship to late mortality is unclear.[22, 23] *Clinical success* is defined as procedural success without the need for urgent repeat PCI or surgical revascularization within the first 30 days of the procedure.[18]

INITIAL CLINICAL RESULTS. Procedural success rates after balloon PTCA have progressively improved over the past 20 years (Table 38-1). An 88 percent angiographic success rate was obtained in patients with multivessel CAD enrolled in the 1988-1991 Bypass Angioplasty Revascularization Investigators (BARI) Trial, but major complications were frequent and included death (1.1 percent), Q wave myocardial infarction (2.1 percent), and CABG (6.3 percent).[26] Major complications after balloon PTCA in other registry series include in-hospital death (0.9 to 3.5 percent), Q wave myocardial infarction (1.0 to 1.7 percent), emergency CABG (2.1 to 6.0 percent) and stroke (<0.5 percent).[33] Minor complications after balloon PTCA include acute or subacute vessel closure requiring urgent repeat balloon PTCA, coronary dissection, sidebranch occlusion, ventricular arrhythmias, vascular access complications, renal insufficiency, coronary perforation, and rarely, cardiac tamponade.

The recent availability of "bailout" coronary stents has reduced the emergency CABG rate after balloon PTCA to less than 1 percent.[34] In one series reporting recent procedural outcomes in 34,752 procedures performed in Northern New England Cardiovascular Group hospitals, adjusted clinical success rates increased from 88.2 percent in 1990 to 1993 to 91.9 percent in 1995 to 1997 ($p < 0.001$).[35] With the combination of balloon PTCA and new devices, higher (95 to 99 percent) procedural success rates are now reported, particularly in women.[36]

Early procedural outcome after balloon PTCA has been correlated with a number of clinical, angiographic, and procedural factors identified in the periprocedural period.[7, 8, 24, 33] *Clinical factors* include age, unstable and Canadian Cardiovascular Society (CCS) Class IV angina, congestive heart failure, cardiogenic shock, renal insufficiency, and preprocedural instability requiring intraaortic balloon pump support, among other factors.[33] *Anatomical variables* include multivessel CAD, presence of thrombus, SVG intervention,

and American College of Cardiology/American Heart Association (ACC/AHA) type C lesion morphology,[16, 33] including chronic total coronary occlusion. *Procedural factors* also affect procedure outcomes, including a higher final percent diameter stenosis, smaller minimal lumen diameter, and the presence of a residual dissection or transstenotic pressure gradient (see Chap. 12 for definitions of ACC/AHA lesion types). Procedural mortality is associated with balloon PTCA of arteries subtending 50 percent or more of the myocardium, a left ventricular ejection fraction less than 25 percent, a more severe preprocedural percent diameter stenosis, multivessel CAD, and female gender, among other factors.[37, 38] These latter factors indicate a greater risk for cardiovascular collapse should abrupt vessel closure occur.[39]

LATE CLINICAL OUTCOME. Clinical events after balloon PTCA are attributable to arterial renarrowing at the PTCA site, progression or instability of atherosclerotic disease at remote sites, or both.[40] These processes can be partially distinguished by the time of occurrence of the event—with angiographic and clinical restenosis generally developing within 6 to 9 months after balloon PTCA[41, 42] and death, myocardial infarction, and progression of atherosclerosis occurring with a low, but constant hazard (1 to 2 percent risk per year) indefinitely after the procedure.

Predictors of higher risk of all-cause late mortality include advanced age,[43] reduced left ventricular function or congestive heart failure,[43] presence of diabetes mellitus,[27, 43] female gender,[44] number of diseased vessels,[43, 45] inoperable disease,[43] or severe concomitant disease.[43] In patients undergoing balloon PTCA, a 95 percent 10-year survival rate was reported in those with single-vessel CAD and an 81 percent 10-year survival rate in those with multivessel CAD.[45] Five-year cardiac mortality rates for patients enrolled in the PTCA Registry were 2.8 percent in patients with single-vessel disease, 6.1 percent in patients with two-vessel disease, and 9.9 percent in patients with three-vessel disease.[43] Higher 9-year mortality rates have also been reported in diabetic patients (35.9 vs. 17.9 percent in nondiabetic patients; $p < 0.01$).[46]

The risk of restenosis after balloon PTCA is influenced by *clinical factors*, such as diabetes mellitus, unstable angina, acute myocardial infarction, and prior restenosis, by *anatomical factors*, such as total occlusions, proximal left anterior descending artery lesions, smaller vessel size, long lesions, and lesions involving an SVG, and by *procedural factors*, such as the final minimal lumen diameter or percent diameter stenosis. Exposure to infectious agents may also predispose to the development of restenosis.[47]

INDICATIONS FOR BALLOON PTCA. A provisional strategy consisting of balloon PTCA with "bailout" (or "provisional") stenting for lesions with abrupt or threatened closure or suboptimal (>40 percent) residual stenosis may be chosen as an alternative to primary stenting in patients with vessel size 2.75 mm or greater and lesion length less than 25 mm, although the advantages of this approach have not been documented in randomized trials. Provisional balloon PTCA may be preferred over primary stenting in small (<2.75 mm) vessels, long (≥25 mm) lesions, anastomotic stenoses in SVGs, and others lesions deemed "high risk" for coronary stenting.

CORONARY ATHERECTOMY

Atherectomy devices provide symptomatic relief in patients with CAD by two primary mechanisms: (1) removal or ablation of the atherosclerotic plaque[48] and (2) improvement in vessel wall compliance by plaque fracture and excision.[49] The primary advantage of atherectomy over balloon PTCA is that a larger final minimal lumen diameter can be

▶ TABLE 38–1. IN-HOSPITAL OUTCOMES ASSOCIATED WITH BALLOON PTCA OVER TIME

VARIABLE	NHLBI-I	NHLBI-II	MAPS	MAPS	BARI	BOAT PTCA ARM	STRESS PTCA ARM	BENESTENT II PTCA ARM	CUTTING BALLOON PTCA ARM
Years of entry	1977–81	1985–86	1986–87	1991	1989–92	1994–95	1991–93	1995–96	1994–96
Number of patients	1155	1802	400	200	915	492	203	413	621
New device use	No	No	No	Yes	No	"Bailout"	"Bailout"	"Bailout"	"Bailout"
Baseline factors									
Mean age (yr)	54	58	58	62	62	58	60	50	58
Women (%)	25	26	29	30	27	24	27	23	23
Diabetes mellitus	9	14	19	25	19	14	16	13	12
Unstable angina (%)	37	49	48	51	63	NA	48	45	64
Multivessel disease (%)	26	53	100	100	100	NA	32	NA	NA
Angiographic success (%)	68	91	NA	92	88	NA	92.6	99	NA
Procedure success (%)	61	78	83.5	90	80	87	89.6	96	94.7
In-hospital complications	NA	NA	NA	NA	NA	3.3	7.9	7.0	5.3
Death (%)	1.2	1.0	1.0	1.0	1.1	0.4	1.5	0	0
Q wave infarction (%)	4.9	4.3	2.0	1.5	2.1	1.2	3.0	1.2	1.0
Emergency CABG (%)	5.8	3.4	5.5	1.0	6.3	2.0	4.0	0.7	NA
Late clinical outcome	5 yr	5 yr	1 yr	1 yr	5.4 yr	1 yr	240 d	12 mo	6 mo
Any event	NA	NA	NA	NA	NA	31.1	23.8	23.2	15.1
Death (%)	4.9	8.3	NA	NA	13.7	1.6	0	1.0	NA
Q wave MI (%)	9.7	9.1	NA	NA	21.3	1.6	0.5	1.9	NA
Revascularization (%)	32.1	38.8	NA	NA	54.5	19.7	15.4	18.9	14.8
Repeat PTCA	22.5	30.9	16.2	13.2	23.2	NA	11.4	9.4	NA
CABG	15.5	13.4	13.4	8.1	20.5	NA	4.5	1.9	NA

CABG = coronary artery bypass graft; MI = myocardial infarction; NA = not available; PTCA = percutaneous transluminal coronary angioplasty.

Data from National Heart, Lung, and Blood Institute (NHLBI) Study I and II[3]; Multivessel Angioplasty Prognosis Study (MAPS) Group[24, 25]; Bypass Angioplasty Revascularization Investigators (BARI)[26–28]; Balloon Versus Optimal Atherectomy Trial (BOAT)[29]; Stent Restenosis Study (STRESS) Investigators[30]; Belgium Netherlands Stent (BENESTENT) II Trial[31]; Cutting Balloon Angioplasty.[32]

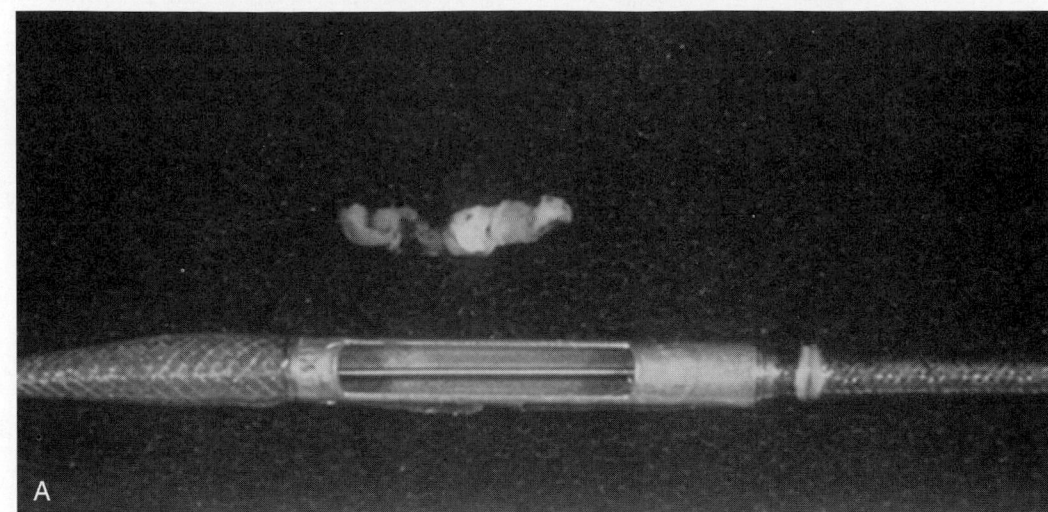

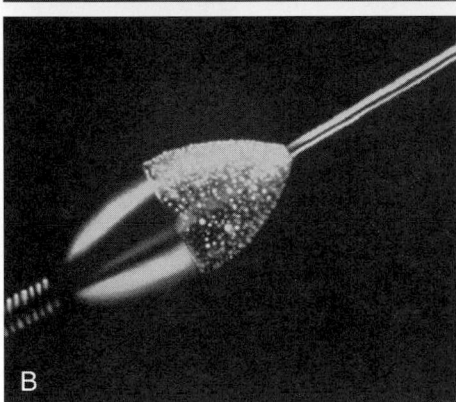

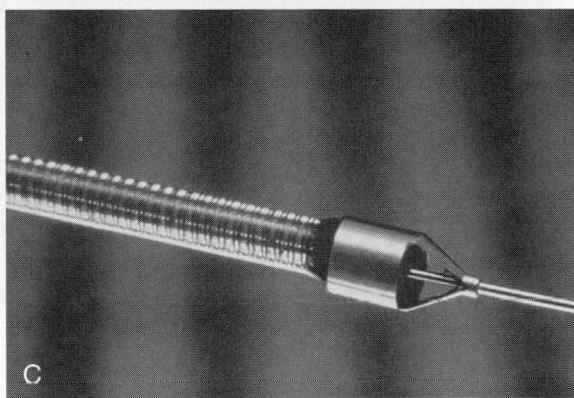

FIGURE 38–1. Atherectomy devices. *A,* Directional coronary atherectomy device with macroscopic tissue resection. *B,* Rotational atherectomy device. *C,* Transluminal extraction catheter.

achieved with atherectomy.[50, 50a] The loss index, defined as the fractional relationship between acute lumen gain and late lumen loss, is largely unchanged with atherectomy, which suggests that these devices do not lessen the degree of arterial injury and subsequent repair.[50] Atherectomy use reached its peak (30 percent of interventional procedures) between 1992 and 1994 but fell dramatically after the clinical availability of coronary stents. It is estimated that 5 to 20 percent of cases currently involve the use of atherectomy devices, alone or in combination with coronary stenting (Fig. 38–1).

Directional Coronary Atherectomy

Directional coronary atherectomy (DCA) was first performed in coronary arteries in 1986 with large (7 French), stiff, prototype atherectomy devices. A clinical study of 873 patients treated with DCA was initiated in 1988 and reported a primary success rate (tissue removal, ≥20 percent reduction in diameter stenosis, and <50 percent residual stenosis after DCA alone) of 85 percent, which increased to 92 percent after adjunct PTCA.[51] Procedural complications included death (0.5 percent), nonfatal Q wave myocardial infarction (0.9 percent), and emergency CABG (4.0 percent). Six-month angiography demonstrated a 42 percent restenosis rate (≥50 percent diameter stenosis). The restenosis rate was lower in de novo than restenotic lesions in both native vessels (30 and 46 percent, respectively) and SVGs (31 and 68 percent, respectively).[51]

Approximately 18 to 20 mg of macroscopic tissue is removed with DCA, although plaque excision accounts for only 70 percent of the lumen gain achieved with DCA.[52, 53] The remaining lumen improvement is achieved through mechanical dilatation by the DCA catheter, balloon PTCA, and to a lesser extent, changes in radial compliance of the vessel by excision of deep wall elastic components.[53] Intra-

vascular ultrasound (IVUS) studies show that a substantial amount (43 to 55 percent cross-sectional narrowing) of atherosclerotic plaque remains even after "optimal DCA."[53–55]

TECHNICAL ASPECTS. The DCA catheter contains a 9-mm, 120-degree cutting window and a contralateral, low–inflation pressure (15 to 45 psi) balloon that forces atherosclerotic plaque into the cutting window. A cup-shaped rotating (2500 rpm) cutter excises macroscopic amounts of atherosclerotic plaque and stores it in a distal collection chamber until its removal. A 6F DCA catheter is recommended for smaller vessels (<3.0 mm) and a 7F DCA device for larger ones (≥3.0 mm). Use of the 5F device is unusual and reserved for subtotal occlusions, calcified vessels, or moderately tortuous vessels; the amount of plaque retrieval with this device is limited.

Large (9.5F to10F) guiding catheters are generally needed for the 5F to 7F DCA catheters. Forceful advancement of the DCA catheter and deep seating of the guiding catheter should be avoided because the stiff guiding catheter may dissect the coronary ostium or proximal portion of the vessel. Tissue removal is achieved by positioning the DCA catheter across the target lesion, inflating the balloon to 10 to 20 psi, and advancing the motor-driven cutter forward slowly. The balloon is deflated after each cut and the device rotated 45 to 90 degrees to reorient it toward the residual plaque. Higher balloon inflation pressures may be used on subsequent cuts to increase the effective working diameter of the device. Adjunct balloon PTCA is often (80 percent) performed to further improve the residual lumen diameter or, less commonly, to treat DCA-induced dissection, although it may have limited incremental benefit on the prevention of restenosis if an "optimal" IVUS-guided DCA result is achieved.[55] An "optimal" DCA result is defined as a final diameter stenosis less than 10 percent, tissue removal, and the avoidance of major clinical complications (death, Q wave myocardial infarction, or emergency CABG).

INITIAL CLINICAL RESULTS. "Optimal" DCA generally results in low (<20 percent) quantitatively determined residual stenosis and a smooth-appearing lumen without dissection; procedural success rates greater than 95 percent have been reported by experienced centers[29, 53, 56, 57] (Table 38–2). "Conservative" atherectomy using smaller DCA devices and no adjunct balloon PTCA results in higher (>25 percent) residual stenosis and more complications and has no benefit over balloon PTCA.[58–60]

Major complications after "optimal" DCA include procedural mortality (<1.0 percent), emergency CABG (<2.0 percent), Q wave myocar-

▶ TABLE 38–2. EARLY AND LATE OUTCOMES AFTER DIRECTIONAL CORONARY ATHERECTOMY IN NATIVE CORONARY ARTERIES

METHOD	CAVEAT PTCA	CAVEAT DCA	C-CAT PTCA	C-CAT DCA	OARS IVUS + DCA	ABACUS DCA	ABACUS DCA + PTCA	BOAT PTCA	BOAT DCA	START Stent	START DCA	SOLD DCA + Stent
Years of entry	1991–92	1991–92	1991–92	1991–92	1993–95	1994–1995	1994–1995	1994–95	1994–95	1995–1997	1995–1997	1996–97
Number of patients	500	512	136	138	199	106	108	492	497	62	60	71
Baseline factors												
Mean age (yr)	59	59	55	58	58	62	60	58	58	62	64	57
Diabetes mellitus (%)	19	19	15	17	17	19	21	14	14	29	22	14
Unstable angina (%)	70	66	52	39	78	30	22	NA	NA	NR	NR	33
Angiographic success (%)	80	89*	91	98	NR		95.1+	NR	NR	NR	NR	NR
Procedure success (%)	76	82+	88	94	98		99.5	87	93‡	NR	NR	96
Reference Diameter (mm)	2.9	2.9	3.13	3.23	3.28	3.24	3.21	3.20	3.25	3.23	3.29	3.27
MLD (mm)												
Baseline	NR	NR	0.89	0.94	1.19	1.04	1.03	1.04	1.07	1.00	1.01	0.87
Final	1.80	2.02*	2.10	2.34*	3.16	2.60	2.88§	2.33	2.82*	2.80	2.89	3.47
Follow-up	NR	NR	1.55	1.61	1.55	1.80	1.85	1.68	1.86‡	1.89	2.18	2.57
Percent diameter stenosis												
Baseline	73	71	71.5	70.6	63.5	68.7	68.0	NR	NR	NR	NR	74
Final	36	29	33	26*	7.1	15.0	10.8§	28.1	14.7*	14.7	12.7	0.4
Follow-up	NR	NR	48.4	48.7	37.0	32.3	33.4	45.6	40.1‡	40.1	32.1	21
Restenosis rate (%)	57	50	43	46	28.9	19.6	23.6	39.8	31.4¶	32.8	15.8	11
Early complications (†)	5	11*	6	5								
Death	0.4	0	0	0	0	0	0	0.4	0	NR	NR	1.4
Q wave MI	2	2	0	0.7	1.5	0.9	0	1.2	2.0	NR	NR	2.8
Emergency CABG	2	3	4.4	1.4	1.0	0	0	2.0	1.0	NR	NR	1.4
Follow-up time		1 yr	6 mo		1 yr		1 yr		1 yr		1 yr	NR
Late clinical events (%)	42.4	38.7	29	29		18.1	21.9	24.8	21.1**	33.9	18.3**	NR
Death	0.6	2.2+	1.6	0.7	1.0	0	0	0.6	0.6	1.6	0	NR
Q wave MI	1.2	2.9	1.6	0	1.5	0.9	0	1.6	2.0	NR	NR	NR
TRL			27.9	28.7	17.8	15.2	21.9	NR	NR	29	15	NR
Repeat PCI	25.9	24.4	23.3	23.5	NR	NR	NR	NR	NR	NR	NR	NR
CABG	9.1	9.3	4.6	5.2	NR	NR	NR	NR	NR	3.2	0	NR

* $p < 0.001$.
+ Optimal angiographic (<30 percent diameter stenosis) result.
‡ $p < 0.005$.
§ $p < 0.01$.
¶ $p < 0.05$.
** Target vessel failure (death, Q wave MI, or target vessel revascularization.

CABG = coronary artery bypass graft; DCA = directional coronary atherectomy; IVUS = intravascular ultrasound; MI = myocardial infarction; MLD = minimal lumen diameter; NR = not reported; PCI = percutaneous coronary intervention; PTCA = percutaneous transluminal coronary angioplasty; TLR = target lesion revascularization.

Data from Coronary Angioplasty Versus Excisional Atherectomy Trial (CAVEAT),[58, 59] C-CAT = Canadian Coronary Atherectomy Trial (C-CAT),[59] Optimal Atherectomy Restenosis Study (OARS),[53] Optimal Atherectomy Trial,[60] Adjunctive Balloon Angioplasty after Intravascular Ultrasound = Guided Optimal Directional Coronary Atherectomy (ABACUS),[55] Balloon vs Optimal Atherectomy Trial (BOAT),[29] Stent Versus Directional Coronary Atherectomy Randomized Trial (START),[61] and Stenting after Optimal Lesion Debulking (SOLD) Registry.[62]

dial infarction, (<1.0 percent), and transient or sustained abrupt vessel closure (2.0 to 4.2 percent).[29, 53, 63] The occurrence of dissection resulting from guide catheter trauma,[64] distal nose cone injury, or guidewire trauma has been reduced with improvements in catheter design and greater operator experience. Other complications include perforation (1.0 percent), sidebranch occlusion (3 percent), vasospasm, "no reflow," and distal plaque embolization (2 percent).[65] The frequency of these complications, particularly atheroembolism, may be higher (13.4 percent) in SVGs.[63] No reflow can be treated with intracoronary agents such as verapamil (100 to 200 μg),[65] diltiazem (500 μg),[66] or nitroprusside (100 to 200 μg). Depending on the definition used, coronary aneurysms after successful DCA have been reported in a few cases.

Frequent (11.5 to 19.0 percent) elevations in creatine kinase isoenzymes (CK-MB) have been reported after DCA.[58, 60] Initial series reported an association between CPK-MB elevations and late mortality,[20, 59] although more recent, prospective studies suggest that clinically silent, low-level CPK-MB elevations may not be independently associated with worse outcomes[67, 68, 68a, 68b]; the causal relationship between periprocedural myocardial necrosis and late mortality may be confounded by the degree of underlying atherosclerosis.[68] The GP IIb/IIIa blocker abciximab reduces the incidence of non-Q-wave myocardial infarction by more than 50 percent in patients undergoing DCA.[69]

LATE CLINICAL OUTCOME. Arterial remodeling, or vessel constriction, between 1 and 6 months after DCA is the major cause of restenosis after this procedure,[54] although varying amounts of intimal hyperplasia may also occur. Significantly ($p < 0.05$) lower angiographic restenosis rates are obtained in patients with discrete, native vessel lesions who undergo "optimal" DCA (31.4 percent) as compared with balloon PTCA (39.8 percent),[29] a finding attributable to the larger final lumen diameter achieved after DCA.[29, 50] "Conservative" atherectomy using smaller DCA devices (without adjunct balloon PTCA) confers no restenosis benefit over balloon PTCA.[58, 60] DCA does not reduce restenosis in de novo lesions located in the body of SVGs[63] and may lead to higher complication rates. Initial concerns that deep adventitial resection results in higher recurrence rates[70] have not been substantiated in larger series.[71]

One small (N = 122) randomized trial has suggested that IVUS-guided "optimal" DCA results in lower angiographic restenosis rates than does stenting (15.8 vs. 33.9 percent; $p = 0.032$),[61] although it is not known whether DCA is better than stenting when IVUS guidance is not performed. DCA has also been used prior to stent implantation for removal of atherosclerotic plaque, which potentially lessens the degree of late lumen loss and restenosis[62, 72]; this effect was independent of the final minimal lumen diameter in one case-matched series.[73] The AMIGO Trial, a large randomized trial comparing DCA followed by stent implantation and stent implantation alone, is under way to evaluate the effect of debulking prior to stenting on the prevention of late restenosis.

INDICATIONS. DCA may be used as an alternative to balloon PTCA to prevent restenosis in patients with de novo lesions in vessels larger than 3.0 mm. DCA may also be used in bifurcation lesions involving a large branch, ostial lesions of the right coronary artery or SVG, and the ostium of the left anterior descending artery, particularly in the case of an acute angle with the origin of the left circumflex. DCA may also be useful for the treatment of in-stent restenosis in larger vessels. Although DCA can be used successfully to rescue failed or suboptimal balloon PTCA, the availability of coronary stents has markedly reduced DCA use in this circumstance. DCA is limited in its ability to remove plaque in the presence of significant (>180 degrees) superficial calcium.[74]

Rotational Atherectomy

The rotational atherectomy (RA) device, or Rotablator (Boston Scientific, Natick, MA), is considered an atherectomy device, although ablation occurs by plaque pulverization rather than by tissue removal. RA relies on differential plaque abrasion in which inelastic tissue (i.e., calcified plaque) is selectively abraded while elastic tissue (i.e., soft plaque) is deflected away from the atherectomy burr.[75] The microparticles generated, 2 to 5 μm in diameter, pass through the coronary microcirculation and are removed by the reticuloendothelial system without interfering with the coronary microcirculation.[75, 76] Lower (140,000 rpm) rotational speeds are associated with less platelet activation and aggregation than are higher (180,000 rpm) speeds.[77] The use of GP IIb-IIIa inhibitors also reduces the degree of platelet aggregation and hypoperfusion associated with

RA.[78] Although coronary flow reserve may be impaired after RA,[79] there is generally no long-term impact on the global left ventricular ejection fraction.

TECHNICAL ASPECTS. The Rotablator device consists of an olive-shaped, stainless steel burr with diamond chips measuring 20 to 50 μm in diameter embedded in its distal portion.[75, 80] The burr is advanced over a 0.009-inch stainless steel guidewire with a 0.017-inch radiopaque platinum coil at its distal tip. A lubricating 4.3F Teflon sheath encases the drive shaft, and a compressed-air turbine rotates it between 140,000 and 200,000 rpm. Burrs for coronary use are available in diameters ranging from 1.25 to 2.50 mm. Current guiding catheter technology allows the passage of 1.25- to 2.15-mm burrs through an 8F guiding catheter, a 2.25- and 2.38-mm burr through a 9F guiding catheter, and a 2.50-mm burr through a 10F guiding catheter.[75]

A prophylactic temporary pacemaker should be positioned prior to RA of right coronary lesions. Because vasodilator administration is routine during this procedure, all patients should be volume-expanded to avoid hypotension after nitrate or calcium channel antagonist use. Two guidewires are available for RA—a floppy guidewire and an extra-support guidewire. The floppy wire minimizes guidewire bias, thereby preventing deep plaque ablation and tissue injury in regions of angulation or vessel tortuosity, and the extra-support guidewire is useful in lesions that require added wire support for burr advancement. After the burr has been advanced just proximal to the lesion in the reference segment, the "platform" speed is adjusted to 150,000 to 180,000 rpm. Short-duration (15 to 30 seconds) burr advancements are recommended, with rapid decelerations of greater then 5000 rpm avoided.[75] Deceleration below 140,000 rpm can lead to inadvertent stalling, burr entrapment, dissection, or vessel occlusion.[75] Two to four passes are made with each burr, with 30 to 60 seconds between passes to allow coronary perfusion.

A stepped-approach (0.50-mm increments up to 2.0 mm, then 0.25-mm increments thereafter) to RA is generally used in larger (>3.0 mm) vessels or for the treatment of diffuse or heavily calcified lesions. Aggressive RA (burr-to-artery ratios of >0.7) techniques do not provide a restenosis advantage over more conservative (burr-to-artery ratio of ≤0.7) methods.[81] Adjunctive balloon PTCA is used in most (82 to 88 percent) cases to reduce residual percent diameter stenosis or to treat coronary dissections.[82–84]

INITIAL CLINICAL RESULTS. RA registries have reported high (88 to 98.6 percent) procedural success rates in complex lesions[82, 83, 85, 86] (Table 38–3). In two large multicenter series, major complications were uncommon after RA but included death (0.31 percent), Q wave myocardial infarction (1 to 2.2 percent), and emergency CABG (0.4 to 0.9 percent).[83, 84] A higher (19 percent) incidence of non-Q-wave myocardial infarction after RA was reported in one study of long (>2 cm) lesions.[89] Other complications include transient or sustained dissection (12 percent), sidebranch occlusion (3 percent), distal embolization (3 percent), and abrupt closure (5 percent).[83] "No reflow" occurs significantly more often after RA (7.7 percent) than after balloon PTCA (0.3 percent) and may be improved with the periprocedural use of intracoronary calcium antagonists[66] or pretreatment with GP IIb-IIIa antagonists.[78] Perforations are rare after RA and may be successfully treated with prolonged balloon inflation.[90] Transient bradycardia and atrioventricular block are occasionally seen during RA, particularly during RA of the right coronary artery.

The procedural outcome in complex lesions may be better after RA than after other methods of PCI. In the Excimer, Rotablator, or Balloon Angioplasty for Complex Lesions (ERBAC) Study, patients with complex native coronary lesions were randomly assigned to treatment with RA, excimer laser angioplasty, or balloon PTCA. Procedure success rates were significantly ($p = 0.016$) higher in patients treated with RA (89 percent) than in those treated with balloon PTCA (80 percent) or excimer laser angioplasty (77 percent); major complication rates did not differ among the three groups.[87]

Predictors of major ischemic complications after RA include female gender; lesions with irregularity, lesions 4 mm or longer, or lesions with outflow obstruction; right coronary artery lesions; angulated (>60 degrees) lesions; and lesions involving a bifurcation or 4 mm or longer.[84] Predictors of "no reflow" include a recent history of myocardial infarction and a right coronary lesion.[84, 91] Larger decelerations (>5000 rpm) are also associated with higher complication rates after RA.[75]

LATE CLINICAL OUTCOME. RA does not appear to reduce restenosis compared with balloon PTCA. Observational studies report high rates of clinical restenosis (38 percent), TLR (36 percent), and angiographic restenosis (31 to 59 percent) (see Table 38–3). In the ERBAC Study, angiographic restenosis at 6 months was similar in patients treated with RA (57 percent), excimer laser angioplasty (59 percent), or balloon PTCA (47 percent).[87] Although smaller burrs were generally used in this study, no restenosis benefit was found in a randomized study of "aggressive" and "conservative" approaches to RA.[81] Predictors of 1-year clinical events after RA include male gender, high risk for surgery, bifurcation lesions, or lesions that are eccentric, long, or highly stenosed.[83] Two series have shown that adjunct stent placement after RA is associated with larger lumen diameter than attained with bal-

▶ TABLE 38–3. EARLY AND LATE OUTCOME AFTER ROTATIONAL CORONARY ATHERECTOMY

VARIABLE	NACI REGISTRY	BEAUMONT RA	ELLIS RA	SETON RA	ERBAC			WASHINGTON HOSPITAL CENTER			DART	
					PTCA	RA	ELCA	RA	Stent	RA + Stent	PTCA	RA
Years of entry	1990–94	1988–91	1989–92	1990–92	1991–1993			1990–1996			1994–1995	
Number of patients	525	104	316	242	222	231	232	147	103	56	219	227
Baseline factors												
Mean age (yr)	65	58	64	63	63	62	62	67	65	67	61	61
Women (%)	46	22	26	24	19	20	22	29	25	25	30	40
Diabetes mellitus (%)	23	NA	24	22	16	15	17	17	27	25	31	33
Unstable angina (%)	53	NA	39	35	12	18	16	37	46	30	41.7	44
Multivessel disease (%)	59	62	59	45	52	59	52	NR	NR	NR	41.6	50.9
Angiographic success (%)	89	96	89.8	95	80	89	77	NR	NR	NR	97.2	96.4
Procedure success (%)	88	NR	NR	94	83.3	90.5	90.5	98.6	98	98.2	94.1	91.6
Early complications (%)	NR		8.9	4.3	3.1	3.2	4.3	0	1	1.8	0	0.4
Death	0.8	0.9	0.3	0	0.9	0.9	0.9	0	1	1.8	0	0
Q wave infarction	1.1	4.4	2.2	3.3	1.8	1.3	1.3	0.68	0.97	0	0	0
Emergency CABG	0.4	1.9	0.9	1.2	0.5	0.9	2.2	0.68	0.97	0	0	0.9
CK-MB >3 × normal	NA	2.7	5.7	NA	NA	NA	NA	14.7	15.4	25.9	NR	NR
Reference diameter (mm)	2.77	3.20	NR	NR	2.80	2.88	2.99	3.20	3.36	3.35*	2.46	2.46
MLD (mm)												
Before RA	0.91	1.0	NR	NR	0.74	0.71	0.74	1.01	1.06	1.12	0.89	0.89
After RA	1.53	1.4	NR	NR	NA	NA	NA	NR	NR	NR	—	NR
After procedure	2.04	2.3	NR	NR	1.88	1.94	1.95	2.29	2.88	3.21*	1.77	1.76
Follow-up	NR	1.4	NR	NR	1.41	1.34	1.24	NR	NR	NR	1.19	1.28
Percent stenosis												
Before RA	70	70	NR	NR	75	76	75	68	68	66	63	63
After RA	44	54	NR	NR	NA	NA	NA	NA	NA	NA	—	NR
After procedure	26	30	NR	NR	35	33	33	27	14	4*	29	28
Follow-up	NR	57	NR	NR	52	56	57	NR	NR	NR	51	48.3
Restenosis rate (%)	NR	51	NR	NR	47	57	59	NR	NR	NR	51	51
Late clinical outcome	1 yr	5 mo		3 mo		1 yr			9 mo		1 yr	
Any MACE (%)	30	NR	NR	NR	36.6	45.9	47.9	NR	NR	NR	24.7	26.0
Death (%)	5	2	NR	4.3	3.7	2.4	1.9	1	2	0	2.3	0.9
Q wave MI (%)	2	0	NR	NR	2.6	2.4	2.4	NA	NA	NA	0	0
Revascularization (%)	34	28	NR	21	15			28	21	15	22.8	24.7
Repeat PTCA	26	28	NR	28	31.9	42.4	46.0	22	18	15	6.8	4.4
CABG	12	8	NR	10	6.3	7.3	7.1	6	3	0	18.7	20.7

* p < 0.001.

CABG = coronary artery bypass graft surgery; ELCA = excimer laser coronary angioplasty; MACE = major adverse cardiac events; MI = myocardial infarction; MLD = minimal lumen diameter; NR = not reported; RA = rotational atherectomy.

Data from New Approaches to Coronary Intervention (NACI) Registry[82]; Beaumont Hospital[83]; Ellis et al.[84]; Seton Medical Center[85]; Excimer Laser, Rotational Atherectomy, and Balloon Angioplasty Comparison (ERBAC) Study[87]; Washington Hospital Center[86]; and Dilation versus Ablation Restenosis Trial (DART).[88]

loon angioplasty alone.[86, 92] The potential benefit of plaque debulking with RA followed by coronary stenting versus stent placement alone is being evaluated in the randomized SPORT trial.

INDICATIONS. RA is indicated in lesions not suitable for balloon PTCA because of excess procedural risk, such as ostial and heavily calcified lesions, selected bifurcation lesions, and lesions that are undilatable with balloon PTCA.[93] RA may also be useful for the treatment of in-stent restenosis,[94] with one registry series suggesting a benefit for RA over balloon PTCA in diffuse lesions.[95] Although procedural success rates are high (97 percent) with the use of RA for in-stent restenosis, clinical recurrence is common (35 percent), and high (49 percent) angiographic restenosis rates have been reported.[96] RA should be avoided in the presence of focal or extensive dissection after balloon PTCA, visible thrombus, or extremely eccentric lesions located on the outer surface of a severe bend. The benefit of RA over balloon PTCA in long lesions is not known.

Transluminal Extraction Atherectomy

The transluminal extraction catheter (TEC) (InterVentional Technologies, San Diego, CA) is an over-the-wire, flexible aspiration device that uses a tip-mounted cutting blade and external vacuum to excise and remove thrombus and soft plaque from native vessels and SVGs.[97] The TEC device is less useful for removing laminated thrombus in large SVGs or for the excision of fibrous or fibrocalcific plaque.

TECHNICAL ASPECTS. The TEC device contains two rotating (750 rpm) stainless steel blades attached to the distal end of the catheter. A hand-held motor drive unit attaches to the proximal end of the cutting catheter, and a vacuum bottle connected to the TEC instrument is used for collection of aspirated atheroma, thrombus, and other debris. A 10F guiding catheter is needed for larger (7.0F and 7.5F) TEC devices, and a 9F guide is used for smaller (5.5F, 6.0F, and 6.5F) ones. A specially designed 300-cm-long, 0.014-inch guidewire with a 2-cm floppy tip terminating in a 0.021-inch ball tip is used to advance the TEC device between two and five times across the lesion. Additional atherectomy or thrombectomy may be performed with larger devices guided by intermittent angiography to assess the residual percent diameter stenosis.

INITIAL CLINICAL RESULTS. The TEC device has been used for large thrombus-containing lesions and as primary or "rescue" treatment of patients with acute myocardial infarction.[98] Procedural success rates up to 94 percent can be achieved with optimal technique.[98] Complications after TEC use include death (0 to 5.9 percent), emergency CABG (0.7 to 3.9 percent), myocardial infarction (2.0 to 7.8 percent), and a need for transfusion (19 percent).[48, 98, 99] Other angiographic complications include sidebranch occlusion (2.7 percent), abrupt closure (2.7 percent), guide catheter dissection (2.2 percent), perforation (2.2 percent), and distal embolization (0.5 to 12.8 percent).[99–103]

The TEC or PTCA in Thrombus-Containing Lesions (TOPIT) Trial, a randomized study of 245 patients with unstable or postinfarction angina and thrombus-containing lesions, was performed to assess the value of TEC and balloon PTCA in these "high-risk" patients.[104] The composite rate of in-hospital major adverse cardiac events (death, myocardial infarction, bailout intervention, or emergent CABG) was 4.5 percent in patients treated with TEC and 11.2 percent in patients treated with balloon PTCA (p = 0.06). A CPK-MB level greater than three times normal occurred significantly (p = 0.03) less often in the TEC group (4.5 percent) than in the balloon PTCA group (15.4 percent). The TEC instrument has also been used in patients with friable SVG lesions with modest (80 to 90 percent) procedural success.[49, 99, 101, 103] Residual stenoses greater than 50 percent and frequent (33 percent) dissections require that adjunctive balloon angioplasty be used in most (90 percent) cases.[49, 99] Use of the TEC device to treat complex native coronary lesions without thrombus has met with more limited (85 to 95 percent) success.[100, 104]

LATE CLINICAL OUTCOME. Extraction atherectomy does not reduce restenosis more than balloon PTCA does. Six-month clinical follow-up after TEC use demonstrated that late cardiac death (1.9 to 11 percent), Q wave myocardial infarction (1.3 to 4 percent), and repeat TLR (25.3 to 34.8 percent) were common,[49, 98, 100] probably related to the frequent treatment of friable SVG lesions in these series. Angiographic restenosis (>50 percent follow-up diameter stenosis) occurred in 52 to 69 percent of lesions treated with the TEC device[49, 99] and late vessel total occlusion was found in 11.9 to 29 percent.[49, 100]

INDICATIONS. TEC atherectomy currently has limited clinical use but may be indicated for the removal of fresh thrombus in SVG and selected native vessel lesions. TEC should not be used for the treatment of dissection caused by other devices, in cases of extreme angulation or calcification, or in vessels less than 2.5 mm in diameter. TEC atherectomy is not useful for routine atherectomy in native vessels or SVG lesions.

ABLATIVE LASER-ASSISTED ANGIOPLASTY

Despite encouraging preclinical studies,[105] laser angioplasty has neither lowered procedural complications nor reduced restenosis in comparison to balloon PTCA.[87, 106–109] Laser angioplasty is now reserved for a small subset of patients with complex lesion morphology unsuitable for therapy with other devices.

TECHNICAL ASPECTS. Light amplification by stimulated emission of radiation (LASER) is the process of creating a high-energy, coherent beam of monochromatic light. Different wavelengths (ranging from 300 nm for ultraviolet light to 1,000 to 2,000 nm for infrared light) are produced, depending on the laser medium used. The xenon chloride (XeCl) excimer laser emits light at 308 nm (in the ultraviolet range), whereas the neodymium yttrium-aluminum-garnet (Nd:YAG) laser emits light above 2000 nm (in the infrared light range). Depending on the laser source, tissue ablation results from either vaporization of tissue (photothermal effects), ejection of debris (photoacoustic effect), or direct breakdown of molecules (photochemical dissociation).[110] Ultraviolet lasers result in atherosclerotic plaque absorption, whereas near-infrared lasers result in thermal energy and photocoagulation (e.g., holmium:YAG). Photoacoustic injury is worsened in the presence of blood and contrast agents.[111]

Two systems are currently available for use in coronary arteries: the XeCl excimer laser coronary angioplasty (ELCA) system and the Ho:YAG laser system. The ELCA system uses a catheter containing a concentric or eccentric array of 61- to 200-mm optical fibers emitting laser light at 308 nm,[110, 112] and the Ho:YAG system has a catheter containing 37 fibers and operates at a wavelength of 2100 nm.[113] A single, slow (0.5 to 1.0 mm/sec) pass of the laser catheter should be performed under fluoroscopic guidance for both systems. The saline flush technique makes certain that all blood and contrast medium are removed from the coronary artery by flushing the guide catheter with 30 ml or more of saline to minimize the degree of photoacoustic injury to the surrounding vessel.[114, 115] After successful laser passage, adjunctive balloon PTCA is needed in most (90 percent) cases to reduce the residual stenosis to below 30 percent.[116–118]

INITIAL CLINICAL RESULTS. Clinical success rates with the ELCA system in complex lesion morphologies have ranged from 84 to 94 percent.[87, 106, 107, 119, 120] Three randomized trials have compared procedural outcomes with laser angioplasty and balloon PTCA. The Laser Angioplasty Versus Angioplasty (LAVA) Trial evaluated 215 patients randomly assigned to treatment with "laser-facilitated balloon angioplasty" using the holmium (TAG) laser system or balloon PTCA.[106] No differences were noted in early or late major clinical events between the two groups, although complications occurred significantly (p = 0.0004) more often in laser-treated patients (18.0 percent) than in balloon PTCA–treated patients (3.1 percent).[106] The ERBAC Trial randomly assigned 620 patients with type B and C lesions to treatment with ELCA, RA, or balloon PTCA.[87] Procedural outcome and complication rates were similar in patients undergoing ELCA or balloon PTCA.[87] The Amsterdam-Rotterdam (AMRO) Trial randomly assigned 308 patients with lesions 10 mm or longer to treatment with ELCA or balloon PTCA.[108] Procedural success rates were similar in patients treated with ELCA (80 percent) and balloon PTCA (79 percent).[108] The late restenosis rate was 51.6 percent in the laser group and 41.3 percent in the balloon-PTCA group.[108]

ELCA has also been used to treat aorto-ostial and shaft SVG lesions, longer (>15 mm) SVG lesions, lesions located in larger (>3.0 mm) friable SVGs, and lesions undilatable with balloon PTCA.[117, 119] Although laser angioplasty has been frequently used in total occlusions,[121] no restenosis benefit was shown with laser angioplasty over balloon PTCA in one study[107] two large registry series have reported the results of ELCA for the treatment of in-stent restenosis[122, 123]; a trend toward reduced clinical events was observed in a nonrandomized series.[123] The ongoing Laser Angioplasty Restenosis Study (LARS) compares late angiographic and clinical outcomes in patients treated with ELCA or balloon PTCA for in-stent restenosis.

LATE CLINICAL OUTCOME. Laser angioplasty does not reduce the occurrence of restenosis, with 47 to 54 percent of patients experiencing symptom recurrence after laser angioplasty.[87, 106, 108, 118, 121] The postprocedural lumen diameter is the most important predictor of restenosis in these series.[118, 120]

INDICATIONS. Laser angioplasty has a limited role in PCI and is reserved for patients with in-stent restenosis, particularly those in SVGs, aorto-ostial SVG lesions, and poten-

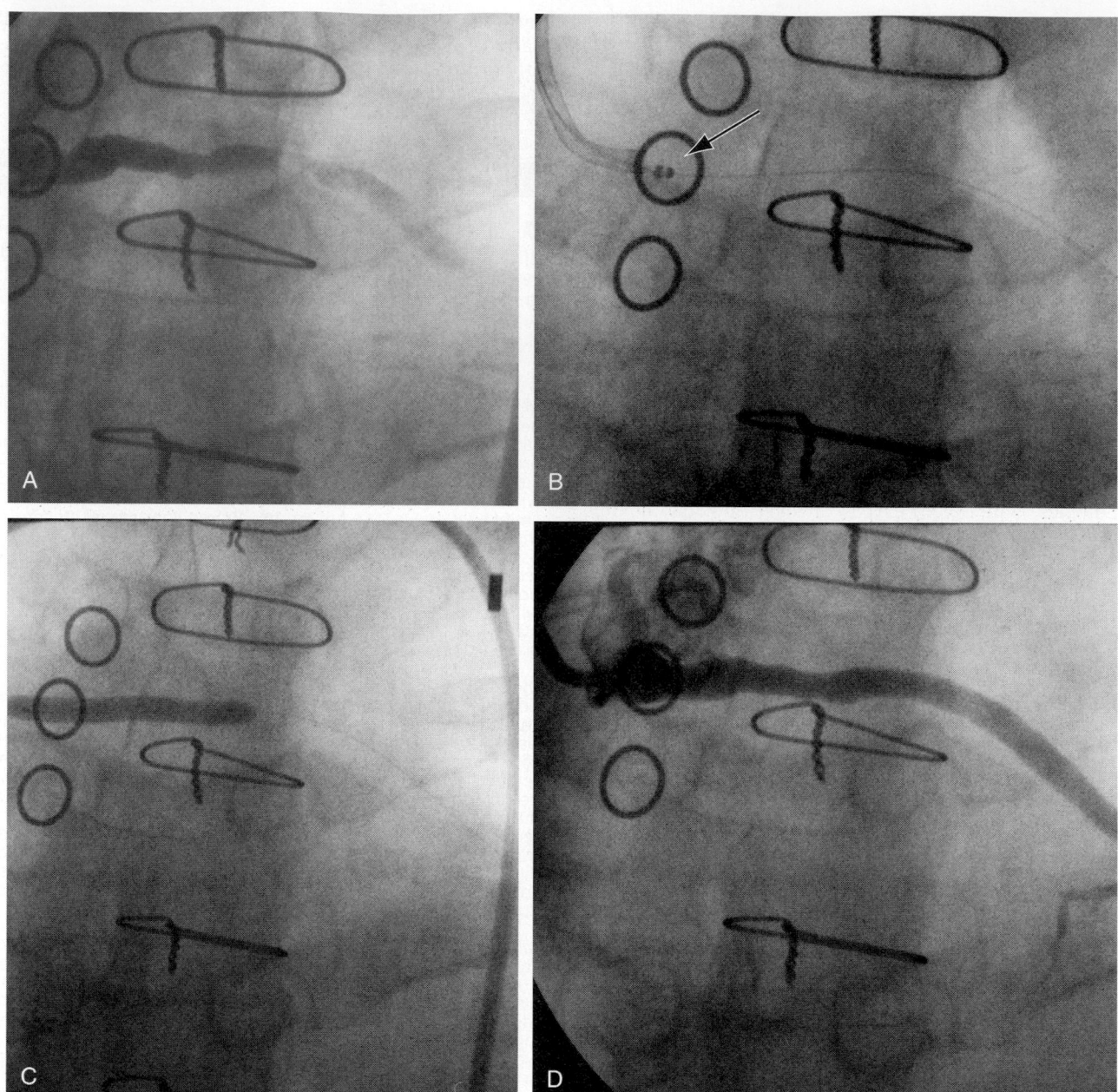

FIGURE 38–2. *A,* Thrombosed saphenous vein graft (SVG) to the obtuse marginal branch in a patient with unstable angina. *B,* An Angiojet thrombectomy catheter was used to remove thrombus within the vessel (arrow). *C,* A 4.0-mm Crown stent was deployed in the proximal segment of the SVG. *D,* Final angiographic result without evidence of distal embolization.

tially, lesions located in friable SVGs. Laser angioplasty should not be used in patients with thrombus or in the presence of severe calcification.

CATHETER-BASED THROMBOLYSIS AND MECHANICAL THROMBECTOMY

Coronary thrombus mediates acute coronary syndromes in native coronary arteries and SVGs.[124] The presence of thrombus within the native vessel or SVG imparts a substantial risk for distal embolization, "no reflow," or other embolic complications during PCI.[125, 126] Embolic complications in patients undergoing PCI of a degenerated SVG may also occur as a result of distal fragmentation of atheromatous debris and fibrointima caused by mechanical contact with the SVG.

CATHETER-BASED THROMBOLYTIC USE. Infusion catheters for intraluminal urokinase administration have been used for the treatment of thrombotic total occlusions in native arteries[127, 128] and SVGs.[129] Recanalization of occluded SVGs was achieved in 69 percent of patients with an average of 3.7 million units of urokinase given by direct catheter-based infusion over a period of 25.4 hours in one study.[129] These favorable results were tempered by a stroke rate of 3 percent and overall mortality rate of 6.5 percent. A randomized study of 469 patients undergoing PCI for unstable angina found that prophylactic use of intracoronary urokinase was associated with a higher (10.2 percent) incidence of abrupt closure (vs. 4.3 percent in placebo-treated patients; $p < 0.05$).[130] This unexpected outcome was possibly caused by plaque hemorrhage and dissection, reduced intimal sealing, or the procoagulant effects of urokinase as a result of platelet activation.

Urokinase may also be delivered directly to the thrombus surface by local drug delivery systems. The Dispatch catheter, an over-the-wire, nondilatation catheter with a 20-mm spiral inflation coil at its tip, has been used to deliver urokinase and has resulted in thrombus dissolution in native coronary and SVG lesions.[131] A hydrogel-coated balloon has been used as a drug delivery system to transfer urokinase locally to the site of thrombotic obstruction.[132] In aggregate, local

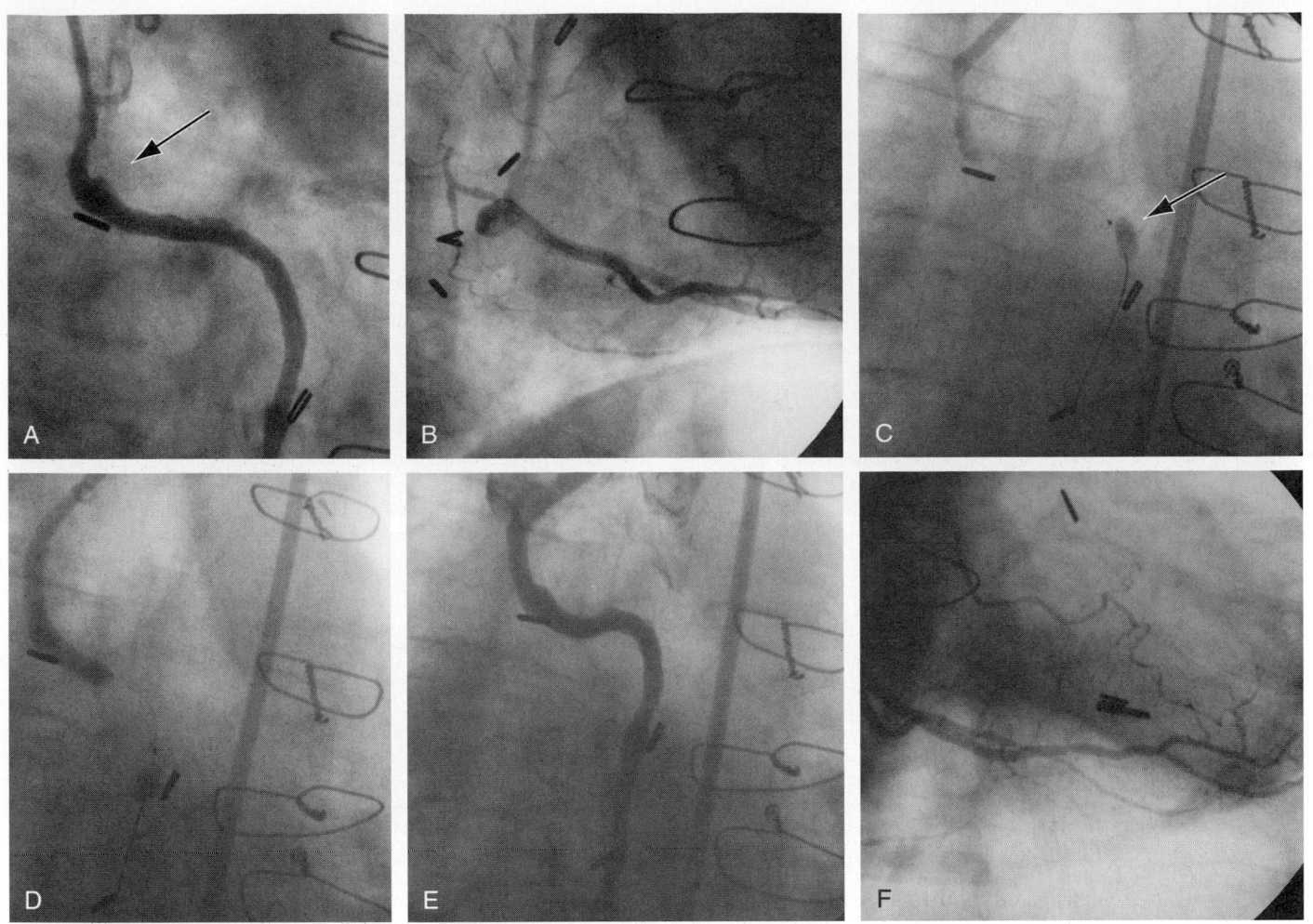

FIGURE 38–3. *A,* Degenerated saphenous vein graft (SVG) to the posterior descending artery with a diffuse stenosis in the proximal segment of the SVG (arrow). *B,* Normal distal perfusion of the SVG with demonstration of secondary and tertiary branches. Positioning of the PercuSurge balloon in the distal portion of the SVG *(C,* arrow) and a 4.0-mm stent in the proximal SVG *(D)* resulted in minimal residual stenosis *(E)* and no evidence of distal embolization *(F).*

thrombolytic therapy has had a limited role in the treatment of patients with unstable angina because of the efficacy of other therapies, such GP IIb-IIIa inhibitors, and the bleeding complications associated with urokinase.

THROMBECTOMY DEVICES. The Cordis Hydrolyzer removes thrombus by Venturi vacuum suction with the use of an external MedRad power injector. Limited European use of this device has been reported in humans in peripheral vessels,[133] hemodialysis shunts,[134] and coronary artery and SVG lesions.[135] Low-frequency (41.9 kHz) intracoronary ultrasound as in the Acolysis system is used therapeutically for thrombolysis.[136] The ATLAS Trial, a randomized clinical trial evaluating use of the Acolysis catheter and abciximab for the treatment of thrombus-containing SVG lesions, is under way.

RHEOLYTIC THROMBECTOMY. The Angiojet (Possis Medical, Inc., Minneapolis, MN) is a 5F catheter with a stainless steel tip connected to a high-pressure flexible cylinder, or hypotube. Saline is injected into the hypotube at the distal tip, where three high-speed saline jets are directed toward the proximal end of the catheter lumen. Venturi suction is created at the catheter tip, and surrounding blood, thrombus, and saline are entrained into the tip opening. The jets fracture the thrombus into small particles and propel the fragments proximally through the catheter lumen, where they are removed from the body. Repeated passes of the Angiojet may be performed until angiography shows no further evidence of improvement in lumen diameter or thrombus burden (Fig. 38–2).

Angiographic thrombus was reduced by 86 percent with the Angiojet in a multicenter registry of 90 patients with acute ischemic syndromes and evidence of intraluminal thrombus.[137] The Angiojet was successfully delivered in all cases, and the overall procedural success rate was 87 percent. Two (2.2 percent) procedure-related deaths occurred within 30 days of the procedure. Other complications included a reduced final TIMI flow grade of less than 3 (4.4 percent), persistent abrupt closure (3.3 percent), and coronary perforation (1.1 percent). The TLR rate was 15.6 percent and the overall target vessel failure rate was 27.5 percent at 1 year. The VEGAS-2 trial randomly assigned 349 patients with angiographic thrombus to treatment with the Angiojet or prolonged intraluminal urokinase consisting of a 250,000-unit bolus over a 30-minute period, followed by urokinase at 20,000 to 240,000 units/hr for 6 to 30 hours.[138] No significant differences were observed in the primary endpoint, target vessel failure, which is defined by at least one of the following: (1) occurrence of a major clinical event, i.e., death, myocardial infarction, or revascularization; (2) failure to achieve less than 50 percent diameter stenosis; (3) presence of final TIMI flow of less than 3; or (4) failure to achieve greater than 20 percent improvement in stenosis severity.[138] The procedure success rate was higher and the complication rate was lower in Angiojet-treated patients.[138]

The Angiojet is currently indicated in patients with moderate to large thrombus-containing native vessels or SVGs prior to definitive therapy with balloon PTCA and stents. The Angiojet is useful for the treatment of recent thrombus, particularly in the setting of acute myocardial infarction or failed thrombolytic therapy. The Angiojet should not be used in small (<2.0 mm) vessels because of the risk of perforation.

DISTAL EMBOLIC PROTECTION DEVICES. Several devices have been developed to prevent (or trap) macroparticulate embolic material from passing into the distal microcirculation during PCI. The PercuSurge Guardwire is a compliant balloon mounted on a hypotube that can function as a 0.014-inch steerable guidewire for catheter transport.[139] Once positioned across the lesion, the balloon is inflated to block the flow of blood in the vessel and PCI is performed over the Guardwire. Liberated debris is trapped by the inflated Guardwire balloon, and an aspiration catheter is used to remove blood and suspended debris. The Guardwire balloon is then deflated and distal flow to the vessel is restored. The aspirated material contains thrombus and macroparticulate atheromatous debris.[139] This device and others are now undergoing clinical evaluation in patients at risk for distal embolization during PCI (Fig. 38–3).

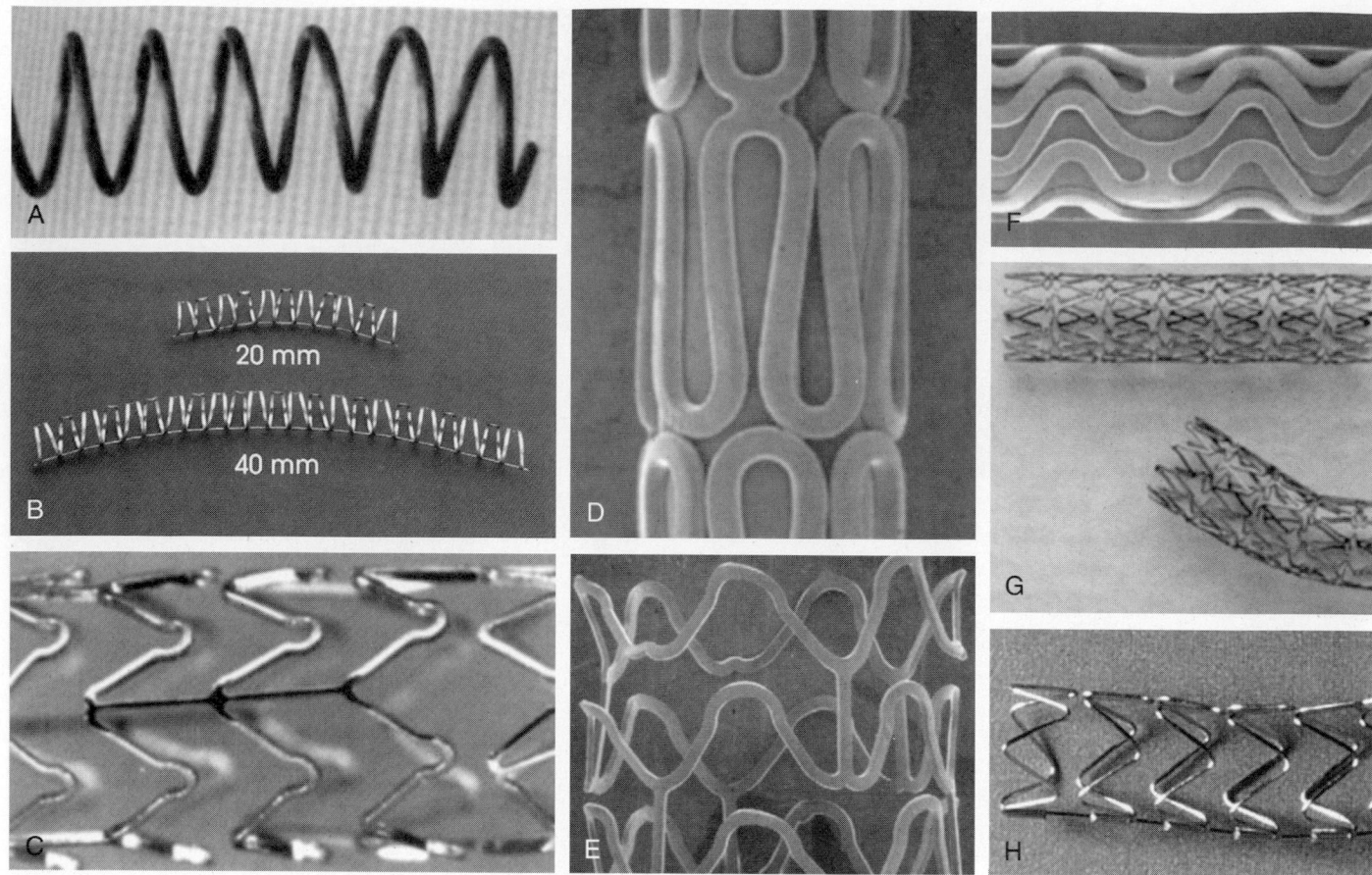

FIGURE 38–4. Representative stents: coil stent proposed by Dotter *(A)*, Gianturco-Roubin stent *(B)*, Guidant Duet stent *(C)*, Medtronic-AVE GFX stent *(D)*, Guidant Multilink stent *(E)*, Cordis Crown *(F)*, Paragon stent *(G)*, and Bard XT stent *(H)*.

CORONARY STENTS

Coronary stents have fundamentally changed the practice of interventional cardiology by reducing early complications and improving late clinical outcomes in a broad array of patients. Charles Dotter introduced the concept of a temporary endoluminal splint to scaffold an occluded peripheral vessel nearly 40 years ago,[140] but the first human coronary implantation was not performed until 1986, when Puel and colleagues[141] and, subsequently, Sigwart and associates[142] deployed self-expanding stents to prevent abrupt closure and reduce restenosis after balloon PTCA. Over the next decade an explosive growth in the use of coronary stents took place as a result of both an expanding number of randomized trials demonstrating benefit in specific lesion subsets and clinicians' empirical satisfaction with the early and late benefits of stents (Fig. 38–4).

Although it is estimated that 50 to 80 percent of PCI procedures now involve the use of at least one stent,[143] the majority of patients receiving a stent do not meet the criteria for currently approved indications. In a series of 700 patients, less than 20 percent would have been candidates for the initial randomized trials demonstrating the benefit of stents.[144] Expanded "off-label" coronary stent use has identified patients at "high-risk" for recurrent symptoms after stenting,[144] such as those with smaller (<2.75 mm) vessels and diffuse (lesions >25 mm) disease. One study has suggested that patients undergoing "off-label" stent use have a risk of angiographic restenosis that is nearly three times higher than observed in patients undergoing stent placement for approved indications.[144] Randomized trials with balloon PTCA in these subsets are ongoing. The re-

sults of randomized trials comparing coronary stenting and balloon PTCA are reviewed (Table 38–4).

Indications

DE NOVO OR RESTENOTIC NATIVE VESSEL LESIONS. At least five randomized trials have shown that coronary stent use in larger (>3.0 mm), de novo native coronary vessels is associated with an improved outcome when compared with balloon PTCA (Fig. 38–5). In the first two of these studies, the Stent Restenosis Study (STRESS) and the Belgium Netherlands Stent (BENESTENT) Trial, Palmaz-Schatz stent placement resulted in a 26 to 31 percent reduction in angiographic restenosis and a 27 to 31 percent lowering of 1-year clinical events when compared with balloon PTCA.[30,][145] A third study, the Stent Versus Angioplasty Restenosis Trial (START), demonstrated similar findings that were maintained up to 4 years after the procedure.[149]

The benefit of stent use over balloon PTCA in restenotic lesions was shown in the Restenosis Stent (REST) Study, a randomized trial of 383 patients with restenosis after balloon PTCA who were randomly assigned to Palmaz-Schatz stent placement or repeat balloon PTCA.[146] Angiographic restenosis (>50 percent follow-up diameter stenosis) was lower (18 percent) in stent-treated patients (vs. 32 percent in balloon PTCA–treated patients; $p = 0.03$); TLR also occurred less often (10 percent) in stent-treated patients (vs. 27 percent in balloon PTCA–treated patients; $p = 0.001$).

ABRUPT OR THREATENED CLOSURE AFTER BALLOON PTCA. Patients in whom periprocedural coronary occlusion develops during balloon PTCA have substantially higher morbidity and mortality than do those in whom this complication does not develop,[4] including death (4 percent),

▶ **TABLE 38–4. EARLY AND LATE OUTCOME IN RANDOMIZED TRIALS OF CORONARY STENT PLACEMENT VERSUS BALLOON PTCA**

VARIABLE	STRESS PTCA	STRESS Stent	BENESTENT PTCA	BENESTENT Stent	BENESTENT II PTCA	BENESTENT II Stent	REST PTCA	REST Stent	SAVED PTCA	SAVED Stent	SICCO PTCA	SICCO Stent
Lesion type	De novo, native		De novo, native		De novo, native		Restenotic, native		SVGs		Chronic occlusion	
Years of entry	1991–93		1991–93		1995–96		1991–96		1993–95		1994–95	
Number of patients	202	205	257	259	410	413	176	178	107	108	59	58
Baseline factors												
Mean age (yr)	60	60	58	57	59	50	60	59	66	66	57	58
Women (%)	27	17	18	20	20	23	18	20	21	18	20	16
Diabetes mellitus (%)	16	15	6	7	11	13	15	20	36	23	NA	NA
Unstable angina (%)	48	47	NA	NA	40	45	22	17	77	82	NA	NA
Multivessel disease (%)	32	36	NA	NA	NA	NA	32	33	NA	NA	NA	NA
Angiographic success (%)	92.6	99.5	98.1	96.9	99	99	93.2	98.9	86	97	NA	NA
Clinical success (%)	89.6	96.1	91.1	92.7	95	96	100	100	69	92	NA	NA
Reference diameter (mm)	2.99	3.03	3.01	2.99	2.93	2.96	3.04	3.01	3.19	3.18	3.17	3.16
Final % stenosis	35	19	33	22	29	16	30	6	32	12	33.5	18.8
Stent use (%)	6.9	96.1	5.1	94.6	13.4	96.6	6.8	98.9	7.0	97	NA	98.3
Early complications	0–14 d		In-hospital		1 Mo		In-hospital		In-hospital		In-hospital	
Death (%)	1.5	0	0	0	0.2	0	0.6	1.1	2	2	0	0
Q wave infarction (%)	3.0	2.9	0.8	1.9	1.0	1.2	0.6	2.8	1	2	NA	NA
Emergency CABG (%)	4.0	2.4	1.6	1.9	0.5	0.7	0.6	1.1	4	2	NA	1.7
Late clinical outcome	15–240 d		7 mos		12 mos		6 mos		240 d		14–180 d	
Death (%)	0	1.5	0.4	0.8	1.0	1.0	1.1	1.1	9	7	0	0
Q wave MI (%)	0.5	1.0	1.6	2.7	1.5	1.9	0.6	2.8	4	5	0	0
Revascularization (%)	15.4	10.2	NA	NA	NA	NA	NA	NA	NA	NA	5.1	5.2
Repeat PTCA	11.4	9.8	20.6	10.0	15.6	9.4	26.6	10.3	16	13	3.4	1.7
CABG	4.5	2.4	2.3	3.1	1.5	1.9	0.6	2.2	12	7	1.7	3.4
Follow-up angiography												
Restenosis (%)	42.1	31.6	32	22	31	16	32	18	47	36	73.7	31.6
Follow-up MLD (mm)	1.56	1.74	1.73	1.82	1.66	1.89	1.85	2.04	1.49	1.73	1.11	1.92
Follow-up % stenosis	49	42	43	38	43	35	47	30	51	46	66	45
Any bleeding complication (%)	4.0	7.3	3.1	13.5	1.0	1.2	1.1	11.2	5	17	0	11

Data from Stent Restenosis Study (STRESS),[30] Belgium Netherlands Stent (BENESTENT) Trial I[145] and II,[31] Restenosis Stent Study (REST),[146] Saphenous Vein Graft De Novo Trial (SAVED),[147] and Stenting in Chronic Coronary Occlusion (SICCO) Trial.[148]

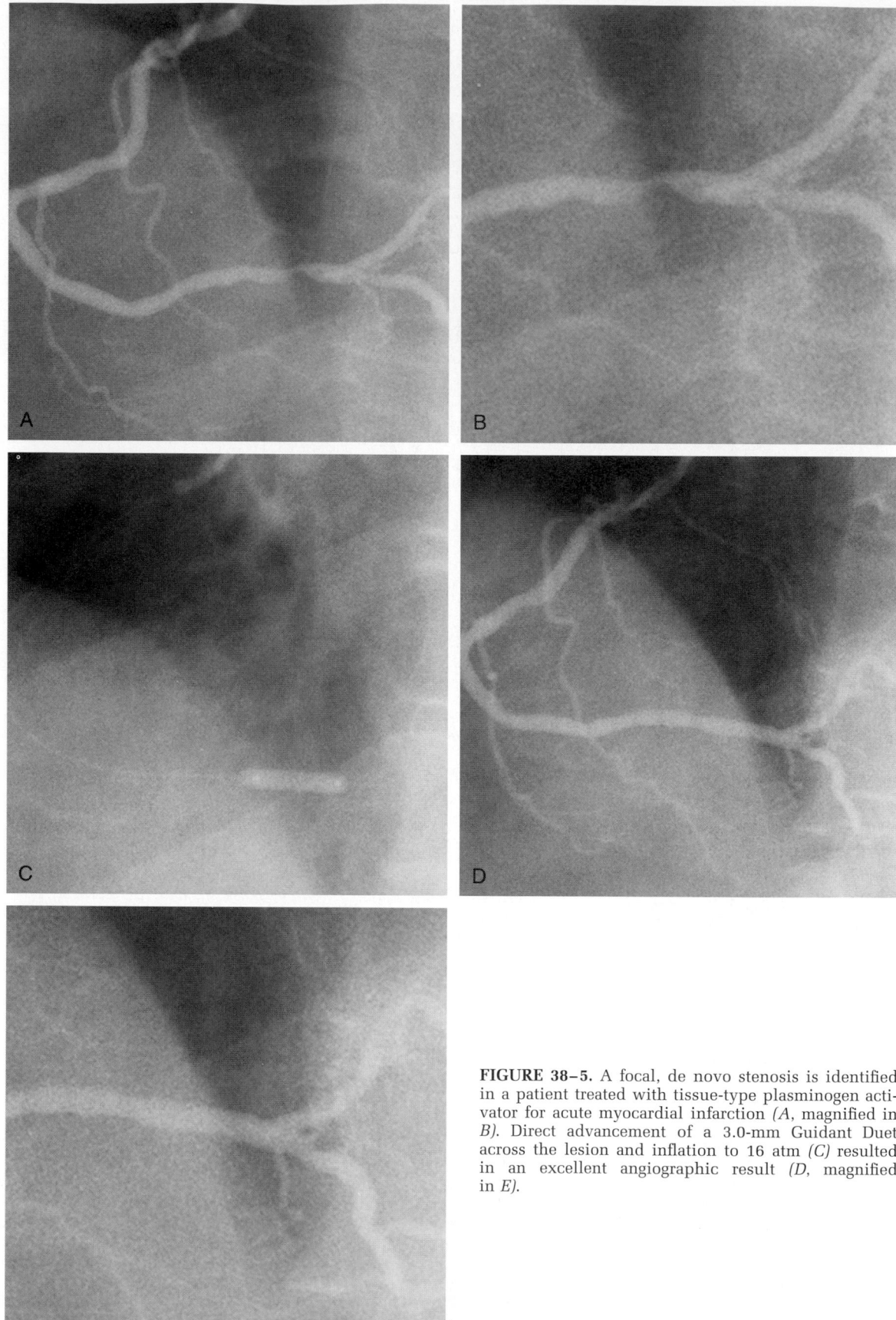

FIGURE 38–5. A focal, de novo stenosis is identified in a patient treated with tissue-type plasminogen activator for acute myocardial infarction *(A, magnified in B)*. Direct advancement of a 3.0-mm Guidant Duet across the lesion and inflation to 16 atm *(C)* resulted in an excellent angiographic result *(D, magnified in E)*.

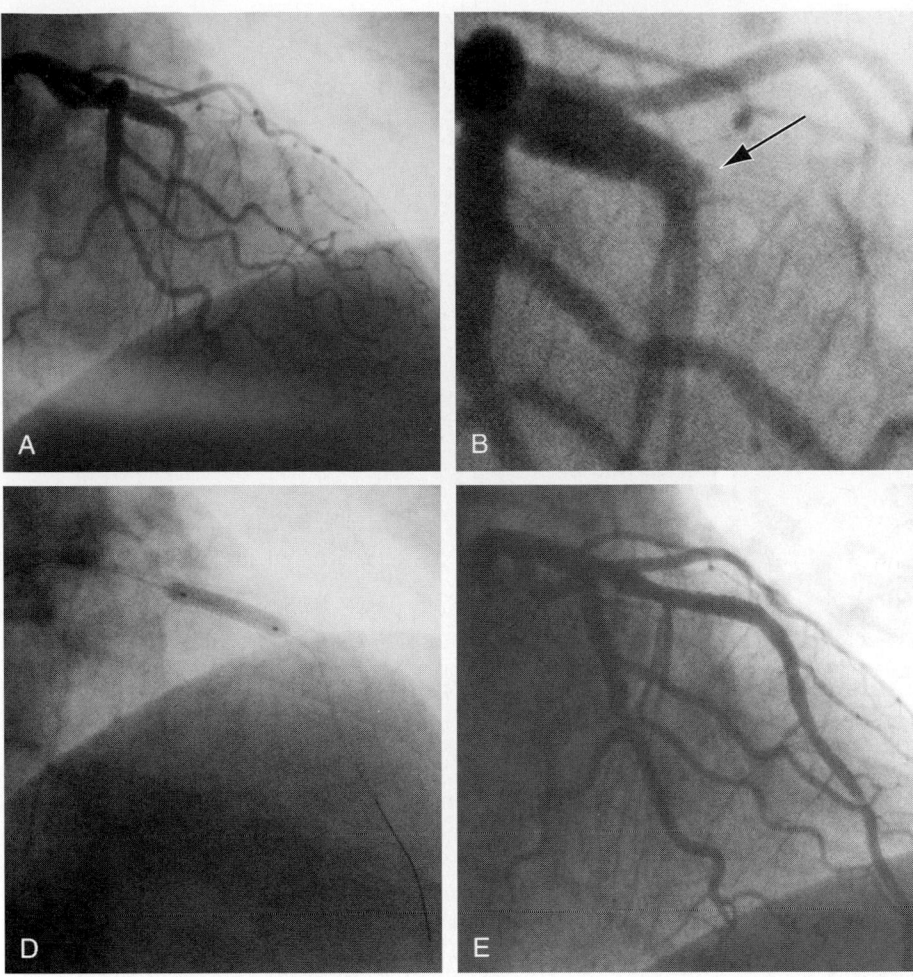

FIGURE 38–6. *A,* Emergency coronary arteriography in a patient with an acute myocardial infarction demonstrates a total occlusion in the midportion of the left anterior descending coronary artery (LAD). *B,* A "nipple" found on a magnified view (arrow) allowed an entry point for the coronary guidewire to pass into the distal segment of the LAD. Reperfusion is reestablished *(C),* and a 3.5-mm stent deployed at the site of occlusion *(D)* resulted in 0% residual stenosis and TIMI 3 flow into the distal part of the vessel *(E).*

myocardial infarction (20 percent), or the need for urgent CABG (7 percent).[4] Self-expanding[141, 142] and balloon-expandable coiled[150] and slotted tube[151] stents were first used to scaffold coronary dissections in patients with balloon PTCA–induced complications. The Trial of Angioplasty and Stents in Canada (TASC II), a randomized evaluation of 43 patients with abrupt closure assigned to primary Palmaz-Schatz stent placement or prolonged autoperfusion balloon PTCA with "bailout" stent placement, showed a higher clinical success rate in stent-treated patients (90 vs. 42 percent).[152] Subsequent attempts to compared prolonged balloon inflation with primary stent placement for abrupt closure were unable to recruit patients[153] given the dramatic effect that stents had on the correction of major coronary dissections and avoidance of emergency CABG. Stents are currently indicated for the treatment of abrupt and threatened closure after balloon or new device PCI.

SAPHENOUS VEIN GRAFTS. Although balloon PTCA of SVG lesions is associated with high (88 percent) procedural success rates,[154] clinical recurrence because of restenosis or progression of disease at other SVG sites is common.[154] Restenosis rates are highest in ostial lesions (58 percent) and in the body of the SVG (52 percent).[154] The Saphenous Vein Graft De Novo (SAVED) Trial randomly assigned 220 patients with de novo SVG lesions to treatment with Palmaz-Schatz stent placement or balloon PTCA alone.[147] Stenting was associated with higher procedural success rates (92 vs. 69 percent in balloon-treated patients; $p <$ 0.001) at the expense of more bleeding events (17 vs. 5 percent in balloon PTCA–treated patients; $p <$ 0.01) attributable to the aggressive anticoagulation regimen used in this study. Although restenosis was not significantly lower in stent-treated patients (37 percent) than in balloon PTCA–

treated patients (46 percent), freedom from significant cardiac events was better in the stent group (73 vs. 58 percent in balloon PTCA–treated patients; $p =$ 0.03).[147] Stents are the preferred therapy in patients with ostial or body SVG lesions. The risk of "no reflow" or distal embolization is higher in patients with severe SVG friability and in those with SVG thrombus.

TOTAL CORONARY OCCLUSIONS. Balloon PTCA of chronic coronary occlusions is associated with reduced (47 to 69 percent) procedural success[155–157] and frequent (45 to 55 percent) recurrence,[158–161] often (19 percent) as total coronary occlusion. Procedural success rates with total occlusion have steadily increased over the past several years, partly as a result of the introduction of hydrophilic guidewires[162] for crossing the occluded segments, but late (6 to 9 months) recurrence rates remain high (Fig. 38–6).

After beneficial results were shown in pilot studies,[163, 164] three randomized trials confirmed the benefit of stent placement over balloon PTCA alone in patients with chronic occlusions.[148, 165, 166] In the Stenting in Chronic Coronary Occlusion (SICCO) Study, 119 patients with successful balloon PTCA of a chronic coronary occlusion were assigned to no further intervention or to Palmaz-Schatz stent placement.[148] Angiographic restenosis occurred less often in stent-treated patients (32 percent) than in patients receiving no further therapy (74 percent) ($p <$ 0.001). TLR was also needed less often in stent-treated patients (22 percent) than in balloon PTCA–treated patients (42 percent) ($p =$ 0.025).[148] This benefit was sustained at late follow-up.[167] In the Gruppo Italiano per lo Studio sullo Stent nelle Occlusioni Coronariche (GISSOC) trial, 110 patients with total occlusions successfully treated by balloon PTCA were assigned to Palmaz-Schatz stent implantation or to no further

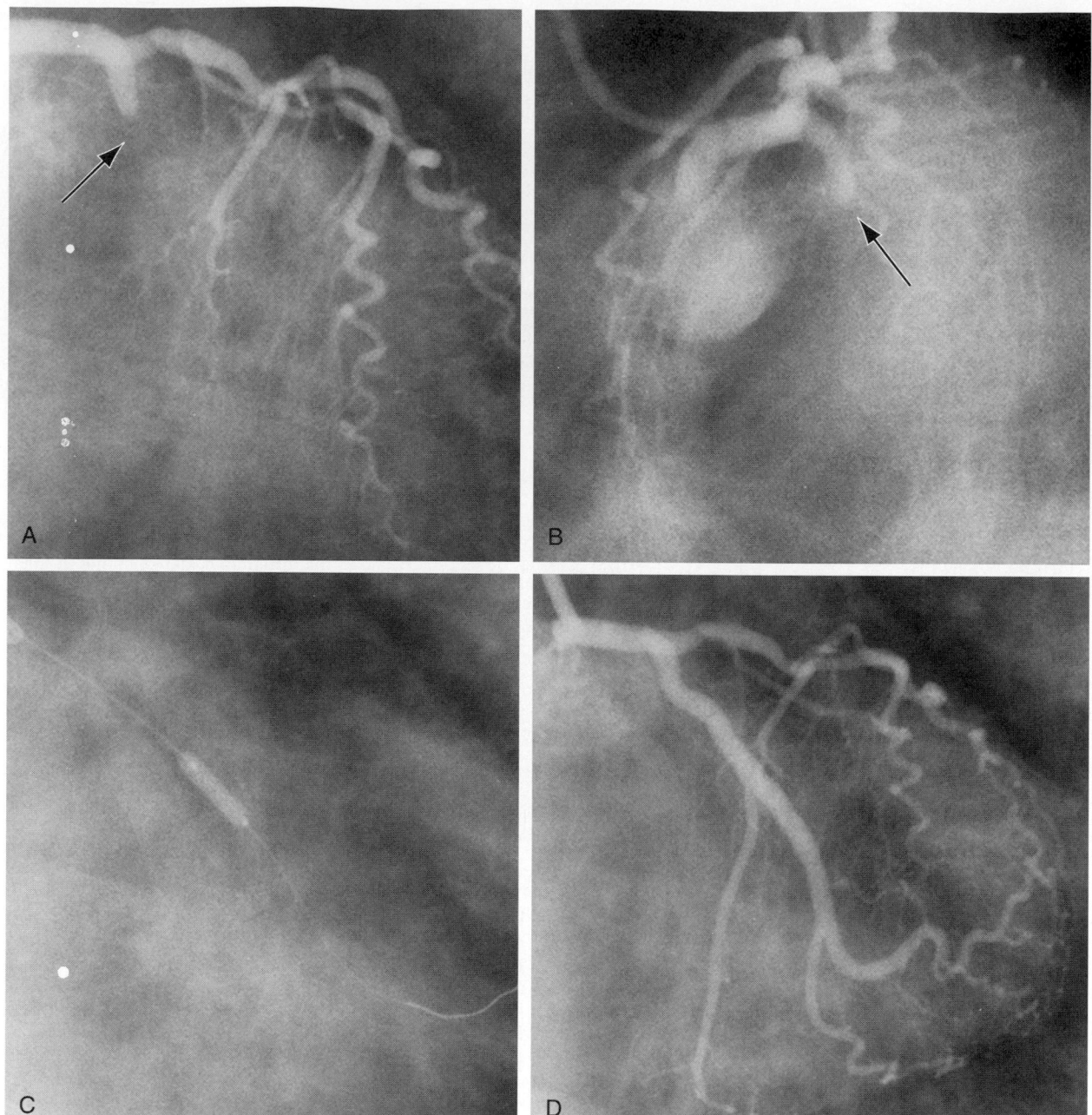

FIGURE 38–7. Acute posterior wall myocardial infarction caused by an acute left circumflex coronary artery in the right anterior oblique *(A, arrow)* and left anterior oblique *(B, arrow)* projection. A 3.0-mm balloon was used to recanalized the vessel *(C)*, and placement of two 3.5-mm S670 stents resulted in an excellent final angiographic result *(D)*.

therapy. Angiographic restenosis occurred less often in stent-treated patients (32 vs. 68 percent in patients without stent placement; $p < 0.001$). Stent-treated patients also had lower rates of reocclusion (8 vs. 34 percent; $p = 0.003$) and TLR (5.3 vs. 22 percent; $p = 0.038$).[165] A third study showed similar benefit with the Wiktor stent.[161]

ACUTE MYOCARDIAL INFARCTION. When compared with thrombolytic therapy, primary balloon PTCA improves TIMI 3 flow rates and reduces the frequency of mortality, reinfarction, and stroke[168–174] (Fig. 38–7). Primary balloon PTCA is limited in some cases by recurrent in-hospital ischemia or reinfarction (10 to 15 percent), restenosis (37 to 49 percent), or late reocclusion (9 to 14 percent).[175] Failed primary balloon PTCA is associated with high (31 percent) in-hospital mortality rates and occurs more often in patients in cardiogenic shock and those with multivessel CAD.[176]

Stent placement may be useful in patients with acute myocardial infarction, either as primary therapy or as a "bailout" for the treatment of coronary dissection or residual stenosis after balloon PTCA. In a pilot multicenter study of 312 patients treated with primary PCI for acute myocardial infarction, stent placement was attempted in all eligible patients, provided that the infarct-related artery was between 3.0 and 4.0 mm, the lesion required only one or two stents, and no large thrombus, major sidebranch jeopardy, or excessive proximal tortuosity or calcification in the infarct-related artery occurred after PTCA.[177] Stenting was performed in 77 percent of patients and was successful in 98 percent, with TIMI 3 flow in 96 percent. Patients treated with stents had low rates of in-hospital death (0.8 percent), reinfarction (1.7 percent), recurrent ischemia (3.8 percent), and predischarge TLR for recurrent ischemia (1.3 percent).[177]

Smaller randomized trials comparing primary stenting and balloon PTCA in patients with acute myocardial infarction have shown a benefit for primary stent placement.[178-182] The Primary Angioplasty in Myocardial Infarction (PAMI) stent trial randomly assigned 900 patients with acute myocardial infarction to treatment with primary balloon PTCA or placement of the Palmaz-Schatz heparin-coated stent.[183] After 6 months, fewer patients in the stent group had angina (11.3 vs. 16.9 percent in the balloon group; $p = 0.02$) or needed TLR (7.7 vs. 17.0 percent in the balloon group; $p < 0.001$). Angiographic restenosis also occurred less often in stent-treated patients (20.3 vs. 33.5 percent in balloon-treated patients; $p < 0.001$).[183]

Based on these results, primary PTCA (and primary or "provisional" stent placement) is indicated as an alternative to thrombolytic therapy in patients with acute myocardial infarction who are seen within 12 hours of symptom onset (or ≥12 hours with persistent symptoms), provided that the door-to-balloon time is less than 90 minutes, the hospital performs more than 200 PCI procedures per year, and the operator meets the ACC/AHA proficiency standards of more than 75 cases per year.[184] Primary PTCA is also indicated in patients in cardiogenic shock, provided that revascularization can be performed within 18 hours of the onset of cardiogenic shock, and in patients who have a contraindication to thrombolytic therapy.[184]

OTHER LESION SUBSETS. It is less clear whether primary stent placement is preferred over balloon PTCA with "bailout" stenting in other lesion subsets.[184a] Although a subset analysis of STRESS suggested an advantage of stenting over balloon PTCA in smaller (<3.0 mm) vessels,[185] other studies have shown a worse outcome when stents are used in this setting.[143] It is not known whether primary stenting (vs. balloon PCA with "bailout" stenting) is preferred in bifurcation lesions, diffuse disease, ostial lesions, or unprotected or protected (Fig. 38–8) left main lesions in patients with patent grafts to one or more left coronary territories.[143] Larger trials in the subsets are ongoing.

Complications

THROMBOSIS. The early use of coronary stents was limited by high (3.5 to 8.6 percent) subacute thrombosis rates[30, 145, 151, 186-188] despite aggressive antithrombotic therapy with aspirin (≥325 mg daily), dipyridamole (225 mg daily), periprocedural dextran 40, and intravenous heparin followed by oral warfarin. Clinical events associated with

subacute thrombosis were profound, virtually always resulting in an untoward outcome (e.g., death, myocardial infarction, or emergency revascularization). Patients at "high-risk" for subacute thrombosis included those with unstable angina, residual proximal or distal dissection, angiographic thrombus or a filling defect, in-laboratory transient or sustained abrupt closure, multiple (more than three) stent implants, smaller (<3.0 mm) vessels, total occlusions, complex (type "C") morphology, left anterior descending or left circumflex lesion location, failed balloon PTCA, or recent (<1 week) myocardial infarction. Anatomical factors after stent deployment (e.g., underdilation of the stent, proximal and distal dissections, poor inflow or outflow obstruction, <3-mm vessel diameter) appeared to play more of a role than did suboptimal anticoagulation regimens in the development of subacute thrombosis in the early stent experience.[189-191] Lower frequencies of subacute stent thrombosis have been achieved with optimal stent deployment.[190]

Prompt vessel recanalization is paramount for the management of subacute thrombosis after stent placement. Although repeat balloon dilatation and, less commonly, CABG are the most prompt and effective methods of establishing reperfusion, intravenous thrombolysis should be used when a catheterization facility is not readily available.[192] Although recanalization can often be achieved after subacute thrombosis within 2 hours of symptom onset, myocardial infarction may still occur.[192]

BLEEDING. Hemorrhagic complications were a major limitation associated with the use of coronary stents,[30, 145, 193, 194] particularly when aggressive anticoagulation regimens that included warfarin (Coumadin) were used. The introduction of reduced anticoagulation regimens has had a profound impact on the reduction of bleeding complications after stent placement. Brachial[195] and radial[196, 197] access sites, percutaneous vascular closure devices, and collagen implants have also reduced bleeding complications with modest success.[198] The safety and efficacy of collagen implants for sealing the femoral puncture site after stent implantation have also been evaluated.[198]

OTHER COMPLICATIONS. Other problems include side-branch occlusion (6 to 14 percent),[199] particularly in bifurcation lesions involving the origin of the sidebranch.[200] The clinical importance of the sidebranch occlusion relates to the size of the sidebranch and extent of myocardium that the sidebranch supplies. Open-cell and coiled stent designs may provide better access to sidebranches than afforded by

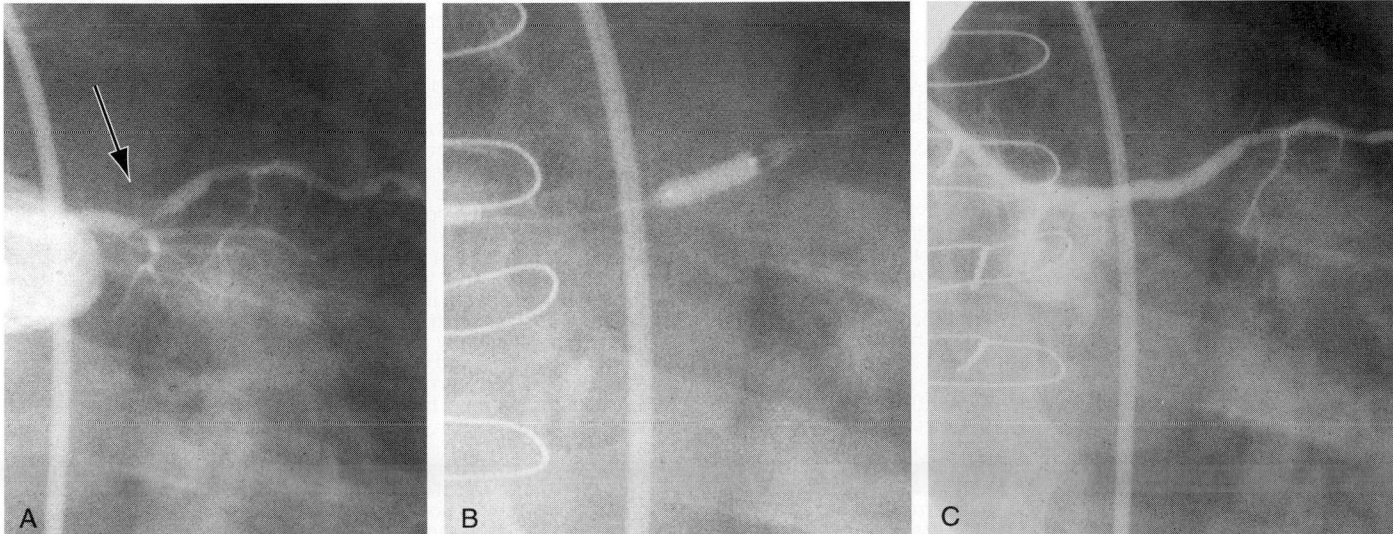

FIGURE 38–8. Complex stenosis involving the distal segment of the left main and proximal segment of the left anterior descending coronary arteries (*A, arrow*). After predilation, placement of a 3.0 × 18 mm NIR stent across the stenosis (*B*) resulted in the final angiographic result (*C*).

the closed-cell, tubular slotted stent designs. Stent dislodgment from the delivery catheter is an uncommon occurrence with second- and third-generation stents with enhanced retention designs, but it may occur more often when stents are "hand-crimped" onto a balloon catheter. Stent embolization within the coronary artery is generally benign.[201] Stent margin dissections can occur during stent deployment or during postdeployment stent dilatation, particularly when stent dilatation strategies are directed at maximizing the internal stent diameter. The availability of shorter (15 mm), noncompliant balloons allows more precise stent dilatation when using high ($\geq$16 atm) pressure, thereby reducing the frequency of edge dissections. Coronary perforation is also an uncommon occurrence after stent deployment, but it may occur during poststent deployment dilatation with an oversized balloon inflated to high pressure. No evidence indicates that higher balloon inflation pressures predispose to higher rates of stent restenosis.

RESTENOSIS. "Very late" (>1 year) restenosis is a rare occurrence after coronary stenting in native coronary arteries. Three-year angiographic and clinical follow-up was obtained in 143 patients (147 lesions) who underwent Palmaz-Schatz stent placement in native coronaries.[202] After 14 months, TLR was necessary in only 2.1 percent of patients, whereas balloon PTCA of a new lesion was required in 7.7 percent of patients. Follow-up coronary angiography showed no further decrease in minimal lumen diameter between 6 months and 1 year (1.95 mm in both groups), as well as a significant ($p < 0.001$) improvement in minimal lumen diameter between 6 months (1.94 mm) and 3 years (2.09 mm).[202] Similar very late improvements in lumen diameter have been reported in two other series,[203, 204] and sustained improvement in the very late (3 to 9 year) clinical outcomes of patients treated with stents has also been reported.[205, 206]

Designs

A number of balloon-expandable and self-expanding stents have become available for clinical use over the past several years (Tables 38–5 and 38–6). Each of these stents varies with respect to its metallic composition, strut design, stent length, delivery and deployment system, and arterial surface coverage, among other factors. One classification system suggested for stent design includes mesh stents, tubular stents, coil stents, ring stents, multidesign stents, and custom-designed stents.[207] Given the proliferation of new stent designs, it is likely that the classification system for stent design will also remain in continuous evolution. A number of stent-versus-stent trials have been used to evaluate the clinical equivalency of these stent designs. Although no stent has proved superior to the Palmaz-Schatz design for the prevention of restenosis in these series, substantial differences in clinical outcome may be found with the various stent designs as their use is expanded beyond the scope of randomized clinical study.[208]

PALMAZ-SCHATZ STENT. The Palmaz-Schatz PS-153 stent (Cordis Corp., Warren, NJ) is a 15-mm, articulated slotted tube composed of 316L stainless steel that is available on a 5F delivery sheath in the United States or as a freestanding stent that is "crimped" onto a conventional balloon outside the United States. The Palmaz-Schatz stent was the first to show superiority over balloon PTCA for the prevention of restenosis[30, 145, 147] and has also been used for the treatment of major dissections and acute and threatened closure.[151, 209] Its slotted tube design imparted high radial compressive strength and yielded symmetrical expansion after deployment. The Palmaz-Schatz stent is no longer used clinically because it is relatively inflexible, is available in only a single 15-mm length, has a 1-mm articulation defect, which is a potential site for restenosis because of protrusion through the articulation site, and lends tenuous access to large sidebranches, among other factors. Because of deformation of the PS-153 at larger expansion diameters, other slotted tube stents, e.g., the P-104, P-154, and PS-204 biliary stents, were used "off-label" for the treatment of large (>4.0 to 5.0 mm) native coronaries and SVGs.[210] Newer stent designs with larger expansion diameters have obviated the need for these stents in current practice.

THE GIANTURCO-ROUBIN STENT. The Gianturco-Roubin (GR) stent was the first stent approved for the treatment of abrupt vessel closure after balloon PTCA.[211] The GR stent is composed of a single 0.006-inch 316L stainless steel wire coiled into a series of interdigitating loops in a "clamshell" design; its 25-mm length provided adequate coverage for lesions up to 20 mm long. The major limitations of the first-generation GR stent were its relative inflexibility, requirement for larger (8F to 9F guides) guiding catheters for 3.5- and 4.0-mm stents, and an inability to precisely localize the position of the stent after deployment. The second-generation GR-II stent, available in 20- and 40-mm lengths, has gold radiopaque markers at both ends of the stent to allow easy visualization of the proximal and distal stent margins. A flat wire design and a central articulation spine prevent stent axial shortening on expansion. The GR-II stent is approved for the treatment of abrupt and threatened closure after balloon PTCA. It has limited use because of high restenosis rates associated with the clinical use of this stent.[212]

THE WIKTOR CORONARY STENT. The Medtronic Wiktor stent is composed of a 0.005-inch tantalum wire arranged in a sinusoidal helical wave. Its radiopacity, preserved access to sidebranches, and flexibility led to its clinical evaluation and subsequent Food and Drug Administration approval for the treatment of abrupt and threatened closure after balloon PTCA.[213] The major disadvantages of the Wiktor stent are its potential for longitudinal elongation and lack of radial scaffolding in ostial lesions. Unraveling of the stent wire may also occur during withdrawal of the balloon catheter, from guide catheter trauma,[214] or after high-pressure balloon dilatation.

THE MULTILINK AND DUET STENTS. The Multilink stent (Guidant Corp., Santa Clara, CA) is a 15-mm balloon-expandable, stainless steel stent designed with multiple rings connected by multiple links. The Multilink stent provides unique longitudinal flexibility, high radial compressive strength, minimal (<5 percent) longitudinal shortening after deployment, and lack of an articulation defect. A low (16.0 percent) restenosis rate was reported in the ASCENT Trial.[215] The DUET stent, a more flexible, radiopaque, next-generation balloon-expandable stent, is approved for the prevention of restenosis in larger (>2.75 mm) native vessels and for the management of abrupt or threatened closure. Strut thickness has been increased from 0.0022 to 0.0055 inches, and to improve stent flexibility, the shape of the ring has been rounded at its apex and the number of articulations between repeating units has been decreased from three articulations per unit to alternating three and two articulations per unit.[207] Edge dissections have been noted after clinical use of the DUET stent and are due to proximal and distal balloon margins up to 1.8 mm beyond the axial stent length and asymmetrical stent expansion as a result of stent compression from "dogboning" of the balloon if the balloon is inflated too rapidly. The TriStar stent with its very short (0.4 mm) balloon margin and a novel centering technology has reduced the frequency of these findings in early clinical experience; this stent was approved for clinical use in the United States in December 1999.

AVE MODULAR STENTS. The Microstent II (Medtronic-Arterial Vascular Engineering, Santa Rosa, CA) is a balloon-expandable stent with 3-mm ring segments arranged in a zigzag design with eight axial struts connected by four crowns. Its major advantages are its marked flexibility in tortuous vessel and through previously deployed stents and its radiopacity for precise positioning in ostial locations or in bifurcation lesions. The Microstent II[216] has been progressively replaced with subsequent generations of the stent, the GFX and GFX-2 and, more recently, the S670 on the discrete balloon. These stents have shortened the repeating subunit from 3 to 2 mm for the GFX and GFX-2 stents and 1.5 mm for the S670 stent; these changes were accompanied by an increase in the number of crowns and laser junction points per unit. The S670 and S660 (for vessels <2.75 mm) are broadly functional stents that are distinguished by their ability to position the stent in distal lesions with proximal tortuosity and through previously stented regions.

THE NIR STENT. The NIR stent (Boston Scientific, Natick, MA) is a balloon-expandable stent composed of 316L stainless steel that is etched from a metal sheet, folded, and welded into its slotted tube design.[207] The NIR stent has seven or nine closed cells around its circumference[207] that impart a unique "transformable geometry" resulting in longitudinal flexibility during stent advancement and radial strength after stent deployment. The NIR stent provides symmetrical arterial scaffolding, and the smooth initial angiographic lumen contour is associated with infrequent late clinical events.[217] An equivalency study comparing the NIR stent with the PS-153 stent demonstrated comparable early and late clinical outcomes, with subsequent clinical approval in the United States.[218] Potential drawbacks of the NIR stent are its radiolucency, closed-cell design that limits access to large sidebranches, and lack of a high-pressure deployment balloon. Each of these issues has been addressed with subsequent NIR stent generations, including the NIR-ON-SOX high-pressure deployment system and the NIR Royal gold-plated stent, which enhances visualization.

THE CROSSFLEX-LC STENT. The first-generation Cordis CrossFlex stent was a 15-mm balloon-expandable stent composed of a 0.005-inch tantalum wire arranged in a single, sinusoidal helical coil. Its major advantage was that it was flexible and radiopaque.[219] The current generation of the CrossFlex-LC is laser-cut from a 316L stainless steel hypotube configured into a dual-spine "S" wave design, now available in a broad range of diameters and stent lengths. Improved

▶ TABLE 38–5. STENT AND STENT FILAMENT CHARACTERISTICS

STENT	MANUFACTURER	STENT DESIGN	STENT MATERIAL	FILAMENT CONFIGURATION	STRUT THICKNESS (inch)	STENT RADIOPACITY	SURFACE COVERAGE (%)	% STENT SHORTENING	EXPANSION METHOD
PS 153	Cordis	ST	316L SS	Diamond shaped	0.0025	Low	<20	2.5–3.5	BE
Crown	Cordis	ST	316L SS	Diamond shaped	0.0027	Low	<20	2.5–3.5	BE
CrossFlex	Cordis	ST	316L SS	Dual-spine S wave design	0.0055	Moderate	12–18	0	BE
Minicrown	Cordis	ST	316L SS	Diamond shaped	0.0025	Low	17	<10	BE
Bx Velocity	Cordis	ST	316L SS	Flex segment	0.0055	Moderate	12–15	<2	BE
GR-II	Cook, Inc	Coil	316L SS	Flat wire coil with interdigitating spine	0.0055	High due to gold markers	16	None	BE
Magic Wallstent	BSC	Mesh	Platinum-cobalt alloy	Braided wire mesh	0.003–0.004	Moderate	14	15–20	SE
Radius	BSC	ST	Nitinol	Zigzag struts constrained by outer sheath	0.0046	Moderate	20	<3	SE
NIR	BSC	ST	316L SS	Multicellular slotted tube design	0.004	Low	12–16	<6	BE
Multilink	Guidant	MC	316L SS	Multiple tubular rings interconnected with "S," "W," and "U" shapes	0.0022	Low	15	2.7	BE
DUET	Guidant	MC	316L SS	Corrugated ring design	0.0055	Moderate	13–16	5.6	BE
TriStar	Guidant	MC	316L SS	Corrugated ring design	0.0025	Moderate	12–18	2.6	BE
Wiktor	Medtronic-AVE	Coil	Tantalum	Single wire	0.005	High	7–9	<5	BE
GFX	Medtronic-AVE	Ring	316L SS	2-mm elliptorectangular sinusoidal rings with welded subunits	0.005	Moderate	20	<2	BE
S670	Medtronic-AVE	Ring	316L SS	Elliptorectangular	0.0055	Moderate	20	3.5	BE
Bard XT	Medtronic-AVE	Ring	316L VM SS	2.1-mm zigzag modules connected by an interdigitating spine	0.0060	Moderate	NA	NA	BE
beStent	Medtronic-AVE	Ring	316L SS	Rectangular serpentine mesh shape with 2 gold markers at each end	0.004 × 0.0035	High	15–18	0	BE
DivYsio	Biocompatibles	MC	316L SS	Interlocking arrowhead	0.0033	Low	NA	NA	BE
Paragon	Tyco, Inc	ST	Martinsitic Nitinol	Flat stent with short ST and interconnected sinusoidal links	0.0072	High	20	1–2	BE

BE = balloon expandable; BSC = Boston-Scientific-SciMed; MC = multicellular; Ring = ringed elements; SE = self-expanding; SS = stainless steel; ST = slotted tube.

▶ TABLE 38–6. CHARACTERISTICS OF NEW CORONARY STENTS

STENT	AVAILABLE DIAMETERS (mm)	IMPLANTABLE LENGTHS (mm)	MINIMUM GUIDE ID (inch)	SHEATH	CROSSING PROFILE (inch)	DEPLOYMENT PRESSURE (atm)	RATED BURST PRESSURE (atm)	BALLOON OVERHANG (mm)
PS-153	3.0, 3.5, 4.0	15	0.084	Yes	0.065	4	8	1.5
Crown	3.0, 3.5, 4.0	15, 22, 30	3.0/3.5 mm—0.064 inch 4.0 mm—0.072 inch	No	0.051–0.057	7	12	1.0
CrossFlex	3.0, 3.5, 4.0	13, 18, 23, 28	0.064	No	0.047–0.054	10	14	1.0
Minicrown	2.25–3.25	11, 15	0.064	No	0.044–0.046	10	18	1.0
Bx Velocity	2.25–5.0	8–33	0.064	No	0.042–0.059	10	16	1.0
GR-II	2.5–5.0	12, 20 40	0.058–0.075 inch	No	0.056–0.073	4–6	NA	2.5
Magic Wallstent	4.0–6.0 for RD of 3.0–5.5	15–47	0.064	Yes	0.056–0.058	NA	NA	NA
Radius	3.0, 3.5, 4.0	14, 20, 31	0.066	Yes	0.056	NA	NA	NA
NIR	2.5, 3.0, 3.5, 4.0	9, 16, 25, 32	0.064	No	0.043–0.049	7	12–14	2.0
Multilink	3.0, 3.5	15, 25	0.072	No	0.058	6	8	2.5
DUET	2.5–4.0	8–38	0.064	No	0.043–0.049	9	16	1.8
TriStar	2.5–4.0	8–38	0.064	No	0.043–0.049	8	16	0.4
Wiktor	3.0–4.5	16	2.5/3.0 mm—0.062 inch 3.5 mm—0.073 inch 4.0 mm—0.086 inch	No	NR	8		
GFX	2.5–4.0	8, 12, 18, 24	0.064	No	0.035	9	9	1.0
S670			0.064	No		8	16	0.4 distal; 0.80 proximal
Bard XT	3.0, 3.5, 4.0	NR	NR	NR	NR	NR	NR	NR
BeStent	3.0, 3.5, 4.0	NR	NR	NR	NR	NR	NR	NR
DivYsio	2.0–4.0	10–28	0.064	No	0.029–0.0473	6	14	1–2
Paragon	3.0, 3.5, 4.0	9–36	0.062	No	0.052	8	16	NR

ID = inner diameter; NR = not reported.

▶ TABLE 38–7. EARLY AND LATE OUTCOME IN RANDOMIZED TRIALS OF STENT-VERSUS-STENT EQUIVALANCY TRIALS IN NATIVE VESSELS

VARIABLE	ASCENT PS-153	ASCENT Multilink	SMART PS-153	SMART MS-II	NIRVANA PS-153	NIRVANA NIR	SCORES PS-153	SCORES Radius	WIN PTCA*	WIN Wallstent	PARAGON PS-153	PARAGON Paragon
Number of patients	522	518	331	330	430	418	551	545	287	299	339	349
Lesion type	Focal <25 mm De novo lesion 3.00–3.75 mm		Focal <25 mm De novo or RS 3.00–4.00 mm		Focal <25 mm De novo or RS 3.00–3.75 mm		Focal <30 mm De novo or RS 2.75–4.25 mm		Focal <35 mm De novo or RS 3.00–5.50 mm		Focal <25 mm De novo or RS 3.00–4.00 mm	
Baseline factors												
Mean age (yr)	61	61	64	63	62	62	62	62	62	63	62	62
Women (%)	31	33	30	31	32	30	32	30	27	28	32	32
Diabetes mellitus (%)	20	19	17	19	22	23	19	22	23	17	21	21
Unstable angina (%)	70	69	69	65	73	75	65	65	68	67	82	81
LAD location (%)	44	42	42	47	40	42	38	40	23	23	45	41
Lesion Length (mm)	11.0	10.9	12.1	11.5	13.3	13.3	13.1	12.8	13.0	17.0	12.2	12.4
ACC/AHA B2 or C (%)	59	63	63	62	65	69	NR	NR	63	67	62.9	69.3
Maximum inflation (%) pressure (atm)	17.1	16.7	17.1	16.6	16.6	15.5	16.7	13.3	11.6	15.0	15.3	14.9
Reference diameter (mm)	2.94	2.95	2.93	2.93	3.03	2.97	3.05	3.06	3.09	3.10	3.05	2.97†
MLD (mm)												
Baseline	1.05	1.05	1.06	1.02	1.08	1.04	0.99	1.01	1.04	1.08	1.07	1.05
Final	2.72	2.77	2.77	2.85	2.79	2.78	2.80	2.86	2.34	2.56	2.83	2.83
Follow-up	1.92	1.96	2.00	1.86	1.90	2.00	1.88	1.88	1.70	1.71	1.93	1.78
Percent diameter stenosis												
Baseline	64	64	64	65	64	65	66.5	67.3	66	65	64.5	64.3
Final	10	8	8	5	8	8	11.8	12.2	26	19	8.9	6.2†
Follow-up	32	35	34	37	37	34	36.1	36.3	46	45	37.8	39.8
Restenosis rate (%)	22.1	16.0	22.9	24.8	22.4	19.3	18.7	24.2	38	38	23.7	29.1
Device success (%)	96.9	98.8	95.2	97.8	97.9	99.5	95.3	98.3‡	60	96	94.1	99.1†
Procedural success (%)	93.9	95.7	94.7	94.1	94.3	95.4	93.5	97.0	96.2	97.0	95.4	92.0
30-Day event rates (%)	6.5	5.0	5.1	6.4	4.4§	4.3	3.1	2.9	5.9	8.4§	4.4	8.0§
Death	1.1	0†	0.3	0.6	0.2	0	0.4	0.4	0.4	0.4	0.3	0.3
Q wave infarction	1.0	0.6	0.6	0.6	0.9	0.5	0.4	0.2	0.4	0	0.3	0.6
Emergency CABG	0.8	0.6	1.2	0.6	0	0.2	0.7	0.9	0.9	0.4	0.3	0.3
Subacute thrombosis	1.8	0.6	0.3	0	0.5	0.5	0.4	0.2	0.7	1.3	0.3	0.6
Follow-up period	9 mo		6 mo		9 mo		9 mo		6 mo		6 mo	
Target vessel failure (%)	16.7	15.1	12.3	14.2	17.2	16.0	20.1	19.3	16.7	17.2	12.4	20.3‡
TLR (%)	9.8	7.7	8.1	8.4	13.4	12.2	10.7	9.5	15.1	13.0	5.9	12.0†
Late clinical events (%)			14.8	16.1							11.2	19.8¶
Death	2.5	1.4	0.3	1.5	1.0	0.9	1.1	1.5	3.5	3.0	0.6	1.1
Q wave MI	1.0	0.6	0.0	0.3	0.7	0.9	0.5	0.7	1.7	2.7	0.3	2.0
CABG	2.9	2.3	1.2	3.0	2.4	3.0	5.3	5.1	1.7	2.7	2.3	2.8
Repeat PCI	6.9	5.4	8.2	6.7	7.2	8.6	11.1	10.3	18.8	19.1	4.1	10.0¶

* Balloon PTCA with "bailout" stenting.
† p < 0.05.
‡ p < 0.005.
§ In = hospital events.
¶ p < 0.01.

ACC/AHA = American College of Cardiology/American Heart Association; CABG = coronary artery bypass graft surgery; LAD = left anterior descending artery; MI = myocardial infarction; MLD = minimal lumen diameter; NR = not reported; PCI = percutaneous coronary intervention; PS = Palmaz-Schatz; RS = restenotic lesion; TLR = target lesion revascularization.

Data from ASCENT,[225] SMART,[225] NIRVANA,[216] Stent Comparative Restenosis (SCORES) Trial,[218] Wallstent in Native Coronary Arteries (WIN) Trial,[222] and Paragon Stent Study.[224]

vessel scaffolding and access to large sidebranches are the major clinical advantages of the CrossFlex-LC over previous iterations of this stent.[220] It can be applied in a broad range of lesion morphologies. The SLAM Trial will compare the results of the CrossFlex-LC and balloon PTCA for the treatment of long lesions.

RADIUS STENT. The Radius stent is a self-expanding, multiple-zig-zag, nitinol stent that has a flexible restraining sheath allowing access to distal lesions, regions of calcification, and vessels distal to previously deployed stents.[207] Proper sizing is essential because the stent will not expand beyond its parent diameter.[207] Once deployed, Radius stents that are slightly larger than the vessel diameter will continue to expand after adjunct balloon PTCA.[221] A limitation of the Radius stent is that it requires precise positioning to avoid distal stent deployment. The Radius stent was approved for use in the United States in native coronary and SVG lesions based on results of the Stent Comparative Restenosis (SCORES) Trial, which demonstrated equivalency to the PS-153 stent in late clinical outcome.[222]

THE MAGIC WALLSTENT. The Magic Wallstent is a self-expanding, wire mesh stent composed of a cobalt-based alloy with a platinum core. The Magic Wallstent is notable for its longitudinal flexibility, but precise localization can be somewhat difficult because of its somewhat unpredictable shortening (up to 20 percent) after deployment. Its major clinical uses are large (>4.0 mm) native vessels, particularly the right coronary artery, and SVGs. Sidebranch access is limited with the use of this stent, and it cannot be expanded beyond its nominal unconstrained diameter.

Stent-Versus-Stent Equivalency Studies

The Palmaz-Schatz PS-153 stent has been the traditional "gold standard" for regulatory-based stent comparisons (Table 38–7). A series of randomized stent-versus-stent equivalency studies were performed to ensure the safety and efficacy of late outcomes associated with newer stent designs.[216, 224] Although these studies were designed to compare freedom from late target vessel failure, i.e., procedure success and freedom from TLR, death, or large myocardial infarction, it is now apparent that selection of stents by interventionists for clinical use is based on a number of secondary factors, including the profile, flexibility, and ease of use of the stent.

Stent equivalency trials have included patients with focal or restenotic native vessel lesions approachable with one or two coronary stents (lesion length <25 mm). In general, lesions were selected for treatment if they were suitable for Palmaz-Schatz stenting, and lesions with angulation greater than 45 degrees, proximal tortuosity, calcification, and thrombus were generally not included. It is likely

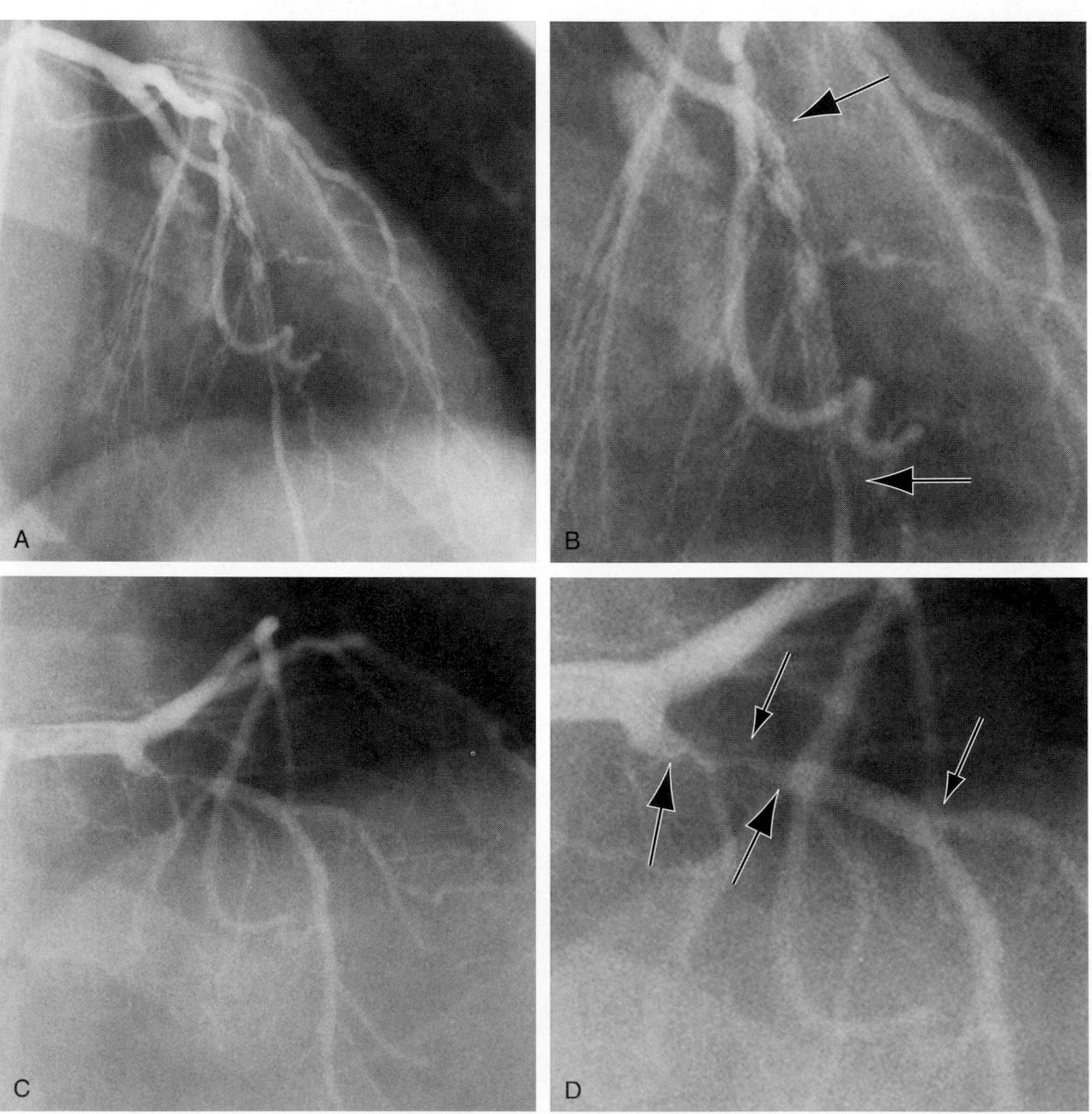

FIGURE 38–9. Two cases of in-stent restenosis. *A*, Diffuse in-stent restenosis in the proximal segment of the left anterior descending artery. A magnified view demonstrates diffuse tissue growth within the axial length of the stent (arrows). *B*, Another case of in-stent restenosis involving the left anterior descending artery (arrow). A focal region of renarrowing (large arrows) is seen in the proximal portion *(C)* and margin *(D)* of the stent (small arrows).

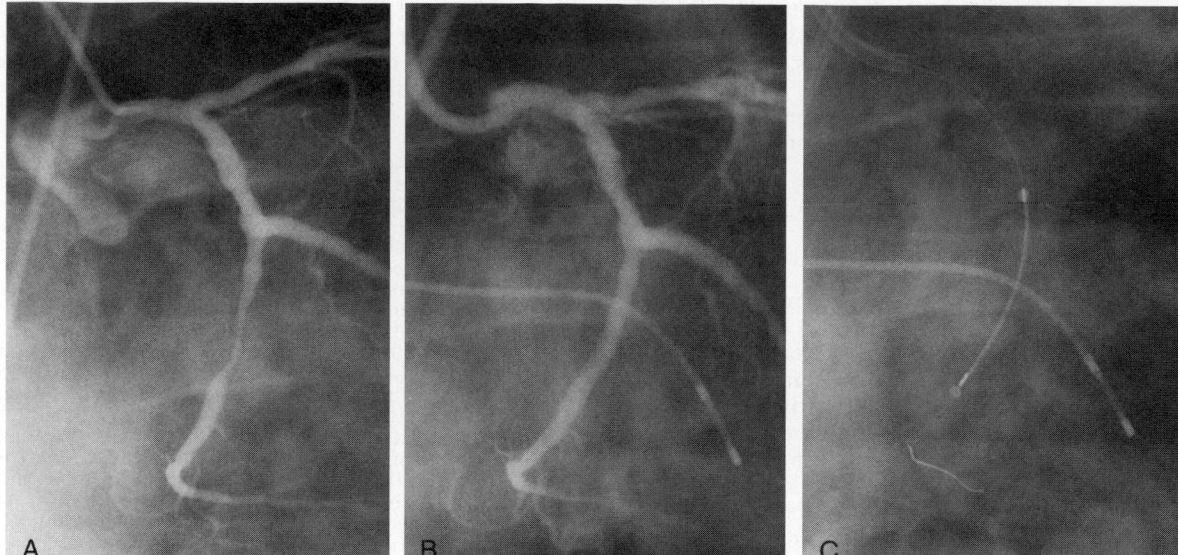

FIGURE 38–10. *A,* Restenosis after coronary stent placement in the midportion of the left circumflex coronary artery. *B,* After rotational atherectomy and balloon angioplasty with a 3.5-mm balloon, an excellent angiographic result is obtained. This patient was enrolled in the randomized Stent and Radiation Therapy (START) Trial, which used catheter-based brachytherapy with strontium-90. *C,* The catheter is positioned (large arrows) and the radiation source train is advanced to the midportion of the circumflex artery (small arrows) to cover the margins of the injured segment by 5 to 10 mm.

that a performance difference may have been shown with the second- and third-generation stents had more complex lesion subsets been included in the studies.

These stent trials have identified a number of multivariable predictors of angiographic restenosis, including patient age, history of diabetes, left anterior descending artery lesion location, small postprocedural minimal lumen diameters, and longer lesion and total stent length. Multivariable predictors of target vessel revascularization (or failure) after stent placement include male gender, presence of thrombus, smaller postprocedural minimal lumen or reference vessel diameters, proximal left anterior descending artery location, longer lesion and total stent length, total number of stents, type C lesions, mandated follow-up angiography, restenotic lesions, or lesion calcification.

In-Stent Restenosis

The mechanism of restenosis after stent placement in virtually all cases is neointimal proliferation within the axial stent length.[225] Recurrence of symptoms may occur in 10 to 20 percent of patients within 12 months after stent implantation; after 6 to 12 months, it appears that contraction of intimal tissue results in slightly larger lumen dimensions over time.[226] Although some patients with multivessel CAD or multiple stent restenoses are best served by referral CABG, the majority of patients with in-stent restenosis can be safety and effectively treated with repeat PCI.[227] The mechanism of benefit of balloon angioplasty relates to both expansion of the stent and extrusion of the tissue through the stent struts and axially along its length.[228] Early tissue recoil may account for loss of 2.0 mm² in nearly 30 percent of patients within 40 minutes of the procedure.[229] Recurrence rates after balloon PTCA for stent restenosis ranged from 11 to 17 percent in two large series,[230, 231] although higher (up to 80 percent) recurrence rates have been reported depending on vessel size, pattern of restenosis (e.g., intrastent, stent margin, or remote disease), and the time to presentation[231a] (Fig. 38–9).

Atheroablation by DCA, RA, or ELCA has been used in patients at "high risk" of recurrence after PCI for in-stent restenosis,[227] but an advantage over conventional balloon PTCA alone has not been demonstrated in a prospective, randomized study. A consecutive registry series of 60 patients with "diffuse" native vessel in-stent restenosis compared early and late outcomes in patients treated with either conventional balloon PTCA or debulking by RA or DCA followed by balloon PTCA.[232] The procedural success rate was 100 percent in both groups, and despite longer lesion lengths in the debulking group (18.4 vs. 13.5 mm in the PTCA-only group; $p = 0.09$), treatment with atherectomy resulted in a lower frequency of postprocedure stenoses (18 vs. 26 percent in the PTCA-only group; $p = 0.01$). One-year repeat TLR was required in 28 percent of patients in the debulking group and 46 percent in the balloon PTCA group ($p = 0.18$). Pending the results of additional randomized studies, it appears that debulking is most useful in patients with diffuse (>15 mm) in-stent restenosis.

Three studies have shown the value of gamma irradiation with iridium-192 in preventing angiographic and clinical recurrence in patients undergoing treatment for in-stent restenosis. In the Scripps Radiation to Inhibit Proliferation after Stent Implantation (SCRIPPS) Trial, 55 patients were randomly assigned to the iridium-192 group or placebo group after treatment of stent restenosis. Angiographic restenosis occurred in 17 percent of the iridium-treated patients and 54 percent of the placebo-treated patients ($p = 0.01$) as a result of a reduction in late lumen loss in the iridium-192 group (0.38 vs. 1.03 mm in placebo-treated patients; $p = 0.03$).[233] These effects have been sustained for up to 3 years after the procedure.[233a] Two other larger studies have shown similar benefits.[234, 235] Studies evaluating results of the use of beta radiation for the treatment of in-stent restenosis are ongoing (Fig. 38–10).

ANTICOAGULATION DURING PERCUTANEOUS CORONARY INTERVENTIONS
(See also Chap. 62)

The safety of PCI has been substantially improved over recent years with the routine use of conventional (e.g., aspirin, ticlopidine, clopidogrel) and novel (e.g., GP IIb-IIIa inhibitors) platelet inhibitors and conventional (e.g., unfractionated heparin, low-molecular-weight heparin [LMWH]) thrombin inhibitors.[236-238] The safety and efficacy of second-generation direct thrombin inhibitors (e.g., hirudin, bivalirudin [Hirulog], argatroban) have also been evaluated in the setting of PCI, but their clinical use is currently limited to the setting of heparin-induced thrombocytopenia syndromes.

Antiplatelet Therapy

ASPIRIN. This agent reduces the frequency of ischemic complications after PCI by 64 to 77 percent.[236, 239] Although the minimum effective aspirin dosage is not known, doses ranging between 80 and 325 mg are generally given 2 or more hours before PCI. The use of dipyridamole provides no incremental value over aspirin alone, so dipyridamole is not currently recommended.[240] Aspirin-intolerant patients may be treated with thienopyridine blockers of platelet adenosine diphosphate (ADP) receptors, such as ticlopidine (250 mg twice daily)[239] or clopidogrel (300-mg loading dose followed by 75 mg daily), but these agents should be given earlier than 24 hours prior to elective PCI to achieve maximum platelet inhibition.[241]

TICLOPIDINE. In patients undergoing stent implantation, ticlopidine, as an adjunct to aspirin, reduces the frequency of 30-day clinical events, including the occurrence of subacute thrombosis.[242, 243] In a clinical trial of 517 patients at "high risk" for stent thrombosis after Palmaz-Schatz stenting, those treated with aspirin plus ticlopidine experienced a 75 percent reduction in early complications in comparison to those who received aspirin plus intravenous heparin plus phenprocoumon.[242] Patients receiving antiplatelet therapy also had an 82 percent lower risk of myocardial infarction and a 78 percent lower need for repeat balloon PTCA than did patients receiving anticoagulation therapy.[242] Bleeding complications were also lower in patients treated with antiplatelet therapy.[242] The Stent Anti-thrombotic Regimen Study (STARS) evaluated the effect of aspirin alone, aspirin plus ticlopidine, and aspirin plus warfarin on the occurrence of 30-day ischemic endpoints in 1653 "low-risk" patients undergoing successful Palmaz-Schatz stent placement.[243] Clinical events, including subacute thrombosis, were reduced by 85 percent in patients treated with aspirin plus ticlopidine.[243]

Ticlopidine has a number of significant side effects in comparison to aspirin, including gastrointestinal distress (20 percent), cutaneous rashes (4.8 to 15 percent), and liver function test abnormalities. Severe, but generally reversible neutropenia and aplastic anemia occur in 1 percent or less of patients. Rare episodes of fatal thrombotic thrombocytopenic purpura have also been reported with ticlopidine.[244] A shorter (10 to 14 days) duration of ticlopidine therapy may reduce the risk of these side effects.[245, 246]

CLOPIDOGREL. This newer thienopyridine inhibitor of ADP-mediated platelet aggregation has also been used in patients undergoing stent placement.[247, 248] The CLASSICS trial showed no difference in clinical efficacy between clopidogrel and ticlopidine, with fewer side effects in patients treated with clopidogrel.[249] Based on randomized studies and single center registries that did not show a difference in outcome with these two agents,[250, 250a] clopidogrel may be used as an alternative to ticlopidine in patients undergoing stent implantation.

GLYCOPROTEIN IIb-IIIa INHIBITORS. Aspirin is only a partial inhibitor of platelet function, and early ischemic events develop in 3.0 to 12.8 percent of aspirin-treated patients undergoing PCI.[5, 6, 9] Thrombin and collagen are potent platelet agonists that can cause ADP and serotonin release and activate GP IIb-IIIa fibrinogen receptors on the platelet surface.[251] Functionally active GP IIb-IIIa activation serves as the "final common pathway" of platelet aggregation by binding fibrinogen and other adhesive proteins that bridge adjacent platelets.[252] A number of intravenous and oral inhibitors of the GP IIb-IIIa receptor have been developed for clinical use.

ABCIXIMAB

The safety and efficacy of abciximab was first evaluated in the Evaluation of 7E3 for the Prevention of Ischemic Complications (EPIC) Trial, a clinical study of 2099 patients at "high risk" for complications after PCI[19] (Table 38-8). "High-risk" criteria included patients with acute myocardial infarction, refractory unstable angina, and "high-risk" clinical and angiographic features. All patients received aspirin 325 mg and a non–weight-adjusted, 10,000- to 12,000-IU heparin bolus prior to PCI and were then randomly assigned to treatment with placebo, a bolus of abciximab 0.25 mg/kg, or the same bolus of abciximab followed by a 12-hour abciximab infusion at 10 μg/min. Bolus and infusion abciximab was associated with a 35 percent reduction in frequency of the composite clinical endpoint, defined as death, nonfatal myocardial infarction, repeat revascularization, or procedural failure (8.3 vs. 12.8 percent in placebo-treated patients; $p = 0.008$).[19] This benefit was greatest in patients with unstable clinical syndromes (acute myocardial infarction and refractory unstable angina).[259, 259a] Pretreatment with abciximab in a randomized trial of 429 patients with acute myocardial infarction was associated with a significant ($p = 0.03$) reduction in the incidence of death, reinfarction, or urgent target vessel revascularization at 30 days in patients treated with abciximab (4.9 percent) versus placebo (10.3 percent). No difference in 6-month restenosis was noted between the two groups.[260]

The Evaluation of PTCA to Improve Long-Term Outcome by Abciximab GP IIb-IIIa Blockade (EPILOG) Trial randomly assigned 2792 "low-risk" patients who were treated with aspirin to standard-dose, weight-adjusted (100 units/kg) heparin and placebo; standard-dose, weight-adjusted heparin and abciximab; or low-dose, weight-adjusted (70 units/kg) heparin. The 30-day composite event rate was significantly ($p < 0.001$) lower in patients treated with abciximab and low-dose (5.2 percent) or standard-dose (5.4 percent) heparin than in patients treated with standard-dose heparin and placebo (11.7 percent).[253] While one study suggested a beneficial effect with abciximab in patients undergoing SVG angioplasty,[261] a larger study failed to demonstrate a convincing reduction in these patients at high risk for macroembolization.[262] "Bailout" abciximab is often given during or just after PCI for the presence of residual dissection, thrombus, or suboptimal results,[263] although its value has not been demonstrated in prospective studies.

The EPISTENT trial randomly assigned 2399 patients with ischemic CAD to stenting plus placebo, stenting plus abciximab, or balloon PTCA plus abciximab.[254] The primary 30-day endpoint, a combination of death, myocardial infarction, or need for urgent revascularization, occurred in 10.8 percent of patients in the stent-plus-placebo group, 5.3 percent of patients in the stent-plus-abciximab group (hazard ratio 0.48; $p < 0.001$), and 6.9 percent of patients in the balloon-plus-abciximab group (hazard ratio 0.63; $p = 0.007$).[254] The occurrence of death and large (CPK-MB more than five times normal) myocardial infarction occurred in 7.8 percent of the placebo group versus 3.0 percent of the stent-plus-abciximab group ($p < 0.001$) and 4.7 percent of the balloon PTCA–plus–abciximab group ($p = 0.01$).[254] No significant differences in bleeding complications were noted among the groups.[254] The need for late revascularization was not significantly ($p = 0.22$) lower in patients receiving stenting plus abciximab (8.7 percent) than in patients receiving stenting plus placebo (10.6 percent).[255] However, a significant ($p = 0.02$) reduction was seen in revascularization in diabetic patients assigned to stenting plus abciximab (8.1 percent) when compared with patients receiving stenting plus placebo (16.6 percent).[255] A pooled analysis also suggests that abciximab may reduce mortality in diabetic patients.[263a]

EPTIFIBATIDE

The effect of eptifibatide (Integrelin) on 30-day clinical events was evaluated in 4010 patients undergoing PCI. The patients were assigned to placebo, an eptifibatide bolus of 135 μg/kg followed by a low-dose eptifibatide infusion at 0.5 μg/kg/min for 20 to 24 hours, or the same eptifibatide bolus and a higher-dose infusion at 0.75 μg/kg/min for 20 to 24 hours.[256] The primary endpoint was a 30-day composite occurrence of death, myocardial infarction, unplanned CABG or repeat PCI, or coronary stenting for abrupt closure. Such events occurred in 11.4 percent of patients in the placebo group versus 9.2 percent in the 135/0.5 eptifibatide group ($p = 0.063$) and 9.9 percent in the eptifibatide 135/0.75 group ($p = 0.22$).[256] In a treatment-received analysis, the eptifibatide 135/0.5 regimen produced a significant reduction in the composite endpoint (9.1 vs. 11.6 percent in placebo-treated patients; $p = 0.035$), but the eptifibatide 135/0.75 regimen produced a less substantial reduction (10.0 vs. 11.6 percent in placebo-treated patients; $p = 0.18$). Eptifibatide treatment did not increase rates of major bleeding or transfusion. It is now recognized that the eptifibatide infusion dosage in the Integrelin to Minimise Platelet Aggregation and Coronary Thrombosis-II (IMPACT-II) Trial was insufficient to provide adequate platelet inhibition. The ongoing randomized ESPRIT Trial will compare a 180-μg/kg double bolus of eptifi-

▶ **TABLE 38–8. EARLY AND LATE OUTCOME IN RANDOMIZED TRIALS OF GLYCOPROTEIN IIb-IIIa INHIBITORS IN PERCUTANEOUS CORONARY INTERVENTION**

| | EPIC | | | EPILOG | | | EPISTENT | | | IMPACT-II | | | RESTORE | |
| | Abciximab | | | Abciximab | | | Abciximab | | | Eptifibatide | | | | |
VARIABLE	Placebo	Bolus	Bolus + Infusion	Placebo + SD Heparin	Abciximab + SD Heparin	Abciximab + LD Heparin	Placebo + Stent	+ Stent	+ PTCA	Placebo	Low Dose	High Dose	Placebo	Tirofiban
Lesion type	High risk			Low risk			Low risk			Low and high risk			High risk	
Years of entry	11/91–11/92			2/95–12.95			7/96–9.97			11/93–11.94			1/95–12.95	
Number of patients	697	695	708	939	918	935	809	794	796	1328	1349	1333	1070	1071
Baseline factors														
Mean age (yr)	61	60	62	60	60	60	59	59	60	60	62	60	59	59
Women (%)	27	28	29	28	27	29	25.5	25	25	25	27	24	28	28
Diabetes mellitus (%)	26	23	23	24	22	23	21.4	20.4	19.6	22	23	23	20	20
Unstable angina (%)	NA	NA	NA	50	46	46	60.4	56.4	54.8	38	38	38	68	67
Stent use (%)	0.6	1.7	0.6	NR	NR	NR	96.0	97.3	19.3	4.5	3.6	4.1	NA	NA
Composite primary endpoint (%)	12.8	11.4	8.3*	11.7	5.4*	5.2*	10.8	5.3*	6.9†	11.4	9.2	9.9	12.2	10.3
Early complications (%)														
Death	1.7	1.3	1.7	0.8	0.4	0.3	0.6	0.3	0.8	1.1	0.5	0.8	0.7	0.8
Q wave infarction	2.3	1.0	3.0	0.8	0.5	0.4	1.4	0.9	1.5	1.6	0.9	1.1	5.7	4.2
Emergency CABG	3.6	2.3	2.4	1.7	0.9	0.4	1.1	0.8	0.6	2.8	1.6	2.0	2.2	1.9
Emergency PTCA	4.5	3.6	0.8*	3.8	1.5†	1.2*	1.2	0.6	1.3	2.8	2.6	2.9	5.4	4.2
Major bleeding (%)	7	11*	14*	3.1	3.5	2.0	2.2	1.5	1.4	4.8	5.1	5.2	3.7	5.3
Follow-up time	3 yr			6 mo			6 mo			6 mo			6 mo	
Late clinical outcome (%)	47.2	47.4	41.1	25.8	22.3	22.8	18.3	13.0	15.5	11.6	10.5	10.1	27.1	24.1
Death	8.6	8.1	6.8	1.7	1.4	1.1	1.2	0.5	1.8	NR	NR	NR	1.4	1.8
Q wave MI	13.6	12.2	10.7	1.6	1.4	1.3	1.5	1.3	2.1	NR	NR	NR	7.6	6.3
Revascularization	40.1	38.6	34.8	19.4	18.4	19.0	10.6	8.7	15.4	NR	NR	NR	NR	NR
Repeat PTCA	NR	NR	NR	NR	NR	NR	NR	NR	NR	NR	NR	NR	17.1	15.7
CABG	NR	NR	NR	NR	NR	NR	NR	NR	NR	NR	NR	NR	6.8	5.5

* p < 0.001.
† p < 0.005.
CABG = coronary artery bypass grafting; LD = low dose; MI = myocardial infarction; PTCA = percutaneous transluminal coronary angioplasty; SD = standard dose.
Data from Evaluation of 7E3 for the Prevention of Ischemic Complications (EPIC) Trial,[19] Evaluation of PTCA to Improve Long-Term Outcome by Abciximab Glycoprotein IIb-IIIa Blockade (EPILOG) Trial,[253] EPISTENT,[254, 255] Integrelin to Minimise Platelet Aggregation and Coronary Thrombosis-II (IMPACT-II),[256] and Randomized Efficacy Study of Tirofiban for Outcomes and Restenosis (RESTORE),[257, 258]

batide followed by a 2.0-μg/kg/min infusion with placebo in lower-risk patients undergoing stent implantation.

TIROFIBAN

The effect of tirofiban, a nonpeptidyl tyrosine derivative, on outcomes after PCI was evaluated in the Randomized Efficacy Study of Tirofiban for Outcomes and Restenosis (RESTORE) Trial, a randomized, double-blind, placebo-controlled study involving 2139 patients undergoing PCI who were seen within 72 hours of an acute coronary syndrome.[257] All patients received aspirin and heparin and were randomly assigned to a tirofiban bolus (10 μg/kg over a 3-minute period) plus infusion (0.15 μg/kg/min) or to a placebo bolus plus infusion for 36 hours after PCI. The primary 30-day composite endpoint was 16 percent lower with tirofiban treatment ($p = 0.160$), although a 38 percent relative reduction in the composite end point was noted at 48 hours ($p = 0.005$) and a 27 percent relative reduction at 7 days ($p = 0.022$).[257] When only urgent or emergency balloon PTCA or CABG were included in the composite endpoint, the 30-day event rates were 10.5 percent for the placebo group and 8.0 percent for the tirofiban group, a relative reduction of 24 percent ($p = 0.052$). Major bleeding tended to be higher in tirofiban-treated patients (5.3 vs. 3.7 percent in the placebo-treated patients; $p = 0.096$), although no difference in bleeding events could be found when using the TIMI criteria[264] for major bleeding.[257] A prospective trial, the TARGET study, will compare clinical outcome in over 4000 patients undergoing PCI treated with either abciximab or tirofiban.

As a class of agents, the GP IIb-IIIa inhibitors (i.e., abciximab, eptifibatide, and tirofiban) have demonstrated benefit in improving clinical outcomes within the first 30 days after PCI. The primary effect of these agents has been on the reduction of ischemic complications, including non-Q-wave myocardial infarction and recurrent ischemia. No consistent evidence indicates that GP IIb-IIIa inhibitors reduce the frequency of restenosis. These agents should be considered for use in all patients undergoing PCI, particularly in those with unstable angina, primary balloon PTCA, or stent placement for acute myocardial infarction, and in other patients at higher risk for ischemic complications after PCI.

Antithrombin Therapy

UNFRACTIONATED HEPARIN (see also Chap. 62). Unfractionated heparin is the most common thrombin inhibitor used during PCI, although other antithrombin III–dependent agents (e.g., LMWH) and antithrombin III–independent agents (e.g., hirudin, bivalirudin, and argatroban) have also been tried. Intravenous heparin is used during PCI to prevent arterial thrombus formation at the site of vessel wall injury and on coronary guidewires and other catheter equipment used for coronary dilatation.[265] Patients with acute coronary syndromes may also benefit from prolonged (>24 hours) heparin therapy alone before PCI[266] or in combination with GP IIb-IIIa inhibitors.[267-269]

Activated partial thromboplastin times have been used to monitor the intensity of anticoagulation *before* and *after* PCI, but these methods have been less useful for monitoring anticoagulation *during* PCI inasmuch as large amounts of heparin are required to prevent thrombus formation during arterial manipulations.[270] "Near-patient" activated clotting time (ACT) monitoring has facilitated heparin dose titration during PCI,[271] although ACT responses have shown marked variability in patients who received a non–weight-adjusted heparin bolus. These differences have been attributed to patient-to-patient differences in heparin sensitivity and clearance, body weight, nitroglycerin use, and coexisting conditions that predispose to heparin resistance (e.g., heparin antibodies, oral contraceptive use, endocarditis, disseminated intravascular coagulation, and placement of an intraaortic balloon pump). Patients with unstable angina and those with complex coronary lesions (irregular borders, overhanging edges, or filling defects) also have higher heparin dosing requirements.[272]

At least two studies have retrospectively related the ACT value to clinical outcome after PCI.[237, 238] Patients who had

complications after PCI in one study had lower mean baseline ACT (HemoTec) values after the initial heparin bolus and at the end of the procedure than did those without complications,[238] although this finding may be confounded because heparin resistance may be a marker of high-risk anatomy.[273] In another study, patients with abrupt closure had a lower mean ACT (Hemochron) at the time of first balloon inflation than did those without this complication (352 vs. 388 seconds; $p < 0.002$).[237] An inverse relationship was shown between in-laboratory ACT values and the probability of abrupt closure ($p = 0.018$).[237] Higher ACT levels[274] and other markers of excess anticoagulation[193] are also independent predictors of bleeding complications after PCI.

More recent studies have also evaluated the safety of lower-dose heparin during PCI. Low-dose bolus heparin at 5000 IU, followed by early (<12 hours) postprocedural sheath removal, in 1375 consecutive patients was associated with infrequent fatal complications (0.3 percent), emergency CABG (1.7 percent), myocardial infarction (3.3 percent), or repeat angioplasty within 48 hours (0.7 percent).[275] In a randomized study of 400 patients assigned to fixed-dose heparin at 15,000 IU or weight-adjusted heparin at 100 IU/kg, clinical outcomes were similar in the two groups (95 percent success rates).[276] Use of the weight-adjusted heparin did result in earlier sheath removal and more rapid transfer to a step-down unit.[276] Lower anticoagulation levels are also needed to avoid bleeding complications during the concomitant administration of agents such as GP IIb-IIIa inhibitors.[253]

The effect of subcutaneous heparin on the reduction in bleeding complications was evaluated in 151 patients treated either with an intravenous heparin infusion at 1000 units/hr for 12 to 18 hours after angioplasty or with subcutaneous heparin at 12,5000 units every 12 hours for three doses and early sheath removal.[277] The rate of ischemic complications was similar in both groups, but the risk of bleeding was significantly lower in the group managed with early (<12 hours) sheath removal and treated with subcutaneous heparin.[277]

Weight-adjusted heparin dosing regimens of 70 to 100 IU/kg or sex-adjusted bolus heparin consisting of 7000 units for women and 8000 units for men is now used in an attempt to avoid "overshooting" the ACT.[278] It is generally recommended that sufficient unfractionated heparin be administered during PCI to achieve an ACT between 250 and 300 seconds with the HemoTec monitor and between 300 and 350 seconds when using the Hemochron monitor.[271] When heparin is not adjusted by weight, the ACT should be monitored frequently and additional, smaller heparin boluses of 2000 to 5000 IU given until the target ACT is achieved. Routine use of intravenous heparin after PCI is no longer indicated because of several randomized studies showing no benefit in reducing ischemic complications and higher access site bleeding complication rates.[279, 280] Early sheath removal is strongly encouraged when the ACT falls to less than 150 to 180 seconds.

LOW-MOLECULAR-WEIGHT HEPARIN (see also Chap. 62). An increasing number of patients with unstable angina are treated with LMWH prior to PCI.[281] Because of the difficulty monitoring anticoagulation levels with LMWH during PCI, conventional dosages of unfractionated heparin are also recommended. In this setting, conventional monitoring methods, such as the ACT, may underestimate the true degree of periprocedural anticoagulation. A pilot randomized trial of 60 patients undergoing PCI and treated with unfractionated heparin or enoxaparin (1 mg/kg intravenously) showed no difference in safety between the two anticoagulants.[282] Routine use of LMWH as the sole anticoagulant during PCI cannot be recommended at this time pending the results of large, multicenter trials evaluating the use of LMWH during PCI.

DIRECT THROMBIN INHIBITORS

A number of direct thrombin inhibitors have been evaluated during PCI. In the Hirudin in a European Trial Versus Heparin in the Prevention of Restenosis after PTCA (HELVETICA) Study,[283] 1141 patients with unstable angina scheduled for PCI were treated with aspirin and randomized to receive a heparin bolus of 10,000 units plus infusion at 15 units/kg/hr for 24 hours; a hirudin bolus of 40 mg plus intravenous infusion at 0.2 mg/kg/hr for 24 hours; or a hirudin bolus of 40 mg, intravenous infusion at 0.2 mg/kg/hr for 24 hours, and subcutaneous infusion of 40 mg twice daily for an additional 3 days. Hirudin use was associated with a 39 percent reduction in early cardiac events ($p = 0.023$), although clinical outcomes were similar 7 months later in the three groups. A recombinant hirudin (lepirudin) bolus of 0.4 mg/kg and infusion at 0.15 mg/kg/hr is approved for use in the United States in patients with heparin-induced thrombocytopenia.

Bivalirudin (Hirulog or AngioMax) was compared with unfractionated heparin in the Hirulog Angioplasty Study, a randomized trial of 4098 patients with postinfarction or unstable angina undergoing coronary angioplasty and then assigned to receive a heparin bolus at 175 units/kg and a 15-unit/kg/hr infusion for 18 to 24 hours or to receive a bivalirudin bolus of 1.0 mg/kg and a 2.5-mg/kg/hr infusion for 4 hours, followed by 0.2 mg/kg/hr for 14 to 20 hours.[284] Although bivalirudin did not reduce the likelihood of in-hospital death, Q wave or non-Q-wave myocardial infarction, or emergency CABG, bivalirudin therapy reduced the likelihood of bleeding complications (odds ratio of 0.4; $p < 0.001$).[284] In the prospectively stratified cohort of 704 patients with post-myocardial infarction angina, bivalirudin resulted in lower rates of major ischemic complications (9.1 vs. 14.2 percent in heparin-treated patients; $p = 0.04$) and lower rates of bleeding (3.0 vs. 11.1 percent in heparin-treated patients; $p < 0.001$).

PHARMACOLOGICAL APPROACHES TO RESTENOSIS

IVUS studies have provided unique insight into the dynamic changes that occur within the vessel wall after PCI and suggest that arterial remodeling[285] and, to a lesser extent, intimal thickening account for most of the lumen renarrowing that occurs after balloon PTCA or coronary atherectomy.[12, 285, 286] In contrast, restenosis after stent implantation is due to intimal thickening within the axial length of the stent and its border in virtually all cases.[225] Conventional pharmacological strategies have not consistently reduced the frequency of angiographic or clinical restenosis indices after PCI (Table 38–9) despite a large number of agents having been tried.[287]

PLATELET INHIBITORS. Randomized studies evaluating the effect of aspirin on restenosis have produced conflicting results, potentially attributable to the varied dosage and duration of aspirin therapy.[236, 288–290] The majority of these studies have shown little, if any sustained effect of aspirin on restenosis prevention, although long-term aspirin at dosages greater than 100 mg daily is recommended after PCI for secondary prevention of cardiac events.[278] Platelet thromboxane A_2 and serotonin receptor antagonists, such as

sulotroban, ketanserin, and prostacyclin, have also been tried without success.[291–295]

Platelet aggregation during PCI may occur as a result of GP IIb-IIIa activation by a number of agonists, which renders the inhibition of a single agonist problematic for the prevention of restenosis. "Final common pathway" GP IIb-IIIa platelet receptor inhibitors provide potent (>80 percent) blockade of platelet aggregation during PCI, irrespective of the platelet agonist. The EPIC study reported a 23 percent reduction in cumulative 6-month clinical events ($p = 0.001$),[296] but these events were primarily related to the prevention of early (<30 day) periprocedural events.[19] Other studies did not show a consistent reduction in clinical or angiographic restenosis with GP IIb-IIIa inhibitors.[258] A subgroup analysis of diabetic patients undergoing stent implantation in EPISTENT demonstrated a reduction in clinical restenosis at 12 months from 22.4 percent in those receiving placebo to 13.7 percent in those receiving abciximab.[297] These findings in diabetic patients require confirmation in future prospective trials.

ANTITHROMBINS. Neither intravenous[279] or subcutaneous[298] unfractionated heparin nor LMWH, including enoxaparin, reviparin, nadroparin, and fraxiparin,[299–301] prevents restenosis after PCI. Antithrombin III–independent thrombin inhibitors such as bivalirudin,[302] hirudin,[283] and long-term warfarin[303] also have had little effect on the prevention of restenosis. It is not known whether local delivery of LMWH will result in a reduction in restenosis after stent placement, although studies evaluating this method of delivery are ongoing.

VASODILATORS. Although calcium channel antagonists may reduce the occurrence of coronary vasospasm early after PCI, diltiazem and verapamil do not prevent restenosis after PCI.[304] Treatment with the nitric oxide donors linsidomine and molsidomine was associated with a modest improvement in the long-term angiographic result after PCI but had no effect on clinical outcome.[305] The improved angiographic result related mostly to a better immediate procedural result because late lumen loss did not differ significantly between groups.[305]

ANTIPROLIFERATIVE AGENTS. Agents thought to interfere with smooth muscle cell migration and proliferation, such as cilazapril[306, 307] and fosinopril,[308] do not reduce the frequency of restenosis after balloon PTCA, although their effect after stent placement is less well studied.[309] Angiopeptin, a nonspecific growth factor inhibitor, has had inconsistent effects on restenosis, related in part to the short half-life and varied administration among studies.[310, 311] Preliminary studies using trapidil, an agent that may antagonize platelet-derived growth factor, have been favorable,[312] but larger studies are needed.

ANTIINFLAMMATORY AGENTS AND ANTIOXIDANTS. Probucol, an anti-antioxidant agent, has been shown to reduce restenosis after balloon angioplasty,[313, 314] primarily as a result of its effect on the prevention of arterial remodeling.[314] In one study, 317 patients undergoing PCI were randomly assigned to either twice-daily placebo; probucol 500 mg; multivitamins consisting of 30,000 IU of beta-carotene, 500 mg of vitamin C, and 700 IU of vitamin E; or both probucol and multivitamins for 4 weeks before and 6 months after PCI. Restenosis rates were 20.7 percent in the probucol group, 28.9 percent in the combined-treatment group, 40.3 percent in the multivitamin group, and 38.9 percent in the placebo group ($p = 0.003$ for probucol vs. no probucol).[314] Probucol, not marketed in the United States, lowers high-density lipoprotein levels. Tranilast, an antiallergic drug used widely in Japan, has been shown to reduce restenosis after successful DCA from 26 percent in patients not treated with tranilast to 11 percent in patients treated with tranilast ($p = 0.03$).[315] A large-scale trial evaluating the effect of tranilast on the prevention of restenosis is ongoing. Other antiinflammatory agents such as dexametha-

▼ **TABLE 38–9. ANGIOGRPAHIC AND CLINICAL ENDPOINTS FOR RESTENOSIS PERCUTANEOUS CORONARY INTERVENTION**

ANGIOGRAPHIC	CLINICAL
Binary	**Binary**
>50% follow-up diameter stenosis	Death
>0.72-mm loss in lumen diameter	Nonfatal myocardial infarction
>20% loss in gain achieved	Revascularization
Continuous	Target vessel failure
Follow-up minimal lumen diameter	Target vessel revascularization
Follow-up % diameter stenosis	Target lesion revascularization
Late lumen loss	Recurrence of angina
Loss index	**Continuous**
	Exercise test duration

sone[316] and colchicines[317] have had limited effect on the prevention of restenosis.

LIPID-LOWERING AGENTS. Several lipid-lowering agents, such as lovastatin,[318, 319] pravastatin,[320] and fluvastatin,[321] have been evaluated as treatment to prevent restenosis after PTCA. While these agents have had limited clinical success in preventing restenosis, lipid reduction therapy is indicated after PCI for the progression of atherosclerosis at remote sites.[322, 323] At least one pilot study has shown that low-density lipoprotein (LDL) apheresis may also reduce restenosis after PCI.[324]

While meta-analysis of several smaller studies suggests a benefit of fish oil on the prevention of restenosis,[325] little evidence supports the routine use of omega-3 fatty acid supplements for preventing restenosis after PTCA[326–329] despite initially encouraging pilot studies.[330–332]

WHY DRUGS HAVE NOT BEEN EFFECTIVE. The limited success in identifying a single pharmacological agent to prevent restenosis after PCI may be related to several factors. Most importantly, our understanding of the pathogenesis of restenosis after PCI has changed dramatically over the past 5 years. Arterial remodeling and contraction of the arterial wall have emerged as important contributors to restenosis after balloon PTCA,[12, 285] although the factors leading to these dynamic changes are not known. Animal models have been poorly predictive of agents that prevent restenosis in clinical studies, possibly because of differences in the pathogenesis of restenosis in different models (i.e., lipid-rich narrowings in hypercholesterolemic rabbits vs. intimal hyperplasia in arteries injured by overexpanded balloons [rats] or stents [pig]). Also, drug dosages higher than the dosage clinically tolerable in humans have been used in the experimental models,[333, 306] and the ineffectiveness of some agents may relate to inadequate drug levels. Given the differences in the pathogenesis of balloon PTCA and stent restenosis, it is possible that agents found ineffective for the prevention of restenosis after balloon PTCA may have value in preventing stent restenosis.

RADIATION THERAPY TO RETARD RESTENOSIS. Emerging data suggest that intracoronary radiotherapy can reduce the intimal hyperplasia in animal models of restenosis.[334–337] Early pilot trials have suggested that both gamma[338] and beta[339] sources prevent restenosis after PCI in native coronary lesions.[340–342] A number of studies are currently ongoing to assess the effect of radiation on the prevention of de novo and restenotic coronary lesions.

INDICATIONS FOR PERCUTANEOUS CORONARY INTERVENTIONS

The major value of coronary revascularization, whether performed by surgical or percutaneous methods, is the relief of symptoms and signs of ischemic CAD caused by obstructive epicardial disease. While two studies have suggested that PCI may reduce mortality and subsequent myocardial infarction risk when compared with medical therapy,[343] these events are better treated with systemic therapies aimed at reducing the extent of atherosclerosis, such as lipid-lowering therapy.[344] In contrast, CABG prolongs life in certain anatomical subsets, such as patients with left main disease, three-vessel CAD, or left anterior descending artery disease with involvement of one or two additional vessels, irrespective of left ventricular function.[345] The risks and benefits of coronary revascularization must be carefully reviewed with the patient and family members, if appropriate, before these procedures are performed. Guidelines for the performance of PCI and CABG have been published by the ACC/AHA.[18, 345]

ASYMPTOMATIC PATIENTS OR THOSE WITH MILD ANGINA. Patients who are asymptomatic or have only mild symptoms are generally best treated with medical therapy, unless one or more significant lesions subtend a large area of viable myocardium confirmed by objective noninvasive testing, the patient prefers to maintain an aggressive life style or has a high-risk occupation, and the procedure can be performed with a high chance of success and low likelihood of complications.[18] Coronary revascularization should not be performed in patients with no or mild symptoms if only a small area of myocardium is at risk, if no objective evidence of ischemia can be found, or if the likelihood of success is low or the chance of complications is high.[18]

PATIENTS WITH MODERATE TO SEVERE ANGINA (see Chap. 37). Patients with CCS Class II to IV angina, particularly those who are refractory to medical therapy, are suitable candidates for coronary revascularization, provided that the lesion subtends a moderate to large area of viable myocardium as determined by noninvasive testing.[18] Patients with recurrent symptoms while receiving medical therapy are candidates for revascularization even if they have a higher risk for an adverse outcome with revascularization.[18] Patients with Class II to IV symptoms should not undergo revascularization without noninvasive evidence of myocardial ischemia or a trial of medical therapy, particularly if only a small region of myocardium is at risk, the likelihood of success is low, or the chance of complications is high.

PATIENTS WITH UNSTABLE ANGINA OR NON-Q-WAVE MYOCARDIAL INFARCTION (see Chap. 36). Cardiac catheterization and coronary revascularization in selected patients with unstable angina or non-Q-wave myocardial infarction may improve the prognosis, although it is less clear whether *routine* angiography and revascularization are indicated in all patients with acute coronary syndromes. The TIMI IIIB trial found no difference in 1-year death or myocardial infarction in patients undergoing routine angiography and those undergoing angiography and revascularization only for recurrent ischemia, although patients treated with an aggressive approach experienced less angina and were rehospitalized less often than those treated with a conservative approach.[346] Patients assigned to early catheterization and revascularization in the Veterans Affairs Non-Q-Wave Infarction Strategies in Hospital (VANQWISH) Trial experienced no reduction in the rate of death or the composite of death and myocardial infarction 1 year later when compared with patients assigned to cardiac catheterization and revascularization only for recurrent ischemia, although the mortality rate was high (>10 percent) in patients undergoing CABG in the aggressive limb.[347] In contrast to these studies, the Fragmin and Fast Revascularization During Instability in Coronary Artery Disease (FRISC II) Study demonstrated a 22 percent reduction ($p = 0.031$) in death or myocardial infarction at 6 months in patients assigned to routine catheterization and revascularization (9.4 percent) versus those assigned to a conservative approach (12.1 percent).[343]

Pending the results of additional trials such as the TACTICS (TIMI-18) Study, early catheterization and coronary revascularization are indicated in patients with acute coronary syndromes at "intermediate" or "high" risk of subsequent death or myocardial infarction.[348] High-risk features include prolonged ongoing (>20 minutes) chest pain, pulmonary edema or worsening mitral regurgitation, dynamic ST segment depression of 1 mm or greater, or hypotension.[348] Intermediate-risk features include angina at rest (>20 minutes) that is relieved with rest or sublingual nitroglycerin, angina associated with dynamic electrocardiographic changes, recent-onset angina with a high likelihood of CAD, pathological Q waves or ST segment depression less than 1 mm in multiple leads, or age older than 65 years.[348] Coronary revascularization is not indicated in patients with unstable angina who do not demonstrate high-risk criteria upon exercise testing after stabilization with medical therapy, patients who do not have objective signs of coronary ischemia, or those in whom revascularization will not improve the quality of life.[348]

PATIENTS WITH ACUTE MYOCARDIAL INFARCTION TREATED WITH THROMBOLYTIC THERAPY (see Chap. 35).

Cardiac catheterization and selective coronary revascularization in patients who have received thrombolytic therapy are indicated in those with recurrent ischemia, in patients with cardiogenic shock or those in whom it later develops, or in those in whom signs of reperfusion fail to develop after thrombolytic administration.[16] Routine coronary revascularization is not indicated within hours to days in patients who are asymptomatic and have no evidence of substantial residual myocardium at risk. Patients in whom recurrent ischemia develops spontaneously or after exercise provocation are candidates for revascularization. In the Danish Trial in Acute Myocardial Infarction (DANAMI) Study, 503 patients with inducible myocardial ischemia after thrombolytic treatment of acute myocardial infarction were assigned to an invasive strategy of coronary revascularization between 2 and 10 weeks after the acute myocardial infarction or to a conservative strategy of revascularization 2 months later.[349] At a 2.4-year follow-up (median), mortality was similar in both groups, although patients treated with the invasive strategy had a lower incidence of acute myocardial infarction (5.6 vs. 10.5 percent; $p = 0.0038$) and a lower incidence of admission for unstable angina (17.9 vs. 29.5 percent; $p < 0.00001$) than did conservatively treated patients.[349]

OPTIONS FOR MEDICAL THERAPY OR CORONARY REVASCULARIZATION
(see also Chap. 37)

In patients with symptomatic CAD, the clinician must decide whether medical therapy or referral for coronary revascularization by PCI or CABG will provide the best prognosis for the individual patient. A number of factors will ultimately affect the decision to undertake one strategy over another, including (1) the patient's general vigor, comorbid conditions, initial symptoms, and personal preferences; (2) the coronary anatomy, number of lesions, and their location and morphology, including the presence of total occlusions; (3) left ventricular function; and (4) whether CABG has already been performed.

PCI VERSUS MEDICAL THERAPY (See Chap. 37)

At least four randomized studies have compared the outcomes of patients assigned to medical therapy or PCI for the treatment of ischemic CAD. In the Veterans Administration Angioplasty Compared to Medicine (ACME) trial, 212 patients with single-vessel coronary disease and stable angina were randomly assigned to medical therapy or balloon PTCA.[350] Although rates of death and myocardial infarction were similar in the two groups, superior symptom control and a better exercise duration were found in patients treated with balloon PTCA.[350] These effects were less pronounced in patients with two-vessel CAD.[351] More recently, the Atorvastatin Versus Revascularization Therapy (AVERT) Trial compared the effect of aggressive lipid lowering with atorvastatin 80 mg daily and coronary angioplasty in 341 patients with asymptomatic or mildly symptomatic (Class I or II) CAD.[352] At an 18-month follow-up, 13 percent of medically treated patients experienced an ischemic event as compared with 21 percent of patients treated with PCI ($p = 0.048$). Although patients in both groups experienced improvement in their angina, more improvement was found at follow-up in patients treated with PCI.[352]

In the second Randomized Intervention Treatment of Angina (RITA-2) Trial, 1018 patients with single-vessel and/or multivessel disease and grade 2 or higher angina were randomly assigned to medical therapy or PCI.[353] Death or definite myocardial infarction occurred significantly ($p = 0.02$) more often in PCI-treated patients (6.3 percent) than in medically treated patients (3.3 percent), primarily attributable to the occurrence of periprocedural myocardial infarction. More angina improvement and better exercise durations were achieved in the

PCI group.[353] These benefits of PTCA were greatest in patients with more severe baseline angina.[353] The authors concluded that in patients with CAD considered suitable for either PCI or medical care, early PCI was associated with greater symptomatic improvement, especially in patients with more severe angina, although these benefits should be weighed against the small excess hazard for periprocedural myocardial infarction.[353]

In the Asymptomatic Cardiac Ischemia Pilot (ACIP) Study, 558 patients with asymptomatic ischemia by stress testing and ambulatory ischemia monitoring were randomly assigned to angina-guided therapy (n = 183), angina plus ischemia-guided therapy (n = 183), or revascularization using PCI or CABG.[348] The incidence of death or myocardial infarction at 2 years was significantly lower ($p < 0.01$) in patients treated with revascularization (4.7 percent) than in patients assigned to angina-guided (12.1 percent) or ischemia-guided (8.8 percent) therapy.

These studies suggest that patients with mild Class I or II angina have a favorable prognosis, whether treated with medical therapy or PCI, although angina relief is greater in patients treated with PCI. A pilot randomized trial suggested that the prognosis is improved with revascularization (PCI or CABG) in patients with Holter monitor–documented ischemia,[354] but these findings will require confirmation in larger studies. Patients with moderate to severe angina, particularly those who have failed medical therapy, should be considered candidates for PCI.

PCI VERSUS CABG (See Chap. 37)

At least nine randomized trials have evaluated the relative value of PCI and CABG in patients with multivessel CAD.[345, 355-362] While these trials were designed to address a critical issue for clinicians managing patients with multivessel CAD, they have had certain unavoidable design limitations, including relatively small sample sizes (127 to 1792 patients), inclusion of both patients with single-vessel and multivessel CAD, low screened-to-recruitment ratios (limiting the generalizability of the study), and limited (1 to 5 years) follow-up. The relatively low, late-term mortality rates (0 to 13.7 percent) and small sample sizes in these studies make it difficult to exclude the *possibility* of a difference between these two strategies (type II error). Not withstanding these limitations, a number of important conclusions can be drawn from these trials.

In the largest randomized trial, BARI, 1792 patients with multivessel CAD were assigned to initial treatment with PCI or CABG. In-hospital Q wave myocardial infarction was significantly ($p < 0.05$) higher in patients assigned to CABG (4.6 percent) than PCI (2.1 percent), although 6.3 percent of PCI-treated patients required emergency CABG for procedure-induced complications. No significant differences were found in long-term survival or freedom from myocardial infarction at 5.4 years' follow-up, although PCI patients had more repeat hospitalization and required more repeat procedures than did CABG patients. One subset was identified in BARI that benefited from CABG over PCI. Diabetic patients assigned to PCI had a significantly ($p = 0.003$) worse survival rate (65.5 percent) than did diabetic patients assigned to CABG (80.6 percent), primarily because of a reduced cardiac mortality rate (20.6 percent in PCI patients vs. 5.8 percent in CABG patients; $p = 0.003$).[26-28] Placement of at least one internal mammary graft was the primary factor contributing to the improved prognosis with CABG in diabetic patients.

A weighted analysis of patients enrolled in the nine randomized trials comparing CABG and PCI for the treatment of single-vessel and multivessel CAD demonstrated similar in-hospital major clinical events, including death (1.3 percent in CABG patients and 1.0 percent in PCI patients) and Q wave myocardial infarction (4.1 percent in CABG patients and 2.3 percent in PCI patients).[345] Late major clinical events were also similar in the two groups and included death (6.5 percent in CABG patients and 7.7 percent in PCI patients) and Q wave myocardial infarction (11.3 percent in CABG patients and 11.0 percent in PCI patients). CABG patients had less frequent recurrence of angina (10.4 percent in CABG patients and 15.5 percent in PCI patients) and fewer repeat revascularization procedures (7.3 percent in CABG patients and 42.3 percent in PCI patients).[345] It should be noted that these trials were completed before the widespread use of stents, GP IIb-IIIa inhibitors, and postprocedural lipid-lowering therapies.

The ultimate choice of the method of revascularization should be made after a frank discussion with the patient about the options of revascularization. In a patient with diffuse involvement of three coronary vessels, particularly in the setting of complex anatomy, including total occlusions, CABG may provide a more definitive long-term benefit, especially if one or more arterial conduits are used. In contrast, in a patient with focal lesions involving two or three large epicardial vessels, multivessel coronary stent placement may be the preferred approach since it is associated with a lower risk of Q wave myocardial infarction and a shorter hospital stay than CABG is. Diabetic patients with diffuse two- or three-vessel CAD are best served with CABG. These recommendations in diabetic patients are supported by preliminary results from the ARTS Trial, a randomized trial of multivessel stenting or CABG in patients with multivessel disease.[363] In all patients with multivessel CAD who are undergoing CABG or PCI, aggressive risk factor modification is warranted, with a target LDL cholesterol of less than 100 mg/dl.[344]

TRAINING STANDARDS AND PROFICIENCY IN INTERVENTIONAL CARDIOLOGY

Standards for core curriculum development and procedural proficiency for interventional cardiology training programs have been established by the ACC[364]; these criteria, coupled with standards for the maintenance of technical competency,[364–366] are now prerequisites for the Certification Examination for Added Qualification in Interventional Cardiology, established by the American Board of Internal Medicine.[367] Proficiency requirements for interventional training have become more rigorous over time, with the minimum case volume for interventional training increasing from 125 to 250 cases as the primary operator[366, 368]; maintenance of proficiency now requires more than 75 cases per year as the primary operator, unless special circumstances are identified.[366] Operator- and hospital-specific procedural outcomes after PCI are also collected by governmental and managed care organizations.

The focus on minimum volume criteria is based on studies that relate procedural outcome after PCI to both hospital and individual operator volumes[369–373] (Tables 38–10 and 38–11). PCI complication rates are higher when the hospital procedural volume is less than 200 to 400 cases per year

or individual operator volume is less than 75 to 100 coronary interventions per year.[369–372] The ACC has recommended that hospitals perform more than 200 to 400 cases per year and individual operators perform more than 75 cases per year.[18, 366] It has been suggested that many interventional cardiologists do not meet these minimal procedural requirements.[373]

Individual institutions need to establish valid methods for peer review, including documentation of procedural success and failure rates of individual operators, minimum volume performance for the hospital and individual operators, quality of the laboratory facility, and training of the support staff. Establishment of an outcomes data base is strongly encouraged for all institutions.[384]

PERCUTANEOUS VALVULOPLASTY
(see also Chap. 46)

Percutaneous valve dilatation has been used as an alternative to definitive surgical repair or replacement in selected patients with symptomatic valvular heart disease. After a decade of experience with these techniques, it is clear that mitral valvuloplasty is a safe and effective alternative to surgical repair in selected patients with mitral stenosis[385] whereas aortic valvuloplasty provides only short-term palliation and should be reserved for inoperable patients

▼ **TABLE 38–10.** RELATIONSHIP BETWEEN HOSPITAL PROCEDURAL VOLUME AND OUTCOME AFTER CORONARY INTERVENTION

STUDY	TIME PERIOD	DATA SOURCE	NUMBER OF PATIENTS	NUMBER OF OPERATORS	CONCLUSIONS	COMMENTS
Hartz et al.[374]	1989–91	Wisconsin Medicare	2091	16	No relationship between volume and outcome	Very low number of cases and hospitals examined
Ritchie et al.[375]	1989	California State	24,883	110	Increased CABG (not death) with <200 cases/yr; finding is valid for both acute MI and non-MI patients	
Jollis et al.[373]	1987–90	MEDPAR	217,836	1194	Death and CABG inversely related to low volume (risk increases with Medicare patient volume [<100–200 total/yr for death, <200–300/yr for CABG])*	
Kimmel et al.[372]	1992–93	SCAI Registry	19,594	48	Fewer major complications for labs with >400 cases/yr	Able to risk-adjust more completely than in other studies
GUSTO IIb[168]	NA	GUSTO	565	59	No difference between 200 and 625 cases/yr vs. >625 cases/yr for acute MI patients	All operators >50 cases per year
O'Neill et al.[376]	NA	PAMI-II	1100	34	No difference between <500, 501–1000, and >1,000 cases/yr for acute MI	
Jollis et al.[373]	1992	Medicare	97,498	984	Incremental decrease in death + CABG as hospital Medicare volume increased from <100, 100–200, and >200 cases/yr	
Tiefenbrunn et al.[377]	NA	Second NRMI	4939	NA	Increased acute MI mortality for hospitals with <25 acute MI cases/yr	
Hannan et al.[370]	1991–94	New York State	62,670	31	Death alone and same-stay CABG increased with caseloads <600/yr	Risk adjusted
Zahn et al.[378]	1992–95	German Hospital Consortium	4625	NA	For patients with acute MI, increased mortality in hospital with <40 acute MI PTCA/yr	No risk adjustment

* Medicare patients usually account for 35 to 50 percent of the total interventional caseload.

CABG = coronary artery bypass graft surgery; MI = myocardial infarction; NRMI = National Registry of Myocardial Infarction; PAMI = Primary Angioplasty Myocardial Infarction Study; PTCA = percutaneous transluminal coronary angioplasty; SCAI = Society for Cardiac Angiography and Intervention.

Modified from Hirshfeld J, Ellis S, Faxon D: American College of Cardiology Clinical Competency Statement: Recommendations for the assessment and maintenance of proficiency in coronary interventional procedures. J Am Coll Cardiol 31:722–743, 1998.

▼ TABLE 38–11. RELATIONSHIP BETWEEN INDIVIDUAL PROCEDURAL VOLUME AND OUTCOME AFTER PERCUTANEOUS CORONARY INTERVENTION 1393

Ch 38

STUDY	TIME PERIOD	DATA SOURCE	NUMBER OF PATIENTS	NUMBER OF OPERATORS	CONCLUSIONS	COMMENTS
Hamad et al.[379]	1986–87	Single center	787	17	Lower success with complex lesions (B–C) for operators with <100 cases/yr and no differences noted for simple lesions	
Shook et al.[371]	1991–94	Single center	2350	38	Higher risk of emergency CABG with operators performing <50 cases/yr, but no difference in mortality	
Ellis et al.[369]	1993–95	High-volume centers	12,941	38	Risk of death and risk of death, MI, or emergency CABG inversely related to caseload but not to years of experience; no volume cut-off, but risk accelerates with less than 100/yr	Able to risk-adjust more completely than other studies
Krone et al.[380]	1992	SCAI data base	7747	122	No differences in <50, 50–99, or >100 cases/yr	Able to risk-adjust more completely than other studies
Bon Tempo et al.[381]	1992–94	Single center	3127	45	Weak trend toward increased risk of abrupt closure and late PTCA with higher-volume operators	No risk adjustment
O'Neill et al.[376]	NA	PAMI-II	1100	NA	No difference for <75 or >75 cases/yr	Selected interventionalists
Jollis et al.[373]	1992	Medicare	97,478	6115	More death + CABG for annual medical volume <50[1]	
McGrath et al.[382]	1990–93	Northern NE Registry	12,033	31	Success and emergency CABG, but not death was related to volume tercile (23–85, 89–143, 153–450)	
Hannan et al.[370]	1991–94	New York State	62,670	NA	Success and emergency CABG increase with annual caseload <75; an operator-hospital caseload interaction affecting outcome also observed	Risk adjusted
Klein et al.[383]	1992–95	Single center	1389	9	Despite performing only an average of 51 PTCA/yr, results (death = 1.0%, CABG = 0.9%) were acceptable when compared with contemporary registry data	

* Medicare patients usually account for 35 to 50 percent of the total interventional caseload.

CABG = coronary artery bypass graft surgery; MI = myocardial infarction; NE = New England; PAMI = Primary Angioplasty Myocardial Infarction Study; PTCA = percutaneous transluminal coronary angioplasty; SCAI = Society for Cardiac Angiography and Intervention.

Modified from Hirshfeld J, Ellis S, Faxon D: American College of Cardiology Clinical Competency Statement: Recommendations for the assessment and maintenance of proficiency in coronary interventional procedures. J Am Coll Cardiol 31:722–743, 1998.

with degenerative calcific aortic stenosis.[385, 386] The indications and contraindications for mitral and aortic valvuloplasty are reviewed in detail elsewhere (see Chap. 46). This chapter focuses on the technical issues, patient selection, and outcomes associated with mitral and aortic valvuloplasty.

Mitral Valvuloplasty (See also Chap. 46)

Percutaneous mitral valvuloplasty (PMV) was first performed in 1984 as an alternative to surgical mitral valve commissurotomy,[387] and later reports confirmed the immediate and long-term benefits of this procedure.[388–390] Although the majority of PMV procedures are performed in developing countries,[389, 391] where rheumatic fever and valvular heart disease continue to be endemic, a few specialized centers in Western countries have developed technical expertise in PMV, and their single[392] and multicenter[393] reports have provided valuable insight into the outcomes associated with PMV.

TECHNICAL ISSUES

A variety of technical approaches may be used for PMV.[385] A transvenous, or anterograde, method is most commonly performed, with a transseptal puncture used to gain access to the left atrium. A wire (or balloon) is then passed across the mitral valve into the left ventricle. Less often, a retrograde, transarterial approach is used to avoid the creation of a large atrial septal defect. Two retrograde methods have been described. In the first, a 0.038-inch exchange wire passed from the right atrium to the left atrium via a transseptal puncture is advanced through the left ventricle into the descending aorta, where it is retrieved with a snare.[394] The mitral valve dilatation balloon is then advanced retrogradely through the descending and ascending aorta into the left ventricle and across the mitral valve.[394] This method has had limited application because it is time consuming, requires advanced technical expertise, and mandates the use of large arterial sheaths. The second retrograde technique involves the use of a specially designed catheter to gain access to the left atrium from the left ventricle while avoiding transseptal puncture.[395–397] Experience with this method is limited except for a few specialized centers.

Two types of balloon approaches are used for PMV.[398] With the double-balloon method, a transseptal puncture is performed and a balloon catheter is advanced across the mitral valve into the left ventricle.[385] Two long exchange wires are then positioned in the left ventricle, and the interatrial septum is dilated with a 6- to 8-mm peripheral dilatation balloon. A combination of two mitral valvuloplasty balloons (trefoil balloon or conventional balloon) are advanced across the mitral valve and inflated.[385] The second technique uses the Inoue balloon,[399, 400] which is a self-positioning, pressure-distensible balloon that allows progressive diameter dilatation by increasing the inflation pressure[385] (Fig. 38–11). A stepwise dilatation technique is performed to minimize the risk of mitral valve rupture and mitral regurgitation. Selection of balloon size is generally based on patient height, body surface area, and diameter of the mitral annulus.

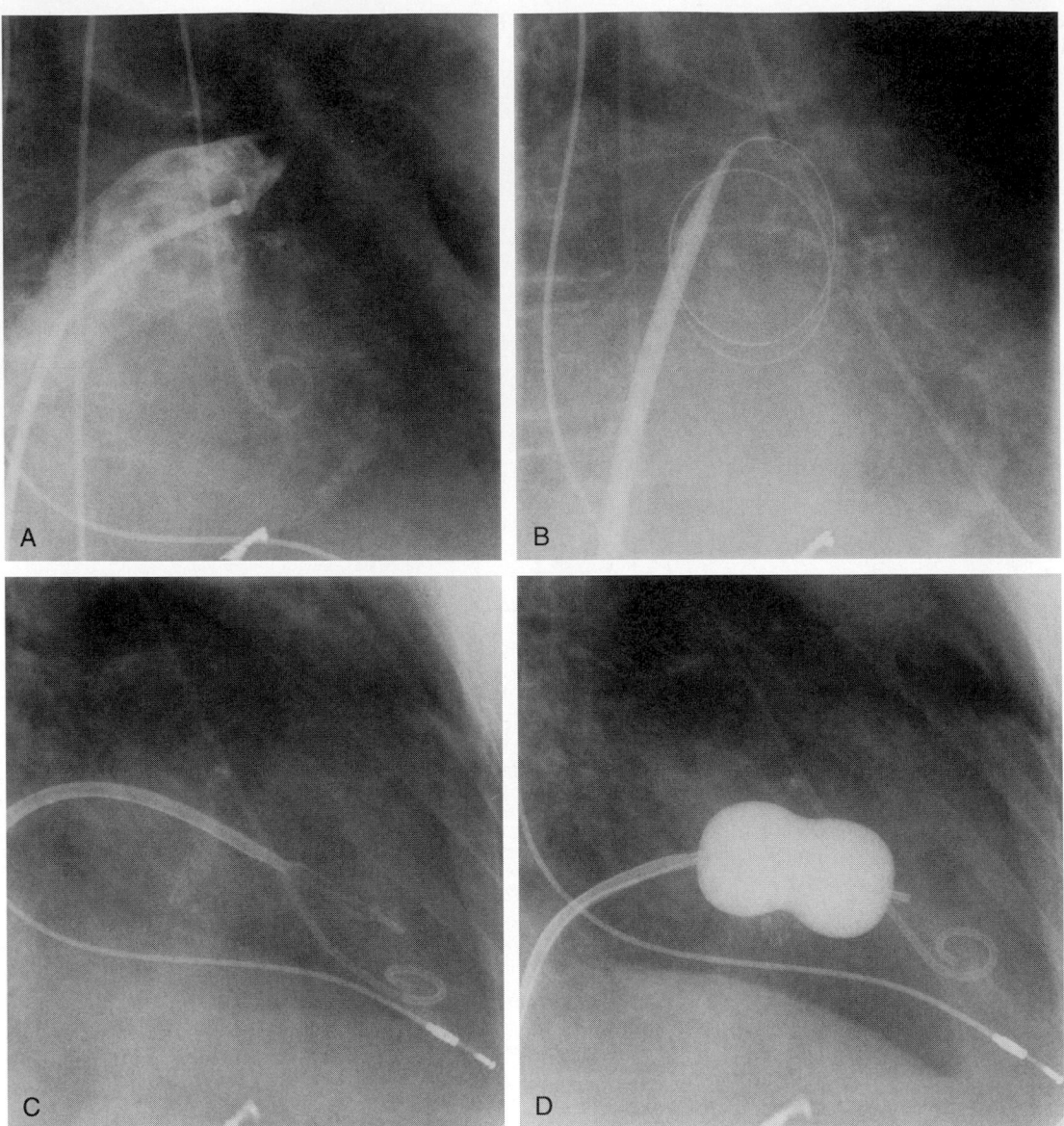

FIGURE 38–11. Mitral valvoloplasty. After transseptal puncture, a Mullins sheath is advanced into the left atrium, as demonstrated by contrast injection *(A)*. An Inoue guidewire is coiled in the left atrium and a Inoue dilator is advanced across the intraatrial septum *(B)*. Advancement of the Inoue balloon dilatation catheter into the left ventricle *(C)* and inflation *(D)* resulted in a successful procedure. (Courtesy of Andrew Eisenhauer, M.D.).

Comparative studies of these two techniques have shown similar clinical success rates,[391, 401] but shorter procedure times and higher disposable costs with the Inoue technique.[391, 401] The Inoue balloon has also been used in patients with severe mitral valve calcification[402] and subvalvular fibrosis[403] with reported success.

HEMODYNAMIC ASSESSMENT

Serial hemodynamic measurements, alone or in combination with echocardiography, may be used to evaluate the result achieved with PMV.[385] An immediate improvement in left atrial mean pressure (and reduction of the transmittal gradient) should be seen, with a gradual decrease in pulmonary artery pressure and an increase in cardiac output.[385] Criteria for termination of the procedure include (1) a mitral valve area larger than 1 cm^2 per square meter of body surface area, (2) complete opening of at least one commissure, or (3) the appearance or an increment in mitral regurgitation.[385] Transesophageal echocardiography may also be performed during the procedure[404–407] and, in particular, may guide the transseptal puncture in patients with obscure cardiac landmarks or skeletal deformity.[408]

PROCEDURE OUTCOME. Procedure success has been related to institutional volume (>25 cases per year), baseline mitral valve area (>0.5 cm^2), and the age of the patient (<70 years).[393] Procedural mortality associated with mitral valvuloplasty ranges from 0 to 3 percent in most series and is primarily related to the development of left ventricular perforation[409] resulting from the transseptal technique or advancement of the guidewire or balloon catheter into the left ventricle[410] or to general patient comorbidity.[411] Cerebral or coronary emboli occur in 0.5 to 5.0 percent of patients and are related to dislodgment of thromboembolic material from the left atrium or air within the dilatation apparatus.[412] Severe mitral regurgitation resulting from rupture of the chordae tendineae or papillary muscle rupture may also occur. Atrial septal defects are commonly (80 percent) seen after PMV, but the magnitude of the left-to-right shunt is generally insignificant.[405] The atrial septal defect also closes in the majority (90 to 100 percent) of cases within 3 months after PMV.[405, 413] Emergency surgery may be required in a minority of cases after PMV. When PMV is required for mitral regurgitation, left ventricular

▼ TABLE 38–12. ECHOCARDIOGRAPHIC ANATOMICAL CLASSIFICATION OF THE MITRAL VALVE IN RELATION TO SUITABILITY FOR PERCUTANEOUS VALVULOPLASTY

POINTS	ECHOCARDIOGRAPHIC VARIABLE
	LEAFLET MOBILITY
1	Highly mobile valve with restriction of only the leaflet tips
2	Midportion and base of leaflets have reduced mobility
3	Valve leaflets move forward in diastole mainly at the base
4	No or minimal forward movement of the leaflets in diastole
	VALVULAR THICKENING
1	Leaflets near normal (4–5 mm)
2	Midleaflet thickening, marked thickening at the margins
3	Thickening extends through the entire leaflets (5–8 mm)
4	Marked thickening of all leaflet tissue (>8–10 mm)
	SUBVALVULAR THICKENING
1	Minimal thickening of chordal structures just below the valve
2	Thickening of the chordae extending up to one-third of chordal length
3	Thickening extending to the distal third of the chordae
4	Extensive thickening and shortening of all chordae extending down to the papillary muscles
	VALVULAR CALCIFICATION
1	A single area of increased echo brightness
2	Scattered areas of brightness confined to leaflet margins
3	Brightness extending into the midportion of the leaflets
4	Extensive brightness through most of the leaflet tissue

Adapted from Wilkins G, Gillam L, Weyman A, et al: Percutaneous balloon dilatation of the mitral valve: An analysis of echocardiographic variables related to outcome and the mechanism of dilatation. Br Heart J 60:299–308, 1988.

rupture, or the development of a left-to-right shunt or as a result of a failed procedure, the mortality rate rises substantially.[414]

LATE OUTCOME. Transthoracic echocardiography may be useful to assess the prognosis after PMV by semiquantitatively scoring leaflet mobility, valvular and subvalvular thickening, and valvular calcification[415, 416] (Table 38–12). In one series of 136 patients undergoing successful PMV, the estimated 5-year mortality rate was 24 percent; the 5-year event rate (i.e., mitral valve replacement, repeat valvuloplasty, or death from cardiac causes) was 49 percent.[392] Multivariable predictors of late events after PMV were a high mitral valve echocardiographic score, an elevated left ventricular end-diastolic pressure, and a worse New York Heart Association (NYHA) functional class ($p = 0.04$).[392] Patients with fewer than two risk factors for early restenosis (echocardiographic score >8, left ventricular end-diastolic pressure >10 mm Hg, or NYHA functional Class IV) had a predicted 5-year event-free survival rate of 60 to 84 percent, whereas patients with two or three risk factors had a predicted 5-year event-free survival rate of only 13 to 41 percent.[392]

Aortic Valvuloplasty (See also Chap. 46)

The most frequent cause of acquired valvular heart disease in Western countries is degenerative calcific aortic stenosis.[385] Percutaneous aortic valvuloplasty (PAV) fractures the calcified aortic leaflets, thereby increasing their flexibility, but its overall effect is modest and hemodynamic improvements are transient (days to weeks).[385] The long-term clinical benefit associated with PAV for calcific aortic stenosis is limited.[417–421]

PAV is generally reserved for adult patients with severe calcific aortic stenosis who have severe comorbidities that preclude aortic valve replacement,[422–424] such as in patients with cardiogenic shock or other significant comorbid conditions, in patients as a "bridge" to definitive surgical correction,[425–428] or in patients with severe left ventricular dysfunction (i.e., "low flow, low gradient") in whom the hemodynamic response to aortic valve replacement cannot be determined.[429, 430] In the absence of these indications, definitive aortic valve replacement rather than PAV should be performed, even in elderly patients.[431] PAV in patients with congenital aortic stenosis is discussed in Chapters 43 and 44.

TECHNICAL ISSUES

The femoral approach is most frequently used for PAV.[385] After crossing the aortic valve with a guidewire, an extra-stiff 0.038-inch wire is inserted into the apex of the left ventricle to stabilize the balloon during inflation. In patients with severe peripheral vascular disease, a brachial approach or anterograde approach using a transseptal puncture can be used to pass a long wire through the left ventricle, across the aortic valve, and into the descending aorta.[385] The interatrium septum is then dilated with a peripheral balloon, and the PAV balloon is then advanced across the aortic valve.

PAV balloons ranging in diameter between 15 and 25 mm and in length between 3 and 5 cm have variable shapes, including a conventional, bifoil, trifoil, and double-sized configuration, with the proximal portion measuring 20 to 23 mm and the distal portion 15 to 18 mm.[385] The size of the balloon should not exceed 1.2 to 1.3 times the diameter of the aortic ring.[385]

HEMODYNAMIC ASSESSMENT

The transaortic valve gradient should be reduced immediately after the procedure, although little change may be noted in cardiac output.[385] After successful dilatation, 25 to 47 percent of patients will obtain a final valve area larger than 1 cm², while 22 to 39 percent of patients achieve a valve area less than 0.7 cm².[385]

PROCEDURAL SUCCESS AND COMPLICATION RATES. The clinical success rate for patients undergoing PAV ranges from 68 to 75 percent.[420, 432–434] Hospital mortality after PAV varies from 3.5 to 13.5 percent, and 20 to 25 percent of patients experience at least one complication during their hospitalization.[385, 433, 435, 436] Complications include a need for vascular access repair, embolic cerebrovascular events, aortic regurgitation, and with the use of oversized balloons, rupture of the aortic ring[434, 437] (Fig. 38–12). Predictors of procedural mortality include the patient's age,[438] NYHA Class,[438] concomitant coronary artery disease,[438] congestive heart failure,[438] lower initial left ventricular systolic pressure,[435, 438] smaller final aortic valve area,[435] lower baseline cardiac output,[434, 435, 438] and the development of procedural complications.[385, 435] Predictors of patient morbidity are depressed left ventricular function, low cardiac output, diffuse coronary disease, and final valve area smaller than 0.7 cm².[385, 432, 439, 440]

The major limitation of PAV is the early recurrence of symptoms in most patients. The estimated incidence of late restenosis is 36 to 80 percent in the first year.[441–444] Determinants of late outcomes after PAV were studied in 205 patients undergoing this procedure.[445] The event-free survival rate, defined as survival without recurrent symptoms, repeated valvuloplasty, or aortic valve replacement, was 18 percent over the 24-month follow-up (range, 1 to 47 months).[445] Significant predictors of event-free survival included the left ventricular ejection fraction, left ventricular and aortic systolic pressure before PAV, and percent reduction in the aortic valve pressure gradient; the pulmonary capillary wedge pressure was inversely associated with event-free survival.[445] Although the predicted event-free survival rate for the entire patient group was 50 percent at 1 year and 25 percent at 2 years, the probability of event-free survival at 1 year varied between 23 and 65 percent when patients were stratified according to three independent predictors: aortic systolic pressure, pulmonary capillary wedge pressure, and percent reduction in the peak aortic valve gradient.[445] The best long-term results after valvuloplasty were observed among patients who would also have been expected to have excellent long-term results after aortic valve replacement.[445] Repeat PAV for symptom recurrence has also been reported.[446]

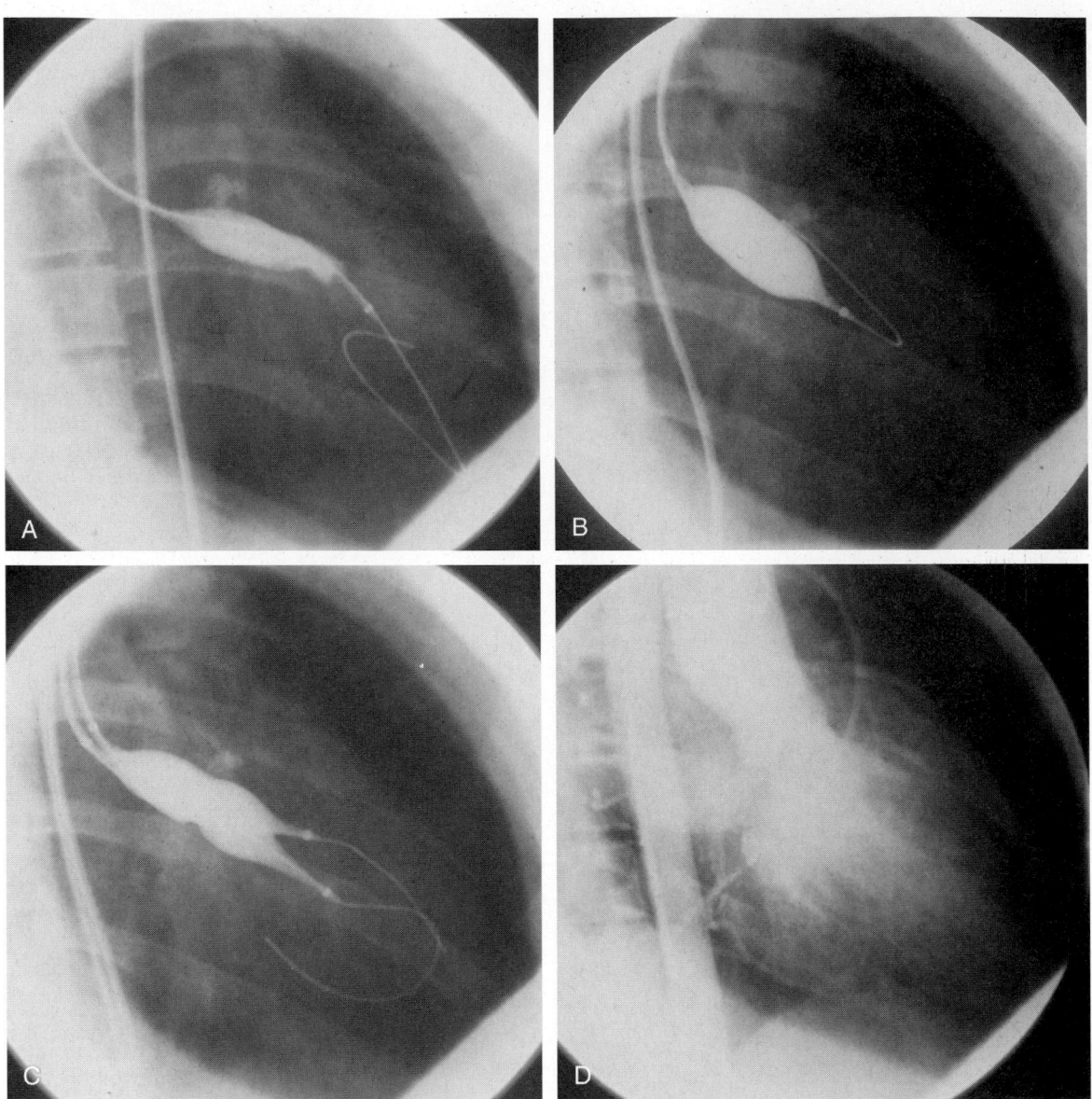

FIGURE 38–12. Aortic valvuloplasty. A 16-mm aortic valvuloplasty balloon is inflated across the aortic valve *(A)* and exchanged for a 24-mm balloon *(B)* because of a persistent gradient. To further improve the aortic gradient, two 16-mm valvuloplasty balloons are advanced across the aortic valve *(C)*. Because of the relative oversizing of the balloons to the aortic ring, aortic regurgitation results *(D)*.

REFERENCES

1. Gruentzig A, Senning A, Siegenthaler W: Nonoperative dilatation of coronary-artery stenosis. Percutaneous transluminal coronary angioplasty. N Engl J Med 301:61–68, 1979.
2. Bourassa MG, Wilson JW, Detre KM, et al: Long-term follow-up of coronary angioplasty: The 1977–1981 National Heart, Lung, and Blood Institute Registry. Eur Heart J 10:36–41, 1989.

BALLOON ANGIOPLASTY

3. Detre K, Holubkov R, Kelsey S, et al: Percutaneous transluminal coronary angioplasty in 1985–1986 and 1977–1981. The National Heart, Lung, and Blood Institute Registry. N Engl J Med 318:265–270, 1988.
4. Detre KM, Holmes DR, Holubkov R, et al: Incidence and consequences of periprocedural occlusion. The 1985–1986 National Heart, Lung, and Blood Institute Percutaneous Transluminal Coronary Angioplasty Registry. Circulation 82:739–750, 1990.
5. Lincoff AM, Popma JJ, Ellis SG, et al: Abrupt vessel closure complicating coronary angioplasty: Clinical, angiographic and therapeutic profile. J Am Coll Cardiol 19:926–935, 1992.
6. de Feyter P, van den Brand M, Jaarman G, et al: Acute coronary artery occlusion during and after percutaneous transluminal coronary angioplasty: Frequency, prediction, clinical course, management and follow-up. Circulation 83:927–936, 1991.
7. Ellis SG, Roubin GS, King SB, et al: Angiographic and clinical predictors of acute closure after native vessel coronary angioplasty. Circulation 77:372–379, 1988.
8. Ellis S, Roubin G, King SB, et al: In-hospital cardiac mortality after acute closure after coronary angioplasty: Analysis of risk factors from 8,207 procedures. J Am Coll Cardiol 11:211–216, 1988.
9. Myler RK, Shaw RE, Stertzer SH, et al: Lesion morphology and coronary angioplasty: Current experience and analysis. J Am Coll Cardiol 19:1641–1652, 1992.
10. Kimmel SE, Berlin JA, Strom BL, et al: Development and validation of simplified predictive index for major complications in contemporary percutaneous transluminal coronary angioplasty practice. The Registry Committee of the Society for Cardiac Angiography and Interventions. J Am Coll Cardiol 26:931–938, 1995.
11. Mintz GS, Pichard AD, Kent KM, et al: Axial plaque redistribution as a mechanism of percutaneous transluminal coronary angioplasty. Am J Cardiol 77:427–430, 1996.
12. Mintz GS, Popma JJ, Pichard AD, et al: Arterial remodeling after coronary angioplasty: A serial intravascular ultrasound study. Circulation 94:35–43, 1996.
13. Roubin GS, Douglas JS, King SB, et al: Influence of balloon size on initial success, acute complications, and restenosis after percutaneous transluminal coronary angioplasty. A prospective randomized study. Circulation 78:557–565, 1988.
14. Serruys PW, di Mario C, Piek J, et al: Prognostic value of intracoronary flow velocity and diameter stenosis in assessing the short- and long-term outcomes of coronary balloon angioplasty: The DEBATE Study

(Doppler Endpoints Balloon Angioplasty Trial Europe). Circulation 96:3369–3377, 1997.

15. Pijls NH, De Bruyne B, Peels K, et al: Measurement of fractional flow reserve to assess the functional severity of coronary-artery stenoses. N Engl J Med 334:1703–1708, 1996.

16. Ryan TJ, Bauman WB, Kennedy JW, et al: Guidelines for percutaneous transluminal coronary angioplasty: A report of the American College of Cardiology/American Heart Association Task Force on Assessment of Diagnostic and Therapeutic Cardiovascular Procedures (Subcommittee on Percutaneous Transluminal Coronary Angioplasty). J Am Coll Cardiol 22:2033–2054, 1993.

17. Faxon DP, Vogel R, Yeh W, et al: Value of visual versus central quantitative measurements of angiographic success after percutaneous transluminal coronary angioplasty. NHLBI PTCA Registry Investigators. Am J Cardiol 77:1067–1072, 1996.

18. Smith S, Dove J, Jacobs A, et al: Americal College of Cardiology/American Heart Association Guidelines for Percutaneous Transluminal Coronary Angioplasty. J Am Coll Cardiol, in press.

19. The EPIC Investigators: Use of a monoclonal antibody directed against the platelet glycoprotein IIb/IIIa receptor in high-risk coronary angioplasty. N Engl J Med 330:956–961, 1994.

20. Califf RM, Abdelmeguid AE, Kuntz RE, et al: Myonecrosis after revascularization procedures. J Am Coll Cardiol 31:241–251, 1998.

21. Abdelmeguid AE, Ellis SG, Sapp SK, et al: Defining the appropriate threshold of creatine kinase elevation after percutaneous coronary interventions. Am Heart J 131:1097–1105, 1996.

22. Costa M, Alamagor Y, Zedek S, et al: The significance of myocardial enzyme release following multivessel stenting or CABG in the ARTS trial (abstract). Circulation 100(Suppl 1):215, 1999.

23. Cutlip D, Ho K, Chauhan M, et al: Predictors of myocardial infarction after coronary stenting and effect on one year mortality (abstract). Circulation 100(Suppl 1):215, 1999.

24. Ellis SG, Vandormael MG, Cowley MJ, et al: Coronary morphologic and clinical determinants of procedural outcome with angioplasty for multivessel coronary disease. Implications for patient selection. Circulation 82:1193–1202, 1990.

25. Ellis SG, Cowley MJ, Whitlow PL, et al: Prospective case-control comparison of percutaneous transluminal coronary revascularization in patients with multivessel disease treated in 1986–1987 versus 1991: Improved in-hospital and 12-month results. Multivessel Angioplasty Prognosis Study (MAPS) Group. J Am Coll Cardiol 25:1137, 1995.

26. The BARI Investigators: Comparison of coronary bypass surgery with angioplasty in patients with multivessel disease. N Engl J Med 335:217–225, 1996.

27. The BARI Investigators: Influence of diabetes on 5-year mortality and morbidity in a randomized trial comparing CABG and PTCA in patients with multivessel disease: The Bypass Angioplasty Revascularization Investigation (BARI). Circulation 96:1761–1769, 1997.

28. The BARI Investigators: Five-year clinical and functional outcome comparing bypass surgery and angioplasty in patients with multivessel coronary disease. A multicenter randomized trial. JAMA 277:715–721, 1997.

29. Baim DS, Cutlip DE, Sharma SK, et al: Final results of the Balloon vs Optimal Atherectomy Trial (BOAT). Circulation 97:322–331, 1998.

30. Fischman DL, Leon MB, Baim DS, et al: A randomized comparison of coronary-stent placement and balloon angioplasty in the treatment of coronary artery disease. Stent Restenosis Study Investigators. N Engl J Med 331:496–501, 1994.

31. Serruys PW, van Hout B, Bonner H, et al: Randomised comparison of implantation of heparin-coated stents with balloon angioplasty in selected patients with coronary artery disease (Benestent II). Lancet 352:673–681, 1998.

32. Bonan R, Roose PL, Suttorp MJ, et al: Cutting balloon randomized trial: Restenosis and revascularization rate (abstract). Circulation 96:I-324, 1997.

33. Block PC, Peterson EC, Krone R, et al: Identification of variables needed to risk adjust outcomes of coronary interventions: Evidence-based guidelines for efficient data collection. J Am Coll Cardiol 32:275–282, 1998.

34. Altmann DB, Racz M, Battleman DS, et al: Reduction in angioplasty complications after the introduction of coronary stents: Results from a consecutive series of 2242 patients. Am Heart J 132:503–507, 1996.

35. McGrath P, Malenka D, Wennberg D, et al: Changing outcomes in percutaneous coronary interventions. J Am Coll Cardiol 34:674–680, 1999.

36. Jacobs AK, Kelsey SF, Yeh W, et al: Documentation of decline in morbidity in women undergoing coronary angioplasty (a report from the 1993–94 NHLBI Percutaneous Transluminal Coronary Angioplasty Registry). National Heart, Lung, and Blood Institute. Am J Cardiol 80:979–984, 1997.

37. O'Conner G, Malenka D, Quiton H, et al: Multivariate prediction of in-hospital mortality after percutaneous coronary interventions in 1994–1996. J Am Coll Cardiol 34:681–691, 1999.

38. Moscucci M, O'Connor G, Ellis S, et al: Validation of risk adjustment models for in-hospital percutaneous transluminal coronary angioplasty on an independent data set. J Am Coll Cardiol 34:692–697, 1999.

39. Ellis SG, Myler RK, King SB, et al: Causes and correlates of death after unsupported coronary angioplasty: Implications for use of angioplasty and advanced support techniques in high-risk settings. Am J Cardiol 68:1447–1451, 1991.

40. Weintraub WS, Ghazzal ZM, Douglas JS, et al: Usefulness of the substitution of nonangiographic end points (death, acute myocardial infarction, coronary bypass and/or repeat angioplasty) for follow-up coronary angiography in evaluating the success of coronary angioplasty in patients with angina pectoris. Am J Cardiol 81:382–386, 1998.

41. Nobuyoshi M, Kimura T, Nosaka H, et al: Restenosis after successful percutaneous transluminal coronary angioplasty: Serial angiographic follow-up of 229 patients. J Am Coll Cardiol 12:616–623, 1988.

42. Serruys P, Luijten H, Beatt K, et al: Incidence of restenosis after successful coronary angioplasty: A time-related phenomenon. A quantitative angiographic study in 342 consecutive patients at 1, 2, 3, and 4 months. Circulation 77:361–371, 1988.

43. Holmes DR, Kip KE, Kelsey SF, et al: Cause of death analysis in the NHLBI PTCA Registry: Results and considerations for evaluating long-term survival after coronary interventions. J Am Coll Cardiol 30:881–887, 1997.

44. Kelsey S, James M, Holubkov A, et al: Results of percutaneous transluminal coronary angioplasty in women: 1985–1986 National Heart, Lung, and Blood Institutes Coronary Angioplasty Registry. Circulation 87:720–727, 1993.

45. King SB, Schlumpf M: Ten-year completed follow-up of percutaneous transluminal coronary angioplasty: The early Zurich experience. J Am Coll Cardiol 22:353–360, 1993.

46. Kip KE, Faxon DP, Detre KM, et al: Coronary angioplasty in diabetic patients. The National Heart, Lung, and Blood Institute Percutaneous Transluminal Coronary Angioplasty Registry. Circulation 94:1818–1825, 1996.

47. Libby P, Egan D, Skarlatos S: Roles of infectious agents in atherosclerosis and restenosis: An assessment of the evidence and need for future research. Circulation 96:4095–4103, 1997.

DIRECTIONAL CORONARY ATHERECTOMY

48. Matar FA, Mintz GS, Farb A, et al: The contribution of tissue removal to lumen improvement after directional coronary atherectomy. Am J Cardiol 74:647–650, 1994.

49. Safian RD, Grines CL, May MA, et al: Clinical and angiographic results of transluminal extraction coronary atherectomy in saphenous vein bypass grafts. Circulation 89:302–312, 1994.

50. Kuntz RE, Baim DS: Defining coronary restenosis. Newer clinical and angiographic paradigms. Circulation 88:1310–1323, 1993.

50a. Bruce CJ, Kuntz RE, Popma JJ, et al: Application of a continuous regression model of restenosis to saphenous vein grafts after successful percutaneous transluminal angioplasty or directional coronary atherectomy. J Am Coll Cardiol 35:619–623, 2000.

51. Baim DS, Hinohara T, Holmes DR, et al: Results of directional coronary atherectomy during multicenter preapproval testing. The US Directional Coronary Atherectomy Investigator Group. Am J Cardiol 72:6E–11E, 1993.

52. Braden GA, Herrington DM, Downes TR, et al: Qualitative and quantitative contrasts in the mechanisms of lumen enlargement by coronary balloon angioplasty and directional coronary atherectomy. J Am Coll Cardiol 23:40–48, 1994.

53. Simonton CA, Leon MB, Baim DS, et al: 'Optimal' directional coronary atherectomy: Final results of the Optimal Atherectomy Restenosis Study (OARS). Circulation 97:332–339, 1998.

54. Lansky AJ, Mintz GS, Popma JJ, et al: Remodeling after directional coronary atherectomy (with and without adjunct percutaneous transluminal coronary angioplasty): A serial angiographic and intravascular ultrasound analysis from the Optimal Atherectomy Restenosis Study. J Am Coll Cardiol 32:329–337, 1998.

55. Suzuki T, Hosokawa H, Katoh O, et al: Effects of adjunctive balloon angioplasty after intravascular ultrasound-guided optimal directional coronary atherectomy: The result of Adjunctive Balloon Angioplasty after Coronary Atherectomy Study (ABACAS) J Am Coll Cardiol 34:1028–1035, 1999.

56. Cohen DJ, Breall JA, Ho KK, et al: Economics of elective coronary revascularization. Comparison of costs and charges for conventional angioplasty, directional atherectomy, stenting and bypass surgery. J Am Coll Cardiol 22:1052–1059, 1993.

57. Baim DS, Kent KM, King SB, et al: Evaluating new devices. Acute (in-hospital) results from the New Approaches to Coronary Intervention Registry. Circulation 89:471–481, 1994.

58. Topol EJ, Leya F, Pinkerton CA, et al: A comparison of directional atherectomy with coronary angioplasty in patients with coronary artery disease. The CAVEAT Study Group. N Engl J Med 329:221–227, 1993.

59. Elliott J, Berdan L, Holmes D, et al: One-year follow-up in the coronary angioplasty versus excisional atherectomy trial (CAVEAT I). Circulation 91:2158–2166, 1995.

60. Adelman AG, Cohen EA, Kimball BP, et al: A comparison of directional atherectomy with balloon angioplasty for lesions of the left anterior descending coronary artery. N Engl J Med 329:228–233, 1993.

61. Tsuchikane E, Sumitsuji S, Awata N, et al: Final results of the STent versus directional coronary Atherectomy Randomized Trial (START). J Am Coll Cardiol 34:1050–1057, 1999.

62. Moussa I, Moses J, Di Mario C, et al: Stenting after optimal lesion debulking (SOLD) registry. Angiographic and clinical outcome. Circulation 98:1604–1609, 1998.

63. Holmes DR, Topol EJ, Califf RM, et al: A multicenter, randomized trial of coronary angioplasty versus directional atherectomy for patients with

saphenous vein bypass graft lesions. CAVEAT-II Investigators. Circulation 91:1966–1974, 1995.

64. Popma JJ, Topol EJ, Hinohara T, et al: Abrupt vessel closure after directional coronary atherectomy. The U.S. Directional Atherectomy Investigator Group. J Am Coll Cardiol 19:1372–1379, 1992.

65. Piana RN, Paik GY, Moscucci M, et al: Incidence and treatment of 'no-reflow' after percutaneous coronary intervention. Circulation 89:2514–2518, 1994.

66. Weyrens FJ, Mooney J, Lesser J, et al: Intracoronary diltiazem for microvascular spasm after interventional therapy. Am J Cardiol 75:849, 1995.

67. Dib N, Cutlip D, Senerchia C, et al: The effect of peri-procedural non-Q-wave MI on late mortality: 3-year follow-up from the Balloon Angioplasty vs. Optimal Atherectomy Trial (BOAT) (abstract). Circulation 100(Suppl 1):779, 1999.

68. Kini A, Marmur J, Kini S, et al: Creatine kinase-MB elevation after coronary intervention correlates with diffuse atherosclerosis, and low-to-medium level elevation has a benign clinical course. J Am Coll Cardiol 34:663–671, 1999.

68a. Saucedo JF, Mehran R, Dangas G, et al: Long-term clinical events following creatine kinase–myocardial band isoenzyme elevation after successful coronary stenting. J Am Coll Cardiol 135:1134–1141, 2000.

68b. Mehran R, Dangas G, Mintz GS, et al: Atherosclerotic plaque burden and CK-MB enzyme elevation after coronary interventions. Intravascular ultrasound study of 2256 patients. Circulation 101:604–610, 2000.

69. Ghaffari S, Kereiakes D, Lincoff A, et al: Platelet glycoprotein IIb/IIIa receptor blockage with abciximab reduces complications in patients undergoing directional coronary atherectomy. Am J Cardiol 82:7–12, 1998.

70. Garratt KN, Holmes DR, Bell MR, et al: Restenosis after directional coronary atherectomy: Differences between primary atheromatous and restenosis lesions and influence of subintimal tissue resection. J Am Coll Cardiol 16:1665–1671, 1990.

71. Holmes DR, Garratt KN, Isner JM, et al: Effect of subintimal resection on initial outcome and restenosis for native coronary lesions and saphenous vein graft disease treated by directional coronary atherectomy. A report from the CAVEAT I and II investigators. Coronary Angioplasty Versus Excisional Atherectomy Trial. J Am Coll Cardiol 28:645–651, 1996.

72. Kiesz R, Rozek M, Mego D, et al: Acute directional coronary atherectomy prior to stenting in complex coronary lesions: ADAPTS Study. Cathet Cardiovasc Diagn 45:105–112, 1998.

73. Moussa I, Krepps E, Collins M: Directional atherectomy prior to stent implantation predicts lower restenosis independent of post-procedural lumen diameter (abstract). Circulation 100(Suppl 1):468, 1999.

ROTATIONAL ATHERECTOMY

74. Mintz GS, Pichard AD, Popma JJ, et al: Preliminary experience with adjunct directional coronary atherectomy after high-speed rotational atherectomy in the treatment of calcific coronary artery disease. Am J Cardiol 71:799–804, 1993.

75. Reisman M: Guide to Rotational Atherectomy. Seattle, Physician's Press, 1997.

76. Friedman H: Mechanical rotary atherectomy: The effects of microparticle embolization on myocardial blood flow and function. J Intervent Cardiol 2:77, 1989.

77. Reisman M, Shuman BJ, Dillard D, et al: Analysis of low-speed rotational atherectomy for the reduction of platelet aggregation. Cathet Cardiovasc Diagn 45:208–214, 1998.

78. Koch KL, vom Dahl J, Kleinhans E, et al: Influence of platelet GPIIb-IIIa receptor antagonist on myocardial hypoperfusion during rotational atherectomy as assessed by myocardial Tc-99 sestamibi scintigraphy. J Am Coll Cardiol 33:998–1004, 1999.

79. Bowers TR, Stewart RE, O'Neill WW, et al: Effect of Rotablator atherectomy and adjunctive balloon angioplasty on coronary blood flow. Circulation 95:1157–1164, 1997.

80. Bertrand ME, Lablanche JM, Leroy F, et al: Percutaneous transluminal coronary rotary ablation with Rotablator (European experience). Am J Cardiol 69:470–474, 1992.

81. Whitlow PL, Cowley MJ, Kuntz RE, et al: Study to determine Rotablator and transluminal angioplasty strategy. Circulation, 92:I-330, 1995.

82. Safian RD, Niazi KA, Strzelecki M, et al: Detailed angiographic analysis of high-speed mechanical rotational atherectomy in human coronary arteries. Circulation 88:961–968, 1993.

83. Brown DL, George CJ, Steenkiste AR, et al: High-speed rotational atherectomy of human coronary stenoses: Acute and one-year outcomes from the New Approaches to Coronary Intervention (NACI) registry. Am J Cardiol 80:60K–67K, 1997.

84. Ellis SG, Popma JJ, Buchbinder M, et al: Relation of clinical presentation, stenosis morphology, and operator technique to the procedural results of rotational atherectomy and rotational atherectomy-facilitated angioplasty. Circulation 89:882–892, 1994.

85. Stertzer S, Rosenblum J, Shaw R, et al: Coronary rotational ablation: Initial experience in 302 procedures. J Am Coll Cardiol 21:287–295, 1993.

86. Hoffmann R, Mintz GS, Kent KM, et al: Comparative early and nine-month results of rotational atherectomy, stents, and the combination of both for calcified lesions in large coronary arteries. Am J Cardiol 81:552–557, 1998.

87. Reifart N, Vandormael M, Krajcar M, et al: Randomized comparison of angioplasty of complex coronary lesions at a single center. Excimer Laser, Rotational Atherectomy, and Balloon Angioplasty Comparison (ERBAC) Study. Circulation 96:91–98, 1997.

88. Brener S, Reifart N, Whitlow PL: The status of three randomized trials: STRATAS, DART, ERBAC. In Serruys PW, Holmes DR (eds): Current Review of Interventional Cardiology. 3rd ed. Philadelphia, Current Medicine, 1997, pp 13–21.

89. Teirstein PS, Warth DC, Haq N, et al: High speed rotational coronary atherectomy for patients with diffuse coronary artery disease. J Am Coll Cardiol 18:1694–1701, 1991.

90. Ellis SG, Ajluni S, Arnold AZ, et al: Increased coronary perforation in the new device era. Incidence, classification, management, and outcome. Circulation 90:2725–2730, 1994.

91. Warth D, Leon MB, O'Neill WW: Rotational atherectomy multicenter registry: Acute results, complication and 6-month angiographic follow-up in 709 patients. J Am Coll Cardiol 24:641–648, 1994.

92. Henneke K, Regar E, Konig A: Impact of target lesion calcification on coronary stent expansion after rotational atherectomy. Am Heart J 137:93, 1999.

93. Brogan WC, Popma JJ, Pichard AD, et al: Rotational coronary atherectomy after unsuccessful coronary balloon angioplasty. Am J Cardiol 71:794–798, 1993.

94. Sharma SK, Duvvuri S, Dangas G, et al: Rotational atherectomy for in-stent restenosis: Acute and long-term results of the first 100 cases. J Am Coll Cardiol 32:1358–1365, 1998.

95. Lee SG, Lee CW, Cheong S, et al: Immediate and long-term outcomes of rotational atherectomy versus balloon angioplasty alone for the treatment of diffuse in-stent restenosis. Am J Cardiol 82:140–143, 1998.

96. von Dahl J, Radke P, Haager P, et al: Clinical and angiographic predictors of recurrent restenosis after percutaneous transluminal rotational atherectomy for treatment of diffuse in-stent restenosis. Am J Cardiol 83:862–867, 1999.

TRANSLUMINAL EXTRACTION ATHERECTOMY

97. Annex BH, Sketch MH Jr, Stack RS, et al: Transluminal extraction coronary atherectomy. Cardiol Clin 12:611–622, 1994.

98. Kaplan BM, Larkin T, Safian RD, et al: Prospective study of extraction atherectomy in patients with acute myocardial infarction. Am J Cardiol 78:383–388, 1996.

99. Popma JJ, Leon MB, Mintz GS, et al: Results of coronary angioplasty using the transluminal extraction catheter. Am J Cardiol 70:1526–1532, 1992.

100. Safian RD, May MA, Lichtenberg A, et al: Detailed clinical and angiographic analysis of transluminal extraction coronary atherectomy for complex lesions in native coronary arteries. J Am Coll Cardiol 25:848–854, 1995.

101. Meany TB, Leon MB, Kramer BL, et al: Transluminal extraction catheter for the treatment of diseased saphenous vein grafts: A multicenter experience. Cathet Cardiovasc Diagn 34:112–120, 1995.

102. Dooris M, Hoffmann M, Glazier S: Comparative results of transluminal extraction atherectomy in saphenous vein graft lesions with and without thrombus. J Am Coll Cardiol 25:1700–1705, 1995.

103. Hong MK, Popma JJ, Pichard AD, et al: Clinical significance of distal embolization after transluminal extraction atherectomy in diffusely diseased saphenous vein grafts. Am Heart J 127:1496–1503, 1994.

104. Kaplan BM Gregory M, Schreiber TL, et al: Transluminal extraction atherectomy versus balloon angioplasty in acute ischemic syndromes. An interim analysis of the Topit Trial (abstract). Circulation 94: I-317, 1996.

LASER ANGIOPLASTY

105. Srinivasan R: Ablation of polymers and biologic tissues by ultraviolet lasers. Science 234:559–565, 1986.

106. Stone GW, de Marchena E, Dageforde D, et al: Prospective, randomized, multicenter comparison of laser-facilitated balloon angioplasty versus stand-alone balloon angioplasty in patients with obstructive coronary artery disease. The Laser Angioplasty Versus Angioplasty (LAVA) Trial Investigators. J Am Coll Cardiol 30:1714–1721, 1997.

107. Appelman Y, Koolen J, Piek J, et al: Excimer laser angioplasty versus balloon angioplasty in functional and total coronary occlusions. Am J Cardiol 78:757–762, 1996.

108. Appelman YE, Piek JJ, Strikwerda S, et al: Randomised trial of excimer laser angioplasty versus balloon angioplasty for treatment of obstructive coronary artery disease. Lancet 347:79–84, 1996.

109. Appelman YE, Piek JJ, Redekop WK, et al: Clinical events following excimer laser angioplasty or balloon angioplasty for complex coronary lesions: Subanalysis of a randomised trial. Heart 79:34–38, 1998.

110. Bonner R, Smith P, Prevosti L, et al: New sources for laser angioplasty: Er:YAG, excimer lasers, and nonlaser hot-tip catheters. In Vogel J, King S (eds): Interventional Cardiology: Future Directions. St Louis, Mosby, 1989, pp 101–108.

111. Clarke RH, Isner JM, Donaldson RF, Jones G 2d: Gas chromatographic-light microscopic correlative analysis of excimer laser photoablation of cardiovascular tissues: Evidence for a thermal mechanism. Circ Res 60:429–437, 1987.

112. Litvack F, Forrester J, Grundfest W, et al: The excimer laser: From basic

science to clinical application. *In* Vogel J, King SB (eds): Interventional Cardiology: Future Directions. St Louis, Mosby, 1989, pp 170–181.

113. Isner J, Pickering J, Mosseri M: Laser-induced dissections: Pathogenesis and implications for therapy. J Am Coll Cardiol 19:1619–1621, 1992.

114. Tcheng JE, Wells LD, Phillips HR, et al: Development of a new technique for reducing pressure pulse generation during 308-nm excimer laser coronary angioplasty. Cathet Cardiovasc Diagn 34:15–22, 1995.

115. Deckelbaum LI, Natarajan MK, Bittl JA, et al: Effect of intracoronary saline infusion on dissection during excimer laser coronary angioplasty: A randomized trial. The Percutaneous Excimer Laser Coronary Angioplasty (PELCA) Investigators. J Am Coll Cardiol 26:1264–1269, 1995.

116. Baumbach A, Bittl JA, Fleck E, et al: Acute complications of excimer laser coronary angioplasty: A detailed analysis of multicenter results. Coinvestigators of the U.S. and European Percutaneous Excimer Laser Coronary Angioplasty (PELCA) Registries. J Am Coll Cardiol 23:1305–1313, 1994.

117. Bittl JA, Sanborn TA, Yardley DE, et al: Predictors of outcome of percutaneous excimer laser coronary angioplasty of saphenous vein bypass graft lesions. The Percutaneous Excimer Laser Coronary Angioplasty Registry. Am J Cardiol 74:144–148, 1994.

118. Bittl JA, Kuntz RE, Estella P, et al: Analysis of late lumen narrowing after excimer laser–facilitated coronary angioplasty. J Am Coll Cardiol 23:1314–1320, 1994.

119. Litvack F, Eigler N, Margolis J, et al: Percutaneous excimer laser coronary angioplasty: Results in the first consecutive 3,000 patients. The ELCA Investigators. J Am Coll Cardiol 23:323–329, 1994.

120. Holmes DR, Mehta S, George CJ, et al: Excimer laser coronary angioplasty: The New Approaches to Coronary Intervention (NACI) experience. Am J Cardiol 80:99K–105K, 1997.

121. Bittl JA, Sanborn TA, Tcheng JE, et al: Clinical success, complications and restenosis rates with excimer laser coronary angioplasty. The Percutaneous Excimer Laser Coronary Angioplasty Registry. Am J Cardiol 70:1533–1539, 1992.

122. Koster R, Hamm CW, Terres W, et al: Treatment of in-stent coronary restenosis by excimer laser angioplasty. Am J Cardiol 80:1424–1428, 1997.

123. Mehran R, Mintz GS, Satler LF, et al: Treatment of in-stent restenosis with excimer laser coronary angioplasty: Mechanisms and results compared with PTCA alone. Circulation 96:2183–2189, 1997.

THROMBECTOMY AND DISTAL PROTECTION DEVICES

124. Fuster V, Badimon L, Badimon J, et al: The pathogenesis of coronary artery disease and the acute coronary syndromes. N Engl J Med 326:242–250, 1992.

125. Liu MW, Douglas JJ, Lembo NJ, et al: Angiographic predictors of a rise in serum creatine kinase (distal embolization) after balloon angioplasty of saphenous vein coronary artery bypass grafts. Am J Cardiol 72:514–517, 1993.

126. Lefkovits J, Holmes DR, Califf RM, et al: Predictors and sequelae of distal embolization during saphenous vein graft intervention from the CAVEAT-II trial. Coronary Angioplasty Versus Excisional Atherectomy Trial. Circulation 92:734–740, 1995.

127. Zidar F, Kaplan B, O'Neill WW, et al: Prospective, randomized trial of prolonged intracoronary urokinase infusion for chronic total occlusions in native coronary arteries. J Am Coll Cardiol 27:1406–1412, 1996.

128. Chapekis AT, George BS, Candela RJ: Rapid thrombus dissolution by continuous infusion of urokinase through an intracoronary perfusion wire prior to and following PTCA: Results in native coronaries and patent saphenous vein grafts. Cathet Cardiovasc Diagn 23:89–92, 1991.

129. Hartmann JR, McKeever LS, O'Neill WW, et al: Recanalization of chronically occluded aortocoronary saphenous vein bypass grafts with long-term low-dose direct infusion of urokinase (Robust): A serial study. J Am Coll Cardiol 27:60–66, 1996.

130. Ambrose JA, Almeida OD, Sharma SK, et al: Adjunctive thrombolytic therapy during angioplasty for ischemic rest angina. Results of the TAUSA Trial. TAUSA Investigators. Thrombolysis and Angioplasty in Unstable Angina trial. Circulation 90:69–77, 1994.

131. Glazier JJ, Kiernan FJ, Bauer HH, et al: Treatment of thrombotic saphenous vein bypass grafts using local urokinase infusion therapy with the Dispatch catheter. Cathet Cardiovasc Diagn 41:261–267, 1997.

132. Glazier JJ, Hirst JA, Kiernan FJ, et al: Site-specific intracoronary thrombolysis with urokinase-coated hydrogel balloons: Acute and follow-up studies in 95 patients. Cathet Cardiovasc Diagn 41:246–253, 1997.

133. Rousseau H, Sapoval M, Ballini P, et al: Percutaneous recanalization of acutely thrombosed vessels by hydrodynamic thrombectomy (Hydrolyser). Eur Radiol 7:935–941, 1997.

134. Overbosch E, Pattynama P, Aarts H, et al: Occluded hemodialysis shunts: Dutch multicenter experience with the Hydrolyser catheter. Radiology 201:485–488, 1996.

135. van Ommen V, van den Bos A, Pieper M, et al: Removal of thrombus from aortocoronary bypass grafts and coronary arteries using the 6 Fr Hydrolyser. Am J Cardiol 79:1012–1016, 1997.

136. Rosenschein U, Roth A, Rassin T, et al: Analysis of coronary ultrasound thrombolysis endpoints in acute myocardial infarction (ACUTE trial). Results of the feasibility phase. Circulation 95:1411–1416, 1997.

137. Popma J, Ramee S, Lansky A, et al: Quantitative changes in thrombus burden after rheolytic thrombectomy in native coronary arteries and saphenous vein grafts (abstract). Circulation 94(Suppl 1):374, 1996.

138. Ramee SR, Bain DS, Popma JJ, et al: A randomized, prospective, multicenter study comparing intracoronary urokinase to rheolytic thrombectomy with the Possis Angiojet catheter for intracoronary thrombus: Final results of the VEGAS-2 trial (abstract). Circulation 98: I-86, 1998.

139. Webb J, Carere R, Virmani R, et al: Retrieval and analysis of particulate debris follow saphenous vein graft intervention. J Am Coll Cardiol 34:461–467, 1999.

CORONARY STENTS

140. Dotter C, Judkins M: Transluminal treatment of atherosclerotic obstruction. Circulation 30:654–670, 1964.

141. Puel J, Joffre F, Rousseau H, et al: Endoprotheses coronariennes auto-expansives dans le prevention des restenoses apres angioplastie transluminale. Arch Mal Coeur 8:1311–1312, 1987.

142. Sigwart U, Puel J, Mirkovitch V, et al: Intravascular stents to prevent occlusion and restenosis after transluminal angioplasty. N Engl J Med 316:701–706, 1987.

143. Kutryk M, Serruys P: Current indications for stenting. *In* Kutryk M, Serruys P (eds): Coronary Stenting. Current Perspectives. London, Martin Dunitz, 1999, pp 139–195.

144. Sawada Y, Nokasa H, Kimura T, et al: Initial and six months outcomes of Palmaz-Schatz stent implantation: STRESS/BENESTENT equivalent vs nonequivalent lesions (abstract). J Am Coll Cardiol 27:252, 1996.

Indications

145. Serruys PW, de Jaegere P, Kiemeneij F, et al: A comparison of balloon-expandable-stent implantation with balloon angioplasty in patients with coronary artery disease. BENESTENT Study Group. N Engl J Med 331:489–495, 1994.

146. Erbel R, Haude M, Hopp H, et al: Coronary-artery stenting compared with balloon angioplasty for restenosis after initial balloon angioplasty. N Engl J Med 339:1672–1678, 1998.

147. Savage MP, Douglas JS Jr, Fischman DL, et al: Stent placement compared with balloon angioplasty for obstructed coronary bypass grafts. Saphenous Vein De Novo Trial Investigators. N Engl J Med 337:740–747, 1997.

148. Sirnes PA, Golf S, Myreng Y, et al: Stenting in Chronic Coronary Occlusion (SICCO): A randomized, controlled trial of adding stent implantation after successful angioplasty. J Am Coll Cardiol 28:1444–1451, 1996.

149. Betriu A, Masotti M, Serra A, et al: Randomized comparison of coronary stent implantation and balloon angioplasty in the treatment of de novo coronary artery lesions (START). J Am Coll Cardiol 34:1498–1506, 1999.

150. Dean LS, George CJ, Roubin GS, et al: Bailout and corrective use of Gianturco-Roubin flex stents after percutaneous transluminal coronary angioplasty: Operator reports and angiographic core laboratory verification from the National Heart, Lung, and Blood Institute/New Approaches to Coronary Intervention Registry. J Am Coll Cardiol 29:934–940, 1997.

151. Schomig A, Kastrati A, Dietz R, et al: Emergency coronary stenting for dissection during percutaneous transluminal coronary angioplasty: Angiographic follow-up after stenting and after repeat angioplasty of the stented segment. J Am Coll Cardiol 23:1053–1060, 1994.

152. Penn I, Ricci D, Brown B, et al: Randomized study of prolonged balloon dilatation in failed angioplasty (PTCA): Preliminary data from the trial of angioplasty and stents in Canada (TASC II) (abstract). Circulation 88(Suppl 1):601, 1993.

153. Keane D, Roubin G, Marco J, et al: GRACE—Gianturco Roubin stent Acute Closure Evaluation: Substrate, challenges, and design of a randomized trial of bailout management. J Intervent Cardiol 7:333–339, 1994.

154. de Feyter PJ, van Suylen RJ, de Jaegere PP, et al: Balloon angioplasty for the treatment of lesions in saphenous vein bypass grafts. J Am Coll Cardiol 21:1539–1549, 1993.

155. Ivanhoe RJ, Weintraub WS, Douglas JS, et al: Percutaneous transluminal coronary angioplasty of chronic total occlusions. Primary success, restenosis, and long-term clinical follow-up. Circulation 85:106–115, 1992.

156. Maiello L, Colombo A, Gianrossi R, et al: Coronary angioplasty of chronic occlusions: Factors predictive of procedural success. Am Heart J 124:581–584, 1992.

157. Stone GW, Rutherford BD, McConahay DR, et al: Procedural outcome of angioplasty for total coronary artery occlusion: An analysis of 971 lesions in 905 patients. J Am Coll Cardiol 15:849–856, 1990.

158. Berger PB, Holmes DR, Ohman EM, et al: Restenosis, reocclusion and adverse cardiovascular events after successful balloon angioplasty of occluded versus nonoccluded coronary arteries. Results from the Multicenter American Research Trial with Cilazapril after Angioplasty to Prevent Transluminal Coronary Obstruction and Restenosis (MARCATOR). J Am Coll Cardiol 27:1–7, 1996.

159. Violaris AG, Melkert R, Serruys PW: Long-term luminal renarrowing after successful elective coronary angioplasty of total occlusions. A quantitative angiographic analysis. Circulation 91:2140–2150, 1995.

160. Bell MR, Berger PB, Bresnahan JF, et al: Initial and long-term outcome of 354 patients after coronary balloon angioplasty of total coronary artery occlusions. Circulation 85:1003–1111, 1992.

161. Ishizaka N, Issiki T, Saeki F, et al: Angiographic follow-up after suc-

cessful percutaneous coronary angioplasty for chronic total coronary occlusion: Experience in 110 consecutive patients. Am Heart J 127:8–12, 1994.

162. Corcos T, Favereau X, Guerin Y, et al: Recanalization of chronic coronary occlusions using a new hydrophilic guidewire. Cathet Cardiovasc Diagn 43:83–90, 1998.

163. Goldberg SL, Colombo A, Maiello L, et al: Intracoronary stent insertion after balloon angioplasty of chronic total occlusions. J Am Coll Cardiol 26:713–719, 1995.

164. Suttorp MJ, Mast EG, Plokker HW, et al: Primary coronary stenting after successful balloon angioplasty of chronic total occlusions: A single-center experience. Am Heart J 135:318–322, 1998.

165. Rubartelli P, Niccoli L, Verna E, et al: Stent implantation versus balloon angioplasty in chronic coronary occlusions: Results from the GISSOC trial. Gruppo Italiano di Studio sullo Stent nelle Occlusioni Coronariche. J Am Coll Cardiol 32:90–96, 1998.

166. Hoher M, Wohrle J, Grebe O, et al: A randomized trial of elective stenting after balloon recanalization of chronic total occlusions. J Am Coll Cardiol 34:722–729, 1999.

167. Sirnes PA, Golf S, Myreng Y, et al: Sustained benefit of stenting chronic coronary occlusion: Long-term clinical follow-up of the Stenting in Chronic Coronary Occlusion (SICCO) study. J Am Coll Cardiol 32:305–310, 1998.

168. The GUSTO IIb Investigators: A clinical trial comparing primary angioplasty with tissue plasminogen activator for acute myocardial infarction. N Engl J Med 336:1621–1628, 1997.

169. Weaver WD, Simes RJ, Betriu A, et al: Comparison of primary coronary angioplasty and intravenous thrombolytic therapy for acute myocardial infarction: A quantitative review. JAMA 278:2093–2098, 1997.

170. Grines CL, Browne KF, Marco J, et al: A comparison of immediate angioplasty with thrombolytic therapy for acute myocardial infarction. The Primary Angioplasty in Myocardial Infarction Study Group. N Engl J Med 328:673–679, 1993.

171. Zijlstra F, de Boer MJ, Hoorntje JC, et al: A comparison of immediate coronary angioplasty with intravenous streptokinase in acute myocardial infarction. N Engl J Med 328:680–684, 1993.

172. Zijlstra F, Beukema WP, van't Hof AW, et al: Randomized comparison of primary coronary angioplasty with thrombolytic therapy in low risk patients with acute myocardial infarction. J Am Coll Cardiol 29:908–912, 1997.

173. Gibbons R, Holmes D, Reeder G, et al: Immediate angioplasty compared with the administration of a thrombolytic agent followed by conservative treatment for myocardial infarction. N Engl J Med 328:685–691, 1993.

174. Michels KB, Yusuf S: Does PTCA in acute myocardial infarction affect mortality and reinfarction rates? A quantitative overview (meta-analysis) of the randomized clinical trials. Circulation 91:476–485, 1995.

175. Brodie BR, Grines CL, Ivanhoe R, et al: Six-month clinical and angiographic follow-up after direct angioplasty for acute myocardial infarction. Final results from the Primary Angioplasty Registry. Circulation 90:156–162, 1994.

176. Bedotto JB, Kahn JK, Rutherford BD, et al: Failed direct coronary angioplasty for acute myocardial infarction: In-hospital outcome and predictors of death. J Am Coll Cardiol 22:690–694, 1993.

177. Stone GW, Brodie BR, Griffin JJ, et al: Prospective, multicenter study of the safety and feasibility of primary stenting in acute myocardial infarction: In-hospital and 30-day results of the PAMI stent pilot trial. Primary Angioplasty in Myocardial Infarction Stent Pilot Trial Investigators. J Am Coll Cardiol 31:23–30, 1998.

178. Rodriquez A, Bernardi V, Fernandez M, et al: In-hospital and late results of coronary stents versus conventional balloon angioplasty in acute myocardial infarction (GRAMI Trial). Am J Cardiol 81:1286–1291, 1998.

179. Saito S, Hosokawa G, Tanaka S, Nakamura S: Primary stent implantation is superior to balloon angioplasty in acute myocardial infarction: Final results of the Primary Angioplasty Versus Stent Implantation in Acute Myocardial Infarction (PASTA) trial. Catheter Cardiovasc Interv 48:262–268, 1999.

180. Antoniucci D, Santoro GM, Bolognese L, et al: A clinical trial comparing primary stenting of the infarct-related artery with optimal primary angioplasty for acute myocardial infarction: Results from the Florence Randomized Elective Stenting in Acute Coronary Occlusions (FRESCO) trial. J Am Coll Cardiol 31:1234–1239, 1998.

181. Suryapranata H, van't Hof AW, Hoorntje JC, et al: Randomized comparison of coronary stenting with balloon angioplasty in selected patients with acute myocardial infarction. Circulation 97:2502–2505, 1998.

182. Rodriquez A, Bernardi V, Fernandex M, et al: In-hospital and late results of coronary stents versus conservative balloon angioplasty in acute myocardial infarction (GRAMI). Am J Cardiol 81:1286–1291, 1998.

183. Grines C, Cox D, Stone G, et al: Coronary angioplasty with or without stent implantation for acute myocardial infarction. N Engl J Med 341:1949–1956, 1999.

184. Ryan T, Antman E, Brooks N, et al: 1999 Update: ACC/AHA guidelines for the management of patients with acute myocardial infarction. J Am Coll Cardiol 34:889–911, 1999.

184a. Saucedo JF, Popma JJ, Kennard ED, et al: Relation of coronary artery size to one-year clinical events after new device angioplasty of native

coronary arteries (a New Approach to Coronary Intervention [NACI] Registry Report). Am J Cardiol 85:166–171, 2000.

185. Savage MP, Fischman DL, Rake R, et al: Efficacy of coronary stenting versus balloon angioplasty in small coronary arteries. Stent Restenosis Study (STRESS) Investigators. J Am Coll Cardiol 31:307–311, 1998.

Stent Complications

186. Roubin GS, Cannon AD, Agrawal SK, et al: Intracoronary stenting for acute and threatened closure complicating percutaneous transluminal coronary angioplasty. Circulation 85:916–927, 1992.

187. Hearn JA, King SB, Douglas JS Jr, et al: Clinical and angiographic outcomes after coronary artery stenting for acute or threatened closure after percutaneous transluminal coronary angioplasty. Initial results with a balloon-expandable, stainless steel design. Circulation 88:2086–2096, 1993.

188. Schomig A, Kastrati A, Mudra H, et al: Four-year experience with Palmaz-Schatz stenting in coronary angioplasty complicated by dissection with threatened or present vessel closure. Circulation 90:2716–2724, 1994.

189. Goldberg S, Colombo A, Nakamura S: The benefit of intracoronary ultrasound on the deployment of Palmaz-Schatz stents. J Am Coll Cardiol 24:996–1003, 1994.

190. Hall P, Colombo A, Almagor Y: Preliminary experience with intravascular ultrasound guided Palmaz-Schatz coronary stenting: The acute and short-term results on a consecutive series of patients. J Intervent Cardiol 7:141–159, 1994.

191. Colombo A, Hall P, Nakamura S, et al: Intracoronary stenting without anticoagulation accomplished with intravascular ultrasound guidance. Circulation 91:1676–1688, 1995.

192. Haude M, Erbel R, Issa H, et al: Subacute thrombotic complications after intracoronary implantation of Palmaz-Schatz stents. Am Heart J 126:15–22, 1993.

193. Popma JJ, Satler LF, Pichard AD, et al: Vascular complications after balloon and new device angioplasty. Circulation 88:1569–1578, 1993.

194. Moscucci M, Mansour KA, Kent KC, et al: Peripheral vascular complications of directional coronary atherectomy and stenting: Predictors, management, and outcome. Am J Cardiol 74:448–453, 1994.

195. Rosenschein U, Ellis SG: Preprocedure warfarinization and brachial approach for elective coronary stent placement—a possible strategy to decrease cost and duration of hospitalization. Cathet Cardiovasc Diagn 25:290–292, 1992.

196. Kiemeneij F, Laarman GJ, de Melker E: Transradial artery coronary angioplasty. Am Heart J 129:1–7, 1995.

197. Kiemeneij F, Laarman GJ, Odekerken D, et al: A randomized comparison of percutaneous transluminal coronary angioplasty by the radial, brachial and femoral approaches: The access study. J Am Coll Cardiol 29:1269–1275, 1997.

198. Bartorelli AL, Sganzerla P, Fabbiocchi F, et al: Prompt and safe femoral hemostasis with a collagen device after intracoronary implantation of Palmaz-Schatz stents. Am Heart J 130:26–32, 1994.

199. Iniguez A, Macaya C, Alfonso F, et al: Early angiographic changes of side branches arising from a Palmaz-Schatz stented coronary segment: Results and clinical implications. J Am Coll Cardiol 23:911–915, 1994.

200. Fischman DL, Savage MP, Leon MB, et al: Fate of lesion-related side branches after coronary artery stenting. J Am Coll Cardiol 22:1641–1646, 1993.

201. Rozenman Y, Burstein M, Hasin Y, et al: Retrieval of occluding unexpanded Palmaz-Schatz stent from a saphenous aorto-coronary vein graft. Cathet Cardiovasc Diagn 34:159–161, 1995.

202. Kimura T, Yokoi H, Nakagawa Y, et al: Three-year follow-up after implantation of metallic coronary-artery stents. N Engl J Med 334:561–566, 1996.

203. Hermiller JB, Fry ET, Peters TF, et al: Late coronary artery stenosis regression within the Gianturco-Roubin intracoronary stent. Am J Cardiol 77:247–251, 1996.

204. Foley JB, White J, Teefy P, et al: Late angiographic follow-up after Palmaz-Schatz stent implantation. Am J Cardiol 76:76–77, 1995.

205. Klugherz B, De Angelo D, Kim B, et al: Three-year clinical follow-up after Palmaz-Schatz stenting. J Am Coll Cardiol 27:1185–1191, 1996.

206. Debbas N, Sigwart U, Eeckhout E, et al: Intracoronary stenting for restenosis: Long-term follow-up: A single center experience. J Invas Cardiol 8:241–248, 1996.

Stent Designs

207. Kutryk M, Serruys P: Stents currently available. In Kutryk M, Serruys P (eds): Coronary Stenting. Current Perspectives. London, Martin Dunitz, 1999, pp 17–86.

208. Escaned J, Goicolea J, Alfonso F, et al: Propensity and mechanism of restenosis in different coronary stent designs. J Am Coll Cardiol 34:1490–1497, 1999.

209. Goy JJ, Eeckhout E, Stauffer JC, et al: Emergency endoluminal stenting for abrupt vessel closure following coronary angioplasty: A randomized comparison of the Wiktor and Palmaz-Schatz stents. Cathet Cardiovasc Diagn 34:128–132, 1995.

210. Wong SC, Popma JJ, Pichard AD, et al: Comparison of clinical and

angiographic outcomes after saphenous vein graft angioplasty using coronary versus 'biliary' tubular slotted stents. Circulation 91:339–350, 1995.

211. George BS, Voorhees WD 3d, Roubin GS, et al: Multicenter investigation of coronary stenting to treat acute or threatened closure after percutaneous transluminal coronary angioplasty: Clinical and angiographic outcomes. J Am Coll Cardiol 22:135–143, 1993.

212. Leon M, Popma J, O'Shaughnessy C, et al: Quantitative angiographic outcomes after Gianturco-Roubin II stent implantation in complex lesion subsets (abstract). Circulation 96(Suppl 1):653, 1997.

213. de Jaegere PP, Serruys PW, Bertrand M, et al: Wiktor stent implantation in patients with restenosis following balloon angioplasty of a native coronary artery. Am J Cardiol 69:598–602, 1992.

214. Chalet Y, Panes F, Chevalier B, et al: Should we avoid ostial implantations of Wiktor stents? Cathet Cardiovasc Diagn 32:376–379, 1994.

215. Baim D, Midei M, Linnemeier T, et al: A randomized trial comparing the Multilink stent to the Palmaz-Schatz stent in de novo lesions. Am J Cardiol, in press.

216. Heuser R, Kuntz R, Lansky A, et al: Six-month clinical and angiographic results of the SMART Trial (abstract). J Am Coll Cardiol 31:64, 1998.

217. Almagor Y, Feld S, Kiemeneij F, et al: First international new intravascular rigid-flex endovascular stent study (FINESS): Clinical and angiographic results after elective and urgent stent implantation. J Am Coll Cardiol 30:847–854, 1997.

218. Baim D, Cutlip D, O'Shaughnessy C, et al: A randomized trial comparing the NIR Stent to the Palmaz-Schatz stent in native coronary lesions. Am J Cardiol, in press.

219. Watson P, Ponde C, Aroney C, et al: Angiographic follow-up and clinical experience with the flexible tantalum Cordis stent. Cathet Cardiovasc Diagn 43:168–173, 1998.

220. Feres F, Sousa E, Londero H, et al: Early results of the SOLACI Registry of a new coil stent (Cross-flex) (abstract). Am J Cardiol 80(Suppl):28, 1997.

221. Kobayashi Y, Teirstein P, Bailey S, et al: Self-expandable stent versus balloon-expandable stent: A serial volumetric analysis by intravascular ultrasound (abstract). J Am Coll Cardiol 31:396, 1998.

222. Han R, Schwatz R, Mann T, et al: Comparative efficacy of self-expanding and balloon expandable stents for the reduction of restenosis (abstract). J Am Coll Cardiol 96:314, 1998.

223. Bilodeau L, Schreiber T, Hilton J, et al: The Wallstent in native coronary arteries (WIN) multicenter randomized trial: In-hospital acute results (abstract). J Am Coll Cardiol 31:80, 1998.

224. Holmes D, Lansky A, Kuntz R, et al: The Paragon stent study: A randomized trial of a new martinsitic nitinol stent versus the Palmaz-Schatz (PS)™ stent for the treatment of complex native coronary arterial lesions. Am J Cardiol, in press.

In-Stent Restenosis

225. Hoffmann R, Mintz GS, Dussaillant GR, et al: Patterns and mechanisms of in-stent restenosis. A serial intravascular ultrasound study. Circulation 94:1247–1254, 1996.

226. Asakura M, Ueda Y, Nanto S, et al: Remodeling of in-stent neointima which became thinner and transparent over 3 years. Circulation 97:2003–2006, 1998.

227. Mintz GS, Hoffmann R, Mehran R, et al: In-stent restenosis: The Washington Hospital Center experience. Am J Cardiol 81:7E–13E, 1998.

228. Mehran R, Mintz GS, Popma JJ, et al: Mechanisms and results of balloon angioplasty for the treatment of in-stent restenosis. Am J Cardiol 78:618–622, 1996.

229. Shiran A, Mintz GS, Waksman R, et al: Early lumen loss after treatment of in-stent restenosis: An intravascular ultrasound study. Circulation 98:200–203, 1998.

230. Reimers B, Moussa I, Akiyama T, et al: Long-term clinical follow-up after successful repeat percutaneous intervention for stent restenosis. J Am Coll Cardiol 30:186–192, 1997.

231. Bauters C, Banos J-L, Van belle E, et al: Six-month angiographic outcomes after successful repeat percutaneous intervention for in-stent restenosis. Circulation 97:318–321, 1998.

231a. Bossi I, Klersy C, Black AJ, et al: In-stent restenosis: Long term outcome and predictors of subsequent target lesion revascularization after repeat balloon angioplasty. J Am Coll Cardiol 35:1569–1576, 2000.

232. Dauerman HL, Baim DS, Cutlip DE, et al: Mechanical debulking versus balloon angioplasty for the treatment of diffuse in-stent restenosis. Am J Cardiol 82:277–284, 1998.

233. Teirstein PS, Massullo V, Jani S, et al: Catheter-based radiotherapy to inhibit restenosis after coronary stenting. N Engl J Med 336:1697–1703, 1997.

233a. Teirstein PS, Massullo V, Jani S, et al: Three-year clinical and angiographic follow-up after intracoronary radiation. Results of a randomized clinical trial. Circulation 101:360–365, 2000.

234. Leon M, Moses J, Lansky A, et al: Intracoronary gamma radiation for the prevention of recurrent in-stent restenosis: Final results from the Gamma-1 Trial (abstract). Circulation 18(Suppl 1):75, 1999.

235. Waksman R, White RL, Chan RC, et al: Intracoronary gamma radiation after angioplasty inhibits recurrence in patients with in-stent restenosis. Circulation, in press.

236. Schwartz L, Bourassa M, Lesperance J, et al: Aspirin and dipyridamole in the prevention of restenosis after percutaneous transluminal coronary angioplasty. N Engl J Med 318:1714–1719, 1988.

237. Narins CR, Hillegass WB Jr, Nelson CL, et al: Relation between activated clotting time during angioplasty and abrupt closure. Circulation 93:667–671, 1996.

238. Ferguson J, Dougherty K, Gaos C, et al: Relation between procedural activated clotting time and outcome after percutaneous transluminal coronary angioplasty. J Am Coll Cardiol 23:1061–1065, 1994.

239. White C, Chaitman B, Lassar T, et al: Antiplatelet agents are effective in reducing the immediate complications of PTCA: Results of the ticlopidine multicenter trial (abstract). Circulation 76(Suppl 4):400, 1987.

240. Lembo NJ, Black AJ, Roubin GS, et al: Effect of pretreatment with aspirin versus aspirin plus dipyridamole on frequency and type of acute complications of percutaneous transluminal coronary angioplasty. Am J Cardiol 65:422–426, 1990.

241. Gregorini L, Marco J, Fajadet J, et al: Ticlopidine and aspirin pretreatment reduces coagulation and platelet activation during coronary dilation procedures. J Am Coll Cardiol 29:13–20, 1997.

242. Schomig A, Neumann FJ, Kastrati A, et al: A randomized comparison of antiplatelet and anticoagulant therapy after the placement of coronary-artery stents. N Engl J Med 334:1084–1089, 1996.

243. Leon M, Baim D, Popma J, et al: A clinical trial comparing three antithrombotic-drug regimens after coronary-artery stenting. N Engl J Med 339:1665–1671, 1998.

244. Bennett C, Weinberg P, Rozenberg-Ben-Dror K, et al: Thrombocytopenic purpura associated with ticlopidine. Ann Intern Med 128:541–544, 1998.

245. Szto G, Linnemeier T, Lewis S: Safety of 10 days of ticlopidine after coronary stenting—a randomized comparison with 30 days: Strategic ALternatives with Ticlopidine in Stenting Study (SALTS) (abstract). J Am Coll Cardiol 31:352, 1998.

246. Berger PB, Bell MR, Hasdai D, et al: Safety of ticlopidine for only 2 weeks after successful coronary stent placement. Circulation 99:248–253, 1999.

247. Coukell AJ, Markham A: Clopidogrel. Drugs 54:745–750, 1997.

248. The CAPRIE Steering Committee: A randomised, blind, trial of clopidogrel versus aspirin in patients at risk of ischemic events (CAPRIE). Lancet 348:1329–1339, 1996.

249. Urban P, Gershuck AH, Rupprecht H-J, et al: Efficacy of ticlopidine and clopidogrel on the rate of cardiac events after stent implantation (abstract). Circulation 100:I-379, 1999.

250. Moussa I, Oetgen M, Roubin G, et al: Effectiveness of clopidogrel and aspirin versus ticlopidine and aspirin in preventing stent thrombosis after coronary stent implantation. Circulation 99:2364–2366, 1999.

250a. Muller C, Buttner HJ, Petersen J, et al: A randomized comparison of clopidogrel and aspirin versus ticlopidine and aspirin after the placement of coronary artery stents. Circulation 101:590–593, 2000.

251. Ruggeri Z: Receptor-specific antiplatelet therapy. Circulation 80:1920–1922, 1989.

252. Phillips D, Charo I, Parise L, et al: The platelet membrane glycoprotein IIb-IIIa complex. Blood 71:831–843, 1988.

253. The EPILOG Investigators: Platelet glycoprotein IIb/IIIa receptor blockade and low-dose heparin during percutaneous coronary revascularization. N Engl J Med 336:1689–1696, 1997.

254. The EPISTENT Investigators: Randomised placebo-controlled and balloon-angioplasty–controlled trial to assess safety of coronary stenting with use of platelet glycoprotein-IIb/IIIa blockade. Lancet 352:87–92, 1998.

255. Lincoff A, Califf R, Moliterno D, et al: Complementary clinical benefits of coronary artery stenting and blockade of platelet glycoprotein IIb/IIIa receptors. N Engl J Med 341:319–327, 1999.

256. The IMPACT-II Investigators: Randomised placebo-controlled trial of effect of eptifibatide on complications of percutaneous coronary intervention: IMPACT-II. Integrilin to Minimise Platelet Aggregation and Coronary Thrombosis-II. Lancet 349:1422–1428, 1997.

257. The RESTORE Investigators: Effects of platelet glycoprotein IIb/IIIa blockade with tirofiban on adverse cardiac events in patients with unstable angina or acute myocardial infarction undergoing coronary angioplasty. Circulation 96:1445–1453, 1997.

258. Gibson CM, Goel M, Cohen DJ, et al: Six-month angiographic and clinical follow-up of patients prospectively randomized to receive either tirofiban or placebo during angioplasty in the RESTORE trial. Randomized Efficacy Study of Tirofiban for Outcomes and Restenosis. J Am Coll Cardiol 32:28–34, 1998.

259. Lincoff AM, Califf RM, Anderson KM, et al: Evidence for prevention of death and myocardial infarction with platelet membrane glycoprotein IIb/IIIa receptor blockade by abciximab (c7E3 Fab) among patients with unstable angina undergoing percutaneous coronary revascularization. J Am Coll Cardiol 30:149–156, 1997.

259a. Neumann F-J, Kastrati A, Schmitt C, et al: Effect of glycoprotein IIb-IIIA receptor blockade with abciximab on clinical and angiographic restenosis rate after the placement of coronary stents following acute myocardial infarction. J Am Coll Cardiol 35:915–921, 2000.

260. Brener SJ, Barr LA, Burchenal JE, et al: Randomized, placebo-controlled trial of platelet glycoprotein IIb/IIIa blockade with primary angioplasty for acute myocardial infarction. Circulation 98:734–741, 1998.

261. Mak KH, Challapalli R, Eisenberg MJ, et al: Effect of platelet glycoprotein IIb/IIIa receptor inhibition on distal embolization during percutaneous revascularization of aortocoronary saphenous vein grafts. Am J Cardiol 80:985–988, 1997.

262. Mathew V, Grill D, Scott C, et al: The influence of abciximab use on clinical outcome after aortocoronary vein graft interventions. J Am Coll Cardiol 34:1163–1169, 1999.

263. Muhlestein JB, Karagounis LA, Treehan S, et al: "Rescue" utilization of abciximab for the dissolution of coronary thrombus developing as a complication of coronary angioplasty. J Am Coll Cardiol 30:1729–1734, 1997.

263a. Bhatt DL, Marso SP, Lincoff AM, et al: Abciximab reduces mortality in diabetics following percutaneous coronary intervention. J Am Coll Cardiol 35:922–928, 2000.

264. Rao T, Pratt C, Berke A, et al: Thrombolysis in Myocardial Infarction (TIMI) trial, phase I: Hemorrhagic manifestations and changes in fibrinogen and the fibrinolytic system in patients treated with recombinant tissue plasminogen activator and streptokinase. J Am Coll Cardiol 11:1–11, 1988.

265. Grayburn P, Willard J, Brincker M, et al: In vivo thrombus formation on a guidewire during intravascular ultrasound imaging: Evidence for inadequate heparinization. Cathet Cardiovasc Diagn 23:141–143, 1991.

266. Laskey MA, Deutsch E, Barnathan E, et al: Influence of heparin therapy on percutaneous transluminal coronary angioplasty outcome in unstable angina pectoris. Am J Cardiol 65:1425–1429, 1990.

267. The CAPTURE Investigators: Randomised placebo-controlled trial of abciximab before and during coronary intervention in refractory unstable angina: The CAPTURE Study. Lancet 349:1429–1435, 1997.

268. The PRISM-PLUS Investigators: Inhibition of the platelet glycoprotein IIb/IIIa receptor with tirofiban in unstable angina and non-Q-wave myocardial infarction. Platelet Receptor Inhibition in Ischemic Syndrome Management in Patients Limited by Unstable Signs and Symptoms (PRISM-PLUS) Study Investigators. N Engl J Med 338:1488–1497, 1998.

269. The PURSUIT Investigators: Inhibition of platelet glycoprotein IIb/IIIa with eptifibatide in patients with acute coronary syndromes. Platelet glycoprotein IIb/IIIa in unstable angina: Receptor suppression using integrilin therapy. N Engl J Med 339:436–443, 1998.

270. Dougherty K, Gaos C, Bush H, et al: Activated clotting times and activated partial thromboplastin times in patients undergoing coronary angioplasty who receive bolus doses of heparin. Cathet Cardiovasc Diagn 26:260–263, 1992.

271. Bowers J, Ferguson J: The use of activated clotting times to monitor heparin therapy during and after interventional procedures. Clin Cardiol 17:357–361, 1994.

272. Marmur J, Merlini P, Sharma S, et al: Thrombin generation in human coronary arteries after percutaneous transluminal balloon angioplasty. J Am Coll Cardiol 24:1484–1491, 1994.

273. Marmur J, Sharma S, Kantrowitz N, et al: Angiographically complex lesions are associated with increased levels of thrombin generation and activity following PTCA (abstract). J Am Coll Cardiol 25:155, 1995.

274. Hillegass W, Narins C, Brott B, et al: Activated clotting time predicts bleeding complications from angioplasty (abstract). J Am Coll Cardiol 23:184, 1994.

275. Koch KT, Piek JJ, de Winter RJ, et al: Early ambulation after coronary angioplasty and stenting with six French guiding catheters and low-dose heparin. Am J Cardiol 80:1084–1086, 1997.

276. Boccara A, Benamer H, Juliard J, et al: A randomized trial of a fixed high dose versus a low weight adjusted low dose of intravenous heparin during coronary angioplasty. Eur Heart J 18:631–635, 1997.

277. Fail PS, Maniet AR, Banka VS: Subcutaneous heparin in postangioplasty management: Comparative trial with intravenous heparin. Am Heart J 126:1059–1067, 1993.

278. Popma JJ, Weitz J, Bittl JA, et al: Antithrombotic therapy in patients undergoing coronary angioplasty. Chest 114(Suppl):728–741, 1998.

279. Ellis S, Roubin G, Wilentz J, et al: Effect of 18- to 24-hour heparin administration for prevention of restenosis after uncomplicated coronary angioplasty. Am Heart J 117:777–782, 1989.

280. Friedman HZ, Cragg DR, Glazier SM, et al: Randomized prospective evaluation of prolonged versus abbreviated intravenous heparin therapy after coronary angioplasty. J Am Coll Cardiol 24:1214–1219, 1994.

281. Cohen M, Demers C, Gurfinkel E, et al: A comparison of low-molecular-weight heparin with unfractionated heparin for unstable coronary artery disease. Efficacy and Safety of Enoxaparin in Non-Q-Wave Coronary Events Study Group. N Engl J Med 337:447–452, 1997.

282. Grines C: Anticoagulation requirements for coronary interventions and the role of low molecular weight heparins. J Invas Cardiol 11:7A–12A, 1999.

283. Serruys PW, Herrman JP, Simon R, et al: A comparison of hirudin with heparin in the prevention of restenosis after coronary angioplasty. Helvetica Investigators. N Engl J Med 333:757–763, 1995.

284. Bittl JA, Strony J, Brinker JA, et al: Treatment with bivalirudin (Hirulog) as compared with heparin during coronary angioplasty for unstable or postinfarction angina. Hirulog Angioplasty Study Investigators. N Engl J Med 333:764–769, 1995.

PHARMACOLOGICAL APPROACHES TO RESTENOSIS

285. Kimura T, Kaburagi S, Tamura T, et al: Remodeling of human coronary arteries undergoing coronary angioplasty or atherectomy. Circulation 96:475–483, 1997.

286. Mintz GS, Popma JJ, Pichard AD, et al: Intravascular ultrasound predictors of restenosis after percutaneous transcatheter coronary revascularization. J Am Coll Cardiol 27:1678–1687, 1996.

287. Lefkovits J, Topol EJ: Pharmacological approaches for the prevention of restenosis after percutaneous coronary intervention. Prog Cardiovasc Dis 40:141–158, 1997.

288. Thornton M, Gruentzig A, Hollman J, et al: Coumadin and aspirin in prevention of recurrence after transluminal coronary angioplasty: A randomized study. Circulation 69:721–727, 1984.

289. Taylor R, Gibbons F, Cope G, et al: Effects of low-dose aspirin on restenosis after coronary angioplasty. Am J Cardiol 68:874–878, 1991.

290. Schwartz L, Lesperance J, Bourassa MG, et al: The role of antiplatelet agents in modifying the extent of restenosis following percutaneous transluminal coronary angioplasty. Am Heart J 119:232–236, 1990.

291. Serruys PW, Rutsch W, Heyndrickx GR, et al: Prevention of restenosis after percutaneous transluminal coronary angioplasty with thromboxane A2-receptor blockade. A randomized, double-blind, placebo-controlled trial. Coronary Artery Restenosis Prevention on Repeated Thromboxane-Antagonism Study (CARPORT). Circulation 84:1568–1580, 1991.

292. Savage M, Goldberg S, Macdonald R, et al: Multi-hospital Eastern Atlantic restenosis trial II: A placebo-controlled trial of thromboxane blockade in the prevention of restenosis following coronary angioplasty. Am Heart J 122:1239–1244, 1991.

293. Serruys PW, Klein W, Tijssen JP, et al: Evaluation of ketanserin in the prevention of restenosis after percutaneous transluminal coronary angioplasty. A multicenter randomized double-blind placebo-controlled trial. Circulation 88:1588–1601, 1993.

294. Knudtson ML, Flintoft VF, Roth DL, et al: Effect of short-term prostacyclin administration on restenosis after percutaneous transluminal coronary angioplasty. J Am Coll Cardiol 15:691–697, 1990.

295. Raizner A, Hollman J, Abukhalil J, et al: Ciprostene for restenosis revisited: Quantitative analysis of angiograms (abstract). J Am Coll Cardiol 21:321, 1993.

296. Topol EJ, Califf RM, Weisman HF, et al: Randomised trial of coronary intervention with antibody against platelet IIb/IIIa integrin for reduction of clinical restenosis: Results at six months. The EPIC Investigators. Lancet 343:881–886, 1994.

297. Marso SP, Linloff AM, Ellis SG, et al: Optimizing the percutaneous interventional outcomes for patients with diabetes mellitus. Results of the EPISTENT (Evaluation of Platelet IIb/IIIa Inhibitor for Stenting Trial) diabetic substudy. Circulation 100:2477, 1999.

298. Brack MJ, Ray S, Chauhan A, et al: The Subcutaneous Heparin and Angioplasty Restenosis Prevention (SHARP) trial. Results of a multicenter randomized trial investigating the effects of high dose unfractionated heparin on angiographic restenosis and clinical outcome. J Am Coll Cardiol 26:947–954, 1995.

299. Faxon DP, Spiro TE, Minor S, et al: Low molecular weight heparin in prevention of restenosis after angioplasty. Results of Enoxaparin Restenosis (ERA) Trial. Circulation 90:908–914, 1994.

300. Karsch KR, Preisack MB, Baildon R, et al: Low molecular weight heparin (reviparin) in percutaneous transluminal coronary angioplasty. Results of a randomized, double-blind, unfractionated heparin and placebo-controlled, multicenter trial (REDUCE trial). Reduction of restenosis after PTCA, early administration of reviparin in a double-blind unfractionated heparin and placebo-controlled evaluation. J Am Coll Cardiol 28:1437–1443, 1996.

301. Lablanche JM, McFadden EP, Meneveau N, et al: Effect of nadroparin, a low-molecular-weight heparin, on clinical and angiographic restenosis after coronary balloon angioplasty: The FACT study. Fraxiparine Angioplastie Coronaire Transluminale. Circulation 96:3396–3402, 1997.

302. Burchenal JE, Marks DS, Tift Mann J, et al: Effect of direct thrombin inhibition with bivalirudin (Hirulog) on restenosis after coronary angioplasty. Am J Cardiol 82:511–515, 1998.

303. Urban P, Buller N, Fox K, et al: Lack of effect of warfarin on the restenosis rate or on clinical outcome after balloon coronary angioplasty. Br Heart J 60:485–488, 1988.

304. O'Keefe JH Jr, Giorgi LV, Hartzler GO, et al: Effects of diltiazem on complications and restenosis after coronary angioplasty. Am J Cardiol 67:373–376, 1991.

305. Lablanche JM, Grollier G, Lusson JR, et al: Effect of the direct nitric oxide donors linsidomine and molsidomine on angiographic restenosis after coronary balloon angioplasty. The ACCORD Study. Angioplastic Coronaire Corvasal Diltiazem. Circulation 95:83–89, 1997.

306. The MERCATOR Investigators: Does the new angiotensin converting enzyme inhibitor cilazapril prevent restenosis after percutaneous transluminal coronary angioplasty? Results of the MERCATOR study: A multicenter, randomized, double-blind placebo-controlled trial. Multicenter European Research Trial with Cilazapril after Angioplasty to Prevent Transluminal Coronary Obstruction and Restenosis (MERCATOR) Study Group. Circulation 86:100–110, 1992.

307. Faxon DP: Effect of high dose angiotensin-converting enzyme inhibition on restenosis: Final results of the MARCATOR Study, a multicenter, double-blind, placebo-controlled trial of cilazapril. The Multicenter American Research Trial with Cilazapril after Angioplasty to Prevent

Transluminal Coronary Obstruction and Restenosis (MARCATOR) Study Group. J Am Coll Cardiol 25:362–369, 1995.

308. Desmet W, Vrolix M, De Scheerder I, et al: Angiotensin-converting enzyme inhibition with fosinopril sodium in the prevention of restenosis after coronary angioplasty. Circulation 89:385–392, 1994.

309. Ellis S, Whitlow P, Franco I, et al: Angiotensin converting enzyme inhibitors may reduce neorevascularization after coronary stenting (abstract). Circulation 100(Suppl 1):468, 1999.

310. Emanuelsson H, Beatt KJ, Bagger JP, et al: Long-term effects of angiopeptin treatment in coronary angioplasty. Reduction of clinical events but not angiographic restenosis. European Angiopeptin Study Group. Circulation 91:1689–1696, 1995.

311. Kent K, Williams D, Cassagneua B, et al: Double blind, controlled trial of the effect of angiopeptin on coronary restenosis following balloon angioplasty (abstract). Circulation 88(Suppl 1):506, 1993.

312. Maresta A, Balducelli M, Cantini L, et al: Trapidil (triazolopyrimidine), a platelet-derived growth factor antagonist, reduces restenosis after percutaneous transluminal coronary angioplasty. Results of the randomized, double-blind STARC study. Studio Trapidil versus Aspirin nella Restenosi Coronarica. Circulation 90:2710–2715, 1994.

313. Yokoi H, Daida H, Kuwabara Y, et al: Effectiveness of an antioxidant in preventing restenosis after percutaneous transluminal coronary angioplasty: The Probucol Angioplasty Restenosis Trial. J Am Coll Cardiol 30:855–862, 1997.

314. Tardif JC, Cote G, Lesperance J, et al: Probucol and multivitamins in the prevention of restenosis after coronary angioplasty. Multivitamins and Probucol Study Group. N Engl J Med 337:365–372, 1997.

315. Kosuga K, Tamai H, Ueda K, et al: Effectiveness of tranilast on restenosis after directional coronary atherectomy. Am Heart J 134:712–718, 1997.

316. Pepine CJ, Hirshfeld JW, Macdonald RG, et al: A controlled trial of corticosteroids to prevent restenosis after coronary angioplasty. M-HEART Group. Circulation 81:1753–1761, 1990.

317. O'Keefe JH Jr, McCallister BD, Bateman TM, et al: Ineffectiveness of colchicine for the prevention of restenosis after coronary angioplasty. J Am Coll Cardiol 19:1597–1600, 1992.

318. Boccuzzi SJ, Weintraub WS, Kosinski AS, et al: Aggressive lipid lowering in postcoronary angioplasty patients with elevated cholesterol (the Lovastatin Restenosis Trial). Am J Cardiol 81:632–636, 1998.

319. Weintraub WS, Boccuzzi SJ, Klein JL, et al: Lack of effect of lovastatin on restenosis after coronary angioplasty. Lovastatin Restenosis Trial Study Group. N Engl J Med 331:1331–1337, 1994.

320. Bertrand ME, McFadden EP, Fruchart JC, et al: Effect of pravastatin on angiographic restenosis after coronary balloon angioplasty. The PREDICT Trial Investigators. Prevention of Restenosis by Elisor after Transluminal Coronary Angioplasty. J Am Coll Cardiol 30:863–869, 1997.

321. Foley DP, Serruys PW: Fluvastatin for the prevention of restenosis after coronary balloon angioplasty: Angiographic and methodological background of the fluvastatin angioplasty restenosis trial. Br J Clin Pract Suppl 1996:40–53, 1996.

322. Lewis SJ, Sacks FM, Mitchell JS, et al: Effect of pravastatin on cardiovascular events in women after myocardial infarction: The cholesterol and recurrent events (CARE) trial. J Am Coll Cardiol 32:140–146, 1998.

323. Weintraub WS, Pederson JP: Atherosclerosis and restenosis: Reflections on the Lovastatin Restenosis Trial and Scandinavian Simvastatin Survival Study (editorial). Am J Cardiol 78:1036–1038, 1996.

324. Daida H, Lee YJ, Yokoi H, et al: Prevention of restenosis after percutaneous transluminal coronary angioplasty by reducing lipoprotein (a) levels with low-density lipoprotein apheresis. Low-Density Lipoprotein Apheresis Angioplasty Restenosis Trial (L-ART) Group. Am J Cardiol 73:1037–1040, 1994.

325. Gapinski JP, Van Ruiswyk JV, Heudebert GR, et al: Preventing restenosis with fish oils following coronary angioplasty. A meta-analysis. Arch Intern Med 153:1595–1601, 1993.

326. Grigg L, Kay T, Valentine P, et al: Determinants of restenosis and lack of effect of dietary supplementation with eicosapentaenoic acid on the incidence of coronary artery restenosis after angioplasty. J Am Coll Cardiol 13:665–672, 1989.

327. Reis G, Sipperly M, McCabe C, et al: Randomised trial of fish oil for prevention of restenosis after coronary angioplasty. Lancet 2:177–181, 1989.

328. Leaf A, Jorgensen MB, Jacobs AK, et al: Do fish oils prevent restenosis after coronary angioplasty? Circulation 90:2248–2257, 1994.

329. Cairns JA, Gill J, Morton B, et al: Fish oils and low-molecular-weight heparin for the reduction of restenosis after percutaneous transluminal coronary angioplasty. The EMPAR Study. Circulation 94:1553–1560, 1996.

330. Dehmer G, Popma J, van den Berg E, et al: Reduction in the rate of early restenosis after coronary angioplasty by a diet supplemented with n-3 fatty acids. N Engl J Med 319:733–740, 1988.

331. Bairati I, Roy L, Meyer F: Double-blind, randomized, controlled trial of fish oil supplements in prevention of recurrence of stenosis after coronary angioplasty. Circulation 85:950–956, 1992.

332. Milner M, Gallino R, Leffingwell A, et al: Usefulness of fish oil supplements in preventing clinical evidence of restenosis after percutaneous transluminal coronary angioplasty. Am J Cardiol 64:294–299, 1989.

333. Powell JS, Muller RK, Baumgartner HR: Suppression of the vascular response to injury: The role of angiotensin-converting enzyme inhibitors. J Am Coll Cardiol 17:137B–142B, 1991.

334. Carter AJ, Laird JR, Bailey LR, et al: Effects of endovascular radiation from a beta-particle–emitting stent in a porcine coronary restenosis model. A dose-response study. Circulation 94:2364–2368, 1996.

335. Waksman R, Robinson KA, Crocker IR, et al: Intracoronary low-dose beta-irradiation inhibits neointima formation after coronary artery balloon injury in the swine restenosis model. Circulation 92:3025–3031, 1995.

336. Waksman R, Robinson KA, Crocker IR, et al: Endovascular low-dose irradiation inhibits neointima formation after coronary artery balloon injury in swine. A possible role for radiation therapy in restenosis prevention. Circulation 91:1533–1539, 1995.

337. Waksman R, Robinson KA, Crocker IR, et al: Intracoronary radiation before stent implantation inhibits neointima formation in stented porcine coronary arteries. Circulation 92:1383–1386, 1995.

338. Condado JA, Waksman R, Gurdiel O, et al: Long-term angiographic and clinical outcome after percutaneous transluminal coronary angioplasty and intracoronary radiation therapy in humans. Circulation 96:727–732, 1997.

339. King SB, Williams DO, Chougule P, et al: Endovascular beta-radiation to reduce restenosis after coronary balloon angioplasty: Results of the beta energy restenosis trial (BERT). Circulation 97:2025–2030, 1998.

340. Condado JA: Basis of endovascular radiation therapy in human coronary arteries. Semin Interv Cardiol 2:115–118, 1997.

341. Jani SK, Massullo V, Steuterman S, et al: Physics and safety aspects of a coronary irradiation pilot study to inhibit restenosis using manually loaded ¹⁹²Ir ribbons. Semin Interv Cardiol 2:119–123, 1997.

342. Williams DO: Radiation vascular therapy: A novel approach to preventing restenosis. Am J Cardiol 81:18E–20E, 1998.

MEDICAL THERAPY OR CORONARY REVASCULARIZATION

343. The FRISC-II Investigators: Invasive compared with non-invasive treatment in unstable coronary artery disease: FRISC II prospective randomised multicentre study. Lancet 354:708–715, 1999.

344. Lansky AJ, Popma JJ, Mintz GS, et al: Lipid-lowering therapy after coronary revascularization: The interventional cardiologist's perspective. Am J Cardiol 81:55E–62E, 1998.

345. Eagle K, Guyton R, Davidoff R, et al: American College of Cardiology/American Heart Association Guidelines for Coronary Artery Bypass Surgery. J Am Coll Cardiol 34:1262–1347, 1999.

346. Anderson H, Cannon C, Stone P, et al: One year results of the Thrombolysis in Myocardial Infarction (TIMI) IIIB clinical trial: A randomized comparison of tissue-type plasminogen activator versus placebo and early invasive versus early conservative strategies in unstable angina and non-Q-wave myocardial infarction. J Am Coll Cardiol 26:1643–1650, 1995.

347. Boden WE, O'Rourke RA, Crawford MH, et al: Outcomes in patients with acute non-Q-wave myocardial infarction randomly assigned to an invasive as compared with a conservative management strategy. Veterans Affairs Non-Q-Wave Infarction Strategies in Hospital (VANQWISH) Trial Investigators. N Engl J Med 338:1785–1792, 1998.

348. Scanlon P, Faxon D, Audet A, et al: American College of Cardiology/American Heart Association guidelines for coronary angiography. J Am Coll Cardiol 33:1756–1824, 1999.

349. Madsen JK, Grande P, Saunamaki K, et al: Danish multicenter randomized study of invasive versus conservative treatment in patients with inducible ischemia after thrombolysis in acute myocardial infarction (DANAMI). DANish trial in Acute Myocardial Infarction. Circulation 96:748–755, 1997.

350. Parisi A, Folland E, Hartigan P: A comparison of angioplasty with medical therapy in the treatment of single-vessel coronary artery disease. Veterans Affairs ACME Investigators. N Engl J Med 326:10–16, 1992.

351. Folland E, Hartigan P, Parisi A: Percutaneous transluminal coronary angioplasty versus medical therapy for stable angina pectoris: Outcomes for patients with double-vessel versus single vessel coronary artery disease in a Veterans Affairs Cooperative randomized trial. J Am Coll Cardiol 1997:1505–1511, 1997.

352. Pitt B, Waters D, Brown W: Aggressive lipid lowering compared with angioplasty in stable coronary artery disease. N Engl J Med 341:70–76, 1999.

353. The RITA-2 Investigators: Coronary angioplasty versus medical therapy: The second Randomised Intervention Treatment of Angina (RITA-2) trial. Lancet 350:461–468, 1997.

354. Davies R, Goldberg A, Forman S: Asymptomatic Cardiac Ischemia Pilot (ACIP) study two-year follow-up: Outcomes of patients randomized to initial strategies of medical therapy versus revascularization. Circulation 95:2037–2043, 1997.

355. Solomon AJ, Gersh BJ: Management of chronic stable angina: Medical therapy, percutaneous transluminal coronary angioplasty, and coronary artery bypass graft surgery. Lessons from the randomized trials. Ann Intern Med 128:216–223, 1998.

356. Pocock S, Henderson R, Rickards A, et al: Meta-analysis of randomized trials comparing coronary angioplasty with bypass surgery. Lancet 346:1184–1189, 1995.

357. King SB, Barnhart HX, Kosinski AS, et al: Angioplasty or surgery for multivessel coronary artery disease: Comparison of eligible registry and randomized patients in the EAST trial and influence of treatment selec-

tion on outcomes. Emory Angioplasty Versus Surgery Trial Investigators. Am J Cardiol 79:1453–1459, 1997.

358. Henderson RA, Pocock SJ, Sharp SJ, et al: Long-term results of RITA-1 trial: Clinical and cost comparisons of coronary angioplasty and coronary-artery bypass grafting. Randomised Intervention Treatment of Angina. Lancet 352:1419–1425, 1998.

359. Rodriquez A, Boullon F, Perez-Balino N, et al: Argentine randomized trial of percutaneous transluminal coronary angioplasty versus coronary artery bypass surgery in multivessel disease (ERACI): In-hospital results and 1-year follow-up. J Am Coll Cardiol 22:1060–1067, 1993.

360. Rodriguez A, Mele E, Peyregne E, et al: Three-year follow-up of the Argentine Randomized Trial of Percutaneous Transluminal Coronary Angioplasty Versus Coronary Artery Bypass Surgery in Multivessel Disease (ERACI). J Am Coll Cardiol 27:1178–1184, 1996.

361. Kurbaan AS, Bowker TJ, Ilsley CD, et al: Impact of postangioplasty restenosis on comparisons of outcome between angioplasty and bypass grafting. Coronary Angioplasty Versus Bypass Revascularisation Investigation (CABRI) Investigators. Am J Cardiol 82:272–276, 1998.

362. Hamm CW, Reimers J, Ischinger T, et al: A randomized study of coronary angioplasty compared with bypass surgery in patients with symptomatic multivessel coronary disease. N Engl J Med 331:1037–1043, 1994.

363. Serruys P, Costa M, Betriu A, et al: The influence of diabetes mellitus in clinical outcome following multivessel stenting or CABG in the ARTS Trial (abstract). Circulation 100(Suppl 1):364, 1999.

TRAINING STANDARDS AND PROFICIENCY

364. Pepine C, Babb J, Brinker J, et al: Training in cardiac catheterization and interventional cardiology. J Am Coll Cardiol 25:1–34, 1995.

365. Committee Members: Society for Cardiac Angiography and Interventions Committee on Training Standards: Core curriculum for adult and pediatric invasive training programs. Cathet Cardiovasc Diagn 37:1–34, 1996.

366. Hirshfeld J, Banas J, Cowley M, et al: American College of Cardiology training statement on recommendations for the structure of an optimal adult interventional cardiology training program. J Am Coll Cardiol, in press.

367. American College of Physicians: Ethics manual. Fourth edition. Ann Intern Med 128:576–594, 1998.

368. Alpert J: Guidelines for Training in Adult Cardiovascular Medicine. Core Cardiology Training Symposium (COCATS). J Am Coll Cardiol 25:1–34, 1995.

369. Ellis SG, Weintraub W, Holmes D, et al: Relation of operator volume and experience to procedural outcome of percutaneous coronary revascularization at hospitals with high interventional volumes. Circulation 95:2479–2484, 1997.

370. Hannan E, Racz M, Ryan T: Coronary angioplasty volume-outcome relationships for hospitals and cardiologists. JAMA 19:892–898, 1997.

371. Shook TL, Sun GW, Burstein S, et al: Comparison of percutaneous transluminal coronary angioplasty outcome and hospital costs for low-volume and high-volume operators. Am J Cardiol 77:331–336, 1996.

372. Kimmel S, Berlin J, Laskey W: The relationship between coronary angioplasty procedure volume and major complications. JAMA 274:1137–1142, 1995.

373. Jollis J, Peterson E, Nelson C: Relationship between physician and hospital coronary angioplasty volume and outcome in elderly patients. Circulation 95:2485–2491, 1997.

374. Hartz A, Kuhn E, Kayser K, et al: Assessing providers of coronary revascularization: A method for peer review organization. Am J Public Health 82:1631–1640, 1992.

375. Ritchie JL, Phillips KA, Luft HS: Coronary angioplasty. Statewide experience in California. Circulation 88:2735–2743, 1993.

376. O'Neill W, Griffin J, Stone G, et al: Operator and institutional volume do not affect procedural outcome of primary angioplasty therapy (abstract). J Am Coll Cardiol 27:13, 1996.

377. Tiefenbrunn AJ, Chandra NC, French WJ, et al: Clinical experience with primary percutaneous transluminal coronary angioplasty compared with alteplase (recombinant tissue-type plasminogen activator) in patients with acute myocardial infarction: A report from the Second National Registry of Myocardial Infarction (NRMI-2). J Am Coll Cardiol 31:1240–1245, 1998.

378. Zahn R, Koch A, Rustige J, et al: Primary angioplasty versus thrombolysis in the treatment of acute myocardial infarction. ALKK Study Group. Am J Cardiol 79:264–269, 1997.

379. Hamad N, Pichard A, Lyle H, et al: A serial trial results of percutaneous transluminal coronary angioplasty by multiple, relatively low frequency operators: 1986–1987 experience. Am J Cardiol 77:1229–1231, 1988.

380. Krone R, Vetrovec G, Noto T, et al: Relation of low, moderate, high volume PTCA operations and outcomes (abstract). Circulation 88(Suppl 1):300, 1993.

381. Bon Tempo C, Sherber H, Sheridan M: Relation of low, moderate, high volume PTCA operations and outcomes (abstract). Cathet Cardiovasc Diagn 35:79, 1995.

382. McGrath P, Wennberg DE, Malenka DJ, et al: Operator volumes and outcomes in 12,988 percutaneous coronary interventions. J Am Coll Cardiol 31:570–576, 1998.

383. Klein LW, Schaer GL, Calvin JE, et al: Does low individual operator

384. Weintraub WS, McKay CR, Riner RN, et al: The American College of Cardiology National Database: Progress and challenges. American College of Cardiology Database Committee. J Am Coll Cardiol 29:459–465, 1997.

coronary interventional procedural volume correlate with worse institutional procedural outcome? J Am Coll Cardiol 30:870–877, 1997.

MITRAL VALVULOPLASTY

385. Vahanian A: Valvuloplasty. In Topol E (ed): Textbook of Cardiovascular Medicine. Philadelphia, Lippincott-Raven, 1998, pp 2155–2175.

386. Cribier A, Savin T, Saoudi N, et al: Percutaneous transluminal valvuloplasty of acquired aortic stenosis in elderly patients: An alternative to valve replacement? Lancet 11:63–76, 1986.

387. Inoue K, Owaki T, Nakamura T, et al: Clinical application of transvenous mitral commissurotomy by a new balloon catheter. J Thorac Cardiovasc Surg 87:394–402, 1984.

388. Carroll J, Feldman T: Percutaneous mitral balloon valvotomy and the new demographics of mitral stenosis. JAMA 270:1731–1736, 1993.

389. Chen CR, Cheng TO, Chen JY, et al: Long-term results of percutaneous balloon mitral valvuloplasty for mitral stenosis: A follow-up study to 11 years in 202 patients. Cathet Cardiovasc Diagn 43:132–139, 1998.

390. Glazier JJ, Turi ZG: Percutaneous balloon mitral valvuloplasty. Prog Cardiovasc Dis 40:5–26, 1997.

391. Abdullah M, Halim M, Rajendran V, et al: Comparison between single (Inoue) and double balloon mitral valvuloplasty: Immediate and short-term results. Am Heart J 123:1581–1588, 1992.

392. Cohen DJ, Kuntz RE, Gordon SP, et al: Predictors of long-term outcome after percutaneous balloon mitral valvuloplasty. N Engl J Med 327:1329–1335, 1992.

393. The National Heart, Lung, and Blood Institute (NHLBI) Valvuloplasty Registry Participants. Multicenter experience with balloon mitral commissurotomy: NHLBI balloon valvuloplasty registry report on immediate and 30-day follow-up results. Circulation 85:448–461, 1992.

394. Babic U, Dorros G, Pejcic P, et al: Percutaneous mitral valvuloplasty: Retrograde, transarterial double-balloon technique utilizing the transseptal approach. Cathet Cardiovasc Diagn 14:229–237, 1988.

395. Stefanidis C, Toutoutzas P: Retrograde non transseptal mitral valvuloplasty. In Topol E (ed): Textbook of Interventional Cardiology. Philadelphia, WB Saunders, 1994, p 1253.

396. Bahl VK, Juneja R, Thatai D, et al: Retrograde nontransseptal balloon mitral valvuloplasty for rheumatic mitral stenosis. Cathet Cardiovasc Diagn 33:331–334, 1994.

397. Bahl VK, Thatai D, Stefanadis C, et al: Retrograde non-transseptal balloon mitral valvuloplasty—an initial experience. Indian Heart J 45:459–462, 1993.

398. Lau KW, Hung JS, Ding ZP, et al: Controversies in balloon mitral valvuloplasty: The when (timing for intervention), what (choice of valve), and how (selection of technique). Cathet Cardiovasc Diagn 35:91–100, 1995.

399. Chen CR, Cheng TO, Chen JY, et al: Percutaneous balloon mitral valvuloplasty for mitral stenosis with and without associated aortic regurgitation. Am Heart J 125:128–137, 1993.

400. Cheng TO, Holmes DR Jr: Percutaneous balloon mitral valvuloplasty by the Inoue balloon technique: The procedure of choice for treatment of mitral stenosis. Am J Cardiol 81:624–628, 1998.

401. Manga P, Landless P, Gebka M: Comparative results of percutaneous balloon mitral valvuloplasty using the Trefoil/Bifoil and Inoue balloon techniques. Int J Cardiol 43:21–25, 1994.

402. Alfonso F, Hernandez R, Banuelos C, et al: Percutaneous mitral valvuloplasty with the Inoue technique in a patient with heavily calcified interatrial septum. Cathet Cardiovasc Diagn 39:82–84, 1996.

403. Benit E, Rocha P, de Geest H, et al: Successful mitral valvuloplasty using the Inoue balloon in a patient with mitral stenosis associated with subvalvular fibrosis and reduced left ventricular inflow cavity: A case report. Cathet Cardiovasc Diagn 22:35–38, 1991.

404. Applebaum RM, Kasliwal RR, Kanojia A, et al: Utility of three-dimensional echocardiography during balloon mitral valvuloplasty. J Am Coll Cardiol 32:1405–1409, 1998.

405. Arora R, Jolly N, Kalra GS, et al: Atrial septal defect after balloon mitral valvuloplasty: A transesophageal echocardiographic study. Angiology 44:217–221, 1993.

406. Arora R, Jolly N, Kalra GS, et al: Role of transesophageal echocardiography during balloon mitral valvuloplasty. Indian Heart J 44:391–394, 1992.

407. Jaarsma W, Visser CA, Suttorp MJ, et al: Transesophageal echocardiography during percutaneous balloon mitral valvuloplasty. J Am Soc Echocardiogr 3:384–391, 1990.

408. Goldstein SA, Campbell AN: Mitral stenosis. Evaluation and guidance of valvuloplasty by transesophageal echocardiography. Cardiol Clin 11:409–425, 1993.

409. Butany J, D'Amati G, Charlesworth D, et al: Fatal left ventricular perforation following balloon mitral valvuloplasty. Can J Cardiol 6:343–347, 1990.

410. Manga P, Singh S, Brandis S: Left ventricular perforation during percutaneous balloon mitral valvuloplasty. Cathet Cardiovasc Diagn 25:317–319, 1992.

411. Joseph G, Chandy ST, Krishnaswami S, et al: Mechanisms of cardiac

perforation leading to tamponade in balloon mitral valvuloplasty. Cathet Cardiovasc Diagn 42:138–146, 1997.

412. Demirtas M, Usal A, Birand A, et al: A serious complication of percutaneous mitral valvuloplasty: Systemic embolism. How can we decrease it? Case history. Angiology 47:285–289, 1996.

413. Nigri A, Alessandri N, Martuscelli E, et al: Clinical significance of small left-to-right shunts after percutaneous mitral valvuloplasty. Am Heart J 125:783–786, 1993.

414. Normandin L, Carrier M, Leclerc Y, et al: Cardiac surgery after failed percutaneous mitral valvuloplasty. Can J Surg 35:155–157, 1992.

415. Wilkins G, Gillam L, Weyman A, et al: Percutaneous balloon dilatation of the mitral valve: An analysis of echocardiographic variables related to outcome and the mechanism of dilatation. Br Heart J 60:299–308, 1988.

416. Eisenberg MJ, Ballal R, Heidenreich PA, et al: Echocardiographic score as a predictor of in-hospital cost in patients undergoing percutaneous balloon mitral valvuloplasty. Am J Cardiol 78:790–794, 1996.

AORTIC VALVULOPLASTY

417. Davidson CJ, Harrison JK, Leithe ME, et al: Failure of balloon aortic valvuloplasty to result in sustained clinical improvement in patients with depressed left ventricular function. Am J Cardiol 65:72–77, 1990.

418. Lieberman EB, Bashore TM, Hermiller JB, et al: Balloon aortic valvuloplasty in adults: Failure of procedure to improve long-term survival. J Am Coll Cardiol 26:1522–1528, 1995.

419. Otto CM, Mickel MC, Kennedy JW, et al: Three-year outcome after balloon aortic valvuloplasty. Insights into prognosis of valvular aortic stenosis. Circulation 89:642–650, 1994.

420. Safian RD, Kuntz RE, Berman AD: Aortic valvuloplasty. Cardiol Clin 9:289–299, 1991.

421. Wang A, Harrison JK, Bashore TM: Balloon aortic valvuloplasty. Prog Cardiovasc Dis 40:27–36, 1997.

422. Alcaino ME, Smith R, Allan RM, et al: Percutaneous aortic valvuloplasty. Med J Aust 156:88–90, 1992.

423. Elliott JM, Tuzcu EM: Recent developments in balloon valvuloplasty techniques. Curr Opin Cardiol 10:128–134, 1995.

424. Eltchaninoff H, Cribier A, Tron C, et al: Balloon aortic valvuloplasty in elderly patients at high risk for surgery, or inoperable. Immediate and mid-term results. Eur Heart J 16:1079–1084, 1995.

425. Bhatia A, Kumar A, Seth A, et al: Successful aortic balloon valvuloplasty in critical aortic stenosis with shock. Cathet Cardiovasc Diagn 29:296–297, 1993.

426. Lieberman EB, Wilson JS, Harrison JK, et al: Aortic valve replacement in adults after balloon aortic valvuloplasty. Circulation 90(Suppl 2):205–208, 1994.

427. Moreno PR, Jang IK, Newell JB, et al: The role of percutaneous aortic balloon valvuloplasty in patients with cardiogenic shock and critical aortic stenosis. J Am Coll Cardiol 23:1071–1075, 1994.

428. Smedira NG, Ports TA, Merrick SH, et al: Balloon aortic valvuloplasty as a bridge to aortic valve replacement in critically ill patients. Ann Thorac Surg 55:914–916, 1993.

429. Blitz LR, Herrmann HC: Hemodynamic assessment of patients with low-flow, low-gradient valvular aortic stenosis. Am J Cardiol 78:657–661, 1996.

430. Nishimura RA, Holmes DR, Michela MA: Follow-up of patients with low output, low gradient hemodynamics after percutaneous balloon aortic valvuloplasty: The Mansfield Scientific Aortic Valvuloplasty Registry. J Am Coll Cardiol 1:828–833, 1991.

431. Bernard Y, Etievent J, Mourand JL, et al: Long-term results of percutaneous aortic valvuloplasty compared with aortic valve replacement in patients more than 75 years old. J Am Coll Cardiol 20:796–801, 1992.

432. Dorros G, Lewin RF, Stertzer SH, et al: Percutaneous transluminal aortic valvuloplasty—the acute outcome and follow-up of 149 patients who underwent the double balloon technique. Eur Heart J 11:429–440, 1990.

433. Kastrup J, Wennevold A, Thuesen L, et al: Short- and long-term survival after aortic balloon valvuloplasty for calcified aortic stenosis in 137 elderly patients. Dan Med Bull 41:362–365, 1994.

434. The Percutaneous Balloon Aortic Valvuloplasty Investigators: Acute and 30-day follow-up results in 674 patients from the NHLBI Balloon Valvuloplasty Registry. Circulation 84:2383–2397, 1991.

435. Holmes DR, Nishimura RA, Reeder GS: In-hospital mortality after balloon aortic valvuloplasty: Frequency and associated factors. J Am Coll Cardiol 17:189–192, 1991.

436. McKay RG: The Mansfield Scientific Aortic Valvuloplasty Registry: Overview of acute hemodynamic results and procedural complications. J Am Coll Cardiol 17:485–491, 1991.

437. Isner JM: Acute catastrophic complications of balloon aortic valvuloplasty. The Mansfield Scientific Aortic Valvuloplasty Registry Investigators. J Am Coll Cardiol 17:1436–1444, 1991.

438. O'Neill WW: Predictors of long-term survival after percutaneous aortic valvuloplasty: Report of the Mansfield Scientific Balloon Aortic Valvuloplasty Registry. J Am Coll Cardiol 17:193–198, 1991.

439. Davidson CJ, Harrison JK, Pieper KS, et al: Determinants of one-year outcome from balloon aortic valvuloplasty. Am J Cardiol 68:75–80, 1991.

440. Legrand V, Beckers J, Fastrez M, et al: Long-term follow-up of elderly patients with severe aortic stenosis treated by balloon aortic valvuloplasty. Importance of haemodynamic parameters before and after dilatation. Eur Heart J 12:451–457, 1991.

441. Bashore TM, Davidson CJ: Follow-up recatheterization after balloon aortic valvuloplasty. Mansfield Scientific Aortic Valvuloplasty Registry Investigators. J Am Coll Cardiol 17:1188–1195, 1991.

442. Feldman T, Glagov S, Carroll JD: Restenosis following successful balloon valvuloplasty: Bone formation in aortic valve leaflets. Cathet Cardiovasc Diagn 29:1–7, 1993.

443. Kale PA, Sathe SV, Rajani RM, et al: Long term results of percutaneous transluminal valvuloplasty in patients with valvular aortic stenosis. Indian Heart J 44:67–70, 1992.

444. Letac B, Cribier A, Eltchaninoff H, et al: Evaluation of restenosis after balloon dilatation in adult aortic stenosis by repeat catheterization. Am Heart J 122:55–60, 1991.

445. Kuntz RE, Tosteson AN, Berman AD, et al: Predictors of event-free survival after balloon aortic valvuloplasty. N Engl J Med 325:17–23, 1991.

446. Kuntz RE, Tosteson AN, Maitland LA, et al: Immediate results and long-term follow-up after repeat balloon aortic valvuloplasty. Cathet Cardiovasc Diagn 25:4–9, 1992.

Chapter 39

Comprehensive Rehabilitation of Patients with Coronary Artery Disease

GERALD F. FLETCHER • KEITH R. OKEN
ROBERT E. SAFFORD

Coronary artery disease (CAD) is the most important public health problem in developed societies. Although the cardiovascular mortality rate for the United States has declined in recent decades, CAD remains the single leading cause of death. Each year, more than 1 million persons in the United States have a myocardial infarction.[1] The economic costs of CAD in the United States are increasing, with estimates of at least $50 billion annually[2] (see Chaps. 1 and 2).

Long-term analysis of case fatality rates for acute myocardial infarction in the community suggests that at least some of the reduction in cardiovascular disease mortality in recent decades can be attributed to the benefits of primary and secondary prevention strategies[3] (see Chap. 32). The American Heart Association has stated that "compelling scientific evidence, including data from recent studies in patients with CAD, demonstrates that comprehensive risk factor interventions extend overall survival, improve the quality of life, decrease the need for interventional procedures such as angioplasty and bypass grafting, and reduce the incidence of subsequent myocardial infarction."[4, 4a] Both genders benefit.[4b]

Comprehensive cardiac rehabilitation and secondary prevention of atherosclerotic cardiovascular disease are complex tasks because of the marked heterogeneity of patients and the numerous factors influencing prognosis and symptoms. Although management by a cardiovascular specialist does confer a survival advantage in patients after myocardial infarction when compared with patients treated by generalists,[5] even cardiologists underuse recommended therapies. Risk factor interventions shown to be effective in clinical trials often do not prove equally effective in community practice, perhaps in part as a result of a paucity of resources, especially nonphysician personnel to facilitate appropriate follow-up of patients. Case management systems with nurses trained to initiate interventions in smoking cessation, exercise training, and pharmacological therapy for hyperlipidemia have proved to be considerably more effective than usual medical care for modification of coronary risk factors after myocardial infarction.[6]

In this chapter, we present the background, science, and implementation of comprehensive rehabilitation in patients with CAD. Principles of secondary prevention are discussed in Chapter 32 and are summarized in Table 39–1. The approach to cardiac rehabilitation and secondary prevention is shown in Table 39–2.

REHABILITATION PROGRAMS

Inpatient Programs

Hospitalization for cardiovascular illnesses or operations now tends to be brief. Consequently, comprehensive, multifaceted inpatient cardiac rehabilitation programs are presently impractical. After initial treatment of an acute coronary syndrome (or following coronary artery bypass surgery) is completed and the patient stabilized, having the patient sit in an armchair should be encouraged, even in the intensive care unit, to minimize the loss of postural reflexes and the onset of orthostatic hypotension resulting from bed rest.[7] Limited range-of-motion exercises are usually safe at this point, except in very unstable patients, and are advisable to minimize deconditioning.[8] Once the patient is moved from the intensive care unit, walking, at first with assistance, should be encouraged as long as the patient is not severely symptomatic. The period of hospitalization is the optimal time to begin long-term pharmacological therapies to improve the patient's risk factor profile, minimize symptoms, and improve long-term event-free survival. Since acute myocardial infarction may result in a transient decline in total and high-density lipoprotein cholesterol,[9, 10] it is important to base initiation of pharmacological therapy for hyperlipidemia on lipid data from prehospital records or from blood drawn at the time of admission.[9]

EDUCATION. It is vital to begin intensive efforts to educate the patient and family regarding the nature of the patient's illness, prognosis, symptoms, medications, and important life style changes. Only one-third of patients maintain risk factor modification long-term.[4] Physicians and paramedical personnel must attempt to influence the patient at a time when concern about heart disease is at its highest. Multimedia approaches are useful adjuncts to verbal and written presentations. Educational efforts must address the need for reinforcement, variations in patient learning styles, and impediments to learning, including anxiety, pain, and sleep deprivation. Dietary guidelines, smoking cessation intervention, and instructions about walking, driving, and resumption of sexual activity[10a] are needed to minimize confusion and anxiety and to foster resumption of a normal life style.

Patients should be taught the proper response to certain symptoms should they arise after discharge, including how

▼ **TABLE 39–1.** GUIDE TO COMPREHENSIVE RISK REDUCTION FOR PATIENTS WITH CORONARY AND OTHER VASCULAR DISEASE

RISK INTERVENTION	RECOMMENDATIONS			
Smoking Goal: Complete cessation	Strongly encourage patient and family to stop smoking. Provide counseling, nicotine replacement, and formal cessation programs as appropriate			
Blood pressure control Goal: ≤140/90 mm Hg	Initiate life style modification—weight control, physical activity, alcohol moderation, and moderate sodium restriction—in all patients with blood pressure >140 mm Hg systolic or 90 mm Hg diastolic Add blood pressure medication, individualized to other patient requirements and characteristics (i.e., age, race, need for drugs with specific benefits) if blood pressure is not <140 mm Hg systolic or 90 mm Hg diastolic in 3 mo or if *initial* blood pressure is >160 mm Hg systolic or >100 mm Hg diastolic			
Lipid management Primary goal LDL <100 mg/dl	Start AHA step II diet in all patients: ≤30% fat, <7% saturated fat, and <200 mg/d cholesterol and promote physical activity Assess fasting lipid profile. In post-MI patients, lipid profile may take 4–6 wk to stabilize. Add drug therapy according to the following guide			
	LDL <100 md/dl	**LDL 100–130 mg/dl**	**LDL >130 mg/dl**	**HDL <35 mg/dl**
Secondary goals HDL >35 mg/dl TG <200 mg/dl	No drug therapy	Consider adding drug therapy to diet, as follows:	Add drug therapy to diet, as follows:	Emphasize weight management and physical activity. Advise smoking cessation If needed to achieve LDL goals, consider niacin, statin, fibrates

	Suggested Drug Therapy		
	TG <200 mg/dl	**TG 200–400 mg/dl**	**TG >400 mg/dl**
	Statin Resin Niacin	Statin Niacin	Consider combined drug therapy (niacin, fibrates, statin)

If LDL goal not achieved, consider combination drug therapy

Weight management	Start intensive diet and appropriate physical intervention, as outlined above, in patients with BMI >25 kg/m² for weight Emphasize need for weight loss especially in patients with hypertension or elevated TG or glucose levels
Antiplatelet agents/ anticoagulants	Start aspirin 80–325 mg/d if not contraindicated Manage warfarin to international normalized ratio of 2–3.5 in post-MI patients not able to take aspirin
ACE inhibitors post-MI	Start early post-MI in stable high-risk patients (anterior MI, previous MI, Killip class II [S₃ gallop, rales, radiographic heart failure]) Continued indefinitely for all with LV dysfunction (ejection fraction ≤40%) or symptoms of failure Use as needed to manage blood pressure or symptoms in all other patients
Beta blockers	Start in high-risk post-MI patients (arrhythmia, LV dysfunction, inducible ischemia) at 5–28 d. Continue 6 mo minimum. Observe usual contraindications Use as needed to manage angina, rhythm, or blood pressure in all other patients
Estrogens	Consider estrogen replacement in all postmenopausal women Individualize recommendation consistent with other health risks

ACE = angiotensin-converting enzyme; AHA = American Heart Association; BMI = body mass index; HDL = high-density lipoprotein; LDL = low-density lipoprotein; LV = left ventricular; MI = myocardial infarction; TG = triglycerides.
Modified from Consensus Panel Statement: Preventing heart attack and death in patients with coronary disease. *Circulation* 92:2–4, 1995.

to access local first-responder systems. Unfortunately, patients with CAD frequently do not seek help at the onset of acute myocardial infarction for multiple reasons. Some patients do not recognize the symptoms of acute myocardial infarction, particularly when they are not severe or consist of chest pressure, dyspnea, or nausea.[11] Other patients simply deny the symptoms in the hope that they will re-

solve.[12, 13] Still others are too embarrassed to seek medical care if the symptoms do not seem typically cardiac for fear of wasting a physician's time because of a "false alarm." Patients who are alone, particularly when they are away from home, may respond more rapidly than if surrounded by the comforts of home and family members.[14] Consequently, education of the family is helpful in minimizing delays. Understanding the emotions of patients as they cope with acute myocardial infarction is important.[15] One should not expect that large amounts of information will be assimilated by most patients during their brief hospitalization. Continued reinforcement of these points at follow-up visits is essential and can be done quite effectively in an outpatient cardiac rehabilitation and secondary prevention setting. Broad areas, including end-of-life care, can be discussed.[15a]

▼ **TABLE 39–2.** TRENDS IN CARDIAC REHABILITATION AND SECONDARY PREVENTION

Aggressive risk factor modification
Primary prevention in families of those with atherosclerotic vascular disease
Home telephone—electrocardiographically monitored cardiac rehabilitation exercise
Home individualized nonmonitored cardiac rehabilitation exercise
Behavior modification and compliance intervention
A greater role in managed and capitated care

Outpatient Programs

Outpatient exercise activity can be accomplished by using different formats, including supervised, nonsupervised, home (group and individual), monitored, and nonmonitored settings.

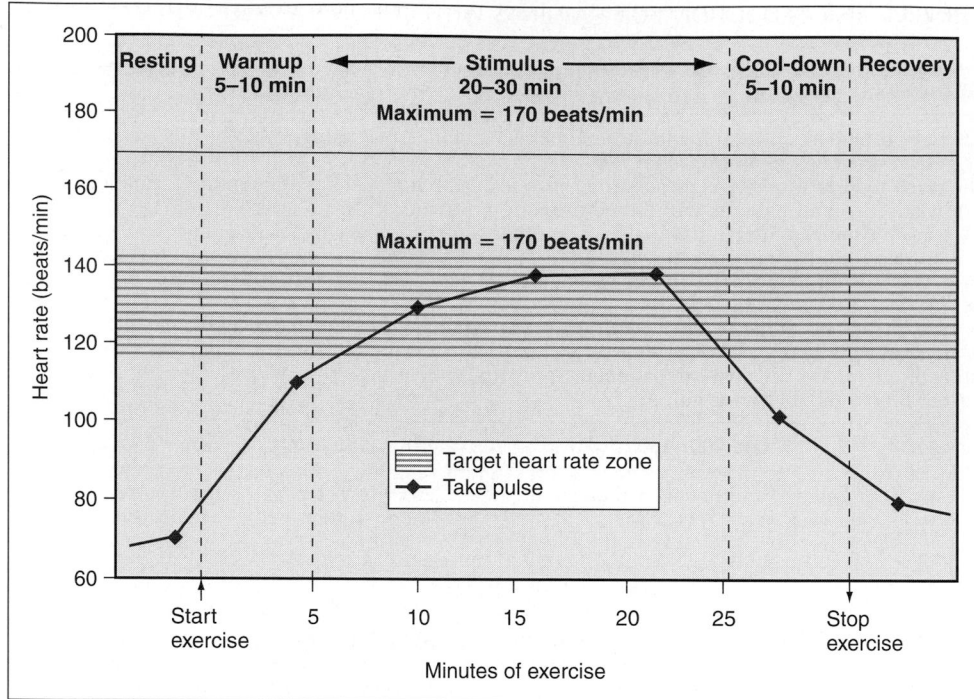

FIGURE 39–1. Format of a typical aerobic exercise training session illustrating the warm-up, stimulus, and cool-down phases along with a representative heart rate response. The target heart rate zone for training corresponds to 70 to 85 percent of the peak heart rate achieved during symptom-limited exercise testing. (From Franklin BA, McCullough PA, Timmis GC: Exercise. *In* Hennekens CH [ed]: Clinical Trials in Cardiovascular Disease. Philadelphia, WB Saunders, 1999, pp 278–295.)

SUPERVISED PROGRAMS. An exercise test and supervision are essential for this type of program.[16] The cardiovascular manifestations that require precautions can vary but usually include ventricular tachycardia, other symptomatic or hemodynamically significant arrhythmias (see Chap. 25), chest discomfort consistent with angina pectoris, exercise-induced ST depression of 2 mm or greater, or a decrease in systolic blood pressure of 20 mm Hg or greater from baseline.

Exercise testing is performed in the usual fashion (see Chap. 6), with the heart rate at which ischemia or arrhythmia is manifested used to determine the training intensity (Fig. 39–1). If the patient continues the exercise test to a high level of effort, a heart rate of 50 to 60 percent of maximum can be used if it falls at least 10 beats/min below the level at which symptoms, ST depression, or arrhythmia occurs. Otherwise, the recommended peak training heart rate is 10 beats/min less than that associated with symptoms, ST depression, or arrhythmia. It is desirable that these patients have medically supervised cardiac rehabilitation and reevaluation to "restratify" them 6 to 12 weeks later. Exercise testing should be repeated at least yearly. These supervised programs are usually conducted in a group hospital or center-based setting and include electrocardiographic (ECG) monitoring until a subject is restratified to low risk.

NONSUPERVISED PROGRAMS. Exercise intensity in these programs should approximate 50 to 80 percent of maximum oxygen consumption ($\dot{V}O_{2max}$), as determined by an exercise test or the estimated metabolic equivalent (MET).[16] If a test is not done initially, a target of 20 beats/min above the resting heart rate is adequate until testing is performed.

The exercise training heart rate should be designated as 50 to 75 percent of the heart rate reserve ([maximal heart rate − resting heart rate] × 50 to 75 percent) plus the resting heart rate. Activities can be prescribed according to the work intensity at which the training heart rate is achieved after 5 to 10 minutes at the same workload (steady state). This intensity may be expressed as watts on an ergometer, speed on a treadmill, or METs. If a patient cannot assess intensity, heart rate counting (manually or with a cardiotachometer) is especially useful. Heart rate counters are widely available and generally accurate for low- to moderate-intensity exercise. However, erroneous readings may occur in patients with irregular rhythms. Group programs may be followed by home programs of various types. Patients can be given an exercise prescription form (Fig. 39–2, Table 39–3).

MD _____

Name _____ Age _____ Starting Date _____

Clinical Status: Normal
Arrhythmia   Angina   CABG   CAD   HTN   MI   PTCA   VR

Note: This prescription is valid only if you remain on the same medications (type and dose), and you are in the same clinical status as on the day your exercise test was conducted.

Contraindications: Angina at rest, fever, illness
Temperature and weather extremes (below 30°F or more than 80° with high humidity)

Activities to avoid: Sudden strenuous lifting or carrying
Exertion that leads to holding your breath

Exercise Type: Aerobic types of exercise that are continuous, dynamic and repetitive in nature

Frequency: _____ times/day _____ days/week

Duration: Total duration of exercise session: _____ min

To be divided as follows:

Warm-up: (light flexibility/stretching routine) _____ min

Aerobic training activity: _____ to _____ min

Cool-down: (slow walking and stretching): _____ min

Intensity:

Target heart rate _____ to _____ beats/min

_____ to _____ beats/10 sec

Perceived exertion should not exceed "somewhat hard"
Re-evaluation

Your next graded exercise test is due: _____
Call our office to schedule an appointment. Phone: _____

Exercise Physiologist _____

FIGURE 39–2. Exercise prescription form. (From Franklin BA, McCullough PA, Timmis GC: Exercise. *In* Hennekens CH [ed]: Clinical Trials in Cardiovascular Disease. Philadelphia, WB Saunders, 1999, pp 278–295.)

▼ **TABLE 39–3.** FUNDAMENTALS IN DEVELOPING AN EXERCISE PRESCRIPTION

Obtain the maximum exercise heart rate—preferably with exercise testing

Designate a target heart rate at a level 60–80% of the maximum heart rate

Begin at a low level (60–70%) and progress over 4–6 wk to the ≤80% level

Exercise activity should be done for 30–60 min, 4–6 times weekly, preferably on most days

Exercise sessions should incorporate aerobic activity, such as walking, jogging, cycling, or water aerobics, with appropriate warm-up and cool-down

Resistance activities such as light weights should be used on a less frequent basis—2–3 times weekly

Home Programs

Strategies for cardiac rehabilitation have changed over recent years. Currently, less emphasis is being placed on office or hospital visits for ECG monitoring and supervised group programs. Many patients are unable to participate in such programs because of travel considerations, expense, or inconvenience. Consequently, more are being managed individually through home programs. These programs involve aggressive coronary risk modification with specific emphasis on smoking cessation, lipid control, blood pressure control, and physical activity.

MONITORED PROGRAMS. Home telephone ECG-monitored programs have been evaluated in several studies. Such monitoring is done by means of a telephone ECG transmitter, in concert with voice transmission, through a standard telephone system. These voice and ECG signals are transmitted, locally or long distance, to a central monitoring station with nurse supervision for interpretation. During these sessions, voice communication may be useful for sharing information, obtaining exercise advice, or discussing safety concerns. The ECG signal is used to document the heart rate and rhythm. A recent study comparing home-monitored exercise with standard hospital-based programs found home programs to be safe and effective in providing rehabilitative exercise.[17, 17a]

UNMONITORED PROGRAMS. Home exercise programs without telephone monitoring are also used by cardiologists and primary care physicians for patients who have been evaluated with an exercise test. Such individual programs should, however, include periodic face-to-face physician counseling. Patients assigned to these programs are predominantly those at low risk as defined by the American Heart Association[16] and show no evidence of left ventricular dysfunction, high-grade arrhythmias, unstable angina pectoris, or other compromising medical problems. An initial exercise test is important for these patients, and some physicians periodically repeat the test to ensure the safety and efficacy of the program, as well as to confirm that the level of exercise training is appropriate.

Exercise Physiology

The circulatory response to exercise involves a complex series of adjustments resulting in a large increase in cardiac output proportional to the increased metabolic demands. These changes ensure that the metabolic needs of exercising muscles are met, that hyperthermia does not occur, and that blood flow to essential organs is protected.

HEART RATE RESPONSE TO EXERCISE. At the transition from rest to strenuous exercise, the heart rate increases rapidly to values of 160 to 180 beats/min. During short periods of maximal exercise, rates as high as 240 beats/min have been recorded. The initial rapid increase is thought to be the result of central command influences or a brisk reflex from muscle mechanoreceptors. The almost instantaneous ac-

celeration in heart rate is due more to vagal withdrawal than an increase in sympathetic tone. Later increases stem from reflex activation of pulmonary stretch receptors, which trigger increased sympathetic tone and additional parasympathetic withdrawal. Increased circulating catecholamines from the adrenal glands play a role as well. It has been shown that during exercise the increase in heart rate accounts for a greater percentage of the increase in cardiac output than does the increase in stroke volume. For instance, stroke volume normally reaches its maximum when cardiac output has increased by only half its maximum. Any further increase in cardiac output occurs by increasing the heart rate alone (Fig. 39–3).

STROKE VOLUME CHANGES WITH EXERCISE. Two physiological mechanisms influence stroke volume. The first involves enhanced cardiac filling secondary to increased venous return, followed by a more forceful contraction (increased preload, Frank-Starling mechanism). The second mechanism involves normal ventricular filling, but with a more forceful contraction secondary to neurohormonal influences that leads to more complete emptying (increased inotropy).

Greater ventricular filling during diastole, or preload, is enhanced by a slower heart rate, increased venous return, and application of the Frank-Starling principle (see Chap. 14). Cardiac output and stroke volume are highest in the supine position. In this position, stroke volume is nearly maximal at rest and increases only slightly during exercise. In the upright position at rest, the diminished venous return to the heart results in smaller stroke volume and cardiac output. During upright exercise, however, stroke volume can approach the maximum stroke volume observed in the recumbent position, usually without an increase in ventricular diastolic dimensions.[18] This effect is achieved in part by increased venous tone and skeletal muscle compression.

DISTRIBUTION OF CARDIAC OUTPUT DURING EXERCISE. During exertion, parasympathetic activity is withdrawn and sympathetic activity is maximal. This shift in activity results in increased release of norepinephrine from sympathetic postganglionic nerve endings. Plasma epinephrine levels are also increased. As a result, the majority of the vascular beds of the body are constricted, except those in the exercising muscles and the coronary and cerebral circulations. Blood flow to the skin increases during light and moderate exercise to facilitate body cooling. Further increases in workload cause a progressive decrease in skin flow as the rising cutaneous sympathetic vascular tone overcomes the thermoregulatory vasodilatory response.[19] The kidneys

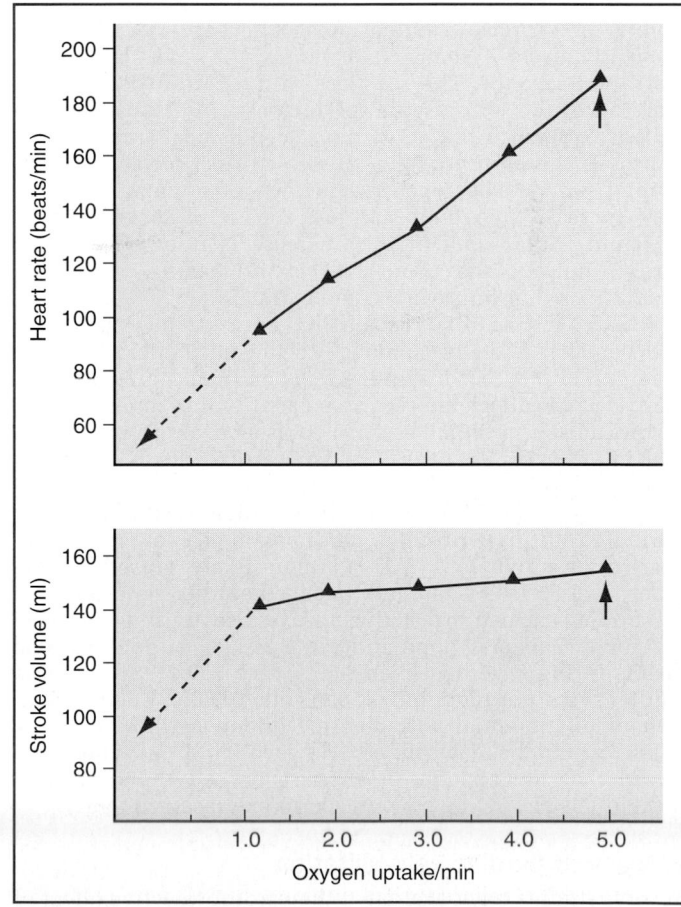

FIGURE 39–3. Graphic display of the relationship of heart rate and stroke volume increase. Of note, stroke volume reaches its maximum when oxygen uptake has increased by only half maximum.

and splanchnic tissue extract 10 to 25 percent of the oxygen delivered. Consequently, considerable reductions in blood flow to these tissues can be tolerated through increased extraction of oxygen from the available blood supply.[20] At rest, the heart extracts about 75 percent of the oxygen in the coronary blood flow. Because of this limited reserve, the increased myocardial oxygen demands during exercise are met mainly by a fourfold increase in coronary blood flow. Cerebral blood flow also increases during exercise by approximately 25 to 30 percent.[21] During maximal exercise, however, cerebral flow may also decrease in association with hyperventilation and respiratory alkalosis.

On cessation of exercise, an abrupt decrease in heart rate and cardiac output occurs secondary to removal of sympathetic drive and reactivation of vagal activity. In contrast, systemic vascular resistance remains lower for some time because of persistent vasodilation in muscles. As a result, arterial pressure falls, often below preexercise levels, for periods of up to 12 hours into recovery.[22] Blood pressure is then stabilized at normal levels by baroreceptor reflexes.

CARDIOVASCULAR RESPONSE TO DIFFERENT TYPES OF EXERCISE. Different types of exercise impose various loads on the cardiovascular system. Isotonic (dynamic) exercise is defined as muscular contraction of large muscle groups that results in movement and primarily places a volume load on the heart. *Isometric* (static) exercise is defined as a constant muscular contraction of smaller muscle groups without movement and results in more pressure than volume load on the heart. Significant increases in both cardiac output and oxygen consumption and a fall in systemic vascular resistance characterize the acute load posed by isotonic exercise. In contrast, isometric exercise acutely increases systemic vascular resistance and blood pressure while producing only minimal changes in cardiac output and oxygen consumption.[23] *Resistance* exercise is a combination of isometric and isotonic exercise that produces muscular contraction with movement, as in free weight lifting. Most activities (such as sports or employment-related activities) usually combine all three types of exercise.

CHRONIC ADAPTATIONS TO EXERCISE. Physical conditioning or exercise training affects the cardiovascular and skeletal muscle systems in a variety of ways to improve work performance. The response of the cardiovascular system to regular exercise is an increase in its capacity to deliver oxygen to the active muscle. Physical training also improves the ability of the muscles to use oxygen. Conditioning induced by repetitive periods of dynamic exercise may increase maximum oxygen consumption twofold to threefold. About half of this increase is due to increased cardiac output, and about half is induced by peripheral adaptations that improve oxygen extraction.[24]

RISKS OF EXERCISE TRAINING. Exercise has both risks and benefits, and the challenge to the physician is to provide guidelines that minimize risks and maximize benefits. Many factors affect the risk associated with exercise. Three of the most important are age, presence of heart disease, and intensity of exercise. Sudden cardiac death is rare in apparently healthy individuals (see Chap. 26). In individuals younger than 35 years, sudden cardiac death is usually attributed to hypertrophic cardiomyopathy or congenital heart disease, whereas CAD is a more likely cause for those older than 35 (see Chap. 59). Selected studies reporting risk of sudden cardiac arrest during exercise training indicate that in the general population, the risk of sudden cardiac death during vigorous exercise is very low.[16] Since these studies were not randomized controlled trials, the contribution of all potential variables to sudden cardiac arrest or death cannot be determined. However, it is generally believed that the benefits of exercise exceed the risks, and individuals should be encouraged to exercise prudently.

Efficacy of Cardiac Rehabilitation

Several studies have evaluated the cardioprotective effect of exercise training in the setting of cardiac rehabilitation programs for survivors of myocardial infarction (see Chap. 35). A review of these trials revealed that cardiovascular rehabilitation programs lead to improved functional capacity

and cardiovascular efficiency, as well as an enhanced sense of well-being.[25] The evidence, however, fell short of indicating that exercise conditioning programs can independently reduce fatal or nonfatal coronary events. Anginal thresholds remain unchanged (Fig. 39–4).

Although more than 4700 patients have been studied in randomized trials of cardiac rehabilitation, most of the individual trials enrolled small numbers of patients and did not have sufficient power to distinguish significant differences between groups.[26] The largest study performed in the United States was the National Exercise and Heart Disease Project, which randomized 651 men who survived myocardial infarction to exercise training or to a control group.[27] The favorable trends seen in both overall mortality and cardiovascular mortality after 3 years in the exercise group failed to reach statistical significance. Recent analysis of the data, however, has revealed that increases in maximum physical work capacity on exercise testing in the study (1-MET increase at each stage) were associated with a reduction in all-cause mortality of 8 to 14 percent for up to 19 years.[28]

Two meta-analyses have examined the effect of cardiovascular rehabilitation. The first combined the results of 10 randomized clinical trials involving over 4300 patients.[29] The rehabilitation programs began 8 weeks to 3 years after myocardial infarction. The duration of the programs ranged from 6 weeks to 4 years. Cardiac rehabilitation resulted in a beneficial effect on mortality but not on nonfatal recurrent myocardial infarction. All-cause mortality was decreased by 24 percent and cardiovascular mortality by 25 percent for patients in the rehabilitation program. The reason for the lack of benefit on recurrent nonfatal myocardial infarction is unclear. The second meta-analysis reported a 20 percent decrease in both overall mortality and cardiovascular mortality.[26] The results were apparent as early as 1 year after randomization and persisted for at least 3 years after infarction. Trials that used a multifactorial approach to risk factor modification showed a greater reduction in mortality than did those that used only exercise training, which suggests that not all of the benefit could be attributed to exercise alone (Fig. 39–5).

Exercise training is the mainstay of cardiac rehabilitation

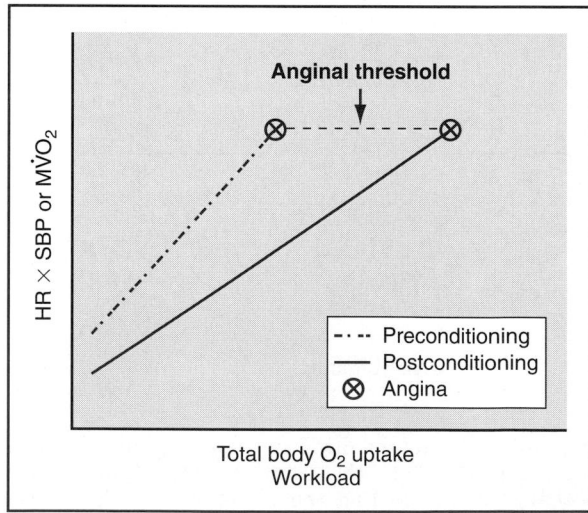

FIGURE 39–4. Effect of physical conditioning on the product of heart rate (HR) × systolic blood pressure (SBP) and on myocardial O_2 consumption ($M\dot{V}O_2$) at submaximal and peak exercise. Peak body O_2 uptake and workload are augmented by exercise. Myocardial O_2 requirements are reduced at a given workload of O_2 uptake, but angina occurs at the same HR × SBP product. (From Franklin BA, McCullough PA, Timmis GC: Exercise. *In* Hennekens CH [ed]: Clinical Trials in Cardiovascular Disease. Philadelphia, WB Saunders, 1999, pp 278–295.)

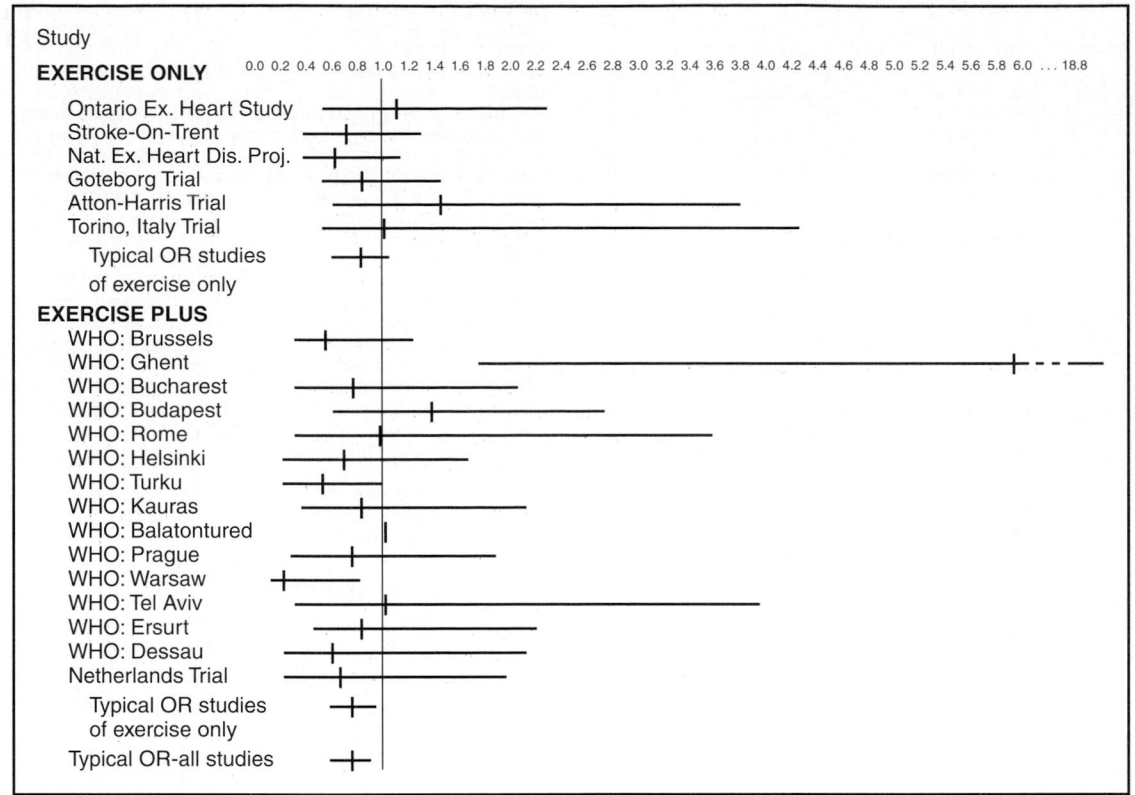

FIGURE 39-5. Chart of effects of pooling from randomized trials of cardiac rehabilitation on the estimate of mortality 3 years after randomization. Short vertical lines indicate point estimates; horizontal lines depict 95 percent confidence intervals. "Exercise Plus" usually refers to the life style and dietary modifications in both the exercise and control groups. (From O'Connor GT, Buring JE, Yusuf S, et al: An overview of randomized trials of rehabilitation with exercise after myocardial infarction. Circulation 80:234, 1989. By permission of the American Heart Association, Inc.)

and can be used with impressive benefits for many cardiac patients.[29a-e] Recent studies using coronary arteriography have shown regression or lack of progression of coronary lesions in patients who performed high-intensity exercise and were also ingesting a low-fat diet.[30, 31] These changes were maintained during a follow-up period of 6 years. High-intensity exercise training has been shown to result in a higher left ventricular ejection fraction in men with CAD than has low-intensity exercise.[32] Other studies report that exercise training programs either have no harmful effects or have significant beneficial effects on ventricular function and/or "remodeling" in subjects with CAD.[33-35]

Cardiac rehabilitation must be carried out simultaneously with an aggressive program to reduce risk factors (secondary prevention), including antiplatelet and antithrombotic therapy, beta blockade, angiotensin-converting enzyme (ACE) inhibition, and statin therapy. Secondary prevention is described in Chapter 32.

Secondary Prevention

ASPIRIN (See Chap. 62). Ensuring that patients seen in the cardiac rehabilitation and secondary prevention center are receiving optimal antiplatelet/anticoagulant therapy is very important. Aspirin in a dose of 81 to 325 mg daily should be used chronically in all patients with CAD who are not intolerant of or allergic to it and who do not have other definite indications for warfarin anticoagulation.[36] An initial dose of 325 mg should be used in acute settings. For those who are unable to take aspirin and do not require warfarin, clopidogrel 75 mg daily is recommended and may be substituted for or added to aspirin in patients with peripheral arterial disease.[37]

BETA BLOCKADE. Beta-adrenergic blocking agents are a "cornerstone" of pharmacological therapy for CAD (see Chap. 37) and should be used within rehabilitation programs whenever possible. Although multiple clinical trials have documented the benefits of beta blockers initiated as a secondary prevention measure during hospitalization for acute myocardial infarction, continued long-term beta blockade remains underused.[38]

Following myocardial infarction, survival of patients who receive beta blockers is greatly improved in comparison to those who do not receive them, predominantly because of fewer sudden deaths. Greater benefit is seen in those with poor left ventricular function.[38] In one study of beta-blocker therapy following acute myocardial infarction, 6 lives were saved per 100 nondiabetic patients treated with beta blockers as opposed to 13 lives saved per 100 diabetics.[39] Because a reduction in heart rate is important, beta blockers with intrinsic sympathomimetic effects should not be used in patients with CAD.

ANGIOTENSIN-CONVERTING ENZYME INHIBITORS. ACE inhibitors are a mainstay in the treatment of patients following myocardial infarction. Heart failure develops in half of all patients seen with acute myocardial infarction.[40] More than 120,000 patients in major clinical trials have been randomized to receive either an ACE inhibitor or placebo in addition to optimal conventional therapy for acute myocardial infarction (see Chap. 35). As a consequence of these studies, ACE inhibitors have been shown to reduce mortality and morbidity during and following myocardial infarction.[41-43]

Most of the benefits associated with early ACE inhibitor use occur during the first week after myocardial infarction, when mortality is the highest.[43] The absolute benefit in mortality reduction is greatest in high-risk groups, such as patients with tachycardia or anterior wall myocardial infarction.[43] In the Trandolapril Cardiac Evaluation (TRACE) Study, trandolapril saved 87 lives per 1000 people treated over a 3-year period. Patients with hypertension and diabetes mellitus benefited the most.[44] Five lives per 1000 are saved in the first week alone if ACE inhibitor therapy is started within the first 36 hours after acute myocardial infarction.[43] Acute, short-term ACE inhibitor therapy was not found to be harmful in any subgroup in a meta-analysis of 100,000 patients with acute myocardial infarction, but hypotension and renal dysfunction were more common side effects in patients older than 75 years.[43] Current recommendations are that ACE inhibitors be continued indefinitely in patients with clinical heart failure or impaired left ventricular systolic dysfunction, but their use may be discontinued after 6 weeks if neither is present.[45] These recommendations should be implemented routinely in the secondary prevention phase of patient care.

ACE inhibitors attenuate the progressive left ventricular dilatation after large, especially anterior myocardial infarction (Fig. 39–6) (see Chap. 35). ACE inhibitors have also been shown to reduce the likelihood of clinical heart failure in patients with asymptomatic left ventricular dysfunction.[47] Large prospective clinical trials are evaluating the potential efficacy of ACE inhibitors in reducing ischemic events

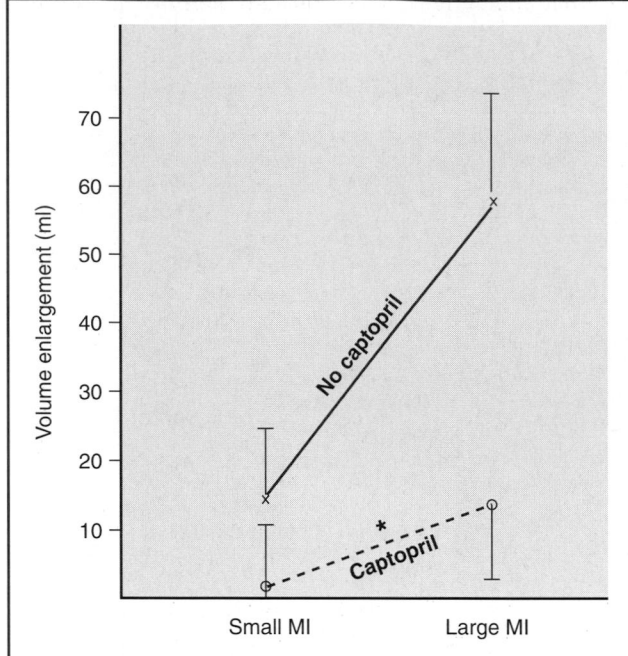

FIGURE 39–6. Attenuation of left ventricular enlargement by captopril therapy after anterior wall myocardial infarction (MI). (Modified from Quigg R, Salyer J, Mohanty PK, Simpson P: Impaired exercise capacity late after cardiac transplantation: Influence of chronotropic incompetence, hypertension, and calcium channel blockers. Am Heart J 136:465–473, 1998.)

and mortality in patients with CAD and preserved left ventricular systolic function (Prevention of Events with Angiotensin-Converting Enzyme Inhibition[48] [PEACE]) and in patients at high risk for CAD[49] (Heart Outcomes Prevention Evaluation [HOPE]). In the HOPE Study, nearly 10,000 patients, most older than 65 years, were randomized to the ACE inhibitor ramipril or to placebo (see Chap. 37). The trial was terminated by the Data and Safety Monitoring Board after 4.5 years because of the clinically important benefit of ramipril therapy.[50] The results of the HOPE Trial suggest that ACE inhibitors can be continued indefinitely in post–myocardial infarction patients with normal left ventricular function.

By blocking the production of angiotensin II and the degradation of bradykinin, ACE inhibitors cause vasodilatation, increased production of nitric oxide, decreased aldosterone secretion (lessening salt and water retention), decreased sympathetic tone, improved endothelial function, reduced left ventricular mass, antiplatelet effects, and reduced blood pressure.[51–54] ACE inhibitors also have an antiischemic effect, with a 25 percent reduction in the risk of subsequent myocardial infarction. Patients in the Survival and Ventricular Enlargement[55] (SAVE) and Studies of Left Ventricular Dysfunction[47] (SOLVD) trials had a reduced need for coronary revascularization and fewer admissions for unstable angina while receiving ACE inhibitor therapy.[47, 51, 55]

ACE inhibitors have important clinical benefits, are easy to use, and are safe, but they are underused.[56, 57] Angiotensin II receptor blockers, which are now more widely used, may be administered to patients in whom ACE inhibitors cause coughing. Both these classes of drugs have similar effects and must be appropriately used in cardiac rehabilitation and secondary prevention programs.

STATIN THERAPY (see Chaps. 31 to 33). A wealth of clinical data strongly support the use of cholesterol reduction therapy for secondary prevention in patients with established CAD. This conclusion results from a large number of well-controlled clinical trials, the most convincing of which used the 3-hydroxy-3-methylglutaryl coenzyme A (HMG-CoA) reductase inhibitors, or statin drugs. The relationship between on-treatment low-density lipoprotein (LDL) cholesterol and the relative risk of coronary heart disease is probably curvilinear, with diminishing returns as LDL cholesterol is reduced.[58, 59] In general, it is recommended that LDL cholesterol be reduced to less than 100 mg/dl.[60] Some have proposed that even a lower goal would be better, a hypothesis that has not yet been tested in clinical trials but will be addressed by the Treat to New Targets (TNT) Study.

Statin therapy is remarkably safe and may exert beneficial effects by several mechanisms other than reduction of LDL cholesterol, including stimulation of endothelial nitric oxide production,[61] as well as antiinflammatory[62] and antithrombotic properties.[63, 64] The survival curves of patients with cardiovascular disease who are taking statins in general diverge quickly (at 6 to 12 months) from those of patients

randomized to placebo in major trials. It is believed that plaque stabilization by reducing LDL core size, inflammation, and thrombosis leads to decreased rates of plaque rupture and fissuring, thereby accounting for a decrease in cardiovascular events and improved survival.[65]

Lipid treatment strategies are progressively being refined. Published studies indicate that nurse-managed facilities can give as good, if not better results than physician-managed facilities.[6] Lipid-lowering therapy is one of the most effective areas of cardiac therapeutics (see Chaps. 33 and 37). When combined with a proper diet and exercise, meaningful improvement in lipids is feasible in most patients, who should not be denied these benefits because they are the cornerstone of modern secondary prevention of CAD.

DIETARY SUPPLEMENTS AND ALTERNATIVE THERAPIES. Nonprescription medications are used widely throughout the United States. In one series of patients undergoing periodic general health examinations, 61 percent were taking dietary supplements. Only half of them reported using these substances on questionnaires completed just before the examination.[66] Because of extensive attention to this subject in the lay press, it is possible that an even higher percentage of patients entering cardiac rehabilitation and secondary prevention might be using dietary supplements. Although plausible biological mechanisms for the beneficial effects of many of these supplements have been proposed, data supporting their use in clinical practice are limited to cohort and retrospective observational studies. Few significant data have been derived from controlled clinical trials.

SMOKING CESSATION. Cigarette smoking increases platelet aggregation, serum fibrinogen, and oxidation of LDL cholesterol. Cessation also reduces high-density lipoprotein cholesterol and induces coronary artery spasm, with consequently decreased coronary and collateral flow reserve as a result of endothelial dysfunction.[67]

The dose-dependent effect of smoking is clearly defined. A 20-year follow-up study of British male physicians found that those who smoked 25 or more cigarettes per day had 2.3 times the relative risk of mortality from coronary heart disease as nonsmokers do.[68]

Patients who continue to smoke after a myocardial infarction have twice the risk of death from recurrent myocardial infarction than those who stop.[69] Many studies, including the Atherosclerosis Risk in Community Study, have shown a substantial increase in the risk of progression of atherosclerosis that is greatest in those who actively smoke, intermediate in those who formerly smoked, and lowest in those who never smoked.[70] Cigarette smoking was believed to be the single most substantial risk factor for progression of disease and a particularly potent factor in patients who had other risk factors such as hypertension or diabetes mellitus. The influence of smoking on disease progression holds for both native vessels[71] and coronary artery bypass grafts.[72]

The cardiovascular benefits of smoking cessation are striking.[73, 74] The risk of myocardial infarction declines quickly after smoking cessation. By 1 year, the risk has declined by approximately one-third from peak values, and by 3 to 4 years after cessation, the risk is equivalent to that of patients who have never smoked. The total cardiovascular mortality rate, however, takes about 10 years to decline to the level of nonsmokers.

Addiction to nicotine is difficult to break. Most patients who are able to terminate the habit have made five or more attempts before they are ultimately successful.[75] Measures such as nicotine replacement, bupropion, and continuous reinforcement by medical professionals are helpful and safe.[75, 76] Patients who smoke more than 20 cigarettes per day, who smoke within 30 minutes of awakening in the morning, or who have significant withdrawal symptoms and relapse within a week of cessation on initial attempts or those who have a current or a past history of a significant psychiatric disorder are generally considered the most difficult to treat.[75]

Unfortunately, success rates at 1 year range from only approximately 6 percent with physician counseling as the sole intervention to 20 to 40 percent with pharmacological interventions. Nonetheless, organized smoking cessation programs appear to be cost-effective and can be implemented in concert with secondary prevention programs. One program that reported a 22 percent smoking cessation rate at 1 year costs approximately $400 per patient (clinic visits plus drug costs). It was estimated that the cost of a net year of life gained (YLG) by the program was $6128, which compares favorably with the cost of pneumococcal vaccine in the elderly ($1500/YLG), treatment of mild to moderate hypertension ($11,300 to $24,400/YLG), heart transplantation ($16,200/YLG), and breast cancer screening ($26,800/YLG).[77]

Fear of weight gain, particularly in women, can be an impediment to smoking cessation. However, exercise improves aerobic capacity and delays weight gain after smoking cessation and can thus be a helpful part of smoking cessation programs.[78] Since a high percentage of patients coming to a cardiac rehabilitation and secondary prevention clinic for advice and follow-up are smokers, it is natural that such clinics would incorporate smoking cessation as a major focus. Evidence-based clinical guidelines from the Agency for Health Care Policy and Research and other professional organizations now define treatment strategies for physicians and health care delivery systems.[79] Because of the importance of the problem, further refinement and proliferation of such guidelines are likely to occur.[80] Smoking cessation is therefore one of the most important components of secondary prevention of CAD and should be aggressively implemented in every patient. Nicotine chewing gum, skin patches, nasal sprays and inhalers, drugs such as mecamylamine and clonidine, serotonergic treatments such as buspirone, antidepressants such as bupropion, and cigarette substitutes are techniques that can be tried.[81]

Heart Failure

Although convincing data indicating that cardiac rehabilitation prolongs life in heart failure patients do not exist, it is clear that rehabilitation is safe and helpful in improving quality of life and exercise tolerance in both medically treated patients and those who have undergone cardiac transplantation.[82, 83] Leg fatigue and exercise intolerance are common symptoms in patients with heart failure (Fig. 39–7). Decreased cardiac reserve as a result of left ventricular systolic dysfunction is important as a cause of exercise intolerance, but the left ventricular ejection fraction and pulmonary capillary wedge pressure actually correlate quite poorly with exercise limitation.[84, 85] Abnormalities of skeletal muscle, including reductions in the number of type I muscle fibers, concentration of aerobic enzymes, and capillary density, as well as changes in contractile muscle proteins, are present in heart failure patients.[86] However, oxygen extraction (utilization) is not impaired.

Rehabilitation exercise programs for heart failure patients typically use aerobic exercises that increase cardiac output, such as treadmill walking and cycling,[87] but these exercises may also increase filling pressure.[88] One study suggested that cardiac rehabilitation was helpful only in patients who had a normal cardiac output response to exercise.[89] In another study, 68 clinically stable patients already receiving maximum medical therapy and awaiting heart transplantation were prescribed a walking program for 6 months. Walking 20 to 30 minutes at moderate intensity for a distance of up to 2 miles, four times a week, led to improved peak exercise tolerance in 38 of the 68 patients. Thirty-one of the 38 responders were subsequently removed from the heart transplant waiting list.[90] A recent randomized Italian study of predominantly men with ischemic cardiomyopathy showed a decreased rate of hospital readmission for heart failure in patients randomized to moderate exercise training (5/50) versus no exercise (14/49) during 14 months of follow-up.[91] Fewer deaths were observed in the exercise group (9/50) than in the nonexercise group (20/49).[92]

An aerobic exercise program in patients who are able to

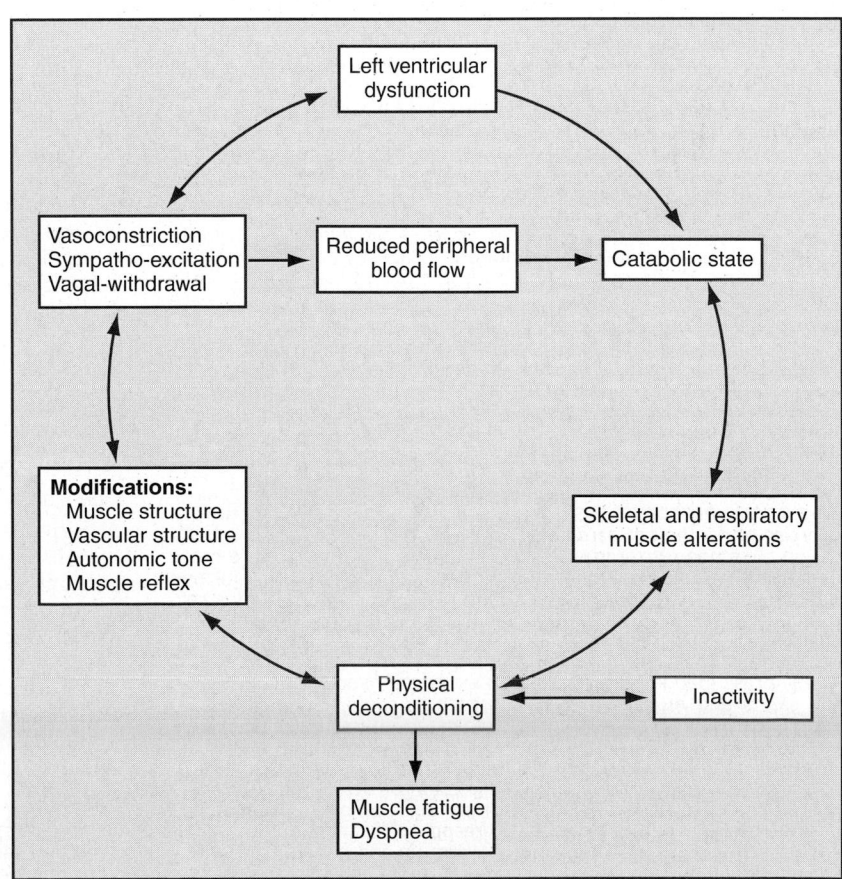

FIGURE 39–7. Peripheral abnormalities leading to physical deconditioning are responsible for some of the exercise intolerance symptoms in chronic heart failure; by reducing physical deconditioning, exercise training is able to partially reverse peripheral and autonomic abnormalities and thus slow or block the vicious cycle. (Modified from Piepoli MF, Flather M, Coats AJ: Overview of studies of exercise training in chronic heart failure: The need for a prospective randomized multicentre European trial. Eur Heart J 19:830–841, 1998.)

tolerate it is an important adjunct to pharmacological therapy for congestive heart failure. Large randomized trials are needed to further define mechanisms of benefit, selection of patients most likely to benefit, optimal modes of training, risks, and costs.[92]

Cardiac Transplantation (see Chap. 20)

Cardiac transplantation is well established as an effective treatment in selected patients with end-stage heart disease. Cardiac rehabilitation following cardiac transplantation is recommended for its salutary effects on functional capacity.[93–95]

In the only currently available randomized trial, 27 cardiac transplant recipients were assigned to participate in a 6-month structured cardiac rehabilitation program or to undergo unstructured therapy at home.[95] Despite spending more time on the transplant waiting list and being more likely to undergo urgent transplantation, the group randomized to structured cardiac rehabilitation manifested greater increases in peak oxygen consumption and workload, as well as a greater reduction in the ventilatory equivalent for carbon dioxide.[95] The structured rehabilitation cohort demonstrated greater exercise capacity at 1 year despite inferior performance 1 month after transplantation. Although exercise training yields significant improvement at 1 year,[95–97] peak oxygen consumption fails to improve further over the ensuing 4 to 5 years,[98, 99] primarily because of limited improvement in chronotropic response beyond the first year.[98, 100]

The impaired chronotropic response of the denervated cardiac allograft is manifested by a high resting heart rate, reduced heart rate reserve, and diminished maximum heart rate during exercise. The allograft is dependent on elevated levels of circulating catecholamines for increases in stroke work and heart rate during exercise.[101] Although biochemical[102] and physiological[103] evidence of reinnervation following human cardiac transplantation is mounting, such reinnervation is usually clinically insignificant.[100, 104]

PERIPHERAL ABNORMALITIES IN OXYGEN TRANSPORT. In addition to chronotropic incompetence and diastolic dysfunction, peripheral abnormalities in oxygen transport/utilization have been reported.[99, 105] These abnormalities may be the result of pretransplantation deconditioning (see Fig. 39–7) or posttransplantation corticosteroid use. Studies in patients with severe heart failure awaiting heart transplantation have demonstrated abnormalities in skeletal muscle morphology and bioenergetics, including reductions in type I fibers, capillary density, and oxidative enzyme activity.[86] Similar findings are seen in patients following transplantation and may contribute to the impaired exercise performance.[106] A longitudinal study of 12 transplant recipients during the first postoperative year suggested improvement in (but not complete normalization of) myocyte fiber cross-sectional area and skeletal muscle enzyme activity commensurate with gains in peak oxygen consumption.[106] Capillary density and fiber-type distribution did not change during follow-up despite 3 months of structured physical rehabilitation.[106] These observations have prompted recommendations for resistance weight training as part of posttransplantation rehabilitation.[93, 94, 107]

In the immediate postoperative phase, rehabilitation is limited to passive and active range of motion.[108] Following extubation, rehabilitation continues with mobilization, progressive ambulation, and incentive spirometry to aid pulmonary toilet. Predischarge exercise testing of patients free of acute allograft rejection or surgical complications has been suggested as a guide for outpatient exercise prescription.[94]

EXERCISE PRESCRIPTIONS IN TRANSPLANT RECIPIENTS. The abnormal exercise physiology of cardiac transplant recipients mandates modification of standard exercise prescriptions. Target heart rates are problematic because of the chronotropic incompetence and diminished heart rate reserve of the denervated allograft. Many authorities recommend the use of Borg[109] ratings of perceived exertion.[93, 94, 108] However, individuals vary considerably in the percentage of maximum heart rate or peak oxygen consumption that they achieve at commonly prescribed levels of perceived exertion.[110] Such variability limits the safety and efficacy of this approach in some patients.[110] Some suggest that exercise training be predicated on fixed-distance/fixed-speed prescriptions fine-tuned by perceived exertion ratings.[110]

The general principles of cardiac rehabilitation, including frequency, intensity, duration, and progression of training, apply to the heart transplantation population. Longer duration of exercise may be appropriate to allow for the delayed response to circulating catecholamines by the denervated allograft. Warm-up and cool-down periods with appropriate stretching before and after exercise are important.

At least 20 minutes of sustained exercise at the prescribed intensity is desirable.

Initiation of supervised rehabilitation will vary according to the preoperative status of the recipient and the postoperative course. Generally, training can start 2 to 6 weeks after surgery[111] and should continue for at least 6 to 8 weeks.[94] Although significant improvement in exercise capacity and strength has been demonstrated with prolonged, home-based training in motivated patients, many programs start with supervised sessions 3 days per week. One study recently demonstrated the benefits of adding supervised aerobic and resistive exercise training to progressive, home-based therapy.[95] Resistive arm training should be deferred for 6 weeks to allow adequate healing of the sternotomy.[111] It should be incorporated thereafter to increase strength and functionality and to improve the skeletal muscle abnormalities of chronic heart failure and mitigate the deleterious muscular effects of immunosuppressive agents. It may also combat the osteoporosis common to this population.

Ideally, initial exercise sessions should be guided by graded exercise test results with a rating of perceived exertion that matches the ventilatory threshold,[97] or 60 to 70 percent of peak oxygen consumption. If rating of perceived exertion alone is used, an initial target of 11 to 13 is appropriate for those debilitated by chronic heart failure or postoperative recovery.[94] The exercise prescription should be advanced as the ventilatory and lactate thresholds, peak oxygen consumption, and maximum heart rate predictably improve with training and postoperative convalescence.[96, 97, 112]

Cardiovascular Rehabilitation in Obese Patients

Weight loss is a key component of cardiovascular rehabilitation in an obese patient.[112a] Exercise training is an important contributor to weight loss, although the effect of exercise is quite variable. It is not clear how much exercise is required to prevent weight gain or weight regain, although it has been suggested that the levels may be much higher than the currently recommended doses of physical activity.[113] Most controlled exercise training studies show only modest weight loss (approximately 2 to 3 kg) in the exercise group. However, when caloric restriction is added to the exercise program, the average weight loss is 8.5 kg, most of which is body fat, while diet alone results in less weight loss (5.1 kg). Over the same study period, those undergoing neither diet nor exercise programming increase weight by an average of 1.7 kg.[114, 115]

These data strongly support a role for both exercise and diet in weight loss programs. Body composition and fat distribution are linked to cardiovascular mortality[114] and are improved by exercise. Physically active men and women have a more favorable waist-to-hip ratio (i.e., less central obesity) than do sedentary individuals.[116] In general, exercise for the obese should be low-impact exercise, such as brisk walking or cycle ergometry, and be performed with greater duration and frequency and less intensity.

One study (unpublished) in obese patients with CAD in a cardiac rehabilitation program compared one group receiving extreme calorie restriction and moderate-intensity exercise with another receiving moderate caloric restriction and high-intensity exercise. The intervention results revealed that the extreme caloric restriction–moderate-intensity exercise group lost significantly more weight over the 6-month study period.

Cardiovascular Rehabilitation in Elderly Patients
(see Chap. 57)

A critical factor in an elderly (≥70 years) person's ability to function independently is mobility, the ability to move without assistance.[117–123a] The overall focus for cardiac rehabilitation and exercise training in the elderly should be to enhance health-related conditioning while simultaneously assisting in the reduction of risk factors for various chronic diseases and improving the overall quality of life. Considerable evidence exists that physical activity, both endurance and resistance-type exercise, can provide for functional independence and overall well-being in older adults.[123b]

Exercise prescription guidelines as described previously are generally appropriate for older participants. As with younger persons, the combination of endurance and resistance exercise is best for achieving health and conditioning goals.[124–128] The exercise capacity of the elderly, both before and after exercise training, is usually lower than that observed in younger persons[117, 129] (Table 39–4). Thus, it is important to recommend activities that require low-level energy expenditure (40 to 50 percent of $\dot{V}O_{2max}$), particularly during the first few weeks of the program. High-intensity exercise training must be recommended with caution in this age group because of the potential for musculoskeletal injury. Those whose exercise duration is limited (<15 minutes per session) because of physical or psychosocial limitations should also attempt to exercise more frequently. Conversely, lengthening the duration of activity to as much as 45 to 60 minutes per session is valuable for increasing caloric expenditure despite lower-intensity exercise.

Cardiovascular Rehabilitation in Patients with Peripheral Vascular Disease (see Chap. 41)

Patients with symptomatic peripheral vascular disease commonly have many traditional risk factors for atherosclerosis and often have severe coexistent CAD that may be symptomatic or clinically silent.[130] Frequently, occult CAD is found in these patients by screening pharmacological stress tests or angiography because exercise is often limited by claudication before the onset of cardiac symptoms. This limited exercise capacity may decrease the diagnostic accuracy of exercise stress testing. CAD is usually the life-limiting illness in these patients.[131] Consequently, aggressive risk factor modification is needed not only to slow the pace of peripheral vascular disease but also to reduce cardiovascular events and the rate of progression of coexisting CAD. Measures to protect the feet and prompt treatment of foot ulcers appear to reduce the risk of amputation.[132]

The initial therapeutic intervention for most patients with intermittent claudication is a walking program. Thirty to 45 minutes of walking performed 4 or more days weekly was reported to increase walking distance by 200 percent or more.[133] However, therapeutic trials in patients with claudication have commonly treated only a small number of patients, are often not randomized, and are difficult to interpret because of a large placebo effect and publication bias.[134–137] A recent meta-analysis of such studies, including only 112 patients, concluded that the increase in pain-free walking distance at the end of an exercise program was 140 meters with a concomitant increase in total walking distance of 180 meters.[134] Thus, although exercise programs are safe and improve physical conditioning, weight control, and hypertension, the magnitude of the treatment effect is not well defined.

Small studies comparing supervised versus home-based training of claudication patients suggest an advantage in favor of the supervised setting.[134, 137, 138] Since the data are so limited at this point, prescription of expensive supervised programs is controversial and cannot yet be recommended on a routine basis.[134] However, in patients who are already enrolled in cardiac rehabilitation programs, where benefit is more readily demonstrable and better documented, treatment of peripheral vascular disease with an exercise program can be an additional benefit.

Peripheral vascular disease usually coexists with CAD. Cardiac rehabilitation programs are beneficial to patients with peripheral vascular disease, and walking improves claudication, but the mode of exercise may need to be altered (treadmill, cycle, or swimming) to limit the likelihood that claudication will prevent a training effect. Secondary preventive measures (smoking cessation, lipid-lowering therapy) are just as important as they are in patients undergoing rehabilitation for CAD alone.

Cardiovascular Rehabilitation in Patients with End-Stage Renal Disease (see Chap. 72)

Cardiovascular disease is the leading cause of morbidity and mortality in patients with end-stage renal disease (ESRD).[139] Although many patients with ESRD are candidates, cardiac rehabilitation is underused in this high-risk cohort.

In one multicenter study of chronic hemodialysis patients, 76 percent manifested ventricular arrhythmias and 69 percent demonstrated supraventricular arrhythmias on 48-hour ambulatory monitoring.[140] Thirty-nine percent manifested multiple episodes of complex ventricular ectopy. The frequency of ventricular arrhythmias increased significantly in the second hour of dialysis and lasted up to 5 hours after dialysis. These findings suggest that close ECG monitoring and avoidance of the early postdialysis period would be prudent in scheduling exercise training sessions.

Several alterations in physiology have an impact on the rehabilitation process. Autonomic insufficiency is common in ESRD and mandates monitoring of supine and standing vital signs and caution with positional changes. Problematic contributing factors include underlying systemic disease (e.g., diabetes mellitus, amyloidosis), antihypertensive medications, aluminum toxicity, and uremia.[141, 142]

Many factors contribute to an imbalance in myocardial oxygen supply and demand in patients with ESRD.[143] Hypertension, increased intravascular volume, diastolic left ventricular dysfunction, valvular heart disease, and left ventricular systolic dysfunction can all contribute to elevated left ventricular end-diastolic pressure and reduced coronary perfusion pressure. Tachycardia-induced shortening of diastolic perfusion time, reduced coronary perfusion pressure, anemia, and dialysis-induced shifts in the hemoglobin oxygen dissociation curve conspire to reduce myocardial oxygen supply. These factors contribute to a propensity for ischemia, including ischemia during exercise training. Coupled with the higher prevalence of silent ischemia in patients with ESRD, these features make supervised, monitored exercise programs prudent for this population.

Many patients with ESRD have reduced exercise capacity[144] as a result of age, malnutrition, comorbidity, deconditioning, immobility, and advanced cardiovascular disease. Fortunately, exercising to target heart rates 50 to 70 percent of those achieved on screening maximum exercise tests achieve improvements in exercise capacity and symptomatology that are similar to those attained with traditional targets of 70 to 85 percent.[93]

Several small studies of dialysis patients free of obvious CAD suggest that intradialysis exercise programs improve quality of life, blood pressure, and some measures of metabolic health.[145–147] The safety of such programs in patients with recent acute coronary events has not been established and cannot be assumed. Limited data suggest potential hemodynamic compromise with exercise in later stages of hemodialysis sessions.[148]

The benefits of exercise training in ESRD patients after major cardiac events should be similar to those derived by others with ESRD and the cardiac rehabilitation population at large. However, profound limitations in exercise capacity may limit the effectiveness of cardiac rehabilitation for some, thus mandating careful selection of rehabilitation candidates and appropriate medical supervision.

PATIENTS WITH CHRONIC OBSTRUCTIVE PULMONARY DISEASE AND CORONARY ARTERY DISEASE

General principles of cardiac rehabilitation are applicable to patients with chronic obstructive pulmonary disease who have suffered a major cardiac event. Those who manifest resting or exercise-induced hypoxia (oxygen saturation less than 88 percent) should receive continuous supplemental oxygen during training sessions. High-risk individuals should be monitored closely in supervised programs and are not candidates for home-based programs.[149] These patients demonstrate less improvement in peak Vo_2 than those participating in cardiac rehabilitation.

Cardiovascular Rehabilitation in Patients with Diabetes Mellitus (see Chap. 63)

Ninety percent of all diabetics manifest insulin resistance as a primary metabolic derangement.[150] These type II diabetics manifest a high prevalence of hypertension, dyslipidemia, abdominal obesity, and endothelial dysfunction, all remedial by weight loss and exercise. Thus cardiac rehabilitation is particularly beneficial in this high-risk population.

In addition to standard pharmacological intervention,

▼ TABLE 39–4. AGE-ASSOCIATED CHANGES IN THE PHYSIOLOGICAL RESPONSE TO AEROBIC EXERCISE

Reduced aerobic capacity—a decline in maximum oxygen consumption of 8–10% per yr in nontrained populations
Reduced maximum heart rate of 1 beat/min/yr
More rapid increase in systolic blood pressure with exercise
Attenuated elevation in left ventricular ejection fraction

comprehensive cardiac rehabilitation is an important intervention for diabetics after major coronary events. Because of the far-ranging benefits of weight loss and exercise on the atherogenic physiology of insulin resistance, this population is particularly well suited for exercise training, behavioral counseling, and risk factor modification. Their increased risk of cardiovascular events suggests that supervised programs may be more appropriate following acute coronary events. Several unique features of this population warrant consideration during exercise training.

The adrenergic response to exercise can exacerbate hyperglycemia in suboptimally treated diabetics. Conversely, patients treated with insulin or sulfonylurea medications can experience hypoglycemia during or after exercise.[151] Monitoring blood sugar before and after exercise is an important tool during exercise training. Results should be used to tailor therapy, educate and reassure patients, and ensure safety during training sessions.[152] If preexercise glucose levels are less than 100 mg/dl, oral glucose should be administered before exercising. Fruit, a starch, or 4 to 5 gm of oral glucose tablets is recommended.[151] Emergency equipment, including glucose tablets or gels and glucagon injection kits, should be readily available to treat hypoglycemic episodes. Recurrent episodes of hypoglycemia should lead to downward adjustment of preexercise sulfonylurea or insulin doses or prompt ingestion of carbohydrate before exercise. Evening exercise sessions can occasionally induce early morning hypoglycemia and necessitate bedtime snacks or a change in the timing of exercise sessions.

To avoid excessive hyperglycemia, exercise should be avoided in the setting of poor glycemic control. If preexercise finger-stick glucose levels exceed 300 mg/dl (or if lesser degrees of hyperglycemia are present in the setting of ketonuria), exercise should be postponed until glycemic control has improved.[151]

DIABETIC NEUROPATHY. Somatic neuropathy puts patients at risk for cutaneous and orthopedic injury during exercise. As many as 22 percent of diabetics with somatic neuropathy and cutaneous foot ulcers have radiographic evidence of foot fractures, often asymptomatic.[153] Screening for sensory deficits, cutaneous lesions, ingrown toenails, or foot deformities is an important part of intake evaluation for exercise rehabilitation programs. Patients with sensory deficits should be coached in regular foot examination before and after exercise. Proper athletic footwear, with orthotics when appropriate, is essential to minimize the risk of injury. Patients with severe neuropathy, including those with Charcot joints, should pursue non–weight-bearing exercises such as swimming, bicycling, rowing, and arm or chair calisthenics.[154]

Exercise training in patients with autonomic neuropathy should be conducted to minimize the adverse consequences of orthostatic hypotension, silent ischemia, and arrhythmia. Patients should be adequately hydrated before exercise. They should avoid exercising after meals or during the morning when orthostatic hypotension is more likely. They should adjust doses or the timing of antihypertensive medications to minimize orthostatic hypotension during or after exercise and avoid vasodilation caused by environmental heat or ethanol ingestion during training sessions. They should use compressive stockings when appropriate and exercise in a supervised setting with ECG monitoring and resuscitative equipment in the early stages after an acute coronary event.[151]

Targets for exercise should be predicated on perceived exertion rather than the heart rate in patients with autonomic neuropathy because of decreased maximum heart rates and resting tachycardia. Moderate levels of perceived exertion should be sought over 2 to 4 weeks of gradual training.[154]

Patients with nonproliferative retinopathy can engage in most forms of exercise with minimal risk of progressive disease. However, most authorities suggest limiting diabetics with severe nonproliferative retinopathy in a similar fashion to those with proliferative disease.[155, 156]

Psychological Factors in Cardiovascular Rehabilitation (see Chap. 70)

RISK FACTORS. The concept that mental stress contributes to CAD pathogenesis or events seems logical. Blood pressure and serum lipids increase with mental stress. Factors promoting thrombosis, decreased endothelial-dependent vasodilation, and paradoxical coronary artery constriction during mental stress have also been identified.[157, 158] However, the type A personality concept and its relationship to CAD remain controversial.[159]

Several studies have indicated that depression often precedes acute myocardial infarction. More commonly, depression begins during hospitalization for the infarction and is first noticed by the patient, family members, and/or caregivers upon the patient's return home.[160] Patients with major depression have a fivefold increase in mortality in the first 6 months following myocardial infarction, and even those with mild depression exhibit increased risk.[161, 162]

PREVENTIVE MEASURES. Cardiac rehabilitation programs improve anxiety and depression in the short term, but proof of long-term benefit is lacking.[163] One 4-month, randomized trial of aerobic exercise, stress management, or standard medical therapy showed a statistically significant 74 percent reduction in cardiac events in the stress management group. Although the patients randomized to the exercise limb improved their aerobic conditioning and lost weight, their risk of cardiac events was not statistically different from that of the standard medical therapy group.[164] However, a meta-analysis of 23 randomized controlled trials concluded that the addition of psychological treatment to standard cardiac rehabilitation programs reduces mortality and morbidity the first 2 years after treatment.[165]

Practical approaches include vigorous measures to encourage and enable patients to return to work[166] because return to work often provides reassurance, helps focus attention away from health problems, and may address the concern that low-income patients have higher mortality after myocardial infarction.[167] Experienced clinicians frequently recount having seen widows or widowers who themselves die shortly after returning home from hospitalization for acute myocardial infarction within months of the death of their spouse. Attempts should also be made to have patients avoid social isolation inasmuch as those living alone after myocardial infarction seem to have higher mortality than those who do not live alone.[168]

Clearly, the cardiac rehabilitation and secondary prevention clinic is most appropriate to address the psychological needs of cardiac patients. These issues need to be dealt with openly and with great sensitivity on the part of all concerned. As the psychological contributions to CAD are better refined, more explicit guidelines will be feasible.

Compliance with Rehabilitation Programs

A recent review of studies regarding physical activity interventions and compliance in health care settings included 12 studies in apparently healthy subjects and 24 randomized studies in patients with cardiovascular disease.[169] Only about half of the programs were successful in increasing physical activity or cardiorespiratory training in their subjects. Characteristics of successful interventions included long-term sustained intervention and multiple contacts, supervised exercise (such as in a cardiac rehabilitation program), provision of exercise equipment, and behavioral approaches. Importantly, the behavioral component fostered subject selection of an enjoyable activity, as well as setting realistic goals, identifying barriers, problem solving, self-monitoring, providing feedback and positive reinforcement, and enhancing social support.[170] Continuing intervention and behavioral approaches have been shown to increase activity levels in CAD patients for as long as 4 to 5 years.[171, 172]

One approach to promote an increase in physical activity is for exercise to begin slowly and then gradually progress to the recommended exercise prescription, with assessment of success and reinforcement provided regularly. Patients can begin at a more moderate intensity, shorter duration, and lower frequency than the ultimate goal. Not only are gradual increases in activity safer for sedentary people and for patients with CAD, but short-term successes may also increase the patient's self efficacy in being physically active.[173] The health care provider can use this positive outcome for feedback and reinforcement. Such an approach requires repeated follow-up visits. The most effective interventions—those with multiple components and a continued maintenance intervention—can be delivered via a model in which physicians provide advice and other members of the health care team provide more in-depth behavioral counseling and follow-up.[174]

For successful implementation of physical activity counseling in a health care setting, a coordinated, multilevel intervention should encompass strategies directed toward the practice environment, patients, and providers.[175] Systematic delivery of a counseling program might be enhanced through the use of encounter forms[176] and case management systems.[177] In addition, achieving greater implementation of physical activity interventions in health care settings will require improved education and training of health professionals and attention to health care policy and reimbursement issues. The cardiac rehabilitation setting is an excellent milieu in which to use the aforementioned modalities to implement physical activity and improve compliance in a motivated population.

Cost-Effectiveness of Cardiac Rehabilitation (see Chap. 2)

A comprehensive economic analysis of cardiac rehabilitation and secondary prevention includes not only the direct costs of the cardiac rehabilitation intervention but also indirect costs and cost savings attributed to treatment benefits. In addition to the expense of the cardiac rehabilitation program and exercise tests, diminished work time while attending the program, transportation, rehospitalization, costs of medical disability, and the medical and pension costs of enhanced longevity must be considered.[178] A number of studies have addressed these issues, but unfortunately, no single study is comprehensive, randomized, and controlled. Furthermore, studies performed in one area or region or in one country are not necessarily relevant in another area or country because of variations in health plans, differences in incentives to return to work, and wide diversity in management "styles" and the availability of revascularization procedures.

One method shown to be effective 3 weeks after myocardial infarction is the performance of an "occupational work evaluation." This intervention consists of an exercise test and advice about exercise with specific recommendations for early return to work in patients stratified by the exercise test to a low-risk category.[179] When compared with a usual care control group, patients randomized to the intervention had an earlier return to work with an average increase in individual earnings of $2100 over a 6-month period. They also realized a decrease of $500 per patient in total medical costs during follow-up.

Several investigations from Sweden and the United States have evaluated the effect of cardiac rehabilitation participation on subsequent rehospitalization and cost. In an American study, the authors investigated the effect of cardiac rehabilitation on subsequent rehospitalization cost in 580 patients over a mean follow-up period of 21 months.[180] In the rehabilitation group, per capita charges for cardiac rehospitalizations were $739 lower than in control patients. The cost difference was explained by both fewer hospitalizations and lower cost per hospitalization in the cardiac rehabilitation intervention group. Of note, admissions for evaluation of chest pain decreased by 42 percent.

The results of three controlled trials from Sweden further support decreased health care cost after cardiac rehabilitation.[181–183] In an initial study of 147 coronary bypass patients, hospital readmissions over a 1-year period were reduced by 62 percent in the comprehensive cardiac rehabilitation group.[183] Another controlled trial of 190 patients 65 years of age or older after myocardial infarction defined the effects of a nurse-managed education program lasting 4 months and low-intensity exercise training of 8 weeks' duration.[182] This program resulted in lower rates of rehospitalization (32 vs. 47 percent) over a 1-year period and significantly fewer visits to the emergency department.

The most detailed economic evaluation to date compared comprehensive cardiac rehabilitation (exercise and risk factor modification) with usual care in 305 nonselected myocardial infarction patients over a 5-year period.[181] In addition to a lower rate of total cardiac events (39 vs. 53 percent), the average total duration of in-hospital care was reduced from 16.1 to 10.7 days in the intervention group. The authors concluded that the actual cost of rehabilitation was balanced over the 5-year period by the decrease in hospital readmissions for cardiovascular disease. They also noted that cardiac rehabilitation patients had a higher 5-year return-to-work rate (43 vs. 38 percent). Increased work productivity (i.e., less disability and sick leave) resulted in $12,250 savings per patient to the Swedish disability system.

Finally, a randomized trial of an 8-week cardiac rehabilitation intervention that focused on anxious or depressed patients after myocardial infarction noted a cost-effectiveness of $9200 per quality-adjusted life year,[184] similar to the cost-effectiveness of well-established medical interventions such as coronary bypass surgery for left main coronary disease and beta-adrenergic blockers after myocardial infarction. It is more cost-effective than other accepted practices such as ACE inhibitors for the treatment of hypertension and lovastatin for hypercholesterolemia.[185] Therefore, limited data support the cost-effectiveness of cardiac rehabilitation in the care of patients after a coronary event.

REFERENCES

1. Gibbons RJ, Chatterjee K, Daley J, et al: ACC/AHA/ACP-ASIM guidelines for the management of patients with chronic stable angina: A report of the American College of Cardiology/American Heart Association Task Force on Practice Guidelines. J Am Coll Cardiol 33:2092–2197, 1999.
2. Gillum RF: Trends in acute myocardial infarction and coronary heart disease death in the United States. J Am Coll Cardiol 23:1273–1277, 1994.
3. Goldberg RJ, Yarzebski J, Lessard D, Gore JM: A two-decades (1975 to 1995) long experience in the incidence, in-hospital and long-term case-fatality rates of acute myocardial infarction: A community-wide perspective. J Am Coll Cardiol 33:1533–1539, 1999.
4. Smith SC Jr, Blair SN, Criqui MH, et al: Preventing heart attack and death in patients with coronary disease. Circulation 92:2–4, 1995.
4a. Kavanagh T, Shepard RJ, Hamm LF, et al: Risk profile and health awareness in male offspring of parents with premature coronary heart disease. J Cardiopulm Rehabil 20:172–179, 1990.
4b. O'Farrel P, Murray J, Huston P, et al: Sex differences in cardiac rehabilitation. Can J Cardiol 16:319–325, 2000.
5. Frances CD, Go AS, Dauterman KW, et al: Outcome following acute myocardial infarction: Are differences among physician specialties the result of quality of care or case mix? Arch Intern Med 159:1429–1436, 1999.
6. DeBusk RF, Miller NH, Superko HR, et al: A case-management system for coronary risk factor modification after acute myocardial infarction. Ann Intern Med 120:721–729, 1994.
7. Convertino V, Hung J, Goldwater D, DeBusk RF: Cardiovascular responses to exercise in middle-aged men after 10 days of bedrest. Circulation 65:134–140, 1982.

8. Dittmer DK, Teasell R: Complications of immobilization and bed rest. Part 1: Musculoskeletal and cardiovascular complications. Can Fam Physician 39:1428–1432, 1435–1437, 1993.

9. Ryder RE, Hayes TM, Mulligan IP, et al: How soon after myocardial infarction should plasma lipid values be assessed? BMJ 289:1651–1653, 1984.

10. Cunningham MJ, Boucher TM, McCabe CH, et al: Changes in total cholesterol and high-density lipoprotein cholesterol in men after coronary artery bypass grafting. Am J Cardiol 60:1393–1394, 1987.

10a. Drory Y, Kravetz S, Weingarten M: Comparison of sexual activity of women and men after a first acute myocardial infarction. Am J Cardiol 85:1283–1287, 2000.

11. Dracup K, Alonzo AA, Atkins JM, et al: The physician's role in minimizing prehospital delay in patients at high risk for acute myocardial infarction: Recommendations from the National Heart Attack Alert Program. Working Group on Educational Strategies to Prevent Prehospital Delay in Patients at High Risk for Acute Myocardial Infarction. Ann Intern Med 126:645–651, 1997.

12. Fields KB: Myocardial infarction and denial. J Fam Pract 28:157–161, 1989.

13. Meischke H, Eisenberg MS, Larsen MP: Prehospital delay interval for patients who use emergency medical services: The effect of heart-related medical conditions and demographic variables. Ann Emerg Med 22:1597–1601, 1993.

14. Alonzo AA: The impact of the family and lay others on care-seeking during life-threatening episodes of suspected coronary artery disease. Soc Sci Med 22:1297–1311, 1986.

15. Alonzo AA, Reynolds NR: The structure of emotions during acute myocardial infarction: A model of coping. Soc Sci Med 46:1099–1110, 1998.

15a. Heffner JE, Barbieri C: End-of-life care preferences of patients enrolled in cardiovascular rehabilitation programs. Chest 117:1474–1481, 2000.

16. Fletcher GF, Balady G, Froelicher VF, et al: Exercise standards. A statement for healthcare professionals from the American Heart Association Writing Group. Circulation 91:580–615, 1995.

17. Ades PA, Pashkow FJ, Fletcher G, et al: A controlled trial of cardiac rehabilitation in the home setting using electrocardiographic and voice transtelephonic monitoring. Am Heart J 139:543–548, 2000.

17a. Brubaker PH, Regeski WJ, Smith MJ, et al: A home-based exercise program after center-based cardiac rehabilitation: effects on blood lipids, body composition, and functional capacity. J Cardiopulm Rehabil 20:50–56, 2000.

EXERCISE PHYSIOLOGY

18. Bevegard S, Holmgren A, Jonsson B: Circulatory studies in well-trained athletes at rest and during heavy exercise, with special reference to stroke volume and the influence of body position. Acta Physiol Scand 57:26, 1963.

19. Rowell LB: Human Cardiovascular Control. New York, Oxford University Press, 1993.

20. Musch TI, Haidet GC, Ordway GA, et al: Training effects on regional blood flow response to maximal exercise in foxhounds. J Appl Physiol 62:1724–1732, 1987.

21. Thomas SN, Schroeder T, Secher NH, Mitchell JH: Cerebral blood flow during submaximal and maximal dynamic exercise in humans. J Appl Physiol 67:744–748, 1989.

22. Pescatello LS, Fargo AE, Leach CN Jr, Scherzer HH: Short-term effect of dynamic exercise on arterial blood pressure. Circulation 83:1557–1561, 1991.

23. Bechuza GR, Lenser MC, Hanson PG, Nagle FJ: Comparison of hemodynamic responses to static and dynamic exercise. J Appl Physiol 53:1589–1593, 1982.

24. Rowell LB: Human cardiovascular adjustments to exercise and thermal stress. Physiol Rev 54:75–159, 1974.

Efficacy of Cardiac Rehabilitation

25. Leon A: Position paper of the American Society of Cardiovascular and Pulmonary Rehabilitation: Scientific evidence of the value of cardiac rehabilitation services with emphasis on patients following myocardial infarction, section I: Exercise conditioning component. J Cardiopulm Rehabil 10:79–87, 1990.

26. O'Connor GT, Buring JE, Yusuf S, et al: An overview of randomized trials of rehabilitation with exercise after myocardial infarction. Circulation 80:234–244, 1989.

27. Brand RJ, Paffenbarger RS Jr, Sholtz RI, Kampert JB: Work activity and fatal heart attack studied by multiple logistic risk analysis. Am J Epidemiol 110:52–62, 1979.

28. Dorn J, Naughton J, Imamura D, Trevisan M: Results of a multicenter randomized clinical trial of exercise and long-term survival in myocardial infarction patients: The National Exercise and Heart Disease Project (NEHDP). Circulation 100:1764–1769, 1999.

29. Oldridge NB, Guyatt GH, Fischer ME, Rimm AA: Cardiac rehabilitation after myocardial infarction. Combined experience of randomized clinical trials. JAMA 260:945–950, 1988.

29a. Kavanagh T: Exercise in cardiac rehabilitation. Br J Sports Med 34:3, 2000.

29b. Carlson JJ, Johnson JA, Franklin BA, VanderLaan RL: Program participation, exercise adherence, cardiovascular outcomes, and program cost of traditional versus modified cardiac rehabilitation. Am J Cardiol 1:17–23, 2000.

29c. Morrin L, Black S, Reid R: Impact of duration in a cardiac rehabilitation program on coronary risk profile and health-related quality of life outcomes. J Cardiopulm Rehabil 20:115, 2000.

29d. Ades PA, Coello CE: Effects of exercise and cardiac rehabilitation on cardiovascular outcomes. Med Clin North Am 84:251–265, 2000.

29e. Leon AS: Exercise following myocardial infarction. Current recommendations. Sports Med 29:301–311, 2000.

30. Schuler G, Hambrecht R, Schlierf G, et al: Myocardial perfusion and regression of coronary artery disease in patients on a regimen of intensive physical exercise and low fat diet. J Am Coll Cardiol 19:34–42, 1992.

31. Niebauer J, Hambrecht R, Velich T, et al: Attenuated progression of coronary artery disease after 6 years of multifactorial risk intervention: Role of physical exercise. Circulation 96:2534–2541, 1997.

32. Oberman A, Fletcher GF, Lee J, et al: Efficacy of high-intensity exercise training on left ventricular ejection fraction in men with coronary artery disease (the Training Level Comparison Study). Am J Cardiol 76:643–647, 1995.

33. Giannuzzi P, Tavazzi L, Temporelli PL, et al: Long-term physical training and left ventricular remodeling after anterior myocardial infarction: Results of the Exercise in Anterior Myocardial Infarction (EAMI) trial. EAMI Study Group. J Am Coll Cardiol 22:1821–1829, 1993.

34. Giannuzzi P, Temporelli PL, Corra U, et al: Attenuation of unfavorable remodeling by exercise training in postinfarction patients with left ventricular dysfunction: Results of the Exercise in Left Ventricular Dysfunction (ELVD) trial. Circulation 96:1790–1797, 1997.

35. Dubach P, Myers J, Dziekan G, et al: Effect of exercise training on myocardial remodeling in patients with reduced left ventricular function after myocardial infarction: Application of magnetic resonance imaging. Circulation 95:2060–2067, 1997.

Secondary Prevention

36. Hirsh J: Aspirin and other platelet-active drugs. Chest 108:2475–2575, 1995.

37. Pepine CJ: Aspirin and newer orally active antiplatelet agents in the treatment of the post-myocardial infarction patient. J Am Coll Cardiol 32:1126–1128, 1998.

38. Deedwania PC, Amsterdam EA, Vagelos RH: Evidence-based, cost-effective risk stratification and management after myocardial infarction. California Cardiology Working Group on Post-MI Management. Arch Intern Med 157:273–280, 1997.

39. Kjekshus J, Gilpin E, Cali G, et al: Diabetic patients and beta-blockers after acute myocardial infarction. Eur Heart J 11:43–50, 1990.

40. Kober L, Torp-Pedersen C, Jorgensen S, et al: Changes in absolute and relative importance in the prognostic value of left ventricular systolic function and congestive heart failure after acute myocardial infarction. TRACE Study Group. Trandolapril Cardiac Evaluation. Am J Cardiol 81:1292–1297, 1998.

41. Garg R, Yusuf S: Overview of randomized trials of angiotensin-converting enzyme inhibitors on mortality and morbidity in patients with heart failure. Collaborative Group on ACE Inhibitor Trials. JAMA 273:1450–1456, 1995.

42. Pfeffer MA: ACE inhibitors in acute myocardial infarction: Patient selection and timing (editorial). Circulation 97:2192–2194, 1998.

43. Indications for ACE inhibitors in the early treatment of acute myocardial infarction: Systematic overview of individual data from 100,000 patients in randomized trials. ACE Inhibitor Myocardial Infarction Collaborative Group. Circulation 97:2202–2212, 1998.

44. Torp-Pedersen C, Kober L: Effect of ACE inhibitor trandolapril on life expectancy of patients with reduced left-ventricular function after acute myocardial infarction. TRACE Study Group. Trandolapril Cardiac Evaluation. Lancet 354:9–12, 1999.

45. Ryan TJ, Anderson JL, Antman EM, et al: ACC/AHA guidelines for the management of patients with acute myocardial infarction. A report of the American College of Cardiology/American Heart Association Task Force on Practice Guidelines (Committee on Management of Acute Myocardial Infarction). J Am Coll Cardiol 28:1328–1428, 1996.

46. Pfeffer MA, Lamas GA, Vaughan DE, et al: Effect of captopril on progressive ventricular dilatation after anterior myocardial infarction. N Engl J Med 319:80–86, 1988.

47. Effect of enalapril on mortality and the development of heart failure in asymptomatic patients with reduced left ventricular ejection fractions. The SOLVD Investigators. N Engl J Med 327:685–691, 1992.

48. Pfeffer MA, Domanski M, Rosenberg Y, et al: Prevention of events with angiotensin-converting enzyme inhibition (the PEACE study design). Prevention of Events with Angiotensin-Converting Enzyme Inhibition. Am J Cardiol 82:25H–30H, 1998.

49. The HOPE (Heart Outcomes Prevention Evaluation) Study: The design of a large, simple randomized trial of an angiotensin-converting enzyme inhibitor (ramipril) and vitamin E in patients at high risk of cardiovascular events. The HOPE study investigators. Can J Cardiol 12:127–137, 1996.

50. Bosch J, Yusuf S, Mann J, et al: Oral presentations of Heart Outcome Prevention Evaluation (HOPE) Study data. In European Society of Cardiology Annual Scientific Sessions. Barcelona, Spain, 1999 (unpublished).

51. Deedwania PC: Anti-ischemic properties of ACE-inhibitors. Cardiologia 41:209–215, 1996.

52. Brown NJ, Vaughan DE: Angiotensin-converting enzyme inhibitors. Circulation 97:1411–1420, 1998.

53. Mancini GB, Henry GC, Macaya C, et al: Angiotensin-converting enzyme inhibition with quinapril improves endothelial vasomotor dysfunction in patients with coronary artery disease. The TREND (Trial on Reversing Endothelial Dysfunction) study. Circulation 94:258–265, 1996.

54. O'Driscoll G, Green D, Maiorana A, et al: Improvement in endothelial function by angiotensin-converting enzyme inhibition in non–insulin-dependent diabetes mellitus. J Am Coll Cardiol 33:1506–1511, 1999.

55. Rutherford JD, Pfeffer MA, Moye LA, et al: Effects of captopril on ischemic events after myocardial infarction. Results of the Survival and Ventricular Enlargement trial. SAVE Investigators. Circulation 90:1731–1738, 1994.

56. Stafford RS, Saglam D, Blumenthal D: National patterns of angiotensin-converting enzyme inhibitor use in congestive heart failure. Arch Intern Med 157:2460–2464, 1997.

57. Philbin EF: Factors determining angiotensin-converting enzyme inhibitor underutilization in heart failure in a community setting. Clin Cardiol 21:103–108, 1998.

58. Grundy SM, Balady GJ, Criqui MH, et al: When to start cholesterol-lowering therapy in patients with coronary heart disease. A statement for healthcare professionals from the American Heart Association Task Force on Risk Reduction. Circulation 95:1683–1685, 1997.

59. Grundy SM: Statin trials and goals of cholesterol-lowering therapy (editorial). Circulation 97:1436–1439, 1998.

60. National Cholesterol Education Program: Second Report of the Expert Panel on Detection, Evaluation, and Treatment of High Blood Cholesterol in Adults (Adult Treatment Panel II). Circulation 89:1333–1445, 1994.

61. Kaesemeyer WH, Caldwell RB, Huang J, Caldwell RW: Pravastatin sodium activates endothelial nitric oxide synthase independent of its cholesterol-lowering actions. J Am Coll Cardiol 33:234–241, 1999.

62. Ridker PM, Rifai N, Pfeffer MA, et al: Inflammation, pravastatin, and the risk of coronary events after myocardial infarction in patients with average cholesterol levels. Cholesterol and Recurrent Events (CARE) Investigators. Circulation 98:839–844, 1998.

63. Rosenson RS, Tangney CC: Antiatherothrombotic properties of statins: Implications for cardiovascular event reduction. JAMA 279:1643–1650, 1998.

64. Szczeklik A, Musial J, Undas A, et al: Inhibition of thrombin generation by simvastatin and lack of additive effects of aspirin in patients with marked hypercholesterolemia. J Am Coll Cardiol 33:1286–1293, 1999.

65. Amsterdam EA, Deedwania PC: A perspective on hyperlipidemia: Concepts of management in the prevention of coronary artery disease. Am J Med 105(Suppl):69–74, 1998.

66. Hensrud DD, Engle DD, Scheitel SM: Underreporting the use of dietary supplements and nonprescription medications among patients undergoing a periodic health examination. Mayo Clin Proc 74:443–447, 1999.

67. Benowitz NL, Gourlay SG: Cardiovascular toxicity of nicotine: Implications for nicotine replacement therapy. J Am Coll Cardiol 29:1422–1431, 1997.

68. Doll R, Peto R: Mortality in relation to smoking: 20 years' observations on male British doctors. BMJ 2:1525–1536, 1976.

69. Cavender JB, Rogers WJ, Fisher LD, et al: Effects of smoking on survival and morbidity in patients randomized to medical or surgical therapy in the Coronary Artery Surgery Study (CASS): 10-year follow-up. CASS Investigators. J Am Coll Cardiol 20:287–294, 1992.

70. Howard G, Wagenknecht LE, Burke GL, et al: Cigarette smoking and progression of atherosclerosis: The Atherosclerosis Risk in Communities (ARIC) Study. JAMA 279:119–124, 1998.

71. Moise A, Theroux P, Taeymans Y, Waters DD: Factors associated with progression of coronary artery disease in patients with normal or minimally narrowed coronary arteries. Am J Cardiol 56:30–34, 1985.

72. Campeau L, Enjalbert M, Lesperance J, et al: The relation of risk factors to the development of atherosclerosis in saphenous-vein bypass grafts and the progression of disease in the native circulation. A study 10 years after aortocoronary bypass surgery. N Engl J Med 311:1329–1332, 1984.

73. Rosenberg L, Kaufman DW, Helmrich SP, Shapiro S: The risk of myocardial infarction after quitting smoking in men under 55 years of age. N Engl J Med 313:1511–1514, 1985.

74. Rosenberg L, Palmer JR, Shapiro S: Decline in the risk of myocardial infarction among women who stop smoking. N Engl J Med 322:213–217, 1990.

75. Dale LC, Hurt RD, Hays JT: Drug therapy to aid in smoking cessation. Tips on maximizing patients' chances for success. Postgrad Med 104:75–78, 83–84, 1998.

76. Mahmarian JJ, Moye LA, Nasser GA, et al: Nicotine patch therapy in smoking cessation reduces the extent of exercise-induced myocardial ischemia. J Am Coll Cardiol 30:125–130, 1997.

77. Croghan IT, Offord KP, Evans RW, et al: Cost-effectiveness of treating nicotine dependence: The Mayo Clinic experience. Mayo Clin Proc 72:917–924, 1997.

78. Marcus BH, Albrecht AE, King TK, et al: The efficacy of exercise as an aid for smoking cessation in women: A randomized controlled trial. Arch Intern Med 159:1229–1234, 1999.

79. The Agency for Health Care Policy and Research Smoking Cessation Clinical Practice Guideline. JAMA 275:1270–1280, 1996.

80. Ockene IS, Miller NH: Cigarette smoking, cardiovascular disease, and stroke: A statement for healthcare professionals from the American Heart Association. American Heart Association Task Force on Risk Reduction. Circulation 96:3243–3247, 1997.

81. Rose JE: Nicotine addiction and treatment. Annu Rev Med 47:493–507, 1996.

HEART FAILURE

82. Piepoli MF, Flather M, Coats AJ: Overview of studies of exercise training in chronic heart failure: The need for a prospective randomized multicentre European trial. Eur Heart J 19:830–841, 1998.

83. Guyatt G: A 75-year-old man with congestive heart failure (clinical conference). JAMA 281:2321–2328, 1999.

84. Franciosa JA, Park M, Levine TB: Lack of correlation between exercise capacity and indexes of resting left ventricular performance in heart failure. Am J Cardiol 47:33–39, 1981.

85. Massie BM: Exercise tolerance in congestive heart failure. Role of cardiac function, peripheral blood flow, and muscle metabolism and effect of treatment. Am J Med 84:75–82, 1988.

86. Duscha BD, Kraus WE, Keteyian SJ, et al: Capillary density of skeletal muscle: A contributing mechanism for exercise intolerance in class II–III chronic heart failure independent of other peripheral alterations. J Am Coll Cardiol 33:1956–1963, 1999.

87. Coats AJ, Adamopoulos S, Radaelli A, et al: Controlled trial of physical training in chronic heart failure. Exercise performance, hemodynamics, ventilation, and autonomic function. Circulation 85:2119–2131, 1992.

88. Faggiano P, D'Aloia A, Gualeni A, Giordano A: Hemodynamic profile of submaximal constant workload exercise in patients with heart failure secondary to ischemic or idiopathic dilated cardiomyopathy. Am J Cardiol 81:437–442, 1998.

89. Wilson JR, Groves J, Rayos G: Circulatory status and response to cardiac rehabilitation in patients with heart failure. Circulation 94:1567–1572, 1996.

90. Stevenson LW, Steimle AE, Fonarow G, et al: Improvement in exercise capacity of candidates awaiting heart transplantation. J Am Coll Cardiol 25:163–170, 1995.

91. Belardinelli R, Georgiou D, Cianci G, Purcaro A: Randomized, controlled trial of long-term moderate exercise training in chronic heart failure: Effects on functional capacity, quality of life, and clinical outcome. Circulation 99:1173–1182, 1999.

92. Coats AJ: Exercise training for heart failure: Coming of age (editorial). Circulation 99:1138–1140, 1999.

93. Wenger NK, Froelicher ES, Smith LK: Cardiac Rehabilitation: Clinical Practice Guideline No 17. Rockville, MD, Public Health Service, October 1995.

94. Pina IL: Exercise training in special populations: Heart failure and post-transplantation patients. In Wenger NK, Smith LK, Froelicher ES, et al (eds): Cardiac Rehabilitation: A Guide to Practice in the 21st Century. 38th ed. Fundamental and Clinical Cardiology. New York, Marcel Dekker, 1999, pp 127–149.

95. Kobashigawa JA, Leaf DA, Lee N, et al: A controlled trial of exercise rehabilitation after heart transplantation. N Engl J Med 340:272–277, 1999.

96. Keteyian S, Shepard R, Ehrman J, et al: Cardiovascular responses of heart transplant patients to exercise training. J Appl Physiol 70:2627–2631, 1991.

97. Ehrman J, Keteyian S, Fedel F, et al: Ventilatory threshold after exercise training in orthotopic heart transplant recipients. J Cardiopulm Rehabil 12:126–130, 1992.

98. Quigg R, Salyer J, Mohanty PK, Simpson P: Impaired exercise capacity late after cardiac transplantation: Influence of chronotropic incompetence, hypertension, and calcium channel blockers. Am Heart J 136:465–473, 1998.

99. Kao AC, Van Trigt P 3rd, Shaeffer-McCall GS, et al: Central and peripheral limitations to upright exercise in untrained cardiac transplant recipients. Circulation 89:2605–2615, 1994.

100. Givertz MM, Hartley LH, Colucci WS: Long-term sequential changes in exercise capacity and chronotropic responsiveness after cardiac transplantation. Circulation 96:232–237, 1997.

101. Quigg RJ, Rocco MB, Gauthier DF, et al: Mechanism of the attenuated peak heart rate response to exercise after orthotopic cardiac transplantation. J Am Coll Cardiol 14:338–344, 1989.

102. Toba M, Ishida Y, Fukuchi K, et al: Sympathetic reinnervation demonstrated on serial iodine-123-metaiodobenzylguanidine SPECT images after cardiac transplantation. J Nucl Med 39:1862–1864, 1998.

103. Stark RP, McGinn AL, Wilson RF: Chest pain in cardiac-transplant recipients. Evidence of sensory reinnervation after cardiac transplantation. N Engl J Med 324:1791–1794, 1991.

104. Lord SW, Brady S, Holt ND, et al: Exercise response after cardiac transplantation: Correlation with sympathetic reinnervation. Heart 75:40–43, 1996.

105. Mettauer B, Lampert E, Petitjean P, et al: Persistent exercise intolerance following cardiac transplantation despite normal oxygen transport. Int J Sports Med 17:277–286, 1996.

106. Bussieres LM, Pflugfelder PW, Taylor AW, et al: Changes in skeletal muscle morphology and biochemistry after cardiac transplantation. Am J Cardiol 79:630–634, 1997.

107. Braith RW, Limacher MC, Leggett SH, Pollock ML: Skeletal muscle strength in heart transplant recipients. J Heart Lung Transplant 12:1018–1023, 1993.
108. Squires RW: Cardiac rehabilitation issues for heart transplantation patients. J Cardiopulm Rehabil 10:159–168, 1990.
109. Borg G: Perceived exertion as an indicator of somatic stress. Scand J Rehabil Med 2:92–98, 1970.
110. Shephard RJ, Kavanagh T, Mertens DJ, Yacoub M: The place of perceived exertion ratings in exercise prescription for cardiac transplant patients before and after training. Br J Sports Med 30:116–121, 1996.
111. Carrel T, Mohacsi P: Optimal timing of rehabilitation after cardiac surgery: The surgeon's view. Eur Heart J 19(Suppl O):38–41, 1998.
112. Daida H, Allison TG, Squires RW, et al: Peak exercise blood pressure stratified by age and gender in apparently healthy subjects. Mayo Clin Proc 71:445–452, 1996.
112a. Brochu M, Poehlman ET, Ades P: Obesity, body fat distribution, and coronary artery disease. J Cardiopulm Rehabil 20:96–108, 2000.

Obese Patients

113. Schoeller DA, Shay K, Kushner RF: How much physical activity is needed to minimize weight gain in previously obese women? Am J Clin Nutr 66:551–556, 1997.
114. Blair SN: Evidence for success of exercise in weight loss and control. Ann Intern Med 119:702–706, 1993.
115. Wood PD, Stefanick ML, Williams PT, Haskell WL: The effects on plasma lipoproteins of a prudent weight-reducing diet, with or without exercise, in overweight men and women. N Engl J Med 325:461–466, 1991.
116. Troisi RJ, Heinold JW, Vokonas PS, Weiss ST: Cigarette smoking, dietary intake, and physical activity: Effects on body fat distribution—the Normative Aging Study. Am J Clin Nutr 53:1104–1111, 1991.

Elderly Patients

117. Elia EA: Exercise and the elderly. Clin Sports Med 10:141–155, 1991.
118. Brown M, Hollozsy JO: Effects of a low intensity exercise program on selected physical performance characteristics of 60- to 71-year-olds. Aging (Milano) 3:129–139, 1991.
119. King AC, Haskell WL, Taylor CB, et al: Group- vs home-based exercise training in healthy older men and women. A community-based clinical trial. JAMA 266:1535–1542, 1991.
120. Shephard RJ: Exercise and aging: Extending independence in older adults. Geriatrics 48:61–64, 1993.
121. Stewart AL, King AC, Haskell WL: Endurance exercise and health-related quality of life in 50–65-year-old adults. Gerontologist 33:782–789, 1993.
122. King AC, Haskell WL, Young DR, et al: Long-term effects of varying intensities and formats of physical activity on participation rates, fitness, and lipoproteins in men and women aged 50 to 65 years. Circulation 91:2596–2604, 1995.
123. Emery CF, Hauck ER, Blumenthal JA: Exercise adherence or maintenance among older adults: 1-year follow-up study. Psychol Aging 7:466–470, 1992.
123a. Marchionni N, Fattirolli F, Fumagalli S, et al: Determinants of exercise tolerance after acute myocardial infarction in older persons. J Am Geriatr Soc 48:146–153, 2000.
123b. Richardson LA, Buckenmeyer PJ, Bauman BD, et al: Contemporary cardiac rehabilitation: patient characteristics and temporal trends over the past decade. J Cardiopulm Rehabil 20:57–64, 2000.
124. Brown M, Holloszy JO: Effects of walking, jogging and cycling on strength, flexibility, speed and balance in 60- to 72-year-olds. Aging (Milano) 5:427–434, 1993.
125. McAuley E: Self-efficacy and the maintenance of exercise participation in older adults. J Behav Med 16:103–113, 1993.
126. Rogers MA, Evans WJ: Changes in skeletal muscle with aging: Effects of exercise training. Exerc Sport Sci Rev 21:365–379, 1993.
127. American College of Sports Medicine, Kenney WL, Humphrey RH, et al: ACSM's Guidelines for Exercise Testing and Prescription. 5th ed. Baltimore, Williams & Wilkins, 1995.
128. American College of Sports Medicine, Roitman JL, Kelsey M: ACSM's Resource Manual for Guidelines for Exercise Testing and Prescription. 3rd ed. Baltimore, Williams & Wilkins, 1998.
129. Williams MA, Maresh CM, Esterbrooks DJ, et al: Early exercise training in patients older than age 65 years compared with that in younger patients after acute myocardial infarction or coronary artery bypass grafting. Am J Cardiol 55:263–266, 1985.

Peripheral Vascular Disease

130. Burek KA, Sutton-Tyrrell K, Brooks MM, et al: Prognostic importance of lower extremity arterial disease in patients undergoing coronary revascularization in the bypass angioplasty revascularization investigation (BARI). J Am Coll Cardiol 34:716–721, 1999.
131. Criqui MH, Langer RD, Fronek A, et al: Mortality over a period of 10 years in patients with peripheral arterial disease. N Engl J Med 326:381–386, 1992.
132. Lavery LA, Armstrong DG, Vela SA, et al: Practical criteria for screen-ing patients at high risk for diabetic foot ulceration. Arch Intern Med 158:157–162, 1998.
133. Ekroth R, Dahllof AG, Gundevall B, et al: Physical training of patients with intermittent claudication: Indications, methods, and results. Surgery 84:640–643, 1978.
134. Girolami B, Bernardi E, Prins MH, et al: Treatment of intermittent claudication with physical training, smoking cessation, pentoxifylline, or nafronyl: A meta-analysis. Arch Intern Med 159:337–345, 1999.
135. Cameron HA, Waller PC, Ramsay LE: Drug treatment of intermittent claudication: A critical analysis of the methods and findings of published clinical trials, 1965–1985. Br J Clin Pharmacol 26:569–576, 1988.
136. Dawson DL, Cutler BS, Meissner MH, Strandness DE Jr: Cilostazol has beneficial effects in treatment of intermittent claudication: Results from a multicenter, randomized, prospective, double-blind trial. Circulation 98:678–686, 1998.
137. Patterson RB, Pinto B, Marcus B, et al: Value of a supervised exercise program for the therapy of arterial claudication. J Vasc Surg 25:312–319, 1997.
138. Regensteiner JG, Meyer TJ, Krupski WC, et al: Hospital vs home-based exercise rehabilitation for patients with peripheral arterial occlusive disease. Angiology 48:291–300, 1997.

End-Stage Renal Disease

139. Brynger H, Brunner FP, Chantler C, et al: Combined report on regular dialysis and transplantation in Europe. X, 1979. Proc Eur Dial Transplant Assoc 17:2–86, 1980.
140. Multicentre, cross-sectional study of ventricular arrhythmias in chronically haemodialysed patients. Gruppo Emodialisi e Patologie Cardiovasculari. Lancet 2:305–309, 1988.
141. Robertson D, Hollister AS, Biaggioni I, et al: The diagnosis and treatment of baroreflex failure. N Engl J Med 329:1449–1455, 1993.
142. Converse RL Jr, Jacobsen TN, Toto RD, et al: Sympathetic overactivity in patients with chronic renal failure. N Engl J Med 327:1912–1918, 1992.
143. Boudoulas H: Coronary arteries. In Leier CV, Boudoulas H (eds): Cardiorenal Diseases and Disorders. 2nd ed. Mt Kisco, NY, Futura, 1992, pp 31–47.
144. Capodaglio EM, Villa G, Jurisic D, Salvadeo A: Levels of sustainable aerobic workload in dialysis patients. Int J Artif Organs 21:391–397, 1998.
145. Lo CY, Li L, Lo WK, et al: Benefits of exercise training in patients on continuous ambulatory peritoneal dialysis. Am J Kidney Dis 32:1011–1018, 1998.
146. Frey S, Mir AR, Lucas M: Visceral protein status and caloric intake in exercising versus nonexercising individuals with end-stage renal disease. J Ren Nutr 9:71–77, 1999.
147. Cappy CS, Jablonka J, Schroeder ET: The effects of exercise during hemodialysis on physical performance and nutrition assessment. J Ren Nutr 9:63–70, 1999.
148. Moore GE, Painter PL, Brinker KR, et al: Cardiovascular response to submaximal stationary cycling during hemodialysis. Am J Kidney Dis 31:631–637, 1998.
149. Wijkstra PJ: Pulmonary rehabilitation at home (editorial). Thorax 51:117–118, 1996.

Diabetes Mellitus

150. National Institute of Diabetes and Digestive and Kidney Diseases: Diabetes Statistics. Bethesda, MD, NIH Publication No 99-3926, 1999.
151. Smith DA, Crandall J: Exercise training in special populations. In Wenger NK, Smith LK, Froelicher ES (eds): Cardiac Rehabilitation: A Guide to Practice in the 21st Century. 38th ed. Fundamental and Clinical Cardiology. New York, Marcel Dekker, 1999, pp 141–149.
152. Gordon NF: The exercise prescription. In Ruderman N, Devlin JT, American Diabetes Association (eds): The Health Professional's Guide to Diabetes and Exercise. Alexandria, VA, American Diabetes Association, 1995, pp 69–82.
153. Cavanaugh PR, Young MJ, Adams JE: Radiographic abnormalities in diabetic feet. In Boulton AJM, Connor H, Cavanagh PR (eds): The Foot in Diabetes. 2nd ed. Chichester, NY, John Wiley & Sons, 1994, pp 165–176.
154. Vinik AI: Neuropathy. In Ruderman N, Devlin JT, American Diabetes Association (eds): The Health Professional's Guide to Diabetes and Exercise. Alexandria, VA, American Diabetes Association, 1995, pp 181–198.
155. American Diabetes Association: Clinical practice recommendations; diabetes mellitus and exercise. Diabetes Care 21(Suppl):40–44, 1998.
156. Aiello L, Cavallevano J, Aiello LP: Retinopathy. In Ruderman N, Devlin JT, American Diabetes Association (eds): The Health Professional's Guide to Diabetes and Exercise. Alexandria, VA, American Diabetes Association, 1995, pp 143–151.

PSYCHOLOGICAL FACTORS

157. Blumenthal JA, Jiang W, Waugh RA, et al: Mental stress–induced ischemia in the laboratory and ambulatory ischemia during daily life.

Association and hemodynamic features. Circulation 92:2102–2108, 1995.

158. Gottdiener JS, Krantz DS, Howell RH, et al: Induction of silent myocardial ischemia with mental stress testing: Relation to the triggers of ischemia during daily life activities and to ischemic functional severity. J Am Coll Cardiol 24:1645–1651, 1994.

159. Friedman M, Thoresen CE, Gill JJ, et al: Alteration of type A behavior and its effect on cardiac recurrences in post myocardial infarction patients: Summary results of the recurrent coronary prevention project. Am Heart J 112:653–665, 1986.

160. Hackett TP, Cassem NH: The psychologic reaction of patients in the pre and post-hospital phases of myocardial infarction. Posgrad Med 57:43–46, 1975.

161. Frasure-Smith N, Lesperance F, Talajic M: Depression following myocardial infarction. Impact on 6-month survival. JAMA 270:1819–1825, 1993.

162. Frasure-Smith N, Lesperance F, Talajic M: Depression and 18-month prognosis after myocardial infarction. Circulation 91:999–1005, 1995.

163. Oldridge N, Guyatt G, Jones N, et al: Effects on quality of life with comprehensive rehabilitation after acute myocardial infarction. Am J Cardiol 67:1084–1089, 1991.

164. Blumenthal JA, Jiang W, Babyak MA, et al: Stress management and exercise training in cardiac patients with myocardial ischemia. Effects on prognosis and evaluation of mechanisms. Arch Intern Med 157:2213–2223, 1997.

165. Linden W, Stossel C, Maurice J: Psychosocial interventions for patients with coronary artery disease: A meta-analysis. Arch Intern Med 156:745–752, 1996.

166. Rost K, Smith GR: Return to work after an initial myocardial infarction and subsequent emotional distress. Arch Intern Med 152:381–385, 1992.

167. Williams RB, Barefoot JC, Califf RM, et al: Prognostic importance of social and economic resources among medically treated patients with angiographically documented coronary artery disease. JAMA 267:520–524, 1992.

168. Case RB, Moss AJ, Case N, et al: Living alone after myocardial infarction. Impact on prognosis. JAMA 267:515–519, 1992.

COMPLIANCE

169. Simons-Morton DG, Calfas KJ, Oldenburg B, Burton NW: Effects of interventions in health care settings on physical activity or cardiorespiratory fitness. Am J Prev Med 15:413–430, 1998.

170. King AC, Blair SN, Bild DE, et al: Determinants of physical activity and interventions in adults. Med Sci Sports Exerc 24(Suppl):221–236, 1992.

171. Haskell WL, Alderman EL, Fair JM, et al: Effects of intensive multiple risk factor reduction on coronary atherosclerosis and clinical cardiac events in men and women with coronary artery disease. The Stanford Coronary Risk Intervention Project (SCRIP). Circulation 89:975–990, 1994.

172. Niebauer J, Hambrecht R, Schlierf G, et al: Five years of physical exercise and low fat diet: Effects on progression of coronary artery disease. J Cardiopulm Rehabil 15:47–64, 1995.

173. McAuley E, Courneya KS, Rudolph DL, Lox CL: Enhancing exercise adherence in middle-aged males and females. Prev Med 23:498–506, 1994.

174. King AC, Sallis JF, Dunn AL, et al: Overview of the Activity Counseling Trial (ACT) intervention for promoting physical activity in primary health care settings. Activity Counseling Trial Research Group. Med Sci Sports Exerc 30:1086–1096, 1998.

175. Lomas J: Diffusion, dissemination, and implementation: Who should do what? Ann N Y Acad Sci 703:226–237, 1993.

176. Logsdon DN, Lazaro CM, Meier RV: The feasibility of behavioral risk reduction in primary medical care. Am J Prev Med 5:249–256, 1989.

177. DeBusk RF, Miller NH, Superko HR, et al: A case-management system for coronary risk factor modification after acute myocardial infarction. Ann Intern Med 120:721–729, 1994.

COST-EFFECTIVENESS

178. Ades PA: Decreased medical costs after cardiac rehabilitation: A case for universal reimbursement. J Cardiopulm Rehabil 13:75–77, 1993.

179. Dennis C, Houston-Miller N, Schwartz RG, et al: Early return to work after uncomplicated myocardial infarction. Results of a randomized trial. JAMA 260:214–220, 1988.

180. Ades PA, Huang D, Weaver SO: Cardiac rehabilitation participation predicts lower rehospitalization costs. Am Heart J 123:916–921, 1992.

181. Levin LA, Perk J, Hedback B: Cardiac rehabilitation—a cost analysis. J Intern Med 230:427–434, 1991.

182. Bondestam E, Breikss A, Hartford M: Effects of early rehabilitation on consumption of medical care during the first year after acute myocardial infarction in patients > or = 65 years of age. Am J Cardiol 75:767–771, 1995.

183. Perk J, Hedback B, Jutterdal S: Cardiac rehabilitation: Evaluation of a long-term programme of physical training for out-patients. Scand J Rehabil Med 21:13–17, 1989.

184. Oldridge N, Furlong W, Feeny D, et al: Economic evaluation of cardiac rehabilitation soon after acute myocardial infarction. Am J Cardiol 72:154–161, 1993.

185. Kupersmith J, Holmes-Rovner M, Hogan A, et al: Cost-effectiveness analysis in heart disease, Part III: Ischemia, congestive heart failure, and arrhythmias. Prog Cardiovasc Dis 37:307–346, 1995.

Chapter 40

Diseases of the Aorta

ERIC M. ISSELBACHER

THE NORMAL AORTA

FUNCTION

Appropriately called "the greatest artery" by the ancients, the aorta is admirably suited for its task. In an average lifetime, this thin but large and remarkably tough vessel must absorb the impact of 2.3 to 3 billion heartbeats while carrying roughly 200 million liters of blood through the body. Arteries can be categorized as either *conductance* or *resistance* vessels. Conductance vessels are conduits for blood, and the aorta is the ultimate conductance vessel.

The aorta is composed of three layers: the thin inner layer, or *intima;* a thick middle layer, or *media;* and a rather thin outer layer, the *adventitia.* The strength of the aorta lies in the media, which is composed of laminated but intertwining sheets of elastic tissue arranged in a spiral manner that affords maximum tensile strength. Indeed, as thin as it is, experimentally the aortic wall can withstand the pressure of thousands of millimeters of mercury without bursting. In contrast to the peripheral arteries, the aortic media contains multiple layers of elastic laminae (see Chap. 30). It is this tremendous accretion of elastic tissue that gives the aorta not only tensile strength but also distensibility and elasticity, which serve a vital circulatory role. The aortic intima is a thin, delicate layer that is lined by endothelium and easily traumatized. The adventitia contains mainly collagen and carries the important vasa vasorum, which nourish the outer half of the aortic wall, including much of the media.

During ventricular systole, the aorta is distended by the force of the blood ejected into it by the left ventricle, and in this manner, part of the kinetic energy generated by the contracting left ventricle is converted into potential energy stored in the aortic wall. Then, during diastole, this potential energy is transformed back into kinetic energy as the aortic walls recoil and propel the blood in the aortic lumen distally into the arterial bed. Thus, the aorta plays an essential role in maintaining forward circulation of the blood in diastole after it is delivered into the aorta by the left ventricle during systole. The pulse wave itself, with its milking effect, is transmitted along the aorta to the periphery at a speed of about 5 meter/sec. This speed is much faster than the velocity of the intraluminal blood itself, which travels at only 40 to 50 cm/sec.

The systolic pressure developing within the aorta is a function of the volume of blood ejected into the aorta, the compliance or distensibility of the aorta, and resistance to blood flow. This resistance is determined primarily by the tone of the peripheral muscular arteries and arterioles and, to a slight extent, by the inertia of the column of blood in the aorta when systole commences.

In addition to its conductance and pumping functions, the aorta also plays a role in indirectly controlling systemic vascular resistance and heart rate. Pressure-responsive receptors, analogous to those in the carotid sinus, lie in the ascending aorta and aortic arch and send afferent signals to the vasomotor center in the brain stem by way of the vagus nerves. An increase in intraaortic pressure causes reflex bradycardia and a reduction in systemic vascular resistance, whereas a decrease in intraaortic pressure increases the heart rate and vascular resistance.

ANATOMICAL CONSIDERATIONS

The aorta is divided anatomically into thoracic and abdominal components. The thoracic aorta is further divided into the *ascending, arch,* and *descending* segments, while the abdominal aorta consists of *suprarenal* and *infrarenal* segments.

The *ascending aorta* is some 5 cm long and has two distinct segments. The lower segment is the *aortic root,* which begins at the level of the aortic valve and extends to the sinotubular junction. This portion of the ascending aorta is the widest and measures about 3.3 cm. The bases of the aortic leaflets are supported by the aortic root, from which the three sinuses of Valsalva bulge outward to allow for full excursion of the aortic valve leaflets during systole. In addition, the two coronary arteries arise from these sinuses of Valsalva. The upper tubular segment of the ascending aorta rises to join the aortic arch. Normally, the ascending aorta sits just to the right of midline, with its proximal portion lying within the pericardial cavity.

The *arch of the aorta* gives rise to all the brachiocephalic arteries. From the ascending aorta it courses slightly leftward in front of the trachea and then proceeds posteriorly to the left of the trachea and esophagus. The pulmonary artery bifurcation and right pulmonary artery lie inferior to the arch, as does the left lung.

The *descending thoracic aorta* begins in the posterior mediastinum to the left of the vertebral column and gradually courses in front of the vertebral column as it descends, where it occupies a position immediately behind the esophagus. Distally, it passes through the diaphragm, usually at the level of the 12th thoracic vertebra.

The point at which the aortic arch joins the descending aorta is called the *aortic isthmus.* The aorta is especially vulnerable to trauma at this site because it is here that the relatively mobile portion of the aorta—the ascending aorta and arch—becomes relatively fixed to the thoracic cage by the pleural reflections, the paired intercostal arteries, and the left subclavian artery. This point is also where coarctations of the aorta are located.

The abdominal aorta continues from the thoracic aorta, gives rise to the mesenteric and renal arteries, and ends at its bifurcation at the level of the fourth lumbar vertebra.

AGING OF THE AORTA

As discussed above, the elastic properties of the aorta are crucial to its normal function. However, the elasticity and distensibility of the aorta decline with age. Such changes occur even in normal healthy adults, and for unknown reasons, these changes occur earlier and are more progressive in men than women.[1] The loss of elasticity and aortic compliance probably accounts for the increase in pulse pressure commonly seen in the elderly. This progressive loss of aortic elasticity with aging is accelerated among those with hypertension when compared with age-matched normotensive controls.[2] Similarly, those with hypercholesterolemia[3] or coronary artery disease show a greater loss of elasticity than do controls.[4] Conversely, among healthy athletes, aortic elasticity is higher than in their age-matched controls.[4]

Histologically, the aging aortic wall exhibits fragmentation of elastin with a concomitant increase in collagen that results in an increased collagen-to-elastin ratio, which contributes to the loss of aortic distensibility observed physiologically.[5] Recent experimental animal data suggest that impairment of vasa vasorum flow to the aortic wall results in stiffening of the aorta with similar histological changes and may therefore be one cause of the degenerative changes seen with age.[6]

In animal models, loss of aortic distensibility directly affects the mechanical performance of the left ventricle, with increases noted in left ventricular systolic pressure and wall tension and in end-diastolic pressure and volume.[7] Furthermore, reduced aortic compliance causes a 20 to 40 percent increase in myocardial oxygen consumption to maintain a given stroke volume.[8] It is therefore likely that over time, the changes in aortic compliance seen with age may cause clinically important alternations in cardiac function.[7]

EXAMINATION OF THE AORTA

Unless the aorta is abnormally enlarged, the only location in which it can be palpated is the abdomen. The ease with which it can be felt depends largely on body habitus and pulse pressure: It is readily felt in thin individuals. It may be quite sensitive to palpation. Auscultation is usually unrevealing in aortic diseases, except for occasional bruits at sites of narrowing of the aorta or its arterial branches. Diseases of the aortic root and proximal ascending aorta sometimes involve the aortic valve, with resultant aortic regurgitation that may be detectable on auscultation. Regurgitant murmurs secondary to root dilatation rather than primary valvular disease are often loudest along the right sternal border.

Chest radiography and fluoroscopy are valuable and simple procedures for assessing the aorta. Normally, the ascending aorta is not visible on the direct anteroposterior chest roentgenogram. The aorta is seen as a "knob" in the superior mediastinum just to the left of the vertebral column. The lateral border of the descending thoracic aorta can often be found to the left of the spine. On the lateral chest roentgenogram, the aortic root and proximal ascending aorta are visible as an indistinct shadow in the middle of the mediastinum arising from the base of the heart. The ascending aorta and arch are best demonstrated in a left anterior oblique projection—a view that should always be included when disease of the thoracic aorta is suspected.

A number of imaging modalities are available for diagnostic examination of the aorta, including aortography, computed tomography (CT), magnetic resonance imaging (MRI), and both transthoracic echocardiography (TTE) and transesophageal echocardiography (TEE). The respective utility of these imaging modalities is discussed below in the context of specific aortic diseases.

AORTIC ANEURYSMS

The term *aortic aneurysm* refers to a pathological dilatation of the normal aortic lumen involving one or several segments. Although perhaps no definition is universally accepted, an aortic aneurysm is best described as a permanent localized dilatation of the aorta having a diameter at least 1.5 times that of the expected normal diameter of that given aortic segment.[9] Aneurysms are usually described in terms of their location, size, morphology, and etiology. The morphology of an aortic aneurysm is typically either *fusiform*, which is the more common shape, or *saccular*. A fusiform aneurysm is fairly uniform in shape, with symmetrical dilatation that involves the full circumference of the aortic wall. The dilatation seen in saccular aneurysms, on the other hand, is more localized and appears as an outpouching of only a portion of the aortic wall. In addition, the aorta may have a *pseudoaneurysm* or *false aneurysm*, which is not actually an aneurysm at all, but rather a well-defined collection of blood and connective tissue outside the vessel wall. This defect may be a consequence of a contained rupture of the aortic wall.

The presence of an aortic aneurysm may be a marker of more diffuse aortic disease. Overall, up to 13 percent of all patients in whom an aortic aneurysm is diagnosed are found to have multiple aneurysms,[10] with up to 25 to 28 percent of those with thoracic aortic aneurysms having concomitant abdominal aortic aneurysms.[11, 12] For this reason, Crawford and Cohen have recommended that a patient in whom an aortic aneurysm is discovered should undergo examination of the entire aorta for the possible presence of other aneurysms.[10]

Abdominal Aortic Aneurysms

Abdominal aortic aneurysms are much more common than thoracic aortic aneurysms. Age is an important risk factor inasmuch as the incidence rises rapidly after 55 years of

age in men and 70 years of age in women,[13] and abdominal aortic aneurysms occur four to five times more frequently in men than women. The incidence of abdominal aneurysms has increased threefold in recent decades, from 8.7 per 100,000 person-years in 1951 to 36.5 to 60 per 100,000 person-years in 1971 to 1980.[14] Because the incidence of abdominal aneurysms of all sizes has increased, it is believed that these data at least in part reflect a true increase in disease incidence. Other factors that may have contributed to the marked rise in the incidence of such aneurysms include the increasing mean age of the population, a greater awareness of the association of aneurysmal disease with other prevalent cardiovascular conditions, and improvements in diagnostic evaluation. The prevalence of abdominal aortic aneurysms in the population 50 years of age and older is at least 3 percent.[15]

ETIOLOGY AND PATHOGENESIS

Although it is now evident that abdominal aortic aneurysms arise as a consequence of multiple interacting factors, classically, atherosclerosis has been considered the common underlying etiology. (See also Chap. 30.) The infrarenal abdominal aorta is most affected by the atherosclerotic process and is similarly the most common site of abdominal aneurysm formation; only a fraction of abdominal aortic aneurysms are suprarenal, with these tending to arise only as an extension of a thoracic (thoracoabdominal) aneurysm. The atherosclerotic process less often involves the thoracic aorta.

Atherosclerotic disease of the aorta may produce either stenotic obstruction, a process that tends to be confined to the infrarenal abdominal aorta, or aneurysmal dilatation; why one process should predominate over the other in any given individual, however, is unknown.[15] Although the mechanism by which atherosclerosis results in aortic aneurysms is obscure, a recent hypothesis may account for the disease's predilection for the infrarenal abdominal aorta over other segments.[16] The media of the infrarenal aorta in humans has no vasa vasorum, and as a consequence, at least the inner media must receive oxygen and nutrients by diffusion from the aortic lumen. Atherosclerotic disease causes thickening of the intima and may thereby compromise the diffusion of such oxygen and nutrients to the medial layer. Exacerbated by increases in aortic wall stress from hypertension, this tissue hypoxia may injure the media and thus initiate a process of degeneration of the media and its elastic elements.[16] The damage produces a weakening of the aortic wall that over time allows the formation of fusiform or, less commonly, saccular dilatation of the aorta. As the aorta then widens, tension in the vessel wall rises in accordance with Laplace's law, which states that tension is proportional to the product of pressure and radius. Further widening results in even greater wall tension, which in turn leads to acceleration of aneurysm enlargement. A vicious circle is thus established in which the dilatation is often rapidly progressive.

Although atherosclerosis certainly contributes to the pathogenesis of abdominal aortic aneurysms, genetic and cellular factors play important roles as well. A genetic predisposition to the development of abdominal aortic aneurysms has been repeatedly suggested by studies of familial incidence, with up to 28 percent of patients who have an abdominal aortic aneurysm having a first-degree relative similarly affected.[17] A report analyzing 313 pedigrees has confirmed the importance of familial factors in the pathogenesis of abdominal aortic aneurysms and supports the hypothesis that abdominal aortic aneurysm might be a predominantly genetic disease.[18] At present, however, few single gene mutations are known to cause aneurysm formation (e.g., Marfan syndrome and Ehlers-Danlos syndrome type IV).[18a] (See also Chap. 56.) It appears likely that the genetic factors involved may be polygenic.

An area of expanding investigation is the role of cellular mechanisms in the pathogenesis of aortic aneurysms. Destruction of the media and its elastic tissue is the striking histological feature of aortic aneurysms when compared with the normal aorta. Experimental evidence indicates excessive activity of proteolytic enzymes in the aortas of affected patients, which may lead to deterioration of structural matrix proteins such as elastin and collagen in the aortic media and thereby promote or perpetuate the formation of aneurysms.[19] Studies have shown that aneurysmal aortas contain elastolytic activity with an active elastase not present in the normal aorta[20] and that other active proteolytic enzymes are present as well. An active inflammatory process may also contribute, given that an abnormal presence of macrophages[21] and elevated levels of cytokines[22] have been demonstrated in aneurysmal aortic tissue.

As a result of flow disturbance through the aneurysmal aortic segment, blood may stagnate along the walls and thus allow the formation of mural thrombus. Such thrombus, as well as atherosclerotic debris, may embolize distally and compromise the circulation of tributary arteries. However, the major risk posed by abdominal aortic aneurysms is that of aneurysm rupture. When rupture does occur, 80 percent rupture into the left retroperitoneum, which may contain the rupture, whereas most of the remainder rupture into the peritoneal cavity and cause uncontrolled hemorrhage and rapid circulatory collapse.[23] Rarely, an aneurysm may rupture into the inferior vena cava, iliac vein, or renal vein.

Clinical Manifestations

The majority of abdominal aortic aneurysms are asymptomatic and discovered incidentally on routine physical examination or on an abdominal roentgenogram[14] or ultrasound scan ordered for other indications. Younger patients (50 years old or less), however, are several times more likely to be symptomatic at the time of diagnosis.[24] Among these patients, pain is the most frequent complaint[14] and is usually located in the hypogastrium or lower part of the back. The pain is usually steady, has a gnawing quality, and may last for hours to days at a time. In contrast to musculoskeletal back pain, aneurysm pain is not affected by movement, although patients may be more comfortable in certain positions, such as with the legs drawn up.

RUPTURED ANEURYSM. Expansion and impending rupture are heralded by the development of new or worsening pain, often of sudden onset. This pain is characteristically constant, severe, and located in the back or lower part of the abdomen, sometimes with radiation into the groin, buttocks, or legs. Actual rupture is associated with abrupt onset of back pain along with abdominal pain and tenderness. Most patients have a palpable, pulsatile abdominal mass, and many are hypotensive when initially seen. However, this familiar triad of abdominal/back pain, a pulsatile abdominal mass, and hypotension—recognized as pathognomonic of a ruptured abdominal aortic aneurysm—is seen in as few as one-third of cases.[25] Moreover, a ruptured aneurysm may mimic other acute abdominal conditions, such as renal colic, diverticulitis, or a gastrointestinal hemorrhage, and may therefore be initially misdiagnosed in as many as 30 percent of cases.[26]

Patients who suffer rupture of an abdominal aortic aneurysm are critically ill. Hemorrhagic shock may ensue rapidly and is manifested by hypotension, vasoconstriction, mottled skin, diaphoresis, mental obtundation, and oliguria and, terminally, by arrhythmias and cardiac arrest. Retroperitoneal hemorrhage may be signaled by hematomas in the flanks and groin. Rupture into the abdominal cavity may result in abdominal distention, whereas rupture into the duodenum is manifested as massive gastrointestinal hemorrhage.

PHYSICAL EXAMINATION. Many aneurysms can be detected on physical examination,[26a] although even large aneurysms may be difficult or impossible to detect in obese individuals.[27] When palpable, a pulsatile mass extending variably from the xiphoid process to the umbilicus may be appreciated. Because of difficulty distinguishing the abdominal aorta from surrounding structures by palpation, the size of an aneurysm tends to be overestimated on physical examination. Moreover, it may be difficult to differentiate a tortuous, ectatic aorta from true aneurysmal dilatation. Aneurysms are often sensitive to palpation and may be quite tender if rapidly expanding or about to rupture. While tender aneurysms should be examined cautiously, no risk is known to be associated with palpation of the abdominal aorta.[27]

Associated occlusive arterial disease is sometimes present in the femoral pulses and distal pulses in the legs and feet. Bruits arising from associated narrowed arteries may be heard over the aneurysm. Occasionally, an arteriovenous fistula may be formed by spontaneous rupture into the inferior vena cava, iliac vein, or renal vein and cause a syndrome of hemodynamic collapse and acute high-output cardiac failure.

DIAGNOSIS AND SIZING. Several diagnostic imaging modalities are currently used for detecting, sizing, and serially monitoring abdominal aortic aneurysms, as well as for precisely defining the aortic anatomy preoperatively. Abdominal ultrasonography is perhaps the most practical way to screen for abdominal aortic aneurysms. It can visualize an aneurysm in the transverse and longitudinal planes, has a sensitivity of nearly 100 percent,[28] and can accurately define aneurysm size to within ±0.3 cm.[29, 30] Its major advantages are that it is inexpensive and noninvasive and does not require the use of a contrast agent. However, ultrasound is limited by its inability to visualize the cephalic or pelvic extent of disease or define the associated mesenteric and renal arterial anatomy. Therefore, it is insufficient for planning operative repair.

Computed tomography is an extremely accurate method for both diagnosing aortic aneurysms (Fig. 40–1) and sizing them to within ±0.2 cm.[31] CT has an advantage over ultrasonography in that it can better define the shape and extent of the aneurysm as well as the local anatomical relationships of the visceral and renal vessels. Its disadvantages are that the procedure is more expensive and less widely available than ultrasonography, and it also requires the use of ionizing radiation and intravenous contrast. Although CT may therefore be less practical than ultrasonography as a screening tool, its high accuracy in sizing aneurysms makes it an excellent modality for serially monitoring changes in aneurysm size.[30] It is important to note that CT measurements of aneurysm size tend to be larger than ultrasound measurements by an average of 0.27 cm.[32] Conventional CT scanning is limited in the preoperative evaluation of abdominal aortic aneurysms because it does not provide information regarding renal or mesenteric arterial occlusive disease. However, newer techniques such as spiral (helical) CT with three-dimensional display of the aorta and its branches[33] provide more comprehensive preoperative evaluation of the anatomy of an abdominal aortic aneurysm.

Aortography has long been the standard imaging modality for the preoperative definition of abdominal aortic aneurysm anatomy. Although it is well recognized that aortography may underestimate aneurysm size in the presence of nonopacified mural thrombus lining the aneurysm walls, it nevertheless remains an excellent technique for defining the suprarenal extent of the aneurysm and any associated iliofemoral disease. It is also excellent for defining renal and mesenteric arterial anatomy. The need for routine preoperative aortography is open to debate,[34] and in fact, many surgeons now use it only selectively.[35] Its disadvantages are that it is expensive, it is an invasive procedure with inherent risks, and it requires the use of intraarterial contrast and ionizing radiation.

Most recently, *magnetic resonance (MR) angiography* has been promoted as an alternative to aortography for the preoperative evaluation of aortic aneurysms.[34] Whereas flowing blood appears as a signal void on conventional spin-echo MRI, with the use of MR angiography blood has a bright appearance and vessels can be displayed in a projective fashion similar to what is seen with traditional angiography. Moreover, because tomographic images are reconstructed to create a three-dimensional image, the aorta may be visualized from a series of projections to facilitate appreciation of anatomical relationships. MR angiography is extremely accurate in determining aneurysm size, and it correctly defines the proximal extent of disease and iliofemoral involvement in greater than 80 percent of cases.[34] The exact role of MR angiography in the evaluation of abdominal aortic aneurysms continues to be investigated.[34, 36]

An important, but unresolved, issue regarding the detection of abdominal aortic aneurysms is the potential place, if any, of screening asymptomatic patients for the presence of aneurysms. At present, no controlled trials of aneurysm screening have provided outcomes data that might be used in guiding any such recommendations. A recent study based on the existing literature suggests that screening men 60 to 80 years of age by physical examination is cost-effec-

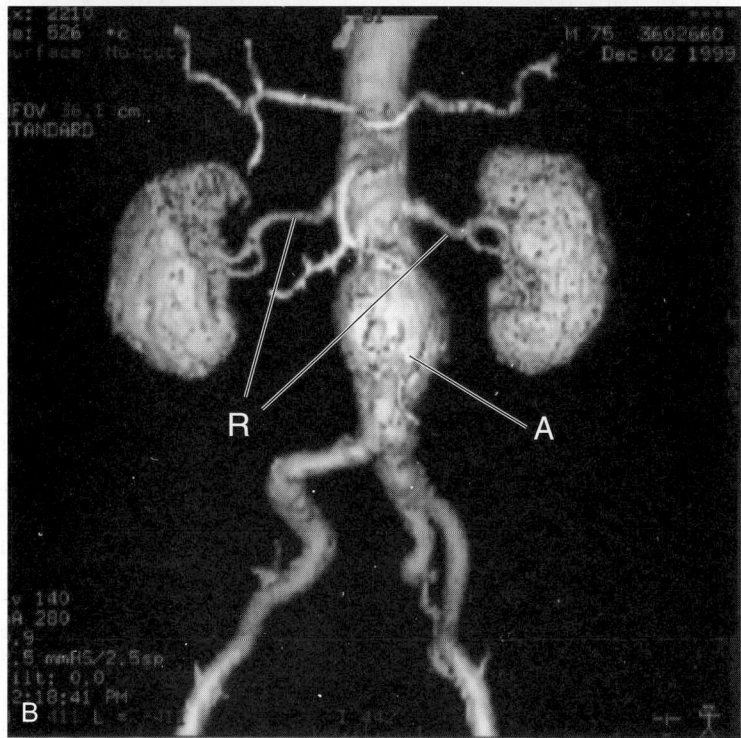

FIGURE 40–1. *A,* Axial contrast-enhanced CT scan showing a 6.6-cm abdominal aortic aneurysm (A) lined with mural thrombus (T). Blistering of the aneurysm (B) is indicative of a weakened aortic wall and suggests impending rupture. *B,* Three-dimensional shaded-surface display of the same CT scan. This anteroposterior projection demonstrates that the aneurysm (A) is infrarenal and displays its anatomical relationship to surrounding structures, including the renal arteries (R) proximally and the aortic bifurcation distally. (Courtesy of John A. Kaufman, M.D., Division of Vascular Radiology, Massachusetts General Hospital, Boston.)

tive, although of small benefit, whereas screening the same population with ultrasonography is at the upper limit of cost-effectiveness and of modest benefit.[37] Repeated screening was found to be not cost-effective. Many authors currently recommend the use of screening ultrasonography only for those at high risk, in particular those with a family history of abdominal aortic aneurysm[17] or those older than 60 years with a history of smoking or hypertension.

NATURAL HISTORY. The paramount concern in managing abdominal aortic aneurysms is their tendency to rupture. Mortality from rupture is quite high: Sixty percent of patients die before receiving medical attention[38] and the operative mortality for those reaching the hospital is approximately 50 percent,[29] for an overall mortality from rupture of 80 percent. In 1950, before the introduction of modern surgical repair, Estes first assessed survival rates for those with abdominal aortic aneurysms[39] and found survival at 3 and 5 years to be 49 percent and 19 percent, respectively, far lower than for age-matched controls, with two-thirds of deaths caused by aneurysm rupture. However, after the introduction of modern surgical repair, it was found that survival among abdominal aortic aneurysm patients undergoing operative repair was significantly higher than among those managed nonoperatively. Surgical repair thus remains the therapy of choice for aneurysms considered to be at risk of rupture.

Darling and colleagues convincingly demonstrated that the risk of rupture increases with aneurysm size.[40] Present estimates suggest that aneurysms smaller than 4.0 cm have a 0 to 2 percent risk of rupture,[41, 42] whereas those larger than 5.0 cm have a 22 percent risk of rupture within 2 years.[42] Because 80 percent of abdominal aortic aneurysms expand over time—with as many as 15 to 20 percent expanding rapidly (>0.5 cm/yr)—the risk of rupture may concomitantly increase with time.

Accordingly, the ability to predict rates of aortic aneurysm expansion would be useful in estimating the risk of future rupture. Although the mean rate of abdominal aortic aneurysm expansion appears to be approximately 0.4 cm/yr,[29] the rates of expansion within a population are extremely variable, and expansion rates even vary within one individual over time. Baseline aneurysm size is perhaps the best predictor of aneurysm expansion rate,[29] with larger aneurysms expanding more rapidly than small ones—probably as a consequence of Laplace's law. A rapid rate of expansion apparently also predicts aneurysm rupture, especially abdominal aneurysms 5.0 cm or greater in diameter.[43] Many surgeons therefore consider both large size and rapid expansion to be indications for repair.

Management

SURGICAL TREATMENT. Debate on the optimal timing of surgical repair in asymptomatic abdominal aortic aneurysms is ongoing. The decision to operate must weigh the natural history of the aneurysm and life expectancy of the patient against the anticipated morbidity and mortality of the proposed surgical procedure. Operative mortality is 4 to 6 percent overall for elective aneurysm repair and as low as 2 percent in low-risk patients. However, operative mortality rises to 19 percent for urgent aortic repair and reaches 50 percent for repair of a ruptured aneurysm.[29, 44] As of this writing, aneurysm size remains the primary indicator for repair of asymptomatic aneurysms, although no clear consensus yet exists regarding the minimum aneurysm diameter that necessitates surgery. Whereas all vascular surgeons would operate for an abdominal aortic aneurysm larger than 6.0 cm in diameter and most for aneurysms larger than 5.0 cm in patients who are reasonable surgical risks, few would operate for an asymptomatic aneurysm smaller than 4.0 cm. The benefit of surgery for asymptomatic aneurysms 4.0 to 5.0 cm in size, however, has not yet been defined. The recommendation of the Society for Vascular Surgery and the International Society for Cardiovascular Surgery is for elective repair of abdominal aortic aneurysms 4.0 cm or larger in diameter,[29] although many other surgeons still consider 5.0 cm or larger to be the indication for surgery.[44a] Prospective controlled multicenter trials currently under way in the United States, Canada, and the United Kingdom should help address the optimal timing of surgery based on aneurysm size.[45, 46]

Surgical repair of abdominal aortic aneurysms consists of opening of the aneurysm and insertion of a synthetic prosthesis, usually fabricated of Dacron or expanded polytetrafluoroethylene (Gore-Tex). Sometimes, a simple tube graft is all that is necessary, although frequently the operation must be carried distally into one or both of the iliac arteries to excise the aneurysm completely. In the case of large aneurysms, much of the aneurysm wall may be left in situ ("intrasaccular approach of Creech"), thereby reducing the need for extensive dissection and thus decreasing aortic cross-clamping time.

A promising new interventional option for the treatment of abdominal aortic aneurysms is the use of percutaneously implanted, expanding endovascular stent-grafts (see Figs. 42–5 and 42–6). The device consists of a collapsible prosthetic tube graft that is inserted remotely (e.g., via the femoral artery), advanced transluminally across the aneurysm under fluoroscopic guidance, and then secured at both its proximal and distal ends with an expandable stent attachment system. For aortic aneurysm repair, the stent-graft serves to bridge the region of the aneurysm, thereby excluding it from the circulation while allowing aortic blood flow to continue distally through the prosthetic stent-graft lumen. In some cases, stent-grafts are bifurcated, with two arms on the distal end designed to extend into the common iliac arteries when these vessels are aneurysmal as well. The rate of successful stent-graft implantation in several recent series ranged from 78 to 94 percent,[47-50] with some outcome variability resulting from differing definitions of procedural success. Despite these promising results, only 30 to 60 percent of patients with abdominal aortic aneurysms have aneurysm anatomy suitable for possible endovascular repair. Moreover, the long-term outcomes of endovascular repair versus conventional surgical repair are not yet known. One of the major technical difficulties associated with the stent-graft technique that has yet to be overcome is the frequent occurrence of *endoleaks,* which are seen angiographically as persistent contrast flow into the aneurysm sac because of failure to completely exclude the aneurysm from the aortic circulation. Such endoleaks, if left untreated, may leave the patient at continued risk for aneurysm expansion or rupture.[51] Therefore, the use of stent-grafts for endovascular repair of abdominal aortic aneurysms is at present limited to a subset of patients, typically older patients or those at high operative risk.[51a]

Assessing Operative Risk (See also Chap. 61). Because patients with abdominal aortic aneurysms, by definition, have vascular disease, their high likelihood of concomitant coronary, renal, and cerebrovascular arterial disease significantly increases the risk of major vascular surgery. Indeed, Hertzer found that half of all perioperative deaths from aneurysm repair are due to myocardial infarction.[52] In addition, routine coronary arteriography in those undergoing aneurysm repair revealed severe correctable coronary artery disease in 31 percent of all patients, including an 18 percent incidence in patients without prior clinical manifestations of coronary disease.[53] Moreover, among those with angiographically significant coronary artery disease, multivessel disease was seen in the majority.[53]

Studies by Boucher and colleagues[54] and Eagle and associates[55] have suggested that dipyridamole-thallium cardiac scanning is an effective means of identifying patients at highest risk for perioperative ischemic events (see also Chaps. 9 and 13). Patients with reversible thallium defects in multiple segments of myocardium are at highest risk,[56] and it is in this subgroup that coronary angiography is likely to be most helpful. The safety of dipyridamole-thallium studies in such patients has been well established. Although exercise thallium scintigraphy is also a useful screening method, many patients with vascular disease fail to achieve an adequate heart rate because of limited exercise capacity. Other techniques shown to be effective for preoperative evaluation of myocardial ischemia include dobutamine stress echocardiography and electrocardiographic exercise testing in patients with a normal baseline electrocardiogram and adequate exercise tolerance.

Selective preoperative evaluation to identify the presence and severity of coronary artery disease in patients with clinical markers of coronary artery disease has been widely advocated,[57] and some further suggest screening those with strong cardiac risk factors despite the absence of clinical evidence of coronary artery disease.[58] Although patients found to have significant correctable coronary artery disease are presumed to benefit from preoperative coronary revascularization with selective coronary artery bypass surgery or angioplasty, at present this conclusion remains unproved.[58] Data available from nonrandomized studies of patients with significant coronary artery disease undergoing vascular surgery do demonstrate lower mortality for those who have undergone coronary bypass surgery.[59] Furthermore, a recent randomized study has demonstrated that the long-term outcome of patients with combined peripheral vascular disease and high-risk coronary artery disease is improved by coronary artery revascularization in those with three-vessel coronary disease.[60] As is the case for coronary artery bypass surgery, no data are yet available to confirm that preoperative coronary angioplasty for significant coronary stenoses decreases the risk from major vascular surgery.

In addition to such preoperative screening and potential coronary revascularization, operative risk secondary to cardiac ischemic events may be further reduced through the use of perioperative invasive hemodynamic monitoring and careful perioperative surveillance for evidence of ischemia. Furthermore, myocardial ischemia and perhaps myocardial infarction may be prevented by using beta-adrenergic blockers perioperatively.[61]

Late Survival. A review by Kiell and Ernst of late survival following abdominal aortic aneurysm repair among almost 2500 patients revealed 1-, 5-, and 10-year survival rates of 93, 63, and 40 percent, respectively.[25] The long-term survival of patients with concomitant coronary artery disease has been found to be approximately 10 percent lower than that for those without overt coronary disease.[62]

MEDICAL MANAGEMENT. Risk factor modification is fundamental in the medical management of abdominal aortic aneurysms. Hypercholesterolemia and hypertension should be carefully controlled. Most patients with abdominal aortic aneurysms are cigarette smokers, and smoking must be discontinued. Beta blockers have long been considered an important therapy for reducing the risk of aneurysm expansion and rupture, and both animal and human studies support such a role. Brophy and coworkers demonstrated that propranolol delays the development of aneurysms in a mouse model prone to spontaneous aortic aneurysms.[63] Interestingly, it appears that the drug's efficacy in this model may have been independent of reductions in blood pressure or diminution of the force of left ventricular ejection (dP/dt) and, instead, may have been the result of changes in connective tissue metabolism and the structure of the aortic wall. In humans, a recent study has shown that the mean rate of abdominal aortic aneurysm expansion was slower in patients treated with beta blockers than in those not treated with beta blockers, with the effect most marked in large aneurysms.[43]

Should one elect to observe an abdominal aortic aneurysm 4.0 cm in size or larger, careful routine follow-up is indicated to detect either rapid expansion ($\geq$0.5 cm/yr) or an increase in size to 5.0 cm or larger, either of which is an indication for surgery.[64] CT scanning every 6 months, perhaps as frequently as every 3 months for those at higher risk, has been advocated as an effective method of follow-up in such patients.[29] CT scanning is preferable to ultrasound for monitoring aneurysm growth because CT measurements of aneurysm size are more accurate.

Thoracic Aortic Aneurysms

Thoracic aortic aneurysms are much less common than aneurysms of the abdominal aorta, and their incidence did not increase over the same 30-year period that saw a marked increase in the incidence of abdominal aortic aneurysms[12] (as noted above). Thoracic aneurysms are classified by the portion of aorta involved, i.e., the ascending, arch, or descending thoracic aorta. This anatomical distinction is important because the etiology, natural history, and treatment of thoracic aneurysms differ for each of these segments. Aneurysms of the descending aorta occur most commonly, followed by aneurysms of the ascending aorta, whereas arch aneurysms occur much less often.[11] In addi-

tion, descending thoracic aneurysms may extend distally to involve the abdominal aorta and create what is known as a *thoracoabdominal aortic aneurysm*. Sometimes, the entire aorta may be ectatic, with localized aneurysms seen at sites in both the thoracic and abdominal aorta.

ETIOLOGY AND PATHOGENESIS. Aneurysms of the ascending thoracic aorta most often result from the process of *cystic medial degeneration* (or *cystic medial necrosis*). Histologically, cystic medial degeneration has the appearance of smooth muscle cell necrosis and elastic fiber degeneration, with the presence in the media of cystic spaces filled with mucoid material. Although these changes occur most frequently in the ascending aorta, in some cases the entire aorta may be similarly affected. The histological changes lead to weakening of the aortic wall, which in turn results in the formation of a fusiform aneurysm. Such aneurysms often involve the aortic root and may consequently result in aortic regurgitation. The term *annuloaortic ectasia* is often used to describe this condition (see below).

Cystic medial degeneration is found in virtually all cases of the Marfan syndrome[65] and may be associated with other connective tissue disorders as well, such as the Ehlers-Danlos syndrome. The Marfan syndrome (see Chap. 56) is an autosomal dominant heritable disorder of connective tissue that has been discovered to be due to mutations in one of the genes for fibrillin, a structural protein that helps direct and orient elastin in the developing aorta.[66] These mutations result in a decrease in the amount of elastin in the aortic wall,[67] together with a loss of elastin's normally highly organized structure. As a consequence, from an early age a marfanoid aorta exhibits markedly abnormal elastic properties and increased systemic pulse wave velocities, and over time the aorta exhibits progressively increasing degrees of stiffness and dilatation.[68]

In patients without the Marfan syndrome, however, it is not possible to recognize the histological diagnosis of cystic medial degeneration prospectively (i.e., without surgery or necropsy).[69] This fact has significantly limited our understanding of medial degeneration and its natural history, and it remains unclear to what extent this syndrome may represent an independent disease process versus a manifestation of another disease state. It has long been suspected that some patients who have annuloaortic ectasia and proven cystic medial degeneration without the classic phenotypic manifestations of the Marfan syndrome may, in fact, have a variation, or *forme fruste*, of the Marfan syndrome,[70] although this theory remains unproved. On the contrary, many patients with ascending thoracic aortic aneurysms appear to have nothing more than idiopathic cystic medial degeneration.

ATHEROSCLEROSIS. Atherosclerotic aneurysms infrequently occur in the ascending aorta and, when they do, tend to be associated with diffuse aortic atherosclerosis. Aneurysms in the aortic arch are often contiguous with aneurysms of the ascending or descending aorta. They may be due to atherosclerotic disease, cystic medial degeneration, syphilis, or other infections. The predominant etiology of aneurysms of the descending thoracic aorta is atherosclerosis.[71] These aneurysms tend to originate just distal to the origin of the left subclavian artery and may be either fusiform or saccular.[72] The pathogenesis of such atherosclerotic aneurysms in the thoracic aorta may be similar to that of abdominal aneurysms but has not been extensively examined.

SYPHILIS. Syphilis was once a common cause of ascending thoracic aortic aneurysm, but today it has become a rarity in most major medical centers[12, 73] as a result of aggressive antibiotic treatment of the disease in its early stages. The latent period from initial spirochetal infection to aortic complications may range from 5 to 40 years but is most commonly 10 to 25 years. During the secondary phase of the disease, spirochetes directly infect the aortic media, most commonly involving the ascending aorta. The muscular and elastic medial elements are destroyed by the infection and inflammatory response and are replaced by fibrous tissue that frequently calcifies. Weakening of the aortic wall from medial destruction results in progressive aneurysmal dilatation. In addition, the infection may spread into the aortic root, and the subsequent root dilatation may result in aortic regurgitation.

INFECTIOUS AORTITIS. This rare cause of aortic aneurysm may result from a primary infection of the aortic wall causing aortic dilatation with the formation of fusiform or saccular aneurysms. More commonly, infected or *mycotic* aneurysms may arise secondarily from an infection occurring in a preexisting aneurysm of another etiology. When an infected aneurysm involves the ascending aorta, it is often the consequence of direct spread from aortic valve bacterial endocarditis.

Several other causes of thoracic aortic aneurysms are discussed in detail elsewhere in this or other chapters, including giant cell arteritis (see Chap. 67), aortic trauma (see Chap. 5), and aortic dissection (p. 1431). Note that the clinical features, natural history, and treatment of thoracic aneurysms discussed below apply specifically to *nondissecting thoracic aortic aneurysms*.

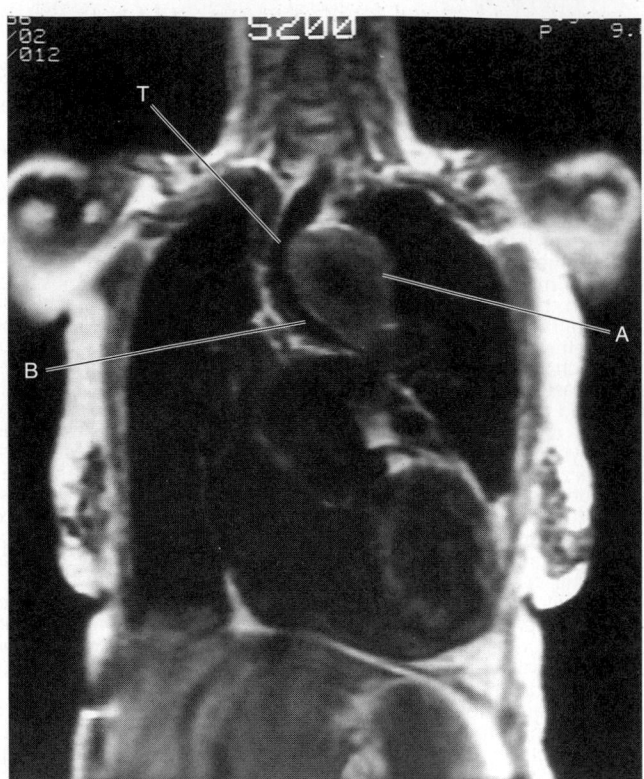

FIGURE 40–2. MRI in the coronal projection of a large thoracic aortic aneurysm in an elderly woman with a complaint of dyspnea and cough. In this view the markedly dilated aortic arch (A) is compressing the trachea (T) and causing rightward tracheal deviation. The aneurysm is also compressing the left main stem bronchus (B). In addition, all four cardiac chambers are dilated, consistent with the patient's known idiopathic dilated cardiomyopathy.

Clinical Manifestations

Forty percent of patients with thoracic aortic aneurysms are asymptomatic at the time of diagnosis,[11] with such aneurysms typically discovered as incidental findings on a routine physical examination or chest roentgenogram. When patients do experience symptoms, the symptoms tend to reflect either a vascular consequence of the aneurysm or a local mass effect. Vascular consequences include aortic regurgitation from dilatation of the aortic root, often associated with secondary congestive heart failure; sinus of Valsalva aneurysms that may rupture into the right side of the heart and cause a continuous murmur and congestive heart failure; and thromboembolism causing stroke, lower extremity ischemia, renal infarction, or mesenteric ischemia.

A local mass effect from an ascending or arch aneurysm may cause superior vena cava syndrome as a result of obstruction of venous return via compression of the superior vena cava or innominate veins. Aneurysms of the arch or descending aorta may compress the trachea (Fig. 40–2) or main stem bronchus and produce tracheal deviation, wheezing, cough, dyspnea (with symptoms that may be positional), hemoptysis, or recurrent pneumonitis. Compression of the esophagus may produce dysphagia, and compression of the recurrent laryngeal nerve may cause hoarseness. Chest pain and back pain occur in 37 and 21 percent, respectively, of nondissecting aneurysms[11] and result from direct compression of other intrathoracic structures or the chest wall or from erosion into adjacent bone. Typically, such pain is steady, deep, boring, and at times extremely severe.

As with abdominal aortic aneurysms, the most worrisome consequence of thoracic aneurysms is leakage or rupture. Rupture is accompanied by the dramatic onset of excruciating pain, usually in the region where less severe pain had previously existed. Rupture occurs most commonly into the left intrapleural space or the intrapericardial space and is manifested as hypotension. The third most common site of rupture is from the descending thoracic aorta into the adjacent esophagus (an aortoesophageal fistula), which causes life-threatening hematemesis.[74] Acute aneurysm expansion, which may herald rupture, can cause similar pain. Thoracic aneurysms may also be accompanied by aortic dissection, as discussed in detail later in this chapter.

DIAGNOSIS AND SIZING. Many thoracic aneurysms are readily visible on chest roentgenograms (Fig. 40–3) and are characterized by widening of the mediastinal silhouette, enlargement of the aortic knob, or displacement of the trachea from the midline. Unfortunately, smaller aneurysms, especially saccular ones, may not be evident on the chest roentgenogram; therefore, this technique cannot exclude the diagnosis of aortic aneurysm.

Aortography is still the preferred modality for the preoperative evaluation of thoracic aortic aneurysms and for precise definition of the anatomy of the aneurysm and great vessels (Fig. 40–4). As for abdominal aortic aneurysms, contrast-enhanced CT scanning is very accurate in detecting and sizing thoracic aortic aneurysms[75] and is useful as a method to monitor aneurysm size (see Fig. 10–49). MRI is also useful in defining thoracic aortic anatomy and detecting aneurysms[76] (see Fig. 40–2) and is of particular utility in patients with preexisting aortic disease. MR angiography may prove especially useful in defining the anatomy of aortic branch vessels.

TTE (Figs. 7–113 and 7–114) is not very accurate for diagnosing thoracic aneurysms and is particularly limited in its ability to examine the descending thoracic aorta. TEE, a far more accurate method for assessing the thoracic aorta, has become widely used for detection of aortic dissection. There has been less experience with TEE, however, in the evaluation of nondissecting thoracic aneurysms. (The advantages and disadvantage of each imaging modality are discussed in greater detail on p. 1437.)

NATURAL HISTORY. Defining the natural history of thoracic aortic aneurysms is complex given the numerous contributing factors. The cause of an aneurysm may affect both its rate of growth and propensity for rupture. The presence or absence of aneurysm symptoms is another important predictor inasmuch as symptomatic patients have a much poorer prognosis than do those without symptoms,[71] in large part because the onset of new symptoms is frequently a harbinger of rupture or death. Moreover, the high preva-

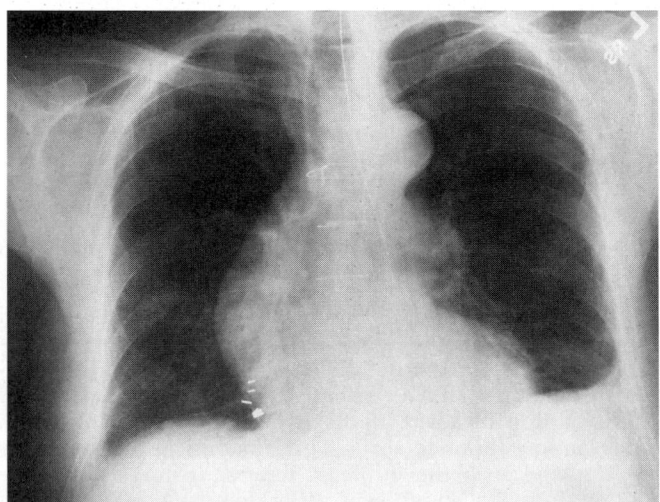

FIGURE 40–3. Chest roentgenogram of a patient with a very large aneurysm of the ascending thoracic aorta. Evident are both marked widening of the mediastinum and an abnormal aortic contour.

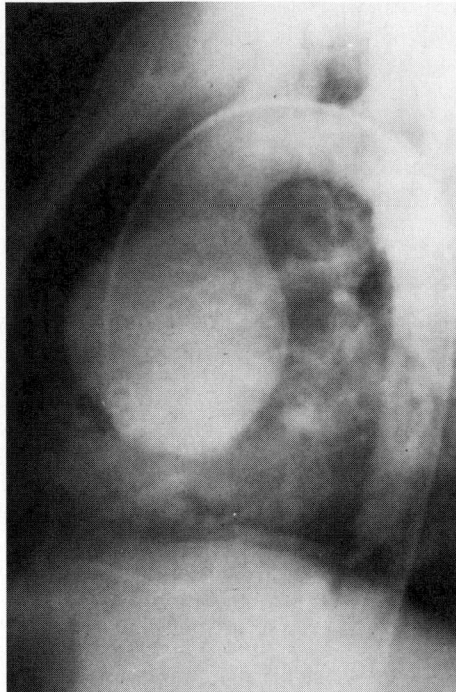

FIGURE 40–4. Lateral aortogram in a man with annuloaortic ectasia and aneurysmal dilation of the ascending thoracic aorta. The bulbous, pear-shaped aortic root can easily be seen. The left ventricle is partially opacified because of aortic regurgitation.

growth. Two additional findings in this series were that no aneurysm smaller than 5.0 cm ruptured during the follow-up period and that the only predictor of survival was initial aneurysm size.

Management

SURGICAL TREATMENT. The optimal timing of surgical repair of thoracic aortic aneurysms remains uncertain for several reasons. First, as noted above, the data available on the natural history of thoracic aneurysms are limited, especially with respect to the outcomes of surgical intervention. Second, with the high incidence of coexisting cardiovascular disease in this population, many patients die of other cardiovascular diseases before their aneurysms ever rupture. Finally, significant risks are associated with thoracic aortic surgery, particularly in the arch and descending aorta, which in many cases may outweigh the potential benefits of aortic repair.

We currently recommend surgery when aneurysms of the ascending thoracic aorta reach 5.5 to 6.0 cm and those of the descending thoracic aorta reach 6.0 cm or larger, or often 7.0 cm or larger in patients at high operative risk. Indications for surgery in patients with smaller aneurysms include a rapid rate of expansion, associated significant aortic regurgitation, or the presence of aneurysm-related symptoms. In patients with the Marfan syndrome, given their higher risk of dissection and rupture, we recommend repair of thoracic aneurysms when they reach only 5.5 cm in size.[81] Surgery should be considered even sooner in Marfan syndrome patients at especially high risk, such as those with rapid and progressive aortic dilatation, those with a family history of the Marfan syndrome plus aortic dissection, or women planning pregnancy.[82] Of course, the aggressiveness with which surgical repair is undertaken in any case should be appropriately influenced by the general condition of the individual patient.

Thoracic aortic aneurysms are generally resected and replaced with a prosthetic sleeve of appropriate size. Cardiopulmonary bypass is necessary for the removal of ascending aortic aneurysms, and partial bypass to support the circulation distal to the aneurysm while the aortic site being repaired is cross-clamped is often advisable when resecting descending thoracic aortic aneurysms.[83] The use of such adjuncts is less important, however, than the nature and extent of the aneurysm in determining the incidence of postoperative complications.[84]

The use of a composite graft consisting of a Dacron tube with a prosthetic aortic valve sewn into one end (the Bentall procedure) is generally the method of choice in treating ascending thoracic aneurysms involving the root and associated with significant aortic regurgitation.[85] The valve and graft are sewn directly into the aortic annulus and the coronary arteries, then reimplanted into the Dacron aortic graft (Fig. 40–5). The operative risk for mortality is about 5 percent.[85] For patients with structurally normal aortic valve leaflets whose aortic regurgitation is secondary to dilatation of the root, David and colleagues have successfully repaired the native valve by either reimplanting it in a Dacron graft or reconstructing the aortic root. In a series of 45 patients, 41 had mild or no aortic regurgitation after this method of aortic valve repair and were stable postoperatively at a mean of 18 months.[86]

Aneurysms of the aortic arch may be successfully excised surgically, but the procedure may be particularly challenging. The brachiocephalic vessels must be removed from the aortic arch before its resection. Then, after interposition of the prosthetic tube graft, the island of native aortic tissue containing the brachiocephalic vessels is reimplanted into the graft and normal cerebral perfusion restored. However, the risk of stroke is significantly increased because of variable periods of cerebral ischemia. The incidence of stroke in recent series is 3 to 7 percent.[87, 88] The

lence of additional cardiovascular disease in these patients may have a dramatic impact on mortality; in fact, next to aneurysm rupture, the most common causes of death in this population are other cardiovascular diseases.[72, 77]

Several small studies of the natural history of thoracic aortic aneurysms have been reported, but the data are far more limited than those available regarding abdominal aortic aneurysms. In the largest modern series, the 1-, 3-, and 5-year survival rates for patients with thoracic aortic aneurysms not undergoing surgical repair were approximately 65, 36, and 20 percent, respectively.[12, 77, 78] Aneurysm rupture occurs in 32 to 68 percent of patients not treated surgically, with rupture accounting for 32 to 47 percent of all patient deaths.[71, 77, 78] Fewer than half of patients with rupture may arrive at the hospital alive[73]; mortality at 6 hours is 54 percent and at 24 hours reaches 76 percent.[73] No apparent association has been made between thoracic aneurysm location and the risk of death from rupture.[77]

Because size is an important predictor of the risk of aneurysm rupture, several studies have examined the rate of expansion of thoracic aortic aneurysms. As with abdominal aneurysms, initial size is the only independent predictor of the rate of thoracic aneurysm growth,[75] although some data also suggest that descending thoracic aneurysms may expand more slowly than others.[79] Dapunt and colleagues monitored 67 patients with thoracic aortic aneurysms by serial CT scanning and found a mean rate of expansion of 0.43 cm/yr.[80] The only independent predictor of rapid expansion (>0.5 cm/yr) was an initial aortic diameter larger than 5.0 cm. Aneurysms that were 5.0 cm or smaller showed mean growth rates of 0.17 cm/yr, whereas those larger than 5.0 cm grew by 0.79 cm/yr. Unfortunately, even when controlling for initial aneurysm size, substantial variation was still seen in individual aneurysm growth rates, thus making such mean growth rates of little value in predicting aneurysm growth for a given patient. More helpful, however, was the finding that growth rates among small aneurysms were more consistent, with only 1 of 25 aneurysms 4.0 cm or smaller at baseline showing rapid

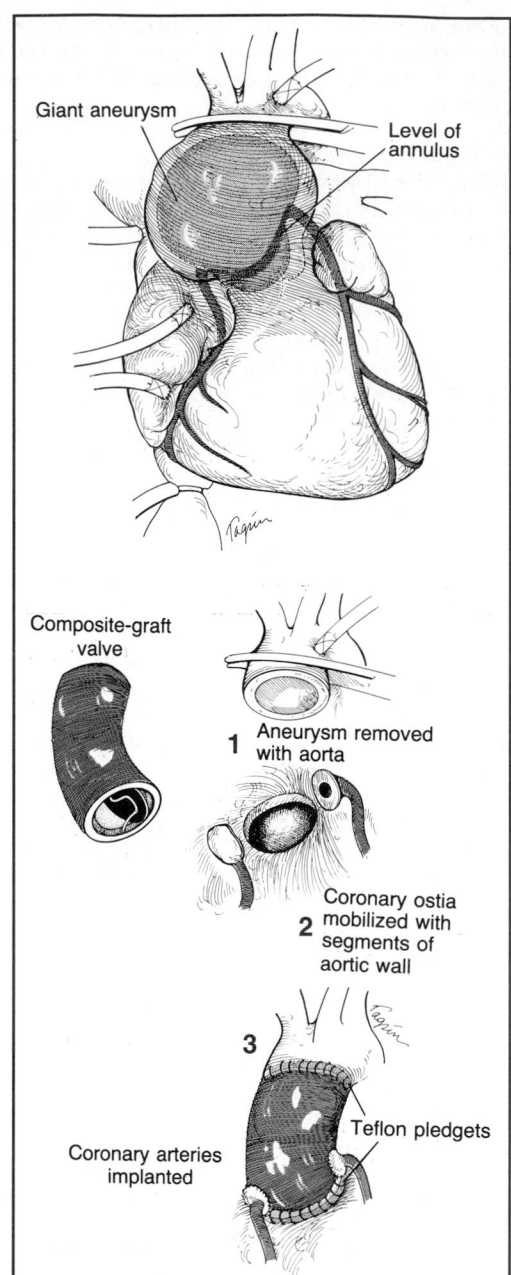

Giant aneurysm

Level of annulus

Composite-graft valve

1 Aneurysm removed with aorta

2 Coronary ostia mobilized with segments of aortic wall

3

Coronary arteries implanted

Teflon pledgets

FIGURE 40–5. Technique for the composite graft replacement of an aneurysm of the ascending aorta. *Top,* The aneurysm is shown involving the sinuses of Valsalva. The patient is maintained on total cardiopulmonary bypass. *Bottom,* The composite graft is shown, with a low-profile, tilting disc aortic prosthesis attached to its inferior end. (1) The aneurysm is resected with the native aortic valve. (2) The coronary ostia have been excised and mobilized with a button of aortic wall. (3) The composite graft has been secured in place with Teflon felt reinforcement for the suture line. The coronary artery ostia are then reimplanted directly into the graft.

standard method for carrying out this operation today is with the use of profound hypothermic circulatory arrest, as reported by Griepp and coworkers in 1975.[89] Some have attempted to add selective cerebral perfusion during aneurysmectomy, but cannulation techniques are difficult. In fact, the incidence of stroke may actually be as high or higher with this method, possibly because of cannulation-induced cerebral emboli.[88, 90] A more recent adjunct for cerebral protection during hypothermic arrest is the use of retrograde cerebral perfusion via a superior vena cava cannula.[87] Not only does this technique provide nutrients and

oxygen to the brain,[91] but it may also serve to flush out both air and particulate matter from the cerebral and carotid arteries that would otherwise embolize. The results of retrograde cerebral perfusion have been quite encouraging, with trends toward lower stroke rates.[92, 93]

More than half of patients undergoing surgical repair of a thoracic aortic aneurysm in Crawford and colleagues' series had multiple aortic segments involved, and almost three-quarters of those with descending thoracic aneurysms had multiple involvement.[94] Such widespread aneurysmal dilatation of the aorta presents a particular challenge to the surgeon and often precludes surgery. However, Crawford and associates have demonstrated that it is possible to successfully replace virtually the entire diseased thoracic and abdominal aorta.[94] A method known as the "elephant trunk" technique, carried out in sequential stages of aortic replacement, has been shown to facilitate such extensive surgical procedures and reduce the associated risks.[92, 95]

Elective surgical repair of ascending and descending thoracic aortic aneurysms is associated with a 90 to 95 percent early survival rate in most centers.[96, 97] Major complications are technical, especially hemorrhage from tearing of the diseased aorta. A catastrophic complication of resection of descending thoracic aortic aneurysms is postoperative paraplegia secondary to interruption of the blood supply to the spinal cord. The incidence of paraplegia ranges from 0 to 17 percent,[83, 84] although most series show an incidence of about 5 to 6 percent.[84, 98, 98a] A number of methods have been proposed to reduce the likelihood of paraplegia, although none has proved to be consistently safe and effective. One of the more promising techniques involves regional hypothermic protection of the spinal cord with epidural cooling during surgical repair of the aorta, which has reduced the frequency of spinal cord complications to 3 percent in one large series by Cambria and colleagues.[99] Other important techniques that may also reduce the risk of spinal cord injury include the reimplantation of patent critical intercostal arteries,[99] cerebrospinal fluid drainage,[100] the use of intraoperative somatosensory evoked potential monitoring,[101] and maintenance of distal aortic perfusion during surgery with the use of atriofemoral bypass.[99] Controlled trials might better clarify the efficacy of such techniques.

An alternative approach to the surgical management of descending thoracic aneurysms is the use of a transluminally placed endovascular stent-graft (see Fig. 42–7). This technique has the advantage of being far less invasive than surgery with potentially fewer postoperative complications and lower morbidity. Dake and coworkers recently reported the results of a large series in which "first-generation" endovascular stent-grafts were implanted in 103 patients with thoracic aortic aneurysms, only 62 (60 percent) of whom were judged to be reasonable candidates for traditional surgical aortic repair.[102] Complete thrombosis of the aortic aneurysm was achieved in 83 percent of patients, but rates of early stroke and paraplegia were 3 and 7 percent, respectively. The authors suggest that with newer and more refined devices together with more precise stent-graft deployment, the overall success rates should rise and complication rates fall. Although still experimental at present, such a device may in the future have an important role in the management of patients who are at risk for aortic rupture but are otherwise poor surgical candidates. Unfortunately, the curvilinear nature of the ascending aorta and arch makes application of similar techniques to aneurysms of these proximal aortic segments far more problematic.

Complications of associated atherosclerosis, such as myocardial infarction, cerebrovascular accidents, and renal failure, often become manifested under the massive physiological stress of aortic surgery. The most frequent causes of early postoperative death are myocardial infarction, congestive heart failure, stroke, renal failure, hemorrhage, respiratory failure, and sepsis. Advanced age, emergency surgery, prolonged aortic cross-clamp time, extent of the aneurysm, diabetes, prior aortic surgery, aneurysm symptoms, and intraoperative hypotension are the most important factors determining perioperative morbidity and mortality. Many patients with atherosclerotic aneurysms are heavy smokers, and pulmonary complications following surgery are common. The left lung may be severely traumatized by compression during resection of large aneurysms of the descending thoracic aorta, a complication that may seriously jeopardize the patient's survival, particularly in the setting of underlying pulmonary disease.

Late deaths are usually associated with cardiac complications, aneurysm rupture, respiratory failure, or stroke.[96] Aneurysm rupture may be due to aneurysm formation at the graft margins or the appearance of new aneurysms at other aortic sites.[11]

MEDICAL MANAGEMENT. The long-term impact of medical therapy on aneurysm growth and survival in patients with typical atherosclerotic thoracic aneurysms has not been examined. However, in a recent report, Shores and colleagues examined the efficacy of beta blockers in adult patients with the Marfan syndrome.[103] They randomized 70 patients to treatment with propranolol versus no beta blocker therapy and monitored them over a 10-year period. The treated group showed a significantly slower rate of aortic dilatation, fewer adverse clinical endpoints (death, aortic dissection, aortic regurgitation, aortic root >6 cm), and significantly lower mortality from the 4-year point onward.[103] Although this study examined only the effect of beta blockade in the Marfan syndrome, it follows logically that medical therapy to reduce dP/dt and control blood pressure is essential to the treatment of thoracic aortic aneurysms, both for those with smaller aneurysms being monitored serially and for patients having undergone aortic aneurysm repair.

Annuloaortic Ectasia

The term *annuloaortic ectasia* was first used by Ellis and colleagues in 1961 to describe a clinicopathological condition seen in a subset of patients with thoracic aortic aneurysms in whom idiopathic dilatation of the proximal aorta and the aortic annulus leads to pure aortic regurgitation.[104] The entity has subsequently been recognized with increasing frequency and makes up about 5 to 10 percent of the population undergoing aortic valve replacement for pure aortic regurgitation. Annuloaortic ectasia is more common in men than women, typically occurring in the fourth, fifth, and sixth decades with progressively more severe aortic regurgitation. Sudden onset of symptoms followed by rapid progression is occasionally seen.

The common pathological feature shared by patients with annuloaortic ectasia is that of cystic medial degeneration of the afflicted aortic wall leading to progressive dilatation. With widening of the aortic root, the valve annulus dilates and the aortic leaflets are pulled apart, thereby resulting in aortic regurgitation despite the fact that the aortic valve leaflets themselves are structurally normal. The weakened aortic walls are also prone to dissection.

Clinically, little distinguishes aortic regurgitation in patients with annuloaortic ectasia from that due to other causes. On physical examination, the diastolic murmur tends to be of greater intensity to the right of the sternum in cases of annuloaortic ectasia and to the left of the sternum in cases of primary aortic regurgitation. Lemon and White found that two features—acute or subacute development of symptoms and the presence of associated chest pain—were more common in patients with annuloaortic ectasia than primary aortic regurgitation.[105]

The chest roentgenogram usually shows a grossly dilated aortic root and ascending aorta with left ventricular enlargement proportional to the degree of aortic regurgitation. Aortographically, annuloaortic ectasia has one of three typical appearances. Most common is a pear-shaped enlargement of the ascending aorta (see Fig. 40–4). Also seen are diffuse symmetrical dilatation and dilatation limited to the aortic root.[105]

Surgical correction is usually undertaken for relief of aortic regurgitation when it is severe and responsible for symptoms of left ventricular failure or when the left ventricle or ascending aorta is increasing in size. In such cases, the aortic valve together with the proximal ascending aorta is usually replaced with a composite prosthetic graft (see Chap. 46).

AORTIC DISSECTION

Acute aortic dissection is an uncommon but potentially catastrophic illness that occurs with an incidence of at least 2000 cases per year in the United States. Early mortality is as high as 1 percent per hour if untreated,[106] but survival may be significantly improved by the timely institution of appropriate medical and/or surgical therapy. Prompt clinical recognition and definitive diagnostic testing are therefore essential in the management of patients with aortic dissection.

Aortic dissection is believed to begin with the formation of a tear in the aortic intima that directly exposes an underlying diseased medial layer to the driving force (or pulse pressure) of intraluminal blood (Fig. 40–6A). This blood penetrates the diseased medial layer and cleaves the media longitudinally, thereby dissecting the aortic wall. Driven by persistent intraluminal pressure, the dissection process extends a variable length along the aortic wall, typically antegrade (driven by the forward force of aortic blood flow) but sometimes retrograde from the site of the intimal tear. The blood-filled space between the dissected layers of the aortic wall becomes the *false lumen.* Shear forces may lead to further tears in the *intimal flap* (the inner portion of the dissected aortic wall) and produce exit sites or additional entry sites for blood flow into the false lumen. Distention of the false lumen with blood may cause the intimal flap to bow into the *true lumen* and thereby narrow its caliber and distort its shape.

It has also been suggested that aortic dissection may begin instead with rupture of the vasa vasorum within the aortic media, i.e., with the development of an intramural hematoma (Fig. 40–6B). Local hemorrhage then secondarily ruptures through the intima layer and creates the intimal tear and aortic dissection. Since in autopsy series as many as 13 percent of aortic dissections do not have an identifiable intimal tear,[107] at least in a minority of cases independent medial hemorrhage does appear to be the primary cause of dissection. On the other hand, one might argue that the lack of an intimal tear in these patients indicates they do not, in fact, have classic aortic dissection, but rather have intramural hematoma of the aorta, a closely related condition (see below).

CLASSIFICATION. Most classification schemes for aortic dissection are based on the fact that the vast majority of aortic dissections originate in one of two locations: (1) the ascending aorta, within several centimeters of the aortic valve, and (2) the descending aorta, just distal to the origin of the left subclavian artery at the site of the ligamentum arteriosum. Sixty-five percent of intimal tears occur in the ascending aorta, 20 percent in the descending aorta, 10 percent in the aortic arch, and 5 percent in the abdominal aorta.[90]

Three major classification systems are used to define the location and extent of aortic involvement, as defined in Table 40–1 and depicted in Figure 40–7: (1) DeBakey types I, II, and III[108]; (2) Stanford types A and B[109]; and (3) the anatomical categories "proximal" and "distal." All three

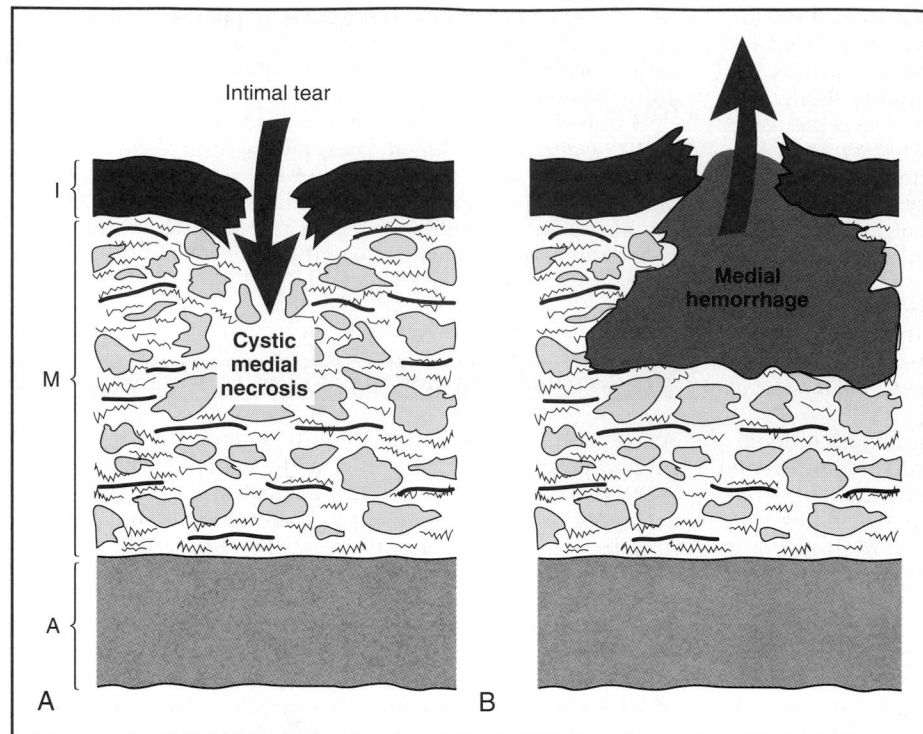

FIGURE 40–6. Proposed mechanism of initiation of aortic dissection.

schemes share the same basic principle of distinguishing aortic dissections with and without ascending aortic involvement for prognostic and therapeutic reasons; in general, surgery is indicated for dissections involving the ascending aorta, whereas medical management is reserved for dissections without ascending aortic involvement. Accordingly, because both DeBakey types I and II involve the ascending aorta, they are grouped together for simplicity in the Stanford (type A) and anatomical (proximal) classification systems. Aortic dissections confined to the abdominal aorta, although quite uncommon, are best categorized as type B or distal dissections. Proximal or type A dissections occur in about two-thirds of cases, with distal dissections composing the remaining third.

In addition to its location, aortic dissection is also classified according to its duration, defined as the length of time from symptom onset to medical evaluation. The mortality from dissection and its risk of progression decrease progres-

sively over time, which makes therapeutic strategies for longstanding aortic dissections quite different from those seen acutely. A dissection present less than 2 weeks is defined as "acute," whereas those present 2 weeks or more are defined as "chronic" because the mortality curve for untreated aortic dissections begins to level off at 75 to 80 percent at this time.[106] At diagnosis, about two-thirds of aortic dissections are acute while the remaining third are chronic.[110]

ETIOLOGY AND PATHOGENESIS. Medial degeneration, as evidenced by deterioration of medial collagen and elastin, is considered to be the chief predisposing factor in most nontraumatic cases of aortic dissection.[69, 87] Therefore, any disease process or other condition that undermines the integrity of the elastic or muscular components of the media

▼ **TABLE 40–1.** COMMONLY USED CLASSIFICATION SYSTEMS TO DESCRIBE AORTIC DISSECTION

TYPE	SITE OF ORIGIN AND EXTENT OF AORTIC INVOLVEMENT
DeBakey	
Type I	Originates in the ascending aorta, propagates at least to the aortic arch and often beyond it distally
Type II	Originates in and is confined to the ascending aorta
Type III	Originates in the descending aorta and extends distally down the aorta or, rarely, retrograde into the aortic arch and ascending aorta
Stanford	
Type A	All dissections involving the ascending aorta, regardless of the site of origin
Type B	All dissections not involving the ascending aorta
Descriptive	
Proximal	Includes DeBakey types I and II or Stanford type A
Distal	Includes DeBakey type III or Stanford type B

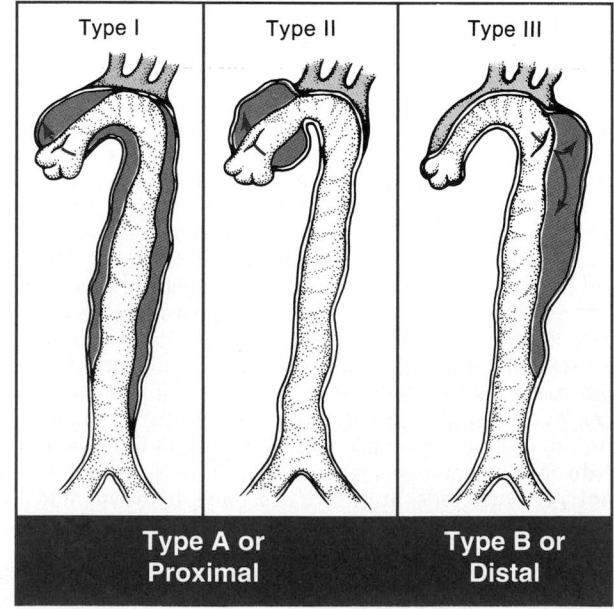

FIGURE 40–7. Commonly used classification systems for aortic dissection. (Refer to Table 40–1 for definitions.)

predisposes the aorta to dissection. Cystic medial degeneration is an intrinsic feature of several hereditary defects of connective tissue, most notably the Marfan and Ehlers-Danlos (see Chap. 56) syndromes. In addition to their propensity for thoracic aortic aneurysms, patients with the Marfan syndrome are indeed at high risk for aortic dissection—especially proximal dissection—at a relatively young age. In fact, the Marfan syndrome accounts for 5 to 9 percent of all aortic dissections.[110–112] (See also Chap. 56.)

In the absence of the Marfan syndrome, histologically classic cystic medial degeneration is identified in only a minority of cases of aortic dissection.[110, 111] Nevertheless, the degree of medial degeneration found in most other cases of aortic dissection still tends to be qualitatively and quantitatively much greater than that expected as part of the aging process. Although the cause of such medial degeneration remains unclear, advanced age and hypertension appear to be two of the most important factors.

The peak incidence of aortic dissection is in the sixth and seventh decades of life, with men affected twice as often as women.[112] A coexisting history of hypertension is found in 72 to 80 percent of cases of aortic dissection.[112] A bicuspid aortic valve is a well-established risk factor for proximal aortic dissection and has historically been found in 7 to 14 percent of all aortic dissections.[110, 111] Interestingly, the risk of aortic dissection appears to be independent of the severity of the bicuspid valve stenosis.[111] Certain other congenital cardiovascular abnormalities predispose the aorta to dissection, including coarctation of the aorta.[111] Aortic dissection has also been reported to occur in association with the Noonan and Turner syndromes.[110, 113] Rarely, aortic dissection complicates arteritis involving the aorta (see Chap. 67), particularly giant cell arteritis.[114] A number of reports describe aortic dissection in association with cocaine abuse among younger men,[115, 116] but no direct causal relationship has yet been established.

An unexplained relationship exists between pregnancy and aortic dissection (see Chap. 65). About half of all aortic dissections in women younger than 40 years occur during pregnancy, typically in the third trimester[117] and also occasionally in the early postpartum period.[118] The increases in blood volume, cardiac output, and blood pressure seen in late pregnancy may contribute to the risk, although this explanation cannot account for postpartum occurrence. Women with the Marfan syndrome and a dilated aortic root are at particular risk for acute aortic dissection during pregnancy,[119] and in some cases, diagnosis of the Marfan syndrome is first made when such women are evaluated for peripartum aortic dissection.

Direct trauma to the aorta may also cause aortic dissection. Blunt trauma tends to cause localized tears, hematomas, or frank aortic transection (see Chap. 51) and only rarely causes classic aortic dissection.[120] Iatrogenic trauma, on the other hand, is associated with true aortic dissection. Both intraarterial catheterization[121] and the insertion of intraaortic balloon pumps[122] may induce aortic dissection, probably from direct trauma to the aortic intima. Cardiac surgery is associated with a very small risk of acute aortic dissection. The majority of these dissections are discovered intraoperatively and repaired at that time, although 20 percent are detected only after a delay.[123] In addition, aortic dissection sometimes occurs late (months to years) after cardiac surgery; in fact, as many as 18 percent of those with acute aortic dissection have a history of prior cardiac surgery.[112] Of cardiac surgical patients, those undergoing aortic valve replacement are at highest risk for aortic dissection as a late complication.[124, 125] von Kodolitsch and colleagues have found that patients with a dilated ascending aorta together with aortic regurgitation or a thinned aortic wall at the time of aortic valve replacement are most likely to have such a late aortic dissection.[126]

SYMPTOMS. Much of the data presented regarding the clinical manifestations of aortic dissection are from the earlier clinical series of Slater and DeSanctis[127] and Spittel and colleagues,[110] as well as from a recent series from the International Registry of Aortic Dissection (IRAD), which studied 464 consecutive patients with acute aortic dissection from 12 international referral centers.[112] By far the most common initial symptom of acute aortic dissection is severe pain, which is found in up to 96 percent of cases,[110, 127, 112] whereas the large majority of those without pain are found to have chronic dissections.[110] The pain is typically severe and of sudden onset[112] and is as severe at its inception as it ever becomes, in contrast to the pain of myocardial infarction, which usually has a crescendo-like onset. In fact, the pain may be all but unbearable in some instances and force the patient to writhe in agony, fall to the ground, or pace restlessly in an attempt to gain relief. Several features of the pain should arouse suspicion of aortic dissection. The quality of the pain as described by the patient is often morbidly appropriate to the actual event, with adjectives such as "tearing," "ripping," "sharp," and "stabbing" frequently used.[112] Another important characteristic of the pain of aortic dissection is its tendency to migrate from its point of origin to other sites, generally following the path of the dissection as it extends through the aorta. However, such migratory pain is described in as few as 17 percent of cases.[112]

The location of pain may be quite helpful in suggesting the location of the aortic dissection because localized symptoms tend to reflect involvement of the underlying aorta. In the series of Spittell and associates, when the location of chest pain was anterior only (or if the most severe pain was anterior), more than 90 percent of patients had involvement of the ascending aorta.[110] Conversely, when the chest pain was interscapular only (or when the most severe pain was interscapular), more than 90 percent of patients had involvement of the descending thoracic aorta (i.e., DeBakey type I or III). The presence of any pain in the neck, throat, jaw, or face strongly predicted involvement of the ascending aorta, whereas pain anywhere in the back, abdomen, or lower extremities strongly predicted involvement of the descending aorta. In rare cases the presenting pain is only pleuritic in nature, due to acute pericarditis that results from hemorrhage into the pericardial space froom the dissected ascending aorta. In such cases the underlying diagnosis may be overlooked if one does not search for other symptoms or signs that might suggest the presence of aortic dissection.

Less common symptoms at initial evaluation, occurring with or without associated chest pain, include congestive heart failure (7 percent), syncope (9 percent), cerebrovascular accident (5 percent),[112] ischemic peripheral neuropathy, paraplegia, and cardiac arrest or sudden death. The presence of acute congestive heart failure in this setting is almost invariably due to severe aortic regurgitation induced by a proximal aortic dissection (discussed below). The occurrence of syncope without focal neurological signs, found in 4 to 5 percent of aortic dissections,[110, 127] may be an ominous sign suggesting a surgical emergency. It is associated most often with rupture of a proximal aortic dissection into the pericardial cavity with resultant cardiac tamponade and, less often, associated with rupture of the descending thoracic aorta into the intrapleural space.[110] On occasion, a patient presents with acute chest pain, and the initial imaging study reveals hemopericardium yet fails to demonstrate an aortic dissection. In such a scenario, unless another diagnosis—such as tumor metastatic to the pericardium—is evident, one must still suspect the presence of acute aortic dissection (or contained aortic rupture). Ideally, such a patient would be taken presumptively to the operating room or, at the very least, immediately undergo additional imaging with other modalities to confirm the diagnosis.[127a]

PHYSICAL FINDINGS. Although extremely variable, findings on physical examination generally reflect the location of aortic dissection and the extent of associated cardiovascular involvement. In some cases, physical findings alone may be sufficient to suggest the diagnosis, whereas in other cases, such pertinent physical findings may be subtle or absent, even in the presence of extensive aortic dissection. Hypertension is seen in 70 percent of those with distal aortic dissection but in only 36 percent with proximal dissection.[112] Hypotension, on the other hand, occurs much more commonly among those with proximal than with distal aortic dissection (25 and 4 percent, respectively).[112, 127] True hypotension is usually the result of cardiac tamponade, acute severe aortic regurgitation, intrapleural rupture, or intraperitoneal rupture. Dissection involving the brachiocephalic vessels may result in "pseudohypotension," an inaccurate measurement of blood pressure caused by compromise or occlusion of the brachial arteries.

The physical findings most typically associated with aortic dissection—pulse deficits, the murmur of aortic regurgitation, and neurological manifestations—are more characteristic of proximal than distal dissection. Reduced or absent pulses in patients with acute chest pain strongly suggest the presence of aortic dissection. Such pulse abnormalities are present in about 50 percent of proximal aortic dissections and occur throughout the arterial tree, but they are seen in only 15 percent of distal dissections, where they usually involve the femoral or left subclavian artery. Impaired pulses—and similarly, visceral ischemia—result from extension of the dissection flap into a branch artery with compression of the true lumen by the false channel, which diminishes blood flow in the aortic true lumen because of narrowing or obliteration by the distended false lumen (occurring most commonly in the descending or abdominal aorta); impaired pulses may also result from proximal obstruction of flow caused by a mobile portion of the intimal flap overlying the branch vessel's orifice. Whichever the cause, the pulse deficits in aortic dissection may be transient, secondary to decompression of the false lumen by distal reentry into the true lumen or secondary to movement of the intimal flap away from the occluded orifice.

Aortic regurgitation is an important feature of proximal aortic dissection, with the murmur of aortic regurgitation detected in 32 percent of cases.[112] When aortic regurgitation is present in patients with distal dissection, it generally antedates the dissection and may be the result of preexisting dilatation of the aortic root from the underlying aortic pathology, such as cystic medial degeneration. The murmur

of aortic regurgitation may wax and wane, the intensity varying directly with the height of the arterial blood pressure. Depending on the severity of the regurgitation, other peripheral signs of aortic incompetence may be present, such as collapsing pulses and a wide pulse pressure. However, in some cases, congestive heart failure secondary to severe acute aortic regurgitation may occur with little or no murmur and no peripheral signs of aortic runoff.

The acute aortic regurgitation associated with proximal aortic dissection, which occurs in one-half to two-thirds of cases,[128] may result from any of several mechanisms as depicted in Figure 40–8. First, the dissection may dilate the aortic root, thereby widening the sinotubular junction from which the aortic leaflets hang so that the leaflets are unable to coapt properly in diastole (incomplete closure). Second, the dissection may extend into the aortic root and detach one or more aortic leaflets from their commissural attachments at the sinotubular junction, thereby resulting in diastolic leaflet prolapse. Not infrequently, both incomplete closure and leaflet prolapse are present at the same time. Finally, in the setting of an extensive or circumferential intimal tear the unsupported intimal flap may prolapse into the left ventricular outflow tract,[129] occasionally appearing as frank intimal intussusception,[130] and produce severe aortic regurgitation.

Neurological manifestations occur in as many as 6 to 19 percent of all aortic dissections[110, 127, 131] but are more common with proximal dissection. Cerebrovascular accidents may occur in 3 to 6 percent when the innominate or left common carotid arteries are directly involved.[131] Less frequently, patients may have altered consciousness or even coma. When spinal artery perfusion is compromised (more common in distal dissection[110]), ischemic spinal cord damage may produce paraparesis or paraplegia.

In a small minority, about 1 to 2 percent of cases,[110, 132] a proximal dissection flap may involve the ostium of a coronary artery and cause acute myocardial infarction. The dissection more often affects the right coronary artery than the left, which explains why these myocardial infarctions tend to be inferior in location.[110] Unfortunately, when secondary myocardial infarction does occur, its symptoms may complicate the clinical picture by obscuring symptoms of the primary aortic dissection. Most worrisome is the possibility that in the setting of electrocardiographic evidence of myocardial infarction, the underlying aortic dissection may go unrecognized. Moreover, the consequences of such a misdiagnosis in the era of thrombolytic therapy can be catastrophic. In a review of the literature, Kamp and colleagues described an early mortality of 71 percent (many from cardiac tamponade) among 21 cases of aortic dissection treated

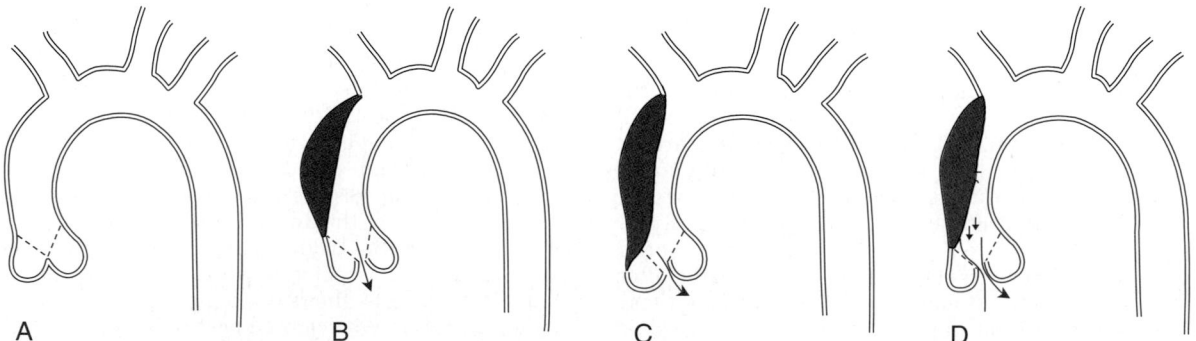

A   B   C   D

FIGURE 40–8. Mechanisms of aortic regurgitation in proximal aortic dissection. *A,* Normal aortic valve anatomy, with the leaflets suspended (dotted lines) from the sinotubular junction. *B,* A type A dissection dilates the ascending aorta, which in turn widens the sinotubular junction from which the aortic leaflets hang so that the leaflets are unable to coapt properly in diastole (incomplete closure). Aortic regurgitation (arrow) results. *C,* A type A dissection extends into the aortic root and detaches an aortic leaflet from its commissural attachment to the sinotubular junction. Diastolic leaflet prolapse results. *D,* In the setting of an extensive or circumferential intimal tear, the unsupported intimal flap may prolapse across the aortic valve and into the left ventricular outflow tract and prevent normal leaflet coaptation.

with thrombolysis.[133] It thus remains essential that when evaluating patients with acute myocardial infarction—particularly inferior infarctions—one carefully consider the possibility of an underlying aortic dissection before thrombolytic or anticoagulant therapy is instituted. Although some physicians feel reassured that performing a chest roentgenogram before the institution of thrombolysis is adequate to exclude the diagnosis of dissection, a blinded study of roentgenogram interpretation in this setting suggests that chest radiography is not sufficient.[134]

Extension of aortic dissection into the abdominal aorta may cause other vascular complications. Compromise of one or both renal arteries occurs in about 5 to 8 percent[131, 135] and may lead to renal ischemia or frank infarction and, eventually, severe hypertension and acute renal failure. Mesenteric ischemia and infarction are also occasional complications of abdominal dissection seen in 3 to 5 percent of cases.[131, 135] In addition, aortic dissection may extend into the iliac arteries and cause diminished femoral pulses (12 percent[131]) and acute lower extremity ischemia. If in such cases the associated chest pain is minimal or absent, the pulse deficit and ischemic peripheral neuropathy may be mistaken for a peripheral embolic event.

Additional clinical manifestations of aortic dissection include the presence of pleural effusions, seen more commonly on the left side. The effusion typically arises secondary to an inflammatory reaction around the involved aorta, but in some cases it may result from hemothorax caused by a transient rupture or leak from a descending dissection. Several rarely encountered clinical manifestations of aortic dissection include hoarseness, upper airway obstruction, rupture into the tracheobronchial tree with hemoptysis, dysphagia, hematemesis from rupture into the esophagus, superior vena cava syndrome, pulsating neck masses, Horner syndrome, and unexplained fever. Other rare findings associated with the presence of a continuous murmur include rupture of the aortic dissection into the right atrium, into the right ventricle, or into the left atrium with secondary congestive heart failure.

A variety of conditions may mimic aortic dissection, including myocardial infarction or ischemia, acute aortic regurgitation without dissection, nondissecting thoracic or abdominal aortic aneurysms, pericarditis, musculoskeletal pain, or mediastinal tumors. Diagnostic confusion may be particularly likely when a patient with chest pain coincidentally has another clinical symptom, physical finding, or chest roentgenographic finding typically associated with aortic dissection.[136]

LABORATORY FINDINGS. Chest roentgenography is included in the discussion of clinical manifestations of aortic dissection rather than the discussion of diagnostic techniques because an abnormal incidental finding on a routine chest roentgenogram may first raise clinical suspicion of aortic dissection. Moreover, although chest roentgenography may help support a diagnosis of suspected aortic dissection, the findings are nonspecific and rarely diagnostic. The results of chest roentgenography therefore add to the other available clinical data used in deciding whether suspicion of aortic dissection warrants proceeding to a more definitive diagnostic study.

The most common abnormality seen on chest radiography in aortic dissection is widening of the aortic silhouette, which appears in 81 to 90 percent of cases.[110, 127] Less often, nonspecific widening of the superior mediastinum is seen. If calcification of the aortic knob is present, separation of the intimal calcification from the outer aortic soft tissue border by more than 1.0 cm—the "calcium sign"—is suggestive, although not diagnostic, of aortic dissection. Comparison of the current chest roentgenogram with a previous study may reveal acute changes in the aortic or mediastinal silhouettes that would otherwise have gone unrecognized (Fig. 40–9). Pleural effusions are common, typically

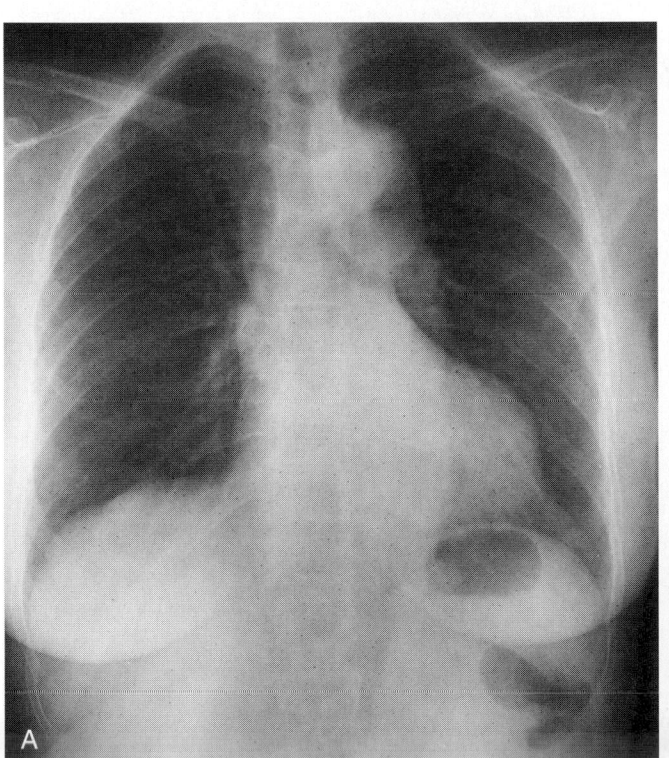
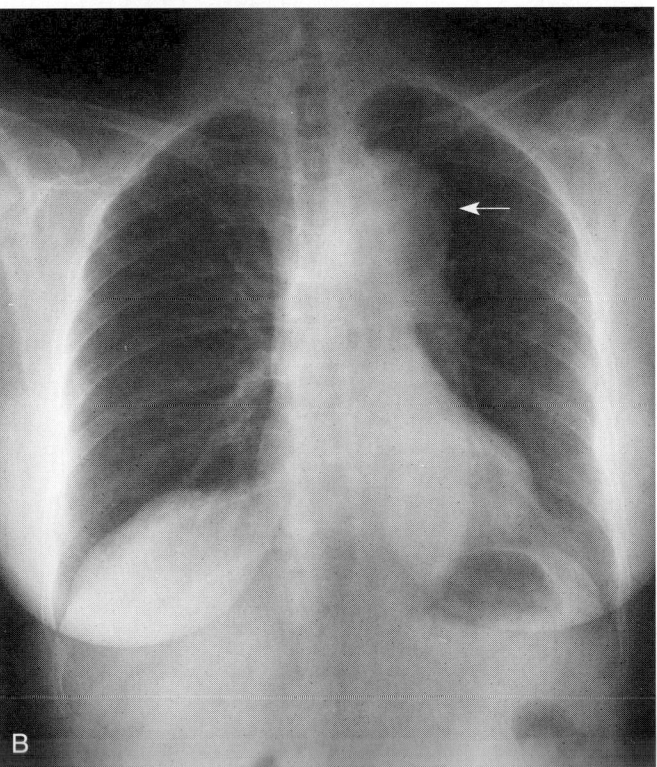

FIGURE 40–9. Chest roentgenogram of a patient with aortic dissection. *A,* The patient's baseline study 3 years before admission shows a normal-appearing aorta. *B,* The chest roentgenogram on admission is remarkable for the interval enlargement of the aortic knob (arrow). The patient was found to have proximal aortic dissection. (From Isselbacher EM, Cigarroa JE, Eagle KA: Aortic dissection. *In* Creager M [ed]: Vascular Disease. *In* Braunwald E [series ed]: Atlas of Heart Diseases. Vol 7. Philadelphia, Current Medicine, 1996.)

occur on the left side, and are more often associated with dissection involving the descending aorta. Although the majority of patients with aortic dissection have one or more of these roentgenographic abnormalities, the remainder, up to 12 percent,[110, 137] have chest roentgenograms that appear unremarkable. Therefore, a normal chest roentgenogram can never exclude the presence of aortic dissection.

Electrocardiographic findings in aortic dissection are nonspecific. One-third of electrocardiograms show changes consistent with left ventricular hypertrophy, while another third are normal. Nevertheless, obtaining an electrocardiogram is diagnostically important for two reasons: (1) in aortic dissection, nonspecific chest pain and the absence of ischemic ST segment and T wave changes on electrocardiogram may argue against the diagnosis of myocardial ischemia and thereby prompt consideration of other chest pain syndromes, including aortic dissection, and (2) in patients with proximal dissection, the electrocardiogram may reveal acute myocardial infarction when the dissection flap has involved a coronary artery.

A promising new biochemical method has recently been introduced that uses serial immunoassays of monoclonal antibodies to smooth muscle myosin heavy chains to detect the presence of acute aortic dissection. In a small prospective study of 27 patients with aortic dissection, the sensitivity and specificity of the assay within the first 12 hours of acute dissection were 90 and 97 percent, respectively.[138] Importantly, the method could also accurately differentiate myocardial infarction from aortic dissection.

Because of the variable extent of aortic, branch vessel, and cardiac involvement occurring with aortic dissection, the signs and symptoms associated with the condition occur sporadically. Consequently, the presence or absence of aortic dissection cannot be diagnosed accurately in most cases on the basis of symptoms and clinical findings alone. In the series of Spittell and associates, of all aortic dissections (without a known diagnosis), the initial clinical diagnosis was aortic dissection in only 62 percent,[110] and the other 38 percent were initially thought to have myocardial ischemia, congestive heart failure, nondissecting aneurysms of the thoracic or abdominal aorta, symptomatic aortic stenosis, pulmonary embolism, and so forth. Among this 38 percent in whom aortic dissection went undiagnosed at initial evaluation, nearly two-thirds had their aortic dissection detected incidentally while undergoing a diagnostic procedure for other clinical questions, and in nearly one-third the aortic dissection remained undiagnosed until necropsy.[110] Given the clinical challenge that detection of aortic dissection presents, physicians should remain vigilant for any risk factors, symptoms, and signs consistent with aortic dissection if a timely diagnosis is to be made.

Diagnostic Techniques

Once the diagnosis of aortic dissection is suspected on clinical grounds, it is essential to confirm the diagnosis both promptly and accurately.[139] The diagnostic modalities cur-

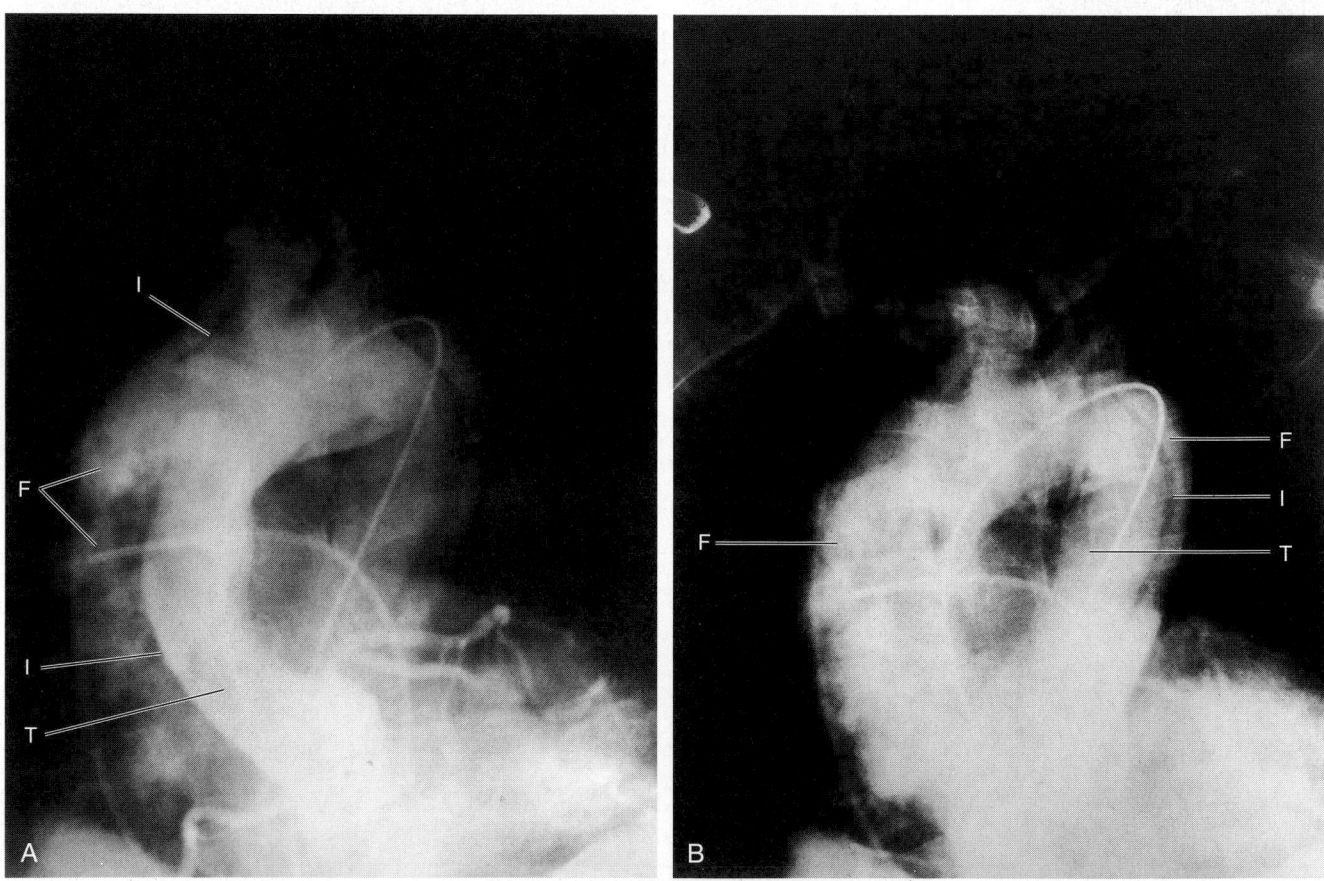

FIGURE 40–10. Thoracic aortogram in the anteroposterior view demonstrating the presence of proximal aortic dissection. *A,* The well-opacified true lumen (T) and the poorly opacified false lumen (F) are separated by an intimal flap (I) that is visible within the ascending aorta as a thin radiolucent line. In addition, the proximal portions of both coronary arteries are well visualized. *B,* In a subsequent aortographic exposure, the false lumen has filled in late and the intimal flap is now clearly visible as it courses distally down the descending aorta. (*A* reprinted, by permission, from Cigarroa JE, Isselbacher EM, DeSanctis RW, Eagle KA: Diagnostic imaging in the evaluation of suspected aortic dissection: Old standards and new directions. N Engl J Med 328:35, 1993. *B* from Isselbacher EM, Cigarroa JE, Eagle KA: Aortic dissection. *In* Creager M [ed]: Vascular Disease. *In* Braunwald E [series ed]: Atlas of Heart Diseases. Vol 7. Philadelphia, Current Medicine, 1996.)

rently available for this purpose include aortography, contrast-enhanced CT, MRI, and TTE or TEE. Each modality has certain advantages and disadvantages with respect to diagnostic accuracy, speed, convenience, risk, and cost, but none is appropriate in all situations.

When comparing the four imaging modalities, one must begin by considering what diagnostic information is needed.[140] First and foremost, the study must confirm or refute the diagnosis of aortic dissection. Second, it must determine whether the dissection involves the ascending aorta (i.e., proximal or type A) or is confined to the descending aorta or arch (i.e., distal or type B). Third, if possible, it should identify a number of the anatomical features of the dissection, including its extent, the sites of entry and reentry, the presence of thrombus in the false lumen, branch vessel involvement by the dissection, the presence and severity of aortic regurgitation, the presence or absence of pericardial effusion, and any coronary artery involvement by the intimal flap. Unfortunately, no single imaging modality provides all of this anatomical detail. The choice of diagnostic modalities should therefore be guided by the clinical scenario and by targeting information that will best assist patient management.

AORTOGRAPHY. Retrograde aortography was the first accurate diagnostic technique for evaluating suspected aortic dissection. The diagnosis of aortic dissection is based on direct angiographic signs, including visualization of two lumina or an intimal flap (considered diagnostic), as in Figure 40–10, or on indirect signs (considered suggestive), such as deformity of the aortic lumen, thickening of the aortic walls, branch vessel abnormalities, and aortic regurgitation.[141] Earnest and colleagues showed that the false lumen was visualized in 87 percent, the intimal flap in 70 percent, and the site of intimal tear in 56 percent of dissections.[142]

Aortography had long been considered the diagnostic standard for the evaluation of aortic dissection because for several decades it was the only accurate method of diagnosing aortic dissection antemortem, although its true sensitivity could not be defined. However, the more recent introduction of alternative diagnostic modalities has shown that aortography is not as sensitive as previously thought. A prospective study by Erbel and colleagues found that for the diagnosis of aortic dissection, the sensitivity and specificity of aortography were 88 and 94 percent, respectively.[143] Furthermore, a series by Bansal and associates found that the sensitivity of aortography was only 77 percent when the definition of aortic dissection included intramural hematoma with noncommunicating dissection.[144] False-negative aortograms occur because of thrombosis of the false lumen, equal and simultaneous opacification of both the true and false lumina,[145] or the presence of an intramural hematoma.

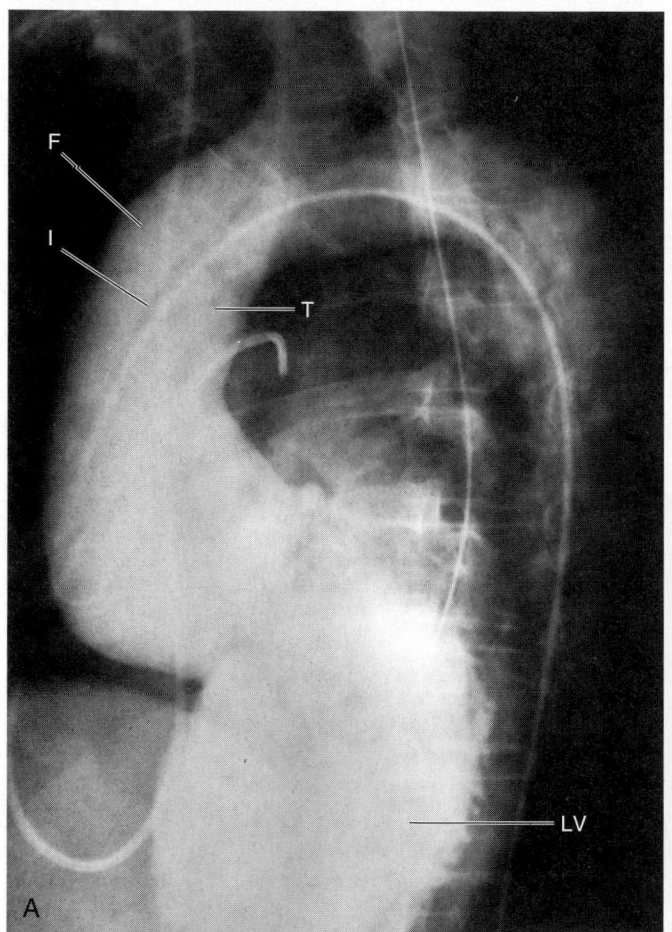
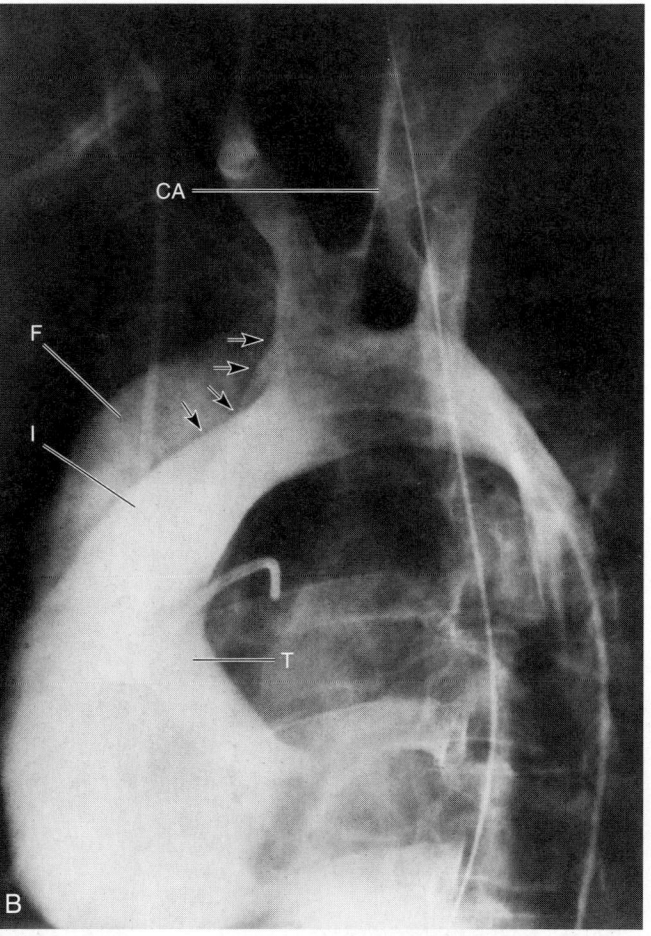

FIGURE 40–11. Aortogram in the left oblique view demonstrating proximal aortic dissection and its associated cardiovascular complications. *A,* The aortic root is dilated. The true lumen (T) and false lumen (F) are separated by the intimal flap (I), which is faintly visible as a radiolucent line following the contour of the pigtail catheter. The abundance of contrast in the left ventricle (LV) is indicative of significant aortic regurgitation (see Fig. 40–8). *B,* The true lumen is better opacified than the false lumen, and two planes of the intimal flap can now be distinguished (arrows). The branch vessels are opacified, along with marked narrowing of the right carotid artery (CA), which suggests that its lumen is compromised by the dissection. (*A* reprinted, by permission, from Cigarroa JE, Isselbacher EM, DeSanctis RW, Eagle KA: Diagnostic imaging in the evaluation of suspected aortic dissection: Old standards and new directions. N Engl J Med 328:35, 1993. *B* from Isselbacher EM, Cigarroa JE, Eagle KA: Aortic dissection. *In* Creager M [ed]: Vascular Disease. *In* Braunwald E [series ed]: Atlas of Heart Diseases. Vol 7. Philadelphia, Current Medicine, 1996.)

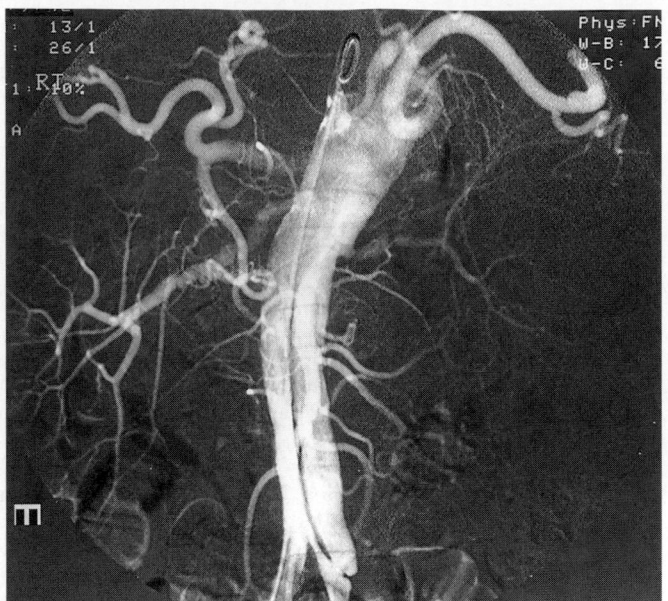

FIGURE 40–12. Digital subtraction angiogram of the abdominal aorta to assess the status of renal perfusion in a patient with distal thoracic aortic dissection. This study confirmed the presence of an intimal flap extending down into the left common iliac artery. The celiac axis, superior mesenteric artery, and right renal artery are widely patent and fill from the true lumen. The left renal artery fills from the false lumen, with the intimal flap involving the ostium of the artery and impairing distal flow. As a consequence, minimal contrast is excreted by the left kidney in comparison to the right.

Important advantages of aortography include its ability to delineate the extent of the aortic dissection, including branch vessel involvement (Figs. 40–11 and 40–12). It is also useful in detecting some of the major complications of aortic dissection, such as the presence of aortic regurgitation (see Fig. 40–11), and often useful in revealing patency of the coronary arteries (see Fig. 40–10). In addition to the limited sensitivity of aortography, other disadvantages are the inherent risks of the invasive procedure, the risks associated with the use of contrast material, and the time needed to complete the study, both in assembling an angi-

ography team and the long duration of the procedure. Finally, aortography requires that potentially unstable patients travel to the angiography suite.

COMPUTED TOMOGRAPHY. In contrast-enhanced CT scanning, aortic dissection is diagnosed by the presence of two distinct aortic lumina, either visibly separated by an intimal flap (Fig. 40–13) or distinguished by a differential rate of contrast opacification. In two large prospective series of patients with suspected aortic dissection, Erbel and colleagues found conventional contrast-enhanced CT scanning to have a sensitivity of 83 percent with a specificity of 100 percent,[143] while Nienaber and coworkers found a sensitivity of 94 percent with a specificity of 87 percent.[146] Spiral (helical) CT scanning, which was introduced more recently and permits three-dimensional display of the aorta and its branches (Fig. 40–14), has improved the accuracy of CT in diagnosing aortic dissection, as well as in defining anatomical features.[147] Indeed, two small series have found that spiral CT scanning has both a sensitivity and specificity for acute aortic dissection of 96 to 100 percent.[148, 149] (See also Figs. 10–48 and 10–49.)

CT scanning has the advantage that unlike aortography, it is noninvasive. However, it does require the use of an intravenous contrast agent. Most hospitals are equipped with a readily accessible CT scanner available on an emergency basis. CT is also helpful in identifying the presence of thrombus in the false lumen and in detecting pericardial effusion. A disadvantage of CT scanning is that the site of intimal tear is rarely identified. CT scanning also cannot reliably detect the presence of aortic regurgitation.

MAGNETIC RESONANCE IMAGING. The use of MRI has particular appeal for diagnosing aortic dissection in that it is entirely noninvasive and does not require the use of intravenous contrast material or ionizing radiation. Furthermore, MRI produces high-quality images in the transverse, sagittal, and coronal planes, as well as in a left anterior oblique view that displays the entire thoracic aorta in one plane (see Figs. 10–28, 10–29, and 10–30). The availability of these multiple views facilitates the diagnosis of aortic dissection and determination of its extent and in many cases reveals the presence of branch vessel involvement. MRI is ideal for the evaluation of patients with preexisting aortic disease, such as those with thoracic aortic aneurysms or prior aortic graft repair, because it provides sufficient

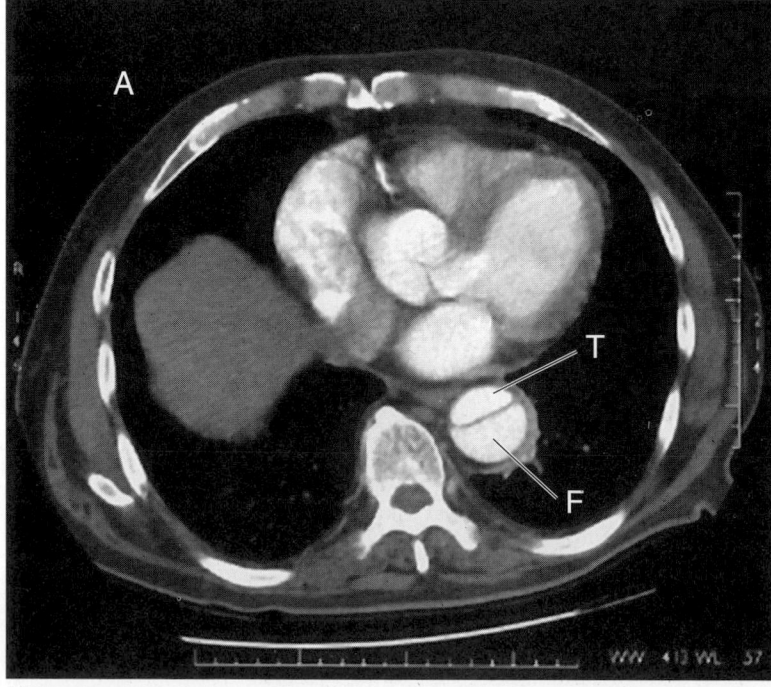

FIGURE 40–13. Contrast-enhanced CT scan of the chest at the level of the left ventricle showing an intimal flap separating the contrast-filled true (T) and false (F) lumina of an aortic dissection of the descending thoracic aorta.

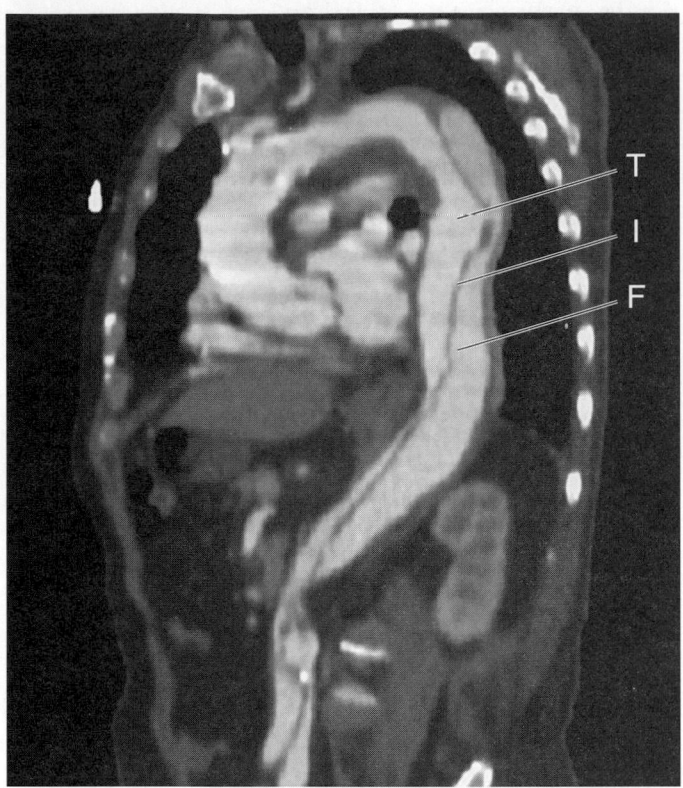

FIGURE 40–14. Reformatted left anterior oblique view of a contrast-enhanced CT angiogram of the thoracic aorta (same patient as in Fig. 40–13) showing aortic dissection of the descending thoracic aorta. The intimal flap originates beyond the left subclavian artery and extends distally well into the abdominal aorta. The true lumen (T) and false lumen (F) are easily distinguished and separated by the dark intimal flap (I).

anatomical detail to distinguish aortic dissection from other aortic pathology.[135]

In the series by Nienaber and colleagues, MRI was used to evaluate 105 patients with suspected aortic dissection and found to have both a sensitivity and specificity of 98 percent,[146] consistent with previous findings.[150, 151] MRI had a sensitivity of 88 percent for identifying the site of intimal tear, 98 percent for the presence of thrombus, and 100 percent for the presence of pericardial effusion. Furthermore, use of the cine-MRI technique in a subset of these patients showed 85 percent sensitivity for detecting aortic regurgitation.

The remarkably high accuracy of MRI has made it the current gold standard for diagnosing the presence or absence of aortic dissection. Still, MRI does have a number of disadvantages. It is contraindicated in patients with pacemakers, certain types of vascular clips, and certain older types of metallic prosthetic heart valves.[152] MRI provides only limited images of branch vessels and does not consistently identify the presence of aortic regurgitation. MR scanners are not available in many hospitals and, when present, may not be readily available on an emergency basis. Many patients with aortic dissection are hemodynamically unstable, often intubated or receiving intravenous antihypertensive medications with arterial pressure monitoring, but MR scanners limit the presence of many monitoring and support devices in the imaging suite and also limit patient accessibility during the lengthy study. Understandably, concern for the safety of unstable patients has led many physicians to conclude that the use of MRI is relatively contraindicated for unstable patients. Notably, despite such concerns, in the studies of Nienaber and colleagues, no complications occurred among their patients with unstable aortic dissection during the performance of MRI.[146, 150]

ECHOCARDIOGRAPHY. Echocardiography is well suited for the evaluation of patients with suspected aortic dissection because it is readily available in most hospitals, it is noninvasive and quick to perform, and the full examination can be completed at the bedside. The echocardiographic finding considered diagnostic of an aortic dissection is the presence of an undulating intimal flap within the aortic lumen that separates the true and false channels. Reverberations and other artifacts can cause linear echodensities within the aortic lumen that mimic aortic dissection; to definitively distinguish an intimal flap from such artifacts, the flap should be identified in more than one view, it should have motion independent of that of the aortic walls or other cardiac structures, and a differential in color Doppler flow patterns should be noted between the two lumina. In cases in which the false lumen is thrombosed, displacement of intimal calcification[143] or thickening of the aortic wall may suggest aortic dissection.

Transthoracic Echocardiography. TTE has a sensitivity of 59 to 85 percent and specificity of 63 to 96 percent for the diagnosis of aortic dissection.[140] Such poor sensitivity significantly limits the general utility of this technique. Furthermore, image quality is often adversely affected by obesity, emphysema, mechanical ventilation, or small intercostal spaces.

Transesophageal Echocardiography. The proximity of the esophagus to the aorta enables TEE to overcome many of the limitations of transthoracic imaging and permits the use of higher frequency ultrasonography, which provides better anatomical detail (Fig. 40–15). The examination is generally performed at the bedside with the patient under sedation or light general anesthesia and typically requires 10 to 15 minutes to complete. The procedure is relatively noninvasive and requires no intravenous contrast or ionizing radiation. Relative contraindications include known esophageal disease (strictures, tumors, and varices), and the required esophageal intubation may not be tolerated in up to 3 percent of patients.[153] The incidence of important side effects (such as hypertension, bradycardia, bronchospasm, or rarely, esophageal perforation) is much less than 1 percent.[153] One important disadvantage of TEE is its limited ability to visualize the distal ascending aorta and proximal arch because of interposition of the air-filled trachea and main stem bronchus.[154]

The results of large prospective studies by Erbel and colleagues[143] and Nienaber and associates[146] demonstrated that the sensitivity of TEE

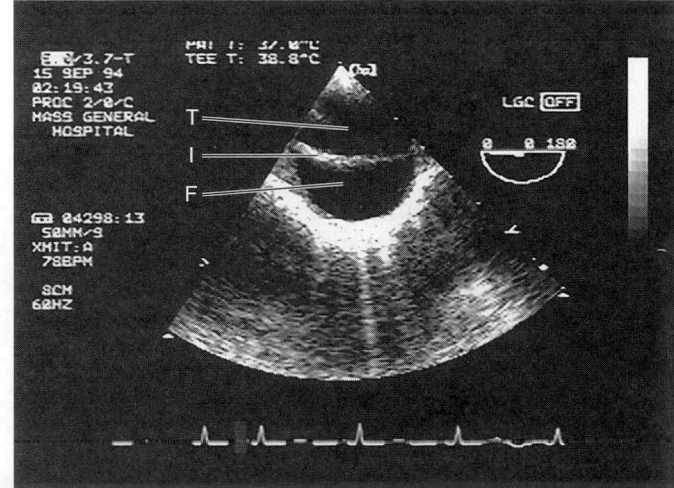

FIGURE 40–15. Cross-sectional transesophageal echocardiogram of the descending thoracic aorta demonstrating aortic dissection. The aorta is dilated. Evident is an intimal flap (I) dividing the true lumen (T) anteriorly and the false lumen (F) posteriorly. The true lumen fills during systole and is therefore seen bowing slightly into the false lumen in this systolic image.

FIGURE 40–16. See color plate 23.

FIGURE 40–17. See color plate 24.

for aortic dissection is 98 to 99 percent. The sensitivity for detecting an intimal tear was 73 percent (Fig. 45–16), and for detecting the presence of thrombus in the false lumen, the sensitivity was 68 percent.[146] Furthermore, TEE detected both aortic regurgitation and pericardial effusion in 100 percent.[146] The specificity of TEE for the diagnosis of aortic dissection was less well defined in these series. Although Erbel and colleagues found the specificity to be as high as 97 percent,[143] Nienaber and coworkers found it to be 77 percent.[146] However, in the latter study the early inexperience of those performing the examinations and the use of monoplane transducers may have contributed to the incidence of false-positives. More recent studies using biplane or multiplane TEE have consistently demonstrated a specificity of 94 to 95 percent.[149, 155]

Several methods have been suggested to reduce the possibility of a false-positive diagnosis by TEE,[140] including the use of multiplane ultrasound transducers to confirm the presence of the intimal flap in multiple planes, the confirmation of two lumina by the demonstration of differential color flow patterns (Fig. 40–17), and the use of M-mode echocardiography to distinguish artifacts.[156] We have proposed that if, in addition to an intimal flap, confirmatory evidence of at least one other echocardiographic feature of aortic dissection is identified, the aortic dissection may be called "definite."[140] If an intimal flap alone is seen (i.e., one that is not considered an artifact) with no other supporting evidence, the diagnosis of dissection should not be considered definitive, and examination with another imaging modality should be performed to exclude the possibility of a false-positive. If this conservative approach were applied to echocardiographic interpretation in the study by Nienaber and colleagues,[146] the specificity of "definite" aortic dissection would have been 100 percent.[140]

In addition to its high sensitivity for detecting aortic dissection, TEE may provide other important information useful to the surgeon. Some surgeons wish to know preoperatively whether the intimal flap involves the ostia of the coronary arteries, but this determination has traditionally required the performance of coronary angiography.[157] Ballal and colleagues performed TEE on 34 patients with aortic dissection, 7 of whom had coronary artery involvement confirmed at surgery.[158] In 6 of these 7 patients, TEE identified the intimal flap extending into the coronary ostia. However, TEE delineates only the very proximal portions of the coronary arteries, so when assessment of coronary atherosclerosis is necessary, coronary angiography is still required (see below).

Among patients with suspected aortic dissection, the diagnosis is excluded in 42 to 68 percent,[150, 159] which yields a group of patients with a chest pain syndrome of unknown etiology. Chan found that among patients determined to not have dissection, TEE detected other aortic abnormalities in 73 percent and evidence of acute myocardial infarction or ischemia in 23 percent.[160] More recently, Armstrong and associates identified such alternative cardiovascular diagnoses by TEE in 66 percent of those found to not have aortic dissection.[137]

INTRAVASCULAR ULTRASONOGRAPHY. One of the more recent developments in the echocardiographic evaluation of aortic dissection has been the use of intravascular ultrasound to define the detailed anatomy of the involved aorta and determine the extent of dissection. The intravascular ultrasound catheter is inserted through an introducer in the femoral artery and positioned within the aortic lumen under fluoroscopic guidance. The aorta is then imaged in a transverse plane through its short axis, which allows visualization of the two lumina and intimal flap.

The most extensive assessment of this technique to date was reported by Yamada and coauthors, who studied 15 patients with previously known chronic aortic dissection and compared the findings of intravascular ultrasound with those of other established imaging modalities.[161] Intravascular ultrasound accurately detected the intimal flap in all segments of the aorta, although it was poor at detecting the sites of intimal tear in the thoracic aorta, probably because of vessel curvature. However, intravascular ultrasound was quite useful in evaluation of the abdominal aorta: It demonstrated the origins of the renal arteries and the distal extent of dissection in all cases and identified the site of intimal tear of the abdominal aorta in 78 percent of cases. Accurate assessment of the abdominal aorta with this technique may have particular relevance given the inability of TEE to image this portion of the aorta. It may also have advantages over TEE in fully imaging the aortic arch.[162] Furthermore, intravascular ultrasound may play an important role in the positioning and deployment of endovascular stenting devices[163] (see below). Nevertheless, the potential future role of intravascular ultrasound in both the evaluation and management of patients with aortic dissection requires further study.

Selecting an Imaging Modality

Each of the four imaging modalities has particular advantages and disadvantages. In selecting among them, one must consider the accuracy as well as the safety and availability of each test. Given its unsurpassed sensitivity and specificity, MRI is considered by most to be the present gold standard for evaluating aortic dissection. The four modalities differ in their ability to detect complications associated with dissection, so the specific diagnostic information sought by the treating physician and/or surgeon should have a bearing on the procedure chosen. A summary of the diagnostic performance of each of the four imaging modalities is presented in Table 40–2.

Both the accessibility of imaging studies and the time required to complete them are key considerations given the high early mortality associated with unoperated proximal aortic dissection. Aortography can only rarely be performed on an emergency basis because it requires assembly of an angiography team at night and is subject to the risks associated with an invasive procedure and use of a contrast agent. MRI, although optimal in its accuracy, is also generally unavailable on an emergency basis and poses the risk of limited patient monitoring and accessibility during the lengthy procedure. CT scanning is more readily available in most emergency departments and is quickly completed. TEE is also readily available in most larger centers and can be completed quickly at the bedside, which makes it ideal for evaluating unstable patients. A practical assessment of the four imaging modalities is summarized in Table 40–3.

In a setting in which all these imaging modalities are available, we believe that TEE should be considered first in the evaluation of suspected aortic dissection in light of its accuracy, safety, speed, and convenience. In many institutions, TEE has indeed become the procedure of

▼ **TABLE 40–2.** DIAGNOSTIC PERFORMANCE OF IMAGING MODALITIES IN THE EVALUATION OF SUSPECTED AORTIC DISSECTION

DIAGNOSTIC PERFORMANCE	ANGIO	CT	MRI	TEE
Sensitivity	++	+++	+++	+++
Specificity	+++	+++	+++	+++
Site of intimal tear	++	+	+++	++
Presence of thrombus	+++	++	+++	+
Presence of aortic insufficiency	+++	−	+	+++
Pericardial effusion	−	++	+++	+++
Branch vessel involvement	+++	++	++	+
Coronary artery involvement	++	−	−	++

+++ = excellent; ++ = good; + = fair; − = not detected.
Angio = angiography; CT = computed tomography; MRI = magnetic resonance imaging; TEE = transesophageal echocardiography.
Modified from Cigarroa JE, Isselbacher EM, DeSanctis RW, Eagle KA: Diagnostic imaging in the evaluation of suspected aortic dissection: Old standards and new directions. N Engl J Med 328:35, 1993.

ADVANTAGES OF STUDY	ANGIO	CT	MRI	TEE
Readily available	Fairly	Quite	Fairly	Very
Quickly performed	Fairly	Quite	Fairly	Very
Performed at the bedside	No	No	No	Yes
Noninvasive	No	Yes	Yes	Yes
No intravenous contrast	No	No	Yes	Yes
Cost	High	Reasonable	Moderate	Reasonable

Angio = angiography; CT = computed tomography; MRI = magnetic resonance imaging; TEE = transesophageal echocardiography.

Modified from Cigarroa JE, Isselbacher EM, DeSanctis RW, Eagle KA: Diagnostic imaging in the evaluation of suspected aortic dissection: Old standards and new directions. N Engl J Med 328:35, 1993.

choice,[137, 155, 164] with surgeons taking patients to the operating room on the basis of echocardiographic findings alone.[165, 166] In institutions where TEE is not readily available, CT scanning is instead the recommended imaging modality for the evaluation of suspected aortic dissection. However, if the diagnosis of aortic dissection is confirmed by CT, after patient transfer to a tertiary care center an additional diagnostic study may be required to more completely define the aortic anatomy before surgery. However, in such instances, the patient may be taken directly to the operating room, where TEE can then be performed to confirm the diagnosis and better define the dissection anatomy without unduly delaying surgery.[165]

Although MRI is less practical than other modalities for the assessment of suspected acute aortic dissection, it is nonetheless well suited for stable or chronic dissections. Given its extraordinary accuracy and high-quality detailed images, we recommend the use of MRI for monitoring patients with aortic dissection, whether treated medically or surgically, as a means of identifying subsequent aneurysm formation, extension of the dissection, or other complications.

Despite its relative disadvantages, aortography still plays an important role when clear definition of the anatomy of the branch vessels is essential for management. Performance of aortography should also be considered when a definitive diagnosis is not made by one or more of the other imaging modalities.

In the final analysis, each institution must determine its own best diagnostic approach to the evaluation of suspected aortic dissection and base it on available human and material resources and the speed with which such resources can be mobilized. It must be emphasized that regardless of which of the four imaging modalities are available at a given institution, the level of skill and experience of those who carry out each diagnostic procedure must, with good reason, also be be considerations in deciding the study of choice.

The Role of Coronary Angiography

The importance of assessing the status of coronary artery patency before surgical repair of acute aortic dissection continues to be controversial. Some surgeons believe that obtaining this information before surgery is essential, whereas others are content to assess the coronaries intraoperatively. Two types of coronary artery involvement must be considered in the setting of aortic dissection. The first is acute proximal coronary narrowing or occlusion as a result of the dissection itself, often caused by occlusion of the coronary ostia by the intimal flap. The second is the possible presence of chronic atherosclerotic coronary artery disease, which although generally independent of the dissection process, may complicate its surgical management.

In some cases, coronary involvement by the intimal flap is self-evident if the electrocardiogram shows evidence of acute myocardial ischemia or infarction. However, should

this acute process not be clinically evident, TEE can effectively define the patency of the proximal coronaries in a majority of cases.[158] Aortography may also reveal such coronary artery involvement. More comprehensive evaluation requires the performance of coronary angiography; however, this study may be risky in patients with aortic dissection and often prolongs the time to aortic repair by several hours. Moreover, catheterization of the coronary arteries is sometimes unsuccessful in patients with proximal dissection and a dilated root, in which case the added procedural delay gains no potential benefit. In addition, such proximal coronary obstructions can usually be readily identified at the time of surgery.

Chronic coronary artery disease is seen in about one-quarter of patients with aortic dissection. Identifying the presence of this underlying coronary disease is beyond the capability of any of the four imaging modalities discussed above. Furthermore, accurately defining such atherosclerotic disease intraoperatively is challenging, although Rizzo and coworkers have suggested probing of the proximal coronaries, epicardial palpation, and angioscopy as possible means to identify coronary stenoses.[165]

The impact of unrecognized coronary artery disease on outcome is not certain. In a 10-year review examining 54 patients undergoing urgent aortic repair, Kern and colleagues found that only 1 of 27 patients with a proximal dissection had a perioperative myocardial infarction; this patient had a prior history of coronary artery disease.[157] In addition, Rizzo and associates observed that of those in whom unrecognized coronary artery disease was discovered at autopsy, none died of coronary ischemia but several died of aortic rupture.[165] Lastly, Penn and colleagues studied 122 consecutive patients undergoing emergency aortic repair and found no difference in in-hospital mortality between those who had preoperative angiography and those who did not.[166a] Accordingly, we and others[157] recommend avoiding preoperative coronary angiography unless a specific indication exists, such as a known history of coronary artery disease, prior coronary artery bypass grafting,[167] or the presence of ischemic electrocardiographic changes. Conversely, Creswell and coauthors reported good outcomes when performing combined aortic repair and coronary artery bypass grafting in patients with underlying coronary artery disease and therefore argue that all stable patients with acute proximal dissection should undergo preoperative coronary angiography.[168] While the debate continues unresolved, the trend in the literature has been a retreat from the routine performance of coronary angiography in acute aortic dissection.

Management

Therapy for aortic dissection is directed at halting progression of the dissecting hematoma because lethal complications arise not from the intimal tear itself but rather from the subsequent course taken by the dissecting aorta, e.g., vascular compromise or aortic rupture. [137] Without treatment, aortic dissection has a high mortality. In a collective review of long-term survival in untreated aortic dissection, more than 25 percent of all patients died within the first 24 hours after the onset of dissection, more than 50 percent died within the first week, more than 75 percent died within 1 month, and more than 90 percent died within 1 year.[169]

The first surgical approach to aortic dissection was a fenestration procedure in which the dissected aorta was incised and a distal communication created between the true and false channels, thereby decompressing the false lumen. This procedure is, in fact, still used by some surgeons in selected cases of dissection involving the descending aorta to relieve limb, renal, or mesenteric ischemia.[170] Definitive surgical therapy was pioneered by DeBakey and colleagues in the early 1950s.[171] Its purpose is to excise the intimal tear, obliterate the false channel by oversewing the aortic edges, reconstitute the aorta directly or with the interposition of a synthetic graft, and in the case of proximal dissection, restore aortic valve competence either by resuspension of the displaced aortic leaflets or by prosthetic aortic valve replacement.

Aggressive medical treatment of aortic dissection was first advocated by Wheat and colleagues.[172] They established reduction of systolic blood pressure and diminution of the force of left ventricular ejection (dP/dt) as the two primary goals of pharmacological therapy. This force is thought to be a major stress acting on the aortic wall that contributes to both the genesis and subsequent propagation of aortic dissection. Originally introduced for patients too ill to withstand surgery, medical therapy is now the initial treatment for virtually all patients with aortic dissection before definitive diagnosis and furthermore serves as the primary long-term therapy in a subset of patients, particularly those with distal dissections.

Immediate Medical Management

All patients in whom acute aortic dissection is strongly suspected should immediately be placed in an acute care setting for hemodynamic stabilization and monitoring of blood pressure, cardiac rhythm, and urine output. Two large-bore intravenous catheters should be inserted for intravenous medications and fluid resuscitation if necessary. An arterial line should be placed, preferably in the right arm so that it remains functional during surgery when the aorta is cross-clamped. However, in cases in which the blood pressure is significantly greater on the left than on the right, the arterial line should be placed on the left. In those with a lower likelihood of dissection who are hemodynamically stable, a automatic blood pressure cuff should suffice.

A central venous or pulmonary arterial line to monitor central venous or pulmonary artery wedge pressure and cardiac output should be considered in patients with hypotension or congestive heart failure. Femoral lines and blood gas studies should be avoided if possible to conserve these sites for bypass cannulation during potential aortic repair. If a femoral line must be placed urgently, the opposite groin site should be protected from needle puncture.

BLOOD PRESSURE REDUCTION. Initial therapeutic goals include the elimination of pain and reduction of systolic blood pressure to 100 to 120 mm Hg (mean of 60 to 75 mm Hg) or the lowest level commensurate with adequate vital organ (cardiac, cerebral, renal) perfusion. Simultaneously, arterial dP/dt, which reflects the force of left ventricular ejection, should be reduced through the use of beta-blocking agents, regardless of whether pain or systolic hypertension is present. The use of long-acting medications should be avoided in patients who are surgical candidates because they may complicate intraoperative arterial pressure management. Pain, which may itself exacerbate hypertension and tachycardia, should be promptly treated with intravenous morphine sulfate.

For the acute reduction of arterial pressure, the potent vasodilator sodium nitroprusside is very effective. It is initially infused at 20 μg/min with the dosage titrated upward, as high as 800 μg/min, according to the blood pressure response. When used alone, however, sodium nitroprusside can actually cause an increase in dP/dt, which in turn may potentially contribute to propagation of the dissection. Therefore, when this drug is used concomitantly achieving adequate beta blockade is essential.

To reduce dP/dt acutely, an intravenous beta blocker should be administered in incremental doses until evidence of satisfactory beta blockade is noted, usually indicated by a heart rate of 60 to 80 beats/min in the acute setting. Because propranolol was the first generally available beta blocker, it has been used most widely in treating aortic dissection. However, it is believed that other noncardioselective beta blockers are equally effective. Propranolol should be administered in intravenous doses of 1 mg every 3 to 5 minutes until the desired effect is achieved, although the maximum initial dose should not exceed 0.15 mg/kg (or approximately 10 mg). To maintain adequate beta blockade, as evidenced by the heart rate, additional propranolol should be given intravenously every 4 to 6 hours, usually in doses somewhat lower than the total initial dose, i.e., 2 to 6 mg.

Labetalol, which acts as both an alpha- and beta-adrenergic receptor blocker, may be especially useful in the setting of aortic dissection because it effectively lowers both dP/dt and arterial pressure. The initial dose of labetalol is 20 mg, administered intravenously over a 2-minute period, followed by additional doses of 40 to 80 mg every 10 to 15 minutes (up to a maximum total dose of 300 mg) until the heart rate and blood pressure have been controlled. Maintenance dosing may then be achieved with a continuous intravenous infusion starting at 2 mg/min and titrating up to 5 to 10 mg/min.

The ultra-short-acting beta blocker esmolol may be particularly useful in patients with labile arterial pressure, especially if surgery is planned, because use of this drug can be abruptly discontinued if necessary. It is administered as a 500 mcg/kg intravenous bolus followed by continuous infusion at 50 mcg/kg/min and titrated up to 200 mcg/kg/min. Esmolol may also be useful as a means to test beta blocker safety and tolerance in patients with a history of obstructive pulmonary disease who may be at uncertain risk for bronchospasm from beta blockade. In such patients, a cardioselective beta blocker, such as atenolol or metoprolol, may be considered.

When contraindications exist to the use of beta blockers—including sinus bradycardia, second- or third-degree atrioventricular block, congestive heart failure, or bronchospasm—other agents to reduce arterial pressure and dP/dt should be considered. Calcium channel antagonists, which are effective in managing hypertensive crisis, are used on occasion in the treatment of aortic dissection. The combined vasodilator and negative inotropic effects of both diltiazem and verapamil make these agents well suited for the treatment of aortic dissection. Moreover, both these agents may be administered intravenously. Nifedipine has the advantage that it can be given immediately by the sublingual route while other medications are being prepared. A key limitation of nifedipine, however, is that it has little negative chronotropic or inotropic effect.

Refractory hypertension may result when a dissection flap compromises one or both of the renal arteries, thereby causing the release of large amounts of renin. In this situation, the most efficacious antihypertensive may be the intravenous angiotensin-converting enzyme (ACE) inhibitor enalaprilat, which is administered initially in doses of 0.625 mg every 4 to 6 hours and the dose then titrated upward.

In the event that a patient with suspected aortic dissection has significant hypotension, rapid volume expansion should be considered given the possible presence of cardiac tamponade or aortic rupture. Before initiating aggressive treatment of such hypotension, however, the possibility of pseudohypotension, which occurs when arterial pressure is being measured in an extremity whose circulation is selectively compromised by the dissection, should be carefully excluded. If vasopressors are absolutely required for refractory hypotension, norepinephrine (Levophed) or phenylephrine (Neo-Synephrine) is preferred. Dopamine should be reserved for improving renal perfusion and used only at very low doses, given that it may raise dP/dt.

Once appropriate medical therapy has been initiated and the patient sufficiently stabilized, a definitive diagnostic study should be promptly undertaken. If a patient remains unstable, TEE is preferred because it can be performed at the bedside in the emergency department or intensive care unit, thereby allowing both monitoring and therapeutic intervention to continue uninterrupted. When a patient with a strongly suspected dissection becomes extremely unstable, aortic rupture or cardiac tamponade is likely and the patient should go directly to the operating room rather than delaying surgery for diagnostic imaging. In such situations, intraoperative TEE can be used both to confirm the diagnosis and to guide surgical repair.

MANAGEMENT OF CARDIAC TAMPONADE. Cardiac tamponade frequently complicates acute proximal aortic dissection and is one of the most common mechanisms of death in these patients. It is often the cause of hypotension when patients have aortic dissection, and pericardiocentesis is commonly performed in this setting in an effort to stabilize patients while they await definitive surgical repair. However, in a retrospective series we found that pericardiocentesis may be harmful rather than beneficial in this setting because it may precipitate hemodynamic collapse and death rather than stabilize the patient as intended.[173] Seven patients in this series were relatively stable initially (six hypotensive, one normotensive). Three of four who underwent successful pericardiocentesis died suddenly between 5 and 40 minutes after the procedure secondary to acute electromechanical dissociation. In contrast, none of the three patients without pericardiocentesis died before surgery. It may be that in such patients the increase in intraaortic pressure that follows pericardiocentesis causes a closed communication between the false lumen and pericardial space to reopen, thereby leading to recurrent hemorrhage and lethal cardiac tamponade.

Therefore, when a patient with acute aortic dissection complicated by cardiac tamponade is relatively stable, the risks of pericardiocentesis probably outweigh the benefits and *every effort should be made to proceed as urgently as possible to the operating room for direct surgical repair of the aorta with intraoperative drainage of the hemopericardium.* However, when patients have electromechanical dissociation or marked hypotension, an attempt to resuscitate the patient with pericardiocentesis is warranted. A prudent strategy in such cases might be to aspirate only enough pericardial fluid to raise blood pressure to the lowest acceptable level.[173]

Definitive Therapy

Despite minor variations from center to center, a reasonable consensus regarding definitive therapy for aortic dissection has evolved over the past several decades. It is universally agreed that surgical therapy is superior to medical therapy for acute proximal dissection.[174, 175] With even limited pro-

gression of a proximal dissection, patients may suffer the potentially devastating consequences of aortic rupture or cardiac tamponade, acute aortic regurgitation, or neurological compromise. Thus, by controlling this risk, immediate surgical repair promises a better outcome. Occasional patients with proximal dissection who refuse surgery or for whom surgery is contraindicated (e.g., by age or prior debilitating illness) may potentially be treated successfully with medical therapy with a 30-day survival rate of up to 42 percent.[112]

Patients suffering acute distal aortic dissection, on the other hand, are generally at lower risk of early death from complications of the dissection than are those with proximal dissection.[128] Furthermore, because patients with distal dissection tend to be older and have a relatively increased prevalence of advanced atherosclerosis or cardiopulmonary disease, their surgical risk is often considerably higher. A large retrospective series involving patients from both Duke and Stanford universities has, by multivariate analysis, shown that medical therapy provides an outcome equivalent to that of surgical therapy in patients with uncomplicated distal dissection.[176] As a consequence, medical therapy for such patients is currently favored by most groups. An important exception is that when distal dissection is complicated by rupture, expansion, saccular aneurysm formation, vital organ or limb ischemia, or continued pain, the results of medical therapy are poor and surgery is therefore recommended.[170, 175]

Patients with chronic aortic dissection have, through self-selection, survived the early period of highest mortality, and whether treated medically or surgically, their subsequent hospital survival rate is approximately 90 percent.[177] Accordingly, medical therapy is recommended for the management of all stable patients with chronic proximal and distal dissection, again unless complicated by rupture, aneurysm formation, aortic regurgitation, arterial occlusion, or extension or recurrence of dissection.

SURGICAL MANAGEMENT. Generally advocated indications for definitive surgical therapy are summarized in Table 40–4. Surgical candidacy should be determined whenever possible at the start of the patient's evaluation because this option guides the selection of diagnostic studies. Surgical risk for all patients is increased by age, comorbid disease (especially pulmonary emphysema), aneurysm leakage, cardiac tamponade, shock, or vital organ compromise as a result of such conditions as myocardial infarction, cerebrovascular accident, and in particular, preexisting renal failure.

Preoperative mortality in patients with acute dissection ranges from 3 percent when surgery is expedited to as high as 20 percent when the preoperative evaluation is more prolonged.[165] These data reinforce the need for prompt di-

▼ **TABLE 40–4. INDICATIONS FOR DEFINITIVE SURGICAL AND MEDICAL THERAPY IN AORTIC DISSECTION**

SURGICAL
Treatment of choice for acute proximal dissection
Treatment for acute distal dissection complicated by the following:
  Progression with vital organ compromise
  Rupture or impending rupture (e.g., saccular aneurysm formation)
  Retrograde extension into the ascending aorta
  Dissection in the Marfan syndrome

MEDICAL
Treatment of choice for uncomplicated distal dissection
Treatment for stable, isolated arch dissection
Treatment of choice for stable chronic dissection (uncomplicated dissection presenting 2 weeks or later after onset)

agnosis and repair to prevent even minimal progression of the dissection, which might lead to further complications.[88]

The usual objectives of definitive surgical therapy include resection of the most severely damaged segment of aorta, excision of the intimal tear when possible, and obliteration of entry into the false lumen by suturing the edges of the dissected aorta both proximally and distally. After resecting the diseased segment containing the intimal tear, typically a segment of the ascending aorta in proximal dissections or the proximal descending aorta in distal dissections, aortic continuity is then reestablished by interposing a prosthetic sleeve graft between the two ends of the aorta (Fig. 40–18).

Importantly, Miller and colleagues have found that the immediate and long-term survival of patients treated surgically was not significantly affected by failure to excise the intimal tear.[174, 178] Some patients with proximal dissection have an intimal tear located in the aortic arch. Because surgical repair of the arch may increase the morbidity and mortality associated with the procedure and because resection of the tear may not necessarily improve mortality,[178a] many authors have elected to not repair the arch if the sole purpose of surgery is resection of the intimal tear.[178] However, with improvements in surgical technique during the last decade, several groups now suggest that even these challenging lesions can be resected with favorable results.[179, 180]

When aortic regurgitation complicates aortic dissection, simple decompression of the false lumen is sometimes all that is required to allow resuspension of the aortic leaflets and restoration of valvular competence. More often, however, preservation of the aortic valve requires approximation of the two layers of dissected aortic wall and resuspension of the commissures with pledgeted sutures. In this setting, the use of intraoperative TEE may be particularly helpful to the surgeon in guiding aortic valve repair.[181] This resuspension technique has had favorable results with a fairly low incidence of recurrent aortic regurgitation in long-term follow-up.[118, 182] Preserving the aortic valve in this fashion may avoid the complications associated with prosthetic valve replacement, especially the requirement for oral anticoagulation, which may pose an added risk in patients prone to future aortic rupture.

Prosthetic aortic valve replacement is sometimes necessary, however, either because attempts at valve repair are unsuccessful or in the setting of preexisting valvular disease or the Marfan syndrome.[182] Many surgeons are aggressive about replacing the aortic valve if it appears that even moderate aortic regurgitation will remain after the leaflets are resuspended and choose to avoid the risk of having to replace the aortic valve at some later date in a second operation through a diseased aorta. When the proximal aorta is fragile or badly torn, most use the Bentall procedure in which a composite prosthetic graft—a prosthetic aortic valve sewn onto the end of a Dacron tube graft—facilitates replacement of both the ascending aorta and aortic valve together (see Fig. 40–5). The coronary arteries are then reimplanted as buttons of aortic tissue into the graft wall. The operative procedure in aortic dissection is technically demanding. The wall of the diseased aorta is often friable, and the repair must be performed with meticulous care. The use of Teflon felt to buttress the wall and prevent sutures from tearing through the fragile aorta is essential (see Fig. 40–18). Determining the sources of vital organ perfusion distal to the surgical site by diagnostic imaging studies may be of critical importance. For example, if one or both renal arteries are supplied by the false lumen and are not going to be directly corrected surgically, the surgeon may leave communication between the true and false channels distal to the site of aortic repair so that renal perfusion is not jeopardized.

COMPLICATIONS. Bleeding, infection, pulmonary failure, and renal insufficiency constitute the most common early complications of surgical therapy. Spinal cord ischemia with paraplegia caused by inadvertent interruption of the blood supply from the anterior spinal or intercostal arteries is an uncommon but dreaded consequence of descending thoracic aortic repair. Late complications include progressive aortic regurgitation if the aortic valve has not been replaced, localized aneurysm formation, and recurrent dissection at the original site or at a secondary site.[178] With modern operative techniques, 30-day surgical survival rates for proximal and distal dissections are 74 and 69 percent, respectively.[112]

NEWER SURGICAL TECHNIQUES. As a modification of more standard operative techniques, several investigators have unified the layers of the dissected aortic wall by using either a fibrin sealant[183] or gelatin-resorcine-formaldehyde glue.[184] After resection of the diseased aortic segment, this glue is used in place of pledgeted sutures to seal the false lumen of the aortic stumps, before implantation of the Dacron prosthesis. The glue not only hardens and reinforces the fragile dis-

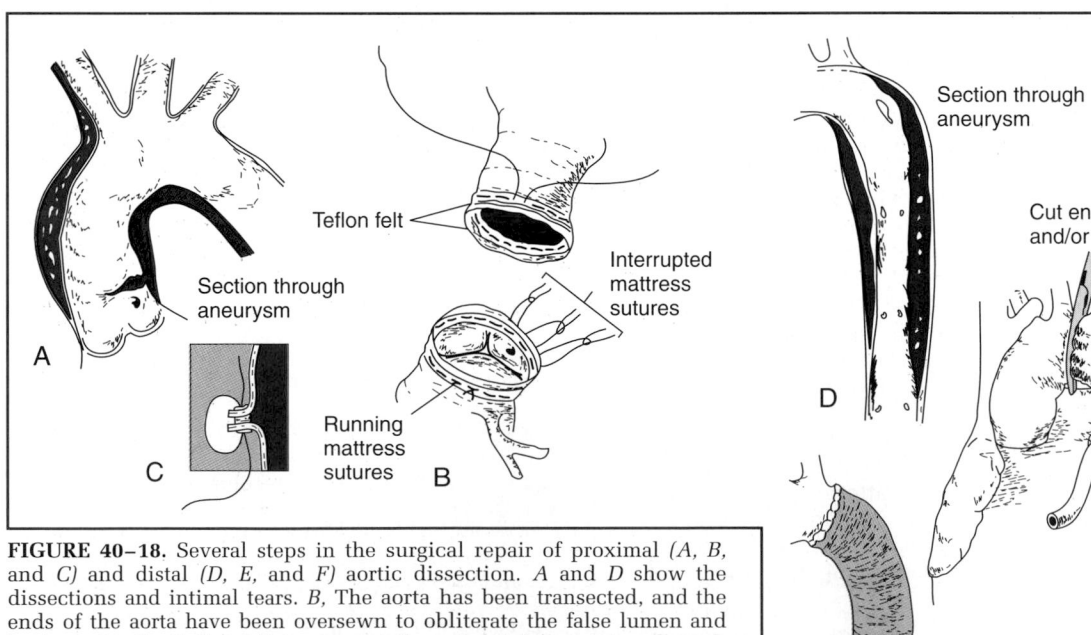

FIGURE 40–18. Several steps in the surgical repair of proximal (*A, B,* and *C*) and distal (*D, E,* and *F*) aortic dissection. *A* and *D* show the dissections and intimal tears. *B,* The aorta has been transected, and the ends of the aorta have been oversewn to obliterate the false lumen and buttressed with Teflon felt to prevent the sutures from tearing through the fragile tissue. *C,* The aortic ends are brought together in such a way that the Teflon is again used to reinforce the suture line between the two ends of the aorta and between the aorta and a sleeve graft, if such a graft is necessary for reconstitution of the aorta. *E,* Resection of a distal dissection, with a Teflon graft interposed in *F.* (*D, E,* and *F* reprinted, by permission, from Austen WG, DeSanctis RW: Surgical treatment of dissecting aneurysm of the thoracic aorta. N Engl J Med 272:1314, 1965.)

sected aortic tissue but may also simplify the operation, facilitate resuspension of the aortic valve, and potentially reduce the incidence of late aortic root aneurysm formation.[183] Another group has used such glue in carrying out direct surgical repair of the aorta without an interposing graft by first suturing the intimal tear, then applying the glue in the false lumen to unify the layers of the dissected aorta, and finally reattaching the free aortic ends. Although early reports show favorable morbidity and mortality with the use of these new techniques,[184] direct comparison with standard operative techniques is needed.

ENDOVASCULAR TECHNIQUES (see also Chap. 42). One of the more promising avenues of investigation is the use of endovascular techniques for treating high-risk patients with aortic dissection. For example, because patients with renal or visceral artery compromise from dissection have operative mortality rates exceeding 50 percent,[185, 186] alternative management strategies are desirable. Two endovascular techniques have been used in many centers to manage patients with acute vascular complications secondary to aortic dissection. The first is balloon fenestration of the intimal flap, which involves crossing an intact intimal flap with a wire, passing a balloon-tipped catheter over the wire, and then expanding the balloon to tear a hole in the intimal flap. The hole acts as a site of reentry to allow blood to flow from the false lumen into the true lumen, thereby decompressing the distended false lumen. The second technique involves percutaneous stenting of an affected arterial branch whose flow has been compromised by the dissection process. Slonim and coauthors reported the use of percutaneous management of ischemic complications of aortic dissection in a series of 22 patients.[186] Sixteen patients were treated with endovascular stents, 3 with balloon fenestration of the intimal flap, and 3 with fenestration in combination with stenting of the aorta or its branches; revascularization with clinical success was achieved in all 22 patients, with excellent long-term outcomes. The utility of aortic intimal flap fenestration in restoring blood flow to hypoperfused organs has also been demonstrated in animal models.[187] In the large IRAD series of acute aortic dissection, 3.2 percent of patients were treated with percutaneous fenestration procedures.[112]

More definitive endovascular techniques have also been introduced. Sutureless intraluminal prostheses placed during cardiopulmonary bypass are intended to improve outcome by decreasing intraoperative and postoperative bleeding complications. These devices have been used successfully with good outcomes in two small series of patients with proximal aortic dissection.[188, 189]

More recently, intraluminal stent-grafts placed percutaneously by the transfemoral catheter technique have been introduced as a potential alternative to aortic repair.[190-192] The purpose of this procedure is to close the site of entry into the false lumen (intimal tear), decompress and promote thrombosis of the false lumen, and relieve any obstruction of branch vessels that may accompany the dissection. It is hoped that this approach will reduce the morbidity and mortality of aortic dissection and reduce the risk of subsequent aneurysm formation. Nienaber and colleagues compared the use of stent-graft placement with standard surgical repair in a group of 24 patients with subacute or chronic type B aortic dissection and a patent false lumen.[191] No procedural complications occurred among the 12 patients undergoing stent-graft treatment, and when compared with the surgical group, the stent-graft group had a significantly shorter hospital stay, lower morbidity, and lower 1-year postprocedural mortality. Dake and colleagues inserted stent-grafts in the descending thoracic aortas of 19 patients with acute aortic dissection and a patent false lumen who suffered from obstruction of branch vessels, acute aortic rupture, or persistent back pain.[192] Endovascular stent-graft deployment was successful in all cases, with complete thrombosis of the false lumen in 79 percent and partial thrombosis in the remaining 21 percent. Restoration of flow to ischemic arterial branches with relief of corresponding symptoms occurred in 76 percent of obstructed branches. The results of these two series are extremely promising, but larger studies with more patients and longer follow-up will be required before stent-graft therapy becomes an accepted therapy for aortic dissection.[193]

DEFINITIVE MEDICAL MANAGEMENT. The indications for definitive medical therapy are summarized in Table 40-4. As discussed above, we prefer medical therapy for stable patients with uncomplicated acute distal dissection given that the 30-day survival rate for those with distal dissection treated medically is 92 percent.[112] However, surgery clearly must be performed in cases of medical management failure, such as in the presence of rupture or impending rupture, progression of the dissection with vital organ compromise, an inability to control pain with medicines, or retrograde progression of a type B dissection into the ascending aorta. Because of the extreme difficulty of surgery to repair the aortic arch when it is involved by the dissection, medical therapy is also usually advocated for distal

dissections that either originate in the arch or extend retrograde into the arch. Operative therapy is again reserved for those with serious complications. Medical therapy is also generally recommended for patients with chronic aortic dissection, whether proximal or distal, unless late complications of the dissection, such as aortic regurgitation or localized aneurysm formation, necessitate surgery.

Severe hypertension is relatively common during the period of hospitalization after acute aortic dissection and may be seen even in patients without a history of significant hypertension. The etiology for this hypertensive response is unclear but it may reflect a marked increase in sympathetic tone triggered by the severe inflammation of the aortic wall that accompanies dissection. While such hypertension often prompts clinicians to order a CT or MR angiogram to rule out renal artery compromise by the dissection, in our experience, renal ischemia is rarely the cause.[194] In most cases, blood pressure begins to fall and becomes more easily controlled about 5 to 7 days after onset of the aortic dissection.

Long-Term Therapy and Late Follow-Up

Late follow-up of patients leaving the hospital with treated aortic dissection shows an actuarial survival rate not much worse than that of individuals of comparable age without dissection. No significant differences are seen among discharged patients when comparing proximal versus distal dissection, acute versus chronic dissection, or medical versus surgical treatment.[128] Five-year survival rates for all these groups are typically 75 to 82 percent.[128, 174, 178] Thus, the initial success of surgical or medical therapy is usually sustained on long-term follow-up. Late complications include aortic regurgitation, recurrent dissection, and aneurysm formation or rupture.

Long-term medical therapy to control hypertension and reduce dP/dt is indicated for all patients who have sustained an aortic dissection, regardless of whether their in-hospital definitive treatment was surgical or medical. Indeed, one study found that late aneurysm rupture after aortic dissection was 10 times more common in patients with poorly controlled hypertension than in those with controlled blood pressure,[195] which dramatically demonstrates the importance of aggressive lifelong antihypertensive therapy. Systolic blood pressure should be maintained at or below 130 mm Hg. The preferred agents are beta blockers or, if contraindicated, other agents with a negative inotropic as well as a hypotensive effect such as verapamil or diltiazem. Pure vasodilators, such as dihydropyridine calcium channel antagonists or hydralazine, may cause an increase in dP/dt and should therefore be used only in conjunction with adequate beta blockade. ACE inhibitors are attractive antihypertensive agents for treating aortic dissection and may be of particular benefit in those with some degree of renal ischemia as a consequence of the dissection.

Up to 29 percent of late deaths following surgery result from rupture of either the dissecting aneurysm or another aneurysm at a remote site. Moreover, the incidence of subsequent aneurysm formation at a site remote from the surgical repair is 17 to 25 percent,[108, 196] with these remote aneurysms accounting for many of the rupture-related deaths. The mean time interval from primary aortic dissection to the appearance of subsequent aneurysms is 18 months, with the majority appearing within 2 years.[196] Many such aneurysms occur from dilatation of the residual false lumen in the more distal aortic segments not resected at the time of surgery. Because the dissected aneurysm wall is relatively thin and consists of only the outer half of the original aortic wall, these aneurysms rupture more frequently than do typical atherosclerotic thoracic aneurysms.[78, 196] Thus, an aggressive approach to treating such late-appearing aneurysms may be indicated.

The high incidence of late aneurysm formation and rupture emphasizes both the diffuse nature of the aortic disease process in this population and the tremendous importance of careful follow-up. The primary goal of long-term surveillance is the early detection of aortic lesions that might require subsequent surgical intervention, such as the appearance of new aneurysms or rapid aneurysm expansion, progression or recurrence of dissection, aortic regurgitation, or peripheral vascular compromise.

Follow-up evaluation of patients after aortic dissection should include careful and repeated physical examinations, periodic chest roentgenograms, and serial aortic imaging with TEE, CT,[175] or MRI.[170, 197] We generally prefer MRI for serially monitoring these patients because it is completely noninvasive and provides excellent anatomical detail that may be exceedingly helpful in evaluating interval changes.[198] Patients are at highest risk immediately after hospitalization and during the first 2 years, with the risk progressively declining thereafter. It is therefore important to have more frequent early follow-up; for example, patients may be seen at 3 and 6 months initially and then return every 6 months for 2 years, after which time they may be reevaluated at 6- to 12-month intervals, depending on the given patient's risk.

Atypical Aortic Dissection

In recent years it has become increasingly clear that in addition to aortic dissection as classically described, two other diseases of the aorta are closely related, *intramural hematoma* of the aorta and *penetrating atherosclerotic ulcer* of the aorta. These two conditions share with aortic dissection many of the predisposing risk factors and initial symptoms, and indeed, both may lead to either classic aortic dissection or aortic rupture. In light of their clinical simi-

larities, it is appropriate to consider classic aortic dissection and its variants collectively among the "acute thoracic aortic syndromes," a category that also includes traumatic aortic transection and rupture, contained rupture (pseudo-aneurysm), or acute expansion of thoracic aortic aneurysms.

INTRAMURAL HEMATOMA. Intramural hematoma is essentially a hemorrhage contained within the medial layer of the aortic wall. Although the pathogenesis of intramural hematoma is still uncertain, rupture of the vasa vasorum is believed to be the initiating event and results in hemorrhage into the outer media and extending into the adventitia.[199] This complication may produce a localized or discrete hematoma, but more often the hemorrhage extends for a variable distance by dissecting along the outer media beneath the adventitia.[200] Intramural hematoma is distinguished from typical aortic dissection by the lack of an associated tear in the intima or direct communication between the media and aortic lumen; hence, some have termed it *aortic dissection without intimal rupture.*[199] Previous pathological studies of what were considered clinically to be aortic dissections have found that 3 to 13 percent did not have an identifiable intimal tear,[106, 107, 201] and it is possible that such cases were in fact actually intramural hematomas. Moreover, it remains uncertain whether intramural hematoma is a distinct pathological entity or instead represents a reversible precursor of classic aortic dissection.

Clinically, intramural hematoma may be indistinguishable from true aortic dissection. In the IRAD series of 464 patients with the clinical diagnosis of acute aortic dissection, 10 percent were found by imaging studies to have an intramural hematoma rather than classic dissection and two-thirds of these intramural hematomas were classified as type B.[112] The majority of patients are elderly with a history of hypertension and typically have extensive aortic atherosclerosis.[202, 203] Almost all patients have the chest and back

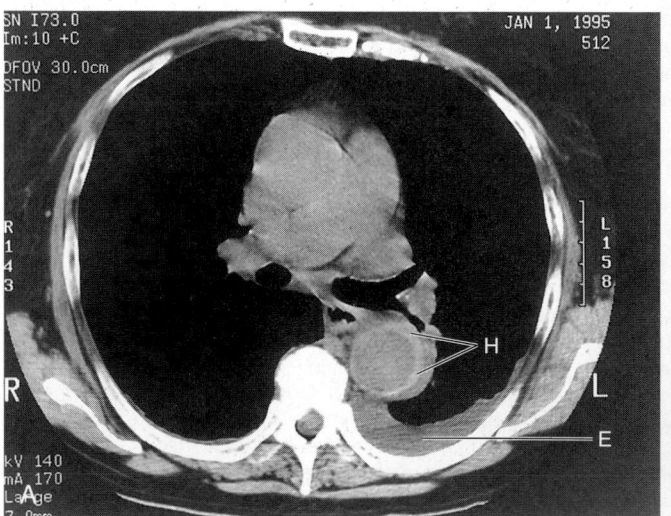
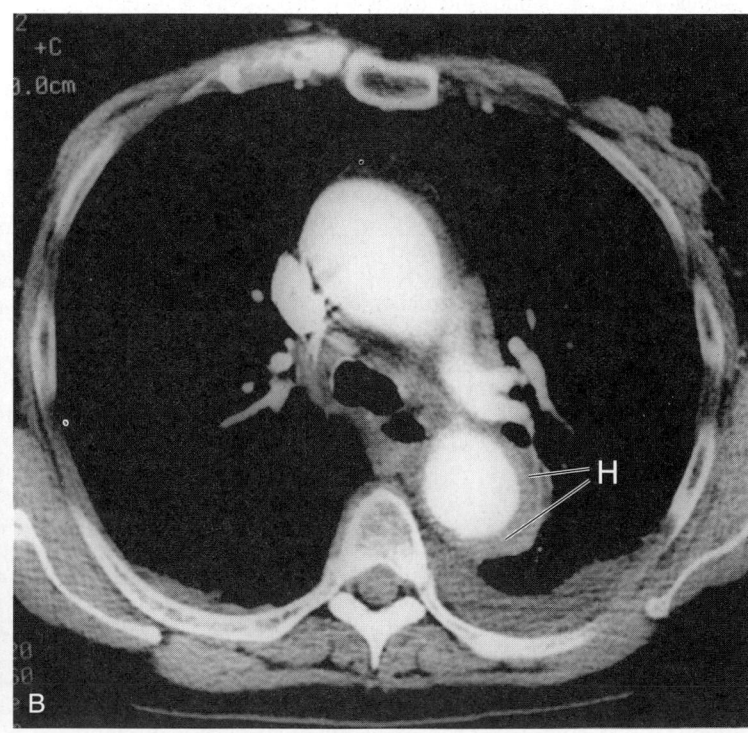

FIGURE 40–19. Intramural hematoma of the descending thoracic aorta. *A,* An axial CT scan without contrast enhancement demonstrates crescentic thickening of the aortic wall that is of increased density (H), consistent with an intramural hematoma of the aorta. A left pleural effusion (E) is also present. *B,* Subsequent contrast-enhanced images of the same patient demonstrating a contrast-filled aortic lumen with dark crescentic thickening of the aortic wall (H) that does not enhance, confirming the presence of an intramural hematoma that does not communicate with the aortic lumen. Note that neither the size nor the shape of the aortic lumen is distorted the way it would typically be in the presence of a classic aortic dissection.

pain symptoms typical of classic aortic dissection. Aortic regurgitation and pulse deficits may be present. One-half of patients may have an associated left pleural effusion[199, 202] that may not appear until several days after the hematoma develops.[199] Pericardial effusion may appear when the ascending aorta is involved.[202]

Intramural hematoma is best diagnosed by CT scanning. On a non–contrast-enhanced CT scan (Fig. 40–19A) it appears as a continuous, crescentic, high-attenuation area along the aortic wall without evidence of an intimal tear, false lumen, or associated intimal atherosclerotic ulcer.[200] This first examination is followed by a contrast-enhanced CT scan (Fig. 40–19B), which demonstrates failure of the intramural hematoma to enhance (appearing as a darker crescentic thickening of the aortic wall), thereby excluding communication with the aortic lumen. In some cases it may be difficult to distinguish intramural hematoma from aortic dissection with thrombosis of the false lumen or from mural thrombus within an aortic aneurysm.[199] However, with an intramural hematoma, the aortic lumen retains its overall size and shape, unlike the case with aortic dissection.

On MRI, an intramural hematoma appears as a crescentic high-intensity area along the aortic wall.[199] On TEE, it is manifested as a continuous crescentic or nearly concentric circular thickening of the aortic wall that in some cases may be difficult to distinguish from severe atherosclerotic thickening of the aortic wall.[204, 205] Aortography, on the other hand, often fails to detect the presence of an intramural hematoma because no contrast escapes the aortic lumen and the intramural hematoma does not usually compress the aortic lumen to produce recognizable aortographic signs such as seen with aortic dissection.[199] In fact, the sensitivity of aortography for detecting intramural hematoma is as low as 19 percent[206]; therefore, while a negative aortogram may exclude the presence of classic aortic dissection, it does not reliably exclude the important variant of intramural hematoma.

The natural history of intramural hematoma is not yet well defined. Involvement of the ascending aorta appears to carry a high risk of death or complications requiring surgical repair, whereas hematomas of the descending aorta have a more favorable prognosis. In a retrospective series, Nienaber and coworkers determined that 13 percent of 195 patients with aortic dissection–like syndromes in fact had intramural hematoma.[204] The actuarial survival rates were similar for the groups with intramural hematoma and overt aortic dissection.[204] Of patients with proximal intramural hematoma, 30-day mortality was 80 percent for those treated medically versus 0 percent for those undergoing early repair. On the other hand, early mortality for distal intramural hematoma was 9 percent and did not differ significantly between medical and surgical treatment.

Intramural hematomas may regress with time or even completely resolve on follow-up imaging.[199] However, should the intramural hematoma completely resolve, the affected portion of the aorta is still at risk for progressive enlargement and fusiform aneurysm formation.[207] Alternatively, intramural hematoma may progress to overt aortic dissection within days[204] to months of initial examination.[200] Nienaber and colleagues found progression to overt dissection, aortic rupture, or cardiac tamponade in one-third of their patients.[204]

The limited data on the natural history of intramural hematoma suggest that it behaves very much like classic aortic dissection and should therefore be treated in a similar fashion. Thus, surgical therapy is best for proximal hematomas, whereas medical therapy is reasonable for distal hematomas. Physicians should have a low threshold, however, for proceeding to surgery in distal disease if symptoms persist or evidence of progression is seen. Medical management should therefore include serial imaging studies to monitor progression or regression of the intramural hematoma.

PENETRATING ATHEROSCLEROTIC ULCER. Penetrating atherosclerotic ulcer, first defined in the literature in 1986 by Stanson and coauthors in 1986,[208] is an ulceration of an atherosclerotic lesion of the aorta that penetrates the internal elastic lamina and allows hematoma formation within the media of the aortic wall (Fig. 40–20). Although such ulcerations occur almost exclusively in the descending thoracic aorta,[209] they may also occur in the arch or rarely in the ascending aorta.[210, 211] The hematoma that results from a penetrating atherosclerotic ulcer usually remains localized or extends several centimeters in length, but a false lumen typically does not develop.[212] However, it has also been suggested that some cases of intramural hematoma of the aorta may in fact be secondary to small penetrating atherosclerotic ulcers that have escaped detection on imaging studies but are later identified at the time of surgery.[213]

Atherosclerotic aortic ulcers penetrate through the media in one-quarter of cases to cause aortic pseudoaneurysms or through the adventitia in 8 percent to cause transmural aortic rupture[210] (Fig. 40–20). Rarely, a penetrating atherosclerotic ulcer may progress to an extensive classic aortic dissection.[211] Over time, penetrating atherosclerotic ulcers frequently lead to the formation of saccular or fusiform aortic aneurysms.[214]

Patients in whom penetrating atherosclerotic ulcers develop tend to be elderly with a history of hypertension and

FIGURE 40–20. Evolution of a penetrating atherosclerotic ulcer of the aorta. Once an intimal ulcer has formed, it may then progress to a variable depth. Penetration through the intima causes a medial hematoma, while penetration through the media leads to the formation of a pseudoaneurysm, and perforation through the adventitial layer results in aortic rupture. (From Stanson AW, Kazmier FJ, Hollier LH, et al: Penetrating atherosclerotic ulcers of the thoracic aorta: Natural history and clinicopathological correlations. Ann Vasc Surg 1:15, 1986.)

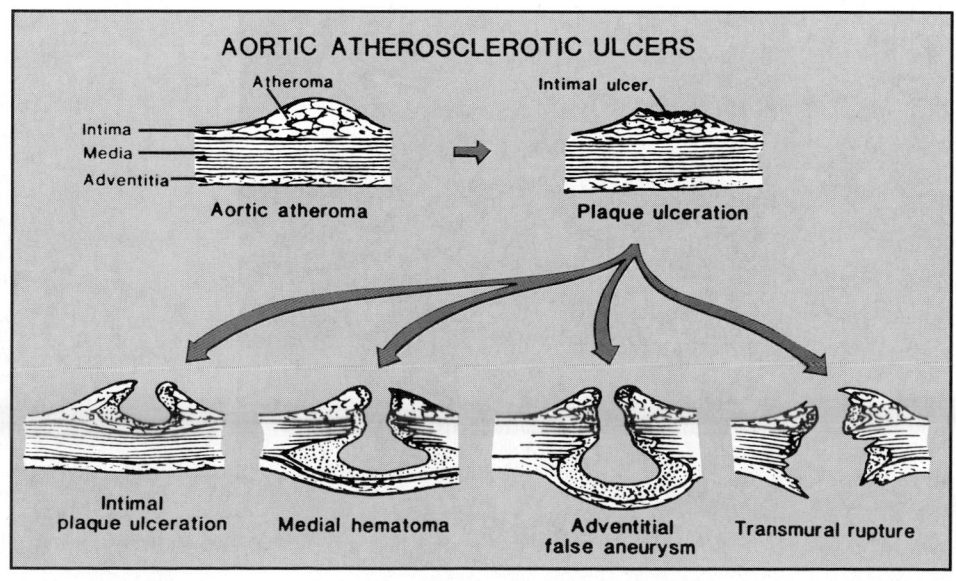

AORTIC ATHEROSCLEROTIC ULCERS

Atheroma — Intimal ulcer

Intima — Media — Adventitia —
Aortic atheroma

Plaque ulceration

Intimal plaque ulceration — Medial hematoma — Adventitial false aneurysm — Transmural rupture

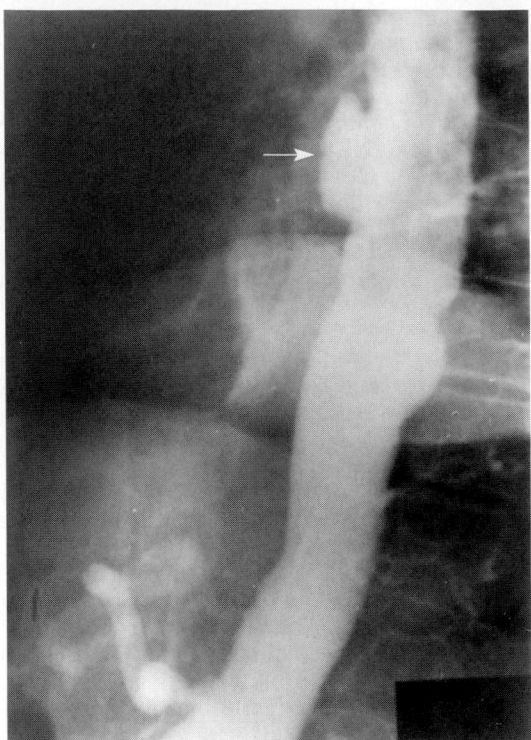

FIGURE 40–21. Thoracic aortogram demonstrating a penetrating atherosclerotic ulcer of the distal end of the descending aorta (arrow). The hematoma of the aortic wall is evident as a localized contrast-filled outpouching of the aorta. The remainder of the aorta is diffusely atherosclerotic.

evidence of other atherosclerotic cardiovascular disease.[209] Initial symptoms include chest and back pain similar to that of aortic dissection, and the majority are hypertensive at initial evaluation.[209] However, since penetrating atherosclerotic ulcers tend to be localized, the vascular compromise or aortic regurgitation that often complicates aortic dissection does not develop.[208]

Chest roentgenograms often demonstrate a dilated descending thoracic aorta as well as left-sided or bilateral pleural effusions.[209] Aortography is the diagnostic standard for detecting a penetrating atherosclerotic ulcer, with the lesion appearing as a contrast-filled outpouching in the descending aorta in the absence of an intimal flap or false lumen[210] (Fig. 40–21). On CT scanning or MRI the lesion appears as a focal ulceration, with thickening of the aortic wall and inward displacement of intimal calcification consistent with intramural hematoma. TEE may identify the presence of a culprit atherosclerotic ulcer in the setting of a visible intramural hematoma,[215] but diagnosis is difficult.[154]

The natural history of a penetrating atherosclerotic ulcer remains largely unclear, and at present no definitive treatment strategy is available. Certainly, patients who are hemodynamically unstable or who have evidence of pseudoaneurysm formation or transmural rupture should undergo urgent surgical repair. Continued or recurrent pain, distal embolization, and progressive aneurysmal dilatation are also indications for surgery.[212] In the near future, transluminal placement of an endovascular stent-graft may become an alternative to surgery in such patients.[216] Those without such complications should be treated with antihypertensive medications and monitored closely with follow-up imaging studies, similar to the management of a patient with a distal aortic dissection.

Aortic Trauma

See Chapter 51.

AORTIC ATHEROMATOUS DISEASE
(see also Chap. 41)

AORTOGENIC ATHEROTHROMBOTIC EMBOLI. The clinical importance of atherosclerotic disease of the aorta has long been recognized inasmuch as atheromatous or fibrinous material, thrombi, or cholesterol particles dislodged from atherosclerotic plaque may cause cerebral or peripheral embolic phenomena.[217] However, assessing the degree of such atherosclerotic disease antemortem has been limited by the inability of the several imaging modalities to directly visualize the aortic intima.[218] Aortography demonstrates the aortic lumen rather than the aortic walls themselves and can thus detect only gross atherosclerotic changes, whereas CT scanning or MRI rarely detects protruding atheromas because the normal pulsatile motion of the aorta may limit definition of the aortic wall on the tomographic images. On the other hand, TEE is uniquely suited to assess atherosclerotic disease of the aorta in real time and has been demonstrated to have greater sensitivity for aortic arch atherosclerosis than is the case with chest roentgenography, aortography, or CT scanning.[218] On echocardiography, mild atherosclerosis appears as intimal thickening, irregularity, and calcification, whereas more severe disease appears as thick plaque with protruding atheromas (Fig. 40–22). In some cases, protruding lesions have highly mobile components that probably represent atheroma with superimposed thrombus.[219]

Risk factors for aortic atherosclerosis include age, hypertension, diabetes,[220] hyperlipidemia,[221] and other vascular disease.[222] Through the use of TEE, the prevalence and extent of macroscopic atherosclerotic disease have now been documented in a variety of patient populations. Atheromatous disease is least common in the ascending aorta, more common in the arch, and most common in the descending thoracic aorta.[223, 224] While aortic atheromas are detected in as few as 2 percent of patients without a history of stroke or known aortic disease, they are found in 38 percent of those with significant carotid artery disease,[225] 60 percent of those with ischemic stroke,[223] and up to 90 percent of those with obstructive coronary artery disease.[226]

In an autopsy series, Amarenco and colleagues found that the presence of ulcerated plaque in the aortic arch was a significant independent risk factor for stroke, particularly cryptogenic stroke,[222] and multiple clinical studies using

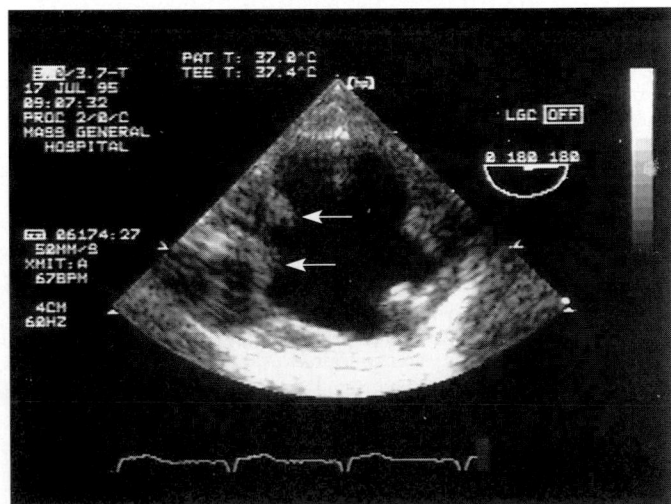

FIGURE 40–22. Cross-sectional transesophageal echocardiogram of the descending thoracic aorta demonstrating extensive atherosclerotic disease. This patient had recently suffered an embolic stoke of uncertain etiology. Multiple atheromatous plaques up to 7 mm in thickness protrude into the aortic lumen. When viewed in real time, two plaques (arrows) had small mobile intraluminal components.

TEE have found an association between aortic atherosclerosis and stroke, as well as other peripheral embolic events.[217, 221, 227] In both retrospective and prospective studies, protruding aortic atheromas are detected in 7 to 8 percent of patients undergoing routine TEE,[217, 228] with about a 33 percent incidence of embolic vascular events over a 2-year follow-up period.[228] The embolic risk is even higher in patients with pedunculated or mobile lesions and those undergoing invasive aortic procedures.[217]

In a prospective case-control study, Amarenco and associates found atherosclerotic plaque measuring 4 mm or greater in the ascending aorta or proximal arch in 14 percent of patients with ischemic stroke as compared with only 2 percent of controls. After adjustment for atherosclerotic risk factors, the odds ratio for stroke was 9.1 for ischemic stroke and 4.7 for cryptogenic stroke, with an even higher risk ratio for complex atheromas than for simple ones.[223] However, the increased risk of stroke was associated only with large atheromas involving the ascending aorta and proximal arch, not with atheromas in the distal arch or descending aorta,[223] thus supporting the hypothesis that atheromas in the ascending aorta and proximal portion of the aortic arch embolize directly into the cerebral circulation and cause ischemic strokes in such patients.[229]

Little is known about the natural history of atheromatous lesions[230] of the aorta, although one prospective trial has demonstrated that individual lesion morphology is dynamic in that mobile components both form on some atheromas and resolve on others during the same time period.[231] At present, therapeutic strategies are limited. Potential approaches for chronic management include the use of antithrombotic[232, 233] or antiplatelet[230] therapy to prevent thrombus formation. In two recent prospective but nonrandomized studies, patients having aortic plaque 4 mm or more in thickness or mobile aortic atheromas on TEE examination were found to have a high rate of recurrent vascular events. Of these study subjects, those subsequently treated with warfarin therapy had a significantly lower rate of recurrent embolic events than did those treated with antiplatelet therapy, which suggests that warfarin may be efficacious in this high-risk population.[234, 235] A prospective randomized trial is clearly needed to confirm the benefits of oral anticoagulant therapy for aortic atheromas. Some investigators have reported the surgical removal, under hypothermic circulatory arrest, of protruding atheromas detected in patients after embolic events.[227] However, this surgery carries the risk of an early adverse outcome, and at present no controlled data suggest that it actually reduces the incidence of future embolization in this population.

CARDIAC SURGERY AND ATHEROEMBOLISM. Perioperative dislodgement with embolization of atherosclerotic material from the aorta is a well-recognized hazard of cardiac surgery and has been increasingly implicated as an important cause of postoperative stroke and other embolic events in these patients. The incidence of cerebral ischemic events after cardiac surgery typically ranges from 1 to 3 percent, with an increased risk among the elderly.[220, 236] In an autopsy series of patients who underwent cardiac surgery, Blauth and colleagues identified atheroemboli in 22 percent of cases.[237] Atheroembolic events occurred in 37 percent of those with severe atherosclerosis of the ascending aorta versus only 2 percent of those without significant ascending aortic atherosclerosis. Moreover, 96 percent of patients with perioperative atheroemboli had severe atherosclerosis of their ascending aorta.[237] Mobile pedunculated lesions appear more prone to embolize.[217]

Mechanisms by which aortic atherosclerotic debris may be dislodged during cardiac surgery include external manipulation of the aorta during palpation,[236] cross-clamping, cannula placement, anastomosis of the bypass grafts to the aorta,[220] and the "sandblasting" effect of the high-velocity jet of blood that exits the aortic cannula and strikes the atherosclerotic intima of the opposite aortic wall.[236, 237] Although surgeons have long relied on direct digital palpation to detect the presence of atherosclerosis in the ascending aorta, this method underestimates the incidence, severity, and extent of atherosclerotic disease.[238] In contrast, ultrasonography is superior for delineating the presence and severity of atherosclerotic disease of the ascending aorta,[217] with intraoperative epi-aortic ultrasound found to be even more sensitive than TEE.[239]

Several studies have examined the potential role of aortic ultrasonography in identifying patients at highest risk for perioperative atheroemboli. In 8 to 17 percent of cases, the ultrasonographic findings led to modifications in surgical technique such as changing the sites of aortic cannulation (with cannulation of the distal aorta or femoral artery instead), cross-clamping, or anastomosis of vein grafts.[220, 236, 238, 240] The results of such procedural modifications have been promising, with several reports showing a trend toward a reduction in stroke rates.

CHOLESTEROL EMBOLIZATION SYNDROME (see also Chap. 41). Cholesterol embolization syndrome is caused by distal showering of cholesterol crystals from ulcerated atheromatous plaque in the aorta or iliac and proximal femoral arteries in patients with diffuse atherosclerosis. These cholesterol crystals then obstruct small peripheral arteries (100 to 300 μm in size), where they cause local tissue ischemia or necrosis and frequently induce a local inflammatory reaction that may contribute to the arteriolar occlusive process.[241]

The precise mechanisms that precipitate cholesterol embolization are unclear. The syndrome is most commonly seen following instrumentation of the aorta, such as with cardiac catheterization, percutaneous transluminal coronary angiography, angiography, or intraaortic balloon pump insertion.[242] The overall incidence following cardiac catheterization was 0.1 percent in the Coronary Artery Surgery Study.[243] Cholesterol embolization may also complicate aortic surgery or cardiopulmonary bypass. At times, cholesterol embolization syndrome may occur spontaneously. Studies have suggested a possible causal relationship between warfarin therapy and such spontaneous cholesterol embolization.[244]

The clinical manifestations depend on the organs affected. Cutaneous manifestations, typically of the lower extremities, are most common and include livedo reticularis, gangrene, cyanosis, and ulceration. Acute onset of pain with digital ischemia and small areas of cutaneous gangrene is often referred to as the "blue toe" or "purple toe syndrome"[244] (see Fig. 41–23). The presence of preserved pedal pulses in the setting of peripheral ischemia distinguishes this syndrome from embolic occlusion of larger arteries.

Acute nonoliguric renal failure with or without hypertension is a common consequence of renal emboli, often seen as a rise in creatinine over several weeks, followed by a slow but progressive worsening of renal function that may become severe and irreversible. Cholesterol embolization to the central nervous system is quite uncommon and may be manifested as focal neurological deficits, amaurosis fugax from retinal emboli, paralysis from spinal cord emboli, or a diffuse encephalopathy. Mesenteric embolization may cause abdominal pain, gastrointestinal bleeding, or pancreatitis. Finally, multiple organ systems may be simultaneously involved and mimic vasculitis or bacterial endocarditis.[241]

When the cholesterol embolization syndrome occurs as the consequence of an invasive procedure, the temporal relationship of events often suggests the diagnosis. In the case of spontaneous embolization, however, recognizing the syndrome remains extremely challenging, and diagnosis in the absence of cutaneous manifestations is especially difficult. An elevated erythrocyte sedimentation rate, eosinophilia, and a reduced complement level are helpful in suggesting the diagnosis, but making a definitive diagnosis requires tissue biopsy. Paraffin-fixed sections reveal needle-shaped clefts in the arteriolar lumina that represent the spaces occupied by cholesterol particles before fixation.

No specific therapy effectively treats cholesterol embolization syndrome. Because cholesterol embolization resembles other atheroembolic phenomena, some have advocated the use of anticoagulant therapy. However, such therapy is typically unsuccessful and may even exacerbate the condition,[245] whereas discontinuing anticoagulation may improve the condition in some cases.[246] Glucocorticoid therapy has also been tried without success. Surgical therapy is generally limited to the amputation of an ischemic or gangrenous extremity. Overall, the prognosis for those suffering cholesterol embolization syndrome is quite poor, with a mortality rate of 38 to 80 percent.[247, 248]

ACUTE AORTIC OCCLUSION

Acute aortic occlusion is an infrequent, but potentially catastrophic, condition with an early mortality of 31 to 52 percent.[249–251] It is caused by either embolic occlusion of the infrarenal aorta at the bifurcation, known as a "saddle embolus," or acute thrombosis of the abdominal aorta. At least 95 percent of aortic emboli originate from the left side of the heart,[250] typically as a thrombus from the left atrium secondary to atrial fibrillation, particularly in the setting of rheumatic mitral stenosis, or from the left ventricle secondary to myocardial infarction, aneurysm, or dilated cardiomyopathy. Less common cardiac sources of emboli include atrial myxoma, prosthetic valve thrombus, and acute bacterial or fungal endocarditis.[252] Primary thrombosis accounts for the remaining 35 to 92 percent of acute aortic occlusions.[249, 250] Seventy-five to 80 percent of thrombotic aortic occlusions occur in the setting of underlying severe aortoiliac occlusive disease and are frequently precipitated by a low-flow state secondary to heart failure or dehydration. In those without aortoiliac occlusive disease, a hypercoagulable state may precipitate thrombosis of an abdominal aortic aneurysm and lead to aortic occlusion.[249, 250]

Acute aortic occlusion is in most cases heralded by the sudden onset of excruciating bilateral lower extremity pain—usually radiating from the midportion of the thigh distally—associated with weakness, numbness, and paresthesias. Nonclassic manifestations include sudden onset of bilateral lower extremity weakness, severe hypertension from renal artery involvement, and abdominal pain from mesenteric ischemia. Persistent ischemia may lead to myonecrosis with secondary hypotension, hyperkalemia, myoglobinuria, and acute tubular necrosis. If perfusion is not reestablished within hours, death is almost inevitable.

DIAGNOSIS. Physical examination reveals cold pale extremities that are cyanotic and often exhibit a mottled, reticulated, and reddish blue appearance that may progress to the blue-black color of gangrene. Pulses are notably absent below the abdominal aorta, and capillary refill is absent. Signs of ischemic neuropathy are present and include symmetrical weakness, loss of all modalities of sensation (usually with demarcation at the level of the midthigh), and diminished or absent deep tendon reflexes. When neurological symptoms predominate, patients are often mistakenly thought to have spinal cord infarction or compression and their ischemic symptoms may initially be overlooked. In fact, as many as 11 to 17 percent of such patients may first undergo neurological or neurosurgical evaluation before the vascular etiology is recognized.[249, 250]

The diagnosis of acute aortic occlusion is confirmed by aortography. While some suggest that all stable patients should undergo the procedure,[249] others advise prompt surgical intervention without angiography if the diagnosis is strongly suspected since added delays increase the likelihood of irreversible ischemic damage to the limbs.[250, 251]

Aortography is desirable in the presence of concomitant abdominal pain, hypertension, or anuria to evaluate the possibility of renal and mesenteric arterial involvement.[250]

MANAGEMENT. Once a clinical diagnosis of acute aortic occlusion is made, intravenous heparin therapy should be initiated while awaiting immediate surgery. A saddle embolus can be removed by using Fogarty balloon-tipped catheters inserted through a transfemoral arterial approach under local anesthesia. If the embolus cannot be retrieved with Fogarty catheters, removal by direct transabdominal aortotomy is undertaken. Patients with thrombotic occlusion generally undergo either direct aortic reconstruction or revascularization with aortofemoral or axillofemoral bypass. Operative mortality for acute aortic occlusion is 31 to 40 percent[250, 251] and as high as 85 percent among those with severe left ventricular dysfunction or a hypercoagulable state.[249] Limb salvage rates are as high as 98 percent.[250, 251] Lifelong anticoagulant therapy is necessary following surgery in almost all cases to prevent recurrent emboli.[253]

AORTOARTERITIS SYNDROMES

See also Chapter 47.

BACTERIAL INFECTIONS OF THE AORTA. Infected aortic aneurysms are rare, with as few as one case per year recently reported from a large medical center.[254] In an effort to avoid confusion with infections truly of fungal origin, the term "infected aneurysm" has gradually replaced the original designation "mycotic aneurysm" used by Osler to define localized dilatation in the wall of the aorta caused by sepsis. While saccular aneurysms are seen most commonly, infections can also cause fusiform and false aneurysms. In a minority of cases, infection may arise in a preexistent aortic aneurysm, typically atherosclerotic ones. Rarely, one may encounter nonaneurysmal bacterial aortitis.[254, 255]

Pathogenesis. Aortic infection may arise by several mechanisms. A septic embolus from bacterial endocarditis was once the most common etiology but has become rare in the era of efficacious antibiotic treatment of septicemia. Contiguous spread of infection from adjacent sites is also infrequently seen. The most common cause of an infected aneurysm is direct deposition of circulating bacteria in a diseased, atherosclerotic, or traumatized aortic intima,[254] after which organisms penetrate the aortic wall through breeches in intimal integrity to cause microbial arteritis. Recent reports suggest that the majority of aortic infections occur in patients with impaired immunity as a consequence of chronic disease, immunosuppressive therapy, or immune deficiency.[254, 256]

Microbiology. Although virtually any organism may infect the aorta, certain bacteria seem to have a proclivity for this site. *Staphylococcus aureus* and *Salmonella* species are consistently the most frequently identified organisms.[257, 258] *Salmonella* commonly infects atherosclerotic arteries[255] but may also adhere to a normal aortic wall and directly penetrate an intact intima.[259] In fact, secondary aortic infection may develop in as many as one-quarter of patients older than 50 years who experience *Salmonella* bacteremia.[259] Other gram-positive organisms, particularly *Pneumococcus*, and gram-negative organisms may also cause infected aortic aneurysms. *Pseudomonas*, *Bacteroides fragilis*, *Campylobacter fetus*, *Neisseria gonorrhoeae*, and fungal infections are seen less often.[254] Aortic infections with unusual organisms are now seen with increasing frequency in the overtly immunocompromised population.[254]

Clinical Manifestations. Most patients with infected aortic aneurysm are febrile, with extremely high fevers and rigors being common. Symptoms may arise from localized expansion of an infected aneurysm, which is palpable in as many as 50 percent of patients and almost always tender.[260] A tender and pulsatile abdominal mass in a febrile patient should therefore be considered an infected aneurysm until proved otherwise.

Leukocytosis and an elevated erythrocyte sedimentation rate are present in most cases. When positive, blood cultures are helpful in suggesting the diagnosis and identifying the pathogen. In any patient with fever of unknown origin and documented *Salmonella* bacteremia, an arterial source of infection should be considered.[255] The absence of positive blood cultures, however, does not exclude the diagnosis of infected aortic aneurysm because cultures have been found to be negative in 25 percent of cases.

Although abdominal ultrasonography may identify the presence of an aortic aneurysm, CT scanning is superior in demonstrating associated pathological findings suggestive of an infectious etiology.[261] However, sometimes the aorta is normal in size when bacterial aortitis is first evaluated, so lack of aneurysmal dilatation does not exclude the diagnosis.[257] In such cases, if a patient's fever, leukocytosis, and pain persist, follow-up imaging should be performed because the aorta may rapidly dilate during the course of the infection. Aortography may also be used to make the diagnosis and is generally performed preoperatively to assist in surgical planning.

The natural history of infected aortic aneurysms is that of expansion and eventual rupture, with extremely rapid progression.[254, 257] *Salmonella* and gram-negative infections have a greater tendency to early rupture and death.[260] Overall mortality from infected aortic aneurysms is over 50 percent despite advances in therapy.[255, 262]

Management. Infected aortic aneurysms are treated with intravenous antibiotics and surgical excision. The standard surgical approach involves resection of the infected aneurysm and infected retroperitoneal tissue, oversewing of the native aorta as stumps, and restoration of distal perfusion by placement of an extraanatomical bypass graft tunneled through unaffected tissue planes to avoid placing a graft in a contaminated region. Antibiotic therapy must be continued postoperatively for at least 6 weeks. Several reports suggest that in selected patients with localized infection and no gross pus, an effective and simpler surgical approach is in situ reconstruction of the aorta with a prosthetic graft.[256, 262]

PRIMARY TUMORS OF THE AORTA

Primary tumors of the aorta are quite rare, with only 47 cases reported in the literature from 1873 to the present. The frequency of such reports has increased significantly over the past decade, probably as a result of improvements in noninvasive imaging techniques. Most are diagnosed in the seventh to eighth decades of life. The thoracic aorta and abdominal aorta are involved with equal frequency. In several cases, aortic tumors have appeared in association with previously inserted Dacron aortic grafts.[263] Histologically, the majority of primary aortic tumors are classified as sarcomas, with the malignant fibrous histiocytoma subtype especially common.

The majority of primary aortic tumors arise in the intima[264] and grow along the intimal surface and into the aortic lumen to form polypoid masses (often with superimposed thrombus), but they tend to not invade the aortic wall. Intimal tumors may be characterized by symptoms of vascular obstruction from narrowing of the aortic lumen or, more typically, by signs and symptoms of peripheral embolization identical to those of atherothrombotic emboli. Emboli are commonly a mixture of tumor and thrombus, and the correct diagnosis may remain obscure until histological analysis of an embolectomy specimen is completed.

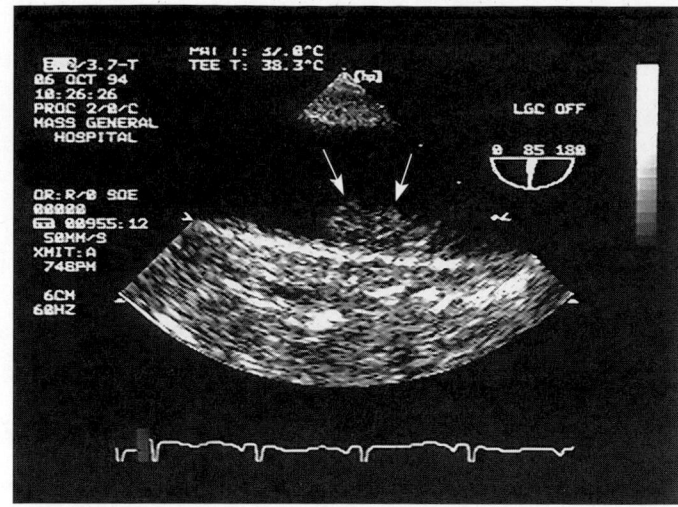

FIGURE 40–23. Transesophageal echocardiogram in a long-axis view of the descending thoracic aorta demonstrating a primary tumor of the aorta (arrows) protruding into the lumen. The tumor, which is 3.5 cm in length, involves the intimal layer but does not appear to be invading any farther into the aortic wall.

Less commonly, aortic tumors arise in the medial or adventitial layers of the aortic wall. Such tumors tend to not invade the aortic lumen but, instead, behave as aggressive mass lesions and cause constitutional symptoms or back pain.

Since primary aortic tumors are so uncommon and their features nonspecific, the diagnosis is rarely considered before surgical exploration or necropsy. However, several imaging modalities may be helpful in suggesting the diagnosis. Aortography demonstrates narrowing of the lumen or an intraluminal filling defect in the presence of an intimal tumor, but it may be negative if the tumor is adventitial.[265] Intraaortic biopsy of an intraluminal aortic mass with intravascular biopsy forceps guided by aortography has been reported.[266, 267] CT scanning can detect intimal tumors but may not easily differentiate these masses from protruding atheromas.[265] MRI may better define both the tumor anatomy and the extent of invasion.[268] Finally, the ability of TEE to image the aortic intima may make it especially useful in the detection of intimal tumors of the thoracic aorta[269] (Fig. 40–23).

Treatment of primary aortic tumors has met with little success. Because the majority of patients initially have metastatic disease, surgical approaches are often only palliative, i.e., to prevent further embolization. Many die secondary to the consequences of multiple emboli to vital organs. Of those undergoing surgical therapy, the large majority die within days to months postoperatively.

Acknowledgment

The author wishes to gratefully acknowledge the contributions of Drs. Kim A. Eagle, Roman W. DeSanctis, and Eve E. Slater to previous versions of this chapter in earlier editions of this text.

REFERENCES

THE NORMAL AORTA

1. Sonesson B, Länne T, Vernersson E, Hansen F: Sex differences in the mechanical properties of the abdominal aorta in human beings. J Vasc Surg 20:959, 1994.
2. Shimojo M, Tsuda N, Iwasaka T, Inada M: Age-related changes in aortic elasticity determined by gated radionuclide angiography in patients with systemic hypertension or healed myocardial infarcts and in normal subjects. Am J Cardiol 68:950, 1991.

3. Dart AM, Lacombe F, Yeoh JK, et al: Aortic distensibility in patients with isolated hypercholesterolemia, coronary artery disease, or cardiac transplant. Lancet 338:270, 1991.

4. Mohiaddin RH, Underwood SR, Bogren HG, et al: Regional aortic compliance studied by magnetic resonance imaging: The effects of age, training and coronary artery disease. Br Heart J 62:90, 1989.

5. Schlatmann TJM, Becker AE: Histologic changes in the normal aging aorta: Implications for dissecting aortic aneurysm. Am J Cardiol 39:13, 1977.

6. Stefanadis C, Vlachopoulos C, Karayannacos P, et al: Effect of vasa vasorum flow on structure and function of the aorta in experimental animals. Circulation 91:2669, 1995.

7. Urschel CW, Covell JW, Sonnenblick EH, et al: Effects of decreased aortic compliance on performance of the left ventricle. Am J Physiol 214:298, 1968.

8. Kelly RP, Tunin R, Kass DA: Effect of reduced aortic compliance on cardiac efficiency and contractile function of in situ canine left ventricle. Circ Res 71:490, 1992.

AORTIC ANEURYSMS

9. Johnston KW, Rutherford RB, Tilson MD, et al: Suggested standards for reporting on arterial aneurysms. J Vasc Surg 13:444, 1991.

10. Crawford ES, Cohen ES: Aortic aneurysm: A multifocal disease. Arch Surg 117:1393, 1982.

11. Pressler V, McNamara JJ: Aneurysm of the thoracic aorta: Review of 260 cases. J Thorac Cardiovasc Surg 89:50, 1985.

12. Bickerstaff LK, Pairolero PC, Hollier LH, et al: Thoracic aortic aneurysms: A population based study. Surgery 92:1103, 1982.

13. Bengtsson H, Bergquist D, Sternby NH: Increasing prevalence of abdominal aortic aneurysms: A necropsy study. Eur J Surg 158:19, 1992.

14. Bickerstaff LK, Hollier LH, Van Peenan HJ, et al: Abdominal aortic aneurysms: The changing natural history. J Vasc Surg 1:6, 1984.

15. Anidjar S, Kieffer E: Pathogenesis of acquired aneurysms of the abdominal aorta. Ann Vasc Surg 6:298, 1992.

16. Holmes DR, Liao S, Parks WC, Thompson RW: Medial neovascularization in abdominal aortic aneurysms: A histopathologic marker of aneurysm degeneration with pathophysiologic implications. J Vasc Surg 21:761, 1995.

17. Webster MW, Ferrell RF, St. Jean PL, et al: Ultrasound screening of first-degree relatives of patients with abdominal aortic aneurysm. J Vasc Surg 13:9, 1991.

18. Verloes A, Sakalihasan L, Koulischer L, Limet R: Aneurysms of the abdominal aorta: Familial and genetic aspects in three hundred thirteen pedigrees. J Vasc Surg 21:646, 1995.

18a. Pepin M, Schwarze U, Superti-Furga A, Byers PH: Clinical and genetic features of Ehlers-Danlos syndrome type IV, the vascular type. J Med 342:673, 2000.

19. Davies MJ: Aortic aneurysm formation: Lessons from human studies and experimental models. Circulation 98:193, 1998.

20. Reilly JM, Brophy CM, Tilson MD: Characterization of an elastase from aneurysmal aorta which degrades intact aortic elastin. Ann Vasc Surg 6:499, 1992.

21. Anidjar S, Dobrin PB, Eichorst M, et al: Correlation of inflammatory infiltrate with the enlargement of experimental aortic aneurysms. J Vasc Surg 16:139, 1992.

22. Pearce WH, Koch AE: Cellular components and features of immune response in abdominal aortic aneurysms. Ann N Y Acad Sci 800:175, 1996.

23. Darling RC: Ruptured arteriosclerotic abdominal aortic aneurysms. Am J Surg 119:397, 1970.

24. Muluk SC, Gertler JP, Brewster DC, et al: Presentation and patterns of aortic aneurysms in young patients. J Vasc Surg 20:880, 1994.

25. Kiell CS, Ernst CB: Advances in the management of abdominal aortic aneurysm. Adv Surg 26:73, 1993.

26. Marston WA, Ahlquist R, Johnson G Jr, Meyer AA: Misdiagnosis of ruptured abdominal aortic aneurysms. J Vasc Surg 16:17, 1992.

26a. Fink HA, Lederle FA, Roth CS, et al: The accuracy of physical examination to detect aortic aneurysms. Arch Intern Med 160:833, 2000.

27. Lederle FA, Simel DL: Does this patient have abdominal aortic aneurysm? JAMA 281:77, 1999.

28. LaRoy LL, Cormier PJ, Matalon TAS, et al: Imaging of abdominal aortic aneurysms. AJR Am J Roentgenol 152:785, 1989.

29. Hollier LH, Taylor LM, Ochsner J: Recommended indications for operative treatment of abdominal aortic aneurysms. Report of a subcommittee of the Joint Council of the Society for Vascular Surgery and of the North American Chapter of the International Society for Cardiovascular Surgery. J Vasc Surg 15:1046, 1992.

30. Ernst CB: Abdominal aortic aneurysm. N Engl J Med 328:1167, 1993.

31. Todd GJ, Nowygrod R, Benvenisty A, et al: The accuracy of CT scanning in the diagnosis of abdominal and thoracoabdominal aortic aneurysms. J Vasc Surg 13:302, 1991.

32. Lederle FA, Wilson SE, Johnson GR, et al: Variability in measurement of abdominal aortic aneurysms. J Vasc Surg 21:945, 1995.

33. Gomes MN, Davros WJ, Zemen RK: Preoperative assessment of abdominal aortic aneurysm: The value of helical and three-dimensional computed tomography. J Vasc Surg 20:367, 1994.

34. Petersen MJ, Cambria RP, Kaufman JA, et al: Magnetic resonance angi-

ography in the preoperative evaluation of abdominal aortic aneurysms. J Vasc Surg 21:891, 1995.

35. Campbell JJ, Bell DD, Gaspar MR: Selective use of arteriography in the assessment of aortic aneurysm repair. Ann Vasc Surg 4:419, 1990.

36. Kandarpa, K, Piwnica-Worms D, Chopra PS, et al: Prospective double-blinded comparison of MR imaging and aortography in the preoperative evaluation of abdominal aortic aneurysms. J Vasc Interv Radiol 3:83, 1992.

37. Frame PS, Fryback DG, Patteson C: Screening for abdominal aortic aneurysm in men ages 60 to 80 years: A cost-effectiveness analysis. Ann Intern Med 179:411, 1993.

38. Ingoldby CJH, Wujanto R, Mitchell JE: Impact of vascular surgery on community mortality from ruptured aortic aneurysm. Br J Surg 73:551, 1986.

39. Estes JE Jr: Abdominal aortic aneurysm: A study of one hundred and two cases. Circulation 2:258, 1950.

40. Darling RC, Messina CR, Brewster DC, Ottinger LW: Autopsy study of unoperated abdominal aortic aneurysms: The case for early resection. Circulation 56(Suppl 2):161, 1977.

41. Ouriel K, Green RM, Donayre C, et al: An evaluation of new methods of expressing aortic aneurysm size: Relationships to rupture. J Vasc Surg 15:12, 1992.

42. Limet R, Sakalihassan N, Adelin A: Determination of the expansion rate and incidence of rupture of abdominal aortic aneurysms. J Vasc Surg 14:540, 1991.

43. Gadowski GR, Pilcher DB, Ricci MA: Abdominal aortic aneurysm expansion rate: Effect of size and beta-adrenergic blockade. J Vasc Surg 19:727, 1994.

44. Katz DJ, Stanley JC, Zelenock GB: Operative mortality rates for intact and ruptured abdominal aortic aneurysms in Michigan: An eleven-year statewide experience. J Vasc Surg 19:804, 1994.

44a. Hallet JW: Management of abdominal aneurysms. Mayo Clin Proc 75: 395, 2000.

45. Lederle FA, Wilson SE, Johnson GR, et al: Design of the Abdominal Aortic Aneurysm Detection and Management Study. J Vasc Surg 20: 296, 1994.

46. Johnston KW, Canadian Society for Vascular Surgery Aneurysm Study Group: Non-ruptured abdominal aortic aneurysm: Six-year follow-up results from the multicenter prospective Canadian aneurysm study. J Vasc Surg 20:163, 1994.

47. Brewster DC, Geller SC, Kaufman JA, et al: Initial experience with endovascular aneurysm repair: Comparison of early results with outcome of conventional open repair. J Vasc Surg 27:992, 1998.

48. Makaroun M, Zajko A, Orons P, et al: The experience of an academic medical center with endovascular treatment of abdominal aortic aneurysms. Am J Surg 176:198, 1998.

49. Blum U, Voshage G, Lammer J, et al: Endoluminal stent-grafts for infrarenal abdominal aortic aneurysms. N Engl J Med 336:13, 1997.

50. Zarins CK, White RA, Schwarten D, et al: AneuRx stent graft versus open surgical repair of abdominal aortic aneurysms: Multicenter prospective clinical trial. J Vasc Surg 29:292, 1999.

51. Wain RA, Marin ML, Ohki T, et al: Endoleaks after endovascular graft treatment of aortic aneurysms: Classification, risk factors, and outcome. J Vasc Surg 27:69, 1998.

51a. Finlayson SR, Birkmeyer JD, Fillinger MF, et al: Should endovascular surgery lower the threshold for repair of abdominal aortic aneurysms? J Vasc Surg 29:973, 1999.

52. Hertzer NR: Fatal myocardial infarction following abdominal aortic aneurysm resection. Three hundred forty-three patients followed 6–11 years postoperatively. Ann Surg 192:671, 1980.

53. Hertzer NR, Beven EG, Young YR, et al: Coronary artery disease in peripheral vascular patients: A classification of 1000 coronary angiograms and results of surgical management. Ann Surg 199:223, 1984.

54. Boucher CA, Brewster DC, Darling RC, et al: Determination of cardiac risk by dipyridamole-thallium imaging before peripheral vascular surgery. N Engl J Med 312:389, 1985.

55. Eagle KA, Singer DE, Brewster DC, et al: Dipyridamole-thallium scanning in patients undergoing vascular surgery. Optimizing preoperative evaluation of cardiac risk. JAMA 257:2185, 1987.

56. Levinson JR, Boucher CA, Coley CM, et al: Usefulness of semiquantitative analysis of dipyridamole-thallium201 redistribution for improving risk stratification before vascular surgery. Am J Cardiol 66:406, 1990.

57. Cambria RP, Brewster DC, Abbott WM, et al: The impact of selective use of dipyridamole-thallium scans and surgical factors on the current morbidity of aortic surgery. J Vasc Surg 15:43, 1992.

58. Gersh BJ, Rihal CS, Rooke TW, Ballard DJ: Evaluation and management of patients with both peripheral vascular and coronary artery disease. J Am Coll Cardiol 18:203, 1991.

59. Hertzer NR, Young JR, Beven EG, et al: Late results of coronary bypass in patients with peripheral vascular disease. II. Five-year survival according to sex, hypertension, and diabetes. Clev Clin J Med 54:15, 1987.

60. Rihal CS, Eagle KA, Mickel MC, et al: Surgical therapy for coronary artery disease among patients with combined coronary artery and peripheral vascular disease. Circulation 91:46, 1995.

61. Pasternack PF, Grossi EA, Bauman FG, et al: Beta blockade to decrease silent myocardial ischemia during peripheral vascular surgery. Am J Surg 158:113, 1989.

62. Reigel MM, Hollier LH, Kazmier FJ, et al: Late survival in abdominal

PLATE 23

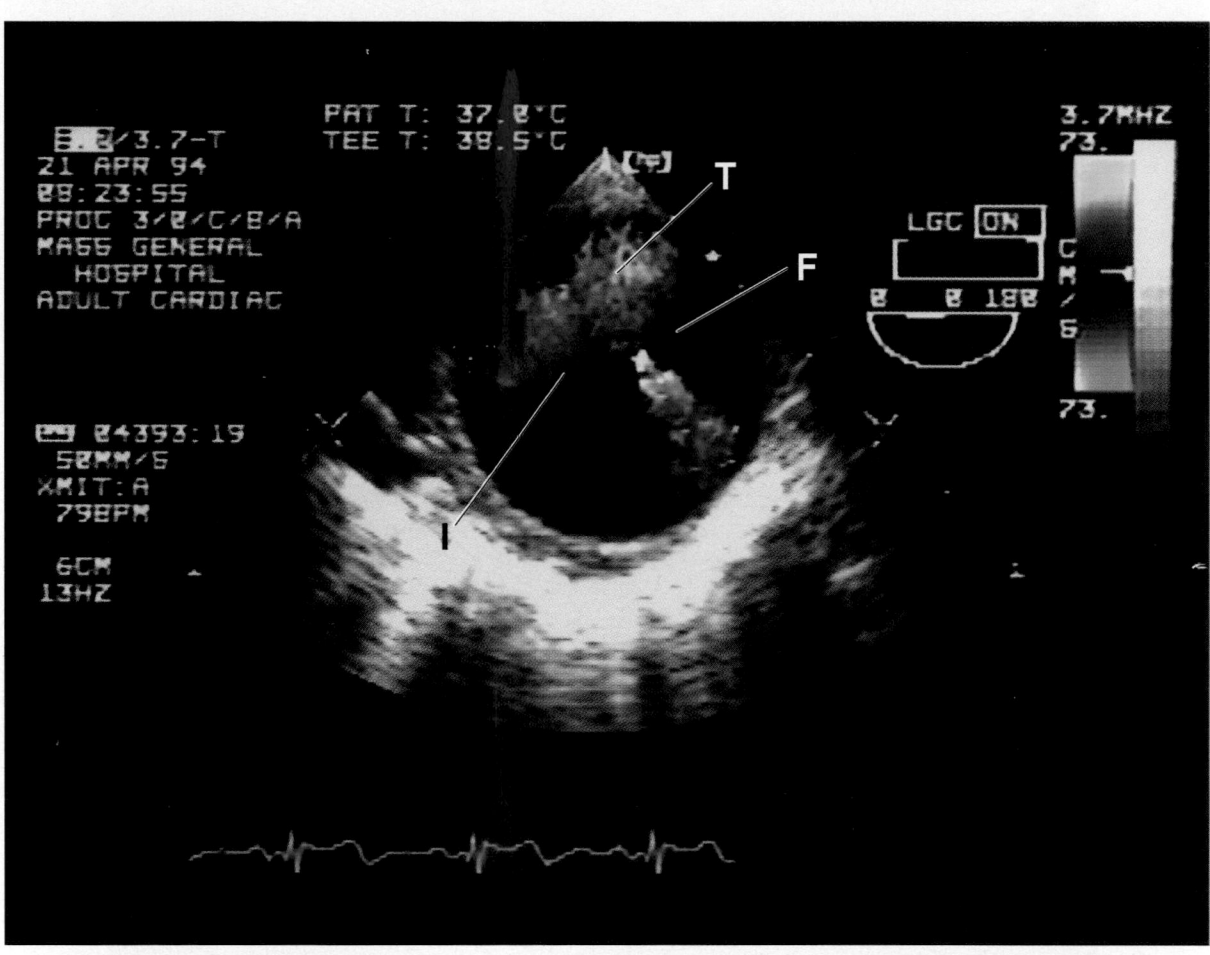

FIGURE 40–16. Cross-sectional transesophageal echocardiogram of a descending aortic dissection demonstrating a site of intimal tear. Blood flow (in orange) is evident in the true lumen (T) during systole, while a narrow jet of high-velocity blood (in blue) crosses into the false lumen (F) through a tear in the intimal flap (I).

PLATE 24

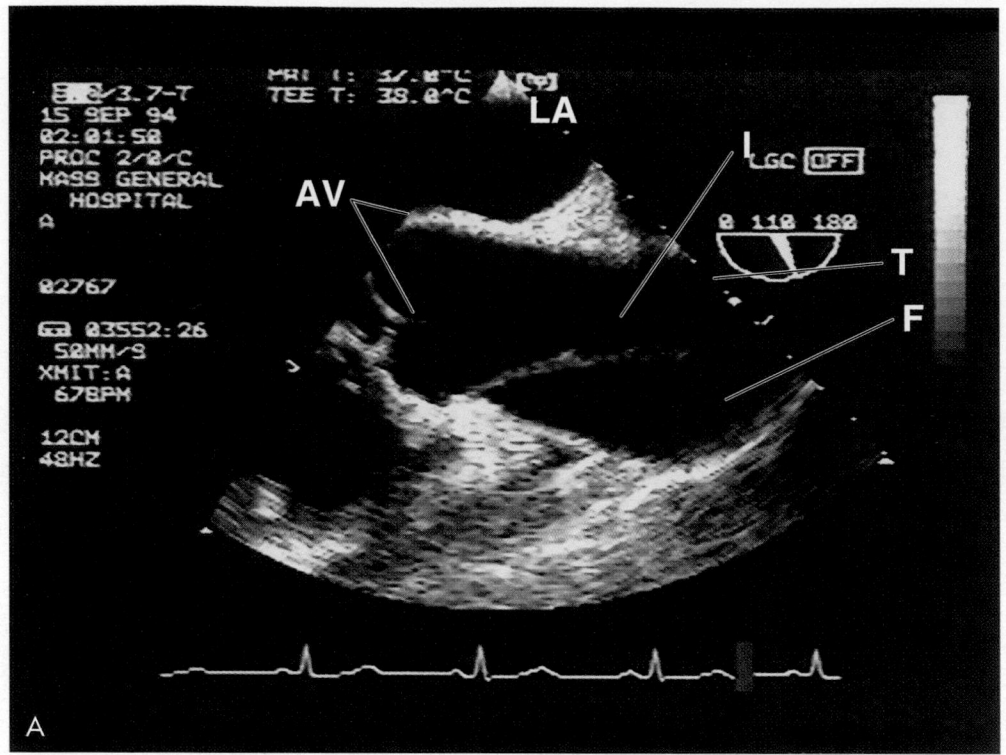

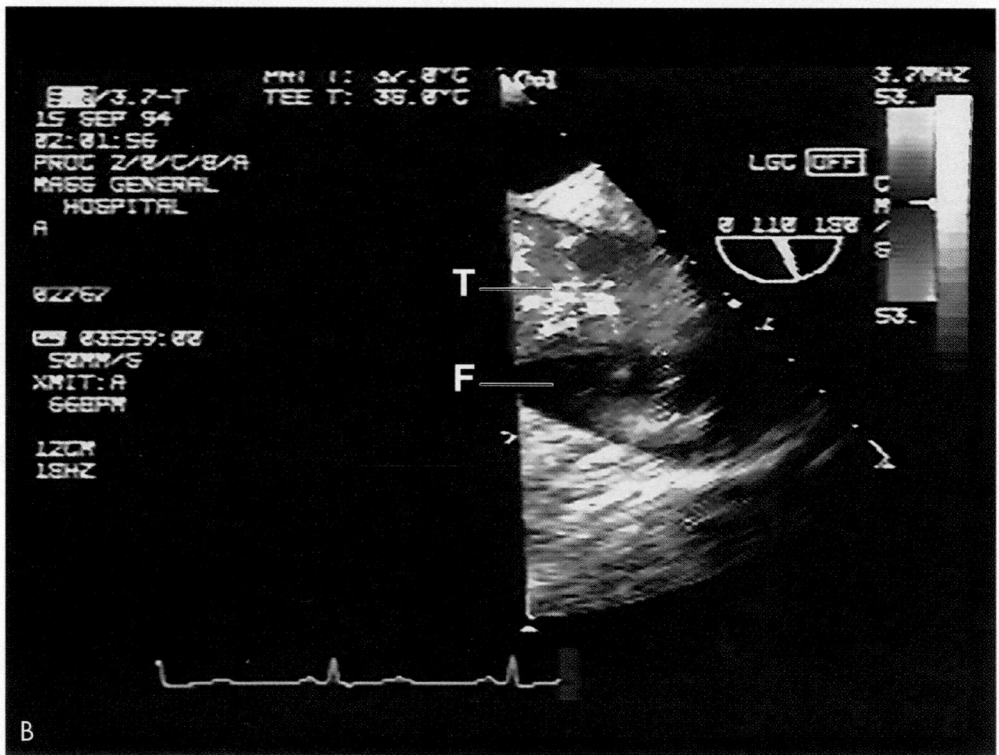

FIGURE 40–17. Transesophageal echocardiogram of the proximal ascending aorta in long-axis view in a patient with proximal aortic dissection. *A*, The left atrium (LA) is closest to the transducer. The aortic valve (AV) is seen on the left in this view, with the ascending aorta extending to the right. Within the proximal aorta is an intimal flap (I) that originates just at the level of the sinotubular junction above the right sinus of Valsalva. The true lumen (T) and the false lumen (F) are separated by the intimal flap. *B*, The addition of color flow Doppler in the same view confirms the presence of two distinct lumina. The true lumen (T) fills completely with brisk blood flow (bright blue color), while at the same time minimal retrograde flow (dark orange) is seen in the false lumen (F).

63. Brophy C, Tilson JE, Tilson MD: Propranolol delays the formation of aneurysms in the male blotchy mouse. J Surg Res 44:687, 1988.

64. Treiman RL, Hartunian SL, Cossman DV, et al: Late results of small untreated abdominal aortic aneurysms. Ann Vasc Surg 5:359, 1991.

65. Pyeritz RE, McKusick VA: The Marfan syndrome: Diagnosis and management. N Engl J Med 300:772, 1979.

66. Milewicz DM: Ultrasonic characterization of the aortic architecture in Marfan patients (editorial). Circulation 91:1272, 1995.

67. Hollister DW, Goodfrey M, Sakai LY, Pyeritz RE: Immunohistologic abnormalities of the microfibrillar-fiber system in the Marfan syndrome. N Engl J Med 323:152, 1990.

68. Jeremy RW, Huang H, Hwa J, et al: Relation between age, arterial distensibility, and aortic dilatation in the Marfan syndrome. Am J Cardiol 74:369, 1994.

69. Marsalese DL, Moodie DS, Lytle BW, et al: Cystic medial necrosis of the aorta in patients without Marfan's syndrome: Surgical outcome and long-term follow up. J Am Coll Cardiol 16:68, 1990.

70. Emanuel R, Ng RA, Marcomichelakis J, et al: Formes frustes of Marfan's syndrome presenting with severe aortic regurgitation. Clinicogenetic study of 18 families. Br Heart J 39:190, 1977.

71. Joyce JW, Fairbairn JF II, Kincaid OW, Juergens JL: Aneurysms of the thoracic aorta. A clinical study with special reference to prognosis. Circulation 29:176, 1964.

72. McNamara JJ, Pressler VM: Natural history of arteriosclerotic thoracic aortic aneurysms. Ann Thorac Surg 26:468, 1978.

73. Johansson G, Markström U, Swedenborg J: Ruptured thoracic aortic aneurysms: A study of incidence and mortality rates. J Vasc Surg 21:985, 1995.

74. Bogey WM Jr, Thomas JH, Hermreck AS: Aortoesophageal fistula: Report of a successfully managed case and review of the literature. J Vasc Surg 16:90, 1992.

75. Masuda, Y, Takanashi K, Takasu J, et al: Expansion rate of thoracic aortic aneurysms and influencing factors. Chest 102:461, 1992.

76. Dinsmore RE, Liberthson RR, Wismer GL, et al: Magnetic resonance imaging of thoracic aortic aneurysms: Comparison with other diagnostic methods. AJR Am J Roentgenol 146:309, 1986.

77. Pressler V, McNamara JJ: Thoracic aortic aneurysm: Natural history and treatment. J Thorac Cardiovasc Surg 79:489, 1980.

78. Crawford ES, DeNatale RW: Thoracoabdominal aortic aneurysm: Observations regarding the natural course of disease. J Vasc Surg 3:578, 1986.

79. Hirose Y, Hamada S, Takamiya M, et al: Aortic aneurysms: Growth rate measured with CT. Radiology 185:249, 1992.

80. Dapunt OE, Galla JD, Sadeghi AM, et al: The natural history of thoracic aortic aneurysms. J Thorac Cardiovasc Surg 107:1323, 1994.

81. Gott VL, Greene PS, Alejo DE, et al: Replacement of the aortic root in patients with Marfan's syndrome. N Engl J Med 340:1307, 1999.

82. Devereux RB, Roman MJ: Aortic disease in Marfan's syndrome. N Engl J Med 340:1358, 1999.

83. Verdant A, Cossette R, Page A, et al: Aneurysms of the descending thoracic aorta: Three hundred sixty-six consecutive cases resected without paraplegia. J Vasc Surg 21:385, 1995.

84. Livesay JJ, Cooley DA, Ventemiglia RA, et al: Surgical experience in descending thoracic aneurysmectomy with and without adjuncts to avoid ischemia. Ann Thorac Surg 39:37, 1985.

85. Gott VL, Gillinov AM, Pyeritz RE, et al: Aortic root replacement: Risk factor analysis of a seventeen-year experience with 270 patients. J Thorac Cardiovasc Surg 109:536, 1995.

86. David TE, Feindel CM, Bos J: Repair of the aortic valve in patients with aortic insufficiency and aortic root aneurysm. J Thorac Cardiovasc Surg 109:345, 1995.

87. Coselli JS, Büket S, Djukanovic B: Aortic arch operation: Current treatment and results. Ann Thorac Surg 59:19, 1995.

88. Svensson LG, Crawford S, Hess KR, et al: Dissection of the aorta and dissecting aortic aneurysms: Improving early and long-term survival results. Circulation 82(Suppl 4):24, 1990.

89. Griepp RB, Stinson EB, Hollingsworth JF, Buehler D: Prosthetic replacement of the aortic arch. J Thorac Cardiovasc Surg 70:1051, 1975.

90. Kitamura M, Hashimoto A, Akimoto T, et al: Operation for type A aortic dissection: Introduction of retrograde cerebral perfusion. Ann Thorac Surg 59:1195, 1995.

91. Usui A, Hotta T, Hiroura M, et al: Retrograde perfusion through a superior vena caval cannula protects the brain. Ann Thorac Surg 53:47, 1992.

92. Safi HJ, Miller CC 3rd, Iliopoulos DC, et al: Staged repair of extensive aortic aneurysm: Improved neurologic outcome. Ann Surg 226:599, 1997.

93. Okita, Y, Takamoto S, Ando M, et al: Mortality and cerebral outcome in patients who underwent aortic arch operations using deep hypothermic circulatory arrest with retrograde cerebral perfusion: No relation of early death, stroke, and delirium to the duration of circulatory arrest. J Thorac Cardiovasc Surg 115:129, 1998.

94. Crawford ES, Coselli JS, Svensson LG, et al: Diffuse aneurysmal disease (chronic aortic dissection, Marfan, and mega aorta syndromes) and multiple aneurysm. Ann Surg 211:521, 1990.

95. Heinemann MK, Buehner B, Jurmann MJ, Borst H-G: Use of the "elephant trunk technique" in aortic surgery. Ann Thorac Surg 60:2, 1995.

96. Crawford ES, Svensson LG, Coselli JS, et al: Surgical treatment of aneurysm and/or dissection of the ascending aorta, transverse aortic arch, and ascending aorta and transverse arch: Factors influencing survival in 717 patients. J Thorac Cardiovasc Surg 98:659, 1989.

97. Coselli JS, Crawford EF: Composite valve-graft replacement of aortic root using separate Dacron tube for coronary artery reattachment. Ann Thorac Surg 47:558, 1989.

98. Hollier LH, Symmonds JB, Pairolero PC, et al: Thoracoabdominal aortic aneurysm repair: Analysis of postoperative morbidity. Arch Surg 123:871, 1988.

98a. Coselli JS, Le Maire SA, Miller CC, et al: Mortality and paraplegia after thoracoabdominal aortic aneurysm repair: A risk factor analysis. Ann Thorac Surg 69:409, 2000.

99. Cambria RP, Davison JK, Zannetti S, et al: Clinical experience with epidural cooling for spinal cord protection during thoracic and thoracoabdominal aneurysm repair. J Vasc Surg 25:234, 1997.

100. Svensson LG, Hess KR, D'Agostino RS, et al: Reduction of neurologic injury after high-risk thoracoabdominal aortic operation. Ann Thorac Surg 66:132, 1998.

101. Galla JD, Ergin MA, Lansman SL, et al: Use of somatosensory evoked potentials for thoracic and thoracoabdominal aortic resections. Ann Thorac Surg 67:1947, 1999.

102. Dake MD, Miller DC, Mitchell RS, et al: The "first generation" of endovascular stent-grafts for patients with aneurysms of the descending thoracic aorta. J Thorac Cardiovasc Surg 116:689, 1998.

103. Shores J, Berger KR, Murphy EA, Pyeritz RE: Progression of aortic dilatation and the benefit of long-term β-adrenergic blockade in Marfan's syndrome. N Engl J Med 330:1335, 1994.

104. Ellis RP, Cooley DA, DeBakey ME: Clinical considerations and surgical treatment of annulo-aortic ectasia. J Thorac Cardiovasc Surg 42:363, 1961.

105. Lemon DK, White CW: Annuloaortic ectasia: Angiographic, hemodynamic, and clinical comparison with aortic valve insufficiency. Am J Cardiol 41:482, 1978.

AORTIC DISSECTION

106. Hirst AE Jr, Johns VJ Jr, Kime SW Jr: Dissecting aneurysm of the aorta: A review of 505 cases. Medicine (Baltimore) 37:217, 1958.

107. Wilson SK, Hutchins GM: Aortic dissecting aneurysms: Causative factors in 204 subjects. Arch Pathol Lab Med 106:175, 1982.

108. DeBakey ME, McCollum CH, Crawford ES, et al: Dissection and dissecting aneurysms of the aorta: Twenty-year follow up of five hundred twenty-seven patients treated surgically. Surgery 92:1118, 1982.

109. Daily PO, Trueblood HW, Stinson EB, et al: Management of acute aortic dissections. Ann Thorac Surg 10:237, 1970.

110. Spittell PC, Spittell JA Jr, Joyce JW, et al: Clinical features and differential diagnosis of aortic dissection: Experience with 236 cases (1980 through 1990). Mayo Clin Proc 68:642, 1993.

111. Larson EW, Edwards WD: Risk factors for aortic dissection: A necropsy study of 161 patients. Am J Cardiol 53:849, 1984.

112. Hagan PG, Nienaber CA, Isselbacher EM, et al: International Registry of Acute Aortic Dissection (IRAD)—new insights into an old disease. JAMA 283:897, 2000.

113. Bordeleau L, Cwinn A, Turek M, et al: Aortic dissection and Turner's syndrome: Case report and review of the literature. J Emerg Med 16:593, 1998.

114. Liu G, Shupak R, Chiu BK: Aortic dissection in giant-cell arteritis. Semin Arthritis Rheum 25:160, 1995.

115. Om A, Porter T, Mohanty PK: Transesophageal echocardiographic diagnosis of acute aortic dissection complicating cocaine abuse. Am Heart J 123:532, 1992.

116. Rashid J, Eisenberg MJ, Topol EJ: Cocaine-induced aortic dissection. Am Heart J 132:1301, 1996.

117. Williams GM, Gott VL, Brawley RK, et al: Aortic disease associated with pregnancy. J Vasc Surg 8:470, 1988.

118. Mazzucotelli J-P, Deleuze PH, Baureton C, et al: Preservation of the aortic valve in acute aortic dissection: Long-term echocardiographic assessment and clinical outcome. Ann Thorac Surg 55:1513, 1993.

119. Elkayam U, Ostzega, E, Shotan A, Mehra A: Cardiovascular problems in pregnant women with the Marfan syndrome. Ann Intern Med 123:117, 1995.

120. Rogers FB, Osler TM, Shackford SR: Aortic dissection after trauma: Case report and review of the literature. J Trauma 41:906, 1996.

121. Ochi M, Yamauchi S, Yajima T, et al: Aortic dissection extending from the left coronary artery during percutaneous coronary angioplasty. Ann Thorac Surg 62:1180, 1996.

122. Jacobs LE, Fraifeld M, Kotler MN, Ioli AW: Aortic dissection following intraaortic balloon insertion: Recognition by transesophageal echocardiography. Am Heart J 124:536, 1992.

123. Still RJ, Hilgenberg AD, Akins CW, et al: Intraoperative aortic dissection. Ann Thorac Surg 53:374, 1992.

124. Albat B, Thevenet A: Dissecting aneurysms of the ascending aorta occurring late after aortic valve replacement. J Cardiovasc Surg 33:272, 1992.

125. von Kodolitsch Y, Simic O, Bregenzer T, et al: Aortic valve replacement as an independent predictive factor for later development of aortic dissection. Z Kardiol 87:604, 1998.

126. von Kodolitsch Y, Simic O, Schwartz A, et al: Predictors of proximal aortic dissection at the time of aortic valve replacement. Circulation 100(Suppl 2):287, 1999.

127. Slater EE, DeSanctis RW: The clinical recognition of dissecting aortic aneurysm. Am J Med 60:625, 1976.

127a. Kim MH, Eagle KA, Isselbacher EM: Bayesian persuasion. Circulation 100:e68, 1999.

128. Doroghazi RM, Slater EE, DeSanctis RW, et al: Long-term survival of patients with treated aortic dissection. J Am Coll Cardiol 3:1026, 1984.

129. Rosenzweig BP, Goldstein S, Sherrid M, Kronzon I: Aortic dissection with flap prolapse into the left ventricle. Am J Cardiol 77:214, 1996.

130. Hudak AM, Konstadt SN: Aortic intussusception: A rare complication of aortic dissection. Anesthesiology 82:1292, 1994.

131. Fann JI, Sarris GE, Mitchell RS, et al: Treatment of patients with aortic dissection presenting with peripheral vascular complications. Ann Surg 212:705, 1990.

132. Glower DD, Speier RH, White WD, et al: Management and long-term outcome of aortic dissection. Ann Surg 214:31, 1991.

133. Kamp TJ, Goldschmidt-Clermont PJ, Brinker JA, Resar JR: Myocardial infarction, aortic dissection, and thrombolytic therapy. Am Heart J 128:1234, 1994.

134. Hartnell GG, Wakeley CJ, Tottle A, et al: Limitations of chest radiography in discriminating between aortic dissection and myocardial infarction: Implications for thrombolysis. J Thorac Imaging 8:152, 1993.

135. Cambria RP, Brewster DC, Moncure AC, et al: Spontaneous aortic dissection in the presence of coexistent or previously repaired atherosclerotic aortic aneurysm. Ann Surg 208:619, 1988.

136. Eagle KA, Quertermous T, Kritzer GA, et al: Spectrum of conditions initially suggesting acute aortic dissection but with negative aortograms. Am J Cardiol 57:322, 1986.

137. Armstrong WF, Bach DS, Carey LM, et al: Clinical and echocardiographic findings in patients with suspected acute aortic dissection. Am Heart J 136:1051, 1998.

138. Suzuki T, Katoh H, Watanabe M, et al: A novel biochemical method for aortic dissection—the results of a prospective study using an immunoassay of smooth muscle myosin heavy chain. Circulation 93:1244, 1996.

139. O'Gara PT, DeSanctis RW: Acute aortic dissection and its variants: Toward a common diagnostic and therapeutic approach. Circulation 92:1376, 1995.

140. Cigarroa JE, Isselbacher EM, DeSanctis RW, Eagle KA: Diagnostic imaging in the evaluation of suspected aortic dissection: Old standards and new directions. N Engl J Med 328:35, 1993.

141. Petasnick JP: Radiologic evaluation of aortic dissection. Radiology 180:297, 1991.

142. Earnest F IV, Muhm JR, Sheedy PF II: Roentgenographic findings in thoracic aortic dissection. Mayo Clin Proc 54:43, 1979.

143. Erbel R, Daniel W, Visser C, et al: Echocardiography in diagnosis of aortic dissection. Lancet 1:457, 1989.

144. Bansal RC, Chandrasekaran K, Ayala K, Smith D: Frequency and explanation of false negative diagnosis of aortic dissection by aortography and transesophageal echocardiography. J Am Coll Cardiol 25:1393, 1995.

145. Mugge A, Daniel WG, Laas J, et al: False-negative diagnosis of proximal aortic dissection by computed tomography or angiography and possible explanations based on transesophageal echocardiographic findings. Am J Cardiol 65:527, 1990.

146. Nienaber CA, von Kodolitsch Y, Nicolas V, et al: Definitive diagnosis of thoracic aortic dissection: The emerging role of noninvasive imaging modalities. N Engl J Med 328:1, 1993.

147. Zeman RK, Berman PM, Silverman PM, et al: Diagnosis of aortic dissection: Value of helical CT with multiplanar reformation and three-dimensional rendering. AJR Am J Roentgenol 164:1375, 1995.

148. Small JH, Dixon AK, Coulden RA, et al: Fast CT for aortic dissection. Br J Radiol 69:900, 1996.

149. Sommer T, Fehske W, Holzknecht N, et al: Aortic dissection: A comparative study of diagnosis with spiral CT, multiplanar transesophageal echocardiography, and MR imaging. Radiology 199:347, 1996.

150. Nienaber CA, Spielmann RP, von Kodolitsch Y, et al: Diagnosis of thoracic aortic dissection: Magnetic resonance imaging versus transesophageal echocardiography. Circulation 85:434, 1992.

151. Kersting-Sommerhoff BA, Higgins CB, White RD, et al: Aortic dissection: Sensitivity and specificity of MR imaging. Radiology 166:651, 1988.

152. Shellock FG, Curtis JS: MR imaging and biomedical implants, materials, and devices: An updated review. Radiology 180:541, 1991.

153. Erbel R, Borner N, Steller D, et al: Detection of aortic dissection by transesophageal echocardiography. Br Heart J 58:45, 1987.

154. Blanchard DG, Kimura BJ, Dittrich HC, DeMaria AN: Transesophageal echocardiography of the aorta. JAMA 272:546, 1994.

155. Keren A, Kim CB, Hu BS, et al: Accuracy of biplane and multiplane transesophageal echocardiography in diagnosis of typical acute aortic dissection and intramural hematoma. J Am Coll Cardiol 28:627, 1996.

156. Evangelista A, Garcia-del-Castillo H, Gonzalez-Alujas T, et al: Diagnosis of ascending aortic dissection by transesophageal echocardiography: Utility of M-mode in recognizing artifacts. J Am Coll Cardiol 27:102, 1996.

157. Kern MJ, Serota H, Callicoat P, et al: Use of coronary arteriography in the preoperative management of patients undergoing urgent repair of the thoracic aorta. Am Heart J 119:143, 1990.

158. Ballal RS, Nanda NC, Gatewood R, et al: Usefulness of transesophageal echocardiography in assessment of aortic dissection. Circulation 84:1903, 1991.

159. Erbel R, Oelert H, Meyer J, et al: Effect of medical and surgical therapy on aortic dissection evaluated by transesophageal echocardiography: Implications for prognosis and therapy. Circulation 87:1604, 1993.

160. Chan, K: Usefulness of transesophageal echocardiography in the diagnosis of conditions mimicking aortic dissection. Am Heart J 122:495, 1991.

161. Yamada E, Matsumura M, Kyo S, Omoto R: Usefulness of a prototype intravascular ultrasound imaging in evaluation of aortic dissection and comparison with aortographic study, transesophageal echocardiography, computed tomography, and magnetic resonance imaging. Am J Cardiol 75:161, 1995.

162. Buck T, Gorge G, Hunold P, Erbel R: Three-dimensional imaging in aortic disease by lighthouse transesophageal echocardiography using intravascular ultrasound catheters. Comparison to three-dimensional transesophageal echocardiography and three-dimensional intra-aortic ultrasound imaging. J Am Soc Echocardiogr 11:243, 1998.

163. White RA, Donayre C, Kopchok G, et al: Intravascular ultrasound: The ultimate tool for abdominal aortic aneurysm assessment and endovascular graft delivery. J Endovasc Surg 4:45, 1997.

164. Banning AP, Ruttley MST, Musumeci F, Fraser AG: Acute dissection of the thoracic aorta: Transesophageal echocardiography is the investigation of choice. BMJ 310:72, 1995.

165. Rizzo RJ, Aranki SF, Aklog L, et al: Rapid noninvasive diagnosis and surgical repair of acute ascending aortic dissection. J Thorac Cardiovasc Surg 108:567, 1994.

166. Simon P, Owen AN, Havel M, et al: Transesophageal echocardiography in the emergency surgical management of patients with aortic dissection. J Thorac Cardiovasc Surg 103:1113, 1992.

166a. Penn MS, Smedira N, Lytle B, Brener SJ: Does coronary angiography before emergency aortic surgery affect in-hospital mortality? J Am Coll Cardiol 35:889, 2000.

167. Gillinov AM, Lytle BW, Kaplon RJ, et al: Dissection of the ascending aorta after previous cardiac surgery: Differences in presentation and management. J Thorac Cardiovasc Surg 117:252, 1999.

168. Creswell LL, Kouchoukos NT, Cox JL, Rosenbloom M: Coronary artery disease in patients with type A aortic dissection. Ann Thorac Surg 59:585, 1995.

169. Anagnostopoulos CE, Prabhakar MJS, Kittle CF: Aortic dissections and dissecting aneurysms. Am J Cardiol 30:263, 1972.

170. Elefteriades JA, Hartleroad J, Gusberg RJ, et al: Long-term experience with descending aortic dissection: The complication-specific approach. Ann Thorac Surg 53:11, 1992.

171. DeBakey ME, Cooley DA, Creech O Jr: Surgical considerations of dissecting aneurysms of the aorta. Ann Surg 142:586, 1955.

172. Wheat MW Jr, Palmer RF, Barley TD, Seelman RC: Treatment of dissecting aneurysms of the aorta without surgery. J Thorac Cardiovasc Surg 50:364, 1965.

173. Isselbacher EM, Cigarroa JE, Eagle KA: Cardiac tamponade complicating proximal aortic dissection: Is pericardiocentesis harmful? Circulation 90:2375, 1994.

174. Miller DC, Stinson EB, Oyer PE, et al: Operative treatment of aortic dissections: Experience with 125 patients over a sixteen-year period. J Thorac Cardiovasc Surg 78:365, 1979.

175. Masuda Y, Yamada Z, Morooka N, et al: Prognosis of patients with medically treated aortic dissections. Circulation 84(Suppl 3):7, 1991.

176. Glower DD, Fann JI, Speier RH, et al: Comparison of medical and surgical therapy for uncomplicated descending aortic dissection. Circulation 82(Suppl 4):39, 1990.

177. Crawford ES, Svensson LG, Coselli JS, et al: Aortic dissection and dissecting aortic aneurysms. Ann Surg 208:254, 1988.

178. Haverich A, Miller DC, Scott WC, et al: Acute and chronic aortic dissections: Determinants of long-term outcome for operative survivors. Circulation 72(Suppl 2):22, 1985.

178a. Sabik JF, Lytle BW, Blackstone EH, et al: Long-term effectiveness of operations for ascending aortic dissections. J Thorac Cardiovasc Surg 119:946, 2000.

179. Crawford ES, Kirklin JW, Naftel DC, et al: Surgery for acute dissection of the ascending aorta. Should the arch be included? J Thorac Cardiovasc Surg 104:46, 1992.

180. Yun KL, Glower DD, Miller DC, et al: Aortic dissection resulting from tear of transverse arch: Is concomitant arch repair warranted? J Thorac Cardiovasc Surg 102:355, 1991.

181. Movsowitz HD, Levine RA, Hilgenberg AD, Isselbacher EM: Transesophageal Echocardiographic description of the mechanisms of aortic regurgitation in acute type A aortic dissection: Implications for aortic valve repair. J Am Coll Cardiol 36:884, 2000.

182. Fann JI, Glower DD, Miller CD, et al: Preservation of aortic valve in type A aortic dissection complicated by aortic regurgitation. J Thorac Cardiovasc Surg 102:62, 1991.

183. Séguin JR, Picard E, Frapier J-M, Chaptal P-A: Aortic valve repair with fibrin glue for type A acute aortic dissection. Ann Thorac Surg 58:304, 1994.

184. Bachet J, Goudot B, Dreyfus G, et al: The proper use of glue: A 20-year experience with the GRF glue in acute aortic dissection. J Card Surg 12(Suppl):243, 1997.

185. Cambria RP, Brewster DC, Gertler J, et al: Vascular complications associated with spontaneous aortic dissection. J Vasc Surg 7:199, 1988.

186. Slonim SM, Nyman U, Semba CP, et al: Aortic dissection: Percutaneous management of ischemic complications with endovascular stents and balloon fenestration. J Vasc Surg 23:241, 1996.

187. Morales DL, Quin JA, Braxton JH, et al: Experimental confirmation of

effectiveness of fenestration in acute aortic dissection. Ann Thorac Surg 66:1679, 1998.

188. Liu DW, Lin PJ, Chang CH: Treatment of acute type A aortic dissection with intraluminal sutureless prosthesis. Ann Thorac Surg 57:987, 1994.

189. Lemole GM, Strong MD, Spagna PM, Karmilowicz MP: Improved results with dissecting aneurysms: Intraluminal sutureless prosthesis. J Thorac Cardiovasc Surg 83:249, 1982.

190. Kato M, Matsuda T, Kaneko M, et al: Outcomes of stent-graft treatment of false lumen in aortic dissection. Circulation 98(Suppl 2):305, 1998.

191. Nienaber CA, Fattori R, Lund G, et al: Nonsurgical reconstruction of thoracic aortic dissection by stent-graft placement. N Engl J Med 340:1539, 1999.

192. Dake MD, Kato N, Mitchell RS, et al: Endovascular stent-graft placement for the treatment of acute aortic dissection. N Engl J Med 340:1546, 1999.

193. Vlahakes G: Catheter-based treatment of aortic dissection. N Engl J Med 340:1585, 1999.

194. Januzzi JL, Movsowitz HD, Choi J, et al: Severe hypertension following type B aortic dissection: A common problem that does not indicate renal ischemia. Submitted for publication.

195. Neya K, Omoto R, Kyo S, et al: Outcome of Stanford type B acute aortic dissection. Circulation 86(Suppl 2):1, 1992.

196. Heinemann M, Laas J, Karck M, Borst HG: Thoracic aortic aneurysms after type A aortic dissection: Necessity for follow-up. Ann Thorac Surg 49:580, 1990.

197. Masani ND, Banning AP, Jones RA, et al: Follow-up of chronic thoracic aortic dissection: Comparison of transesophageal echocardiography and magnetic resonance imaging. Am Heart J 131:1156, 1996.

198. Laissy J-P, Blanc F, Soyer P, et al: Thoracic aortic dissection: Diagnosis with transesophageal echocardiography versus MR imaging. Radiology 194:331, 1995.

199. Yamada T, Tada S, Harada J: Aortic dissection without intimal rupture: Diagnosis with MR imaging and CT. Radiology 168:347, 1988.

200. Lui RC, Menkis AH, McKenzie FN: Aortic dissection without intimal rupture: Diagnosis and management. Ann Thorac Surg 53:886, 1992.

201. Gore I: Pathogenesis of dissecting aneurysm of the aorta. Arch Pathol 53:142, 1952.

202. Mohr-Kahaly S, Erbel R, Kearney P, et al: Aortic intramural hematoma visualized by transesophageal echocardiography: Findings and prognostic implications. J Am Coll Cardiol 23:658, 1994.

203. Robbins RC, McManus RP, Mitchell RS, et al: Management of patients with intramural hematoma of the thoracic aorta. Circulation 88:1, 1993.

204. Nienaber CA, von Kodolitsch Y, Petersen B, et al: Intramural hemorrhage of the thoracic aorta. Circulation 92:1465, 1995.

205. Harris KM, Braverman AC, Gutierrez FR, et al: Transesophageal echocardiographic and clinical features of aortic intramural hematoma. J Thorac Cardiovasc Surg 114:619, 1997.

206. Vilacosta I, San Roman JA, Ferreiros J, et al: Natural history and serial morphology of aortic intramural hematoma: A novel variant of aortic dissection. Am Heart J 134:495, 1997.

207. Sueyoshi E, Matsuoka Y, Sakamoto I, et al: Fate of intramural hematoma of the aorta: CT evaluation. J Comput Assist Tomogr 21:931, 1997.

208. Stanson AW, Kazmier FJ, Hollier LH, et al: Penetrating atherosclerotic ulcers of the thoracic aorta: Natural history and clinicopathological correlations. Ann Vasc Surg 1:15, 1986.

209. Kazerooni EA, Bree RL, Williams DM: Penetrating atherosclerotic ulcers of the descending thoracic aorta: Evaluation with CT and distinction from aortic dissection. Radiology 183:759, 1992.

210. Movsowitz HD, Lampert C, Jacobs LE, Kotler MN: Penetrating atherosclerotic aortic ulcers. Am Heart J 128:1210, 1994.

211. Benitez RM, Gurbel PA, Chong H, Rajasingh C: Penetrating atherosclerotic ulcer of the aortic arch resulting in extensive and fatal dissection. Am Heart J 129:821, 1995.

212. Braverman AC: Penetrating atherosclerotic ulcers of the aorta. Curr Opin Cardiol 9:591, 1994.

213. Muluk SC, Kaufman JA, Torchiana DF, et al: Diagnosis and treatment of thoracic aortic intramural hematoma. J Vasc Surg 24:1022, 1996.

214. Harris JA, Bis KG, Glover JL, et al: Penetrating atherosclerotic ulcers of the aorta. J Vasc Surg 19:90, 1994.

215. Movsowitz HD, David M, Movsowitz C, et al: Penetrating atherosclerotic ulcers: The role of transesophageal echocardiography in the diagnosis and clinical management. Am Heart J 126:745, 1993.

216. Murgo S, Dussaussois L, Golzarian J, et al: Penetrating atherosclerotic ulcer of the descending thoracic aorta: Treatment by endovascular stent-graft. Cardiovasc Intervent Radiol 21:454, 1998.

AORTIC ATHEROMATOUS DISEASE

217. Karalis DG, Chandraskeran C, Victor MF, et al: Recognition and embolic potential of intraaortic atherosclerotic debris. J Am Coll Cardiol 17:73, 1991.

218. Toyoda K, Yasaka M, Nagata S, Yamaguchi T: Aortogenic embolic stroke: A transesophageal echocardiography approach. Stroke 23:1056, 1992.

219. Kronson I, Tunick PA: Atheromatous disease of the thoracic aorta: Pathological and clinical implications. Ann Intern Med 126:629, 1997.

220. Davila-Roman VG, Barzilai B, Wareing TH, et al: Intraoperative ultrasonographic evaluation of the ascending aorta in 100 consecutive patients undergoing cardiac surgery. Circulation 84(Suppl 3):47, 1991.

221. Mitusch R, Stierle U, Tepe C, et al: Systemic embolism in aortic arch atheromatosis. Eur Heart J 15:1373, 1994.

222. Amarenco P, Duyckaerts C, Tzourio C, et al: The prevalence of ulcerated plaques in the aortic arch in patients with stroke. N Engl J Med 326:221, 1992.

223. Amarenco P, Cohen A, Tzourio C, et al: Atherosclerotic disease of the aortic arch and the risk of ischemic stroke. N Engl J Med 331:1474, 1994.

224. Royce C, Royce A, Blake D, Grigg L:. Assessment of thoracic aortic atheroma by echocardiography: A new classification and estimation of risk of dislodging atheroma during three surgical techniques. Ann Thorac Cardiovasc Surg 4:72, 1998.

225. Demopoulos LA, Tunick PA, Bernstein NE, et al: Protruding atheromas of the aortic arch in symptomatic patients with carotid artery disease. Am Heart J 129:40, 1995.

226. Fazio GP, Redberg RF, Winslow T, Schiller NB: Transesophageal echocardiographically detected atherosclerotic aortic plaque is a marker for coronary artery disease. J Am Coll Cardiol 21:144, 1993.

227. Tunick PA, Culliford AT, Lamparello PJ, Kronzon I: Atheromatosis of the aortic arch as an occult source of multiple systemic emboli. Ann Intern Med 114:391, 1991.

228. Tunick PA, Rosensweig BP, Katz ES, et al: High risk for vascular events in patients with protruding aortic atheromas: A prospective study. J Am Coll Cardiol 23:1085, 1994.

229. Jones EF, Kalman JM, Calafiore P, et al: Proximal aortic atheroma: An independent risk factor for cerebral ischemia. Stroke 26:218, 1995.

230. Kistler JP: The risk of embolic stroke: Another piece of the puzzle. (editorial). N Engl J Med 331:1517, 1994.

231. Montgomery DH, Ververis JJ, McGorisk G, et al: Natural history of severe atheromatous disease of the thoracic aorta: A transesophageal echocardiographic study. J Am Coll Cardiol 27:95, 1996.

232. Freedberg RS, Tunick PA, Culliford AT, et al: Disappearance of a large intraaortic mass in a patient with prior systemic embolization. Am Heart J 125:1445, 1993.

233. Bansal RC, Pauls GL, Shankel SW: Blue digit syndrome: Transesophageal echocardiography identification of thoracic aortic plaque—related thrombi and successful outcome with warfarin. J Am Soc Echocardiogr 6:319, 1993.

234. Dressler FA, Craig WR, Castello R, Labovitz AJ: Mobile aortic atheroma and systemic emboli: Efficacy of anticoagulation and influence of plaque morphology on recurrent stroke. J Am Coll Cardiol 31:134–138, 1998.

235. Ferrari E, Vidal R, Chevallier T, Baudouy M: Atherosclerosis of the thoracic aorta and aortic debris as a marker of poor prognosis: Benefit of oral anticoagulants. J Am Coll Cardiol 33:1317, 1999.

236. Katz ES, Tunick PA, Rusinek H, et al: Protruding atheromas predict stroke in elderly patients undergoing cardiopulmonary bypass: Experience with intraoperative transesophageal echocardiography. J Am Coll Cardiol 20:70, 1992.

237. Blauth CI, Cosgrove DM, Webb BW, et al: Thromboembolism from the ascending aorta: An emerging problem in cardiac surgery. J Thorac Cardiovasc Surg 103:1104, 1992.

238. Wareing TH, Davila-Roman VG, Barzilai B, et al: Management of the severely atherosclerotic aorta during cardiac operation: A strategy for detection and treatment. J Thorac Cardiovasc Surg 103:453, 1992.

239. Davila-Roman VG, Phillips KJ, Daily BB, et al: Intraoperative transesophageal echocardiography and epiaortic ultrasound for assessment of atherosclerosis of the thoracic aorta. J Am Coll Cardiol 28:942, 1996.

240. Duda AM, Letwin LB, Sutter FP, Goldman SM: Does routine use of aortic ultrasonography decrease the stroke rate in coronary artery bypass surgery? J Vasc Surg 21:98, 1995.

241. Om A, Ellahham S, DiSciascio G: Cholesterol embolism: An underdiagnosed clinical entity. Am Heart J 124:1321, 1992.

242. Keeley EC, Grines CL: Scraping of aortic debris by coronary guiding catheters: A prospective evaluation of 1,000 cases. J Am Coll Cardiol 32:1861, 1998.

243. Davis K, Kennedy JW, Kemp HG Jr, et al: Complications of coronary arteriography from the collaborative study of coronary artery surgery (CASS). Circulation 59:1105, 1979.

244. Hyman BT, Landas SK, Ashman RF, et al: Warfarin-related purple toes syndrome and cholesterol microembolization. Am J Med 82:1233, 1987.

245. Arora RR, Magun AM, Grossman M, Katz J: Cholesterol embolization syndrome after intravenous tissue plasminogen activator for acute myocardial infarction. Am Heart J 126:225, 1993.

246. Bruns FJ, Segel DP, Apler S: Control of cholesterol embolization by discontinuation of anticoagulant therapy. Am J Med Sci 275:105, 1978.

247. Blankenship JC, Butler M, Garbes A: Prospective assessment of cholesterol embolization in patients with acute myocardial infarction treated with thrombolytic vs. conservative therapy. Chest 107:662, 1995.

248. Fine MJ, Kapoor W, Falanga V: Cholesterol crystal embolization: A review of 221 cases in the English literature. Angiology 38:769, 1987.

249. Babu SC, Shah PM, Nitahara J: Acute aortic occlusion: Factors that influence outcome. J Vasc Surg 21:567, 1995.

250. Dossa CD, Shepard AD, Reddy DJ, et al: Acute aortic occlusion: A 40-year experience. Arch Surg 129:603, 1994.

251. Tapper SS, Jenkins JM, Edwards WH, et al: Juxtarenal aortic occlusion. Ann Surg 215:443, 1992.

252. Light JT, Hendrickson M, Sholes WM, et al: Acute aortic occlusion secondary to *Aspergillus* endocarditis in an intravenous drug abuser. Ann Vasc Surg 5:271, 1991.

253. Busuttil RW, Keehn G, Milliken J, et al: Aortic saddle embolus: A twenty-two year experience. Ann Surg 197:698, 1983.

254. Gomes MN, Choyke PL, Wallace RB: Infected aortic aneurysms: A changing entity. Ann Surg 215:435, 1992.

255. Katz SG, Andros G, Kohl RD: *Salmonella* infections of the abdominal aorta. Surg Gynecol Obstet 175:102, 1992.

256. Pasic M, Carrel T, von Segesser L, Turina M: In situ repair of mycotic aneurysm of the ascending aorta. J Thorac Cardiovasc Surg 105:321, 1993.

257. Oz MC, Brener BJ, Buda JA, et al: A ten-year experience with bacterial aortitis. J Vasc Surg 10:439, 1989.

258. Moneta GL, Talylor LM, Yeager RA, et al: Surgical treatment of infected aortic aneurysms. Am J Surg 175:396, 1998.

259. Cohen OS, O'Brien TF, Schoenbaum SC, Mederos AA: The risk of endothelial infection in adults with *Salmonella* bacteremia. Ann Intern Med 89:931, 1978.

260. Jarrett F, Darling RC, Mundth ED, Austen WG: The management of infected arterial aneurysms. J Cardiovasc Surg 17:361, 1977.

261. Vogelzang RL, Sohaey R: Infected aortic aneurysms: CT appearance. J Comput Assist Tomogr 12:109, 1988.

262. Robinson JA, Johansen K: Aortic sepsis: Is there a role for in situ graft reconstruction? J Vasc Surg 13:677, 1991.

263. Fyfe BS, Quintana CS, Kaneka M, Griepp RB: Aortic sarcoma four years after Dacron graft insertion. Ann Thorac Surg 58:1752, 1994.

264. Khan A, Jilani F, Kaye S, Greenberg BR: Aortic wall sarcoma with tumor emboli and peripheral ischemia: Case report with review of literature. Am J Clin Oncol 20:73, 1997.

265. Navarra G, Occhionorelli S, Mascoli F, et al: Primary leiomyosarcoma of the aorta: Report of a case and review of the literature. J Cardiovasc Surg 35:33, 1994.

266. Ronaghi AH, Roberts AC, Rosenkrantz H: Intraaortic biopsy of a primary aortic tumor. J Vasc Interv Radiol 5:777, 1994.

267. Settmacher U, Heise M, Dette K, et al: Primary malignant intraluminal tumor of the aorta. Langenbecks Arch Chir 382:138, 1997.

268. Higgins R, Posner MC, Moosa HH, et al: Mesenteric infarction secondary to tumor emboli from primary aortic sarcoma. Cancer 68:1622, 1991.

269. Cziner DG, Freedberg RS, Tunick PA, et al: Transesophageal echocardiographic diagnosis of a primary intraaortic tumor. Am Heart J 125:1189, 1993.

Chapter 41

Peripheral Arterial Diseases

MARK A. CREAGER • PETER LIBBY

▼ Peripheral Arterial Disease

The term *peripheral arterial disease* (PAD) generally refers to atherosclerosis when it obstructs the blood supply to the lower or upper extremities. Other nomenclature includes peripheral arterial occlusive disease and arteriosclerosis obliterans, although the latter term has fallen into disuse. The term *peripheral vascular disease* should be avoided when referring specifically to PAD since it fails to convey the nature of the problem and is more appropriately used to designate a group of diseases affecting blood vessels, including PAD, vasculitis, vasospasm, venous thrombosis, venous insufficiency, and lymphatic disorders.

Traditionally, cardiologists have devoted most of their efforts to diagnosis and treatment of arterial disease in the coronary tree. While diseases of the aorta have often been accorded a place in cardiology training and practice, focus on disease of the peripheral arteries has lagged. PAD is a strong marker of risk for major cardiovascular events since it is frequently associated with coronary and cerebral atherosclerosis. Moreover, symptoms of PAD, including intermittent claudication, jeopardize quality of life and independence for many patients. In contrast to coronary artery afflictions, PAD is commonly underdiagnosed and undertreated. Thus, practitioners of cardiology have increasing interest in the diagnosis and management of PAD. This chapter aims to provide a framework for an approach to the diagnosis and management of patients with PAD.

EPIDEMIOLOGY

The prevalence of PAD depends on the population studied, the diagnostic method used, and whether symptoms are included to derive estimates. Most epidemiologic studies have used a noninvasive measurement, the ankle/brachial index (ABI), to diagnose PAD. The ABI is the ratio of ankle to brachial systolic blood pressure and is described in greater detail on p. 1464. In relatively large population-based studies conducted in the United States, Europe, and the Middle East, the prevalence of PAD based on an abnormal ABI ranged from 4.6 to 19.1 percent (Table 41–1).[1–7] In a free-living population participating in a lipid research clinic protocol, PAD was detected in less than 3 percent of those younger than 60 but in more than 20 percent of those 75 years and older and was 27 percent more prevalent in men than women.[1] In other studies, however, the prevalence was similar or greater in women.[2, 5] Taking these aggregate data into consideration, approximately 8 to 10 million individuals in the United States have PAD.

The prevalence of symptomatic disease in these populations can be assessed by questionnaires specifically designed to elicit symptoms of intermittent claudication. Estimates have varied depending on the age and gender of the population but generally indicate that only one-third to one-half of patients with PAD have symptoms of claudication. In the Whitehall Study of 18,388 male civil servants living in London and aged 40 to 64 years, approximately 1 percent were thought to have claudication.[8] Other estimates of claudication range from 1.6 to 4.5 percent of a population typically older than 40 years.[1, 3, 5, 6, 9–11] In the Edinburgh Artery Study of 1592 subjects aged 55 to 74 years, 116 new cases of claudication developed over a 5-year period, for an incidence of claudication of 15.5 per 1000 patient-years.[12] The prevalence and incidence of claudication increase with age (Fig. 41–1) and are greater in men than in women in most, but not all studies.[1–3, 5, 11, 13–15] In the Framingham Study of 5209 subjects aged 35 to 84 years, the 2-year incidence of claudication was 7.1 per 1000 for men and 3.6 per 1000 for women.[16]

Less information is available regarding the incidence of critical limb ischemia. In a prospective 7-year study of hospitals in northern Italy, the incidence of critical limb ischemia was 450 per million population per year, and the incidence of amputation was 112 per million per year.[17] Similarly, the Vascular Surgery Society of Great Britain estimated the incidence of critical limb ischemia in Britain and Ireland at 400 cases per million population per year. In Denmark, approximately 250 per million population per year underwent amputation because of critical limb ischemia.[18]

Contribution of Risk Factors

The well-known modifiable risk factors associated with coronary atherosclerosis also contribute to atherosclerosis of the peripheral circulation. Cigarette smoking, diabetes mellitus, dyslipidemia, hypertension, and hyperhomocysteinemia increase the risk of PAD (Table 41–2).

SMOKING. Data derived from several observational studies (including the Edinburgh Artery Study, the Framingham

▼ TABLE 41–1. PREVALENCE OF PERIPHERAL ARTERIAL DISEASE

STUDY/LOCATION	POPULATION (No.)	AGE (yr)	PREVALENCE (%)
San Diego[1]	613	38–82	11.7
Jerusalem Lipid Research Clinic Prevalence Study[2]	1592	≥35	4.6
Edinburgh Artery Study[3]	1592	55–74	9.0
Cardiovascular Health Study[4]	5084	≥65	12.4
Rotterdam Study[5]	7715	≥55	19.1
Limburg PAOD Study[6]	3650	40–78	12.4
Strong Heart Study[7]	4549	45–74	5.3

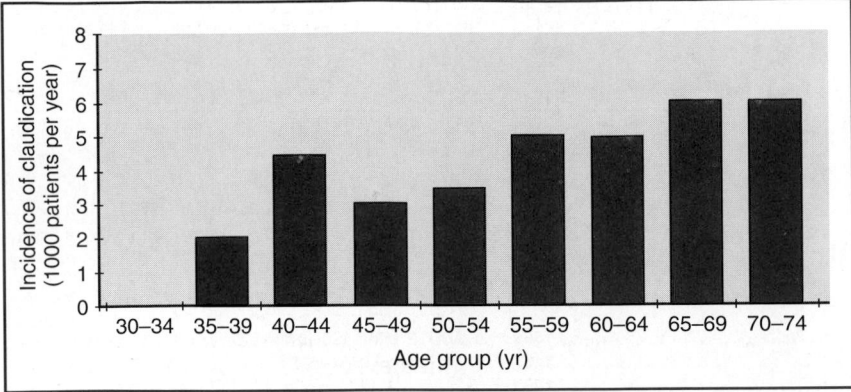

FIGURE 41-1. Age-related incidence of intermittent claudication derived from large population-based studies. (From Dormandy JA, Rutherford RB: Management of peripheral arterial disease [PAD]. TASC Working Group. J Vasc Surg 31[Suppl]:1-296, 2000.)

Heart Study, and the Cardiovascular Health Study, among others) indicate a twofold to fivefold increased risk of PAD in smokers.[2, 4, 10, 11, 14, 19, 20, 31] In the Whitehall Study, approximately 84 percent of patients with claudication were current smokers or ex-smokers,[8] and in another large recent study, 90 percent of patients with PAD were current or former smokers.[32] Progression of disease to critical limb ischemia and limb loss is more likely to occur in patients who continue to smoke than in those who stop.[33] Smoking may even increase the risk of development of PAD more than it does coronary artery disease.[19, 34]

DIABETES MELLITUS. In patients with diabetes mellitus, PAD is often extensive and severe, and these patients have a greater propensity for vascular calcification. Involvement of the femoral and popliteal arteries is similar to that of nondiabetic persons, but distal disease affecting the tibial and peroneal arteries occurs more frequently. The risk of development of PAD increases threefold to fourfold in patients with diabetes mellitus.[4, 14, 16, 19, 21] In the Framingham cohort, glucose intolerance contributed more as a risk factor for claudication than it did for coronary artery disease or stroke.[34]

LIPID DISORDERS. Abnormalities in lipid metabolism are also associated with an increased prevalence of PAD. Elevations in total or low-density lipoprotein (LDL) cholesterol increased the risk of PAD and claudication in some studies but not in others.[2, 10, 13, 14, 35] In a large Israeli study involving 10,059 men aged 40 to 65 years, the odds ratio for development of claudication was 1.35 for each increase in serum cholesterol of 50 mg/dl.[10] Similar observations were made in the Framingham Heart Study, in which the odds ratio for claudication was 1.2 for each 40-mg/dl increase in total cholesterol.[14] In a cohort of patients participating in a lipid research clinic protocol, however, LDL cholesterol was not associated with PAD based on a multiple logistic regression analysis that included cigarette smoking, blood pressure, glucose, and obesity. Hypertriglyceridemia independently predicts risk for PAD.[36, 37] Increased levels of lipoprotein (a) impart a twofold increased risk of PAD, with

higher levels associated with a greater risk for critical limb ischemia.[38]

HYPERTENSION. Hypertension increased the risk of claudication 2.5-fold in men and 4-fold in women in the Framingham Heart Study,[16] and the risk increased proportionally with the severity of hypertension.[14, 16] Similarly, in the Edinburgh Artery Study, elevations in systolic blood pressure correlated with PAD. However, this finding has not been consistently shown in all epidemiological studies. In the British Whitehall Study and a large Finnish study, hypertension was not found to be associated with claudication.[8, 13]

HYPERHOMOCYSTEINEMIA. Hyperhomocysteinemia increases the risk of atherosclerosis by approximately twofold to threefold.[28-30] In a meta-analysis of studies relating homocysteine to atherosclerotic disease, the odds ratio for PAD in patients with increased homocysteine levels was 6.8.[30] High levels of homocysteine have been detected in 30 to 40 percent of patients with PAD.[39, 40] Prospective studies have not consistently confirmed a relationship of hyperhomocysteinemia with cardiovascular events, however (see Chap. 31). Plasma levels of B complex vitamins, including folate, cobalamin, and pyridoxal 5'-phosphate, all inversely relate to the plasma homocysteine concentration, and patients taking B vitamin supplements have a lower risk of vascular disease.[29]

FIBRINOGEN. An increase in fibrinogen is also associated with an increased risk of PAD.[11, 22-24, 41] The Edinburgh Artery Study noted a 35 percent increased risk for PAD over 5 years for each 0.70-gm/liter increase in fibrinogen.[25, 26] Patients with PAD have elevated levels of C-reactive protein, a serological marker of systemic inflammation. In the Physicians' Health Study, the relative risk of development of PAD among men in the highest quartile for C-reactive protein concentration was 2.1[27] (see also Chap. 31).

The risk of PAD and intermittent claudication developing increases progressively with the burden of contributing factors. In the Framingham Heart Study, the occurrence of claudication in men whose risk factor was smoking versus nonsmoking was 2.6 versus 0.8 per 8 years per 1000 population.[16] In male smokers who were also hypertensive, hypercholesterolemic, and diabetic, the risk was 44.3 per 8 years per 1000 (Fig. 41-2).[16] Similar observations have been made in women.

PATHOBIOLOGY

Heterogeneity of Blood Vessels in Different Circulatory Beds

Atherosclerosis preferentially affects certain locations in the circulation. As discussed in Chapter 30, atheromatous lesions tend to form at flow dividers and branch points in arteries and usually spare veins. In the last several years, progress has been made in understanding the link between hydrodynamics of the circulation, the cellular and molecu-

▼ **TABLE 41-2.** RISK OF PERIPHERAL ARTERIAL DISEASE IN PERSONS WITH MODIFIABLE RISK FACTORS

RISK FACTOR	ESTIMATED RELATIVE RISK
Cigarette smoking[2, 4, 10, 19, 20]	2.0-5.0
Diabetes mellitus[4, 14, 16, 19, 21]	3.0-4.0
Hypertension[14, 16, 19]	1.1-2.2
Hypercholesterolemia (per 40- to 50-mg/dl increase in total cholesterol)[10, 14]	1.2-1.4
Fibrinogen (per 0.7-gm/liter increase in fibrinogen)[22-26]	1.35
C-reactive protein[27]	2.1
Hyperhomocysteinemia[28-30]	2.0-3.2

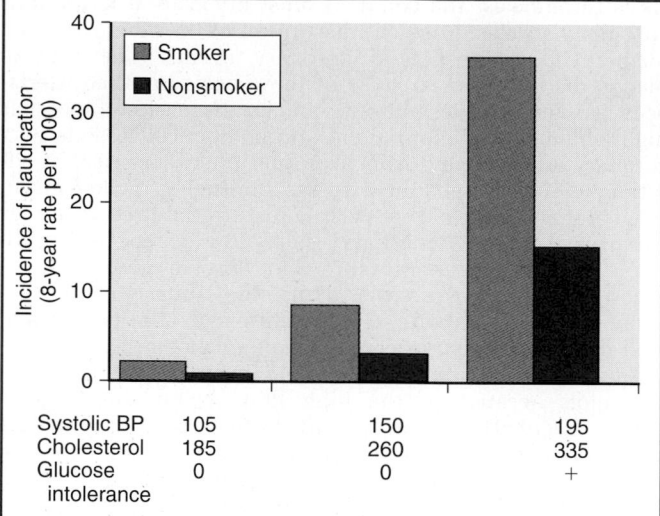

Systolic BP	105	150	195
Cholesterol	185	260	335
Glucose intolerance	0	0	+

FIGURE 41-2. The incidence of intermittent claudication in the Framingham Heart Study in smokers and nonsmokers is compounded by an increased burden of risk factors. (From Murabito JM, D'Agostino RB, Silbershatz H, et al: Intermittent claudication. A risk profile from The Framingham Heart Study. Circulation 96: 44–49, 1997. By permission of the American Heart Association, Inc.)

 amples illustrate how the common precursor of endothelial cells shows molecular diversity early in life that depends on its location in the circulation.

SMOOTH MUSCLE CELLS DERIVE FROM MULTIPLE, LOCAL SOURCES DURING DEVELOPMENT

In contrast to endothelial cells, which derive from a common precursor, smooth muscle cells can arise from many sources. After endothelial cells form tubular anlage, or rudimentary, precursor of blood vessels, they recruit the cells that will become smooth muscle, or pericytes (smooth muscle–like cells associated with microvessels). In the descending aorta and arteries of the lower half of the body, regional mesoderm serves as the source of smooth muscle precursors. Mesodermal cells in somites give rise to the smooth muscle cells that invest much of the distal aorta and its branches. In arteries of the upper part of the body, however, smooth muscle cells actually derive from a completely different germ layer, neuroectoderm rather than mesoderm. Before the neural tube closes, neuroectodermal cells migrate and become the precursors of smooth muscle cells in the ascending aorta and some of its branches, including the carotid arteries.[45] Smooth muscle cells in the coronary arteries are derived from mesoderm, but in a special way. The precursors of coronary artery smooth muscle cells arise from a structure known as the proepicardial organ.[46, 47]

As in the case of endothelial cells, smooth muscle cells show molecular heterogeneity early during development. For example, the promoter of a characteristic smooth muscle gene known as SM22 drives gene expression in venous but not arterial smooth muscle cells during embryogenesis.[48] Much of the localization of structures in embryos depends on a family of genes known as homeobox genes. Deletion of a pair of homeobox genes known as Prx1/Prx2 that are involved in mesenchymal pattern development causes selective impairment in development of the great vessels and the ductus arteriosus while sparing morphogenesis of other vessels.[49] Transcription factors also play an important role in determining the phenotype of cells. A specific transcription factor known as dHAND signals the recruitment of mesenchyme by endothelial cells in an anatomically heterogeneous manner during development. In particular, dHAND regulation selectively participates in the recruitment of mesenchyme in upper body blood vessels versus those of the more caudal portions of the embryo.[50]

CLINICAL IMPLICATIONS OF VASCULAR DEVELOPMENTAL BIOLOGY. Far from being of mere theoretical concern, the developmental biology of the arterial tree has important clinical implications regarding issues that arise in daily practice. The distinct embryonic origins of smooth muscle cells in various arteries may help explain why some regions of the arterial tree are particularly prone to atheroma formation. While local hydrodynamics doubtless controls the expression of genes that protect against or promote atherogenesis (see Chap. 30), the cellular substrate acted on by biomechanical forces varies as described above.

Intimal cushions, which consist of expanded regions populated by smooth muscle cells and extracellular matrix (Fig. 41–3), develop in very interesting regions of the arterial tree early in life. Two regions of intimal cushion formation of particular consequence for cardiologists are the proximal left anterior descending coronary artery and the carotid siphon.[51, 52] The intimal cushion in the proximal left anterior descending coronary artery begins to form even during intrauterine life. It progresses rapidly in early postnatal life and leads to intimal cushions in the proximal left anterior coronary artery in all humans by 2 years of age.[51] It remains unclear to what extent lineage differences versus local hemodynamic forces contribute to the formation of these intimal cushions in arteries prone to the development of atherosclerosis. These cushions of smooth muscle and connective tissue form the "soil" in which atheromatous lesions can grow in later life.[53]

HETEROGENEITY IN VASCULAR FUNCTIONS. The functions of blood vessels differ in various regions of the circulation as evidenced by the preferential effects of many vasoactive drugs commonly used in the practice of cardiology on selected vascular beds. Nitrates dilate both arteries and veins, whereas other vasodilators, such as hydralazine, act primarily as arterial vasodilators. The well-recognized differences in clinical outcomes of saphenous vein and internal mammary artery bypass grafts furnish another exam-

lar mechanisms of atherosclerosis, and the atheroprotective functions of vascular wall cells. Chapter 30 discusses the focality of atherosclerosis in terms of local hemodynamic differences. However, questions remain: Are blood vessels intrinsically different in different regions of the circulation? Do regional variations in the propensity for atherosclerosis merely depend on the external hemodynamic forces that impinge on them? Indeed, vessels in different beds have distinct morphology, physiology, and pharmacology and therefore intrinsic heterogeneity. Recent work has elucidated the biological basis of differences among blood vessels. This section will consider, in turn, new information regarding the development of blood vessels related to arterial heterogeneity, differences in functions of blood vessels depending on the circulatory bed, and finally, whether the mechanisms leading to clinical manifestations of arterial disease vary from one circulatory bed (e.g., the coronary circulation) to another and in different arteries (e.g., the carotid or the distal aorta).

DEVELOPMENTAL BIOLOGY OF HETEROGENEITY AMONG BLOOD VESSELS

Endothelial cells have a common origin but acquire bed-specific characteristics during development. The endothelial cells that form the inner lining of all blood vessels arise during embryogenesis from regions known as the blood islands located on the embryo's periphery. Angioblasts, which are predecessors of endothelial cells, share this site with the precursors of blood cells. Despite arising from the same site, cells display considerable heterogeneity even during embryological and early postnatal development. Although presumably derived from a common precursor, the signals that endothelial cells encounter during vessel development differ. As rudimentary blood vessels begin to form, endothelial precursors interact with the surrounding cells. This interchange permits spatial and temporal gradients of various stimuli and their receptors on endothelial cells, which leads to heterogeneity of this cell type in the adult.

Differential expression of endothelial genes in various types of blood vessels depend on transcriptional regulation by the local environment. For example, the promoter region of the gene that encodes von Willebrand factor directs expression of brain and heart microvessels in the endothelium but not in larger arteries.[42] Indeed, coculture of endothelial cells with cardiac myocytes, but not other cell types, could selectively activate a von Willebrand factor gene promoter construct. Likewise, endothelial nitric oxide synthase gene activity in the heart shows bed-specific regulation.[43] A recently recognized family of tyrosine kinase receptors known as EPH and their ligands known as epherins display heterogeneous expression in arterial versus venous endothelial cells during development.[44] These ex-

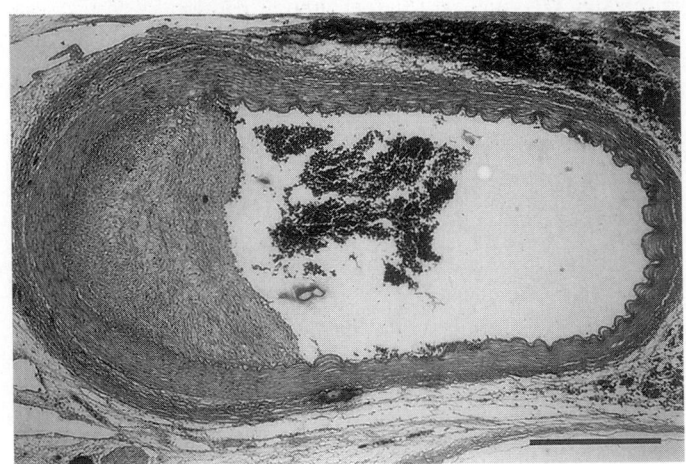

FIGURE 41–3. An intimal cushion shown in a cross section through the internal carotid artery of a 10-week-old male infant. Areas where intimal cushions form in early life are prone to the development of atheroma more commonly in later years. The bar shows 0.5 mm. (From Weninger WJ, Muller GB, Reiter C, et al: Intimal hyperplasia of the infant parasellar carotid artery: A potential developmental factor in atherosclerosis and SIDS. Circ Res 85: 970–975, 1999. By permission of the American Heart Association, Inc.)

ple of clinically relevant heterogeneity among vessels. Internal mammary arteries release more nitric oxide than do saphenous veins. In addition, saphenous veins produce more vasoconstrictor endothelial-derived cyclooxygenase products than do internal mammary arteries. Such differences may help explain the superior clinical outcomes with internal mammary grafts versus autologous venous bypass grafts.[54]

Indeed, the reactions of blood vessels or vascular cells from various regions of the circulation sometimes differ directionally. The pulmonary vasoconstrictive versus systemic vasodilator response to hypoxia and the disparate response of the cerebral versus the systemic arterial circulation to carbon dioxide are commonly encountered examples. Neuroectoderm-derived smooth muscle cells in upper body blood vessels grow in response to transforming growth factor-beta; however, mesenchymal-derived smooth muscle cells from lower body arteries actually show growth inhibition when exposed to this mediator.[55] Perhaps, the different embryonic origins of smooth muscle cells in the ascending versus the descending aorta explain why certain gene defects express themselves primarily in the ascending aorta. In Marfan syndrome, for example, the fibrillin mutation characteristically involves the ascending aorta first (see also Chap. 56). Likewise, in Williams syndrome, elastin is genetically defective throughout the body, yet the vascular phenotype of these patients is localized to the supervalvular portion of the ascending aorta.[45]

Heterogeneity of the Clinical Manifestations of Arterial Disease

The Pathobiological Determinants of Atherosclerosis in Youth (PDAY) study collected arterial specimens from Americans younger than 35 years who died of non-cardiac causes. This study found that fatty streaks and raised arterial lesions initially localize in the dorsal portion of the abdominal aorta. Involvement of the thoracic aorta with fatty streaks or early atheroma follows lesion formation in the abdominal aorta. The PDAY data suggest that the formation of coronary atheroma actually lags behind the development of fatty lesions in the aorta.[56, 57]

The most dreaded clinical consequence of atherosclero-

sis is thrombosis, the cause of most myocardial infarctions and many strokes. Physical disruption of the atherosclerotic plaque causes most fatal coronary events. The role of plaque disruption as a cause of thrombosis in other arterial beds has received less attention. The discussion above has highlighted the developmental and anatomical reasons why coronary arteries may differ from peripheral arteries. In addition, the hemodynamic stresses impinging on lesions in the coronary versus the peripheral arterial tree differ as well. Notably, most coronary artery flow occurs during diastole, whereas peak pressure and flow in peripheral arteries occur during systole. Thus, the underlying mechanism of the thrombotic complications of atheroma might well differ in coronary versus peripheral arteries.

In the aorta, mural thrombi seldom develop into occlusive clots because of the high flow. Nonetheless, aortic plaque frequently ruptures, and aortic thrombi are recognized as a clinically important source of embolic disease (Fig. 41–4). Plaque in the aorta encounters high "hoop" (circumferential) stress as a result of the large radius, according to the Laplace relationship. This difference may account for the prevalence of disrupted plaque in an atherosclerotic aorta. Recent evidence suggests that plaque rupture also underlies symptoms of carotid arterial disease. In one study, histopathological evaluation of carotid artery specimens removed by endarterectomy revealed plaque rupture in 74 percent of symptomatic versus only 32 percent of asymptomatic patients.[58] The degree of stenosis was similar in both symptomatic and asymptomatic individuals in this study. Ulcerated plaque with superimposed thrombus was found in six of seven occluded internal carotid arteries in a neuropathological autopsy series.[59] Features

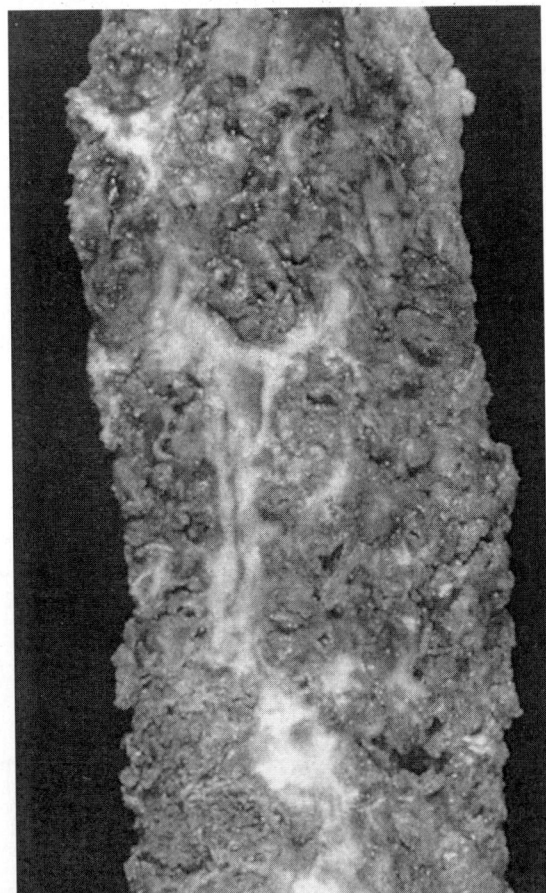

FIGURE 41–4. Atherosclerotic aorta of a patient with atheroemboli. Multiple protruding, shaggy atheromas with superimposed mural thrombi are present. (Courtesy of R.M. Mitchell, M.D., Ph.D., Department of Pathology, Brigham and Women's Hospital, Boston.)

associated with vulnerability of coronary plaque, including foam cells and thinning of the fibrous cap, are more frequent in symptomatic than in asymptomatic carotid plaque.[58] As in unstable coronary plaque, inflammatory cells infiltrate and are activated (determined by expression of the histocompatibility antigen HLA-DR). The proportion of active inflammatory cells is consistently higher in ruptured plaque than in asymptomatic carotid plaque with a similar degree of stenosis.[60]

An independent line of clinical evidence supports a commonality in the mechanisms of complication shared by carotid and coronary arteries. A recent large study dichotomized patients with symptomatic carotid artery lesions into those with and those without irregularity of the carotid lesion by angiography. Over 10 years of follow-up, those with irregular carotid lesions had a greater than twofold higher cumulative incidence of non–stroke-related vascular death (mostly caused by coronary events) than did those with smooth lesions.[61] Nonvascular deaths and the risk factors assessed in this study did not differ between groups. Similar mechanisms are likely to account for acute thromboses in peripheral arteries, although detailed investigations are not available. Despite the considerable biological and functional heterogeneity among arterial beds, the mechanisms causing the most important clinical manifestations appear to be similar.

PATHOPHYSIOLOGY OF LIMB ISCHEMIA

Pathophysiological considerations in patients with PAD must take into account the balance of the circulatory supply of nutrients to the skeletal muscle and the oxygen and nutrient demand of skeletal muscle (Table 41–3).

FACTORS REGULATING BLOOD SUPPLY (see also Chap. 34)

The primary determinant of inadequate blood supply to the extremity is a flow-limiting lesion of a conduit artery. Flow through an artery is directly proportional to perfusion pressure and inversely proportional to vascular resistance. If atherosclerosis causes a stenosis, flow through the artery is reduced as described in the Poiseuille equation, in which $Q = \frac{\Delta P \pi r^4}{8 \eta l}$, where ΔP is the pressure gradient across the stenosis, r is the radius of the residual lumen, η is blood viscosity, and l is the length of the vessel affected by the stenosis. As the severity of a stenotic lesion increases, flow becomes progressively reduced. The pressure gradient across the stenosis increases in a nonlinear manner, thus emphasizing the importance of a stenosis at high blood flow rates. Usually, a blood pressure gradient exists at rest if the stenosis reduces luminal diameter by more than 50 percent because kinetic energy is lost as turbulence develops.[62] A stenosis that does not cause a pressure gradient at rest may cause a gradient during exercise, when blood flow rises consequent to higher cardiac output and decreased vascular resistance. Thus, as flow through a stenosis increases, distal perfusion pressure is not maintained. Also, as the metabolic demand of exercising muscle outstrips its blood supply, local metabolites, including adenosine, nitric oxide, potassium, and hydrogen ion, accumulate and peripheral resistance vessels dilate.

▼ TABLE 41–3. PATHOPHYSIOLOGICAL CONSIDERATIONS IN PERIPHERAL ARTERIAL DISEASE

Factors regulating blood supply to limb
  Flow-limiting lesion (stenosis severity, inadequate collaterals)
  Impaired vasodilation (decreased nitric oxide and reduced responsiveness to vasodilators)
  Accentuated vasoconstriction (thromboxane, serotonin, angiotensin II, endothelin, norepinephrine)
  Abnormal rheology (reduced red blood cell deformability, increased leukocyte adhesiveness, platelet aggregation, microthombosis, increased fibrinogen)
Altered skeletal muscle structure and function
  Axonal denervation of skeletal muscle
  Loss of type II, glycolytic fast twitch fibers
  Increased mitochondrial enzymatic activity

This response results in a further drop in perfusion pressure since the stenosis limits flow. In addition, intramuscular pressure rises during exercise and may exceed the arterial pressure distal to an occlusion and cause blood flow to cease.[62] Flow through collateral blood vessels is usually adequate to meet the resting metabolic needs of skeletal muscle tissue, but it is not enough during exercise.

Functional abnormalities in vasomotor reactivity may also interfere with blood flow. The vasodilator capability of both conduit and resistance vessels is impaired in patients with peripheral atherosclerosis. Normally, arteries dilate in response to pharmacological and biochemical stimuli, such as acetylcholine, serotonin, thrombin, or bradykinin, as well as in response to shear stress induced by increases in blood flow. This vasodilator response results from the release of biologically active substances from the endothelium, particularly nitric oxide (see also Chap. 34). The vascular relaxation of a conduit vessel that occurs after a flow stimulus, such as that induced by exercise, may facilitate the delivery of blood to exercising muscles in healthy persons. Vasodilation subsequent to flow or pharmacological stimuli does not occur in the atherosclerotic femoral arteries and calf resistance vessels of patients with PAD.[63] This failure of vasodilation might prevent an increase in nutritive blood supply to exercising muscle since endothelium-derived nitric oxide has been shown to contribute to hyperemic blood volume following an ischemic stimulus.[63, 64] Preliminary studies have suggested that L-arginine, the precursor for endothelium-derived nitric oxide, increases muscle blood flow and improves claudication distance in patients with PAD, further supporting the contention that endothelium-dependent vasodilation is abnormal in these individuals.[65, 66] It is not known whether vasodilator function with respect to prostacyclin, adenosine, or ion channels is abnormal in peripheral atherosclerotic arteries. Endogenous vasoconstrictor substances such as prostanoids and other lipid mediators, thrombin, serotonin, angiotensin II, endothelin, and norepinephrine may interfere with vasodilation.

SKELETAL MUSCLE STRUCTURE AND METABOLIC FUNCTION

Electrophysiological and histopathological examination has found evidence of partial axonal denervation of skeletal muscle in legs affected by PAD.[67] Type I, oxidative slow-twitch fibers are preserved, but type II, or glycolytic, fast twitch fibers are lost in the skeletal muscle of patients with PAD.[68] Loss of type II fibers is associated with decreased muscle strength and reduced exercise capacity.[68] Within skeletal muscle, metabolism shifts to anaerobic earlier during exercise and it persists longer after cessation of exercise. Patients with claudication have increased lactate release and accumulation of acylcarnitines during exercise, indicative of ineffective oxidative metabolism.[69, 70] Yet, mitochondrial enzymatic activity is increased in the skeletal muscle of patients with claudication, possibly reflecting a metabolic adaptation to the reduced blood supply.[71, 72]

Pathophysiology of Critical Limb Ischemia

Abnormalities in the microcirculation contribute to the pathophysiology of critical limb ischemia. The number of perfused skin capillaries is reduced in patients with severe limb ischemia.[73] Other potential causes of decreased capillary perfusion in this condition include reduced red cell deformability, increased leukocyte adhesivity, platelet aggregates, fibrinogen, microthrombosis, excessive vasoconstriction, and interstitial edema (Fig. 41–5).[74–76] Intravascular pressure may also be decreased because precapillary arterioles are dilated as a result of locally released vasoactive metabolites.[77]

CLINICAL FEATURES

Symptoms

INTERMITTENT CLAUDICATION. The two cardinal symptoms of PAD are intermittent claudication and pain at rest. The term *claudication* is derived from the Latin word *claudicare*, to limp. Intermittent claudication is characterized by pain, ache, a sense of fatigue, or other discomfort that occurs in the affected leg during exercise, particularly walking, and resolves with rest. Claudication occurs when skeletal muscle oxygen demand during effort exceeds the blood supply and results from activation of local sensory recep-

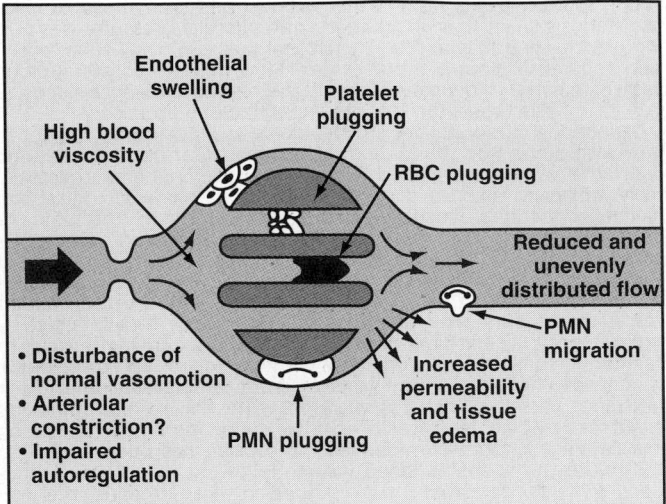

Endothelial
swelling

Platelet
plugging

High blood
viscosity

RBC plugging

Reduced and
unevenly
distributed flow

PMN
migration

• Disturbance of
normal vasomotion
• Arteriolar
constriction?
• Impaired
autoregulation

PMN plugging

Increased
permeability
and tissue
edema

FIGURE 41–5. Schematic representation of potential pathophysiological mechanisms that lead to microvascular obstruction in patients with critical limb ischemia. (From Second European Consensus Document on chronic critical leg ischemia. Circulation 84[Suppl 4]:1–26, 1991. By permission of the American Heart Association, Inc.)

tors by the accumulation of lactate or other metabolites. The location of the symptom often relates to the site of the most proximal stenosis. Buttock, hip, or thigh claudication is typical of patients with obstruction of the aorta and iliac arteries. Calf claudication occurs in patients with femoral and popliteal artery stenoses. The gastrocnemius muscle consumes more oxygen during ambulation than do other muscle groups in the leg and hence causes the most frequent symptom reported by patients. Ankle or pedal claudication occurs in patients with tibial and peroneal artery disease. Similarly, stenoses of the subclavian, axillary, and brachial arteries may cause shoulder, biceps, or forearm claudication, respectively. Symptoms should resolve several minutes following cessation of effort. Calf and thigh pain that occurs at rest, such as nocturnal cramps, should not be confused with claudication and is not a symptom of PAD. The history obtained from claudicants should note the distance walked, speed, and incline that precipitates claudication to evaluate disability and to provide a baseline qualitative measure with which to determine stability, improvement, or deterioration during subsequent encounters with the patient. Symptoms other than claudication can limit functional capacity.[78] Patients with PAD walk more slowly and have less walking endurance than do patients without PAD.[79, 80]

Several questionnaires have been developed to assess the presence and severity of claudication. The Rose Questionnaire was initially developed to diagnose both angina and intermittent claudication in epidemiological surveys.[81] It queries whether pain develops in either calf with walking and whether it occurs at rest, while walking at an ordinary or hurried pace, or when walking uphill. Several modifications of this questionnaire have been made, including the Edinburgh Claudication Questionnaire and the San Diego Claudication Questionnaire,[82, 83] which are both more sensitive and specific in comparison to a physician's diagnosis of intermittent claudication based on walking distance, walking speed, and nature of the symptoms. A more recently validated instrument, the Walking Impairment Questionnaire, asks a series of questions and assigns a point score based on walking distance, walking speed, and nature of the symptoms.[84]

Limb claudication may occasionally result from nonatherosclerotic causes of arterial occlusive disease (Table 41–4). Several of these causes are discussed later in the chapter and include arterial embolism; vasculitides such as

thromboangiitis obliterans (TAO), Takayasu arteritis, or giant cell arteritis; aortic coarctation; fibromuscular dysplasia; irradiation; and extravascular compression secondary to arterial entrapment or an adventitial cyst (see also Chap. 67).

Several nonvascular causes of exertional leg pain should be considered in patients with symptoms suggestive of intermittent claudication (Table 41–4). Lumbosacral radiculopathy resulting from degenerative joint disease, spinal stenosis, and herniated discs may cause pain in the buttock, hip, thigh, calf, and/or foot with walking, often after very short distances or even with standing.[85, 86] The term *neurogenic pseudoclaudication* has been used to describe this symptom. Lumbosacral spine disease and PAD each affect the elderly, and as such, both may be present in the same individual. Arthritis of the hips and knees also provokes leg pain with walking. Typically, the pain is localized to the affected joint and may be elicited on physical examination by palpation and range-of-motion maneuvers. Rarely, skeletal muscle disorders such as myositis can cause exertional leg pain. Muscle tenderness, abnormal neuromuscular examination findings, elevated skeletal muscle enzymes, and a normal pulse examination should distinguish myositis from PAD. McArdle syndrome, characterized by a deficiency of skeletal muscle phosphorylase, can cause symptoms mimicking the claudication of PAD. Patients with chronic venous regurgitation may complain of leg discomfort with exertion, a condition designated venous claudication.[87–89] Venous hypertension during exercise increases resistance and limits blood flow. In the case of venous insufficiency, the elevated extravascular pressure caused by interstitial edema further diminishes capillary perfusion. A physical examination demonstrating peripheral edema, venous stasis pigmentation, and occasionally, venous varicosities will identify this unusual cause of exertional leg pain.

REST PAIN. Pain at rest occurs in patients with critical limb ischemia in whom the resting metabolic needs of the tissue are not adequately met by the available blood supply. Typically, patients complain of pain or paresthesias in the foot or toes of the affected extremity. This discomfort is worsened by leg elevation and improved by leg dependency, as might be anticipated by the respective effects of gravity on perfusion pressure. The pain may be particularly severe at sites of skin fissuring, ulceration, or necrosis. Of-

▼ **TABLE 41–4. DIFFERENTIAL DIAGNOSIS OF EXERTIONAL LEG PAIN**

VASCULAR CAUSES
Atherosclerosis
Thrombosis
Embolism
Vasculitis
   Thromboangiitis obliterans
   Takayasu arteritis
   Giant cell arteritis
Aortic coarctation
Fibromuscular dysplasia
Irradiation
Extravascular compression
   Arterial entrapment (e.g., popliteal artery entrapment, thoracic outlet syndrome)
   Adventitial cysts

NONVASCULAR CAUSES
Lumbosacral radiculopathy
   Degenerative arthritis
   Spinal stenosis
   Herniated disc
Arthritis
   Hip, knees
Venous insufficiency
Myositis
McArdle syndrome

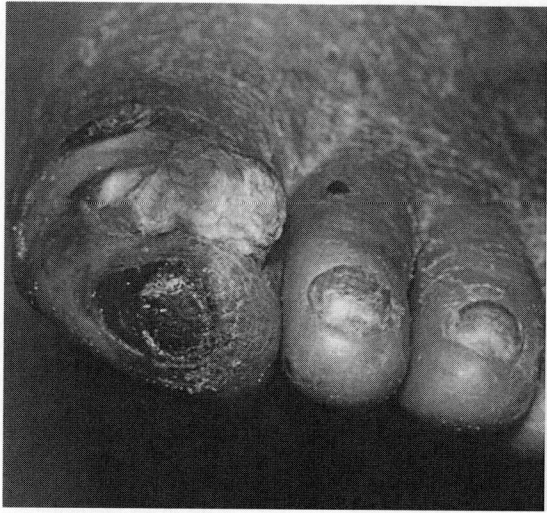 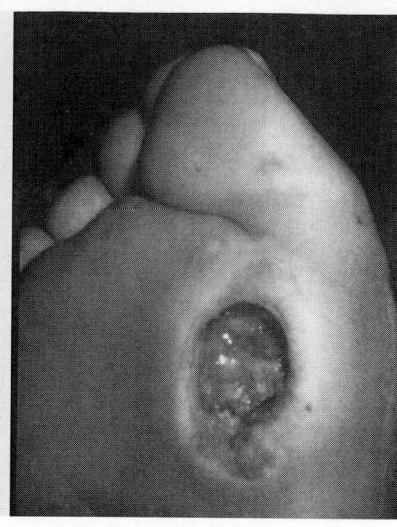

FIGURE 41–6. *Left,* Typical arterial ulcer. It is a discrete, circumscribed, necrotic ulcer located on the great toe. *Right,* Trophic ulcer in a patient with diabetes mellitus located on the volar surface of the foot beneath the head of the first metatarsal bone, a typical area of pressure; its base has granulation tissue.

ten, the skin is very sensitive, and even the weight of bedclothes or sheets elicits pain. Patients may sit on the edge of the bed and dangle their legs to alleviate the discomfort. However, patients with ischemic or diabetic neuropathy may have little or no pain despite the presence of severe ischemia.

Critical limb and digital ischemia may result from arterial occlusions other than those caused by atherosclerosis. Such conditions include vasculitides such as TAO, connective tissue disorders such as systemic lupus erythematosus and scleroderma, vasospasm, atheromatous embolism, and acute arterial occlusion caused by thrombosis or embolism. Many of these disorders are discussed later in this chapter. Acute gouty arthritis, trauma, and sensory neuropathy such as that caused by diabetes mellitus, lumbosacral radiculopathy, and reflex sympathetic dystrophy can cause foot pain. Leg ulcers also occur in patients with venous insufficiency and sensory neuropathy, particularly that related to diabetes. These ulcers are easily distinguished from arterial ulcers, which are described below. A venous ulcer is usually located near the medial malleolus, its border is irregular, and its base is pink with granulation tissue. The pain accompanying venous ulcers is milder than that of arterial ulcers. Neurotrophic ulcers occur with pressure or trauma, usually on the sole of the foot. These ulcers are deep, frequently infected, and not usually painful because of the loss of sensation (Fig. 41–6, right panel).

Physical Findings

A careful vascular examination includes palpation of pulses and auscultation of accessible arteries for bruits. Pulses that are readily palpable in healthy individuals include the brachial, radial, and ulnar arteries of the upper extremity and the femoral, popliteal, dorsalis pedis, and posterior tibial arteries of the lower extremities. The aorta also can be palpated in asthenic persons. A decreased or absent pulse provides insight into the location of arterial stenoses. For example, a normal right femoral pulse but absent left femoral pulse suggests the presence of left iliofemoral arterial stenosis. A normal femoral artery pulse but absent popliteal artery pulse would indicate a stenosis in the superficial femoral artery or proximal popliteal artery. Similarly, disease of the anterior and posterior tibial arteries may be inferred when the popliteal artery pulse is present but the dorsalis pedis and posterior tibial pulses, respectively, are not palpable. Bruits are often indicative of accelerated blood flow velocity and turbulence at sites of stenosis. A stethoscope should be used to auscultate the supraclavicular and infraclavicular fossae for evidence of subclavian artery stenosis; the abdomen, flank, and pelvis for evidence

of stenoses in the aorta and its branch vessels; and each groin for evidence of femoral artery stenoses. Pallor may be elicited on the soles of the feet of some patients with PAD by performing a maneuver in which the feet are elevated above the level of the heart and the calf muscles are exercised by repeated dorsiflexion and plantar flexion of the ankle. The legs are then placed in the dependent position and the time to the onset of hyperemia and venous distention is measured. Each of these parameters is dependent on the rate of blood flow, which is influenced by the severity of the stenosis and the adequacy of collateral vessels.

Muscle atrophy may be apparent in the legs of patients with chronic aortoiliac disease. Additional signs of chronic low-grade ischemia include hair loss, thickened and brittle toenails, smooth and shiny skin, and subcutaneous fat atrophy of the digital pads. The skin is cool in patients with severe limb ischemia, and they may have petechiae, persistent cyanosis or pallor, dependent rubor, pedal edema resulting from prolonged dependency, skin fissures, ulceration, or gangrene. Arterial ulcers typically have a pale base with irregular borders and usually involve the tips of the toes or the heel of the foot or develop at sites of pressure (Fig. 41–6, left panel). These ulcers vary in size and may be as small as 3 to 5 mm.

Categorization of PAD

Patients with PAD may be classified according to the severity of the symptoms and abnormalities detected on physical examination. Categorization of the clinical manifestations of PAD improves communication among professionals caring for these patients and provides a structure for defining guidelines for therapeutic intervention. The traditional scheme described by Fontaine classified patients in one of four stages progressing from asymptomatic to critical limb ischemia (Table 41–5). A contemporary, more descriptive classification has been adopted by several professional vascular societies and includes asymptomatic patients, three

▼ **TABLE 41–5. FONTAINE CLASSIFICATION OF PERIPHERAL ARTERIAL DISEASE**

STAGE	SYMPTOMS
I	Asymptomatic
II	Intermittent claudication
IIa	Pain free, claudication walking >200 meters
IIb	Pain free, claudication walking <200 meters
III	Rest and nocturnal pain
IV	Necrosis, gangrene

▼ **TABLE 41-6. CLINICAL CATEGORIES OF CHRONIC LIMB ISCHEMIA**

GRADE	CATEGORY	CLINICAL DESCRIPTION
	0	Asymptomatic, not hemodynamically correct
I	1	Mild claudication
	2	Moderate claudication
	3	Severe claudication
II	4	Ischemic rest pain
	5	Minor tissue loss: nonhealing ulcer, focal gangrene with diffuse pedal ulcer
III	6	Major tissue loss extending above the transmetatarsal level, functional foot no longer salvageable

Adapted from Rutherford RB, Baker JD, Ernst C, et al: Recommended standards for reports dealing with lower extremity ischemia: Revised version. J Vasc Surg 26:517–538, 1997.

grades of claudication, and three grades of critical limb ischemia ranging from rest pain alone to minor and major tissue loss (Table 41–6).[90]

DIAGNOSTIC TESTS

Segmental Pressure Measurement

One of the most useful and simplest noninvasive tests to evaluate the presence and severity of stenoses in the peripheral arteries is the measurement of systolic blood pressure along selected segments of each extremity. In the lower extremities, pneumatic cuffs are placed on the upper and lower portions of the thigh, on the calf, above the ankle, and often over the metatarsal area of the foot. Likewise, in the upper extremity, pneumatic cuffs are placed on the upper part of the arm over the biceps, on the forearm below the elbow, and at the wrist. Systolic blood pressure at each respective limb segment can be measured by first inflating the pneumatic cuff to suprasystolic pressure and then determining the pressure at which blood flow occurs during cuff deflation. The onset of flow can be assessed by placing a Doppler ultrasound flow probe over an artery distal to the cuff. In the lower extremities, it is most convenient to place the Doppler probe on the foot over the posterior tibial artery as it courses inferior and posterior to the medial malleolus or over the dorsalis pedis artery on the dorsum of the metatarsal arch. In the upper extremities, the Doppler probe can be placed over the brachial artery in the antecubital fossa or over the radial and ulnar arteries at the wrist.

Left ventricular contraction creates the kinetic energy for blood pressure, which is maintained throughout the large and medium-sized vessels. Systolic blood pressure in the more distal vessels may be higher than that in the aorta and proximal vessels because of reflection of blood pressure waves.[91] Stenosis can cause loss of pressure energy as a result of increased frictional forces and turbulence at the site of the stenosis. Approximately 90 percent of the cross-sectional area of the aorta must be narrowed before a pressure gradient develops. In smaller vessels such as the iliac and femoral arteries, a 70 to 90 percent decrease in cross-sectional area will cause a resting pressure gradient sufficient to decrease systolic blood pressure distal to the stenosis. Taking into consideration the precision of this noninvasive method and the variability in blood pressure over even short periods, a blood pressure gradient in excess of 20 mm Hg between successive cuffs is generally used as evidence of arterial stenosis in the lower extremity, whereas a 10-mm Hg gradient between sequential cuffs in

the upper extremity is indicative of stenosis (Table 41–7). Systolic blood pressure in the toes and fingers approximates 60 percent of the systolic blood pressure at the ankle and wrist, respectively, as additional pressure energy is lost in the smaller distal vessels.

Ankle/Brachial Index

Determination of the ABI furnishes a simplified application of leg segmental blood pressure measurements that can readily be used at the bedside. The ABI is the ratio of systolic blood pressure measured at the ankle to systolic blood pressure at the brachial artery. A pneumatic cuff placed around the ankle is inflated to suprasystolic pressure and subsequently deflated while the onset of flow is detected with a Doppler ultrasound probe placed over the dorsalis pedis and posterior tibial arteries, thus denoting ankle systolic blood pressure. Brachial artery systolic pressure can be assessed in routine manner by using either a stethoscope to listen for the first Korotkoff sound or a Doppler probe to listen for the onset of flow during cuff deflation. A normal ABI should be 1.0 or greater. However, in view of the variability intrinsic to sequential blood pressure measurements, an ABI less than 0.90 is considered abnormal and is 95 percent sensitive for angiographically verified peripheral arterial stenosis.[15, 92] The ABI is often used to gauge the severity of PAD. Patients with symptoms of leg claudication often have ABIs ranging from 0.5 t0 0.8, and patients with critical limb ischemia usually have an ABI less than 0.5. In patients with skin ulcerations, ankle pressure less than 55 mm Hg predicts poor ulcer healing.[93, 94]

One limitation of leg blood pressure recordings is that they cannot be used reliably in patients with calcified vessels, as might occur in persons with diabetes mellitus or renal insufficiency. The calcified vessel cannot be compressed during inflation of the pneumatic cuff, and therefore the Doppler probe indicates continuous blood flow, even when the mercury manometer records pressure in excess of 250 mm Hg.

PULSE VOLUME RECORDING

The pulse volume recording graphically illustrates the volumetric change in a segment of the limb that occurs with each pulse. Plethysmographic instruments, typically with strain gauges or pneumatic cuffs, are used to transduce volumetric changes in the limb that can be displayed on a graphic recorder. These transducers are strategically placed along the limb to record the pulse volume in its different segments, such as the thigh, calf, ankle, metatarsal region, and toes, or the upper part of the arm, forearm, and fingers. The normal pulse volume contour is influenced by both local arterial pressure and vascular wall distensibility and resembles a blood pressure waveform. It

▼ **TABLE 41-7. LEG SEGMENTAL PRESSURE MEASUREMENTS (mm Hg) IN A PATIENT WITH BILATERAL CALF CLAUDICATION**

Brachial artery		152/84
	RIGHT LEG	**LEFT LEG**
Upper thigh	160	162
Lower thigh	110	140
Calf	108	100
Ankle	64	78
A/B index	0.42	0.51

The right leg has pressure gradients between upper and lower parts of the thigh and between the calf and ankle. These gradients are indicative of stenoses in the superficial femoral artery and in the tibioperoneal arteries. The left leg has pressure gradients between the upper and lower parts of the thigh, between the lower part of the thigh and calf, and between the calf and ankle. These gradients are indicative of stenoses in the superficial femoral and popliteal arteries and in the tibioperoneal arteries.

A/B = ankle/brachial.

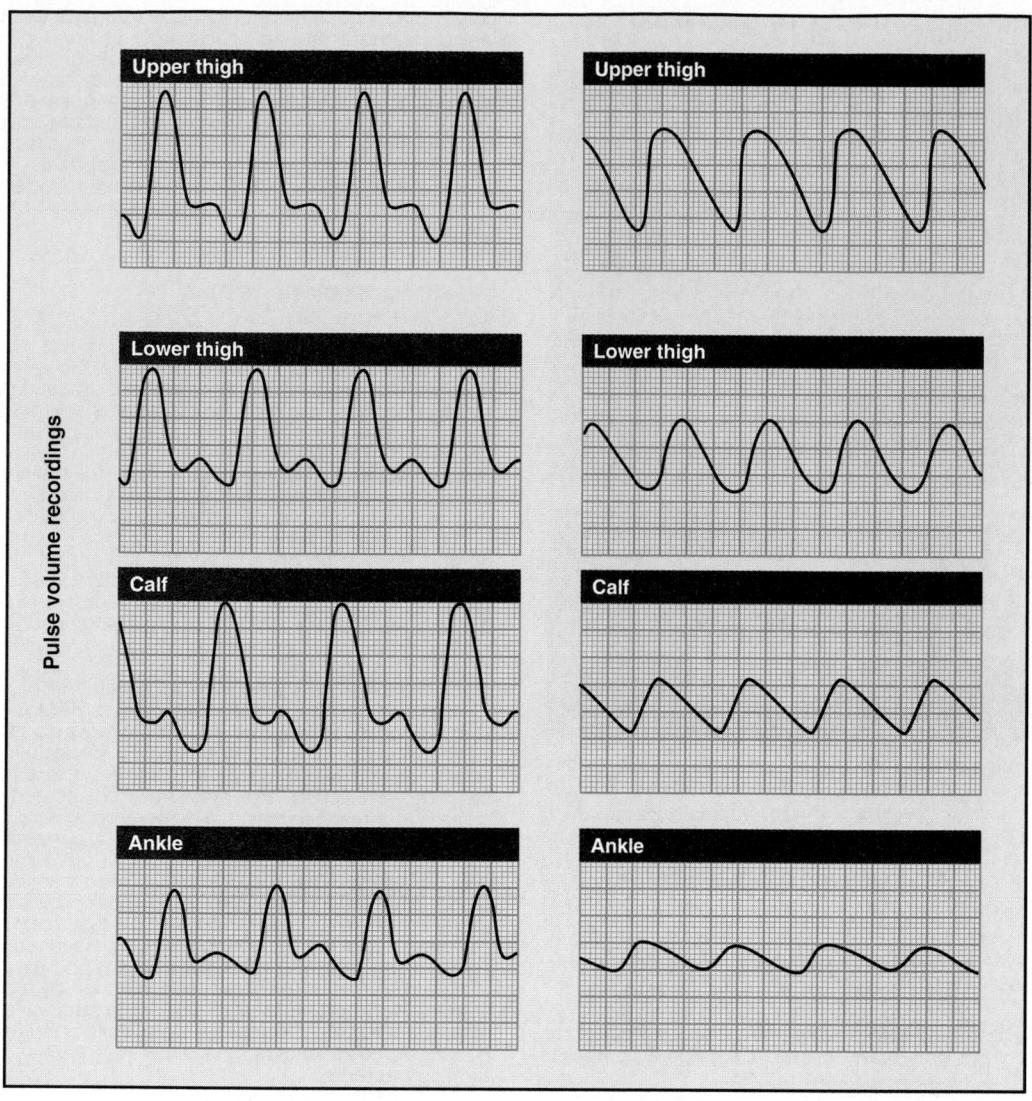

FIGURE 41–7. *Left panel,* Normal pulse volume recordings from the upper part of the thigh, lower part of the thigh, calf, and ankle showing a characteristic waveform consisting of a rapid systolic upstroke, a sharp peak, a dicrotic notch, and a concave downslope. *Right panel,* Abnormal pulse volume recordings showing a slower rate of rise, absence of a dicrotic notch, decreased amplitude, and slower descent.

comprises a sharp systolic upstroke that rises rapidly to a peak, a dicrotic notch, and a concave downslope that drops off gradually toward baseline (Fig. 41–7).[94, 95] The contour of the pulse wave changes distal to a stenosis, with loss of the dicrotic notch, a slower rate of rise, a more rounded peak, and a slower descent. The amplitude becomes lower with increasing severity of disease, and the pulse wave may not be recordable at all in a critically ischemic limb.[94] Segmental analysis of the pulse wave may indicate the location of an arterial stenosis, which is likely to be found in the artery between a normal and abnormal pulse volume recording. The pulse volume wave also provides information regarding the integrity of blood flow when blood pressure measurements cannot be accurately obtained because of noncompressible vessels.

DOPPLER ULTRASOUND

Continuous-wave and pulsed-wave Doppler systems transmit and receive high-frequency ultrasound signals. The Doppler frequency shift caused by moving red blood cells is proportional to the velocity of blood flow. Typically, the perceived frequency shift is between 1 and 20 kHz and is within the audible range of the human ear. Therefore, placement of a Doppler probe along an artery enables the examiner to hear whether blood flow is present and the vessel is patent. Processing and graphically recording the Doppler signal permit more detailed analysis of the frequency components.

Doppler instruments can be used with or without gray-scale imaging to evaluate an artery for the presence of stenoses. The Doppler probe is positioned at approximately a 60-degree angle over the common femoral, superficial femoral, popliteal, dorsalis pedis, and posterior tibial arteries. A normal Doppler waveform has three components: a rapid forward flow component during systole, transient flow reversal during early diastole, and a slow antegrade component dur-

ing late diastole. The Doppler waveform becomes altered if the probe is placed distal to an arterial stenosis and is characterized by deceleration of systolic flow, loss of the early diastolic reversal, and diminished peak frequencies. Arteries in a limb with critical ischemia may not show any Doppler frequency shift. As with pulse volume recordings, change from a normal to an abnormal Doppler waveform as the artery is interrogated more distally provides inferential evidence of the location of a stenosis.[95, 96]

DUPLEX ULTRASOUND IMAGING

Duplex ultrasound imaging provides a direct, noninvasive means of assessing both the anatomical characteristics of peripheral arteries and the functional significance of arterial stenoses. The methodology incorporates gray-scale B-mode ultrasound imaging, pulsed Doppler velocity measurements, and color coding of the Doppler shift information (Fig. 41–8). Real-time ultrasound scanners emit and receive high-frequency sound waves, typically ranging from 2 to 10 mHz, to construct an image. The acoustic properties of the vascular wall differ from those of the surrounding tissue, which enables them to be imaged easily. Atherosclerotic plaque may be present and visible on gray-scale images (Fig. 41–9). Pulsed-wave Doppler systems emit ultrasound beams at precise times and can therefore sample the reflected ultrasound waves at specific depths, which enables the examiner to sample the blood cell velocity within the lumen of the artery. By positioning the pulsed Doppler beam at a known angle, blood flow velocity is calculated according to the equation $Df = 2VF\cos\theta/C$, where Df is the frequency shift, V is the velocity, F is the frequency of the transmitted sound, θ is the angle between the transmitted sound and the velocity vector, and C is the velocity of sound in tissue. For optimal measurements, the angle of the pulsed Doppler beam should be less than 60 degrees. With color Doppler, the frequency shift infor-

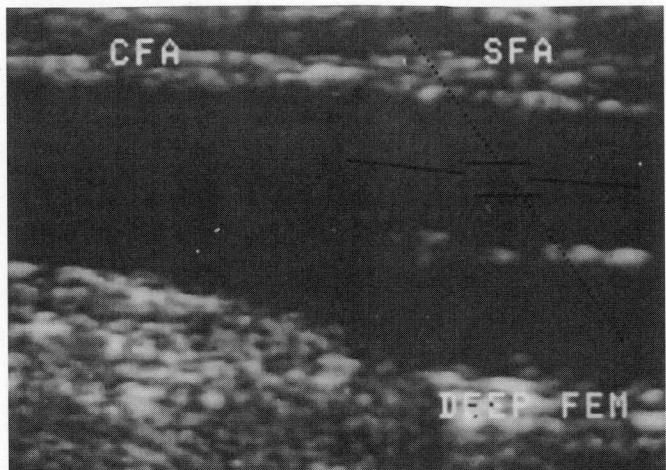

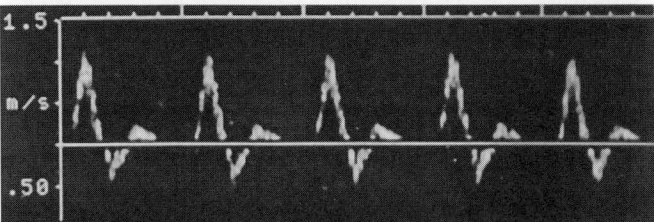

FIGURE 41–8. Duplex ultrasound of the common femoral artery bifurcation into the superficial and deep femoral arteries. The *upper* image shows a normal gray-scale image of the artery in which the intima is not thickened and the lumen is widely patent. The *lower* image is a recording of the pulsed Doppler velocity sampled from the superficial femoral artery. The triphasic profile is apparent, the envelope is thin, and the peak systolic velocity is within normal limits.

color. Pulsed Doppler velocity measurements can be made along the length of the artery and particularly at areas of flow abnormalities suggested by the color images. A twofold or greater increase in peak systolic velocity at the site of an atherosclerotic plaque indicates a 50 percent or greater diameter stenosis (Fig. 41–9).[97, 98] A threefold increase in velocity is suggestive of a 75 percent or greater stenosis. No Doppler signal is obtained if the artery is occluded. With contrast angiography used as a reference standard, the specificity and sensitivity of duplex ultrasound imaging for identifying sites of arterial stenoses are approximately 95 and 80 to 85 percent, respectively.[97–101]

TREADMILL EXERCISE TESTING

Treadmill exercise testing is used to evaluate the clinical significance of peripheral arterial stenoses and to provide objective evidence of the patient's walking capacity. The initial claudication distance is defined as the point at which symptoms of claudication first develop, and the absolute claudication distance is the point at which the patient is no longer able to continue walking because of severe leg discomfort. This standardized and more objective measurement of walking capacity supplements the patient's history and thus provides quantitative assessment of the patient's disability, as well as a metric that can be monitored after therapeutic interventions.

Treadmill exercise protocols use a motorized treadmill that incorporates fixed or progressive speeds and angles of incline.[102–104] A fixed workload test usually maintains a constant grade of 12 percent and speed of 1.5 to 2.0 mph. A progressive, or graded, treadmill protocol typically maintains a constant speed of 2 mph while gradually increasing the grade by 2 percent every 2 to 3 minutes.[102, 103] Reproducibility of repeated treadmill tests is reportedly better with progressive-grade than with constant-grade protocols.[103, 105]

Treadmill testing provides a means to determine whether arterial stenoses contribute to the patient's symptoms of exertional leg pain. During exercise, blood flow through a stenosis increases as vascular resistance falls in the exercising muscle. According to Poiseuille's law, described previously, the pressure gradient across the stenosis increases in a manner that is directly proportional to flow. Thus, ankle and brachial systolic blood pressures are measured under resting conditions before treadmill exercise, within 1 minute after exercise, and repeatedly until baseline values are reestablished. Normally, the blood pressure increase that occurs during exercise should be the same in both the upper and lower extremities, with maintenance of constant ABI of 1.0 or greater. In the presence of peripheral arterial stenosis, the ABI decreases because the increase in blood pressure that is observed in the arm is not matched by a comparable increase in ankle blood pressure. A 25 percent or greater decrease in ABI after exercise in a patient whose walking capacity is limited by claudication is considered diagnostic and implicates PAD as a cause of the patient's symptoms.

Many patients with PAD also have coronary atherosclerosis. The addition of cardiac monitoring to the exercise protocol may provide adjunctive information regarding the presence of myocardial ischemia. A workload sufficient to increase myocardial oxygen demand and provoke myocardial ischemia may not be achieved in patients whose exercise capacity is limited by claudication. Nonetheless, electrocardiographic change, particularly during low levels of treadmill exercise, may provide evidence of severe coronary artery disease.

mation within the entire field sampled by the ultrasound beam can be superimposed on the gray-scale image to provide a composite real-time display of flow velocity within the vessel.

Color-assisted duplex ultrasound imaging is an effective means of localizing peripheral arterial stenoses. Normal arteries have laminar flow with the highest velocity at the center of the artery. The representative color image is usually homogeneous, with relatively constant hue and intensity. In the presence of an arterial stenosis, blood flow velocity increases through the narrowed lumen. As the velocity increases, progressive desaturation of the color display can be noted, and flow disturbance distal to the stenosis causes changes in hue and

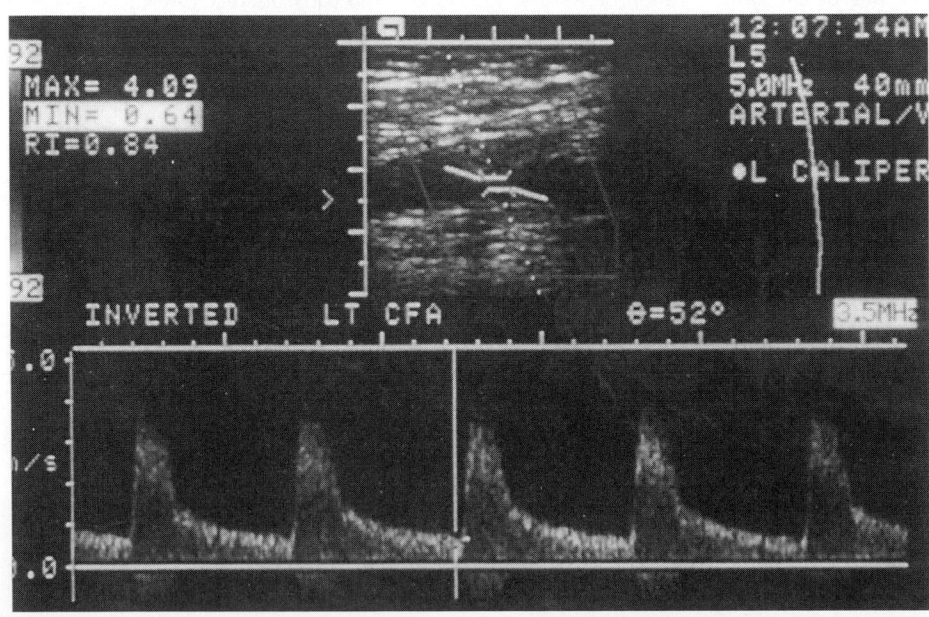

FIGURE 41–9. Duplex ultrasound of the common femoral artery. The *upper* image shows a gray-scale image of the artery in which plaque is present and encroaching on the lumen. The *lower* image is a recording of the pulsed Doppler velocity sampled from the common femoral artery. The peak velocity of 350 cm/sec is elevated. These features are consistent with significant stenosis.

Magnetic Resonance Angiography

(see also Chaps. 10 and 42)

Magnetic resonance angiography (MRA) is a noninvasive means to visualize the aorta and the peripheral arteries. A detailed description of the instrumentation and technique is beyond the scope of this chapter. Resolution of the vascular anatomy with gadolinium-enhanced MRA approaches that of conventional contrast digital subtraction angiography (Fig. 41–10). Comparative studies have reported sensitivities of 93 to 100 percent and specificities of 96 to 100 percent for the aorta, iliac, femoral-popliteal, and tibial-peroneal arteries.[106–109] Its current utility may be greatest for the evaluation of symptomatic patients to assist decision-making prior to performance of an endovascular intervention or in patients at risk for renal, allergic, or other complications during conventional angiography. As the technology improves, MRA may play a greater role in the preoperative evaluation of patients with PAD.

Contrast Angiography

Conventional angiography with a radioiodinated or other contrast agent is indicated for evaluation of arterial anatomy prior to a revascularization procedure. It is used occasionally when the diagnosis is in doubt. Most contemporary angiography laboratories use digital subtraction techniques after the intraarterial administration of contrast to enhance resolution. A retrograde transfemoral catheterization technique is generally used to evaluate the aorta and the pe-

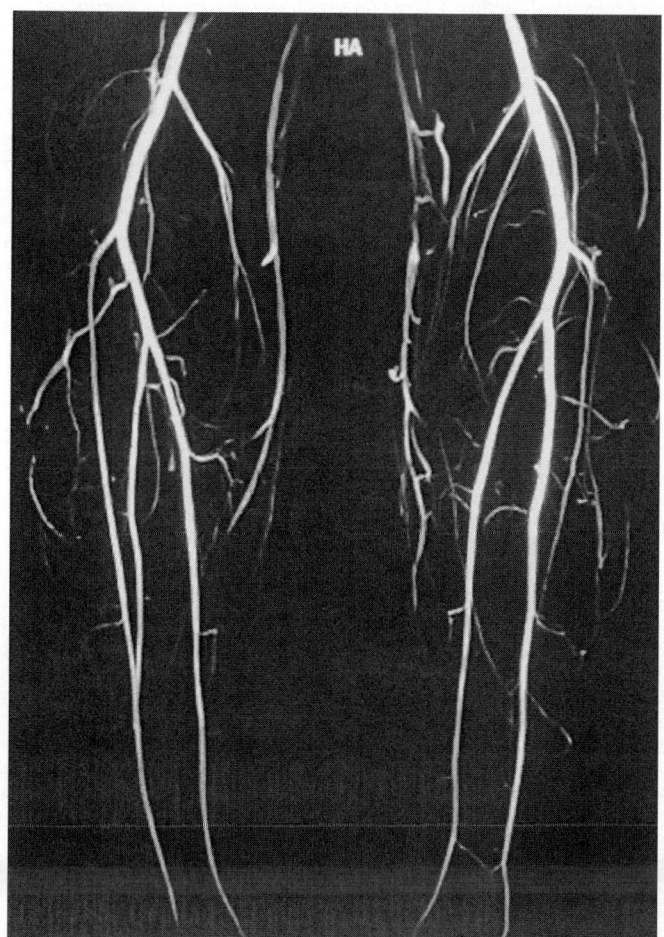

FIGURE 41–10. Gadolinium-enhanced two-dimensional magnetic resonance angiogram of both legs from the knee to above the ankle. Resolution of the popliteal and crural arteries is excellent.

ripheral arteries. Injection of the radiocontrast material into the aorta permits visualization of the aorta and iliac arteries, and injection of contrast into the iliofemoral segment of the involved leg permits optimal visualization of the femoral, popliteal, tibial, and peroneal arteries (Fig. 41–11). In patients with aortic occlusion, catheterization of the femoral arteries is not feasible. The aorta can be approached by brachial or axillary artery cannulation or, if necessary, directly by a translumbar approach.

PROGNOSIS

The prognosis of patients with PAD is affected by an increased risk for adverse cardiovascular events, as well as the risk of limb loss (Fig. 41–12).[110] Patients with PAD frequently have concomitant coronary artery disease and cerebrovascular disease.[32, 111] The relative prevalence of each depends, in part, on the diagnostic criteria used to establish the diagnosis of each of these entities. In the Clopidogrel vs. Aspirin in Patients at Risk of Ischemic Events (CAPRIE) Trial, 21 percent of the patients with PAD had a history of myocardial infarction and 26 percent had angina. In the Cardiovascular Health Study, patients with abnormal ABIs were twice as likely to have a history of myocardial infarction, angina, congestive heart failure, or cerebrovascular ischemia as those with normal ABIs.[4] Approximately 15 to 25 percent of patients with PAD have significant carotid artery stenoses by duplex ultrasound.[112, 113] Epidemiological studies have found that the risk of death from cardiovascular causes is increased 2.5- to 6-fold in patients with PAD and the annual mortality rate is 4.3 to 4.9 percent.[4, 8, 12, 13, 32, 114–120] The risk of death is greatest in those with the most severe PAD, and mortality correlates with decreasing ABI (Fig. 41–13).[121, 122] Approximately 25 percent of patients with critical limb ischemia die within 1 year, and the 1 year mortality rate in patients who have undergone amputation may be as high as 45 percent.[114, 123]

Angiographic progression of PAD occurs in over 60 percent of patients studied 5 years after the initial diagnosis.[124] Worsening symptoms develop in approximately 25 percent of patients with claudication.[110, 125] Clinical progression to critical limb ischemia occurs in 7.5 to 8.0 percent of patients with claudication in the first year after diagnosis and approximately 2.2 percent each year thereafter.[12, 125] Both smoking and diabetes mellitus independently predict progression of disease.[33, 120, 126, 127] Of patients with PAD, those with diabetes mellitus have a 21 percent risk of major amputation as compared with 3 percent in non-diabetic persons.[127]

TREATMENT

The goals of therapy for PAD include a reduction in cardiovascular morbidity and mortality and improvement in quality of life by decreasing symptoms of claudication, eliminating rest pain, and preserving limb viability. Therapeutic considerations therefore include risk factor modification and antiplatelet therapy to reduce the risk of adverse cardiovascular events, such as myocardial infarction, stroke, and death. Symptoms of claudication can improve with pharmacotherapy or exercise rehabilitation, whereas optimal management of critical limb ischemia often includes endovascular interventions or surgical reconstruction to improve blood supply and maintain limb viability.

Risk Factor Modification (see also Chaps. 32 and 33)
Lipid-lowering therapy reduces the risk of adverse cardiovascular events in patients with coronary artery disease.

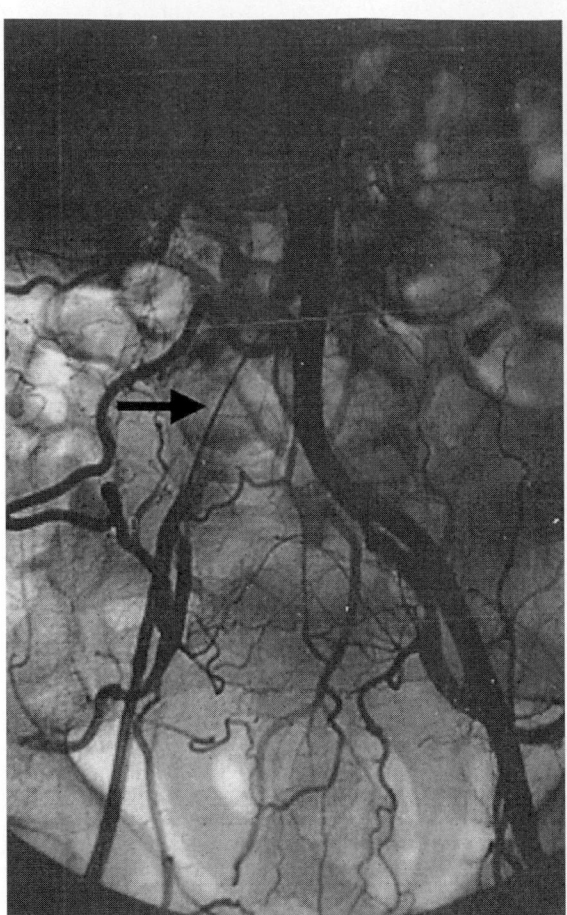
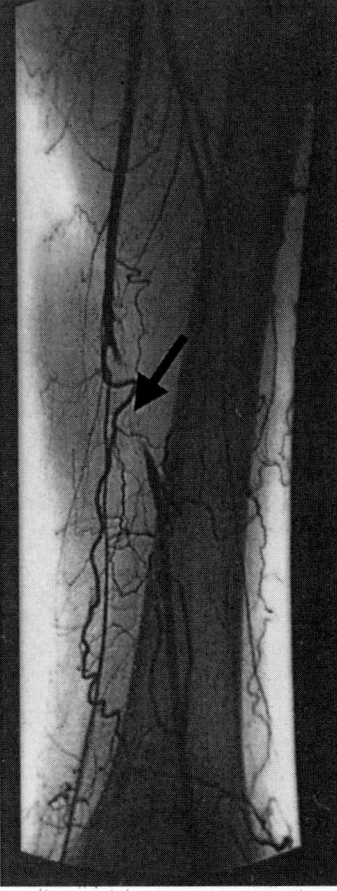

FIGURE 41–11. Angiogram of a patient with an ischemic right foot. *Left,* Complete occlusion of the right common iliac artery (arrow). *Right,* A 99 percent stenosis in the midportion of the superficial femoral artery with reconstitution via collaterals.

Secondary prevention trials, which include the Scandinavian Simvastatin Survival Study (4S), Cholesterol and Recurrent Events (CARE), and the Long-Term Intervention with Pravastatin in Ischemic Disease (LIPID), documented a reduced risk of nonfatal myocardial infarction or death from coronary artery disease by 24 to 34 percent (see also Chap. 33).[128–130] No studies to date, however, have prospectively evaluated the effect of lipid-lowering therapy with 3-hydroxy-3-methylglutaryl coenzyme A (HMG CoA) reduc-

tase inhibitors on these cardiovascular outcomes in patients with PAD. Pending such studies, recommendations for lipid-lowering therapy for patients with PAD are the same as recommendations for those with coronary artery disease. The National Cholesterol Education Program has advised that patients with atherosclerosis and hypercholesterolemia be treated with diet and drug therapy to achieve a target LDL cholesterol of 100 mg/dl or less.[131] Several clinical trials have found that lipid-lowering therapy with diet, niacin,

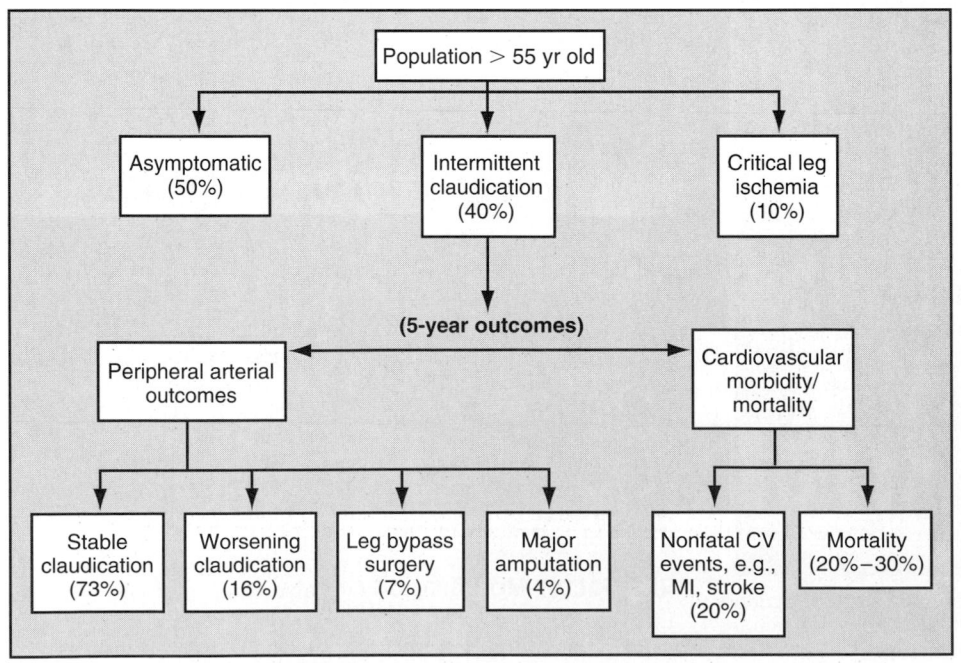

FIGURE 41–12. A schema of the natural history of patients with peripheral arterial disease emphasizing both the potential outcome of the affected limb and the cardiovascular prognosis. (From Weitz JI, Byrne J, Clagett GP, et al: Diagnosis and treatment of chronic arterial insufficiency of the lower extremities: A critical review. Circulation 94:3026–3049, 1996. By permission of the American Heart Association, Inc.)

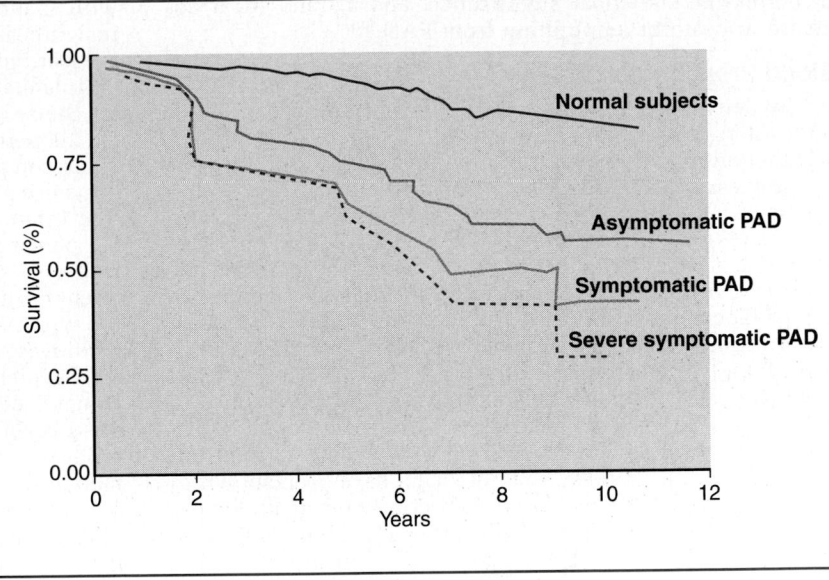

FIGURE 41–13. Survival rates of patients with peripheral arterial disease (PAD) derived from a population-based study. PAD was diagnosed by measuring the ankle/brachial index. Just the presence of PAD, even in the absence of symptoms, was associated with decreased survival. Survival was poorest in patients with symptoms. (Reprinted, by permission, from Criqui M, Langer RD, Fronek A, et al: Mortality over a period of 10 years in patients with peripheral arterial disease. N Engl J Med 326:381–386, 1992.)

binding resins, or clofibrate reduces the progression of femoral artery atherosclerosis.[132, 133] In one study, the addition of probucol to cholestyramine did not affect femoral atherosclerosis.[134] Lipid-lowering therapy may also reduce the incidence or severity of claudication. The Program on the Surgical Control of the Hyperlipidemias (POSCH) found that partial ileal bypass surgery, a surgical procedure that lowers cholesterol levels, reduced the incidence of intermittent claudication or critical limb ischemia by 34 percent and reduced the risk of development of an abnormal ABI by 44 percent.[135] A post hoc analysis of the 4S found that simvastatin reduced the risk of new or worsening claudication by 38 percent in comparison to placebo (Fig. 41–14).[136]

Smoking Cessation

Prospective trials examining the benefits of smoking cessation are lacking. However observational evidence unequivocally supports the notion that cigarette smoking increases the risk of atherosclerosis and its clinical sequelae. In patients with PAD, survival rates are better in nonsmokers than in those who have smoked or continue to smoke, and those who discontinue smoking have approximately twice the 5-year survival rate of those who continue to smoke.[137, 138] In one study of patients with PAD, the 10-year rate of myocardial infarction was 53 percent in smokers and 11 percent in nonsmokers.[33] Smoking cessation also lowers the risk for critical limb ischemia.[33]

Treatment of Diabetes (see also Chap. 63)

Aggressive treatment of diabetes decreases the risk for microangiopathic events such as nephropathy and retinopathy; however, only limited data support the benefit of aggressive treatment of diabetes on the clinical manifestations of atherosclerosis. In the Diabetes Control and Complications Trial (DCCT), which involved patients with type I diabetes mellitus, post hoc analysis found that intensive insulin therapy versus usual care caused a nonsignificant 42 percent reduction in cardiovascular events, including a 22 percent reduction in events related to PAD.[139] The United Kingdom Prospective Diabetes Study (UKPDS) of patients with type II diabetes mellitus found that intensive treatment with sulfonylureas or insulin was associated with

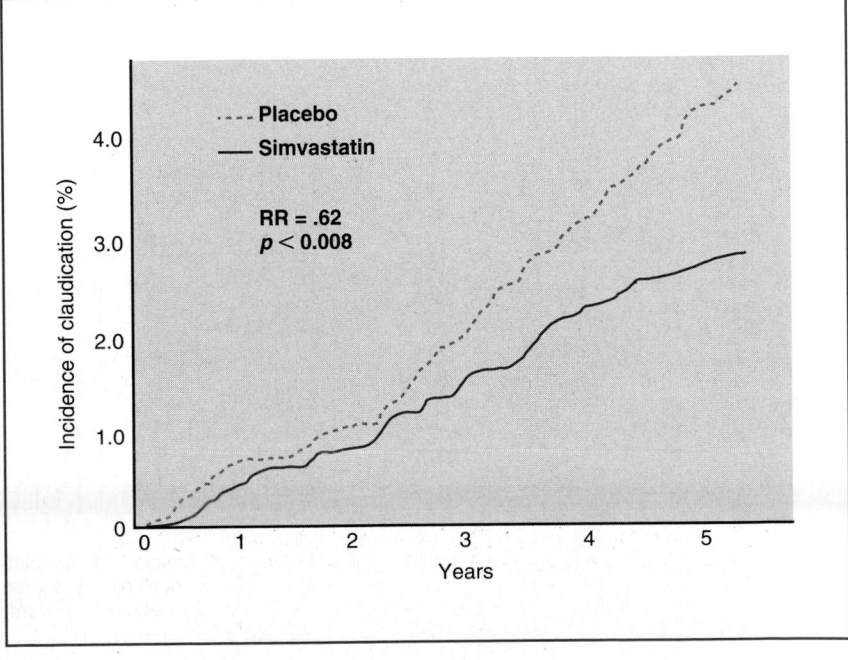

FIGURE 41–14. In the Scandinavian Simvastatin Survival Study, lipid-lowering therapy with simvastatin reduced the incidence of new or worsening claudication. (Adapted from Pedersen TR, Kjekshus J, Pyorala K, et al: Effect of simvastatin on ischemic signs and symptoms in the Scandinavian Simvastatin Survival Study (4S). Am J Cardiol 81:333–335, 1998.)

a 16 percent reduction in myocardial infarction, a finding of borderline statistical significance, and a trend for a decrease in death or amputation from PAD.[140]

Blood Pressure Control

Antihypertensive therapy reduces the risk of stroke, coronary artery disease, and vascular death.[141] It is not known whether antihypertensive therapy prevents the development or progression of PAD. It is conceivable, however, that treatment of hypertension may decrease perfusion pressure to extremities that are already compromised by peripheral arterial stenoses. In addition, concern has been raised regarding the potential adverse affects of beta-adrenergic receptor blockers on peripheral blood flow and symptoms of claudication or critical limb ischemia. Beta blockers have been found to worsen claudication in some trials, but not in others.[142–146] A meta-analysis that included 11 studies of beta blocker therapy in patients with intermittent claudication found no significant impairment in walking capacity in comparison to placebo.[147] Beta blockers have been shown to reduce the risk of myocardial infarction and death in patients with coronary artery disease, a problem affecting many patients with PAD.[148, 149] Thus, if clinically indicated for other conditions, these drugs should not be withheld in patients with PAD. The balance of evidence would support treatment of hypertension in patients with PAD according to established clinical guidelines (see Chap. 29).[150]

Angiotensin-converting enzyme (ACE) inhibitors have been shown to reduce coronary events in patients with left ventricular dysfunction.[151, 152] In the Heart Outcomes Prevention Evaluation (HOPE) Study, the ACE inhibitor ramipril decreased the risk of vascular death, myocardial infarction, or stroke by 22 percent. Forty-four percent of the patients enrolled in the HOPE Trial had evidence of PAD as manifested by an ABI of less than 0.9. Ramipril reduced cardiovascular events in patients with PAD to a comparable degree as in those without PAD.[153]

Antiplatelet Therapy

Substantial evidence supports the use of antiplatelet agents to reduce adverse cardiovascular outcome in patients with atherosclerosis. A meta-analysis that included approximately 70,000 high-risk patients with atherosclerosis, including those with acute and prior myocardial infarction, stroke, and transient cerebrovascular ischemia, as well as other high-risk groups such as those with PAD, found that antiplatelet therapy was associated with a 27 percent odds reduction for subsequent vascular death, myocardial infarc-

tion, or stroke (see also Chap. 62).[154] Of the 3295 patients with claudication included in this analysis, a statistically insignificant 18 percent reduction was noted in the risk of myocardial infarction, stroke, or death after 27 months of antiplatelet therapy.[155] The Swedish Ticlopidine Multicenter Study (STIMS) found that ticlopidine reduced mortality by 29 percent in patients with claudication. The CAPRIE Trial compared the efficacy of clopidogrel and aspirin in preventing ischemic events in patients with recent myocardial infarction, recent ischemic stroke, or PAD. Overall, an 8.7 percent relative risk reduction for myocardial infarction, ischemic stroke, or vascular death was seen in the group treated with clopidogrel.[32] Notably, of the 6452 patients in the PAD subgroup, clopidogrel treatment reduced adverse cardiovascular events by 23.8 percent.

Antiplatelet therapy also prevents occlusion in the peripheral circulation after revascularization procedures (Fig. 41–15). Of approximately 3000 patients with peripheral arterial procedures analyzed by the Antiplatelet Trialists Collaboration, the odds reduction for arterial or graft occlusion by antiplatelet therapy, primarily aspirin or aspirin plus dipyridamole, was 43 percent.[155] Ticlopidine also improves the long-term patency of peripheral saphenous vein bypass grafts.[156] Several studies have suggested that ticlopidine improves claudication or reduces the need for reconstructive vascular surgery, but these observations require confirmation in additional clinical trials.[157, 158]

Pharmacotherapy

The development of effective pharmacotherapy for treating symptoms of PAD has lagged substantially behind that for treating coronary artery disease. A report of 75 trials that included 33 drugs for the treatment of intermittent claudication found that approximately 75 percent of the trials were flawed by lack of a placebo control or blinded randomization, inappropriate endpoints, or small sample size.[159] Published consensus guidelines for conducting clinical trials of pharmacological agents for the treatment of patients with PAD should provide common ground for the objective evaluation of new drugs.[160, 161] Most studies of vasodilator therapy have failed to demonstrate any efficacy in patients with intermittent claudication.[162] Several pathophysiological explanations may account for the failure of vasodilator therapy in PAD. During exercise, resistance vessels distal to a stenosis dilate in response to ischemia. Vasodilators would have minimal, if any, effect on these endogenously dilated vessels but would decrease resistance in other vessels and thereby create a relative steal phenome-

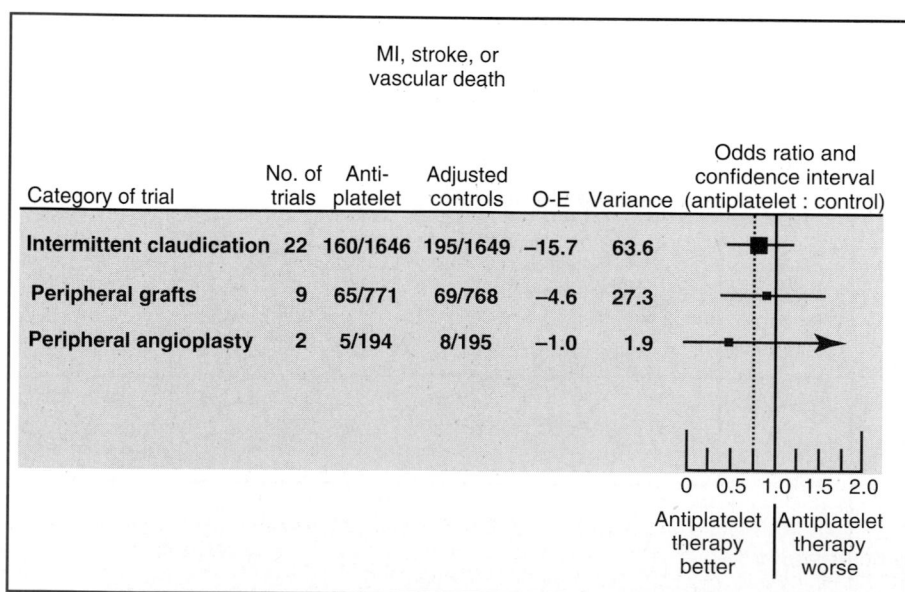

Category of trial	No. of trials	Anti-platelet	Adjusted controls	O-E	Variance	MI, stroke, or vascular death — Odds ratio and confidence interval (antiplatelet : control)
Intermittent claudication	22	160/1646	195/1649	−15.7	63.6	
Peripheral grafts	9	65/771	69/768	−4.6	27.3	
Peripheral angioplasty	2	5/194	8/195	−1.0	1.9	

0 0.5 1.0 1.5 2.0

Antiplatelet therapy better | Antiplatelet therapy worse

FIGURE 41–15. Effect of antiplatelet therapy on arterial occlusion in patients with peripheral arterial disease based on the Antiplatelet Trialists' Collaboration. The odds ratios are shown for patients with claudication, infrainguinal bypass grafts, and percutaneous transluminal angioplasty. (From Antiplatelet Trialists' Collaboration. Collaborative overview of randomised trials of antiplatelet therapy—I: Prevention of death, myocardial infarction, and stroke by prolonged antiplatelet therapy in various categories of patients. BMJ 308: 81–106, 1994.)

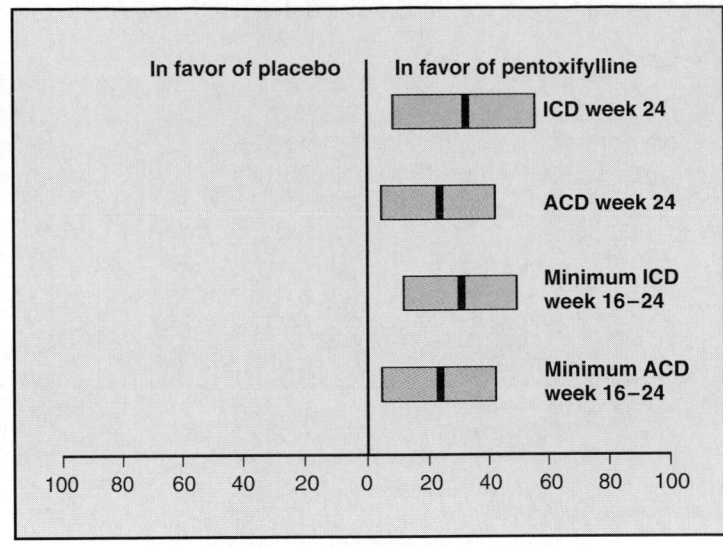

FIGURE 41–16. Effect of pentoxifylline on claudication distance based on a pooled analysis of two studies. ICD = initial claudication distance; ACD = absolute claudication distance. Number of patients = 278. (Data from Porter JM, Cutler BS, Lee BY, et al: Pentoxifylline efficacy in the treatment of intermittent claudication: Multicenter controlled double-blind trial with objective assessment of chronic occlusive arterial disease patients. Am Heart J 104:66–72, 1982; Lindgärde F, Labs KH, Rössner M: The pentoxifylline experience: Exercise testing reconsidered. Vasc Med 1:145–154, 1996; Lindgärde F, Jelnes R, Björkman H, et al: Conservative drug treatment in patients with moderately severe chronic occlusive peripheral arterial disease. Scandinavian Study Group. Circulation 80:1549–1556, 1989.)

non that reduces blood flow and perfusion pressure to the affected leg. Moreover, in contrast to their effects on myocardial oxygen consumption in patients with coronary artery disease (because of afterload reduction), vasodilators do not reduce skeletal muscle oxygen demand.

In the United States, the Food and Drug Administration (FDA) has approved two drugs, pentoxifylline (Trental) and cilostazol (Pletal), for treating claudication in patients with PAD. Additional drugs have been approved by licensing bodies in Europe, Asia, and South America.

PENTOXIFYLLINE. Pentoxifylline is a xanthine derivative that is used to treat patients with intermittent claudication. Its action is thought to be mediated via its hemorrheological properties, including its ability to decrease blood viscosity and improve erythrocyte flexibility.[163] It also has antiinflammatory and antiproliferative effects.[164, 165] Two prospective multicenter trials found that pentoxifylline increased absolute claudication distance after 24 weeks of treatment by approximately 20 percent (Fig. 41–16).[166–168] Two meta-analyses of randomized placebo-controlled trials of pentoxifylline found that it increased initial claudication distance by approximately 20 to 30 meters and absolute claudication distance by approximately 45 to 50 meters.[169, 170] Another meta-analysis, however, concluded that the quality of reported data precluded a reliable estimate of pentoxifylline's efficacy.[171]

CILOSTAZOL. This quinolinone derivative inhibits phosphodiesterase III, thereby decreasing cyclic adenosine monophosphate degradation and increasing its concentration in platelets and blood vessels. Although cilostazol inhibits platelet aggregation and causes vasodilation in experimental animals, its mechanism of action in patients with PAD is not known.[172, 173] Several trials have reported that cilostazol improves absolute claudication distance by 40 to 50 percent in comparison to placebo (Fig. 41–17).[174, 175] Quality-of-life measures, as assessed by the Medical Outcomes Scale (SF-36) and the Walking Impairment Questionnaire, also improved. In addition, one study found that absolute walking distance improves more with cilostazol than with either pentoxyfilline or placebo, with the latter two having equivalent efficacy.[176] An advisory from the FDA has stated that cilostazol should not be used in patients with congestive heart failure since other phosphodiesterase III inhibitors have been shown to decrease survival in these patients.[177, 178] The effect of cilostazol on cardiac morbidity and mortality is not known.

OTHER DRUGS. Many other drugs are under investigation for the treatment of either claudication or critical limb ischemia, including serotonin (5-hydroxytryptamine) antagonists, calcium channel blockers, L-arginine, carnitine derivatives, vasodilator prostaglandins, and angiogenic growth factors. One serotonin antagonist, ketanserin, did not improve claudication distance in a multicenter trial,[179] whereas another, naftidrofuryl, has been reported to improve symptoms of claudication in some trials and is currently available for use in Europe.[180, 181] L-Arginine, the precursor for endothelium-derived nitric oxide, was found to improve claudication distance after 3 weeks of intravenous therapy.[65] Propionyl L-carnitine, a cofactor for fatty acid metabolism, has also been reported to improve claudication, particularly in patients whose baseline maximum walking distance is less than 250 meters.[182, 183]

Therapy with vasodilator prostaglandins has been investigated in patients with intermittent claudication and in those with critical limb ischemia. Intravenous administration of prostaglandin E_1 (PGE₁) or its precursor improved claudication distance in preliminary trials.[65, 184] Phase III studies with oral prostacyclin derivatives in patients with intermittent claudication are in progress or have been completed recently, and the results are pending. In a large trial of 1560 patients with critical limb ischemia, PGE₁ administered intravenously for up to 28 days reduced the composite endpoint of death, major amputation, persistence of critical limb ischemia, acute myocardial infarction, and stroke at the time of hospital discharge from 73 to 64 percent, but its effect on this outcome was not significantly different from that of placebo at the 6-month time point.[185] Most of the benefit of PGE₁ in this trial was related to recovery from leg ischemia.

The therapeutic use of angiogenic growth factors has engendered considerable enthusiasm. Administration of basic fibroblast growth factor (bFGF) and vascular endothelial growth factor (VEGF) as protein or gene therapy increases collateral blood vessel development, capil-

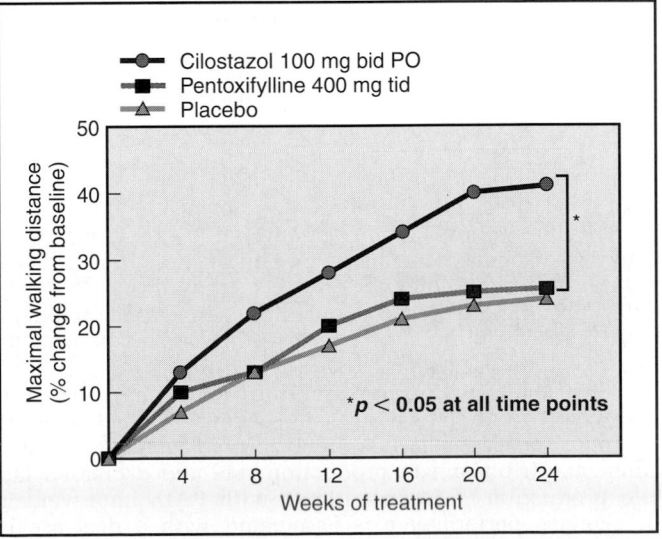

FIGURE 41–17. Effect of cilostazol versus pentoxifylline and placebo on maximal walking distance. (From Dawson DL, Cutler BS, Hiatt WR, et al: A comparison of cilostazol and pentoxifylline for treating intermittent claudication. Am J Med, in press.)

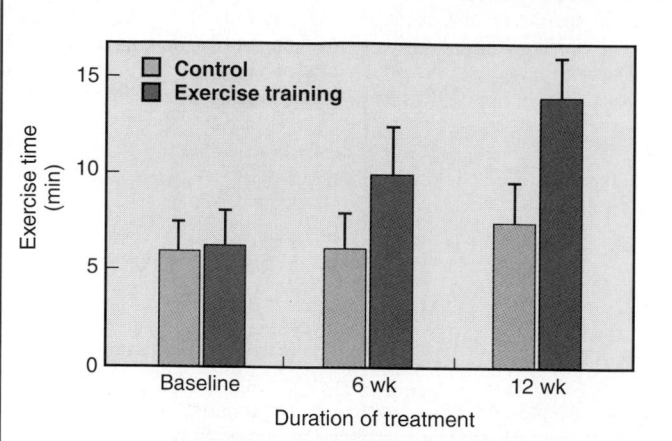

FIGURE 41–18. Effect of supervised exercise training on peak treadmill exercise time in patients with intermittent claudication. (Adapted from Hiatt WR, Regensteiner JG, Hargarten ME, et al: Benefit of exercise conditioning for patients with peripheral arterial disease. Circulation 81:602–609, 1990.)

lary number, and blood flow in experimental models of hindlimb ischemia.[186-191] Gene transfer of human plasmid phVEGF165 by an intra-arterial catheter–based technique or by intramuscular injection into the ischemic extremity improved collateral blood vessel development in small case series.[192, 193] Placebo-controlled clinical trials of angiogenic growth factors in patients with either claudication or critical limb ischemia are in progress.

Exercise

Supervised exercise rehabilitation programs improve symptoms of claudication in patients with PAD (Fig. 41–18).[194] A meta-analysis of 21 controlled studies of exercise rehabilitation found that a supervised exercise program increased the average distance walked to the onset of claudication by 179 percent and the maximal distance walked by 122 percent.[195] The greatest benefit occurred when sessions were at least 30 minutes in duration at least three times per week for 6 months and when walking was used as the mode of exercise. In a randomized study, exercise training resulted in greater improvement in maximal walking distance than did percutaneous transluminal angioplasty (PTA).[196]

The mechanisms through which exercise training improves claudication are not known. Studies in experimental models of hindlimb ischemia have suggested that regular exercise increases the development of collateral blood vessels.[197-199] Expression of angiogenic factors is increased by exercise, particularly in hypoxic tissue.[200-202] Exercise training has been shown to improve endothelium-dependent vasodilation of coronary arteries in patients with coronary atherosclerosis and in the peripheral circulation of patients with congestive heart failure.[203-205] However, improvement in calf blood flow commensurate with improvement in walking distance has not been demonstrated in patients with claudication following exercise training.[194, 206, 207] To date, imaging studies demonstrating increased collateral blood vessels following exercise training in patients with PAD have not been reported.

The benefits of exercise training in patients with PAD may result from changes in skeletal muscle function, such as increased muscle mitochondrial enzyme activity and adenosine triphosphate production rate and decreased lactate production.[208, 209] In patients with PAD, improvement in exercise performance is associated with a decrease in plasma and skeletal muscle short-chain acylcarnitine concentrations, which indicate improvement in oxidative metabolism, as well as increased peak oxygen consumption.[194, 210] Training may also enhance biomechanical per-

formance and enable patients to walk more efficiently with less energy expenditure.

Percutaneous Transluminal Angioplasty and Stents (see also pp. 1485–1488)

PTA and stent placement are being increasingly used in the management of patients with PAD, particularly those with disabling claudication and critical limb ischemia. Various endpoints have served to indicate the efficacy of these interventions, including the ABI, vessel patency by duplex ultrasound or conventional angiography, relief of symptoms, and limb salvage. In general, the efficacy of percutaneous interventions is better for treatment of stenoses than occlusions and when targeting vessels with good runoff (i.e., patent distal vessels) as opposed to poor runoff.[15, 211-213]

Iliac artery PTA alone is associated with 4- to 5-year patency rates of approximately 60 to 80 percent.[211, 214, 215] Iliac artery stent placement yields 4- to 5-year patency rates that range from 70 to 95 percent.[216-218] A meta-analysis of six iliac PTA studies comprising 1300 patients and eight iliac stent placement studies involving 816 patients found that the long-term patency rate was greater with stent placement than with PTA alone (Fig. 41–19).[219] Overall, stent placement reduced late failure by 39 percent. The Dutch Iliac Stent Trial Group found that primary PTA followed by selective stent placement was more cost-effective than primary stent placement.[220, 221] Clinical success at 2 years was 78 percent for primary stent placement and 77 percent for selective stent placement. Quality of life improved comparably in each group.[221, 222] In a study comparing stent placement with surgery in patients with aortoiliac disease, the long-term patency rate was less in those who received stents.[223]

The overall efficacy of PTA of the femoral-popliteal arteries is less than that of the iliac arteries.[213, 216, 224-227] Several large institutional series have found that primary patency rates 1, 3, and 5 years after femoral-popliteal PTA average 60, 50, and 45 percent, respectively.[224, 226-228] A life table based on a meta-analysis of seven femoral-popliteal PTA studies yielded a 5-year patency rate of approximately 45 percent.[229] An analysis comparing femoral-popliteal PTA with bypass surgery suggested that PTA was more cost-effective than surgery in patients with claudication who had either stenoses or occlusions and in patients with critical limb ischemia who had stenoses. Surgery, however, was more cost-effective than PTA in patients with critical limb ischemia who had arterial occlusions.[229, 230]

PTA of the tibial and peroneal arteries is technically more difficult and associated with a poorer outcome than is endovascular treatment of more proximal lesions,[213] possibly because most series included patients with critical limb ischemia who were considered high risk for bypass surgery. Long-term success appears to be greater in those with focal stenoses in whom distal perfusion is restored.[231-234]

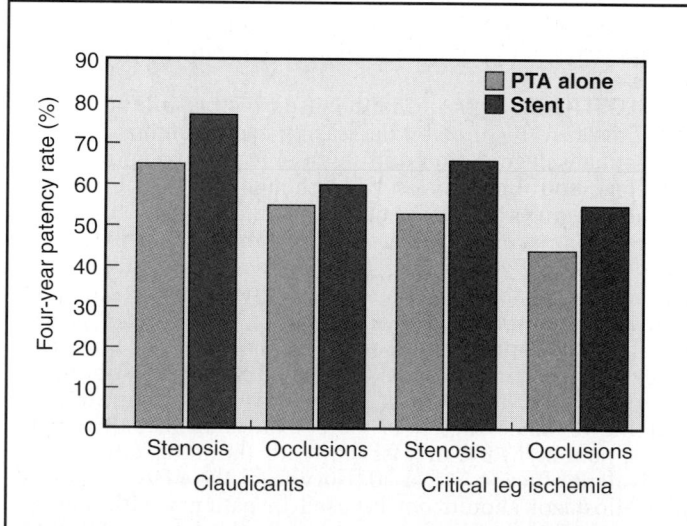

FIGURE 41–19. Four-year patency rate after percutaneous transluminal angioplasty (PTA) alone or stent placement for iliac artery lesions based on a meta-analysis of six iliac PTA studies and eight iliac stent studies. (From Bosch JL, Hunink MG: Meta-analysis of the results of percutaneous transluminal angioplasty and stent placement for aortoiliac occlusive disease. Radiology 204:87–96, 1997.)

count the anatomical location of the arterial lesions and the presence of comorbid conditions. The surgical procedure is planned after angiographic identification of the arterial obstruction to ensure sufficient arterial inflow to and outflow from the graft to maintain patency. Preoperative evaluation to assess the risk of vascular surgery should be performed since many of these patients have coexisting coronary artery disease. Guidelines for this evaluation have been established and are beyond the scope of this chapter (see Chap. 61).[241]

Aortobifemoral bypass is the most frequent operation for patients with aortoiliac disease. Typically, a knitted or woven prosthesis made of Dacron or polytetrafluoroethylene (PTFE) is anastomosed proximally to the aorta and distally to each common femoral artery (Fig. 41–20).[242] Occasionally, the iliac artery is used for the distal anastomosis to maintain antegrade flow into at least one hypogastric artery. A recent meta-analysis of aortic bifurcation grafts in 23 studies reported from 1970 to 1996 noted that 5- and 10-year limb patency rates were 91 and 87 percent for claudicants, respectively, and 88 and 82 percent for patients with critical limb ischemia, respectively.[243] Among the more recent series in this analysis, operative morbidity and mortality rates were 8.3 and 3.3 percent, respectively.[243]

Extraanatomical surgical reconstructive procedures for aortoiliac disease include axillobifemoral bypass, iliobifemoral bypass, and femorofemoral bypass. These bypass grafts, made of Dacron or PTFE, circumvent the aorta and iliac arteries and are generally used in high-risk patients with critical limb ischemia.[244, 245] Long-term patency rates are inferior to those of aortobifemoral bypass procedures. A recent Veteran's Administration Cooperative Study that included 340 femoro-femoral bypass procedures and 79 axillofemoral or axillobifemoral bypass operations performed primarily in patients with critical limb ischemia reported a 5-year primary patency rate of approximately 50 percent. In other series, 5-year patency rates for axillobifemoral bypass operations have been reported to range from 50 to 70 percent, and those for femorofemoral bypass grafts have ranged from 70 to 80 percent.[246-249] The operative mortality for extraanatomical bypass procedures is 3 to 5 percent, which reflects, in part, the serious comorbid conditions and advanced atherosclerosis of many of the patients who undergo these procedures.

Reconstructive surgery for infrainguinal arterial disease includes femoropopliteal, femorotibial, or femoroperoneal artery bypass. *In situ* or reversed autologous saphenous veins or synthetic grafts made of PTFE are used for the infrainguinal bypass. Patency rates for autologous saphenous vein bypass grafts are superior to those seen with PTFE grafts.[250-252] Also, patency rates are better for grafts in which the distal anastomosis is placed in the popliteal artery above the knee versus below the knee.[250,251,253-255] Five-year primary patency rates for femoropopliteal reconstruction in claudicants are approximately 80 and 75 percent for autogenous vein or PTFE grafts, respectively, and in patients with critical limb ischemia they are approximately 65 and 45 percent, respectively.[229, 253-256] For femoral below-knee bypass, including tibioperoneal artery reconstruction, five-year patency rates for saphenous vein grafts in patients with claudication or critical limb ischemia are comparable to those of femoropopliteal above-knee grafts and range from 60 to 80 percent,[229,244,251,253-255,257] whereas 5-year patency rates for PTFE grafts in the infrapopliteal position are considerably inferior, approximating 65 percent in claudicants and 33 percent in patients with critical limb ischemia.[229,244,250] Operative mortality for infrainguinal bypass operations based on recent series is 1 to 2 percent.[258-261]

Graft stenoses may result from technical errors at the time of surgery, such as retained valve cuffs or intimal flap or valvutome injury; from fibrous intimal hyperplasia, usually within 6 months of surgery; or from atherosclerosis, usually occurring within the vein graft at least 1 to 2 years after surgery.[255, 262] Institution of graft surveillance protocols using color-assisted duplex ultrasonography has enabled the identification of graft stenoses, thereby prompting graft revision and avoiding complete graft failure.[263-267] Several studies have reported improved graft outcome as a result of routine ultrasound surveillance.[263, 266]

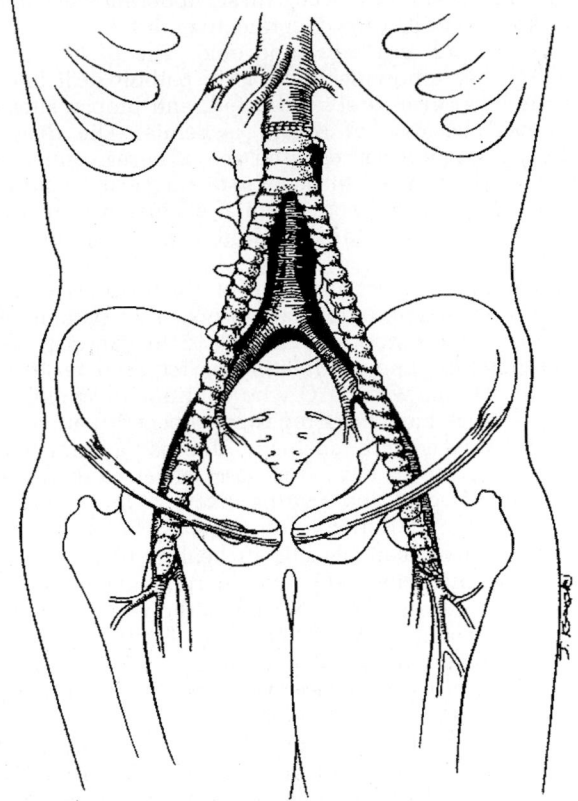

FIGURE 41–20. Schematic of an aortobifemoral bypass. The infrarenal aorta has been transected and stapled closed. The proximal end of the graft is anastomosed end to end with the aorta. The distal limbs are anastomosed to the common femoral arteries via retroperitoneal tunnels. (From Whittemore AD, Mannick JA: Principles of vascular surgery. *In* Loscalzo J, Creager MA, Dzau VJ (eds): Vascular Medicine. 2nd ed. Boston, Little, Brown, 1996, pp 675–702.)

Limb salvage rates at 1 and 2 years ranged from 50 to 75 percent.[233, 235-237]

Innominate and subclavian artery PTA and stent placement are considered for localized lesions in patients with arm claudication or vertebrobasilar insufficiency secondary to subclavian steal. Initial success is achieved in approximately 80 to 90 percent of cases, and the 1-year patency rate averages 85 percent.[238-240]

Complications occur in approximately 4 to 6 percent of endovascular interventions and usually relate to the severity of arterial disease and the complexity of the procedure.[15] Local complications include thrombosis, dissection, hematoma, and pseudoaneurysm, and occasionally these complications require surgical repair.

Peripheral Arterial Surgery

Surgical revascularization is generally indicated to improve quality of life in patients with disabling claudication who are receiving maximal medical therapy and to relieve rest pain and preserve limb viability in patients with critical limb ischemia. The specific operation must take into ac-

Vasculitis (see also Chap. 67)

THROMBOANGIITIS OBLITERANS

TAO is a segmental vasculitis that affects the distal arteries, veins, and nerves of the upper and lower extremities. It typically occurs in young persons who smoke. A patient with characteristics of TAO was described initially by von Winiwater in 1879.[268] Leo Buerger coined the term "throm-

boangiitis obliterans" and described its pathology in 11 amputated limbs.[269]

PATHOLOGY AND PATHOGENESIS. TAO primarily affects the medium and small vessels of the arms, including the radial, ulnar, palmar, and digital arteries, and their counterparts in the legs, including the tibial, peroneal, plantar, and digital arteries. The cerebral, coronary, renal, mesenteric, aortoiliac, and pulmonary arteries may also be involved.[270-273] The pathology is characterized by an occlusive, highly cellular thrombus composed of polymorphonuclear leukocytes forming microabscesses and, occasionally, multinucleated giant cells.[274-275] The inflammatory infiltrate may also affect the vascular wall, but the internal elastic membrane remains intact. In the chronic phase of the disease, the thrombus becomes organized and the vascular wall becomes fibrotic.

The precise cause of TAO is not known. Tobacco use or exposure is present in virtually every patient.[274, 276-278] Potential immunological mechanisms include increased cellular sensitivity to type I and type III collagen or the presence of anti–endothelial cell antibodies.[279,280] Decreased endothelium-dependent vasodilation to acetylcholine has been observed in both the affected and unaffected limbs of patients with TAO, which raises the possibility that reduced bioavailability of nitric oxide contributes to the disorder.[281]

CLINICAL FINDINGS. The prevalence of TAO is greater in Asia than North America or Western Europe. In the United States, TAO occurs in approximately 13 per 100,000 population.[282-284] Most patients with TAO have symptoms before 45 years of age, and 75 to 90 percent are men.[284, 285]

Patients may have claudication of the hands, forearms, feet, or calves. The majority of patients with TAO have pain at rest and digital ulcerations. Often, more than one extremity is affected. Raynaud phenomenon occurs in approximately 45 percent of patients, and superficial thrombophlebitis, which may be migratory, occurs in approximately 40 percent of patients.[285]

The radial, ulnar, dorsalis pedis, and posterior tibial pulses may be absent if the corresponding vessel is involved. The clinical characteristics of critical limb ischemia and ischemic digital ulceration were described earlier in this chapter. The Allen test is abnormal in two-thirds of patients.[285] To perform this test, both the radial and ulnar arteries are compressed while the hand is clenched and then opened.[286] This activity causes palmar blanching. Release of compression from either pulse should normally produce palmar erythema if the palmar arches are patent. If they are occluded, pallor persists on the side where compression is maintained. Discrete, tender, erythematous subcutaneous cords, indicating a superficial thrombophlebitis, may be present on the distal aspects of the extremities.

DIAGNOSIS. No specific laboratory tests, other than biopsy, can be used to diagnose TAO. Most tests, therefore, are required to exclude other diseases that might have similar clinical features, including autoimmune diseases such as scleroderma or systemic lupus erythematosus, hypercoagulable states, diabetes, or acute arterial occlusion secondary to embolism. The erythrocyte sedimentation rate and acute phase reactants, such as C-reactive protein, are usually normal. Serum immunological markers, including antinuclear antibodies, rheumatoid factor, and antiphospholipid antibodies, should not be present, and serum complement levels should be normal. If clinically indicated, a proximal source of embolism should be excluded by cardiac and vascular ultrasound or by arteriography. Arteriography of an affected limb supports the diagnosis of TAO if the patient has segmental occlusion of small- and medium-sized arteries, absence of atherosclerosis, and corkscrew collaterals circumventing the occlusion (Fig. 41–21). These same

findings, however, may occur in scleroderma, systemic lupus erythematosus, mixed connective tissue disease, and antiphospholipid antibody syndrome. The pathognomonic test is a biopsy showing the classic pathological findings. Biopsy is otherwise rarely indicated, and biopsy sites may fail to heal because of severe ischemia. The diagnosis, therefore, is usually based on an age of onset younger than 45 years, a history of tobacco use, physical examination demonstrating distal limb ischemia, exclusion of other diseases, and if necessary, angiographic demonstration of typical lesions.[287-289]

TREATMENT. The cornerstone of treatment is cessation of tobacco use. Amputation rarely ensues in patients without gangrene who stop smoking.[290, 291] In contrast, one or more amputations may ultimately be required in 40 to 45 percent of patients with TAO who continue to smoke.

Several drugs have been reported to benefit patients with TAO. The prostacyclin analogue iloprost administered 6 hours per day for 28 days was more effective than aspirin in relieving rest pain and healing ulcers.[292] In a multicenter trial, however, oral iloprost administered for 8 weeks was no more effective than placebo in healing ulcers, although it was somewhat more effective in relieving pain at low doses.[293] A naked plasmid DNA encoding vascular endothelial growth factor (phVEGF165) was intramuscularly injected into seven limbs of six patients with TAO, with subsequent healing of ulcers in three to five limbs and relief of rest pain in two others.[294]

Vascular reconstructive surgery is not usually a viable option because of the segmental nature of this disease and involvement of distal vessels. An autogenous saphenous vein bypass graft can be considered if a target vessel for the distal anastomosis is available. Long-term patency rates are better in ex-smokers than smokers.[295, 296]

TAKAYASU ARTERITIS AND GIANT CELL ARTERITIS
See Chapter 67.

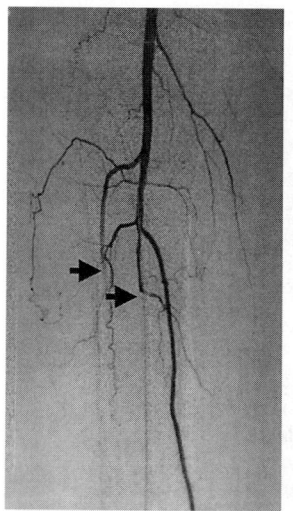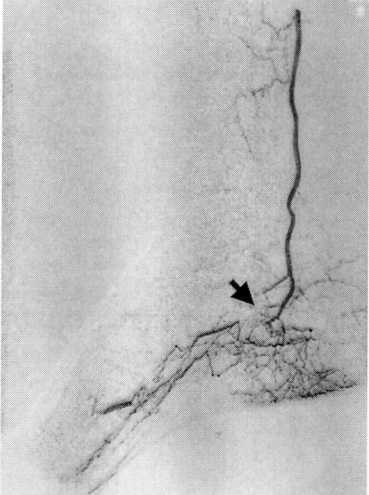

FIGURE 41–21. Angiogram of a young woman with thromboangiitis obliterans. *Left,* Occlusion of the anterior tibial arteries (arrows). *Right,* Occlusion of the distal portion of the posterior tibial artery (arrow) with bridging collaterals.

Acute Limb Ischemia

Acute limb ischemia occurs when blood flow to the arm or leg is suddenly reduced by arterial occlusion. Perfusion is inadequate to meet the metabolic needs of the tissue, and limb viability is jeopardized. The clinical features of patients with acute limb ischemia are related to the location of the arterial occlusion and the resulting decrease in blood flow. Depending on the severity of ischemia, patients may note disabling claudication or pain at rest. Pain may develop over a short period and is manifested in the affected extremity distal to the site of obstruction. It is not necessarily confined to the foot or toes or to the hand or fingers as is usually the case in chronic limb ischemia. Concurrent ischemia of peripheral nerves causes sensory loss and motor dysfunction.

Physical examination findings may include absence of pulses distal to the occlusion, cool skin, pallor, delayed capillary return and venous filling, diminished or absent sensory perception, and muscular weakness or paralysis. This constellation of symptoms and signs is often recalled as the five P's: pain, pulselessness, pallor, paresthesias, and paralysis.

Prognosis

Comorbid cardiovascular disorders are usually present in patients with acute limb ischemia and may even be responsible for the event. As such, the long-term prognosis is limited in this population. Five-year survival rates after acute limb ischemia caused by thrombosis approximate 45 percent and after embolism are less than 20 percent.[297] The 1-month survival rate in persons older than 75 years with acute limb ischemia approximates 40 percent.[298] The risk of limb loss depends on the severity of the ischemia and the time elapsed before a revascularization procedure is undertaken. Amputation rates are approximately 6 percent if revascularization is performed within 12 hours of the onset of symptoms, 12 percent if performed between 12 and 24 hours, and 20 percent if delayed for more than 24 hours after symptom onset.[299]

A classification scheme that takes into consideration the severity of ischemia and viability of the limb, along with related neurological findings and Doppler signals, has been developed by the Society for Vascular Surgery and the International Society for Cardiovascular Surgery (Table 41–8). A viable limb, category I, is not immediately threatened, has neither sensory nor motor abnormalities, and has blood flow detectable by Doppler. Threatened viability, category II, indicates that the severity of ischemia will cause limb loss unless the blood supply is restored promptly. The category is subdivided into marginally and immediately threat-

ened limbs, the latter characterized by pain, sensory deficits, and muscular weakness. Arterial blood flow cannot be detected by Doppler. Irreversible limb ischemia leading to tissue loss and requiring amputation, category III, is characterized by loss of sensation, paralysis, and the absence of Doppler-detected blood flow in both arteries and veins distal to the occlusion.

Pathogenesis

The causes of acute limb ischemia include arterial embolism, thrombosis in situ, dissection, and trauma.[300] Most arterial emboli arise from thrombotic sources in the heart. Atrial fibrillation complicating valvular heart disease, congestive heart failure, coronary artery disease, and hypertension accounts for approximately 50 percent of cardiac emboli to the limbs. Other sources include rheumatic or prosthetic cardiac valves, ventricular thrombus resulting from myocardial infarction or left ventricular aneurysm, paradoxical embolism of venous thrombi through the intraatrial or intraventricular communications, and cardiac tumors such as left atrial myxomas. Aneurysms of the aorta or peripheral arteries may harbor thrombi that subsequently embolize to more distal arterial sites, usually lodging at branch points where the artery decreases in size.

Thrombosis in situ occurs in atherosclerotic peripheral arteries, infrainguinal bypass grafts, and peripheral artery aneurysms, as well as in normal arteries of patients with hypercoagulable states. In patients with peripheral atherosclerosis, thrombosis in situ may complicate plaque rupture and cause acute arterial occlusion and limb ischemia in a manner analogous to what occurs in coronary arteries in patients with acute myocardial infarction. Thrombosis complicating popliteal artery aneurysms is a much more common complication than rupture and may account for 10 percent of cases of acute limb ischemia in elderly men.[15, 301] Acute thrombotic occlusion of a normal artery is unusual but may occur in patients with procoagulant disorders such as antiphospholipid antibody syndrome, activated protein C resistance (factor V Leiden), deficiency of protein C or S, heparin-induced thrombocytopenia, essential thrombocythemia, and hyperhomocysteinemia. One of the most common causes of acute limb ischemia is thrombotic occlusion of an infrainguinal bypass graft, as discussed previously.

Diagnostic Tests

The history and physical examination usually establish the diagnosis of acute limb ischemia. Time available for diagnostic tests is often limited, and urgent revascularization

▼ TABLE 41–8. CLINICAL CATEGORIES OF ACUTE LIMB ISCHEMIA (MODIFIED FROM THE SVS/ISCVS CLASSIFICATION)

| CATEGORY | DESCRIPTION/PROGNOSIS | FINDINGS | | DOPPLER SIGNALS | |
		Sensory Loss	Muscle Weakness	Arterial	Venous
I. Viable	Not immediately threatened	None	None	Audible	Audible
II. Threatened					
a. Marginally	Salvageable if promptly treated	Minimal (toes) or none	None	(Often) inaudible	Audible
b. Immediately	Salvageable with immediate revascularization			(Usually) inaudible	Audible
III. Irreversible	Major tissue loss or permanent nerve damage inevitable	Profound, anesthetic	Profound, paralysis (rigor)	Inaudible	Inaudible

SVS/ISCVS = Society for Vascular Surgery/International Society for Cardiovascular Surgery.
Adapted from Rutherford RB, Baker JD, Ernst C, et al: Recommended standards for reports dealing with lower extremity ischemia: Revised version. J Vasc Surg 26:517–538, 1997.

▼ TABLE 41–9. COMPARISON OF CATHETER-DIRECTED THROMBOLYSIS AND SURGICAL REVASCULARIZATION IN TREATMENT OF LIMB ISCHEMIA

STUDY	RESULTS AT	CATHETER-DIRECTED THROMBOLYSIS			SURGICAL REVASCULARIZATION		
		Patients (No.)	Limb Salvage (%)	Mortality (%)	Patients (No.)	Limb Salvage (%)	Mortality (%)
Rochester[312]	12 mo	57	82	16	57	82	42
STILE[313]	6 mo	246	88.2	6.5	141	89.4	8.5
TOPAS[314]	12 mo	144	82.7	13.3	54	81.1	15.7

From Dormandy JA, Rutherford RB: Management of peripheral arterial disease (PAD). TASC Working Group. J Vasc Surg 31(Suppl):1–296, 2000.

procedures should not be delayed if limb viability is immediately threatened. The pressure in the affected limb and corresponding ABI can be measured if flow is detectable by Doppler ultrasound. A Doppler probe can be used to detect the presence of blood flow in peripheral arteries, particularly when pulses are not palpable. Color-assisted duplex ultrasonography can be used to determine the site of occlusion. It is particularly applicable for evaluation of the patency of infrainguinal bypass grafts. Contrast arteriography demonstrates the site of occlusion and provides an anatomical guide for revascularization.

Treatment

Analgesic medications should be administered to reduce pain. For patients with acute leg ischemia, the bed should be positioned such that the feet are lower than chest level, thereby increasing limb perfusion pressure via gravitational effects. Proper bed positioning can be accomplished by putting blocks under the posts at the head of the bed. Effort

should be made to reduce pressure on the heels, on bony prominences, and between the toes by appropriate placement of soft material on the bed, such as sheepskin, and between the toes, such as lamb's wool. The room should be kept warm to prevent cold-induced cutaneous vasoconstriction.

Heparin is administered intravenously as soon as the diagnosis of acute limb ischemia is made.[15] The dose should be sufficient to increase the partial thromboplastin time by 1.5 to 2.5 times control values to prevent thrombus propagation or recurrent embolism. It is not known whether low-molecular-weight heparin would be as effective as unfractionated heparin in patients with acute limb ischemia.

Catheter-directed intraarterial thrombolysis is an initial treatment option for patients with category I and IIa acute limb ischemia if they have no contraindication to thrombolysis.[15, 302] Catheter-based thrombolysis can also be considered for patients with more severe limb ischemia who are considered high risk for surgical intervention. Long-term

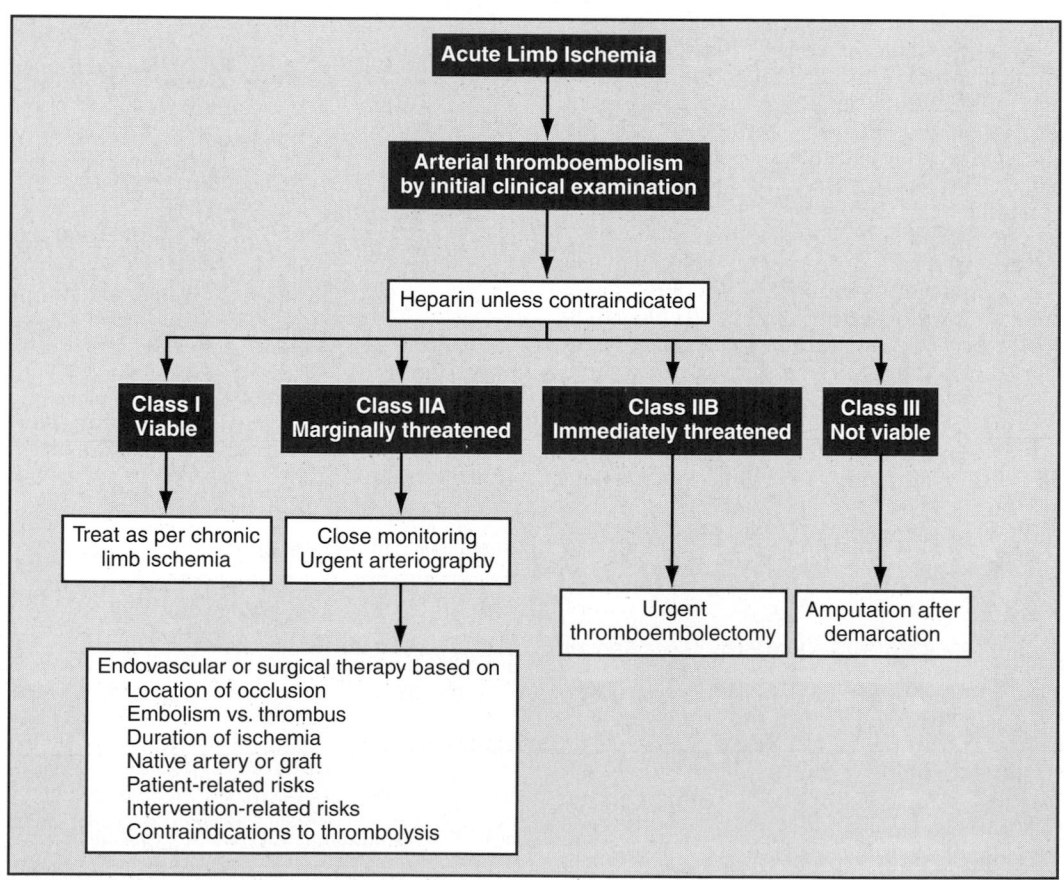

FIGURE 41–22. Management algorithm for treatment of acute limb ischemia. (Adapted from Dormandy JA, Rutherford RB: Management of peripheral arterial disease [PAD]. TASC Working Group. J Vasc Surg 31[Suppl]:1–296, 2000.)

patency after thrombolysis is greater in patients with category I and II critical limb ischemia than in those with category III, in native arteries than in grafts, and in vein grafts than in prosthetic grafts.[303-305] Identification and repair of a graft stenosis after successful thrombolysis improve long-term graft patency.[306,307] Thrombolytic regimens have used streptokinase, urokinase, recombinant tissue-type plasminogen activator (rt-PA), and reteplase. Outcome has varied among the published reports, but small studies have suggested that initial success in achieving graft patency is greater with urokinase than with streptokinase and greater with rt-PA than with urokinase.[306, 308] The duration of catheter-based thrombolytic therapy should generally be less than 48 hours to achieve optimal benefit and limit the risk of bleeding.

Surgical revascularization is indicated for patients with category IIb and early category III acute limb ischemia.[15] The surgical procedure depends on the nature and location of the arterial occlusion. Thromboembolectomy is the procedure of choice, particularly in patients whose acute limb ischemia is due to systemic embolism.[242, 309-311] After completion of an embolectomy procedure, angiography should be performed to search for residual thrombus, which can be treated with repeated passage of the balloon embolectomy catheter or by intraoperative thrombolysis. If thromboembolectomy is neither feasible nor successful, surgical reconstruction to bypass the occluded area should be performed. These techniques were discussed previously in this chapter.

Three prospective randomized trials have compared the benefits and risks of thrombolysis and surgical reconstruction in patients with acute limb ischemia (Table 41–9). In the first of these, often referred to as the Rochester Trial, 114 patients with acute arterial occlusion secondary to thrombosis or embolism and involving either native arteries or bypass grafts were randomized to intraarterial urokinase or surgical revascularization.[312] After 1 year of follow-up, limb salvage rates were 82 percent in each group; however, the survival rate was only 58 percent in the group randomized to surgery versus 84 percent in the group receiving thrombolysis. The higher mortality rate in the surgical treatment group was attributed to cardiopulmonary complications.

The Surgery versus Thrombolysis for Ischemia of the Lower Extremity (STILE) trial compared thrombolysis with either rt-PA or urokinase to surgery after native artery or graft occlusion in patients with limb ischemia of less than 6 months' duration. The trial was stopped prematurely after enrollment of 393 patients. The composite outcome of death, ongoing or recurrent ischemia, major amputation, and major morbidity occurred in 62 percent of the group randomized to thrombolysis as compared with 36 percent of those randomized to surgery. Of patients who had symptoms for less than 14 days, however, amputation-free survival at 6 months was greater in patients treated with thrombolysis than in those treated with surgery.[313] In the Thrombolysis or Peripheral Arterial Study (TOPAS), intraarterial thrombolysis with urokinase was compared with surgery in 554 patients with acute limb ischemia of less than 14 days. Amputation-free survival rates at 6 and 12 months were 72 and 65 percent, respectively, in the thrombolysis group, and 75 and 70 percent, respectively, in the surgery group.[314] Taken together, the findings from these trials would suggest that catheter-based thrombolysis is an appropriate initial option in patients with category I and IIa acute limb ischemia of less than 7 days' duration, whereas surgical revascularization would be more appropriate for those with category IIb and early category III acute limb ischemia and in those whose symptoms have been present for more than 7 days (Fig. 41–22).

▼ Atheroembolism (see also Chap. 40)

Atheroembolism refers to the occlusion of arteries resulting from detachment and embolization of atheromatous debris, including fibrin, platelets, cholesterol crystals, and calcium fragments. Other terms include atherogenic embolism and cholesterol embolism. Atheroemboli originate most frequently from shaggy protruding atheromas of the aorta and less frequently from atherosclerotic branch arteries. The atheroemboli typically occlude small downstream arteries and arterioles of the extremities, brain, eyes, kidneys, or mesentery.[315]

The prevalence of atheroembolism in the general population is not known. Most affected individuals are men older than 60 who have clinical evidence of atherosclerosis.[316-318] The Dutch National Pathology Information System reported an incidence of atheroemboli of 6.2 patients per million per year, and atheroemboli were present in 0.3 percent of autopsy cases.[316] In autopsy series of persons older than 60 years, the incidence of atheroembolism has ranged from 0.8 to 2.4 percent.[319, 320] Atheroembolism accounted for 5 to 10 percent of acute renal failure encountered in a nephrology consulting service and was found in 1 percent of renal biopsy specimens obtained from patients with an unexplained decline in renal function.[321, 322]

Pathogenesis

The risk of atheroembolism is greatest in patients with aortic atherosclerosis characterized by large protuding atheromas (see Fig. 41–4). A strong association is observed between large aortic plaque identified by ultrasound and previous embolic disease.[323, 324] Similarly, identification of large protruding atheromas by transesophageal echocardiography predicts future embolic events.[323, 325, 326] Approximately 50 percent of atheroemboli involve vessels in the lower extremities.

Catheter manipulation is responsible for a large proportion of atheroemboli.[327-332] Similarly, surgical manipulation of the aorta during cardiac or vascular operations may precipitate atheroembolism in 2 to 3 percent of patients.[333, 334] It remains controversial whether anticoagulants or thrombolytic drugs contribute to atheroembolism.[335-338] In the Stroke Prevention and Atrial Fibrillation (SPAF) Study, atheroembolism occurred in 0.7 percent per patient-year in those assigned to adjusted-dose warfarin.[339] In the French Study of Aortic Plaques in Stroke Group, in no patient receiving warfarin did clinical evidence of atheroembolism develop.[326] Muscle biopsies at the time of coronary artery bypass surgery in patients with recent myocardial infarction detected atheroemboli in 14 percent of patients who received thrombolysis and in 10 percent of those who did not.[340] Atheroembolism may entail an inflammatory component inasmuch as cholesterol crystals can activate complement in vitro.[341] Hypocomplementemia can occur in patients with atheroembolism, an indication of complement activation in vivo.[315]

Clinical Findings

The most notable clinical features of atheroembolism to the extremities include painful cyanotic toes resulting in the appelation "blue toe syndrome" (Fig. 41–23). Livedo reticularis occurs in approximately 50 percent of patients.[342] Local areas of erythematous or violaceous discoloration may be present on the lateral aspects of the feet, on the soles, and also on the calves.[315, 343] Other findings include digital and foot ulcerations, nodules, purpura, and petechiae.[342] Pedal pulses are typically present since the emboli tend to lodge in the more distal digital arteries and arterioles. Symptoms and signs indicating additional organ involvement with atheroemboli should be sought. Hollenhorst plaque may be seen with funduscopic examination in patients with visual loss secondary to retinal ischemia or infarction. Renal involvement manifested by increased blood pressure and azotemia commonly occurs in patients with

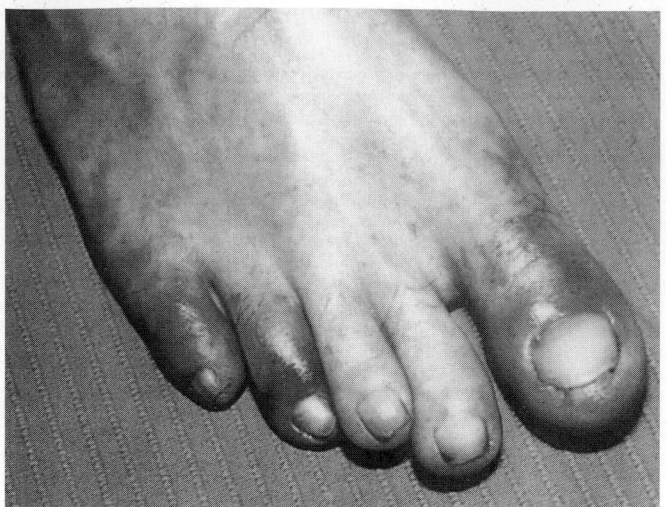

FIGURE 41–23. Atheroemboli to the foot: "blue toe syndrome." Cyanotic discoloration of the first, fourth, and fifth toes is apparent as well as localized areas of violaceous discoloration along the lateral aspect of the foot. (From Halperin JL, Creager MA: Arterial occlusive diseases of the extremities. *In* Loscalzo J, Creager MA, Dzau VJ (eds): Vascular Medicine. 2nd ed. Boston, Little, Brown, 1996, pp 825–852.)

peripheral atheroemboli.[344] Patients may also have evidence of mesenteric or bladder ischemia and splenic infarction.

The clinical setting and findings are usually sufficient to diagnose atheroembolism. However, some of the manifestations of atheroemboli may be present with other diseases. As discussed previously, critical limb ischemia occurs in patients with severe peripheral atherosclerosis, and acute limb ischemia is a consequence of thrombembolism, each of which would be characterized by an abnormal pulse examination. Vasculitides secondary to connective tissue diseases, infections, drugs, polyarteritis nodosa, or cryglobulinemia, for example, may be characterized by multisystem organ damage and cutaneous findings of purpura, ulcers, and digital ischemia, similar to findings that result from atheroemboli (see also Chap. 67). Procoagulant disorders such as antiphospholipid antibody syndrome, heparin-induced thrombocytopenia, and myeloproliferative disorders such as essential thrombocythemia can cause digital artery thrombosis with resultant digital ischemia, cyanosis, and ulceration.

Diagnostic Tests

Laboratory studies that are consistent with atheroembolism include an elevated erythrocyte sedimentation rate, eosinophilia, and eosinophiluria.[344] Other findings may include anemia, thrombocytopenia, hypocomplementemia, and azotemia. Imaging of the aorta with ultrasound, magnetic resonance angiography, or computed tomography may identify sites of severe atherosclerosis and shaggy atheroma indicative of a source for atheroemboli (see Fig. 40–22). The only definitive test for atheroembolism is pathological confirmation by skin or muscle biopsy. Pathognomonic findings include elongated needle-shaped clefts in small arteries that are caused by cholesterol crystals, often accompanied by inflammatory infiltrates composed of lymphocytes and possibly giant cells and eosinophils, intimal thickening, and perivascular fibrosis.[315]

Treatment

No definitive treatment is known for atheroembolism. Analgesics should be administered for pain. Local foot care should be provided as described previously for patients with critical limb ischemia. It may be necessary to excise or amputate necrotic areas.

These patients are subject to recurrent atheroembolic events. Risk factor modification such as lipid-lowering therapy and smoking cessation may have favorable effects on the overall outcome from atherosclerosis, but it is not known whether such intervention will prevent recurrent atheroembolism. The use of antiplatelet drugs to prevent recurrent atheroembolism has been advocated by some and refuted by others.[345,346] It is reasonable, however, to administer antiplatelet agents even in the absence of strong clinical evidence of efficacy since these agents will prevent other adverse cardiovascular events in patients with atherosclerosis. The use of warfarin is also controversial, and some have even suggested that anticoagulants precipitate atheroemboli.[323, 336, 347] Others have found that warfarin reduces atheroembolic events, particularly in patients with mobile aortic atheroma.[338]

Surgical removal of the source should be considered in patients with atheroembolism, particularly those in whom it recurs. Surgical procedures include excision and replacement of affected portions of the aorta, endarterectomy, and bypass operations.[348] Operative intervention is targeted to the site of the aorta or the iliac or femoral arteries where an aneurysm has formed or where obvious shaggy friable atherosclerotic plaque is present. Oftentimes, the aorta is diffusely affected by severe atherosclerosis and it is not possible to identify the precise segment that is responsible for atheroembolism. In addition, many of these patients are elderly and have coexisting coronary artery disease, which increases the risk associated with major vascular operations.

REFERENCES

EPIDEMIOLOGY

1. Criqui MH, Fronek A, Barrett-Connor E, et al: The prevalence of peripheral arterial disease in a defined population. Circulation 71:510–515, 1985.
2. Gofin R, Kark JD, Friedlander Y, et al: Peripheral vascular disease in a middle-aged population sample. The Jerusalem Lipid Research Clinic Prevalence Study. Isr J Med Sci 23:157–167, 1987.
3. Fowkes FG, Housley E, Cawood EH, et al: Edinburgh Artery Study: Prevalence of asymptomatic and symptomatic peripheral arterial disease in the general population. Int J Epidemiol 20:384–392, 1991.
4. Newman AB, Siscovick DS, Manolio TA, et al: Ankle-arm index as a marker of atherosclerosis in the Cardiovascular Health Study. Cardiovascular Heart Study (CHS) Collaborative Research Group. Circulation 88:837–845, 1993.
5. Meijer WT, Hoes AW, Rutgers D, et al: Peripheral arterial disease in the elderly: The Rotterdam Study. Arterioscler Thromb Vasc Biol 18:185–192, 1998.
6. Hooi JD, Stoffers HE, Kester AD, et al: Risk factors and cardiovascular diseases associated with asymptomatic peripheral arterial occlusive disease. The Limburg PAOD Study. Peripheral Arterial Occlusive Disease. Scand J Prim Health Care 16:177–182, 1998.
7. Fabsitz RR, Sidawy AN, Go O, et al: Prevalence of peripheral arterial disease and associated risk factors in American Indians: The Strong Heart Study. Am J Epidemiol 149:330–338, 1999.
8. Smith GD, Shipley MJ, Rose G: Intermittent claudication, heart disease risk factors, and mortality. The Whitehall Study. Circulation 82:1925–1931, 1990.
9. Stoffers HE, Rinkens PE, Kester AD, et al: The prevalence of asymptomatic and unrecognized peripheral arterial occlusive disease. Int J Epidemiol 25:282–290, 1996.
10. Bowlin SJ, Medalie JH, Flocke SA, et al: Epidemiology of intermittent claudication in middle-aged men. Am J Epidemiol 140:418–430, 1994.
11. Bainton D, Sweetnam P, Baker I, et al: Peripheral vascular disease: Consequence for survival and association with risk factors in the Speedwell prospective heart disease study. Br Heart J 72:128–132, 1994.
12. Leng GC, Lee AJ, Fowkes FG, et al: Incidence, natural history and cardiovascular events in symptomatic and asymptomatic peripheral arterial disease in the general population. Int J Epidemiol 25:1172–1181, 1996.
13. Reunanen A, Takkunen H, Aromaa A: Prevalence of intermittent claudication and its effect on mortality. Acta Med Scand 211:249–256, 1982.
14. Murabito JM, D'Agostino RB, Silbershatz H, et al: Intermittent claudication. A risk profile from The Framingham Heart Study. Circulation 96:44–49, 1997.

15. Dormandy JA, Rutherford RB: Management of peripheral arterial disease (PAD). TASC Working Group. J Vasc Surg 31(Suppl):1–296, 2000.
16. Kannel WB, McGee DL: Update on some epidemiologic features of intermittent claudication: The Framingham Study. J Am Geriatr Soc 33: 13–18, 1985.
17. Catalano M: Epidemiology of critical limb ischaemia: North Italian data. Eur J Med 2:11–14, 1993.
18. Ebskov LB, Schroeder TV, Holstein PE: Epidemiology of leg amputation: The influence of vascular surgery. Br J Surg 81:1600–1603, 1994.
19. Fowkes FG, Housley E, Riemersma RA, et al: Smoking, lipids, glucose intolerance, and blood pressure as risk factors for peripheral atherosclerosis compared with ischemic heart disease in the Edinburgh Artery Study. Am J Epidemiol 135:331–340, 1992.
20. Criqui MH, Browner D, Fronek A, et al: Peripheral arterial disease in large vessels is epidemiologically distinct from small vessel disease. An analysis of risk factors. Am J Epidemiol 129:1110–1119, 1989.
21. Hiatt WR, Hoag S, Hamman RF: Effect to diagnostic criteria on the prevalence of peripheral arterial disease. The San Luis Valley Diabetes Study. Circulation 91:1472–1479, 1995.
22. Ernst E, Resch KL: Fibrinogen as a cardiovascular risk factor: A meta-analysis and review of the literature. Ann Intern Med 118:956–963, 1993.
23. Smith FB, Lowe GD, Lee AJ, et al: Smoking, hemorheologic factors, and progression of peripheral arterial disease in patients with claudication. J Vasc Surg 28:129–135, 1998.
24. Lassila R, Peltonen S, Lepantalo M, et al: Severity of peripheral atherosclerosis is associated with fibrinogen and degradation of cross-linked fibrin. Arterioscler Thromb 3:1738–1742, 1993.
25. Lowe GD, Fowkes FG, Dawes J, et al: Blood viscosity, fibrinogen, and activation of coagulation and leukocytes in peripheral arterial disease and the normal population in the Edinburgh Artery Study. Circulation 87:1915–1920, 1993.
26. Smith FB, Lee AJ, Hau, CM, et al: Plasma fibrinogen, haemostatic factors and prediction of peripheral arterial disease in the Edinburgh Artery Study. Blood Coagul Fibrinolysis 11:43–50, 2000.
27. Ridker PM, Cushman M, Stampfer MJ, et al: Plasma concentration of C-reactive protein and risk of developing peripheral vascular disease. Circulation 97:425–428, 1998.
28. Clarke R, Daly L, Robinson K, et al: Hyperhomocysteinemia: An independent risk factor for vascular disease. N Engl J Med 324:1149–1155, 1991.
29. Graham IM, Daly LE, Refsum HM, et al: Plasma homocysteine as a risk factor for vascular disease. The European Concerted Action Project. JAMA 277:1775–1781, 1997.
30. Boushey CJ, Beresford SA, Omenn GS, et al: A quantitative assessment of plasma homocysteine as a risk factor for vascular disease. Probable benefits of increasing folic acid intakes. JAMA 274:1049–1057, 1995.
31. Kannel WB, Shurtleff D: The Framingham Study. Cigarettes and the development of intermittent claudication. Geriatrics 28:61–68, 1973.
32. A randomised, blinded, trial of clopidogrel versus aspirin in patients at risk of ischaemic events (CAPRIE). CAPRIE Steering Committee. Lancet 348:1329–1339, 1996.
33. Jonason T, Bergstrom R: Cessation of smoking in patients with intermittent claudication. Effects on the risk of peripheral vascular complications, myocardial infarction and mortality. Acta Med Scand 221:253–260, 1987.
34. Gordon T, Kannel W B: Predisposition to atherosclerosis in the head, heart, and legs. The Framingham study. JAMA 221:661–666, 1972.
35. Criqui MH, Denenberg JO, Langer RD, et al.: The epidemiology of peripheral arterial disease: Importance of identifying the population at risk. Vasc Med 2:221–226, 1997.
36. Smith I, Franks PJ, Greenhalgh RM, et al: The influence of smoking cessation and hypertriglyceridaemia on the progression of peripheral arterial disease and the onset of critical ischaemia. Eur J Vasc Endovasc Surg 11:402–408, 1996.
37. Senti M, Nogues X, Pedro-Botet J, et al: Lipoprotein profile in men with peripheral vascular disease. Role of intermediate density lipoproteins and apoprotein E phenotypes. Circulation 85:30–36, 1992.
38. Cheng SW, Ting AC, Wong J: Lipoprotein (a) and its relationship to risk factors and severity of atherosclerotic peripheral vascular disease. Eur J Vasc Endovasc Surg 14:17–23, 1997.
39. Takahashi M, Yui Y, Yasumoto H, et al: Lipoproteins are inhibitors of endothelium-dependent relaxation of rabbit aorta. Am J Physiol 258: H1–H8, 1990.
40. Taylor LM Jr, DeFrang RD, Harris EJ Jr, et al: The association of elevated plasma homocyst(e)ine with progression of symptomatic peripheral arterial disease. J Vasc Surg 13:128–136, 1991.
41. Kannel WB: Epidemiology of cardiovascular disease in the elderly: An assessment of risk factors. Cardiovasc Clin 22:9–22, 1992.

PATHOBIOLOGY

42. Aird WC, Edelberg JM, Weiler-Guettler H, et al: Vascular bed–specific expression of an endothelial cell gene is programmed by the tissue microenvironment. J Cell Biol 138:1117–1124, 1997.
43. Guillot PV, Guan J, Liu L, et al: A vascular bed–specific pathway. J Clin Invest 103:799–805, 1999.
44. Adams RH, Wilkinson GA, Weiss C, et al: Roles of ephrinB ligands and EphB receptors in cardiovascular development: Demarcation of arterial/venous domains, vascular morphogenesis, and sprouting angiogenesis. Genes Dev 13:295–306, 1999.
45. Bergwerff M, Verberne ME, DeRuiter MC, et al: Neural crest cell contribution to the developing circulatory system: Implications for vascular morphology? Circ Res 82:221–231, 1998.
46. Mikawa T, Gourdie RG: Pericardial mesoderm generates a population of coronary smooth muscle cells migrating into the heart along with ingrowth of the epicardial organ. Dev Biol 174:221–232, 1996.
47. Mikawa T, Fischman DA: Retroviral analysis of cardiac morphogenesis: Discontinuous formation of coronary vessels. Proc Natl Acad Sci U S A 89:9504–9508, 1992.
48. Li L, Liu Z, Mercer B, et al: Evidence for serum response factor–mediated regulatory networks governing SM22alpha transcription in smooth, skeletal, and cardiac muscle cells. Dev Biol 187:311–321, 1997.
49. Bergwerff M, Gittenberger-de Groot AC, Wisse LJ, et al: Loss of function of the Prx1 and Prx2 homeobox genes alters architecture of the great elastic arteries and ductus arteriosus. Virchows Arch 436:12–19, 2000.
50. Yamagishi H, Olson EN, Srivastava D: The basic helix-loop-helix transcription factor, dHAND, is required for vascular development. J Clin Invest 105:261–270, 2000.
51. Ikari Y, McManus BM, Kenyon J, et al: Neonatal intima formation in the human coronary artery. Arterioscler Thromb Vasc Biol 19:2036–2040, 1999.
52. Weninger WJ, Muller GB, Reiter C, et al: Intimal hyperplasia of the infant parasellar carotid artery: A potential developmental factor in atherosclerosis and SIDS. Circ Res 85:970–975, 1999.
53. Schwartz SM: The intima: A new soil. Circ Res 85:877–879, 1999.
54. Yang ZH, von Segesser L, Bauer E, et al: Different activation of the endothelial L-arginine and cyclooxygenase pathway in the human internal mammary artery and saphenous vein. Circ Res 68:52–60, 1991.
55. Topouzis S, Majesky MW: Smooth muscle lineage diversity in the chick embryo. Two types of aortic smooth muscle cell differ in growth and receptor-mediated transcriptional responses to transforming growth factor-beta. Dev Biol 178:430–445, 1996.
56. Rainwater DL, McMahan CA, Malcom GT, et al: Lipid and apolipoprotein predictors of atherosclerosis in youth: Apolipoprotein concentrations do not materially improve prediction of arterial lesions in PDAY subjects. The PDAY Research Group. Arterioscler Thromb Vasc Biol 19: 753–761, 1999.
57. Strong JP, Malcom GT, Oalmann MC, et al: The PDAY Study: Natural history risk factors, and pathobiology. Pathobiological Determinants of Atherosclerosis in Youth. Ann N Y Acad Sci 811:226–235, 1997.
58. Carr S, Farb A, Pearce WH, et al: Atherosclerotic plaque rupture in symptomatic carotid artery stenosis. J Vasc Surg 23:755–765, 1996.
59. Lammie GA, Sandercock PA, Dennis MS: Recently occluded intracranial and extracranial carotid arteries. Relevance of the unstable atherosclerotic plaque. Stroke 30:1319–1325, 1999.
60. Carr SC, Farb A, Pearce WH, et al: Activated inflammatory cells are associated with plaque rupture in carotid artery stenosis. Surgery 122: 757–763, 1997.
61. Rothwell PM, Villagra R, Gibson R, et al: Evidence of a chronic systemic cause of instability of atherosclerotic plaques. Lancet 355:19–24, 2000.

PATHOPHYSIOLOGY OF LIMB ISCHEMIA

62. Coffman JD: Pathophysiology of obstructive arterial disease. Herz 13: 343–350, 1988.
63. Liao JK, Bettmann MA, Sandor T, et al: Differential impairment of vasodilator responsiveness of peripheral resistance and conduit vessels in humans with atherosclerosis. Circ Res 68:1027–1034, 1991.
64. Tagawa T, Imaizumi T, Endo T, et al: Role of nitric oxide in reactive hyperemia in human forearm vessels. Circulation 90:2285–2290, 1994.
65. Böger RH, Bode-Böger SM, Thiele W, et al: Restoring vascular nitric oxide formation by L-arginine improves the symptoms of intermittent claudication in patients with peripheral arterial occlusive disease. J Am Coll Cardiol 32:1336–1344, 1998.
66. Schellong SM, Böger RH, Burchert W, et al: Dose-related effect of intravenous L-arginine on muscular blood flow of the calf in patients with peripheral vascular disease: A $H_2^{15}O$ positron emission tomography study. Clin Sci (Colch) 93:159–165, 1997.
67. England JD, Regensteiner JG, Ringel SP, et al: Muscle denervation in peripheral arterial disease. Neurology 42:994–999, 1992.
68. Regensteiner JG, Wolfel EE, Brass EP, et al: Chronic changes in skeletal muscle histology and function in peripheral arterial disease. Circulation 87:413–421, 1993.
69. Sorlie D, Myhre K, Mjos OD: Exercise- and post-exercise metabolism of the lower leg in patients with peripheral arterial insufficiency. Scand J Clin Lab Invest 38:635–642, 1978.
70. Hiatt WR, Wolfel EE, Regensteiner JG, et al: Skeletal muscle carnitine metabolism in patients with unilateral peripheral arterial disease. J Appl Physiol 73:346–353, 1992.
71. Bylund AC, Hammarsten J, Holm J, et al: Enzyme activities in skeletal muscles from patients with peripheral arterial insufficiency. Eur J Clin Invest 6:425–429, 1976.
72. Lundgren F, Dahllof AG, Schersten T, et al: Muscle enzyme adaptation in patients with peripheral arterial insufficiency: Spontaneous adaptation, effect of different treatments and consequences on walking performance. Clin Sci 77:485–493, 1989.

73. Bollinger A, Hoffmann U, Franzeck UK: Microvascular changes in arterial occlusive disease: Target for pharmacotherapy. Vasc Med 1:50–54, 1996.
74. Nash GB, Thomas PR, Dormandy JA: Abnormal flow properties of white blood cells in patients with severe ischaemia of the leg. BMJ 296:1699–1701, 1988.
75. Neumann FJ, Waas W, Diehm C, et al: Activation and decreased deformability of neutrophils after intermittent claudication. Circulation 82:922–929, 1990.
76. Second European Consensus Document on chronic critical leg ischemia. Circulation 84(Suppl 4):1–26, 1991.
77. Ubbink DT, Jacobs MJ, Tangelder GJ, et al: Posturally induced microvascular constriction in patients with different stages of leg ischaemia: Effect of local skin heating. Clin Sci (Colch) 81:43–49, 1991.

CLINICAL FEATURES

78. McDermott MM, Mehta S, Greenland P: Exertional leg symptoms other than intermittent claudication are common in peripheral arterial disease. Arch Intern Med 159:387–392, 1999.
79. McDermott MM, Fried L, Simonsick E, et al: Asymptomatic peripheral arterial disease is independently associated with impaired lower extremity functioning: The Women's Health and Aging Study. Circulation 101:1007–1012, 2000.
80. McDermott MM, Liu K, Guralnik JM, et al: The ankle brachial index independently predicts walking velocity and walking endurance in peripheral arterial disease. J Am Geriatr Soc 46:1355–1362, 1998.
81. Rose GA: The diagnosis of ischaemic heart pain and intermittent claudication in field surveys. Bull World Health Organ 27:648–658, 1962.
82. Leng GC, Fowkes FG: The Edinburgh Claudication Questionnaire: An improved version of the WHO/Rose Questionnaire for use in epidemiological surveys. J Clin Epidemiol 45:1101–1109, 1992.
83. Criqui MH, Denenberg JO, Bird CE, et al.: The correlation between symptoms and non-invasive test results in patients referred for peripheral arterial disease testing. Vasc Med 1:65–71, 1996.
84. Regensteiner JG, Steiner JF, Panzer RJ, et al: Evaluation of walking impairment by questionnaire in patients with peripheral arterial disease. J Vasc Med Biol 2:142–152, 1990.
85. Hawkes CH, Roberts GM: Neurogenic and vascular claudication. J Neurol Sci 38:337–345, 1978.
86. Alvarez JA, Hardy RH Jr: Lumbar spine stenosis: A common cause of back and leg pain. Am Fam Physician 57:1825–1834, 1839–1840, 1998.
87. Killewich LA, Martin R, Cramer M, et al: Pathophysiology of venous claudication. J Vasc Surg 1:507–511, 1984.
88. Qvarfordt P, Eklof B, Ohlin P, et al: Intramuscular pressure, blood flow, and skeletal muscle metabolism in patients with venous claudication. Surgery 95:191–195, 1984.
89. Walker RT, Woodyer AB, Dormandy JA: Venous claudication. A report of 15 cases and a review of the literature. Int Angiol 4:365–367, 1985.

TESTING FOR PAD

90. Rutherford RB, Baker JD, Ernst C, et al: Recommended standards for reports dealing with lower extremity ischemia: Revised version. J Vasc Surg 26:517–538, 1997.
91. Nichols WW, O'Rourke MF: Wave reflections. In Nichols WW, O'Rourke MF (eds): McDonald's Blood Flow in Arteries. 3rd ed. Sevenoaks, Kent, UK, Edward Arnold, 1990, pp 251–269.
92. Yao JS: New techniques in objective arterial evaluation. Arch Surg 106:600–604, 1973.
93. Carter SA: The relationship of distal systolic pressures to healing of skin lesions in limbs with arterial occlusive disease, with special reference to diabetes mellitus. Scand J Clin Lab Invest Suppl 128:239–243, 1973.
94. Raines JK, Darling RC, Buth J, et al: Vascular laboratory criteria for the management of peripheral vascular disease of the lower extremities. Surgery 79:21–29, 1976.
95. Creager MA: Clinical assessment of the patient with claudication: The role of the vascular laboratory. Vasc Med 2:231–237, 1997.
96. Gale SS, Scissons RP, Salles-Cunha SX, et al: Lower extremity arterial evaluation: Are segmental arterial blood pressures worthwhile? J Vasc Surg 27:831–838, 1998.
97. Ranke C, Creutzig A, Alexander K: Duplex scanning of the peripheral arteries: Correlation of the peak velocity ratio with angiographic diameter reduction. Ultrasound Med Biol 18:433–440, 1992.
98. Sacks D, Robinson ML, Marinelli DL, et al: Peripheral arterial Doppler ultrasonography: Diagnostic criteria. J Ultrasound Med 11:95–103, 1992.
99. Koelemay MJ, den Hartog D, Prins MH, et al: Diagnosis of arterial disease of the lower extremities with duplex ultrasonography. Br J Surg 83:404–409, 1996.
100. Pemberton M, London NJ: Colour flow duplex imaging of occlusive arterial disease of the lower limb. Br J Surg 84:912–919, 1997.
101. Whelan JF, Barry MH, Moir JD: Color flow Doppler ultrasonography: Comparison with peripheral arteriography for the investigation of peripheral vascular disease. J Clin Ultrasound 20:369–374, 1992.
102. Gardner AW, Skinner JS, Cantwell BW, et al: Progressive vs single-stage treadmill tests for evaluation of claudication. Med Sci Sports Exerc 23:402–408, 1991.
103. Labs KH, Nehler MR, Roessner M, et al: Reliability of treadmill testing in peripheral arterial disease: A comparison of a constant load with a graded load treadmill protocol. Vasc Med 4:239–246, 1999.
104. Gardner AW, Skinner JS, Vaughan NR, et al: Comparison of three progressive exercise protocols in peripheral vascular occlusive disease. Angiology 43:661–671, 1992.
105. Chaudhry H, Holland A, Dormandy J: Comparison of graded versus constant treadmill test protocols for quantifying intermittent claudication. Vasc Med 2:93–97, 1997.
106. Poon E, Yucel EK, Pagan-Marin H, et al: Iliac artery stenosis measurements: Comparison of two-dimensional time-of-flight and three-dimensional dynamic gadolinium-enhanced MR angiography. AJR Am J Roentgenol 169:1139–1144, 1997.
107. Ho KY, de Haan MW, Kessels AG, et al: Peripheral vascular tree stenoses: Detection with subtracted and nonsubtracted MR angiography. Radiology 206:673–681, 1998.
108. Quinn SF, Sheley RC, Semonsen KG, et al: Aortic and lower-extremity arterial disease: Evaluation with MR angiography versus conventional angiography. Radiology 206:693–701, 1998.
109. Rofsky NM, Johnson G, Adelman MA, et al: Peripheral vascular disease evaluated with reduced-dose gadolinium-enhanced MR angiography. Radiology 205:163–169, 1997.

PROGNOSIS OF PAD

110. Weitz JI, Byrne J, Clagett GP, et al: Diagnosis and treatment of chronic arterial insufficiency of the lower extremities: A critical review. Circulation 94:3026–3049, 1996.
111. Ness J, Aronow WS: Prevalence of coexistence of coronary artery disease, ischemic stroke, and peripheral arterial disease in older persons, mean age 80 years, in an academic hospital–based geriatrics practice. J Am Geriatr Soc 47:1255–1256, 1999.
112. Klop RB, Eikelboom BC, Taks AC: Screening of the internal carotid arteries in patients with peripheral vascular disease by colour-flow duplex scanning. Eur J Vasc Surg 5:41–45, 1991.
113. Alexandrova NA, Gibson WC, Norris JW, et al: Carotid artery stenosis in peripheral vascular disease. J Vasc Surg 23:645–649, 1996.
114. Criqui M, Langer RD, Fronek A, et al: Mortality over a period of 10 years in patients with peripheral arterial disease. N Engl J Med 326:381–386, 1992.
115. Newman AB, Sutton-Tyrrell K, Vogt MT, et al: Morbidity and mortality in hypertensive adults with a low ankle/arm blood pressure index. JAMA 270:487–489, 1993.
116. Newman AB, Tyrrell KS, Kuller LH: Mortality over four years in SHEP participants with a low ankle-arm index. J Am Geriatr Soc 45:1472–1478, 1997.
117. Kornitzer M, Dramaix M, Sobolski J, et al: Ankle/arm pressure index in asymptomatic middle-aged males: An independent predictor of ten-year coronary heart disease mortality. Angiology 46:211–219, 1995.
118. Vogt MT, Cauley JA, Newman AB, et al: Decreased ankle/arm blood pressure index and mortality in elderly women. JAMA 270:465–469, 1993.
119. Vogt MT, McKenna M, Anderson SJ, et al: The relationship between ankle-arm index and mortality in older men and women. J Am Geriatr Soc 41:523–530, 1993.
120. Dormandy JA, Murray GD: The fate of the claudicant—a prospective study of 1969 claudicants. Eur J Vasc Surg 5:131–133, 1991.
121. McKenna M, Wolfson S, Kuller L: The ratio of ankle and arm arterial pressure as an independent predictor of mortality. Atherosclerosis 87:119–128, 1991.
122. Howell MA, Colgan MP, Seeger RW, et al: Relationship of severity of lower limb peripheral vascular disease to mortality and morbidity: A six-year follow-up study. J Vasc Surg 9:691–696, 1989.
123. Luther M: The influence of arterial reconstructive surgery on the outcome of critical leg ischaemia. Eur J Vasc Surg 8:682–689, 1994.
124. Coran AG, Warren R: Arteriographic changes in femoropopliteal arteriosclerosis obliterans. A five year follow-up study. N Engl J Med 274:643, 1966.
125. Jelnes R, Gaardsting O, Hougaard Jensen K, et al: Fate in intermittent claudication: Outcome and risk factors. BMJ 293:1137–1140, 1986.
126. Jonason T, Ringqvist I: Changes in peripheral blood pressures after five years of follow-up in non-operated patients with intermittent claudication. Acta Med Scand 220:127–132, 1986.
127. McDaniel MD, Cronenwett JL: Basic data related to the natural history of intermittent claudication. Ann Vasc Surg 3:273–277, 1989.

TREATMENT OF PAD

128. Randomised trial of cholesterol lowering in 4444 patients with coronary heart disease: The Scandinavian Simvastatin Survival Study (4S). Lancet 344:1383–1389, 1994.
129. Pfeffer MA, Sacks FM, Moye LA, et al: Cholesterol and Recurrent Events: A secondary prevention trial for normolipidemic patients. CARE Investigators. Am J Cardiol 76:98C–106C, 1995.
130. Prevention of cardiovascular events and death with pravastatin in patients with coronary heart disease and a broad range of initial cholesterol levels. The Long-Term Intervention with Pravastatin in Ischaemic Disease (LIPID) Study Group. N Engl J Med 339:1349–1357, 1998.

131. Summary of the second report of the National Cholesterol Education Program (NCEP) Expert Panel on Detection, Evaluation, and Treatment of High Blood Cholesterol in Adults (Adult Treatment Panel II). JAMA 269:3015–3023, 1993.

132. Blankenhorn DH, Azen SP, Crawford DW, et al: Effects of colestipol-niacin therapy on human femoral atherosclerosis. Circulation 83:438–447, 1991.

133. Duffield RG, Lewis B, Miller NE, et al: Treatment of hyperlipidaemia retards progression of symptomatic femoral atherosclerosis. A randomised controlled trial. Lancet 2:639–642, 1983.

134. Walldius G, Erikson U, Olsson AG, et al: The effect of probucol on femoral atherosclerosis: the Probucol Quantitative Regression Swedish Trial (PQRST). Am J Cardiol 74:875–883, 1994.

135. Buchwald H, Bourdages HR, Campos CT, et al: Impact of cholesterol reduction on peripheral arterial disease in the Program on the Surgical Control of the Hyperlipidemias (POSCH). Surgery 120:672–679, 1996.

136. Pedersen TR, Kjekshus J, Pyorala K, et al: Effect of simvastatin on ischemic signs and symptoms in the Scandinavian Simvastatin Survival Study (4S). Am J Cardiol 81:333–335, 1998.

137. Faulkner KW, House AK, Castleden WM: The effect of cessation of smoking on the accumulative survival rate of patients with symptomatic peripheral vascular disease. Med J Aust 1:217–219, 1983.

138. Lassila R, Lepantalo M: Cigarette smoking and the outcome after lower limb arterial surgery. Acta Chir Scand 154:635–640, 1988.

139. Effect of intensive diabetes management on macrovascular events and risk factors in the Diabetes Control and Complications Trial. Am J Cardiol 75:894–903, 1995.

140. UK Prospective Diabetes Study (UKPDS) Group. Intensive blood-glucose control with sulphonylureas or insulin compared with conventional treatment and risk of complications in patients with type 2 diabetes (UKPDS 33). Lancet 352:837–853, 1998.

141. Collins R, Peto R, MacMahon S, et al: Blood pressure, stroke, and coronary heart disease. Part 2. Short-term reductions in blood pressure: Overview of randomized drug trials in their epidemiological context. Lancet 335:827–838, 1990.

142. Frohlich ED, Tarazi RC, Dustan HP: Peripheral arterial insufficiency. A complication of beta-adrenergic blocking therapy. JAMA 208:2471–2472, 1969.

143. Rodger JC, Sheldon CD, Lerski RA, et al: Intermittent claudication complicating beta-blockade. BMJ 1:1125, 1976.

144. Hiatt WR, Stoll S, Nies AS: Effect of beta-adrenergic blockers on the peripheral circulation in patients with peripheral vascular disease. Circulation 72:1226–1231, 1985.

145. Roberts DH, Tsao Y, McLoughlin GA, et al: Placebo-controlled comparison of captopril, atenolol, labetalol, and pindolol in hypertension complicated by intermittent claudication. Lancet 2:650–653, 1987.

146. Solomon SA, Ramsay LE, Yeo WW, et al: Beta blockade and intermittent claudication: Placebo controlled trial of atenolol and nifedipine and their combination BMJ 303:1100–1104, 1991.

147. Radack K, Deck C: Beta-adrenergic blocker therapy does not worsen intermittent claudication in subjects with peripheral arterial disease. A meta-analysis of randomized controlled trials. Arch Intern Med 151:1769–1776, 1991.

148. Goldstein S: Propranolol therapy in patients with acute myocardial infarction: The Beta-Blocker Heart Attack Trial. Circulation 67(Suppl 1):53–57, 1983.

149. Freemantle N, Cleland J, Young P, et al: Beta blockade after myocardial infarction: Systematic review and meta regression analysis. BMJ 318:1730–1737, 1999.

150. The sixth report of the Joint National Committee on Prevention, Detection, Evaluation, and Treatment of High Blood Pressure. Arch Intern Med 157:2413–2446, 1997.

151. Rutherford JD, Pfeffer MA, Moye LA, et al: Effects of captopril on ischemic events after myocardial infarction. Results of the Survival and Ventricular Enlargement trial. SAVE Investigators. Circulation 90:1731–1738, 1994.

152. Yusuf S, Pepine CJ, Garces C, et al: Effect of enalapril on myocardial infarction and unstable angina in patients with low ejection fractions. Lancet 340:1173–1178, 1992.

153. Yusuf S, Sleight P, Pogue J, et al: Effects of an angiotensin-converting-enzyme inhibitor, ramipril, on cardiovascular events in high-risk patients. The Heart Outcomes Prevention Evaluation Study Investigators. N Engl J Med 342:145–153, 2000.

154. Antiplatelet Trialists' Collaboration. Collaborative overview of randomised trials of antiplatelet therapy—I: Prevention of death, myocardial infarction, and stroke by prolonged antiplatelet therapy in various categories of patients. BMJ 308:81–106, 1994.

155. Antiplatelet Trialists' Collaboration. Collaborative overview of randomized trials of antiplatelet therapy—II: Maintenance of vascular graft or arterial patency by antiplatelet therapy. BMJ 308:159–168, 1994.

156. Becquemin JP: Effect of ticlopidine on the long-term patency of saphenous-vein bypass grafts in the legs. Etude de la Ticlopidine apres Pontage Femoro-Poplite and the Association Universitaire de Recherche en Chirurgie. N Engl J Med 337:1726–1731, 1997.

157. Balsano F, Coccheri S, Libretti A, et al: Ticlopidine in the treatment of intermittent claudication: A 21-month double-blind trial. J Lab Clin Med 114:84–91, 1989.

158. Janzon L, Bergqvist D, Boberg J, et al: Prevention of myocardial infarction and stroke in patients with intermittent claudication; effects of

ticlopidine. Results from STIMS, the Swedish Ticlopidine Multicentre Study. J Intern Med 227:301–308, 1990.

159. Cameron HA, Waller PC, Ramsay LE: Drug treatment of intermittent claudication: A critical analysis of the methods and findings of published clinical trials, 1965–1985. Br J Clin Pharmacol 26:569–576, 1988.

160. Hiatt WR, Hirsch AT, Regensteiner JG, et al: Clinical trials for claudication. Assessment of exercise performance, functional status, and clinical end points. Vascular Clinical Trialists. Circulation 92:614–621, 1995.

161. Labs KH, Dormandy JA, Jaeger KA, et al: Transatlantic Conference on Clinical Trial Guidelines in Peripheral Arterial Disease: Clinical trial methodology. Basel PAD Clinical Trial Methodology Group. Circulation 100:e75–e81, 1999.

162. Coffman JD: Drug therapy: Vasodilator drugs in peripheral vascular disease. N Engl J Med 300:713–717, 1979.

163. Angelkort B, Spurk P, Habbaba, A, et al: Blood flow properties and walking performance in chronic arterial occlusive disease. Angiology 36:285–292, 1985.

164. Hansen PR, Holm AM, Qi JH, et al: Pentoxifylline inhibits neointimal formation and stimulates constrictive vascular remodeling after arterial injury. J Cardiovasc Pharmacol 34:683–689, 1999.

165. Chen YM, Wu KD, Tsai TJ, et al: Pentoxifylline inhibits PDGF-induced proliferation of and TGF-beta–stimulated collagen synthesis by vascular smooth muscle cells. J Mol Cell Cardiol 31:773–783, 1999.

166. Porter JM, Cutler BS, Lee BY, et al: Pentoxifylline efficacy in the treatment of intermittent claudication: Multicenter controlled double-blind trial with objective assessment of chronic occlusive arterial disease patients. Am Heart J 104:66–72, 1982.

167. Lindgärde F, Labs KH, Rössner M: The pentoxifylline experience: Exercise testing reconsidered. Vasc Med 1:145–154, 1996.

168. Lindgärde F, Jelnes R, Björkman H, et al: Conservative drug treatment in patients with moderately severe chronic occlusive peripheral arterial disease. Scandinavian Study Group. Circulation 80:1549–1556, 1989.

169. Hood SC, Moher D, Barber GG: Management of intermittent claudication with pentoxifylline: Meta-analysis of randomized controlled trials. CMAJ 155:1053–1059, 1996.

170. Girolami B, Bernardi E, Prins MH, et al: Treatment of intermittent claudication with physical training, smoking cessation, pentoxifylline, or nafronyl: A meta analysis. Arch Intern Med 159:337–345, 1999.

171. Radack K, Wyderski RJ: Conservative management of intermittent claudication. Ann Intern Med 113:135–146, 1990.

172. Ikeda Y: Antiplatelet therapy using cilostazol, a specific PDE3 inhibitor. Thromb Haemost 82:435–438, 1999.

173. Tanaka T, Ishikawa T, Hagiwara M, et al: Effects of cilostazol, a selective cAMP phosphodiesterase inhibitor on the contraction of vascular smooth muscle. Pharmacology 36:313–320, 1988.

174. Money SR, Herd JA, Isaacsohn JL, et al: Effect of cilostazol on walking distances in patients with intermittent claudication caused by peripheral vascular disease. J Vasc Surg 27:267–274, 1998.

175. Beebe HG, Dawson DL, Cutler BS, et al: A new pharmacological treatment for intermittent claudication: Results of a randomized, multicenter trial. Arch Intern Med 159:2041–2050, 1999.

176. Dawson DL, Cutler BS, Hiatt WR, et al: A comparison of cilostazol pentoxifylline for treating intermittent claudication. Am J Med, in press.

177. Packer M, Carver JR, Rodeheffer RJ, et al: Effect of oral milrinone on mortality in severe chronic heart failure. The PROMISE Study Research Group. N Engl J Med 325:1468–1475, 1991.

178. Cohn JN, Goldstein SO, Greenberg BH, et al: A dose-dependent increase in mortality with vesnarinone among patients with severe heart failure. Vesnarinone Trial Investigators. N Engl J Med 339:1810–1816, 1998.

179. PACK Claudication Substudy. Randomized placebo-controlled, double-blind trial of ketanserin in claudicants. Changes in claudication distance and ankle systolic pressure. Circulation 80:1544–1548, 1989.

180. Barradell LB, Brogden RN: Oral naftidrofuryl. A review of its pharmacology and therapeutic use in the management of peripheral occlusive arterial disease. Drugs Aging 8:299–322, 1996.

181. Lehert P, Riphagen FE, Gamand S: The effect of naftidrofuryl on intermittent claudication: A meta-analysis. J Cardiovasc Pharmacol 16(Suppl):81–86, 1990.

182. Brevetti G, Perna S, Sabba C, et al: Propionyl-L-carnitine in intermittent claudication: Double-blind, placebo-controlled, dose titration, multicenter study. J Am Coll Cardiol 26:1411–1416, 1995.

183. Brevetti G, Diehm C, Lambert D: European multicenter study on propionyl-L-carnitine in intermittent claudication. J Am Coll Cardiol 34:1618–1624, 1999.

184. Belch JJ, Bell PR, Creissen D, et al: Randomized, double-blind, placebo-controlled study evaluating the efficacy and safety of AS-013, a prostaglandin E1 prodrug, in patients with intermittent claudication. Circulation 95:2298–2302, 1997.

185. The ICAI Study Group. Ischemia Cronica degli Arti Inferiori. Prostanoids for chronic critical leg ischemia. A randomized, controlled, open-label trial with prostaglandin E1. Ann Intern Med 130:412–421, 1999.

186. Baffour R, Berman J, Garb JL, et al: Enhanced angiogenesis and growth of collaterals by in vivo administration of recombinant basic fibroblast growth factor in a rabbit model of acute lower limb ischemia: Dose-response effect of basic fibroblast growth factor. J Vasc Surg 16:181–191, 1992.

187. Takeshita S, Pu LQ, Stein LA, et al: Intramuscular administration of vascular endothelial growth factor induces dose-dependent collateral

artery augmentation in a rabbit model of chronic limb ischemia. Circulation 90(Suppl 2):228–234, 1994.

188. Takeshita S, Zheng LP, Brogi E, et al: Therapeutic angiogenesis. A single intraarterial bolus of vascular endothelial growth factor augments revascularization in a rabbit ischemic hind limb model. J Clin Invest 93:662–670, 1994.

189. Takeshita S, Tsurumi Y, Couffinahl T, et al: Gene transfer of naked DNA encoding for three isoforms of vascular endothelial growth factor stimulates collateral development in vivo. Lab Invest 75:487–501, 1996.

190. Yang HT, Deschenes MR, Ogilvie RW, et al: Basic fibroblast growth factor increases collateral blood flow in rats with femoral arterial ligation. Circ Res 79:62–69, 1996.

191. Tsurumi Y, Kearney M, Chen D, et al: Treatment of acute limb ischemia by intramuscular injection of vascular endothelial growth factor gene. Circulation 96(Suppl 2):382–388, 1997.

192. Isner JM, Pieczek A, Schainfeld R, et al: Clinical evidence of angiogenesis after arterial gene transfer of phVEGF165 in patient with ischaemic limb. Lancet 348:370–374, 1996.

193. Baumgartner I, Pieczek A, Manor O, et al: Constitutive expression of phVEGF165 after intramuscular gene transfer promotes collateral vessel development in patients with critical limb ischemia. Circulation 97:1114–1123, 1998.

194. Hiatt WR, Regensteiner JG, Hargarten ME, et al: Benefit of exercise conditioning for patients with peripheral arterial disease. Circulation 81:602–609, 1990.

195. Gardner AW, Poehlman ET: Exercise rehabilitation programs for the treatment of claudication pain. A meta-analysis. JAMA 274:975–980, 1995.

196. Perkins JM, Collin J, Creasy TS, et al: Exercise training versus angioplasty for stable claudication. Long and medium term results in a prospective, randomised trial. Eur J Vasc Endovasc Surg 11:409–413, 1996.

197. Yang HT, Ogilvie RW, Terjung RL: Training increases collateral-dependent muscle blood flow in aged rats. Am J Physiol 268:H1174–H1180, 1995.

198. Coffman JD: Peripheral collateral blood flow and vascular reactivity in the dog. J Clin Invest 45:923–931, 1966.

199. Conrad MC: Effects of therapy on maximal walking time following femoral ligation in the rat. Circ Res 41:775–778, 1977.

200. Hoppeler H: Vascular growth in hypoxic skeletal muscle. Adv Exp Med Biol 474:277–286, 1999.

201. Breen EC, Johnson EC, Wagner H, et al: Angiogenic growth factor mRNA responses in muscle to a single bout of exercise. J Appl Physiol 81:355–361, 1996.

202. Gustafsson T, Puntschart A, Kaijser L, et al: Exercise-induced expression of angiogenesis-related transcription and growth factors in human skeletal muscle. Am J Physiol 276:H679–H685, 1999.

203. Hambrecht R, Wolf A, Gielen S, et al: Effect of exercise on coronary endothelial function in patients with coronary artery disease. N Engl J Med 342:454–460, 2000.

204. Hambrecht R, Fiehn E, Weigl C, et al: Regular physical exercise corrects endothelial dysfunction and improves exercise capacity in patients with chronic heart failure. Circulation 98:2709–2715, 1998.

205. Hornig B, Maier V, Drexler H: Physical training improves endothelial function in patients with chronic heart failure. Circulation 93:210–214, 1996.

206. Larsen OA, Lassen NA: Effect of daily muscular exercise in patients with intermittent claudication. Lancet 2:1093–1096, 1966.

207. Ekroth R, Dahllof AG, Gundevall B, et al: Physical training of patients with intermittent claudication: Indications, methods, and results. Surgery 84:640–643, 1978.

208. Holloszy JO, Coyle EF: Adaptations of skeletal muscle to endurance exercise and their metabolic consequences. J Appl Physiol 56:831–838, 1984.

209. Wibom R, Hultman E, Johansson M, et al: Adaptation of mitochondrial ATP production in human skeletal muscle to endurance training and detraining. J Appl Physiol 73:2004–2010, 1992.

210. Hiatt WR, Regensteiner JG, Wolfel EE, et al.: Effect of exercise training on skeletal muscle histology and metabolism in peripheral arterial disease. J Appl Physiol 81:780–788, 1996.

211. Johnston KW: Iliac arteries: Reanalysis of results of balloon angioplasty. Radiology 186:207–212, 1993.

212. Motarjeme A, Gordon GI, Bodenhagen K: Thrombolysis and angioplasty of chronic iliac artery occlusions. J Vasc Interv Radiol 6(Suppl):66–72, 1995.

213. Pentecost MJ, Criqui MH, Dorros G, et al: Guidelines for peripheral percutaneous transluminal angioplasty of the abdominal aorta and lower extremity vessels. A statement for health professionals from a special writing group of the Councils on Cardiovascular Radiology, Arteriosclerosis, Cardio-Thoracic and Vascular Surgery, Clinical Cardiology, and Epidemiology and Prevention, the American Heart Association. Circulation 89:511–531, 1994.

214. Gupta AK, Ravimandalam K, Rao VR, et al: Total occlusion of iliac arteries: Results of balloon angioplasty. Cardiovasc Intervent Radiol 16:165–177, 1993.

215. Tegtmeyer CJ, Hartwell GD, Selby JB, et al: Results and complications of angioplasty in aortoiliac disease. Circulation 83(Suppl 1):53–60, 1991.

216. Henry M, Amor M, Ethevenot G, et al: Palmaz stent placement in iliac and femoropopliteal arteries: Primary and secondary patency in 310 patients with 2–4-year follow-up. Radiology 197:167–174, 1995.

217. Sullivan TM, Childs MB, Bacharach JM, et al: Percutaneous transluminal angioplasty and primary stenting of the iliac arteries in 288 patients. J Vasc Surg 25:829–838, 1997.

218. Martin EC, Katzen BT, Benenati JF, et al: Multicenter trial of the Wallstent in the iliac and femoral arteries. J Vasc Interv Radiol 6:843–849, 1995.

219. Bosch JL, Hunink MG: Meta-analysis of the results of percutaneous transluminal angioplasty and stent placement for aortoiliac occlusive disease. Radiology 204:87–96, 1997.

220. Tetteroo E, van der Graaf Y, Bosch JL, et al: Randomised comparison of primary stent placement versus primary angioplasty followed by selective stent placement in patients with iliac-artery occlusive disease. Dutch Iliac Stent Trial Study Group. Lancet 351:1153–1159, 1998.

221. Bosch JL, Tetteroo E, Mali WP, et al: Iliac arterial occlusive disease: Cost-effectiveness analysis of stent placement versus percutaneous transluminal angioplasty. Dutch Iliac Stent Trial Study Group. Radiology 208:641–648, 1998.

222. Bosch JL, van der Graaf Y, Hunink MG: Health-related quality of life after angioplasty and stent placement in patients with iliac artery occlusive disease: Results of a randomized controlled clinical trial. The Dutch Iliac Stent Trial Study Group. Circulation 99:3155–3160, 1999.

223. Ballard JL, Bergan JJ, Singh P, et al: Aortoiliac stent deployment versus surgical reconstruction: Analysis of outcome and cost. J Vasc Surg 28:94–101, 1998.

224. Hunink MG, Donaldson MC, Meyerovitz MF, et al: Risks and benefits of femoropopliteal percutaneous balloon angioplasty. J Vasc Surg 17:183–192, 1993.

225. Matsi PJ, Manninen HI: Complications of lower-limb percutaneous transluminal angioplasty: A prospective analysis of 410 procedures on 295 consecutive patients. Cardiovasc Intervent Radiol 21:361–366, 1998.

226. Capek P, McLean GK, Berkowitz HD: Femoropopliteal angioplasty. Factors influencing long-term success. Circulation 83(Suppl 1):70–80, 1991.

227. Johnston KW: Femoral and popliteal arteries: Reanalysis of results of balloon angioplasty. Radiology 183:767–771, 1992.

228. Matsi PJ, Manninen HI, Vanninen RL, et al: Femoropopliteal angioplasty in patients with claudication: Primary and secondary patency in 140 limbs with 1–3-year follow-up. Radiology 191:727–733, 1994.

229. Hunink MG, Wong JB, Donaldson MC, et al: Patency results of percutaneous and surgical revascularization for femoropopliteal arterial disease. Med Decis Making 14:71–81, 1994.

230. Hunink MG, Wong JB, Donaldson MC, et al.: Revascularization for femoropopliteal disease. A decision and cost-effectiveness analysis. JAMA 274:165–171, 1995.

231. Bakal CW, Sprayregen S, Scheinbaum K, et al: Percutaneous transluminal angioplasty of the infrapopliteal arteries: Results in 53 patients. AJR Am J Roentgenol 154:171–174, 1990.

232. Bakal CW, Cynamon J, Sprayregen S: Infrapopliteal percutaneous transluminal angioplasty: What we know. Radiology 200:36–43, 1996.

233. Matsi PJ, Manninen HI, Suhonen MT, et al: Chronic critical lower-limb ischemia: Prospective trial of angioplasty with 1–36 months follow-up. Radiology 188:381–387, 1993.

234. Dorros G, Jaff MR, Murphy KJ, et al: The acute outcome of tibioperoneal vessel angioplasty in 417 cases with claudication and critical limb ischemia. Cathet Cardiovasc Diagn 45:251–256, 1998.

235. Brown KT, Moore ED, Getrajdman GI, et al: Infrapopliteal angioplasty: Long-term follow-up. J Vasc Interv Radiol 4:139–144, 1993.

236. Durham JR, Horowitz JD, Wright JG, et al: Percutaneous transluminal angioplasty of tibial arteries for limb salvage in the high-risk diabetic patient Ann Vasc Surg 8:48–53, 1994.

237. Lofberg AM, Lorelius LE, Karacagil S, et al: The use of below-knee percutaneous transluminal angioplasty in arterial occlusive disease causing chronic critical limb ischemia. Cardiovasc Intervent Radiol 19:317–322, 1996.

238. Sullivan TM, Gray BH, Bacharach JM, et al: Angioplasty and primary stenting of the subclavian, innominate, and common carotid arteries in 83 patients. J Vasc Surg 28:1059–1065, 1998.

239. Mathias KD, Luth I, Haarmann P: Percutaneous transluminal angioplasty of proximal subclavian artery occlusions. Cardiovasc Intervent Radiol 16:214–218, 1993.

240. Millaire A, Trinca M, Marache P, et al: Subclavian angioplasty: Immediate and late results in 50 patients. Cathet Cardiovasc Diagn 29:8–17, 1993.

241. Eagle KA, Brundage BH, Chaitman BR, et al: Guidelines for perioperative cardiovascular evaluation for noncardiac surgery. Report of the American College of Cardiology/American Heart Association Task Force on Practice Guidelines (Committee on Perioperative Cardiovascular Evaluation for Noncardiac Surgery). J Am Coll Cardiol 27:910–948, 1996.

242. Brewster DC: Clinical and anatomical considerations for surgery in aortoiliac disease and results of surgical treatment. Circulation 83(Suppl 1):42–52, 1991.

243. de Vries SO, Hunink MG: Results of aortic bifurcation grafts for aortoiliac occlusive disease: A meta-analysis. J Vasc Surg 26:558–569, 1997.

244. Whittemore AD, Mannick JA: Principles of Vascular Surgery. In Loscalzo J, Creager MA, Dzau VJ (eds): Vascular Medicine. 2nd ed. Boston, Little, Brown, 1996, pp 675–702.

245. Biancari F, Lepantalo M: Extra-anatomic bypass surgery for critical leg ischemia. A review. J Cardiovasc Surg (Torino) 39:295–301, 1998.

246. McKinsey JF: Extra-anatomic reconstruction. Surg Clin North Am 75:731–740, 1995.

247. Dick LS, Brief DK, Alpert J, et al: A 12-year experience with femoro-femoral crossover grafts. Arch Surg 115:1359–1365, 1980.

248. Schneider JR, McDaniel MD, Walsh DB, et al: Axillofemoral bypass: Outcome and hemodynamic results in high-risk patients. J Vasc Surg 15:952–962, 1992.

249. Harrington ME, Harrington EB, Haimov M, et al: Axillofemoral bypass: Compromised bypass for compromised patients. J Vasc Surg 20:195–201, 1994.

250. Veith FJ, Gupta SK, Ascer E, et al: Six-year prospective multicenter randomized comparison of autologous saphenous vein and expanded polytetrafluoroethylene grafts in infrainguinal arterial reconstructions. J Vasc Surg 3:104–114, 1986.

251. Veterans Administration Cooperative Study Group 141. Comparative evaluation of prosthetic, reversed, and in situ vein bypass grafts in distal popliteal and tibial-peroneal revascularization. Arch Surg 123:434–438, 1988.

252. Illig KA, Green RM: Prosthetic above-knee femoropopliteal bypass. Semin Vasc Surg 12:38–45, 1999.

253. Taylor LM Jr, Edwards JM, Porter JM: Present status of reversed vein bypass grafting: Five-year results of a modern series. J Vasc Surg 11:193–205, 1990.

254. Donaldson MC, Mannick JA, Whittemore AD: Femoral-distal bypass with in situ greater saphenous vein. Long-term results using the Mills valvulotome. Ann Surg 213:457–464, 1991.

255. Bergamini TM, Towne JB, Bandyk DF, et al: Experience with in situ saphenous vein bypasses during 1981 to 1989: Determinant factors of long-term patency. J Vasc Surg 13:137–147, 1991.

256. Abbott WM, Green RM, Matsumoto T, et al: Prosthetic above-knee femoropopliteal bypass grafting: Results of a multicenter randomized prospective trial. Above-Knee Femoropopliteal Study Group. J Vasc Surg 25:19–28, 1997.

257. Mannick JA, Whittemore AD, Donaldson MC: Clinical and anatomic considerations for surgery in tibial disease and the results of surgery. Circulation 83(Suppl 1):81–85, 1991.

258. Gentile AT, Lee RW, Moneta GL, et al: Results of bypass to the popliteal and tibial arteries with alternative sources of autogenous vein. J Vasc Surg 23:272–279, 1996.

259. Belkin M, Knox J, Donaldson MC, et al: Infrainguinal arterial reconstruction with nonreversed greater saphenous vein. J Vasc Surg 24:957–962, 1996.

260. Alexander JJ, Wells KE, Yuhas JP, et al: The role of composite sequential bypass in the treatment of multilevel infrainguinal arterial occlusive disease. Am J Surg 172:118–122, 1996.

261. Londrey GL, Bosher LP, Brown PW, et al: Infrainguinal reconstruction with arm vein, lesser saphenous vein, and remnants of greater saphenous vein: A report of 257 cases. J Vasc Surg 20:451–456, 1994.

262. Donaldson MC, Mannick JA, Whittemore AD: Causes of primary graft failure after in situ saphenous vein bypass grafting. J Vasc Surg 15:113–118, 1992.

263. Lundell A, Lindblad B, Bergqvist D, et al: Femoropopliteal-crural graft patency is improved by an intensive surveillance program: A prospective randomized study. J Vasc Surg 21:26–33, 1995.

264. Bandyk DF, Seabrook GR, Moldenhauer P, et al: Hemodynamics of vein graft stenosis. J Vasc Surg 8:688–695, 1988.

265. Gentile AT, Mills JL, Gooden MA, et al: Identification of predictors for lower extremity vein graft stenosis. Am J Surg 174:218–221, 1997.

266. Mattos MA, van Bemmelen PS, Hodgson KJ, et al: Does correction of stenoses identified with color duplex scanning improve infrainguinal graft patency? J Vasc Surg 17:54–64, 1993.

267. Buth J, Disselhoff B, Sommeling C, et al. Color-flow duplex criteria for grading stenosis in infrainguinal vein grafts. J Vasc Surg 14:716–726, 1991.

VASCULITIS

268. von Winiwater F: Ueber eine eighenthumliche Form von Endarteritis und Endophlebitis mit Gangran des Fusses. Arch Klin Chir 23:202–226, 1879.

269. Buerger L: Thromboangiitis obliterans: A study of the vascular lesions leading to presenile spontaneous gangrene. Am J Med Sci 136:567–580, 1908.

270. Harten P, Muller-Huelsbeck S, Regensburger D, et al: Multiple organ manifestations in thromboangiitis obliterans (Buerger's disease). A case report. Angiology 47:419–425, 1996.

271. Donatelli F, Triggiani M, Nascimbene S, et al: Thromboangiitis obliterans of coronary and internal thoracic arteries in a young woman. J Thorac Cardiovasc Surg 113:800–802, 1997.

272. Lie JT: Visceral intestinal Buerger's disease. Int J Cardiol 66(Suppl 1):249–256, 1998.

273. Michail PO, Filis KA, Delladetsima JK, et al: Thromboangiitis obliterans (Buerger's disease) in visceral vessels confirmed by angiographic and histological findings. Eur J Vasc Endovasc Surg 16:445–448, 1998.

274. Olin JW, Lie JT: Thromboangiitis obliterans (Buerger's disease). In Loscalzo J, Creager M A, Dzau VJ (eds): Vascular Medicine. ed 2. Boston, Little, Brown, 1996, pp 1033–1049.

275. Olin JW: Thromboangiitis obliterans (Buerger's disease). N Engl J Med, in press.

276. Olin JW, Melia M, Young JR, et al: Prevalence of atherosclerotic renal artery stenosis in patients with atherosclerosis elsewhere. Am J Med 88:46N–51N, 1990.

277. Papa M, Bass A, Adar R, et al.: Autoimmune mechanisms in thromboangiitis obliterans (Buerger's disease): The role of tobacco antigen and the major histocompatibility complex. Surgery 111:527–531, 1992.

278. Lie J T: Thromboangiitis obliterans (Buerger's disease) and smokeless tobacco (letter). Arthritis Rheum 31:812–813, 1988.

279. Adar R, Papa MZ, Halpern Z, et al: Cellular sensitivity to collagen in thromboangiitis obliterans. N Engl J Med 308:1113–1116, 1983.

280. Eichhorn J, Sima D, Lindschau C, et al: Antiendothelial cell antibodies in thromboangiitis obliterans. Am J Med Sci 315:17–23, 1998.

281. Makita S, Nakamura M, Murakami H, et al: Impaired endothelium-dependent vasorelaxation in peripheral vasculature of patients with thromboangiitis obliterans (Buerger's disease). Circulation 94(Suppl 2):211–215, 1996.

282. Lie JT: Thromboangiitis obliterans (Buerger's disease) revisited. Pathol Annu 23:257–291, 1988.

283. Lie JT: The rise and fall and resurgence of thromboangiitis obliterans (Buerger's disease). Acta Pathol Jpn 39:153–158, 1989.

284. Lie JT: Thromboangiitis obliterans (Buerger's disease) in women. Medicine (Baltimore) 66:65–72, 1987.

285. Olin JW, Young JR, Graor RA, et al: The changing clinical spectrum of thromboangiitis obliterans (Buerger's disease). Circulation 82(Suppl 4):3–8, 1990.

286. Allen EV: Thromboangiitis obliterans. Methods of diagnosis of chronic occlusive arterial lesions distal to the wrist with illustrative cases. Am J Med Sci 178:237–244, 1929.

287. Mills JL, Porter JM: Buerger's disease (thromboangiitis obliterans). Ann Vasc Surg 5:570–572, 1991.

288. Shionoya S: Diagnostic criteria of Buerger's disease. Int J Cardiol 66(Suppl 1):243–245, 1998.

289. Papa MZ, Rabi I, Adar R: A point scoring system for the clinical diagnosis of Buerger's disease. Eur J Vasc Endovasc Surg 11:335–339, 1996.

290. Olin JW: Thromboangiitis obliterans (Buerger's disease). In Rutherford RB(ed): Vascular Surgery. 4th ed. Philadelphia, WB Saunders, 2000, pp 350–364.

291. Shigematsu H, Shigematsu K: Factors affecting the long-term outcome of Buerger's disease (thromboangiitis obliterans). Int Angiol 18:58–64, 1999.

292. Fiessinger JN, Schafer M: Trial of iloprost versus aspirin treatment for critical limb ischaemia of thromboangiitis obliterans. The TAO Study. Lancet 335:555–557, 1990.

293. Oral iloprost in the treatment of thromboangiitis obliterans (Buerger's disease): A double-blind, randomised, placebo-controlled trial. The European TAO Study Group. Eur J Vasc Endovasc Surg 15:300–307, 1998.

294. Isner JM, Baumgartner I, Rauh G, et al: Treatment of thromboangiitis obliterans (Buerger's disease) by intramuscular gene transfer of vascular endothelial growth factor: Preliminary clinical results. J Vasc Surg 28:964–973, 1998.

295. Sayin A, Bozkurt AK, Tuzun H, et al: Surgical treatment of Buerger's disease: Experience with 216 patients. Cardiovasc Surg 1:377–380, 1993.

296. Sasajima T, Kubo Y, Inaba M, et al: Role of infrainguinal bypass in Buerger's disease: An eighteen-year experience. Eur J Vasc Endovasc Surg 13:186–192, 1997.

ACUTE LIMB ISCHEMIA

297. Aune S, Trippestad A: Operative mortality and long-term survival of patients operated on for acute lower limb ischaemia. Eur J Vasc Endovasc Surg 15:143–146, 1998.

298. Braithwaite BD, Davies B, Birch PA, et al: Management of acute leg ischaemia in the elderly. Br J Surg 85:217–220, 1998.

299. Panetta T, Thompson JE, Talkington CM, et al: Arterial embolectomy: A 34-year experience with 400 cases. Surg Clin North Am 66:339–353, 1986.

300. Elliott JP Jr, Hageman JH, Szilagyi E, et al: Arterial embolization: Problems of source, multiplicity, recurrence, and delayed treatment. Surgery 88:833–845, 1980.

301. Anton GE, Hertzer NR, Beven EG, et al: Surgical management of popliteal aneurysms. Trends in presentation, treatment, and results from 1952 to 1984. J Vasc Surg 3:125–134, 1986.

302. Working Party on Thrombolysis in the Management of Limb Ischemia. Thrombolysis in the management of lower limb peripheral arterial occlusion—a consensus document. Am J Cardiol 81:207–218, 1998.

303. McNamara TO, Bomberger RA: Factors affecting initial and 6 month patency rates after intraarterial thrombolysis with high dose urokinase. Am J Surg 152:709–712, 1986.

304. McNamara TO, Gardner KR, Bomberger RA, et al: Clinical and angiographic selection factors for thrombolysis as initial therapy for acute lower limb ischemia. J Vasc Interv Radiol 6(Suppl):36–47, 1995.

305. Sullivan KL, Gardiner GA Jr, Kandarpa, K, et al: Efficacy of thrombolysis in infrainguinal bypass grafts. Circulation 83(Suppl 1):99–105, 1991.

306. Gardiner GA Jr, Harrington DP, Koltun W, et al: Salvage of occluded arterial bypass grafts by means of thrombolysis. J Vasc Surg 9:426–431, 1989.

307. Isner JM, Rosenfield K: Redefining the treatment of peripheral artery disease. Role of percutaneous revascularization. Circulation 88:1534–1557, 1993.

308. Meyerovitz MF, Goldhaber SZ, Reagan K, et al: Recombinant tissue-type plasminogen activator versus urokinase in peripheral arterial and graft occlusions: A randomized trial. Radiology 175:75–78, 1990.
309. Pemberton M, Varty K, Nydahl S, et al: The surgical management of acute limb ischaemia due to native vessel occlusion. Eur J Vasc Endovasc Surg 17:72–76, 1999.
310. Wyffels PL, DeBord JR: Increased limb salvage. Distal tibial/peroneal artery thrombectomy/embolectomy in acute lower extremity ischemia. Am Surg 56:468–475, 1990.
311. Fogarty TJ, Chin AK, Olcott CT, et al: Combined thrombectomy and dilation for the treatment of acute lower extremity arterial thrombosis. J Vasc Surg 10:530–533, 1989.
312. Ouriel K, Shortell CK, DeWeese JA, et al: A comparison of thrombolytic therapy with operative revascularization in the initial treatment of acute peripheral arterial ischemia. J Vasc Surg 19:1021–1030, 1994.
313. The STILE trial. Results of a prospective randomized trial evaluating surgery versus thrombolysis for ischemia of the lower extremity. Ann Surg 220:251–266, 1994.
314. Ouriel K, Veith FJ, Sasahara AA: A comparison of recombinant urokinase with vascular surgery as initial treatment for acute arterial occlusion of the legs. Thrombolysis or Peripheral Arterial Surgery (TOPAS) Investigators. N Engl J Med 338:1105–1111, 1998.

ATHEROEMBOLISM

315. Coffman JD: Atheromatous embolism. Vasc Med 1:267–273, 1996.
316. Moolenaar W, Lamers CB: Cholesterol crystal embolization in the Netherlands. Arch Intern Med 156:653–657, 1996.
317. Lie JT: Cholesterol atheromatous embolism. The great masquerader revisited. Pathol Annu 27:17–50, 1992.
318. Fine MJ, Kapoor W, Falanga V: Cholesterol crystal embolization: A review of 221 cases in the English literature. Angiology 38:769–784, 1987.
319. Kealy WF: Atheroembolism. J Clin Pathol 31:984–989, 1978.
320. Cross SS: How common is cholesterol embolism? J Clin Pathol 44:859–861, 1991.
321. Mayo RR, Swartz RD: Redefining the incidence of clinically detectable atheroembolism. Am J Med 100:524–529, 1996.
322. Jones DB, Iannaccone PM: Atheromatous emboli in renal biopsies. An ultrastructural study. Am J Pathol 78:261–276, 1975.
323. Kronzon I, Tunick PA: Atheromatous disease of the thoracic aorta: Pathologic and clinical implications. Ann Intern Med 126:629–637, 1997.
324. Spittell PC, Seward JB, Hallett JW Jr: Mobile thrombi in the abdominal aorta in cases of lower extremity embolic arterial occlusion: Value of extended transthoracic echocardiography. Am Heart J 139:241–244, 2000.
325. Tunick PA, Rosenzweig BP, Katz ES, et al: High risk for vascular events in patients with protruding aortic atheromas: A prospective study. J Am Coll Cardiol 23:1085–1090, 1994.
326. The French Study of Aortic Plaques in Stroke Group. Atherosclerotic disease of the aortic arch as a risk factor for recurrent ischemic stroke. N Engl J Med 334:1216–1221, 1996.
327. Davis K, Kennedy JW, Kemp HG Jr, et al: Complications of coronary arteriography from the Collaborative Study of Coronary Artery Surgery (CASS). Circulation 59:1105–1112, 1979.
328. Ramirez G, O'Neill WM Jr, Lambert R, et al: Cholesterol embolization: A complication of angiography. Arch Intern Med 138:1430–1432, 1978.
329. Drost H, Buis B, Haan D, et al: Cholesterol embolism as a complication of left heart catheterisation. Report of seven cases. Br Heart J 52:339–342, 1984.
330. Colt HG Begg RJ, Saporito JJ, et al: Cholesterol emboli after cardiac catheterization. Eight cases and a review of the literature. Medicine (Baltimore) 67:389–400, 1988.
331. Thadhani RI, Camargo CA Jr, Xavier RJ, et al: Atheroembolic renal failure after invasive procedures. Natural history based on 52 histologically proven cases. Medicine (Baltimore) 74:350–358, 1995.
332. Nasser TK, Mohler ER, 3rd, Wilensky RL, et al: Peripheral vascular complications following coronary interventional procedures. Clin Cardiol 18:609–614, 1995.
333. Sharma PV, Babu SC, Shah PM, et al: Changing patterns of atheroembolism. Cardiovasc Surg 4:573–579, 1996.
334. Kolh PH, Torchiana DF, Buckley MJ: Atheroembolization in cardiac surgery. The need for preoperative diagnosis. J Cardiovasc Surg (Torino) 40:77–81, 1999.
335. Hyman BT, Landas SK, Ashman RF, et al: Warfarin-related purple toes syndrome and cholesterol microembolization. Am J Med 82:1233–1237, 1987.
336. Bols A, Nevelsteen A, Verhaeghe R: Atheromatous embolization precipitated by oral anticoagulants. Int Angiol 13:271–274, 1994.
337. Shapiro LS: Cholesterol embolization after treatment with tissue plasminogen activator (letter). N Engl J Med 321:1270, 1989.
338. Dressler FA, Craig WR, Castello R, et al: Mobile aortic atheroma and systemic emboli: Efficacy of anticoagulation and influence of plaque morphology on recurrent stroke. J Am Coll Cardiol 31:134–138, 1998.
339. Blackshear JL, Zabalgoitia M, Pennock, G, et al: Warfarin safety and efficacy in patients with thoracic aortic plaque and atrial fibrillation. SPAF TEE Investigators. Stroke Prevention and Atrial Fibrillation. Transesophageal echocardiography. Am J Cardiol 83:453–455, 1999.
340. Blankenship JC, Butler M, Garbes A: Prospective assessment of cholesterol embolization in patients with acute myocardial infarction treated with thrombolytic vs conservative therapy. Chest 107:662–668, 1995.
341. Seifert PS, Hugo F, Tranum-Jensen J, et al: Isolation and characterization of a complement-activating lipid extracted from human atherosclerotic lesions. J Exp Med 172:547–557, 1990.
342. Falanga V, Fine MJ, Kapoor WN: The cutaneous manifestations of cholesterol crystal embolization. Arch Dermatol 122:1194–1198, 1986.
343. Dahlberg PJ, Frecentese DF, Cogbill TH: Cholesterol embolism: Experience with 22 histologically proven cases. Surgery 105:737–746, 1989.
344. Rosman HS, Davis TP, Reddy D, et al: Cholesterol embolization: Clinical findings and implications. J Am Coll Cardiol 15:1296–1299, 1990.
345. Morris-Jones W, Preston FE, Greaney M, et al: Gangrene of the toes with palpable peripheral pulses. Ann Surg 193:462–466, 1981.
346. Comerford JA, Broe PJ, Wilson IA, et al: Digital ischaemia and palpable pedal pulses. Br J Surg 74:493–494, 1987.
347. Kakolyris S, Giatromanolaki A, Koukourakis M, et al: Assessment of vascular maturation in non–small cell lung cancer using a novel basement membrane component, LH39: Correlation with p53 and angiogenic factor expression. Cancer Res 59:5602–5607, 1999.
348. Bojar RM, Payne DD, Murphy RE, et al: Surgical treatment of systemic atheroembolism from the thoracic aorta. Ann Thorac Surg 61:1389–1393, 1996.

Chapter 42

Extracardiac Vascular Interventions

SHAUN L. W. SAMUELS · MICHAEL D. DAKE

The exciting development and widespread use of endovascular procedures for managing extracardiac vascular disease are explained by several factors, including rising health care costs, advances in percutaneous catheter technology, and a high level of acceptance by patients of nonoperative interventions for the management of arterial occlusive disease, aneurysms, arterial hemorrhage, neoplastic disease, arterial-venous malformations, and venous disease. In this chapter we provide a review of the experience for each general topic along with the limitations and complications of these procedures. The application of various endovascular techniques, including percutaneous transluminal angioplasty (PTA), stents, and stent-grafts, to this wide spectrum of vascular disease is also addressed. It is beyond the scope of this presentation to discuss percutaneous procedures directed at dialysis access lesions, bypass graft stenoses, abnormalities affecting variant native anatomy, and uncommon causes of vascular disease.

Over the past decade a consensus has evolved regarding the indications and benefits of percutaneous treatment of extracardiac vascular disease. There is now a tremendous enthusiasm and potential for further growth of percutaneous endovascular therapies based on the ease, safety, short recuperation, and long-term results associated with these procedures.

ARTERIAL INTERVENTIONS

From the time of the great Charles Dotter, the father of interventional therapy, on, the focus of this therapy has been trained in on the problem of arterial occlusive disease. Atherosclerotic disease is the leading cause of death in the United States, and its presence in the heart reflects its presence elsewhere. The heart serves as a microcosm of the treatment of atherosclerosis in the periphery. The tools of the trade are essentially the same, and hence no detailed description of stents, thrombolytic agents, mechanical thrombectomy devices, or angioplasty balloons is provided in this chapter (see Chap. 38). Whether in the coronary or extracardiac circulations, the bane of successful intervention is restenosis. For the most part, the approaches to restenosis in the coronary arteries should apply to the periphery. The early results of brachytherapy in the coronaries are promising.[1] Coated stents, local drug therapy, and gene therapy also deserve careful evaluation.

Iliac Interventions

If there is an ideal substrate for percutaneous intervention, it is the iliac artery. The iliac is a large vessel, it is close to the puncture site, and the surgical alternative to iliac interventions is usually a major operation. For all the apparent simplicity of percutaneous treatment, however, closer inspection reveals layers of complexity that make definitive answers about the specifics of the role of iliac intervention elusive. Thus, a brief primer on unresolved issues in the iliacs includes, but is not limited to: (1) surgery versus percutaneous intervention in complex iliac occlusions; (2) primary stenting versus secondary stenting for PTA failure; (3) the role of lesion morphology (i.e., eccentricity, degree of calcification, and tortuosity) in decision-making between PTA and stenting; (4) efficacy of treatment in stenoses versus occlusions; (5) the importance or lack thereof in maintaining the patency of the hypogastrics during interventions; (6) the role of thrombolysis in chronic occlusions; (7) the choice of stent from among a now dizzying variety; (8) the acceptable residual pressure gradient after iliac intervention; (9) the appropriate length of stent for a given lesion length; (10) the maximum lesion length that is appropriate for percutaneous therapy; (11) the optimum strategy for treating lesions at the aortic bifurcation; and (12) the conditions that make it appropriate to treat an iliac lesion through contralateral access. All of these issues have very practical implications on the daily decision-making facing an interventionalist who, in essentially every case involving treatment of the iliac segment, must address each of them in determining the appropriate therapy.

Rarely can the solutions to these problems be found in the literature. More often, one is left to confront them armed only with one's experience and the conflicting dogmas of various experts. Although iliac angioplasty/stenting is technically among the more straightforward arterial interventions, the issues surrounding such a seemingly well-explored territory reveal large gaps in our knowledge. As in many areas, the rapidity of technology development, the multiple competitive stent technologies, the plethora of variables to be controlled, and the many specific questions needing to be answered have conspired to make controlled, randomized studies of percutaneous iliac intervention daunting. At the same time, the absence of such trials will always provide ammunition to the skeptics who dismiss percutaneous iliac therapy as a quick fix.

Iliac angioplasty has been shown safe and effective (Fig. 42-1), with impressive patencies, based on several studies.[2-4] The evidence for the efficacy of iliac stent placement also has been established through the many large series that have been published to date.[5-18] Lack of standardized reporting and vast differences in technique, stents employed, and lesion type have made it difficult to draw conclusions from these studies (Table 42-1). Bosch and Hunink[19] published a meta-analysis of iliac angioplasty and stent placement in an attempt to consolidate the findings of many series to yield meaningful information. It serves both as a

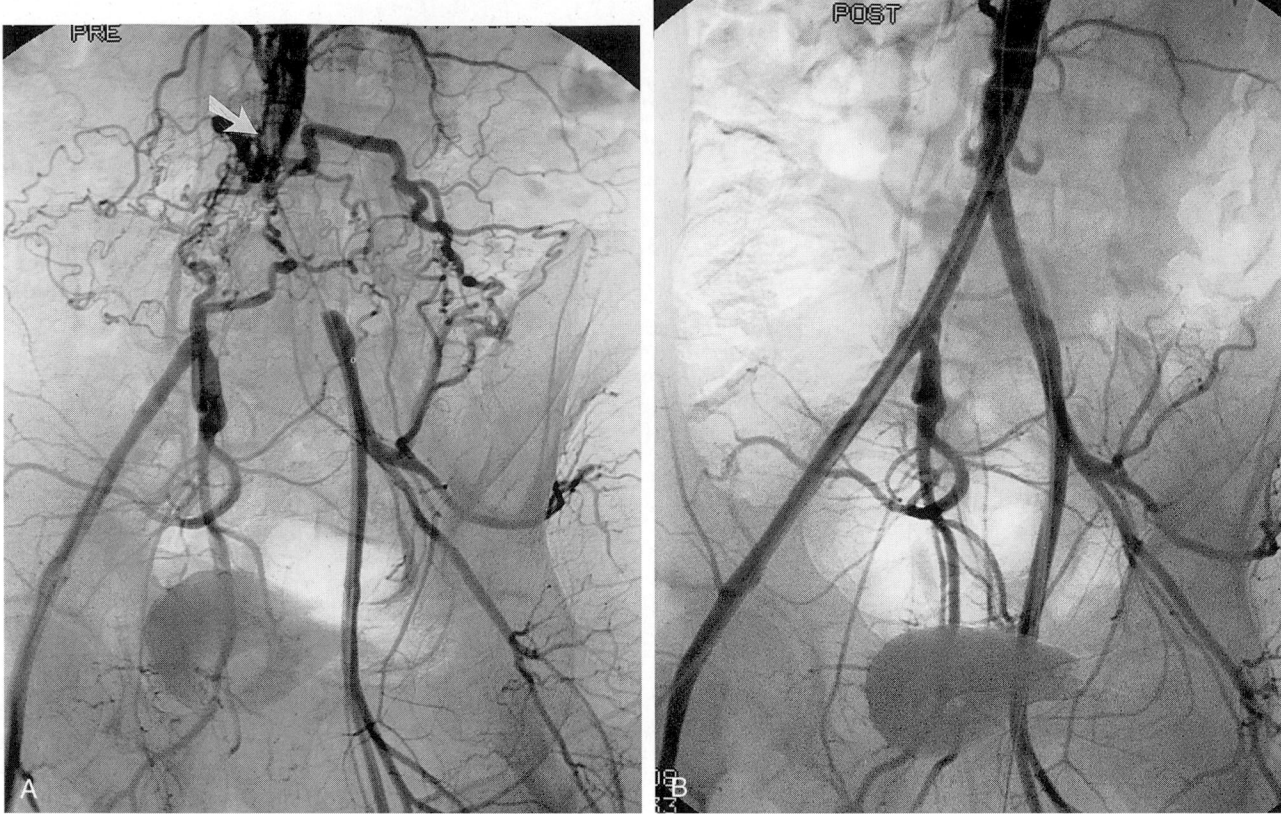

FIGURE 42–1. Iliac artery stent placement. *A,* Initial pelvic arteriogram demonstrates bilateral common iliac artery occlusions in a 52-year-old man with severe bilateral lower extremity claudication. *B,* After bilateral Palmaz stent (Johnson and Johnson, Miami Lakes, FL) placement, final arteriogram demonstrates restoration of normal-caliber common iliac arteries without residual stenosis. No pressure gradient was present after intervention.

useful review of studies done to that date and as a reasonable comparison of PTA with stent placement in the iliacs. The conclusion that there is a 39 percent reduction of late failure with stent placement as opposed to PTA gave comfort to those who intuitively believed that primary stent placement was a superior strategy. Those hopes were deflated by a later cost-effectiveness analysis by the same group[20] based on their meta-analysis[19] and an additional randomized trial of iliac PTA versus stent by the same group.[21] The cost-effectiveness evaluation[20] reveals that PTA with selective stent placement is a more cost-effective strategy than primary stent placement. This conclusion is based on stent and balloon costs in Holland, which the investigators acknowledge is higher than those in the United States. The findings are also based on patients being treated for claudication who are found to have stenotic disease rather than an occlusion. These caveats provide a glimmer of hope for proponents of the primary stent strategy in the United States.

Femoropopliteal Interventions

It is reasonable to question whether atherosclerotic disease of the superficial femoral artery (SFA) should be treated at all. This consideration has enormous implications: approximately 1 million people in the United States develop claudication each year.[22] The vessel may occlude and be asymptomatic in about 10 percent of those who progress to occlusion,[22, 23] or it may result in mild claudication, which improves with walking.[24] The profunda femoris artery shoulders the burden as a collateral in the case of SFA occlusion. The natural history of femoropopliteal (FP) dis-

ease is well documented.[23, 24] In the tabulations of McDaniel and Cronenwett,[23] the 5-year outcome for claudicators is as follows: mortality, 29 percent; need for operation, 25 percent; improved or stable, 55 percent; claudication worse, 16 percent; and amputation, 4 percent. Similar numbers have been confirmed in other published reports.[25] The high mortality in this population reflects the role of peripheral vascular disease as a marker for generalized atherosclerosis. These data, culled from a large number of first-rate studies that for the most part preceded the era of percutaneous therapy, are hardly compelling when used to support arguments for intervention in this population. A walking program may be as effective as more aggressive approaches,[24, 26] although the study of Price and associates[26] found that at 6 years the results of PTA and an exercise program were equivalent in their lack of benefit to the patient. The message has emerged that conservative therapy is appropriate for patients with stable claudication. Intervention is usually warranted for patients with progressive claudication, severe life-style limitation, or critical ischemia (rest pain, tissue loss); it is this population that gives rise to the debate over appropriate treatment.

Approaching the field of PTA of the FP segment invites confusion. A wide array of reports have come from many quarters with disparate results. Reporting methods and definitions vary. The word "patency", for example, takes on all shades of meaning, prompting some authors to discuss at considerable length what is meant by the term. PTA in the FP segment has been accepted by most, albeit begrudgingly by some, as a useful tool in the treatment of chronic lower extremity ischemia. The appropriate use of this procedure remains an issue clouded by the glaring disparity in quoted patency rates in the literature.

▶ TABLE 42–1. RESULTS OF ILIAC ARTERY STENT PLACEMENT

AUTHOR	REFERENCE	YEAR	NO. PATIENTS	LESIONS TREATED	PERCENT WITH OCCLUSIONS	TECHNICAL SUCCESS (%)	ABI PRE	ABI POST	MEAN LESION LENGTH (cm)	STENT USED	PRIMARY PATENCY AT 2 YEARS (%)	CUMULATIVE PATENCY AT 2 YEARS (%)
Murphy, T*	14	1998	65	90	31	97	0.62	0.9	5.6	P,W	69	80
Tetteroo	21	1998	143	187	9	NA	0.78	NA	NA	P	NA	71.3
Reyes	18	1997	59	61	100	92	0.51	0.9	10	W	73	88
Dyet	17	1997	72	72	100	93	NA	NA	6.7	A	85	85
Vorwerk	6	1996	109	118	0	100	0.58	0.92	3	W	88	93
Spoval	8	1996	95	101	43	99	0.71	0.93	NA	W	65	87
Murphy, T	13	1996	66	94	41	91	0.51	0.76	6.5	W	53	82
Henry	5	1995	184	184	9	100	0.57	0.98	3.15	P	91	96
Vorwerk	16	1995	127	103	100	79	0.48	0.89	5.1	W	83	90
Martin	9	1995	140	171	9	97	0.64	0.86	3.3	W	71	86
Murphy	10	1995	83	108	21.4	100	NA	NA	4	P	87.5[†]	97.5[†]
Vorwerk	7	1992	125	125	50	98	NA	NA	4	W	NA	86.5
Palmaz	12	1992	486	567	13.5	NA	0.62	0.8	3.2	P	NA	NA

* Data from this series partially included in reference 13.
† At latest follow-up interval.
A = all types; ABI = ankle-brachial index; NA = not available; P = Palmaz; W = Wallstent

Fortunately, the amassed body of experience is large enough to allow reasonable conclusions about indications for FP PTA. An exhaustive analysis of PTA and surgical revascularization is provided by Hunink and coworkers,[27] who set out to establish when PTA and when bypass surgery is the preferred method of FP level revascularization. This analysis in turn was based on data from a prior meta-analysis by the same investigators[28] that summarized the results of 7 series of PTA and 10 series of bypass surgery to determine patency rates. The metric used to evaluate outcome in this study is the quality-adjusted life-year (QALY). The data were deemed appropriate or not based on the reporting methods used, and only those studies adhering to the chosen reporting criteria were included. Several large series, therefore, were excluded.[29] Using a theoretical model, the authors determined that, for a 65-year-old man with life style–limiting claudication or chronic critical ischemia (tissue loss or rest pain) and a *stenotic* lesion in the FP segment, PTA was the more cost-effective strategy. For the same cohort with claudication and an *occlusion*, PTA was also the optimal strategy. For chronic critical ischemia and FP occlusion, bypass surgery is the optimal initial strategy. The population is narrowly defined and the results based on assumptions, but the methods employed in this analysis were stringent. This generalized conclusion notwithstanding, application of such rules in individual patients, with a host of medical and social factors influencing treatment choices, may be extremely difficult.

The degree to which anatomical and technical factors sway one in choosing a method of revascularization cannot be overestimated. The larger series include subgroup analyses of impressive specificity. For example, the series by Capek and colleagues[30] breaks down the data in terms of presenting symptoms, risk factors, lesion number and distribution, lesion length and severity, lesion characteristics (calcification, eccentricity, irregularity), and runoff status. Life table analyses are performed on several variables. Those factors having a statistically significant impact on outcome included presence of other vascular disease, diabetes, severity of presenting symptoms, eccentricity of lesion, degree of stenosis, and lesion length. The effect of lesion length is further subdivided, with all the permutations, among lesions of 0 to 2 cm, 2 to 5 cm, 5 to 10 cm, and larger than 10 cm. Comparisons among all these groups reveal a significant difference in outcome between lesions 0 to 2 cm and those larger than 10 cm and between those 2 to 5 cm and those larger than 10 cm. Given the multiplicity of factors analyzed, it is striking that the greatest statistical significance ($p < 0.001$) was found for presence of a palpable pulse at the conclusion of the procedure as a predictor of good outcome. This finding is highly reassuring to those of us for whom the first move after performing SFA PTA is to check for a pedal pulse by physical examination. Interestingly, if technical failures are omitted from the numbers for interventional treatment of FP occlusions, there is no statistical difference in patency between stenosis and occlusion. The 5-year patency of 42 percent for FP PTA is comparable with other recent large series,[31, 32] in which secondary patencies range from 38 to 45 percent. The complication rate for FP PTA is about 10 percent.[25, 33] Of these, only about 2 percent require surgical intervention and 0.2 percent result in death.[25] The specific techniques of PTA are rarely a focus of various studies, although differences in technique may account for the wide variation in patency. Proper balloon sizing and balloon length are important factors in angioplasty success, but they are seldom described in sufficient detail to be of use to the reader. In addition, some adjunctive techniques, such as prolonged balloon inflation to improve the result following suboptimal initial PTA, have been published.[34]

The role of stents in the FP segment is uncertain. One large study by Henry and associates[5] reported a 4-year secondary patency rate of 95 percent for SFA stents. These results have not been duplicated by others.[9, 35] The consensus appears to be that stents are only warranted for salvage in the FP segment for a PTA failure.[9]

Infrapopliteal Interventions

Anatomy, the limitations of technology, and a misplaced sense of futility have until recently kept the infrapopliteal vessels beyond the reach of the interventionist. Anatomy continues to be an obstacle, whereby occlusion of the main conduit, the FP segment, thwarts efforts to treat lesions below the knee. As for equipment limitations, the balloon technology has improved immensely and multiple low-profile, highly flexible balloon catheters are now available on long shafts to access the trifurcation vessels. Digital angiography provides excellent anatomical detail and superb real-time fluoroscopic guidance enhanced by angiographic image overlay ("roadmapping"); and steerable guidewires, with liberal use of intraarterial vasodilators, have allowed access to the ankle and beyond.

The nihilistic attitude adopted by some when treating infrapopliteal disease does not hold up to scrutiny. Usually called on in a last ditch effort at limb salvage, after surgery has been ruled out or failed, tibial angioplasty is performed on a skewed population of those with the most severe critical ischemia, facing imminent amputation, and frequently having the most significant comorbid conditions. Such heroic interventions are occasionally doomed to failure by the underlying anatomy but attempted nonetheless, the interventionalist responding to pressure from the referring surgeon or from the patient to salvage the limb. In spite of these obstacles, many series report an impressive limb salvage rate given the circumstances. Saab and coworkers[36] reported on 14 tibial PTA procedures with technical success in 10, of which seven patients were spared amputation. Bakal and colleagues,[37] in a series of 53 patients, achieved a successful clinical response in 67 percent of patients overall, 85 percent of whom were diabetic, and in 97 percent of patients in whom straight line flow to the foot was restored through PTA. The series of Matsi and colleagues[38] had a technical success rate of 83 percent of 84 limbs treated for tibial disease, with a limb salvage rate of 63 percent at 2 years among those in whom one to three calf vessel runoff was restored. Schwarten reported a 2-year limb salvage rate of 83 percent in his series of 96 patients.[39] His series imposed restrictions on suitability for angioplasty: a maximum of five lesions and a maximum occlusion length of 5 cm. Other large series[40, 41] also report respectable limb salvage rates.

There are those who still challenge the appropriateness of infrapopliteal angioplasty.[42, 43] A vigorous defense is delivered by Bakal and coworkers,[44] who offer an excellent review of the literature and rebuttal of the juxtaposed submission by Fraser and associates.[42] There is agreement that uniform reporting standards and improved patient selection would aid in analysis of the published data and that a controlled randomized trial would be helpful in determining the cost-effectiveness of PTA versus surgery for infrapopliteal disease. Such trials are more easily designed than done, as partisans of one modality or the other often have little enthusiasm for enrolling patients.

Aortic Interventions

The large caliber of the aorta can mask significant atherosclerotic disease. Stenotic disease, resulting in a pressure gradient, is therefore uncommon, especially in a location not contiguous with the aortic bifurcation.

Reasonable concerns about angioplasty or stenting the infrarenal abdominal aorta, where vessel rupture could be rapidly fatal, have not been validated by the few series thus far published. Hallisey and coworkers[45] reported a series of 14 patients in which 100 percent technical success was achieved, with clinical success in 93 percent and no significant complications.

Infrarenal aortic stent placement was reported in a small series by Long and colleagues,[46] also achieving a 0 percent morbidity rate. The clinical success in the series of seven patients was more difficult to deduce because of associated iliac segment disease. Comparison of aortic PTA and stenting was made through analysis of a subgroup of the SCVIR Transluminal Angioplasty and Revascularization (STAR) registry.[47] Stent placement, at least in the short term, bestowed no clinical benefit in the retrospective analysis of 25 patients.

Renal Artery Interventions

(See also Chap. 48)

Several aspects of renovascular disease (RVD) make its treatment unique among those discussed here. The outcome measures are systemic physiological parameters (blood pressure, serum creatinine concentration) rather than improvement of a specific symptom. As paired organs, often with multiple arteries feeding each, the kidneys may play a sort of anatomical shell game, through which it may be difficult to determine which kidney or which artery is the culprit in a hypertensive patient. To complicate matters, renal artery stenosis (RAS) has a domino effect, whereby the stenotic lesion provokes a humoral response leading to hypertension and this hypertension proceeds to nephropathy in the seemingly uninvolved kidney. Furthermore, in addition to eliciting a hyperreninemic response, decreased blood flow to the kidney causes a separate ischemic nephropathy, leading to a loss of glomeruli and renal mass. Ischemia often causes shrinkage of the affected kidney. It is these secondary effects of RAS that probably lead to the occasionally tepid responses to interventional therapy. The damage to the kidney has already been done, and the intervention merely retards further deterioration. On the other hand, somewhat mysteriously, patients with severe RAS, involving one or both kidneys, may be normotensive and have normal function. Other factors, such as renal size, differential function, and the importance of nonatherosclerotic stenosis (fibromuscular dysplasia, Takayasu's arteritis), further distinguish RAS from stenotic disease elsewhere in the arterial system.

RVD is common, occurring in 27 percent of the population evaluated arteriographically for atherosclerotic disease in the lower extremities, in whom RVD was unexpected.[48] Given the prevalence of hypertension and the aging population, this subgroup constitutes a large cohort. Furthermore, the rapid progression of disease with deterioration of renal function is documented in the same study.[48] Aortorenal bypass surgery produces good clinical results, but at the cost of relatively high morbidity, length of hospital stay, and cost.

Renal angioplasty and stent placement have emerged as elegant solutions to the problems imposed by RVD (Fig. 42–2). Numerous studies have been done to date supporting the effectiveness of percutaneous intervention for RAS.[49–63] The results of several of the more recent series on renal artery stent placement may be found in Table 42–2. Many of the findings of these studies have also been summarized in the excellent review article by Rees and associates,[64] which also includes data from the U.S. multicenter trial of stents in renal arteries. The data presented therein are striking: the technical success for renal stent placement approaches 100 percent benefit; achieved in 61 percent of patients treated for hypertension and improvement or stabilization of renal function in 70 percent of patients after stenting. The beneficial effects of stent placement on azotemia are particularly well displayed in a series by Harden and associates,[51] in which reciprocal serum creatinine plots dramatically flatten at the time of stent placement. One recent trial deemed the effectiveness of renal artery angio-

plasty vs. antihypertensive drug therapy similar.[64a] However, the follow-up of these patients was limited to 12 months, the use of stents does not reflect current practice, and there was a high degree of "cross-over" to PTCA from the drug-treated group, tempering the ability to generalize these results.[64b, 64c]

With regard to the issue of angioplasty versus stenting, a recent randomized study by van de Ven and colleagues[65] suggests that primary renal artery stenting is a superior strategy for ostial atherosclerotic RAS when compared to angioplasty with selective stent placement for angioplasty failure. The relative roles of angioplasty and stent placement in *nonostial* atherosclerotic RAS are not as clear-cut and probably favor initial angioplasty with selective stenting. One recent retrospective analysis[66] comparing renal PTA, renal stenting, and aortorenal bypass surgery provides evidence that percutaneous therapy is more cost effective and that PTA is probably the procedure of choice in nonostial RAS. In renal stent procedures, the complication rate hovers around 20 percent, including both major and minor complications.[67] The complication rate depends, however, on operator experience.[64] Aspects of this procedure aided by operator experience include exercising judgment in case selection, choice of access, what procedure to perform, and when to desist.

In summary, it stands to reason that improvement of renal blood flow is desirable, not only to improve function and ameliorate hypertension but also to spare renal parenchyma. It can be argued that early intervention for RAS may be warranted even *before* azotemia has occurred and in normotensive patients. Although this is far from proven, and renal intervention in the absence of these known indications is often eschewed, delaying renal artery interventions until clear end-organ damage has been done seems analogous to allowing asymptomatic patients with carotid disease to progress to stroke before action is taken. Clearly, the timing of intervention in this context warrants careful study.

Visceral Artery Interventions

Occlusive disease of the visceral vessels does not often lead to mesenteric ischemia, owing primarily to the redundancy in the system. Multiple collateral pathways exist among the celiac artery, superior mesenteric artery (SMA), and inferior mesenteric artery (IMA). When mesenteric ischemia does occur, it is rarely thought of a priori because the symptoms mimic those of peptic ulcer disease and because the frequent accompanying weight loss usually precipitates a work-up for malignancy. A careful history, however, usually reveals that patients maintain their appetites but experience such excruciating pain after eating that they avoid food altogether.

Patients with the classic symptoms and endoscopic evidence of bowel ischemia have a high likelihood of having significant stenotic disease of at least two of three mesenteric vessels on angiography.[68] If a single vessel is involved, however, it is usually the SMA, which is almost invariably involved when patients have confirmed visceral ischemia. It should be noted that both computed tomographic angiography and magnetic resonance angiography are of sufficient quality to be used as screening tests for stenotic disease of the visceral vessels. Surgical treatment of this disease has a high incidence of morbidity, given the patients' generally advanced age and diffuse atherosclerotic disease. Mateo and coworkers[69] reported an 8 percent mortality rate and a 45 percent complication rate among 85 patients in their series. These were similar to numbers reported by Kihara and colleagues.[70]

The common refrain is again sounded that less invasive

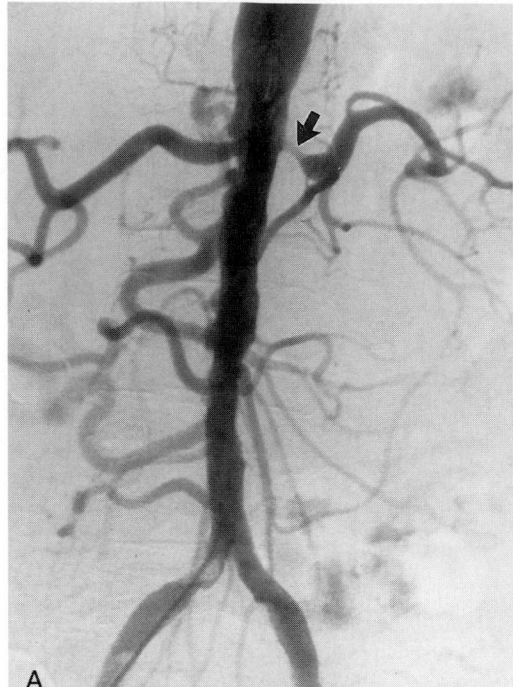

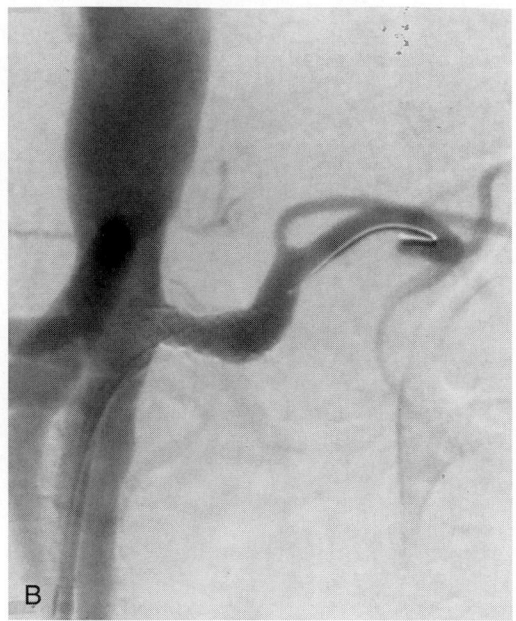

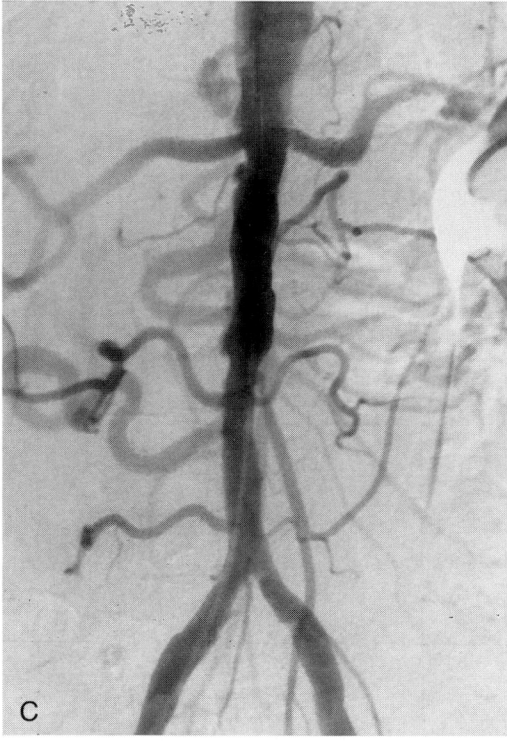

FIGURE 42–2. Renal artery stent placement. *A,* Initial renal arteriogram demonstrates a critical left renal artery ostial stenosis in a 48-year-old man with renal insufficiency and hypertension. *B,* Arteriogram obtained after stent placement demonstrates no significant residual stenosis. No pressure gradient was detectable after stent placement. *C,* The patient also received a stent in the right renal artery and was able to be taken off dialysis with a creatinine level stabilized in the 3 to 4 mg/dl range.

therapy should go a long way toward improving on these high rates of surgical morbidity (Fig. 42–3). To that end, several series of both angioplasty[68, 71–74] and stent placement (Table 42–3)[75] in the visceral vessels have demonstrated a high degree of technical success and clinical effectiveness. The complication rate and the mortality rate are not inconsequential, although both are lower than that presented in surgical series. A skewing of the populations can be seen as a result of patient selection, with patients undergoing percutaneous therapy if deemed poor operative candidates. This is the case in the series by Allen and associates, for example. The results of percutaneous therapy might well have been even more impressive were all patients with mesenteric ischemia, irrespective of comorbidities, given that option.

Supraaortic Interventions

The treatment of occlusive disease of the brachiocephalic vessels has followed the typical progression from surgical management, to PTA, to stent placement, all within the past decade. Percutaneous intervention has been advocated as the primary treatment for symptomatic subclavian artery stenosis or occlusion.[76, 77] Treatment of common carotid lesions is somewhat more problematic, especially when combined with carotid endarterectomy at the bifurcation.[78] The treatment of carotid bifurcation lesions by stent placement is addressed below. The innominate artery tends to be included in reports of subclavian artery intervention,[78] although separate reports of innominate stenting contain excellent results.[79, 80]

▶ TABLE 42-2. RESULTS OF RENAL ARTERY STENT PLACEMENT IN SEVERAL RECENT SERIES

AUTHOR	REFERENCE	YEAR	PATIENTS	ARTERIES TREATED	STENT TYPE	OSTIAL LESIONS (%)	TECHNICAL SUCCESS (%)	HYPERTENSION CURE (%)	HYPERTENSION BENEFIT (%)	AZOTEMIA IMPROVED (%)	AZOTEMIA STABILIZED (%)	MAJOR COMPLICATIONS (%)	30-DAY MORTALITY (%)
Rodriguez-Lopez	59	1999	108	125	P	66	97.6	11	68	0	100	1.6	1.6
Rees	64	1999	123	296	P	80	98	3	61	37	37	NA	2.7
Xue	66	1999	39	45	P/W	23	93	10	72	35	50	15	0
Dorros	61	1998	163	202	P	NA	99	1	42	35	36	14	1.8
Tuttle	62	1998	129	148	P	100	98	0	55	15	81	4.1	3.1
Rundback	50	1998	45	54	P	80	94	NA	NA	17.5	52.5	4.4	4.4
Harden	51	1997	32	33	P	NA	100	NA	67	34	34	18.6	3.1
Boisclair	58	1997	33	35	P	54	100	6	67	41	35	21	0
Blum	60	1997	68	74	P	100	100	16	78	0	100	0	0
Henry	54	1996	59	64	P	53	100	18	75	20	NA	3.4	0
van de Ven	49	1995	24	28	P	100	100	0	69	36	64	8.3	0
Hennequin	57	1994	21	21	W	33	100	14	86	17	50	19	0

The follow-up intervals for the various outcome parameters are highly variable and are omitted here for clarity. Interested readers may find this information in the individual cited references.
NA = not available; P = Palmaz; W = Wallstent

▶ TABLE 42-3. RESULTS OF INTERVENTION FOR VISCERAL ISCHEMIA

AUTHOR	REFERENCE	YEAR	PATIENTS	TECHNICAL SUCCESS (%)	CLINICAL SUCCESS (%)	PRIMARY PATENCY (%)	SECONDARY PATENCY (%)	MEAN FOLLOW-UP (mo)	MAJOR COMPLICATIONS (%)	DEATHS (%)
Hallisey	71	1995	16	88	75	75	75	28	0	6
Matsumoto	68	1995	19	79	80	83	92	25	16	0
Maspes	73	1998	23	90	77	88	100	27	0	0
Allen	72	1996	19	95	79	NA	92	39	5	5
Sheeran*	75	1999	12	92	NA	74	83	16	0	8

* Stent study.
NA = not available.

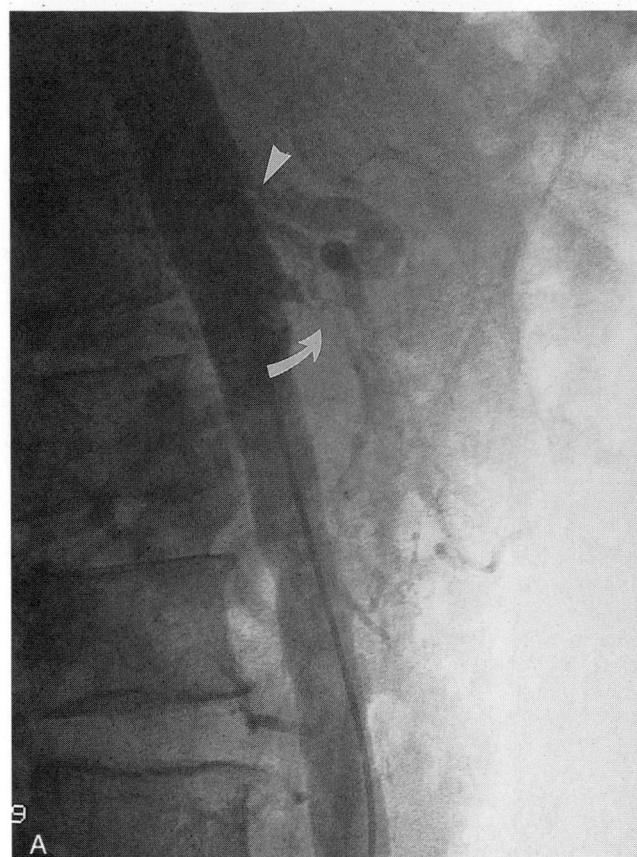
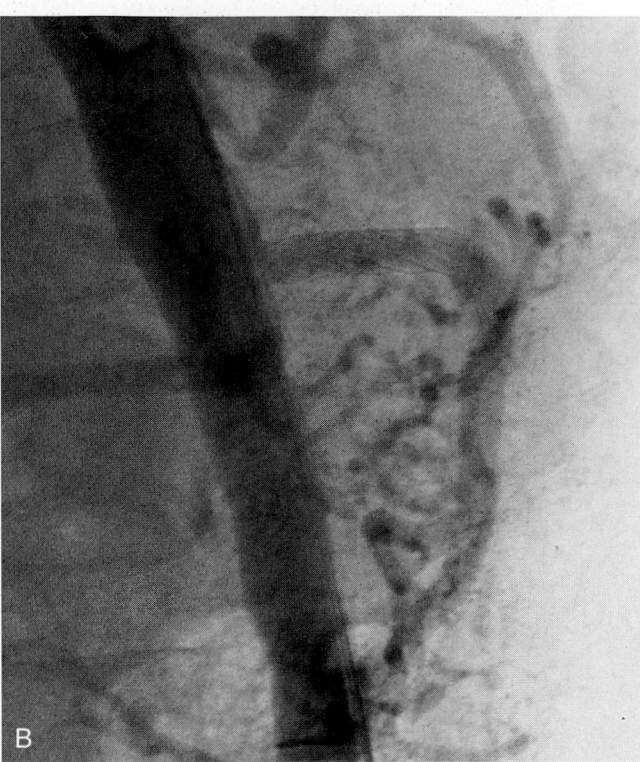

FIGURE 42–3. Recanalization and stent placement for superior mesenteric artery (SMA) occlusion in a 78-year-old man with recent 30-lb. weight loss, severe postprandial pain, and food avoidance. *A,* Lateral abdominal aortogram demonstrates occlusion of the SMA 4 mm beyond its origin. Faint reconstitution of the SMA can be seen (arrowhead). Severe stenosis at the origin of the celiac axis can also be seen (curved arrow). *B,* After recanalization and primary stent placement, antegrade flow in the SMA has been restored without significant residual stenosis. The patient's symptoms resolved immediately, and he gained back much of the weight he lost.

Crucial to patient selection in the treatment of subclavian occlusive disease is establishing the presence of symptoms referable to the lesion. When proximal subclavian occlusion occurs it is often asymptomatic. In such cases, intervention is not warranted. Upper extremity claudication and vertebrobasilar insufficiency are the most common presenting symptoms.[78, 81, 82, 82a] Technique for recanalization of occlusions may involve femoral and/or brachial access. Results of PTA alone in the subclavian show a clinical success rate of 68 to 92 percent.[76, 82, 83] For subclavian stent placement, clinical success ranged from 83 to 100 percent.[78, 84–86a] The much-feared complication of embolization into the vertebral artery has only rarely occurred in these series. Some protection from this is naturally afforded by the delay in reversal of flow in the vertebral artery after antegrade subclavian flow is reestablished.

A separate and expanding indication for left subclavian intervention follows the advent of left internal mammary artery (LIMA) coronary artery bypass grafting (CABG). Several case reports and small series have been published describing the syndrome of coronary steal and its treatment by percutaneous therapy, with generally excellent results.[87–95]

Common carotid artery interventions are uncommon and are usually done in conjunction with planned carotid bifurcation surgery to guarantee adequate postoperative inflow. PTA or stenting of the proximal common carotid is most frequently performed intraoperatively with direct carotid puncture. In this fashion the technical difficulty introduced by navigating from the groin is obviated and distal control

of the vessel may be obtained to prevent embolization at the time of intervention.

Vertebral artery PTA and stenting are rarely performed. The single small series in the literature does, however, demonstrate an adjunctive role for vertebral artery stenting.[96]

Carotid Interventions

One look at the inside of a carotid bifurcation gives one a good idea why surgeons are skeptical about carotid angioplasty and stenting. The plaque is usually an ulcerated, pockmarked, craggy mess, with friable wisps of thrombus and tenuously attached fronds of atheroma. The suggestion that someone should pass a large-caliber catheter through this figurative minefield, inflate a balloon, and then deploy a stent over the path of destruction seems unthinkable. Contrary to expectation, however, this procedure is feasible and unexpectedly safe (Fig. 42–4). As with most procedures in interventional radiology, what remains to be seen is how well it works, and for how long.

Few areas have provoked more controversy. Editorials concerning carotid interventions flood the literature.[97–109] Several things about carotid interventions specifically make it a hotbed of controversy. Compare it, for example, to iliac interventions. Unlike iliac percutaneous interventions, those in the carotid eliminate the need for an operation of very *low* morbidity and mortality.[110–113] As opposed to aortofemoral surgery, hospital stays for carotid surgery are gen-

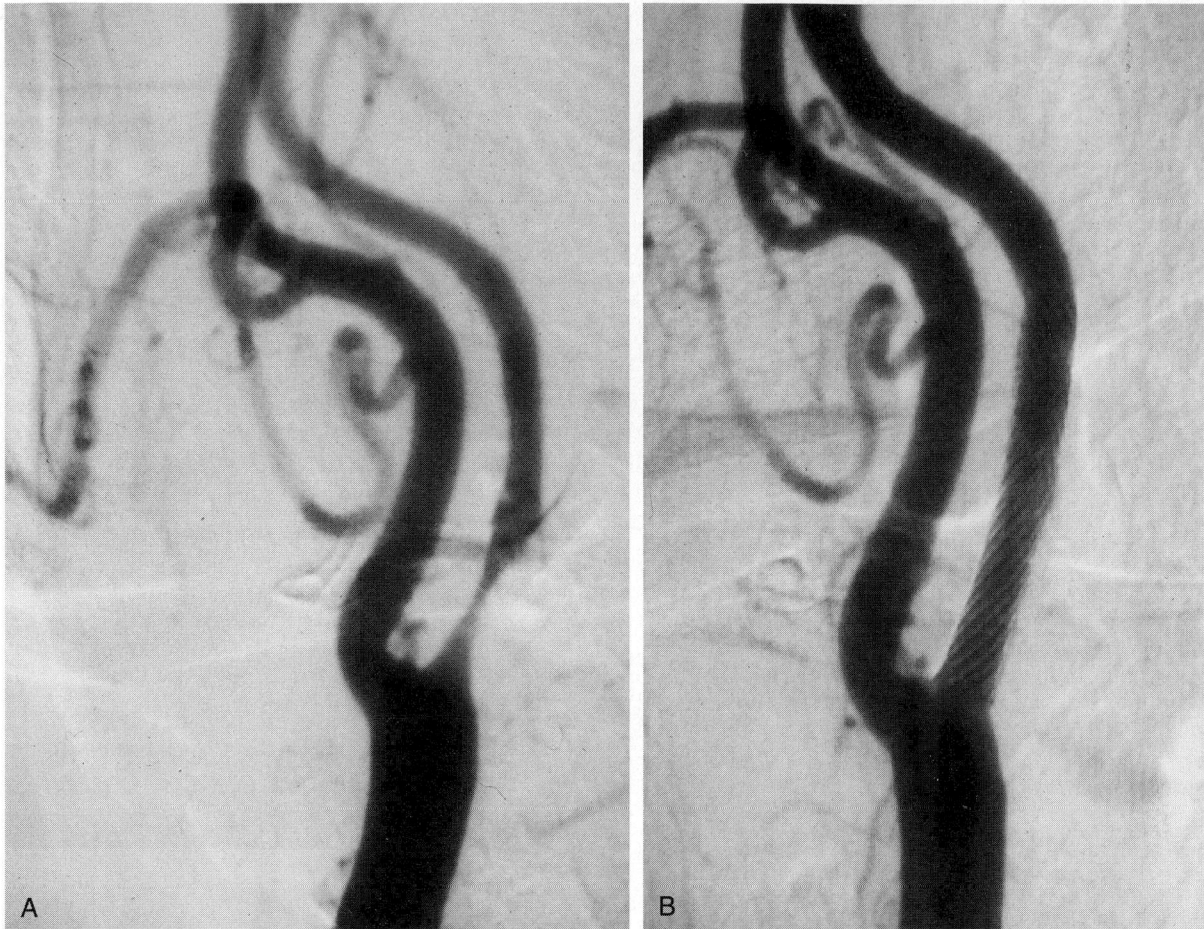

FIGURE 42–4. Internal carotid artery stent placement. *A,* Common carotid arteriogram identifies smooth concentric narrowing of the proximal internal carotid artery in a patient with a history of two neurologic episodes corresponding to the distribution of this vessel. *B,* After placement of a self-expanding Wallstent, no residual stenosis is noted.

erally short. In the iliacs, intervention does not burn any surgical bridges. In the carotid, stent placement makes surgery at the very least difficult and perhaps impossible. Emboli precipitated by iliac interventions can usually be managed percutaneously and rarely have long-term sequelae. In the carotid, emboli can be catastrophic, for obvious reasons. Fear of downstream embolization has led, in fact, to a burgeoning industry in various filtering or blocking devices deployed distal to the carotid bifurcation during interventions to trap emboli.

Careful scrutiny of the carotid endarterectomy trials[112, 113] reveals that a large number of patients were excluded from them for a variety of comorbid conditions. It is often precisely these patients who are offered carotid stent placement, and it is therefore not surprising that the complication rate may be higher in this population. Furthermore, stent technology is evolving, techniques are improving, and operator skills have been honed. As a result, it stands to reason that results of carotid stent placement will only improve. There have been few recent innovations in carotid surgery. At the same time, those series that have involved carotid stents in high-risk patients have demonstrated favorable results, certainly better than those of the medical alternative.[114–116] One aborted randomized trial,[117] in which 5 of 7 patients suffered strokes in the early stent experience, is difficult to reconcile with the superb results published in other series.[118, 119] Clinical and angiographic criteria may help in selecting patients at risk for complications of carotid interventions.[119a] In one large series, Yadav and colleagues treated 126 carotid arteries in 107 consecutive patients. The patients were often in a risk category that would have excluded them from the North American Symptomatic Carotid Endarterectomy Trial (NASCET)[112] or Asymptomatic Carotid Atherosclerosis Study (ACAS)[113] by virtue of their carotid arterial anatomy and/or preexisting medical conditions. Despite this relatively high risk group, the overall 30-day stroke plus death rate was 9.3 percent, and the major stroke plus death rate was 2.8 percent. These numbers compare favorably with surgical complication rates sufficiently well to justify further investigation.

A randomized trial of carotid stenting versus carotid endarterectomy has recently been funded by the National Institutes of Health. The Carotid Revascularization Endarterectomy versus Stent (CREST) trial has enrolled sites and will soon be under way. Such a controlled, randomized trial should help clarify the role of percutaneous carotid intervention, an issue that involves hundreds of thousands of patients each year and has huge repercussions as a major health care concern.

Disease of the Aorta

Aortic Dissection (See also Chap. 40)

There is currently much discussion among vascular interventionalists over the percutaneous therapy for aortic dissection, an unusual but potentially devastating complication of arterial disease. Even the most vehement naysayers concerning endovascular therapies must acknowledge the inroads interventionalists have made on the management of aortic dissection. Surgical results in this disease are mediocre; and although medical control of hypertension is of great importance still in preventing extension of the dissection, current data support the role of interventional treatment of the ischemic complications. Aortic dissection frequently causes acute ischemia in the renal, mesenteric, and lower extremity vascular beds.

The largest series published to date is that of Slonim and associates,[120] in which 40 patients were treated for ischemic complications of aortic dissection by stent placement and/or percutaneous balloon fenestration of the dissection flap. Ninety-three percent were successfully revascularized, although 25 percent died within 30 days, most often due to irreversible ischemic damage acquired before revascularization. These results were closely matched by those of Williams and colleagues.[121]

The latest innovation in the treatment of acute aortic dissection is the use of stent-grafts to cover the primary entry tear.[122] In one series of 19 patients, 76 percent had restoration of flow to the ischemic bed by placement of the stent-graft alone and there was 100 percent technical success in stent-graft placement.

INTERVENTIONS FOR ANEURYSMAL DISEASE

The covered stent, or stent-graft, represents the next great area of promise in minimally invasive therapy. At present, it cannot be referred to as *percutaneous* therapy, because currently available devices require a cutdown for arterial access. However, with the technology advancing at a rapid pace, minification of the equipment to percutaneously manageable sizes is inevitable. The current reservations over this approach involve the training of individuals who should place stent-grafts and technical limitations of current devices. Increasingly, case reports of late endoleaks (see later) have called into question the long-term viability of the technology in its current form. As in other arenas of vascular intervention, more comparative data will be required to evaluate the role of surgical and interventional approaches to abdominal aortic aneurysm treatment.

ABDOMINAL AORTIC ANEURYSM. Abdominal aortic aneurysm (AAA) is a significant health care issue in terms of the prevalence of the problem and the expense to treat it (see Chap. 40). As the population ages, and for unknown other reasons, the incidence of AAA is increasing.[123, 124] Standard therapy, open surgical excision of the aneurysm, is well tolerated in most patients, but significant morbidity occurs in a large percentage of patients.[125] The pressure applied by increased health care costs has driven physicians to seek less invasive, less morbid, and less costly procedures to meet this demand. The standard set by surgical treatment, however, is a high one, and surgeons have had about 40 years to perfect their craft.

The patent literature on endoluminal aneurysm repair dates to 1979, but it was not until Parodi's first series in humans that interest broadened in this approach.[126] Recognizing the aforementioned pressures and the presence of an untapped market, industry and vascular specialists have moved rapidly to address the need. As a result, a daunting profusion of devices has become available. Stiff competition has emerged to enroll patients in trials of various devices. The lay press has entered the fray, and many patients

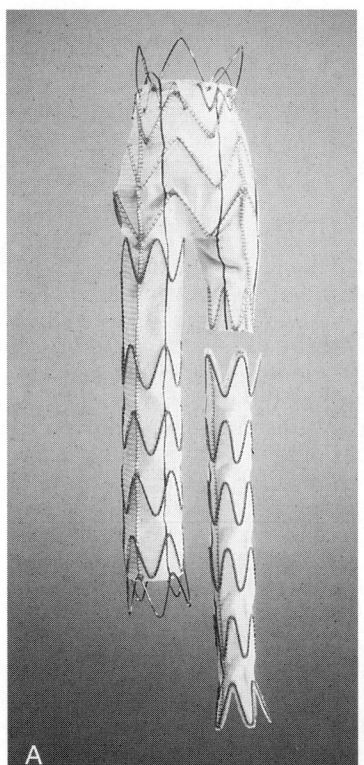
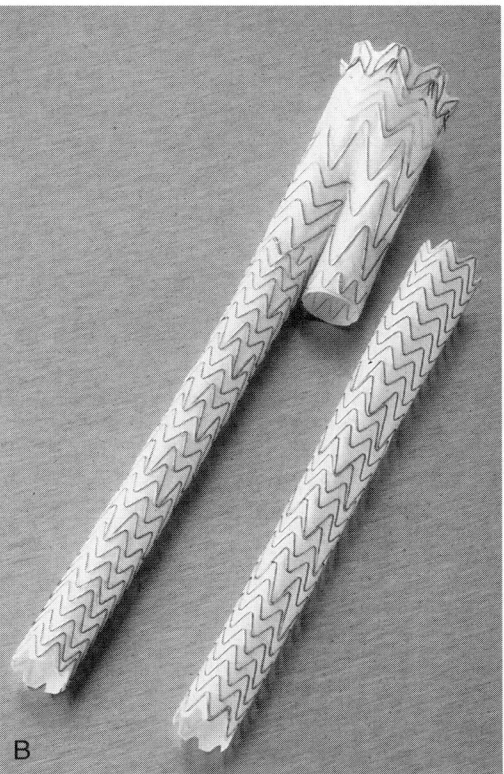
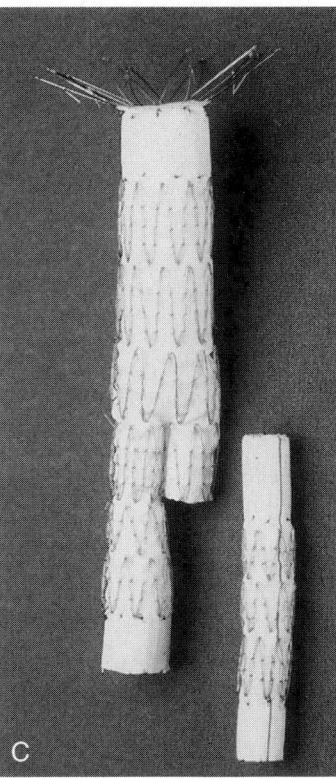

FIGURE 42–5. Modular, bifurcated endovascular grafts for the treatment of abdominal aortic aneurysm. *A,* Talent endograft (World Medical, Inc./AVE Inc., Sunrise, FL) is constructed with a series of serpentine nitinol self-expandable springs attached to a polyester surgical graft by a continuous series of polyester sutures. The Talent system allows for transrenal fixation of the device using a proximal bare stent design. This may help to secure the position of the endograft in patients with short (less than 15 mm) infrarenal aneurysm necks. *B,* Excluder endograft (W. L. Gore and Associates, Inc., Sunnyvale, CA) is composed of thin-wall polytetrafluoroethylene graft material that lines a self-expanding nitinol stent exoskeleton. The modular bifurcated design includes proximal hooks to provide enhanced fixation to the proximal neck and a polytetrafluoroethylene cuff to prevent leaks. *C,* Zenith prosthesis (Cook, Inc., Bloomington, IN) is constructed with a series of Z-stents and polyester graft material. This device utilizes a proximal uncovered stent framework with hooks to secure attachment of the endograft to the aortic wall and allow treatment of relatively short proximal aneurysm necks.

express interest in innovative and less invasive alternatives to surgery.

Whereas open surgical repair has stood the test of time, current follow-up of endoluminal repair is necessarily shorter, with measures of effectiveness given for 2-year, rather than 10-year, follow-up. However, prolonged follow-up of patients with endoluminal AAA repair will help establish the utility of such procedures with time.

The natural history of untreated AAA is fairly well documented,[127] and its unpredictability has led to a gradual, but stepwise, reduction in the size of an aneurysm at which elective repair should be recommended.[128] With the advent of a new technology that promises greatly decreased morbidity, the bar may be lowered farther. The issue remains, however, to what extent the placement of an endoluminal graft alters the long-term natural history of AAA. A new array of problems has accompanied the emergence of endoluminal aneurysm repair, problems only recognizable because of the superb imaging capabilities of computed tomography, ultrasonography, and digital subtraction angiography.

Aneurysm elongation, widening of the infrarenal neck, increasing tortuosity, persistence of collaterals through the IMA and lumbars, and incomplete apposition of the proximal and/or distal fixation of a device, all can be determined with serial imaging, and the information has identified a new problem: the "endoleak." Endoleaks are continued flow within the aneurysm sac, external to the device, after endoluminal repair. The degree to which an endoleak may

be tolerated is unknown currently, although it is the object of intense scrutiny.[129-138] Endoleaks may resolve spontaneously, but they may also persist,[139] and the specter of continued rupture risk looms in such situations. Unfortunately, even when aneurysm size decreases after stent-graft repair, there is still a risk of rupture.[140]

DEVICES AVAILABLE FOR AORTIC ENDOLUMINAL REPAIR. Appreciation of the rarity of having a distal aneurysm neck has dictated the terms of stent-graft design. The two major categories of devices are (1) aortounilateral iliac with contralateral blocker and (2) bifurcated. Most of the commercially developed devices are bifurcated (Fig. 42–5). Most are composed of either polyester or polytetrafluoroethylene (PTFE), with a fully supported endoskeleton of either nitinol or stainless steel. The main exception is the EGS (Endovascular Technologies, Menlo Park, CA) device, that incorporates self-expanding metallic cuffs with radially arrayed hooks at the fixation points and is not fully supported. Some evidence has been published that suggests advantages to a system that is fully supported[141] (Fig. 42–6). Each device, used under a U.S. Food and Drug Administration (FDA)–approved protocol or on a compassionate use basis, has its own set of imaging criteria to determine which patients have anatomy suitable for inclusion, primarily focusing on infrarenal neck length, diameter, and angulation, as well as diameter and tortuosity of the iliac arteries.

DEVICE INTRODUCTIONS. Devices all require introduction through a sheath, usually 18 to 24 French. This is

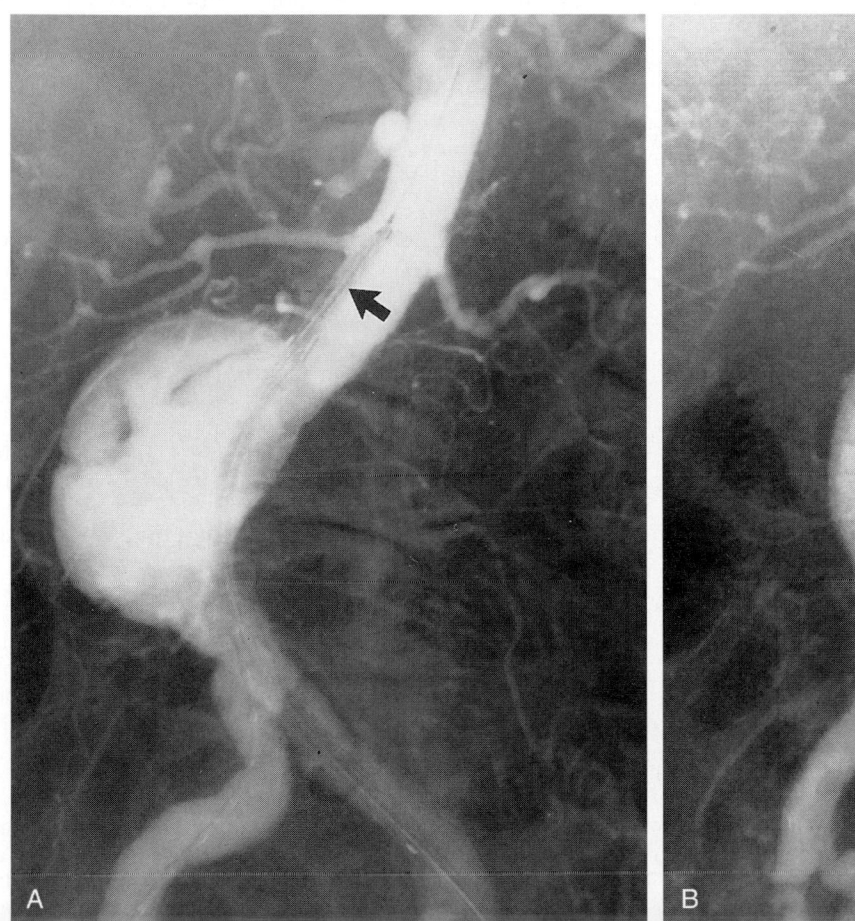
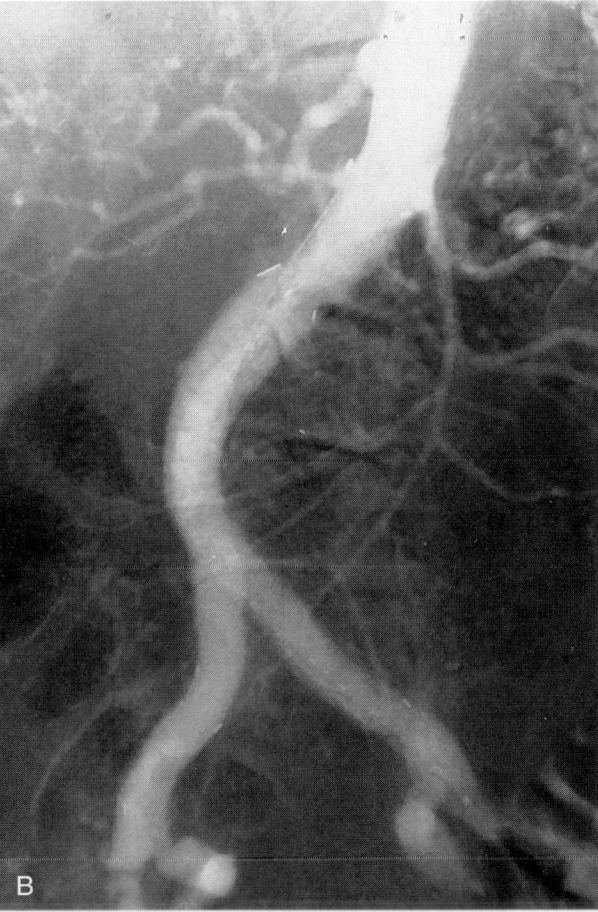

FIGURE 42–6. Endovascular stent-graft management of an abdominal aortic aneurysm. *A,* Abdominal aortogram demonstrates a large eccentric infrarenal abdominal aortic aneurysm before stent-graft deployment. An Excluder (W. L. Gore and Associates, Inc., Sunnyvale, CA) constrained on its delivery catheter (arrow) is located in the abdominal aorta before deployment. *B,* Completion abdominal aortogram after placement of the modular, bifurcated stent-graft demonstrates good flow through the prosthesis without evidence of an endoleak into the aneurysm sac.

done by femoral cutdown, although modifications of technique involving iliac or direct aortic access are sometimes necessary. Procedures are performed under general or spinal anesthesia, either in the operating room or in the angiography suite equipped with operating room–quality air. Combined suites are being built in many centers. Correct positioning of the device is critical, requiring both knowledge of the underlying anatomy and the characteristics of the particular device's deployment. Malpositioning of the device may lead to occlusion of the renal arteries or caudal placement too near the aneurysm sac, the latter necessitating addition of extender cuffs. Open repair, for the most part, does not impose the same anatomical constraints on selection of aneurysm.

All currently available devices, because of the similarity of their construction, have similar shortcomings. None of the devices can be repositioned after deployment. Most of them have a self-expanding metal frame that springs into place, often very rapidly and without opportunity to alter the position during deployment. Many of the devices flare proximally during placement, creating a potential "windsock" effect, through which aortic flow pushes against the briefly occlusive, partially opened stent-graft. This tends to push the device caudally, and this displacement may result in a suboptimal final position. Although some of the devices can be partially pulled back during deployment, none can be significantly advanced once deployment has begun. Therefore, correction of this caudal shift during placement requires additional devices, as mentioned earlier. Reports of material failure and device migration have surfaced,[134, 138, 140, 142] and this may in part result from the somewhat awkward juxtaposition of the graft and metallic components, which do not lend themselves easily to bonding. In addition, sutures holding the two components together must endure significant cumulative stress for years, perhaps decades, after implantation. Anatomical constraints have eliminated many patients from being considered for endoluminal repair. Inadequate infrarenal aneurysm proximal neck is invoked most frequently, and devices most often require 1.5 to 2.0 cm of relatively normal caliber aorta to facilitate sealing.[143, 144] Until devices can be designed that duplicate the security of a surgically constructed suture line, these limitations will continue to cast doubt on the long-term effectiveness of the technology as it stands.

RESULTS. Despite the above reservations, endoluminal AAA repair displays promising results.[139, 145–153] Irrespective of the particular product involved, technical success rate is high, aneurysm exclusion is achieved 80 to 95 percent of the time, and conversion to open repair is rare. Complications are not uncommon, however. Numerous case reports and small series of various complications have emerged,[131, 132, 134, 135, 154–156] and some of these report relatively late sequelae. The degree to which these late complications affect patients with stent-graft AAA repair will determine which device or devices, if any, will prove superior and guide the development of second generation stent-graft systems.

THORACIC ANEURYSMS (see also Chap. 40). Open repair of thoracic aortic aneurysms is a major surgical undertaking with an attendant high morbidity and mortality rate. This fact, coupled with the development of stent-graft technology,[126, 157, 158] has led inexorably to the application of stent-graft technology to thoracic aneurysm repair.

As in most stent-graft applications, the underlying lesional anatomy imposes great challenges. In the case of thoracic aortic aneurysms, it is the frequent juxtaposition of the aneurysm to the left subclavian artery that restricts the use of the device, or forces adjunctive surgical transposition of the left subclavian to left carotid (Fig. 42–7). Furthermore, the large caliber of the thoracic aorta in general challenges the limits of deliverability, because one can only percutaneously introduce devices through sheaths up to about 30 French. Moreover, the natural curvature of the aortic arch and proximal descending thoracic aorta must be accommodated by the device, which in its current incarnations contains a metal skeleton limited in its ability to handle such curves. Finally, there is concern about the occlusion of intercostal arteries, anastomoses from which may supply the spinal cord.

Despite these potential pitfalls, the procedure has been used with success in several series.[159–161a] In the largest of these, Mitchell and colleagues report the results of 103 patients receiving stent-grafts for treatment of aneurysms of the descending thoracic aorta.[159] Sixty percent of these patients were not deemed operative candidates. Primary success was achieved in 73 percent of patients, and secondary success occurred in another 12 percent, but only 53 percent of patients were free of treatment failure at 3.7 years. Complications were common, and major perioperative morbidity occurred in 31 patients. Paraplegia occurred in 3 patients, and was associated with concomitant or preceding abdominal aortic aneurysm repair. There was one conversion to open repair in the series, and 5 patients required late operative intervention for persistent endoleaks. The patient population offered endoluminal repair was obviously a skewed one, with coexistent disease severe enough to exclude well over half from consideration for open surgery. Nonetheless, the results underscore the challenge of treating this disease for the reasons outlined earlier and that the technology must undergo further refinement if it is to become the mainstay of treatment. In a more selected patient population, the results were much better.[161]

Stent-grafts have also been used with success in the treatment of mycotic aneurysms of the thoracic aorta[162] and in patients with acute rupture of the thoracic aorta, even in those with traumatic rupture.[163]

ILIAC ANEURYSMS

Isolated iliac aneurysms are uncommon. When they occur, however, they may be very dangerous, with an unpredictable course. They are not easily detected on physical examination, and rupture may not be discovered until it is too late because the diagnosis was not considered. Even in elective cases the mortality of open surgical repair is relatively high; and in emergency cases it is about 50 percent.[164, 165]

Several investigators have now demonstrated that stent-graft repair of isolated iliac artery aneurysms is feasible.[166–169] All studies demonstrated 100 percent technical success with the exception of a single patient in the series by Quinn and coworkers,[168] the single failure attributed to marked tortuosity of the iliac artery. All but one patient has achieved complete aneurysm exclusion in these series, although the follow-up periods are generally short. Complications in all series were rare.

Stent-grafts have also been used to exclude isolated internal iliac aneurysms.[170] The outflow of the internal iliac artery is coil embolized, and the origin of the internal iliac is then occluded by placement of a stent-graft across it, from the common to external iliac artery. This approach effectively excludes the aneurysm by shutting off both inflow and outflow.

OTHER APPLICATIONS OF STENT-GRAFTS

Stent-grafts have been used in a variety of clinical applications beyond those discussed earlier. The repair of aneurysms and arteriovenous fistulas in the region of the subclavian artery[171, 172] has proven successful. In fact, the first report of placement of a covered stent in a patient documented use of a silicone-coated balloon expandable stent in the subclavian artery.[173] Marin and associates[172] have also reported on repair of femoral pseudoaneurysms with stent-grafts. Autologous vein-stent combinations have also been used for the treatment of internal carotid pseudoaneu-

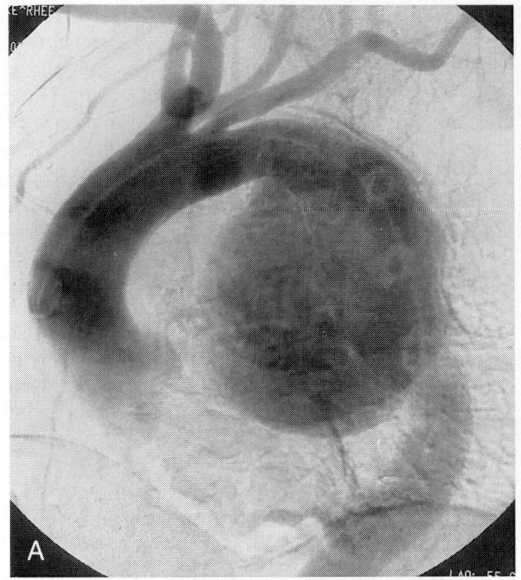

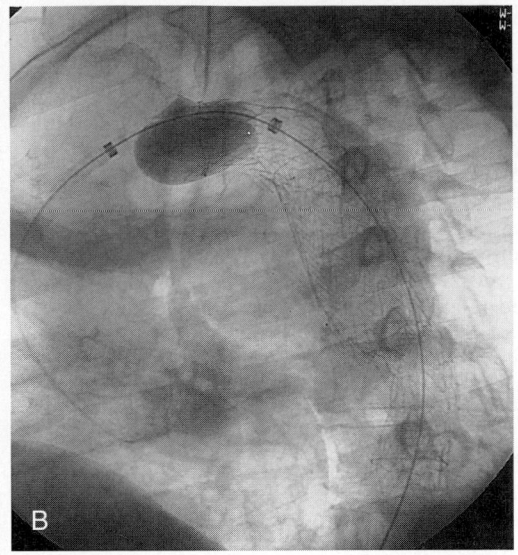

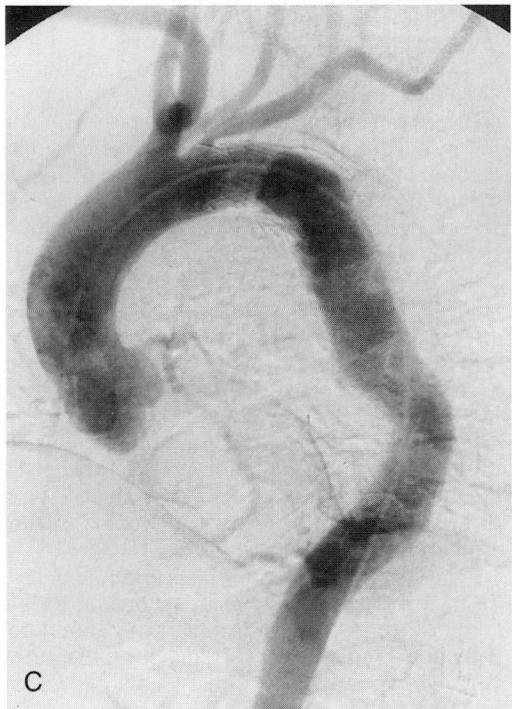

FIGURE 42-7. Stent-graft placement for treatment of a fusiform aneurysm involving the descending thoracic aorta. *A,* Thoracic aortogram in a left anterior oblique projection shows a large aneurysm of the proximal descending thoracic aorta associated with a relatively short proximal neck distal to the left subclavian artery. *B,* After placement of a thoracic Excluder (W. L. Gore and Associates, Inc., Sunnyvale, CA), a balloon is inflated within the proximal aspect of the device to fully expand the prosthesis within the proximal neck and smooth out any graft wrinkles. *C,* Similar left anterior oblique projection of a thoracic aortogram after stent-graft placement shows no further filling of the aneurysm sac and good positioning of the device.

rysm[174] and pseudoaneurysm of the SMA.[175] Covered stents have been used with reasonable success in transjugular intrahepatic portosystemic shunt (TIPS) treatment of patients with complications of portal hypertension, a procedure associated with considerable restenosis.[176]

VENOUS INTERVENTIONS

The conventional wisdom regarded venous interventions with considerable skepticism. The venous endothelium was considered too delicate, the flow too slow, and the walls of the veins too flimsy for seemingly crude techniques applied to the more robust arterial circulation. Surgeons learned this lesson long ago. It is with surprise, then, that vascular specialists have found that the veins can prove quite responsive to interventions. Especially surprising are the results seen in aggressive treatment of lower extremity deep venous thrombosis (DVT). Important roles are also played by interventionalists in treating upper extremity venous

thrombosis and in the management of superior vena cava (SVC) syndrome. As on the arterial side, it appears that the size of the conduit and restoration of in-line, anatomical flow channels are the crucial factors in maintaining patency.

LOWER EXTREMITY VENOUS INTERVENTIONS. Lower extremity deep venous thrombosis (LEDVT) is a common disease. Pulmonary embolus (PE) is the most dangerous consequence of LEDVT. However, the post-thrombotic syndrome, resulting in chronic pain and leg swelling, causes considerable morbidity and a decrease in quality of life. Although warfarin anticoagulation can limit PE, it does little to alter the course of post-thrombotic syndrome. The presence of clot within the veins eventually leads to inflammation and scarring, causing permanent damage to the venous valves and rendering them incompetent. It is the aim of more aggressive therapy of LEDVT to intervene before the onset of irreversible valve damage, and thereby salvage venous valve function.

Thrombolysis. The mainstay of this more aggressive therapy is thrombolysis. Lysis potentially clears the vein of clot, restores flow, and hence aborts the cycle of events leading to valve damage. Furthermore, many patients who develop LEDVT have an underlying anatomical lesion leading to thrombosis. Lysis of clot uncovers these lesions, which may then be treated by stenting. Semba and Dake published the first large series using lytic agents for the treatment of iliofemoral DVT and produced excellent results,[177] and this prompted the creation of a national venous registry. The preliminary results of that registry, representing 287 patients subjected to lysis, have confirmed the efficacy of this more aggressive approach to LEDVT.[178] What has emerged is an understanding of the importance of early treatment of DVT. Patients in whom evidence of chronic DVT was found demonstrated less complete lysis and less impressive patency rates than those with acute DVT.[178] The overall 1-year primary patency was 60 percent. Following these patients for several years will be necessary to establish the impact of treatment on the development of post-thrombotic syndrome. Fatal complications occurred in 2 of 287 patients (<1 percent), and 6 patients had pulmonary emboli.

INTERVENTIONS FOR PAGET-SCHROETTER SYNDROME.
Effort vein thrombosis, or Paget-Schroetter syndrome, occurs as a result of mechanical trauma to the subclavian vein at the thoracic outlet. It can occur at any age but has a predilection for young, athletic individuals. A developmental anomaly resulting in impingement on the vein may be present.[179] The natural history of the disorder is typically one of chronic venous obstruction with development of a painful, swollen extremity.

A multidisciplinary approach to its management has emerged, in which thrombolysis is performed in the acute setting and surgical decompression is performed after a variable interval of oral anticoagulation.[180–183] PTA of the subclavian vein may prove a useful adjunct as well.[180, 181] Other studies, however, found no benefit to PTA in this setting.[184] The role of stent placement in this region is controversial. An emerging consensus that stenting is to be avoided has arisen from experience with stent fracture in this region. Encouraging results of stent placement for Paget-Schroetter syndrome, however, have been reported.[185, 186]

INTERVENTIONS IN SUPERIOR VENA CAVA SYNDROME.
Obstruction of the superior vena cava (SVC) is most frequently a result of malignant disease invading the mediastinum (see also Chap. 69). To an increasing extent, however, benign causes are responsible, especially obstruction secondary to multiple central venous catheter placements. Not all patients with SVC obstruction are symptomatic. When symptoms do occur, however, they are dramatic: intense facial and upper extremity swelling gives patients a gargoyle-like appearance, which is intensely uncomfortable and unsettling not only to the patient but to the family as well. Patients also suffer from intense headaches, exacerbated while supine, making sleep difficult. Cognitive dysfunction occasionally occurs because of progressive brain edema brought on by venous obstruction. Although patients with malignant SVC syndrome generally have a short life expectancy, the quality of that life is abysmal if the obstruction is untreated. It is in that spirit that aggressive palliative therapy is offered.

Radiation therapy has been the mainstay of treatment for malignant SVC syndrome. The occasionally slow response to radiation and the achievement of maximum radiation dosages without relief have prompted a gradual shift away from brachytherapy to initial percutaneous interventional therapy when it is available. Although some small series of surgical treatment of malignant SVC syndrome report excellent results,[187] such interventions are proposed with curative intent, only applicable in a small minority of patients with malignant mediastinal involvement with tumor.

SVC stent placement has been demonstrated in numerous reports to provide rapid relief of symptoms of SVC syndrome[188, 189] (Fig. 42–8). The largest series in the literature was produced by Kee and coworkers,[188] in which a series of 59 patients, 16 of whom had a benign etiology, presented with SVC syndrome. Occlusion of the SVC was found in 31 of these patients, of whom 28 underwent catheter directed thrombolysis before stent placement. In patients with malignant disease, the clinical patency rate was 93 percent; and in those with benign disease, it was 85 percent. Relief of symptoms is often instantaneous and dramatic. Even in patients with a short life expectancy, SVC stent placement greatly improves the quality of their remaining time. In patients with benign disease, patency is comparable to surgery, with less morbidity. In institutions where expertise is available, stent placement is a reasonable first choice in the treatment of SVC syndrome.

Venous Filtration (See also Chap. 52)

Inferior vena cava (IVC) filter placement is one of the more common venous interventions. The utility of such devices would be even broader pending development of temporary and/or retrievable filters, the applications of which could be far reaching in trauma and perioperative management.

IVC FILTERS.
Although there remains some uncertainty about the indications for IVC filter placement, there is general agreement on the core indications: (1) contraindication to anticoagulation; (2) failure of anticoagulation; (3) complication of anticoagulation; and (4) free-floating iliocaval thrombus. The use of filters for prophylaxis against PE in the absence of documented DVT is controversial. Four filter designs are in wide use in the United States, all with purported advantages relative to other designs. Each has been subjected to scrutiny through both single center experiences[190–194] and review articles.[195, 196]

The major advantage of the Simon Nitinol filter (Nitinol Medical Technologies, Woburn, MA) is its flexibility and low profile (9F), allowing introduction through an antecubital vein.[193] This is particularly useful in patients with coagulopathy or on anticoagulation, in whom the risk of bleeding is higher. Antecubital veins are easily compressed, and there is less risk of clinically significant hematoma than in a jugular or femoral puncture.

The Vena Tech LGM (B. Braun Vena Tech, Evanston, IL) filter is the easiest to place, according to the manufacturer's advertising and in the opinion of many interventionalists. Questions have been raised about the rate of caval occlusion with Vena Tech filters,[194] which have been addressed in later publications.[192] Filter retraction has also been reported.[192]

The Bird's Nest Filter (Cook, Bloomington, IN) can be deployed in IVCs up to 40 mm in diameter, significantly larger than the 28-mm maximum of the other filters. It is also typically less expensive than the other filters. Arguably, a Bird's Nest Filter designed for jugular access is appropriate for treating any patient requiring a filter.

The titanium Greenfield filter (Medi-Tech/Boston Scientific, Watertown, MA) is the more sleek offspring of the earlier stainless steel Greenfield filter (Medi-Tech/Boston Scientific, Watertown, MA). The latest incarnation of this filter allows for delivery over the wire, although this apparently offers no advantage over standard deployment.[191]

All filters are reasonably effective in their primary function of preventing PE, with recurrent PE rates ranging from 1 to 5 percent.[195] The rate of development of caval thrombus is difficult to accurately ascertain but appears to be on the order of 5 to 25 percent.[195]

The introduction of an effective temporary filter would go a long way toward solving the problem of filter placement for prophylaxis. To date, no temporary filters are approved, although some are undergoing trials. Experimental results with one retrievable filter are encouraging.[197]

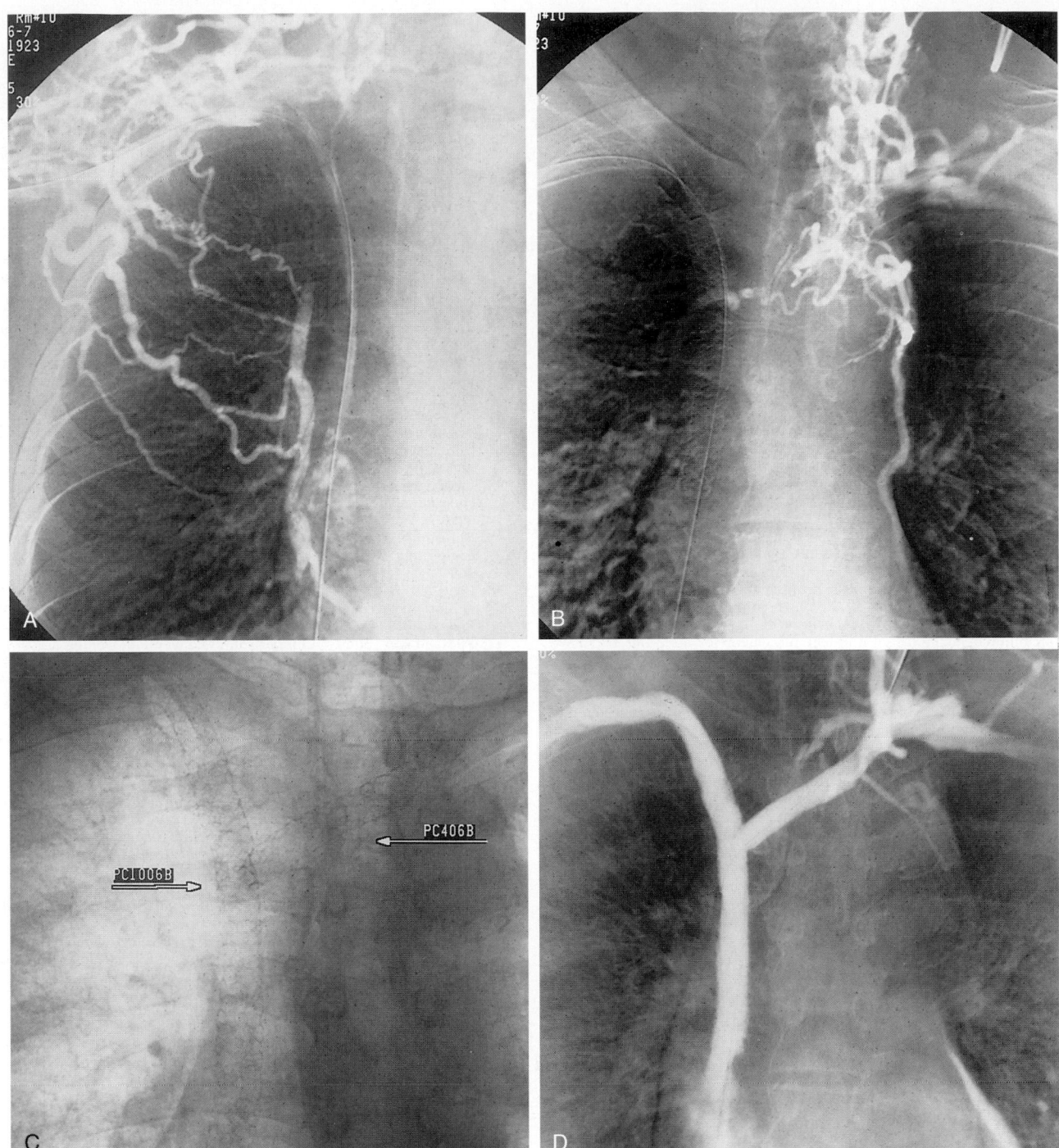

FIGURE 42–8. Endovascular stent placement for management of venous obstruction in a 68-year-old man with symptoms of superior vena cava syndrome. *A,* Right arm venogram demonstrates obstruction of the right subclavian and brachiocephalic veins with a highly developed collateral network that includes chest wall veins. *B,* Left internal jugular venogram identifies occlusion of the left jugular system and brachiocephalic vein. *C,* Chest radiograph demonstrates a series of balloon expandable stents (Corinthian, Cordis, Inc., Miami, FL) placed in the right subclavian, right brachiocephalic, left brachiocephalic, and superior vena cava. *D,* Bilateral upper extremity venogram performed after stent placement demonstrates reestablished flow within the previously occluded mediastinal veins. Full expansion of the stented segments is apparent, and a paucity of collateral flow is evident.

REFERENCES

PERIPHERAL VASCULAR INTERVENTION

1. Lansky AJ, Popma JJ, Massullo V, et al: Quantitative angiographic analysis of stent restenosis in the Scripps Coronary Radiation to Inhibit Intimal Proliferation Post Stenting (SCRIPPS) Trial. Am J Cardiol 84: 410–414, 1999.
2. Motarjeme A, Gordon GI, Bodenhagen K: Thrombolysis and angioplasty of chronic iliac artery occlusions. J Vasc Interv Radiol 6(6 Pt 2 Su): 66S–72S, 1995.
3. Johnston KW: Iliac arteries: Reanalysis of results of balloon angioplasty. Radiology 186:207–212, 1993.
4. Gupta AK, Ravimandalam K, Rao VR, et al: Total occlusion of iliac arteries: Results of balloon angioplasty. Cardiovasc Intervent Radiol 16: 165–177, 1993.
5. Henry M, Amor M, Ethevenot G, et al: Palmaz stent placement in iliac and femoropopliteal arteries: Primary and secondary patency in 310 patients with 2-4-year follow-up. Radiology 197:167–174, 1995.
6. Vorwerk D, Gunther RW, Schurmann K, Wendt G: Aortic and iliac stenoses: Follow-up results of stent placement after insufficient balloon angioplasty in 118 cases. Radiology 198:45–48, 1996.

7. Vorwerk D, Gunther RW: Stent placement in iliac arterial lesions: Three years of clinical experience with the Wallstent. Cardiovasc Intervent Radiol 15:285–290, 1992.

8. Sapoval MR, Chatellier G, Long AL, et al: Self-expandable stents for the treatment of iliac artery obstructive lesions: Long-term success and prognostic factors. AJR Am J Roentgenol 166:1173–1179, 1996.

9. Martin EC, Katzen BT, Benenati JF, et al: Multicenter trial of the wallstent in the iliac and femoral arteries. J Vasc Interv Radiol 6:843–849, 1995.

10. Murphy KD, Encarnacion CE, Le VA, Palmaz JC: Iliac artery stent placement with the Palmaz stent: Follow-up study. J Vasc Interv Radiol 6:321–329, 1995.

11. Mendelsohn FO, Santos RM, Crowley JJ, et al: Kissing stents in the aortic bifurcation. Am Heart J 136:600–605, 1998.

12. Palmaz JC, Laborde JC, Rivera FJ, et al: Stenting of the iliac arteries with the Palmaz stent: Experience from a multicenter trial. Cardiovasc Intervent Radiol 15:291–297, 1992.

13. Murphy TP, Webb MS, Lambiase RE, et al: Percutaneous revascularization of complex iliac artery stenoses and occlusions with use of Wallstents: Three-year experience. J Vasc Interv Radiol 7:21–27, 1996.

14. Murphy TP, Khwaja AA, Webb MS: Aortoiliac stent placement in patients treated for intermittent claudication. J Vasc Interv Radiol 9:421–428, 1998.

15. Blum U, Gabelmann A, Redecker M, et al: Percutaneous recanalization of iliac artery occlusions: Results of a prospective study. Radiology 189:536–540, 1993.

16. Vorwerk D, Guenther RW, Schurmann K, et al: Primary stent placement for chronic iliac artery occlusions: Follow-up results in 103 patients. Radiology 194:745–749, 1995.

17. Dyet JF, Gaines PA, Nicholson AA, et al: Treatment of chronic iliac artery occlusions by means of percutaneous endovascular stent placement. J Vasc Interv Radiol 8:349–353, 1997.

18. Reyes R, Maynar M, Lopera J, et al: Treatment of chronic iliac artery occlusions with guide wire recanalization and primary stent placement. J Vasc Interv Radiol 8:1049–1055, 1997.

19. Bosch JL, Hunink MG: Meta-analysis of the results of percutaneous transluminal angioplasty and stent placement for aortoiliac occlusive disease [published erratum appears in Radiology 205:584, 1997]. Radiology 204:87–96, 1997.

20. Bosch JL, Tetteroo E, Mali WP, Hunink MG: Iliac arterial occlusive disease: Cost-effectiveness analysis of stent placement versus percutaneous transluminal angioplasty. Dutch Iliac Stent Trial Study Group. Radiology 208:641–648, 1998.

21. Tetteroo E, van der Graaf Y, Bosch JL, et al: Randomised comparison of primary stent placement versus primary angioplasty followed by selective stent placement in patients with iliac-artery occlusive disease. Dutch Iliac Stent Trial Study Group. Lancet 351:1153–1159, 1998.

22. Weitz JI, Byrne J, Clagett GP, et al: Diagnosis and treatment of chronic arterial insufficiency of the lower extremities: A critical review. Circulation 94:3026–3049, 1996.

23. McDaniel MD, Cronenwett JL: Basic data related to the natural history of intermittent claudication. Ann Vasc Surg 3:273–277, 1989.

24. Hertzer NR: The natural history of peripheral vascular disease: Implications for its management. Circulation 83(2 Suppl):I12–I19, 1991.

25. Pentecost MJ, Criqui MH, Dorros G, et al: Guidelines for peripheral percutaneous transluminal angioplasty of the abdominal aorta and lower extremity vessels: A statement for health professionals from a special writing group of the Councils on Cardiovascular Radiology, Arteriosclerosis, Cardio-Thoracic and Vascular Surgery, Clinical Cardiology, and Epidemiology and Prevention, the American Heart Association. Circulation 89:511–531, 1994.

26. Price JF, Leng GC, Fowkes FG: Should claudicants receive angioplasty or exercise training? Cardiovasc Surg 5:463–470, 1997.

27. Hunink MG, Wong JB, Donaldson MC, et al: Revascularization for femoropopliteal disease: A decision and cost-effectiveness analysis. JAMA 274:165–171, 1995.

28. Hunink MG, Wong JB, Donaldson MC, et al: Patency results of percutaneous and surgical revascularization for femoropopliteal arterial disease. Med Decis Making 14:71–81, 1994.

29. Jeans WD, Armstrong S, Cole SE, et al: Fate of patients undergoing transluminal angioplasty for lower-limb ischemia. Radiology 177:559–564, 1990.

30. Capek P, McLean GK, Berkowitz HD: Femoropopliteal angioplasty: Factors influencing long-term success. Circulation 83(2 Suppl):I70–I80, 1991.

31. Johnston KW: Femoral and popliteal arteries: Reanalysis of results of balloon angioplasty [see comments]. Radiology 183:767–771, 1992.

32. Hunink MG, Donaldson MC, Meyerovitz MF, et al: Risks and benefits of femoropopliteal percutaneous balloon angioplasty. J Vasc Surg 17:183–192; discussion 192–194, 1993.

33. Matsi PJ, Manninen HI: Complications of lower-limb percutaneous transluminal angioplasty: A prospective analysis of 410 procedures on 295 consecutive patients. Cardiovasc Intervent Radiol 21:361–366, 1998.

34. Manninen HI, Soder HK, Matsi PJ, et al: Prolonged dilation improves an unsatisfactory primary result of femoropopliteal artery angioplasty: Usefulness of a perfusion balloon catheter. J Vasc Interv Radiol 8:627–632, 1997.

35. Vroegindeweij D, Vos LD, Tielbeek AV, et al: Balloon angioplasty combined with primary stenting versus balloon angioplasty alone in femoropopliteal obstructions: A comparative randomized study. Cardiovasc Intervent Radiol 20:420–425, 1997.

36. Saab MH, Smith DC, Aka PK, et al: Percutaneous transluminal angioplasty of tibial arteries for limb salvage. Cardiovasc Intervent Radiol 15:211–216, 1992.

37. Bakal CW, Sprayregen S, Scheinbaum K, et al: Percutaneous transluminal angioplasty of the infrapopliteal arteries: Results in 53 patients. AJR Am J Roentgenol 154:171–174, 1990.

38. Matsi PJ, Manninen HI, Suhonen MT, et al: Chronic critical lower-limb ischemia: Prospective trial of angioplasty with 1–36 months follow-up. Radiology 188:381–387, 1993.

39. Schwarten DE: Clinical and anatomical considerations for nonoperative therapy in tibial disease and the results of angioplasty. Circulation 83(2 Suppl):I86–I90, 1991.

40. Bull PG, Mendel H, Hold M, et al: Distal popliteal and tibioperoneal transluminal angioplasty: Long-term follow-up. J Vasc Interv Radiol 3:45–53, 1992.

41. Varty K, Bolia A, Naylor AR, et al: Infrapopliteal percutaneous transluminal angioplasty: A safe and successful procedure. Eur J Vasc Endovasc Surg 9:341–345, 1995.

42. Fraser SC, al-Kutoubi MA, Wolfe JH: Percutaneous transluminal angioplasty of the infrapopliteal vessels: The evidence [see comments]. Radiology 200:33–36, 1996.

43. Treiman GS, Treiman RL, Ichikawa L, Van Allan R: Should percutaneous transluminal angioplasty be recommended for treatment of infrageniculate popliteal artery or tibioperoneal trunk stenosis? [see comments]. J Vasc Surg 22:457–463; discussion 464–465, 1995.

44. Bakal CW, Cynamon J, Sprayregen S: Infrapopliteal percutaneous transluminal angioplasty: What we know [comment]. Radiology 200:36–43, 1996.

45. Hallisey MJ, Meranze SG, Parker BC, et al: Percutaneous transluminal angioplasty of the abdominal aorta. J Vasc Interv Radiol 5:679–687, 1994.

46. Long AL, Gaux JC, Raynaud AC, et al: Infrarenal aortic stents: Initial clinical experience and angiographic follow-up. Cardiovasc Intervent Radiol 16:203–208, 1993.

47. Westcott MA, Bonn J: Comparison of conventional angioplasty with the Palmaz stent in the treatment of abdominal aortic stenoses from the STAR registry. SCVIR Transluminal Angioplasty and Revascularization. J Vasc Interv Radiol 9:225–231, 1998.

RENAL ARTERIAL INTERVENTIONS

48. Hansen KJ: Prevalence of ischemic nephropathy in the atherosclerotic population. Am J Kidney Dis 24:615–621, 1994.

49. van de Ven PJ, Beutler JJ, Kaatee R, et al: Transluminal vascular stent for ostial atherosclerotic renal artery stenosis [see comments]. Lancet 346:672–674, 1995.

50. Rundback JH, Gray RJ, Rozenblit G, et al: Renal artery stent placement for the management of ischemic nephropathy. J Vasc Interv Radiol 9:413–420, 1998.

51. Harden PN, MacLeod MJ, Rodger RS, et al: Effect of renal-artery stenting on progression of renovascular renal failure [see comments]. Lancet 349:1133–1136, 1997.

52. Hoffman O, Carreres T, Sapoval MR, et al: Ostial renal artery stenosis angioplasty: Immediate and mid-term angiographic and clinical results. J Vasc Interv Radiol 9:65–73, 1998.

53. Joffre F, Rousseau H, Bernadet P, et al: Midterm results of renal artery stenting. Cardiovasc Intervent Radiol 15:313–318, 1992.

54. Henry M, Amor M, Henry I, et al: Stent placement in the renal artery: Three-year experience with the Palmaz stent. J Vasc Interv Radiol 7:343–350, 1996.

55. Raynaud AC, Beyssen BM, Turmel-Rodrigues LE, et al: Renal artery stent placement: Immediate and midterm technical and clinical results. J Vasc Interv Radiol 5:849–858, 1994.

56. Rodriguez-Perez JC, Plaza C, Reyes R, et al: Treatment of renovascular hypertension with percutaneous transluminal angioplasty: Experience in Spain. J Vasc Interv Radiol 5:101–109, 1994.

57. Hennequin LM, Joffre FG, Rousseau HP, et al: Renal artery stent placement: Long-term results with the Wallstent endoprosthesis [see comments]. Radiology 191:713–719, 1994.

58. Boisclair C, Therasse E, Oliva VL, et al: Treatment of renal angioplasty failure by percutaneous renal artery stenting with Palmaz stents: Midterm technical and clinical results. AJR Am J Roentgenol 168:245–251, 1997.

59. Rodriguez-Lopez JA, Werner A, Ray LI, et al: Renal artery stenosis treated with stent deployment: Indications, technique, and outcome for 108 patients. J Vasc Surg 29:617–624, 1999.

60. Blum U, Krumme B, Flugel P, et al: Treatment of ostial renal-artery stenoses with vascular endoprostheses after unsuccessful balloon angioplasty [see comments]. N Engl J Med 336:459–465, 1997.

61. Dorros G, Jaff M, Mathiak L, et al: Four-year follow-up of Palmaz-Schatz stent revascularization as treatment for atherosclerotic renal artery stenosis. Circulation 98:642–647, 1998.

62. Tuttle KR, Chouinard RF, Webber JT, et al: Treatment of atherosclerotic ostial renal artery stenosis with the intravascular stent [see comments]. Am J Kidney Dis 32:611–622, 1998.

63. Pattynama PM, Becker GJ, Brown J, et al: Percutaneous angioplasty for

atherosclerotic renal artery disease: Effect on renal function in azotemic patients. Cardiovasc Intervent Radiol 17:143–146, 1994.

64. Rees CR: Stents for atherosclerotic renovascular disease. J Vasc Interv Radiol 10:689–705, 1999.

64a. van Jaarsveld BC, Krijnen P, Pieterman H, et al: The effect of balloon angioplasty on hypertension in atherosclerotic renal-artery stenosis. N Engl J Med 342:1007–1014, 2000.

64b. Ritz E, Mann JFE: Renal angioplasty for lowering blood pressure. N Engl J Med 342:1042–1043, 2000.

64c. Lim ST, Rosenfield K: Renal artery stent placement: Indications and results. Curr Interv Cardiol Rep 2:130–139, 2000.

65. van de Ven PJ, Kaatee R, Beutler JJ, et al: Arterial stenting and balloon angioplasty in ostial atherosclerotic renovascular disease: A randomised trial. Lancet 353:282–286, 1999.

66. Xue F, Bettmann MA, Langdon DR, Wivell WA: Outcome and cost comparison of percutaneous transluminal renal angioplasty, renal arterial stent placement, and renal arterial bypass grafting. Radiology 212:378–384, 1999.

67. Beek FJ, Kaatee R, Beutler JJ, et al: Complications during renal artery stent placement for atherosclerotic ostial stenosis. Cardiovasc Intervent Radiol 20:184–190, 1997.

VISCERAL ARTERY INTERVENTION

68. Matsumoto AH, Tegtmeyer CJ, Fitzcharles EK, et al: Percutaneous transluminal angioplasty of visceral arterial stenoses: Results and long-term clinical follow-up. J Vasc Interv Radiol 6:165–174, 1995.

69. Mateo RB, O'Hara PJ, Hertzer NR, et al: Elective surgical treatment of symptomatic chronic mesenteric occlusive disease: Early results and late outcomes. J Vasc Surg 29:821–831; discussion 832, 1999.

70. Kihara TK, Blebea J, Anderson KM, et al: Risk factors and outcomes following revascularization for chronic mesenteric ischemia. Ann Vasc Surg 13:37–44, 1999.

71. Hallisey MJ, Deschaine J, Illescas FF, et al: Angioplasty for the treatment of visceral ischemia. J Vasc Interv Radiol 6:785–791, 1995.

72. Allen RC, Martin GH, Rees CR, et al: Mesenteric angioplasty in the treatment of chronic intestinal ischemia. J Vasc Surg 24:415–421; discussion 421–423, 1996.

73. Maspes F, Mazzetti di Pietralata G, Gandini R, et al: Percutaneous transluminal angioplasty in the treatment of chronic mesenteric ischemia: Results and 3 years of follow-up in 23 patients. Abdom Imaging 23:358–363, 1998.

74. Levy PJ, Haskell L, Gordon RL: Percutaneous transluminal angioplasty of splanchnic arteries: An alternative method to elective revascularisation in chronic visceral ischaemia. Eur J Radiol 7:239–242, 1987.

SUPRAAORTIC INTERVENTIONS

75. Sheeran SR, Murphy TP, Khwaja A, et al: Stent placement for treatment of mesenteric artery stenoses or occlusions [In Process Citation]. J Vasc Interv Radiol 10:861–867, 1999.

76. Millaire A, Trinca M, Marache P, et al: Subclavian angioplasty: Immediate and late results in 50 patients. Cathet Cardiovasc Diagn 29:8–17, 1993.

77. Al-Mubarak N, Liu MW, Dean LS, et al: Immediate and late outcomes of subclavian artery stenting. Catheter Cardiovasc Interv 46:169–172, 1999.

78. Sullivan TM, Gray BH, Bacharach JM, et al: Angioplasty and primary stenting of the subclavian, innominate, and common carotid arteries in 83 patients. J Vasc Surg 28:1059–1065, 1998.

79. Ruebben A, Tettoni S, Muratore P, et al: Feasibility of intraoperative balloon angioplasty and additional stent placement of isolated stenosis of the brachiocephalic trunk. J Thorac Cardiovasc Surg 115:1316–1320, 1998.

80. Iannone LA, Toon RS, Rayl KL: Percutaneous transluminal angioplasty of the innominate artery combined with carotid endarterectomy. Am Heart J 126:1466–1469, 1993.

81. Criado FJ, Queral LA: Carotid-axillary artery bypass: A ten-year experience. J Vasc Surg 22:717–722; discussion 722–723, 1995.

82. Mathias KD, Luth I, Haarmann P: Percutaneous transluminal angioplasty of proximal subclavian artery occlusions. Cardiovasc Intervent Radiol 16:214–218, 1993.

82a. Eisenhauer AC: Subclavian and innominate revascularization: Surgical therapy versus catheter-based intervention. Curr Interv Cardiol Rep 2:101–110, 2000.

83. Romanowski CA, Fairlie NC, Procter AE, Cumberland DC: Percutaneous transluminal angioplasty of the subclavian and axillary arteries: Initial results and long term follow-up. Clin Radiol 46:104–107, 1992.

84. Lyon RD, Shonnard KM, McCarter DL, et al: Supra-aortic arterial stenoses: Management with Palmaz balloon-expandable intraluminal stents. J Vasc Interv Radiol 7:825–835, 1996.

85. Sueoka BL: Percutaneous transluminal stent placement to treat subclavian steal syndrome. J Vasc Interv Radiol 7:351–356, 1996.

86. Queral LA, Criado FJ: The treatment of focal aortic arch branch lesions with Palmaz stents. J Vasc Surg 23:368–375, 1996.

86a. Hilfiker PR, Razavi MK, Kee ST, et al: Stent-graft therapy for subclavian artery aneurysms and fistulas: Single-center mid-term results. J Vasc Interv Radiol 11:578–584, 2000.

87. Crowe KE, Iannone LA: Percutaneous transluminal angioplasty for sub-

clavian artery stenosis in patients with subclavian steal syndrome and coronary subclavian steal syndrome. Am Heart J 126:229–233, 1993.

88. Holmes JR, Crane R: Coronary steal through a patent internal mammary artery graft: Treatment by subclavian angioplasty. Am Heart J 125:1166–1167, 1993.

89. Perrault LP, Carrier M, Hudon G, et al: Transluminal angioplasty of the subclavian artery in patients with internal mammary grafts. Ann Thorac Surg 56:927–930, 1993.

90. Mufti SI, Young KR, Schulthesis T: Restenosis following subclavian artery angioplasty for treatment of coronary-subclavian steal syndrome: Definitive treatment with Palmaz-stent placement. Cathet Cardiovasc Diagn 33:172–174, 1994.

91. Kugelmass AD, Kim D, Kuntz RE, et al: Endoluminal stenting of a subclavian artery stenosis to treat ischemia in the distribution of a patent left internal mammary graft. Cathet Cardiovasc Diagn 33:175–177, 1994.

92. Hallisey MJ, Rees JH, Meranze SG, et al: Use of angioplasty in the prevention and treatment of coronary-subclavian steal syndrome. J Vasc Interv Radiol 6:125–129, 1995.

93. FitzGibbon GM, Keon WJ: Coronary subclavian steal: A recurrent case with notes on detecting the threat potential. Ann Thorac Surg 60:1810–1812, 1995.

94. Marques KM, Ernst SM, Mast EG, et al: Percutaneous transluminal angioplasty of the left subclavian artery to prevent or treat the coronary-subclavian steal syndrome. Am J Cardiol 78:687–690, 1996.

95. Rabah MM, Gangadharan V, Brodsky M, Safian RD: Unstable coronary ischemic syndromes caused by coronary-subclavian steal. Am Heart J 131:374–378, 1996.

EXTRACRANIAL CAROTID INTERVENTION

96. Storey GS, Marks MP, Dake M, et al: Vertebral artery stenting following percutaneous transluminal angioplasty. Technical note. J Neurosurg 84:883–887, 1996.

97. Thompson JE: Carotid angioplasty—a reserved position [editorial]. Cardiovasc Surg 5:459–460, 1997.

98. Clagett GP, Barnett HJ, Easton JD: The carotid artery stenting versus endarterectomy trial (CASET) [editorial]. Cardiovasc Surg 5:454–456, 1997.

99. Hobson RW II, Brott T, Ferguson R, et al: CREST: Carotid revascularization endarterectomy versus stent trial [editorial]. Cardiovasc Surg 5:457–458, 1997.

100. Bettmann MA, Katzen BT, Whisnant J, et al: Carotid stenting and angioplasty: A statement for healthcare professionals from the Councils on Cardiovascular Radiology, Stroke, Cardiothoracic and Vascular Surgery, Epidemiology, and Prevention, and Clinical Cardiology, American Heart Association. Stroke 29:336–338, 1998.

101. Baker W: CREST: A moral and ethical conundrum [editorial]. Cardiovasc Surg 5:461–462, 1997.

102. Dorros G: Stent-supported carotid angioplasty: Should it be done, and, if so, by whom? A 1998 perspective. Circulation 98:927–930, 1998.

103. Ferguson GG: Angioplasty for carotid disease: No. Arch Neurol 53:698–700, 1996.

104. Ferguson RD, Ferguson JG: Carotid angioplasty: In search of a worthy alternative to endarterectomy. Arch Neurol 53:696–698, 1996.

105. Yao JS: Angioplasty and stenting for carotid lesions: An argument against. Adv Surg 32:245–54, 1999.

106. Mathias KD: Angioplasty and stenting for carotid lesions: An argument for. Adv Surg 32:225–243, 1999.

107. Becker GJ: Should metallic vascular stents be used to treat cerebrovascular occlusive diseases? [editorial; comment]. Radiology 191:309–312, 1994.

108. Beebe HG: Scientific evidence demonstrating the safety of carotid angioplasty and stenting: Do we have enough to draw conclusions yet? [see comments]. J Vasc Surg 27:788–790, 1998.

109. Beebe HG, Kritpracha B: Carotid stenting versus carotid endarterectomy: Update on the controversy. Semin Vasc Surg 11:46–51, 1998.

110. Lawhorne TW Jr, Brooks HB, Cunningham JM: Five hundred consecutive carotid endarterectomies: Emphasis on vein patch closure. Cardiovasc Surg 5:141–144, 1997.

111. Hertzer NR, O'Hara PJ, Mascha EJ, et al: Early outcome assessment for 2228 consecutive carotid endarterectomy procedures: The Cleveland Clinic experience from 1989 to 1995. J Vasc Surg 26:1–10, 1997.

112. Beneficial effect of carotid endarterectomy in symptomatic patients with high-grade carotid stenosis. North American Symptomatic Carotid Endarterectomy Trial Collaborators [see comments]. N Engl J Med 325:445–453, 1991.

113. Endarterectomy for asymptomatic carotid artery stenosis. Executive Committee for the Asymptomatic Carotid Atherosclerosis Study [see comments]. Jama 273:1421–1428, 1995.

114. Al-Mubarak N, Roubin GS, Gomez CR, et al: Carotid artery stenting in patients with high neurologic risks. Am J Cardiol 83:1411–1413, A8–A9, 1999.

115. Mathur A, Roubin GS, Gomez CR, et al: Elective carotid artery stenting in the presence of contralateral occlusion. Am J Cardiol 81:1315–1317, 1998.

116. Abrahamsen J, Roeder OC, Justesen P, Enevoldsen E: Percutaneous transluminal angioplasty in selected patients with severe carotid artery

stenoses: The results of a consecutive series of 24 patients. Eur J Vasc Endovasc Surg 16:438–442, 1998.

117. Naylor AR, Bolia A, Abbott RJ, et al: Randomized study of carotid angioplasty and stenting versus carotid endarterectomy: A stopped trial. J Vasc Surg 28:326–334, 1998.

118. Yadav JS, Roubin GS, Iyer S, et al: Elective stenting of the extracranial carotid arteries [see comments]. Circulation 95:376–381, 1997.

ENDOLUMINAL REPAIR OF AORTIC AND OTHER ANEURYSMS

119. Wholey MH, Wholey M, Bergeron P, et al: Current global status of carotid artery stent placement [see comments]. Cathet Cardiovasc Diagn 44:1–6, 1998.

119a. Qureshi AI, Luft AR, Janardhan V, et al: Identification of patients at risk for periprocedural neurological deficits associated with carotid angioplasty and stenting. Stroke 31:376–382, 2000.

120. Slonim SM, Miller DC, Mitchell RS, et al: Percutaneous balloon fenestration and stenting for life-threatening ischemic complications in patients with acute aortic dissection. J Thorac Cardiovasc Surg 117:1118–1126, 1999.

121. Williams DM, Lee DY, Hamilton BH, et al: The dissected aorta: Percutaneous treatment of ischemic complications—principles and results. J Vasc Interv Radiol 8:605–625, 1997.

122. Dake MD, Kato N, Mitchell RS, et al: Endovascular stent-graft placement for the treatment of acute aortic dissection [see comments]. N Engl J Med 340:1546–1552, 1999.

123. Melton LJD, Bickerstaff LK, Hollier LH, et al: Changing incidence of abdominal aortic aneurysms: A population-based study. Am J Epidemiol 120:379–386, 1984.

124. Bengtsson H, Bergqvist D, Sternby NH: Increasing prevalence of abdominal aortic aneurysms: A necropsy study. Eur J Surg 158:19–23, 1992.

125. Johnston KW: Multicenter prospective study of nonruptured abdominal aortic aneurysm: II. Variables predicting morbidity and mortality. J Vasc Surg 9:437–447, 1989.

126. Parodi JC, Palmaz JC, Barone HD: Transfemoral intraluminal graft implantation for abdominal aortic aneurysms. Ann Vasc Surg 5:491–499, 1991.

127. Ernst CB: Abdominal aortic aneurysm [see comments]. N Engl J Med 328:1167–1172, 1993.

128. Brown PM, Pattenden R, Vernooy C, et al: Selective management of abdominal aortic aneurysms in a prospective measurement program. J Vasc Surg 23:213–220; discussion 221–222, 1996.

129. Kato N, Semba CP, Dake MD: Embolization of perigraft leaks after endovascular stent-graft treatment of aortic aneurysms. J Vasc Interv Radiol 7:805–811, 1996.

130. Khilnani NM, Sos TA, Trost DW, et al: Embolization of backbleeding lumbar arteries filling an aortic aneurysm sac after endovascular stent-graft placement. J Vasc Interv Radiol 7:813–817, 1996.

131. Lumsden AB, Allen RC, Chaikof EL, et al: Delayed rupture of aortic aneurysms following endovascular stent grafting. Am J Surg 170:174–178, 1995.

132. Nasim A, Thompson MM, Sayers RD, et al: Late failure of endoluminal abdominal aortic aneurysm repair due to continued aneurysm expansion. Br J Surg 83:810–811, 1996.

133. Walker SR, Halliday K, Yusuf SW, et al: A study on the patency of the inferior mesenteric and lumbar arteries in the incidence of endoleak following endovascular repair of infra-renal aortic aneurysms. Clin Radiol 53:593–595, 1998.

134. Bohm T, Soldner J, Rott A, Kaiser WA: Perigraft leak of an aortic stent graft due to material fatigue. AJR Am J Roentgenol 172:1355–1357, 1999.

135. Dorffner R, Thurnher S, Polterauer P, et al: Treatment of abdominal aortic aneurysms with transfemoral placement of stent-grafts: Complications and secondary radiologic intervention. Radiology 204:79–86, 1997.

136. Schurink GW, Aarts NJ, Wilde J, et al: Endoleakage after stent-graft treatment of abdominal aneurysm: Implications on pressure and imaging—an in vitro study. J Vasc Surg 28:234–241, 1998.

137. Schurink GW, Aarts NJ, van Bockel JH: Endoleak after stent-graft treatment of abdominal aortic aneurysm: A meta-analysis of clinical studies. Br J Surg 86:581–587, 1999.

138. Krohg SrK, Brekke M, Drolsum A, Kvernebo K: Periprosthetic leak and rupture after endovascular repair of abdominal aortic aneurysm: The significance of device design for long-term results. J Vasc Surg 29:1152–1158, 1999.

139. Zarins CK, White RA, Schwarten D, et al: AneuRx stent graft versus open surgical repair of abdominal aortic aneurysms: Multicenter prospective clinical trial. J Vasc Surg 29:292–305; discussion 306–308, 1999.

140. Alimi YS, Chakfe N, Rivoal E, et al: Rupture of an abdominal aortic aneurysm after endovascular graft placement and aneurysm size reduction. J Vasc Surg 28:178–183, 1998.

141. Silberzweig JE, Marin ML, Hollier LH, et al: Aortoiliac aneurysms: Endoluminal repair—clinical evidence for a fully supported stent-graft. Radiology 209:111–116, 1998.

142. Maleux G, Rousseau H, Otal P, et al: Modular component separation and reperfusion of abdominal aortic aneurysm sac after endovascular repair of the abdominal aortic aneurysm: A case report. J Vasc Surg 28:349–352, 1998.

143. Armon MP, Yusuf SW, Latief K, et al: Anatomical suitability of abdominal aortic aneurysms for endovascular repair. Br J Surg 84:178–180, 1997.

144. D'Ayala M, Hollier LH, Marin ML: Endovascular grafting for abdominal aortic aneurysms. Surg Clin North Am 78:845–862, 1998.

145. Mialhe C, Amicabile C, Becquemin JP: Endovascular treatment of infrarenal abdominal aneurysms by the Stentor system: Preliminary results of 79 cases. Stentor Retrospective Study Group. J Vasc Surg 26:199–209, 1997.

146. Hausegger KA, Mendel H, Tiessenhausen K, et al: Endoluminal treatment of infrarenal aortic aneurysms: Clinical experience with the Talent stent-graft system. J Vasc Interv Radiol 10:267–274, 1999.

147. Chuter TA, Risberg B, Hopkinson BR, et al: Clinical experience with a bifurcated endovascular graft for abdominal aortic aneurysm repair. J Vasc Surg 24:655–666, 1996.

148. Chuter TA, Gordon RL, Reilly LM, et al: Abdominal aortic aneurysm in high-risk patients: Short- to intermediate-term results of endovascular repair. Radiology 210:361–365, 1999.

149. Kato N, Dake MD, Semba CP, et al: Treatment of aortoiliac aneurysms with use of single-piece tapered stent-grafts. J Vasc Interv Radiol 9(1 Pt 1):41–49, 1998.

150. Edwards WH Jr, Naslund TC, Edwards WH Sr, et al: Endovascular grafting of abdominal aortic aneurysms: A preliminary study. Ann Surg 223:568–573; discussion 573–575, 1996.

151. Lawrence-Brown MM, Hartley D, MacSweeney ST, et al: The Perth endoluminal bifurcated graft system—development and early experience. Cardiovasc Surg 4:706–712, 1996.

152. Uflacker R, Robison JG, Brothers TE, et al: Abdominal aortic aneurysm treatment: Preliminary results with the Talent stent-graft system. J Vasc Interv Radiol 9:51–60, 1998.

153. May J, White GH, Yu W, et al: Concurrent comparison of endoluminal versus open repair in the treatment of abdominal aortic aneurysms: Analysis of 303 patients by life table method. J Vasc Surg 27:213–220; discussion 220–221, 1998.

154. Jaeger HJ, Mathias KD, Gissler HM, et al: Rectum and sigmoid colon necrosis due to cholesterol embolization after implantation of an aortic stent-graft. J Vasc Interv Radiol 10:751–755, 1999.

155. Chuter TA, Reilly LM, Kerlan RK, et al: Endovascular repair of abdominal aortic aneurysm: Getting out of trouble. Cardiovasc Surg 6:232–239, 1998.

156. Jacobowitz GR, Lee AM, Riles TS: Immediate and late explantation of endovascular aortic grafts: The endovascular technologies experience. J Vasc Surg 29:309–316, 1999.

157. Laborde JC, Parodi JC, Clem MF, et al: Intraluminal bypass of abdominal aortic aneurysm: Feasibility study. Radiology 184:185–190, 1992.

158. Mirich D, Wright KC, Wallace S, et al: Percutaneously placed endovascular grafts for aortic aneurysms: Feasibility study. Radiology 170:1033–1037, 1989.

159. Mitchell RS, Miller DC, Dake MD, et al: Thoracic aortic aneurysm repair with an endovascular stent graft: The "first generation". Ann Thorac Surg 67:1971–1974; discussion 1979–1980, 1999.

160. Ehrlich M, Grabenwoeger M, Cartes-Zumelzu F, et al: Endovascular stent graft repair for aneurysms on the descending thoracic aorta. Ann Thorac Surg 66:19–24; discussion 24–25, 1998.

161. Dake MD, Miller DC, Semba CP, et al: Transluminal placement of endovascular stent-grafts for the treatment of descending thoracic aortic aneurysms. N Engl J Med 331:1729–1734, 1994.

161a. Grabenwoger M, Hutschala D, Ehrlich MP, et al: Thoracic aortic aneurysms: Treatment with endovascular self-expandable stent grafts. Ann Thorac Surg 69:441–445, 2000.

162. Semba CP, Sakai T, Slonim SM, et al: Mycotic aneurysms of the thoracic aorta: Repair with use of endovascular stent-grafts. J Vasc Interv Radiol 9:33–40, 1998.

163. Semba CP, Kato N, Kee ST, et al: Acute rupture of the descending thoracic aorta: Repair with use of endovascular stent-grafts. J Vasc Interv Radiol 8:337–342, 1997.

164. Richardson JW, Greenfield LJ: Natural history and management of iliac aneurysms. J Vasc Surg 8:165–171, 1998.

165. Krupski WC, Selzman CH, Floridia R, et al: Contemporary management of isolated iliac aneurysms. J Vasc Surg 28:1–11; discussion 11–13, 1998.

166. Razavi MK, Dake MD, Semba CP, et al: Percutaneous endoluminal placement of stent-grafts for the treatment of isolated iliac artery aneurysms. Radiology 197:801–804, 1995.

167. Marin ML, Veith FJ, Lyon RT, et al: Transfemoral endovascular repair of iliac artery aneurysms. Am J Surg 170:179–182, 1995.

168. Quinn SF, Sheley RC, Semonsen KG, et al: Endovascular stents covered with pre-expanded polytetrafluoroethylene for treatment of iliac artery aneurysms and fistulas. J Vasc Interv Radiol 8:1057–1063, 1997.

169. Gasparini D, Lovaria A, Saccheri S, et al: Percutaneous treatment of iliac aneurysms and pseudoaneurysms with Cragg Endopro System 1 stent-grafts. Cardiovasc Intervent Radiol 20:348–352, 1997.

170. Cynamon J, Marin ML, Veith FJ, et al: Endovascular repair of an internal iliac artery aneurysm with use of a stented graft and embolization coils. J Vasc Interv Radiol 6:509–512, 1995.

171. May J, White G, Waugh R, et al: Transluminal placement of a prosthetic graft-stent device for treatment of subclavian artery aneurysm. J Vasc Surg 18:1056–1059, 1993.

172. Marin ML, Veith FJ, Panetta TF, et al: Transluminally placed endovascular stented graft repair for arterial trauma [see comments]. J Vasc Surg 20:466–472; discussion 472–473, 1994.

173. Becker GJ, Benenati JF, Zemel G, et al: Percutaneous placement of a balloon-expandable intraluminal graft for life-threatening subclavian arterial hemorrhage. J Vasc Interv Radiol 2:225–229, 1991.

174. Marotta TR, Buller C, Taylor D, et al: Autologous vein-covered stent repair of a cervical internal carotid artery pseudoaneurysm: Technical case report. Neurosurgery 42:408–412; discussion 412–413, 1998.

175. McGraw JK, Patzik SB, Gale SS, et al: Autogenous vein-covered stent for the endovascular management of a superior mesenteric artery pseudoaneurysm. J Vasc Interv Radiol 9:779–782, 1998.

VENOUS INTERVENTIONS

176. Sze DY, Vestring T, Liddell RP, et al: Recurrent TIPS failure associated with biliary fistulae: Treatment with PTFE-covered stents [In Process Citation]. Cardiovasc Intervent Radiol 22:298–304, 1999.

177. Dake MD, Semba CP: Thrombolytic therapy in venous occlusive disease. J Vasc Interv Radiol 6(6 Pt 2 Su):73S–77S, 1995.

178. Mewissen MW, Seabrook GR, Meissner MH, et al: Catheter-directed thrombolysis for lower extremity deep venous thrombosis: Report of a national multicenter registry. Radiology 211:39–49, 1999.

179. Makhoul RG, Machleder HI: Developmental anomalies at the thoracic outlet: An analysis of 200 consecutive cases. J Vasc Surg 16:534–542; discussion 542–545, 1992.

180. Sheeran SR, Hallisey MJ, Murphy TP, et al: Local thrombolytic therapy as part of a multidisciplinary approach to acute axillosubclavian vein thrombosis (Paget-Schroetter syndrome). J Vasc Interv Radiol 8:253–260, 1997.

181. Machleder HI: Evaluation of a new treatment strategy for Paget-Schroetter syndrome: Spontaneous thrombosis of the axillary-subclavian vein. J Vasc Surg 17:305–315; discussion 316–317, 1993.

182. Molina JE: Surgery for effort thrombosis of the subclavian vein. J Thorac Cardiovasc Surg 103:341–346, 1992.

183. Urschel HC Jr, Razzuk MA: Improved management of the Paget-Schroetter syndrome secondary to thoracic outlet compression. Ann Thorac Surg 52:1217–1221, 1991.

184. Lee MC, Grassi CJ, Belkin M, et al: Early operative intervention after thrombolytic therapy for primary subclavian vein thrombosis: An effective treatment approach. J Vasc Surg 27:1101–1107; discussion 1107–1108, 1998.

185. Meier GH, Pollak JS, Rosenblatt M, et al: Initial experience with venous stents in exertional axillary-subclavian vein thrombosis. J Vasc Surg 24:974–981; discussion 981–983, 1996.

186. Cohen GS, Braunstein L, Ball DS, Domeracki F: Effort thrombosis: Effective treatment with vascular stent after unrelieved venous stenosis following a surgical release procedure. Cardiovasc Intervent Radiol 19:37–39, 1996.

187. Dartevelle PG, Chapelier AR, Pastorino U, et al: Long-term follow-up after prosthetic replacement of the superior vena cava combined with resection of mediastinal-pulmonary malignant tumors [see comments]. J Thorac Cardiovasc Surg 102:259–265, 1991.

188. Kee ST, Kinoshita L, Razavi MK, et al: Superior vena cava syndrome: Treatment with catheter-directed thrombolysis and endovascular stent placement. Radiology 206:187–193, 1998.

189. Hochrein J, Bashore TM, O'Laughlin MP, Harrison JK: Percutaneous stenting of superior vena cava syndrome: A case report and review of the literature. Am J Med 104:78–84, 1998.

190. Wojtowycz MM, Stoehr T, Crummy AB, et al: The Bird's Nest inferior vena caval filter: Review of a single-center experience. J Vasc Interv Radiol 8:171–179, 1997.

191. Johnson SP, Raiken DP, Grebe PJ, et al: Single institution prospective evaluation of the over-the-wire Greenfield vena caval filter. J Vasc Interv Radiol 9:766–773, 1998.

192. Crochet DP, Brunel P, Trogrlic S, et al: Long-term follow-up of Vena Tech-LGM filter: Predictors and frequency of caval occlusion. J Vasc Interv Radiol 10:137–142, 1999.

193. Engmann E, Asch MR: Clinical experience with the antecubital Simon nitinol IVC filter. J Vasc Interv Radiol 9:774–778, 1998.

194. Millward SF, Peterson RA, Moher D, et al: LGM (Vena Tech) vena caval filter: Experience at a single institution. J Vasc Interv Radiol 5:351–356, 1994.

195. Ferris EJ, McCowan TC, Carver DK, McFarland DR: Percutaneous inferior vena caval filters: Follow-up of seven designs in 320 patients [see comments]. Radiology 188:851–856, 1993.

196. Grassi CJ: Inferior vena caval filters: Analysis of five currently available devices. AJR Am J Roentgenol 156:813–821, 1991.

197. Vorwerk D, Schmitz-Rode T, Schurmann K, et al: Use of a temporary caval filter to assist percutaneous iliocaval thrombectomy: Experimental results. J Vasc Interv Radiol 6:737–740, 1995.

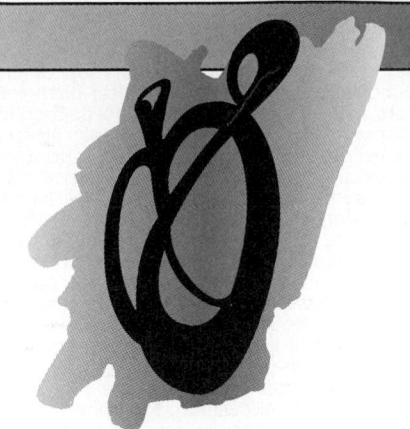

▼ PART V

DISEASES OF THE HEART, PERICARDIUM, AND PULMONARY VASCULAR BED

Chapter 43

Congenital Heart Disease in Infancy and Childhood

WILLIAM F. FRIEDMAN · NORMAN SILVERMAN

▼ General Considerations

DEFINITION

Congenital cardiovascular disease is defined as an *abnormality in cardiocirculatory structure or function that is present at birth, even if it is discovered much later.*[1a, b] Congenital cardiovascular malformations usually result from altered embryonic development of a normal structure or failure of such a structure to progress beyond an early stage of embryonic or fetal development. The aberrant patterns of flow created by an anatomical defect may, in turn, significantly influence the structural and functional development of the remainder of the circulation. For instance, the presence in utero of mitral atresia may prohibit normal development of the left ventricle, aortic valve, and ascending aorta. Similarly, constriction of the fetal ductus arteriosus may result directly in right ventricular dilatation and tricuspid regurgitation in the fetus and newborn, it may contribute importantly to the development of pulmonary arterial aneurysms in the presence of ventricular septal defect (VSD) and absent pulmonic valve, or, further, it may result in an alteration in the number and caliber of fetal and newborn pulmonary vascular resistance vessels.

POSTNATAL EVENTS. These may markedly influence the clinical presentation of a specific "isolated" malformation. Infants with Ebstein's malformation of the tricuspid valve may improve dramatically as the magnitude of tricuspid regurgitation diminishes with normal fall in pulmonary vascular resistance after birth; infants with hypoplastic left heart syndrome or interrupted aortic arch may not exhibit circulatory collapse; and infants with pulmonic atresia or severe stenosis may not become cyanotic until normal spontaneous closure of a patent ductus arteriosus occurs. Ductal constriction many days after birth also may be a central factor in some infants in the development of coarctation of the aorta. Still later in life, patients with a VSD may experience spontaneous closure of the abnormal communication or may develop right ventricular outflow tract obstruction and/or aortic regurgitation or pulmonary vascular obstructive disease. These selected examples serve to emphasize that anatomical and physiological changes in the heart and circulation may continue indefinitely from prenatal life in association with any specific congenital cardiocirculatory lesion.

Certain congenital defects are not apparent on gross inspection of the heart or circulation. Examples include the electrophysiological pathways for ventricular preexcitation or interruptions in the cardiac conduction system giving rise to paroxysmal supraventricular tachycardia or congenital complete heart block, respectively. Similarly, abnormalities in the development of myocardial autonomic innervation or in the ultrastructure of myocardial cells may ultimately prove to contribute to asymmetrical septal hypertrophy and left ventricular outflow tract obstruction. These examples make clear that occasional difficulties arise in distinguishing between congenital anomalies that are readily apparent at or shortly after birth and lesions that may have as their basis a subtle or undetectable abnormality that is present at birth.

INCIDENCE. The true incidence of congenital cardiovascular malformations is difficult to determine accurately, partly because of the difficulties in definition discussed earlier. About 0.8 percent of live births are complicated by a cardiovascular malformation.[1] This figure does not take into account what may be the two most common cardiac anomalies: the congenital, nonstenotic bicuspid aortic valve[2] and the leaflet abnormality associated with mitral valve prolapse.[3] Moreover, the widely quoted 0.8 percent incidence figure fails to include small preterm infants, almost all of whom have persistent patent ductus arteriosus. Further, if the calculations were to include stillbirths and abortuses, the incidence would be greatly increased. Cardiac malformations occur 10 times more often in stillborn than in liveborn babies, and many early spontaneous abortions are associated with chromosomal defects (see Chap. 56).[1] Thus, it is clear that past statistical analyses have seriously *underestimated* the incidence of congenital heart disease.

Precise data concerning the frequency of individual congenital lesions also are lacking, and the results of many analyses differ, depending on the source (living or dead) and the selection of the study population. Table 43–1 is a compilation from both clinical and pathological studies that approximates the frequency of occurrence of specific cardiovascular malformations.[4–6]

Considered in toto, children with congenital heart disease are predominantly male. Moreover, specific defects may show a definite gender preponderance; patent ductus

▼ **TABLE 43–1. RELATIVE FREQUENCY OF OCCURRENCE OF CARDIAC MALFORMATIONS AT BIRTH**

DISEASE	PERCENTAGE
Ventricular septal defect	30.5
Atrial septal defect	9.8
Patent ductus arteriosus	9.7
Pulmonic stenosis	6.9
Coarctation of the aorta	6.8
Aortic stenosis	6.1
Tetralogy of Fallot	5.8
Complete transposition of the great arteries	4.2
Persistent truncus arteriosus	2.2
Tricuspid atresia	1.3
All others	16.5

Data based on 2310 cases.

arteriosus, Ebstein's anomaly of the tricuspid valve, and atrial septal defect are more common in *females,* whereas valvular aortic stenosis, coarctation of the aorta, hypoplastic left heart, pulmonary and tricuspid atresia, and transposition of the great arteries are more common in *males.*[7]

Extracardiac anomalies occur in about 25 percent of infants with significant cardiac disease,[10] and their presence may significantly increase mortality. The extracardiac anomalies often are multiple, in part involving the musculoskeletal system; one-third of infants with both cardiac and extracardiac anomalies have some established syndrome.

ETIOLOGY

Malformations appear to result from an interaction between multifactorial genetic and environmental systems too complex to allow a single specification of cause[8]; in most instances, a causal factor cannot be identified. However, the explosion of new genetic research suggests that genetic causes are far more common than thought previously.[8, 9] Maternal rubella, ingestion of thalidomide and isotretinoin early during gestation, and chronic maternal alcohol abuse are environmental insults known to interfere with normal cardiogenesis in humans.[10, 11] *Rubella syndrome* consists of cataracts, deafness, microcephaly, and, either singly or in combination, patent ductus arteriosus, pulmonic valvular and/or arterial stenosis, and atrial septal defect. *Thalidomide* exposure is associated with major limb deformities and, occasionally, with cardiac malformations without predilection for a specific lesion. Tricuspid valve anomalies are associated with ingestion of *lithium* during pregnancy. The *fetal alcohol syndrome* consists of microcephaly, micrognathia, microphthalmia, prenatal growth retardation, developmental delay, and cardiac defects. The latter—often defects of the ventricular septum—occur in about 45 percent of affected infants. *Maternal lupus erythematosus* during pregnancy has been linked to congenital complete heart block. Animal experiments have incriminated hypoxia, deficiency or excess of several vitamins, intake of several categories of drugs, and ionizing irradiation as teratogens capable of causing cardiac malformations. The precise relation of these animal teratogens to human malformations is not clear.

The genetic aspects of congenital heart disease are discussed extensively in Chapter 56. A single gene mutation may be causative in the familial forms of atrial septal defect with prolonged atrioventricular (AV) conduction, mitral valve prolapse, VSD, congenital heart block, situs inversus, pulmonary hypertension, and the syndromes of Noonan, LEOPARD, Ellis-van Creveld, and Kartagener. The genes responsible for several defects have either been mapped (e.g., long QT syndrome, Holt-Oram syndrome) or identified (e.g., Marfan syndrome, hypertrophic cardiomyopathy, supravalvular aortic stenosis). Contiguous gene defects on the long arm of chromosome 22 likely underlie the conotruncal malformations of the DiGeorge and velocardiofacial syndromes.[12] Table 43–2 provides a partial list of syndromes in which cardiovascular anomalies may be manifestations of the pleiotropic effects of single genes or examples of gross chromosomal defects. At present, less than 15 percent of all cardiac malformations can be accounted for by chromosomal aberrations or genetic mutations or transmission.

The finding that, with some exceptions, only one of a pair of monozygotic twins is affected by congenital heart disease indicates that the vast majority of cardiovascular malformations are not inherited in a simple manner.[13] However, this observation may have led, in the past, to an underestimation of genetic contribution, because most recent twin studies reveal more than double the incidence of

SYNDROME	MAJOR CARDIOVASCULAR MANIFESTATIONS	MAJOR NONCARDIAC ABNORMALITIES
Heritable and Possibly Heritable/(Genetic Locus)		
Ellis-van Creveld	Single atrium or atrial septal defect	Chondrodystrophic dwarfism, nail dysplasia, polydactyly
TAR (thrombocytopenia—absent radius)	Atrial septal defect, tetralogy of Fallot	Radial aplasia or hypoplasia, thrombocytopenia
Holt-Oram	Atrial septal defect (other defects common) (12q21–q3)	Skeletal upper limb defect, hypoplasia of clavicles
Kartagener	Dextrocardia	Situs inversus, sinusitis, bronchiectasis
Laurence-Moon-Biedl-Bardet	Variable defects	Retinal pigmentation, obesity, polydactyly
Noonan	Pulmonic valve dysplasia, cardiomyopathy (usually hypertrophic) (12Q24)	Webbed neck, pectus excavatum, cryptorchidism
Tuberous sclerosis	Rhabdomyoma, cardiomyopathy (type 1–9q, type 2–16p)	Phakomatosis, bone lesions, hamartomatous skin lesions
Multiple lentigines (LEOPARD)	Pulmonic stenosis	Basal cell nevi, broad facies, rib anomalies, deafness
Rubinstein-Taybi	Patent ductus arteriosus (others) (16p13.3)	Broad thumbs and toes, hypoplastic maxilla, slanted palpebral fissures
Familial deafness	Arrhythmias, sudden death	Sensorineural deafness
Weber-Osler-Rendu	Arteriovenous fistulas (lung, liver, mucous membranes) (9q33–4)	Multiple telangiectasias
Apert	Ventricular septal defect (10q26)	Craniosynostosis, midfacial hypoplasia, syndactyly
Crouzon	Patent ductus arteriosus, aortic coarctation (10q26, 4p16.3)	Ptosis with shallow orbits, craniosynostosis, maxillary hypoplasia
Hypertrophic cardiomyopathy	Asymmetric septal hypertrophy (locus heterogeneity, 14q11.2–12, 1q32, 15.q22, 11p11.2, and others)	Family history of sudden death
Incontinentia pigmenti	Patent ductus arteriosus	Irregular pigmented skin lesions, patchy alopecia, hypodontia
Alagille (arteriohepatic dysplasia)	Peripheral pulmonic stenosis, pulmonic stenosis (20p12)	Biliary hypoplasia, vertebral anomalies, prominent forehead, deep-set eyes
Catch-22 (DiGeorge)	Interrupted aortic arch, tetralogy of Fallot, truncus arteriosus (22q11)	Thymic hypoplasia or aplasia, parathyroid aplasia or hypoplasia, abnormal facies
Shprintzen (velocardiofacial)	Ventricular septal defect, tetralogy of Fallot, right aortic arch (22q11.2)	Cleft palate, prominent nose, slender hands, learning disability
Williams	Supravalvular aortic stenosis, peripheral pulmonic stenosis (7q11.23)	Mental deficiency, elfin facies, loquacious personality, hoarse voice
Long Q-T (Jervell and Lange-Nielsen, Romano-Ward)	Long QT interval, ventricular arrhythmias (11p15.5, 7q35, 3p21) 21q22	Family history of sudden death, congenital deafness (not in Romano-Ward)
Friedreich's ataxia	Cardiomyopathy and conduction defects (9q)	Ataxia, speech defect, degeneration of spinal cord dorsal columns
Muscular dystrophy	Cardiomyopathy	Pseudohypertrophy of calf muscles, weakness of trunk and proximal limb muscles
Cystic fibrosis	Cor pulmonale (7q)	Pancreatic insufficiency, malabsorption, chronic lung disease
Sickle cell anemia	Cardiomyopathy, mitral regurgitation (11p)	Hemoglobin SS
Conradi-Hünermann	Ventricular septal defect, patent ductus arteriosus	Asymmetrical limb shortness, early punctate mineralization, large skin pores
Cockayne	Accelerated atherosclerosis	Cachectic dwarfism, retinal pigment abnormalities, photosensitivity dermatitis
Progeria	Accelerated atherosclerosis	Premature aging, alopecia, atrophy of subcutaneous fat, skeletal hypoplasia
Connective Tissue Disorders		
Cutis laxa	Peripheral pulmonic stenosis	Generalized disruption of elastic fibers, diminished skin resilience, hernias
Ehlers-Danlos	Arterial dilatation and rupture, mitral regurgitation (2q31)	Hyperextensible joints, hyperelastic and friable
Marfan	Aortic dilatation, aortic and mitral incompetence (15q21.1)	Gracile habitus, arachnodactyly with hyperextensibility, lens subluxation
Osteogenesis imperfecta	Aortic incompetence (7, 17)	Fragile bones, blue sclerae
Pseudoxanthoma elasticum	Peripheral and coronary arterial disease	Degeneration of elastic fibers in skin, retinal angioid streaks

Table continued on following page

▼ TABLE 43–2. SYNDROMES WITH ASSOCIATED CARDIOVASCULAR INVOLVEMENT *Continued*

SYNDROME	MAJOR CARDIOVASCULAR MANIFESTATIONS	MAJOR NONCARDIAC ABNORMALITIES
Inborn Errors of Metabolism		
Pompe disease	Glycogen storage disease of heart	Acid maltase deficiency, muscle weakness
Homocystinuria	Aortic and pulmonary artery dilatation, intravascular thrombosis	Cystathionine β-synthase deficiency, lens subluxation, osteoporosis
Mucopolysaccharidoses: Hurler; Hunter	Multivalvular and coronary and great artery disease; cardiomyopathy	Hurler: Deficiency of α-L-iduronidase, corneal clouding, coarse features, growth and mental retardation
		Hunter: Deficiency of L-idurano-sulfate sulfatase, coarse facies, clear cornea, growth and mental retardation
Morquio; Scheie; Maroteaux-Lamy	Aortic regurgitation	Morquio: Deficiency of *N*-acetylhexosamine sulfate sulfatase, cloudy cornea, severe bone changes involving vertebrae and epiphyses
		Scheie: Deficiency of α-L-iduronidase, cloudy cornea, normal intelligence, peculiar facies
		Maroteaux-Lamy: Deficiency of arylsulfatase B, cloudy cornea, osseous changes
Chromosomal Abnormalities		
Trisomy 21 (Down syndrome)	Endocardial cushion defect, atrial or ventricular septal defect, tetralogy of Fallot	Hypotonia, hyperextensible joints, mongoloid facies, mental retardation
Trisomy 13(D)	Ventricular septal defect, right ventricle patent ductus arteriosus, double-outlet right ventricle	Single midline intracerebral ventricle with midfacial defects, polydactyly, nail changes, mental retardation
Trisomy 18(E)	Congenital polyvalvular dysplasia, ventricular septal defect, patent ductus	Clenched hand, short sternum, low arch dermal ridge pattern on fingertips, mental retardation
Cri du chat (short-arm deletion-5)	Ventricular septal defect	Cat cry, microcephaly, antimongoloid slant of palpebral fissues, mental retardation
XO (Turner)	Coarctation of aorta, bicuspid aortic valve, aortic dilatation	Short female, broad chest, lymphedema, webbed neck
XXXY and XXXXX	Patent ductus arteriosus	XXXY: Hypogenitalism, mental retardation, radial-ulnar synostosis
		XXXXX: Small hands, incurving of fifth fingers, mental retardation
Sporadic Disorders		
VATER association	Ventricular septal defect	Vertebral anomalies, anal atresia, tracheoesophageal fistula, radial and renal anomalies
CHARGE association	Tetralogy of Fallot (other defects common)	Colobomas, choanal atresia, mental and growth deficiency, genital and ear anomalies
Cornelia de Lange	Ventricular septal defect	Micromelia, synophrys, mental and growth deficiency
Teratogenic Disorders		
Rubella	Patent ductus arteriosus, pulmonic valvular and/or arterial stenosis, atrial septal defect	Cataracts, deafness, microcephaly
Alcohol	Ventricular septal defect (other defects)	Microcephaly, growth and mental deficiency, short palpebral fissures, smooth philtrum, thin upper lip
Dilantin	Pulmonic stenosis, aortic stenosis, coarctation, patent ductus arteriosus	Hypertelorism, growth and mental deficiency, short phalanges, bowed upper lip
Thalidomide	Variable	Phocomelia
Lithium	Ebstein's anomaly, tricuspid atresia	None

Modified from Friedman WF, Child JS: Congenital heart disease. *In* Fauci A,, Braunwald E, Isselbacher KJ, et al (eds): Harrison's Principles of Internal Medicine. 14th ed. New York, McGraw-Hill, 1998, p 1300. © 1998 The McGraw-Hill Companies, Inc.

heart defects in monozygotic twins but usually in only one of the pair.[14] Family studies indicate a 2-fold to 10-fold increase in the incidence of congenital heart disease in siblings of affected patients or in the offspring of an affected parent. Malformations often are concordant or partially concordant within families.[15, 16] Because the incidence of congenital heart disease in the offspring or siblings of an index patient is only 2 to 10 percent, it is seldom wise to discour-

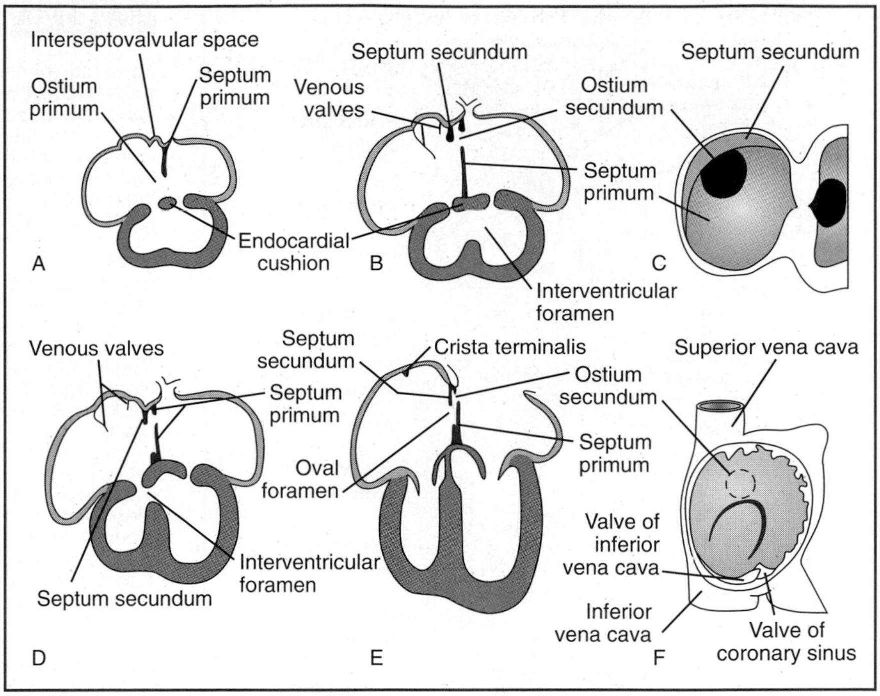

FIGURE 43–1. Diagrammatic representation of the atrial septa at 30 days *(A)*, at 33 days *(B)*, at 33 days (seen from the right side) *(C)*, at 37 days *(D)*, and in the newborn *(E)*; the newborn atrial septum viewed from the right *(F)*. (From Clark EB, Van Mierop LHS: Development of the cardiovascular system. *In* Adams FH, Emmanouilides GC, Riemenschneider TA, et al [eds]: Moss' Heart Disease in Infants, Children, and Adolescents. 4th ed. Baltimore, © Williams & Wilkins, 1989.)

age the parents of one affected child from having additional children if either parent is free of a cardiovascular anomaly.[1] Moreover, the low recurrence rate and the increasing possibilities for effective treatment for nearly all cardiac lesions usually justify a positive approach to family counseling. When two or more members of the family are affected, the recurrence risk may be quite high, and a pedigree should be obtained before further counseling. If a dominant or recessive mendelian pattern is established, the mendelian laws apply, and the risk of recurrence in each pregnancy is equal.

PREVENTION

The feasibility of preventive programs depends on what is learned in the future about the 85 percent or more of cardiovascular anomalies for which no cause currently is known. Strict animal testing of new drugs that may be teratogenic when taken during pregnancy may be expected to reduce the chances of another thalidomide tragedy. In this regard, the dictum cannot be emphasized too strongly that no medication should be taken during pregnancy without prior consultation with a physician. Physicians who deal with pregnant women should be aware of known teratogens as well as drugs that may have a functional rather than a structural damaging influence on the fetal and newborn heart and circulation, and they should recognize that for many drugs, information about their teratogenic potential is inadequate. Similarly, appropriate radiological equipment and techniques for reducing gonadal and fetal radiation exposure should always be used to reduce the potential hazards of this likely cause of birth defects.

Detection of abnormal chromosomes in fetal cells obtained from amniotic fluid or chorionic villus biopsy (see Chap. 56) may predict cardiac malformation as one component of the multisystem involvement that may exist in such syndromes as Down, Turner's, or trisomy 13–15 (D1) or 16–18 (E). Similarly, identification in such cells of the enzyme disorders observed in the mucopolysaccharidoses, homocystinuria, or type II glycogen storage disease may allow one to predict the ultimate presence of cardiac disease. Finally, immunization of children with rubella vaccine will avoid the effects of maternal rubella and its cardiac consequences.

Although fetal echocardiography may allow the identification of congenital heart disease, it is not yet clear if this modality will improve survivability.[17, 18] It is apparent, however, that a prenatal diagnosis of serious cardiac disease has resulted in a decision by some families to terminate pregnancies.

EMBRYOLOGY

NORMAL CARDIAC DEVELOPMENT. Correlation of anatomical features of malformed hearts and embryonic cardiac morphology allows a developmental analysis of various anomalies.[19] Detailed accounts of the normal development of the cardiovascular system are provided elsewhere.[20] In brief, during the first month of gestation, the primitive, straight cardiac tube is formed, comprising the sinuatrium, the primitive ventricle, the bulbus cordis, and the truncus arteriosus in series, from cephalad to caudad. In the second month of gestation, this tube doubles over on itself to form two parallel pumping systems, each with two chambers and a great artery. The two atria develop from the sinuatrium, the AV canal is divided by the endocardial cushions into tricuspid and mitral orifices, and the right and left ventricles develop from the primitive ventricle and bulbus cordis. Differential growth of myocardial cells causes the straight cardiac tube to bear to the right, and the bulboventricular portion of the tube doubles over on itself, bringing the ventricles side by side. Migration of the AV canal to the right and of the ventricular septum to the left serves to align each ventricle with its appropriate AV valve. At the distal end of the cardiac tube, the bulbus cordis divides into a subaortic muscular conus and a subpulmonic muscular conus; the subpulmonic conus elongates and the subaortic conus resorbs, allowing the aorta to move posteriorly and connect with the left ventricle.

ABNORMAL DEVELOPMENT. A host of anomalies may result from defects in this basic developmental pattern. Thus, double-inlet left ventricle is observed if the tricuspid orifice does not align over the right ventricle. The various types of persistent truncus arteriosus result from failure of the truncus to divide into the main pulmonary artery and aorta. Double-outlet anomalies of the right ventricle are produced by failure of either the subpulmonic or subaortic conus to resorb, whereas resorption of the subpulmonic instead of the subaortic conus may be central to transposition of the great arteries.

THE ATRIA. The primitive sinuatrium is separated into right and left atria by the downgrowth from its roof of the septum primum toward the AV canal, thereby creating an inferior intraatrial ostium primum opening (Fig. 43–1). Numerous perforations form in the anterosuperior portion of the septum primum as the septum secundum begins to develop to the right of the former. The coalescence of these perforations forms the ostium secundum. The septum secundum completely separates the atrial chambers except for a central opening—the fossa ovalis—which is covered by tissue of the septum primum, forming the valve of the foramen ovale.

Fusion of the endocardial cushions anteriorly and posteriorly divides the AV canal into tricuspid and mitral inlets (Fig. 43–2). The inferior portion of the atrial septum, the superior portion of the ventricular septum, and portions of the septal leaflets of both the tricuspid and mitral valves are formed from the endocardial cushions. The integrity of the atrial septum depends on growth of the septum primum and septum secundum and proper fusion of the endocardial cushions. Atrial septal defects and various degrees of endocardial cushion defect are the result of developmental deficiencies of this process.

THE VENTRICLES. Partitioning of the ventricles occurs as cephalic growth of the main ventricular septum results in its fusion with the endocardial cushions and the infundibular or conus septum. Defects in the ventricular septum may occur owing to a deficiency of septal substance; malalignment of septal components in different planes, preventing their fusion; or an overly long conus, keeping the septal components apart. Isolated defects probably result from the first

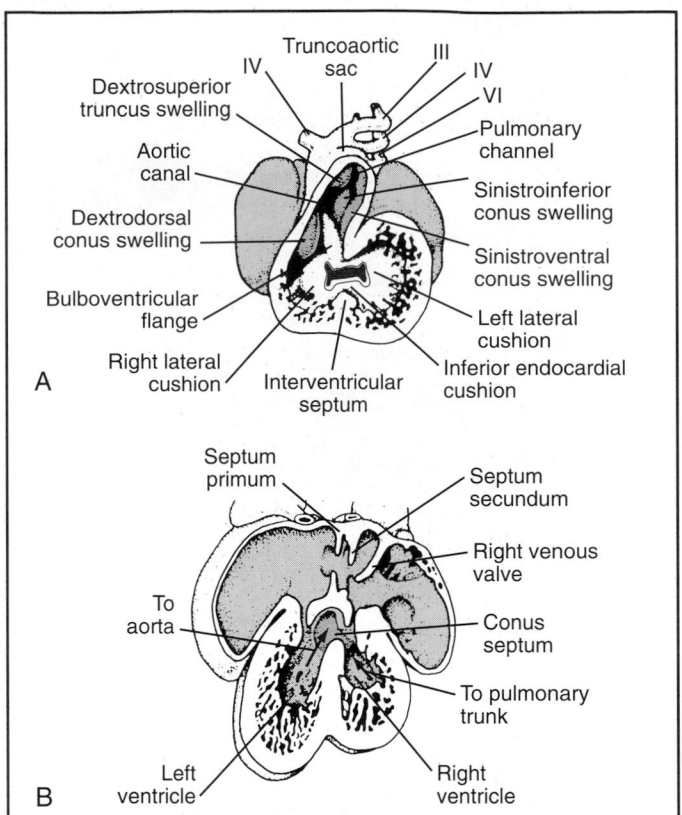

FIGURE 43–2. Frontal section through the heart of a 9-mm embryo *(A)* and 15-mm embryo *(B)*. At 9 mm, development of the cushions in the atrioventricular canal is noted, and the truncus and conus swellings are visible. At 15 mm, the conus septum is completed; note the septation in the atrial region. (From Clark EB, Van Mierop LHS: Development of the cardiovascular system. *In* Adams FH, Emmanouilides GC, Riemenschneider TA, et al [eds]: Moss' Heart Disease in Infants, Children, and Adolescents. 4th ed. Baltimore, © Williams & Wilkins, 1989.)

mechanism, whereas the latter two appear to generate the ventricular defects in tetralogy of Fallot and transposition complexes.

THE LUNGS. These structures arise from the primitive foregut and are drained early in embryogenesis by channels from the splanchnic plexus to the cardinal and umbilicovitelline veins. An outpouching from the posterior left atrium forms the common pulmonary vein, which communicates with the splanchnic plexus, establishing pulmonary venous drainage to the left atrium. The umbilicovitelline and anterior cardinal vein communications atrophy as the common pulmonary vein is incorporated into the left atrium. Anomalous pulmonary venous connections to the umbilicovitelline (portal) venous system or to the cardinal system (superior vena cava) result from failure of the common pulmonary vein to develop or establish communications to the splanchnic plexus. Cor triatriatum results from a narrowing of the common pulmonary vein–left atrial junction.

THE GREAT ARTERIES. The truncus arteriosus is connected to the dorsal aorta in the embryo by six pairs of aortic arches. Partition of the truncus arteriosus into two great arteries is a result of the fusion of tissue arising from the back wall of the vessel and the truncus septum. Rotation of the truncus coils the aorticopulmonary septum and creates the normal spiral relation between the aorta and pulmonary artery. Semilunar valves and their related sinuses are created by absorption and hollowing out of tissue at the distal side of the truncus ridges. Aorticopulmonary septal defect and persistent truncus arteriosus represent various degrees of partitioning failure.

Although the six aortic arches appear sequentially, portions of the arch system and dorsal aorta disappear at different times during embryogenesis (Fig. 43–3). The first, second, and fifth sets of paired arches regress completely. The proximal portions of the sixth arches become the right and left pulmonary arteries, and the distal left sixth arch becomes the ductus arteriosus. The third aortic arch forms the connection between the internal and external carotid arteries, and the left fourth arch becomes the arterial segment between the left carotid and subclavian arteries; the proximal portion of the right subclavian artery forms from the right fourth arch. An abnormality in regression of the arch system in a number of sites can produce a wide variety of arch anomalies, whereas a failure of regression usually results in a double aortic arch malformation.

FETAL AND TRANSITIONAL CIRCULATIONS

Although the illness created by the presence of a cardiac malformation is almost always recognized only after an affected baby is born, important effects on the circulation have existed from early in pregnancy until the time of delivery. Thus, knowledge of the changes in cardiocirculatory structure, function, and metabolism that accompany development is central to a systematic comprehension of congenital heart disease.

FETAL CIRCULATORY PATHWAYS. Dynamic alterations occur in the circulation during the transition from fetal to neonatal life when the lungs take over the function of gas exchange from the placenta. The single fetal circulation consists of parallel pulmonary and systemic pathways (Fig. 43–4) in contrast to the two-circuit system in the newborn and adult, in whom the pulmonary vasculature exists in series with the systemic circulation. Prenatal survival is not endangered by major cardiac anomalies as long as one side of the heart can drive blood from the great veins to the aorta; in the fetus, blood can bypass the nonfunctioning lungs both proximal and distal to the heart.

Oxygenated blood returns from the placenta through the umbilical vein and enters the portal venous system. A variable amount of this stream bypasses the hepatic microcirculation and enters the inferior vena cava by way of the ductus venosus. Inferior vena caval blood flows from the ductus venosus, hepatic vein, and lower body venous drainage, which is summarily deflected to a significant extent across the foramen ovale into the left atrium. Almost all superior vena caval blood passes directly through the tricuspid valve, entering the right ventricle. Most of the blood that reaches the right ventricle bypasses the high-resistance, unexpanded lungs and passes through the ductus arteriosus into the descending aorta. The right ventricle contributes about 55 percent and the left 45 percent to the total fetal cardiac output. The major portion of blood ejected from the left ventricle supplies the brain and upper body, with lesser flow to the coronary arteries; the balance passes across the aortic isthmus to the descending aorta, where it joins with the large stream from the ductus arteriosus before flowing to the lower body and placenta.

FETAL PULMONARY CIRCULATION. In fetal life, pulmonary arteries and arterioles are surrounded by a fluid medium, have relatively thick walls and small lumina, and resemble comparable arteries in the systemic circulation. The low pulmonary blood flow in the fetus (7 to 10 percent of the total cardiac output) is the result of high pulmonary vascular resistance. Fetal pulmonary vessels are highly reactive to changes in oxygen tension or in the pH of blood perfusing them as well as to a number of other physiological and pharmacological influences.

EFFECTS OF CARDIAC MALFORMATIONS ON THE FETUS. Although fetal somatic growth may be unimpaired, the hemodynamic effects in utero of many cardiac malformations may alter the development and structure of the fetal heart and circulation.[22] Thus, anomalous pulmonary venous connection in utero may result in underdevelopment of the left atrium and left ventricle, and premature closure of the foramen ovale may result in hypoplasia of the left ventricle. Moreover, postnatally, the caliber of the aortic isthmus may be reduced in the presence of lesions in utero that create left ventricular hypertrophy, such as aortic stenosis, and impede filling because of reduced compliance of that chamber. It may also be reduced in the presence of a lesion that interferes with left ventricular filling directly (e.g., mitral stenosis) or indirectly by diverting a proportion of left ventricular output away from the ascending aorta while increasing right ventricular output and ductus arteriosus flow (e.g., AV septal defect with left ventricular–right atrial shunt or aortic or subaortic stenosis with VSD). Similarly, obstruction in utero to right ventricular outflow is associated with an increase in proximal aortic flow and diameter and almost never with aortic coarctation. Ebstein's malformation of the tricuspid valve is more commonly recognized in the fetus than ex utero. Death with severe hydrops in utero or early in postnatal life may account for a much lower frequency of this lesion in data gathered after birth. The anomaly, which produces fetal AV valvar regurgitation, a large right-to-left atrial shunt, and ineffective pulmonary flow compromising pulmonary vasculature development, is one of the most significant causes of fetal hydrops, heart failure, and loss. Similar tricuspid valve hemodynamic consequences can also occur in pulmonary atresia with intact ventricular septum.[17, 21] In these and other examples, it is important to recognize that malformations compatible with fetal survival may nonetheless result in abnormal development of the circulation in utero and also affect circulatory adjustments after birth.[23]

FUNCTION OF THE FETAL HEART. Compared with the adult heart, the fetal and newborn heart is unique with respect to its ultrastructural appearance[24] its mechanical and biochemical properties,[25–30] and autonomic innervation.[31] During late fetal and early neonatal development, there is maturation of the excitation-contraction coupling process[32, 33] and the biochemical composition of the heart's energy-utilizing myofibrillar proteins and of adenosine triphosphate and creatine phosphate energy-producing proteins.[29] Moreover, fetal and neonatal myocardial cells are small in diameter and reduced in density, so that the young heart contains relatively more noncontractile mass (pri-

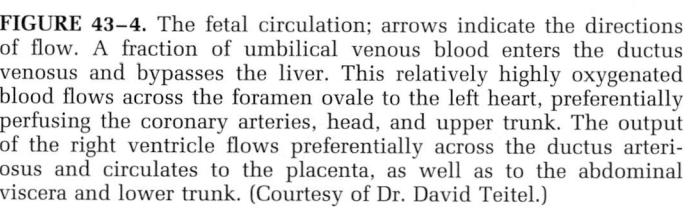

FIGURE 43–3. Transformation of the aortic arches and dorsal aorta into the definitive vascular pattern is a process of fusion and segmental resorption of the paired first to sixth branchial arches with the paired dorsal aorta. (From Castañcda A, Jonas RΛ, Mayer JE Jr, et al: Cardiac Surgery of the Neonate and Infant. Philadelphia, WB Saunders, 1994, p 398.)

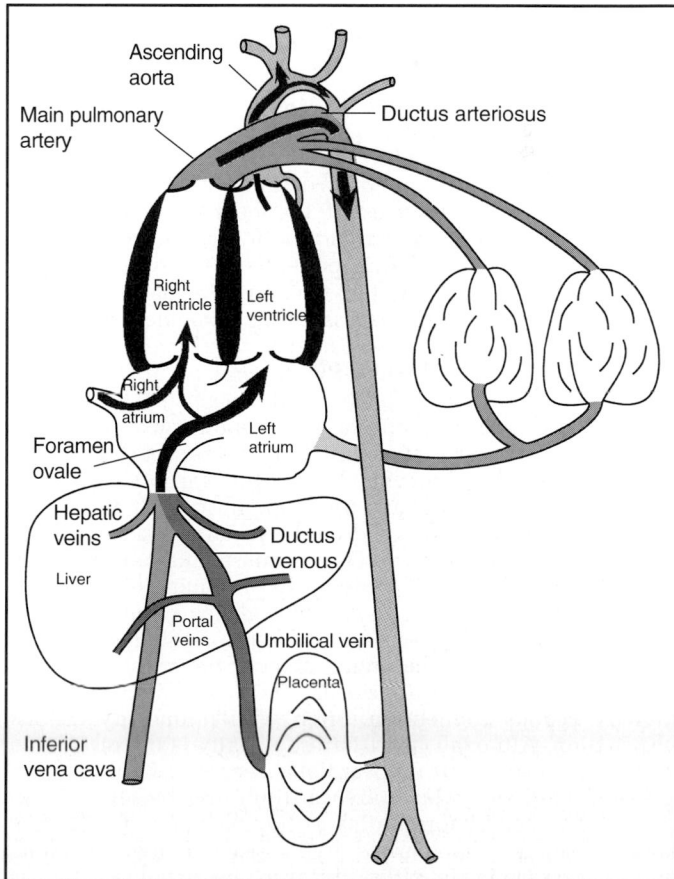

FIGURE 43–4. The fetal circulation; arrows indicate the directions of flow. A fraction of umbilical venous blood enters the ductus venosus and bypasses the liver. This relatively highly oxygenated blood flows across the foramen ovale to the left heart, preferentially perfusing the coronary arteries, head, and upper trunk. The output of the right ventricle flows preferentially across the ductus arteriosus and circulates to the placenta, as well as to the abdominal viscera and lower trunk. (Courtesy of Dr. David Teitel.)

marily mitochondria, nuclei, and surface membranes) than later in postnatal life. As a result, force generation and the extent and velocity of shortening are decreased, and stiffness and water content of ventricular myocardium are increased in the fetal and early newborn periods.

The diminished function of the young heart is reflected in its limited ability to increase cardiac output in the presence of either a volume load or a lesion that increases resistance to emptying.[34] Although functional integrity of efferent and afferent cardiac autonomic pathways exists early in life, fetal and newborn myocardium lacks the complete development of sympathetic but not cholinergic innervation. Thus, adaptation to cardiocirculatory stress in fetal or early newborn life may be less effective than in adulthood.

CHANGES AT BIRTH. The fundamental change that normally occurs at birth is a division of the single parallel fetal circulation into separate, independent circulations. Inflation of the lungs at the first inspiration produces a marked reduction in pulmonary vascular resistance, owing partly to the sudden suspension in air of fetal pulmonary vessels previously supported by fluid media. The reduced extravascular pressure assists new vessels to open and already patent vessels to enlarge. The rapid decrease in pulmonary vascular resistance is related more importantly to vasodilatation owing to the increase in oxygen tension to which pulmonary vessels are exposed rather than to physical expansion of alveoli with gas. Defining the role of nitric oxide in the mediation of changes in pulmonary vascular tone in these events is of great interest.[35] Pulmonary arterial pressure falls, and pulmonary blood flow increases greatly. Systemic vascular resistance rises when clamping of the umbilical cord removes the low-resistance placental circulation. Increased pulmonary blood flow increases the return of blood to the left atrium and raises left atrial pressure, which in turn closes the foramen ovale.

The shift in oxygen dependence from the placenta to the lungs produces a sudden increase in arterial blood oxygen tension, which, in concert with alterations in the local prostaglandin milieu, initiates constriction of the ductus arteriosus.[36] Pulmonary pressure falls further as the ductus constricts. In healthy mature infants, the ductus arteriosus is profoundly constricted at 10 to 15 hours and is closed functionally by 72 hours, with total anatomical closure following within a few weeks by a process of thrombosis, intimal proliferation, and fibrosis. Preterm infants have a high incidence of persistent patency of the ductus arteriosus because of an immaturity of those mechanisms responsible for constriction. In surviving preterm infants, the ductus arteriosus spontaneously closes within 4 to 12 months of birth.

The ductus venosus, ductus arteriosus, and foramen ovale remain potential channels for blood flow after birth. Thus, persistent patency of the ductus venosus may mask the most marked signs of pulmonary venous obstruction in infants with total anomalous pulmonary venous connection below the diaphragm. Similarly, lesions producing right or left atrial volume or pressure overload may stretch the foramen ovale and render incompetent the flap valve mechanism for its closure. Anomalies that depend on patency of the ductus arteriosus for preserving pulmonary or systemic blood flow remain latent until the ductus arteriosus constricts. A common example is the rapid intensification of cyanosis observed in infants with tetralogy of Fallot when the magnitude of pulmonary hypoperfusion is unmasked by spontaneous closure of the ductus arteriosus. Moreover, increasing evidence shows that ductal constriction is a key factor in the postnatal development of coarctation of the aorta. Finally, it should be recognized that because the ductus arteriosus is potentially patent after birth and the pulmonary resistance vessels are hyperreactive, hypoxic pulmonary vasoconstriction of diverse causes may result in a right-to-left shunt through the ductus.

 # Pathological Consequences of Congenital Cardiac Lesions

CONGESTIVE HEART FAILURE

Although the basic mechanisms of cardiac failure, as outlined in Chapter 16, are similar for all ages, pediatric cardiologists should clearly recognize that the common causes, time of onset, and often the approach to treatment vary with age.[37, 38] The development of fetal echocardiography has allowed the diagnosis of intrauterine cardiac failure.[21, 39] The cardinal findings of fetal heart failure are scalp edema, ascites, pericardial effusion, and decreased fetal movements. Although abnormalities in several organ systems may result in nonimmunological fetal hydrops, cardiac causes include a host of structural, functional, rhythm, and metabolic disturbances of the heart. Infants younger than 1 year and having cardiac malformations account for 80 to 90 percent of pediatric patients who develop congestive failure. Moreover, cardiac decompensation in an infant is a medical emergency necessitating immediate treatment if the patient is to be saved.

CAUSES OF HEART FAILURE. In preterm infants, especially less than 1500-gm birth weight, persistent patency of the ductus arteriosus is the most common cause of cardiac decompensation, and other forms of structural heart disease are rare.[40] In full-term newborns, the earliest important causes of heart failure are the hypoplastic left heart and coarctation of the aorta syndromes, sustained tachyarrhythmia, cerebral or hepatic arteriovenous fistula, and myocarditis. Among the lesions commonly producing heart failure beyond age 1 to 2 weeks, when diminished pulmonary vascular resistance allows substantial left-to-right shunting, are VSD and atrioventricular septal defects, transposition of the great arteries, truncus arteriosus, and total anomalous pulmonary venous connection, often with pulmonary venous obstruction. Although heart failure usually is the result of a structural defect or of myocardial disease, it should be recognized that the newborn myocardium may be severely depressed by such abnormalities as hypoxemia and acidemia, anemia, septicemia, marked hypoglycemia, hypocalcemia, and polycythemia. In older children, heart failure often is

due to acquired disease (see Chap. 45) or is a complication of open-heart surgical procedures. In the acquired category are rheumatic and endomyocardial diseases, infective endocarditis, hematological and nutritional disorders, and severe cardiac arrhythmias.

CLINICAL MANIFESTATIONS IN THE INFANT. The clinical expression of cardiac decompensation in infants consists of distinctive signs of pulmonary and systemic venous congestion and altered cardiocirculatory performance that resemble, but often are not identical to, those of older children or adults (Table 43–3).[37, 41] These reflect the interplay between the hemodynamic burden and adaptive responses. Common symptoms and signs are feeding difficulties and failure to gain weight and grow, tachypnea, tachycardia, pulmonary rales and rhonchi, liver enlargement, and cardiomegaly. Less frequent manifestations include peripheral edema, ascites, pulsus alternans, gallop rhythm, wheezing, and inappropriate sweating. Pleural and pericardial effusions are exceedingly rare. The distinction between left and right heart failure is less obvious in infants than in older children or adults because most lesions that create a left ventricular pressure or volume overload also result in left-to-right shunting of blood through the foramen ovale and/or patent ductus arteriosus as well as pulmonary hypertension owing to elevated pulmonary venous pressures. Conversely, aug-

▼ **TABLE 43–3.** FEATURES OF HEART FAILURE IN INFANTS

Poor feeding and failure to thrive
Respiratory distress—mainly tachypnea
Rapid heart rate (160 to 180 beats/min)
Pulmonary rales or wheezing
Cardiomegaly and pulmonary edema on radiogram
Hepatomegaly (peripheral edema unusual)
Gallop sounds
Color—ashen pale or faintly cyanotic
Excessive perspiration
Diminished urine output

mented filling or elevated pressure of the right ventricle in infants reduces left ventricular compliance disproportionately when compared with older children or adults and gives rise to signs of both systemic and pulmonary venous congestion.[37]

Fatigue and dyspnea on exertion express themselves as a feeding problem in infants. Characteristically, the respiratory rate in heart failure is rapid (50 to 100 breaths/min). In the presence of left ventricular failure, interstitial pulmonary edema reduces pulmonary compliance and results in tachypnea and retractions. Excessive pulmonary blood flow by way of significant left-to-right shunts may further decrease lung compliance. Moreover, upper airway obstruction may be produced by selective enlargement of cardiovascular structures. In patients with large left-to-right shunts and left atrial and main pulmonary artery enlargement, the left main stem bronchus may be compressed, resulting in emphysematous expansion of the left upper or lower lobe or left lower lobe collapse.[42] Respiratory distress with grunting, flaring of the alae nasi, and intercostal retractions is observed when failure is severe and especially when pulmonary infection precipitates cardiac decompensation, which often is the case. Under these circumstances, pulmonary rales may be due to the infection, failure, or both. A resting heart rate with little variability is also characteristic of heart failure. Hepatomegaly is common in infants in failure, although liver tenderness is uncommon. Cardiomegaly may be assessed roentgenographically, but it must be recognized that in normal newborn infants, the cardiac diameter may be as much as 60 percent of the thoracic diameter, and the large thymus gland in infants occasionally interferes with evaluation of heart size. Two-dimensional and Doppler echocardiography provide a reliable estimate of cardiac performance and chamber dimensions, and values may be compared with data derived from normal infants.[43-45]

Cardiac decompensation may progress with extreme rapidity in the first hours and days of life, producing a clinical picture of advanced cardiogenic shock and a profoundly obtunded infant. The presence of marked hepatomegaly and gross cardiomegaly usually allows distinction from noncardiac causes of diminished systemic perfusion.

CYANOSIS

Cyanosis is produced by reduced hemoglobin in cutaneous vessels in excess of approximately 3 gm/dl (see p. 1539). Peripheral cyanosis usually reflects an abnormally great extraction of oxygen from normally saturated arterial blood, commonly the result of peripheral cutaneous vasoconstriction. Central cyanosis is a result of arterial blood oxygen unsaturation, most often in patients with congenital heart disease caused by shunting of systemic venous blood into the arterial circuit. Infants especially (as compared with adults) may appear cyanotic when in heart failure because of both peripheral and central factors[46]; the latter may include severe impairment of pulmonary function that commonly exists with alveolar hypoventilation, ventilation-perfusion inequality, or impaired oxygen diffusion.

In patients with central cyanosis owing to arterial oxygen unsaturation, the degree of cutaneous discoloration depends on the absolute amount of reduced hemoglobin, the magnitude of the right-to-left shunt relative to systemic flow, and the oxyhemoglobin saturation of venous blood. The last of these depends in turn on the tissue extraction of oxygen. Cyanosis commonly appears or intensifies with physical activity or exercise as the saturation of systemic venous blood declines concurrent with an increase in right-to-left shunting across a defect as peripheral vascular resistance decreases. Oxygen transfer to the tissues is affected

by shifts in the oxygen-hemoglobin dissociation relation, which may be altered by blood pH and levels of red blood cell 2,3-diphosphoglycerate concentration.

CLUBBING AND POLYCYTHEMIA/ERYTHROCYTOSIS. Prominent accompaniments of arterial hypoxemia are polycythemia and clubbing of the digits. The latter is associated with an increased number of capillaries with increased blood flow through extensive arteriovenous aneurysms and an increase of connective tissue in the terminal phalanges of the fingers and toes. Polycythemia is a physiological response to chronic hypoxemia that stimulates erythrocytosis. The extremely high hematocrits observed in patients with arterial oxygen unsaturation cause a progressive increase in blood viscosity. Because the relationship is nonlinear between hematocrit and blood viscosity, relatively small increases beyond packed blood cell volumes of 60 percent result in large increases in viscosity. Also, the apparent viscosity of blood increases in the microcirculation, where lower shear rates exist, an increasingly important factor as the hematocrit exceeds 70 percent.

Both the hematocrit and the circulating whole blood volume are increased in polycythemia accompanying cyanotic congenital heart disease; the hypervolemia is the result of an increase in red blood cell volume. The augmented red blood cell volume provoked by hypoxemia provides an increased oxygen-carrying capacity and enhanced oxygen supply to the tissues. The compensatory polycythemia often is of such severity that it becomes a liability and produces such adverse physiological effects as hyperviscosity, cellular aggregation, and thrombotic lesions in diverse organs and a hemorrhagic diathesis.[47] In this regard, oral steroid contraceptives are contraindicated in adolescent cyanotic females because of the enhanced risk of cerebral thrombosis.

Management. Red blood cell volume reduction and replacement with plasma or albumin (erythropheresis) lower blood viscosity and increase systemic blood flow and systemic oxygen uptake; they thus may be helpful in the treatment of patients with severe hypoxic polycythemia (hematocrit $\geq$ 65 percent). A final hematocrit of 55 to 63 percent should be achieved; the higher level is necessary in patients with low initial oxygen saturation to avoid a severe reduction in arterial oxygen content. Acute phlebotomy without fluid replacement is contraindicated.

CEREBRAL AND PULMONARY COMPLICATIONS. Cerebrovascular accidents and brain abscesses occur particularly in cyanotic patients with substantial arterial desaturation.[48, 49] *Cerebral thrombosis* is most common before age 2 years in severely cyanotic children, even in the presence of relatively low hematocrits, and occurs especially in a clinical setting in which oxygen requirements are raised by fever or, if blood viscosity is increased, dehydration.

Brain Abscess. This is an important complication of cyanotic heart disease.[49] Such abscesses are rare before 18 months of age and commonly are of insidious onset marked by headache, low-grade fever, vomiting, and a change in personality. Seizures or paralysis less frequently herald the onset of a brain abscess. Abscess must be suspected in any cyanotic child with focal neurological signs. Morbidity and mortality are related inversely to oxygen saturation levels. Brain abscess is thought to occur in about 2 percent of the population with cyanotic congenital heart disease; a mortality rate of 30 to 40 percent often is related to delay in diagnosis and treatment.

Paradoxical Embolus. This is a rare complication of cyanotic heart disease, usually observed only at necropsy.[50] Emboli arising in systemic veins may pass directly to the systemic circulation, because right-to-left intracardiac shunts allow venous blood to bypass the normal filtering action of the lungs.

Retinopathy. Dilated tortuous vessels progressing to papilledema and retinal edema occasionally are observed in cyanotic patients and appear to be related to decreased arterial oxygen saturation and/or to erythrocytosis but not to hypercapnia.

Hemoptysis. This is an uncommon but major complication in cyanotic patients with congenital heart disease; it occurs most often in the presence of pulmonary vascular obstructive disease or in patients with an extensive bronchial collateral circulation or pulmonary venous congestion.[51] Massive hemoptysis almost always represents rupture of a dilated bronchial artery.

SQUATTING. After exertion, patients with cyanotic heart disease, especially tetralogy of Fallot, typically assume a squatting posture to obtain relief from breathlessness.[52] Squatting appears to improve arterial oxygen saturation by increasing systemic vascular resistance, thereby diminishing the right-to-left shunt, and by the pooling of markedly desaturated blood in the lower extremities. In addition, systemic venous return, and therefore pulmonary blood flow, may increase.

HYPOXIC SPELLS. Hypercyanotic or hypoxemic spells commonly complicate the clinical course in younger children with certain types of cyanotic heart disease, especially tetralogy of Fallot.[52] The spells occur commonly in the morning and are characterized by anxiety, hyperpnea, and a sudden marked increase in cyanosis; they are the result of an abrupt reduction in pulmonary blood flow. Unless terminated, the hypercyanotic episodes may lead to convulsions and may even be fatal. The sudden reduction in pulmonary blood flow may be precipitated by fluctuations in arterial P_{CO_2} and pH, a sudden fall in systemic or increase in pulmonary vascular resistance, or an acute increase in the severity of right ventricular outflow tract obstruction, either by augmented contraction of the hypertrophied muscle in the right ventricular outflow tract or by a decrease in right ventricular cavity volume owing to tachycardia.

Treatment. This consists of oxygen administration, placing the child in the knee-chest position, and administration of morphine sulfate. Additional medications that may prove of value include intravenous administration of sodium bicarbonate to correct the accompanying acidemia, alpha-adrenoceptor stimulants such as phenylephrine hydrochloride (Neo-Synephrine) or methoxamine to raise peripheral resistance and diminish right-to-left shunting, and beta-adrenoceptor blocking agents, which reduce cardiac sympathetic tone, depress cardiac contractility directly, and increase ventricular volume by reducing heart rate.

ACID-BASE IMBALANCE

Disturbances in blood gas and acid-base equilibrium are noted particularly in infants with either congestive heart failure or cyanosis.[53] Large-volume left-to-right shunts, especially with pulmonary edema, may be associated with moderate respiratory acidemia and a lowering of arterial oxygen tensions, reflecting an increase in the alveolar-arterial oxygen tension gradient and ventilation-perfusion imbalance. Interference with carbon dioxide transport implies moderate to severe failure in these infants. Lesions associated with a reduced systemic cardiac output, such as severe coarctation of the aorta or critical aortic stenosis in infancy, often present as cardiac failure complicated by a severe metabolic acidemia and relatively high values of arterial oxygen tension. The latter finding, even in the presence of right-to-left shunting across a patent ductus arteriosus, is a result of diminished systemic perfusion and an elevated pulmonary-systemic blood flow ratio.

Respiratory acidemia and depressed levels of oxygen tension are observed in infants with obstruction to pulmonary venous return and right-to-left atrial shunting. Many infants with severe hypoxemia caused by lesions such as transposition of the great arteries or pulmonic atresia show metabolic acidemia and marked reductions in carbon dioxide tension secondary to hyperventilation, resulting from hypoxic stimulation of peripheral chemoreceptors.

IMPAIRED GROWTH

Impaired growth and physical development and delayed onset of adolescence are common features of many cyanotic and, to a lesser extent, acyanotic forms of congenital heart disease.[54, 55] Mental development seldom is affected. The severity of growth disturbance depends on the anatomical lesion and its functional effect. Most children with mild defects grow normally. Weight gain is commonly slower than linear growth in acyanotic patients with large left-to-right shunts, whereas in cyanotic congenital heart disease, height and weight usually parallel each other. Boys appear to be more retarded in growth than girls, especially in the second decade of life. Skeletal maturity (i.e., bone age) is delayed in cyanotic children in relation to the severity of hypoxemia.

In some children, prenatal factors such as intrauterine infection and chromosomal or other hereditary and nonhereditary syndromes are responsible for growth retardation. In other patients, extracardiac malformations may contribute to poor weight gain and linear growth. Additional explanations for the mechanisms of growth interference have implicated malnutrition as a result of anorexia and inadequate nutrient and caloric intake, hypermetabolic state, acidemia and cation imbalance, tissue hypoxemia, diminished peripheral blood flow, chronic cardiac decompensation, malabsorption or protein loss, recurrent respiratory infections, and endocrine or genetic factors. In some instances, the underdevelopment is influenced little by operative correction of the underlying cardiac anomaly.

Among factors that may be responsible for persistent growth retardation postoperatively are age at operation, hemodynamically significant residual lesions, and sequelae or complications of operation. As a general rule, it is unwise preoperatively to guarantee to the parents of a child with heart disease that surgery will result in accelerated growth and development.

PULMONARY HYPERTENSION
(See also Chap. 53)

Pulmonary hypertension is a common accompaniment of many congenital cardiac lesions, and the status of the pulmonary vascular bed often is the principal determinant of the clinical manifestations, the course, and whether surgical treatment is feasible.[56] Increases in pulmonary arterial pressure result from elevations of pulmonary blood flow and/or resistance, the latter sometimes caused by an increase in vascular tone but usually the result of underdevel-

opment and/or obstructive, obliterative structural changes within the pulmonary vascular bed.[57–59]

Pulmonary vascular resistance normally falls rapidly immediately after birth, owing to onset of ventilation and subsequent release of hypoxic pulmonary vasoconstriction. Subsequently, the medial smooth muscle of pulmonary arterial resistance vessels thins gradually. This latter process often is delayed by several months in infants with large aorticopulmonary or ventricular communications, at which time levels of pulmonary vascular resistance are still somewhat elevated. In patients with high pulmonary arterial pressure from birth, failure of normal growth of the pulmonary circulation may occur, and anatomical changes in the pulmonary vessels in the form of proliferation of intimal cells and intimal and medial thickening often progress, so that in an older child or adult vascular resistance ultimately may become fixed by obliterative changes in the pulmonary vascular bed. The causes of pulmonary vascular obstructive disease remain unknown, although increased pulmonary arterial blood pressure, elevated pulmonary venous pressure, polycythemia, systemic hypoxia, acidemia, and the nature of the bronchial circulation all have been implicated. Quite likely, injury to pulmonary vascular endothelial cells initiates a cascade of events that involve the release or activation of factors that alter the extracellular matrix, induce hypertrophy, cause proliferation of vascular smooth muscle cells, and promote connective tissue protein synthesis. Considered together, these may permanently alter vessel structure and function.[60, 61]

Many patients with pulmonary vascular obstruction have a cardiac anomaly that places them at particular risk early in life, precluding survival to adulthood. Patients at particularly high risk for the development of significant pulmonary vascular obstruction are those with certain forms of cyanotic congenital heart disease, such as complete transposition of the great arteries with or without VSD or patent ductus arteriosus, single ventricle without pulmonary stenosis, double-outlet right ventricle, and truncus arteriosus.[62] Other conditions in which pulmonary vascular obstruction appears to progress rapidly include large VSD, as well as the less common conditions of unilateral pulmonary artery absence, congenital left-to-right shunts in an environment of high altitude or in association with the Down syndrome of trisomy 21, and complete AV canal defects, even those unassociated with a chromosomal anomaly.

MECHANISMS OF DEVELOPMENT. Intimal damage appears to be related to shear stresses because endothelial cell damage occurs at high-flow shear rates. A reduction in pulmonary arteriolar lumen size due to either thickened medial muscle or vasoconstriction increases the velocity of flow. Shear stress also increases as blood viscosity rises; therefore, infants with hypoxemia and high hematocrits as well as increased pulmonary blood flow are at increased risk of developing pulmonary vascular disease. In patients with left-to-right shunts, pulmonary arterial hypertension, if not present in infancy or childhood, may never occur or may not develop until the third or fourth decade or later. Once developed, intimal proliferative changes with hyalinization and fibrosis are not reversible by repair of the underlying cardiac defect. In severe pulmonary vascular obstructive disease, arteriovenous malformations may develop and predispose to massive hemoptysis.

Most vexing is the variability among patients with the same or similar cardiac lesions in both the time of appearance and rate of progression of their pulmonary vascular obstructive process. Although genetic influences may be operative (an example is the apparent acceleration of pulmonary vascular disease in patients with congenital heart disease and trisomy 21), evidence is now accumulating for important prenatal and postnatal modifiers of the pulmonary vascular bed that appear, at least in part, to be lesion dependent. Thus, a quantitative variability exists in the pulmonary vascular bed related to the *number*, not just the size and wall structure, of arterial vessels within the pulmonary circulation.[63, 64]

Modeling of the blood vessels occurs proximal to and within terminal bronchioles (preacinar and intraacinar vessels, respectively) continuously from before birth. The intraacinar vessels, in particular, increase in size and number from late fetal life throughout childhood, with minimal muscularization of their walls. The ensuing increase in the cross-sectional area of the pulmonary arterial circulation allows the cardiac output to rise substantially without an increase in pulmonary arterial pressure. If, however, the presence of a cardiac lesion interferes with the normal growth and multiplication of these most peripheral arteries, the resulting elevation of pulmonary vascular resistance may first be related to failure of the intraacinar pulmonary circulation to develop fully, and then secondarily to the morphological changes of obliterative vascular disease—medial thickening, intimal proliferation, hyalinization and fibrosis, angiomatoid and plexiform lesions, and ultimately, arterial necrosis.[59]

In essence, the morphometric framework adds an important dimension—that of growth and development of the pulmonary circulation—to the traditional view of pulmonary vascular obstructive disease occurring primarily as a result of anatomical changes in the individual pulmonary arterioles. Research attention currently focuses on the cellular and molecular biology of the vessel wall and abnormalities in endothelial cell–smooth muscle interactions in pulmonary hypertension.

ASSESSMENT OF THE PATIENT WITH PULMONARY HYPERTENSION. It is important to understand the difficulties that exist with standard methods of assessing the severity of pulmonary vascular obstructive disease. Clinical and electrocardiographic (ECG) observations do not distinguish between reversible and irreversible elevations in pulmonary vascular resistance. Echocardiography and Doppler interrogation of the heart may enable one to diagnose the presence of pulmonary hypertension but do not provide an accurate estimate of pressure or a reliable calculation of pulmonary vascular resistance. The pulmonary systolic pressure is predicted from the velocity of tricuspid regurgitation using the modified Bernoulli equation, which is susceptible to error if the right atrial pressure is elevated. The mean pulmonary regurgitant velocity can also be relatively predictive of the mean pulmonary artery pressure. Thus, hemodynamic measurements at cardiac catheterization are the mainstay in assessing the pulmonary vascular bed, especially its reactivity. The premium on accuracy is high because the presence, degree, and reactivity of pulmonary vascular obstruction determine the feasibility and long-term outcome of operation. Surgery must not be offered to patients with severe, fixed pulmonary vascular obstruction, even when the cardiac defect is anatomically correctable. Such patients either do not survive operation or, if they do, are not benefited and more often than not are harmed.

The aims of hemodynamic study are to quantify and compare the pulmonary and systemic flows and resistances and to determine the reactivity of the pulmonary vascular bed in patients with pulmonary hypertension. Because resistance to pulmonary blood flow cannot be measured directly, it is calculated from the ratio of pressure gradient to flow across the pulmonary bed according to Poiseuille's equation, which refers to steady flow of a newtonian fluid through straight, rigid tubes. There are potential errors in applying the equation and errors inherent in the methods of measurement. Furthermore, it is not possible in every patient to catheterize the pulmonary artery; when this is the case, pulmonary venous wedge pressures may be used, but they are not always reliable indicators of pulmonary artery pressure, and the moment of hemodynamic evaluation may not be representative of potentially variable states of the pulmonary circulation. Nonetheless, a practical index of pulmonary vascular resistance can be established from measurements of pulmonary and systemic arterial pressures and calculated flows. One can then determine whether administration of drugs or oxygen or nitric oxide reduces the pulmonary vascular resistance, implying that the resistance is not fixed and therefore may decrease or at least not progress after successful operation.[65] A reduction in calculated pulmonary vascular resistance in response to oxygen or nitric oxide inhalation or pharmacological intervention does not preclude coexisting anatomical pulmonary vascular disease but does imply a component of potentially reversible vasoconstriction contributing to the high resistance.

OTHER DIAGNOSTIC METHODS. Because of the aforementioned shortcomings, additional methods have been developed to study the morphology of the small pulmonary arteries in patients with pulmonary hypertension. An example is the use of high-resolution magnification for *pulmonary wedge angiography* to determine the presence and extent of obstructive pulmonary vascular changes.[66] Pulmonary wedge angiograms, assessed quantitatively, appear to correlate well with both hemodynamic findings and histological observations of the structural state of the pulmonary vascular bed. Of additional interest is the current practical application of morphometric structural analyses that attempt to identify for operation patients whose postoperative pulmonary hemodynamics might be expected to improve, if not normalize.[67] Thus, preoperative or intraoperative *lung biopsy* has been proposed for patients with equivocal hemodynamic data to aid in determining whether to proceed with operation in reasonable anticipation of postoperative regression of elevated pulmonary vascular resistance.[68]

THE MORPHOMETRIC APPROACH. Decisions on optimal timing of operations often are difficult because of the varying rates of development of pulmonary vascular disease in different patients with the same anomaly and because evaluation of pulmonary vascular resistance and reactivity in the catheterization laboratory is a less than perfect science. Preoperative lung biopsy using the Heath-Edwards criteria has enjoyed little popularity, especially because sampling errors may result from the scatter of different grades of lesion in different parts of the lung. Accordingly, it is attractive to seek an alternative method that would obviate these problems. In this regard, application of a morphometric approach holds promise because the described changes in pulmonary vessel morphological characteristics are more uniformly distributed throughout the lung and, importantly, lend themselves to quantification.

Three abnormalities have been identified as anatomical markers of elevated pulmonary vascular resistance: (1) an excessive and premature extension of vascular smooth muscle into intraacinar pulmonary arteries, (2) failure of preacinar arterial wall thickness to regress normally, and (3) failure of pulmonary arteries to grow and proliferate normally during postnatal development. Frozen-section lung biopsy provides a firmer basis for judgment of whether reparative or palliative operation should proceed. The technique has proved useful in patients with univentricular hearts or tricuspid atresia in determining the feasibility of a Fontan procedure and in patients with lesions known to exhibit early and rapidly progressive pulmonary vascular disease such as complete transposition of great arteries, complete AV canal defect, and nonrestrictive VSD.[68, 69]

CLINICAL MANIFESTATIONS OF PULMONARY HYPERTENSION. When this condition is associated with a large left-to-right shunt, the clinical manifestations reflect the specific malformation responsible. When pulmonary vascular resistance is elevated and a significant right-to-left shunt exists, the patient is cyanotic, and polycythemia and clubbing are noted. A dominant *a* wave in the jugular venous pulse may be seen, reflecting vigorous right atrial contraction caused by diminished compliance of the right ventricle. In some instances there are large systolic *c-v* waves, which suggest tricuspid regurgitation. A prominent right ventricular parasternal lift and palpable systolic expansion of the pulmonary artery are present. A soft pulmonary systolic ejection murmur preceded by an ejection sound and followed by a markedly accentuated pulmonic component of the second heart sound often is audible on auscultation; an early diastolic decrescendo blowing murmur of pulmonary regurgitation may be heard. If right ventricular failure and dilatation supervene, the systolic murmur of tricuspid regurgitation may be audible at the lower left sternal border. Right ventricular enlargement may be evident on the chest roentgenogram and ECG. The former examination also reveals a conspicuously enlarged pulmonary artery, prominent hilar pulmonary vascular markings, and attenuated peripheral vessels. The presence of pulmonary hypertension is suggested by analysis of Doppler waveforms of right and left ventricular ejection. The site of the underlying defect may be localized by means of two-dimensional and Doppler echocardiography and/or cardiac catheterization and angiocardiography. Pressures in the right side of the heart are essentially identical to systemic pressures in cyanotic patients if the shunt is at the ventricular or aorticopulmonary levels, but they usually are lower than systemic pressures in patients with an intraatrial shunt. Efforts continue to identify a specific treatment for obstructive pulmonary vascular disease.[70, 71]

This fact underscores the importance of efforts to define the optimal age at operation to provide the highest probability of postoperative normalization of the pulmonary vascular bed. It is important to emphasize that almost all congenital cardiovascular defects are amenable to surgical repair in infancy, and it is likely that the surgical art will progress to the point that virtually all patients with lesions associated with pulmonary hypertension will be operated on within the first 3 to 18 months of life. When this goal is reached without increased operative mortality, the incidence of postoperative pulmonary vascular obstruction may well achieve the status of a bygone concern.

OTHER CONSEQUENCES OF CONGENITAL HEART DISEASE

INFECTIVE ENDOCARDITIS (see also Chap. 47). Infective endocarditis is uncommon before age 2 years and thereafter most often affects children with tetralogy of Fallot (especially after systemic-pulmonary anastomosis), VSD, aortic stenosis, and patent ductus arteriosus. Postsurgical patients with prosthetic heterograft or homograft valves or conduits are at particular risk. Infants and children with normal cardiac anatomy are at increased risk now that the use of central venous catheters is routine, and drug addiction in adolescents is an emerging risk factor.[72]

A causative organism can be isolated in about 90 percent of children, usually either alpha streptococci (usually *Streptococcus viridans*) or *Staphylococcus aureus*, although uncommon organisms may also be identified.[73-75] Fungal endocarditis is quite rare in the pediatric age group. Mortality appears to be highest when coagulase-positive *Staphylococcus* is the offending organism and when the endocarditis involves the left, rather than the right, side of the heart. Most recent data suggest 75 to 80 percent overall survival. Factors predisposing to endocarditis may be identified in about one-third of cases. These include cardiovascular surgery with infection during the perioperative period, respiratory tract infections, and ear, nose, throat, and dental procedures. Less often, contamination during a surgical procedure or cardiac catheterization or an infection involving the skin, genitourinary tract, or other organ system has been the cause.

Although routine antimicrobial prophylaxis is recommended for all children with congenital heart disease and for the majority of patients after operative repair of the lesion,[74, 74a] it should be recognized that many different microbes are responsible for the disease and that an effective preventive approach ultimately may center on active immunization rather than antibiotics. Antibiotic prophylaxis currently is recommended for all dental procedures known to induce gingival or mucosal bleeding, including cleaning, oral trauma, and other procedures such as tonsillectomy, gastrointestinal surgery, genitourinary surgery, and incision and drainage of infected tissue (Table 43–4). The risk of endocarditis is undoubtedly related both to the magnitude of bacteremia and to the type of underlying heart disease. Because infection on a prosthetic heart valve or conduit may be devastating, combinations of antibiotics given parenterally are advisable in these patients.

CHEST PAIN (see also Chap. 3). *Angina pectoris* is an uncommon symptom of cardiac disease in infants and children, occurring in association with anomalous pulmonary origin of a coronary artery or, occasionally, in association with severe aortic stenosis, pulmonic stenosis, or pulmonary hypertension owing to pulmonary vascular obstruction. Cardiac pain in infants with anomalous coronary artery usually takes the form of irritability and crying during feeding or straining at bowel movement. In children with severe or right ventricular outflow tract obstruction, chest pain commonly follows effort and is identical to angina observed in adults. Cardiac pain associated with *pulmonary vascular obstruction* may be anginal in nature but often is evanescent and pleuritic in type. Atypical forms of chest pain associated with the syndrome of *mitral valve prolapse* are much less usual in children than in adults. A sensation of chest discomfort or cardiac awareness frequently is interpreted as pain by the parents of children with cardiac arrhythmias. Careful questioning serves to identify palpitations rather than pain as the symptom and often elicits an additional history of anxiety, pallor, and sweating. Pain caused by *pericarditis* is commonly of acute onset and associated with fever, and it can be identified by specific physical, roentgenographic, and echocardiographic findings.

Most commonly, chest pain in children is *musculoskeletal* in origin and may be reproduced on upper extremity movement or by palpation; chest wall pain often is the result of *costochondritis*.[75] Finally,

TABLE 43–4. PROPHYLACTIC ANTIBIOTICS FOR PROTECTION FROM BACTERIAL ENDOCARDITIS

PROPHYLACTIC REGIMENS FOR DENTAL, ORAL, RESPIRATORY TRACT, OR ESOPHAGEAL PROCEDURES*,†

Standard General Prophylaxis for Patients at Risk
Amoxicillin: adults, 2.0 gm (children, 50 mg/kg) PO 1 hr before procedure.

Unable to Take Oral Medications
Ampicillin: adults, 2.0 gm (children, 50 mg/kg) IM or IV within 30 min before procedure.

Amoxicillin/Ampicillin/Penicillin-Allergic Patients
Clindamycin: Adults, 600 mg (children, 20 mg/kg) PO 1 hr before procedure.
or
Cephalexin* or cefadroxil‡: adults, 2.0 gm (children, 50 mg/kg) PO 1 hr before procedure.
or
Azithromycin or clarithromycin: Adults, 500 mg (children, 15 mg/kg) PO 1 hr before procedure.

Amoxicillin/Ampicillin/Penicillin-Allergic Patients Unable to Take Oral Medications
Clindamycin: adults, 600 mg (children, 20 mg/kg) IV within 30 min before procedure.
or
Cefazolin: adults, 1.0 gm (children, 25 mg/kg) IM or IV within 30 min before procedure.

PROPHYLACTIC REGIMENS FOR GENITOURINARY/ GASTROINTESTINAL PROCEDURES†

High-Risk Patients
Ampicillin plus gentamicin: ampicillin (adults, 2.0 gm; children, 50 mg/kg) plus gentamicin 1.5 mg/kg (for both adults and children, not to exceed 120 mg) IM or IV within 30 min before starting procedure. 6 hr later, ampicillin (adults, 1.0 gm; children, 25 mg/kg) IM or IV, or amoxicillin (adults, 1.0 gm; children, 25 mg/kg) PO.

High-Risk Patients Allergic to Ampicillin/Amoxicillin
Vancomycin plus gentamicin: vancomycin (adults, 1.0 gm; children, 20 mg/kg) IV over 1–2 hr plus gentamicin 1.5 mg/kg (for both adults and children, not to exceed 120 mg) IM or IV. Complete injection/infusion within 30 min before starting procedure.

Moderate-Risk Patients
Amoxicillin: adults, 2.0 gm (children, 50 mg/kg) PO 1 hr before procedure.
or
Ampicillin: adults, 2.0 gm (children, 50 mg/kg) IM or IV within 30 min before starting procedure.

Moderate-Risk Patients Allergic to Ampicillin/Amoxicillin
Vancomycin: adults, 1.0 gm (children, 20 mg/kg) over 1–2 hr. Complete infusion within 30 min before starting procedure.

*Follow-up dose no longer recommended.
†Total children's dose should not exceed adult dose.
‡Cephalosporins should not be used in patients with immediate-type hypersensitivity reaction to penicillins.
Adapted from Prevention of Bacterial Endocarditis: Recommendations by the American Heart Association by the Committee on Rheumatic Fever, Endocarditis, and Kawasaki Disease. JAMA 277:1794–1801, 1997. Circulation 96:358–366, 1997. Copyright 1997 American Medical Association.

children, like adults, may suffer chest pain of nonspecific form owing to *anxiety*, with or without hyperventilation; a history often is elicited of a family member or friend who had recently died of or suffered myocardial infarction.

SYNCOPE (see also Chap. 27). Syncope is an unusual feature of heart disease in children; its presence suggests specific diagnoses, the most common being an arrhythmia. The symptom is observed in patients with long QT syndrome and in children with complete AV block that is less often of congenital origin than a sequela of cardiac operation. Syncope caused by abrupt episodes of either bradycardia or tachycardia occurs in association with the sick sinus syndrome. The latter is most commonly produced in children after surgical procedures that involve the region of the sinoatrial node, e.g., atrial septal defect closure or Mustard's venous switch procedure for transposition of the great arteries. Syncope is an occasional but ominous symptom if associated with severe aortic stenosis, pulmonary vascular obstruction, or a left atrial myxoma that transiently occludes left ventricular inflow.[76]

In children with an anatomically normal heart, transient episodes of vasovagally mediated hypotension and bradycardia (neurocardiogenic syncope) may be diagnosed by autonomic function testing and head-upright tilt-table testing (see Chap. 27). The latter is especially helpful in assessing the adequacy of prophylactic therapy, usually by volume expansion (e.g., salt and fludrocortisone), or by beta-adrenergic blockade or alpha-adrenergic agonist or serotonin reuptake inhibitor therapy.[77]

SUDDEN DEATH (see also Chap. 24). The sudden infant death syndrome is not likely due to a cardiac cause but rather to pulmonary and/or central nervous system causes. In contrast to adults, children seldom die suddenly and unexpectedly of cardiovascular disease.[78]

Arrhythmias, hypoxemia, and coronary insufficiency secondary to left ventricular outflow tract obstruction are the most frequent causes of death. Sudden death most often is reported in patients with postoperative heart disease or dilated cardiomyopathy. It is also observed in patients with aortic stenosis or hypertrophic obstructive cardiomyopathy, primary pulmonary hypertension, Eisenmenger's syndrome of pulmonary vascular obstruction, myocarditis, congenital complete heart block, primary endocardial fibroelastosis, anomalies of the coronary arteries, and cyanotic congenital heart disease with pulmonic stenosis or atresia. A relation exists between strenuous exercise and sudden death in patients with aortic stenosis or obstructive cardiomyopathy, thus providing justification for restricting patients with these lesions from gymnastic activities and strenuous competitive sports.[79]

Congenital long QT syndrome is most often inherited as an autosomal dominant trait and is associated with malignant arrhythmias. It is characterized by a prolonged Q-T interval in the surface ECG, syncope, seizures, and sudden death caused by ventricular tachyarrhythmias. On a molecular level, a great many mutations in four ion channel genes have thus far been identified in these patients[80] (see chaps. 23 and 25).

The High-Risk Infant with Congenital Heart Disease

Without prompt recognition, accurate diagnosis, and treatment, about one-third of all infants born with congenital heart disease die in the first months of life. Heart failure and cyanosis are the two cardinal signs in high-risk infants with heart disease, and this section provides an approach to the management of each.

HEART FAILURE

Care of infants with heart failure must include careful consideration of the underlying structural or functional disturbance. The general aims of treatment are to achieve an increase in cardiac performance, augment peripheral perfusion, and decrease pulmonary and systemic venous congestion.[37] It must be emphasized, however, that under many conditions medical management cannot control the effects of the abnormal loads imposed by a host of congenital cardiac lesions. Under these circumstances, cardiac diagnosis and interventional catheter or operative intervention may be urgently required. Thus, initial therapy is aimed at stabilizing an infant's condition for diagnostic ultrasonography or hemodynamic or angiocardiographic study as soon as possible. In almost all situations, the decision to intervene surgically or to continue medical management requires a definitive anatomical diagnosis.

RESERVE MECHANISMS IN THE NEONATAL HEART

Pediatricians in particular should be aware of the important concept of cardiac reserve because it is in this regard that important differences exist between the young heart (of the preterm or newborn infant) and the fully developed heart of the older child, adolescent, and adult (Fig. 43-5).

Clinicians have long recognized the unique fragility and lability of the neonatal circulation in response to disease states and various physiological stimuli. Moreover, it often is apparent that newborns may exhibit suboptimal therapeutic responses to drugs such as digitalis, which directly stimulate cardiac contractility. The age dependence of these observations has its basis in the reduced ability of the hearts of premature and full-term newborns, when compared with the hearts and circulation of older children or adults, to call on a functional reserve capacity to adapt to stress.[37, 81, 82]

Studies from our and other laboratories have shown that structural, functional, biochemical, and pharmacological properties of the young heart differ considerably from those of its older counterpart.[21-34] The young heart contains fewer myofilaments to generate force with and to shorten during contraction. In addition, the chamber stiffness of the young heart's ventricles is greater than that later in life.

PRELOAD RESERVE. Any increase in ventricular filling or volume in the small, young heart results in a disproportionately greater rise in

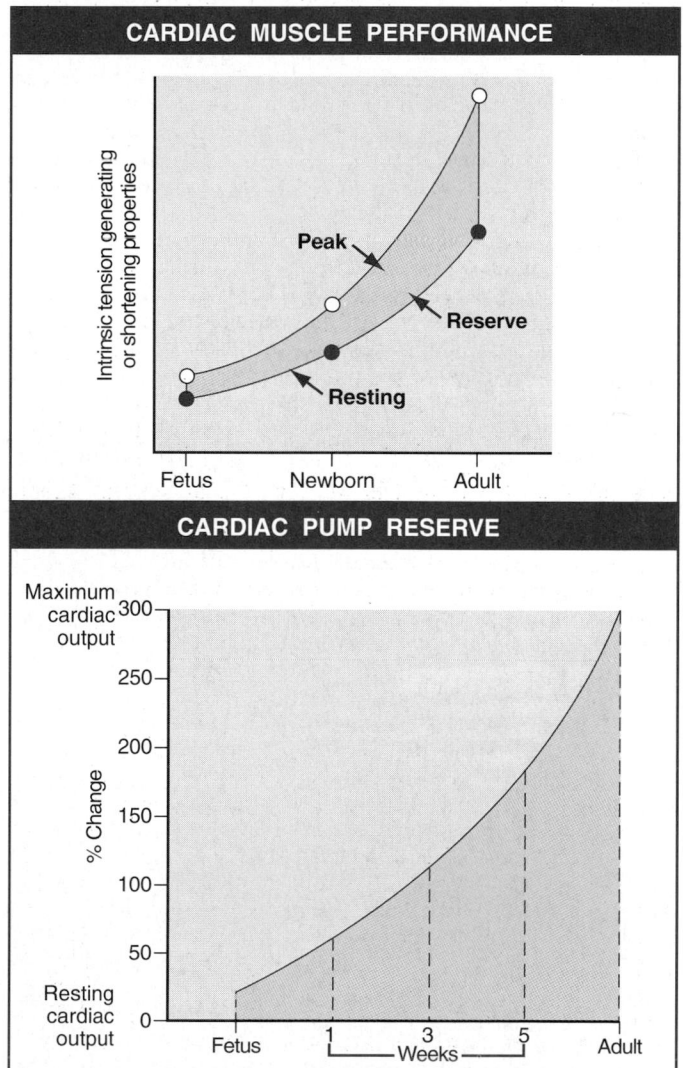

FIGURE 43-5. Schema of reduced cardiac reserve in fetal and newborn hearts compared with an adult's. In a newborn infant, resting cardiac muscle performance *(top panel)* is close to the peak of ventricular function because of limitations in diastolic, systolic, and heart rate reserve. Similarly, pump reserve *(bottom panel)* early in life is limited by these factors, as well as by a much higher resting cardiac output relative to body weight, compared with an adult.

ventricular wall tension or stress. Similarly, it takes a smaller increase in ventricular filling to reach the limits of assistance given to cardiac pump and muscle function by stretching the myofilaments; that is, *preload or diastolic reserve is limited.*

The young heart generates relatively less force; it cannot generate the same ventricular systolic pressure or wall tensions, or obtain the same stroke volume augmentation from any initial stretch, as can the older heart. With these facts in mind, it must be remembered that the oxygen consumption of a normal newborn is considerably higher than later in life; accordingly, a newborn at rest has a much higher cardiac output per square meter than a child or adult. Thus, even in the absence of stress, the young heart must function near peak performance just to satisfy the normal demands of the peripheral tissues. Because newborn cardiac performance at rest is so close to its ceiling, or limits of function, little *systolic reserve* is available to adapt to an acute or chronic stress such as pressure or volume load from an obstructive lesion or left-to-right circulatory shunt, respectively, or asphyxia.

HEART RATE RESERVE. This consists of the ability of the heart to change its rate of pumping to raise the level of cardiac output. In this regard, newborns also are limited because in this age group the intrinsic heart rate normally is high. In addition, heart failure per se raises the frequency of contraction even further, primarily as a result of high circulating levels of catecholamines. In this sense, a newborn's heart rate also is closer than a child's or adult's to its ceiling, or upper limits of effectiveness. Furthermore, increases in heart rate occur largely at the expense of diastolic filling time. Thus, at very rapid heart rates, there is a disproportionately diminished diastolic time and therefore diminished time for perfusion of the myocardium by its own coronary arterial system. In addition, rapid heart rates result in elevated myocardial energy expenditure and increased myocardial demand for oxygen. The sum of these considerations indicates that newborn *heart rate reserve* is reduced.

TREATMENT (see also Chap. 18). Table 43–5 lists supportive and pharmacological measures in the treatment of newborns with heart failure. The supportive measures are designed to increase tissue oxygen supply, decrease tissue oxygen consumption, and correct metabolic abnormalities. Digitalis glycosides, preload reduction with certain diuretic agents, and afterload reduction with angiotensin-converting enzyme inhibitors provide the most important elements of medical therapy, but it is important to recognize that the

▼ **TABLE 43–5. TREATMENT OF CONGESTIVE HEART FAILURE**

GENERAL INTERVENTIONS
Rest (occasional sedation)
Semi-Fowler's position
Temperature and humidity control
Oxygen
Decrease sodium load
Avoid aspiration
Treat infection, if present
 	
SPECIFIC INTERVENTIONS
Preload manipulation
  Move ventricular function curve up by volume infusion to increase venous return
  Move ventricular function curve down with diuretics, venodilators
Afterload reduction
  Facilitate ventricular emptying by reducing wall tension
  Reduce blood viscosity
  Drugs, arteriolar dilators, mechanical counterpulsation
Inotropic stimulation
  Improve physical and metabolic milieu: pH, PaO_2, glucose, calcium, hemoglobin
  Inotropic drugs: digitalis, catecholamines, dobutamine, dopamine, levodopa
Heart rate
  Control rhythm disturbances with pacing, drugs
Other
  Mechanical ventilation
  Prostaglandin manipulation
  Peritoneal dialysis
 	
INTERVENTIONAL CATHETER-DIRECTED THERAPY or SURGERY (may include transplantation)

▼ **TABLE 43–6. DIURETIC AND DIGITALIS DOSAGES FOR INFANTS**

PREPARATION	DOSAGE AND ROUTE OF ADMINISTRATION
Furosemide	IV, 1 mg/kg/dose; PO, 2–6 mg/kg/d
Ethacrynic acid	IV, 1 mg/kg/dose; PO, 2–3 mg/kg/d
Hydrochlorothiazide	PO 2–5 mg/kg/d
Spironolactone	PO 1–3 mg/kg/d
Triamterene	PO 2–4 mg/kg/d
Digoxin	
Elixir	0.05 mg/ml
Parenteral	0.10 mg/ml

	DOSE AND ROUTE*	
AGE AND WEIGHT	**Acute Digitalization**	**Maintenance**
Prematures <1.5 kg	10–20 µg/kg IV TDD: ½, ¼, ¼ of dose q8h	4 µg/kg/d IV (may increase to 4 µg/kg q12hr at age 1 mo)
1.5–2.5 kg	Same as above	4 µg/kg q12hr IV
Full-term newborns	30 µg/kg IV, TDD	4–5 µg/kg q12hr IV
Infants (1–12 mo)	35 µg/kg IV, TDD	5–10 µg/kg q12hr IV
>12 mo	40 µg/kg IV, TDD (maximum 1.0 mg)	5–10 µg/kg q12hr IV
Older children (>20 kg)	1.0–2.0 mg IV, TDD over 48 hr	0.125–0.250 mg IV qd

*PO = Oral dose approximately 20 percent greater than IV dose except in "older children." In older children, IV = oral dose.
TDD = Total digitalizing dose.

dosage regimen of drugs administered to young patients must be adjusted to take into account the age and size of the patient and the maturity-dependent pharmacological properties of cardioactive drugs. Because this is especially true in early infancy, Table 43–6 provides the dosages of digoxin and diuretics commonly used for infants.

Digitalis and Diuretics. Digoxin is the glycoside used exclusively to treat pediatric patients in most cardiac centers because it is readily absorbed, available in convenient dosage form, and excreted rapidly from the body. The efficacy and safety of digitalis remain topics of debate, although on balance, continued use is warranted. Premature infants are more sensitive to digitalis than are full-term newborns, who, in turn, are more sensitive than older infants. Infants absorb and excrete digoxin as well as adults do, and their relative distribution of the glycoside to different body tissues is also similar. The prevailing dose schedules for digoxin produce higher serum concentrations in infants than would be considered optimal for adults.[83] The basis for the higher digitalis requirement in infancy is unclear, although it may relate to an age-dependent alteration in the sensitivity of the myocardium per se to the glycosides. In this regard, infants tolerate higher serum digoxin concentrations than adults without developing signs of toxicity. In adults, the usual therapeutic concentrations of digoxin are less than 2 ng/ml blood, and toxicity commonly occurs above that level. In contrast, in infants, therapeutic levels of digoxin range from 1 to 5 ng/ml (mean = 3.5), and toxicity is associated with concentrations in excess of 3 ng/ml. Older children have therapeutic and toxic levels similar to those of adults.[84]

A restricted fluid intake (65 ml/kg/day) and a low-sodium diet (1 to 2 mEq/kg/day) should accompany diuretic therapy in the most seriously ill infants with heart failure. Furosemide is the agent of choice when the rapid elimination of excess salt and water is needed. Hydrochlorothiazide, occasionally in conjunction with spironolactone or triamterene to reduce potassium loss and sodium retention, is convenient for long-term therapy.

▼ **TABLE 43–7.** DOSAGE REGIMENS: INOTROPIC AGENTS

DRUG	DOSE	COMMENTS
Epinephrine (Adrenalin)	0.05–1.0 μg/kg/min IV	May cause hypertension and cardiac arrhythmias; inactivated in alkaline solution
Isoproterenol (Isuprel)	0.05–0.5 μg/kg/min IV	May decrease coronary blood flow; results in peripheral and pulmonary vasodilation
Norepinephrine (Levophed)	0.05–0.5 μg/kg/min IV	Causes significant vasoconstriction
Dobutamine (Dobutrex)	2–10 μg/kg/min IV (max 40 μg/kg/min)	No direct effect on renal perfusion, little or no peripheral vasodilatation or tachycardia
Dopamine (Intropin)	2–20 μg/kg/min IV (max 50 μg/kg/min)	Significant renal vasodilatation
	2–5 μg/kg/min	Inotropic ± heart rate acceleration
	5–8 μg/kg/min	Significant heart rate acceleration
	>8 μg/kg/min	±Vasoconstriction
	>10 μg/kg/min	Significant vasoconstriction
	15–20 μg/kg/min	
Levodopa	40–80 mg/kg/d PO; maximum single dose 1 gm q6h	Administer with pyridoxine 0.7 mg/kg/d (maximum 25 mg) and metoclopramide 0.1 mg/kg/dose, 1 hr before levodopa dose
	(Above dose/effect relations speculative in neonates)	
Amrinone	Dose schedule not well established for infants and children	May cause thrombocytopenia, hepatic and gastrointestinal disturbance, fever, and arrhythmias
	40–75 μg/kg/min IV for 2–3 min, then maintenance at 3–10 μg/kg/min; Dose not to exceed 10 mg/kg/24 hr	
Milrinone	Dose schedule not established for infants and children	See Amrinone
	Adults: bolus 50 μg/kg maintenance 0.375–0.75 μg/kg/min	

Modified from Friedman WF, George BL: New concepts and drugs in the treatment of congestive heart failure. Pediatr Clin North Am 31:1197, 1984.

Other Pharmacological Approaches. These may prove to be of significant benefit in selected instances in which digitalis and diuretics are relatively ineffective. In situations in which cardiac decompensation is not the result of an obstructive lesion, catecholamines may be used temporarily to alleviate cardiac failure while the patient is awaiting more definitive operative treatment (Table 43–7).[81] In infants with the coarctation of the aorta syndrome, in whom ductal constriction unmasks the aortic branch point, producing aortic narrowing, or with aortic arch interruption, heart failure may be reversed dramatically by intravenous infusion of prostaglandin E$_1$ (0.03 to 0.1 mg/kg/min), which results in dilatation of the ductus arteriosus and relief of the obstruction.[85] Conversely, in preterm infants in whom patent ductus arteriosus is responsible for profound cardiopulmonary deterioration, constriction of the ductus arteriosus may be accomplished by inhibition of prostaglandin synthesis with the nonsteroidal anti-inflammatory agent indomethacin (0.2 mg/kg intravenously).[86, 87]

Vasodilator therapy also is used in infants or children with heart disease in whom preload or afterload alterations may be expected to improve cardiac performance (Table 43–8).[81, 88] Moreover, treatment of severe cardiac failure often requires combining inotropic and afterload-reducing agents (see Chap. 18). Combinations of dopamine, dobutamine, and nitroprusside have been used extensively and effectively in the pediatric population, primarily in the setting of low cardiac output after open-heart surgery.[89, 90] Use of oral afterload-reducing agents, e.g., hydralazine or captopril, in association with digoxin is worthwhile in the long-term therapy of outpatients with congestive cardiomyopathy and/or significant mitral or aortic regurgitation.[88]

Rapid developments in molecular biology have begun to revolutionize our understanding of cardiovascular regulation, both before and after birth and at all ages. As knowledge is gained about the mechanisms responsible for the variability of gene expression in the heart, it is apparent that the future holds the opportunity for clinicians to mod-

▼ **TABLE 43–8.** DOSAGE REGIMENS: VASODILATORS IN INFANTS AND CHILDREN

DRUG	DOSE AND ROUTE OF ADMINISTRATION	COMMENTS
Nitroglycerin	0.5–20 μg/kg/min IV (max 60 μg/kg/min IV)	Dosage schedule for IV and other routes of administration not well established for children
Hydralazine (Apresoline)	0.5 mg/kg/d PO q6–8hr (max 200 mg/d or 7 mg/kg/d)	May cause tachycardia, gastrointestinal symptoms, neutropenia, lupus-like syndrome
	1.5 μg/kg/min IV or 0.1–0.5 mg/kg/dose IV q6hr (max 2 mg/kg q6hr)	
Captopril (Capoten)	0.1–0.4 mg/kg/dose PO given q6–24hr as needed	May cause neutropenia/proteinuria
Enalopril (Vasotec)	0.1 mg/kg/24 hr PO; increase as needed over 2 wk (max 0.5 mg/kg/24 hr IV: 0.01 mg/kg/dose q8–24 hr)	
Nitroprusside (Nipride)	0.5–8 μg/kg/min IV	May result in thiocyanate or cyanide toxicity if used in high doses or for prolonged periods; light sensitive
Prazosin (Minipress)	1st dose: 5 μg/kg PO (max 25 μg/kg/dose q6hr)	Initial dose used to elevate hypotensive effects; orthostatic hypotension, attenuation of hemodynamic effects may occur

Modified from Friedman WF, George BL: New concepts and drugs in the treatment of congestive heart failure. Pediatr Clin North Am 31:1197, 1984.

ify gene expression in ways that will importantly enhance the heart's ability to respond to both the heart failure state and those diseases that are responsible for the abnormalities leading to cardiac disease.[91]

CYANOSIS (See also p. 1617)

Cyanosis in infants often presents as a diagnostic emergency, necessitating prompt detection of the underlying cause. The schema in Figure 43–6 outlines a general approach to diagnosis. The cardiologist must distinguish between three types of cyanosis—peripheral, differential, and central—while recognizing that cyanosis may accompany diseases of the central nervous, hematological, respiratory, and cardiac systems.

PERIPHERAL CYANOSIS. Peripheral cyanosis (normal arterial oxygen saturation and widened arteriovenous oxygen differences) usually indicates stasis of blood flow in the periphery. The level of reduced hemoglobin in the capillaries of the skin usually exceeds 3 gm/100 dl. The most prominent causes of peripheral cyanosis in newborns are autonomically controlled alterations in the cutaneous distribution of capillary blood flow (acrocyanosis) and septicemia associated with evidence of a low cardiac output, i.e., hypotension, weak pulse, and cold extremities. In many instances, peripheral cyanosis is clearly the result of a cold environment or high hemoglobin content. When cyanosis is caused by the former, vasodilatation produced by immersing the extremity in warm water for several minutes reverses the cyanosis.

CENTRAL CYANOSIS. Oxygen unsaturation in central cyanosis may result from inadequately oxygenated pulmonary venous blood, in which case inhalation of 100 percent oxygen may diminish or clear the discoloration (discussed later). Conversely, in instances in which cyanosis is due to an intracardiac or extracardiac right-to-left shunt, pulmonary venous blood is fully saturated, and inhalation of 100 percent oxygen usually does not improve the infant's color. It is necessary to qualify the latter statement because oxygen may act directly in infants with elevated pulmonary vascular resistance to dilate the pulmonary blood vessels and thus reduce the magnitude of the venoarterial shunt. Central cyanosis also may be due to the replacement of normal by abnormal hemoglobin, as in methemoglobinemia.

Several factors influence the oxygen saturation produced at any given arterial Po_2. These include temperature, pH, ratio of fetal to adult hemoglobin, and erythrocyte concentration of 2,3-diphosphoglycerate. For example, fetal hemoglobin has a higher affinity for oxygen than does adult hemoglobin and therefore would be more highly saturated at any given Po_2. Thus, determination of the systemic arterial oxygen tension may provide a more accurate picture of the underlying pathophysiology than simply measuring the oxygen saturation.[46, 92]

DIFFERENTIAL CYANOSIS. Differential cyanosis virtually always indicates the presence of congenital heart disease, often with patency of the ductus arteriosus and coarctation of the aorta as components of the abnormal anatomical complex. If the upper part of the body is pink and the lower part of the body blue, coarctation of the aorta or interruption of the aortic arch is probable, with oxygenated blood supplying the upper body and desaturated blood supplying the lower body by way of right-to-left flow through the ductus arteriosus. The latter also occurs in patients with patent ductus arteriosus and markedly elevated pulmonary vascular resistance. A patient with transposition of the great arteries and coarctation of the aorta with retrograde flow through a patent ductus arteriosus demonstrates the reverse situation, i.e., the lower part of the body is pink and the upper part blue. Simultaneous determinations of oxygen saturation in the temporal or right brachial artery and the femoral artery are helpful in confirming the presence of differential cyanosis.

Differentiating Between Pulmonary and Cardiac Causes of Cyanosis

The distinction between respiratory signs and symptoms arising from cyanotic cardiac disease and those associated with a primary pulmonary disorder is an important challenge to the cardiologist.[41] Upper airway obstruction precipitates cyanosis by producing alveolar hypoventilation owing to reduced pulmonary ventilation. Mechanical obstruction may occur from the nares to the carina, and the important diagnostic possibilities among congenital abnormalities are choanal atresia, vascular ring, laryngeal web, and tracheomalacia. Acquired causes include vocal cord paresis, obstetrical injury to the cricothyroid cartilage, and

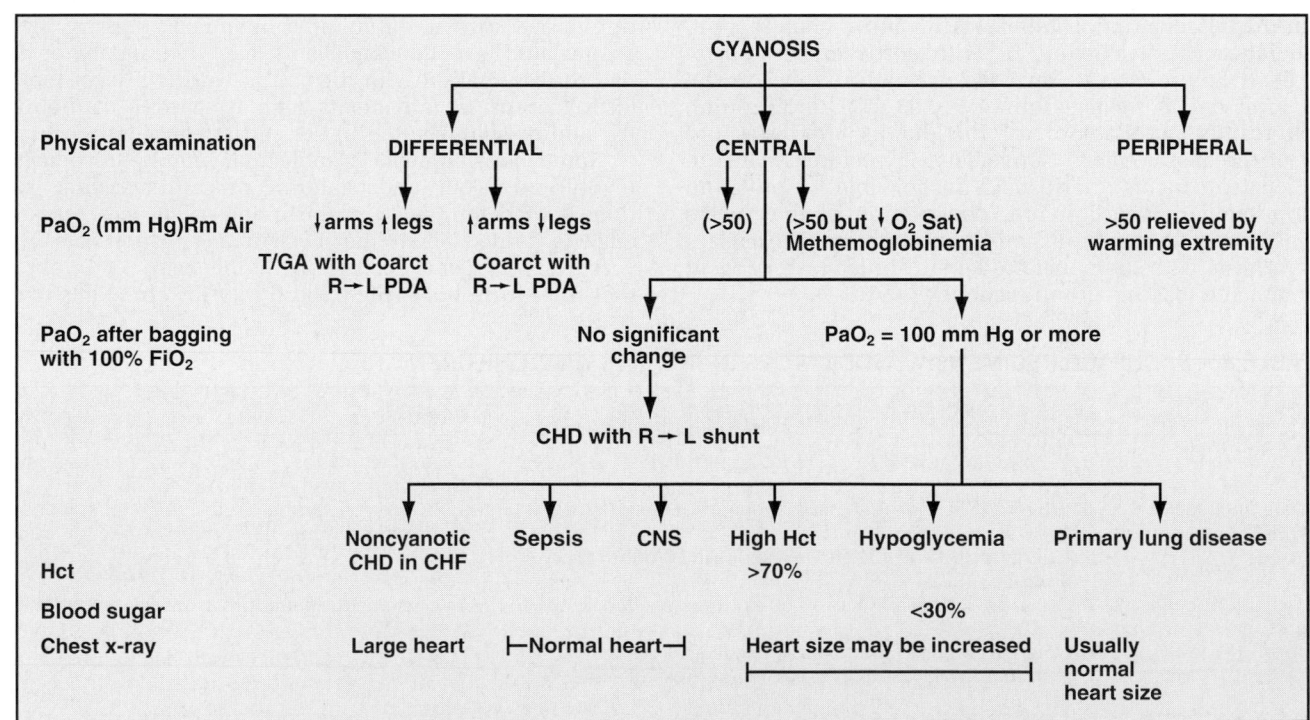

FIGURE 43–6. Flow chart for the evaluation of cyanotic infants. Tests to be done are listed at the left. The response to each of these tests leads along the line to the proper diagnostic category. CHD = congenital heart disease; CHF = congestive heart failure; CNS = central nervous system; Hct = hematocrit; PDA = patent ductus arteriosus; T/GA = transposition of great arteries; Coarct = coarctation; Rm = room. (From Kirkpatrick SE, Friedman WF, Pitlick P, et al: Differential diagnosis of congenital heart disease in the newborn—University of California, San Diego, School of Medicine, and University Hospital, San Diego [Specialty Conference]. West J Med 128:127, 1978.)

▼ TABLE 43–9. ARTERIAL BLOOD GAS PATTERNS IN VARIOUS DISORDERS CAUSING CYANOSIS IN INFANTS

PATTERN	pH	Po₂	Pco₂	RESPONSE TO O₂	VENOUS pH	SUGGESTED CONDITION
1	↓	↓↓	↑	↑↑	↓	Hyaline membrane or other pulmonary parenchymal disease
2	↓	↓	↑↑↑	↑	↓	Hypoventilation
3	—	↓	—	↑	—	Venous admixture
4	↓	↓↓	—	—↑	↓	Decreased or ineffective pulmonary blood flow
5	↓↓↓	↓	—↑	—↑	↓↓↓↓	Systemic hypoperfusion

— = no effect. For description of patterns, see pp. 1524ff.

foreign body. Structural abnormalities in the lungs resulting from intrapulmonary disease are more frequently a basis for cyanosis among newborns than is upper airway obstruction. Hyaline membrane disease, atelectasis, or pneumonitis causing inflammation, collapse, and fluid accumulation in the alveoli results in reduction of the oxygenation of blood reaching the systemic circulation.

Successfully distinguishing among these various causes of cyanosis depends on interpretation of the respiratory pattern, the cardiac physical examination, evaluation of arterial blood gases (Table 43–9), and interpretation of the ECG, chest radiograph, and echocardiogram.

RESPIRATORY PATTERNS. The key to differential diagnosis at the bedside commonly is the proper evaluation of the pattern of respiration. Term infants normally exhibit a progressive reduction in respiratory rate during the first day of life from 60 to 70 breaths/min to 35 to 55 breaths/min. Moreover, mild intercostal retractions and minimal expiratory grunting disappear within several hours of birth. An increased depth of respiration in the presence of cyanosis but without other signs of respiratory distress often is associated with congenital cardiac disease in which inadequate pulmonary blood flow is the most important functional component.

Apnea. The most important variations from normal respiratory patterns are apnea, bradypnea, and tachypnea. Intermittent apneic episodes are common in premature infants with central nervous system immaturity or disease. In addition, higher centers may be depressed as a result of severe hypoxemia, acidemia, or administration of pharmacological agents to mother or baby. The association of apneic episodes, lethargy, hypotonicity, and a reduction of spontaneous movement most often points to intracranial disease as an underlying cause.

Tachypnea. Diverse conditions result in tachypnea in the newborn period. Tachypnea in the presence of intrinsic pulmonary disease with upper or lower airway obstruction usually is accompanied by flaring of the alae nasi, chest-wall retractions, and grunting. In contrast, tachypnea associated with intense cyanosis in the absence of obvious respiratory distress suggests the presence of cyanotic congenital heart disease. In general, highest respiratory rates (80 to 110 breaths/min) occur in association with primary lung disease, not heart disease. Initial chest radiography frequently is diagnostic, especially if the problem is aspiration, mucous plug, adenomatoid malformation, lobar emphysema, diaphragmatic hernia, pneumothorax, lung agenesis, pulmonary hemorrhage, or an abnormal thoracic cage configuration. Choanal atresia may be precluded by passing a feeding tube through the nares, and the more common types of esophageal atresia and tracheoesophageal fistula may be excluded by passing the tube farther into the stomach.

CARDIAC EXAMINATION. Specific findings on cardiovascular examination may direct attention to a cardiac cause of cyanosis. Peripheral perfusion is poor in the presence of severe primary myocardial disease or the hypoplastic left heart syndrome. In contrast, peripheral pulses are bounding and the dorsalis pedis and palmar pulses are easily palpable in infants with patent ductus arteriosus, truncus arteriosus, or aorticopulmonary window. A marked discrepancy between upper and lower extremity blood pressures helps to identify infants with coarctation of the aorta. Inspection and palpation of the precordium allow an overall estimate of cardiac activity. A thrill in the suprasternal notch and/or over the precordium occasionally may be felt in infants with patent ductus arteriosus, critical aortic stenosis, or coarctation of the aorta. Characterization of the second heart sound may be of help because it often is single in infants with a hypoplastic left heart complex, pulmonary atresia with or without an intact ventricular septum, or truncus arteriosus. Wide splitting of the second heart sound may occur in infants with total anomalous pulmonary venous return. Ejection sounds often are detectable in infants with persistent truncus arteriosus and occasionally with critical aortic or pulmonic stenosis. The presence of a third heart sound is normal, but a gallop rhythm may provide a clue to myocardial failure. Wide splitting of the first and second heart sounds may produce the characteristically rhythmic auscultatory cadence of Ebstein's anomaly of the tricuspid valve (see Chaps. 25 and 44). The presence of a cardiac murmur may point clearly to underlying cardiac disease, but the absence of a murmur does not preclude a cardiac malformation. Moreover, cardiac murmurs of specific anomalies often are atypical in the newborn period. However, certain cardiac murmurs such as the decrescendo holosystolic murmur of tricuspid regurgitation in Ebstein's anomaly or the transient tricuspid regurgitation of infancy may point clearly to an accurate diagnosis. Auscultation of the head and abdomen may detect the murmur of an arteriovenous malformation at those sites in infants who present with findings of severe heart failure.

BLOOD GAS AND pH PATTERNS. Arterial blood gas analysis may be a reliable method of evaluating cyanosis, suggesting the type of altered physiology, and assessing responses to therapeutic maneuvers.[53] Specimens for blood gas analysis should be obtained in room air and in 100 percent oxygen. Stick capillary samples from the patient's warmed heel may be used, although determinations obtained by arterial puncture are preferable for evaluation of oxygenation because they are less susceptible to alterations in regional blood flow in critically ill infants. Sampling of right radial or temporal arterial blood is preferable because these sites are proximal to flow through a ductus arteriosus and do not reflect right-to-left ductal shunting, as would a sample from the descending aorta obtained by means of an umbilical artery catheter. A trial of continuous positive airway pressure may improve oxygenation in infants with either hyaline membrane disease or pulmonary edema.

Arterial blood gas patterns in various pathophysiological conditions are listed in Table 43–9. Pattern 1 typically is observed in infants with ventilation-perfusion abnormalities resulting from primary respiratory disease, often associated with elevated pulmonary vascular resistance and venoarterial shunting across a patent foramen ovale or patent ductus arteriosus. Pulmonary hypoventilation with carbon dioxide retention produces pattern 2. In the presence of a lesion causing obligatory venous admixture, such as total anomalous pulmonary venous connection (pattern 3), the response to oxygen may reflect an increase in pulmonary venous return secondary to a fall in pulmonary vascular resistance. Pattern 4 typically is seen in infants with a cardiac malformation that results in reduced pulmonary blood flow. Oxygen administration in these infants does not alter the arterial PO_2. The alterations of pattern 5 are observed when systemic hypoperfusion is the principal hemodynamic problem. In these babies, the arteriovenous oxygen difference is high, and the acidemia may be progressive and unrelenting.

ELECTROCARDIOGRAM (see also Chap. 5). ECG is less helpful in suggesting a diagnosis of heart disease in premature and newborn infants than in older children. Right ventricular hypertrophy is a normal finding in neonates, and the range of normal voltages is wide. However, specific observations can offer major clues to the presence of a cardiovascular anomaly. A counterclockwise, superiorly oriented frontal QRS loop with absent or reduced right ventricular forces suggests the diagnosis of tricuspid atresia. In contrast, when the QRS axis is normal but left ventricular forces predominate, the diagnosis of pulmonic atresia must be considered. The counterclockwise, superior QRS orientation also is observed in infants with an endocardiac cushion defect and in some with double-outlet right ventricle; right ventricular forces in these babies are increased.

The initial septal vector should be assessed from the ECG. Q waves often are not clearly seen in the lateral precordial leads in the first 72 hours of life. A leftward, posteriorly directed septal vector giving rise to Q waves in the right precordial leads is abnormal and suggests the presence of marked right ventricular hypertrophy, single ventricle, or inversion of the ventricles. T wave alterations may be seen on a normal neonatal ECG and may be of no particular consequence. By 72 hours of age, however, the T waves should be inverted in V_3 and V_1 and upright in the lateral precordium; persistently upright T waves in the right precordial leads are a sign of right ventricular hypertrophy. Depressed or flattened T waves in the lateral precordium may suggest subendocardial ischemia and a left heart outflow tract obstructive lesion, electrolyte disturbance, acidosis, or hypoxemia. An ECG pattern of myocardial infarction suggests a diagnosis of anomalous pulmonary origin of the coronary artery. Finally, rhythm disturbances such as complete heart block or supraventricular tachycardia (see Chap. 25) can be detected readily by ECG.

RADIOGRAPHIC EXAMINATION (see also Chap. 8). Chest radiography often is useful in differentiating between respiratory and cardiac causes of cyanosis in the newborn period. Determination of a normal cardiac and abdominal situs aids in ruling out several kinds of complex cyanotic cardiac malformations associated with asplenia or polysplenia with abdominal heterotaxy and dextrocardia. The distinct appearance of pulmonary parenchymal disease, such as the classic reticulogranular pattern of hyaline membrane disease, may allow a specific radiological diagnosis. In those premature infants with a large ductus arteriosus, the radiographic appearance often evolves from the typical findings of hyaline membrane disease to increased pulmonary vascular markings and finally to perihilar and generalized pulmonary edema.

Most important, the pediatric cardiologist depends heavily on the evaluation of pulmonary vascular markings to categorize neonatal congenital cardiac malformations according to function. In the presence of cyanosis, diminished pulmonary vascular markings call attention to the group of anomalies that includes tetralogy of Fallot, pulmonic stenosis with intact ventricular septum, pulmonic atresia, tricuspid atresia, and Ebstein's malformation of the tricuspid valve. Reduced pulmonary blood flow is responsible for the systemic arterial desaturation in these babies.

Increased pulmonary vascular markings in cyanotic infants are associated with lesions in which an obligatory admixture of systemic venous and pulmonary venous blood occurs. The more common anomalies in this category include transposition of the great arteries, hypoplastic left heart syndrome, truncus arteriosus, and total anomalous pulmonary venous drainage.

As mentioned earlier, overall heart size in normal newborn infants is greater than in older children, and cardiothoracic ratios up to 0.60 are within normal limits. The thymus shadow occasionally obscures the cardiac silhouette and prohibits accurate estimation of heart size. An enlarged heart on x-ray examination suggests a cardiac disorder. However, in the presence of severe respiratory difficulties with an increase in carbon dioxide tension and a decrease in both pH and arterial oxygen tension, cardiomegaly may be only moderate. A right aortic arch suggests the presence of either tetralogy of Fallot or persistent truncus arteriosus. An ovoid heart with a narrow base associated with increased pulmonary vascular marking is typical of transposition of the great arteries. A boot-shaped heart with concavity of the pulmonary outflow tract suggests tetralogy of Fallot, pulmonic atresia, or tricuspid atresia.

LABORATORY STUDIES IN CONGENITAL HEART DISEASE

FETAL ECHOCARDIOGRAPHY (see also Chap. 7). Ultrasound technology now allows examination of human fetal cardiac development and function in utero.[39, 93–95] Diagnostic-quality images of the fetal heart in utero can be obtained as early as 16 weeks of gestation. Cardiac structures are imaged primarily by cross-sectional echocardiography and augmented by a combination of range-gated pulsed Doppler ultrasonography, Doppler color flow imaging, and M-mode echocardiography. Analysis of the structure and function of the fetal heart during the second and third trimesters of pregnancy has allowed cardiologists to counsel prospective parents and, in a number of instances, to formulate management plans for pregnancy, delivery, and the immediate postnatal period. Using fetal echocardiography, major forms of congenital heart disease have been diagnosed in utero and cardiac rhythm abnormalities have been detected, permitting direct efforts at transplacental therapy. In particular, it has been established that a high incidence of cardiac pathology exists in the presence of nonimmune fetal hydrops. It appears clear that hydrops fetalis often represents end-stage fetal cardiac decompensation (Fig. 43–7). AV

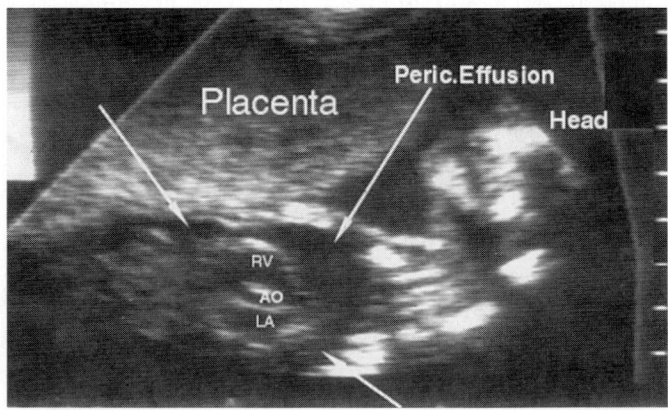

FIGURE 43–7. Fetal echocardiogram taken transabdominally through the uterus and the placenta shows a fetus lying with its head to the right hand side of the figure and demonstrates a pericardial (Peric) effusion (arrows). The right ventricle (RV), the aorta (AO), and the left atria (LA) are seen within the cardiac silhouette.

valve insufficiency often causes fetal right ventricular volume overload and systemic venous hypertension, leading to hydrops fetalis.

Pulsed Doppler and color flow mapping ultrasound examination of the fetus importantly supplement the echocardiographic findings in identifying the responsible defects, such as Ebstein's malformation of the tricuspid valve, atrial isomerism with AV septal defects, and the absent pulmonary valve and hypoplastic left heart syndromes.

Fetal cardiac ultrasonography is of special importance in analyzing disturbances of fetal cardiac rhythm, which usually are first suspected on the basis of auscultatory findings. Transabdominal ECG cannot identify atrial depolarization and is of limited value in the analysis of cardiac arrhythmias in utero. However, M-mode recordings of cardiac motion versus time allow conclusions about electrical events in the fetal heart, as they are reflected by the mechanical responses that are recorded echocardiographically. Supraventricular tachyarrhythmias are a common cause of nonimmune fetal hydrops (Fig. 43–8). Detection is of practical use in the treatment of these patients because the arrhythmia is treatable with the use of various antiarrhythmic drugs, such as digoxin, procainamide, propranolol, and flecainide, administered to the mother and reaching the fetus transplacentally or, rarely, under sonographic guidance, by injecting drugs, such as amiodarone, into the umbilical vein.[96]

ECHOCARDIOGRAPHY IN THE NEONATE. Echocardiography is of immense value in differentiating between heart disease and lung disease in newborns.[97, 97a] Indeed, it has become the standard for the diagnosis of virtually all cardiovascular malformations. A great many infants are now referred directly after ultrasound study for operative repair, without intervening cardiac catheterization. Echocardiographic diagnoses that often can be made with certainty include coarctation of the aorta, interruption of the aortic arch, patent ductus arteriosus, hypoplastic left heart syndrome, aortic valve stenosis, membranous and fibromuscular subvalvular aortic stenosis, aortic coarctation, hypertrophic cardiomyopathy, cor triatriatum, total anomalous pulmonary venous connection, atrial septal defect, tricuspid atresia, Ebstein's anomaly of the tricuspid valve, valvular pulmonic stenosis, AV septal defect, single ventricle, double-outlet right ventricle, transposition of the great arteries, and patent ductus arteriosus. The echocardiogram provides suggestive and often conclusive evidence for tetralogy of Fallot, truncus arteriosus, and pulmonary atresia with an intact ventricular septum, as well as pulmonary atresia with a VSD and a patent ductus arteriosus.

Doppler ultrasonography (see Chap. 7) supplements the two-dimensional echocardiographic examination by its ability to quantify valve gradients, cardiac output, blood flow patterns in the cardiac chambers and great arteries, and often shunt size.[98, 99] For example, the pulmonary-systemic blood flow ratio can be calculated by multiplying the square of the ratio of the great vessel diameters by the ratio of the peak systolic flow velocities, the pulmonary variable being the numerator in each ratio. The coupling of Doppler ultrasonographic techniques with the two-dimensional echocardiogram, and the representation in color of abnormalities in flow, volume, and direction (see Chap. 7), greatly improve diagnostic accuracy. Magnetic resonance imaging (see Chap. 10) can also be useful.[99a]

DIAGNOSTIC CARDIAC CATHETERIZATION (see also Chap. 11). If certain cardiac anomalies are identified by noninvasive studies or if a clear-cut differentiation cannot be made between cardiac and pulmonary disease, heart catheterization and angiocardiography may be necessary to define the underlying state precisely. However, fewer cardiac catheterizations have been performed in infants and children of all ages since the beginning of aggressive pursuit of preoperative diagnoses by noninvasive imaging modalities, particularly two-dimensional Doppler flow echocardiography.[99, 100] Hemodynamic study of newborn infants carries a small but distinct risk.[101] As a general rule, cardiac catheterization is not performed unless the information sought is central to treatment of the infant. Most infants with serious heart disease require therapeutic intervention, and thus catheterization should be performed only when surgical support is readily available. Cardiac catheterization is often performed in newborns who experience congestive heart failure in the first days after birth if the cause is an anatomical abnormality rather than an arrhythmia or a metabolic disturbance. Preferably, medical measures will have been instituted to stabilize the clinical state before a hemodynamic study is performed.

Some newborns with cyanotic congenital heart disease require prompt cardiac catheterization because of the considerable risk of rapid deterioration. Under these circumstances, hemodynamic and angiographic studies may not only provide the anatomical diagnosis required before emergency operation but also allow the opportunity for therapeutic maneuvers such as balloon atrial septostomy to facilitate intercirculatory mixing in patients with complete transposition of the great arteries or to augment interatrial shunting in patients with a restrictive patent foramen ovale and either tricuspid, pulmonic, or mitral atresia or total anomalous pulmonary venous connection. Selective intravenous infusion of low doses of prostaglandin E_1 (0.05 to 0.1 μg/kg/min) has been used before and at cardiac catheterization for the emergency palliation of ductus-dependent cardiac lesions such as pulmonary atresia, aortic coarctation, and interruption of the aortic arch. Because a patent ductus arteriosus maintains pulmonary and systemic blood flow, respectively, in these infants, dilatation of the ductus with vasodilatory prostaglandins may retard their clinical deterioration. Thus, prostaglandin E_1 infusion has been shown to be an effective short-term measure to correct hypoxemia and acidemia and to improve the preoperative and intraoperative status of infants who require surgical relief of the congenital cardiac lesion that is causing pulmonary or systemic hypoperfusion.

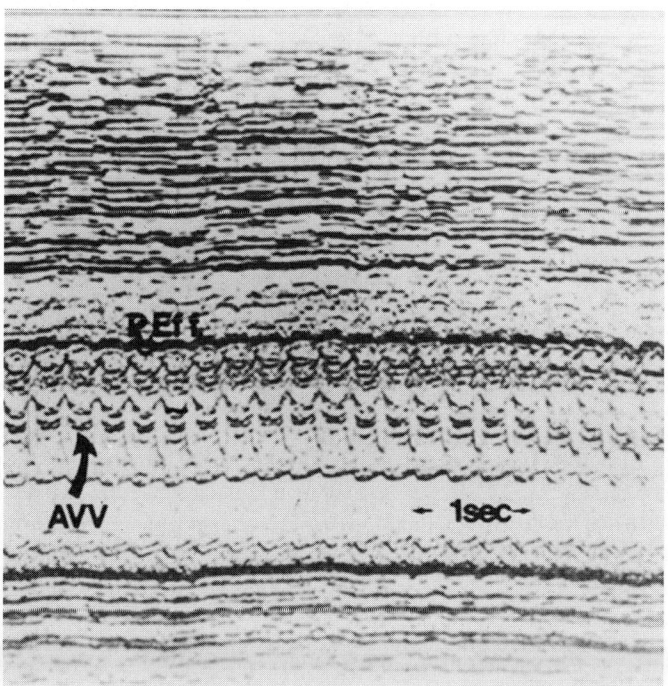

FIGURE 43–8. M-mode echocardiogram at 35 weeks' gestation, showing fetal supraventricular tachycardia and pericardial effusion (PEff). The tracing, taken at the midventricular level, allows the heart rate to be calculated from atrioventricular valve (AVV) motion (250 beats/min). (Courtesy of Dr. Charles Kleinman.)

THERAPEUTIC CATHETERIZATION (see also Chap. 38). Balloon atrial septostomy was the first catheter intervention that proved useful in treating congenital heart disease, and it remains the standard initial palliation in infants with complete transposition of the great arteries unless the arterial switch operation is performed imminently.[102] Many additional transcatheter techniques are now used successfully to treat congenital heart disease. These include knife blade atrial septostomy; umbrella or coil closure of patent ductus arteriosus; self-expanding and centering Amplatzer occluding device, or buttoned or modified clamshell or umbrella device closure of atrial septal defect; balloon-expandable intravascular stents for peripheral pulmonary artery and selected postoperative stenoses; and balloon and coil embolization of large systemic pulmonary artery collateral vessels and arteriovenous fistulas.[103–105] Other procedures that have expanded the role of the cardiac catheter from a diagnostic tool to a therapeutic instrument include transvenous or transarterial pacemaker insertion and retrieval of foreign bodies from the cardiovascular system. Transluminal balloon angioplasty currently is used principally in pediatrics for dilation of pulmonic and aortic valve stenoses, native and recoarctation of the aorta, and peripheral pulmonary artery stenosis. Questions about transluminal angioplasty in native neonatal coarctation, tetralogy of Fallot, and congenital subaortic and mitral stenoses remain unresolved. Finally, electrode catheter radiofrequency ablative techniques for the treatment of tachycardias are now performed routinely in centers with pediatric electrophysiology programs.[106]

ELECTROPHYSIOLOGICAL STUDIES (see also Chap. 23). The cardiac catheterization laboratory also is being used with increasing frequency to define the anatomical and physiological diagnoses of arrhythmias, thus facilitating an accurate prognosis and providing a rational basis for pharmacological, catheter ablation, or surgical treatment.[107–109] Catheter ablation approaches to tachyarrhythmias are now standard pediatric procedures (see Chaps. 23 and 25). The invasive electrophysiological approach provides unique information that cannot be obtained noninvasively. This includes determination of conduction times of individual components of the conducting system and measurement of refractory periods for structures such as the AV node, His bundle, and bundle branches. In addition, one can determine the origin or anatomical circuit, sustaining mechanisms, and possible perturbations that terminate the arrhythmia. This last maneuver is particularly important because it may enable the planning of effective drug treatment. It also may determine the advisability of catheter ablation, pacemaker control, or surgical treatment of the rhythm disturbance.

▼ Specific Cardiac Defects

Many classifications of congenital cardiovascular lesions have been proposed on the basis of hemodynamic, anatomical, and radiographic factors. Although the groups overlap, the following arrangement of cardiac anomalies is used in this chapter: (1) communications between the systemic and pulmonary circulations without cyanosis (left-to-right shunts), (2) obstructing valvular and vascular lesions with or without associated right-to-left shunt, (3) abnormalities in the origins of the great arteries and veins (the transposition complexes), (4) malpositions of the heart and cardiac apex, and (5) miscellaneous anomalies.

LEFT-TO-RIGHT SHUNTS

Atrial Septal Defect

(See also p. 1593)

MORPHOLOGY. Atrial septal defect is one of the most commonly recognized congenital cardiac anomalies in adults but is very rarely diagnosed and even less commonly results in disability in infants.[110] The anatomical sites of interatrial defects are shown in Figure 43–9. Defects of the sinus venosus type are high in the atrial septum near the entry of the superior vena cava and may be created by a deficiency in the wall that normally separates the pulmonary veins from the right lung and the superior vena cava and right atrium, thereby also resulting in partial anomalous pulmonary venous drainage.[111] The atrial septal defect most often involves the fossa ovalis, is midseptal in location, and is of the ostium secundum type. This type of defect is a true deficiency of the atrial septum and should not be confused with a patent foramen ovale. Embryologically, the left side of the atrial septum is derived from the septum primum, which possesses an opening—the interatrial ostium secundum (see Fig. 43–1). The ostium secundum lies forward and superior to the position of the foramen ovale. The latter is formed by the septum secundum and occupies the right side of the atrial septum. Tissue of the septum primum lying to the left of the foramen ovale

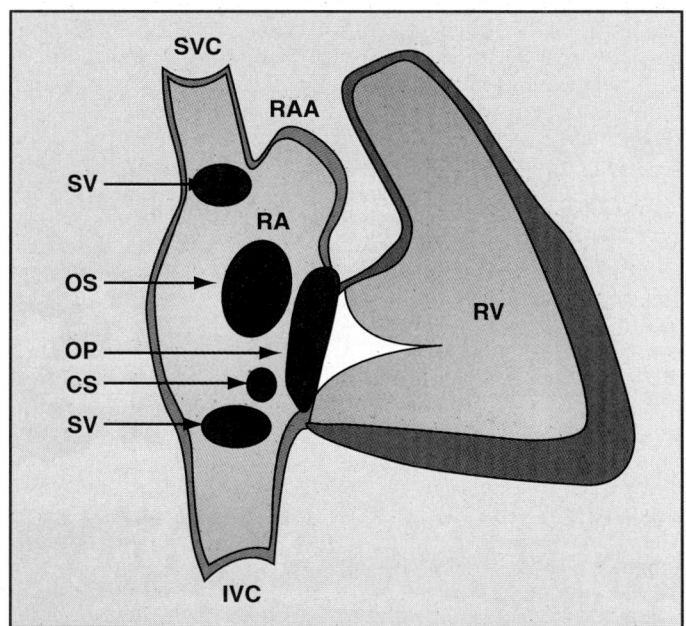

FIGURE 43–9. Diagrammatic representation of open right atrium (RA) and right ventricle (RV) showing the position of the various types of interatrial communications. The superior vena cava (SVC), inferior vena cava (IVC), and right atrial appendage (RAA) define the areas of the right atrium. There are five potential spaces of interatrial communication. The classic ostium secundum (OS) atrial septal lies within the fossa ovalis. The second most frequent defect is an ostium primum (OP) atrial communication, followed by the superior vena caval type of sinus venosus (SV) defect lying posteriorly within the right atrium at the junction of the SVC and pulmonary veins. An IVC sinus venosus (SV) defect lies at the junction of the right atrium with the IVC. The last communication is through the coronary sinus (CS).

serves as a flap valve that usually becomes fused postnatally with the side of the foramen ovale, yielding an anatomically closed or sealed foramen. "Probe patency," or an incomplete seal of the foramen ovale, occurs in about 25 percent of adults. A widely patent foramen ovale may be considered an acquired form of atrial septal defect that occurs especially when a disproportion exists between the size of the foramen ovale and the effective length of its valve. Enlargement of the foramen ovale per se is commonly associated with obstructive lesions on the right side of the heart, whereas a short valve relative to the size of the foramen often attends large-volume left-to-right shunts in which left atrial dilatation is prominent.

Ostium primum atrial septal anomalies are a form of AV septal defect and are dealt with in the next section. Lutembacher's syndrome is a designation applied to the rare combination of atrial septal defect and mitral stenosis, which is almost invariably the result of acquired rheumatic valvulitis.[112] Ten to 20 percent of patients with ostium secundum atrial septal defect also have prolapse of the mitral valve as an associated anomaly.[113]

HEMODYNAMICS. The magnitude of the left-to-right shunt through an atrial septal defect depends on the size of the defect, the relative compliance of the ventricles, and the relative resistance in both the pulmonary and the systemic circulation.[114] In patients with a small atrial septal defect or patent foramen ovale, the left atrial pressure may exceed the right by several millimeters of mercury, whereas the mean pressures in both atria are nearly identical when the defect is large. Left-to-right shunting occurs predominantly in late ventricular systole and early diastole with some augmentation during atrial contraction. The shunt results in diastolic overloading of the right ventricle and increased pulmonary blood flow. During the first few days and weeks of life, pulmonary resistance falls and systemic resistance rises, facilitating right ventricular emptying and impeding left ventricular emptying; the left-to-right shunt rises. Early in infancy, left-to-right flow through even a large interatrial communication commonly is limited by both the reduced chamber compliance of the thick neonatal right ventricle and the elevated pulmonary and reduced systemic vascular resistance of the neonate. The pulmonary vascular resistance commonly is normal or low in older infants or children with atrial septal defect, and the volume load usually is well tolerated, even though pulmonary blood flow may be two to five times greater than systemic. A transient and small right-to-left shunt occurring with the onset of left ventricular contraction and especially during respiratory periods of decreasing intrathoracic pressure is common in patients with ostium secundum defect, even in the absence of pulmonary hypertension.

CLINICAL FINDINGS. Patients with atrial septal defect usually are asymptomatic early in life, although occasional reports describe congestive heart failure and recurrent pneumonia in infancy.[110] Children with atrial septal defect may experience undue fatigue and exertional dyspnea. They tend to be somewhat underdeveloped physically and prone to respiratory infection. Atrial arrhythmias, pulmonary arterial hypertension, development of pulmonary vascular obstruction, and heart failure are exceedingly uncommon in the pediatric age range, in contrast to their common appearance in adults with atrial septal defect. In the former group, diagnosis often is entertained after detection of a heart murmur on routine physical examination prompts a more extensive cardiac evaluation. Small defects, less than 4 to 8 mm, have a modest probability of spontaneous closure.[115]

Physical Examination. Common findings include a prominent right ventricular cardiac impulse and palpable pulmonary artery pulsation. The first heart sound is normal or split, with accentuation of the tricuspid valve closure sound. Increased flow across the pulmonic valve is responsible for a midsystolic pulmonary ejection murmur. After the normal postnatal decline in pulmonary vascular resistance, the second heart sound is split widely and is relatively fixed in relation to respiration in patients with normal pulmonary pressures and low pulmonary vascular impedance because of a delay in pulmonic valve closure. With pulmonary hypertension, the splitting interval is a function of the electromechanical intervals of each ventricle; wide splitting occurs with shortening of the left and/or lengthening of the right ventricular electromechanical interval.[116] If the shunt is large, increased blood flow across the tricuspid valve is responsible for a mid-diastolic rumbling murmur at the lower left sternal border. In patients with associated prolapse of the mitral valve, an apical holosystolic or late systolic murmur radiating to the axilla often is heard, but a midsystolic click may be difficult to discern. Moreover, left ventricular precordial overactivity usually is absent because mitral regurgitation is mild in most patients.

In teenage patients, the physical findings may be altered when an increase in pulmonary vascular resistance results in diminution of the left-to-right shunt. Both the pulmonary and the tricuspid murmurs decrease in intensity, whereas the pulmonic component of the second heart sound becomes accentuated and the two components of the second heart sound may fuse; a diastolic murmur of pulmonic incompetence appears. Cyanosis and clubbing accompany development of a right-to-left shunt.

Electrocardiogram. In patients with an ostium secundum defect, the ECG usually shows right-axis deviation, right ventricular hypertrophy, and rSR′ or rsR′ pattern in the right precordial leads with a normal QRS duration (Fig. 43–10; see also Fig. 44–1). It is not clear whether the delay in right ventricular activation is a manifestation of right ventricular volume overload or a true conduction delay in the right bundle branch and peripheral Purkinje system. An early notch (triphasic "crochetage") pattern on the R wave in inferior limb leads is as sensitive an indicator of atrial defect as incomplete right bundle branch block.[117] Left-axis

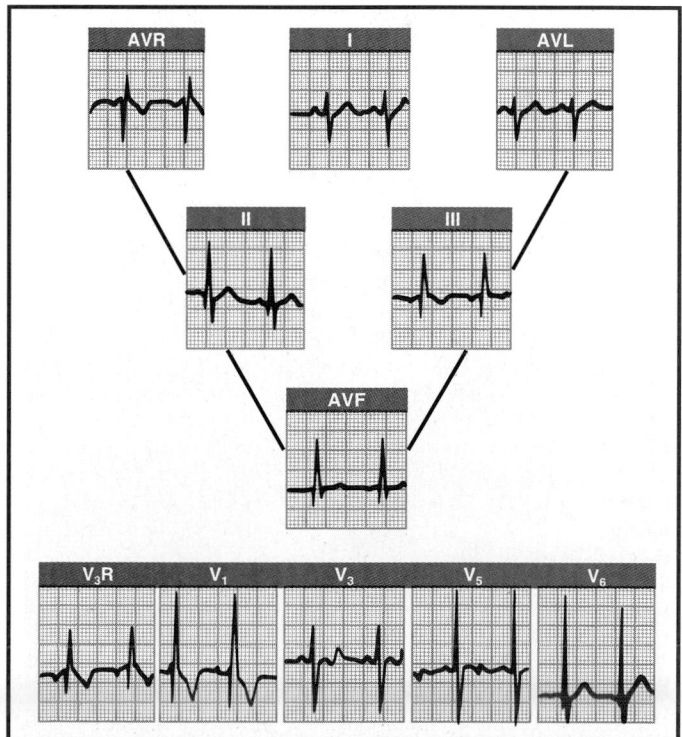

FIGURE 43–10. Typical electrocardiographic tracing in secundum atrial septal defect showing right-axis deviation, rSR′ in the right pericordial leads, and right ventricular hypertrophy. (Courtesy of Dr. Delores A. Danilowicz.)

deviation of the P wave in the frontal plane (manifested by a negative P wave in lead III) suggests the presence of a sinus venosus rather than an ostium secundum type of atrial septal defect. Left-axis deviation and superior orientation and counterclockwise rotation of the QRS loop in the frontal plane suggest the presence of either an ostium primum defect or a secundum atrial septal defect in association with mitral valve prolapse. Prolongation of the PR interval may be seen with all types of atrial septal defects; the prolonged internodal conduction time may be related to both the increased size of the atrium and the increased distance for internodal conduction produced by the defect itself.[117]

Chest Roentgenogram (see Fig. 44–2). This usually reveals enlargement of the right atrium and ventricle, dilatation of the pulmonary artery and its branches, and increased pulmonary vascular markings. Dilatation of the proximal portion of the superior vena cava occasionally is noted in patients with a sinus venosus defect. Left atrial dilatation is extremely rare but may be observed when significant mitral regurgitation exists.

Echocardiographic Features. These include pulmonary arterial and right ventricular dilatation and anterior systolic (paradoxical) or "flat" interventricular septal motion if significant right ventricular volume overload is present.[98] The defect may be visualized directly by two-dimensional echo imaging, particularly from a subcostal view of the interatrial septum (Fig. 43–11; also see Chap. 7). Transesophageal color-coded Doppler echocardiography and color flow provides excellent visualization of defects of the atrial septum.[118, 119] Associated mitral valve prolapse also may be identified by echocardiographic examination (see Chap. 7). Findings on ultrafast computed tomographic (CT) scanning are discussed in Chapter 10.

Two-dimensional echocardiography, supplemented by conventional or color-coded Doppler flow and/or contrast echocardiography, has supplanted cardiac catheterization as the confirmatory test for atrial septal defect.[120] Cardiac catheterization is then used if inconsistencies exist in the clinical data or if significant pulmonary hypertension is suspected.

Cardiac Catheterization. Diagnosis may be readily confirmed by passage of the catheter across the atrial defect. The site at which the catheter crosses, if high in the cardiac silhouette, may suggest a sinus venosus defect; if midseptal, a patent foramen ovale or ostium secundum defect; or, if low, a primum defect.[121] Serial determinations of the oxygen saturation or indicator dilution curve techniques may be used to estimate the magnitude of the shunt. In the absence of pulmonary hypertension, pressures on the right side of the heart often are normal, despite a large shunt. When a high oxygen saturation is found in the superior vena cava or when the catheter enters pulmonary veins directly from the right atrium, a sinus venosus defect is likely, and indicator dilution curves and selective angiography aid in identifying the number and location of the anomalous veins. *Partial anomalous pulmonary venous connection,* although usually associated with sinus venosus defect, may accompany secundum defects. Selective left ventricular angiography identifies prolapse of the mitral valve and allows assessment of the magnitude of mitral regurgitation that may be present in such patients.[128]

MANAGEMENT. In contrast to adults, children with sinus venosus or secundum types of atrial septal defect seldom require treatment for heart failure or antiarrhythmic medications for atrial fibrillation or supraventricular tachycardia. Respiratory tract infections should be treated promptly. Although the risk of infective endocarditis is low, antibiotics should be administered prophylactically before dental procedures.

Operative or Transcatheter Repair. This should be advised for all patients with uncomplicated atrial septal defects and evidence of significant left-to-right shunting, i.e., with pulmonary-systemic flow ratios exceeding about 1.5:1.0. Ideally, this should be carried out in those 2 to 4 years of age. Rarely, an atrial septal aneurysm is seen in association with a secundum-type atrial septal defect.[122] Such patients may experience spontaneous closure and may be monitored more conservatively until an older age before advising operation. Whether by median sternotomy or by minimally invasive transxiphoid techniques,[123] the defect is closed by suture or with a patch of prosthetic material with the patient on cardiopulmonary bypass. Earlier surgical repair is definitive treatment for the small number of infants and young children with significant symptoms or congestive failure. The surgical mortality rate is less than 1 percent, and results usually are excellent. Although the mitral valve may be examined directly at operation, it seldom is necessary in childhood to attempt plication or replacement of a ballooning or prolapsing mitral valve.

Operation should *not* be carried out in patients with small defects and trivial left-to-right shunts (pulmonary-systemic flow ratio ≤ 1.5:1.0) or in those with severe pulmonary vascular disease (pulmonary-systemic resistance ratio ≥ 0.7:1.0) without a significant left-to-right shunt.[124] Although still investigational, considerable experience exists with transcatheter closure by a variety of occluding devices using fluoroscopic or transesophageal echocardiographic imaging guidance[125–127] (Fig. 43–12). Limitations include difficulties in centering the device, the size of the sheath delivery system, the need to have more than a 4-mm separation between the edges of the defect and other important cardiac structures, and the inability to close defects whose stretched diameter exceeds 22 mm.

Subtle evidence of left ventricular dysfunction may be observed preoperatively at cardiac catheterization in children with isolated large atrial septal defects but without overt left or right ventricular failure.[128] Thus, decreased left ventricular stroke volume and cardiac output have been observed in children with both low and normal left ventricular end-diastolic volumes. In routine catheterization studies carried out on patients whose atrial septal defects were closed during preadolescence or later, a residual reduced cardiac output response to intense upright exercise in the absence of residual shunts, arrhythmias, or pulmonary arterial hypertension has been observed.[129] Normal myocardial function is preserved in patients in whom the defects were closed in early childhood.[130]

Electrophysiological Abnormalities. Intracardiac electrophysiological studies reveal a high incidence of intrinsic

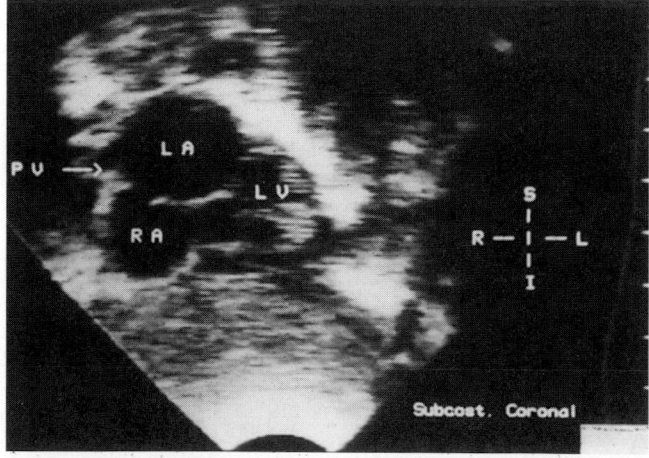

FIGURE 43–11. Subcostal coronal view showing a secundum atrial septal defect between the left atrium (LA) and the right atrium (RA). The right upper pulmonary vein (PV) is seen entering the left atrium. This view is posterior to the major portion of the ventricles; the left ventricle (LV) is seen, but only a small portion of the right ventricle (unlabeled) is apparent. I = inferior; L = left; R = right; S = superior.

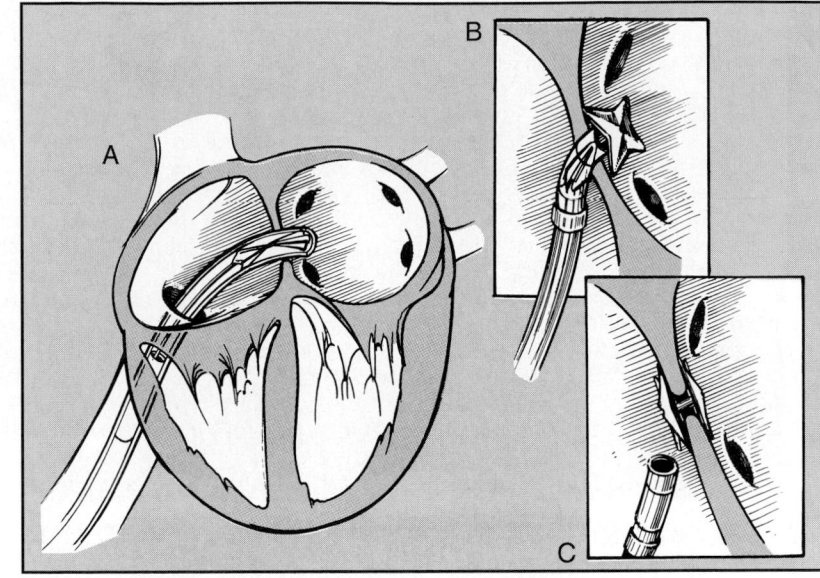

FIGURE 43-12. Clamshell umbrella occlusion of an ostium secundum atrial septal defect. A long sheath is positioned in the left atrium *(A)*. *B,* The distal umbrella arms are opened in the left atrium and the umbrella and sheath are pulled back together to the atrial septum. *C,* The proximal set of arms is then delivered on the right atrial side of the atrial septum. The correct position of the device is confirmed by fluoroscopy, angiography, and echocardiography before the device is released. (From Castañeda A, Jonas AR, Mayer JE Jr, et al: Cardiac Surgery of the Neonate and Infant. Philadelphia, WB Saunders, 1994, p 136.)

dysfunction of the sinoatrial and AV nodes, which persists after surgical repair. These intrinsic nodal abnormalities are more common in sinus venosus than in ostium secundum defects[131] but occur in both varieties. There also is evidence that the type of venous cannulation at the time of operative repair may contribute to the incidence and severity of arrhythmias observed at long-term follow-up.[132]

Atrioventricular Septal Defect
(See also p. 1596)

AV septal defects account for 4 to 5 percent of congenital heart defects and comprise a range of malformations characterized by various degrees of incomplete development of the inferior portion of the atrial septum, the inflow portion of the ventricular septum, and the AV valves (see Figs. 43-1 and 44-3). These anomalies also have been called endocardial cushion defects and AV canal defects. The basic defect is a deficiency of the AV septum, which separates the left ventricular inlet from the right atrium; it causes anomalies that range in severity from a small ostium primum atrial defect to a complete AV septal malformation that also involves defects in the interventricular septum and the mitral and tricuspid valves. The latter often are abnormal to various degrees, with five or six leaflets of variable size present, and variability also in the completeness of their commissures. AV septal defects are often encountered in association with other congenital abnormalities, such as asplenia or polysplenia syndromes, trisomy 21 (Down syndrome), and Ellis-van Creveld syndrome of ectodermal dysplasia and polydactyly.

Ostium Primum Defect (Partial AV Canal)

Ostium primum atrial septal defects lie immediately adjacent to the AV valves, either of which may be deformed and incompetent. Most often, only the anterior or septal leaflet of the mitral valve is displaced, and it commonly is cleft; the tricuspid valve usually is not involved. A cleft often is considered to be present in the mitral valve, although it is likely that the valve is in fact a trileaflet structure, with the cleft representing an abnormal commissure. The interatrial defect often is large, and the size of the left-to-right interatrial shunt in these patients is controlled by the same factors that exist in patients with ostium secundum atrial septal defect. Moreover, the clinical features are quite similar and principally consist of right ventricular precordial hyperactivity, a wide and persistently split sec-

ond heart sound, a right ventricular outflow tract systolic ejection murmur, and a mid-diastolic tricuspid flow rumble. The murmurs of AV valve regurgitation may be audible if either valve is significantly abnormal; however, serious AV valve regurgitation usually is absent. In the occasional patient, mitral regurgitation is substantial and creates prominent signs of left ventricular overload.

Chest roentgenography usually reveals right atrial and ventricular cardiomegaly, prominence of the right ventricular outflow tract, and increased pulmonary vascular markings. The *ECG findings* (see Fig. 44-4) are characteristic and show a right ventricular conduction defect accompanied by left anterior division block, left-axis deviation, and superior orientation and counterclockwise rotation of the QRS loop in the frontal plane (see Chap. 5). Hemodynamic factors do not appear to be important in producing the characteristic ECG appearance. Rather, the superior QRS vector in patients with a shortened H-V interval appears to be related to early activation of the posterobasal left ventricular wall; in other patients with a normal conduction time between the bundle of His and the ventricles, the counterclockwise superior inscription of the frontal plane vector appears to be related to late activation of the anterolateral left ventricular wall.[133] A prolonged P-R interval is observed in many patients with an ostium primum atrial septal defect; prolonged internodal conduction may be related to displacement of the AV node in a posteroinferior direction in some patients and/or to the enlarged right atrium.

ECHOCARDIOGRAPHY. Two-dimensional echocardiography is considered the standard for the diagnosis of all forms of AV septal defect (see Chap. 7). Important features include enlargement of both the right ventricle and the pulmonary artery, systolic anterior ventricular septal motion, prolonged mitral-septal apposition in diastole, and various abnormalities in mitral valve motion.[134] The defect is clearly visualized from the precordial apical and subxiphoid positions, with the latter views best demonstrating the relation between the atrial defect, the AV valves, and the interventricular septum (Fig. 43-13). Doppler color flow enhances these relations. Interatrial septal tissue is absent in the region of the crest of the interventricular septum; the trileaflet configuration of the mitral valve also may be identified. The subxiphoid long-axis view of the left ventricular outflow tract exhibits the gooseneck deformity in a manner similar to that with a right anterior oblique left ventricular angiogram. Echocardiography is particularly useful for detecting and characterizing double-orifice mitral valve, an association in about 3 percent of patients with ostium primum atrial defect. It also allows detection of

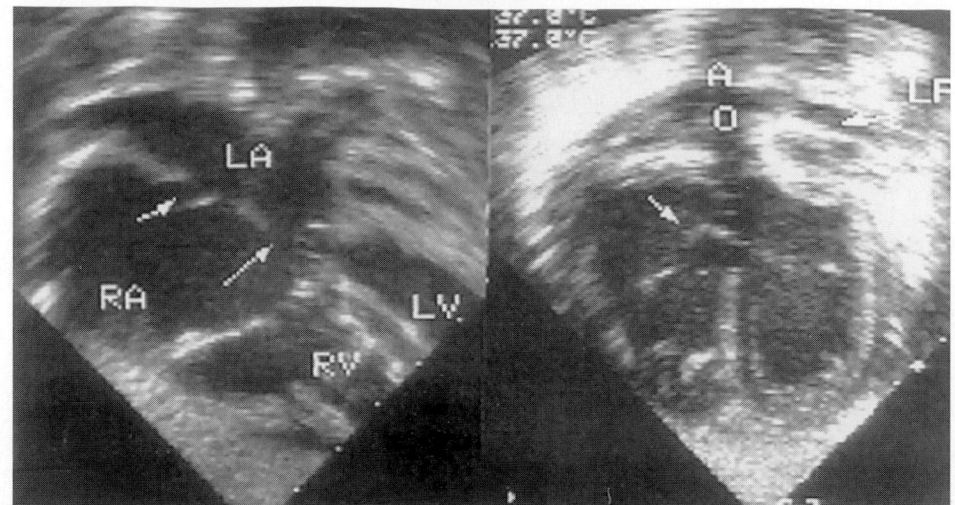

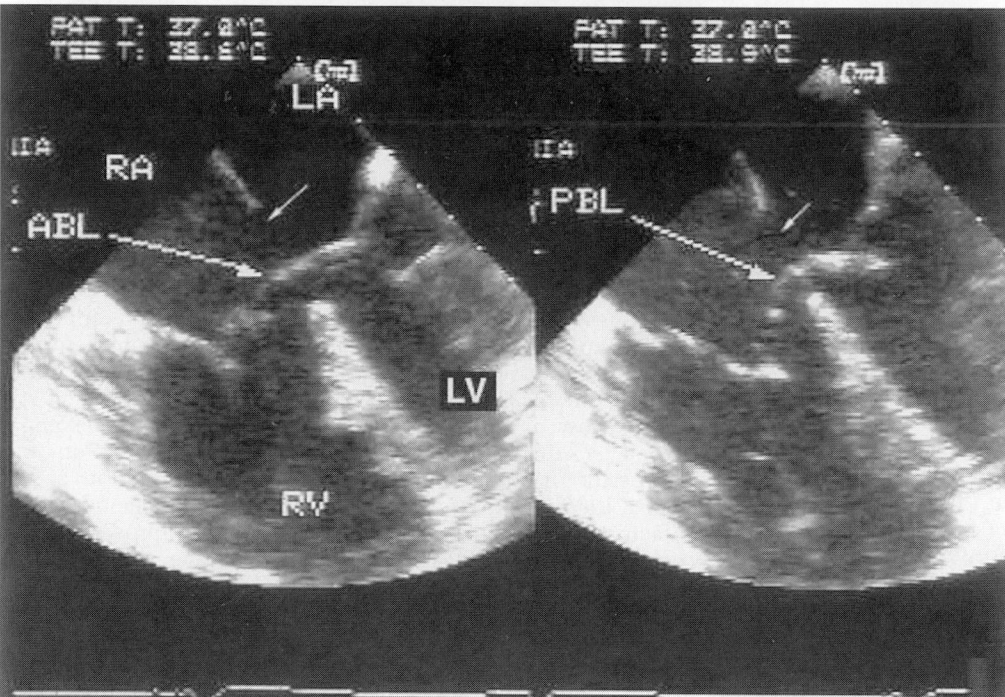

FIGURE 43–13. *Top panel,* Transesophageal echocardiogram taken from a subcostal transgastric plane in a patient with tetralogy of Fallot and type C complete atrioventricular septal defect. A secundum atrial septal defect (upper smaller arrow) is also seen in the left panel, and the ostium primum component of the complete atrioventricular canal is seen below (larger lower arrow). The right frame shows the complete atrioventricular septal defect with the anterosuperior bridging leaflet (arrow) straddling between the left and right ventricles (LV, RV) without attaching to the interventricular septum. The left pulmonary artery (LP) is seen behind the ascending aorta (AO). *Bottom panel,* Four-chamber transesophageal plane demonstrates a communication above the anterior and bridging leaflets (ABL and PBL) in the right- and left-hand frames, respectively. The small arrow indicates the typical position of an ostium primum atrial septal defect lying immediately below the rim of the atrial septum and above the valve tissue. LA = left atrium; RA = right atrium.

single left ventricular papillary muscle, hypoplasia of the left ventricle, and coarctation of the aorta, seen especially in symptomatic infants with an ostium primum atrial defect but without trisomy 21.[135] The *angiographic features* resemble those in the complete form of AV septal defect and are discussed later.

Complete AV Septal Defect

MORPHOLOGY. The complete form of the AV septal defect includes, in addition to the ostium primum atrial septal defect, a VSD in the posterior basal inlet portion of the ventricular septum and a common AV orifice.[136] The common AV valve usually has six leaflets: left superior and inferior, left and right lateral, and right superior and inferior. The left and right superior leaflets together often are referred to as the "anterior" bridging leaflet. No attachment exists between the left superior and inferior leaflets and the right superior and inferior leaflets. The left superior leaflet may cross the crest of the ventricular septum to reside partially on the right ventricular side. A classification of complete AV canal defect into types A, B, and C reflects the variability and the degree of anterior leaflet bridging of the ventricular septum (see Fig. 43–13). Thus, in type A,

the anterior leaflet is almost entirely committed to the left ventricle and is attached by chordae tendineae to the crest of the ventricular septum. In type C there is marked rightward displacement of the anterior bridging leaflet, which floats freely over the crest of the ventricular septum and is not attached to it by chordae tendineae. In type B, chordal attachments extend medially to an anomalous papillary muscle adjacent to the septum in the right ventricle.

A high incidence (about 35 percent) of additional cardiovascular lesions exists in patients with common AV canal. Principal among those associated with type C are tetralogy of Fallot, double-outlet right ventricle, transposition of the great arteries, and asplenia and polysplenia syndromes. Moreover, the type A complete AV septal anomaly commonly is seen in patients with Down syndrome.

The designation *unbalanced atrioventricular canal* is applied to the condition in which one ventricle is hypoplastic and the other receives most of the common AV valve. Subaortic obstruction may be due to abnormal features of the left side of the common AV valve or to hypoplasia of the left ventricle. The left-sided (mitral) component may also be the site of a potential form of double-orifice mitral stenosis postoperatively.

DIAGNOSIS. Patients with common AV septal defects present clinically before age 1 year with a history of frequent respiratory infections and poor weight gain. Heart failure in infancy is extremely common. The *physical findings* are similar to those observed in patients with ostium primum atrial septal defect but may include as well the holosystolic, lower left sternal border murmur of an interventricular communication and/or the decrescendo, holosystolic apical murmur of mitral regurgitation. The ECG features of complete AV canal defects resemble those in the partial ostium primum variety of AV septal anomalies (see Fig. 43–10). *Radiographically,* the usual findings are generalized cardiomegaly and engorged pulmonary vessels.

Two-dimensional echocardiography is diagnostic (see Chap. 7).[134] Apical and subcostal views are used to determine the size of the septal defects, the commitment of valve tissue and chordal attachments to the ventricles, ventricular size, the magnitude of AV valve insufficiency, and the anatomy of the left ventricular outflow tract. The subcostal oblique coronal view is often best to evaluate the commitment of AV valve tissue to each ventricle. Patterns of shunting and the number and magnitude of regurgitant jets are best evaluated by using pulsed, continuous-wave, and color flow Doppler imaging. On *hemodynamic study,* patients with persistent common AV canal invariably have elevated pulmonary arterial pressures; after age 2 years, a significant number of these patients have progressively severe pulmonary vascular obstructive disease.

Diagnosis also is reliably established by selective left ventricular *angiocardiography* using rapid injection of relatively large quantities of contrast material.[137] The findings include an absence of the AV septum and a deficiency of the inlet portion of the ventricular septum, with elongation of the left ventricular outflow tract in relation to the inflow tract. The aortic valve is elevated and displaced anteriorly relative to the AV valves, changing the relation between the anterior components of the left AV valve and the aorta, which produces a pathognomonic gooseneck deformity seen angiographically in diastole.

MANAGEMENT. In patients with complete AV canal, cardiac decompensation should be controlled initially. Even with an adequate response to medical therapy early in life, operation should be considered before age 6 months because infants with a complete form of the AV septal defect are at high risk of obstructive pulmonary vascular disease. The level of major shunting should be determined by echocardiographic-Doppler data, or less often during initial hemodynamic and angiographic studies, because if it is mainly at the ventricular level, pulmonary artery banding occasionally may be advised for intractable heart failure and failure to thrive. Often, however, there is a significant left ventricular–right atrial shunt either directly or indirectly by way of mitral regurgitation and left-to-right interatrial shunting, which will be unaffected by pulmonary artery banding and requires complete surgical correction.

Surgical Repair. Operative repair of uncomplicated primum defects is, for the most part, simple and yields good results. Left AV valve regurgitation and subaortic stenosis can be late complications amenable to reoperation. In most centers, primary repair in patients who have intractable heart failure, growth failure, or severe pulmonary hypertension is the preferred approach at any age.[138] Mild to moderate regurgitation often persists after surgical repair, particularly if significant AV valve incompetence existed preoperatively.[139] Rarely, if left AV leaflet tissue is remarkably deficient or deformed, mitral valve replacement may be required. Advances in the surgical approach to complex forms of AV septal defects have greatly improved the outlook for patients born with this malformation.[140, 141] These include better reconstruction of the mitral valve (Fig. 43–14) and more precise preoperative detection of such anatomical features as additional muscular VSDs, malalign-

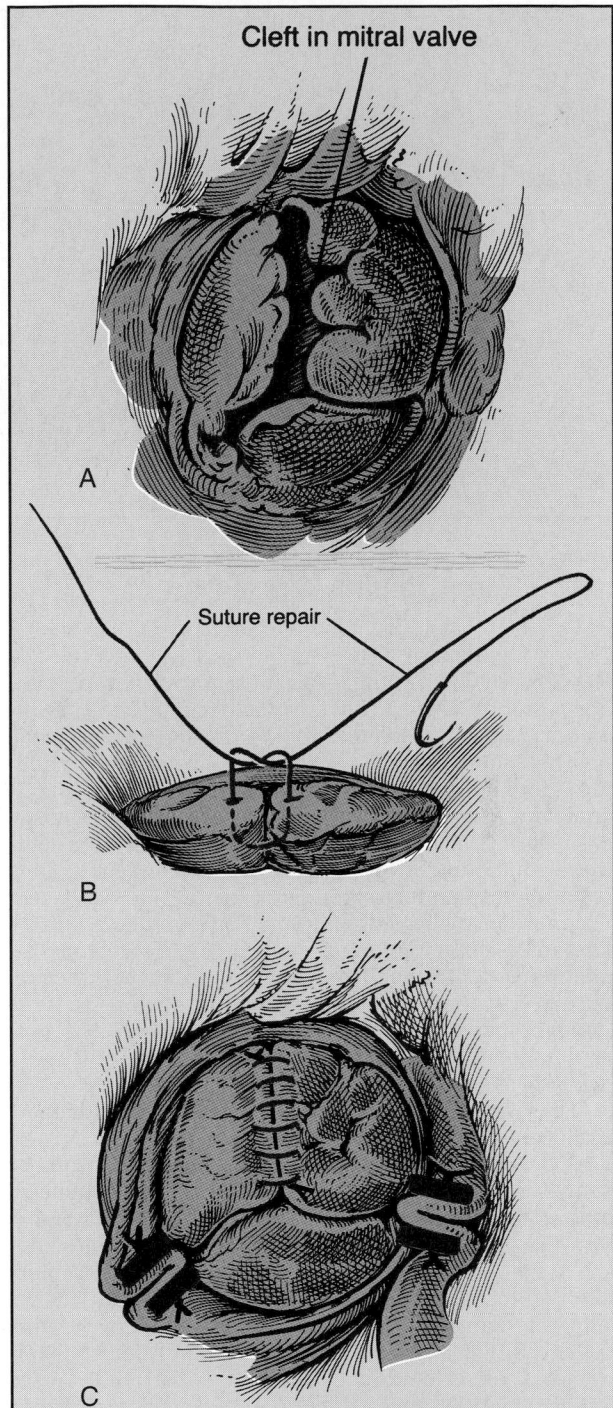

FIGURE 43–14. A suture technique is illustrated for repair of a cleft mitral valve *(A).* Absolute alignment of the cleft in all its dimensions is of critical importance with placement of the sutures where the edges naturally coapt *(B). C,* The cleft repair is accompanied by annuloplasty. (From Castañeda A, Jonas RA, Mayer JE Jr, et al: Cardiac Surgery of the Neonate and Infant. Philadelphia, WB Saunders, 1994, p 174.)

ment of the complete AV septum, and left ventricular hypoplasia. Operative improvement is primarily related to a clearer understanding of the anatomy of this complex lesion and to the ability to reconstruct the left AV valve, often by splitting of papillary muscles and shortening of chordae tendineae, with or without annuloplasty. Many surgeons prefer to close the septal defects with a single patch rather than separating ventricular and atrial patches. Suture placement is avoided in the region of the AV node and the bundle of His.

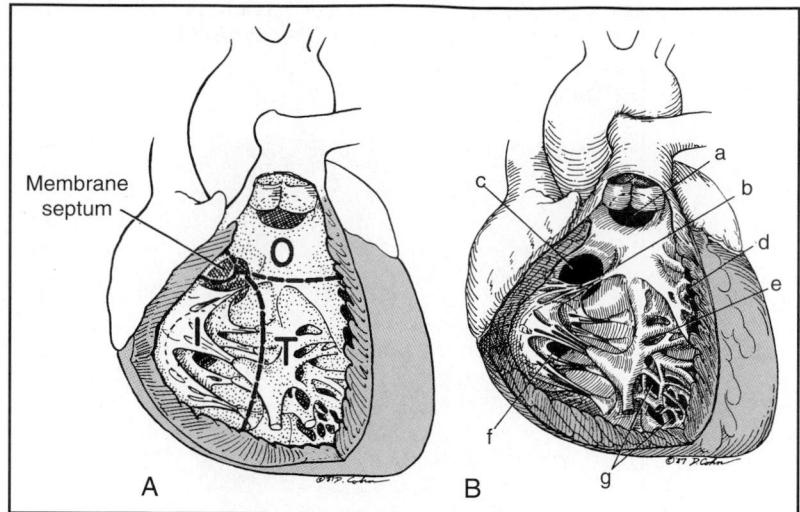

FIGURE 43–15. *A,* The four components of the ventricular septum viewed from the right ventricular side. I = inlet component, which extends from tricuspid annulus to attachments of the tricuspid valve; T = trabecular septum, which extends from the inlet out to the apex and up to the smooth-walled outlet; O = outlet septum or infundibular septum, which extends up to the pulmonary valve and membranous septum. *B,* The anatomical position of ventricular septal defects. a = outlet defect; b = papillary muscle of the conus; c = perimembranous defect; d = marginal muscular defects; e = central muscular defects; f = inlet defect; g = apical muscular defects. (From Graham TP Jr, Gutgesell HP: Ventricular septal defects. *In* Emmanouilides GC, Riemenschneider TA, Allen HD, et al [eds]: Moss and Adams' Heart Disease in Infants, Children, and Adolescents. 5th ed. Baltimore, © Williams & Wilkins, 1994, p 724.)

Ventricular Septal Defect

(See also p. 1595)

MORPHOLOGY. Among the most prevalent of cardiac malformations, defects of the ventricular septum occur commonly, both as isolated anomalies and in combination with other anomalies. The ventricular septum is made up of four compartments: the membranous septum, the inlet septum, the trabecular septum, and the outlet, or infundibular, septum. Defects result from a deficiency of growth or a failure of alignment or fusion of component parts. Defects most commonly are classified as occurring in or adjacent to one or more of the septal components (Fig. 43–15).[142, 143]

The most common defects occur in the region of the membranous septum and are referred to as *paramembranous* or *perimembranous defects* because they are larger than the membranous septum itself and are associated with a muscular defect at a portion of their perimeter. They also are known as infracristal, subaortic, or conoventricular defects. These perimembranous defects also can be defined by their adjacent areas as inlet, trabecular, or outlet. A second type of defect is one with an entirely muscular rim. Such muscular defects also can be defined as inlet, trabecular, central, apical, marginal or Swiss cheese, or outlet and vary greatly in size, shape, and number. A third type of defect occurs when the outlet septum is deficient and commonly is referred to as supracristal, subpulmonary, outlet, infundibular, or conoseptal. Because the aortic and pulmonary valves are in fibrous continuity, this type of defect also may be referred to as doubly committed subarterial. A septal deficiency of the site of the AV septum characterizes defects called AV septal, AV canal, or inlet septal defects.

The other feature of any defect may be a malalignment of the septal components. Either the inlet or the outlet septum can be malaligned. Malalignment of the inlet septum produces either mitral or tricuspid valve override and/or straddle. Malalignment of the outlet septum can be to the right or the left of the trabecular septum; when to the left of the trabecular septum, the VSD is characteristic of tetralogy of Fallot, double-outlet ventricle, truncus arteriosus, and, in some cases, transposition of the great arteries.

ECHOCARDIOGRAPHY. Two-dimensional and Doppler color flow mapping identify the type of defect in the ventricular septum (Fig. 43–16).[144–146] Perimembranous VSDs are identified by septal dropout in the area adjacent to the septal leaflet of the tricuspid valve and below the right border of the aortic annulus. The subaortic or anterior malalignment type of VSD appears just below the posterior semilunar valve cusps, entirely superior to the tricuspid valve. The subpulmonary VSD appears as echo dropout

within the outflow septum and extending to the pulmonary annulus. One or two of the aortic cusps may be seen to be protruding through the defect into the right ventricular outflow tract. The inlet AV septal–type of VSD extends from the fibrous annulus of the tricuspid valve into the muscular septum and often is entirely beneath the septal tricuspid leaflet. Muscular defects may appear anywhere throughout the ventricular septum and may be either large and single or small and multiple. Anatomical localization of all VSDs is facilitated by coupling two-dimensional ultrasound images (see Chap. 7) with a Doppler system and by superimposing a color-coded direction and velocity of blood flow on the real-time images.

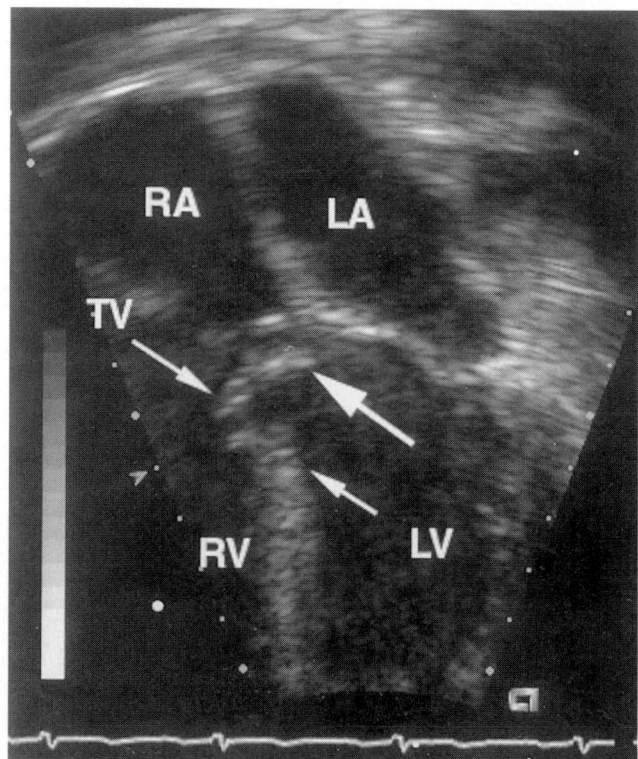

FIGURE 43–16. Four-chamber echocardiographic view in anatomical position demonstrates the ventricular septal defect (arrows within the left ventricular [LV] cavity). The tricuspid valve (TV) is adjacent to the ventricular septal defect and billows into the right ventricle (RV), a feature consistent with typical tricuspid tissue tags associated with perimembranous ventricular septal defect (formerly called ventricular septal aneurysm). LA = left atrium; RA = right atrium.

Pulmonary and systemic blood flow can be calculated from arterial velocity profiles and cross-sectional areas of the great vessels.[147] Calculation of pulmonary/systemic flow ratios is reasonably accurate. Detection of jets within the right ventricle allows determination of right ventricular pressure by subtracting the product using the Bernoulli equation, which gives the pressure difference, from the systemic systolic blood pressure. Continuous-wave Doppler has been helpful in determining the right ventricular pressure from tricuspid regurgitation, which is found fairly often with VSDs. Many other techniques of Doppler measurement have been used with varying success in efforts to determine pulmonary arterial pressure accurately.

PATHOPHYSIOLOGY. The functional disturbance caused by a VSD depends primarily on its size and the status of the pulmonary vascular bed rather than on the location of the defect. A small VSD with high resistance to flow permits only a small left-to-right shunt. A large interventricular communication allows a large left-to-right shunt only if there is no pulmonic stenosis or high pulmonary vascular resistance because these factors also determine shunt flow. Resistance to left ventricular emptying also affects shunt flow because it is an important factor in determining left ventricular pressure. Large defects allow both ventricles to function hemodynamically as a single pumping chamber with two outlets, equalizing the pressure in the systemic and pulmonary circulations. In such patients, the magnitude of the left-to-right shunt varies inversely with pulmonary vascular resistance. The natural history of VSDs has a wide spectrum, ranging from spontaneous closure to congestive cardiac failure and death in early infancy. Within this spectrum are possible development of pulmonary vascular obstruction, right ventricular outflow tract obstruction, aortic regurgitation, and infective endocarditis.[148–151]

Infants

It is unusual for a VSD to cause difficulties in the immediate postnatal period, although congestive heart failure during the first 6 months of life is a frequent occurrence. Early diagnosis is helpful to ensure more careful observation of the affected infant.[148] The examining physician usually suspects the diagnosis because of a harsh systolic murmur at the lower left sternal border. The ECG and chest roentgenogram findings are within normal limits in the immediate neonatal period because appreciable left-to-right shunting occurs only after the pulmonary vascular resistance decreases as the pulmonary vessels lose their fetal characteristics. It is desirable to monitor these infants closely.

A VSD that either decreases in size or closes completely during the first year of life presents no problems to the practicing physician. Spontaneous closure occurs by age 3 years in about 45 percent of patients born with VSD; occasional patients, however, do not experience spontaneous closure until age 8 to 10 years or even later.[152] Closure is more common in patients born with a small VSD; nonetheless, about 7 percent of infants with a large defect and congestive heart failure early in life also may experience spontaneous closure. Partial rather than complete closure is common in patients with both large and small VSDs. Anatomically, reduction of the VSD often is based on adherence of the tricuspid valve to the defect, hypertrophy of septal muscle, or ingrowth of fibrous tissue. Rarely, closure of the VSD is the result of prolapse of an aortic cusp or infective endocarditis.[150] Some defects close when an aneurysm forms in the ventricular septum (see Fig. 43–16). On auscultation, a click may be heard in early systole as the aneurysm tenses toward the right; the septal aneurysm may be detected by echocardiography as an anterior systolic bulge in the right ventricular outflow tract. A persistent minute VSD is not life threatening unless infective endocarditis develops. With proper precautions (see Chap. 47), the incidence of this complication is less than 1 percent.

If a moderate or large defect maintains its size after birth, the net left-to-right shunt increases during the first month of life as pulmonary vascular resistance falls. *Physical examination* during this time usually reveals a thrill along the lower left sternal border, and the holosystolic murmur of flow across the interventricular defect is accompanied by a low-pitched diastolic rumble at the apex, reflecting increased flow across the mitral valve. *Chest roentgenograms* reveal increased pulmonary vascular markings; evidence of left or biventricular hypertrophy may be observed on the ECG. Infants with a large left-to-right shunt tend to fare poorly, with recurrent upper and lower respiratory tract infections, failure to gain weight, and congestive heart failure. Congestive heart failure may be severe and intractable despite intensive medical management.

MANAGEMENT. We currently recommend primary intracardiac repair of the VSD at any age rather than surgical banding of the pulmonary artery[153] to reduce pulmonary blood flow and alleviate heart failure. An exception is made for the rare infant with multiple VSDs and a sievelike septum, who is at higher risk for complications after operative repair. Operation usually is deferred, along with debanding of the pulmonary artery, until the child reaches 3 to 5 years. Primary closure of the VSD, preferably through the right atrium, may be performed in infancy using cardiopulmonary bypass, profound hypothermia and cardiocirculatory arrest, or a combination of the two techniques. Mortality approaches zero in major centers if the defect is isolated and uncomplicated but approaches 10 percent if many anomalies are present.[154]

Fortunately, medical treatment often is successful in controlling congestive heart failure. Nevertheless, these infants should be referred for cardiac catheterization to evaluate pulmonary vascular resistance and to detect associated defects that may require operation, such as patent ductus arteriosus and coarctation of the aorta.

Children

Beyond the first year of life, a variable clinical picture emerges in children with VSD.[148, 155] If a small defect is present, the child usually is asymptomatic, the ECG usually appears normal, and the chest roentgenogram shows normal or only a mild increase in pulmonary vascular markings. Effort intolerance and fatigue are associated with moderate left-to-right shunts. These children exhibit cardiomegaly with a forceful left ventricular impulse and a prominent systolic thrill along the lower left sternal border. The second heart sound normally is split, with moderate accentuation of the pulmonic component; a third heart sound and rumbling diastolic murmur that reflects increased flow across the mitral valve are audible at the cardiac apex. The characteristic murmur resulting from flow across the defect is harsh and holosystolic, is best heard along the third and fourth interspaces to the left of the sternum, and is widely transmitted over the precordium. A basal midsystolic ejection murmur due to increased flow across the pulmonic valve also may be heard. The ECG reveals left or combined ventricular hypertrophy, and the chest roentgenogram and CT scan (see Chap. 5) show cardiomegaly, left atrial enlargement, and vascular engorgement.

PULMONARY HYPERTENSION. It is of utmost importance to identify patients who may develop irreversible pulmonary vascular obstructive disease (Eisenmenger's reaction).[155–158] Retrospective analyses of children who develop this complication indicate that infants with systemic or near systemic pressures in the pulmonary artery at the time of initial hemodynamic study are most at risk. If early primary closure is not recommended, recatheterization before age 18 months and a second determination of pulmonary vascular resistance should be performed in these patients to decide whether surgical intervention is obligatory to prevent development of fixed obliterative changes in the pulmonary vessels.

Mechanisms. It is likely that numerous factors are involved in the development of pulmonary vascular disease (see Chap. 53). The anatomically large VSD allows some or all of the systemic pressure to be transmitted to the pulmonary arteries, thereby retarding regression of their muscular media. Medial hypertrophy in the first months of life is responsible for higher pulmonary vascular resistance than would be anticipated for the amount of pulmonary blood flow. The shearing forces created by the high velocity of flow through narrowed pulmonary arterioles cause endothelial damage that is progressive.

Although an elevation in left atrial pressure may contribute to the rise in pulmonary vascular resistance, it is not an essential factor because pulmonary venous pressures can be low in patients who later develop pulmonary vascular disease. Nonetheless, pulmonary venous hypertension also may contribute to pulmonary arterial vasoconstriction and thus to increased shear forces. In this same regard, pulmonary vasoconstriction enhancing the risk of pulmonary vascular obstruction also may be caused by hypoxia due to either high altitude or lung disease. At high altitudes, large VSDs have higher pulmonary vascular resistances and smaller shunts than at low altitudes.

Clinical Features. If a child who previously had a loud murmur and thrill associated with poor growth suddenly has a growth spurt, fewer respiratory infections, and a diminution of the intensity of the cardiac murmur and disappearance of the thrill, he or she may be developing severe obliterative changes in the pulmonary vascular bed. An increase in intensity of the second heart sound, a reduction in heart size on the chest roentgenogram, and more pronounced right ventricular hypertrophy on the ECG also are noted. These changes occur because the increased pulmonary vascular resistance causes a decrease in the left-to-right shunt. If these changes are suspected, cardiac catheterization should be repeated; if they are confirmed, prompt surgical repair is indicated before an inoperable predominant right-to-left shunt ensues. If operation is performed before age 2 years, pulmonary vascular resistance may be expected to fall to normal levels.[158]

In older patients, the degree to which pulmonary vascular resistance is elevated before operation is a critical factor determining prognosis. If the pulmonary vascular resistance is one-third or less of the systemic value, progressive pulmonary vascular disease after operation is unusual. However, if a moderate-to-severe increase in pulmonary vascular resistance exists preoperatively, either no change or progression of pulmonary vascular disease is common postoperatively. Moreover, the presence of increased pulmonary vascular resistance results in a higher immediate postoperative mortality rate for surgical closure of VSD. These observations make it clear that a large VSD should be approached surgically very early in life when pulmonary vascular disease is still reversible or has not yet developed (Fig. 43–17).

RIGHT VENTRICULAR OUTFLOW TRACT OBSTRUCTION. With time, the clinical picture changes in 5 to 10 percent of patients with VSD and a moderate to large left-to-right shunt early in life. It begins to resemble more closely the tetralogy of Fallot (see Chap. 44); i.e., subvalvular right ventricular outflow tract obstruction develops owing to progressive hypertrophy of the crista supraventricularis. Depending on the severity of the latter process, it ultimately may result in reduced blood flow and a right-to-left shunt across the VSD. As right ventricular outflow tract obstruction develops, the holosystolic murmur is replaced by the crescendo-decrescendo ejection systolic murmur of pulmonic stenosis, and the pulmonary closure sound becomes softer. Right ventricular hypertrophy is evident on the ECG, and the chest roentgenogram shows a reduction in pulmonary vascular markings and a smaller heart size with a right ventricular configuration. Infun-

dibular hypertrophy may progress quite rapidly within the first year of life, but the typical evolution to a clinical picture of cyanotic tetralogy of Fallot often takes 1 to 4 years. In those infants who develop right ventricular outflow obstruction, the incidence of spontaneous closure or reduction in size of a VSD is low.

VENTRICULAR SEPTAL DEFECT WITH AORTIC REGURGITATION. This well-described complication of VSD occurs in about 5 percent of patients.[159] It usually is noted after age 5 years when a physician detects the early diastolic blowing murmur and wide pulse pressure of aortic regurgitation while monitoring a patient with a VSD. The diagnosis is readily confirmed by Doppler echocardiography. In such patients, aortic regurgitation may become the predominant hemodynamic abnormality. It is of interest that VSD with aortic regurgitation is rare in Europe and the United States, with an incidence of about 4 percent of all cases of isolated VSD, whereas in Japan the incidence is substantially higher (about 10 percent). In the Japanese, in particular, aortic regurgitation is the result of herniation of an aortic leaflet (usually the right coronary) through a subpulmonic supracristal VSD. In these patients, closure of the VSD may be all that is required to relieve aortic regurgitation. In many patients, however, especially in the Western world, the VSD is below the infundibular septum (crista supraventricularis). Although aortic leaflet herniation, especially of the right or noncoronary cusp, may occur in some of these patients, aortic regurgitation often results from a primary abnormality of the valve, usually one defective commissure. In the latter situation, plication of the elongated leaflet may lessen but not abolish the aortic regurgitation; in some patients, prosthetic valve replacement may be necessary to provide hemodynamic relief.

In most patients with VSD and aortic regurgitation, the VSD is small to moderate in size, and mild right ventricular outflow tract obstruction exists. The latter is caused by either subpulmonic infundibular stenosis or projection of the herniated aortic cusp into the right ventricular outflow tract. The distinction between types of VSD with aortic regurgitation usually can be made by two-dimensional and Doppler echocardiography and by selective left ventricular angiocardiography to define the site of the interventricular communication in combination with retrograde aortography to assess the anatomy and competence of the aortic valve.[160]

Management. Treatment of patients with VSD and aortic regurgitation is controversial. In patients with a large, hemodynamically significant left-to-right shunt, repair of the VSD is indicated, but aortic regurgitation is repaired only if at least moderate aortic regurgitation exists. If a supracristal VSD without aortic regurgitation is identified at cardiac catheterization in early childhood, a sensible argument for prophylactic closure of the VSD can be put forth to prevent the potential complication of aortic valve incompetence. In the presence of moderate or severe aortic regurgitation, valvuloplasty is preferred to valve replacement,[161] in recognition of the fact that the severity of aortic regurgitation may increase in subsequent years and that reoperation with valve replacement may be necessary. Operation should probably be deferred in asymptomatic patients with a subcristal VSD and an insignificant left-to-right shunt when aortic regurgitation is not severe. If the defect is supracristal in the same clinical setting, its closure may not alleviate the mild degree of aortic incompetence but may retard its progression.

OTHER FORMS OF VENTRICULAR DEFECT. Unusual forms of VSD include numerous muscular defects and left ventricular–right atrial communications. Defects in the muscular ventricular septum frequently are several small fenestrations that produce a large net left-to-right shunt.[151] Their recognition is a necessary preliminary to successful operation because incomplete repair may result in postoperative cardiac failure and death. A shunt from the left ventricle to right atrium may occur with a VSD in the most superior portion of the ventricular septum because the tricuspid valve is lower than the mitral valve. The clinical, ECG, and radiological findings in these patients do not differ appreciably from those in patients with a simple VSD, although right atrial enlargement may provide a clue to correct diagnosis of left ventricular–right atrial communication.[162]

The pathophysiology of a single or common ventricle may resemble that of a large VSD, although these defects are dissimilar embryologically. The single chamber frequently is the morphological left ventricle; malposition of the great arteries is common. No cyanosis may be detectable if selective streaming and increased pulmonary blood flow rather than complete mixing occurs. Pulmonary hypertension invariably is present unless pulmonic stenosis exists. It is imperative to differentiate a single ventricle from a large VSD by echocardiography and angiography because the operative approaches to the former malformation require the atriopulmonary Fontan's connection.

MANAGEMENT. It is rarely necessary to restrict the activities of a child with an isolated VSD. Infective bacterial endocarditis is always a threat, and antibiotic prophylaxis for dental procedures and minor surgery is indicated (see Table 43–4, p. 1516).[163] Respiratory infections require prompt evaluation and treatment. These children should be seen at least once or twice yearly to detect changes in the clinical picture that suggest the development of pulmonary vascular obliterative changes.

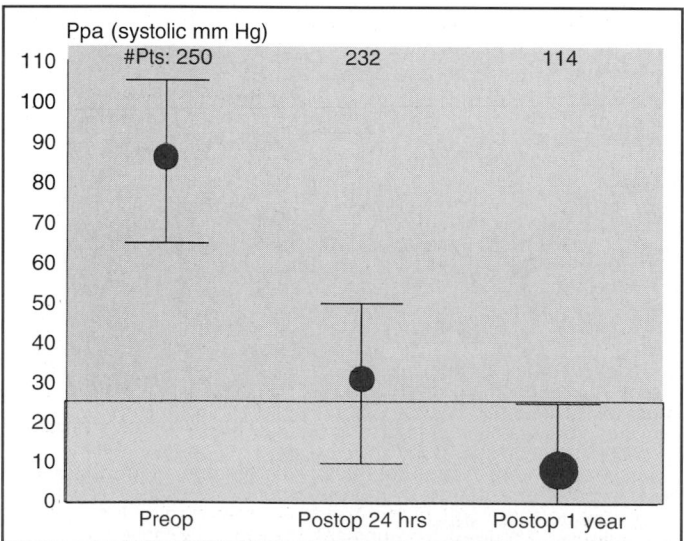

FIGURE 43–17. Early and late postoperative changes of pulmonary artery pressure after closure of ventricular septal defects in infants. (From Castañeda A, Jonas RA, Mayer JE Jr, et al: Cardiac Surgery of the Neonate and Infant. Philadelphia, WB Saunders, 1994, p 200.)

SURGICAL TREATMENT. When clinical findings suggest a moderate shunt but no pulmonary hypertension, elective hemodynamic evaluation should be undertaken before age 3 years. Of prime importance in the hemodynamic evaluation is determination of pressure and blood flow in the pulmonary artery.[164] Surgical treatment is not recommended for children who have normal pulmonary arterial pressures with small shunts (pulmonary-systemic flow ratios of less than 1.5 to 2.0:1).[165] In such patients, the remaining risk of infective endocarditis does not exceed the risk of operation. Moreover, although the inherent risk of operation is small, the possibility of postoperative heart block, infection, or other complications of operation and cardiopulmonary bypass dictates a conservative approach when the cardiac defect may be well tolerated for life.

In some centers, the use of intraoperative transesophageal echocardiography has provided accurate assessment of patch integrity and the presence of additional muscular defects after termination of cardiopulmonary bypass.[166, 167]

With larger shunts, elective operation may be advised before the child enters school, thus minimizing any subsequent distinction of these patients from their normal classmates. Total assessment of the psychosocial dynamics of the family and child is helpful in determining the proper age for elective operation in each patient.

Under investigation is transcatheter closure by umbrella or clamshell occluder devices inserted by crossing the ventricular defect to guide a venous catheter through a long sheath and, ultimately, placing the device across the ventricular septum from the right ventricular side.[168–170] The use of such devices is limited to defects in the apical muscular septum, well distanced from the semilunar and AV valves.

Complete heart block is the most significant surgically induced conduction system abnormality, occurring immediately after surgery in fewer than 1 percent of patients. Late-onset complete heart block occasionally is a problem, especially in the 10 to 25 percent of patients whose postoperative ECG findings show complete right bundle branch block with left anterior hemiblock. When the latter ECG pattern is observed in patients with transient complete heart block in the early postoperative period, electrophysiological studies should be conducted at postoperative cardiac catheterization. Patients presenting postoperatively with right bundle block and left anterior hemiblock appear to fall into two populations, defined by either peripheral damage to the conduction system or damage to the bundle of His or its proximal branches. The former has not been associated with transient postoperative complete heart block, and these patients usually have a benign course. Trifascicular damage may be demonstrated in the latter population by a prolonged H-V interval, which implies a higher risk of complete heart block later in life. Although prophylactic use of permanent pacemakers in asymptomatic patients with evidence of trifascicular damage is not currently recommended, this group certainly requires careful follow-up and continued study.

Treadmill exercise studies of patients who preoperatively had normal or only moderately elevated pulmonary vascular resistance and essentially normal postoperative cardiac catheterization data may uncover late abnormalities in circulatory function.[171] Despite normal cardiac output at rest, an impaired cardiac output response to exercise is noted in some. Moreover, despite normal pulmonary arterial pressure at rest, markedly abnormal increases in pulmonary arterial pressure may be noted during exercise. These findings may be related to abnormal left ventricular function after closure of the VSD and/or to persistent pathological changes in the pulmonary arterioles or to abnormal pulmonary vascular reactivity.[172] A direct relation exists between age at operation and the magnitude of the pulmonary arterial pressure response to intense exercise, suggesting that early operation may prevent permanent impairment of the functional capacity of the myocardium and pulmonary vascular bed.

A child who has already developed pulmonary vascular obstruction and a net right-to-left shunt across the VSD may occasionally come to medical attention (see also p. 1614). Symptoms may consist of exertional dyspnea, chest pain, syncope, and hemoptysis; the right-to-left shunt leads to cyanosis, clubbing, and polycythemia. Little can currently be offered to this group of patients other than continuing support to the patient and family.

Patent Ductus Arteriosus

(See also Chap. 44)

The ductus arteriosus normally exists in the fetus as a widely patent vessel connecting the pulmonary trunk and the descending aorta just distal to the left subclavian artery (see Fig. 43–4, p. 1511). In a fetus, most of the output of the right ventricle bypasses the unexpanded lungs by way of the ductus arteriosus and enters the descending aorta, where it travels to the placenta, the fetal organ of oxygenation.

It was earlier assumed that during fetal life the ductus arteriosus is a passively open channel that constricted postnatally by means of undefined molecular mechanisms in response to the abrupt rise in arterial Po_2 accompanying the first breath of life.[173] Even in utero, the lumen of the ductus arteriosus may be influenced by vasoactive substances, particularly prostaglandins.[86, 87, 174–176] Thus, inhibition of prostaglandin synthesis causes profound constriction of the ductus arteriosus in the mammalian fetus that may be reversed by administration of vasodilatory E-type prostaglandins. Initial contraction and functional closure of the ductus arteriosus shortly after birth is related both to the sudden increase in the partial pressure of oxygen that accompanies ventilation and to changes in the synthesis and metabolism of vasoactive eicosanoids. Intimal proliferation and fibrosis proceed more gradually, so that anatomical closure may take as long as several weeks for completion.[177]

The ductus arteriosus is a unique structure after birth because its patency may, on the one hand, result in cardiac decompensation but may, on the other hand, provide the only life-sustaining conduit to preserve systemic or pulmonary arterial blood flow in the presence of certain cardiac malformations.[178] Appreciable left-to-right shunting across the patent ductus arteriosus frequently complicates the clinical course of infants born prematurely.[179] The ductal shunt has been implicated specifically in the deterioration of pulmonary function in infants with the respiratory distress syndrome; in these infants severe congestive heart failure often is unresponsive to digitalis and diuretics.[87]

A distinction should be made between patency of the ductus arteriosus in a *preterm* infant, who lacks the normal mechanisms for postnatal ductal closure because of immaturity, and a full-term newborn, in whom patency of the ductus is a true congenital malformation, probably related to a primary anatomical defect of the elastic tissue within the wall of the ductus.[177] In the former circumstance, delayed spontaneous closure of the ductus may be anticipated if the infant does not succumb to the cardiopulmonary difficulties caused by the ductus itself or to some lethal complication of prematurity, such as hyaline membrane disease, intraventricular hemorrhage, or necrotizing enterocolitis. In a similar manner, some full-term newborns have persistent patency of the ductus arteriosus for weeks or months because their relative hypoxemia contributes to vasodilatation of the channel. In the latter category are infants born at high altitude; those born with congenital malformations causing hypoxemia, such as pulmonary atresia with or without VSD; or those born with malformations in which ductal flow supplies the systemic circulation, such as hypoplastic left heart syndrome, interruption of the aortic arch, or some examples of coarctation of the aorta syndrome.

In the clinical settings in which the ductus preserves pulmonary blood flow, the essentially inevitable spontaneous closure of the vessel is associated with profound clinical deterioration. The latter may be reversed medically within the first 4 to 5 days of life by infusion of prostaglandin E_1 intravenously. By dilating the constricted ductus arteriosus, a temporary increase occurs in arterial blood oxygen tension and oxygen saturation and correction of acidemia.[178] These infants can then undergo operative repair or a palliative systemic-pulmonary anastomosis, under more optimal circumstances. Pharmacological dilation of the ductus arteriosus also is effective in preoperative restoration of systemic blood flow and alleviation of heart failure, especially in infants with aortic coarctation or hypoplastic left heart syndrome, and in infants with complete transposition of the great arteries in whom intercirculatory mixing is augmented.

PREMATURE INFANTS. In most, if not all, preterm infants less than 1500-gm birth weight, persistence of a patent ductus arteriosus is prolonged, and in about one-third of these infants a large aorticopulmonary shunt is responsible for significant cardiopulmonary deterioration.[180, 181] Radiographic, echocardiographic, and Doppler ultrasound signs of significant left-to-right shunting usually precede the appearance of physical findings suggesting ductal patency. A significant increase in the cardiothoracic ratio is seen on sequential roentgenograms, as well as increased pulmonary arterial markings progressing to perihilar and generalized pulmonary edema. Serial echocardiographic evaluations that demonstrate increases in left ventricular end-diastolic and left atrial dimensions, especially when correlated with the aforementioned radiographic signs, are highly suggestive of a large shunt. Two-dimensional and Doppler echocardiography directly visualize and define the flow characteristics of the ductus arteriosus with great accuracy.[182]

Clinical Findings. These include bounding peripheral pulses, an infraclavicular and interscapular systolic murmur (occasionally a continuous murmur), precordial hyperactivity, hepatomegaly, and either multiple episodes of apnea and bradycardia or respiratory dependence. Cardiac catheterization carries a high risk in preterm infants and seldom is indicated unless the diagnosis is obscure.

Treatment. Treatment of preterm infants with a patent ductus arteriosus varies with the magnitude of shunting and the severity of hyaline membrane disease because the ductus may contribute importantly to mortality in the respiratory distress syndrome. Intervention in an asymptomatic infant with a small left-to-right shunt is unnecessary because the patent ductus arteriosus almost invariably undergoes spontaneous closure and does not require late surgical ligation and division. Those infants who demonstrate unmistakable signs of a significant ductal left-to-right shunt during the course of the respiratory distress syndrome often are unresponsive to medical measures to control congestive heart failure and require closure of the patent ductus arteriosus to survive. These infants are best treated within the first 2 to 7 days of life by pharmacological inhibition of prostaglandin synthesis with indomethacin to constrict and close the ductus[179, 183–185]; surgical ligation is required in the estimated 10 percent of infants who are unresponsive to indomethacin.[186] Early intervention is advised to reduce the likelihood of necrotizing enterocolitis and of bronchopulmonary dysplasia related to prolonged respirator and oxygen dependence. Less often, indications for pharmacological or surgical closure of the ductus consist of life-threatening episodes of apnea and bradycardia or a prolonged failure to gain weight and grow.

FULL-TERM INFANTS AND CHILDREN. In full-term newborns and older infants and children, patency of the ductus arteriosus occurs particularly in girls and in the offspring of pregnancies complicated by first-trimester rubella. Although most frequent in isolated form, the anomaly may coexist with other malformations, particularly coarctation of the aorta, VSD, pulmonic stenosis, and aortic stenosis. Flow across the ductus is determined by the pressure relation between the aorta and the pulmonary artery and by the cross-sectional area and length of the ductus itself.[187] Pulmonary pressures most commonly are normal, and a persistent gradient and shunt from aorta to pulmonary artery exist throughout the cardiac cycle.

Physical examination reveals a characteristic thrill and a continuous machinery murmur, with a late systolic accentuation at the upper left sternal border. The left atrium and left ventricle enlarge to accommodate the increased pulmonary venous return, and flow murmurs across the mitral and aortic valves may be detected. With significant left-to-right shunting, the runoff of blood through the ductus causes a widened systemic pulse pressure and bounding peripheral pulses. The hemodynamic abnormality is reflected in the ECG by left ventricular and occasionally left atrial hypertrophy, and in the chest roentgenogram by left atrial and ventricular enlargement, prominent ascending aorta and pulmonary artery, and pulmonary vascular engorgement (see Chaps. 8 and 44).

The clinical diagnosis may be difficult when the findings do not conform to the classic presentation. As mentioned earlier, disappearance of the diastolic component of the murmur is common in premature infants because pulmonary arterial diastolic pressures are higher at that age. In older patients, both heart failure and pulmonary hypertension are associated with a reduction in the pressure gradient across the ductus arteriosus and result in atypical systolic murmurs. When severe pulmonary vascular obstructive disease results in reversal of flow through the ductus and preferential shunting of unoxygenated blood to the descending aorta, the toes, rather than the fingers, may show cyanosis and clubbing.

Full-term infants with patent ductus arteriosus may survive for a number of years, although a large defect occasionally results in heart failure and pulmonary edema early in life. The leading causes of death in older children are infective endocarditis and heart failure. Beyond the third

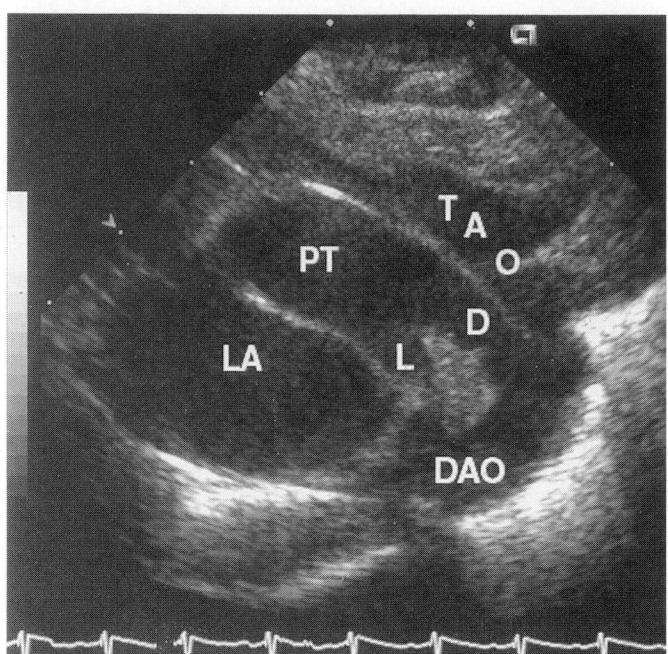

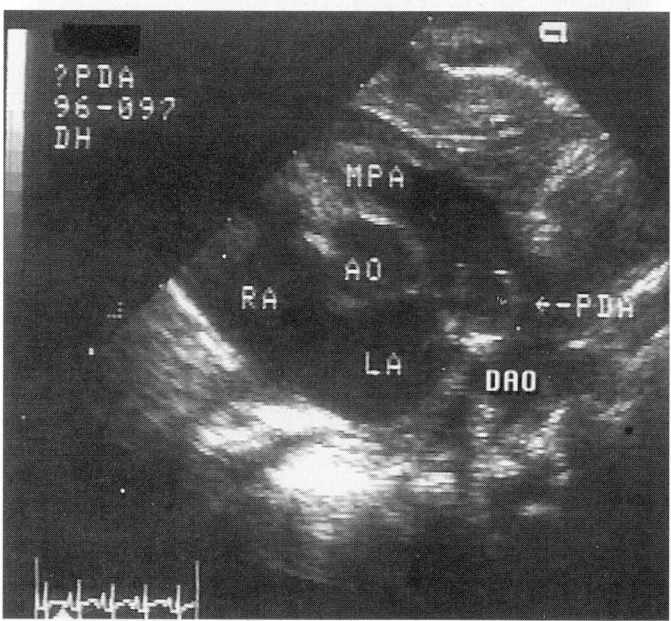

FIGURE 43–18. *Top panel,* High parasternal view of a patent ductus arteriosus in the sagittal plane demonstrating the classic position of a ductus arteriosus (D) lying between the pulmonary trunk (PT) and the descending aorta (DAO). The transverse aorta (TAO) giving rise to vessels to the head and neck is seen lying above the pulmonary trunk. The left atrium (LA) is seen inferiorly. The pulmonary trunk appears continuous with a wide patent ductus into the descending aorta just above the origin of the left pulmonary artery (L). *Bottom panel,* Patent ductus arteriosus (PDA) in a conventional parasternal short-axis view arising from the main pulmonary artery (MPA). The left pulmonary artery lies immediately to the right of the ductus and the left pulmonary artery lies adjacent to the ascending aorta (AO). The ductus is continuous with the descending aorta (DAO). The AO lies between the MPA anteriorly, the right atrium (RA) and LA posteriorly, and the right pulmonary artery laterally to the left.

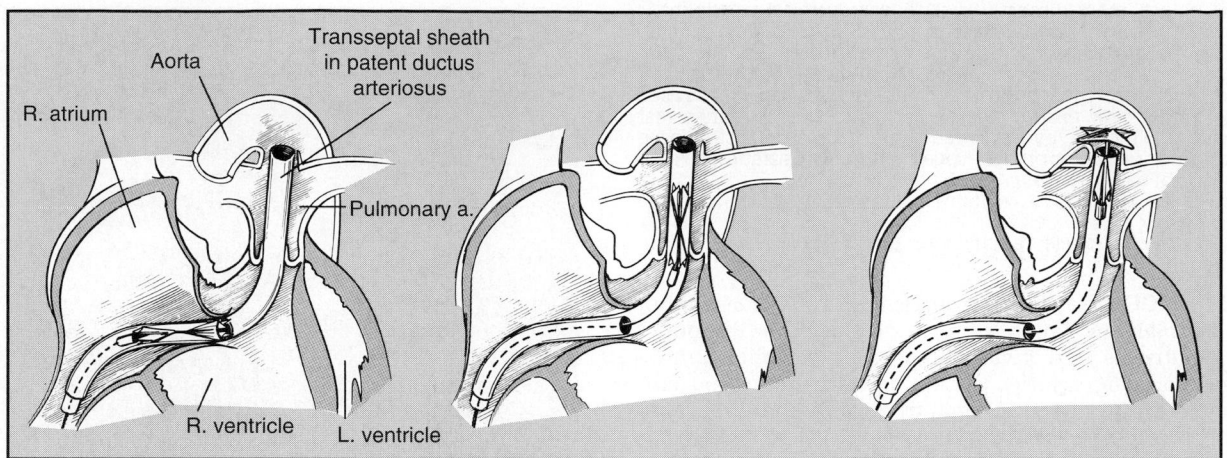

FIGURE 43-19. Transcatheter closure of a patient ductus arteriosus is illustrated using the Rashkind double-umbrella technique. The catheter approaches the ductus via a long sheath advanced from the femoral vein. The *right panel* shows expansion of the distal umbrella. (From Castañeda A, Jonas RA, Mayer JE Jr, et al: Cardiac Surgery of the Neonate and Infant. Philadelphia, WB Saunders, 1994, p 136.)

decade of life, severe pulmonary vascular obstruction has been known to cause aneurysmal dilatation, calcification, and rupture of the ductus.[188]

The patent ductus can be directly visualized by two-dimensional echocardiography (Fig. 43-18); range-gated pulsed Doppler echocardiography shows the characteristic flow abnormalities across the ductus, as well as a continuous flow disturbance in the pulmonary artery. Cardiac catheterization may be indicated when additional lesions or pulmonary vascular obstruction is suspected.

Management. In the absence of severe pulmonary vascular disease with predominant right-to-left shunting, the anatomical presence of a patent ductus usually is considered sufficient indication for closure. Ligation or division of the ductus carries a low risk, whether performed electively in an asymptomatic child or at any age if symptoms are present. The operative risk is reduced if heart failure can be compensated by medical measures before surgery. Operation should be deferred for several months in patients treated successfully for infective endarteritis because the ductus may remain somewhat edematous and friable. Rarely, when the infection does not subside with intensive antibiotic treatment, surgical ligation may be necessary to eradicate the infection.

Although strictly speaking still investigational, substantial experience exists with transcatheter closure of the patent ductus using various approaches, including coils, buttons, plugs, and umbrellas, with each occluder device introduced through a relatively large-diameter sheath from the femoral vein (Fig. 43-19)[189-195] (see Chap. 44). The approach is especially feasible in patients who weigh more than 10 kg and who have neither a long tubular ductus nor a ductus with a long, narrow aortic end. In experienced hands, initial occlusion is successful in 85 to 90 percent of patients; reocclusion adds 5 to 7 percent to the overall success rate. Potential complications in 5 to 10 percent of patients include embolization of the device, endocarditis, and hemolysis. Ductal closure by manually invasive surgery or thoracoscopy will undoubtedly undergo future evaluation.[196, 197]

Aorticopulmonary Septal Defect

Aorticopulmonary window or fenestration, partial truncus arteriosus, and aortic septal defect are other designations applied to this relatively uncommon anomaly. Septation of the aortopulmonary trunk occurs by fusion of the conotruncal ridges (see Fig. 43-2). The right and left sixth aortic arches, destined to become the pulmonary arteries, join the pulmonary artery to complete great artery develop-

ment (see Fig. 43-5). Congenital defects between the ascending aorta and the pulmonary artery result from faulty development of this area during embryonic life. The typical aortopulmonary septal defect results because of incomplete fusion of the distal aortopulmonary septum.[198] Malalignment of the conotruncal ridges results in unequal partitioning of the aortopulmonary trunk, which may result in partial or complete fusion of the right pulmonary artery to the aorta.

The usual defect consists of a communication between the aorta and pulmonary artery just above the semilunar valves. Persistent patency of the ductus arteriosus is an associated lesion in 10 to 15 percent of cases. Less common accompanying cardiovascular lesions include VSD, aortic origin of the right pulmonary artery, aortic arch interruption, coarctation of the aorta, and right aortic arch. Aorticopulmonary septal defects usually are large and are accompanied by severe pulmonary arterial hypertension and early-onset pulmonary vascular obstruction.

PHYSICAL EXAMINATION. The pulses typically are bounding, like those of a large patent ductus arteriosus. The murmur, however, seldom is continuous, and a basal systolic murmur is most common. Cardiomegaly is present, and pulmonary hypertension is reflected in a loud and palpable sound of pulmonary valve closure. Aorticopulmonary septal defect should be suspected whenever a large shunt into the pulmonary artery is demonstrated at catheterization. Diagnosis of the anomaly and its distinction from patent ductus and persistent truncus arteriosus usually can be done by two-dimensional echocardiography. Identification of the aortopulmonary window and associated malformations may also employ hemodynamic study and selective angiocardiography with the injection of contrast material into the left ventricle and/or the root of the aorta (Fig. 43-20). Although some patients may survive to adulthood with uncorrected aorticopulmon-

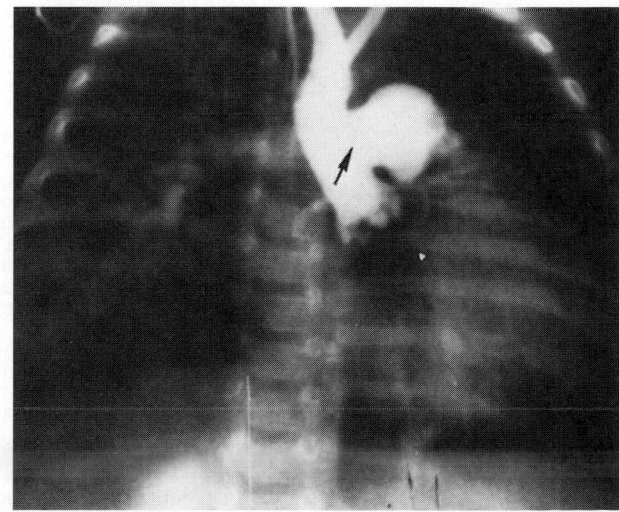

FIGURE 43-20. Aortic root injection of contrast material in the frontal view produces simultaneous opacification of the aorta and pulmonary artery through a large aorticopulmonary septal defect (arrow). (Courtesy of Dr. Robert White.)

ary septal defect, most die early in life unless surgical treatment is undertaken. Rarely, transcatheter closure by insertion of an occluding device may be feasible in infants with a small aortopulmonary window.[199] As a general rule, operative correction is indicated in all symptomatic infants when the diagnosis is made. Elective repair is advised at 3 to 6 months.[200, 201] Profound hypothermic total circulatory arrest or total cardiopulmonary bypass is required, and the defect is closed by way of a transaortic approach, usually with a prosthetic or xenograft pericardial patch.

Persistent Truncus Arteriosus

MORPHOLOGY. Persistent truncus arteriosus is a rare but serious anomaly in which a single vessel forms the outlet of both ventricles and gives rise to the systemic, pulmonary, and coronary arteries.[202] The defect results from failure of septation of the embryonic truncus by the infundibular truncal ridges (see Fig. 43–4, p. 1511). It is always accompanied by a VSD, frequently with a right-sided aortic arch. The VSD is due to the absence or underdevelopment of the distal portion of the pulmonary infundibulum. The truncal valve usually is tricuspid but is quadricuspid in about one-third of patients and rarely can be bicuspid. Truncal valve regurgitation and truncal valve stenosis are each seen in 10 to 15 percent of patients. There may be a single coronary artery, displacement of the coronary ostia (usually the left ostium posteriorly), or a single posterior descending coronary artery arising from the right coronary or, less often, from the left circumflex artery, especially in patients with a single coronary artery.[203]

Truncus malformations can be classified either anatomically according to the mode of origin of pulmonary vessels from the common trunk or from a functional point of view, based on the magnitude of blood flow to the lungs. In the common type (type I) of truncus arteriosus malformation, a partially separate pulmonary trunk of variable length exists because of the presence of an incompletely formed aorticopulmonary septum. The pulmonary trunk usually is very short and gives rise to left and right pulmonary arteries. When the aorticopulmonary septum is absent, there is no discrete main pulmonary artery component, and both pulmonary artery branches arise directly from the truncus.

In type II, each pulmonary artery arises separately but close to the other from the posterior aspect of the truncus (Fig. 43–21). In type III, each pulmonary artery arises from the lateral aspect of the truncus. Less commonly, one pulmonary artery branch may be absent, with collateral arteries supplying the lung that does not receive a pulmonary artery branch from the truncus. Truncus arteriosus malformation should not be confused with "pseudotruncus arteriosus," which is the severe form of tetralogy of Fallot with pulmonary atresia in which the single aorta arises from the heart accompanied by a remnant of atretic pulmonary artery.

HEMODYNAMICS. Pulmonary blood flow is governed by the size of the pulmonary arteries and the pulmonary vascular resistance. In infancy, pulmonary blood flow is usually excessive because pulmonary vascular resistance is not greatly increased. Thus, despite an obligatory admixture of systemic and pulmonary venous blood in the common trunk, only minimal cyanosis is present. Rarely, pulmonary blood flow is restricted by hypoplastic or stenotic pulmonary arteries arising from the truncus. Pulmonary vascular obstruction usually does not restrict pulmonary blood flow before 1 year of age.[204]

CLINICAL FEATURES. Infants with truncus arteriosus usually present with mild cyanosis coexisting with the cardiac findings of a large left-to-right shunt. Symptoms of heart failure and poor physical development usually appear in the first weeks or months of life. The most frequent physical findings include cardiomegaly, a systolic ejection sound accompanied by a thrill, a loud single second heart sound, a harsh systolic murmur, and a low-pitched mid-diastolic rumbling murmur and bounding pulses. Truncus arteriosus often is a measure of the *DiGeorge's syndrome* (see Table 43–2); thus, facial dysmorphism, a high incidence of extracardiac malformations (particularly of the limbs, kidneys, and intestines), atrophy or absence of the thymus gland, T-lymphocyte deficiency, and predilection to infection also may be features of clinical presentation.[205] Evidence suggests that genetically induced embryonic abnormalities in the cardiac neural crest play a major part in creation of the cardiovascular malformation as well as the other components of the syndrome[206] (see Chap. 56).

Truncal valve incompetence is suggested by the presence of a diastolic decrescendo murmur at the base of the heart. The physical findings are different if pulmonary blood flow is restricted by either high pulmonary vascular resistance or pulmonary arterial stenosis: Cyanosis is prominent, congestive failure is rare, and only a short systolic ejection may be audible, occasionally accompanied by continuous murmurs posteriorly of bronchial collateral flow.

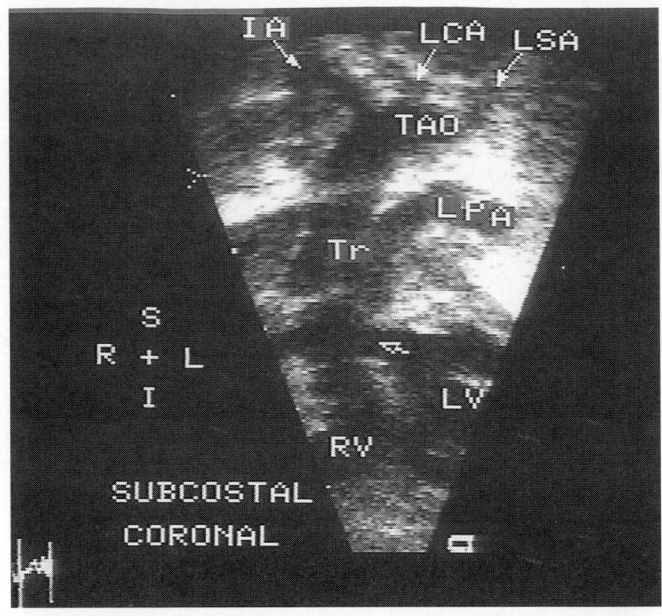

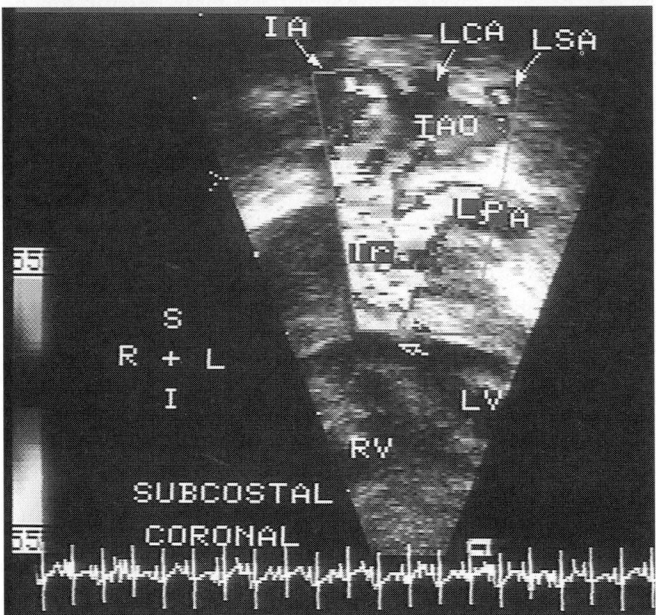

FIGURE 43–21. *Top,* Subcostal coronal view of truncus arteriosus (Tr). The truncal valve lies above the ventricular septal defect (open arrow), which appears above the left ventricle (LV) and right ventricle (RV). The Tr is seen dividing into the transverse aortic arch (TAO), which gives rise to the vessels supplying the head and neck: the innominate artery (IA), the left carotid artery (LCA), and the left subclavian artery (LSA). *Bottom,* Doppler color flow image showing the superimposition of color flow into the truncus arteriosus, left pulmonary artery, transverse aorta, and branches to the head and neck.

ELECTROCARDIOGRAPHY AND RADIOGRAPHY. Left ventricular hypertrophy alone or in combination with right ventricular hypertrophy is present electrocardiographically when a prominent left-to-right shunt exists; right ventricular hypertrophy is observed in patients with restricted pulmonary blood flow. The radiographic findings depend on the hemodynamic circumstances. Gross cardiomegaly with left or combined ventricular enlargement, left atrial enlargement, and a small or absent main pulmonary artery segment with pulmonary vascular engorgement are the usual radiographic features. A right aortic arch is common (25 to 30 percent of patients). When pulmonary blood flow is reduced, both heart size and pulmonary vascular markings are less prominent.

The *echocardiographic* features of truncus arteriosus (see Fig. 43–21) include a large truncal root overriding the ventricular septum and an outlet VSD. Additionally seen are truncal valve abnormalities with a variable number of cusps and leaflets, often thickened with rolled edges, an increase in the right ventricular dimension, and mitral valve–truncal root continuity. Differentiation between truncus arteriosus and tetralogy of Fallot by ultrasonography may be difficult unless either the separate origin of the pulmonary arteries or a single trunk from the ascending portion of a single arterial root can be identified. The origin of the pulmonary arteries is detected from various imaging planes, including high short-axis views, scanning superiorly from the truncal valve, or from a subcostal view (see Fig. 43–21). Diagnosis should be suspected at cardiac catheterization if the catheter fails to enter the central pulmonary arteries from the right ventricle. Selective angiocardiography and retrograde aortography are necessary to establish a precise diagnosis and to reveal the common trunk arising from the heart and the origin of the pulmonary arteries from the truncus.[207]

The early fatal course as well as early development of pulmonary vascular obstructive disease in patients surviving infancy is responsible for the poor prognosis associated with truncus arteriosus. In infants and young children with large left-to-right shunts, surgical banding of one or both pulmonary arteries to reduce pulmonary flow has been used with little success. Corrective operation is indicated before age 3 months to avoid the development of severe pulmonary vascular obstructive disease.[208]

SURGICAL TREATMENT. Operation consists of closure of the VSD, leaving the aorta arising from the left ventricle; the pulmonary arteries are excised from their truncus origin, and a valve-containing prosthetic conduit or aortic homograft valve conduit is used to establish continuity between the right ventricle and the pulmonary arteries (Fig. 43–22). Truncal valve insufficiency is a challenging problem and may require valve replacement or more moderate plastic repair to correct prolapse and improve central cusp coaptation. Important risk factors for perioperative death are severe truncal valve regurgitation, interrupted aortic arch, coronary artery anomalies, and age at operation greater than 100 days.[209, 210] Patients with only one pulmonary artery are especially prone to early development of severe pulmonary vascular disease but otherwise are not at increased risk from surgery.

With truncus arteriosus defects, the possible inequalities of pressure and flow between the two pulmonary arteries often make precise calculation of pulmonary resistance difficult. Corrective operation may be performed in patients with at least one adequate pulmonary artery having low distal pressure or arteriolar resistance. Conversely, significant systemic arterial desaturation in a patient with two pulmonary arteries and with neither pulmonary artery stenosis nor a previous pulmonary artery band signifies that high pulmonary vascular resistance exists and that the condition is probably inoperable. It is not yet clear how often and at what age the conduit between the right ventricle and pulmonary artery must be replaced with a larger prosthesis because of either growth of the patient, in whom a small conduit causes eventual obstruction, heterograft valve degeneration, or obstruction created by neointimal proliferation within a prosthetic conduit.[211] When operation is carried out within a conduit in the first year of life, conduit replacement often is required within 3 to 5 years.

Coronary Arteriovenous Fistula

Coronary arteriovenous fistula (see also Chap. 44) is an unusual anomaly that consists of a communication between one of the coronary arteries and a cardiac chamber or vein. The right coronary artery, or its branches, is the site of the fistula in about 55 percent of cases; the left coronary artery is involved in about 35 percent, and both coronary arteries in 5 percent. Connections between the coronary system and a cardiac chamber appear to represent persistence of embryonic intertrabecular spaces and sinusoids. Most of these fistulas drain into the right ventricle, right atrium, or coronary sinus; fistulous communication to the pulmonary artery, left atrium, or left ventricle is much less frequent. The shunt through the fistula most often is of small magnitude, and myocardial blood flow is not compromised.[212] Rarely, spontaneous closure may occur. Potential complications include pulmonary hypertension and congestive heart failure if a large left-to-right shunt exists, bacterial endocarditis, rupture or thrombosis of the fistula or an associated arterial aneurysm, and myocardial ischemia distal to the fistula due to decreased coronary blood flow.

Most pediatric patients are asymptomatic and are referred because of a cardiac murmur that is loud, superficial, and continuous at the lower or midsternal border. The site of maximal intensity of the murmur is related to the site of drainage and usually is different from the second left intercostal space—the classic site of the continuous murmur of

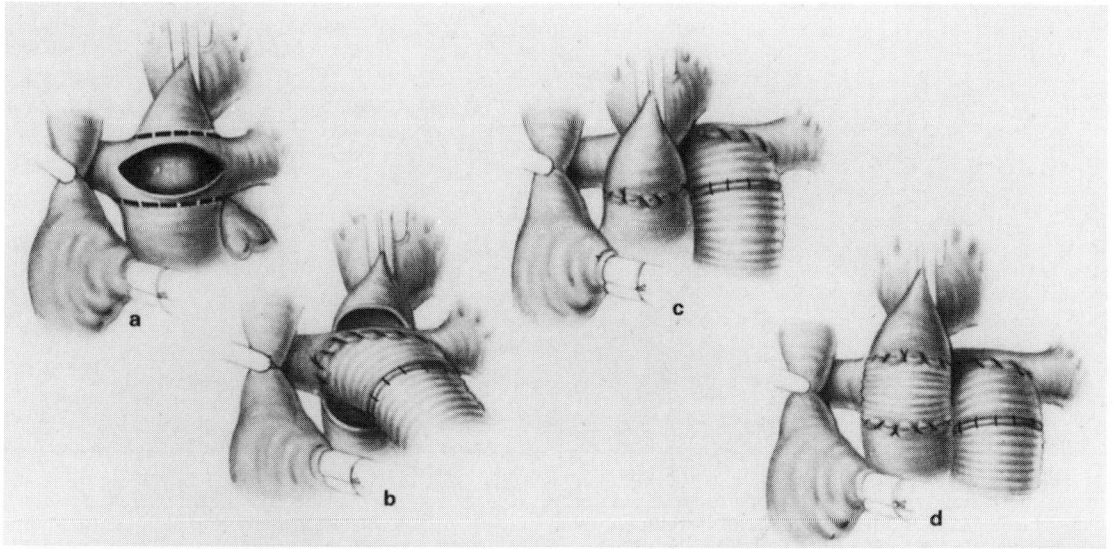

FIGURE 43–22. Operative correction of truncus arteriosus, type III. The pulmonary arteries arise separately from the truncus. An anterior incision is made, and a segment of aorta containing the orifices of both pulmonary arteries is excised from the truncus (a). The cuff of tissue containing the two pulmonary arteries is anastomosed to an extracardiac valved conduit (b). Aortic continuity is restored by direct suture (c) or by interposing a preclotted graft (d). The diagram does not show closure of the ventricular septal defect. (From Stark J, deLaval M: Surgery for Congenital Heart Defects. New York, Grune & Stratton, 1983, p 420.)

persistent ductus arteriosus—except when the fistula drains into the pulmonary artery or right ventricle. In the latter situation, the murmur is louder in diastole than in systole because of compression of the fistula by contracting myocardium. The ECG and chest roentgenogram findings often are normal and seldom show selective chamber enlargement or myocardial ischemia. A significantly enlarged feeding coronary artery can usually be detected by two-dimensional echocardiography. The entire course and site of entry of the AV fistula can be traced by combining two-dimensional echocardiography and Doppler color flow mapping and imaging techniques. The shunt entry site is characterized by a continuous turbulent systolic and diastolic flow pattern (see Chaps. 7 and 44).[212, 213] Multiplane transesophageal echocardiography also accurately defines the origin, course, and drainage site of the fistula.

Standard retrograde thoracic aortography, balloon occlusion angiography of the aortic root with a 45-degree caudal tilt of the frontal camera ("laid-back" aortogram),[214] or coronary arteriography can be used reliably to identify the size and anatomical features of the fistulous tract, which can be closed preferably by transcatheter coil embolization or suture obliteration in most cases.[215, 216] In the presence of a large left-to-right shunt and symptoms of heart failure, the decision to operate is clearly justified. The fistula most often is closed in asymptomatic patients to prevent future symptoms or complications, such as infective endocarditis. The prognosis after successful closure of a coronary artery–cardiac chamber fistula is excellent.

Anomalous Pulmonary Origin of the Coronary Artery

This rare malformation occurs in about 0.4 percent of patients with congenital cardiac anomalies. In almost all patients, the left coronary artery originates from the posterior sinus of the pulmonary artery.[217]

In unusual cases that have been reported, the right coronary artery, or the entire coronary artery system, originates from the main pulmonary trunk. Embryologically, the distal coronary artery system is formed by 9 weeks from solid angioblastic buds that extend through-

out the epicardium to form the major coronary artery branches. Proximally, the coronary network forms a ring around the truncus arteriosus, joining with coronary buds from the primitive aortic sinuses as the truncus partitions to form the great arteries. The varieties of anomalous pulmonary origin of the coronary artery are the result of displacement in this proximal process.

PATHOPHYSIOLOGY. During fetal life, pulmonary artery pressure is slightly greater than aortic pressure, and perfusion of the left coronary artery is antegrade (Fig. 43-23A). After birth, when pulmonary artery pressure falls below aortic pressure, perfusion of the left coronary artery from the pulmonary artery ceases, and the direction of flow in the anomalous vessel reverses. Blood flows from the aorta to the right coronary artery, then through collateral channels to the left coronary artery, and finally to the pulmonary artery (Fig. 43-23B). In effect, the left coronary artery behaves as a fistulous communication between the aorta and pulmonary artery. If adequate collateral channels exist or develop between the two coronary artery circulations, total myocardial perfusion through the right coronary artery increases (Fig. 43-23C). In 10 to 15 percent of patients, myocardial ischemia never develops because extensive intercoronary collaterals allow survival to adolescence or adulthood. In fact, if collateral blood flow is considerable, patients may develop the clinical manifestations of a large arteriovenous shunt and a continuous or diastolic murmur.

By far the most common clinical presentation is that of an infant who suffers a myocardial infarction and develops congestive heart failure.[218] The infant syndrome usually becomes manifested at age 2 to 4 months with angina-like symptoms that may be misinterpreted as colic. Feeding and defecation often are accompanied by dyspnea, irritability and crying, pallor, diaphoresis, and occasional loss of consciousness. Older children or adults usually present with a continuous murmur or with mitral regurgitation resulting from dysfunction of ischemic or infarcted papillary muscles. In some instances, the coronary anomaly is unsuspected until a previously well adolescent or adult experiences angina, heart failure, or sudden death.

DIAGNOSIS. The diagnosis of anomalous origin of the coronary artery is supported by ECG demonstration of deep Q waves in association with ST segment alterations and T wave inversions in leads I, aV_L, V_5, and V_6 (Fig. 43-24). These findings greatly assist the differentiation of this anomaly from myocarditis and dilated cardiomyopathy.[219] Chest roentgenograms show moderate to severe enlargement of the left atrium and ventricle. Echocardiography with Doppler color flow mapping has replaced cardiac catheterization as the standard method of diagnosis. The pulmonary

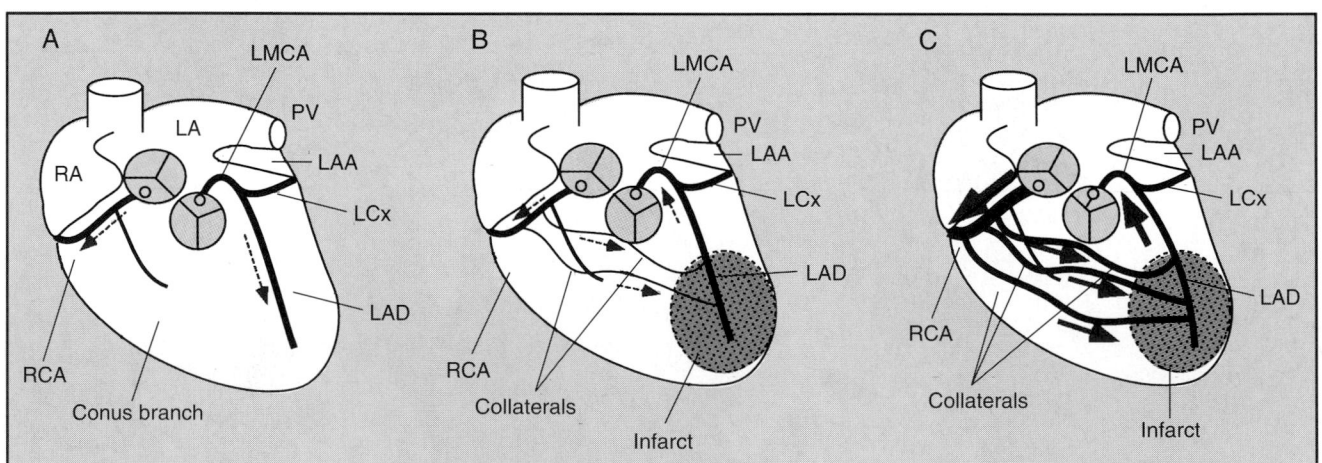

FIGURE 43–23. Anomalous origin of the left main coronary artery from the pulmonary artery. *A,* In a fetus, both right and left coronary arteries receive forward flow from their respective great arteries. *B,* Soon after birth, before collaterals are well developed, there may be an anterolateral infarct and slight retrograde flow from the left coronary artery to the pulmonary artery. *C,* After collaterals have enlarged, there is high flow in the enlarged right coronary artery and the collaterals and significant retrograde flow into the pulmonary artery. Dotted arrows indicate direction and approximate magnitude of flow in the right and left coronary arteries and the collaterals between them. PV = pulmonary vein; LA = left atrium; LAA = left atrial appendage; RA = right atrium; LMCA = left main coronary artery; LCx = left circumflex coronary artery; LAD = left anterior descending coronary artery; RCA = right coronary artery. (From Hoffman JIE: *In* Emmanouilides GC, Riemenschneider TA, Allen HD, et al [eds]: Moss and Adams' Heart Disease in Infants, Children, and Adolescents. 5th ed. Baltimore, © Williams & Wilkins, 1994, p 776.)

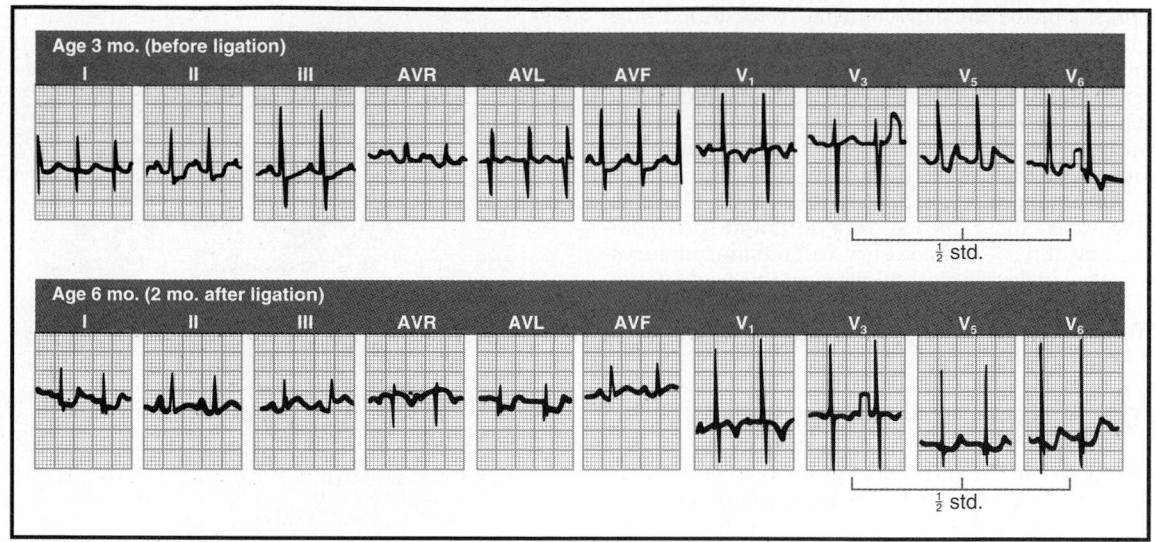

FIGURE 43-24. Typical electrocardiogram of an infant with anomalous left coronary artery before *(above)* and after *(below)* ligation of the anomalous left coronary artery. Note the abnormal Q waves in I, AVL, and V$_6$. (Courtesy of Dr. Delores A. Danilowicz.)

origin of the anomalous left coronary artery is visualized from long- or short-axis views. Color flow mapping demonstrates retrograde flow in the left coronary system and an abnormal flow jet from the left coronary artery into the pulmonary trunk. Moreover, detection of anterograde flow in the left coronary system helps to preclude the diagnosis.[221] Color flow mapping of the jet from the origin of the left coronary artery as it enters the pulmonary artery is diagnostic. Detection of anterograde diastolic flow in the left coronary system virtually precludes this diagnosis.[220] If the echocardiographic diagnosis is unequivocal, coronary arteriography or aortography is not required to make the diagnosis. The origin of the anomalous left coronary artery occasionally may be visualized echocardiographically from long- or short-axis views of the pulmonary artery.[221] Absence of the left coronary artery from its usual origin in the left sinus of Valsalva does not distinguish this lesion from single coronary artery. Color flow Doppler examination may also reveal associated mitral regurgitation. Ischemia or infarction is suggested by the echocardiographic findings of segmental wall motion abnormalities, particularly involving the anterolateral free wall of the left ventricle. Electron beam CT after intravenous contrast infection may accurately define the malformation (see Chap. 10). Stress thallium scintigraphy shows a characteristic defect of the anterolateral wall of the left ventricle. Positron emission

tomography reveals both the perfusion defect and its metabolic consequences (Fig. 43–25).

Aortography or coronary angiography demonstrates the retrograde drainage of the coronary vessel into the pulmonary artery. It should be recognized that ventricular arrhythmias may complicate the course of hemodynamic study. The magnitude of shunting into the pulmonary artery may be determined by oximetry, indicator-dilution curves, or angiography.

MANAGEMENT. *Medical treatment* is indicated in infants with myocardial infarction for congestive heart failure, arrhythmias, and cardiogenic shock. In patients with a small left-to-right shunt or no shunt at all, the prognosis is exceedingly poor with conservative management, justifying an attempt to reestablish a two–coronary artery system. The *operations* that have been used include reimplanting the left coronary artery into the aortic root, surgically creating an aortopulmonary window and a tunnel to convey blood from the window across the back of the pulmonary trunk to the origin of the anomalous left coronary artery, with reconstruction of the anterior wall of the pulmonary trunk, and anastomosis of the left coronary artery with the subclavian artery or with the aorta by means of a graft.[222, 223] If clinical deterioration occurs in infants with a sizable left-to-right shunt into the pulmonary artery, simple ligation of the left coronary artery at its origin prevents retrograde flow

FIGURE 43-25. Positron emission tomography (PET) transaxial images depict myocardial perfusion and glucose metabolism in a 7-month-old infant with anomalous origin of the left coronary artery (LCA) from the pulmonary artery. The ammonia (NH$_3$) scan demonstrates hypoperfusion *(left panel)*, whereas the fluorodeoxyglucose scan shows increased glucose metabolism *(right panel)* in the anterior lateral left ventricular wall (arrows) in the region perfused by the LCA. Under fasting conditions, normal myocardium has minimal glucose (FDG) uptake, whereas in this figure, hypoperfused myocardium preferentially metabolizes glucose. The "mismatch" pattern in this figure indicates ischemic but viable myocardium. This patient underwent reimplantation of the LCA with subsequent complete recovery of cardiac function and normalization of PET perfusion and metabolism. RV = right ventricle; LV = left ventricle; IVS = interventricular septum.

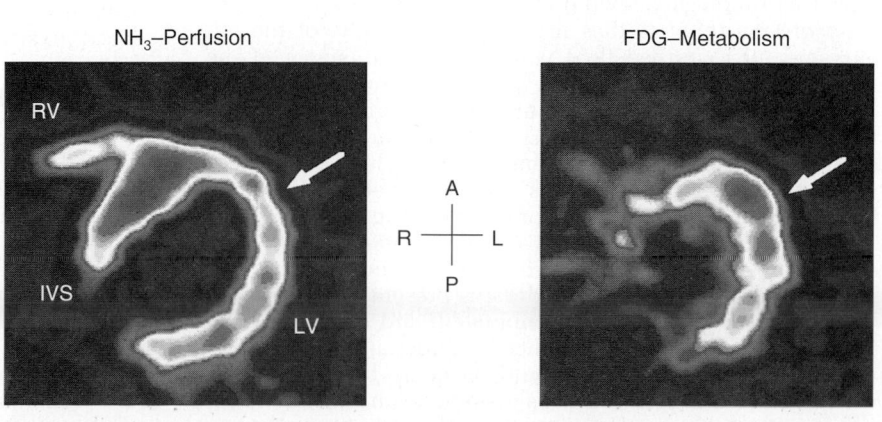

and allows perfusion of the left ventricle with blood supplied through anastomoses with the right coronary artery. If medical management stabilizes the infant with significant intercoronary collaterals, operation may be postponed to allow the patient to grow, because increased size of the vessels enhances the likelihood of successful reimplantation or coronary arterial bypass surgery. The outcome of surgery and ultimate prognosis are significantly influenced by the degree of myocardial damage suffered preoperatively.[224] Uncommonly, it is necessary to consider aneurysmectomy or mitral valve replacement. Cardiac transplantation has been suggested as an option only if recovery of myocardial function is poor.

Aortic Sinus Aneurysm and Fistula

Congenital aneurysm of an aortic sinus of Valsalva, particularly the right coronary sinus, is an uncommon anomaly that occurs three times more often in males than in females. The malformation consists of a separation, or lack of fusion, between the media of the aorta and the annulus fibrosis of the aortic valve.[225] The receiving chamber of the aorticocardiac fistula usually is the right ventricle, but occasionally, when the noncoronary cusp is involved, the fistula drains into the right atrium.

Five to 15 percent of aneurysms originate in the posterior or noncoronary sinus; seldom is the left aortic sinus involved. Associated anomalies are common and include bicuspid aortic valve, VSD, and coarctation of the aorta.

The deficiency in the aortic media appears to be congenital. Reports in infants are exceedingly rare[226] and are infrequent in children, because progressive aneurysmal dilatation of the weakened area develops but may not be recognized until the third or fourth decade of life, when rupture into a cardiac chamber occurs.

An *unruptured aneurysm* usually does not produce a hemodynamic abnormality, although pressure on the intracardiac conduction system by an unruptured aneurysm may be a rare cause of complete AV block; rarely, myocardial ischemia may be caused by coronary arterial compression. Rupture is often of abrupt onset, causes chest pain, and creates continuous arteriovenous shunting and volume loading of both right and left heart chambers, which results in heart failure. An additional complication is infective endocarditis, which may originate either on the edges of the aneurysm or on those areas in the right side of the heart that are traumatized by the jetlike stream of blood flowing through the fistula.

DIAGNOSIS. The presence of this anomaly should be suspected in a patient with a history of chest pain of recent onset, symptoms of diminished cardiac reserve, bounding pulses, and a loud superficial continuous murmur accentuated in diastole when the fistula opens into the right ventricle, as well as a thrill along the right or left lower parasternal border. The *physical findings* can be difficult to distinguish from those produced by a coronary arteriovenous fistula. *Electrocardiography* shows biventricular hypertrophy, and chest roentgenography demonstrates generalized cardiomegaly. Two-dimensional and pulsed Doppler *echocardiographic* studies may detect the walls of the aneurysm and disturbed flow within the aneurysm or at the site of perforation, respectively.[227] *Transesophageal echocardiography* may provide more precise information than the transthoracic approach. *Cardiac catheterization* reveals a left-to-right shunt at the ventricular or, less commonly, the atrial level; the diagnosis may be established definitively by retrograde thoracic aortography (Fig. 43–26).

MANAGEMENT. Preoperative medical management consists of measures to relieve cardiac failure and to treat coexistent arrhythmias or endocarditis, if present. At operation, the aneurysm is closed and amputated, and the aortic wall is reunited with the heart, either by direct suture or with a prosthesis.[228] Every effort should be made to preserve the aortic valve in children because patch closure of the defect combined with prosthetic valve replacement greatly enhances the risk of operation in small patients.

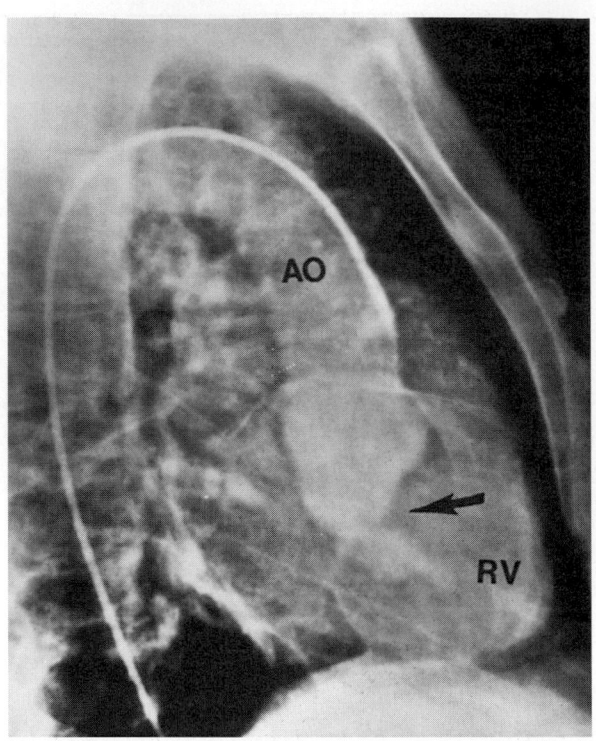

FIGURE 43–26. A retrograde aortogram shows the fistulous connection between the noncoronary sinus of Valsalva and the right ventricle (RV) (arrow). AO = aorta. (Courtesy of Dr. Robert White.)

VALVULAR AND VASCULAR LESIONS WITH OR WITHOUT RIGHT-TO-LEFT SHUNT

Aortic Arch Obstruction

The conventional anatomical and clinical divisions into preductal and postductal coarctation or infantile and adult types, respectively, are misleading because the anatomical localization is inaccurate and the age dependence of the clinical presentation does not hold true (i.e., the adult type often is seen in the first weeks of life). A spectrum of anatomical lesions exists, causing obstruction of the aortic arch or proximal portion of the descending aorta. These range from a localized coarctation or constriction of the lumen, most commonly located just distal to the origin of the left subclavian artery and closely related to the attachment of the ductus arteriosus with the aorta, to diffuse narrowing or interruption of a portion of the aortic arch. In this chapter, aortic arch obstruction is divided into three types: (1) localized juxtaductal coarctation, (2) hypoplasia of the aortic isthmus, and (3) aortic arch interruption. *Pseudocoarctation* is used synonymously with "kinking" or "buckling" of the aorta, which is a subclinical form of localized juxtaductal coarctation of the aorta.

Localized Juxtaductal Coarctation
(See also p. 1600)

MORPHOLOGY. This lesion consists of a localized shelf-like thickening and infolding of the media of the posterolateral aortic wall opposite the ductus arteriosus; the wall of the aorta into which the ductus or ligamentum arteriosum inserts is not involved.[229] Juxtaductal coarctation occurs two to five times more commonly in males than in females, and there is a high degree of association with gonadal dysgenesis (Turner's syndrome) and bicuspid aortic valve.[230] Other common associated anomalies include VSD and mitral stenosis or regurgitation. The most important extracardiac anomaly is aneurysm of the circle of Willis.

PATHOGENESIS. Juxtaductal coarctation is probably related to an abnormality in the pattern of ductus arteriosus blood flow in utero, which in turn may be the result of associated intracardiac anomalies.[230, 231] Thus, in fetal life, blood flow through the aortic isthmus constitutes only 12 to 17 percent of the total cardiac output, whereas blood flow through the ductus arteriosus exceeds that across the aortic valve. The dorsal aortic wall directly opposite the ductus arteriosus resembles morphologically the apex of a normal branch point of the aorta if ductal flow pathways in utero diverge, with some flow directed cephalad into the aortic isthmus and the remainder proceeding into the descending aorta. The aortic branch point is identical histologically to the posterior shelf of juxtaductal aortic coarctation. A divergence of ductal flow is fostered by the presence of lesions in the fetus that create an imbalance between left and right ventricular outputs, with right-sided flow predominating (e.g., bicuspid aortic valve, mitral valve anomaly). In the absence of an anomaly fostering augmented ductal flow, a branch point may be created by an alteration in the angle at which the ductus arteriosus meets the aorta, pointing the ductal stream directly against the posterior aortic wall rather than obliquely down into the descending aorta. Cardiac anomalies that cause augmented ascending aortic blood flow (e.g., pulmonic atresia or stenosis, tetralogy of Fallot) prevent development of a branch point and indeed are almost never seen in association with juxtaductal coarctation of the aorta.

During fetal life, the posterior aortic shelf is not obstructive because blood may pass readily from the ascending aorta to the descending aorta by traversing the anterior aortic segment and the aortic end of the ductus arteriosus. Postnatally, however, when the ductus undergoes obliteration at its aortic end, the shelflike projection of the posterior aortic wall unmasks the obstruction to aortic flow (Fig. 43–27). After pharmacological interventions that dilate the ductus arteriosus (prostaglandin E_1 infusion), the pressure difference may be obliterated across the site of coarctation because the fetal flow pattern is reestablished.[178, 232]

The pathogenesis of juxtaductal coarctation already described explains the prevalence of associated intracardiac anomalies that foster reduced ascending aortic flow and augmented ductus arteriosus flow in utero, as well as the absence of associated intracardiac anomalies in which the converse flow conditions exist in utero. The dependence of aortic obstruction on constriction of the ductus arteriosus postnatally explains the variable onset after birth of the clinical manifestations of coarctation, as well as the dramatic alleviation of the obstruction produced pharmacologically by dilatation of the ductus arteriosus.

CLINICAL FINDINGS. The manifestations of juxtaductal coarctation of the aorta depend on the prominence of the posterolateral aortic shelf, which determines the intensity of obstruction, and on the rapidity with which obstruction develops.

NEONATES AND INFANTS. Rapid, severe obstruction in infancy is a prominent cause of left ventricular failure and systemic hypoperfusion. Substantial left-to-right shunting across a patent foramen ovale and pulmonary venous hypertension secondary to heart failure cause pulmonary arterial hypertension. Because little or no aortic obstruction existed during fetal life, the collateral circulation in the newborn period is often poorly developed. In these infants, peripheral pulses characteristically are weak throughout the body until left ventricular function is improved with medical management; a significant pressure difference then develops between the arms and the legs, allowing detection of a pulse discrepancy. Cardiac murmurs are nonspecific in infancy and commonly are derived from associated lesions.

The *ECG* shows the right-axis deviation and right ventricular hypertrophy; the *chest radiograph* shows generalized cardiomegaly and pulmonary arterial and venous engorgement. Two-dimensional and Doppler echocardiography provide an accurate noninvasive assessment of the anatomy and physiology in most patients. Hemodynamic study also allows delineation of the site and extent of aortic obstruction and detection of associated cardiac malformations. Most infants with early-onset severe heart failure respond poorly to medical management, and balloon angioplasty, surgical excision of the coarctation, or a subclavian flap angioplasty often is required. We prefer an operation consisting of excision of the area of coarctation and extended end-to-end repair or end-to-side anastomosis with absorbable sutures to allow remodeling of the aorta with time.[233]

Aortic obstruction may develop slowly in infants in whom the posterolateral aortic shelf is not prominent at birth and in whom ductus arteriosus constriction is gradual. In these babies, compensatory myocardial hypertrophy and an extensive collateral circulation have time to develop. If the obstruction does not intensify and cardiac failure does not occur by age 6 or 9 months, circulatory compensation is likely until adult life.

CHILDREN. Most children with isolated juxtaductal coarctation are asymptomatic. Complaints of headache, cold extremities, and claudication with exercise may be noted, although attention usually is directed to the cardiovascular system by detection of a heart murmur of upper extremity hypertension on routine physical examination. Mechanical factors rather than those of renal origin play the primary role in the production of hypertension. Absent, markedly diminished, or delayed pulsations in the femoral arteries and a low or unobtainable arterial pressure in the lower extremities with hypertension in the arms are the basic clues to the diagnosis. A midsystolic murmur over the anterior chest, back, and spinous processes is most frequent, becoming continuous if the lumen is sufficiently narrowed to result in a high-velocity jet across the lesion throughout the cardiac cycle. Additional systolic and continuous murmurs over the lateral thoracic wall may reflect increased flow through dilated and tortuous collateral vessels.

ECG reveals left ventricular hypertrophy of various degrees, depending on the height of arterial pressure above the obstruction and the patient's age. Combined with right ventricular hypertrophy, this usually implies a complicated lesion. *Chest roentgenograms* (see Chaps. 8 and 44) can show a dilated left subclavian artery high on the left mediastinal border and a dilated ascending aorta. Indentation of the aorta at the site of coarctation and prestenotic and poststenotic dilatation (the "3" sign) along the left premediastinal shadow is almost pathognomonic. Poststenotic dilation also may be detected by indentation of the barium-filled esophagus. Notching of the ribs, an important radiographic sign, is due to erosion by dilated collateral vessels, increases with age, and usually becomes apparent between the 4th and 12th years of life. The aortic coarctation may be visualized directly by two-dimensional echocardiography from high parasternal or suprasternal notch views with short focused transducers and from the subxiphoid window with extended focal range transducers (Fig. 43–28). Doppler examination reveals a flow disturbance and high-velocity jet at the site of obstruction and provides a reasonable estimate of the transcoarctation pressure gradient.[234, 235] CT, magnetic resonance imaging[235, 236] (Fig. 43–29 and Chap. 10), or cardiac catheterization and aortography (see Fig. 44–7, p. 1601) also accurately localizes the site of

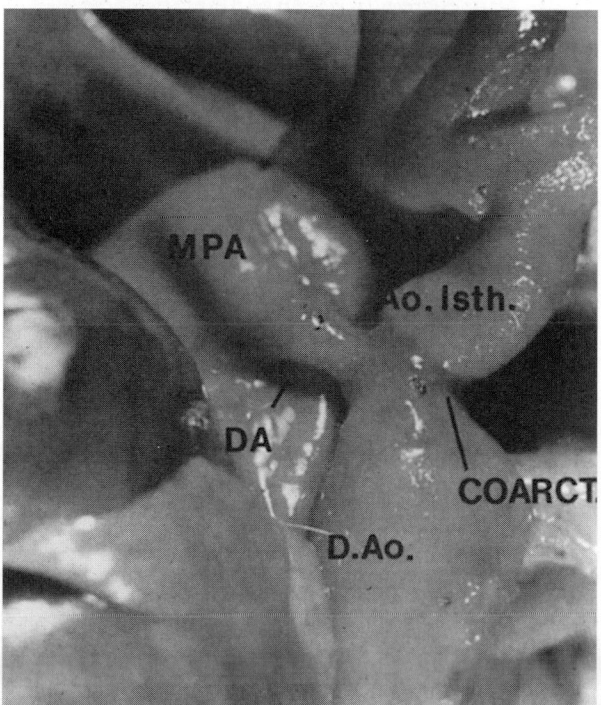

FIGURE 43–27. Juxtaductal coarctation (COARCT) unmasked by constriction of the ductus arteriosus (DA). MPA = main pulmonary artery; D.Ao. = descending aorta; Ao.Isth. = aortic isthmus. (Courtesy of Dr. Norman Talner.)

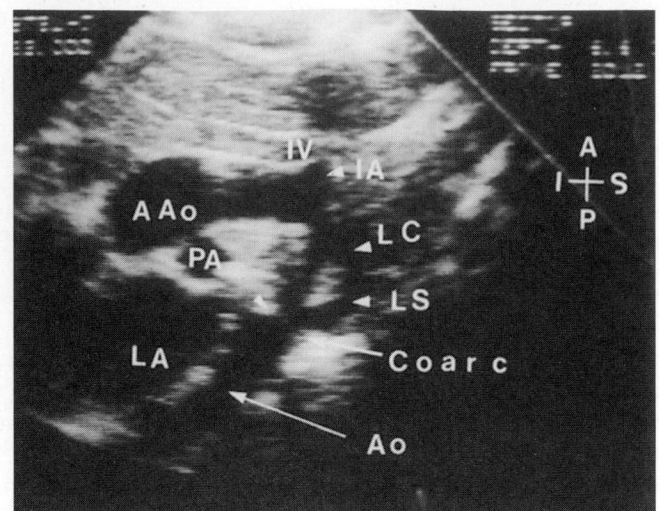

FIGURE 43–28. Aortic coarctation (Coarc) is visualized from the suprasternal notch. The aorta (Ao) can be traced from the ascending aorta (AAo). The aortic arch is somewhat narrowed, and the relationship of the left subclavian artery (LS) to the coarctation is identified clearly. LA = left atrium; PA = pulmonary artery; IA = innominate artery; LC = left carotid artery.

obstruction, determines the length of coarctation, and, particularly, identifies associated malformations. Preoperative catheterization is avoided for selected patients with typical clinical and two-dimensional and Doppler echocardiographic findings.[237] Intravascular ultrasonography provides interesting morphological images suitable especially for comparison with postoperative status.[238]

MANAGEMENT. Controversy exists about the role of balloon angioplasty (see Chap. 38), with or without balloon-expandable stents, in the treatment of native coarctation, especially in neonates.[239–241a] There is concern about residual pressure gradients, aneurysm formation, aortic dissection and rupture, and femoral arterial complications, especially late after angioplasty. It is clear that angioplasty can effectively reduce obstruction in many patients, albeit with an unpredictable late outcome.

An extended end-to-end anastomosis with resection of the aortic isthmus and ductal tissue yields a low mortality and a low rate of recoarctation. It is now the procedure of

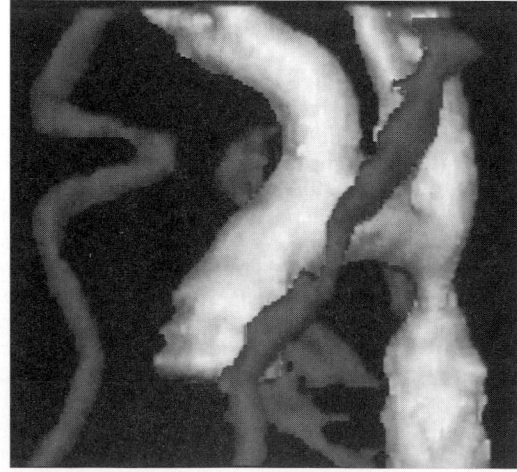

FIGURE 43–29. Three-dimensional computer reconstruction of magnetic resonance images in a child with discrete coarctation and numerous large collateral vessels, displayed in a lateral projection. Dilated brachiocephalic and internal mammary arteries are evident. (Courtesy of Dr. W. James Parks, The Children's Heart Center, Emory University, Atlanta, GA.)

choice at many centers.[242] Subclavian flap aortoplasty, particularly in neonates and infants, or surgical resection and end-to-end anastomosis of uncomplicated juxtaductal coarctation of the aorta can be accomplished with excellent results in most patients[243]; some surgeons prefer an onlay patch across the site of obstruction. In children who are asymptomatic, it is preferable to delay surgery until age 4 to 6 years, at which time coarctation seldom recurs. Paradoxical hypertension of short duration often is noted in the immediate postoperative period, a phenomenon much less common after balloon angioplasty.[244–247] A resetting of carotid baroreceptors and increased catecholamine secretion appears to be responsible for the initial phase of postoperative systemic hypertension, with a later, second phase of prolonged elevation of systolic and particularly diastolic blood pressure related to activation of the renin-angiotensin system. A necrotizing panarteritis of the small vessels of the gastrointestinal tract of uncertain cause occasionally complicates the course of recovery.

The risk of recurrent narrowing after repair of coarctation in infancy is 5 to 10 percent. Such narrowing is best detected by magnetic resonance imaging or Doppler ultrasonography.[235] This problem is treated most effectively by transcutaneous balloon angioplasty,[248, 248a, 249] which may be expected to markedly reduce but not entirely abolish the pressure differences across the site of recoarctation.

In those patients who survive the first 2 years of life, complications of juxtaductal coarctation are uncommon before the second or third decade. The chief hazards to patients with coarctation result from severe hypertension and include the development of cerebral aneurysms and hemorrhage, hypertensive encephalopathy, rupture of the aorta, left ventricular failure, and infective endocarditis. Systemic hypertension in the absence of residual coarctation has been observed in resting or exercise-stressed patients postoperatively and appears to be related to the duration of preoperative hypertension.[250] Lifelong observation is desirable because of the late onset of hypertension in some postoperative patients.[251]

Hypoplasia of the Aortic Arch

MORPHOLOGY. The aortic isthmus, the portion of the aorta between the left subclavian artery and the ductus arteriosus, normally is narrowed in the fetus and newborn. The lumen of the aortic isthmus is about two-thirds that of the ascending and descending portions of the aorta until age 6 to 9 months, when the physiological narrowing disappears.[252] Pathological tubular hypoplasia of the aortic arch usually is noted in the aortic isthmus and often is referred to as preductal or infantile coarctation of the aorta.[253] Associated major cardiac malformations occur in virtually all such infants and include large VSD, AV septal defect, transposition of the great arteries, the Taussig-Bing type of anomaly, and double-outlet right ventricle. The VSD most often is subpulmonary, lying within the substance of the infundibular septum. Thus, muscle persists between the aortic and pulmonary valve leaflets, and when it is displaced leftward, it produces subaortic stenosis. Persistent patency of the ductus arteriosus commonly coexists, and right-to-left flow across the ductus arteriosus usually provides filling of the descending aorta. The adequacy of blood flow to the lower body depends on the degree of aortic hypoplasia, the caliber of the ductus arteriosus, and the relationship between pulmonary and systemic vascular resistance. Substantial right-to-left shunting through a wide-open ductus arteriosus minimizes the arterial blood pressure difference between the upper and lower body.

CLINICAL FINDINGS. Differential cyanosis of the toes and feet with normal color of the fingers and hands may be difficult to discern because intracardiac left-to-right shunting and pulmonary edema attenuate the differences in oxygen saturation in the ascending and descending aorta. Clinical deterioration is associated with ductal constriction or a decline in pulmonary vascular resistance. Moreover, the clinical presentation often is dictated by the hemodynamic effects of complex associated intracardiac malformations. Infants most often present with findings of a large left-to-right intracardiac shunt, pulmonary hypertension, and marked cardiac decompensation. Although tubular hypoplasia is detectable by two-dimensional echocardiography, cardiac catheterization may be required to evaluate the full extent of intracardiac and extracardiac lesions. Surgical repair of aortic

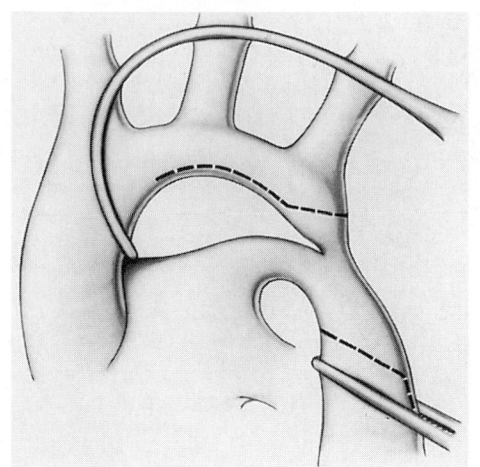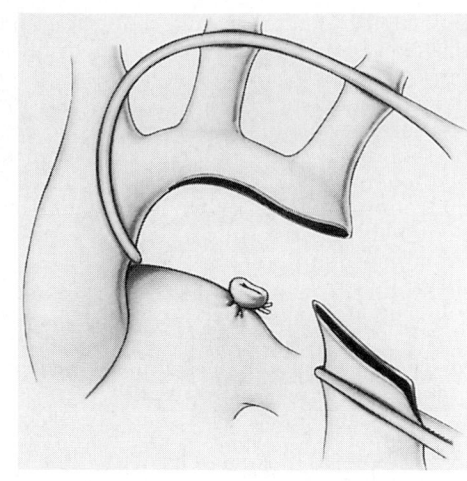

FIGURE 43–30. An extended repair of aortic coarctation is used in the presence of a hypoplastic aortic arch. The broken lines in the *left panel* delineate resection sites of the coarcted segment. In the *right panel*, the ductus arteriosus has been ligated and the incisions are extended to the undersurface of the aortic arch and onto the distal aorta. When the suture line is completed, the reconstruction of the arch is generally excellent. (From Stark J, deLaval M: Surgery for Congenital Heart Defects. 2nd ed. Philadelphia, WB Saunders, 1994, p 292.)

arch hypoplasia usually must be accompanied by operative palliation or correction of associated intracardiac lesions. An extended end-to-end anastomosis (Fig. 43–30), classic or reversed subclavian flap angioplasty, patch aortography, and bypass grafting are among the operative approaches to correct long segment narrowing.[247] Recoarctation is common and often necessitates transcatheter balloon aortoplasty and/or a second operation later in life to relieve anastomotic stenosis.[247, 248]

AORTIC ARCH INTERRUPTION

Aortic arch interruption is a rare and usually lethal anomaly; unless treated surgically, almost all infants die within the first month of life.[254] Interruptions distal to the left subclavian artery (type A) occur with almost equal frequency to interruptions distal to the left common carotid artery (type B); interruptions distal to the innominate artery (type C) are extremely uncommon. The right subclavian artery often is of variable origin, frequently arising from the descending aortic segment distal to the interruption. The clinical presentation resembles that in tubular hypoplasia or severe juxtaductal coarctation of the aorta with a patent ductus arteriosus.

Virtually all patients have associated intracardiac anomalies. A patent ductus arteriosus almost always connects the main pulmonary artery with the descending aorta. With rare exceptions, patients with interrupted aortic arch have either a VSD (80 to 90 percent of cases) or an aorticopulmonary window (10 to 20 percent). Because the ductus arteriosus provides lower body blood flow, its spontaneous constriction results in profound clinical deterioration. The latter may be temporarily ameliorated by prostaglandin E$_1$ infusion. The VSD most often is subpulmonic, lying within the substance of the infundibular septum. Thus, muscle persists between the aortic and pulmonary valve leaflets; when the muscle is displaced leftward, it produces subaortic stenosis.[255] Other complex intracardiac malformations, such as transposition of the great arteries, aortopulmonary window, and truncus arteriosus, are common.

CLINICAL FEATURES. An association is frequent with the genetic 22q11 deletion of DiGeorge's syndrome, a constellation of cardiac, parathyroid, thymic, and facial anomalies attributed to disruption of the interaction of premigratory neural crest cells with endodermal pharyngeal pouch cells. In this syndrome, thymic hypoplasia or aplasia is accompanied by immunological and hypocalcemia problems.[256, 257] The major clinical problem is severe congestive heart failure as a consequence of volume overload of the left ventricle resulting from an associated intracardiac left-to-right shunt and of pressure overload imposed by systemic hypertension.

Management. The perioperative clinical condition of most patients can be improved by intensive medical management with mechanical ventilation, inotropic support, and prostaglandin infusion. Various forms of palliative operative techniques have fair to poor results. There has been increasing success with complete primary repair in infancy as the procedure of choice.[258] Greater mortality is associated when a two-stage approach with initial arch repair and pulmonary artery banding is followed by later repair of the intracardiac lesion. Recurrent narrowing at the aortic suture line can be treated by balloon angioplasty or reoperation.

Congenital Valvular Aortic Stenosis

(See also p. 1599)

MORPHOLOGY. Congenital valvular aortic stenosis is a relatively common anomaly, estimated to occur in 3 to 6 percent of patients with congenital cardiovascular defects.

However, it must be appreciated that the true incidence of the malformation is probably grossly underestimated because the congenital bicuspid aortic valve may be undetected in early life and becomes stenotic and of clinical significance only in adult life, at a time when it may be indistinguishable from the acquired forms of aortic stenosis. Congenital valvular aortic stenosis occurs much more frequently in males than in females, with the gender ratio approximating 4:1. Associated cardiovascular anomalies have been noted in as many as 20 percent of patients.[259] Patent ductus arteriosus and coarctation of the aorta occur most frequently with valvular aortic stenosis; all three of these lesions may coexist (see also Chap. 44).

The basic malformation consists of thickening of valve tissue with various degrees of commissural fusion. The valve most commonly is the bicuspid, with a single fused commissure and an eccentrically place orifice. A third commissure, incomplete or rudimentary, is sometimes apparent. Less commonly, the valve has three fused cusps with a stenotic central orifice. In some patients, the stenotic aortic valve is unicuspid and dome shaped, with no or one lateral attachment to the aorta at the level of the orifice. In infants and young children with severe aortic stenosis, the aortic valve ring may be relatively underdeveloped. This lesion forms a continuum with the hypoplastic left heart syndrome and the aortic atresia and hypoplasia complexes. Secondary calcification of the valve is extremely rare in childhood, but the dynamics of blood flow associated with the congenitally deformed aortic valve ultimately lead to thickening of the cusps and calcification in adult life. When the obstruction is hemodynamically significant, concentric hypertrophy of the left ventricular wall and dilatation of the ascending aorta occur.

HEMODYNAMICS (see also Chaps. 11 and 46). The hemodynamic abnormalities produced by obstruction to left ventricular outflow are discussed in Chapter 46. A peak systolic gradient exceeding 75 mm Hg in association with a normal cardiac output or an effective aortic orifice less than 0.5 cm^2/m^2 body surface area is considered to reflect critical or severe obstruction to left ventricular outflow.[259] The normal outflow orifice approximates 2.0 cm^2/m^2 body surface area; areas of 0.5 to 0.8 cm^2/m^2 signify moderate obstruction; when the area is larger than 0.8 cm^2/m^2, the obstruction is considered to be mild.

The resting cardiac output and stroke volume usually are within normal limits. During exercise, most children with critical stenosis show an elevation of the cardiac output and an associated elevation in the transvalvular pressure gradient.[260] When left ventricular failure occurs, cardiac output decreases and left atrial, left ventricular end-diastolic, and pulmonary vascular pressures increase.

Studies of left ventricular performance in children with aortic stenosis often reveal supernormal pump function, as indicated by increases in ejection fraction and circumferential fiber shortening.[261] Despite high left ventricular systolic pressures, left ventricular wall stress appears to be lower than normal throughout systole, presumably because increases in wall thickness provide overcompensation for the pressure overload. Undoubtedly, a spectrum exists, from well-compensated patients at one end, who have supernormal pump function and normal contractile function, to patients with heart failure at the opposite end, who have both impaired pump function and a reduced contractile state.

While pressure overload hypertrophy can preserve systolic function, it can also result in abnormal left ventricular early diastolic filling.[262] Thus, clinical studies seeking to analyze the determinants of left ventricular filling by a separate assessment of dynamic (elastic recoil, ventricular relaxation rate, and atrial driving pressure) and static (chamber stiffness and left ventricular hypertrophy) determinants suggest that diastolic function most importantly varies according to the severity of left ventricular hypertrophy and systolic function. Studies of children suggest that hypertrophy is a more important factor than excessive wall stress and depressed ejection performance in accounting for abnormal diastolic filling.

The blood supply to the myocardium may be significantly compromised in infants and children with aortic stenosis, despite normal patency of the coronary arteries.[263] Coronary blood flow and arterial oxygen content are critical determinants of oxygen supply to the myocardium. Because intramyocardial compressive forces are greatest in the subendocardium, blood flow to that region of the left ventricle is entirely diastolic in the presence of elevated left ventricular systolic pressure. In patients with left ventricular outflow tract obstruction, coronary vasodilatation may give an inadequate response to an increase in the demands of the myocardium for oxygen at rest or with exercise. When subendocardial vessels are maximally dilated, the coronary artery driving pressure and the duration of diastole determine the magnitude of subendocardial flow. When the duration of systolic ejection lengthens across the stenotic orifice, diastole is shortened, especially at high heart rates. Moreover, a reduction occurs in coronary driving pressure if left ventricular end-diastolic pressure is high or if aortic diastolic pressure is low, e.g., with aortic regurgitation or heart failure. In patients with severe aortic stenosis, the redistribution of flow away from the subendocardium and the ischemia that results in that portion of ventricular muscle may be estimated by relating the diastolic pressure–time index (DPTI) (i.e., the area between the aortic and left ventricular pressures in diastole) to the systolic pressure–time index (SPTI) (a measure of myocardial oxygen demands). Inadequate subendocardial oxygen delivery has been shown to exist when the ratio [DPTI × arterial oxygen content/SPTI] falls below 10.[263]

NEONATES AND INFANTS

Reports exist of cardiac dysfunction and even nonimmunological fetal hydrops fetalis in association with severe aortic stenosis.[264-266] The hydrops can be the result of in utero left ventricular myocardial infarction or profound left ventricular systolic and diastolic dysfunction. Balloon dilation using coronary balloon catheters has been attempted via transabdominal echo-guided needle puncture of the fetal left ventricle. This approach is not established, and it is doubtful that it will become a management option.

Fortunately, isolated aortic valvular stenosis seldom causes symptoms in infancy.[267] This lesion, however, occasionally can be responsible for profound and intractable heart failure, even in fetal life. Despite normal coronary arterial anatomy, infarction of left ventricular papillary muscles may occur, resulting in an acquired form of mitral valvular regurgitation that intensifies the heart failure state. In addition, endocardial fibroelastosis may result from limited subendocardial oxygen delivery, and myocardial degeneration may be significant. Symptomatic infants with isolated valvular aortic stenosis are irritable, pale, and hypotensive and present with tachycardia, cardiomegaly, and pulmonary congestion manifested by dyspnea, tachypnea, subcostal retractions, and diffuse rales. Cyanosis may be observed secondary to pulmonary venous desaturation. The systolic murmur in infants often is atypical; it is best heard at the apex or along the lower left sternal border and may be confused with that caused by a VSD. In infants with heart failure, the murmur occasionally may be absent or extremely soft, becoming louder when myocardial contractility is improved with digitalis and other medical measures. Infants with heart failure frequently have a poor response to medical management.

The *ECG findings* may not be characteristic; left ventricular hypertrophy and/or strain as well as right atrial enlargement and right ventricular hypertrophy may be detected shortly after birth.[267] The latter signs of right heart involvement result from both pulmonary hypertension secondary to elevated left ventricular diastolic and left atrial pressures and from volume loading of the right ventricle caused by left-to-right shunting across the foramen ovale. Survival past the early neonatal period does not preclude subsequent difficulties, and clinical deterioration may recur with the onset of physiological anemia.

Management

Congenital aortic stenosis must be considered a medical emergency in a seriously ill newborn, and echocardiography, and sometimes cardiac catheterization and angiocardiography, may be indicated in the first 24 hours of life. Two-dimensional echocardiographic studies show a severe immobility of the aortic valve, with little or no systolic opening, poststenotic dilation of the aorta, left ventricular hypertrophy, right ventricular enlargement, and a severely disturbed Doppler-determined pattern of ascending aortic flow velocity. The echo-Doppler examination must also identify associated intracardiac and extracardiac anomalies, one of the most important of which is severe aortic arch obstruction.

Dilation of the ductus arteriosus with prostaglandin E₁ infusion may provide transitional support of the systemic circulation. In many centers, expeditious balloon aortic valvuloplasty follows the echo-Doppler examination in infants who are unstable and markedly symptomatic.[268-272] A number of approaches have been reported for performing this procedure, including the use of a carotid artery cutdown, which thus far does not appear to result in any abnormalities of the carotid pulse or any neurological sequelae. A transumbilical technique of balloon valvuloplasty can be performed quickly, safely, and effectively with preservation of the femoral artery. Because of a high risk of iliofemoral artery complications in infants with the transfemoral route to valvuloplasty, when this route is used it is advisable to use double-balloon techniques to allow insertion of small valvuloplasty catheters. The complications of balloon valvuloplasty are related to the small size and young age of the patient. Accordingly, if arterial access is a problem, and in infants younger than 1 month, surgical valvotomy remains a satisfactory option. Open repair under direct vision is the preferred type of operation.

Hemodynamic findings in neonates and infants frequently include left-to-right shunting at the atrial level, elevated left atrial and left ventricular end-diastolic pressures, and a small pressure drop across the aortic valve as a result of markedly reduced cardiac output. Right-to-left shunting across a patent ductus arteriosus is encountered occasionally. The lesion may be distinguished from the hypoplastic left heart syndrome echocardiographically and angiographically by the presence of normal or enlarged left ventricular cavity and normal or dilated ascending aorta.[273, 274] Establishment of the diagnosis and prompt catheter valvuloplasty or surgical valvotomy are justified because prolonged periods of stabilization are uncommon with medical therapy. Poor myocardial performance resulting from endocardial fibroelastosis, subendocardial ischemia, reduced left ventricular compliance, and inadequate relief of obstruction with or without aortic insufficiency are some of the factors accounting for high mortality and morbidity after catheter-directed treatment or operation.

At the extreme end of the spectrum of critical valvar aortic stenosis in newborns are patients with many small left-sided structures; in these patients, the adverse effects of small inflow, outflow, and/or cavity size of the left ventricle appear to be cumulative.[274] It is in this group that traditional treatment by aortic valvuloplasty or valvotomy, which is a two-sided ventricle repair, may be less effective than a multistaged Norwood approach.[274] The latter consists of an initial single-ventricle repair in which the main pulmonary artery is anastomosed to the aorta with creation of a systemic-to-pulmonary arterial shunt, followed later by a Fontan-type operation that creates an atriopulmonary connection, with or without a prior superior cava–pulmonary connection. The single-ventricle repair results in functional sacrifice of the left ventricle and the right ventricle supporting the systemic circulation without a pulmonary ventricle.

CHILDREN

Congenital aortic stenosis may be responsible for severe obstruction to left ventricular outflow in the absence of clinical symptoms of diminished cardiac reserve that are so frequent in other forms of congenital heart disease.[275] Most children with congenital aortic stenosis grow and develop normally and are asymptomatic. Attention usually is called to these children when a murmur is detected on routine examination. When symptoms occur, those noted most commonly are undue fatigue, exertional dyspnea, angina pectoris, and syncope. Less often described are abdominal pain, profuse sweating, and epistaxis. A symptomatic child usually has critical stenosis. There is a distinct threat of sudden death in patients with severe obstruction[276] (see Chap. 26). Although the precise cause is poorly understood, ventricular arrhythmias, perhaps initiated by acute myocardial ischemia, are probably the most common inciting event. It has been speculated that an abrupt rise in intracavity left ventricular systolic pressure elicits a reflex hypotensive syncope that promotes acute ischemia and ventricular fibrillation. Bacterial endocarditis occurs in about 4 percent of patients with congenital valvular aortic stenosis.[277]

DIAGNOSIS

Physical Findings. When the magnitude of obstruction is significant, a left ventricular lift usually is palpable, and a precordial systolic thrill often is palpated over the base of the heart with transmission to the jugular notch and along the carotid arteries; presystolic expansion often is palpable. The obstruction usually is mild if neither a left ventricular lift nor a thrill is present.

Opening of the aortic valve produces a systolic aortic ejection sound that typically is present at the cardiac apex when the valve is mobile, particularly in patients with mild to moderate stenosis. A delay in closure of the stenotic aortic valve leads to a single or a closely split second heart sound, and paradoxical splitting may be present. A fourth heart sound normally is associated with severe obstruction. A loud, harsh, rhomboid-shaped systolic murmur starts after completion of left ventricular isometric contraction and is best heard at the base of the heart. The murmur, like the thrill, radiates to the suprasternal notch and carotid vessel as well as to the apex. An early diastolic blowing murmur of aortic regurgitation is present in some patients, but unless the valve leaflets have been eroded by bacterial endocarditis, the regurgitation usually is not hemodynamically significant; uncommonly, in patients with a congenitally bicuspid valve, aortic regurgitation may be severe and may predominate.

Electrocardiography. ECG signs of left ventricular hypertrophy tend to vary with the severity of obstruction, although a normal or near-normal ECG does not preclude severe aortic stenosis, and excessive left ventricular voltages may be observed in children with mild obstruction.[275] The lack of close correlation between the ECG and the transvalvular pressure gradient emphasizes the potential hazard of relying on the ECG in patient care. The most reliable index of the severity of obstruction is the presence of a left ventricular "strain pattern," consisting of left ventricular hypertrophy combined with ST segment depressions and T wave inversion in the left precordial leads (Fig. 43–31).

Roentgenography. Overall heart size is normal or the degree of enlargement is slight in most children with congenital valvular aortic stenosis. Concentric left ventricular hypertrophy accompanies moderate or severe obstruction and is manifested by rounding of the cardiac apex in the frontal projection and posterior displacement in the lateral view.

Echocardiography. Two-dimensional and Doppler echocardiography are the current methods of choice for defining the anatomy and the hemodynamic severity of valvular aortic stenosis.[278, 279] Real-time cross-sectional echocardiography reveals impaired mobility of cusp tissue, an alteration in the phasic movement of the aortic valve with reduced lateral and increased superior excursions of valve echoes, and an increase in the internal aortic root dimension beyond the level of the valve annulus.[259] Imaging of the valve must be performed many times in order to display the

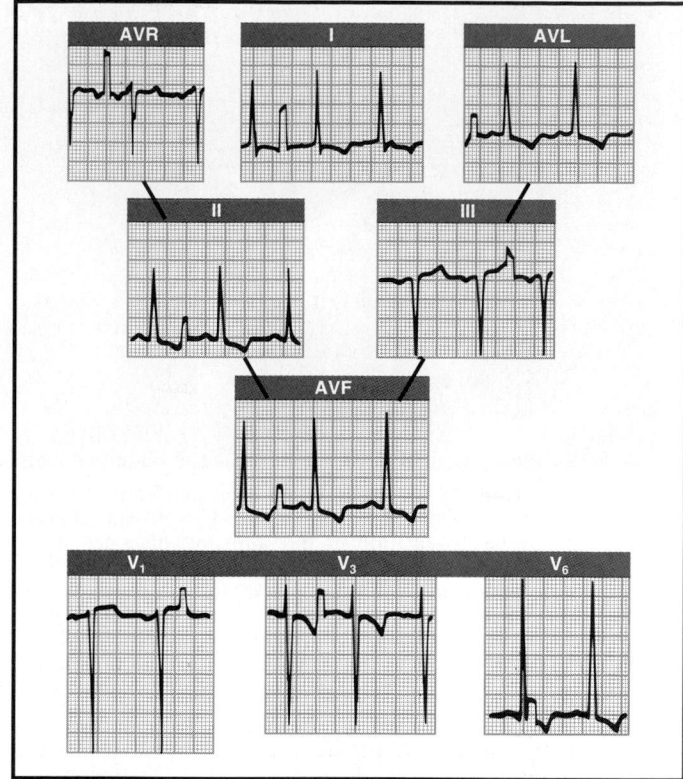

FIGURE 43–31. Electrocardiogram in congenital aortic stenosis. This tracing shows left ventricular hypertrophy and the typical left ventricular "strain" pattern (V_6). (Courtesy of Dr. Delores A. Danilowicz.)

valve through the long axis of the left ventricular outflow tract and then through a plane parallel to the valve annulus. The long-axis view of the left ventricular outflow tract allows evaluation of the valve mobility and cusp separation; it is the best view for demonstrating doming of the aortic valve. The parasternal short-axis view bisects the face of the valve, demonstrating the anatomy of the commissures (Fig. 43–32).

The echocardiogram also reveals associated left ventricular hypertrophy and the presence of endocardial fibroelastosis (seen as bright endocardial echoes). Further, measurements of mitral valve diameter, left ventricular end-diastolic dimension, and left ventricular cross-sectional area serve to distinguish those infants with critical aortic stenosis from those with a hypoplastic left ventricle.[274] Among these calculations suggesting the latter are an end-diastolic volume less than 20 ml/m², an inflow dimension of 25 mm, a narrow ventricular aortic junction less than 5 mm, or a small mitral orifice less than 9 mm. Pulsed-wave Doppler echocardiography allows inspection of the pattern of flow velocity within the circulation. This technique detects the altered and disturbed turbulence of flow in patients with aortic stenosis. A highly accurate noninvasive approach to quantifying the severity of obstruction combines continuous-wave Doppler flow analysis with the cross-sectional echocardiographic determination of the area of the orifice.[280] A simplified Bernoulli equation uses the measurement of the maximum velocity of the aortic jet and time-averaged pressure drop obtained from planimetry of the maximal velocity spectral reading. A simpler estimate of the transvalvular gradient (in mm Hg) may be calculated as four times the square of the peak Doppler velocity (m/sec).

The Doppler method records a peak instantaneous pressure difference, which may differ importantly from the gradient recorded by a cardiac catheter, which is a peak-to-peak pressure difference.[281] Doppler mean gradient is more

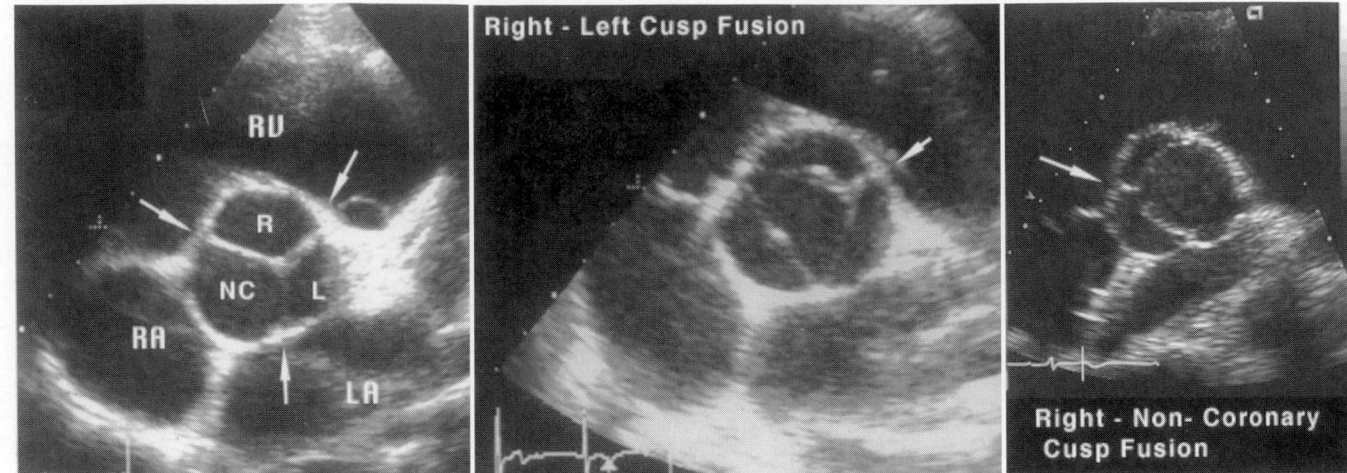

FIGURE 43–32. Standard short-axis view of aortic cusps in the closed position in a patient with a bicuspid aortic valve. *Left frame,* The right (R) and noncoronary (NC) left (L) cusps are seen within the aortic root. The arrows indicate the points of adherence of the cusps to the aortic wall. The right ventricle (RV) is seen anteriorly; the right atrium (RA), and left atrium (LA) are seen posteriorly. *Middle frame,* Same patient, with open valve leaflets in systole, shows fusion between the right and left coronary cusps. The fused raphe (arrow) between these cusps is typical of a bicuspid aortic valve. *Right frame,* Taken in systole from another patient with a bicuspid aortic valve, this frame demonstrates similar features but with a fused raphe (arrow) between the right and noncoronary cusps.

accurate than the instantaneous gradient when compared with the pressures found at cardiac catheterization. Management decisions often depend on estimation of the severity of obstruction, and all pressure gradient estimations depend on flow velocity across the valve, which may be confounded by low cardiac output or concomitant valvar regurgitation. Thus, an important argument can be made that the determination of the stenotic valve systolic area is often more important than calculation of a systolic gradient.[279–281]

The most widely accepted technique for correcting the gradient for flow is to use the continuity equation, which measures the flow velocity ratio across the aortic valve and therefore corrects for high and low flow rates. The continuity equation presumes that for flow in a series, the product of mean velocity and cross-sectional area is constant at all points in the flow circuit. In patients with aortic stenosis, the area of the left ventricular outflow tract is determined by two-dimensional echocardiography, the flow velocity of the outflow tract by pulsed-wave Doppler, and the flow velocity immediately above the valve by continuous-wave Doppler, all of which, taken together, allow determination of the valve area by the continuity equation: Aortic valve area: $[(area)LVOT \times V(LVOT)]/(V)AV$ (obtained by converting the diameter to area and assuming that it is circular); $(V)LVOT$ = peak outflow tract velocity, and $(V)AV$ = peak velocity across the aortic valve.

Transesophageal two-dimensional echocardiographic determination of aortic valve area has been applied in adults with aortic stenosis.[282] The approach offers considerably better resolution of cardiac anatomy than does conventional transthoracic two-dimensional echocardiography and may also prove to be more accurate in estimating pressure gradients and aortic valve areas. The approach is applicable to older children but has not yet been reported in young children in sufficient detail to make specific recommendations.

Diagnostic Cardiac Catheterization. Cardiac catheterization is now rarely used to establish the site and severity of obstruction to left ventricular outflow because the malformation is readily diagnosed and the evaluation of the intensity of stenosis is accurate by echo-Doppler examination.[283] Instead, catheterization is undertaken when therapeutic interventional transcatheter balloon aortic valvuloplasty is indicated.

During the catheterization procedure, cardiac output is measured by the indicator-dilution, thermodilution, or Fick technique. Retrograde left heart catheterization allows withdrawal pressure recordings across the site of stenosis, and left ventricular angiocardiography can be carried out, permitting an evaluation of the size of the left ventricular cavity, the thickness of the wall, the competence of the mitral valve, the patency of the coronary arteries, and the diameter of the aortic root and ascending aorta. If aortic insufficiency is thought to be present, cineaortography is performed with injection of contrast material into the aortic root. The severity of aortic insufficiency can be assessed qualitatively by cineaortography and quantitatively by ventriculography, with calculation of regurgitant volume by subtraction of net forward flow (calculated by the Fick method) from angiographically determined total forward flow. The typical angiocardiographic features of valvar stenosis are thickening of the aortic cusps, poststenotic dilation of the ascending aorta, and, occasionally, a jet of contrast material entering the ascending aorta through a central or eccentric narrowed valve orifice (Fig. 43–33). The leaflets of the bicuspid valve are domed in systole, and a central jet corresponds to the orifice of the stenotic valve. In contrast, the stenotic orifice of the unicommissural valve can be visualized by the systolic jet in contact with the posterior wall of the aorta, with leaflet tissue and valve motion seen only anteriorly.[259]

Balloon Valvuloplasty. Balloon dilatation may be indicated in any infant or child who has a clinical diagnosis of aortic stenosis and in whom the clinical examination, roentgenogram, resting or exercise ECG, or Doppler echocardiogram suggests the possibility of severe obstruction.[284] Even in the absence of such findings, balloon valvuloplasty may be performed if symptoms that might be related to aortic stenosis exist, such as dizziness, fainting, or angina.

We prefer to catheterize the left side of the heart via a retrograde approach by femoral percutaneous puncture. The goals of the study are to analyze the severity of obstruction and assess the function of the left ventricle. In most centers, balloon valvuloplasty is recommended if the severity of the aortic stenosis would otherwise require surgical treatment—that is, a peak systolic pressure gradient exceeding 70 mm Hg measured in the basal state or a calculated effective orifice less than 0.5 cm²/m² of body surface area. In the

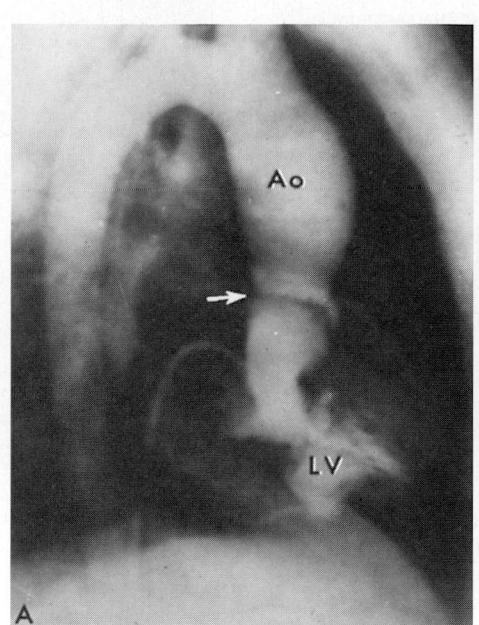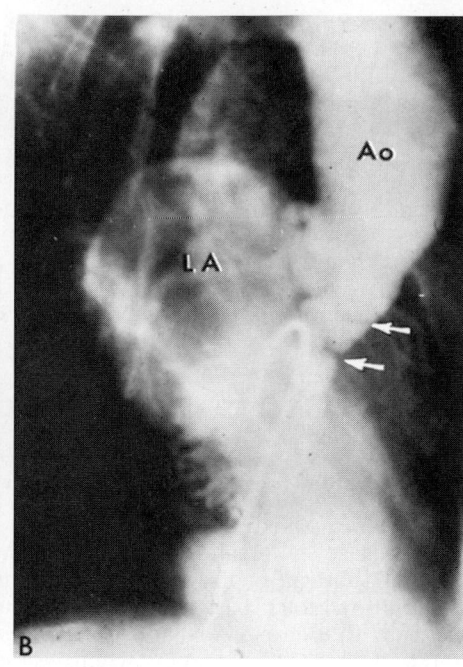

FIGURE 43–33. *A,* Left ventricular angiocardiogram obtained by the transseptal method in a patient with congenital valvular aortic stenosis. Ao = poststenotic dilatation of the aorta; LV = left ventricle. Arrow denotes the thickened valve cusp. *B,* Selective angiocardiogram in a patient with discrete subvalvular stenosis (bottom arrow). Associated mitral regurgitation is evident from the reflux of contrast material into an enlarged left atrium (LA). The aortic valve (top arrow) is normal, and the right coronary artery is visualized. (From Friedman WF, Kirkpatrick SE: Congenital aortic stenosis. *In* Adams FH, Emmanouilides GC, Riemenschneider TA, et al: Moss' Heart Disease in Infants, Children, and Adolescents. 4th ed. Baltimore, © Williams & Wilkins, 1989.)

presence of symptoms or left ventricular strain pattern on the ECG or an abnormal exercise ECG, there is less rigid regard to the hemodynamic assessment of the severity of stenosis. Further, some centers go forward with balloon valvuloplasty with peak systolic gradients greater than or equal to 50 mm Hg. There is general agreement that there be no significant aortic regurgitation (less than grade 2 of 4) and that other associated cardiac anomalies be absent, except aortic coarctation.

Balloon dilatation of the aortic valve began in the mid-1980s; truly long-term follow-up studies are not yet available. Early studies and our experience suggest that the diameter of the balloon should not exceed that of the aortic valve ring. Most centers prefer a balloon with a diameter 80 to 100 percent that of the aortic annulus or at least 1 mm smaller than it. The expected hemodynamic result is a reduction in the catheterization-measured peak-to-peak ejection gradient of about 60 to 70 percent. The appearance of aortic regurgitation or its progression is the major complication of valvuloplasty, although the aortic regurgitation is mild in the great majority of patients.[284] Significant aortic regurgitation appears to accompany the development of aortic valve prolapse, which is likely due to tearing of the valve cusp or its raphe or partial detachment of the valve from the valve ring, all of which undermine the support mechanism of the valve. In those patients whose balloon valvuloplasty has resulted in very significant aortic regurgitation, valve surgery may be required to either replace the valve or repair a tear in the valve. Other complications from balloon aortic valvuloplasty include bleeding, arrhythmias, cerebral vascular accidents, iliofemoral arterial complications, injury to the mitral valve, and, rarely beyond infancy, death.[284]

Natural History. Congenital aortic stenosis frequently is a progressive disorder, even early in life, in a significant fraction of patients presenting initially with mild obstruction.[285–287] Thus, clinical deterioration may be anticipated because of an intensification in the severity of stenosis rather than the development of significant aortic regurgitation. Progression of obstruction usually is the result of the increase in cardiac output that occurs concurrently with increased body growth. Less often, a decrease in the area of the orifice is an added factor in the intensification of obstruction. The onset of symptoms or changes in the phonocardiogram or graphic pulse tracings, chest roentgenograms, ECGs, or vectorcardiograms cannot be depended on to indicate progressive obstruction in the individual patient; Doppler echocardiography is most reliable.

MANAGEMENT. A malformed aortic valve is a potential site of bacterial infection; antibiotic prophylaxis is recommended for all patients, regardless of the severity of obstruction. Strict avoidance of strenuous physical activity is advised if severe aortic stenosis is present. Participation in competitive sports also should probably be restricted in patients with milder degrees of obstruction. Digitalis should be administered to patients who have symptoms of diminished cardiac reserve and also should be considered for patients with left ventricular hypertrophy, even if they are not in heart failure.

Surgery. Percutaneous balloon aortic valvuloplasty is a useful palliation to delay open valvulotomy, the Ross procedure (see below), or valve replacement. For those patients in whom balloon valvuloplasty is unsuccessful, operation is carried out under direct vision after institution of cardiopulmonary bypass, and the fused commissures are opened. When this is done precisely and judiciously, the commissural incision enlarges the valve orifice and does not result in significant aortic regurgitation.[288] When operation is performed in childhood, a mortality rate of less than 2 percent can be expected.[289] Among the factors influencing the indications, techniques, and results of operation are the patient's age, the nature of the valvar deformity, and the experience of the surgical team.

Long-term follow-up studies indicate that aortic valvotomy is a safe and effective means of palliative treatment with excellent relief of symptoms.[289, 290] Aortic insufficiency can occasionally be progressive and require valve replacement. Moreover, after commissurotomy, the valve leaflets remain somewhat deformed, and it is likely that further degenerative changes, including calcification, will lead to significant stenosis in later years.[259] Thus, prosthetic valve replacement is required in approximately 35 percent of patients within 15 to 20 years of the original operation. Because the valve is not rendered normal, antibiotic prophylaxis is indicated in postoperative patients, even if the systolic pressure gradient has been abolished. For those patients eventually requiring aortic valve replacement, the surgical options include replacement with a prosthetic aortic valve, an aortic homograft, or a pulmonary autograft in the aortic position. Accumulating evidence shows that the pulmonary autograft may ultimately be preferable to the aortic homograft for aortic reconstruction, and many surgeons prefer the procedure to palliative surgical valvotomy as the initial operation of choice. In the pulmonary autograft, called the Ross procedure, the patient's pulmonary valve is removed and used to replace the diseased aortic valve, and the right ventricular outflow tract is reconstructed with a pulmnary valve allograft.[291-294] We consider it likely that the Ross procedure will emerge as the approach of choice in the future. Neither homografts nor autografts require anticoagulation. There is a finite incidence of valve degeneration of approximately 2 percent per patient per year with the former, whereas primary tissue failure has not been observed among pulmonary autografts.

Discrete Subaortic Stenosis

(See also p. 1599)

This malformation accounts for 8 to 10 percent of all cases of congenital aortic stenosis and occurs twice as frequently in males as in females. The lesion consists of a membranous diaphragm or fibrous ring encircling the left ventricular outflow tract or a long fibromuscular narrowing just beneath the base of the aortic valve. Subaortic stenosis is rarely diagnosed in infancy, when it is usually the result of a malalignment VSD with deviation posteriorly of the outlet septum into the left ventricular outflow tract, often associated with coarctation of the aorta or interruption of the aortic arch.

Distinction of subvalvular from valvular aortic stenosis is extremely difficult by means of clinical findings alone.[259] Rarely, a systolic ejection sound is heard, and the diastolic murmur of aortic regurgitation is more common than it is in valvular aortic stenosis. Dilatation of the ascending aorta is common, but valvular calcification is not observed.

Echocardiography is useful in differentiating between valvular and subvalvular stenosis (see Chap. 7).[295] The criterion for diagnosis of the latter is demonstration of a localized subvalvar discrete ridge or long segment narrowing in the left ventricular outflow tract. Further, because of the possibility of recurrence of subvalvular aortic stenosis, careful postoperative follow-up echocardiography is required. Two-dimensional echocardiographic studies from the apical two-chamber and left parasternal and subxiphoid long-axis views demonstrate persistent, prominent echoes in the subaortic left ventricle in both systole and diastole (Fig. 43–34). Doppler sampling proximal to the aortic valve shows increased flow velocity.[295] Most important, echocardiography also can identify hypertrophic subaortic stenosis when it coexists with fixed subaortic stenosis and can differentiate between the two forms of obstruction.

Definitive distinction between valvular and subvalvular obstruction is also provided by transesophageal Doppler echocardiography[296] and by recording pressure tracings as a catheter is withdrawn across the outflow tract and valve, or by localizing the site of obstruction with selective left ventricular angiocardiography (see Fig. 43–33).

Mild degrees of aortic valvular regurgitation commonly are observed in patients with discrete subaortic stenosis and appear to be caused by thickening of the valve and impaired mobility of the cusps secondary to the trauma created by the high-velocity jet passing through the subaortic diaphragm. Further deformation of these abnormal valve cusps by the vegetations of bacterial endocarditis often results in severe aortic regurgitation.

MANAGEMENT. Because of the likelihood of both progressive obstruction and aortic regurgitation, the presence of even mild or moderate subaortic stenosis warrants consideration of elective operation.[297-299] Reports describe transluminal balloon dilation for discrete subaortic stenosis, but it is unlikely that this palliative approach will be an acceptable alternative, since the relief of obstruction is not

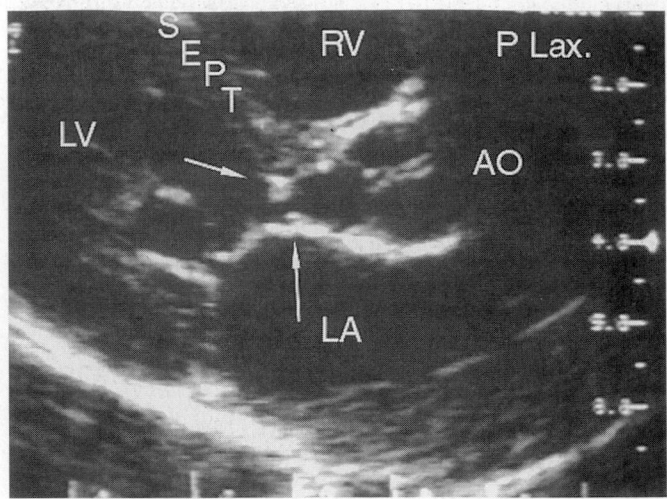

FIGURE 43–34. Parasternal long axis (P Lax.) view of membranous subaortic stenosis. The ventricular septum (SEPT), right ventricle (RV), left ventricle (LV), and left atrium (LA), as well as the aorta (AO), are seen. The arrows indicate the attachments of the subvalvar membrane to the septum anteriorly and to the mitral valve posteriorly.

likely to be as complete or as long as in those patients undergoing surgical resection.

The risks of operation in patients with discrete subaortic stenosis and valvular aortic stenosis are essentially the same. Surgical treatment of discrete subaortic stenosis has evolved from simply excising the membrane or fibrous ridge to adding a generous ventricular myotomy and myectomy to the membranectomy.[300] Operation may be expected to improve the hemodynamic state substantially; it frequently is totally curative.

Evidence indicates that muscle resection combined with membrane excision lowers the risk of reoperation for recurrent subaortic stenosis.[301] Discrete membranous subaortic stenosis may tend to recur after operation, although we and others consider these recurrences to be often related, at least in part, to incomplete removal of the lesion at initial operation. Intraoperative echocardiography has been used as an adjunct to operation to enable immediate assessment of the adequacy of relieving obstruction. Studies have suggested that abnormal flow patterns may predispose to pathological proliferation of subvalvar aortic tissue, which reinforces the requirement that careful echocardiographic and surgical exploration of the outflow tract, even well below the subvalvar stenosis, be undertaken to detect and resect structures that cause turbulence.[302] For patients with recurrent obstruction, operation may consist of repeat resection plus creation of an outlet VSD extending up to but not across the aortic valve. This iatrogenic VSD is patched on the right side to further enlarge the subaortic area. For patients in whom the aortic valve cannot be repaired, the Ross pulmonary valve autograft procedure is used.[303]

UNCOMMON FORMS OF SUBAORTIC STENOSIS

COMBINED VALVULAR AND SUBVALVULAR STENOSIS. In some patients, valvular and subvalvular aortic stenosis coexist with hypoplasia of the aortic valve ring and thickened valve leaflets, producing a tunnel-like narrowing of the left ventricular outflow tract. Additional findings often include a small ascending aorta. The subvalvular fibrous process usually extends onto the aortic valve cusps and almost always makes contact with the ventricular aspect of the anterior mitral leaflet at its base. The presence of "tunnel stenosis" may be suspected echocardiographically or angiographically from the appearance of the outflow tract and the aortic root. Operative treatment often is complicated by the need for an aortoventriculoplasty, consisting of prosthetic or homograft replacement of the aortic valve as well as enlarging the aortic annulus, proximal aorta, and left ventricular outlet tract (the Kono-Rastan operation). The *modified* Kono-Rastan operation preserves the native aortic valve if the annulus is normal or near normal. Alternatively, a conal enlargement technique may be used.[304, 305]

Various anatomical lesions other than a discrete membrane or ridge may produce subaortic stenosis.[306-308] Among these are abnormal adherence of the anterior leaflet of the mitral valve to the left septal surface, and the presence in the left ventricular outflow tract of accessory endocardial cushion tissue. In some patients with an AV canal, the part of the ventricular septum that contributes to the wall of the left ventricular outflow tract is deficient, and the ventricular aspect of the anterior leaflet of the common AV valve is adherent to the posterior edge of the deficient septum, resulting in a narrow left ventricular outflow tract. Malalignment of the conoventricular septum, resulting in an inferior VSD, produces a leftward superior deviation and insertion of the conal septum, obstructing left ventricular outflow. In patients with a single ventricle and an outflow chamber, the bulboventricular foramen serves as a potential site of aortic outflow obstruction. Additionally, rarer causes of subaortic stenosis include redundant dysplastic left AV valve tissue in patients with congenitally corrected transposition of the great arteries and anomalous muscle bundles of the left ventricular outflow tract.

MUSCULAR SUBAORTIC STENOSIS. A muscular type of subaortic stenosis may result from a convergence of all the mitral chordae into one or two fused papillary muscles; a "parachute" deformity of the mitral valve is produced, and it is often seen in association with supravalvular stenosis of the left atrium and coarctation of the aorta. In some of these patients, discrete membranous subvalvular aortic obstruction also has been noted.

In patients with VSD, muscular subaortic stenosis has been shown to develop after surgical banding of the pulmonary artery, possibly as a result of hypertrophy of the conal septum or crista supraventricularis encroaching on the left ventricular outflow tract above the septal defect.

Subaortic muscular hypertrophy secondary to diffuse involvement of the myocardium by glycogen storage disease (Pompe's disease) is an extremely rare cause of obstruction to left ventricular outflow. A positive family history, symptoms of muscle weakness, heart failure in infancy, and the characteristic ECG findings of a short PR interval, high-voltage QRS and T waves, and left ventricular hypertrophy warrant skeletal muscle biopsy or fibroblast culture, permitting an antemortem diagnosis.

The last, relatively uncommon form of subaortic stenosis to be mentioned occurs infrequently in patients with congenitally corrected transposition of the great arteries; in these patients, an anomalous muscle bundle in the subaortic area of the arterial ventricle obstructs outflow.

Supravalvular Aortic Stenosis

Supravalvular aortic stenosis is a congenital narrowing of the ascending aorta that may be localized or diffuse, originating at the superior margin of the sinuses of Valsalva just above the levels of the coronary arteries.

The clinical picture of supravalvular obstruction usually differs in major respects from that observed in the other forms of aortic stenosis. Chief among these differences is the association of supravalvular aortic stenosis with idio-pathic infantile hypercalcemia, a disease that occurs in the first years of life and may be associated with deranged vitamin D metabolism.[309-312]

It is helpful to classify patients according to their clinical presentation into nonfamilial, sporadic cases with normal facies and intelligence; autosomal dominant familial cases with normal facies and intelligence; and the Williams syndrome with abnormal facial appearance and mental retardation (Fig. 43–35). In contrast to the other forms of aortic stenosis, no gender predilection is noted in any of these three categories.

WILLIAMS SYNDROME. The designations supravalvular aortic stenosis syndrome or Williams syndrome or Williams-Beuren syndrome[310, 310a] have been applied to the distinctive picture produced by coexistence of the cardiac and multiple-system disorders. Beyond infancy in these patients, a challenge with vitamin D or calcium loading tests unmasks abnormalities in the regulation of circulating 25-hydroxyvitamin D. Unanimity of opinion about the exact relation between Williams syndrome and calcium metabolism does not exist[311, 312].

Infants with Williams syndrome often exhibit feeding difficulties, failure to thrive, and gastrointestinal problems in the form of vomiting, constipation, and colic. The entire spectrum of clinical manifestations includes auditory hyperacusis, inguinal hernia, a hoarse voice, and a typical personality that is outgoing and engaging. Other manifestations of this syndrome include mental retardation, "eifin facies" (see Fig. 43–32), narrowing of peripheral systemic and pulmonary arteries, strabismus, and abnormalities of dental development consisting of microdontia, enamel hypoplasia, and malocclusion[312a].

Many medical conditions can complicate the course of Williams syndrome,[312b] including systemic hypertension, gastrointestinal problems, and urinary tract abnormalities. Particularly in an older child or adult, progressive joint limitation and hypertonia may become a problem. Adult patients are usually handicapped by their developmental disabilities.

Williams syndrome was previously considered to be nonfamilial. Interestingly, a number of families in which parent-to-child transmission of Williams syndrome has occurred have now been identified. These are not families with autosomal dominant supravalvular aortic stenosis whose members are normal in appearance and intelligence. All of these families show a parent and child to be affected with Williams syndrome, including one instance of male-to-male transmission. This supports autosomal dominant inheritance as the likely pattern, with most cases of Williams syndrome probably occurring as the result of a new mutation. New information indicates that a genetic defect for supravalvular aortic stenosis is located in the same chromosomal subunit as elastin on chromosome 7.[312b, 313] Elastin is an important component of the arterial wall, but precisely how mutations in elastin genes cause the phenotypes of supravalvular aortic stenosis is not known for certain. The various aspects of Williams syndrome may represent a contiguous gene deletion syndrome (see Chap. 56).

FAMILIAL AUTOSOMAL DOMINANT PRESENTATION. Most commonly, supravalvular aortic stenosis is a feature of the distinctive Williams syndrome described earlier.[312a, 312b] However, the aortic anomaly and pe-

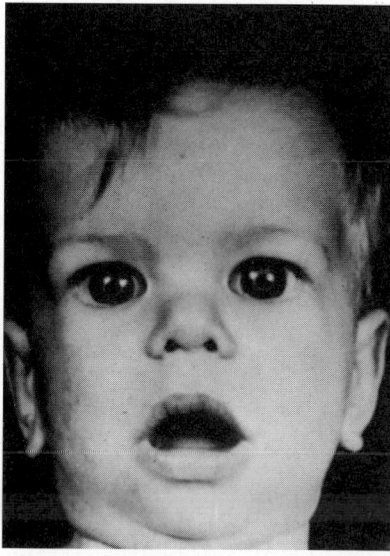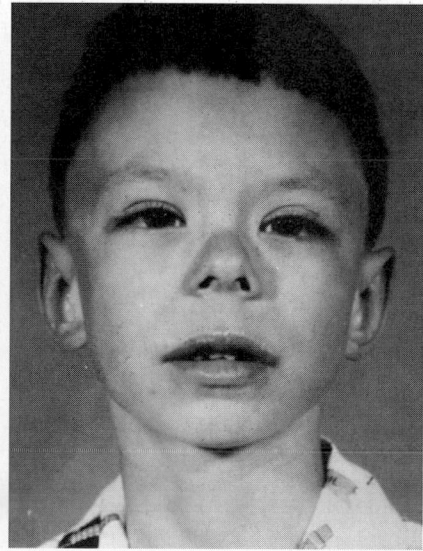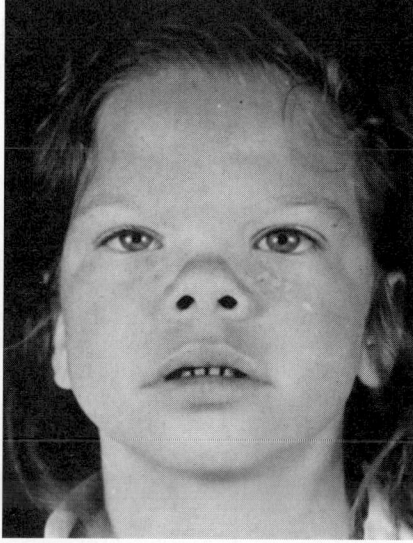

FIGURE 43–35. Typical elfin facies in three patients with supravalvular aortic stenosis. (From Friedman WF, Kirkpatrick SE: Congenital aortic stenosis. *In* Adams FH, Emmanouilides GC, Riemenschneider TA, et al: [eds]: Moss' Heart Disease in Infants, Children, and Adolescents. 4th ed. Baltimore, © Williams & Wilkins, 1989.)

ripheral pulmonary arterial stenosis are also found in familial and sporadic forms *unassociated* with the other features of the syndrome. Thus, affected patients have normal intelligence and are normal in facial appearance. Genetic studies suggest that when the anomaly is familial, it is transmitted as autosomal dominant with variable expression. Some family members may have peripheral pulmonary stenosis either as an isolated lesion or in combination with the supravalvular aortic anomaly.

Linkage analyses in two unrelated families with autosomal dominant supravalvular aortic stenosis were performed. Linkage was identified between the supravalvular aortic stenosis phenotype and polymorphic markers on the long arm of chromosome 7. These findings indicate that the gene for supravalvular aortic stenosis is located in the same chromosomal subunit as elastin. Further, a family has been identified as having autosomal dominant supravalvular aortic stenosis and a balanced translocation, which disrupts the elastin gene and cosegregates with the disease in this family, also supporting the hypothesis that mutations in the elastin gene may cause supravalvular aortic stenosis.[314] Hemizygosity at the elastin locus is likely responsible for the vascular pathology in Williams syndrome, although it is unlikely that elastin deletions account for all features of the syndrome. Because the deletions responsible for Williams syndrome extend well beyond the elastin locus, it is probable that the syndrome is a contiguous gene disorder.

MORPHOLOGY. Three anatomical types of supravalvular aortic stenosis are recognized, although some patients may have findings of more than one type. Most common is the hourglass type, in which marked thickening and disorganization of the aortic media produce a constricting annular ridge at the superior margin of the sinuses of Valsalva. The membranous type is the result of a fibrous or fibromuscular semicircular diaphragm with a small central opening stretched across the lumen of the aorta. Uniform hypoplasia of the ascending aorta characterizes the hypoplastic type.[315]

Because the coronary arteries arise proximal to the site of outflow obstruction in supravalvular aortic stenosis, they are subjected to the elevated pressure that exists within the left ventricle. These vessels often are dilated and tortuous, and premature coronary arteriosclerosis has been observed. Moreover, if the free edges of some or all of the aortic cusps adhere to the site of supravalvular stenosis, coronary artery inflow may be reduced. The formation of thoracic aortic aneurysms has been described in several patients.

CLINICAL FEATURES. Patients with Williams syndrome are mentally retarded and resemble one another in their facial features. The typical appearance is similar to that of the elfin facies observed in the severe form of idiopathic infantile hypercalcemia and is characterized by a high prominent forehead, stellate or lacy iris patterns, epicanthal folds, underdeveloped bridge of the nose and mandible, overhanging upper lip, strabismus, and anomalies of dentition (see Fig. 43–35). Recognition of this distinctive appearance, even in infancy, should alert the physician to the possibility of underlying multisystem disease. In addition, a positive family history in a patient with a normal appearance and clinical signs suggesting left ventricular outflow obstruction should lead to the suspicion of either supravalvular aortic stenosis or hypertrophic obstructive cardiomyopathy.

Patients with supravalvular aortic obstruction appear to be subject to the same risks of unexpected sudden death [in some of whom myocardial infarction has been found at autopsy[316]] and endocarditis as those with valvular aortic stenosis. Studies of the natural history of the principal vascular lesions in these patients[317]—supravalvular aortic stenosis and peripheral pulmonary artery stenosis—indicate that the aortic lesion is usually progressive, with an increase in the intensity of obstruction related often to poor growth of the ascending aorta. In contrast, the patients with pulmonary branch stenosis, whether or not associated with the aortic lesion, tend to show no change or a reduction in right ventricular pressure with time.

With few exceptions, the major *physical findings* resemble those observed in patients with valvular aortic stenosis. Among these exceptions are accentuation of aortic valve closure due to elevated pressure in the aorta proximal to the stenosis, an infrequent systolic ejection sound, and the especially prominent transmission of a thrill and murmur into the jugular notch and along the carotid vessels. Found uncommonly is an early diastolic, decrescendo, blowing murmur of aortic regurgitation caused by the fusion of one or more cusps to the area of stenosis. The narrowing of the peripheral pulmonary arteries that often coexists in these patients frequently produces a late systolic or continuous murmur that may help to distinguish this anomaly from valvular aortic stenosis. This differentiation is reinforced by the frequent finding of a significant disparity between the arterial pressures in the upper extremities in supravalvular aortic stenosis; the systolic pressure in the right arm tends to be the higher than in the left and occasionally exceeds that in the femoral arteries. The disparity in pulses may relate to the tendency of a jet stream to adhere to a vessel wall (Coanda effect) and selective streaming of blood into the innominate artery.[318, 319]

ECG usually reveals left ventricular hypertrophy when obstruction is severe. Biventricular or even right ventricular hypertrophy may be found if significant narrowing of peripheral pulmonary arteries coexists. Radiographically, in contrast to valvular and discrete subvalvular aortic stenosis, poststenotic dilation of the ascending aorta seldom is seen. The sinuses of Valsalva usually are dilated, and the ascending aorta and aortic arch appear small or of normal size.

Echocardiography is the most valuable technique for localizing the site of obstruction to the supravalvular area (Fig. 43–36). Most often the sinuses of Valsalva are dilated, and the ascending aorta and arch appear small or of normal size. A useful ratio can be constructed of the measurements of the aortic annulus and the sinotubular junction, in which the latter is always less than the former in patients with supravalvular stenosis, a finding not present in normal persons.[320] Intraluminal ultrasound imaging has also been used to visualize the vascular pathology in Williams syndrome.[321] Doppler examination and retrograde aortic catheterization can determine the degree of hemodynamic abnormality.[322]

Because of the nature of the anatomical defect, we do not think that transcatheter balloon angioplasty,[323] with or without stenting, is an effective treatment option. For several reasons, depending primarily on the anatomical variant of the lesion, supravalvular aortic stenosis may be less amenable to operative treatment than either valvular or discrete subvalvular stenosis. The lumen of the aorta at the supravalvular level may be widened by the insertion of an oval- or diamond-shaped fabric prosthesis or pericardial symmetric aortoplasty in those patients with a normal or near-normal ascending aorta. If the aorta is markedly hypoplastic, however, this operation merely displaces the pressure gradient distally without abolishing the obstruction.

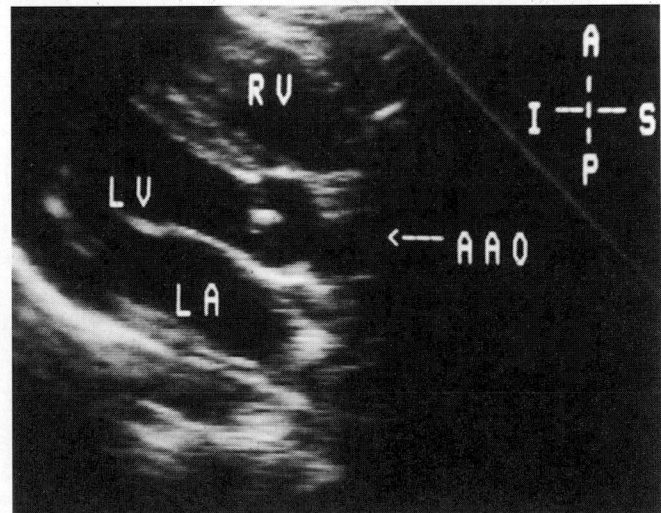

FIGURE 43–36. Supravalvar aortic stenosis is seen in a parasternal long-axis view. The constriction is distal to the sinuses of Valsalva in the ascending aorta (AAO). RV = right ventricle; LV = left ventricle; LA = left atrium.

Under these circumstances, repair may require replacement or widening of the entire hypoplastic aorta with an appropriate prosthesis.[324-327]

Hypoplastic Left Heart Syndrome

This designation is used to describe a group of closely related cardiac anomalies characterized by underdevelopment of the left cardiac chambers, atresia or stenosis of the aortic and/or the mitral orifices, and hypoplasia of the aorta.[327] These anomalies are an especially common cause of heart failure in the first week of life. The left atrium and ventricle often exhibit *endocardial fibroelastosis*. Pulmonary venous blood traverses a patent foramen ovale, and a dilated and hypertrophied right ventricle acts as the systemic, as well as pulmonary, ventricle; the systemic circulation receives blood by way of a patent ductus arteriosus (Fig. 43–37).

The diagnosis should be considered in infants, particularly boys, with the sudden onset of heart failure, systemic hypoperfusion, and nonspecific murmur. *ECG* frequently reveals right-axis deviation, right atrial and ventricular enlargement, and ST and T wave abnormalities in the left precordial leads. Chest roentgenography may show only slight enlargement shortly after birth, but with clinical deterioration there are marked cardiomegaly and increased pulmonary venous and arterial vascular markings. The *echocardiographic* findings usually are diagnostic (Fig. 43–38). The aortic root is usually diminutive, less than 4 to 5 mm in diameter at the level of the sinuses of Valsalva and narrowed farther above. The left ventricle is frequently absent or is a small slit with a diminutive mitral valve. The endocardium is often thickened, consistent with endocardial fibroelastosis or papillary muscle infarction, features usually more suggestive of aortic stenosis. Indeed, distinction from the latter is pivotal to determine if a biventricular, rather than a Fontan, approach is feasible. Ultrasound study also determines the extent of patency of the interatrial communication; substantial restriction is predictive of

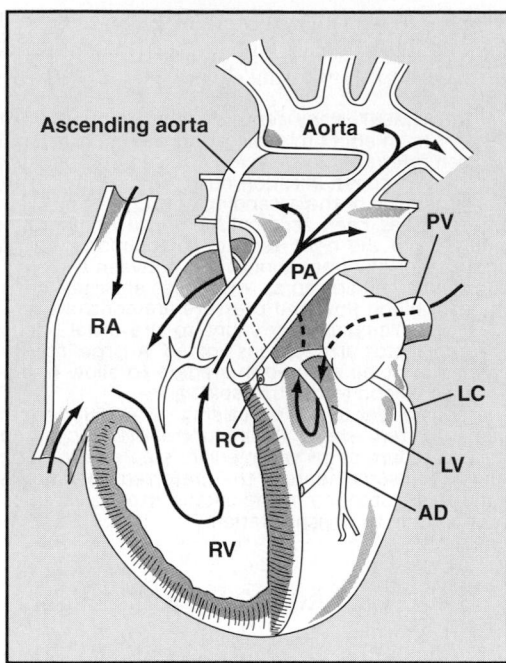

FIGURE 43–37. Hypoplastic left heart with aortic hypoplasia, aortic valve atresia, and a hypoplastic mitral valve and left ventricle. RA = right atrium; RV = right ventricle; RC = right coronary artery; PA = pulmonary artery; PV = pulmonary vein; LC = left coronary artery; LV = left ventricle; AD = anterior descending coronary artery. (From Neufeld HN, Adams P Jr, Edwards JE, et al: Diagnosis of aortic atresia by retrograde aortography. Circulation 25:278, 1962.)

severe pulmonary edema and death. *Retrograde aortography* shows hypoplasia of the ascending aorta.

MANAGEMENT. Medical therapy directed at cardiac decompensation, hypoxemia, and metabolic acidemia seldom prolongs survival beyond the first days of life.[328] Constriction of the patent ductus arteriosus and limited flow

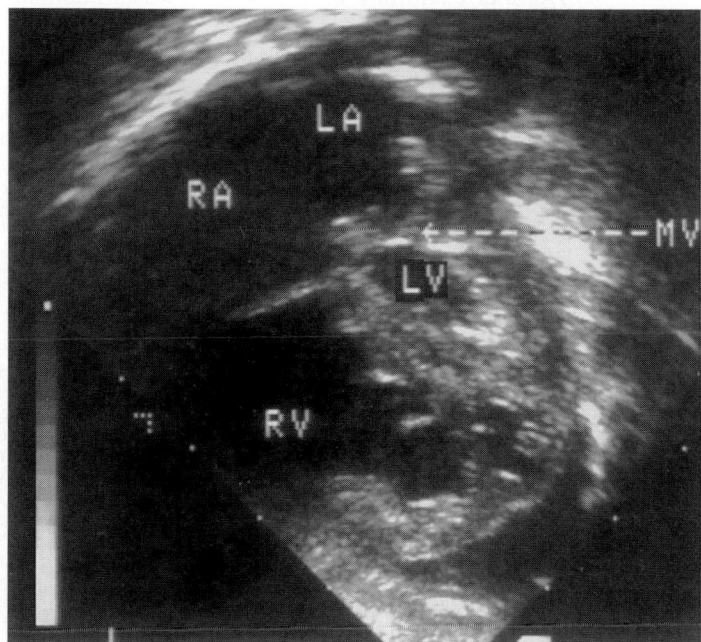
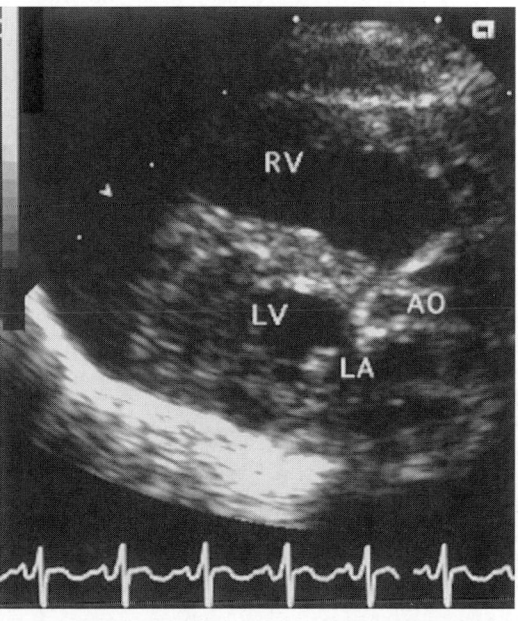

FIGURE 43–38. *Left,* Four-chamber view of hypoplastic left heart syndrome demonstrating the right ventricle (RV) anteriorly, considerably larger than the diminutive left ventricle (LV) seen posteriorly. A small mitral valve (MV) separates the left atrium (LA) from the left ventricle. The apex of the heart is formed by the right ventricle. *Right,* Parasternal long-axis view demonstrating the discrepant relative sizes between the right ventricle and the left heart chambers. The aorta (AO) is diminutive and measures approximately 4 mm in diameter. The larger pulmonary valve plate is seen anteriorly. A small platelike mitral valve (MV, dashed arrow) is seen between the left atrium and left ventricle.

through a restrictive patent foramen ovale are the principal factors responsible for early death. Prostaglandin E_1 infusion is effective in maintaining ductal patency.

SURGICAL TREATMENT. Many centers are attempting staged surgical management in an effort to provide long-term palliation.[329, 330] The first stage, often referred to as *Norwood procedure*, consists of creating an unobstructed communication between the right ventricle and aorta and enlargement of the ascending aorta. The right ventricular-aortic connection has been accomplished with homograft or prosthetic conduits from the right ventricle or pulmonary trunk to the descending aorta, or by direct connection between the proximal pulmonary trunk and ascending aorta, which also enlarges the ascending aorta. Pulmonary blood flow and pressure are controlled by a tubed interposition systemic-pulmonary shunt to the distal pulmonary artery. The patent ductus arteriosus is ligated. A large interatrial communication also must be ensured in stage 1 to allow free access of pulmonary venous blood to the tricuspid valve.

Most surgeons prefer to perform a stage 2 modified superior vena cava-pulmonary artery shunt (bidirectional Glenn operation) or a hemi-Fontan procedure as an intermediate step before a Fontan correction (stage 3). In some centers, the preferred operation is cardiac transplantation.[331, 332] Stenting of the ductus arteriosus can be used as an ambulatory bridge to transplantation.[333]

Congenital Aortic Regurgitation

Congenital aortic valve regurgitation is a rare isolated congenital cardiac lesion.[334, 345] Aortic regurgitation most often occurs in association with congenital valvular aortic stenosis in which the valve commissures are fused, inhibiting cusp mobility; subvalvular aortic stenosis in which the aortic ring is dilated and the valve cusps are deformed; coarctation of the aorta when the aortic ring is dilated and the aortic valve is bicuspid; VSD; and endocardial fibroelastosis. Aortic valve regurgitation may accompany various complex cardiac anomalies and also may accompany aortic sinus aneurysm or be secondary to dilatation of the ascending aorta in patients with Marfan syndrome, Turner syndrome, cystic medial necrosis, or osteogenesis imperfecta, in which the aortic lesions are manifestations of the underlying connective tissue disorder.

Severe aortic regurgitation also may occur through channels other than the aortic valve.[336] Thus, aortic–left ventricular tunnel is a rare anomaly that must be distinguished from congenital aortic valve regurgitation, because the approach to management of the former usually does not include consideration for prosthetic valve replacement. The aortic–left ventricular tunnel is an abnormal channel beginning in the ascending aorta above the right coronary orifice and ending in the left ventricle below the right aortic cusp. The channel usually passes behind the right ventricular infundibulum and through the ventricular septum.

Echocardiography, Doppler studies, and aortography combine to establish a precise diagnosis. Exercise testing[337] and magnetic resonance velocity mapping[338] are useful to assess the severity of the lesion. In infants and children with congenital aortic regurgitation, the severity of regurgitation increases with time, and valve replacement rather than plication is almost always necessary to correct the lesion. Operation should be deferred until symptoms, signs, and noninvasive assessment dictate its necessity.[339] Conversely, closure of an aortic–left ventricular communication is advisable before progressive dilation of the aortic annulus creates secondary changes in the aortic valve itself, which may necessitate aortic valve replacement.

Pulmonary Vein Atresia and Stenosis

Pulmonary vein atresia is a rare anomaly in which the pulmonary veins do not connect with the heart or with a major systemic vein. The lesion is incompatible with life, but infants may survive for days, probably because communications exist between the pulmonary veins and the bronchial or esophageal veins and allow limited egress for pulmonary venous blood. Pulmonary vein stenosis may occur as a focal stenosis at the atrial junction or generalized hypoplasia of one or more pulmonary veins. The incidence of associated cardiac malformations is extremely high, including atrial septal defect, tetralogy of Fallot, tricuspid and mitral atresia, and endocardial cushion defect. The severe pulmonary vein obstruction imposed by pulmonary vein abnormalities causes severe cyanosis, congestive cardiac failure, and early death. Focal stenosis of one or more pulmonary veins at the atrial junction, recognized by two-dimensional echocardiography, magnetic resonance imaging, or angiography, may be relieved surgically. Results of transcutaneous balloon angioplasty have been disappointing.

Cor Triatriatum

In this malformation, failure of resorption of the common pulmonary vein results in a left atrium divided by an abnormal fibromuscular diaphragm into a posterosuperior chamber receiving the pulmonary veins and an anteroinferior chamber giving rise to the left atrial appendage and leading to the mitral orifice.[340] The communication between the divided atrial chambers may be large, small, or absent, depending on the size of the opening in the subdividing diaphragm, which determines the degree of obstruction to pulmonary venous return. Elevations of both pulmonary venous pressure and pulmonary vascular resistance result in severe pulmonary artery hypertension.

The diagnosis is established by two-dimensional or transesophageal echocardiography[341, 342]; cardiac catheterization and angiography are necessary only if major associated cardiac anomalies are suspected. The obstructive membrane is visualized in the parasternal long- and short-axis and four-chamber (Fig. 43–39) views and can be distinguished from a supravalvular mitral ring[343] by its position superior to the left atrial appendage, which forms part of the distal chamber. Also present are diastolic fluttering of the mitral leaflets and high-velocity flow detected by Doppler examination in the distal atrial chamber and at the mitral orifice.

The diagnosis should be suspected at cardiac catheterization if the pulmonary arterial wedge pressure is higher than a simultaneous left atrial pressure. The diagnosis also may be established by visualizing the obstructing lesion angiographically. Although rare, the malformation is important to recognize because it may be easily correctable at operation.[344]

Congenital Mitral Stenosis

Anatomical types of mitral stenosis include the parachute deformity of the valve, in which shortened chordae tendineae converge and insert into a single large papillary muscle; thickened leaflets with shortening and fusion of the chordae tendineae; an anomalous arcade of obstructing papillary muscles; accessory mitral valve tissue; and a supravalvular circumferential ridge of connective tissue arising at the base of the atrial aspect of the mitral leaflets.[345, 346] Associated cardiac defects are common, including endocardial fibroelastosis, coarctation of the aorta, patent ductus arteriosus, and left ventricular outflow tract obstruction. Two-dimensional echocardiography, combined with Doppler studies, often provides a complete analysis of the anatomy and function of congenital left ventricular inflow lesions.[346] The clinical and hemodynamic consequences of isolated congenital mitral stenosis are similar to those of acquired mitral obstruction, with modifications imposed by coexisting anomalies.

The prognosis is poor; symptoms attributable to pulmonary vein obstruction usually begin in infancy, and the majority of patients expire before age 1 year unless catheter balloon dilation or operation is successful.[347, 348] Conduit bypass of the mitral valve and prosthetic valve replacement are required if a reparative operation is not possible.[349, 350] The use of a porcine bioprosthesis is contraindicated because of its rapid degeneration in an infant or young child.

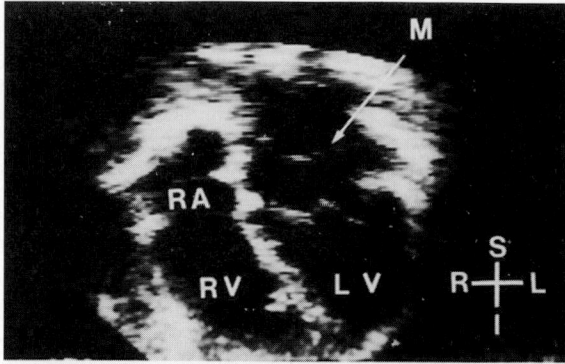

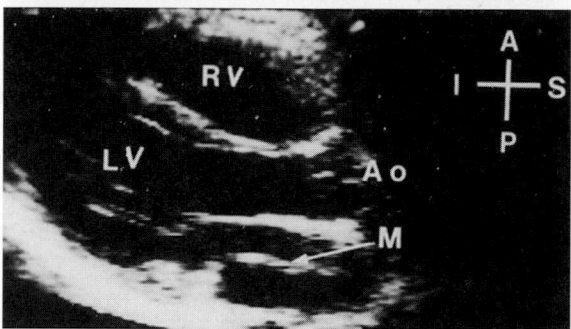

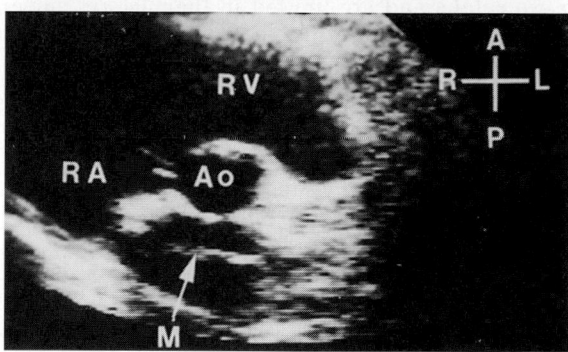

FIGURE 43–39. Echocardiograms demonstrating the membrane (M) of cor triatriatum. The apical four-chamber view *(top panel)* shows the membrane lying within the left atrial chamber. The atrial appendage is distal to the membrane, and the pulmonary veins drain into the proximal portion. The parasternal long-axis view *(center panel)* shows the membrane posterior to the aortic root (Ao) and mitral valve, dividing the left atrium into two chambers. In the parasternal short-axis view *(bottom panel)*, the membrane is within the left atrium close to the posterior aortic root. RA = right atrium; RV = right ventricle; LV = left ventricle.

Congenital Mitral Regurgitation

The syndrome of *mitral valve prolapse* is discussed in Chapter 46. This condition usually is quite benign in children.[351, 352] However, occasional difficulties exist with infective endocarditis, arrhythmias, atypical chest pain, and sudden death. *Isolated congenital mitral regurgitation* of hemodynamic significance is an unusual lesion in infants and children.

MORPHOLOGY. Congenital malformations of the mitral valve producing insufficiency most often are encountered in association with endocardial cushion defect, congenitally corrected transposition of the great arteries, endocardial fibroelastosis, anomalous pulmonary origin of the coronary artery, congenital subaortic stenosis, hypertrophic obstructive cardiomyopathy, and coarctation of the aorta. Mitral valve dysfunction also is common in various metabolic disorders (e.g., the mucopolysaccharidoses), primary and secondary cardiomyopathies, connective tissue disease (e.g., rheumatoid arthritis, Marfan's syndrome, Ehlers-Danlos syndrome, pseudoxanthoma elasticum), and rheumatic and nonrheumatic inflammatory diseases of the myocardium.[353]

The various anatomical lesions that result in isolated congenital mitral regurgitation include prolapse of one or both mitral leaflets, cleft or perforated mitral leaflet, inadequate leaflet tissue, double orifice of the mitral valve, anomalous insertion of chordae tendineae (anomalous mitral arcade), redundant leaflet tissue, displacement inferiorly of the ring of the inferior leaflet into the left ventricle, and abnormal length of the chordae tendineae.

CLINICAL FINDINGS. The clinical, echocardiographic, and hemodynamic findings in patients with isolated congenital mitral incompetence resemble those observed in acquired mitral regurgitation. Mitral annuloplasty (which is preferred) and prosthetic valve replacement are procedures reserved for infants and children who are at least moderately symptomatic despite comprehensive medical treatment, often with repeated episodes of pulmonary infection or with cardiac failure with anorexia and retarded growth and development.[353] Operative candidates are shown by echocardiographic, Doppler, hemodynamic, and angiographic studies to have pulmonary hypertension, a regurgitant fraction in excess of 50 percent, and a marked increase in left ventricular end-diastolic volume.

Pulmonary Arteriovenous Fistula

Abnormal development of the pulmonary arteries and veins in a common vascular complex is responsible for this rare congenital anomaly (see also Chap. 44). A variable number of pulmonary arteries communicate directly with branches of the pulmonary veins; in some cases, the fistula receives systemic arterial branches.[354] Most patients have an associated Weber-Osler-Rendu syndrome; additional associated problems include bronchiectasis and other malformations of the bronchial tree, as well as absence of the right lower lobe. Venoarterial shunting depends on the extent of the fistulous communications and may result in cyanosis and secondary polycythemia. Paradoxical emboli and brain abscess may cause major neurological deficits.

Patients with hereditary hemorrhagic telangiectasis often are anemic owing to repeated blood loss and may have less obvious cyanosis. Systolic and continuous murmurs are audible over areas of the fistula. Rounded opacities of various sizes in one or both lungs on chest roentgenogram may suggest the presence of the lesion. Pulmonary angiography reveals the site and extent of the abnormal communication. Unless the lesions are widespread throughout both lungs, surgical treatment aimed at removing the lesions with preservation of healthy lung tissue commonly is indicated to avoid the complications of massive hemorrhage, bacterial endocarditis, and rupture of arteriovenous aneurysms. Pulmonary arteriovenous fistulas may also be acquired and the result of surgical creation of cavopulmonary shunts.[355]

Transcatheter balloon or plug or coil occlusion embolotherapy may prove to be the therapeutic procedure of choice.[356]

Peripheral Pulmonary Artery Stenosis

Stenosis of the pulmonary artery may occur as single or numerous lesions located anywhere from the main pulmonary trunk to the smaller peripheral arterial branches.[357] Associated defects are observed in most patients and include pulmonic valvular stenosis, VSD, tetralogy of Fallot, and supravalvular aortic stenosis.

ETIOLOGY. The most important cause of significant pulmonary artery stenoses producing symptoms in newborns is intrauterine rubella infection.[358] Diagnosis is facilitated in these infants by finding elevations of the IgM fraction and rubella antibody titer. Other cardiovascular malformations commonly found in association with congenital rubella include patent ductus arteriosus, pulmonic valve stenosis, and atrial septal defect. Generalized systemic arterial stenotic lesions also may be a feature of the rubella embryopathy, often involving large and medium-sized vessels such as the aorta and coronary, cerebral, mesenteric, and renal arteries. Cardiovascular lesions are but one manifestation of intrauterine rubella infection because cataracts, microphthalmia, deafness, thrombocytopenia, hepatitis, and blood dyscrasias also are common. Thus, the clinical picture in infants with rubella syndrome depends on the severity of the cardiovascular lesions and the associated abnormalities of other organs and systems.

Peripheral pulmonary stenosis also often is associated with supravalvular aortic stenosis in patients with the familial form of the latter anomaly or in patients with Williams syndrome.

MORPHOLOGY. Obstruction within the pulmonary arterial tree may be classified into four types: (1) stenosis of the main pulmonary trunk or the main left or right branch; (2) narrowing at the bifurcation of the pulmonary artery, extending into both right and left branches; (3) numerous sites of peripheral branch stenosis; and (4) a combination of main and peripheral stenosis. Pulmonary artery obstruction may be produced by localized narrowing, diffuse constrictions, or, rarely, a membrane or diaphragm. Poststenotic dilatation is usual when the stenosis is localized but may be absent or minimal with elongated constriction. It should be recognized that a physiological branch pulmonary artery stenosis often is present in normal newborns in whom both right and left main pulmonary arteries are small and arise almost perpendicular from a large main pulmonary artery.[359] The branch vessels increase in size with growth and become less angulated in their takeoff from the main pulmonary artery.

CLINICAL FINDINGS. The degree of obstruction is the principal determinant of clinical severity; the type of obstruction determines the feasibility of direct surgical relief. The clinical features vary; most infants and children are asymptomatic.[360] An ejection systolic murmur heard at the upper left sternal border and well transmitted to the axillae and back is most common. The presence of an ejection sound suggests that pulmonic valve stenosis coexists. The pulmonic component of the second heart sound may be slightly accentuated but occasionally is extremely loud if multiple peripheral stenoses exist. A continuous murmur is audible, especially in patients with main or branch stenosis and particularly if an associated cardiovascular anomaly produces increased pulmonary blood flow. ECG shows right ventricular hypertrophy when obstruction is severe; left-axis deviation with counterclockwise orientation of the frontal QRS vector is common in the rubella syndrome and when the lesion coexists with supravalvular aortic stenosis. Mild or moderate stenosis usually produces normal findings on chest roentgenogram; detectable differences in vascularity between regions of the lungs or dilated pulmonary artery segments are uncommon. When obstruction is bilateral and severe, right atrial and ventricular enlargement may be observed.

Diagnosis. This is confirmed by observing pressure gradients within the pulmonary arterial system at cardiac catheterization; digital subtraction and/or selective pulmonary angiography defines the exact location, extent, and distribution of the lesion (Fig. 43–40). Mild to moderate unilateral or bilateral stenosis does not require surgical relief; numerous stenotic areas are not amenable to correction, even with intraoperative balloon angioplasty. Well-localized obstruction of severe degree in the main pulmonary artery or its

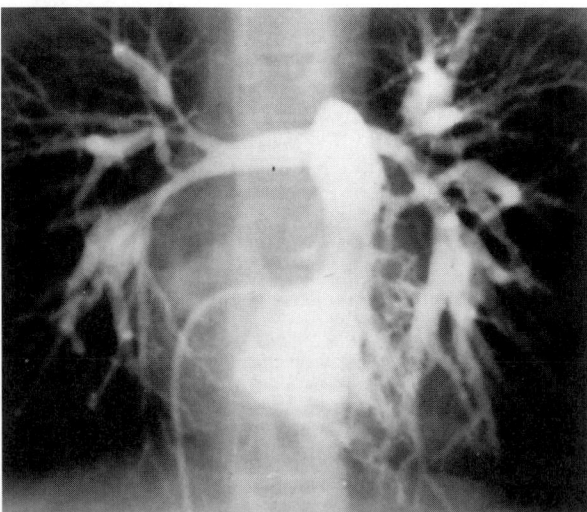

FIGURE 43–40. Right ventricular angiocardiogram showing numerous sites of peripheral pulmonic stenosis and poststenotic dilatation of the peripheral pulmonic arteries.

major branches may be alleviated by percutaneous transcatheter balloon angioplasty (see Chap. 38),[361] often accompanied by endovascular stent implantation[362, 363] or with a patch graft or bypassed with a tubular conduit. The natural history of peripheral pulmonary stenosis is not clear. Obstruction may increase by discrepant growth between a stenotic area and normal portions of the pulmonary artery tree, or as a result of an increase in cardiac output, especially during adolescence. Rarely, hypertrophy of right ventricular infundibular muscle is progressive and results in hypercyanotic spells.

Pulmonic Stenosis with Intact Ventricular Septum (See also p. 1602)

Valvular pulmonic stenosis, resulting from fusion of the valve cusps during mid- to late intrauterine development, is the most common form of isolated right ventricular obstruction and occurs in about 7 percent of patients with congenital heart disease. Hypertrophy of the septal and parietal bands narrowing the right ventricular infundibulum often accompanies the pulmonic valve lesion, especially if it is severe. Fused cusps of varying thickness and rigidity form a fibrous dome in the severest forms. Pulmonic valve dysplasia, especially common in patients with Noonan's syndrome (see Chap. 56), produces obstruction in the absence of adherent leaflets because leaflets are thickened, rigid, and myxomatous and are limited in their lateral movement because of the presence of tissue pads within the pulmonic valve sinuses.[364]

NEONATES AND INFANTS. The clinical presentation and course of circulation in a newborn with pulmonic stenosis depends on the severity of obstruction and the degree of development of the right ventricle and its outflow tract, the tricuspid valve, and the pulmonary arterial tree. The greater the degree of pulmonic valve stenosis, the more closely the manifestations resemble those observed with pulmonary atresia and intact ventricular septum. Severe pulmonic stenosis is characterized by cyanosis caused by right-to-left shunting through the foramen ovale, cardiomegaly, and diminished pulmonary blood flow in the absence of persistent patency of the ductus arteriosus. Hypoxemia and metabolic acidemia rather than right ventricular failure are the main clinical disturbances in symptomatic neonates and can be alleviated temporarily by infusion of prostaglandin E_1 to dilate the ductus arteriosus and increase pulmonary blood flow. Distinction of these babies from those with tetralogy of Fallot or tricuspid or pulmonary atresia usually is possible because infants with tetralogy usually do not have roentgenographic evidence of cardiomegaly; infants with tricuspid and pulmonary atresia show a preponderance of left ventricular forces by ECG, in contrast to the right ventricular hypertrophy usually observed with critical pulmonic stenosis in the absence of right ventricular hypoplasia.

Combined two-dimensional echocardiographic and continuous-wave Doppler examination (see Chap. 7) characterizes the anatomical valve abnormality and its severity and has essentially eliminated the requirement for cardiac catheterization and angiographic studies to establish a precise diagnosis (Fig. 43–41).[365, 366]

Balloon Valvuloplasty. Balloon dilatation of the pulmonary valve is the therapeutic procedure of choice,[365–370] but a pulmonary valvotomy and systemic-to-pulmonary arterial shunt may be necessary in infants with underdevelopment of the right ventricular cavity.[371] In this group, success has been achieved by modification of balloon valvuloplasty with predilation initially using a coronary dilatation catheter to facilitate introduction of a definitive balloon catheter. Transcatheter balloon valvuloplasty can be expected to reduce but not abolish the pressure difference in neonates with mobile doming valves. Sustained relief of the severe obstruction is usual, and so is good growth of the right ventricle. This approach is of lesser efficacy in those patients with dysplastic valves and is contraindicated if valve dysplasia is associated with annular hypoplasia.[372]

CHILDREN. The clinical profile of patients with valvular pulmonic stenosis beyond infancy usually is distinctive.[373] The severity of obstruction is the most important determinant of the clinical course. In the presence of a normal cardiac output, a peak systolic transvalvular pressure gradient between 50 and 80 mm Hg or a peak systolic right ventricular pressure between 75 and 100 mm Hg is considered to be indicative of moderate stenosis; levels below and above that range are classified as mild and severe, respectively. Most patients with mild pulmonic stenosis are asymptomatic, and the condition is discovered during routine examination. In patients with more significant obstruction, the severity of stenosis may increase with time. Progres-

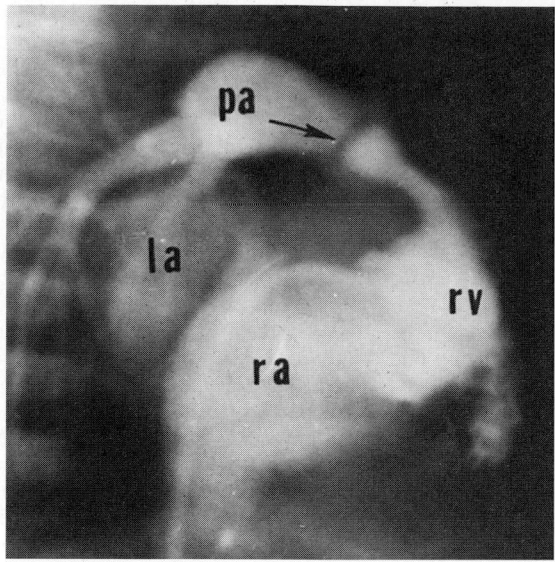 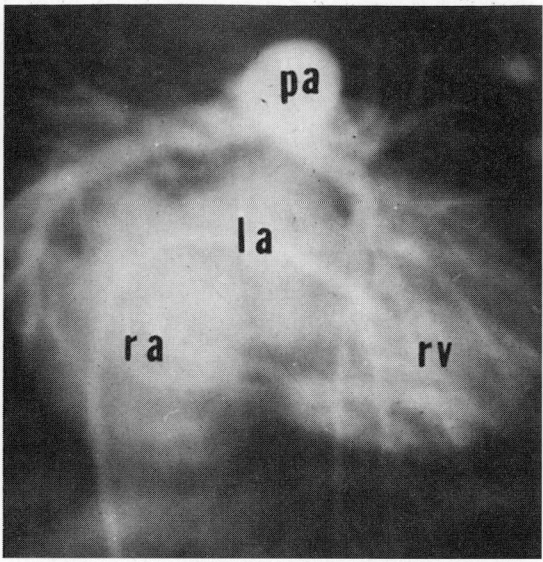

FIGURE 43–41. Right ventriculogram in an infant with critical pulmonic stenosis shows the thickened, nonmobile pulmonic valve (arrow) in the lateral projection *(left)*. Both the lateral and frontal *(right)* projections show regurgitation of contrast material across the tricuspid valve into the right atrium (ra), with subsequent shunting across the foramen ovale to the left atrium (la). rv = right ventricle; pa = pulmonary artery. (Courtesy of Dr. Norman Talner).

sion may be relative and reflect disproportional physical growth of the patient, infundibular narrowing due to progressive hypertrophy of the right ventricular outflow tract, or fibrosis of the valve cusps. Symptoms, when present, vary from mild exertional dyspnea and mild cyanosis to signs and symptoms of heart failure, depending on the degree of obstruction and the level of myocardial compensation. Exertional fatigue, syncope, and chest pain are related to an inability to augment pulmonary blood flow during exercise in some patients with moderate or severe obstruction.

PHYSICAL EXAMINATION. The severity of obstruction often is suggested by the physical findings. Right ventricular hypertrophy reduces compliance of that chamber, and a forceful right atrial contraction is necessary to augment right ventricular filling. Prominent *a* waves in the jugular venous pulse, a fourth heart sound, and, occasionally, presystolic pulsations of the liver reflect a vigorous atrial contraction and suggest the presence of severe stenosis. Cardiomegaly and a right ventricular parasternal lift accompany moderate or severe obstruction. A systolic thrill is palpable along the upper left sternal border in all but the mildest forms of stenosis. The first heart sound is normal and is followed by a systolic ejection sound at the upper left sternal edge produced by sudden opening of the stenotic valve; an ejection sound is not heard in patients with pulmonic valve dysplasia. The ejection sound typically is louder during expiration; when it is inaudible or occurs less than 0.08 second from the onset of the Q wave on ECG, severe obstruction is suggested. Right ventricular ejection is prolonged in patients with moderate or severe stenosis, and the sound of pulmonic valve closure is delayed and soft. The characteristic feature of valvular pulmonic stenosis on auscultation is a harsh, diamond-shaped systolic ejection murmur heard best at the upper left sternal border. The systolic murmur becomes louder and its crescendo occurs later in systole, obscuring the aortic component of the second sound with more severe degrees of valvular obstruction because these patients have a greater prolongation of right ventricular systole. The holosystolic decrescendo murmur of tricuspid regurgitation may accompany severe pulmonic stenosis, especially in the presence of congestive heart failure. Cyanosis, reflecting venoarterial shunting through a patent foramen ovale, is absent with mild stenosis and infrequent with moderate obstruction. Cyanosis may not be apparent in patients with severe obstruction if the atrial septum is intact.

ELECTROCARDIOGRAPHY. This technique may be helpful in assessing the degree of obstruction to right ventricular output.[374] In mild cases, the ECG often appears normal, whereas moderate and severe stenoses are associated with right-axis deviation and right ventricular hypertrophy. In the latter patients between ages 2 and 20 years, an estimate of right ventricular pressure can be made by multiplying the height of the R wave in lead V_{4R} or V_1 by 5. A tall QR wave in the right precordial leads with T wave inversion and ST segment suppression (right ventricular "strain") reflects severe stenosis. When an rSR′ pattern is observed in lead V_1 (20 percent of patients), lower right ventricular pressures are found than in patients with a pure R wave of equal amplitude. High-amplitude P waves in leads II and V_1 indicating right atrial enlargement are associated with severe stenosis.

CHEST ROENTGENOGRAPHY. In patients with mild or moderate pulmonic stenosis, chest roentgenography often shows a heart of normal size and normal pulmonary vascularity (see Chap. 8). Poststenotic dilatation of the main and left pulmonary arteries often is evident. Right atrial and right ventricular enlargement are observed in patients with severe obstruction and resultant right ventricular failure. The pulmonary vascularity may be reduced in patients with severe stenosis, right ventricular failure, and/or a venoarterial shunt at the atrial level.

ECHOCARDIOGRAPHY. Reliable localization of the site of obstruction and assessment of its severity are obtained by combined continuous-wave or pulsed-wave Doppler and two-dimensional echocardiography[375] (see Chap. 7 and Fig. 43–42). The latter usually shows prominent pulmonary valve echoes with restricted systolic motion as well as poststenotic dilation of the main pulmonary artery and its branches. In contrast to these findings in classic valvular pulmonic stenosis, patients with a dysplastic valve show thickened and immobile leaflets with hypoplasia of the pulmonary valve annulus and absent poststenotic dilatation of the pulmonary artery. Parasternal and subcostal views are required to detect most accurately maximal pulmonary artery blood flow velocity, which is converted to a pressure difference across the valve using a modified Bernoulli equation (pressure difference [mm Hg] = 4 × the squared peak Doppler velocity [m/sec]) (Fig 43–42). A semiquantitative estimation of pulmonary and tricuspid regurgitation can be

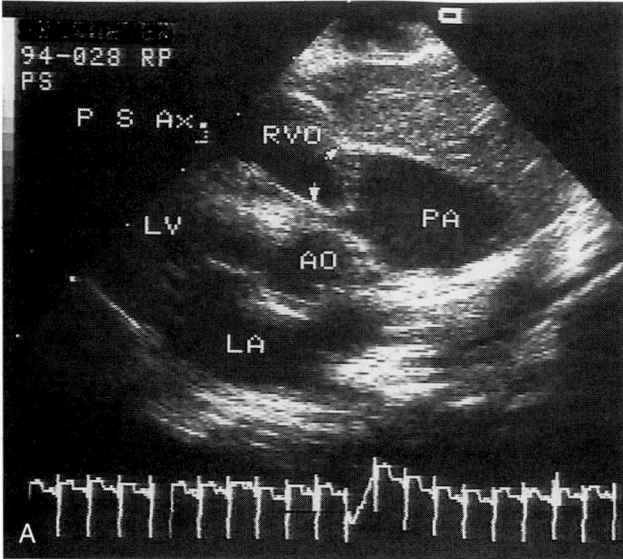

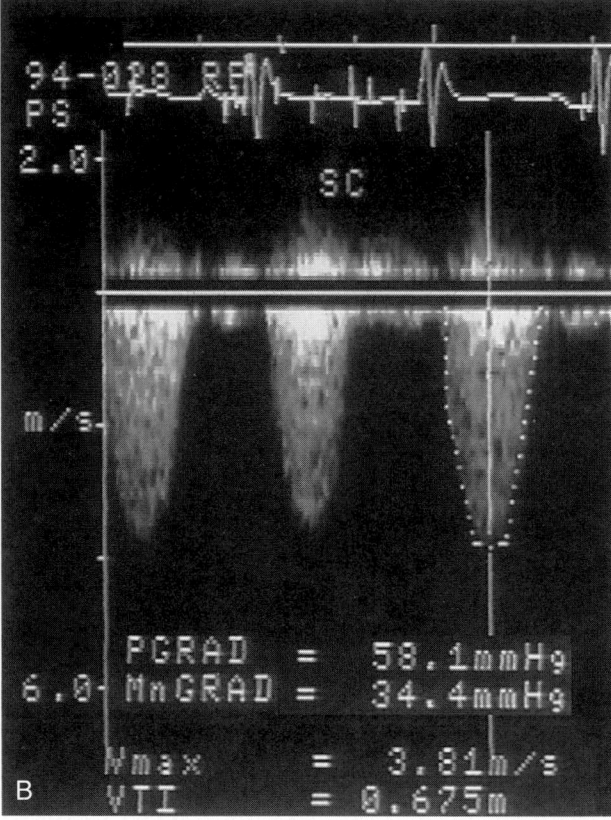

FIGURE 43–42. *A,* Severe valvular pulmonic stenosis seen from a parasternal short-axis view. The thickened pulmonary valve can be seen lying between the right ventricular outflow tract (RVO) and a dilated pulmonary artery (PA). The arrows are at the annulus of the pulmonary valve; the thickened, domed valve can be identified clearly. LV = left ventricle; AO = aorta; LA = left atrium. *B,* Doppler ultrasound from the subcostal (SC) transducer position. The velocity signal is approximately 3.8 m/sec at its height; predicted peak gradient (PGRAD) is 58 mm Hg, predicted mean gradient (MnGRAD) is 34 mm Hg.

obtained. The peak systolic velocity of the tricuspid regurgitant jet provides a reliable indirect measurement of the severity of obstruction because the reverse gradient between the right ventricle and right atrium allows derivation of the ventricular peak systolic pressure. The constant value of 14 is used for right atrial pressure in the calculation.

CARDIAC CATHETERIZATION AND ANGIOCARDIOGRA-PHY. These techniques are now used only rarely to estab-

lish or preclude other diagnostic possibilities. The usual indication for cardiac catheterization is to provide definitive therapy for the lesion. Cardiac catheterization, however, may also localize the site of obstruction, evaluate its severity, and document the coexistence of additional cardiac malformations. The resting cardiac output usually is normal, even in cases of severe stenosis, and most children show the ability to increase cardiac output with exercise.[376] Right ventricular dysfunction occurs especially when venoarterial shunting is significant and produces systemic arterial desaturation. In patients with critical stenosis, care must be taken during hemodynamic study that the cardiac catheter does not dangerously occlude the stenotic valve opening. The angiographic appearance of a typical valvular pulmonic stenosis differs from that of a dysplastic valve. The former is thickened and domed during systole, returning to normal configuration in diastole. Poststenotic dilatation of the main pulmonary trunk and sometimes of the left pulmonary artery is usual. The leaflets of the dysplastic valve are not fused anatomically but are thickened and immobile, creating little change in the angiographic picture during the cardiac cycle. Moreover, a small annulus and narrow sinuses of Valsalva are common accompaniments of valve dysplasia. With either type of valve, systolic narrowing of the right ventricular infundibulum usually is associated with moderate or severe obstruction.

NATURAL HISTORY. Mild and moderate pulmonic valve stenoses have a generally favorable course; uncommonly, progression occurs in the severity of obstruction, particularly in infancy.[377] Serial hemodynamic studies reveal unchanged pressure gradients over 4- to 8-year intervals in three-fourths of patients. Equal percentages of the remainder have an increase or a decrease in the severity of obstruction; significant increases in the pressure gradient occur especially in children with a gradient in excess of 50 mm Hg at initial examination.[373]

MANAGEMENT. Percutaneous transluminal balloon valvuloplasty (see Chap. 38) is the initial procedure of choice in patients with typical pulmonary valve stenosis and moderate to severe degrees of obstruction (Fig. 43–43).[372] This approach provides palliative improvement with the great likelihood that the improvement is permanent. In these same patients, *surgical relief* also can be accomplished at extremely low risk.[378] The valve is approached through an incision in the pulmonary arterial trunk, and resection of infundibular muscle, if necessary, may be accomplished through the pulmonic valve. Reoperation or subsequent balloon valvuloplasty is seldom required. In patients with a dysplastic valve, in whom transcatheter valvuloplasty is ineffective, the thickened valve tissue is removed and a patch often is required to widen the annulus and proximal main pulmonary artery. In children with mild pulmonic valve stenosis, prophylaxis against infective endocarditis is recommended; these patients need not restrict their physical activities. After relief of stenosis, cardiac performance as judged by exercise testing improves in children in whom postoperative resolution of right ventricular hypertrophy is expected. In contrast, myocardial fibrosis can explain a lack of improvement in adults.[379]

Pulmonic Atresia with Intact Ventricular Septum

MORPHOLOGY. This anomaly is an uncommon and highly lethal cause of neonatal cyanosis that may respond well to aggressive medical and surgical treatment.[380, 381] In almost all infants, the pulmonic valve is atretic; in the majority, both the valve ring and the main pulmonary artery are hypoplastic. The right ventricular infundibulum may occasionally be atretic or extremely narrowed. Right ventricular cavity size and configuration span the spectrum from a diminutive right ventricular chamber, often with tricuspid stenosis, to a large right ventricle, frequently with tricuspid regurgitation (Fig. 43–44). In most infants, the right ventricle is hypoplastic, and sinusoidal com-

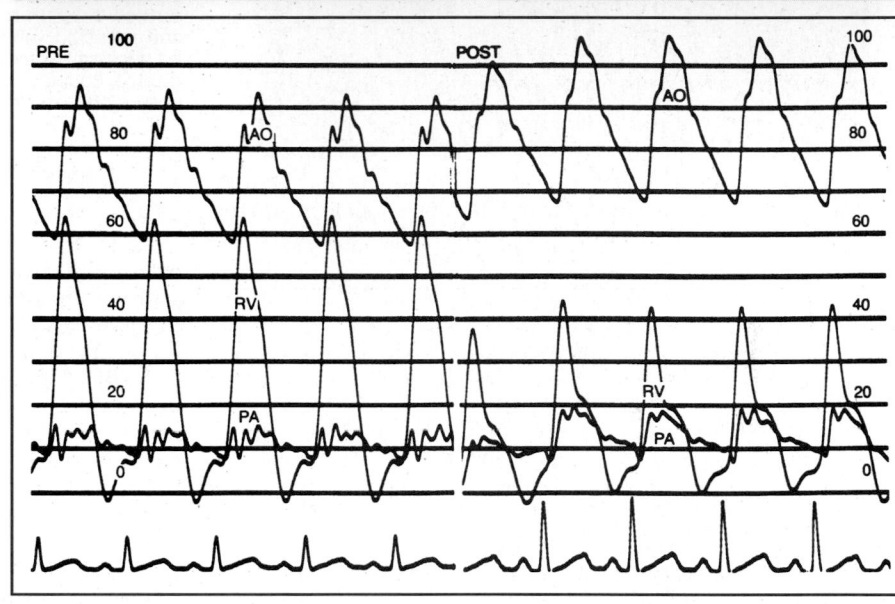

FIGURE 43–43. Right ventriculogram (RV) in the lateral projection *(top left)* from a patient with valvular pulmonic stenosis. The pulmonary valve (PV) is thickened and domes in systole. Poststenotic dilatation of the pulmonary artery (PA) is seen. At the *top right,* successful balloon valvuloplasty shows almost complete disappearance of the stenotic waist (arrow). The *bottom panel* shows the pre- *(left)* and post- *(right)* valvuloplasty hemodynamics, showing a reduction from moderately severe to mild pulmonic stenosis. AO = aorta. (Courtesy of Dr. Thomas G. DiSessa.)

munications exist in half the patients between the right ventricular cavity and the coronary circulation.[382, 383]

The intramyocardial sinusoids may end blindly or communicate with coronary arteries. Further, these communications may be nu-

merous and may feed both the left and right coronary systems, or they may be fed via a single dilated vessel. The proximal coronary arteries in some patients may be atrophic, proximal to a communication between the sinusoids and the distal coronary artery, particularly

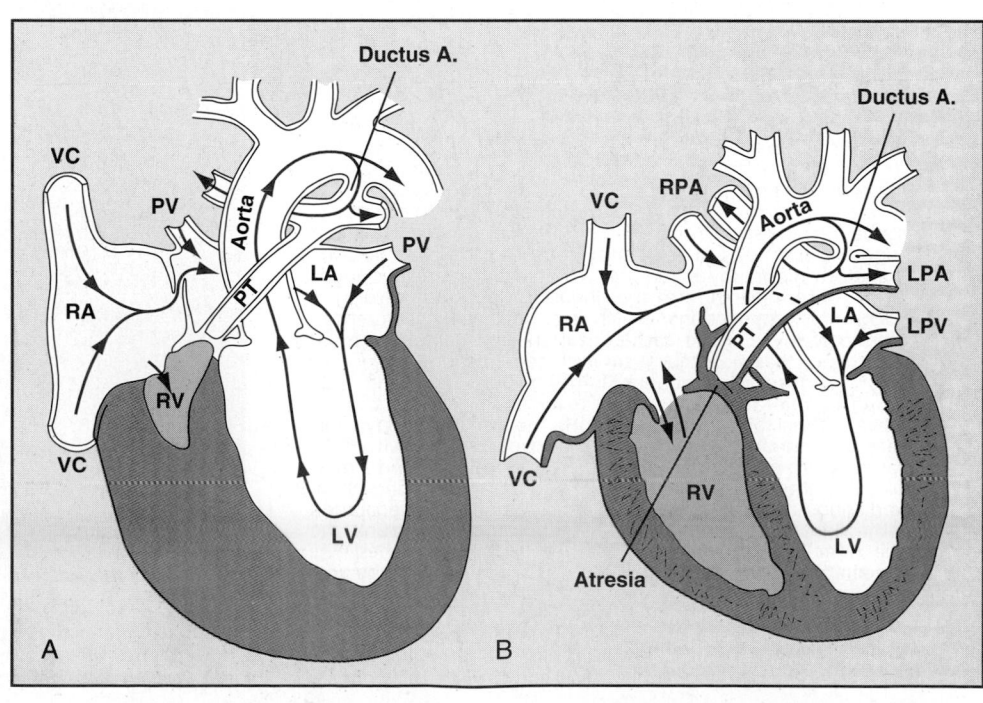

FIGURE 43–44. Pulmonic atresia with intact ventricular septum. With a competent tricuspid valve, the right ventricular chamber is diminutive *(A)*; significant tricuspid regurgitation is associated with a normal or large right ventricular cavity *(B)*. VC = vena cava; RA = right atrium; RV = right ventricle; PT = pulmonary trunk; PV = pulmonary vein; LA = left atrium; LV = left ventricle; Ductus A. = ductus arteriosus; LPA = left pulmonary artery; RPA = right pulmonary artery; LPV = left pulmonary vein. (From Edwards JE: Congenital malformations of the heart and great vessels. *In* Gould SE [ed]: Pathology of the Heart. 2nd ed, 1960. Courtesy of Charles C Thomas, Publisher, Ltd., Springfield, Illinois.)

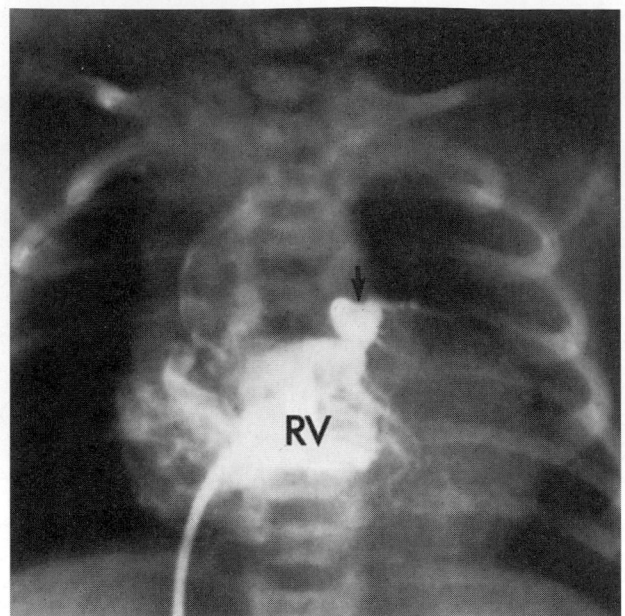

FIGURE 43–45. Right ventricular angiocardiogram in the frontal projection in a 1-day-old infant with an atretic pulmonic valve (arrow). The cavity of the right ventricle (RV) is small and eccentrically shaped. (Courtesy of Dr. Robert Freedom.)

in hearts with severe hypoplasia of the right ventricle. In these circumstances, the distal coronary vessels are supplied by communications with the right ventricle, and the coronary circulation therefore is right ventricle dependent. In this group, decompression of the right ventricle by a surgical procedure would be associated with a high risk of myocardial ischemia and death.[384, 385]

Because the pulmonic valve is imperforate and completely obstructed, systemic venous blood returning to the heart bypasses the right ventricle through an interatrial communication. Right ventricular output does not contribute to the effective cardiac output and is proportional to the magnitude of tricuspid regurgitation and the size and extent of the sinusoidal communications with the coronary arterial tree. The blood supply to the lungs is derived from the bronchial circulation and from flow through a persistently patent ductus arteriosus. The size and patency of the ductus arteriosus are critical determinants in postnatal survival; ductus closure results in death. Reduced pulmonary blood flow by way of a partially constricted ductus arteriosus results in profound hypoxemia, tissue hypoxia, and metabolic acidemia.

DIAGNOSIS. The diagnosis is suggested by roentgenographic findings of pulmonary hypoperfusion and the ECG observation of a normal QRS axis, absent or diminished right ventricular forces, and/or dominant left ventricular forces. In the minority of infants with marked tricuspid regurgitation, the right ventricle and right atrium are massively enlarged. The echocardiogram in the usual infant shows a small right ventricular cavity and diminutive or absent pulmonic valve echoes.[386] Doppler examination shows continuous retrograde flow to the pulmonary artery and/or its branches through a patent ductus arteriosus, which usually is narrow and tortuous. Only if tricuspid valve echoes are imaged by ultrasound examination can tricuspid atresia be distinguished from pulmonic atresia.

Although the diagnosis of this entity can be made by echocardiography, angiocardiography is required to assess treatment options because key determinants are the identification and nature of ventriculocoronary connections, which are not well characterized by echocardiography. Cardiac catheterization is usually performed on an emergency basis. Because survival depends on patency of the ductus arteriosus, intravenous infusion of prostaglandin E₁, (0.05 to 0.1 μg/kg/min) may dramatically reverse clinical deterioration and improve arterial blood gases and pH. The usual hemodynamic findings are right atrial and right ventricular hypertension, with right ventricular pressure often greater than systemic pressure, and a massive right-to-left interatrial shunt. Selective angiocardiography establishes the diagnosis and allows evaluation of the degree of separation between the right ventricular infundibular and pulmonary trunk, the size of the right ventricular cavity and the pulmonary arteries (Fig. 43–45), the anatomy and function of the tricuspid valve, and the anatomical and functional details of the coronary circulation.

MANAGEMENT. Initial stabilization is usually required in infants, necessitating infusion of prostaglandin E₁ to dilate the ductus arteriosus and measures to correct metabolic acidosis. The rare infant with membranous pulmonary atresia may be a candidate for balloon val-

votomy. Initial surgical considerations focus on whether the patient is a candidate for a biventricular or univentricular (Fontan) repair (Fig. 43–45).[384, 387–389] The angiographic delineation of coronary artery anatomy determines the feasibility of early decompression of the right ventricle, because this approach is contraindicated when there are ventriculocoronary connections with part or all of the coronary circulation right ventricle dependent. Patients in this latter group cannot undergo operation that decompresses the right ventricle and are ultimately candidates for a lateral tunnel Fontan procedure, after initial palliation by balloon atrial septostomy followed by a systemic-pulmonary artery shunt.[390]

At the other end of the spectrum, babies with only mild hypoplasia of the right ventricle and tricuspid valve are candidates for a transventricular closed pulmonary valvotomy, followed later by balloon angioplasty or repeat surgical valvotomy. Ultimately, the size of the tricuspid valve and right ventricle, and occasionally the presence of coronary artery obstructive lesions in association with right ventricle to coronary artery fistulas, will dictate whether patients will be candidates for two-ventricle repair or whether a less corrective procedure such as the Fontan operation will be the most definite surgical option.[387] In infants with moderate right ventricular hypoplasia, a biventricular repair is preferred, often using a homograft valve in the outflow tract. In this group, the smaller the size of the right ventricle and tricuspid valve, the more likely a partial biventricular repair will be necessary, relieving the outflow tract obstruction with insertion of a valve, coupled with a bidirectional cavopulmonary (Glenn) shunt to ensure obligatory pulmonary blood flow.

Intraventricular Right Ventricular Obstruction

Infundibular pulmonic stenosis with an intact ventricular septum and the presence of anomalous muscle bundles are the two principal causes of intraventricular right ventricular obstruction (Fig. 43–46).[391]

SUBPULMONIC INFUNDIBULAR STENOSIS. This anomaly usually occurs at the proximal portion of the infundibulum and consists of a fibrous band at the junction of the right ventricular cavity and outflow tract. The clinical manifestations, course, and prognosis of infundibular stenosis are similar to those of valvular stenosis, although the former diagnosis is suggested by the absence of a systolic ejection

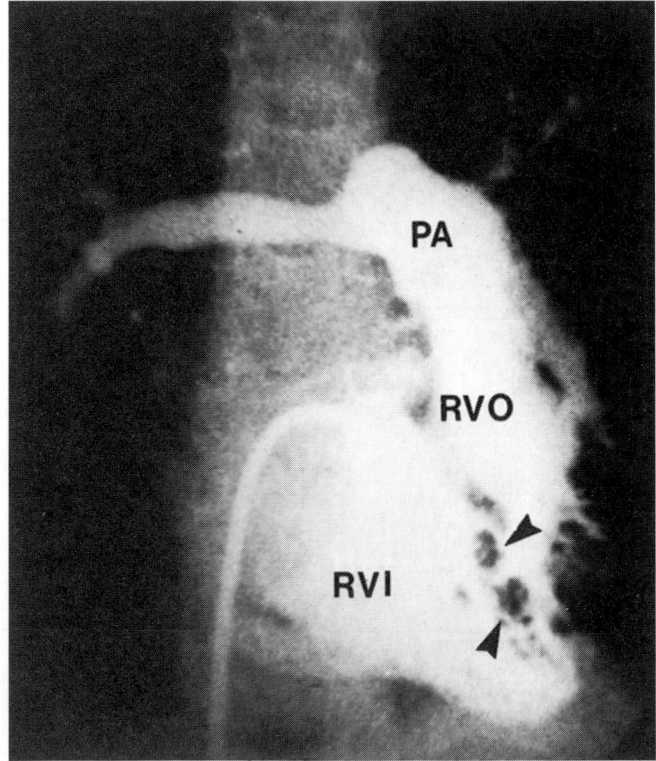

FIGURE 43–46. Intraventricular right ventricular obstruction. The right ventricular inflow (RVI) and outflow (RVO) tracts are separated by bands (arrowheads), creating intraventricular right ventricular obstruction. PA = pulmonary artery.

sound and a systolic murmur lower along the left sternal border. Doppler echocardiography, withdrawal pressure tracings, and selective right ventricular angiocardiography permit localization of the site of obstruction and assessment of its extent and severity. Surgical treatment consists of resection of the fibrotic narrowed area and hypertrophied muscle. It may occasionally be necessary to widen the outflow tract with a pericardial or prosthetic patch.

ANOMALOUS MUSCLE BUNDLES. A two-chambered right ventricle is formed by right ventricular obstruction due to anomalous muscle bundles; most of the patients have an associated malalignment or perimembranous VSD, and about 5 percent have subaortic stenosis.[392] Aberrant hypertrophied muscle bands, occasionally in association with a VSD, traverse the right ventricular cavity, extending from its anterior wall to the crista supraventricularis and/or the portion of the adjacent interventricular septum. The anomalous pyramid-shaped muscle mass obstructs blood flow through the body of the right ventricle and produces a proximal high-pressure inflow chamber and a distal low-pressure chamber. Thus, this type of obstruction is distinguishable from that in tetralogy of Fallot, in which hypertrophied infundibular muscle protrudes into but does not cross the cavity of the right ventricle.

The clinical, ECG, and chest roentgenographic findings resemble those observed in pulmonic valvular or subvalvular infundibular obstruction, although the systolic thrill and murmur may be displaced lower along the left sternal border. Progressive obstruction occurs in some patients. The diagnosis may be established by two-dimensional echocardiography.[393] Selective right ventricular angiocardiography provides the most accurate diagnosis and reveals a filling defect in the midportion of the right ventricle; this defect often does not change significantly with systole and diastole.

Management. The treatment for anomalous muscle bundles consists of surgical removal.[394] In the absence of preoperative recognition of the anomaly, the surgeon should be alerted to the correct diagnosis by the presence of a dimple during contraction on the ordinarily smooth anterior surface of the right ventricle and/or the inability to view the tricuspid valve through a longitudinal ventriculotomy because of the presence of the abnormal muscle mass.

Tetralogy of Fallot

DEFINITION. The overall incidence of this anomaly approaches 10 percent of all forms of congenital heart disease, and it is the most common cardiac malformation responsible for cyanosis after 1 year of age. The four components of this malformation are (1) VSD, (2) obstruction to right ventricular outflow, (3) overriding of the aorta, and (4) right ventricular hypertrophy. The basic anomaly is the result of an anterior deviation of the septal insertion of the infundibular ventricular septum from its usual location in the normal heart between the limbs of the trabecular septum. The interventricular malalignment defect usually is large, approximating the aortic orifice in size, and is located high in the septum just below the right cusp of the aortic valve, separated from the pulmonic valve by the crista supraventricularis. The aortic root may be displaced anteriorly and straddle or override the septal defect, but as in a normal heart, it lies to the right of the origin of the pulmonary artery. In most cases, no dextroposition of the aorta exists; overriding of the aorta is a phenomenon secondary to the subaortic location of the VSD.

HEMODYNAMICS. The degree of obstruction to pulmonary blood flow is the principal determinant of the clinical presentation.[395] The site of obstruction is variable[396]; infundibular stenosis is the only major obstruction in about 50 percent of patients and coexists with valvular obstruction in another 20 to 25 percent (Fig. 43–47). Supravalvular and peripheral pulmonary arterial narrowing may be observed, and unilateral absence of a pulmonary artery (usually the left) is found in a small number of patients. Circulation to the abnormal lung is accomplished by bronchial and other collateral arteries.[397, 398] Atresia of the pulmonic valve, infundibulum, or main pulmonary artery is occasionally referred to as "pseudotruncus arteriosus." True truncus arteriosus with absent pulmonary arteries (type 4) differs from

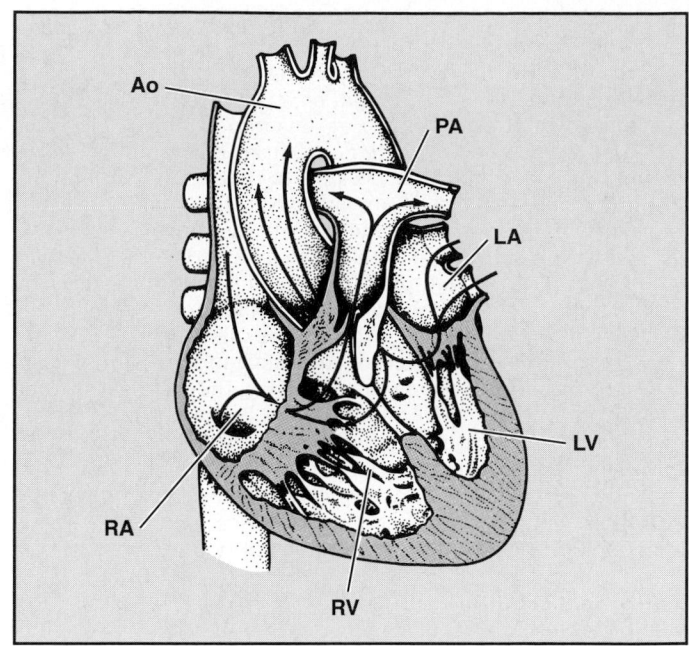

FIGURE 43–47. Tetralogy of Fallot with infundibular and valvular pulmonic stenosis. The arrows indicate direction of blood flow. A substantial right-to-left shunt exists across the ventricular septal defect. RA = right atrium; LA = left atrium; RV = right ventricle; LV = left ventricle; Ao = aorta; PA = pulmonary artery.

tetralogy of Fallot, in which pulmonary artery branches are present but are fed by a patent ductus arteriosus and/or bronchial arteries (see Fig. 43–50). A right-sided aortic knob, aortic arch, and descending aorta occur in about 25 percent of patients with tetralogy of Fallot. The coronary arteries may have surgically important variations[399]: The anterior descending artery may originate from the right coronary artery; a single right coronary artery may give off a left branch that courses anterior to the pulmonary trunk; a single left coronary artery may give off a right branch that crosses the infundibulum of the right ventricle. Enlargement of the infundibulum branch of the right coronary artery often presents a problem with respect to a right ventriculotomy.

Associated cardiac anomalies exist in about 40 percent of patients. Major associated cardiac anomalies include patent ductus arteriosus, numerous (usually muscular) VSDs, and complete AV septal defects. Localized single or multiple peripheral pulmonary arterial stenotic lesions are common; rarely, the right or left pulmonary artery may arise anomalously from the ascending aorta. Infrequently, aortic valve regurgitation results from aortic cusp prolapse. Associated extracardiac anomalies are present in 20 to 30 percent of patients.

The relation between the resistance of blood flow from the ventricles into the aorta and into the pulmonary vessels has a major role in determining the hemodynamic and clinical picture.[400] Thus, the severity of obstruction to right ventricular outflow is of fundamental significance. When right ventricular outflow tract obstruction is severe, the pulmonary blood flow is markedly reduced, and a large volume of unsaturated systemic venous blood is shunted from right to left across the VSD. Severe cyanosis and polycythemia occur, and symptoms and sequelae of systemic hypoxemia are prominent. At the opposite end of the spectrum, the term "acyanotic" or "pink" tetralogy of Fallot often is used to describe an interventricular communication and a milder degree of obstruction to right ventricular outflow with little or no venoarterial shunting. In many infants and children, the obstruction to right ventricular outflow is mild but progressive, so that early in life pulmonary exceeds systemic blood flow and the symptoms resemble those produced by a simple VSD.

CLINICAL MANIFESTATIONS. Few children with tetralogy of Fallot remain asymptomatic or acyanotic (see Chap. 44). Most are cyanotic from birth or develop cyanosis before age 1 year. In general, the earlier the onset of systemic hypoxemia, the more likely the possibility that severe pulmonary outflow tract stenosis or atresia exists. Dyspnea with exertion, clubbing, and polycythemia is common. When resting after exertion, children with tetralogy characteristically assume a squatting posture. The latter may be obvious even in infancy; many cyanotic infants prefer to lie in a knee-chest position. Spells of intense cyanosis related to a sudden increase in renoarterial shunting and a reduction in pulmonary blood flow most often have their onset between 2 and 9 months of age and constitute an important threat to survival.[401, 402] The attacks are not restricted to patients with severe cyanosis; they are most common in the morning after awakening and are characterized by hyperpnea and increasing cyanosis that progresses to limpness and syncope and occasionally terminates in convulsions, a cerebrovascular accident, and death.

Physical Examination. This reveals variable degrees of underdevelopment and cyanosis. Clubbing of the terminal digits may be prominent after the first year of life. The heart is not hyperactive or enlarged; a right ventricular impulse and systolic thrill often are palpable along the left sternal border. An early systolic ejection sound that is aortic in origin may be heard at the lower left sternal border and apex; the second heart sound is single, the pulmonic component rarely being audible. A systolic ejection murmur is produced by flow across the narrowed right ventricular infundibulum or pulmonic valve. The intensity and duration of the murmur vary inversely with the severity of obstruction—the opposite of the relation that exists in patients with pulmonic stenosis and an intact ventricular septum. Polycythemia, decreased systemic vascular resistance, and increased obstruction to right ventricular outflow may all be responsible for a decrease in intensity of the murmur; with extreme outflow tract stenosis or pulmonic atresia and during an attack of paroxysmal hypoxemia, no murmur or only a very short, faint murmur may be detected. A continuous murmur faintly audible over the anterior or posterior chest reflects flow through enlarged bronchial collateral vessels. A loud continuous murmur of flow through a patent ductus arteriosus occasionally may be heard at the upper left sternal border.

LABORATORY EXAMINATIONS. The *ECG* ordinarily shows right ventricular and, less frequently, right atrial hypertrophy. In a patient with acyanotic tetralogy, combined ventricular hypertrophy may be noted initially, progressing to right ventricular hypertrophy as cyanosis develops. *Roentgenographic* examination characteristically reveals a normal-sized boot-shaped heart (coeur en sabot) with prominence of the right ventricle and a concavity in the region of the underdeveloped right ventricular outflow tract and main pulmonary artery. The pulmonary vascular markings are typically diminished, and the aortic arch and knob may be on the right side; the ascending aorta usually is large. A uniform, diffuse, fine reticular pattern of vascular markings is noted in the presence of prominent collateral vessels.

Echocardiography. Findings include aortic enlargement, aortic-septal discontinuity, and aortic overriding of the ventricular septum.[403] Two-dimensional echocardiography (see Chap. 7) shows the right ventricular outflow tract to be narrowed and in a more horizontal orientation than normal. The main pulmonary artery and its branches are mildly to severely hypoplastic. The usual ventricular septal malalignment defect lies superior to the tricuspid valve and immediately below the aortic valve cusps. These findings are best displayed in views of the long axis of the right ventricular outflow tract, which are the subxiphoid short

axis and the high transverse parasternal echo windows. Echo views that show the anteroposterior coordinates best indicate the overriding of the aorta; these are the parasternal long-axis, apical two-chamber, and subxiphoid views (Fig. 43–48). The echocardiographic examination also reveals the origin of the main pulmonary artery from the right ventricle, as well as continuity of the main pulmonary artery with its right and left branches, and is accurate for diagnosing coronary abnormalities,[404, 405] although the latter are identified best by angiography. Delineation or complex pulmonary vascular abnormalities may require combined angiography and advanced CT[406] (see Chaps. 10 and 11). Combined angiography and three-dimensional CT has been shown to be useful for assessing systemic-to-pulmonary collaterals. The demonstration of mitral-semilunar valve continuity helps to distinguish tetralogy from double-outlet right ventricle with pulmonic stenosis, in which discontinuity of the mitral valve echo and the aortic cusp echo is a critical feature.

Cardiac Catheterization and Angiocardiography (Fig. 43–49). Despite the accuracy of noninvasive approaches, many centers still consider invasive study necessary to confirm the diagnosis; assess the magnitude of right-to-left shunting; provide details of additional muscular VSDs, if present; evaluate the architecture of the right ventricular outflow tract, pulmonic valve, and annulus and the morphology and caliber of the main branches of the pulmonary arteries; and analyze the anatomy of the coronary arteries. *Axial cineangiography,* using the sitting-up projection, greatly facilitates evaluation of the pulmonary outflow tract and arteries.[137] Preoperative assessment of tetralogy with pulmonic atresia must include delineation of the arterial supply to both lungs by selective catheterization and visualization of bronchial collateral arteries with late serial filming; pulmonary arteries may be opacified only after the bronchial collateral arteries have cleared of contrast material (Fig. 43–50). A patient with pulmonic atresia should not be ruled out as a candidate for surgical correction unless an inadequate pulmonary arterial supply to the lungs is clearly demonstrated.[397] Rarely, injection of contrast through a catheter in the pulmonary venous capillary wedge position is required to assess the possibility that anatomical pulmonary arteries are present. CT may visualize central pulmonary arteries when conventional angiography cannot.

MANAGEMENT. Among the factors that may complicate the management of tetralogy are iron deficiency anemia,

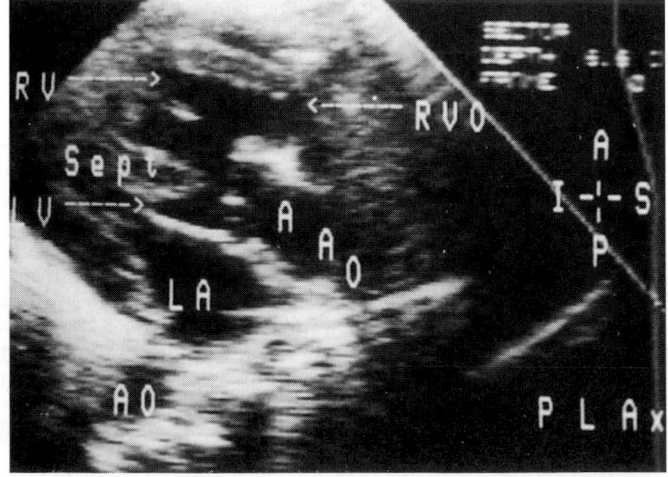

FIGURE 43–48. Tetralogy of Fallot in a parasternal long-axis (PLAx) view, which demonstrates the aorta overriding the ventricular septum (Sept). RV = right ventricle; RVO = right ventricular outflow tract; LV = left ventricle; LA = left atrium; AO = aorta; AAO = ascending aorta.

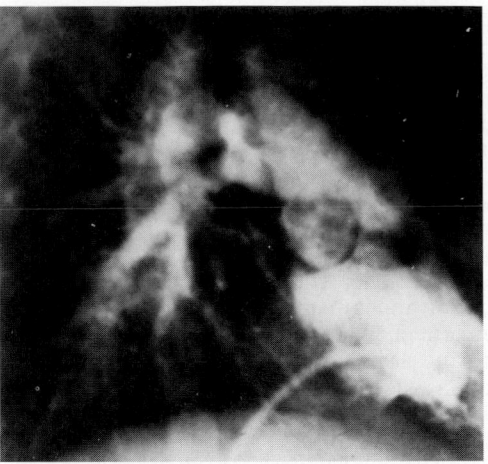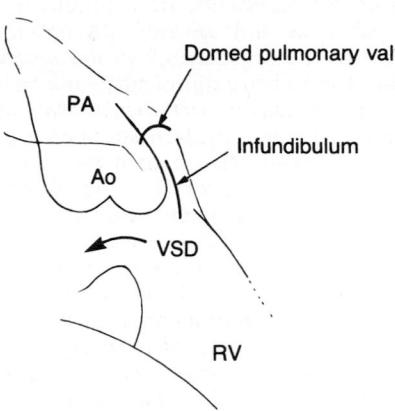

FIGURE 43–49. Lateral view of a right ventriculogram in a child with tetralogy of Fallot showing simultaneous opacification of the pulmonary artery (PA) and aorta (Ao). PV = pulmonic valve; VSD = ventricular septal defect; RV = right ventricle.

infective endocarditis, paradoxical embolism, polycythemia, coagulation disorders, and cerebral infarction or abscess. Paroxysmal hypercyanotic spells may respond quickly to oxygen, placing the child in the knee-chest position, and morphine. If the spell persists, metabolic acidosis develops from prolonged anaerobic metabolism, and infusion of sodium bicarbonate may be necessary to interrupt the attack. Vasopressors, beta-adrenoceptor blockade, or general anesthesia occasionally may be necessary.[402]

Total Surgical Correction. This operation is advisable ultimately for almost all patients with tetralogy of Fallot. Early definitive repair, even in infancy, is currently advocated in most centers that are experienced in intracardiac surgery in infants.[407–409] Successful early correction appears to prevent the consequences of progressive infundibular obstruction and acquired pulmonic atresia, delayed growth and development, and complications secondary to hypoxemia and polycythemia with bleeding tendencies. The anatomy of the right ventricular outflow tract and the size of the pulmonary arteries, rather than the age or size of the infant or child, are the most important determinants in assessing candidacy for primary repair; a transannular patch may be used in infants with severe outflow narrowing.[410] Marked hypoplasia of the pulmonary arteries is a relative contraindication for early corrective operation.

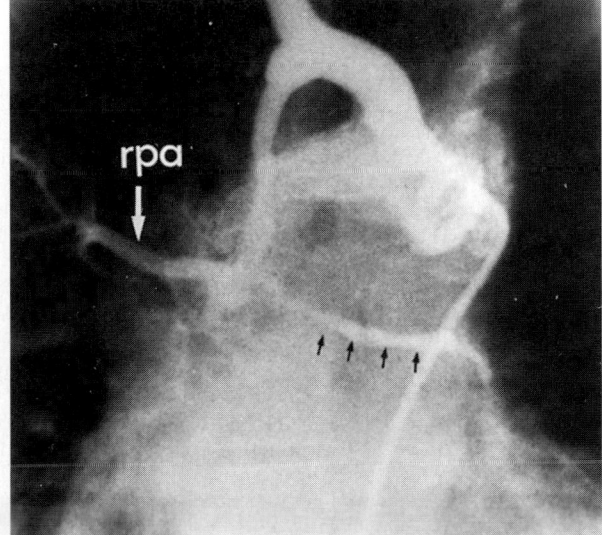

FIGURE 43–50. Selective systemic collateral bronchial arteriogram demonstrates gull-wing configuration of the hypoplastic right pulmonary artery (rpa) and left pulmonary artery (arrows) in a patient with tetralogy of Fallot and pulmonic atresia. (Courtesy of Dr. Robert Freedom.)

Palliative Surgery. When marked hypoplasia of the pulmonary arteries exists, a palliative operation designed to increase pulmonary blood flow is recommended and usually consists in the smallest infants of a systemic–pulmonary arterial anastomosis.[411] A transventricular infundibulectomy or valvulotomy is an alternative palliative procedure that may be considered. Balloon dilatation of the pulmonary valve may afford palliation in selected infants.[412] Total correction can then be carried out at a lower risk later in childhood. The palliative procedures relieve hypoxemia caused by diminished pulmonary blood flow and reduce the stimulus to polycythemia. Because pulmonary venous return is augmented, the left atrium and ventricle are stimulated to enlarge their capacity in anticipation of total correction. In the most severe forms of tetralogy of Fallot with pulmonic atresia, the goals of operation include establishment of nonstenotic continuity between the right ventricle and pulmonary arteries, closure of the intracardiac shunt, and interruption of surgically created shunts or major collateral arteries to the lungs. Transcatheter coil occlusion of significant aorta-pulmonary collateral vessels as well as of modified Blalock-Taussig shunts and ascending aorta to pulmonary artery interposition grafts can be used before corrective operation.[413, 414] When atresia is confined to the infundibulum or pulmonic valve, repair may be accomplished by infundibular resection and reconstruction of the outflow tract with a pericardial patch. If a long segment of pulmonary arterial atresia exists, a valve-containing conduit is inserted from the right ventricle to the distal pulmonary artery.[415] The presence of a single pulmonary artery in the hilus of either lung is a prerequisite for repair of pulmonic atresia. Prior unifocalization to incorporate several systemic to pulmonary artery collaterals into a neopulmonary artery may be required in selected patients.[416] A conduit also may be necessary in less severe forms of right ventricular outflow tract obstruction when an anomalous coronary artery crosses the right ventricular outflow tract.

Postoperative Complications. Various complications are common in the postoperative period after palliative or corrective operation. Mild to moderate left ventricular decompensation may be secondary to the sudden increase in pulmonary venous return; various degrees of pulmonic valvular regurgitation increase right ventricular cavity size further. Patients with progressive pulmonary insufficiency and severe right ventricular dilatation are candidates for prosthetic pulmonary valve insertion.[417]

Bleeding problems are common, especially in older polycythemic patients (see Chap. 44). Complete right bundle branch block or the pattern of left anterior hemiblock often is seen, but disabling dysrhythmias are infrequent.[418, 419] Restricted pulmonary arterial flow is the greatest cause of early and late mortality and poor late results.[420] After convalescence from intracardiac repair, symptoms of hypoxemia and severe exercise intolerance are relieved even in the presence of some residual right ventricular outflow tract obstruction, pulmonic valve incompetence, and/or cardiomegaly. However, cardiovascular performance at rest or during exercise may remain below normal,[421-423] and major complications, such as trifascicular block, complete heart block, ventricular arrhythmias, and sudden death, may rarely occur many years after surgical treatment.[419]

Late ventricular arrhythmias are rare in patients with successful early correction of the malformation unless complex or numerous operations were performed. Because widespread use of ambulatory ECG monitoring has resulted in greater detection of ventricular arrhythmias, usually isolated ventricular extrasystoles or nonsustained tachycardia, some have suggested that the asymptomatic patients in this category should have pharmacological suppression of their arrhythmias. It would appear that both ventricular depolarization and repolarization abnormalities contribute to the pathogenesis of ventricular arrhythmias after repair of the anomaly (see Chaps. 25 and 44). Most studies, however, do not support the use of potentially dangerous long-term antiarrhythmic treatment for asymptomatic postoperative patients, and a large-scale long-term follow-up study is indicated before prophylactic therapeutic options can be established definitively (see Chap. 23).

Congenital Absence of the Pulmonic Valve

PATHOLOGY AND PATHOGENESIS. In the majority of cases of this rare malformation, the lesion is associated with a VSD, a narrowed obstructive annulus of the pulmonic valve, and marked aneurysmal dilatation of the pulmonary arteries. The combination of anomalies often is referred to as tetralogy of Fallot with absent pulmonic valve. The obstructing lesion principally consists of underdeveloped, primitive valve tissue within a hypoplastic annulus; infundibular obstruction and the VSD do not differ from classic tetralogy of Fallot. Reports indicate that deletion within chromosome 22 is common in patients with this anomaly.[424]

The massively dilated pulmonary arteries often are the major determinant of the clinical course because they frequently result in upper airway obstruction and severe respiratory distress in infancy.[425] Smaller intrapulmonary bronchi may also be compressed by abnormally branching distal pulmonary arteries, and in some cases the number of bronchial generations or alveolar multiplications is reduced.[426] Poststenotic pulmonary artery aneurysms develop in utero, and their size and location appear to be related to the magnitude of pulmonic regurgitation in fetal life, the orientation of the right ventricular infundibulum to the right or left, and the size of the ductus arteriosus.[427]

CLINICAL AND LABORATORY FINDINGS. The *clinical* features often are distinctive, with an early onset of severe respiratory distress caused by tracheobronchial compression accompanied by a systolic ejection and a widely transmitted low-pitched, decrescendo diastolic murmur at the upper left sternal border. In the absence of pulmonary complications, cyanosis is commonly mild. *Roentgenographically*, the heart is moderately enlarged; hyperinflated lung fields are observed, with large hilar densities representing the aneurysmally dilated pulmonary arteries. The *echocardiographic* features are similar to those seen in classic tetralogy of Fallot, in addition to massive dilatation of the main pulmonary artery and branch pulmonary arteries. Remnants of pulmonary cusps may be visible. Right ventricular dilatation is produced by significant pulmonary regurgitation; the latter is identified by retrograde diastolic flow in the pulmonary arteries and right ventricle at Doppler examination. These findings may be detected before birth (Fig. 43–51). Definitive diagnosis is established by cardiac catheterization and selective angiocardiography. Magnetic resonance imaging is a complementary diagnostic modality and is particularly useful for demonstrating bronchial morphology and the severity of bronchial obstruction.[428]

NATURAL HISTORY AND MANAGEMENT. Prognosis is related to the intensity of upper airway obstruction; pulmonary complications are the usual cause of death in infancy. If survival beyond infancy is accomplished, the respiratory symptoms usually diminish, probably because of maturational changes in the structure of the tracheobronchial tree. The surgical approach in infancy often is unsatisfactory; various procedures have been attempted, ranging from aneurysmorrhaphy to pulmonary artery suspension to transection and reanastomosis of pulmonary artery segments to homograft insertion.[429] Also suggested are ligation of the main pulmonary artery and creation of a systemic-pulmonary shunt, as well as primary repair of the VSD with pulmonary arterial plication. In older patients, the stenotic annulus

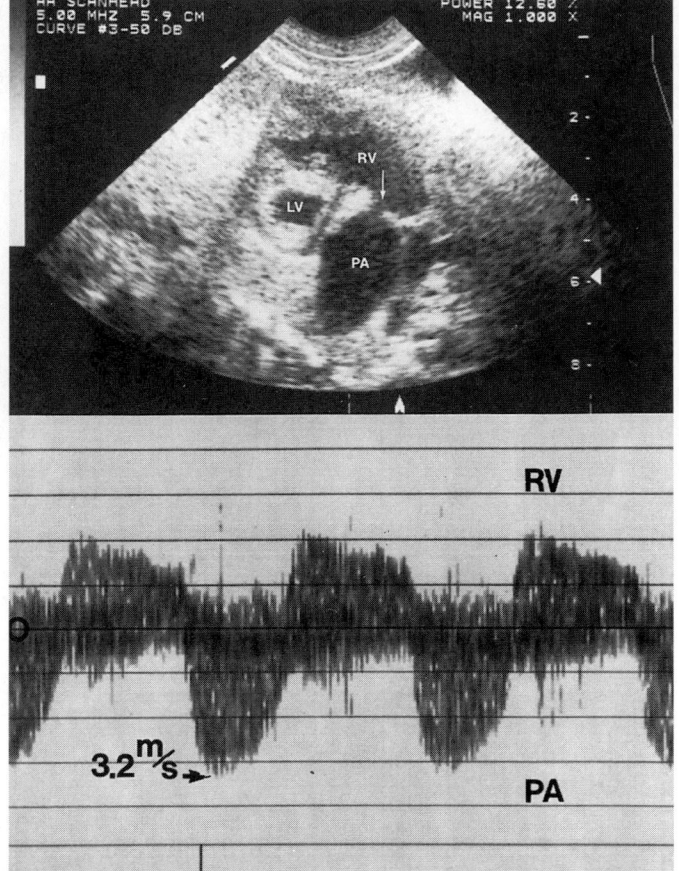

FIGURE 43–51. Two-dimensional *(top panel)* and Doppler *(lower panel)* echocardiogram of a 30-week-gestation fetus with tetralogy of Fallot and an absent pulmonary valve. The pulmonary artery (PA) is aneurysmally dilated, and the right ventricle (RV) is also dilated. The arrow points to the stenotic pulmonary valve annulus. Pulmonary valve leaflets are not detectable. The Doppler study at the level of the pulmonary valve annulus demonstrates to-and-fro flow with increased forward velocity in systole. LV = left ventricle. (Courtesy of Dr. James C. Huhta.)

may be widened with a patch and the VSD closed. It seldom is necessary to replace the pulmonic valve.

Tricuspid Atresia

MORPHOLOGY. This anomaly is characterized by absence of the tricuspid orifice, an interatrial communication, hypoplasia of the right ventricle, and the presence of a communication between the systemic and pulmonary circulations, usually a VSD.[430] Thus formed is a univentricular AV connection, consisting of a left-sided mitral valve between the morphological left atrium and left ventricle. Unequal division of the AV canal by fusion of the right-sided endocardial cushions has been proposed as the embryological fault. Patients may be subdivided into those with normally related great arteries (70 to 80 percent of cases) and those with dextro- or D-transposition of the great arteries; further classification depends on the presence of pulmonic stenosis or atresia and the absence or size of the VSD (Fig. 43–52). Additional cardiovascular malformations often are present, especially in patients with D-transposition of the great arteries, and include persistent left superior vena cava, patent ductus arteriosus, coarctation of the aorta, and juxtaposition of the atrial appendages.

PATHOPHYSIOLOGY. The association with other cardiac malformations determines whether or not pulmonary blood

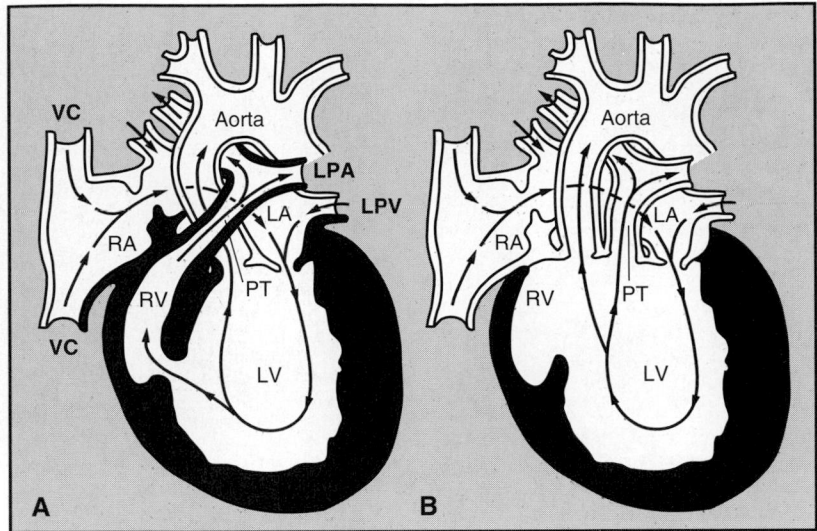

FIGURE 43–52. *A,* Tricuspid atresia with normally related great arteries, a small ventricular septal defect, diminutive right ventricular chamber, and narrowed outflow tract. *B,* An example of tricuspid atresia and complete transposition of the great arteries in which the left ventricular chamber is essentially a common ventricle, with the aorta arising from an infundibular component (RV) of the common ventricle. VC = vena cava; RA = right atrium; LA = left atrium; RV = right ventricle; LV = left ventricle; LPV = left pulmonary vein; LPA = left pulmonary artery; PT = pulmonary trunk. (Modified from Edwards JE, Burchell HB: Congenital tricuspid atresia: Classification. Med Clin North Am 33:1177, 1949.)

flow is decreased, normal, or increased and therefore the degree of systemic hypoxemia.[431] The clinical picture usually is dominated by symptoms resulting from greatly diminished pulmonary blood flow with severe cyanosis. Cyanosis results from an obligatory admixture of systemic and pulmonary venous blood in the left atrium, and its intensity primarily depends on the magnitude of pulmonary blood flow. Heart failure, rather than cyanosis, is the predominant problem in infants with torrential pulmonary blood flow, which results when D-transposition of the great arteries, a VSD, and an unobstructed pulmonary outflow tract coexist. If these patients survive infancy, they are at risk for pulmonary vascular obstructive disease; a favorable response to pulmonary arterial banding is common early in life.

CLINICAL FEATURES. The diagnosis is easily established in the vast majority of infants with tricuspid atresia and pulmonary hypoperfusion. The *ECG* findings of left-axis deviation, right atrial enlargement, and left ventricular hypertrophy in a cyanotic infant strongly suggest tricuspid atresia. *Echocardiography* reveals a small or absent right ventricle, large left ventricle, and absent tricuspid valve echoes (Fig. 43–53; see also Chap. 7); further, it may demonstrate the relation of the great arteries unless pulmonic atresia is present. Color flow and pulsed Doppler echocardiography reveal the abnormal flow patterns; apical and subxiphoid cross-sectional views best reveal the atretic tricuspid orifice. Seen *roentgenographically* are diminished pulmonary vascular markings and a concavity in the region of the cardiac silhouette usually occupied by the main pulmonary artery. The right atrial shadow may be prominent unless left-sided juxtaposition of the atrial appendages exists, which produces a straight and flattened right heart border.

CARDIAC CATHETERIZATION AND ANGIOGRAPHY. The right ventricle cannot be entered directly from the right atrium. When the great arteries are related normally, pulmonary blood flow is found to be derived from shunting through a VSD or by way of a patent ductus arteriosus; the latter and the bronchial collaterals are the source of pulmonary flow if the ventricular septum is intact. In complete transposition, the pulmonary artery fills directly from the left ventricle and the aorta indirectly through a VSD and the hypoplastic right ventricle. Because complete admixture exists in the left atrium of pulmonary and systemic venous return, the degree of systemic arterial hypoxemia depends on the pulmonary-systemic flow ratio. Right atrial angiography does not opacify the right ventricle unless by way of a VSD. Selective left ventricular *angiography* permits identification of the hypoplastic right ventricle, the size and location of the VSD, the type of pulmonary obstruction, the relation between the great arteries, and the size of the distal pulmonary arterial tree.

MANAGEMENT. *Balloon atrial septostomy* in those infants with a restrictive interatrial communication and palliative operations designed to increase pulmonary blood flow (systemic arterial—or venous—pulmonary artery anastomosis) are capable of producing clinical improvement of significant duration in patients with diminished blood flow.[431]

Functional correction of the anomaly has been accomplished in children older than 12 months by an intraatrial cavopulmonary baffle (lateral tunnel Fontan) (Fig. 43–54) or connection of the left pulmonary artery to the superior vena cava and inferior vena cava to the right pulmonary artery.[432] An adjustable snare around the atrial septal defect or a fenestrated cavocaval baffle with later transcatheter closure appears to prevent acute increases in systemic venous pressure, improve cardiac output, and enhance surgical survival.[433, 434] In patients with tricuspid atresia and complete transposition of the great arteries, subaortic obstruction can be anticipated when the VSD becomes restrictive, also referred to as an obstructive bulboventricular foramen. In most patients, the subaortic tissue must be resected, or preferably, a main pulmonary artery to ascending aorta anastomosis (Damus-Stansel-Kaye procedure) is performed at the time of the Fontan operation.[435] Candidates for these corrective procedures must have normal pulmonary vascular resistance and a mean pulmonary artery pressure less than 15 mm Hg, pulmonary arteries of adequate size, pulmonary vascular resistance less than 3 units/m² and good left ventricular function.[436] The postoperative period usually is characterized transiently by a superior vena cava syndrome with right heart failure, edema, ascites, and hepatomegaly. Long-term results have been generally good, but late management issues after Fontan operation are concerned with ventricular dysfunction,

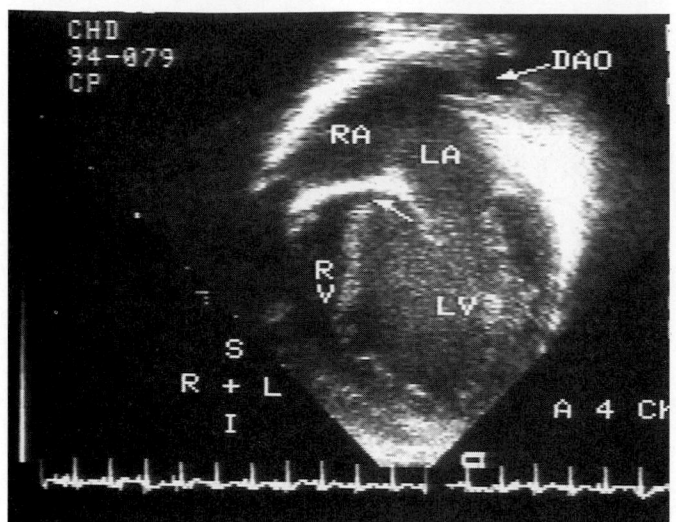

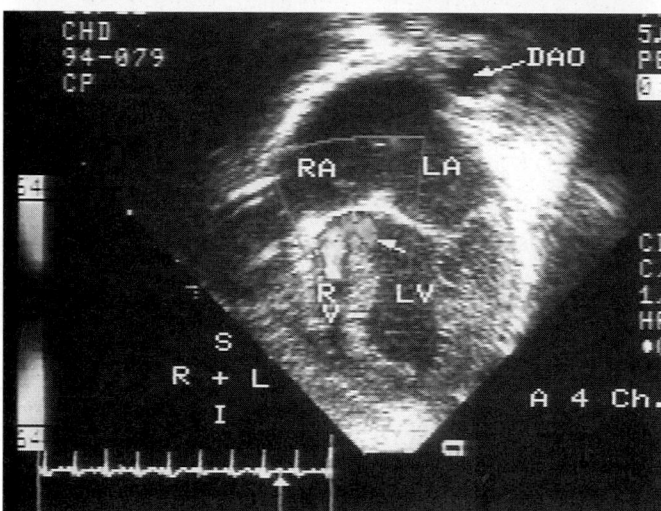

FIGURE 43–53. Apical four-chamber views of a patient with tricuspid atresia. In these views, the right atrium (RA) and left atrium (LA) can be seen above, and the small right ventricle (RV) and large left ventricle (LV) can be seen below. *Top,* Diastole with the mitral valve in the open position. Note the intense tissue echoes from the right atrioventricular groove between the right atrium (RA) and right ventricle (RV), indicating absence of the tricuspid valve. The descending aorta (DAO) can be identified posterior to the left atrium (LA). *Bottom,* Doppler color flow map of the same patient taken toward end-systole, showing the passage of blood across the ventricular septal defect (arrow).

atrial ventricular valve regurgitation, atrial arrhythmia, cyanosis, thromboembolism, and protein-losing enteropathy.[437, 438] Late postoperative exercise studies show subnormal exercise tolerance.[439] Late atrial arrhythmias can be a consequence of adverse preoperative hemodynamic function or the type of surgical correction (see Chap. 25).[440]

Ebstein Anomaly of the Tricuspid Valve

(See also p. 1603)

This malformation is characterized by a downward displacement of the tricuspid valve into the right ventricle due to anomalous attachment of the tricuspid leaflets (Fig. 43–55; see also (Fig. 44–8).[441] Case-control studies suggest that maternal exposure in the first trimester to lithium carbonate, used in the management of manic-depressive psychosis, is associated with a greatly increased risk of this anomaly in exposed offspring.[442] Tricuspid valve tissue is dysplastic, and a variable portion of the septal and inferior

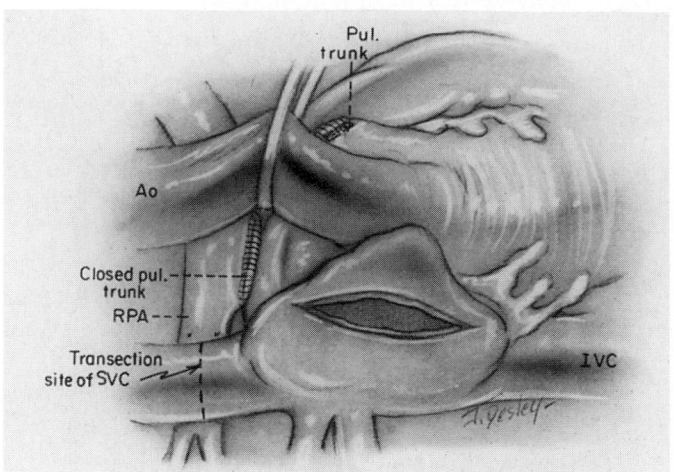

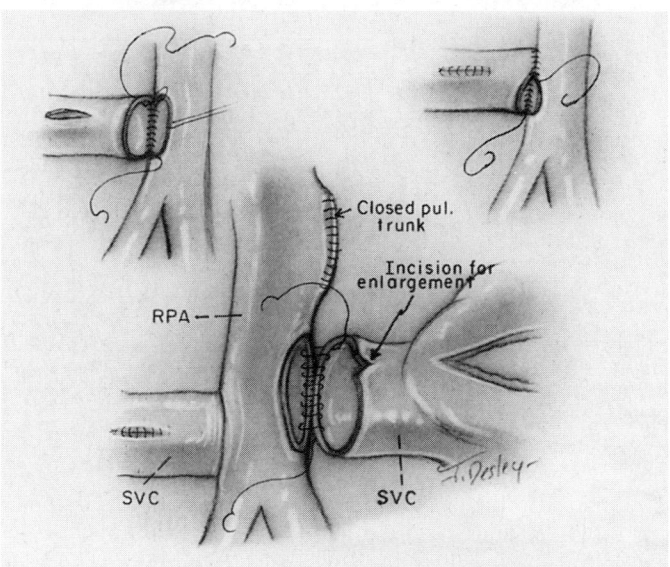

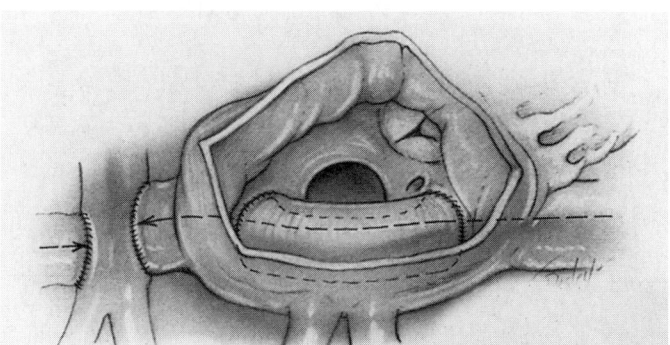

FIGURE 43–54. Fontan operation by total cavopulmonary connection. *Top,* The pulmonary trunk has been divided close to the pulmonary valve, and both ends have been closed. The right atrium is opened, and a pump sump sucker is placed across the foramen orale and into the left atrium (not shown). Marking stitches are placed at the proposed site of transection of the superior vena cava (SVC) and at the proposed sites of the two longitudinal incisions on the superior and inferior aspects of the right pulmonary artery (RPA). *Middle,* The anastomosis is made between the distal end of the divided superior vena cava and the incision in the superior aspect of the right pulmonary artery. The cardiac end of the superior vena cava is rarely enlarged; anastomosis is made to an incision in the inferior aspect of the right pulmonary artery. *Bottom,* A tunnel is created from a cylinder of either Dacron, Gore-Tex, or pericardium connecting the inferior vena cava (IVC) to the atrial orifice of the superior vena cava. The right pulmonary veins drain behind the tunnel. Ao = aorta. (From Kirklin, JW, Barratt-Boyes BG: Cardiac Surgery. 2nd ed. New York, Churchill Livingstone, 1993, p 1068.)

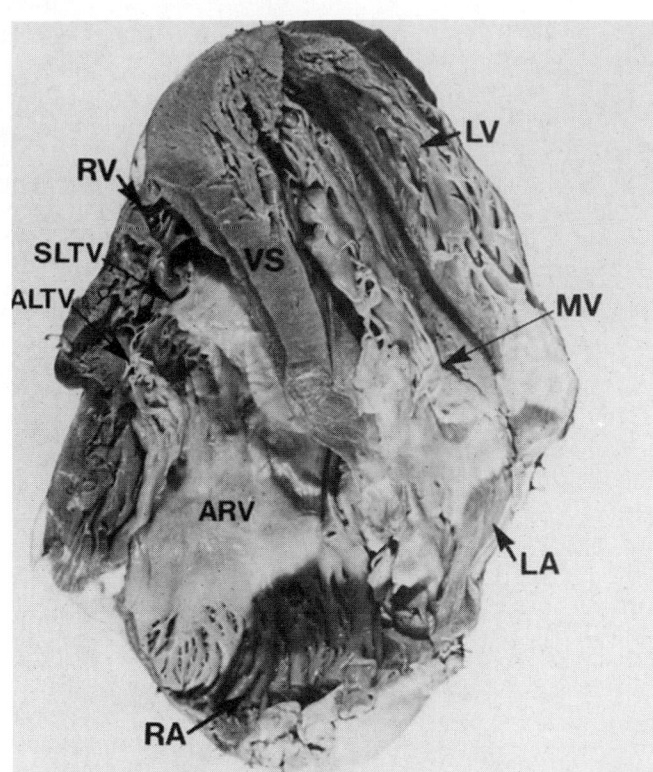

FIGURE 43–55. Anatomical specimen of Ebstein's anomaly of the tricuspid valve, cut in the same plane as an apical four-chamber echocardiographic view (see Fig. 43–56). The septal and anterior leaflets of the tricuspid valve (SLTV, ALTV) are displaced into the right ventricle (RV), producing a large atrialized right ventricle (ARV). VS = ventricular septum; RA = right atrium; LA = left atrium; MV = mitral valve; LV = left ventricle. (Courtesy of Dr. Thomas DiSessa.)

cusps adheres to the right ventricular wall some distance away from the AV junction. Because of the abnormally situated tricuspid orifice, a portion of the right ventricle lies between the AV ring and the origin of the valve, which is continuous with the right atrial chamber. This proximal segment is "atrialized," and a distal, functionally small ventricular chamber exists. The degree of impairment of right ventricular function depends primarily on the extent to which the right ventricular inflow portion is atrialized and on the magnitude of tricuspid valve regurgitation.

CLINICAL MANIFESTATIONS. These are variable because the spectrum of pathology varies widely and because of the presence of associated malformations.[443, 444] If the tricuspid valve is severely deformed, neonatal heart failure or even fetal hydrops and intrauterine death may occur.[445] At the other end of the spectrum, patients with a mildly deformed tricuspid valve may remain symptom free well into adulthood. The severity of symptoms also depends on the presence or absence of associated malformations. An interatrial communication consisting of a patent foramen ovale or an ostium secundum atrial septal defect is present in more than half the cases. The most common important associated defect is pulmonic stenosis or atresia. Other coexistent anomalies may include an ostium primum type of atrial septal defect and VSD alone or in combination with other lesions. The Ebstein lesion commonly is observed in association with congenitally corrected transposition of the great arteries, in which the tricuspid valve is in the left AV orifice. The usual manifestations in infancy are cyanosis, a cardiac murmur, and severe congestive heart failure. The magnitude of tricuspid regurgitation in neonates is enhanced because the pulmonary vascular resistance is normally high early in life.[446] In this regard, newborn infants with Ebstein anomaly and massive tricuspid regurgitation

must be distinguished by two-dimensional and Doppler echocardiography from those with organic pulmonary atresia and the presence of elevated perinatal pulmonary vascular resistance.

The tricuspid regurgitation in infants with Ebstein anomaly may lessen substantially, and cyanosis may disappear early in life as pulmonary vascular resistance falls, only to occur at a later age when right ventricular dysfunction and/or paroxysmal arrhythmias develop. In some infants with Ebstein malformation, cyanosis is suddenly intensified as the degree of pulmonary hypoperfusion is unmasked by spontaneous closure of a patent ductus arteriosus.[447]

Beyond infancy, the onset of symptoms is insidious; the most common complaints are exertional dyspnea, fatigue, and cyanosis. About 25 percent of patients suffer episodes of paroxysmal atrial tachycardia. A prominent systolic pulsation of the liver and a large *v* wave in the jugular venous pulse accompany the systolic thrill and murmur of tricuspid regurgitation. Wide splitting of the first and second heart sounds and prominent third and fourth heart sounds may produce a characteristically rhythmic auscultatory cadence with a triple, quadruple, and quintuple combination of sounds.

LABORATORY FINDINGS. The ECG abnormalities commonly fall into two categories—those with a right bundle branch block pattern and those with a Wolff-Parkinson-White (WPW) pattern (see Chap. 25). The ECG presentation in the latter is always from a right-sided accessory pathway, resembling left bundle branch block with predominant S waves in the right precordial leads. The presence of a WPW pattern increases the risk of supraventricular paroxysmal tachycardia (WPW syndrome).[448] The ECG most often shows giant P waves, a prolonged PR interval (in the absence of WPW), and prolonged terminal QRS depolarization, producing variable degrees of right bundle branch block. These distinctive findings help to distinguish Ebstein's anomaly from other forms of right ventricular dysplasia (see Chaps. 25 and 48), whose presenting problem often is an arrhythmia. *Roentgenographic* studies (see Chap. 8) usually demonstrate an enlarged right atrium, a small right ventricle, and a pulmonary artery with reduced pulsations; the pulmonary vascularity can be reduced if a large right-to-left shunt is present.

Echocardiographic Findings. Echocardiography clearly defines the features of Ebstein malformation.[449] The apical four-chamber plane shows the downward displacement of the attachment of the septal leaflet of the tricuspid valve, a finding overemphasized in the literature. The most important valvar displacement is that of the posterior or mural leaflet of the tricuspid valve, which is not well seen in the four-chamber view but rather in the subcostal view in infants and smaller children and in the parasternal long-axis or apical two-chamber view in older children and adults (Fig. 43–56). Subcostal echocardiography also defines the dysplasia of the leaflets of the valve, the right atrial dilatation, and the displacement of the entire tricuspid valve into the right ventricle. An additional challenge posed by the malformation, especially important for operative repair, is to determine whether the valvular attachment of the anterosuperior tricuspid leaflet is attached to the underlying myocardium. Echocardiographic identification of the chordae tendineae informs the surgeon of the need for freeing the valve during annuloplasty.

Doppler color flow imaging defines the degree of tricuspid regurgitation. Mapping determines the magnitude of regurgitation and the site of origin well within the body of the right ventricle. In addition, the presence of valvular stenosis (or nonopening) is determined by Doppler, particularly in neonates in whom patent ductus arteriosus supported systemic pressure may hold the pulmonary valve leaflets shut, simulating pulmonary atresia. The faint detection of pulmonary regurgitation by Doppler flow mapping aids differentiation of these two entities.

Invasive Study. These are rarely necessary. When *cardiac catheterization* is performed, the intracavitary ECG recorded just proximal to the tricuspid valve shows a right ventricular type of complex, while the pressure recorded is that of the right atrium. A right-to-left atrial shunt is normally present. The hemodynamic findings depend on the degree of tricuspid regurgitation. The cardiac muscle is unusually irritable, and a high incidence of significant arrhythmias during catheterization has been noted. Selective right ventricular *angiocardiography* shows the position of the displaced tricuspid valve, the size of the right ventricle, and the configuration of the outflow portion of the right ventricle.

MANAGEMENT. Ebstein anomaly may be compatible with a relatively long and active life, with most patients surviving into the third decade of life[450] (see Chap. 44). In

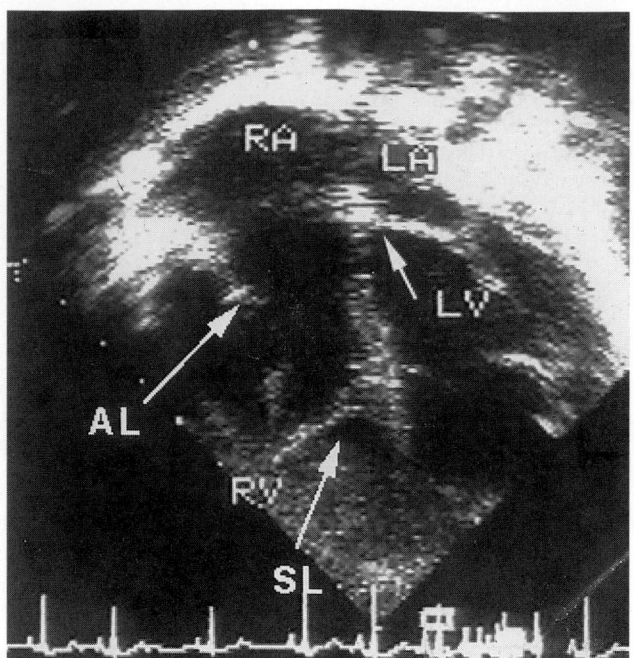

FIGURE 43-56. Apical four-chamber view of Ebstein's malformation in anatomical orientation. The left atrium (LA) and right atrium (RA) are seen above, and the right ventricle (RV) and left ventricle (LV) are seen below. Arrows point to the anterior leaflet of the tricuspid valve (AL) and septal leaflet (SL). The space between the septal attachment of the tricuspid valve and the mitral valve arrows is enlarged. This area between the true right atrium and the atrioventricular valve indicates the area of atrialized right ventricle.

symptomatic infants with severe cardiomegaly, the initial surgical approach is similar to that in patients with tricuspid atresia, creating a systemic pulmonary shunt, and at a later age the Fontan approach, which necessitates suture or pericardial patch closure of the tricuspid valve. Consideration may be given in some of these patients to creating a bidirectional Glenn shunt from the superior vena cava to the pulmonary arteries, to divert systemic venous return from the right atrium and to increase pulmonary blood flow. In older patients, significant benefit has resulted from reconstruction of the tricuspid valve, closure of the atrial septal defect, plication of the free wall of the right ventricle, posterior tricuspid annuloplasty, and a reduction in right atrial size.[443, 455] Because late results of this latter approach are encouraging, we now recommend operation for all symptomatic patients and even asymptomatic patients if their heart size is increasing significantly.[451-454] Some surgeons have sought to minimize postoperative tricuspid regurgitation by inserting a bioprosthetic valve if tricuspid valve tissue is inadequate for a good result.[456] In patients with a preexcitation syndrome (see Chap. 25) that is producing life-threatening rhythm disturbances, the accessory conduction pathways are either catheter ablated or surgically divided (see Chap. 23).[457]

TRANSPOSITION COMPLEXES

The term *transposition* identifies a group of malformations that have in common an abnormal relation between the cardiac chambers and great arteries. In this chapter the term is used to include both anomalous insertion of the pulmonary veins and cardiac malpositions.

Complete Transposition of the Great Arteries (See also p. 1609)

MORPHOLOGY. This is a common and potentially lethal form of heart disease in newborns and infants.[458] The malformation consists of the origin of the aorta arising from the morphological right ventricle and that of the pulmonary artery from the morphological left ventricle. With rare exceptions, there is no fibrous continuity between the aortic and mitral valves. The origin of the aorta usually is to the right and anterior to the main pulmonary artery but may be lateral to it. Thus, dextro- or D-transposition is a term often used interchangeably with complete transposition. In other classifications, the anomaly is described as concordant AV and discordant ventriculoarterial connections. The embryogenesis of complete transposition of the great arteries is controversial. The consensus is that the ventricular origins of the great arteries are reversed after development of a straight rather than a spiral infundibulotruncal septum. Transposition appears to result from a transfer of the pulmonary artery, instead of the aorta, from the heart tube's outlet zone to the left ventricle.[459] The latter can result from maldevelopment of the infundibulum or from a combination of both infundibulum maldevelopment and truncal malseptation; the former results if the subpulmonary rather than the subaortic infundibulum is absorbed.

The anatomical arrangement results in two separate and parallel circulations. Some communication between the two circulations must exist after birth to sustain life; otherwise, unoxygenated systemic venous blood is directed inappropriately to the systemic circulation and oxygenated pulmonary venous blood is directed to the pulmonary circulation. Almost all patients have an interatrial communication (Fig. 43-57; see also Fig. 44-17). Two-thirds have a patent ductus arteriosus, and about one-third have an associated VSD. Complete transposition occurs more frequently in the offspring of diabetic mothers and more often in males than in females. Without treatment, about 30 per cent of these infants die within the first week of life, 50 percent within the first month, 70 percent within 6 months, and 90 percent

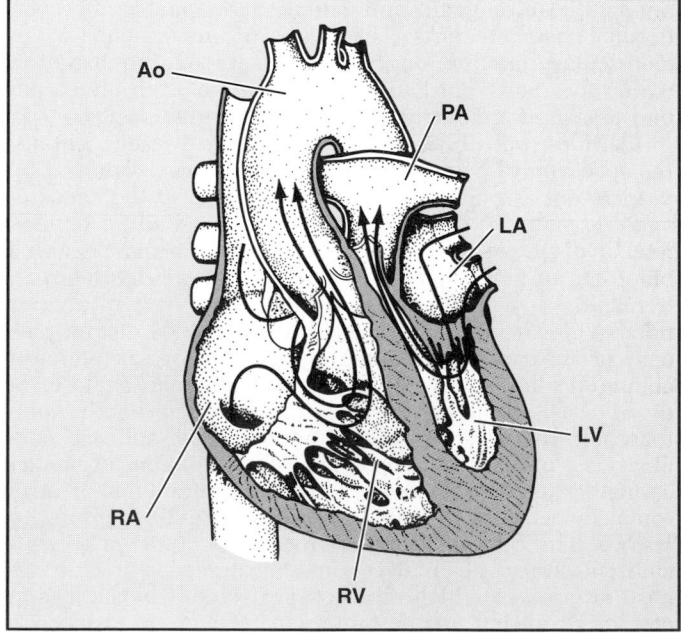

FIGURE 43-57. Complete transposition of the great arteries. Intercirculatory mixing occurs only at the atrial level. RA = right atrium; LA = left atrium; RV = right ventricle; LV = left ventricle; Ao = aorta; PA = pulmonary artery.

within the first year.[458] Those who live beyond infancy have, as a general rule, either an isolated large atrial septal defect or a single ventricle, or VSD and pulmonic stenosis. Current aggressive medical and surgical approaches to this group of patients have transformed the prognosis for an infant with this malformation from hopeless to very good.

HEMODYNAMICS. The *clinical course* is determined by the degree of tissue hypoxia, the ability of each ventricle to sustain an increased workload in the presence of reduced coronary arterial oxygenation, the nature of the associated cardiovascular anomalies, and the anatomical and functional status of the pulmonary vascular bed.[460] A bidirectional shunt is always present because continuous unidirectional shunting would result in progressive depletion of the circulating volume in either the pulmonary or the systemic vascular bed.

A major determinant of the systemic arterial oxygen saturation is the amount of blood exchanged between the two circulations by intercirculatory shunts. The net volume of blood passing left to right from the pulmonary to the systemic circulation represents the anatomical left-to-right shunt and is in fact the effective systemic blood flow (i.e., the amount of oxygenated pulmonary venous return reaching the systemic capillary bed). Conversely, the volume of blood passing right to left from the systemic to the pulmonary circulation constitutes the anatomical right-to-left shunt and is in fact the effective pulmonary blood flow (i.e., the net volume of unsaturated systemic venous return perfusing the pulmonary capillary bed).

The net volume exchange between the two circulations per unit time is equal. The magnitude of the intercirculatory mixing volume is modified by the number of intercirculatory communications that exist, the presence of associated obstructive intracardiac and extracardiac anomalies, the extent of the bronchopulmonary circulation, and the relation between pulmonary and systemic vascular resistance. For example, in newborns with an intact ventricular septum and a constricted or closed patent ductus arteriosus, inadequate mixing through a small patent foramen ovale often is the cause of severe hypoxemia. If a large interatrial communication or a VSD exists, systemic arterial oxygen saturation is influenced more importantly by the pulmonary-systemic blood flow relation than by the adequacy of mixing; augmented pulmonary blood flow produces a higher systemic arterial saturation if the left ventricle can sustain a high-output state without the intervention of congestive heart failure and pulmonary edema. The systemic arterial oxygen saturation is low, despite adequate intercirculatory mixing sites, if pulmonary blood flow is reduced by left ventricular outflow tract obstruction or increased pulmonary vascular resistance.

Pulmonary Vascular Changes. Infants with complete transposition of the great arteries are particularly susceptible to the early development of *pulmonary vascular obstructive disease*.[460] Moderately severe morphological alterations develop in the pulmonary vascular bed by the age of 6 to 12 months in many infants and by 2 years in almost all patients with an associated large VSD or large patent ductus arteriosus in the absence of obstruction to left ventricular outflow. Advanced pulmonary vascular disease is also noted within this same time frame in 15 to 30 percent of patients without a patent ductus arteriosus and with an intact ventricular septum. Systemic arterial hypoxemia, increased pulmonary blood flow, and pulmonary hypertension contribute to the development of pulmonary vascular obstruction in these patients, as they do in other forms of congenital heart disease. Among the additional factors implicated in the accelerated and more widespread pulmonary vascular obstruction found in patients with complete transposition is the presence of extensive bronchopulmonary anastomotic channels, which enter the pulmonary vascular bed proximal to the pulmonary capillary bed; thus, oxygen tension is reduced at the precapillary level, causing pulmonary vasoconstriction.[461]

Beyond the early neonatal period, many patients have an abnormal distribution pattern of pulmonary blood flow, with preferential flow to the right lung. The asymmetrical distribution of pulmonary blood flow in these individuals results from an abnormal rightward inclination of the main pulmonary artery in the transposition malformation that favors flow from the main to the right pulmonary artery. Persistently increased pulmonary blood flow to the right lung would be expected to contribute to pulmonary vascular obstructive changes within the lung; in the left pulmonary vascular bed, thrombotic changes may occur because of the combination of reduced flow and polycythemia. Finally, it should be recognized that a prenatal alteration in pulmonary vascular smooth muscle may exist because blood perfusing the fetal lungs in complete transposition of great arteries has a higher than normal PO_2 and may serve to dilate pulmonary vessels in utero. Postnatally, such vessels may have an enhanced capacity to constrict in response to vasoactive stimuli and suffer anatomical, obliterative changes.

CLINICAL FINDINGS. Average birth weight and size of infants born with complete transposition of the great arteries are greater than normal. The usual clinical manifestations are dyspnea and cyanosis from birth, progressive hypoxemia, and congestive heart failure. Early in postnatal life, the clinical manifestations and course are influenced principally by the magnitude of intercirculatory mixing. The most severe cyanosis and hypoxemia are observed in infants who have only a small patent foramen ovale or ductus arteriosus and an intact ventricular septum and in whom mixing is inadequate, or in those infants with relatively reduced pulmonary blood flow because of left ventricular outflow tract obstruction.[462] With a large persistent patent ductus arteriosus or a large VSD, cyanosis may be minimal and heart failure is the usual dominant problem after the first few weeks of life.[458] It should be recognized that a patent ductus arteriosus is present in about half of newborn infants with transposition, although it closes functionally and anatomically soon after birth in almost all cases. If the ductus arteriosus remains open, better mixing of the venous and arterial circulations usually is at the expense of pulmonary artery hypertension.[463]

Cardiac murmurs are of little diagnostic significance and are absent or insignificant in about 30 to 50 percent of infants with complete transposition of the great arteries and an intact ventricular septum. In infants with a large persistent patent ductus arteriosus, fewer than half exhibit physical signs typical of ductus arteriosus, such as continuous murmur, bounding pulses, or a prominent mid-diastolic rumble. Moreover, *differential cyanosis* caused by reversed pulmonary-to-systemic shunting across the ductus arteriosus is difficult to detect because of generalized arterial desaturation. In those infants with a large VSD, a pansystolic murmur usually emerges within the first 7 to 10 days of life. In newborns with transposition and severe pulmonic stenosis or atresia, the clinical findings are similar to those in infants with tetralogy of Fallot.

ELECTROCARDIOGRAPHY AND ROENTGENOGRAPHY. The most usual *ECG findings* include right-axis deviation, right atrial enlargement, and right ventricular hypertrophy, reflecting that the right ventricle is the systemic pumping chamber. Combined ventricular hypertrophy may be present in those patients with a large VSD and elevated pulmonary blood flow. Isolated left ventricular hypertrophy is encountered rarely in patients with a VSD and a hypoplastic right ventricle, in many of whom the tricuspid valve is displaced abnormally and straddles a VSD. In the first days of life, the chest radiograph may appear normal, particularly in infants with an intact ventricular septum. Thereafter, roentgenographic findings often are highly suggestive of the diagnosis,[464] and consist of (1) progressive cardiac enlargement in early infancy; (2) a characteristic oval or egg-shaped cardiac configuration in the anteroposterior view, and a narrow vascular pedicle created by superimposition of the aortic and pulmonary artery segments; and (3) increased pulmonary vascular markings (Fig. 43–58). A right aortic arch is seen in about 4 percent of infants with an intact ventricular septum and 11 percent of infants with VSD.

CT scanning and magnetic resonance imaging (see Chap. 10) are also capable of establishing the diagnosis.

ECHOCARDIOGRAPHY. Two-dimensional echocardiography is the procedure of choice in the diagnosis of complete transposition of the great arteries and the detection of significant associated cardiac anomalies[465] (Figs. 43–59 and 43–60; see also Fig. 44–21). Indeed, prenatal detection, leading to early management, favorably modifies neonatal morbidity and mortality.[465] Postnatally, in sagittal cross sections, the aorta is observed to ascend retrosternally, in contrast to the normal posterior sweep of the pulmonary artery. With transverse short-axis cross-sectional imaging, the diagnosis is confirmed by demonstrating that the anterior great artery (the aorta) is to the right of the posterior great artery (pulmonary) or that the two arteries are visualized side by side (see Fig. 43–59). Moreover, from subcostal views (see Fig. 43–60), the course of the two great arteries may be traced to delineate their ventricle of origin, demonstrating that the anterior rightward vessel (aorta) originates from the right ventricle and the posterior leftward vessel (pulmonary artery) originates from the left ventricle (see Fig. 43–60). In addition, echocardiography allows sensitive demonstration of the proximal coronary artery position, branching, and course. The intramural proximal course of a coronary artery has also been recognized.[467, 468] Echocardiography also readily identifies associated defects. VSDs may be localized to the membranous, AV, and trabecular muscular septa, and malalignment types of VSDs may be identified if the infundibular septum is shifted either anteriorly or posteriorly.[469] A subaortic obstruction may be created by anterior shifting of the infundibular septum, whereas a posterior shift may narrow the subpulmonary area. The nature of left ventricular outflow tract obstruction may be further identified as a fixed obstruction caused by a fibromuscular ridge or as a dynamic obstruction caused by deviation of the interven-

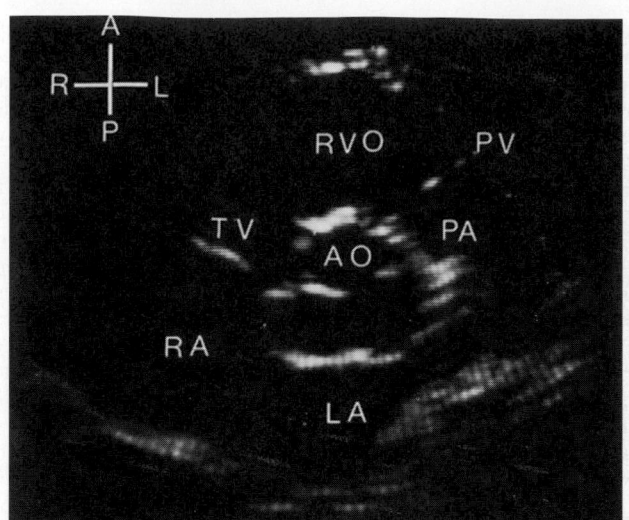

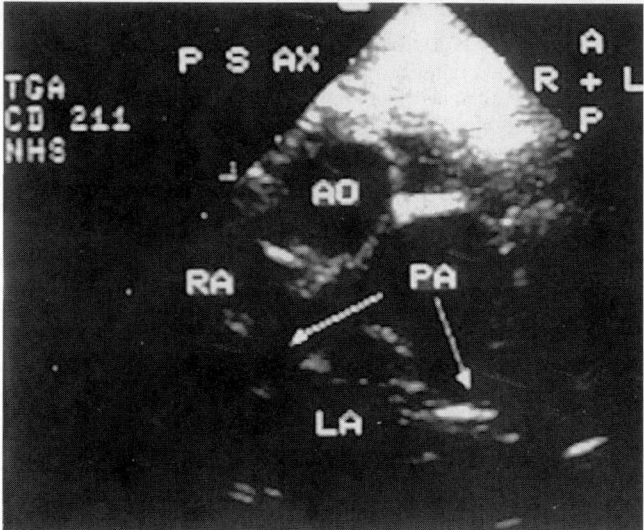

FIGURE 43–59. *Top,* A two-dimensional echocardiographic short-axis scan demonstrates normal great artery relations. The right ventricular outflow tract (RVO) wraps around the aorta (AO) in a clockwise direction. The pulmonic valve (PV) is to the left of the aortic valve. *Bottom,* Parasternal short-axis (P S AX) view showing the aorta (AO) anteriorly and the pulmonary artery (PA) posteriorly bifurcating into its left and right branches (arrow). LA = left atrium; RA = right atrium; TV = tricuspid valve.

tricular septum toward the left ventricular cavity and the apposition between a thickened interventricular septum and systolic anterior motion of the mitral valve.

Ultrasound imaging has become a standard procedure to guide catheter placement and manipulation during balloon atrial septostomy[470] and to assess the anatomical adequacy of the septostomy. Because echocardiography so clearly delineates the arterial transposition, the coronary arteries, and associated anomalies, many infants may proceed to surgery without prior cardiac catheterization.

CARDIAC CATHETERIZATION. The major abnormal hemodynamic findings include right ventricular pressure at systemic levels and either a high or low left ventricular pressure, depending on pulmonary blood flow, pulmonary vascular resistance, and the presence or absence of left ventricular outflow tract obstructive lesions. Oxygen saturation in the aorta is lower than that in the pulmonary artery. Application of the Fick principle to the calculation of pulmonary and systemic blood flow rates in these patients is an important source of error. Assumed values of oxygen consumption are unreliable in severely hypoxemic infants.

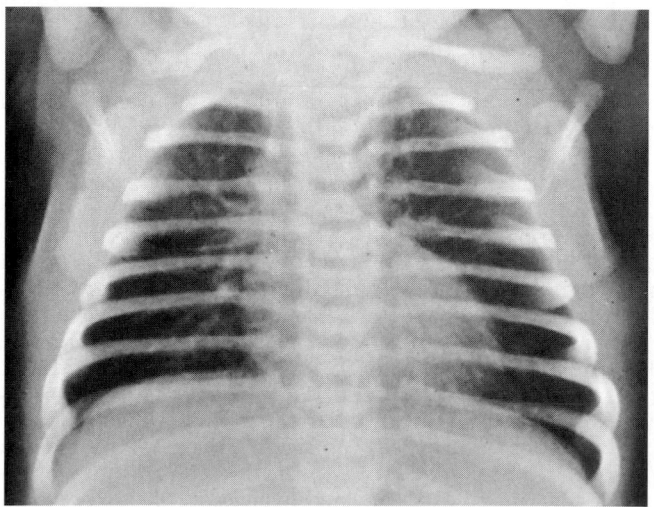

FIGURE 43–58. Chest roentgenogram in a 4-day-old infant with complete transposition of the great arteries showing an oval-shaped heart with a narrow base and increased pulmonary vascular markings.

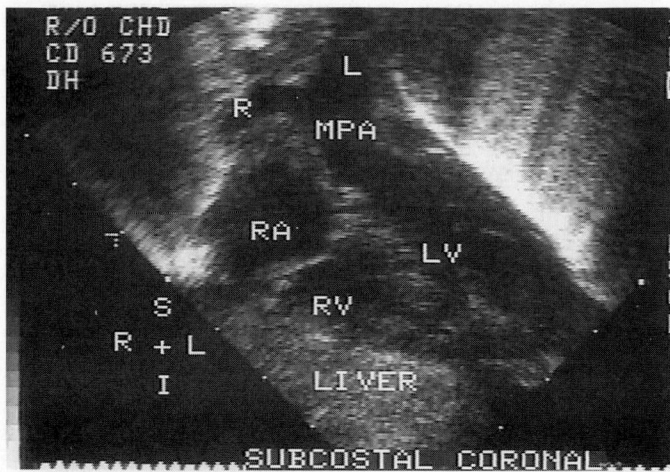

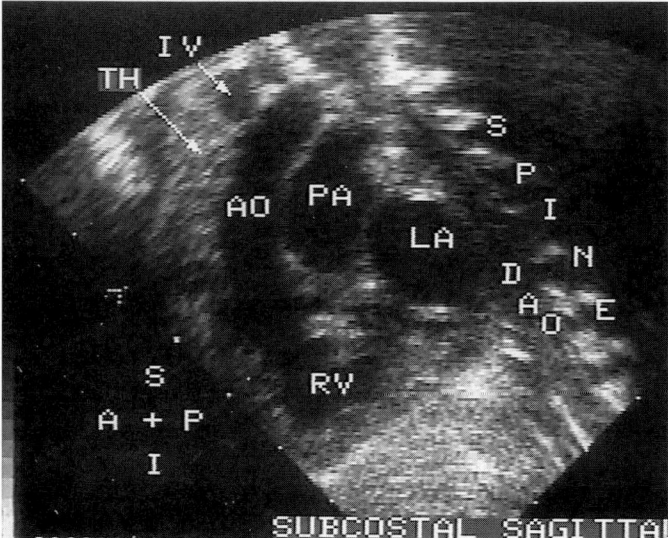

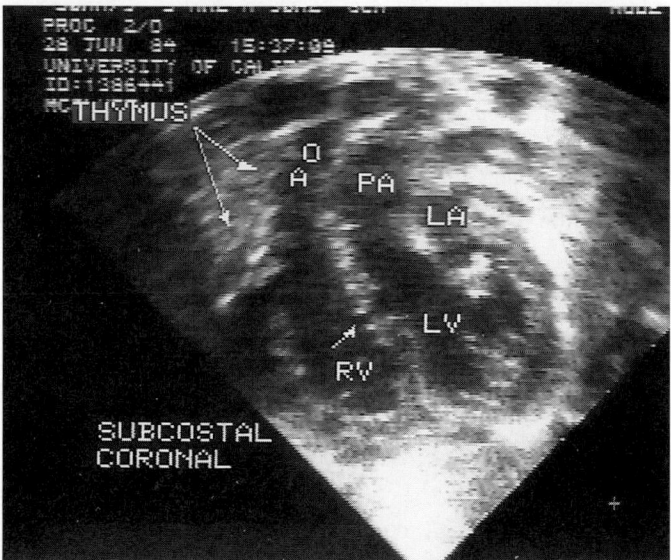

Moreover, because systemic and particularly pulmonary arteriovenous oxygen differences may be quite reduced, small errors in oxygen saturation values result in large errors in flow calculations. Furthermore, because bronchial collaterals enter the pulmonary circuit at the precapillary level, a true mixed pulmonary artery saturation cannot be sampled; pulmonary blood flow is therefore overestimated when one uses a sample from the central pulmonary artery, and pulmonary vascular resistance values often are underestimated.

Infants who have simple, complete transposition of the great arteries and who present in the first few weeks of life to a center prepared to correct the anomaly by the arterial switch operation (discussed later) often are taken to the operating room shortly after two-dimensional echocardiography and Doppler examination are performed.[21] In these cases, transcatheter balloon atrial septostomy is not performed unless a delay is expected in taking the patient to the operating room. In essentially all other patients, under echocardiographic or fluoroscopic guidance at cardiac catheterization, balloon septostomy is the initial approach to the patient.

The diagnostic portion of the cardiac catheterization allows confirmation of the anatomical derangement of the great arteries and establishes the presence of associated lesions; in newborns, unless prompt arterial switch repair is planned, it should always be accompanied by a palliative balloon atrial septostomy, which serves to enlarge the interatrial communication and improve oxygenation. In older neonates, usually beyond age 3 weeks, thickening of the atrial septum may preclude satisfactory balloon septostomy. In those instances, transcatheter blade septostomy is the preferred approach to palliation. Two-dimensional echocardiography, with or without fluoroscopy, may be used as the imaging mode for both balloon and blade creation of an atrial septal defect.[471] Subcostal four-chamber and sagittal views image cardiac anatomy and catheter position during the procedure, substantially reducing radiation dose.

Both the diagnostic and the palliative procedures can be performed by percutaneous entry into the femoral vein, umbilical vein catheterization, or direct cutdown into the femoral or saphenous vein. The catheter passes easily across the foramen ovale into the left atrium and left ventricle and may be manipulated into the pulmonary artery by means of a flow-directed balloon-guided catheter or by manipulation of a standard catheter bent in the form of a J loop within the left ventricle, with the tip pointed posteriorly to the pulmonary artery. When a large VSD is present, the catheter can often be manipulated directly across it from the right ventricle into the pulmonary artery.

ANGIOGRAPHY. This is diagnostic and demonstrates that the anteriorly placed aorta arises from the right ventricle and that the posteriorly placed pulmonary artery in continuity with the mitral valve arises from the left ventricle. The status of the ductus arteriosus and the site and size of a VSD can be well visualized by angiography. Interventricular defects posterior and inferior to the crista supraventricularis occur in about half of these patients; less often, the defects are anterior and superior to the crista supraventricularis or are of the AV septal type.[472] Various lesions may be

FIGURE 43-60. Composite subcostal views of transposition of the great arteries. *Top,* Subcostal coronal view showing the main pulmonary artery (MPA) arising directly from the left ventricle (LV) and dividing into the right (R) and left (L) pulmonary arteries. The right atrium (RA) and right ventricle (RV) lie adjacent in this view to the liver. *Middle,* The scan plane has been rotated 90 degrees clockwise (note the change in spatial orientation and the position of the spine). The thymus (TH) is seen anteriorly, and the innominate vein (IV) lies anterior to the aortic arch (indicated by arrows, respectively). The right ventricle (RV) lies anteriorly above the diaphragm and behind the thymus and gives rise to the aorta (AO), its arch, and the descending aorta (DAO). The main pulmonary artery (PA) lies in the crux of the aortic arch. *Bottom,* An intermediate subcostal view, lying oblique in a plane between the top two panels. The entire ventriculoarterial connection is imaged in this plane, showing the right ventricle connecting to the aortic arch, a small ventricular septal defect indicated by the small arrow, and the pulmonary artery (PA) arising from the left ventricle (LV). The left atrium (LA) can be seen below the pulmonary artery.

identified as the cause of left ventricular outflow tract obstruction, including ventricular septal hypertrophy with systolic anterior movement of the mitral valve, discrete or tunnel fibromuscular subpulmonic stenosis, valvular and supravalvular stenosis, and, rarely, an aneurysm of the membranous ventricular septum or redundant tricuspid valve tissue protruding through a VSD.

Both angiographic and echocardiographic imaging may be required to detect the coronary arterial patterns seen in patients with complete transposition of the great arteries.[467, 468, 473, 474] In the majority, the left coronary artery originates in the left sinus and the right coronary artery originates in the posterior sinus, with a single ostium above both the left and the posterior sinus. In almost 20 percent of patients, the left circumflex artery arises as a branch of the right coronary artery; a single coronary artery is present in about 6 percent; in 3 to 4 percent of patients, either the right coronary and anterior descending arteries originate in the left sinus, with the left circumflex originating in the posterior sinus, or two ostia are present above one sinus, one giving rise to the right and the other to the left coronary artery. To avoid the danger of excision during transfer of the coronary arteries as part of the arterial switch corrective operation, the intramural course of the left coronary artery or the left anterior descending coronary artery should be identified, a finding in up to 5 percent of patients. An intramural course should be assumed when the vessel has an aberrant origin from the right sinus or when it is in intimate relationship with the commissure between the right and left sinuses and courses between the great arteries.

MANAGEMENT

Medical Treatment. This often is of limited help but should be vigorous because both functional and anatomical corrections of the malformation achieve good results. Conservative measures include the use of oxygen, digitalis, diuretics, iron (if an associated iron-deficiency anemia is present), and intravenous sodium bicarbonate for severe hypoxemic metabolic acidosis. Dilatation of the ductus arteriosus by prostaglandin E_1 in the early neonatal period both augments pulmonary blood flow and enhances intercirculatory mixing.

Atrial Septostomy. Creation or enlargement of an interatrial communication is the simplest procedure for providing increased intracardiac mixing of systemic and pulmonary venous blood; this is preferably achieved by rupturing the valve of the foramen ovale by balloon catheter during transseptal catheterization of the left side of the heart (Rashkind procedure) or by blade septostomy. Surgical atrial septectomy seldom is required. The balloon should be inflated to a diameter of about 15 mm before pull-back to the right atrium. Salutary results consist of a fall in left atrial pressure, equalization of mean left and right atrial

pressures, and an increase in the systemic arterial oxygen saturation. When the foramen ovale is stretched by the balloon without accomplishing rupture of the septum primum valve of the fossa ovalis, the improvement in oxygenation is short lived. Infusion or reinfusion intravenously of prostaglandin E_1 (0.05 to 0.1 mg/kg/min) has been shown to improve systemic oxygenation temporarily in the latter situation by dilating the ductus arteriosus and thereby facilitating intercirculatory mixing. Although balloon atrial septostomy usually is successful in stabilizing the infant's condition and allowing survival in the neonatal period, the initial rise in systemic arterial oxygen saturation to 65 to 75 percent often is not sustained beyond 6 to 9 months of age.

SURGICAL TREATMENT

The development of *corrective operations* for infants born with transposition of the great arteries has greatly improved prognosis.[475] It has also been suggested that prenatal detection of the anomaly reduces neonatal morbidity and mortality.

ARTERIAL SWITCH OPERATION. A one-stage anatomical correction is the approach of choice in major centers that care for infants with congenital heart disease.[475-479] In this operation, both coronary arteries are transposed to the posterior artery; the aorta and pulmonary arteries are transected, contraposed, and anastomosed (Jatene operation) (Fig. 43-61; see also Fig. 44-18). The arterial switch anatomical correction may be complicated by coronary ostial stenosis, acquired supravalvular aortic and/or pulmonary stenosis, and pulmonic and/or aortic incompetence. The major advantages of the arterial switch procedure, when compared with the atrial switch procedure, are restoration of the left ventricle as the systemic pump and the potential for long-term maintenance of sinus rhythm.[480]

Within the first month of life or rarely two,[477] the arterial switch operation may be performed as a single-stage repair. In such patients, the origin and branching patterns of the coronary arteries are reliably defined preoperatively by two-dimensional echocardiography. One of the main limiting factors for success in the arterial switch procedure is proper relocation of the coronary arteries. Thus, it is particularly important to know the precise variations in coronary arterial anatomy. In approximately 5 percent of the patients, the arteries follow an intramural course, requiring reroofing to allow coronary transfer.[458] Most centers consider that in infants beyond age 1 month it is necessary to prepare the left ventricle to withstand the systemic pressure that is produced after switching the great arteries, because if the ventricular septum is intact, left ventricular pressure and left ventricular wall thickness diminish normally in relation to the postnatal reduction in pulmonary artery pressure. In these infants, a two-stage approach is used, the first of which consists of banding the pulmonary artery; the arterial switch is performed soon thereafter, in some centers as early as 1 to 2 weeks later.[481]

In the unusual infant with an intact ventricular septum and a significant patent ductus arteriosus, an early neonatal arterial switch corrective operation with closure of the ductus is indicated. The optimal management of a large VSD is a one-stage intraarterial switch anatomical correction as early in life as possible.

In some patients, after early arterial repair of transposition of the great arteries, abnormally enlarged bronchial arteries are identified at postoperative catheterization, and they explain continuous murmurs or persistent cardiomegaly. When these vessels are large enough to produce a volume load to the systemic ventricle, catheter-directed coli embolization is indicated.[482] Follow-up studies after the arterial switch operation have demonstrated good left ventricular function

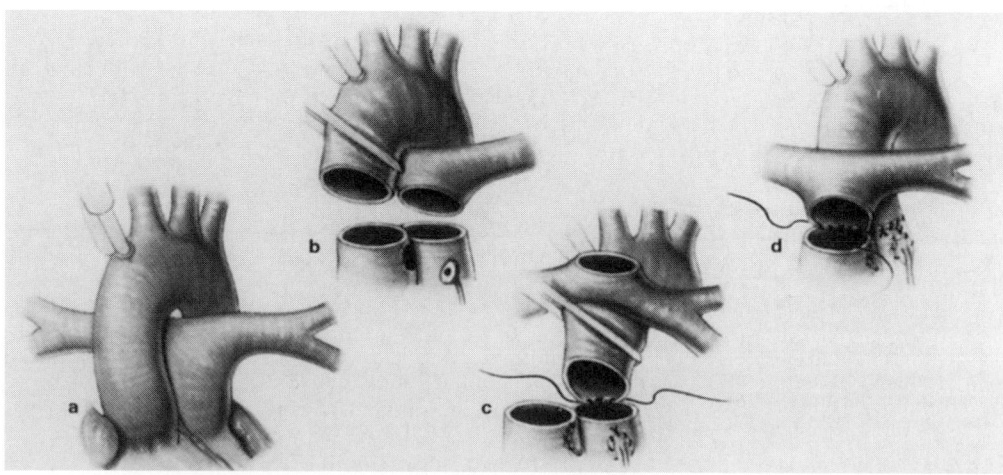

FIGURE 43–61. Complete transposition of the great arteries, corrected by a modified arterial switch operation (a). The aorta and pulmonary artery are transected, and the orifices of the coronary arteries are excised with a rim of adjacent aortic wall (b). The aorta is brought under the bifurcation of the pulmonary artery, and the proximal pulmonary artery and the aorta are anastomosed without necessitating graft interposition. The coronary arteries are transferred to the pulmonary artery (c). The mobilized pulmonary artery is directly anastomosed to the proximal aortic stump (d). (From Stark J, deLaval M: Surgery for Congenital Heart Defects. New York, Grune & Stratton, 1983, p 379.)

and normal exercise capacity.[483, 484] Potential sequelae of the operation include supravalvular pulmonary stenosis (which may be treated by either reoperation or balloon angioplasty), supravalvular aortic stenosis, and neoaortic regurgitation, usually mild. Long-term patency and growth of the coronary arteries appear satisfactory.[485-487] Infants with transposition of the great arteries plus a VSD and left ventricular outflow tract obstruction may require a systemic–pulmonary artery anastomosis when a pronounced diminution in pulmonary blood flow exists. A later corrective procedure for these patients bypasses the left ventricular outflow obstruction and uses an intracardiac ventricular baffle connecting the left ventricle to the aorta and an extracardiac prosthetic conduit between the right ventricle and the distal end of a divided pulmonary artery (Rastelli procedure).[488] An alternative approach (Lecompte procedure) couples an intraventricular tunnel and the arterial switch operation, avoiding the use of an extracardiac conduit.[489]

ATRIAL (VENOUS) SWITCH OPERATION. This correction, by either the Mustard or Senning techniques, diverts systemic venous return into the left ventricle through the mitral valve and thence through the left ventricle and pulmonary artery, while the pulmonary venous blood is diverted through the tricuspid and right ventricle to the aorta. Because midterm results of atrial switch procedures disclosed numerous problems involving late right ventricular failure, tricuspid insufficiency, and arrhythmias, most centers have abandoned the use of the atrial switch approach in favor of the more anatomical arterial switch operation.[490-496]

After physiological correction by atrial switch, postoperative complications are directly related to the intraatrial repair (shunts across the intraatrial patch and obstruction to either systemic or pulmonary venous return or both). There is a high incidence of early and late postoperative dysrhythmias that are more likely to have their basis in injury to the sinoatrial node and/or its arterial supply than in disruption of internodal tracts or damage to the AV node.[491] Tricuspid regurgitation is a less common complication of operation and may in some patients be related to a preexisting abnormality of the tricuspid valve, whereas in most it is related to right ventricular dysfunction. Although assessment of right ventricular contractility is difficult, the right ventricular pump function appears to be impaired before Mustard operation and does not return to normal after successful surgery.[496] It seems likely that the right ventricle can perform as a systemic pumping chamber for the duration of a normal life span.[492]

In patients with significant pulmonary vascular obstructive disease, the risk associated with definitive repair (anatomical correction or intraatrial baffle and closure of the ventricular septal defect) is great. In this group of patients, a "palliative" Mustard or Senning procedure leaving the ventricular septal defect open often provides good, short-term, symptomatic improvement by increasing arterial oxygen tension and reducing the stimulus to progressive polycythemia.[497]

Congenitally Corrected Transposition of the Great Arteries (See also p. 1612)

This term is applied to two distinctly different anomalies: anatomically corrected transposition or malposition of the great arteries and physiologically corrected levo- or L-transposition of the great arteries.

DEFINITION. Invariably, the term *congenitally corrected L-transposition* is applied to the heart in which a functional correction of the circulation exists by virtue of the relation between the ventricles and great arteries.[499, 500] Corrected or L-transposition occurs when the primitive cardiac tube loops to the left instead of to the right during embryogenesis. The anatomical right ventricle comes to lie on the left and receives oxygenated blood from the left atrium; this blood is ejected into an anteriorly placed, left-sided aorta. The anatomical left ventricle lies to the right and connects the right atrium to a posteriorly placed pulmonary artery. Thus, there are both ventriculoarterial and AV discordant connections, with ventricular inversion. This arrangement of the great arteries and ventricles (in contrast to the uncorrected, complete, or D-transposition) permits functional correction, so that systemic venous blood passes into the pulmonary trunk while arterialized pulmonary venous blood flows into the aorta. In a heart with congenitally corrected transposition, the venae cavae and coronary sinus drain into a right atrium that is normal in position and structure.

MORPHOLOGY. Anatomically corrected malposition of the great arteries is a rare form of congenital heart disease in which the great arteries are abnormally related to each other and to the ventricles but arise, nonetheless, above the anatomically correct ventricles.[498] Because of this, the term *malposition* rather than *transposition* is preferable. The anomaly results from either leftward looping of the ventricular segment of the embryonic heart tube in the situs solitus heart or from rightward looping in the situs inversus heart. In this unusual malformation, the aorta is anterior and to the left (levo- or L-malposition) and the pulmonary artery is posteromedial and to the

right, presumably because of a subaortic conus that causes mitral-aortic discontinuity.

When no other defect exists, the circulation proceeds normally. When an associated lesion prompts ochocardiographic examination, the diagnosis is indicated by the finding of AV concordance in association with wide mitral-aortic discontinuity with an anteriorly placed aorta. At cardiac catheterization, the diagnosis of the abnormal relation between the great arteries may be made by biplane angiocardiography. Anomalies commonly associated with anatomically corrected malposition of the great arteries include VSD, left juxtaposition of the atrial appendages, tricuspid atresia or stenosis, and valvular and subvalvular pulmonic stenosis.

PHYSIOLOGY. Venous blood flows from the right atrium, designated as the "venous atrium," across an AV valve that has the structure of a normal mitral valve and into the right-sided "venous ventricle" (Fig. 44–22). The venous ventricle, however, has the morphological characteristics of a normal left ventricle; i.e., its interior lining is trabeculated, it has no crista supraventricularis, and the AV valve is in continuity with the posteriorly placed semilunar valve. It ejects blood into the pulmonary trunk, which arises posterior to the ascending aorta. Oxygenated blood returns from the lungs to the left atrium, which is normal in position and structure; from there it flows into the left-sided "arterial ventricle" across an AV valve that has the structure of a normal tricuspid valve. The interior lining of the arterial ventricle has the morphological characteristics of a normal right ventricle (i.e., it has coarse trabeculations and a crista supraventricularis), and the tricuspid AV valve is not in continuity with the anteriorly placed semilunar valve. The arterial ventricle ejects blood into the aorta, which arises anterior to the pulmonary trunk. In addition to inversion of the cardiac ventricles, there is inversion of the conduction system and coronary arteries. Commonly associated anatomical lesions include atrial and ventricular septal defects, often accompanied by valvular or subvalvular pulmonary stenosis; single ventricle with an outlet chamber with or without pulmonic stenosis; left AV valve regurgitation, usually because of an Ebstein's malformation of the left-sided tricuspid valve; and abnormalities of visceral and atrial situs.[499]

CLINICAL MANIFESTATIONS. The clinical presentation, course, and prognosis of patients with congenital functionally corrected transposition vary, depending on the nature and severity of the complicating intracardiac anomalies.[500] Patients in whom corrected transposition exists as an isolated anomaly present no functional alterations and have no symptoms.[501] Asymptomatic children with an increase in the size of the systemic ventricle, due to significant left-to-right shunting or tricuspid regurgitation, usually develop symptoms of systemic ventricular dysfunction by the third or fourth decade.[500-503] The natural history of the anomaly and the ability of the right ventricle to perform systemic work are determined primarily by the nature and severity of the associated cardiac defects.[502]

The *physical findings* in congenitally corrected transposition are those of the associated lesions with two exceptions: (1) a single accentuated second heart sound usually is present in the second left intercostal space, representing closure of the aortic valve lying lateral and anterior to the pulmonic valve; and (2) there is a high incidence of cardiac dysrhythmias.

LABORATORY EXAMINATION. Because of the inversion of the heart's conduction system, the *ECG* can provide important clues in the diagnosis. An abnormal direction of initial (septal) depolarization from right to left causes leftward, anterior, and superior orientation of the initial QRS forces and reversal of the precordial Q wave pattern (Q waves are present in the right precordial leads and absent in the left). Two AV nodes, one posterior and one anterior, are present in some patients.[504] In addition to inversion of the conduction system, the His bundle is elongated because of the greater distance between the AV node and the base of the ventricular septum. The His bundle is located beneath the pulmonic valve in the position of mitral pulmonary continuity; thus, it is subject to significant excursions during mitral valve closure. The anterior "accessory" AV node may be connected directly with an aberrantly located penetrating portion of the His bundle. This arrangement may be a causal factor in the arrhythmias and AV conduction disturbances commonly observed in these patients. First-degree AV block occurs in about 50 percent and complete AV block occurs in 10 to 15 percent of patients. Other degrees of AV dissociation may be observed, as well as paroxysmal supraventricular tachycardia and ventricular extrasystoles. In some patients, Kent bundle connections provide the anatomical substrate for preexcitation.[504]

Roentgenographic examination characteristically reveals absence of the normal pulmonary artery segment and a smooth convexity of the left supracardiac border produced by the displaced ascending aorta (see Chap. 8). The latter may be visualized by radionuclide scintillation scans of the central circulation. The main pulmonary trunk is medially displaced and absent from the cardiac silhouette; the right pulmonary hilus often is prominent and elevated compared with the left, producing a right-sided waterfall appearance.

Two-dimensional echocardiography seeks to identify the morphology of each ventricle by defining the characteristics of the inflow and outflow tracts and papillary and trabecular muscle morphology, ventricular shape, and great artery position.[505] By tracing the great arteries back to their ventricles of origin in subxiphoid and parasternal short-axis planes, one would find that the anterior leftward great artery (the aorta) arises from the left-sided ventricle and is not in continuity with the left-sided AV valve. The great arteries exit the heart in parallel fashion; the position, origin, and branching pattern of the great arteries are observed in subxiphoid and suprasternal views, and the anteroposterior and right-left positions of the great arteries can be seen from the parasternal short-axis view. Because the ventricular septum lies in the anteroposterior plane parallel to the echo beam, it may not be visualized from a left parasternal view. In apical-basal or subxiphoid four-chamber echocardiographic views, the right and left ventricular morphology and the inverted position of the AV valves may be ascertained correctly. The latter views also demonstrate the level of attachment of the AV valves and allow detection of inferior displacement of the left-sided tricuspid valve when Ebstein's anomaly coexists.

At *cardiac catheterization*, the diagnosis should be suspected when the venous catheter enters a posterior and midline main pulmonary trunk. Retrograde arterial catheter passage establishes the typical position of the ascending aorta at the upper left cardiac border. Hemodynamic abnormalities depend on the lesions associated with corrected transposition. Selective *angiocardiography* allows visualization of the transposed great arteries and morphological differentiation of the two ventricles (Fig. 43–62). The ventricles usually lie side by side, with the ventricular septum oriented in an anteroposterior direction. Selective aortography demonstrates the inverted coronary arterial pattern that is invariably present in corrected transposition. The competence of the left AV valve may be determined by injection of contrast material into the arterial ventricle.[506] When a left-sided Ebstein's malformation exists, the leaflets are displaced distal to the true valve annulus. The level of the annulus may be determined by visualization of the circumflex branch of the left coronary artery, which courses posteriorly in the AV groove.

Specific problems have attended operative repair of the lesions associated with congenitally corrected transposition, owing primarily to the course of the conduction AV system and the coronary arterial pattern.[507, 508] The inversion of the coronary arterial system occasionally may limit and preclude an incision into the venous ventricle, thereby interfering with exposure of intracardiac defects in the usual manner. The disadvantage in approaching intracardiac anomalies using an incision in the morphological right ventricle is that this is the systemic ventricle. When significant pulmonary stenosis exists within a VSD, a valved extracardiac conduit often is a required part of the surgical repair. Surgical risks are especially high in patients in whom significant regurgitation exists from the arterial ventricle to the arterial atrium. In these patients, annuloplasty or, more usually, valve replacement is required. In all operative approaches, if complete heart block has been present intermittently or permanently preoperatively or intraoperatively, permanent epicardial atrial and ventricular pacemaker leads are implanted.

The disappointing results with traditional techniques of repair have led to more anatomical forms of surgical correction in which the morphological left ventricle supports the systemic circulation, rather than leaving the morphological right ventricle and tricuspid valve in the systemic circulation. Thus, the so-called double-switch procedure promises to decrease the development and significance of tricuspid valve regurgitation as well as the incidence of surgical complete heart block. In this procedure, an arterial switch operation establishes ventriculoarterial concordance and the systemic and pulmonary venous returns are rerouted by either the Mustard or Senning technique. If a VSD is present, it can be closed in the usual manner. When pulmonary stenosis is present in association with a ventricular defect, the performance of an arterial switch procedure is precluded, but the left ventricle can be routed to the aorta via a prosthetic baffle within the right ventricle to channel the VSD to the aortic valve. The outflow tract of the right ventricle can then be reconstructed by placement of a conduit from the right ventricle to the pulmonary artery bifurcation, and a venous switch procedure completes the operation.

Double-Outlet Right Ventricle

MORPHOLOGY. Other designations applied to this lesion include origin of both great arteries from the right ventricle, partial transposition, complete transposition of the aorta and levoposition of the pulmonary artery, complete dextroposition of the aorta, and the Taussig-Bing complex. This is an extremely heterogeneous category of malformations in which an abnormal relation exists between the aorta and the pulmonary trunk, which arise wholly or in large part from the right ventricle.[509]

DEFINITIONS. A uniform definition or classification of double-outlet right ventricle does not exist. To some, double-outlet right ventricle means origin of one great artery and at least 50 percent of the other over the right ventricle; others require the presence of bilateral conus muscle between both great arteries and the AV annulus. One or both great arteries may arise from an infundibular chamber; there may be considerable variability in the amount of subarterial conus muscle. Thus, the semilunar valves may lie side by side, or with the pulmonary valve more anterior and superior, or with a more anterior and superior aortic valve. Commonly, neither semilunar valve is in fibrous continuity with either AV valve, and a VSD is usually present and represents the only outlet from the left ventricle. The VSD is of the malalignment type because the infundibular septum is positioned abnormally.

When the amount of conus muscle beneath the two great arteries varies, the VSD commonly is positioned beneath the more posterior semilunar valve, which in fact usually overrides the interventricular septum through this VSD. The amount of conus muscle underneath the valve determines the position of the semilunar root in relation to the ventricles below. Thus, double-outlet right ventricle resides within the spectrum of conotruncal abnormalities ranging from tetralogy of Fallot to transposition of the great arteries. The VSD occasionally extends beneath both great arteries and is referred to as doubly committed. In some instances, the VSD is remote from both great arteries, or is considered uncommitted, in which case the defect often lies in the inlet or muscular portion of the interventricular septum.

ASSOCIATED LESIONS. More than half of patients with double-outlet right ventricle have associated anomalies of the right AV valves.[509, 510] Mitral atresia associated with a hypoplastic left ventricle is common; less often observed are tricuspid stenosis, Ebstein's anomaly of the tricuspid valve, complete AV septal defect, and overriding or straddling of either AV valve. Aortic coarctation may be associated with double-outlet right ventricle, particularly when the subaortic area is narrowed by malalignment of the infundibular septum. Double-outlet right ventricle also may be a component of the many cardiovascular anomalies of the splenic dysgenesis or heterotaxy syndromes. An increased incidence of the anomaly occurs in infants with the trisomy 18 syndrome.

The pathological features in most patients include side-by-side pulmonic and aortic valves and discontinuity between the mitral and aortic valves. The latter exists because muscular infundibulum is usual beneath both semilunar valves. The VSD may be remote from or closely related to one or both semilunar valves (Fig. 43–63). When the interventricular defect is subpulmonic, with or without a straddling pulmonary trunk, the complex is designated Taussig-Bing. In most patients, the interventricular septal defect is below the crista supraventricularis and is subaortic in location. Least often, the defect ei-

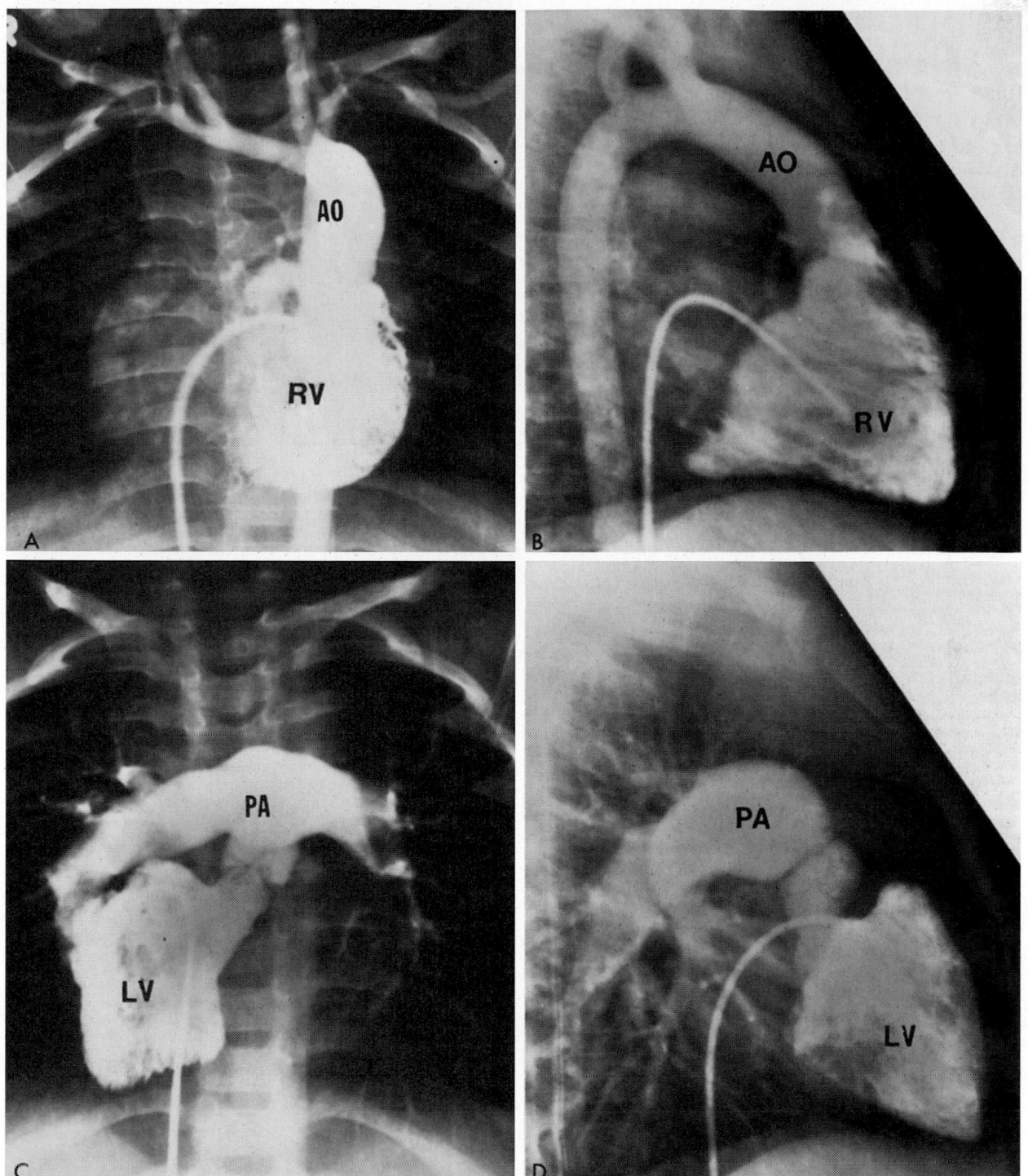

FIGURE 43–62. Congenitally corrected (levo-)transposition of the great arteries in a 4-year-old boy. *A,* Anteroposterior ventriculogram in left-sided ventricle with mesocardia. The morphological right ventricle (RV) is left sided, indicating an L-ventricular loop (inverted ventricles in situs solitus). The aorta (AO) originates above the morphological right ventricle and is thus transposed and in classic levo-transposition. *B,* Lateral ventriculogram in left-sided ventricle (same frame as *A).* The aorta originates anteriorly above the morphological right ventricle (RV). *C,* Anteroposterior ventriculogram in right-sided morphological left ventricle (LV). The transposed pulmonary artery (PA) arises from this ventricle, and the ventricular septum appears intact. Pulmonic valve thickening is also evident. The aorta *(A)* is to the left of the pulmonary artery. Note that the ventricular septum in the L-ventricular loop is visualized best in the anteroposterior views. *D,* Lateral ventriculogram in right-sided ventricle (same frame as *C).* The pulmonary artery is posterior to the aorta, and supravalvular pulmonic narrowing is seen. (From Freedom RM, Harrington DP, White RI Jr, et al: The differential diagnosis of levo-transposed or malposed aorta: An angiocardiographic study. Circulation 50:1040, 1974.)

ther is remote from both semilunar valves (uncommitted) or underlies both (doubly committed).

CLINICAL MANIFESTATIONS. The clinical and physiological picture is determined by the size and location of the VSD and the presence or absence of pulmonic stenosis. In the Taussig-Bing form of double-outlet right ventricle, the malformation resembles physiologically and clinically complete transposition with VSD and pulmonary hypertension. When the VSD is subaortic, the stream of blood from the left

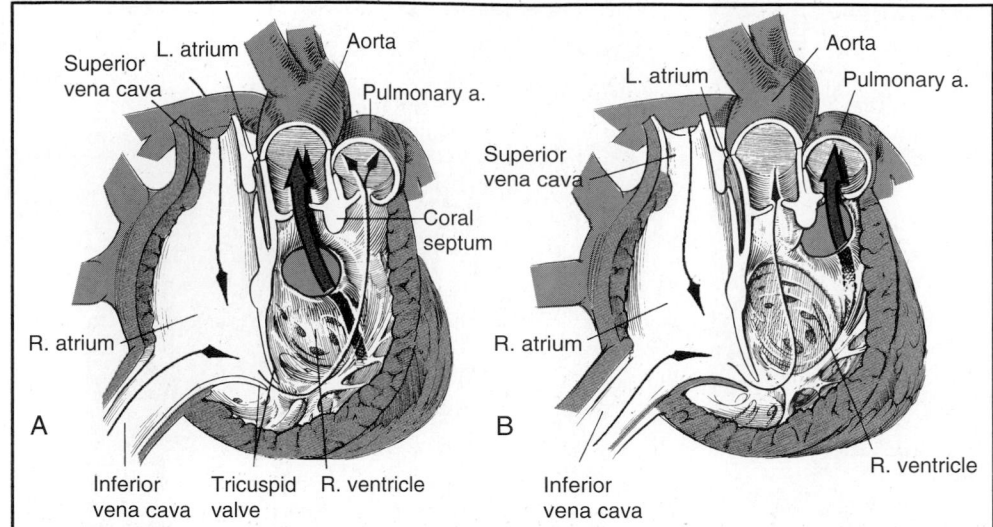

FIGURE 43–63. Double-outlet right ventricle with side-by-side relation of great arteries is illustrated in both panels. *A,* A subaortic ventricular septal defect below the crista supraventricularis favors delivery of left ventricular blood to the aorta. *B,* Subpulmonary location of the ventricular septal defect above the crista favors streaming to the pulmonary trunk. (From Castañeda A, Jonas RA, Mayer JE Jr, et al: Cardiac Surgery of the Neonate and Infant. Philadelphia, WB Saunders, 1994, p 446.)

ventricle is directed preferentially to the aorta. Thus, there may be little or no detectable cyanosis, and these patients usually clinically resemble those with an isolated large VSD and pulmonary hypertension.

The most important determinant of the natural history in both these types of double-outlet right ventricle is the progression of pulmonary vascular obstruction. In contrast, when there is pulmonary outflow tract obstruction, which often is severe and found commonly in these patients in whom the VSD is subaortic, clinical findings are similar to those of cyanotic tetralogy of Fallot. In some patients, especially without pulmonic stenosis, the ECG shows a superiorly oriented counterclockwise frontal plane QRS loop in addition to right ventricular hypertrophy.[511] The pattern appears to result from relative hypoplasia of the anterosuperior left bundle and preferential activation of the posteroinferior left ventricular wall. The presence of the latter ECG pattern in patients with double-outlet right ventricle should alert one to the possibility of a coexistent AV septal defect or abnormality of the mitral valve.

DIAGNOSIS. Two-dimensional *echocardiography* may reliably distinguish double-outlet right ventricle from other lesions causing cyanosis, such as tetralogy of Fallot and transposition of the great arteries.[512, 513] The three key imaging features are origin of both great arteries from the anterior right ventricle, mitral-semilunar valve discontinuity, and absence of left ventricular outflow other than the VSD. The relative anteroposterior positions of the great arteries can be determined from the parasternal short-axis view. The parasternal long-axis view shows the position of the more posterior semilunar root relative to the interventricular septum and anterior mitral leaflet and is the best view for demonstrating the presence of subarterial conus muscle. Subxiphoid views best demonstrate the position of both great arteries over the ventricles. Each great artery is displayed on long- and short-axis subxiphoid sweeps.

In reporting echocardiographic results, it is imperative to state each component's anatomical feature, i.e., the position of both great arteries, the presence and amount of infundibulum under each semilunar valve, the anatomy of both subpulmonary and subaortic outflow tracts, the position and size of the associated VSD, and the presence of all other associated lesions, particularly AV valve anomalies and coarctation of the aorta.

In each of the different types of double-outlet right ventricle, precise delineation of the malformation also depends on careful angiocardiographic analysis. The diagnosis can be established with confidence when the angiographic findings include simultaneous opacification of both great vessels from the right ventricle, aortic and pulmonic valves at the same transverse level, and separation of the aortic valve from the aortic leaflet of the mitral valve by the crista supraventricularis (Fig. 43–64). The position of the VSD and the relation between the great arteries must be defined to plan surgical procedures appropriately.

Experience is growing with the application of transesophageal echocardiography in analyzing the complex anatomical and spatial relationships encountered in double-outlet right ventricle, requiring a biplane or multiplane format for adequate assessment.

SURGICAL TREATMENT. The goals of operative treatment are to establish left ventricle–to-aorta continuity, create adequate right ventricle–to-pulmonary continuity, and repair associated lesions.[510] Because of the complexity of intracardiac repair of these anomalies, many centers prefer to give palliation to infants, attempting reparative surgery after the age of 1 to 2 years. In double-outlet right ventricle with subaortic VSD, repair is accomplished by creating an intraventricular baffle that conducts left ventricular blood to the aorta. When the VSD is subpulmonic, repair is accomplished by closure of the VSD and arterial switch.[510, 514] When the VSD is doubly

committed, i.e., both subaortic and subpulmonic, operation consists of creating an intraventricular baffle that conducts left ventricular blood to the aorta. The type of double-outlet right ventricle in which the VSD is remote and uncommitted to either semilunar orifice may be approached by a venous switch operation, permitting the right ventricle to eject into the aorta, followed by placement of a conduit between the left ventricle and the pulmonary trunk. Alternatively, some patients may be candidates for a cavopulmonary shunt or a modified Fontan procedure, particularly if additional findings include a common AV orifice, hypoplastic ventricles, a straddling tricuspid valve, or a straddling mitral valve.[515]

Double-Outlet Left Ventricle

One of the rarest cardiac anomalies consists of the origin of both great arteries from the morphological left ventricle. Conal musculature or an infundibulum usually is absent or deficient beneath the orifices of both semilunar valves.[516] The spectrum of associated malformations is broad. VSD and valvular or subvalvular pulmonic stenosis has been present in most patients. Supportive diagnostic information is provided by magnetic resonance imaging. Echocardiographic[517] and angiocardiographic assessment of the spatial relations of the origins of the great arteries are essential to an accurate diagnosis and to evaluating the possibility of operative repair. In most patients, the latter consists of closure of the VSD and placement of a right ventricle–pulmonary artery conduit.

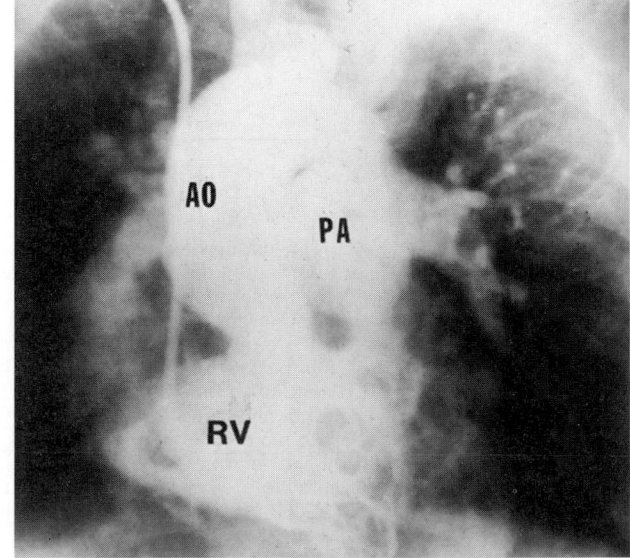

FIGURE 43–64. Simultaneous opacification of both great arteries from a right ventricular injection of contrast material in a patient with double-outlet right ventricle (RV). The aortic and pulmonic valves are at the same transverse level. AO = aorta; PA = pulmonary artery. (Courtesy of Dr. Robert White.)

Total Anomalous Pulmonary Venous Connection

This anomaly has been estimated to account for 1 to 3 percent of all cases of congenital heart disease and 2 percent of deaths therefrom in the first year of life.[518] The anomaly is the result of persistence during embryogenesis of communications between the pulmonary portion of the foregut plexus and the cardinal or umbilicovitelline system of veins, resulting in the connection of all the pulmonary veins either to the right atrium directly or to the systemic veins and their tributaries. Because all venous blood returns to the right atrium, an interatrial communication is an integral part of this malformation. Additional major cardiac malformations occur in about 30 percent of patients. Among these are common atrium, atrial isomerism, single ventricle, truncus arteriosus, and anomalies of the systemic veins. Extracardiac malformations, particularly of the alimentary, endocrine, and genitourinary systems, are present in 25 to 30 percent of cases.

MORPHOLOGY. The anatomical varieties of total anomalous pulmonary venous connection may be subdivided, depending on the level of the abnormal drainage (Fig. 43–65). Table 43–10 provides average figures of the distribution of the sites of anomalous connection.[578] The anomalous connection usually is supradiaphragmatic and to the left brachiocephalic vein, right atrium, coronary sinus, or superior vena cava. In about 13 percent, particularly in males, the distal site of connection is below the diaphragm. In this situation, a common trunk originates from the confluence of pulmonary veins and descends in front of the esophagus, penetrating the diaphragm through the esophageal hiatus. The anomalous trunk then connects into the portal vein or one of its tributaries, the ductus venosus, or, rarely, to one

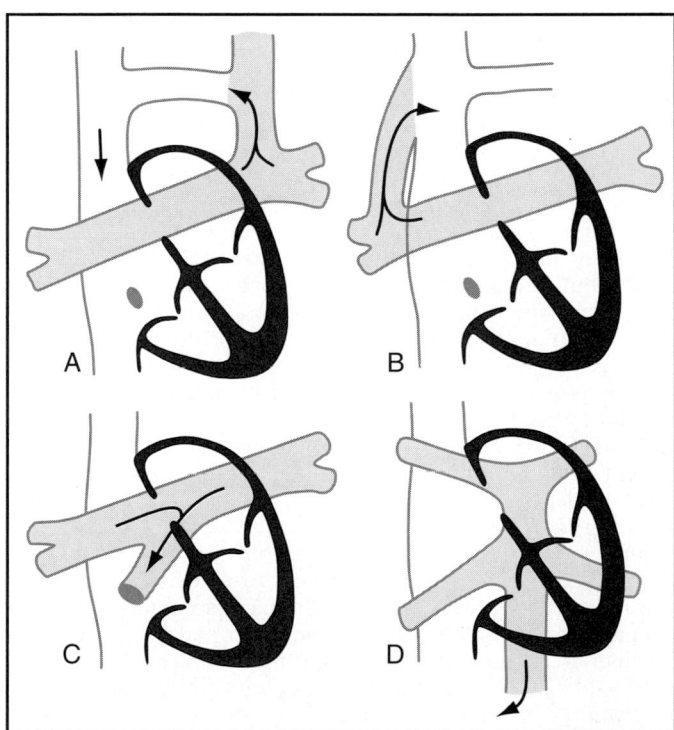

FIGURE 43–65. Anatomical types of total anomalous pulmonary venous return: supracardiac, in which the pulmonary veins drain either via the vertical vein to the anomalous vein *(A)* or directly to the superior vena cava with the orifice close to the orifice of the azygos vein *(B)*. *C,* Drainage directly into the right atrium or into the coronary sinus. *D,* Infracardiac drainage via a vertical vein into the portal vein or the inferior vena cava. (From Stark I, deLeval M: Surgery for Congenital Heart Defects. 2nd ed. Philadelphia, WB Saunders, 1994, p 330.)

Connection to right atrium	15%
Connection to common cardinal system	
(Right) superior vena cava	11%
Azygos vein	1%
Connection to left common cardinal system	
Left innominate vein	36%
Coronary sinus	16%
Connection to umbilicovitelline system	
Portal vein	6%
Ductus venosus	4%
Inferior vena cava	2%
Hepatic vein	1%
Multiple sites	7%
Unknown	1%

of the hepatic veins. In rare cases, various combinations of anomalous connection occur, with drainage to several levels.

HEMODYNAMICS. The physiological consequences and, accordingly, the clinical picture depend on the size of the interatrial communication and on the magnitude of the pulmonary vascular resistance. When the interatrial communication is small, systemic blood flow is markedly limited.[519] Right atrial and systemic venous pressures are elevated, and hepatic enlargement and peripheral edema are present. The size of the interatrial communication also is an important determinant in the development in utero and postnatally of the left atrium and left ventricle. Left atrial cavity size usually is somewhat reduced, whereas left ventricular volumes may be reduced or normal. The magnitude of pulmonary blood flow and therefore the ratio of oxygenated to unoxygenated blood that returns to the right atrium are a function of pulmonary vascular resistance. The arterial oxygen saturation, which ranges from markedly reduced to normal values, is inversely related to the pulmonary vascular resistance. In this regard, in most patients, the principal determinant of pulmonary pressures and resistance is related less to augmented pulmonary blood flow and pulmonary arteriolar vascular obstruction than to the presence and intensity of pulmonary venous obstruction.[520, 521]

Obstruction to pulmonary venous return and pulmonary venous hypertension are invariably present in patients with infradiaphragmatic anomalous pulmonary venous connection and in many with a subdiaphragmatic pathway. In the former type, pulmonary venous obstruction results from the length and narrowness of the common pulmonary venous trunk, compression at the esophageal hiatus of the diaphragm, constriction at the subdiaphragmatic site of insertion, or pulmonary venous return that must pass first through the portal-hepatic circulation before returning to the right atrium. When venous obstruction occurs in supradiaphragmatic types of drainage, constriction may exist at the entrance site of the anomalous veins into the systemic venous circulation, and/or the anomalous venous channel may be kinked or situated abnormally and compressed between the left pulmonary artery and left bronchus.[520] The presence of a small, restrictive patent foramen ovale occasionally results in pulmonary venous obstruction. Pulmonary vascular obstructive disease is rare during infancy, although exceptions have been reported. In patients without pulmonary venous obstruction, the risk of developing Eisenmenger reaction is comparable with that in patients with an atrial septal defect.

CLINICAL MANIFESTATIONS. The majority of patients with total anomalous pulmonary venous connection have symptoms during the first year of life, and 80 percent die before age 1 year if left untreated.[518] The few who remain asymptomatic have a relatively good prognosis; once the condition is detected, operation may be elected later in childhood. Symptomatic infants with total anomalous pulmonary venous connection present with signs of heart failure and/or cyanosis. Infants with pulmonary venous obstruction present with the early onset of severe dyspnea, pulmonary edema, cyanosis, and right heart failure. Cardiac murmurs often are not prominent. In the unobstructed forms of total anomalous pulmonary venous connection, the characteristic physical findings include right ventricular precordial overactivity and minimal cyanosis unless congestive heart failure intervenes. Multiple heart sounds often are audible, consisting of a first heart sound followed by an ejection sound; a fixed, widely split second heart sound with an accentuated pulmonic component; and a third and often a fourth heart sound. A soft systolic ejection murmur is usual along the left sternal border, and a mid-diastolic murmur of flow across the tricuspid valve commonly is audible at the lower left sternal border.

LABORATORY FINDINGS. The *ECG* shows right-axis deviation and right atrial and right ventricular hypertrophy. *Roentgenograms* of the chest reveal increased pulmonary blood flow; the right atrium and ventricle are dilated and hypertrophied, and the pulmonary artery segment is enlarged (Fig. 43–66). In addition, the specific site of anomalous connection may cause a characteristic appearance of the cardiac silhouette. Thus, in patients with total anomalous pulmonary venous connection to the left brachiocephalic vein, the superior vena cava on the right, left brachiocephalic vein superiorly, and vertical vein on the left produce a cardiac shadow that resembles a snowman or figure eight. The upper right cardiac border may be prominent when the anomalous connection is to the right superior vena cava.

Echocardiography demonstrates marked enlargement of the right ventricle and a small left atrium.[522] The objective of ultrasound imaging in these patients is to confirm the clinical diagnosis and to locate the site of connection of the common pulmonary vein. Doppler flow and color mapping enhance the capability of identifying all the pulmonary veins and their drainage sites and help to assess the presence of obstruction within individual pulmonary veins and along the vertical vein.[523, 524] An echo-free space representing the common pulmonary venous chamber may occasionally be seen to lie behind the left atrium on ultrasound examination. The use of echocardiography has supplanted cardiac catheterization in preoperative diagnosis in patients without atrial isomerism or single-ventricle hearts. Diagnostic echocardiographic findings include an absence of pulmonary vein connections and a small left atrium in the presence of right-to-left bulging of the septum primum at the foramen ovale. Positive diagnosis is made by identifying pulmonary venous connection to the systemic veins, coronary sinus, or right atrium rather than to the left atrium. All four pulmonary veins and their connections must be identified to diagnose mixed types accurately. There is no standard echocardiographic method for tracing pulmonary venous pathways because of their diverse anatomical positions, although transesophageal studies can importantly assist in this regard.[524]

An infradiaphragmatic total anomalous pulmonary venous connection usually connects to the portal venous system but can connect to the hepatic veins. Doppler is used to distinguish between the abdominal vessels. Thus, the flow pattern in the inferior vena cava is phasic, nearly continuous, and toward the heart, in contrast to flow in the descending aorta, which has a laminar profile in systole in a direction away from the heart. Flow in the common pulmonary vein resembles that of the inferior vena cava except that its direction is away from the heart. Although not often used, especially in infants, magnetic resonance imaging may also delineate the site of connections of the various types of total anomalous pulmonary venous return.

At *cardiac catheterization,* those patients found to have systemic arterial saturations below 70 percent and pulmonary artery pressure at or above systemic levels are likely to have pulmonary venous obstruction. Variations in oxygen saturation in the systemic venous circulation may be helpful. In the subdiaphragmatic type, a step-up may not be apparent in inferior vena caval oxygen saturations obtained by way of femoral vein cannulation because of the contribution of highly oxygenated renal venous blood to the caval stream. In contrast, sampling of the hepatic or portal vein by way of a catheter inserted through the umbilical vein yields diagnostically higher oxygen saturations, indicating anomalous return to those vessels. If the cardiac catheter can be manipulated directly into the anomalous trunk through its site of connection, selective injection of contrast material into the common channel provides anatomical definition of the pulmonary venous tree. If the pulmonary veins cannot be entered directly, selective right and left main pulmonary artery injection of contrast material often is more helpful than is injection into a main pulmonary artery because many infants have a persistent patent ductus arteriosus through which the contrast agent flows right to left. Moreover, the drainage from both lungs must be outlined clearly to preclude a mixed type of anomalous venous drainage. Pulmonary venous obstruction may be detected by noting a pressure difference between the pulmonary artery wedge pressure and the right atrium.

MANAGEMENT. Corrective surgery for sick infants should be performed as soon as possible, usually on the basis of two-dimensional and Doppler echocardiography, avoiding the additional stress of invasive diagnostic study. Before age 1 month, survival greater than 75 percent is anticipated. Infants with the worst prognosis are those in whom individual pulmonary vein sizes are smallest, which are measurements that can be made preoperatively by echocardiogram. Unless a child has pulmonary vascular disease, results of operation for total anomalous pulmonary venous connection in patients beyond infancy are generally good.[525, 526] The procedure consists of creating an anastomosis between the common pulmonary venous channel and left atrium and closing the atrial defect and the anomalous venous pathway. Improved results of operation in infancy require that postoperative pulmonary venous hypertension be averted by construction of a generally large anastomosis with or without enlargement of the left atrium. Normal hemodynamics and cardiac function have been demonstrated after surgical correction.

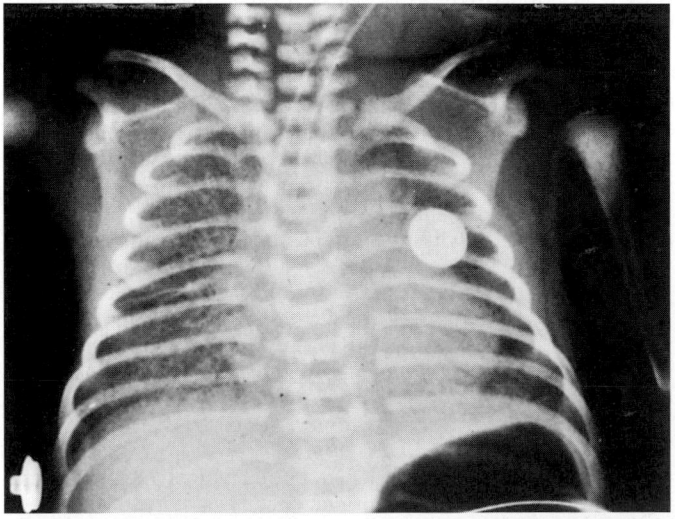

FIGURE 43–66. Chest roentgenogram in an infant with total anomalous pulmonary venous connection below the diaphragm shows normal overall heart size but a diffuse pattern of pulmonary venous hypertension in both lung fields.

Partial Anomalous Pulmonary Venous Connection

In this condition, one or more of the pulmonary veins, but not all, are connected to the right atrium or to one or more of its venous tributaries. An atrial septal defect, particularly one of the sinus venosus type, commonly accompanies this anomaly; the usual connection involves the veins of the right upper and middle lobes and the superior vena cava.[518] Exclusive of atrial septal defects, major additional cardiac malformations occur in about 20 percent of patients: these include VSD, tetralogy of Fallot, and various complex anomalies.

In the absence of associated anomalies, the physiological disturbance is determined by the number of anomalous veins and their site of connection, the presence and size of an atrial septal defect, and the state of the pulmonary vascular bed.[527] In the usual patient with isolated partial pulmonary venous connection, the hemodynamic state and physical findings are similar to those in atrial septal defect. Rarely, venous drainage of the right lung is into the inferior vena cava. This condition often is associated with hypoplasia of the right lung, dextroposition of the heart, pulmonary parenchymal abnormalities, and anomalous system supply to the lower lobe of the right lung from the abdominal aorta or its main branches. This complex has been designated the *scimitar syndrome* because of the characteristic roentgenographic finding of a crescent-like shadow in the right lower lung field that is produced by the anomalous venous channel.[528]

Transesophageal echocardiography is highly diagnostic of partial anomalous pulmonary venous connection and can obviate catheterization and angiography.[524] At *cardiac catheterization,* partial anomalous pulmonary venous connection to the coronary sinus, azygos vein, or superior vena cava may be identified by careful and frequent oximetry sampling. Oximetry is of limited value when the anomalous connection is to the inferior vena cava because of both reduced flow through the right lung and the contribution to the vena caval stream of highly oxygenated blood from the renal veins. Selective angiography is most helpful in cases in which the anomalous veins connect far away from the right atrium. Surgical repair offers definitive therapy at low risk if pulmonary vascular obliterative disease has not yet developed.

Malpositions of the Heart and Cardiac Apex

Positional anomalies of the heart are conditions in which the cardiac apex is located in the right side of the chest (dextrocardia) or is centrally located (mesocardia), or in which the heart is in its normal location in the left side of the chest but the position of the viscera is abnormal (isolated levocardia). Such hearts commonly are abnormal with respect to chamber localization and great artery attachments: associated complex intracardiac and extracardiac lesions are common.

Problems of terminology abound in the literature describing these complex cardiac anomalies, although sensible and uniform systems of classification are available.[529, 530]

ANATOMICAL FEATURES. Defining the cardiac anatomy in instances of cardiac malposition requires a description of three cardiac segments—the visceroatrial situs, the ventricular loop, and the conotruncus (the atria, ventricles, and great arteries, respectively). In addition to defining positional interrelation, the description of the malposed heart also must include the connections of the ventricles to the atria and great arteries as well as chamber identification, both morphologically and functionally.

DIAGNOSIS. To accomplish accurate diagnosis may require a synthesis of findings from noninvasive tests such as two-dimensional echocardiography, CT, and magnetic resonance imaging,[531] as well as hemodynamic and cineangiographic findings obtained at cardiac catheterization. Expert echocardiographers analyze, separately and independently of adjacent segments, each cardiac segment (atria, AV canal, ventricles, infundibulum, and great arteries) in terms of both situs and alignments.[532, 533]

In general, the determination of the body situs indicates the position of the atria. The visceral situs usually can be determined by the location of the stomach bubble and liver on a routine roentgenogram and of the inferior vena cava by means of echocardiography or the position of a cardiac catheter or by means of a CT or venous or radioisotope angiocardiogram. Atrial anatomy is best investigated noninvasively by using subxiphoid long- and short-axis and apical four-chamber echocardiographic views. Venous contrast injections may be useful to define systemic venous connections.

Situs solitus is the normal arrangement of viscera and atria, with the right atrium right sided and the left atrium left sided. Situs solitus is further characterized by a trilobed right lung and eparterial bronchus (i.e., the right upper lobe bronchus passes above the right pulmonary artery), a bilobed left lung and hyparterial bronchus (i.e., the left bronchus passes below the left pulmonary artery), the major lobe of the liver on the right, a left-sided stomach and spleen, and right-sided venae cavae. *Situs inversus* is a mirror image of normal.

Situs ambiguus or visceral heterotaxy refers to an anatomically uncertain or indeterminate body configuration. The latter often is seen in association with congenital asplenia, which resembles bilateral right-sidedness (right isomerism), and congenital polysplenia, which resembles bilateral left-sidedness (left isomerism).[530–535]

ASPLENIA (RIGHT ISOMERISM). Cardiac anomalies commonly associated with asplenia include anomalous systemic venous connection, atrial septal or complete endocardial cushion defect, common ventricle, transposition of the great arteries, severe pulmonic stenosis or atresia, and anomalous pulmonary venous connection usually infradiaphragmatic or to the superior vena cava–atrium junction. Polysplenia (left isomerism) commonly is associated with absence of the hepatic portion of the inferior vena cava with azygos continuation, bilateral superior venae cavae, anomalous pulmonary venous connection, and atrial septal defect (either ostium secundum or endocardial cushion). Pulmonic stenosis and double-outlet right ventricle are each observed in about 25 percent of cases. It is important to recognize these complex syndromes to distinguish them from forms of cyanotic heart disease that may be more amenable to corrective surgical therapy. In many of these patients, improvement results from palliation by modifications of the Fontan procedure, despite anomalies of systemic and pulmonary venous return in association with single ventricle anatomy.[536, 537] Diagnosis is suggested by a symmetrical liver shadow roentgenographically and, in asplenia, by the presence of Howell-Jolly and Heinz bodies in red blood cells demonstrated on blood smear, and it is confirmed by a negative or abnormal radioactive spleen scan.

Once the type of visceral situs is defined, it is necessary to describe the bulboventricular loop. The primitive cardiac tube normally bends to the right (D-loop), and thus the anatomical right ventricle is brought to the right of the anatomical left ventricle. An L-loop brings the morphological right ventricle left-sided relative to the morphological left ventricle. The L-loop is normal in the presence of situs inversus, but in situs solitus it is synonymous with inverted ventricles.

VENTRICULAR MORPHOLOGY. The number, morphology, and size of the ventricles can be ascertained by using various echocardiographic views. The morphological features of each ventricle also can be identified angiographically. The anatomical right ventricle is equipped with a tricuspid valve, is highly trabeculated, and contains the septal band of the single papillary muscle; its infundibulum lies anterior to and superiorly beyond the outlet of the left ventricle. The anatomical right ventricle usually connects with whichever of the two great arteries is the more anterior. The anatomical left ventricle is smooth walled and contains an outlet that lies posterior to the right ventricular infundibulum; its entrance is guarded by a bicuspid mitral valve, the anterior leaflet of which is normally in continuity with elements of the semilunar valve at its outlet. On echocardiographic examination, the insertion of the AV valves assists identification of the ventricle. The tricuspid valve is more apically situated than the mitral valve and is attached to the ventricular septum by papillary muscles, whereas the mitral valve is not. The right ventricular apical musculature is coarse and contains a moderator band of muscle.

GREAT ARTERIES. The great arteries are described in terms of their positional interrelations and their ventricular connections. Each outflow tract and semilunar valve should be examined in both long- and short-axis echocardiographic views.[533] The ventriculoarterial alignments may be determined by direct visualization from the subxiphoid window. The relation between the great arteries can best be demonstrated noninvasively using parasternal short-axis echocardiographic views, which display the semilunar roots. The aortic arch and brachiocephalic arteries are seen well using suprasternal notch views. The pulmonary artery is seen from high parasternal or suprasternal notch short-axis sections. The ventricular attachments may be normal or may form the anomalies of double-outlet right or left ventricle or transposition. The arterial interrelations are described as D (dextro), in which the ascending aorta sweeps toward the right and lies to the right of the main pulmonary artery; L (levo), in which the ascending aorta sweeps toward the left and lies to the left of the main pulmonary artery; or A (antero), which is the rare situation in which the aorta lies directly in front of the pulmonary artery. The D, L, and A descriptions of the aorticopulmonary artery interrelations should not be confused with the D- or L-loop designation of the ventricular interrelations.[530]

Using segmental sets composed of descriptive units of visceroatrial situs/ventricular loop/great artery relations greatly simplifies expression of the type of cardiac anatomy present in cardiac malposition. For example, the normal heart in a patient with situs inversus and dextrocardia is referred to as inversus/L loop/L normal; complete transposition of the great arteries in a patient with situs inversus is referred to as inversus/L loop/L transposition; functionally corrected transposition in a patient with situs solitus is referred to as solitus/L loop/L transposition; dextrocardia and functionally corrected transposition is designated solitus/D loop/D transposition with dextrocardia.

After the cardiac chambers are diagnosed functionally (arterial and venous), the positional and morphological relations are understood, and the presence of associated anomalies is established, the principles of medical and surgical treatment apply to these cardiac malpositions as they do to normally located hearts.[536]

Congenital Pericardial Defects

Isolated pericardial defects (see Chap. 50) are rare. They most commonly occur in males and usually are left sided, although they may be right sided, diaphragmatic, or total.[538] The anomaly is produced by deficient formation of the pleuropericardial membrane or, if diaphragmatic, defective formations of the septum transversum. Associated congenital anomalies of the heart and lungs occur in about 30 percent of cases. Most patients with the isolated defect are asymptomatic. Nonspecific anterior chest pain may be the result of torsion of the great arteries due to absence of the stabilizing forces of the left pericardium.

With complete absence of the left pericardium, a conspicuous apical impulse may be noted to be shifted leftward to the anterior or midaxillary line. ECG changes may be related to levoposition of the heart; a leftward displacement of the QRS transition in the precordial leads and vertical or right-axis deviation are usual. The diagnosis may be suggested by chest roentgenograms. With complete left pericardial absence, the heart is levo-posed, and the aortic knob, pulmonary artery, and ventricles form three prominent left heart border convexities.

A partial left pericardial defect may be suspected on the basis of various degrees of prominence of the pulmonary artery and/or the left atrial appendage. Echocardiographic findings often mimic those observed in patients with right ventricular volume overload (enlarged right ventricle and abnormal ventricular septal motion), probably owing to the altered cardiac position and motion with the thorax.[539] Other echocardiographic clues include lateral extension of the left atrial appendage as it herniates through the pericardial defect; this is best seen in short-axis views. The anomaly can be definitively diagnosed by CT or magnetic resonance imaging.[540] Cardiac catheterization is of little diagnostic value.

Complete absence of the left pericardium requires no treatment. Partial defects, however, may impose serious risks, including herniation and strangulation of the ventricles or left atrial appendage with left-sided defects or the possibility of a superior vena cava obstructive syndrome with right-sided defects.[541] In the diaphragmatic type, cardiac compression by abdominal contents requires surgical repair. Partial left or right defects may be closed with a patch of mediastinal pleura.

Single Atrium

Single or common atrium is a rare, isolated defect. The anomaly consists of an absent atrial septum, usually with a cleft in the anteromedial leaflet of the mitral valve and, occasionally, with a cleft tricuspid valve as well. The lesion may be one component of the Ellis-van Creveld syndrome (see Table 43–2) or of the complex cardiac anomalies in patients with asplenia or polysplenia.

Single atrium may be suspected clinically by the presence of cardiac murmurs of an atrial septal defect and mitral regurgitation associated with mild cyanosis, roentgenographic evidence of cardiac enlargement and increased pulmonary blood flow, and ECG features of AV septal defect. An absence of echoes from any part of the atrial septum is the essential feature of two-dimensional echocardiographic examination, which also may show a cleft anterior mitral leaflet, increased right ventricular end-diastolic dimension, paradoxical ventricular septal motion, and a dilated, pulsatile pulmonary trunk. Angiographically, the absence of the atrial septum produces a large, globe-shaped single atrial structure. Selective left ventricular angiocardi-

ography shows the characteristic gooseneck appearance seen in the various forms of AV septal defect. In the absence of pulmonary vascular obstructive disease, surgical correction is indicated by means of a prosthetic patch.

Single Ventricle (Univentricular Atrioventricular Connection)

Hearts with univentricular AV connection constitute a family of complex lesions in which both AV valves or a common AV valve open into a single ventricular chamber.[542] Terminology is varied, and the anomaly often is referred to as a double-inlet, single, or common ventricle, which is imprecise but useful shorthand for the entity. The definition excludes examples of tricuspid or mitral atresia. Single ventricle is almost always accompanied by abnormal great artery positional relations; the incidence of L-malposition of the great arteries is about equal to that of D-malposition. Associated anomalies are common and include, in particular, pulmonic valvular or subvalvular stenosis, subaortic stenosis, total or partial anomalous pulmonary venous connection, and coarctation of the aorta.

MORPHOLOGY. In about 80 percent of patients, the single ventricle morphologically resembles a left ventricular chamber that is separated from an infundibular outlet chamber by a bulboventricular septum.[543] The opening is variously called the bulboventricular foramen and VSD. The infundibular chamber is considered to represent developmentally the outflow tract of the right ventricle. The usual AV connection is transposition; when the heart is left sided, the connection is usually L-transposition, whereas it is usually D-transposition when the heart is right sided. When the great arteries are malposed, the infundibulum lying anteriorly at the basal position of the single ventricle communicates with the aorta and may be in one of two positions: noninverted (D-malposition), when it is situated at the right basal aspect of the heart, or inverted (L-malposition), when it is located at the left base of the heart. In the unusual situation in which the great arteries are normally related, the infundibulum communicates with the pulmonary trunk.[542] *Double-inlet left ventricle* is a term used synonymously to describe the most frequently encountered single ventricular chamber that has the anatomical characteristics of the left ventricle. Less commonly, the single ventricular chamber resembles a right ventricle (double-inlet right ventricle) or contains features suggestive of both ventricles or neither one; the latter two situations occasionally have been designated common ventricle and single ventricle of the primitive type, respectively.

CLINICAL FINDINGS. Depending on the associated anomalies, the clinical presentation of single ventricle mimics other conditions in which cyanosis and decreased or increased pulmonary blood flow coexist, e.g., tetralogy of Fallot or tricuspid atresia in the former instance or complete transposition of the great arteries and double-outlet right ventricle in the latter. The *ECG* in double-inlet left ventricle without inversion of the infundibulum (D-malposition) usually shows features of left ventricular hypertrophy. with infundibular inversion (L-malposition) the electrical forces are directed anteriorly and rightward, as they are in ventricular inversion without associated defects. In patients with the more primitive types of common or single ventricle, a repetitious rS pattern is seen in all the precordial ECG leads. *Chest roentgenographic* findings resemble those observed in patients with complete (dextro-) transposition of the great arteries or functionally corrected (levo-) transposition of the great arteries without features distinctive of single ventricle.

ECHOCARDIOGRAPHY. Two-dimensional and Doppler echocardiography are extremely important to demonstrate ventricular anatomy and to recognize associated intra- and extracardiac anomalies (Fig. 43–67). A segmental approach should be used for accurate and complete echocardiographic evaluation. Thus, precise details are required of the basic anatomy of atrial and visceral situs, location of the cardiac apex, the extracardiac course of the great arteries, and systemic and pulmonary venous connections.

In those patients in whom two separate AV valves communicate with the single ventricular chamber, *echocardiography* (see Chap. 7) suggests the correct diagnosis when echoes are visualized from the two valves without an intervening interventricular septum. In the absence of ventricular septal echoes when the two valves are not visualized simultaneously, they may be identified separately with a careful long-axis sweep of the ventricle. It is possible to detect the presence of a small outflow chamber anterior to the AV valves by using subcostal or parasternal short-axis views and a plane orthogonal to the long-axis plane (see Fig. 43–63).

The single ventricle with a single AV valve is suspected when the excursion of echoes from the single valve located posteriorly in the ventricular chamber is of large amplitude. Enhanced assessment of the AV valve in patients with single ventricle is provided by Doppler echocardiography.[544] Magnetic resonance imaging provides valuable information complementary to echocardiographic study. Selective ventriculography is necessary to delineate with certainty the anatomical type of single ventricle and to diagnose the associated great artery interrelations and the presence or absence of additional lesions.

SURGICAL TREATMENT. Modifications of Fontan approach are generally applied to patients with all types of anatomical and functional single ventricle.[545-547] Surgical outcome is related to the creation of an unobstructed pathway from the systemic veins to the pulmonary arteries, low pulmonary vascular resistance, and a compliant, well-functioning ventricle. In most centers, Fontan procedure is divided into two stages, an initial superior vena cava–pulmonary artery anastomosis (bidirectional Glenn shunt or hemi-Fontan procedure: Fig. 43–68), followed later by completion of the Fontan procedure directing flow from the inferior vena cava to the amalgamation of the superior vena cava and the branch pulmonary arteries. At first-stage operation, prior systemic-pulmonary shunts are eliminated and any areas of distortion or narrowing of the pulmonary arteries are repaired, particularly if a prior pulmonary artery banding was performed to limit pulmonary blood flow.

At our center, the complete Fontan procedure is accompanied by placement of a snare around the atrial septal defect to control its size postoperatively,[548] whereas in other centers, fenestrations in the atrial baffle may be used.[549-552] These procedures appear to reduce significantly postoperative morbidity from pericardial effusions and significantly improve survival. Results of early bidirectional cavopulmonary shunting in young infants are encouraging. The objective of this approach early in life is to yield a more suitable Fontan candidate while reducing ventricular volume overload and repeated palliative procedures. Subaortic stenosis, a common occurrence in patients with univentricular heart and malposed great arteries, occurs as a result of a restrictive bulboventricular foramen (VSD) or as a consequence of ventricular hypertrophy from a previous pulmonary banding operation.

The *Damus-Kaye-Stansel operation*, consisting of anastomosis of the pulmonary artery to the ascending aorta, is a generally successful approach to this problem.[552] After operation, all patients need continued close surveillance.[553-556] Complications include thromboembolic phenomena and atrial arrhythmias. Survivors generally lead active lives with exercise levels less than normal but relevant to ordinary daily life.

VASCULAR RINGS

MORPHOLOGY. The normal development of the aortic arch system is described earlier (see Fig. 43–3). The term *vascular ring* is used for those aortic arch or pulmonary artery malformations that exhibit an abnormal relation with the esophagus and trachea, causing compression, dysphagia, and/or respiratory symptoms.[557] The most common and serious vascular ring is produced by a double aortic arch in which both the right and left fourth embryonic aortic arches persist. In the most common type of double aortic arch, there is a left ligamentum arteriosum or ductus arteriosus and both arches are patent, the right being larger than the left. A right aortic arch with a left ductus or ligamentum arteriosum connecting the left pulmonary artery and the upper part of the descending aorta and with an anomalous right subclavian artery arising from the left descending aorta are additional important vascular ring arrangements.

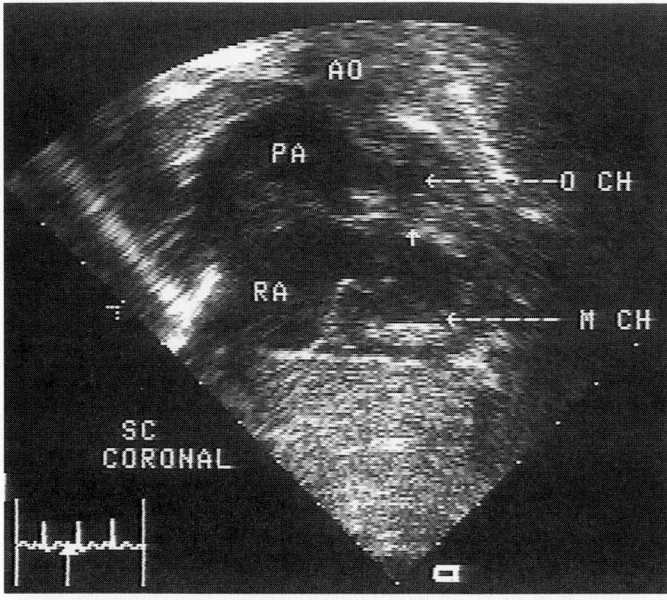

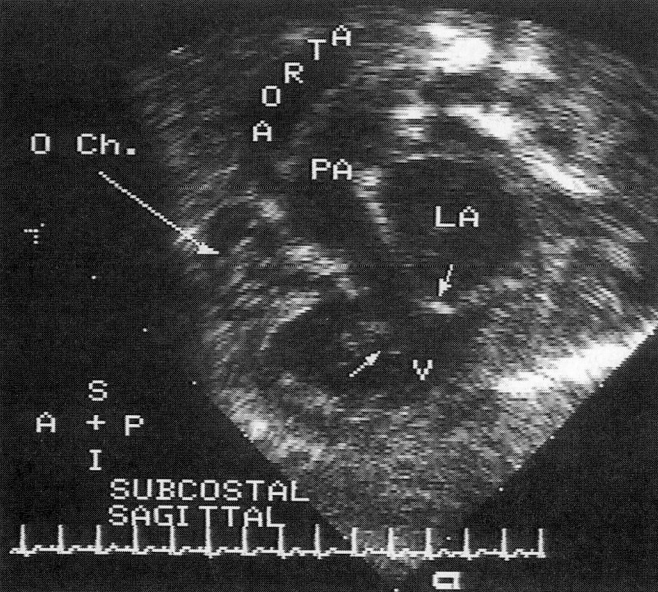

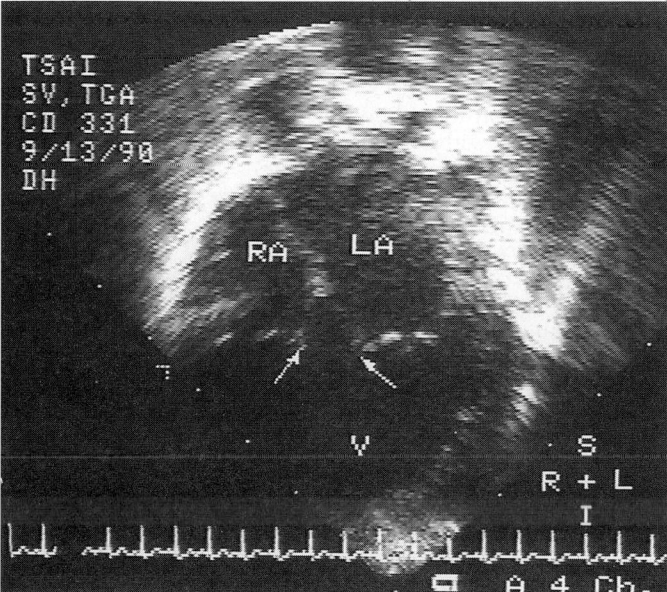

FIGURE 43–67. Echo images of a double-inlet left ventricle type of univentricular heart. *Top,* Subcostal coronal view shows the right atrium (RA) giving rise to a tricuspid valve guarding entry into a main chamber (M CH) of left ventricular morphology from which the pulmonary artery (PA) arises. The arrow indicates the small ventricular septal defect (bulboventricular foramen) entering into an outflow chamber (O CH), which gives rise to the aorta (AO). *Middle,* Orthogonal subcostal sagittal equivalent to the top frame. The left atrium (LA) is seen above the main chamber of left ventricular morphology (V). The arrows indicate the origin of the left and right atrioventricular valves within the same ventricular chamber. The pulmonary artery (PA) arises from the main chamber, and the long narrow bulboventricular foramen is shown to enter the outlet chamber (O Ch.), with its connection to the aorta. *Bottom,* Apical four-chamber view shows the right atrium (RA) and the left atrium (LA) with their corresponding valves (arrows) entering into the common large ventricle (V).

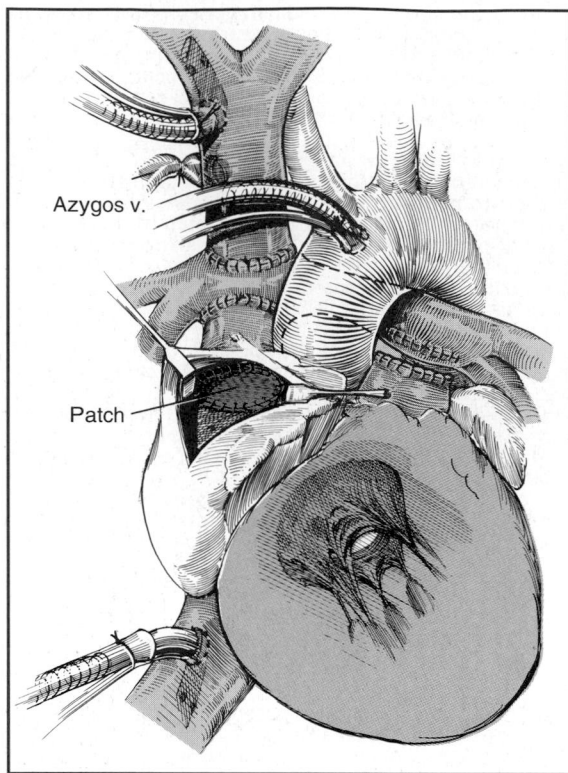

Azygos v.

Patch

FIGURE 43–68. A bidirectional cavopulmonary artery shunt with patch occlusion of the superior vena cava right atrial junction (hemi-Fontan procedure) using direct cannulation of the superior and inferior venae cavae and a single arterial cannula. The main pulmonary artery is shown divided and oversewn, but in some cases it may be allowed to remain patent. Connections are made between both ends of the divided superior vena cava and the pulmonary artery. A subsequent Fontan operation involves only removal of the patch at the junction of the superior vena cava and the right atrium and placement of the intraatrial baffle to divert the inferior vena caval blood up to the superior vena cava orifice. (From Castañeda A, Jonas RA, Mayer JE Jr, et al: Cardiac Surgery of the Neonate and Infant. Philadelphia, WB Saunders, 1994, p 263.)

The latter anomaly frequently exists in cases of tetralogy of Fallot and otherwise uncomplicated coarctation of the aorta. An unusual cause of tracheal compression is the vascular sling created by an anomalous left pulmonary artery that arises from a rightward, elongated pulmonary trunk and courses between the trachea and esophagus before it branches normally within the left lung.[558] This arrangement commonly is associated with other cardiac and extracardiac anomalies.

CLINICAL FINDINGS. The symptoms produced by vascular rings depend on the tightness of anatomical constriction of the trachea and esophagus and consist principally of respiratory difficulties, cyanosis (associated especially with feeding), stridor, and dysphagia. The ECG appears normal unless associated cardiovascular anomalies are present. The barium esophagogram is a useful screening procedure. Prominent posterior indentation of the esophagus is observed in the common vascular ring arrangements, although the pulmonary artery vascular sling produces an anterior indentation. Unusual and rare aortic arch anomalies may create rings that impinge on the trachea but do not compress the esophagus and are detected not by this simple radiographic procedure but rather by bronchoscopy. Selective contrast angiography delineates the anatomy of the aorta and its branches or the course of the main pulmonary arteries. CT and magnetic resonance imaging offer excellent imaging alternatives.[559]

MANAGEMENT. The severity of symptoms and the anatomy of the malformation are the most important factors in determining treatment. Patients, particularly infants, with respiratory obstruction require prompt surgical intervention. Operative repair of the double aortic arch requires division of the minor arch (usually the left).[560] A reported 10 to 20 percent operative mortality is related, in part, to problems in postoperative respiratory care, especially when there is coexistent residual anatomical tracheal narrowing. Patients with a right aortic arch and a left ductus or ligamentum arteriosum require division of the ductus or ligamentum and/or ligation and division of the left subclavian artery, which is the posterior component of the ring. Video-assisted thoracoscopy holds promise as an alternative to open thoracotomy for management.[561] Operation seldom is indicated for patients with an aberrant right subclavian artery derived from a left aortic arch and left descending aorta. In patients with a pulmonary artery vascular sling, operation consists of detachment of the left pulmonary artery at its origin and anastomosis to the main pulmonary artery directly or by way of a conduit of its proximal end brought anterior to the trachea.[560] Some patients with persistent respiratory symptoms require postoperative evaluation of residual anatomical obstruction, tests of pulmonary function, and bronchodilator therapy.[562]

CONGENITAL ARRHYTHMIAS

This classification refers to arrhythmias that are present in infancy, whose causes, when known, relate to a structural malformation or defect of the conduction system or to an acquired prenatal condition such as myocarditis, hypoxia acidosis, or transplacental passage of a drug or substance from mother to fetus. In these latter examples, the substrate for the postnatal expression of the rhythm disturbance existed before birth and the arrhythmia is therefore designated congenital. Complete heart block and supraventricular and ventricular tachycardias are the most common important congenital arrhythmias.[563] The electrophysiological and ECG features of these arrhythmias are discussed elsewhere (see Chaps. 23 and 25).

Congenital Complete Heart Block

The AV node and the His bundle originate during fetal development as separate structures and later join together. Anatomical studies have shown the basic lesion in congenital complete heart block to consist of discontinuity between the atrial musculature and the AV node or the His bundle, if the AV node is absent. The anatomical interruption occasionally can be situated between the AV node and the main His bundle or within the bundle itself.[564] No cause is known for the vast majority of cases of congenital heart block in infants, who usually have otherwise anatomically normal hearts. However, fetal myocarditis, idiopathic hemorrhage and necrosis involving conduction tissue, and degeneration and fibrosis related in some instances to the transplacental passage of anti-SSA/Ro-SSB/La antibodies and other immune complexes from mothers with systemic lupus erythematosus all are entities capable of causing congenital heart block.[565] It is not clear if medical treatment in high-risk pregnancies aimed at reducing antibody titers will modify immunopathologic damage to the fetus. Less often, congenital heart block can be associated with various forms of congenital heart disease, the most common malformation being congenitally corrected transposition of the great arteries.[566]

Detection of consistent fetal bradycardia (heart rate 40 to 80 beats/min) by auscultation, fetal echocardiography (Fig. 43–69), or electronic monitoring allows anticipation of the correct diagnosis. A newborn, especially with a ventricular

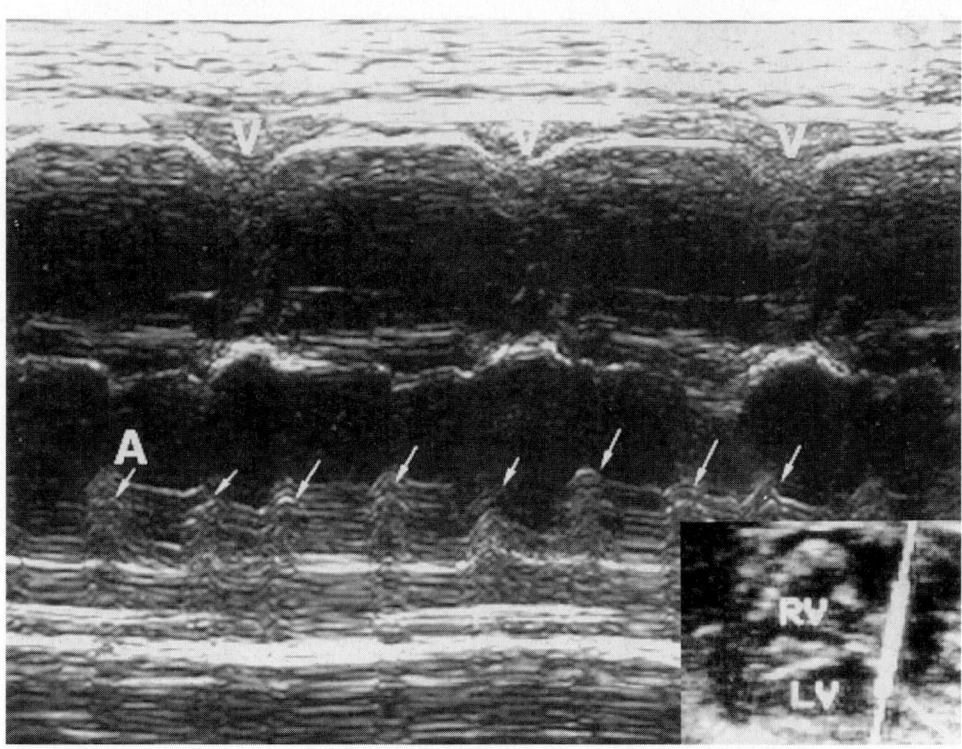

FIGURE 43-69. M-mode recording taken from the four-chamber fetal reference image shown in the lower right corner. The image is inverted, with the M-mode reference from fetal left ventricle (LV) through to the right atrium. In the M-mode, the ventricle is seen above (V) and the atrium (A) is seen below. The ventricular rate is approximately 48 beats/min, whereas the atrial rate is approximately 150 beats/min. There were no structural cardiac abnormalities. The mother had lupus erythematosus.

rate less than 50 beats/min and atrial rate in excess of 150 beats/min, is at highest risk; the presence of an associated cardiovascular anomaly greatly lessens the chances of survival. Treatment is not required for asymptomatic infants. Digitalization is recommended for infants in congestive heart failure, irrespective of complete heart block. Isoproterenol and other sympathomimetic drugs and atropine do not have permanent or beneficial effect. Congestive heart failure and Stokes-Adams attacks require pacemaker treatment at any age, including transvenous or transatrial placement of endocardial leads in older children or permanent epicardial pacemaker insertion in infants and small children.[567, 568] Various problems can be anticipated after pacemaker implantation related to growth of the patient, which stresses the electrical lead system; the fragility of the lead system in a physically active young patient; and the limited life span of the pulse generator. Patients who have congenital complete heart block and who survive infancy usually remain asymptomatic until late in childhood or adolescence.[569]

Supraventricular Tachycardia

Paroxysmal tachycardia of supraventricular origin can have its origin in utero or in the immediate postnatal period. The most frequent arrhythmias producing symptoms are paroxysmal supraventricular tachycardia with or without ventricular preexcitation, atrial flutter, and junctional tachycardia. The arrhythmia can cause intrauterine cardiac failure and hydrops fetalis[570, 571]; its detection and persistence prenatally should prompt consideration of administration of digitalis or, if that fails, of propranolol, quinidine, flecainide, or amiodarone to the mother if amniocentesis indicates surfactant deficiency and fetal lung immaturity, because early delivery is not indicated if the baby will have hyaline membrane disease. Experience with antiarrhythmic drugs, delivered by umbilical venous infusion, is limited.[96] Cesarean delivery or induced labor may be indicated if the fetus is close to term. No cause is recognized for the disorder in the majority of infants. Transplacental passage of long-acting thyroid stimulators (LATSs) and immune gamma-2-globulin from hyperthyroid mothers, hypoglycemia, and Eb-

stein's anomaly of the tricuspid valve occasionally are causative. WPW syndrome (see Chaps. 23 and 25) is present in 10 to 50 percent of infants with supraventricular tachycardia.[572] Symptoms produced by the tachyarrhythmia after birth are subtle and often remain undetected until signs of heart failure have been present for 24 to 36 hours. Conversion to normal sinus rhythm usually is accomplished by administration of digitalis or adenosine, direct-current cardioversion, transesophageal atrial pacing, or a diving reflex elicited by covering the face with an ice-cold wet washcloth for 4 to 5 seconds.[573-577] Conversion should be followed by digitalization on a prophylactic basis. Common practice consists of digitalis treatment for 9 to 12 recurrence-free months followed by its abrupt cessation.[578] Recurrence of tachycardia, particularly in those infants with ventricular preexcitation, is not uncommon; maintenance of normal rhythm may require administration, alone or in combination, of digitalis, phenytoin sodium, flecainide, sotalol, and amiodarone.[573] The rate of recurrence falls substantially between ages 2 and 10 years, with a slight rise during adolescence. In general, the prognosis is excellent.

ELECTROPHYSIOLOGICAL STUDIES. Beyond infancy, patients whose condition is refractory to medical treatment are candidates for electrophysiological catheter evaluation, which facilitates differentiation of a causative ectopic anatomical focus within the atria from accessory conduction pathways (see Chap. 23).[579, 580] If the tachyarrhythmia is refractory to pharmacological therapy, it should be treated definitively by radiofrequency catheter ablation of accessory pathways (see Chaps. 23 and 25). This procedure has become the primary treatment modality for most symptomatic rhythm disturbances in children. The results are excellent, with success exceeding 90% and very low complication rates.[576, 580, 581] Among the advantages of this approach is that successful ablation represents a cure; the heart is left structurally normal, and the cause of the arrhythmia is eliminated. Further, the need for antiarrhythmic agents with the concomitant risk of side effects or proarrhythmia is eliminated.

ATRIAL FLUTTER (see Chaps. 23 and 25). Uncommonly, atrial flutter is the cause of supraventricular tachycardia,[582] especially in newborn infants with hydrops fetalis, whose intrauterine tachyarrhythmia is an alternation between supraventricular tachycardia with WPW syndrome and atrial flutter. Another common clinical setting for atrial flutter is in infants younger than 6 months with an otherwise normal heart, who show frequent premature atrial complexes. In infants, classic flutter waves may not be present on a surface ECG or rhythm strip; detection may require recordings of transesophageal atrial electrograms. Acute treatment with electrical conversion or transesophageal overdrive pacing effectively terminates the rhythm disturbance.[583] If synchronized direct-current electrocardioversion is used, standby pacing should be available; if overdrive pacing is used, the same pacing catheter can be used to pace the heart in the event of asystole. Long-term drug treatment with digitalis, digitalis plus quinidine, or amiodarone may uncommonly be required.

Junctional automatic tachycardia is characterized by a narrow QRS complex and AV dissociation, with the ventricular rate faster than the normal atrial rate. Ventricular dysfunction and congestive heart failure occur early, and the rhythm disturbance usually is not convertible to sinus rhythm by any medical treatment. When the latter fails and because sudden death is a risk, catheter ablation can be used to eliminate the tachycardia focus. Pacemaker implantation may be necessary if heart block results (see Chap. 25).

VENTRICULAR TACHYCARDIA. Ventricular tachycardia is defined as three or more consecutive premature ventricular complexes (see Chap. 25). The definition, however, fails to identify a high-risk group. Infants or children who meet this criterion but seldom require treatment and seem to be at little risk have no symptoms and no evidence of anatomical heart disease. Potentially serious ventricular tachycardia in the newborn is associated with QT prolongation, mitral valve prolapse, and Marfan's syndrome. In these settings, the tachycardia is potentially life threatening and always merits treatment.[563]

Numerous genes causing long QT syndrome have been identified, confirming that the defects occurs in a transmembrane ion channel in most patients (see Chaps. 23 and 25).[584] The two most effective treatments are beta blockade and high thoracic left sympathectomy, which reduce the incidence of syncope and sudden death without affecting the QT interval. Trials of gene-specific therapy directed at the involved ion channel may be anticipated in the future.[584] Implantable defibrillators can be life saving in patients at risk for torsades de pointes and ventricular fibrillation.

The treatment of ventricular tachycardia (see Chap. 23) consists of intravenous administration of lidocaine, followed by direct-current electrical cardioversion. In the absence of QT prolongation but in the presence of mitral prolapse or other cardiac abnormalities, long-term treatment should be undertaken of multiform premature ventricular complexes, couplets, or ventricular tachycardia. In infants and children unresponsive to conventional or investigational antiarrhythmic drugs, consideration should be given to pacemaker implantation, cardiac sympathetic denervation, and perhaps implantation of a defibrilator.[585]

REFERENCES

1. Hoffman JIE: Congenital heart disease. Pediatr Clin North Am 37:45, 1990.
1a. Brickner ME, Hillis LD, Lange RA: Congenital heart disease in adults: I. N Engl J Med 342:256–263, 2000.
1b. Brickner ME, Hillis LD, Lange RA: Congenital heart disease in adults: II. N Engl J Med 342:334–342, 2000.
2. Roberts WC: Anatomically isolated aortic valvular disease: The case against its being of rheumatic etiology. Am J Cardiol 49:151, 1970.
3. Warth DC, King ME, Cohen JM, et al: Prevalence of mitral valve prolapse in normal children. J Am Coll Cardiol 5:1173, 1985.
4. Fontana RS, Edwards JE: Congenital Cardiac Disease: A Review of 357 Cases Studied Pathologically. Philadelphia, WB Saunders, 1962.
5. Bankl H: Congenital Malformations of the Heart and Great Vessels: Synopsis of Pathology, Embryology and Natural History. Baltimore-Munich, Urban & Schwarzenberg, 1977.
6. Gerlis LM: Covert congenital cardiovascular malformations discovered in an autopsy series of nearly 5000 cases. Cardiovasc Pathol 5:11, 1996.
7. Samanek M: Boy:girl ratio in children born with different forms of cardiac malformation: A population-based study. Pediatr Cardiol 15:53, 1994.
8. Clark EB, Gibson WT: Congenital cardiovascular malformations: An intersection of human genetics and developmental biology. Prog Pediatr Cardiol 9:199, 1999.
9. Goldmuntz E, Clark BJ, Mitchell LE, et al: Frequency of 22q11 deletions in patients with conotruncal defects. J Am Coll Cardiol 32:492, 1998.
10. Greenwood RD: Cardiovascular malformations associated with extracardiac anomalies and malformation syndromes. Clin Pediatr 23:145, 1984.
11. Ouelette EM, Rossett HL, Rossman MP, Wiener L: Adverse effects on offspring of maternal alcohol abuse during pregnancy. N Engl J Med 297:528, 1977.
12. Farrell MJ, Stadt H, Wallis KT, et al: HIRA, a DiGeorge syndrome candidate gene, is required for cardiac outflow tracts septation. Circ Res 84:127, 1999.
13. Noonan J: Twins, conjoined twins, and cardiac defects. Am J Dis Child 132:17, 1978.
14. Burn J: Consequences of chromosome 22q11.2 deletions. Circulation 90:II–ID, 1994.
15. Corone P, Bonaiti C, Feingold J, et al: Familial congenital heart disease: How are the various types related? Am J Cardiol 51:942, 1983.
16. Whittemore R, Wells, JA, Castellsague X: A second-generation study of 427 probands with congenital heart defects and their 837 children. J Am Coll Cardiol 23:1459, 1994.
17. Daubeney PEF, Sherland GK, Cook AC, et al: Pulmonary atresia with intact ventricular septum: Impact of fetal echocardiography on incidence at birth and postnatal outcome. Circulation 98:562, 1998.
18. Kumar RK, Newburger JW, Gauvreau K, et al: Comparison of outcome when hypoplastic left heart syndrome and transposition of the great arteries are diagnosed prenatally versus when diagnosis of these two conditions is made only postnatally. Am J Cardiol 83:1649, 1999.
19. Angelini P: Embryology and congenital heart disease. Tex Heart Inst J 22:1, 1995.
20. Anderson RH, Ashley GT: Anatomic development of the cardiovascular system. In Davies J, Dobbing J (eds): Scientific Foundations of Paediatrics. London, Heinemann, 1974, p 165.
21. Tworetzky W, McElhinney DB, Reddy VM, et al: Echocardiography as the definitive diagnostic modality for the preoperative evaluation of complex congenital heart defects. J Am Coll Cardiol 31(Suppl A):427A, 1998.
22. Rudolph AM: Congenital Diseases of the Heart. Chicago, Year Book Medical Publishers, 1974.
23. Hornberger LK, Sanders SP, Rein AJ, et al: Left heart obstructive lesions and left ventricular growth in the midtrimester fetus. A longitudinal study. Circulation 92:1531, 1995.
24. Sheldon CA, Friedman WF, Sybers HD: Scanning electron microscopy of fetal and neonatal lamb cardiac cells. J Mol Cell Cardiol 8:853, 1976.
25. McPherson RA, Kramer MF, Covell JW, Friedman WF: A comparison of the active stiffness of fetal and adult cardiac muscle. Pediatr Res 10:660, 1976.
26. Friedman WF: The intrinsic physiologic properties of the developing heart. Prog Cardiovasc Dis 15:87, 1972.
27. Huynh TV, Wetzel GT, Friedman WF, Klitzner TS: Developmental changes in membrane Ca²⁺ and K⁺ currents in fetal, neonatal, and adult heart cells. Circ Res 70:508, 1992.
28. Chen F, Wetzel GT, Friedman WF, Klitzner TS: ATP sensitive potassium channels in isolated neonatal and adult rabbit ventricular myocytes. Pediatr Res 32:230, 1992.
29. Ingwall JS, Kramer MF, Woodman D, Friedman WF: Maturation of energy metabolism in the lamb: Changes in myosin ATPase and creatine kinase activities. Pediatr Res 15:1128, 1981.
30. Friedman WF: Physiological properties of the developing heart. In Paediatric Cardiology. Vol 6. New York, Churchill Livingstone, 1987, p 3.
31. Geis WP, Tatooles CJ, Priola DV, Friedman WF: Factors influencing neurohumoral control of the heart and newborn. Am J Physiol 228:1685, 1975.
32. Klitzner TS, Friedman WF: Excitation contraction coupling in developing mammalian myocardium. Pediatr Res 23:428, 1988.
33. Klitzner TS, Friedman WF: A diminished role for the sarcoplasmic reticulum in newborn myocardial contraction. Pediatr Res 26:98, 1989.
34. Romero TE, Friedman WF: Limited left ventricular response to volume overload in the neonatal period. Pediatr Res 33:910, 1979.
35. Finer NN, Etches PC, Kamstra B, et al: Inhaled nitric oxide in infants referred for extracorporeal membrane oxygenation: Dose response. J Pediatr 124:302, 1994.
36. Friedman WF, Printz MP, Kirkpatrick SE, Hoskins EJ: The vasoactivity of the fetal lamb ductus arteriosus studied in utero. Pediatr Res 17:331, 1983.

PATHOLOGICAL CONSEQUENCES

37. Friedman WF, George BL: Medical progress—treatment of congestive heart failure by altering loading conditions of the heart. J Pediatr 106:697, 1985.
38. Artman M, Parrish MD, Graham TP Jr: Congestive heart failure in childhood and adolescence: Recognition and management. Am Heart J 105:471, 1983.
39. Meijboom EJ, Van Engelen AD, Van de Beek EW, et al: Fetal arrhythmias. Curr Opin Cardiol 9:97, 1994.
40. Milne MJ, Sung RYT, Fok TF, Crozier IG: Doppler echocardiographic assessment of shunting via the ductus arteriosus in newborn infants. Am J Cardiol 64:102, 1989.
41. Sahn DJ, Friedman WF: Difficulties in distinguishing cardiac from pulmonary disease in the neonate. Pediatr Clin North Am 20:293, 1973.
42. Stanger P, Lucas RV Jr, Edwards JE: Anatomic factors causing respiratory distress in acyanotic congenital cardiac disease: Special reference to bronchial obstruction. Pediatrics 43:760, 1969.
43. DiSessa TG, Friedman WF: Echocardiographic evaluation of cardiac performance. In Friedman WF, Higgins CB (eds): Pediatric Cardiac Imaging. Philadelphia, WB Saunders, 1984, p 219.
44. Mercier JC, DiSessa TG, Jarmakani J, Friedman WF: Two dimensional echocardiographic assessment of left ventricular volumes and ejection fraction. Circulation 65:962, 1982.
45. Huwez FU, Houston AB, Watson J, et al: Age and body surface area related normal upper and lower limits of M mode echocardiographic measurements and left ventricular volume and mass from infancy to early adulthood. Br Heart J 72:276, 1994.

46. Teitel D, Rudolph AM: Perinatal oxygen delivery and cardiac function. Adv Pediatr 32:321, 1985.
47. Rosenthal A, Nathan DG, Marty AT, et al: Acute hemodynamic effects of red cell volume reduction, polycythemia of cyanotic congenital heart disease. Circulation 42:297, 1970.
48. Voigt GC, Wright JR: Cyanotic congenital heart disease and sudden death. Am Heart J 87:773, 1974.
49. Fischbein CA, Rosenthal A, Fischer EG, et al: Risk factors for brain abscess in patients with congenital heart disease. Am J Cardiol 34:97, 1974.
50. Corrin C: Paradoxical embolism. Br Heart J 26:549, 1964.
51. Haroutunian LM, Neill CA: Pulmonary complications of congenital heart disease: Hemoptysis. Am Heart J 84:540, 1972.
52. Guntheroth WG, Morgan BC, Mullens GL: Physiologic studies of paroxysmal hyperpnea in cyanotic congenital heart disease. Circulation 31:70, 1965.
53. Talmer NS: Congestive heart failure in the infant. Pediatr Clin North Am 18:1011, 1971.
54. Gingell RI, Hornung MG: Growth problems associated with congenital heart disease in infancy. In Lebenthal E (ed): Textbook of Gastroenterology and Nutrition in Infancy. New York, Raven Press, 1989, p 639.
55. Salzer HR, Haschke F, Wimmer M, et al: Growth and nutritional intake of infants with congenital heart disease. Pediatr Cardiol 10:17, 1989.
56. Friedman WF, Heiferman MF, Perloff JK: Late postoperative pulmonary vascular disease—clinical concerns. In Engle MA, Perloff JK (eds): Congenital Heart Disease After Surgery. New York, York Medical Publishers, 1983, p 151.
57. Rabinovitch M: Structure and function of the pulmonary vascular bed: An update. Cardiol Clin 7:227, 1989.
58. Rabinovitch M, Keane JF, Norwood WI: Vascular structure and lung biopsy tissue correlated with pulmonary hemodynamic findings after repair of congenital heart defects. Circulation 69:655, 1984.
59. Heath D, Edwards JE: The pathology of hypertensive pulmonary vascular disease. Circulation 18:533, 1958.
60. Burchenal JEB, Loscalzo J: Endothelial dysfunction and pulmonary hypertension. Primary Cardiol 20:28, 1994.
61. Celermajer DS, Dollery C, Burch M, Deanfield JE: Role of endothelium in the maintenance of low pulmonary vascular tone in normal children. Circulation 89:2041, 1994.
62. Niwa K, Perloff JK, Kaplan S, et al: Eisenmenger syndrome in adults: Ventricular septal defect, truncus arteriosus, univentricular heart. J Am Coll Cardiol 34:223, 1999.
63. Rabinovitch M, Reid LM: Quantitative structural analysis of the pulmonary vascular bed in congenital heart defects. In Engle MA (ed): Pediatric Cardiovascular Disease. Philadelphia, FA Davis, 1981, p 149.
64. Friedman WF: Proceedings of the National Heart, Lung and Blood Institute Pediatric Cardiology Workshop: Pulmonary Hypertension. Pediatr Res 20:8, 1986.
65. Kovalchin JP, Mott AR, Rosen KL, et al: Nitric oxide for the evaluation and treatment of pulmonary hypertension in congenital heart disease. Tex Heart Inst J 24:308, 1997.
66. Rabinovitch M, Keane JF, Fellows KE, et al: Quantitative analysis of the pulmonary wedge angiogram in congenital heart defects. Circulation 63:152, 1981.
67. Rabinovitch M, Castaneda AR, Reid L: Lung biopsy with frozen section as a diagnostic aid in patients with congenital heart defects. Am J Cardiol 47:77, 1981.
68. Yamaki S, Abe A, Tabayashi K, et al: Inoperable pulmonary vascular disease in infants with congenital heart disease. Ann Thorac Surg 66:1565, 1998.
69. Rabinovitch M: Pathophysiology of pulmonary hypertension. In Emmanouilides GC, Riemenschneider TA, Allen HD, et al (eds): Moss and Adams' Heart Disease in Infants, Children, and Adolescents. 5th ed. Baltimore, Williams & Wilkins, 1995, p 1659.
70. Rosenzweig EB, Kerstein D, Barst RJ: Long-term prostacyclin for pulmonary hypertension with associated congenital heart defects. Circulation 99:1858, 1999.
71. Barst RJ: Recent advances in the treatment of pulmonary artery hypertension. Am Coll Cardiol Curr J Rev 7:60, 1998.
72. Awadallah SM, Kavey RE, Byrum CJ, et al: The changing pattern of infective endocarditis in childhood. Am J Cardiol 68:90, 1991.
73. Roberts GJ, Holzel HS, Sury MRJ, et al: Dental bacteremia in children. Pediatr Cardiol 18:24, 1997.
74. Dajani AS, Taubert KA, Wilson W, et al: Prevention of bacterial endocarditis: Recommendations by the American Heart Association. Circulation 96:358, 1997.
74a. Bayer AS, Bolger AF, Taubert KA, et al: Diagnosis and management of infective endocarditis and its complications. Circulation 98:2936, 1998.
75. Selbst SM, Ruddy RM, Clark BJ, et al: Pediatric chest pain: A prospective study. Pediatrics 82:319, 1988.
76. Driscoll DJ, Jacobsen SJ, Porter CJ, Wollan PC: Syncope in children and adolescents. J Am Coll Cardiol 29:1039, 1997.
77. Grubb BP, Samoil D, Kosinski D, et al: Use of sertraline hydrochloride in the treatment of refractory neurocardiogenic syncope in children and adolescents. Am Coll Cardiol 24:490, 1994.
78. Gillette PC, Garson A: Sudden cardiac death in the pediatric population. Circulation 85:1, 1992.
79. Maron BJ, Gohman TE, Aeppli D: Prevalence of sudden cardiac death during competitive sports activities in Minnesota high school athletes. J Am Coll Cardiol 32:1881, 1998.
80. Ackerman MJ: The long QT syndrome: Ion channel diseases of the heart. Mayo Clin Proc 73:250, 1998.

APPROACH TO THE HIGH-RISK INFANT

81. Friedman WF, George BL: New concepts and drugs in the treatment of congestive heart failure. Pediatr Clin North Am 31:1197, 1984.
82. Anderson PAW: Maturation in cardiac contractility. Cardiol Clin 7:209, 1989.
83. Park MK: Use of digoxin in infants and children, with specific emphasis on dosage. J Pediatr 108:871, 1986.
84. Hauptman PJ, Kelly RA: Digitalis. Circulation 99:1265, 1999.
85. Lewis AB, Freed MD, Heymann MA, et al: Diagnosis and management of infective endocarditis and its complications. Circulation 98:2936, 1998.
86. Friedman WF, Kurlinski J, Jacob J, et al: Inhibition of prostaglandin and prostacyclin synthesis in clinical management of PDA. Semin Perinatol 4:125, 1980.
87. Friedman WF: Patent ductus arteriosus in respiratory distress syndrome. Pediatr Cardiol 4(Suppl 2):3, 1983.
88. Brunner-La Rocca HP, Vaddadi G, Esler MD: Recent insight into therapy of congestive heart failure: Focus on ACE inhibition and angiotensin-II antagonism. J Am Coll Cardiol 33:1163, 1999.
89. Harada K, Tamura M, Ito T, et al: Effects of low-dose dobutamine on left ventricular diastolic filling in children. Pediatr Cardiol 17:220, 1996.
90. Mendelsohn AM, Johnson CE, Brown CE, et al: Hemodynamic and clinical effects of oral levodopa in children with congestive heart failure. J Am Coll Cardiol 30:237, 1997.
91. Colucci WS: Molecular and cellular mechanisms of myocardial failure. Am J Cardiol 80(11A):15L, 1997.
92. Snyder JV: Assessment of systemic oxygen transport. In Snyder JV (ed): Oxygen Transport in the Clinically Ill. Chicago, Year Book, 1987, p 179.
92a. Kleinman CS, Donnerstein RL: Ultrasonic assessment of cardiac function in the intact human fetus. J Am Coll Cardiol 5:84S, 1985.
93. Silverman NH, Kleinman CS, Rudolph AM, et al: Fetal atrioventricular valve insufficiency associated with nonimmune hydrops: A two-dimensional echocardiographic and pulsed Doppler ultrasound study. Circulation 72:825, 1985.
94. Allan LD, Sharland GK, Millburn A, et al: Prospective diagnosis of 1,006 consecutive cases of congenital heart disease in the fetus. J Am Coll Cardiol 23:1452, 1994.
95. Hornberger LK, Bromley B, Lichter E, Benacerraf BR: Development of severe aortic stenosis and left ventricular dysfunction with endocardial fibroelastosis in a second trimester fetus. J Ultrasound Med 15:651, 1996.
96. Gembruch U, Manz M, Bald R, et al: Repeated intravascular treatment with amiodarone in a fetus with refractory supraventricular tachycardia and hydrops fetalis. Am Heart J 118:1335, 1989.
97. Tworetzky W, McElhinney DB, Brook MM, et al: Echocardiographic diagnosis alone for the complete repair of major congenital heart defects. J Am Coll Cardiol 33:228, 1999.
97a. Balestrini L, Fleishman C, Lanzoni L, et al: Real-time 3-dimensional echocardiography evaluation of congenital heart disease. J Am Soc Echocardiogr 13:171–176, 2000.
98. Silverman NH, Schmidt KG: The current role of Doppler echocardiography in the diagnosis of heart disease in children. Cardiol Clin 7:265, 1989.
99. Cloez JL, Schmidt KG, Birk E, Silverman NH: Determination of pulmonary systemic blood flow ratio in children by simplified Doppler echocardiographic method. J Am Coll Cardiol 11:825, 1988.
99a. de Roos A, Roest AA: Evaluation of congenital heart disease by magnetic resonance imaging. Eur Radiol 10:2–6, 2000.
100. Beekman RP, Filippini LHPM, Meijboom EJ: Evolving usage of pediatric cardiac catheterization. Curr Opin Cardiol 9:721, 1994.
101. Stanger P, Heymann MA, Tarnoff H, et al: Complications of cardiac catheterization of neonates, infants and children. Circulation 50:595, 1974.
102. Allen HD, Driscoll DJ, Fricker FJ, et al: Guidelines for pediatric therapeutic cardiac catheterization. Circulation 84:2248, 1991.
103. Shim D, Lloyd TR, Crowley DC, Beekman RH: Neonatal cardiac catheterization: A 10-year transition from diagnosis to therapy. Pediatr Cardiol 20:131, 1999.
104. Mullins CE: History of pediatric interventional catheterization: Pediatric therapeutic cardiac catheterizations. Pediatr Cardiol 19:3, 1998.
105. Moore JW: Advances in pediatric interventional catheterization. Prog Pediatr Cardiol 6:93, 1996.
106. Kugler JD, Danford DA, Deal BJ: Radiofrequency catheter ablation for tachyarrhythmias in children and adolescents. N Engl J Med 330:1481, 1994.
107. Zipes DP, Akthar M, Denes P, et al: Guidelines for clinical intracardiac electrophysiologic studies: A report of the American College of Cardiology/AHA Task Force on assessment of diagnostic and therapeutic cardiovascular procedures. J Am Coll Cardiol 14:1827, 1989.
108. Klitzner TS, Wetzel GT, Saxon LA, Stevenson WG: Radiofrequency ablation: A new era in the management of pediatric arrhythmias. Am J Dis Child 147:769, 1993.
109. Van Hare GF, Lesh MD, Stanger P: Radiofrequency catheter ablation of supraventricular arrhythmias in patients with congenital heart disease: Results and technical considerations. J Am Coll Cardiol 22:883, 1993.

110. Hunt CE, Lucas RV Jr: Symptomatic atrial septal defect in infancy. Circulation 42:1042, 1973.

111. Van Praagh S, Carrera ME, Sanders SP, et al: Sinus venosus defects: Unroofing of the right pulmonary veins—anatomic and echocardiographic findings and surgical treatment. Am Heart J 128:365, 1994.

112. Bashi VV, Ravikumar E, Jairaj PS, et al: Coexistent mitral valve disease with left-to-right shunt at the atrial level: Clinical profile, hemodynamics, and surgical considerations in 67 consecutive patients. Am Heart J 114:1406, 1987.

113. Leachman RD, Cokkinos DV, Cooley DA: Association of ostium secundum atrial septal defects with mitral valve prolapse. Am J Cardiol 38:167, 1976.

114. Levin AR, Spach MS, Boineau JP et al: Atrial pressure flow dynamics and atrial septal defects (secundum type). Circulation 37:476, 1968.

115. Helgason H, Jonsdottir G: Spontaneous closure of atrial septal defects. Pediatr Cardiol 20:195, 1999.

116. O'Toole JD, Reddy I, Curtiss EI, Shaver JA: The mechanism of splitting the second heart sound in atrial septal defect. Circulation 41:1047, 1977.

117. Heller J, Hagège AA, Besse B, et al: "Crochetage" (notch) on R wave in inferior limb leads: A new independent electrocardiographic sign of atrial septal defect. J Am Coll Cardiol 27:877, 1996.

118. Konstantinides S, Kasper W, Geibel A, et al: Detection of left-to-right shunt in atrial septal defect by negative contrast echocardiography: A comparison of transthoracic and transesophageal approach. Am Heart J 126:909, 1993.

119. Pascoe RD, Oh JK, Warnes CA, et al: Diagnosis of sinus venosus atrial septal defect with transesophageal echocardiography. Circulation 94:1049, 1996.

120. Shub C, Tajik AJ, Seward JB, et al: Surgical repair of uncomplicated atrial septal defect without "routine" preoperative cardiac catheterization. J Am Coll Cardiol 6:49, 1985.

121. Taketa RM, Sahn DJ, Simon AL, et al: Catheter positions in congenital cardiac malformations. Circulation 51:749, 1975.

122. Brand A, Keren A, Branski D, et al: Natural course of atrial septal aneurysm in children and the potential for spontaneous closure of associated septal defect. Am J Cardiol 64:996, 1989.

123. Black MD, Freedom RM: Minimally invasive repair of atrial septal defects. Ann Thorac Surg 65:765, 1998.

124. Steele PM, Fuster V, Cohen M, et al: Isolated atrial septal defect with pulmonary vascular obstructive disease—long term follow up and prediction of outcome after surgical correction. Circulation 76:1037, 1987.

125. Thanopoulos B, Laskari CV, Tsaousis GS, et al: Closure of atrial septal defects with the Amplatzer occlusion device: Preliminary results. J Am Coll Cardiol 31:1110, 1998.

126. Formigari R, Santoro G, Rossetti L, et al: Comparison of three different atrial septal defect occlusion devices. Am J Cardiol 82:690, 1998.

127. Rao PS: Transcatheter closure of atrial septal defect: Are we there yet? J Am Coll Cardiol 31:1117, 1998.

128. Levin AR, Liebson PR, Ehlers KH, Daimant B: Assessment of left ventricular function in atrial septal defect. Pediatr Res 9:894, 1975.

129. Epstein SE, Beiser GD, Goldstein RE, et al: Hemodynamic abnormalities in response to mild and intense upright exercise following operative correction of an atrial septal defect or tetralogy of Fallot. Circulation 42:1065, 1973.

130. Murphy JG, Gersh BJ, McGoon MD, et al: Long term outcome after surgical repair of isolated atrial septal defect. N Engl J Med 323:1645, 1990.

131. Bink-Boelkens MTE, Bergstra A, Landsman MLJ: Functional abnormalities of the conduction system in children with an atrial septal defect. Int J Cardiol 20:263, 1988.

132. Bink-Boelkens MTE, Meuzelaar KJ, Eygelaar A: Arrhythmias after repair of secundum atrial septal defect: The influence of surgical modification. Am Heart J 115:629, 1988.

133. Jacobsen JR, Gillette PC, Corbett BN, et al: Intracardiac electrography in endocardial cushion defects. Circulation 54:599, 1976.

134. Minich LA, Snider AR, Bove EL, et al: Echocardiographic evaluation of atrioventricular orifice anatomy in children with atrioventricular septal defect. J Am Coll Cardiol 19:149, 1992.

135. DeBia SEL, DiCommo V, Ballerini L, et al: Prevalence of left-sided obstructive lesions in patients with atrial ventricular canal without Down's syndrome. J Thorac Cardiovasc Surg 91:467, 1986.

136. Suzuki K, Ho SY, Anderson RH, et al: Morphometric analysis of atrioventricular septal defect with common valve orifice. J Am Coll Cardiol 31:217, 1998.

137. Elliott LP, Bargeron LM Jr, Green CE: Angled angiography: General approach and findings. In Friedman WF, Higgins CB (eds): Pediatric Cardiac Imaging. Philadelphia, WB Saunders, 1984, p 1.

138. Najm HK, Williams WG, Chuaratanaphong S, et al: Primum atrial septal defect in children: Early results, risk factors, and freedom from reoperation. Ann Thorac Surg 66:829, 1998.

139. Meisner H, Guenther T: Atrioventricular septal defect. Pediatr Cardiol 19:276, 1998.

140. Najm HK, Coles JG, Endo M, et al: Complete atrioventricular septal defects: Results of repair, risk factors, and freedom from reoperation. Circulation 96(Suppl II):II-311, 1997.

141. Michielon G, Stellin G, Rizzoli G, Casarotto DC: Repair of complete common atrioventricular canal defects in patients younger than four months of age. Circulation 96(Suppl II):II-316, 1997.

142. Soto B, Ceballos R, Kirklin JW: Ventricular septal defects: A surgical viewpoint. J Am Coll Cardiol 14:1291, 1989.

143. Hagler DJ, Edwards WD, Seward JB, Tajik AJ: Standardized nomenclature of the ventricular septum and venticular septal defects, with applications for two-dimensional echocardiography. Mayo Clin Proc 60:741, 1985.

144. Baker EJ, Leung MP, Anderson RH, et al: The cross-sectional anatomy of ventricular septal defects: A reappraisal. Br Heart J 69:339, 1988.

145. Helmcke F, Souza A, Nanda NC, et al: Two-dimensional and color Doppler assessment of ventricular septal defect of congenital origin. Am J Cardiol 63:1112, 1989.

146. Pieroni DR, Nishimura RA, Bierman FZ, et al: Second natural history study of congenital heart defects: Ventricular septal defect: Echocardiography. Circulation 87:1, 1993.

147. Sabry AF, Reller MD, Silberbach GM, et al: Comparison of four Doppler echocardiographic methods for calculating pulmonary-to-systemic shunt flow ratios in patients with ventricular septal defect. Am J Cardiol 75:611, 1995.

148. Friedman WF, Pitlick PT: Ventricular septal defect in infancy—University of California, San Diego (Specialty Conference). West J Med 120:295, 1974.

149. Van Den Heuvel F, Timmers T, Hess J: Morphological, haemodynamic, and clinical variables as predictors for management of isolated ventricular septal defect. Br Heart J 73:49, 1995.

150. Kidd L, Driscoll DJ, Gersony WM, et al: Second natural history study of congenital heart defects: Results of treatment of patients with ventricular septal defects. Circulation 87:1, 1993.

151. Friedman WF, Mehrizi A, Pusch AL: Multiple muscular ventricular septal defects. Circulation 32:35, 1964.

152. Krovetz LJ: Spontaneous closure of ventricular septal defect. Am J Cardiol 81:100, 1998.

153. Kirklin JW, Barrett-Boyes BJ (eds): Cardiac Surgery. 2nd ed. New York, Churchill Livingstone, 1993, p 798.

154. Carotti A, Marino B, Bevilacqua M, et al: Primary repair of isolated ventricular septal defect in infancy guided by echocardiography. Am J Cardiol 79:1498, 1997.

155. Neutze JM, Ishikawa T, Clarkson PM, et al: Assessment and follow up of patients with ventricular septal defect and elevated pulmonary vascular resistance. Am J Cardiol 63:327, 1989.

156. Gheen KM, and Reeves JT: Effects of size of ventricular septal defect and age on pulmonary hemodynamics at sea level. Am J Cardiol 75:66, 1995.

157. Hislop A, Haworth SG, Shinebourne EA, Reid L: Quantitative structural analysis of pulmonary vessels in isolated ventricular septal defect in infancy. Br Heart J 37:1014, 1975.

158. DuShane JW, Kirklin JW: Late results of the repair of ventricular septal defect on pulmonary vascular disease. In Kirklin JW (ed): Advances in Cardiovascular Surgery. New York, Grune & Stratton, 1973, p 9.

159. Rhodes LA, Keane JF, Keane JP, et al: Long-term follow up (up to 43 years) of ventricular septal defect with audible aortic regurgitation. Am J Cardiol 66:340, 1990.

160. Wang JK, Lue HC, Wu MH, et al: Assessment of ventricular septal defect with aortic valvar prolapse by means of echocardiography and angiography. Cardiol Young 4:44, 1994.

161. Tohyama K, Satomi G, Momma K: Aortic valve prolapse and aortic regurgitation association with subpulmonic ventricular septal defect. Am J Cardiol 79:1285, 1997.

162. Leung MP, Mok CK, Lo RNS, Lau KC: An echocardiographic study of perimembranous ventricular septal defect with left ventricular to right atrial shunting. Br Heart J 55:45, 1986.

163. Gersony WM, Hayes CJ: Bacterial endocarditis in patients with pulmonary stenosis, aortic stenosis, or ventricular septal defect: Natural history study. Circulation 56(Suppl):1, 1977.

164. deLeval M: Ventricular septal defects. In Stark J, deLeval M (eds): Surgery for Congenital Heart Defects. New York, Grune & Stratton, 1983, p 271.

165. Waldman JD: Why not close a small ventricular septal defect? Ann Thorac Surg 56:1011, 1993.

166. Kumar K, Lock JE, Geva T: Apical muscular ventricular septal defects between the left ventricle and the right ventricular infundibulum: Diagnostic and interventional considerations. Circulation 95:1207, 1997.

167. Tee SDC, Shiota T, Weintraub R, et al: Evaluation of ventricular septal defect by transesophageal echocardiography: Intraoperative assessment. Am Heart J 127:585, 1994.

168. Rigby M, Redington AN: Primary transcatheter umbrella closure of perimembranous ventricular septal defect. Br Heart J 72:368, 1994.

169. Sideris EB, Walsh KP, Haddad JL, et al: Occlusion of congenital ventricular septal defects by the buttoned device. Heart 77:276, 1997.

170. Thanopoulos BD, Tsaousis GS, Konstadopoulou GN, et al: Transcatheter closure of muscular ventricular septal defects with the Amplatzer ventricular septal defect occluder: Initial clinical applications in children. J Am Coll Cardiol 33:1395, 1999.

171. Otterstad JE, Simonsen S, Erikssen J: Hemodynamic findings at rest and during mild supine exercise in adults with isolated uncomplicated ventricular septal defects. Circulation 71:650, 1985.

172. Graham TP Jr, Atwood GF, Boucek RJ Jr, et al: Right ventricular volume characteristics in ventricular septal defect. Circulation 54:800, 1976.

173. Heymann MA, Rudolph AM: Control of the ductus arteriosus. Physiol Rev 55:62, 1975.

174. Friedman WF, Printz MP, Kirkpatrick SE, Hoskins EJ: The vasoactivity of the fetal lamb ductus arteriosus studied in utero. Pediatr Res 17:331, 1983.

175. Skidgel RA, Friedman WF, Printz MP: Prostaglandin biosynthetic activities of the fetal lamb ductus arteriosus, other blood vessels and fetal lung. Pediatr Res 18:12, 1984.

176. Printz MP, Skidgel RA, Friedman WF: Studies of pulmonary prostaglandin biosynthetic and catabolic enzymes as factors in ductus arteriosus patency and closure: Evidence for a shift in products with gestational age. Pediatr Res 18:19, 1984.

177. Gittenberger-DeGroot AC: Persistent ductus arteriosus: Most probably a primary congenital malformation. Br Heart J 39:610, 1977.

178. Freed MD, Hegmann AB, Lewis AB, et al: Prostaglandin E₁ in infants with ductus arteriosus dependent congenital heart disease. Circulation 64:899, 1981.

179. Friedman WF, Hirschklau MJ, Printz MP, et al: Pharmacologic closure of patent ductus arteriosus in the premature infant. N Engl J Med 295:526, 1976.

180. Douidar SM, Richardson J, Snodgrass WR: Use of indomethacin in ductus closure: An updated evaluation. Dev Pharmacol Ther 11:196, 1988.

181. Shimada S, Kasai T, Konishi M, et al: Effects of patent ductus arteriosus on left ventricular output and organ blood flows in preterm infants with respiratory distress syndrome treated with surfactant. J Pediatr 125:270, 1994.

182. Hiraishi S, Horiguchi Y, Misawa H, et al: Noninvasive Doppler echocardiographic evaluation of shunt flow dynamics of the ductus arteriosus. Circulation 75:1146, 1987.

183. Merritt TA, Harris JP, Roghmann K: Early closure of the patent ductus arteriosus in very low birth weight infants: A controlled trial. J Pediatr 99:281, 1981.

184. Yeh TF, Achanti B, Patel H, Pildes RS: Indomethacin therapy in premature infants with patent ductus arteriosus—determination of therapeutic plasma levels. Dev Pharmacol Ther 12:169, 1989.

185. Gersony WM, Peckham GJ, Ellison RC, et al: Effects of indomethacin in premature infants with patent ductus arteriosus: Results of a national collaborative study. J Pediatr 102:895, 1983.

186. Wagner HR, Ellison RC, Zierler S, et al: Surgical closure of patent ductus arteriosus in 268 preterm infants. J Thorac Cardiovasc Surg 87:870, 1984.

187. Jarmakini MM, Graham TP Jr, Canent RV Jr, et al: Effect of site of shunt on left heart volume characteristics in children with ventricular septal defect and patent ductus arteriosus. Circulation 40:411, 1969.

188. Bessenger FB Jr, Blieden LC, Edwards JE: Hypertensive pulmonary vascular disease associated with patent ductus arteriosus. Circulation 52:157, 1975.

189. Prieto LR, DeCamillo DM, Conrad DJ, et al: Comparison of cost and clinical outcome between transcatheter coil occlusion and surgical closure of isolated patent ductus arteriosus. Pediatrics 101:1020, 1998.

190. Shim D, Beekman RH: Transcatheter management of patent ductus arteriosus. Pediatr Cardiol 19:67, 1998.

191. Ing FF, Sommer RJ: The snare-assisted technique for transcatheter coil occlusion of moderate to large patent ductus arteriosus: Immediate and intermediate results. J Am Coll Cardiol 33:1710, 1999.

192. Rao PS, Kim SH, Choi JY, et al: Follow-up results of transvenous occlusion of patent ductus arteriosus with the buttoned device. J Am Coll Cardiol 33:820, 1999.

193. Gray DT, Walker AM, Fyler DC, et al: Examination of the early "learning curve" for transcatheter closure of patent ductus arteriosus using the Rashkind occluder. Circulation 90:36, 1994.

194. Masura J, Walsh KP, Thanopoulus B, et al: Catheter closure of moderate to large-sized patent ductus arteriosus using the new Amplatzer duct occluder: Immediate and short-term results. J Am Coll Cardiol 31:878, 1998.

195. Singh TP, Morrow WR, Walters HL, et al: Coil occlusion versus conventional surgical closure of patent ductus arteriosus. Am J Cardiol 79:1283, 1997.

196. Hines MH, Bensky AS, Hammon JW, et al: Video-assisted thoracoscopic ligation of patent ductus arteriosus: Safe and outpatient. Ann Thorac Surg 66:853, 1998.

197. Le Bret E, Folliguet TA, Laborde F: Videothoracoscopic surgical interruption of patent ductus arteriosus. Ann Thorac Surg 64:1492, 1997.

198. Kutsche LM, Van Mierop LHS: Anatomy and pathogenesis of aorticopulmonary septal defect. Am J Cardiol 59:443, 1987.

199. Tulloh RMR, Rigby ML: Transcatheter umbrella closure of aorto-pulmonary window. Heart 77:479, 1997.

200. DiBella I, Gladstone DJ: Surgical management of aortopulmonary window. Ann Thorac Surg 65:768, 1998.

201. McElhinney DB, Reddy VM, Tworetzky W, et al: Early and late result after repair of aortopulmonary septal defect and associated anomalies in infants <6 months of age. Am J Cardiol 81:195, 1998.

202. Crupi G, Macartney FJ, Anderson RH: Persistent truncus arteriosus: A study of 66 autopsy cases with special reference to definition and morphogenesis. Am J Cardiol 40:569, 1977.

203. Suzuki A, Ho SY, Anderson RH, Deanfield JE: Coronary arterial and sinusal anatomy in hearts with a common arterial trunk. Ann Thorac Surg 48:792, 1989.

204. Juaneda E, Haworth SG: Pulmonary vascular disease in children with truncus arteriosus. Am J Cardiol 54:1314, 1984.

205. Farrell MJ, Stadt H, Wallis KT, et al: HIRA, a DiGeorge syndrome candidate gene, is required for cardiac outflow tracts septation. Circ Res 84:127, 1999.

206. Poelmann RE, Mikawa T, Gittenberger-de Groot AC: Neural crest cells in outflow tract septation of the embryonic chicken heart: Differentiation and apoptosis. Dev Dyn 212:373, 1998.

207. Yoshizato T, Julsrud PR: Truncus arteriosus revisited: An angiographic demonstration. Pediatr Cardiol 11:36, 1990.

208. Williams JM, de Leeuw M, Black MD, et al: Factors associated with outcomes of persistent truncus arteriosus. J Am Coll Cardiol 34:545, 1999.

209. Imamura M, Drummond-Webb JJ, Sarris GE, Mee RBB: Improving early and intermediate results of truncus arteriosus repair. A new technique of truncal valve repair. Ann Thorac Surg 67:1142, 1999.

210. Urban AE, Sinzobahamvya N, Brecher AM, et al: Truncus arteriosus: Ten-year experience with homograft repair in neonates and infants. Ann Thorac Surg 66:S183, 1998.

211. Heinemann MK, Hanley FL, Fenton KN, et al: Fate of small homograft conduits after early repair of truncus arteriosus. Ann Thorac Surg 55:1409, 1993.

212. Lin FC, Chang HJ, Chem MS, et al: Multiplane transesophageal echocardiography in the diagnosis of congenital coronary artery fistula. Am Heart J 130:1236, 1995.

213. Cox ID, Heald SC, Murday AJ: Value of transesophageal echocardiography in surgical ligation of coronary artery fistulas. Heart 76:181, 1996.

214. Hofbeck M, Wild F, Singer H: Improved visualisation of a coronary artery fistula by the "laid-back" aortogram. Br Heart J 70:272, 1993.

215. Zuppiroli A, Mori F, Santoro G, Dolara A: Coronary arteriovenous aneurysmatic fistula draining into the right atrium. Circulation 98:1946, 1998.

216. Sherwood MC, Rockenmacher S, Colan SD, Geva T: Prognostic significance of clinically silent coronary artery fistulas. Am J Cardiol 83:407, 1999.

217. Angelini P: Normal and anomalous coronary arteries: Definitions and classification. Am Heart J 117:418, 1989.

218. Hurwitz RA, Caldwell RL, Girod DA, et al: Clinical and hemodynamic course of infants and children with anomalous left coronary artery. Am Heart J 118:1176. 1989.

219. Johnsrude CL, Perry JC, Cecchin F, et al: Differentiating anomalous left main coronary artery originating from the pulmonary artery in infants from myocarditis and dilated cardiomyopathy by electrocardiogram. Am J Cardiol 75:71, 1995.

220. Karr SS, Parness IA, Spevak PJ, et al: Diagnosis of anomalous left coronary artery by Doppler color flow mapping: Distinction from other causes of dilated cardiomyopathy. J Am Coll Cardiol 19:1271, 1992.

221. Hamada S, Yoshimura N, Takamiya M: Noninvasive imaging of anomalous origin of the left coronary artery from the pulmonary artery. Circulation 97:219, 1998.

222. Vouhe PR, Tamisier D, Sidi D, et al: Anomalous left coronary artery from the pulmonary artery: Results of isolated aortic reimplantation. Ann Thorac Surg 54:621, 1992.

223. Francois K, Provenier F, Jordaens L, Van Nooten GJ: Anomalous origin of the left coronary artery from the pulmonary artery. Ann Thorac Surg 56:1168, 1993.

224. Schwartz ML, Jonas RA, Colan SD: Anomalous origin of left coronary artery from pulmonary artery: Recovery of left ventricular function after dual coronary repair. J Am Coll Cardiol 30:547, 1997.

225. Boutefeu JM, Morat PR, Hahn C, Hauf E: Aneurysms of the sinus of Valsalva: Report of seven cases in review of the literature. Am J Med 65:18, 1978.

226. Perry LW, Martin GR, Galioto FM, Midgley FM: Rupture of congenital sinus of Valsalva aneurysm in a newborn. Am J Cardiol 68:1255, 1991.

227. Holdright DR, Brecker S, Sheppard M: Ruptured aneurysm of the aortic sinus of Valsalva—difficulties in establishing the diagnosis. Cardiol Young 5:75, 1995.

228. Barragry TP, Ring WS, Moller JH, Lillehei CW: 15 to 30 year follow up of patients undergoing repair of ruptured congenital aneurysms of the sinus of Valsalva. Ann Thorac Surg 46:515, 1988.

229. Hutchins GM: Coarctation of the aorta explained as a branch point of the ductus arteriosus. Am J Pathol 63:203, 1971.

230. Prandstraller D, Mazzanti L, Picchio FM, et al: Turner's syndrome: Cardiologic profile according to the different chromosomal patterns and long-term clinical follow-up of 136 nonpreselected patients. Pediatr Cardiol 20:108, 1999.

231. Talner NS, Berman MA: Postnatal development of obstruction in coarctation of the aorta: Role of the ductus arteriosus. Pediatrics 56:562, 1975.

232. Heymann MA, Berman W Jr, Rudolph AM, Whitman V: Dilatation of the ductus arteriosus by prostaglandin E₁ in aortic arch abnormalities. Circulation 59:169, 1979.

233. Vitullo DA, DeLeon SY, Graham LC, et al: Extended end-to-end repair and enlargement of the entire arch in complex coarctation. Ann Thorac Surg 67:528, 1999.

234. Van Son JAM, Skotnicki SH, Van Asten WN, et al: Quantitative assessment of coarctation in infancy by Doppler spectral analysis. Am J Cardiol 63:1282, 1989.

235. Mendelsohn AM, Banerjee A, Donnelly LF, Schwartz DC: Is echocardi-

ography or magnetic resonance imaging superior for precoarctation angioplasty evaluation? Cathet Cardiovasc Diagn 42:26, 1997.

236. Pitlick PT, Anthony CL, Moore P, et al: Three-dimensional visualization of recurrent coarctation of the aorta by electron-beam tomography and MRI. Circulation 99:3086, 1999.

237. George B, DiSessa TG, Williams RG, et al: Coarctation repair without cardiac catheterization in infants. Am Heart J 114:1421, 1987.

238. DeGroff CG, Rice MJ, Reller MD, et al: Intravascular ultrasound can assist angiographic assessment of coarctation of the aorta. Am Heart J 128:836, 1994.

239. Fletcher S, Nihill MR, Grifka RG, et al: Balloon angioplasty of native coarctation of the aorta: Midterm follow-up and prognostic factors. J Am Coll Cardiol 25:730, 1995.

240. Rao PS: Stents in treatment of aortic coarctation. J Am Coll Cardiol 30: 1853, 1997.

241. Ebeid MR, Prieto LR, Latson LA: Use of balloon-expandable stents for coarctation of the aorta: Initial results and intermediate-term follow-up. J Am Coll Cardiol 30:1847, 1997.

241a. Cheung YF, Sanatani S, Leung MP, et al: Early and intermediate-term complications of self-expanding stents limit its potential application in children with congenital heart disease. J Am Coll Cardiol 35:1007–1015, 2000.

242. Backer CL, Mavroudis C, Zias EA, et al: Repair of coarctation with resection and extended end-to-end anastomosis. Ann Thorac Surg 66:1365, 1998.

243. Merrill WH, Hoff SJ, Stewart JR, et al: Operative risk factors and durability of repair of coarctation of the aorta in the neonate. Ann Thorac Surg 58:399, 1994.

244. Choy M, Rocchini AP, Beekman RH, et al: Paradoxical hypertension after repair of coarctation of the aorta in children: Balloon angioplasty versus surgical repair. Circulation 75:1186, 1987.

245. Siblini G, Rao PS, Nouri S, et al: Long-term follow-up results of balloon angioplasty of postoperative aortic recoarctation. Am J Cardiol 81:61, 1998.

246. Fawzy, ME, Sivanandam V, Galal O, et al: One- to ten-year follow-up results of balloon angioplasty of native coarctation of the aorta in adolescents and adults. J Am Coll Cardiol 30:1542, 1997.

247. Ovaert C, Benson LN, Nykanen D, Freedom RM: Transcatheter treatment of coarctation of the aorta: A review. Pediatr Cardiol 19:27, 1998.

248. Mühler EG, Neuerburg JM, Rüben A, et al: Evaluation of aortic coarctation after surgical repair: Role of magnetic resonance imaging and Doppler ultrasound. Br Heart J 70:285, 1993.

248a. Yetman AT, Nykanen D, McCrindle BW, et al: Balloon angioplasty of recurrent coarctation: A 12-year review. J Am Coll Cardiol 30:811, 1997.

249. Hijazi AM, Geggel RL: Balloon angioplasty for postoperative recurrent coarctation of the aorta. J Interven Cardiol 8:509, 1995.

250. Seirafi PA, Warner KG, Geggel RL, et al: Repair of coarctation of the aorta during Infancy minimizes the risk of late hypertension. Ann Thorac Surg 66:1378, 1998.

251. Johnson MC, Gutierrez FR, Sekarski DR, et al: Comparison of ventricular mass and function in early versus late repair of coarctation of the aorta. Am J Cardiol 73:698, 1994.

252. Van Woezik EVM, Kline HW, Krediet P: Normal internal calibers of ostia, great arteries and aortic isthmus in children. Br Heart J 39:860, 1977.

253. Bharati S, Lev M: The surgical anatomy of the heart in tubular hypoplasia of the transverse aorta (preductal coarctation). J Thorac Cardiovasc Surg 91:79, 1986.

254. Kocis KC, Midgley FM, Ruckman RN: Aortic arch complex anomalies: 2-year experience with symptoms, diagnosis, associated cardiac defects, and surgical repair. Pediatr Cardiol 18:127, 1997.

255. Apfel HD, Levenbraun J, Quaegebeur JM, Allan LD: Usefulness of preoperative echocardiography in predicting left ventricular outflow obstruction after primary repair of interrupted aortic arch with ventricular septal defect. Am J Cardiol 82:470, 1998.

256. Lewin MB, Lindsay EA, Jurecic V, et al: A genetic etiology for interruption of the aortic arch type B. Am J Cardiol 80:493, 1997.

257. Buck SH, Graham TP Jr, Lawton AR: DiGeorge syndrome: Implications for aortic arch obstruction. Prog Pediatr Cardiol 3:94, 1994.

258. Matsuki O, Yagihara T, Yamamoto F, et al: One-stage repair for intracardiac malformations associated with interrupted aortic arch or aortic coarctation in the first year of life. Cardiol Young 5:15, 1995.

259. Friedman WF: Congenital aortic stenosis. In Emmanoulides GC, Riemenschneider TA, Allen HD, et al (eds): Moss and Adams' Heart Disease in Infants, Children, and Adolescents. 5th ed. Baltimore, Williams & Wilkins, 1994, p 1087.

260. Driscoll DJ, Wolfe RR, Gersony WM, et al: Cardiorespiratory responses to exercise of patients with aortic stenosis, pulmonary stenosis, and ventricular septal defect. Circulation 87(Suppl I):I, 1993.

261. Graham TP, Louis BJ, Jarmakani JM, et al: Left heart volume and mass quantification in children with left ventricular pressure overload. Circulation 41:203, 1970.

262. Villari B, Hess OM, Kaufmann P, et al: Effect of aortic valve stenosis (pressure overload) and regurgitation (volume overload) on left ventricular systolic and diastolic function. Am J Cardiol 69:927, 1992.

263. Lewis AL, Heymann MA, Stanger P, et al: Evaluation of subendocardial ischemia in valvar aortic stenosis in children. Circulation 49:978, 1974.

264. Strasburger JF, Kugler JD, Cheatham JP, McManus BM: Nonimmuno-

265. McCaffrey FM, Sherman FS: Prenatal diagnosis of severe aortic stenosis. Pediatr Cardiol 18:276, 1997.

266. Mielke G, Mayer R, Hassberg D, Breuer J: Sequential development of fetal aortic valve stenosis and endocardial fibroelastosis during the second trimester of pregnancy. Am Heart J 133:607, 1997.

267. Lakier JB, Lewis AB, Heymann MA, et al: Isolated aortic stenosis of the neonate: Natural history and hemodynamic considerations. Circulation 50:801, 1974.

268. Magee AG, Nykanen D, McCrindle BW, et al: Balloon dilation of severe aortic stenosis in the neonate: Comparison of anterograde and retrograde catheter approaches. J Am Coll Cardiol 30:106, 1997.

269. Hawkins JA, Minich LL, Tani LY, et al: Late results and reintervention after aortic valvotomy for critical aortic stenosis in neonates and infants. Ann Thorac Surg 65:1758, 1998.

270. Egito ES, Moore P, O'Sullivan J, et al: Transvascular balloon dilation for neonatal critical aortic stenosis: Early and midterm results. J Am Coll Cardiol 29:442, 1997.

271. Rhodes LA, Colan SD, Perry SB, et al: Predictors of survival in neonates with critical aortic stenosis. Circulation 84:2325, 1991.

272. Weber HS, Mart CR, Kupferschmid J, et al: Transcarotid balloon valvuloplasty with continuous transesophageal echocardiographic guidance for neonatal critical aortic valve stenosis: An alternative to surgical palliation. Pediatr Cardiol 19:212, 1998.

273. Rhodes LA, Colan SD, Perry SB, et al: Predictors of survival in neonates with critical aortic stenosis. Circulation 84:2325, 1991.

274. Kovalchin JP, Brook MM, Rosenthal GL, et al: Echocardiographic hemodynamic and morphometric predictors of survival after two-ventricle repair in infants with critical aortic stenosis. J Am Coll Cardiol 32:237, 1998.

275. Braunwald E, Goldblatt A, Aygen MM, et al: Congenital aortic stenosis. I. Clinical and hemodynamic findings in 100 patients. Circulation 27:426, 1963.

276. Nishimura RA, Pieroni DR, Bierman FZ, et al: Second natural history study of congenital heart defects: Aortic stenosis: Echocardiography. Circulation 87:1, 1993.

277. Gersony WM, Hayes CJ, Driscoll DJ, et al: Bacterial endocarditis in patients with aortic stenosis, pulmonary stenosis, or ventricular septal defect. Circulation 87(Suppl I):I, 1993.

278. Parsons NK, Moreau GA, Graham TP Jr, et al: Echocardiographic estimation of critical left ventricular size in infants with isolated aortic valve stenosis. J Am Coll Cardiol 18:1049, 1991.

279. Bengur AR, Snider AR, Meliones JM, Vermilion RP: Doppler evaluation of aortic valve area in children with aortic stenosis. J Am Coll Cardiol 18:1499, 1991.

280. Gutgesell HP, French M: Echocardiographic determination of aortic and pulmonary valve areas in subjects with normal hearts. Am J Cardiol 68:773, 1991.

281. Beekman RH, Rocchini AP, Gillon JH et al: Hemodynamic determinants of the peak systolic left ventricular–aortic pressure gradient in children with valvar aortic stenosis. Am J Cardiol 69:813, 1992.

282. Tribouilloy C, Shen WF, Pelrier M, et al: Quantitation of aortic valve area in aortic stenosis with multiplane transesophageal echocardiography: Comparison with monoplane transesophageal approach. Am Heart J 128:526, 1994.

283. Shah PM, Graham BM: Management of aortic stenosis: Is cardiac catheterization necessary? Am J Cardiol 67:1031, 1991.

284. McCrindle BW, for the Valvuloplasty and Angioplasty of Congenital Anomalies (VACA) Registry Investigators: Independent predictors of immediate results of percutaneous balloon aortic valvotomy in childhood. Am J Cardiol 77:286, 1996.

285. El-Said G, Galioto FJ, Mullens CE, McNamara DG: Natural hemodynamic history of congenital aortic stenosis in childhood. Am J Cardiol 30:6, 1972.

286. Friedman WF, Modlinger J, Morgan J: Serial hemodynamic observations in asymptomatic children with valvar aortic stenosis. Circulation 43:91. 1971.

287. Cohen LS, Friedman WF, Braunwald E: Natural history of mild congenital aortic stenosis elucidated by serial hemodynamic studies. Am J Cardiol 30:1, 1972.

288. DeBoer BA, Robbins RC, Maron BJ, et al: Late results of aortic valvotomy for aortic valvular aortic stenosis. Ann Thorac Surg 50:69, 1990.

289. Keane JF, Driscoll DJ, Gersony WM, et al: Second natural history study of congenital heart defects. Circulation 87(Suppl I):I, 1993.

290. Kitchiner D, Sreeram N, Malaiya N, et al: Long-term follow-up of treated clinical aortic stenosis. Cardiol Young 5:9, 1995.

291. Jones TK, Lupinetti FM: Comparison of Ross procedures and aortic valve allografts in children. Ann Thorac Surg 66:5170, 1998.

292. Oury JH, Hiro SP, Maxwell JM, et al: The Ross procedure: Current registry results. Ann Thorac Surg 66:S162, 1998.

293. Chambers JC, Somerville J, Stone S, Ross DN: Pulmonary autograft procedure for aortic valve disease: Long-term results of the pioneer series. Circulation 96:2206, 1997.

294. Jaggers J, Harrison JK, Bashore TM, et al: The Ross procedure: Shorter hospital stay, decreased morbidity, and cost effective. Ann Thorac Surg 65:1553, 1998.

295. Frommelt MA, Snider AR, Bove EL, Lupinetti FM: Echocardiographic

assessment of subvalvular aortic stenosis before and after operation. J Am Coll Cardiol 19:1018, 1992.

296. Mugge A, Daniel WG, Wolpers HG, et al: Improved visualization of discrete subvalvular aortic stenosis by transesophageal color-coded Doppler echocardiography. Am Heart J 117:474, 1989.

297. Choi JY, Sullivan ID: Fixed subaortic stenosis: Anatomical spectrum and nature of progression. Br Heart J 65:280, 1991.

298. DeVries AG, Hess J, Witsenburg M, et al: Management of fixed subaortic stenosis: A retrospective study of 57 cases. J Am Coll Cardiol 19: 1013, 1992.

299. Brauner R, Laks H, Drinkwater DC Jr, et al: Benefits of early surgical repair in fixed subaortic stenosis. J Am Coll Cardiol 30:1835, 1997.

300. Serraf A, Zoghby J, Lacour-Gayet F, et al: Surgical treatment of subaortic stenosis: A seventeen-year experience. J Thorac Cardiovasc Surg 117:669, 1999.

301. Drinkwater DC, Laks H: Surgery for subvalvular aortic stenosis. Prog Pediatr Cardiol 3:189, 1994.

302. Gewillig M, Daenen W, Dumoulin M, Van Der Hauwaert L: Rheologic genesis of discrete subvalvular aortic stenosis: A Doppler echocardiographic study. J Am Coll Cardiol 19:818, 1992.

303. Williams WG: Surgical management of subaortic stenosis: Resection vs. modified Kono vs. Ross. Prog Pediatr Cardiol 9:23, 1998.

304. Frommelt PC, Lupinetti FM, Bove EL: Aortoventriculoplasty in infants and children. Circulation 86:II, 1992.

305. DeLeon SY, Iobawi MN, Robertson DA, et al: Conal enlargement for diffuse subaortic stenosis. J Thorac Cardiovasc Surg 102:814, 1991.

306. McElhinney DB, Reddy VM, Silverman NH, Hanley FL: Accessory and anomalous atrioventricular valvar tissue causing outflow tract obstruction: Surgical implications of a heterogeneous and complex problem. J Am Coll Cardiol 32:1741, 1998.

307. Ow EP, DeLeon SY, Freeman JE, et al: Recognition and management of accessory mitral tissue causing severe subaortic stenosis. Ann Thorac Surg 57:952, 1994.

308. Reeder GS, Danielson GK, Seward JB, et al: Fixed subaortic stenosis in atrioventricular canal defect: A Doppler echocardiographic study. J Am Coll Cardiol 20:386, 1992.

309. Garcia RC, Friedman WF, Kaback MM, Rowe RD: Idiopathic hypercalcemia and supravalvular aortic stenosis: Documentation of a new syndrome. N Engl J Med 271:117, 1964.

310. Friedman WG, Roberts WC: Vitamin D and the subvalvular aortic stenosis syndrome: The transplacental effects of vitamin D on the aorta of the rabbit. Circulation 34:77, 1966.

310a. Zalzstein E, Moes CAF, Musewe NN, Freedom RM: Spectrum of cardiovascular anomalies in Williams-Beuren syndrome. Pediatr Cardiol 12:219, 1991.

311. Friedman WF: Vitamin D embryopathy. Adv Teratol 3:85, 1968.

312. Friedman WF, Mills LF: The relationship between vitamin D and the craniofacial and dental anomalies of the supraventricular aortic stenosis syndrome. Pediatrics 43:12, 1969.

312a. Morris CA, Demsey SA, Leonard CO, et al: Natural history of Williams syndrome: Physical characteristics. J Pediatr 113:318, 1988.

312b. Friedman WF: Supravalvar aortic stenosis. Prog Pediatr Cardiol 3:133, 1994.

313. Li DY, Toland AE, Boak BB, et al: Elastin point mutations cause an obstructive, vascular disease supravalvular aortic stenosis. Hum Mol Genet 6:1021, 1997.

314. Keating MT: Genetic approaches to cardiovascular disease, supravalvular aortic stenosis, Williams syndrome, and long-QT syndrome. Circulation 92:142, 1995.

315. Zalzstein E, Moes CAF, Musewe NN, Freedom RM: Spectrum of cardiovascular anomalies in Williams-Beuren syndrome. Pediatr Cardiol 12: 219, 1991.

316. Conway EE, Noonan J, Marion RW, Steeg CN: Myocardial infarction leading to sudden death in the Williams syndrome: Report of three cases. J Pediatr 117:593, 1990.

317. Wren C, Oslizlok P, Bull C: Natural history of supravalvular aortic stenosis and pulmonary artery stenosis. J Am Coll Cardiol 15:1625, 1990.

318. French JW, Guntheroth WG: An explanation of asymmetric upper extremity blood pressure in supravalvular aortic stenosis: The Coanda effect. Circulation 42:31, 1970.

319. Goldstein RE, Epstein SE: Mechanism of elevated innominate artery pressures in supravalvular aortic stenosis. Circulation 42:23, 1970.

320. Masura J, Bzduch J, Lolan M, et al: Diagnosis of supravalvular aortic stenosis by means of two-dimensional echocardiography (in Slovak). Bratisl Lek Listy 90:895, 1989.

321. Rein AJJT, Preminger TJ, Perry SB, et al: Generalized anteriopathy in Williams syndrome: An intravascular ultrasound study. J Am Coll Cardiol 21:1727, 1993.

322. Brand A, Keren A, Reifen RM, et al: Echocardiographic and Doppler findings in the Williams syndrome. Am J Cardiol 63:633, 1989.

323. de Lezo JS, Pan M, Romero M, et al: Tailored stent treatment for severe supravalvular aortic stenosis. Am J Cardiol 78:1081, 1996.

324. Permut LC, Laks H: Surgery for valvar and supravalvar aortic stenosis. Prog Pediatr Cardiol 3:177, 1994.

325. Kitchiner D, Jackson M, Walsh K, et al: Prognosis of supravalve aortic stenosis in 81 patients in Liverpool (1960–1993). Heart 75:396, 1996.

326. Hazekamp MG, Kappetein AP, Schoof PH, et al: Brom's three-patch technique for repair of supravalvular aortic stenosis. J Thorac Cardiovasc Surg 118:252, 1999.

327. Sade RM, Crawford FA Jr, Fyfe DA: Symposium on hypoplastic left heart syndrome. J Thorac Cardiovasc Surg 91:937, 1986.

328. Rychik J, Rome JJ, Collins MH, et al: The hypoplastic left heart syndrome with intact atrial septum: Atrial morphology, pulmonary vascular histopathology and outcome. J Am Coll Cardiol 34:554, 1999.

329. Bove EL: Current status of staged reconstruction hypoplastic left heart syndrome. Pediatr Cardiol 19:308, 1998.

330. Gutgesell HP, Massaro TA: Management of hypoplastic left heart syndrome in a consortium of university hospitals. Am J Cardiol 76:809, 1995.

331. Bailey LL, Gundry SR: Hypoplastic left heart syndrome. Pediatr Clin North Am 37:137, 1990.

332. Bartram U, Grünenfelder J, Van Praagh R: Causes of death after the modified Norwood procedure: A study of 122 postmortem cases. Ann Thorac Surg 64:1795, 1997.

333. Slack MC, Kirby WC, Towbin JA, et al: Stenting of the ductus arteriosus in the hypoplastic left heart syndrome as an ambulatory bridge to cardiac transplantation. Am J Cardiol 74:636, 1994.

334. Donofrio MT, Engle MA, O'Loughlin JE, et al: Congenital aortic regurgitation: Natural history and management. J Am Coll Cardiol 20:336, 1992.

335. Folliguet TA, Laborde F, Macé L, et al: Aortic insufficiency associated with complex cardiac anomalies. Cardiol Young 5:125, 1995.

336. Hovaguimian H, Cobanoglu A, Starr A: Aortico-left ventricular tunnel: A clinical review and new surgical classification. Ann Thorac Surg 45: 106, 1988.

337. Goforth D, James FW, Kaplan S, Donner R: Maximal exercise in children with aortic regurgitation: An adjunct to noninvasive assessment of disease severity. Am Heart J 108:1306, 1984.

338. Sondergaard L, Lindvig K, Hildebrandt P, et al: Quantification of aortic regurgitation by magnetic resonance velocity mapping. Am Heart J 125: 1081, 1993.

339. Cheitlin MD: Finding 'just the right moment' for operative intervention in the asymptomatic patient with moderate to severe aortic regurgitation. Circulation 97:518, 1998.

340. Marin-Garcia J, Tandon R, Lucas RV Jr, Edwards JE: Cor triatriatum: Study of 20 cases. Am J Cardiol 35:59, 1975.

341. Shuler CO, Fyfe DA, Sade R, Crawford FA: Transesophageal echocardiographic evaluation of cor triatriatum in children. Am Heart J 129: 507, 1995.

342. Burton DA, Chin A, Weinberg PM, Pigott JD: Identification of cor triatriatum dexter by two-dimensional echocardiography. Am J Cardiol 59: 409, 1987.

343. Tulloh RMR, Bull C, Elliott MJ, Sullivan ID: Supravalvar mitral stenosis: Risk factors for recurrence or death after resection. Br Heart J 73: 164, 1995.

344. Oglietti J, Cooley DA, Izquierdo JP, et al: Cor triatriatum: Operative results in 25 patients. Ann Thorac Surg 35:415, 1983.

345. Ruckman RN, Van Praagh R: Anatomic types of congenital mitral stenosis: Report of 49 autopsy cases with consideration of diagnosis and surgical implications. Am J Cardiol 42:592 1978.

346. Banerjee A, Kohl T, Silverman NH: Echocardiographic evaluation of congenital mitral valve anomalies in children. Am J Cardiol 76:1284, 1995.

347. Patel JJ, Munclinger MJ, Mitha AS, Patel M: Percutaneous balloon dilatation of the mitral valve in critically ill young patients with intractable heart failure. Br Heart J 73:555, 1995.

348. Tulloh RMR, Bull C, Elliott MJ, Sullivan ID: Supravalvular mitral stenosis: Risk factors for recurrence or death after resection. Br Heart J 73: 164, 1995.

349. Mazzera E, Corno A, Di Donato R, et al: Surgical bypass of the systemic atrioventricular valve in children by means of a valve conduit. J Thorac Cardiovasc Surg 96:321, 1988.

350. Zweng TN, Bluett MK, Mosca R, et al: Mitral valve replacement in the first 5 years of life. Ann Thorac Surg 47:720, 1989.

351. Freed LA, Levy D, Levine RA, et al: Prevalence and clinical outcome of mitral-valve prolapse. N Engl J Med 341:1, 1999.

352. Nishimura RA, McGoon MD: Perspectives on mitral-valve prolapse. N Engl J Med 341:48, 1999.

353. Carpentier A: Congenital malformations of the mitral valve. In Stark J, deLeval M (eds): Surgery for Congenital Heart Defects. New York, Grune & Stratton, 1983, p 467.

354. Gonzalez VR, Pieper WM, Kap-herr, SH: Pulmonary arteriovenous fistula in childhood. Z Kinderchir 40:101, 1985.

355. Bernstein HS, Ursell PC, Brook MM, et al: Fulminant development of pulmonary arteriovenous fistulas in an infant after total cavopulmonary shunt. Pediatr Cardiol 17:46, 1996.

356. Grady RM, Sharkey AM, Bridges ND: Transcatheter coil embolisation of a pulmonary arteriovenous malformation in a neonate. Br Heart J 71: 370, 1994.

357. D'Cruz IA, Agustssou MM, Bicoff JP, et al: Stenotic lesions of the pulmonary arteries: Clinical hemodynamic findings in 84 cases. Am J Cardiol 13:441, 1964.

358. Venables AW: The syndrome of pulmonary stenosis complicating maternal rubella. Br Heart J 27:49, 1965.

359. Du ZD, Roguin N, Barak M, et al: Doppler echocardiographic study of the pulmonary artery and its branches in 114 normal neonates. Pediatr Cardiol 18:38, 1997.

360. Eldredge WJ, Tingelstad JB, Robertson LW, et al: Observations on the

natural history of pulmonary artery coarctation. Circulation 45:404, 1972.

361. Kan JS, Marvin WJ Jr, Bass JL, et al: Balloon angioplasty–branch pulmonary artery stenosis: Results from the valvuloplasty and angioplasty of congenital anomalies registry. Am J Cardiol 65:798, 1990.

362. Shaffer KM, Mullins CE, Grifka RG, et al: Intravascular stents in congenital heart disease: Short- and long-term results from a large single-center experience. J Am Coll Cardiol 31:661, 1998.

363. O'Laughlin MP: Catheterization treatment of stenosis and hypoplasia of pulmonary arteries. Pediatr Cardiol 19:48, 1998.

364. Burch M, Sharland M, Shinebourne E, et al: Cardiologic abnormalities in Noonan syndrome: Phenotypic diagnosis and echocardiographic assessment of 118 patients. J Am Coll Cardiol 22:1189, 1993.

365. Kovalchin JP, Forbes TJ, Nihill MR, Geva T: Echocardiographic determinants of clinical course in infants with critical and severe pulmonary valve stenosis. J Am Coll Cardiol 29:1095, 1997.

366. Rowland DG, Hammill WW, Allen HD, Gutgesell HP: Natural course of isolated pulmonary valve stenosis in infants and children utilizing Doppler echocardiography. Am J Cardiol 79:344, 1997.

367. Gournay V, Piechaud JF, Delogu A, et al: Balloon valvotomy for critical stenosis or atresia of pulmonary valve in newborns. J Am Coll Cardiol 26:1725, 1995.

368. Fedderly RT, Beekman RH: Balloon valvuloplasty for pulmonary valve stenosis. J Interven Cardiol 8:451, 1995.

369. Tabatabaei H, Boutin C, Nykanen DG, et al: Morphologic and hemodynamic consequences after percutaneous balloon valvotomy for neonatal pulmonary stenosis: Medium-term follow-up. J Am Coll Cardiol 27:473, 1996.

370. Rome JJ: Balloon pulmonary valvuloplasty. Pediatr Cardiol 19:18, 1998.

371. Srinivasan V, Konyer A, Broda JJ, Subramanian S: Critical pulmonary stenosis in infants less than three months of age: A reappraisal of closed transventricular pulmonary valvotomy. Ann Thorac Surg 34:46, 1982.

372. Fedderly RT, Lloyd TR, Mendelsohn AM, et al: Determinants of successful balloon valvotomy in infants with critical pulmonary stenosis or membranous pulmonary atresia with intact ventricular septum. J Am Coll Cardiol 25:460, 1995.

373. Lange PE, Onnasch GW, Heintzen PH: Valvular pulmonary stenosis: Natural history and right ventricular function in infants and children. Eur Heart J 6:706, 1985.

374. Mahra-Pour M, Whitney A, Liebman J, et al: Quantification of the Frank and MacFee-Parungao orthogonal electrocardiogram in valvular pulmonic stenosis: Correlation with hemodynamic measurements. J Electrocardiol 12:69, 1979.

375. Nishimura RA, Pieroni DR, Bierman FZ, et al: Second natural history of congenital heart defects. Pulmonary stenosis: Echocardiography. Circulation 87:1, 1993.

376. Krabill KA, Wang Y, Einzig S, Moller JH: Rest and exercise hemodynamics in pulmonary stenosis: Comparison of children and adults. Am J Cardiol 56:360, 1985.

377. Wennevold A, Jacobsen JR: Natural history of valvular pulmonary stenosis in children below the age of two years: Long-term follow-up with serial heart catheterizations. Eur J Cardiol 8:371, 1978.

378. Hayes CJ, Gersony WM, Driscoll DJ, et al: Second natural history study of congenital heart defects: Results of treatment of patients with pulmonary valvar stenosis. Circulation 87:1, 1993.

379. Steinberger J, Moller JH: Exercise testing in children with pulmonary valvar stenosis. Pediatr Cardiol 20:27, 1999.

380. Laks H, Billingsley AM: Advances in the treatment of pulmonary atresia with intact ventricular septum: Palliative and definitive repair. Cardiol Clin 7:387, 1989.

381. Coles JG, Freedman RM, Lightfoot NE, et al: Long-term results in neonates with pulmonary atresia and intact ventricular septum. Ann Thorac Surg 47:213, 1989.

382. Oosthoek PW, Moorman AF, Sauer U, Gittenberger-de Groot AC: Capillary distribution in the ventricles of hearts with pulmonary atresia and intact ventricular septum. Circulation 91:1790, 1995.

383. Daliento L, Scognamiglio R, Thiene G, et al: Morphologic and functional analysis of myocardial status in pulmonary atresia with intact ventricular septum—an angiographic, histologic and morphometric study. Cardiol Young 2:361, 1992.

384. Freedom RM, Wilson G, Trusler G, et al: Pulmonary atresia and intact ventricular septum: A review of the anatomy, myocardium and factors influencing right ventricular growth and guidelines for surgical intervention. Scand J Thorac Cardiovasc Surg 17:1, 1983.

385. Black MD, Shuria V, Freedom RM: Direct neonatal ventriculo-arterial connections (REV): Early results and future implications. Ann Thorac Surg 67:1137, 1999.

386. Hanseus K, Bjorkhom G, Lundstrom NR, Laurin S: Cross-sectional echocardiographic measurements of right ventricular size and growth in patients with pulmonary atresia and intact ventricular septum. Pediatr Cardiol 12:135, 1991.

387. Mair DD, Juisrud PR, Puga FJ, Danielson GK: The Fontan procedure for pulmonary atresia with intact ventricular septum: Operative and late results. J Am Coll Cardiol 29:1359, 1997.

388. Hanley FL, Sade RM, Blackstone EH, et al: Outcomes in neonatal pulmonary atresia with intact ventricular septum: A multi-institutional study. J Thorac Cardiovasc Surg 105:406, 1993.

389. Laks H, Pearl J M, Drinkwater DC, et al: Partial biventricular repair of pulmonary atresia with intact ventricular septum: Use of an adjustable atrial septal defect. Circulation 86:II, 1992.

390. Leung MP, Lo RNS, Cheung H, at al: Balloon valvuloplasty after pulmonary valvotomy for babies with pulmonary atresia and intact ventricular septum. Ann Thorac Surg 53:664, 1992.

391. Alva C, Ho SY, Lincoln CR, et al: The nature of the obstructive muscular bundles in double-chambered right ventricle. J Thorac Cardiovasc Surg 117:1180, 1999.

392. Ward CJB, Colham JAG, Patterson MWH, Sandor GGS: The trilogy of double-chambered right ventricle, perimembranous ventricular septal defect and subaortic narrowing—a more common association than previously recognized. Cardiol Young 5:140, 1995.

393. Wong PC, Sanders SP, Jonas RA, et al: Pulmonary valve–moderator band distance and association with development of double-chambered right ventricle. Am J Cardiol 68:1681, 1991.

394. Ford DK, Bollaboy CA, Derkac WM, et al: Transatrial repair of double-chambered right ventricle. Ann Thorac Surg 46:412, 1988.

395. Pinsky WW, Arciniegas E: Tetralogy of Fallot. Pediatr Clin North Am 37:179, 1990.

396. Soto B, McConnell ME: Tetralogy of Fallot: Angiographic and pathological correlation. Semin Thorac Cardiovasc Surg 2:12, 1990.

397. Barbero-Marcial M, Jatene AD: Surgical management of the anomalies of the pulmonary arteries in the tetralogy of Fallot with pulmonary atresia. Semin Thorac Cardiovasc Surg 2:93, 1990.

398. Hiraishi S, Misawa H, Hirota H, et al: Noninvasive quantitative evaluation of the morphology of the major pulmonary artery branches in cyanotic congenital heart disease. Angiocardiographic and echocardiographic correlative study. Circulation, 89:1306, 1994.

399. Carvalho JS, Silva CMC, Rigby ML, et al: Angiographic diagnosis of anomalous coronary artery in tetralogy of Fallot. Br Heart J 70:75, 1993.

400. Feldt RH, Liao P, Puga FJ: Clinical profile and natural history of pulmonary atresia and ventricular septal defect. Prog Pediatr Cardiol 1:18, 1992.

401. Morgan BC, Guntheroth WG, Blume RS, Fyler DC: A clinical profile of paroxysmal hyperpnea in cyanotic congenital heart disease. Circulation 31:66, 1965.

402. Shaddy RE, Viney J, Judd VE, McGough EC: Continuous intravenous phenylephrine infusion for treatment of hypoxemic spells in tetralogy of Fallot. J Pediatr 114:468, 1989.

403. McConnell ME: Echocardiography in classical tetralogy of Fallot. Semin Thorac Cardiovasc Surg 2:2, 1990.

404. Santoro G, Marino B, Di Carlo D, et al: Echocardiographically guided repair of tetralogy of Fallot. Am J Cardiol 73:808, 1994.

405. Jureidini SB, Appleton RS, Nouri S: Detection of coronary artery abnormalities in tetralogy of Fallot by two-demensional echocardiography. J Am Coll Cardiol 14:960, 1989.

406. Le Bret E, Mace L, Dervanian P, et al: Combined angiography and three-dimensional computed tomography for assessing systemic-to-pulmonary collaterals in pulmonary atresia with ventricular septal defect. Circulation 98:2930, 1998.

407. Castaneda AR: Classical repair of tetralogy of Fallot: Timing, technique, and results. Semin Thorac Cardiovasc Surg 2:70, 1990.

408. Groh MA, Meliones JN, Bove E, at al: Repair of tetralogy of Fallot in infancy: Effect of pulmonary artery size on outcome. Circulation 84(Suppl III):206, 1991.

409. Munkhammar P, Cullen S, Jogi P, et al: Early age at repair prevents restrictive right ventricular (RV) physiology after surgery for tetralogy of Fallot (TOF): Diastolic RV function after TOF repair in infancy. J Am Coll Cardiol 32:1083, 1998.

410. Kirklin JW, Blackstone EH, Jonas RA, et al: Morphologic and surgical determinants of outcome events after repair of tetralogy of Fallot and pulmonary stenosis. J Thorac Cardiovasc Surg 103:706, 1992.

411. Rosankranz ER: Modified Blalock-Taussig shunts in the treatment of tetralogy of Fallot. Semin Thorac Cardiovasc Surg 2:27, 1990.

412. Sluysmans T, Neven B, Rubay J, et al: Early balloon dilatation of the pulmonary valve in infants with tetralogy of Fallot. Circulation 91:1506, 1995.

413. Lane GK, Lucas VW, Sklansky MS, et al: Percutaneous coil occlusion of ascending aorta to pulmonary shunts. Am J Cardiol 81:1389, 1998.

414. Murthy KS, Rao SG, Niak SK, et al: Evolving surgical management for ventricular septal defect, pulmonary atresia, and major aortopulmonary collateral arteries. Ann Thorac Surg 67:760, 1999.

415. Chan KC, Fyfe DA, McKay CA, et al: Right ventricular outflow reconstruction with cryopreserved homografts in pediatric patients: Intermediate-term follow-up with serial echocardiographic assessment. J Am Coll Cardiol 24:483, 1994.

416. Hopkins RA, Imperato DA, Cockerman JT, Shapiro SR: Use of pulmonary arterial unifocalization into cryopreserved homograft pulmonary arterial bifurcation grafts to facilitate complete correction of pulmonary atresia with ventricular septal defect, nonconfluent (absent) central pulmonary arteries and multiple major aortopulmonary collateral arteries. Cardiol Young 5:217, 1995.

417. Warner KG, Anderson JE, Fulton DR, et al: Restoration of the pulmonary valve reduces right ventricular volume overload after previous repair of tetralogy of Fallot. Circulation 88:189, 1993.

418. Gatzoulis MA, Till JA, Redington AN: Depolarization-repolarization inhomogeneity after repair of tetralogy of Fallot: The substrate for malignant ventricular tachycardia? Circulation 95:401, 1997.

419. Bricker JT: Sudden death in tetralogy of Fallot: Risks, markers, and causes. Circulation 92:158, 1995.

420. Oku H, Shirotani H, Sunakawa A, Yokoyama T: Postoperative long-term results in total correction of tetralogy of Fallot: Hemodynamics and cardiac function. Ann Thorac Surg 41:413, 1986.

421. Hayabuchi Y, Matsuoka S, Kubo M, Kuroda Y: Usefulness of color kinesis imaging for evaluation of regional right ventricular wall motion in patients with surgically repaired tetralogy of Fallot. Am J Cardiol 82:1224, 1998.

422. Singh GK, Greenberg SB, Yap YS, et al: Right ventricular function and exercise performance late after primary repair of tetralogy of Fallot with the transannular patch in infancy. Am J Cardiol 81:1378, 1998.

423. Rhodes J, Dave A, Pulling MC, et al: Effective pulmonary artery stenoses on the cardiopulmonary response to exercise following the repair of tetralogy of Fallot. Am J Cardiol 81:1217, 1998.

424. Johnson MC, Strauss AW, Dowton SB, et al: Deletion within chromosome 22 is common in patients with absent pulmonary valve syndrome. Am J Cardiol 76:66, 1995.

425. Fouron JC: Tetralogy of Fallot with absent pulmonary valve: Clarification of a complex malformation and of its therapeutic challenge. Circulation 82:1531, 1990.

426. Milanesi O, Talenti E, Pallegrino PA, Thiene G: Abnormal pulmonary artery branching in tetralogy of Fallot with absent pulmonary valve. Int J Cardiol 6:375, 1984.

427. Fischer DR, Neches WH, Beerman LB, et al: Tetralogy of Fallot with absent pulmonic valve: Analysis of 17 patients. Am J Cardiol 53:1433, 1984.

428. Frank H, Salzer U, Popow C, et al: Magnetic resonance imaging of absent pulmonary valve syndrome. Pediatr Cardiol 17:35, 1996.

429. Kron IL, Johnson AM, Carpenter MA, et al: Treatment of absent pulmonary valve syndrome with homograft. Ann Thorac Surg 46:579, 1988.

430. Rigby ML, Carvalho JS, Anderson RH, Redington A: The investigation and diagnosis of tricuspid atresia. Int J Cardiol 27:1, 1990.

431. Sade RM, Fyfe DA: Tricuspid atresia: Current concepts in diagnosis and treatment. Pediatr Clin North Am 7:151, 1990.

432. Laks H, Ardehali A, Grant PW, et al: Modification of the Fontan procedure. Superior vena cava to left pulmonary artery connection and inferior vena cava to right pulmonary artery connection with adjustable atrial septal defect. Circulation 91:2943, 1995.

433. Bridges ND, Mayer JE, Lock JE, et al: Effect of baffle fenestration on outcome of the modified Fontan operation. Circulation 86:1762, 1992.

434. Kuhn MA, Jarmakani JM, Laks H, et al: Effect of late postoperative atrial septal defect closure on hemodynamic function in patients with a lateral tunnel Fontan procedure. J Am Coll Cardiol 26:259, 1995.

435. Carter T, Mainwaring RD, Lamberti JJ: Damus-Kaye-Stansel procedure: Midterm follow-up and technical considerations. Ann Thorac Surg 58:1603, 1994.

436. Graham TP: Appropriate and borderline indications for Fontan surgery—when not to proceed. Prog Pediatr Cardiol 9:29, 1998.

437. Main DD, Puga FJ, Danielson GK: Late functional status of survivors of the Fontan procedure performed during the 1970s. Circulation 86:II, 1992.

438. Driscoll DJ, Offord KP, Feldt RH, et al: Five- to fifteen-year follow-up after Fontan operation. Circulation 85:469, 1992.

439. Driscoll DJ, Durongpisitkul K: Exercise testing after the Fontan operation. Pediatr Cardiol 20:57, 1999.

440. Gewillig M, Wyse RK, de Leval MR, Deanfield JE: Early and late arrhythmias after the Fontan operation: Predisposing factors and clinical consequences. Br Heart J 67:72, 1992.

441. Gussenhoven EJ, Stewart PA, Becker AE, et al: "Offsetting" of the septal tricuspid leaflet in normal hearts and in hearts with Ebstein's anomaly. Am J Cardiol 53:172, 1984.

442. Zalzstein E, Koran G, Einarson T, Freedom RM: A case control study on the association between first trimester exposure to lithium and Ebstein's anomaly. Am J Cardiol 65:817, 1990.

443. Mair DD: Ebstein's anomaly: Natural history and management. J Am Coll Cardiol 19:1047, 1992.

444. Celermajer DS, Bull C, Till JA, et al: Ebstein's anomaly: Presentation and outcome from fetus to adult. J Am Coll Cardiol 23:170, 1994.

445. Oberhoffer R, Cook AC, Lang D, et al: Correlation between echocardiographic and morphological investigations of lesions of the tricuspid valve diagnosed during fetal life. Br Heart J 68:580, 1992.

446. Boucek RJ Jr, Graham TP Jr, Morgan JP, et al: Spontaneous resolution of massive congenital tricuspid insufficiency. Circulation 54:795, 1976.

447. Yetman AT, Freedom RM, McCrindle BW: Outcome in cyanotic neonates with Ebstein's anomaly. Am J Cardiol 81:749, 1998.

448. Kastor JA, Goldreier BN, Josephson ME, et al: Electrophysiologic characteristics of Ebstein's anomaly of the tricuspid valve. Circulation 52:987, 1975.

449. Silverman NH: Pediatric Echocardiography. Baltimore, Williams & Wilkins, 1993, p 327.

450. Hong YM, Moller JH: Ebstein's anomaly: A long-term study of survival. Am Heart J 125:1419, 1993.

451. Chauvaud SM, Mihaileanu SA, Gaer JAR, Carpentier AC: Surgical treatment of Ebstein's malformation: The Hôpital Broussals experience. Cardiol Young 6:4, 1996.

452. Danielson GK, Driscoll DJ, Mair DD, et al: Operative treatment of Ebstein's anomaly. J Thorac Cardiovasc Surg 104:1195, 1992.

453. Starnes VA, Pitlick PT, Bernstein D, et al: Ebstein's anomaly appearing in the neonate. J Thorac Cardiovasc Surg 101:1082, 1991.

454. Marianeschi SM, McElhinney DB, Reddy VM, et al: Alternative approach to the repair of Ebstein's malformation: Intracardiac repair with ventricular unloading. Ann Thorac Surg 66:1546, 1998.

455. MacLelian-Tobert SG, Driscoll DJ, Mottram CD, et al: Exercise tolerance in patients with Ebstein's anomaly. J Am Coll Cardiol 29:1615, 1997.

456. Kiziltan HT, Theodoro DA, Warnes CA, et al: Late results of bioprosthetic tricuspid valve replacement in Ebstein's anomaly. Ann Thorac Surg 66:1539, 1998.

457. Cappato R, Schiutar M, Weiss C, et al: Radiofrequency current catheter ablation of accessory atrioventricular pathways in Ebstein's anomaly. Circulation 94:376, 1996.

458. Paul NH, Wernodsky G: Transposition of the great arteries. In Emmanoulides GC, Riemenschneider TA, Allen HD, et al (eds): Moss and Adams' Heart Disease in Infants, Children and Adolescents. 5th ed. Baltimore, Williams & Wilkins, 1994, p 1154.

459. Anderson RH, Henry GW, Becker AE: Morphologic aspects of complete transposition. Cardiol Young 1:41, 1991.

460. Lakier JB, Stanger P, Heymann MA, et al: Early onset of pulmonary vascular obstruction in patients with aortopulmonary transposition and intact ventricular septum. Circulation 51:875, 1975.

461. Aziz KU, Paul MH, Rowe RD: Bronchopulmonary circulation in D-transposition of the great arteries: Possible role and genesis of accelerated pulmonary vascular disease. Am J Cardiol 39:432, 1977.

462. Chiu I, Anderson RH, Macartney FJ, et al: Morphologic features of an intact ventricular septum susceptible to subpulmonary obstruction in complete transposition. Am J Cardiol 53:1633, 1984.

463. Waldman JD, Paul MH, Newfeld EA, et al: Transposition of the great arteries with intact ventricular septum and patent ductus arteriosus. Am J Cardiol 39:232, 1977.

464. Tonkin IL, Kelley MJ, Bream PR, Elliott LP: The frontal chest film as a method of suspecting transposition complexes. Circulation 53:1016, 1976.

465. Rigby ML, Chan K-Y: The diagnostic evaluation of patients with complete transposition. Cardiol Young 1:26, 1991.

466. Bonnet D, Coltri A, Butera G, et al: Detection of transposition of the great arteries and fetuses reduces neonatal morbidity and mortality. Circulation 99:916, 1999.

467. Pasquini L, Parness IA, Colan SD, et al: Diagnosis of intramural coronary artery in transposition of the great arteries using two-dimensional echocardiography. Circulation 88:1136, 1993.

468. Chiu IS, Chu SH, Wang JK, et al: Evolution of coronary artery pattern according to short-axis aortopulmonary rotation: A new categorization for complete transposition of the great arteries. J Am Coll Cardiol 26:250, 1995.

469. Pasquini L, Sanders SP, Parness IA, et al: Conal anatomy in 119 patients with D-loop transposition of the great arteries and ventricular septal defect: An echocardiographic and pathologic study. J Am Coll Cardiol 21:1712, 1993.

470. Jamjureeruk V, Sangtawesin C, Layangool T: Balloon atrial septostomy under two-dimensional echocardiographic control: A new outlook. Pediatr Cardiol 18:197, 1997.

471. Lin AE, DiSessa TG, Williams RG, et al: Balloon and blade atrial septostomy facilitated by two-dimensional echocardiography. Am J Cardiol 57:273, 1986.

472. Moene RJ, Oppanheimer-Dekker A, Wenink ACG, et al: Morphology of ventricular septal defect in complete transposition of the great arteries. Am J Cardiol 55:1566, 1985.

473. Amato JJ, Zelen J, Bushong J: Coronary arterial patterns in complete transposition—classification in relation to the arterial switch procedure. Cardiol Young 4:329, 1994.

474. Sim EKW, van Son JAM, Edwards WD, et al: Coronary artery anatomy in complete transposition of the great arteries. Ann Thorac Surg 57:690, 1994.

475. Gulgesell HP, Massaro TA, Kron LL: The arterial switch operation for transposition of the great arteries in a consortium of university hospitals. Am J Cardiol 74:959, 1994.

476. Planche C, Lacour-Gayet F, Serraf A: Arterial switch. Pediatr Cardiol 19:297, 1998.

477. Foran JP, Sullivan ID, Elliott MJ, de Leval MR: Primary arterial switch operation for transposition of the great arteries with intact ventricular septum in infants older than 21 days. J Am Coll Cardiol 31:883, 1998.

478. Blume ED, Altmann K, Mayer JE, et al: Evolution of risk factors influencing early mortality of the arterial switch operation. J Am Coll Cardiol 33:1702, 1999.

479. Soongswang J, Adatia I, Newman C, et al: Mortality in potential arterial switch candidates with transposition of the great arteries. J Am Coll Cardiol 32:753, 1998.

480. Villafane J, White S, Elbl F, et al: An electrocardiographic midterm follow up study after anatomic repair of transposition of the great arteries. Am J Cardiol 66:350, 1990.

481. Boutin C, Jonas RA, Sanders SP, et al: Rapid two-stage arterial switch operation: Acquisition of left ventricular mass after pulmonary artery banding in infants with transposition of the great arteries. Circulation 90:1304, 1994.

482. Wernovsky G, Bridges ND, Mandell VS: Enlarged bronchial arteries after early repair of transposition of the great arteries. J Am Coll Cardiol 21:465, 1993.

483. Massin M, Hovels-Gurich H, Dabritz S, et al: Results of the Bruce treadmill test in children after arterial switch operation for simple transposition of the great arteries. Am J Cardiol 81:56, 1998.

484. Soongswang J, Adatia I, Newman C, et al: Mortality in potential arterial

switch candidates with transposition of the great arteries. J Am Coll Cardiol 32:753, 1998.

485. Bonhoeffer P, Bonnet D, Piechaud JF, et al: Coronary artery obstruction after the arterial switch operation for transposition of the great arteries in newborns. J Am Coll Cardiol 29:202, 1997.

486. Bengel FM, Hauser M, Duvernoy CS, et al: Myocardial blood flow and coronary flow reserve late after anatomical correction of transposition of the great arteries. J Am Coll Cardiol 32:1955, 1998.

487. Weindling SN, Wernovsky G, Colan SD, et al: Myocardial perfusion, function and exercise tolerance after the arterial switch operation. J Am Coll Cardiol 23:424, 1994.

488. Corno A, George B, Pearl J, Laks H: Surgical options for complex transposition of the great arteries. J Am Coll Cardiol 14:742, 1989.

489. Lecomple Y, Neveux JY, Leca F, et al: Reconstruction of the pulmonary outflow tract without prosthetic conduit. J Thorac Cardiovasc Surg 87:727, 1982.

490. Gelatt M, Hamilton RM, McCrindle BW, et al: Arrhythmia and mortality after the Mustard procedure: A 30-year single-center experience. J Am Coll Cardiol 29:194, 1997.

491. Van Hare, GF, Lesh MD, Ross BA, et al: Mapping and radiofrequency ablation of intraatrial reentrant tachycardia after the Senning or Mustard procedure for transposition of the great arteries. Am J Cardiol 77:985, 1996.

492. Wilson NJ, Clarkson PM, Barratt-Boyes BG, et al: Long-term outcome after the Mustard repair for simple transposition of the great arteries: 28-year follow-up. J Am Coll Cardiol 32:758, 1998.

493. Merrill WH, Stewart JR, Hammon JW Jr, et al: The Senning operation for complete transposition: Mid-term physiologic, electrophysiologic, and functional results. Cardiol Young 1:80, 1991.

494. Hochreiter C, Snyder MS, Borer JS, et al: Right and left ventricular performance 10 years after Mustard repair of transposition of the great arteries. Am J Cardiol 74:478, 1994.

495. Reybrouck T, Gewillig M, Dumoulin M, et al: Cardiorespiratory exercise performance after Senning operation for transposition of the great arteries. Br Heart J 70:175, 1993.

496. Hurwitz RA, Caldwell RL, Girod DA, Brown J: Right ventricular systolic function in adolescents and young adults after Mustard operation for transposition of the great arteries. Am J Cardiol 77:294, 1996.

497. Corno AF, Parisi F, Marino B, et al: Palliative Mustard operation: An expanded horizon. Eur J Cardiothorac Surg 1:144, 1987.

498. Colli AM, De Leval M, Somerville J: Anatomically corrected malposition of the great arteries. Am J Cardiol 55:1367, 1985.

499. Freedom RM: Congenitally corrected transposition of the great arteries: Definitions and pathologic anatomy. Prog Pediatr Cardiol 10:3, 1999.

500. Webb CL: Congenitally corrected transposition of the great arteries: Clinical features, diagnosis, and prognosis. Prog Pediatr Cardiol 10:17, 1999.

501. Presbitero P, Somerville J, Rabajoli F, et al: Corrected transposition of the great arteries without associated defects in adult patients: Clinical profile and follow up. Br Heart J 74:57, 1995.

502. Cowley CG, Rosenthal A: Congenitally corrected transposition of the great arteries: The systemic right ventricle. Prog Pediatr Cardiol 10:31, 1999.

503. Roffi M, de Marchi SF, Seiler C: Congenitally corrected transposition of the great arteries in an 80 year old woman. Heart 79:622–623, 1998.

504. Fischbach PS, Law IH, Serwer GS: Congenitally corrected L-transposition of the great arteries: Abnormalities of atrioventricular conduction. Prog Pediatr Cardiol 10:37, 1999.

505. Meissner MD, Panidis IP, Eshaghpour E, et al: Corrected transposition of the great arteries: Evaluation by two-dimensional and Doppler echocardiography. Am Heart J 111:599, 1986.

506. Freedom RM, Harrington DP, White RI Jr: The differential diagnosis of levotransposed or malposed aorta: An angiocardiographic study. Circulation 50:1040, 1974.

507. Bove EL: Congenitally corrected transposition of the great arteries: Surgical options for biventricular repair. Prog Pediatr Cardiol 10:43, 1999.

508. Sharma R, Bhan A, Juneja R, et al: Double switch for congenitally corrected transposition of the great arteries. Eur J Cardiothorac Surg 15:276, 1999.

509. Hagler DJ: Double-outlet right ventricle. In Emmanouilides GC, Riemenschneider TA, Allen HD, et al (eds): Moss and Adams' Heart Disease in Infants, Children and Adolescents. 5th ed. Baltimore, Williams & Wilkins, 1995, p 1246.

510. Kleinert S, Sano T, Weintraub RG, et al: Anatomic features and surgical strategies in double-outlet right ventricle. Circulation 96:1233, 1997.

511. Goitein KJ, Neches WH, Park SC, et al: Electrocardiogram in double chamber right ventricle. Am J Cardiol 45:604, 1980.

512. Roberson DA, Silverman NH: Malaligned outlet septum with subpulmonary ventricular septal defect and abnormal ventriculoarterial connection: A morphologic spectrum defined echocardiographically. J Am Coll Cardiol 16:459, 1990.

513. Ewing S, Silverman NH: Echocardiographic diagnosis of single coronary artery in double-outlet right ventricle. Am J Cardiol 77:535, 1996.

514. Kirklin JW, Pacifico AD, Blackstone EH, et al: Current risks and protocols for operations for double-outlet right ventricle. J Thorac Cardiovasc Surg 92:913, 1986.

515. Day R, Laks H, Milgalter E, et al: Partial biventricular repair for double-outlet right ventricle with left ventricular hypoplasia. Ann Thorac Surg 49:1003, 1990.

516. Van Praagh R, Weinberg PM, Srebro JP: Double-outlet left ventricle. In Adams FH, Emmanouilides GC, Riemenschneider TA, et al (eds): Moss and Adams' Heart Disease in Infants, Children, and Adolescents. 4th ed. Baltimore, Williams & Wilkins, 1989, p 461.

517. Marino B, Bevilacqua M: Double-outlet left ventricle: Two-dimensional echocardiographic diagnosis. Am Heart J 123:1075, 1992.

518. Krabill KA, Lucas RV Jr: Abnormal pulmonary venous connections. In Emmanouilides GC, Riemenschneider TA, Allen HD, et al (eds): Moss and Adams' Heart Disease in Infants, Children, and Adolescents. 5th ed. Baltimore, Williams & Wilkins, 1995, p 838.

519. Ward KE, Mullins CE, Huhta JC, et al: Restrictive interatrial communication in total anomalous pulmonary venous connection. Am J Cardiol 57:1131, 1986.

520. Wang JK, Lue HC, Wu MH, et al: Obstructed total anomalous pulmonary venous connection. Pediatr Cardiol 14:28, 1993.

521. Patton WL, Momenah T, Gooding CA, Silverman NH: The vascular vise causing TAPVR type I to radiographically mimic TAPVR type III. Pediatr Radiol 29:323, 1999.

522. Chin AJ, Sanders SP, Sherman F, et al: Accuracy of subcostal two-dimensional echocardiography in prospective diagnosis of total anomalous pulmonary venous connection. Am Heart J 113:1153, 1987.

523. Van Hare GF, Schmidt KG, Cassidy SC, et al: Color Doppler flow mapping in the ultrasound diagnosis of total anomalous pulmonary venous connection. J Am Soc Echocardiog 1:341, 1988.

524. Ammash NM, Seward JB, Warnes CA, et al: Partial anomalous pulmonary venous connection: Diagnosis by transesophageal echocardiography. J Am Coll Cardiol 29:1351, 1997.

525. Caldarone CA, Najm HK, Kadletz M, et al: Surgical management of total anomalous pulmonary venous drainage: Impact of coexisting cardiac anomalies. Ann Thorac Surg 66:1521, 1998.

526. Lamb RK, Qureshi SA, Wilkinson JL, et al: Total anomalous pulmonary venous drainage: 17-year surgical experience. J Thorac Cardiovasc Surg 96:368, 1988.

527. Van Meter C Jr, LeBlanc JG, Culpepper WS III, Ochsner JL: Partial anomalous pulmonary venous return. Circulation 82(Suppl IV):195, 1990.

528. Gao YA, Burrows PE, Benson LN, et al: Scimitar syndrome in infancy. J Am Coll Cardiol 22:873, 1993.

529. Stanger P, Rudolph AM, Edwards JE: Cardiac malpositions: An overview based on a study of 65 necropsy specimens. Circulation 56:159, 1977.

530. Van Praagh R: Diagnosis of complex congenital heart disease: Morphologic-anatomic method and terminology. Cardiovasc Intervent Radiol 7:115, 1984.

531. Niwa K, Uchishiba M, Aotsuka H, et al: Systemic diagnostic method using magnetic resonance imaging to analyze viscero-bronchial-cardiovascular anomalies in pediatric patients with congenital heart disease. Int J Angiol 5:70, 1996.

532. Silverman NH: An ultrasonic approach to the diagnosis of cardiac situs, connections, and malposition. In Friedman WF, Higgins CB (eds): Pediatric Cardiac Imaging. Philadelphia, WB Saunders, 1984, p 188.

533. Atkinson DE, Drant S: Diagnosis of heterotaxy syndrome by fetal echocardiography. Am J Cardiol 82:1147, 1998.

534. Anderson C, Devine WA, Anderson RH, et al: Abnormalities of the spleen in relation to congenital malformations of the heart: Survey of necropsy findings in children. Br Heart J 63:122, 1990.

535. Phoon CK, Neill CA: Asplenia syndrome—risk factors for early unfavorable outcome. Am J Cardiol 73:1235, 1994.

536. Hashmi A, Abu-Sulaiman R, McCrindle BW, et al: Management and outcomes of right atrial isomerism: A 26-year experience. J Am Coll Cardiol 31:1120, 1998.

537. Culbertson CB, George BL, Day RW, et al: Factors influencing survival of patients with heterotaxy syndrome undergoing the Fontan procedure. J Am Coll Cardiol 20:678, 1992.

538. Gehlman HR, Van Ingen GJ: Symptomatic congenital complete absence of the left pericardium: Case report and review of the literature. Eur Heart J 10:670, 1989.

539. Rowland TW, Twible EA, Norwood WI Jr, Keane JF: Partial absence of the left pericardium: Diagnosis by two-dimensional echocardiography. Am J Dis Child 136:628, 1982.

540. Gassner I, Judmaier W, Fink C, et al: Diagnosis of congenital pericardial defects on magnetic resonance imaging. Br Heart J 74:60, 1995.

541. Jones JW, McManus BM: Fatal cardiac strangulation by congenital partial pericardial defect. Am Heart J 107:183, 1984.

542. Anderson RH, Macartney FJ, Tynan M, et al: Univentricular atrioventricular connection: The single ventricle trap unsprung. Pediatr Cardiol 4:273, 1983.

543. Julsrud PR, Weigel TJ, Edwards WD: Angiographic determination of ventricular morphology: Correlation with pathology in 36 hearts with single functional ventricles. Pediatr Cardiol 18:208, 1997.

544. Moak JP, Gersony WM: Progressive atrioventricular valvular regurgitation in single ventricle. Am J Cardiol 59:656, 1987.

545. Mair DD, Hagler DJ, Julsrud PR, et al: Early and late results of the modified Fontan procedure for double-inlet left ventricle: The Mayo Clinic experience. J Am Coll Cardiol 18:1727, 1991.

546. Calderon-Colmenero J, Ramirez S, Rijlaarsdam M, et al: Use of bidirectional cavopulmonary shunt in patients under one year of age. Cardiol Young 5:28, 1995.

547. de Leval MR: The Fontan circulation: What have we learned? What to expect? Pediatr Cardiol 19:316, 1998.

548. Kuhn MA, Jarmakani JM, Laks H, et al: Effect of late postoperative atrial septal defect closure on hemodynamic function in patients with a lateral tunnel Fontan procedure. J Am Coll Cardiol 26:259, 1995.

549. Shu DT, Quaegebeur JM, Ing FF, et al: Outcome after the single-stage, nonfenestrated Fontan procedure. Circulation 96(Suppl II):II-335, 1997.

550. Thompson LD, Petrossian E, McElhinney DB, et al: Is it necessary to routinely fenestrate an extracardiac Fontan? J Am Coll Cardiol 34:539, 1999.

551. Takeda M, Shimada M, Sekiguchi A, Ishizawa A: Long-term results of the fenestrated Fontan operation. Progress of patients with patent fenestrations. Jpn J Thorac Cardiovasc Surg 47:432–439, 1999.

552. Broekhuis E, Brizard CP, Mee RB, et al: Damus-Kaye-Stansel connections in children with previously transected pulmonary arteries. Ann Thorac Surg 67:519, 1999.

553. Jacobs MI, Norwood WI: Fontan operation: Influence of modifications on morbidity and mortality. Ann Thorac Surg 58:945, 1994.

554. Gewillig M, Wyse RK, De Leval MR, et al: Early and late arrhythmias after the Fontan operation: Predisposing factors and clinical consequences. Br Heart J 67:72, 1992.

555. Parikh SR, Hurwitz RA, Caldwell RL, Girod DA: Ventricular function in the single ventricle before and after Fontan surgery. Am J Cardiol 67:1390, 1991.

556. Rosenthal M, Bush A, Deanfield J, Redington A: Comparison of cardiopulmonary adaptation during exercise in children after the atriopulmonary and total cavopulmonary connection Fontan procedures. Circulation 91:372, 1995.

557. Stevenson O, Soderlund S, Thoren C, Wallgren G: Arterial anomalies causing compression of the trachea and/or the esophagus. Acta Paediatr Scand 60:81, 1971.

558. Erickson LC, Cocalis MW, George L: Partial anomalous pulmonary artery: New evidence on the development of the pulmonary artery sling. Pediatr Cardiol 17:319, 1996.

559. Azarow KS, Pearl RH, Hoffman MA, et al: Vascular ring: Does magnetic resonance imaging replace angiography? Ann Thorac Surg 53:882, 1992.

560. deLeval M: Vascular rings. In Stark J, deLeval M (eds): Surgery for Congenital Heart Defects. New York, Grune & Stratton, 1983, p 227.

561. Burke RP, Rosenfeld HM, Wernovsky G, Jonas RA: Video-assisted thoracoscopic vascular ring division in infants and children. J Am Coll Cardiol 25:943, 1995.

562. Anand R, Dooley KJ, Williams WH, et al: Follow-up of surgical correction of vascular anomalies causing tracheobronchial compression. Pediatr Cardiol 15:58, 1994.

563. Perry JC, Garson A Jr: Diagnosis and treatment of arrhythmias. Adv Pediatr 36:177, 1989.

564. Anderson RH, Wenick ACG, Losekoot TG, Becker AE: Congenitally complete heart block. Circulation 56:90, 1977.

565. Buyon JP, Hiebert R, Copel J, et al: Autoimmune-associated congenital heart block: Demographics, mortality, morbidity and recurrence rates obtained from a national neonatal lupus registry. J Am Coll Cardiol 31:1658, 1998.

566. Michaelsson M: Congenital complete atrioventricular block. Progr Pediatr Cardiol 4:1, 1995.

567. Gregoratos G, Cheitlin MD, et al: ACC/AHA guidelines for implantation of cardiac pacemakers and antiarrhythmia devices. J Am Coll Cardiol 31:1175, 1998.

568. Kertesz NJ, Fenrich AL, Friedman RA: Congenital complete atrioventricular block. Tex Heart Inst J 24:301, 1997.

569. Michaelsson M, Engle MA: Congenital complete heart block: An international study of the natural history. Cardiovasc Clin 4:65, 1982.

570. Simpson JM, Milbum A, Yates RW, et al.: Outcome of intermittent tachyarrhythmias in the fetus. Pediatr Cardiol 18:78, 1997.

571. Kleinman CS, Donnerstein RL, DeVore GR, et al: Fetal echocardiography for evaluation of in utero congestive heart failure. N Engl J Med 306:568, 1982.

572. Deal BJ, Keane JF, Gillette PC, Gardon A Jr: Wolff-Parkinson-White syndrome and supraventricular tachycardia during infancy: Management and follow-up. J Am Coll Cardiol 5:130, 1985.

573. Klitzner TS, Friedman WF: Cardiac arrhythmias: The role of pharmacologic intervention. Cardiol Clin 7:299, 1989.

574. Paul T, Pfammatter JP: Adenosine: An effective and safe antiarrhythmic drug in pediatrics. Pediatr Cardiol 18:118, 1997.

575. Drago F, Mazza A, Guccione P, et al: Amiodarone used alone or in combination with propranolol: A very effective therapy for tachyarrhythmias in infants and children. Pediatr Cardiol 19:445, 1998.

576. Kugler JD, Danford DA: Management of infants, children, and adolescents with paroxysmal supraventricular tachycardia. J Pediatr 129:324, 1996.

577. Kortesz NJ, Friedman RA, Fenrich AL, Garson A: Current management of the infant and child with supraventricular tachycardia. Cardiol Rev 6:221, 1998.

578. Lernier MS, Schaffer MS: Neonatal supraventricular tachycardia: Predictors of successful treatment withdrawal. Am Heart J 133:130, 1997.

579. Zipes DP, Akhtar M, Denes P, et al: Guidelines for clinical intracardiac electrophysiologic studies: A report of the American College of Cardiology/American Heart Association Task Force on Assessment of Diagnostic and Therapeutic Cardiovascular Procedures. J. Am Coll Cardiol 14:1827, 1989.

580. Klitzner TS, Wetzel GT, Saxon LA, et al: Radiofrequency ablation: A new era in the treatment of pediatric arrhythmias. Am J Dis Child 147:769, 1993.

581. Tanel RE, Walsh EP, Triedman JK, et al: Five-year experience with radiofrequency catheter ablation: Implications for management of arrhythmias in pediatric and young adult patients. J Pediatr 131:878, 1997.

582. Mendelsohn A, Dick M, Serwer GA: Natural history of isolated atrial flutter in infancy. J Pediatr 119:386, 1991.

583. Dick M, Scott WA, Serwer GS, et al: Acute termination of supraventricular tachyarrhythmias in children by transesophageal atrial pacing. Am J Cardiol 61:925, 1988.

584. Compton SJ, Lux RL, Ramsey MR, et al: Genetically defined therapy of inherited long-QT syndrome. Circulation 94:1018, 1996.

585. Garson A Jr, Dick M II, Fournier A, et al: The long QT syndrome in children: An international study of 287 patients. Circulation 87:1866, 1993.

Chapter 44

Congenital Heart Disease in Adults

JUDITH THERRIEN • GARY D. WEBB

Adult patients with congenital heart defects are a growing patient population.[1–1b] There are about 1 million affected Americans in the year 2000, compared with an estimated 300,000 in 1980, and 1.4 million are anticipated in 2020. About half of these patients are at significant risk of premature mortality, reoperation, or future complications of their conditions and their treatments.

One of the special challenges in this field is that there are about 100 separate main diagnostic groups. Each patient may have one or more of such diagnoses. The cardiologist may meet these patients in the office, the emergency department, the hospital, or the diagnostic laboratories. Dealing appropriately with these patients is a challenge. For many patients, especially those with "high-risk conditions," the preferred method is to have them seen by an expert. At present, there are not enough such individuals or facilities to make this possible. The cardiologist may then need access to educational material as a reminder of the anatomy, the clinical issues, the treatments, and expected residua and sequelae for the specific patient needing informed attention.[2]

This chapter has been written for the practicing cardiologist to provide the essential information to draw on when seeing such patients. The information here is fully compatible with the only existing expert recommendations for the care of adult patients with congenital cardiac defects.[2] These and further guidelines are/will be available on the Internet at www.cachnet.org and at www.library.utoronto.ca/nevil_thomas/. For congenital cardiac defects not included in this chapter, such as anomalous origin of coronary arteries,[2a] see Chapter 43.

GENERAL PRINCIPLES

All patients should have been taught in adolescence about their condition, their future outlook, and the possibility of further surgery and complications, and they also should have been advised about their responsibilities in ensuring self-care and professional surveillance. This is not always the case, and staff in adult clinics may have to take the patient through this process. Patients may wish to continue their own education through Internet sites or to join a chat line or listserver.

Some of the most important data in the files of adult patients with congenital heart defects are prior operative reports. Heart catheterization reports may be important as well. These should all be obtained. They may be invaluable when clinical questions arise. Those patients believed to be

at significant risk of future complications, future surgery, and premature death should be monitored life long.

Congenital heart disease in the adult is not a simple continuation of the childhood experience. The patterns of many lesions change in adult life. Arrhythmias are more frequent and of a different character. Cardiac chambers often enlarge, and ventricles tend to develop systolic dysfunction. Bioprosthetic valves, prone to quick failure in childhood, last longer when implanted at an older age. The patient is planning or involved in a career and may need advice on types of work to avoid. The comorbidities that tend to develop in adult life often become an important factor needing attention.

As a result, the needs of these patients are often best met by a physician or a team familiar with both pediatric and adult cardiology issues. Surgery and interventional catheterization procedures should usually be performed at centers with adequate surgical and institutional volumes of congenital heart cases at any age.[3] Diagnostic heart catheterizations, electrophysiological studies, and even magnetic resonance imaging (MRI)[3a] and other imaging of complex cases are best done where qualified staff have relevant training, experience, and equipment. Patient care in the ideal world should be multidisciplinary. Skilled cardiology and echocardiography skills are essential, but other individuals with special training, experience, and interest should also be accessible. This includes nurses, reproductive health staff, mental health professionals,[3b] anesthesiologists, medical imaging technicians, respiratory consultants, and others. Beyond the issues raised by individual lesions, these patients may also wish to have normal sex lives and to have children.

Pregnancy

Many female patients will need confirmation that they can safely carry a pregnancy. The literature offers guidance for certain lesions,[3] but, for many, certain principles can be reasonable guides.[4] Maternal risks for pregnancy include pulmonary hypertension, obstructive lesions, ventricular dysfunction, heart failure, and ascending aortic aneurysms (mainly in patients with Marfan syndrome). In severe cases, termination and sometimes sterilization may be recommended to protect the mother. Fetal risks are high in the presence of maternal cyanosis and medication exposure (e.g., warfarin and angiotensin-converting enzyme [ACE] inhibitors).

Delivery should usually be vaginal unless there is an obstetrical reason for cesarean section. Women at moderate and high risk for pregnancy should usually be evaluated and treated in a high-risk pregnancy unit. The staff in such units will know how to obtain templates for the management of specific patients with lesions of concern.

Patients will wish advice on contraception and on recurrence risks of congenital heart disease in their offspring. Referral to a geneticist may be helpful. As a rule, the recurrence risk is 3 to 4 percent, compared with the risk in the general population of 0.8 percent (range, 0.5–1.2 percent).[5, 6] In some patients, such as those with chromosome 22 microdeletion or Marfan syndrome, the risk is 50 percent.

Cardiac Arrhythmias (see also Chap. 25)

These are a major clinical challenge in adult congenital heart patients. They are the most frequent reason for emergency department visits/admissions. They are usually chronically recurrent and may worsen or become less responsive to treatment with time.[7] Treatment options are often limited and of limited efficacy.

Atrial flutter and, to a lesser degree, atrial fibrillation are most common. Atrial flutter tends to reflect right atrial, and atrial fibrillation left atrial, abnormalities. Atrial flutter in such patients is often atypical in appearance and behavior and is better called intraatrial reentrant tachycardia. We will use the simpler term. Recognition of atrial flutter may be difficult, and the observer will need to be vigilant in recognizing 2:1 conduction masquerading as sinus rhythm. Recurrence is likely and should not be assumed to represent failure of the management strategy. The conditions in which atrial flutter is most likely are Mustard/Senning repairs of transposition of the great arteries (TGA),[8, 9] repaired or unrepaired atrial septal defects (ASDs), repaired tetralogy of Fallot, Ebstein's anomaly of the tricuspid valve, and Fontan operation. Atrial flutter may reflect hemodynamic deterioration in patients who have had Mustard/Senning, tetralogy of Fallot, or Fontan repairs. Its arrival is usually associated with more symptoms and functional limitation.

The pharmaceutical agents most commonly used in therapy are warfarin, beta blockers, amiodarone, sotalol, propafenone, and digoxin. As a rule, patients with good ventricular function can receive sotalol or propafenone, whereas those with depressed ventricular function should receive amiodarone. Other therapies, including pacemakers, ablative procedures, and innovative surgery, are being both applied and refined. Sustained ventricular tachycardia or ventricular fibrillation occur less often, usually in the setting of ventricular dilation and scarring. Although sudden death is common in several conditions, the mechanism is poorly understood.

SPECIFIC CARDIAC DEFECTS

Atrial Septal Defect

(See also Chap. 43)

ASDs are the most common congenital cardiac malformation first diagnosed in adults.

ANATOMY. Four types of ASDs occur: ostium primum, ostium secundum, sinus venosus, and coronary sinus. Ostium primum is discussed later (see Atrioventricular Septal Defect). Ostium secundum defects occur from either excessive resorption of the septum primum or from deficient growth of the septum secundum and are occasionally associated with anomalous pulmonary venous drainage (<10 percent). Sinus venosus/superior vena cava (SVC) type defect occurs inferior to the orifice of the SVC, giving rise to an SVC connected to both atria and always associated with anomalous pulmonary venous drainage (usually from the right lung). Sinus venosus/inferior vena cava (IVC) type defects abut the junction of the IVC, inferior to the fossa ovalis. Coronary sinus septal defects are rare and arise from

an opening in the wall of the distal portion of the coronary sinus, allowing left-to-right atrial shunting (see Fig. 43–9). In any type of ASD, the degree of left-to-right atrial shunting depends on the size of the defect and the relative diastolic filling properties of the two ventricles. Any condition causing reduced left ventricular compliance (e.g., systemic hypertension, cardiomyopathy or myocardial infarction) or increased left atrial pressure (e.g., mitral stenosis and/or regurgitation) will tend to increase the left-to-right shunt.

NATURAL HISTORY OF THE UNOPERATED PATIENT. A significant shunt ($Qp/Qs > 1.5/1.0$) probably causes symptoms over time, and symptomatic patients become progressively more limited as they age. Effort dyspnea is seen in about 30 percent of patients by the third decade and over 75 percent of patients by the fifth decade. Supraventricular arrhythmias (atrial fibrillation or flutter) and right-sided heart failure develop by age 40 in about 10 percent of patients. The development of pulmonary hypertension, although probably not as common as originally thought, can occur at an early age. Life expectancy is probably reduced, although not nearly as severely as was quoted in an early article. Data regarding the natural history of ASD should be interpreted carefully because much of the data relates predominantly to sicker patients and the follow-up information was often inadequate.[10]

CLINICAL MANIFESTATIONS. The most common symptoms are exercise intolerance (dyspnea and fatigue) and palpitations (usually from atrial fibrillation, less often atrial flutter or sick sinus syndrome). Paradoxical embolism resulting in transient ischemic attack or cerebrovascular accident can call the diagnosis to attention. Right ventricular failure can be the presenting symptom in older patients. The presence of cyanosis should alert one to the possibility of shunt reversal and Eisenmenger syndrome (see p. 1614) or, alternatively, to a prominent eustachian valve directing IVC flow to the left atrium through a secundum or sinus venosus/IVC ASD. On examination, there is "left atrialization" of the jugular venous pressure (a wave = v wave). A hyperdynamic right ventricular impulse can be felt at the left sternal border at the end of expiration or in the subxiphoid area on deep inspiration. A dilated pulmonary artery trunk can be palpated in the second left intercostal space. A wide and fixed split S_2 is the auscultatory hallmark of ASD. A systolic ejection murmur, usually grade 2, is best heard at the second left intercostal space, and a mid-diastolic rumble, from increased flow through the tricuspid valve, can be present at the left lower sternal border. When right ventricular failure ensues, a holosystolic murmur of tricuspid regurgitation is usual.

DIAGNOSTIC TESTING

Electrocardiogram. Sinus rhythm or atrial fibrillation/flutter may occur. The QRS axis is normal or rightward in secundum ASD (see Fig. 43–10). Negative P waves in the inferior leads indicate a low atrial pacemaker and are often seen in sinus venosus/SVC type defects, which are located in the area of the sinoatrial node rendering it deficient. Partial to complete right bundle branch block can prolong the QRS duration (Fig. 44–1).

Chest Radiography. The classic radiographic features are cardiomegaly (from right atrial and ventricular enlargement), dilated central pulmonary arteries with pulmonary plethora indicating increased pulmonary flow, and a small aortic knuckle (Fig. 44–2).

Echocardiography (see Figs. 7–81 and 43–11). Transthoracic echocardiography (TTE) documents the type(s) and size (defect diameter) of the ASD(s) and the direction(s) of the shunt and perhaps can determine the presence or absence of anomalous pulmonary venous return. The functional importance of the defect can be estimated by the size of the right ventricle, the presence or absence of right ventricular volume overload (paradoxical motion of the septum), and the calculation of pulmonary artery blood flow

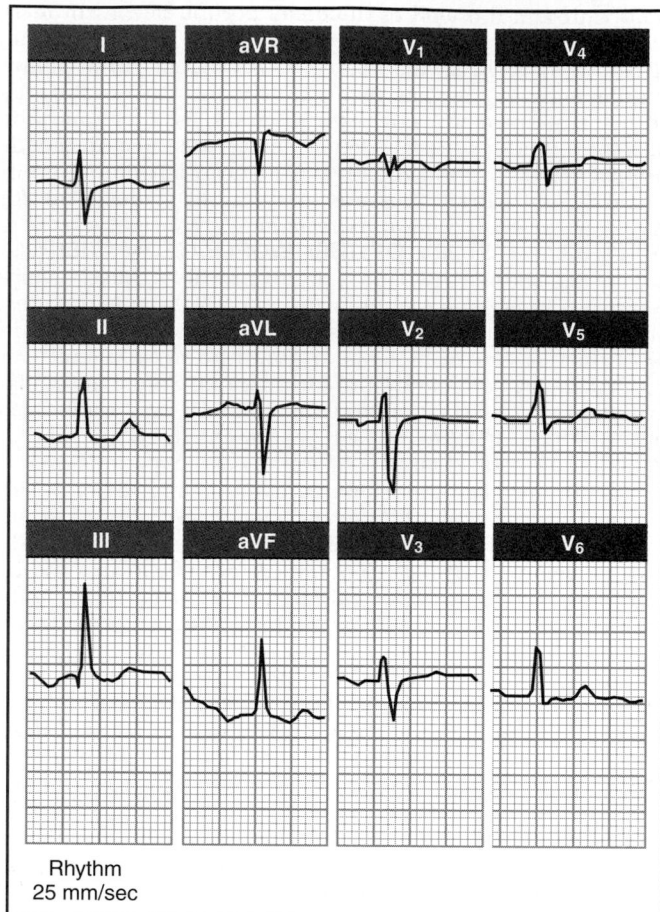

FIGURE 44–1. Typical electrocardiogram of a sinus venosus atrial septal defect of the superior vena cava type showing low atrial rhythm, mild right-axis deviation, and right bundle branch block.

relative to systemic blood flow (Qp/Qs). Indirect measurement of the pulmonary artery pressure can be obtained from the Doppler velocity of the tricuspid regurgitation jet. Transesophageal echocardiography (TEE) permits better visualization of the interatrial septum and may be required when device closure is contemplated or assessment of pulmonary venous drainage is incomplete (see Fig. 43–11).

Catheterization. Cardiac catheterization may be required when the hemodynamic significance of an ASD is questioned or when assessment of pulmonary artery pressures and resistances is needed.

Open-Lung Biopsy. Open-lung biopsy should only be considered when the reversibility of the pulmonary hypertension is uncertain from hemodynamic data (see section on Eisenmenger syndrome).

INDICATIONS FOR INTERVENTION. Hemodynamically "nonsignificant" ASDs (Qp/Qs < 1.5) do not require closure, with the possible exception of trying to prevent paradoxical emboli.[11] "Significant" ASDs (Qp/Qs > 1.5, or ASDs associated with right ventricular volume overload) require closure when symptoms are present.[12–14] In the absence of symptoms, indications for closure are somewhat controversial. In patients younger than age 40 years, "significant" ASDs should probably be closed, although this practice has been challenged by some.[15] The proper therapeutic strategy for asymptomatic patients > 40 years old with "significant" ASDs is still disputed. For patients with pulmonary hypertension (pulmonary artery pressure [PAP] > two thirds of systemic arterial blood pressure [SABP], or pulmonary arteriolar resistance more than two thirds of systemic arteriolar resistance), closure can be recommended if there is a net left-to-right shunt of at least 1.5:1, evidence of pulmonary artery reactivity when challenged with a pulmo-

nary vasodilator (e.g., oxygen or nitric oxide), or evidence on lung biopsy that pulmonary arterial changes are potentially reversible (see Chap. 53).

Transvenous pacing should be avoided when possible in patients with ASDs, because paradoxical emboli can occur. For the same reason, venous thromboemboli from any site are potential sources of systemic emboli. If a source of paradoxical embolism is found, anticoagulation and/or ASD closure may be recommended.

INTERVENTIONAL OPTIONS AND OUTCOMES

Device Closure. The use of devices to close ASDs percutaneously under fluoroscopy and TEE guidance[16] is gaining popularity. Indications for device closure are the same as for surgical closure but selection criteria are stricter. This technique is available mainly for patients with single secundum ASD with a stretched diameter of less than 50 percent of the diameter of the biggest available device and with adequate septal margin for proper device support. Anomalous pulmonary venous drainage or proximity of the defect to the atrioventricular (AV) valves, coronary sinus, or systemic venous drainage precludes the use of this technique. It is a safe and effective procedure in experienced hands, with major complications (e.g., device embolization, atrial perforation) occurring in less than 1 percent of patients and echo closure achieved in 85 percent or more of patients. Using "older" devices, silent residual shunts, more than half of which are trivial or mild, are still seen in 19 to 53 percent of patients at 6 to 12 months' follow-up.[17] Long-term follow-up data are not available.[17] Notwithstanding, device closure can be attractive to a patient wishing to avoid the consequences of surgery (general anesthesia, pain, and a scar) or to a patient believed to be at high surgical risk (see Fig. 43–12).

Surgery. Surgical closure of ASDs can be performed by primary suture closure or using an autologous pericardial

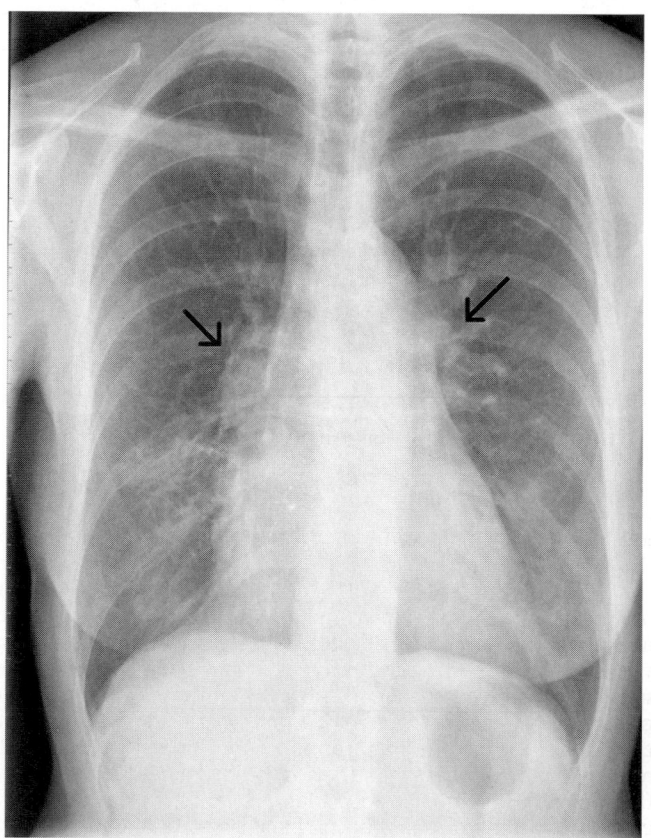

FIGURE 44–2. Chest radiograph in an adult with ostium secundum atrial septal defect. Arrows point to the enlarged right and left pulmonary arteries. Note the increase in peripheral pulmonary perfusion.

or synthetic patch. The procedure is usually performed through a midline sternotomy, but the availability of an inframammary or minithoracotomy approach to a typical secundum ASD should be made known to potentially interested patients. Surgical mortality in the adult without pulmonary hypertension should be less than 1 percent with a low morbidity related mainly to the development of perioperative arrhythmias (atrial flutter/fibrillation or junctional rhythm).[12, 18] Surgical closure of an ASD improves functional status and exercise capacity in symptomatic patients[12] and improves survival, especially when patients are operated on at an earlier age.[13, 15] The incidence of late congestive heart failure is probably also reduced.[13] However, surgical closure of ASD does not prevent atrial fibrillation/flutter or stroke[13] especially when patients are operated on after the age of 40 years.[12] The role of a concomitant Cox/Maze procedure (see Chaps. 23 and 25) in patients older than the age of 40 years with a prior history of atrial flutter/fibrillation is unclear.[19] Patients with persistent atrial fibrillation should undergo anticoagulation.

Follow-Up. Patients who have had surgical or device repair as adults, with or without elevated pulmonary artery pressures at the time of operation, patients with atrial arrhythmias preoperatively or postoperatively, and patients with ventricular dysfunction preoperatively should remain under long-term cardiology surveillance.

Isolated Ventricular Septal Defect
(see also Chap. 43)

Ventricular septal defects (VSDs) are the second most common congenital malformation of the heart, accounting for approximately 20 percent of all congenital cardiac malformations. Surgical repair of large defects and spontaneous closure of smaller defects during childhood decrease the overall incidence of VSDs in adulthood.

ANATOMY. The ventricular septum is composed of a muscular septum that can be divided into three major components (inlet, trabecular, and outlet) and a small membranous septum lying just underneath the aortic valve. VSDs are classified into three main categories according to their location and margins. *Muscular* VSDs are bordered entirely by myocardium and can be trabecular, inlet, or outlet in location. *Membranous* VSDs often have inlet, outlet, or trabecular extension and are bordered in part by fibrous continuity between the leaflets of an AV valve and an arterial valve. *Doubly committed subarterial* or *outlet* VSDs are situated in the outlet septum and are bordered by fibrous continuity of the aortic and pulmonary valves (see Fig. 43–15). In this section, we will deal with VSDs occurring in isolation from major associated cardiac anomalies.

NATURAL HISTORY OF THE UNOPERATED PATIENT. A *restrictive* VSD is defined as a defect that produces a significant pressure gradient between the left ventricle and the right ventricle, is accompanied by a small (<1.5/1.0) shunt, and does not cause significant hemodynamic derangement. A *moderately restrictive* VSD is accompanied by a moderate shunt (Qp/Qs = 1.5–2.5/1.0) and will pose a hemodynamic burden on the left ventricle. This will lead to left atrial and ventricular dilation and dysfunction as well as a variable increase in pulmonary vascular resistance. Important atrial arrhythmias and, less often, ventricular arrhythmias can occur. A large or *nonrestrictive* VSD results initially in left ventricular volume overload early in life with a progressive rise in pulmonary artery pressure. In turn, this leads to higher pulmonary vascular resistance and eventually irreversible pulmonary vascular changes and systemic pulmonary pressures, the so-called Eisenmenger syndrome (see p. 1614).

Spontaneous closure of a perimembranous VSD (from tricuspid leaflet tissue apposition) or of a small muscular

VSD during adulthood is uncommon (<10 percent). Small VSDs pose an ongoing and relatively high risk of endocarditis.[20] Perimembranous or outlet VSDs can be associated with progressive aortic valve regurgitation due to prolapse of the aortic cusp(s) into the defect. Late development of subaortic and subpulmonary stenosis has also been reported.[21]

CLINICAL MANIFESTATIONS. Most adult patients with a small *restrictive* VSD are asymptomatic. Physical examination reveals a harsh or high-frequency holosystolic murmur, usually grade 3 to 4/6, heard with maximal intensity at the left sternal border in the third or fourth intercostal space. Patients with a *moderately restrictive* VSD often present with dyspnea in adult life. Physical examination typically reveals a displaced cardiac apex with a similar holosystolic murmur as well as an apical diastolic rumble and third heart sound (S_3) at the apex from the increased flow through the mitral valve. Patients with large *nonrestrictive* VSDs are discussed in the section on Eisenmenger syndrome.

DIAGNOSTIC TESTING
Electrocardiogram. The ECG mirrors the size of the shunt and the degree of pulmonary hypertension. Small *restrictive* VSDs usually produce a normal tracing. *Moderate-sized* VSDs produce a broad, notched P wave characteristic of left atrial overload as well as signs of left ventricular volume overload, namely, deep Q and tall R waves with tall T waves in lead V_5 and V_6, and often atrial fibrillation. Large VSDs will produce right ventricular hypertrophy with right axis deviation (see section on Eisenmenger syndrome, p. 1614).

Chest Radiography. The chest radiograph reflects the magnitude of the shunt as well as the degree of pulmonary hypertension. A moderate-sized shunt causes signs of left ventricular dilation with some pulmonary plethora. A large-sized shunt will over time produce pulmonary hypertension with enlarged central pulmonary arteries and peripheral pruning (see section on Eisenmenger syndrome, p. 1614).

Echocardiography (see also Chap. 43). TTE can identify the location, size, and hemodynamic consequences of the VSD as well as any associated lesions (aortic regurgitation, right ventricular outflow tract obstruction [RVOTO], or left ventricular outflow tract obstruction [LVOTO]).

INDICATIONS FOR INTERVENTION. The presence of a significant VSD (the symptomatic patient; Qp/Qs > 1.5/1.0; pulmonary artery systolic pressure > 50 mm Hg; increased left ventricular and left atrial size, or deteriorating left ventricular function) in the absence of irreversible pulmonary hypertension warrants surgical closure.

If severe pulmonary hypertension is present (defined as pulmonary arteriolar resistance greater than two thirds of systemic arteriolar resistance), surgical closure can be safely undertaken if there is a net left-to-right shunt of at least 1.5/1.0, strong evidence of pulmonary reactivity when challenged with a pulmonary vasodilator (oxygen, nitric oxide), or lung biopsy evidence that pulmonary artery changes are reversible.

Other relative indications for VSD closure include the presence of a perimembranous or outlet VSD with more than mild aortic regurgitation and a history of endocarditis, especially if recurrent.[22]

INTERVENTIONAL OPTIONS
Surgery. Surgical closure, by direct suture closure or with a Dacron patch, has been used for over 50 years with low perioperative mortality—even in adults—and a very high closure rate.[6]

Device Closure. Successful transcatheter device closure of trabecular (muscular) and perimembranous VSDs has been reported.[23] Trabecular VSDs have proven more amenable to this technique because of their relatively straightforward anatomy and muscular rim to which the device attaches well. The closure of perimembranous VSDs is technically more challenging and should be considered experimental.

INTERVENTIONAL OUTCOMES. For patients with good to excellent functional class and good left ventricular function before surgical closure, life expectancy after surgical correction is close to normal. The risk of progressive aortic regurgitation is markedly reduced after surgery, as is the risk of endocarditis, unless a residual VSD persists. Intraventricular conduction disturbances are slightly increased after surgical closure and may be responsible for the slight increase in risk of sudden death encountered in this patient population.[24]

FOLLOW-UP. Yearly cardiac evaluation is suggested for patients with associated cardiac lesions (RVOTO, LVOTO, aortic regurgitation) not undergoing surgical repair, Eisenmenger syndrome patients, and adults with significant atrial or ventricular arrhythmias. Cardiac surveillance is also recommended for patients who had late repair of moderate or large defects, which are often associated with left ventricular impairment and elevated pulmonary artery pressure at the time of surgery. Residual patch or device leaks are seldom hemodynamically important but can predispose to endocarditis. Maintenance of good dental hygiene and antibiotic prophylaxis in these patients is very important.

Atrioventricular Septal Defect

(see also Chap. 43)

Unlike secundum ASDs, unoperated atrioventricular septal defects (AVSDs) are seldom first diagnosed in adults.

ANATOMY. AVSDs comprise a spectrum of anomalies caused by abnormal development of the endocardial cushions, which may give rise to partial, intermediate, or complete AVSDs (Table 44–1). In AVSD, the AV valves are fundamentally abnormal, being derived from five leaflets (a right anterosuperior leaflet, a right inferior leaflet, a superior bridging leaflet, an inferior bridging leaflet, and a left mural leaflet). This arrangement may result in separate but

▼ **TABLE 44–1. DEFINITIONS OF TYPES OF ATRIOVENTRICULAR SEPTAL DEFECTS (AVSD)**

PARTIAL AVSD
Ostium primum ASD
Two separate AV valves
"Cleft" left AV valve
Intact ventricular septum
Rarely, no ASD with only a "cleft" in the left AV valve
Associated anomalies: Down syndrome (<10%), unroofed coronary sinus, left superior vena cava, and patent ductus arteriosus

INTERMEDIATE AVSD
Primum ASD
Restrictive VSD
Separate, abnormal AV valves

COMPLETE AVSD
Contiguous primum ASD
Nonrestrictive VSD
Common AV valve
   Rastelli type A: Superior bridging leaflet with a cleft with chordal attchment to the crest of the ventricular septum
   Rastelli type B: Superior bridging leaflet with a cleft with chordal attachment to a papillary muscle in the right ventricle
   Rastelli type C: Superior bridging leaflet without a cleft and with no chordal attachment. The superior bridging leaflet is therefore "free floating." Associated anomalies include Down syndrome (>90%).

   ASD = Atrial septal defect; AV = atrioventricular; VSD = ventricular septal defect.

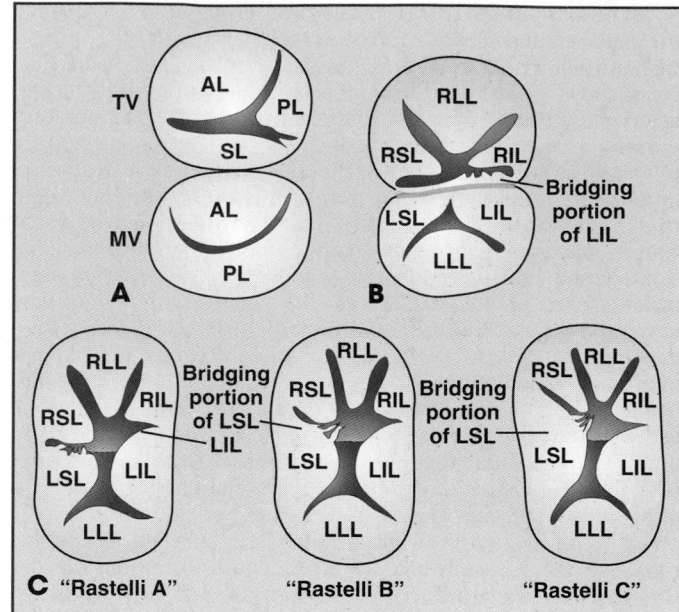

FIGURE 44–3. Right- and left-sided atrioventricular valve in normal heart *(A)*, partial atrioventricular septal defect *(B)*, and complete atrioventricular septal defect *(C)*. Rastelli type A: Superior bridging leaflet (RSL and LSL) has a cleft with ventricular septal attachment. Rastelli type B: Superior bridging leaflet has a cleft with right papillary muscle attachment. Rastelli type C: Superior bridging leaflet has no cleft and no attachment. TV = tricuspid valve; MV = mitral valve; AL = anterior leaflet; PL = posterior leaflet; SL = septal leaflet; RSL = right superior (bridging) leaflet; RLL = right lateral (anterosuperior) leaflet; RIL = right inferior (bridging) leaflet; LSL = left superior (bridging) leaflet; LLL = left lateral (mural) leaflet; LIL = left inferior (bridging) leaflet. (From Kirklin JW, Barratt-Boyes BG: Cardiac Surgery. 2nd ed. New York, Churchill Livingstone, 1993.)

abnormal right and left AV valves (primum and intermediate AVSD) or a common valve (complete AVSD) (Fig. 44–3). The left AV valve is invariably abnormal, having a "cleft" at the conjunction of the superior and inferior bridging leaflets. Rarely, a double orifice left (mitral) AV valve is also encountered. The "unwedged" anteriorly located aorta, coupled to an apically displaced left AV valve (at the same level as the right AV valve), gives rise to an elongated left ventricular outflow tract, often characterized as a "gooseneck deformity." AVSD may occur in association with Down syndrome, tetralogy of Fallot, and other forms of complex congenital heart disease, including univentricular hearts.

NATURAL HISTORY OF THE UNOPERATED PATIENT

Partial and Intermediate AVSD. Patients with partial and intermediate AVSDs have a course similar to that of patients with large secundum ASDs, with the caveat that symptoms may appear sooner when significant mitral regurgitation occurs through the cleft left AV valve. Patients are usually asymptomatic until their third or fourth decade, but progressive symptoms related to congestive heart failure, atrial arrhythmias, complete heart block, and variable degrees of pulmonary hypertension develop in virtually all of them by the fifth decade.

Complete AVSD. Most patients with complete defects have had surgical repair in infancy. Some patients may have had palliative surgery in the past with pulmonary artery bands and have variable degrees of pulmonary vascular obstructive disease. When presenting de novo, most adults have established pulmonary vascular disease (see Eisenmenger Syndrome). Patients with Down syndrome have a propensity to develop pulmonary hypertension at an even earlier age than do other patients with AVSD.

Clinical Manifestations. Clinical presentation depends on the presence and size of the ASD, on the VSD, and on the competence of the left AV valve. A large left-to-right shunt gives rise to symptoms of heart failure (dyspnea or fatigue on exertion) or, worse, pulmonary vascular disease (exertional syncope, cyanosis). Severe chronic left or right AV valve insufficiency leads to pulmonary congestion, hepatic congestion, and peripheral edema. Palpitations from atrial arrhythmias are very common. Down syndrome is seen in 35 percent of patients with AVSD. Almost all have the complete form. Cardiac findings on physical examination for patients with partial AVSD are similar to those of patients with secundum ASD, with the important addition of a prominent left ventricular apex and holosystolic murmur when significant left AV valve regurgitation is present. The murmur of left AV valve regurgitation can sometimes be heard radiating to the left sternal border if the regurgitant jet is directed into the right atrium (the Gerbode defect). Intermediate AVSDs resemble partial AVSD with the addition of a holosystolic VSD murmur heard best at the left sternal border, sometimes difficult to differentiate from a left AV valve regurgitant murmur. Complete AVSDs have a single first heart sound (S$_1$) (common AV valve), a mid-diastolic murmur from augmented AV valve inflow, and findings of pulmonary hypertension and/or a right-to-left shunt.

DIAGNOSTIC TESTING

Electrocardiogram. Because of the posteriorly located AV node and hence the closer proximity of the left posterior fascicle, most patients have first-degree AV block and left-axis deviation from late left anterior fascicular depolarization. Complete AV block and/or atrial fibrillation/flutter can be present in older patients. Partial or complete right bundle branch block is usually associated with right ventricular dilation (Fig. 44–4).

Chest Radiography. Cardiomegaly and pulmonary plethora are the rule with an enlarged left atrium commonly present.

Echocardiography. Echocardiography is essential to document the type of AVSD; assess the magnitude and direction of intracardiac shunting, the degree of AV valve regurgitation, the presence/absence of subaortic stenosis; and estimate pulmonary artery pressure (Fig. 43–13). The lack of "offsetting" between the left and right AV valves (the right AV valve being apically displaced in normal hearts) is readily seen in the four-chamber view and is the echocardiographic hallmark of AVSD (Fig. 44–5). TEE may be needed to further define the underlying anatomy of the defect (Rastelli type, see Table 44–1) and associated lesions (e.g., double orifice mitral valve) if unclear after TTE.

Cardiac Catheterization. Heart catheterization to determine the severity of pulmonary vascular disease, the presence and magnitude of intracardiac shunts, and the severity of subaortic stenosis may be necessary. The typical "goose neck" deformity of the left ventricular outflow tract is readily demonstrated on angiography.

Open-Lung Biopsy. This should only be considered when the reversibility of the pulmonary hypertension is uncertain from the hemodynamic data (see Eisenmenger Syndrome, p. 1614).

INDICATIONS FOR INTERVENTION. The patient with an unoperated or newly diagnosed AVSD and significant hemodynamic defects, manifested by atrial arrhythmias and impaired ventricular function or right ventricular volume overload, requires surgical repair. Equally, patients with symptoms, reversible pulmonary hypertension, or signifi-

FIGURE 44–5. See color plate 25.

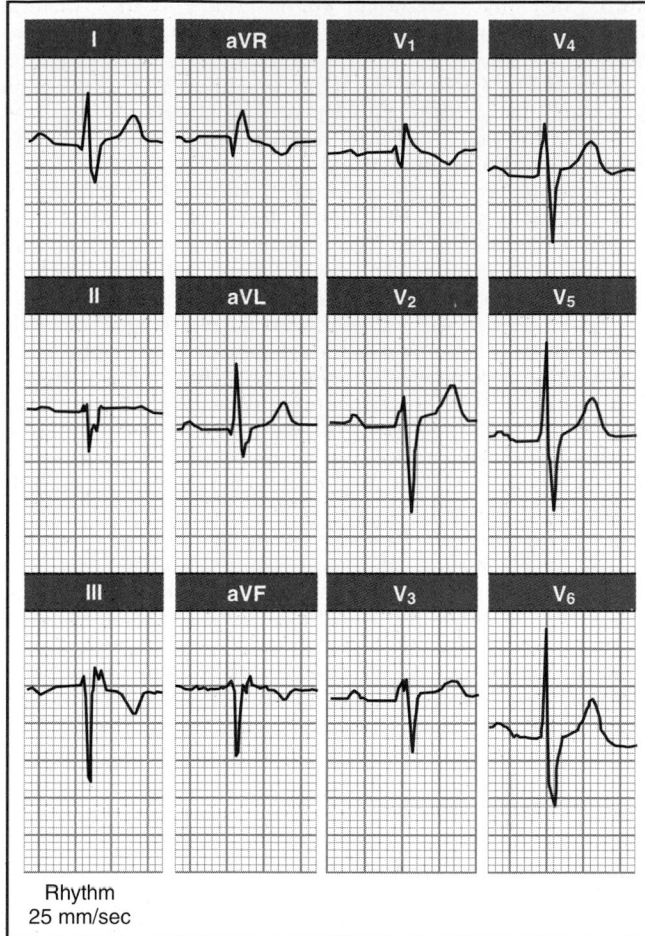

FIGURE 44–4. Typical electrocardiogram of partial atrioventricular septal defect shows first-degree atrioventricular block, left-axis deviation, and complete right bundle branch block.

cant subaortic obstruction (peak gradient of at least 50 mm Hg at rest) require surgical intervention.

INTERVENTIONAL OPTIONS

Partial AVSD. Pericardial patch closure of the primum ASD with concomitant suture (±annuloplasty) of the "cleft" left AV valve is usually performed. When "mitral" valve repair is not possible, "mitral" valve replacement may be necessary.

Intermediate/Complete AVSD. The "staged approach" (pulmonary artery banding followed by intracardiac repair) has been supplanted by primary intracardiac repair. The goals of intracardiac repair are ventricular and atrial septation with adequate mitral and tricuspid reconstruction. Both "single" and "double" patch techniques to close atrial and ventricular septal defects have been described with comparable results.[25] "Tricuspidization" of the left AV "mitral" valve (making a trileaflet left AV valve) at the time of surgery has been advocated by some,[26, 27] but a bileaflet repair is preferred by most.[28, 29] Patch augmentation of the tissue-deficient "bridging leaflets" forming the mitral valve is sometimes performed.[30] Occasionally, left AV valve replacement is necessary when valve repair is not possible. In patients with complete heart block, endocardial transvenous pacing should be avoided when intraatrial or intraventricular communications are present, because paradoxical emboli may occur.

INTERVENTIONAL OUTCOMES. Surgical mortality in adults with partial AVSDs varies between 0 and 6 percent with 5- and 10-year survivals of 87 percent and 72 percent, respectively.[31–32a] The worst outcome occurs in patients with pulmonary arterial hypertension, severe AV valve regurgitation, and an enlarged heart.[32b] Improvement in functional class after surgical repair is the rule.[31, 32] Postoperative complications include patch dehiscence or residual septal defects (1 percent), the development of complete heart block (3 percent), late atrial fibrillation/flutter, left AV valve dysfunction, and progressive or de novo subaortic stenosis. Recurrent left AV valve regurgitation is the principal cause of late morbidity after surgical repair of AVSDs, necessitating reoperation in at least 10 percent of patients.[28, 29, 31–33] Left AV stenosis from overly zealous cleft suturing may occur. The development or progression of subaortic stenosis after AVSD surgery occurs in about 5 percent of cases.[34] The morphological features of AVSD (the long, narrow left ventricular outflow tract) promote actual or potential subaortic stenosis. Subaortic stenosis can be discrete or tunnel-like, and surgical repair is often necessary. An operation tailored to the underlying cause of obstruction has been advocated because of the high risk of recurrence after surgical resection[34] (see Subaortic Stenosis, p. 1599).

FOLLOW-UP. All patients require periodic follow-up by a cardiologist because of the possibility of progressive AV valve regurgitation (or stenosis), the development of subaortic stenosis, significant atrial arrhythmias, or progression of the commonly present first-degree AV block. Particular attention should be paid to those patients with pulmonary hypertension, severe AV valve regurgitation, and an enlarged heart.

Patent Ductus Arteriosus

(see also Chap. 43)

The incidence of isolated persistent patency of the ductus arteriosus has been estimated at 1:2000 to 1:5000 births, or about 10 to 12 percent of all varieties of congenital heart disease.

ANATOMY. The ductus arteriosus derives from the left sixth primitive aortic arch and connects the proximal left pulmonary artery to the descending aorta, just distal to the left subclavian artery. Occasionally, the ductus fails to close at birth and presents as a potential clinical problem.

NATURAL HISTORY OF THE UNOPERATED PATIENT. Physiological consequences of a patent ductus arteriosus (PDA) depend on the degree of left-to-right shunting, which is determined by both the size of the duct and the difference between systemic and pulmonary vascular resistances.[35] A small ductus accompanied by a small shunt does not cause significant hemodynamic derangement but may predispose to endarteritis, especially if accompanied by an audible murmur.[2] A moderate-sized duct and shunt pose a volume load on the left atrium and ventricle with resultant left ventricular dilation and dysfunction and eventual atrial fibrillation. A large duct results initially in left ventricular volume overload, with a progressive rise in pulmonary artery pressure leading to high pulmonary vascular resistance and eventually irreversible pulmonary vascular changes and systemic pulmonary pressures (see Eisenmenger Syndrome, p. 1614).

CLINICAL MANIFESTATIONS. Patients with *silent* PDAs are asymptomatic, and the PDAs are detected by nonclinical means, usually echocardiography. A small audible duct usually causes no symptoms but may rarely present as an endovascular infection. Physical examination reveals a grade 1–2 continuous murmur, peaking in late systole, and best heard in the first or second left intercostal space. Patients with a moderate-sized duct may present with dyspnea or palpitations from atrial arrhythmias. A louder

continuous "machinery" murmur in the first or second left intercostal space is typically accompanied by a wide systemic pulse pressure from aortic diastolic runoff into the pulmonary trunk and signs of left ventricular volume overload, such as a displaced left ventricular apex and sometimes a left-sided S_3. With a moderate degree of pulmonary hypertension, the diastolic component of the murmur disappears, leaving a systolic murmur. Adults with a large uncorrected PDA eventually present with Eisenmenger syndrome physiology (see p. 1614).

DIAGNOSTIC TESTING

Electrocardiogram. The ECG reflects the size and degree of shunting occurring through the duct. A small duct produces a normal ECG. A moderate-sized duct may show left ventricular volume overload with broad, notched P waves together with deep Q waves, tall R waves, and peaked T waves in V_5 and V_6. A large duct produces findings of right ventricular hypertrophy (see Eisenmenger syndrome, p. 1614).

Chest Radiography. A small duct produces a normal chest radiograph. A moderate-sized duct causes moderate cardiomegaly with left-sided heart enlargement and increased pulmonary perfusion. A large duct produces right ventricular hypertrophy and enlarged central pulmonary arteries with peripheral pruning (see Eisenmenger syndrome, p. 1614).

Echocardiography. This will determine the presence, size, and degree of shunting and the physiological consequences of the shunt. Suprasternal and parasternal short-axis views will best identify the duct. In the absence of Eisenmenger physiology, color flow Doppler shows a jet that travels on the lateral wall of the main pulmonary artery toward the pulmonary valve in systole and diastole (Fig. 44–6; see also Fig. 43–18). Direction and timing of the flow as well as the Doppler-derived gradient obtained from the jet provide estimates of the pulmonary artery pressure.

INDICATIONS FOR INTERVENTION. Closure of a clinically detectable PDA, in the absence of irreversible pulmonary hypertension, is usually recommended to avoid its associated morbidity and premature mortality. The risk of endarteritis in a patient with a *silent* PDA is considered negligible, and closure of such ducts is not recommended for that reason.[2] In the presence of pulmonary hypertension (PAP > two thirds of SAP, or pulmonary arteriolar resistance > two thirds of systemic arteriolar resistance), PDA closure should be carried out if there is a net pulmonary/systemic blood flow greater than 1.5/1.0, evidence of pulmonary artery reactivity when challenged with a pulmonary vasodilator (e.g., oxygen, nitric oxide), or lung biopsy evidence that pulmonary arterial changes are potentially reversible (Heath-Edwards grade II or less). Contraindications to ductal closure include irreversible pulmonary hypertension or active endarteritis.[2]

INTERVENTIONAL OPTIONS AND OUTCOMES

Transcatheter Treatment. Over the past 20 years, the efficacy and safety of transcatheter device closure for ducts less than 8 mm has been established,[36–38] with complete ductal closure achieved in more than 85 percent of patients by 1 year after device placement at a mortality rate of less than 1 percent. The avoidance of general anesthesia, thoracotomy, postoperative pain, and prolonged convalescence makes transcatheter closure a very attractive modality. In centers with appropriate resources and experience, transcatheter device occlusion should be the method of choice for ductal closure (see Chap. 43, Fig. 43–19).

Surgical Treatment. Surgical closure, by ductal ligation and/or division, has been performed for over 50 years with a marginally greater closure rate than device closure but somewhat greater morbidity and mortality. Immediate clinical closure (no shunt audible on physical examination) is achieved in more than 95 percent of patients.[39] Surgical mortality in adults is 1.0 to 3.5 percent and relates to the presence of pulmonary artery hypertension and the difficult

FIGURE 44–6. See color plate 25.

ductal morphology (calcified or aneurysmal) often seen in adults. Surgical closure of a duct should be reserved for patients with larger ducts (> 8 mm diameter) or at centers without access to interventional expertise. Emerging procedures such as muscle-sparing minithoracotomy and video-assisted thoracoscopic surgery may further broaden therapeutic surgical choices in the future.

FOLLOW-UP. Patients with a silent PDA do not require follow-up. Patients with device occlusion or after surgical closure should be examined periodically for possible recanalization. Silent residual shunts may be found by TTE. The risk of late endarteritis from a clinically silent residual shunt after device implantation or surgical closure is unclear,[40, 41] and the clinical management of such patients remains problematic. Until long-term follow-up data become available, it may be prudent to continue antibiotic endocarditis prophylaxis in such patients.[36, 40, 41]

Bicuspid Aortic Valve
(see also Chap. 43)

The bicuspid aortic valve remains the most common congenital malformation of the heart (1–2 percent of the population). This lesion accounts for approximately half the cases of surgically important isolated aortic stenosis in adults.

ANATOMY. A bicuspid aortic valve consists of two cusps, often of unequal size, the larger usually containing a false raphe. There is a male preponderance of 4:1. It usually occurs in isolation but is associated with other abnormalities in 20 percent, the most common being coarctation of the aorta and PDA. There is also a high prevalence of aortic root enlargement in patients with bicuspid aortic valve that occurs irrespective of altered hemodynamics or age.[42–42b]

NATURAL HISTORY OF THE UNOPERATED PATIENT. Patients with a bicuspid aortic valve may not experience any problems, although there is always the risk of endocarditis. Mild aortic stenosis from bicuspid aortic valve commonly progresses as the patient ages, but the rate is variable.[43] Late aortic stenosis from calcification of the valve in the sixth decade is common. Other patients can develop aortic regurgitation, aneurysmal aortic root dilation, and possibly aortic dissection.[44]

DIAGNOSTIC TESTING
Electrocardiogram. The ECG ranges from normal to showing marked left ventricular hypertrophy from severe aortic stenosis or regurgitation. (see Fig. 43–31).
Chest Radiography. Dilation of the ascending aorta is common. Valvar calcification can sometimes be detected. The left ventricle is enlarged in proportion to the degree of aortic regurgitation.
Echocardiography. This permits identification of the bileaflet aortic valve and quantification of the severity of obstruction and/or regurgitation. It also provides information on left ventricular size and function as well as aortic root size. Concomitant defects such as coarctation or dissection of the aorta should be sought (see Fig. 43–32).

INDICATIONS FOR INTERVENTION. Bicuspid aortic valves require intervention for stenosis when symptoms (exertional dyspnea, angina, presyncope or syncope) are present. Intervention for asymptomatic "critical" aortic stenosis (valve area < 0.6 cm²) is debatable. Patients with moderate or severe regurgitation associated with deteriorating ventricular function, a dilating ventricle, or symptoms are surgical candidates. Prophylactic surgery for proximal aortic dilation (> 55 mm) seems better than waiting for the aorta to dissect or rupture, although there is no agreement on the diameter at which referral for surgery is appropriate.

INTERVENTIONAL OPTIONS. Bicuspid aortic stenosis can be treated with balloon valvuloplasty if the valve is noncal-

cified.[45] Other treatment options include open aortic valvotomy or valve replacement using a mechanical valve, a biological valve, or a pulmonary autograft. The pulmonary autograft (Ross procedure), introduced by Donald Ross in 1967, consists of replacing the aortic valve with the patient's pulmonary valve and implanting a homograft in the pulmonary position. The advantages of this procedure—avoidance of anticoagulation and much reduced risk of thromboembolism—need to be weighed against the greater technical complexity of the procedure, the risk of early and late autograft dysfunction, and homograft failure.[46, 47] The choice of intervention depends on the availability and skills of the team involved and the preference of the patient. Aortic valve repair has been reported for aortic regurgitation from a prolapsing aortic valve leaflet. Short-term results are promising, but long-term data are awaited.[48]

FOLLOW-UP. All patients, treated and untreated, require skilled follow-up, the frequency being determined by the severity of the pathology.

Subaortic Stenosis
(see also Chap. 43)

ANATOMY. Subvalvar LVOTO can be either *discrete* (most common) or *tunnel* shaped. Discrete obstruction is due to a membranous ridge or fibromuscular narrowing partially or completely encircling the left ventricular outflow tract beneath the base of the aortic valve.[49] Tunnel-like obstruction is produced by a fibromuscular channel that involves a long segment of the left ventricular outflow tract and is usually associated with a small aortic root. Rarely, abnormal insertion of the mitral valve or an accessory mitral leaflet will cause subvalvar obstruction. Subvalvar LVOTO can also be seen after repair of AVSD (see p. 1596). The concurrence of subvalvar LVOTO, coarctation, and mitral stenosis (parachute mitral valve and supramitral ring) is known as Shone syndrome. VSD is sometimes associated with subvalvar LVOTO.

NATURAL HISTORY OF THE UNOPERATED PATIENT. Subvalvar LVOTO, discrete or tunnel-like, usually progresses at variable rate, resulting in left ventricular hypertrophy and the development of symptoms.[50] It is often associated with progressive aortic regurgitation (up to 60 percent of cases) from a bicuspid aortic valve or an otherwise normal valve damaged by the subvalvar jet of blood. Aortic regurgitation in this setting is seldom more than moderate. These patients are particularly vulnerable to endocarditis.

CLINICAL MANIFESTATIONS. Patients can be asymptomatic or can present with angina, syncope, or heart failure. On examination, the pulse pressure may be diminished if the obstruction is severe. A_2 may be normal or diminished depending on the severity of the stenosis. A systolic ejection murmur may be heard at the mid-left sternal edge in cases of tubular stenosis and in the second right intercostal space in cases of discrete stenosis. A blowing diastolic murmur from concomitant aortic regurgitation is often present. A systolic ejection click is not present in subvalvar aortic stenosis, and the systolic murmur does not radiate to the carotid arteries.[51]

DIAGNOSTIC TESTING
Electrocardiogram. Left ventricular hypertrophy may be present.
Chest Radiography. An inconspicuous cardiac silhouette and ascending aorta are the rule unless LVOTO is associated with a bicuspid aortic valve (see bicuspid valve/ascending aortopathy) or significant aortic regurgitation.
Echocardiography. Two-dimensional echocardiography permits identification of the morphology of the obstruction and any associated anomalies (e.g., bicuspid aortic valve, VSD, coarctation, or mitral inflow obstruction).[52] The sever-

ity of LVOTO can be determined by continuous-wave Doppler and the severity of aortic regurgitation by Doppler and color flow imaging.

Angiography. An angiogram to assess the severity of obstruction may be needed when noninvasive means are not adequate.

INDICATIONS FOR INTERVENTION. Whereas patients with symptomatic subvalvar LVOTO require intervention, indications for intervention in asymptomatic patients are less well defined. A resting peak-to-peak angiographic gradient greater than 50 mm Hg as well as progressive or moderate to severe aortic regurgitation have been used as criteria for intervention.[6] Some advocate earlier relief of subvalvar obstruction to minimize early aortic valve damage and prevent progressive regurgitation.[53]

INTERVENTIONAL OPTIONS

Surgical. For discrete obstruction, membranectomy with concomitant myomectomy or myotomy is usually performed. For tunnel-like obstruction, the left ventricular outflow tract often requires surgical augmentation using the modified Konno procedure (aortoventriculoplasty with aortic valve sparing).[54] In patients with significant aortic stenosis or moderate/severe aortic regurgitation, the Konno procedure (aortoventriculoplasty with aortic valve replacement) or the Konno-Ross procedure (aortoventriculoplasty with pulmonary autograft)[55] for younger patients or those with a contraindication to anticoagulation should be performed. Left ventricular apex-to-aorta valved conduits, bypassing the LVOTO, have been used in the past, but the long-term durability is unacceptable and the procedure has largely been abandoned.

Transcatheter. Transluminal balloon dilation of discrete subaortic stenosis has been described with good short- and intermediate-term results,[56] but long-term data have not been reported. At present, a surgical approach is still recommended.

INTERVENTIONAL OUTCOMES. Complications related to surgery include complete AV block, creation of VSD, or mitral valve regurgitation from intraoperative damage to the mitral valve apparatus. Long-term complications include recurrence of fibromuscular subvalvar LVOTO (up to 20 percent), particularly with tunnel-like obstruction or following isolated membranectomy for discrete obstruction. Clinically important aortic regurgitation is also not uncommon (up to 25 percent of patients).

FOLLOW-UP. Particular attention should be paid to patients with recurrent subvalvar stenosis or patients with an associated bicuspid aortic valve or progressive aortic regurgitation because they are most likely to require eventual surgery. Patients with bioprosthetic aortic valves in the aortic position (after the Konno procedure) or the pulmonic position (after the Konno-Ross procedure) need close follow-up. Reoperation is required in up to 25 percent of patients in the 20 years[57, 58] after surgical repair. Endocarditis prophylaxis should be used for prosthetic valves or in the presence of any residual lesions.

Coarctation of the Aorta

(see also Chap. 43)

This left-sided obstructive lesion occurs most frequently in males, with a sex ratio approaching 3:1.

ANATOMY. Coarctation of the aorta is a narrowing usually in the region of the ligamentum arteriosum (see Fig. 43–27). It may be discrete or associated with hypoplasia of the aortic arch and isthmus. The specific anatomy, severity, and degree of hypoplasia proximal to the coarctation are highly variable. "Complex" coarctation is used to describe coarctation in the presence of other important intracardiac anomalies (e.g., VSD, LVOTO, and mitral stenosis) and is usually detected in infancy. "Simple" coarctation refers to

coarctation in the absence of such lesions. It is the most common form detected de novo in adults. Associated abnormalities include bicuspid aortic valve in 50 to 85 percent of cases, intracranial aneurysms (most commonly of the circle of Willis), and acquired intercostal artery aneurysms. One definition of "significant" coarctation is one with a gradient greater than 20 mm Hg across the coarctation site at angiography with or without proximal systemic hypertension. A second definition of "significant" coarctation requires the presence of proximal hypertension in the company of echocardiographic or angiographic evidence of aortic coarctation. Of note, if there is an extensive collateral circulation, there may be minimal or no pressure gradient and acquired aortic atresia.

NATURAL HISTORY OF THE UNOPERATED PATIENT. A significant coarctation causes a pressure load proximally with consequent left ventricular hypertrophy and ultimately heart failure. Most patients will develop systemic hypertension, typically during childhood, and are at risk of premature coronary artery disease. The mean survival of patients with untreated coarctation is 35 years, with 75 percent mortality by 50 years of age.[59] Death in patients who do not undergo repair is usually due to heart failure (usually beyond 30 years of age), coronary artery disease, aortic rupture/dissection, concomitant aortic valve disease, infective endarteritis/endocarditis, or cerebral hemorrhage.[59]

CLINICAL MANIFESTATIONS. Patients may be asymptomatic or present with minimal symptoms of epistaxis, headache, leg weakness on exertion, or more serious symptoms of congestive heart failure, angina, aortic stenosis, aortic dissection, or unexplained intracerebral hemorrhage. Leg claudication is rare unless there is concomitant abdominal aortic coarctation (Somerville J, personal communication, 1998). A thorough clinical examination reveals upper limb systemic hypertension as well as a differential systolic blood pressure of at least 10 mm Hg (brachial > popliteal artery pressure). Radial-femoral pulse delay is evident unless significant aortic regurgitation coexists. Auscultation may reveal an interscapular systolic murmur emanating from the coarctation site and a widespread crescendo-decrescendo systolic murmur throughout the chest wall from intercostal collateral arteries. Fundoscopic examination can reveal "corkscrew" tortuosity of retinal arterioles.[60]

DIAGNOSTIC TESTING

Electrocardiogram. Left ventricular hypertrophy is common. Concomitant left atrial enlargement may be present.

Chest Radiography. Prestenotic and poststenotic dilation of the aorta gives the "3 sign" appearance on a chest radiograph. Rib notching appearing as sclerotic scalloping on the inferior surface of ribs number 3 through 8 from dilated intercostal arteries may be present, usually bilaterally, unless the left or right subclavian artery arises aberrantly below the coarctation, giving rise to unilateral right-sided or left-sided rib notching, respectively.

Echocardiography. The coarctation site can be visualized from the suprasternal view and its severity assessed by Doppler mode (see Fig. 43–28). A peak gradient greater than 20 mm Hg, especially if accompanied by continuous forward flow during diastole in the descending or abdominal aorta, suggests significant aortic coarctation. In addition, the echocardiographer should evaluate other cardiac lesions—notably aortic, mitral, or subaortic abnormality and the status of left ventricular function.

Angiography. Angiography with hemodynamic measurements can be done to assess the location, type, and severity of coarctation and to determine the presence/absence of collaterals or aneurysm formation. Associated stenoses in other great vessels (carotids and subclavian arteries) can also be detected by this modality. Coronary angiography should be performed if surgery is planned because of the risk of premature coronary artery disease in these patients.

Magnetic Resonance Imaging (MRI). MRI (two-dimensional and velocity mapping) provides as good anatomical and hemodynamic details as angiography and may obviate the need for angiography, unless coronary artery disease needs to be excluded.

INDICATIONS FOR INTERVENTION. All patients with significant coarctation or re-coarctation (arm > leg systolic pressure difference ≥ 10 mm Hg; radial-femoral pulse delay; peak transcoarctation gradient > 20 mm Hg at angiography) including those with long-standing hypertension (regardless of age), whether symptomatic or asymptomatic, warrant intervention to reduce or eliminate the gradient.[59]

INTERVENTIONAL OPTIONS

Surgical. Surgical techniques include end-to-end repair, subclavian flap plasty, patch repair, interposed graft, or bypass graft and varies according to the underlying anatomy of the coarctation.[61] Patients with significant aortic valve stenosis may also require valve surgery that may or may not be done at the same time as coarctation repair. If lesions are operated on separately, the more severe lesion should be dealt with first.

Transcatheter. Balloon dilation with or without stent insertion in patients with native coarctation and re-coarctation has been performed with good immediate and medium-term results in children and adolescents.[62-64] However, it should still be considered experimental in the adult population and should only be performed in centers and by individuals with expertise in this domain (Fig. 44–7).

INTERVENTIONAL OUTCOMES

Surgical. After surgical repair of simple coarctation, the obstruction is usually relieved with minimal mortality (<1 percent). Paraplegia due to spinal cord ischemia is uncommon (0.4 percent) and may occur in patients who do not have well-developed collateral circulation. The prevalence of recoarctation reported in the literature varies widely, from 7 to 60 percent depending on the definition used, the length of follow-up, and the age at surgery.[65] The appropriateness of the surgical repair for a given anatomy is probably the main factor dictating the chance of recoarctation, rather than the type of surgical repair itself.[66] True aneurysm formation at the site of coarctation repair is also a well-recognized entity with a reported incidence between 2 and 27 percent.[67] Aneurysms are particularly common after

Dacron patch aortoplasty and usually occur in the native aorta opposite the patch. Late dissection at the repair site is rare but false aneurysms, usually at the suture line, can occur.

Prior hypertension resolves in up to 50 percent of patients but may recur later in life, especially if the intervention is performed at an older age. In some of these patients this may be "essential hypertension," but a hemodynamic basis should be sought and blood pressure control attained. Systolic hypertension is also common with exercise and may be related to residual arch hypoplasia or more likely to increased renin and catecholamine activity from residual functional abnormality of the precoarctation vessels.[69, 70] Late cerebrovascular events occur, notably in those patients undergoing repair as adults and in those with residual hypertension. Endocarditis/endarteritis can occur at the coarctation site or on intracardiac lesions; and if this occurs at the coarctation site, embolic manifestations are restricted to the legs.

Long-term follow-up after surgical correction of coarctation of the aorta still reveals an increased incidence of premature cardiovascular disease and death.

Transcatheter. After balloon dilation, aortic dissection, restenosis, and aneurysm formation at the site of coarctation have all been documented.[62-64] These complications may well be reduced if stents are used. The significance of aneurysm formation is unknown,[68] and longer-term data are needed.

FOLLOW-UP. All patients should have follow-up every 1 to 3 years. Particular attention should be directed toward residual hypertension, heart failure, or intracardiac disease, such as an associated bicuspid aortic valve, which can become stenotic or regurgitant later in life, or an ascending aortopathy (due to cystic medial necrosis) sometimes seen in the presence of bicuspid aortic valve. Complications at the site of repair such as restenosis and aneurysm formation should also be sought using clinical examination, chest radiography, echocardiography, or, preferably, MRI.[68a] Patients with Dacron patch repair should probably undergo an MRI or spiral computed tomographic (CT) examination every 3 to 5 years or so to detect subclinical aneurysm formation. Hemoptysis from a leaking/ruptured aneurysm is a serious complication requiring immediate investigation

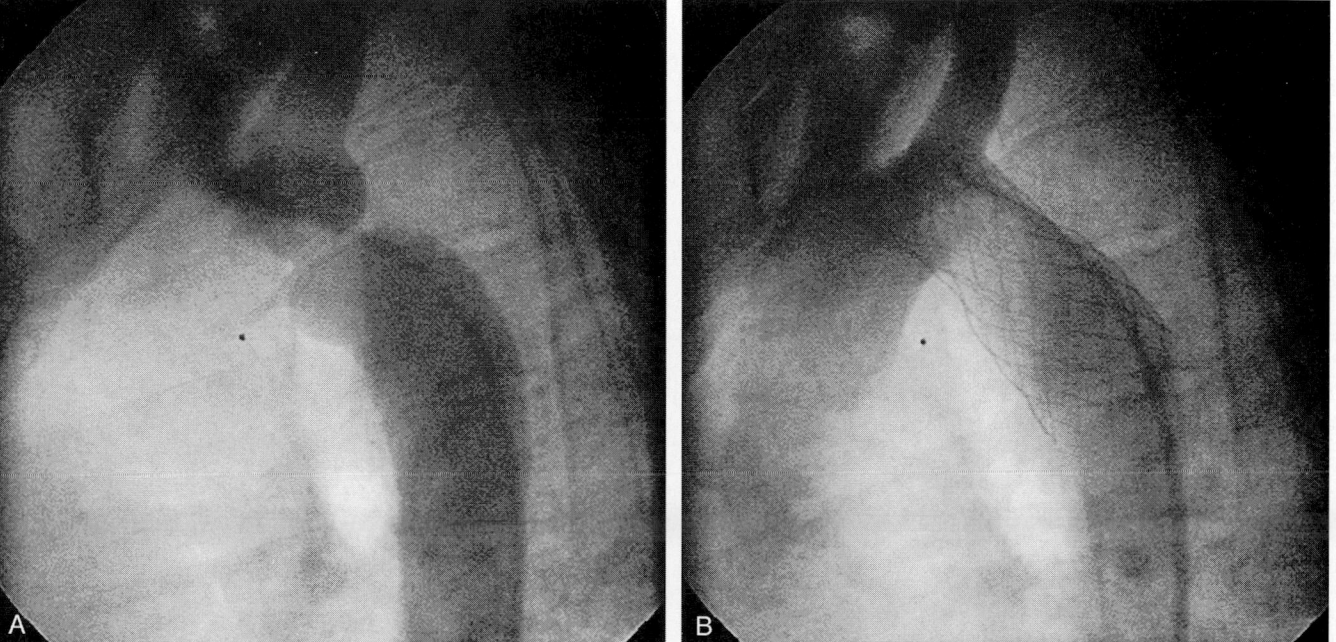

FIGURE 44–7. Angiograms of coarctation of the thoracic aorta *(A)* and transcatheter stent placement in the treatment of coarctation of the aorta *(B)*.

and surgery. New or unusual headaches should raise the possibility of berry aneurysm. Endocarditis prophylaxis is recommended for any residual turbulent flow.

Right Ventricular Outflow Tract Obstruction

(see also Chap. 43)

Right ventricular outflow tract obstruction (RVOTO) can occur at supravalvar, valvar, and subvalvar levels.

ANATOMY. *Supravalvar* RVOTO seldom occurs in isolation. It may occur in tetralogy of Fallot, Williams syndrome, Noonan syndrome, VSD, or arteriohepatic dysplasia (Alagille syndrome) (Table 44–2). *Branch* pulmonary artery stenosis may occur in the setting of congenital rubella syndrome and tetralogy of Fallot. *Subvalvar* (infundibular) RVOTO usually occurs in combination with other lesions, particularly ventricular septal defect, as part of tetralogy of Fallot, or in association with subaortic stenosis. The *"double-chambered right ventricle"* is different from infundibular RVOTO. It consists of a midcavity obstruction, often from a prominent moderator band, and may be associated with a small VSD. *Valvar* RVOTO (pulmonic stenosis) is the most common form of RVOTO. It is almost always congenital in origin. It usually occurs as an isolated anomaly but it can be part of a syndrome (see Table 44–2). Typically, the stenotic pulmonic valve is a thin, pliable, dome-shaped structure, with a narrow opening at its apex. In 15 percent of cases, the stenotic valve is dysplastic with thickened and immobile cusps. The severity of stenosis is classified by the level of the peak systolic pressure gradient (Table 44–3).

NATURAL HISTORY OF THE UNOPERATED PATIENT. *Supravalvar* RVOTO can progress in severity and should be monitored. *Subvalvar* (infundibular and double-chamber) RVOTO often progresses in severity, causing worsening right ventricular hypertrophy, symptoms, and critical gradients requiring surgical repair. Patients with trivial and mild *valvar* RVOTO rarely become worse with time.[71] Moderate valvar RVOTO can progress in 20 percent of unoperated

▼ **TABLE 44–2. SYNDROMES ASSOCIATED WITH PULMONARY VALVE STENOSIS**

Williams Syndrome
Cardiac: Pulmonary stenosis, pulmonary artery stenosis, supravalvar aortic stenosis
CNS: Mental retardation, "cocktail personality"
Facies: Small chin, large mouth, upturned and blunt nose, wide-set eyes, broad forehead, baggy cheeks, and malformed teeth
Other: Infantile hypercalcemia, short stature

Noonan Syndrome
Cardiac: Dysplastic pulmonary stenosis, hypertrophic cardiomyopathy, atrial septal defect
CNS: Mental retardation (1 in 3 patients)
Facies: Short webbed neck, low-set ears, low posterior hair line, high-arched palate, micrognathia, eye abnormality (ptosis/hypertelorism)
Other: Short stature; thoracic, penile, and testicular abnormality

Congenital Rubella
Cardiac: Pulmonary stenosis, pulmonary artery stenosis, patent ductus arteriosus
CNS: Mental retardation, hypotonia, hearing loss
Facies: Cataracts, retinopathy

Alagille Syndrome
Cardiac: Pulmonary stenosis, pulmonary arterial stenosis
Facies: Prominent overhanging forehead, deep-set eyes, small pointed chin

▼ **TABLE 44–3. HEMODYNAMIC SEVERITY GRADING FOR RIGHT VENTRICULAR OUTFLOW TRACT OBSTRUCTION (PEAK GRADIENT)**

Trivial	<25 mm Hg
Mild	25–49 mm Hg
Moderate	50–79 mm Hg
Severe or critical	>80 mm Hg

patients, especially as adults because of calcification of the valve, and may require intervention.[71] Some of these patients can also become symptomatic, particularly in later life, because of atrial arrhythmias resulting from right ventricular pressure overload and tricuspid regurgitation. Patients with severe valvar RVOTO will have had valvotomy (balloon or surgical) to survive to adult life. Long-term survival in patients with repaired pulmonic valvar stenosis is similar to that of the general population, with excellent to good functional class at long-term follow-up in the vast majority of patients.[71]

CLINICAL MANIFESTATIONS. Patients with isolated mild to moderate RVOTO of any type are usually asymptomatic. Patients with severe RVOTO may present with exertional fatigue, dyspnea, lightheadedness, and chest discomfort (right ventricular angina). Physical examination may reveal a prominent jugular a wave, a right ventricular lift, and possibly a thrill in the second left interspace. Auscultation reveals a normal S_1, a split second heart sound (S_2) with a diminished pulmonic component (P_2) (unless the obstruction is supravalvular in which case the intensity of the P_2 does not change), and a systolic ejection murmur best heard in the second left intercostal space. When the pulmonic valve is thin and pliable, a systolic ejection click, which decreases on inspiration, is heard. As the severity of stenosis progresses, the interval between the S_1 and the systolic ejection click becomes shorter, the S_2 becomes widely split, the P_2 diminishes or disappears (but remains the same if the obstruction is supravalvular), and the systolic ejection murmur lengthens and peaks later in systole, often extending beyond the aortic component of the S_2 (A_2). An ejection click seldom occurs with dysplastic pulmonic stenosis or subvalvar or supravalvar RVOTO. Typically, the systolic murmur of subvalvar stenosis is located lower on the left chest (third to fifth intercostal space) and that of supravalvular stenosis (pulmonary artery/branches stenosis) has a wide thoracic distribution. Mild cyanosis may be present when a patent foramen ovale or ASD permits right-to-left shunting.

DIAGNOSTIC TESTING

Electrocardiogram. A peaked P wave consistent with right atrial overload and evidence of right ventricular hypertrophy may be present.

Chest Radiography. Dilation of the main and left pulmonary arteries is the radiographic hallmark of valvar pulmonary stenosis. Pulmonary valvar calcification occasionally is seen. Dilation of the pulmonary trunk is not a feature of subvalvar and supravalvar RVOTO. Peripheral pulmonary vascular markings may be diminished when RVOTO is severe.

Echocardiography. Echocardiography is useful to document the level(s) of obstruction and quantitate the severity (see Fig. 43–42). Associated abnormalities such as ASD, PDA, VSD, and tetralogy of Fallot can be identified.

Diagnostic Catheterization. Cardiac catheterization can be useful to assess the hemodynamics and severity of obstruction as well as to delineate the extent and site of pulmonary artery branch stenoses.

INDICATIONS FOR INTERVENTION. Intervention is recommended when the peak gradient across the right ventricular outflow tract is more than 50 mm Hg at rest[2, 72] or when the patient is symptomatic. Intervention may be indicated occasionally for other reasons (e.g., a person with a lesser degree of obstruction who wishes to play vigorous sports, scuba dive, or become pregnant). An associated ASD should be closed at the time of intervention.

INTERVENTIONAL OPTIONS

Balloon Valvuloplasty. Balloon valvuloplasty is the treatment of choice for valvar RVOTO. It is a highly effective procedure that can be carried at low risk.[73]

Surgical Valvotomy. Surgical valvotomy may be required for pulmonary stenosis when the valve is calcified or dysplastic.[74] Pulmonary valvectomy or pulmonary valve replacement is seldom performed.

Relief of peripheral pulmonary stenosis can be accomplished by balloon dilation with or without stent placement.

Relief of obstruction in a double-chambered right ventricle is accomplished by surgical resection of right ventricular muscle bands.

INTERVENTIONAL OUTCOMES

Balloon Valvuloplasty. The prognosis and outcomes of pulmonic valvuloplasty compare favorably with those of surgical valvotomy.[75] A 55 to 75 percent immediate reduction in transvalvular gradient is the rule, and usually the benefit persists at up to 9 years of follow-up. After pulmonic valvuloplasty, dynamic RVOTO from residual subvalvular hypertrophy is sometimes seen but usually regresses by 3 to 12 months and can be treated with a beta blocker in the meantime.[76] Severe pulmonic regurgitation as a consequence of valvuloplasty is rare. The results of balloon dilation for dysplastic pulmonary valves are less satisfactory.[74]

Surgical Valvotomy. The long-term results of surgical pulmonary valvotomy are well known and excellent. Relief of valvar RVOTO is usually permanent, but residual obstruction can progress. Significant pulmonary regurgitation is reportedly more frequent after surgery and can become severe enough to warrant re-intervention.

Subvalvar and supravalvar RVOTO seldom recur after adequate intervention.

FOLLOW-UP. Patients with moderate or greater RVOTO require annual monitoring because intervention or re-intervention may be required. After intervention, severe pulmonic regurgitation associated with reduced exercise capacity, arrhythmias, or evidence of deteriorating right ventricular function may necessitate pulmonary valve replacement.

Ebstein Anomaly

(see also Chap. 43)

ANATOMY. Ebstein anomaly results from apical displacement of the septal, posterior, or (rarely) anterior leaflet of the tricuspid valve, resulting in "atrialization" (functioning as an atrial chamber) of the inflow tract of the right ventricle and consequently a variably small functional right ventricle (Figs. 7–89, and 44–55). Varying degrees of tricuspid regurgitation (or in exceptional cases tricuspid stenosis) result from this abnormal tricuspid leaflet morphology with consequent further right atrial enlargement. Infundibular dilation can also be present. Associated anomalies include patent foramen ovale or ASD in approximately 50 percent of patients, accessory conduction pathways in 25 percent, and, occasionally, varying degrees of RVOTO, VSD, coarctation of the aorta, PDA, or mitral valve disease.

Natural History of the Unoperated Patient. The natural history of patients with Ebstein anomaly depends on its severity.[77] Adults with Ebstein anomaly can remain asymptomatic throughout their life if the anomaly is mild—survival to the ninth decade has been reported. With moderate tricuspid valve deformity and dysfunction, patients will usually develop symptoms during late adolescence or young adult life.

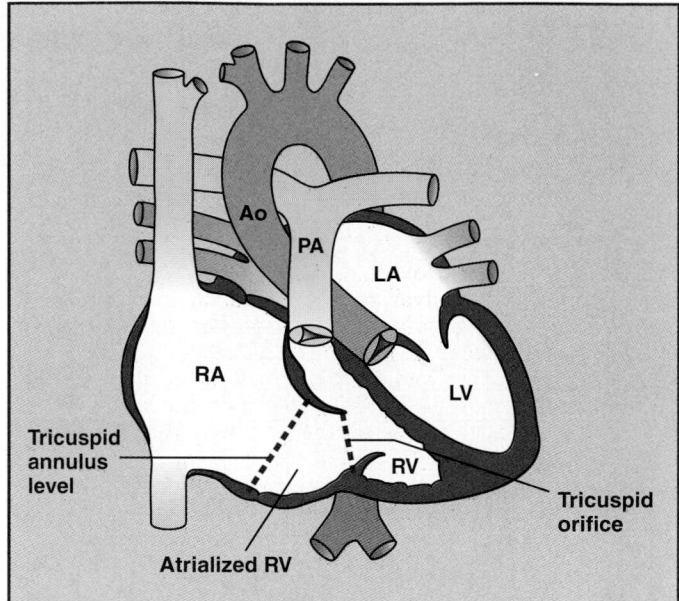

FIGURE 44–8. Diagrammatic representation of Ebstein anomaly. RA = right atrium; RV = right ventricle; LA = left atrium; LV = left ventricle; Ao = aorta; PA = pulmonary artery. (From Mullins CE, Mayer DC: Congenital Heart Disease: A Diagrammatic Atlas. New York, Wiley-Liss, 1988.)

Clinical Manifestations. Most adult patients present with exercise intolerance (dyspnea and fatigue), palpitations of supraventricular origin, or cyanosis from a right-to-left shunt at the atrial level.[1] Occasionally, a paradoxical embolus resulting in a transient ischemic attack or cerebrovascular accident can call attention to the diagnosis. End-stage right-sided cardiac failure from severe tricuspid regurgitation and right ventricular dysfunction is possible. Sudden death (presumed to be arrhythmic in nature) is known to occur.[78] Physical examination reveals an unimpressive jugular venous pressure because of the large and compliant right atrium and atrialized right ventricle, a widely split S_1 with a loud tricuspid component (the "sail sound"), a widely split S_2 from the right bundle branch block, and a right-sided S_3. A holosystolic murmur increasing on inspiration from tricuspid regurgitation is best heard at the lower left sternal border. Cyanosis from a right-to-left shunt at the atrial level may or may not be present.[79]

DIAGNOSTIC TESTING

Electrocardiogram. The ECG presentation of Ebstein anomaly varies widely. Low voltage is typical. Peaked P waves in lead II and V_1 reflect right atrial enlargement. The PR interval is usually prolonged, but a short PR interval and a delta wave from early activation through an accessory pathway can be present. An rsr′ pattern consistent with right ventricular conduction delay is typically seen in lead V_1 (Fig. 44–9). Atrial flutter and fibrillation are common. Alternatively, the ECG may be normal.

Chest Radiography. A rightward convexity from an enlarged right atrium and atrialized right ventricle coupled with a leftward convexity from a dilated infundibulum give the heart a "water bottle" appearance on a chest radiograph. Cardiomegaly, highly variable in degree, is the rule. The aorta and the pulmonary trunk are inconspicuous. The pulmonary vasculature is usually normal to reduced.

Echocardiography. The diagnosis of Ebstein anomaly can often be made by echocardiography. Apical displacement of the septal leaflet of the tricuspid valve by 8 mm/m² or more, combined with an elongated sail-like appearance of the anterior leaflet, confirms the diagnosis[80] (Figs. 44–10, 7–90, and 43–56). The size of the atrialized portion of the right ventricle (identified between the tricuspid annulus and the ventricular attachment of the tricuspid valve leaf-

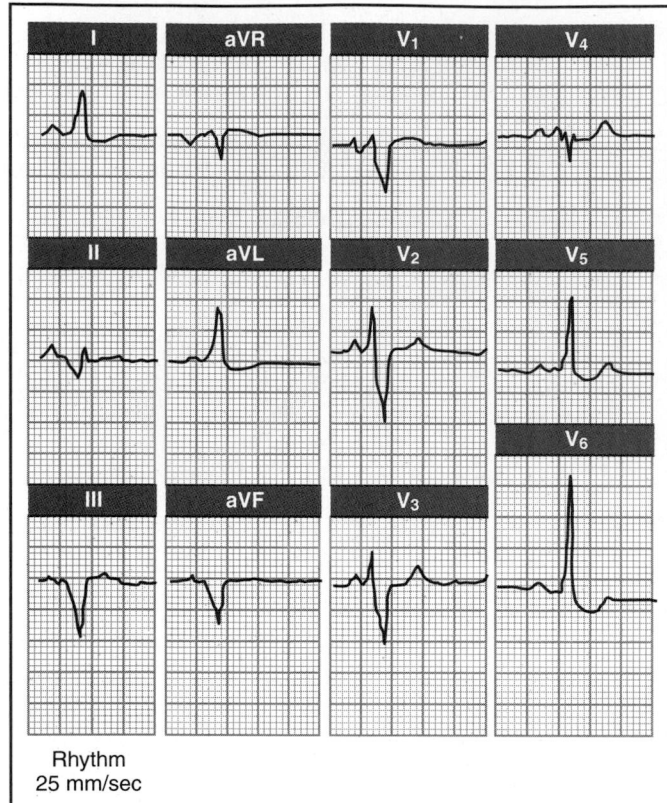

FIGURE 44–9. Electrocardiogram typical of Ebstein anomaly. Accessory pathway exemplified by the short PR interval, delta wave, and wide QRS complex. Note the peaked P wave in V_2 representing right atrial overload.

functional right ventricle [because of size or function], and/or chronic supraventricular arrhythmias), a bidirectional cavopulmonary connection can be added to reduce right ventricular preload (see Glen procedure, Chap. 43).[83] Occasionally, a Fontan operation may be the best option in patients with tricuspid stenosis and/or hypoplastic right ventricle (see Fontan operation, p. 1607). Concomitant right atrial maze procedure at the time of surgery should be considered in patients with chronic atrial flutter/fibrillation.[84] If an accessory pathway is present, it should be mapped and obliterated either at the time of surgical repair or preoperatively in the catheter laboratory (see Chaps. 23 and 25). An atrial communication, if present, should be closed.

INTERVENTIONAL OUTCOMES. With satisfactory valve repair, with or without plication of the atrialized right ventricle or bidirectional cavopulmonary connection, the medium-term prognosis is excellent.[81, 82] Late arrhythmias can occur. With valve replacement, results are less satisfactory. Valve re-replacement may be necessary because of a failing bioprosthesis or thrombosed mechanical valve. Long-term anticoagulation with mechanical valves is mandatory. Complete heart block after tricuspid valve replacement can occur.

FOLLOW-UP. All patients with Ebstein anomaly should have regular follow-up, the frequency dictated by the severity of their disease. Particular attention should be paid to patients with cyanosis, cardiomegaly, worsening right ventricular function, and important atrial arrhythmias. Patients with tricuspid regurgitation after tricuspid valve repair need close follow-up, as do patients with recurrent atrial arrhythmias, degenerating bioprostheses, or dysfunctional mechanical valves.

lets) and the systolic performance of the functional right ventricle can be determined. The degree of tricuspid regurgitation (and more rarely stenosis) can be assessed. Associated defects such as ASDs as well as the presence and direction of shunting can also be identified.

Angiography. Heart catheterization is required mainly when concomitant coronary artery disease is suspected. When performed, selective right ventricular angiography shows the extent of tricuspid valve displacement, the size of the functional right ventricle, and configuration of its outflow tract.

INDICATIONS FOR INTERVENTION. Indications for intervention include deteriorating functional capacity (NYHA ≥ Class III), progressive cyanosis, right-sided heart failure, and the occurrence of paradoxical emboli. Recurrent supraventricular arrhythmias not controlled by medical or ablation therapy (see Chap. 23) and asymptomatic cardiomegaly (cardiothoracic ratio > 65 percent) are relative indications.[78, 81]

INTERVENTIONAL OPTIONS. Tricuspid valve repair when feasible is preferable to tricuspid valve replacement. The feasibility of tricuspid valve repair depends primarily on the experience and skill of the surgeon, as well as on the adequacy of the anterior leaflet of the tricuspid valve to form a monocusp valve.[81, 82] Tricuspid valve repair is possible when the edges of the anterior leaflet of the tricuspid valve are not severely tethered down to the myocardium and when the functional right ventricle is of adequate size (>35 percent of the total right ventricle). If the tricuspid valve cannot be repaired, valve replacement with either a bioprosthetic or mechanical tricuspid valve is necessary. It is controversial whether the atrialized portion of the right ventricle should be plicated at the time of surgery to reduce the risk of atrial arrhythmias. For "high-risk" patients (those with severe tricuspid regurgitation, an inadequate

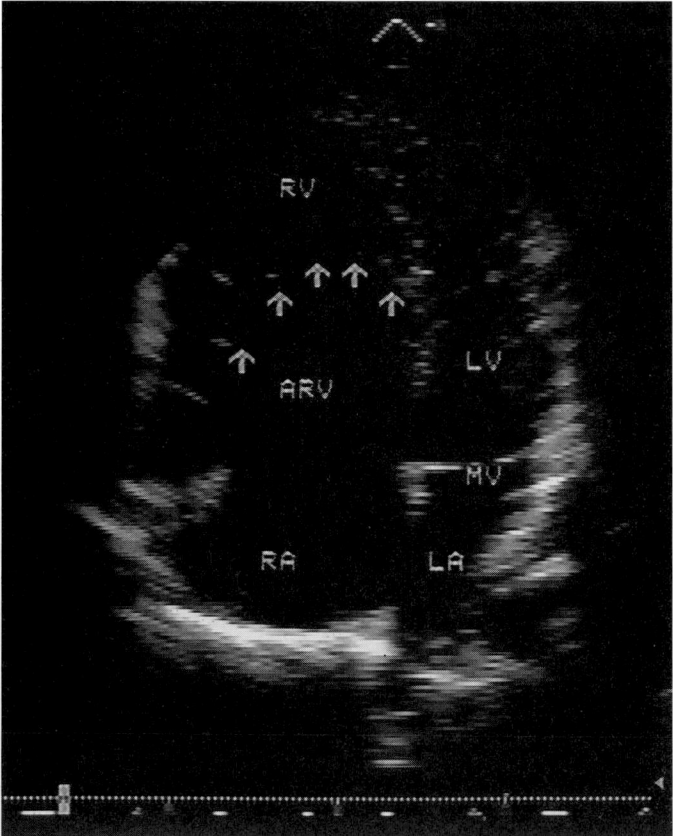

FIGURE 44–10. Four-chamber view, transthoracic echocardiogram of Ebstein anomaly. Multiple arrows point at the apically displaced tricuspid valve. RA = right atrium; ARV = atrialized right ventricle; RV = functional right ventricle; LA = left atrium; MV = mitral valve; LV = left ventricle.

Tetralogy of Fallot

(see also Chap. 43)

Tetralogy of Fallot is the most common form of cyanotic congenital heart disease after 1 year of age, with an incidence approaching 10 percent of all forms of congenital heart disease.

ANATOMY. The defect is due to anterocephalad deviation of the outlet septum resulting in four features: (1) nonrestrictive VSD; (2) overriding aorta (but < 50 percent); (3) RVOTO, which may be infundibular, valvar, or (usually) a combination of both, with or without supravalvar or branch pulmonary artery stenosis; and (4) consequent right ventricular hypertrophy. The so-called pentalogy of Fallot also has an ASD. Accompanying features can include additional VSDs, anomalous coronary arteries, right-sided aortic arch, PDA, aortic root dilation, aortic regurgitation, and aortopulmonary collaterals (Figs. 44–11 and 43–47).

NATURAL HISTORY OF THE UNOPERATED PATIENT. To reach adulthood, most patients will have had surgery, either palliative or, more commonly, reparative. A few patients however will present as adults with uncorrected tetralogy of Fallot. Natural survival into the fourth decade is rare (approximately 3 percent).

SURGICAL PROCEDURES. These are usually done in childhood.

Palliation. Palliative procedures in tetralogy of Fallot serve to increase pulmonary blood flow. The types of palliative procedures include the Blalock-Taussig shunt (classic or modified—subclavian artery to pulmonary artery end-to-side shunt or interposition graft), Waterston shunt (ascending aorta to right pulmonary artery shunt), Potts shunt (descending aorta to left pulmonary artery shunt), or a central interposition tube graft (see shunt procedure, Chap. 43). The Brock procedure (infundibular resection), pulmonary valvotomy, or right ventricle to pulmonary artery conduit without VSD closure or with fenestrated closure were occasionally performed.

Repair. Reparative surgery involves closing the VSD with a Dacron patch and relieving the RVOTO. The latter

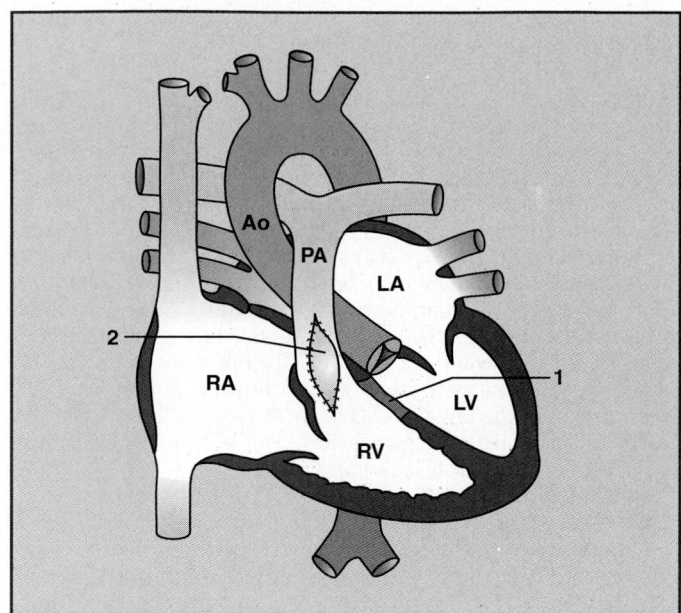

FIGURE 44–12. Diagrammatic representation of the surgical repair of tetralogy of Fallot. Patch closure of ventricular septal defect (1); right ventricular outflow/main pulmonary artery outflow patch (transannular patch) (2). RA = right atrium; RV = right ventricle; LA = left atrium; LV = left ventricle; Ao = aorta; PA = pulmonary artery. (From Mullins CE, Mayer DC: Congenital Heart Disease: A Diagrammatic Atlas. New York, Wiley-Liss, 1988.)

may involve resection of infundibular muscle and insertion of a right ventricular outflow tract or transannular patch—a patch across the pulmonary valve annulus that disrupts the integrity of the pulmonary valve and causes important pulmonary regurgitation (Fig. 44–12). Occasionally, the pulmonic valve is replaced with a pericardial monocusp valve. When an anomalous coronary artery crosses the right ventricular outflow tract and precludes transection of the latter, an extracardiac conduit is placed between the right ventricle and pulmonary artery, bypassing the RVOTO. A patent foramen ovale or secundum ASD is closed. Additional treatable lesions such as muscular VSDs, PDA, and aortopulmonary collaterals should also be addressed at the time of surgery or in the catheterization laboratory.

CLINICAL MANIFESTATIONS

Unoperated. The pathophysiology varies depending on the degree of RVOTO. With mild obstruction, the presentation is of increased pulmonary blood flow and minimal cyanosis, the so-called pink, or acyanotic, tetralogy of Fallot. This is a rare presentation in adults. Progressive cyanosis from worsening RVOTO along with cerebrovascular accidents, endocarditis, supraventricular arrhythmias, and aortic regurgitation are the most common presenting features. On physical examination, the length and loudness of the systolic murmur are inversely related to the severity of the RVOTO. As the RVOTO increases toward occlusion, the right ventricular blood flow is directed through the VSD into the aorta and the pulmonic stenosis murmur becomes shorter and softer.[85] P_2 is faint and delayed in patients with mild cyanosis and inaudible with severe cyanosis. An ejection sound from aortic dilation and a diastolic murmur from consequent aortic regurgitation can be heard. Central cyanosis and clubbing are present to varying degrees.

Palliated. Progressive cyanosis with its complications (see p. 1608) can result from worsening RVOTO, gradual stenosis and occlusion of palliative aorto-pulmonary shunts, or development of pulmonary hypertension (sometimes seen after Waterston or Potts shunts). Left ventricular dilation and failure from long-standing left-to-right shunting can also occur. On physical examination, central cyanosis

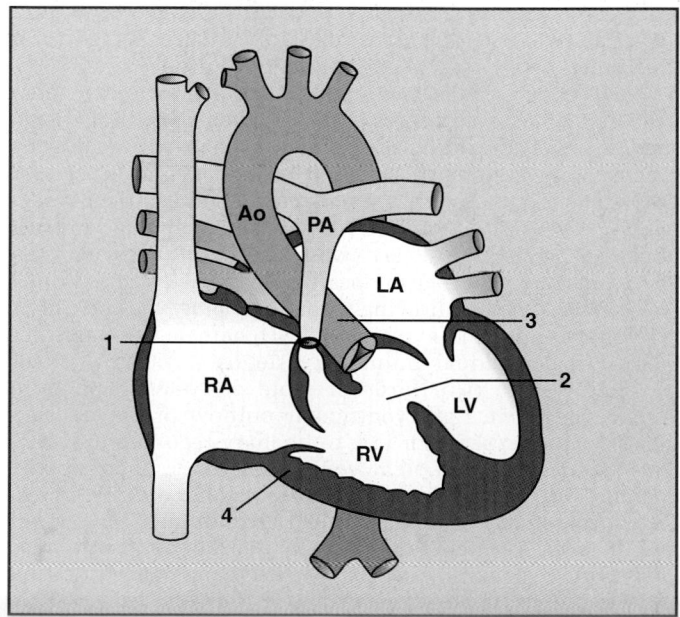

FIGURE 44–11. Diagrammatic representation of tetralogy of Fallot. 1, Pulmonary stenosis; 2, ventricular septal defect; 3, overriding aorta; 4, right ventricle hypertrophy. RA = right atrium; RV = right ventricle; LA = left atrium; LV = left ventricle; Ao = aorta; PA = pulmonary artery. (From Mullins CE, Mayer DC: Congenital Heart Disease: A Diagrammatic Atlas. New York, Wiley-Liss, 1988.)

and clubbing invariably are present. Continuous murmurs should be sought to assess shunt patency.

Repaired. After intracardiac repair, over 85 percent of patients are asymptomatic on follow-up. Palpitations from atrial and ventricular tachycardias, with or without dizziness or syncope, and dyspnea from progressive right ventricular dilation secondary to chronic pulmonary regurgitation or severe residual RVOTO occur in 10 to 15 percent of patients at 20 years after initial repair.[86] An ascending aortic aneurysm and progressive aortic regurgitation from a dilated aortic root can also be present. Physical examination may reveal a parasternal right ventricular lift from right ventricular dilation, a normal S_1, but a soft and delayed P_2 with a low-pitched diastolic murmur from pulmonary regurgitation at the left sternal border. A systolic ejection murmur from RVOTO, a high-pitched diastolic murmur from aortic regurgitation, and a holosystolic murmur from a VSD patch leak can also be heard.

DIAGNOSTIC TESTING
Electrocardiogram

Unoperated. Right ventricular hypertrophy with right-axis deviation is the rule. Right bundle branch block can be present.

Palliated. A prominent R wave in V_5 to V_6 can be present and represents left ventricular hypertrophy.

Repaired. Complete right bundle branch block after repair is the rule. QRS width reflects the degree of right ventricular dilation[87] (Fig. 44–13).

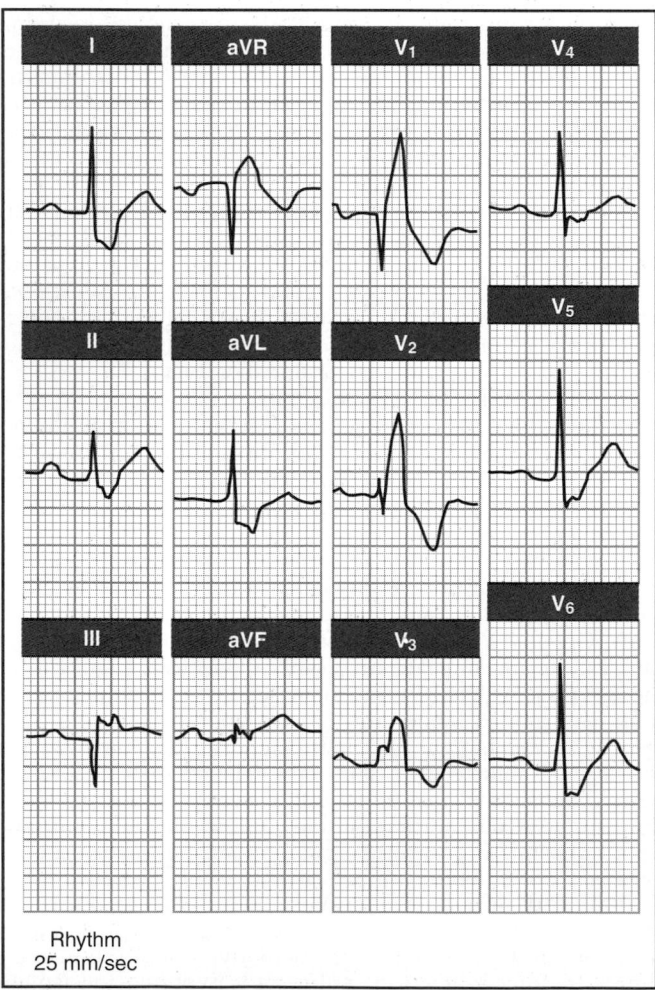

Rhythm
25 mm/sec

FIGURE 44–13. Electrocardiogram of tetralogy of Fallot after surgical repair. Note the wide right bundle branch block (160 msec). First-degree atrioventricular block is also present.

Chest Radiography

Unoperated. The distinctive "coeur en sabot" or "boot-shaped heart" configuration results from a small main pulmonary artery and a hypertrophied right ventricle coupled to a small to normal-sized left ventricle. Pulmonary vascularity is reduced. A right-sided aortic arch in present in 25 percent.

Palliated. Increased pulmonary blood flow with rib notching on the side of the shunt (Blalock-Taussig) or evidence of unilateral pulmonary hypertension (Waterston or Potts shunt) may be seen.

Repaired. Cardiomegaly from right ventricular dilation can be present, along with dilation of the ascending aorta.

Echocardiography

Unoperated. The malaligned, nonrestrictive VSD and overriding aorta (<50 percent override) are readily identified in the left parasternal long-axis or four-chamber views. Additional muscular VSDs should be sought on two-dimensional and color flow Doppler. The presence and degree of RVOTO (infundibular, valvar, and/or pulmonary arterial stenosis) are best assessed using two-dimensional and Doppler modes (see Figs. 7–86 and 43–48).

Palliated. Aortopulmonary shunts can be detected from a suprasternal view, by color flow and Doppler mode, as turbulent flow entering the right or left pulmonary artery.

Repaired. Residual pulmonary stenosis and regurgitation, residual VSD, right and left ventricular sizes and function, aortic root size, and the degree of aortic regurgitation should be assessed (Fig. 44–14).

Catheterization

Unrepaired/Palliated. Cardiac catheterization should be performed before surgical repair in patients in whom the presence of an anomalous coronary artery, significant aortopulmonary collaterals, additional muscular VSDs, peripheral pulmonary artery stenosis, and pulmonary hypertension have not been excluded by other modalities.

Repaired. Complete heart catheterization including coronary angiography (for patients with risk factors for coronary artery disease) should be done if surgical re-intervention is planned or when adequate assessment of the hemodynamics is not obtainable by noninvasive means.

INDICATIONS FOR INTERVENTION

Unoperated. For unoperated adults, surgical repair is still recommended because the results are gratifying and the operative risk is comparable to pediatric series (provided there is no serious coexisting morbidity).[88]

Palliated. Palliation was seldom intended as a permanent treatment strategy, and most of these patients should undergo surgical repair. In particular, palliated patients with increasing cyanosis and erythrocytosis (from gradual shunt stenosis or development of pulmonary hypertension), left ventricular dilation, or aneurysm formation in the shunt should undergo intracardiac repair with takedown of the shunt unless irreversible pulmonary hypertension has developed.

Repaired. The following situations *may* warrant intervention after repair: a residual VSD with a shunt greater than 1.5/1.0; residual pulmonary stenosis with right ventricular pressure two thirds or more of systemic pressure (either the native right ventricular outflow or valved conduit if one is present); or free pulmonary regurgitation associated with important right ventricular enlargement and/or dysfunction, exercise intolerance, or sustained arrhythmias. The development of major cardiac arrhythmias, most commonly atrial flutter/fibrillation or sustained ventricular tachycardia, usually reflects hemodynamic deterioration and should be treated accordingly.[87] Surgery is necessary for significant aortic regurgitation associated with symp-

FIGURE 44–14. See color plate 25.

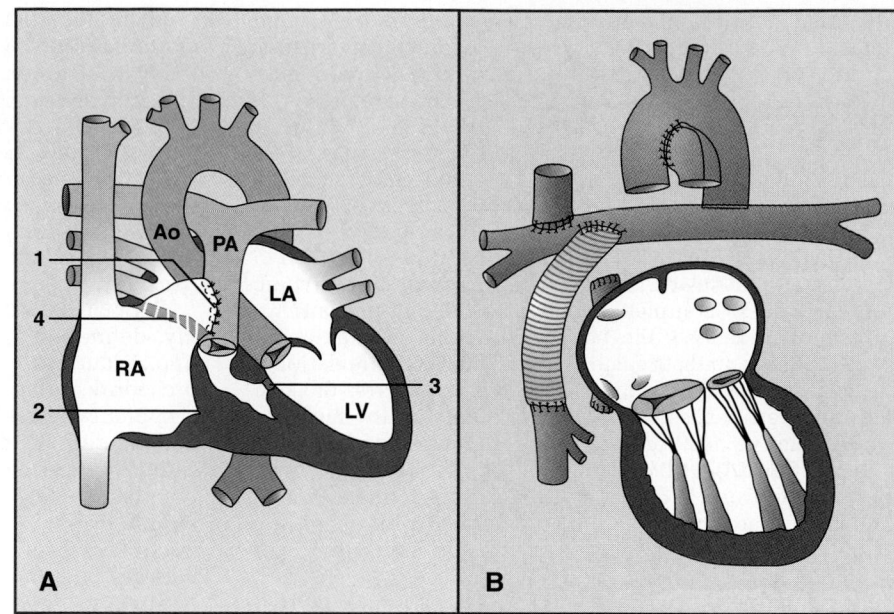

FIGURE 44–15. Modifications of the Fontan operation. *A*, Direct atriopulmonary connection (1) for tricuspid valve atresia (2); ventricular septal defect, oversewn (3); patch closure of atrial septal defect (4). RA = right atrium; LA = left atrium; LV = left ventricle; Ao = aorta; PA = pulmonary artery. (From Mullins CE, Mayer DC: Congenital Heart Disease: A Diagrammatic Atlas. New York, Wiley-Liss, 1988.) *B*, Extracardiac conduit made of a Dacron graft bypassing the right atrium, connecting the inferior vena cava to the inferior aspect of the right pulmonary artery. Superior vena cava is anastomosed to the superior aspect of the right pulmonary artery. (From Marcelletti C: Inferior vena cava–pulmonary artery extracardiac conduit: A new form of right heart bypass. J Thorac Cardiovasc Surg 100:228–232, 1990.)

toms and/or progressive left ventricular dilation and perhaps for aortic root enlargement of 55 mm or more in diameter.[89] Rapid enlargement of a right ventricular outflow tract aneurysm or evidence of infection or false aneurysm needs surgical attention.

INTERVENTIONAL OPTIONS

Surgery. Reoperation is necessary in 10 to 15 percent of patients after reparative surgery over a 20-year follow-up, mainly due to long-term complications of the RVOT.[86] For persistent RVOTO, resection of residual infundibular stenosis or placement of an RV outflow or transannular patch, with or without pulmonary arterioplasty, can be performed. Occasionally, an extracardiac valved conduit may be necessary. Pulmonary valve replacement (either homograft or xenograft) often is used to treat severe pulmonary regurgitation. Concomitant tricuspid valve annuloplasty may be performed for moderate or severe tricuspid regurgitation. Concomitant cryoablation should be performed at the time of surgery for patients with either preexisting atrial or ventricular arrhythmias.[86, 90]

Interventional. Significant branch pulmonary artery stenosis can be managed with balloon dilation and usually stent insertion.

INTERVENTIONAL OUTCOMES.

The overall survival of patients who have had initial operative repair is excellent, provided the VSD has been closed and the RVOTO has been relieved. A 25-year survival of more than 94 percent has been reported.[91, 95, 97] Pulmonary valve replacement for chronic pulmonary regurgitation or RVOTO after initial intracardiac repair can be done safely with a mortality rate of 1 percent.[97] Pulmonic valve replacement, when performed for significant pulmonary regurgitation, leads to an improvement in functional class and may lead to improvement in right ventricular dimension and function.[93, 93a] Death, however, can occur from congestive heart failure or can be sudden, presumably arrhythmic, from either ventricular tachycardia or complete heart block. Ventricular tachycardia can arise at the site of the right ventriculotomy, from VSD patch suture lines, or from the right ventricular outflow tract. Patients at high risk for sudden death include those with right ventricular dilation and a QRS duration of 180 milliseconds or more on their ECG.[87, 94] The reported incidence of sudden death is approximately 5 percent, which accounts for approximately one third of late deaths over 20 years of follow-up.[91, 95]

FOLLOW-UP. All patients should have expert cardiology follow-up every 1 to 2 years.[96, 97]

Post-Fontan Procedure

SURGICAL PROCEDURES. Since its description for the surgical management of tricuspid atresia in 1971, the Fontan procedure has become the definitive palliative surgical treatment when a biventricular repair is not feasible (e.g., for pulmonary atresia with intact ventricular septum or univentricular hearts). The principle is diversion of the systemic venous return directly to the pulmonary arteries without passing through a subpulmonary ventricle. Over the years, many modifications of the original procedure have been described and performed, namely, direct atriopulmonary connection (Fig. 44–15A), total cavopulmonary connection (see Chap. 43, Fig. 43–54), and extracardiac tunnel/conduit (see Fig. 44–15B). Fenestration (5 mm diameter) of the Fontan circuit into the left atrium is sometimes performed at the time of surgery in "high-risk" patients, permitting right-to-left shunting and decompression of the Fontan circuit. A right atrium to right ventricular conduit for tricuspid atresia is sometimes performed when right ventricular size and function are adequate.

FONTAN POSTOPERATIVE HISTORY. Patient selection is of utmost importance and has a major impact on clinical outcome. Long-term survival in "ideal candidates" (see Table 44–4)[98] is 81 percent at 10 years,[99] compared with 60 to 71 percent in "all comers."[100] Death occurs mostly from congestive heart failure and atrial arrhythmias. The Fontan procedure remains a palliative, not curative, procedure.

CLINICAL MANIFESTATIONS. The majority of patients (≥90 percent) present with functional Class I to II at 5 years follow-up after a Fontan procedure.[99, 101] Progressive deterioration of functional status with time is the rule.[99, 100] Supraventricular arrhythmias such as atrial tachycardia, flutter, and fibrillation are common. Physical examination in an otherwise uncomplicated patient will reveal an ele-

▼ **TABLE 44–4. IDEAL CANDIDATES FOR THE FONTAN PROCEDURE**

Preoperative mean pulmonary artery pressure ≤15 mm Hg
Pulmonary resistance ≤4 units/m²
Pulmonary artery–aortic diameter ratio ≥0.75
Systemic ventricular ejection fraction ≥60%
Systemic atrioventricular regurgitation ≤ mild

vated, usually nonpulsatile jugular venous pulse (10 cm above the sternal angle, needed to provide the hydrostatic pressure to drive cardiac output through the pulmonary circulation), a quiet apex, a normal S_1, and a single S_2 (the pulmonary artery having been tied off). A heart murmur should not be present, and its identification suggests the presence of systemic AV valve regurgitation or subaortic obstruction. Generalized edema may be a sign of protein-losing enteropathy (see Protein-Losing Enteropathy).

DIAGNOSTIC TESTING

Electrocardiogram. Sinus rhythm, atrial flutter, junctional rhythm, or complete heart block may be present. The QRS complex reflects the basic underlying cardiac anomaly. In patients with tricuspid atresia, left-axis deviation is the norm. In patients with univentricular hearts, the conduction pattern varies widely and depends on the morphology and relative position of the rudimentary chamber.

Chest Radiography. Mild bulging of the right lower heart border from a dilated right atrium is often seen in patients with atriopulmonary connection. A prominent inferior vena cava is sometimes visualized (Somerville J, personal communication, 1998).

Echocardiography. The presence or absence of right atrial stasis, thrombus, patency of a fenestration, and Fontan circuit obstruction should be sought. SVC/IVC biphasic and pulmonary artery triphasic flow pattern that varies with respiration suggests unobstructed flow in the Fontan circuit, whereas a mean gradient between the Fontan circuit and the pulmonary artery of 2 mm Hg or more may represent significant obstruction. Assessment of the pulmonary venous flow pattern is important in detecting pulmonary vein (PV) obstruction (right PV > left PV) sometimes caused by an enlarged right atrium (often 80 by 60 mm or so in adults with atriopulmonary connections). Concomitant assessment of systemic ventricular function and AV valve regurgitation can be readily accomplished. TEE may be required if there is inadequate visualization of the Fontan anastomosis or to exclude thrombus in the right atrium.[102]

Diagnostic Catheterization. Complete heart catheterization is advised if surgical re-intervention is planned or if adequate assessment of the hemodynamics is not obtained by noninvasive means.

MRI. MRI may be needed as a complement to or replacement for TEE and sometimes even heart catheterization if the Fontan circuit cannot be assessed otherwise.

COMPLICATIONS AND SEQUELAE

Arrhythmia. Atrial flutter/fibrillation is common (15–20 percent at 5 years follow-up)[103, 104] and increases with duration of follow-up.[103, 105] Atrial flutter/fibrillation carries significant morbidity, can be associated with profound hemodynamic deterioration, and needs prompt medical attention (see later). The combination of atrial incisions and multiple suture lines at the time of Fontan surgery combined with increased right atrial pressure and size probably explains the high incidence of atrial arrhythmias in such patients. Patients at greater risk for atrial tachyarrhythmias are those who were operated on at an older age, with poor ventricular function, systemic AV valve regurgitation, or increased pulmonary artery pressure.[103, 105] It has been suggested that the exclusion of the right atrium from elevated systemic venous pressure (as in total cavopulmonary connection [TCPC] or extracardiac conduit) leads to a decrease in the incidence of atrial arrhythmias.[106, 107] This apparent benefit may, however, be due exclusively to the shorter length of follow-up in this group of patients.[103] Sinus node dysfunction and complete heart block can occur and require pacemaker insertion (see later).

Thrombosis and Stroke. The reported incidence of thromboembolic complications in the Fontan circuit varies from 6 to 25 percent, depending on the diagnostic method used and the length of follow-up.[108] Thrombus formation may relate to the presence of supraventricular arrhythmias, right atrial dilation, right atrial "smoke," and the presence of artificial material used to construct the Fontan circuit[112] (Fig. 44–16). Accordingly, a similar incidence of thrombus formation had been reported for all types of Fontan circuits.[107] Systemic arterial embolism in patients with and without a fenestrated Fontan has also been reported. Protein C deficiency has been reported in these patients and may explain in part their propensity to thromboembolism.[108, 109]

Protein-Losing Enteropathy. Protein-losing enteropathy, defined as severe loss of serum protein into the intestine, occurs in 4 to 13 percent of patients after a Fontan procedure.[110] Patients present with generalized edema, ascites, pleural effusion, or chronic diarrhea.[110] Protein-losing enteropathy is thought to result principally from chronically elevated systemic venous pressure causing intestinal lymphangiectasia with consequent loss of albumin, protein, lymphocytes, and immunoglobulin into the gastrointestinal tract. The diagnosis is confirmed by finding low serum albumin and protein, low plasma alpha$_1$-antitrypsin level and lymphocyte counts, and, most important, a high alpha$_1$-antitrypsin stool clearance. It carries a dismal prognosis, with a 5-year survival of 46 to 59 percent.[110]

Right Pulmonary Vein Compression/Obstruction. Right pulmonary vein obstruction/compression can occur from the enlarged right atrium or atrial baffle bulging into the left atrium and can lead to increased pulmonary artery pressure with further dilation of the right atrium.

Fontan Obstruction. Stenosis/partial obstruction of the Fontan connection leads to exercise intolerance, atrial tachyarrhythmias, and right-sided heart failure. Sudden total obstruction can present as sudden death.

Ventricular Dysfunction and Valvar Regurgitation. Progressive deterioration of systemic ventricular function, with or without progressive AV valve regurgitation, is common. Patients with morphological systemic right ventricles tend to fare less well than those with morphological left ventricles.

Hepatic Dysfunction. Mildly raised hepatic transaminase levels from hepatic congestion are frequent but seldom clinically important.

Cyanosis. Worsening cyanosis may relate to worsening of ventricular function, the development of venous collat-

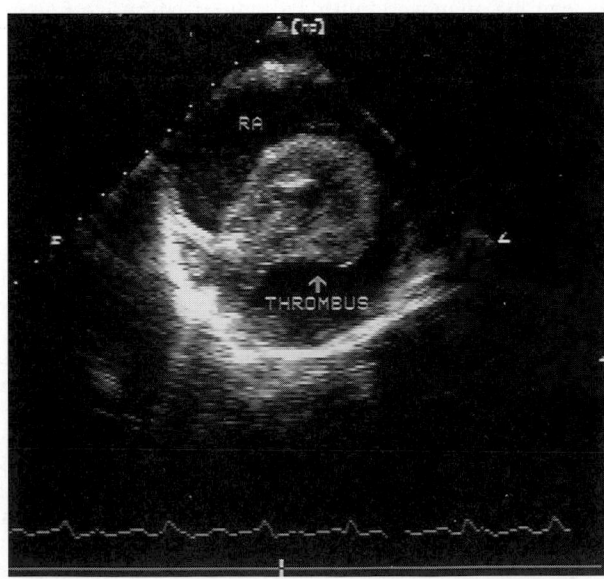

FIGURE 44–16. Transesophageal echocardiogram of a large thrombus located in the right atrium of a patient with a right atrium to pulmonary artery Fontan connection. RA = right atrium.

eral channels draining to the left atrium, or the development of pulmonary arteriovenous malformations (especially if a classic Glenn procedure (see Chap. 43) remains as part of the Fontan operation).

TREATMENT OPTIONS

Arrhythmias. Atrial tachyarrhythmias are very difficult to manage, and should quickly raise the thought of long-term warfarin therapy. When atrial flutter/fibrillation are present, an underlying hemodynamic cause should *always* be sought, and, in particular, evidence for obstruction of the Fontan circuit needs to be sought. Prompt attempts should be made to restore sinus rhythm. Antiarrhythmic medications, alone or combined with an antitachycardia pacing device, and radiofrequency catheter ablation techniques have had limited success.[111] Surgical conversion from an atriopulmonary Fontan to a total cavopulmonary connection with concomitant atrial cryoablation therapy at the time of surgery has been reported with good short-term success.[112, 112a] Pacemaker insertion for sinus node dysfunction and/or complete heart block may be necessary. Endovenous ventricular pacing through the coronary sinus is possible, but epicardial AV sequential pacing should be employed whenever possible.[113]

Anticoagulant Therapy. The use of prophylactic long-term anticoagulation is contentious.[114] It is recommended that patients with a history of documented arrhythmias, fenestration in the Fontan connection, or spontaneous contrast ("smoke") in the right atrium on echocardiography be anticoagulated. For established thrombus, thrombolytic therapy versus surgical removal of the clot and conversion of the Fontan circuit have been described.

Protein-Losing Enteropathy. Treatment modalities include a low-fat, high-protein, medium-chain triglyceride diet to reduce intestinal lymphatic production; albumin infusions to increase intravascular osmotic pressure; and/or the introduction of diuretics, afterload reducing agents, and positive inotropic agents to lower central venous pressure. Catheter-based interventions such as balloon dilation of pathway obstruction or creation of an atrial fenestration[115] as well as surgical interventions from conversion or takedown of the Fontan circuit to cardiac transplantation[116] have also been advocated. Newer treatment modalities include subcutaneous heparin,[117] octreotide treatment,[118] and prednisone therapy.[119]

Right Pulmonary Vein Compression/Obstruction. When hemodynamically significant, Fontan conversion to a total cavopulmonary connection or extracardiac conduit may be recommended.[120, 121]

Fontan Obstruction. Surgical revision for obstructed right atrium–pulmonary artery, SCV/IVC-pulmonary artery, or right atrium–right ventricle connection is recommended. Alternatively, balloon angioplasty with or without stenting may be used when appropriate and feasible.

Ventricular Failure and Valvar Regurgitation. ACE inhibitors are of unproven benefit and do not appear to enhance exercise capacity.[122] Patients with systemic AV valve regurgitation may require AV valve repair or replacement. Cardiac transplantation should also be considered.

Cyanosis. In the setting of a fenestrated Fontan, surgical or preferably transcatheter closure of the fenestration can be attempted. Pulmonary arteriovenous fistulas from a classic Glenn may be improved by surgical conversion to a bidirectional Glenn connection.[123]

FOLLOW-UP. Close and expert follow-up is recommended with particular attention to ventricular function and systemic AV valve regurgitation. The development of atrial tachyarrhythmia should instigate a search for possible obstruction at the Fontan anastomosis, right pulmonary vein obstruction, or thrombus within the right atrium.

ANATOMY. In patients with complete TGA, the connections between the atria and ventricles are concordant and the connections between ventricles and great arteries are discordant. Consequently, the pulmonary and systemic circulations are connected in parallel rather than the normal in-series connection. In one circuit, systemic venous blood passes to the right atrium, the right ventricle, and then to the aorta. In the other, pulmonary venous blood passes through the left atrium and ventricle to the pulmonary artery. The aorta arises from the morphological right ventricle and usually lies anterior and to the right of the pulmonary artery, whereas the pulmonary artery arises from the morphological left ventricle (Fig. 44–17 and see Fig. 43–57). This situation is incompatible with life unless mixing of the two circuits occurs.

Approximately two thirds of patients have no major associated abnormalities ("simple" transposition) and one third have associated abnormalities ("complex" transposition). The most common associated abnormalities are VSD and pulmonary/subpulmonary stenosis.

NATURAL HISTORY OF THE UNOPERATED PATIENT. Survival before surgical repair is dependent on mixing of the circulations at one level or another, whether natural (VSD, ASD, PDA) or by intervention (Blalock-Hanlon atrial septectomy or Rashkind balloon atrial septostomy). Unoperated (simple) transposition is a lethal condition, with 90 percent mortality by 1 year. Nearly all patients seen as adults will have had surgical intervention (atrial switch, arterial switch, or Rastelli operation—see later), with the exception perhaps of patients with a large VSD who may survive into adulthood without intervention and present with pulmonary vascular disease.

SURGICAL PROCEDURES

Atrial Switch. The most common surgical procedure in patients who are currently adults is the atrial switch operation. Patients will have had either a Mustard or a Senning procedure. Blood is redirected at the atrial level using a

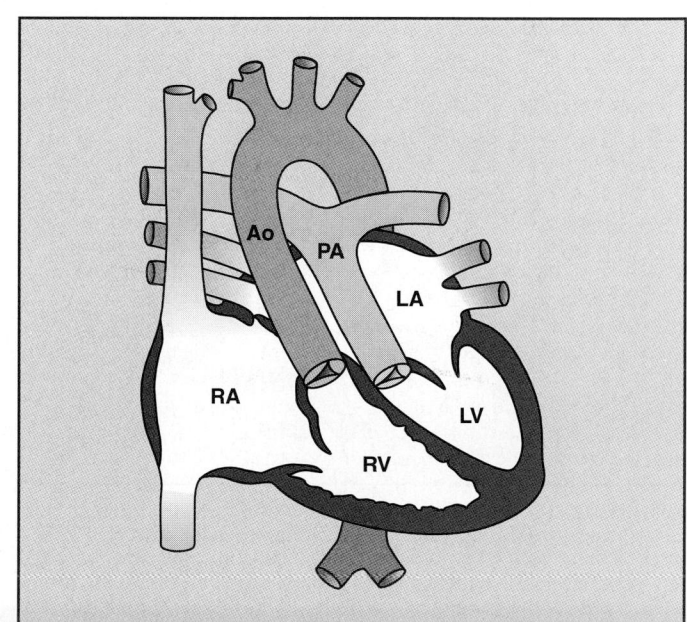

FIGURE 44–17. Diagrammatic representation of complete transposition of the great arteries. RA = right atrium; RV = right ventricle; LA = left atrium; LV = left ventricle; Ao = aorta; PA = pulmonary artery. (From Mullins CE, Mayer DC: Congenital Heart Disease: A Diagrammatic Atlas. New York, Wiley-Liss, 1988.)

baffle made of Dacron or pericardium (Mustard operation) or atrial flaps (Senning operation), achieving physiological correction. Systemic venous return is diverted through the mitral valve into the subpulmonary morphological left ventricle, and the pulmonary venous return is rerouted through the tricuspid valve into the subaortic morphological right ventricle. By virtue of this repair, the morphological right ventricle is left to support the systemic circulation (Fig. 44–18).

Arterial Switch. The atrial switch operation has gradually been supplanted by the arterial switch operation (Jatene) since the late 1970s, but few of these patients have yet become adults. Blood is redirected at the great artery level by switching the aorta and pulmonary arteries (often using the Lecompte maneuver) such that the morphological left ventricle becomes the subaortic ventricle and supports the systemic circulation and the morphological right ventricle becomes the subpulmonary ventricle (see Chap. 43, Fig. 43–61). The coronary arteries, with a sleeve of surrounding tissue, are translocated to the proximal neoaorta (formerly the proximal pulmonary artery), with the loss of tissue from the former coronary ostia of the neopulmonary artery (formerly the aorta) made good with pericardial patches.

Rastelli Procedure. Patients (<10 percent of all TGA patients) who have VSD and pulmonary/subpulmonary stenosis may have been corrected by the Rastelli operation. This procedure consists of redirecting the blood at the ventricular level with the left ventricle tunneled to the aorta through the VSD and a valved conduit placed from the right ventricle to the pulmonary artery. By virtue of this procedure, the left ventricle supports the systemic circulation.

Palliative Atrial Switch. Uncommonly, in patients with a large VSD and established pulmonary vascular disease, a palliative atrial switch operation will be done to improve oxygenation. The VSD is left open or enlarged at the time of atrial baffle surgery. These patients resemble patients

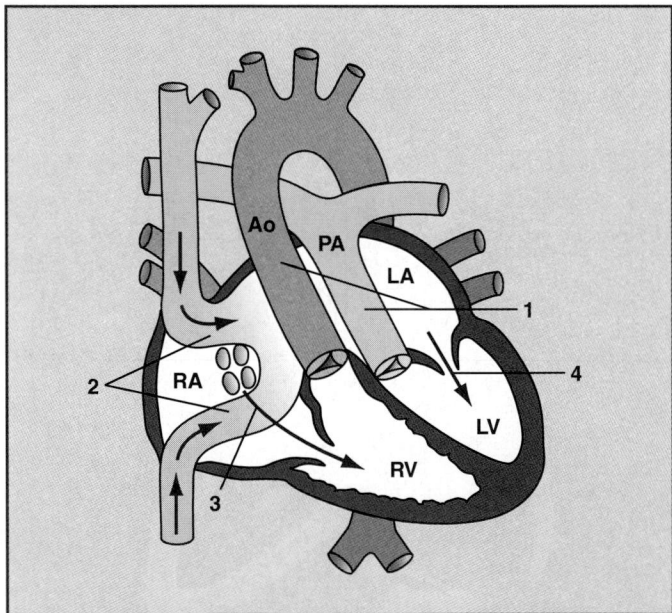

FIGURE 44–18. Diagrammatic representation of atrial switch surgery (Mustard/Senning procedure). Superior vena cava (SVC) and inferior vena cava (IVC) blood is redirected into the morphological left ventricle (LV), which pumps blood into the pulmonary artery (PA), whereas the pulmonary venous blood flow is rerouted to the morphological right ventricle (RV), which empties into the aorta (Ao). RA = right atrium; LA = left atrium; 1 = transposition of the great arteries; 2 = atrial baffles; 3 = pulmonary vein blood flow through tricuspid valve to RV; 4 = IVC and SVC blood flow through mitral valve to LV. (From Mullins CE, Mayer DC: Congenital Heart Disease: A Diagrammatic Atlas. New York, Wiley-Liss, 1988.)

with Eisenmenger VSDs and should be managed as such (see p. 1614).

POSTOPERATIVE CLINICAL PICTURE
Atrial Switch. After atrial baffle surgery, most patients who reach adulthood are in NYHA Classes I and II.[124, 125] Over 25 years of follow-up, some will present with symptoms of congestive heart failure (2–15 percent) despite objective evidence of moderate or severe systemic right ventricular dysfunction in up to 40 percent of patients.[129–131] More than mild systemic tricuspid regurgitation is present in 10 to 40 percent,[125] exacerbating right ventricular dysfunction. Palpitations or near-syncope/syncope from rhythm disturbances is common. Atrial flutter occurs in 20 percent of patients by age 20,[9, 124–126] and progressive sinus node dysfunction is seen in half of the patients by that time.[9, 125, 126] These rhythm disturbances are thought to be a consequence of direct and indirect atrial and sinus node damage at the time of atrial baffle surgery.

Shortened life expectancy is the rule with 70 to 80 percent survival at 20 to 30 years follow-up.[8, 9, 124] Patients with "complex" TGA in general fare much worse than "simple" TGA.[89, 91] Sudden cardiac death is the clinical presentation in about 5 percent of these patients[8, 9, 127] and may relate to systemic right ventricular dysfunction,[8, 125] the presence of atrial flutter,[8, 128] and pulmonary hypertension.[125] Significant pulmonary vascular disease can develop over time and relates to older age at the time of atrial switch operation, particularly in patients with a substantial VSD, as well as in those with long-standing left-to-right shunts through a baffle leak. Rarely, cyanosis can be the presenting symptom due to atrial baffle leak with right-to-left shunting. Superior vena cava or inferior vena cava baffle obstruction often goes undetected because collateral drainage through the azygos vein prevents systemic venous congestion. Pulmonary baffle obstruction causes elevated pulmonary artery pressure, and patients can present with dyspnea and pulmonary venous congestive features. Physical examination of a patient whose condition is otherwise uncomplicated reveals a right ventricular parasternal lift, a normal S_1, a single S_2 (P_2 is not heard because its posterior location), a holosystolic murmur from tricuspid regurgitation if present (best heard at the left lower sternal border, but not increasing with inspiration), and a right-sided S_3 when severe systemic ventricular dysfunction is present.

Arterial Switch. Data on clinical presentation in adults who have undergone the arterial switch procedure are lacking, because most patients have not yet reached adulthood. Clinical arrhythmia promises to be less of a problem in this group of patients.[129] Concerns about the development of supra-neopulmonary artery stenosis, ostial coronary artery disease, and progressive neoaortic valve regurgitation remain to be addressed over the long term.[129a] Cardiac examination in uncomplicated patients is normal.

Rastelli Procedure. Progressive right ventricular to pulmonary artery conduit obstruction can cause exercise intolerance or right ventricular angina. Left ventricular tunnel obstruction can present as dyspnea or syncope. Physical examination in uncomplicated patients reveals, in contrast to atrial switches, no right ventricular lift, an ejection systolic murmur from the conduit, and two components to the S_2.

DIAGNOSTIC TESTING
Electrocardiogram. Atrial flutter, sinus bradycardia, or junctional rhythm, in the absence of a right atrial overload pattern, with evidence of right ventricular hypertrophy and right axis deviation is characteristically present in patients after the atrial switch procedure (Fig. 44–19). The ECG is typically normal in patients after the arterial switch procedure. The ECG typically shows right bundle branch block after a Rastelli procedure.

Chest Radiography. On the posteroanterior film, a narrow vascular pedicle with an oblong cardiac silhouette ("egg on its side") is typically seen in patients after the

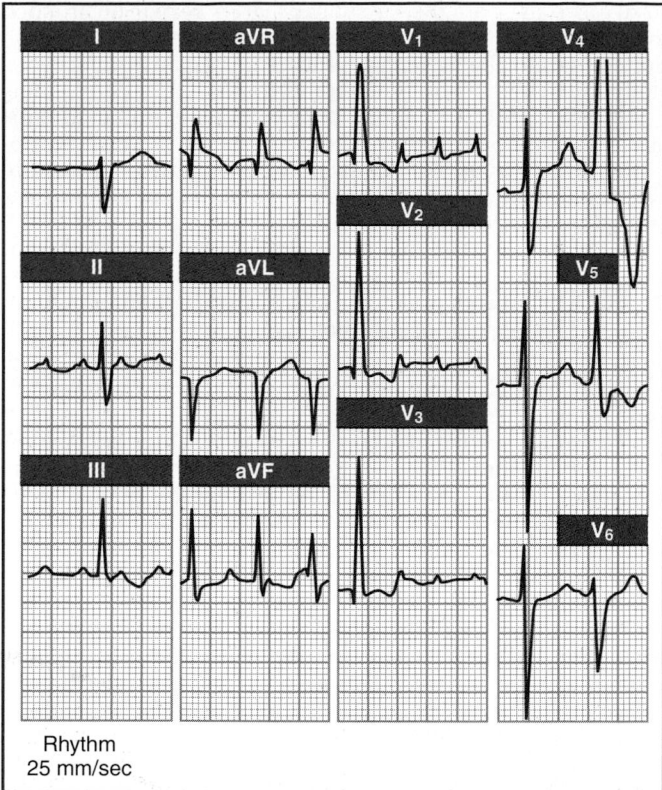

FIGURE 44-19. Electrocardiogram of a patient with complete transposition of the great arteries after an atrial switch procedure. Note the atrial flutter at 200 beats/min, the right ventricular hypertrophy, and the right-axis deviation. There is an incidental ventricular premature beat.

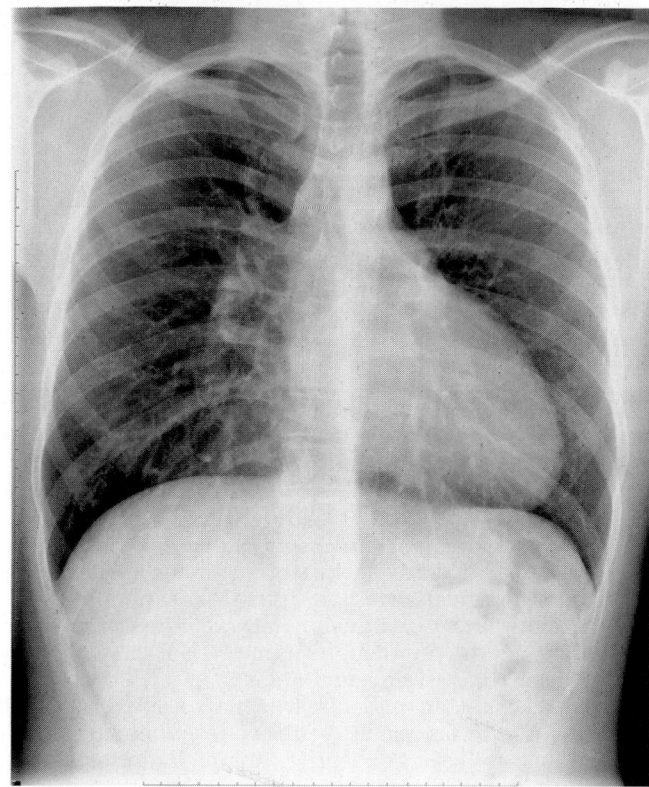

FIGURE 44-20. Chest radiograph of an adult with complete transposition of the great arteries after a Mustard procedure. Note the narrow mediastinum with the "egg-on-its-side" configuration of the cardiac silhouette.

atrial switch procedure (Fig. 44-20). On the lateral view, the anterior aorta is seen to fill the retrosternal air space. For the arterial switch, normal mediastinal borders are present despite the Lecompte maneuver. After the Rastelli procedure, the chest radiograph is normal unless the conduit becomes calcified or a nonhomograft prosthesis is employed.

Echocardiography. After the atrial switch procedure, parallel great arteries are the hallmark of TGA. They are best visualized from a long parasternal view (running side-by-side) or from a short parasternal view (seen en face, with the aorta anterior and rightward) (Fig. 44-21). Qualitative assessment of systemic right ventricular function, the degree of tricuspid regurgitation, and the presence or absence of subpulmonic left ventricular obstruction (dynamic or fixed) is possible. Assessment of baffle leak or obstruction is best done using color and Doppler flow imaging. Normal baffle flow should be phasic in nature and varies with respiration, with a peak velocity less than 1 m/sec.[130] After arterial switch, neoaortic valve regurgitation, supra-neopulmonary valve stenosis, and segmental wall motion abnormality from ischemia due to coronary ostial stenosis should be sought. In patients who have undergone the Rastelli operation, left ventricular to aorta tunnel obstruction as well as right ventricular to pulmonary artery conduit degeneration (stenosis/regurgitation) must be sought.

Diagnostic Cardiac Catheterization. Diagnostic cardiac catheterization may be required for assessing the presence or severity of systemic/pulmonary baffle obstruction, baffle leak, and pulmonary hypertension; coronary ostial stenosis; or tunnel or conduit obstruction when not diagnosed by noninvasive means.

INDICATIONS FOR RE-INTERVENTION. After the atrial switch procedure, severe symptomatic right ventricular dysfunction *may* warrant surgical treatment in the form of

"two-stage arterial switch" procedure (see Two-Stage Arterial Switch)[131-133] or cardiac transplantation. Tricuspid valve replacement can be performed for severe systemic (tricuspid) AV valve regurgitation providing right ventricular function is adequate.[128] Baffle leak resulting in a significant left-to-right shunt (>1.5/1.0), any right-to-left shunt, or symptoms requires surgical or transcatheter closure. SVC or IVC pathway obstruction may require intervention. SVC ste-

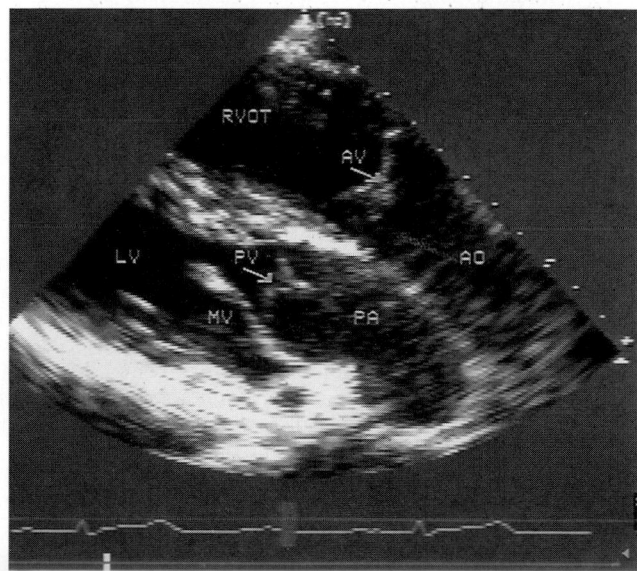

FIGURE 44-21. Left parasternal transthoracic echocardiogram of a patient with complete transposition of the great arteries shows the typical arrangement of the great arteries in parallel. AO = aorta; AV = aortic valve; RVOT = right ventricular outflow tract; PA = pulmonary artery; PV = pulmonary valve; LV = left ventricle; MV = mitral valve.

nosis is usually benign, whereas IVC stenosis may be life threatening. Balloon dilation of SVC or IVC stenosis is an option, but success is limited in adults. Pathway obstruction after the Senning operation is usually more amenable to balloon dilation and stenting. Pulmonary venous obstruction, although usually seen early and reoperated on in childhood, may present in adulthood. Consideration for the "two-stage arterial switch" procedure in these patients is warranted (see Two-Stage Arterial Switch).[134–135] Symptomatic bradycardia warrants permanent pacemaker implantation, whereas tachyarrhythmias may require catheter ablation, antitachycardia pacemaker device, or medical therapy. After an atrial switch, transvenous pacing leads must traverse the upper limb of the baffle to enter the morphological left ventricle. Active fixation is required because coarse trabeculation is absent in the morphological left ventricle. Transvenous pacing should be avoided in patients with residual intracardiac communications because paradoxical emboli can occur.

After an arterial switch procedure, significant RVOTO at any level (peak gradient > 50 mm Hg or RV/LV pressure ratio >0.6) may require surgical or catheter augmentation of the right ventricular outflow tract. Myocardial ischemia from coronary artery obstruction may require coronary artery bypass grafting, preferably with arterial conduits. Significant neoaortic valve regurgitation[136] may warrant aortic valve replacement. In patients who have had the Rastelli operation, significant right ventricle-to-pulmonary artery conduit stenosis (peak gradient > 50 mm Hg) or significant regurgitation necessitates conduit replacement. Subaortic obstruction across the left ventricle-to-aorta tunnel necessitates left ventricle-to-aorta baffle reconstruction. A significant residual VSD (shunt > 1.5/1.0) may require surgical closure.[137] Patients with clinical deterioration and a palliative atrial switch should be considered for lung or heart-lung transplantation.

INTERVENTIONAL OPTIONS

Medical Therapy. The role of afterload reduction with ACE inhibitors to preserve systemic right ventricular function is as yet unknown. In light of the effects of these drugs on dysfunctional systemic left ventricles, it seems logical to assume that similar beneficial effects on systemic right ventricles may occur.

Two-Stage Arterial Switch. Patients with symptomatic, severe systemic (right) ventricular dysfunction with or without severe systemic (tricuspid) AV valve regurgitation, following an atrial switch procedure, may require consideration of a conversion procedure to an arterial switch ("two-stage arterial switch") or heart transplantation. The "two-stage arterial switch" or "switch-conversion" procedure consists of banding the pulmonary artery in the first stage, to induce morphological pulmonary left ventricular hypertrophy and "train" the left ventricle to support systemic pressure. Once left ventricular systolic pressure is more than 75 percent of systemic pressure and the left ventricular mass is considered adequate, in the second stage, the atrial baffles and the pulmonary band are taken down, the atrial septum is reconstructed, and the great arteries are switched, leaving the morphological left ventricle as the systemic ventricle. This procedure, however, is still experimental in adults, with little data available to assess its short- and long-term efficacy.[133]

Cardiac Transplantation. Heart transplantation should be considered as an alternative, given its relatively good 5- to 10-year survival.[7]

FOLLOW-UP. Regular follow-up by physicians with special expertise in adult congenital heart disease is recommended.

Atrial Switch. Serial follow-up of systemic right ventricular function is warranted. Echocardiography, radionuclide angiography, and MRI can be used.[138, 139] ACE inhibitors are often recommended empirically for moderate to severe right ventricular dysfunction and may be helpful to all

atrial switch patients. Asymptomatic baffle obstruction should be sought with echocardiography or MRI. Regular Holter monitoring is recommended to diagnose unacceptable bradyarrhythmias or tachyarrhythmias.

Arterial Switch. Regular follow-up with echocardiography is recommended.

Rastelli Procedure. Regular follow-up with echocardiography is warranted given the inevitability of conduit degeneration over time.

Congenitally Corrected Transposition of the Great Arteries (see also Chap. 43)

ANATOMY. Congenitally corrected TGA is a rare condition, accounting for less than 1 percent of all congenital heart disease. In congenitally corrected TGA, the connections of both the atria to ventricles and of the ventricles to the great arteries are discordant. Systemic venous blood passes from the right atrium through a mitral valve to the left ventricle and then to the right-sided posteriorly located pulmonary artery. Pulmonary venous blood passes from the left atrium through a tricuspid valve to the right ventricle and then to an anterior, left-sided aorta (Fig. 44–22). The circulation is thus "physiologically" corrected but the morphological right ventricle supports the systemic circulation. Associated anomalies occur in up to 95 percent of patients and consist of VSD (75 percent), pulmonary or subpulmonary stenosis (75 percent), and left-sided (tricuspid and often "Ebstein-like") valve anomalies (>75 percent).[140]

Because of the inherently abnormal conduction system (anterior origin of the AV node and anterior course of the His bundle [anterior to the pulmonary artery and down the morphological left ventricular side of the septum]), 5 percent of patients with congenitally corrected TGA are born with congenital complete heart block. Congenitally corrected transposition may exist in the setting of univentricular heart.

NATURAL HISTORY OF THE UNOPERATED PATIENT. Patients with no associated abnormalities ("isolated" congenitally corrected TGA) can survive until the seventh or eighth

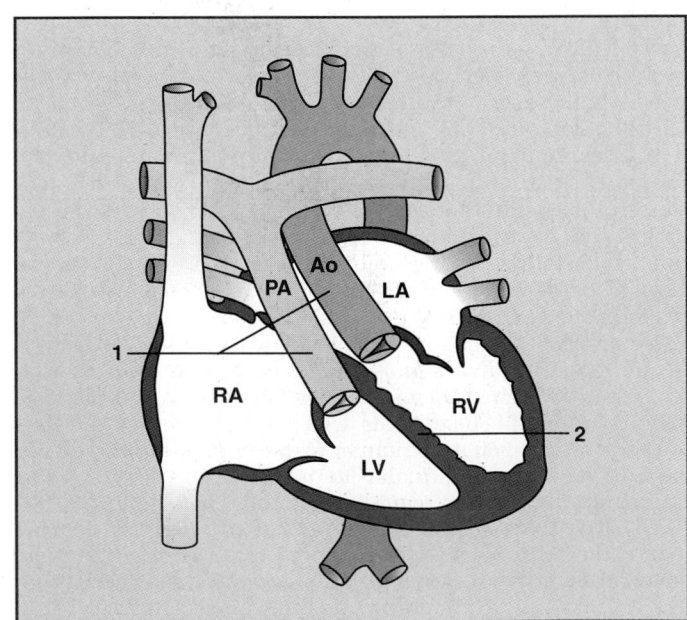

FIGURE 44–22. Diagrammatic representation of congenitally corrected transposition of the great arteries. AV and VA discordance (1). Note intact ventricular septum (2). RA = right atrium; RV = right ventricle; LA = left atrium; LV = left ventricle; Ao = aorta; PA = pulmonary artery. (From Mullins CE, Mayer DC: Congenital Heart Disease: A Diagrammatic Atlas. New York, Wiley-Liss, 1988.)

decade and can go unrecognized until cardiac problems arise.[141] Progressive systemic (tricuspid) AV valve regurgitation and systemic (right) ventricular dysfunction tend to occur from the fourth decade onward, whereas atrial tachyarrhythmias are more common from the fifth decade onward.[142] In addition to those born with congenital complete heart block, acquired complete AV block continues to develop at a rate of 2 percent per year. Patients with associated anomalies (VSD, pulmonary stenosis, left-sided [tricuspid] valve anomaly) often have undergone surgical palliation (systemic-to-pulmonary artery shunt for cyanosis) or repair of the associated anomalies (see surgical procedures).

SURGICAL PROCEDURES

"Classic" Repair. VSD patch closure for hemodynamically significant VSD, left ventricular to pulmonary artery valved conduit insertion for significant pulmonary valvar or subvalvar stenosis, and systemic tricuspid valve replacement for significant regurgitation may have been performed. VSD patch closure is carried out with a particular attention to avoid the anterior conduction system (coursing anterior to the VSD). In isolated pulmonary/subpulmonary stenosis, direct enlargement of the outflow tract and valve is seldom possible and a pulmonary (morphological left) ventricle to pulmonary artery conduit is required. Patients who have undergone this "classic" repair continue to have a morphological right ventricle supporting the systemic circulation.

CLINICAL MANIFESTATIONS

Unoperated. Patients with no associated defects (1 percent of all such patients) can be asymptomatic until late adulthood. Dyspnea, exercise intolerance from developing congestive heart failure, and palpitations from supraventricular arrhythmias may arise in the fifth or sixth decade. Patients with well-balanced VSD/pulmonary stenosis can present with paradoxical emboli or cyanosis, especially if pulmonary stenosis is severe. Physical examination of a patient whose condition is otherwise uncomplicated reveals a somewhat more medial apex due to the side-by-side orientation of the two ventricles. The A_2 is often palpable in the second left intercostal space due to the anterior and leftward location of the aorta. A single S_2 (A_2) is heard, with P_2 being silent due to its posterior location. The murmur of an associated VSD or of left AV valve regurgitation may be heard. The murmur of pulmonary stenosis will radiate upward and to the right given the rightward direction of the main pulmonary artery. If there is complete heart block, cannon a waves with an S_1 of variable intensity are present.

"Classic" Repair. The majority of patients are in functional Class I at 5 to 10 years after surgery[143, 144] despite the common development of tricuspid regurgitation and systemic right ventricular dysfunction after surgical repair (>30 percent of patients at 3 years after surgery).[143, 145, 146] Dyspnea, exercise intolerance, and palpitations from supraventricular arrhythmia can occur in the fourth decade.[147] Complete heart block may complicate surgery in an additional 25 percent.[6–8, 144–146] Physical examination reflects the basic cardiac malformation with or without residual coexisting anomalies.

DIAGNOSTIC TESTING

Electrocardiogram. Complete AV block can be present in up to 40 percent of adults. A delta wave from a left-sided accessory bypass tract (associated with "Ebstein-like" anomaly of the left-sided AV valve) can be seen. The presence of Q wave in leads V_1 and V_2 combined with an absent Q wave in leads V_5 and V_6 is typical and reflects the initial right-to-left septal depolarization occurring in the setting of "ventricular inversion" (Fig. 44–23). This should not be mistaken for evidence of previous anterior myocardial infarction.

Chest Radiography. Because of the unusual position of the great vessels (pulmonary artery to the right and aorta to the left), the pulmonary trunk is inconspicuous and an ab-

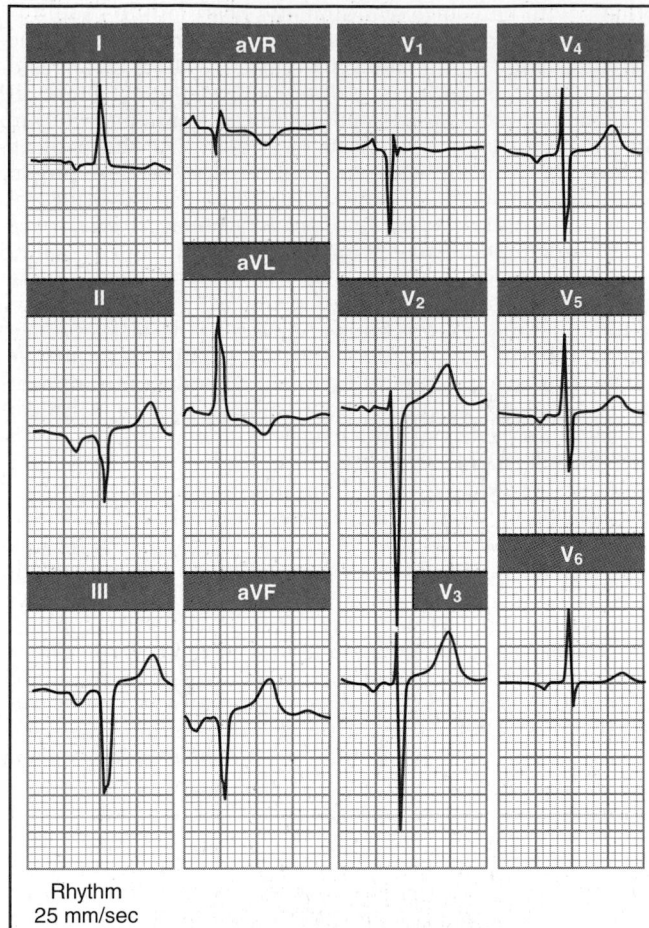

FIGURE 44–23. Electrocardiogram of a patient with congenitally corrected transposition of the great arteries. Note the presence of Q wave in V_1 and the absence of Q wave in V_{5-6}. Low atrial rhythm and left-axis deviation are also present.

normal bulge along the left side of the cardiac contour reflects the left-sided ascending aorta rising to the aortic knuckle. A shallow indentation or "septal notch" can be seen above the left hemidiaphragm reflecting the apical portion of the interventricular groove (Fig. 44–24).

Echocardiography. Echocardiography permits the identification of the basic malformation as well as any associated anomalies. The morphological pulmonary left ventricle is characterized by its smooth endocardial surface and is guarded by a bileaflet AV (mitral) valve with no direct septal attachment. The morphological systemic right ventricle is recognized by its apical trabeculation and moderator band and is guarded by a trileaflet apically displaced AV valve (tricuspid valve) with direct attachment to the septum (Fig. 44–25). "Ebstein-like" malformation of the left (tricuspid) AV valve is defined by excessive (>8 mm/m²) apical displacement of the left (tricuspid) AV valve, with or without dysplastic features.

Diagnostic Cardiac Catheterization. This may be required to assess the hemodynamic significance or consequences of associated anomalies.

INDICATION FOR INTERVENTION OR RE-INTERVENTION. If moderate or severe systemic (tricuspid) AV valve regurgitation develops, valve replacement is usually required. Left AV valve replacement should be performed before systemic right ventricular function deteriorates, namely at an ejection fraction of 45 percent or more.[148] When tricuspid regurgitation is associated with poor systemic (right) ventricular function, the "double switch" procedure (see Double Switch Procedure) should perhaps be considered.[131, 149–152]

Patients with end-stage symptomatic heart failure should be referred for cardiac transplantation. The presence of a hemodynamically significant VSD (Qp/Qs > 1.5:1.0) or residual VSD with significant native or postsurgical (conduit) pulmonary outflow tract stenosis (peak gradient >50 mm Hg) may require surgical correction. Left AV valve replacement at the time of VSD and pulmonary stenosis surgery should be considered if concomitant left AV valve regurgitation is present.[153] Complete AV block may require pacemaker implantation for symptoms, progressive or profound bradycardia, poor exercise heart rate response, or cardiac enlargement. The optimal pacing modality is DDD. Active fixation electrodes are required, owing to the lack of apical trabeculation in the morphological pulmonary left ventricle. Transvenous pacing should be avoided if there are intracardiac shunts because paradoxical emboli may occur. Epicardial leads are preferred under these circumstances.[154]

INTERVENTIONAL OPTIONS

Medical Therapy. ACE inhibitor therapy for patients with systemic ventricular dysfunction is recommended. The role of afterload reduction with an ACE inhibitor to preserve systemic right ventricular function is as yet unknown. The results of clinical trials are awaited.

Classic Repair. Tricuspid valve replacement for significant regurgitation is preferable to tricuspid valve repair. Valve repair is usually unsuccessful because of the abnormal, often "Ebstein-like" anatomy of the valve.

Double Switch Procedure. This procedure has been successfully performed in children. It should be considered for patients with severe tricuspid regurgitation and systemic ventricular dysfunction. Its purpose is to relocate the left ventricle into the systemic circulation and the right ventricle into the pulmonary circulation, achieving "anatomical" correction. An atrial switch procedure (Mustard or Senning) together with either an arterial switch procedure (when pulmonary stenosis is not present, see Chap. 43) or a Rastelli-type repair, the so-called Ilbawi procedure (left ventricle tunneled to aorta and right ventricular to pulmonary artery valved conduit when VSD and pulmonary stenosis are present), can be performed after adequate left ventricu-

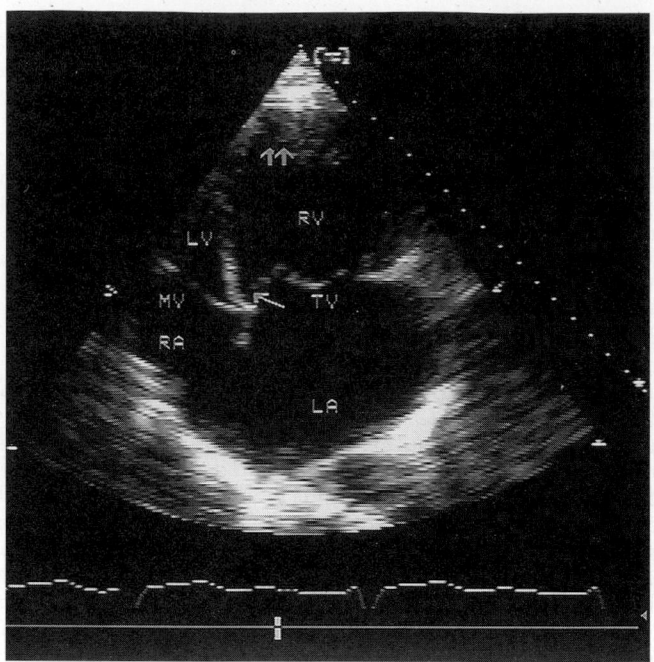

FIGURE 44–25. Transthoracic echocardiographic picture of a patient with congenitally corrected transposition of the great arteries. *A*, Single arrow points to the normally apically displaced left-sided tricuspid valve. Double arrows point to the left-sided right ventricular trabeculations. RA = right atrium; MV = mitral valve; LV = right-sided morphologic left ventricle; LA = left atrium; TV = tricuspid valve; TR = tricuspid regurgitation; RV = left-sided morphologic right ventricle.

lar retraining, leaving the regurgitant tricuspid valve and failing right ventricle on the pulmonary side.

Cardiac Transplantation. Patients with deteriorating systemic (right) ventricular function should be treated aggressively with medical therapy but may need to be considered for transplantation.

INTERVENTIONAL OUTCOMES

"Classic" Repair. After "classic" surgical repair, median survival of patients reaching adulthood is 40 years.[143–145, 147, 155] Usual causes of death are sudden (presumed arrhythmic) or, more commonly, progressive systemic right ventricular dysfunction with systemic (tricuspid) AV valve regurgitation. The major predictor of poor outcome is the presence of left AV (tricuspid) valve regurgitation.[155] Reoperation is common (15–25 percent), with left AV valve replacement usually being the primary reason.[143, 144, 146, 147]

Double Switch Procedure. Data in adults using the "double switch" procedure is lacking, and this procedure should be considered experimental in this patient population.

FOLLOW-UP. All patients should have at least annual cardiology follow-up with an expert in the care of adult patients with congenital cardiac defects. Regular assessment of systemic (tricuspid) AV valve regurgitation by serial echocardiographic studies and systemic ventricular function by echocardiography, MRI, or radionuclide angiography should be done. Holter recording may be useful if paroxysmal atrial arrhythmias or transient complete AV block is suspected.

Eisenmenger Syndrome

(see also Chaps. 43 and 53)

DEFINITION. Eisenmenger syndrome, a term coined by Paul Wood, is defined as pulmonary vascular obstructive disease that develops as a consequence of a large preexisting left-to-right shunt such that pulmonary artery pressures

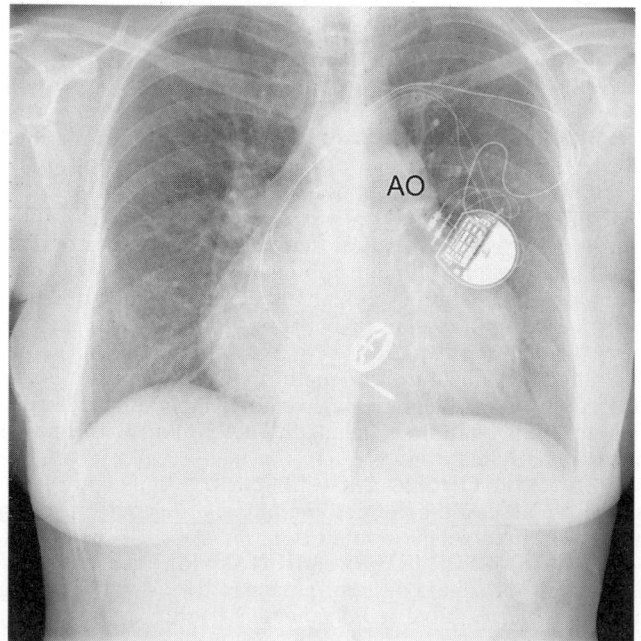

FIGURE 44–24. Chest radiograph of a patient with congenitally corrected transposition of the great arteries. Note the left-sided ascending aorta (AO), transvenous pacemaker and mechanical left-sided (tricuspid) atrioventricular valve, and enlarged right atrium.

approach systemic levels and the direction of the flow becomes bidirectional or right to left. Congenital heart defects that can result in Eisenmenger syndrome include "simple" defects such as ASD, VSD, and PDA as well as more "complex" defects such as AVSD, truncus arteriosus, aortopulmonary window, and univentricular heart. The high pulmonary vascular resistance is usually established in infancy (by age 2 years, except in ASD) and sometimes is present from birth.

NATURAL HISTORY OF THE UNOPERATED PATIENT. Patients with defects that allow free communication between the pulmonary and systemic circuits at the aortic or ventricular levels usually have a fairly healthy childhood and gradually become progressively cyanotic during their second or third decade. Exercise intolerance (dyspnea and fatigue) is proportional to the degree of hypoxemia or cyanosis. In the absence of complications, these patients generally have an excellent to good functional capacity up to their third decade[156, 157] and thereafter usually experience a slowly progressive decline in their physical abilities. Most patients survive to adulthood,[157, 158] with a reported 77 percent and 42 percent survival rate at 15 and 25 years of age.[157]

Complications from Eisenmenger syndrome tend to occur from the third decade onward. Congestive heart failure, the most serious complication, usually occurs after age 40.[156] The most common modes of death are sudden death (30 percent), congestive heart failure (25 percent), and hemoptysis (15 percent). Pregnancy, perioperative mortality after noncardiac surgery, and infectious causes (brain abscesses and endocarditis) account for most of the remainder.[156, 157]

CLINICAL MANIFESTATIONS. Patients can present with the following complications: those related to their cyanotic state (see p. 1617); palpitations in nearly half the patients (atrial fibrillation/flutter—35 percent, ventricular tachycardia—10 percent); hemoptysis in about 20 percent; pulmonary thromboembolism, angina, syncope, and endocarditis in about 10 percent; and congestive heart failure.[156] Hemoptysis is usually due to bleeding bronchial vessels or pulmonary infarction. Physical examination reveals central cyanosis and clubbing of the nail beds. Patients with Eisenmenger PDA can have pink nail beds on the right (± left) hand and cyanosis and clubbing of both feet (± the left hand), so-called "differential cyanosis." This occurs because venous blood shunts through the ductus and enters the aorta distal to the right subclavian artery. The jugular venous pressure in Eisenmenger syndrome patients can be normal or elevated—especially with prominent v waves when tricuspid regurgitation is present. Signs of pulmonary hypertension—a right ventricular heave, palpable and loud P_2, and a right-sided S_4—are typically present. In many patients, a pulmonary ejection click and a soft and scratchy systolic ejection murmur, attributable to dilation of the pulmonary trunk, and a high-pitched decrescendo diastolic murmur of pulmonary regurgitation (Graham Steele) are audible. Peripheral edema is absent until right-sided heart failure ensues.

DIAGNOSTIC TESTING

Electrocardiogram. Peaked P waves consistent with right atrial overload and evidence of right ventricular hypertrophy with right axis deviation are the rule. Atrial arrhythmias can be present (Fig. 44–26).

Chest Radiography. Dilated central pulmonary arteries with "pruning" of the peripheral pulmonary vasculature are the radiographic hallmarks of Eisenmenger syndrome (Fig. 44–27). Pulmonary artery calcification may be seen and is diagnostic of long-standing pulmonary hypertension. Eisenmenger syndrome due to VSD or PDA usually has a normal or slightly increased cardiothoracic ratio. Eisenmenger syndrome due to an ASD typically has a large cardiothoracic ratio due to right atrial and ventricular dilation, along with

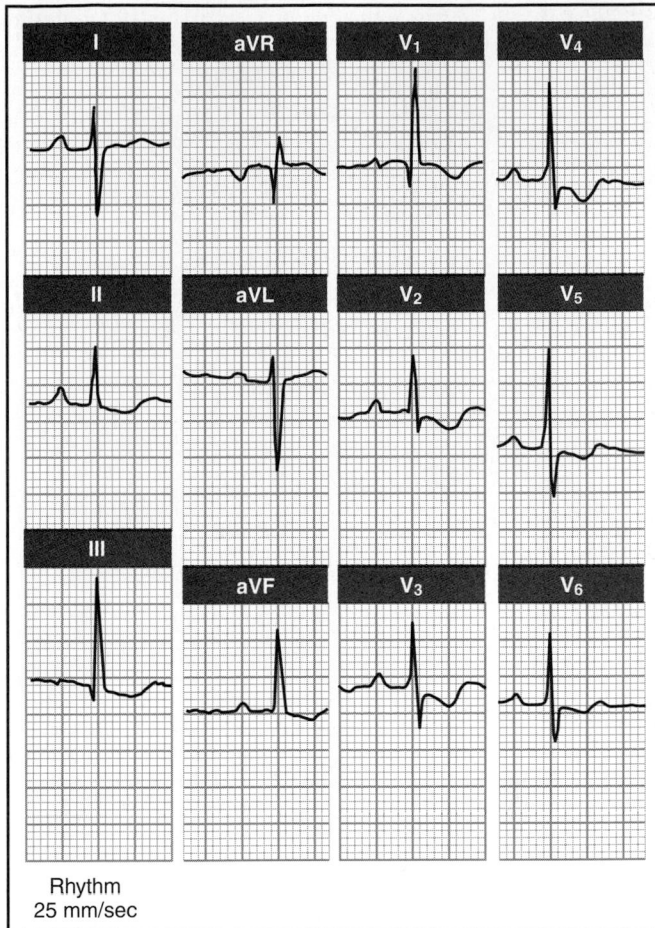

Rhythm
25 mm/sec

FIGURE 44–26. ECG of a patient with Eisenmenger syndrome due to a VSD. Note the peaked P wave in lead II, right ventricular hypertrophy, and right-axis deviation.

an inconspicuous aorta. Calcification of the duct may be seen in Eisenmenger PDA.

Echocardiography. The intracardiac defect should be seen readily along with bidirectional shunting. Evidence of pulmonary hypertension will be found. Assessment of pulmonary right ventricular function adds prognostic value.

Catheterization. Cardiac catheterization not only provides direct measurement of the pulmonary artery pressure, documenting the existence of severe pulmonary hypertension, but also may allow assessment of reactivity of the pulmonary vasculature. Administration of pulmonary arterial vasodilators (O_2, nitric oxide, prostaglandin I_2) can discriminate between patients in whom surgical repair is contraindicated and those with reversible pulmonary hypertension who may benefit from surgical repair. Radiographic contrast material may cause hypotension and worsening cyanosis and should be used cautiously.

Open-Lung Biopsy. Open-lung biopsy should only be considered when the reversibility of the pulmonary hypertension is uncertain from the hemodynamic data. An expert opinion will determine the severity of the changes, usually using the Heath-Edwards classification.

INDICATIONS FOR INTERVENTION. The underlying principle of clinical management in patients with Eisenmenger syndrome is to avoid any factors that may destabilize the delicately balanced physiology. In general, an approach of nonintervention is recommended. The main interventions, therefore, are directed toward preventing complications (e.g., flu shots to reduce the morbidity of respiratory infections) or to restore the physiological balance (e.g., iron replacement for iron deficiency; antiarrhythmic management of atrial arrhythmias; digoxin and diuretics for right-sided

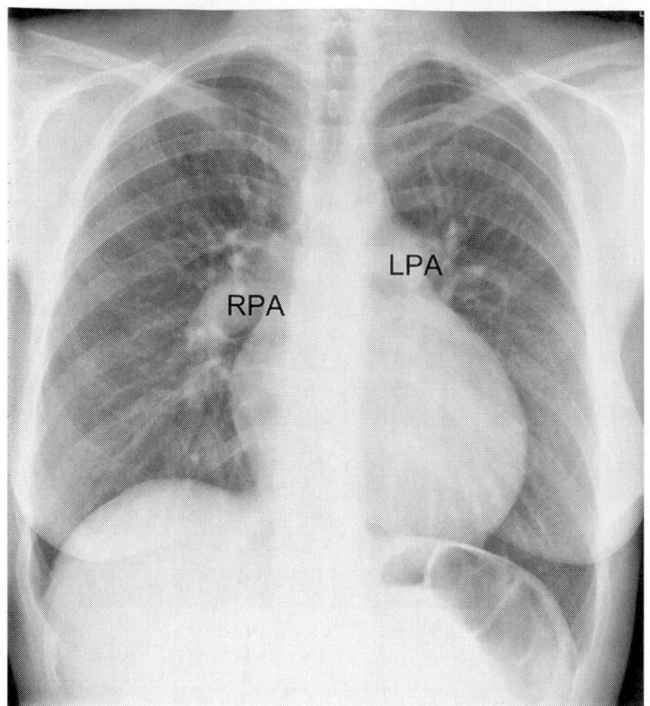

FIGURE 44–27. Typical chest radiograph of a patient with Eisenmenger syndrome due to a ventricular septal defect. Note the enlarged central pulmonary arteries and the peripheral pruning of the pulmonary vasculature. *A,* Posteroanterior view. LPA = left pulmonary artery; RPA = right pulmonary artery.

heart failure). As a general rule, the first episode of hemoptysis should be considered an indication for hospital admission and investigation. Bed rest should be implemented; and, although usually self-limiting, each such episode should be regarded as potentially life threatening, and a treatable cause sought. When patients are severely incapacitated from severe hypoxemia or congestive heart failure, the main intervention available is lung (plus repair of the cardiac defect) or heart-lung transplantation. This is generally reserved for individuals without contraindications who are thought to have a 1-year survival of less than 50 percent. Such assessment is fraught with difficulty because of the unpredictability of the time course of the disease and the risk of sudden death.

Noncardiac surgery should be performed only when absolutely necessary because of its high associated mortality.[156, 159] Eisenmenger syndrome patients are particularly vulnerable to alterations in hemodynamics induced by anesthesia or surgery, such as minor decrease in systemic vascular resistance that can increase right-to-left shunting and possibly potentiate cardiovascular collapse. Local anesthesia should be used whenever possible. Avoidance of prolonged fasting and especially dehydration, the use of antibiotic prophylaxis when appropriate,[160] and careful intraoperative monitoring (sometimes with an arterial line ± a central venous line to allow early detection of sudden pressure and volume changes during surgery) are recommended.[159, 161] The choice of general versus epidural-spinal anesthesia is controversial. An experienced cardiac anesthetist with an understanding of Eisenmenger syndrome physiology should administer anesthesia. Additional risks of surgery include excessive bleeding, postoperative arrhythmias, and deep venous thrombosis with paradoxic emboli. An "air filter" or "bubble trap" should be used for any intravenous lines. Early ambulation is recommended.[159, 161] Postoperative care in an intensive care unit setting is optimal.

INTERVENTIONAL OPTIONS AND OUTCOMES
Oxygen. In a small prospective nonrandomized study of 15 children with pulmonary vascular disease, chronic administration of oxygen (12 hours a day for up to 5 years) resulted in an increased survival in the treatment group (n = 9).[162] The impact of supplemental oxygen on survival in adult patients with Eisenmenger syndrome has never been studied, and its role is unclear. Chronic oxygen therapy can perhaps help raise oxygen saturation and reduce symptoms, but this should be counterbalanced with the potential effect of mucosal dehydration and increased incidence of epistaxis. Supplemental oxygen during commercial air travel is often recommended, but the scientific basis for this recommendation is lacking.[163]

Transplantation. Lung transplant may be undertaken in association with repair of existing cardiovascular defect(s). Alternatively, heart-lung transplantation may be required if the intracardiac anatomy is not correctable. The outcome of transplantation in these patients is generally less satisfactory than for transplant recipients without Eisenmenger syndrome. The 1-year survival rate for adults undergoing lung transplantation with primary intracardiac repair is 70 to 80 percent, and less than 50 percent of patients are alive 4 years after transplantation.[164, 165] The outcome after heart-lung transplantation is not better, with a 1-year survival rate of 60 to 80 percent and a 10-year survival rate of less than 30 percent.[164] These options, however sobering, may be relatively attractive to individuals who are confronting death and have an intolerable quality of life.

INVESTIGATIONAL THERAPY
Calcium Channel Blockers. The chronic use of nifedipine in a small group of patients with Eisenmenger syndrome demonstrated a small but significant increase in exercise tolerance[166] and a decrease in pulmonary vascular resistance, especially in children.[167] This therapy is still considered investigational and should only be prescribed in a clinical research setting.

ACE Inhibitors. Data available on a highly selected group of 10 patients with cyanotic congenital heart disease showed no change in oxygen saturation despite a subjective improvement in functional capacity.[168] Proponents of the use of ACE inhibitors in these patients argue that, by decreasing systemic vascular resistance, one improves the cardiac output and thus oxygen delivery. The counter argument is that these agents are potentially dangerous because they lower systemic vascular resistance without changing pulmonary vascular resistance and lead to an increase in right-to-left shunting. The use of this medication remains highly experimental and again should only be administered within the boundaries of a study trial guided by rigorous monitoring.

Prostacyclin. A recent study of chronic prostacyclin administration in such patients showed improvement in hemodynamics (lower pulmonary vascular resistance and increased cardiac output) and a somewhat increased exercise capacity.[169] Further research in this field is needed before recommendations on the use of prostaglandins in these patients can be made.

Pulmonary Artery Banding. Pulmonary artery banding in one patient with biopsy-proven irreversible pulmonary vascular changes led to regression of pulmonary vascular changes, which made surgical closure of the defects possible.[170] Further data regarding this revolutionary practice are awaited.

FOLLOW-UP. Patient education is critical. Avoidance of over-the-counter medications, dehydration, smoking, high-altitude exposure, and excessive physical activity should be stressed. Avoidance of pregnancy is of paramount importance (see Chap. 65). Annual flu shots and use of endocarditis prophylaxis together with proper skin hygiene (avoidance of nail biting) are recommended. A yearly assessment of complete blood cell count and uric acid, creatinine, and ferritin levels should be done to monitor treatable causes of deterioration.

Medical Management of Cyanotic Congenital Heart Disease

PATHOPHYSIOLOGY OF CYANOSIS. Patients with cyanotic congenital heart lesions, either unoperated or palliated, have chronic hypoxemia as a result of persistent systemic venous to arterial shunting. Ensuing physiological adaptive mechanisms to enhance oxygen delivery include, among others, an increase in red blood cell mass to improve systemic oxygen transport. Erythropoietin production is stimulated as a result of exposure of renal oxygen sensors to hypoxemia. Red blood cell production is enhanced, oxygen content (hemoglobin × O_2 saturation) increases, and oxygen delivery (cardiac output × O_2 saturation) is reestablished, albeit at the cost of a higher hematocrit. Erythrocytosis, in the setting of chronic cyanotic congenital heart disease, is thus an adaptive physiological mechanism.[171]

HYPERVISCOSITY SYNDROME. Symptoms of hyperviscosity include headaches, altered mentation, visual disturbances, tinnitus, paresthesias, fatigue, dizziness, and myalgias.[171] These symptoms can be mild, moderate, or severe. They usually present in patients with an elevated hematocrit (>65 percent) or can present at a hematocrit less than 65 percent if the patient is iron deficient. The patient usually experiences the same hyperviscosity symptoms each time (e.g., headache, visual disturbances, fatigue), and they must be relieved by phlebotomy to qualify as hyperviscosity symptoms.

An increased hematocrit level, in the absence of symptoms, does not constitute an indication for phlebotomy. Repeated phlebotomy under these circumstances will lead to iron deficiency, and perhaps cerebral arterial events. Dehydration secondary to excessive heat, illness, fever, diarrhea, or vomiting can be the cause of hyperviscosity symptoms and should be managed appropriately with volume replacement.

If dehydration or iron deficiency is not the cause of hyperviscosity symptoms, phlebotomy becomes the treatment of choice. Removal of 500 ml of blood over 30 to 45 minutes preceded by or simultaneous with a 500- to 1000-ml volume replacement with normal saline (or dextran for patients with congestive heart failure) can usually be performed in an outpatient setting. The goal of phlebotomy is symptom control. The patient having phlebotomy is at risk of iron deficiency. As a rule, iron supplementation should be prescribed.

IRON DEFICIENCY AND REPLACEMENT. Iron deficiency is an important and common finding in cyanotic adults. The etiology can be multifactorial and includes excessive bleeding from hemoptysis, epistaxis, or excessive menses, but by far the most distressing cause is inappropriate phlebotomy. Microcytosis from iron deficiency results in an increase in whole blood viscosity because microspheres are much less deformable than the normal biconcave disc-shaped iron-replete red blood cell.

In contrast to normocytic erythrocytosis, which seldom causes symptoms at hematocrit levels less than 65 percent, iron deficiency can present as hyperviscosity symptoms at hematocrit levels well below 65 percent. The treatment of choice in this case is iron repletion and not phlebotomy. If iron deficiency is confirmed, supplemental iron should be administered until a rise in hematocrit is registered, or until the iron-replete state has been achieved. Intravenous iron preparations are an alternative for patients intolerant of oral iron supplementation.[171]

HEMOSTATIC ABNORMALITIES. Hemostatic abnormalities have been documented in cyanotic patients with erythrocytosis.[171] Any bleeding tendency is usually mild and superficial, leading to easy bruising, petechiae, or mucosal bleeding. However, at times, bleeding can be moderate, with epistaxis or hemoptysis, or can even be life threatening, particularly in the postoperative setting. An increase in prothrombin time (PT) and partial thromboplastin time (PTT) from decreased levels of factors V, VII, VIII, and X, from quantitative and qualitative platelet disorders, and from increased fibrinolytic activity have all been described.

The management of a bleeding diathesis can be subdivided into two clinical categories: spontaneous bleeding and perioperative prevention. Spontaneous, superficial bleeding usually is self-limited. Avoidance of aspirin, nonsteroidal antiinflammatory drugs, and heparin is an important prophylactic measure. The treatment of severe spontaneous bleeding is dictated by the specific hemostatic disturbances. Platelet transfusions, fresh-frozen plasma, vitamin K, and cryoprecipitate have all been used.

It is recommended that cyanotic patients facing major surgery undergo prophylactic phlebotomy if the hematocrit level is greater than 65 percent to minimize hemostatic abnormalities intraoperatively and postoperatively. Isovolumetric phlebotomy of 500 ml can be performed every 24 hours until the hematocrit levels decrease below 65 percent. Blood that has been withdrawn should be kept for autologous transfusion if needed.

CEREBROVASCULAR EVENTS. Cerebrovascular events including stroke secondary to thrombosis or embolus have been recognized as a complication of cyanosis in adults with congenital heart disease. The risk of stroke caused by cerebral arterial thrombosis has usually been seen in patients with iron deficiency and not iron-replete erythrocytosis.[172, 173] Cerebral hemorrhage can occur due to hemostatic defects and is most often observed after the use of often dangerous anticoagulant therapy. Patients with right-to-left shunts can also be at risk for paradoxical emboli. Focal brain injury can provide a nidus for brain abscess if bacteremia supervenes. Brain abscess patients can present with headaches with fever and focal neurological findings or seizures.[174] It follows from the previous discussion that prophylactic phlebotomy has no place in the prevention of cerebral arterial thrombosis. Avoidance of microcytosis is of paramount importance.[172, 173] Meticulous attention should be paid to the use of air filters in peripheral intravenous lines to avoid paradoxical emboli through a right-to-left shunt.[174] Anticoagulants should usually be avoided in chronically cyanotic cardiac patients. In the uncommon patient with atrial fibrillation or a mechanical prosthesis, a risk-benefit dilemma must be addressed.

RENAL DYSFUNCTION. Renal dysfunction can present as proteinuria, hyperuricemia, and, rarely, overt renal failure.[175] Hyperuricemia, commonly observed in patients with cyanotic congenital heart disease, is caused mainly by increased reabsorption of uric acid rather than by overproduction from erythrocytosis. Fortunately, urate nephropathy, uric acid nephrolithiasis, and gouty arthritis are rare. Asymptomatic hyperuricemia need not be treated. Acute gouty arthritis responds to intravenous colchicine. Corticosteroid therapy is a viable alternative. Nonsteroidal antiinflammatory drugs should be avoided, given the baseline hemostatic anomalies in these patients. Symptomatic hyperuricemia and chronic gouty arthritis can be treated with probenecid or sulfinpyrazone, which are uricosuric agents, or with allopurinol, which decreases uric acid production. Most diuretics are relatively contraindicated because they reduce renal tubular secretion of uric acid and may aggravate existing hyperuricemia.

ARTHRALGIA. Hypertrophic osteoarthropathy is thought to be the mechanism responsible for the arthralgias affecting up to one third of patients with cyanotic congenital heart disease. In patients with right-to-left shunting, megakaryocytes released from the bone marrow can bypass the lung. The entrapment of megakaryocytes in the systemic arterioles and capillaries induces the release of platelet-derived growth factor, promoting local cell proliferation.

New osseous formation with periostitis ensues and gives rise to arthralgia and bony pain.[175] Arthralgias can be managed with salsalate, a nonacetylated analog of aspirin. This medication does not appear to interfere with platelet function and, therefore, is an ideal antiinflammatory medication for patients with bleeding tendencies.

FOLLOW-UP. Patients with cyanotic congenital heart disease should be followed regularly by experts. Hemoglobin levels, mean corpuscular volume, ferritin, renal function, and uric acid should be checked at least annually to avoid treatable causes of deterioration. Annual flu shots are recommended. Avoidance of unnecessary phlebotomies and anticoagulant therapy is key. Smoking is to be strongly discouraged because it impairs oxygen-carrying capacity and worsens oxygen delivery.

REFERENCES

1. Perloff JK: Congenital heart disease in adults: A new cardiovascular subspecialty. Circulation 84:1881–1890, 1991.
1a. Brickner ME, Hillis LD, Lange RA: Congenital heart disease in adults [first of two parts]. N Engl J Med 342:256–263, 2000.
1b. Brickner ME, Hillis LD, Lange RA: Congenital heart disease in adults [second of two parts]. N Engl J Med 342:334–342, 2000.
2. Connelly MS, Webb GD, Somerville J, et al: Canadian Consensus Conference on Adult Congenital Heart Disease 1996. Can J Cardiol 14:395–452, 1998.
2a. Taylor AM, Thorne SA, Rubens MB, et al: Coronary artery imaging in grown up congenital heart disease: Complementary role of magnetic resonance and x-ray coronary angiography. Circulation 101:1670–1678, 2000.
3. Weiss BM, Zemp L, Seifert B, Hess OM: Outcome of pulmonary vascular disease in pregnancy: A systematic overview from 1978 through 1996. J Am Coll Cardiol 31:1650–1657, 1998.
3a. Chung T: Assessment of cardiovascular anatomy in patients with congenital heart disease by magnetic resonance imaging. Pediatr Cardiol 21:18–26, 2000.
3b. Horner T, Liberthson R, Jellinek MS: Psychosocial profile of adults with complex congenital heart disease. Mayo Clin Proc 75:31–36, 2000.

MEDICAL MANAGEMENT OF CYANOTIC CONGENITAL HEART DISEASE

4. Siu SC, Sermer M, Harrison DA, et al: Risk and predictors for pregnancy-related complications in women with heart disease. Circulation 96:2789–2794, 1997.
5. Siu S, Chitayat D, Webb G: Pregnancy in women with congenital heart defects: What are the risks? Heart 81:225–226, 1999.
6. Burn J, Brennan P, Little J, et al: Recurrence risks in offspring of adults with major heart defects: Results from first cohort of British collaborative study. Lancet 351:311–316, 1998.
7. Lamour JM, Addonizio LJ Mancini DM, et al: Outcome after orthotopic heart transplantation in adults with congenital heart disease. Circulation 100[suppl I]:I-97, 1999.
8. Gewillig M, Cullen S, Mertens B, et al: Risk factors for arrhythmia and death after Mustard operation for simple transposition of the great arteries. Circulation 84:187–192, 1991.
9. Gelatt M, Hamilton RM, McCrindle BW, et al: Arrhythmia and mortality after the Mustard procedure: A 30-year single-center experience. J Am Coll Cardiol 29:194–201, 1997.

ATRIAL SEPTAL DEFECT

10. Ward C: Secundum atrial septal defect: Routine surgical treatment is not of proven benefit. Br Heart J 71:219–223, 1994.
11. Di Tullio M, Sacco RL, Gopal A, et al: Patent foramen ovale as a risk factor for cryptogenic stroke. Ann Intern Med 117:461–465, 1992.
12. Gatzoulis MA, Freeman MA, Siu SC, et al: Atrial arrhythmia after surgical closure of atrial septal defects in adults. N Engl J Med 340:839–846, 1999.
13. Konstantinides S, Geibel A, Olschewski M, et al: A comparison of surgical and medical therapy for atrial septal defect in adults. N Engl J Med 333:469–473, 1995.
14. Helber U, Baumann R, Seboldt H, et al: Atrial septal defect in adults: Cardiopulmonary exercise capacity before and 4 months and 10 years after defect closure. J Am Coll Cardiol 29:1345–1350, 1997.
15. Shah D, Azhar M, Oakley CM, et al: Natural history of secundum atrial septal defect in adults after medical or surgical treatment: A historical prospective study. Br Heart J 71:224–228, 1994.
16. Rao PS, Sideris EB, Hausdorf G, et al: International experience with secundum atrial septal defect occlusion by the buttoned device. Am Heart J 128:1022–1035, 1994.
17. Boutin C, Musewe NN, Smallhorn JF, et al: Echocardiographic follow-up of atrial septal defect after catheter closure by double-umbrella device. Circulation 88:621–627, 1993.
18. Horvath KA, Burke RP, Collins JJ Jr, Cohn LH: Surgical treatment of adult atrial septal defect: Early and long-term results. J Am Coll Cardiol 20:1156–1159, 1992.
19. Sandoval N, Velasco VM, Orjuela H, et al: Concomitant mitral valve or atrial septal defect surgery and the modified Cox-maze procedure. Am J Cardiol 77:591–596, 1996.

ISOLATED VENTRICULAR SEPTAL DEFECT

20. Freed MD: Infective endocarditis in the adult with congenital heart disease. Cardiol Clin 11:589–602, 1993.
21. Neumayer U, Stone S, Somerville J: Small ventricular septal defects in adults. Eur Heart J 19:1573–1582, 1998.
22. Trusler GA, Williams WG, Smallhorn JF, Freedom RM: Late results after repair of aortic insufficiency associated with ventricular septal defect. J Thorac Cardiovasc Surg 103:276–281, 1992.
23. Sideris EB, Walsh KP, Haddad JL, et al: Occlusion of congenital ventricular septal defects by the buttoned device. "Buttoned device" Clinical Trials International Register. Heart 77:276–279, 1997.
24. Kidd L, Driscoll DJ, Gersony WM, et al: Second natural history study of congenital heart defects: Results of treatment of patients with ventricular septal defects. Circulation 87:38–51, 1993.

ATRIOVENTRICULAR SEPTAL DEFECT

25. Mavroudis C, Backer CL: The two-patch technique for complete atrioventricular canal. Semin Thorac Cardiovasc Surg 9:35–43, 1997.
26. Ashraf MH, Amin Z, Sharma R, Subramanian S: Atrioventricular canal defect: Two-patch repair and tricuspidization of the mitral valve. Ann Thorac Surg 55:347–350; discussion 350–351, 1993.
27. Carpentier A: Surgical anatomy and management of mitral component of atrioventricular canal defects. In Paediatric Cardiology. Edinburgh, Churchill Livingstone, 1978, pp 477–490.
28. Pearl JM, Laks H: Intermediate and complete forms of atrioventricular canal. Semin Thorac Cardiovasc Surg 9:8–20, 1997.
29. Michielon G, Stellin G, Rizzoli G, et al: Left atrioventricular valve incompetence after repair of common atrioventricular canal defects. Ann Thorac Surg 60:s604–s609, 1995.
30. van Son JA, Van Praagh R, Falk V, Mohr FW: Pericardial patch augmentation of the tissue-deficient mitral valve in common atrioventricular canal. J Thorac Cardiovasc Surg 112:1117–1119, 1996.
31. Burke RP, Horvath K, Landzberg M, et al: Long-term follow-up after surgical repair of ostium primum atrial septal defects in adults. J Am Coll Cardiol 27:696–699, 1996.
32. Bergin ML, Warnes CA, Tajik AJ, Danielson GK: Partial atrioventricular canal defect: Long-term follow-up after initial repair in patients > or = 40 years old. J Am Coll Cardiol 25:1189–1194, 1995.
32a. Gatzoulis MA, Hechter S, Webb GD, Williams WG: Surgery for partial atrioventricular septal defect in the adult. Ann Thorac Surg 67:504–510, 1999.
32b. Kameyama T, Ando F, Okamoto F, et al: Long term follow up of atrioventricular valve function after repair of atrioventricular septal defect. Ann Thorac Cardiovasc Surg. 5:101–106, 1999.
33. Bando K, Turrentine MW, Sun K, et al: Surgical management of complete atrioventricular septal defects: A twenty-year experience. J Thorac Cardiovasc Surg 110:1543–1552, 1995.
34. Van Arsdell GS, Williams WG, Boutin C, et al: Subaortic stenosis in the spectrum of atrioventricular septal defects: Solutions may be complex and palliative. J Thorac Cardiovasc Surg 110:1534–1541, 1995.

PATENT DUCTUS ARTERIOSUS

35. Perloff JK: Patent ductus arteriosus. In The Clinical Recognition of Congenital Heart Disease. Philadelphia, WB Saunders, 1999, pp 467–489.
36. Harrison DA, Benson LN, Lazzam C, et al: Percutaneous catheter closure of the persistently patent ductus arteriosus in the adult. Am J Cardiol 77:1094–1097, 1996.
37. Landzberg MJ, Bridges ND, Perry SB, et al: Transcatheter occlusion: The treatment of choice for the adult with a patent ductus arteriosus. Circulation 84(Suppl II):67. 1999.
38. Sievert H, Ensslen R, Fach A, et al: Transcatheter closure of patent ductus arteriosus with the Rashkind occluder: Acute results and angiographic follow-up in adults. Eur Heart J 18:1014–1018, 1997.
39. Sorensen KE, Kristensen B, Hansen OK: Frequency of occurrence of residual ductal flow after surgical ligation by color-flow mapping. Am J Cardiol 67:653–654, 1991.
40. Houston AB, Gnanapragasam JP, Lim MK, et al: Doppler ultrasound and the silent ductus arteriosus. Br Heart J 65:97–99, 1991.
41. Hosking MC, Benson LN, Musewe N, et al: Transcatheter occlusion of the persistently patent ductus arteriosus: Forty-month follow-up and prevalence of residual shunting. Circulation 84:2313–2317, 1991.

BICUSPID AORTIC VALVE

42. Hahn RT, Roman MJ, Mogtader AH, Devereux RB: Association of aortic dilation with regurgitant, stenotic and functionally normal bicuspid aortic valves. J Am Coll Cardiol 19:283–288, 1992.
42a. De Sa M, Moshkovitz Y, Butany J, David TE: Histologic abnormalities of the ascending aorta and pulmonary trunk in patients with bicuspid aortic valve disease: Clinical relevance to the Ross procedure. J Thorac Cardiovasc Surg 118:588–594, 1999.
42b. Nistri S, Sorbo MD, Marin M, et al: Aortic root dilatation in young men with normally functioning bicuspid aortic valves. Heart 82:19–22, 1999.
43. Kitchiner D, Jackson M, Walsh K, et al: The progression of mild congenital aortic valve stenosis from childhood into adult life. Int J Cardiol 42:217–223, 1993.
44. Burks JM, Illes RW, Keating EC, Lubbe WJ: Ascending aortic aneurysm and dissection in young adults with bicuspid aortic valve: Implications for echocardiographic surveillance. Clin Cardiol 21:439–443, 1998.
45. Bahl VK, Chandra S, Goswami KC, Manchanda SC: Balloon aortic valvuloplasty in young adults by antegrade, transseptal approach using Inoue balloon. Cathet Cardiovasc Diagn 44:297–301, 1998.
46. Elkins RC, Lane MM, McCue C: Pulmonary autograft reoperation: Incidence and management. Ann Thorac Surg 62:450–455, 1996.
47. Niwaya K, Knott-Craig CJ, Lane MM, et al: Cryopreserved homograft valves in the pulmonary position: Risk analysis for intermediate-term failure. J Thorac Cardiovasc Surg 117:141–146, 1999.
48. Cosgrove DM, Rosenkranz ER, Hendren WG, et al: Valvuloplasty for aortic insufficiency. J Thorac Cardiovasc Surg 102:571–576, 1991.

SUBAORTIC STENOSIS

49. Somerville J: Fixed subaortic stenosis—a frequent misunderstood lesion. Int J Cardiol 8:145–148, 1999.
50. Choi JY, Sullivan ID: Fixed subaortic stenosis: Anatomical spectrum and nature of progression. Br Heart J 65:280–286, 1991.
51. Perloff JK: Congenital aortic stenosis; congenital aortic regurgitation. In The Clinical Recognition of Congenital Heart Disease. Philadelphia, WB Saunders, 1999, pp 91–131.
52. Cabrera A, Galdeano JM, Zumalde J, et al: Fixed subaortic stenosis: The value of cross-sectional echocardiography in evaluating different anatomical patterns. Int J Cardiol 24:151–157, 1989.
53. Brauner R, Laks H, Drinkwater DCJ, et al: Benefits of early surgical repair in fixed subaortic stenosis. J Am Coll Cardiol 30:1835–1842, 1997.
54. Vouhe PR, Ouaknine R, Poulain H, et al: Diffuse subaortic stenosis: Modified Konno procedures with aortic valve preservation. Eur J Cardiothor Surg 7:132–136, 1999.
55. Reddy VM, Rajasinghe HA, Teitel DF, et al: Aortoventriculoplasty with the pulmonary autograft: The "Ross-Konno" procedure. J Thorac Cardiovasc Surg 111:158–165, 1996.
56. Suarez dL, Pan M, Medina A, et al: Immediate and follow-up results of transluminal balloon dilation for discrete subaortic stenosis. J Am Coll Cardiol 18:1309–1315, 1991.
57. Delius RE, Samyn MM, Behrendt DM: Should a bicuspid aortic valve be replaced in the presence of subvalvar or supravalvar aortic stenosis? Ann Thorac Surg 66:1337–1342, 1998.
58. Brauner R, Laks H, Drinkwater DCJ, et al: Benefits of early surgical repair in fixed subaortic stenosis. J Am Coll Cardiol 30:1835–1842, 1997.

COARCTATION OF THE AORTA

59. Campbell M: Natural history of coarctation of the aorta. Br Heart J 32:633–640, 1970.
60. Perloff JK: Coarctation of the aorta. In The Clinical Recognition of Congenital Heart Disease. Philadelphia: WB Saunders, 1999, pp 132–169.
61. Messmer BJ, Minale C, Muhler E, von Bernuth G: Surgical correction of coarctation in early infancy: Does surgical technique influence the result? Ann Thorac Surg 52:594–600, 1991.
62. Ebeid MR, Prieto LR, Latson LA: Use of balloon-expandable stents for coarctation of the aorta: Initial results and intermediate-term follow-up. J Am Coll Cardiol 30:1847–1852, 1997.
63. Yetman AT, Nykanen D, McCrindle BW, et al: Balloon angioplasty of recurrent coarctation: A 12-year review. J Am Coll Cardiol 30:811–816, 1997.
64. McCrindle BW, Jones TK, Morrow WR, et al: Acute results of balloon angioplasty of native coarctation versus recurrent aortic obstruction are equivalent. Valvuloplasty and Angioplasty of Congenital Anomalies (VACA) Registry Investigators. J Am Coll Cardiol 28:1810–1817, 1996.
65. Behl PR, Sante P, Blesovsky A: Isolated coarctation of the aorta: surgical treatment and late results: Eighteen years' experience. J Cardiovasc Surg 29:509–517, 1988.
66. Trinquet F, Vouhe PR, Vernant F, et al: Coarctation of the aorta in infants: Which operation? Ann Thorac Surg 45:186–191, 1988.
67. Hehrlein FW, Mulch J, Rautenburg HW, et al: Incidence and pathogenesis of late aneurysms after patch graft aortoplasty for coarctation. J Thorac Cardiovasc Surg 92:226–230, 1986.
68. Shaddy RE, Boucek MM, Sturtevant JE, et al: Comparison of angioplasty and surgery for unoperated coarctation of the aorta. Circulation 87:793–799, 1993.
68a. Therrien J, Thorne SA, Wright A, et al: Repaired coarctation: A "cost-effective" approach to identify complications in adults. J Am Coll Cardiol 35:997–1002, 2000.
69. Ross RD, Clapp SK, Gunther S, et al: Augmented norepinephrine and renin output in response to maximal exercise in hypertensive coarctectomy patients. Am Heart J 123:1293–1299, 1992.
70. Guenthard J, Zumsteg U, Wyler F: Arm-leg pressure gradients on late follow-up after coarctation repair: Possible causes and implications. Eur Heart J 17:1572–1575, 1996.

RIGHT VENTRICULAR OUTFLOW TRACT OBSTRUCTION

71. Hayes CJ, Gersony WM, Driscoll DJ, et al: Second natural history study of congenital heart defects: Results of treatment of patients with pulmonary valvar stenosis. Circulation 87:28–37, 1993.
72. Lock JE, Perry S, Beane JF: Profiles in congenital heart disease. In Cardiac Catheterisation, Angiography and Intervention. Philadelphia, Lea & Febiger, 1999, pp 654–675.
73. Teupe CH, Burger W, Schrader R, Zeiher AM: Late (five to nine years) follow-up after balloon dilation of valvular pulmonary stenosis in adults. Am J Cardiol 80:240–242, 1997.
74. McCrindle BW: Independent predictors of long-term results after balloon pulmonary valvuloplasty. Valvuloplasty and Angioplasty of Congenital Anomalies (VACA) Registry Investigators. Circulation 89:1751–1759, 1994.
75. O'Connor BK, Beekman RH, Lindauer A, Rocchini A: Intermediate-term outcome after pulmonary balloon valvuloplasty: Comparison with a matched surgical control group. J Am Coll Cardiol 20:169–173, 1992.
76. Fawzy ME, Galal O, Dunn B, et al: Regression of infundibular pulmonary stenosis after successful balloon pulmonary valvuloplasty in adults. Cathet Cardiovasc Diagn 21:77–81, 1990.

EBSTEIN ANOMALY

77. Celermajer DS, Bull C, Till JA, et al: Ebstein's anomaly: Presentation and outcome from fetus to adult. J Am Coll Cardiol 23:170–176, 1994.
78. Gentles TL, Calder AL, Clarkson PM, Neutze JM: Predictors of long-term survival with Ebstein's anomaly of the tricuspid valve. Am J Cardiol 69:377–381, 1992.
79. Perloff JK: Ebstein's anomaly of the tricuspid valve. In The Clinical Recognition of Congenital Heart Disease. Philadelphia, WB Saunders, 1999, pp 467–489.
80. Ammash NM, Warnes CA, Connolly HM, et al: Mimics of Ebstein's anomaly. Am Heart J 134:508–513, 1997.
81. Augustin N, Schmidt-Habelmann P, Wottke M, et al: Results after surgical repair of Ebstein's anomaly. Ann Thorac Surg 63:1650–1656, 1997.
82. Hetzer R, Nagdyman N, Ewert P, et al: A modified repair technique for tricuspid incompetence in Ebstein's anomaly. J Thorac Cardiovasc Surg 115:857–868, 1998.
83. Chauvaud S, Fuzellier JF, Berrebi A, et al: Bi-directional cavopulmonary shunt associated with ventriculo and valvuloplasty in Ebstein's anomaly: Benefits in high risk patients. Eur J Cardiothorac Surg 13:514–519, 1998.
84. Theodoro DA, Danielson GK, Porter CJ, Warnes CA: Right-sided maze procedure for right atrial arrhythmias in congenital heart disease. Ann Thorac Surg 65:149–153, 1998.

TETRALOGY OF FALLOT

85. Perloff JK: Ventricular septal defect with pulmonary stenosis. In The Clinical Recognition of Congenital Heart Disease. Philadelphia, WB Saunders, 1999, pp 467–489.
86. Oechslin EN, Harrison DA, Harris L, et al: Reoperation in adults with repair of Tetralogy of Fallot: Indications and outcomes. J Thorac Cardiovasc Surg 118:245–251, 1999.
87. Gatzoulis MA, Till JA, Somerville J, Redington AN: Mechanoelectrical interaction in tetralogy of Fallot: QRS prolongation relates to right ventricular size and predicts malignant ventricular arrhythmias and sudden death. Circulation 92:231–237, 1995.
88. Nollert G, Fischlein T, Bouterwek S, et al: Long-term results of total repair of tetralogy of Fallot in adulthood: 35 years follow-up in 104 patients corrected at the age of 18 or older. Thorac Cardiovasc Surg 45:178–181, 1997.
89. Bonow RO, Lakatos E, Maron BJ, Epstein SE: Serial long-term assessment of the natural history of asymptomatic patients with chronic aortic regurgitation and normal left ventricular systolic function. Circulation 84:1625–1635, 1991.
90. Downar E, Harris L, Kimber S, et al: Ventricular tachycardia after surgical repair of tetralogy of Fallot: Results of intraoperative mapping studies. J Am Coll Cardiol 20:648–655, 1992.
91. Nollert G, Fischlein T, Bouterwek S, et al: Long-term survival in patients with repair of tetralogy of Fallot: 36-year follow-up of 490 survivors of the first year after surgical repair. J Am Coll Cardiol 30:1374–1383, 1997.

92. Yemets IM, Williams WG, Webb GD, et al: Pulmonary valve replacement late after repair of tetralogy of Fallot. Ann Thorac Surg 64:526–530, 1997.

93. d'Udekem Y, Rubay J, Shango-Lody P, et al: Late homograft valve insertion after transannular patch repair of tetralogy of Fallot. J Heart Valve Dis 7:450–454, 1998.

93a. Therrien J, Sui CS, McLaughlin PR, et al: Pulmonary valve replacement in adults late after repair of tetralogy of Fallot: Are we operating too late? J Am Coll Cardiol 35(Suppl A):509A, 1999.

94. Berul CI, Hill SL, Geggel RL, et al: Electrocardiographic markers of late sudden death risk in postoperative tetralogy of Fallot children. J Cardiovasc Electrophysiol 8:1349–1356, 1997.

95. Murphy JG, Gersh BJ, Mair DD, et al: Long-term outcome in patients undergoing surgical repair of tetralogy of Fallot. N Engl J Med 329:593–599, 1993.

96. Rosenthal A: Adults with tetralogy of Fallot—repaired, yes; cured, no (editorial; comment). N Engl J Med 329:655–656, 1993.

97. Waien SA, Liu PP, Ross BL, et al: Serial follow-up of adults with repaired tetralogy of Fallot. J Am Coll Cardiol 20:295–300, 1992.

POST-FONTAN PROCEDURE

98. Choussat A, Fontan F, Besse P, et al: Selection criteria for Fontan's procedure. In Paediatric Cardiology. New York, Churchill-Livingstone, 1999, pp 559–566.

99. Fontan F, Kirklin JW, Fernandez G, et al: Outcome after a "perfect" Fontan operation. Circulation 81:1520–1536, 1990.

100. Gentles TL, Mayer JEJ, Gauvreau K, et al: Fontan operation in five hundred consecutive patients: Factors influencing early and late outcome. J Thorac Cardiovasc Surg 114:376–391, 1997.

101. Gates RN, Laks H, Drinkwater DC Jr, et al: The Fontan procedure in adults. Ann Thorac Surg 63:1085–1090, 1997.

102. Stumper O, Sutherland GR, Geuskens R, et al: Transesophageal echocardiography in evaluation and management after a Fontan procedure. J Am Coll Cardiol 17:1152–1160, 1991.

103. Fishberger SB, Wernovsky G, Gentles TL, et al: Factors that influence the development of atrial flutter after the Fontan operation. J Thorac Cardiovasc Surg 113:80–86, 1997.

104. Durongpisitkul K, Porter CJ, Cetta F, et al: Predictors of early- and late-onset supraventricular tachyarrhythmias after Fontan operation. Circulation 98:1099–1107, 1998.

105. Peters NS, Somerville J: Arrhythmias after the Fontan procedure. Br Heart J 68:199–204, 1992.

106. Amodeo A, Galletti L, Marianeschi S, et al: Extracardiac Fontan operation for complex cardiac anomalies: Seven years' experience. J Thorac Cardiovasc Surg 114:1020–1030, 1997.

107. Shirai LK, Rosenthal DN, Reitz BA, et al: Arrhythmias and thromboembolic complications after the extracardiac Fontan operation. J Thorac Cardiovasc Surg 115:499–505, 1998.

108. Kaulitz R, Luhmer I, Bergmann F, et al: Sequelae after modified Fontan operation: Postoperative haemodynamic data and organ function. Heart 78:154–159, 1997.

109. Jahangiri M, Shore D, Kakkar V, et al: Coagulation factor abnormalities after the Fontan procedure and its modifications. J Thorac Cardiovasc Surg 113:989–992; discussion 992–993. 1997.

110. Mertens L, Hagler DJ, Sauer U, et al: Protein-losing enteropathy after the Fontan operation: An international multicenter study. PLE study group. J Thorac Cardiovasc Surg 115:1063–1073, 1998.

111. Balaji S, Johnson TB, Sade RM, et al: Management of atrial flutter after the Fontan procedure. J Am Coll Cardiol 23:1209–1215, 1994.

112. Mavroudis C, Backer CL, Deal BJ, Johnsrude CL: Fontan conversion to cavopulmonary connection and arrhythmia circuit cryoblation. J Thorac Cardiovasc Surg 115:547–556, 1998.

112a. Deal BJ, Mavroudis C, Backer CL, et al: Impact of arrhythmia circuit cryoablation during Fontan conversion for refractory atrial tachycardia. Am J Cardiol 83:563–568, 1999.

113. Fishberger SB, Wernovsky G, Gentles TL, et al: Long-term outcome in patients with pacemakers following the Fontan operation. Am J Cardiol 77:887–889, 1996.

114. Monagle P, Cochrane A, McCrindle B, et al: Thromboembolic complications after Fontan procedures—the role of prophylactic anticoagulation. J Thorac Cardiovasc Surg 115:493–498, 1998.

115. Rychik J, Rome JJ, Jacobs ML: Late surgical fenestration for complications after the Fontan operation. Circulation 96:33–36, 1997.

116. Sierra C, Calleja F, Picazo B, Martinez-Valverde A: Protein-losing enteropathy secondary to Fontan procedure resolved after cardiac transplantation. J Pediatr Gastroenterol Nutr 24:229–230, 1997.

117. Kelly AM, Feldt RH, Driscoll DJ, Danielson GK: Use of heparin in the treatment of protein-losing enteropathy after Fontan operation for complex congenital heart disease. Mayo Clin Proc 73:777–779, 1998.

118. Bac DJ, Van Hagen PM, Postema PT, et al: Octreotide for protein-losing enteropathy with intestinal lymphangiectasia (letter). Lancet 345:1639, 1995.

119. Therrien J, Webb GD, Gatzoulis MA: Reversal of protein losing enteropathy with prednisone therapy in adult patients with modified Fontan operations: Long-term palliation or bridge to cardiac transplantation? Heart 82:241–243, 1999.

120. McElhinney DB, Reddy VM, Moore P, Hanley FL: Revision of previous Fontan connections to extracardiac or intraatrial conduit cavopulmonary anastomosis. Ann Thorac Surg 62:1276–1282, 1996.

121. Kreutzer J, Keane JF, Lock JE, et al: Conversion of modified Fontan procedure to lateral atrial tunnel cavopulmonary anastomosis. J Thorac Cardiovasc Surg 111:1169–1176, 1996.

122. Kouatli AA, Garcia JA, Zellers TM, et al: Enalapril does not enhance exercise capacity in patients after Fontan procedure. Circulation 96:1507–1512, 1997.

123. Shah MJ, Rychik J, Fogel MA, et al: Pulmonary AV malformations after superior cavopulmonary connection: Resolution after inclusion of hepatic veins in the pulmonary circulation. Ann Thorac Surg 63:960–963, 1997.

COMPLETE TRANSPOSITION OF THE GREAT ARTERIES

124. Wilson NJ, Clarkson PM, Barratt-Boyes BG, et al: Long-term outcome after the Mustard repair for simple transposition of the great arteries: 28-year follow-up. J Am Coll Cardiol 32:758–765, 1998.

125. Puley G, Siu S, Connelly M, et al: Arrhythmia and survival in patients > 18 years of age after the Mustard procedure for complete transposition of the great arteries. Am J Cardiol 83:1080–1084, 1999.

126. Myridakis DJ, Ehlers KH, Engle MA: Late follow-up after venous switch operation (Mustard procedure) for simple and complex transposition of the great arteries. Am J Cardiol 74:1030–1036, 1994.

127. Ing FF, Mullins CE, Rose M, et al: Transcatheter closure of the patient ductus arteriosus in adults using the Gianturco coil. Clin Cardiol 19:875–879, 1996.

128. Warnes CA, Somerville J: Transposition of the great arteries: late results in adolescents and adults after the Mustard procedure. Br Heart J 58:148–155, 1987.

129. Rhodes LA, Wernovsky G, Keane JF, et al: Arrhythmias and intracardiac conduction after the arterial switch operation. J Thorac Cardiovasc Surg 109:303–310, 1995.

129a. Haas F, Wottke M, Popper H, Meisner H: Long-term survival and functional follow-up in patients after the arterial switch operation. Ann Thorac Surg 68:1692–1697, 1999.

130. Mahoney LT, Knoedel DL, Skorton DJ: Echocardiographic postoperative assessment of patients with transposition of the great arteries. Echocardiography 12:545–557. 1999.

131. Helvind MH, McCarthy JF, Imamura M, et al: Ventriculo-arterial discordance: Switching the morphologically left ventricle into the systemic circulation after 3 months of age. Eur J Cardiothorac Surg 14:173–178, 1998.

132. Cochrane AD, Karl TR, Mee RB: Staged conversion to arterial switch for late failure of the systemic right ventricle. Ann Thorac Surg 56:854–862, 1993.

133. van Son JA, Reddy VM, Silverman NH, Hanley FL: Regression of tricuspid regurgitation after two-stage arterial switch operation for failing systemic ventricle after atrial inversion operation. J Thorac Cardiovasc Surg 111:342–347, 1996.

134. De Jong PL, Bogers AJ, Witsenburg M, Bos E: Arterial switch for pulmonary venous obstruction complicating Mustard procedure. Ann Thorac Surg 59:1005–1007, 1995.

135. Cetta F, Bonilla JJ, Lichtenberg RC, et al: Anatomic correction of dextro-transposition of the great arteries in a 36-year-old patient. Mayo Clin Proc 72:245–247, 1997.

136. Jenkins KJ, Hanley FL, Colan SD, et al: Function of the anatomic pulmonary valve in the systemic circulation. Circulation 84(Suppl III):III173–III179, 1991.

137. Vouhe PR, Tamisier D, Leca F, et al: Transposition of the great arteries, ventricular septal defect, and pulmonary outflow tract obstruction: Rastelli or Lecompte procedure? J Thorac Cardiovasc Surg 103:428–436, 1992.

138. Lorenz CH, Walker ES, Graham TP Jr, Powers TA: Right ventricular performance and mass by use of cine MRI late after atrial repair of transposition of the great arteries. Circulation 92(Suppl II):II233–II239, 1995.

139. Wilson NJ, Neutze JM, Rutland MD, Ramage MC: Transthoracic echocardiography for right ventricular function late after the Mustard operation. Am Heart J 131:360–367, 1996.

CONGENITALLY CORRECTED TRANSPOSITION OF THE GREAT ARTERIES

140. Van Praagh R, Papagiannis J, Grunenfelder J, et al: Pathologic anatomy of corrected transposition of the great arteries: Medical and surgical implications. Am Heart J 135:772–785, 1998.

141. Ikeda U, Kimura K, Suzuki O, et al: Long-term survival in "corrected transposition." Lancet 337:180–181, 1991.

142. Presbitero P, Somerville J, Rabajoli F, et al: Corrected transposition of the great arteries without associated defects in adult patients: Clinical profile and follow up. Br Heart J 74:57–59, 1995.

143. Sano T, Riesenfeld T, Karl TR, Wilkinson JL: Intermediate-term outcome after intracardiac repair of associated cardiac defects in patients with atrioventricular and ventriculoarterial discordance. Circulation 92(Suppl II):II272–II278, 1995.

144. Szufladowicz M, Horvath P, de Leval M, et al: Intracardiac repair of lesions associated with atrioventricular discordance. Eur J Cadiothorac Surg 10:443–448, 1996.

145. Voskuil M, Hazekamp MG, Kroft LJ, et al: Postsurgical course of patients with congenitally corrected transposition of the great arteries. Am J Cardiol 83:558–562, 1999.

146. Termignon JL, Leca F, Vouhe PR, et al: "Classic" repair of congenitally corrected transposition and ventricular septal defect. Ann Thorac Surg 62:199–206, 1996.

147. Connelly MS, Liu PP, Williams WG, et al: Congenitally corrected transposition of the great arteries in the adult: Functional status and complications [see comments]. J Am Coll Cardiol 27:1238–1243, 1996.

148. van Son JA, Danielson GK, Huhta JC, et al: Late results of systemic atrioventricular valve replacement in corrected transposition. J Thorac Cardiovasc Surg 109:642–652, 1995.

149. Imai Y: Double-switch operation for congenitally corrected transposition. Adv Cardiac Surg 9:65–86, 1997.

150. Karl TR, Weintraub RG, Brizard CP, et al: Senning plus arterial switch operation for discordant (congenitally corrected) transposition. Ann Thorac Surg 64:495–502, 1997.

151. Yagihara T, Kishimoto H, Isobe F, et al: Double switch operation in cardiac anomalies with atrioventricular and ventriculoarterial discordance. J Thorac Cardiovasc Surg 107:351–358, 1994.

152. Stumper O, Wright JG, De Giovanni JV, et al: Combined atrial and arterial switch procedure for congenital corrected transposition with ventricular septal defect. Br Heart J 73:479–482, 1995.

153. Horvath P, Szufladowicz M, de Leval MR, et al: Tricuspid valve abnormalities in patients with atrioventricular discordance: Surgical implications. Ann Thorac Surg 57:941–945, 1994.

154. Silka MJ, Rice MJ: Paradoxic embolism due to altered hemodynamic sequencing following transvenous pacing. Pacing Clin Electrophysiol 14:499–503, 1991.

155. Prieto LR, Hordof AJ, Secic M, et al: Progressive tricuspid valve disease in patients with congenitally corrected transposition of the great arteries. Circulation 98:997–1005, 1998.

EISENMENGER SYNDROME

156. Daliento L, Somerville J, Presbitero P, et al: Eisenmenger syndrome: Factors relating to deterioration and death. Eur Heart J 19:1845–1855, 1998.

157. Saha A, Balakrishnan KG, Jaiswal PK, et al: Prognosis for patients with Eisenmenger syndrome of various aetiology. Int J Cardiol 45:199–207, 1994.

158. Vongpatanasin W, Brickner ME, Hillis LD, Lange RA: The Eisenmenger syndrome in adults. Ann Intern Med 128:745–755, 1998.

159. Ammash NM, Connolly HM, Abel MD, Warnes CA: Noncardiac surgery in Eisenmenger syndrome. J Am Coll Cardiol 33:222–227, 1999.

160. Dajani AS, Taubert KA, Wilson W, et al: Prevention of bacterial endocarditis: Recommendations by the American Heart Association. JAMA 277:1794–1801, 1997.

161. O'Kelly SW, Hayden-Smith J: Eisenmenger's syndrome: Surgical perspectives and anaesthetic implications. Br J Hosp Med 51:150–153, 1994.

162. Bowyer JJ, Busst CM, Denison DM, Shinebourne EA: Effect of long term oxygen treatment at home in children with pulmonary vascular disease. Br Heart J 55:385–390, 1986.

163. Harinck E, Hutter PA, Hoorntje TM, et al: Air travel and adults with cyanotic congenital heart disease. Circulation 93:272–276, 1996.

164. Hosenpud JD, Novick RJ, Bennett LE, et al: The Registry of the International Society for Heart and Lung Transplantation: Thirteenth official report—1996. J Heart Lung Transplant 15:655–674, 1996.

165. Bridges ND, Mallory GB Jr, Huddleston CB, et al: Lung transplantation in children and young adults with cardiovascular disease. Ann Thorac Surg 59:813–820; discussion 820–821, 1995.

166. Wong CK, Yeung DW, Lau CP, et al: Improvement of exercise capacity after nifedipine in patients with Eisenmenger syndrome complicating ventricular septal defect. Clin Cardiol 14:957–961, 1991.

167. Wimmer M, Schlemmer M: Long-term hemodynamic effects of nifedipine on congenital heart disease with Eisenmenger's mechanism in children. Cardiovasc Drugs Ther 6:183–186, 1992.

168. Hopkins WE, Kelly DP: Angiotensin-converting enzyme inhibitors in adults with cyanotic congenital heart disease. Am J Cardiol 77:439–440, 1996.

169. Rosenzweig EB, Kerstein D, Barst RJ: Long-term prostacyclin for pulmonary hypertension with associated congenital heart defects. Circulation 99:1858–1865, 1999.

170. Batista RJ, Santos JL, Takeshita N, et al: Successful reversal of pulmonary hypertension in Eisenmenger complex. Arq Bras Cardiol 68:279–280, 1997.

171. Perloff JK, Rosove MH, Child JS, Wright GB: Adults with cyanotic congenital heart disease: Hematologic management. Ann Intern Med 109:406–413, 1988.

172. Perloff JK, Marelli AJ, Miner PD: Risk of stroke in adults with cyanotic congenital heart disease. Circulation 87:1954–1959, 1993.

173. Ammash N, Warnes CA: Cerebrovascular events in adult patients with cyanotic congenital heart disease. J Am Coll Cardiol 28:768–772, 1999.

174. Perloff JK, Marelli A: Neurological and psychosocial disorders in adults with congenital heart disease. Heart Dis Stroke 1:218–224, 1992.

175. Perloff JK: Systemic complications of cyanosis in adults with congenital heart disease: Hematologic derangements, renal function, and urate metabolism. Cardiol Clin 11:689–699, 1993.

Chapter 45

Acquired Heart Disease in Children

STEVEN D. COLAN · JANE W. NEWBURGER

The purpose of this chapter is to review cardiac diseases acquired in childhood. Congenital cardiac defects are discussed in Chapters 43 and 44, while neurological diseases that affect the heart are described in Chapter 71. Here we focus on cardiomyopathies, Kawasaki disease, hypertension, and hyperlipidemias.

CARDIOMYOPATHIES (see also Chap. 48)

This diverse group of disorders has historically been understood to represent "heart muscle diseases of unknown etiology,"[1] clearly excluding secondary processes such as hypertension, ischemic heart disease, and valvar and congenital heart disease. In addition, the World Health Organization definition also specifically excluded myocardial disease related to a known systemic disorder. Clinical practice does not concur with these exclusions, and secondary forms of cardiomyopathy are referred to as "anthracycline cardiomyopathy," "infectious cardiomyopathy," and other descriptive terms. Even etiologies that were intended to be specifically excluded have been incorporated under names such as "ischemic cardiomyopathy" and "cardiomyopathy of overload," a term that embodies the clinically familiar concept of load-induced myocyte dysfunction. Cardiomyopathy is now more familiarly taken to imply a disease process involving the heart muscle that results in intrinsic myocardial dysfunction, subcategorized as primary and secondary forms. Classification of the cardiomyopathies as dilated, hypertrophic, and restrictive has fared the test of time somewhat better, although this terminology clearly has problems as well. The mixture of morphology and physiology inherent within this classification is unquestionably problematic because many overlapping cases are encountered. Furthermore, it is clear that the same etiology can be manifested as dilated cardiomyopathy (DCM) in some patients and as hypertrophic cardiomyopathy (HCM) in others and that individual patients can transition between the two. Although this effort at categorization is merely a general, descriptive approach that cannot be relied on for unambiguous classification, it nonetheless provides a clinically useful framework and will be used in this presentation.

Dilated Cardiomyopathy

(see also Chap. 48)

DCM has numerous etiologies, clinical manifestations, and outcomes that vary depending on both the pathogenesis and host response. Multiple associations have been described in children, but most cases remain idiopathic. Although the true frequency of the various causes of DCM is currently unknown, improved methods of diagnosis have enabled determination of the cause for a progressively larger proportion of the previously idiopathic cases. Between one-third and one-half of cases are thought to be familial.[2] Inflammatory heart disease caused by viral myocarditis or an abnormal immunologic response to viral infection is believed to be a common cause, but problems in confirming this diagnosis beyond the acute stage have hampered determination of the true incidence. Progress in molecular identification of viral presence in diseased human heart tissue[3] has created new opportunities to define the relationship between viral infections and myocarditis.

It is generally assumed clinically that the primary functional change at the myofiber level in DCM is depression of contractile function. Despite how commonly this assumption is believed, several groups have shown that isolated cardiac muscle harvested from patients with end-stage heart failure is capable of normal force-generating capacity under ideal conditions and low stimulation frequencies,[4] even when force generation deteriorates at higher stimulation frequencies.[5] In contrast, diastolic abnormalities are a constant property of failing heart muscle.[6] The molecular event or events that account for myocardial failure remain elusive, although many metabolic abnormalities have been described. Numerous abnormalities often coexist, and their relative importance is not known. Although most investigators have sought a single final pathway to contractile dysfunction, this approach may not be correct. Since DCM appears as the end result of many quite different processes, it is likely that numerous metabolic disturbances may have contractile dysfunction as the final common manifestation. Clarification of the disease-specific pathogenesis of contractile failure has no doubt been hampered by our very limited ability to determine etiology.

Clinical Features and Diagnostic Evaluation

Regardless of the underlying cause of the ventricular dysfunction, the congestive cardiomyopathies have a similar mode of expression. Older children experience exercise intolerance, dyspnea on exertion, tachycardia, palpitations, abdominal distention, syncope or near-syncope, and occasionally, cardiovascular collapse and sudden death. Although many symptoms parallel those seen in adults, primary complaints of peripheral edema and paroxysmal nocturnal dyspnea are uncommon in children. Infants are generally recognized on the basis of respiratory distress, abdominal distention, and poor feeding, but occasionally the process is subacute and failure to thrive is present at the time of diagnosis. Secondary cardiomyopathies can manifest a broad spectrum of noncardiac abnormalities, depending on the nature of the primary disorder.

PHYSICAL FINDINGS. Physical findings depend on the severity of clinical compromise. Patients with mild ventricular dysfunction can have reduced exercise capacity but no abnormal physical findings. Congestive heart failure is nearly always accompanied by tachypnea and tachycardia. Peripheral cyanosis is noted only in the presence of severe compromise. Peripheral pulses are often weak and can be difficult to palpate because of narrow pulse pressure and occasionally hypotension. Cool extremities and poor capillary refill can be noted, particularly in infants. Intercostal retractions are a common finding in infants and young children, but in contrast to adults, pulmonary auscultation rarely reveals rales, even when frank pulmonary edema is present on chest radiographs. Wheezing can be heard at all ages because of attenuated airway relaxation, a process that appears to result from the generalized desensitization of beta-adrenergic receptors that is characteristic of congestive heart failure.[7] Hepatomegaly is a seminal finding and can be massive in infants but changes rapidly in response to therapy. Neck vein distention and peripheral edema are almost never observed in infants but become more common with age. The cardiac impulse is often displaced laterally and is frequently diffuse. Gallop rhythm with a third heart sound is common, as is a murmur of mitral regurgitation.

LABORATORY DATA. Cardiomegaly, pulmonary venous congestion, pulmonary edema, atelectasis, and pleural effusions are common radiographic findings. The electrocardiogram (ECG) shows sinus tachycardia in most patients. Nonspecific ST-T wave changes and left ventricular hypertrophy are noted in about half of patients,[8] with atrial and right ventricular hypertrophy in 25%. Just under 50% of patients have arrhythmias on initial evaluation, including atrial fibrillation and flutter, ventricular ectopic beats, and nonsustained ventricular tachycardia on Holter recording. DCM must be differentiated from tachycardia-induced cardiomyopathy, a process that can have similar features but responds to arrhythmia control with complete recovery.[9]

Echocardiography. Diagnostic findings on echocardiography are a dilated left ventricle with diminished systolic performance. Dysfunction is global, although moderate regional variation in wall motion is usually present. Quantitative assessment of systolic and diastolic functional parameters and ventricular morphology is diagnostically and prognostically useful. Pericardial effusions are frequent. Intracardiac thrombi have been reported in as many as 23% of children, although rarely in infants.[10] Color flow and spectral Doppler examinations are useful for assessment of mitral regurgitation, as well as diastolic function. The echocardiogram is equally critical for excluding valvar and structural cardiac disease. Anomalous origin of the left main coronary artery from the pulmonary artery can be reliably recognized through the combined use of imaging and color flow Doppler.[11]

Cardiac Catheterization. This procedure is performed primarily for endomyocardial biopsy. Occasionally, the possibility of a coronary anomaly remains in doubt, in which case coronary arteriography is mandatory. Assessment of hemodynamics is rarely useful for patient management unless the clinical findings are discrepant from the echocardiographic findings, but hemodynamic evaluation has important prognostic implications and is needed if organ transplantation is considered. Biopsy findings in idiopathic DCM are nonspecific and demonstrate myocyte hypertrophy and variable amounts of fibrosis without evidence of inflammatory infiltrates. The primary importance of biopsy is detection of known causes of DCM, including histological or polymerase chain reaction evidence of myocarditis, infiltrative or mitochondrial disorders, cytoskeletal protein defects,[12] and endocardial fibroelastosis (EFE).[10] Numerous rare disorders can be diagnosed only by tissue analysis. A finding of inflammatory heart disease justifies a delay in consideration of transplantation because myocarditis in children is generally associated with a more favorable prognosis,[10] including the potential for complete recovery. The safety of transvenous biopsy has been amply demonstrated,

and extensive experience in its use has been gained through routine application in cardiac transplant recipients. The highest risk is noted in infants,[13] in whom perforation by the stiff biopsy catheters is a recognized complication. However, this patient group is exactly the one in which the results can be most helpful, with the risk-benefit ratio shifted in favor of the test, even in this age group.

DIFFERENTIAL DIAGNOSIS. In children and infants with DCM the differential diagnosis is complex because of the imposing array of possible rare disorders. An ordered and logical algorithm for diagnostic evaluation based on standard and widely available laboratory screening tests has been published[14] and has led to targeted specific testing for particular disorders of metabolism. This field is rapidly evolving as new enzymatic disorders are recognized and must be incorporated within this algorithm.[14a-c] Certain disorders, such as the mitochondrial disorders,[15, 15a-c] can be particularly difficult to diagnose because of tissue-selective and heterogeneous expression related to either tissue-specific isoenzyme or to unbalanced segregation of mutated and wild-type mitochondrial DNA. The defect is biochemically manifested when a certain threshold of mutated mitochondrial DNA is reached. The situation is rendered even more complex by the age-dependent accumulation of mitochondrial DNA deletions that appear to have no causal relation to DCM.[16]

Treatment

In the absence of an identifiable cause, treatment is supportive, nonspecific, and targeted at controlling the symptoms of congestive heart failure. The severity of clinical compromise determines the level of support needed. Critically ill children will generally require mechanical ventilation and inotropic support. Management at centers that have extracorporeal membrane oxygenator and ventricular assist device support available is advised for these patients. Some patients can experience sufficient recovery within a period of days to permit withdrawal of mechanical myocardial support, and the method can at times be used as a bridge to transplantation.[17] Once the patient is stabilized, or in patients who are not critically compromised at the time of initial assessment, oral therapy with digoxin, angiotensin-converting enzyme (ACE) inhibitors, and diuretics remains the mainstay of treatment. Recent data in adults indicate a 30% reduction in deaths when spironolactone is included in the diuretic scheme.[18] This medication is well tolerated in children, and despite the absence of specific data in this age group, these results are fairly compelling for its use. No consensus has been reached regarding which of these agents to institute first in children who do not require multidrug therapy, but asymptomatic ventricular dysfunction is often managed with ACE inhibitors alone because of the absence of significant reported risk.

Arrhythmias are common in children with DCM,[8] and their management is not substantially different from that of adults. Data concerning the utility of ventricular stimulation protocols are rare in children, but the available data suggest that it is useful in risk stratification but not clearly effective in guiding therapy.[19] Intermittent infusion of inotropes such as dobutamine, a common practice in the management of children with severe chronic congestive heart failure, has been based on practice in adult clinics. Although the results in adult studies are mixed, with some trials reporting that survival can be adversely affected, most studies continue to note symptomatic improvement.[20] Intermittent inotrope infusion appears to be a reasonable alternative to achieve stabilization and symptom control in patients awaiting transplantation.

Carnitine deficiency and disorders of carnitine transport can result in DCM and HCM, and in some cases, dietary carnitine supplementation can lead to dramatic cardiac and clinical improvement. In an attempt to avoid delays in therapy, it is not uncommon for clinicians to initiate empirical carnitine supplementation prior to biochemical confirmation of this disorder. In fact, cardiomyopathy is not a prominent feature of myopathic carnitine deficiency, in which skeletal muscle weakness and recurrent metabolic crises dominate. In addition to potentially obscuring diagnostic evaluation, other inborn errors of metabolism have been described that are manifested as DCM but deteriorate rapidly in response to carnitine supplementation.[21] Plasma carnitine concentrations and fatty acid metabolism byproducts should be evaluated in all infants with cardiomyopathy of unknown etiology, but empirical therapy is not advised.

Children with DCM are at risk for intracardiac thrombus formation and systemic embolization. Intracardiac thrombi were seen in 46 to 84 percent of children at autopsy, but their relationship to premorbid findings is unclear since one of these studies documented no intracardiac thrombi during life.[22] Clinical series report the presence of intracardiac thrombi in 0 to 23 percent.[10, 22, 23] Comparison of these studies indicates an age-related trend toward a higher incidence, but none of the series have been large enough to draw firm conclusions. Guidelines for antithrombotic therapy are derived from and parallel those in adults.

Mitral valve regurgitation is common in DCM and in some instances can be moderate or more pronounced in severity. Clinical improvement in symptoms, ventricular function, and survival after mitral valvuloplasty has, however, been reported in patients with DCM.[24, 25] The repair represents a form of afterload reduction, with a fall in wall stress consequent to ventricular remodeling. In patients with moderate to severe mitral regurgitation associated with DCM, valve repair should be seriously considered, but valve replacement generally entails excessive risk.

Several forms of therapy are currently investigational in children. Two recent large and favorable experiences with beta blockers in adults with congestive heart failure[26, 26a] have not been adequately replicated in children. There is ample theoretical justification for their use, and preliminary results in children have been reported,[27] but data on risk-benefit analysis, appropriate dosing schedule, and patient selection criteria are limited. The combination of an ACE inhibitor and beta blocker has been found to result in a synergistic effect in adult patients with asymptomatic dysfunction,[28] an issue that has not been addressed in children. Trials of angiotensin II receptor antagonist[29] use in children have not been reported. Early reports of potential benefits of growth hormone therapy in adults with DCM[30] have not been confirmed in children. Patients with DCM often have markedly asynchronous ventricular activation resulting in a diminished peak force of contraction.[30a] Biventricular DDD pacing with optimized atrioventricular synchrony can improve ventricular performance and has been tried as a therapeutic modality in several small series of adult patients.[31, 31a] Again, no data are available in children. The recent advent of ventricular volume reduction surgery as a means of afterload reduction in patients with end-stage DCM has been attempted in a few children,[32] but the numbers are too few to draw any conclusions. This procedure improves systolic function at the expense of further impairing diastolic function,[33, 33a] with an unpredictable net impact on overall cardiac function. Infants and children with DCM have a marked dominance of systolic dysfunction with less evidence of diastolic dysfunction than is generally noted in adult studies, thus suggesting that they might indeed benefit from this procedure.

Predictors of Outcome

Negative predictors of outcome in children with DCM include the severity of dysfunction, spherical ventricular shape, coexistence of right ventricular dysfunction, familial cardiomyopathy, tissue diagnosis of EFE, persistent cardiomegaly, and persistent congestive heart failure. Tissue diagnosis of myocarditis has been associated with a better out-

come. Ventricular size and mass at initial evaluation have not been found to be predictive of outcome. Younger age at diagnosis has been reported to be associated with a better outcome by some groups,[34] has been associated with a worse outcome by other groups,[35] and in other series has not been found to be a significant factor.[36] One motivation for defining factors predictive of outcome is to facilitate early recommendation for cardiac transplantation. It is therefore disturbing that so little agreement has been found in the many studies to date. Given the heterogeneity of the disorder itself and the small number of patients included in many series, it is likely that the patient samples are quite dissimilar. Entry criteria have also varied substantially among these studies, with specific inclusion of myocarditis in some but exclusion in others. Many of the variables are likely to have a real association with outcome, but the relationship is weak. The fact that commonly used measures of ventricular performance are only weakly predictive of survival severely limits their utility in decisions concerning transplantation.

OUTCOME. Survival statistics for infants (Fig. 45–1) and older children (Fig. 45–2) with idiopathic DCM have varied, with 1-, 2-, 5-, and 10-year survival rates of 41 to 94 percent, 20 to 88 percent, 34 to 86 percent, and 52 to 84 percent, respectively, having been reported. In those who survive, nearly half have full normalization of ventricular function, 25 percent have improved but abnormal function, and 25 percent have persistently severely depressed function.[37] Recovery of function is generally complete within the first year, but occasional patients experience continued late improvement.[10, 38]

Infective Myocarditis (see also Chap. 48)

Myocardial inflammatory diseases are an important cause of DCM in children. Myocarditis cannot be reliably distinguished from other forms of DCM on clinical grounds alone because both the acute and chronic forms have symptoms and functional consequences related to the severity of ventricular dysfunction. A significant number of cases of myocarditis have manifestations that are subclinical and associated with ECG changes or arrhythmias, and in a significant number the myocarditis can be occult or cause sudden death.[39] Nearly all the organisms that cause common infectious illnesses in children can also cause myocarditis,[40] although fewer have been associated with the manifestations of DCM. In addition, myocarditis can occur as a hypersensitivity or toxic reaction and is associated with a number of important systemic diseases such as rheumatic fever.

Management of myocarditis is similar to management of other forms of DCM in that etiology-specific therapy is not generally available. Considerable evidence indicates that the immune response and autoimmunity may play a central role in the acute and chronic myocardial damage,[41] thus suggesting a role for immunosuppressive therapy. Small, uncontrolled trials of corticosteroid therapy in children with evidence of myocarditis[42, 43] have reported favorable outcomes. Similar to trials of these and other immunosuppressive agents in adults, these uncontrolled studies in a disease with a high rate of spontaneous resolution are impossible to interpret. In some centers, administration of high-dose intravenous gamma globulin to children with findings indicative of acute myocarditis has led to improved survival and more rapid recovery of function.[44]

Endocardial Fibroelastosis

(see also Chap. 48)

Diffuse thickening of the left ventricular endocardium secondary to proliferation of fibrous and elastic tissue is an

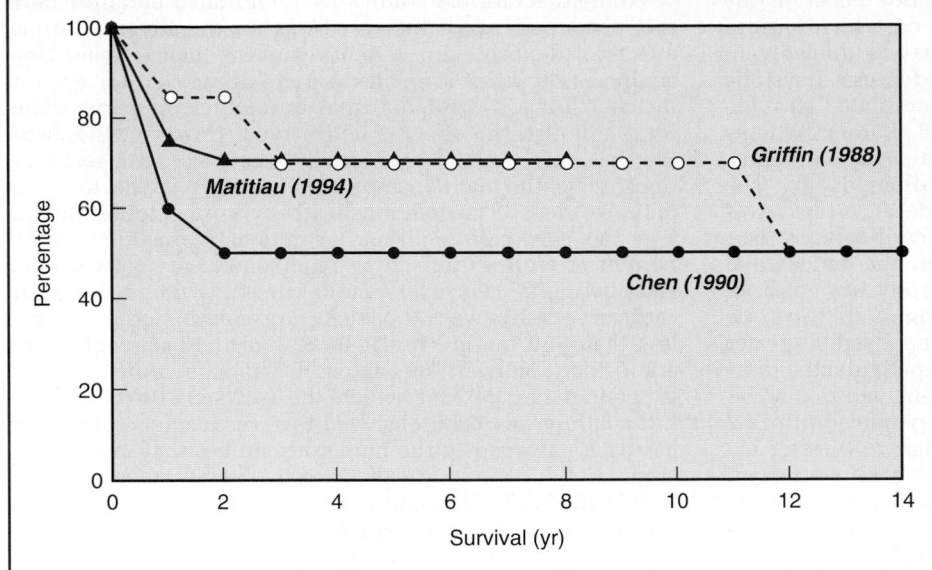

FIGURE 45–1. Survival in infants with idiopathic dilated cardiomyopathy. *Chen (1990):* Chen S, Nouri S, Balfour I, et al: Clinical profile of congestive cardiomyopathy in children. J Am Coll Cardiol 15:189, 1990; *Griffin (1988):* Griffin ML, Hernandez A, Martin TC, et al: Dilated cardiomyopathy in infants and children. J Am Coll Cardiol 11:139, 1988; *Matitiau (1994):* Matitiau A, Perez-Atayde A, Sanders SP, et al: Infantile dilated cardiomyopathy: Relation of outcome to left ventricular mechanics, hemodynamics, and histology at the time of presentation. Circulation 90:1310, 1994.

uncommon but nonspecific response to a variety of inciting agents. The finding was at one time thought to represent a specific disease, but as emphasized by Lurie,[45] it is now clear that EFE represents a final common pathway for many different myocardial stressors. An association with mumps virus infection has been suspected for many years, a theory supported by detection of the mumps virus genome in the myocardium of infants and children.[46] This proposed etiology for a significant proportion of cases is further supported by the observed fall in EFE incidence coincident with implementation of widespread vaccination. Despite the reduction in frequency, this histological finding continues to be reported in association with a wide variety of cardiac diseases, including prenatal and postnatal left ventricular outflow tract obstruction, numerous other forms of congenital heart disease, and many forms of DCM and HCM, as well as being a focal finding in adults with various cardiac disorders.[47] Among the various associations, no single theme emerges, which supports the interpretation that EFE represents a nonspecific tissue response. The pathophysiology of the response is of interest inasmuch as it can provide clues to pathways of injury shared by various diseases.

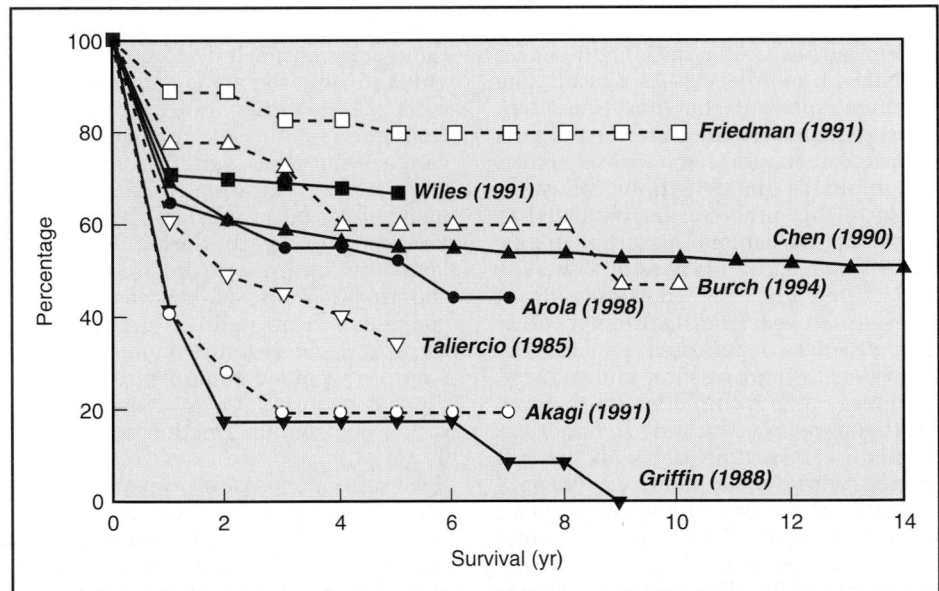

FIGURE 45–2. Survival in children with idiopathic dilated cardiomyopathy. *Akagi (1991):* Akagi T, Benson LN, Lightfoot NE, et al: Natural history of dilated cardiomyopathy in children. Am Heart J 121:1502, 1991; *Arola (1998):* Arola A, Tuominen J, Ruuskanen O, et al: Idiopathic dilated cardiomyopathy in children: Prognostic indicators and outcome. Pediatrics 101:369, 1998; *Burch (1994):* Burch M, Siddiqi SA, Celermajer DS, et al: Dilated cardiomyopathy in children: Determinants of outcome. Br Heart J 72:246, 1994; *Chen (1990):* Chen S, Nouri S, Balfour I, et al: Clinical profile of congestive cardiomyopathy in children. J Am Coll Cardiol 15:189, 1990; *Friedman (1991):* Friedman RA, Moak JP, Garson A Jr: Clinical course of idiopathic dilated cardiomyopathy in children. J Am Coll Cardiol 18:152, 1991; *Griffin (1988):* Griffin ML, Hernandez A, Martin TC, et al: Dilated cardiomyopathy in infants and children. J Am Coll Cardiol 11:139, 1988; *Taliercio (1985):* Taliercio CP, Seward JB, Driscoll DJ, et al: Idiopathic dilated cardiomyopathy in the young: Clinical profile and natural history. J Am Coll Cardiol 6:1126, 1985; *Wiles (1991):* Wiles HB, McArthur PD, Taylor AB, et al: Prognostic features of children with idiopathic dilated cardiomyopathy. Am J Cardiol 68:1372, 1991.

Clinically, more than 80 percent of cases occur in the first year of life, with features dependent on which form of the disease is manifested. Most patients have a dilated ventricle with increased wall thickness and depressed systolic function. The clinical manifestations of the dilated form are similar to findings in other types of DCM. Rarely, patients have a contracted form characterized by a small left ventricle and a clinical picture of restrictive cardiomyopathy. The diagnosis of EFE is most commonly made at autopsy. Although EFE is often suspected on echocardiography (see Chap. 7) when the ultrasound signal from the endocardial surface is unusually strong, echocardiography has not been found to be a reliable diagnostic technique.[48] EFE can be recognized on endomyocardial biopsy, and despite greater involvement of the left ventricle in many patients, the diagnosis can frequently be confirmed on right ventricular biopsy. An autopsy series found that most patients with EFE had right ventricular involvement, although to a lesser extent than on the left,[49] but the diagnostic accuracy of endomyocardial biopsy of the right ventricle has not been systematically tested. The purpose of the diagnosis is primarily for prognosis since in some clinical situations the finding of EFE has been associated with a poor outcome. For example, in case series of DCM, EFE is often identified as one of the risk factors for death.[10, 23] Nevertheless, in a group of patients with idiopathic EFE, the 4-year survival rate was 77 percent, which is not worse than rates reported in other forms of DCM.

Doxorubicin Cardiomyopathy

(see Chaps. 48 and 69)

The anthracycline antibiotics include a number of valuable antitumor agents, with doxorubicin (Adriamycin) in particular having the broadest spectrum of antitumor activity of the available cancer chemotherapeutic agents. Thousands of children have received doxorubicin over the past 30 years for several of the most common pediatric oncological disorders, including acute lymphocytic leukemia. A dramatic improvement in long-term survival after childhood cancer has occurred during the same time interval. As a result, late residua from therapy often represent the most important clinical problem for these patients. Among these residua is doxorubicin-associated cardiomyopathy, the consequences of which continue to unfold as the length of follow-up increases. The magnitude of this problem has escalated to the point that for many pediatric centers, doxorubicin cardiomyopathy accounts for the majority of cases of DCM.

CLINICAL FEATURES. Clinically, the most significant problems relate to a chronic, dose-related cardiomyopathy. Historically, cardiomyopathy was manifested by left ventricular dysfunction, elevated filling pressure, and reduced cardiac output 2 to 4 months after completion of therapy. The myocardial insult is often delayed for a period after the last dose of the drug because of a time delay in the full cytotoxic effect of the drug, with a mean latency between 3 and 8 weeks. More recently, new onset of congestive heart failure has been described in patients years after completion of therapy.[50] As a group, these patients manifest a low incidence of depressed contractility. The dominant abnormality is elevated afterload related to inadequate hypertrophy in the absence of significant dilation.[50, 51] Total cumulative dose, age at the time of doxorubicin therapy, and duration since completion of therapy each relate to the incidence of cardiac abnormalities. Excess afterload is a particular risk for young children; it appears gradually and is manifested as inadequate myocardial growth when compared with the rate of somatic growth. This form of doxorubicin-mediated cardiac injury appears to represent impaired growth capacity of the myocardium, a problem of particular importance to a small child.

Numerous clinical studies have identified certain factors that place patients at increased risk for the adverse cardiac effects of doxorubicin. Patients younger than 4 years have an increased risk.[50] Females are at higher risk on a dose-matched basis.[52, 53] Mediastinal irradiation increases toxicity,[54] although the effect is not marked. However, the factor that has been consistently found to bear the strongest relationship to the incidence of cardiotoxicity is the total cumulative dose. The relationship between the total cumulative dose of doxorubicin and symptomatic cardiotoxicity is nonlinear, with an inflection point somewhere between 400 and 600 mg/m². For example, in one study the incidence of cardiomyopathy was 7 percent in subjects who received less than 550 mg/m², but it increased to 18 percent in the group that received 700 mg/m².[55] Although some variation is seen in the dose at which the incidence of congestive heart failure has been observed to rise, this general pattern has been observed in the numerous studies that have examined it.

PREVENTION. Recognition of the dose-related nature of early-onset congestive heart failure has resulted in nearly universal limitation of the cumulative dose to less than 350 to 450 mg/m², which successfully reduces this complication to 1 percent or less. Although late toxicity also appears to be dose related, doses as low as 90 to 220 mg/m² still represent a measurable risk,[50, 51] with no "safe" dose having been demonstrated. In addition to uniform dose reduction for all patients, alternative means of toxicity reduction that have been reported include dosing regimens designed to reduce peak serum levels (such as continuous infusion), coadministration of agents aimed at providing cardioprotection, and programmed dose reduction as dictated by one of several monitoring programs. Numerous agents with the potential to reduce doxorubicin cardiotoxicity have been tried in animal and human trials, but at present the most promising is dexrazoxane (ICRF-187). Dexrazoxane has a plausible mechanism of action (iron chelation),[56] evidence of reduced early and late toxicity in animals, and promising early results in clinical trials in children.[57]

Cardiac monitoring programs that attempt to detect cardiotoxicity on an individual basis, thereby permitting individual dosing regimens and dose reduction in patients with evidence of cardiac injury, are both widely used and highly contentious.[58, 59] Although the means used to detect myocardial injury has varied from study to study, in other regards the monitoring programs that have been recommended are quite similar. The basic approach is to evaluate patients periodically during doxorubicin therapy and to delay or discontinue treatment with the drug in patients with abnormal test results. It is generally agreed that the onset of congestive heart failure justifies cessation of doxorubicin therapy. However, the more typical scenario is a patient who has received some fraction of the intended cumulative dose of doxorubicin, at which time an asymptomatic drop in left ventricular function is detected. For patients treated by set protocols, if the fall in function exceeds some predefined criteria, cessation of anthracycline therapy is advised. This approach is advocated to minimize adverse cardiac outcomes.[58] However, opponents of published criteria voice concern that the impact of these programs on overall outcome has not been addressed.[59] Fundamentally, it is important to recognize that administration of anthracyclines is intrinsically a compromise between cancer cure and cardiac injury such that any reduction in the total cumulative dose decreases the antitumor effect. Even a reduction in cumulative dose from 270 to 180 mg/m² has been shown to have a detectable impact on the cancer cure rate.[51] Similarly, cardiotoxicity is a progressive phenomenon, with mild but detectable injury even at very low doses.[50, 51] Evaluation of the success of any cardiac monitoring program must include a decision regarding what severity of cardiac injury is unacceptable to achieve the desired antitumor effect. At perhaps the most simplistic level, dose reduction in response to a monitoring program should result in verifiable net improvement in survival. However, at present the benefits of serial cardiac assessment for doxorubicin-induced cardiomyopathy as a means of dose adjustment remain enticing but unproven.

Hypertrophic Cardiomyopathy

(see Chap. 48)

HCM is defined as the presence of ventricular hypertrophy without an identifiable hemodynamic cause such as hypertension, valvular heart disease, catecholamine-secreting tumors, hyperthyroidism, or any other condition that could secondarily stimulate cardiac hypertrophy. It is clear that HCM represents a heterogeneous group of disorders, and this diversity is more apparent in childhood than at any other age. These disorders can be subdivided into primary and secondary forms, where the primary form is a familial disorder ("familial HCM") typically devoid of findings outside of the heart. Secondary forms include diseases such as Friedreich ataxia, where ventricular hypertrophy is common but not the dominant clinical manifestation (see Chap. 71), and others such as glycogenosis type IX, in which a systemic disorder has primarily or exclusively cardiac manifestations.

Familial Hypertrophic Cardiomyopathy

CLINICAL DESCRIPTION. In about half of affected patients, it is possible to elicit a history of another family member with familial HCM or a family history of sudden death at a young age. Although many young patients are asymptomatic, the full spectrum of symptoms associated with this disease can be present from early childhood. Limitation of exercise capacity because of either dyspnea or chest pain is often the primary and most disabling symptom in familial HCM. As a group, exercise performance is impaired, even when asymptomatic patients are included.[60] Chest pain, which is an extremely unusual finding in most forms of heart disease in children, is common in children with familial HCM and can have characteristics of angina; however, the chest pain is often atypical in that it occurs at rest, has a variable threshold of onset, and is at times prolonged. Infants with familial HCM often have clinical features more typical of congestive heart failure, with a history of tachypnea, hepatomegaly, and poor feeding and growth. Palpitations are common in adults but rarely noted by children. Syncope occurs in 15 to 25 percent of adult subjects. Although syncope is less common in childhood, it is strongly associated with the risk of sudden death.

PHYSICAL FINDINGS. Most children and young adults are remarkably healthy, with a frequent predilection for athletics. Although many physical findings have been described in this disease, most relate to dynamic ventricular outflow obstruction and are absent in subjects without obstruction. Therefore, a completely normal physical examination in a healthy patient who may be quite athletic does not exclude the presence of this potentially fatal disorder, an observation that has led some observers to suggest echocardiographic screening as part of an evaluation prior to sports participation. The apical and parasternal cardiac impulses are often augmented but rarely displaced. Hepatomegaly is common in infants but is generally not seen beyond this age. In the presence of outflow obstruction, a bisferious carotid pulse can be encountered that corresponds to the "spike-and-dome" aortic pulse contour of patients with dynamic outflow obstruction. Parasternal and carotid systolic thrills are frequent in patients with left or right ventricular outflow obstruction. The murmur of dynamic left ventricular outflow obstruction can be noted, and it rises in intensity with physiological maneuvers that lower preload or afterload or increase contractility. Very loud systolic murmurs are usually found in subjects with subpulmonary stenosis, which is more common in infants and children. The murmur of mitral regurgitation is frequent in patients with subaortic stenosis, although diffi-

cult to separate from the outflow murmur. Aortic regurgitation can be heard but is less commonly encountered than in discrete subaortic stenosis.

ELECTROCARDIOGRAM AND HOLTER RECORDING. Although the vast majority of patients with familial HCM and obstruction to left ventricular outflow have an abnormal ECG, about 25 percent of patients without obstruction have a normal ECG. The most common abnormalities are left ventricular hypertrophy, ST segment and T wave abnormalities, and abnormal Q waves. Atrial fibrillation develops in approximately 15 percent of adults with familial HCM but is unusual in children. Symptomatic ventricular tachycardia on Holter recording or induced at electrophysiology study appears to identify a high-risk subgroup.[61] Although syncope is a risk factor for sudden death,[62] the presence of asymptomatic ventricular tachycardia on Holter recording is not a risk factor.[63] In children, ventricular arrhythmias on Holter recording are less frequent than in adults.

ECHOCARDIOGRAM. The echocardiogram permits noninvasive assessment of ventricular size, wall thickness, systolic and diastolic function, outflow obstruction, and valvar insufficiency. Localized hypertrophy of the anterior septum is seen in 10 to 15 percent of patients, and 20 to 35 percent of patients have involvement of both anterior and posterior portions of the septum. At least 50 percent of patients have involvement of the anterolateral free wall in addition to the septum. The incidence of isolated involvement of the posterior and apical portions of the septum or anterolateral free wall without hypertrophy of the anterior septum is as much as 20 percent. The reported incidence of concentric hypertrophy is quite variable but can be as much as 20 percent. The anatomical pattern has not proved to be predictive of outcome but is a primary determinant of outflow obstruction and is an important factor in surgical planning.[64]

EXERCISE TESTING. Quantitative assessment of functional capacity is useful for documenting clinical status, as well as for objectively assessing the response to therapeutic interventions. High-grade arrhythmias are elicited in some patients and have a negative prognostic implication. A hypotensive response to exercise appears to represent a risk for sudden death,[65] but more definitively, a normal exercise blood pressure response identifies a low-risk cohort.[66] Children and young adults with thallium scintigraphic evidence of ischemia have been reported to be at increased risk of sudden death.[67] Unfortunately, ECG changes with exercise are an unreliable marker of ischemia because they occur with equal frequency in patients with and without inducible ischemia.

CATHETERIZATION. The hemodynamic findings in familial HCM depend on the presence or absence of obstruction. The right ventricle can be involved, particularly in infants and children, and can demonstrate outflow gradients and elevated diastolic pressure. In infants, the septum often impinges on right ventricular outflow, and right ventricular cavity obliteration in systole can be noted. Myocardial bridges, i.e., muscle bands overlying epicardial coronary arteries, are congenital and sufficiently common (having been observed in 20 to 66 percent of hearts) that they are considered an anatomical variant rather than a congenital anomaly.[68] Despite angiographic evidence of systolic compression of the underlying coronary artery, little evidence supports the hypothesis that myocardial bridges can be associated with ischemia. Compression of the coronary artery by myocardial bridges has been detected angiographically in 30 percent of adults with familial HCM,[69] with no evidence of adverse impact on outcome. In a recent provocative report of a relationship between sudden death and the presence of myocardial bridging in children with familial HCM, Yetman and associates suggested that surgical unroofing of the coronary artery can prevent sudden death.[70] These authors describe delayed diastolic filling of the affected coronary artery as a mechanism for ischemia. It is unclear why myocardial bridges would have a greater impact on children than has been described in adults, so further confirmation is required before myocardial bridging can be accepted as an adverse risk factor worthy of surgical intervention.

DIFFERENTIAL DIAGNOSIS. Ultimately, the diagnosis of familial HCM depends on molecular identification of the offending gene or the abnormal gene product. Until this test is available on a commercial basis, reliance on current, less than perfect diagnostic tools is necessary. Although echocardiographic identification of hypertrophy is the primary diagnostic modality in current clinical use, familial HCM with an associated risk of sudden death can be present even in the absence of hypertrophy. Surprisingly, when a genotyped population is investigated, the usual ECG and echocardiographic criteria accurately detect disease in only 83 percent of adults and only 50 percent of children.[71] Under these circumstances, the need for alternative diagnostic modalities is apparent. Endomyocardial biopsy is useful for excluding other causes of HCM, including mitochondrial disorders and storage diseases, and is therefore recommended in infants and young children. However, the primary histological abnormality of focal myocardial disarray is not unique to familial HCM and cannot be reliably detected on biopsy specimens.

Although isolated case reports have described HCM in association with many disorders, in a number of disorders HCM is seen with sufficient frequency to indicate that it is an intrinsic element of the disease (Table 45–1). Patients with Friedreich ataxia have a 25 to 50 percent incidence of HCM, with clinical characteristics quite different from those of familial HCM (see also Chap. 71). HCM is seen in up to 20 to 30 percent of patients with Noonan syndrome,[72] with findings similar to those in familial HCM. Although the risk of congestive heart failure is more common than in familial HCM, there is also at least some risk of sudden death.[73] Infants of diabetic mothers and neonates exposed to corticosteroids often have transient biventricular hypertrophy, sometimes with outflow tract obstruction and occasionally causing symptoms. Finally, many genetic disorders are often accompanied by cardiac hypertrophy. Generally, HCM in infants is associated with unique problems in the differential diagnosis. In various series, diseases other than familial HCM have accounted for 30 to 70 percent of HCM cases in patients younger than 2 years.[73] Hypertrophy with depressed function is rare in familial HCM and highly suggestive of a metabolic or mitochondrial disorder.[74] Myocardial biopsy is often necessary to distinguish among these disorders, is recommended in all patients younger than 2 years, and can be particularly helpful in children with symmetrical hypertrophy or depressed function who have no family history of familial HCM.[74] Mitochondrial disorders present a particular problem in diagnosis because of variable and often tissue-specific involvement.

Differentiation between physiological hypertrophy secondary to athletic participation and pathological hypertrophy in familial HCM is a frequent and important problem in children and young adults. The cardiac response to chronic, intense exercise has been well characterized and includes dilation and hypertrophy with preservation of myocardial contractility. The hypertrophic response is most intense in sports that elicit a marked rise in blood pressure during exercise, such as rowing, wrestling, and power lifting. Wall thickness greater than 13 mm, as occasionally found in athletes, and the not infrequent

▼ **TABLE 45–1. CONDITIONS OTHER THAN FAMILIAL HYPERTROPHIC CARDIOMYOPATHY ASSOCIATED WITH HYPERTROPHIC CARDIOMYOPATHY**

Syndromes
  Beckwith-Wiedemann syndrome
  Cardiac-facial-cutaneous syndrome
  Costello syndrome
  Friedreich ataxia
  Lentiginosis (LEOPARD syndrome)
  Noonan syndrome
Secondary forms
  Anabolic steroid therapy and abuse
  Infant of diabetic mother
  Prenatal and postnatal corticosteroid therapy
Metabolic disorders
  Carnitine deficiency (carnitine palmitoyltransferase II deficiency, carnitine-acylcarnitine translocase deficiency)
  Fucosidosis type 1
  Glycogenoses types II, III, and IX (Pompe disease, Forbes disease, phosphorylase kinase deficiency)
  Glycolipid lipidosis (Fabry disease)
  I cell disease
  Lipodystrophy, total
  Mannosidosis
  Mitochondrial disorders (multiple forms)
  Mucopolysaccharidoses types I, II, and V (Hurler syndrome, Hunter syndrome, Scheie syndrome)
  Selenium deficiency

LEOPARD = lentigenes (multiple), electrocardiographic conduction abnormalities, ocular hypertelorism, pulmonary stenosis, abnormal genitalia, retardation of growth, and sensorineural deafness.

occurrence of mild left ventricular hypertrophy in patients with familial HCM result in a significant incidence of diagnostic ambiguity. ECG has not been particularly helpful in differentiation because of the frequent presence of ECG abnormalities in athletes.[75] Echocardiographic and clinical features that increase the probability of familial HCM include (1) a family history of HCM or early sudden death, (2) significant regional differences in hypertrophy, (3) diastolic dysfunction, (4) abnormal ultrasonic myocardial reflectivity, (5) absence of deconditioning-induced regression of hypertrophy, and (6) abnormalities in coronary flow reserve.[76] Ultimately, differentiation by available techniques is simply not possible in some subjects.

MANAGEMENT

The therapeutic options available in children are not fundamentally different from those in adults (see Chap. 48). Although safety data from small series are available for most of these alternatives, no sufficiently large studies have independently addressed efficacy in infants or children. Chest pain and dyspnea are often relieved by propranolol, but improved exercise capacity is seen less often, and side effects such as fatigue and depression are often encountered. Calcium channel blockers can also reduce dyspnea and chest pain, and an increase in exercise capacity usually occurs. Although older patients with congestive heart failure can be intolerant of these drugs, pediatric tolerance has been excellent, even in neonates.[73] While several retrospective studies report a reduced risk of sudden death,[73, 77, 78] definitive controlled trials to support this finding are not available.

Each of the several interventions used to reduce outflow obstruction in adults with familial HCM and subaortic stenosis (surgery, asynchronous pacing, and septal ablation) are also available to children, but additional technical considerations affect the risk-benefit ratio. Often, clinicians attach too much significance to the presence or absence of outflow obstruction, as discussed by Criley.[79] Outflow obstruction is present in less than half of patients with familial HCM and is not predictive of outcome, with symptomatic patients without obstruction faring more poorly than those who have gradients. The magnitude of outflow obstruction is unrelated to the occurrence of ventricular tachycardia or risk of sudden death. Surgical or pharmacological reduction in the outflow gradient in symptomatic patients is usually associated with a reduction in symptoms, although the incidence of sudden death is not improved. In general, dynamic outflow obstruction is not a negative prognostic factor, and interventions aimed at reducing the gradient are justified only inasmuch as symptomatic benefit can be anticipated.

SEPTAL MYOTOMY-MYECTOMY. In symptomatic HCM with subaortic stenosis, this procedure results in symptomatic improvement in nearly all patients despite the fact that symptoms are generally not correlated with the presence and degree of obstruction. Results in children have been similar to those reported in adults.[80] Although occasional studies have reported improved survival, most have documented no change. Consequently, surgery should be considered for relief of symptoms in patients with intractable and debilitating symptoms in spite of maximum medical therapy. Intervention based on gradient alone cannot be recommended.

ASYNCHRONOUS VENTRICULAR PACING. This technique has emerged as an effective method of symptomatic treatment in some patients with left ventricular outflow tract obstruction.[81] Studies in small cohorts of children with outflow obstruction who were symptomatic despite medical therapy have reported symptomatic improvement, reduced outflow obstruction, and improved exercise tolerance.[82, 83] Controlled studies in adults found that only about 60 percent of patients improved, in two-thirds of these the benefit appeared to reflect a placebo effect, and an adverse effect on symptoms was seen in 5 percent.[84] Pacemaker implantation is associated with a significant incidence of complications,[85] particularly in growing children. Based on current information, dual-chamber pacing can be considered as an alternative to surgical or transcatheter septal reduction in patients with obstructive HCM who are symptomatic despite maximum medical therapy.

EXERCISE RESTRICTION. Avoidance of strenuous exercise is generally recommended for patients with familial HCM. The rationale for this restriction is based on the observations that sudden death is the usual cause of death in familial HCM and has a higher than expected association with exercise,[86] and that familial HCM is believed to be the most common cause of sudden death in young, competitive athletes.[87] Nevertheless, the basis for this recommendation has several serious weaknesses.[88] The true incidence of familial HCM in athletes who experience sudden death is uncertain since genetic confirmation was not available and diagnosis was based on morphological criteria that cannot unequivocally differentiate familial HCM from physiological hypertrophy. It is clear that some patients with familial HCM tolerate intense, competitive athletic participation without symptoms or sudden death.[89] Population studies have documented the

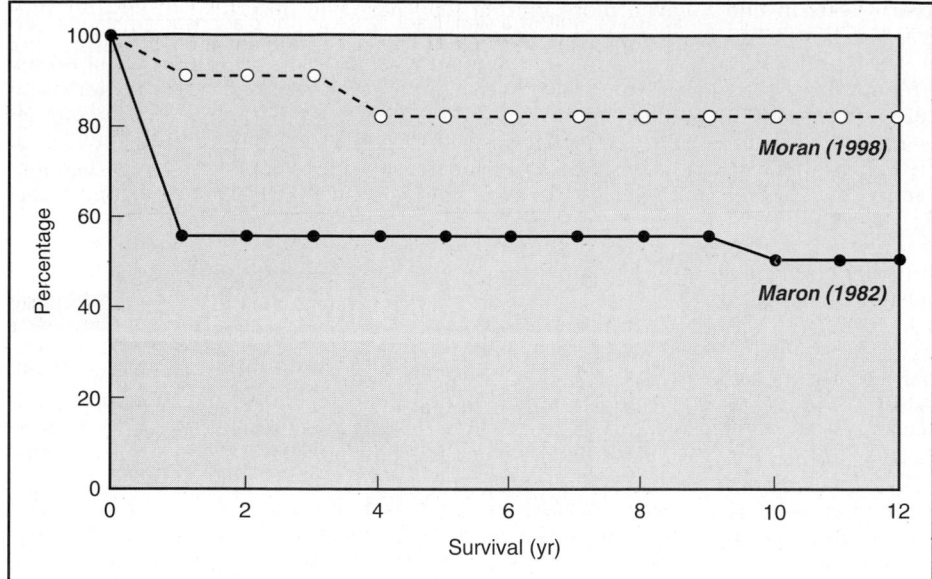

FIGURE 45-3. Survival in infants with hypertrophic cardiomyopathy. *Maron (1982):* Maron BJ, Tajik AJ, Ruttenberg HD, et al: Hypertrophic cardiomyopathy in infants: Clinical features and natural history. Circulation 65:7, 1982; *Moran (1998):* Moran AM, Colan SD: Verapamil therapy in infants with hypertrophic cardiomyopathy. Cardiol Young 8:310, 1998.

apparent paradox that although patients with coronary artery disease who regularly participate in low- and high-level exertion have a transient increase in the risk for sudden death during intense exercise, these individuals experience an overall reduction in the risk for sudden death (see Chap. 26).[90] In addition, patients who do not exercise regularly have an exaggerated risk of sudden death during exercise. Studies have not been conducted to determine whether athletic participation increases the overall risk for sudden death; it has not been shown that survival is improved in those who do not exercise, nor is the level of exercise that represents a safe limit known. Detraining and social stigmatization are particularly difficult problems for an adolescent who is excluded from the usual school activities and peer interactions. Competitive team sports elicit an emotional overlay that appears to increase the risk associated with the sport itself, in addition to demanding more intense exercise. Certain activities such as weightlifting are associated with high levels of circulating catecholamines that can predispose to arrhythmias and elicit a marked stimulus to eccentric cardiac hypertrophy. However, little evidence indicates that moderate aerobic-type exercise is a significant risk in these patients, and it does provide measurable hemodynamic and psychological benefits.

RISK STRATIFICATION. Many prognostic factors for sudden death have been reported, but few have been confirmed. It is likely that the availability of genotyping will permit genetic risk stratification (see Fig. 48–11), but at present, four major risk factors have been identified: a family history of sudden death, exercise-induced hypotension, syncope, and symptomatic nonsustained ventricular tachycardia on Holter recording. Patients free of all risk factors are considered to be at low risk, and interventions (other than for symptoms such as chest pain or exercise intolerance) are not indicated. With two or more risk factors or with syncope alone in children, risk is considered high and aggressive management such as with an implantable cardioverter-fibrillator is recommended (see Chaps. 23 to 25). No consensus has been reached on management of intermediate-risk patients. Additional negative prognostic factors such as evidence of ischemia on exercise thallium testing, marked QT dispersion, and myocardial bridging can also be useful in management decisions for these patients.[91]

CLINICAL COURSE. The clinical course of familial HCM is highly age dependent. HCM in infancy appears to carry a worse prognosis than in older age groups. Symptomatic infants generally manifest congestive heart failure and cyanosis and have been reported to have a particularly poor

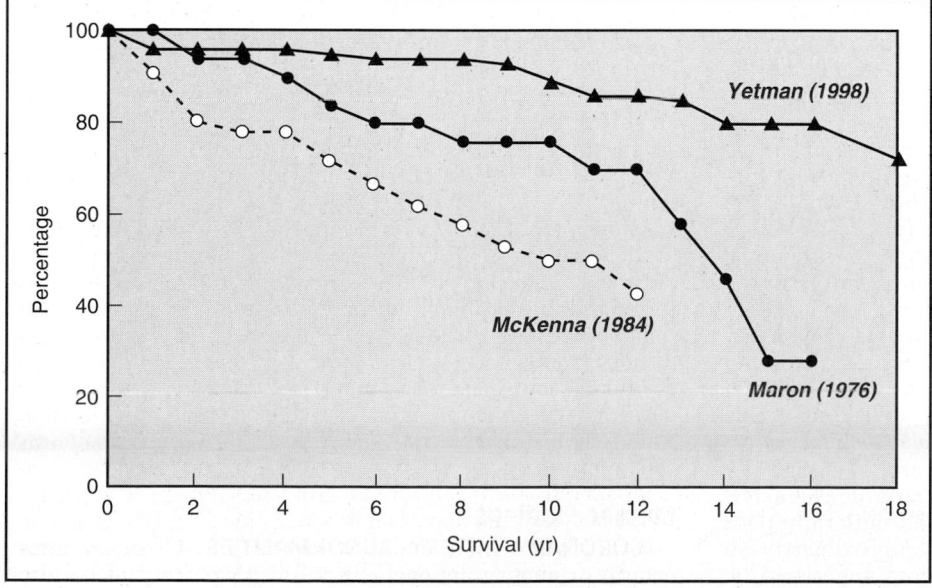

FIGURE 45-4. Survival in children with hypertrophic cardiomyopathy. *Maron (1976):* Maron BJ, Henry WL, Clark CE, et al: Asymmetric septal hypertrophy in childhood. Circulation 53:9, 1976; *McKenna (1984):* McKenna WJ, Deanfield JE: Hypertrophic cardiomyopathy: An important cause of sudden death. Arch Dis Child 59:971, 1984; *Yetman (1998):* Yetman AT, Hamilton RM, Benson LN, et al: Long-term outcome and prognostic determinants in children with hypertrophic cardiomyopathy. J Am Coll Cardiol 32:1943, 1998.

outlook, with 9 of 11 dying within the first 5 years in one series[92] and 10 of 19 dying in the first year of life in another.[93] However, some series have noted survival not dissimilar to that in older children, with reported survival rates of 100 percent at 6 years[94] and 85 percent at 12 years,[73] probably representing differences related to small series and the numerous etiologies of HCM in this age group. The reported survival in several series of HCM in infants (Fig. 45–3) and older children (Fig. 45–4) illustrate the diversity of results in these several series. Ventricular hypertrophy can develop during childhood or adolescence, and ECG abnormalities can precede its appearance, but new appearance in a previously normal adult has not been described. The severity of hypertrophy can progress during periods of accelerated somatic growth, particularly during adolescence,[95] whereas in adults, progression does not appear to be a feature of the disease. Importantly, the increase in magnitude of hypertrophy that is sometimes seen does not have prognostic importance and does not justify an alteration in management.[96] Regression of hypertrophy is not generally considered a characteristic of the disease, although it has occasionally been reported in children.[97]

Systolic function is nearly always normal or hyperdynamic and generally does not change over time unless transition to a thin-walled congestive cardiomyopathy occurs, a transformation rarely observed during childhood[97] and invariably associated with a grim prognosis. In patients with obstruction, the pressure gradient is also generally stable in adult subjects, although progression does occur in children and adolescents.[98] Sudden death in patients referred to tertiary care centers is seen annually in 3 to 5 percent of adults and 6 to 8 percent of children.[99] Recent population studies indicate a much lower annual mortality (0.1 to 1 percent), which indicates a major referral bias in these statistics.[100] Asymptomatic adults appear to be at even lower risk,[101] although a similar relationship to symptoms has not been demonstrated in children. While improved survival has been reported with medical and surgical interventions, the studies are invariably retrospective and usually rely on historical controls. Definitive evidence of improved survival with any available therapy has not yet appeared.

Restrictive Cardiomyopathy

(see also Chap. 48)

Restrictive cardiomyopathy is the least common form of cardiomyopathy and is quite rare among children. With the exception of occasional case reports, only four series in children with a total of 36 patients (8 patients in each of three studies[102–104] and 12 in the other[105]) have appeared. Clinical characteristics have been similar to those in adults, with a pattern of normal ventricular size and function, severe elevation in diastolic filling pressure, and marked atrial dilation. Numerous secondary causes of restrictive cardiomyopathy have been described in adults, but the pediatric cases have been uniformly idiopathic despite tissue analysis in nearly all, although several cases were familial. Differentiation from many of the secondary causes, such as myocardial noncompaction (persistence of embryonic or "spongy" myocardium[106]), can be made on morphological criteria. Tissue analysis is generally undertaken given the dismal prognosis of the disease and the desire to exclude any potentially treatable disorder. Methods of differentiation between restrictive cardiomyopathy and constrictive pericarditis have not been specifically investigated in children, primarily because constrictive pericarditis is virtually never encountered in children. The most striking characteristic of the reports in children has been the uniformly poor prognosis, with a 1-year survival rate of approximately 50 percent in all four series. Survival therefore appears to be

even more limited than has been described in adults. Anticoagulation is recommended because a 25 percent incidence of thromboembolism has been seen in children. Therapy is otherwise nonspecific and usually of very limited benefit. The onset of irreversible elevation in pulmonary vascular resistance can occur within 1 to 4 years in these patients, and early cardiac transplantation is therefore recommended to avoid the need for heart and lung transplantation.[105]

KAWASAKI DISEASE

Kawasaki disease is an acute vasculitis of unknown etiology that occurs predominantly in infants and young children. Kawasaki first described the illness in Japanese in 1967,[107] but the entity is now recognized in both endemic and community-wide epidemic forms in children of all races throughout the world. Features of Kawasaki disease include fever, bilateral nonexudative conjunctivitis, erythema of the lips and oral mucosa, changes in the extremities, rash, and cervical lymphadenopathy. Coronary artery aneurysms or ectasia develop in approximately 15 to 25 percent of untreated children with the disease and may lead to myocardial infarction, sudden death, or chronic coronary artery insufficiency.[108] In the United States, acquired heart disease in children is now caused more commonly by Kawasaki disease than by acute rheumatic fever (see Chap. 66).[109] The cause of Kawasaki disease remains unknown.

Clinical Features

The clinical criteria put forth in Kawasaki's first English language description of the disease are still in use today.[107] A child with Kawasaki disease must have fever lasting 5 or more days without another reasonable explanation and satisfy at least four of the following criteria: (1) bilateral, nonexudative conjunctival injection; (2) at least one of the following: mucous membrane changes, injected or fissured lips, injected pharynx, or "strawberry tongue"; (3) at least one of the following extremity changes: erythema of the palms or soles, edema of the hands or feet, or periungual desquamation; (4) polymorphous exanthem; and (5) acute nonsuppurative cervical lymphadenopathy (at least one node 1.5 cm or larger in diameter). An additional category of "atypical Kawasaki disease" includes patients with only four criteria and coronary artery abnormalities by echocardiography.[110] None of the clinical features of Kawasaki disease is pathognomonic. For this reason, the diagnosis of Kawasaki disease requires exclusion of other illnesses that might mimic its clinical features, including streptococcal and staphylococcal toxin–mediated illness; infection with adenovirus, enterovirus, and measles; and systemic allergic reactions to various medications. Many symptoms and signs apart from the diagnostic criteria are frequently present in children with Kawasaki disease and include arthralgias, arthritis, urethritis, aseptic meningitis, diarrhea, vomiting, and abdominal pain.

The conventional diagnostic criteria should be viewed as guidelines; they are especially useful in preventing overdiagnosis but may result in failure to recognize incomplete forms of illness. Signs and symptoms of Kawasaki disease may be particularly subtle or absent in infants younger than 6 months, a subgroup at high risk for coronary lesions. The frequent occurrence of coronary artery involvement among children with incomplete criteria suggests that echocardiography should be performed in all children with prolonged, unexplained fever and some signs of Kawasaki disease.

Cardiac Findings

CORONARY ARTERY ABNORMALITIES. Coronary artery ectasia or aneurysms occur in 15 to 25 percent of children with Kawasaki disease who do not receive treatment with intravenous gamma globulin (IVIG) in the acute phase.[111, 112] Dilatation of coronary arteries (Japanese Ministry of Health criteria)[113] may be detected by echocardiography beginning 7 days after the first appearance of fever, with the coronary diameter usually peaking around 4 weeks after illness onset. In general, clinical and laboratory indices of greater inflammation are associated with a higher likelihood of aneurysm development.

MYOCARDITIS. Myocarditis has been demonstrated in autopsy and myocardial biopsy studies to be a universal feature of early Kawasaki disease. With high-dose IVIG treatment, myocardial function improves rapidly, i.e., within days, in patients with acute Kawasaki disease.[114] When myocardial dysfunction occurs after the acute phase of the disease, it is usually secondary to ischemia or infarction, with or without mitral regurgitation.

With the use of endomyocardial biopsy, myocardial abnormalities have been detected in all time periods after disease onset; their severity was unrelated to the presence of coronary artery abnormalities. In addition, electron microscopic examination of endomyocardial biopsy specimens has demonstrated histological abnormalities late after Kawasaki disease.[115] Assessment of the full impact of Kawasaki disease on heart function and structure must await follow-up of these children into later adult life.

VALVAR REGURGITATION. Mitral regurgitation may result from transient papillary muscle dysfunction, myocardial infarction, or valvulitis. Kato and colleagues reported mitral regurgitation in 1.0 percent of patients in their series.[116] The appearance of mitral regurgitation after the acute stage is usually secondary to myocardial ischemia, although late-onset valvulitis unrelated to ischemia has been documented.

Aortic regurgitation has been documented angiographically by Nakano and colleagues in approximately 5 percent of children with Kawasaki disease and was attributed to valvulitis.[117] Others have observed a much lower incidence of aortic regurgitation in the acute phase.[116] Late-onset aortic regurgitation has been reported as a rare finding after Kawasaki disease and may be associated with the need for aortic valve replacement.

Laboratory Data

GENERAL TESTS. Laboratory findings in acute Kawasaki disease reflect the marked degree of systemic inflammation. Common initial findings include anemia, leukocytosis with a left shift, elevation of acute phase reactants, and mild elevation of liver transaminase levels. Thrombocytosis usually peaks in the third to fourth week after the onset of fever. Urinalysis may reveal the presence of white cells on microscopic examination. Since the white cells are mononuclear rather than polymorphonuclear, the dipstick test for nonspecific esterase activity (i.e., neutrophil enzyme) is usually negative. Examination of cerebrospinal fluid reveals a mild mononuclear cell pleocytosis with normal glucose and normal to mildly elevated protein.[118]

ELECTROCARDIOGRAPHY. The ECG in acute Kawasaki disease may show mild abnormalities consistent with myocarditis, most commonly a prolonged PR interval and nonspecific ST and T wave changes.

TWO-DIMENSIONAL ECHOCARDIOGRAPHY. Two-dimensional echocardiography has high sensitivity and specificity for proximal vessels of the right and left coronary arterial trees (see Chap. 7). The initial echocardiogram should be obtained as soon as the diagnosis of Kawasaki disease is suspected.[110] Longitudinal echocardiographic follow-up should begin 10 to 14 days after the onset of illness, when early coronary dilation will first be noticed in the majority of children in whom aneurysms are destined to develop. In the absence of significant coronary dilation, cardiac ultrasound may be repeated approximately 6 to 8 weeks after

illness onset. Follow-up of patients with coronary dilation should be adapted to their clinical course and the severity of their lesions.

Echocardiographers often find it difficult to reach an agreement on the exact configuration and extent of any given coronary artery lesion as seen by two-dimensional echocardiography. In 1984, the Japanese Ministry of Health established criteria for coronary artery abnormalities in Kawasaki disease.[113] These criteria classify coronary arteries as abnormal if the internal lumen diameter is greater than 3 mm in children younger than 5 years or greater than 4 mm in children at least 5 years of age, if the internal diameter of a segment measures at least 1.5 times that of an adjacent segment, or if the coronary artery lumen is clearly irregular. Current statistics on the prevalence of coronary dilation secondary to Kawasaki disease are based on these criteria. Recently, de Zorzi and colleagues showed, in patients with Kawasaki disease whose coronary arteries are classified as "normal" by Japanese Ministry of Health criteria, that body surface area–adjusted coronary dimensions are larger than expected in the acute, convalescent, and late phases.[119] Thus, the Japanese Ministry of Health criteria may underestimate the true prevalence of coronary dilation following Kawasaki disease. Figure 45–5A to C depicts normal left main, left anterior descending, and right coronary artery size, respectively, according to body surface area.

CORONARY ARTERIOGRAPHY. Selective coronary arteriography can provide definitive delineation of coronary artery anatomy. This technique is especially useful for visualization of coronary artery stenoses or distal coronary artery lesions that are difficult to define by two-dimensional echocardiography.

Based on the coronary artery classification system used in the Coronary Artery Surgery Study,[120] Takahashi and colleagues defined coronary artery aneurysms imaged at angiography as either localized or extensive.[121] Localized aneurysms, i.e., confined to one arterial segment, are further classified as either fusiform (spindle shaped) or saccular (showing abrupt transition from the normal to the dilated state, e.g., spherical, dumbbell shaped, triangular, or sacklike). Extensive aneurysms involve more than one segment and may be either ectatic (uniformly dilated) or segmented (having multiple dilated segments joined by normal or stenotic segments). Coronary aneurysms in early Kawasaki disease usually occur in the proximal segments of the major coronary vessels; aneurysms that occur distally are almost always associated with proximal coronary abnormalities.

Aneurysms can also occur in arteries outside the coronary system, most commonly the subclavian, brachial, axillary, iliac, or femoral vessels and occasionally the abdominal aortic and renal arteries.[112] For this reason, abdominal aortography and subclavian arteriography are often performed in patients undergoing coronary arteriography for Kawasaki disease.

Treatment

ASPIRIN. Aspirin has been a standard therapy for Kawasaki disease because of its antiinflammatory and antithrombotic effects, but it does not reduce the prevalence of coronary artery aneurysms.[122] Therapy with aspirin is usually initiated at the time of initial assessment in a dose of 80 to 100 mg/kg/day divided into four doses. Once fever has resolved, the dose is lowered to an antiplatelet regimen of 3 to 5 mg/kg/day orally for up to 6 to 8 weeks. For children in whom coronary aneurysms develop, aspirin (with or without anticoagulation or other antiplatelet agents) may be continued indefinitely.

INTRAVENOUS GAMMA GLOBULIN THERAPY. Although its exact mechanism of action remains unknown, IVIG administered in the acute phase of Kawasaki disease reduces the prevalence of coronary artery abnormalities.[122–123] Patients should be treated with IVIG 2 gm/kg in a single

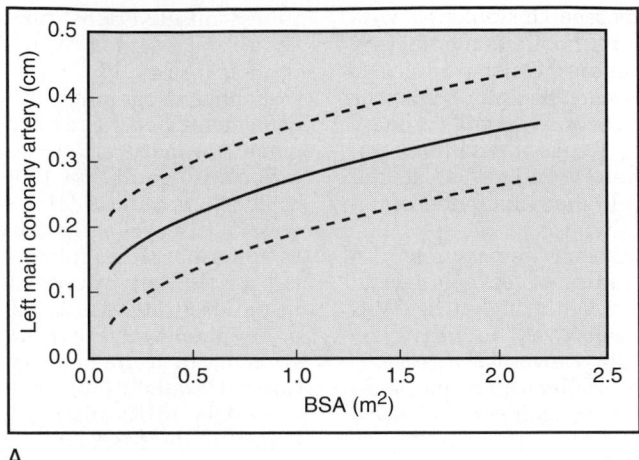

A

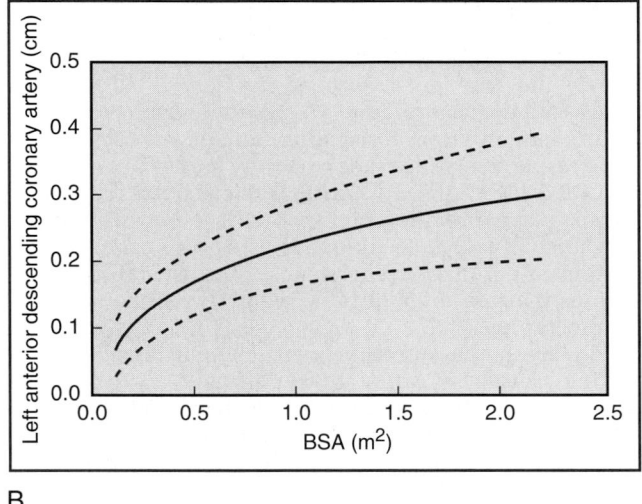

B

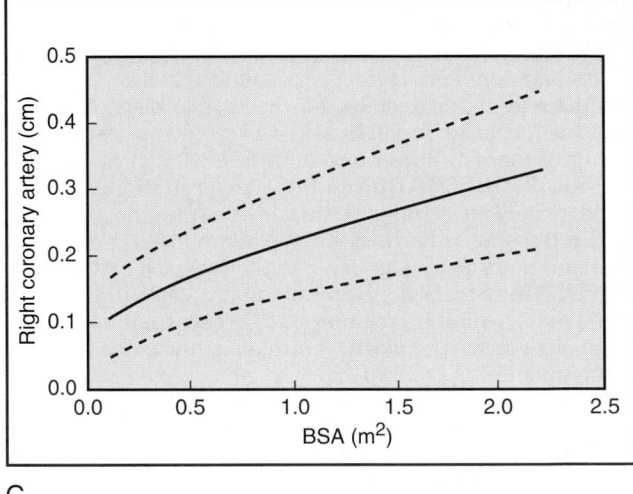

C

FIGURE 45–5. Mean and 95% prediction limits for size of the left main coronary artery *(A)*, left anterior descending coronary artery *(B)*, and proximal right coronary artery *(C)* according to body surface area for children younger than 18 years, as derived from 152 normal children at Children's Hospital, Boston.

infusion, together with aspirin.[110] Ideally, this therapy should be instituted within the first 10 days of illness (optimally by day 7 of illness), but it should be administered after the 10th day of illness to any child with persistent fever[124] or with aneurysms and ongoing signs of inflammation. Even when treated with high-dose IVIG regimens within the first 10 days of illness, however, approximately 5 percent of children with Kawasaki disease experience at least transient coronary artery dilation, and giant aneurysms develop in 1 percent.[125] Most experts recommend retreatment with IVIG 2 gm/kg in patients with persistent or recrudescent fever 48 to 72 hours after initial therapy.

CORTICOSTEROIDS. The subgroup of patients with Kawasaki disease resistant to IVIG therapy is at greatest risk for the development of coronary artery aneurysms and long-term sequelae of the disease.[126, 127] Although one early study showed a detrimental effect of steroid use in Kawasaki disease,[128] others have suggested that steroids may be beneficial in the prevention of coronary artery aneurysms.[129, 130] Further studies are needed to assess the risks and benefits of steroid administration in Kawasaki disease.

OTHER THERAPIES DURING THE ACUTE PHASE. High-dose pentoxifylline, a vasodilator and inhibitor of platelet aggregation and neutrophil activation, has been shown in one study to reduce the incidence of coronary artery aneurysms.[131] Case reports suggest that plasmapheresis may produce dramatic improvement in severe Kawasaki disease[132]; however, it is a technically complex intervention in young children and should be reserved for those who remain desperately ill despite multiple doses of IVIG and intravenous methylprednisolone.

ANTITHROMBOTIC THERAPY. Paradoxically, the risk of coronary artery thrombosis is greatest *after* the acute phase subsides, when well-established coronary vasculitis occurs concomitantly with marked elevation of the platelet count and a hypercoagulable state. As above, low-dose aspirin (3 to 5 mg/kg/day given as a single dose) is the mainstay of antithrombotic therapy in Kawasaki disease. Other antiplatelet agents, such as clopidogrel or dipyridamole, may be substituted for aspirin when salicylates are contraindicated. For children without evidence of coronary artery ectasia or aneurysms, antiplatelet therapy is usually discontinued approximately 2 months after illness onset.

Children with coronary artery abnormalities require long-term antithrombotic therapy, usually with low-dose aspirin. The risk of coronary thrombosis and myocardial infarction is especially great in children with rapidly increasing coronary dimensions or with giant aneurysms during the subacute phase.[133, 134] During this period, some investigators advocate treatment with systemic heparin, together with an antiplatelet agent. For chronic antithrombotic therapy, therapeutic options include antiplatelet therapy with aspirin, with or without dipyridamole or another inhibitor of antiplatelet aggregation; anticoagulant therapy with warfarin; or a combination of anticoagulant and antiplatelet therapy, usually warfarin plus aspirin. No prospective data exist to guide the clinician in choosing the optimal regimen. The most common regimen for patients with giant aneurysms is low-dose aspirin together with warfarin, with the international normalized ratio maintained at 2.0:2.5. Some physicians substitute low-molecular-weight heparin for warfarin, although this therapy requires subcutaneous injections twice daily.

THROMBOLYTIC THERAPY. Despite the use of antithrombotic agents, myocardial infarction secondary to thrombotic occlusion of coronary aneurysms can develop in some children, especially those with giant aneurysms. Sometimes, coronary artery thrombus can be detected in asymptomatic patients by two-dimensional echocardiography. Because no large trials of thrombolytic therapy have been performed in children, the choice of thrombolytic agent for the treatment of infants and children with coronary thrombosis is derived from studies in adults with coronary thrombosis. Although effective in adults, the use of immediate coronary angioplasty has not been reported in children with Kawasaki disease and coronary artery thrombosis.

SURGICAL MANAGEMENT. Surgical management in Kawasaki disease consists primarily of coronary artery bypass grafts for obstructive lesions.[134a] However, indications for coronary bypass graft procedures in children have not been established. Such surgery should be considered when reversible ischemia is present on stress-imaging tests, the myocardium to be perfused through the graft is still viable, and no appreciable lesions are present in the artery peripheral to the planned graft site.

The earliest coronary artery bypass operations in children with Kawasaki disease were performed with autologous saphenous veins or veins obtained from parents. However, the late results with this technique have been relatively unsatisfactory, especially in very young children. Kitamura and coworkers reported improved results with the use of internal mammary artery grafts in pediatric patients.[135] The diameter and length of internal mammary grafts increase with the general somatic growth of the child, as opposed to the tendency of saphenous vein grafts to shorten somewhat over time. In children younger than 7 years, the arterial graft patency rate 90 months after surgery was 70 percent. Children who were older than 8 years at the time of coronary arterial grafting appeared to have even better long-term patency than seen in younger children; by 90 months after surgery, the arterial graft patency rate was 84 percent. Of note, 8 years after internal mammary artery grafting to the left anterior descending coronary artery, 98.7 percent of patients in the series of Kitamura and colleagues were still alive.

INTERVENTIONAL CARDIAC CATHETERIZATION TECHNIQUES. Although results over the first decade after surgery are encouraging, graft patency in later adult life after coronary artery bypass grafting in childhood is still unknown. When it is preferable to delay the time until surgery, percutaneous transluminal coronary angioplasty (PTCA) may be performed in the stenotic coronary arteries of children with Kawasaki disease[136, 137] (Fig. 45–6). PTCA is not as effective in patients with Kawasaki disease as in adults with atherosclerotic coronary artery disease because the stenotic lesions in long-term Kawasaki disease are very stiff and often associated with marked calcifications, especially many years after illness onset. The relatively high balloon pressures necessary under these circumstances can lead to late aneurysm formation.[137] Intravascular ultrasound imaging has been found to be a useful tool for evaluating internal morphology before and after PTCA.[136] Once calcification and stenosis have become severe, rotational ablation techniques may be necessary for the success of coronary angioplasty.

CARDIAC TRANSPLANTATION. Cardiac transplantation has been performed in a small number of patients with severe ischemic heart disease resulting from Kawasaki dis-

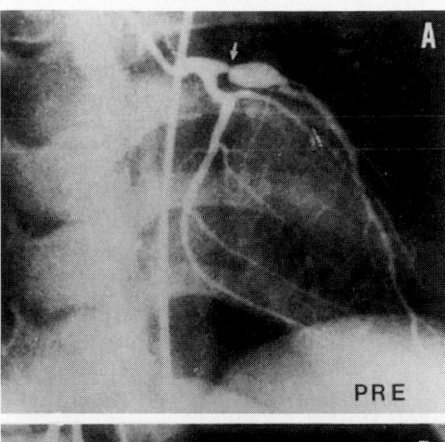
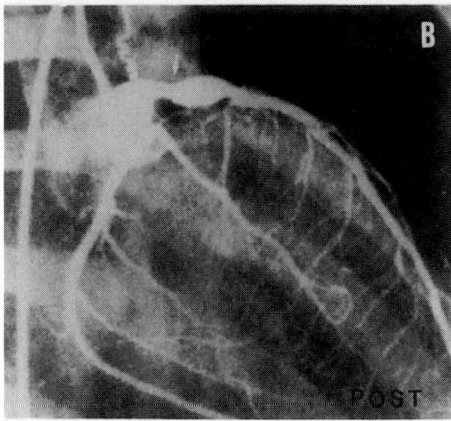
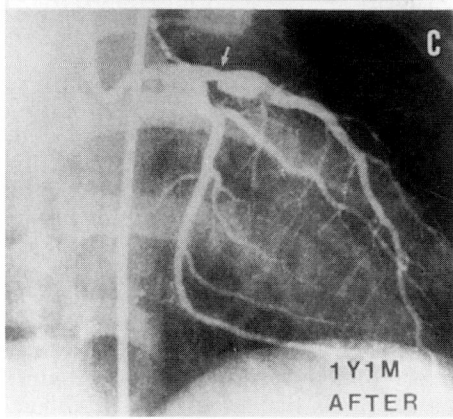

FIGURE 45–6. Left coronary arteriograms. *A,* Localized stenosis can be seen at a site just proximal to the aneurysm of the left anterior descending artery. *B,* The stenosis was dilated by conventional percutaneous transluminal coronary angioplasty (PTCA). *C,* Follow-up angiography performed 13 months after the initial PTCA revealed no significant restenoses. Pre = pre-PTCA; POST = post-PTCA. (From Ino T, Akimoto K, Ohkubo M, et al: Application of percutaneous transluminal angioplasty to coronary arterial stenosis in Kawasaki disease. Circulation 93:1711, 1996. By permission of the American Heart Association, Inc.)

ease.[138] This procedure should be considered only for individuals with severe, irreversible myocardial dysfunction and coronary lesions for which interventional catheterization procedures or coronary artery bypass is not feasible.

Clinical Course

REGRESSION AND EVOLUTION OF CORONARY LESIONS. Coronary artery lesions resulting from Kawasaki disease change dynamically with time. Angiographic resolution 1 to 2 years after disease onset has been observed in approximately half to two-thirds of vessels with coronary aneurysms.[121, 139] The likelihood of resolution of the aneurysm appears to be determined in large measure by the initial size of the aneurysm, with smaller aneurysms having a greater likelihood of regression.[133] Takahashi and coauthors reported other factors positively associated with regression of aneurysms, including age younger than 1 year, saccular (rather than fusiform) aneurysm morphology, and aneurysm location in a distal coronary segment.[121] Vessels that do not undergo apparent resolution of abnormalities may show persistence of aneurysmal morphology, development of stenosis or occlusion, or abnormal tortuosity.

PATIENTS WITH PERSISTENT CORONARY ARTERY ABNORMALITIES. Whereas aneurysm size tends to diminish over time, stenotic lesions secondary to marked myointimal proliferation are frequently progressive.[112] In the series of Kato and coworkers, stenotic lesions were recognized within 2 years from disease onset in about half of the patients in whom coronary stenoses ultimately developed, but the prevalence of stenosis continued to rise almost linearly over time.[139] Kamiya and colleagues have also reported a steady increase in the presence of coronary artery stenoses with increasing duration since illness onset; the highest rate of progression to stenosis occurred among patients whose aneurysms were large.[140]

The worst prognosis occurs in children with so-called giant aneurysms, i.e., those with a maximum diameter greater than 8 mm.[141] In these aneurysms, thrombosis is promoted by sluggish blood flow within the massively dilated vascular space, together with frequent development of stenotic lesions at the proximal or distal end of the aneurysms.

Myocardial infarction caused by thrombotic occlusion in an aneurysmal and/or stenotic coronary artery is the principal cause of death in Kawasaki disease.[111] The highest risk of myocardial infarction occurs in the first year after disease onset, and most fatal attacks are associated with obstruction either in the left main coronary artery or in both the right main and left anterior descending coronary arteries.[111] Serial stress tests and myocardial imaging are mandatory in the management of patients with Kawasaki disease and significant coronary artery disease to determine the need for coronary angiography and for surgical or transcatheter intervention.

Late cardiac sequelae of Kawasaki disease may first become apparent in adulthood. Burns and associates identified 74 patients in the English and Japanese literature with Kawasaki disease in childhood whose first symptoms of coronary artery disease occurred in young adulthood.[142] A history of a Kawasaki-like illness in childhood should be sought in patients with coronary aneurysms in the absence of generalized atherosclerotic disease. However, adult patients may be unable to recall an illness that occurred so early in life.

PATIENTS WITH SPONTANEOUS REGRESSION OF ANEURYSMS. Approximately half of vascular segments with coronary artery aneurysms show angiographic regression of the aneurysms. This regression usually occurs by myointimal proliferation, although more rarely the mechanism of regression can be organization and recanalization of a thrombus. Pathological examination reveals fibrous intimal thickening despite normal coronary artery diameter. Similarly, transluminal (intravascular) ultrasound of regressed coronary aneurysms shows marked symmetrical or asymmetrical myointimal thickening.[143] Regressed coronary artery aneurysms not only are histopathologically abnormal but also show reduced vascular reactivity.[144, 144a]

KAWASAKI DISEASE WITHOUT DETECTABLE CORONARY LESIONS. Although coronary artery aneurysms produce the most serious sequelae of Kawasaki disease, vascular inflammation during the acute stage of the illness is diffuse. Generalized endothelial dysfunction has been suggested by the observation that plasma 6-ketoprostaglandin F_1 remains generally undetectable over an observation period of 8 weeks after the onset of Kawasaki disease.[145] In addition,

Kawasaki disease produces altered lipid metabolism that persists beyond clinical resolution of the disease.[146] Histological data concerning the long-term status of coronary arteries in children who never had demonstrable abnormalities are few and difficult to interpret.[147]

Some investigators in Japan have studied coronary physiology in the population without aneurysms. Among children with a history of Kawasaki disease but with normal epicardial coronary arteries, Muzik and colleagues found lower myocardial flow reserve and higher total coronary resistance than in normal controls.[148] Children without a history of coronary aneurysms have also been reported to have abnormal endothelium-dependent brachial artery reactivity.[149] Data are conflicting regarding impairment in long-term endothelium-dependent relaxation of the epicardial coronary arteries among children with Kawasaki disease in whom coronary artery dilation was never detected.[150, 151]

From a purely clinical perspective, children without known cardiac sequelae during the first month after diagnosis of Kawasaki disease appear to return to their previous, usually excellent state of health, without signs or symptoms of cardiac impairment.[139] Meaningful knowledge about long-term myocardial function, late-onset valvar regurgitation, and coronary artery status in this population must await their careful surveillance over the coming decades.

SYSTEMIC HYPERTENSION

Hypertension is well recognized as a major risk factor for cardiovascular disease, including stroke, myocardial infarction, congestive heart failure, and renal failure. Because the precursors of these processes are likely to arise early in life, evaluation and treatment of pediatric hypertension are important. Estimates of significant hypertension in childhood have ranged from 0.26 to 2.0 percent.[152] The most common causes of hypertension change during childhood, with secondary causes of hypertension predominating in the youngest patients and those in whom systemic hypertension is the most severe. For many years, pediatricians focused solely on identification and treatment of secondary forms of hypertension, such as renal parenchymal disease and renal artery stenosis.[152] With recommendations for routine measurement of blood pressure during well-child visits to the pediatrician, as well as the publication of national norms for blood pressure in children, essential hypertension has been increasingly recognized, especially in adolescents with mild to moderate elevation of blood pressure. Children with higher blood pressure are more likely to have first-degree relatives with histories of hypertension, and the tracking correlation of blood pressure from childhood into young adult life is relatively high. Nonetheless, the sensitivities and predictive values for childhood blood pressure are only modest as a screening test for adult blood pressure.[153]

DEFINITION. The distribution of blood pressure in the normal pediatric population is shown in Tables 45-2 and 45-3. The National High Blood Pressure Education Program has recommended that blood pressure between the 90th and 95th percentiles be considered high-normal or borderline hypertension. Hypertension is defined as average systolic or diastolic blood pressure greater than or equal to the 95th percentile for sex, age, and height on at least three separate occasions. Thus, elevation of blood pressure must be sustained to establish a diagnosis of hypertension. Ideally, blood pressure should be measured with a standard sphygmomanometer, blood pressure cuff, and stethoscope. Many centers currently use automated oscillometric blood pressure monitoring devices for ease of use and elimination of interobserver variability. In addition, 24-hour ambulatory

▼ TABLE 45–2. BLOOD PRESSURE LEVELS FOR THE 90TH AND 95TH PERCENTILES OF BLOOD PRESSURE FOR BOYS AGED 1 TO 17 YEARS BY PERCENTILES OF HEIGHT

1635

Ch 45

AGE (yr)	BLOOD PRESSURE PERCENTILE*	SYSTOLIC BLOOD PRESSURE BY PERCENTILE OF HEIGHT (mm Hg)†							DIASTOLIC BLOOD PRESSURE BY PERCENTILE OF HEIGHT (mm Hg)†						
		5%	10%	25%	50%	75%	90%	95%	5%	10%	25%	50%	75%	90%	95%
1	90th	94	95	97	98	100	102	102	50	51	52	53	54	54	55
	95th	98	99	101	102	104	106	106	55	55	56	57	58	59	59
2	90th	98	99	100	102	104	105	106	55	55	56	57	58	59	59
	95th	101	102	104	106	108	109	110	59	59	60	61	62	63	63
3	90th	100	101	103	105	107	108	109	59	59	60	61	62	63	63
	95th	104	105	107	109	111	112	113	63	63	64	65	66	67	67
4	90th	102	103	105	107	109	110	111	62	62	63	64	65	66	66
	95th	106	107	109	111	113	114	115	66	67	67	68	69	70	71
5	90th	104	105	106	108	110	112	112	65	65	66	67	68	69	69
	95th	108	109	110	112	114	115	116	69	70	70	71	72	73	74
6	90th	105	106	108	110	111	113	114	67	68	69	70	70	71	72
	95th	109	110	112	114	115	117	117	72	72	73	74	75	76	76
7	90th	106	107	109	111	113	114	115	69	70	71	72	72	73	74
	95th	110	111	113	115	116	118	119	74	74	75	76	77	78	78
8	90th	107	108	110	112	114	115	116	71	71	72	73	74	75	75
	95th	111	112	114	116	118	119	120	75	76	76	77	78	79	80
9	90th	109	110	112	113	115	117	117	72	73	73	74	75	76	77
	95th	113	114	116	117	119	121	121	76	77	78	79	80	80	81
10	90th	110	112	113	115	117	118	119	73	74	74	75	76	77	78
	95th	114	115	117	119	121	122	123	77	78	79	80	80	81	82
11	90th	112	113	115	117	119	120	121	74	74	75	76	77	78	78
	95th	116	117	119	121	123	124	125	78	79	79	80	81	82	83
12	90th	115	116	117	119	121	123	123	75	75	76	77	78	78	79
	95th	119	120	121	123	125	126	127	79	79	80	81	82	83	83
13	90th	117	118	120	122	124	125	126	75	76	76	77	78	79	80
	95th	121	122	124	126	128	129	130	79	80	81	82	83	83	84
14	90th	120	121	123	125	126	128	128	76	76	77	78	79	80	80
	95th	124	125	127	128	130	132	132	80	81	81	82	83	84	85
15	90th	123	124	125	127	129	131	131	77	77	78	79	80	81	81
	95th	127	128	129	131	133	134	135	81	82	83	83	84	85	86
16	90th	125	126	128	130	132	133	134	79	79	80	81	82	82	83
	95th	129	130	132	134	136	137	138	83	83	84	85	86	87	87
17	90th	128	129	131	133	134	136	136	81	81	82	83	84	85	85
	95th	132	133	135	136	138	140	140	85	85	86	87	88	89	89

* Blood pressure percentile was determined by a single measurement.
† Height percentile was determined by standard growth curves.

From National Heart, Lung and Blood Institute: Update on the 1987 Task Force Report on High Blood Pressure in Children and Adolescents: A working group report from the National High Blood Pressure Education Program. Pediatrics 98:649, 1996. Copyright American Academy of Pediatrics 1996.

blood pressure monitoring has been used when "white coat" hypertension is suspected and for management of known hypertension.[154, 155, 155a]

EVALUATION. Evaluation of an asymptomatic child or adolescent with hypertension should focus on potential etiologies. The family history should be carefully probed for hypertension, premature cardiovascular disease, and renal disease, medical conditions, or drugs. In adolescents, the possibility of substance abuse should always be considered. The physical examination should be directed toward signs of definable causes of hypertension, as well as toward its sequelae.

Many adolescents whose blood pressure is at or just greater than the 95th percentile have family histories of hypertension and are overweight, but they have an otherwise negative history and physical examination.[152] For such patients, a work-up that includes urinalysis, urine culture, and electrolyte, serum creatinine (noting that normal values vary according to age), and blood urea nitrogen levels may be sufficient.[156] Such patients would also usually benefit from a lipid profile to exclude other risk factors for premature cardiovascular disease.[152] When children or adolescents with borderline high blood pressure are not obese and have no family history of hypertension, renal Doppler ultrasound provides a first-line screen for renovascular hypertension, parenchymal integrity, and hydronephrosis.

For patients in whom blood pressure is well above the 95th percentile, secondary causes of hypertension should be pursued aggressively, with targeting of conditions believed to be most likely on the basis of age (Table 45–4) or targeting of findings on initial assessment. Most children with secondary hypertension (60 to 80 percent) have renal parenchymal disease,[156] commonly reflux nephropathy, pyelonephritis, and obstructive uropathy. Less common renal etiologies include glomerulonephritis, nephrotic syndrome, congenital renal dysplasia, renal damage following hemolytic-uremic syndrome, and polycystic disease.[156] Renal parenchymal disease can be assessed with imaging studies, including renal ultrasonography, voiding cystourethrography, or renal scintiscanning.

Renovascular hypertension has been reported in 8 to 10 percent of children with secondary hypertension.[156, 157] In such patients, hypertension may be caused by stenosis of a main renal artery or by segmental renal artery stenoses in one or both kidneys.[156] Methods of evaluation of renovascular hypertension vary in different centers and include renal scanning before and after captopril challenge, intravenous digital subtraction angiography, captopril radionuclide renography, Doppler sonography, computed tomographic angiography, and magnetic resonance angiography. Conventional angiography and intraarterial digital subtraction angiography remain the gold standard for the diagnosis of renovascular hypertension and should be considered for children with severe, persistent hypertension without other findings, greatly elevated plasma renin activity, a bruit, or a solitary kidney and severe hypertension.[156]

▼ TABLE 45–3. BLOOD PRESSURE LEVELS FOR THE 90TH AND 95TH PERCENTILES OF BLOOD PRESSURE FOR GIRLS AGED 1 TO 17 YEARS BY PERCENTILES OF HEIGHT

AGE (yr)	BLOOD PRESSURE PERCENTILE*	SYSTOLIC BLOOD PRESSURE BY PERCENTILE OF HEIGHT (mm Hg)†							DIASTOLIC BLOOD PRESSURE BY PERCENTILE OF HEIGHT (mm Hg)†						
		5%	10%	25%	50%	75%	90%	95%	5%	10%	25%	50%	75%	90%	95%
1	90th	97	98	99	100	102	103	104	53	53	53	54	55	56	56
	95th	101	102	103	104	105	107	107	57	57	57	58	59	60	60
2	90th	99	99	100	102	103	104	105	57	57	58	58	59	60	61
	95th	102	103	104	105	107	108	109	61	61	62	62	63	64	65
3	90th	100	100	102	103	104	105	106	61	61	61	62	63	63	64
	95th	104	104	105	107	108	109	110	65	65	65	66	67	67	68
4	90th	101	102	103	104	106	107	108	63	63	64	65	65	66	67
	95th	105	106	107	108	109	111	111	67	67	68	69	69	70	71
5	90th	103	103	104	106	107	108	109	65	66	66	67	68	68	69
	95th	107	107	108	110	111	112	113	69	70	70	71	72	72	73
6	90th	104	105	106	107	109	110	111	67	67	68	69	69	70	71
	95th	108	109	110	111	112	114	114	71	71	72	73	73	74	75
7	90th	106	107	108	109	110	112	112	69	69	69	70	71	72	72
	95th	110	110	112	113	114	115	116	73	73	73	74	75	76	76
8	90th	108	109	110	111	112	113	114	70	70	71	71	72	73	74
	95th	112	112	113	115	116	117	118	74	74	75	75	76	77	78
9	90th	110	110	112	113	114	115	116	71	72	72	73	74	74	75
	95th	114	114	115	117	118	119	120	75	76	76	77	78	78	79
10	90th	112	112	114	115	116	117	118	73	73	73	74	75	76	76
	95th	116	116	117	119	120	121	122	77	77	77	78	79	80	80
11	90th	114	114	116	117	118	119	120	74	74	75	75	76	77	77
	95th	118	118	119	121	122	123	124	78	78	79	79	80	81	81
12	90th	116	116	118	119	120	121	122	75	75	76	76	77	78	78
	95th	120	120	121	123	124	125	126	79	79	80	80	81	82	82
13	90th	118	118	119	121	122	123	124	76	76	77	78	78	79	80
	95th	121	122	123	125	126	127	128	80	80	81	82	82	83	84
14	90th	119	120	121	122	124	125	126	77	77	78	79	79	80	81
	95th	123	124	125	126	128	129	130	81	81	82	83	83	84	85
15	90th	121	121	122	124	125	126	127	78	78	79	79	80	81	82
	95th	124	125	126	128	129	130	131	82	82	83	83	84	85	86
16	90th	122	122	123	125	126	127	128	79	79	79	80	81	82	82
	95th	125	126	127	128	130	131	132	83	83	83	84	85	86	86
17	90th	122	123	124	125	126	128	128	79	79	79	80	81	82	82
	95th	126	126	127	129	130	131	132	83	83	83	84	85	86	86

* Blood pressure percentile was determined by a single reading.
† Height percentile was determined by standard growth curves.
From National Heart, Lung and Blood Institute: Update on the 1987 Task Force Report on High Blood Pressure in Children and Adolescents: A working group report from the National High Blood Pressure Education Program. Pediatrics 98:649, 1996. Copyright American Academy of Pediatrics 1996.

Coarctation of the aorta (see Chap. 43), a common cause of hypertension in the first year of life, is present in one-third of infants with hypertension but accounts for only 2 percent of cases of secondary hypertension in childhood and adolescence.[156] This cause of hypertension is easily detected on physical examination by careful measurement of upper and lower extremity blood pressures, together with palpation of radial and femoral pulses. Since 80 percent of patients with coarctation have an associated bicuspid aortic valve, physical examination often includes a constant early systolic ejection click at the apex and base. A soft early to midsystolic ejection murmur is frequently heard over the left lateral aspect of the chest, and older children with collateral circulation may have continuous murmurs over the back. The diagnosis of coarctation of the aorta may be confirmed by two-dimensional echocardiography or, in an older child or adolescent, by magnetic resonance imaging (MRI). After the coarctation is repaired, a residual gradient may either remain or recur, sometimes necessitating late procedures such as balloon dilation or stenting of the aorta. Some patients require chronic antihypertensive medication after adequate repair of coarctation.

More rarely, hypertension can be caused by endocrine disorders.[158] Pheochromocytoma alone causes approximately 0.5 to 2.0 percent of cases of secondary hypertension in children.[159] Most children with pheochromocytoma (88 percent) have sustained rather than episodic hypertension, and many have extraadrenal or multiple tumors (31 and 32 percent, respectively).[156] Elevation of urinary catecholamine levels in a 24-hour urine collection or elevation of plasma catecholamines points to a diagnosis of pheochromocytoma (or other types of neural crest tumor). Definitive diagnosis is made with MRI (T_2 weighted or gadolinium-labeled diethylenetriaminepentaacetic acid [DTPA] enhanced) or with meta-iodobenzylguaninine (MIBG) scanning.[156, 160, 161] Pheochromocytomas are removed surgically, after the hypertension is controlled.[159, 162, 163] Other endocrine causes of secondary hypertension (e.g., excess glucocorticoids or mineralocorticoids, hyperthyroidism) may be pursued if the history, physical examination, or screening tests are suggestive.

Hypertension may rarely be associated with abnormalities of the central nervous system (CNS). These abnormalities may be primary (e.g., brain tumors, familial dysautonomia) or secondary (e.g., hypercalcemia or lead poisoning). Because hypertension of CNS origin may have a fulminant manifestation, CNS-mediated causes of hypertension should always be considered by the clinician.[156, 164]

MANAGEMENT. All children with blood pressure consistently above the 90th percentile should be introduced to nonpharmacological therapies, including a diet rich in fruits, vegetables, and low-fat dairy products, reduced in-

TABLE 45–4. MOST COMMON CAUSES OF SECONDARY HYPERTENSION, BY AGE

AGE GROUP	CAUSE
Newborn	Renal artery or venous thrombosis
	Renal artery stenosis
	Congenital renal abnormalities
	Coarctation of the aorta
	Bronchopulmonary dysplasia
First year	Coarctation of the aorta
	Renovascular disease
	Renal parenchymal disease
	Iatrogenic (medication, volume)
	Tumor
Infancy to 6 yr	Renal parenchymal disease
	Renovascular disease
	Coarctation of the aorta
	Endocrine causes*
	Iatrogenic*
	Essential hypertension*
Age 6–10 yr	Renal parenchymal disease
	Renovascular disease
	Essential hypertension
	Coarctation of the aorta
	Endocrine causes*
	Iatrogenic*
Age 12–18 yr	Essential hypertension
	Iatrogenic
	Renal parenchymal disease*
	Endocrine causes*
	Coarctation of the aorta*

* Uncommon for category.

From Swinford RD, Ingelfinger JR: Evaluation of hypertension in childhood diseases. In Barratt TM, Avner ED, Harmon WD (eds): Pediatric Nephrology. 4th ed. Baltimore, Lippincott Williams & Wilkins, 1999, p 1007.

take of saturated fat,[165] and for obese children, weight modification. Children and their families should also be counseled regarding the benefits of aerobic physical activity and the hazards of smoking.[152] Treatment with medications should be instituted for patients with severe hypertension or evidence of end-organ damage (e.g., increased left ventricular mass by two-dimensional echocardiography). In addition, pharmacological treatment of hypertension should be guided by the presence of other cardiovascular risk factors (e.g., childhood diabetes, chronic renal disease).

When drugs are prescribed for children and adolescents with hypertension, the goal is to reduce blood pressure to below the 95th percentile for age, gender, and height.[152] Drug therapy should aim at prescribing the simplest regimen with the fewest adverse side effects. All antihypertensive medications should be individualized to the patient's medical history (including the etiology of the hypertension), severity of hypertension, response to therapy, and occurrence of side effects.[152] Thiazide diuretics and beta blockers have been used for years in children and adolescents and continue to have a role in the treatment of hypertension. Since publication of the Report of the Second Task Force on Blood Pressure Control in Children in 1987,[166] newer antihypertensive agents have come into common use in pediatric patients. These medications include ACE inhibitors and calcium channel blockers.[167] Use of the other classes of antihypertensive agents (e.g., central alpha-adrenergic agonists, alpha-adrenergic blocking drugs, direct vasodilators) is only rarely indicated in pediatric cardiology practice. Long-term clinical trials have not examined the benefits and risks of antihypertensive therapy in children and adolescents. Until such data are available, when choosing the optimal antihypertensive medication, physicians should draw on the adult experience.

Abnormalities in plasma lipoproteins are an important cause of premature coronary artery disease. Because epidemiological and pathological observations have introduced the concept that the process of atherosclerosis begins early in life and progresses to cardiovascular morbidity and mortality in later life, efforts to prevent clinical disease have centered around the modification of plasma lipid concentrations in childhood and adolescence.[168]

RATIONALE FOR LIPID MODIFICATION IN CHILDHOOD. The rationale for modification of cholesterol in childhood is based on postmortem and epidemiological data. In 1953, Enos and colleagues first reported that postmortem examination showed advanced lesions in the coronary arteries of young American soldiers killed in the Korean war.[169] The Pathobiological Determinants of Atherosclerosis in Youth (PDAY) Study, a multiinstitutional study of atherosclerosis in 15- to 34-year-old males and females, demonstrated that the conditions predicting risk of coronary heart disease in adults are also associated with the extent and severity of atherosclerosis in youth.[170] Recently, this group reported on the ubiquity of fatty streaks in the abdominal aortas and the frequency of fibrous plaques in the aortas and coronary arteries in the 15- to 19-year-old age group.[171] Other autopsy studies have shown that antemortem low-density lipoprotein (LDL) and total cholesterol are highly associated with aortic fatty streaks in subjects aged 7 to 24 years.[172] Recently, Berenson and associates reported that serum concentrations of total cholesterol, triglycerides, LDL cholesterol (LDL-C), and high-density lipoprotein cholesterol (HDL-C) were strongly associated with the extent of lesions in the aorta and coronary arteries at autopsy in young persons who died of various causes, principally trauma.[173] Among these subjects, greater numbers of cardiovascular risk factors were directly associated with increased severity of asymptomatic coronary and aortic atherosclerosis.[173]

Epidemiological investigations in children across and within different populations have provided further evidence of the importance of cholesterol in pediatrics. In cross-population studies, children from countries with a high incidence of coronary artery disease in adults have higher cholesterol levels than do children from countries where adults have a low incidence of coronary artery disease. Within populations, elevated levels of total cholesterol and LDL-C in children have been associated with coronary artery disease in their adult relatives. In a study of the progeny of individuals with premature coronary artery disease, half had abnormal lipid profiles.[174]

The importance of monitoring lipid levels in childhood is further supported by evidence that children and adolescents with severe dyslipidemia are more likely than the general population to have abnormal lipid profiles as they grow older. Furthermore, long-term prospective studies have shown a strong association between cholesterol levels in young adult life and later risk of cardiovascular disease.[175]

SCREENING FOR DYSLIPIDEMIAS. The distribution of fasting lipid and lipoprotein levels in children and adolescents is displayed in Table 45–5. The value of selective versus universal screening strategies for hyperlipidemia in childhood has been controversial. The National Cholesterol Education Program (NCEP) has advocated a selective screening strategy in which high-risk children older than 2 years are targeted for cholesterol screening.[176] High-risk children are defined as those whose parents or grandparents, at 55 years of age or younger, underwent diagnostic coronary arteriography and were found to have coronary atherosclerosis or suffered a documented myocardial infarction, angina pectoris, peripheral vascular disease, cerebro-

▼ TABLE 45–5. FASTING LIPID AND LIPOPROTEIN LEVELS (mg/dl) IN CHILDREN BY AGE

	MALES			FEMALES		
	5%	50%	95%	5%	50%	95%
Cholesterol						
0–4 yr	114	155	203	112	156	200
5–9 yr	121	160	203	126	164	205
10–14 yr	119	158	202	124	160	201
15–19 yr	113	150	197	120	158	203
Triglycerides						
0–4 yr	29	56	98	34	64	112
5–9 yr	30	56	101	32	60	105
10–14 yr	32	66	125	37	75	131
15–19 yr	37	78	148	39	75	132
HDL cholesterol						
5–9 yr	38	56	74	36	53	73
10–14 yr	37	55	74	37	52	70
15–19 yr	30	46	63	35	52	74
LDL cholesterol						
5–9 yr	63	93	129	68	100	140
10–14 yr	64	100	140	68	97	132
15–19 yr	62	94	130	59	96	137

HDL = high-density lipoprotein; LDL = low-density lipoprotein.
Data from Lipid Research Clinics: Population Studies Data Book, Vol 1, The Prevalence Study. Bethesda, MD, Department of Health and Human Services, Publication (NIH) 80-1527.

vascular disease, or sudden cardiac death; those whose parent(s) have a total cholesterol level of 240 mg/dl or higher; those for whom the health history of a parent or grandparent is unknown; or those whose personal health includes risk factors (e.g., diabetes). In such a selective screening strategy, adult cardiologists should refer the children of their patients with premature atherosclerotic cardiovascular disease for cholesterol testing and follow-up.

Some experts continue to recommend universal screening based on the observation that almost half of children with elevated cholesterol levels would be missed if screening were performed only on children with a positive family history.[177, 178] Moreover, a family history does not selectively identify the most severely affected children.[178] The relationship of parental history to children's lipid profiles appears to be associated with race.[177] Specifically, the Bogalusa Heart Study found that white children with a parental history of heart attack or diabetes were significantly more likely than black children to have elevated levels of total cholesterol and LDL-C, whereas in black children, a parental history of cardiovascular disease was more likely to be associated with low levels of HDL-C than in white children. Only 40 percent of white children and 21 percent of black children with elevated levels of LDL-C had a parent with a history of vascular diseases.[173]

The NCEP formulated recommendations for the management of hypercholesterolemia in children.[176] When children or adolescents have a documented history of premature cardiovascular disease in a parent or grandparent, the initial test should be a fasting lipoprotein analysis. Random screening in the nonfasting state should always include both a total cholesterol and HDL-C level because total cholesterol alone is a poor screening test in childhood.[179]

SECONDARY CAUSES. Dyslipidemia most commonly results from a combination of genetic and dietary factors, but it can also be secondary to other systemic disorders. Indeed, the lipid profile can be affected by the use of medications and by endocrine and metabolic disorders, obstructive liver disease, or renal disease. Viral and bacterial infections, so common in childhood, can have profound effects on the lipid profile in the month after the onset of infection. In the first year of life, the most common causes of secondary hyperlipidemia are congenital biliary atresia and glycogen storage disease. Endocrine disorders (e.g., hypothyroidism and diabetes mellitus) and renal disease are the most common secondary causes later in childhood. Especially in adolescents, exogenous causes, such as medications, smoking, or alcohol, can affect the lipid profile. Secondary causes are usually evident from a careful review of the medical history and use of medications, together with a physical examination. When a secondary cause is not apparent, it may be appropriate to measure blood levels of thyroid-stimulating hormone, perform liver function tests, and obtain a urinalysis.

MANAGEMENT. Because atherosclerosis is a continuous process throughout life, expert panels have suggested guidelines to reduce the risk of cardiovascular disease beginning in childhood. With the rationale that symptomatic adult coronary heart disease might be prevented or retarded by lowering of the LDL-C level in childhood and adolescence, the NCEP published guidelines for detection and management of childhood hyperlipidemia in a 1991 Report of the Expert Panel on Blood Cholesterol Levels in Children and Adolescents.[176] The NCEP expert panel recommended initial nonpharmacological intervention in hyperlipidemic children, including diet modification. To lower the average population cholesterol levels, a so-called prudent diet was recommended for all children older than 2 years. In addition to providing adequate nutrients and calories to maintain ideal body weight, this diet restricts total fat calories to 30 percent or less, saturated fat calories to 40 percent or less, and cholesterol intake to 300 mg/day or less. Indeed, the long-term safety, efficacy, and acceptability of lower fat diets in high-risk pubertal children have been demonstrated in the Dietary Intervention Study in Children (DISC).[180]

In children with severe familial hyperlipidemia, LDL-C rarely decreases by more than 15 percent with diet management alone. The NCEP guidelines recommended pharmacological therapy with bile acid sequestrants (cholestyramine or colestipol) for children older than 10 years who despite diet modification had an LDL-C level of 190 mg/dl or higher or a level of 160 mg/dl or higher with a family history of premature cardiovascular disease or with two other cardiovascular disease risk factors. Tonstad and coworkers studied 72 children in a randomized, placebo-controlled trial of cholestyramine and found only modest reductions (<20 percent) in LDL-C.[181] Furthermore, the inconvenience and unpalatability of bile acid sequestrants have limited the compliance and hence the usefulness of these agents in later childhood and adolescence.[182] In the pediatric population, alternative therapies with nicotinic acid are also poorly tolerated,[182, 183] and fibric acid derivatives have been associated with significant transaminase elevations.[181]

Since formulation of the NCEP guidelines, hydroxymethylglutaryl coenzyme A (HMG-CoA) reductase inhibitors (statins) have become the most widely used cholesterol-lowering agents in adults and have been shown to be effective in reducing mortality and morbidity from coronary heart disease in both primary and secondary prevention trials. In children, investigations of the use of HMG-CoA reductase inhibitors have included both early observational studies[182, 184] and short-term therapeutic trials in heterozygous familial dyslipidemias. In a placebo-controlled study, Knipscheer and colleagues treated 72 patients aged 8 to 16 years with pravastatin in doses ranging from 5 to 20 mg/day.[185] LDL-C fell by 23 to 32 percent and no adverse effects were observed. Lambert and associates performed a multicenter 8-week trial in which 69 adolescent boys (weight >27 kg) were randomized to four doses of lovastatin ranging from 10 to 40 mg/day after a 4-week placebo period; LDL-C was reduced 21 to 36 percent in a dose-response relationship.[186] Increases in HDL-C and apolipoprotein A1 were also observed. Neither serious clinical adverse events nor important elevations in serum transaminases or creatine kinase values were found. Most recently, in a randomized, placebo-controlled trial in 132 adolescent boys aged 10 to 17 years with familial hyperlipidemia, Stein and coauthors reported that lovastatin was effective in lowering LDL-C.[187] Comprehensive clinical and biochemical data on growth, hormonal, and nutritional status indicated no significant differences between the groups treated with lovastatin and placebo. Although HMG-CoA reductase inhibitor treatment of hyperlipidemic children and adolescents has been demonstrated to have short-term safety and efficacy in lowering the serum lipid profile, it is unknown whether such treatment affects preclinical disease in this age group.

Antioxidant vitamins may also have a role in the treatment of dyslipidemic children and adolescents. In a recent study in children with familial hyperlipidemia, impaired brachial vasoreactivity was improved after therapy with vitamin E and vitamin C.[188]

ASSESSMENT OF PRECLINICAL ATHEROSCLEROSIS. Assessment of the effect of treatment of hyperlipidemia in childhood on vascular health is hampered by the long latency until occurrence of clinical disease. Therefore, the effects of therapies on preclinical markers of atherosclerosis are important. Methods of assessment of preclinical atherosclerosis that have been demonstrated to relate to risk factors in children include brachial artery flow–mediated dilation,[189, 189a] carotid intimal-medial thickness,[190, 191] and coronary artery calcification on electron beam computed tomography.[192]

REFERENCES

CARDIOMYOPATHIES

1. Report of the WHO/ISFC Task Force on the definition and classification of cardiomyopathies. Br Heart J 44:672, 1980.
2. Crispell KA, Wray A, Ni H, et al: Clinical profiles of four large pedigrees with familial dilated cardiomyopathy: Preliminary recommendations for clinical practice. J Am Coll Cardiol 34:837, 1999.
3. Katsuragi M, Yutani C, Mukai T, et al: Detection of enteroviral genome and its significance in cardiomyopathy. Cardiology 83:4, 1993.
4. Bristow MR, Minobe W, Rasmussen R, et al: Beta-adrenergic neuroeffector abnormalities in the failing human heart are produced by local rather than systemic mechanisms. J Clin Invest 89:803, 1992.
5. Böhm M, La Rosée K, Schmidt U, et al: Force-frequency relationship and inotropic stimulation in the nonfailing and failing human myocardium: Implications for the medical treatment of heart failure. Klin Wochenschr 70:421, 1992.
6. Del Monte F, O'Gara P, Poole-Wilson PA, et al: Cell geometry and contractile abnormalities of myocytes from failing human left ventricle. Cardiovasc Res 30:281, 1995.
7. Borst MM, Beuthien W, Schwencke C, et al: Desensitization of the pulmonary adenylyl cyclase system: A cause of airway hyperresponsiveness in congestive heart failure? J Am Coll Cardiol 34:848, 1999.
8. Friedman RA, Moak JP, Garson A Jr: Clinical course of idiopathic dilated cardiomyopathy in children. J Am Coll Cardiol 18:152, 1991.
9. Fishberger SB, Colan SD, Saul JP, et al: Myocardial mechanics before and after ablation of chronic tachycardia. Pacing Clin Electrophysiol 19: 42, 1996.
10. Matitiau A, Perez-Atayde A, Sanders SP, et al: Infantile dilated cardiomyopathy: Relation of outcome to left ventricular mechanics, hemodynamics, and histology at the time of presentation. Circulation 90:1310, 1994.
11. Karr SS, Parness IA, Spevak PJ, et al: Diagnosis of anomalous left coronary artery by Doppler color flow mapping: Distinction from other causes of dilated cardiomyopathy. J Am Coll Cardiol 19:1271, 1992.
12. Li DX, Tapscoft T, Gonzalez O, et al: Desmin mutation responsible for idiopathic dilated cardiomyopathy. Circulation 100:461, 1999.
13. Webber SA, Boyle GJ, Jaffe R, et al: Role of right ventricular endomyocardial biopsy in infants and children with suspected or possible myocarditis. Br Heart J 72:360, 1994.
14. Schwartz ML, Cox GF, Lin AE, et al: Clinical approach to genetic cardiomyopathy in children. Circulation 94:2021, 1996.
14a. Bennett MJ, Rinaldo P, Straiss AW: Inborn errors of mitochondrial fatty acid oxidation. Crit Rev Clin Lab Sci 37:1, 2000.
14b. Infante JP, Huszagh VA: Secondary carnitine deficiency and impaired docosahexaenoic (22:6n-3) acid synthesis: a common denominator in the pathophysiology of diseases of oxidative phosphorylation and β-oxidation. FEBS Lett 468:1, 2000.
14c. Pierpont MEM, Breningstall GN, Stanley CA, Singh A: Familial carnitine transporter defect: A treatable cause of cardiomyopathy in children. Am Heart J 139:S96, 2000.
15. Strauss AW: Defects of mitochondrial proteins and pediatric heart disease. Prog Pediatr Cardiol 6:83, 1996.
15a. Jarreta D, Orús J, Barrientos A, et al: Mitochondrial function in heart muscle from patients with idiopathic dilated cardiomyopathy. Cardiovasc Res 45:860, 2000.
15b. Wallace DC: Mitochondrial defects in cardiomyopathy and neuromuscular disease. Am Heart J 139:S70, 2000.
15c. Winter SC, Buist NRM: Cardiomyopathy in childhood, mitochondrial dysfunction, and the role of L-carnitine. Am Heart J 139:S63, 2000.
16. Remes AM, Hassinen IE, Ikäheimo MJ, et al: Mitochondrial DNA deletions in dilated cardiomyopathy: A clinical study employing endomyocardial sampling. J Am Coll Cardiol 23:935, 1994.
17. Reddy M, Hanley FL: Mechanical support of the myocardium. In Chang AC, Hanley FL, Wernovsky G, et al (eds): Pediatric Cardiac Intensive Care. Baltimore, Williams & Wilkins, 1998, p 345.
18. Pitt B, Zannad F, Remme WJ, et al: The effect of spironolactone on morbidity and mortality in patients with severe heart failure. Randomized Aldactone evaluation study investigators. N Engl J Med 341:709, 1999.
19. Alexander ME, Walsh EP, Saul JP, et al: Value of programmed ventricular stimulation in patients with congenital heart disease. J Cardiovasc Electrophysiol 10:1033, 1999.
20. Oliva F, Latini R, Politi A, et al: Intermittent 6-month low-dose dobutamine infusion in severe heart failure: DICE Multicenter Trial. Am Heart J 138:247, 1999.
21. Östman-Smith I, Brown G, Johnson A, et al: Dilated cardiomyopathy due to type II X-linked 3-methylglutaconic aciduria: Successful treatment with pantothenic acid. Br Heart J 72:349, 1994.
22. Akagi T, Benson LN, Lightfoot NE, et al: Natural history of dilated cardiomyopathy in children. Am Heart J 121:1502, 1991.
23. Arola A, Tuominen J, Ruuskanen O, et al: Idiopathic dilated cardiomyopathy in children: Prognostic indicators and outcome. Pediatrics 101: 369, 1998.
24. Cooper HA, Gersh BJ: Treatment of chronic mitral regurgitation. Am Heart J 135:925, 1998.
25. Chen FY, Adams DH, Aranki SF, et al: Mitral valve repair in cardiomyopathy. Circulation 98(Suppl 2):124–127, 1998.
26. Kim MH, Devlin WH, Das SK, et al: Effects of β-adrenergic blocking therapy on left ventricular diastolic relaxation properties in patients with dilated cardiomyopathy. Circulation 100:729, 1999.
26a. Cirillo W, Decanini R, Coelho OR, et al: Effects of metoprolol CR in patients with ischemic and dilated cardiomyopathy—the randomized evaluation of strategies for left ventricular dysfunction pilot study. Circulation 101:378, 2000.
27. Shaddy RE: β-Blocker therapy in young children with congestive heart failure under consideration for heart transplantation. Am Heart J 136: 19, 1998.
28. Exner DV, Dries DL, Waclawiw MA, et al: Beta-adrenergic blocking agent use and mortality in patients with asymptomatic and symptomatic left ventricular systolic dysfunction: A post hoc analysis of the studies of left ventricular dysfunction. J Am Coll Cardiol 33:916, 1999.
29. Sander GE, McKinnie JJ, Greenberg SS, et al: Angiotensin-converting enzyme inhibitors and angiotensin II receptor antagonists in the treatment of heart failure caused by left ventricular systolic dysfunction. Prog Cardiovasc Dis 41:265, 1999.
30. Johnson MR, Gheorghiade M: Growth hormone therapy in patients with congestive heart failure: Need for further research. Am Heart J 137:989, 1999.
30a. Curry CW, Nelson GS, Wyman BT, et al: Mechanical dyssynchrony in dilated cardiomyopathy with intraventricular conduction delay as depicted by 3D tagged magnetic resonance imaging. Circulation 101:E2, 2000.
31. Kass DA, Chen CH, Curry C, et al: Improved left ventricular mechanics from acute VDD pacing in patients with dilated cardiomyopathy and ventricular conduction delay. Circulation 99:1567, 1999.
31a. Kerwin WF, Botvinick EH, O'Connell JW, et al: Ventricular contraction abnormalities in dilated cardiomyopathy: Effect of biventricular pacing to correct interventricular dyssynchrony. J Am Coll Cardiol 35:1221, 2000.
32. Del Nido PJ: Editorial: Partial left ventriculectomy for dilated cardiomyopathy in children. J Thorac Cardiovasc Surg 117:918, 1999.
33. Ratcliffe MB, Hong J, Salahieh A, et al: The effect of ventricular volume reduction surgery in the dilated, poorly contractile left ventricle: A simple finite element analysis. J Thorac Cardiovasc Surg 116:566, 1998.
33a. Popovic Z, Miric M, Gradinac S, et al: Partial left ventriculectomy improves left ventricular end systolic elastance in patients with idiopathic dilated cardiomyopathy. Heart 83:316, 2000.
34. Burch M, Siddiqi SA, Celermajer DS, et al: Dilated cardiomyopathy in children: Determinants of outcome. Br Heart J 72:246, 1994.
35. Pongpanich B, Isaraprasart S: Congestive cardiomyopathy in infants and children. Clinical features and natural history. Jpn Heart J 27:11, 1986.
36. Lewis AB, Chabot M: Outcome of infants and children with dilated cardiomyopathy. Am J Cardiol 68:365, 1991.
37. Ciszewski A, Bilinska ZT, Lubiszewska B, et al: Dilated cardiomyopathy in children: Clinical course and prognosis. Pediatr Cardiol 15:121, 1994.

38. Lewis AB: Late recovery of ventricular function in children with idiopathic dilated cardiomyopathy. Am Heart J 138:334, 1999.

Infective Cardiomyopathy

39. Nakagawa M, Sato A, Okagawa H, et al: Detection and evaluation of asymptomatic myocarditis in schoolchildren—report of four cases. Chest 116:340, 1999.
40. Psani B, Taylor DO, Mason JW: Inflammatory myocardial diseases and cardiomyopathies. Am J Med 102:459, 1997.
41. Luppi P, Rudert WA, Zanone MM, et al: Idiopathic dilated cardiomyopathy—a superantigen-driven autoimmune disease. Circulation 98:777, 1998.
42. Chan KY, Iwahara M, Benson LN, et al: Immunosuppressive therapy in the management of acute myocarditis in children: A clinical trial. J Am Coll Cardiol 17:458, 1991.
43. Balaji S, Wiles HB, Sens MA, et al: Immunosuppressive treatment for myocarditis and borderline myocarditis in children with ventricular ectopic rhythm. Br Heart J 72:354, 1994.
44. Drucker NA, Colan SD, Lewis AB, et al: Gamma-globulin treatment of acute myocarditis in the pediatric population. Circulation 89:252, 1994.

Endocardial Fibroelastosis

45. Lurie PR: Endocardial fibroelastosis is not a disease. Am J Cardiol 62:468, 1988.
46. Ni JY, Bowles NE, Kim YH, et al: Viral infection of the myocardium in endocardial fibroelastosis—molecular evidence for the role of mumps virus as an etiologic agent. Circulation 95:133, 1997.
47. Kuboki K, Ohkawa S, Chida K, et al: Torsades de pointes in a case of hypertrophic cardiomyopathy with special reference to the pathologic findings of the heart including the conduction system. Jpn Heart J 40:233, 1999.
48. Mahle WT, Weinberg PM, Rychik J: Can echocardiography predict the presence or absence of endocardial fibroelastosis in infants <1 year of age with left ventricular outflow obstruction? Am J Cardiol 82:122, 1998.
49. Angelov A, Kulova A, Gurdevsky M: Endocardial fibroelastosis. Clinicopathological study of 38 cases. Pathol Res Pract 178:384, 1984.

Doxorubicin Cardiomyopathy

50. Lipshultz SE, Colan SD, Gelber RD, et al: Late cardiac effects of doxorubicin therapy for acute lymphoblastic leukemia in childhood. N Engl J Med 324:808, 1991.
51. Sorensen K, Levitt G, Bull C, et al: Anthracycline dose in childhood acute lymphoblastic leukemia: Issues of early survival versus late cardiotoxicity. J Clin Oncol 15:61, 1997.
52. Lipshultz SE, Lipsitz SR, Mone SM, et al: Female sex and drug dose as risk factors for late cardiotoxic effects of doxorubicin therapy for childhood cancer. N Engl J Med 332:1738, 1995.
53. Ewer MS, Jaffe N, Ried H, et al: Doxorubicin cardiotoxicity in children: Comparison of a consecutive divided daily dose administration schedule with single dose (rapid) infusion administration. Med Pediatr Oncol 31:512, 1998.
54. Pihkala J, Saarinen UM, Lundstrom U, et al: Myocardial function in children and adolescents after therapy with anthracyclines and chest irradiation. Eur J Cancer 32A:97, 1996.
55. Von Hoff DD, Layard MW, Basa P, et al: Risk factors for doxorubicin-induced congestive heart failure. Ann Intern Med 91:710, 1979.
56. Wiseman LR, Spencer CM: Dexrazoxane. A review of its use as a cardioprotective agent in patients receiving anthracycline-based chemotherapy. Drugs 56:385, 1998.
57. Schiavetti A, Castello MA, Versacci P, et al: Use of ICRF-187 for prevention of anthracycline cardiotoxicity in children: Preliminary results. Pediatr Hematol Oncol 14:213, 1997.
58. Steinherz LJ, Graham T, Hurwitz R, et al: Guidelines for cardiac monitoring of children during and after anthracycline therapy: Report of the Cardiology Committee of the Children's Cancer Study Group. Pediatrics 89:942, 1992.
59. Lipshultz SE, Sanders SP, Goorin AM, et al: Monitoring for anthracycline cardiotoxicity. Pediatrics 93:433, 1994.

Hypertrophic Cardiomyopathy

60. Jones S, Elliott PM, Sharma S, et al: Cardiopulmonary responses to exercise in patients with hypertrophic cardiomyopathy. Heart 80:60, 1998.
61. Fananapazir L, Chang AC, Epstein SE, et al: Prognostic determinants in hypertrophic cardiomyopathy: Prospective evaluation of a therapeutic strategy based on clinical, Holter, hemodynamic, and electrophysiological findings. Circulation 86:730, 1992.
62. Nienaber CA, Hiller S, Spielmann RP, et al: Syncope in hypertrophic cardiomyopathy: Multivariate analysis of prognostic determinants. J Am Coll Cardiol 15:948, 1990.
63. Spirito P, Rapezzi C, Autore C, et al: Prognosis of asymptomatic patients with hypertrophic cardiomyopathy and nonsustained ventricular tachycardia. Circulation 90:2743, 1994.

64. Lewis JF, Maron BJ: Hypertrophic cardiomyopathy characterized by marked hypertrophy of the posterior left ventricular free wall: Significance and clinical implications. J Am Coll Cardiol 18:421, 1991.
65. Maki S, Ikeda H, Muro A, et al: Predictors of sudden cardiac death in hypertrophic cardiomyopathy. Am J Cardiol 82:774, 1998.
66. Olivotto I, Maron BJ, Montereggi A, et al: Prognostic value of systemic blood pressure response during exercise in a community-based patient population with hypertrophic cardiomyopathy. J Am Coll Cardiol 33:2044, 1999.
67. Dilsizian V, Bonow RO, Epstein SE, et al: Myocardial ischemia detected by thallium scintigraphy is frequently related to cardiac arrest and syncope in young patients with hypertrophic cardiomyopathy. J Am Coll Cardiol 22:796, 1993.
68. Yamaguchi M, Tangkawattana P, Hamlin RL: Myocardial bridging as a factor in heart disorders: Critical review and hypothesis. Acta Anat (Basel) 157:248, 1996.
69. Kitazume H, Kramer JR, Krauthamer D, et al: Myocardial bridges in obstructive hypertrophic cardiomyopathy. Am Heart J 106:131, 1983.
70. Yetman AT, McCrindle BW, MacDonald C, et al: Myocardial bridging in children with hypertrophic cardiomyopathy—a risk factor for sudden death. N Engl J Med 339:1201, 1998.
71. Charron P, Dubourg O, Desnos M, et al: Diagnostic value of electrocardiography and echocardiography for familial hypertrophic cardiomyopathy in genotyped children. Eur Heart J 19:1377, 1998.
72. Noonan J, O'Connor W: Noonan syndrome: A clinical description emphasizing the cardiac findings. Acta Paediatr Jpn 38:76, 1996.
73. Moran AM, Colan SD: Verapamil therapy in infants with hypertrophic cardiomyopathy. Cardiol Young 8:310, 1998.
74. Goldstein JD, Shanske S, Bruno C, et al: Maternally inherited mitochondrial cardiomyopathy associated with a C-to-T transition at nucleotide 3303 of mitochondrial DNA in the tRNA(Leu(UUR)) gene. Pediatr Dev Pathol 2:78, 1999.
75. Bjornstad H, Storstein L, Meen HD, et al: Electrocardiographic findings of repolarization in athletic students and control subjects. Cardiology 84:51, 1994.
76. Manolas J, Kyriakidis M, Anastasakis A, et al: Usefulness of noninvasive detection of left ventricular diastolic abnormalities during isometric stress in hypertrophic cardiomyopathy and in athletes. Am J Cardiol 81:306, 1998.
77. Seiler C, Hess OM, Schoenbeck M, et al: Long-term follow-up of medical versus surgical therapy for hypertrophic cardiomyopathy: A retrospective study. J Am Coll Cardiol 17:634, 1991.
78. Pelliccia F, Cianfrocca C, Romeo F, et al: Hypertrophic cardiomyopathy: Long-term effects of propranolol versus verapamil in preventing sudden death in "low-risk" patients. Cardiovasc Drugs Ther 4:1515, 1990.
79. Criley JM: Unobstructed thinking (and terminology) is called for in the understanding and management of hypertrophic cardiomyopathy. J Am Coll Cardiol 29:741, 1997.
80. Theodoro DA, Danielson GK, Feldt RH, et al: Hypertrophic obstructive cardiomyopathy in pediatric patients: Results of surgical treatment. J Thorac Cardiovasc Surg 112:1589, 1996.
81. O'Rourke RA: Cardiac pacing. An alternative treatment for selected patients with hypertrophic cardiomyopathy and adjunctive therapy for certain patients with dilated cardiomyopathy. Circulation 100:786, 1999.
82. Alday LE, Bruno E, Moreyra E, et al: Mid-term results of dual-chamber pacing in children with hypertrophic obstructive cardiomyopathy. Echocardiogr J Cardiovasc Ultrasound Allied Tech 15:289, 1998.
83. Rishi F, Hulse JE, Auld DO, et al: Effects of dual-chamber pacing for pediatric patients with hypertrophic obstructive cardiomyopathy. J Am Coll Cardiol 29:734, 1997.
84. Nishimura RA, Trusty JM, Hayes DL, et al: Dual-chamber pacing for hypertrophic cardiomyopathy: A randomized, double-blind, crossover trial. J Am Coll Cardiol 29:435, 1997.
85. Kiviniemi MS, Pirnes MA, Eränen HJK, et al: Complications related to permanent pacemaker therapy. Pacing Clin Electrophysiol 22:711, 1999.
86. Semsarian C, Richmond DR: Sudden cardiac death in familial hypertrophic cardiomyopathy: An Australian experience. Aust N Z J Med 29:368, 1999.
87. Maron BJ, Shirani J, Poliac LC, et al: Sudden death in young competitive athletes. Clinical, demographic, and pathological profiles. JAMA 276:199, 1996.
88. Shephard RJ: The athlete's heart: Is big beautiful? Br J Sports Med 30:5, 1996.
89. Maron BJ, Klues HG: Surviving competitive athletics with hypertrophic cardiomyopathy. Am J Cardiol 73:1098, 1994.
90. Kohl HW, Powell KE, Gordon NF, et al: Physical activity, physical fitness, and sudden cardiac death. Epidemiol Rev 14:37, 1992.
91. Yetman AT, Hamilton RM, Benson LN, et al: Long-term outcome and prognostic determinants in children with hypertrophic cardiomyopathy. J Am Coll Cardiol 32:1943, 1998.
92. Maron BJ, Tajik AJ, Ruttenberg HD, et al: Hypertrophic cardiomyopathy in infants: Clinical features and natural history. Circulation 65:7, 1982.
93. Suda K, Kohl T, Kovalchin JP, et al: Echocardiographic predictors of poor outcome in infants with hypertrophic cardiomyopathy. Am J Cardiol 80:595, 1997.
94. Schaffer MS, Freedom RM, Rowe RD: Hypertrophic cardiomyopathy presenting before 2 years of age in 13 patients. Pediatr Cardiol 4:113, 1983.

95. Maron BJ, Spirito P: Implications of left ventricular remodeling in hypertrophic cardiomyopathy. Am J Cardiol 81:1339, 1998.

96. Eidem BW, Lindor NM, Driscoll DJ: Resolution of neonatal hypertrophic cardiomyopathy in an infant with an affected mother. Pediatr Cardiol 20:208, 1999.

97. Ino T, Nishimoto K, Okubo M, et al: Apoptosis as a possible cause of wall thinning in end-stage hypertrophic cardiomyopathy. Am J Cardiol 79:1137, 1997.

98. Panza JA, Maris TJ, Maron BJ: Development and determinants of dynamic obstruction to left ventricular outflow in young patients with hypertrophic cardiomyopathy. Circulation 85:1398, 1992.

99. McKenna WJ: The natural history of hypertrophic cardiomyopathy. Cardiovasc Clin 19:135, 1988.

100. Maron BJ, Casey SA, Poliac LC, et al: Clinical course of hypertrophic cardiomyopathy in a regional United States cohort. JAMA 281:650, 1999.

101. Takagi E, Yamakado T, Nakano T: Prognosis of completely asymptomatic adult patients with hypertrophic cardiomyopathy. J Am Coll Cardiol 33:206, 1999.

Restrictive Cardiomyopathy

102. Lewis AB: Clinical profile and outcome of restrictive cardiomyopathy in children. Am Heart J 123:1589, 1992.

103. Cetta F, O'Leary PW, Seward JB, et al: Idiopathic restrictive cardiomyopathy in childhood: Diagnostic features and clinical course. Mayo Clin Proc 70:634, 1995.

104. Neudorf U, Bolte A, Lang D, et al: Diagnostic findings and outcome in children with primary restrictive cardiomyopathy. Cardiol Young 6:44, 1996.

105. Denfield SW, Rosenthal G, Gajarski RJ, et al: Restrictive cardiomyopathies in childhood. Tex Heart Inst J 24:38, 1997.

106. Hook S, Ratliff NB, Rosenkranz E, et al: Isolated noncompaction of the ventricular myocardium. Pediatr Cardiol 17:43, 1996.

KAWASAKI DISEASE

107. Kawasaki T: Acute febrile mucocutaneous syndrome with lymphoid involvement with specific desquamation of the fingers and toes in children [Japanese]. Jpn J Allergy 116:178, 1967.

108. Dajani AS, Taubert KA, Gerber MA, et al: Diagnosis and therapy of Kawasaki disease in children. Circulation 87:1776, 1993.

109. Taubert KA, Rowley AH, Shulman ST: Seven-year national survey of Kawasaki disease and acute rheumatic fever. Pediatr Infect Dis J 13:704, 1994.

110. Dajani AS, Taubert KA, Gerber MA, et al: Diagnosis and therapy of Kawasaki disease in children. Circulation 87:1776, 1993.

111. Kato H, Ichinose E, Kawasaki T: Myocardial infarction in Kawasaki disease: Clinical analyses in 195 cases. J Pediatr 108:923, 1986.

112. Suzuki A, Kamiya T, Kuwahara N, et al: Coronary arterial lesions of Kawasaki disease: Cardiac catheterization findings of 1100 cases. Pediatr Cardiol 7:3, 1986.

113. Research Committee on Kawasaki Disease: Report of Subcommittee on Standardization of Diagnostic Criteria and Reporting of Coronary Artery Lesions in Kawasaki Disease. Tokyo, Ministry of Health and Welfare, 1984.

114. Moran AM, Newburger JW, Sanders SP, et al: Abnormal myocardial mechanics in Kawasaki syndrome: Rapid response to gamma-globulin. Am Heart J 139:217–223, 2000.

115. Takahashi M, Shimada H, Billingham ME, et al: Electron microscopic findings of myocardial biopsy correlated with perfusion scan and coronary angiography in chronic Kawasaki syndrome: Myocellular ischemia possibly due to microvasculopathy. In Kato H (ed): Kawasaki Disease. Proceedings of the 5th International Kawasaki Disease Symposium, Fukuoka, Japan, May 22–25, 1995. Amsterdam, The Netherlands, Elsevier, 1995, p 401.

116. Kato H, Sugimura T, Akagi T, et al: Long-term consequences of Kawasaki Disease. A 10- to 21-year follow-up study of 594 patients. Circulation 94:1379, 1996.

117. Nakano H, Nojima K, Saito A, et al: High incidence of aortic regurgitation following Kawasaki disease. J Pediatr 107:59, 1985.

118. Dengler LD, Capparelli EV, Bastian JF, et al: Cerebrospinal fluid profile in patients with acute Kawasaki disease. J Pediatr Infect Dis 17:478, 1998.

119. de Zorzi A, Colan SD, Gauvreau K, et al: Coronary artery dimensions may be misclassified as normal in Kawasaki disease. J Pediatr 133:254, 1998.

120. National Heart, Lung, and Blood Institute Coronary Artery Surgery Study: A multicenter comparison of the effects of randomized medical and surgical treatment of mildly symptomatic patients with coronary artery disease, and a registry of consecutive patients undergoing coronary angiography. Circulation 63(Suppl 1):1–81, 1981.

121. Takahashi M, Mason W, Lewis AB: Regression of coronary aneurysms in patients with Kawasaki syndrome. Circulation 75:387, 1987.

122. Durongpisitkul K, Gururaj VJ, Park JM, et al: The prevention of coronary artery aneurysm in Kawasaki disease: A meta-analysis on the efficacy of aspirin and immunoglobulin treatment. Pediatrics 96:1057, 1995.

123. Newburger JW, Takahasha M, Burns JC, et al: The treatment of Kawsaki syndrome with intravenous gamma globulin. N Engl J Med 315:341, 1986.

124. Marasini M, Pongiglione G, Gazzolo D, et al: Late intravenous gamma globulin treatment in infants and children with Kawasaki disease and coronary artery abnormalities. Am J Cardiol 68:796, 1991.

125. Dajani AS, Taubert KA, Takahashi M, et al: Guidelines for long-term management of patients with Kawasaki disease. Report from the Committee on Rheumatic Fever, Endocarditis, and Kawasaki Disease, Council on Cardiovascular Disease in the Young, American Heart Association. Circulation 89:916, 1994.

126. Newburger JW, Takahashi M, Beiser AS, et al: A single intravenous infusion of gamma globulin as compared with four infusions in the treatment of acute Kawasaki syndrome. N Engl J Med 324:1633, 1991.

127. Burns JC, Capparelli EV, Brown JA, et al: Intravenous gamma globulin treatment and retreatment in Kawasaki disease. US/Canadian Kawasaki Syndrome Study Group. Pediatr Infect Dis J 17:1144, 1998.

128. Kato H, Koike S, Yokoyama T: Kawasaki disease: Effect of treatment on coronary artery involvement. Pediatrics 63:175, 1979.

129. Newburger JW: Treatment of Kawasaki disease: Corticosteroids revisited (editorial). J Pediatr 135:411, 1999.

130. Wright DA, Newburger JW, Baker A, et al: Treatment of immune globulin–resistant Kawasaki disease with pulsed doses of corticosteroids. J Pediatr 128:146, 1996.

131. Matsubara T, Yabuta K, Furukawa S: Immunoregulation and pentoxifylline therapy during acute Kawasaki disease. In Kato H (ed): Kawasaki Disease. Proceedings of the 5th International Kawasaki Disease Symposium, Fukuoka, Japan, May 22–25, 1995. Amsterdam, The Netherlands, Elsevier, 1995, p 237.

132. Villain E, Kachaner J, Sidi D, et al: [Trial of prevention of coronary aneurysm in Kawasaki's using plasma exchange or infusion of immunoglobulins.] Arch Fr Pediatr 44:79, 1987.

133. Fujiwara T, Fujiwara H, Hamashima Y: Size of coronary aneurysm as a determinant factor of the prognosis in Kawasaki disease: Clinicopathologic study of coronary aneurysms. Prog Clin Biol Res 250:519, 1987.

134. Tatara K, Kusakawa S: Long-term prognosis of giant coronary aneurysm in Kawasaki disease: An angiographic study. J Pediatr 111:705, 1987.

134a. Yoshikawa Y, Yagihara T, Kameda Y, et al: Result of surgical treatments in patients with coronary-arterial obstructive disease after Kawasaki disease. Eur J Cardiothorac Surg 17:515, 2000.

135. Kitamura S, Kameda Y, Seki T, et al: Long-term outcome of myocardial revascularization in patients with Kawasaki coronary artery disease. J Thorac Cardiovasc Surg 107:663, 1994.

136. Ino T, Akimoto K, Ohkubo M, et al: Application of percutaneous transluminal coronary angioplasty to coronary arterial stenosis in Kawasaki disease. Circulation 93:1709, 1996.

137. Sugimura T, Yokoi H, Sato N, et al: Interventional treatment for children with severe coronary artery stenosis with calcification after long-term Kawasaki disease. Circulation 96:3928, 1997.

138. Checchia PA, Pahl E, Shaddy RE, et al: Cardiac transplantation for Kawasaki disease. Pediatrics 100:695, 1997.

139. Kato H, Sugimura T, Akagi T, et al: Long-term consequences of Kawasaki disease: A 10- to 21-year follow-up study of 594 patients. Circulation 94:1379, 1996.

140. Kamiya T, Suzuki A, Ono Y, et al: Angiographic follow-up study of coronary artery lesion in the cases with a history of Kawasaki disease—with a focus on the follow-up more than ten years after the onset of the disease. In Kato H (ed): Kawasaki Disease. Proceedings of the 5th International Kawasaki Disease Symposium, Fukuoka, Japan, May 22–25, 1995. Amsterdam, The Netherlands, Elsevier, 1995, p 569.

141. Fujiwara T, Fujiwara H, Hamashima Y: Frequency and size of coronary arterial aneurysm at necropsy in Kawasaki disease. Am J Cardiol 59:808, 1987.

142. Burns JC, Shike H, Gordon JB, et al: Sequelae of Kawasaki disease in adolescents and young adults. J Am Coll Cardiol 28:253, 1996.

143. Sugimura T, Kato H, Inoue O, et al: Intravascular ultrasound of coronary arteries in children. Assessment of the wall morphology and the lumen after Kawasaki disease. Circulation 89:258, 1994.

144. Sugimura T, Kato H, Inoue O, et al: Vasodilatory response of the coronary arteries after Kawasaki disease: Evaluation by intracoronary injection of isosorbide dinitrate. J Pediatr 121:684, 1992.

144a. Iemura M, Ishii M, Sugimura T, et al: Long term consequences of regressed coronary aneurysms after Kawasaki disease: Vascular wall morphology and function. Heart 83:307, 2000.

145. Fulton DR, Meissner C, Peterson MB: Effects of current therapy of Kawasaki disease on eicosanoid metabolism. Am J Cardiol 61:1323, 1988.

146. Newburger JW, Burns JC, Beiser AS, et al: Altered lipid profile after Kawasaki syndrome. Circulation 84:625, 1991.

147. Fujiwara T, Fujiwara H, Nakano H: Pathological features of coronary arteries in children with Kawasaki disease in which coronary arterial aneurysm was absent at autopsy. Circulation 78:345, 1988.

148. Muzik O, Paridon SM, Singh TP, et al: Quantification of myocardial blood flow and flow reserve in children with a history of Kawasaki disease and normal coronary arteries using positron emission tomography. J Am Coll Cardiol 28:757, 1996.

149. Dhillon R, Clarkson P, Donald AE, et al: Endothelial dysfunction late after Kawasaki disease. Circulation 94:2103, 1996.

150. Mitani Y, Okuda Y, Shimpo H, et al: Impaired endothelial function in

epicardial coronary arteries after Kawasaki disease. Circulation 96:454, 1997.

151. Yamakawa R, Ishii M, Sugimura T, et al: Coronary endothelial dysfunction after Kawasaki disease: Evaluation by intracoronary injection of acetylcholine. J Am Coll Cardiol 31:1074, 1998.

SYSTEMIC HYPERTENSION

152. National Heart, Lung, and Blood Institute: Update on the 1987 Task Force Report on High Blood Pressure in Children and Adolescents: A working group report from the National High Blood Pressure Education Program. Pediatrics 98:649, 1996.
153. Bartosh SM, Aronson AJ: Childhood hypertension. An update on etiology, diagnosis, and treatment. Pediatr Clin North Am 46:235, 1999.
154. Reusz GS, Hobor M, Tulassay T, et al: 24 hour blood pressure monitoring in healthy and hypertensive children. Arch Dis Child 70:90, 1994.
155. Harshfield GA, Alpert BS, Pulliam DA, et al: Ambulatory blood pressure recordings in children and adolescents. Pediatrics 94:180, 1994.
155a. Sorof JM, Portman RJ: Ambulatory blood pressure monitoring in the pediatric patient. J Pediatr 136:578, 2000.
156. Swinford RD, Ingelfinger JR: Evaluation of hypertension in childhood diseases. In Barratt TM, Avner ED, Harmon EW (eds): Pediatric Nephrology. 4th ed. Baltimore, Lippincott Williams & Wilkins, 1999, p 1007.
157. Sinaiko AR: Childhood hypertension. In Laragh GH, Brenner BM (eds): Hypertension: Pathophysiology, Diagnosis, and Management. New York, Raven, 1995, p 209.
158. Rodd CJ, Sockalosky JJ: Endocrine causes of hypertension in children. Pediatr Clin North Am 40:149, 1993.
159. Deal JE, Sever PS, Barratt TM, et al: Phaeochromocytoma: Investigation and management of 10 cases. Arch Dis Child 65:269, 1990.
160. Schmedtje JF, Sax S, Poole JL, et al: Imaging methods in diagnosis of pheochromocytoma. Bildgeb Chir 122:438, 1997.
161. Boraschi P, Braccini G, Grassi L, et al: Incidentally discovered adrenal masses: Evaluation with gadolinium enhancement and fat-suppressed MR imaging at 0.5. Eur J Radiol 24:245, 1997.
162. Perel Y, Schlumberger M, Marguerite G, et al: Pheochromocytoma and paraganglioma in children: A report of 24 cases of the French Society of Pediatric Oncology. Pediatr Hematol Oncol 14:413, 1997.
163. Spear RM, Deshpande JK, Davis PJ: Systemic disorders in pediatric anesthesia. In Motoyama EK, Davis PJ (eds): Smith's Anesthesia for Infants and Children. St. Louis, Mosby, 1990, p 779.
164. Phillips SJ, Whisnant JP: Hypertension and the brain. The National High Blood Pressure Education Program. Arch Intern Med 152:938, 1992.
165. Appel LJ, Moore TJ, Obarzanek E, et al: A clinical trial of the effects of dietary patterns on blood pressure. N Engl J Med 336:1117, 1997.
166. National Heart, Lung, and Blood Institute: Report of the Task Force on Blood Pressure Control in Children. Pediatrics 79:1, 1987.
167. Drugs for hypertension. Med Lett 41:2328, 1999.

HYPERLIPIDEMIA

168. Berenson GS, Srinivasan S, Bao W, et al: Association between multiple cardiovascular risk factors and atherosclerosis in children and young adults. N Engl J Med 338:1650, 1998.
169. Enos WF, Holmes RH, Beyer J: Coronary disease among United States soldiers killed in action in Korea. JAMA 152:1090, 1953.
170. Strong JP, for the Pathobiological Determinants of Atherosclerosis in Youth (PDAY) Research Group: Natural history and risk factors for early human atherogenesis. Clin Chem 41:134, 1995.
171. Strong JP, Malcom GT, McMahan CA, et al: Prevalence and extent of atherosclerosis in adolescents and young adults: Implications for prevention from the Pathobiological Determinants of Atherosclerosis in Youth Study. JAMA 281:727, 1999.

172. Newman WPI, Freedman DS, Voors AW, et al: Relation of serum lipoprotein levels and systolic blood pressure to early atherosclerosis. N Engl J Med 314:138, 1986.
173. Berenson GS, Srinivasan SR, Bao W, et al: Association between multiple cardiovascular risk factors and atherosclerosis in children and young adults. N Engl J Med 338:1650, 1998.
174. Lee J, Lauer RM, Clarke WR: Lipoproteins in the progeny of young men with coronary artery disease. Children with increased risk. Pediatrics 78:330, 1986.
175. Klag MJ, Ford DE, Mead LA, et al: Serum cholesterol in young men and subsequent cardiovascular disease. N Engl J Med 328:313, 1993.
176. National Cholesterol Education Program: Report of the Expert Panel on Blood Cholesterol Levels in Children and Adolescents. Bethesda, MD, National Heart, Lung, and Blood Institute, NIH Publication 91-2732, 1991.
177. Dennison BA, Kikuchi DA, Srinivasan SR, et al: Parental history of cardiovascular disease as an indication for screening for lipoprotein abnormalities in children. J Pediatr 115:186, 1989.
178. Griffin TC, Christoffel KK, Binns HJ, et al: Family history evaluation as a predictive screen for childhood hypercholesterolemia. Pediatrics 84:365, 1989.
179. Neufeld EJ, Newburger JW: How should children with hypercholesterolemia be managed? Choices Cardiol 7:233, 1993.
180. The Writing Group for the DISC Collaborative Research Group: Efficacy and safety of lowering dietary intake of fat and cholesterol in children with elevated low-density lipoprotein cholesterol: The Dietary Intervention Study in Children (DISC). JAMA 18:1429, 1995.
181. Tonstad S, Knudtzon J, Siversten M, et al: Efficacy and safety of cholestyramine therapy in peripubertal and prepubertal children with familial hypercholesterolemia. J Pediatr 129:42, 1996.
182. Stein EA: Treatment of familial hypercholesterolemia with drugs in children. Arteriosclerosis 9(Suppl 1):145–151, 1989.
183. Colletti RB, Neufeld EJ, Roff NK, et al: Niacin treatment of hypercholesterolemia in children. Pediatrics 92:78, 1993.
184. Ducobu J, Brasseur D, Chaudron JM, et al: Simvastatin use in children. Lancet 339:1488, 1992.
185. Knipscheer HC, Boelen CC, Kastelein JJP, et al: Short-term efficacy and safety of pravastatin in 72 children with familial hypercholesterolemia. Pediatr Res 39:867, 1996.
186. Lambert M, Lupien PJ, Gagne C, et al: Treatment of familial hypercholesterolemia in children and adolescents: Effect of lovastatin. Pediatrics 97:619, 1996.
187. Stein EA, Illingsworth DR, Kwiterovich PO Jr, et al: Efficacy and safety of lovastatin in adolescent males with heterozygous familial hypercholesterolemia. A randomized controlled trial. JAMA 281:137–144, 1999.
188. Mietus-Snyder M, Malloy MJ: Endothelial dysfunction occurs in children with two genetic hyperlipidemias: Improvement with antioxidant vitamin therapy. J Pediatr 133:35, 1998.
189. Sorensen KE, Celermajer DS, Georgakopoulis D, et al: Impairment of endothelium-dependent dilatation is an early event in children with familial hypercholesterolemia and is related to lipoprotein(a). J Clin Invest 93:50, 1994.
189a. Leeson CP, Whincup PH, Cook DL, et al: Cholesterol and arterial distensibility in the first decade of life: A population based study. Circulation 101:1533, 2000.
190. Pauciullo P, Arcangelo I, Renata S, et al: Increased intima-media thickness of the common carotid artery in hypercholesterolemic children. Arterioscler Thromb 7:1075, 1994.
191. Tonstad S, Joakimsen O, Stensland-Bugge E, et al: Risk factors related to carotid intima-media thickness and plaque in children with familial hypercholesterolemia and control subjects. Arterioscler Thromb Vasc Biol 16:984, 1996.
192. Mahoney LT, Burns TL, Stanford W, et al: Coronary risk factors measured in childhood and young adult life are associated with coronary artery calcification in young adults: The Muscatine Study. J Am Coll Cardiol 27:277, 1996.

Chapter 46
Valvular Heart Disease

EUGENE BRAUNWALD

Mitral Stenosis

ETIOLOGY AND PATHOLOGY

The predominant cause of mitral stenosis (MS) is rheumatic fever[1] (see Chap. 66), and rheumatic involvement is present in 99 percent of stenotic mitral valves excised at the time of mitral valve replacement.[2] Approximately 25 percent of all patients with rheumatic heart disease have pure MS, and an additional 40 percent have combined MS and mitral regurgitation (MR).[3-5] Two thirds of all patients with rheumatic MS are female.

Rheumatic fever results in four forms of fusion of the mitral valve apparatus leading to stenosis: (1) commissural, (2) cuspal, (3) chordal, and (4) combined.[3-5] Thickening of the commissures alone occurs in 30 percent of patients, of the cusps alone in 15 percent, and of the chordae tendineae alone in 10 percent; in the remaining patients, thickening of more than one of these structures is involved. Characteristically, mitral valve cusps fuse at their edges, and fusion of the chordae tendineae results in thickening and shortening of these structures. The leaflets exhibit fibrous obliteration and revascularization. The stenotic mitral valve is typically funnel-shaped, and the orifice is frequently shaped like a "fish mouth" or buttonhole, with calcium deposits in the valve leaflets sometimes extending to involve the valve ring, which may become quite thick (Fig. 46–1). The thickened leaflets may be so adherent and rigid that they cannot open or shut, reducing or rarely even abolishing the first heart sound (S_1) and leading to combined MS and MR. When rheumatic fever results exclusively or predominantly in contraction and fusion of the chordae tendineae, with little fusion of the valvular commissures, dominant MR results.[6]

A debate continues about whether the anatomical changes in severe MS result from a smoldering rheumatic process or whether, once the valve has been deformed by the initial episode, the constant trauma produced by the turbulent blood flow leads to progressive fibrosis, thickening, and calcification of the valve apparatus.[7] Probably both processes are involved. Enlargement of the left atrium and resultant elevation of the left main stem bronchus, calcification of the left atrial wall, development of mural thrombi, and obliterative changes in the pulmonary vascular bed (see Chap. 53) may all result from chronic rheumatic MS.

Far less frequently, MS is congenital in etiology, and this form is observed almost exclusively in infants and young children (see Chap. 43). Very rarely, MS is a complication of malignant carcinoid, systemic lupus erythematosus, rheumatoid arthritis,[8] the mucopolysaccharidoses of the Hunter-Hurler phenotype,[9] Fabry disease, and Whipple disease. Amyloid deposits may occur on rheumatic valves and contribute to the obstruction to left atrial emptying.[10] Methysergide therapy is an unusual but documented cause of MS.[11] Atrial septal defect is associated with MS, generally of rheumatic origin, in Lutembacher syndrome (see Chap. 43). Obstruction to left atrial outflow may be caused by a left atrial tumor, particularly myxoma (see Chap. 49); ball-valve thrombus in the left atrium (usually associated with MS)[12]; infective endocarditis with large vegetations; and a congenital membrane in the left atrium, i.e., cor triatriatum (see Chap. 43). These conditions may simulate MS. Although calcification of the mitral annulus usually causes MR, MS may result when subvalvular or intravalvular extension is extensive.

PATHOPHYSIOLOGY

In normal adults, the cross-sectional area of the mitral valve orifice is 4 to 6 cm². When the orifice is reduced to approximately 2 cm², which is considered to represent *mild* MS, blood can flow from the left atrium to the left ventricle only if propelled by a small, although abnormal, pressure gradient. When the mitral valve opening is reduced to 1 cm², which is considered to represent *critical* MS,[13] a left atrioventricular pressure gradient of approximately 20 mm Hg (and, therefore, in the presence of a normal left ventricular diastolic pressure, a mean left atrial pressure of approximately 25 mm Hg) is required to maintain normal car-

1643

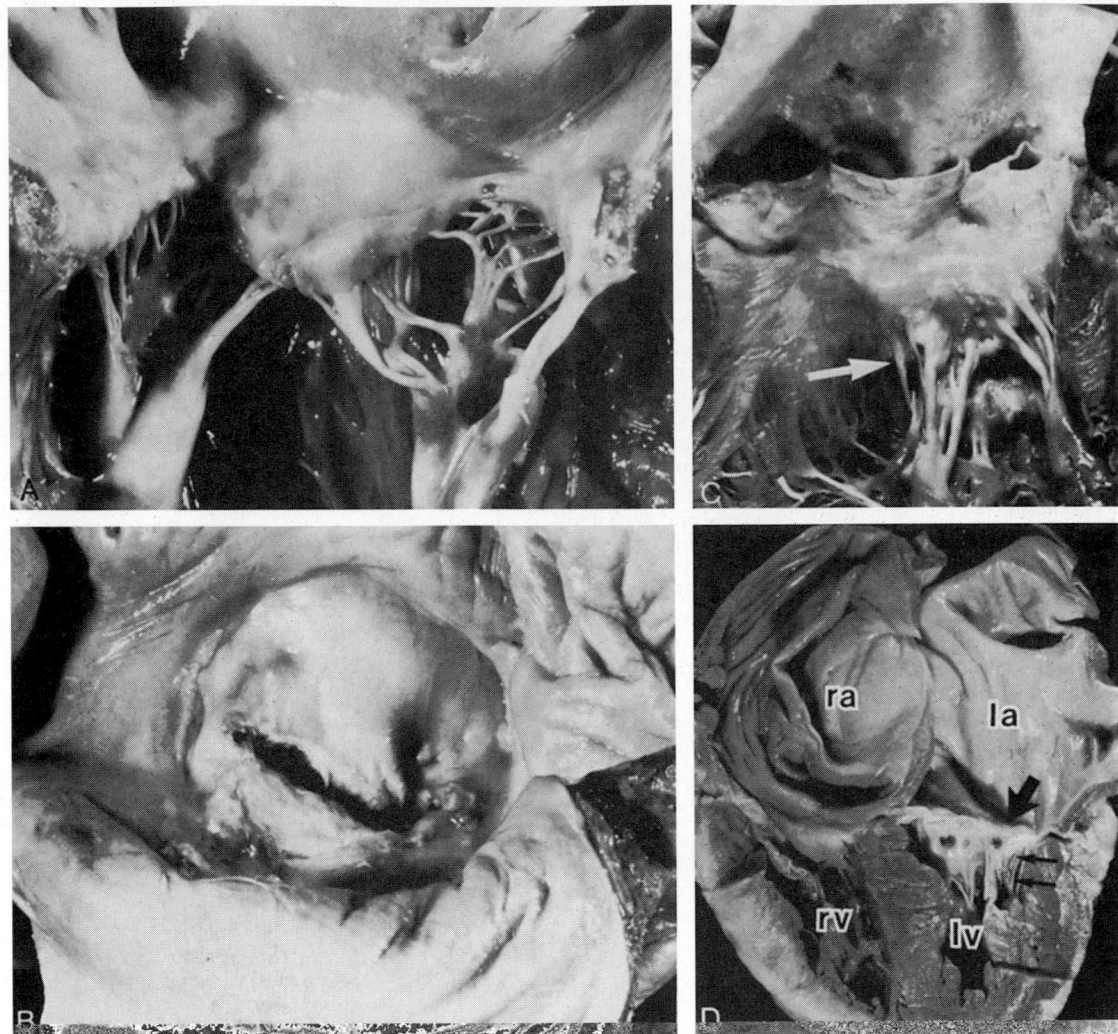

FIGURE 46–1. Rheumatic mitral stenosis. *A,* Moderate valvular changes including diffuse leaflet fibrosis, commissural fusion, and chordal thickening and fusion. In another patient, an atrial view (*B*) and subvalvular and aortic aspects (*C*) show prominent subvalvular involvement; severe subvalvular distortion is evident (arrow). *D,* Severe rheumatic mitral stenosis with specimen shown in apical four-chamber echocardiographic view, demonstrating small left ventricle (lv) and enlarged left atrium (la), right ventricle (rv), and right atrium (ra). Note the calcified stenotic valve (arrow) and prominent subvalvular changes (double arrows). (*A* and *D* from Schoen FJ, St. John Sutton M: Contemporary issues in the pathology of valvular heart disease. Hum Pathol 18:568, 1987.)

diac output at rest (Fig. 46–2; see also Fig. 11–14). The elevated left atrial pressure, in turn, raises pulmonary venous and capillary pressures, resulting in exertional dyspnea. The first bouts of dyspnea in patients with MS are usually precipitated by exercise, emotional stress, sexual intercourse, infection, or atrial fibrillation, all of which increase the rate of blood flow across the mitral orifice and result in further elevation of the left atrial pressure.[14, 15]

In order to assess the severity of obstruction of the mitral valve (and, for that matter, of any valve), both the transvalvular pressure gradient and the transvalvular flow rate must be measured (see Chap. 11).[16] The latter is a function not only of the cardiac output but also of the heart rate. An increase in heart rate shortens diastole proportionately more than systole and diminishes the time available for flow across the mitral valve. Therefore, at any given level of cardiac output, tachycardia augments the transmitral valvular pressure gradient and elevates left atrial pressures further.[17] This explains the sudden occurrence of dyspnea and pulmonary edema in previously asymptomatic patients with MS who develop atrial fibrillation with a rapid ventricular rate. It also accounts for the equally rapid improvement in these patients when the ventricular rate is

slowed by cardiac glycosides, beta-blocking agents, and/or heart-rate-slowing calcium antagonists, even when the transvalvular flow rate per minute remains constant. Hydraulic considerations dictate that at any given orifice size the transvalvular pressure gradient is a function of the square of the transvalvular flow rate.[18] Thus, a doubling of flow rate quadruples the pressure gradient, so that a stress such as exercise in patients with moderate or severe MS causes a marked elevation of left atrial pressure.[19] Pregnancy, hypervolemia, and hyperthyroidism all increase mitral valve flow and thereby the transvalvular pressure gradient.

Atrial contraction augments the presystolic transmitral valvular gradient by approximately 30 percent in patients with MS. Withdrawal of atrial transport when atrial fibrillation develops reduces cardiac output by about 20 percent.

Although the Gorlin formula (see Chap. 11) has been the benchmark for evaluating stenotic valvular orifices since 1951,[18] there is increasing evidence that valvular orifices are not rigid and that, in fact, as transvalvular flow increases, the orifice becomes distended. Accordingly, it has been proposed that stenosis can also be expressed as valvular resistance, the quotient of the mean transvalvular pressure gradient and the mean transvalvular flow.[20]

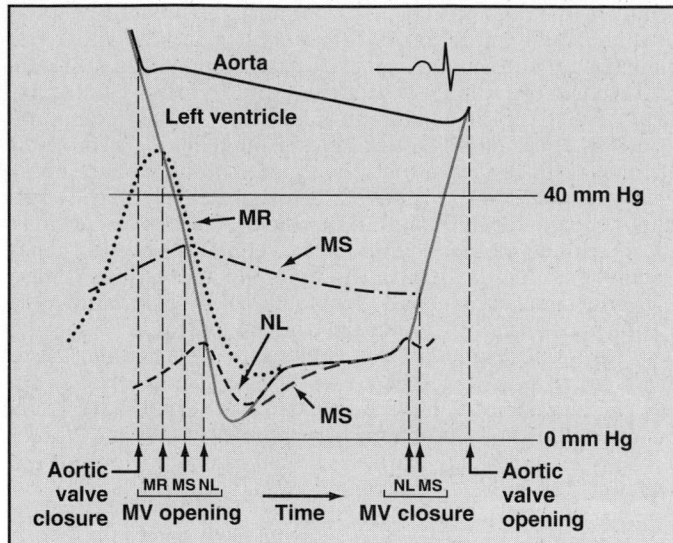

FIGURE 46-2. Schematic relationship of left ventricular, aortic, and pulmonary arterial wedge (PAW) pressures. Note that the higher the left atrial *v* wave, the earlier the pressure crossover and the earlier the mitral valve (MV) opening. The higher left atrial end-diastolic pressure with severe mitral stenosis (MS) also results in later closure of the mitral valve. PAW pressures are shown in severe mitral regurgitation (MR), mitral stenosis (MS), and normal (NL). The left ventricular diastolic pressure in mitral stenosis rises slowly, denoting the absence of a rapid filling wave. (From Braunwald E, Turi ZG: Pathophysiology of mitral valve disease. *In* Wells FC, Schapiro LM [eds]: Mitral Valve Disease. London, Butterworths, 1996.)

Intracardiac and Intravascular Pressures

LEFT ATRIAL AND RIGHT HEART PRESSURES. In patients with MS and sinus rhythm, mean left atrial pressure is elevated, and the left atrial pressure pulse generally exhibits a prominent atrial contraction (*a*) wave and a gradual pressure decline after mitral valve opening (*y* descent). In patients with mild to moderate MS without elevated pulmonary vascular resistance, pulmonary arterial pressure may be normal or only minimally elevated at rest but rises during exercise. However, in patients with severe MS and those in whom the pulmonary vascular resistance is significantly increased, pulmonary arterial pressure is elevated when the patient is at rest. In very rare patients with extremely elevated pulmonary vascular resistance, pulmonary arterial pressure may exceed systemic arterial pressure. Further elevations of left atrial and pulmonary vascular pressures occur during exercise and/or tachycardia. With moderately elevated pulmonary arterial pressure (systolic pressure 30 to 60 mm Hg), right ventricular performance is usually maintained.[21] However, a greater elevation of pulmonary arterial pressure represents a serious impedance to emptying of the right ventricle. During exercise, patients with MS and severe pulmonary hypertension commonly fail to exhibit normal elevation of the right ventricular ejection fraction.

LEFT VENTRICULAR DIASTOLIC PRESSURE. This pressure is normal in patients with isolated MS; however, coexisting MR, aortic valve lesions, systemic hypertension, ischemic heart disease, and cardiomyopathy may all be responsible for elevations of left ventricular diastolic pressure. In approximately 85 percent of patients with isolated MS, the left ventricular end-diastolic volume is within the normal range, whereas it is reduced in the remaining patients.[22] In approximately 25 percent of patients with isolated MS, the ejection fraction and other ejection indices of systolic performance (see Chap. 15) are below normal, most

likely resulting in part from chronic reduction in preload and elevated afterload.[23] Regional hypokinesis is common,[24] perhaps caused by extension of the scarring process from the mitral valve into the adjacent posterior basal myocardium or by associated ischemic heart disease. Leftward displacement of the interventricular septum secondary to more rapid early filling of the right ventricle may be responsible for a reduction of left ventricular compliance (left ventricular stiffening).[25] The left ventricular mass is normal or slightly reduced.[22]

The bulk of available evidence suggests that other than the posterior basal myocardium, left ventricular contractility is normal or only slightly impaired in the majority of patients with isolated MS.[26] Most patients with MS have a normal elevation of ejection fraction and a reduction of end-systolic volume during exercise.[27] Associated ischemic heart disease may, however, be responsible for myocardial dysfunction.[28]

PULMONARY HYPERTENSION. Pulmonary hypertension in patients with MS results from (1) passive backward transmission of the elevated left atrial pressure; (2) pulmonary arteriolar constriction, which presumably is triggered by left atrial and pulmonary venous hypertension (reactive pulmonary hypertension); and (3) organic obliterative changes in the pulmonary vascular bed, which may be considered to be a complication of longstanding and severe MS[29] (see Chap. 53). In time, severe pulmonary hypertension results in right-sided heart failure, with dilatation of the right ventricle and its annulus and secondary tricuspid and sometimes pulmonic regurgitation. These changes in the pulmonary vascular bed may also exert a protective effect; the elevated precapillary resistance makes the development of symptoms of pulmonary congestion less likely by tending to prevent blood from surging into the pulmonary capillary bed and damming up behind the stenotic mitral valve, although this protection occurs at the expense of a reduced cardiac output. In patients with severe MS, pulmonary vein–bronchial vein shunts occur.[30] Their rupture may cause hemoptysis. Patients with severe MS manifest a reduction in pulmonary compliance, an increase in the work of breathing, and a redistribution of pulmonary blood flow from the base to the apex.

CLINICAL AND HEMODYNAMIC FEATURES. At any given severity of stenosis, the clinical picture is dictated largely by the levels of cardiac output and pulmonary vascular resistance. The response to a given degree of mitral obstruction may be characterized at one end of the hemodynamic spectrum by a normal cardiac output and a high left atrioventricular pressure gradient or, at the opposite end of the spectrum, by a markedly reduced cardiac output and low transvalvular pressure gradient. Thus, in some patients with moderately severe MS (mitral valve area = 1.0 to 1.5 cm²), cardiac output at rest may be normal and rises normally during exertion. In these patients, the high transvalvular pressure gradient causes marked elevation of left atrial and pulmonary capillary pressures. This leads to severe pulmonary congestion during exertion. In contrast, in the majority of patients with severe MS, cardiac output rises subnormally during exertion, thus reducing the pulmonary venous pressure and the severity of symptoms of pulmonary congestion more than would be the case if the cardiac output rose normally. In patients with severe MS (mitral valve area ≤ 1.0 cm²), particularly when pulmonary vascular resistance is elevated, cardiac output is usually depressed at rest and may fail to rise at all during exertion. These patients frequently have severe weakness and fatigue secondary to a low cardiac output.

LEFT ATRIAL CHANGES. The combination of mitral valve disease and atrial inflammation secondary to rheumatic carditis causes (1) left atrial dilatation, (2) fibrosis of the atrial wall, and (3) disorganization of the atrial muscle bundles. The last leads to disparate conduction velocities and inhomogeneous refractory periods. Premature atrial activation, due either to an automatic focus or to reentry, may stimulate the left atrium during the vulnerable period and thereby precipitate atrial fibrillation. The development of this arrhythmia correlates independently with the severity of the MS and the height of the left atrial pressure.[31] Atrial fibrillation is often episodic at first, but then becomes more persistent. Atrial fibrillation per se causes diffuse atrophy of atrial muscle, further atrial enlargement,[32] and further inhomogeneity of refractoriness and conduction. These changes, in turn, lead to irreversible atrial fibrillation.

History

The principal symptom of MS is exertional dyspnea, largely the result of reduced pulmonary compliance. Dyspnea may be accompanied by cough and wheezing. Vital capacity is reduced, presumably owing to the presence of engorged pulmonary vessels and interstitial edema. Patients who have critical obstruction to left atrial emptying and dyspnea with ordinary activity (New York Heart Association [NYHA] Class III) generally have orthopnea as well and are at risk of experiencing attacks of frank pulmonary edema. The latter may be precipitated by effort, emotional stress, respiratory infection, fever, sexual intercourse, pregnancy, or atrial fibrillation with a rapid ventricular rate or other tachyarrhythmia. Indeed, pulmonary edema may be caused by any condition that increases flow across the stenotic mitral valve, either by increasing total cardiac output or by reducing the time available for blood flow across the mitral orifice to occur. In patients with a markedly elevated pulmonary vascular resistance, right ventricular function is often impaired.[33]

HEMOPTYSIS. Wood has differentiated between several kinds of *hemoptysis* complicating MS.[14]

1. Sudden hemorrhage (previously called "pulmonary apoplexy"). Although the hemorrhage is often profuse, it is only rarely life-threatening.[34] It results from the rupture of thin-walled, dilated bronchial veins,[30] usually as a consequence of a sudden rise in left atrial pressure. With persistence of pulmonary venous hypertension, the walls of these veins thicken appreciably. This form of hemoptysis tends to disappear as MS progresses.
2. Blood-stained sputum associated with attacks of paroxysmal nocturnal dyspnea.
3. Pink, frothy sputum characteristic of acute pulmonary edema with rupture of alveolar capillaries.
4. Pulmonary infarction, a late complication of MS associated with heart failure.
5. Blood-stained sputum complicating chronic bronchitis. The edematous bronchial mucosa in patients with chronic MS increases the likelihood of chronic bronchitis, which is a common complication of MS, particularly in Great Britain.

CHEST PAIN. A small percentage, perhaps 15 percent, of patients with MS experience chest discomfort that is indistinguishable from angina pectoris.[14] This symptom may be caused by severe right ventricular hypertension secondary to the pulmonary vascular disease or by concomitant coronary atherosclerosis.[28] Rarely, chest pain may be secondary to coronary obstruction caused by coronary embolization.[35] In many patients, however, a satisfactory explanation for the chest pain cannot be uncovered even after complete hemodynamic and angiographic studies.

SYSTEMIC EMBOLISM.[36, 36a] Before the advent of surgical treatment, this serious complication of MS developed in at least 20 percent of patients at some time during the course of their disease.[37] Before the era of anticoagulant therapy and surgical treatment, approximately 25 percent of all fatalities in patients with mitral valve disease were secondary to systemic embolism. The tendency for development of systemic embolization correlates directly with the patient's age and the size of the left atrial appendage and inversely with the cardiac output; 80 percent of patients with MS in whom systemic emboli develop are in atrial fibrillation. When embolization occurs in patients in sinus rhythm, the possibility of transient atrial fibrillation or underlying infective endocarditis should be considered. There is no simple correlation between the incidence of embolism on the one hand and the size of the mitral orifice on the other. Indeed, embolism may be the first symptom of MS and may occur in patients with mild MS even before the development of dyspnea.

Because thrombi are found in the left atrium at operation in only a minority of patients with a history of recent embolism, it is likely that only fresh clots are discharged. Approximately half of all clinically apparent emboli are found in the cerebral vessels. Coronary embolism may lead to myocardial infarction and/or angina pectoris, and renal emboli may be responsible for the development of systemic hypertension. Emboli are recurrent and multiple in approximately 25 percent of patients who develop this complication. Rarely, massive thrombosis develops in the left atrium, resulting in a pedunculated ball-valve thrombus, which may suddenly aggravate obstruction to left atrial outflow when a specific body position is assumed or may cause sudden death.[12] Similar consequences occur in patients with free-floating thrombi in the left atrium. These two conditions are usually characterized by variability in the physical findings, often on a positional basis. They are very hazardous and require surgical treatment, often as an emergency.

INFECTIVE ENDOCARDITIS (see also Chap. 47). This complication tends to occur *less frequently* on rigid, thickened, calcified valves and is therefore more common in patients with mild MS than those with severe MS.

OTHER SYMPTOMS. Compression of the left recurrent laryngeal nerve by a greatly dilated left atrium, enlarged tracheobronchial lymph nodes, and a dilated pulmonary artery may cause hoarseness (Ortner syndrome).[38] A history of repeated hemoptysis is common in patients with pulmonary hemosiderosis. Systemic venous hypertension, hepatomegaly, edema, ascites, and hydrothorax are all signs of severe MS with elevated pulmonary vascular resistance and right-sided heart failure.

Physical Examination[39, 40]

Patients with severe MS, a low cardiac output, and systemic vasoconstriction may exhibit the so-called *mitral facies,* characterized by pinkish-purple patches on the cheeks.[14] The *arterial pulse* is usually normal, but in patients with a reduced stroke volume, the pulse may be small in volume. The *jugular venous pulse* usually exhibits a prominent *a* wave in patients with sinus rhythm (see Fig. 4-5) and elevated pulmonary vascular resistance. In patients with atrial fibrillation, the *x* descent of the jugular venous pulse disappears, and there is only one crest, a prominent *v* or *c-v* wave, per cardiac cycle. *Palpation* of the cardiac apex usually reveals an inconspicuous left ventricle; the presence of either a palpable presystolic expansion wave or an early diastolic rapid filling wave speaks strongly against serious MS. A readily palpable, tapping S_1 suggests that the anterior mitral valve leaflet is pliable. When the patient is in the left lateral recumbent position, a diastolic thrill of MS may be palpable at the apex. Often a right ventricular lift is felt in the left parasternal region in patients with pulmonary hypertension. A markedly enlarged right ventricle may displace the left ventricle posteriorly and produce a prominent apex beat that can be confused with a left ventricular lift. A loud pulmonic closure sound (P_2) may be palpable in the second left intercostal space in patients with MS and pulmonary hypertension.

AUSCULTATION. The auscultatory features of MS (Fig. 46-3; see also Figs. 4-16*B* and 4-34) include an accentuated S_1 with prolongation of the Q-S_1 interval, correlating with the level of the left atrial pressure. Accentuation of S_1 occurs when the mitral valve leaflets are flexible.[41] It is caused, in part, by the rapidity with which left ventricular pressure rises at the time of mitral valve closure as well as by the wide closing excursion of the leaflets.[42] Marked calcification and/or thickening of the mitral valve leaflets reduces the amplitude of S_1, probably because of diminished motion of the leaflets. As pulmonary arterial pressure rises, P_2 at first becomes accentuated and widely transmitted and can often be readily heard at both the mitral and the aortic areas. With further elevation of pulmonary arterial pressure,

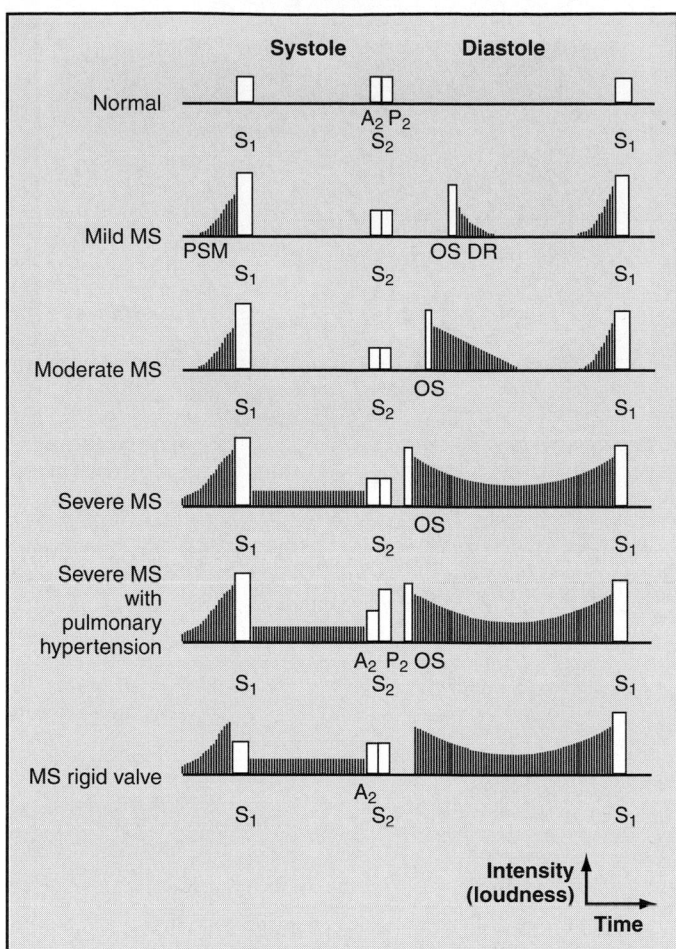

FIGURE 46–3. The classic auscultatory signs of MS in patients in sinus rhythm. These include a presystolic murmur, a loud S_1, an opening snap (OS), and a mid-diastolic murmur (DR, low-pitched, decrescendo diastolic rumble). These signs may be accentuated at or at times may only be heard by placing the patient in the left lateral decubitus position. These signs are helpful in assessing the severity of MS; as MS becomes more severe, the S_2-OS interval is shortened, and the length of the mid-diastolic rumble is increased. (From Kawanishi DT, Rahimtoola SH: Mitral stenosis. *In* Rahimtoola SH [ed]: Valvular Heart Disease. Atlas of Heart Diseases, vol. 11. Braunwald E, series ed. Philadelphia, Current Medicine, 1997, pp 8.1–8.24.)

splitting of S_2 narrows because of reduced compliance of the pulmonary vascular bed, and this shortens the "hangout interval." Finally, S_2 becomes single and accentuated. Other signs of severe pulmonary hypertension include a nonvalvular pulmonic ejection sound that diminishes during inspiration, owing to dilatation of the pulmonary artery; a systolic murmur of tricuspid regurgitation; a Graham Steell murmur of pulmonic regurgitation; and an S_4 originating from the right ventricle. An S_3 originating from the left ventricle is absent in patients with MS unless significant mitral or aortic regurgitation coexists.

The *opening snap* (OS) of the mitral valve is caused by a sudden tensing of the valve leaflets after the valve cusps have completed their opening excursion. The OS occurs when the movement of the mitral dome into the left ventricle suddenly stops.[42] It is most readily audible at the apex, using the diaphragm of the stethoscope. The OS can usually be differentiated from P_2 because the OS occurs later, unless right bundle branch block is present. The mitral valve cannot be totally rigid if it produces an OS, which is usually accompanied by an accentuated S_1. Calcification confined to the tip of the mitral valve leaflets does not

preclude an OS, although calcification of both the body and the tip does. The mitral OS follows A_2 by 0.04 to 0.12 second; this interval varies inversely with the left atrial pressure.[41] A short A_2-OS interval is a reliable indicator of severe MS.

The Diastolic Murmur of MS. This murmur is a low-pitched, rumbling murmur, best heard at the apex, with the bell of the stethoscope and with the patient in the left lateral recumbent position. When this murmur is soft, it is limited to the apex, but when louder, it may radiate to the left axilla or the lower left sternal area. Although the intensity of the diastolic murmur is not closely related to the severity of stenosis, the *duration* of the murmur is a guide to the severity of mitral valve narrowing. The murmur persists for as long as the left atrioventricular pressure gradient exceeds approximately 3 mm Hg. The murmur usually commences immediately after the OS. In mild MS, the early diastolic murmur is brief, but in the presence of sinus rhythm it resumes in presystole. In severe MS, the murmur is holodiastolic.

The *diastolic rumbling murmur* of MS may be masked by the presence of a thick chest wall, pulmonary emphysema, and a low cardiac output with a low flow rate across the mitral valve. This murmur may be sharply localized and thus missed unless palpation is used to detect the apex of the left ventricle and to pinpoint the area at which auscultation should be carried out. In so-called "silent" MS, there is usually marked right ventricular enlargement. Consequently, the right ventricle occupies the cardiac apex, the left ventricle is rotated posteriorly, and cardiac output is reduced, so that the murmur either is not audible at all or can be heard only in the mid- or posterior axillary line. Auscultation of the murmur is facilitated by placing the patient in the left lateral position and auscultating during expiration after having the patient do a few sit-ups, walk up a flight of stairs, or other maneuvers described later.

DYNAMIC AUSCULTATION (See also Chap. 4). The diastolic murmur and OS of MS are often reduced during inspiration and augmented during expiration,[39, 40] which is the opposite of what occurs when these findings are secondary to tricuspid stenosis (see p. 1690). During inspiration, the A_2-OS interval widens, and three sequential sounds (A_2, P_2, and OS) may be audible. Sudden standing and the resultant reduction of venous return lower the left atrial pressure and widen the A_2-OS interval; this maneuver is useful in distinguishing an A_2-OS combination from a split S_2, which narrows on standing. In contrast, the A_2-OS interval is significantly narrowed during exercise as left atrial pressure rises. The diastolic rumbling murmur of MS is reduced during the strain of a Valsalva maneuver and in any condition in which transmitral valve flow rate declines. Amyl nitrite inhalation, coughing, isometric or isotonic exercise, and sudden squatting are all useful in accentuating a faint or equivocal murmur of MS.

DIFFERENTIAL DIAGNOSIS. The *Carey-Coombs murmur* of acute rheumatic fever is a sign of active mitral valvulitis and can be confused with the murmur of MS. The Carey-Coombs murmur is a soft early diastolic murmur, usually varies from day to day, and is higher pitched than the diastolic rumbling murmur of established MS. In pure, severe MR—indeed in any condition in which flow across a nonstenotic mitral valve is increased—there may also be a short diastolic murmur following an S_3. *Left atrial myxoma* may produce auscultatory findings similar to those in rheumatic valvular MS (see Chap. 49).

A high-frequency early systolic murmur is audible along the lower left sternal border in one-third of patients with MS. This should be distinguished from the apical (often holosystolic or late systolic) murmur of MR. In addition, a *pansystolic murmur of tricuspid regurgitation* and an S_3 originating from the right ventricle may be audible in the 4th intercostal space in the left parasternal region in patients with severe MS. These signs, which are secondary to pulmonary hypertension, may be confused with the findings of MR. However, the inspiratory augmentation of the murmur and of the S_3 and the prominent v wave in the jugular venous pulse aid in establishing that the murmur originates from the tricuspid valve. A high-pitched decrescendo diastolic murmur along the left sternal border in patients with MS and pulmonary hypertension is usually due to aortic regurgitation but occasionally represents a Graham Steell murmur of pulmonary regurgitation. The latter, when present, characteristically increases during inspiration.

LABORATORY EXAMINATION

ELECTROCARDIOGRAPHY (See also Chap. 5). The electrocardiogram (ECG) is relatively insensitive for detecting mild MS, but it does show characteristic changes in moderate or severe obstruction.[43] Left atrial enlargement (P-wave duration in lead II ≥ 0.12 sec and/or a P-wave axis between +45 and −30 degrees) is a principal ECG feature of MS and is found in 90 percent of patients with significant MS and sinus rhythm.[44] The ECG signs of left atrial enlargement correlate more closely with left atrial volume than with left atrial pressure and often regress following successful valvotomy.[14] Atrial fibrillation usually develops in the presence of preexisting ECG evidence of left atrial enlargement and is related to the size of the chamber, the extent of fibrosis of the left atrial myocardium, the duration of atriomegaly, and the age of the patient.

Whether or not there is ECG evidence of right ventricular hypertrophy depends largely on the height of right ventricular systolic pressure. Approximately half of all patients with right ventricular systolic pressures between 70 and 100 mm Hg manifest the ECG criteria for right ventricular hypertrophy, including both a mean QRS axis greater than 80 degrees in the frontal plane and an R:S ratio greater than 1.0 in lead V_1. Other patients with this degree of pulmonary hypertension have no frank evidence of right ventricular hypertrophy, but the R:S ratio fails to increase from the right to the midprecordial leads. When right ventricular systolic pressure is greater than 100 mm Hg in patients with isolated or predominant MS, ECG evidence of right ventricular hypertrophy is found quite consistently.

The QRS axis in the frontal plane correlates roughly with the severity of valve obstruction and with the level of pulmonary vascular resistance in patients with pure MS. Thus, a mean frontal axis between 0 and +60 degrees suggests that the mitral valve area is greater than 1.3 cm², whereas an axis more than 60 degrees suggests that the valve area is less than 1.3 cm². In patients in whom pulmonary vascular resistance exceeds 650 dyne·sec·cm⁻⁵, the mean axis is usually greater than +110 degrees. In patients whose pulmonary artery systolic pressure approaches systemic levels, the mean axis averages +150 degrees.[45]

RADIOLOGICAL FINDINGS (See also Figs. 8–7B and 8–25). Although their cardiac silhouette may be normal in the frontal projection, patients with hemodynamically significant MS almost invariably have evidence of left atrial enlargement on the lateral and left anterior oblique views. Extreme left atrial enlargement rarely occurs in pure MS; when it is present, MR is usually severe. Enlargement of the pulmonary artery, right ventricle, and right atrium (as well as the left atrium) is commonly seen in patients with severe MS. Occasionally, calcification of the mitral valve is evident on the chest roentgenogram, but, more commonly, fluoroscopy is required to detect valvular calcification.

Radiological changes in the lung fields indirectly reflect the severity of MS. Interstitial edema, an indication of severe obstruction, is manifested as Kerley B lines (dense, short, horizontal lines most commonly seen in the costophrenic angles). This finding is present in 30 percent of patients with resting pulmonary arterial wedge pressures less than 20 mm Hg and in 70 percent of patients with pressures greater than 20 mm Hg. Severe, longstanding mitral obstruction often results in Kerley A lines (straight, dense lines up to 4 cm in length running toward the hilum) as well as the findings of pulmonary hemosiderosis and rarely of parenchymal ossification. Pulmonary edema is seldom evident.

ANGIOGRAPHY. Angiograms exposed in the right and left anterior oblique projections afford the best views of the mitral valve. Although contrast material should ideally be injected into the left atrium, it is often possible to achieve good visualization of the left side of the heart by injecting a large volume of contrast material into the main pulmonary artery. Such angiograms provide an assessment of left atrial size, may demonstrate thickening and reduced motion of the valve leaflets, and outline large intraluminal thrombi.[46] Left ventriculography makes possible simultaneous assessment of left ventricular contractile function and of the subvalvular mitral apparatus. However, echocardiography has largely superseded angiography in the evaluation of patients with MS or suspected MS.

ECHOCARDIOGRAPHY (See also Chap. 7). This is now the cornerstone of the diagnostic assessment of patients with MS. Two-dimensional transthoracic or transesophageal

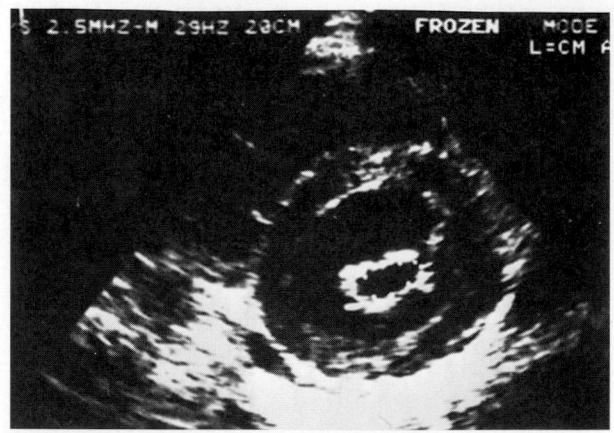

FIGURE 46–4. Two-dimensional transthoracic parasternal short-axis view of the mitral valve orifice during diastole, demonstrating the echocardiographic method of mitral valve area calculation. The innermost border of the mitral orifice was planimetered with the use of a light-pen system to obtain the area (in cm²). (Reproduced with permission from Smith MD et al: Comparative accuracy of two-dimensional echocardiography and Doppler pressure half-time methods in assessing severity of mitral stenosis in patients with and without prior commissurotomy. Circulation 73:100, 1986. Copyright 1986 American Heart Association.)

echocardiograms of a thickened, calcified, stenotic rheumatic valve demonstrate increased acoustic impedance and fusion of the mitral valve leaflets and poor leaflet separation in diastole (Fig. 46–4). The leaflets fail to close normally in mid-diastole and may not reopen widely during atrial contraction when sinus rhythm is present. The left atrium is usually enlarged, and in isolated MS the left ventricular cavity is normal or reduced in size. Two-dimensional echocardiography (see Figs. 7–47 to 7–52) may be helpful in recognizing left atrial thrombus preoperatively and in assessing mitral valve calcification and left ventricular contractility.[47] With progressive thickening and fibrosis of the leaflets, the orifice becomes fixed and can then often be imaged directly and measured. Two-dimensional echocardiography also provides information on the pliability of the leaflets, the extent of valvular calcification, thickening of the subvalvular apparatus, and fusion and retraction of the chordae tendineae, as well as calcification of the mitral annulus. This technique allows determination of left ventricular size and function and can also evaluate the aortic valve. The two-dimensional echocardiogram is helpful in determining whether the patient with MS is a suitable candidate for balloon mitral valvuloplasty (see p. 1651). Transesophageal two-dimensional echocardiography provides images of the mitral valve that are superior to those obtained by transthoracic imaging and is more sensitive in detecting left atrial thrombus. Pedunculated and free-floating thrombi are also usually readily detected by this technique. Transesophageal echocardiography is necessary when the transthoracic signal is inadequate.

Doppler echocardiography is the most accurate noninvasive technique available for quantifying the severity of MS[47] (see Fig. 7–51) and for estimating pulmonary arterial pressure.[48, 49] Color flow Doppler imaging can enhance the accuracy of the Doppler data by determining whether MR, aortic regurgitation, and other valvular abnormalities coexist. The pulmonary arterial pressure also can be estimated from the tricuspid regurgitation velocity signal.

In a patient with MS, a detailed echocardiographic examination, including two-dimensional echocardiography (transthoracic or transesophageal), a Doppler study, and color flow Doppler imaging, can usually provide sufficient information to develop a therapeutic plan without the need for cardiac catheterization (see below).[50]

MANAGEMENT

Medical Treatment

Patients with MS due to rheumatic heart disease should receive penicillin prophylaxis for beta-hemolytic streptococcal infections and prophylaxis for infective endocarditis (see Chaps. 47 and 66). Anemia and infections should be treated promptly and aggressively in patients with valvular heart disease. Adolescents and young adults with severe valvular heart disease should be advised to avoid entering occupations requiring strenuous exertion. Asymptomatic patients with moderate MS should be reevaluated yearly.[51] Heavy exertion is contraindicated in symptomatic patients.

In symptomatic patients with mitral valve disease, considerable improvement occurs with the administration of oral diuretics and the restriction of sodium intake. Digitalis glycosides do not alter the hemodynamics and usually do not benefit patients with MS and sinus rhythm,[52] but these drugs are of value in slowing the ventricular rate in patients with atrial fibrillation and in treating patients with right-sided heart failure. Hemoptysis is managed by measures designed to reduce pulmonary venous pressure, including sedation, assumption of the upright position, and aggressive diuresis. Beta-blocking agents and rate-slowing calcium antagonists may increase exercise capacity by reducing heart rate in patients with sinus rhythm[53] and especially in patients with atrial fibrillation.

Anticoagulant therapy is helpful in preventing venous thrombosis and pulmonary embolism in patients who have experienced one or more previous pulmonary embolic episodes; in patients who are at high risk of systemic embolization, i.e., with persistent or transient atrial fibrillation (especially elderly patients > 70 years of age); and in those with previous systemic emboli. Treatment with warfarin, to maintain the international normalized ratio (INR) between 2.0 and 3.0, is indicated.[54] However, no firm evidence exists that anticoagulant therapy reduces the incidence of pulmonary or systemic embolism in patients in sinus rhythm in whom such episodes have not previously occurred.

TREATMENT OF ARRHYTHMIAS. Frequent premature atrial contractions often presage atrial fibrillation. The administration of antiarrhythmic agents (see Chap. 23) may be effective in preventing this complication. However, once atrial fibrillation has developed, these agents may be ineffective in restoring sinus rhythm because of the pathological changes that occur in the atrium secondary to the arrhythmia itself. After electrical cardioversion, sinus rhythm can often be maintained with antiarrhythmic agents, especially in young patients with mild MS but without marked left atrial enlargement who have been in atrial fibrillation less than 6 months and who are maintained on adequate doses of quinidine.

Immediate treatment of atrial fibrillation should include intravenous heparin followed by oral warfarin. The ventricular rate should be slowed with intravenous digoxin and a beta-blocking agent or rate-slowing calcium antagonist. An effort should be made to reestablish sinus rhythm by a combination of pharmacological treatment and cardioversion. If cardioversion is planned in a patient who has had atrial fibrillation for more than 24 hours before the procedure, anticoagulation with warfarin for more than three weeks is indicated. Alternatively, if a transesophageal echocardiogram shows no atrial thrombus, immediate cardioversion can be carried out using intravenous heparin.[55] Paroxysmal atrial fibrillation and repeated conversions, spontaneous or induced, carry the risk of embolization. In patients who cannot be converted or maintained in sinus rhythm, digitalis should be used to maintain the ventricular rate at rest at approximately 60 beats/min. If this is not possible, small doses of a beta-blocking agent, such as atenolol (25 mg daily), may be added. Multiple repeat cardioversions are *not* indicated if the patient fails to sustain sinus rhythm while on adequate doses of an antiarrhythmic. Patients with chronic atrial fibrillation who undergo open mitral valve repair or replacement may undergo the Cox maze procedure (atrial compartment operation). More than 80 percent of patients undergoing this procedure can be maintained in sinus rhythm postoperatively[56] and can regain normal atrial function.[57]

NEED FOR CATHETERIZATION. There has been considerable debate concerning the need for routine cardiac catheterization in determining whether valvotomy is indicated.[51]

A careful clinical evaluation and noninvasive assessment, particularly using two-dimensional and Doppler echocardiography, can provide sufficient information to permit an informed decision in the majority of patients. Preoperative catheterization is recommended for the following patients with MS: (1) patients who have a discrepancy between clinical and echocardiographic findings; hemodynamic measurements during exercise are often useful in these patients; (2) patients who have associated chronic obstructive pulmonary disease in whom it is important to determine the contribution of MS to the symptoms; (3) patients in whom left atrial myxoma should be excluded; (4) patients who have angina pectoris or angina-like chest pain in whom associated coronary artery disease must be excluded; and (5) men over 40 years of age and women over 50 years of age who have risk factors for coronary artery disease or a positive stress test and in whom surgery is planned; it is important to ascertain whether or not bypass grafting is indicated for those patients at risk of having coexisting coronary artery disease. Critical narrowing of one or more coronary vessels occurs in approximately 25 percent of all adults with severe MS. This finding is more common in men over 45 years of age who have angina and risk factors for coronary artery disease.[28]

Natural History

The development of effective surgical treatment has obscured our understanding of the natural history of MS (Fig. 46–5) and, for that matter, of all valvular lesions. Although few meaningful data are available, it appears that in temperate zones, such as the United States and Western Europe, patients who develop acute rheumatic fever have an asymptomatic period of approximately 15 to 20 years before symptoms of MS develop. It then takes approximately 5 to 10 years for most patients to progress from mild disability (i.e., early NYHA Class II) to severe disability (i.e., NYHA Class III or IV). The progression is much more rapid in patients in tropical and subtropical areas,[58] in Polynesians, and in Alaskan Inuit. Both economic and genetic conditions may play a role. In India, critical MS may be present in children as young as 6 to 12 years old. In North America and Western Europe, however, symptoms develop

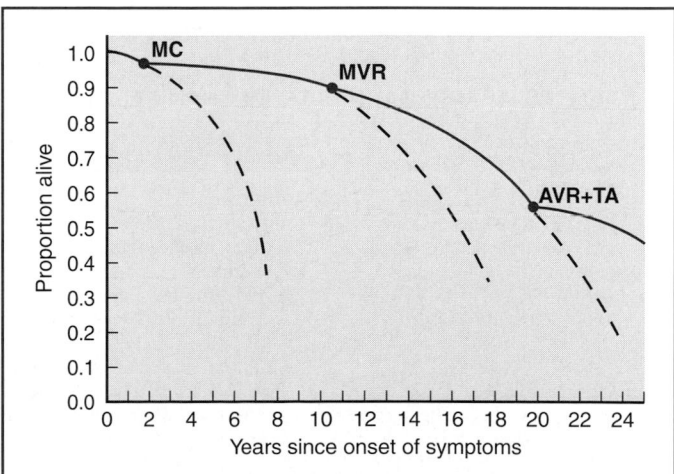

FIGURE 46–5. Schematic representation of the subsequent life history after the initial development of symptoms in a large group of patients with mitral stenosis. The colored solid circles and colored lines indicate a surgical procedure. The dashed lines represent estimated survival of patients who are not receiving the surgical procedure. MC = mitral commissurotomy; MVR = mitral valve replacement; TA = tricuspid annuloplasty; AVR = aortic valve replacement. (From Kirklin JW, Barratt-Boyes BG [eds]: Cardiac Surgery. New York, John Wiley and Sons, 1986, p 328.)

more slowly and occur most commonly between the ages of 45 and 65.[51] Two echocardiographic studies have reported hemodynamic progression in patients with MS who had not undergone surgery[59, 60]; there was considerable interpatient variability, but on average the mitral valve area decreased by 0.09 cm²/yr.

In the *presurgical era,* Olesen found 62 percent 5-year survival rates and 38 percent 10-year survival rates among medically treated patients with MS in NYHA Class III but only 15 percent 5-year survival rates among patients in Class IV.[61] Among asymptomatic patients with MS treated medically, 40 percent deteriorated or died within 10 years. Among mildly symptomatic patients (NYHA Class II), the comparable number was 80 percent.[62] In medically treated patients with MS or with combined MS and MR, Munoz and associates found a 45 percent 5-year survival rate.[63] In a comparable group of patients who underwent mitral valvotomy, the 5-year survival rate was substantially better. Horstkotte et al. reported a 5-year survival rate of 44 percent in patients with symptomatic MS who refused valvotomy (Fig. 46–6).[64]

Valvotomy

Indications

Patients with MS who are asymptomatic or minimally symptomatic frequently remain so for years. However, once moderate symptoms develop (NYHA Class II), if the stenosis is not relieved mechanically, the disease may progress relatively rapidly, as already discussed (Table 46–1). Valvotomy (percutaneous balloon mitral valvuloplasty [BMV] or surgical valvotomy) should therefore be carried out in symptomatic patients with moderate to severe MS (i.e., a mitral valve orifice area < approximately 1.0 cm²/m² body surface area [BSA] or <1.5 to 1.7 cm² in normal-sized adults). It is also indicated in patients with mild stenosis (orifice area 1.0 to 1.5 cm²/m² who are symptomatic during ordinary activity and who develop pulmonary arterial systolic pressures exceeding 60 mm Hg or mean pulmonary capillary wedge pressures exceeding 25 mm Hg during exercise.[51]

Treatment must be individualized. For instance, mechanical relief of obstruction might well be deferred in a retired, mildly symptomatic, sedentary septuagenarian with a mitral valve orifice of 0.8 cm²/m² BSA. On the other hand, a 30-year-old laborer whose family's economic well-being depends on his continued physical exertion might be an excellent candidate for mechanical relief of obstruction, although his mitral valve orifice size is 1.2 cm²/m² BSA. Some years ago, I saw a 33-year-old woman with MS who

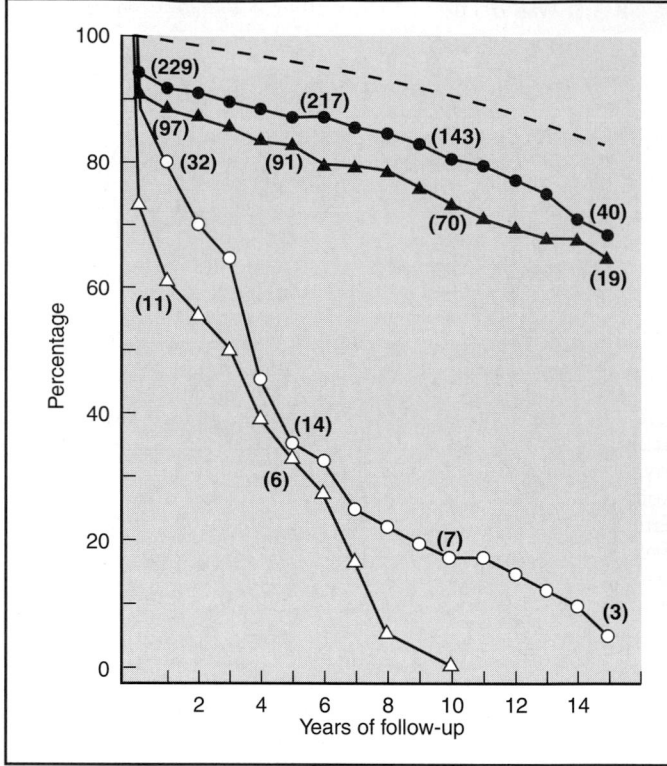

FIGURE 46–6. Natural history of 159 patients with isolated mitral stenosis (open circles) or mitral regurgitation (open triangles) who were not operated upon (even though the operation was indicated) compared with patients treated with valve replacement for mitral stenosis (solid circles) or mitral regurgitation (solid triangles). The expected survival rate in the absence of mitral valve disease is indicated by the upper curve (dashed line). (From Horstkotte D, Niehues R, Strauer BE: Pathomorphological aspects, aetiology, and natural history of acquired mitral valve stenosis. Eur Heart J 12(Suppl):55–60, 1991.)

had had hemoptysis and pulmonary edema during the second trimester of a pregnancy 2 years previously. She then became asymptomatic but wished to have another child. Hemodynamic study showed a pulmonary artery wedge pressure of 17 mm Hg and a mitral orifice area of 1.7 cm²/m² BSA. This patient underwent prophylactic BMV

▼ **TABLE 46–1. APPROACHES TO MECHANICAL RELIEF OF MITRAL STENOSIS**

APPROACH	ADVANTAGES	DISADVANTAGES
Closed surgical valvotomy	Inexpensive Relatively simple Good hemodynamic results in selected patients Good long-term outcome	No direct visualization of valve Only feasible with flexible, noncalcified valves Contraindicated if MR > 2+ Surgical procedure with general anesthesia
Open surgical valvotomy	Visualization of valve allows directed valvotomy Concurrent annuloplasty for MR is feasible	Best results with flexible, noncalcified valves Surgical procedure with general anesthesia
Valve replacement	Feasible in all patients regardless of extent of valve calcification or severity of MR	Surgical procedure with general anesthesia Effect of loss of annular-papillary muscle continuity on LV function Prosthetic valve Chronic anticoagulation
Balloon mitral valvotomy	Percutaneous approach Local anesthesia Good hemodynamic results in selected patients Good long-term outcome	No direct visualization of valve Only feasible with flexible, noncalcified valves Contraindicated if MR > 2+

LV = left ventricular; MR = mitral regurgitation.
From Otto CM: Valvular Heart Disease. Philadelphia, WB Saunders, 1999, p 261.

because it was deemed that another pregnancy would have resulted in serious symptoms. However, there is no evidence that valvotomy improves the prognosis of patients with no or only slight functional impairment. Therefore, valvotomy is *not* ordinarily indicated in patients who are entirely asymptomatic. Because of the high rate of recurrence, mechanical relief of obstruction is also indicated in patients with MS who have had a previous systemic embolism, even if they are otherwise asymptomatic and even though there is no *definitive* evidence that the incidence of recurrent emboli will be significantly reduced. Anticoagulants should be administered to such patients up to the time of the procedure.

Balloon Mitral Valvotomy (See also Chap. 38)

This percutaneous technique consists of advancing a small balloon flotation catheter across the interatrial septum (after transseptal puncture), enlarging the opening, advancing a large (23 to 25 mm) hourglass-shaped balloon (the Inoue balloon), and inflating it within the orifice. Alternatively, two smaller (12 to 18 mm) balloons may be employed.[65] Commissural separation and fracture of nodular calcium appear to be the mechanisms responsible for improvement in valvular function. In several series, the hemodynamic results of BMV have been quite favorable (Fig. 46–7), with reduction of the transmitral pressure gradient from an average of approximately 18 mm Hg to 6 mm Hg, a small (average 20 percent) increase in cardiac output, and an average doubling of the calculated mitral valve area from 1.0 to 2.0 cm². Although the double-balloon technique may result in a slightly greater valve opening, the clinical outcomes of the two approaches are similar.[66] Improvement in exercise tolerance has paralleled the favorable hemodynamic changes.

Results are especially impressive in younger patients without valvular thickening or calcification. Elevated pulmonary vascular resistance declines rapidly, although usually not completely.[67, 67a] The reported mortality rate has ranged from 1 to 2 percent. Complications include cerebral emboli and cardiac perforation, each in approximately 1

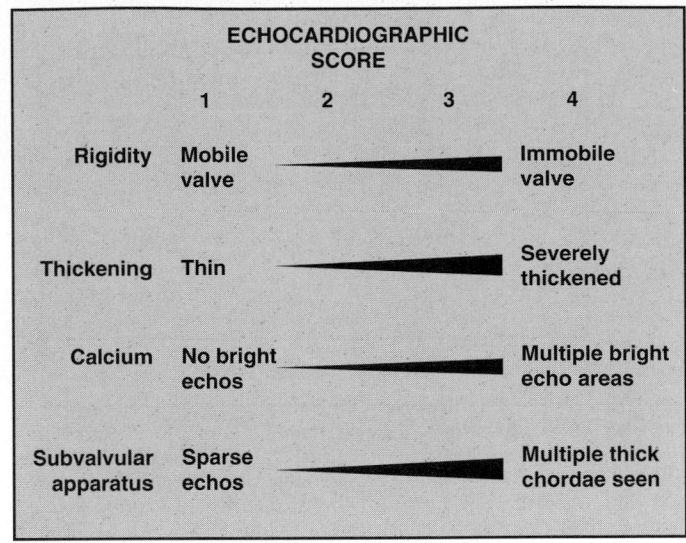

FIGURE 46–8. Determination of echocardiographic score. Leaflet rigidity, thickening, calcification, and the amount of subvalvular disease are graded 0 to 4, depending on the severity of the abnormality. The sum of the four factors equals the echocardiographic score. (From Block PC: Mitral balloon valvotomy: Why, when and how? Cardiol Rev 2:19, 1994.)

percent of patients, and the development of MR severe enough to require operation in another 2 percent (approximately 15 percent develop lesser, but still undesirable, degrees of MR). Approximately 5 percent of patients are left with a small residual atrial septal defect, but this closes or decreases in size in the majority. Rarely, the defect is large enough to cause right-sided heart failure. Results are surgeon-dependent and patients should be referred to experienced teams.[68, 69, 69a]

The indications for BMV are the same as those for valvotomy (discussed below). A combination of significant symptoms and documented MS generally serves as the indication. Detailed two-dimensional and Doppler echocardiographic studies are indicated before a decision is made. Left atrial thrombus must be excluded by echocardiography.

An echocardiographic scoring system developed by Wilkins and colleagues[70] has been found to be particularly valuable in patient selection and has been widely adopted. Leaflet rigidity, leaflet thickening, valvular calcification, and subvalvular disease are each scored from 0 to 4 (Fig. 46–8). Rigid, thickened valves with extensive subvalvular fibrosis and calcification lead to suboptimal results. A score of 8 or less is usually associated with an excellent immediate and long-term result, whereas scores exceeding 8 are associated with less impressive results (Fig. 46–9), including the risk of development of MR.[71] Fluoroscopically visible calcium[72] and coexisting MR[73] are additional important predictors of an adverse outcome.[72] Transesophageal echocardiography provides a precise assessment of mitral valve structure and function and evaluation of accompanying MR and left atrial thrombus (a contraindication to BMV).[74] It also provides an accurate assessment of outcome. Three-dimensional echocardiography has also been found to be useful in assessing indications for BMV.[75] The findings on echocardiography affect the outcome of both open and closed surgical valvotomy in a similar manner. A trial in which patients with severe MS were randomized to undergo either BMV or open surgical valvotomy resulted in similar clinical results from the two techniques. Indeed, after 3 years, mitral valve area was greater in the balloon catheter–treated group.[76] In patients with favorable anatomical findings, survival without functional disability or need for surgery or repeat BMV

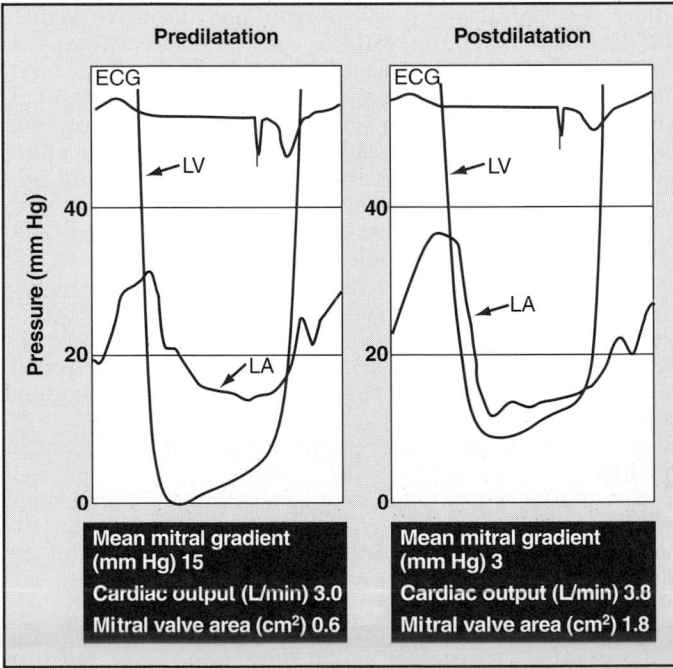

FIGURE 46–7. Simultaneous left atrial (LA) and left ventricular (LV) pressure before and after balloon mitral valvotomy in a patient with severe mitral stenosis. (Courtesy of Raymond G. McKay, M.D.)

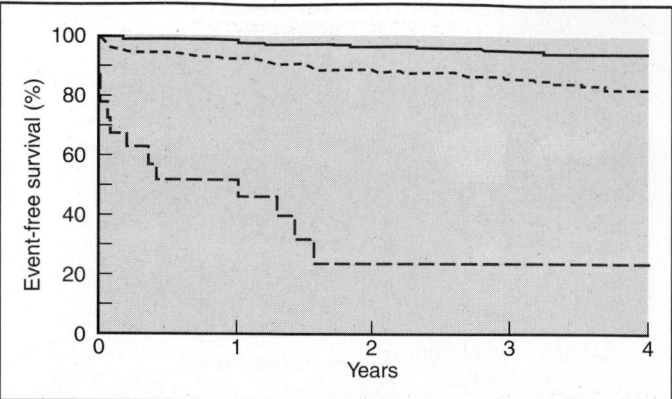

FIGURE 46–9. Event-free survival after balloon mitral valvotomy for 736 patients enrolled in the Balloon Valvuloplasty Registry who were stratified by baseline echocardiographic morphology score: less than 8 (solid line), 8 to 12 (short-dashed line), or more than 12 (long-dashed line); P < 0.0001. (From Dean LS, Mickel MC, Bonan R, et al: Four-year follow-up of patients undergoing percutaneous balloon mitral commissurotomy: A report from the National Heart, Lung and Blood Institute Balloon Valvuloplasty Registry. J Am Coll Cardiol 28:1452, 1996.)

is 70 percent at 7 years.[77–79] Excellent results have also been reported in children[80] and adolescents[81] in developing nations, where patients tend to be younger. These young patients usually have quite pliable valves, which are ideal for BMV.[82]

Percutaneous BMV is the procedure of choice in patients who have symptomatic, hemodynamically severe stenosis with an echocardiographic score of 8 or less and without left atrial thrombus.[69] The lower cost and morbidity are obvious advantages. BMV can also be the initial procedure in patients with symptomatic, severe MS and less favorable valves (echocardiographic score > 8 and/or dense calcification on fluoroscopic examination).[65, 72] However, the failure rate is considerable in these patients, and they may require surgical treatment, most often mitral valve replacement. BMV also has acceptable results in patients with accompanying mild or moderate aortic regurgitation[74, 83] and in those with mitral restenosis after surgical valvotomy.[84] It may also be used in patients with less favorable valves who are unsuitable for surgery because of very high risk.[85] These include very elderly, frail patients; patients with associated severe ischemic heart disease; patients in whom MS is complicated by pulmonary, renal, or neoplastic disease; women of childbearing age in whom valve replacement is undesirable; and pregnant women with MS.[86, 87] BMV is contraindicated in patients with severe mitral or aortic regurgitation and should probably not be used in patients with stenotic bioprosthetic valves.[85]

Because the cost of the balloon catheter is deemed high in countries with restricted financial resources, a reusable metallic valvulotome has been devised. Early results are at least as good as those achieved with balloon catheters.[88]

Surgical Valvotomy

Three operative approaches are available for the treatment of rheumatic MS: (1) closed mitral valvotomy using a transatrial or transventricular approach[89–91]; (2) open valvotomy, i.e., valvotomy carried out under direct vision with the aid of cardiopulmonary bypass; and (3) mitral valve replacement (see Table 46–1).

CLOSED MITRAL VALVOTOMY. This procedure is performed without cardiopulmonary bypass but with the aid of a transventricular dilator. It is an effective operation, provided that MR, atrial thrombosis, or valvular calcification is not serious and that chordal fusion and shortening are not severe. Echocardiography is useful in selecting suitable can-

didates for this procedure by identifying patients without valvular calcification or dense fibrosis. If possible, closed mitral valvotomy should be carried out with "pump standby"; if the surgeon is unable to achieve a satisfactory result, the patient can be placed on cardiopulmonary bypass and the valvotomy carried out under direct vision or the valve replaced.

On average, the mitral valve area is increased by 1.0 cm², with only 20 to 30 percent of patients requiring mitral valve replacement within 15 years.[92] In one large series,[90] the hospital mortality rate was 1.5 percent, and 0.3 percent of patients developed severe MR. Marked symptomatic improvement occurred in 86 percent of survivors. The actuarial survival rate was 89.5 percent after 18 years. Patients undergoing closed valvotomy for restenosis had a 6.7 percent mortality rate. Long-term follow-up has shown that the results are best if the operation is carried out before chronic atrial fibrillation and/or heart failure has occurred, but complication rates are higher when valves are calcified and/or severely thickened.[89]

Closed mitral valvotomy is rarely used in the United States today, having been replaced by BMV, which is of similar effectiveness in patients who are candidates for closed mitral valvotomy. Closed mitral valvotomy is more popular in developing nations, where the expense of open-heart surgery and even of balloon catheters for BMV is an important factor and where patients with mitral valve disease are younger and therefore have more pliable valves. But even in these nations, closed mitral valvotomy is being displaced by BMV.

OPEN VALVOTOMY. Most surgeons in North America and Western Europe now prefer to carry out *direct-vision* or *open valvotomy*.[92–94] This operation is most frequently performed in patients with MS whose mitral valves are too distorted or calcified for BMV. Cardiopulmonary bypass is established, and in order to obtain a dry, quiet heart, body temperature is usually lowered, the heart is arrested, and the aorta is occluded intermittently. Thrombi are removed from the left atrium and its appendage, and the latter is often amputated in order to remove a potential source of postoperative emboli. The commissures are incised, and, when necessary, fused chordae tendineae are separated, the underlying papillary muscle is split, and the valve leaflets are debrided of calcium. Mild or even moderate MR may be corrected. Left atrial and ventricular pressures are measured after bypass has been discontinued to confirm that the valvotomy has, in fact, been effective. When it has not been effective, another attempt can be made. When repair is not possible—most commonly owing to severe distortion and calcification of the valve and subvalvular apparatus with accompanying regurgitation that cannot be corrected—mitral valve replacement should be carried out (see p. 1653).[95] In patients with atrial fibrillation, conversion to sinus rhythm is done at the completion of the operation. In a series of open mitral valve reconstructive procedures for MS at Brigham and Women's Hospital, the actuarial probability of survival at 10 years was 95 percent. The annual reoperation rate was 1.7 percent.[93] A survival rate of 75 percent over 20 years after surgical repair of MS has been reported.[96]

The mortality rate after mitral valvotomy, whether open or closed, ranges from 1 to 3 percent, depending on the condition of the patient and the skill and experience of the surgical team.[93] Five-year survival rates are 90 to 96 percent, and event-free survival rates are 72 to 94 percent.[96, 97] In general, open valvotomy provides better hemodynamic relief of mitral valve obstruction than does the closed procedure,[94, 98] and the risk of dislodging thrombi from the atrium or calcium from the mitral valve is also less.[93] Left atrial size, the need for mitral or tricuspid annuloplasty, and the presence of left atrial thrombus are all "risk factors" for a less than optimal outcome after open mitral valvotomy.[95] Although a contemporary control series of medically and surgically treated patients is not available (nor is it likely ever to be), valvotomy appears to prolong survival substantially in patients with MS (see Fig. 46–6).

MITRAL RESTENOSIS. Mitral valvotomy, whether percutaneous or operative and whether open or closed, is *palliative* rather than curative, and even when successful, this procedure merely "turns the clock back." (The generally more effective open valvotomy turns the clock back further than does the closed valvotomy or BMV.) Thus, successful valvotomy does not result in a normal mitral valve but rather in one resembling the valve as it existed perhaps a decade earlier. Because the valve is not normal postoperatively, turbulent flow usually persists in the paravalvular region, and the resultant trauma may well play a role in restenosis. These changes are analogous to the gradual development of obstruction in a congenitally bicuspid aortic valve and are *not* usually the result of recurrent rheumatic fever.

On clinical grounds alone, i.e., based on the reappearance of symptoms, the incidence of "restenosis" has been estimated to range widely (from 2 to 60 percent).[99] Approximately 10 percent of patients who have undergone surgical mitral valvotomy require reoperation within 5 years, but that number increases to 60 percent by 10 years.[100] Recurrence of symptoms is usually *not* due to restenosis but may be due to one or more of the following conditions: (1) an inadequate first operation with residual stenosis; (2) the presence or development of MR, either at operation or as a consequence of infective endocarditis; (3) the progression of aortic valve disease; and (4) the development of coronary artery disease. True restenosis occurs in less than 20 percent of patients who are followed for 10 years.[51] In a study of 18 patients who had undergone successful surgical valvotomy in whom the size of the mitral orifice was estimated using two-dimensional echocardiography, no change in the mitral valve area occurred over a 10- to 14-year period in 13 patients (72 percent), whereas in true restenosis developed in 5 patients (28 percent).[100] Others have estimated the rate of true restenosis to be approximately 10 percent within 6 years.[101]

Thus, in properly selected patients, mitral valvotomy, however performed—balloon angioplasty, closed or open valvotomy—is a low-risk procedure that results in a significant increase in the size of the mitral orifice and favorably alters the clinical course of an otherwise progressive disease. Pulmonary arterial pressure falls promptly and decisively when mitral obstruction is effectively relieved.[102, 103] The majority of patients maintain clinical improvement for 10 to 15 years of follow-up. When a second procedure is required because of symptomatic deterioration, the valve is usually calcified and more seriously deformed than at the time of the first operation, and adequate reconstruction may not be possible. Accordingly, mitral valve replacement (MVR) is often necessary at that time.

INDICATIONS FOR MITRAL VALVE REPLACEMENT. This procedure is often required in patients with combined MS and moderate or severe MR; in those with extensive com-

▼ **TABLE 46–2. OPERATIVE MORTALITY RATES FOLLOWING VALVE REPLACEMENT AND REPAIR**

OPERATIVE CATEGORY	NUMBER	OPERATIVE MORTALITY (%)
AVR (isolated)	26,317	4.3
MVR (isolated)	13,936	6.4
Multiple valve replacement	3,840	9.6
AVR + CAB	22,713	8.0
MVR + CAB	8,788	15.3
Multiple valve replacement + CAB	1,424	18.8
AVR + any valve repair	938	7.4
MVR + any valve repair	1,266	12.5
Aortic valve repair	597	5.9
Mitral valve repair	4,167	3.0
Tricuspid valve repair	144	13.9
AVR + aortic aneurysm repair	1,723	9.7

AVR = aortic valve replacement; CAB = coronary artery bypass; MVR = mitral valve replacement.

Modified from Jamieson WRE, Edwards FH, Schwartz M, et al: Risk stratification for cardiac valve replacement. National Cardiac Surgery Database. Ann Thorac Surg 67:943, 1999.

missural calcification, severe fibrosis, and subvalvular fusion; and in those who have undergone previous valvotomy. The operative mortality rate following isolated MVR ranges from 3 to 8 percent in most centers and averaged 6.4 percent in the large database of 13,936 such operations for patients with MS and/or MR reported in the Society of Thoracic Surgeons National Database[104] (Table 46–2). As described later (see p. 1701), mechanical deterioration of bioprosthetic valves may occur. Also, the hazards of lifelong anticoagulant treatment in patients with mechanical prostheses must be considered. Therefore, the threshold for operation should be higher in patients in whom preoperative evaluation suggests that valve replacement may be required than in patients in whom valvotomy alone appears to be indicated.

MVR is indicated in two groups of patients with MS whose valves are not suitable for valvotomy: (1) those with a mitral valve area less than 1.5 cm^2 in NYHA Class III or IV; and (2) those with severe MS (mitral valve area < 1.0 cm^2), NYHA Class II, and severe pulmonary hypertension (pulmonary artery systolic pressure >70 mm Hg).[51] Since the operative mortality risk may be quite high (10 to 20 percent) in patients in NYHA Class IV, operation should be carried out before patients reach this stage if possible. On the other hand, such patients should not be denied operation unless they have comorbid conditions that preclude surgery or a satisfactory outcome. (The results of MVR are discussed on p. 1663).

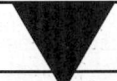

Mitral Regurgitation

ETIOLOGY AND PATHOLOGY

The mitral valve apparatus involves the mitral leaflets *per se,* chordae tendineae, papillary muscles, and mitral annulus. Abnormalities of any of these structures may cause MR.[104a] The major causes of MR include rheumatic heart disease, infective endocarditis, collagen-vascular disease, cardiomyopathy, and ischemic heart disease (Table 46–3). The mitral valve prolapse syndrome, an important cause of MR, is discussed in a separate section (see p. 1665). A less common cause is use of certain appetite suppressant drugs.

ABNORMALITIES OF VALVE LEAFLETS. MR due to predominant involvement of the valve leaflets occurs in patients with chronic rheumatic heart disease. However, in contrast to MS, this lesion is more frequent in men than in women. It is a consequence of shortening, rigidity, deformity, and retraction of one or both mitral valve cusps and is associated with shortening and fusion of the chordae tendineae and papillary muscles. Infective endocarditis can cause MR by perforating valve leaflets (see Chap. 47); vegetations can prevent leaflet coaptation, and valvular retraction during the healing phase of endocarditis can cause MR. Destruction of the mitral valve leaflets can also occur

▼ TABLE 46–3. CAUSES OF ACUTE AND CHRONIC MITRAL REGURGITATION

ACUTE
Mitral Annulus Disorders
 Infective endocarditis (abscess formation)
 Trauma (valvular heart surgery)
 Paravalvular leak due to suture interruption (surgical technical problems or infective endocarditis)
Mitral Leaflet Disorders
 Infective endocarditis (perforation or interfering with valve closure by vegetation)
 Trauma (tear during percutaneous balloon mitral valvotomy or penetrating chest injury)
 Tumors (atrial myxoma)
 Myxomatous degeneration
 Systemic lupus erythematosus (Libman-Sacks lesion)
Rupture of Chordae Tendineae
 Idiopathic, e.g., spontaneous
 Myxomatous degeneration (mitral valve prolapse, Marfan syndrome, Ehlers-Danlos syndrome)
 Infective endocarditis
 Acute rheumatic fever
 Trauma (percutaneous balloon valvotomy, blunt chest trauma)
Papillary Muscle Disorders
 Coronary artery disease (causing dysfunction and rarely rupture)
 Acute global left ventricular dysfunction
 Infiltrative diseases (amyloidosis, sarcoidosis)
 Trauma
Primary Mitral Valve Prosthetic Disorders
 Porcine cusp perforation (endocarditis)
 Porcine cusp degeneration
 Mechanical failure (strut fracture)
 Immobilized disc or ball of the mechanical prosthesis
CHRONIC
Inflammatory
 Rheumatic heart disease
 Systemic lupus erythematosus
 Scleroderma
Degenerative
 Myxomatous degeneration of mitral valve leaflets (Barlow click-murmur syndrome, prolapsing leaflet, mitral valve prolapse)
 Marfan syndrome
 Ehlers-Danlos syndrome
 Pseudoxanthoma elasticum
 Calcification of mitral valve annulus
Infective
 Infective endocarditis affecting normal, abnormal, or prosthetic mitral valves
Structural
 Ruptured chordae tendineae (spontaneous or secondary to myocardial infarction, trauma, mitral valve prolapse, endocarditis)
 Rupture or dysfunction of papillary muscle (ischemia or myocardial infarction)
 Dilatation of mitral valve annulus and left ventricular cavity (congestive cardiomyopathies, aneurysmal dilatation of the left ventricle)
 Hypertrophic cardiomyopathy
 Paravalvular prosthetic leak
Congenital
 Mitral valve clefts or fenestrations
 Parachute mitral valve abnormality in association with:
  Endocardial cushion defects
  Endocardial fibroelastosis
  Transposition of the great arteries
  Anomalous origin of the left coronary artery

 Data from Jutzy KR, Al-Zaibag M: Acute mitral and aortic valve regurgitation. *In* Al-Zaibag M, Duran CMG (eds): Valvular Heart Disease. New York, Marcel Dekker, 1994, pp 345–382 (top portion); and Haffajee CI: Chronic mitral regurgitation. *In* Dalen JE, Alpert JS (eds): Valvular Heart Disease. 2nd ed. Boston, Little, Brown and Co, 1987, p 112 (lower portion).

in patients with penetrating and nonpenetrating trauma (see Chap. 51).

ABNORMALITIES OF THE MITRAL ANNULUS

Dilatation. In a normal adult, the mitral annulus measures approximately 10 cm in circumference. It is soft and flexible, and contraction of the surrounding left ventricular muscle during systole causes the annular constriction that contributes importantly to valve closure. MR secondary to dilatation of the mitral annulus can occur in any form of heart disease characterized by dilatation of the left ventricle, especially dilated cardiomyopathy. Left ventricular submitral aneurysm has been reported as a cause of annular MR in sub-Saharan Africa. It appears to be due to a congenital defect in the posterior portion of the annulus. Diagnosis by transesophageal echocardiography[105] and surgical repair have been reported.

Calcification. Idiopathic (degenerative) calcification of the mitral annulus is one of the most common cardiac abnormalities found at autopsy; in most hearts it is of little functional consequence. However, when severe, it may be an important cause of MR,[106] and, in contrast to MR secondary to rheumatic fever, it is more common in women than in men. The development of degenerative calcification of the mitral annulus is accelerated by systemic hypertension, aortic stenosis, and diabetes, as well as by an intrinsic defect in the fibrous skeleton of the heart, as occurs in the Marfan and Hurler syndromes. In these two syndromes, the mitral annulus is not only calcified but also dilated, further contributing to MR. The incidence of mitral annular calcification is also increased in patients who have chronic renal failure with secondary hyperparathyroidism.[107] The annulus may also become thick, rigid, and calcified secondary to rheumatic involvement; when this process is severe, it also can interfere with valve closure.

With severe annular calcification, a rigid, curved bar or ring of calcium encircles the mitral orifice (see Fig. 8–20), and calcific spurs may project into the adjacent left ventricular myocardium.[108] The calcification may immobilize the basal portion of the mitral leaflets, preventing their normal excursion in diastole and coaptation in systole, and aggravating the MR that results from loss of the normal sphincteric action of the mitral ring. Rarely, obstruction to left ventricular filling may occur when severe calcification encroaches on or protrudes into the mitral orifice. In patients with severe calcification, the conduction system may be invaded by calcium, leading to atrioventricular and/or intraventricular conduction defects.[108] Calcification of the aortic valve cusps is an associated finding in approximately 50 percent of patients with severe mitral annular calcification, but this rarely causes aortic stenosis. Occasionally, calcific deposits extend into the coronary arteries.

ABNORMALITIES OF THE CHORDAE TENDINEAE. Such abnormalities are important causes of MR. Lengthening and rupture of the chordae tendineae are cardinal features of the mitral valve prolapse syndrome (see p. 1666). The chordae may be congenitally abnormal; rupture may be spontaneous ("primary")[109] or may occur as a consequence of infective endocarditis, trauma, rheumatic fever, or, rarely, osteogenesis imperfecta or relapsing polychondritis.[110] In most patients, no cause for chordal rupture is apparent other than increased mechanical strain. Chordae to the posterior leaflet rupture more frequently than those to the anterior leaflet. Patients with idiopathic rupture of mitral chordae tendineae frequently exhibit pathological fibrosis of the papillary muscles. It is possible that the dysfunction of the papillary muscles may cause stretching and ultimately rupture of the chordae tendineae. Chordal rupture may also result from acute left ventricular dilatation, regardless of the cause. Depending on the number of chordae involved in rupture and the rate at which rupture occurs, the resultant MR may be mild, moderate, or severe and acute, subacute, or chronic.

INVOLVEMENT OF THE PAPILLARY MUSCLES. Diseases of the left ventricular papillary muscles are a frequent cause of MR.[111] Because these muscles are perfused by the terminal portion of the coronary vascular bed, they are particularly vulnerable to ischemia, and any disturbance in coronary perfusion may result in papillary muscle dysfunction. When ischemia is transient, it results in temporary papillary muscle dysfunction and may cause transient episodes of MR that are sometimes associated with attacks of angina pectoris. When ischemia of papillary muscles is severe and prolonged, it causes papillary muscle dysfunction and scarring, as well as chronic MR. The posterior papillary muscle, which is supplied by the posterior descending branch of the right coronary artery, becomes ischemic and infarcted more frequently than does the anterolateral papillary muscle; the latter is supplied by diagonal branches of the left anterior descending coronary artery and often by marginal branches from the left circumflex artery as well. Ischemia of the papillary muscles is caused most commonly by coronary atherosclerosis, but it may also occur in patients with severe anemia, shock, coronary arteritis of any cause, or an anomalous left coronary artery. MR occurs frequently in patients with healed myocardial infarcts[112] and is caused by dyskinesis of the left ventricular myocardium at the base of a papillary muscle. MR has been reported in patients who are taking certain appetite suppressant drugs.[112a]

Left ventricular dilatation of any cause, including ischemia, can alter the spatial relationships between the papillary muscles and the chordae tendineae and thereby result in MR.[113] Although *necrosis of a papillary muscle* is a frequent complication of myocardial infarction,[114] frank rupture is far less common; the latter is usually fatal because of the extremely severe MR that it produces (see Chap. 35). However, rupture of one or two of the apical heads of a papillary muscle results in a lesser degree of MR and thus makes survival possible, usually following surgical therapy (see Chap. 35).

Some degree of MR is found in approximately 30 percent of patients with coronary artery disease who are being considered for coronary artery bypass surgery. In these patients, MR is secondary to ischemic damage to the papillary muscles and/or dilatation of the mitral valve ring. In most of these patients, MR is mild; however, in the small percentage with severe MR (3 percent in one large series of patients with coronary artery disease proved by coronary arteriography), it is associated with a poor prognosis.[115] The incidence and severity of regurgitation vary inversely with the left ventricular ejection fraction and directly with the left ventricular end-diastolic pressure. MR occurs in approximately 20 percent of patients following acute myocardial infarction and, even when mild, is associated with a higher risk of adverse outcomes.[112]

Various other disorders of the papillary muscles may also be responsible for the development of MR (see Table 46–3). These include congenital malposition of the muscles; absence of one papillary muscle, resulting in the so-called parachute mitral valve syndrome; and involvement or infiltration of the papillary muscles by a variety of processes, including abscesses, granulomas, neoplasms, amyloidosis, and sarcoidosis.

Other causes of MR, discussed in greater detail elsewhere, include mitral valve prolapse (see p. 1665), obstructive cardiomyopathy (see Chap. 48), the hypereosinophilic syndrome,[116] endomyocardial fibrosis,[117] trauma affecting the leaflets[118] and/or papillary muscles[119] (see Chap. 51), Kawasaki disease[120] (see Chap. 45), left atrial myxoma (see Chap. 49), and various congenital anomalies, including cleft anterior leaflet[121] and ostium secundum atrial septal defect (see Chap. 43).[122]

Because the regurgitant mitral orifice is functionally in parallel with the aortic valve, the impedance to ventricular emptying is reduced in patients with MR. Consequently, MR enhances left ventricular emptying. Almost 50 percent of the regurgitant volume is ejected into the left atrium before the aortic valve opens. The volume of MR flow depends on a combination of the instantaneous size of the regurgitant orifice and the (reverse) pressure gradient between the left ventricle and the left atrium.[19, 123–125] Both the orifice size and the pressure gradient are labile. Left ventricular systolic pressure, and therefore the left ventricular–left atrial gradient, depends on systemic vascular resistance,[123] and in patients in whom the mitral annulus has normal flexibility, the cross-sectional area of the mitral annulus may be altered by many interventions. Thus, increase of both preload and afterload and depression of contractility increase left ventricular size and enlarge the mitral annulus and thereby the regurgitant orifice.[125] When ventricular size is reduced by treatment with positive inotropic agents, diuretics, and particularly vasodilators, the volume of regurgitant flow declines, as reflected in the height of the v wave in the left atrial pressure pulse and in the intensity and duration of the systolic murmur. Pharmacological reductions of systemic vascular resistance and left ventricular filling pressure reduce the volume of regurgitant flow by means of a reduction in the regurgitant orifice area.[126] Conversely, left ventricular dilatation, regardless of cause, may increase MR.

LEFT VENTRICULAR COMPENSATION. The left ventricle initially compensates for the development of *acute* MR in part by emptying more completely and in part by increasing preload, i.e., by use of the Frank-Starling principle. As regurgitation, particularly severe regurgitation, becomes chronic, the left ventricular end-diastolic volume increases and the end-systolic volume returns to normal. By means of the Laplace principle (which states that myocardial wall tension is related to the product of intraventricular pressure and radius), the increased ventricular end-diastolic volume increases wall tension to normal or supranormal levels in the so-called chronic compensated stage of severe MR.[127] The resultant increase in left ventricular end-diastolic volume and mitral annular diameter may create a vicious circle in which "MR begets more MR." In patients with chronic MR, both left ventricular end-diastolic volume and mass are increased; i.e., typical volume overload (eccentric) hypertrophy develops. The degree of hypertrophy is usually proportionate to the degree of left ventricular dilatation, so that the ratio of left ventricular mass to end-diastolic volume is normal (see Fig. 16–5). The eccentric ventricular hypertrophy that accompanies the elevated end-diastolic volume of chronic MR is secondary to new sarcomeres laid down in parallel. A shift to the right (greater volume at any pressure) occurs in the left ventricular diastolic pressure-volume curve in patients with chronic MR (Fig. 46–10C). With decompensation chamber stiffness increases, raising the diastolic pressure at any volume[128] (see Fig. 46–10D).

In most patients with severe primary MR, compensation is maintained for years, but ultimately the prolonged hemodynamic overload leads to myocardial decompensation. End-systolic volume, preload, and afterload all rise, whereas ejection fraction and stroke volume decline. A depressed ratio of phosphocreatine/adenosine triphosphate has been reported in patients with MR and severe decompensation.[129] It is not clear whether this is the cause or a marker of heart failure in these patients.

In canine experiments which compared the *acute* effects of equally severe MR and aortic regurgitation (AR) on the left ventricle, left ventricular end-diastolic pressure, volume, and radius increased with

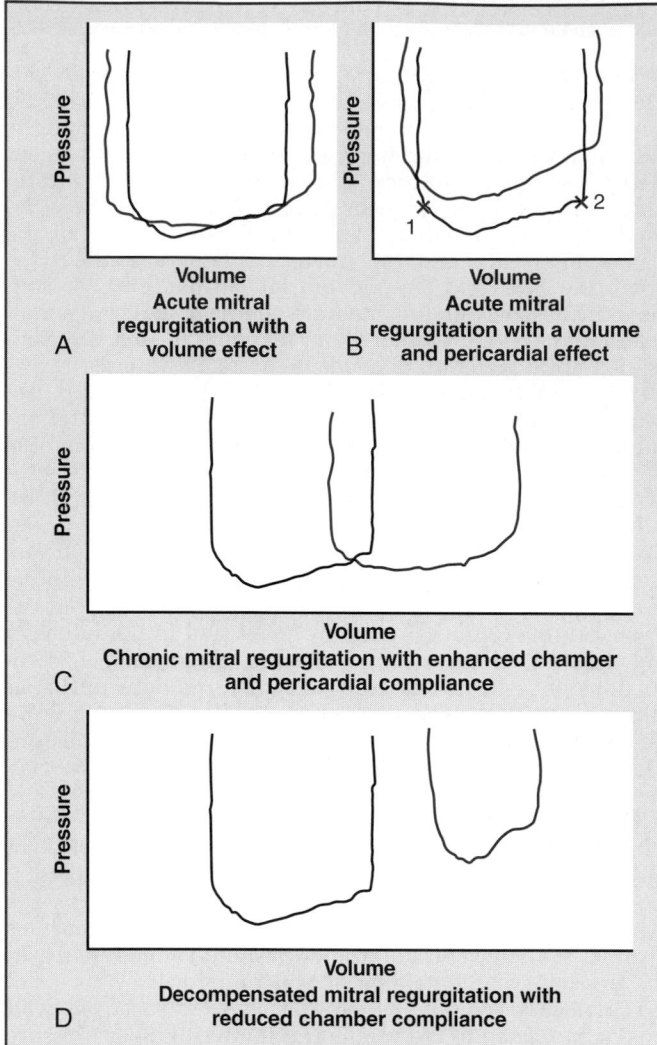

FIGURE 46–10. Left ventricular diastolic pressure-volume relationships in volume overload. *A,* A moderate acutely applied volume overload from MR. There is modest chamber enlargement at end-diastole with little increase in end-diastolic pressure and a leftward shift of the diastolic pressure-volume relationship due to a smaller end-systolic chamber size achieved from the hyperdynamic chamber performance. *B,* A major upward shift represents a higher pressure for a wide range of chamber volumes. This is acute pericardial restraint and a right-left ventricular interaction effect. These two mechanisms come into play when the acute MR is so severe that the total intrapericardial volume increases to the point of stretching the noncompliant pericardial sac. *C,* This is the classic rightward shift of compensated volume overload lesions—mitral, tricuspid, and aortic regurgitation being the most common (red line). With little change in wall thickness, the chamber is greatly enlarged, with myocardial cell slippage allowing a reduction in chamber stiffness and growth of the pericardium allowing increased intracavitary volumes to exist with a normal low pericardial pressure. *D,* Chamber stiffness increases when decompensation occurs in volume overload (red line). Often the myocardium has become myopathic and fibrotic. End-diastolic pressure volume and end-systolic volume have risen. ×1 = end-systolic pressure and volume; ×2 = end-diastolic pressure and volume in the normal subject.

both lesions, but far *less so* with MR.[130] Peak left ventricular wall tension rose markedly when AR was induced but either did not change greatly or actually declined with MR. Because *acute* MR reduces both late systolic ventricular pressure and radius, left ventricular wall tension declines markedly (and proportionately to a greater extent than left ventricular pressure), permitting a reciprocal increase in both the extent and the velocity of myocardial fiber shortening. The ratio of wall thickness to ventricular radius is lower and the fractional shortening of myocardium is greater in patients with MR

than in those with AR.[131] Thus, the reduced left ventricular afterload allows a greater proportion of the contractile energy of the myocardium to be expended in shortening than in tension development and explains how the left ventricle can adapt to the load imposed by MR.

A large volume of induced experimentally MR produces only slightly increased myocardial oxygen consumption (MVo$_2$) because myocardial fiber shortening, which is elevated in patients with MR, is not one of the principal determinants of MVo$_2$.[132] One of these determinants, mean left ventricular wall tension, may actually be reduced in patients with MR, whereas the other two, contractility and heart rate, may be little affected. These experimental observations correlate with the low incidence of clinical manifestations of myocardial ischemia in patients with severe MR compared with the much higher incidence occurring in those with aortic stenosis and AR, conditions in which MVo$_2$ is augmented.

ASSESSMENT OF MYOCARDIAL CONTRACTILITY IN MITRAL REGURGITATION. Because the ejection phase indices of myocardial contractility are inversely correlated with afterload, patients with early MR (with reduced left ventricular afterload) often exhibit elevations in ejection phase indices of myocardial contractility, such as ejection fraction (EF), fractional fiber shortening (FS), and velocity of circumferential fiber shortening (VCF).[133] However, by the time patients become seriously symptomatic, EF, FS, and mean VCF have usually declined to *normal* or *below normal* levels. As MR persists, the reduction in afterload, which increases myocardial fiber shortening and the earlier-mentioned ejection phase indices, is opposed by the impairment of myocardial function characteristic of severe chronic diastolic overload. However, even in patients with overt heart failure secondary to MR, the EF and FS may be only modestly reduced.[133a] Therefore, *normal* values for the ejection phase indices of myocardial performance in patients with acute MR may actually reflect impaired myocardial function,[134] whereas moderately reduced values (e.g., EF of 40 to 50 percent) generally signify severe, often irreversible, impairment of contractility. An EF of less than 35 percent in patients with severe MR usually represents advanced myocardial dysfunction; such patients are high operative risks and may not experience marked improvement following mitral valve replacement (see p. 1663).[127]

END-SYSTOLIC VOLUME. Preoperative myocardial contractility is an important determinant of the risk of operative death, of cardiac failure perioperatively, and of the level of left ventricular function postoperatively. Therefore, it is not surprising that the end-systolic pressure/volume (or stress/dimension) relation has emerged as a useful index for evaluating left ventricular function in patients with MR.[135] Indeed, the simple measurement of end-systolic volume has been found to be more useful as a predictor of outcome than the EF, end-diastolic volume, or end-diastolic pressure.[136] Patients with severe MR who had a normal preoperative end-systolic volume (< 40 ml/m²) retained normal left ventricular function postoperatively, whereas a marked increase in the end-systolic volume (> 80 ml/m²) signified a high perioperative mortality rate and residual left ventricular dysfunction. An end-systolic volume of 55 ml/m² appears to discriminate between patients who do well after surgical correction (<55 ml/m²) and those who are at risk of irreversible dysfunction (>55 ml/m²). Patients with MR and a modest increase in end-systolic volume (40 to 80 ml/m²) usually tolerate operation satisfactorily but may have reduced left ventricular function postoperatively.

A closely related variable, the end-systolic diameter, determined by echocardiography, is a reliable noninvasive predictor of outcome (survival without severe heart failure) following mitral valve replacement. The outcome is excellent until the end-systolic diameter exceeds approximately 45 mm or 26 mm/m² (Fig. 46–11).[137]

HEMODYNAMICS. Effective (forward) *cardiac output* is usually depressed in severely symptomatic patients with MR, whereas *total* left ventricular output (the sum of forward and regurgitant flow) is usually elevated until quite late in the patient's course. The cardiac output achieved during exercise, not the regurgitant volume, is the principal determinant of functional capacity.[138] The atrial contraction (*a*) wave in the left atrial pressure pulse is usually not as prominent in MR as in MS, but the *v* wave is often much taller (see Fig. 11–5) because it is inscribed during ventricular systole, when the left atrium is being filled with blood from the pulmonary veins as well as from the left ventricle. Occasionally, backward transmission of the tall *v* wave into

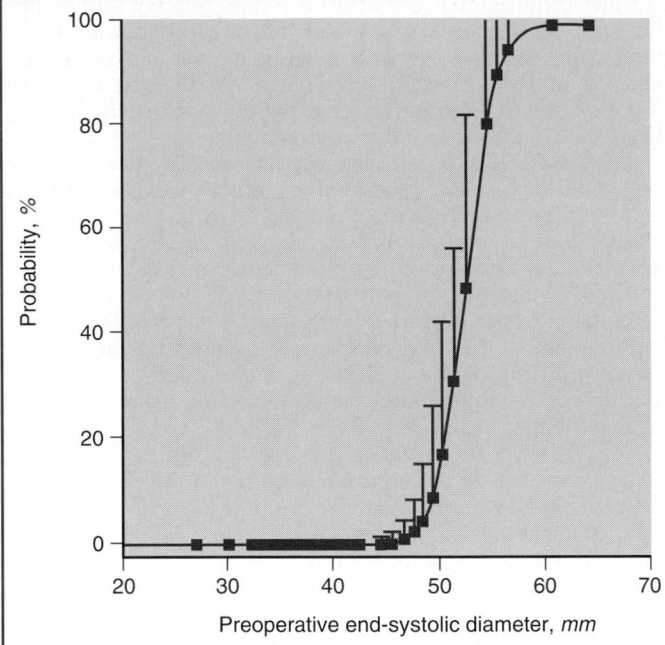

FIGURE 46–11. The probability of postoperative death or persistence of severe heart failure in patients with mitral regurgitation plotted against preoperative echocardiographic end-systolic diameter. As end-systolic diameter exceeded 45 mm, the incidence of a poor postoperative outcome increased abruptly. (Reproduced with permission from Wisenbaugh T, et al: Prediction of outcome after valve replacement for rheumatic mitral regurgitation in the era of chordal preservation. Circulation 89:191, 1994. Copyright 1994 American Heart Association.)

the pulmonary arterial bed may result in an early diastolic "pulmonary arterial *v* wave."[139] In patients with pure MR, the *y* descent in the pulmonary capillary pressure pulse is particularly rapid as the distended left atrium empties rapidly during early diastole. However, in patients with combined MS and MR, the *y* descent is gradual. Although a left atrioventricular pressure gradient persisting throughout diastole signifies the presence of significant associated MS, a brief early diastolic gradient may occur in patients with isolated, severe MR as a result of the rapid flow of blood across a normal-sized mitral orifice early in diastole.[140]

LEFT ATRIAL COMPLIANCE

The compliance of the left atrium (and pulmonary venous bed) is an important determinant of the hemodynamic[141] and clinical picture in patients with severe MR. Three major subgroups of patients with severe MR based on left atrial compliance have been identified[130, 142, 143] (Fig. 46–12) and are characterized as follows:

NORMAL OR REDUCED COMPLIANCE. In this subgroup, there is little enlargement of the left atrium but marked elevation of the mean left atrial pressure, particularly of the *v* wave,[144, 145] and pulmonary congestion is a prominent symptom. Severe MR usually develops acutely, as occurs with rupture of the chordae tendineae, infarction of one of the heads of a papillary muscle, or perforation of a mitral leaflet as a consequence of trauma or endocarditis. In patients with acute MR, the left atrium initially operates on the steep portion of its pressure-volume curve with a marked rise in pressure for a small increase in volume. Sinus rhythm is usually present; after the passage of weeks or a few months, the left atrial wall becomes hypertrophied, is capable of contracting vigorously, and facilitates left ventricular filling. The thicker atrium is less compliant than normal, which further increases the height of the *v* wave. Thickening of the walls of the pulmonary veins and proliferative changes in the pulmonary arteries, as well as marked elevations of pulmonary vascular resistance and pulmonary artery pressure, usually develop over the course of 6 to 12 months after the onset of acute, severe MR.

MARKEDLY INCREASED COMPLIANCE. At the opposite end of the spectrum from patients in the first group are those with severe, longstanding MR with massive enlargement of the left atrium and normal or only slightly elevated left atrial pressure.[143] The atrial wall contains only a small remnant of muscle surrounded by fibrous tissue. Longstanding MR in these patients has altered the physical prop-

erties of the left atrial wall and thereby displaced the atrial pressure-volume curve to the right, allowing a normal or almost normal pressure to exist in a greatly enlarged left atrium. Pulmonary arterial pressure and pulmonary vascular resistance may be normal or only slightly elevated at rest. Atrial fibrillation and a low cardiac output are almost invariably present.[143]

MODERATELY INCREASED COMPLIANCE. This, the most common subgroup, consists of patients between the ends of the spectrum represented by the first and second groups. These patients have severe, chronic MR and exhibit variable degrees of enlargement of the left atrium, associated with significant elevation of the left atrial pressure.

CLINICAL MANIFESTATIONS

History

The nature and severity of symptoms in patients with chronic MR are functions of its severity, rate of progression, the level of pulmonary arterial pressure, and the presence of associated valvular, myocardial, or coronary artery dis-

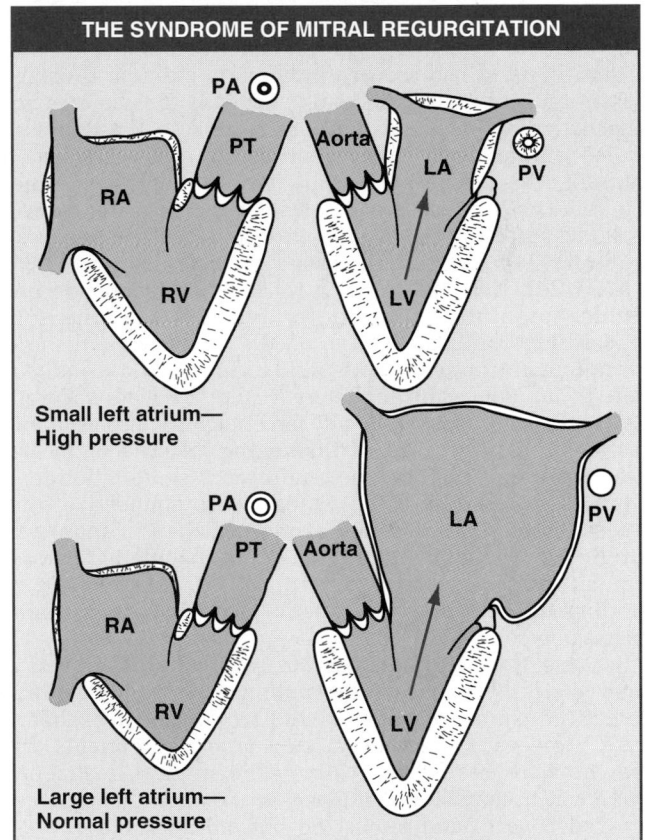

FIGURE 46–12. Diagram depicting the two extremes of the spectrum in pure mitral regurgitation. When severe mitral regurgitation appears suddenly in individuals with previously normal or near-normal hearts (top), the left atrium (LA) is relatively small and the high pressure within it is reflected back into the pulmonary vessels and right ventricle (RV). The anatomical indicator of this latter physiological event is severe hypertrophy of the left atrial and right ventricular walls and marked intimal proliferation and medial hypertrophy of the pulmonary arteries (PA), arterioles, and veins (PV). At the other extreme, in patients with severe chronic mitral regurgitation (bottom), the left atrial cavity is of giant size and its wall is thin. It is thus able to "absorb" the left ventricular (LV) pressure without reflecting it back into the pulmonary vessels or right ventricle. As a consequence, pulmonary vessels remain normal, and the right ventricular wall does not thicken. PT = pulmonary trunk; RA = right atrium. (From Roberts WC, et al: Nonrheumatic valvular cardiac disease. A clinicopathologic survey of 27 different conditions causing valvular dysfunction. *In* Likoff W [ed]: Cardiovascular Clinics. Vol. 5, No. 2, Valvular Heart Disease. Philadelphia, F.A. Davis Co, 1973, p 403.)

ease. Because symptoms usually do not develop in patients with chronic MR until left ventricular decompensation occurs, the time interval between the initial attack of rheumatic fever (if one has occurred) and the development of symptoms tends to be longer in these patients than in those with MS and often exceeds two decades. Hemoptysis and systemic embolization are less common in patients with isolated or predominant MR than in those with MS. The development of atrial fibrillation affects the course adversely but perhaps not as dramatically as in MS. On the other hand, chronic weakness and fatigue secondary to a low cardiac output are more prominent features in MR.

The majority of patients with MR of rheumatic origin have only mild disability, unless regurgitation progresses as a result of chronic rheumatic activity, infective endocarditis, or rupture of the chordae tendineae. However, the indolent course of MR may be deceptive. By the time that symptoms secondary to a reduced cardiac output and/or pulmonary congestion become apparent, serious and sometimes even irreversible left ventricular dysfunction may have developed.

In patients with severe, chronic MR who have a greatly enlarged left atrium and relatively mild left atrial hypertension (patients with increased left atrial compliance [second subgroup], described earlier), pulmonary vascular resistance does not usually rise markedly. Instead, the major symptoms, fatigue and exhaustion, are related to the depressed cardiac output. Right-sided heart failure, characterized by congestive hepatomegaly, edema, and ascites, is prominent in patients with acute MR, elevated pulmonary vascular resistance, and pulmonary hypertension. Angina pectoris is rare unless coronary artery disease coexists.

NATURAL HISTORY. This is variable and depends on a combination of the volume of regurgitation, the state of the myocardium, and the cause of the underlying disorder. Asymptomatic patients with mild primary MR usually remain in a stable state for many years.[146] Severe regurgitation develops in only a small percentage of these patients, most commonly because of intervening infective endocarditis or rupture of the chordae tendineae. Regurgitation tends to progress more rapidly in patients with connective tissue diseases, such as the Marfan syndrome, than in those with chronic MR of rheumatic origin. Acute rheumatic fever is a frequent cause of isolated, severe MR in adolescents in developing nations, and these patients often have a rapidly progressive course.

Because the natural history of severe MR has been altered greatly by surgical intervention, it is difficult now to predict the course of patients who receive medical therapy alone. However, in an unselected group of patients with MR who were treated medically before surgical treatment of severe MR became commonplace, approximately 80 percent survived 5 years and almost 60 percent survived 10 years after the diagnosis was established.[147] Patients with combined MS and MR had a poorer prognosis, with only 67 percent surviving 5 years and 30 percent surviving 10 years after diagnosis. Munoz and colleagues[63] found that medically treated patients with severe MR had a 5-year survival rate of 45 percent, whereas Horstkotte and associates[64] reported a 5-year survival of only 30 percent in patients who were candidates for but who declined operation (see Fig. 46–6).

Physical Examination

Palpation of the arterial pulse is helpful in differentiating aortic stenosis from MR, both of which may produce a prominent systolic murmur at the base of the heart. The carotid arterial upstroke is sharp in severe MR[148] and delayed in aortic stenosis; the volume of the pulse may be normal or reduced in the presence of heart failure. The cardiac impulse, like the arterial pulse, is brisk and hyperdynamic. It is displaced to the left, and a prominent left ventricular filling wave is frequently palpable. Systolic expansion of the enlarged left atrium may result in a late systolic thrust in the parasternal region, which may be confused with right ventricular enlargement.

AUSCULTATION. With severe, chronic MR due to defective valve cusps, S_1, produced by mitral valve closure, is usually diminished. Wide splitting of S_2 is common and results from the shortening of left ventricular ejection and an earlier A_2 as a consequence of reduced resistance to left ventricular outflow. In patients with MR who have severe pulmonary hypertension, P_2 is louder than A_2. The abnormal increase in the flow rate across the mitral orifice during the rapid filling phase is often associated with an S_3, which should not be interpreted as a feature of heart failure in these patients.

The *systolic murmur* is the most prominent physical finding; it must be differentiated from the systolic murmur of aortic stenosis, tricuspid regurgitation, and ventricular septal defect. In most patients with severe MR, the systolic murmur commences immediately after the soft S_1 and continues beyond and may obscure the A_2 because of the persisting pressure difference between the left ventricle and left atrium after aortic valve closure. The holosystolic murmur of chronic MR is usually constant in intensity, blowing, high-pitched, and loudest at the apex with radiation to the left axilla and left infrascapular area; however, radiation toward the sternum or the aortic area may occur with abnormalities of the posterior leaflet. The murmur shows little change even in the presence of large beat-to-beat variations of left ventricular stroke volume, as occur in atrial fibrillation. This contrasts with most midsystolic (ejection) murmurs, such as in aortic stenosis, which vary greatly in intensity with stroke volume and therefore with the duration of diastole.[149] There is little correlation between the intensity of the systolic murmur and the severity of MR. Indeed, in patients with severe MR due to left ventricular dilatation, acute myocardial infarction, or paraprosthetic valvular regurgitation, or in those who have marked emphysema, obesity, chest deformity, or a prosthetic heart valve, the systolic murmur may be barely audible or even absent, a condition referred to as "silent MR."[150]

The murmur of MR may be holosystolic, late systolic, or early systolic. When the murmur is confined to late systole, the regurgitation is usually mild and may be secondary to prolapse of the mitral valve or to papillary muscle dysfunction. These causes of MR are frequently associated with a normal S_1 because initial closure of the mitral valve cusps may be unimpaired. The late systolic murmur of papillary muscle dysfunction is particularly variable; it may become accentuated or holosystolic during acute myocardial ischemia and often disappears when ischemia is relieved. The response of a mid- to late systolic murmur to a number of maneuvers, as described on page 1668, helps to establish the diagnosis of mitral valve prolapse. When the left atrial *v* wave is markedly elevated in acute MR, the murmur may diminish or disappear in late systole as the reverse pressure gradient declines (see Fig. 4–29). A short, low-pitched diastolic murmur following S_3 may be audible in patients with severe MR, even without accompanying MS.

DYNAMIC AUSCULTATION. The holosystolic murmur of rheumatic MR varies little during respiration. However, sudden standing and amyl nitrite inhalation usually diminish the murmur (Table 46–4), whereas squatting augments it. The murmur is reduced during the strain of the Valsalva maneuver and shows a left-sided response (i.e., a transient overshoot that occurs six to eight beats following release of the strain). The murmur of MR is usually intensified by isometric exercise, differentiating it from the systolic murmurs of valvular aortic stenosis and hypertrophic obstructive cardiomyopathy, both of which are reduced by this intervention. The murmur of MR caused by left ventricular dilatation *decreases* in intensity and duration following

INTERVENTION	HYPERTROPHIC OBSTRUCTIVE CARDIOMYOPATHY	AORTIC STENOSIS	MITRAL REGURGITATION	MITRAL VALVE PROLAPSE
Valsalva	↑	↓	↓	↑ or ↓
Standing	↑	↑ or unchanged	↓	↑
Handgrip or squatting	↓	↓ or unchanged	↑	↓
Supine position with legs elevated	↓	↑ or unchanged	Unchanged	↓
Exercise	↑	↑ or unchanged	↓	↑
Amyl nitrite	↑ ↑	↑	↓	↑
Isoproterenol	↑ ↑	↑	↓	↑

↑ ↑ = Markedly increased.
Modified from Paraskos JA: Combined valvular disease. *In* Dalen JE, Alpert JS (eds): Valvular Heart Disease. 2nd ed. Boston, Little, Brown and Co, 1987, p 365.

effective therapy with cardiac glycosides, diuretics, rest, and particularly vasodilators.

DIFFERENTIAL DIAGNOSIS. The holosystolic murmur of MR resembles that produced by a ventricular septal defect. However, the latter is usually loudest at the sternal border rather than the apex and is usually accompanied by a parasternal, rather than an apical, thrill. The murmur of MR may also be confused with that of tricuspid regurgitation, which is usually heard best along the left sternal border, is augmented during inspiration, and is accompanied by a prominent *v* wave and *y* descent in the jugular venous pulse.

When the chordae tendineae to the posterior leaflet of the mitral valve rupture, the regurgitant jet is often directed anteriorly, so that it impinges on the atrial septum adjacent to the aortic root and causes a systolic murmur that is most prominent at the base of the heart. This murmur can be confused with that of aortic stenosis. On the other hand, when the chordae tendineae to the anterior leaflet rupture, the jet is usually directed to the posterior wall of the left atrium, and the murmur may be transmitted to the spine or even to the top of the head.[151]

Patients with rheumatic disease of the mitral valve exhibit a spectrum of abnormalities, ranging from pure MS to pure MR. The presence of an S_3, a rapid left ventricular filling wave and left ventricular impulse on palpation, and a soft S_1 all favor predominant MR. In contrast, an accentuated S_1, a prominent opening snap (OS) with a short A_2-OS interval, and a soft, short systolic murmur all point to predominant MS. Elucidation of the predominant valvular lesion may be complicated by the presence of a holosystolic murmur of tricuspid regurgitation in patients with pure MS and pulmonary hypertension; this murmur may sometimes be heard at the apex when the right ventricle is greatly enlarged and may therefore be mistaken for the murmur of MR.

LABORATORY EXAMINATION

ELECTROCARDIOGRAPHY. The principal ECG findings are left atrial enlargement[44, 152] and atrial fibrillation. ECG evidence of left ventricular enlargement occurs in about one-third of patients with severe MR. Approximately 15 percent of patients exhibit ECG evidence of right ventricular hypertrophy, a change that reflects the presence of pulmonary hypertension of sufficient severity to counterbalance the hypertrophied left ventricle of MR.

RADIOLOGICAL FINDINGS (see Fig. 8–18D). Cardiomegaly with left ventricular enlargement, and particularly with left atrial enlargement, is a common finding in patients with chronic, severe MR.[153] However, there is little correlation between left atrial size and pressure. Interstitial edema with Kerley B lines is frequently seen in patients with acute MR or with progressive left ventricular failure.

In patients with combined MS and MR, overall cardiac enlargement and particularly left atrial dilatation are prominent findings. However, it is often difficult to determine which lesion is predominant from the plain chest roentgenogram because distinguishing between right and left ventricular enlargement may not be possible. Predominant MS is suggested by relatively mild cardiomegaly (principally straightening of the left cardiac border) and significant changes in the lung fields, whereas predominant MR is more likely when the heart is greatly enlarged and the changes in the lungs are relatively inconspicuous. Chronic MR is almost always the dominant lesion when the left atrium is aneurysmally dilated. *Calcification of the mitral annulus,* an important cause of MR in the elderly, is most prominent in the posterior third of the cardiac silhouette. The lesion is best visualized on chest films exposed in the lateral or right anterior oblique projections, in which it appears as a dense, coarse, C-shaped opacity (see Fig. 8–20).

ECHOCARDIOGRAPHY (See also Chap. 7). In patients with severe MR, *two-dimensional echocardiography* shows enlargement of the left atrium and left ventricle, with increased systolic motion of both chambers. The underlying cause of the regurgitation, e.g., rupture of chordae tendineae, mitral valve prolapse (see Fig. 7–57), a flail leaflet[154] (see Figs. 7–55 and 7–56), vegetations (see Chap. 47), and left ventricular dilatation (see Fig. 7–54) can often be determined on the transthoracic echocardiogram. It may also show calcification of the mitral annulus as a band of dense echoes between the mitral apparatus and the posterior wall of the heart.[155] This technique is also useful for estimating the hemodynamic consequences of MR[155a, 155b]; in patients with left ventricular dysfunction, end-diastolic and end-systolic volumes are increased and the ejection fraction and shortening rate may decline.

Doppler echocardiography in MR characteristically reveals a high-velocity jet in the left atrium during systole. The severity of the regurgitation is a function of the distance from the valve that the jet can be detected (see Fig. 7–53) and the size of the left atrium. Both color flow Doppler imaging and pulsed techniques correlate well with angiographic methods in estimating the severity of MR.[156] Other methods of assessing the severity of MR include measurement of the area of the mitral jet (≥8 cm² indicates severe MR). However, color flow jet areas are significantly influenced by the cause of the regurgitation and jet eccentricity, thus limiting the accuracy of this approach.[157] The vena contracta, defined as the narrowest cross-sectional areas of the regurgitant jet as mapped by color flow Doppler echocardiography, predicts the severity of MR[158–160] (Fig. 46–13). Reversal of flow in the pulmonary veins during systole[161] and a high peak mitral inflow velocity[162] are also useful signs of severe MR.

Transesophageal echocardiography (see Fig. 7–55) is superior to transthoracic echocardiography in assessing the detailed anatomy of the regurgitant mitral valve. Therefore, this technique is useful when the transthoracic image is suboptimal and when determining whether valve repair is feasible or whether MVR is necessary.[163, 164] Also, angiographic grading of MR correlates better with color flow mapping obtained by the transesophageal than by the transthoracic technique.[165] Three-dimensional transthoracic echocardiography and three-dimensional color Doppler[166] have also been reported to help elucidate the mechanism of MR.

RADIONUCLIDE ANGIOGRAPHY (see also Chap. 9). Gated blood pool nuclear imaging or first-pass angiography may reveal an increased end-diastolic volume; the regurgitant fraction can be estimated from the ratio of left ventricular to right ventricular stroke volume. In patients with MR and impaired left ventricular function, the ejection fraction fails to rise normally during exercise. Radionuclide angiograms are useful for interval follow-up. Progressive increases in ventricular end-diastolic and/or end-systolic volume often suggest that surgical treatment is necessary (discussed later).

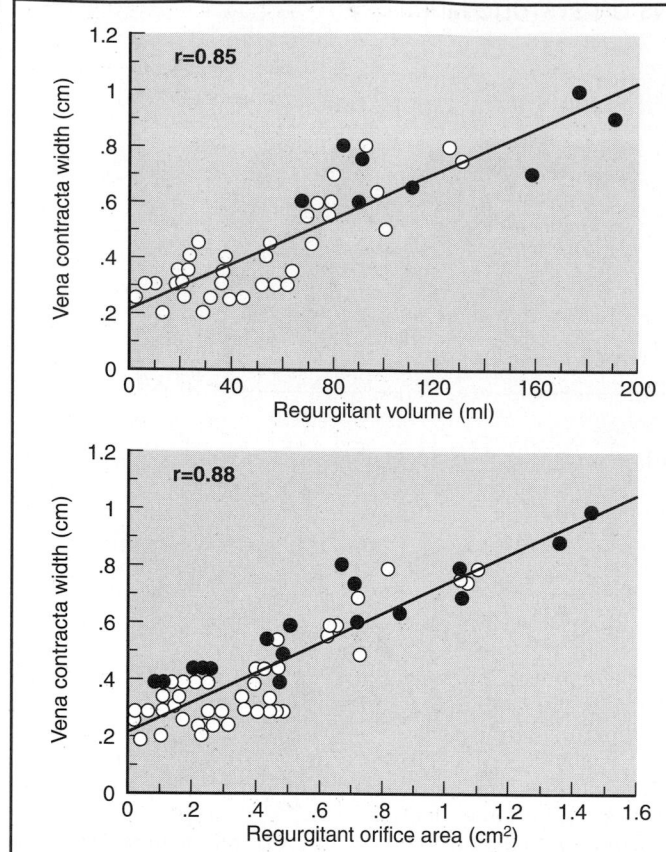

FIGURE 46–13. Linear regression plot showing good correlation between biplane vena contracta width and regurgitant volume. (From Hall SA, Brickner E, Willen DL, et al: Assessment of mitral regurgitation severity by Doppler color flow mapping of the vena contracta. Circulation 95:636, 1997.)

LEFT VENTRICULAR ANGIOCARDIOGRAPHY. The prompt appearance of contrast material in the left atrium following its injection into the left ventricle indicates the presence of MR.[167] The injection should be rapid enough to permit left ventricular opacification but slow enough to avoid the development of premature ventricular contractions, which can induce spurious regurgitation.

The regurgitant volume can be determined from the difference between the total left ventricular stroke volume, estimated by angiocardiography, and the simultaneous measurement of the effective forward stroke volume by the Fick method. In patients with severe MR, the regurgitant volume may approach, and in rare instances may even exceed, the effective forward stroke volume. Qualitative but clinically useful estimates of the severity of MR may be made by cineangiographic observation of the degree of opacification of the left atrium and pulmonary veins following the injection of contrast material into the left ventricle.

The cause of the regurgitation (e.g., prolapse of the mitral valve) and a flail leaflet can often be distinguished by angiography. MR secondary to rheumatic heart disease is characterized angiographically by a central regurgitant jet and by thickened leaflets that exhibit reduced motion. In regurgitation due to other causes, particularly dilatation or calcification of the mitral annulus or ruptured chordae tendineae and papillary muscles, the systolic jet may be eccentric, and the valves consist of thin filaments that display excessive motion.

MAGNETIC RESONANCE IMAGING. This study (see Fig. 10–24) is the most accurate technique for measuring regurgitant flow and provides measurements that correlate well with quantitative Doppler imaging.[168, 169] It is also the most accurate noninvasive technique that can provide measurement of ventricular end-diastolic and end-systolic volumes and ventricular mass.

Acute Mitral Regurgitation

The causes of acute MR are shown at the top of Table 46–3. They are diverse and represent acute manifestations of disease processes that may, under other circumstances, cause chronic MR. Especially important causes of acute MR are infective endocarditis with disruption of valve leaflets or rupture of chordae tendineae, ischemic dysfunction or rupture of a papillary muscle, and malfunction of a prosthetic valve.

One major hemodynamic difference between acute and chronic MR derives from the differences in left atrial compliance, as discussed on page 1657 and as illustrated in Figure 46–12. Acute, severe MR causes a marked reduction of forward stroke volume, a slight reduction of end-systolic volume, and an increase in end-diastolic volume. Patients who develop acute, severe MR usually have a normal-sized left atrium (normal or reduced left atrial compliance [first subgroup], see p. 1657). The left atrial pressure rises abruptly, which often leads to pulmonary edema, marked elevation of pulmonary vascular resistance, and right-sided heart failure.

Because the v wave is markedly elevated in patients with acute, severe MR, the reverse pressure gradient between the left ventricle and left atrium declines at the end of systole, and the murmur may be decrescendo rather than holosystolic, ending well before A_2 (see Fig. 4–29). It is usually lower pitched and softer than the murmur of chronic MR. A left-sided S_4 is frequently found.[130] Pulmonary hypertension, which is common in patients with acute MR, may increase the intensity of P_2 and the murmurs of pulmonary and tricuspid regurgitation, and a right-sided S_4 may also develop. In patients with severe, acute MR, a v wave (late systolic pressure rise) in the pulmonary artery pressure pulse (see Fig. 11–5) may rarely cause premature closure of the pulmonary valve, an early P_2, and paradoxical splitting of S_2. Acute MR, even if severe, often does not increase overall cardiac size, as seen on the chest roentgenogram, and may produce only mild left atrial enlargement despite marked elevation of left atrial pressure. In addition, the echocardiogram may show little increase in the internal diameter of either the left atrium or the left ventricle, but increased systolic motion of the left ventricle is prominent.

MANAGEMENT

Medical Treatment

This includes all of the measures used in the treatment of cardiac dysfunction, as outlined in Chapter 18. Afterload reduction is of particular benefit in the management of both the acute and the chronic forms of MR.[170, 171] By reducing the impedance to ejection into the aorta, the volume of blood regurgitating into the left atrium is reduced. In addition, decreasing left ventricular volume reduces the regurgitant orifice.[172] Mean left atrial pressure and, in particular, the elevated v wave both decline. Afterload reduction with intravenous nitroprusside may be lifesaving in patients with acute MR due to rupture of the head of a papillary muscle that occurs during an acute myocardial infarction. It may permit stabilization of the patient's condition and thereby allow coronary arteriography and surgery to be performed with the patient in optimal condition. In patients with acute MR who are hypotensive, an inotropic agent such as dobutamine should be administered with the nitroprusside. Intraaortic balloon counterpulsation may be necessary to stabilize the patient as preparations for surgery are made.

When surgical treatment is contraindicated in patients with severe, chronic MR, chronic afterload reduction with an angiotensin converting enzyme inhibitor[170, 171, 173, 173a] or oral hydralazine may improve the clinical status. However, definitive randomized trials documenting the efficacy of these agents are not available. In addition to diuretics, digitalis glycosides are indicated in patients with severe MR

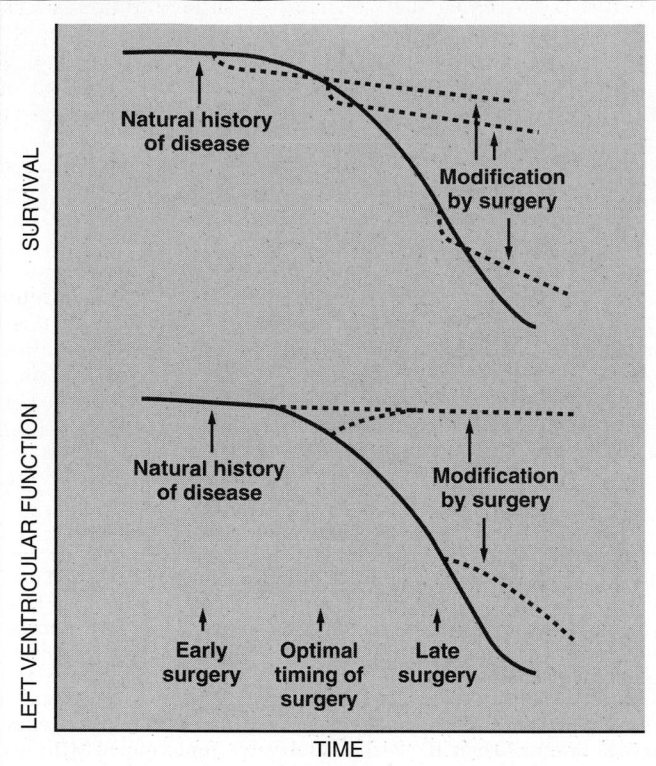

FIGURE 46-14. Schematic representation of the concept of optimal timing of valve replacement surgery. Early surgery yields low operative mortality and preservation of ventricular function. However, because of a finite postoperative risk of prosthesis-associated complications (the major determinant of the slope of the postoperative survival curve in either early or optimally timed surgery), postoperative risk exceeds that of pure medical treatment at this early phase of the disease. In contrast, if surgery is done too late, operative mortality is increased and ventricular function may progressively deteriorate after surgery. Thus, following late surgery, postoperative survival is primarily determined by both prosthesis-associated complications and congestive heart failure. Optimal timing of surgery balances the risks of maintaining medical management with the new risks associated with postoperative complications. With optimally timed surgical intervention, operative mortality is relatively low, ventricular function is almost completely preserved, and postoperative risk is determined, as in early surgery, predominantly by the risk of prosthesis-associated complications. (From Schoen FJ, St. John Sutton M: Contemporary issues in the pathology of valvular disease. Hum Pathol 18:568, 1987.)

and clinical evidence of heart failure and are particularly helpful in patients with established atrial fibrillation. The latter should also receive anticoagulants. As do all patients with valvular lesions, patients with MR require appropriate prophylaxis to prevent infective endocarditis (see Chap. 47).

Surgical treatment should be considered for patients with functional disability despite optimal medical management and/or for patients with only mild symptoms but with progressively deteriorating left ventricular function as documented by noninvasive studies. Two-dimensional or transesophageal echocardiography with Doppler echocardiography and color flow Doppler imaging provide detailed assessment of mitral valve structure and function. However, left heart catheterization, left ventricular angiocardiography, and coronary arteriography are indicated for the following: (1) in evaluating a discrepancy between echocardiographic findings and the clinical picture; (2) in detecting and assessing the severity of any associated valvular lesions; and (3) in determining the presence and assessing the extent of coronary artery disease.

Without surgical treatment, the prognosis for patients with MR and heart failure is poor (see Fig. 46-6). When operative treatment is being considered, the chronic and often slowly but relentlessly progressive nature of MR must be weighed against the immediate risks and long-term uncertainties attendant upon surgery, especially mitral valve replacement (MVR) (Fig. 46-14). Surgical mortality depends on the patient's clinical and hemodynamic status (particularly the function of the left ventricle); on the presence of comorbid conditions such as renal, hepatic, or pulmonary disease; and on the skill and experience of the surgical team[104] (see Table 46-2). The decision to replace or to reconstruct the valve (Fig. 46-15) is of critical importance. Replacement involves the operative risk, as well as the risks of thromboembolism and anticoagulation in patients receiving mechanical prostheses, of late valve deterioration in patients receiving bioprostheses (see p. 1696), and of late

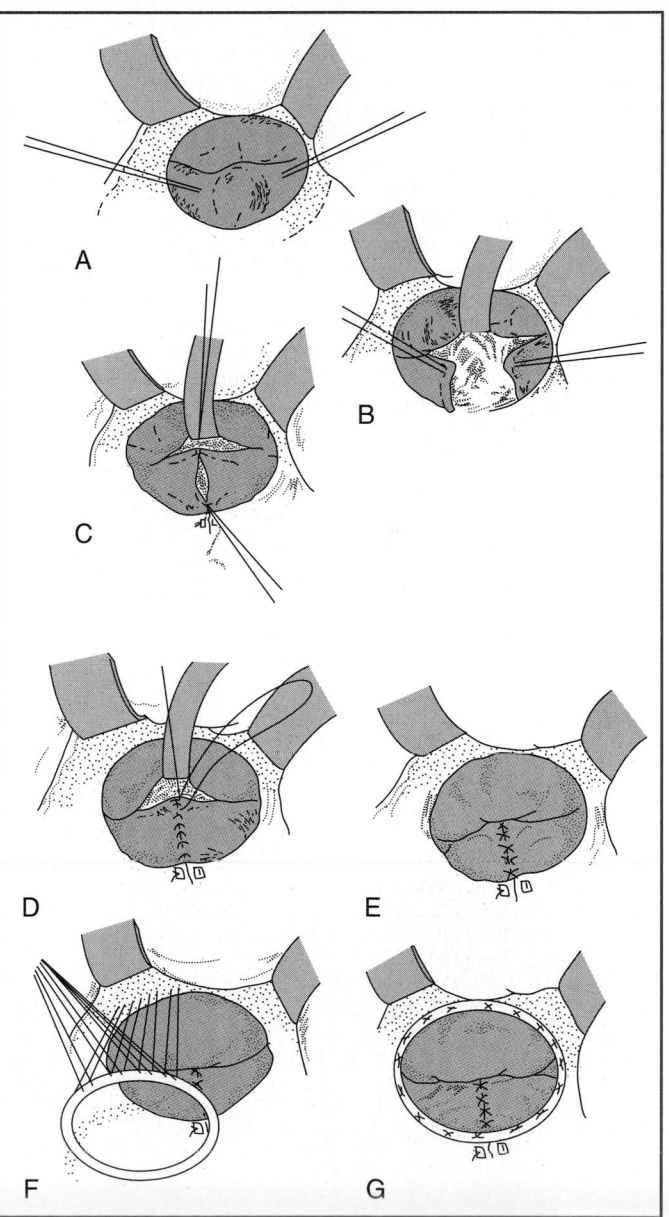

FIGURE 46-15. Valve repair techniques for quadrilateral resection of the posterior leaflet of the mitral valve. (From Cohn LH, DiSesa VJ, Couper GS, et al: Mitral valve repair for myxomatous degeneration and prolapse of the mitral valve. J Thorac Cardiovasc Surg 98: 987, 1989.)

mortality, especially in patients with associated coronary artery disease who require coronary artery bypass grafting (see Table 46–2). Surgical mortality does not depend significantly on *which* of the currently used tissue or mechanical valve prostheses is selected.

The reconstructive procedure consists of annuloplasty, often with the use of a rigid (Carpentier) or a flexible prosthetic (Duran) ring (Fig. 46–16) or with reconstruction of the valve[174–179] (see Fig. 46–15). Prolapsed valves causing severe MR are usually treated with resection of the prolapsing segment and plication of the annulus (see p. 1671). Replacing,[180] reimplanting, elongating, or shortening of chordae tendineae; splitting the papillary muscles; and repairing the subvalvular apparatus have been successful in selected patients with pure or predominant MR.[175] Reconstruction of the mitral valve is most often successful in (1) children and adolescents with pliable valves; (2) adults with MR secondary to mitral valve prolapse[18]; (3) annular dilatation; (4) papillary muscle secondary to ischemia, dysfunction, or rupture; or (5) chordal rupture and perforation of a mitral leaflet due to infective endocarditis. These procedures are less likely to be successful in older patients with the rigid, calcified, deformed valves of rheumatic heart disease or those with severe subvalvular chordal thickening and major loss of leaflet substance. Many of the latter patients require MVR, which is also usually the procedure of choice for patients with badly scarred mitral valves who have previously undergone MVR. Young patients in developing countries who have severe rheumatic MR in the absence of active carditis may undergo successful repair.

Ischemic MR following acute myocardial infarction may be managed by reattaching the papillary muscle to adjacent myocardium or by valve replacement. Ischemic MR secondary to severe annular dilatation may be treated by direct or ring annuloplasty.[176–177a] Episodic MR due to transient ischemia is often eliminated by coronary revascularization, whereas severe, chronic MR secondary to fibrotic infarcted papillary muscle usually requires valve replacement.

Although MVR with a mechanical or bioprosthesis has been used successfully in treating MR for almost four decades,[181] there has been some dissatisfaction with the results of this operation. First, left ventricular function often deteriorates following this procedure, contributing to early and late mortality and late disability. The increase in afterload

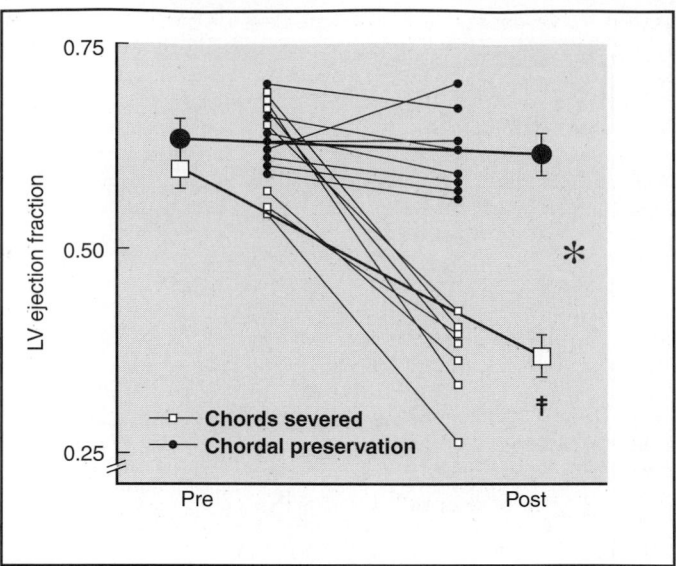

FIGURE 46–17. Preoperative (PRE) and postoperative (POST) left ventricular (LV) ejection fractions for patients undergoing MVR with chordae tendineae severed (open squares) or with chordae tendineae preserved (closed circles). MVR with chords severed resulted in decreased ejection fraction, but MVR with chords preserved did not. ‡, $P < 0.05$ for comparing PRE and POST status with chords severed. *, No significant difference with chords preserved. (From Rozich JD et al: Mitral valve replacement with and without chordal preservation in patients with chronic mitral regurgitation; mechanisms for differences in postoperative ejection performance. Circulation 86:1718, 1992.)

consequent to abolishing the low impedance leak was first believed to be responsible, but now it is clear that the loss of annular–chordal–papillary muscle continuity interferes with left ventricular function in patients who have undergone MVR. This does not occur after mitral valve reconstruction.[180] Indeed, animal experiments have shown convincingly that the normal function of the mitral valve apparatus "primes" the left ventricle for normal contraction and that contraction is prevented when operation causes discontinuity of this apparatus. There is evidence from animal experiments[182] and from human patients[183–185] that preservation of the papillary muscle and its chordal attachments to the mitral annulus is beneficial to postoperative left ventricular function, after both mitral valve reconstruction and in MVR (Fig. 46–17). Thus, preservation of these tissues, whenever possible, is now considered a critical feature of MVR.[186]

A second disadvantage of MVR results from the prosthesis itself. This includes thromboembolism or hemorrhage associated with mechanical prostheses, late mechanical dysfunction of bioprostheses, and the risk of infective endocarditis with all prostheses (see p. 1697). For these reasons, increasing efforts are being made to reconstruct the mitral valve whenever possible, especially in patients with isolated or predominant MR.[187–190] These procedures have been widely employed in Europe since the early 1960s and are now frequently being used by surgeons in the United States as well. The Society of Thoracic Surgeons National Database Committee reported a 3 percent mortality rate in 4167 patients undergoing isolated mitral valve repair[104] (see Table 46–2).

Intraoperative transesophageal color flow Doppler mapping is extremely useful in assessing the adequacy of mitral valve repair. In the minority of patients with persistent severe MR in whom the operative results are unsatisfactory, the problem can usually be corrected immediately, or, if necessary, the valve can be replaced. Left ventricular outflow tract obstruction due to systolic anterior motion of the

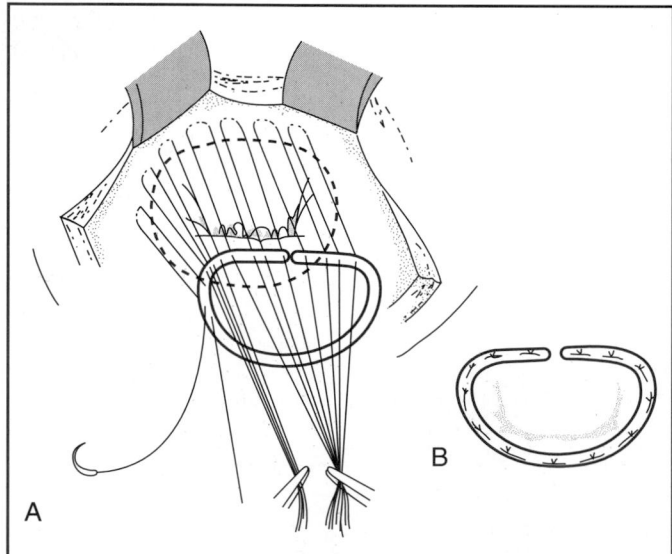

FIGURE 46–16. Insertion of an annuloplasty ring. (Reproduced with permission from Galloway AC, Colvin SB, Baumann FG, et al: Current concepts of mitral valve reconstruction for mitral insufficiency. Circulation 78:1087, 1988. Copyright 1989 American Heart Association.)

mitral valve occurs in 5 to 10 percent of patients following mitral valve repair. The causes are not clear; but they may include excess valvular tissue with severe leaflet redundancy and/or an interventricular septum bulging into a small left ventricle.[191, 192] These complications may also be recognized intraoperatively by transesophageal echocardiography. Treatment with volume loading and beta-blocking agents is often helpful. The obstruction usually disappears with time; if it does not, reoperation and re-repair or MVR may be necessary.

Progressive decrease in the prevalence of rheumatic heart disease (involving severely damaged valves that often are not suitable for reconstructive surgery) and a simultaneous increase in degenerative causes of MR (including mitral valve prolapse and rupture of chordae tendineae) as well as in ischemic MR are increasing the number of patients in whom reconstruction is carried out.[193] In many centers in the United States, approximately two-thirds of all patients requiring operation for pure or predominant MR now receive reconstructive procedures, and the remainder undergo MVR. However, mitral valve repair is technically a more demanding procedure than is MVR, with a distinct learning curve for the surgeon. Furthermore, some regurgitant valves, particularly those that are thickened, severely deformed, calcified, and partly stenotic, are not suitable for reconstruction, and patients with these valves require MVR.[193a, 193b]

Minimally invasive surgical techniques (Fig. 46-18) utilizing a small, low, asymmetrical sternotomy or anterior thoracotomy[194] and percutaneous cardiopulmonary bypass,[195, 195a] although quite demanding technically, have been found to be less traumatic and can be employed for both valve repair and replacement. This approach has been reported to reduce cost, improve cosmetic results, and shorten the recovery time.[196] However, it also is technically difficult and is successfully performed by only a minority of cardiac surgeons.

SURGICAL RESULTS. Mortality rates of 3 to 9 percent are now common in many centers for patients with pure or predominant MR (NYHA Class II or III) who undergo elective isolated MVR.[137, 197, 198] The Society of Thoracic Surgeons National Database Committee reported an overall operative mortality rate of 6.4 percent in 13,936 patients undergoing isolated MVR; this compares with 4.3 percent for isolated aortic valve replacement and 3 percent for isolated mitral valve repair. The combination of MVR and repair of another valve was associated with a mortality rate of 12.5 percent and of MVR with coronary artery bypass grafting of 8 percent. The mortality rate is higher (up to 25 percent) in older patients with severe left ventricular dysfunction, especially when MR is secondary to myocardial ischemia, when pulmonary or renal function is impaired, or when the operation must be carried out as an emergency. Age *per se* is no barrier to successful surgery; MVR can be performed in patients older than 75 years of age if their general health status is adequate; however, surgery in these patients has a higher risk than in younger patients.[184]

Surgical treatment substantially improves survival in patients with symptomatic MR. Preoperative factors such as age less than 60 years, NYHA Class II, a cardiac index exceeding 2.0 liters/min/m², a left ventricular end-diastolic pressure less than 12 mm Hg, and a normal ejection fraction and end-systolic volume all correlate with excellent immediate and long-term survival rates. Both preoperative end-systolic diameter (see Fig. 46-11) and ejection fraction (Fig. 46-19) are important predictors of short-term and long-term outcome. Excellent survival is observed in patients with end-systolic diameters less than 45 mm and ejection fractions of 60 percent or more. Intermediate outcomes are seen in patients with end-systolic diameters between 45 and 52 mm and ejection fractions between 50 and

60 percent. Poor outcomes are associated with values beyond these limits.

A large proportion of operative survivors have improved clinical status, quality of life, and exercise tolerance following valve replacement or repair. Severe pulmonary hypertension is reduced, and left ventricular end-diastolic volume and mass decrease. Depressed contractile function improves, especially if the papillary muscles and chordal attachment to the annulus remain intact. However, patients with MR who have marked left ventricular dysfunction preoperatively sometimes remain symptomatic with a depressed ejection fraction despite a technically satisfactory surgical procedure. Indeed, progressive left ventricular dysfunction and death from heart failure may occur in adults. Recovery of left ventricular function is much better in children.[199] Long-term survival in patients with predominant MR who undergo MVR may be poorer than in those with pure MS or with mixed stenotic and regurgitant lesions, presumably because left ventricular dysfunction may be quite advanced and largely irreversible by the time patients with pure MR develop serious symptoms.[200] Ten-year survival was 76 percent in patients in NYHA-Class I or II versus 48 percent in patients in Class III or IV.[200] Thus, every effort should be made to operate on patients before they develop serious symptoms. However, even though operating on patients with MR is clearly desirable before they develop marked left ventricular dysfunction[201] and despite the limitations of the results of surgical treatment, operation is still indicated in the majority of these patients because conservative therapy has little to offer.

The cause of MR also plays an important role in the outcome following surgical treatment.[202] In patients in whom mitral dysfunction is secondary to ischemic heart disease, the 5-year survival rate is about 40 percent, whereas in patients with rheumatic MR it is approximately 75 percent. Occlusive coronary artery disease coexisting with, but not the primary cause of, mitral dysfunction requires simultaneous coronary artery bypass grafting and mitral valve repair or replacement and is associated with decreased perioperative and long-term postoperative survival (Fig. 46-20). However, some improvement resulting from mitral valve repair or replacement can be expected even in patients with MR secondary to ischemic heart disease who did not respond to medical treatment and now have congestive heart failure, as long as the cardiac index exceeds 1.8 liters/min/m² and the ejection fraction is greater than 30 percent. When left ventricular dysfunction is more severe, however, the risk of perioperative death becomes very high.[203]

SURGICAL TREATMENT OF ACUTE MITRAL REGURGITATION. Emergency surgical treatment may be required for patients with acute left ventricular failure caused by acute MR secondary to myocardial infarction and rupture of the head of a papillary muscle, by trauma to the mitral valve, or by infective endocarditis. Emergency surgery is associated with higher mortality rates than is elective surgery for chronic MR. However, unless patients with acute, severe MR and heart failure are treated aggressively, a fatal outcome is almost certain. If patients with MR secondary to acute myocardial infarction can be stabilized by medical treatment, it is preferable to defer operation until 4 to 6 weeks after the infarction. Vasodilator treatment may be useful during this period. However, medical management should not be prolonged if multisystem (renal and/or pulmonary) failure develops. Intraaortic balloon counterpulsation may be required to stabilize the patient preoperatively. Surgical mortality rates are also higher in patients with acute MR and refractory heart failure (NYHA Class IV), in those in whom a previously implanted prosthetic valve must be replaced because of thromboembolism or valve dysfunction, and in those with active infective endocarditis (of either a natural or a prosthetic valve). Despite the higher

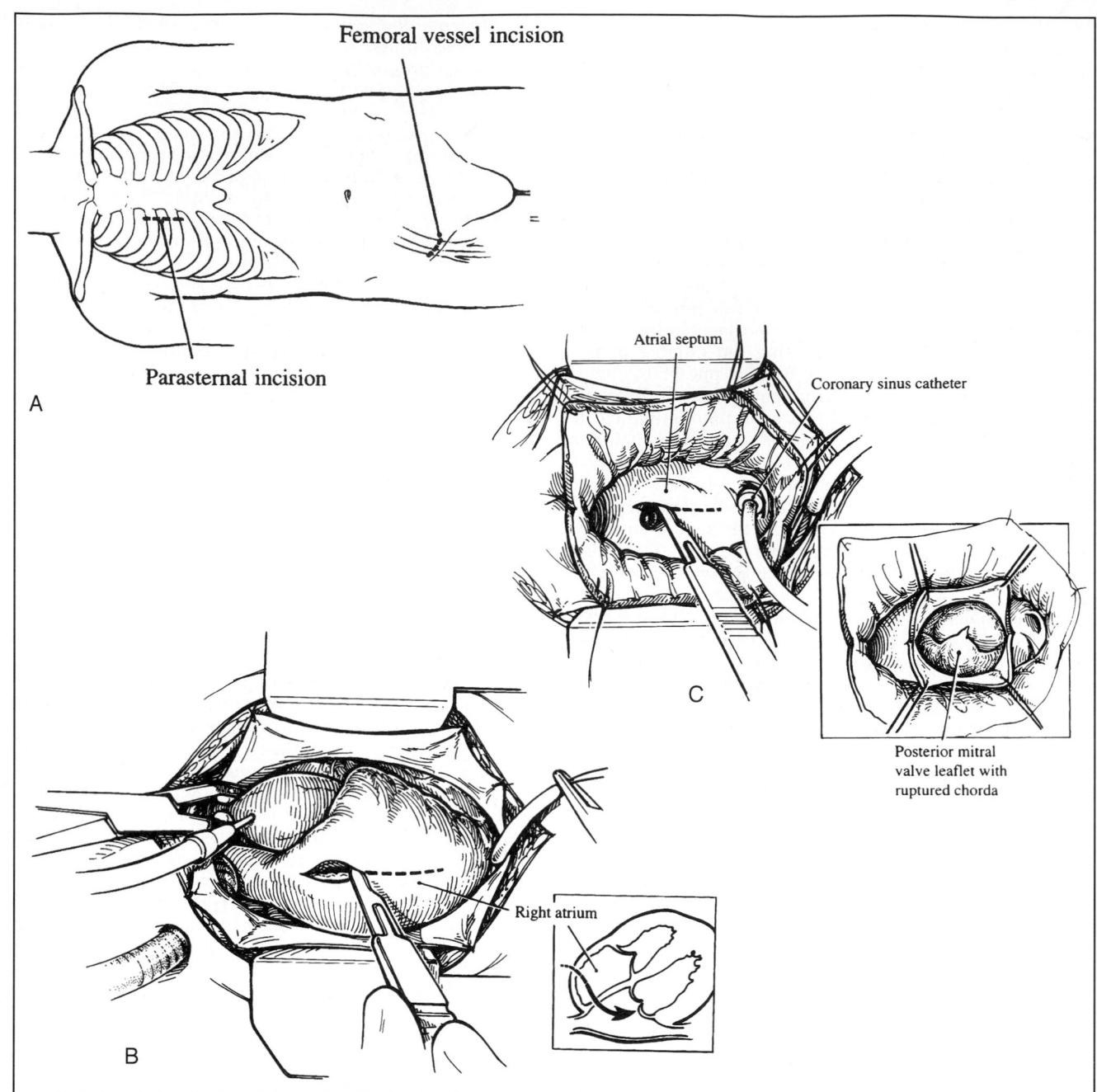

FIGURE 46–18. *A,* Minimally invasive right parasternal incision: A 5- to 7-cm incision is made, resecting a small portion of the third and fourth costal cartilages. Cannulation of the groin vessels (femoral artery and vein) has been performed frequently but has been revised to allow for minimal wound and vascular complications. The groin incision is placed parallel to the groin crease and is only 5 cm long. The artery and vein are exposed, and, after heparinization, the vein is cannulated using a pursestring and a 25- to 27-French wire reinforced Biomedicus catheter over a wire and then a dilator. The arterial cannula may be introduced by a small transverse cut downward. *B,* With the minimally invasive approach, a right atrial incision is used after exclusion of both the inferior and the superior vena cava, and the valve is approached through the septum (insert). *C,* When the right atrium is incised, an incision is made in the atrial septum through the fossae ovalis. Retraction sutures, on both the right atrium and the atrial septum, of 2-0 silk, are then used to elevate the septum and to keep the left atrium open. The mitral valve will then be exposed (insert). (From Byrne JG, et al: Minimally invasive direct access mitral valve surgery. Semin Thorac Cardiovasc Surg 11:212, 1999.)

surgical risks, the efficacy of early operation has been established in patients with infective endocarditis complicated by medically uncontrollable congestive heart failure and/or recurrent emboli (see Chap. 47). Because fungal endocarditis responds poorly to medical management, the practice now is to recommend valve replacement in these patients *before* the onset of heart failure or embolization.

INDICATIONS FOR OPERATION. The threshold for surgical treatment of MR is declining for several reasons. These include the reductions in operative mortality, the improvements in both mitral valve reconstructive procedures and procedures involving prosthetic valves, and the recognition of the poor long-term results in many patients whose MR is corrected only after a long history of im-

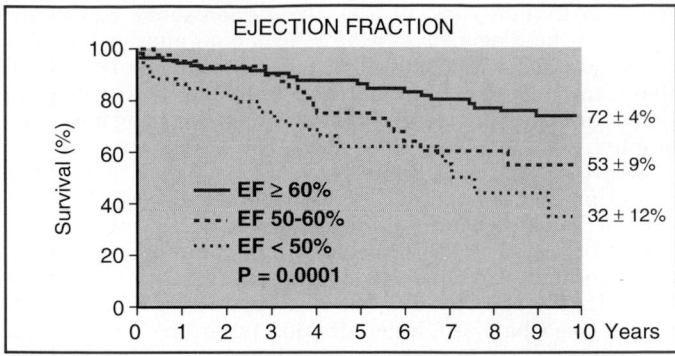

FIGURE 46–19. Graph of the late survival of of patients who underwent surgical correction of MR according to preoperative echocardiographic ejection fraction (EF). (Reproduced with permission from Enriquez-Sarano M, et al: Echocardiographic prediction of survival after surgical correction of organic mitral regurgitation. Circulation 90:833, 1994. Copyright 1994 American Heart Association.)

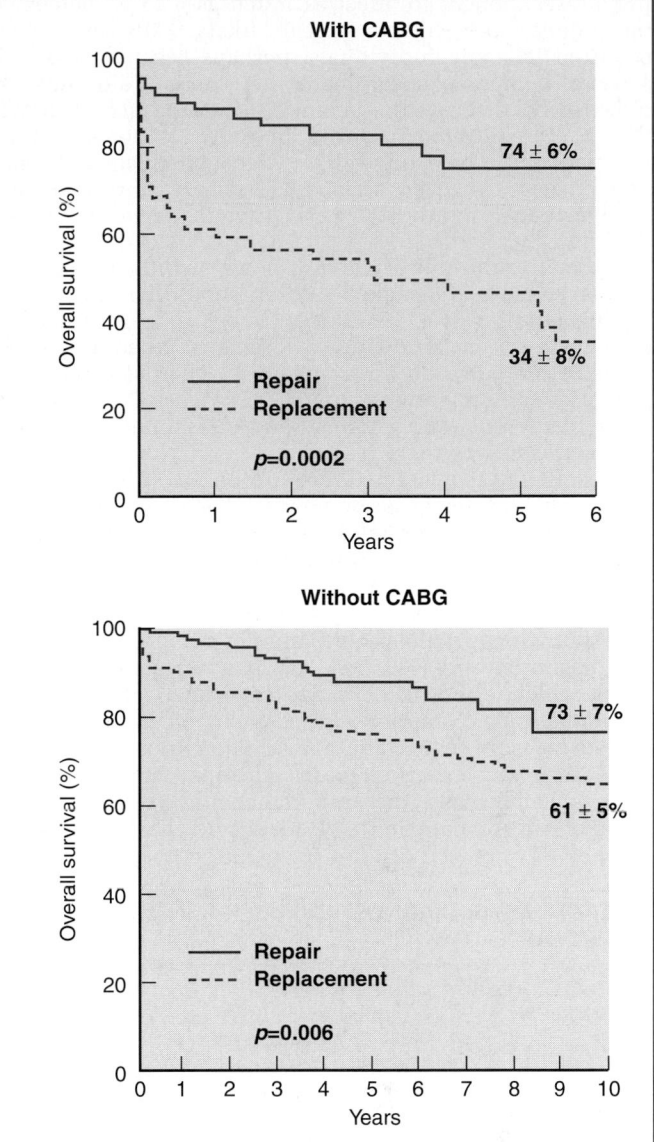

FIGURE 46–20. Plots of overall survival compared for repair and replacement groups for patients who had (left) or did not have (right) associated coronary artery bypass grafting (CABG). Note that the outcome is better with repair than with replacement in both groups and that the outcome is worse in patients who underwent CABG and MVR. (From Enriquez-Sarano M, Schaff HV, Orszulak TA, et al: Valve repair improves the outcome of surgery for mitral regurgitation: A multivariate analysis. Circulation 91:1022, 1995.)

paired left ventricular function, atrial fibrillation, or pulmonary hypertension.

A detailed echocardiographic examination should be carried out to assess the likelihood that mitral valve repair, rather than replacement, is possible. In addition, the difference in outcome between these procedures should be weighed when deciding whether or not to proceed. Asymptomatic patients (NYHA Class I) should be considered for mitral valve reconstruction only if they have left ventricular dysfunction (ejection fraction ≤60 percent and/or left ventricular end-systolic diameter ≥45 mm). Class I patients with normal left ventricular function should be followed clinically and by echocardiography every 6 to 12 months. Rarely, they _may_ be considered for operation if atrial fibrillation or pulmonary hypertension is present. At times, a careful history and performance of an exercise test often reveal that these patients are not truly asymptomatic.[204, 205] Patients with severe MR who are asymptomatic, who perform well on an exercise test, and who have excellent ventricular function (ejection fraction > 70 percent, end-systolic diameter <40 mm, end-systolic volume <40 ml/m²) can be followed by echocardiography every 6 to 12 months. However, operation may be considered even in asymptomatic patients if they are less than 70 years of age, if they are likely to be candidates for mitral valve repair, and if ventricular function (as reflected by end-systolic diameter and ejection fraction) shows _progressive_ deterioration. If valve replacement is likely to be necessary, a higher threshold for clinical and hemodynamic impairment should be employed than if valve reconstruction is contemplated. Because of the higher operative mortality, older patients (>75 years of age) should, in general, undergo surgery only if they are symptomatic.

Patients with severe MR and moderate or severe symptoms (NYHA Classes II, III, and IV) should generally be considered for surgery. One exception is a patient in whom echocardiography suggests that MVR will be required and whose ejection fraction is less than 30 percent. Because of the high risk of operation in these patients, medical therapy is usually advised, but the outcome is poor in any event. However, when mitral valve repair appears possible, even patients with serious left ventricular dysfunction may be considered for operation.[206–208]

Mitral Valve Prolapse Syndrome

ETIOLOGY AND PATHOLOGY

DEFINITION. The mitral valve prolapse (MVP) syndrome has been given many names, including the systolic click-murmur syndrome, Barlow syndrome, billowing mitral cusp syndrome, myxomatous mitral valve syndrome, floppy valve syndrome, and redundant cusp syndrome.[209–213] It is a variable clinical syndrome that results from diverse pathogenic mechanisms of one or more portions of the mitral valve apparatus, valve leaflets, chordae tendineae, papillary muscle, and valve annulus. The MVP syndrome is one of the most prevalent cardiac valvular abnormalities and was previously thought to affect as much as 5 to 10 percent of the population.[212] It now appears likely that overdiagnosis occurred in many individuals, perhaps because of the absence of rigorous echocardiographic criteria. Using such criteria (to be discussed), a community-based study showed that MVP syndrome occurred in only 2.4 percent of the population.[202] The syndrome is twice as frequent in females as in males. However, serious MR occurs more frequently in elderly males with MVP than in young females with this disorder.

Normally, the mitral valve billows slightly into the left atrium, and an exaggerated finding should be termed "billowing mitral valve." A "floppy valve" is regarded as an extreme form of billowing. MR occurs when the leaflet edges of the valve do not coapt. With chordal rupture, the prolapsed mitral valve is "flail." Obviously, these conditions blend into one another, and it is often difficult to distinguish among them.

Perloff and coworkers have proposed specific clinical criteria for the diagnosis of MVP.[213] They have divided the findings into three groups (Table 46-5): (1) major criteria, the presence of one or more of which establishes the diagnosis of MVP; (2) minor criteria, the presence of which cannot be discounted and should raise the suspicion of MVP but which by themselves are not sufficient to establish the diagnosis; and (3) other findings not shown in Table 46-5, which, although often present in patients with MVP, are nonspecific. Superior displacement of the mitral valve leaflets by more than 2 mm above the annulus is an important diagnostic criterion.[202] In addition, Marks and colleagues emphasized the importance of systolic displacement of one or both mitral leaflets into the left atrium in the *parasternal view* in the two-dimensional echocardiogram in the diagnosis of MVP.[214] Such an approach avoids overdiagnosis, which may occur with posterior bowing of the mitral valve on M-mode echocardiography and even in the four-chamber view on two-dimensional echocardiography.

ETIOLOGY. Most frequently, MVP occurs as a primary condition that is not associated with other diseases.[211] However, it has also been reported to be associated with many conditions.[212, 215-229] MVP occurs quite commonly in heritable disorders of connective tissue that increase the size of the mitral leaflets and apparatus, including Marfan syndrome (see Chap. 56), Ehlers-Danlos syndrome[224] (see Chap. 56), osteogenesis imperfecta, pseudoxanthoma elasticum,[225] periarteritis nodosa, myotonic dystrophy,[218] von Willebrand disease,[217] hyperthyroidism,[216] and congenital malformations such as Ebstein anomaly of the tricuspid valve, atrial septal defect of the ostium secundum variety, the Holt-Oram syndrome, and hypertrophic cardiomyopathy.[51] There may be a higher incidence of MVP in patients with an asthenic habitus[226] and various congenital thoracic deformities, including "straight back syndrome," pectus excavatum, and a shallow chest.[220, 222] These associations have not been proved using rigorous echocardiographic criteria, and, with the exception of connective tissue disorders, it is not clear how many of these are chance associations.

PATHOLOGY (Fig. 46-21). Findings include myxomatous proliferation of the mitral valve, in which the spongiosa component of the valve (i.e., the middle layer of the leaflet composed of loose, myxomatous material) is unusually prominent,[227, 227a] and the quantity of acid mucopolysaccharide is increased. Electron microscopy shows a haphazard arrangement of cells with disruption and with fragmentation of collagen fibrils (Fig. 46-22). The concordance between inadequate production of type III collagen and echocardiographic findings of MVP in patients with type IV Ehlers-Danlos syndrome suggests that this collagen abnormality may be responsible in patients with this syndrome.[228] Although the majority of patients with MVP exhibit myxomatous degeneration of the valve, postinflammatory changes may also be responsible for prolapse.[229]

In mild cases, the valvular myxoid stroma is enlarged on histological examination, but the leaflets are grossly normal. However, with increasing quantities of myxoid stroma, the leaflets become grossly abnormal, redundant, and prolapsed. Regions of endothelial disruption are common and are possible sites of endocarditis or thrombus formation.[230] The severity of MR depends on the extent of the prolapse. The cusps of the mitral valve, the chordae tendineae, and the annulus may all be affected by myxomatous proliferation. Degeneration of collagen within the central core of the chordae tendineae is primarily responsible for chordal rupture, which often occurs and may intensify the severity of MR. Increased chordal tension resulting from the enlarged area of the valve cusps may play a contributory role.[231] Myxomatous changes in the annulus may result in annular dilatation and calcification, contributing to the severity of MR.

Myxomatous proliferation, although most commonly affecting the mitral valve, has also been described in the tricuspid, aortic, and pulmonic valves, particularly in patients with the Marfan syndrome, and may lead to regurgitation of these valves as well as the mitral valve.

The MVP syndrome can coexist with rheumatic MS, and it may develop following mitral valvotomy. Ischemic heart disease and MVP are both common disorders and sometimes coexist. MVP may also occur secondary to papillary muscle dysfunction. In some patients, MVP has been documented to develop for the first time *following* myocardial infarction.[232] It has been proposed that MVP may *cause* myocardial ischemia by increasing tension on the base of the involved muscle. During systole, the tips of the papillary muscles move basally instead of apically.

▼ **TABLE 46-5. DIAGNOSTIC CRITERIA IN MITRAL VALVE PROLAPSE**

MAJOR CRITERIA
Auscultation
  Mid- to late systolic clicks and late systolic murmur or "whoop" alone or in combination at the cardiac apex
Two-dimensional echocardiogram
  Marked superior systolic displacement of mitral leaflets (≥ 2 mm above annulus) with coaptation point at or superior to annular plane
  Mild to moderate superior systolic displacement of mitral leaflets with:
    Chordal rupture
    Doppler mitral regurgitation
    Annular dilatation
Echocardiogram plus auscultation
  Mild to moderate superior systolic displacement of mitral leaflets with:
    Prominent mid- to late systolic clicks at the cardiac apex
    Apical late systolic or holosystolic murmur in the young patient
    Late systolic "whoop"

MINOR CRITERIA
Auscultation
  Loud S$_1$ with an apical holosystolic murmur
Two-dimensional echocardiogram
  Isolated mild to moderate superior systolic displacement of the posterior mitral leaflet
  Moderate superior systolic displacement of both mitral leaflets
Echocardiogram plus history of:
  Mild to moderate superior systolic displacement of mitral leaflets with:
    Focal neurologic attacks or amaurosis fugax in the young patient
    First-degree relatives with major criteria

Modified from Perloff JK, Child JS, Edwards JE: New guidelines for the clinical diagnosis of mitral valve prolapse. Am J Cardiol 57:1124, 1986.

CLINICAL MANIFESTATIONS

The MVP syndrome appears to exhibit a strong hereditary component[209, 232] and in some patients is transmitted as an

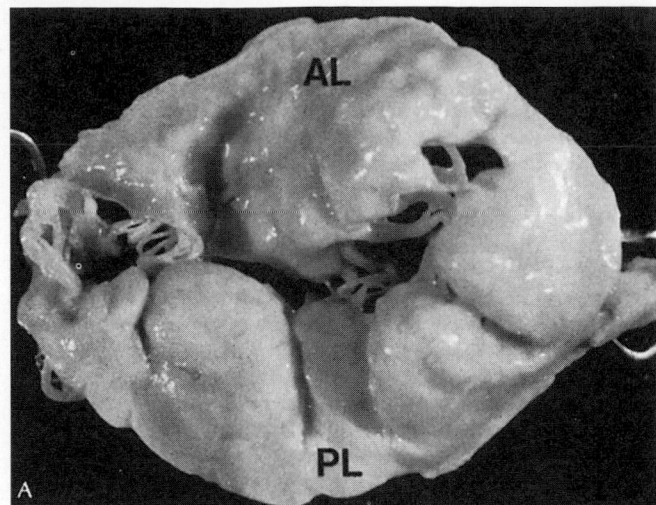

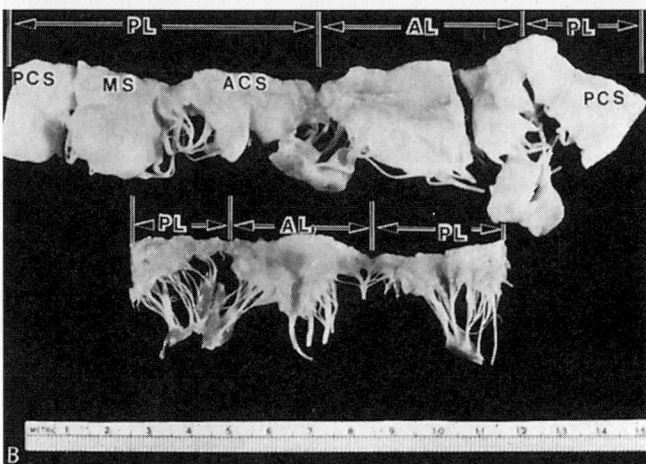

FIGURE 46–21. *A,* Myxomatous mitral valve, atrial view, from a patient with severe mitral regurgitation. The surface area of the valve is increased, with increased folding of the valve surface. The widths of the anterior leaflet (AL) and the posterior leaflet (PL) are almost equal. Individual scallops of the posterior leaflet are enlarged and redundant. *B,* Comparison of an excised myxomatous mitral valve from a patient who had severe mitral regurgitation (top) with a normal mitral valve from a patient who died of noncardiac causes (bottom), showing the increased surface area of both anterior leaflets (AL) and posterior leaflets (PL) of the myxomatous valve with enlarged and redundant posterior leaflet scallops, enlarged mitral annulus, and elongated chordae tendineae. PCS = posteromedial commissural scallops; MS = middle scallop; ACS = anterolateral commissural scallop. (From Boudoulas H, Wooley CF: Mitral valve prolapse and the mitral valve prolapse syndrome. *In* Yu P, Goodwin J [eds]: Progress in Cardiology. Philadelphia, Lea and Febiger, 1986.)

autosomal dominant trait with varying penetrance. The clinical presentations of the MVP syndrome are diverse.[213] The condition has been observed in patients of all ages and in both sexes. Despite the overestimation of the prevalence in the population referred to earlier, MVP is the most common cause of isolated MR requiring surgical treatment in the United States.[211] Echocardiographic evidence of MVP has been found in more than 90 percent of patients with the Marfan syndrome[233] and in many of their first-degree relatives.

History

A large majority of patients with MVP are asymptomatic and remain so throughout their lives[234] (Fig. 46–23). In many cases, otherwise asymptomatic patients with MVP suffer from undue anxiety, perhaps precipitated by their

having been informed of the presence of heart disease. Boudoulas and colleagues have called attention to an "MVP syndrome" with a characteristic systolic nonejection click and various nonspecific symptoms, such as fatigability, palpitations, postural orthostasis, and neuropsychiatric symptoms, as well as symptoms of autonomic dysfunction.[235] How, and even whether, these symptoms relate to the presence of MVP is not clear. It has been suggested that many of the symptoms are related to dysfunction of the autonomic nervous system, with increased excretion of catecholamines that occurs frequently in the MVP syndrome.[236, 237]

Patients may complain of syncope, presyncope, palpitations, chest discomfort, and, when MR is severe, symptoms of diminished cardiac reserve. Chest discomfort may be typical of angina pectoris but is more often atypical in that

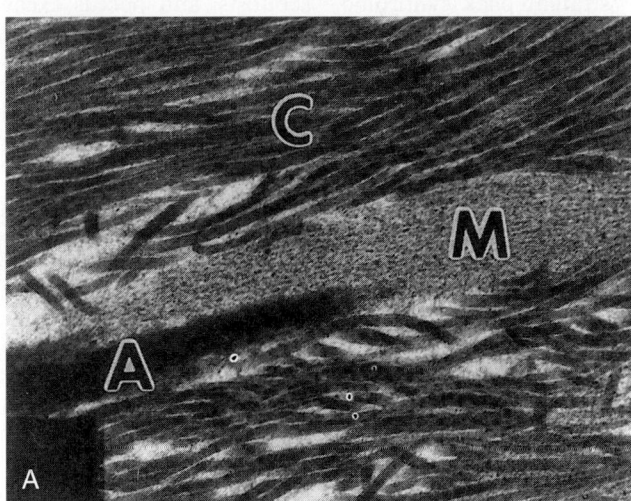

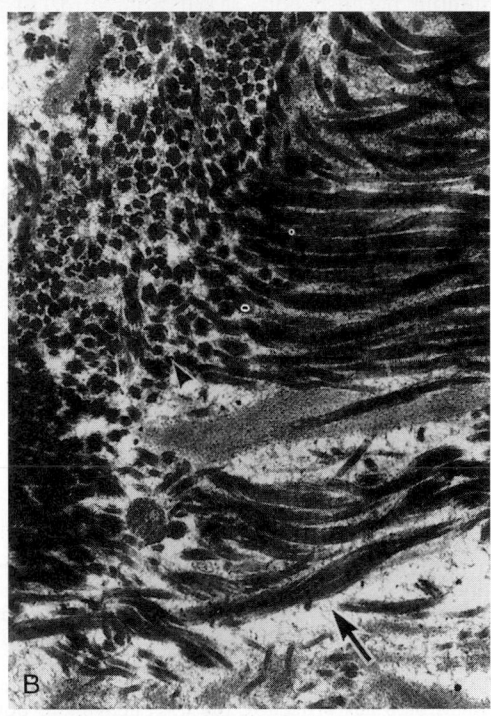

FIGURE 46–22. Electron micrographs of mitral valve. *A,* Normal mitral valve: Elastic fiber is composed of amorphous component (A), associated with microfibrils (M) oriented in parallel. Collagen fibrils (C) are compactly arranged (Kajikawa stain; original magnification 22,000). *B,* Prolapsed mitral valve. Collagen fibrils show spiraling appearance in longitudinal section (arrow) and flower-like appearance (arrowhead) in transverse section (Kajikawa stain; original magnification 27,000). (From Tamura K, Fukuda Y, Ishizaki M, et al: Abnormalities in elastic fibers and other connective-tissue components of floppy mitral valve. Am Heart J 129:1149, 1995.)

it is prolonged, not clearly related to exertion, and punctuated by brief attacks or severe stabbing pain at the apex. The discomfort may be secondary to abnormal tension on papillary muscles. In patients with MVP and severe MR, the symptoms of the latter (fatigue, dyspnea, and exercise limitation, see p. 1658) are present. Patients with MVP and arrhythmias (to be discussed) may have symptoms related to the latter.

Physical Examination

The body weight is often low, and the habitus may be asthenic. Blood pressure is usually normal or low; orthostatic hypotension may be present. As already mentioned, patients with MVP have a higher than expected prevalence of "straight back syndrome," scoliosis, and pectus excavatum.[222] MR ranges from nonexistent to severe.

The auscultatory findings are best elicited with the diaphragm of the stethoscope. The patient should be examined in the supine, left decubitus, and sitting positions. The physical findings unique to the MVP syndrome are detected by auscultation and can be corroborated by phonocardiography. The most important is a nonejection systolic click at least 0.14 second after S_1 (see Fig. 4–30).[237a] This can be differentiated from a systolic ejection click by phonocardiography because it occurs *after* the beginning of the carotid pulse upstroke. Occasionally, multiple mid- and late systolic clicks are audible, most readily along the lower left sternal border. The clicks are believed to be produced by sudden tensing of the elongated chordae tendineae and of the prolapsing leaflets. They are often, although not invariably, followed by a mid- to late crescendo systolic murmur that continues to A_2. This murmur is similar to that produced by papillary muscle dysfunction, which is readily understandable because both result from mid- to sys-

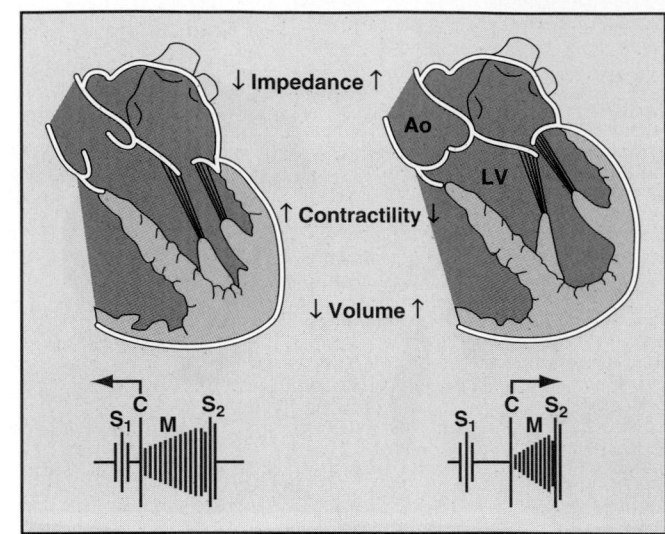

FIGURE 46–24. Dynamic auscultation in MVP. Any maneuver that decreases left ventricular (LV) volume (e.g., decreased venous return, tachycardia, decreased outflow impedance, increased contractility) will worsen the mismatch in size between the enlarged mitral valve and LV chamber, resulting in prolapse earlier in systole and movement of the click (C) and murmur (M) toward the first heart sound (S_1). Conversely, maneuvers that increase LV volume (e.g., increased venous return, bradycardia, increased outflow impedence, decreased contractility) will delay the occurrence of prolapse, resulting in movement of the click and murmur toward the second heart sound. (S_2). Ao = aorta. (From Prabhu SD, O'Rourke RA: Mitral valve prolapse. *In* Rahimtoola SH (ed): Valvular Heart Disease. Atlas of Heart Diseases. Vol. 11. Braunwald E, series ed. Philadelphia: Current Medicine, 1997, pp 10.1–10.18 Adapted from O'Rourke RA, Crawford MH: The systolic click-murmur syndrome: Clinical recognition and management. Curr Probl Cardiol 1: 9, 1976.)

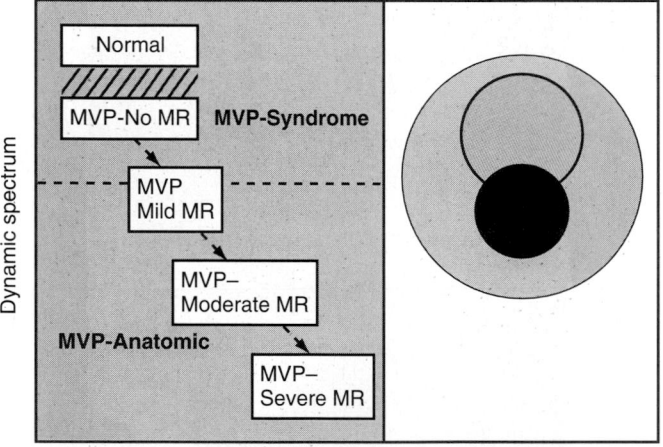

FIGURE 46–23. *Left panel,* The dynamic spectrum and progression of mitral valve prolapse (MVP) are shown. A subtle gradation exists between the normal mitral valve and valves that produce mild MVP without mitral regurgitation (no MR). Progression from the level MVP–no MR to another level may or may not occur. Most of the MVP syndrome cases occupy the area above the dotted line, whereas progressive mitral valve dysfunction cases occupy the area below the dotted line. *Right panel,* The large circle represents the total number of patients with MVP. Patients with MVP may be symptomatic or asymptomatic. Symptoms may be directly related to mitral valve dysfunction (black circle) or to autonomic dysfunction (pink circle). Certain patients with symptoms directly related to mitral valve dysfunction may present with and continue to have symptoms secondary to autonomic dysfunction. (From Boudoulas H, Wooley CF: Mitral Valve Prolapse and the Mitral Valve Prolapse Syndrome. Mount Kisco, NY, Futura Publishing Co, Inc, 1988.)

tolic MR. In general, the duration of the murmur is a function of the severity of the MR. When the murmur is confined to the latter portion of systole, MR usually is not severe. However, as MR becomes more severe, the murmur commences earlier and ultimately becomes holosystolic.

It is important to emphasize the variability of the physical findings in the MVP syndrome. Some patients exhibit both a midsystolic click and a mid- to late systolic murmur; others present with only one of these two findings; still others have only a click on one occasion and only a murmur on another, both on a third examination, and no abnormality at all on a fourth. Conditions other than MVP cause midsystolic clicks; these include tricuspid valve prolapse, atrial septal aneurysms, and extracardiac causes.

DYNAMIC AUSCULTATION. The auscultatory (and phonocardiographic) findings are exquisitely sensitive to physiological and pharmacological interventions, and recognition of the changes induced by these interventions is of great value in the diagnosis of the MVP syndrome (Fig. 46–24; see also Tables 4–4 and 46–4). The mitral valve begins to prolapse when the reduction of left ventricular volume during systole reaches a critical point at which the valve leaflets no longer coapt; at that instant, the click occurs and the murmur commences. Any maneuver that decreases left ventricular volume, such as a reduction of impedance to left ventricular outflow, a reduction in venous return, tachycardia, or an augmentation of myocardial contractility, results in an earlier occurrence of prolapse during systole. As a consequence, the click and onset of the murmur move closer to S_1. When prolapse is severe and/or left ventricular size is markedly reduced, prolapse may begin with the onset of systole. As a consequence, the click may not be audible, and the murmur may be holosystolic. On the other hand, when left ventricular volume is augmented by an increase in the impedance to left ventricular emptying, an increase in venous return, a reduction of myocardial contractility, or bradycardia, both the click and the onset of the murmur will be delayed.

During the straining phase of the Valsalva maneuver, upon sudden standing, and early during the inhalation of amyl nitrite, cardiac size decreases, and both the click and the onset of the murmur occur earlier in systole. In contrast, a sudden change from the standing to the supine position, leg-raising, squatting, maximal isometric exercise, and, to a lesser extent, expiration will delay the click and the onset of the murmur. During the overshoot phase of the Valsalva maneuver (i.e., six to eight cycles following release) and with prolongation of the R-R interval, either following a premature contraction or in atrial fibrillation, the click and onset of the murmur are usually delayed, and the intensity of the murmur is reduced. Maneuvers that elevate arterial pressure, such as isometric exercise, increase the intensity of the click and murmur. In general, when the onset of the murmur is delayed, both its duration and intensity are diminished, reflecting a reduction in the severity of MR.

The response to several interventions may be helpful in differentiating hypertrophic obstructive cardiomyopathy (HOCM) from MVP. During the strain of the Valsalva maneuver, the murmur of HCM increases in intensity, whereas the murmur of MVP becomes longer but usually not louder. The murmur of HCM becomes louder after amyl nitrite inhalation, whereas that of MVP does not. Following a premature beat, the murmur of HCM increases in intensity and duration, whereas that due to MVP usually remains unchanged or decreases.

LABORATORY EXAMINATION

ELECTROCARDIOGRAPHY

The ECG is usually normal in asymptomatic patients with MVP. In a minority of asymptomatic patients and in many symptomatic patients, the ECG shows inverted or biphasic T waves and nonspecific ST segment changes in leads II III, and a$_{vf}$ and occasionally in the anterolateral leads as well.

ARRHYTHMIAS. A spectrum of arrhythmias have been observed. These include atrial and ventricular premature contractions and supraventricular and ventricular tachyarrhythmias,[238, 239, 239a] as well as bradyarrhythmias due to sinus node dysfunction or varying degrees of atrioventricular block. The mechanism of the arrhythmias is not clear. Diastolic depolarization of muscle fibers in the anterior mitral leaflet in response to stretch has been demonstrated experimentally, and the abnormal stretch of the prolapsed leaflet may be of pathogenetic significance. Wit and associates have shown that mitral valve leaflets contain atrium-like muscle fibers in continuity with left atrial myocardium.[240] It is possible that mechanical stimulation of these fibers generates slow-response action potentials and sustained rhythmic action that penetrates the cardiac chambers.[240]

Paroxysmal supraventricular tachycardia is the most common sustained tachyarrhythmia in patients with MVP and may be related to what may be an increased incidence of left atrioventricular bypass tracts.[238] The incidence of MVP among patients with the Wolff-Parkinson-White syndrome is increased.[241] There is also an increased association between MVP and prolongation of the QT interval, and this association may play a role in the pathogenesis of serious ventricular arrhythmias.[238] Patients with MVP have an increased incidence of abnormal late potentials on signal-averaged ECGs, as well as reduced heart rate variability.[239]

MITRAL VALVE PROLAPSE AND SUDDEN DEATH. The relation between the MVP syndrome and sudden death is not clear. However, the best evidence suggests that MVP increases the risk of sudden death slightly,[209, 242, 243, 243a] especially in patients with severe MR or severe valvular deformity. The immediate cause of the sudden, unexpected death is probably ventricular fibrillation.[244] Kligfield and Devereux have identified the following as potential risks for sudden death in patients with MVP: the presence of severe MR, complex ventricular arrhythmias, QT interval prolongation, and a history of syncope and palpitations.[238]

ECHOCARDIOGRAPHY (See also Chap. 7). Echocardiography plays a key role in the diagnosis of MVP and has been most useful in the delineation of this syndrome[244a] (see Figs. 7–57 and 7–58). The most common finding on M-mode echocardiography is abrupt posterior movement of the posterior leaflet or of both mitral leaflets in midsystole with the leaflet interface greater than 2 mm posterior to the

C-D line. This movement occurs simultaneously with the systolic click. A second finding is pansystolic posterior prolapse of one or both leaflets, giving rise to a U- or hammock-shaped configuration 3 mm or more posterior to the C-D segment.

To establish the diagnosis, the two-dimensional echocardiogram must show that one or both mitral valve leaflets billow by at least 2 mm into the left atrium during systole in the long-axis view (Fig. 46–25).[202, 245, 246] Thickening of the involved leaflet to greater than 5 mm supports the diagnosis. This finding is also helpful in identifying patients at significant risk for developing severe MR or infective endocarditis.[214] The mitral annular diameter is often abnormally increased.[245, 247] Transesophageal echocardiography provides additional details regarding the mitral valve apparatus, such as rupture of chordae tendineae. In MR secondary to MVP, the echocardiogram provides valuable information regarding left ventricular function.

The variability in physical findings in this syndrome, already commented upon, extends to the echocardiogram.[247, 248] Thus, some patients have a systolic click with or without a murmur and show no evidence of MVP on the echocardiogram. Conversely, the echocardiographic findings of MVP may be observed in patients without a click or murmur. Others have both the typical echocardiographic and auscultatory features. The echocardiographic findings of MVP have been reported to occur in a large number of first-degree relatives of patients with established MVP. Two-dimensional echocardiography has also revealed prolapse of the tricuspid and aortic valves in approximately 20 percent of patients with MVP.[249] Conversely, however, prolapse of the tricuspid and aortic

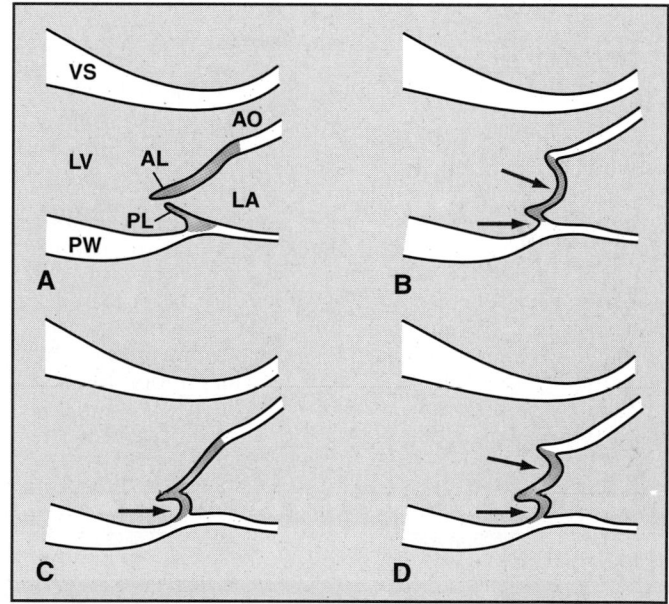

FIGURE 46–25. Diagram of parasternal view of two-dimensional echocardiography in normal subject and in patient with MVP. *A,* Normal parasternal long-axis view at end-diastole immediately preceding mitral valve closure. Labeled are the anterior leaflet (AL), posterior leaflet (PL), ventricular septum (VS), posterior wall (PW), aorta (AO), left atrium (LA), and left ventricle (LV). Systolic prolapse may be predominantly anterior leaflet (*B,* arrows), predominantly posterior (*C,* arrow), or both (*D,* arrows). The presence of leaflet thickening, leaflet redundancy, chordal elongation, and annular dilatation should also be assessed on the two-dimensional study. Color flow and pulsed-wave Doppler studies are used to determine the presence and extent of mitral regurgitation, an important supporting finding in borderline cases. (From Prabhu SD, O'Rourke RA: Mitral valve prolapse. *In* Rahimtoola SH (ed): Valvular Heart Disease. Atlas of Heart Diseases. Vol. 11. Braunwald E, series ed. Philadelphia: Current Medicine, 1997, pp 10.1–10.18.)

valves occurs *uncommonly* in patients without prolapse of the mitral valve.[249]

Doppler echocardiography frequently reveals mild MR that is not always associated with an audible murmur. Color flow Doppler echocardiography is useful in identifying the location and severity of the regurgitant jets. MR is moderate or severe in about 10 percent of patients with MVP, most commonly in men over the age of 50.[247]

STRESS SCINTIGRAPHY. The differential diagnosis between two common conditions—MVP associated with atypical chest pain and ECG abnormalities and primary coronary artery disease associated with MVP—may be aided by exercise electrocardiography. However, myocardial perfusion scintigraphy using thallium-201 or sestamibi during pharmacological exercise stress (see Chap. 9) is more specific. When findings are normal, i.e., when there is no evidence of stress-induced regional myocardial ischemia, the diagnosis of MVP unrelated to ischemic heart disease is favored.[250]

ANGIOGRAPHY. The configuration of the left ventriculogram during systole is helpful in confirming the diagnosis of MVP. The right anterior oblique projection is most useful for defining the posterior leaflet of the mitral valve, and the left anterior oblique projection is most useful for studying the anterior leaflet. The most helpful sign is extension of the mitral leaflet tissue inferiorly and posteriorly to the point of attachment of the mitral leaflets to the mitral annulus.[251] Angiography may also reveal scalloped edges of the leaflets, reflecting redundancy of tissue. Other abnormalities noted on angiography of some patients with MVP include dilatation, decreased systolic contraction, and calcification of the mitral annulus and poor contraction of the basal portion of the left ventricle.[252]

NATURAL HISTORY

The outlook for children with MVP is excellent; a large majority remain asymptomatic for many years without any change in clinical or laboratory findings[209, 234, 253, 253a] (see Fig. 46–23). Zuppiroli and associates monitored 316 patients with MVP for an average of more than 8 years; 70 percent were women and 29 percent had familial MVP.[234] Serious complications (cardiac death, need for cardiac surgery, acute infective endocarditis, or cerebral embolic events) occurred at a rate of only 1 per 100 patient years.[234]

Progressive MR with gradual increase in left atrial and left ventricular size, atrial fibrillation, pulmonary hypertension, and the development of congestive heart failure is the most frequent serious complication,[234, 254] occurring in about 15 percent of patients over a 10- to 15-year period. The incidence of this complication is significantly greater in patients with both murmurs and clicks than in those with an isolated click. In many patients, rupture of chordae tendineae is responsible for the precipitation and/or intensification of the MR. Severe MR occurs more frequently in men older than 50 years of age with MVP and in patients with thickened (>5 mm diameter) mitral valve leaflets.[243, 254–256] Patients with the MVP syndrome are also at risk of developing infective endocarditis.[257, 257a] Although the incidence of infective endocarditis appears to be extremely low in patients with only a midsystolic click, it increases in patients with a systolic murmur. The incidence is higher in men than in women and in those more than 50 years of age. Infective endocarditis often aggravates the severity of MR and therefore the need for surgical treatment.

Acute hemiplegia, transient ischemic attacks, cerebellar infarcts, amaurosis fugax, and retinal arteriolar occlusions have been reported to occur more frequently in patients with the MVP syndrome, suggesting that cerebral emboli are unusually common in this condition.[258, 259, 259a] It has been proposed that these neurological complications are associated with loss of endothelial continuity and tearing of the endocardium overlying the myxomatous valve, which initiates platelet aggregation and the formation of mural platelet–fibrin complexes.[258] Although it has been proposed that embolization secondary to MVP may be a significant cause for unexplained strokes in young people without cerebrovascular disease, a large case-controlled study showed no association between MVP and ischemic neurological events in persons under 45 years of age.[260]

MANAGEMENT (Table 46–6)

Patients with the physical findings of MVP (and those without such findings who have been given the diagnosis) should have two-dimensional and color flow Doppler echocardiography. This procedure should also be performed in first-degree relatives of patients with MVP.[51] The diagnosis of MVP requires definitive echocardiographic findings, and overdiagnosis and incorrect "labeling" have been a major problem with this condition. *Asymptomatic patients* (or those whose principal complaint is anxiety), with no arrhythmias evident on a routine extended ECG tracing and without evidence of MR, have an excellent prognosis. They should be reassured about the favorable prognosis and be encouraged to engage in normal life styles, but should have follow-up examinations every every 3 to 5 years. This should include a two-dimensional echocardiogram and a color flow Doppler study.

Patients with a long systolic murmur may show progression of MR and should be evaluated more frequently, at intervals of approximately 12 months. *Endocarditis prophylaxis* is advisable for patients with a typical click and systolic murmur and in those with only a click and characteristic echocardiographic features of MVP. Prophylaxis does *not* appear to be necessary for patients with a midsystolic

▼ **TABLE 46–6. MATCHING RISK AND MANAGEMENT IN PATIENTS WITH MITRAL VALVE PROLAPSE**

RISK LEVEL	PATIENTS	MANAGEMENT
Lowest	Patients without mitral regurgitant murmurs or regurgitation revealed by Doppler echocardiography, especially women younger than age 45	Reassurance; prophylactic antibiotics not clearly necessary and if used should not include medication with risk of allergic reactions; reevaluation and echocardiography at moderate intervals (5 years)
Moderate	Patients with intermittent or persistent mitral murmurs and mild regurgitation revealed by Doppler echocardiography	Antibiotic prophylaxis with erythromycin or amoxicillin; treatment of even mild established hypertension; reevaluation and echocardiography more frequently (2 to 3 years)
High	Patients with moderate or severe mitral regurgitation	Antibiotic prophylaxis with amoxicillin (unless allergic); optimization of afterload (arterial pressure); reevaluation with Doppler echocardiography and other tests if needed annually; consider valve repair or replacement for exertional dyspnea or decline of left ventricular function into low-normal range

From Devereux RB: Recent developments in the diagnosis and management of mitral valve prolapse. Curr Opin Cardio 10:107, 1995. Modified from Devereux RB, Kligfield P: Mitral valve prolapse. *In* Rakel R: Current Therapy. Philadelphia, WB Saunders, 1992, pp 237, 241.

click without a systolic murmur or without typical echocardiographic findings (see also Chap. 47).[261]

Patients with a history of palpitations, lightheadedness, dizziness, or syncope or those who have ventricular arrhythmias or QT prolongation on a routine ECG should undergo ambulatory (24-hour) ECG monitoring and/or exercise ECG to detect arrhythmias. Because of the risk, albeit very low, of sudden death,[238] electrophysiologic studies may be carried out to characterize arrhythmias if they exist. Beta-adrenergic blockers are useful in the treatment of palpitations secondary to frequent premature ventricular contractions and for self-terminating episodes of supraventricular tachycardia. These drugs may also be useful in the treatment of chest discomfort, both in patients with associated coronary artery disease and in those with normal coronary vessels in whom the symptoms may be due to regional ischemia secondary to MVP. Radiofrequency ablation of atrioventricular bypass tracts is useful for frequent or prolonged episodes of supraventricular tachycardia.

Aspirin should be given to patients with MVP who have had a documented focal neurological event and in whom no other cause, such as a left atrial thrombus or atrial fibrillation, is apparent. Treatment with an angiotensin-converting enzyme inhibitor has been reported to reduce the severity of MR in patients with MVP.[171]

Patients with MVP and severe MR should be treated similarly to other patients with severe MR (see p. 1661) and may require mitral valve surgery. Reconstructive surgery without valve replacement is usually possible (see Fig. 46-15).[179a, 211, 261a] Therefore, the threshold for surgical treatment in these patients is lower than in patients with MR in whom MVR may be necessary. Approximately 50 percent of all mitral valve reconstructions for MR are now carried out in patients with MVP. Among 252 such patients operated upon at the Brigham and Women's Hospital, resection of the most deformed leaflet segment and insertion of an annuloplasty ring to reduce the dilated annulus was the most commonly employed procedure. Rupture of the chordae tendineae to the anterior leaflet could sometimes be treated by chordal transfer from the posterior leaflet. In other patients, shortening of the chordae tendineae and/or papillary muscle was necessary. The operative mortality was 2 percent; structural valve degeneration occurred in 15 percent of patients at 5 years. Chordal replacement with polytetrafluoroethylene sutures has been reported to enhance mitral valve repair in patients with MVP.[210]

Coronary arteriography should be performed in patients with angina pectoris on effort and/or ischemic ECG changes or those with abnormalities on a stress myocardial perfusion scan. Treatment should take into account both the responsiveness of symptoms to medical management and the coronary anatomy.

Although this discussion has focused attention on complications of the MVP syndrome, it should not be forgotten that, on the whole, this is a benign condition and that the *vast majority* of patients with this syndrome remain asymptomatic for their entire lives and require, at most, observation every few years and reassurance.

Aortic Stenosis

ETIOLOGY AND PATHOLOGY

Obstruction to left ventricular outflow is localized most commonly at the aortic valve and is discussed in this section. However, obstruction may also occur above the valve (supravalvular stenosis) or below the valve (discrete subvalvular aortic stenosis [see Chap. 43]), or it may be caused by hypertrophic obstructive cardiomyopathy (see Chap. 48). Valvular aortic stenosis (AS) *without accompanying mitral valve disease* is more common in men than in women and very rarely occurs on a rheumatic basis. Instead, isolated AS is usually either congenital or degenerative in origin[262, 263] (Figs. 46-26 and 46-27).

CONGENITAL AORTIC STENOSIS (See also Chaps. 43 and 44). Congenital malformations of the aortic valve may be unicuspid, bicuspid, or tricuspid, or there may be a dome-shaped diaphragm. *Unicuspid valves* produce severe obstruction in infancy and are the most frequent malformations found in fatal valvular AS in children under the age of 1 year. Congenitally *bicuspid valves* may be stenotic with commissural fusion at birth, but more often they are not responsible for serious narrowing of the aortic orifice during childhood. Their abnormal architecture induces turbulent flow, which traumatizes the leaflets and leads to fibrosis, increased rigidity, calcification of the leaflets, and narrowing of the aortic orifice in adulthood[264] (Fig. 46-28). Infective endocarditis may develop on a congenitally bicuspid valve, which then becomes regurgitant. Rarely, a congenitally bicuspid valve is purely regurgitant in the absence of antecedent infection.

A third form of a congenitally malformed valve is *tricuspid*, with the cusps of unequal size and some commissural fusion. Although many of these valves retain normal function throughout life, it has been postulated that the turbulent flow produced by the mild congenital architectural

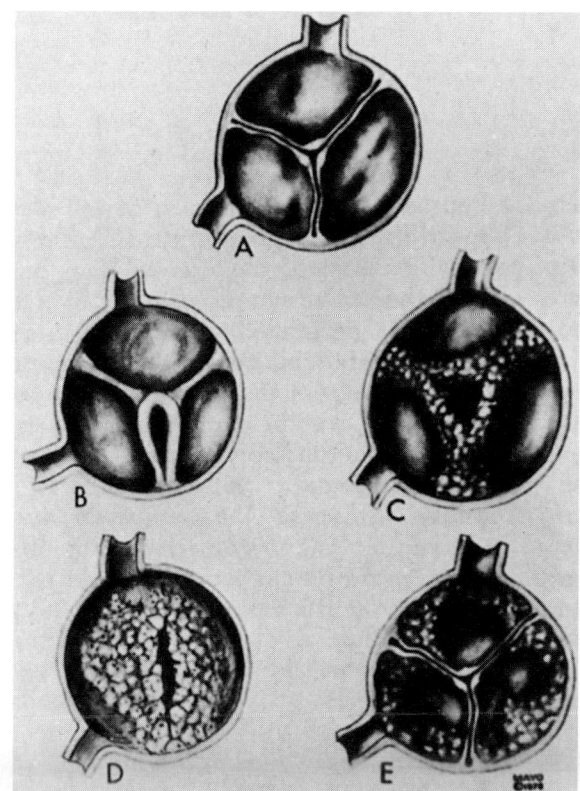

FIGURE 46-26. Types of aortic valve stenosis. *A,* Normal aortic valve. *B,* Congenital aortic stenosis. *C,* Rheumatic aortic stenosis. *D,* Calcific aortic stenosis. *E,* Calcific senile aortic stenosis. (From Brandenburg RO, et al: Valvular heart disease—When should the patient be referred? Pract Cardiol 5:50, 1979.)

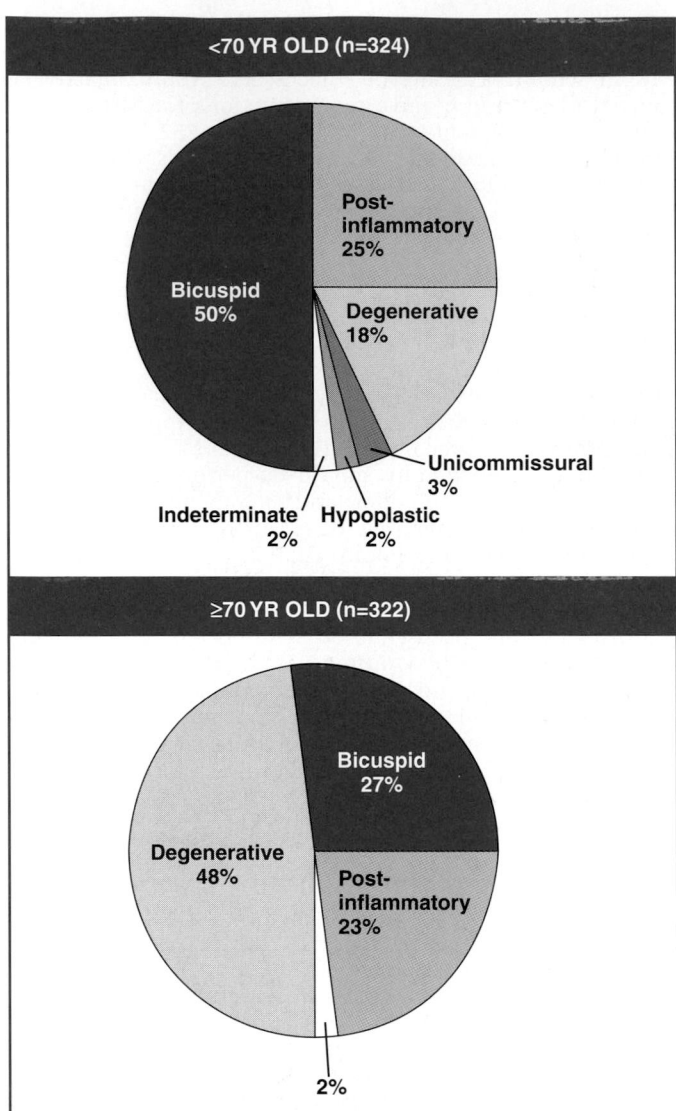

FIGURE 46–27. Causes of aortic stenosis, shown for two age groups. Among patients younger than 70 years (*top*), calcification of congenitally bicuspid valves accounted for half of the surgical cases. In contrast, in those 70 years of age or older (*bottom*), degenerative calcification accounted for almost half of the cases. (From Passik CS, et al: Temporal changes in the causes of aortic stenosis: A surgical pathologic study of 646 cases. Mayo Clin Proc 62:119, 1987.)

abnormality may lead to fibrosis and ultimately to calcification and stenosis. Tricuspid stenotic aortic valves in adults may be congenital, rheumatic, or degenerative in origin.

ACQUIRED AORTIC STENOSIS. Rheumatic AS results from adhesions and fusions of the commissures and cusps and vascularization of the leaflets of the valve ring, leading to retraction and stiffening of the free borders of the cusps. Calcific nodules develop on both surfaces, and the orifice is reduced to a small round or triangular opening. As a consequence, the rheumatic valve is often regurgitant as well as stenotic.[262] The heart frequently exhibits other stigmata of rheumatic disease, especially mitral valve involvement. With the decline in rheumatic fever in industrialized nations, rheumatic AS is decreasing in frequency.

Age-related degenerative calcific (formerly termed senile) AS is now the most common cause of AS in adults and the most frequent reason for aortic valve replacement in patients with AS.[265] It appears to result from years of normal mechanical stress on a valve that sometimes exhibits inflammatory changes with infiltration of macrophages and T

lymphocytes. The cusps are immobilized, and the stenosis is caused by deposits of calcium along the flexion lines at their bases. Immunohistochemical evidence of *Chlamydia pneumoniae* has been found in early lesions of age-related degenerative AS.[266] In a population-based echocardiographic study, 2 percent of persons 65 years of age or older had frank calcific AS, whereas 29 percent exhibited age-related aortic valve sclerosis without stenosis, defined by Otto and colleagues as irregular thickening of the aortic valve leaflets detected by echocardiography without significant obstruction and believed to represent a milder and/or earlier disease process.[265] This form of AS may be accompanied by calcifications of the mitral annulus and coronary arteries but rarely by aortic regurgitation. Both diabetes mellitus and hypercholesterolemia are risk factors for the development of age-related AS or degenerative calcific AS.[267, 268] It has been suggested that the hypercholesterolemia accelerates age-related degenerative changes in the aortic root and valve.[269] In turn, it has been noted that age-related aortic valve sclerosis and calcific AS are associated with traditional risk factors for atherosclerosis such as cigarette smoking, a history of hypertension, and low high-density-lipoprotein cholesterol values.[270] Not surprisingly, age-related aortic valve sclerosis is associated with an increased risk of cardiovascular death and mycoardial infarction.[265] In *atherosclerotic* aortic valve stenosis, severe atherosclerosis involves the aorta and other major arteries; this form of AS occurs most frequently in patients with severe hypercholesterolemia and is observed in children with homozygous type II hyperlipoproteinemia.[271]

Calcific AS is observed in a number of other conditions, including Paget disease of bone[272] and end-stage renal disease.[273] *Rheumatoid involvement* of the valve is a rare cause of AS and results in nodular thickening of the valve leaflets and involvement of the proximal portion of the aorta. *Ochronosis* with alkaptonuria is another rare cause of AS.[274]

Roberts studied hearts with AS obtained at autopsy from patients between 15 and 65 years of age and found that almost 40 percent had tricuspid aortic valves.[275] Because thickening of the mitral valve and a history of acute rheumatic fever were present in 50 percent of these patients, it is likely that the AS was rheumatic in etiology; in the remainder, it was either congenital or degenerative in origin. In 90 percent of hearts examined at autopsy in patients with AS who were older than 65 years of age, the valves were tricuspid, with nodular calcific deposits on the aortic aspects of the cusps, but without commissural fusion,[275] indicative of age-related degenerative calcific AS.

Hemodynamically significant AS leads to severe concentric left ventricular hypertrophy,[276] with heart weights as great as 1000 gm. The interventricular septum often bulges into and encroaches on the right ventricular cavity. When left ventricular failure supervenes, the ventricle dilates, the left atrium enlarges, and changes secondary to backward failure occur in the pulmonary vascular bed, the right side of the heart, and the systemic venous bed.

PATHOPHYSIOLOGY (Fig. 46–29)

The left ventricle responds to *sudden* severe obstruction to outflow by dilatation and reduction of stroke volume.[277] However, in adults with AS, the obstruction usually develops and increases gradually over a prolonged period. In infants and children with congenital AS, the valve orifice shows little change as the child grows, thereby intensifying the relative obstruction quite gradually. Left ventricular function can be well maintained in experimentally produced, gradually developing subcoronary AS in animals. In the experimental model, as well as in children and adults

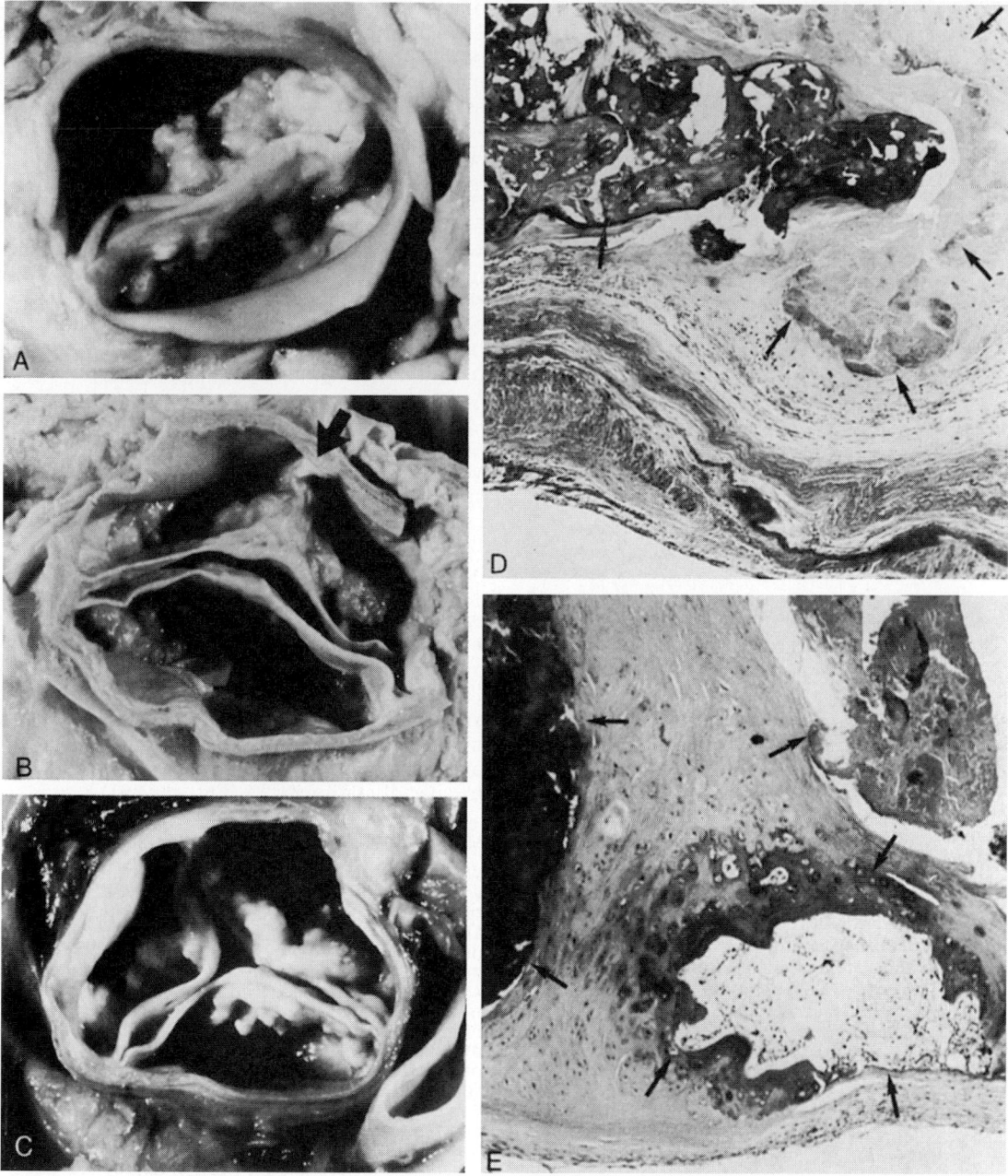

FIGURE 46–28. Calcific aortic stenosis. *A,* Congenitally bicuspid aortic valve, characterized by two equal cusps with basal mineralization. *B,* Congenitally bicuspid aortic valve having two unequal cusps, the larger with a central raphe (arrow). *C,* Otherwise anatomically normal tricuspid aortic valve in an elderly patient, characterized by isolated cusps with calcification localized to basilar aspect; cuspal free edges are not involved. *D* and *E,* Photomicrographs of calcific deposits in calcific aortic stenosis; deposits are rimmed by arrows (hematoxylin and eosin, original magnification ×15). *D,* Deposits with underlying cusp largely intact; transmural calcific deposits are shown in *E.* (*A* and *C* from Schoen FJ, St. John Sutton M: Contemporary issues in the pathology of valvular heart disease. Hum Pathol 18:568, 1987.)

with chronic, severe AS, left ventricular output is maintained by the presence of left ventricular hypertrophy, which may sustain a large pressure gradient across the aortic valve for many years without a reduction in cardiac output, left ventricular dilatation, or the development of symptoms. Critical obstruction to left ventricular outflow is usually characterized by (1) a peak systolic pressure gradient exceeding 50 mm Hg in the presence of a normal cardiac output or (2) an effective aortic orifice (calculated by the Gorlin formula [see Chap. 11]) less than about 0.8 cm² in an average-sized adult, i.e., 0.5 cm²/m² of body surface area (less than approximately one-fourth of the normal aortic orifice of 3.0 to 4.0 cm²). An aortic valve orifice of 1.0 to 1.5 cm² is considered moderate stenosis, and an orifice of

1.5 to 2.0 cm² is referred to as mild stenosis (see Fig. 11–13).

As contraction of the left ventricle becomes progressively more isometric, the left ventricular pressure pulse exhibits a rounded, rather than flattened, summit. The elevated left ventricular end-diastolic pressure, which is characteristic of severe AS, often reflects diminished compliance of the hypertrophied left ventricular wall.[278, 279]

In patients with severe AS, large *a* waves usually appear in the left atrial pressure pulse because of the combination of enhanced contraction of a hypertrophied left atrium and diminished left ventricular compliance. Atrial contraction plays a particularly important role in filling of the left ventricle in AS. It raises left ventricular end-diastolic pressure

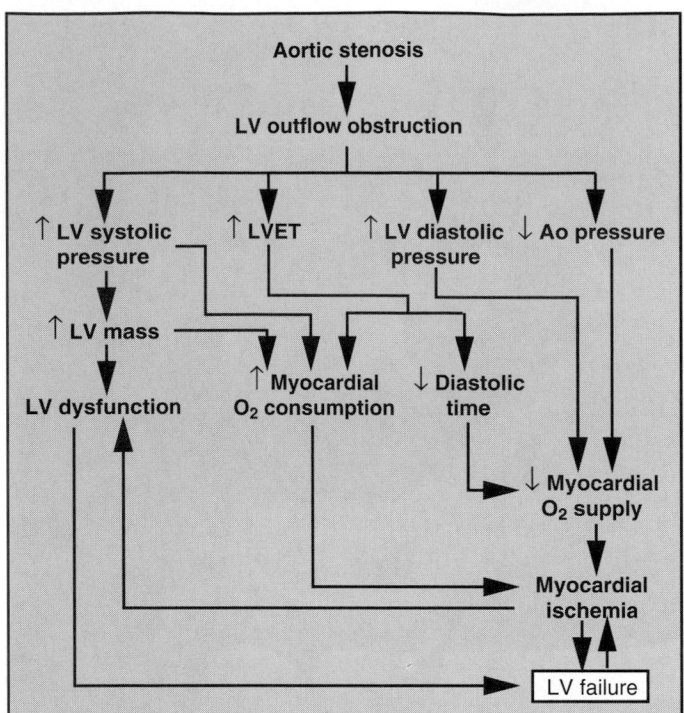

FIGURE 46–29. Pathophysiology of aortic stenosis. Left ventricular (LV) outflow obstruction results in an increased LV systolic pressure, increased left ventricular ejection time (LVET), increased left ventricular diastolic pressure, and decreased aortic (Ao) pressure. Increased LV systolic pressure with LV volume overload increases LV mass, which may lead to LV dysfunction and failure. Increased LV systolic pressure, LV mass, and LVET increase myocardial oxygen (O_2) consumption. Increased LVET results in a decrease of diastolic time (myocardial perfusion time). Increased LV diastolic pressure and decreased Ao diastolic pressure decrease coronary perfusion pressure. Decreased diastolic time and coronary perfusion pressure decrease myocardial O_2 supply. Increased myocardial O_2 consumption and decreased myocardial O_2 supply produce myocardial ischemia, which further deteriorates LV function ($\uparrow$ = increased, $\downarrow$ = decreased). (From Boudoulas H, Gravanis MB: Valvular heart disease. In Gravanis MB: Cardiovascular Disorders: Pathogenesis and Pathophysiology. St. Louis, CV Mosby Co, 1993, p 64.)

without causing a concomitant elevation of mean left atrial pressure.[280] This "booster pump" function of the left atrium prevents the pulmonary venous and capillary pressures from rising to levels that would produce pulmonary congestion, while at the same time maintaining left ventricular end-diastolic pressure at the elevated level necessary for

effective contraction of the hypertrophied left ventricle. Loss of appropriately timed, vigorous atrial contraction, as occurs in atrial fibrillation or atrioventricular dissociation, may result in rapid clinical deterioration in patients with severe AS.

Although the *cardiac output* at rest is within normal limits in the majority of patients with severe AS, it often fails to rise normally during exertion. Late in the course of the disease, the cardiac output, stroke volume, and therefore the left ventricular–aortic pressure gradient all decline, whereas the mean left atrial, pulmonary capillary, pulmonary arterial, right ventricular systolic and diastolic, and right atrial pressures rise, often sequentially. As a consequence of pulmonary hypertension and/or bulging of the hypertrophied septum into the right ventricular cavity, the *a* wave in the right atrial pressure pulse becomes prominent.

Left ventricular end-diastolic volume usually remains normal until late in the course of severe AS, but left ventricular mass increases in response to the chronic pressure overload, resulting in an increase in the mass/volume ratio. However, the increase in mass may not be as great as that seen with aortic regurgitation (AR) or combined AS and AR.

Gender differences in the response of the left ventricle to AS have been reported.[281–283] Women more frequently exhibit normal or even supernormal ventricular performance and a smaller, thicker-walled, concentrically hypertrophied left ventricle with diastolic dysfunction (to be discussed) and normal or even subnormal systolic wall stress. Men more frequently have eccentric left ventricular hypertrophy, excessive systolic wall stress, systolic dysfunction, and ventricular dilatation[284–286] (Fig. 46–30).

MYOCARDIAL FUNCTION IN AORTIC STENOSIS

When the aorta is suddenly constricted in experimental animals, left ventricular pressure rises, wall stress increases significantly, and both the extent and the velocity of shortening decline. As pointed out in Chapter 16, the development of ventricular hypertrophy is one of the principal mechanisms by which the heart adapts to such an increased hemodynamic burden. The increased systolic wall stress induced by AS leads to parallel replication of sarcomeres and concentric hypertrophy (see Fig. 16–4). The increase in left ventricular wall thickness is often sufficient to counterbalance the increased pressure, so that peak systolic wall tension returns to normal or remains normal if the obstruction develops slowly.[287] An inverse correlation between wall stress and ejection fraction has been described in patients with AS.[288] This suggests that the depressed ejection fraction and velocity of fiber shortening that occur in *some* patients are a consequence of inadequate wall thickening,[289] resulting in "afterload mismatch."[290] In others, the lower ejection fraction is secondary to a true depression of contractility; in this group, surgical treatment is less effective.[291] Thus, both increased afterload and altered contractility are operative to varying extents in depressing left ventricular performance.[281, 282] In order to evaluate myocardial function in patients with AS, the ejec-

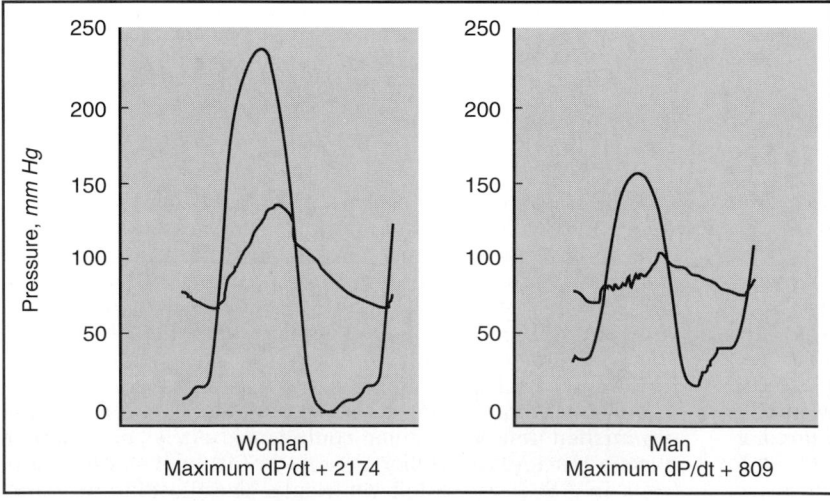

FIGURE 46–30. The difference in pressure-generating capabilities of the left ventricle in an 83-year-old woman and a 60-year-old man with a similar degree of aortic stenosis is shown. dP/dt = rate of pressure increase. (Reproduced with permission from Carroll JD, Carroll EP, Felman T, et al: Sex-associated differences in left ventricular function in aortic stenosis of the elderly. Circulation 86:1099, 1992. Copyright 1992 American Heart Association.)

tion phase indices, such as ejection fraction and myocardial fiber shortening, should be related to the existing wall tension.

DIASTOLIC PROPERTIES (see also Chap. 15). Although ventricular hypertrophy is a key adaptive mechanism to the pressure load imposed by AS, it has an adverse pathophysiological consequence; i.e., it increases diastolic stiffness. As a result, greater intracavitary pressure is required for ventricular filling.[278, 279, 292] Some patients with AS manifest an increase in stiffness of the left ventricle (increased *chamber stiffness*) due simply to increased muscle mass with no alteration in the diastolic properties of each unit of myocardium (normal *muscle stiffness*); others exhibit increases in both chamber and muscle stiffness. This increased stiffness, however produced, contributes to the elevation of ventricular diastolic filling pressure at any level of ventricular diastolic volume[293, 294] and may be responsible for flash pulmonary edema in patients with AS. Diastolic dysfunction may revert toward normal as hypertrophy regresses following relief of AS.[279]

CARDIAC STRUCTURE. An increase in the total collagen volume of the myocardium and in the orthogonal collagen fiber network in AS has been reported.[295, 296] This likely contributes to the altered diastolic properties just discussed. An inverse correlation between the left ventricular ejection fraction and myocardial fiber diameter has been reported.[297] Changes in the myocardial ultrastructure in patients with severe AS include unusually large nuclei, loss of myofibrils, accumulation of mitochondria, large cytoplasmic areas devoid of contractile material, and proliferation of fibroblasts and collagen fibers in the interstitial space. The depression of myocardial function that occurs late in the course of the disease may well be related to these morphological alterations. In adults with AS, both myocardial cellular hypertrophy and relative and absolute increases in connective tissue occur.

ISCHEMIA. In patients with AS, coronary blood flow at rest is elevated in absolute terms but is normal when corrections are made for myocardial mass.[298] There may be inadequate myocardial oxygenation in patients with severe AS, even in the absence of coronary artery disease. The hypertrophied left ventricular muscle mass, the increased systolic pressure, and the prolongation of ejection all elevate myocardial oxygen consumption. The abnormally heightened pressure compressing the coronary arteries may exceed the coronary perfusion pressure, and the shortening of diastole interferes with coronary blood flow,[299, 300] thus leading to an imbalance between myocardial oxygen supply and demand. Myocardial perfusion is also impaired by the relative decrease in myocardial capillary density as myocardial mass increases and by the elevation of left ventricular end-diastolic pressure, which lowers the aortic–left ventricular pressure gradient in diastole (i.e., the coronary perfusion pressure gradient). This underperfusion may be responsible for the development of subendocardial ischemia, especially during tachycardia. Marcus and associates have demonstrated a reduction in the velocity of coronary blood flow during reactive hyperemia in patients with severe AS,[301] and this may correlate with the angina pectoris commonly observed in these patients.

Myocardial ischemia in patients with severe AS and normal coronary arteries may be secondary to high systolic and diastolic stresses caused by inadequate ventricular hypertrophy and the reduced coronary flow reserve just described.[302, 303] Metabolic evidence of myocardial ischemia, i.e., lactate production, can be demonstrated when myocardial oxygen needs are stimulated by exercise or by isoproterenol in patients with AS, even in the absence of coronary artery narrowing.

CLINICAL MANIFESTATIONS

History

In the natural history of adults with AS, a long latent period exists during which there is gradually increasing obstruction and an increase in the pressure load on the myocardium while the patient remains asymptomatic.[304] The cardinal manifestations of acquired AS, which commence most commonly in the fifth or sixth decades of life, are angina pectoris, syncope, exertional dyspnea, and ultimately heart failure.[305]

Angina occurs in approximately two-thirds of patients with critical AS (about half of whom have associated significant coronary artery obstruction).[306] It usually resembles the angina observed in patients with coronary artery disease, in that it is commonly precipitated by exertion and relieved by rest. In patients without coronary artery disease, angina results from the combination of the increased oxygen needs of the hypertrophied myocardium and the reduction of oxygen delivery secondary to the excessive compression of coronary vessels[298, 301–303] (see Ischemia, just

discussed). In patients with coronary artery disease, angina is caused by a combination of the epicardial coronary artery obstruction and the earlier-described oxygen imbalance characteristic of AS. Rarely, angina results from calcium emboli to the coronary vascular bed.[307]

Syncope is most commonly due to the reduced cerebral perfusion that occurs during exertion when arterial pressure declines consequent to systemic vasodilation in the presence of a fixed cardiac output. Syncope has also been attributed to malfunction of the baroreceptor mechanism in severe AS[277], as well as to a vasodepressor response to a greatly elevated left ventricular systolic pressure during exercise.[308] Premonitory symptoms of syncope are common. Exertional hypotension may also be manifested as "graying out" spells or dizziness on effort. Syncope at rest may be due to transient ventricular fibrillation,[309] from which the patient recovers spontaneously; to transient atrial fibrillation with loss of the atrial contribution to left ventricular filling, which causes a precipitous decline in cardiac output; or to transient atrioventricular block due to extension of the calcification of the valve into the conduction system. Exertional dyspnea with orthopnea, paroxysmal nocturnal dyspnea, and pulmonary edema reflect varying degrees of pulmonary venous hypertension. These are relatively late symptoms in patients with AS, and their presence for more than 5 years should suggest the possibility of associated mitral valvular disease.

Gastrointestinal bleeding, either idiopathic or due to angiodysplasia (most commonly of the right colon) or other vascular malformations, occurs more often in patients with calcific AS than in persons without this condition; it may cease after aortic valve replacement.[310] Infective endocarditis is a greater risk in younger patients with milder valvular deformity than in older patients with rocklike calcific aortic deformities. Cerebral emboli resulting in stroke or transient ischemic attacks may be due to microthrombi on thickened bicuspid valves.[311] Calcific AS may cause embolization of calcium to various organs, including the heart, kidneys, and brain. Abrupt loss of vision has been reported when calcific emboli occlude the central retinal artery.[307, 312]

Because cardiac output is usually well maintained for many years in patients with severe AS, marked fatigability, debilitation, peripheral cyanosis, and other clinical manifestations of a low cardiac output are usually not prominent until quite late in the course of the disease. Other late findings in patients with isolated AS include atrial fibrillation, pulmonary hypertension, and systemic venous hypertension. Although AS may be responsible for sudden death, this usually occurs in patients who had previously been symptomatic (see Chap. 26).

In patients in whom the obstruction remains unrelieved, the prognosis is poor once these symptoms are manifested. Survival curves show that the interval from the onset of symptoms to the time of death is approximately 2 years in patients with heart failure, 3 years in those with syncope, and 5 years in those with angina (Fig. 46–31).

Physical Examination (Table 46–7)

The arterial pulse characteristically rises slowly and is small and sustained (pulsus parvus et tardus) (see Fig. 4–8B).[313, 314] In the late stage of AS, systolic and pulse pressures are both reduced. However, in patients with mild AS with associated AR and in older patients with an inelastic arterial bed, both systolic and pulse pressures may be normal or even increased. A systolic pressure exceeding 200 mm Hg is rare in patients with critical AS. The anacrotic notch and coarse systolic vibrations are felt most readily in the carotid arterial pulse, producing the so-called carotid shudder. Simultaneous palpation of the apex and carotid arteries reveals a lag in the latter in patients with

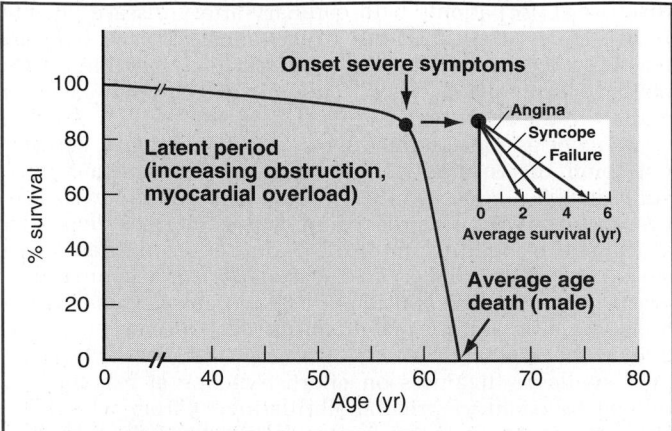

FIGURE 46-31. Natural history of aortic stenosis without operative treatment. (Reproduced with permission from Ross J Jr, Braunwald E: Aortic stenosis. Circulation 38[Suppl V]:61, 1968. Copyright 1968 American Heart Association.)

severe AS.[315] Although left ventricular alternans occurs commonly in patients who have AS with left ventricular dysfunction,[316] obstruction of the aortic valve may prevent its recognition in the peripheral arterial pulse. The jugular venous pulse usually shows prominent a waves, reflecting reduced right ventricular compliance consequent to hypertrophy of the ventricular septum.[317] With pulmonary hypertension and secondary right ventricular failure and tricuspid regurgitation, v or c-v waves may become prominent.

The cardiac impulse is sustained and becomes displaced inferiorly and laterally with left ventricular failure. Presystolic distention of the left ventricle (i.e., a prominent precordial a wave) is often both visible and palpable. A hyperdynamic left ventricle suggests concomitant aortic and/or mitral regurgitation. A systolic thrill is usually best appreciated when the patient leans forward during full expiration. It is palpated most readily in the second left intercostal space on either side of the sternum or in the suprasternal notch and is frequently transmitted along the carotid arteries. A systolic thrill is quite specific for severe AS.

Rarely, right ventricular failure with systemic venous congestion, hepatomegaly, and edema precedes left ventricular failure. This is probably caused by the so-called Bernheim effect, which results when the hypertrophied ventricular septum bulges into and encroaches on the right ventricular cavity and leads to impairment of right ventricular filling. In such cases, the jugular venous pressure is elevated, and the a wave is prominent.

AUSCULTATION (See Table 46-7). S_1 is normal or soft and S_4 is prominent, presumably because atrial contraction is vigorous and the mitral valve is partially closed during presystole.[318] S_2 may be single because calcification and immobility of the aortic valve make A_2 inaudible, because P_2 is buried in the prolonged aortic ejection murmur, or because prolongation of left ventricular systole makes A_2 coincide with P_2. Paradoxical splitting of S_2, which suggests associated left ventricular dysfunction, may also occur. In patients with left ventricular failure and secondary pulmonary hypertension, P_2 may become accentuated. When the aortic valve is rigid, which is the usual finding in adults with severe AS, A_2 may be inaudible, but when the valve is flexible, as may occur in patients with congenital AS, A_2 may be snapping and accentuated.

An aortic ejection sound occurs simultaneous with the halting upward movement of the aortic valve (see Fig. 4-15). Like an audible A_2, this sound is dependent on mobility of the valve cusps and disappears when they become severely calcified. Thus, it is common in children with congenital AS but is rare in adults with acquired calcific AS and rigid valves. The ejection sound occurs approximately 0.06 second after the onset of S_1.

The *systolic murmur* of AS is usually late peaking and heard best at the base of the heart but is often well transmitted both along the carotid vessels and to the apex. Cessation of the murmur before A_2 is usually helpful in differentiating it from a pansystolic mitral murmur. However, the systolic murmur may be mistaken for a pansystolic murmur because it may end with S_2, which represents pulmonic valve closure, whereas the pansystolic murmur is soft or even inaudible. In patients with calcified aortic valves, the systolic murmur is loudest at the base of the heart, but high-frequency components selectively radiate to the apex (the so-called Gallavardin phenomenon [see Fig. 4-24]), where it may actually be more prominent and where it may be mistaken for the murmur of MR. Frequently, there is a

▼ TABLE 46-7. DIFFERENTIAL DIAGNOSIS OF AORTIC STENOSIS: PHYSICAL FINDINGS

TYPE OF STENOSIS	MAXIMUM MURMUR AND THRILL	AORTIC EJECTION SOUND	AORTIC COMPONENT OF SECOND SOUND	REGURGITANT DIASTOLIC MURMUR	ARTERIAL PULSE
Acquired nonrheumatic or rheumatic	Second right sternal border to neck; may be at apex in the aged	Uncommon	Decreased or absent	Common	Delayed upstroke; anacrotic notch; ± small amplitude
Hypertrophic subaortic	Fourth left sternal border to apex (± regurgitant systolic murmur at apex)	Rare	Normal or decreased	Very rare	Brisk upstroke, sometimes bisferiens
Congenital valvular	Second right sternal border to neck (along left sternal border in some infants)	Very common in children, disappearing with decrease in valve mobility with age	Normal or increased in children; decreased with decreased in valve mobility with age	Uncommon in children; not uncommon in adults	Delayed upstroke; anacrotic notch; ± small amplitude
Congenital subvalvular	Discrete: like valvular; tunnel: left sternal border	Rare	Not helpful (normal, increased, decreased, or absent)	Almost all	
Congenital supravalvular	First right sternal border to neck and sometimes to medial aspect of right arm; occasionally greater in neck than in chest	Rare	Normal or decreased	Uncommon	Rapid upstroke in right carotid, delayed in left carotid; right arm pulse pressure greater than left

From Levinson GE: Aortic stenosis. *In* Dalen JE, Alpert JS (eds): Valvular Heart Disease. 2nd ed. Boston, Little, Brown and Co, 1987, p 202.

"quiet area" between the base and apex where the murmur is diminished in intensity, supporting the erroneous impression that the apical and basal murmurs have different origins. In general, the more severe the stenosis, the longer the duration of the murmur and the more likely that it peaks later in systole.[320]

Patients with degenerative aortic sclerosis may have severe valvular calcification; however, obstruction may be mild or absent because the commissural fusion characteristic of congenital and rheumatic AS is not present.[92] The nonfused, calcified cusps vibrate freely, resulting in a softer and more musical murmur that is more prominent at the apex than the murmur of congenital or rheumatic AS. High-pitched decrescendo diastolic murmurs secondary to aortic regurgitation are common in many patients with dominant AS.

When the left ventricle fails and the stroke volume falls, the systolic murmur of AS becomes softer; rarely, it disappears altogether. The slow rise in the arterial pulse is more difficult to recognize. Stated simply, with left ventricular failure, the clinical picture changes from typical AS to that of severe left ventricular failure with a low cardiac output. Thus, occult AS may be a cause of intractable heart failure, and critical AS should be ruled out by echocardiography in patients with severe heart failure of unknown cause because operative treatment may be life-saving and may result in substantial clinical improvement.[321]

DYNAMIC AUSCULTATION (see Table 46-4). The intensity of the systolic murmur varies from beat to beat when the duration of diastolic filling varies, as in atrial fibrillation or following a premature contraction. This characteristic is helpful in differentiating AS from MR, in which the murmur is usually unaffected. The murmur of valvular AS is augmented by squatting, which increases stroke volume. It is reduced in intensity during the strain of the Valsalva maneuver and when standing, which reduce transvalvular flow.[322] Findings on physical examination including a delay in the carotid upstroke, a loud, long systolic murmur, and a single S_2 all correlate with severe stenosis.[323]

LABORATORY EXAMINATION

ELECTROCARDIOGRAPHY. The principal ECG change is left ventricular hypertrophy (Fig. 5-19), which is found in approximately 85 percent of patients with severe AS. The absence of left ventricular hypertrophy does not exclude the presence of critical AS, and the correlation between the absolute ECG voltages in precordial leads and the severity of obstruction is poor in adults but is quite good in children with congenital AS. T wave inversion and ST segment depression in leads with upright QRS complexes are common. ST segment depressions greater than 0.2 mV in patients with AS (left ventricular "strain") suggest that severe ventricular hypertrophy is present. Occasionally, a "pseudoinfarction" pattern is present, characterized by a loss of r waves in the right precordial leads. There is evidence of left atrial enlargement in more than 80 percent of patients with severe, isolated AS. The principal manifestation is prominent late negativity of the P wave in lead V_1 rather than an increased duration in lead II, suggesting hypertrophy rather than dilatation. Atrial fibrillation is an uncommon and late sign of pure AS, and its presence in a patient who does not appear to have end-stage aortic disease should suggest coexisting mitral valvular disease.

The extension of calcific infiltrates from the aortic valve into the conduction system may cause various forms and degrees of atrioventricular and intraventricular block in 5 percent of patients with calcific AS.[324] Such conduction defects are more common in patients who have associated mitral annular calcification.

RADIOLOGICAL FINDINGS. (See Figs. 8-8, 8-19, and 8-20). Routine radiological examination may be normal in patients with critical AS. The heart is usually of normal size or slightly enlarged, with a rounding of the left ventricular border and apex, unless regurgitation or left ventricular failure is present and causes substantial cardiomegaly. Poststenotic dilatation of the ascending aorta is a common finding. Calcification of the aortic valve is found in almost all adults with hemodynamically significant AS.[325] It is more readily detected on fluoroscopy or echocardiography than on roentgenography. The absence of calcium in the aortic valve region on careful fluoroscopic examination in a patient older than 35 years of age essentially rules out severe valvular AS. The converse is not true, however, and in patients over the age of 65 with degenerative AS, severe calcification of the

aortic valve may occur with no or only mild obstruction. The left atrium may be slightly enlarged in patients with severe AS, and there may be radiological signs of pulmonary venous hypertension. However, when left atrial enlargement is marked, the presence of associated mitral valvular disease should be suspected.

ANGIOGRAPHY. There is some hazard associated with the rapid injection of a large volume of contrast material into a high-pressure left ventricle, and therefore this procedure is usually not advisable in patients with AS and critical obstruction. Angiographic studies of the left ventricle and aortic valve in these patients are best performed by injecting contrast material into the pulmonary artery and filming in the 30-degree right anterior oblique and 60-degree left anterior oblique projections. These examinations often make it possible to ascertain the number of cusps of the stenotic valve and to demonstrate doming of a thickened valve and a systolic jet.

ECHOCARDIOGRAPHY (see also Chap. 7 and Figs. 7-60 to 7-63). The normal range of opening of the aortic valve is 1.6 to 2.6 cm. Two-dimensional transthoracic echocardiography is helpful in detecting valvular calcification, in outlining the valve leaflets, and sometimes in determining the severity of the stenosis by imaging the orifice.[326] The orifice may be more clearly defined by transesophageal echocardiography, which offers a precise short-axis view of the aortic valve.[327] Multiplanar transesophageal echocardiography is particularly useful.[328] Two-dimensional echocardiography is invaluable in detecting associated mitral valve disease and in assessing left ventricular systolic performance, diastolic function, dilatation, and hypertrophy. Doppler echocardiography allows calculation of the left ventricular–aortic pressure gradient[329] using a modified Bernoulli (continuity) equation (see Fig 7-25). The gradients noninvasively determined by this method correlate well with those determined by left-heart catheterization.[329, 330] Color flow Doppler imaging is helpful in detecting and determining the severity of aortic regurgitation (which coexists in approximately 75 percent of patients with predominant AS) and in estimating pulmonary artery pressure.[331] Indeed, in a large majority of patients the echocardiographic examination provides the information obtained by cardiac catheterization (except for the status of the coronary arteries).[329] Echocardiography has become the most important laboratory technique for evaluating and following patients with AS and selecting them for operation.

NATURAL HISTORY

In contrast to MS, which leads to symptoms almost immediately after its development, patients with severe AS may be asymptomatic for many years despite the presence of severe obstruction.[304, 306] The systolic pressure gradient may exceed 150 mm Hg, and the peak left ventricular systolic pressure may reach approximately 300 mm Hg with relatively little increase in overall heart size on radiological examination and with normal left ventricular end-diastolic and end-systolic volumes.

Patients with severe, chronic AS tend to be free of cardiovascular symptoms until relatively late in the course of the disease. Thus, there is a long latent period during which mortality and morbidity are very low.[51] In Rapaport's report, 40 percent of patients treated medically survived for 5 years and 20 percent for 10 years after diagnosis.[147] In another series of patients with hemodynamically significant valvular AS treated medically, the 5-year survival rate was 64 percent. However, obstruction is progressive and often insidious, with the aortic valve area decreasing by an average of 0.12 cm^2/year in one study.[331] When symptoms develop, the valve area is, on average, 0.6 cm^2.[332] Once patients with AS develop angina pectoris or syncope, the average survival is 1 to 3 years[333-335] (see Fig. 46-31). In an analysis of elderly patients with severe AS and symptoms of heart failure who declined surgery, 50 percent had died by 18 months of follow-up; the ejection fraction correlated inversely with survival.[336] Among symptomatic patients with severe AS, the outlook is poorest when the left ventricle has failed and the cardiac output and transvalvular gradient are both low.

Asymptomatic patients have an excellent prognosis.[92, 337, 338] Sudden death, like syncope, in patients with severe AS may be due to cerebral hypoperfusion followed by arrhythmia. Although severe AS is a potentially lethal disease, death (even when sudden) usually occurs in *symptomatic* patients. A number of authors who have followed asymptomatic patients with critical AS have found that sudden death is extremely rare in this group. Of 229 asymptomatic patients with critical AS, only 5 (2 percent) died suddenly (certainly not higher than the mortality from operation).[51, 337]

MANAGEMENT

Medical Treatment

Patients with known severe AS who are asymptomatic should be advised to report promptly the development of any symptoms possibly related to AS. Patients with critical obstruction should be cautioned to avoid vigorous athletic and physical activity. However, such restrictions do not apply to patients with mild obstruction. The need for infective endocarditis prophylaxis should be explained (see Chap 47). Because of the gradual increase in the severity of obstruction, noninvasive assessment of this finding by Doppler echocardiography should be carried out at intervals. Doppler-derived gradients have been shown to increase by 4 to 8 mm Hg per year.[92] In patients with mild obstruction, this measurement should be repeated every 2 years. In asymptomatic patients with severe obstruction, repeat echocardiography should be carried out every 6 to 12 months, with particular attention to detecting changes in left ventricular function. Exercise stress testing should be avoided in symptomatic patients, but may be carried out in asymptomatic patients to detect limited exercise capacity.

Symptomatic patients with severe AS are usually operative candidates, as medical therapy has little to offer. However, medical therapy may be necessary in patients who are considered to be inoperable (usually because of comorbid conditions that preclude surgery.) Digitalis glycosides are indicated if the ventricular volume is increased or the ejection fraction is reduced. Although diuretics are beneficial when there is abnormal accumulation of fluid, they must be used with caution because hypovolemia may reduce the elevated left ventricular end-diastolic pressure, lower cardiac output, and produce orthostatic hypotension. Beta-adrenergic blockers can depress myocardial function and induce left ventricular failure and should be avoided in patients with AS.

Atrial flutter or fibrillation occurs in fewer than 10 percent of patients with severe AS, perhaps because of the late occurrence of left atrial enlargement in this condition. When such an arrhythmia is observed in a patient with AS, the possibility of associated mitral valvular disease should be considered. When atrial fibrillation occurs, the rapid ventricular rate may cause angina pectoris. The loss of the atrial contribution to ventricular filling and a sudden fall in cardiac output may cause serious hypotension. Therefore, atrial fibrillation should be treated promptly, usually with cardioversion, and a search for previously unrecognized mitral valvular disease should be undertaken. Adults with severe AS who are being considered for surgical therapy should undergo coronary arteriography. Left-heart catheterization is also indicated if there is a discrepancy between the clinical picture and the echocardiographic findings.[50]

Surgical Treatment

INDICATIONS FOR OPERATION.

Children. The indications for surgery, as well as the techniques and results of operation, depend on the patient's age, the type of valvular deformity, and the function of the left ventricle. In children and adolescents with noncalcific congenital AS, who most commonly have bicuspid aortic valves, simple commissural incision under direct vision usually leads to substantial hemodynamic improvement with low risk (i.e., a mortality rate of less than 1 percent) (see Chap. 43).[339] Therefore, this procedure (or now, more commonly, balloon aortic valvuloplasty) is indicated not only in symptomatic patients but also in asymptomatic children and adolescents with severe AS, which is often defined as a calculated effective orifice less than 0.8 cm² or 0.5 cm²/m² body surface area (BSA). Despite the salutary hemodynamic results following this procedure, the valve is not rendered entirely normal anatomically. The turbulent blood flow through the valve may subsequently lead to further deformation, calcification, the development of regurgitation, and restenosis after 10 to 20 years, probably requiring reoperation and valve replacement later.

Adults. In most adults with calcific AS, satisfactory long-term valvular function cannot usually be restored even by careful sculpturing procedures under direct vision, and valve replacement is the surgical treatment of choice. Aortic valve replacement (AVR) (Fig. 46–32) should, in general, be performed in adults who have hemodynamic evidence of severe obstruction (aortic valve orifice <0.8 to 0.9 cm² or <0.5 to 0.6 cm²/m² BSA) and whose symptoms are believed to result from AS. AVR should also be carried out in asymptomatic patients with *progressive* left ventricular dysfunction or a hypotensive response to exercise.[340] Although a prospective randomized controlled study has not been done, the long-term mortality in asymptomatic patients with critical AS and left ventricular dysfunction who undergo operation appears to be lower than that in medically treated patients who do not undergo operation.[51] As prosthetic valves and surgical skills continue to improve, it is likely that patients with severe AS will become candidates for operation at progressively earlier stages in the natural history of their disease.[340a] At the present time, however, I do *not* recommend prophylactic replacement of a critically narrow calcific aortic valve in *asymptomatic* adults unless they have progressive left ventricular dysfunction.

AVR is also indicated in patients with severe stenosis who are undergoing another cardiovascular operation (e.g., coronary artery bypass grafting or surgery on the aorta or another heart valve).[51] Surgical risk is higher in patients with impaired left ventricular function[340] (EF < 35 percent). However, since their prognosis is very poor without operation and some patients even in this group have clinical and functional recovery following AVR,[341, 341a] the procedure should generally be offered to these patients. Even octogenarians with left ventricular dysfunction can have improved survival after AVR.[342, 343, 343a] Exceptions are patients with advanced congestive heart failure or left ventricular dysfunction that can be related to previous myocardial infarction.

RESULTS. Successful replacement of the aortic valve results in substantial clinical and hemodynamic improvement in patients with AS, aortic regurgitation, or combined lesions.[343] In patients without frank left ventricular failure, the operative risk ranges from 2 to 5 percent in most centers, and in patients under 70 years of age, the operative risk has been reported to be as low as 1 percent.[344] The Society of Thoracic Surgeons National Database Committee reported an overall operative mortality rate of 4.3 percent in 26, 317 patients undergoing isolated AVR, 8.0 percent in 22,713 patients undergoing AVR and coronary artery by-

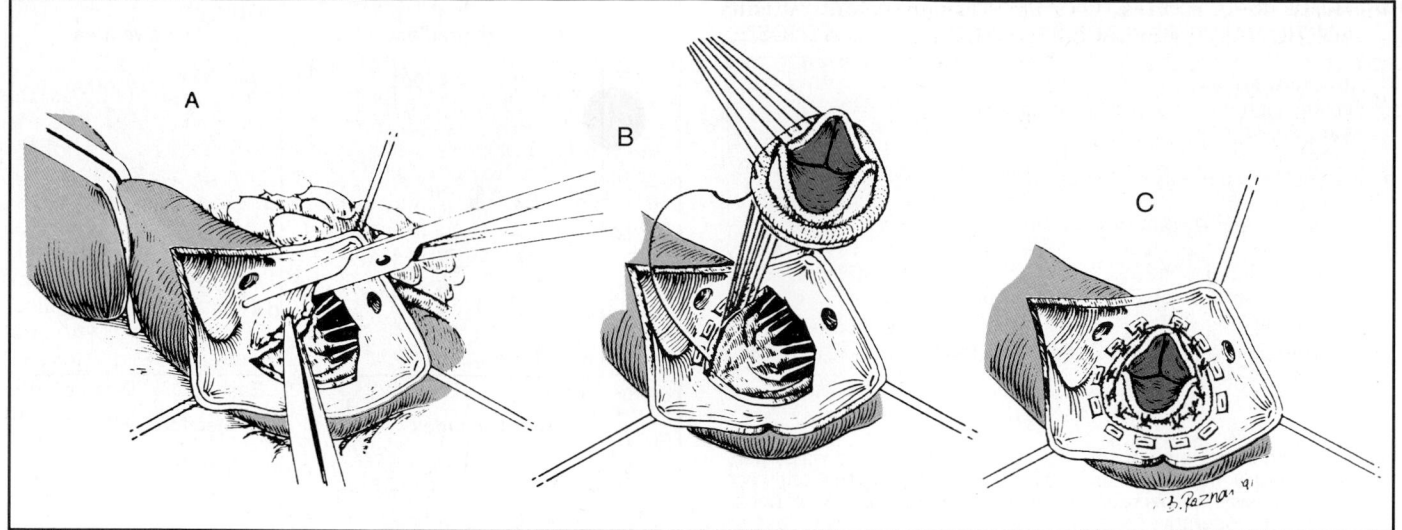

FIGURE 46–32. Interrupted suture technique for aortic valve replacement. *A,* The aortic valve is excised, leaving 1 or 2 mm of annular tissue as a sewing cuff. *B,* Pledgetted Tyeron mattress sutures (2-0) are placed with the pledget on the aortic side. Sutures are placed in the aortic ring and passed directly onto the prosthetic valve sewing ring held at a distance. *C,* After all sutures are placed, the valve is lowered in place and the sutures tied. The valve is then inspected for proper function and fit. (From Albertucci M, Karp RB: Prosthetic valve replacement. *In* Al-Zaibag M, Duran CMG [eds]: Valvular Heart Disease. New York, Marcel Dekker, 1994, pp 601–634.)

pass grafting, 7.4 percent in 938 patients undergoing AVR and repair of another valve, and 9.7 percent in 1723 patients undergoing AVR and aortic aneurysm repair[104] (see Table 46–2).

Risk factors causing a higher mortality rate include a high NYHA class, impairment of left ventricular function, advanced age, and the presence of associated coronary artery disease. The 10-year actuarial survival rate of hospital survivors in surgically treated patients is approximately 85 percent.[345, 345a] Risk factors for late death include higher preoperative NYHA class, advanced age, concomitant untreated coronary artery disease, preoperative impaired left ventricular function, preoperative ventricular arrhythmias, and associated significant aortic regurgitation.

Symptoms of pulmonary congestion (exertional dyspnea) and of myocardial ischemia (angina pectoris) are relieved in almost every patient. Hemodynamic results of AVR are also impressive; elevated end-diastolic and end-systolic volumes show significant reduction. Impaired ventricular performance returns to normal more frequently in patients with AS than in those with aortic or mitral regurgitation. Diastolic function is improved as well.[278, 279] However, the finding that the strongest predictor of postoperative left ventricular dysfunction is preoperative dysfunction[346, 347] suggests that patients should, if possible, be operated on *before* left ventricular function becomes seriously impaired. The increased left ventricular mass is reduced toward (but not to) normal within 18 months after AVR in patients with AS.[348, 349] When patients were restudied 5 years postoperatively, left ventricular mass usually had returned to normal.[350, 350a] Myocyte hypertrophy regresses as well. Diastolic dysfunction returns to normal long after systolic dysfunction.[351]

When operation is carried out in patients with critical AS, frank left ventricular failure, a depressed ejection fraction, or a low cardiac output (and hence a reduced transaortic pressure gradient[351a, 351b]), the operative risk is higher, and the mortality rate ranges from 8 to 20 percent, depending on the skill of the surgical team and the severity of heart failure.[341a] Obviously, performing surgery before heart failure develops is desirable, but emergency operation, even in patients with heart failure, is sometimes life-saving. In view of the extremely poor prognosis of such patients who are treated medically, unless serious comorbid conditions

exist that preclude surgery, there is usually little choice but to advise immediate mechanical relief of obstruction, i.e., balloon angioplasty (see below) or urgent AVR. Since many symptomatic patients with calcific AS are elderly, particular attention must be directed to the adequacy of hepatic, renal, and pulmonary functions. However, the results of AVR are often quite satisfactory in patients older than 70 or even 80 years of age.[352] Therefore, advanced age per se, while adding to the risk, should not be considered a contraindication to operation.

In patients with AS and obstructive coronary artery disease (a relatively common combination), AVR and myocardial revascularization should be performed together.[353, 353a] Although the risk of AVR is increased when accompanied by coronary artery bypass grafting (see Table 46–2),[104] the surgical risk increases even more when severe coronary artery disease is left untreated. The ability to avoid serious myocardial ischemia in the perioperative period is a major factor that has served to reduce operative mortality in these patients. Characteristics of patients that have been shown to increase the risk of AVR, as reported in different series, are shown in Table 46–8.

There has been increasing interest in performing AVR through a very small incision, generally a transverse sternotomy, so-called "minimally invasive surgery." Although the advantages (shorter hospital stay, less tissue damage, better cosmetic results) are clear, the procedure is technically demanding and the mortality rate may actually be higher than when a standard approach is employed.[354, 354a]

BALLOON AORTIC VALVULOPLASTY (See also Chap. 38)

Balloon aortic valvuloplasty (BAV) represents an increasingly attractive alternative to aortic valvotomy in children, adolescents, and young adults with congenital noncalcific AS (see Chap. 43),[355, 356] but its value is limited in adults with calcific AS. A series of balloon dilation catheters are advanced along a guidewire positioned at the left ventricular apex. Fracture of calcified nodules, separation of fused commissures, and stretching of the aortic valve ring are responsible for the relief of obstruction.[355, 357, 358] Although the response of adult patients with calcific AS varies considerably, BAV initially results in relief of obstruction in most patients[359–362] (Fig. 46–33). The valve area in these patients initially increased from 0.5 to 0.8 cm², and the mean transvalvular gradient declined from approximately 55 to 29 mm Hg. Left ventricular ejection fraction tends to rise in patients with depressed left ventricular function who undergo BAV. In a report of a multicenter registry involving 674 seriously ill, elderly patients (average age 78

▼ **TABLE 46–8. PREDICTORS OF POOR OUTCOME AFTER AORTIC VALVE REPLACEMENT FOR AORTIC STENOSIS**

Advanced age (>70 yr)
Female gender
Emergent surgery
Coronary artery disease
Previous coronary artery bypass grafting surgery
Hypertension
Left ventricular dysfunction (ejection fraction <45% or 50%)
Heart failure
Atrial fibrillation
Concurrent mitral valve replacement or repair
Renal failure

Adapted from Otto CM: Valvular Heart Disease. Philadelphia, WB Saunders, 1999, p 203.

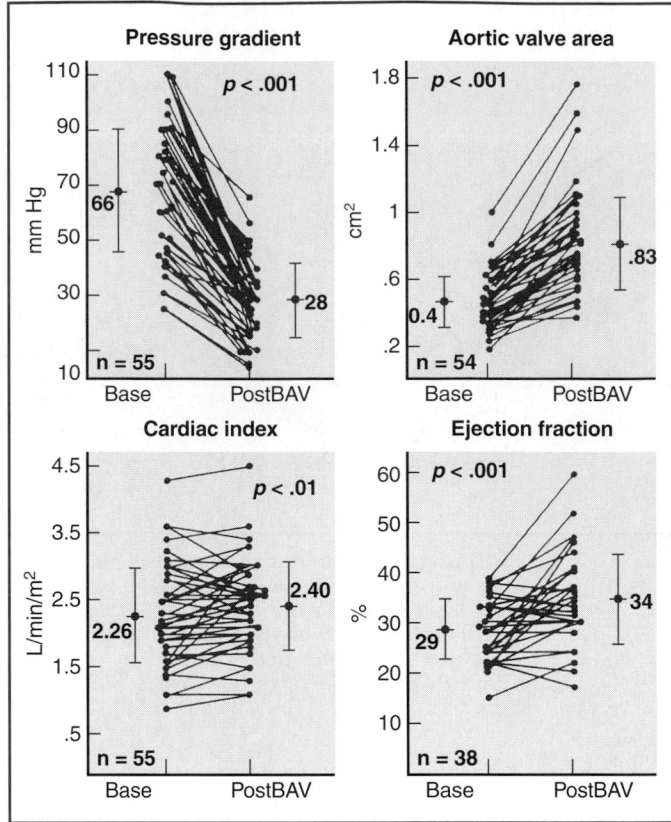

FIGURE 46–33. Plots of changes in pressure gradient, valve area, cardiac index, and ejection fraction at baseline (Base) after balloon aortic valvuloplasty (BAV). (Reproduced with permission from Berland J et al: Percutaneous balloon valvuloplasty in patients with severe aortic stenosis and low ejection fraction. Circulation 79: 1189, 1989. Copyright 1989 American Heart Association.)

years) treated at 24 centers, the procedural mortality rate was 3 percent, the 30-day mortality rate was 14 percent, and the one-year mortality rate was 45 percent. Better survival was seen in patients with higher preoperative pressure gradients, in those with better preserved left ventricular systolic function, and in women. In addition to the procedural mortality, another 6 percent of patients developed serious complications such as myocardial perforation, myocardial infarction, and severe aortic regurgitation.[363]

The major disadvantage of BAV in adults with critical calcified AS is restenosis due to scarring, which occurs in about 50 percent of patients within 6 months. Symptoms lessen in severity in the majority of patients but recur in approximately 30 percent by 6 months.

Although the overall intermediate-term results (6 to 12 months) of BAV have been disappointing, largely because of restenosis, the procedure does have a role in the management of severe calcific AS in patients who are not surgical candidates. Indications include: (1) patients with cardiogenic shock due to critical AS,[364] (2) patients with critical AS who require an urgent noncardiac operation, (3) patients with severe heart failure who are at extremely high operative risk as a "bridge" to AVR, (4) pregnant women with critical AS,[365] (5) patients with severe comorbid conditions that preclude surgery, and (6) patients with critical AS who refuse surgical treatment. However, in adults with calcified AS, BAV is *not* a substitute for surgery (as balloon mitral valvuloplasty may be in patients with MS [see p. 1651]).

▼ Aortic Regurgitation

ETIOLOGY AND PATHOLOGY

Aortic regurgitation (AR) may be caused by primary disease of the aortic valve leaflets and/or the wall of the aortic root (Fig. 46–34). Among patients with *pure* AR who undergo valve replacement, the percentage with aortic root disease has been increasing steadily during the past few decades and now accounts for more than 50 percent of all such patients.[262]

Valvular Disease

Rheumatic fever is a common cause of primary disease of the aortic valve that leads to regurgitation[92, 366] (Fig. 46–35). The cusps become infiltrated with fibrous tissues and retract, a process that prevents cusp apposition during diastole and usually leads to regurgitation into the left ventricle through a defect in the center of the valve.[5] The associated fusion of the commissures may restrict the opening of the valve, resulting in combined AS and AR; some associated mitral valve involvement is also common. Other primary valvular causes of AR include calcific AS in the elderly, in

which some degree (usually mild) of AR is present in 75 percent of patients; *infective endocarditis* (see Chap. 47), in which the infection may destroy or cause perforation of a leaflet, or the vegetations may interfere with proper coaptation of the cusps; and *trauma* that results in a tear of the ascending aorta, in which loss of commissural support can cause prolapse of an aortic cusp. Although the most common complication of a congenitally *bicuspid valve* in adults is stenosis, incomplete closure and/or prolapse of a bicuspid valve may also cause isolated regurgitation or a combination of stenosis and regurgitation.[367–369] Progressive AR may occur in patients with a large ventricular septal defect as well as in patients with membranous subaortic stenosis (see Chap. 43) and as a complication of radiofrequency catheter ablation.[370] Progressive regurgitation may also occur in patients with myxomatous proliferation of the aortic valve.[371] An increasingly common cause of valvular AR is structural deterioration of a bioprosthetic valve (see p. 1701).

Less common causes of AR include various forms of congenital AR, such as unicommissural and quadricuspid valves, or rupture of a congenitally fenestrated valve,[372] particularly in the presence of hypertension.[373] Other less com-

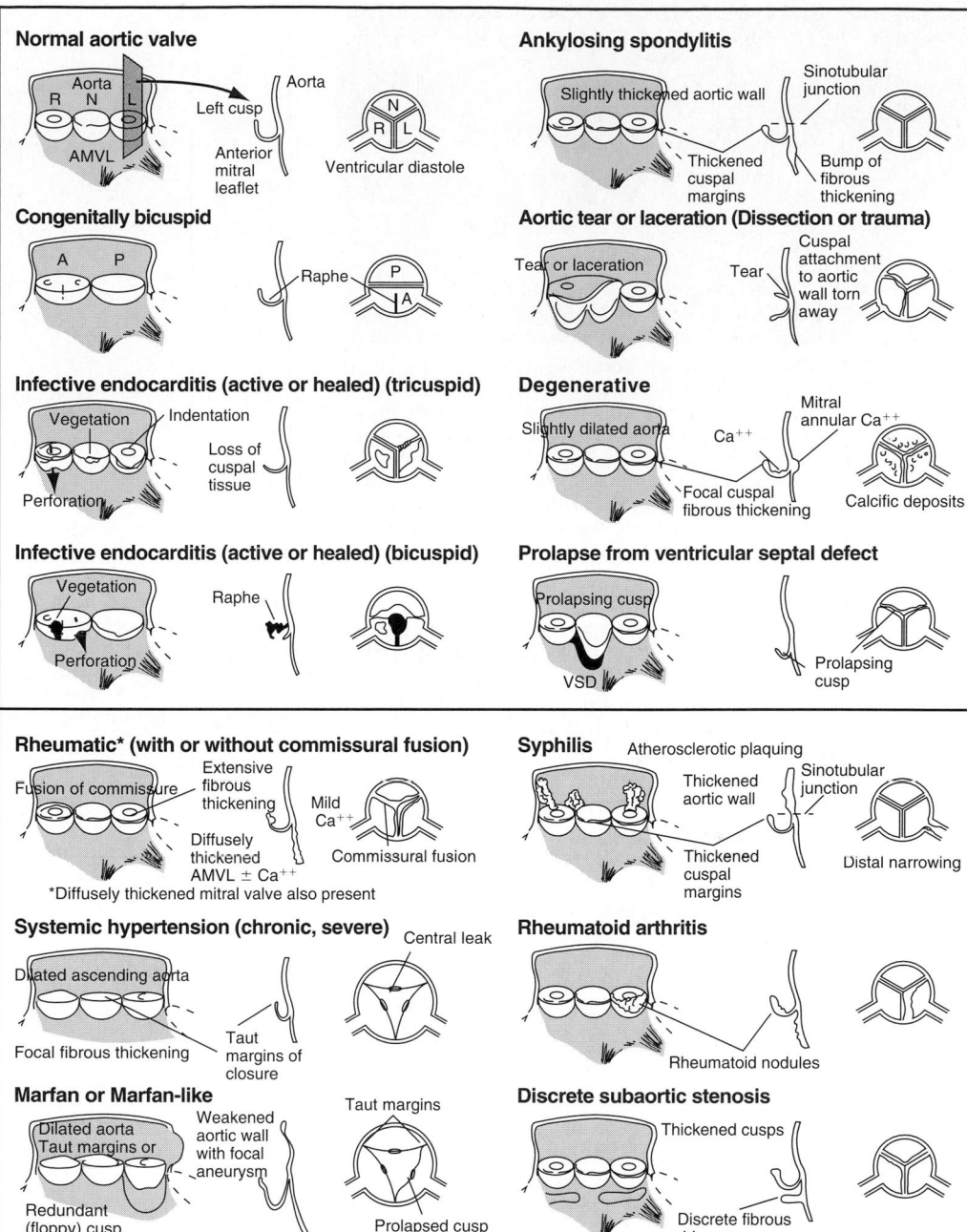

FIGURE 46–34. Diagram of various causes of pure aortic regurgitation. (From Waller BF: Rheumatic and nonrheumatic conditions producing valvular heart disease. *In* Frankl WS, Brest AN [eds]: Cardiovascular Clinics. Valvular Heart Disease: Comprehensive Evaluation and Management. Philadelphia, FA Davis Co, 1986, pp 30–31.)

mon causes of AR occur in association with systemic lupus erythematosus, rheumatoid arthritis, ankylosing spondylitis,[374] Jaccoud arthropathy, Takayasu disease, Whipple disease,[375] Crohn disease,[376] and, in the past, use of certain anorectic drugs. Isolated congenital AR is an uncommon lesion on necropsy studies, but, when present, is usually associated with a bicuspid valve.[377]

Aortic Root Disease (See also Chap. 40)

AR secondary to marked dilatation of the ascending aorta is now more common than primary valve disease in patients undergoing AVR for pure AR.[262] The conditions responsible for aortic root disease include age-related (degenerative) aortic dilatation, cystic medial necrosis of the aorta (either isolated or associated with classic Marfan syndrome), aortic dissection, osteogenesis imperfecta, syphilitic aortitis, ankylosing spondylitis, the Behçet syndrome, psoriatic arthritis,

arthritis associated with ulcerative colitis, relapsing polychondritis, the Reiter syndrome, giant cell arteritis, and systemic hypertension,[378-381] as well as the ingestion of some appetite suppressant drugs.[381a]

When the aortic annulus becomes greatly dilated, the aortic leaflets separate, and AR may ensue. Dissection of the diseased aortic wall may occur and aggravate the AR. Dilatation of the aortic root may also have secondary effects on the aortic valve because dilatation causes tension and bowing of the individual cusps, which may thicken, retract, and become too short to close the aortic orifice. This leads to intensification of the AR, further dilating the ascending aorta and thus leading to a vicious circle in which, as is the case for MR, "regurgitation begets regurgitation."

AR, regardless of its cause, produces dilatation and hypertrophy of the left ventricle, dilatation of the mitral valve ring, and sometimes hypertrophy and dilatation of the left atrium. Endocardial pockets frequently develop in the left ventricular cavity at sites of impact of the regurgitant jet.

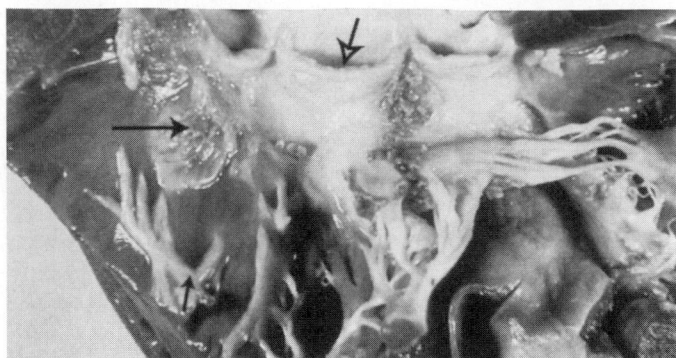

FIGURE 46–35. Chronic rheumatic aortic regurgitation with cuspal fibrosis, thickening, and retraction, with a jet lesion consisting of endocardial fibrosis (large arrow) and a "pocket" (small arrow) below the valve. Warty, small vegetations resulting from acute rheumatic fever are on the aortic valve edge, the aortic and mitral valve leaflets, and the chordae tendinae (open arrow). (From Rozich JD, et al: Mitral valve replacement with and without chordal preservation in patients with chronic mitral regurgitation: Mechanisms for differences in postoperative ejection performance. Circulation 86:7718, 1992.)

PATHOPHYSIOLOGY (Fig. 46–36)

In contrast to MR, in which a fraction of the left ventricular stroke volume is ejected into the low-pressure left atrium, in AR the entire left ventricular stroke volume is ejected

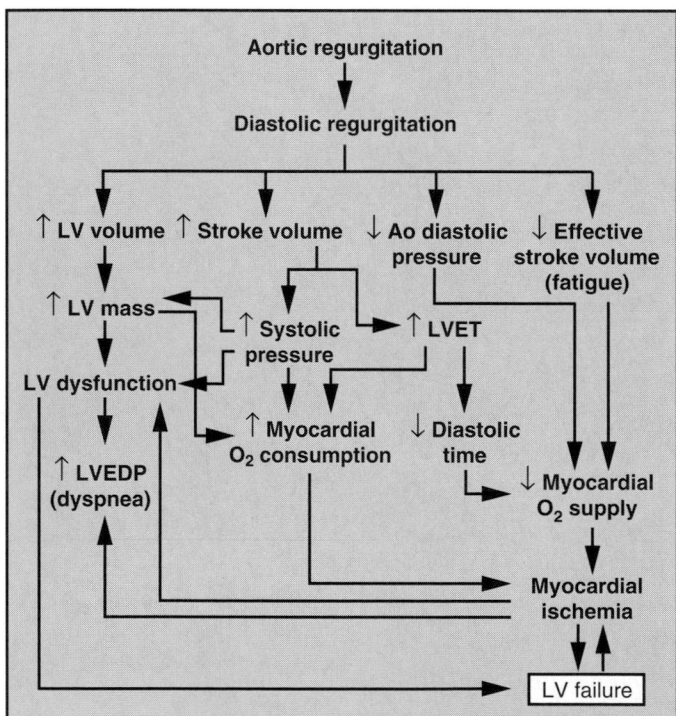

FIGURE 46–36. Pathophysiology of aortic regurgitation. Aortic regurgitation results in an increased left ventricular (LV) volume, increased stroke volume, increased aortic (Ao) systolic pressure, and decreased effective stroke volume. Increased LV volume results in an increased LV mass, which may lead to LV dysfunction and failure. Increased LV stroke volume increases systolic pressure and prolongation of left ventricular ejection time (LVET). Increased LV systolic pressure results in a decrease in diastolic time. Decreased diastolic time (myocardial perfusion time), diastolic aortic pressure, and effective stroke volume reduce myocardial O_2 supply. Increased myocardial O_2 consumption and decreased myocardial O_2 supply produce myocardial ischemia, which further deteriorates LV function ($\uparrow$ = increased, $\downarrow$ = decreased). (From Boudoulas H, Gravanis MB: Valvular heart disease. *In* Gravanis MB: Cardiovascular Disorders: Pathogenesis and Pathophysiology. St. Louis, CV Mosby Co, 1993, p 64.)

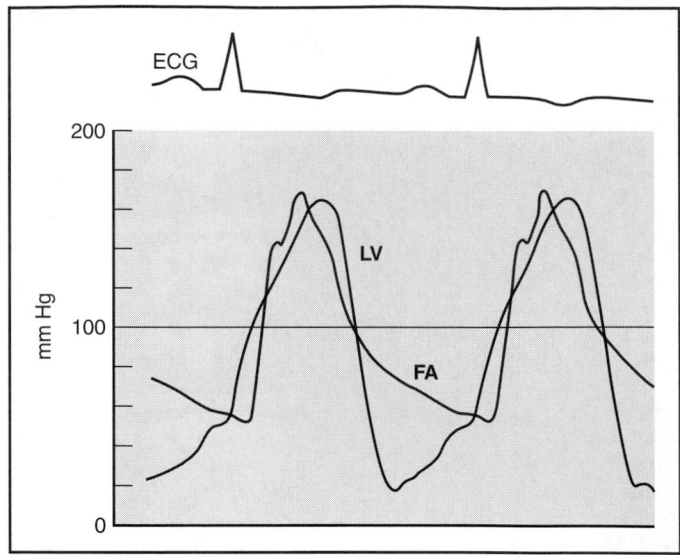

FIGURE 46–37. Pressure curves obtained from a 63-year-old man with symptoms of left ventricular failure and a loud decrescendo diastolic murmur. The femoral arterial (FA) pressure tracing demonstrates a widened pulse pressure of 115 mm Hg and equalization with left ventricular (LV) pressure late in diastole. The LV pressure curve exhibits a steady pressure increase throughout diastole, culminating in a markedly elevated end-diastolic pressure of 45 mm Hg. These findings are indicative of severe aortic regurgitation.

into a high-pressure chamber, i.e., the aorta (although the low aortic diastolic pressure does facilitate ventricular emptying during early systole). In MR, especially acute MR, the reduction of wall tension (i.e., reduced afterload) allows more complete systolic emptying; in AR the increase in left ventricular end-diastolic volume (i.e., increased preload) provides hemodynamic compensation.[382, 383]

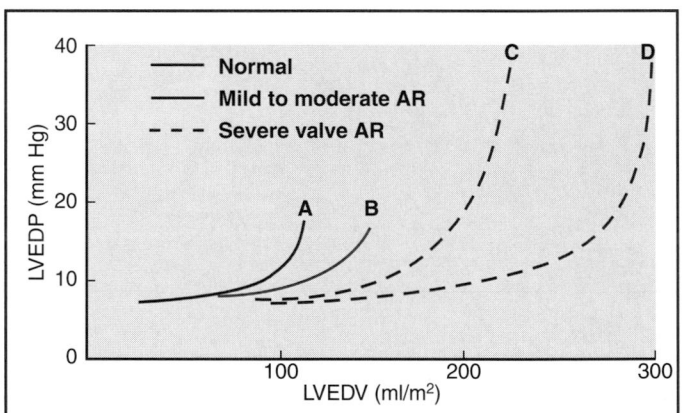

FIGURE 46–38. Left ventricular (LV) diastolic pressure-volume (P-V) curve relationships: effects of chronic valve regurgitation. When the AR is mild to moderate, the LV end-diastolic volume (LVEDV) is increased moderately, the LV diastolic P-V curve is moved to the right (curve B) of normal (curve A) and the LV end-diastolic pressure (LVEDP) is usually normal. In severe AR, the LV diastolic P-V curves are moved to the right (curves C and D). If the LV systolic pump function is normal, the LVEDV can be quite large without significant elevation of LVEDP (curve C). However, if the LVEDV increases further, the LVEDP will be increased. If LV systolic pump dysfunction supervenes, the LV diastolic P-V curve relationships are moved even further to the right (curve D) with quite marked LV dilatation and increases in LVEDP. (From Rahimtoola SH: Aortic valve regurgitation. *In* Rahimtoola SH (ed): Valvular Heart Disease. Atlas of Heart Diseases. Vol. 11. Braunwald E, series ed. Philadelphia, Current Medicine, 1997, pp 7.1–7.26 Adapted from Rahimtoola SH: Management of heart failure in valve regurgitation. Clin Cardiol 15(Suppl I):322–327, 1992.)

Severe AR may occur with a normal effective forward stroke volume and a normal ejection fraction (forward plus regurgitant stroke volume/end-diastolic volume), together with an elevated left ventricular end-diastolic volume, pressure, and stress[384] (Fig. 46–37). In accord with Laplace's law (which indicates that wall tension is related to the product of the intraventricular pressure and radius divided by wall thickness), left ventricular dilatation also increases the left ventricular systolic tension required to develop any level of systolic pressure. The volume overload leads to eccentric hypertrophy, with replication of sarcomeres in series and elongation of myocytes and myocardial fibers. In compensated AR, there is sufficient wall thickening so that the ratio of ventricular wall thickness to cavity radius remains normal. This maintains or returns end-diastolic wall stress to normal levels.[385] AR contrasts with AS, in which there is pressure overload (concentric) hypertrophy with replication of sarcomeres largely in parallel and an increased ratio of wall thickness to radius. In AR, left ventricular mass is usually greatly increased, often to levels even higher than in isolated AS,[276] and sometimes exceeding 1000 g. As AR persists and increases in severity over time, wall thickening fails to keep pace with the hemodynamic load and end-systolic wall stress rises.[386, 387] At this point, the ejection fraction falls.

Patients with severe chronic AR have the largest end-diastolic volumes of those with any form of heart disease (resulting in so-called cor bovinum). However, end-diastolic pressure is not uniformly elevated (i.e., left ventricular compliance is often increased [Fig. 46–38]).[388]

In the more severe cases of AR, the regurgitant flow may exceed 20 liters/min, so that the total left ventricular output at rest approaches 25 liters/min, a level that can be achieved acutely only by a trained endurance runner during maximal exercise. Thus, the adaptive response to gradually increasing, chronic AR permits the ventricle to function as an effective high-compliance pump, handling a large stroke volume, often with little increase in filling pressure. During exercise, peripheral vascular resistance declines, and with an increase in heart rate, diastole shortens and the regurgitation per beat decreases,[389, 390] facilitating an increment in effective (forward) cardiac output without substantial increases in end-diastolic volume and pressure. The ejection fraction and related ejection phase indices are often within normal limits, both at rest and during exercise, even though myocardial function, as reflected in the slope of the end-systolic pressure-volume relationship, is depressed.

LEFT VENTRICULAR FUNCTION. As the left ventricle decompensates, interstitial fibrosis increases, compliance declines, and left ventricular end-diastolic pressure and volume rise (Fig. 46–39). In advanced stages of decompensation, left atrial, pulmonary artery wedge, pulmonary arterial, right ventricular, and right atrial pressures rise and the effective (forward) cardiac output falls, at first during exercise[390] and then at rest. The normal decline in end-systolic volume or the rise in ejection fraction fails to occur during exercise. Symptoms of heart failure, particularly those secondary to pulmonary congestion, develop.

MYOCARDIAL ISCHEMIA. When *acute* AR is induced experimentally, myocardial oxygen requirements rise substantially,[132] secondary to an increase in wall tension. In patients with chronic, severe AR, total myocardial oxygen requirements are also augmented by the increase in left ventricular mass. Because the major portion of coronary blood flow occurs during diastole, when arterial pressure is lower than nor-

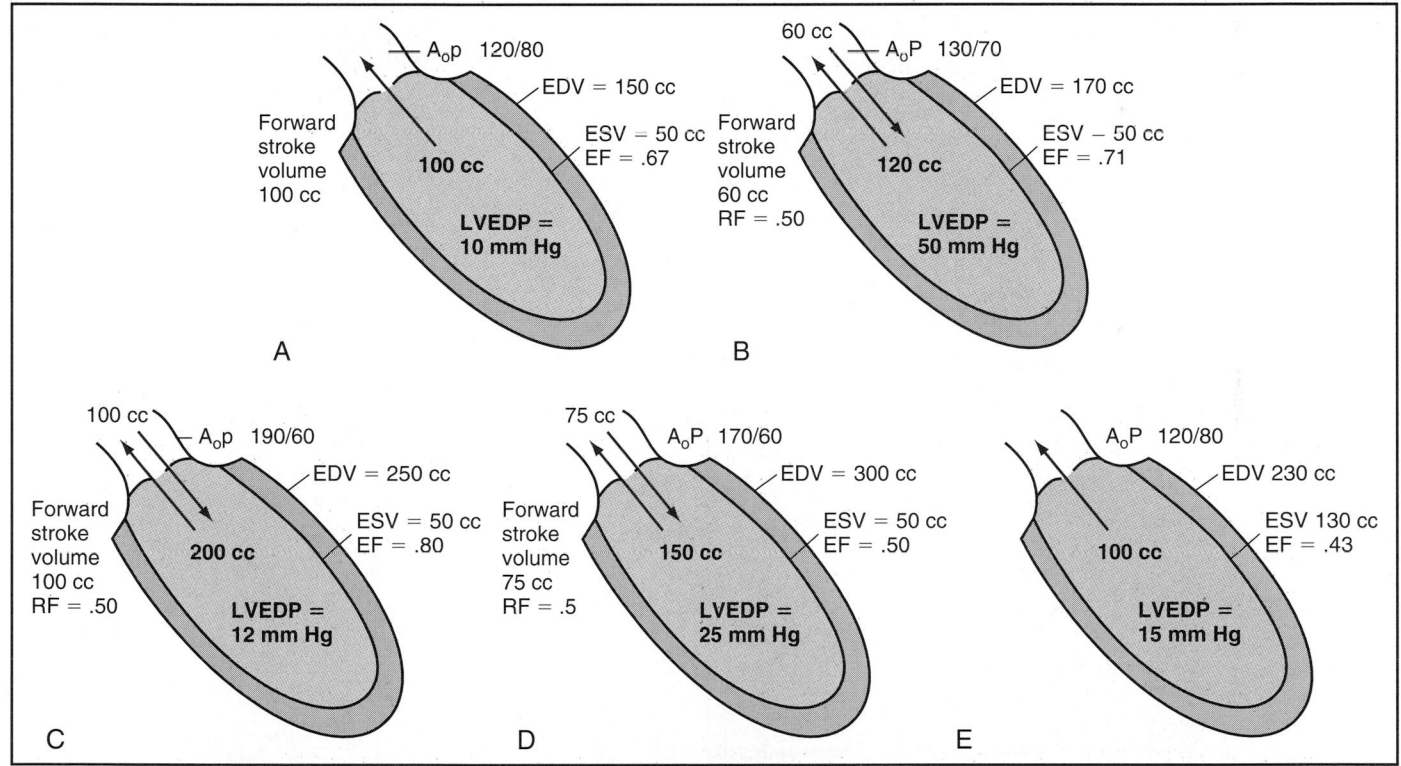

FIGURE 46–39. Hemodynamics of aortic regurgitation. *A,* Normal conditions. *B,* The hemodynamic changes that occur in severe acute aortic regurgitation. Although total stroke volume is increased, forward stroke volume is reduced. Left ventricular end-diastolic pressure rises dramatically. *C,* Hemodynamic changes occurring in chronic compensated aortic regurgitation are shown. Eccentric hypertrophy produces increased end-diastolic volume, which permits an increase in total as well as forward stroke volume. The volume overload is accommodated and left ventricular filling pressure is normalized. Ventricular emptying and end-systolic volume remain normal. *D,* In chronic decompensated aortic regurgitation, impaired left ventricular emptying produces an increase in end-systolic volume and a fall in ejection fraction, total stroke volume, and forward stroke volume. There is further cardiac dilatation and re-elevation of left ventricular filling pressure. *E,* Immediately following valve replacement, preload estimated by end-diastolic volume decreases, as does filling pressure. End-systolic volume also is decreased, but to a lesser extent. The result is an initial fall in ejection fraction. Despite these changes, elimination of regurgitation leads to an increase in forward stroke volume. AoP = aortic pressure; EDV = end-diastolic volume; ESV = end-systolic volume; EF = ejection fraction; LVEDP = left ventricular end-diastolic pressure; RF = regurgitant fraction. (From Carabello BA: Aortic regurgitation: Hemodynamic determinants of prognosis. *In* Cohn LH and DiSesa VJ [eds]: Aortic Regurgitation: Medical and Surgical Management. New York, Marcel Dekker, Inc, 1986.)

mal in AR, coronary perfusion pressure is reduced. Studies in experimentally induced AR have shown a reduction in coronary flow reserve with a change in forward coronary flow from diastole to systole.[391] The result—a combination of increased oxygen demand and reduced supply—sets the stage for the development of myocardial ischemia, especially during exercise.[392] Thus, patients with severe AR exhibit a reduction of coronary reserve,[393] which may be responsible for myocardial ischemia, which in turn may play a role in the deterioration of left ventricular function.

Acute Aortic Regurgitation

Acute AR is caused most commonly by infective endocarditis, aortic dissection, or trauma. In contrast to the pathophysiological events in chronic AR just described, in which the left ventricle is able to adapt to the increased hemodynamic load, in acute AR the regurgitant volume fills a ventricle of normal size that cannot accommodate the combined large regurgitant volume and inflow from the left atrium.[394] Because the ability of total stroke volume to rise acutely is limited, forward stroke volume declines. The sudden increase in left ventricular filling causes the left ventricular diastolic pressure to rise rapidly above left atrial pressure during early diastole,[382] causing the mitral valve to close prematurely in diastole (Fig. 46–40).[395] Premature closure of the mitral valve protects the pulmonary venous bed from backward transmission of the greatly elevated end-diastolic pressure unless it is accompanied by diastolic mitral regurgitation.[396] Premature closure of the mitral valve, together with tachycardia that also shortens diastole, reduces the time interval during which the mitral valve is open. Left ventricular and aortic *systolic* pressures exhibit little change. Because aortic diastolic pressure cannot decline below the elevated left ventricular end-diastolic pressure, the systemic arterial pulse pressure widens relatively little.

History

CHRONIC AORTIC REGURGITATION. In patients with chronic, severe AR, the left ventricle gradually enlarges while the patient remains asymptomatic or almost so.[397] Symptoms of reduced cardiac reserve or myocardial ischemia develop, most often in the fourth or fifth decade and usually only *after* considerable cardiomegaly and myocardial dysfunction have occurred. The principal complaints of exertional dyspnea, orthopnea, and paroxysmal nocturnal dyspnea usually develop gradually. Angina pectoris is prominent late in the course; nocturnal angina may be troublesome and is often accompanied by diaphoresis that occurs when the heart rate slows and arterial diastolic pressure falls to extremely low levels. Patients with severe AR often complain of an uncomfortable awareness of the heartbeat, especially on lying down, and disagreeable thoracic pain due to pounding of the heart against the chest wall. Tachycardia, occurring with emotional stress or exertion, may cause troubling palpitations and head pounding. Premature ventricular contractions are particularly distressing because of the great heave of the volume-loaded left ventricle during the postpremature beat. These complaints may be present for many years before symptoms of overt left ventricular dysfunction develop.

ACUTE AORTIC REGURGITATION. In light of the limited ability of the left ventricle to tolerate acute, severe AR, patients with this valvular lesion often develop clinical manifestations of sudden cardiovascular collapse, including weakness, severe dyspnea, and hypotension secondary to the reduced stroke volume and elevated left atrial pressure.

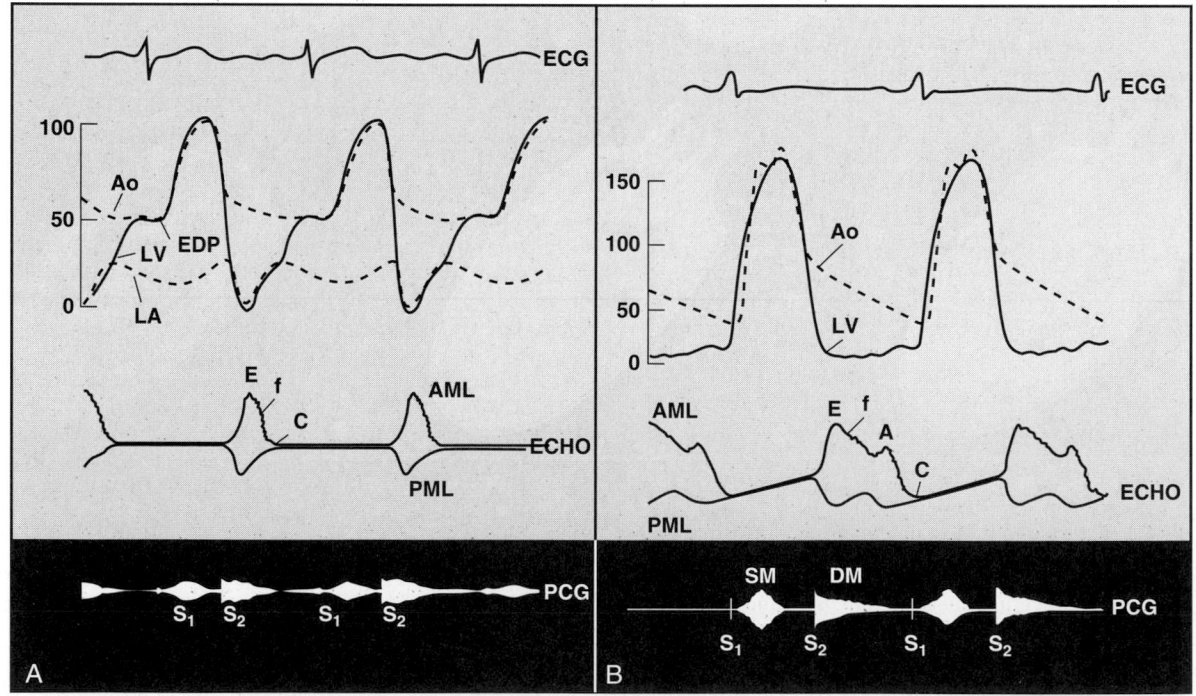

FIGURE 46–40. Schematic representations contrasting the hemodynamic, echocardiographic (ECHO), and phonocardiographic (PCG) manifestations of acute severe (*A*) and chronic severe (*B*) aortic regurgitation. Ao = aorta; LV = left ventricle; LA = left atrium; EDP = end-diastolic pressure; f = flutter of anterior mitral valve leaflet; AML = anterior mitral valve leaflet; PML = posterior mitral valve leaflet; SM = systolic murmur; DM = diastolic murmur; C = closure point of mitral valve. (From Morganroth J et al: Acute severe aortic regurgitation. Ann Intern Med 87:225, 1977.)

Physical Examination (See also Chap. 4)

In patients with chronic, severe AR, the head frequently bobs with each heartbeat (*de Musset sign*),[398] and the pulses are of the "water-hammer" or collapsing type with abrupt distention and quick collapse (*Corrigan pulse*). The arterial pulse is often prominent and can be best appreciated by palpation of the radial artery with the patient's arm elevated. A *bisferiens pulse* may be present (see Fig. 4–8C) and is more readily recognized in the brachial and femoral arteries than in the carotid arteries. A variety of auscultatory findings provide confirmation of a wide pulse pressure. *Traube sign* (also known as "pistol shot sounds"[399]) refers to booming systolic and diastolic sounds heard over the femoral artery, *Müller sign* consists of systolic pulsations of the uvula, and *Duroziez sign* consists of a systolic murmur heard over the femoral artery when it is compressed proximally and a diastolic murmur when it is compressed distally. Capillary pulsations, i.e., *Quincke sign,* can be detected by pressing a glass slide on the patient's lip or by transmitting a light through the patient's fingertips.

Systolic arterial pressure is elevated, and diastolic pressure is abnormally low. *Hill sign* refers to popliteal cuff systolic pressure exceeding brachial cuff pressure by more than 60 mm Hg. Korotkoff sounds often persist to zero even though intraarterial pressure rarely falls below 30 mm Hg. The point of change in Korotkoff sounds, i.e., the muffling of these sounds in phase IV, correlates with the diastolic pressure. As heart failure develops, peripheral vasoconstriction may occur and arterial diastolic pressure may rise. This finding should not be interpreted as the presence of mild AR.

The apical impulse is diffuse and hyperdynamic and is displaced laterally and inferiorly; there may be systolic retraction over the parasternal region. A rapid ventricular filling wave is often palpable at the apex (as is a *systolic thrill*), at the base of the heart or suprasternal notch, and over the carotid arteries, resulting from the augmented stroke volume. In many patients, a carotid shudder is palpable or may be recorded.[400]

CHRONIC AORTIC REGURGITATION. The PR interval may be prolonged, causing a soft S_1. A_2 may be normal or accentuated when AR is due to disease of the aortic root, but is soft or absent when the valve is causing AR. P_2 may be obscured by the early diastolic murmur. Thus, S_2 may be absent or single or exhibit narrow or paradoxical splitting. A systolic ejection sound, presumably related to abrupt distention of the aorta by the augmented stroke volume, is frequently audible. An S_3 gallop correlates with an increased left ventricular end-diastolic volume. Its development may be a sign of impaired left ventricular function, which is useful in identifying patients with severe regurgitation who are candidates for surgical treatment.

The aortic regurgitant murmur, the principal physical finding of AR,[401] is one of high frequency that begins immediately after A_2. It may be distinguished from the murmur of pulmonic regurgitation by its earlier onset, i.e., immediately after A_2 rather than after P_2, and usually by the presence of a widened pulse pressure. The murmur is heard best with the diaphragm of the stethoscope while the patient is sitting up and leaning forward, with the breath held in deep exhalation. In severe AR, the murmur reaches an early peak and then has a dominant decrescendo pattern throughout diastole.

The severity of the regurgitation correlates better with the *duration* than with the *intensity* of the murmur. In mild AR, the murmur may be limited to early diastole and is typically high pitched and blowing. In severe AR, the murmur is holodiastolic and may have a rough quality. When the murmur is musical ("cooing dove" murmur), it usually signifies eversion or perforation of an aortic cusp. In pa-

tients with severe AR and left ventricular decompensation, equilibration of aortic and left ventricular pressures in late diastole (see Fig. 46–40) abolishes this component of the regurgitant murmur. When regurgitation is caused by primary valvular disease, the diastolic murmur is heard best along the left sternal border in the 3rd and 4th intercostal spaces. However, when it is due mainly to dilatation of the ascending aorta, the murmur is often more readily audible along the right sternal border.

A mid- and late diastolic apical rumble, the *Austin Flint murmur,* is common in severe AR and may occur in the presence of a normal mitral valve. This murmur appears to be created by rapid antegrade flow across a mitral orifice that is narrowed by the rapidly rising left ventricular diastolic pressure caused by severe aortic reflux impinging on the anterior leaflet of the mitral valve.[402] The Austin Flint murmur may be difficult to differentiate from that due to MS, but the presence of an opening snap and a loud S_1 in MS and the absence of these findings in AR are helpful clues. As the left ventricular end-diastolic pressure rises, the Austin Flint murmur commences and terminates earlier, and in acute AR with premature diastolic closure of the mitral valve, the presystolic portion of the Austin Flint murmur is eliminated. A short midsystolic murmur, caused by the increased ejection rate and stroke volume, may be audible at the base of the heart and transmitted to the carotid vessels. It may be higher pitched and less rasping than the murmur of AS but is often accompanied by a systolic thrill.

DYNAMIC AUSCULTATION. The diastolic murmur of AR may be accentuated when the patient sits up and leans forward or by interventions that raise the arterial pressure, such as squatting or isometric exercise. The intensity of the murmur is reduced by interventions that lower the systolic pressure, such as inhalation of amyl nitrite or the strain of the Valsalva maneuver. The Austin Flint murmur, like the murmur of AR, is augmented by isometric exercise and administration of vasopressors and is reduced by amyl nitrite inhalation.[403]

ACUTE AORTIC REGURGITATION. Patients with acute, severe AR appear gravely ill, with tachycardia, severe peripheral vasoconstriction and cyanosis, and sometimes pulmonary congestion and edema.[394, 404] The peripheral signs of AR are often not impressive and certainly not as dramatic as in patients with chronic AR. Duroziez murmur, Traube sign over the peripheral arteries, and bisferiens pulses are usually *absent* in acute AR. The normal or only slightly widened pulse pressure may lead to serious underestimation of the severity of the valvular lesion. The left ventricular impulse is normal or nearly so, and the rocking motion of the chest characteristic of chronic AR is not apparent. S_1 may be soft or absent because of premature closure of the mitral valve,[405] and the sound of mitral valve closure in mid- or late diastole is occasionally audible. However, closure of the mitral valve may be incomplete, and diastolic mitral regurgitation may occur.[395] Evidence of pulmonary hypertension, with an accentuated P_2, S_3, and S_4, is frequently present. The early diastolic murmur of acute AR is lower pitched and shorter than that of chronic AR, because as left ventricular diastolic pressure rises, the (reverse) pressure gradient between the aorta and the left ventricle is rapidly reduced. A systolic murmur is common, resulting in "to and fro" sounds. The Austin Flint murmur, if present, is brief and ceases when left ventricular pressure exceeds left atrial pressure in diastole.

LABORATORY EXAMINATION

ELECTROCARDIOGRAM. *Chronic,* severe AR results in left axis deviation and a pattern of left ventricular diastolic volume overload, characterized by an increase in initial forces (prominent Q waves in leads I, aVL, and V_3 through V_6) and a relatively small r wave in lead V_1 (Fig. 46–41). With the passage of time, these initial forces diminish, but the

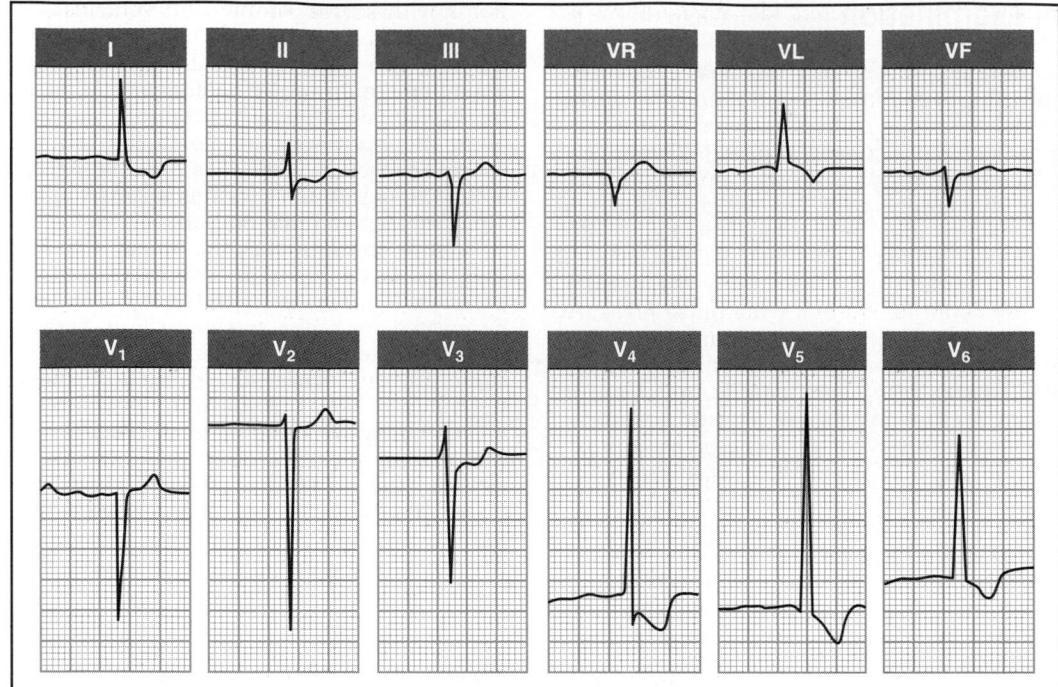

FIGURE 46–41. Atrial fibrillation and left ventricular hypertrophy in a patient with chronic AR. The most prominent features are the gross increase in precordial voltage ($RV_5 + SV_2 = 70$ mm) and the marked anterolateral ST/T wave changes (leads I, aVL, and V_4 through V_6). The patient had aortic regurgitation and normal coronary arteries and was not taking digitalis. (Normal standardization, i.e., 1 mV = 10 mm.) (From Hall RJ, Julian DG: Diseases of the Cardiac Valves. New York, Churchill Livingstone, 1989, p 39.)

total QRS amplitude increases (Fig. 5–20). The T waves may be tall and upright in the left precordial leads early in the course, but, more commonly they are inverted, with ST segment depressions. A left ventricular "strain" pattern correlates with the presence of dilatation and hypertrophy.[92, 406] Left intraventricular conduction defects occur late in the course and are usually associated with left ventricular dysfunction. The ECG is not an accurate predictor of the severity of AR or cardiac weight. When AR is caused by an inflammatory process, prolongation of the PR interval may be present.[407]

In *acute* AR, the ECG may or may not show left ventricular hypertrophy, depending upon the severity and duration of the regurgitation. However, nonspecific ST segment and T wave changes are common.

RADIOLOGICAL FINDINGS (See Figs. 8–4, 8–8, and 8–24.) Cardiac size is a function of the duration and severity of regurgitation and the state of left ventricular function. In acute AR, there may be minimal cardiac enlargement, but marked enlargement is a common finding in chronic AR. Typically, the left ventricle enlarges in an inferior and leftward direction, causing a significant increase in the long axis (see Fig. 8–24) but sometimes causing little or no increase in the transverse diameter of the heart. Calcification of the aortic valve is uncommon in patients with pure AR but is often present in patients with combined AS and AR. Distinct left atrial enlargement in the absence of heart failure suggests associated mitral valve disease. Dilatation of the ascending aorta is usually more marked than in AR and may involve the entire aortic arch, including the aortic knob. Severe aneurysmal dilatation of the aorta suggests that aortic root disease (e.g., the Marfan syndrome, cystic medial necrosis, or annuloaortic ectasia) is responsible for the AR. Linear calcifications in the wall of the ascending aorta are seen in syphilitic aortitis but are nonspecific and are observed in degenerative disease as well.

For angiographic assessment of AR, contrast material should be injected rapidly (i.e., 25 to 35 ml/sec) into the aortic root, and filming should be carried out in the right and left anterior oblique projections. Opacification may be improved by filming during a Valsalva maneuver. In acute AR, there is only a slight increase in ventricular end-diastolic volume, but with the passage of time both the end-diastolic volume and the thickness of the ventricular wall increase, usually in parallel.

ECHOCARDIOGRAPHY (See Figs. 7–64 to 7–67). This technique is helpful in identifying the cause of AR. The echocardiogram may show thickening of the valve cusps, prolapse of the valve, a flail leaflet, vegetations, or dilatation of the aortic root.[379] Two-dimensional studies are useful for the measurement of left ventricular end-diastolic and end-systolic dimensions, volumes, shortening fraction, ejec-

tion fraction, and mass. These measurements, when made serially, are of great value in selecting the optimal time for surgical intervention (see p. 1688). Although transthoracic imaging is usually satisfactory, transesophageal echocardiography often provides more detail.

In acute AR, the echocardiogram reveals a reduction in amplitude of the opening movement, premature closure and delayed opening of the mitral valve.[408] Left ventricular end-diastolic dimensions are not markedly increased, and fractional shortening is normal. This contrasts with the findings in chronic AR, in which end-diastolic dimensions and wall motion are increased. Occasionally, with equilibration of aortic and left ventricular pressures in diastole, premature opening of the aortic valve may be detected.[409]

High-frequency fluttering of the anterior leaflet of the mitral valve during diastole is an important echocardiographic finding in both acute and chronic AR; however, it does not develop when the mitral valve is rigid, as occurs with rheumatic involvement. This sign, which, unlike the Austin Flint murmur, occurs even in mild AR, results from the movement imparted to the anterior leaflet of the mitral valve by the jet of blood regurgitating from the aorta.

Doppler echocardiography and color flow Doppler imaging are the most sensitive and accurate noninvasive techniques in the assessment of AR.[410–413a] They readily detect mild degrees of AR that may be inaudible on physical examination. Both the aortic regurgitant orifice size and the aortic regurgitant flow can be estimated. Serial studies permit determination of the progression of regurgitation and its effect on the left ventricle.

RADIONUCLIDE IMAGING (See Chap. 9). Radionuclide angiography provides an accurate noninvasive assessment of the severity of AR by allowing determination of the regurgitant fraction and of the left ventricular/right ventricular stroke volume ratio.[414] This technique is nonspecific because the ratio is increased by the presence of associated MR and reduced by tricuspid or pulmonary regurgitation. However, in the absence of these complicating lesions, a left ventricular/right ventricular stroke volume ratio of 2.0

or more denotes severe AR. Radionuclide angiography is also of value in the assessment of left ventricular function in patients with AR.[415] Serial measurements are useful in the early detection of deterioration of left ventricular function.

MAGNETIC RESONANCE IMAGING (see Fig. 10–23). This technique provides accurate measurements of regurgitant volumes and of ventricular end-systolic and diastolic volumes and allows calculation of the regurgitant orifice and of ventricular mass.[416] Although expensive, nuclear magnetic resonance imaging is the most accurate noninvasive technique for assessing the patient with AR (see Chap. 10).

MANAGEMENT

The management of severe AR must take account of the natural history. Since this differs in patients with chronic and acute AR, the two disorders are presented separately.

NATURAL HISTORY OF CHRONIC AORTIC REGURGITATION. Moderately severe or even severe chronic AR may be associated with a generally favorable prognosis for many years. Approximately 75 percent of patients survive for 5 years and 50 percent for 10 years after diagnosis.[147] However, as is the case for AS, once the patient becomes symptomatic, the downhill course becomes progressive. Congestive heart failure, punctuated by episodes of acute pulmonary edema, and sudden death may occur, usually in previously symptomatic patients who have considerable left ventricular dilatation. Without surgical treatment, death usually occurs within 4 years after the development of angina pectoris and within 2 years after the onset of heart failure. In a multivariate analysis of patients with severe or moderately severe AR diagnosed by Doppler echocardiography, Dujardin and colleagues found that the following were associated with a poor outcome: advanced age, progressive symptoms, atrial fibrillation, and end-systolic diameter >25 mm/m² BSA.[417] Gradual deterioration of left ventricular function may occur even during the asymptomatic period; it is therefore important to intervene surgically before these changes have become irreversible.[418] A review of multiple studies on the natural history of chronic AR has been described by Bonow and associates[51] (Table 46–9).

ACUTE AORTIC REGURGITATION. Since early death due to left ventricular failure is frequent in patients with *acute, severe* AR despite intensive medical management, prompt surgical intervention is indicated. Even a normal ventricle cannot sustain the burden of acute, severe volume overload; therefore, the risk of *acute* AR is much greater than that of chronic AR.[394, 404] While the patient is being prepared for surgery, treatment with an intravenous positive

▼ **TABLE 46–9. NATURAL HISTORY OF AORTIC REGURGITATION**

Asymptomatic patients with normal LV systolic function:	
• Progression to symptoms and or LV dysfunction	<6%/yr
• Progression to asymptomatic LV dysfunction	<3.5%/yr
• Sudden death	<0.2%/yr
Asymptomatic patients with LV systolic dysfunction:	
• Progression to cardiac symptoms	>25%/yr
Symptomatic patients:	
• Mortality rate	>10%/yr

LV = left ventricular.
From Bonow RO, Carabello B, de Leon AC Jr, et al: ACC/AHA Guidelines for the management of patients with valvular heart disease. J Am Coll Cardiol 32:1486, 1998.

inotropic agent (dopamine or dobutamine) and/or a vasodilator (nitroprusside) may be necessary. The agent and dosage should be selected on the basis of arterial pressure (see Chap. 21). Beta-blocking agents and intraaortic balloon counterpulsation are contraindicated. In hemodynamically stable patients with acute AR secondary to active infective endocarditis, operation may be deferred to allow 5 to 7 days of intensive antibiotic therapy. However, AVR should be undertaken at the earliest sign of hemodynamic instability or if echocardiographic evidence of diastolic closure of the mitral valve develops.[419]

Medical Treatment

Patients with mild or moderate AR who are asymptomatic with normal or only minimally increased cardiac size require no therapy but should be followed clinically and by echocardiography every 12 or 24 months. These patients should also receive antibiotic prophylaxis for infective endocarditis. Asymptomatic patients with chronic, severe AR and normal left ventricular function should be examined at intervals of approximately 6 months. In addition to clinical examination, serial echocardiographic assessments of left ventricular size and ejection fraction should be made. Left-heart catheterization and aortography are useful in patients whose noninvasive test results are inconclusive or discordant with clinical findings.[51] As is the case for patients with other valvular lesions, adult surgical candidates who may need coronary artery bypass grafting should undergo coronary arteriography.

Patients with limitations of cardiac reserve and/or left ventricular dysfunction secondary to AR should not engage in vigorous sports or heavy exertion. Systemic arterial diastolic hypertension, if present, should be treated because it increases the regurgitant flow; however, beta-blocking agents should be used with great caution. Atrial fibrillation and bradyarrhythmias are poorly tolerated and should be prevented if possible. If these arrhythmias occur, they must be treated promptly and vigorously. Even though nitroglycerin and other nitrates are not as helpful in relieving anginal pain in patients with AR as they are in patients with coronary artery disease or AS, they are worth a trial. Although patients with left ventricular failure secondary to AR require prompt surgical treatment, they respond, at least temporarily, to treatment with digitalis glycosides, salt restriction, and diuretics.

The response to vasodilator therapy is often impressive. Hemodynamic studies have shown beneficial effects of intravenous hydralazine,[420] sublingual nifedipine,[421] felodipine,[421a] as well as oral prazosin.[422] Vasodilator therapy may be particularly helpful in stabilizing patients with acute lesions or those with decompensated chronic AR who are awaiting operation. However, because of the high incidence of side effects of hydralazine, attention has focused on calcium antagonists and angiotensin-converting enzyme (ACE) inhibitors.[423] In a comparison of digoxin with nifedipine in asymptomatic patients with severe AR, nifedipine delayed the need for operation as the result of development of symptoms or of left ventricular dysfunction.[424] In children with severe AR, therapy with an ACE inhibitor for one year has been reported to reverse ventricular dilatation and left ventricular wall stress.[425]

Thus, vasodilator therapy is indicated for patients with chronic, severe AR under the following circumstances: (1) as short-term therapy to improve the hemodynamic profile in the presence of heart failure while preparing for AVR; (2) as chronic therapy for patients in whom AVR is not possible; (3) as therapy for asymptomatic patients; and (4) as therapy for patients with left ventricular dysfunction after AVR.[51]

Surgical Treatment

INDICATIONS FOR OPERATION. Because of their excellent prognosis in the short and medium term, operative correction should be deferred in patients with chronic, severe AR who are asymptomatic, have good exercise tolerance, *and* have an ejection fraction greater than 50 percent *without* severe left ventricular dilatation (i.e., an end-diastolic diameter <70 mm and an end-systolic diameter <50 mm). Similarly, in the absence of obvious contraindications or serious comorbidity, surgical treatment is advisable for symptomatic patients with severe AR. Between these two ends of the clinical-hemodynamic spectrum are many patients in whom it may be quite difficult to balance the immediate risks of operation and the continuing risks of an implanted prosthetic valve on the one hand against the hazards of allowing a severe volume overload to damage the left ventricle on the other.[426–428]

Since severe symptoms (NYHA Class III or IV) and left ventricular dysfunction with an ejection fraction less than 40 percent are independent risk factors for poor postoperative survival, surgery should be carried out in NYHA Class II patients before severe left ventricular dysfunction has developed.[51] Even after successful correction of AR, patients with severe left ventricular dysfunction may have persistent cardiomegaly and depressed left ventricular function.[429–431] Such patients often exhibit histological changes in the left ventricle, including massive fiber hypertrophy and increased interstitial fibrous tissue. Therefore, it is highly desirable to operate on patients *before* irreversible left ventricular changes have occurred.

Because AR has complex effects on both preload and afterload, the selection of appropriate indices of ventricular contractility to identify patients for operation is challenging. The relationship between end-systolic wall stress and ejection fraction or percent fractional shortening is a useful measurement.[136] However, in the absence of such measurements, *serial* changes in ventricular end-diastolic and end-systolic volumes or dimensions can be used to detect *relative* deterioration of ventricular function. Although left ventricular end-diastolic volume and the ejection phase indices such as ejection fraction and ventricular fraction shortening are strongly influenced by loading conditions, they are nonetheless useful empirical predictors of postoperative function.

Serial echocardiograms or radionuclide ventriculograms should be obtained to detect changes in left ventricular size and function in asymptomatic patients with severe AR. Both techniques allow repeated evaluation of ejection fraction and end-systolic volume (or dimensions) both at rest and during exercise. Impaired left ventricular function at *rest* is the basis for selecting patients for operation; normal left ventricular function at rest with failure of the ejection fraction to rise normally with *exercise* is not considered an indication for surgery *per se,* but is an early warning sign that portends impaired function at rest.[432]

Bonow and colleagues have reported that asymptomatic patients with severe AR but normal left ventricular function have an excellent prognosis and do not warrant prophylactic operation (see Table 46–9).[427] Less than 4 percent of patients per year require operation because of the development of symptoms of left ventricular dysfunction. The end-systolic diameter determined by two-dimensional echocardiography is valuable in predicting outcome in asymptomatic patients. Patients with severe AR and an end-systolic diameter less than 40 mm almost invariably remain stable and can be followed without immediate surgery. However, patients with an end-systolic diameter greater than 55 mm (see Fig. 46–43), an end-systolic volume greater than 55 ml/m², an end-diastolic volume greater than 200 ml/m², or an ejection fraction less than 50 percent have an increased risk of death secondary to left ventricular dysfunction if they are not operated upon. Furthermore, Bonow and coworkers found that patients with *prolonged* left ventricular dysfunction had poor postoperative survival.[430]

In *summary,* the following considerations apply to the selection of patients with chronic AR for surgical treatment. Operation should be *deferred* in asymptomatic patients with normal and stable left ventricular function and should be *recommended* in symptomatic patients. In asymptomatic patients with left ventricular dysfunction, a decision should be based not on a single abnormal measurement but rather on several observations of depressed performance and impaired exercise tolerance, carried out at intervals of 2 to 4 months. If evidence of left ventricular dysfunction is borderline or is not consistent, continued close follow-up is indicated. If abnormalities are progressive or consistent (i.e., the left ventricular ejection fraction declines to 50 to 55 percent, the left ventricular end-systolic diameter rises to >55 mm, or the left ventricular end-systolic volume increases to >55 ml/m² [the "55 rule"[124]]), operation should be strongly considered even in asymptomatic patients. The threshold for operation may be lower when the surgeon believes that AVR will not be necessary (to be discussed), but this prediction may be difficult. Symptomatic patients with severe AR who have normal, mildly depressed, or moderately depressed left ventricular function should be operated upon. Patients with severely impaired left ventricular function (ejection fraction < 25 percent) are at high surgical risk and have a guarded prognosis even after suc-

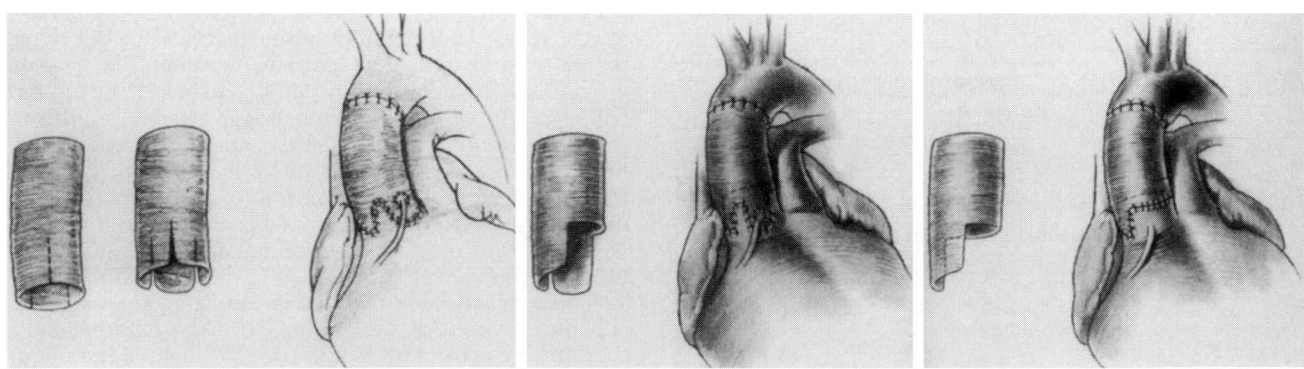

FIGURE 46–42. Repair of the aortic valve in patient with severe AR. Conduit tailoring in the supravalvular position. The conduit is cut to replace three (*left*), two (*middle*), or one (*right*) individual sinuses. The aortic aneurysm is replaced and the valve is spared. (From David TE, Feindel CM, Bos J: Repair of the aortic valve in patients with aortic insufficiency and aortic root aneurysm. J Thorac Cardiovasc Surg 109: 345, 1995.)

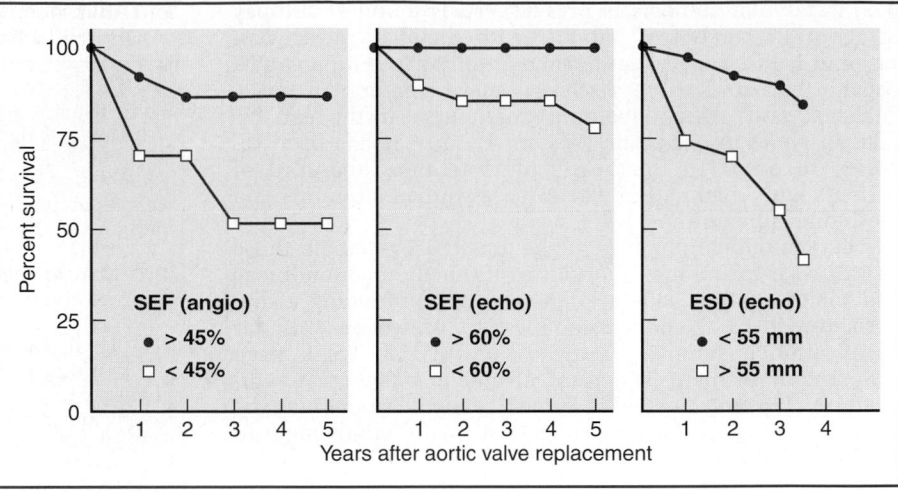

FIGURE 46–43. Relation of preoperative ventricular function to postoperative survival. Data of Greves and colleagues (*left*) and those of Bonow and associates (*right*) show remarkable agreement: Both groups incorporated limits clearly in the abnormal range. Cunha and coworkers (*center*) selected a limit that was well within normal range. These and other published data indicate that preoperative ventricular function is an important determinant of postoperative survival. SEF = systolic ejection fraction; ESD = echocardiographically measured dimension at end-systole; angio = angiography; echo = echocardiography. (From Errichetti A et al: Is valve replacement indicated in asymptomatic patients with aortic stenosis or aortic regurgitation? *In* Cheitlin M [ed]: Dilemmas in Clinical Cardiology. Philadelphia, FA Davis Co, 1990, p 204.)

cessful AVR. Their outlook is also poor when they receive medical therapy, and their management should be considered on an individual basis.

The indications for surgery in patients with severe AR secondary to aortic root disease are similar to those in patients with primary valvular disease. However, progressive expansion of the aortic root and/or a diameter greater than 50 mm by echocardiography with any degree of regurgitation is also an indication for surgery in patients with aortic root disease.

OPERATIVE PROCEDURES. Because an increasing proportion of patients with severe, isolated AR coming to operation now have primary aortic root rather than primary valvular disease, an increasing number can be treated surgically by correcting the dilated aortic root.[433] One of two annuloplasty procedures may be employed—an encircling suture of the aorta or a subcommissural annuloplasty. Aneurysmal dilatation of the ascending aorta requires excision, replacement with a graft that includes a prosthetic valve, and reimplantation of the coronary arteries.[434]

AVR is required for a large majority of patients with severe AR due to primary valve disease (as opposed to aortic root disease) and for many patients with combined AS and AR. In some patients with aortic root disease, the native valve can be spared when the aortic root is replaced (Fig. 46–42). Because the aortic annulus in patients with severe AR is usually not as narrow as it is in patients with AS, a larger prosthetic valve can be inserted, and mild postoperative obstruction to left ventricular outflow is less of a problem than it is in some patients with AS (to be discussed). Occasionally, when a leaflet has been torn from its attachments to the aortic annulus by trauma, surgical replacement without repair may be possible. In patients with AR secondary to prolapse of an aortic leaflet, aortic cusp resuspension or cusp resection may be employed.

When AR is caused by leaflet perforation resulting from healed infective endocarditis, a pericardial patch can be used for repair.[435, 436]

In general, the risks and results of AVR in patients with AR are similar to those in patients with AS (see p. 1679), with a large percentage of patients exhibiting striking improvement in symptoms. Reductions in heart size and in left ventricular diastolic volume and mass occur in the majority of patients. Exceptions are patients who are in Class NYHA III or IV heart failure and/or patients who have severe left ventricular dysfunction preoperatively.[433] As is true for patients with AS, the operative risk of AVR for patients with AR depends on the general condition of the patient, the state of left ventricular function, and the skill and experience of the surgical team.[437] The mortality rate ranges from 3 to 8 percent in most medical centers (see Table 46–2). A late mortality of approximately 5 to 10 percent per year is observed in survivors who had marked cardiac enlargement and/or prolonged left ventricular dysfunction preoperatively (Fig. 46–43). Follow-up studies have shown both early rapid and then slower long-term reductions of ventricular mass, ejection fraction, myocyte hypertrophy, and ventricular fibrous content following relief of AR.[296, 350] By extending the indications for operation to symptomatic patients with normal left ventricular function as well as to asymptomatic patients with left ventricular dysfunction, both early and late results are improving.[437] With the continued improvement of surgical techniques and results, it will likely become possible to extend the recommendation for operative treatment to asymptomatic patients with severe regurgitation and normal cardiac function. However, given the risks of operation and the long-term complications of presently available prosthetic valves, I believe that the time for such a policy has not yet arrived.

Tricuspid, Pulmonic, and Multivalvular Disease

TRICUSPID STENOSIS

Etiology and Pathology

Tricuspid stenosis (TS) is almost always rheumatic in origin.[7] Other causes of obstruction to right atrial emptying are unusual and include congenital tricuspid atresia (see Chap. 43); right atrial tumors, which may produce a clinical picture suggesting rapidly progressive TS[438] (see Chap. 49); and the carcinoid syndrome (see Chap. 48), which more

frequently produces tricuspid regurgitation. Rarely, obstruction to right ventricular inflow can be due to endomyocardial fibrosis, tricuspid valve vegetations,[438a] a pacemaker lead,[438b] or extracardiac tumors.

The majority of patients with rheumatic tricuspid valve disease present with tricuspid regurgitation or a combination of stenosis and regurgitation. Isolated rheumatic TS is uncommon and *almost* never occurs as an isolated lesion but generally accompanies mitral valve disease.[51, 439] In many patients with TS, the aortic valve is also involved (i.e., trivalvular stenosis is present). TS is found at autopsy in about 15 percent of patients with rheumatic heart disease but is of clinical significance in only about 5 percent.[92] Organic tricuspid valve disease is more common in India, Pakistan, and other developing nations near the equator than in North America or Western Europe; it has been reported to occur in the hearts of more than one-third of patients with rheumatic heart disease studied at autopsy on the Indian subcontinent.[440]

The anatomical changes of rheumatic TS resemble those of MS, with fusion and shortening of the chordae tendineae and fusion of the leaflets at their edges, producing a diaphragm with a fixed central aperture. However, valvular calcification is rare. As is the case with MS, TS is more common in women. The right atrium is often greatly dilated in TS, and its walls are thickened. There may be evidence of severe passive congestion, with enlargement of the liver and spleen.

Pathophysiology

A diastolic pressure gradient between the right atrium and ventricle—the hemodynamic expression of TS—is augmented when the transvalvular blood flow increases during inspiration or exercise and is reduced when the blood flow declines during expiration. A relatively modest diastolic pressure gradient (i.e., a mean gradient of only 5 mm Hg) is usually sufficient to elevate mean right atrial pressure to levels that result in systemic venous congestion and, unless sodium intake has been restricted or diuretics have been given, is associated with jugular venous distention, ascites, and edema.

In patients with sinus rhythm, the right atrial a wave may be very tall and may even approach the level of the right ventricular systolic pressure. Resting cardiac output is usually markedly reduced and fails to rise during exercise. This accounts for the normal or only slightly elevated left atrial, pulmonary arterial, and right ventricular systolic pressures, despite the presence of accompanying mitral valvular disease.

A *mean* diastolic pressure gradient across the tricuspid valve as low as 2 mm Hg is sufficient to establish the diagnosis of TS. However, exercise, deep inspiration, and the rapid infusion of fluids or the administration of atropine may greatly enhance a borderline pressure gradient in a patient with TS. Therefore, when this diagnosis is suspected, right atrial and ventricular pressures should be recorded simultaneously, using two catheters or a single catheter with a double lumen, with one lumen opening on either side of the tricuspid valve. The effects of respiration on any pressure difference should be examined.

Clinical Manifestations (Table 46–10)

HISTORY. The low cardiac output characteristic of TS causes fatigue, and patients often complain of discomfort due to hepatomegaly, swelling of the abdomen, and anasarca. The severity of these symptoms, which are secondary to an elevated systemic venous pressure, is out of proportion to the degree of dyspnea. Some patients complain of a fluttering discomfort in the neck, caused by giant a waves in the jugular venous pulse. Despite the coexistence of MS, the symptoms characteristic of this valvular lesion (i.e., severe dyspnea, orthopnea, and paroxysmal nocturnal dyspnea) are usually mild or absent in the presence of severe TS because the latter prevents surges of blood into the pulmonary circulation behind the stenotic mitral valve. Indeed, the *absence* of symptoms of pulmonary congestion in a patient with obvious MS should suggest the possibility of TS.

▼ **TABLE 46–10. CLINICAL AND LABORATORY FEATURES OF RHEUMATIC TRICUSPID STENOSIS**

HISTORY
Long history
Progressive fatigue, edema, anorexia
Minimal orthopnea, paroxysmal nocturnal dyspnea
Rheumatic fever in two-thirds of patients
Female preponderance
Pulmonary edema and hemoptysis are rare

PHYSICAL FINDINGS
Signs of multivalvular involvement
Wasting
Peripheral cyanosis
Neck vein distention, with prominent v waves
Right ventricular lift
Associated murmurs of mitral and aortic valve disease
Holosystolic murmur maximal at lower left sternal border, accentuating with inspiration
Hepatic pulsation
Ascites, peripheral edema

LABORATORY FINDINGS
Normal sinus rhythm is frequently present with large a waves in the neck veins
Absent right ventricular lift
Auscultation reveals a diastolic rumble at lower left sternal border, increasing in intensity with inspiration
Electrocardiogram shows tall right atrial P waves and no right ventricular hypertrophy
Chest roentgenogram shows a dilated right atrium without an enlarged pulmonary artery segment

Modified from Ockene IS: Tricuspid valve disease. *In* Dalen JE, Alpert JS (eds): Valvular Heart Disease. 2nd ed. Boston, Little, Brown and Co, 1987, pp 356, 390.

PHYSICAL EXAMINATION. Because of the high frequency with which MS occurs in patients with TS and the similarity in the physical findings between the two valvular lesions, the diagnosis of TS is commonly missed. The physical findings are mistakenly attributed to MS, which is more common and may be more obvious. Therefore, a high index of suspicion is required to detect the tricuspid valvular lesion. In the presence of sinus rhythm, the a wave in the jugular venous pulse is tall, and a presystolic hepatic pulsation is often palpable. The y descent is slow and barely appreciable. The lung fields are clear, and despite engorged neck veins and the presence of ascites and anasarca, the patient may be comfortable while lying flat. Thus, the diagnosis of TS may be suspected from inspection of the jugular venous pulse in a patient with MS but without clinical evidence of pulmonary hypertension. This suspicion is strengthened when a diastolic thrill is palpable at the lower left sternal border, particularly if the thrill appears or becomes more prominent during inspiration.

The auscultatory findings of the accompanying MS are usually prominent and often overshadow the more subtle signs of TS. A tricuspid opening snap (OS) may be audible but is often difficult to distinguish from a mitral OS. However, the tricuspid OS usually follows the mitral OS and is localized to the lower left sternal border, whereas the mitral OS is usually most prominent at the apex and radiates more widely. The diastolic murmur of TS is also commonly heard best along the lower left parasternal border in the 4th intercostal space and is usually softer, higher pitched, and shorter in duration than the murmur of MS. The presystolic component of the TS murmur has a scratchy quality and a crescendo-decrescendo configuration that diminishes before S_1.[439] The diastolic murmur and OS of TS are both augmented by maneuvers that increase transtricuspid valve flow, including inspiration, the Mueller maneuver, assumption of the right lateral decubitus position, leg raising, inhalation of amyl nitrite, squatting, and isotonic exercise. They are reduced during expiration or the strain of the Valsalva maneuver and return to control levels immediately (i.e., within two to three beats) after Valsalva release.

Laboratory Examination

ELECTROCARDIOGRAM. In the absence of atrial fibrillation in a patient with valvular heart disease, TS is suggested by the presence of ECG evidence of right atrial enlargement (see Chap. 5). The P wave amplitude in leads II and V_1 exceeds 0.25 mV. Because most patients with TS have mitral valvular disease, the ECG signs of biatrial enlargement are commonly found. The amplitude of the QRS complex in lead V_1 may be reduced by the dilated right atrium.

RADIOLOGICAL FINDINGS. The key radiological finding is marked cardiomegaly with conspicuous enlargement of the right atrium (i.e., prominence of the right heart border), which extends into a dilated superior vena cava and azygos vein, but without conspicuous dilatation of the pulmonary artery. The vascular changes in the lungs characteristic of mitral valvular disease may be masked, with little or no interstitial edema or vascular redistribution, but left atrial enlargement may be present.

Angiography carried out following injection of contrast material into the right atrium and filming in the 30-degree right anterior oblique projection characteristically shows thickening and decreased mobility of the leaflets, a diastolic jet through the constricted orifice, and thickening of the normal atrial wall.

ECHOCARDIOGRAM (See also Chap. 7). The echocardiographic changes of the tricuspid valve in TS resemble those observed in the mitral valve in MS (see pp. 1648 and 1695). Two-dimensional echocardiography characteristically shows diastolic doming of the leaflets (especially the anterior tricuspid valve leaflet), thickening and restricted motion of the other leaflets, reduced separation of the tips of the leaflets,[441] and a reduction in diameter of the tricuspid orifice (Fig. 46–44). Transesophageal echocardiography allows added delineation of the details of valve structure.[442] Doppler echocardiography shows a prolonged slope of antegrade flow and compares well with cardiac catheterization in the quantification of TS and in the assessment of associated tricuspid regurgitation.[443, 443a]

Management

Although the fundamental approach to the management of severe TS is surgical treatment, intensive sodium restriction and diuretic therapy may diminish the symptoms secondary to the accumulation of excess salt and water. A preparatory period of diuresis may diminish hepatic congestion and thereby improve hepatic function sufficiently to diminish the risks of subsequent operation.

Most patients with TS have coexisting valvular disease that requires surgery. In patients with combined TS and MS, the former must *not* be corrected alone because pulmonary congestion or edema may ensue. Surgical treatment of TS should be carried out at the time of mitral valve repair or replacement in patients with TS in whom the mean diastolic pressure gradient exceeds 5 mm Hg and the tricuspid orifice is less than approximately 2.0 cm². The final decision concerning surgical treatment is often made at the operating table.[444]

Because TS is almost always accompanied by some TR, simple finger fracture valvotomy may not result in significant hemodynamic improvement but may merely substitute severe regurgitation for stenosis. However, open valvotomy in which the stenotic tricuspid valve is converted into a functionally bicuspid valve may result in substantial improvement. The commissures between the anterior and septal leaflets and between the posterior and septal leaflets are opened. It is not advisable to open the commissure between the anterior and posterior leaflets for fear of producing severe regurgitation. If open valvotomy does not restore reasonably normal valve function, the tricuspid valve may have to be replaced.[445–447a] A large porcine bioprosthesis

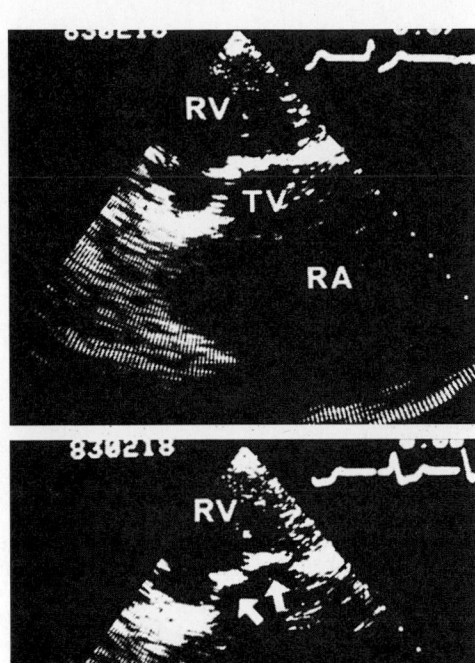

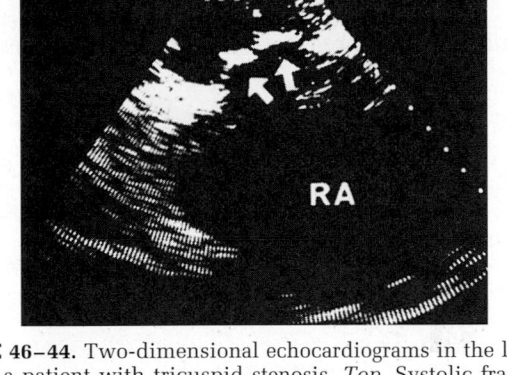

FIGURE 46–44. Two-dimensional echocardiograms in the long-axis view in a patient with tricuspid stenosis. *Top,* Systolic frame. *Bottom,* Diastolic frame that shows doming of both leaflets of the tricuspid valve (TV) (arrows). RA = right atrium; RV = right ventricle. (From Shimada R et al: Diagnosis of tricuspid stenosis by M-mode and two-dimensional echocardiography. Am J Cardiol 53: 164, 1984.)

(see p. 1704) is preferred to a mechanical prosthesis in the tricuspid position because of the high risk of thrombosis of the latter[447] and the longer durability of bioprostheses in the tricuspid than in the mitral or aortic positions.[448–451] The feasibility of tricuspid balloon valvuloplasty has been demonstrated, and this procedure may be combined with mitral balloon valvuloplasty.[452]

TRICUSPID REGURGITATION

Etiology and Pathology
(Table 46–11)

The most common cause of tricuspid regurgitation (TR) is not intrinsic involvement of the valve itself (i.e., primary TR) but rather *dilatation of the right ventricle* and of the tricuspid annulus causing secondary (functional) TR. This may be a complication of right ventricular failure of any cause. It is observed in patients with right ventricular hypertension secondary to any form of cardiac or pulmonary vascular disease, most commonly mitral valve disease.[452–455] In general, a systolic right ventricular systolic pressure greater than 55 mm Hg will cause functional TR.[51] TR can also occur secondary to right ventricular infarction,[456] congenital heart disease (see Chap. 43) (e.g., pulmonic stenosis and pulmonary hypertension secondary to Eisenmenger syndrome), primary pulmonary hypertension, and, rarely, cor pulmonale. In infants, TR may complicate right ventricular failure secondary to neonatal pulmonary diseases and pulmonary hypertension with persistence of

▼ TABLE 46–11. CAUSES AND MECHANISMS OF PURE TRICUSPID REGURGITATION

CAUSES

Anatomically ABNORMAL valve
  Rheumatic
  Nonrheumatic
    Infective endocarditis
    Ebstein anomaly
    Floppy (prolapse)
    Congenital (non-Ebstein)
    Carcinoid
    Papillary muscle dysfunction
    Trauma
    Connective tissue disorders (Marfan)
    Rheumatoid arthritis
    Radiation injury
Anatomically NORMAL valve (functional)
  Elevated right ventricular systolic pressure (dilated annulus)

MECHANISMS

Condition	Leaflet Area	Annular Circumference	Leaflet Insertion
Floppy	↑	↑	Normal
Ebstein anomaly	↑	↑	Abnormal
Pulmonary/right ventricular systolic hypertension	Normal	↑	Normal
Papillary muscle dysfunction	Normal	Normal	Normal
Carcinoid	↓/Normal	Normal	Normal
Rheumatic	↓/Normal	Normal	Normal
Infective endocarditis	↓/Normal	Normal	Normal

Modified from Waller BF: Rheumatic and nonrheumatic conditions producing valvular heart disease. *In* Frankl WS, Brest AN (eds): Cardiovascular Clinics. Valvular Heart Disease: Comprehensive Evaluation and Management. Philadelphia, FA Davis Co, 1989, pp 35, 95.

the fetal pulmonary circulation.[457] In all of these cases, TR reflects the presence of, and in turn aggravates, severe right ventricular failure. Functional TR may diminish or disappear as the right ventricle decreases in size with the treatment of heart failure. TR can also occur as a consequence of dilatation of the annulus in the Marfan syndrome, in which right ventricular dilatation secondary to pulmonary hypertension is not present.

A variety of disease processes can affect the tricuspid valve apparatus *directly* and lead to regurgitation (primary TR).[457] Thus, organic TR may occur on a congenital basis, as part of *Ebstein anomaly,* in atrioventricular canal, and when the tricuspid valve is involved in the formation of an aneurysm of the ventricular septum,[458] or in corrected transposition of the great arteries,[459] or it may occur as an isolated congenital lesion.[457] Rheumatic fever may involve the tricuspid valve directly.[92] When this occurs, it usually causes scarring of the valve leaflets and/or chordae tendineae, leading to limited leaflet mobility and either isolated TR or a combination of TR and TS. Rheumatic involvement of the mitral, and often aortic, valves coexist.

TR or the combination of TR and TS is an important feature of the *carcinoid syndrome* (Fig. 46–45), which leads to focal or diffuse deposits of fibrous tissue on the endocardium of the valvular cusps and cardiac chambers and on the intima of the great veins and coronary sinus[460–463] (see Chap. 48). The white, fibrous carcinoid plaques are most extensive on the right side of the heart, where they are usually deposited on the ventricular surfaces of the tricuspid valve and cause the cusps to adhere to the underlying right ventricular wall, thereby producing TR. Endomyocardial fibrosis with shortening of the tricuspid leaflets and chordae tendineae is an important cause of TR in tropical Africa (see Chap. 48). TR may result from prolapse of the

tricuspid valve caused by myxomatous changes in the valve and chordae tendineae; prolapse of the mitral valve is usually present in these patients as well.[464, 465] Prolapse of the tricuspid valve occurs in about 20 percent of all patients with mitral valve prolapse. Tricuspid valve prolapse may also be associated with atrial septal defect. Other causes of TR include penetrating and nonpenetrating trauma,[460] dilated cardiomyopathy,[467] infective endocarditis[468] (particularly staphylococcal endocarditis in narcotics addicts), and following surgical excision of the tricuspid valve in patients with infective endocarditis that is unresponsive to medical management.[469] Less common causes of TR[470] include cardiac tumors (particularly right atrial myxoma), transvenous pacemaker leads, repeated endomyocardial biopsy in a transplanted heart,[471] endomyocardial fibrosis, methysergide-induced valvular disease,[472] administration of fenfluramine-phentermine,[473] and systemic lupus erythematosus involving the tricuspid valve.[474]

Clinical Manifestations

HISTORY. In the absence of pulmonary hypertension, TR is generally well tolerated. However, when pulmonary hypertension and TR coexist, cardiac output declines, and the manifestations of right-sided heart failure become intensified.[475] Thus, the symptoms of TR result from a reduced cardiac output and from ascites, painful congestive hepatomegaly, and massive edema. Occasionally, patients have throbbing pulsations in the neck, which intensify on effort and are due to jugular venous distention; and systolic pulsations of the eyeballs have also been described.[476] In the many patients with TR who have mitral valve disease, the symptoms of the latter usually predominate. Symptoms of pulmonary congestion may abate as TR develops, but they are replaced by weakness, fatigue, and other manifestations of a depressed cardiac output.

PHYSICAL EXAMINATION. Evidence of weight loss and cachexia, cyanosis, and jaundice are often present on inspection in patients with severe TR. Atrial fibrillation is common. There is jugular venous distention,[477] the normal

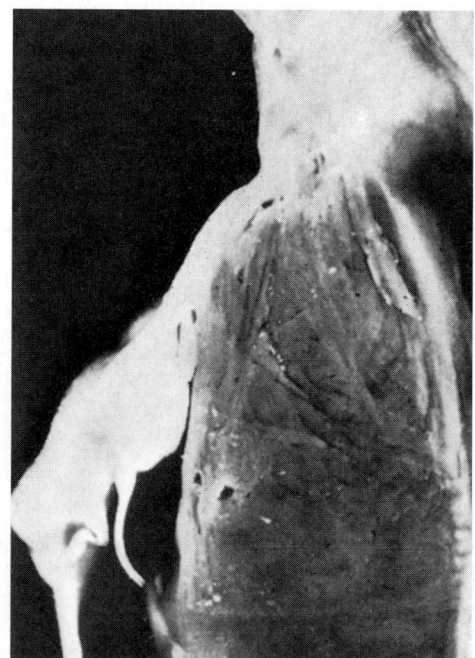

FIGURE 46–45. Septal tricuspid leaflet thickened by carcinoid plaques and fused to underlying ventricular septum. (From Callahan JA et al: Echocardiographic features of carcinoid heart disease. Am J Cardiol 50:766, 1982.)

x and x' descents disappear, and a prominent systolic wave, i.e., a c-v wave (or s wave), is apparent (see Fig. 4–5). The descent of this wave, the y descent, is sharp and becomes the most prominent feature of the venous pulse (unless there is coexisting TS, in which case it is slowed). A venous systolic thrill and murmur in the neck may be present in patients with severe TR.[478] The right ventricular impulse is hyperdynamic and thrusting in quality. Systolic pulsations of an enlarged, tender liver are commonly present initially. However, in patients with chronic TR and congestive cirrhosis, the liver may become firm and nontender. Ascites and edema are frequent.

Auscultation. This usually reveals an S_3 originating from the right ventricle, which is accentuated by inspiration. When TR is associated with and secondary to pulmonary hypertension, P_2 is accentuated as well. When TR occurs in the presence of pulmonary hypertension, the systolic murmur is usually high-pitched, pansystolic, and loudest in the 4th intercostal space in the parasternal region but occasionally is loudest in the subxiphoid area. When TR is mild, the murmur may be short. When TR occurs in the absence of pulmonary hypertension (e.g., in infective endocarditis or following trauma), the murmur is usually of low intensity and limited to the first half of systole. When the right ventricle is greatly dilated and occupies the anterior surface of the heart, the murmur may be prominent at the apex and difficult to distinguish from that produced by MR.

The response of the systolic murmur to respiration and other maneuvers is of considerable aid in establishing the diagnosis of TR (see Table 4–4). The murmur is characteristically augmented during inspiration (Carvallo sign). However, when the failing ventricle can no longer increase its stroke volume in the recumbent or sitting positions, the inspiratory augmentation may be elicited by standing. The murmur also increases during the Mueller maneuver (forced inspiration against a closed glottis), exercise, legraising, and hepatic compression. It demonstrates an immediate overshoot after release of the Valsalva strain but is reduced in intensity and duration in the standing position and during the strain of the Valsalva maneuver. Increased atrioventricular flow across the tricuspid orifice in diastole may cause a short early diastolic flow rumble in the left parasternal region following S_3. Tricuspid valve prolapse, like mitral valve prolapse, causes nonejection systolic clicks and late systolic murmurs. However, in tricuspid valve prolapse, these findings are more prominent at the lower left sternal border. With inspiration, the clicks occur later, and the murmurs intensify and become shorter in duration.

Laboratory Examination

ELECTROCARDIOGRAM. This is usually nonspecific and characteristic of the lesion causing TR. Incomplete right bundle branch block, Q waves in lead V_1, and atrial fibrillation are commonly found.

RADIOLOGICAL FINDINGS. In patients with functional TR, marked cardiomegaly is usually evident, and the right atrium is prominent. Evidence of elevated right atrial pressure may include distention of the azygos vein and the presence of a pleural effusion. Ascites with upward displacement of the diaphragm may be present. Systolic pulsations of the right atrium may be present on fluoroscopy.

ECHOCARDIOGRAM (See Figs. 7–68 and 7–69). The goal of echocardiography is to detect TR, estimate its severity, and assess pulmonary arterial pressure and right ventricular function.[443a] In patients with TR secondary to dilation of the tricuspid annulus, the right atrium, right ventricle, and tricuspid annulus are all usually greatly dilated on echocardiography.[479, 480] There is evidence of right ventricular diastolic overload with paradoxical motion of the ventricular septum similar to that observed in atrial septal defect. Exaggerated motion and delayed closure of the tricuspid valve are evident in patients with Ebstein anomaly. Prolapse of the tricuspid valve due to myxomatous degeneration may be evident on echocardiography.[465, 466] Echocardiographic indications of tricuspid valve abnormalities, especially TR by Doppler examination, can be detected in the majority of patients with carci-

noid heart disease.[463] In patients with TR due to endocarditis, echocardiography may reveal vegetations on the valve or a flail valve. Transesophageal echocardiography enhances detection of TR.

Contrast Echocardiography. This involves rapid injection of saline indocyanine green dye or sanicated human albumin (Albunex)[481] into an antecubital vein while a two-dimensional echocardiogram is recorded[482] (see Chap. 7). The injection produces microcavities that are readily visible on echocardiography and normally travel as a bolus through the circulation. In TR, these microcavities can be seen to travel back and forth across the tricuspid orifice and to pass into the inferior vena cava and hepatic veins during systole.

Pulsed Doppler Echocardiography. This reveals systolic flow from the right ventricle to the right atrium and is a sensitive technique for detecting and quantifying[483, 484] TR. Reverse flow can also be recorded in the inferior vena cava and hepatic veins. The peak velocity of TR flow is useful in the noninvasive estimation of right ventricular (and pulmonary arterial) systolic pressure. Color flow Doppler imaging is a sensitive and specific method for assessing TR and is helpful in selecting patients for surgical treatment and in evaluating postoperative results.

HEMODYNAMIC FINDINGS. The right atrial and right ventricular end-diastolic pressures are often elevated in TR, whether the condition is due to organic disease of the tricuspid valve or is secondary to right ventricular systolic overload. The right atrial pressure tracing usually reveals absence of the x descent and a prominent v or c-v wave ("ventricularization" of the atrial pressure). Absence of these findings essentially excludes moderate or severe TR.[485] As the severity of TR increases, the contour of the right atrial pressure pulse increasingly resembles that of the right ventricular pressure pulse (Fig. 46–46). A rise or no change in right atrial pressure on deep inspiration, rather than the usual fall, is a characteristic finding. Determination of the pulmonary arterial (or right ventricular) systolic pressure may be helpful in deciding whether the TR is primary (i.e., due to disease of the valve or its supporting structures) or functional (i.e., secondary to right ventricular dilatation). A pulmonary arterial or right ventricular systolic pressure less than 40 mm Hg favors a primary cause, whereas a pressure greater than 55 mm Hg suggests that TR is secondary. Intermediate values are not helpful. Diagnosis and quantitative assessment of TR can be aided in many instances by right ventriculography.[486]

Management

TR in the absence of pulmonary hypertension usually is well tolerated and may not require surgical treatment. In-

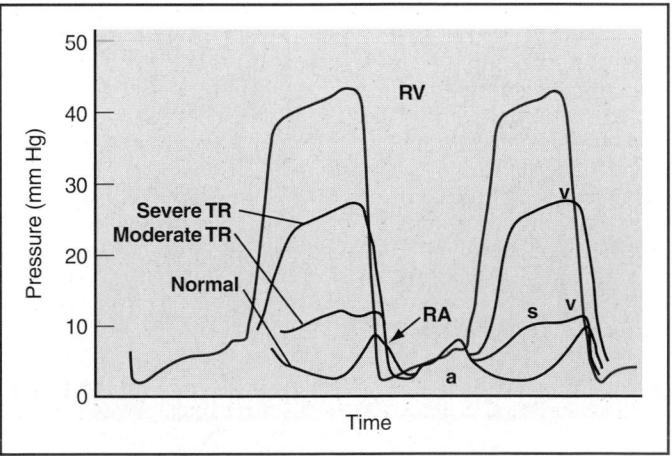

FIGURE 46–46. Appearance of right atrial (RA) pressure contour in patients with severe tricuspid regurgitation (TR), moderate TR, and no TR (normal). Note the regurgitant systolic ("s") wave that blends with the normal filling ("v") wave in severe TR. The resultant RA pressure waveform resembles a right ventricular (RV) pressure recording. (From Grossman W [ed]: Cardiac Catheterization and Angiography. 5th ed. Philadelphia, Lea and Febiger, 1996.)

deed, both human patients and experimental animals with normal pulmonary arterial pressure may tolerate total excision of the tricuspid valve as long as right ventricular systolic pressure is normal. Dilatation of the right side of the heart usually occurs months or years after tricuspid valvectomy (usually carried out for acute infective endocarditis). *Surgical treatment* of acquired regurgitation secondary to annular dilatation was greatly improved when Carpentier introduced the concept of suturing the annulus to a prosthetic ring.[487] Annuloplasty without insertion of a prosthetic ring (the so-called DeVega annuloplasty) has also been found to be effective in patients with annular dilatation. This technique is now widely employed.[444, 475, 488-490]

At the time of mitral valve surgery in patients with TR secondary to pulmonary hypertension, the severity of the regurgitation should be assessed by palpation of the tricuspid valve. In addition, it should be determined whether the TR is secondary to pulmonary hypertension, in which case the valve is normal, or whether it is secondary to rheumatic fever. Patients with mild TR usually do not require surgical treatment[491]; pulmonary vascular pressures decline following successful mitral valve surgery, and the mild TR tends to disappear. Excellent results have been reported in patients with moderate TR with the use of suture annuloplasty of the posterior (unsupported) portion of the annulus. Patients with severe TR and primary rheumatic tricuspid valve disease with commissural fusion require valvotomy and ring annuloplasty.[488] The latter is also employed for TR secondary to annular dilatation. A surgical mortality rate of 13.9 percent has been reported (see Table 46-2).[104] If these procedures do not provide a good functional result at the operating table (as assessed by transesophageal echocardiography), valve replacement using a large porcine mitral heterograft may be required.

When organic disease of the tricuspid valve (Ebstein anomaly or carcinoid heart disease[449]) causes TR severe enough to require surgery, valve replacement is usually needed. The risk of thrombosis of mechanical prostheses is greater in the tricuspid than in the mitral or aortic positions, presumably because pressure and flow rates are lower in the right side of the heart. For this reason, the artificial valve of choice for the tricuspid position in adults is a large porcine heterograft.[450, 451] Anticoagulants are not required, and a graft durability of more than 10 years has been established.

In treating the difficult problem of tricuspid endocarditis in heroin addicts (see Chap. 47), total excision of the tricuspid valve *without immediate replacement* can generally be tolerated by these patients, who usually do not have associated pulmonary hypertension. When antibiotic therapy is unsuccessful, valvular replacement frequently results in reinfection or continued infection. Therefore, diseased valvular tissue should be excised to eradicate the endocarditis, and antibiotic treatment can then be continued. Initially, most patients tolerate loss of the tricuspid valve without great difficulty. Later, right ventricular dysfunction usually occurs. A bioprosthetic valve may therefore be inserted 6 to 9 months after valve excision and control of the infection.

PULMONIC VALVE DISEASE

Etiology and Pathology

PULMONIC STENOSIS. The *congenital* form is the most common cause of pulmonic stenosis (PS).[492] Manifestations in children are discussed in Chapter 43 and in adults in Chapter 44. *Rheumatic* inflammation of the pulmonic valve is very uncommon, is usually associated with involvement of other valves, and rarely leads to serious deformity. However, in one study, a high incidence of significant pulmonic valve involvement secondary to rheumatic fever was reported in Mexico City, perhaps related to the pulmonary hypertension that occurs at high altitudes and the resultant greater stress on the pulmonic valve.[493] *Carcinoid* plaques, similar to those involving the tricuspid valve, are often present in the outflow tract of the right ventricle of patients with malignant carcinoid. The plaques result in constriction of the pulmonic valve ring, retraction and fusion of the valve cusps, and either PS or the combination of PS and pulmonic regurgitation (Fig. 46-47).[494, 495] Obstruction in the region of the pulmonic valve may be extrinsic to the valve apparatus and may be produced by cardiac tumors or by aneurysm of the sinus of Valsalva.[496]

Management of congenital PS focuses on balloon dilation (see Chaps. 38, 43, and 44).

PULMONIC REGURGITATION. By far the most common cause of pulmonic regurgitation (PR) is dilatation of the valve ring secondary to pulmonary hypertension (of any etiology) or to dilatation of the pulmonary artery, either idiopathic[497, 498] or consequent to a connective tissue disorder such as the Marfan syndrome. The second most common cause of PR is infective endocarditis.[499] Less frequently, PR is iatrogenic and is induced at the time of surgical treatment of congenital PS or tetralogy of Fallot.[499a] PR may also result from various lesions that directly affect the pulmonic valve. These include congenital malformations, such as absent, malformed, fenestrated, or supernumerary leaflets. These anomalies may occur as isolated lesions[500] but more often are associated with other congenital anomalies,[501] particularly tetralogy of Fallot, ventricular septal defect, and pulmonic valvular stenosis. Less common causes include trauma, carcinoid syndrome,[494] rheumatic involvement, injury produced by a pulmonary artery flow-directed catheter,[502] syphilis, and chest trauma.[503]

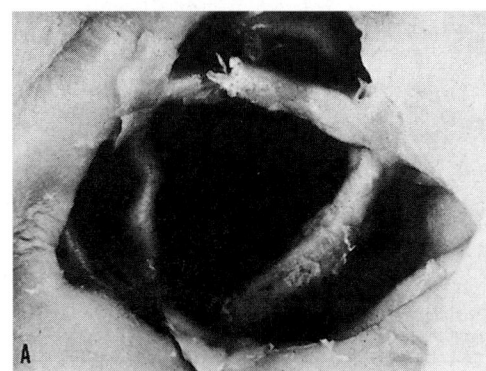

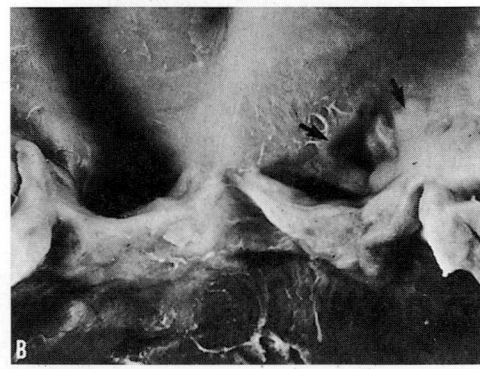

FIGURE 46-47. Carcinoid heart disease; pulmonary valve viewed from above (*A*) and opened (*B*). The thickened and retracted cusps result in valvular incompetence. The constricted annulus results in valvular stenosis. Carcinoid plaques (arrows) extend onto the pulmonary trunk. (From Callahan, JA et al: Echocardiographic features of carcinoid heart disease. Am J Cardiol 50:767, 1982.)

Clinical Manifestations

Like TR, isolated PR causes right ventricular volume overload and may be tolerated for many years without difficulty unless it complicates, or is complicated by, pulmonary hypertension. In this case, PR is usually accompanied by and aggravates right ventricular failure. Patients with PR caused by infective endocarditis who develop septic pulmonary emboli and pulmonary hypertension often exhibit severe right ventricular failure.[503] In most patients, the clinical manifestations of the primary disease are severe and usually overshadow the PR, which often results only in incidental auscultatory findings. *Physical examination* reveals a hyperdynamic right ventricle that produces palpable systolic pulsations in the left parasternal area and an enlarged pulmonary artery that often results in systolic pulsations in the 2nd left intercostal space. Sometimes systolic and diastolic thrills are felt in the same area. A tap reflecting pulmonic valve closure is usually easily palpable in the 2nd intercostal space in patients with pulmonary hypertension and secondary PR.

AUSCULTATION. P_2 is not audible in patients with congenital absence of the pulmonic valve; however, this sound is accentuated in patients with PR secondary to pulmonary hypertension. There may be wide splitting of S_2 caused by prolongation of right ventricular ejection accompanying the augmented right ventricular stroke volume.[501] A nonvalvular systolic ejection click due to the sudden expansion of the pulmonary artery by the augmented right ventricular stroke volume frequently initiates a midsystolic ejection murmur, most prominent in the 2nd left intercostal space. An S_3 and S_4 originating from the right ventricle are often audible, most readily in the 4th intercostal space at the left parasternal area, and are augmented by inspiration.

In the absence of pulmonary hypertension, the diastolic murmur of PR is low pitched and usually heard best at the 3rd and 4th left intercostal spaces adjacent to the sternum (see Fig. 4-37).[504] The murmur commences when pressures in the pulmonary artery and right ventricle diverge, approximately 0.04 second after P_2. It is diamond-shaped in configuration and brief, reaching a peak intensity when the gradient between these pressures is maximal and ending with equilibration of the pressures. The murmur becomes louder during inspiration.

The Graham Steell Murmur. When systolic pulmonary arterial pressure exceeds approximately 55 mm Hg, dilatation of the pulmonic annulus results in a high-velocity regurgitant jet that is responsible for the Graham Steell murmur of PR. (Doppler ultrasonography reveals pulmonary regurgitation at much lower pulmonary arterial pressures.) The Graham Steell murmur is a high-pitched, blowing, decrescendo murmur beginning immediately after P_2 and is most prominent in the left parasternal region in the 2nd to 4th intercostal spaces. Thus, although it resembles the murmur of AR, it is usually accompanied by severe pulmonary hypertension, i.e., an accentuated P_2 or fused S_2, an ejection sound, and a systolic murmur of TR, and not by a widened arterial pulse pressure. Sometimes a low-frequency presystolic murmur is present, i.e., a right-sided Austin Flint murmur originating from the mitral valve.[505]

The Graham Steell murmur of PR secondary to pulmonary hypertension usually increases in intensity with inspiration, exhibits little change after amyl nitrite inhalation or vasopressor administration, is diminished during the Valsalva strain, and returns to baseline intensity almost immediately after release of the Valsalva strain. This murmur resembles and may be confused with the diastolic blowing murmur of AR. However, indicator dilution studies[506] and aortography have established that a diastolic blowing murmur along the left sternal border in patients with rheumatic heart disease and pulmonary hypertension (even in the *absence* of peripheral signs of AR) is usually due to AR rather than PR.

Laboratory Examination

ELECTROCARDIOGRAM. In the absence of pulmonary hypertension, PR often results in an ECG that reflects right ventricular diastolic overload, i.e., an rSr (or rsR) configuration in the right precordial leads. PR secondary to pulmonary hypertension is usually associated with ECG evidence of right ventricular hypertrophy.

RADIOLOGICAL FINDINGS. Both the pulmonary artery and the right ventricle are usually enlarged, but these signs are nonspecific. Fluoroscopy may demonstrate pronounced pulsation of the main pulmonary artery. PR can be diagnosed by observing opacification of the right ventricle following injection of contrast material into the main pulmonary artery (Fig. 46-48). The diagnosis is supported by noting

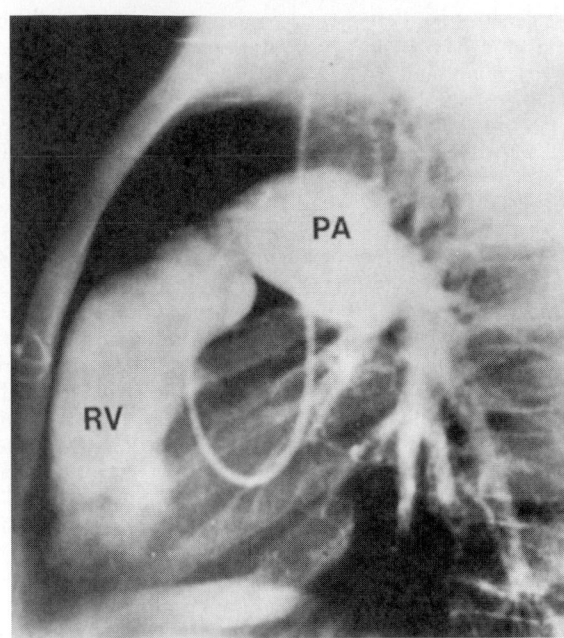

FIGURE 46-48. Pulmonic valvular regurgitation. Contrast material has been injected into the main pulmonary artery (PA) and regurgitates back into an enlarged right ventricle (RV). (Reproduced with permission from Carlsson E et al: The radiological diagnosis of cardiac valvular insufficiency. Circulation 55:921, 1977. Copyright 1977, American Heart Association.)

superimposition of the pulmonary arterial and right ventricular pressure curves during mid- and late diastole. Indicator dilution studies with injections into the pulmonary artery and sampling from the right ventricle,[507] as well as intracardiac phonocardiography, can also be helpful in establishing the diagnosis in mild cases.

ECHOCARDIOGRAM. Two-dimensional echocardiography shows right ventricular dilatation and, in patients with pulmonary hypertension, right ventricular hypertrophy as well. Right ventricular function can be estimated. Abnormal motion of the septum characteristic of volume overload of the right ventricle in diastole and/or septal flutter[508] may be evident. The motion of the pulmonic valve may point to the cause of the PR. Absence of *a* waves and systolic notching of the posterior leaflet suggest pulmonary hypertension; large *a* waves indicate pulmonic stenosis. PR can be detected by contrast echocardiography. The pulsed Doppler technique is also extremely accurate in detecting PR and in helping to estimate its severity. Abnormal Doppler signals in the right ventricular outflow tract with velocity sustained throughout diastole are generally observed in patients in whom PR is caused by dilatation of the valve ring secondary to pulmonary hypertension. When the velocity falls during diastole, the pulmonary artery pressure is usually normal, and the regurgitation is caused by an abnormality of the valve itself.[509]

Management

PR alone is seldom severe enough to require specific treatment. Cardiac glycosides are useful in the management of right ventricular dilatation or failure. Treatment of the primary condition, such as infective endocarditis, or the lesion responsible for the pulmonary hypertension, such as surgery for mitral valvular disease, often ameliorates the PR. Surgical treatment directed specifically at the pulmonic valve (e.g., in patients in whom surgical correction of tetralogy of Fallot has caused severe PR[509a]) is required only occasionally because of intractable right heart failure. Under such circumstances, valve replacement may be carried out,[510, 510a, 510b] preferably with a porcine bioprosthesis or a pulmonary allograft.[499a]

Multivalvular involvement is caused most frequently by rheumatic fever, and various clinical and hemodynamic syndromes can be produced by different combinations of valvular abnormalities. The Marfan syndrome and other connective tissue disorders may cause multivalve prolapse and dilatation, resulting in multivalvular regurgitation. Degenerative calcification of the aortic valve may be associated with degenerative mitral annular calcification and cause AS and MR. Different pathological conditions may affect two valves in the same patient, such as infective endocarditis on the aortic valve causing AR and ischemia causing MR. Development of PR and TR secondary to dilatation of the pulmonic valve ring and tricuspid annulus, as a consequence of pulmonary hypertension secondary to mitral and/or aortic valvular disease, was discussed previously, as was the combination of organic rheumatic tricuspid and mitral valvular disease.

In patients with multivalvular disease, the clinical manifestations depend on the relative severities of each of the lesions. When the valvular abnormalities are of approximately equal severity, clinical manifestations produced by the more proximal (upstream) of the two valvular lesions (i.e., the mitral valve in patients with combined mitral and aortic valvular disease and the tricuspid valve in patients with combined tricuspid and mitral valvular disease) are generally more prominent than those produced by the distal lesion. Thus, the proximal lesion tends to mask the distal lesion.

It is important to recognize multivalvular involvement preoperatively because failure to correct all significant valvular disease at the time of operation increases mortality considerably. In patients with multivalvular disease, the relative severity of each lesion may be difficult to estimate by clinical examination and noninvasive techniques because one lesion may mask the manifestations of the other. For this reason, patients suspected of having multivalvular involvement and who are being considered for surgical treatment should undergo right- and left-cardiac catheterization and angiography. These studies are in addition to careful clinical examination and a noninvasive workup, with emphasis on two-dimensional and Doppler echocardiography. If there is any question concerning the presence of significant AS in patients undergoing mitral valve surgery, the aortic valve should be inspected because overlooking this condition can lead to a high perioperative mortality. Similarly, it is useful to palpate the tricuspid valve at the time of mitral valve surgery.

MITRAL STENOSIS AND AORTIC REGURGITATION

Approximately two-thirds of patients with severe MS have an early blowing diastolic murmur along the left sternal border with a normal pulse pressure. In about 90 percent of these patients, the murmur is due to mild or moderate AR and is usually of little clinical importance. However, approximately 10 percent of patients with MS have severe rheumatic AR,[511] which can generally be recognized by the usual signs of AR (i.e., a widened pulse pressure, left ventricular dilatation and increased wall motion on echocardiography, and signs of left ventricular enlargement on radiological and ECG examinations).

In keeping with the general observation that a proximal lesion may mask a distal lesion, significant AR may be missed in patients with severe MS.[512] The widened pulse pressure, in particular, may be absent. On the other hand, MS may be missed or, conversely, may be falsely diagnosed on clinical examination of patients with obvious AR. An accentuated S_1 and an opening snap in a patient with AR should suggest the possibility of mitral valvular disease. However, an Austin Flint murmur is often inappropriately considered to be the diastolic rumbling murmur of MS. These two murmurs may be distinguished at the bedside by means of amyl nitrite inhalation, which diminishes the Austin Flint murmur but augments the murmur of MS; isometric handgrip and squatting augment both the diastolic murmur of AR and the Austin Flint murmur. Echocardiography, particularly pulsed Doppler echocardiography, is of decisive value in detecting MS and MR.

Since double-valve replacement is associated with increased short-term and long-term risk,[114, 512a] balloon mitral valvotomy can be the first procedure. If this causes left ventricular dilatation, aortic valve replacement can follow. Alternatively, open mitral valvotomy and aortic valve replacement can be performed at the same time.[51]

MITRAL STENOSIS AND AORTIC STENOSIS

The left ventricle of a patient with these two lesions is usually small, stiff, and hypertrophied. When severe MS and AS coexist, the former masks many of the manifestations of the latter.[513] The cardiac output tends to be reduced more than in patients with isolated AS. The reduced cardiac output lowers both the transaortic valvular pressure gradient and the left ventricular systolic pressure, diminishes the incidence of angina pectoris, and retards the development of aortic valvular calcification and left ventricular hypertrophy.[514] On the other hand, clinical manifestations associated with MS, such as pulmonary congestion and hemoptysis, atrial fibrillation, and systemic embolization, occur more frequently in patients with coexisting MS and AS than in those with isolated AS.

On physical examination, an S_4, (which is common in patients with pure AS) is usually not present. The midsystolic murmur characteristic of AS may be reduced in intensity and duration because the stroke volume is reduced by the MS. The ECG may fail to demonstrate left ventricular hypertrophy, but left atrial enlargement is common. The chest roentgenogram is usually typical of MS except that calcium may be present in the region of the aortic valve. The two-dimensional and Doppler echocardiograms are of the greatest value because stenosis of both valves may be evident. However, the low cardiac output characteristic of the combined lesions may reduce the transvalvular pressure gradients estimated by Doppler echocardiography.

It is vital to recognize the presence of hemodynamically significant aortic valvular disease (i.e., stenosis and/or regurgitation) preoperatively in patients who are to undergo mitral valvotomy. This procedure may be hazardous because it can impose a sudden hemodynamic load on the left ventricle that had previously been protected by the MS and may lead to acute pulmonary edema. Balloon mitral valvotomy and aortic valve replacement may be the treatment of choice.

AORTIC STENOSIS AND MITRAL REGURGITATION

This combination of lesions is usually caused by rheumatic heart disease, although AS may be congenital and MR may be due to mitral valve prolapse. The combination of severe AS and MR is a hazardous one, but fortunately it is relatively uncommon. Obstruction to left ventricular outflow augments the volume of MR flow,[123] whereas the presence of MR diminishes the ventricular preload necessary for maintenance of the left ventricular stroke volume in patients with AS. The result is a reduced forward cardiac output and marked left atrial and pulmonary venous hypertension. The development of atrial fibrillation (due to left atrial enlargement) has an adverse hemodynamic effect in the presence of AS. The physical findings may be confusing because it may be difficult to recognize two distinct systolic murmurs. On echocardiography and roentgenography, the left atrium and ventricle are usually larger than in isolated AS. In patients with severe AS and MR, both valves must usually be treated surgically by aortic valve replacement and, if possible, by mitral valve repair.

AORTIC REGURGITATION AND MITRAL REGURGITATION

This relatively frequent combination of lesions[515] may be caused by rheumatic heart disease, by prolapse of both the aortic and the mitral valves due to myxomatous degeneration,[516] or by dilatation of both annuli in patients with connective tissue disorders. The left ventricle is usually greatly dilated. The clinical features of AR usually predominate, and it is sometimes difficult to determine whether the MR is due to organic involvement of this valve or to dilatation of the mitral valve ring secondary to left ventricular enlargement. When both valvular leaks are severe, this combination of lesions is poorly tolerated. The normal mitral valve ordinarily serves as a "backup" to the aortic valve, and premature (diastolic) closure of the mitral valve limits the volume of reflux that occurs in patients with acute AR.[382] With severe combined regurgitant lesions, regardless of the cause of the mitral lesion, blood may reflux from the aorta through both chambers of the left side of the heart into the pulmonary veins. Physical and laboratory examinations usually show evidence of both lesions. An S_3 and a brisk arterial pulse are frequently present. The relative severity of each lesion can be assessed best by Doppler echocardiography and contrast angiography. This combination of lesions leads to severe left ventricular dilatation.

MR that occurs in patients with AR secondary to left ventricular dilatation often regresses following aortic valve replacement alone. If severe, the MR may be corrected by annuloplasty at the time of aortic valve replacement. An intrinsically normal mitral valve that is regurgitant because of a dilated annulus should not be replaced.

Surgical Treatment of Multivalvular Disease

Combined aortic and mitral valve replacement is usually associated with a higher risk and poorer survival than is replacement of either of the valves alone.[517, 517a] The operative risk of double-valve replacement is about 70 percent higher than it is for single-valve replacement. The Society of Thoracic Surgeons National Database Committee reported an overall operative mortality rate of 9.6 percent for multiple (usually double) valve replacement in 3840 patients, compared with 4.3 percent and 6.4 percent for isolated aortic valve replacement and mitral valve replacement, respectively[104] (see Table 46–2). Kirklin and Barrat-Boyes reported a 5-year survival rate of 63 percent after double-valve replacement compared with 80 percent for single-valve replacement.[517] The long-term survival depends strongly on the preoperative functional status. Patients operated on for combined AR and MR have poorer outcomes than patients receiving double-valve replacement for any of the other combinations of lesions, presumably because both AR and MR may produce irreversible left ventricular damage. Mitral repair or balloon valvotomy in combination with aortic valve replacement is preferable to double-valve replacement and should be carried out whenever possible. Risk factors that reduce long-term survival after double-valve replacement include advanced age, higher NYHA class, greater left ventricular enlargement, and accompanying ischemic heart disease requiring coronary artery bypass grafting.

Given the higher risks, a higher threshold is required for multivalvular versus single-valve surgery. Thus, patients are generally advised not to undergo multivalvular surgery until they reach late NYHA Class II or Class III. Despite a detailed noninvasive and invasive workup, the decision to treat more than one valve is often made by palpation or by direct inspection at the operating table.

THREE-VALVE DISEASE. Hemodynamically significant disease involving the mitral, aortic, and tricuspid valves is uncommon. Patients with trivalvular disease may present in advanced heart failure with marked cardiomegaly, and surgical correction of all three valvular lesions is imperative. However, triple-valve replacement is a long and complex operation. Early in the experience with this procedure, the mortality rate was 20 percent for patients in NYHA Class III and 40 percent for patients in Class IV. More recently, the mortality rate has declined, but, nevertheless, triple-valve replacement should be avoided if possible. In many patients with trivalvular disease, it is possible to replace the aortic valve, repair the mitral valve, and perform a tricuspid annuloplasty or valvuloplasty.

Patients who survive triple-valve replacement surgery usually show substantial clinical improvement during the early postoperative period,[517b, 518, 518a] and postoperative catheterization studies show marked reductions in pulmonary arterial and capillary pressures. However, some patients die of arrhythmias or congestive heart failure in the late postoperative period despite three normally functioning prostheses.[519] The cause of cardiac failure in this situation is not known, but it may be related to intraoperative myocardial ischemia, microemboli from the multiple prostheses, or continued subclinical episodes of rheumatic myocarditis.

When multiple prosthetic valves must be inserted, it is logical to select either two bioprostheses or two mechanical prostheses for the left side of the heart. If the patient is to be exposed to the hazards of anticoagulants for one mechanical prosthesis, it seems unreasonable to add the potential risks of early failure of a bioprosthesis. However, if two mechanical prostheses are selected for the left side of the heart, the use of a bioprosthesis in the tricuspid position is suggested.

▼ Prosthetic Cardiac Valves

The first successful replacements of cardiac valves in the human were accomplished by Nina Braunwald and colleagues,[520] Harken and coworkers,[521] and Starr and Edwards[522] in 1960. Two major groups of artificial (prosthetic) valves are currently available in models designed for both the atrioventricular (mitral and tricuspid) and the aortic positions: mechanical prostheses and bioprostheses (tissue valves).[523]

MECHANICAL PROSTHESES

Mechanical prosthetic valves are classified into two major groups: caged-ball and tilting-disc valves. The *Starr-Edwards* caged-ball valve, the oldest prosthetic valve in continuous use (Figs. 46–49 and 46–50), has the longest record of predictable performance of any artificial valve.[523–525] The poppet is made of silicone rubber, the cage of Stellite alloy, and the sewing ring of Teflon/polypropylene cloth. A disadvantage is its bulky cage design. Therefore, the Starr-Edwards valve is not suitable for the mitral position in patients with a small left ventricular cavity or for the aortic position in those with a small aortic annulus or a valve–aortic arch composite graft. In a small number of patients, this valve induces hemolysis, which may be greatly exaggerated and become clinically important if a perivalvular leak develops. When they are of small size, the Starr-Edwards valve may cause mild obstruction, and the incidence of thromboembolism is slightly higher than with the tilting-disc valve.[526]

Several types of disc valves are widely employed; these are less bulky, have a lower profile than the caged-ball valve, and are therefore superior hemodynamically. The *St. Jude* bileaflet valve (see Fig. 46–49D), currently the most widely used prosthesis worldwide (Table 46–12), is coated with pyrolytic carbon and has two semicircular discs that pivot between open and closed positions without the need for supporting struts. It has favorable flow characteristics and causes a lower transvalvular pressure gradient at any outer diameter and cardiac output than the caged-ball or single-leaflet tilting valves.[527] The St. Jude valve appears to have particularly favorable hemodynamic characteristics in the smaller sizes; therefore, it is especially useful in children. Thrombogenicity in the mitral position *may* be less than that associated with other prosthetic valves. However, as with other mechanical prostheses, lifelong anticoagulation is needed.[528] A variation of the St. Jude valve, the *Carbomedics* prosthesis[529] (see Fig. 46–49E), is also a bileaflet valve composed of pyrolytic carbon with a titanium housing that can be rotated so as to avoid interference with disc excursion by subvalvular tissue.

The *Omniscience* valve (see Fig. 46–49B), the successor to the *Lillehei-Kaster* pivoting-disc valve, consists of a titanium valve housing with a polyester knit sewing ring in which a pyrolytic disc is suspended. In the open position, the disc swings to an angle of 80 degrees, providing a large central flow orifice.[530] A closely related valve is the *Medtronic-Hall* valve[531] (see Fig. 46–49C), which has a Teflon sewing ring and titanium housing; its thin, carbon-coated pivoting disc has a central perforation that allows improved hemodynamics. Thrombogenicity appears to be quite low (less than one episode per 100 patient-years in the mitral position[532]), and mechanical performance is excellent over the long term. Both the bileaflet and the tilting-disc valves

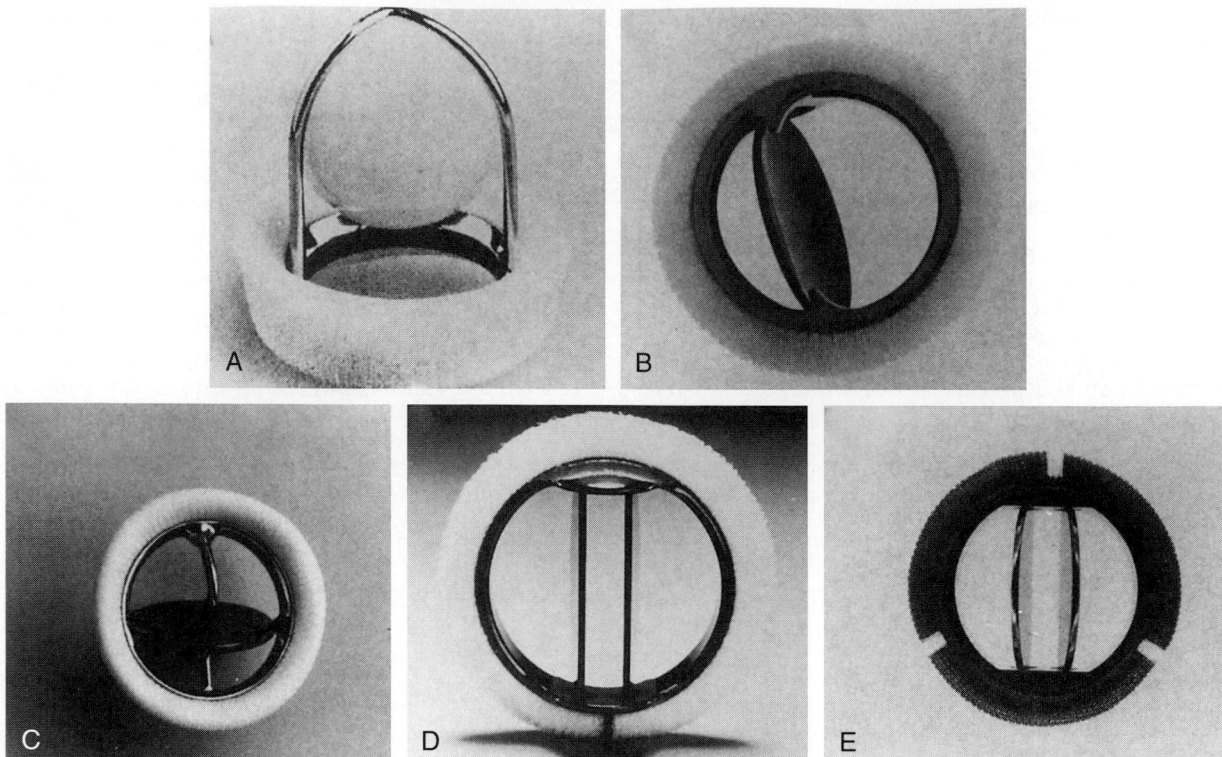

FIGURE 46–49. *A,* The Starr-Edwards caged ball valve. *B,* The Omniscience valve. *C,* The Medtronic-Hall valve. *D,* The St. Jude bileaflet valve. *E,* The Carbomedics bileaflet valve. (From Cohn, LH: Aortic valve prostheses. Cardiol Rev 2:219, 1995.)

are associated with small (~5–10 ml/beat) obligatory (normal) regurgitation.[92] All have distinctive auscultatory features (Fig. 46–51).

DURABILITY AND THROMBOGENICITY. All mechanical prosthetic valves have an excellent record of durability, up to 40 years for the Starr-Edwards valve. In the mitral position, perivalvular regurgitation appears to occur more frequently with mechanical than with tissue valves.[533] However, patients with any *mechanical* prosthesis, regardless of design or site of placement, require long-term anticoagulation and aspirin administration because of the hazard of thromboembolism, which is greatest in the first postoperative year. Without anticoagulants and aspirin, the incidence of thromboembolism is three- to sixfold higher than when proper doses of these medications are administered. Very rarely, thrombosis of the mechanical valve occurs. This

may be a fatal event, but when nonfatal, it interferes with prosthetic valve function.

Warfarin should begin about 2 days after operation, and the international normalized ratio (INR) should be in the range of 2.0 to 3.0 for patients with the bileaflet disc and the Medtronic-Hall valve in the aortic position. The INR should be between 2.5 and 3.5 for patients at higher risk for thrombosis (e.g., atrial fibrillation, previous thromboembolism) as well as for patients with other mechanical valves in the aortic position and for *all* valves in the mitral position (see also p. 1722 and Chap. 62).[51] This relatively conservative approach reduces the risk of anticoagulant hemorrhage but does not appear to be associated with a greater frequency of thromboembolism than an INR of 3.0 to 4.0, which was used in the past.[534–536] Antiplatelet agents without anticoagulants do not provide adequate protection.

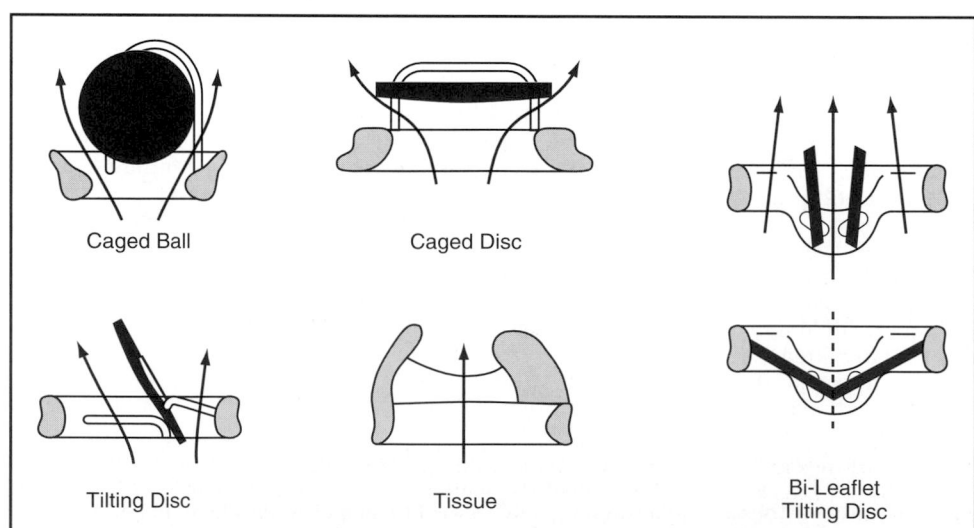

Caged Ball

Caged Disc

Tilting Disc

Tissue

Bi-Leaflet Tilting Disc

FIGURE 46–50. Designs and flow patterns of major categories of prosthetic heart valves: caged-ball, caged-disc, tilting-disc, bileaflet tilting-disc, and bioprosthetic (tissue) valves. Whereas flow in mechanical valves must course along both sides of the occluder, bioprostheses have a central flow pattern. (Reproduced by permission from Schoen FJ et al: Bioengineering aspects of heart valve replacement. Ann Biomed Eng 10:97, 1982. Copyright 1983, Pergamon Press Limited, 1983; and from Schoen FJ: Pathology of cardiac valve replacement. *In* Morse D, Steiner RM, Fernandez J [eds]: Guide to Prosthetic Cardiac Valves. New York, Springer-Verlag, 1985, p. 209. Copyright 1985 Springer-Verlag, Inc.)

TYPE	MANUFACTURER	MODEL	YEAR OF FIRST CLINICAL USE	IMPLANTS* (thousands)
Mechanical				
Ball	Baxter-Edwards	Starr-Edwards	1965	200
Disc	Medtronic	Medtronic-Hall	1977	178
	Medical Inc.	Omniscience	1978	48
	Alliance	Monostrut	1982	94
Bileaflet	St. Jude	St. Jude	1977	580
	Baxter-Edwards	Duromedics	1982†	20
	CarboMedics	CarboMedics	1986	110
Biological				
Porcine	Medtronic	Hancock Standard	1970	177
		Hancock MO	1978	32
	Baxter-Edwards	CE Standard	1971	400
		CE SupraAnnular	1982	45
	St. Jude	Toronto Stentless (TSP)	1991	5
	Medtronic	Free Style Stentless	1992	5
Pericardial	Baxter-Edwards	CE	1982	35
Homograft	Noncommercial‡		1962	12
	Cryolife‡		1984	14
Autologous	Noncommerical‡	Pulmonary autograft	1967	2

*Approximate number of implants through part or all of 1994.
†Discontinued in 1988.
‡Does not require FDA approval for clinical use.
CE = Carpentier-Edwards; FDA = Food and Drug Administration; MO = modified orifice.
Adapted from Grunkemeier G, Starr A, Rahimtoola SH: Replacement of heart valves. *In* O'Rourke RA (ed): The Heart: Update I. New York, McGraw-Hill Publishing Co; 1996, pp 98–123. From Bonow RO, Carabello B, de Leon AC Jr, et al: ACC/AHA Guidelines for the management of patients with valvular heart disease. J Am Coll Cardiol 32:1486, 1998.

However, the addition of aspirin, 80 to 150 mg daily, together with warfarin may reduce the risk of thromboembolism and should be given to all patients with prosthetic valves.

Prosthetic valve thrombosis should be suspected by the sudden appearance of dyspnea and muffled sounds or new murmurs on auscultation (see Fig. 46–51). This serious complication is diagnosed by transesophageal two-dimensional and Doppler echocardiography. Treatment consists of infusion of a thrombolytic agent for 24 to 72 hours, heparin, and aspirin. Surgery is required for nonresponders and for patients with mobile thrombi.[537]

It must be recognized that (1) the administration of warfarin carries its own mortality and morbidity, i.e., serious hemorrhage, estimated at 0.2 and 2.2 episodes per 100 pa-

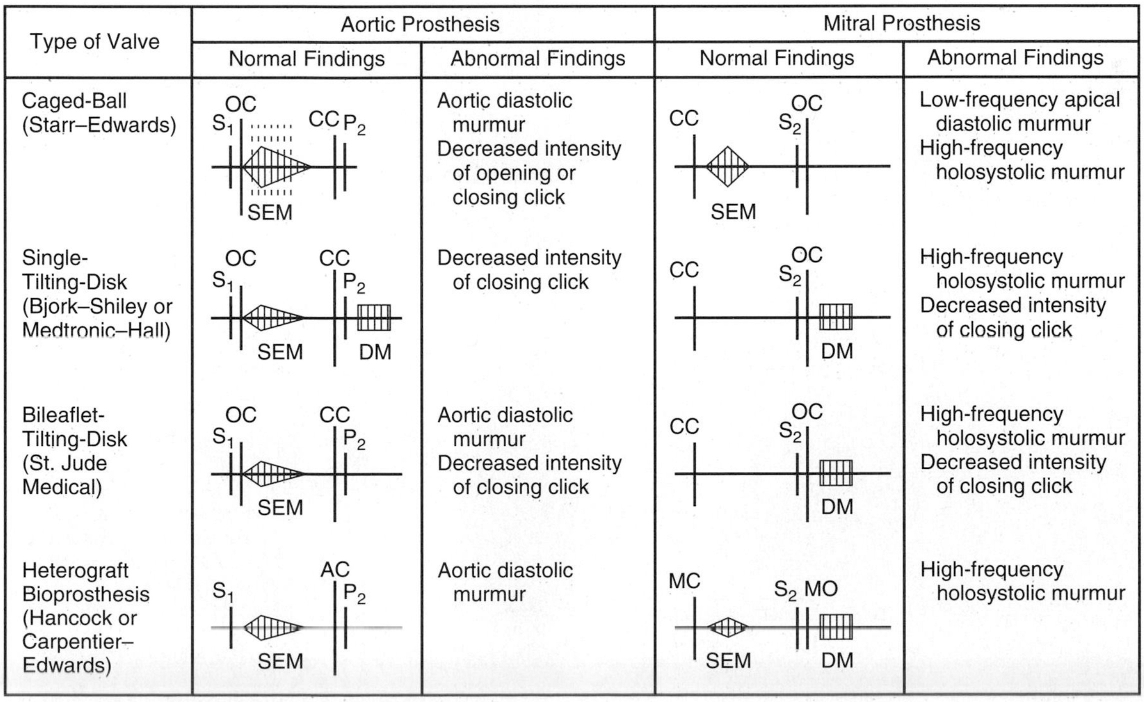

FIGURE 46–51. Auscultatory characteristics of various prosthetic valves in the aortic and mitral positions, with schematic diagrams of normal findings and descriptions of abnormal findings. OC = opening click; CC = closing click; SEM = systolic ejection murmur; DM = diastolic murmur; AC = aortic closure; MC = mitral valve closure; MO = mitral opening. (From Vongpatanasin W, Hillis LD, Lange RA: Prosthetic heart valves. N Engl J Med 335:407, 1996.)

tient-years, respectively; and (2) despite treatment with anticoagulants, the incidence of thromboembolic complications with the best mechanical prosthesis is still about 0.2 fatal complications and 1.0 to 2.0 nonfatal complications per 100 patient-years for aortic valves and 2.0 to 3.0 nonfatal complications for mitral valves.[538] Valve thrombosis, a particularly hazardous complication, occurs at an incidence of about 0.1 percent per year in the aortic position and 0.35 percent per year in the mitral position. Thrombosis of mechanical prostheses in the tricuspid position is quite high, and for this reason bioprostheses are preferred at this site. The incidence of embolization in patients who have experienced repeated emboli from a prosthetic valve despite anticoagulants may be reduced by replacement with a tissue valve.

Mechanical prostheses regularly cause mild hemolysis,[538] but this is not severe enough to be of clinical importance unless the patient develops periprosthetic regurgitation.

TISSUE VALVES

Tissue valves (bioprostheses) have been developed primarily to overcome the risk of thromboembolism that is inherent in all mechanical prosthetic valves and the attendant hazards and inconvenience of permanent anticoagulant therapy.[539a] The first tissue valves to be widely used were chemically sterilized aortic homografts (allografts) obtained from cadavers. However, these had a high incidence of breakdown within 3 years, and antibiotic-treated, cryopreserved, frozen, irradiated homografts were then developed. These homografts are more durable, but, although they have many desirable properties, their use has been restricted by the problems inherent in their procurement (to be discussed).

PORCINE HETEROGRAFTS. Stented porcine aortic heterografts were developed for both the mitral and the aortic positions and have been in wide clinical use since 1965.[523] The semirigid stents facilitate implantation and maintain the three-dimensional relationship between the leaflets.[92] Three porcine heterografts are widely used today.[523, 540–543a] The *Hancock* valve (Fig. 46–52A) is fixed and preserved in glutaraldehyde and is mounted on a Dacron cloth-covered flexible polypropylene strut. In the smaller aortic models, the right coronary cusp is replaced by a posterior cusp from another valve to reduce obstruction resulting from the septal shelf of the valve. The *Carpentier-Edwards* valve (Fig. 46–52B) is pressure-fixed, preserved in glutaraldehyde, and mounted on a Teflon-covered Eljgiloy strut so as to minimize the septal shelf. The *Intact* valve is also glutaraldehyde-treated but at a fixation pressure of zero and with toluidine in an attempt to inhibit calcium deposition. The hemodynamic profiles of the porcine heterografts are similar to those of comparably sized low-profile mechanical prostheses.[541, 544]

During the first 3 postoperative months, while the sewing ring becomes endothelialized, the thromboembolic rate is high enough that anticoagulation is extremely desirable. Thereafter, anticoagulants are not required for porcine valves in the aortic position, and the thromboembolic rate is approximately 1 to 2 episodes per 100 patient-years

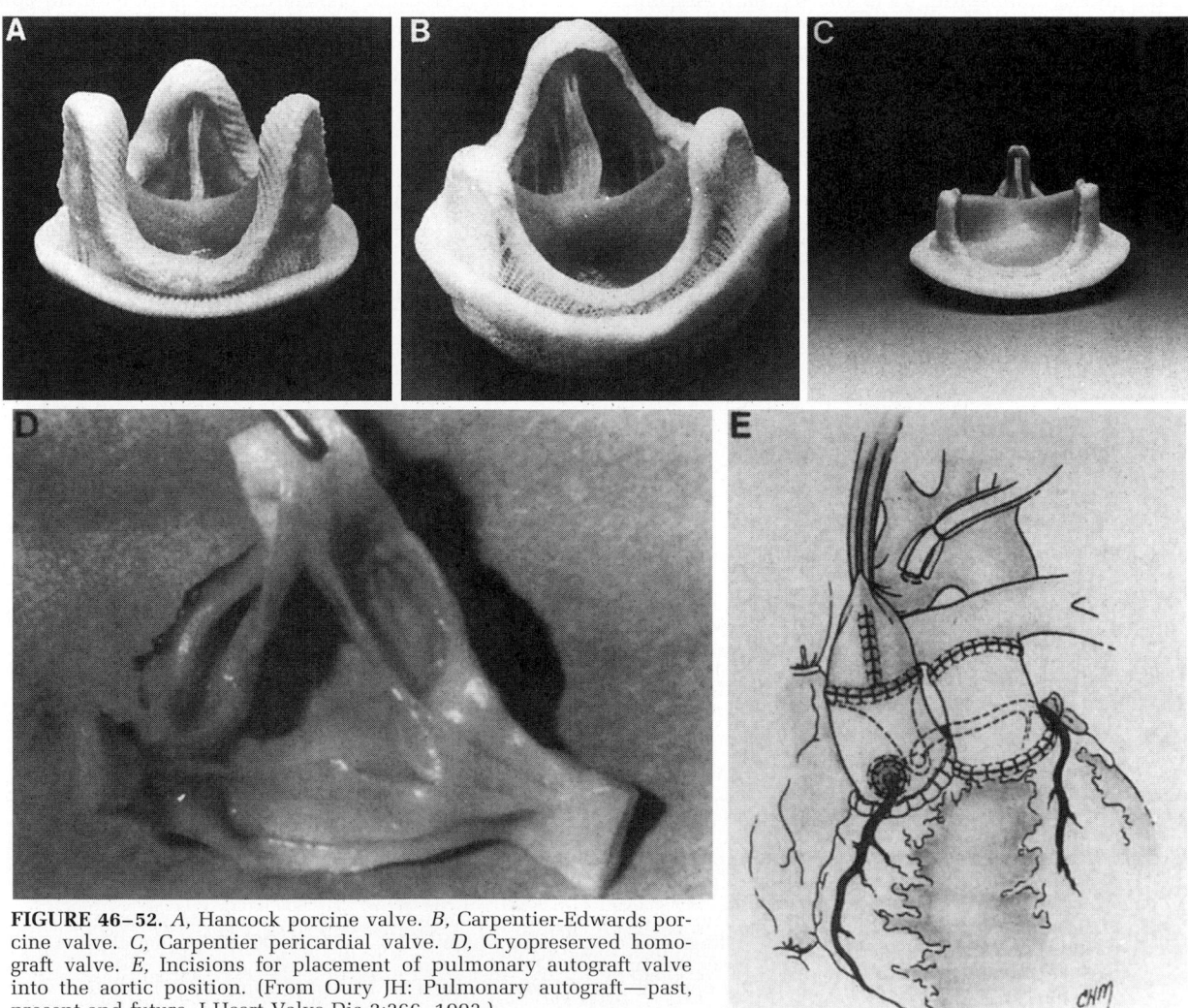

FIGURE 46–52. *A,* Hancock porcine valve. *B,* Carpentier-Edwards porcine valve. *C,* Carpentier pericardial valve. *D,* Cryopreserved homograft valve. *E,* Incisions for placement of pulmonary autograft valve into the aortic position. (From Oury JH: Pulmonary autograft—past, present and future. J Heart Valve Dis 2:366, 1993.)

without these drugs.[545, 546] When these valves have been placed in the mitral position in patients who are in sinus rhythm, who do not have heart failure or thrombus in the left atrium or the left atrial appendage, and who do not have a history of embolism preoperatively, anticoagulants are not needed after the first 3 postoperative months, and the thromboembolic rate is also approximately 1 to 2 episodes per 100 patient-years. This rate is comparable to that observed in patients with the St. Jude or other mechanical valves who are receiving anticoagulants and are therefore subject to the risks of hemorrhage. It is unlikely that any mitral valve replacement can be associated with a thromboembolic rate much below 0.5 episode per 100 patient-years because some of the emboli in patients with longstanding mitral disease are derived from the left atrium rather than from the valve itself.[546] In patients undergoing mitral valve replacement (MVR) with a bioprosthesis who have experienced a previous embolism, in whom thrombus is found in the left atrium at operation, or who remain in atrial fibrillation postoperatively (approximately one-third of all patients receiving MVR), the hazard of thromboembolism and the need for anticoagulants persist. This negates the principal advantage of the tissue valves, and mechanical prostheses would appear to be preferable to bioprostheses in these patients.

The major problem with porcine bioprostheses is their limited durability (Fig. 46–53). Cuspal tears, degeneration, fibrin deposition, disruption of the fibrocollagenous structure, perforation, fibrosis, and calcification sufficiently severe to require reoperation begin to appear in some patients in the fourth or fifth postoperative year, and by 10 years the rate of primary tissue failure averages 30 percent. It then accelerates, and by 15 years postoperatively the actuarial *freedom* from bioprosthetic primary tissue failure has

ranged from 30 to 60 percent in several series. Structural valve deterioration is more frequent in patients with bioprostheses in the mitral than in the aortic position, presumably because of the higher closing pressure. With the passage of time, even more of these valves will likely fail, and essentially all valves implanted into patients less than 60 years of age may have to be replaced ultimately.[547] Fortunately, however, these valves usually do not fail suddenly (as is often the case for structural failure or thrombosis of mechanical prostheses). Re-replacement of a bioprosthetic valve should be carried out when significant and/or progressive structural deterioration is evident but before operation becomes an emergency. The second operation, when carried out on an elective basis, may be associated with a surgical mortality rate of 10 to 15 percent.

Color Doppler echocardiography with two-dimensional imaging is extremely helpful in the early detection of bioprosthetic valve malfunction. Transesophageal echocardiography is more sensitive than transthoracic imaging in detecting bioprosthetic valve deterioration. Even patients without new murmurs or other physical findings of valve dysfunction should have routine echocardiographic studies to look for early bioprosthetic valve dysfunction every year for 5 to 6 years after valve replacement and every 6 months after that.

The time after implantation at which tissue valves fail varies inversely with age[543a] (Fig. 46–54). Valve failure is prohibitively rapid in children and in adults under 35 to 40 years of age. Therefore, bioprostheses are *not* advisable in these age groups. On the other hand, degeneration is rare when these valves are implanted into patients over 70 years of age.[547] Bioprostheses also have extremely limited durability in patients with chronic renal failure and hypercalcemia related to secondary hyperparathyroidism.

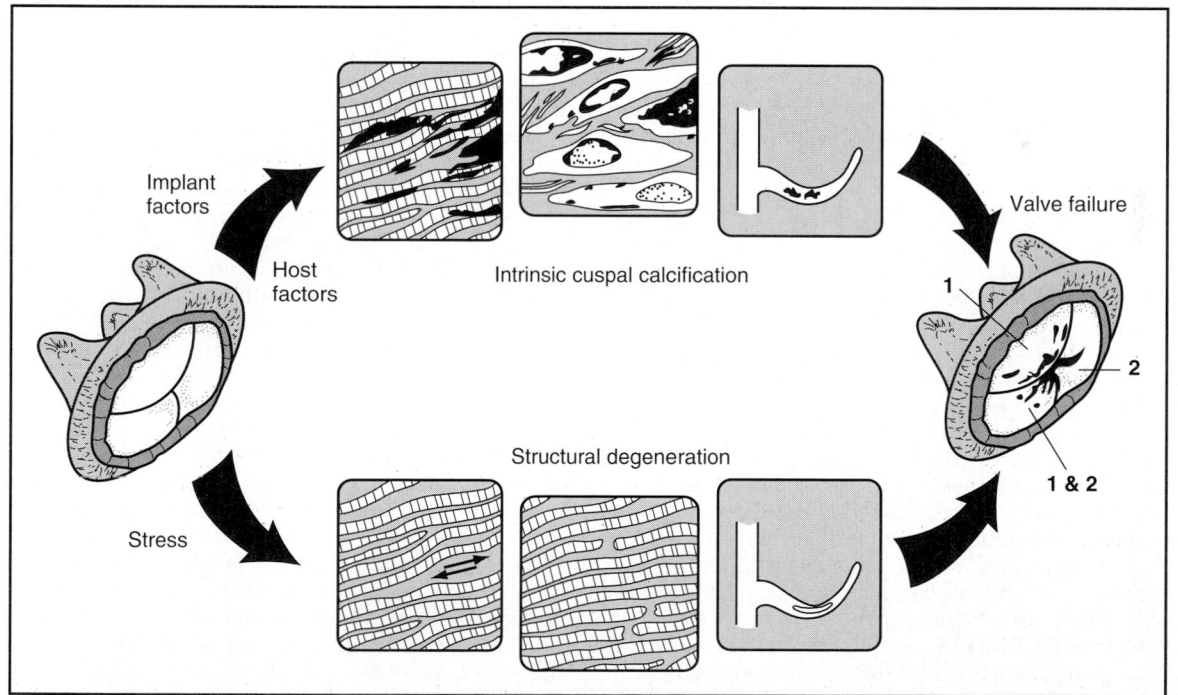

FIGURE 46–53. Unified model for bioprosthetic heart valve failure relating isolated tissue processes of mineralization and collagen degeneration to gross clinical failures. Such failures have calcification with cuspal stiffening (1), cuspal defects without calcific deposits (2), or cuspal tears associated with mineralization (1 and 2). These processes may occur independently or they may be synergistic. Specifically, implant and host factors interact to induce the collagen-oriented and cell-oriented calcific deposits noted ultrastructurally. The deposits predominate in the central portions of valve cusps, particularly at flexion points such as the commissures (Pathway 1). Stress causes shear between and fracture of collagen fibers, which may create gross cuspal defects (Pathway 2). Although dynamic mechanical activity is not a prerequisite for calcification, stress may promote (i.e., accelerate) this process by means of unknown mechanisms. (Amended from Schoen FJ, Levy RJ: Bioprosthetic heart valve failure: Pathology and pathogenesis. Cardiol Clin 2:717, 1984.)

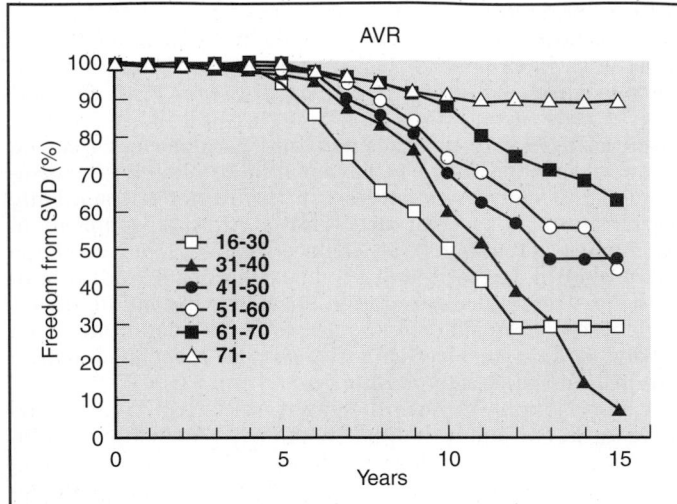

FIGURE 46–54. Estimates of freedom from structural valve deterioration (SVD) for patients undergoing porcine aortic valve replacement (AVR) are stratified according to age. (From Fann JI, Miller DC, Moore KA, et al: Twenty-year clinical experience with porcine bioprostheses. Ann Thorac Surg 62:1301, 1996. Reprinted with permission from the Society of Thoracic Surgeons.)

Prosthetic valve endocarditis is a serious, often grave illness (see Chap. 47).

STENTLESS PORCINE XENOGRAFTS. Since the stent adds to the obstruction and thereby increases stress on the leaflets, stentless valves have been developed for the aortic position[548] and are now being used increasingly, especially in patients with small aortic roots.[549] These include the Toronto SPV stentless valve (St. Jude Medical valve),[550] the Edwards stentless valve,[551] and the Medtronic freestyle valve.[548] It is hoped that the slightly improved hemodynamics provided by the stentless valves will translate into better long-term durability than that of valves mounted on stents.

HOMOGRAFT (ALLOGRAFT) AORTIC VALVES. These are harvested from cadavers, often along with kidneys, usually within 24 hours of donor death. They are sterilized with antibiotics and cryopreserved for long periods at −196°C (see Fig. 46–52D). They are inserted directly, usually in the aortic position, *without* being placed into a prosthetic stent. Their hemodynamics are superior to those of stented porcine valves. Like porcine xenografts, their thrombogenicity is low, but cryopreserved valves appear to have a similar rate of structural deterioration.[552, 552a] Perhaps this rate is reduced with the use of freshly harvested valves and approximate matching of donor's and patient's ages. Homograft aortic valves are indicated for patients with native or prosthetic valve endocarditis, but they are difficult to use when the aortic root and ascending aorta are greatly enlarged. Availability is often limited.[553]

PULMONARY AUTOGRAFTS. In this operation, the Ross procedure, the patient's own pulmonary valve and adjacent main pulmonary artery are removed and used to replace the diseased aortic valve and often the neighboring aorta, with reimplantation of the coronary arteries into the graft[554] (see Fig. 46–52E). A human pulmonary or aortic homograft is then inserted into the pulmonary position. The autograft is nonthrombogenic.[555] In children and adolescents, there is evidence that the autograft grows along with the patient. The risk of endocarditis is very low, anticoagulants are not required, and, perhaps most important, the long-term durability appears to be excellent.[556] Although the pulmonary autograft is the replacement valve of choice in children, adolescents, and younger adults who have a long (>20-year) life expectancy, its use has been limited because the operation is technically much more complex than a simple aortic valve replacement. The procedure should be carried out only by experienced surgeons.

PERICARDIAL AUTOGRAFTS. The patient's own pericardium is inserted into a frame on the operating table (the Carpentier-Edwards Perimount pericardial bioprosthesis) and is inserted into either the aortic or the mitral position. Long-term durability appears to be excellent; in 267 patients undergoing isolated aortic valve replacement, the 14-year actuarial freedom of need for re-replacement because of structural valve dysfunction was 85 percent (94 percent in patients > 65 years of age).[557] Good results have also been reported for this valve in the mitral position, in which the results are also exceptional in older patients. However, there is a greater risk for the development of stenosis in the mitral position.[558]

HEMODYNAMICS OF VALVE REPLACEMENTS

The most commonly used prosthetic valves, i.e., mechanical prostheses and stented porcine xenografts, have an effective in vitro orifice size that is *smaller* than the normal valve at the same site. (Unstented, i.e., free, homografts and pulmonary autografts do not have this problem.) After implantation, tissue ingrowth and endothelialization reduce the size of the effective orifice even more. Therefore, the prosthetic valves that are currently available must be considered to be mildly stenotic. However, postoperative hemodynamic measurements of the mechanical prostheses show reasonably good function, with effective mitral valve orifice areas averaging 1.7 to 2.0 cm^2 and mitral valve gradients of 4 to 8 mm Hg at rest. The cloth-covered Starr-Edwards valve appears to be intrinsically slightly more stenotic than the Medtronic-Hall or Omniscience tilting-disc valves. The bileaflet St. Jude and Carbomedics valves, in turn, may be slightly superior to the Medtronic-Hall or Omniscience valve. In hemodynamic studies, the stented porcine mitral valves behave in a manner similar to mechanical prosthetic valves of the same diameter. *Serious* hemodynamic obstruction of an artificial valve in the mitral position is quite uncommon, unless the valve (most commonly the Starr-Edwards valve) is placed into a small left ventricular cavity or into an unusually small mitral annulus or the prosthesis chosen is of inappropriate size.

The problem of prosthetic valve stenosis may be more serious in patients who undergo aortic valve replacement for AS. The annulus into which the prosthesis is inserted in these patients is usually smaller than it is in patients with AR, and the surgeon may be forced to select an artificial valve of relatively small size. As a consequence, aortic valve replacement, may not abolish obstruction in patients with AS but may merely convert severe to mild or moderate obstruction. When the smaller models of the stented porcine xenograft or mechanical prosthesis are placed into the aortic position, effective orifice areas of about 1.1 to 1.3 cm^2 are common. In such patients, peak transvalvular gradients as high as 40 mm Hg during exercise have been recorded. The poor late results observed in a minority of patients undergoing replacement of stenotic aortic valves may possibly be related to the moderate stenosis of the prosthesis. In patients with AS who do not exhibit clinical improvement postoperatively, it is important to evaluate the function of both the prosthetic valve and the left ventricle. Rarely, reoperation to correct a malfunctioning prosthesis may be necessary.

SELECTION OF AN ARTIFICIAL VALVE
(Table 46–13)

Most comparisons of mechanical and bioprosthetic valves indicate similar overall results in terms of early and late mortality, prosthetic valve endocarditis and other complications, and the need for reoperation, at least for the first 5 years postoperatively. As indicated, there appear to be no significant differences insofar as hemodynamics are concerned, except that patients with an unusually small left ventricular cavity or mitral or aortic annulus may have better results with the low-profile (tilting-disc) St. Jude or Carbomedics prosthesis or a tissue valve.[559] Patients with a small aortic annulus may be better candidates for unstented homografts, heterografts, or pulmonary autografts.

The major task in selecting an artificial valve is to weigh the advantage of durability and the disadvantages of the risks of thromboembolism and anticoagulant treatment inherent in mechanical prostheses on the one hand with the advantage of low thrombogenicity and the disadvantage of abbreviated durability of bioprostheses on the other. Hammermeister and associates[560] have compared the outcome in 575 men who were randomized to replacement of the mitral or the aortic valve with either mechanical or a bioprosthetic valve. There was no difference in survival or in the probability of developing a valve-related complication, including endocarditis, valve thrombosis, and systemic embolism, in patients receiving either a mechanical or a bioprosthetic valve. The rate of structurally related valve failure requiring reoperation (which is associated with about twice the mortality of the initial procedure) was much higher in patients receiving tissue as opposed to mechanical valves. As anticipated, anticoagulant-related bleeding was higher in patients receiving mechanical valves. Patients with mechanical valves also had a higher incidence of perivalvular regurgitation in the mitral position. In the Edinburgh randomized trial, which also compared a mechanical with a porcine xenograft valve,[561] actuarial survival rates tended to be better and the freedom from all valve-related adverse events was significantly better with mechanical valves. Retrospective cohort analyses are in agreement with the results of these trials.[562–564] Therefore, mechanical prostheses, usually of the bileaflet variety, are the valves of choice in the majority of patients under 65 years of age.

However, the following groups of patients should receive bioprostheses: (1) patients with coexisting disease who are prone to hemorrhage and who therefore tolerate anticoagulants poorly, such as those with bleeding disorders, intestinal polyposis, and angiodysplasia; (2) patients who are likely to be noncompliant with permanent anticoagulant treatment, who are unwilling to take anticoagulants on a regular basis, or who live in developing nations and cannot be monitored; (3) patients over the age of 65 years in whom bioprosthetic valves deteriorate very slowly, who are unlikely to outlive their bioprostheses, and who because of their age may also be at greater risk of hemorrhage while taking anticoagulants; (4) patients with a small aortic annulus in whom an unstented (free) bioprosthetic graft may provide superior hemodynamics; and (5) younger patients (< 40 years of age), especially women wishing to bear children, who require aortic valve replacement and in whom a pulmonary autograft may be preferable. However, the technical difficulties associated with the last procedure must be taken into account.

Special Situations

PREGNANCY (see also Chap. 65). Women with artificial valves can tolerate the hemodynamic burden of pregnancy well, but the hypercoagulable state of pregnancy increases the risk of thromboembolism in pregnant patients with mechanical prostheses. Anticoagulation must not be interrupted, although an increased risk of fatal fetal hemorrhage occurs in women in whom anticoagulants are continued. There is also a risk of fetal malformation caused by the probable teratogenic effect of warfarin. Although these problems represent rationales for the use of tissue valves in all women of childbearing age,[565, 566] their limited durability in young adults makes their use unacceptable. Therefore, unless a pulmonary autograft can be employed (for patients who require aortic valve replacement), every effort should be made to defer valve replacement until after childbirth. In pregnant women with critical MS or AS, balloon valvuloplasty should be considered, and, if at all possible, mitral valve repair instead of replacement should be undertaken for patients with MR. Women of childbearing potential who have a mechanical prosthesis should be counseled against pregnancy. When a woman who already has a mechanical prosthetic valve becomes pregnant, the risk to the fetus if the mother receives oral anticoagulants appears to be lower than the risk to the mother if anticoagulants are discontinued. Therefore, coumarin derivatives should be continued and the INR maintained between 2.0 and 3.0 until 2 weeks before expected delivery, at which time the patient should be switched to intravenous heparin.[564] Heparin should be discontinued at the onset of labor but may be restarted, along with coumarin, several hours after delivery. Alternatively, warfarin may be briefly interrpted at the 38th week of gestation and planned cesarean section carried out.[567]

NONCARDIAC SURGERY. When noncardiac surgery is required in patients with prosthetic valves who are receiving anticoagulants, the risk is minimal when the anticoagulant is stopped 1 to 3 days preoperatively and for a similar period postoperatively. It may be desirable, however, to protect the patient with low-molecular-weight dextran during the perioperative period and to resume anticoagulation rapidly with intravenous heparin.

PATIENTS DESTINED TO RECEIVE ANTICOAGULANTS. Patients with earlier implantation of a mechanical prosthesis, chronic atrial fibrillation with an enlarged left atrium, a history of thromboembolism, or a thrombus in the left atrium at operation and who therefore are destined to receive anticoagulants should receive a mechanical valve prosthesis because the potential advantage of a tissue valve is negated.

CHILDREN AND PATIENTS RECEIVING CHRONIC HEMODIALYSIS. The high incidence of bioprosthetic valve failure in children and adolescents[568, 569] and in patients on chronic hemodialysis virtually prohibits their use in these

▼ **TABLE 46–13. VALVE SELECTION FOR AN INDIVIDUAL PATIENT**

RELATIVE INDICATIONS FOR A MECHANICAL VALVE
Long expected lifetime (age < 40 years)
Previous dysfunctional tissue valve
Anticoagulation required anyway
Double valve replacement
Composite graft (aortic root + valve) needed
Renal failure, dialysis

RELATIVE INDICATIONS FOR A BIOPROSTHESIS
Short expected lifetime (age ≥ 65 years)
Unreliable anticoagulant risk
Previous thrombosed valve
Anticoagulant intolerance
Pregnancy anticipated

From Grunkemeier GL, Rahimtoola SH, Starr A: Prosthetic heart valves. *In* Rahimtoola SH (ed): Valvular Heart Disease. Atlas of Heart Diseases. Vol 11. Braunwald E, series ed. Philadelphia, Current Medicine, 1977, pp 13.1–13.27.

groups. In young adults between the ages of 25 and 35 years, the failure of bioprosthetic valves is somewhat higher than it is in older adults; this serves as a relative, but not an absolute, contraindication to their use in this age group.

In children, a mechanical prosthesis (generally the St. Jude valve) with its favorable hemodynamics is preferred despite the disadvantages inherent in the need for anticoagulants in this age group.[570] Similarly, mechanical valve prostheses should be used in patients with chronic renal failure and/or hypercalcemia. Alternatively, if an experienced surgical team is available and the patient requires an aortic valve replacement, a pulmonary autograft may be employed.

TRICUSPID POSITION. The risk of thrombosis for all valves is highest in the tricuspid position because of the lower pressures and velocity of blood flow. This complication appears to be highest for tilting-disc valves, intermediate for caged-ball valves, and lowest for bioprostheses, which are the valves of choice as tricuspid replacements. Fortunately, bioprostheses exhibit a much slower rate of mechanical deterioration in the tricuspid position than in the mitral or aortic positions.

R E F E R E N C E S

MITRAL STENOSIS

1. Waller BE: Rheumatic and nonrheumatic conditions producing valvular heart disease. Cardiovasc. Clin. 16:3, 1986.
2. Olson LJ, Subramanian R, Ackerman DM, et al: Surgical pathology of the mitral valve: A study of 712 cases spanning 21 years. Mayo Clin Proc 62:22, 1987.
3. Dare A, Harrity P, Tazelaar H, et al: Evaluation of surgically excised mitral valves: Revised recommendations, based on changing operative procedures in the 1990s. Hum Pathol 24:1286, 1993.
4. Waller B, Howard J, Fess S: Pathology of mitral valve stenosis and pure mitral regurgitation—part I. Clin Cardiol 17:330, 1994.
5. Schoen EJ and St John Sutton M: Contemporary pathologic considerations in valvular disease. In Virmani R, Atkinson JB, Feuoglio JJ (eds): Cardiovascular Pathology. Philadelphia, WB Saunders Co, 1991, p 334.
6. Wells FC, Shapiro LM (eds): Mitral Valve Disease. 2nd ed. London, Butterworths, 1996, 204 pp.
7. Dalen JE and Alpert JS (eds): Valvular Heart Disease. 2nd ed. Boston, Little, Brown and Co, 1987, 600 pp.
8. Bortolotti U, Valente M, Agozzino L, et al: Rheumatoid mitral stenosis requiring valve replacement. Am Heart J 107:1049, 1984.
9. Fischer TA, Lehr HA, Nixdorff U: Combined aortic and mitral stenosis in mucopolysaccharidosis type I-S (Ulrich-Scheie syndrome). Heart 81:97, 1999.
10. Ladefoged C, Rohr N: Amyloid deposits in aortic and mitral valves. Virchows Arch (A) 404:301, 1984.
11. Misch, KA: Development of heart valve lesions during methysergide therapy. Br Med J 2:365, 1974.
12. Wrisley D, Giambartolomei A, Lee I, Brownlee W: Left atrial ball thrombus: Review of clinical and echocardiographic manifestations with suggestions for management. Am Heart J 121:1784, 1991.
13. Kwanishi DT and Rahimtoola SH: Mitral stenosis. In Rahimtoola, SH (ed): Valvular Heart Disease and Endocarditis. Atlas of Heart Diseases. Vol 11. Braunwald E (series ed) Philadelphia Current Medicine, 1996.
14. Wood P: An appreciation of mitral stenosis. Br Med J 1:1051, 1113, 1954.
15. Kawanishi DT and Rahimtoola SH: Mitral stenosis. In Rahimtoola, S.H. (ed.): Valvular Heart Disease and Endocarditis. Atlas of Heart Diseases. Vol 11. Braunwald E (series ed): Philadelphia, Current Medicine, 1996.
16. Grossman W: Profiles in valvular heart disease. In Baim DS, Grossman W (eds): Cardiac Catheterization, Angiography and Interventions. 6th ed. Baltimore, Lippincott, Williams and Wilkins, 2000.
17. Leavitt JL, Coats MH, Falk RH: Effects of exercise on transmitral gradient and pulmonary artery pressure in patients with mitral stenosis or a prosthetic mitral valve: A Doppler echocardiographic study. J Am Coll Cardiol 17:1520, 1991.
18. Gorlin R, Gorlin SG: Hydraulic formula for calculation of the area of stenotic mitral valve, other cardiac valves and central circulatory shunts. Am Heart J 41:1, 1951.
19. Braunwald E, Turi ZG: Pathophysiology of mitral valve disease. In Wells FC, Shapiro LM (eds): Mitral Valve Disease. 2nd ed. London, Butterworths, 1996, pp 28–36.
20. Ford LE, Feldman T, Carroll JD: Valve resistance. Circulation 89:893, 1994.
21. Wroblewski E, Spann JF, Bove AA: Right ventricular performance in mitral stenosis. Am J Cardiol 47:51, 1981.
22. Kennedy JW: The use of quantitative angiocardiography in mitral valve disease. In Duran C, Angell WW, Johnson AD, Oury JH (eds): Recent Progress in Mitral Valve Disease. London, Butterworths, 1984, pp 149–159.
23. Gash AK, Carabello BA, Cepin D, Spann JF: Left ventricular ejection performance and systolic muscle function in patients with mitral stenosis. Circulation 67:148, 1983.
24. Colle JP, Rahal S, Ohayon J, et al: Global left ventricular function and regional wall motion in pure mitral stenosis. Clin Cardiol 7:573, 1984.
25. Gaasch WH and Folland ED: Left ventricular function in rheumatic mitral stenosis. Eur Heart J 12(Suppl B):66, 1991.
26. Mohan JC, Khalilullah M, Arora R: Left ventricular intrinsic contractility in pure rheumatic mitral stenosis. Am J Cardiol 64:240, 1989.
27. Johnston DL, Kotsuk WJ: Left and right ventricular function during symptom-limited exercise in patients with isolated mitral stenosis. Chest 89:186, 1986.
28. Reis RN, Roberts WC: Amounts of coronary arterial narrowing by atherosclerotic plaques in clinically isolated mitral valve stenosis: Analysis of 76 necropsy patients older than 30 years. Am J Cardiol 57:1117, 1986.
29. Haworth SG, Hall SM, Patel M: Peripheral pulmonary vascular and airway abnormalities in adolescents with rheumatic mitral stenosis. Int J Cardiol 18:405, 1988.
30. Babic UU, Popovic Z, Grujicic S, et al: Systemic and pulmonary flow in mitral stenosis: Evidence for a bronchial vein shunt. Cardiology 78:311, 1991.
31. Moreyra AE, Wilzon AC, Deac R, et al: Factors associated with atrial fibrillation in patients with mitral stenosis: A cardiac catheterization study. Am Heart J 135:138–45, 1998.
32. Keren G, Etzion T, Sherez J, et al: Atrial fibrillation and atrial enlargement in patients with mitral stenosis. Am Heart J 114:1146, 1987.
33. Leatham A: Assessment of mitral valve function: clinical presentation, assessment and prognosis. In Wells FC, Shapiro LM (eds): Mitral Valve Disease. 2nd ed. London, Butterworths, 1996, pp 37–46.
34. Scarlat A, Bodner G, and Liron M: Massive haemoptysis as the presenting symptom in mitral stenosis. Thorax 41:413, 1986.
35. Baxter, RH, Reid JM, McGuiness JB, Stevenson JG: Relation of angina to coronary artery disease in mitral and aortic valve disease. Br Heart J 40:918, 1978.
36. Nielson GH, Galea EG, Houssack KF: Thromboembolic complications of mitral valve disease. Aust NZ J Med 8:372, 1978.
36a. Chiang CW, Lo SK, Ko YS, et al: Predictors of systemic embolism in patients with mitral stenosis. A prospective study. Ann Intern Med 128:885, 1998.
37. Chiang CW, Lo SK, Kuo CT, et al: Noninvasive predictors of systemic embolism in mitral stenosis: An echocardiographic and clinical study of 500 patients. Chest 106:396, 1994.
38. Sharma NGK, Kapoor CP, Mahambre L, Borkar MP: Ortner's syndrome. J Indian Med Assoc 60:427, 1973.
39. Horwitz LD and Groves BM (eds): Signs and Symptoms in Cardiology. Philadelphia, JB Lippincott, 1985, 506 pp.
40. Abrams J: Mitral stenosis. In Essentials of Cardiac Physical Diagnosis. Philadelphia, Lea and Febiger, 1987, pp 275–306.
41. Longhini C, Baracca E, Aggio S, et al: The first heart sound in mitral stenosis. Acta Cardiol (Brux) 46:73, 1991.
42. Barrington WW, Boudoulas J, Bashore T, et al: Mitral stenosis: Mitral dome excursion and M₁ and the mitral opening snap—the concept of reciprocal heart sounds. Am Heart J 115:1280, 1988.
43. Saunders JL, Calatayud JB, Schultz KJ, et al: Evaluation of ECG criteria for P-wave abnormalities. Am Heart J 74:757, 1967.
44. Cooksey JD, Dunn, M, Massie E: Clinical Vectorcardiography and Electrocardiography. 2nd ed. Chicago, Year Book Medical Publishers, 1977, p 272.
45. Donoso E, Jick S, Braunwald E, et al: The spatial vectorcardiogram in mitral valve disease. Am Heart J 53:760, 1957.
46. Parker BM, Friedenberg MJ, Templeton AW, Burford TH: Preoperative angiocardiographic diagnosis of left atrial thrombi in mitral stenosis. N Engl J Med 273:136, 1965.
47. Shapiro LM: Echocardiography of the mitral valve. In Wells FC, Shapiro LM (eds): Mitral Valve Disease. 2nd ed. London, Butterworths, 1996, pp 47–50.
48. Sagie A, Freitas N, Chen MH, et al: Echocardiographic assessment of mitral stenosis and its associated valvular lesions in 205 patients and lack of association with mitral valve prolapse. J Am Soc Echocardiogr 10:141, 1997.
49. Faletr F, Pezzano JA, Fusc R, et al: Measurement of mitral valve area in mitral stenosis: Four echocardiographic methods compared with direct measurement of anatomic orifices. J Am Coll Cardiol 28:1190, 1996.
50. Popovic AD, Thomas JD, Neskovic AN, et al: Time-related trends in the preoperative evaluation of patients with valvular stenosis. Am J Cardiol 80:1464, 1997.
51. Bonow RO, Carabello B, de Leon AC Jr: ACC/AHA Guidelines for the management of patients with valvular heart disease. J Am Coll Cardiol 32:1486, 1998.
52. Beiser GD, Epstein SE, Braunwald E, et al: Studies on digitalis. XVIII. Effects of ouabain on the hemodynamic response to exercise in patients with mitral stenosis in normal sinus rhythm. N Engl J Med 278:131, 1968.
53. Klein HO, Sareli P, Schamroth CL, et al: Effects of atenolol on exercise capacity in patients with mitral stenosis with sinus rhythm. Am J Cardiol 56:598, 1985.

54. Prystowsky EN, Benson DW Jr, Fuster V, et al: Management of patients with atrial fibrillation: A Statement for Healthcare Professionals. From the Subcommittee on Electrocardiography and Electrophysiology. Circulation 93:1262, 1996.

55. Manning WJ, Silverman DI, Keighley CS, et al: Transesophageal echocardiographically facilitated early cardioversion from atrial fibrillation using short-term anticoagulation: final results of a prospective 4.5 year study. J Am Coll Cardiol 25:1354, 1995.

56. Kosakai Y, Kawaguchi AT, Isobe F, et al: Cox maze procedure for chronic atrial fibrillation associated with mitral valve disease. J Thorac Cardiovasc Surg 108:1049, 1994.

57. Shyu KG, Cheng JJ, Chen JJ, et al: Recovery of atrial function after atrial compartment operation for chronic atrial fibrillation in mitral valve disease. J Am Coll Cardiol 24:392, 1994.

58. Joswig BC, Glover MU, Handler JB, et al: Contrasting progression of mitral stenosis in the Malayans versus American-born Caucasians. Am Heart J 104:1400, 1982.

59. Gordon SP, Douglas PS, Come PC, et al: Two-dimensional and Doppler echocardiographic determinants of the natural history of mitral valve narrowing in patients with rheumatic mitral stenosis: Implications for followup. J Am Coll Cardiol 19:968, 1992.

60. Sagie A, Freitas N, Padial LR, et al: Doppler echocardiographic assessment of long-term progression of mitral stenosis in 103 patients: Valve area and right heart disease. J Am Coll Cardiol 28:472, 1996.

61. Olesen KH: The natural history of 271 patients with mitral stenosis under medical treatment. Br Heart J 24:349, 1962.

62. Rowe JC, Bland EF, Sprague HB, White PD: The course of mitral stenosis without surgery: Ten- and twenty-year perspectives. Ann Intern Med 52:741, 1960.

63. Munoz S, Gallardo J, Diaz-Gorrin JR, Medina O: Influence of surgery on the natural history of rheumatic mitral and aortic valve disease. Am J Cardiol 35:234, 1975.

64. Horstkotte D, Niehues R, Strauer BE: Pathomorphological aspects, aetiology and natural history of acquired mitral valve stenosis. Eur Heart J 12(Suppl):55, 1991.

65. Chen CR, Chang TO, Chen JY, et al: Percutaneous balloon mitral valvuloplasty for mitral stenosis with and without associated aortic regurgitation. Am Heart J 125:128, 1993.

66. Leon MN, Harrell LC, Simosa HF, et al: Comparison of immediate and long-term results of mitral balloon valvuloplasty with the double-balloon versus Inoue techniques. Am J Cardiol 83:1356, 1999.

67. Fawzy ME, Mimish L, Sivanandam V, et al: Immediate and long-term effect of mitral balloon valvotomy on severe pulmonary hypertension in patients with mitral stenosis. Am Heart J 131:89, 1996.

67a. Gomez-Hospital JA, Cequier A, Romero PV, et al: Partial improvement in pulmonary function after successful percutaneous balloon mitral valvotomy. Chest 117:643, 2000.

68. Orrange E, Kawanishi DT, Lopez BM, et al: Actuarial outcome after catheter balloon commissurotomy in patients with mitral stenosis. Circulation 95:382, 1997.

69. Palacios IF, Tuzeu ME, Weyman AE, et al: Clinical follow-up of patients undergoing percutaneous mitral balloon valvotomy. Circulation 91:671, 1995.

69a. Hamasaki N, Nosaka H, Kimura T, et al: Ten-years clinical follow-up following successful percutaneous transvenous mitral commissurotomy: Single-center experience. Cathet Cardiovasc Intervent 49:284, 2000.

70. Wilkins GT, Weyman AE, Abascal VM, et al: Percutaneous mitral valvotomy: An analysis of echocardiographic variables related to outcome and the mechanism of dilatation. Br Heart J 60:299, 1988.

71. Padial LR, Abascal VM, Moreno PR, et al: Echocardiography can predict the development of severe mitral regurgitation after percutaneous mitral valvuloplasty by the Inoue technique. Am J Cardiol 83:1210, 1999.

72. Tuzcu EM, Block PC, Griffin B, et al: Percutaneous mitral balloon valvotomy in patients with calcific mitral stenosis: Immediate and long-term outcome. J Am Coll Cardiol 23:1604, 1994.

73. Zhang HP, Yen GS, Allen JW, et al: Comparison of late results of balloon valvotomy in mitral stenosis with versus without mitral regurgitation. Am J Cardiol 81:51, 1998.

74. Mazur W, Parilak LD, Kaluza G, et al: Balloon valvuloplasty for mitral stenosis. Curr Opin Cardiol 14:95, 1999.

75. Applebaum R, Kasliwal R, Kanojia A, et al: Utility of three-dimensional echocardiography during balloon mitral valvuloplasty. J Am Coll Cardiol 32:1405, 1998.

76. Reyes VP, Raju BS, Wynne J, et al: Percutaneous balloon valvuloplasty compared with open surgical commissurotomy for mitral stenosis. N Engl J Med 331:961, 1994.

77. Hernandez R, Banuelos C, Alfonso F, et al: Long-term clinical and echocardiographic follow-up after percutaneous mitral valvuloplasty with the Inoue balloon. Circulation 99:1580, 1999.

78. Meneveau N, Schiele F, Sernde MF, et al: Predictors of event-free survival after percutaneous mitral commissurotomy. Heart 80:359, 1998.

79. Orrange SE, Kawanishi DT, Lopez BM, et al.: Actuarial outcome after catheter balloon commissurotomy in patients with mitral stenosis. Circulation 95:382, 1997.

80. Joseph PK, Bhat A, Francis B, et al: Percutaneous transvenous mitral commissurotomy using an Inoue balloon in children with rheumatic mitral stenosis. Int J Cardiol 62:19, 1997.

81. Zaki A, Salama M, El Masry M, Elhendy A: Five-year follow-up after percutaneous balloon mitral valvuloplasty. Am J Cardiol 83:735, 1999.

82. Kothari SS, Kamath P, Juneja R, et al: Percutaneous transvenous mitral commissurtomy using Inoue balloon in children less than 12 years. Cathet Cardiovasc Diagn 43:408, 1998.

83. Chen C-R and Cheng TO: Percutaneous balloon mitral valvuloplasty by the Inoue technique: A multicenter study of 4832 patients in China. Am Heart J 129:1197, 1995.

84. Serra A, Bonan R, Lefevre T, et al: Balloon mitral commissurotomy for mitral restenosis after surgical commissurotomy. Am J Cardiol 71:1311, 1993.

85. Casale PN, Whitlow P, Currie PJ, et al: Transesophageal echocardiography in percutaneous balloon valvuloplasty for mitral stenosis. Cleve Clin J Med 56:597, 1989.

86. Ben Farat M, Gamra H, Betbout F, et al: Percutaneous balloon mitral commissurotomy during pregnancy. Heart 77:564, 1997.

87. Iung B, Cormier B, Elias J, et al: Usefulness of percutaneous balloon commissurotomy for mitral stenosis during pregnancy. Am J Cardiol 73:398, 1994.

88. Cribier A, Elchaninoff H, Koning R, et al: Percutaneous mechanical mitral commissurotomy with a newly designed metallic valvulotome: Immediate results of the initial experience in 153 patients. Circulation 99:793, 1999.

89. Gautam PC, Coulshed N, Epstein EJ, et al: Preoperative clinical predictors of long-term survival in mitral stenosis: Analysis of 200 cases followed for up to 27 years after closed mitral valvotomy. Thorax 41:401, 1986.

90. English T: Closed mitral valvotomy. In Wells FC, Shapiro LM (eds): Mitral Valve Disease. 2nd ed. London, Butterworths, 1996, pp 107–113.

91. de Vivie ER, Hellberg K: Closed transventricular mitral commissurotomy. In Ionescu MI, Cohn LH (eds): Mitral Valve Disease: Diagnosis and Treatment. London, Butterworths, 1985, pp 139–152.

92. Otto CM (ed): Valvular Heart Disease. Philadelphia, WB Saunders, 1999, 468 pp.

93. Cohn LH, Allred EN, Cohn LA, et al: Long-term results of open mitral valve reconstruction for mitral stenosis. Am J Cardiol 55:731, 1985.

94. Farhat MB, Boussadia H, Gandjbakhch I, et al: Closed versus open mitral commissurotomy in pure noncalcific mitral stenosis: Hemodynamic studies before and after operation. J Thorac Cardiovasc Surg 99:639, 1990.

95. Kirklin JW, Barrat-Boyes BG: Mitral commissurotomy. In Kirklin JW, Barrat-Boyes BG: Cardiac Surgery. 2nd ed. New York, Churchill-Livingstone, 1993, p 444.

96. Cohen DJ, Kuntz RE, Gordon SPF, et al: Predictors of long-term outcome after percutaneous balloon mitral valvuloplasty. N Engl J Med 327:1329, 1992.

97. Hickey MS, Blackstone EH, Kirklin JW, Dean LS: Outcome probabilities and life history after surgical mitral commissurotomy: Implications for balloon commissurotomy. J Am Coll Cardiol 17:29, 1991.

98. Gross RJ, Cunningham JN Jr, Snively SL, et al: Long-term results of open radical mitral commissurotomy: Ten year follow-up study of 202 patients. Am J Cardiol 47:821, 1981.

99. Aora R, Khalilullah M, Gupta MP, Padmavati S: Mitral restenosis. Incidence and epidemiology. Indian Heart J 30:265, 1978.

100. Heger JJ, Wann LS, Weyman AE, et al: Long-term changes in mitral valve area after successful mitral commissurotomy. Circulation 59:443, 1979.

101. Higgs LM, Glancy DL, O'Brien KP, et al: Mitral restenosis: An uncommon cause of recurrent symptoms following mitral commissurotomy. Am J Cardiol 26:34, 1970.

102. Braunwald E, Braunwald NS, Ross J Jr, Morrow AG: Effects of mitral valve replacement on the pulmonary vascular dynamics of patients with pulmonary hypertension. N Engl J Med 273:509, 1965.

103. Foltz BD, Hessel EA, Ivey TD: The early course of pulmonary artery hypertension in patients undergoing mitral valve replacement with cardioplegic arrest. J Thorac Cardiovasc Surg 88:238, 1984.

104. Jamieson WRE, Edwards FH, Schwartz M, et al: Risk stratification for cardiac valve replacement. National Cardiac Surgery Database. Ann Thorac Surg 67:943, 1999.

MITRAL REGURGITATION

104a. Carabello B: Mitral regurgitation. In Rahimtoola SH (ed): Valvular Heart Disease and Endocarditis. Atlas of Heart Diseases. Vol. 11. Braunwald E (series ed). Philadelphia, Current Medicine, 1996.

105. Essop MR, Skoularigis J, Sareli P: Transesophageal echocardiography in congenital submitral aneurysm. Am J Cardiol 71:481, 1993.

106. Mann JM, Davies MJ: The pathology of the mitral valve. In Wells FC, and Shapiro LM (eds): Mitral Valve Disease. 2nd ed. London, Butterworths, 1996, pp. 16–27.

107. Nestico PF, DePace NL, Kotler MN, et al: Calcium phosphorus metabolism in dialysis patients with and without mitral anular calcium. Analysis of 30 patients. Am J Cardiol 51:497, 1983.

108. Mellino M, Salcedo EE, Lever HM, et al: Echographic-quantified severity of mitral annulus calcification: Prognostic correlation to related hemodynamic, valvular, rhythm, and conduction abnormalities. Am Heart J 103:222, 1982.

109. Scott-Jupp W, Barnett NL, Gallagher PJ, et al: Ultrastructural changes in spontaneous rupture of mitral chordae tendineae. J Pathol 133:185, 1981.

110. Otasevic P, Pavlovski K, Popovic AD: Isolated mitral regurgitation complicating relapsing polychondritis. Int J Cardiol 60:213, 1997.

111. Godley RW, Wann LS, Rogers EW, et al: Incomplete mitral leaflet closure in patients with papillary muscle dysfunction. Circulation 63:565, 1981.

112. Lamas GA, Mitchell GF, Flaker GC, et al: Clinical significance of mitral regurgitation after acute myocardial infarction: Survival and Ventricular Enlargement Investigators. Circulation 96:827, 1997.

112a. Weissman NJ, Tighe JF Jr, Gottdiener JS, Gwynne JT: An assessment of heart-valve abnormalities in obese patients taking dexfenfluramine, sustained-release dexfenfluramine, or placebo. N Engl J Med 339:725, 1998.

113. Ballester M, Jajoo J, Rees S, et al: The mechanism of mitral regurgitation in a dilated left ventricle. Clin Cardiol 6:333, 1983.

114. Tcheng JE, Jackman JD, Nelson CL, et al: Outcome of patients sustaining acute ischemic mitral regurgitation during myocardial infarction. Ann Intern Med 117:18, 1992.

115. Hickey M St J, Smith LR, Muhlbaier LH, at al: Current prognosis of ischemic mitral regurgitation: Implications for future management. Circulation 78 (Suppl. I):I51, 1988.

116. Gottdiener JS, Maron BJ, Schooley RT, et al: Two-dimensional echocardiographic assessment of the idiopathic hypereosinophilic syndrome. Anatomic basis of mitral regurgitation and peripheral embolization. Circulation 67:572, 1983.

117. Metras D, Ouezzin-Coulibaly A, Ouattara K, et al: Endomyocardial fibrosis masquerading as rheumatic mitral incompetence. A report of six surgical cases. J Thorac Cardiovasc Surg 86:753, 1983.

118. Mazzucco A, Rizzoli G, Faggian G, et al: Acute mitral regurgitation after blunt chest trauma. Arch Intern Med 143:2326, 1983.

119. Jolly DT: Traumatic rupture of a papillary muscle of the mitral valve due to blunt thoracic trauma. Can Fam Phys 29:1960, 1983.

120. Gidding SS, Shulman ST, Ibawi M, et al: Mucocutaneous lymph node syndrome (Kawasaki disease): Delayed aortic and mitral insufficiency secondary to active valvulitis. J Am Coll Cardiol 7:894, 1986.

121. DiSegni E, and Edwards JE: Cleft anterior leaflet of the mitral valve with intact septa. A study of 20 cases. Am J Cardiol 51:919, 1983.

122. Nagata S, Nimura Y, Sakakibara H, et al: Mitral valve lesion associated with secundum atrial septal defect. Analysis of real-time two-dimensional echocardiography. Br Heart J 49:151, 1983.

123. Braunwald E, Welch GH Jr, Sarnoff SJ: Hemodynamic effects of quantitatively varied experimental mitral regurgitation. Circ Res 5:539, 1957.

124. Carabello BA, Crawford FA Jr: Valvular heart disease. N Engl J Med 337:32, 1997.

125. Yellin EL, Yoran C, Frater RWM, Sonnenblick EH: Dynamics of acute experimental mitral regurgitation. In Ionescu MI, Cohn LH (eds): Mitral Valve Disease: Diagnosis and Treatment. London, Butterworths, 1985, pp 11–26.

126. Rosario LB, Stevenson LW, Solomon SD, et al: The mechanism of decrease in dynamic mitral regurgitation during heart failure treatment: Importance of reduction in the regurgitant orifice size. J Am Coll Cardiol 32:1819, 1998.

127. Kontos GJ Jr, Schaff HV, Gersh BJ, Bove AA: Left ventricular function in subacute and chronic mitral regurgitation: Effect on function early postoperatively. J Thorac Cardiovasc Surg 98:163, 1989.

128. Corin WJ, Murakami T, Monrad ES, et al: Left ventricular passive diastolic properties in chronic mitral regurgitation. Circulation 83:797, 1991.

129. Conway MA, Bottomley PA, Ouwerkerk R, et al: Mitral regurgitation: Impaired systolic function, eccentric hypertrophy, and increased severity are linked to lower phosphocreatine/ATP ratios in humans. Circulation 97:1716, 1998.

130. Braunwald E: Mitral regurgitation: Physiological, clinical and surgical considerations. N Engl J Med 281:425, 1969.

131. Nwasokwa O, Camesas A, Weg I, Bodenheimer MM: Differences in left ventricular adaptation to chronic mitral and aortic regurgitation. Chest 95:106, 1989.

132. Braunwald E: Control of myocardial oxygen consumption: Physiologic and clinical considerations. Am J Cardiol 27:416, 1971.

133. Ross J Jr: Left ventricular function and the timing of surgical treatment in valvular heart disease. Ann Intern Med 94:498, 1981.

133a. Timmis SB, Kirsh MM, Montgomery DG, Starling MR: Evaluation of left ventricular ejection fraction as a measure of pump performance in patients with chronic mitral regurgitation. Cathet Cardiovasc Intervent 49:290, 2000.

134. Enriquez-Sarano M, Tajik AK, Schaff HV, et al: Echocardiographic prediction of survival after surgical correction of organic mitral regurgitation. Circulation 90:830, 1994.

135. Ramanthan KB, Knowles J, Connor MJ, et al: Natural history of chronic mitral insufficiency: Relation of peak systolic pressure/end-systolic volume ratio to morbidity and mortality. J Am Coll Cardiol 3:1412, 1984.

136. Borow K, Green LH, Mann T, et al: End-systolic volume as a predictor of postoperative left ventricular performance in volume overload from valvular regurgitation. Am J Med 68:655, 1980.

137. Wisenbaugh T, Skudicky D, Sareli P: Prediction of outcome after valve replacement for rheumatic mitral regurgitation in the era of chordal preservation. Circulation 89:191, 1994.

138. Leung DY, Griffin BP, Snader CE, et al: Determinant of functional capacity in chronic mitral regurgitation unassociated with coronary artery disease or left ventricular dysfunction. Am J Cardiol 79:914, 1997.

139. Grose R, Strain J, Cohen MV: Pulmonary arterial v waves in mitral regurgitation. Clinical and experimental observations. Circulation 69:214, 1984.

140. Schofield PM: Invasive investigation of the mitral valve. In Wells FC, Shapiro LM (eds): Mitral Valve Disease. 2nd ed. London, Butterworths, 1996, pp 84–91.

141. Pape LA, Price JM, Alpert JS, et al: Relation of left atrial size to pulmonary capillary wedge pressure in severe mitral regurgitation. Cardiology 78:297, 1991.

142. Braunwald E, Awe WC: The syndrome of severe mitral regurgitation with normal left atrial pressure. Circulation 27:29, 1963.

143. Roberts WC, Braunwald E, Morrow AG: Acute severe mitral regurgitation secondary to ruptured chordae tendineae. Clinical, hemodynamic and pathologic considerations. Circulation 33:58, 1966.

144. Cohen LS, Mason DT, Braunwald E: Significance of an atrial gallop sound in mitral regurgitation: A clue to the diagnosis of ruptured chordae tendineae. Circulation 35:112, 1966.

145. Rippe JM, Howe JP III: Acute mitral regurgitation. In Dalen JE, Alpert JS (eds): Valvular Heart Disease. 2nd ed. Boston, Little, Brown and Co, 1987, pp 151–176.

146. Rosen SF, Borer JS, Hochreiter C, et al: Natural history of the asymptomatic patient with severe mitral regurgitation secondary to mitral valve prolapse and normal right and left ventricular performance. Am J Cardiol 74:374, 1994.

147. Rapaport E: Natural history of aortic and mitral valve disease. Am J Cardiol 35:221, 1975.

148. Elkins RC, Morrow AG, Vasko JS, Braunwald E: The effects of mitral regurgitation on the pattern of instantaneous aortic blood flow. Clinical and experimental observations. Circulation 36:45, 1967.

149. Karliner JS, O'Rourke RA, Kearney DJ, Shabetai R: Haemodynamic explanation of why the murmur of mitral regurgitation is independent of cycle length. Br Heart J 35:397, 1973.

150. Schreiber TL, Fisher J, Mangla A, Miller D: Severe "silent" mitral regurgitation: A potentially reversible cause of refractory heart failure. Chest 96:242, 1989.

151. Merendino KA, and Hessel EA: The murmur on top of the head in acquired mitral insufficiency. JAMA 199:392, 1967.

152. Morris JJ, Estes EH, Whalen RE, et al: P wave analysis in valvular heart disease. Circulation 29:242, 1964.

153. Priest EA, Finlayson JK, Short DS: The x-ray manifestations in the heart and lungs of mitral regurgitation. Prog Cardiovasc Dis 5:219, 1962.

154. Himelman RB, Kusumoto F, Oken K, et al: The flail mitral valve: Echocardiographic findings by precordial and transesophageal imaging and Doppler color flow mapping. J Am Coll Cardiol 17:272, 1991.

155. Nair CK, Aronow WS, Sketch MH, et al: Clinical and echocardiographic characteristics of patients with mitral annular calcification. Am J Cardiol 51:992, 1983.

155a. Heinle SK, Grayburn PA: Doppler echocardiographic assessment of mitral regurgitation. Coron Artery Dis 11:11, 2000.

155b. Armstrong GP, Griffin BP: Exercise echocardiographic assessment in severe mitral regurgitation. Coron Artery Dis 11:23, 2000.

156. Dujardin KS, Enriquez-Sarano M, Bailey KR, et al: Grading of mitral regurgitation by quantitative Doppler echocardiography: Calibration by left ventricular angiography in routine clinical practice. Circulation 96:3409, 1996.

157. Krivokapich J: Echocardiography in valvular heart disease. Curr Opin Cardiol 9:158, 1994.

158. Zhou X, Jones M, Shiota T, et al: Vena contracta imaged by Doppler color flow mapping predicts the severity of eccentric mitral regurgitation better than color jet area: A chronic animal study. J Am Coll Cardiol 30:1393, 1997.

159. Hall SA, Brickner ME, Willett DL, et al: Assessment of mitral regurgitation severity by Doppler color flow mapping of the vena contracta. Circulation 95:636, 1997.

160. Mele D, Vandervoort P, Palacios I, et al: Proximal jet size by Doppler color flow mapping predicts severity of mitral regurgitation. Circulation 91:746, 1995.

161. Enriquez-Sarano M, Dujardin KS, Tribouilloy CM, et al: Determinants of pulmonary venous flow reversal in mitral regurgitation and its usefulness in determining the severity of regurgitation. Am J Cardiol 83:535, 1999.

162. Thomas L, Foster E, Schiller NB: Peak mitral inflow velocity predicts mitral regurgitation severity. J Am Coll Cardiol 31:174, 1998.

163. Shyu K, Lei M, Hwang J: Morphologic characterization and quantitative assessment of mitral regurgitation with ruptured chordae tendineae by transesophageal echocardiography. Am J Cardiol 70:1152, 1992.

164. Smith MD, Cassidy JM, Gurley JC, et al: Echo Doppler evaluation of patients with acute mitral regurgitation: Superiority of transesopageal echocardiography with color flow imaging. Am Heart J 129:967, 1995.

165. Bach D-S, Deeb GM, Bolling SF: Accuracy of intraoperative transesophageal echocardiography for estimating the severity of functional mitral regurgitation. Am J Cardiol 76:508, 1995.

166. De Simone R, Glombitza G, Vahl CF, et al: Three dimensional color Doppler: a clinical study in patients with mitral regurgitation. J Am Coll Cardiol 33:1646, 1999.

167. Wexler L, Silverman JF, DeBusk RF, Harrison DC: Angiographic features of rheumatic and nonrheumatic mitral regurgitation. Circulation 44:1080, 1971.

168. Manzara CC, Pennell DJ, Underwood SR: Assessment of the mitral valve by magnetic resonance imaging. In Wells FC, Shapiro LM (eds): Mitral Valve Disease. 2nd ed. London, Butterworths, 1996, pp 71–83.

169. Kizilbash AM, Hundley WG, Willett DL, et al: Comparison of quantitative Doppler with magnetic resonance imaging for assessement of the severity of mitral regurgitation. Am J Cardiol 81:792, 1998.

170. Shimoyama H, Sabbah HN, Roman H, et al: Effects of long-term therapy with enalapril on severity of functional mitral regurgitation in dogs with moderate heart failure. J Am Coll Cardiol 25:768, 1995.

171. Tischler MD, Rowan M, LeWinter MM: Effect of enalapril therapy on left ventricular mass and volumes in asymptomatic chronic, severe, mitral regurgitation secondary to mitral valve prolapse. Am J Cardiol 82:242, 1998.

172. Yoran C, Yellin EL, Becker RM, et al: Mechanism of reduction of mitral regurgitation with vasodilator therapy. Am J Cardiol 43:773, 1979.

173. Schon HR, Schroter G, Barthel P, Schomig A: Quinapril therapy in patients with chronic mitral regurgitation. J Heart Valve Dis 3:303, 1994.

173a. Host U, Kelbaek H, Hildebrant P, et al: Effect of ramipril on mitral regurgitation secondary to mitral valve prolapse. Am J Cardiol 80:655, 1997.

174. Chauvaud S, Fuzellier JF, Houel R, et al: Reconstructive surgery in congenital mitral valve insufficiency (Carpentier's techniques): Long-term results. J Thorac Cardiovasc Surg 115:84, 1998.

175. Wells FC: Conservation and surgical repair of the mitral valve. In Wells FC, Shapiro LM (eds): Mitral Valve Disease. 2nd ed. London, Butterworths, 1996, pp 114–134.

176. Bolling SF, Pagani FD, Deeb GM, Bach DS: Intermediate-term outcome of mitral reconstruction in cardiomyopathy. J Thorac Cardiovasc Surg 115:381, 1998.

177. Chen FY, Adams DH, Aranki SF, et al: Mitral valve repair in cardiomyopathy. Circulation 98:III124, 1998.

177a. von Oppell UO, Stemmet F, Braink J, et al: Ischemic mitral valve repair surgery. Heart Valve Dis 9:64, 2000.

178. Cooper HA and Gersh BJ: Treatment of chronic mitral regurgitation. Am Heart J 135:925, 1998.

179. Odell JA, Orszulak TA: Surgical repair and reconstruction of valvular lesions. Curr Opin Cardiol 10:135, 1995.

179a. Phillips MR, Daly RC, Schaff HV, et al: Repair of anterior leaflet mitral valve prolapse: Chordal replacement versus chordal shortening. Ann Thorac Surg 69:25, 2000.

180. Frater RWM, Vetter O, Zussa C, Dahm M: Chordal replacement in mitral valve repair. Circulation 82(Suppl IV):125, 1990.

181. Colon R, Frazier OH: Mitral valve replacement techniques. In Wells FC, Shapiro LM (eds): Mitral Valve Disease. 2nd ed. London, Butterworths, 1996, pp 135–147.

182. Nakano K, Swindler MM, Spinale FB, et al: Depressed contractile function due to canine mitral regurgitation improves after correction of the volume overload. J Clin Invest 87:2077, 1991.

183. Duran CM, Gometza B, Saad E: Valve repair in rheumatic mitral disease: An unsolved problem. J Cardiovasc Surg 9(Suppl):282, 1994.

184. Enriquez-Sarano M, Schaff HV, Orszulak TA, et al: Valve repair improves the outcome of surgery for mitral regurgitation. Circulation 91:1022, 1995.

185. Corin WJ, Sutsch G, Murakami T, et al: Left ventricular function in chronic mitral regurgitation. Preoperative and postoperative comparison. J Am Coll Cardiol 25:113, 1995.

186. Reardon MJ, David TE: Mitral valve replacement with preservation of the subvalvular apparatus. Curr Opin Cardiol 14:104, 1998.

187. Enriquez-Sarano M, Scaff HV, Orszulak TA, et al: Valve repair improves the outcome of surgery for mitral regurgitation: A multivariate analysis. Circulation 91:1022, 1995.

188. Espada R, Westaby S: New developments in mitral valve repair. Curr Opin Cardiol 13:80, 1998.

189. Smedira NG, Selman R, Cosgrove DM, et al: Repair of anterior prolapse: Chordal transfer is superior to chordal shortening. J Thorac Cardiovasc Surg 117:287, 1996.

190. Lee EM, Shapiro LM, Wells FC: Midterm results of mitral valve repair with the Sculptor annuloplasty ring. Ann Thorac Surg 63:1340, 1997.

191. Lee KS, Stewart WJ, Lever HM, et al: Mechanism of outflow tract obstruction causing failed mitral valve repair: Anterior displacement of leaflet coaptation. Circulation 88:24, 1993.

192. Lee KS, Stewart WJ, Lever HM, et al: Mechanism of outflow tract obstruction causing failed mitral valve repair, anterior displacement of leaflet coaptation. Circulation 88:1124, 1993.

193. Ling LH, Enriquez-Sarano M, Seward JB, et al: Early surgery in patients with mitral regurgitation due to flail leaflets: A long-term outcome study. Circulation 96:1819, 1997.

193a. Grossi EA, Galloway AC, Miller JS, et al: Valve repair versus replacement for mitral insufficiency: When is a mechanical valve still indicated? J Thorac Cardiovasc Surg 115:389, 1998.

193b. Byrne JG, Aranki SF, Cohn LH: Repair versus replacement of mitral valve for treating severe ischemic mitral regurgitation. Coron Artery Dis 11:31, 2000.

194. Loulmet DF, Carpentier A, Cho PW, et al: Less invasive techniques for mitral valve surgery. J Thorac Cardiovasc Surg 115:772, 1998.

195. Schwartz DS, Ribakove GH, Grossi EA, et al: Minimally invasive mitral valve replacement: Port-access technique, feasibility, and myocardial functional preservation. J Thorac Cardiovasc Surg 113:1022, 1997.

195a. Byrne JG, Mitchell ME, Adams DH, et al: Minimally invasive direct access mitral valve surgery. Sem Thorac Cardiovasc Surg 11:212, 1999.

196. Letsou GV, Reardon MJ: Minimally invasive valve surgery. Curr Opin Cardiol 13:105, 1998.

197. Wisenbaugh T, Skucicky D, Sarelli P: Prediction of outcome after valve replacement for rheumatic mitral regurgitation in the era of chordal preservation. Circulation 89:191, 1994.

198. Lee SJK, Bay KS: Mortality risk factors associated with mitral valve replacement: A survival analysis of 10 year follow-up data. Can J Cardiol 7:11, 1991.

199. Krishnan US, Gersony WW, Berman-Rosenzweig E, Apfel HD: Late left ventricular function after surgery for children with chronic symptomatic mitral regurgitation. Circulation 96:4280, 1997.

200. Tribouilloy CM, Enriquez-Sarano M, Schaff HV, et al: Impact of preoperative symptoms on survival after surgical correction of organic mitral regurgitation: Rationale for optimizing surigical indications. Circulation 99:400, 1999.

201. Peterson KL: The timing of surgical intervention in chronic mitral regurgitation. Cathet Cardiovasc Diagn 9:433, 1983.

202. Freed LA, Levy D, Levine RA, et al: Prevalence and clinical outcome of mitral-valve prolapse. N Engl J Med 341:1, 1999.

203. Akins CW, Hilgenberg AD, Buckley MJ, et al: Mitral valve reconstruction versus replacement for degenerative ischemic mitral regurgitation. Ann Thorac Surg 58:668, 1994.

204. Gaasch WH, and Aurigemma GP: Is corrective surgery ever indicated in the asymptomatic patient with mitral regurgitation? Cardiol Rev 2:138, 1994.

205. Treasure T: Timing of surgery in chronic mitral regurgitation. In Wells FC, Shapiro LM: Mitral Valve Disease. 2nd ed. London, Butterworths, 1996, pp 187–196.

206. Bolling SF, Deeb GM, Brunsting LA, Bach DS: Early outcome of mitral valve reconstruction in patients with end-stage cardiomyopathy. J Thorac Cardiovasc Surg 109:676, 1995.

207. Bach DS, Bolling SF: Early improvement in congestive heart failure after correction of secondary mitral regurgitation in end-stage cardiomyopathy. Am Heart J 129:1165, 1995.

208. Bach DS, Bolling SF: Improvement following corrrection of secondary mitral regurgitation in end-stage cardiomyopathy with mitral annuloplasty. Am J Cardiol 78:966, 1996.

MITRAL VALVE PROLAPSE SYNDROME

209. Devereux RB: Recent developments in the diagnosis and management of mitral valve prolapse. Curr Opin Cardiol 10:107, 1995.

210. David TE, Omran A, Armstrong S, et al: Long-term results of mitral valve repair for myxomatous disease with and without chordal replacement with expanded polytetrafluoroethylene sutures. J Thorac Cardiovasc Surg 115:1279, 1998.

211. Cohn LH, Couper GS, Aranki SF, et al: Long-term results of mitral valve reconstruction for the regurgitating myxomatous mitral valve. J Thorac Cardiovasc Surg 107:143, 1994.

212. Devereux RB, Hawkins I, Kramer-Fox R, et al: Complications of mitral valve prolapse: Disproportionate occurrence in men and older patients. Am J Med 81:751, 1986.

213. Perloff JK, Child JS, Edwards JE: New guidelines for the clinical diagnosis of mitral valve prolapse. Am J Cardiol 57:1124, 1986.

214. Marks AR, Choong CY, Sanfilippo AJ, et al: Identification of high-risk and low-risk subgroups of patients with mitral valve prolapse. N Engl J Med 320:1031, 1989.

215. Goldhaber SZ, Brown WD, St John Sutton MG: High frequency of mitral valve prolapse and aortic regurgitation among asymptomatic adults with Down's syndrome. JAMA 258:1793, 1987.

216. Noah MS, Sulimani RA, Famuyiwa FO, et al: Prolapse of the mitral valve in hyperthyroid patients in Saudi Arabia. Int J Cardiol 19:217, 1988.

217. Froom P, Margulis T, Grenadier E, et al: Von Willebrand factor and mitral valve prolapse. Thromb Haemost 60:230, 1988.

218. Streib EW, Meyers DG, Sun SF: Mitral valve prolapse in myotonic dystrophy. Muscle Nerve 8:650, 1985.

219. Johnson GL, Humphries LL, Shirley PB, et al: Mitral valve prolapse in patients with anorexia nervosa and bulimia. Arch Intern Med 146:1525, 1986.

220. Waite P, McCallum CA: Mitral valve prolapse in craniofacial skeletal deformities. Oral Surg Oral Med Oral Pathol 61:15, 1986.

221. Comens SM, Alpert MA, Sharp GC, et al: Frequency of mitral valve prolapse in systemic lupus erythematosus, progressive systemic sclerosis and mixed connective tissue disease. Am J Cardiol 63:59, 1989.

222. Chan FL, Chen WW, Wong PHC, Chow, JSF: Skeletal abnormalities in mitral valve prolapse. Clin Radiol 34:207, 1983.

223. Lu-Li S, Guang-Gen C, Ru-Lian L: Valve prolapse in Behçet's disease. Br Heart J 54:100, 1985.

224. Cabeen WR, Jr, Reza MJ, Kovick RB, Stern MS: Mitral valve prolapse and conduction defects in Ehlers-Danlos syndrome. Arch Intern Med 137:1227, 1977.

225. Lebwohl MG, Distefano D, Prioleau PG, et al: Pseudoxanthoma elasticum and mitral valve prolapse. N Engl J Med 307:228, 1982.

226. Zema MJ, Chiaramida S, DeFilipp GJ, et al: Somatotype and idiopathic mitral valve prolapse. Cathet Cardiovasc Diagn 8:105, 1982.

227. Malcolm AD: Mitral valve prolapse associated with other disorders. Causal coincidence, common link, or fundamental genetic disturbance? Br Heart J 53:353, 1985.

227a. Becker AE, Davies MJ: Pathomorphology of mitral valve prolapse. In Boudoulas H, Wooley CF (eds): Mitral Valve: Floppy Mitral Valve,

Mitral Valve Prolapse, Mitral Valvular Regurgitation. 2nd ed. Armonk, NY, Futura, 2000, pp 91–114.

228. Jaffe AS, Geltman EM, Rodey GE, Uitto J: Mitral valve prolapse: A consistent manifestation of Type IV Ehlers-Danlos syndrome. The pathogenetic role of the abnormal production of Type III collagen. Circulation 64:121, 1981.

229. Tomaru T, Uchida Y, Mohri N, et al: Postinflammatory mitral and aortic valve prolapse: A clinical and pathological study. Circulation 76:68, 1987.

230. Stein PD, Wang C-H, Riddle JM, et al: Scanning electron microscopy of operatively excised severely regurgitant floppy mitral valves. Am J Cardiol 64:392, 1989.

231. Baker PB, Bansal G, Boudoulas H, et al: Floppy mitral valve chordae tendineae: Histopathologic alterations. Hum Pathol 19:507, 1988.

232. Devereux RB, Kramer-Fox R, Kligfield P: Mitral valve prolapse: Causes, clinical manifestations, and management. Arch Intern Med 111:305, 1989.

233. Pan CW, Chen CC, Wang SP, et al: Echocardiographic study of cardiac abnormalities in families of patients with Marfan's syndrome. J Am Coll Cardiol 6:1016, 1985.

234. Zuppiroli A, Rinaldi M, Kramer-Fox R, et al: Natural history of mitral valve prolapse. Am J Cardiol 75:1028, 1995.

235. Boudoulas H, Kolibash AJ, Jr, Baker P, et al: Mitral valve prolapse and the mitral valve prolapse syndrome: A diagnostic classification and pathogenesis of symptoms. Am Heart J 118:796, 1989.

236. Davies AO, Mares A, Pool JL, Taylor AA: Mitral valve prolapse with symptoms of beta-adrenergic hypersensitivity. Beta₂-adrenergic receptor supercoupling with desensitization on isoproterenol exposure. Am J Med 82:193, 1987.

237. Gaffney FA, Bastian BC, Lane LB, et al: Abnormal cardiovascular regulation in the mitral valve prolapse syndrome. Am J Cardiol 52:316, 1983.

237a. Fontana MF: Mitral valve prolapse and floppy mitral valve: Physical examination. In Boudoulas H, Wooley CF (eds): Mitral Valve: Floppy Mitral Valve, Mitral Valve Prolapse, Mitral Valvular Regurgitation. 2nd ed. Armonk, NY, Futura, 2000, pp 283–304.

238. Kligfield P, Hochreiter C, Niles N, et al: Relation of sudden death in pure mitral regurgitation with and without mitral valve prolapse to repetitive ventricular arrhythmias and right and left ventricular ejection fraction. Am J Cardiol 60:397, 1987.

239. Stein KM, Borer JS, Hochreiter C, et al: Prognostic value and physiological correlates of heart rate variability in chronic severe mitral regurgitation. Circulation 88:127, 1993.

239a. Schaal SF: Mitral valve prolapse: Cardiac arrhythmias and electrophysiological correlates. In Boudoulas H, Wooley CF (eds): Mitral Valve: Floppy Mitral Valve, Mitral Valve Prolapse, Mitral Valvular Regurgitation. 2nd ed. Armonk, NY, Futura, 2000, pp 409–430.

240. Wit AL, Fenoglio JJ, Hordof AJ, Reemtsma K: Ultrastructure and transmembrane potentials of cardiac muscle in the human anterior mitral valve leaflet. Circulation 59:1283, 1979.

241. Gallagher JJ, Gilbert M, Svenson RH: Wolff-Parkinson-White syndrome. The problem, evaluation and surgical correction. Circulation 57:767, 1975.

242. Davies MJ, Moore BP, Braimbridge MV: The floppy mitral valve: Study of incidence, pathology, and complications in surgical, necropsy, and forensic material. Br Heart J 40:468, 1978.

243. Nishimura RA, McGoon MD, Shub C, et al: Echocardiographically documented mitral valve prolapse: long-term followup. N Engl J Med 313:1305, 1985.

243a. Boudoulas H, Wooley CF: Floppy mitral valve/Mitral valve prolapse: Sudden death. In Boudoulas H, Wooley CF (eds): Mitral Valve: Floppy Mitral Valve, Mitral Valve Prolapse, Mitral Valvular Regurgitation. 2nd ed. Armonk, NY, Futura, 2000, pp 431–448.

244. Pocock WA, Bosman CK, Chesler E, et al: Sudden death in primary mitral valve prolapse. Am Heart J 107:378, 1984.

244a. Malkowski MJ, Pearson AC: The echocardiographic assessment of the floppy mitral valve: An integrated approach. In Boudoulas H, Wooley CF (eds): Mitral Valve: Floppy Mitral Valve, Mitral Valve Prolapse, Mitral Valvular Regurgitation. 2nd ed. Armonk, NY, Futura, 2000, pp 231–252.

245. Levine RA, Stathogiannis E, Newell JB, et al: Reconsideration of echocardiographic standards for mitral valve prolapse: Lack of association between leaflet displacement isolated to the apical four chamber view and independent echocardiographic evidence of abnormality. J Am Coll Cardiol 11:1010, 1988.

246. Langholz D, Mackin WJ, Wallis DE, et al: Transesophageal echocardiographic assessment of systolic mitral leaflet displacement among patients with mitral valve prolapse. Am Heart J 135:197, 1998.

247. Panidis IP, McAllister M, Ross J, Mintz GS: Prevalence and severity of mitral regurgitation in the mitral valve prolapse syndrome: A Doppler echocardiographic study of 80 patients. J Am Coll Cardiol 7:975, 1986.

248. Weissman NJ, Pini R, Roman MJ, et al: In vivo mitral valve morphology and function in mitral valve prolapse. Am J Cardiol 73:1080, 1994.

249. Rodger JC, Morley P: Abnormal aortic valve echoes in mitral prolapse. Echocardiographic features of floppy aortic valve. Br Heart J 47:337, 1982.

250. Klein GJ, Kostuk WJ, Boughner DR, Chamberlain MJ: Stress myocardial imaging in mitral leaflet prolapse syndrome. Am J Cardiol 42:746, 1978.

251. Cohen MV, Shah PK, Spindola-Franco H: Angiographic-echocardiographic correlation of mitral valve prolapse. Am Heart J 97:43, 1979.

252. Cipriano PR, Kline SA, Baltaxe HA: An angiographic assessment of left

ventricular function in isolated mitral valvular prolapse. Invest Radiol 15:293, 1980.

253. Mills P, Rose J, Hollingsworth J, et al: Long-term prognosis of mitral valve prolapse. N Engl J Med 297:13, 1977.

253a. Boudoulas H, Kolibash AJ, Wooley CF: Floppy mitral valve, mitral valve prolapse, mitral valvular regurgitation: Natural history. In Boudoulas H, Wooley CF (eds): Mitral Valve: Floppy Mitral Valve, Mitral Valve Prolapse, Mitral Valvular Regurgitation. 2nd ed. Armonk, NY, Futura, 2000, pp 503–540.

254. Wilcken DEL, Hickey AJ: Lifetime risk for patients with mitral prolapse of developing severe valve regurgitation requiring surgery. Circulation 78:10, 1988.

255. Duren DR, Becker AE, Dunning AJ: Long-term follow-up of idiopathic mitral valve prolapse in 300 patients: A prospective study. J Am Coll Cardiol 11:42, 1988.

256. Fakuda N, Oki T, Iuchi A, et al: Predisposing factors for severe mitral regurgitation in idiopathic mitral valve prolapse. Am J Cardiol 76:503, 1995.

257. Danchin N, Briancon S, Mathieu P, et al: Mitral valve prolapse as a risk factor for infective endocarditis. Lancet 1:743, 1989.

257a. Koletar SL: Mitral valve prolapse and infective endocarditis. In Boudoulas H, Wooley CF (eds): Mitral Valve: Floppy Mitral Valve, Mitral Valve Prolapse, Mitral Valvular Regurgitation. 2nd ed. Armonk, NY, Futura, 2000, pp 371–386.

258. Schnee MA, Bucal AA: Fatal embolism in mitral valve prolapse. Chest 83:285, 1983.

259. Barletta GA, Gagliardi R, Benvenuti L, Fantini F: Cerebral ischemic attacks as a complication of aortic and mitral valve prolapse. Stroke 16:219, 1985.

259a. Slivka AP, Walz ET: Cerebral ischemia in mitral valve prolapse. In Boudoulas H, Wooley CF (eds): Mitral Valve: Floppy Mitral Valve, Mitral Valve Prolapse, Mitral Valvular Regurgitation. 2nd ed. Armonk, NY, Futura, 2000, pp 393–404.

260. Gilon D, Buonanno FS, Joffe MM, et al: Lack of evidence of an association between mitral-valve prolapse and stroke in young patients. N Engl J Med 341:8, 1999.

261. Hickey AJ, MacMahon SW, Wilcken DEL: Mitral valve prolapse and bacterial endocarditis: When is antibiotic prophylaxis necessary? Am Heart J 109:431, 1985.

261a. Reul RM, Cohn LH: Surgical reconstruction of the complicated floppy mitral valve. In Boudoulas H, Wooley CF (eds): Mitral Valve: Floppy Mitral Valve, Mitral Valve Prolapse, Mitral Valvular Regurgitation. 2nd ed. Armonk, NY, Futura, 2000, pp 455–480.

AORTIC STENOSIS

262. Dare AJ, Veinot JP, Edwards WD, et al: New observations on the etiology of aortic valve disease. Hum Pathol 24:1330, 1993.

263. Rahimtoola SH: Aortic stenosis. In Rahimtoola SH (ed): Valvular Heart Disease and Endocarditis. Atlas of Heart Diseases. Vol. 11. Braunwald E (Series ed) Philadelphia, Current Medicine, 1996.

264. Braunwald E, Goldblatt A, Aygen MM, et al: Congenital aortic stenosis: Clinical and hemodynamic findings in 100 patients. Circulation 27:426, 1963.

265. Otto CM, Lind BK, Kitzman DW, et al: Association of aortic valve sclerosis with cardiovascular mortality and morbidity in the elderly. N Engl J Med 341:142, 1999.

266. Juvonen J, Juvonen T, Laurilia A, et al: Can degenerative aortic valve stenosis be related to persistent Chlamydia pneumoniae infection? Ann Intern Med 128:741, 1998.

267. Deutscher S, Rockette HE, Krishnaswami V: Diabetes and hypercholesterolemia among patients with calcific aortic stenosis. J Chron Dis 37:407, 1984.

268. Wilmshurst PT, Stevenson RN, Griffiths H, Lord JR: A case-control investigation of the relation between hyperlipidemia and calcific aortic valve stenosis. Heart 78:475, 1997.

269. Ralladis L, Naoumova RP, Thompson GR, Nihoyannopoulos P: Extent and severity of atherosclerotic involvement of the aortic valve and root in familial hypercholesterolemia. Heart 80:583, 1998.

270. Stewart BF, Siscovick D, Lind BK, et al: Clinical factors associated with calcific aortic valve disease. J Am Coll Cardiol 29:630, 1997.

271. Kawaguchi A, Miyatake K, Yutani C, et al: Characteristic cardiovascular manifestations in homozygous and heterozygous familial hypercholesterolemia. Am Heart J 137:410, 1999.

272. Hultgren HN: Osteitis deformans (Paget's disease) and calcific disease of the heart valves. Am J Cardiol 81:1461, 1998.

273. Maher ER, Young G, Smyth-Walsh B, et al: Aortic and mitral valve calcification in patients with end stage renal diseases. Lancet I:875, 1987.

274. Hangaishi M, Taguchi J, Ikari Y, et al: Aortic valve stenosis in alkaptonuria. Circulation 98:1148, 1998.

275. Roberts WC: Valvular, subvalvular and supravalvular aortic stenosis. Morphologic features. Cardiovasc Clin 5:97, 1973.

276. Kennedy JW, Twiss RD, Blackmon JR: Quantitative angiography. III. Relationships of left ventricular pressure volume and mass in aortic valve disease. Circulation 38:838, 1968.

277. Carabello BA: Aortic stenosis. Cardiol Rev 1:59, 1993.

278. Hess OM, Villari B, Krayenbuehl H: Diastolic dysfunction in aortic stenosis. Circulation 87:IV-73, 1993.

279. Villari B, Vassalli G, Monrad ES, et al: Normalization of diastolic dys-

function in aortic stenosis late after valve replacement. Circulation 91: 2353, 1995.

280. Braunwald E, Frahm CJ: Studies on Starling's law of the heart. IV. Observations on the hemodynamic functions of the left atrium in man. Circulation 24:633, 1961.

281. Carroll JD, Carroll EP, Feldman T, et al: Sex-associated differences in left ventricular function in aortic stenosis of the elderly. Circulation 86: 1099, 1992.

282. Morris JJ, Schaff HV, Mullany CJ, et al: Gender differences in left ventricular functional response to aortic valve replacement. Circulation 90:II-183, 1994.

283. Legget ME, Kuusisto J, Healy NL, et al: Gender differences in left ventricular function at rest and with exercise in asymptomatic aortic stenosis. Am Heart J 131:94, 1996.

284. Douglas PS, Otto CM, Mickel MC, et al: Gender differences in left ventricular geometry and function in patients undergoing balloon dilation of the aortic valve or isolated aortic stenosis. Br Heart J 73:548, 1995.

285. Legget ME, Kuusisto J, Healy NL, et al: Gender differences in left ventricular function at rest and with exercise in asymptomatic aortic stenosis. Am Heart J 131:94, 1996.

286. Douglas PS, Berko B, Lesh M, Reichek N: Alterations in diastolic function in response to progressive left ventricular hypertrophy. J Am Coll Cardiol 13:461, 1989.

287. Brouwer CB, Verwers FA, Alpert JS, Goldberg RJ: Isolated aortic stenosis: Analysis of clinical and hemodynamic subsets. J Appl Cardiol 4: 565, 1989.

288. Krayenbuehl HP, Hess OM, Ritter M, et al: Left ventricular systolic function in aortic stenosis. Eur Heart J 9(Suppl E):19, 1988.

289. Gunther S, Grossman W: Determinants of ventricular function in pressure overload hypertrophy in man. Circulation 59:679, 1979.

290. Ross J Jr: Afterload mismatch and preload reserve: A conceptual framework for the analysis of ventricular function. Prog Cardiovasc Dis 18: 255, 1976.

291. Carabello BA, Green LH, Grossman W, et al: Hemodynamic determinants of prognosis of aortic valve replacement in critical aortic stenosis and advanced congestive heart failure. Circulation 62:42, 1980.

292. Movsowitz C, Kussmaul WG, Laskey WK: Left ventricular diastolic response to exercise in valvular aortic stenosis. Am J Cardiol 77:275, 1996.

293. Dineen E, Brent BN: Aortic valve stenosis: Comparison of patients to those without chronic congestive heart failure. Am J Cardiol 57:419, 1986.

294. Fifer MA, Borow KM, Colan SD, Lorel; BH: Early diastolic left ventricular function in children and adults with aortic stenosis. J Am Coll Cardiol 5:1147, 1985.

295. Villari B, Campbell SE, Hess OM, et al: Influence of collagen network on left ventricular systolic and diastolic function in aortic valve disease. J Am Coll Cardiol 22:1477, 1993.

296. Krayenbuehl HP, Hess OM, Monrad ES, et al: Left ventricular myocardial structure in aortic valve disease before, intermediate, and later after aortic valve replacement. Circulation 79:744, 1989.

297. Schwarz F, Flameng W, Schaper J, et al: Myocardial structure and function in patients with aortic valve disease and their relation to postoperative results. Am J Cardiol 41:661, 1978.

298. Bertrand ME, LaBlanche JM, Tilmant PY, et al: Coronary sinus blood flow at rest and during isometric exercise in patients with aortic valve disease. Mechanism of angina pectoris in presence of normal coronary arteries. Am J Cardiol 47:199, 1981.

299. Smucker ML, Tedesco CL, Manning SB: Demonstration of an imbalance between coronary perfusion and excessive load as a mechanism of ischemia during stress in patients with aortic stenosis. Circulation 78: 573, 1988.

300. Matsuo S, Tsuruta M, Hayano M, et al: Phasic coronary artery flow velocity determined by Doppler flowmeter catheter in aortic stenosis and aortic regurgitation. Am J Cardiol 62:917, 1988.

301. Marcus ML, Dot DD, Hiratzka LF, et al: Decreased coronary reserve. A mechanism for angina pectoris in patients with aortic stenosis and normal coronary arteries. N Engl J Med 307:1362, 1982.

302. Julius BK, Spillmann M, Vassalli G, et al: Angina pectoris in patients with aortic stenosis and normal coronary arteries. Circulation 95:892, 1997.

303. Gould KL: Why angina pectoris in aortic stenosis? Circulation 95:790, 1997.

304. Oakley CM: Management of valvular stenosis. Curr Opin Cardiol 10: 117, 1995.

305. Kennedy KD, Nishimura RA, Holmes DR, et al: Natural history of moderate aortic stenosis. J Am Coll Cardiol 17:313, 1991.

306. Hakki AH, Kimbiris D, Iskandrian AS, et al: Angina pectoris and coronary artery disease in patients with severe aortic valvular disease. Am Heart J 100:441, 1980.

307. Holley KE, Bahn RC, McGoon DC, Mankin HT: Spontaneous calcific embolization associated with calcific aortic stenosis. Circulation 27:197, 1963.

308. Schwartz LS, Goldfischer J, Sprague GJ, Schwartz SP: Syncope and sudden death in aortic stenosis. Am J Cardiol 23:647, 1969.

309. Grech ED, Ramsdale DR: Exertional syncope in aortic stenosis: Evidence to support inappropriate left ventricular baroreceptor response. Am Heart J 121:603, 1991.

310. Love JW: The syndrome of calcific aortic stenosis and gastrointestinal

bleeding: Resolution following aortic valve replacement. J Thorac Cardiovasc Surg 83:779, 1982.

311. Pleet AB, Massey EW, Vengrow ME: TIA, stroke, and the bicuspid aortic valve. Neurology 31:1540, 1981.

312. Brockmeier LB, Adolph RJ, Gustin BW, et al: Calcium emboli to the retinal artery in calcific aortic stenosis. Am Heart J 101:32, 1981.

313. Wood P: Aortic stenosis. Am. J. Cardiol. 1:553, 1958.

314. Fowler NO: Aortic stenosis. In Fowler NO: Diagnosis of Heart Disease. New York, Springer-Verlag, 1991, pp 134–145.

315. Abrams J: Aortic stenosis. In Essentials of Cardiac Physical Diagnosis. Philadelphia, Lea and Febiger, 1987, pp 205–224.

316. Cooper T, Braunwald E, Morrow AG: Pulsus alternans in aortic stenosis: Hemodynamic observations in 50 patients studied by left heart catheterization. Circulation 18:64, 1958.

317. Perloff JK: Clinical recognition of aortic stenosis. The physical signs and differential diagnosis of the various forms of obstruction to left ventricular outflow. Prog Cardiovasc Dis 10:323, 1968.

318. Goldblatt A, Aygen MM, Braunwald E: Hemodynamic-phonocardiographic correlations of the fourth heart sound in aortic stenosis. Circulation 26:92, 1962.

319. Morton BC: Natural history and management of chronic aortic valve disease. Can Med Assoc J 126:477, 1982.

320. Forssell G, Jonasson R, Orinius E: Identifying severe aortic valvular stenosis by bedside examination. Acta Med Scand 218:397, 1985.

321. Dymond DS, Wolf FG, Schmidt DH: Severe left ventricular dysfunction in critical aortic stenosis: Reversal following aortic valve replacement. Postgrad Med J 59:781, 1983.

322. Delman AJ, Stein E: Valvular aortic stenosis. In Dynamic Cardiac Auscultation and Phonocardiography. Philadelphia, WB Saunders Co, 1979, p 795.

323. Munt B, Legget ME, Kraft CD, et al: Physical examination in valvular aortic stenosis: Correlation with stenosis severity and prediction of clinical outcome. Am Heart J 137:298, 1999.

324. Nair CK, Aronow WS, Stokke K, et al: Cardiac conduction defects in patients older than 60 years with aortic stenosis and without mitral annular calcium. Am J Cardiol 53:169, 1984.

325. Szamosi A, Wassberg B: Radiologic detection of aortic stenosis. Acta Radiol Diagn 24:201, 1983.

326. Okura H, Yoshida K, Hozumi T, et al: Planimetry and transthoracic two-dimensional echocardiography in noninvasive assessment of aortic valve area in patients with valvular aortic stenosis. J Am Coll Cardiol 30:753, 1997.

327. Hoffmann R, Flachskampf FA, Hanrath P: Aortic stenosis using multiplane transesophageal echocardiography. J Am Coll Cardiol 22:529, 1993.

328. Kim KS, Maxted W, Nanda NC, et al: Comparison of multiplane and biplane transesophageal echocardiography in the assessment of aortic stenosis. Am J Cardiol 79:436, 1997.

329. Leborgne L, Tribouilloy C, Otmani A, et al: Comparative value of Doppler echocardiography and cardiac catheterization in the decision to operate on patients with aortic stenosis. Int J Cardiol 65:163, 1998.

330. Baumgartner H, Stefenelli T, Niederberger J, et al: "Overestimation" of catheter gradients by Doppler ultrasound in patients with aortic stenosis: a predictable manifestation of pressure recovery. J Am Coll Cardiol 33:1655, 1999.

331. Otto CM, Burwarsh IG, Legget ME, et al: A prospective study of asymptomatic valvular aortic stenosis: Clinical, echocardiographic, and exercise predictors of outcome. Circulation 95:2262, 1997.

332. Otto CM, Nishimura RA, Davis KB, et al: Balloon Valvuloplasty Registry Echocardiographers: Doppler echocardiographic findings in adults with severe symptomatic valvular aortic stenosis. Am J Cardiol 68:1477, 1991.

333. Ross J Jr, Braunwald E: The influence of corrective operations on the natural history of aortic stenosis. Circulation 37(Suppl V):61, 1968.

334. Frank S, Johnson A, Ross J Jr: Natural history of valvular aortic stenosis. Br Heart J 35:41, 1973.

335. Iivanainian AM, Lindroos M, Tilvis R, et al: Natural history of aortic valve stenosis of varying severity in the elderly. Am J Cardiol 78:97, 1996.

336. Aronow WS, Ahn C, Kronson I, Nanna M: Prognosis of congestive heart failure in patients aged 62 years with unoperated severe valvular aortic stenosis. Am J Cardiol 72:846, 1993.

337. Braunwald E: On the natural history of severe aortic stenosis. J Am Coll Cardiol 15:1018, 1990.

338. Pellikka PA, Nishimura RA, Bailey KR, Tajik AJ: The natural history of adults with asymptomatic hemodynamically significant aortic stenosis. J Am Coll Cardiol 15:1012, 1990.

339. Kirklin JW, Barratt-Boyes BG: Congenital aortic stenosis. In Cardiac Surgery. 2nd ed. New York, Churchill-Livingstone, 1993, pp 1195–1238.

340. Blitz LR, Gorman M, Herrmann HC: Results of aortic valve replacement for aortic stenosis with relatively low transvalvular pressure gradients. Am J Cardiol 81:358, 1998.

340a. Braunwald E: Aortic valve replacement: An update at the turn of the millenium. Eur Heart J 21:1032–1033, 2000.

341. Connolly HM, Oh JK, Orszulak TA, et al: Aortic valve replacement for aortic stenosis with severe left ventricular dysfunction. Prognostic indicators. Circulation 95:2395, 1997.

341a. Powell DE, Tunick PA, Rosenzweig BP, et al: Aortic valve replacement in patients with aortic stenosis and severe left ventricular dysfunction. Arch Intern Med 160:1337, 2000.

342. Monrad ES, Hess OM, Murakami T, et al: Abnormal exercise hemodynamics in patients with normal systolic function late after aortic valve replacement. Circulation 77:613, 1988.

343. Wong JB, Salem DN, Pauker SG: You're never too old. N Engl J Med 328:971, 1993.

343a. Jolobe O: Surgery for aortic stenosis in severely symptomatic patients older than 80 years: Experience in a single UK centre. Heart 83:583, 2000.

344. Kirklin JW, Barratt-Boyes BG: Aortic valve disease. In Cardiac Surgery. 2nd ed. New York, Churchill-Livingstone, 1993, pp 491–571.

345. Carabello BA: Timing of valve replacement in aortic stenosis: Moving closer to perfection. Circulation 95:2241, 1997.

345a. Kvidal P, Bergstrom R, Horte LG, Stahle E: Observed and relative survival after aortic valve replacement. J Am Coll Cardiol 35:747, 2000.

346. Lund O: Preoperative risk evaluation and stratification of long-term survival after valve replacement for aortic stenosis. Circulation 82:124, 1990.

347. Hwang MH, Hammermeister KE, Oprian C, et al: Preoperative identification of patients likely to have left ventricular dysfunction after aortic valve replacement. Participants in the Veterans Administration Cooperative Study on Valvular Heart Disease. Circulation 80(Suppl I):165, 1989.

348. Bech-Hanssen P, Caidahl K, Wahl B, et al: Influence of aortic valve replacement, prosthesis type, and size on functional outcome and ventricular mass in patients with aortic stenosis. J Thorac Cardiovasc Surg 118:57, 1999.

349. De Paulis R, Sommariva L, Colagrande L, et al: Regression of left ventricular hypertrophy after aortic valve replacement for aortic stenosis with different valve substitutes. J Thorac Cardiovasc Surg 116:590, 1998.

350. Monrad ES, Hess OM, Murakami T, et al: Time course of regression of left ventricular hypertrophy after aortic valve replacement. Circulation 77:1345, 1988.

350a. Khan SS, Siegel RJ, DeRobertis MA, et al: Regression of hypertrophy after Carpentier-Edwards pericardial aortic valve replacement. Ann Thorac Surg 69:531, 2000.

351. Villari B, Campbell SE, Schneider J, et al: Sex-dependent differences in left ventricular function and structure in chonic pressure overload. Eur Heart J 16:1410, 1995.

351a. Connolly HM, Oh JK, Schaff HV, et al: Severe aortic stenosis with low transvalvular gradient and severe left ventricular dysfunction: result of aortic valve replacement in 52 patients. Circulation 101:1940, 2000.

351b. Rahimtoola SH: Severe aortic stenosis with low systolic gradient: The good and bad news. Circulation 101:1892, 2000.

352. Culliford AT, Galloway AC, Colvin SB, et al: Aortic valve replacement for aortic stenosis in persons aged 80 years and over. Am J Cardiol 67:1256, 1991.

353. Iung B, Drissi MF, Michel P-L, et al: Prognosis of valve replacement for aortic stenosis with or without coexisting coronary heart disease: A comparative study. J Heart Valve Dis 2:430, 1993.

353a. Gall S Jr, Lowe JE, Wolfe WG, et al: Efficacy of the internal mammary artery in combined aortic valve replacement coronary artery bypass grafting. J Thorac Surg 69:524, 2000.

354. Cohn LH: Minimally invasive aortic valve surgery: technical considerations and results with the parasternal approach. J Card Surg 13:302, 1998.

354a. Bouchard D, Perrault LP, Carrier M, et al: Ministernotomy for aortic valve replacement: A study of the preliminary experience. Can J Surg 43:39–42, 2000.

355. Bahl VK, Chandra S, Goswami KC: Combined mitral and aortic valvuloplasty by antegrade transseptal approach using Inoue baloon catheter. Int J Cardiol 63:313, 1998.

356. Galal O, Rao PS, Al-Fadley F, Wilson AD: Follow-up result of balloon aortic valvuloplasty in children with special reference to causes of late aortic insufficiency. Am Heart J 133:418, 1997.

357. Safian RD, Mandell VS, Thurer RE, et al: Postmortem and intraoperative balloon valvuloplasty of calcific aortic stenosis in elderly patients: Mechanisms of successful dilation. J Am Coll Cardiol 9:655, 1987.

358. Beatt KJ: Balloon dilatation of the aortic valve in adults: A physician's view. Br Heart J 63:207, 1990.

359. Nishimura RA, Holmes DR Jr, Michela MA, et al: Follow-up of patients with low output, low gradient hemodynamics after percutaneous balloon aortic valvuloplasty: The Mansfield Scientific Aortic Valvuloplasty Registry. J Am Coll Cardiol 17:828, 1991.

360. Otto CM, Mickel MC, Kennedy JW, et al: Three-year outcome after balloon aortic valvuloplasty: Insights into prognosis of valvular aortic stenosis. Circulation 89:642, 1994.

361. Elliott JM, Tuzcu EM: Recent developments in balloon valvuloplasty techniques. Curr Opin Cardiol 10:128, 1995.

362. Acar P, Aggoun Y, Saliba Z, et al: Effect of balloon dilatation on aortic stenosis assessed by 3-dimensional echocardiographic reconstruction. Circulation 99:2598, 1999.

363. Holmes DR Jr, Nishimura RA, Reeder GS: In-hospital mortality after balloon aortic valvuloplasty: Frequency and associated factors. J Am Coll Cardiol 17:189, 1991.

364. Moreno PR, Jang I-K, Newell JB, et al: The role of percutaneous aortic balloon valvuloplasty in patients with cardiogenic shock and critical aortic stenosis. J Am Coll Cardiol 23:1071, 1994.

365. Angel JL, Chapman C, Knuppel RA: Percutaneous balloon aortic valvuloplasty in pregnancy. Obstet Gynecol 72:438, 1988.

AORTIC REGURGITATION

366. Rahimtoola SH: Aortic regurgitation. In Rahimtoola SH (ed): Valvular Heart Disease and Endocarditis. Atlas of Heart Diseases. Vol. 11. St. Louis, CV Mosby Co, 1996.

367. Frahm CJ, Braunwald E, Morrow AG: Congenital aortic regurgitation. Clinical and hemodynamic findings in four patients. Am J Med 31:63, 1961.

368. Roberts WC, Morrow AG, McIntosh CL, et al: Congenitally bicuspid aortic valve causing severe, pure aortic regurgitation without superimposed infective endocarditis. Am J Cardiol 47:206, 1981.

369. Stewart WJ, King ME, Gillam LD, et al: Prevalence of aortic valve prolapse with bicuspid aortic valve and its relation to aortic regurgitation: A cross-sectional echocardiographic study. Am J Cardiol 54:1277, 1984.

370. Olsson A, Darpo B, Bergfeldt L, Rosenqvist M: Frequency and long-term followup of valvar insufficiency caused by retrograde aortic radiofrequency catheter ablation procedures. Heart 81:292, 1999.

371. Tonnemacher D, Reid C, Kawanishi D, et al: Frequency of myxomatous degeneration of the aortic valve as a cause of isolated aortic regurgitation severe enough to warrant aortic valve replacement. Am J Cardiol 60:1194, 1987.

372. Morain SV, Casanegra P, Maturana G, Dubernet J: Spontaneous rupture of a fenestrated aortic valve. Surgical treatment. J Thorac Cardiovasc Surg 73:716, 1977.

373. Waller BF, Kishel JC, Roberts WC: Severe aortic regurgitation from systemic hypertension. Chest 82:365, 1982.

374. Demoulin JC, Lespagnard J, Bertholet M, Soumagne D: Acute fulminant aortic regurgitation in ankylosing spondylitis. Am Heart J 105:859, 1983.

375. Bostwick DG, Bensch KG, Burke JS, et al: Whipple's disease presenting as aortic insufficiency. N Engl J Med 305:995, 1981.

376. Burdick S, Tresch DD, Komokowski RA: Cardiac valvular dysfunction associated with Crohn's disease in the absence of ankylosing spondylitis. Am. Heart J. 118:174, 1989.

377. Darvill FR Jr: Aortic insufficiency of unusual etiology. JAMA, 184:753, 1963.

378. Emanuel R, Ng RAL, Marcomichelakis J, et al: Formes frustes of Marfan's syndrome presenting with severe aortic regurgitation. Clinicogenetic study of 18 families. Br Heart J 39:190, 1977.

379. Roldan CA, Chavez J, Wiest PW, et al: Aortic root disease and valve disease associated with ankylosing spondylitis. J Am Coll Cardiol 32:1397, 1998.

380. Heppner RL, Babitt HI, Blanchine JW, Warbasse JR: Aortic regurgitation and aneurysm of sinus of Valsalva associated with osteogenesis imperfecta. Am J Cardiol 31:654, 1973.

381. Esdah J, Hawkins D, Gold P, et al: Vascular involvement in relapsing polychondritis. Can Med Assoc J 116:1019, 1977.

381a. Khan MA, Herzog CA, St Peter JV, et al: The prevalence of cardiac valvular insufficiency assessed by transthoracic echocardiography in obese patients treated with appetite-suppressant drugs. N Engl J Med 339:713, 1998.

382. Welch GH Jr, Braunwald E, Sarnoff SJ: Hemodynamic effects of quantitatively varied experimental aortic regurgitation. Circ Res 5:546, 1957.

383. Wisenbaugh T, Spann JF, Carabello BA: Differences in myocardial performance and load between patients with similar amounts of chronic aortic versus chronic mitral regurgitation. J Am Coll Cardiol 3:916, 1984.

384. Borow KM, Marcus RH: Aortic regurgitation: The need for an integrated physiologic approach. J Am Coll Cardiol 17:898, 1991.

385. Grossman W, Jones D, McLaurin LP: Wall stress and patterns of hypertrophy in the human left ventricle. J Clin Invest 56:56, 1975.

386. Bonow RO, Lakatos E, Maron BJ, Epstein SE: Serial long-term assessment of the natural history of asymptomatic patients with chronic aortic regurgitation and normal left ventircular systolic function. Circulation 84:1625, 1991.

387. Starling MR, Kirsh MM, Montgomery DG, Gross MD: Mechanisms for left ventricular systolic dysfunction in aortic regrgitation: Importance for predicting the functional response to aortic valve replacement. J Am Coll Cardiol 18:887, 1991.

388. Scognamiglio R, Roelandt J, Fasoli G, et al: Relation between myocardial contractility, hypertrophy and pump performance in patients with chronic aortic regurgitation: An echocardiographic study. Int J Cardiol 6:473, 1984.

389. Kawanishi DT, McKay CR, Chandraratna AN, et al: Cardiovascular response to dynamic exercise in patients with chronic symptomatic mild-to-moderate and severe aortic regurgitation. Circulation 73:62, 1986.

390. Massie BM, Kramer BL, Loge D, et al: Ejection fraction response to supine exercise in asymptomatic aortic regurgitation: Relation to simultaneous hemodynamic measurements. J Am Coll Cardiol 5:847, 1985.

391. Ardehall A, Segal J, Cheitlin MD: Coronary blood flow reserve in acute aortic regurgitation. J Am Coll Cardiol 25:1387, 1995.

392. Uhl GS, Boucher CA, Oliveros RA, Murgo, JP: Exercise-induced myocardial oxygen supply-demand imbalance in asymptomatic or mildly symptomatic aortic regurgitation. Chest 80:686, 1981.

393. Nitenberg A, Foult J-M, Antony I, et al: Coronary flow and resistance reserve in patients with chronic aortic regurgitation, angina pectoris, and normal coronary arteries. J Am Coll Cardiol 11:478, 1988.

394. Benotti JR: Acute aortic insufficiency. In Dalen JE and Alpert JS (eds):

Valvular Heart Disease. 2nd ed. Boston, Little, Brown and Co, 1987, pp 319–352.

395. Downes TR, Nomeir A-M, Hackshaw BT, et al: Diastolic mitral regurgitation in acute but not chronic aortic regurgitation: Implications regarding the mechanism of mitral valve closure. Am Heart J 117:1106, 1989.

396. Eusebio J, Louie EK, Edwards DC, et al: Alterations in transmitral flow dynamics in patients with early mitral valve closure and aortic regurgitation. Am. Heart J. 128:941, 1994.

397. Iskandrian AS, Hakki AH, Manno B, et al: Left ventricular function in chronic aortic regurgitation. J Am Coll Cardiol 1:1374, 1983.

398. Sapira JD: Quincke, DeMusset, Duroziez and Hill: Some aortic regurgitations. South Med J 74:459, 1981.

399. Boudoulas H, Triposkiadis F, Dervenagas J, et al: Mechanisms of pistol shot sounds in aortic regurgitation. Acta Cardiol 46:139, 1991.

400. Alpert JS, Veiweg WVR, Hagan AD: Incidence and morphology of carotid shudders in aortic valve disease. Am Heart J 92:435, 1976.

401. Choudhry NK, Etchells EE: Does this patient have aortic regurgitation? JAMA 281:2231, 1999.

402. Fortuin NJ, Craige E: On the mechanism of the Austin Flint murmur. Circulation 45:558, 1972.

403. Delman AJ, Stein E: Aortic regurgitation. In Dynamic Cardiac Auscultation and Phonocardiography. Philadelphia, WB Saunders Co, 1979, pp 811–824.

404. Perloff JK: Acute severe aortic regurgitation: Recognition and management. J Cardiovasc Med 8:209, 1983.

405. Spring DA, Folts JD, Young WP, Rowe GG: Premature closure of the mitral and tricuspid valves. Circulation 45:663, 1972.

406. Chen J, Okin PM, Roman MJ, et al: Combined rest and exercise electrocardiographic repolarization findings in relation to structural and functional abnormalities in asymptomatic aortic regurgitation. Am Heart J 132:343, 1996.

407. Roberts WC, Day PJ: Electrocardiographic observations in clinically isolated, pure, and chronic, severe aortic regurgitation: Analysis of 30 necropsy patients aged 19 to 65 years. Am J Cardiol 55:431, 1985.

408. Meyer T, Sareli P, Pocock WA, et al: Echocardiographic and hemodynamic correlates of diastolic closure of mitral valve and diastolic opening of aortic valve in severe regurgitation. Am J Cardiol 59:1144, 1987.

409. Weaver WF, Wilson CS, Rourke T, Caudill CC: Middiastolic aortic valve opening in severe acute aortic regurgitation. Circulation 55:112, 1977.

410. Zarauza J, Ares M, Vilchez FG, et al: An integrated approach to the quantification of aortic regurgitation by Doppler echocardiography. Am Heart J 136:1030, 1998.

411. Tribouilloy CM, Enriquez-Sarano M, Fett SL, et al: Application of the proximal flow convergence method to calculate the effective regurgitant orifice area in aortic regurgitation. J Am Coll Cardiol 32:1032, 1998.

412. Reimold SC, Maier SE, Fleischmann KE, et al: Dynamic nature of the aortic regurgitant orifice area during diastole in patients with chronic aortic regurgitation. Circulation 89:2085, 1994.

413. Shiota T, Jones M, Agler DA, McDonald RW: New echo cardiographic windows for quantitative determination of aortic regurgitation volume using color Doppler flow convergence and vena contracta. Am J Cardiol 83:1064, 1999.

413a. Evangelista A, del Castillo HG, Calvo F, et al: Strategy for optimal aortic regurgitation quantification by Doppler echocardiography: Agreement among different methods. Am Heart J 139:773, 2000.

414. Manyari DE, Nolewajka AJ, Kostuk WJ: Quantitative assessment of aortic valvular insufficiency by radionuclide angiography. Chest 81:170, 1982.

415. Dehmer GJ, Firth EG, Hillis LD, et al: Alterations in left ventricular volumes and ejection fraction at rest and during exercise in patients with aortic regurgitation. Am J Cardiol 48:17, 1981.

416. Globits S, Higgins CB: Assessment of valvular heart disease by magnetic resonance imaging. Am Heart J 129:369, 1995.

417. Dujardin KS, Enriquez-Sarano M, Schaff HV et al: Mortality and morbidity of aortic regurgitation in clinical practice: A long-term follow-up study. Circulation 99:1851, 1999.

418. Klodas E, Enriquez-Sarano M, Tajik AJ, et al: Aortic regurgitation complicated by extreme left ventricular dilatation: Long-term outcome after surgical correction. J Am Coll Cardiol 27:670, 1996.

419. Sareli P, Klein HO, Schamroth CL, et al: Contribution of echocardiography and immediate surgery to the management of severe aortic regurgitation from active infective endocarditis. Am J Cardiol 57:413, 1986.

420. Elkayam U, McKay CR, Weber L, et al: Favorable effects of hydralazine on the hemodynamic response to isometric exercise in chronic severe aortic regurgitation. Am J Cardiol 54:1603, 1984.

421. Fioretti P, Benussi B, Scardi S, et al: Afterload reduction with nifedipine in aortic insufficiency. Am J Cardiol 49:1728, 1982.

421a. Sondergaard L, Aldershvile J, Hildebrandt P, et al: Vasodilatation with felodipine in chronic asymptomatic aortic regurgitation. Am Heart J 139:667, 2000.

422. Jebavy P, Koudelkova E, Henzlova M: Unloading effects of prazosin in patients with chronic aortic regurgitation. Am Heart J 105:567, 1983.

423. Rothlisberger C, Sareli P, Wisenbaugh T: Comparison of single dose nifedipine and captopril for chronic severe aortic regurgitation. Am J Cardiol 71:799, 1993.

424. Scognamiglio R, Rahimtoola SH, Fasoli G, et al: Nifedipine in asymptomatic patients with severe aortic regurgitation and normal left ventricular function. N Engl J Med 331:689, 1994.

425. Alehan D, Ozkutlu S: Beneficial effects of 1-year captopril therapy in children with chronic aortic regurgitation who have no symptoms. Am Heart J 135:598, 1998.

426. Bonow RO: Asymptomatic aortic regurgitation: Indications for operation. J Cardiovasc Surg 9(Suppl):170, 1994.

427. Bonow RO, Lakatos E, Maron BJ, Epstein SE: Serial long-term assessment of the natural history of asymptomatic patients with chronic aortic regurgitation and normal left ventricular systolic function. Circulation 84:1625, 1991.

428. Klodas E, Enriquez-Sarano M, Tajik AJ, et al: Optimizing timing of surgical correction in patients with severe aortic regurgitation: Role of symptoms. J Am Coll Cardiol 30:746, 1997.

429. Taniguchi K, Nakano S, Matsuda H, et al: Depressed myocardial contractility and normal ejection performance after aortic valve replacement in patients with aortic regurgitation. J Thorac Cardiovasc Surg 98: 258, 1989.

430. Borow KM: Surgical outcome in chronic aortic regurgitation: A physiologic framework for assessing preoperative predictors. J Am Coll Cardiol 10:1165, 1987.

431. Tornos MO, Olona M, Permanyer-Miralda G, et al: Heart failure after aortic valve replacement for aortic regurgitation: Prospective 20-year study. Am Heart J 136:681, 1998.

432. Borer JS, Hochreiter C, Herrold EM, et al: Prediction of indications for valve replacement among asymptomatic or minimally symptomatic patients with chronic aortic regurgitation and normal left ventricular performance. Circulation 97:525, 1998.

433. Odell JA, Orszulak TA: Surgical repair and reconstruction of valvular lesions. Curr Opin Cardiol 10:135, 1995.

434. David TE: Aortic valve repair in patients with Marfan syndrome and ascending aorta aneurysms due to degenerative disease. J Cardiovasc Surg 9(Suppl):182, 1994.

435. Cosgrove M, Rosenkranz ER, Hendren WG, et al: Valvuloplasty for aortic insufficiency. J Thorac Cardiovasc Surg. 102:571, 1991.

436. Duran CMG: Conservative valve surgery. In Al-Zaibag M, Duran CMG (eds): Valvular Heart Disease. New York, Marcel Dekker, 1994, p 569.

437. Turina J, Millincic J, Seifert B, Turina M: Valve replacement in chronic aortic regurgitation. True predictors of survival after extended follow-up. Circulation 98:III100, 1998.

TRICUSPID, PULMONIC, AND MULTIVALVULAR DISEASE

438. Ananthasubramaniam K, Farha A: Primary right atrial angiosarcoma mimicking acute pericarditis, pulmonary embolism, and tricuspid stenosis. Heart 81:556, 1999.

438a. Hagers Y, Koole M, Schoors D, Van Camp G: Tricuspid stenosis: A rare complication of pacemaker-related endocarditis. J Am Soc Echocardiogr 13:66, 2000.

438b. Heaven DJ, Henein MY, Sutton R: Pacemaker lead related to tricuspid stenosis: A report of two cases. Heart 83:351, 2000.

439. Wooley CF, Fontana ME, Kilman JW, Ryan JM: Tricuspid stenosis: Atrial systolic murmur, tricuspid opening snap and right atrial pressure pulse. Am J Med 78:375, 1985.

440. Ewy GA: Tricuspid valve disease. In Chatterjee K, Cheitlin MD, Karliner J, et al (eds): Cardiology: An Illustrated Text Reference, Vol. 2. Philadelphia, JB Lippincott, 1991, p 991.

441. Ribeiro PA, Al-Zaibag M, Sawyer W: A prospective study comparing the haemodynamic with the cross-sectional echocardiographic diagnosis of rheumatic tricuspid stenosis. Eur Heart J 10:120, 1989.

442. Lundin L, Landelius J, Adren B, Oberg K: Transesophageal echocardiography improves the diagnostic value of cardiac ultrasound in patients with carcinoid heart disease. Br Heart J 64:190, 1990.

443. Fawzy ME, Mercer EN, Dunn B, et al: Doppler echocardiography in the evaluation of tricuspid stenosis. Eur Heart J 10:985, 1989.

443a. Ha JW, Chung N, Jang Y, Rim SJ: Tricuspid stenosis and regurgitation: Doppler and color flow echocardiography and cardiac catheterization findings. Clin Cardiol 23:51, 2000.

444. Kirklin JW, Barratt-Boyes BG: Tricuspid valve disease. In Kirklin JW, Barratt-Boyes BG: Cardiac Surgery. 2nd ed. New York, Churchill-Livingstone, 1993, pp 589–608.

445. Guerra F, Bertolotti U, Thiene G, et al: Long-term performance of the Hancock porcine bioprosthesis in the tricuspid position. A review of 45 patients with 14-year follow-up. J Thorac Cardiovasc Surg 99:838, 1990.

446. Throburn CW, Morgan JJ, Shanahan MX, Chang VP: Long-term results of tricuspid valve replacement and the problem of prosthetic valve thrombosis. Am J Cardiol 51:1128, 1983.

447. Boskovic D, Elezovic I, Boskovic D, et al: Late thrombosis of the Bjork-Shiley tilting disc valve in the tricuspid position. J Thorac Cardiovasc Surg 91:1, 1986.

447a. Del Campo C, Sherman JR: Tricuspid valve replacement: Results comparing mechanical and biological prostheses. Ann Thorac Surg 69:1295, 2000.

448. Treasure T: Which prosthetic valve should we choose? Curr Opin Cardiol 10:144, 1995.

449. Robiolio PA, Rigolin VH, Harrison JK, et al: Predictors of outcome of tricuspid valve replacement in carcinoid heart disease. Am J Cardiol 75:485, 1995.

450. Jegaden OL, Perinetti M, Barthelet M, et al: Long-term results of porcine bioprostheses in the tricuspid position. Cardiothorac Surg 6:256, 1992.

451. McGrath LB, Chen C, Bailey BM, et al: Early and late phase events following bioprosthetic tricuspid valve replacement. J Cardiovasc Surg 7:245, 1992.

452. Bahl VK, Chandra S, Mishra S: Concurrent balloon dilatation of mitral and tricuspid stenosis during pregnancy using an Inoue balloon. Int J Cardiol 59:199, 1997.

453. Shafie MZ, Hayat N, Majid OA: Fate of tricuspid regurgitation after closed valvotomy for mitral stenosis. Chest 88:870, 1985.

454. Cohen SR, Sell JE, McIntosh CL, Clark RE: Tricuspid regurgitation in patients with acquired, chronic, pure mitral regurgitation. 1. Prevalence, diagnosis, and comparison of preoperative clinical and hemodynamic features in patients with and without tricuspid regurgitation. J Thorac Cardiovasc Surg 94:481, 1987.

455. Morrison DA, Ovitt T, Hammermeister KE: Functional tricuspid regurgitation and right ventricular dysfunction in pulmonary hypertension. Am J Cardiol 62:108, 1988.

456. Vatterott PJ, Nishimura RA, Gersh BJ, Smith HC: Severe isolated tricuspid insufficiency in coronary artery disease. Int J Cardiol 14:295, 1987.

457. Sakai K, Inoue Y, Osawa M: Congenital isolated tricuspid regurgitation in an adult. Am Heart J 110:680, 1985.

458. Esaghpour E, Kawai N, Linhart JW: Tricuspid insufficiency associated with aneurysm of the ventricular septum. Pediatrics 61:586, 1978.

459. Prieto LR, Hordof AJ, Secic M, et al: Progressive tricuspid valve disease in patients with congenitally corrected transposition of the great arteries. Circulation 98:997, 1998.

460. Ohri SK, Schofield JB, Hodgson H, et al: Carcinoid heart disease: Early failure of an allograft valve replacement. Ann Thorac Surg 58:1161, 1994.

461. Lundin L, Norheim I, Landelius J, et al: Carcinoid heart disease: Relationship of circulating vasoactive substances to ultrasound-detectable cardiac abnormalities. Circulation 77:264, 1988.

462. Connolly HM, Nishimura RA, Smith HC, et al: Outcome of cardiac surgery for carcinoid heart diease. J Am Coll Cardiol 25:410, 1995.

463. Pellika PA, Tajik AJ, Khandheria BK, et al: Carcinoid heart disease: Clinical and echocardiographic spectrum in 74 patients. Circulation 87:1188, 1993.

464. Jackson D, Gibbs HR, Zee-Cheng CS: Isolated tricuspid valve prolapse diagnosed by echocardiography. Am J Med 80:281, 1986.

465. Schlamowitz RA, Gross S, Keating E, et al: Tricuspid valve prolapse: A common occurrence in the click-murmur syndrome. J Clin Ultrasound 10:435, 1982.

466. Gayet C, Pierre B, Delahaye J-P, et al: Traumatic tricuspid insufficiency: An underdiagnosed disease. Chest 92:429, 1987.

467. Dickerman SA and Rubler S: Mitral and tricuspid valve regurgitation in dilated cardiomyopathy. Am J Cardiol 63:629, 1989.

468. Ginzton LE, Siegel RJ, Criley JM: Natural history of tricuspid valve endocarditis: A two-dimensional echocardiographic study. Am J Cardiol 49:1853, 1982.

469. Arbulu A and Asfaw I: Tricuspid valvulectomy without prosthetic replacement. Ten years of clinical experience. J Thorac Cardiovasc Surg. 82:684, 1981.

470. Paniagua D, Aldrich HR, Lieberman EH, et al: Increased prevalence of significant tricuspid regurgitation in patients with transvenous pacemaker leads. Am J Cardiol 82:1130, 1998.

471. Reynertson MD, Kundur R, Mullen GM, et al: Asymmetry of right ventricular enlargement in response to tricuspid regurgitation. Circulation 100:465, 1999.

472. Mason JW, Billingham ME, Friedman JP: Methysergide-induced heart disease: A case of multivalvular and myocardial fibrosis. Circulation 56:889, 1977.

473. Jick H, Vasilakis C, Weinrauch LA, et al: A population-based study of appetite suppressant drugs and the risk of cardiac valve regurgitation. N Engl J Med 339:719, 1998.

474. Laufer J, Frand M, Milo S: Valve replacement for severe tricuspid regurgitation caused by Libman-Sachs endocarditis. Br Heart J 48:294, 1982.

475. Pellegrini A, Columbo T, Donatelli E, et al: Evaluation and treatment of secondary tricuspid insufficiency. Eur J Cardiothorac Surg 6:288, 1992.

476. Allen SJ, Naylor D: Pulsation of the eyeballs in tricuspid regurgitation. Can Med Assoc J 133:119, 1985.

477. Abrams J: Tricuspid regurgitation. In Essentials of Cardiac Physical Diagnosis. Philadelphia, Lea and Febiger, 1987, pp 375–400.

478. Amidi M, Irwin JM, Salerni R, et al: Venous systolic thrill and murmur in the neck: A consequence of severe tricuspid insufficiency. J Am Coll Cardiol 7:942, 1986.

478a. Naschitz JE, Goldstein L, Zuckerman E, et al: Benign course of congestive cirrhosis associated with tricuspid regurgitation: Does pulsatility protect against complications of venous hypertension? J Clin Gastroenterol 30:213, 2000.

479. Come PC, Riley MF: Tricuspid annular dilatation and failure of tricuspid leaflet coaptation in patients with tricuspid regurgitation. Am J Cardiol 55:599, 1985.

480. Popp RL: When is tricuspid regurgitation important? Cardiol Rev 2:183, 1994.

481. Kemp WE Jr, Kerins DM, Shyr Y, Byrd BF 3rd: Optimal Albunex dosing for enhancement of Doppler tricuspid regurgitation spectra. Am J Cardiol 79:232, 1997.

482. Meltzer RS, van Hoogenhuyze D, Serruys PW, et al: Diagnosis of tricuspid regurgitation by contrast echocardiography. Circulation 63:1093, 1981.

483. Grossmann G, Giesler M, Stein M, et al: Quantification of mitral and tricuspid regurgitation by the proximal flow convergence method using two-dimensional colour Doppler and colour Doppler M-mode: Influence of the mechanism of regurgitation. Int J Cardiol 66:299, 1998.

484. Suzuki Y, Kambara H, Kadota K, et al: Detection and evaluation of tricuspid regurgitation using a real-time, two-dimensional, color-coded, Doppler flow imaging system: Comparison with contrast two-dimensional echocardiography and right ventriculography. Am J Cardiol 57:811, 1986.

485. Pitts WR, Lange RA, Cigarroa JE, Hillis LD: Predictive value of prominent right atrial V waves in assessing the presence and severity of tricuspid regurgitation. Am J Cardiol 83:617, 1999.

486. Cheitlin M, MacGregor JS: Acquired tricuspid and pulmonary valve disease. In Rahimtoola SH (ed): Valvular Heart Disease and Endocarditis. Atlas of Heart Diseases. Vol. 11. Braunwald E (section ed). Philadelphia, Current Medicine, 1996.

487. Lambertz H, Minale C, Flachskampf FA, et al: Long-term follow-up after Carpentier tricuspid valvuloplasty. Am Heart J 117:615, 1989.

488. Duran CM: Tricuspid valve surgery revisited. J Card Surg 9:242, 1994.

489. Sugimoto T, Okada M, Ozaki N, et al: Long-term evaluation of treatment for functional tricuspid regurgitation with regurgitant volume: characteristic differences based on primary cardiac lesion. J Thorac Cardiovasc Surg 117:463, 1999.

490. Bajzer CT, Stewart WJ, Cosgrove DM, et al: Tricuspid valve surgery and intraoperative echocardiography: Factors affecting survival, clinical outcome, and echocardiographic success. J Am Coll Cardiol 32:1023, 1998.

491. Cohn LH: Tricuspid regurgitation secondary to mitral valve disease: When and how to repair. J Cardiovasc Surg 9(Suppl):237, 1994.

492. Kirshenbaum HD: Pulmonary valve disease. In Dalen JE and Alpert JS (eds): Valvular Heart Disease. 2nd ed. Boston, Little, Brown and Co, 1987, pp 403–438.

493. Vela JE, Conteras R, Sosa FR: Rheumatic pulmonary valve disease. Am J Cardiol 23:12, 1969.

494. Altrichter PM, Olson LJ, Edwards WD, et al: Surgical pathology of the pulmonary valve: A study of 116 cases spanning 15 years. Mayo Clin Proc 64:1352, 1989.

495. Ohri SK, Schofield JB, Hodgson H, et al: Carcinoid heart disease: Early failure of an allograft valve replacement. Ann Thorac Surg 58:1161, 1994.

496. Seymour J, Emanuel R, Patterson N: Acquired pulmonary stenosis. Br Heart J 30:776, 1968.

497. Brayshaw JR, Perloff JK: Congenital pulmonary insufficiency complicating idiopathic dilatation of the pulmonary artery. Am J Cardiol 10:282, 1962.

498. Runco V, Levin HS: The spectrum of pulmonic regurgitation. In Physiologic Principles of Heart Sounds and Murmurs. American Heart Association Monograph No 46, 1975, p 175.

499. Cassling RS, Rogler WC, McManus BM: Isolated pulmonic valve infective endocarditis: A diagnostically elusive entity. Am Heart J 109:558, 1985.

499a. Balaguer JM, Byrne JG, Cohn LH: Orthotopic pulmonic valve replacement with a pulmonary homograft as an interposition graft. J Card Surg 11:417, 1996.

500. Collins NP, Braunwald E, Morrow AG: Isolated congenital pulmonic valvular regurgitation. Am J Med 28:159, 1960.

501. Jacoby WJ, Tucker DH, Sumner RG: The second heart sound in congenital pulmonary valvular insufficiency. Am Heart J 69:603, 1965.

502. O'Toole JD, Wurtzbacher JJ, Wearner NE, Jain AC: Pulmonary valve injury and insufficiency during pulmonary-artery catheterization. N Engl J Med 301:1167, 1979.

503. DePace NL, Nestico PF, Iskandrian AS, Morganroth J: Acute severe pulmonic valve regurgitation: Pathophysiology, diagnosis and treatment. Am Heart J 108:567, 1984.

504. Bousvaros GA, Deuchar DC: The murmur of pulmonary regurgitation which is not associated with pulmonary hypertension. Lancet 2:962, 1961.

505. Green EW, Agruss NS, Adolph RJ: Right-sided Austin Flint murmur. Documentation by intracardiac phonocardiography, echocardiography and postmortem findings. Am J Cardiol 32:370, 1973.

506. Braunwald E, Morrow AG: A method for detection and estimation of aortic regurgitant flow in man. Circulation 17:505, 1958.

507. Collins NP, Braunwald E, Morrow AG: Detection of pulmonic and tricuspid valvular regurgitation by means of indicator solutions. Circulation 20:561, 1959.

508. Van Meurs-Van Woezik H, McGhie J, Roelandt J: Septal flutter in pulmonary insufficiency. J Cardiovasc Ultrasonogr 3:159, 1984.

509. Miyatake K, Okamoto M, Kinoshita N, et al: Pulmonary regurgitation studied with the ultrasonic pulsed Doppler technique. Circulation 65:969, 1982.

509a. Helbing WA, de Roos A: Optimal imaging in assessment of right ventricular function in tetralogy of Fallot with pulmonary regurgitation. Am J Cardiol 82:1561, 1998.

510. Emery RW, Landes RG, Moller JH, Nicoloff DM: Pulmonary valve replacement with a porcine aortic heterograft. Ann Thorac Surg 27:148, 1979.

510a. Conte S, Jashari R, Eyskens B, et al: Homograft valve insertion for pulmonary regurgitation late after valveless repair of right ventricular outflow tract obstruction. Eur J Cardiothorac Surg 15:143, 1999.

510b. Balaguer JM, Byrne JG, Cohn LH: Orthotopic pulmonic valve replacement with a pulmonary homograft as an interposition graft. J Card Surg 11:417, 1996.

511. Segal J, Harvey WP, Hufnagel CA: Clinical study of one hundred cases of severe aortic insufficiency. Am J Med 21:200, 1956.

512. Gash AK, Carabello BA, Kent RL, et al: Left ventricular performance in patients with coexistent mitral stenosis and aortic insufficiency. J Am Coll Cardiol 3:703, 1984.

512a. John S, Ravikumar E, John CN, Bashi VV: 25-year experience with 456 combined mitral and aortic valve replacement for rheumatic heart disease. Ann Thorac Surg 69:1167, 2000.

513. Zitnik RS: The masking of aortic stenosis by mitral stenosis. Am Heart J 69:22, 1965.

514. Schattenberg TT, Titus JL, Parkin TW: Clinical findings in acquired aortic valve stenosis. Effect of disease of other valves. Am Heart J 73: 322, 1967.

515. Melvin DB, Tecklenberg PL, Hollingsworth JF, et al: Computer-based analysis of preoperative and postoperative prognostic factors in 100 patients with combined aortic and mitral valve replacement. Circulation 48(Suppl III):58, 1973.

516. Rippe JM: Multiple floppy valves. An echocardiographic syndrome. Am J Med 66:817, 1979.

517. Kirklin JW, Barratt-Boyes BG: Combined aortic and mitral valve disease with or without tricuspid valve disease. In Cardiac Surgery. 2nd ed. New York, Churchill-Livingstone, 1993, pp 573–588.

517a. Nitter-Hauge S and Horstkotte D: Management of multivalvular heart disease. Eur Heart J 8:643, 1987.

517b. Coll-Mazzei JV, Jegaden O, Janody P, et al: Results of triple valve replacement: Perioperative mortality and long-term results. J Cardiovasc Surg 28:369, 1987.

518. Michel PL, Houdart E, Ghanem G, et al: Combined aortic mitral and tricuspid surgery: Results in 78 patients. Eur Heart J 8:457, 1987.

518a. MacManus Q, Grunkemeier G, Starr A: Late results of triple valve replacement: A 14-year review. Ann Thorac Surg 25:402, 1978.

519. Vatterott PJ, Gersh BJ, Fuster V, et al: Long-term followup (2–20 years) of patients with triple valve replacement. J Am Coll Cardiol 1(Abs):586, 1983.

PROSTHETIC CARDIAC VALVES

520. Braunwald NS, Cooper TS, Morrow AG: Complete replacement of the mitral valve. J Thorac Cardiovasc Surg 40:1, 1960.

521. Harken DE, Soroff MS, Taylor MC: Partial and complete prostheses in aortic insufficiency. J Thorac Cardiovasc Surg 40:744, 1960.

522. Starr A, Edwards ML: Mitral replacement: Clinical experience with a ball-valve prosthesis. Ann Surg 154:726, 1961.

523. Grunkemeier GL, Starr A, Rahimtoola SH: Performance of prosthetic heart valves. In Rahimtoola SH (ed): Valvular Heart Disease and Endocarditis. Atlas of Heart Diseases. Vol. 11. Braunwald, E (series ed). Philadelphia, Current Medicine, 1996.

524. Grunkemeier GL and Starr A: Twenty-five year experience with Starr-Edwards heart valves: Follow-up methods and results. Can J Cardiol 4: 381, 1988.

525. Pilegaard HK, Lund O, Nielsen TT, et al: Twenty-two-year experience with aortic valve replacement: Starr-Edwards ball valves versus disc valves. Texas Heart Inst J 18:24, 1991.

526. Cohn LH: Aortic valve prosthesis. Cardiol Rev 2:219, 1994.

527. Nair C, Mohiuddin SM, Hilleman DE, et al: Ten-year results with the St. Jude medical prosthesis. Am J Cardiol 65:217, 1990.

528. Burckhardt D, Streibel D, Vogt S, et al: Heart valve replacement with St. Jude medical valve prosthesis: Long-term experience in 743 patients in Switzerland. Circulation 78(Suppl I):I18, 1988.

529. Van Rijk Zwikker GL, Delemarre BJ, Huysman HA: The orientation of the bi-leaflet Carbomedics valve in the mitral position determines left ventriclar spatial flow patterns. Eur J Cardiothorac Surg 10:513, 1996.

530. Stewart S, Cianciotta D, Hicks GL, DeWeese JA: The Lillehei-Kaster aortic valve prosthesis. J Thorac Cardiovasc Surg 95:1023, 1988.

531. Starek PJK, Beaudet RL, Hall K-V: The Medtronic-Hall valve: Development and clinical experience. In Crawford FA (ed): Cardiac Surgery: Current Heart Valve Prostheses. Vol. 1. Philadelphia, Hanley and Belfus, 1987, pp 223–236.

532. Beaudet RL, Nakhle G, Beaulieu CR, et al: Medtronic-Hall prosthesis: Valve related deaths and complications. Can J Cardiol 4:376, 1988.

533. Hammermeister KE, Sethi GK, Henderson WG, et al: A comparison of outcomes in men 11 years after heart-valve replacement with a mechanical valve or bioprosthesis. N Engl J Med 328:1289, 1993.

534. Cannegieter SC, Rosendaal FR, Wintzen AR, et al: Optimal oral anticoagulant therapy in patients with mechanical heart valves. N Engl J Med 333:11, 1995.

535. Acar J, Iung B, Boissel JP, et al: AREVA, multicenter randomized comparison of low-dose versus standard-dose anticoagulation in patients with mechanical prosthetic heart valves. Circulation 94:2107, 1996.

536. Meschengieser SS, Fondevila CG, Frontroth J, et al: Low-intensity oral anticoagulation plus low-dose aspirin versus high-intensity oral anticoagulation alone: A randomized trial in patients with mechanical prosthetic heart valves. J Thorac Cardiovasc Surg 113:910, 1997.

537. Lengyel M, Fuster V, Keltai M, et al: Guidelines for management of left-sided prosthetic valve thrombosis: a role for thrombolytic therapy. Consensus Conference on Prosthetic Valve Thrombosis. J Am Coll Cardiol 30:1521, 1997.

538. Skoularigis J, Essop MR, Skucicky D, et al: Frequency and severity of intravascular hemolysis after left-sided cardiac valve replacement with Medtronic-Hall, St. Jude Medical Prostheses and influence of prosthetic type, position, size and number. Am J Cardiol 71:587, 1993.

539. Turina, J, Hess OM, Turina M, Krayenbuehl HP: Cardiac bioprosthesis in the 1990s. Circulation 88:775, 1993.

539a. Schoen FJ, Levy RJ: Tissue heart valves: current challenges and future research perspectives. J Biomed Mater Res 47:439, 1999.

540. Glower DD, White WD, Hatton CF, et al: Determinants of reoperation after 960 valve replacements with Carpentier-Edwards prostheses. J Thorac Cardiovasc Surg 107:381, 1994.

541. Grunkemeier GL, Bodnar E: Comparison of structural valve failure among different "models" of homograft valves. J Heart Valve Dis 3:556, 1994.

542. Barratt-Boyes BG and Christie GW: What is the best bioprosthetic operation for the small aortic root? Allograft, autograft, porcine, pericardial? Stented or unstented? J Cardiovasc Surg 9(Suppl):158, 1994.

543. Bloomfield P, Wheatley DJ, Prescott RJ, Miller HC: Twelve-year comparison of a Bjork-Shiley mechanical heart valve with porcine bioprostheses. N Engl J Med 324:573, 1991.

543a. Cohn LH, Collins JJ, Rizzo RJ, et al: Twenty-year follow-up of the Hancock modified orifice porcine aortic valve. Ann Thorac Surg 66:S30, 1998.

544. Khuri SF, Folland ED, Sethi GK, et al: Six month postoperative hemodynamics of the Hancock heterograft and the Bjork-Shiley prosthesis: Results of a Veterans' Administration cooperative prospective randomized trial. J Am Coll Cardiol 12:8, 1988.

545. Cohn LH, Collins JJ, DiSesa VJ, et al: Fifteen-year experience with 1678 Hancock porcine bioprosthetic heart valve replacements. Ann Surg 210: 435, 1989.

546. Janusz MT, Jamieson WRE, Burr LH, et al: Thromboembolism risks and role of anticoagulants in patients in chronic atrial fibrillation following mitral valve replacement with porcine bioprostheses. J Am Coll Cardiol 1:587, 1983.

547. Jamieson WRE, Tyers GFO, Janusz MT, et al: Age as a determinant for selection of porcine bioprostheses for cardiac valve replacement: Experience with Carpentier-Edwards standard bioprosthesis. Can J Cardiol 7: 181, 1991.

548. Westaby S, Jin XY, Katsumata T, Arifi A: Valve replacement with a stentless bioprosthesis: Versatility of the porcine aortic root. J Thorac Cardiovasc Surg 116:477, 1998.

549. Hvass U, Palatianos GM, Frassani R, et al: Multicenter study of stentless valve replacement in the small aortic root. J Thorac Cardiovasc Surg 117:267, 1999.

550. David TE, Bos J, Rakowski H: Aortic valve replacement with the Toronto SPV bioprosthesis. J Heart Valve Dis 1:244, 1992.

551. Konertz W, Hamann P, Schwammenthal E, et al: Aortic valve replacement with stentless xenografts. J Heart Valve Dis 1:249, 1992.

552. Kirklin JK, Smith D, Novick W: Long-term function of cryopreserved aortic homografts: A ten year study. J Thorac Cardiovasc Surg 106:154, 1993.

552a. Lund O, Chandrasekaran V, Grocott-Mason R, et al: Primary aortic valve replacement with allografts over twenty-five years; valve related and procedure-related determinants of outcome. J Thorac Cardiovasc Surg 117:77, 1999.

553. Doty DB, Michielon G, Wang N-D, et al: Replacement of the aortic valve with cryopreserved aortic allograft. Ann Thorac Surg 56:228, 1993.

554. Chambers JC, Somerville J, Stone S, Ross DN: Pulmonary autograft procedure for aortic valve disease: long-term results of the pioneer series. Circulation 96:2206, 1997.

555. Santini F, Dyke C, Edwards S, et al: Pulmonary autograft versus homograft replacement of the aortic valve: A prospective randomized trial. J Thorac Cardiovasc Surg 113:894, 1997.

556. Elkins RC, Knott-Craig CJ, Ward KE, Lane MM: The Ross operation in children: 10-year experience. Ann Thorac Surg 65:496, 1998.

557. Frater RWM, Cosgrove CM, et al: Long-term durability and patient functional status of the Carpentier-Edwards Perimount Pericardial Bioprosthesis in the aortic position. J Heart Valve Dis 7:48, 1998.

558. Aupart MR, Neville PH, Hammami S, et al: Carpentier-Edwards pericardial valves in the mitral position: Ten-year follow-up. J Thorac Cardiovasc Surg 113:492, 1997.

559. Nashef SAM, Sethia B, Turner MA, et al: Bjork-Shiley and Carpentier-Edwards valves: A comparative analysis. J Thorac Cardiovasc Surg 93: 394, 1987.

560. Hammermeister LE, Sethi GK, Henmderson WG, et al: A comparison of outcomes in men 11 years after heart valve replacement with a mechanical valve or bioprosthesis. Veterans Affairs Cooperative Study on Valvular Heart Disease. N Engl J Med 328:1289, 1993.

561. Bloomfield P, Wheatley DJ, Prescott RJ, Miller HC: Twelve year comparison of a Bjork-Shiley mechanical heart valve with porcine bioprostheses. N Engl J Med 324:573, 1991.

562. Peterseim DS, Cen YY, Cheruvu S, et al: Long-term outcome after biologic versus mechanical aortic valve replacement in 841 patients. J Thorac Cardiovasc Surg 117:890, 1999.

563. Cohen G, David TE, Ivanov J, et al: The impact of age, coronary artery disease, and cardiac comorbidity on late survival after bioprosthetic aortic valve replacement. J Thorac Cardiovasc Surg 117:273, 1999.

564. Hammond GI, Geha AS, Klopf GS, Hashim SW: Biological versus mechanical valves: Analysis of 1116 valves inserted in 1012 adult patients

565. Sareli P, England MJ, Berk MR, et al: Maternal and fetal sequelae of anticoagulation during pregnancy in patients with mechanical heart valve prostheses. Am J Cardiol 63:1462, 1989.

566. Vitale N, De Feo M, De Santo LS, et al: Dose-dependent fetal complications of warfarin in pregnant women with mechanical heart valves. J Am Coll Cardiol 33:1637, 1999.

567. Elkayam U: Pregnancy through a prosthetic heart valve. J Am Coll Cardiol 33:1642, 1999.

(top of first column)
with a 4818 patient-year and a 5327 valve-year followup. J Thorac Cardiovasc Surg 93:182, 1987.

568. John S: Valve replacement in the young patients with rheumatic heart disease: Review of a twenty year experience. J Thorac Cardiovasc Surg 99:631, 1990.

569. Selwyn L, Rao S, Mardin MK, et al: Prosthetic valves in children and adolescents. Am Heart J 121:557, 1991.

570. Gardner TJ: Anticoagulants for children requiring heart valve replacement. In Dunn JM (ed): Cardiac Valve Disease in Children. New York, Elsevier, 1988, p 359.

GUIDELINES

MANAGEMENT OF VALVULAR HEART DISEASE

Thomas H. Lee

Guidelines for management of patients with valvular heart disease were published by an American College of Cardiology/American Heart Association (ACC/AHA) committee in 1998.[1] As is the case for other ACC/AHA guidelines, the indications for various tests and procedures are divided into classes:

Class I: Conditions for which there is evidence and/or general agreement that a given procedure or treatment is useful and effective.

Class II: Conditions for which there is conflicting evidence and/or a divergence of opinion about the usefulness/efficacy of a procedure or treatment.

Class IIa: Weight of evidence/opinion is in favor of usefulness/efficacy.

Class IIb: Usefulness/efficacy is less well established by evidence/opinion.

Class III: Conditions for which there is evidence and/or general agreement that the procedure/treatment is not useful/effective and in some cases may be harmful.

Some material from these guidelines is presented elsewhere in this book. Guidelines for prevention and treatment of infective endocarditis are summarized in Chapter 47 and its guidelines. Guidelines for management of anticoagulation in pregnancy are included in the appendix to Chapter 65. Recommendations for prevention of recurrence of rheumatic fever are included in the appendix to Chapter 66.

The guidelines emphasize that the decision to use echocardiography to evaluate patients with cardiac murmurs should be influenced by the patient's symptomatic status and the physical examination. Additional reassurance that a murmur is clinically insignificant may be drawn from other clinical tests, such as the electrocardiogram and chest roentgenogram, if these tests are normal. Echocardiography is considered inappropriate (Class III) for evaluation of murmurs that experienced observers consider innocent or functional. In contrast, echocardiography is considered appropriate even in asymptomatic patients with murmurs suggesting significant valvular disease or in patients with other signs or symptoms of cardiovascular disease (Table 46–G–1).

Mitral Stenosis

Transthoracic echocardiography is endorsed in the ACC/AHA guidelines as a valuable test for diagnosis and follow-up of patients with mitral stenosis. The ACC/AHA guidelines do not endorse routine use of transesophageal echocardiography for evaluation of mitral valve morphology, but do note a potential role (Class IIa) for detection of left atrial thrombus in patients being considered for percutaneous balloon mitral valvotomy or cardioversion.

Anticoagulation is endorsed for patients with mitral stenosis who have a history of atrial fibrillation or a prior embolic event. The ACC/AHA panel is not strongly supportive of anticoagulation on the basis of a left atrial dimension ≥ 55 mm in patients in sinus rhythm. Surgical therapy with valvotomy, valve repair, or valve replacement is indicated for patients with moderate or severe mitral stenosis (valve ≤ 1.5 cm²) and NYHA functional class III or IV, with the choice of the procedure dictated by the anatomical findings. Balloon valvotomy is also endorsed for patients who are NYHA functional class II. For patients with mild or no symptoms of mitral stenosis, balloon valvotomy is considered appropriate (Class IIa) in the presence of pulmonary hypertension and in the absence of left atrial thrombus or moderate to severe mitral regurgitation.

Mitral Regurgitation

Echocardiography is considered appropriate for the diagnosis of acute or chronic mitral regurgitation, as well as in annual or semiannual surveillance of left ventricular function in patients with severe mitral regurgitation, even if the patients are asymptomatic. Serial use of chest roentgenograms and electrocardiograms is considered to be of less value. In asymptomatic patients with mild mitral regurgitation and no evidence of left ventricular enlargement or dysfunction, the guidelines recommend yearly evaluations to detect worsening symptomatic status, but do not support annual echocardiography. Transesophageal echocardiography is considered most appropriate for intraoperative guidance and when transthoracic studies are inadequate.

Cardiac catheterization is usually performed before surgery in patients with mitral regurgitation. Coronary angiography is not considered routinely necessary in the ACC/AHA guidelines for patients younger than age 35 years who have no clinical suspicion of coronary artery disease. Left ventriculography and hemodynamic assessment are appropriate when noninvasive studies do not provide definitive information about the severity of mitral regurgitation or left ventricular dysfunction or the need for surgery.

Surgery is considered appropriate for patients with acute symptomatic mitral regurgitation and for those with chronic severe mitral regurgitation and symptoms of congestive heart failure, even if they have normal left ventricular function. Even if patients are asymptomatic, surgery is appropriate when they have mild or more severe left ventricular dysfunction (i.e., ejection fraction 50 to 60 percent and end-systolic dimension 50 to 55 mm).

Mitral Valve Prolapse

Recommendations on use of echocardiography for patients with mitral valve prolapse were adopted from the recommendations of an earlier ACC/AHA task force on echocardiography.[2] These guidelines emphasize that the diagnosis of mitral valve prolapse should be made by physical examination and that echocardiography is primarily appropriate for evaluation of mitral regurgitation and ventricular compensation. Echocardiography is also appropriate for *excluding* the diagnosis of mitral valve prolapse in patients who have been given the diagnosis inappropriately. Serial use of echocardiography in stable patients with mild or no regurgitation is discouraged.

Antibiotic prophylaxis is considered appropriate for patients with the characteristic click-murmur complex or with echocardiographic evidence of mitral value prolapse with regurgitation. (Additional information on the use of antibiotic prophylaxis is included in the guidelines to Chapter 47.) Daily aspirin therapy is recommended for patients who have had cerebral transient ischemic attacks and for patients younger than age 65 years who have atrial fibrillation without other complicating factors. Warfarin therapy is recommended for poststroke patients and for older patients with atrial fibrillation.

Aortic Stenosis

Doppler echocardiography is considered a highly appropriate test for diagnosis and assessment of aortic stenosis and for evaluation of left

Text continued on page 1720

Indication	Class I	Class IIa	Class IIb	Class III
Echocardiography in asymptomatic patients with cardiac murmurs	1. Diastolic or continuous murmurs 2. Holosystolic or late systolic murmurs 3. Grade 3 or greater midsystolic murmurs	1. Murmurs associated with abnormal physical findings on cardiac palpation or auscultation 2. Murmurs associated with an abnormal ECG or chest roentgenogram	—	1. Grade 2 or softer midsystolic murmur identified as innocent or functional by an experienced observer 2. To detect "silent" AR or MR in patients without cardiac murmurs; then recommend endocarditis prophylaxis
Echocardiography in symptomatic patients with cardiac murmurs	1. Symptoms or signs of congestive heart failure, myocardial ischemia, or syncope 2. Symptoms or signs consistent with infective endocarditis or thromboembolism	Symptoms or signs likely due to noncardiac disease with cardiac disease not excluded by standard cardiovascular evaluation	—	Symptoms or signs of noncardiac disease with an isolated midsystolic "innocent" murmur
Transesophageal echocardiography in patients with MS	—	1. Assess for presence or absence of left atrial thrombus in patients being considered for percutaneous balloon mitral valvotomy or cardioversion 2. Evaluate mitral valve morphology and hemodynamics when transthoracic echocardiographic data are suboptimal	—	Routine evaluation of mitral valve morphology and hemodynamics when complete transthoracic echocardiographic data are satisfactory
Anticoagulation in patients with MS	1. Patients with paroxysmal or chronic atrial fibrillation 2. Patients with a prior embolic event	—	1. Patients with severe MS and left atrial dimension ≥55 mm by echocardiography	All other patients with MS
Cardiac catheterization in patients with MS	Perform percutaneous balloon mitral valvotomy in properly selected patients	1. Assess severity of MR in patients being considered for percutaneous balloon mitral valvotomy when clinical and echocardiographic data are discordant 2. Assess pulmonary artery, left atrial, and LV diastolic pressures when symptoms and/or estimated pulmonary arterial pressure is discordant with the severity of MS by 2-D and Doppler echocardiography 3. Assess hemodynamic response of pulmonary arterial and left atrial pressures to stress when clinical symptoms and resting hemodynamics are discordant.	—	1. Assess mitral valve hemodynamics when 2-D and Doppler echocardiographic data are concordant with clinical findings

Table continued on following page

Indication	Class I	Class IIa	Class IIb	Class III
Percutaneous balloon mitral valvotomy	1. Symptomatic patients (NYHA functional Class II, III, or IV), moderate or severe MS (mitral valve area ≤1.5 cm²), and valve morphology favorable for percutaneous balloon valvotomy in the absence of left atrial thrombus or moderate to severe MR	1. Asymptomatic patients with moderate or severe MS (mitral valve area ≤1.5 cm²)* and valve morphology favorable for percutaneous balloon valvotomy who have pulmonary hypertension (pulmonary arterial systolic pressure >50 mm Hg at rest or 60 mm Hg with exercise) in the absence of left atrial thrombus or moderate to severe MR 2. Patients with NYHA functional Class III–IV symptoms, moderate or severe MS (mitral valve area ≤1.5 cm²),* and a nonpliable calcified valve who are at high risk for surgery in the absence of left atrial thrombus or moderate to severe MR	1. Asymptomatic patients with moderate or severe MS (mitral valve area ≤1.5 cm²) and valve morphology favorable for percutaneous balloon valvotomy who have new onset of atrial fibrillation in the absence of left atrial thrombus or moderate to severe MR 2. Patients in NYHA functional Class III–IV, moderate or severe MS (mitral valve area ≤1.5 cm²), and a nonpliable calcified valve who are low-risk candidates for surgery	Patients with mild MS.
Mitral valve repair for MS	Patients with NYHA functional Class III–IV symptoms, moderate or severe MS (mitral valve area ≤1.5 cm²), and valve morphology favorable for repair if percutaneous balloon mitral valvotomy is not available	—	Patients with NYHA functional Class I symptoms, moderate or severe MS (mitral valve area ≤1.5 cm²), and valve morphology favorable for repair who have had recurrent embolic events on adequate anticoagulation	1. Patients with NYHA functional Class I–IV symptoms and mild MS
Mitral valve replacement for MS	Patients with moderate or severe MS (mitral valve area ≤1.5 cm²) and NYHA functional Class III–IV symptoms who are not considered candidates for percutaneous balloon valvotomy or mitral valve repair	1. Patients with severe MS (mitral valve area ≤1.0 cm²) and severe pulmonary hypertension (pulmonary arterial systolic pressure >60 to 80 mm Hg) with NYHA functional Class I–II symptoms who are not considered candidates for percutaneous balloon valvotomy or mitral valve repair	—	—
Coronary angiography in patients with MR	1. When mitral valve surgery is contemplated in patients with angina or previous myocardial infarction 2. When mitral valve surgery is contemplated in patients with one or more risk factors for CAD 3. When ischemia is suspected as an etiologic factor in MR	—	To confirm noninvasive tests in patients not suspected of having CAD	When mitral valve surgery is contemplated in patients aged <35 years in whom there is no clinical suspicion of CAD
Left ventriculography and hemodynamic measures in patients with MR	1. When noninvasive tests are inconclusive regarding severity of MR, LV function, or the need for surgery 2. When there is a discrepancy between clinical and noninvasive findings regarding severity of MR	—	—	Patients in whom valve surgery is not contemplated

Indication	Class I	Class IIa	Class IIb	Class III
Mitral valve surgery in patients with non-ischemic severe MR	1. Patients with acute symptomatic MR in whom repair is likely 2. Patients with NYHA functional Class II, III, or IV symptoms with normal LV function, defined as ejection fraction >60% and end-systolic dimension <45 mm 3. Symptomatic or asymptomatic patients with mild LV dysfunction, ejection fraction 50% to 60%, and end-systolic dimension 45 to 50 mm 4. Symptomatic or asymptomatic patients with moderate LV dysfunction, ejection fraction 30% to 50%, and/or end-systolic dimension 50 to 55 mm	1. Asymptomatic patients with preserved LV function and atrial fibrillation 2. Asymptomatic patients with preserved LV function and pulmonary hypertension (pulmonary arterial systolic pressure >50 mm Hg at rest or >60 mm Hg with exercise) 3. Asymptomatic patients with ejection fraction 50% to 60% and end-systolic dimension <45 mm, and asymptomatic patients with ejection fraction >60% and end-systolic dimension 45 to 55 mm 4. Patients with severe LV dysfunction (ejection fraction <30% and/or end-systolic dimension >55 mm) in whom chordal preservation is highly likely	1. Asymptomatic patients with chronic MR with preserved LV function in whom mitral valve repair is highly likely 2. Patients with MVP and preserved LV function who have recurrent ventricular arrhythmias despite medical therapy	Asymptomatic patients with preserved LV function in whom significant doubt about the feasibility of repair exists
Antibiotic endocarditis prophylaxis for patients with MVP undergoing procedures associated with bacteremia	1. Patients with characteristic systolic click-murmur complex 2. Patients with isolated systolic click and echocardiographic evidence of MVP and MR	Patients with isolated systolic click, echocardiographic evidence of high-risk MVP	—	Patients with isolated systolic click and equivocal or no evidence of MVP
Aspirin and oral anticoagulants in patients with MVP	1. Aspirin therapy for transient ischemic attacks 2. Warfarin therapy for patients aged ≥65 years in atrial fibrillation with hypertension, MR, or history of heart failure 3. Aspirin therapy for patients aged <65 years in atrial fibrillation with no history of MR, hypertension, or heart failure 4. Warfarin therapy for poststroke patients	1. Warfarin therapy for patients with transient ischemic attacks despite aspirin therapy 2. Aspirin therapy for poststroke patients with contraindications to anticoagulants	1. Aspirin therapy for patients in sinus rhythm with echocardiographic evidence of high-risk MVP	
Cardiac catheterization in patients with aortic stenosis	1. Coronary angiography before aortic valve replacement in patients at risk for CAD 2. Assessment of severity of aortic stenosis in symptomatic patients when aortic valve replacement is planned, when noninvasive tests are inconclusive, or when there is a discrepancy with clinical findings regarding severity of aortic stenosis or need for surgery	—	Assessment of severity of aortic stenosis before aortic valve replacement when noninvasive tests are adequate and concordant with clinical findings and coronary angiography is not needed	Assessment of LV function and severity of aortic stenosis in asymptomatic patients when noninvasive tests are adequate

Table continued on following page

Indication	Class I	Class IIa	Class IIb	Class III
Aortic valve replacement in patients with aortic stenosis	1. Symptomatic patients with severe aortic stenosis 2. Patients with severe aortic stenosis undergoing coronary artery bypass surgery 3. Patients with severe aortic stenosis undergoing surgery on the aorta or other heart valves	1. Patients with moderate aortic stenosis undergoing coronary artery bypass surgery or surgery on the aorta or other heart valves 2. Asymptomatic patients with severe aortic stenosis and: a. LV systolic dysfunction, or b. Abnormal response to exercise (e.g., hypotension)	1. Asymptomatic patients with severe aortic stenosis and: a. Ventricular tachycardia, or b. Marked or excessive LV hypertrophy, or c. Valve area <0.6 cm^2	Prevention of sudden death in asymptomatic patients with none of the findings listed in Class II
Aortic balloon valvotomy in adults with aortic stenosis	—	A "bridge" to surgery in hemodynamically unstable patients who are at high risk for AVR	1. Palliation in patients with serious comorbid conditions 2. Patients who require urgent noncardiac surgery	An alternative to AVR
Vasodilator therapy for patients with chronic aortic regurgitation	1. Chronic therapy in patients with severe regurgitation who have symptoms and/or LV dysfunction, when surgery is not recommended because of additional cardiac or noncardiac factors 2. Long-term therapy in asymptomatic patients with severe regurgitation who have LV dilatation but normal systolic function 3. Long-term therapy in asymptomatic patients with hypertension and any degree of regurgitation 4. Long-term ACE inhibitor therapy in patients with persistent LV systolic dysfunction after AVR 5. Short-term therapy to improve hemodynamic profile of patients with severe heart failure symptoms and severe LV dysfunction before AVR	—	—	1. Long-term therapy in asymptomatic patients with mild to moderate aortic regurgitation and normal LV systolic function 2. Long-term therapy in asymptomatic patients with LV systolic dysfunction who are otherwise candidates for valve replacement 3. Long-term therapy in symptomatic patients with either normal LV function or mild to moderate LV systolic dysfunction who are otherwise candidates for valve replacement
Cardiac catheterization in patients with chronic AR	1. Coronary angiography before AVR in patients at risk for CAD 2. Assessing severity of regurgitation when noninvasive tests are inconclusive or discordant with clinical findings regarding severity of regurgitation or need for surgery 3. Assessing LV function when noninvasive tests are inconclusive or discordant with clinical findings regarding LV dysfunction and need for surgery in patients with severe AR	—	Assessing LV function and severity of regurgitation before AVR when noninvasive tests are adequate and concordant with clinical findings and coronary angiography is not needed	Assessing LV function and severity of regurgitation in asymptomatic patients when noninvasive tests are adequate

Indication	Class I	Class IIa	Class IIb	Class III
Aortic valve replacement in patients with chronic severe AR	1. Patients with NYHA functional Class III or IV symptoms and preserved LV systolic function, defined as normal ejection fraction at rest (ejection fraction ≥50%) 2. Patients with NYHA functional Class II symptoms and preserved LV systolic function (ejection fraction ≥50% at rest) but with progressive LV dilatation or declining ejection fraction at rest on serial studies or declining effort tolerance on exercise testing 3. Patients with Canadian Heart Association functional Class II or greater angina with or without CAD 4. Asymptomatic or symptomatic patients with mild to moderate LV dysfunction at rest (ejection fraction 25% ro 49%) 5. Patients undergoing coronary artery bypass surgery or surgery on the aorta or other heart valves	1. Patients with NYHA functional Class II symptoms and preserved LV systolic function (ejection fraction ≥50% at rest) with stable LV size and systolic function on serial studies and stable exercise tolerance 2. Asymptomatic patients with normal LV systolic function (ejection fraction >50%) but with severe LV dilatation (diastolic dimension >75 mm or end-systolic dimension >55 mm; consider lower threshold values for patients of small stature	1. Patients with severe LV dysfunction (ejection fraction <25%) 2. Asymptomatic patients with normal systolic function at rest (ejection fraction >50%) and progressive LV dilatation when the degree of dilatation is moderately severe (end-diastolic dimension 70 to 75 mm, end-systolic dimension 50 to 55 mm) 3. Asymptomatic patients with normal systolic function at rest (ejection fraction >50%) but with decline in ejection fraction during exercise radionuclide angiography	1. Asymptomatic patients with normal systolic function at rest (ejection fraction >50%) but with decline in ejection fraction during stress echocardiography 2. Asymptomatic patients with normal systolic function at rest (ejection fraction >50%) and LV dilatation when degree of dilatation is not severe (end-diastolic dimension <70 mm, end-systolic dimension <50 mm)
Recommendations for surgery for patients with TR	Annuloplasty for severe TR and pulmonary hypertension in patients with mitral valve disease requiring mitral valve surgery	1. Valve replacement for severe TR secondary to diseased/abnormal tricuspid valve leaflets not amenable to annuloplasty or repair 2. Valve replacement or annuloplasty for severe TR with mean pulmonary arterial pressure <60 mm Hg when symptomatic	Annuloplasty for mild TR in patients with pulmonary hypertension secondary to mitral valve disease requiring mitral valve surgery	Valve replacement or annuloplasty for TR with pulmonary arterial systolic pressure <60 mm Hg with a normal mitral valve in asymptomatic patients or in symptomatic patients who have not had a trial of diuretic therapy
Follow-up strategy in patients with prosthetic heart valves	1. History, physical exam, ECG, chest roentgenogram, echocardiogram, CBC, serum chemistries, and INR (if indicated) at first postoperative outpatient evaluation (this evaluation should be performed 3 to 4 weeks after hospital discharge) 2. Radionuclide angiography or magnetic resonance imaging to evaluate LV function if echocardiography is unsatisfactory 3. Routine follow-up visits at yearly intervals with earlier reevaluations for change in clinical status		Routine serial echocardiograms at time of annual follow-up visit in absence of change in clinical status	Routine serial fluoroscopy

Table continued on following page

TABLE 46–G–1. MANAGEMENT OF VALVULAR HEART DISEASE IN ADULTS *Continued*

Indication	Class I	Class IIa	Class IIb	Class III
Valve replacement with a mechanical prosthesis	Patients with expected long life spans Patients with a mechanical prosthetic valve already in place in a different position than the valve to be replaced	1. Patients in renal failure, on hemodialysis, or with hypercalcemia (Class II rather than IIa) 2. Patients requiring warfarin therapy because of risk factors for thromboembolism 3. Patients ≤65 years for AVR and ≤70 years for MVR	Valve re-replacement for thrombosed biological valve	Patients who cannot or will not take warfarin therapy
Valve replacement with a bioprosthesis	1. Patients who cannot or will not take warfarin therapy 2. Patients ≥65 years needing AVR who do not have risk factors for thromboembolism	1. Patients considered to have possible compliance problems with warfarin therapy 2. Patients >70 years needing MVR who do not have risk factors for thromboembolism	1. Valve re-replacement for thrombosed mechanical valve 2. Patients <65 years	1. Patients in renal failure, on hemodialysis, or with hypercalcemia 2. Adolescent patients who are still growing

* In centers with expertise in cardiac magnetic resonance imaging, cardiac MRI may be used in place of radionuclide angiography for these indications.

AR = atrial regurgitation; AVR = aortic valve replacement; CAD = coronary artery disease; CBC = complete blood count; 2-D = two-dimensional; ECG = electrocardiogram; INR = international normalized ratio; LV = left ventricle; MR = mitral regurgitation; MS = mitral stenosis; MVP = mitral valve prolapse; MVR = mitral valve replacement; NYHA = New York Heart Association; TR = tricuspid regurgitation.

ventricular function in patients with this condition. The ACC/AHA guidelines note that yearly echocardiograms may be helpful for management of asymptomatic patients with severe aortic stenosis, but recommend an interval of 2 years for echocardiography in asymptomatic patients with moderate aortic stenosis and 5 years for asymptomatic patients with mild stenosis.

The guidelines indicate that exercise testing of asymptomatic patients can be performed safely and can provide useful information; however, the need for supervision by an experienced physician with close monitoring of blood pressure and electrocardiographic findings is emphasized. Recommendations from the Task Force on Acquired Valvular Heart Disease of the 26th Bethesda Conference address the issue of participation in competitive athletics.[3] These guidelines recommend that patients with severe aortic stenosis be advised to limit such activity to relatively low levels.

Coronary angiography is considered appropriate in the ACC/AHA guidelines for patients with possible coronary artery disease and may be needed to assess the severity of stenosis in symptomatic patients when other data are inconclusive. The guidelines discourage catheterization solely for the purpose of confirming information available from noninvasive tests.

Aortic valve replacement is indicated for virtually all symptomatic patients with severe aortic stenosis, and the ACC/AHA guidelines are generally supportive (Class IIa) of this procedure for asymptomatic patients with severe aortic stenosis, and left ventricular systolic dysfunction or exertional hypotension (see Table 46–G–1). However, valve replacement for asymptomatic patients is otherwise discouraged. Aortic balloon valvotomy is given qualified support only as a "bridge" to surgery in hemodynamically unstable patients who cannot undergo immediate aortic valve replacement.

Aortic Regurgitation

Doppler echocardiography is a highly appropriate test for diagnosis and serial assessment of patients with aortic regurgitation. For new patients in whom the chronic nature of the lesion is uncertain, the guidelines support repeating the physical examination and echocardiogram 2 to 3 months after the initial evaluation to ensure that rapid progression is not underway. Asymptomatic patients with mild aortic regurgitation, normal left ventricular function, and little or no left ventricular dilatation can be seen on an annual basis, and echocardiography can be performed every 2 to 3 years in the absence of changes in symptoms. However, the guidelines support echocardiography every 6 to 12 months for patients with severe aortic regurgitation and significant left ventricular dilatation, such as an end-diastolic dimension greater than 60 mm. For patients with even more advanced left ventricular dilatation, echocardiography as often as every 4 to 6 months is endorsed.

Exercise testing is considered appropriate for assessment of functional capacity in patients in whom the history is not definitive, but the impact of this test on management is not otherwise strongly supported by the ACC/AHA guidelines. Radionuclide angiography is endorsed as an alternative to echocardiography for assessment of left ventricular volume and function. However, the ACC/AHA guidelines emphasize that there is no need for serial testing using both techniques.

The ACC/AHA guidelines consider vasodilator therapy appropriate for patients with aortic regurgitation who have hypertension or left ventricular dysfunction, even if the patients are asymptomatic. However, the guidelines do not endorse vasodilator therapy for normotensive patients with normal left ventricular function and mild aortic regurgitation. The guidelines emphasize that vasodilator therapy is *not* an alternative to surgery for patients who are appropriate candidates for valve replacement.

Cardiac catheterization is not routinely needed to confirm the diagnosis or assess the severity of aortic regurgitation when echocardiographic studies are adequate. The most common appropriate indication for cardiac catheterization is the performance of coronary angiography before surgery. Aortic valve replacement is considered clearly appropriate in patients with severe (NYHA functional Class III or IV) symptoms, progressive left ventricular dilatation, mild-to-moderate left ventricular dysfunction, or declining exercise tolerance. The guidelines are not supportive of surgery solely because of a decline in ejection fraction during exercise.

Other Valvular Diseases

Tricuspid valve annuloplasty is an appropriate procedure for patients with severe tricuspid regurgitation and pulmonary hypertension who are undergoing surgery for mitral valve disease, but is inappropriate for patients whose pulmonary arterial systolic pressure does not exceed 60 mm Hg or more.

Valvular Disease in Young Adults

For adolescents and young adults with aortic stenosis, ACC/AHA guidelines reflect a lower threshold for exercise testing and cardiac catheterization to assess the risk of participation in athletics (Table 46–G–2). In this population, balloon valvotomy is an effective and appropriate option. Since this procedure has little morbidity and mortality, the indications for intervention are more liberal in younger patients than in older adults. The indications for management of chronic aortic regurgitation and mitral valvular disease are similar to those for older adult patients (see Table 46–G–1). Pulmonic valvotomy is considered an appropriate intervention for patients who have symptomatic pulmonic stenosis and for asymptomatic patients with a peak valve gradient greater than 50 mm.

Indication	Class I	Class IIa	Class IIb	Class III
Mitral valve surgery in adolescent or young adult with congenital MR with severe MR	1. NYHA functional Class III or IV symptoms 2. Asymptomatic patients with LV systolic dysfunction (ejection fraction ≤60%)	NYHA functional Class II symptoms with preserved LV systolic function if valve repair rather than replacement is likely	Asymptomatic patients with preserved LV systolic function in whom valve replacement is highly likely.	—
Mitral valve surgery in adolescent or young adult with congenital mitral stenosis	Symptomatic patients (NYHA functional Class III or IV) and mean mitral valve gradient >10 mm Hg on Doppler echocardiography.	1. Mildly symptomatic patients (NYHA functional Class II) and mean mitral valve gradient >10 mm Hg on Doppler echocardiography. 2. Systolic pulmonary arterial pressure 50 to 60 mm Hg with a mean mitral valve gradient ≥10 mm Hg.	New-onset atrial fibrillation or multiple systemic emboli while receiving adequate anticoagulation.	—
Diagnostic evaluation of adolescent or young adult with aortic stenosis	1. ECG* 2. Echo-Doppler study*	1. Graded exercise test† 2. Cardiac catheterization† for evaluation of gradient	Chest roentgenogram*	Coronary arteriography without history suggestive of concomitant CAD
Aortic balloon valvotomy in adolescent or young adult (≤21 years) with normal cardiac output	1. Symptoms of angina, syncope, and dyspnea on exertion, with catheterization peak gradient ≥50 mm Hg‡ 2. Catheterization peak gradient >60 mm Hg 3. New-onset ischemic or repolarization changes on ECG at rest or with exercise (ST depression, T wave inversion over left precordium) with a catheterization peak gradient >50 mm Hg)‡	Catheterization peak gradient >50 mm Hg if patient wants to play competitive sports or desires to become pregnant		Catheterization peak gradient <50 mm Hg without symptoms or ECG changes
Aortic valve surgery (replacement with mechanical valve, homograft, or pulmonary autograft) in adolescent or young adult with chronic aortic regurgitation	1. Onset of symptoms 2. Asymptomatic patients with LV systolic dysfunction (ejection fraction <50%) on serial studies 1 to 3 months apart 3. Asymptomatic patients with progressive LV enlargement (end-diastolic dimension >4 SD above normal)	—	1. Moderate aortic stenosis (gradient >40 mm Hg) (peak-to-peak gradient at cardiac catheterization) 2. Onset of ischemic or repolarization abnormalities (ST depression, T wave inversion) over left precordium at rest.	
Intervention in adolescent or young adult with pulmonic stenosis (balloon valvotomy or surgery)	1. Patients with exertional dyspnea, angina, syncope, or presyncope 2. Asymptomatic patients with normal cardiac output (estimated clinically or determined by catheterization) and right ventricular to pulmonary arterial peak gradient >50 mm Hg	Asymptomatic patients with normal cardiac output (estimated clinically or determined by catheterization) and right ventricular to pulmonary arterial peak gradient 40 to 49 mm Hg	Asymptomatic patients with normal cardiac output (estimated clinically or determined by catheterization) and right ventricular to pulmonary arterial peak gradient 30 to 39 mm Hg	Asymptomatic patients with normal cardiac output (estimated clinically or determined by catheterization) and right ventricular to pulmonary arterial peak gradient <30 mm Hg

* Yearly if echo-Doppler gradient >36 mm Hg (velocity ≥3 m/s). Every 2 years if echo-Doppler gradient <36 mm Hg (peak velocity <3 m/s).
† If echo-Doppler gradient >36 mm Hg (velocity >3 m/s) and patient interested in athletic participation or if clinical findings and echo-Doppler are disparate.
‡ If gradient <50 mm Hg, other causes of symptoms should be explored.
ECG = electrocardiogram; LV = left ventricle; MR = mitral regurgitation; SD = standard deviation.
Bonow RO, Carabello B, de Leon AC Jr., et al: ACC/AHA guidelines for the management of patients with valvular heart disease: executive summary. A report of the American College of Cardiology/American Heart Association Task Force on Practice Guidelines (Committee on Management of Patients With Valvular Heart Disease). Circulation. 98:1949–1984, 1998.

TABLE 46–G–3. AMERICAN COLLEGE OF CARDIOLOGY/AMERICAN HEART ASSOCIATION RECOMMENDATIONS FOR APPROPRIATE (CLASS I) ANTITHROMBOTIC THERAPY IN PATIENTS WITH PROSTHETIC HEART VALVES

Indication	Medication	Target	Class
1. First 3 months after valve replacement	Warfarin	INR 2.5 to 3.5	I
2. ≥3 months after valve replacement:			
a. Mechanical valve:			
(1). AVR and no risk factors*			
Bileaflet valve or Medtronic-Hall valve	Warfarin	INR 2.0 to 3.0	I
(2). Other disc valves or Starr-Edwards valve	Warfarin	INR 2.5 to 3.5	I
(3). AVR plus risk factors*	Warfarin	INR 2.5 to 3.5	I
(4). MVR	Warfarin	INR 2.5 to 3.5	I
b. Bioprosthesis:			
(1). AVR and no risk factors*	Aspirin	80 to 100 mg/day	I
(2). AVR and risk factors*	Warfarin	INR 2.0 to 3.0	I
(3). MVR and no risk factors*	Aspirin	80 to 100 mg/day	I
(4). MVR and risk factors*	Warfarin	INR 2.5 to 3.5	I

* Risk factors: Atrial fibrillation, left ventricular dysfunction, previous thromboembolism, hypercoagulable conditions.
AVR = aortic valve replacement; INR = international normalized ratio; MVR = mitral valve replacement.

Patients with Prosthetic Heart Valves

The ACC/AHA guidelines recommend that INR be maintained between 2.0 and 3.0 for patients with bileaflet mechanical valves and Medtronic-Hall valves and between 2.5 and 3.5 for other disc valves and Starr-Edwards valves (Table 46–G–3). Aspirin therapy is considered appropriate for patients with aortic or mitral valve bioprostheses and no risk factors for thromboembolism.

The guidelines indicate that hospital admission to administer heparin before noncardiac surgery or dental care is usually unnecessary. They recommend that heparin be reserved for patients who have had a recent thrombosis or embolism, those with demonstrated thrombotic problems when previously off therapy, those with a Björk-Shiley valve, and those with three or more risk factors for thromboembolism.

After prosthetic valve implantation, asymptomatic patients need be seen only at 1-year intervals (see Table 46–G–1). Routine serial echocardiograms are not strongly endorsed (Class IIb).

The ACC/AHA guidelines offer general recommendations to guide the selection of bioprosthetic versus mechanical valves. Bioprostheses are considered *inappropriate* for patients in renal failure, on hemodialysis, or with hypercalcemia, or for adolescent patients who are still growing.

References

1. Bonow RO, Carabello B, de Leon AC Jr., et al: ACC/AHA guidelines for the management of patients with valvular heart disease: Executive summary. A report of the American College of Cardiology/American Heart Association Task Force on Practice Guidelines (Committee on Management of Patients With Valvular Heart Disease). Circulation 98:1949–1984, 1998.
2. Cheitlin MD, Alpert JS, Armstrong WF, et al: ACC/AHA guidelines for the clinical application of echocardiography: A report of the American College of Cardiology/American Heart Association Task Force on Practice Guidelines (Committee on Clinical Application of Echocardiography). Circulation 95: 1686–1744, 1997.
3. Cheitlin MD, Douglas PS, Parmley WW: 26th Bethesda conference: Recommendations for determining eligibility for competition in athletes with cardiovascular abnormalities. Task Force 2: Acquired valvular heart disease. J Am Coll Cardiol 24:874–880, 1994.

Chapter 47

Infective Endocarditis

ADOLF W. KARCHMER

DEFINITION

Infective endocarditis (IE) is a microbial infection of the endothelial surface of the heart. The characteristic lesion, the vegetation, is a variably sized amorphous mass of platelets and fibrin in which abundant microorganisms and scant inflammatory cells are enmeshed. Heart valves are most commonly involved; however, infection may occur at the site of a septal defect or on chordae tendineae or mural endocardium. Infection of arteriovenous shunts, arterioarterial shunts (patent ductus arteriosus), or coarctation of the aorta, although actually an endarteritis, is clinically and pathologically similar to IE. Many species of bacteria and fungi, mycobacteria, rickettsiae, chlamydiae, and mycoplasmas cause IE; nevertheless, streptococci, staphylococci, enterococci, and fastidious gram-negative coccobacilli cause the majority of cases of IE.

The terms *acute* and *subacute* are often used to describe IE. Acute IE presents with marked toxicity and progresses over days to several weeks to valvular destruction and metastatic infection. In contrast, subacute IE evolves over weeks to months with only modest toxicity and rarely causes metastatic infection. Acute IE is caused typically, although not exclusively, by *Staphylococcus aureus,* whereas the subacute syndrome is more likely caused by viridans streptococci, enterococci, coagulase-negative staphylococci, or gram-negative coccobacilli.

EPIDEMIOLOGY

The incidence of IE remained relatively stable from 1950 through 1987 at about 4.2 per 100,000 patient-years. During the early 1980's, the yearly incidence of IE per 100,000 population was 2.0 in the United Kingdom and Wales and 1.9 in the Netherlands.[1] A higher incidence was noted from 1984 through 1990; 5.9 and 11.6 episodes per 100,000 population were reported from Sweden and Metropolitan Philadelphia, respectively.[2, 3] Injection drug abuse accounted for approximately half of the cases in Philadelphia. Endocarditis usually occurred more frequently in men; gender-derived ratios range from 1.6 to 2.5. The age-specific incidence of endocarditis increased progressively after 30 years of age and exceeded 15 to 30 cases per 100,000 person-years in the sixth through eighth decades of life.[2] From 55 to 75 percent of patients with native valve endocarditis (NVE) have predisposing conditions: rheumatic heart disease, congenital heart disease, mitral valve prolapse, degenerative heart disease, asymmetrical septal hypertrophy, or intravenous drug abuse.[24, 5] From 7 to 25 percent of cases involve prosthetic valves.[2, 3] Predisposing conditions cannot be identified in 25 to 45 percent of patients. The nature of predisposing conditions and, in part, the microbiology of IE correlate with the age of patients (Table 47–1).

CHANGE IN PATIENTS WITH IE. Changes in the epidemiology of IE appear incontestable despite the hazard of referral bias in available data. As a consequence of changes in both the frequency of predisposing conditions encountered in patients with IE as well as the increasing age of the population at risk for IE, the median age of patients has gradually increased from 30 to 40 years of age in the preantibiotic and early antibiotic eras to 47 to 69 years in recent decades.[2, 4, 5] Rheumatic fever with subsequent rheumatic heart dis-

ease in children and young adults has been markedly reduced in developed countries. Acquired valvular disease emerges as a risk for IE as patients enjoy greater longevity. Additionally, during their later years, many of these patients require valve replacement, which places them at greater risk for endocarditis. The increasing life span of the general population results in the emergence of degenerative heart disease as a major substrate for IE. Finally, nosocomial endocarditis presents with increased frequency among the elderly, who experience high rates of hospitalization for underlying illnesses.[6] In recent decades, only the increasing role of intravenous (IV) drug abuse as predisposition for IE and the high IE risk in children and young adults surviving after correction of complex congenital heart disease favor the occurrence of infection in younger patients.[2, 7]

CHANGES IN THE MICROBIOLOGY OF IE. Coagulase-negative staphylococci, previously a minor cause of NVE, are an important cause of prosthetic valve endocarditis (PVE) and nosocomial IE.[8] *S. aureus* is the predominant cause of IE among IV drug abusers, particularly of infection involving the tricuspid valve. In addition, *Pseudomonas aeruginosa,* other gram-negative bacilli, and *Candida* species, unusual causes of NVE in other settings, are important causes of IE in drug abusers. Even in series not biased by inclusion of large numbers of cases

▼ TABLE 47–1. PREDISPOSING CONDITIONS AND MICROBIOLOGY OF NATIVE VALVE ENDOCARDITIS

	CHILDREN (%)		ADULTS (%)	
	Neonates	2 mo–15 yr	15–60 yr	>60 yr
Predisposing Conditions				
RHD		2–10	25–30	8
CHD	28	75–90*	10–20	2
MVP		5–15	10–30	10
DHD			Rare	30
Parenteral drug abuse			15–35	10
Other			10–15	10
None	72†	2–5	25–45	25–40
Microbiology				
Streptococci	15–20	40–50	45–65	30–45
Enterococci		4	5–8	15
S. aureus	40–50	25	30–40	25–30
Coagulase-negative staphylococci	10	5	3–5	5–8
GNB	10	5	4–8	5
Fungi	10	1	1	Rare
Polymicrobial	4		1	Rare
Other			1	2
Culture negative	4	0–15	3–10	5

*50% of cases follow surgery and may involve implanted devices and foreign material.

†Often tricuspid valve IE.

RHD = rheumatic heart disease; CHD = congenital heart disease; MVP = mitral valve prolapse; DHD = degenerative heart disease; GNB = gram-negative bacteria, frequently *Haemophilus* species, *Actinobacillus actinomycetemcomitans, Cardiobacterium hominis.*

1723

associated with drug abuse, *S. aureus* causes an increasing proportion of cases and rivals viridans streptococci.[2, 9] IE caused by enterococci, which are associated with genitourinary tract manipulations, and by *Streptococcus bovis*, which is associated with gastrointestinal malignancy and colonic polyps, occurs more frequently in the elderly, the population likely to experience these precipitating conditions.

PATIENT GROUPS

CHILDREN. The incidence of IE among hospitalized children ranges from 1 in 4500 to 1 in 1280.[10] In the Netherlands, IE was noted in 1.7 and 1.2 per 100,000 male and female children younger than 10 years, respectively.[1] IE has been noted in neonates with increasing frequency. Among neonates, IE typically involves the tricuspid valve of structurally normal hearts and is associated with very high mortality rates. It is likely that many of these episodes arise as a consequence of infected IV and right-heart catheters as well as cardiac surgery.[10, 11]

The vast majority of children with IE occurring after the neonatal period have identifiable structural cardiac abnormalities (see Table 47–1). In some series, rheumatic heart disease was an infrequent predisposition for IE (≤4 percent).[11, 12] Congenital heart abnormalities, particularly those involving the aortic valve; ventricular septal defects; tetralogy of Fallot; and other complex structural anomalies associated with cyanosis are found in 75 to 90 percent of cases. Of children with IE on congenital defects, 50 percent develop infection after cardiac surgery; in these children, infection frequently involves prosthetic valves, valved conduits, or synthetic patches.[7, 11, 12] Secundum atrial septal defects are not associated with an increased risk for IE nor is patent ductus arteriosus or pulmonic stenosis after repair.[7] Since 1990, mitral valve prolapse has been recognized to predispose to IE in children; it, generally in association with a regurgitant murmur, was the predisposing cardiac abnormality in 15 percent and 5 percent of cases in two series.[12]

Endocarditis among neonates is caused primarily by *S. aureus*, coagulase-negative staphylococci, and group B streptococci.[10] Occasionally, infection is caused by gram-negative bacilli and *Candida* species.[10, 11] Among older children, streptococci, the predominant cause, account for at least 40 percent of cases, and *S. aureus* occurring as a nosocomial or community-acquired acute infection is the second most common cause of IE.[10–12] *Streptococcus pneumoniae*, a common cause of bacteremia in children, is nevertheless an uncommon cause of IE. *S. aureus* and *S. pneumoniae* may involve normal or abnormal valves, present as acute fulminant IE, cause rapid valve destruction and heart failure, and often result in death.[10]

The clinical features and echocardiographic findings of IE in children are similar to those noted among adults with NVE or PVE, respectively.[10] In contrast, IE among neonates is more cryptic; the clinical picture is dominated by bacteremia, and classical signs of IE are rare.[10]

ADULTS. Mitral valve prolapse (MVP) has emerged as a prominent predisposing structural cardiac abnormality and in adults accounts for 7 to 30 percent of NVE in cases not related to drug abuse or nosocomial infection.[1, 4, 5] The frequency of MVP in IE is not entirely a direct reflection of risk but rather arises because of the high frequency of the lesion in the general population, 2 to 4 percent of healthy persons and 20 percent among young women.

The relative risk of endocarditis among patients with MVP ranges from 3.5 to 8.2. This increased risk of endocarditis is largely confined to patients with both prolapse and a mitral regurgitation murmur. Risk is also increased among men and patients older than 45 years. Valve redundancy and thickened leaflets (>5 mm) by echocardiography also identify a population at increased risk for IE (see Chap. 46). Among patients with MVP and a systolic murmur, the incidence of IE is 52 per 100,000 person-years, compared with a rate of 4.6 per 100,000 person-years among those with prolapse and no murmur or among the general population. The microbiology of IE engrafted on MVP is similar to that of NVE that is not associated with drug abuse. Similarly, the mortality rate of 14 percent approximates that of NVE in general.

Rheumatic heart disease was the predisposing cardiac lesion for IE in 20 to 25 percent of cases in the 1970's and 1980's.[13] In reports from hospitals in North America and Europe in the 1980's, rheumatic heart disease predisposed to IE in only 7 and 18 percent of cases.[2, 4, 5, 9] In patients with rheumatic heart disease, endocarditis occurs most frequently on the mitral valve, a site at which women are more commonly infected. The aortic valve is the next most common site for IE; infection in this setting occurs more commonly in men.

Congenital heart disease is the substrate for IE in 10 to 20 percent of younger adults and 8 percent of older adults. Among adults, the common predisposing lesions are patent ductus arteriosus, ventricular septal defect, and bicuspid aortic valve, the latter particularly found among older men (>60 years).[2, 9]

In settings where NVE among adults is not skewed dramatically by infection occurring among IV drug abusers and nosocomial disease, the microbiology is notably similar to that shown in Table 47–1.[2, 9] *Coxiella burnetii*, an uncommon cause of IE in the United States, caused 3 percent of all cases in the United Kingdom from 1976 to 1985 and is a prominent cause of IE in France.[14] *Bartonella* species have emerged as a significant cause of IE, accounting for 3 percent of cases in one report.[15]

INTRAVENOUS DRUG ABUSERS. The risk for IE among IV drug abusers, 2 to 5 percent per patient-year, is estimated to be severalfold greater than that of patients with rheumatic heart disease or prosthetic valves.[16] In one study, IE was diagnosed in 74 (6.4 percent) of 1150 IV drug abusers who were hospitalized during 12 months. In metropolitan Philadelphia, 5.3 of a total of 11.6 cases of IE per 100,000 population was attributed to injection drug abuse.[3] From 65 to 80 percent of cases of IE in this population occurs in men, and the average age of patients ranges from 27 to 37 years.[17–20]

Endocarditis occurring in IV drug abusers has a unique propensity to infect right heart valves.[16, 17, 20] On postmortem examination of 80 addicts with active or healed IE involving 103 valves, evidence of infection was seen on the tricuspid valve in 44 percent, the mitral valve in 43 percent, the aortic valve in 40 percent, and the pulmonic valve in 3 percent. Because mortality rates are higher in patients with left-sided versus right-sided IE, this distribution is undoubtedly skewed. In clinical series, distribution of valve involvement is tricuspid in 46 to 78 percent, mitral in 32 to 24 percent, and aortic in 8 to 19 percent (as many as 16 percent of patients have infection at multiple sites).[18] In IV drug abusers, the valves were normal before infection in 75 to 93 percent of patients.[16–18] The remaining patients have preexisting aortic or mitral valve abnormalities, resulting primarily from rheumatic heart disease, congenital heart disease, or prior episodes of IE. IV drug abuse is a risk factor for recurrent NVE.

The microbiology of IE occurring in IV drug abusers is unique in several respects (Table 47–2). In contrast to NVE among adults in general, *S. aureus* causes more than 50 percent of these infections overall and 60 to 70 percent of those involving the tricuspid valve. The well-established predilection for *S. aureus* to infect normal as well as abnormal left heart valves is noted in addicts. Although the phenomenon of *S. aureus* infection of normal tricuspid valves is not unique to addicts, the high frequency is characteristic.[16, 21] Streptococcal and enterococcal infection of previously abnormal mitral or aortic valves in addicts is comparable to that noted generally in NVE. In contrast, infection of right and left heart valves by *P. aeruginosa* and other gram-negative bacilli and left heart valves by fungi occurs with increased frequency among drug abusers. In addition, unusual organisms, some of which are likely related to injection of contaminated materials, cause endocarditis in these patients, e.g., *Corynebacterium* species, *Lactobacillus*, *Bacillus cereus*, and nonpathogenic *Neisseria* species. Polymicrobial endocarditis occurs with increased frequency in IV drug abusers.

The clinical manifestations of IE in IV drug abusers depend on the valve(s) involved and, to a lesser degree, on the infecting organism. Tricuspid valve endocarditis, particularly when caused by *S. aureus*, presents with pleuritic

▼ **TABLE 47–2. MICROBIOLOGY OF ENDOCARDITIS ASSOCIATED WITH INTRAVENOUS DRUG ABUSE**

	NUMBER OF CASES (%)		
	Endocarditis In Drug Addicts*		
	Right-Sided† N = 346	Left-Sided† N = 204	Total‡ N = 675
Streptococci§	17 (5)	31 (15)	80 (12)
Enterococci	7 (2)	49 (24)	59 (9)
Staphylococcus aureus	267 (77)	47 (23)	396 (57)
Gram-negative bacilli¶	17 (5)	26 (13)	45 (7)
Fungi (predominantly Candida species)	—	25 (12)	26 (4)
Polymicrobial/miscellaneous	28 (8)	20 (10)	49 (7)
Culture negative	10 (3)	6 (3)	20 (3)

*Ten patients with right- and left-sided IE are counted twice.
†Data from references 16, 17, 136.
‡Data from references 9, 16–18, 136.
§Includes viridans streptococci, *Streptococcus bovis*, other nongroup A groupable streptococci, *Abiotrophia* species (nutritionally variant streptococci).
¶*P. aeruginosa, S. marcescens*, and Enterobacteriaceae.

chest pain, shortness of breath, cough, and hemoptysis. In 65 to 75 percent of patients, chest roentgenograms reveal abnormalities due to septic pulmonary emboli. Murmurs of tricuspid regurgitation are noted in less than half of these patients. Infection of the aortic or mitral valve in addicts clinically resembles IE seen in other patients. That caused by *S. aureus* generally presents as acute endocarditis with marked systemic toxicity. Symptoms and signs of left heart failure, neurologic injury, systemic emboli, metastatic infections, and the classical peripheral stigmata of IE are strongly associated with left-sided endocarditis.[16, 18]

Infection with human immunodeficiency virus (HIV) has been noted in 27 to 73 percent of IV drug abusers with IE[18-20] (see Chap. 68). Among drug abusers with IE, HIV serostatus does not significantly modify the clinical presentation, microbiology, complications, and overall survival. However, among HIV-infected drug abusers with IE, the risk of death is increased among those with a CD4 count less than 200/mm[3, 19, 20]

PROSTHETIC VALVE ENDOCARDITIS. Epidemiologic studies suggest that prosthetic valve endocarditis (PVE) comprises 10 to 30 percent of all cases of IE in developed countries.[19] In metropolitan Philadelphia, 0.94 cases of IE per 100,000 population involved prosthetic valves.[3] The cumulative incidence of PVE estimated actuarially has ranged from 1.4 to 3.1 percent at 12 months and 3.2 to 5.7 percent at 5 years.[22-26] The risk of PVE over time, however, is not uniform. The risk is greatest during the initial 6 months after valve surgery (particularly during the initial 5 to 6 weeks) and thereafter declines to a lower but persistent risk (0.2 to 0.35 percent per year).[22-27]

PVE has been called "early" when symptoms begin within 60 days of valve surgery and "late" with onset thereafter. These terms were established to distinguish early PVE that arose as a complication of valve surgery from late infection that was more likely community acquired. In fact, many cases with onset between 60 days and 1 year after surgery are likely to be nosocomial and, despite their delayed presentation, derive from events during the surgical admission.[28] Studies to identify risk factors for PVE have not resulted in a coherent picture. Data suggest that, during the initial months after valve implantation, mechanical prostheses are at greater risk of infection than bioprosthetic valves but that after 12 months the risk of infection of bioprostheses exceeds that of mechanical valves.[23-27] Patients with antecedent NVE, particularly if the disease is active, are at increased risk for PVE.[23, 24-27]

Microbiology. The microbiology of PVE is relatively predictable and reflects in part the presumed nosocomial or community acquisition of infection (Table 47–3). Coagulase-negative staphylococci, which when speciated are primarily *Staphylococcus epidermidis,* are the predominant causes of PVE diagnosed within 60 days after surgery. *S. aureus,* gram-negative bacilli, diphtheroids (particularly *Corynebacterium jeikeium*), and fungi (particularly *Candida* species) are also common causes of PVE during this period.

Occasional cases of nosocomial PVE caused by *Legionella* species, atypical mycobacteria, mycoplasma, and fungi other than *Candida* have been reported. The spectrum and frequency of microorganisms causing PVE that occurs between 2 and 12 months after cardiac surgery and within the initial 60 postoperative days are similar. More than 80 percent of the coagulase-negative staphylococci from either of these periods are resistant to methicillin and all other beta-lactam antibiotics. In contrast, 30 percent or fewer of the coagulase-negative staphylococci causing PVE with onset more than 1 year after valve surgery are methicillin resistant.[25, 28] PVE with onset 1 year or more postoperatively presumably results from transient bacteremia arising from dental, gastrointestinal, and genitourinary manipulations; breaks in the skin barrier; and intercurrent infections.[27, 28] Consequently, the microbiology of these cases resembles that in community-acquired NVE in nonaddicts: streptococci, *S. aureus,* enterococci, and fastidious gram-negative coccobacilli (*Haemophilus* species, *Actinobacillus actinomycetemcomitans, Cardiobacterium hominis, Eikenella,* and *Kingella*–the so-called HACEK group). Coagulase-negative staphylococci cause about 10 percent of these cases of PVE.

Pathology. The intracardiac pathology of PVE differs notably from the largely leaflet-confined pathology of NVE. Infection on mechanical prostheses commonly extends beyond the valve ring into the annulus and periannular tissue as well as the mitral-aortic intravalvular fibrosa, resulting in ring abscesses, septal abscesses, fistulous tracts, and dehiscence of the prosthesis with hemodynamically significant paravalvular regurgitation (Fig. 47–1). In autopsy experience with 74 patients, which is clearly biased toward the

▼ **TABLE 47–3. MICROBIOLOGY OF PROSTHETIC VALVE ENDOCARDITIS 1975–1994**

	NUMBER OF CASES (%)*		
	Time Of Onset After Valve Surgery		
	<2 mo N = 144	2–12 mo N = 31	>12 mo N = 194
Streptococci†	2 (1)	3 (9)	61 (31)
Pneumococci	—	—	—
Enterococci	12 (8)	4 (12)	22 (11)
Staphylococcus aureus	32 (22)	4 (12)	34 (18)
Coagulase-negative staphylococci	47 (33)	11 (32)	22 (11)
Fastidious gram-negative coccobacilli (HACEK group)‡	—	—	11 (6)
Gram-negative bacilli	19 (13)	1 (3)	11 (6)
Fungi, Candida species	12 (8)	4 (12)	3 (1)
Polymicrobial/miscellaneous	4 (3)	2 (6)	9 (5)
Diphtheroids	9 (6)	—	5 (3)
Culture negative	7 (5)	2 (6)	16 (8)

*Data from references 9 and 133.
†Includes viridans streptococci, *Streptococcus bovis*, other nongroup A groupable streptococci, *Abiotrophia* species (nutritionally variant streptococci).
‡Includes *Haemophilus* species, *Actinobacillus actinomycetemcomitans, Cardiobacterium hominis, Eikenella* species, and *Kingella kingae.*
Adapted from Karchmer AW: Infections of prosthetic valves and intravascular devices. *In* Mandell GL, Bennett JE, Dolin R (eds): Principles and Practice of Infectious Diseases. 5th ed. New York, Churchill Livingstone, 2000.

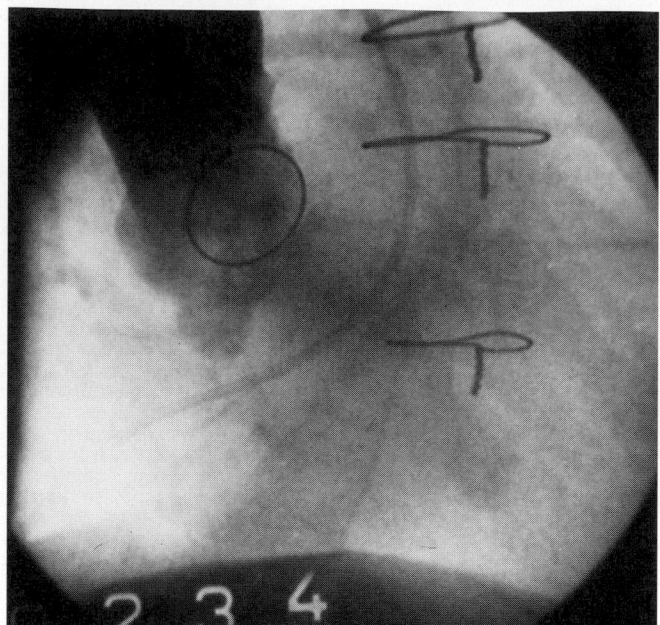

FIGURE 47-1. *S. epidermidis* infection of a bioprosthetic aortic valve 3 months after surgery. Contrast material injected supravalvularly fills a paravalvular abscess and regurgitates into the left ventricle.

most severe pathology, annular invasion was noted in 85 percent, myocardial abscess in 32 percent, and valve obstruction by vegetation overgrowth, a phenomenon of PVE at the mitral site, in 19 percent.[28] Erosion through the aortic annulus to cause pericarditis occurred in 5 percent[28] (Fig. 47-2). In clinical series encompassing 85 patients, the rate of annulus invasion was 42 percent, myocardial abscess 14 percent, valve obstruction 4 percent, and pericarditis 2 percent.[28] Bioprosthetic valve IE may result in invasive disease, comparable to that noted when PVE involves mechanical valves, as well as leaflet destruction (see Fig. 47-1). Among 85 patients with bioprosthetic PVE, 29 (59 percent) of 49 with infection within a year after surgery had invasive disease, in contrast to only 9 (25 percent) of 36 patients with infection occurring more than 1 year postoperatively.[28] In surgically treated bioprosthetic IE, invasion was confirmed in 15 of 19 cases (79 percent), with onset in the initial 12 months after surgery but in only 22 of 71 bioprostheses (31 percent) when infection began more than 12 months after surgery.[29] Fernicola and Roberts, at surgery or autopsy, noted annular invasion in 4 of 5 bioprosthetic infections with onset within 60 days of surgery and in 17

of 32 infected bioprostheses with presentation occurring more than 60 days after surgery.[30] Aortic site and clinical onset within a year of valve surgery were significantly correlated with an increased risk of invasive infection.

Signs and symptoms in patients developing PVE within 60 days of cardiac surgery may be obscured by surgery or other postoperative complications. Peripheral signs of endocarditis (5 to 14 percent) and central nervous system emboli (10 percent) occur less frequently in these patients than in those with PVE occurring later after surgery. Among patients with later-onset PVE, congestive heart failure occurs in 40 percent, cerebrovascular complications in 26 to 28 percent, and peripheral signs in 15 to 28 percent.[28, 31, 32]

NOSOCOMIAL ENDOCARDITIS. Hospital-acquired endocarditis unrelated to concurrent cardiac surgery comprises 5 to 29 percent of all cases of IE in various series.[4-6, 33] Nosocomial IE has involved abnormal native cardiac valves, normal valves including the tricuspid, and prosthetic valves and occurs with similar frequency among patients with NVE and PVE (unrelated to valve surgery).[1, 4] Infected intravascular devices and catheters give rise to 45 to 65 percent of the bacteremia that results in nosocomial IE.[6, 33] Other sources of bacteremia include genitourinary and gastrointestinal tract instrumentation or surgery. Right-sided endocarditis was found in 5 and 7 percent of patients with central venous catheters extending into or near the right atrium and those with flow-directed pulmonary artery catheters, respectively. The onset of nosocomial IE is usually acute, and although a changing murmur may be heard, other classical signs of endocarditis are infrequent.[33] Mortality rates among these patients, many of whom are elderly and have serious underlying diseases, are high (40 to 56 percent).[6, 33]

Microbiology. Gram-positive cocci are the predominant cause of nosocomial IE. Among 45 episodes from two series, *S. aureus* caused 44 percent, coagulase-negative staphylococci 22 percent, enterococci 18 percent, and streptococci and *Candida* species and gram-negative bacilli each 4 percent. One patient (2 percent) had negative cultures.[6] In a meta-analysis, the mean rate of endocarditis or other deep-seated *S. aureus* infections after catheter-related bacteremia was 6.1 percent (95 percent confidence interval 2.0 to 10.2 percent).[34] When patients with *S. aureus* catheter-related bacteremia were studied with transesophageal echocardiography (TEE), 16 of 69 (23 percent) were found to have IE.[35] Accordingly, patients with catheter-related *S. aureus* bacteremia should be studied by transthoracic echocardiography (TTE) and, if IE is not diagnosed, should be evaluated by TEE.

Catheter-associated *S. aureus* bacteremia occurs with sufficient frequency to be the predominant predisposing factor for nosocomial IE.[6, 34-36] IE complicates 0.85 to 3.1 percent of cases of nosocomial enterococcal bacteremia; although the risk of nosocomial enterococcal IE is increased in patients with abnormal valves, it remains small, relative to that for nosocomial *S. aureus* bacteremia.[6] Among 115 patients who had prosthetic valves and who experienced a nosocomial bacteremia that was not indicative of PVE, 18 (15.6 percent) subsequently developed PVE that was the apparent consequence of the bacteremia. *S. aureus* and *S. epidermidis* were the most common organisms in these cases of PVE, although gram-negative bacilli and fungi also caused episodes of PVE.[37] Bacteremia persisting for days before treatment or for 72 hours or more after removal of an infected catheter and initiation of treatment, especially in patients with abnormal heart valves or prosthetic valves, suggests the diagnosis of IE.[6, 33, 36]

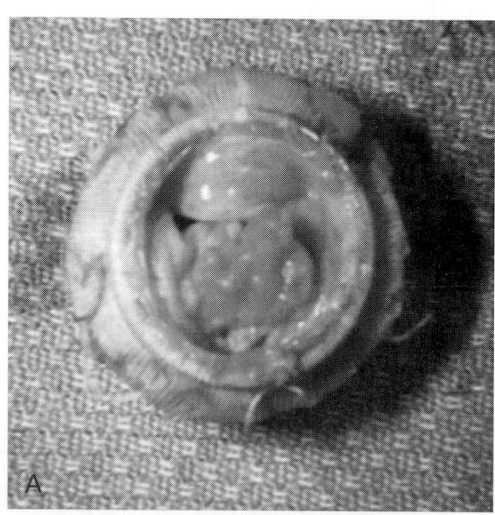
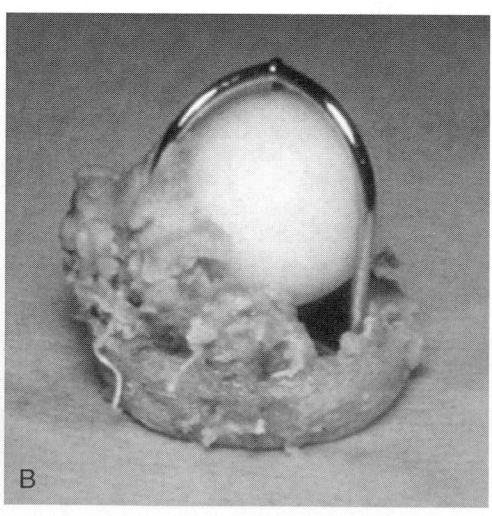

FIGURE 47-2. *A,* A large vegetation caused by *Candida albicans* partially occludes the orifice of a bioprosthetic valve removed from the mitral position. (From Karchmer AW: Infections of prosthetic heart valves. *In* Korzeniowski OM [ed]: Cardiovascular Infection, vol. x, Atlas of Infectious Diseases. Philadelphia, Current Medicine; with permission.) *B,* A Starr-Edwards prosthesis removed from the aortic position, where this large vegetation due to *Aspergillus* infection partially obstructed the outflow tract but also allowed regurgitation by preventing valve closure.

Etiological Microorganisms

VIRIDANS STREPTOCOCCI. These streptococci, which cause 30 to 65 percent of NVE cases unrelated to drug abuse, are normal inhabitants of the oropharynx, characteristically produce alpha-hemolysis when grown on sheep blood agar, and are usually nontypable using Lancefield's system. Using earlier taxonomy, the species causing streptococcal NVE were distributed as follows: *Streptococcus mitior* (31 percent of cases), *Streptococcus sanguis* (24 percent), *S. bovis* (27 percent), *Streptococcus mutans* (7 percent), *Streptococcus milleri* (4 percent), *Streptococcus faecalis* (now *Enterococcus faecalis*) (7 percent), and *Streptococcus salivarius* and other species (2 percent). Another study, adjusted for the new taxonomy, has reported a similar distribution of streptococci causing IE.[38] Nutritional variant organisms that require media supplemented with either pyridoxal hydrochloride or L-cysteine for growth and were previously speciated as *Streptococcus adjacens* or *Streptococcus defectivus*, cause 5 percent of streptococcal NVE. These organisms have been reclassified into a new genus, *Abiotrophia*.[39]

The viridans streptococci, other than the nutritionally variant organisms, had been in general highly susceptible to penicillin (minimum inhibitory concentration [MIC] ≤ 0.1 μg/ml for 83 percent) and are killed in an enhanced manner (synergistically) by penicillin plus gentamicin.[39] Viridans streptococci isolated from blood, although not specifically from patients with IE, have demonstrated increased resistance to penicillin (penicillin MIC > 0.12 μg/mL).[40] This finding raises the concern that strains causing IE may also be less susceptible to penicillin than in the past. *Abiotrophia* species, previously called *S. adjacens* and *S. defectivus*, appear more resistant to penicillin (MIC > 0.12 μg/ml in more than 30 percent of strains).[39] Although penicillin-aminoglycoside synergy was not demonstrated in vitro with *S. adjacens* and *S. defectivus*, in therapy of experimental endocarditis caused by these organisms, penicillin-aminoglycoside combinations were more effective than penicillin alone; also, therapy with vancomycin alone was comparable to that with the penicillin-aminoglycoside combination.[39]

STREPTOCOCCUS BOVIS AND OTHER STREPTOCOCCI. *S. bovis,* part of the gastrointestinal tract normal flora, causes 27 percent of the episodes of streptococcal NVE. Although superficially resembling the enterococci, this species can be easily distinguished by its biochemical characteristics. The distinction is important because *S. bovis* is highly penicillin susceptible, in contrast to the relative penicillin resistance of enterococci. *S. bovis* NVE is frequently associated with coexistent colonic polyps or malignancy.[41]

Group A streptococci, which can infect normal valves, cause rare episodes of endocarditis. Among IV drug abusers, group A streptococci have caused tricuspid valve IE similar to that noted with *S. aureus*. Group B organisms, *Streptococcus agalactiae*, are part of the normal flora of the mouth, genital tract, and gastrointestinal tract. Group B streptococci infect normal and abnormal valves and cause a morbid NVE syndrome with a high incidence of systemic emboli and septic musculoskeletal complications (arthritis, diskitis, osteomyelitis).[42] The organisms' failure to produce fibrinolysin may result in large vegetations and a high rate of systemic emboli. Endocarditis caused by this organism may be associated with villous adenomas and colonic neoplasms. Group G streptococci also produce a destructive, highly morbid left-sided NVE. The *S. milleri* group, now divided into three species—*Streptococcus intermedius, Streptococcus constellatus,* and *Streptococcus anginosus*—are highly pyogenic organisms that cause destructive infections similar to those caused by *S. aureus* and accounted for 2 to 5 percent of streptococcal NVE cases.[38]

STREPTOCOCCUS PNEUMONIAE. Although pneumococcal bacteremia occurs frequently, *S. pneumoniae* accounts for only 1 to 3 percent of NVE cases. When causing IE, *S. pneumoniae* frequently involves a previously normal aortic valve and progresses rapidly with valve destruction, myocardial abscess formation, and acute congestive heart failure (CHF).[43] The mortality rate among medically treated patients exceeded 60 percent but was 32 percent among those undergoing medical-surgical therapy.[43] Alcoholism is a risk factor for pneumococcal IE, and concurrent pneumonia or meningitis is common. Pneumococci that are resistant to penicillin and ceftriaxone are increasingly common causes of infection, particularly in children. These strains remain susceptible to vancomycin. In the future, these penicillin-resistant strains are likely to cause sporadic cases of IE; therefore, vancomycin might be included in the therapy of suspected pneumococcal IE until definitive susceptibility results for the isolate become available.[44]

ENTEROCOCCI. *E. faecalis* and *Enterococcus faecium* cause 85 percent and 10 percent of cases of enterococcal IE, respectively. Enterococci are part of the normal gastrointestinal flora and cause genitourinary tract infection. Enterococci account for 5 to 15 percent of cases of NVE and a similar percentage of PVE cases (see Tables 47–2 and 47–3).[9, 28, 45] Cases occur in young women as a consequence of genitourinary tract manipulation or infection and in older predominantly male patients, who have the urinary tract as a likely portal of entry. Enterococci infect either normal or previously abnormal valves and present as either acute or subacute IE.[45]

Enterococci are overtly resistant to cephalosporins, semisynthetic penicillinase-resistant penicillins (oxacillin and nafcillin), and therapeutic concentrations of aminoglycosides. Most enterococci are inhibited by modest concentrations of the cell wall–active antibiotics—penicillin, ampicillin, vancomycin, and teicoplanin (not licensed in the United States). Bactericidal antienterococcal activity can be achieved by combining an inhibitory cell wall–active agent and an appropriate aminoglycoside. This bactericidal activity called *synergy*, is essential for optimal treatment of enterococcal IE.[45] Strains of enterococci that are highly resistant to penicillin and ampicillin, resistant to vancomycin, and highly resistant to all aminoglycosides have been identified as causes of nosocomial infections.[45, 46]

STAPHYLOCOCCI. The coagulase-positive staphylococci are a single species, *S. aureus*. Of the 13 species of coagulase-negative staphylococci that colonize humans, one, *S. epidermidis*, has emerged as an important pathogen in the setting of implanted devices and hospitalized patients. Coagulase-negative staphylococci on the surface of foreign devices have altered phenotypes, including increased resistance to the bactericidal effects of many antibiotics.[47, 48]

Antibiotic Resistance. In excess of 90 percent of *S. aureus* cases, whether acquired in the hospital or community, produce beta-lactamase and thus are resistant to penicillin, ampicillin, and the ureido-penicillins. These organisms are, however, susceptible to the penicillinase-resistant beta-lactam antibiotics (oxacillin, nafcillin, cefazolin, and other first-generation cephalosporins). Methicillin-resistant strains of *S. aureus* are increasingly prevalent in nosocomial settings and among selected, nonhospitalized populations (IV drug abusers, nursing home residents) and must be considered when selecting initial empirical therapy for IE in patients from these groups.[17, 49] Coagulase-negative staphylococci frequently produce beta-lactamase; furthermore, strains causing community-acquired infections are frequently methicillin susceptible, whereas those causing nosocomial infections, including IE, are commonly methicillin resistant.[50] Coagulase-negative staphylococci may not always phenotypically express methicillin resistance (a property called *heteroresistance*). Consequently, special testing may be required to detect this resistance.[49, 50] Staphylococci, including most strains that are resistant to methicillin, remain susceptible to vancomycin and telcoplanin.[49]

Clinical Features. *S. aureus* is a major cause of IE in all population groups (see Tables 47–1 and 47–2). *S. aureus* IE is characterized by a highly toxic febrile illness, frequent focal metastatic infection, and a 30 to 50 percent rate of central nervous system complications.[49] A cerebrospinal fluid polymorphonuclear pleocytosis, with or without *S. aureus* cultured from the cerebrospinal fluid, is common.[49] Heart murmurs are heard in 30 to 45 percent of patients on initial evaluation and are ultimately heard in 75 to 85 percent as a consequence of intracardiac damage. The mortality rate in nonaddicts with left-sided *S. aureus* endocarditis ranges from 16 to 46 percent overall and increases in those over 50 years of age, in those with significant underlying diseases, and when IE is complicated by a major neurologic event valve dysfunction or CHF.[49, 51, 52] Among addicts, left-sided *S. aureus* IE resembles that in nonaddicts. In contrast, in patients with IE limited to the tricuspid valve, complications and mortality rates are only 2 to 4 percent.[18] Tricuspid staphylococcal IE occasionally results in overwhelming septic pulmonary emboli, pyopneumothorax, and severe respiratory insufficiency.

Coagulase-Negative Staphylococci. These are a major cause of PVE, particularly during the initial year after valve surgery, an important cause of nosocomial IE, and the cause of 3 to 8 percent of NVE cases, usually in the setting of prior valve abnormalities (see Tables 47–1 and 47–2.[49, 50] The vast majority of coagulase-negative staphylococci causing PVE, when speciated, are *S. epidermidis*.[49] In contrast, when infection involves native valves, only 50 percent of isolates are *S. epidermidis*.[49, 50] *Staphylococcus lugdunensis*, a coagulase-negative species, has caused highly destructive, often fatal NVE and PVE.[53] *S. lugdunensis* IE is usually community acquired, and the organism is often susceptible to many antistaphylococcal antibiotics, including penicillin.[53]

GRAM-NEGATIVE BACTERIA. Organisms of the so-called HACEK group, which are part of the upper respiratory tract and oropharyngeal flora, infect abnormal cardiac valves, causing subacute NVE, and cause PVE that occurs a year or more after valve surgery.[54] In NVE, the HACEK organisms have been associated with large vegetations and a high incidence of systemic emboli.[54] These organisms are fastidious and slow growing; when they are suspected, blood cultures should be incubated for 3 weeks. *Haemophilus* species, primarily *H. aphrophilus* followed by *H. parainfluenzae* and *H. influenzae*, account for 0.5 to 1.0 percent of all IE.

P. aeruginosa is the gram-negative bacillus that most commonly causes endocarditis. The proclivity of *P. aeruginosa*, as opposed to Enterobacteriaceae, to cause IE correlates with its resistance to the bactericidal activity of human sera and its adherence to cardiac valves and platelet-fibrin thrombi. Pseudomonal IE involves normal and abnormal valves on both sides of the heart and often causes valve destruction and heart failure.[54]

The Enterobacteriaceae, despite causing frequent episodes of bacteremia, are implicated in only sporadic cases of IE.

Neisseria gonorrhoeae, a common cause of IE during the preantibiotic era, rarely causes endocarditis today.[55, 56] Gonococci, similar to pneumococci, infect the aortic valve of young patients, resulting in valve destruction abscess formation, and a probable need for valve replacement.[53, 54, 55, 56] Penicillinase production and intrinsic resistance to penicillin are common among gonococci; however, all strains remain susceptible to ceftriaxone.

OTHER ORGANISMS. *Corynebacterium* species, often called diphtheroids, although often contaminants in blood cultures, cannot be ignored when isolated from multiple blood cultures. Prolonged incubation of blood cultures is often required to isolate these slow-growing, fastidious organisms from patients with IE. They are an important cause of PVE occurring during the initial year after valve surgery and a surprisingly common cause of endocarditis involving abnormal valves.[28, 56, 57] *Listeria monocytogenes*, a small gram-positive rod, causes occasional cases of IE involving abnormal left heart valves and prosthetic devices.[56] *Bartonella quintana*, *Bartonella elizabethae*, and *Bartonella henselae* have caused IE and can be isolated from blood cultures by prolonged incubation (2 weeks) followed by blind subculturing to fresh chocolate agar or sheep blood agar, which is in turn incubated for 2 to 3 weeks in 5 to 8 percent carbon dioxide.[58, 59] In the absence of special efforts in culturing, or serologic testing, many cases would have been "culture negative."[15, 58, 59] *Tropheryma whippelii*, the cause of Whipple's disease, has caused a cryptic afebrile form of IE with associated arthralgias but without diarrhea. The diagnosis has been established by examination of valve tissue by polymerase chain reaction and by microscopic identification of the organism in periodic acid–Schiff (PAS) or silver-stained vegetations.[60]

The rickettsia *C. burnetii* infects humans after inhalation of desiccated materials from infected animals or contact with infected parturient animals. At variable intervals after acute infection by *C. burnetii* (Q fever), persons with abnormal mitral or aortic valves who have not been able to eradicate the organism develop subacute IE with typical manifestations and often with valve dysfunction causing heart failure.[14] The diagnosis is typically based on high IgG and IgA antibody titers to phase I *C. burnetii* antigens. The organism can be demonstrated in excised cardiac valves by immunohistological or Gimenez staining.[14] *Chlamydia psittaci*, the agent of psittacosis, has caused occasional episodes of subacute IE and has resulted in hemodynamically significant valve damage.

FUNGI. *Candida albicans*, nonalbicans *Candida* species, *Torulopsis glabrata*, and *Aspergillus* species are the most common of the many fungal organisms identified as causing IE. Fungal endocarditis arises in specific settings. Valve replacement cardiac surgery and IV drug abuse are major predispositions. The most frequent fungi causing PVE are *C. albicans*, *Aspergillus* species, and nonalbicans *Candida* species, whereas addiction-associated fungal IE is most commonly caused by nonalbicans *Candida* species, particularly *C. parapsilosis*.[61–64] Fungal IE resulting from prolonged IV antimicrobial therapy and parenteral alimentation is caused predominantly by *C. albicans* and *T. glabrata*. Patients who are severely immunodepressed occasionally experience IE caused by *Candida* species, *Aspergillus* species, or opportunistic mycelia fungi. Blood cultures frequently are positive when *Candida* species or *T. glabrata* causes IE but rarely yield organisms when IE is caused by mycelial organisms. Bulky vegetations, which embolize frequently, are common in fungal IE. Removal and careful microbiological evaluation of an embolic vegetation may provide an etiological diagnosis in fungal IE.[61, 62]

PATHOGENESIS

The interactions between the human host and selected microorganisms that culminate in IE involve the vascular endothelium, hemostatic mechanisms, the host immune system, gross anatomic abnormalities in the heart, surface properties of microorganisms, and peripheral events that initiate bacteremia. Each component of these interactions is in itself complex, influenced by many factors and not fully elucidated. The rarity of endocarditis and endarteritis in the presence of frequent transient asymptomatic and symptomatic bacteremia indicates that the intact endothelium is resistant to infection. Endothelial damage results in platelet-fibrin deposition, which in turn is more receptive to colonization by bacteria than is the intact endothelium. It is hypothesized that platelet-fibrin deposition occurs spontaneously in persons vulnerable to endocarditis and that these deposits, called nonbacterial thrombotic endocarditis (NBTE), are the sites at which microorganisms adhere during bacteremia to initiate IE.[65] The relative uniformity of organisms causing IE, as contrasted with the variety of organisms causing overt and asymptomatic bacteremia, and the infectiousness of specific organisms in animal models of endocarditis indicate that certain microorganisms are advantaged in their ability to colonize and infect NBTE. The events after colonization that lead to IE entail survival and multiplication of microorganisms and the accrual of vegetation, as well as complex host-pathogen interactions.[66]

DEVELOPMENT OF NONBACTERIAL THROMBOTIC ENDOCARDITIS. Two major mechanisms appear pivotal in the formation of NBTE: endothelial injury and a hypercoagulable state. NBTE has been found in 1.3 percent of patients at autopsy and is more common with increasing age. These lesions have also been noted frequently in patients with malignancy, disseminated intravascular coagulation, uremia, burns, systemic lupus erythematosus, valvular heart disease, and intracardiac catheters.[66] The platelet-thrombin deposits are found at the valve closure-contact line on the atrial surfaces of the mitral and tricuspid valves and on the ventricular surfaces of the aortic and pulmonic valves, the sites of infected vegetations in patients with IE.

Three hemodynamic circumstances may injure the endothelium, initiating NBTE: (1) a high-velocity jet impacting endothelium, (2) flow from a high- to a low-pressure chamber, and (3) flow across a narrow orifice at high velocity. Flow through a narrowed orifice, as a consequence of Venturi's effect, deposits bacteria maximally at the low-pressure sink immediately beyond an orifice or at the site where a jet stream impacts a surface. These are the same sites where NBTE forms as a result of hemodynamic circumstances. The superimposition of NBTE formation and preferential deposition of bacteria help to explain the distribution of infected vegetations.[67]

CONVERSION OF NBTE TO IE. Bacteremia is the initiating event that ultimately converts NBTE to IE. The frequency and magnitude of bacteremia associated with daily activities and health care procedures appear related to specific mucosal surfaces and skin, the density of colonizing bacteria, the disease state of the surface, and the extent of the local trauma. Bacteremia rates are highest for events that traumatize the oral mucosa, particularly the gingiva, and progressively decrease with procedures involving the genitourinary tract and the gastrointestinal tract.[68] A diseased mucosal surface—particularly one that is infected—is associated with an increased risk of bacteremia.

Although IE develops when circulating microorganisms are deposited at a site of NBTE, the coincidence of bacteremia and NBTE does not uniformly result in IE. To cause IE, the organism must be able to persist and propagate on the endothelium. This requires resistance to host defenses. The complement-mediated bactericidal activity of serum limits the ability of susceptible aerobic gram-negative bacilli to cause IE. Only strains resistant to the bactericidal activity of serum, e.g., selected *E. coli*, *P. aeruginosa*, and *Serratia marcescens*, cause IE with significant frequency or are virulent in the rabbit model of endocarditis.[66] The precise role of granulocytes in eradicating early colonizing organisms is not clear. Platelet-released microbicidal material has been shown to eliminate recently adherent, susceptible viridans streptococci from valves in experimental endocarditis, and the resistance of *S. aureus* to these peptides correlates with ability of strains to cause endocarditis in animal models as well as IE and intravascular infection in patients.[68–71]

The adherence of microorganisms to the NBTE is a pivotal early event in the development of IE. Those organisms that most frequently cause endocarditis adhere more vigorously in vitro to cardiac valves than do organisms that rarely cause IE. Many mechanisms promote this adherence, including the surface carbohydrates of bacteria. Bacteremic streptococci that produce extracellular dextran cause endocarditis more frequently than do strains that do not produce dextran. Dextran on the surface of streptococci can be shown to mediate adherence to platelet fibrin lattices and injured valves. Dextran production, however, is not universal among the major microbial causes of IE; thus, other mechanisms of adherence are likely.

Fibronectin has been identified as an important factor in this process. Fibronectin has been identified in lesions on heart valves and is produced by endothelial cells, platelets, and fibroblasts in response to vascular injury; a soluble form binds to exposed subendothelial collagen. Receptors for fibronectin are present on the surface of *S. aureus*; viridans streptococci; groups A, C, and G streptococci; enterococci; *S. pneumoniae;* and *C. albicans.* Fibronectin has numerous binding domains and thus can bind simultaneously to fibrin, collagen, cells, and microorganisms and can serve to facilitate adherence of bacteria to the valve at the site of injury or NBTE. Clumping factor (or fibrinogen-binding surface protein) of *S. aureus* also mediates the binding of these organisms to platelet fibrin thrombin and to aortic valves in models of endocarditis.[72] The glycocalyx or slime on the surface of *S. epidermidis* does not appear to function as an adhesin but may render organisms more virulent by virtue of enhancing their ability to avoid eradication by host defenses.[73]

The mechanism by which virulent organisms colonize and infect intact valvular endothelium is less clearly understood. Endothelial cells in monolayers in vitro can phagocytize *S. aureus* and *Candida.* Multiplication of the organism intracellularly results in cell death, which in turn disrupts the endothelial surface and initiates formation of platelet-fibrin deposits. Alternatively, fibronectin may facilitate the adherence of *S. aureus* to intact endothelium.

After adherence to the NBTE or endothelium, persistence and multiplication result in a complex dynamic process during which the infected vegetation increases in size by platelet-fibrin aggregation, microorganisms are shed into the blood, and vegetation fragments embolize. Staphylococci and streptococci promote platelet aggregation and growth of the vegetation. Surface antigens that promote platelet adhesion (class I antigen) and aggregation (class II antigen that functionally mimics a platelet interactive domain of collagen) are expressed by *S. aureus.* Strains of *S. sanguis* with the aggregation antigen cause more severe endocarditis in the rabbit model than do antigen-negative strains.[74] Fibrin deposition is enhanced by tissue factor (a tissue thromboplastin that binds to factor VII) elaborated by endothelial cells, fibroblasts, or monocytes interacting with bacteria.[75] The persistence of this cycle results in the clinical syndrome of IE.

PATHOPHYSIOLOGY

Aside from the constitutional symptoms of infection, which are likely mediated by cytokines, the clinical manifestations of IE result from (1) the local destructive effects of intracardiac infection; (2) the embolization of bland or septic fragments of vegetations to distant sites, resulting in infarction or infection; (3) the hematogenous seeding of remote sites during continuous bacteremia; and (4) an antibody response to the infecting organism with subsequent tissue injury due to deposition of preformed immune complexes or antibody-complement interaction with antigens deposited in tissues.

The intracardiac consequences of IE range from trivial, characterized by an infected vegetation with no attendant tissue damage, to catastrophic, when infection is locally destructive or extends beyond the valve leaflet. Distortion or perforation of valve leaflets, rupture of chordae tendineae, and perforations or fistulas between major vessels and cardiac chambers or between chambers themselves as a consequence of burrowing infection may result in CHF that is progressive (Fig. 47–3).[76, 77] Infection, particularly that involving the aortic valve or prosthetic valves, may extend into paravalvular tissue and result in abscesses and persistent fever due to antibiotic-unresponsive infection, disruption of the conduction system with electrocardiographic conduction abnormalities and clinically relevant arrhythmias, or purulent pericarditis.[78] Large vegetations, particularly at the mitral valve, can result in functional valvular stenosis and hemodynamic deterioration.[28, 79] In general, intracardiac complications involving the aortic valve evolve more rapidly than those associated with the mitral valve; nevertheless, the progression is highly variable and unpredictable in individual patients.

Embolization of fragments from vegetations is clinically evident in 11 to 43 percent of patients.[9, 67, 80, 81] However, pathologic evidence of emboli at autopsy is found more frequently (45 to 65 percent). Emboli from left-sided IE produce symptoms by infection or infarction at the site of lodgment. Although not demonstrated in all studies, pooled data suggest that larger vegetations (>10 mm) are associated with a higher frequency of emboli, as are hypermobile vegetations and those attached to the mitral valve, particularly the anterior leaflet.[82, 83] Pulmonary emboli, which are often

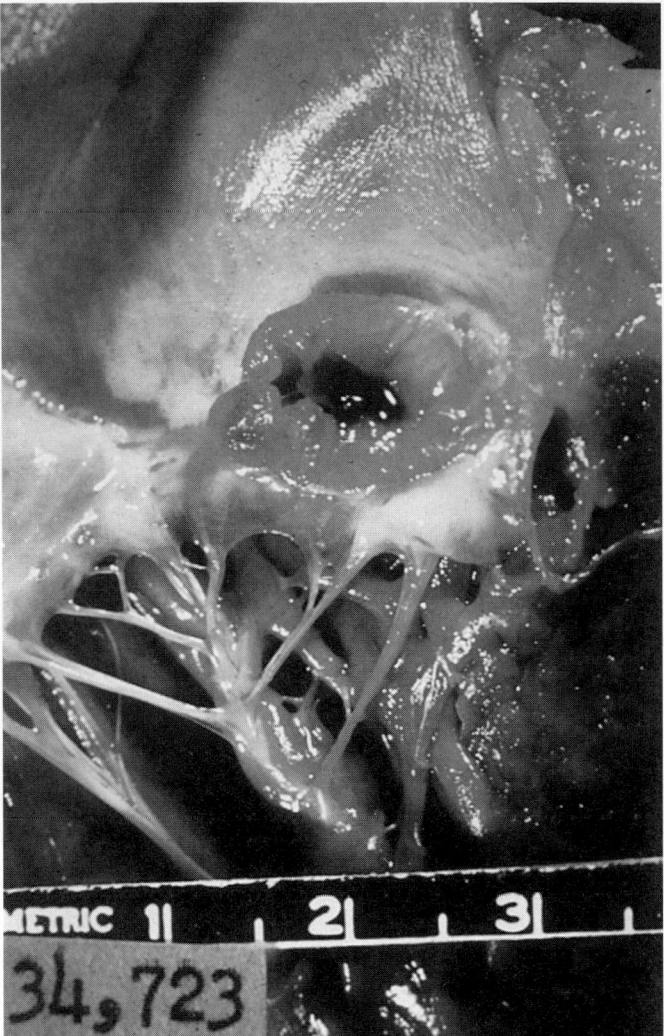

FIGURE 47–3. A normal valve with a large, bulky vegetation caused by *Staphylococcus aureus* infection. Clot is present centrally in the vegetation, obscuring a valve fenestration.

septic, occur in 66 to 75 percent of IV drug abusers with tricuspid valve IE (Fig. 47–4).[16, 18]

The persistent bacteremia of IE, with or without septic emboli, may result in metastatic infection. These infections may present as local signs and symptoms or as persistent fever during therapy.[78, 84] IE caused by virulent organisms, particularly *S. aureus* or beta-hemolytic streptococci, is complicated more frequently by metastatic infection than is that due to avirulent bacteria, e.g., viridans streptococci. Virtually any organ or tissue may be hematogenously infected. Metastatic abscesses are often small and miliary. Metastatic infection assumes particular importance when the required therapy is more than the antibiotics indicated for IE or when these infections constitute a focus that engenders relapse.[84]

The humoral and cell-mediated arms of the immune system are stimulated in patients with IE. Antibodies to the infecting organism in the three major classes—IgM, IgG, and IgA—with functional capacity including opsonization, agglutination, and complement fixation have been noted. Additionally, hypergammaglobulinemia and cryoglobulinemia have been noted. Cellular responses are suggested by activated circulating macrophages and splenomegaly.

Circulating immune complexes in high titer have been detected in most patients with bacteremic IE and PVE. The frequency and titer of the circulating immune complexes are highest in IE of long duration, in the presence of extravalvular manifestation, and in right-sided IE. Although circulating immune complex titers fall with effective antibiotic therapy, titers are not widely used to monitor therapy. Immune complexes are clinically relevant when, with complement, they de-

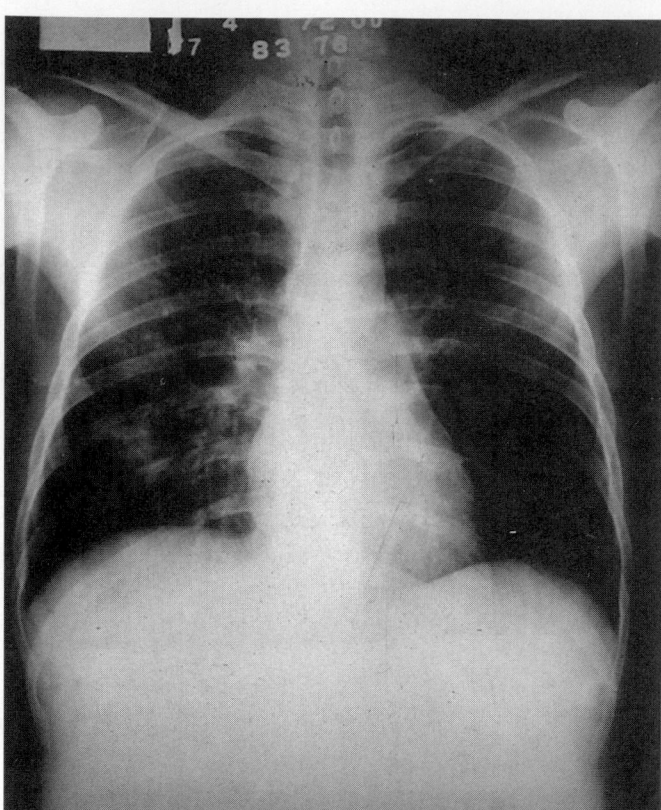

FIGURE 47–4. Infiltrates in the right and left midlung fields caused by septic pulmonary emboli arising from *Staphylococcus aureus* tricuspid valve infective endocarditis in an intravenous drug abuser.

posit subepithelially along the glomerular basement membrane to cause diffuse or focal glomerulonephritis.[67] Histological examination of affected glomeruli stained with fluorescent-labeled antibody to human globulin reveals a "lumpy-bumpy" pattern. The immunoglobulin eluted from the glomerular lesions reacts with bacterial antigens. Rheumatological manifestations of IE and some peripheral manifestations of IE, such as Osler's nodes, have been attributed to local deposition of immune complexes.[67] Osler's nodes, however, have also been associated with septic embolization in *S. aureus* IE.

Rheumatoid factor (an IgM antibody directed against IgG) is present in half of the patients with IE of greater than 6 weeks' duration.[67] The titer of rheumatoid factor decreases slowly with effective antimicrobial therapy.

CLINICAL FEATURES

The interval between the presumed initiating bacteremia and the onset of symptoms of IE is estimated to be less than 2 weeks in more than 80 percent of patients with NVE. Interestingly, in some patients with intraoperative or perioperative infection of prosthetic valves, the incubation period may be prolonged (2 to 5 or more months).[28]

Fever is the most common symptom and sign in patients with IE (Table 47–4). Fever may be absent or minimal in the elderly or in those with CHF, severe debility, or chronic renal failure and occasionally in patients with NVE caused by coagulase-negative staphylococci.[50, 85]

Heart murmurs are noted in 80 to 85 percent of patients with NVE and are emblematic of the lesion predisposing to IE. Murmurs are commonly not audible in patients with tricuspid valve IE. Similarly, in acute NVE due to *S. aureus,* murmurs are heard in only 30 to 45 percent of patients on initial evaluation but are ultimately noted in 75 to 85 percent. The new or changing murmurs (alterations unrelated to heart rate or cardiac output but rather regurgitant murmurs indicative of valve dysfunction) are relatively in-

▼ **TABLE 47–4.** CLINICAL FEATURES OF INFECTIVE ENDOCARDITIS

SYMPTOMS	PERCENT	SIGNS	PERCENT
Fever	80–85	Fever	80–90
Chills	42–75	Murmur	80–85
Sweats	25	Changing/new murmur	10–40
Anorexia	25–55		
Weight loss	25–35	Neurological abnormalities†	30–40
Malaise	25–40		
Dyspnea	20–40	Embolic event	20–40
Cough	25	Splenomegaly	15–50
Stroke	13–20	Clubbing	10–20
Headache	15–40	Peripheral manifestation	
Nausea/vomiting	15–20		
Myalgia/arthralgia	15–30	Osler's nodes	7–10
Chest pain*	8–35	Splinter hemorrhage	5–15
Abdominal pain	5–15		
Back pain	7–10	Petechiae	10–40
Confusion	10–20	Janeway's lesion	6–10
		Retinal lesion/Roth's spots	4–10

*More common in intravenous drug abusers.
†Central nervous system.

frequent in subacute NVE and are more prevalent in acute IE and PVE.[28, 86] They frequently are important harbingers of CHF.

Enlargement of the spleen is noted in 15 to 50 percent of patients and is more common in subacute IE of long duration.

The classical peripheral manifestations of IE are encountered less frequently today and are absent in IE restricted to the tricuspid valve.[4, 16] *Petechiae* (Fig. 47–5), the most common of these manifestations, are found on the palpebral conjunctiva, the buccal and palatal mucosa, and the extremities. They are not specific for endocarditis even on the conjunctiva. *Splinter or subungual hemorrhages* (Fig. 47–6) are dark red, linear, or occasionally flame-shaped streaks in the nail bed of the fingers or toes. Distal lesions are likely due to trauma, whereas the more proximal ones are more likely related to IE. *Osler's nodes* are small, tender subcutaneous nodules that develop in the pulp of the digits or occasionally more proximally in the fingers and persist for hours to several days. These too are not pathognomonic for

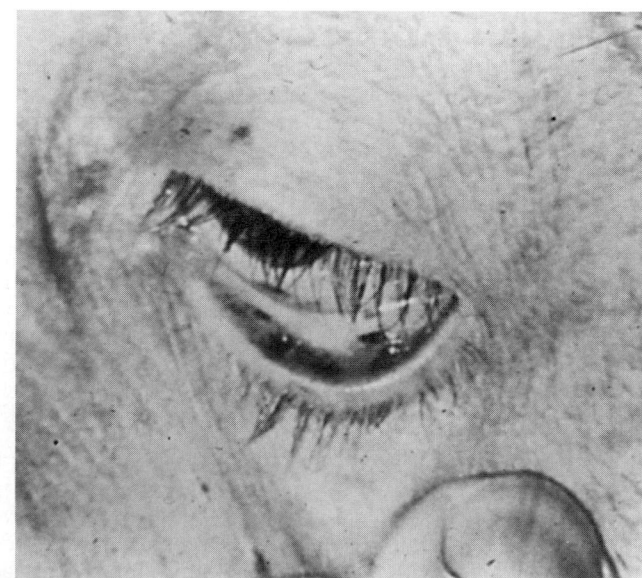

FIGURE 47–5. Conjunctival petechiae in a patient with infective endocarditis. (From Kaye D: Infective Endocarditis. Baltimore, University Park Press, 1976.)

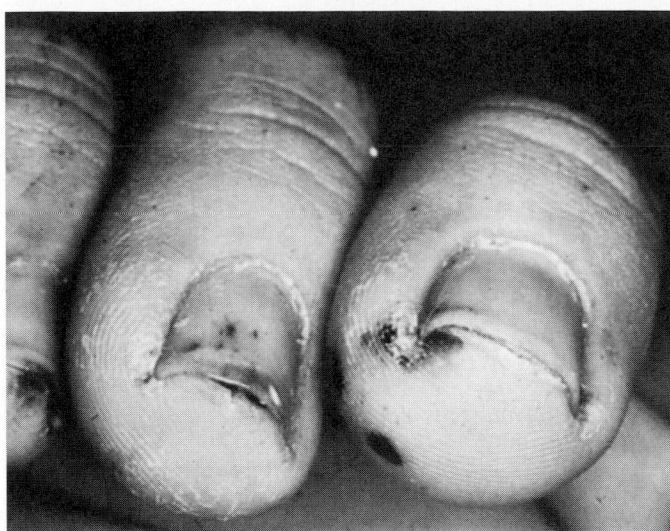

FIGURE 47-6. Subungual hemorrhages (splinter hemorrhages) and digital petechiae in a patient with infective endocarditis. (From Korzeniowski OM, Kaye D: Infective endocarditis. *In* Braunwald E [ed]: Heart Disease. 4th ed. Philadelphia, WB Saunders, 1992.)

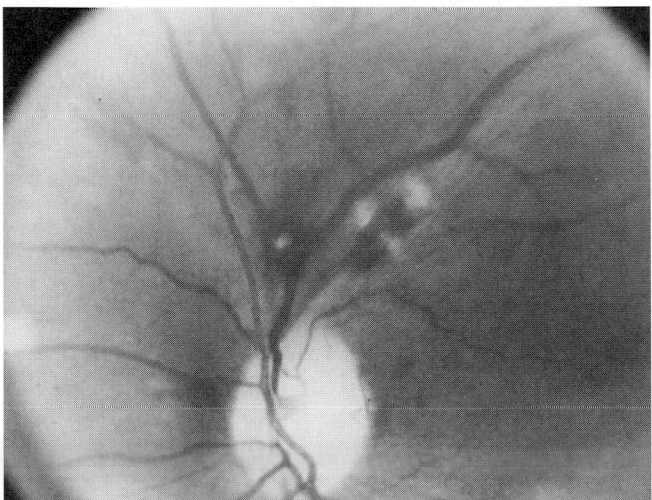

FIGURE 47-7. Roth spot (retinal hemorrhage with a clear center) in a patient with infective endocarditis. (From Korzeniowski OM, Kaye D: Infective endocarditis. *In* Braunwald E [ed]: Heart Disease. 4th ed. Philadelphia, WB Saunders, 1992.)

IE.[86] Janeway's lesions are small erythematous or hemorrhagic macular nontender lesions on the palms and soles and are the consequence of septic embolic events. Roth's spots (Fig. 47-7), oval retinal hemorrhages with pale centers, are infrequent findings in patients with IE. They have been noted in patients with collagen vascular disease and hematologic disorders, including severe anemia.

Musculoskeletal symptoms, unrelated to focal infection, are relatively common in patients with IE. These include arthralgias and myalgias, occasional true arthritis with nondiagnostic but inflammatory synovial fluid findings, and prominent back pain without evidence of vertebral body, disc space, or sacroiliac joint infection.[86] In patients with arthritis or back pain, focal infection must be precluded because additional therapy may be required.

Systemic emboli are among the most common clinical sequelae of IE, occurring in up to 40 percent of patients, and are frequent subclinical events found only at autopsy.[9, 67, 80, 81] Emboli often antedate diagnosis. Although embolic events may occur during or after antimicrobial therapy, the incidence decreases promptly during administration of ef-

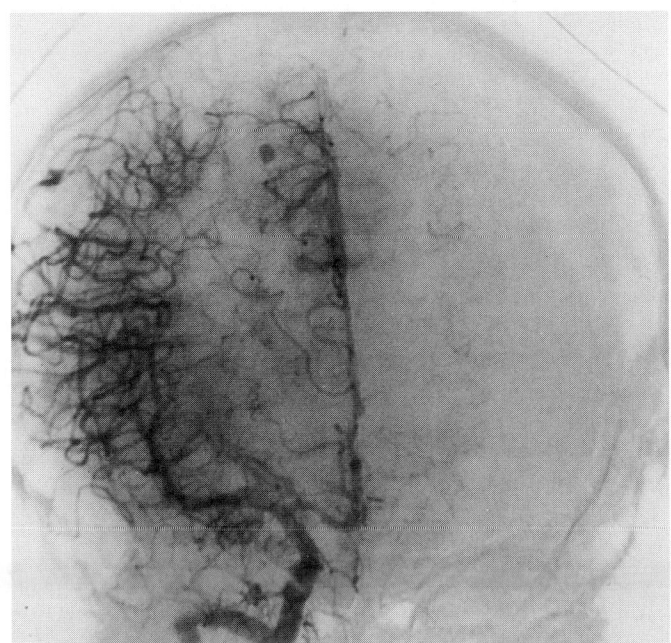

FIGURE 47-8. An irregular mycotic aneurysm of the middle cerebral artery lies laterally on the cerebral cortex. A second aneurysm is projected just lateral to the anterior cerebral artery.

fective antibiotic therapy.[85, 87] Embolic splenic infarction may cause left upper quadrant abdominal pain and left shoulder pain. Renal emboli may occur asymptomatically or with flank pain and may cause gross or microscopic hematuria. Embolic stroke syndromes, predominantly involving the middle cerebral artery territory, occur in 15 to 20 percent of patients with NVE and PVE.[28, 88] Coronary artery emboli are common findings at autopsy but rarely result in transmural infarction. Emboli to the extremities may produce pain and overt ischemia, and those to mesenteric arteries may cause abdominal pain, ileus, and guaiac-positive stools.

Neurological symptoms and signs occur in 30 to 40 percent of patients with IE, are more frequent when IE is caused by *S. aureus,* and are associated with increased mortality rates.[80, 86, 89, 90] Embolic stroke is the most common and clinically important of the neurological manifestations. Intracranial hemorrhage occurs in 5 percent of patients with IE. Bleeding results from rupture of a mycotic aneurysm, rupture of an artery due to septic arteritis at the site of embolic occlusion, or hemorrhage into an infarct.[91] Mycotic aneurysms, with or without rupture, occur in 2 to 10 percent of patients with IE; approximately half of these involve intracranial arteries (Fig. 47-8). Cerebritis with microabscesses complicates IE caused by invasive pathogens such as *S. aureus,* but large brain abscesses are rare.[88] Purulent meningitis complicates some episodes of IE caused by *S. aureus* or *S. pneumoniae,* but more typically the cerebrospinal fluid has an aseptic profile.[43, 89] Other neurological manifestations include severe headache (a potential clue to a mycotic aneurysm), seizure, and encephalopathy.

CHF complicating IE is primarily the result of valve destruction or distortion or rupture of chordae tendineae. Intracardiac fistulas, myocarditis, or coronary artery embolization may occasionally contribute to the genesis of CHF, as obviously can underlying cardiac disease. In the absence of surgery to correct valvular dysfunction, CHF, particularly that due to aortic insufficiency, is associated with very high mortality rates.[76]

Renal insufficiency as a result of immune complex–mediated glomerulonephritis occurs in less than 15 percent of patients with IE. Azotemia as a result of this process may develop or progress during initial therapy; it usually improves with continued administration of effective antibiotic therapy.[86] Focal glomerulonephritis and embolic renal infarcts cause hematuria but rarely result in azotemia. Renal dysfunction in patients with IE is most commonly a manifestation of impaired hemodynamics or toxicities associated with antimicrobial therapy (interstitial nephritis or aminoglycoside-induced injury).

DIAGNOSIS

The symptoms and signs of endocarditis are often constitutional and, when localized, often result from a complication of IE rather than reflect the intracardiac infection itself (see Table 47–4). Consequently, if physicians are to avoid overlooking the diagnosis of IE, a high index of suspicion must be maintained. The diagnosis must be investigated when patients with fever present with one or more of the cardinal elements of IE: a predisposing cardiac lesion or behavior pattern, bacteremia, embolic phenomenon, and evidence of an active endocardial process. Because patients with prosthetic heart valves are always at risk for PVE, the presence of fever or new prosthesis dysfunction at any time warrants considering this diagnosis. In patients at risk for endocarditis, concurrent illnesses or iatrogenic events may create clusters of symptoms and signs that superficially mimic IE and require careful consideration to arrive at a correct diagnosis. Even when the illness seems typical of endocarditis, the definitive diagnosis requires positive blood cultures or positive cultures (or histology or polymerase chain reaction recovery of a microorganism's DNA) from the vegetation or embolus. There are many culture-negative mimics of IE: atrial myxoma, acute rheumatic fever, systemic lupus erythematosus or other collagen-vascular disease, marantic endocarditis, the antiphospholipid syndrome, carcinoid syndrome, renal cell carcinoma with increased cardiac output, and thrombotic thrombocytopenic purpura.

When used judiciously over the entire evaluation sequence, i.e., not limited to initial findings, published criteria provide a sensitive and specific approach to the diagnosis of IE (Table 47–5).[92, 94] Erroneous rejection of the diagnosis of endocarditis is unlikely. When using these diagnostic criteria to guide therapy, patients who are categorized with possible endocarditis should be treated as if they have IE. This management philosophy, however, may lead to the treatment of individuals as possible IE patients who are not likely to have the infection.[96] Requiring at least one major criterion or three minor criteria to designate possible endocarditis may reduce this potential for overdiagnosis.[94]

To use bacteremia due to coagulase-negative staphylococci or diphtheroids (organisms that may cause IE but more often contaminate blood cultures) to support the diagnosis of endocarditis, blood cultures must be persistently positive or the organisms recovered in several sporadically positive cultures must be proved to represent a single clone.[92]

Inclusion of echocardiographic evidence of endocardial infection in these criteria recognizes the high sensitivity of two-dimensional echocardiography with color Doppler, especially if multiplanar TEE and TTE are combined, and the relative infrequency of false-positive studies when experienced operators use specific definitions for vegetations.[94, 97, 98] Although the sensitivity of TEE to detect vegetations in patients with suspected infective endocarditis is 82 to 94 percent (or higher if a follow-up study is performed), a negative study result does not preclude the diagnosis or the need for therapy if the clinical suspicion is high.[98] The likelihood of a false-negative result can be reduced to 5 to 10 percent if TEE is repeated, especially if the study is biplanar or multiplanar.[94, 98] Thus, these studies help to preclude the diagnosis when the clinical suspicion is

▼ **TABLE 47–5. DIAGNOSIS OF INFECTIVE ENDOCARDITIS**

Definitive Infective Endocarditis

Pathological criteria

Microorganisms: demonstrated by culture or histology in a vegetation, *or* in a vegetation that has embolized, *or* in an intracardiac abscess, *or*

Pathological lesions: vegetation or intracardiac abscess present, confirmed by histology showing active endocarditis

Clinical criteria, using specific definitions listed below

Two major criteria, *or*

One major and three minor criteria, *or*

Five minor criteria

Possible Infective Endocarditis

Findings consistent with infective endocarditis that fall short of definite endocarditis but are not rejected

Rejected

Firm alternative diagnosis for manifestations of endocarditis, *or*

Sustained resolution of manifestations of endocarditis, with antibiotic therapy for 4 days or less, *or*

No pathological evidence of infective endocarditis at surgery or autopsy, after antibiotic therapy for 4 days or less

Criteria for Diagnosis of Infective Endocarditis

Major Criteria

Positive blood culture

Typical microorganism for infective endocarditis from two separate blood cultures

Viridans streptococci, *Streptococcus bovis,* HACEK group *or*

Community-acquired *Staphylococcus aureus* or enterococci in the absence of a primary focus, *or*

Persistently positive blood culture, defined as recovery of a microorganism consistent with infective endocarditis from:

Blood cultures drawn more than 12 hr apart, *or*

All of three or a majority of four or more separate blood cultures, with first and last drawn at least 1 hr apart

Evidence of endocardial involvement

Positive echocardiogram

Oscillating intracardiac mass, on valve or supporting structures, *or* in the path of regurgitant jets, *or* on implanted material, in the absence of an alternative anatomical explanation, *or*

Abscess, *or*

New partial dehiscence of prosthetic valve, *or*

New valvular regurgitation (increase or change in preexisting murmur not sufficient)

Minor Criteria

Predisposition: predisposing heart condition *or* intravenous drug use

Fever ≥38.0°C (100.4°F)

Vascular phenomena: major arterial emboli, septic pulmonary infarcts, mycotic aneurysm, intracranial hemorrhage, conjunctival hemorrhages, Janeway's lesions

Immunological phenomena: glomerulonephritis, Osler's nodes, Roth's spots, rheumatoid factor

Microbiological evidence: positive blood culture but not meeting major criterion as noted previously* *or* serologic evidence of active infection with organism consistent with infective endocarditis

Echocardiogram: consistent with infective endocarditis but not meeting major criterion

*Excluding single positive cultures for coagulase-negative staphylococci and organisms that do not cause endocarditis.

Adapted from Durack DT, Lukes AS, Bright DK: New criteria for diagnosis of infective endocarditis: Utilization of specific echocardiographic findings. Am J Med 96:200, 1994.

low.[94, 98] Nevertheless, when the clinical suspicion is high, even these highly sensitive tests cannot preclude the diagnosis. These guidelines are vulnerable to misidentifying as culture-negative IE the vegetations that complicate marasmus, malignancy, cryptic collagen-vascular disease, or the antiphospholipid antibody syndrome.

A microbial cause of IE is established by recovering the infecting agent from the blood or by identifying it in surgically removed vegetations or embolic material. In detecting the bacteremia of IE there is no advantage to obtaining blood cultures in relationship to fever nor from arterial blood (as opposed to venous blood). In patients who have not received prior antibiotics and who will ultimately have blood culture–positive IE, it is likely that 95 to 100 percent of all cultures obtained will be positive and that one of the first two cultures will be positive in at least 98 percent of patients. Prior antibiotic therapy is a major cause of blood culture–negative IE, particularly when the causative microorganism is highly antibiotic susceptible. At least 35 percent of cases of culture-negative IE can be attributed to prior antimicrobial therapy.[99] After subtherapeutic antibiotic exposure, the time required for reversion to positive cultures is directly related to the duration of antimicrobial therapy and the susceptibility of the causative agent; days to a week or more may be required.

OBTAINING BLOOD CULTURES. Three separate sets of blood cultures, each from a separate venipuncture, obtained over 24 hours, are recommended to evaluate patients with suspected endocarditis.[94] Each set should include two flasks, one containing an aerobic medium and the other containing thioglycollate broth (anaerobic medium) into which at least 10 ml of blood should be placed. For optimal processing, the laboratory should be advised that endocarditis is a possible diagnosis and which, if any, unusual bacteria are suspected (*Legionella* species, *Bartonella* species, HACEK organisms). If a clinically stable patient has received an antimicrobial agent during the past several weeks, it is prudent to delay therapy so that repeat cultures can be obtained on successive days. If fungal endocarditis is suspected, blood cultures should be obtained using the lysis-centrifugation method. The laboratory should be asked to save the organism causing endocarditis until successful therapy has been completed. Serologic tests are occasionally used to make the presumptive etiological diagnosis of endocarditis caused by *Brucella* species, *Legionella* species, *Bartonella* species, *C. burnetii,* or *Chlamydia* species. By special techniques, including polymerase chain reaction, these agents and others that are difficult to recover in blood culture can be identified in or recovered from blood or vegetations.[14, 58–60, 94, 100, 101]

Laboratory Tests

Many other tests are inevitably performed in the evaluation of patients with suspected IE.[102] Hematological parameters are commonly abnormal. Anemia, with normochromic normocytic red blood cell indices, a low serum iron level, and low serum iron-binding capacity, is found in 70 to 90 percent of patients. Anemia worsens with increased duration of illness and thus in acute IE may be absent. In subacute IE, the white blood cell count is usually normal; in contrast, a leukocytosis with increased segmented granulocytes is common in acute IE. Thrombocytopenia occurs only rarely.

The *erythrocyte sedimentation rate* (ESR) is elevated (average approximately 55 mm/hr) in almost all patients with IE; the exceptions are those with CHF, renal failure, or disseminated intravascular coagulation. Other tests often indicate immune stimulation or inflammation (see Pathophysiology): circulating immune complexes, rheumatoid factor, quantitative immune globulin determinations, cryoglobulins, and C-reactive protein. Although the results of these tests parallel disease activity, the tests are costly and not efficient ways to diag-

nose IE or monitor response to therapy. Measurement of circulating immune complexes and complement may be useful in evaluating for azotemia due to diffuse immune complex glomerulonephritis.[102]

The *urinalysis* result is often abnormal, even when renal function remains normal. Proteinuria and microscopic hematuria are noted in 50 percent of patients. Urinalysis has a standard role in the evaluation of azotemia.

Serological tests are used to evaluate blood culture–negative IE (see Diagnosis). The presence or absence of antibodies to ribitol teichoic acids from staphylococci does not distinguish uncomplicated *S. aureus* bacteremia from that associated with IE or other deep-seated infection.

Echocardiography (See also Chap. 7)

Evaluation of patients with clinically suspected IE by this technique frequently allows morphological confirmation of infection and increasingly aids in decisions about management.[97, 98] Echocardiography should not be used as a screening test for IE in unselected patients with positive blood cultures or in patients with fevers of unknown origin when the clinical probability is low.[94, 95] Nevertheless, echocardiographic evaluation should be performed in all patients with clinically suspected IE, including those with negative blood cultures.[94] Although many patients with NVE involving the aortic or mitral valve can be imaged adequately by TEE using biplane or multiplane technology with incorporated color flow and continuous as well as pulsed Doppler is the state of the art.[94, 99, 103] TEE allows visualization of smaller vegetations and provides improved resolution compared with TTE. Not only is TEE the preferred approach in patients with clinically suspected IE in whom TTE is suboptimal, it is also the procedure of choice for imaging the pulmonic valve, patients with PVE (especially at the mitral site), and patients who are at high risk for intracardiac complications or those with signs of persistent or invasive infection despite adequate antimicrobial therapy.[94, 97, 103–105]

A decision analysis evaluation of echocardiography for diagnosis of IE involving native valves suggests that, assuming the diagnostic enhancement of TEE over TTE is 15 percent, the most cost-effective strategy (yielding optional quality adjusted life years) is 1) if prior probability of IE is less than 2 percent, treat for bacteremia without echocardiography; 2) if prior probability is 2 to 4 percent, use TTE; 3) if prior probability is 5 to 45 percent, use TEE in lieu of TTE, which would be followed by TEE if negative. If the prior probability of IE is greater than 45 percent, therapy without echocardiography is cost effective, although studies may still be desirable to evaluate for complications and other risks.[105a]

The sensitivity of TTE for the detection of vegetations in NVE is less than 65 percent, although its specificity is excellent. In contrast, in proven NVE, the sensitivity for vegetation detection of TEE was 100 and 90 percent, and in clinically suspected NVE, it ranged from 82 to 94 percent (see Diagnosis).[98] In patients with PVE, TTE is limited by the shadowing effect of mitral valve prostheses. The sensitivity of TEE for detecting vegetations in PVE involving mechanical or bioprosthetic devices ranged from 82 to 96 percent, whereas that of TTE was from 36 to 16 percent.[104–106]

Despite the sensitivity of TEE in detecting vegetations in patients with proven IE, echocardiography does not itself provide a definite diagnosis. Vegetations and valve dysfunction may be demonstrated, but determination of causality requires clinical or direct anatomical and microbiological confirmation. Infectious vegetations cannot be distinguished from marantic lesions, nor can vegetations be distinguished from thrombus or pannus on prostheses. Furthermore, it is usually not possible to distinguish active from healed vegetations in NVE.[97, 107] Thickened valves, ruptured chordae or valves, valve calcification, and nodules may be mistaken for vegetations, indicating the specificity limitations of echocardiography.[97]

Valve dysfunction due to tissue disruption or large obstructing vegetations can be visualized and quantitated by echocardiogram with Doppler.[82, 97] Some degree of regurgitation by Doppler is almost universal early in the course of NVE and PVE and does not necessarily predict subsequent hemodynamic deterioration.[97] Extension of infection beyond the valve leaflet into surrounding tissue is an ominous step in the progression of IE. It can result in abscesses in various areas of the annulus or adjacent structures, mycotic aneurysms of the sinus of Valsalva or mitral valve, intracardiac fistulas, and purulent pericarditis. Myocardial abscesses are more readily detected by TEE than TTE in patients with NVE or PVE.[104–106] The sensitivity and specificity for abscess detection were 28 percent and 98 percent for TTE, compared with 87 percent and 95 percent for TEE. Other studies have reported similar findings, especially in recognizing subaortic invasive disease.[108]

The natural history of vegetations during therapy is variable. On repeat echocardiogram 3 weeks to 3 months after initiation of ultimately effective antimicrobial therapy, 29 percent of 41 initial vegetations were no longer detectable. Of the 29 vegetations that remained detectable, 58 percent were unchanged, 24 percent were smaller, and 17 percent were larger. Mobility and extent (valves involved) of vegetations were unchanged in 86 and 65 percent, respectively. The evolution of these vegetations was not related to the duration of therapy or initial vegetation size, nor did it predict late complications of IE.[107, 108] In another study among patients, not all of whom were responding to therapy, persistence or increase in vegetation size during therapy was associated with an increased rate of complications. Accordingly, changes in vegetations must be interpreted in a clinical context and do not in themselves reflect the efficacy of therapy.

Stratification of patients into groups that are at high and low risk for CHF, systemic embolization, need for surgical intervention, and death based on the presence or absence of vegetations remains controversial.[82, 94, 97] The heterogeneous nature of the patients examined, the technologies used, and the lack of correlation with other features of IE, as well as the increasing ability to visualize vegetations in most patients with IE using TEE, undermine this debate. Although not demonstrated in all individual studies, pooled data from two-dimensional echocardiographic studies suggest that patients with larger vegetations (>10 mm in diameter) are at increased risk for embolic complications (20 percent versus 40 percent).[82, 97] This increased risk appears to be associated with large vegetations involving the mitral valve, particularly the anterior leaflet, and with the mobility of vegetations.[94, 97] The correlation of aortic or mitral valve vegetation size, extent, mobility, and site with CHF, need for surgical intervention, and mortality (other than that associated with embolic events) has not been fully established.[94, 97]

Among patients with right-sided IE, visualization of vegetations by TTE has been correlated with prolonged fever during therapy and increased right ventricular end-diastolic dimensions. These findings were not related to vegetation size, nor did the presence of vegetations or their size predict the failure of medical therapy and a need for surgical intervention.

MAGNETIC RESONANCE IMAGING. This technique has identified paravalvular extension of infection, aortic root aneurysms, and fistulas; however, its utility relative to echocardiography has not been established.

SCINTIGRAPHY. Efforts to identify vegetations and intracardiac abscess in patients with IE and in animal models have used scintigraphy with gallium-67 citrate, indium-111–labeled granulocytes, and indium-111–labeled platelets. These efforts have not been sufficiently sensitive or anatomically localizing to be useful clinically.[109]

TREATMENT

Two major objectives must be achieved to treat IE effectively. The infecting microorganism in the vegetation must be eradicated. Failure to accomplish this results in relapse of infection. Also, invasive, destructive intracardiac and focal extracardiac complications of infection must be resolved if morbidity and mortality are to be minimized. The second objective often exceeds the capacity of effective antimicrobial therapy and requires cardiac or other surgical intervention.

Bacteria in vegetations multiply to population densities approaching 10^9 to 10^{10} organisms per gram of tissue, become metabolically dormant, and are difficult to eradicate. Clinical experience and animal model experiments suggest

that optimal therapy should use bactericidal antibiotics or antibiotic combinations rather than bacteriostatic agents. Additionally, antibiotics reach the central areas of avascular vegetations by passive diffusion. To reach effective antibiotic concentrations in vegetations, high serum concentrations must be achieved, and penetration by some agents is limited even then. Parenteral antimicrobial therapy is used whenever feasible in order to achieve suitable serum antibiotic concentrations and to avoid the potentially erratic absorption of orally administered therapy. Treatment is continued for prolonged periods to ensure eradication of dormant microorganisms.

In selecting antimicrobial therapy for patients with IE, one must consider the ability of potential agents to kill the causative organism as well as the MIC and minimum bactericidal concentration (MBC) of these antibiotics for the organism. The MIC is the lowest concentration that inhibits growth, and the MBC is the lowest concentration that decreases a standard inoculum of organisms 99.9 percent during 24 hours. For the vast majority of streptococci and staphylococci, the MIC and MBC of penicillins, cephalosporins, or vancomycin are the same or differ by only a factor of two to four. Organisms for which the MBC for these antibiotics is 10-fold or greater than the MIC are occasionally encountered. This phenomenon has been termed *tolerance*.[110] Most of the tolerant strains are simply killed more slowly than nontolerant strains, and with prolonged incubation (48 hours) their MICs and MBCs are similar. Enterococci exhibit what superficially appears to be tolerance when tested against penicillins and vancomycin; however, these organisms are, in fact, not killed by these agents but are merely inhibited, even after longer incubation times. Enterococci can be killed by the combined activity of selected penicillins or vancomycin and an aminoglycoside. This enhanced antibiotic activity of the combination against enterococci, if of sufficient magnitude, is called *synergy* or a *synergistic bactericidal* effect.[45, 110] A similar effect can be seen with these combinations against streptococci and staphylococci; this effect overcomes tolerance.[110]

A synergistic bactericidal effect is required for optimal therapy of enterococcal endocarditis and has been used to achieve more effective therapy or effective short-course therapy of IE caused by other organisms. Tolerance in streptococci or staphylococci has been associated with reduced eradication of organisms from vegetations in animal model experiments.[111, 112] However, this finding in organisms causing endocarditis has not been correlated with decreased cure rates or delayed responses to treatment with penicillins, cephalosporins, or vancomycin. Accordingly, the presence of tolerance in streptococci or staphylococci has not required combination therapy, and, in fact, regimens are designed using the MICs of these organisms.[113]

The regimens recommended for the treatment of IE caused by specific organisms are designed to provide high concentrations of antibiotics in serum, also deep in vegetations. Concentrations that exceed the organism's MIC throughout most, if not all, of the interval between doses are recommended. Although antibiotic concentrations in vegetations of patients with IE have been measured infrequently, the success of the recommended regimens suggests that this goal has been achieved. Accordingly, for optimal therapy, it is important that the recommended regimens be followed carefully.

Antimicrobial Therapy for Specific Organisms

The antimicrobial therapy for endocarditis should not only eradicate the causative agent but should do so while causing little or no toxicity. Therapy for a given patient requires modification to accommodate end-organ dysfunction, existing allergies, and other anticipated toxicities. With the exception of staphylococcal endocarditis, the antimicrobial regimens recommended for the treatment of NVE and PVE are similar, although more prolonged treatment is often advised for PVE.[28, 113]

PENICILLIN-SUSCEPTIBLE VIRIDANS STREPTOCOCCI OR STREPTOCOCCUS BOVIS. Four regimens provide highly effective, comparable therapy for patients with endocarditis caused by penicillin-susceptible streptococci and *S. bovis* (Table 47–6). The 4-week regimens yield bacteriologic cure rates of 98 percent among patients who complete therapy. Treatment with the synergistic combination of penicillin plus gentamicin for 2 weeks is as effective in selected cases as treatment with the 4-week regimens. The combination regimen is recommended for patients who have uncomplicated native valve endocarditis and who are not at increased risk for aminoglycoside toxicity. Patients with endocarditis caused by nutritionally variant streptococci, endocarditis involving a prosthetic valve, or endocarditis complicated by a mycotic aneurysm, myocardial abscess, perivalvular infection, or an extracardiac focus of infection should not be treated with this short-course regimen. From 2 to 8 percent of viridans streptococci and *S. bovis* causing endocarditis are highly resistant to streptomycin (MIC > 2000 μg/ml) and are not killed synergistically by penicillin plus streptomycin. These highly streptomycin-resistant strains are, however, killed synergistically by penicillin plus gentamicin. Consequently, unless a causative streptococcus can be evaluated to preclude high-level resistance to streptomycin, gentamicin is recommended for use in the short-course combination regimen.[114] Ceftriaxone 2 gm once daily plus either gentamicin (3 mg/kg) or netilmicin (4 mg/kg) given as a single daily dose for 14 days has effectively treated endocarditis caused by penicillin-susceptible

▼ TABLE 47–7. TREATMENT FOR NATIVE VALVE ENDOCARDITIS DUE TO STRAINS OF VIRIDANS STREPTOCOCCI AND *STREPTOCOCCUS BOVIS* RELATIVELY RESISTANT TO PENICILLIN G (MINIMUM INHIBITORY CONCENTRATION >0.1 μg/ml AND <0.5 μg/ml)

1735

Ch 47

ANTIBIOTIC	DOSAGE AND ROUTE*	DURATION (WK)
Aqueous penicillin G *plus*	18 million units/24 hr IV either continuously or every 4 hr in 6 equally divided doses	4
Gentamicin	1 mg/kg IM or IV every 8 hr	2
Vancomycin	30 mg/kg/24 hr IV in two equally divided doses, not to exceed 2 gm/24 hr unless serum levels are monitored	4

*Dosages are for patients with normal renal function; see Table 47–6 footnote.

Modified from Wilson WR, Karchmer AW, Dajani AS, et al: Antibiotic treatment of adults with infective endocarditis due to streptococci, enterococci, staphylococci, and HACEK microorganisms. JAMA 274:1706, 1995. Copyright 1995 American Medical Association.

streptococci.[115, 116] Nevertheless, experience with single daily doses of aminoglycosides in the treatment of IE is limited, and these regimens are not currently recommended. The *Abiotrophia* species, previously called nutritionally variant streptococci, *S. adjacens* and *S. defectivus,* are generally more resistant to penicillin than are other viridans streptococci.[39] Patients with endocarditis caused by these organisms are treated with regimens recommended for enterococcal endocarditis (see Table 47–8); however, outcome remains unsatisfactory.

For the treatment of streptococcal endocarditis in patients with a history of immediate allergic reactions (urticarial or anaphylactic reactions) to a penicillin or cephalosporin antibiotic, vancomycin is recommended (see Table 47–6). Patients with other forms of penicillin allergy (delayed maculopapular skin rash) may be treated cautiously with the ceftriaxone regimen (see Table 47–6) or with cefazolin, 2 gm IV every 8 hours for 4 weeks.

For patients with PVE caused by penicillin-susceptible streptococci, treatment with 6 weeks of penicillin is recommended, with gentamicin given during the initial 2 weeks.[28]

RELATIVELY PENICILLIN-RESISTANT STREPTOCOCCI. Four weeks of high-dose parenteral penicillin plus an aminoglycoside (primarily gentamicin for the reasons noted previously) during the initial 2 weeks is recommended for treatment of patients with endocarditis caused by streptococci with MICs for penicillin between 0.2 and 0.5 μg/ml (Table 47–7). Patients who cannot tolerate penicillin because of immediate hypersensitivity reactions can be treated with vancomycin alone. For those with nonimmediate penicillin hypersensitivity, effective treatment can be accomplished with either vancomycin alone or by adding gentamicin to the initial 2 weeks of the ceftriaxone regimen (see Table 47–6). Patients with endocarditis caused by streptococci that are highly resistant to penicillin (MIC > 0.5 μg/ml) should be treated with one of the regimens recommended for enterococcal endocarditis (see Table 47–8).

STREPTOCOCCUS PYOGENES, STREPTOCOCCUS PNEUMONIAE, AND GROUPS B, C, AND G STREPTOCOCCI. Endocarditis caused by these streptococci has been either refractory to antibiotic therapy or associated with extensive valvular damage. Penicillin G in a dose of 3 million units IV every 4 hours for 4 weeks is recommended for the treatment of group A streptococcal and pneumococcal endocarditis. Pneumococci that are relatively resistant (MIC > 0.1

▼ TABLE 47–6. TREATMENT FOR NATIVE VALVE ENDOCARDITIS DUE TO PENICILLIN-SUSCEPTIBLE VIRIDANS STREPTOCOCCI AND *STREPTOCOCCUS BOVIS* (MINIMUM INHIBITORY CONCENTRATION ≤0.1 μg/ml)*

ANTIBIOTIC	DOSAGE AND ROUTE†	DURATION (WK)
Aqueous penicillin G	12–18 million units/24 hr IV either continuously or every 4 hr in six equally divided doses	4
Ceftriaxone	2 gm once daily IV or IM	4
Aqueous penicillin G *plus*	12–18 million units/24 hr IV either continuously or every 4 hr in six equally divided doses	2
Gentamicin	1 mg/kg IM or IV every 8 hr	2
Vancomycin	30 mg/kg/24 hr IV in two equally divided doses, not to exceed 2 gm/24 hr unless serum levels are monitored	4

*For nutritionally variant streptococci (*Streptococcus adjacens, Streptococcus defectivus*), see Table 47–8.

†Dosages given are for patients with normal renal function. Vancomycin and gentamicin doses must be reduced for treatment of patients with renal dysfunction. Vancomycin and gentamicin doses are calculated using ideal body weight (men = 50 kg + 2.3 kg per inch over 5 feet; women = 45.5 kg + 2.3 kg per inch over 5 feet).

Modified from Wilson WR, Karchmer AW, Dajani AS, et al: Antibiotic treatment of adults with infective endocarditis due to streptococci, enterococci, staphylococci, and HACEK microorganisms. JAMA 274:1706, 1995. Copyright 1995 American Medical Association.

µg/ml to 1.0 µg/ml) and highly resistant (MIC > 1.0 µg/ml) to penicillin are widely distributed and likely to cause sporadic cases of endocarditis. Treatment with ceftriaxone plus vancomycin may be preferable until the penicillin susceptibility of the infecting strain is confirmed.[44] IE caused by group G, C, or B streptococci is more difficult to treat than that caused by penicillin-susceptible viridans streptococci. Consequently, the addition of gentamicin to the first 2 weeks of a 4-week regimen using high doses of penicillin is often advocated[42] (see Table 47–7). Early cardiac surgery to correct intracardiac complications is needed in almost half of these cases; prompt intervention may improve outcome.[42]

BACTEREMIA. Sustained bacteremia is typical of IE. In evaluating positive blood cultures, sustained bacteremia (persisting over >1 hour) should be distinguished from transient bacteremia. When several blood cultures obtained over 24 hours or more are positive, the diagnosis of IE must be considered. The identity of the organism is also helpful in determining the intensity with which the diagnosis is entertained. Organisms can be divided into those that commonly cause IE, those that rarely cause IE, and the intermediate-behaving organisms, e.g., enterococci and *S. aureus*, which, when in the blood, may or may not indicate IE. Finally, the presence or absence of alternative sources for the bacteremia aids in the assessment of bacteremia. These considerations are embodied in the diagnostic criteria for IE (see Table 47–5).[90, 92]

Among patients with *S. aureus* bacteremia, the risk of IE has been greatest in those with community-acquired infection, those who lack a peripheral site of infection, those who are IV drug abusers, those who have evidence of valvular disease, and those who are diabetic with chronic cutaneous infections. Screening of patients with community-acquired *S. aureus* bacteremia using TTE demonstrated 20 percent of the patients to have either occult IE or valve lesions predisposing to IE.[93] Early studies have suggested that *S. aureus* catheter-associated bacteremia leads to IE in only 6.1 percent of patients.[34] IE was noted in 23 percent of 69 patients with catheter-associated *S. aureus* bacteremia.[35] In an additional study, 50 percent of patients with *S. aureus* IE had an intravascular catheter or a hemodialysis graft as the presumed source of infection.[52] In both of these studies, TTE was not sufficiently sensitive, and TEE was frequently required to diagnose IE. Thus, it is prudent to use TTE to evaluate patients with catheter-associated *S. aureus*, who appear to be at moderate clinical risk of having IE and to use TEE if that is negative or not diagnostic.[51, 94, 95] Patients with *S. aureus* bacteremia who have known underlying valvular heart disease, have a new significant heart murmur, or have persistent fever or bacteremia for 3 days or more after removal of the presumed primary focus of infection (intravascular catheter or drainage of an abscess) and initiation of therapy are at high risk for IE and require full echocardiographic evaluation.[36, 93]

ENTEROCOCCI. Optimal therapy for enterococcal endocarditis requires synergistic bactericidal interaction of an antimicrobial targeted against the bacterial cell wall (penicillin, ampicillin, or vancomycin) and an aminoglycoside that is able to exert a lethal effect (primarily streptomycin or gentamicin). High-level resistance, defined as the inability of high concentrations of streptomycin (2000 µg/ml) or gentamicin (500 to 2000 µg/ml) to inhibit the growth of an enterococcus, is predictive of the agent's inability to exert this lethal effect and participate in the bactericidal synergistic interaction in vitro and in vivo.[45, 46] The standard regimens recommended for the treatment of enterococcal endocarditis (Table 47–8) are designed to achieve bactericidal synergy. Synergistic combination therapy has resulted in cure rates of approximately 85 percent, compared with 40 percent with single-agent, nonbactericidal treatment.[45]

▼ **TABLE 47–8. STANDARD THERAPY FOR ENDOCARDITIS DUE TO ENTEROCOCCI***

ANTIBIOTIC	DOSAGE AND ROUTE†	DURATION (WK)
Aqueous penicillin G	18–30 million units/24 hr IV given continuously or every 4 hr in six equally divided doses	4–6
plus		
Gentamicin	1 mg/kg IM or IV every 8 hr	4–6
Ampicillin	12 gm/24 hr IV given continuously or every 4 hr in six equally divided doses	4–6
plus		
Gentamicin	1 mg/kg IM or IV every 8 hr	4–6
Vancomycin‡	30 mg/kg/24 hr IV in two equally divided doses not to exceed 2 gm/24 hr unless serum levels are monitored	4–6
plus		
Gentamicin	1 mg/kg IM or IV every 8 hr	4–6

*All enterococci causing endocarditis must be tested for antimicrobial susceptibility in order to select optimal therapy. These regimens are for treatment of endocarditis caused by enterococci that are susceptible to vancomycin or ampicillin and not highly resistant to gentamicin. These may also be used for treatment of endocarditis caused by penicillin-resistant (MIC > 0.5) viridans streptococci and nutritionally variant streptococci (*S. defectivus, S. adjacens*), or enterococcal PVE.

†Dosages are for patients with normal renal function. See Table 47–6, footnote.

‡Cephalosporins are not alternatives to penicillin/ampicillin in penicillin-allergic patients.

Modified from Wilson WR, Karchmer AW, Dajani AS, et al: Antibiotic treatment of adults with infective endocarditis due to streptococci, enterococci, staphylococci, and HACEK microorganisms. JAMA 274:1706, 1995. Copyright 1995 American Medical Association.

Some authorities prefer gentamicin doses of 1.5 mg/kg every 8 hours; however, because this dose may be associated with an increased frequency of nephrotoxicity, others advocate doses of 1 mg/kg every 8 hours. Peak serum gentamicin concentrations of approximately 5 µg/ml and 3.5 µg/ml are sought with these doses, respectively. In the absence of high-level resistance to streptomycin in a causative strain, streptomycin, 7.5 mg/kg intramuscularly (IM) or IV, every 12 hours, to achieve a peak serum concentration of approximately 20 µg/ml, can be substituted for gentamicin in the standard regimens. For patients allergic to penicillin, the vancomycin-aminoglycoside regimen (Table 47–8) is recommended; alternatively, patients can be desensitized to penicillin. Desensitization may be desirable when preexisting renal dysfunction favors avoiding the potentially more nephrotoxic vancomycin-aminoglycoside combination. Cephalosporins are not effective in the treatment of enterococcal endocarditis. Therapy is administered for 4 to 6 weeks, with the longer course used to treat patients with IE that was symptomatic for more than 3 months, with complicated disease, and with enterococcal PVE. During treatment, careful clinical follow-up of patients and aminoglycoside levels is required to prevent nephrotoxicity and ototoxicity.

Previously, 40 percent of enterococci demonstrated high-level resistance to streptomycin, and none was highly resistant to gentamicin. Furthermore, penicillin, ampicillin, and vancomycin inhibited all enterococci at concentrations achieved in the serum with standard IV doses. Accordingly, one of the standard regimens could be selected for treatment with confidence that bactericidal synergy would be achieved. Antimicrobial resistance among enterococci is now complex and cannot be predicted without in vitro testing. High-level resistance to gentamicin has been noted in 25 percent of *E. faecalis* and 50 percent of *E. faecium* infections, and resistance to penicillin, ampicillin, and vancomycin has become commonplace, especially in *E. faecium* infections. Resistance to these antibiotics is most common among enterococci isolated from hospitalized or previously hospitalized persons.

Nevertheless, all enterococci causing endocarditis must be evaluated carefully in order to select effective therapy (Table 47–9). The strain causing endocarditis must be tested for high-level resistance to both streptomycin and gentamicin, as well as to determine its susceptibility to penicillin, ampicillin, and vancomycin. If the strain is either resistant to achievable serum concentrations of the cell wall–active agent or highly resistant to the aminoglycosides, synergy and optimal therapy cannot be obtain with a standard regimen that includes the inactive antimicrobial. Furthermore, high-level resistance to gentamicin predicts resistance to all other aminoglycosides except

streptomycin. These susceptibility data allow selection of a bacteri- **1737**
cidal synergistic regimen, if one is possible, or alternative treatment
(see Table 47–9).[46]

Ch 47

▼ **TABLE 47–9.** STRATEGY FOR SELECTING THERAPY FOR ENTEROCOCCAL ENDOCARDITIS CAUSED BY STRAINS RESISTANT TO COMPONENTS OF THE STANDARD REGIMEN 1

I. Ideal therapy includes a cell wall–active agent plus an effective aminoglycoside to achieve bactericidal synergy
II. Cell wall–active antimicrobial
   A. Determine MIC for ampicillin and vancomycin; test for beta-lactamase production (nitrocefin test)
   B. If ampicillin and vancomycin susceptible, use ampicillin
   C. If ampicillin resistant (MIC ≥ 16 μg/ml) and vancomycin susceptible, use vancomycin
   D. If beta-lactamase produced, use vancomycin or consider ampicillin-sulbactam
   E. If ampicillin resistant and vancomycin resistant (MIC ≥ 16 μg/ml), consider teicoplanin*
   F. If ampicillin resistant and highly resistant to vancomycin and teicoplanin (MIC ≥ 256 μg/ml), see IV C, D
III. Aminoglycoside to be used with cell wall–active antimicrobial
   A. If no high level resistance to streptomycin (MIC < 2000 μg/ml) or gentamicin (MIC < 500–2000 μg/ml), use gentamicin or streptomycin
   B. If high-level resistance to gentamicin (MIC > 500–2000 μg/ml), test streptomycin. If no high-level resistance to streptomycin, use streptomycin
   C. If high-level resistance to gentamicin and streptomycin, omit aminoglycoside therapy; use prolonged therapy (8–12 wk) with cell wall–active antimicrobial if the organism is susceptible (see II A–E) or alternative therapy (see IV C,D)
IV. Alternative regimens and approaches
   A. Single drug therapy (see III C) and surgical intervention
   B. Consider ampicillin, vancomycin (or teicoplanin), and gentamicin (or streptomycin) based on absence of high-level resistance
   C. Consider quinupristin/dalfopristin therapy for infective endocarditis due to susceptible *Enterococcus faecium* and surgical intervention
   D. Consider suppressive therapy with chloramphenicol or tetracycline and surgical intervention
   E. Treatment with fluoroquinolones, rifampin, or trimethoprim-sulfamethoxazole of questionable efficacy

MIC = minimum inhibitory concentration.
*Not approved by the Food and Drug Administration for use in the United States; may be available by compassionate-use protocol.

STAPHYLOCOCCI. More than 90 percent of coagulase-positive and coagulase-negative staphylococci are penicillin resistant. Methicillin resistance is common among coagulase-negative staphylococci and is a less frequent but important characteristic among *S. aureus*. Methicillin-resistant strains are resistant to all beta-lactam antibiotics but usually remain susceptible to vancomycin. Although staphylococci are killed by cell wall–active antibiotics, the bactericidal effects of these agents can be enhanced by aminoglycosides. Combinations of semisynthetic penicillinase-resistant penicillins or vancomycin with rifampin do not result in predictable bactericidal synergism; nevertheless, rifampin has unique activity against staphylococcal infections that involve foreign material.[28, 117] Staphylococcal infections involving prosthetic heart valves are treated differently from native valve endocarditis caused by the same species (Table 47–10).[28, 50, 113]

STAPHYLOCOCCAL NATIVE VALVE ENDOCARDITIS. The semisynthetic penicillinase-resistant penicillins are the cornerstones of the treatment of endocarditis caused by methicillin-susceptible staphylococci. When patients have a penicillin allergy that does not induce urticaria or anaphylaxis, a first-generation cephalosporin can be used. The synergistic interaction of beta-lactam antibiotics with an aminoglycoside has not increased the cure rates for staphylococcal endocarditis; however, treatment with these combinations has modestly accelerated the eradication of staphylococci in vegetations and from the blood. To achieve this potential benefit, gentamicin may be added to beta-lactam antibiotic therapy for *S. aureus* during the initial 3 to 5 days of treatment.[113] More prolonged administration of gentamicin has been associated with nephrotoxicity and should be avoided. The role for combination therapy is less well defined in NVE caused by coagulase-negative staphylococci; pooled data suggest improved cure rates with combination therapy.[50] In IV drug addicts, Methicillin-susceptible *S. aureus* endocarditis that is apparently uncomplicated and limited to the right heart valves has been effectively treated with 2 weeks of semisynthetic penicillinase-resistant penicillin (but not vancomycin) plus an aminoglycoside (doses as noted in Table 47–10).[118] However, some patients with right-sided *S. aureus* endocarditis remain febrile and toxic for a significant portion or the entire 2 weeks of combina-

▼ **TABLE 47–10.** TREATMENT FOR STAPHYLOCOCCAL ENDOCARDITIS IN THE ABSENCE OF PROSTHETIC MATERIAL

ANTIBIOTIC	DOSAGE AND ROUTE*	DURATION (WK)
Methicillin-Susceptible Staphylococci†		
Nafcillin or oxacillin	2 gm IV every 4 hr	4–6
With optional addition of gentamicin	1 mg/kg IM or IV every 8 hr	3–5 days
Cefazolin (or other first-generation cephalosporins in equivalent dosages)‡	2 gm IV every 8 hr	4–6
With optional addition of gentamicin	1 mg/kg IM or IV every 8 hr	3–5 days
Vancomycin‡	30 mg/kg/24 hr IV in two equally divided doses, not to exceed 2 gm/24 hr unless serum levels are monitored	4–6
Methicillin-Resistant Staphylococci		
Vancomycin	30 mg/kg/24 hr IV in two equally divided doses, not to exceed 2 gm/24 hr unless serum levels are monitored	4–6

*Dosages are for patients with normal renal function. See Table 47–6, footnote.
†For treatment of endocarditis due to penicillin-susceptible staphylococci (minimum inhibitory concentration ≤0.1 μg/ml), aqueous penicillin G (18–24 million units/24 hr) can be used for 4–6 wk instead of nafcillin or oxacillin.
‡Cefazolin, other first-generation cephalosporins, or vancomycin may be used in selected penicillin-allergic patients.
Modified from Wilson WR, Karchmer AW, Dajani AS, et al: Antibiotic treatment of adults with infective endocarditis due to streptococci, enterococci, staphylococci, and HACEK microorganisms. JAMA 274:1706, 1995. Copyright 1995 American Medical Association.

tion therapy. Hence, clinical judgment must be exercised when this abbreviated regimen is used. Therapy should be extended in those patients who remain febrile after 1 week of treatment or who develop signs suggesting left-sided infection.

Endocarditis caused by methicillin-resistant staphylococci requires treatment with vancomycin (see Table 47–10). Trimethoprim-sulfamethoxazole treatment of right-sided endocarditis caused by *S. aureus* susceptible to this antimicrobial has been only moderately successful.[119] Truly suitable alternatives to vancomycin are not available. Teicoplanin, a glycopeptide antibiotic similar to vancomycin but not available in the United States, has been considered a possible alternative; however, some strains of *S. aureus* have become resistant to teicoplanin.[120] If the methicillin-resistant strain is susceptible to gentamicin, the aminoglycoside can be used in combination with vancomycin to enhance activity against these organisms. However, the frequency of renal toxicity may also be increased by this combination. The addition of rifampin to vancomycin for treatment of methicillin-resistant *S. aureus* NVE has not been beneficial. Right-sided endocarditis caused by methicillin-resistant *S. aureus* is not treated with a 2-week regimen.

STAPHYLOCOCCAL PROSTHETIC VALVE ENDOCARDITIS. Staphylococcal infections of prosthetic heart valves should be treated with two or preferably three antibiotics in combination. Rifampin provides unique antistaphylococcal activity when infection involves foreign bodies.[117] However, rifampin-resistant staphylococci rapidly emerge when rifampin is used alone or in combination with vancomycin to treat staphylococcal PVE.[28] Consequently, staphylococcal PVE is treated with two antimicrobials plus rifampin.[28] I prefer to delay rifampin therapy briefly until treatment with two effective antistaphylococcal agents is begun.

For PVE caused by methicillin-resistant staphylococci, treatment is initiated with vancomycin plus gentamicin, with rifampin added if the organism is susceptible to gentamicin. If the organism is resistant to gentamicin, an alternative aminoglycoside to which the organism is susceptible should be sought. Alternatively, for treatment of PVE caused by an organism resistant to all aminoglycosides, a quinolone to which it is susceptible may be used in lieu of an aminoglycoside.[28] For treatment of PVE caused by methicillin-susceptible staphylococci, a semisynthetic penicillinase-resistant penicillin should be substituted for vancomycin in the combination regimen (Table 47–11).

Patients with a nonimmediate penicillin allergy can be treated with a first-generation cephalosporin in lieu of the semisynthetic penicillin. PVE caused by coagulase-negative staphylococci that occurs within the initial year after valve placement is often complicated by perivalvular extension of infection, and valve replacement surgery is often required to eradicate infection and maintain suitable valve function.[28] Patients with *S. aureus* PVE have frequent intracardiac complications and exceptionally high mortality rates. Cure of *S. aureus* PVE is significantly more likely if early surgical intervention is combined with appropriate combination antimicrobial therapy.[121, 122]

HAEMOPHILUS PARAINFLUENZAE, HAEMOPHILUS APHROPHILUS, ACTINOBACILLUS ACTINOMYCETEMCOMITANS, CARDIOBACTERIUM HOMINIS, EIKENELLA CORRODENS, AND KINGELLA KINGAE (HACEK ORGANISMS). Endocarditis caused by the HACEK group has in the past been treated with ampicillin administered alone or in combination with gentamicin. Occasional HACEK organisms that are ampicillin resistant by virtue of beta-lactamase production have been isolated. Given the marked susceptibility of both beta-lactamase–producing and non-beta-lactamase–producing HACEK strains to third-generation cephalosporins, ceftriaxone or a comparable third-generation cephalosporin is recommended for treatment of NVE or PVE caused by these organisms (Table 47–12).[113] For endocarditis caused by strains that do not produce beta-lactamase, ampicillin combined with gentamicin can be used in lieu of ceftriaxone (see Table 47–12).

OTHER PATHOGENS. Antimicrobial therapy for patients with IE caused by unusual organisms is based on limited clinical experience

and data from animal models and in vitro studies. Therapeutic regimens for most of these infections are beyond the scope of this chapter: in fact, physicians are urged to review the published experience with a specific causative agent as well as to seek assistance from experienced infectious disease consultants when treating these infections. Among the more common of the unusual agents causing endocarditis are *P. aeruginosa*, *Candida* species, and *Corynebacterium* species. The preferred treatment for endocarditis caused by *P. aeruginosa* is an antipseudomonal penicillin (ticarcillin or piperacillin) plus high doses of tobramycin (8 mg/kg/d IM or IV in divided doses every 8 hours to achieve peak serum concentrations of 15 μg/ml). Endocarditis caused by *P. aeruginosa* is often both destructive and poorly responsive to antibiotic therapy. As a result, many patients with *P. aeruginosa* endocarditis require cardiac surgery.

Amphotericin at full doses, often combined with 5-fluorocytosine, is recommended for treatment of *Candida* endocarditis. Several patients with *Candida* NVE and PVE without intracardiac complications are reported to have been cured by prolonged treatment with fluconazole.[123, 124] Nevertheless, surgical intervention shortly after beginning amphotericin treatment remains the standard treatment for *Candida* endocarditis.[125, 126] Prolonged or indefinite finuconazole administration has been advocated for patients treated either medically or surgically [124–126]

▼ **TABLE 47–11. TREATMENT OF STAPHYLOCOCCAL ENDOCARDITIS IN THE PRESENCE OF A PROSTHETIC VALVE OR OTHER PROSTHETIC MATERIAL**

ANTIBIOTIC	DOSAGE AND ROUTE*	DURATION (WK)
Regimen for Methicillin-Resistant Staphylococci		
Vancomycin	30 mg/kg/24 hr IV in two equally divided doses,	≥6
plus	not to exceed 2 gm/24 hr unless serum levels are monitored	
Rifampin *and*	300 mg PO every 8 hr	≥6
gentamicin†	1.0 mg/kg IM or IV every 8 hr	2
Regimen for Methicillin-Susceptible Staphylococci		
Nafcillin or oxacillin	2 gm IV every 4 hr	≥6
plus		
Rifampin *and*	300 mg PO every 8 hr	≥6
gentamicin†	1.0 mg/kg IM or IV every 8 hr	2

*Dosages are for patients with normal renal function. See Table 47–6, footnote.

†Use during initial 2 wk of treatment. If strain is gentamicin resistant, see text for alternatives.

Modified from Wilson WR, Karchmer AW, Dajani AS, et al: Antibiotic treatment of adults with infective endocarditis due to streptococci, enterococci, staphylococci, and HACEK microorganisms. JAMA 274:1706, 1995. Copyright 1995 American Medical Association.

▼ **TABLE 47–12. TREATMENT FOR ENDOCARDITIS DUE TO HACEK MICROORGANISMS***

ANTIBIOTIC	DOSAGE AND ROUTE†	DURATION (WK)
Ceftriaxone‡	2 gm once daily IV or IM	4
Ampicillin	12 gm/24 hr IV given continuously or every 4 hr in six equally divided doses	4
plus		
Gentamicin	1 mg/kg IM or IV every 8 hr	4

*HACEK microorganisms are *Haemophilus parainfluenzae*, *Haemophilus aphrophilus*, *Actinobacillus actinomycetemcomitans*, *Cardiobacterium hominis*, *Eikenella corrodens*, and *Kingella kingae*.

†Dosages are for those with normal renal function. See Table 47–6, footnote.

‡Cefotaxime or ceftizoxime in comparable doses may be substituted for ceftriaxone.

Modified from Wilson WR, Karchmer AW, Dajani AS, et al: Antibiotic treatment of adults with infective endocarditis due to streptococci, enterococci, staphylococci, and HACEK microorganisms. JAMA 274:1706, 1995. Copyright 1995 American Medical Association.

The antimicrobial susceptibility of corynebacteria causing endocarditis must be carefully evaluated. Many remain susceptible to penicillin, vancomycin, and aminoglycosides. Strains susceptible to aminoglycosides are killed synergistically by penicillin in combination with an aminoglycoside. *C. jelkeium*, although often resistant to penicillin and aminoglycosides, is killed by vancomycin. NVE or PVE caused by *Corynebacterium* species can be treated with the combination of penicillin plus an aminoglycoside or vancomycin, contingent on the susceptibilities of the causative strain.[55]

The Enterobacteriaceae (*E. coli* and *Klebsiella*, *Enterobacter*, *Serratia*, and *Proteus* species) are highly susceptible to third-generation cephaloporins, imipenem, and aztreonam. One of these antimicrobial agents in high doses is combined with an aminoglycoside to treat IE caused by Enterobacteriaceae.

Coxiella burnetii IE is difficult to eradicate. Prolonged therapy (at least 4 years) using doxycycline (100 mg twice daily) or another tetracycline combined with a quinolone has been advocated. Treatment with doxycycline combined with hydroxychloroquine for 18 to 48 months (mean 31 months, median 26 months) may be as effective as longer courses of doxycycline plus a quinolone.[127] Surgery is important in effective treatment.

CULTURE-NEGATIVE ENDOCARDITIS. Special studies to diagnose IE caused by fastidious bacteria and other organisms must be performed (see Diagnosis). Thereafter, unless clinical or epidemiologic clues suggest an etiological diagnosis, the recommended treatment for culture-negative NVE is ampicillin plus gentamicin (see standard regimen for enterococcal endocarditis, Table 47–8); because in the absence of confounding antibiotic therapy enterococci and staphyclococci are unlikely causes of culture-negative NVE, ceftriaxone could be used in this regimen instead of ampicillin. For patients with culture-negative PVE, vancomycin is added to this regimen.[28, 128] Mortality rates are lower for patients who have culture-negative endocarditis and who received antibiotics before obtaining blood cultures and those who become afebrile during the initial week of antimicrobial treatment.[96, 128] Marantic endocarditis should be carefully considered when treating patients for culture-negative IE. Surgical intervention should be considered for those who do not fully respond to empirical antimicrobial therapy. If surgical intervention is undertaken, a detailed microbiological and pathological examination of excised material must be performed to establish an etiologic diagnosis.

TIMING THE INITIATION OF ANTIMICROBIAL THERAPY. Current cost-containment pressures frequently result in initiation of antimicrobial therapy for suspected endocarditis immediately after blood cultures have been obtained. This practice is appropriate in the treatment of patients with acute IE that is highly destructive and rapidly progressive and of patients presenting with hemodynamic decompensation requiring urgent or emergent surgical intervention. Immediate therapy may have a favorable impact on outcome in these patients. In contrast, precipitous initiation of therapy in hemodynamically stable patients with suspected subacute endocarditis does not prevent early complications and may, by compromising subsequent blood cultures, obscure the etiological diagnosis of endocarditis. In these latter patients, it is prudent to delay antibiotic therapy briefly pending the results of the initial blood cultures. If these cultures are not positive promptly, this delay provides an important opportunity to obtain additional blood cultures without the confounding effect of empirical treatment. This opportunity is particularly important when patients have received antibiotics recently.

MONITORING THERAPY FOR ENDOCARDITIS. Patients must be carefully monitored during therapy and for several months thereafter. Failure of antimicrobial therapy, myocardial or metastatic abscess, emboli, hypersensitivity to antimicrobial agents, and other complications of therapy (catheter-related infection, thrombophlebitis) or intercurrent illness may be manifested by persistent or recurrent fever. Adverse reactions occur in 33 percent of patients treated for IE with beta-lactam antimicrobials, especially penicillin and ampicillin. The reactions include fever, rash, and neutropenia;

they are increasingly frequent after 15 days of therapy.[129] Clinical events may indicate a need for potentially life-saving revision of antimicrobial therapy or adjunctive surgical therapy.

The serum bactericidal titer (SBT), the highest dilution of the patient's serum during therapy that in vitro kills 99.9 percent of a standard inoculum of the patient's infecting organism, has been used to assess the adequacy of antimicrobial therapy. The SBT has correlated poorly with outcome of therapy because it has been performed in a non-standardized manner and because of the marked impact of complications on outcome. Peak and trough titers of at least 1:64 or 1:32 and 1:32, respectively, obtained with a standardized SBT method, correlate with bacteriological cure. When using regimens considered optimal on the basis of clinical experience, monitoring therapy with this test is not recommended.[113] The SBT may be useful when treating patients with endocarditis caused by organisms for which optimal therapy is not established or when using unconventional antimicrobial regimens.

The serum concentration of vancomycin or aminoglycosides should be measured periodically. This allows dose adjustment to ensure optimal therapy and avoid adverse events. Additionally, renal function should be monitored in patients receiving these two antimicrobials, and the complete blood count should be checked at least weekly in patients receiving high-dose beta-lactam antibiotics or vancomycin.

Repeat blood cultures should be obtained during the initial days of therapy or if fever persists to determine if the bacteremia has been controlled. In patients with recrudescent fever after treatment, prompt cultures are essential to assess possible relapse of endocarditis.

OUTPATIENT ANTIMICROBIAL THERAPY. Technical advances allowing safe administration of complex antimicrobial regimens, combined with well-developed home care systems that provide supplies and monitor outpatient treatment, make it feasible to treat patients with endocarditis on an outpatient basis. Doing so can significantly reduce the cost of therapy. However, only those patients who have responded to initial therapy and are free of fever, who are not experiencing threatening complications, who will be compliant with therapy, and who have a home situation that is physically suitable should be considered for outpatient treatment. Furthermore, patients being treated at home must be apprised of the potential complications of endocarditis, instructed to seek advice promptly when encountering unexpected or untoward clinical events, and have assiduous clinical and laboratory monitoring. Finally, outpatient therapy must not result in compromises of antimicrobial therapy leading to suboptimal treatment.

Surgical Treatment of Intracardiac Complications

Cardiac surgical intervention has an increasingly important role in the treatment of intracardiac complications of endocarditis. Retrospective data suggest that mortality is unacceptably high when these complications are treated with antibiotics alone, whereas mortality is reduced when treatment combines antibiotics and surgical intervention.[76, 130, 131] Accordingly, these complications have become indications for cardiac surgery (Table 47–13).

VALVULAR DYSFUNCTION. Medical therapy of NVE that is complicated by moderate to severe (New York Heart Association Class III and IV) CHF due to new or worsening valvular dysfunction results in mortality rates of 50 to 90 percent. Survival rates for a similar group of patients treated with antibiotics and cardiac surgery are 60 to 80 percent.[76, 130, 131] Although survival rates among surgically treated patients with PVE complicated by valvular dysfunction and CHF are 45 to 85 percent, few PVE patients with these complications are alive at 6 months when treated with antibiotics alone.[28, 29] Worsening aortic valve incompetence is associated with more severe and more rapidly progressive CHF than is mitral valve incompetence. Hence, patients with aortic valve endocarditis not only account for

▼ TABLE 47–13. CARDIAC SURGERY IN PATIENTS WITH INFECTIVE ENDOCARDITIS

Indications
Moderate to severe congestive heart failure due to valve dysfunction
Unstable prosthesis
Uncontrolled infection despite optimal antimicrobial therapy
Unavailable effective antimicrobial therapy: endocarditis due to fungi, *Brucellae, Pseudomonas aeruginosa* (aortic or mitral valves)
Staphylococcus aureus PVE with an intracardiac complication
Relapse of PVE after optimal therapy

Relative Indications*
Perivalvular extension of infection, intracardiac fistula
Poorly responsive *S. aureus* NVE (aortic or mitral valves)
Relapse of NVE after optimal antimicrobial therapy
Culture-negative NVE or PVE with persistent fever (≥10 d)
Large (>10 mm diameter) hypermobile vegetation (with or without prior arterial embolus)
Endocarditis due to highly antibiotic-resistant enterococci

PVE = prosthetic valve endocarditis; NVE = native valve endocarditis.

*Surgery commonly required for optimal outcome.

the majority of surgically treated patients but also require surgery on a more urgent basis when heart failure supervenes. Severe mitral valve insufficiency, nevertheless, results in inexorable heart failure and ultimately requires surgical intervention. Doppler echocardiography and color flow mapping indicating significant valvular regurgitation during the initial week of endocarditis treatment do not reliably predict those patients who will require valve replacement during active endocarditis. Alternatively, despite the absence of significant valvular regurgitation on early echocardiography, marked CHF may still develop. Decisions about surgical intervention should not be made solely on the basis of echocardiographic findings but rather by integrating clinical data during careful serial monitoring. On occasion, very large vegetations on the mitral valve, particularly a mitral valve prosthesis, result in significant obstruction and require surgery.[28]

UNSTABLE PROSTHESES. Dehiscence of an infected prosthetic valve is a manifestation of perivalvular infection and often results in hemodynamically significant valvular dysfunction. Surgical intervention is recommended for PVE patients with these complications.[28, 130] The risk of invasive infection is increased among patients with onset of PVE within the year after valve implantation and those with infection of an aortic valve prosthesis. Endocarditis in these patients is often caused by invasive antimicrobial-resistant organisms; consequently, the benefit of combined medical-surgical therapy is enhanced further. Patients who appear clinically stable but who have overtly unstable and hypermobile prostheses, a finding indicative of dehiscence in excess of 40 percent of the circumference, are likely to experience progressive valve instability and warrant surgical treatment. Occasional patients with PVE caused by noninvasive, highly antibiotic-susceptible organisms, e.g., streptococci, despite a favorable clinical course during antibiotic therapy, late in treatment experience minor valve dehiscence without prosthesis instability or hemodynamic deterioration. Surgical treatment of these patients can be deferred unless clear indications arise.

UNCONTROLLED INFECTION OR UNAVAILABLE EFFECTIVE ANTIMICROBIAL THERAPY. Surgical intervention has improved the outcome of several forms of endocarditis when maximal antibiotic therapy fails to eradicate infection or, in some instances, even to suppress bacteremia. Amphotericin B is inadequate therapy for fungal endocarditis, in-

cluding that caused by *Candida* species, and surgical intervention is recommended shortly after initiation of full doses of antifungal therapy. Endocarditis caused by some gram-negative bacilli, e.g., *P. aeruginosa, Achromobacter xylosoxidans,* may not be eradicated by maximum tolerable antibiotic therapy and may require surgical excision of the infected tissue to achieve cure. Similarly, standard therapy of endocarditis caused by *Brucella* species includes surgery because medical therapy is rarely successful.[94] Surgical intervention is recommended when patients with enterococcal endocarditis caused by a strain resistant to synergistic bactericidal therapy do not respond to initial therapy or relapse. Perivalvular invasive infection is in some instances a form of ineradicable infection. Relapse of PVE after optimal antimicrobial therapy reflects invasive disease or the difficulty in eradicating infection involving foreign devices. Patients with relapse of PVE are treated surgically.[28] In contrast, patients with NVE that relapses, unless it is associated with a highly resistant microorganism or demonstrable perivalvular infection, often are treated again with an intensified, prolonged course of antimicrobial therapy.[132]

S. AUREUS PROSTHETIC VALVE ENDOCARDITIS. Among 129 patients who had *S. aureus* PVE and who were culled from large retrospective general series of PVE, the crude mortality rate for those treated with antibiotics alone and with antibiotics plus surgery was 73 and 25 percent, respectively.[51, 122, 133, 134] The overall mortality rate in 33 cases of *S. aureus* PVE treated at a single institution was 42 percent.[122] In these latter cases, when a multivariate model was used for analysis to adjust for confounding variables, the presence of intracardiac complications was associated with a 13.7-fold increased risk of death, and surgical intervention during active disease was accompanied by a 20-fold reduction in mortality. These data suggest that surgical treatment can improve outcome. Although the occurrence of central nervous system emboli is often considered to limit the opportunity for surgical intervention, in fact, appropriately timed surgery remains the preferred treatment. Thus, surgical intervention is recommended for *S. aureus* PVE with intracardiac complication and may benefit even those patients with uncomplicated *S. aureus* PVE.[122, 133]

PERIVALVULAR INVASIVE INFECTION. NVE at the aortic site and PVE are most commonly associated with perivalvular invasion with abscess or intracardiac fistula formation.[28] Invasive infection occurs in 10 to 14 percent of patients with NVE and 45 to 60 percent of those with PVE.[28] Persistent, otherwise unexplained fever despite appropriate antimicrobial therapy or pericarditis in patients with aortic valve endocarditis suggests infection extending beyond the valve leaflet.[78] New-onset and persistent electrocardiographic conduction abnormalities, although not a sensitive indicator of perivalvular infection (28 percent), are relatively specific (85 to 90 percent).[135] TEE is superior to TTE for detecting invasive infection in patients with NVE and PVE. Doppler and color flow Doppler or contrast two-dimensional echocardiography optimally define fistulas. Patients who have IE and in whom an abscess is suspected but not detected by an initial and repeat TEE should undergo magnetic resonance imaging, including magnetic resonance angiography. Cardiac catheterization adds little to these imaging studies and is not recommended unless coronary angiography is needed.

In patients with endocarditis complicated by perivalvular extension of infection, cardiac surgery should be considered to debride invasive infection, ablate abscesses, and reconstruct anatomical damage. Surgery is warranted in patients with invasive disease that significantly disrupts cardiac structures, that is associated with CHF, that results in instability of a prosthetic valve, or that renders infection uncontrolled (persistent fever). However, it is likely that increasingly sensitive imaging techniques will elucidate invasive infections that do not require immediate surgery. Sporadic case reports of medically treated invasive infection suggest that these infections will be small, structurally nonsignificant abscesses in which the cavity is open to the circulatory stream.

LEFT-SIDED *S. AUREUS* ENDOCARDITIS. Because this infection is difficult to control, highly destructive, and associated with high mortality, some investigators have suggested that these patients should be considered for surgical treatment when the response to antimicrobial therapy is not prompt and complete. Additionally, patients with *S. aureus* NVE (aortic or mitral valve) and vegetations that are visible by TTE are at increased risk for arterial emboli and death and should be considered for surgery.[52] In contrast, IV drug abusers with *S. aureus* endocarditis limited to the tricuspid or pulmonary valves often experience prolonged fever during antimicrobial therapy; nevertheless, the vast majority of these patients respond to antimicrobial therapy and do not require surgery.[136]

UNRESPONSIVE CULTURE-NEGATIVE ENDOCARDITIS. Patients who have culture-negative endocarditis and who experience unexplained persistent fever during empirical antimicrobial therapy, particularly those with PVE, should be considered for surgical intervention. If endocarditis is not marantic, persistent fever in these patients is likely to represent either unrecognized perivalvular infection or ineffective antimicrobial therapy.

LARGE VEGETATIONS (>10 mm) AND THE PREVENTION OF SYSTEMIC EMBOLI. Systemic embolization was increased in patients with vegetations greater than 10 mm versus those with smaller or no detectable vegetations, 33 percent versus 19 percent.[82] Larger mitral valve vegetations (>10 mm), particularly those on the anterior mitral valve leaflet, are uniquely associated with systemic emboli. Although a relationship may exist between vegetation characteristics—including size, mobility, and extent (number of leaflets involved)—and embolic complications, the implications for surgical intervention are not clear. Yet to be performed are multivariate analyses examining the relationship between outcome or the need for surgical intervention and variables including not only vegetation characteristics but also valve dysfunction, perivalvular invasion by infection, organism, and infection site. Nevertheless, some researchers have concluded that vegetation characteristics alone might warrant surgery to prevent arterial emboli. This recommendation can be questioned, as can the recommendation for valve surgery after two major arterial emboli.[94]

In deciding to intervene in the therapy of IE with cardiac surgery to prevent arterial emboli, many factors must be considered carefully. The rate of systemic or cerebral emboli in patients with NVE and PVE decreases during the course of effective antibiotic therapy.[87, 137] Additionally, it is not clear that surgical intervention reduces the frequency of systemic emboli.[76, 130] Finally, the risks of morbidity and mortality caused by cerebral and coronary emboli, the major events to be prevented, must be compared with the immediate and long-term risks of valve replacement surgery. The latter include perioperative mortality, recrudescent endocarditis on the prosthesis, thromboembolic complications, early and late valve dysfunction requiring repeat valve replacement, the hazards of warfarin anticoagulation (including its contraindication during pregnancy), and the risk and morbidity of late-onset PVE.[128] Vegetation size alone is rarely an indication for surgery. The clinical findings and echocardiographic evidence for other intracardiac complications must be weighed against the immediate and remote hazards of cardiac surgery, including the possibility of valve preservation by vegetectomy and valve repair, when recommending therapy.[82, 94] Thus, the risk for systemic embolization as related to vegetation size or prior systemic embolus is not an independent indication for sur-

gical intervention but is only one of many factors to be considered when planning treatment.[87, 94, 137]

TECHNIQUES FOR REPAIR OF INTRACARDIAC DEFECTS. New surgical techniques to address severe tissue destruction in NVE and PVE have been developed. Although these are beyond the scope of this discussion, examples include valve composite graft replacement of the aortic root, use of sewing skirts attached to the prostheses, and homograft replacement of the aortic valve and root with coronary artery reimplantation.[138, 139] Furthermore, repair of the mitral valve in patients with acute or healed endocarditis avoids the need for insertion of prosthetic materials and the associated hazards.[140] Although tricuspid valvulectomy without valve replacement has been advocated for treatment of uncontrolled tricuspid valve infection in IV drug abusers at high risk of recidivism and recurrent endocarditis, the likelihood of refractory right-heart failure with time after valvulectomy makes tricuspid valve repair preferable. Cardiac transplantation has been used to salvage an occasional patient with refractory endocarditis.

TIMING OF SURGICAL INTERVENTION. When endocarditis is complicated by valvular regurgitation and significant impairment of cardiac function, surgical intervention before the development of severe intractable hemodynamic dysfunction is recommended, regardless of the duration of antimicrobial therapy.[130, 141] Postoperative mortality correlates with the severity of preoperative hemodynamic dysfunction; consequently, this approach is justified.[94] In patients who have valvular dysfunction and in whom infection is controlled and cardiac function is compensated, surgery may be delayed until antimicrobial therapy has been completed. However, if infection is not controlled, surgery should be performed promptly. Similarly, if a patient who requires valve replacement in the near future has a large vegetation, indicating a high risk for systemic embolization, early cardiac surgery is appropriate.

To avoid worsening of neurological status or death in patients who have sustained recent neurological injury, the timing of surgical intervention may require modification. Among patients who have had a nonhemorrhagic embolic stroke, exacerbation of cerebral dysfunction occurs during cardiac surgery in 44 percent of cases when the interval between the stroke and surgery is 7 days or less, in 17 percent when the interval is 8 to 14 days, and in 10 percent or less when more than 2 weeks has elapsed. After hemorrhagic intracerebral events, the risk for neurological worsening or death with cardiac surgery persists at 20 percent even after 1 month.[142]

Thus, when the response of IE to antimicrobial therapy and hemodynamic status permit, delaying cardiac surgery for 2 to 3 weeks after a significant embolic infarct and at least a month after intracerebral hemorrhage (with prior repair of a mycotic aneurysm) has been recommended.[142, 143] In another study of patients with nonhemorrhagic focal cerebral lesions or encephalopathy, those undergoing cardiac surgery without delay experienced no greater mortality or neurological deterioration than did those treated medically. This study suggests that the improved outcomes reported with delayed surgery may simply reflect selection of hardier patients and that more prompt cardiac surgery in patients with nonhemorrhagic cerebral complications, if required, is reasonable and potentially beneficial.[144] Contrast-enhanced cerebral tomography is recommended as the initial study of choice to detect intracerebral hemorrhage with subsequent magnetic resonance angiography or standard cerebral angiography to further evaluate hemorrhagic lesions for a leaking mycotic aneurysm.[143, 145] It is prudent to evaluate the cerebral vasculature in patients who have sustained an embolic infarct or who have persistent headaches before cardiac surgery. If a mycotic aneurysm is found, the timing of cardiac surgery should be reconsidered and prostheses that require postoperative anticoagulant therapy should be avoided.[94]

DURATION OF ANTIMICROBIAL THERAPY AFTER SURGICAL INTERVENTION. Inflammatory changes and bacteria are commonly found in vegetations removed from patients who have received most or all of the standard antibiotic therapy recommended for endocarditis caused by the specific microorganism. If valve cultures are negative, this does not indicate that antimicrobial therapy has failed or that a full course of antibiotic therapy is needed postoperatively. The duration of antimicrobial therapy after surgery depends on the length of preoperative therapy, the antibiotic susceptibility of the causative organism, the presence of paravalvular invasive infection, and the culture status of the vegetation. In general, for endocarditis caused by relatively antibiotic-resistant organisms with negative cultures of operative specimens, preoperative plus postoperative therapy should at least equal a full course of recommended therapy; for those patients with positive intraoperative cultures, a full course of therapy should be given postoperatively. Patients with PVE should receive a full course of antimicrobial therapy postoperatively when organisms are seen in resected material.[28]

Treatment of Extracardiac Complications

SPLENIC ABSCESS. Three to 5 percent of patients with IE develop a splenic abscess.[80] Although splenic defects can be identified by ultrasonography and computed tomography, these tests usually cannot discriminate between abscess and infarct. Persistent fever and progressive enlargement of the lesion during antimicrobial therapy suggest that it is an abscess; this can be confirmed by percutaneous needle aspiration. Successful therapy of splenic abscesses generally requires drainage, which can often be accomplished by percutaneous placement of a catheter.[84] In patients with endocarditis complicated by numerous splenic abscesses or in whom percutaneous drainage is unsuccessful, splenectomy is required.[84, 94] Splenic abscesses should be effectively treated before valve replacement surgery. If they are not effectively treated before cardiac surgery, splenectomy should be performed as soon thereafter as surgical risks permit.[94]

MYCOTIC ANEURYSMS AND SEPTIC ARTERITIS. From 2 to 10 percent of patients with endocarditis have mycotic aneurysms; in 1 to 5 percent, the aneurysms involve cerebral vessels.[88] Cerebral mycotic aneurysms occur at the branch points in cerebral vessels, are generally located distally over the cerebral cortex, and are found most commonly in branches of the middle cerebral artery. The aneurysms arise either from occlusion of vessels by septic emboli with secondary arteritis and vessel wall destruction or from bacteremic seeding of the vessel wall through the vasa vasorum. *S. aureus* is commonly implicated in the former and viridans streptococci in the latter.[91] Many patients with mycotic aneurysms or septic arteritis present with devastating intracranial hemorrhage. Focal deficits from embolic events, persistent focal headache, or sterile meningeal irritation (cerebrospinal fluid pleacytosis) may be premonitory symptoms. Cerebral angiography is required to evaluate patients with subarachnoid hemorrhage, and this or magnetic resonance angiography has been recommended for patients experiencing premonitory symptoms, especially if cardiac surgery or anticoagulant therapy is planned.[88, 94] Mycotic aneurysms may resolve during antimicrobial therapy[94]; however, when anatomically feasible, aneurysms that have ruptured should be repaired surgically. Aneurysms that have not leaked should be monitored angiographically during antimicrobial therapy. Surgery should be considered for a single lesion that enlarges during or after antimicrobial therapy. Anticoagulant therapy should be avoided in patients with a persisting mycotic aneurysm. Although persistent stable aneurysms may rupture after completion of standard antimicrobial therapy, there is no accurate estimation of risk for late rupture, and recommendations for surgical intervention are arbitrary. Nevertheless, prevailing opinion favors, whenever possible without serious neurological injury, the resection of single aneurysms that persist after therapy. The potential existence of occult aneurysms in patients without neurological symptoms or in those who have had a nondiagnostic angiographic evaluation is not considered a contraindication to anticoagulant therapy after completion of antimicrobial therapy.

Extracranial mycotic aneurysms should be managed as outlined for cerebral aneurysms. Those that leak, are expanding during therapy, or persist after therapy should be repaired. Particular attention should be given to aneurysms that involve intraabdominal arteries, rupture of which could result in life-threatening hemorrhage.[94]

ANTICOAGULANT THERAPY. Patients with PVE involving devices that would usually warrant maintenance anticoagulation are continued on anticoagulant therapy.[28] Prothrombin times should be maintained at 1.5 times the control (INR = 3.0). Anticoagulation is not initiated as prophylaxis against thromboembolism in patients with PVE involving devices that do not usually require this therapy. Among patients with NVE, no evidence shows that anticoagulant therapy prevents embolization, and in some instances it may contribute to intracranial hemorrhage, particularly in the presence of a recent cerebral infarct or a mycotic aneurysm.[88] Anticoagulant therapy in patients with NVE is limited to those patients for whom there is a clear indication for this therapy and for whom there is not a known increased risk for intracranial hemorrhage. If central nervous system complications occur in patients who have IE and who are receiving anticoagulant therapy, anticoagulation should be reversed immediately.[28]

Response to Therapy and Outcome

Within a week after initiation of effective antimicrobial therapy, almost 75 percent of patients with IE, including those with PVE, are afebrile and 90 percent have defervesced by the end of the second week of treatment.[47, 137, 28, 76, 146] The duration of fever during therapy is longer in patients with IE due to *S. aureus, P. aeruginosa,* and culture-negative IE as well as IE characterized by microvascular phenomena and major embolic complications.[76, 146] Persistence or recurrence of fever more than 7 to 10 days after initiation of antibiotic therapy identified patients with increased mortality rates and with complications of infection or therapy.[28, 78, 146] Those patients with prolonged or recurrent fever should be evaluated for intracardiac complications, focal extracardiac septic complications, intercurrent nosocomial infections, recurrent pulmonary emboli (patients with right-sided IE), drug-associated fever, additional underlying illnesses, and, if appropriate, in-hospital substance abuse.

Blood cultures should be repeated in search of persistent bacteremia or the presence of additional pathogens, e.g., previously unrecognized polymicrobial IE. The antimicrobial susceptibility of the causative organism should be reevaluated, as should the adequacy of antibiotic therapy. Drug reactions have accounted for fever in 17 to 28 percent of these patients.[78, 124] Drug fever attributed to the antimicrobial therapy itself may warrant revision of treatment if a suitable alternative is available. In the absence of effective alternative therapy, treatment can be continued despite drug fever if the antimicrobial is not causing significant end-organ toxicity. In 33 to 45 percent of patients, persistent fever was associated with significant intracardiac complications, many of which required surgical intervention.[76]

Many clinical and laboratory features of IE are slow to resolve despite effective antimicrobial therapy. Systemic emboli occur during the early weeks of treatment, although with decreasing frequency.[87] The increased ESR and anemia may not correct until after therapy has been completed.

Mortality rates for large series of NVE treated between 1975 and 1993 range from 16 to 27 percent.[1, 4, 5, 9, 134] Death due to IE has been associated with increased age (>65 to 70 years old), underlying diseases, infection involving the aortic valve, development of CHF, renal failure, and central nervous system complications.[1, 5] The treatment of heart failure due to valve dysfunction by early surgical intervention has decreased the mortality associated with CHF, but subsequently, neurological events and septic complications, e.g., uncontrolled infection and myocardial abscess, have accounted for a larger proportion of deaths and have been associated with high mortality rates.[80]

Mortality rates among patients with IE caused by viridans streptococci and *S. bovis* have ranged from 4 to 16 percent.[1, 4, 9] Higher mortality rates are reported with left-sided NVE caused by other organisms: enterococci, 15 to 25 percent[1, 4, 9]; *S. aureus,* 25 to 47 percent[1, 4, 9, 50, 73]; nonviridans streptococci (groups B, C, and G), 13 to 50 percent[42, 147]; *C. burnetti,* 5 to 37 percent[31, 114, 124]; *P. aeruginosa,* Enterobacteriaceae, and fungi, greater than 50 percent.[54, 61]

In a retrospective study of patients with NVE with either Class III or IV heart failure (New York Heart Association) or invasive uncontrolled infection, only 9 percent of patients treated surgically died, compared with 51 percent of those treated with antibiotics alone.[76] Mortality rates among patients who have NVE, particularly involving the aortic valve, and who were treated surgically have ranged from 5 to 26 percent, with rates toward the high end of this range reported more frequently.[148-150] Severity of heart failure, abscess, *S. aureus* infection, and decreased renal function (possibly related to heart failure) have been associated with increased postoperative mortality.[150] Nevertheless, survival rates of 85 percent can be achieved when patients with paravalvular abscesses undergo meticulous débridement and reconstructive cardiac surgery.[151]

Outcome for patients with PVE, as contrasted with NVE, has been less desirable. Before 1980, mortality rates among patients with onset less than 60 days after surgery and later-onset PVE averaged 70 and 45 percent, respectively. With the recognition that PVE was frequently complicated by invasive infection and that patients would benefit from surgical intervention, mortality rates have decreased to 33 to 45 percent, with lower rates in later-onset cases.[28, 151] Long-term survival was adversely affected by the presence of moderate or severe heart failure at discharge. Survival rates after aggressive surgery for PVE ranged from 75 to 85 percent and were not related to time of onset after cardiac surgery.[29, 139]

Among patients with NVE (nonaddicts) discharged after medical or medical-surgical therapy, long-term survival was 88 percent at 5 years and 81 percent at 10 years.[134] Among patients treated surgically for NVE, survival at 5 years ranged from 70 to 80 percent.[138, 149] Among patients with PVE treated surgically, survival rates at 4 to 6 years range from 50 to 82 percent.[29, 139]

RELAPSE AND RECURRENCE. Relapse of IE usually occurs within 2 months of discontinuing antibiotic treatment. Of patients who have NVE caused by penicillin-susceptible viridans streptococci and who receive a recommended course of therapy, less than 2 percent suffer relapse. From 8 to 20 percent of patients with enterococcal IE experience relapse after standard therapy.[132] Patients with IE caused by S. aureus, Enterobacteriaceae, or fungi are more likely to experience overt failure of therapy rather than relapse; nevertheless, 4 percent of patients with S. aureus IE suffer relapse.[132] Relapse of fungal endocarditis at long intervals after treatment has been reported. Relapse occurs in 10 percent of patients with PVE overall and in 6 to 15 percent of those treated surgically.[131]

Among nonaddicts with an initial episode of NVE or PVE, 4.5 to 7 percent experience one or more additional episodes.[132, 134] Among these patients, recurrent IE shares the clinical, microbiological, and response to therapy noted

in primary episodes of IE. IV drug abuse is now the most common predisposition for recurrent IE (43 percent of patients).

PREVENTION

During bacteremia provoked by daily activities, infections, or health care procedures, bacteria adhere to and colonize the platelet fibrin aggregates, NBTE, that have formed on the valve endothelium as a consequence of preexisting congenital or acquired cardiac disease. If the adherence and the subsequent multiplication of bacteria at this site exceed the capacity of host defenses for bacterial eradication, IE results. Although many bacteria enter the bloodstream, those uniquely suited to adhere to NBTE cause the majority of cases of endocarditis. These organisms and the cardiac abnormalities vulnerable to IE are evident from reported cases. Events that predispose to bacteremia by organisms causing endocarditis have been identified. By identifying the patients at risk, the causative bacteria, and the events that induce bacteremia, strategies for prevention of some episodes of IE have been formulated and are routinely recommended even in the absence of supporting clinical trials.[152–154]

Viridans streptococci, the most common cause of NVE and late-onset PVE, are the primary target for prophylaxis used in conjunction with procedures involving the oral cavity, respiratory tract, or esophagus. Procedures involving the genitourinary and gastrointestinal tracts commonly precede the development of enterococcal endocarditis. Accordingly, the prophylaxis for endocarditis used in conjunction with procedures involving these mucosal surfaces is targeted against enterococci. When incision and drainage of infected skin or soft tissue infections are undertaken, prophylaxis is focused on S. aureus.

Procedures for which IE prophylaxis is recommended or not recommended have been identified by the American Heart Association and others (Table 47–14).[152–155] Although prophylaxis is advised for all at-risk patients who undergo dental procedures that cause gingival bleeding, extractions

▼ TABLE 47–14. PROCEDURES FOR WHICH PROPHYLAXIS AGAINST ENDOCARDITIS IS CONSIDERED

PROPHYLAXIS RECOMMENDED	PROPHYLAXIS NOT RECOMMENDED
Dental procedures known to induce gingival or mucosal bleeding, including professional cleaning and scaling Tonsillectomy or adenoidectomy Surgery involving gastrointestinal or upper respiratory mucosa Bronchoscopy with rigid bronchoscope Sclerotherapy for esophageal varices Esophageal dilation Endoscopic retrograde cholangiography with biliary obstruction Gallbladder surgery Cytoscopy, urethral dilation Urethral catheterization if urinary infection is present Urinary tract surgery, including prostate surgery Incision and drainage of infected tissue*	Dental procedures not likely to cause bleeding, such as adjustment of orthodontic appliances and simple fillings above the gum line Intraoral injection or local anesthetic (nonintraligamentary) Shedding of primary teeth Tympanostomy tube insertion Endotracheal tube insertion Bronchoscopy with flexible bronchoscope, with or without biopsy† Transesophageal echocardiography Cardiac catheterization, coronary angioplasty Pacemaker implantation Gastrointestinal endoscopy, with or without biopsy† Incision or biopsy of scrubbed skin Cesarean section Vaginal hysterectomy† Circumcision In the absence of infection: urethral catheterization, dilatation and curettage, uncomplicated vaginal delivery, therapeutic abortion, insertion or removal of intrauterine device, sterilization procedures, laparoscopy†

*Antibiotic prophylaxis should be directed against the most likely endocarditis-associated pathogen(s), often staphylococci.
†In patients at highest risk, physicians may elect to use prophylaxis for these procedures.
Adapted from Dajani AS, Taubert KA, Wilson W, et al: Prevention of bacterial endocarditis: Recommendations of the American Heart Association from the Committee on Rheumatic Fever, Endocarditis, and Kawasaki Disease, Council on Cardiovascular Disease in the Young. JAMA 277:1794, 1997; and from Durack DT: Prevention of endocarditis. N Engl J Med 332:38, 1995.

▼ TABLE 47–15. RELATIVE RISK OF INFECTIVE ENDOCARDITIS ASSOCIATED WITH PREEXISTING CARDIAC DISORDERS

RELATIVELY HIGH RISK	INTERMEDIATE RISK	VERY LOW OR NEGLIGIBLE RISK*
Prosthetic heart valves†	Mitral valve prolapse with regurgitation (murmur) or thickened valve leaflets	Mitral valve prolapse without regurgitation (murmur) or thickened valve leaflets
Previous infective endocarditis†	Pure mitral stenosis	Trivial valvular regurgitation on echocardiography without structural abnormality
Cyanotic congenital heart disease†	Tricuspid valve disease	
Patent ductus arteriosus	Pulmonary stenosis	
Aortic regurgitation	Asymmetrical septal hypertrophy	Isolated atrial septal defect (secundum)
Aortic stenosis	Bicuspid aortic valve or calcific aortic sclerosis with minimal hemodynamic abnormality	Arteriosclerotic plaques
Mitral regurgitation		Coronary artery disease
Mitral stenosis and regurgitation		Cardiac pacemaker, implanted defibrillators
Ventricular septal defect	Degenerative valvular disease in elderly patients	Surgically repaired intracardiac lesions, with minimal or no hemodynamic abnormality, more than 6 mo after operation (atrial septal defect, ventricular septal defect, patent ductus arteriosus, pulmonary stenosis)
Coarctation of the aorta	Surgically repaired intracardiac lesions with minimal or no hemodynamic abnormality, less than 6 mo after operation	
Surgically repaired intracardiac lesion with residual hemodynamic abnormality or prosthetic device		
Surgically constructed systemic-pulmonary shunts†		Prior coronary bypass graft surgery
		Prior Kawasaki's disease or rheumatic fever without valvular dysfunction

*Prophylaxis against endocarditis not recommended.
†Lesions considered at highest risk for endocarditis.
Adapted from Durack DT: Prevention of infective endocarditis. N Engl J Med 332:38, 1995; and Dajani AS, Taubert KA, Wilson W, et al: Prevention of bacterial endocarditis: Recommendations of the American Heart Association from the Committee on Rheumatic Fever, Endocarditis, and Kawasaki Disease, Council on Cardiovascular Disease in the Young. JAMA 277:1794, 1997. Copyright 1997 American Medical Association.

are the most strongly associated with subsequent IE.[154] Because endocarditis has been reported only rarely in association with other gastrointestinal endoscopic procedures with or without biopsy, prophylaxis is not routinely recommended in this situation. Prophylaxis is not recommended with routine cardiac catheterization or TEE.[152, 155]

Based on the frequency of a lesion among patients with endocarditis compared with the general population, lesions have been assigned to high, intermediate, low, and negligible risk categories (Table 47–15).[7, 13, 155–157, 157a] Rheumatic heart disease currently is a less common predisposition for IE in most of the developed countries; however, the attack rate of IE among persons with rheumatic valvular disease approaches that with prosthetic valves and suggests that these lesions entail a high risk also.[158]

The risk of IE for patients with mitral valve prolapse and the resulting role of prophylaxis among these patients have been controversial. Mitral valve prolapse has been identified frequently among patients with IE. However, the risk of endocarditis among patients with mitral valve prolapse and a murmur of mitral regurgitation is still relatively low. It is 5- to 10-fold higher than that in the general population but 100-fold less than that among patients with rheumatic valvular heart disease.[158] As a result, mitral valve prolapse with a murmur of mitral regurgitation or mitral valve thickening and prolapse defines a patient with an intermediate risk for IE and one for whom prophylaxis against endocarditis is recommended.

GENERAL METHODS. The incidence of IE can be significantly reduced by total surgical correction of some congenital lesions that otherwise predispose patients to IE, e.g., patent ductus arteriosus, ventricular septal defect, and pulmonary stenosis.[7, 157] The incidence of IE remains high among patients who have undergone surgical correction of other major congenital defects, especially those involving a stenotic aortic valve.[7] Patients with persisting as well as many corrected congenital lesions and those with acquired valvular heart disease who remain at risk for IE should be given written material about their predisposing lesion, their risk for endocarditis, and the recommended antibiotic prophylaxis.

Maintenance of attentive oral hygiene which decreases the frequency of bacteremia that accompanies daily activities (chewing, brushing teeth), may be a more important preventive than procedure-focused chemoprophylaxis.[156] Oral hygiene should be addressed before prosthetic valves are placed electively.

Among patients at risk for IE, some activities or procedures likely to induce bacteremia should be avoided. Oral irrigating devices, which may produce bacteremia even in patients with normal gingiva, are not recommended. Similarly, the use of central intravascular catheters and urinary catheters should be minimized. Infections associated with bacteremia must be treated promptly and if possible eradicated before the involved tissues are incised or manipulated.[153]

CHEMOPROPHYLAXIS. The widely promulgated recommendations of antimicrobial prophylaxis for endocarditis are based on circumstantial evidence supplemented by studies of prophylaxis using animal models. Studies suggest that prophylactic antibiotics prevent endocarditis by inhibiting growth of the bacteria adherent to NBTE sufficiently to allow their subsequent complete elimination by host defenses.[155, 159] Experimental studies that mimic single-dose amoxicillin prophylaxis in humans suggest adequate margins of efficacy are present after a single prophylactic dose. Nevertheless, because a more sustained inhibitory effect can be achieved through a postprocedure dose of antibiotics this is recommended for patients in the high-risk group.[152, 160]

Clinical studies supporting the efficacy of antibiotic prophylaxis for endocarditis are limited. A retrospective study of patients who had prosthetic valves and who underwent dental and surgical procedures suggested that antibiotic prophylaxis prevented PVE.[161] However, a large case-control study failed to identify dental procedures as a risk for IE among persons with valvular abnormalities and questioned the benefit of antibiotic prophylaxis for these procedures.[162] Additionally, failures of antibiotic prophylaxis unrelated to resistant bacteria have been noted.[155]

Risk-benefit and cost-benefit analyses have raised significant questions about antibiotic prophylaxis for patients with mitral valve prolapse. Unless both the cost and risks of prophylaxis are very low, the cost per case of IE prevented is high and mortality or morbidity may not be reduced. From a population perspective, prophylaxis in low-

▼ **TABLE 47–16. REGIMENS FOR PROPHYLAXIS AGAINST ENDOCARDITIS: USE WITH GENITOURINARY AND GASTROINTESTINAL (EXCEPT ESOPHAGEAL) PROCEDURES**

SETTING	ANTIBIOTIC	REGIMEN*
High-risk patients	Ampicillin plus gentamicin	Ampicillin 2.0 gm IV/IM plus gentamicin 1.5 mg/kg within 30 min of procedure, repeat ampicillin 1.0 gm IV/IM or give amoxicillin 1.0 gm PO 6 hr later
High-risk, penicillin-allergic patients	Vancomycin plus gentamicin	Vancomycin 1.0 gm IV over 1–2 hr plus gentamicin 1.5 mg/kg IM/IV infused or injected 30 min before procedure. No second dose recommended
Moderate-risk patients	Amoxicillin or ampicillin	Amoxicillin 2.0 gm PO 1 hr before procedure or ampicillin 2.0 gm IM/IV 30 min before procedure
Moderate-risk, penicillin-allergic patients	Vancomycin	Vancomycin 1.0 gm IV infused over 1–2 hr and completed within 30 min of procedure

*Dosing for children: ampicillin 50 mg/kg IV/IM, vancomycin 20 mg/kg IV, gentamicin 1.5 mg/kg IV/IM (children's doses should not exceed adult doses).

Adapted from Dajani AS, Taubert KA, Wilson W, et al: Prevention of bacterial endocarditis: Recommendations by the American Heart Association from the Committee on Rheumatic Fever, Endocarditis, and Kawasaki Disease, Council on Cardiovascular Disease in the Young. JAMA 277:1794–1801, 1997.

to intermediate-risk settings may not be cost or risk beneficial, and prophylaxis might be reserved for patients who have high-risk cardiac lesions and who are undergoing high-risk procedures.[162]

Even if antibiotic prophylaxis is effective as well as safe and inexpensive, only a small percentage of the cases are preventable. For example, only 55 to 75 percent of patients with NVE have preexisting endocarditis-prone valvular disease, and many are not aware of the lesion before the onset of NVE.[4, 5, 155, 156] Additionally, among patients with IE, only a small fraction (5 percent) had both a known valve lesion and a procedure within 30 days of onset of IE that would have warranted prophylaxis.[156] Nevertheless, the morbidity and mortality associated with IE are used to justify prophylaxis (Table 47–16; see Table 43–4) in patients who have high- and intermediate-risk cardiac lesions (see Table 47–15) and who are to undergo bacteremia-inducing procedures (see Table 47–14). Penicillin-resistant flora may emerge among patients who are receiving continuous penicillin for prevention of rheumatic fever or repetitive courses of antibiotics for serial dental procedures. Consequently, a nonpenicillin prophylaxis regimen is preferred for these patients. Initiation of prophylaxis several days before a procedure encourages the emergence of antibiotic-resistant organisms at the mucosal site and is not recommended.

REFERENCES

EPIDEMIOLOGY

1. van der Meer JTM, Thompson J, Valkenburg IIA, Michel MF: Epidemiology of bacterial endocarditis in the Netherlands. I. Patient characteristics. Arch Intern Med 152:1863, 1992.
2. Hogevik H, Olaison L, Andersson R, et al: Epidemiologic aspects of infective endocarditis in an urban population: A 5-year prospective study. Medicine 74:324–339, 1995.
3. Berlin JA, Abrutyn E, Strom BL, et al: Incidence of infective endocarditis in the Delaware Valley, 1988–1990. Am J Cardiol 76:933–936, 1995.
4. Watanakunakorn C, Burkert T: Infective endocarditis at a large community teaching hospital, 1980–1990: A review of 210 episodes. Medicine 72:90, 1993.
5. Kazanjian P: Infective endocarditis: Review of 60 cases treated in community hospitals. Infect Dis Clin Pract 2:41, 1993.
6. Fernandez-Guerrero ML, Verdejo C, Azofra J, de Gorgolas M: Hospital-acquired infectious endocarditis not associated with cardiac surgery: An emerging problem. Clin Infect Dis 20:16, 1995.
7. Morris CD, Reller MD, Menashe VD: Thirty-year incidence of infective endocarditis after surgery for congenital heart defect. JAMA 279:599–603, 1998.
8. van der Meer JTM, van Wijk W, Thompson J, et al: Awareness of need and actual use of prophylaxis: Lack of patient compliance in the prevention of bacterial endocarditis. J Antimicrob Chemother 29:187, 1992.
9. Sandre RM, Shafran SD: Infective endocarditis: Review of 135 cases over 9 years. Clin Infect Dis 22:276–286, 1996.

PATIENT GROUPS

10. Stull TL, LiPuma JJ: Endocarditis in children. In Kaye D (ed): Infective Endocarditis. 2nd ed. New York, Raven Press, 1992, p 313.
11. Baltimore RS: Infective endocarditis in children. Pediatr Infect Dis J 11: 907, 1992.
12. Normand J, Bozio A, Etienne J, et al: Changing patterns and prognosis of infective endocarditis in childhood. Eur Heart J 16(Suppl B):28, 1995.
13. Michel PL, Acar J: Native cardiac disease predisposing to infective endocarditis. Eur Heart J 16(Suppl B):2, 1995.
14. Stein A, Raoult D: Q fever endocarditis. Eur Heart J 16(Suppl B):19, 1995.
15. Raoult D, Fournier PE, Drancourt M, et al: Diagnosis of 22 new cases of Bartonella endocarditis. Ann Intern Med 125:646–652, 1996.
16. Sande MA, Lee BL, Mills J, et al: Endocarditis in intravenous drug users. In Kaye D (ed): Infective Endocarditis. 2nd ed. New York, Raven Press, 1992, p 345.
17. Levine DP, Crane LR, Zervos MJ: Bacteremia in narcotic addicts at the Detroit Medical Center. II. Infectious endocarditis: A prospective comparative study. Rev Infect Dis 8:374, 1986.
18. Mathew J, Addai T, Anand A, et al: Clinical features, site of involvement, bacteriologic findings, and outcome of infective endocarditis in intravenous drug users. Arch Intern Med 155:1641–1648, 1995.
19. Pulvirenti JJ, Kerns E, Benson C, et al: Infective endocarditis in injection drug users: Importance of human immunodeficiency virus serostatus and degree of immunosuppression. Clin Infect Dis 22:40–45, 1996.
20. Ribera E, Miro JM, Cortes E, et al: Influence of human immunodeficiency virus 1 infection and degree of immunosuppression in the clinical characteristics and outcome of infective endocarditis in intravenous drug users. Arch Intern Med 158:2043–2050, 1998.
21. Clifford CP, Eykyn SJ, Oakley CM: Staphylococcal tricuspid valve endocarditis in patients with structurally normal hearts and no evidence of narcotic abuse. Q J Med 87:755, 1994.
22. Rutledge R, Kim J, Applebaum RE: Actuarial analysis of the risk of prosthetic valve endocarditis in 1,598 patients with mechanical and bioprosthetic valves. Arch Surg 120:469, 1985.
23. Ivert TSA, Dismukes WE, Cobbs CG, et al: Prosthetic valve endocarditis. Circulation 69:223, 1984.
24. Arvay A, Lengyel M: Incidence and risk factors of prosthetic valve endocarditis. Eur J Cardiothorac Surg 2:340, 1988.
25. Calderwood SB, Swinski LA, Waternaux CM, et al: Risk factors for the development of prosthetic valve endocarditis. Circulation 72:31, 1985.
26. Agnihotri AK, McGiffin DC, Galbraith AJ, O'Brien MF: Surgery for acquired heart disease. J Thorac Cardiovasc Surg 110:1708–1724, 1995.
27. Horskotte D, Piper C, Niehues R, et al: Late prosthetic valve endocarditis. Eur Heart J 16(Suppl B):39, 1995.
28. Karchmer AW, Gibbons GW: Infections of prosthetic heart valves and vascular grafts. In Bisno AL, Waldvogel FA (eds): Infections Associated with Indwelling Devices. 2nd ed. Washington, DC, American Society for Microbiology, 1994, p 213.
29. Lytle BW, Priest BP, Taylor PC, et al: Surgery for acquired heart disease: Surgical treatment of prosthetic valve endocarditis. J Thorac Cardiovasc Surg 111:198–210, 1996.
30. Fernicola DJ, Roberts WC: Frequency of ring abscess and cuspal infection in active infective endocarditis involving bioprosthetic valves. Am J Cardiol 72:314–323, 1993.
31. Chastre J, Trouillet JL: Early infective endocarditis on prosthetic valves. Eur Heart J 16(Suppl B):32, 1995.
32. Douglas JL, Cobbs CG: Prosthetic valve endocarditis. In Kaye D (ed): Infective Endocarditis. 2nd ed. New York, Raven Press, 1992, p 375.
33. Sobel JD: Nosocomial infective endocarditis. In Kaye D (ed): Infective Endocarditis, 2nd ed. New York, Raven Press, 1992, p 361.
34. Jernigan JA, Farr BM: Short-course therapy of catheter-related Staphylo-

coccus aureus bacteremia: A meta-analysis. Ann Intern Med 119:304, 1993.

35. Fowler VG Jr, Li J, Corey GR, et al: Role of echocardiography in evaluation of patients with *Staphylococcus aureus* bacteremia: Experience in 103 patients. J Am Coll Cardiol 30:1072–1078, 1997.

36. Raad II, Sabbagh MF: Optimal duration of therapy for catheter-related *Staphylococcus aureus* bacteremia: A study of 55 cases and review. Clin Infect Dis 14:75, 1992.

37. Fang G, Keys TF, Gentry LO, et al: Prosthetic valve endocarditis resulting from nosocomial bacteremia: A prospective, multicenter study. Ann Intern Med 119:560, 1993.

Etiologic Microorganisms

38. Douglas CWI, Heath J, Hampton KK, Preston FE: Identity of viridans streptococci isolated from cases of infective endocarditis. J Med Microbiol 39:179, 1993.

39. Bouvet A: Human endocarditis due to nutritionally variant streptococci: *Streptococcus adjacens* and *Streptococcus defectivus.* Eur Heart J 16(Suppl B):24, 1995.

40. Doern GV, Ferraro MJ, Brueggeman AB, Ruoff KL: Emergence of high rates of antimicrobial resistance among viridans group streptococci in the United States. Antimicrob Agents Chemother 40:891–894, 1996.

41. Ballet M, Gevigney G, Gare JP, et al: Infective endocarditis due to *Streptococcus bovis:* A report of 53 cases. Eur Heart J 16:1975–1980, 1995.

42. Baddour LM, Infectious Diseases Society of America Emerging Infections Network: Infective endocarditis caused by β-hemolytic streptococci. Clin Infect Dis 26:66–71, 1998.

43. Aronin SI, Mukherjee SK, West JC, Cooney EL: Review of pneumococcal endocarditis in adults in the penicillin era. Clin Infect Dis 26:165–171, 1998.

44. Whitby S, Pallera A, Schaberg DR, Bronze MS: Infective endocarditis caused by *Streptococcus pneumoniae* with high-level resistance to penicillin and cephalosporin. Clin Infect Dis 23:1176–1177, 1996.

45. Eliopoulos, GM: Enterococcal endocarditis. In Kaye, D. (ed.): Infective Endocarditis. 2nd ed. New York, Raven Press, 1992, p. 209.

46. Eliopoulos GM: Aminoglycoside resistant enterococcal endocarditis. Infect Dis Clin North Am 7:117, 1993.

47. Chuard C, Vaudaux P, Waldvogel FA, Lew DP: Susceptibility of *Staphylococcus aureus* growing on fibronectin-coated surfaces to bactericidal antibiotics. Antimicrob Agents Chemother 37:625, 1993.

48. Anwar H, Strap JL, Costerton JW: Establishment of aging biofilms: Possible mechanism of bacterial resistance to antimicrobial therapy. Antimicrob Agents Chemother 36:1347, 1992.

49. Karchmer AW: Staphylococcal endocarditis. In Kaye D (ed): Infective Endocarditis. 2nd ed. New York, Raven Press, 1992, p 225.

50. Whitener C, Caputo GM, Weitekamp MR, Karchmer AW: Endocarditis due to coagulase-negative staphylococci: Microbiologic, epidemiologic, and clinical considerations. Infect Dis Clin North Am 7:81, 1993.

51. Roder BL, Wandall DA, Frimodt-Moller N, et al: Clinical features of *Staphylococcus aureus* endocarditis: A 10-year experience in Denmark. Arch Intern Med 159:462–469, 1999.

52. Fowler VG Jr, Sanders LL, Kong LK, et al: Infective endocarditis due to *Staphylococcus aureus:* 59 prospectively identified cases with follow-up. Clin Infect Dis 28:106–114, 1999.

53. Vandenesch F, Etienne J, Reverdy ME, Eykyn SJ: Endocarditis due to *Staphylococcus lugdunensis:* Report of 11 cases and review. Clin Infect Dis 17:871, 1993.

54. Hessen MT, Abrutyn E: Gram-negative bacterial endocarditis. In Kaye D (ed): Infective Endocarditis. 2nd ed. New York, Raven Press, 1992, p 251.

55. Siller KA, Johnson WD Jr: Unusual bacterial causes of endocarditis. In Kaye D (ed): Infective Endocarditis. 2nd ed. New York, Raven Press, 1992, p 265.

56. Berbari EF, Cockerill FR III, Steckelberg J: Infective endocarditis due to unusual or fastidious microorganisms. Mayo Clin Proc 72:532–542, 1997.

57. Petit AIC, Bok JW, Thompson J, et al: Native-valve endocarditis due to CDC coryneform group ANF-3: Report of a case and review of corynebacterial endocarditis. Clin Infect Dis 19:897, 1994.

58. Drancourt M, Mainardi JL, Brouqui P, et al: *Bartonella (Rochalimaea) quintana* endocarditis in three homeless men. N Engl J Med 332:419, 1995.

59. Spach DH, Kanter AS, Daniels NA, et al: *Bartonella (Rochalimaea)* species as a cause of apparent "culture-negative" endocarditis. Clin Infect Dis 20:1044, 1995.

60. Gubler JGH, Kuster M, Dutly F, et al: Whipple endocarditis without overt gastrointestinal disease: Report of four cases. Ann Intern Med 131:112–116, 1999.

61. Rubinstein E, Lang R: Fungal endocarditis. Eur Heart J 16(Suppl B):84, 1995.

62. Moyer DV, Edwards JE Jr: Fungal endocarditis. In Kaye D (ed): Infective Endocarditis. 2nd ed. New York, Raven Press, 1992, p 299.

63. Melgar GR, Nasser RM, Gordon SM, et al: Fungal prosthetic valve endocarditis in 16 patients. An 11 year experience in a tertiary care hospital. Medicine 76:94–103, 1997.

64. Gilbert HM, Peters ED, Lang SJ, Hartman BJ: Successful treatment of fungal prosthetic valve endocarditis: Case report and review. Clin Infect Dis 22:348–354, 1996.

65. Weinstein L, Schlesinger JJ: Pathoanatomic, pathophysiologic and clinical correlations in endocarditis (first of two parts). N Engl J Med 291:832, 1974.

66. Livornese LL Jr, Korzeniowski OM: Pathogenesis of infective endocarditis. In Kaye D (ed): Infective Endocarditis. 2nd ed. New York, Raven Press, 1992, p 19.

67. Weinstein L, Schlesinger JJ: Pathoanatomic, pathophysiologic and clinical correlations in endocarditis (second of two parts). N Engl J Med 291:1122, 1974.

68. Dankert J, van der Werff J, Zaat SAJ, et al: Involvement of bactericidal factors from thrombin-stimulated platelets in clearance of adherent viridans streptococci in experimental infective endocarditis. Infect Immun 63:663, 1995.

69. Bayer AS, Cheng D, Yeaman MR, et al: In vitro resistance to thrombin-induced platelet microbicidal protein among clinical bacteremic isolates of *Staphylococcus aureus* correlates with an endovascular infectious source. Antimicrob Agents Chemother 42:3169–3172, 1998.

70. Sullam PM, Frank U, Yeaman MR, et al: Effect of thrombocytopenia on the early course of streptococcal endocarditis. J Infect Dis 168:910, 1993.

71. Yeaman MR, Puentes SM, Norman DC, Bayer AS: Partial characterization and staphylocidal activity of thrombin-induced platelet microbicidal protein. Infect Immun 60:1202, 1992.

72. Moreillon P, Entenza J, Francioli P, et al: Role of *Staphylococcus aureus* coagulase and clumping factor in pathogenesis of experimental endocarditis. Infect Immun 63:4738–4743, 1995.

73. Shiro H, Muller E, Gutierrez N, et al: Transposition mutants of *Staphylococcus epidermidis* deficient in elaboration of capsular polysaccharide/adhesin and slime are avirulent in a rabbit model of endocarditis. J Infect Dis 169:1042, 1994.

74. Herzberg MC, MacFarlane GD, Gong K, et al: The platelet interactivity phenotype of *Streptococcus sanguis* influences the course of experimental endocarditis. Infect Immun 60:4809, 1992.

75. Bancsi MJLMF, Thompson J, Bertina RM: Stimulation and monocyte tissue expression in an in vitro model of bacterial endocarditis. Infect Immun 52:5669, 1994.

76. Croft CH, Woodward W, Elliott A, et al: Analysis of surgical versus medical therapy in active complicated native valve infective endocarditis. Am J Cardiol 51:1650, 1983.

77. Watanabe G, Haverich A, Speier R, et al: Surgical treatment of active infective endocarditis with paravalvular involvement. J Thorac Cardiovasc Surg 107:171, 1994.

78. Blumberg EA, Robbins N, Adimora A, Lowy FD: Persistent fever in association with infective endocarditis. Clin Infect Dis 15:983, 1992.

79. Douglas JL, Dismukes WE: Surgical therapy of infective endocarditis on natural valves. In Kaye D (ed): Infective Endocarditis. 2nd ed. New York, Raven Press, 1992, p 397.

80. Mansur AJ, Grinberg M, Lamos da Luz P, Bellotti G: The complications of infective endocarditis: A reappraisal in the 1980's. Arch Intern Med 152:2428, 1992.

81. Steckelberg JM, Murphy JG, Wilson WR: Management of complications of infective endocarditis. In Kaye D (ed): Infective Endocarditis. 2nd ed. New York, Raven Press, 1992, p 435.

82. Aragam JR, Weyman AE: Echocardiographic findings in infective endocarditis. In Weyman AE, (ed): Principles and Practice of Echocardiography. 2nd ed. Philadelphia, Lea & Febiger, 1994, p 1178.

83. Rohman S, Erbel R, George G, et al: Clinical relevance of vegetation localization by transesophageal echocardiography in infective endocarditis. Eur Heart J 13:446–452, 1992.

84. Allan JD Jr: Splenic abscess: Pathophysiology, diagnosis, and management. In Remington JS, Swartz MN (eds): Current Clinical Topics in Infectious Diseases. Boston, Blackwell Scientific Publications, 1994, p 23.

CLINICAL FEATURES

85. Werner GS, Schulz R, Fuchs JB, et al: Infective endocarditis in the elderly in the era of transesophageal echocardiography: Clinical features and prognosis compared with younger patients. Am J Med 100:90–97, 1996.

86. Bush LM, Johnson CC: Clinical syndrome and diagnosis. In Kaye D (ed): Infective Endocarditis. 2nd ed. New York, Raven Press, 1992, p 99.

87. Steckelberg JM, Murphy JG, Ballard D, et al: Emboli in infective endocarditis: The prognostic value of echocardiography. Ann Intern Med 114:635, 1991.

88. Kanter MC, Hart RG: Neurologic complications of infective endocarditis. Neurology 41:1015, 1991.

89. Roder BL, Wandall DA, Espersen F, et al: Neurologic manifestations in *Staphylococcus aureus* endocarditis: A review of 260 bacteremic cases in nondrug addicts. Am J Med 102:379–386, 1997.

90. Gagliardi JP, Nettles RE, McCarty DE, et al: Native valve infective endocarditis in elderly and younger adult patients: Comparison of clinical features and outcomes with use of the Duke criteria and the Duke endocarditis data base. Clin Infect Dis 26:1165–1168, 1998.

91. Masuda J, Yutani C, Waki R, et al: Histopathological analysis of the mechanisms of intracranial hemorrhage complicating infective endocarditis. Stroke 23:843, 1992.

DIAGNOSIS

92. Durack DT, Lukes AS, Bright DK: New criteria for diagnosis of infective endocarditis: Utilization of specific echocardiographic findings. Am J Med 96:200, 1994.
93. Mortara LA, Bayer AS: Staphylococcus aureus bacteremia and endocarditis: New diagnostic and therapeutic concepts. Infect Dis Clin North Am 7:53, 1993.
94. Bayer AS, Bolger AF, Taubert KA, et al: Diagnosis and management of infective endocarditis and its complications. Circulation 98:2936–2948, 1998.
95. Lindner JR, Case RA, Dent JM, et al: Diagnostic value of echocardiography in suspected endocarditis: An evaluation based on the pretest probability of disease. Circulation 93:730, 1996.
96. Sekeres MA, Abrutyn E, Berlin JA, et al: An assessment of the usefulness of the Duke criteria for diagnosis of active infective endocarditis. Clin Infect Dis 24:1185–1190, 1997.
97. Mugge A: Echocardiographic detection of cardiac valve vegetations and prognostic implications. Infect Dis Clin North Am 7:877, 1993.
98. Sochowski RA, Chan KL: Implication of negative results on a monoplane transesophageal echocardiographic study in patients with suspected infective endocarditis. J Am Coll Cardiol 21:216, 1993.
99. Hoen B, Selton-Suty C, Lacassin F, et al: Infective endocarditis in patients with negative blood cultures: Analysis of 88 cases from a one-year nationwide survey in France. Clin Infect Dis 20:501, 1995.
100. Shapiro DS, Kenney SC, Johnson M, et al: Brief report: Chlamydia psittaci endocarditis diagnosed by blood culture. N Engl J Med 326:1192, 1992.
101. Goldenberger D, Kunzli A, Vogt P, et al: Molecular diagnosis of bacteria endocarditis by broad-range PCR amplification and direct sequencing. J Clin Microbiol 35:2733–2739, 1992.
102. Kaye KM, Kaye D: Laboratory findings including blood cultures. In Kaye D (ed): Infective Endocarditis. 2nd ed. New York, Raven Press, 1992, p 117.
103. Daniel WG, Mugge A: Transesophageal echocardiography. N Engl J Med 332:1268, 1995.
104. Vered Z, Mossinson D, Peleg E, et al: Echocardiographic assessment of prosthetic valve endocarditis. Eur Heart J 16(Suppl B):63, 1995.
105. Morguet AJ, Werner GS, Andreas S, Kreuzer H: Diagnostic value of transesophageal compared with transthoracic echocardiography in suspected prosthetic valve endocarditis. Herz 20:390–398, 1995.
105a. Heidenreich PA, Masoudi FA, Maini B, et al: Echocardiography in patients with suspected endocarditis: A cost-effectiveness analysis. Am J Med 107:198, 1999.
106. Daniel WG, Mugge A, Grote J, et al: Comparison of transthoracic and transesophageal echocardiography for detection of abnormalities of prosthetic and bioprosthetic valves in the mitral and aortic positions. Am J Cardiol 71:210, 1993.
107. Vuille C, Nidorf M, Weyman AE, Picard MH: Natural history of vegetations during successful medical treatment of endocarditis. Am Heart J 128:1200, 1994.
108. Karalis DG, Bansal RC, Hauck AJ, et al: Transesophageal echocardiographic recognition of subaortic complications in aortic valve endocarditis: Clinical and surgical implications. Circulation 86:353, 1992.
109. Sokil AB: Cardiac imaging in infective endocarditis. In Kaye D (ed): Infective Endocarditis. 2nd ed. New York, Raven Press, 1992, p 125.

TREATMENT

110. Scheld WM, Sande MA: Endocarditis and intravascular infections. In Mandell GL, Bennett JE, Dolin R (eds): Mandel, Douglas and Bennett's Principles and Practice of Infectious Diseases. 4th ed. New York, Churchill Livingstone, 1995, p 740.
111. Entenza JM, Caldelari I, Glauser MP, et al: Importance of genotypic and phenotypic tolerance in the treatment of experimental endocarditis due to Streptococcus gordonii. J Infect Dis 175:70–76, 1997.
112. Enzler MJ, Fluckiger U, Glauser MP, Moreillon P: Antibiotic treatment of experimental endocarditis due to methicillin-resistant Staphylococcus epidermidis. J Infect Dis 170:100–109, 1994.
113. Wilson WR, Karchmer AW, Dajani AS, et al: Antibiotic treatment of adults with infective endocarditis due to streptococci, enterococci, staphylococci, and HACEK microorganisms. JAMA 274:1706, 1995.

Antimicrobial Therapy

114. Roberts SA, Lang SDR, Ellis-Pegler RB: Short-course treatment of penicillin-susceptible viridans streptococcal infective endocarditis with penicillin and gentamicin. Infect Dis Clin Pract 2:191, 1993.
115. Francioli P, Ruch W, Stamboulian D: The International Infective Endocarditis Study Treatment of streptococcal endocarditis with a single daily dose of ceftriaxone and netilmicin for 14 days: A prospective multicenter study. Clin Infect Dis 21:1406–1410, 1995.
116. Sexton DJ, Tenenbaum MJ, Wilson WR, et al: Ceftriaxone once daily for four weeks compared with ceftriaxone plus gentamicin once daily for two weeks for treatment of endocarditis due to penicillin-susceptible streptococci. Clin Infect Dis 27:1470–1474, 1998.
117. Chuard C, Herrmann M, Vaudaux P, et al: Successful therapy of experimental chronic foreign-body infection due to methicillin-resistant

118. Torres-Tortosa M, de Cueto M, Vergara A, et al: Prospective evaluation of a two-week course of intravenous antibiotics in intravenous drug addicts with infective endocarditis. Eur J Clin Microbiol Infect Dis 13:559, 1994.
119. Markowitz N, Quinn EL, Saravolatz LD: Trimethoprim-sulfamethoxazole compared with vancomycin for the treatment of Staphylococcus aureus infection. Ann Intern Med 117:390, 1992.
120. Mainardi JL, Shlaes DM, Goering RV, et al: Decreased teicoplanin susceptibility of methicillin-resistant strains of Staphylococcus aureus. J Infect Dis 171:1646, 1995.
121. Sett SS, Hudon MPJ, Jamieson WRE, Chow AW: Prosthetic valve endocarditis: Experience with porcine bioprostheses. J Thorac Cardiovasc Surg 105:428, 1993.
122. John MVD, Hibberd PL, Karchmer AW, et al: Staphylococcus aureus prosthetic valve endocarditis: Optimal management and risk factors for death. Clin Infect Dis 26:1302–1309, 1998.
123. Venditti M, DeBernardis F, Micozzi A, et al: Fluconazole treatment of catheter-related right-sided endocarditis caused by Candida albicans and associated endophthalmitis and folliculitis. Clin Infect Dis 14:422, 1992.
124. Nguyen MH, Nguyen ML, Yu VL, et al: Candida prosthetic valve endocarditis: Prospective study of six cases and review of the literature. Clin Infect Dis 22:262–267, 1996.
125. Muehrcke DD: Fungal prosthetic valve endocarditis. Sem Thor Cardiovasc Surg 7:20, 1995.
126. Nasser RM, Melgar GR, Longworth DL, Gordon SM: Incidence and risk of developing fungal prosthetic valve endocarditis after nosocomial candidemia. Am J Med 103:25, 1997.
127. Raoult D, Houpikian P, Tissot Dupont H, et al: Treatment of Q fever endocarditis: Comparison of 2 regimens containing doxycycline and ofloxacin or hydroxychloroquine. Arch Intern Med 159:167–173, 1999.
128. Tunkel AR, Kaye D: Endocarditis with negative blood cultures. N Engl J Med 326:1215, 1992.
129. Olaison L, Berlin L, Hogevik H, Alestig K: Incidence of β-lactam-induced delayed hypersensitivity and neutropenia during treatment of infective endocarditis. Arch Intern Med 159:607–615, 1999.

Surgical Treatment of Intracardiac Complications

130. Alsip SG, Blackstone EH, Kirklin JW, Cobbs CG: Indications for cardiac surgery in patients with active infective endocarditis. Am J Med 78(Suppl 6B):138, 1985.
131. Al Jubair K, Al Fagih M, Ashmeg A, et al: Cardiac operations during active endocarditis. J Thorac Cardiovasc Surg 104:487, 1992.
132. Santoro J, Ingerman M: Response to therapy: Relapses and reinfections. In Kaye D (ed): Infective Endocarditis. 2nd ed. New York, Raven Press, 1992, p 423.
133. Karchmer AW: Infections of prosthetic valves and intravascular devices. In Mandell GL, Bennett JE, Dolin R (eds): Principles and Practice of Infectious Diseases. New York, Churchill Livingstone, 2000.
134. Tornos MP, Permanyer-Miralda G, Olona M, et al: Long-term complications of native valve infective endocarditis in non-addicts: A 15-year follow-up study. Ann Intern Med 117:567, 1992.
135. Blumberg EA, Karalis DA, Chandrasekaran K, et al: Endocarditis-associated paravalvular abscess. Do clinical parameters predict the presence of abscess? Chest 107:898–903, 1995.
136. Hecht SR, Berger M: Right-sided endocarditis in intravenous drug users: Prognostic features in 102 episodes. Ann Intern Med 17:560, 1992.
137. Davenport J, Hart RG: Prosthetic valve endocarditis 1976–1987: Antibiotics, anticoagulation, and stroke. Stroke 21:993, 1990.
138. McGiffin DC, Galbraith AJ, McLachian GJ, et al: Aortic valve infection: Risk factors for death and recurrent endocarditis after aortic valve replacement. J Thorac Cardiovasc Surg 104:511, 1992.
139. Jault F, Gandjbakheh I, Chastre JC, et al: Prosthetic valve endocarditis with ring abscesses: Surgical management and long-term results. J Thorac Cardiovasc Surg 105:1106, 1993.
140. Hendren WG, Morris AS, Rosenkranz ER, et al: Mitral valve repair for bacterial endocarditis. J Thorac Cardiovasc Surg 103:124, 1992.
141. Reinhartz O, Herrmann M, Redling F, Zerkowski HR: Timing of surgery in patients with acute infective endocarditis. J Cardiovasc Surg 37:397–400, 1996.
142. Eishi K, Kawazoe K, Kuriyama Y, et al: Surgical management of infective endocarditis associated with cerebral complications: Multicenter retrospective study in Japan. J Thorac Cardiovasc Surg 110:1745–1755, 1995.
143. Gillinov AM, Shah RV, Curtis WE, et al: Valve replacement in patients with endocarditis and acute neurologic deficit. Ann Thorac Surg 61:1125–1130, 1996.
144. Parrino PE, Kron IL, Ross SD, et al: Does a focal neurologic deficit contraindicate operation in a patient with endocarditis? Ann Thorac Surg 67:59–64, 1999.
145. Huston JH III, Nichols DA, Luetmer PH, et al: Blinded prospective evaluation of sensitivity of MR angiography to known intracranial aneurysms: Importance of aneurysm size. Am J Neuroradiol 15:1607–1614, 1994.

146. Lederman MM, Sprague L, Wallis RS, Ellner JJ: Duration of fever during treatment of infective endocarditis. Medicine 71:52, 1992.
147. Roberts RB: Streptococcal endocarditis: The viridans and beta hemolytic streptococci. *In* Kaye D (ed): Infective Endocarditis. 2nd ed. New York, Raven Press, 1992, p 191.
148. Acar J, Michel PL, Varenne O, et al: Surgical treatment of infective endocarditis. Eur Heart J 16(Suppl B):94, 1995.
149. Amrani M, Schoevaerdts JC, Eucher P, et al: Extension of native aortic valve endocarditis: Surgical considerations. Eur Heart J 16(Suppl B): 103, 1995.
150. Mullany CJ, Chua YL, Schaff HV, et al: Early and late survival after surgical treatment of culture-positive active endocarditis. Mayo Clin Proc 70:517, 1995.
151. d'Udekem Y, David TE, Feindel CM, et al: Long-term results of operation for paravalvular abscess. Ann Thorac Surg 62:48–53, 1996.

PREVENTION

152. Dajani AS, Taubert KA, Wilson W, et al: Prevention of bacterial endocarditis: Recommendations by the American Heart Association, from the Committee on Rheumatic Fever, Endocarditis, and Kawasaki Disease, Council on Cardiovascular Diseases in the Young. JAMA 277: 1794–1801, 1997.
153. Leport C, Horstkotte D, Burckhardt D, Group of Experts of the International Society for Chemotherapy: Antibiotic prophylaxis for infective endocarditis from an international group of experts towards a European consensus. Eur Heart J 16(Suppl B):126, 1995.
154. Hay DR, Chambers ST, Ellis-Pegler RB, et al: Prevention of infective endocarditis associated with dental treatment and other medical interventions. N Z Med J 105:192, 1992.
155. Durack DT: Prevention of infective endocarditis. N Engl J Med 332:38, 1995.
156. van der Meer JTM, Thompson J, Valkenburg HA, Michel MF: Epidemiology of bacterial endocarditis in the Netherlands. II. Antecedent procedures and use of prophylaxis. Arch Intern Med 152:1869, 1992.
157. DeGevigney G, Pop C, Delahaye JP: The risk of infective endocarditis after cardiac surgical and interventional procedures. Eur Heart J 16(Suppl B):7, 1995.
157a. Spirito P, Rapezzi C, Bellone P, et al: Infective endocarditis hypertrophic cardiomyopathy. Circulation 99:2132, 1999.
158. Steckelberg JM, Wilson WR: Risk factors for infective endocarditis. Infect Dis Clin North Am 7:9, 1993.
159. Blatter M, Francioli P: Endocarditis prophylaxis: From experimental models to human recommendation. Eur Heart J 16(Suppl B):107, 1995.
160. Fluckiger U, Moreillon P, Blaser J, et al: Simulation of amoxicillin pharmacokinetics in humans for the prevention of streptococcal endocarditis in rats. Antimicrob Agents Chemother 38:2846, 1994.
161. Horstkotte D, Friedrichs W, Pippert H, et al: Nutzen der endokarditis-prophylaxe bei patienten mit prothetischen herzklappen. Kardiologie 75:8, 1986.
162. Strom BL, Abrutyn E, Berlin JA, et al: Dental and cardiac risk factors for infective endocarditis: A population-based, case-control study. Ann Intern Med 129:761–769, 1998.

GUIDELINES

PREVENTION, EVALUATION, AND MANAGEMENT OF INFECTIVE ENDOCARDITIS

THOMAS H. LEE

Guidelines for antibiotic prophylaxis were issued by the American Heart Association (AHA) in 1997.[1] These guidelines represented a major departure from prior recommendations by emphasizing that most cases are not attributable to an invasive procedure. According to these guidelines, patients with preexisting cardiac disease should be divided into high-, moderate-, and negligible-risk categories on the basis of their potential outcomes if endocarditis were to develop (see Table 47–15). For dental work, for example, antibiotic prophylaxis is recommended only for patients who have high- and moderate-risk cardiac conditions and who are undergoing high-risk procedures (Table 47–G–1). For nondental procedures, endocarditis prophylaxis is recommended only for high-risk patients undergoing high-risk procedures (see Table 47–15); this strategy is considered optional for medium-risk patients. Antibiotic regimens are described in Table 47–16.

The 1998 American College of Cardiology/American Heart Association (ACC/AHA) guidelines for patients with valvular heart disease[2] endorse the earlier guidelines from the AHA, with a few caveats (Table 47–G–2). The ACC/AHA guidelines recommend antibiotic prophylaxis for patients with hypertrophic cardiomyopathy only when latent or resting obstruction is a factor. In addition, the ACC/AHA committee expressed concern that an increased risk for endocarditis may exist for some patients with mitral valve prolapse without regurgitation; hence, this group was not willing to state that antibiotic prophylaxis was inappropriate for such patients. Instead, the ACC/AHA guidelines indicate that this issue must be addressed by using clinical judgment in individual cases. Finally, the ACC/AHA guidelines specified that antibiotic prophylaxis was not necessary for patients with physiological mitral regurgitation in the absence of a murmur.

INDICATIONS FOR ECHOCARDIOGRAPHY

Echocardiography is strongly supported in virtually all patients with suspected or known infective endocarditis, but the 1997 ACC/AHA guidelines on echocardiography[3] do *not* recommend transesophageal echocardiography (TEE) as the initial test of choice in the diagnosis of native valve endocarditis (see Table 47–G–2). Instead, the guidelines urge use of TEE when specific questions are not adequately addressed by the initial transthoracic echocardiography (TTE) evaluation, such as when the TTE study is of poor quality, when the TTE is nondiagnostic despite a high clinical suspicion of endocarditis, when a prosthetic valve is involved, when there is a high suspicion such as in

TABLE 47–G–1. DENTAL PROCEDURES AND ENDOCARDITIS PROPHYLAXIS

Endocarditis Prophylaxis Recommended for Patients with High- and Moderate-Risk Cardiac Conditions (see Table 47–15)
Dental extractions
Periodontal procedures including surgery, scaling and root planing, probing, and recall maintenance
Dental implant placement and reimplantation of avulsed teeth
Endodontic (root canal) instrumentation or surgery only beyond the apex
Subgingival placement of antibiotic fibers or strips
Initial placement of orthodontic bands but not brackets
Intraligamentary local anesthetic injections
Prophylactic cleaning of teeth or implants when bleeding is anticipated

Endocarditis Prophylaxis Not Recommended
Restorative dentistry* (operative and prosthodontic) with or without retraction cord†
Local anesthetic injections (nonintraligamentary)
Intracanal endodontic treatment; postplacement and build-up
Placement of rubber dams
Postoperative suture removal
Placement of removable prosthodontic or orthodontic appliances
Taking of oral impressions
Fluoride treatments
Taking of oral radiographs
Orthodontic appliance adjustment
Shedding of primary teeth

*This includes restoration of decayed teeth (filling cavities) and replacement of missing teeth.

†Clinical judgment may indicate antibiotic use in selected circumstances that may create significant bleeding.

From Dajani AS, Taubert KA, Wilson W, et al: Prevention of bacterial endocarditis: Recommendations by the American Heart Association. Circulation 96:358–366, 1997.

Indication	Class I*	Class IIa†	Class IIb‡	Class III§
Antibiotic endocarditis prophylaxis for patients with mitral valve prolapse undergoing procedures associated with bacteremia	1. Patients with characteristic systolic click-murmur complex 2. Patients with isolated systolic click and echocardiographic evidence of MVP and MR	1. Patients with isolated systolic click, echocardiographic evidence of high-risk MVP		1. Patients with isolated systolic click and equivocal or no evidence of MVP
Echocardiography in infective endocarditis: Native valves (from 3)	1. Detection and characterization of valvular lesions, their hemodynamic severity, and/or ventricular compensation¶ 2. Detection of vegetations and characterization of lesions in patients with congenital heart disease in whom infective endocarditis is suspected 3. Detection of associated abnormalities (e.g., abscesses, shunts)¶ 4. Reevaluation studies in complex endocarditis (e.g., virulent organism, severe hemodynamic lesion, aortic valve involvement, persistent fever or bacteremia, clinical change, or symptomatic deterioration) 5. Evaluation of patients with high clinical suspicion of culture-negative endocarditis¶	1. Evaluation of bacteremia without a known source¶ 2. Risk stratification in established endocarditis¶	1. Routing reevaluation in uncomplicated endocarditis during antibiotic therapy	1. Evaluation of fever and nonpathological murmur without evidence of bacteremia
Echocardiography in infective endocarditis: Prosthetic valves (from 3)	1. Detection and characterization of valvular lesions, their hemodynamic severity, and/or ventricular compensation¶ 2. Detection of associated abnormalities (e.g., abscesses, shunts)¶ 3. Reevaluation in complex endocarditis (e.g., virulent organism, severe hemodynamic lesion, aortic valve involvement, persistent fever or bacteremia, clinical change, or symptomatic deterioration) 4. Evaluation of suspected endocarditis and negative cultures¶ 5. Evaluation of bacteremia without a known source¶	1. Evaluation of persistent fever without evidence of bacteremia or new murmur¶	1. Routine reevaluation in uncomplicated endocarditis during antibiotic therapy¶	1. Evaluation of transient fever without evidence of bacteremia or new murmur
Surgery for native valve endocarditis (criteria also apply to repaired mitral and aortic allograft or autograft valves)	1. Acute AF or MR with heart failure 2. Acute AF with tachycardia and early closure of the mitral valve 3. Fungal endocarditis 4. Evidence of annular or aortic abscess, sinus or aortic true or false aneurysm 5. Evidence of valve dysfunction and persistent infection after a prolonged period (7 to 10 days) of appropriate antibiotic therapy, as indicated by presence of fever, leukocytosis, and bacteremia, provided there are no noncardiac causes of infection	1. Recurrent emboli after appropriate antibiotic therapy 2. Infection with gram-negative organisms or organisms with a poor response to antibiotics in patients with evidence of valve dysfunction	1. Mobile vegetations >10 mm	1. Early infections of the mitral valve that can likely be repaired 2. Persistent pyrexia and leukocytosis with negative blood cultures

Table continued on following page

Indication	Class I*	Class IIa†	Class IIb‡	Class III§
Surgery for prosthetic valve endocarditis (criteria exclude repaired mitral and aortic allograft or autograft valves)	1. Early prosthetic valve endocarditis (first 2 months or less after surgery) 2. Heart failure with prosthetic valve dysfunction 3. Fungal endocarditis 4. Staphylococcal endocarditis not responding to antibiotic therapy 5. Evidence of paravalvular leak, annular or aortic abscess, sinus or aortic true or false aneurysm, fistula formation, or new-onset conduction disturbances 6. Infection with gram-negative organisms or organisms with a poor response to antibiotics	1. Persistent bacteremia after a prolonged course (7 to 10 days) of appropriate antibiotic therapy without noncardiac causes of bacteremia 2. Recurrent peripheral embolus despite therapy	1. Vegetation of any size on or near the prosthesis	

* Procedure or treatment is beneficial, useful, and effective.
† Weight of evidence in favor of usefulness/efficacy.
‡ Usefulness/efficacy less well established.
§ Procedure or treatment not considered useful or effective.
¶ Transesophageal echocardiography may provide incremental value in addition to information obtained by transthoracic imaging.
AF = atrial fibrillation; MR = mitral regurgitation; MVP = mitral valve prolapse.

a patient with staphylococcus bacteremia, or in an elderly patient with valvular abnormalities that make diagnosis difficult.

Diagnosis of prosthetic valve endocarditis with TTE is more difficult than diagnosis of endocarditis of native valves. Thus, the ACC/AHA guidelines suggest a lower threshold for performance of TEE in patients with prosthetic valves and suspected endocarditis (see Table 47–G–2).

SURGERY FOR ACTIVE ENDOCARDITIS

The ACC/AHA guidelines for valvular heart disease support performance of surgery for patients with life-threatening congestive heart failure or cardiogenic shock due to active endocarditis. Indications for surgery for patients with stable endocarditis are considered less clear (see Table 47–G–2).

REFERENCES

1. Dajani AS, Taubert KA, Wilson W, et al: Prevention of bacterial endocarditis: Recommendations by the American Heart Association. Circulation 96:358–366, 1997.
2. Bonow RO, Carabello B, de Leon AC Jr, et al: ACC/AHA guidelines for the management of patients with valvular heart disease: Executive summary. A report of the American College of Cardiology/American Heart Association Task Force on Practice Guidelines (Committee on Management of Patients with Valvular Heart Disease). Circulation 98:1949–1984, 1998.
3. Cheitlin MD, Alpert JS, Armstrong WF, et al: ACC/AHA guidelines for the clinical application of echocardiography: A report of the American College of Cardiology/American Heart Association Task Force on Practice Guidelines (Committee on Clinical Application of Echocardiography). Circulation 95:1686–1744, 1997.

Chapter 48

The Cardiomyopathies and Myocarditides

JOSHUA WYNNE · EUGENE BRAUNWALD

The cardiomyopathies constitute a group of diseases in which the dominant feature is direct involvement of the heart muscle itself. They are distinctive because they are *not* the result of pericardial, hypertensive, congenital, valvular, or ischemic diseases. Although the diagnosis of cardiomyopathy requires the exclusion of these etiological factors, the features of cardiomyopathy are often sufficiently distinctive—both clinically and hemodynamically—to allow a definitive diagnosis to be made.[1] With increasing awareness of this condition, along with improvements in diagnostic techniques, cardiomyopathy is being recognized as a significant cause of morbidity and mortality.[2] Whether the result of improved recognition or of other factors, the incidence and prevalence of cardiomyopathy appear to be increasing.[2] Although coronary artery disease is the most common cause of congestive heart failure (accounting for about two thirds of all cases), we avoid using the term *cardiomyopathy* in this setting, because the primary problem is in the coronary arteries and not the heart muscle itself.

▼ **TABLE 48–1. CLASSIFICATION OF THE CARDIOMYOPATHIES**

DISORDER	DESCRIPTION
Dilated cardiomyopathy	Dilatation and impaired contraction of the left or both ventricles. Caused by familial/genetic, viral and/or immune, alcoholic/toxic, or unknown factors, or is associated with recognized cardiovascular disease.
Hypertrophic cardiomyopathy	Left and/or right ventricular hypertrophy, often asymmetrical, which usually involves the interventricular septum. Mutations in sarcoplasmic proteins cause the disease in many patients.
Restrictive cardiomyopathy	Restricted filling and reduced diastolic size of either or both ventricles with normal or near-normal systolic function. Is idiopathic or associated with other disease (e.g., amyloidosis, endomyocardial disease).
Arrhythmogenic right ventricular cardiomyopathy	Progressive fibrofatty replacement of the right, and to some degree left, ventricular myocardium. Familial disease is common.
Unclassified cardiomyopathy	Diseases that do not fit readily into any category. Examples include systolic dysfunction with minimal dilatation, mitochondrial disease, and fibroelastosis.
Specific Cardiomyopathies	
Ischemic cardiomyopathy	Presents as dilated cardiomyopathy with depressed ventricular function not explained by the extent of coronary artery obstructions or ischemic damage.
Valvular cardiomyopathy	Presents as ventricular dysfunction that is out of proportion to the abnormal loading conditions produced by the valvular stenosis and/or regurgitation.
Hypertensive cardiomyopathy	Presents with left ventricular hypertrophy with features of cardiac failure due to systolic or diastolic dysfunction.
Inflammatory cardiomyopathy	Cardiac dysfunction as a consequence of myocarditis.
Metabolic cardiomyopathy	Includes a wide variety of causes, including endocrine abnormalities, glycogen storage disease, deficiencies (such as hypokalemia), and nutritional disorders.
General systemic disease	Includes connective tissue disorders and infiltrative diseases such as sarcoidosis and leukemia.
Muscular dystrophies	Includes Duchenne, Becker-type, and myotonic dystrophies.
Neuromuscular disorders	Includes Friedreich ataxia, Noonan syndrome, and lentiginosis.
Sensitivity and toxic reactions	Includes reactions to alcohol, catecholamines, anthracyclines, irradiation, and others.
Peripartal cardiomyopathy	First becomes manifest in the peripartum period, but it is likely a heterogeneous group.

Derived from Richardson P, McKenna W, Bristow M, et al: Report of the 1995 World Health Organization/International Society and Federation of Cardiology Task Force on the Definition and Classification of Cardiomyopathies. Circulation 93:841, 1996. Copyright 1996, American Heart Association.

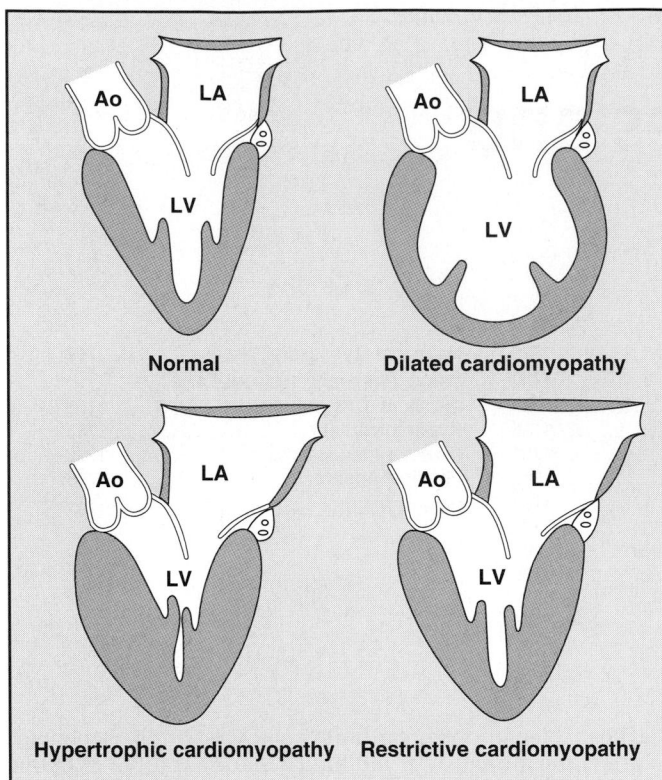

Normal

Dilated cardiomyopathy

Hypertrophic cardiomyopathy

Restrictive cardiomyopathy

FIGURE 48–1. Diagram comparing three morphologic types of cardiomyopathies of unknown cause. Ao = aorta; LA = left atrium; LV = left ventricle. (From Waller BF: Pathology of the cardiomyopathies. J Am Soc Echocardiogr 1:4, 1988.)

FIGURE 48–2. See color plate 26.

A variety of schemes have been proposed for classifying the cardiomyopathies. The most widely recognized classification is that promulgated jointly by the World Health Organization (WHO) and the International Society and Federation of Cardiology (ISFC) (Table 48–1).[3] In the WHO/ISFC classification, the cardiomyopathies are classified based on their predominant pathophysiological features; other diseases that affect the myocardium that are associated with a specific cardiac disorder or are part of a generalized systemic disorder are termed *specific cardiomyopathies* (in the previous WHO/ISFC classification, they were termed *specific heart muscle diseases*).[3]

Three basic types of functional impairment have been described (Fig. 48–1; Table 48–2): (1) *dilated* (DCM, formerly called congestive), the most common form, accounting for 60 percent of all cardiomyopathies[4] and characterized by ventricular dilatation, contractile dysfunction, and often symptoms of congestive heart failure (Fig. 48–2); (2) *hypertrophic* (HCM), recognized by inappropriate left ventricular hypertrophy, often with asymmetrical involvement of the interventricular septum, with preserved or enhanced contractile function until late in the course; and (3) *restrictive* (RCM), the least common form in western countries, marked by impaired diastolic filling and in some cases with endocardial scarring of the ventricle. Two other forms of cardiomyopathy are recognized: *arrhythmogenic right ventricular cardiomyopathy* and *unclassified;* the latter includes fibroelastosis, systolic dysfunction with minimal dilatation, and mitochondrial involvement.[3] The distinction

▼ TABLE 48–2. FUNCTIONAL CLASSIFICATION OF THE CARDIOMYOPATHIES

	DILATED	RESTRICTIVE	HYPERTROPHIC
Symptoms	Congestive heart failure, particularly left sided	Dyspnea, fatigue	Dyspnea, angina pectoris
	Fatigue and weakness	Right-sided congestive heart failure	Fatigue, syncope, palpitations
	Systemic or pulmonary emboli	Signs and symptoms of systemic disease: amyloidosis, iron storage disease, etc.	
Physical Examination	Moderate to severe cardiomegaly: S_3 and S_4	Mild to moderate cardiomegaly: S_3 or S_4	Mild cardiomegaly
			Apical systolic thrill and heave; brisk carotid upstroke
	Atrioventricular valve regurgitation, especially mitral	Atrioventricular valve regurgitation; inspiratory increase in venous pressure (Kussmaul sign)	S_4 common
			Systolic murmur that increases with Valsalva maneuver
Chest Roentgenogram	Moderate to marked cardiac enlargement, especially left ventricular	Mild cardiac enlargement	Mild to moderate cardiac enlargement
	Pulmonary venous hypertension	Pulmonary venous hypertension	Left atrial enlargement
Electrocardiogram	Sinus tachycardia	Low voltage	Left ventricular hypertrophy
	Atrial and ventricular arrhythmias	Intraventricular conduction defects	ST segment and T wave abnormalities
	ST segment and T wave abnormalities	Atrioventricular conduction defects	Abnormal Q waves
	Intraventricular conduction defects		Atrial and ventricular arrhythmias
Echocardiogram	Left ventricular dilatation and dysfunction	Increased left ventricular wall thickness and mass	Asymmetrical septal hypertrophy (ASH)
	Abnormal diastolic mitral valve motion secondary to abnormal compliance and filling pressures	Small or normal-sized left ventricular cavity	Narrow left ventricular outflow tract
		Normal systolic function	Systolic anterior motion (SAM) of the mitral valve
		Pericardial effusion	Small or normal-sized left ventricle

	DILATED	RESTRICTIVE	HYPERTROPHIC
Radionuclide Studies	Left ventricular dilatation and dysfunction (RVG)	Infiltration of myocardium (^{201}Tl) Small or normal-sized left ventricle (RVG) Normal systolic function (RVG)	Small or normal-sized left ventricle (RVG) Vigorous systolic function (RVG) Asymmetrical septal hypertrophy (RVG or ^{201}Tl)
Cardiac Catheterization	Left ventricular enlargement and dysfunction Mitral and/or tricuspid regurgitation Elevated left- and often right-sided filling pressures Diminished cardiac output	Diminished left ventricular compliance "Square root sign" in ventricular pressure recordings Preserved systolic function Elevated left- and right-sided filling pressures	Diminished left ventricular compliance Mitral regurgitation Vigorous systolic function Dynamic left ventricular outflow gradient

RVG = Radionuclide ventriculogram; ^{201}Tl = thallium-201.

▼ TABLE 48-3. CLINICAL INDICATIONS FOR ENDOMYOCARDIAL BIOPSY

DEFINITE
Monitoring of cardiac allograft rejection
Monitoring of anthracycline cardiotoxicity

POSSIBLE
Detection and monitoring of myocarditis
Diagnosis of secondary cardiomyopathies
Differentiation between restrictive and constrictive heart disease

UNCERTAIN
Unexplained, life-threatening ventricular tachyarrhythmias
Acquired immunodeficiency syndrome
Formulation of prognosis in idiopathic dilated cardiomyopathy

From Mason JW, O'Connell JB: Clinical merit of endomyocardial biopsy. Circulation 79:971, 1989. Copyright 1989, American Heart Association.

between the three major functional categories is not absolute, and often there is overlap; in particular, patients with HCM also have increased wall stiffness (as a consequence of the myocardial hypertrophy) and thus present some of the features of an RCM.[3] Late in their course, ventricular dilation and systolic heart failure, bearing some resemblance to DCM, may occur.

Examples of *specific cardiomyopathies* include ischemic cardiomyopathy, valvular cardiomyopathy, hypertensive cardiomyopathy, and inflammatory cardiomyopathy (myocarditis with cardiac dysfunction) (see Table 48-1).[3] Most forms of specific cardiomyopathy are characterized by the DCM pattern. The term *ischemic cardiomyopathy* (see Chap. 37) has been used to describe the condition in which coronary artery disease causes multiple infarctions, diffuse fibrosis, and/or severe ischemia that leads to left ventricular dilatation with congestive heart failure; it may or may not be associated with angina pectoris.[5]

Endomyocardial Biopsy

Evaluation of some patients suspected of suffering from a cardiomyopathy has been facilitated by the use of endomyocardial biopsy.[6] Using a flexible bioptome, the clinician may obtain tissue samples from the right ventricle (and left ventricle when required) through a transvenous (or transarterial) approach with ease and safety (see Chap. 11). The availability of disposable transfemoral bioptomes has further facilitated endomyocardial biopsy. Two-dimensional echocardiography may help guide the placement of the bioptome and reduce or eliminate radiation exposure.[7] Endomyocardial biopsy results in a small tissue sample (average size 1 to 2 mm), and multiple samples (usually four or more) are required because pronounced topographical variations may be found within the myocardium. Which patients should be subjected to biopsy remains controversial, but there is general agreement that biopsy may be of benefit in certain specific situations (Table 48-3).[6] There is little debate as to its clinical utility in detecting infiltrative disorders of the myocardium and in monitoring for anthracycline cardiotoxicity and cardiac transplant rejection.

Although on occasion endomyocardial biopsy may identify a specific etiological agent in an individual patient with cardiac disease of uncertain cause (Table 48-4), the clinical utility of routine biopsy in cardiomyopathy is limited (particularly because no definitive pattern has been found in DCM) (Fig. 48-3).[8, 9] It has been estimated that a specific etiological diagnosis is obtained by biopsy in fewer than 10 percent of patients with cardiomyopathy and a treatable disease is found in only about 2 percent.[6]

DALLAS CRITERIA. Interpretation of biopsy specimens had been plagued by a high degree of interobserver variability; the adoption of a generally accepted set of histological definitions, the *Dallas criteria*, has improved agreement.[10] It is hoped that newer immunohistochemical and molecular biological techniques (such as the polymerase chain reaction or in situ hybridization techniques to detect viral infection of the heart) may expand further the diagnostic utility of endomyocardial biopsy.[10-12]

▼ TABLE 48-4. SPECIFIC DIAGNOSES THAT CAN BE CONFIRMED BY MYOCARDIAL BIOPSY

Cardiac allograft rejection	Fabry disease of the heart	Henoch-Schönlein purpura
Myocarditis	Carcinoid disease	Rheumatic carditis
Giant cell myocarditis	Irradiation injury	Chagasic cardiomyopathy
Doxorubicin cardiotoxicity	Glycogen storage disease	Chloroquine cardiomyopathy
Cardiac amyloidosis	Cardiac tumors of cardiac origin	Lyme carditis
Cardiac sarcoidosis	Cardiac tumors of noncardiac origin	Carnitine deficiency cardiomyopathy
Cardiac hemochromatosis	Kearns-Sayre syndrome	Right ventricular lipomatosis
Endocardial fibrosis	Cytomegalovirus infection	Hypereosinophilic syndrome
Endocardial fibroelastosis	Toxoplasmosis	

From Mason JW, O'Connell JB: Clinical merit of endomyocardial biopsy. Circulation 79:971, 1989. Copyright 1989, American Heart Association.

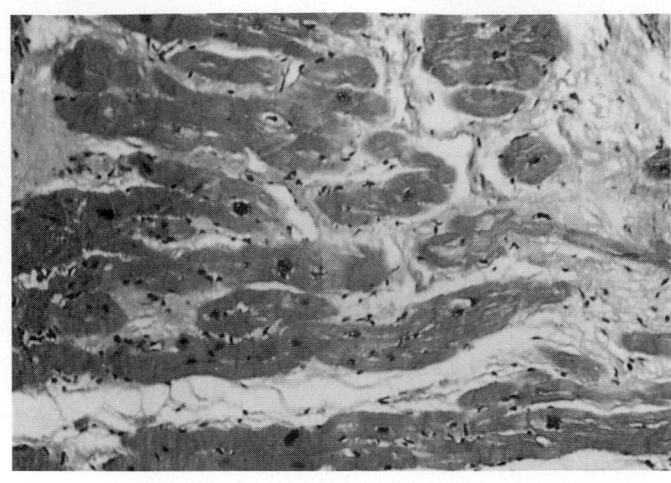 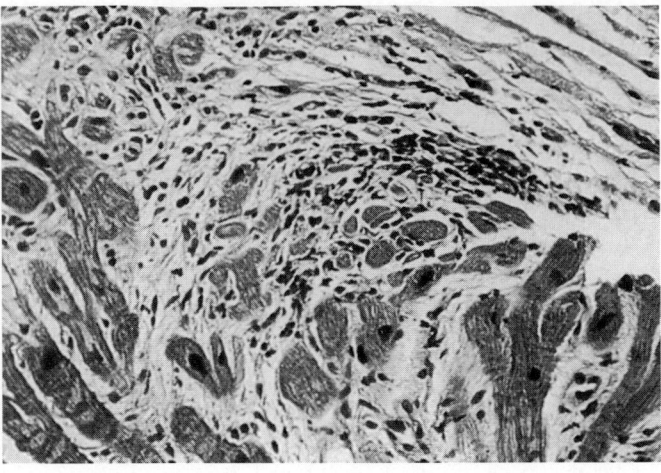

A   B

FIGURE 48–3. Histological specimens obtained by right ventricular endomyocardial biopsy. *A,* Idiopathic dilated cardiomyopathy with varying degrees of interstitial fibrosis and myocyte hypertrophy (trichrome stain, 210×). *B,* Myocarditis with dense focal area of mononuclear cell infiltrate adjacent to necrotic and degenerating myocytes, with irregular myocytic hypertrophy and dense interstitial fibrosis (hematoxylin-eosin, 210×). (From Dec GW, Fuster V: Idiopathic dilated cardiomyopathy. N Engl J Med 331:1564, 1994. Copyright 1994, Massachusetts Medical Society.)

Dilated Cardiomyopathy

IDIOPATHIC DILATED CARDIOMYOPATHY

Dilated cardiomyopathy is a syndrome characterized by cardiac enlargement and impaired systolic function of one or both ventricles (see Fig. 48–2). Although it was formerly called congestive cardiomyopathy, the term *dilated cardiomyopathy* is now preferred because the earliest abnormality usually is ventricular enlargement and systolic contractile dysfunction, with the signs and symptoms of congestive heart failure often (but not invariably) developing later. In an occasional patient, the predominant finding is that of contractile dysfunction with only a mildly dilated left ventricle. In the WHO/ISFC classification scheme, this variant of DCM is placed in the unclassified cardiomyopathy group. Conversely, apparently normal elite athletes may demonstrate considerable ventricular enlargement with *normal* systolic performance. It is presumed that this is a physiological adaptation to intense athletic training and does not appear to represent a disease state, although the long-term consequences are not fully known.[13]

The incidence of DCM is reported to be 5 to 8 cases per 100,000 population per year and appears to be increasing, although the true figure likely is higher as a consequence of underreporting of mild or asymptomatic cases.[14] It occurs almost three times more frequently in blacks and males as in whites and females, and this difference does not appear to be related solely to differing degrees of hypertension, cigarette smoking, or alcohol use.[2, 15, 16] Survival in blacks and males appears to be worse than in whites and females.[17]

Although the cause is not definable in many cases, more than 75 specific diseases of heart muscle can produce the clinical manifestations of DCM. It is likely that this condition represents a final common pathway that is the end result of myocardial damage produced by a variety of cytotoxic, metabolic, immunological, familial, and infectious mechanisms. Alcohol, for example, may lead to severe cardiac dysfunction and may produce clinical, hemodynamic, and pathological findings identical to those present in idiopathic DCM (see p. 1758).

NATURAL HISTORY. The natural history of DCM is not well established. Many patients have minimal or no symptoms, and the progression of the disease in these patients is unclear, although there is some evidence that the long-term prognosis is not good.[18] Nevertheless, in symptomatic patients the course usually is one of progressive deterioration, with one quarter of newly diagnosed patients referred to major medical centers dying within a year and half dying within 5 years, although a minority improve, with a reduction in cardiac size and longer survival.[14] Recent data suggest that in patients with mild dilatation not referred to a medical center the prognosis may be more favorable, no doubt reflecting at least in part earlier diagnosis and perhaps more effective treatment options now available in the community.[1, 19, 20] About a fourth of patients with recent-onset DCM improve spontaneously, even some sick enough initially to be considered for cardiac transplantation.[21] In some patients clinical and functional improvement may occur years after initial presentation.

PROGNOSIS. A variety of clinical predictors of patients at enhanced risk of dying of DCM have been identified, including the presence of a protodiastolic (S_3) gallop, ventricular arrhythmias, advanced age, and specific endomyocardial biopsy features.[22] However, the predictive reliability of any single feature is not high,[23] and it may be difficult to predict with any accuracy the clinical course and outcome in an individual patient.[14, 20] Nevertheless, greater ventricular enlargement and worse dysfunction tend to correlate with poorer prognosis,[16, 22, 24] particularly if the right ventricle is dilated and dysfunctional as well.[25]

Cardiopulmonary exercise testing also can provide prognostic information (see Chap. 6). Marked limitation of exercise capacity manifested by reduced maximal systemic oxygen uptake (especially when below 10 to 12 ml/kg/min) is a reliable predictor of mortality and is used widely as an indicator for consideration of cardiac transplantation.[14, 16] It has been suggested that specific endomyocardial biopsy morphological findings (such as loss of intracellular myofilaments) may offer some predictive information regarding prognosis.[14, 26]

Pathology

MACROSCOPIC EXAMINATION. This reveals enlargement and dilatation of all four cardiac chambers; the ventricles are more dilated than the atria (see Fig. 48–2). Although the thickness of the ventricular wall is increased in some cases, the degree of hypertrophy often is less than might be expected given the severe dilatation present.[14] The development of left ventricular hypertrophy appears to have a protective or beneficial role in DCM, presumably because it reduces systolic wall stress and thus protects against further cavity dilatation. The cardiac valves are intrinsically normal, and intracavitary thrombi, particularly in the ventricular apex, are common.[14] The coronary arteries usually are normal. The right ventricle is preferentially involved in some cases of DCM, sometimes on a familial basis.

HISTOLOGICAL EXAMINATION. Microscopic study reveals extensive areas of interstitial and perivascular fibrosis, particularly involving the left ventricular subendocardium (see Fig. 48–3). Small areas of necrosis and cellular infiltrate are seen on occasion, but these typically are not prominent features. There is marked variation in myocyte size; some myocardial cells are hypertrophied, and others are atrophied. No viruses or other etiological agents have been identified with any regularity in tissue from patients with DCM. Particularly disappointing has been the failure to identify any immunological, histochemical, morphological, ultrastructural, or microbiological marker that might be used to establish the diagnosis of idiopathic DCM or to clarify its cause.

Etiology

About a fourth of the cases of congestive heart failure in the United States are due to idiopathic DCM[27]; most of the remainder are caused by the sequelae of coronary artery or hypertensive heart disease. It is likely that idiopathic DCM represents a common expression of myocardial damage that has been produced by a variety of as yet unestablished myocardial insults. Although the cause(s) remain unclear, interest has centered on three possible basic mechanisms of damage: (1) familial and genetic factors; (2) viral myocarditis and other cytotoxic insults; and (3) immunological abnormalities (Figs. 48–4 and 48–5).[14, 28]

Familial linkage of DCM occurs more commonly than often is appreciated. In 20 percent or more of patients, a first-degree relative also shows evidence of DCM, suggesting that familial transmission is relatively frequent.[20, 29–33] Some asymptomatic relatives of patients with DCM have subclinical left ventricular enlargement and/or dysfunction that may progress to overt symptomatic DMC.[29] Most familial cases demonstrate autosomal dominant transmission; six chromosomal loci have been identified, and more are likely to be found.[34] However, the disease is genetically quite heterogeneous[32] and autosomal recessive[35] and X-linked inheritance[36] have been found. One form of familial X-linked DCM is due to a deletion in the promoter region and the first exon of the gene that codes for the protein dystrophin, a component of the cytoskeleton of myocytes.[37, 38] This has fueled speculation that a resulting deficiency of cardiac dystrophin is the cause of the associated DCM (see also Chap. 21). Mutations involving mitochondrial DNA have been reported as well.[39–41]

Whether any of the patients without apparent familial linkage has a genetic predisposition to DCM remains un-

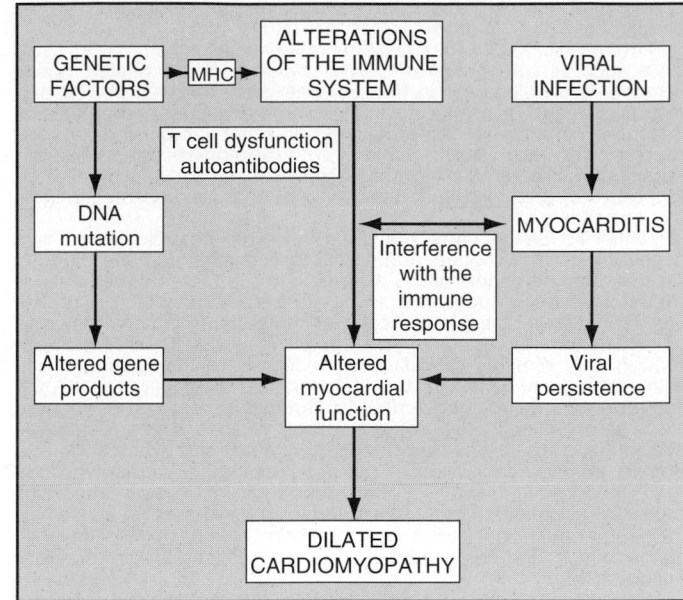

FIGURE 48–5. Hypotheses to explain the pathogenesis of dilated cardiomyopathy. MHC = myosin heavy chain. (From Mestroni L, Krajinovic M, Severini GM, et al: Familial dilated cardiomyopathy. Br Heart J 72:S35, 1994.)

known. There is great interest in using molecular genetic techniques to identify markers of disease susceptibility in asymptomatic carriers at risk for the eventual development of overt clinical DCM.[36, 42] An example of such a marker may be the angiotensin-converting enzyme DD genotype that is found with increased frequency in DCM patients.[43] One intriguing familial metabolic deficiency is that of carnitine, with improvement occurring in the myopathy with carnitine repletion.[44]

SEQUELA OF VIRAL MYOCARDITIS. Wide speculation exists that an episode of subclinical viral myocarditis initiates an autoimmune reaction that culminates in the development of full-blown DCM.[27, 45] Although this hypothesis is inviting, it remains largely unsupported[46]; it has been estimated that only about 15 percent of patients with myocarditis progress to DCM. In some patients who exhibit the clinical features of DCM, endomyocardial biopsy reveals evidence of an inflammatory myocarditis (see Fig. 48–3B). The reported frequency of evidence of an inflammatory infiltrate in DCM varies widely and undoubtedly depends largely on patient selection and the criteria used for diagnosis; using rigorous criteria, only about 10 percent (or less) of patients with DCM have biopsy evidence of myocarditis.[6] Other evidence favoring the concept that DCM is a postviral disorder includes the presence of high antibody viral titers, viral-specific RNA sequences, and apparent viral particles in patients with "idiopathic" DCM.[47] On the other hand, the more rigorous technique of polymerase chain reaction generally has not confirmed the presence of viral remnants in the myocardium of most cardiomyopathy patients,[48] although data are conflicting.[49, 50]

AUTOIMMUNITY. Abnormalities of both humoral and cellular immunity have been found in patients with DCM,[28, 51, 52] although the findings have not been completely reproducible. There is speculation that antibodies might be the *result* of myocardial damage, rather than the cause.[53] There appears to be an association with specific HLA Class II antigens (particularly DR4), suggesting that abnormalities of immunoregulation may play a role in DCM.[31, 54] Circulating antimyocardial antibodies to a variety of antigens (including the myosin heavy chain, the beta adrenoreceptor, the muscarinic receptor, laminin, and mitochondrial proteins) have been identified.[28, 55–57] Additional evidence for the significance of circulating antimyocardial antibodies comes from the demonstration of short-term clinical improvement in the manifestations of heart failure in a small number of patients treated with immunoadsorption and elimination of anti-beta₁-adrenergic receptor antibodies.[58, 58a, 58b] Abnormalities of various T cells, including cytotoxic T cells, suppressor T lymphocytes, and natural killer cells, have been found in some studies.[14, 59] These immunological abnormalities may be the consequence of prior viral myocarditis.[59] It has been postulated that viral components may be incorporated into the cardiac sarcolemma, only to serve as an antigenic source that directs the immune response to attack the myocardium. Nevertheless, the pre-

FIGURE 48–4. See color plate 26.

cise role of either humoral or cellular immunomodulation in the pathogenesis of DCM remains unestablished.[14]

PROINFLAMMATORY CYTOKINES. A variety of proinflammatory cytokines such as tumor necrosis factor-alpha (and the related tumor necrosis factor-alpha converting enzyme) are expressed in DCM and may play a role in producing contractile dysfunction; whether viral infection, autoimmune abnormalities, or other factors induce their expression is unknown.[60, 61] Similarly, the vasoconstrictor peptide endothelin is increased in decompensated DCM and has been implicated as a cause of the heightened vascular tone that accompanies congestive heart failure.[62]

OTHER POTENTIAL CAUSES. A variety of other possible causes have been proposed, although none is accepted as *the* cause of DCM. Thus, endocrine abnormalities as well as the effects of chemicals or toxins have been suggested as possible etiological factors. It has been suggested that microvascular hyperreactivity (spasm) may lead to myocellular necrosis and scarring, with resultant heart failure, although this remains speculative.[5] Apoptosis, or programmed cell death, has been demonstrated in the hearts of patients with DCM and arrhythmogenic right ventricular cardiomyopathy, although there is some controversy regarding the veracity of these findings in DCM.[63] Even if true, the significance of this finding, and whether it is a primary or secondary event in the development of cardiomyopathy, remains unclear. From a clinical standpoint, the more important causes of nonidiopathic DCM include alcohol and cocaine abuse, human immunodeficiency virus (HIV) infection[64] (see Chap. 68), metabolic abnormalities, and the cardiotoxicity of anticancer drugs (especially doxorubicin).

ABNORMALITIES OF THE SYMPATHETIC NERVOUS SYSTEM. Several abnormalities of the sympathetic nervous system have been demonstrated in DCM, but they appear to be the result rather than the cause of the disease.[14, 65] A reduction in density of membrane-associated beta adrenoreceptors[66] is believed to be a consequence of the development of anti-beta-adrenoreceptor autoantibodies. An alteration in the signal transmission pathway by which the beta adrenoreceptors stimulate the contractile apparatus (the G-protein system) has been found as well. Inhibition of this system is enhanced in DCM patients, perhaps accounting for their depressed contractile function. An increase of the subunits of the inhibitory guanine nucleotide-binding protein (G_i) has been reported to occur in the membranes of myocytes from failing hearts.[67] This increase in G_i is associated with a striking reduction of basal adenylate cyclase activity and of the positive inotropic effects of isoproterenol and the phosphodiesterase inhibitor milrinone. These findings suggest that the increase of G_i might contribute to the reduced effects of endogenous catecholamines in DCM. The precise cause of contractile dysfunction at the cellular level in patients with DCM remains speculative. Although there are demonstrable abnormalities of cellular metabolism and calcium handling by cardiomyopathic tissue,[5, 68–70] the significance of these findings is not yet clear.[62]

Clinical Manifestations

HISTORY. Symptoms usually develop gradually in patients with DCM. Some patients are asymptomatic and yet have left ventricular dilatation for months or even years. This dilatation may be recognized clinically only later when symptoms develop or when routine chest roentgenography demonstrates cardiomegaly. A relatively small number of patients develop symptoms of heart failure for the first time after recovery from what appears to be a systemic viral infection. In still others, severe heart failure develops acutely during an episode of myocarditis; although some recovery occurs, chronic manifestations of diminished cardiac reserve persist and heart failure reappears months or years later. It is important to question the patient and family carefully about alcohol consumption, because excessive alcohol consumption is a major cause of DCM, and its cessation may result in substantial clinical improvement.[14] Although patients of any age may be affected, the disease is most common in middle age and is more frequent in men than in women.

The most striking symptoms of DCM are those of left ventricular failure. Fatigue and weakness due to diminished cardiac output are common. Right-sided heart failure is a late and ominous sign and is associated with a particularly poor prognosis. Chest pain occurs in about one third of patients and may suggest concomitant ischemic heart disease.[1, 14] The demonstrated reduction in the vasodilator reserve of the coronary microvasculature in DCM suggests that subendocardial ischemia may play a role in the genesis of chest pain that occurs despite angiographically normal coronary arteries.[71] Chest pain secondary to pulmonary embolism and abdominal pain secondary to congestive hepatomegaly are frequent in the late stages of illness.

PHYSICAL EXAMINATION (See also Chaps. 4 and 17). Examination usually reveals variable degrees of cardiac enlargement and findings of congestive heart failure. The systolic blood pressure is usually normal or low, and the pulse pressure is narrow, reflecting a diminished stroke volume. *Pulsus alternans* (see Fig. 17–5) is common when severe left ventricular failure is present. Cheyne-Stokes breathing may be present and is associated with a poor prognosis.[72] The jugular veins are distended when right-sided heart failure appears, but on initial presentation most patients do not have evidence of this.[14] Prominent *a* and *v* waves may be visible. Grossly pulsatile jugular veins with prominent regurgitant waves indicate the presence of tricuspid valvular regurgitation; this is usually a late and often ominous finding. The liver may be engorged and pulsatile. Peripheral edema and ascites are present when right-sided heart failure is advanced.

The precordium usually reveals left and, occasionally, right ventricular impulses, but the heaves are not sustained as they are in patients with ventricular hypertrophy. The apical impulse is usually displaced laterally, reflecting left ventricular dilatation. A presystolic *a* wave may be palpable on occasion and is generated in a similar manner as a presystolic (S_4) gallop heard on auscultation. The second heart sound (S_2) is usually normally split, although paradoxical splitting may be detected in the presence of left bundle branch block, an electrocardiographic (ECG) finding that is not unusual in DCM. If pulmonary hypertension is present, the pulmonary component of S_2 may be accentuated and the splitting may be narrow. Presystolic gallop sounds (S_4) are almost universally present and often precede the development of overt congestive heart failure.[14] Ventricular gallops (S_3) are the rule once cardiac decompensation occurs, and a summation gallop is heard when there is concomitant tachycardia.

Systolic murmurs are common and are usually due to mitral or, less commonly, tricuspid valvular regurgitation.[14] Mitral regurgitation results from enlargement and abnormal motion of the mitral annulus; ventricular dilatation with resultant distortion of the geometry of the subvalvular apparatus ("papillary muscle dysfunction") plays a lesser role. Gallop sounds and regurgitant murmurs can often be elicited or intensified by isometric handgrip exercise with its attendant enhancement of systemic vascular resistance and impedance to left ventricular outflow. Systemic emboli resulting from dislodgement of intracardiac thrombi from the left atrium and ventricle and pulmonary emboli that originate in the venous system of the legs are common late complications.

NONINVASIVE LABORATORY EXAMINATIONS. To identify potentially reversible causes of DCM, several basic screening biochemical tests are indicated, including determination of levels of serum phosphorus (hypophosphatemia), serum calcium (hypocalcemia), and serum creatinine and urea nitrogen (uremia), thyroid function studies (hypothyroidism and hyperthyroidism), and iron studies (hemochromatosis). It is prudent to test for HIV as well, because this infection is an important and often unrecognized cause of congestive heart failure[64] (see Chap. 68). The chest roentgenogram usually reveals generalized cardiomegaly and pulmonary vascular redistribution; interstitial and alveolar edema are less common on initial presentation.[14] Pleural effusions may be present, and the azygos vein and superior vena cava may be dilated when right-sided heart failure supervenes.

Electrocardiography. The ECG often shows sinus tachycardia when heart failure is present. The entire spectrum of atrial and ventricular tachyarrhythmias may be seen. Poor R wave progression and intraventricular conduction abnormalities, especially left bundle branch block, are common.[14] Anterior Q waves may be present when there is extensive left ventricular fibrosis, even without a discrete myocardial scar or evidence of coronary artery disease.[14] ST segment and T wave abnormalities are common, as are P wave changes, especially left atrial abnormality. Ambulatory monitoring demonstrates the ubiquity of ventricular arrhythmias, with about half of monitored patients with DCM exhibiting nonsustained ventricular tachycardia.[14] There is no consensus that complex or frequent ventricular arrhythmias predict sudden (presumably arrhythmic) death, although they do appear to predict *total* mortality.[73] Perhaps ventricular arrhythmias as detected on ambulatory monitoring are a marker for the extent of myocardial damage in DCM and therefore are associated with sudden death without necessarily being its cause. In occasional cases, particularly in children, recurrent and/or incessant supraventricular or ventricular tachyarrhythmias may actually be the cause (rather than the result) of ventricular dysfunction.[74, 75] In those cases, restoration of sinus rhythm or slowing of the heart rate may reverse the cardiomyopathy.[76, 77]

Echocardiography. Two-dimensional and Doppler forms of echocardiography are useful in assessing the degree of impairment of left ventricular function and for excluding concomitant valvular or pericardial disease (see Fig. 7–99).[20] In addition to examining all four cardiac valves for evidence of structural or functional abnormalities, echocardiography allows evaluation of the size of the ventricular cavity and thickness of the ventricular walls. A pericardial effusion may be demonstrated on occasion. Doppler studies are useful in delineating the severity of mitral (and tricuspid) regurgitation. Patients with a pattern of left ventricular filling on Doppler studies that simulates that seen with RCM appear to have more advanced disease.[78] Combining echocardiography with dobutamine infusion may identify patients with left ventricular dysfunction due to coronary artery disease by demonstrating provocable differences in regional wall motion and thus distinguish them from patients with idiopathic DCM.[79] It has been suggested that thallium-201 imaging may be helpful in distinguishing left ventricular enlargement caused by DCM from that caused by coronary artery disease,[80] although there is not complete agreement on this point.[14, 81] Scanning with gallium or antimyosin antibody (see Chap. 9) may help to identify patients more likely to have evidence of myocarditis on biopsy, although whether this finding is useful clinically is not yet established.[14, 82]

Radionuclide Ventriculography. Like echocardiography, radionuclide ventriculography reveals increased end-diastolic and end-systolic left ventricular volumes, reduced ejection fraction in one or both ventricles, and wall motion abnormalities (see Chap. 9); it is used most commonly when echocardiography is technically suboptimal.[14] Like echocardiography, it may demonstrate segmental wall motion abnormalities in DCM even in the absence of coronary artery disease, the disease process that most commonly produces regional dysfunction. In most patients it is not necessary to carry out serial studies or batteries of noninvasive tests to follow patients with DCM and evaluate their response to treatment; adjustments in pharmacological therapies usually are made based on routine bedside clinical features and symptomatic response.

CARDIAC CATHETERIZATION AND ANGIOCARDIOGRAPHY. Only certain patients with DCM require cardiac catheterization (particularly those with chest pain and a suspicion of ischemic disease or patients thought to have a treatable systemic disease such as sarcoidosis or hemochromatosis, where myocardial biopsy is an important part of the catheterization procedure).[14] When cardiac catheterization is carried out, the left ventricular end-diastolic, left atrial, and

pulmonary artery wedge pressures usually are elevated. Modest degrees of pulmonary arterial hypertension are common. Advanced cases may demonstrate right ventricular dilatation and failure as well, with resultant elevation of the right ventricular end-diastolic, right atrial, and central venous pressures.

Left ventriculography demonstrates enlargement of this chamber, typically with diffuse reduction in wall motion. Segmental wall motion abnormalities are not uncommon and may simulate the angiographic findings in ischemic heart disease. However, prominent localized wall motion disturbances are more characteristic of ischemic heart disease, whereas diffuse global dysfunction is more typical of DCM. The ejection fraction is reduced and the end-systolic volume is increased as a result of the impairment of left ventricular contractility. Sometimes left ventricular thrombi may be visualized within the left ventricle as intracavitary filling defects. Mild mitral regurgitation is often present. On occasion, it may be difficult to distinguish left ventricular dilatation secondary to severe mitral regurgitation due to intrinsic mitral valve disease from DCM with secondary mitral regurgitation.

Coronary arteriography usually reveals normal vessels, although coronary vasodilatory capacity may be impaired[83, 84]; in some cases this may relate to marked elevation of the left ventricular filling pressures.[85] This examination may be of particular value in excluding coronary artery disease in patients with abnormal Q waves on the ECG or regional left ventricular wall motion abnormalities on noninvasive evaluation (although noninvasive testing, including electron-beam computed tomography [CT], may be sufficiently reliable to exclude important coronary artery disease without resorting to arteriography).[86] Coronary arteriography, when necessary, thus helps to distinguish between myocardial infarction as a result of obstructive coronary artery disease and extensive localized myocardial fibrosis secondary to severe DCM in the absence of coronary artery obstruction.

Management

Because the cause of idiopathic DCM, by definition, is unknown, specific therapy is not possible.[27] Treatment, therefore, is for heart failure, as discussed in Chapters 18 and 21.

Many of the therapeutic approaches are directed at modifying the results of the long-term activation of two interrelated neurohormonal/autocrine-paracrine systems, the adrenergic and renin-angiotensin systems.[87] Physical, dietary, and pharmacological interventions may help to control symptoms; regular physical exercise (as tolerated) increases exercise capacity by improving endothelial dysfunction and augmenting blood flow in skeletal muscles.[88] Only cardiac transplantation (see Chap. 20) and specific pharmacological therapy (the vasodilators enalapril or hydralazine plus nitrates, the beta-adrenoceptor blocker carvedilol, and the aldosterone receptor blocker spironolactone) have been shown to prolong life.[14, 27, 89-91]

BETA-ADRENERGIC RECEPTOR BLOCKADE. Because of evidence that activation of the adrenergic system may have deleterious cardiac effects (rather than being an important compensatory mechanism as traditionally thought), beta-adrenoceptor blockade has been suggested as treatment for DCM (see Chaps. 18 and 21).[78, 92] Results to date generally have been favorable, with evidence of improved symptoms, exercise capacity, and left ventricular function and a suggestion that survival has been improved.[14, 93-97a] Beta-adrenoceptor blockade has been surprisingly well tolerated, with infrequent aggravation of heart failure (which, on occasion, may be profound). The mechanism of beneficial action of beta-adrenoceptor blockers is unknown but may relate to (1) negative chronotropic effect with reduced myocardial oxygen demand, (2) reduced myocardial damage due to catecholamines, (3) improved diastolic relaxation (both early active and late passive properties), (4) inhibition of sympathetically mediated vasoconstriction, (5) increase ("upregulation") in myocardial beta-adrenoceptor density, (6) improved calcium handling at slower heart rates, (7) modulation of postreceptor inhibitory G proteins, and/or (7) a direct effect on myocyte and interstitial growth, with attendant inhibition of the remodeling process (remodeling refers to the change in ventricular shape, size, and geometry that occurs after myocyte dysfunction).[90, 92, 98-100] Modulation of the remodeling process has also been implicated in the successful use of growth hormone in a small number of patients with DCM.[101]

Beta-adrenergic blocker therapy is now accepted as part of the four-drug approach (along with digoxin, vasodilators and diuretics) advocated for all suitable patients with symptomatic congestive heart failure (see Chap. 21). Patients with advanced heart failure or in a decompensated state should not ordinarily be given a beta-adrenergic blocker for fear of worsening the failure.[102] Recent data indicate that carvedilol (a beta-adrenoceptor blocker with alpha-adrenoceptor blocking and antioxidant effects) substantially reduces mortality in DCM.[90] It remains unestablished whether carvedilol has additional clinical benefits beyond those found with the other beta-adrenergic blockers, although some patients appear to respond more favorably.[103, 104]

CALCIUM ANTAGONISTS. Because of the possible link between DCM, microvascular circulatory abnormalities, and abnormal myocardial calcium handling, there has been interest in the use of calcium antagonists. These agents have generally been well tolerated when used in DCM patients, although myocardial depression is an important potential side effect of the calcium antagonists as a group. Unfortunately, combining a calcium antagonist with traditional standard therapy (digoxin, diuretics, and vasodilator) does not appear to have substantial clinical benefit, nor does it reduce further the mortality in DCM.[105] At present, the routine use of calcium antagonists in DCM is considered nonstandard and not first-line therapy.[106]

ANTIARRHYTHMICS. Although there is no definitive evidence that antiarrhythmic agents prolong life or prevent sudden death in DCM,[14, 73, 107] it may be appropriate to use them in the treatment of symptomatic arrhythmias. Because of the adverse effects of most available agents, many of which depress myocardial contractility and have a proarrhythmic effect (see Chap. 23), treatment should be individualized, with both efficacy and toxicity carefully monitored. Unfortunately, electrophysiological testing is of limited utility in DCM because it is positive in a minority of patients at risk,[14, 108] the lack of inducibility of ventricular tachyarrhythmias does not identify a low-risk group, and pharmacological suppression of provoked arrhythmias does not necessarily predict freedom from recurrences.[109] The recording of late potentials by the signal-averaged ECG has appeared to be of benefit in assessing the risk of death in some studies, although this has not been a universal finding and awaits further confirmation.[110, 111] The implantable cardioverter-defibrillator (ICD) (see Chap. 24) should be considered in appropriate candidates with symptomatic ventricular tachyarrhythmias.[112, 113] Even patients with unexplained syncope and no demonstrated tachyarrhythmia (even during electrophysiological testing) may profit from the insertion of an ICD.

ANTICOAGULANTS. There is a lack of agreement as to the appropriateness and usefulness of chronic anticoagulant therapy in DCM to protect against pulmonary and especially systemic emboli.[114, 115] Even in the absence of controlled clinical trials demonstrating their efficacy,[116] we believe that the available observational data support the use of anticoagulants in good-risk patients with DCM and heart failure.[114, 117] There is general agreement that anticoagulants should be used in the presence of atrial fibrillation, if the patient has previously had a stroke, and when there is visible thrombus on echocardiography. Oral warfarin is used to achieve a prolongation of the prothrombin time of 2.0 to 3.0 international normalized ratio.

IMMUNOSUPPRESSIVES. In those patients with chronic heart failure secondary to DCM and lymphocytic infiltrate on myocardial biopsy, treatment with corticosteroids and immunosuppressive agents had been advocated in the past. Unfortunately, such therapy does not appear to have a clinically important effect on symptoms, exercise performance, or ejection fraction (in more than just the short term) and may be associated with significant complications.[118] Routine clinical use of immunosuppressive therapy thus cannot be recommended at present.

DUAL CHAMBER PACING. This has been used in some patients with DCM and intact atrioventricular conduction in an attempt to change the sequence of ventricular depolarization, reduce functional mitral regurgitation, and thus improve clinical status; some symptomatic and hemodynamic improvement has been reported, especially in patients with intraventricular conduction delay or those with disturbed timing of atrioventricular mechanical activation.[119, 120] In a small number of patients followed short term, biventricular or left ventricular pacing appeared to be preferable to traditional right ventricular pacing.[120a] However, the data to date are largely anecdotal and equivocal, and demonstration of long-term benefit is lacking.[109, 121]

SURGICAL TREATMENT. Mitral annuloplasty or replacement of regurgitant valves has been attempted in some patients with DCM and prominent atrioventricular valvular regurgitation. The results of operation are usually less than satisfactory because of the degree of preexisting cardiac dysfunction and damage, although some patients have shown some degree of symptomatic improvement, at least over the intermediate term.[122] In appropriately selected patients, cardiac transplantation (see Chap. 20) may be an attractive alternative to medical therapy, with a 5-year survival rate of about 75 percent. Surgical translocation of the latissimus dorsi muscle to wrap around the heart and augment cardiac performance (dynamic cardiomyoplasty) appears to have benefited some patients who are not otherwise suitable candidates for cardiac transplantation.[53, 123] Excision of part of the left ventricle (partial ventriculotomy) has been proposed as an additional surgical alternative to cardiac transplantation[124]; the lack of a randomized control trial demonstrating efficacy has limited the widespread adoption of the procedure.

ALCOHOLIC CARDIOMYOPATHY

Chronic excessive consumption of alcohol may be associated with congestive heart failure, hypertension, cerebrovascular accidents, arrhythmias, and sudden death; it is the major cause of secondary, nonischemic DCM in the western world and accounts for upward of one third of all cases of DCM.[125] It is estimated that two thirds of the adult population use alcohol to some extent, and more than 10 percent are heavy users.[126] Therefore, it is not surprising that alcoholic cardiomyopathy is a major problem. Ceasing alcohol consumption early in the course of alcoholic cardiomyopathy may halt the progression of or even reverse left ventricular contractile dysfunction, unlike nonalcoholic cardiomyopathy, which often is marked by progressive clinical deterioration.[9, 127]

The consumption of alcohol may result in myocardial damage by three basic mechanisms: (1) a presumed direct toxic effect of alcohol or its metabolites; (2) nutritional effects, most commonly in association with thiamine deficiency that leads to beriberi heart disease (see Chap. 17); and (3) rarely, toxic effects due to additives in the alcoholic beverage (cobalt) (see p. 1759).[9, 128] There had been speculation that alcohol caused myocardial damage only through dietary deficiencies, but it is now clear that alcoholic cardiomyopathy occurs in the absence of nutritional deficiencies.[125, 126, 129]

Typical Oriental beriberi (see Chap. 17) may coexist with alcoholic cardiomyopathy, although it is no longer noted with any frequency.[130] The distinguishing features of each include peripheral vasodilatation and high-output heart failure, often right sided, in the former and reduced contractility with typically left-sided low-output failure in the latter.[125, 130]

Alcohol results in acute as well as chronic depression of myocardial contractility and may produce reversible cardiac dysfunction even when ingested by normal nonalcoholic individuals. What is responsible for the transition from the reversible acute effects to permanent myocardial damage remains unclear.[126]

The precise mechanisms of cardiac depression produced by alcohol are undetermined, but a direct toxic effect on striated muscle is likely (particularly because alcoholics often demonstrate concomitant skeletal myopathy and cardiomyopathy).[125, 126] In acute studies, alcohol and its metabolite acetaldehyde have been shown to interfere with a number of membrane and cellular functions that involve the transport and binding of calcium, mitochondrial respiration, myocardial lipid metabolism, myocardial protein synthesis, and signal transduction.[126] Studies in isolated ferret papillary muscles have shown that ethanol in concentrations similar to those occurring in intoxicated humans depresses myocardial contractility by interfering with excitation-contraction coupling through inhibition of the interaction between calcium and the myofilaments.[126] There are data supporting the role of free radical damage and defects in protein synthesis in the genesis of alcohol-induced myocardial damage.[126] The role that other associated electrolyte imbalances (hypokalemia, hypophosphatemia, hypomagnesemia) may play in alcohol-mediated damage has not been settled.

PATHOLOGY. The gross and microscopic pathological findings are nonspecific and similar to those observed in idiopathic DCM, with interstitial fibrosis, myocytolysis, evidence of small vessel coronary artery disease, and myocyte hypertrophy.[125, 131] Electron microscopy shows enlarged and disorganized mitochondria, with large glycogen-containing vacuoles.[126]

Clinical Manifestations

Alcoholic cardiomyopathy most commonly occurs in men 30 to 55 years of age who have been heavy consumers of whisky, wine, or beer, usually for more than 10 years. Female alcoholics who develop cardiomyopathy appear to have a lower cumulative lifetime dose of alcohol than men.[127] Although alcoholic cardiomyopathy may be observed in the homeless, malnourished, "skid row" alcoholic man, many patients are well-nourished individuals of middle and even upper socioeconomic status without liver disease or peripheral neuropathy. Accordingly, unless a high index of suspicion is maintained, it may be easy to miss a history of alcohol abuse.[132] Persistent questioning of the patient and particularly the relatives of patients with unexplained cardiomegaly or cardiomyopathy is often required to elicit a history of alcoholism.

It is frequently possible to demonstrate mild depression of cardiac function in chronic alcoholics even before cardiac dysfunction becomes clinically manifest. Abnormalities of both systolic function (reduced ejection fraction) and diastolic function (increased myocardial wall stiffness) have been demonstrated in alcoholic patients without cardiac symptoms by a variety of invasive and noninvasive techniques.[132a] Although overt alcoholic liver disease and cardiac involvement usually do not occur together, even cirrhotic patients without signs or symptoms of heart disease have demonstrable evidence of asymptomatic myocardial disease.

The development of symptoms may be insidious, although some patients have acute and florid left-sided congestive heart failure. A paroxysm of atrial fibrillation is a relatively frequent initial presenting finding. More advanced cases demonstrate findings of biventricular failure, with left ventricular dysfunction usually dominating. Dyspnea, orthopnea, and paroxysmal nocturnal dyspnea frequently are observed. Palpitations may be present and usually are due to supraventricular tachyarrhythmias. Syncope may be seen as well and may be the result of supraventricular, or more likely ventricular, tachyarrhythmias. Angina pectoris does not occur unless there is concomitant coronary artery disease or aortic stenosis, although atypical chest pain may be seen.

PHYSICAL EXAMINATION. The cardiac findings resemble those seen in idiopathic DCM (see p. 1756). Examination usually reveals a narrow pulse pressure, often with an elevated diastolic pressure secondary to excessive peripheral vasoconstriction. There is cardiomegaly, and protodiastolic (S_3) and presystolic (S_4) gallop sounds are common. An apical systolic murmur of mitral regurgitation often is found. The severity of right-sided heart failure varies, but jugular venous distention and peripheral edema are common. A concomitant skeletal muscle myopathy involving the shoulder and pelvic girdle is a frequent finding, and the degree of muscle weakness and histological abnormality in the skeletal muscles parallels that in the heart.[125]

LABORATORY EXAMINATION. The chest roentgenogram in advanced cases demonstrates considerable cardiac enlargement, pulmonary congestion, and pulmonary venous hypertension (see Chap. 8). Pleural effusions often are seen. ECG abnormalities are common and frequently are the only indication of alcoholic heart disease during the preclinical phase. Alcoholic patients without other evidence of heart disease often are seen after developing palpitations, chest discomfort, or syncope, typically after a binge of alcohol consumption on a weekend, particularly during the year-end holiday season. This is dubbed the "holiday heart syndrome." The most common arrhythmia observed is atrial fibrillation, followed by atrial flutter and frequent ventricular premature contractions. Alcohol consumption may predispose to atrial flutter or fibrillation, even in nonalcoholics. Hypokalemia may play a role in the genesis of some of these arrhythmias. Supraventricular arrhythmias are also frequently observed in patients with overt alcoholic cardiomyopathy. Sudden unexpected death is not uncommon in young adult alcoholics, and it is likely that ventricular fibrillation is responsible.

Atrioventricular conduction disturbances (most commonly first-degree heart block), bundle branch block, left ventricular hypertrophy, poor R wave progression across the precordium, and repolarization abnormalities are common ECG findings. Prolongation of the QT interval is noted frequently. ST segment and T wave changes are often restored to normal within several days after cessation of alcohol consumption.

The hemodynamic findings observed at cardiac catheterization and the assessment of left ventricular function by noninvasive methods (echocardiography and isotope angiography) resemble those found in idiopathic DCM.

MANAGEMENT. The natural history of alcoholic cardiomyopathy depends on the drinking habits of the patient. Total abstinence in the early stages of the disease may lead to resolution of the manifestations of congestive heart failure and a return of heart size toward normal, although patients with severe heart failure may show no improvement in function or prognosis.[9, 133] Continued alcohol consumption leads to further myocardial damage and fibrosis, with the development of refractory congestive heart failure. Death may be due to arrhythmia, heart block, or systemic or pulmonary embolism, in addition to myocardial failure.

The key to the long-term treatment of alcoholic cardiomyopathy is immediate and total abstinence as early in the course of the disease as possible. This may be quite effective in improving the signs and symptoms of congestive heart failure.[133] The reversibility of alcoholic myocardial depression is supported by the demonstration of a reduction of myocardial uptake of labeled monoclonal antimyosin antibodies (a marker of myocyte damage) in alcoholics who stop drinking.[82] The prognosis in patients who continue to drink is poor, particularly if they have been symptomatic for a long time. Prolonged bed rest is thought to result in functional improvement, although its major benefit may simply be the decreased alcohol consumption.

The management of acute episodes of congestive heart failure is similar to that of idiopathic DCM (see p. 1757). For patients with severe congestive heart failure, it is prudent to administer thiamine on the chance that beriberi may be contributing to the heart failure.[130] Whether to use chronic anticoagulation (as is often considered in idiopathic DCM) is a difficult question; we usually do not prescribe warfarin unless there are unequivocal and pressing indications because of the risk of bleeding due to noncompliance, trauma, and over-anticoagulation due to hepatic dysfunction.

COBALT CARDIOMYOPATHY

A previously unrecognized syndrome of severe congestive heart failure appeared in the mid 1960s, first in Canada and subsequently in the United States and Europe.[129] The disease was found in people who drank a particular brand of beer to which cobalt sulfate had been added as a foam stabilizer. Since cobalt was removed from the process, no more cases of the disease have been reported. On very rare occasions occupational exposure to cobalt may result in myocardial damage and attendant congestive heart failure.[129, 134]

ARRHYTHMOGENIC RIGHT VENTRICULAR CARDIOMYOPATHY (See also Chap. 25)

This unique cardiomyopathy (which is also called arrhythmogenic right ventricular dysplasia [ARVD]) is marked by myocardial cell loss with partial or total replacement of right ventricular muscle by adipose and fibrous tissue; apoptosis appears to be a principal cause of the cell death (Fig. 48–6).[135, 136] ARVD is associated with reentrant ventricular tachyarrhythmias of right ventricular origin (producing a left bundle branch block configuration of the QRS complex) and the risk of sudden death.[137, 138] In about one third of the cases there is autosomal dominant inheritance of the disease, and several distinct genetic mutations have been reported.[137, 139] One variant, found on the Greek island

FIGURE 48–6. See color plate 27.

of Naxos, is inherited as a recessive trait but with a high degree of penetrance.[138]

ARVD appears to be distinct from *Uhl disease,* which is marked by extreme thinning of the ventricular wall.[138, 140] The diagnosis is based on a constellation of clinical, ECG, histological, and echocardiographic findings.[137] Typical clinical features include male predominance, normal physical examination, inverted T waves in the right precordial ECG leads, symptoms of palpitations and syncope, and a risk of sudden death.[137, 141, 142] In some patients with ventricular arrhythmias of no evident cause, clinically subtle right ventricular dysplasia may be etiological.[143]

Noninvasive and invasive evaluation demonstrate a dilated, poorly contractile right ventricle, usually with a normal left ventricle, although some degree of left ventricular dysfunction has been seen.[138, 141, 144] Magnetic resonance imaging (MRI) shows promise for identifying patients with this condition.[145] Antiarrhythmic therapy, especially with beta-adrenoceptor blockers, sotalol, or amiodarone, often is effective in controlling the arrhythmias.[140] The arrhythmias may be related to abnormalities of regional right ventricular sympathetic innervation, or impaired presynaptic catecholamine reuptake, as has been demonstrated by noninvasive scintigraphy.[146] Cryo- or catheter-based radiofrequency ablation of the presumed arrhythmogenic focus has been successful in resolving the ventricular arrhythmia in some patients unresponsive to or intolerant of antiarrhythmic drug therapy.[147, 148] Insertion of an ICD or cardiac transplantation is reserved for recalcitrant cases.[140]

Hypertrophic Cardiomyopathy

Although first described over a century ago, the unique features of HCM were not studied systematically until the late 1950s.[148–154] The characteristic finding was inappropriate myocardial hypertrophy that occurred in the absence of an obvious cause for the hypertrophy (e.g., aortic stenosis or systemic hypertension), often predominantly involving the interventricular septum of a nondilated left ventricle that showed hyperdynamic systolic function (Fig. 48–7; see also Fig. 48–13).[152, 153] A distinctive clinical feature was soon recognized in some patients with HCM—a dynamic pressure gradient in the subaortic area that divided the left ventricle into a high-pressure apical region and a lower-pressure subaortic region (Fig. 48–8). Although subsequent

studies have shown that only a minority of patients (perhaps a fourth)[155] demonstrate this outflow gradient, its unique features attracted much attention and led to a myriad of terms (more than 75) used to describe the disease (among the more popular terms were *idiopathic hypertrophic subaortic stenosis [IHSS]* and *muscular subaortic stenosis*).[156] The term *hypertrophic cardiomyopathy* (HCM) is now preferred because most patients do not have an outflow gradient or "stenosis" of the left ventricular outflow tract.[153] Because hypertrophy typically occurs in the absence of a pressure gradient, the characteristic distinguishing feature of HCM is myocardial hypertrophy that is out of proportion to the hemodynamic load.

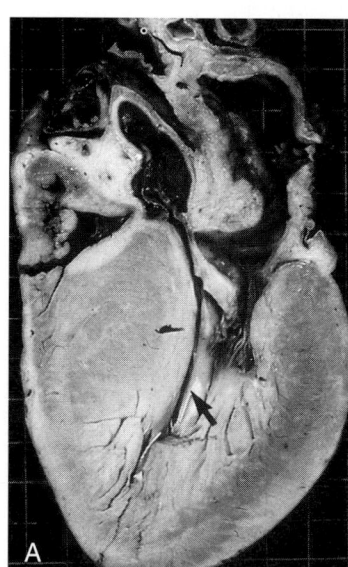

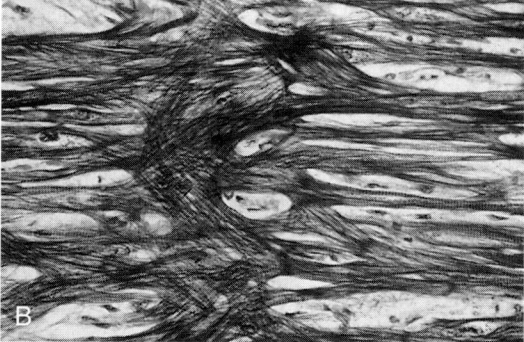

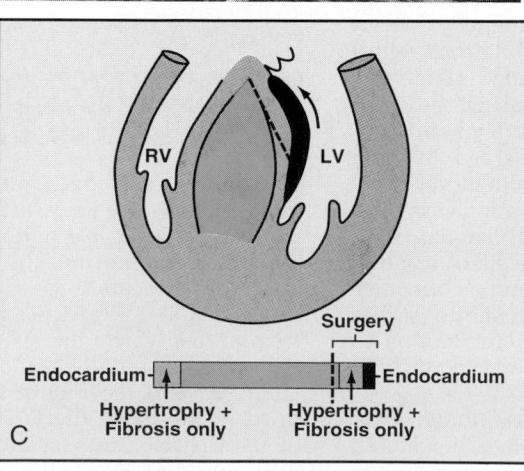

FIGURE 48–7. *A,* Pathological findings in a patient with hypertrophic cardiomyopathy who had a left ventricular outflow tract gradient during life. The heart is opened in the longitudinal plane. This patient had mitral regurgitation that was due partially to abnormal insertion of an anomalous papillary muscle (arrow) onto the ventricular surface of the anterior mitral leaflet. (Modified from Wigle ED, Sasson Z, Henderson MA, et al: Hypertrophic cardiomyopathy: The importance of the site and the extent of hypertrophy. A review. Prog Cardiovasc Dis 28:1, 1985.) *B,* Histological specimen of a patient with hypertrophic cardiomyopathy showing myofibrillar disarray. In the central area the myofibrils cross each other in a disorganized manner, but in adjacent areas on each side the appearance is more normal, with parallel arrays of myofibrils. (PTHA stain, 240×.) (From Davies MJ, McKenna WJ: Hypertrophic cardiomyopathy: An introduction to pathology and pathogenesis. Br Heart J 72:S2, 1994.) *C,* Diagrammatic representation showing usual location of myocyte disarray in interventricular septum in hypertrophic cardiomyopathy. This explains why disarray is usually deep or absent in septectomy specimen, and why endomyocardial biopsy (3-mm maximum dimension) is also unlikely to sample a zone of disarray. RV = right ventricle, LV = left ventricle. (From Tazelaar HD, Billingham ME: The surgical pathology of hypertrophic cardiomyopathy. Arch Pathol Lab Med 111:257, 1987.)

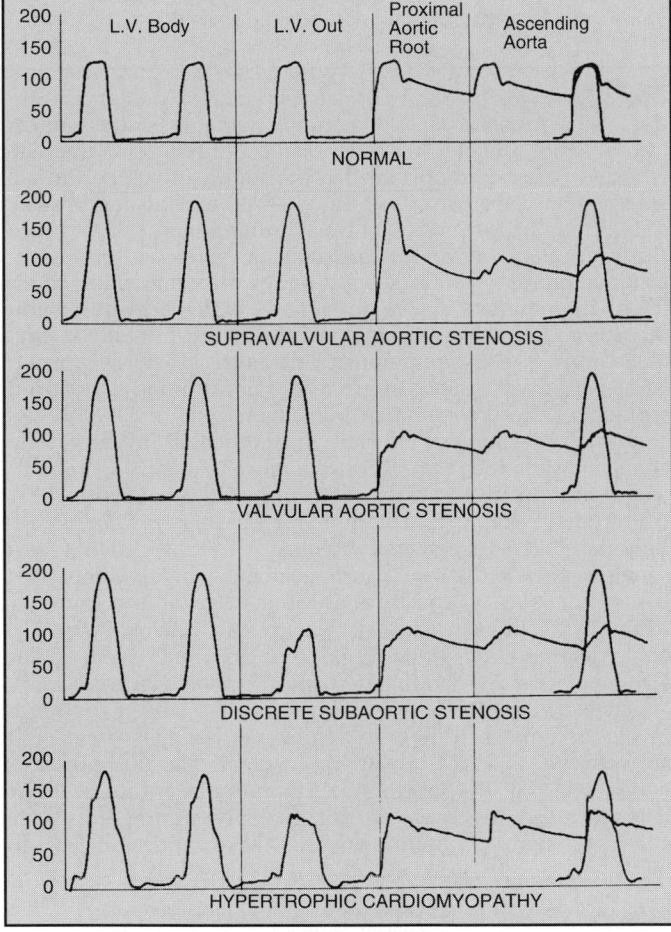

FIGURE 48–8. Left-sided heart pressures in various conditions. In each horizontal panel there is an idealized depiction of the pressure tracing that would be obtained as a catheter is withdrawn from the left ventricular body through the left ventricular outflow tract into the proximal aortic root. On the far right is a superimposition of the pressures in the left ventricular body and in the aorta. The vertical lines bound the regional catheter position within the heart during withdrawal. All forms of discrete stenosis (supravalvular, valvular, and subvalvular) have delayed aortic upstroke rates downstream from the stenosis. Only in hypertrophic cardiomyopathy is the aortic upstroke rate rapid and parallel to the left ventricular pressure. L.V. = left ventricular; Out = outflow tract. (From Criley JM, Siegel RJ: Subaortic stenosis revisited: The importance of the dynamic pressure gradient. Medicine 72:412, 1993.)

MACROSCOPIC EXAMINATION. This typically discloses a marked increase in myocardial mass, and the ventricular cavities are small (see Fig. 48–7A).[157, 158] The left ventricle is usually more involved in the hypertrophic process than is the right. The atria are dilated and often hypertrophied, reflecting the high resistance to filling of the ventricles caused by diastolic dysfunction and the effects of atrioventricular valve regurgitation. The pattern and extent of left ventricular hypertrophy in HCM vary greatly from patient to patient, and a characteristic feature is heterogeneity in the amount of hypertrophy evident in different regions of the left ventricle.[153, 157, 158] A feature found in most patients with HCM is disproportionate involvement of the interventricular septum and anterolateral wall compared with the posterior segment of the free wall of the left ventricle.[153, 157] When hypertrophy is largely localized to the anterior septum, the process has been called asymmetrical septal hypertrophy (ASH). A wide variety of other patterns of hypertrophy may be seen, and about 30 percent of patients show only localized and relatively mild hypertrophy in a single region of the ventricle.[153] The differentiation of the "physiological" hypertrophy that occurs in some highly trained male athletes from that seen in HCM may be difficult; athletes may demonstrate left ventricular wall thicknesses up to 16 mm in the absence of HCM (normal < 12 mm).[159] Additional features that may permit differentiation of the two are the abnormal response of Doppler ultrasound-derived indices of diastolic function in response to isometric handgrip and the identification of HCM in a relative.[153, 160] Some patients with HCM have substantial hypertrophy in unusual locations, such as the posterior portion of the septum, the posterobasal free wall, and the midventricular level.[157]

The degree of hypertrophy is dynamic in most patients; although prominent hypertrophy may be found in infants, the typical patient develops hypertrophy during adolescence.[153] Development of the morphological features of HCM is unusual after the age of about 18 years,[153] although when it occurs it is seen especially with a mutation of cardiac myosin-binding protein C (where hypertrophy may occur at any time during adult life).[161, 162] There usually is an inverse relationship between the extent of hypertrophy

The physiological characteristics of HCM differ substantially from those of DCM (Table 48–5). The most characteristic pathophysiological abnormality in HCM is *diastolic* rather than systolic dysfunction (see Chap. 15). Thus, HCM is characterized by abnormal stiffness of the left ventricle with resultant impaired ventricular filling. This abnormality in diastolic relaxation produces increased left ventricular end-diastolic pressure with resulting pulmonary congestion and dyspnea, the most common symptoms in HCM, despite typically hyperdynamic left ventricular systolic function. The overall prevalence of HCM is low, although probably higher than thought previously; it is found in about 0.2 percent (1 in 500) of the general population and in 0.5 percent of unselected patients referred for an echocardiographic examination.[152] It may be the most common genetically transmitted cardiac disorder.[153]

▼ **TABLE 48–5. DIFFERENCES IN SYSTOLIC AND DIASTOLIC FUNCTION IN DILATED (CONGESTIVE) AND HYPERTROPHIC CARDIOMYOPATHY**

	DILATED CARDIO-MYOPATHY	HYPERTROPHIC CARDIOMYOPATHY
Left ventricular volume		
End-diastolic	Increased	Normal
End-systolic	Markedly increased	Decreased
Left ventricular mass	Increased	Markedly increased
Mass/volume ratio	Decreased	Increased
Systolic function		
Ejection fraction	Decreased	Normal or increased
Myocardial shortening	Decreased	Increased
Wall stress	Increased	Decreased
Diastolic function		
Chamber stiffness	Decreased	Increased
Myocardial stiffness	Increased	Increased

From Chatterjee K: Pathophysiology of cardiomyopathy. *In* Giles TD, Sander GE (eds): Cardiomyopathy. Middleton, MA, PSG Publishing Co, 1988, p 65.

in HCM and age. Whether this is due to premature death of younger patients with greater hypertrophy or progressive reduction in the extent of hypertrophy is unknown.[153, 157]

Other morphological abnormalities include enlargement and elongation of the mitral valve leaflets and anomalous papillary muscle insertion directly into the anterior mitral valve leaflet.[153]

APICAL HCM. A variant with predominant involvement of the apex is common in Japan and is estimated to represent a fourth of Japanese HCM patients.[163] In other parts of the world, apical HCM is much less common. Typical features include a characteristic spadelike configuration of the left ventricle during angiographic study (although some patients with this variant do not demonstrate this abnormality),[164] giant negative T waves in the precordial ECG leads, the absence of an intraventricular pressure gradient, mild symptoms, and a generally benign course (Fig. 48–9).[157, 165]

HCM may on occasion present in the elderly and often demonstrates unique features, including an especially small left ventricular cavity but with relatively mild hypertrophy.[166] Other findings include marked anterior displacement of the mitral valve, extensive submitral (annular) calcification in some patients, a left ventricular outflow gradient, and the late appearance of severe and progressive symptoms.[167]

Gross cardiac morphological features similar to those in HCM may be seen in infants of diabetic mothers and in patients with hyperparathyroidism, neurofibromatosis, generalized lipodystrophy, lentiginosis, pheochromocytoma, Friedreich ataxia, and Noonan syndrome.[168] Rarely, the findings may be simulated by amyloid, glycogen storage disease, or tumor involvement of the septum.[169]

HISTOLOGY. Microscopic findings in HCM are distinc-

FIGURE 48–10. See color plate 28.

tive, with myocardial hypertrophy and gross disorganization of the muscle bundles resulting in a characteristic whorled pattern; abnormalities are found in the cell-to-cell arrangement (disarray) (see Fig. 48–7B) and disorganization of the myofibrillar architecture within a given cell.[157] Fibrosis is usually prominent and may be extensive enough to produce grossly visible scars. Foci of disorganized cells are often interspersed between areas of hypertrophied but otherwise normal-appearing muscle cells. Interstitial (matrix) connective tissue elements are increased.[157] Disarray in HCM patients is found in grossly hypertrophied myocardial segments as well as relatively normal segments.[170] Although abnormally arranged cardiac muscle cells initially were considered specific for HCM, it is now recognized that they may be found in a variety of acquired and congenital heart conditions.[157] What is unique about the disarray in HCM is its ubiquity and frequency. Almost all HCM patients have some degree of disarray, and most have involvement of 5 percent or more of the myocardium; in general, a fourth or more of the myocardium demonstrates disarray.[153] In contrast, disarray in non-HCM patients (when it occurs) usually involves only about 1 percent of the myocardium.[157]

Abnormal intramural coronary arteries, with a reduction in the size of the lumen and thickening of the vessel wall, are common in HCM, occurring in more than 80 percent of patients.[155, 157] The prominence of abnormal intramural coronary arteries in areas of extensive myocardial fibrosis is consistent with the hypothesis that these abnormalities may

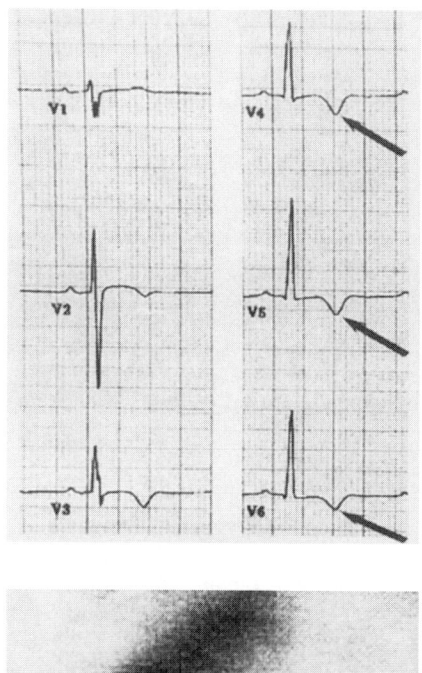
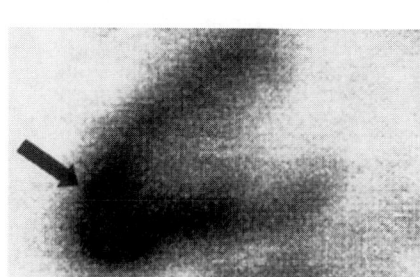
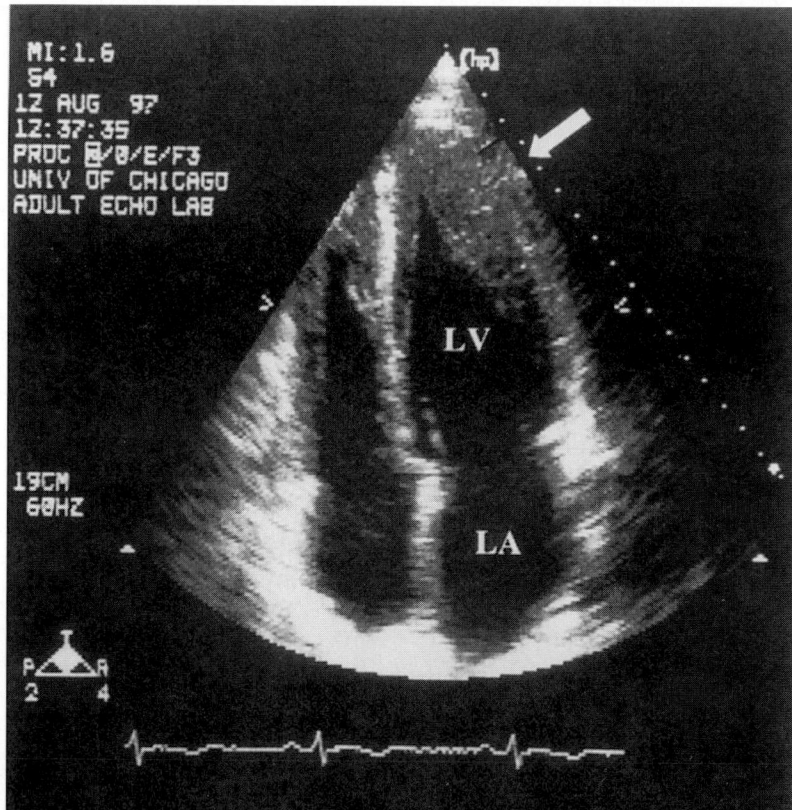

FIGURE 48–9. Findings in apical hypertrophic cardiomyopathy. *Top left,* Electrocardiogram showing prominent T wave inversion (arrows). *Bottom left,* Thallium-201 scan demonstrating increased apical myocardial uptake (arrow). *Right,* Two-dimensional echocardiogram (apical view) showing apical hypertrophy and "ace-of-spades" configuration. LA = left atrium; LV = left ventricle. (From Reddy V, Korcarz C, Weinert L, et al: Apical hypertrophic cardiomyopathy. Circulation 98:2354, 1998. Copyright 1998, American Heart Association.)

be responsible for the development of myocardial ischemia.[153]

Etiology

GENETICS OF HYPERTROPHIC CARDIOMYOPATHY (see also Chap. 56). Familial HCM occurs as an autosomal dominant mendelian-inherited disease at least 50 percent of the time.[166, 171, 172] It is thought that some if not all of the sporadic forms of the disease are due to spontaneous mutations.[171, 173] At least eight different genes, all encoding sarcomeric polypeptides, are associated with HCM (Fig. 48-10). Over 125 different mutations have been discovered thus far. It is clear that not all of the genetic defects have been identified yet.[172] Most of the mutations are of the missense type. Familial HCM thus is a genetically heterogeneous disease (i.e., it can be caused by genetic defects at more than one locus).[174] However, the genetic heterogeneity does *not* appear to explain the clinical variability.

The genetic basis of HCM was first reported in 1989 by Seidman and her collaborators, who reported the existence of a disease gene located on chromosome 14q11-12.[175] Subsequently they found this to be the gene encoding for beta cardiac myosin heavy chain (MHC). Sequencing of this gene in one family with HCM revealed that the abnormality was caused by a gene duplication in which the alpha and beta MHC genes were fused and present in an extra copy. In the second family, there was a point mutation in the beta MHC sequence that altered the myosin's arginine to glutamine. Both of these mutations affect the polypeptides crucial to the structure of myofibrils and might be responsible for the myocyte and myofibrillar disarray characteristic of familial HCM. Other disease loci that have been identified include chromosome 1g3 (encoding troponin T); chromosome 19p13 (encoding troponin I); chromosome 15q2 (encoding alpha-tropomyosin); chromosome 11p11 (encoding myosin-binding protein C); chromosomes 3p21 and 12q23 (encoding essential and regulatory myosin light chains); and chromosome 15q11-14 (encoding actin).[166, 172, 176, 176a] There is an (as yet) unidentified mutation on chromosome 7q3 that has been found in a large Irish family with HCM and the Wolff-Parkinson-White syndrome.[177]

It is estimated that about 30 percent of familial HCM is due to mutations of the cardiac MHC gene, 15 percent is caused by mutations of the cardiac troponin T gene, less than 3 percent is due to mutations of the tropomyosin gene, and the remainder is due to mutations of other genes.[178] It now appears that HCM is genetically transmitted in most patients as an autosomal dominant trait with disease loci on one of at least eight different chromosomes (chromosomes 1, 3, 7, 11, 12, 14, 15, and 19).[166] The cause of HCM in the remainder of patients is unknown. Morphological evidence of the disease is found in about one fourth of the first-degree relatives of a patient with HCM; in many of the relatives the disease is milder than in the propositus, the degree of hypertrophy is less and is more localized, and outflow gradients usually are lacking. Symptoms often are absent or minimal, and the disease is detected only by echocardiography.

Thus, there is wide variation in the phenotypical expression of a specific mutation of a given gene, with variability in clinical symptoms and the degree as well as time course of appearance of hypertrophy.[179-181] Of particular interest are mutations of the troponin T gene that typically result in only modest (or no) hypertrophy but indicate a poor prognosis and a high risk of sudden death (although at least one mutation has a favorable prognosis).[166, 178, 182] Conversely, certain genes and mutations are associated with more favorable prognoses (Fig. 48-11).[183, 184] In some patients with an abnormal gene and no echocardiographic evidence of HCM, the ECG is abnormal. Therefore, otherwise unexplained abnormalities of the ECG in first-degree relatives of patients with HCM may be indicative of a carrier or preclinical state. Unfortunately, genetic testing is not yet easily available for routine clinical use and remains largely a research tool.

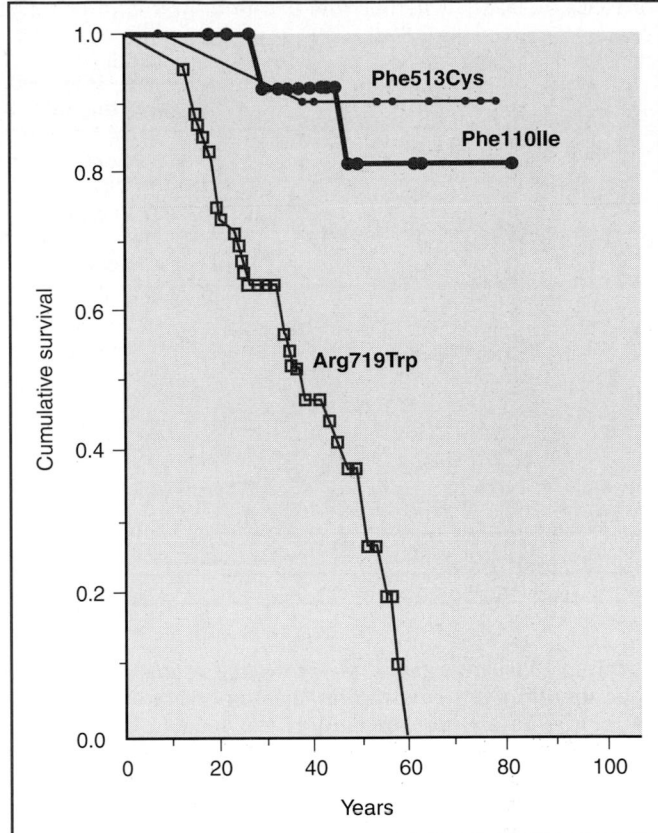

FIGURE 48-11. Kaplan-Meier product-limit curves for survival of individuals with hypertrophic cardiomyopathy and three gene mutations. Survival was good in patients with Phe110Ile mutation in the troponin T gene and similar to that for benign Phe513Cys beta-cardiac myosin heavy chain gene mutation. A significant difference ($p = 0.0002$) in the life expectancy was observed in individuals with Phe110Ile versus malignant Arg719Trp mutation in the beta-cardiac myosin heavy chain gene. (From Anan R, Shono H, Kisanuki A: Patients with familial hypertrophic cardiomyopathy caused by a Phe110Ile missense mutation in the cardiac troponin T gene have variable cardiac morphologies and a favorable prognosis. Circulation 98:391, 1998. Copyright 1998, American Heart Association.)

Pathophysiology

SYSTOLE. Since the initial descriptions of HCM, the feature that has attracted the greatest attention is the dynamic pressure gradient across the left ventricular outflow tract (Figs. 48-8 and 48-12). Although this pressure gradient was initially attributed to a muscular sphincter action in the subaortic region or was believed by some to be an artifact,[156] it is now considered to be related to further narrowing of an already small outflow tract (narrowed by the prominent septal hypertrophy and possibly abnormal location of the mitral valve) by systolic anterior motion of often elongated mitral valve leaflets against the hypertrophied septum.[154, 157]

There continues to be considerable controversy about the cause and significance of the outflow gradient.[156, 185] Central to the disagreement is whether there is true obstruction to left ventricular ejection or whether the pressure gradient is simply the consequence of vigorous ventricular

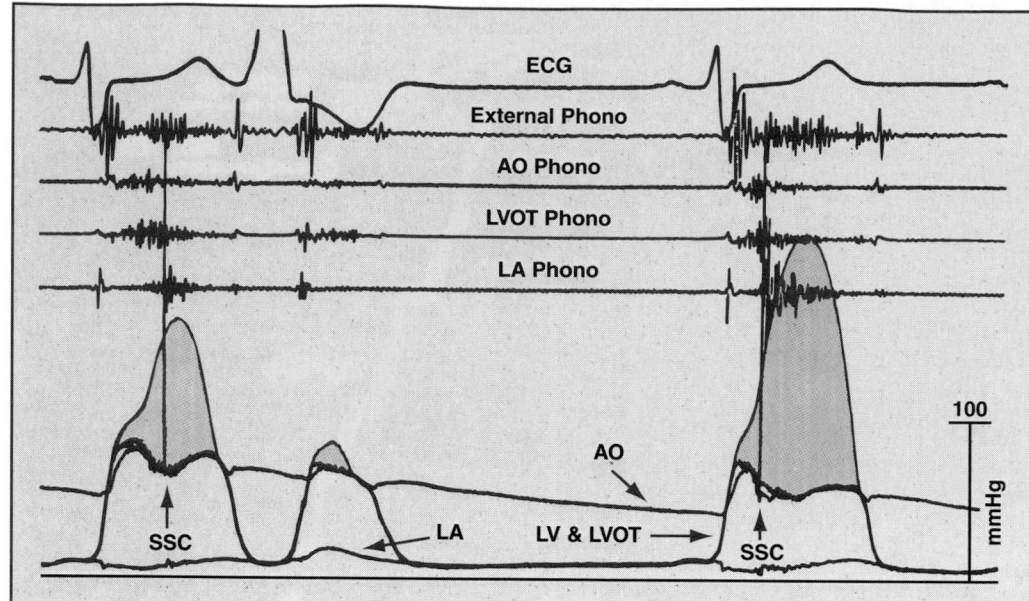

FIGURE 48–12. Hypertrophic cardiomyopathy with intracardiac pressure and phonocardiographic (phono) recordings from aorta (AO), left ventricle (LV), left ventricular outflow tract (LVOT), and left atrium (LA). Note the marked accentuation of the murmur and gradient (shaded) (in the third cycle) after a premature ventricular contraction with failure of the aortic pulse pressure to rise in the post premature ventricular contraction beat (Brockenbrough-Braunwald sign). ECG = electrocardiogram; SSC = systolic anterior motion of the mitral valve septal contact. (From Murgo JP: Systolic ejection murmurs in the era of modern cardiology: What do we really know? J Am Coll Cardiol 32:1596, 1998.)

emptying. Most now favor the view that a true mechanical impediment to left ventricular ejection occurs when outflow gradients are present and is the result of distal portions of the mitral valve apparatus moving anteriorly across the outflow tract and contacting the ventricular septum in mid systole.[153] It is likely that the mitral valve is displaced anteriorly because of Venturi effects and as a result of the increased ejection velocities produced by the abnormal left ventricular outflow tract orientation and geometry.[185]

DIASTOLE. Most patients with HCM demonstrate abnormalities of diastolic function (see Chap. 15) at rest or with stress, whether or not a pressure gradient is present and whether or not they are symptomatic.[160, 186] These abnormalities of global diastolic filling are largely independent of the extent and distribution of myocardial hypertrophy; patients with mild and apparently localized hypertrophy may demonstrate prominent diastolic dysfunction, suggesting that the myopathic process occurs in ventricular regions that are not macroscopically hypertrophied.[163] Others have found that diastolic filling varies in different regions of the left ventricle and is influenced by the thickness of the septum.[187] Diastolic dysfunction in turn leads to increased filling pressure despite a normal or small left ventricular cavity and appears to result from abnormalities of left ventricular relaxation and distensibility. Early diastolic filling is impaired when relaxation is prolonged, perhaps related to abnormal calcium kinetics, subendocardial ischemia, or the abnormal loading conditions found in HCM.[188] Late diastolic filling is altered when left ventricular distensibility is impaired; as a consequence, filling pressures rise. HCM may cause abnormal distensibility of the ventricle because of fibrosis or cellular disorganization.[189]

MYOCARDIAL ISCHEMIA. Myocardial ischemia is common and multifactorial in HCM (Table 48–6).[190] Major

causes include impaired vasodilator reserve (perhaps related to the thickened and narrowed small intramural coronary arteries found in HCM)[191]; increased oxygen demand, especially in patients with outflow gradients; and elevated filling pressures with resultant subendocardial ischemia.[157, 190, 192–194] In children, compression of intramyocardial segments of the left anterior descending coronary artery (so-called myocardial bridge) may predispose to myocardial ischemia and sudden death.[195]

Clinical Manifestations

SYMPTOMS. The majority of patients with HCM are asymptomatic or only mildly symptomatic[152] and often are identified during screening of relatives of a patient with HCM. Unfortunately, the first clinical manifestation of the disease in such individuals may be sudden death. The disease is identified most often in adults in their 30s and 40s; it occurs more often than is commonly suspected in elderly patients. The condition has been observed at necropsy in stillborns and both clinically and pathologically in octogenarians. The importance of recognizing this disorder in children at the earliest possible time is highlighted by the higher mortality rate in younger patients; death is often sudden and unexpected. When HCM is first diagnosed in older patients, several features are distinctive and are in contrast to findings in younger patients: generally mild degrees of left ventricular hypertrophy; frequent demonstration of outflow gradients; and appearance of marked symptoms late in life (typically after age 55).[167] A particularly high index of suspicion of this condition must be maintained to make the clinical diagnosis in the elderly because their symptoms may easily be confused with those due to coronary artery or aortic valve disease. Because syncope and sudden death have been associated with competitive sports and severe exertion in patients with HCM, it is important to diagnose this condition so that these activities may be proscribed. The disease is slightly more common in men, although women may be more likely to be severely disabled and may initially present at a younger age than men.[196]

The clinical picture varies considerably, ranging from the asymptomatic relative of a patient with recognized HCM who has a slightly abnormal echocardiogram but no other overt manifestation of the disease to the patient with incapacitating symptoms. A general relationship exists be-

▼ **TABLE 48–6. PROPOSED CAUSES OF ISCHEMIA IN HYPERTROPHIC CARDIOMYOPATHY DESPITE NORMAL EPICARDIAL CORONARY ARTERIES**

Increased muscle mass
Inadequate capillary density
Elevated diastolic filling pressures
Abnormal intramural coronary arteries
Impaired vasodilatory reserve
Systolic compression of arteries
Enhanced myocardial oxygen demand (increased wall stress)

tween the extent of hypertrophy and the severity of symptoms, but the relationship is not absolute, and some patients have severe symptoms with only mild and apparently localized hypertrophy, and vice versa.[157] A complex interaction occurs between left ventricular hypertrophy, the left ventricular pressure gradient, diastolic dysfunction, and myocardial ischemia, which accounts for the great variability in symptoms from patient to patient.

The most common symptom is *dyspnea,* occurring in up to 90 percent of symptomatic patients, which is largely a consequence of the elevated left ventricular diastolic (and therefore left atrial and pulmonary venous) pressure, which results principally from impaired ventricular filling owing to diastolic dysfunction.[157] Angina pectoris (found in about three fourths of symptomatic patients), fatigue, presyncope, and syncope are also common. Palpitations, paroxysmal nocturnal dyspnea, overt congestive heart failure, and dizziness are found less frequently, although severe congestive heart failure culminating in death may be seen. Exertion tends to exacerbate many of the symptoms.[197] A variety of mechanisms may contribute to the production of angina pectoris (see Table 48-6). It is at least in part the result of an imbalance between oxygen supply and demand as a consequence of the greatly increased myocardial mass. Abnormalities of the small coronary arteries may contribute to myocardial ischemia, particularly during exertion, and perhaps 20 percent of older patients with HCM may have concurrent atheromatous obstructive coronary artery disease. Transmural infarction may occur in the absence of narrowing of the extramural coronary arteries.[157] Impaired diastolic relaxation may produce subendocardial ischemia as a result of prolonged maintenance of wall tension with a concomitant slower-than-normal decrease in the impedance to coronary blood flow. Syncope may result from inadequate cardiac output with exertion or from cardiac arrhythmias. It occurs most commonly in young patients with small left ventricular chamber size and evidence of ventricular tachycardia on ambulatory monitoring.[198] Near-syncopal ("graying out") spells that occur in the erect posture and that can be relieved by immediately lying down are common. However, in contrast to valvular aortic stenosis, syncope or near-syncope may not be an ominous finding in adult patients with HCM; some patients have a history of such episodes dating back many years without clinical deterioration.[152] In children and adolescents, however, presyncope and syncope identify patients at increased risk of sudden death (see Natural History).

PHYSICAL EXAMINATION. This may be normal in asymptomatic patients without gradients, particularly those with the apical variant of HCM, save for a left ventricular lift and a loud S_4, but findings are usually prominent in patients with a left ventricular outflow tract pressure gradient. The apical precordial impulse is often displaced laterally and is usually abnormally forceful and diffuse.[196] Because of decreased left ventricular compliance, a prominent presystolic apical impulse that results from forceful atrial systole often is present. This may result in a double apical impulse as a result of the prominent *a* wave.[154] A more characteristic but less frequently recognized abnormality is a triple apical beat, the third impulse consisting of a late systolic bulge that occurs when the heart is almost empty and is performing near-isometric contraction.[196] The jugular venous pulse may demonstrate a prominent *a* wave, reflecting diminished right ventricular compliance secondary to massive hypertrophy of the ventricular septum.[159] The carotid pulse typically rises briskly and then declines in midsystole as the gradient develops, followed by a secondary rise.[196] This may be appreciated on physical examination but can be demonstrated more clearly by means of indirect carotid pulse tracings.

Auscultation. The S_1 is normal and is often preceded by an S_4 that corresponds to the apical presystolic im-

pulse.[196] The S_2 usually is normally split. In some patients, however, it is narrowly split and in others, particularly those with severe outflow gradients, paradoxical splitting may be noted.[154] An S_3 may be present but does not have the same ominous significance as in patients with valvular aortic stenosis. Systolic ejection sounds relating to rapid acceleration of blood flow may be found on occasion. The auscultatory hallmark of HCM associated with an outflow gradient is a systolic murmur that typically is harsh and crescendo-decrescendo in configuration (Fig. 4-46); it usually commences well after S_1 and is best heard between the apex and the left sternal border.[196] It often radiates well to the lower sternal border, the axillae, and base of the heart but not into the neck vessels. In patients with large gradients, the murmur usually reflects both left ventricular outflow tract turbulence and concomitant mitral regurgitation.[154] Accordingly, the murmur is often more holosystolic and blowing at the apex and in the axillae (due to mitral regurgitation) and midsystolic and harsher along the lower sternal border (due to turbulent flow across the narrowed outflow tract).[196]

The systolic murmur is labile in intensity and duration, and a variety of maneuvers may be used to augment or suppress it (Table 48-7).[154] A diastolic rumbling murmur, reflecting increased transmitral flow, may occur in patients with marked mitral regurgitation. The murmur of aortic regurgitation is observed in about 10 percent of patients, although mild aortic regurgitation can be demonstrated by Doppler echocardiography in one third.[199] It may develop after operation to correct the outflow gradient or following infective endocarditis.

Differentiation from Valvular Aortic Stenosis. It is important to emphasize the features of physical examination that permit differentiation of HCM from fixed orifice obstruction, most commonly due to valvular aortic stenosis (see Chap. 46). The character of the carotid pulse and features of the murmur are most useful in this regard. Because there is obstruction to left ventricular emptying from the

▼ TABLE 48-7. EFFECTS OF INTERVENTIONS ON OUTFLOW GRADIENT AND SYSTOLIC MURMUR IN HYPERTROPHIC CARDIOMYOPATHY

	CONTRACTILITY	PRELOAD	AFTER-LOAD
Increase in Gradient and Murmur			
Valsalva maneuver (during strain)	—	↓	↓
Standing	—	↓	—
Postextrasystole	↑	↑	—
Isoproterenol	↑	↓	↓
Digitalis	↑	↓	—
Amyl nitrite	— then ↑	↓ then ↑	↓
Nitroglycerin	—	↓	↓
Exercise	↑	↓	↑
Tachycardia	↑	↓	—
Hypovolemia	↑	↓	↓
Decrease in Gradient and Murmur			
Mueller maneuver	—	↑	↑
Valsalva overshoot	—	↑	↑
Squatting	—	↑	↑
Alpha-adrenoceptor stimulation (phenylephrine)	—	—	↑
Beta-adrenoceptor blockade	↓	↑	—
General anesthesia	↓	—	—
Isometric handgrip	—	—	↑

↑ = increase; ↓ = decrease; — = no major change.

beginning of systole with fixed valvular stenosis, the carotid upstroke is slowed and of low amplitude (pulsus parvus et tardus).[200] With HCM, initial ejection of blood from the left ventricle is actually enhanced, and therefore the arterial upstroke is brisk. The murmur of HCM, as opposed to that of aortic stenosis, can be reliably identified by its increase with the Valsalva maneuver and during standing from a squatting position, and its decrease during squatting from a standing position, passive leg elevation, and hand grip (see Table 48–7).[196] Other features that may be helpful but are of considerably less significance are the location of the murmur (it radiates along the carotid arteries in valvular aortic stenosis but not in HCM) and the location of the systolic thrill when present (most prominent in the second right intercostal space in valvular aortic stenosis and in the fourth interspace along the left sternal border in HCM).

ELECTROCARDIOGRAM. This is usually abnormal in HCM[201] and invariably so in symptomatic patients with left ventricular outflow tract gradients.[157] Entirely normal ECGs are seen in only 15 to 25 percent of patients and usually are found in the presence of only localized left ventricular hypertrophy.[202] The most common abnormalities are ST segment and T wave abnormalities, followed by evidence of left ventricular hypertrophy, with QRS complexes that are tallest in the midprecordial leads.[157] Progressive ECG evidence of hypertrophy may develop over time. Giant negative T waves in the midprecordial leads of Japanese patients are characteristic of HCM involving the apex[203] (see p. 1762), but such a pattern may be found in whites with HCM involving segments other than the apex. Prominent Q waves are relatively common, occurring in 20 to 50 percent of patients. The Q wave abnormalities often involve the inferior (II, III, aV_F) and/or precordial (V_2–V_6) leads. The cause of the Q waves remains unestablished; although they do not correlate simply with the degree of septal hypertrophy,[157] they may relate to the balance of electrical forces emanating from the left versus the right ventricle.[154] A variety of other ECG abnormalities may occur, including abnormal electrical axis (usually left-axis deviation) and P wave abnormalities (usually left atrial abnormality). Accessory atrioventricular pathways have been found in HCM, although they are uncommon.[204] Clinically significant abnormalities of atrioventricular conduction are uncommon but may cause syncope.[205]

ARRHYTHMIAS. Although hemodynamic or ischemic mechanisms may play roles in the death of patients with HCM (particularly the young),[206] many deaths, particularly those that are known to have been sudden, likely are due to an arrhythmia.[207, 208] Because of the systolic and diastolic abnormalities in this disorder, rhythm disturbances are less well tolerated.

Ventricular arrhythmias are common in patients with HCM, occurring in more than three fourths of patients undergoing continuous ambulatory ECG monitoring. Runs of nonsustained ventricular tachycardia are found in about one fourth of patients with HCM, although sustained monomorphic tachycardia is uncommon.[207] In some it is a harbinger of subsequent sudden death; however, its overall predictive value in identifying patients at high risk for sudden death is limited. Treadmill testing may expose arrhythmias that are not present at rest, although continuous ambulatory monitoring is superior in detecting repetitive ventricular tachyarrhythmias.

Supraventricular tachycardia may be found in one fourth to one half of patients.[207] Atrial fibrillation occurs in about 10 percent of patients (often those with no gradient and mild hypertrophy), and the resultant loss of the atrial contribution to the filling of a hypertrophied, stiff ventricle may result in clinical deterioration.[157, 209] Treatment is often effective in controlling symptoms and restoring sinus rhythm; if this is done, long-term survival usually is not jeopardized.[210] The signal-averaged ECG has not proved to be helpful in identifying patients at increased risk of sustained or lethal ventricular arrhythmia, although additional studies are necessary.[211] Reduced heart rate variability on ambulatory monitor recordings, a predictor of increased sudden death risk after myocardial infarction, appears to be less useful in risk stratification in HCM patients.[212]

ELECTROPHYSIOLOGICAL TESTING. The role of electrophysiological studies in identifying HCM patients at increased risk of sudden death is controversial; despite earlier enthusiasm, it is now generally believed that it is of limited predictive value.[152, 157] These studies may identify a variety of abnormalities in HCM patients; they induce polymorphic ventricular tachycardia in many patients with HCM, but such a response is generally believed to be nonspecific and does not identify high-risk patients.[152] Unfortunately, unlike its utility in ischemic heart disease, the predictive value of the more typical inducible sustained ventricular arrhythmias during electrophysiological testing is low in HCM. Aggressive stimulation protocols are required to induce a sustained arrhythmia in high-risk HCM patients, often resulting in arrhythmias in low-risk patients as well.[208] Tilt-table testing has not been particularly useful in identifying the cause of syncope in HCM; neurally mediated syncope is uncommon in this setting and true positive tests are uncommon, but false-positive tests are frequent and significantly limit the usefulness of the test.[213]

CHEST ROENTGENOGRAM. The findings on radiographic examination are variable; the cardiac silhouette may range from normal to markedly increased, and in most cases of apparent "cardiomegaly" the enlarged cardiac silhouette is the result of left ventricular hypertrophy and/or left atrial enlargement.[157] Left atrial enlargement is observed frequently, especially when significant mitral regurgitation is present.[154] Aortic root enlargement and valvular calcification are not seen unless associated diseases are present, although calcification of the mitral annulus is common in HCM.

ECHOCARDIOGRAPHY. Because echocardiography combines the attributes of high resolution and no known risk, it has been widely used in the evaluation of HCM. It is useful in the study of patients with suspected HCM and also in the screening of relatives of HCM patients. The echocardiogram is of value in identifying and quantifying morphological features (i.e., distribution of septal hypertrophy), functional aspects (e.g., hypercontractile left ventricle), and (when combined with Doppler recordings) hemodynamic findings (e.g., magnitude of outflow gradient). (See Figs. 7–99, 7–100, and 7–101.)

Left Ventricular Hypertrophy. The cardinal echocardiographic feature of HCM is left ventricular hypertrophy. Although the characteristic feature is hypertrophy of the septum and anterolateral free wall, the echocardiogram is useful in identifying involvement of other left ventricular locations, including portions of the free wall and the apex.[157, 170, 214] Considerable variability exists in the degree and pattern of hypertrophy; in most patients, there is variation in the extent of hypertrophy from one left ventricular region to another.[157] Maximal hypertrophy of the septum often occurs midway between the base and apex of the left ventricle. The finding of a thickened septum that is at least 1.3 to 1.5 times the thickness of the posterior wall when measured in diastole just before atrial systole has been the time-honored criterion for the diagnosis of ASH. The septum not only is relatively thicker than the posterior wall but is typically at least 15 mm in thickness (normal 11 mm). Although the average wall thickness detected on echocardiography is about 20 mm (i.e., almost twice normal), there is great variation, ranging from very mild hypertrophy (13 to 15 mm) to massive hypertrophy (50 mm).[159]

An unusual echocardiographic pattern consisting of a ground-glass appearance has been noted in portions of the hypertrophied myocardium in some patients with HCM. Even when abnormalities are not apparent on visual inspection, quantitative texture analysis often identifies them in both nonhypertrophied (but presumably abnormal) and hypertrophied regions of the ventricle and can be used to distinguish HCM patients from those with secondary hypertrophy.[215] It has been speculated that this pattern may be related to the abnormal cellular architecture and myocardial fibrosis that has been noted in pathological studies.[216]

Outflow Tract Obstruction. A second echocardiographic feature often found in HCM in addition to left ventricular hypertrophy is narrowing of the left ventricular outflow tract, which is formed by the interventricular septum anteriorly and the anterior leaflet of the mitral valve posteriorly. The mitral valve leaflets are abnormally large and elongated and are associated with abnormal left ventricular outflow tract geometry that culminates in the production of a pressure gradient.[214, 217, 218] This abnormal geometry is causally related to the mitral regurgitation that accompanies an outflow gradient; the degree of mitral regurgitation correlates with the extent of anterior and posterior leaflet malcoaptation.[219] When HCM is associated with a pressure gradient, there is abnormal systolic anterior motion of the anterior leaflet, and occasionally the posterior leaflet of the mitral valve.[214] A close relationship exists between the degree of systolic anterior motion and the magnitude of the outflow gradient. Prolonged interventricular septal contact of the mitral apparatus is limited to HCM with resting pressure gradients, and a close temporal relationship exists between the onset of the pressure gradient and the onset of septal apposition of the mitral apparatus.

MECHANISMS OF SYSTOLIC ANTERIOR MOTION. Three explanations have been offered for systolic anterior motion: (1) the mitral valve is *pulled* against the septum by contraction of abnormally oriented papillary muscles and elongated leaflets[220]; (2) the mitral valve is *pushed* against the septum (perhaps by the left ventricular posterior wall) because of its abnormal position in the outflow tract; and (3) the mitral valve is drawn toward the septum because of the lower pressure that occurs as blood is ejected at a high velocity through a narrowed outflow tract (Venturi effect).[221] In a minority of cases (less than 15 percent), one or both papillary muscles insert anomalously directly into the anterior mitral leaflet, causing a long area of midventricular narrowing that results in an intraventricular pressure gradient.

Systolic anterior motion of the mitral valve and dynamic left ventricular gradients are not pathognomonic of HCM but may be found in a variety of other conditions, including hypercontractile states, left ventricular hypertrophy, transposition of the great arteries, and infiltration of the septum. Even mild degrees of left ventricular hypertrophy may be associated with systolic anterior motion and outflow gradients, particularly under conditions of enhanced sympathetic tone. In many cases in conditions other than HCM, systolic anterior motion is due to buckling of the chordae tendineae rather than to movement of the anterior mitral valve leaflet as occurs in HCM (although the chordae tendineae and papillary muscles may contribute to systolic anterior motion in HCM).

Other Echocardiographic Findings. The following may be present: (1) a small left ventricular cavity; (2) reduced septal motion and thickening during systole, particularly of the upper septum (presumably because of the disarray of the myofibrillar architecture and abnormal contractile function)[222]; (3) normal or increased motion of the posterior wall; (4) a reduced rate of closure of the mitral valve in mid diastole secondary to a decrease in left ventricular compliance or abnormal transmittal diastolic flow; (5) mitral valve prolapse; and (6) partial systolic closure or, more commonly, coarse systolic fluttering of the aortic valve related to turbulent blood flow in the outflow tract. MRI studies have shown that regional left ventricular function and the degree of local hypertrophy are inversely related and the hypertrophied septum typically is hypokinetic.[222, 223] The echocardiographic findings that accompany a left ventricular outflow tract gradient (systolic anterior motion and aortic valve partial closure) may be quite labile, and provocative measures such as the Valsalva maneuver, pharmacologically induced vasodilatation with amyl nitrite, stimulation of contractility with isoproterenol, or an induced premature ventricular contraction may be required to precipitate the findings.[150, 224] Abnormalities of diastolic function (see Chap. 15) may be demonstrated by echocardiography and Doppler recordings in about 80 percent of patients with HCM, independent of the presence or absence of a systolic pressure gradi-

ent.[157] Because the septum typically is hypokinetic, the rate of left ventricular filling is determined primarily by the rate of free wall thinning. Little relationship exists between the extent of hypertrophy and the severity of abnormalities of diastolic function. Doppler ultrasonography has confirmed the virtual ubiquity of mitral regurgitation when an outflow pressure gradient is present[157] and has accurately measured the magnitude of the outflow tract gradient.[155] Doppler color flow imaging reveals mitral regurgitation, most prominent in late systole, accompanying the appearance of turbulent flow in the left ventricular outflow tract. Recordings from the left ventricular outflow tract support the concept that true obstruction to flow occurs and accounts for the pressure gradient.[155]

RADIONUCLIDE SCANNING. Thallium-201 myocardial imaging, particularly when tomographic imaging (single-photon emission computed tomography [SPECT]) is performed (see Chap. 9), permits direct determination of the relative thicknesses of the septum and free wall and may be of particular value when technical constraints limit the reliability of echocardiographic evaluation in a given patient with presumed HCM. Reversible thallium defects, presumably indicative of ischemia, are common findings in HCM in the absence of obstructive coronary artery disease.[225] They are common in adult patients with HCM and in those young patients with a history of sudden death or syncope, suggesting that myocardial ischemia is an important factor and probably a mechanism of demise in younger patients.[226] Fixed defects, probably indicative of myocardial scarring, occur primarily in patients with impaired systolic function. Gated radionuclide ventriculography with blood pool labeling permits the evaluation of not only the size but also the motion of the septum and left ventricle. As with the echocardiogram, abnormal diastolic filling of the ventricle has been observed in patients with HCM (both with and without gradients) by computer analysis of the blood pool scan.[227] Because of the ease and availability of transthoracic and transesophageal echocardiography, this technique is not widely used in the evaluation of HCM.

Hemodynamics and Angiography

CARDIAC CATHETERIZATION. Heart catheterization is not required for the diagnosis of HCM, because noninvasive evaluation almost always suffices; it is reserved for situations where concomitant coronary artery disease is a consideration, or when invasive modalities of therapy (e.g., pacemaker, surgery) are being considered.[154] It discloses diminished diastolic left ventricular compliance and in some patients a systolic pressure gradient within the body of the left ventricle (see Fig. 48–8), which is separated from a subaortic chamber by the thickened septum and the anterior leaflet of the mitral valve that abuts the septum (see Fig. 48–12).[155] The pressure gradient may be quite labile and may vary between 0 and 175 mm Hg in the same patient under different conditions (see later). The arterial pressure tracing may demonstrate a "spike and dome" configuration similar to the carotid pulse recording.[155] As a consequence of diminished left ventricular compliance, the mean and particularly the *a* wave in the left atrial pressure pulse and the left ventricular end-diastolic pressures are usually elevated. Artifactual outflow gradients may occur if the left ventricular catheter becomes entrapped in the trabeculae of a markedly hypertrophied left ventricle.[156] Proper technique and choice of catheters with side holes should clarify the mechanism of such gradients. Cardiac output may be depressed in patients with long-standing severe gradients, but in the majority of patients it is normal; occasionally it is elevated.

Hemodynamic abnormalities in HCM are not limited to the left side of the heart. Approximately one fourth of patients demonstrate pulmonary hypertension, which is usually mild but in some cases may be moderate to severe. This is due (at least in part) to elevated mean left atrial pressures as a consequence of diminished left ventricular compliance. A pressure gradient in the right ventricular outflow tract occurs in approximately 15 percent of patients who have obstruction to left ventricular outflow[196, 228] and appears to result from markedly hypertrophied right ventricular tissue.[229] Right atrial and right ventricular end-diastolic pressures may be slightly elevated.

LABILITY OF GRADIENT. A feature characteristic of HCM is the variability and lability of the left ventricular outflow gradient (see Table 48–7).[149, 150, 230] A given patient may demonstrate a large outflow gradient on one occasion but have none at another time. In some patients without a resting gradient, it may be temporarily provoked. Three basic mechanisms are involved in the production of dynamic gradients, all of which act by reducing ventricular volume and presumably accentuate the apposition of the anterior mitral leaflet against the septum[150]: (1) increased contractility, (2) decreased preload, and (3) decreased afterload. In a minority of patients with HCM, the gradient is midventricular and may be intensified by increased contractility, which exerts a direct muscular sphincter action.[154, 155] The stimuli that provoke or intensify left ventricular outflow tract gradients in HCM generally improve myocardial performance in normal subjects and in patients with most other forms of heart disease. Conversely, reductions in contractility or increases in preload or afterload, which increase left ventricular dimensions, reduce or abolish the left ventricular outflow gradient.

Alterations in the magnitude of the gradient are reflected by changes in the findings on physical examination, noninvasive tests, and left-sided heart catheterization. *This dynamic characteristic of HCM distinguishes it from the discrete forms of obstruction to ventricular outflow.* An increase in the gradient usually results in a louder murmur, a longer ejection period with a more characteristic spike and dome configuration in the carotid pulse, and more flagrant echocardiographic evidence of systolic anterior motion of the anterior mitral leaflet. In some patients, the intensity of the murmur may *not* track with the gradient, perhaps because in many cases the murmur reflects mitral regurgitation (at least in part).[154]

A number of bedside procedures may be useful in the evaluation of suspected HCM.[154] Perhaps the most helpful is sudden standing from a squatting position. Squatting results in an increase in venous return and an increase in aortic pressure, which increases ventricular volume, diminishing the gradient and decreasing the intensity of the murmur. Sudden standing has the opposite effects and results in accentuation of the gradient and the murmur.

VALSALVA MANEUVER. This is another useful bedside technique for eliciting or exacerbating the gradient. After a transient increase in arterial pressure that usually lasts for four or five cardiac cycles after the onset of the strain and coincident with an increase in heart rate, the arterial systolic and pulse pressures and ventricular volume decline and the gradient (and murmur) increases. After release of the strain, a compensatory overshoot of arterial pressure and venous return with cardiac slowing occur, all of which increase ventricular volume and reduce the magnitude of the gradient and the murmur. Occasional patients may show paradoxical attenuation of the systolic murmur despite an increase in the pressure gradient, presumably related to a critical reduction in stroke volume. Inhalation of amyl nitrite also intensifies the murmur and the abnormality of the arterial pulse. The murmur of HCM is attenuated by passive leg elevation, hand grip, and sudden squatting from a standing position.

Postextrasystolic Changes. One of the most potent stimuli for enhancing the gradient is *postextrasystolic potentiation* (see Chap. 14), which may occur after a spontaneous premature contraction or be induced by mechanical stimulation with a catheter.[231] The resultant increase in contractility in the beat after the extrasystole is so marked that it outweighs the otherwise salutary effect of increased ventricular filling caused by the compensatory pause and produces an increase in the gradient and often of the murmur as well. A characteristic change often occurs in the directly recorded arterial pressure tracing, which, in addition to displaying a more marked spike and dome configu-

ration, exhibits a pulse pressure that fails to increase as expected or actually decreases (the so-called Brockenbrough-Braunwald phenomenon) (see Fig. 48–12). This is one of the more reliable signs of dynamic obstruction of the left ventricular outflow tract. In some patients, the postextrasystolic murmur is attenuated despite an increase in the outflow gradient, apparently because in this setting the murmur (a hybrid of outflow tract turbulence and mitral regurgitation) is mirroring to a greater degree changes in the severity of mitral regurgitation rather than changes in the outflow tract gradient.

POSITIVE INOTROPIC AGENTS. Digitalis glycosides and the beta-adrenoceptor agonist isoproterenol augment the gradient because they increase myocardial contractility, whereas nitroglycerin and amyl nitrite exaggerate the gradient by decreasing arterial pressure and ventricular volume. The ingestion of alcoholic beverages may exacerbate the outflow pressure gradient by producing systemic vasodilatation.[232] Hypovolemia (as a result of hemorrhage or overly aggressive diuresis) may also provoke overt obstruction to left ventricular outflow. The intensity of the murmur and the left ventricular outflow gradient may be decreased by beta-adrenoceptor blockade, although the effect of the latter is often not dramatic and is of greatest hemodynamic benefit in protecting against the *increase* in the gradient that may be provoked by exercise. In most patients the severity of mitral regurgitation and the intensity of the apical blowing regurgitant murmur vary with the degree of obstruction of left ventricular outflow.

ANGIOGRAPHY. Left ventriculography shows a hypertrophied ventricle; when an outflow gradient is present, the anterior leaflet of the mitral valve moves anteriorly during systole and encroaches on the outflow tract. Associated with this motion of the leaflet is mitral regurgitation, which is a constant finding in patients with gradients. The left ventricular cavity is often small, and systolic ejection is typically vigorous, resulting in virtual obliteration of the cavity at end systole (Fig. 48–13), although the apparent hypercontractile state may relate more to reduced afterload (low end-systolic wall stress) than to enhanced inotropy. The papillary muscles are often prominent and may fill the left ventricular cavity in late systole. In patients with apical involvement, the extensive hypertrophy may convey a spadelike configuration to the left ventricular angiogram.[165]

It may be helpful to supplement angiographic evaluation of the left ventricle with simultaneous right ventriculography in a cranially angulated left anterior oblique projection to obtain optimal visualization of the size, shape, and configuration of the interventricular septum. The left septal surface either is flat or bulges into the left ventricular cavity at its mid or lower portion, in contrast to the normal findings of the septum curving toward the right ventricle.

In patients older than 45 years of age, obstructive coronary artery disease may be present, although the symptoms of ischemic pain are indistinguishable from those of patients with normal coronary angiograms and HCM. The left anterior descending and septal perforator coronary arteries may demonstrate phasic narrowing and associated abnormalities of flow during systole.[233]

Natural History

The clinical course in HCM is varied; in many patients symptoms are absent or mild, remain stable, and in some instances improve over a period of 5 to 10 years. The annual mortality is about 3 percent in adults seen in large referral centers[234] but probably is closer to 1 percent when all patients with HCM are included.[235–237] The risk of sudden death is higher in children, perhaps as high as 6 percent per year.[171] Clinical deterioration (aside from sudden death) usually is slow. Although symptoms are unrelated to the severity or even the presence of a gradient,[157] the percentage of severely symptomatic patients does increase with age. The onset of atrial fibrillation may lead to an increase in symptoms, although counterintuitively often it appears to be well tolerated.[210] Conversion to sinus rhythm by pharmacological or electrical cardioversion should be

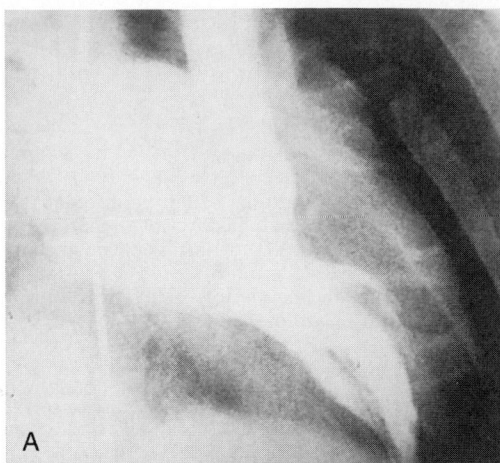

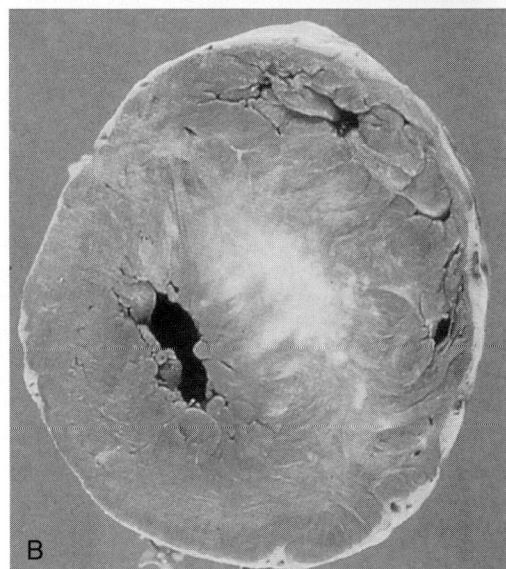

FIGURE 48–13. *A,* Left ventriculogram in the right anterior oblique view showing the typical appearance of hypertrophic cardiomyopathy with a very small end systolic cavity, hypertrophied papillary muscles, and associated severe mitral regurgitation. *B,* Postmortem transverse section through the heart at the level of the ventricles in a case of sudden death in hypertrophic cardiomyopathy. There is marked left ventricular hypertrophy particularly affecting the interventricular septum (approximately 4.5 cm) with associated fibrosis and virtual obliteration of the left and right ventricular cavities. (From Davies MK: Images in cardiology. Hypertrophic cardiomyopathy. Br Heart J 74:527, 1995.)

attempted, although maintenance of sinus rhythm may be difficult.[157] Patients who develop atrial fibrillation ordinarily are started on long-term therapy with oral anticoagulants.

Progression of HCM to left ventricular dilatation and dysfunction without a gradient (i.e., DCM) occurs in 10 to 15 percent of patients.[157, 238] It appears to result, at least in part, from wall thinning and scar formation as a consequence of myocardial ischemia caused by small vessel coronary artery disease and abnormal coronary vasodilator reserve (Fig. 48–14).[157] It is more likely to occur in patients with marked septal hypertrophy and generally is associated with a poor prognosis. The extent of left ventricular hypertrophy in adults usually remains stable over time, although a majority of children demonstrate increasing degrees of hypertrophy (often considerable) and many adults demonstrate a very gradual degree of regression of hypertrophy over time (Fig. 48–15).[239] In some children, the findings of HCM may develop despite a previous normal echocardiogram; this is not common in adults, but it may be seen in

particular with the cardiac myosin-binding protein C mutation.[161, 166] Its occurrence emphasizes that a single normal echocardiogram does *not* exclude HCM in a child or adolescent; cellular disarray and the attendant risk of sudden death may be present even in the absence of left ventricular hypertrophy. A marker for the later appearance of clinical HCM may be an initially abnormal ECG demonstrating increased QRS voltage.

SUDDEN DEATH. Death is most often sudden in HCM and may occur in previously asymptomatic patients, in individuals who were unaware they had the disease, and in patients with an otherwise stable course (Fig. 48–16). There is great difficulty in identifying those patients at particular risk of sudden death[240, 240a]; nevertheless, the features that most reliably identify high-risk patients include young age (< 30 years) at diagnosis, a family history of HCM with sudden death (so-called malignant family history), an abnormal blood pressure response to exercise (presumably related to subendocardial ischemia[241]), and genetic abnormalities associated with increased prevalence of sudden death.[152, 234, 242, 242a] The presence or severity of an outflow tract gradient, the degree of functional limitation, and symptoms in general do not correlate with the risk of death.[208, 234] A history of syncope is ominous in children but less so in adults. In the latter, nonsustained ventricular tachycardia (NSVT) on 48-hour electrocardiographic monitoring has some predictive value for subsequent sudden

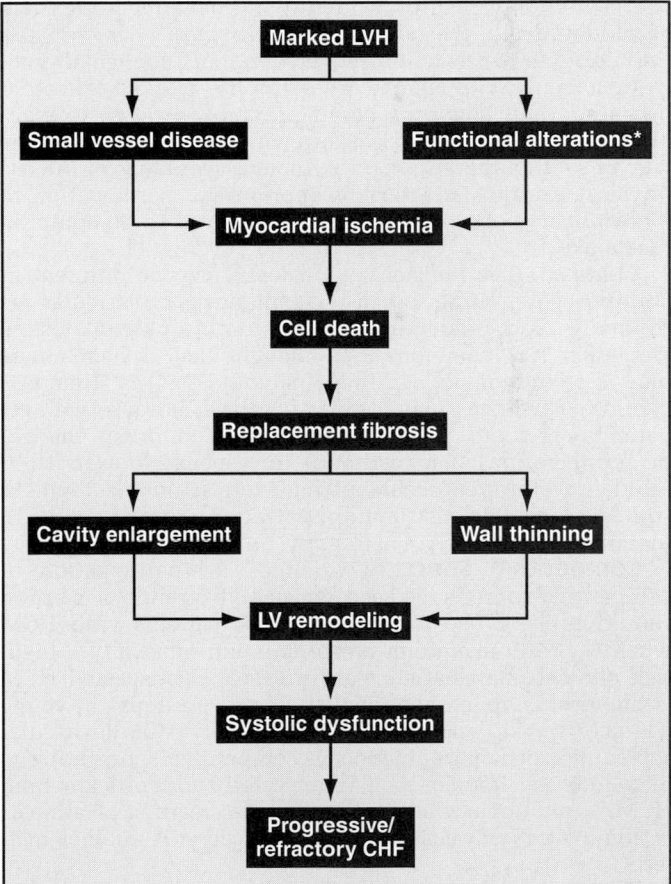

FIGURE 48–14. Hypothetical model for the pathogenesis of the end-stage phase of hypertrophic cardiomyopathy. Asterisk designates the following possibilities: (1) enhanced myocardial oxygen requirements and reduced myocardial capillary density relative to marked left ventricular (LV) hypertrophy (LVH) and (2) increased diastolic wall tension and coronary vascular resistance resulting from abnormal LV relaxation and impaired filling. CHF = congestive heart failure. (From Maron BJ, Spirito P: Implications of left ventricular remodeling in hypertrophic cardiomyopathy. Am J Cardiol 81:1339–1344, 1998.)

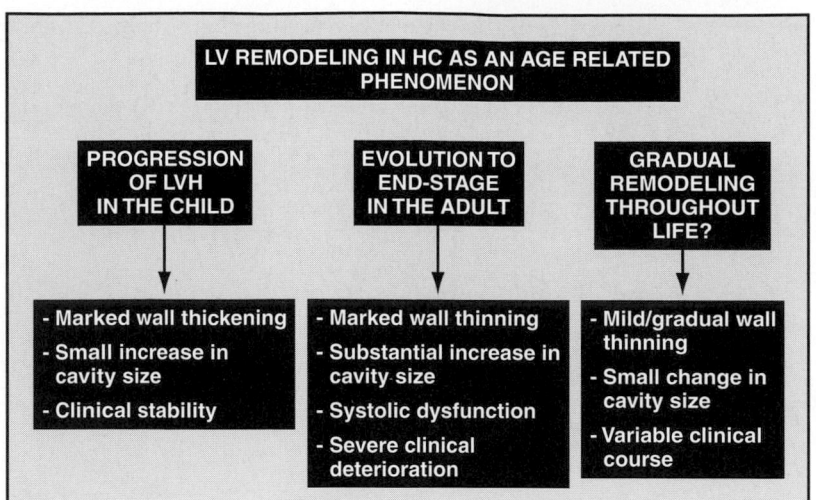

FIGURE 48–15. Patterns of left ventricular (LV) remodeling in the natural history of hypertrophic cardiomyopathy (HC). LVH = left ventricular hypertrophy. (Reprinted from Maron BJ, Spirito P: Implications of left ventricular remodeling in hypertrophic cardiomyopathy. Am J Cardiol 81:1339–1344, 1998.)

death, although most patients (more than 75 percent) with NSVT do *not* die suddenly.[243] The absence of NSVT is a stronger predictor of a good prognosis than is the presence of NSVT of a bad one.[207] It is presumed, but not established, that sudden death is due to a ventricular arrhythmia, although atrial arrhythmias may play a role in sensitizing the heart so that ventricular arrhythmias appear subsequently.[242]

Despite the difficulty in identifying patients at high risk of sudden death, the *absence* of a variety of characteristics (including the absence of severe symptoms, malignant family history, NSVT, marked hypertrophy, marked left atrial dilatation, and abnormal blood pressure response to exercise) identifies a low-risk group who require little in the way of routine therapy.[152, 244] Although avoidance of intense physical exertion is probably appropriate, participation in recreational sports activities is not believed to be contraindicated.[152]

Children. The mechanism of death may be different in children with HCM, because spontaneous ventricular arrhythmias and inducibility on electrophysiological testing are much less common. It is thought that ischemia may play a prominent role in these patients.[226, 245, 246] Hemodynamic mechanisms may also be involved, because younger patients are more likely to demonstrate abnormal changes in peripheral vascular resistance in response to exercise.[247] Sudden death often occurs during exercise but also demonstrates a circadian distribution, with clustering of deaths in the morning and early evening.[248]

Competitive Sports. Guidelines for participation in competitive sports have been developed; strenuous exertion should probably be proscribed in all patients with HCM whether or not symptoms are prominent, especially if high-risk clinical characteristics are present. Unsuspected HCM is the most common abnormality found at autopsy in young competitive athletes who die suddenly. Cardiovascular screening before participation in competitive sports appears to reduce the frequency of unexpected sudden death from HCM,[142] although whether large-scale screening of athletes is administratively feasible or cost effective is another matter.[249]

Why some athletes with HCM die suddenly and others are able to continue to compete without limitation or death is not known.[250] It has been speculated that the extent and severity of myocardial disarray may play an important role in determining prognosis, although this is not a finding that is ordinarily or easily obtainable in a living patient! Patients with marked hypertrophy are at increased risk.[251] Sudden death is unlikely, however, in asymptomatic or mildly symptomatic patients with mild hypertrophy.[252]

Bradyarrhythmias and disease of the atrioventricular conduction system may also play a role in sudden death.

Management

Management of patients with HCM is directed toward alleviation of symptoms, prevention of complications, and reduction in the risk of death (Fig. 48–17). Whether asymptomatic patients should receive drug therapy is not established because no adequate controlled studies are available.[152, 157] Digitalis glycosides should generally be avoided unless atrial fibrillation or systolic dysfunction develops. Diuretics were previously thought to be contraindi-

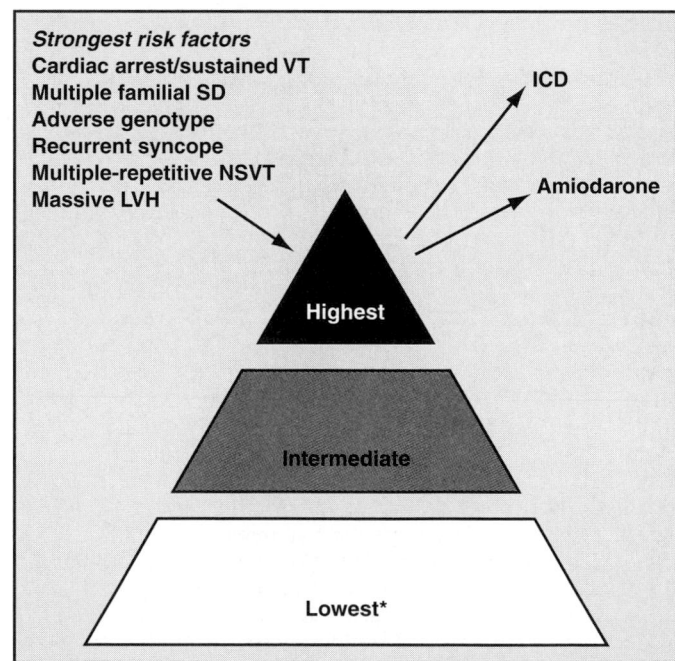

FIGURE 48–16. Assessment of risk of sudden cardiac death (SD) in overall hypertrophic cardiomyopathy (HCM) population. Treatment for prevention of sudden death is limited to the small subset perceived to be at the highest risk. Asterisk indicates asymptomatic individuals with mild left ventricular hypertrophy (LVH) and without ventricular tachycardia (VT) on Holter monitoring, hypotensive blood pressure response to exercise, and family history of premature HCM-related death. ICD = internal cardioverter-defibrillator; NSVT = nonsustained VT. (From Maron BJ: Hypertrophic cardiomyopathy. Lancet 350:127–133. © by The Lancet Ltd. 1997.)

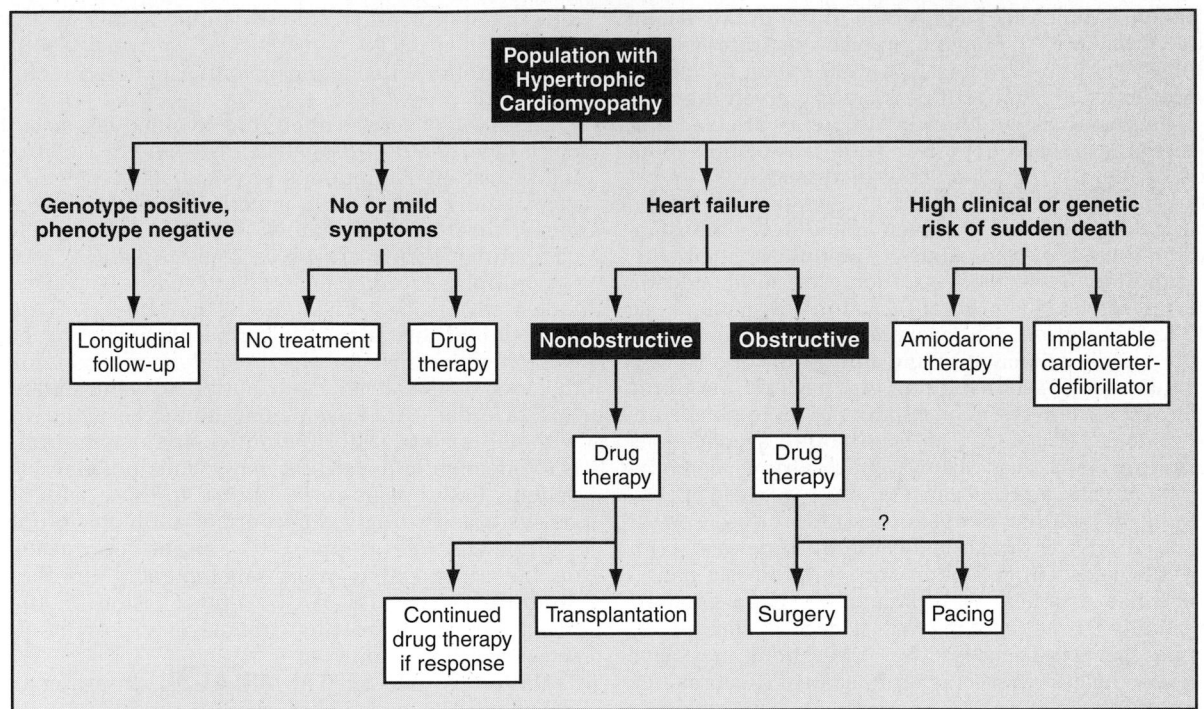

FIGURE 48–17. The principal clinical presentations of hypertrophic cardiomyopathy and corresponding treatment strategies. The size of the arrows indicates the approximate proportion of patients with hypertrophic cardiomyopathy in each subgroup. The dashed arrow indicates the present uncertainties regarding the size of this subgroup, and the question mark indicates the uncertainties regarding the therapeutic efficacy of pacing. (Modified from Spirito P, Seidman C, McKenna W, et al: The management of hypertrophic cardiomyopathy. N Engl J Med 336:775, 1997. Copyright 1997, Massachusetts Medical Society.)

cated to avoid precipitating or worsening the outflow gradient. More recent experience indicates that cautious use of diuretics often helps reduce symptoms of pulmonary congestion, particularly when they are combined with beta-adrenergic blockers or calcium antagonists.[154, 253] Beta-adrenergic agonists may improve diastolic filling but should not be used because they may produce ischemia and usually worsen the outflow gradient. The vast majority of patients with HCM require only medical management; invasive interventions are needed in only 5 to 10 percent of patients, and then only in those patients with outflow gradients who remain severely symptomatic despite optimal medical therapy.[152]

BETA-ADRENOCEPTOR BLOCKERS. These drugs are the mainstay of medical therapy of HCM. With their use, angina, dyspnea, and presyncope may all be improved. In patients with resting or provocable gradients beta-adrenoceptor blockade may prevent the increase in outflow obstruction that accompanies exertion, although resting gradients are largely unchanged.[152] The drugs reduce the determinants of myocardial oxygen consumption and thus angina pectoris and perhaps exert an antiarrhythmic action as well. Angina pectoris generally responds more favorably to treatment with a beta-adrenoceptor blocker than does dyspnea. It has been suggested that beta-adrenoceptor blockade may prevent sudden death, and accordingly some use prophylactic beta-adrenoceptor blockade therapy in asymptomatic patients. However, its efficacy for this purpose has not been established.[155, 171] Beta-adrenoceptor blockade also blunts the heart's chronotropic response, thus limiting the demand for increased myocardial oxygen delivery. Beta-adrenoceptor blockade previously was thought to have a beneficial effect on diastolic ventricular filling, but it now appears that any benefit is simply the consequence of a slower heart rate.[155] The overall clinical response to beta-adrenoceptor blockade is variable, and only about one third

to two thirds of patients experience symptomatic improvement.[155] One small blinded trial of beta-adrenoceptor blocker therapy found that nadolol improved symptoms more than placebo or a calcium antagonist but did not improve exercise capacity.[254] If beta-adrenoceptor blockers are discontinued, they probably should be withdrawn slowly to avoid rebound adrenergic hypersensitivity.

CALCIUM ANTAGONISTS. These are an alternative to beta-adrenoceptor blockade in the management of HCM; most of the experience has been with verapamil, with more limited use of nifedipine, diltiazem, and amlodipine.[155, 157] No clear consensus exists as to whether therapy should be initiated first with a beta-adrenoceptor blocker or a calcium antagonist, although verapamil often is effective in improving symptoms in patients who have failed beta-adrenoceptor blockade.[157] Exercise performance in particular may be improved when patients are changed from a beta-adrenoceptor blocker to verapamil. Both the hypercontractile systolic function and the abnormalities of diastolic filling may be related to abnormal calcium kinetics, and drugs that block the inward transport of calcium across the myocardial cell membrane may be able to rectify both abnormalities.

Verapamil has been the most widely used calcium antagonist in this condition.[157] Its use was suggested, at least in part, by the observation that it produces a protective and beneficial effect in the hereditary cardiomyopathy of the Syrian hamster, a condition marked by intracellular calcium overload in which propranolol is ineffective.[255] Although the vasodilator effects of verapamil should not be helpful in HCM, it appears that by depressing myocardial contractility, verapamil can decrease the left ventricular outflow gradient when given intravenously or orally. Perhaps more important from a symptomatic point of view, verapamil improves diastolic filling in HCM, at least in part by reducing asynchronous regional diastolic performance.[155, 157] It also improves regional myocardial blood flow in some patients, which may contribute to the improvement in diastolic behavior.[256] Verapamil appears to improve diastolic filling by improving relaxation rather than by changing left ventricular diastolic stiffness; at any given diastolic volume, filling pressure is reduced. Although variable clinical responses have been reported with verapamil, about two thirds or more of patients show increased exercise capacity and an improved symptomatic status. Sustained symptomatic improvement has been noted with the long-term administration of verapamil in ambulatory patients, although important adverse effects, including sudden death, have been observed in a small fraction of patients so treated.[152] Complications with verapamil include suppression of sinus node automaticity and inhibition of atrioventricular conduction, vasodilatation, and negative inotropic effects. These side effects may culminate in hypotension, pulmonary edema, and death; antiarrhythmic agents, especially quinidine, may exacerbate the deleterious hemodynamic effects of verapamil. Because of these adverse effects, it has been suggested that verapamil should not be used, or should be used only with extreme caution, in patients with high left ventricular filling pressure or symptoms of paroxysmal nocturnal dyspnea or orthopnea.[152] Unfortunately, these are usually the patients in greatest need of therapy.

Nifedipine has also been used in HCM, and it may have theoretical advantages over verapamil because it causes less depression of atrioventricular conduction. This may be counteracted by its more potent vasodilator action. Its effect on diastolic function have been inconsistent.[155] Nifedipine may alleviate the chest pain in HCM patients. Combined administration of nifedipine and propranolol may be of benefit in some patients, particularly those with outflow gradients. However, it should be recognized that the potent vasodilator effects of nifedipine may lead to systemic hypotension and an increase in the outflow gradient,[152] and in high doses it may depress left ventricular function. *Diltiazem* has also shown beneficial effects in HCM, producing improved diastolic function, although like verapamil and nifedipine it has caused an increase in the outflow gradient and a worrisome elevation of pulmonary capillary pressure.[155, 257]

The combination of a beta-adrenoceptor blocker and a calcium antagonist may be effective in patients responding inadequately to monotherapy, although there are only anecdotal reports of the superiority of combination therapy.[152, 258]

OTHER DRUGS. Disopyramide, an antiarrhythmic drug that alters calcium kinetics, has produced symptomatic improvement and abolition of the pressure gradient in patients with HCM, presumably as a consequence of depression of left ventricular systolic performance as well as a peripheral vasoconstrictor effect.[259] It does not appear to have significant effects on diastolic function,[259] although this issue has not been entirely resolved.[260] Long-term experience with disopyramide is limited, particularly in asymptomatic patients and those without outflow gradients, although the initial benefits appear to decrease with time.[152]

Beta-adrenoceptor blockers, calcium antagonists, and the conventional antiarrhythmic agents do not appear to suppress serious ventricular arrhythmias or reduce the frequency of supraventricular arrhythmias. However, amiodarone is effective in the treatment of both supraventricular and ventricular tachyarrhythmias in HCM.[243] Although there is some belief that amiodarone improves prognosis in HCM, only limited and inconclusive data are available.[152, 153, 261] Amiodarone may also improve symptoms and exercise capacity, although its putative beneficial effects on diastolic ventricular function are controversial.[155] Experience with sotalol, although limited, has been generally favorable; in addition to its antiarrhythmic effects on supraventricular and ventricular arrhythmias, its beta-adrenoceptor blocking effects are beneficial.[262] We do not favor empirical use of

amiodarone (or other antiarrhythmic agents for that matter) in unselected HCM patients, and we worry about possible proarrhythmic effects and potential toxicity, including sudden death.[213, 214, 236]

Strenuous exercise should be avoided because of the risk of sudden death; almost half of deaths in HCM occur during or just after strenuous physical activity.[263] Even though many individuals with subclinical HCM exercise vigorously, the threat of sudden death is sufficiently real that competitive sports are proscribed in patients with marked hypertrophy or other factors believed to be associated with increased risk (see Figs. 48–16 and 48–17). Atrial fibrillation should usually be pharmacologically or electrically converted because of the hemodynamic consequences of the loss of the atrial contribution to ventricular filling in this disorder. Anticoagulants should be given to patients with chronic atrial fibrillation when no contraindication exists. Infective endocarditis may occur in about 5 percent of patients but appears to be limited to those with an outflow gradient; accordingly, appropriate antibiotic prophylaxis is indicated in this group.[157, 264] The infection usually occurs on the aortic valve or mitral apparatus, on the endocardium, or at the site of the contact lesion on the septum; thus, chronic endocardial trauma may provide a nidus for subsequent infection.

DEVICES AND SEPTAL ABLATION. Insertion of a dual-chamber DDD pacemaker may be useful in some patients with an outflow gradient and severe symptoms, especially the elderly,[265–268] but it is likely that no more than 10 percent of HCM patients are candidates. Symptoms generally are improved, and the gradient is reduced by an average of about 25 percent, although better symptomatic and hemodynamic results appear to follow surgery (Fig. 48–18).[157] Benefits have been described even after termination of pacing, suggesting a modification of myocardial properties.[265] The long-term utility of pacing, however, is not known at present, and a substantial placebo effect has been demonstrated.[267, 269–271a] The benefit of its use in patients without a resting outflow gradient is even more equivocal; it usually improves symptoms and exercise capacity, but there is no improvement or even worsening of various hemodynamic variables and pharmacological therapy usually needs to be reinstituted.[272] Therefore, its use in this setting generally is not recommended at present.

In high-risk patients (especially the minority of HCM patients with sustained monomorphic ventricular tachycardia) or those with aborted sudden death, an ICD should be inserted,[242, 273] although an ICD may be less beneficial in HCM than in other conditions with aborted sudden death.[274]

A number of patients with severe obstruction have derived benefit at least over the short-term from intentional infarction of a portion of the interventricular septum by the infusion of alcohol into a selectively catheterized septal artery, with reduction of the outflow gradient and improvement in symptoms (Fig. 48–19).[275, 276]

SURGICAL TREATMENT. A number of surgical procedures aimed at reducing the outflow gradient have been developed. They are most commonly used in the markedly symptomatic patient with a gradient at rest above 50 mm Hg who has not responded well to medical management.[157, 277, 278]

Myectomy. The most widely used operation for HCM consists of excising a portion of the hypertrophied septum using a transaortic approach (the operation has been called the Morrow procedure, named after the cardiac surgeon who developed the technique).[279] Left transventricular as well as combined transaortic and left ventricular approaches have also been used successfully. Operative management is facilitated by intraoperative echocardiography, and operative mortality is now less than 5 percent[280]; large centers have reported mortalities of 3 percent or less.[157, 228,

PLATE 25

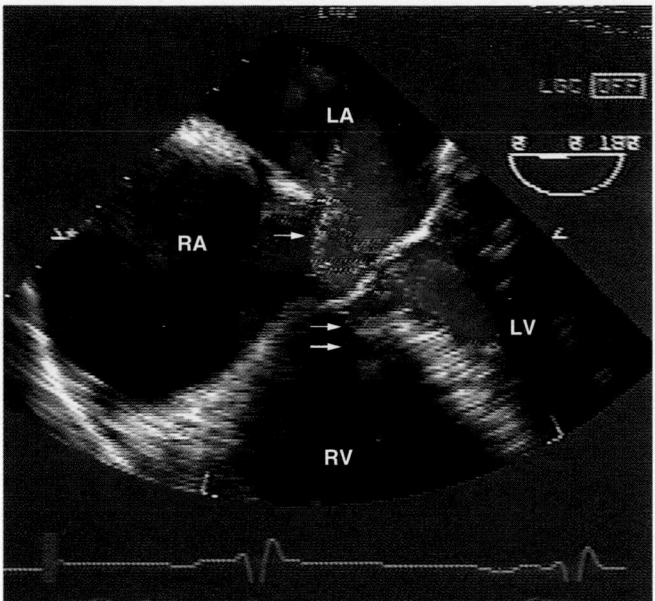

FIGURE 44–5. Transesophageal echocardiogram of intermediate atrioventricular septal defect illustrates the lack of offsetting between the left-sided and right-sided atrioventricular valves. Single arrow points at the primum atrial septal defect; double arrows point at the restrictive ventricular septal defect. RA = right atrium; LA = left atrium; RV = right ventricle; LV = left ventricle.

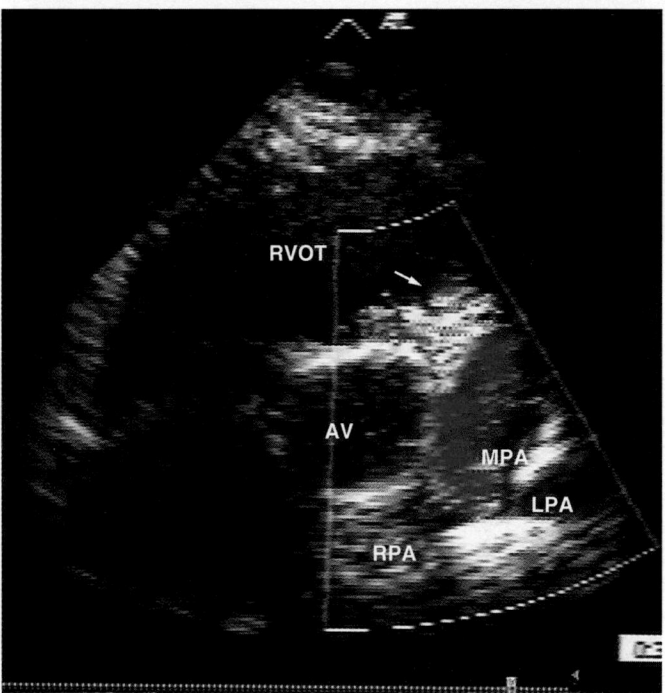

FIGURE 44–14. Transthoracic echocardiogram of severe pulmonary regurgitation as exemplified by the broad base, nonturbulent flow in diastole (arrow) originating from as far as the right and left pulmonary arteries. RVOT = right ventricular outflow tract; AV = aortic valve; MPA = main pulmonary artery; LPA = left pulmonary artery; RPA = right pulmonary artery.

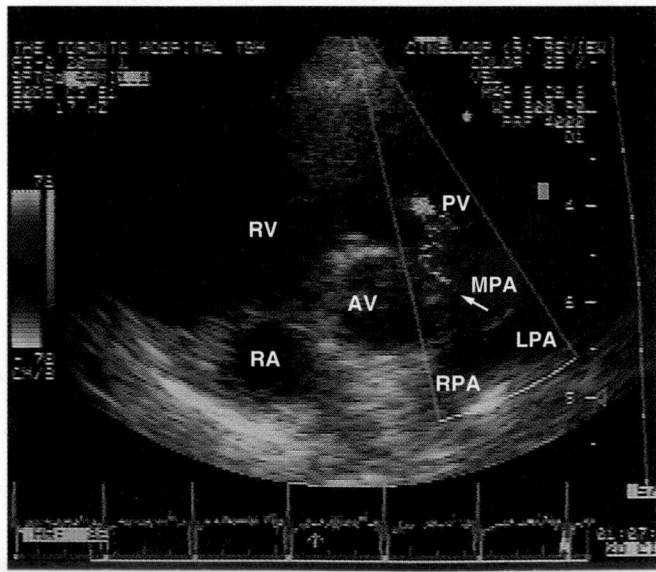

FIGURE 44–6. Short-axis left parasternal transthoracic echocardiogram of systolic flow traveling toward the pulmonary valve (arrow) in the main pulmonary artery from a patent ductus arteriosus. RV = right ventricle; RA = right atrium; AV = aortic valve; PV = pulmonary valve; MPA = main pulmonary artery; LPA = left pulmonary artery; RPA = right pulmonary artery.

PLATE 26

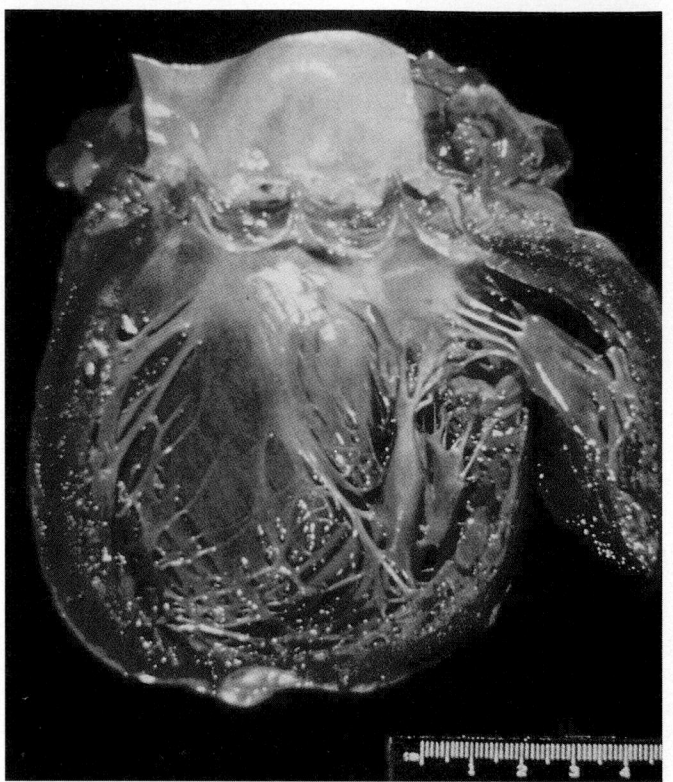

FIGURE 48–2. Gross pathology of dilated cardiomyopathy. Prominent ventricular dilatation is apparent in this heart, which has been opened so that the interior of the left ventricle can be seen. Wall thickness is normal, but the shape of the heart has become more globular. (From Kasper EK, Hruban RH, Baughman KL: Idiopathic dilated cardiomyopathy. *In* Abelmann WH, Braunwald E [eds.]: Atlas of Heart Diseases. Vol 2. Cardiomyopathies, Myocarditis, and Pericardial Disease. Philadelphia, Current Medicine, 1995, pp 3.1–3.18.)

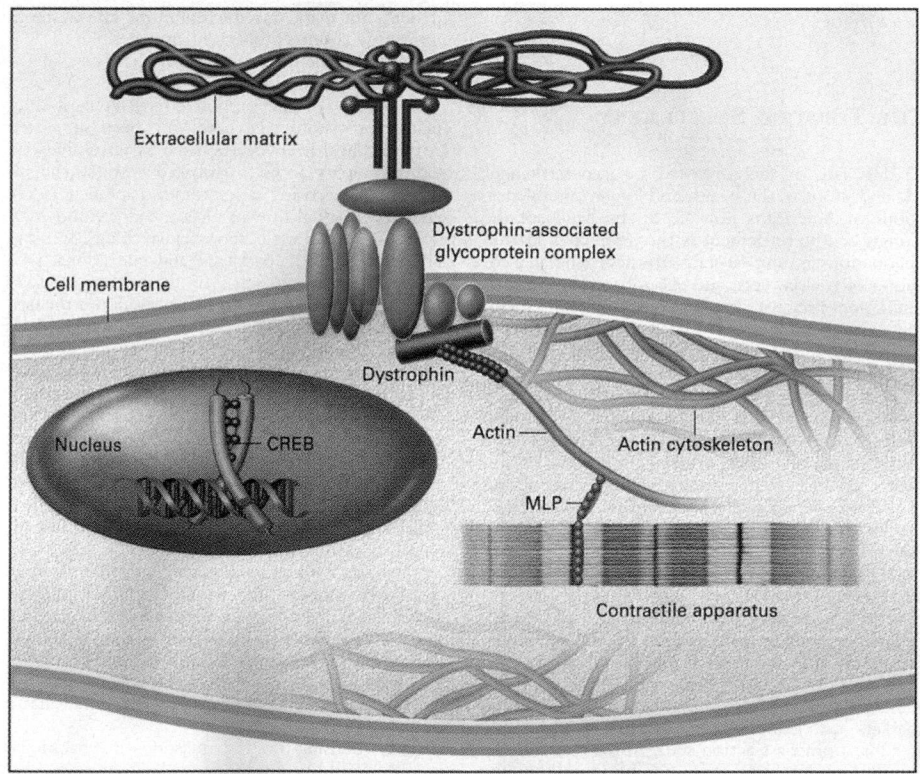

FIGURE 48–4. Diagram showing the cardiac myocyte and the molecules that have been implicated in dilated cardiomyopathy. The actin cytoskeleton is linked to the extracellular matrix by dystrophin and the dystrophin-associated glycoprotein complex. Linkage of the actin cytoskeleton to the contractile apparatus is hypothesized to occur through the muscle LIM (Lin-11, Isl-1, Mec-3) protein (MLP). A nuclear transcription factor, cyclic AMP response-element binding protein (CREB), is shown binding to a cyclic AMP response element in the myocyte DNA. Mutations in dystrophin and other members of the dystrophin-associated glycoprotein complex, as well as in MLP and CREB, have all been shown to result in dilated cardiomyopathy in mice or humans. (From Leiden JD: The genetics of dilated cardiomyopathy: Emerging clues to the puzzle. N Engl J Med 337:1080, 1997. Copyright 1997, Massachusetts Medical Society.)

PLATE 27

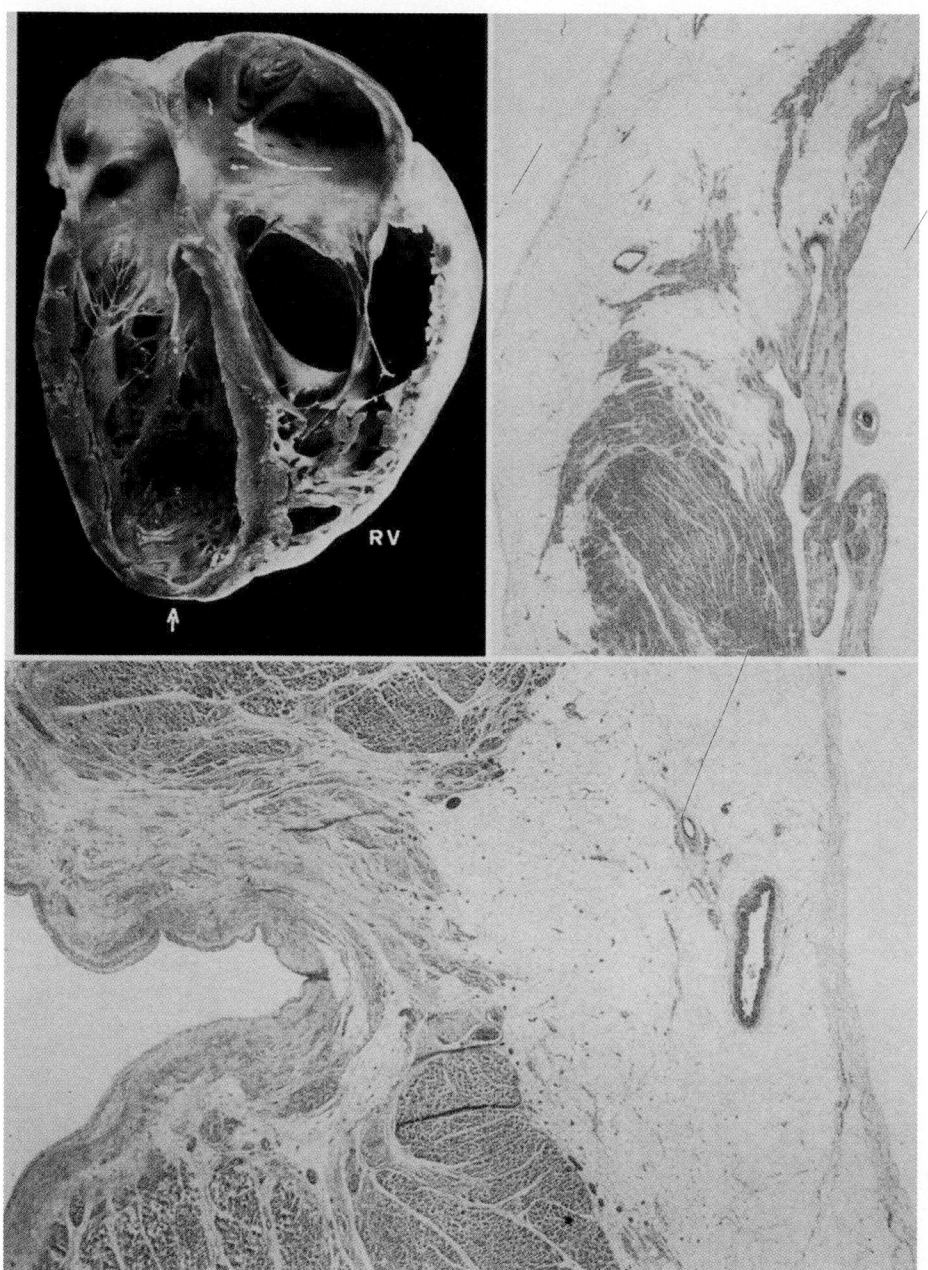

FIGURE 48–6. *Top left,* Postmortem pathological section of heart (four-chamber) in a patient with right ventricular cardiomyopathy (arrhythmogenic right ventricular dysplasia) and biventricular involvement. Severe widespread fatty infiltration of right ventricular (RV) wall is present; an apical aneurysm is present at the left ventricular level (arrow). *Top right,* Histological section at level of RV inflow (hematoxylin-eosin, × 2.5). Severe transmural fibrofatty infiltration of RV wall is present, compatible with RV dysplasia. *Bottom,* Histological section at the level of the left ventricle (outflow) (hematoxylin-eosin, ×2.5) shows focal severe fibrofatty infiltration with myocellular atrophy, compatible with left ventricular involvement. (From Pinamonti B, Pagnan L, Bussani R, et al: Right ventricular dysplasia with biventricular involvement. Circulation 98:1943–1945, 1998. Copyright 1998, American Heart Association.)

PLATE 28

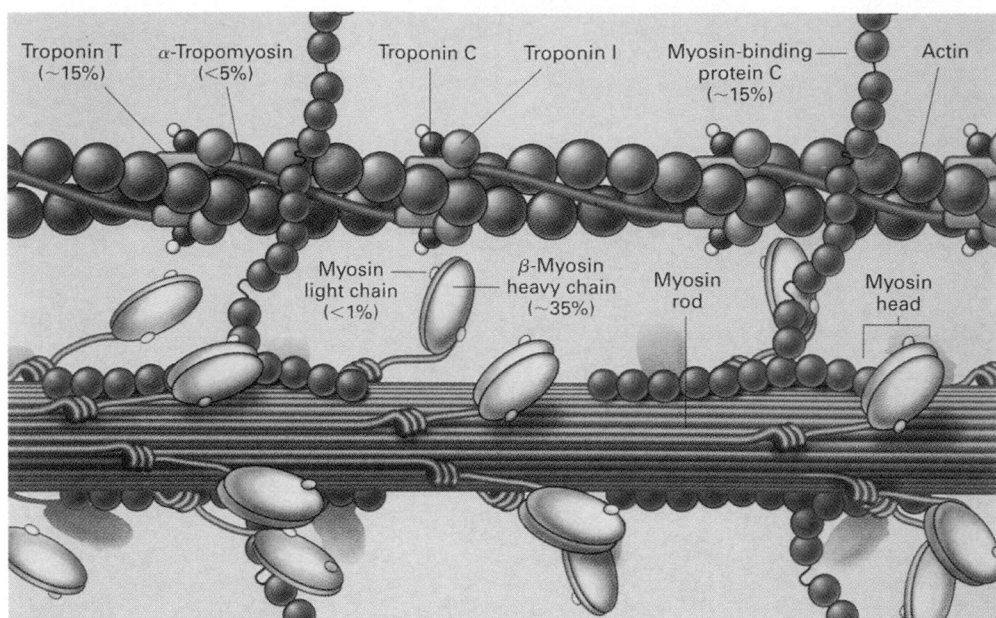

FIGURE 48–10. Cartoon showing components of the sarcomere and mutations in hypertrophic cardiomyopathy. Cardiac contraction occurs when calcium binds the troponin complex (subunits C, I, and T) and alpha-tropomyosin. Actin stimulates ATPase activity in the globular myosin head and results in the production of force along actin filaments. Cardiac myosin-binding protein C binds myosin and modulates contraction. In hypertrophic cardiomyopathy, mutations may impair these and other protein interactions, result in ineffectual contraction, and produce hypertrophy. Percentages represent the estimated frequency with which a mutation causes hypertrophic cardiomyopathy. (From Spirito P, Seidman C, McKenna WJ, et al: The management of hypertrophic cardiomyopathy. N Engl J Med 336: 775, 1997. Copyright 1997, Massachusetts Medical Society.)

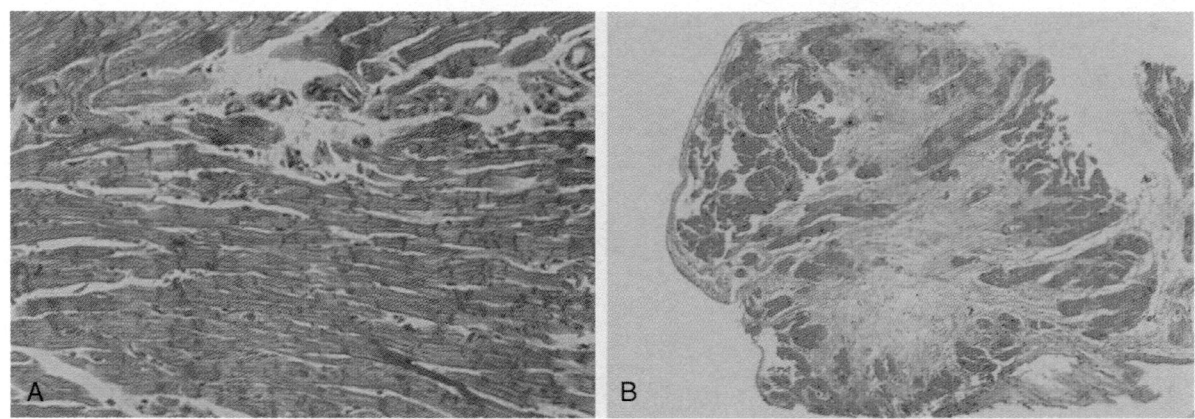

FIGURE 48–21. Endomyocardial biopsy specimens from patients with idiopathic restrictive cardiomyopathy. *A*, This histologic specimen (hematoxylin-eosin, ×250) shows myocytes with slight hypertrophy but is otherwise normal. *B*, Another specimen (hematoxylin-eosin, ×40), from another patient, shows marked interstitial fibrosis, which may also occur in idiopathic restrictive cardiomyopathy. (From Kushwaha SS, Fallon JT, Fuster V: Restrictive Cardiomyopathy. N Engl J Med 336:267, 1997. Copyright 1997, Massachusetts Medical Society.)

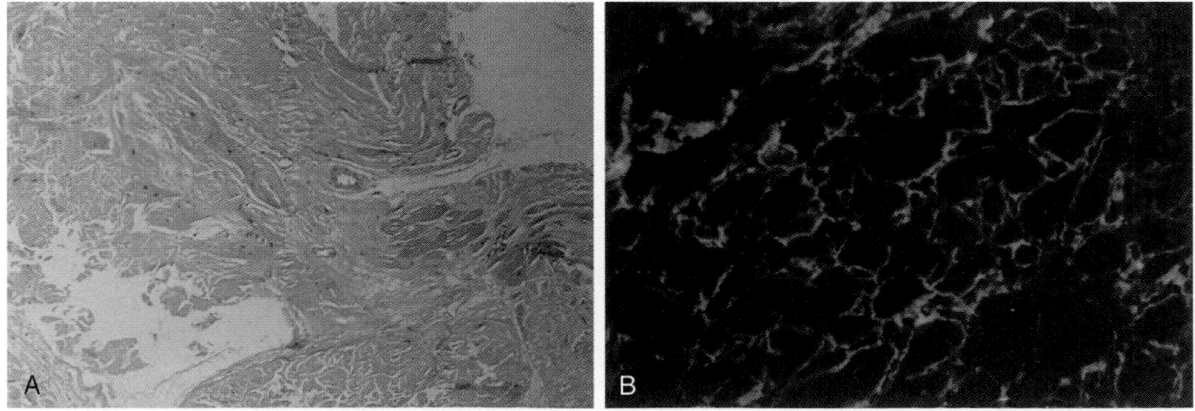

FIGURE 48–23. Endomyocardial biopsy specimens from patients with cardiac amyloidosis. *A*, This histologic section (hematoxylin and eosin, ×250) shows interstitial deposition of amyloid fibrils in a specimen from the right ventricle. *B*, Immunofluorescent stain (×400) shows lambda light chains. (From Kushwaha SS, Fallon JT, Fuster V: Restrictive cardiomyopathy. N Engl J Med 336:267, 1997. Copyright 1997, Massachusetts Medical Society.)

PLATE 29

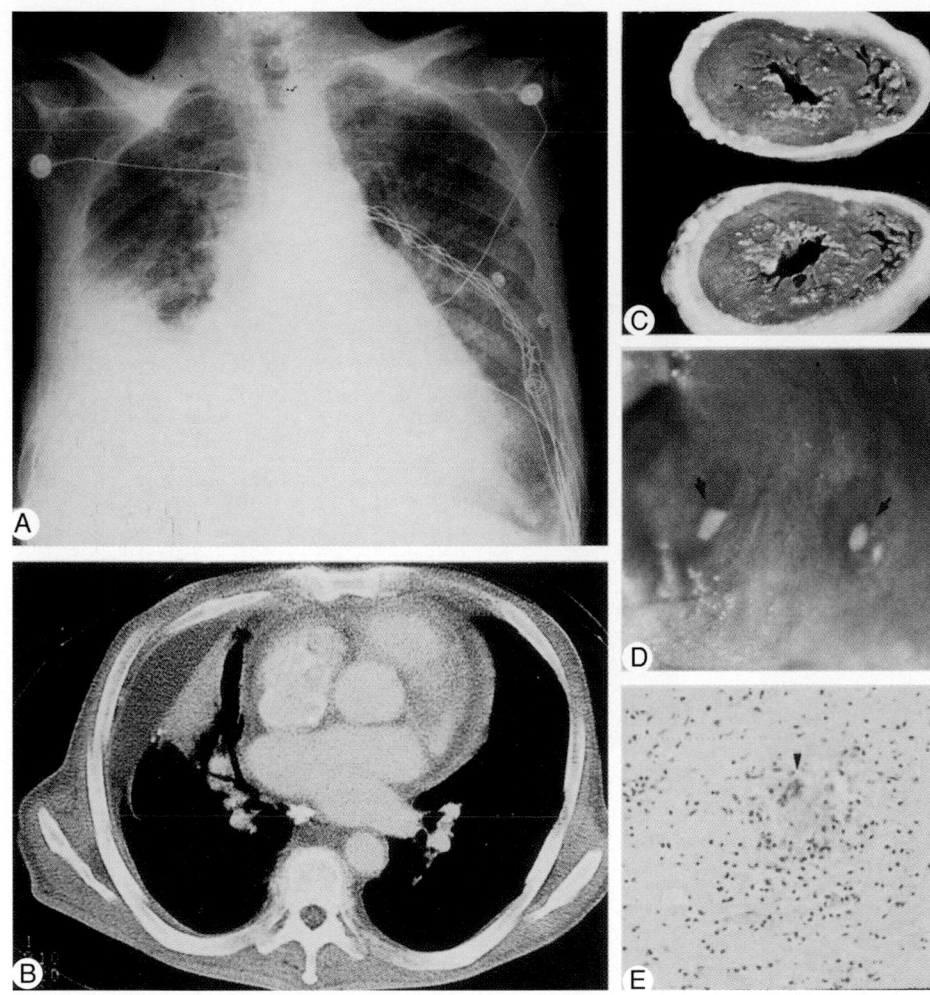

FIGURE 48–31. Findings in cardiac tuberculosis. *A,* Chest radiograph reveals right-sided pleural effusion, cardiomegaly, and borderline perihilar edema. *B,* CT of chest confirmed right-sided pleural effusion and also reveals pericardial effusion and pericardial thickening. *C,* Cross section of heart shows thickened pericardium. *D,* Close examination of apical myocardium (arrow) reveals myocardial tubercles. *E,* Histology shows the presence of granulomas (arrowhead) with giant cells. (From Dhar SC, Hayes S, Cercek B, et al: Images in cardiovascular medicine: Cardiac tuberculosis. Circulation 98:730, 1998. Copyright 1998, American Heart Association.)

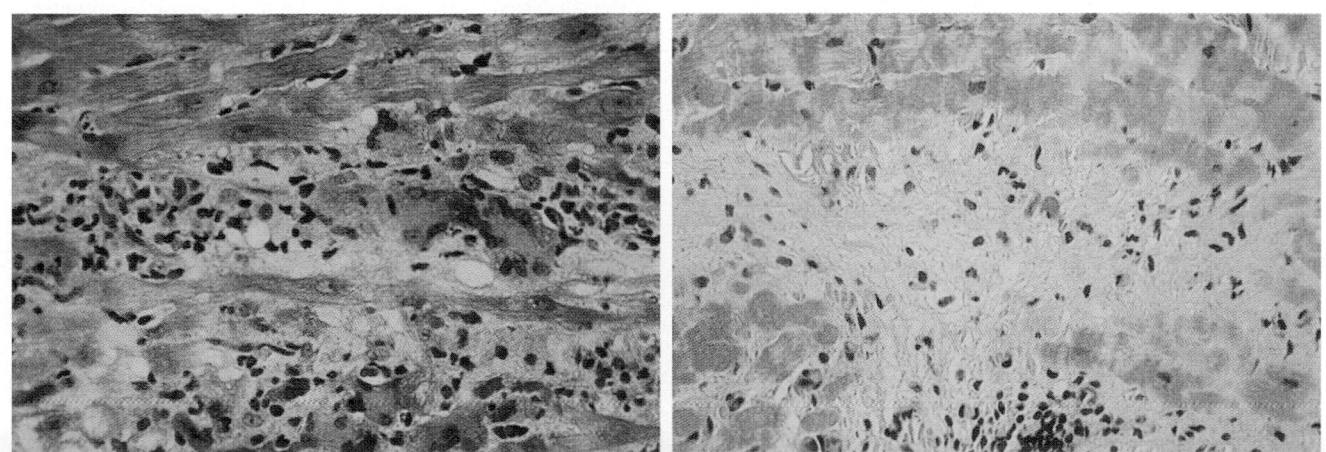

FIGURE 48–35. Endomyocardial biopsy findings in giant-cell myocarditis. *Left,* Active giant-cell myocarditis. Initial pretreatment biopsy showed several giant cells and a mixed lymphocyte-eosinophilic infiltrate (hematoxylin-eosin; original magnification, ×250). *Right,* Healing giant-cell myocarditis. Biopsy after therapy showed interstitial fibrosis with residual mononuclear cells but no giant cells or myocyte necrosis (hematoxylin-eosin; original magnification, ×250). (From Levy NT, Olson LJ, Weyand C, et al: Histologic and cytokine response to immunosuppression in giant-cell myocarditis. Ann Intern Med 128:648, 1998.)

PLATE 30

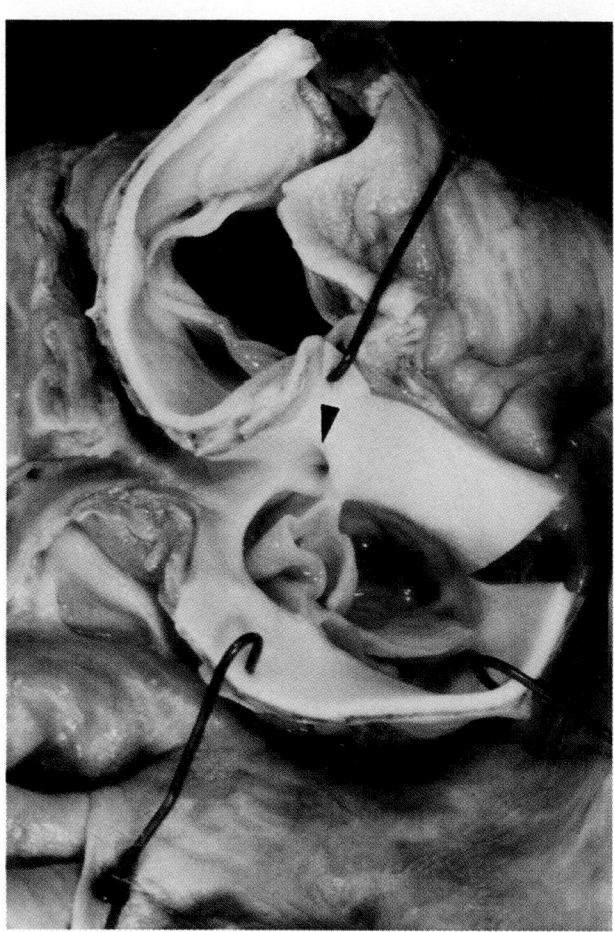

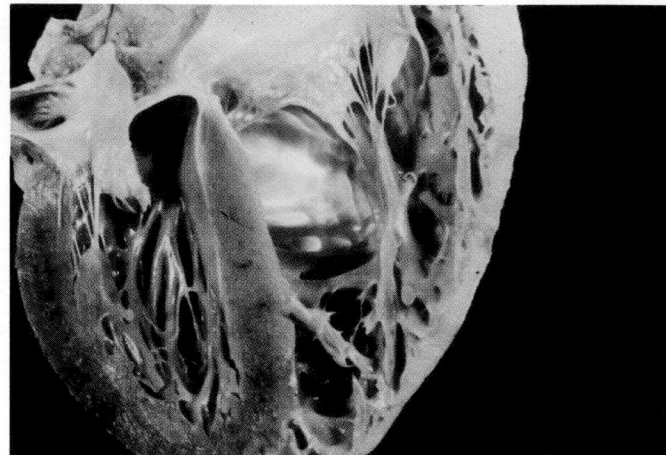

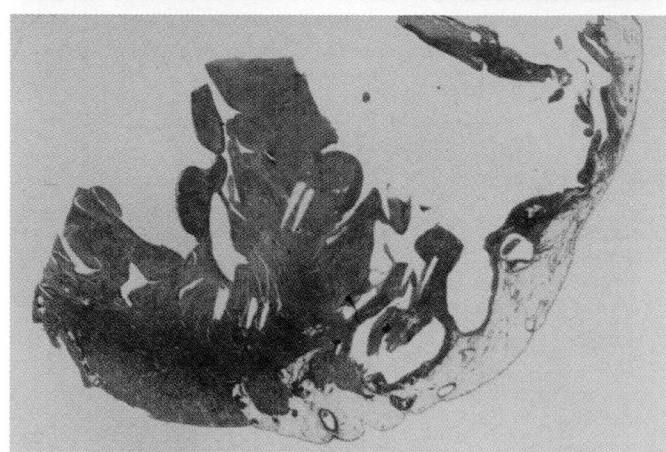

FIGURE 59–4. View of the aortic root in wrong sinus origin of the right coronary artery from the left sinus of Valsalva in a 22-year-old man who died suddenly during a soccer match. Incision has been carried out into the right sinus of Valsalva, but no coronary ostium was found. Both the anomalous right coronary artery (arrowhead) and the left main coronary artery originate from the left sinus of Valsalva. The left main trunk has been opened and divides into anterior descending and left circumflex branches. (From Basso C, Corrado D, Thiene G: Cardiovascular causes of sudden death in young individuals including athletes. Cardiol Rev 7:127–135, 1997.)

FIGURE 59–6. Arrhythmogenic right ventricular cardiomyopathy in a 25-year-old man who died suddenly at rest. *Top panel,* Heart specimen is sectioned in a four-chamber plane viewed from the posterior aspect. Fatty replacement of the anterior right ventricular free wall and infundibulum is demonstrated by transillumination. *Bottom panel,* Macrohistological section confirming that fatty replacement of myocytes is confined to the right ventricular wall, sparing the ventricular septum and left ventricular free wall. Heidenhain trichrome stain ×3. (Reproduced with permission from Basso C, Corrado D, Rossi L, Thiene G: Arrhythmogenic right ventricular cardiomyopathy/dysplasia. *In* Nava A, Rossi L, Thiene G [eds]: Morbid Anatomy. Amsterdam, Elsevier Publishers, 1997, pp 71–86.)

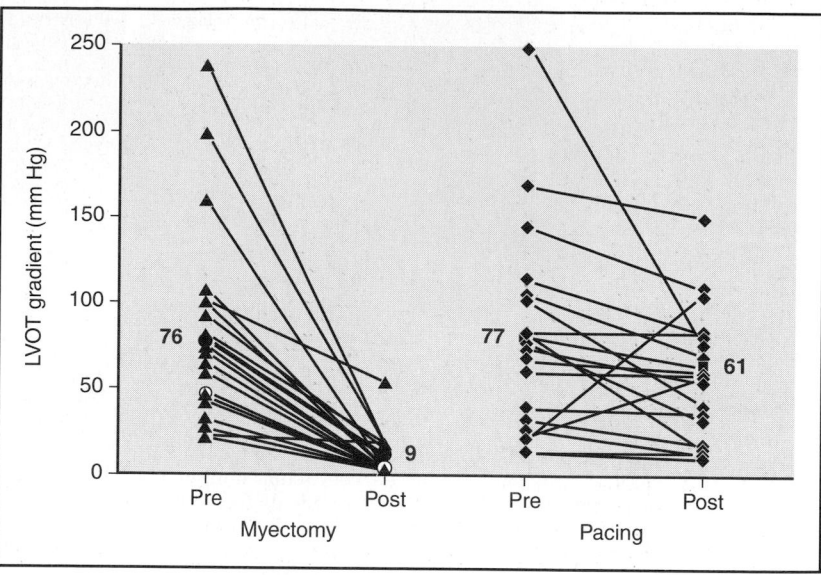

FIGURE 48–18. Change in Doppler ultrasound–derived resting left ventricular outflow tract (LVOT) gradient from baseline (pre) to follow-up assessment (post) in patients with hypertrophic cardiomyopathy undergoing surgery or pacemaker insertion. Both groups (surgical myectomy, *left;* dual-chamber pacing, *right*) show significant reductions in resting gradient (*p* < 0.05). (From Ommen SR, Nishimura RA, Squires RW, et al: Comparison of dual-chamber pacing versus septal myectomy for the treatment of patients with hypertrophic obstructive cardiomyopathy. J Am Coll Cardiol 34:191, 1999.)

[281, 282] Operation often relieves the obstruction (Figs. 48–18 and 48–20) as well as the mitral regurgitation.[281] The reduction in the left ventricular systolic pressure produced by the operation leads to reduced evidence of postoperative myocardial ischemia on thallium stress testing.[283] Patients older than the age of 65 as well as younger than the age of

10 years have undergone successful operations; the operative risk is higher in older patients.[282, 284]

Surgery results in long-term improvement in symptoms and exercise capacity in most patients.[281, 282, 285, 286] Occasional patients experience myocardial damage and fibrosis as a consequence of the procedure.[283] Significant aortic re-

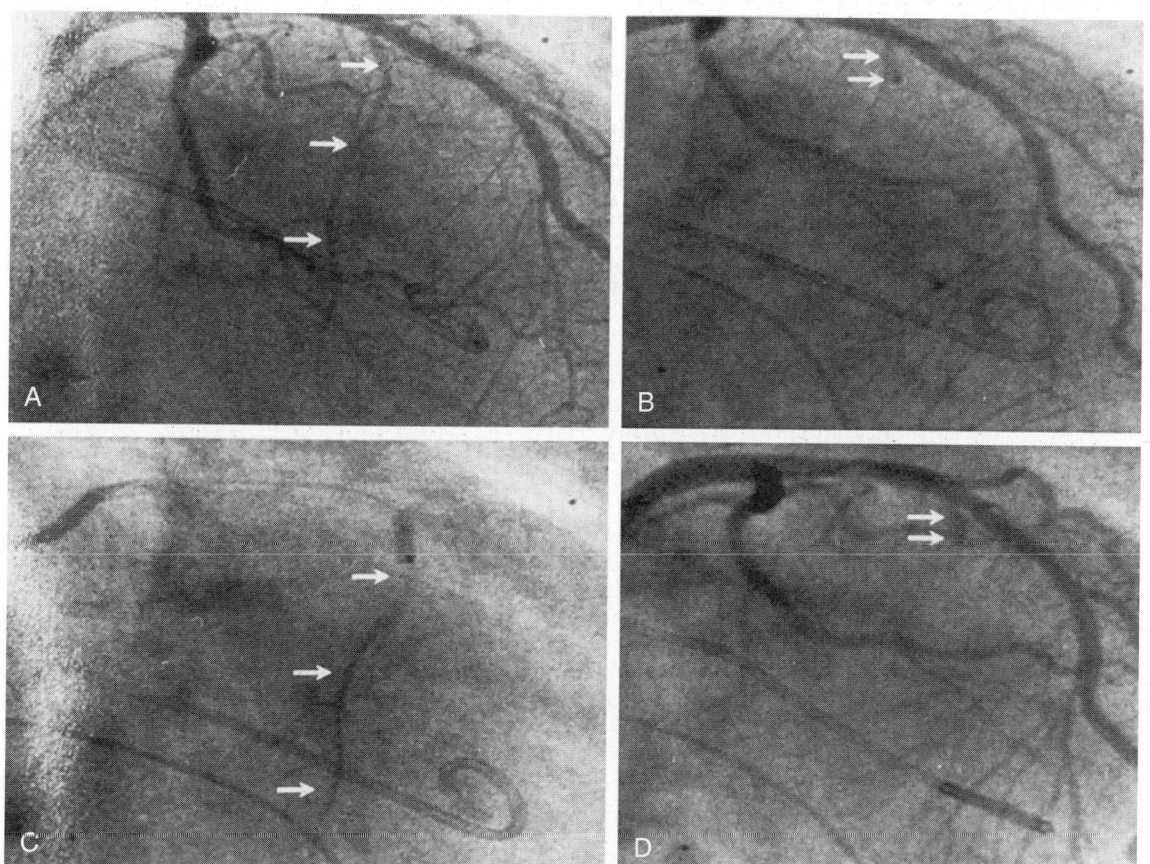

FIGURE 48–19. Coronary angiograms in a patient with hypertrophic cardiomyopathy undergoing percutaneous septal ablation. *A,* Identification of target vessel in right anterior oblique view (arrows). *B,* Balloon inflation in proximal part of target vessel. *C,* Injection of contrast dye to define perfusion area and to exclude reflux into other vessels. *D,* Final visualization of vessel stump after completed percutaneous occlusion of vessel. (From Faber L, Seggewiss H, Gleichmann U: Percutaneous transluminal septal myocardial ablation in hypertrophic obstructive cardiomyopathy: Results with respect to intraprocedural myocardial contrast echocardiography. Circulation 98:2415, 1999. Copyright 1999, American Heart Association.)

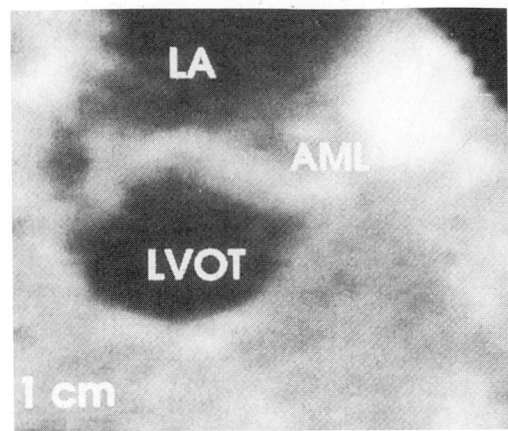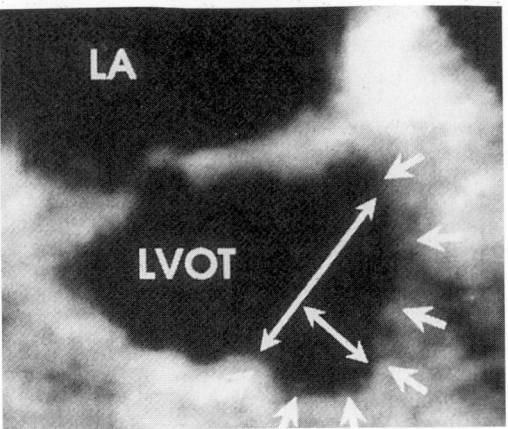

FIGURE 48–20. Three-dimensional transesophageal echocardiographic images before (*left*) and after (*right*) surgical myectomy of the left ventricular outflow tract (LVOT) in a patient with hypertrophic cardiomyopathy. The maximal width and depth of the myectomy trough are marked by large arrows. Small arrows indicate limits of myectomy trough. LA = left atrium. (From Franke A, Schondube FA, Kuhl HP, et al: Quantitative assessment of the operative results after extended myectomy and surgical reconstruction of the subvalvular mitral apparatus in hypertrophic obstructive cardiomyopathy using dynamic three-dimensional transesophageal echocardiography. J Am Coll Cardiol 31:1641, 1998.)

gurgitation is an uncommon complication of the transaortic valve approach, occurring in less than 4 percent of patients.[287] Myotomy-myectomy may be combined with other necessary operative procedures (particularly coronary artery bypass grafting), although the surgical risk is increased.[280] There has been recent enthusiasm for combining septal myotomy-myectomy with plication of the anterior leaflet of the mitral valve and reconstruction of the submitral valvular apparatus.[288]

Mitral Valve Replacement. Although this procedure or mitral valve repair is performed in fewer centers than myotomy-myectomy, the long-term results also have been favorable, with symptomatic benefit and an improvement in

hemodynamics.[289] The rationale for this operation is that it abolishes obstruction by preventing systolic anterior motion of the mitral valve. It appears to be of particular value in patients with less than severe (< 18 mm) hypertrophy of the upper septum or other atypical septal morphology, in those with previous myotomy-myectomy with persistent severe symptoms and obstruction, and in patients with intrinsic mitral valve disease. In appropriate candidates not responding to maximal standard medical and surgical therapy, cardiac transplantation may be considered; this usually is required only for patients who have entered the dilated phase of HCM and have intractable symptoms of congestive heart failure.[290]

Restrictive and Infiltrative Cardiomyopathies

Of the three major functional categories of the cardiomyopathies (dilated, hypertrophic, and restrictive), restrictive cardiomyopathy (RCM) is the least common form in Western countries, although nonidiopathic forms of RCM such as endomyocardial disease (Table 48–8) are common in specific geographical regions of the world.[291, 292] The hallmark of the RCMs is abnormal diastolic function; the ventricular walls are excessively rigid and impede ventricular filling. Systolic function, on the other hand, often is unimpaired, even in many cases with extensive infiltration of the myocardium.[291, 293, 294] Thus, RCM bears some functional resemblance to constrictive pericarditis, which is also characterized by normal or nearly normal systolic function but abnormal ventricular filling (see Chap. 50).[291] Differentiation of the two conditions is mandatory because of the potential for successful surgical treatment of constriction.[292, 295]

A variety of specific pathological processes may result in restrictive cardiomyopathy, although the cause often remains unknown. Myocardial fibrosis (Fig. 48–21), infiltration, or endomyocardial scarring is usually responsible for the abnormal diastolic behavior; in the idiopathic variety there often is histological evidence of myocyte hypertrophy.[291, 296] Myocardial involvement with amyloid is a common cause of RCM, although it can be caused by a variety of other conditions (see Table 48–8).[291, 292]

Some patients may manifest the clinical features of an RCM and yet exhibit the pathological findings of left ventricular hypertrophy and fibrosis[294]; certainly ventricular hypertrophy, especially HCM, can cause diminished ventricular compliance, but not RCM per se. RCM on occasion is inherited; in such cases there may be an associated skeletal muscle disease.[291]

HEMODYNAMICS. The clinical and hemodynamic features of restrictive heart disease simulate those of chronic constrictive pericarditis; endomyocardial biopsy, CT and radionuclide angiography may be particularly useful in differentiating the two diseases by demonstrating myocardial scarring or infiltration (biopsy) or thickening of the pericardium (CT and MRI).[292, 297] With the use of these modalities, exploratory thoracotomy should rarely be required; nevertheless, if the differentiation between constriction and restrictive cardiomyopathy cannot be established with certainty, surgical exploration is in order.[291] The characteristic hemodynamic feature in both conditions is a deep and rapid early decline in ventricular pressure at the onset of diastole, with a rapid rise to a plateau in early diastole

---

FIGURE 48–21. See color plate 28.

▼ TABLE 48–8. CLASSIFICATION OF TYPES OF RESTRICTIVE CARDIOMYOPATHY ACCORDING TO CAUSE

Myocardial
Noninfiltrative
Idiopathic cardiomyopathy*
Familial cardiomyopathy
Hypertrophic cardiomyopathy
Scleroderma
Pseudoxanthoma elasticum
Diabetic cardiomyopathy

Infiltrative
Amyloidosis*
Sarcoidosis*
Gaucher disease
Hurler disease
Fatty infiltration

Storage Diseases
Hemochromatosis
Fabry disease
Glycogen storage disease

Endomyocardial
Endomyocardial fibrosis*
Hypereosinophilic syndrome
Carcinoid heart disease
Metastatic cancers
Radiation*
Toxic effects of anthracycline*
Drugs causing fibrous endocarditis
   (serotonin, methysergide, ergotamine, mercurial agents, busulfan)

   * This condition is more likely than the others to be encountered in clinical practice.
   From Kushwaha S, Fallon JT, Fuster V: Restrictive cardiomyopathy. N Engl J Med 336:267, 1997. Copyright 1997, Massachusetts Medical Society.

(although this finding is absent in some patients with RCM).[291] This dip and plateau has been termed the *square root sign* (see Chap. 50) and is manifested in the atrial pressure tracing as a prominent *y* descent followed by a rapid rise and plateau. The *x* descent may also be rapid, and the combination results in the characteristic M or W waveform in the atrial pressure tracing.[291] The *a* wave is prominent and often is of the same amplitude as the *v* wave. Both systemic and pulmonary venous pressures are elevated, although patients with restrictive heart disease typically have left ventricular filling pressures that exceed right ventricular filling pressure by more than 5 mm Hg; this difference is accentuated by exercise, fluid challenge, and Valsalva maneuver (although not all patients demonstrate this finding).[291, 298]

In this respect they differ from patients with constrictive pericarditis, in whom diastolic pressures are similar in both ventricles, usually differing by no more than 5 mm Hg. The pulmonary artery systolic pressure is often greater than 50 mm Hg in patients with RCM but is lower in constrictive pericarditis.[291] Furthermore, the plateau of the right ventricular diastolic pressure is usually at least one third of the peak right ventricular systolic pressure in patients with constrictive pericarditis, whereas it is frequently lower in RCM.[291]

CLINICAL MANIFESTATIONS. Exercise intolerance is frequent because of the inability of patients with RCM to increase their cardiac output by tachycardia without further compromising ventricular filling. Weakness and dyspnea are often prominent. Exertional chest pain may be prominent in some patients but is usually absent. Particularly in advanced cases, the central venous pressure is elevated, with attendant peripheral edema, enlarged liver, ascites,

and anasarca. *Physical examination* may reveal jugular venous distention and an S_3, S_4, or both. An inspiratory increase in venous pressure may be seen. However, in contrast to constrictive pericarditis, the apex impulse is usually palpable in RCM.[291]

LABORATORY STUDIES. Various ancillary laboratory findings in addition to endomyocardial biopsy, CT and MRI[297] (see Chap. 10) may be useful in distinguishing between constrictive and restrictive disease. Although pericardial calcification is neither absolutely sensitive nor specific for constrictive pericarditis (see Chap. 50), its presence in a patient in whom the differential diagnosis rests between RCM and constrictive pericarditis lends strong support to the latter diagnosis. The echocardiogram may demonstrate thickening of the left ventricular wall and an increase of left ventricular mass in patients with infiltrative disease causing RCM. The pattern of filling of the left ventricle differs in the two conditions, as can be demonstrated by transthoracic and transesophageal Doppler ultrasonography.[291, 295, 299] In patients with RCM, there is increased early left ventricular filling velocity, decreased atrial filling velocity, and decreased isovolumetric relaxation time.[291]

The prognosis in RCM is variable; usually it is one of relentless symptomatic progression and high mortality.[295, 299a] No specific therapy (other than symptomatic) is available (excepting the cardiomyopathy due to iron overload which is improved by removal of the iron and amyloidosis, in which some patients appear to benefit from alkylating-based chemotherapy).[295]

AMYLOIDOSIS

ETIOLOGY AND TYPES. Amyloidosis is a disease complex that results from deposition of unique twisted beta-pleated sheet fibrils formed from various proteins by several different pathogenic mechanisms.[300] Amyloid may be found in almost any organ, but clinically evident disease does not appear unless infiltration is extensive. Several classification systems have been used to characterize the different clinical presentations of amyloidosis. The condition with the traditional designation of primary amyloidosis is now known to be caused by the production of an amyloid protein composed of portions of immunoglobulin light chain (designated *AL*) by a monoclonal population of plasma cells, often as a consequence of multiple myeloma. Secondary amyloidosis is due to the production of a nonimmunoglobulin protein termed *AA*.[300]

Familial Amyloidosis. This condition, inherited as an autosomal dominant trait, results from the production of a variant prealbumin protein termed *transthyretin;* more than 50 different point mutations have been described so far.[301, 302] It generally occurs in one of three clinical presentations: progressive neuropathy, cardiomyopathy, or nephropathy. Senile systemic amyloidosis is due to the production of either an atrial natriuretic-like protein or transthyretin[300] and is becoming increasingly common as the average age of the population increases. It is four times as common in blacks as in whites.[303] Scattered deposits of amyloid localized to the aorta or atria are virtually ubiquitous in individuals older than the age of 80.[292, 300] Small deposits of amyloid may often be found in the pulmonary vessels or the vessels of other organs as well.

Cardiac Amyloidosis

Involvement of the heart is a common finding and is the most frequent cause of death in amyloidosis associated with an immunocyte dyscrasia.[304] Clinically apparent heart disease is present in one third of patients, although the heart is virtually always involved when studied pathologically. In secondary amyloidosis, on the other hand, clinically significant cardiac involvement is uncommon; the myocardial deposits are typically small and perivascular and usually do not result in significant myocardial dysfunction.[300] Familial amyloidosis is associated with overt cardiac involvement in about one fourth of the afflicted patients, usually late in the course of the disease.[305] The clinical course is usually dominated by neurological or renal dysfunction, although death is due to heart failure or arrhythmia about half the time.[305] Cardiac involvement in senile amyloidosis varies from small atrial deposits that do not result in functional impairment to extensive ventricular involvement with resultant cardiac failure.[302]

Cardiac amyloidosis occurs more commonly in men than in women, and it is rare before the age of 30 years. Even in the familial form, the onset of clinical cardiac disease usually does not occur before the age of 35 years and generally occurs much later in life.[305]

PATHOLOGY. The pathological findings often include mild atrial enlargement, usually without significant ventricular dilatation. The walls of both ventricles are typically firm, rubbery, noncompliant, and thickened. Amyloid is present between the myocardial fibers, often with extensive deposition in the papillary muscles. Endocardial involvement of the atria and ventricles is frequent. Amyloidosis often results in focal thickening of or deposits on the cardiac valves, but these abnormalities do not appear to interfere with valvular function other than to produce murmurs. The intramural coronary arteries and veins frequently contain amyloid deposits in the media and adventitia, occasionally compromising the lumina of the vessels.[293, 301]

CLINICAL MANIFESTATIONS. Involvement of the cardiovascular system by amyloidosis occurs in four general forms:

1. The most common presentation of cardiac amyloidosis is that of RCM.[291] Right-sided findings dominate the clinical presentation; peripheral edema is a prominent finding, whereas paroxysmal nocturnal dyspnea and orthopnea are absent.[292] Amyloid infiltration of the myocardium results in increased stiffness of the myocardium, producing the characteristic diastolic dip and plateau (square root sign) in the ventricular pressure pulse that may simulate constrictive pericarditis. In contrast to the accelerated early left ventricular diastolic filling found in constrictive pericarditis, cardiac amyloidosis is marked by an impaired rate of early diastolic filling.

2. A second common presentation is congestive heart failure due to systolic dysfunction.[302] Hemodynamic evidence of restriction of ventricular filling may not be prominent in these patients. In some patients amyloid deposition in the atria may be responsible for loss of atrial transport function despite the maintenance of electrical "sinus" rhythm, with the production of congestive heart failure.[306] The course of this form of the disease is often one of relentless progression, usually poorly responsive to treatment. Angina pectoris occurs on occasion despite angiographically normal coronary arteries.[293]

3. Orthostatic hypotension occurs in about 10 percent of cases. Although most likely due to amyloid infiltration of the autonomic nervous system or of blood vessels, amyloid deposition in the heart and adrenals may contribute to the pathogenesis of this variant. Hypovolemia as a result of the nephrotic syndrome secondary to renal amyloidosis may aggravate the postural hypotension.[305]

4. An abnormality of cardiac impulse formation and conduction is the fourth and least common mode of presentation and may result in arrhythmias and conduction disturbances. Sudden death, presumably arrhythmic in origin, is relatively common and may be preceded by episodes of syncope.[305, 307]

PHYSICAL EXAMINATION. This often reveals congestive heart failure, especially right sided[292]; a systolic murmur due to atrioventricular valvular regurgitation may be present. Jugular venous distention, a protodiastolic gallop, hepatomegaly, peripheral edema, and a narrow pulse pressure are found in patients presenting with RCM. An S_4 is uncommon, presumably due to amyloid infiltration of the atrium with attendant reduced systolic function of the atrial myocardium.[306] Patients typically are normotensive or hypotensive; even previously hypertensive individuals usually have a fall in blood pressure as the disease progresses.

NONINVASIVE TESTING. The chest roentgenogram usually shows cardiomegaly in patients with systolic dysfunction, although heart size may be normal in patients with the restrictive form.[92] Pulmonary congestion may be prominent in patients with congestive heart failure. The ECG is often abnormal; the most characteristic feature (but often absent) is diffusely diminished voltage.[292] Myocardial infarction is often simulated because of small or absent R waves in right precordial leads or, less frequently, by Q waves in the inferior leads.[300] Arrhythmias, particularly atrial fibrillation, are common, although they rarely are the presenting feature of cardiac amyloidosis. Complex ventricular arrhythmias are found frequently in patients with cardiac amyloidosis and may be a harbinger of sudden death.[301] Various forms of atrioventricular conduction defects are often seen and may be associated with increased mortality, although significant infra-Hisian block may only be apparent on electrophysiological testing.[305, 308] Abnormalities of atrioventricular conduction appear to be particularly common in familial amyloidosis with polyneuropathy.[305] Sinus node involvement is common, and the clinical and ECG features of the sick sinus syndrome may be present (see Chap. 25).

Echocardiography (see Fig. 7–103). In advanced cases this most commonly reveals increased thickness of the walls of the ventricles, small ventricular chambers, dilated atria, and thickening of the interatrial septum (Fig. 48–22),[309] although the findings are more prominent in the familial than in the primary (AL) form.[293] Left ventricular dysfunction may be seen, especially in advanced cases, but systolic function often is surprisingly normal.[293] Early preclinical unsuspected cardiac involvement may be detectable only by echocardiography or Doppler ultrasonography.[291] Although the cardiac valves may be thickened, they usually move normally.[302] A pericardial effusion is common but rarely results in tamponade. The appearance of the thickened cardiac walls is often distinctive on two-dimensional echocardiography, demonstrating a granular sparkling texture, presumably due to the amyloid deposit.[309] In some cases the pattern of increased wall thickness is nonuniform and may resemble HCM. Echocardiographic demonstration of thick left ventricular walls with concomitant low voltage on the ECG appears to distinguish cardiac amyloidosis from pericardial disease or left ventricular hypertrophy, and this distinctive voltage/mass ratio is characteristic of myocardial infiltration by amyloid.[309] Doppler ultrasonography and radionuclide ventriculography routinely demonstrate abnormalities of diastolic function, and, by estimating the degree of cardiac involvement by amyloid, provide prognostic information.[310] MRI may be of some help by using tissue characterization signatures to identify myocardial infiltration.[311]

Nuclear Imaging. *Scintigraphy* with technetium-99m pyrophosphate is often strongly positive with prominent amyloid involvement, although in some patients it is falsely negative.[309, 312] Positive scans tend to correlate with extensive cardiac involvement. Scanning with indium-labeled antimyosin antibody may also detect cardiac amyloid involvement.[313] Scanning with specialized agents has shown sympathetic denervation in patients with cardiac amyloidosis.[312]

DIAGNOSIS. Whereas two or three decades ago the clinical diagnosis of systemic amyloidosis was made correctly ante mortem in about one fourth of cases, with more recent clinical awareness of the disease and the utilization of *biopsy techniques* the diagnosis is now made before death in the majority of patients. An abdominal fat aspirate has been the single most useful diagnostic procedure, combining the attributes of ease of performance, sensitivity, and safety.[292] Biopsy of rectum, gingiva, bone marrow, liver, kidney, and various other tissues has also been used. Endomyocardial biopsy of the right or left ventricles may be

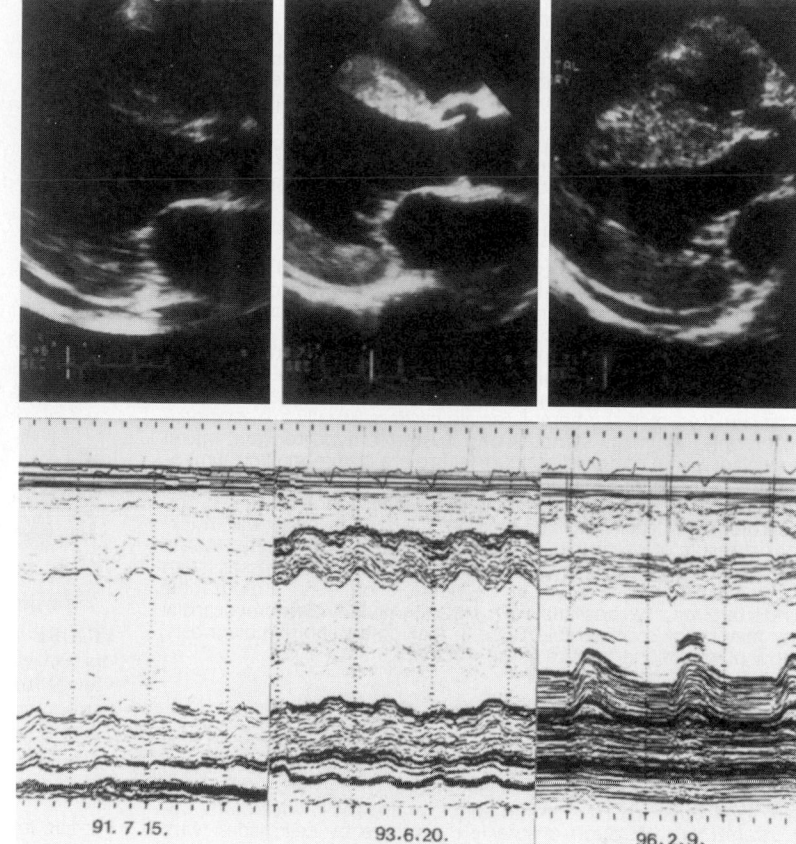

FIGURE 48–22. Serial echocardiographic findings in a patient developing cardiac amyloidosis. *Top,* Serial two-dimensional echocardiographic findings. Note the thickening of all myocardial walls and valves. *Bottom,* Serial M-mode echocardiography shows gradual increase of interventricular septal, left ventricular posterior wall, and right ventricular wall thickness. The date of the study is shown at the bottom (year.month.day). (From Youn H, Chae JS, Lee KY, et al: Images in cardiovascular medicine: Amyloidosis with cardiac involvement. Circulation 97:2093, 1998. Copyright 1998, American Heart Association.)

FIGURE 48–23. See color plate 28.

helpful in establishing the diagnosis of cardiac amyloidosis (Fig. 48–23) if the abdominal fat aspirate is negative.[292] Immunohistochemical staining of tissue samples is important to distinguish systemic senile, familial, and primary forms of amyloidosis in otherwise equivocal presentations, because prognosis and management differ in the various forms.[302, 314]

MANAGEMENT. The treatment of cardiac amyloidosis is generally unsatisfactory, although there has been some improvement in survival and functional state with the use of alkylating agents in primary (AL) amyloidosis.[302, 315, 316] Digitalis glycosides should be used with caution because patients with cardiac amyloidosis appear to be particularly sensitive to digitalis preparations, and the use of ordinary doses may lead to serious arrhythmias; this may relate to selective binding of digoxin to amyloid fibrils in the myocardium.[292] Similarly, nifedipine binds to amyloid fibrils; its use and that of the other calcium antagonists may lead to exacerbation of congestive heart failure symptoms due to an enhanced negative inotropic effect.[292, 317] Insertion of a permanent pacemaker may be beneficial in the short term in patients with symptomatic conducting system disease.[318] Careful use of low doses of diuretics and vasodilators may afford some symptomatic benefit, but there is a risk of hypotension and hypoperfusion with use of these agents.[291] In patients with atrial standstill due to amyloid infiltration, anticoagulation may be appropriate even in the absence of atrial arrhythmias, because there is some risk of thrombus formation, presumably as a consequence of stasis in the atrium.[306]

Autologous stem cell transplantation is being used with increasing frequency in primary (AL) amyloidosis, but the long-term benefit, especially in patients with cardiac involvement, is not known.[319] A small number of patients have undergone cardiac transplantation, with poor long-term results (39 percent survival at 4 years in one study) due to progressive amyloidosis in other organs or recurrence in the transplanted heart, although a few carefully selected patients have shown long-term survival and functional improvement.[291, 320] An heroic alternative approach for the familial form of cardiac amyloidosis is simultaneous heart and liver transplantation because the circulating transthyretin in these patients is produced in the liver and can be corrected with liver transplantation.[301, 302] No therapy is effective for the senile form, but survival is about 10 times longer than in the primary form (60 vs. 6 months).[314]

INHERITED INFILTRATIVE DISORDERS CAUSING RESTRICTIVE CARDIOMYOPATHY

The intramyocardial accumulation or infiltration of an abnormal metabolic product typically produces a restrictive picture with impaired diastolic ventricular filling. Systolic impairment may be seen as well but is not invariably found. A variety of infiltrative diseases, often inherited, may result in this hemodynamic picture, including the glycogenoses, the mucopolysaccharidoses, Fabry disease, and Gaucher disease.

FABRY DISEASE

Fabry disease (angiokeratoma corporis diffusum universale) is an X-linked recessive disorder of glycosphingolipid metabolism due to a deficiency of the lysosomal enzyme alpha-galactosidase A that is caused by one of more than four dozen mutations.[321] Some mutations result in no detectable alpha-galactosidase A activity and widespread manifestations throughout the body, whereas others produce some degree of enzyme activity with attendant atypical variants of Fabry disease with involvement limited solely to the myocardium.[322] The disease is characterized by an intracellular accumulation of a neutral glycolipid, with prominent involvement of the skin and kidneys as well as the myocardium in the classic form. *Histological examination* often reveals widespread involvement of the myocardium, vascular endothelium, conducting tissues, and valves, particularly the mitral valve. The major clinical manifestations of the disease result from the accumulation of the glycolipid substrate in endothelial cells, with eventual occlusion of small arterioles. The accumulation of the glycolipid occurs in the lysosomes of the cardiac tissues and is responsible for the multiple cardiovascular manifestations of Fabry disease (Fig. 48-24).

CARDIAC FINDINGS. These typically include angina and myocardial infarction caused by accumulation of lipid moieties in coronary endothelial cells, but coronary arteries are usually angiographically normal. There is increased left ventricular wall thickness simulating HCM, left ventricular dysfunction and failure due to lipid accumulation in myocytes, and mitral regurgitation (due to deposition in valvular fibroblasts).[323] Symptomatic cardiovascular involvement occurs eventually in most affected males, whereas female carriers usually are asymptomatic or only minimally symptomatic. Systemic hypertension, mitral valve prolapse, and congestive heart failure are common clinical manifestations. ECG abnormalities may include a short PR interval, atrioventricular block, and ST segment and T wave abnormalities.[323] The echocardiogram usually reveals increased left ventricular wall thickness as a result of glycolipid deposition, which may simulate HCM.[323] Differentiation from other hypertrophic or restrictive processes (such as cardiac amyloidosis) may not be possible on echocardiographic grounds but may be possible with MRI (Fig. 48-25). Endomyocardial biopsy may be of considerable value in making a definitive diagnosis, as is low plasma alpha-galactosidase A activity.

GAUCHER DISEASE

Gaucher disease is an uncommon inherited disorder of glycosyl ceramide metabolism. It is secondary to a deficiency of the enzyme beta-glucosidase and results in accumulation of cerebrosides in the spleen, liver, bone marrow, lymph nodes, brain, and myocardium. Diffuse interstitial infiltration of the left ventricle by cells laden with cerebroside produces reduced left ventricular compliance and cardiac output. Clinical evidence of cardiac involvement is uncommon, but when present it is characterized by left ventricular dysfunction, hemorrhagic pericardial effusion, increased left ventricular wall mass, and thickening of the left-sided valves.[324] Liver transplantation may produce a reduction in tissue infiltration by cerebrosides.[325]

HEMOCHROMATOSIS (See also Chap. 69)

Hemochromatosis is characterized by excessive deposition of iron in a variety of parenchymal tissues (heart, liver, gonads, and pancreas). It may occur (1) as a familial (autosomal recessive) or idiopathic disorder; (2) in association with a defect in hemoglobin synthesis resulting in ineffective erythropoiesis; (3) in chronic liver disease; and (4) with excessive oral or parenteral intake of iron (or blood transfusions) over many years.[326, 327] Although patients who have iron deposits in the myocardium almost always have deposits in other organs (e.g., liver, spleen, pancreas, bone marrow), the severity of myocardial involvement varies widely and only roughly parallels that in other organs.

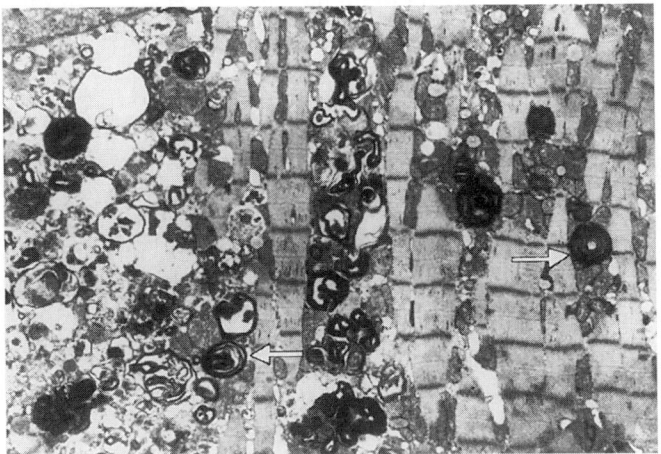

FIGURE 48-24. Electron microscopy of cardiac tissue in Fabry disease, showing complex concentric lamellar bodies (arrow) (original magnification 2000×). (From Cantor WJ, Butany J, Iwanochko M, Liu P: Restrictive cardiomyopathy secondary to Fabry's disease. Circulation 98:1457, 1998. Copyright 1998, American Heart Association.)

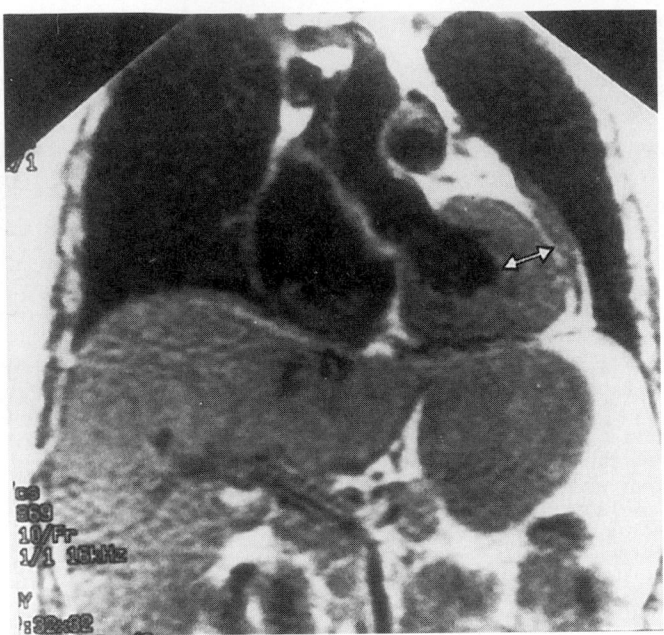

FIGURE 48-25. Cardiac MRI (T1-weighted spin echo) in Fabry disease, showing marked ventricular thickening (arrow). Coronal view. (From Cantor WJ, Butany J, Iwanochko M, Liu P: Restrictive cardiomyopathy secondary to Fabry's disease. Circulation 98:1457, 1998. Copyright 1998, American Heart Association.)

Cardiac involvement leads to a mixed DCM/RCM with both systolic and diastolic dysfunction, often with associated arrhythmias.[326, 328-330] Myocardial damage is thought to be due to direct tissue toxicity of the free iron moiety rather than simply to tissue infiltration.[326] Although cirrhosis and hepatocellular carcinoma are the most common causes of death, cardiac mortality is an important additional concern (especially in the group of patients—usually men—who present at a young age).[327]

PATHOLOGICAL FINDINGS. These consist of a dilated heart with thickened ventricular walls. Myocardial iron deposits are found within the sarcoplasmic reticulum and are most common in the subepicardial region, followed by the subendocardial region, and are least common in the midmyocardial wall.[326] They are more extensive in ventricular than in atrial myocardium. Involvement of the cardiac conducting system is common. Myocardial degeneration and fibrosis may also occur.

The severity of myocardial dysfunction is proportional to the quantity of iron present in the myocardium.[331] Extensive deposits of cardiac iron (particularly those grossly visible at postmortem examination) are invariably associated with cardiac dysfunction.

CLINICAL MANIFESTATIONS. These vary widely, depending on the extent of myocardial involvement. Some patients remain asymptomatic despite echocardiographic evidence of myocardial involvement, which is expressed initially as increased left ventricular wall thickness and later as chamber enlargement and contractile dysfunction.[331] In such cases, a variety of noninvasive techniques (CT and especially MRI) may demonstrate early subclinical myocardial involvement in which treatment is most effective (Fig. 48-26).[226, 332] Symptomatic cardiac involvement is usually associated with ECG abnormalities, including ST segment and T wave abnormalities, as well as supraventricular arrhythmias[331]; these ECG changes correlate with the degree of iron deposit in the heart.

Cardiac involvement usually is evident from the clinical and echocardiographic features; endomyocardial biopsy may be useful to confirm (but not exclude) the diagnosis.[327] The diagnosis is aided by finding an elevated plasma iron level, a normal or low total iron-binding capacity, and markedly elevated values for serum ferritin, urinary iron, liver iron, and especially saturation of transferrin.[327] Repeated phlebotomies or the use of the chelating agent desferrioxamine may be clinically beneficial.[326, 333]

GLYCOGEN STORAGE DISEASES

Adult patients may demonstrate cardiac involvement in these diseases; in type III (glycogen debranching enzyme deficiency), cardiac involvement is found only in patients with deficient enzyme in muscle tissue.[334] Cardiac involvement is marked most commonly by apparent left ventricular hypertrophy on the ECG and echocardiogram.[169, 334, 335]

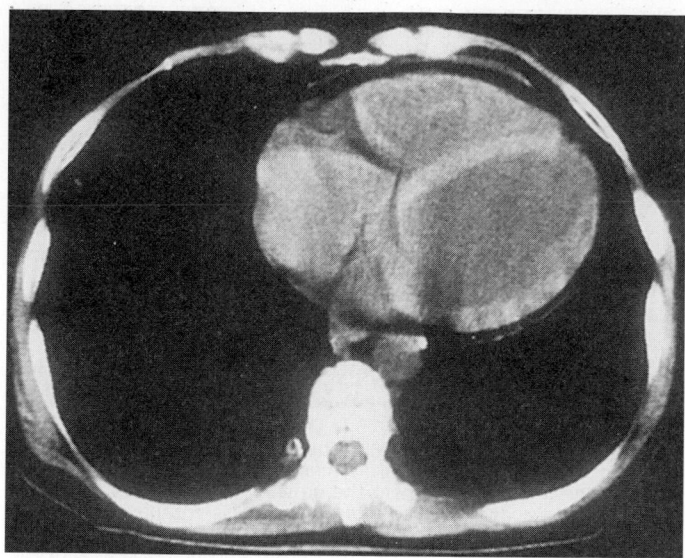

FIGURE 48-26. Standard-plane CT of chest without contrast medium enhancement at level of seventh thoracic vertebra in a patient with cardiac hemochromatosis. Gated scanning was not used, and scanning speed was one scan per 4 seconds. Right ventricle (*top*), left ventricle (*bottom*), and left atrium were scanned at this level. Left ventricular wall and part of right ventricular wall could be identified as a high-density area as a result of iron deposition in the myocardium. (From Niwano S, Yokoyama J, Niwano H, et al: Images in cardiovascular medicine: Iron deposition in myocardium documented on standard computed tomography in cardiac hemochromatosis. Circulation 97:2371, 1998. Copyright 1998, American Heart Association.)

involvement.[337] Syncope is common and may reflect paroxysmal arrhythmias or conduction disturbances.[336] Atrial and ventricular arrhythmias, especially ventricular tachycardia, are observed frequently.[336] Although cor pulmonale as a consequence of pulmonary sarcoidosis accounts for some of the symptoms of heart failure, many symptoms are caused by direct myocardial involvement by granulomas and scar tissue, and patients show the clinical features of RCM and/or DCM[336] Symptoms of myocardial sarcoid may be present for variable lengths of time; however, the disease may progress rapidly to death, and in some patients the interval from the onset of cardiac symptoms to death is measured in months. In others, survival may be considerably longer.[336]

Cardiac dysfunction is often severe and progressive. Occasionally, patients with extensive involvement develop overt left ventricular aneurysms. Pericardial effusions are not uncommon.[341]

The physical examination may reveal findings of extracardiac sarcoid or may be totally normal. A systolic murmur reflecting mitral regurgitation is common. This appears to be more the result of left ventricular dilatation than of direct sarcoid involvement of the papillary muscles.

The ECG frequently is abnormal and most commonly demonstrates T wave abnormalities. Sarcoidosis appears to have an affinity for involvement of the atrioventricular junction and bundle of His, and thus varying degrees of intraventricular or atrioventricular block are common.[336, 340] With extensive myocardial involvement, pathological Q waves may appear and simulate myocardial infarction (Fig. 48-27). Characteristic echocardiographic features include left ventricular dilatation and dysfunction, often with regional wall motion abnormalities suggestive of ischemic heart disease[336]; wall thinning and increased echogenicity

Sarcoidosis

Sarcoidosis is a granulomatous disorder of unknown cause, characterized by multisystem involvement. Infiltration of the lungs, reticuloendothelial system, and skin usually dominates the clinical picture, but virtually any tissue may be affected. The most important manifestation results from pulmonary involvement. This often leads to diffuse fibrosis that may result in fatal right-sided heart failure. Primary cardiac involvement is not often recognized clinically, although it may be demonstrated at autopsy in 20 to 30 percent of cases, most of which demonstrate generalized sarcoidosis.[336]

Clinical manifestations of sarcoid heart disease are present in less than 5 percent of patients, although myocardial involvement may result in heart block, congestive heart failure, ventricular arrhythmias, and sudden death.[337, 338] Myocardial sarcoidosis may have restrictive as well as congestive features because cardiac infiltration by sarcoid granulomas results not only in increased stiffness of the ventricular wall but in diminished systolic contractile function as well. Myocardial sarcoidosis typically affects young or middle-aged adults of either gender; there usually is evidence of generalized sarcoidosis.[336]

PATHOLOGY. The typical pathological feature of sarcoidosis is the presence of noncaseating granulomas, which occur in many organs. They infiltrate the myocardium and may eventually form fibrotic scars.[336] The granulomas may involve any region of the heart, although the left ventricular free wall and the interventricular septum are the most common sites, and extensive granulomas and scar tissue in the cephalad portion of the interventricular septum are constant findings in patients with abnormalities of the conduction system.[339] Cardiac infiltration may range from a few scattered lesions to extensive involvement. Because of the variable cardiac involvement, myocardial biopsy may be positive in only about half of the patients, and therefore a negative biopsy by no means excludes the diagnosis.[336] Transmural involvement is common, and large portions of the ventricular wall may be replaced by scar tissue, which may lead to aneurysm formation. Although involvement of small coronary artery branches may be found in sarcoidosis, the larger conductance vessels are uninvolved.[336]

CLINICAL MANIFESTATIONS. Sudden death is the most feared and unfortunately one of the more common manifestations of cardiac sarcoidosis.[336, 340] Conduction disturbances and congestive heart failure are common manifestations of symptomatic involvement in nonfatal cases, but many patients are asymptomatic despite extensive cardiac

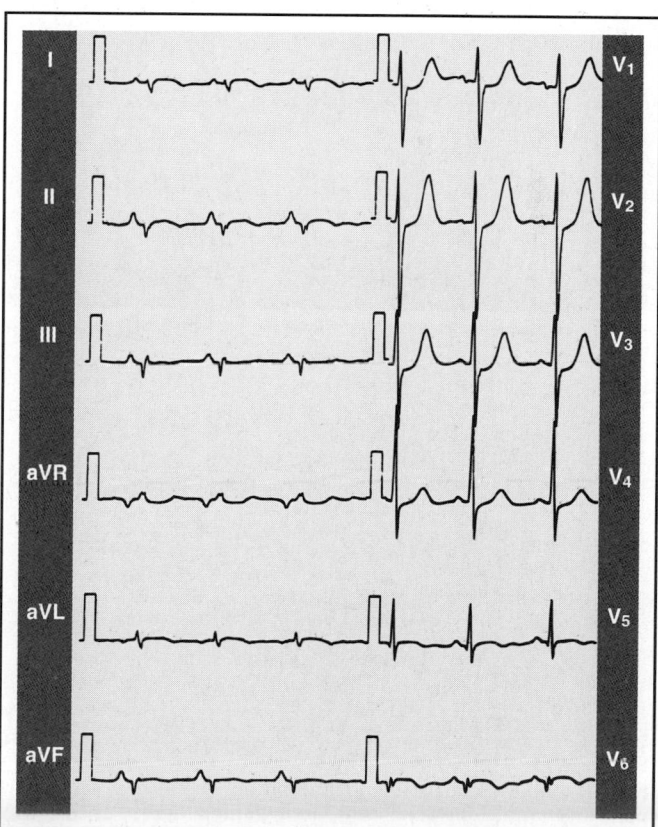

FIGURE 48-27. Electrocardiogram in patient with cardiac sarcoidosis shows abnormal Q wave in leads II, III, and aVF and ST segment elevation in V_5 and V_6. (From Shindo T, Kurihara H, Ohishi N, et al: Images in cardiovascular medicine: Cardiac sarcoidosis. Circulation 97: 1306, 1998. Copyright 1998, American Heart Association.)

are sometimes observed (Fig. 48–28). A small to moderate-sized pericardial effusion is seen in about 20 percent.[341]

DIAGNOSIS. In many cases the diagnosis may be suspected in patients with bilateral hilar lymphadenopathy on chest roentgenogram in whom there is clinical or ECG evidence of myocardial disease. Endomyocardial biopsy may be useful in establishing the diagnosis, although the nonuniform involvement of the heart by sarcoidosis means that a negative biopsy does not exclude the diagnosis. The echocardiogram demonstrates diffuse and often regional left ventricular wall motion abnormalities in patients with clinical cardiac involvement (see Fig. 48–28). Myocardial imaging with thallium-201 or technetium-99m sestimibi may be helpful in demonstrating segmental perfusion defects that result from sarcoid infiltration of the myocardium.[337, 342, 343] Imaging may also indicate the presence of right ventricular hypertrophy in patients with right ventricular overload due to pulmonary fibrosis and pulmonary hypertension. Uptake of technetium pyrophosphate, gallium, and labeled antimyosin antibody may aid in the diagnosis, as may MRI.[336, 343–347]

MANAGEMENT. The treatment of myocardial sarcoidosis is difficult.[340] Arrhythmias are often refractory to antiarrhythmic drugs. Permanent pacing may be helpful in patients with involvement of the atrioventricular conduction system. Although the matter is not settled, corticosteroids may be of some benefit in treating the conduction disturbances, arrhythmias, and myocardial dysfunction of sar-

coidosis.[336, 348] It has been suggested that further benefit may be derived from the addition of hydroxychloroquine, methotrexate, or cyclophosphamide.[340] Because the risk of sudden death appears to be greatest in patients with extensive myocardial involvement, it may be reasonable to attempt to halt the progression of the disease with corticosteroids before irreversible fibrosis occurs. Insertion of an ICD may be considered in appropriate patients at high risk of sudden death.[349] Heart or heart-lung transplantation has been used in selected patients with intractable heart failure, although recurrent sarcoid involvement of the transplanted heart can occur.[291]

ENDOMYOCARDIAL DISEASE

DEFINITION AND PATHOGENESIS. Endomyocardial disease (EMD) is a common form of restrictive cardiomyopathy that typically is found in a geographical distribution near the equator.[350] It is most frequent in equatorial Africa and is encountered with less frequency in South America, Asia, and nontropical countries, including the United States.[351] It is marked by intense endocardial fibrotic thickening of the apex and subvalvular regions of one or both ventricles that results in obstruction to inflow of blood into the respective ventricle, thus producing restrictive physiology. For many years it had been thought that there are two variants of the disease, one occurring principally in tropical countries (termed *endomyocardial fibrosis* [EMF] or Davies disease) and the other in temperate countries (Löffler's endocarditis parietalis fibroplastica or hypereosinophilic syndrome).[292] However, despite the pathological similarities,[352] there are important contrasts in clinical presentation that challenge the concept of a single disease process.[353] In addition to the geographical differences, the temperate form of the disease is a more aggressive and rapidly progressive disorder, affecting principally males, and is associated with hypereosinophilia, thromboembolic phenomena, and generalized arteritis. EMF, conversely, shows no gender predilection, occurs in younger patients, and is not associated with an intense eosinophilia.[292]

DIFFERENCES BETWEEN LÖFFLER ENDOCARDITIS AND EMF. Part of the thesis that Löffler endocarditis and EMF are different phases of a single disease is based on a theory of pathogenesis involving the toxic effect of eosinophils on the heart.[354] Under this formulation, an initial hypereosinophilia of whatever cause results in damage to the myocardium that produces the first phase of EMD: a necrotic phase, marked by an intense myocarditis, rich in eosinophils, and with an associated arteritis (i.e., Löffler endocarditis).[354] This initial phase occurs within the first few months of illness. It may be followed by a thrombotic stage, occurring about a year after initial presentation, during which the myocarditis has receded, nonspecific thickening of the myocardium is beginning, and there is a variable degree of superimposed thrombus formation.[354] The putative last stage is one of fibrosis, presenting all of the features of EMF. The three stages—necrotic, thrombotic, and fibrotic—have been defined on the basis of postmortem material, and it is not suggested by proponents of the unified pathogenesis hypothesis that each patient with advanced disease (manifested by EMF) has necessarily passed through the earlier phases.

ROLE OF EOSINOPHILS. The possible role of eosinophils in the production of the cardiac abnormalities has intrigued investigators for years.[354, 355] Eosinophils may damage tissues by direct invasion or by the release of toxic substances. The presence of degranulated eosinophils in the peripheral blood of patients with Löffler endocarditis suggests that the protein constituents of the eosinophil's granule may be cardiotoxic, first producing the necrotic phase of EMD, followed by the thrombotic and fibrotic phases after the disappearance of the initial eosinophilia.[353]

There is now, however, increasing speculation that this continuum occurs only in the temperate countries, and the endemic EMF found in tropical countries is a distinct and separate disease, because a link with eosinophilia has been difficult to document, despite the frequency of parasitic diseases.[292, 356–358] Other etiological factors have been implicated (Fig 48–29); the fibrosis of tropical EMF has been linked to the higher levels of cerium and lower concentrations of magnesium that apparently are found in endemic areas.[356, 359, 360]

Because the clinical manifestations of EMD demonstrate geographical and clinical differences, Löffler endocarditis and EMF are discussed separately, even though they could be part of the same disease continuum.

Löffler Endocarditis: The Hypereosinophilic Syndrome

Marked eosinophilia of any cause may be associated with endomyocardial disease. The typical patient who presents

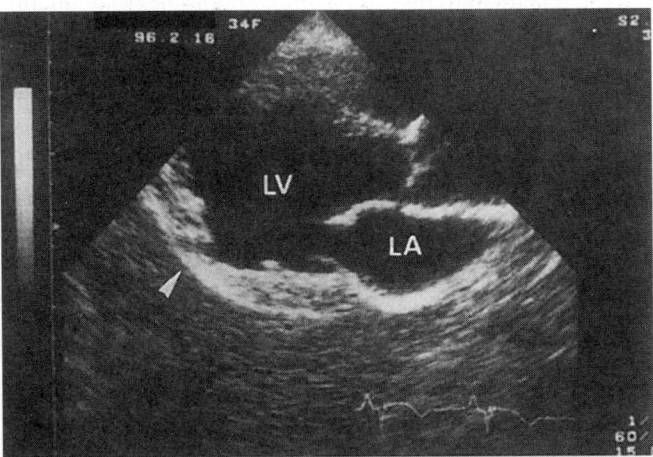
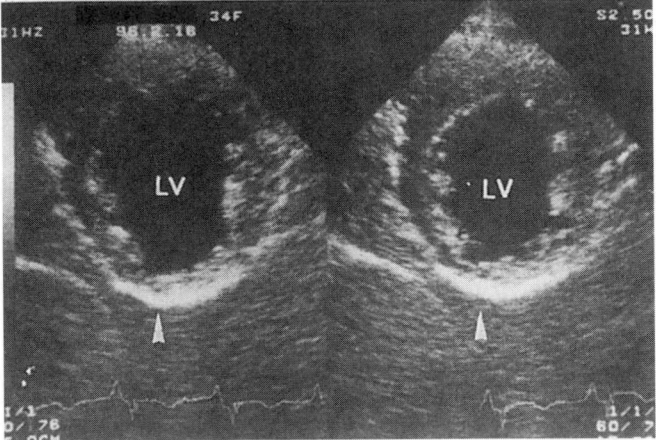

FIGURE 48–28. Echocardiographic findings in cardiac sarcoidosis. *Top,* Parasternal long-axial echocardiographic view. Arrows show wall thinning and increased echogenicity of inferior wall. *Bottom,* Parasternal short-axial view showing end-diastolic (*lower left*) and end-systolic (*lower right*) phases. These is impaired systolic shortening. Arrows show increased echogenicity. (From Shindo T, Kurihara H, Ohishi N, et al: Images in cardiovascular medicine. Cardiac sarcoidosis. Circulation 97:1306, 1998. Copyright 1998, American Heart Association.)

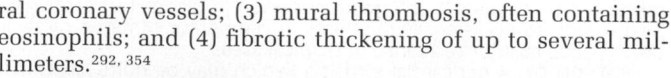

Pathogenesis of Löffler's syndrome

Allergic reaction → Autoimmune disease

Parasitic and protozoal infections → Malignancy → Idiopathic

↓

Overproduction of cytotoxic eosinophils

↓

Infiltration of myocardium by eosinophils

↓

Degranulation of eosinophilic granules

↓

Tissue damage by major basic and cationic proteins

Necrotic phase

↓

Acute pericarditis, myocarditis, or endocarditis

Thrombotic phase

↓

Formation of intramural thrombi adjacent to the injured endocardium

Fibrotic phase

↓

Localized or extensive replacement fibrosis

FIGURE 48–29. The pathogenesis of Löffler syndrome. Tissue damage is caused by major basic and cationic proteins derived from cytotoxic eosinophils. These cytotoxic proteins may stay in the myocardium for a prolonged period and produce continuous tissue damage. In the fibrotic phase, various types of heart diseases, such as endomyocardial fibrosis, dilated cardiomyopathy, atrioventricular block, or valvular regurgitation can be seen according to the site of the most dominant involvement. (From Hirota Y: Restrictive cardiomyopathy, cardiac amyloidosis, and hypereosinophilic heart disease. *In* Abelmann WH, Braunwald E [eds]: Atlas of Heart Diseases. Vol 2. Cardiomyopathies, Myocarditis, and Pericardial Disease. Philadelphia, Current Medicine, 1995.)

with Löffler endocarditis is a man in his fourth decade who lives in a temperate climate and has the hypereosinophilic syndrome (i.e., persistent eosinophilia with 1500 eosinophils/mm[3] for at least 6 months or until death, with evidence of organ involvement).[292, 354, 361] Cardiac involvement in the hypereosinophilic syndrome is the rule, occurring in more than three fourths of patients.[362] Hypereosinophilia and cardiac involvement are also seen in the Churg-Strauss syndrome, which is differentiated by asthma or allergic rhinitis and a necrotizing vasculitis.[292] The cause of the eosinophilia in most patients with Löffler endocarditis is unknown, although in some it may be the result of leukemia, or it may be reactive (i.e., secondary to various parasitic, allergic, granulomatous, hypersensitivity, or neoplastic disorders).[355]

PATHOLOGY. In the hypereosinophilic syndrome, a variety of organs are usually involved besides the heart, including the lungs, bone marrow, and brain.[354] Cardiac involvement is often biventricular, with mural endocardial thickening of the inflow portions and apex of the ventricles.[292] Histological findings include variable degrees of (1) an acute inflammatory eosinophilic myocarditis involving the myocardium and endocardium; (2) thrombosis, fibrinoid change, and inflammatory reaction involving small intramu-

ral coronary vessels; (3) mural thrombosis, often containing eosinophils; and (4) fibrotic thickening of up to several millimeters.[292, 354]

CLINICAL MANIFESTATIONS. The principal clinical features include weight loss, fever, cough, rash, and congestive heart failure. Although early cardiac involvement may be asymptomatic, overt cardiac dysfunction occurs in more than half of the patients and may be right and/or left sided.[362] Cardiomegaly, often without overt symptoms of congestive heart failure, may be present, and the murmur of mitral regurgitation is common.[354] Systemic embolism is frequent and may lead to neurological and renal dysfunction. Death is usually due to congestive heart failure, often with associated renal, hepatic, or respiratory dysfunction.[292]

LABORATORY EXAMINATION. The chest roentgenogram may reveal cardiomegaly and pulmonary congestion or, less commonly, pulmonary infiltrates. The ECG most commonly shows nonspecific ST segment and T wave abnormalities.[292] Arrhythmias, especially atrial fibrillation, and conduction defects, particularly right bundle branch block, may also be present.

The echocardiogram commonly demonstrates localized thickening of the posterobasal left ventricular wall, with absent or markedly limited motion of the posterior leaflet of the mitral valve.[292] There may be obliteration of the apex by thrombus. Enlargement of the atria may be seen, along with Doppler ultrasound evidence of atrioventricular regurgitation. Systolic function often is well preserved, in keeping with the restrictive picture seen in this condition.

The hemodynamic consequences of the dense endocardial scarring seen in Löffler endocarditis are those of an RCM, with abnormal diastolic filling due to increased stiffness of the ventricles and a reduction in the size of the ventricular cavity by organized thrombus.[354] Atrioventricular valvular regurgitation may occur because of involvement of the supporting apparatus of the mitral or tricuspid valves.[362] *Cardiac catheterization* reveals markedly elevated ventricular filling pressures, and there may be evidence of tricuspid or mitral regurgitation. A characteristic feature on angiocardiography is largely preserved systolic function with obliteration of the apex of the ventricles.[354] The diagnosis is often confirmed by percutaneous endomyocardial biopsy, but the biopsy is not invariably positive.

MANAGEMENT. Medical therapy during the course of early Löffler endocarditis and surgical therapy during the later phases of fibrosis may have a positive effect on symptoms and survival. Corticosteroids appear to have a beneficial effect on acute myocarditis[363] and together with cytotoxic drugs (hydroxyurea in particular) may improve survival substantially.[291, 354] A limited number of patients not responding to standard therapy have responded to treatment with interferon.[355, 361] Routine cardiac therapy with digitalis, diuretics, afterload reduction, and anticoagulation as indicated are adjuncts in the management of these patients.[354] Surgical therapy (see p. 1782) appears to offer significant palliation of symptoms once the fibrotic stage has been reached.[292, 354]

Endomyocardial Fibrosis

Endomyocardial fibrosis occurs most commonly in tropical and subtropical Africa, particularly Uganda and Nigeria. It is characterized by fibrous endocardial lesions of the inflow of the right or left ventricle or both and often involves the atrioventricular valves, resulting in regurgitation.[356] It is a relatively frequent cause of heart failure and death in equatorial Africa, accounting for 10 to 20 percent of deaths due to heart disease.[353]

Although most prominent in Africa, it is also found in tropical and subtropical regions in the rest of the world, typically within 15 degrees of the equator,[350] including India,[360] Brazil, Colombia, and Sri Lanka.[353] EMF is most common in specific ethnic groups, notably the Rwanda tribe in Uganda, and in people of low socioeconomic status.[364] The disease is equally frequent in both genders, and, although most common in children and young adults, its reported age range is 4 to 70 years.[351] It is most common in blacks, but cases have been reported occasionally in whites in temperate climates, rarely in the absence of prior residence in tropical areas.

PATHOLOGY. A pericardial effusion, which may be quite large, may be present. The heart is normal in size or slightly enlarged, but massive cardiomegaly does not occur. The right atrium is often dilated, and in patients with severe right ventricular involvement there may be massive enlargement of this chamber. Indentation of the right border of the heart above the apex as a result of apical scarring may occur.

Combined right and left ventricular disease occurs in about half the cases, with pure left ventricular involvement occurring in 40 percent and pure right ventricular involvement in the remaining 10 percent of patients who are examined post mortem.[352] When affected, the right ventricle exhibits extensive dense fibrous thickening of the inflow tract and apex, with involvement of the papillary muscles and chordae tendineae. Involvement of the right ventricle may lead to obliteration of the apex, with a mass of thrombus and fibrous tissue filling the cavity.[352] The tricuspid valve is often distorted by the fibrous process involving the supporting structures. Right atrial thrombi occur commonly. Left ventricular involvement is similar, with fibrosis extending from the apex up the inflow portion of the left ventricle to the posterior mitral valve leaflet. The anterior leaflet of the mitral valve and the outflow portion of the left ventricle are usually spared. Thrombi often overlie the endocardial lesions, and widely distributed endocardial calcific deposits may occur.[353] The epicardial coronary arteries are free of obstructive lesions.

HISTOLOGIC FINDINGS. Microscopically, the involved endocardium demonstrates a thick layer of collagen tissue on top of a layer of loosely arranged connective tissue.[351] Septa composed of fibrous and granulation tissue extend for variable distances into the myocardium.[353] Interstitial edema is often present, but there is no prominent cellular infiltration. Small patches of fibroelastosis may occur in both ventricular outflow tracts beneath the semilunar valves but are thought to be a secondary phenomenon due to local trauma rather than a result of the basic pathological process. The intramural coronary arteries may show medial degeneration and fibrosis and fibrin deposits.[353]

CLINICAL MANIFESTATIONS. Because EMF may involve both ventricles or either ventricle selectively, symptoms vary. Left-sided involvement results in symptoms of pulmonary congestion, whereas predominant right-sided disease may present features of an RCM and therefore simulate constrictive pericarditis. There is often regurgitation of one or both atrioventricular valves. The onset of the disease is usually insidious, but it is sometimes ushered in by an acute febrile illness. Rarely, the disease appears to stabilize; although survival for up to 12 years has been observed, EMF is usually relentlessly progressive.[292] Death is due to progressive myocardial failure, often associated with pulmonary congestion, infection, or infarction, or sudden, unexpected cardiovascular collapse, presumably arrhythmic in origin. Survival appears to be unrelated to the site of predominant involvement (right or left ventricle), although patients presenting in advanced right-sided failure have a worse prognosis than other patients.[292]

RIGHT VENTRICULAR EMF. Pure or predominant right ventricular involvement is characterized by fibrous obliteration of the right ventricular apex that diminishes the capacity of this chamber.[352] The fibrosis often extends to the supporting apparatus of the tricuspid valve,[365] resulting in tricuspid regurgitation. Clinical manifestations in patients with right-sided involvement include an elevated jugular venous pressure, a prominent *v* wave, and a rapid *y* descent. A protodiastolic gallop sound may be heard along the lower sternal border, reflecting right ventricular dysfunction.[352] The liver is usually large and pulsatile, and ascites, splenomegaly, and peripheral edema are common. Pulmonary congestion is not present in the absence of left-sided involvement, and the pulmonary artery and pulmonary capillary wedge pressures are normal. A pericardial effusion, which is sometimes quite large, may be present. The right atrium is often enlarged, sometimes massively so.

Laboratory Findings. The ECG is usually abnormal, with diminished QRS voltage (probably resulting from the presence of a pericardial effusion), ST segment and T wave abnormalities, and findings suggestive of right-sided enlargement, especially a qR pattern in lead V_1.[351] The chest roentgenogram demonstrates cardiac enlargement, usually with gross prominence of the right atrium and a pericardial effusion. Calcification in the walls of the right or, less commonly, the left ventricle may be seen.[353] Echocardiography may demonstrate right ventricular thickening, obliteration of the apex, dilated atrium, strong echoes emanating from the endocardial surface, and abnormal septal motion in patients with tricuspid regurgitation.[352, 357, 366] At angiography the right ventricular apex is characteristically not visualized because of obliteration by the fibrous endocardium, but tricuspid regurgitation, right atrial enlargement, and filling defects in the right atrium due to intraatrial thrombi are sometimes seen.[351] Early angiographic changes that may be present before advanced disease develops include a change in the endocardial appearance, small apical filling defects, and mild tricuspid regurgitation.

LEFT VENTRICULAR EMF. With predominant *left-sided* involvement, the endomyocardial fibrosis invades the apex of the ventricle and usually the chordae tendineae or the posterior mitral valve leaflet as well, leading to mitral regurgitation.[367] The murmur may be confined to late systole, as is characteristic of the papillary muscle dysfunction type of murmur, or it may be pansystolic. Findings of pulmonary hypertension may be prominent. A protodiastolic gallop is commonly heard.

Laboratory Findings. The ECG usually shows T wave abnormalities. QRS voltage may be diminished in the presence of a pericardial effusion, although left ventricular hypertrophy may be present.[292] There may be findings of left atrial abnormality. As with right-sided involvement, atrial fibrillation often is present. Echocardiographic features include thickening and reduced motion of the posterobasal wall and posterior mitral leaflet, increased echoreflectivity of the endocardium, preserved systolic wall motion in the presence of apical obliteration, dilated atrium, and Doppler ultrasound evidence of mitral regurgitation.[292] Cardiac catheterization often reveals pulmonary hypertension, with elevated left ventricular filling pressures and a reduced cardiac index.[367] The left ventriculogram usually shows mitral regurgitation, and a filling defect due to an intracavitary thrombus within the ventricle may be seen on occasion. Coronary arteriography does not reveal obstructive disease.

BIVENTRICULAR EMF. This form of EMF occurs more frequently than either isolated right- or left-sided disease.[351] If there is more than minimal right ventricular involvement, severe pulmonary hypertension does not occur and the right-sided findings dominate the clinical presentation. Typical patients with biventricular involvement may have the features of right ventricular EMF, with only a mitral regurgitant murmur to suggest left ventricular involvement. Systemic embolization may occur in up to 15 percent of patients; infective endocarditis is even less frequent and is found in less than 2 percent.

DIAGNOSIS. This is based on the presence in an individual of the typical clinical and laboratory features, particularly angiography, from the appropriate geographical area. Eosinophilia is usually not a prominent feature and when present may reflect associated parasitic infestation. Endomyocardial biopsy may occasionally be helpful in establishing the diagnosis. However, this risks dislodging a mural thrombus, with resultant embolization. Left-sided biopsy is *not* recommended. In addition, because the disease is often focal, the biopsy may miss the pathological process, particularly if a right ventricular biopsy is performed in a patient with isolated left-sided disease.

MANAGEMENT. The medical treatment of EMF is often difficult and not particularly effective. In patients with advanced disease, the outlook is poor, with a 35 to 50 percent 2-year mortality. Substantially better survival may be seen in less symptomatic patients who have milder forms of the disease. Digitalis glycosides may be helpful in controlling the ventricular rate in patients with atrial fibrillation,[292] but the response of congestive symptoms is disappointing, and the development of atrial fibrillation is a poor prognostic sign.[368] Diuretics are not particularly helpful in the treatment of ascites.[292] Once endomyocardial disease has reached the fibrotic stage, surgery offers the possibility of symptomatic improvement and is the treatment of choice.[369] Operative excision of the fibrotic endocardium and replacement of the mitral and/or tricuspid valves have led to substantial symptomatic improvement, especially with predominant left-sided involvement.[291, 370] Mitral valve repair, rather than replacement, can be accomplished in some patients.[371] Postoperative catheterization has provided objective evidence of hemodynamic improvement with a reduction in ventricular filling pressures, an increase in cardiac output, and normalization of the angiographic appearance. Operative mortality has been high, running between 15 and 25 percent in the larger series,[291, 292, 369] although it appears to be lower if valve replacement can be avoided.[371] Long-term results suggest that surgery is at best palliative, with recurrent fibrosis, continued functional limitation, and cumulative mortality limiting the overall success of an operative approach.[369]

Endocardial Fibroelastosis (See Chap. 45)

Carcinoid Heart Disease (See also Chap. 46)

ETIOLOGY. The carcinoid syndrome is caused by a metastasizing carcinoid tumor and is characterized by cutaneous flushing, diarrhea, bronchoconstriction, and endocardial plaques composed of a unique type of fibrous tissue. The vasomotor, bronchoconstrictor, and cardiac manifestations are undoubtedly related to circulating humoral substances secreted by the tumor,[372] although the precise substance(s) responsible remains to be elucidated.[373] Virtually all patients develop diarrhea and flushing, and cardiac abnormalities are found on echocardiography in more than half; clinically apparent and severe right-sided disease is seen in a fourth of patients.[372, 374]

Sixty to 90 percent of tumors arise in the small bowel and appendix, and the rest originate in other areas of the gastrointestinal tract and bronchus.[372] Carcinoid tumors of the ileum are the most likely to metastasize, with involvement of the regional lymph nodes and liver. Usually only carcinoid tumors that invade the liver result in carcinoid heart disease.[372] The cardiac lesions may be related to large circulating quantities of serotonin, bradykinin, or other substances secreted by the tumor, which usually are inactivated by the liver, lungs, and brain.[375] Hepatic metastases apparently allow large quantities of tumor products to reach the heart.[374] The preferential right-sided involvement presumably is related to inactivation of the offending humoral substance(s) by the lungs. In 5 to 10 percent of cases, significant left-sided valvular disease develops,[376] related in most to passage of blood directly from the right to the left side of the heart through a patent foramen ovale, or less commonly by tumor involvement of the lungs.[372]

PATHOLOGY. The characteristic pathological findings are fibrous plaques that involve the "downstream" aspect of the tricuspid and pulmonic valves, the endocardium of the cardiac chambers, and the intima of the venae cavae, pulmonary artery, and coronary sinus (see Figs. 46–45 and 46–47). The fibrous tissue in the plaques results in structural and functional distortion of the valves, leading to both stenosis and regurgitation.[372] Histologically, the plaques consist of deposits of fibrous tissue located superficially on the endocardium, often with extension into the underlying layers. Identical morphological features have been found in some patients treated with the anorectic drugs fenfluramine and dexfenfluramine.[374] Ultrastructural and immunohistochemical studies have demonstrated that the plaques are composed of smooth muscle cells embedded in a stroma rich in acid mucopolysaccharides and collagen. Metastatic involvement of the myocardium itself is rare.[372]

CLINICAL MANIFESTATIONS. Physical examination usually reveals a systolic murmur along the left sternal border, produced by tricuspid regurgitation; in some cases, there may be a concomitant murmur of pulmonic stenosis and/or regurgitation.[372]

The chest roentgenogram is normal in half of the patients, but it may reveal enlargement of the heart and pleural effusions or nodules; the pulmonary artery trunk is typically of normal size, without evidence of poststenotic dilatation as occurs in congenital pulmonic stenosis. No specific ECG pattern is diagnostic of carcinoid heart disease.[372] Right atrial enlargement may be seen on occasion, but ECG evidence of right ventricular hypertrophy usually is lacking. Nonspecific ST segment and T wave abnormalities and sinus tachycardia are the most common findings, although severely symptomatic patients usually have low QRS voltage.[377] Echocardiography may reveal tricuspid and/or pulmonary valve thickening, along with right atrial and right ventricular dilatation; small pericardial effusions are present in a minority.[372]

The hemodynamic findings most commonly encountered are those of tricuspid regurgitation and occasionally pulmonic stenosis. A rare patient with the carcinoid syndrome demonstrates a hyperkinetic state (which may lead to high-output heart failure) but without the typical cardiac lesions; in one patient this was caused by profound vasodilatation by substance P.[378]

MANAGEMENT. In patients with mild congestive heart failure therapy includes digitalis and diuretics. Symptomatic improvement and improved survival have been noted with the use of somatostatin analogs.[374, 375] Balloon valvuloplasty of the right-sided valves has produced symptomatic improvement in some patients with stenotic tricuspid or pulmonary valves,[379] although others have developed recurrent symptoms despite "successful" valvuloplasty.[380] Surgical replacement of the tricuspid valve and pulmonic valvotomy or valvectomy may result in symptomatic improvement in severely symptomatic patients with serious valvular dysfunction, although the operative mortality is high (35 percent in one series).[377] Surgery may improve the functional status and survival of patients with carcinoid heart disease, but patients older than the age of 60 years have a very high surgical mortality (reportedly over 50 percent).[376] The long-term mortality remains high regardless of treatment modality, with half the patients dead within 1 to 2 years.[372, 377]

Obesity and Heart Disease (See Chap. 64)

Diabetic Cardiomyopathy (See Chap. 63)

▼ Myocarditis

Myocarditis is considered to be present when the heart is involved in an inflammatory process, often caused by an infectious agent. The inflammation may involve the myocytes, interstitium, vascular elements, and/or pericardium; involvement of the latter structure is discussed in Chapter 50.

Etiology

Myocarditis has been described during and after a wide variety of viral, rickettsial, bacterial, protozoal, and metazoal diseases; indeed, virtually any infectious agent may produce cardiac inflammation (Table 48–9). Infectious agents cause myocardial damage by three basic mechanisms: (1) invasion of the myocardium, (2) production of a myocardial toxin (e.g., diphtheria), and (3) immunologically mediated myocardial damage.[381] The principal mechanism of cardiac involvement in viral myocarditis is believed to be a cell-mediated immunological reaction to new cell surface changes or a new antigen related to the virus, and not merely the result of cell damage caused by viral replication.[382, 383] Additional evidence for an immune-mediated mechanism is the demonstration of a marked increase in major histocompatibility complex antigen expression in the biopsy specimens from patients with myocarditis.[384] Antibodies against intracellular components may also play a role.[385] Such cross-reactivity of antibodies to both virus and myocardial proteins (termed *molecular mimicry*) may play a role in producing immune-mediated myocardial damage.[386] Patients with ongoing myocarditis (unlike those with resolved myocarditis) have myocytes that express intercellular adhesion molecule-1 (ICAM-1), and it is speculated that the persistent expression of ICAM-1 may play a role in continued myocardial inflammation. Thus, the ultimate impact of the immune response associated with viral infection is a result of the balance between its protective and deleterious effects.[386] Although the term is often mistakenly used to indicate myocardial inflammation solely due to an infective agent, myocarditis may also be caused by allergic reactions and pharmacological agents, as well as occurring during the course of some systemic diseases such as vasculitis.

Myocarditis may be an acute or a chronic process and may occur during the peripartum period (see Chap. 65).[387] In North America, viruses (especially enteroviruses) are believed to be the most common agents producing myocarditis,[388] whereas in South America, Chagas disease (produced by *Trypanosoma cruzi*) is far more common. The identifica-

▼ **TABLE 48–9. INFECTIOUS CAUSES OF MYOCARDITIS**

Viral
Adenovirus
Arbovirus (dengue fever, yellow fever)
Arenavirus (Lassa fever)
Coxsackievirus
Cytomegalovirus
Echovirus
Encephalomyocarditis virus
Epstein-Barr virus
Hepatitis B
Herpesvirus
Human immunodeficiency virus-1
Influenza virus
Mumps virus
Poliomyelitis virus
Rabies
Respiratory syncytial virus
Rubella virus
Rubeola virus
Vaccinia virus
Varicella virus
Variola virus

Bacterial
Brucellosis
Clostridia
Diphtheria
Francisella (tularemia)
Gonococcus
Haemophilus
Legionella
Meningococcus
Mycobacterium (tuberculosis, avium-intracellulare, leprae)
Mycoplasma
Pneumococcus
Psittacosis
Salmonella
Staphylococcus
Streptococcus
Tropheryma whippelii (Whipple disease)

Fungal
Actinomyces
Aspergillus
Blastomyces
Candida
Coccidioides
Cryptococcus
Histoplasma
Nocardia
Sporothrix

Rickettsial
Rocky Mountain spotted fever
Q fever
Scrub typhus
Typhus

Spirochetal
Borrelia (Lyme disease and relapsing fever)
Leptospira
Syphilis

Helminthic
Cysticercus
Echinococcus
Schistosoma
Toxocara (visceral larva migrans)
Trichinella

Protozoal
Entamoeba
Leishmania
Trypanosoma (Chagas disease)
Toxoplasmosis

From Pisani B, Taylor D, Mason J: Inflammatory myocardial disease and cardiomyopathies. Am J Med 102:459, 1997.

tion of the specific etiological agent responsible for infective myocarditis usually rests on the associated extracardiac findings because the cardiovascular signs and symptoms are often nonspecific. The histological findings vary, depending on the stage of the disease, the mechanism of myocardial damage, and the specific etiological agent. Myocardial involvement may be focal or diffuse; it appears that myocarditis may begin as a focal process but then spread to involve the myocardium diffusely over a period of several weeks.[389] The clinical consequences depend to a large extent on the size and distribution of the myocarditic lesions. However, a single small lesion may have profound consequences if it is located within the cardiac conducting system. The histological findings are usually nonspecific (except for some parasitic and granulomatous forms of myocarditis), and with certain exceptions (see p. 1753) myocardial biopsy seldom elucidates the specific etiological agent.

Clinical Manifestations

The clinical expression of myocarditis ranges from the asymptomatic state associated with limited and focal inflammation to fulminant fatal congestive heart failure due to diffuse myocarditis.[27] In some patients, otherwise unexplained ventricular arrhythmias may be due to silent myocarditis.[390] An initial episode of viral myocarditis, perhaps unrecognized and forgotten, may be the initial event that eventually culminates in an "idiopathic" DCM.[10] In experimental animals, the structural and functional myocardial alterations that follow viral myocarditis may persist well beyond the stage of viral replication and myocardial inflammatory response, and the late changes resemble those of DCM.

The outcome after viral myocarditis is quite variable,[27, 390a] perhaps related to differing genetic susceptibility of individual patients. In most patients, the event is entirely self-limited and often unrecognized.[388, 391] More overt myocarditis may result in acute congestive heart failure.[338] In others, unrecognized myocarditis may be the cause of arrhythmias in what appears to be a structurally normal heart.[392] Some patients with chest pain and angiographically normal coronary arteries may have had subclinical myocarditis at some point in the past. Most intriguing is the possibility that viral myocarditis may culminate in DCM, presumably as a consequence of viral-mediated immunological cardiac damage.[391]

Although transient ECG abnormalities suggesting myocardial involvement are noted in many patients with infectious disease, most patients do not have other clinical manifestations of myocarditis. It is postulated that these ECG changes reflect subclinical myocardial involvement. That unrecognized myocardial involvement occurs with systemic infections is supported by histological evidence of unsuspected myocarditis found during routine postmortem examinations; this occurs about 1 percent of the time.[338] Some degree of myocardial involvement, often subepicardial in location, also frequently occurs in patients with acute pericarditis.

Because myocardial involvement is subclinical in most acute infectious diseases, the majority of patients have no specific complaints referable to the cardiovascular system; the presence of myocarditis is often inferred from ST segment and T wave abnormalities on the ECG. From a clinical viewpoint, myocardial involvement is associated with nonspecific symptoms including fatigue, dyspnea, palpitations, and precordial discomfort.[338] Chest pain usually reflects associated pericarditis, but precordial discomfort suggestive of myocardial ischemia is occasionally observed. In some cases, the clinical presentation (with chest pain, ECG abnormalities, increased muscle enzyme levels in the blood, and regional wall motion abnormalities) may simulate an acute myocardial infarction.[393, 394]

PHYSICAL EXAMINATION. Tachycardia is usual and may be out of proportion to the temperature elevation. The S_1 is often muffled, and a protodiastolic gallop may be present. A transient apical systolic murmur may appear,[338] but diastolic murmurs are rare. Clinical evidence of congestive heart failure occurs only in the more severe cases. The heart is usually normal in size in the clinically silent cases, but it may be dilated in patients with congestive heart failure. Pulmonary and systemic emboli may occur.

LABORATORY FINDINGS. ECG abnormalities are usually transient and occur far more frequently than does clinical myocardial involvement. The most common changes are abnormalities of the ST segment and T wave, but atrial and, in particular, ventricular arrhythmias, artrioventricular and intraventricular conduction defects, and, rarely, Q waves may be seen.[395] Complete artrioventricular block is usually transient and resolves without sequelae, but it is occasionally a cause of sudden death in patients with myocarditis. Intraventricular conduction abnormalities are associated with more severe myocardial damage and a worse prognosis.[396] On radiological examination, heart size may range from normal to markedly enlarged, and pulmonary congestion may be present in patients with fulminant disease. Blood levels of myocardial enzymes (serum transaminases, creatine kinase) may be normal or elevated, reflecting the absence or presence of variable degrees of clinically detectable myocardial necrosis; cardiac troponin levels are more sensitive to myocardial damage and may be detected when other enzymes are not elevated.[397] Echocardiography demonstrates some degree of left ventricular dysfunction (surprisingly often regional in nature) in many patients with clinical myocarditis, although wall motion may be normal. Other findings may include increased wall thickness, left ventricular thrombi, and abnormal diastolic filling despite normal systolic function.[398] Radionuclide scanning after the administration of gallium-67, indium-111 antimyosin antibody, or technetium-99m pyrophosphate may identify inflammatory and necrotic changes characteristic of myocarditis, as may MRI (Fig. 48–30).[338, 399]

DIAGNOSIS. This is often predicated on the identification of the associated systemic illness and its characteristic features.[10] The diagnosis of viral myocarditis is supported by the identification of the virus in stool, throat washings, blood, myocardium, or pericardial fluid or by a distinct (usually fourfold) increase in virus-neutralizing antibody, complement-fixation, or hemagglutination inhibition titers, but cultures usually are negative and serological tests nondiagnostic.[338, 400] Even in fatal cases, isolation of virus from the myocardium at necropsy is unusual.[401] Endomyocardial biopsy frequently is used to confirm the diagnosis of myocarditis.[10] A borderline or negative biopsy does not exclude the diagnosis, and, if clinically indicated, a repeat biopsy may be appropriate and diagnostic.[338] Molecular biological techniques such as the polymerase chain reaction (using tissue obtained by endomyocardial biopsy or samples obtained from other sites) offer promise as a way of rapidly and confidently diagnosing acute myocarditis.[11, 402] Coronary arteriography is not usually required nor is its use routinely recommended. It may, in fact, provide confusing information; some patients with myocarditis are discovered

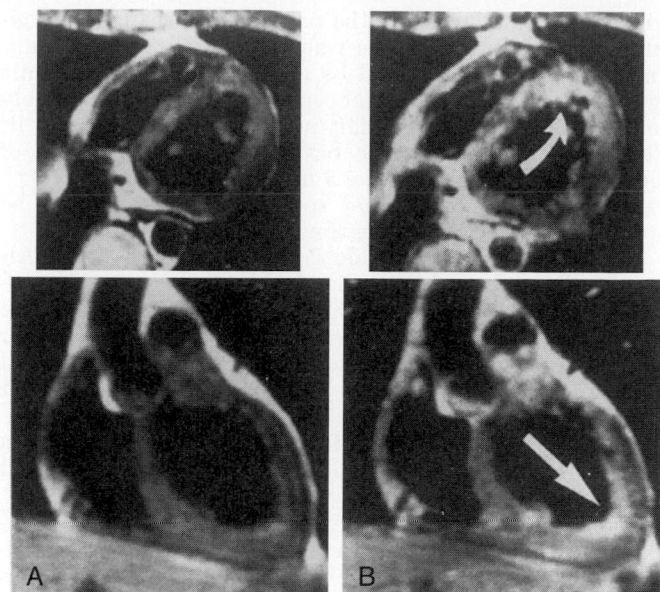

FIGURE 48–30. *A,* Precontrast T1-weighted transaxial (*upper*) and coronal (*lower*) magnetic resonance (MR) images through the left ventricle in case with myocarditis. *B,* Postcontrast MR images at the same levels after contrast injection. Note enhancement of the myocardial signal in the septum and apical region (arrows). (From Matsouka H, Hamada M, Honda T, et al: Evaluation of acute myocarditis and pericarditis by Gd-DTPA enhanced magnetic resonance imaging. E Heart J 15:283, 1994.)

to have coincidental coronary artery disease that is not playing a significant role in their illness.[403]

PATHOLOGY. Patients with myocarditis demonstrate a wide spectrum of gross and histological changes, reflecting the range of disease seen clinically. Grossly, the hearts in acute cases are flabby, with focal hemorrhages; in chronic cases, the hearts are enlarged and hypertrophied. The histological hallmark of myocarditis is an inflammatory myocardial infiltrate, with associated evidence of myocyte damage.[338] The inflammatory infiltrate may be composed of a variety of cell types, including polymorphonuclear cells, lymphocytes, macrophages, plasma cells, eosinophils, and/or giant cells. In bacterial myocarditis, polymorphonuclear cells predominate; in viral infections, lymphocytes predominate; and in hypersensitivity myocarditis, eosinophils are seen in abundance. In some cases, morphological changes are absent and evidence of inflammation is provided by immunohistologic techniques.[12] Routine histological examination of the heart rarely provides a specific diagnosis, although in some instances electron microscopic and immunofluorescent techniques may allow elucidation of a specific cause.

Management

Therapy is often supportive and is usually directed at the more prominent systemic manifestations of the disease.[27] The demonstration of a particular predilection for involvement of the artrioventricular conducting system in some forms of myocarditis suggests that patients with suspected myocarditis should be observed closely for any evidence of conduction abnormality. Bed rest (or at least restricted activity) is advisable because exercise in experimental animals with myocarditis is deleterious.[338] Because myocarditis often occurs in young adults, it is important to limit their athletic activities; it is recommended that athletes abstain from sports for a 6-month convalescent period, and until heart size and function have returned to normal. Congestive heart failure responds to routine management, including digitalization and diuresis,[338] although patients with myocarditis appear to be particularly sensitive to digitalis and toxicity should be watched for. Significant symptomatic arrhythmias should be treated with antiarrhythmic agents, although beta-adrenoceptor blockers are probably best avoided in view of their negative inotropic action (it should be noted that there have been too few reports of their use in humans to make a firm recommendation).[338, 404] Participation in athletic and sporting activities should be proscribed until arrhythmias have resolved.

The use of corticosteroids is controversial.[27, 381, 405] Although these agents were previously thought to be proscribed in acute viral myocarditis (because increased tissue necrosis and viral replication have been demonstrated after their use in experimental myocarditis), their use in a small number of patients has not been associated with similar dire short-term consequences.[391] A randomized trial of immunosuppression in myocarditis found no improvement in left ventricular ejection fraction or survival, however, and they are generally believed to be of limited value.[118, 406] Nonsteroidal antiinflammatory agents—indomethacin, salicylates, and ibuprofen, along with cyclosporine—are contraindicated during the acute phase of viral myocarditis (the first 2 weeks) because they increase myocardial damage in animal models.[381, 400] On the other hand, nonsteroidal antiinflammatory agents appear to be safe in the late phase of myocarditis. High-dose intravenous gamma globulin appears to be associated with more rapid resolution of left ventricular dysfunction and perhaps improved survival, at least in children (and in a small number of adults who have been so treated).[407, 408] In experimental models of myocarditis, the converting enzyme inhibitor captopril has beneficial effects in the acute phase of myocarditis; human data are not yet available.[338, 409]

It is hoped that effective antiviral agents, immunosuppressive agents, or immunomodulating agents for treating viral myocarditis will become available for clinical use.[118, 410, 411] Antibiotics may be employed with benefit in infections caused by atypical pneumonia and psittacosis.

VIRAL MYOCARDITIS

Approximately two dozen viruses may be associated with clinical evidence of myocarditis (see Table 48–9).[338] The myocarditis characteristically develops after a latent period of several weeks after the initial systemic infection, suggesting involvement of an immunological mechanism.[412] In animals, a variety of factors appears to enhance susceptibility to myocardial damage, including radiation, malnutrition, corticosteroids, exercise, and previous myocardial injury. Viral myocarditis may be particularly virulent in infants[388] and in pregnant women.

HUMAN IMMUNODEFICIENCY VIRUS (See Chap. 68)

COXSACKIEVIRUS. Both coxsackieviruses A and B may produce myocarditis, although infection with coxsackievirus B is more common; this agent is the most frequent cause of viral myocarditis, causing more than half the cases.[413] The myocardium appears to be particularly susceptible to the effects of this virus because of the apparent affinity of myocardial membrane receptors for the viral particles. Necropsy often demonstrates a pericardial effusion, pericarditis, cardiac enlargement, and a predominantly mononuclear inflammatory infiltrate, with necrosis of the atrial and ventricular myocardium. In some cases, focal myocardial necrosis simulating myocardial infarction is seen, despite normal coronary arteries.[414]

Although most infections are benign, self-limited, and subclinical, coxsackieviral myocarditis appears to be particularly virulent in the neonate and child (see Chap. 45).[415] In most infections in adults, the other clinical manifestations of viral involvement, such as pleurodynia, myalgia, upper respiratory tract symptoms, and arthralgias, predominate. Severe cases in the adult are characterized by myopericardial involvement with pleuritic or pericarditic chest pain, palpitations, and fever. Many patients with overt myocardial involvement develop congestive heart failure with cardiomegaly and pulmonary edema.[415]

The *electrocardiogram* is virtually always abnormal, with ST segment and T wave abnormalities and arrhythmias, often ventricular in

origin; artrioventricular conduction disturbances are common. *Echocardiography* may reveal diffuse and regional left ventricular wall motion abnormalities that usually improve or disappear over time.

Most patients recover completely within weeks,[415] although the ECG and ventricular function may require months to return to normal. Rarely, coxsackieviral myocarditis is fatal in adults. Some patients become symptomatic after resolution of the infection, and they may present years later with DCM.[416]

Treatment. This is symptomatic; despite occasional postmortem evidence of intracardiac thrombi, anticoagulation should probably be avoided because of the risk of a hemorrhagic pericardial effusion. Bed rest is indicated during the acute course of myocarditis, but no convincing evidence exists that a period of prolonged rest after apparent resolution of the acute process is useful. Heart failure and cardiac arrhythmias are treated in the usual fashion.

CYTOMEGALOVIRUS. Unrecognized infection with cytomegalovirus (CMV) is extremely common in childhood, and the majority of the adult population have antibodies to CMV.[417] Primary infection after the age of 35 years is uncommon, and generalized infection usually occurs only in immunosuppressed patients with neoplastic disease, after transplantation, and with HIV infection.[418] The cardiovascular manifestations in adults are generally limited to asymptomatic and transient ECG abnormalities. Symptomatic cardiac involvement is rare, although a hemorrhagic pericardial effusion or myocarditis with left ventricular dysfunction and attendant congestive heart failure may occur.[419] The diagnosis of CMV myocarditis may be suggested by the presence of viral inclusions in myocardial biopsy specimens and confirmed by the detection of viral DNA in the myocardium.[418] Although fatalities are unusual, when they do occur, histological examination of the heart may reveal focal lymphocytic infiltration and fibrosis.

DENGUE. Although previous dengue epidemics often were associated with symptomatic cardiac involvement, more recent outbreaks have been associated with fewer apparent cardiac complications.[420, 421] The major clinical feature is hypotension due to a capillary leak syndrome. Nonspecific ECG repolarization abnormalities are common but typically benign and transient.[421] Transient ventricular arrhythmias may be seen on occasion.

VIRAL HEPATITIS. Clinical cardiac involvement in hepatitis is rare; an occasional patient may develop fulminant myocarditis with congestive heart failure, hypotension, and death.[422] There are contested data implicating hepatitis C viral infection as an etiological factor in at least some cases of DCM.[423–425] The characteristic pathological changes are minute foci of necrosis of isolated muscle bundles, often surrounded by lymphocytes and a diffuse serous inflammation.[422] The ventricles may be dilated, with petechial hemorrhages. Hemorrhage into the myocardium may be a conspicuous finding.[422] Myocardial damage may be produced indirectly through an immune-mediated mechanism or directly by viral invasion of the heart.[422]

Symptomatic myocarditis is generally observed in the first to third week of illness. Patients may have dyspnea, palpitations, and anginal chest pain; fatalities have been reported.[422] ECG changes, including bradycardia, ventricular premature beats, and ST segment and T wave abnormalities, may be seen during the course of hepatitis.[422] These abnormalities are usually transient and asymptomatic, although congestive heart failure, cardiomegaly, and sudden death have been reported.[422]

INFECTIOUS MONONUCLEOSIS. Cardiac involvement in infectious mononucleosis is extremely rare, although nonspecific ST segment and T wave abnormalities may be seen. In rare cases, pericarditis and myocarditis (even simulating a myocardial infarction) may be present.[426]

INFLUENZA. Although clinically apparent myocarditis is rare in influenza, the presence of preexisting cardiovascular disease greatly increases the risk of morbidity and mortality.[427] During epidemics, 5 to 10 percent of infected patients may experience cardiac symptoms.[10] Postmortem findings in fatal cases include biventricular dilatation, with evidence of a mononuclear infiltrate, especially in perivascular areas.[427]

Cardiac involvement typically occurs within 1 to 2 weeks of the onset of the illness and may be severe, sometimes contributing to mortality. The clinical manifestations include dyspnea, palpitations, anginal chest pain, arrhythmia, and heart failure; there may be concomitant involvement of the pericardium.[428] Sinus tachycardia or, less commonly, sinus bradycardia may be seen. The ECG may show transient ST segment and T wave abnormalities, conduction defects, and even complete atrioventricular block; death may be associated with massive hemorrhagic pulmonary edema due to viral or bacterial involvement of the lungs.

LASSA FEVER. Lassa fever, a major cause of death in West Africa that is caused by an arenavirus, often is associated with ECG abnormalities[429] that may represent subclinical myocardial involvement. More than half the patients demonstrate nonspecific repolarization changes and low voltage.[429] Pericardial involvement may occur. Pathological findings include myocardial congestion, edema, and a mononuclear cellular infiltrate. In most cases, however, the putative cardiac involvement does not appear to play a major clinical role.[429]

MUMPS. Myocardial involvement during the course of mumps is rarely recognized.[430] The hearts of only a few patients with mumps have undergone postmortem examination, and they have been found to be both dilated and hypertrophied. Histologically, there is diffuse interstitial fibrosis, with infiltration of mononuclear cells and areas of focal necrosis.[430, 430a] There is speculation that prior mumps myocarditis may be involved in the development of endocardial fibroelastosis.[431] Cardiac involvement is usually unrecognized clinically, and the diagnosis of myocarditis is based on nonspecific ECG changes.[430] Transient ST segment and T wave abnormalities are most common, but extrasystoles and atrioventricular conduction block may occur.[430] Tachycardia, a transient apical systolic murmur, and protodiastolic gallop may be present.

POLIOMYELITIS. Myocarditis occurs in about 5 to 10 percent of epidemic poliomyelitis and is a frequent finding in fatal cases, occurring in half or more of all patients dying with this disease; death may be sudden.[12] Although myocardial involvement is usually focal and minimal in extent, some patients with bulbar disease succumb early in the course of the illness, often with cardiovascular collapse.[432] These patients all have viral infection of the medulla and severe systemic vasoconstriction that leads to pulmonary edema. Myocarditis appears to contribute to the heart failure.[432] The ECG is frequently abnormal, with ST segment and T wave abnormalities, prolongation of the PR and QT intervals, extrasystoles, tachycardia, and atrial fibrillation. Treatment is symptomatic, with aggressive support of pulmonary function; tracheostomy and prolonged mechanical ventilatory support may be required. Fortunately, this disease has been largely eliminated by immunization.

RESPIRATORY SYNCYTIAL VIRUS. Although respiratory syncytial virus is an important cause of respiratory disease, particularly in children, it rarely results in cardiac involvement.[433] Congestive heart failure, pericardial effusion, arrhythmias, cardiogenic shock, and complete heart block have been seen on occasion.[433, 434]

RUBELLA AND RUBEOLA. Congenital cardiovascular lesions may develop in the offspring when rubella is contracted by the mother during the first trimester of pregnancy, with persistent ductus arteriosus and pulmonary artery maldevelopment as prominent anomalies. Rare cases of postgestational myocarditis occur, with attendant conduction defects and heart failure.[435]

Overt myocarditis is rare in rubeola, although transient ECG abnormalities, including prolongation of the PR interval, ST segment and T wave changes, atrioventricular conduction abnormalities, and ventricular tachycardia, have been reported.[436] Congestive heart failure occurs on rare occasions, and its appearance is a poor prognostic sign, often indicating a fatal outcome. Histological examination of the heart in fatal cases has revealed evidence of myocarditis characterized predominantly by a perivascular lymphocytic infiltrate.[436]

VARICELLA. Clinical myocarditis is a rare finding in varicella, although unsuspected myocarditis is common in fatal varicella. Occasionally, a patient may develop overt clinical evidence of myocarditis with congestive heart failure.[437] Histological findings include rare but characteristic intranuclear inclusion bodies within the myocardial cells, along with interstitial edema, cellular infiltrates, and myonecrosis.[437] The ECG may show conduction abnormalities, including complete heart block; sudden death occurs rarely.

VARIOLA AND VACCINIA. Cardiac involvement after smallpox is rare, although several cases of myocarditis associated with acute cardiac failure and death have been reported. Myocarditis with pericardial effusion and congestive heart failure has also been observed as a complication of smallpox vaccination; an immunological mechanism has been suggested, and dramatic responses to corticosteroids have been reported.[438] The histological changes include a mixed mononuclear infiltrate, with interstitial edema and occasional degenerating or necrotic muscle bundles.

RICKETTSIAL MYOCARDITIS

The rickettsial diseases are frequently associated with evidence of myocardial involvement, but usually it is subclinical. Transient ST segment and T wave alterations are commonly observed. The circulatory collapse that may accompany these diseases is largely a manifestation of abnormalities of the peripheral vascular bed, but a myocardial component may also be present. The basic histopathological process is a vasculitis, with a periarterial interstitial infiltrate.

Q FEVER. Endocarditis is the most common cardiac manifestation of infection with *Rickettsia burnetii* (Q fever).[439] Myocarditis is not a prominent feature,[439a] although dyspnea and chest pain, perhaps reflecting associated pericarditis, occur frequently. The ECG may demonstrate transient ST segment and T wave changes as well as paroxysmal ventricular arrhythmias. Abnormalities of the immune system have been implicated in the pathogenesis of the disease.

ROCKY MOUNTAIN SPOTTED FEVER. Clinical evidence of myocarditis is more common than often appreciated in Rocky Mountain spotted fever (caused by *R. rickettsii*), and the heart is often involved in the multisystem damage that occurs as the result of a widespread vasculitis.[440] Unsuspected left ventricular dysfunction is common, and echocardiographic evidence of dysfunction may persist in some patients.

SCRUB TYPHUS. Myocarditis is common during the course of scrub typhus (tsutsugamushi disease, caused by *R. tsutsugamushi*), espe-

cially in fatal cases.[441] The histological findings are those of a focal panvasculitis involving the small blood vessels. Myocardial necrosis is unusual, but hemorrhage into the heart and subepicardial petechiae may occur.[441] Clinical evidence of myocardial involvement typically is not severe and is usually not associated with residual cardiac damage. The ECG may show nonspecific ST segment and T wave abnormalities, as well as first-degree atrioventricular block.[441] A protodiastolic gallop and apical systolic murmur suggestive of mitral regurgitation are occasionally found.

BACTERIAL MYOCARDITIS

BRUCELLOSIS. Cardiac involvement in the course of brucellosis is uncommon, usually consisting of endocarditis. Myocardial involvement, when it occurs, is manifested by T wave abnormalities and prolongation of atrioventricular conduction. An occasional patient develops fulminant myocarditis, with a lymphocytic and polymorphonuclear infiltrate.[442]

CLOSTRIDIAL INFECTION. Cardiac involvement is common in patients with clostridial infections with multiple organ involvement. The myocardial damage results from the toxin elaborated by the bacteria, but the precise actions of the toxin remain to be elucidated.[443] The pathological findings are distinctive, with gas bubbles present in the myocardium. Areas of degenerated muscle fibers are apparent, but an inflammatory infiltrate is usually absent.[443] *Clostridium perfringens* may cause myocardial abscess formation, with myocardial perforation and resultant purulent pericarditis.

DIPHTHERIA. Myocardial involvement is one of the more serious complications of diphtheria and occurs in up to one fourth of cases.[443a] Indeed, myocardial involvement is the most common cause of death in this infection, and half of the fatal cases demonstrate cardiac involvement.[444] Cardiac damage is due to the liberation by the diphtheria bacillus of a toxin that inhibits protein synthesis by interfering with the transfer of amino acids from soluble RNA to polypeptide chains under construction. The toxin appears to have a particular affinity for the cardiac conducting system.

Pathological Findings. These include a flabby and dilated heart with a myocardium that has a "streaky" appearance. Microscopic examination reveals characteristic fatty infiltration of the myocytes,[444] often with an interstitial inflammatory infiltrate, myocytolysis, and hyaline necrosis of muscle fibers. With time, fibrosis and hypertrophy of the remaining myocardial cells develop. The conduction system is often involved.

Clinical Manifestations. Signs of cardiac dysfunction typically appear at the end of the first week of the illness. Cardiomegaly and severe congestive heart failure are often present. A protodiastolic gallop and pulmonary congestion may be prominent features. Elevation of the serum transaminase levels may be seen; a high level is associated with a poor prognosis. Sudden circulatory failure and death may occur. Many patients develop ST segment and T wave abnormalities, but atrial and ventricular arrhythmias and conduction defects may also occur.[444] Persistently abnormal ECGs are common after diphtheritic myocarditis, as are cardiomegaly and symptoms of reduced cardiac reserve. Some patients recover fully.

Because of the serious effects of the toxin on the myocardium, antitoxin should be administered as rapidly as possible.[444] Antibiotic therapy is of less urgency. Overt congestive heart failure may be resistant to therapy with cardiac glycosides. The development of complete atrioventricular block is an ominous complication, and mortality is high despite insertion of a transvenous pacemaker.

LEGIONNAIRES DISEASE. Although pneumonia, rhabdomyolysis, renal failure, and hepatic as well as central nervous system involvement are common with *Legionella pneumophila*, overt cardiac involvement is not.[445] Occasional ECG changes may be noted, consisting primarily of ST segment and T wave abnormalities; ventricular arrhythmias may be seen. Rarely, pericardial effusion, myocarditis with evidence of myocardial necrosis, or congestive heart failure may be seen.[445]

MENINGOCOCCAL INFECTION. Myocardial involvement is common during the course of fatal meningococcal infections but is less commonly recognized in the usual case. Pathological findings include hemorrhagic myocardial lesions, occasionally associated with intracellular organisms. An interstitial myocarditis composed of lymphocytes, plasma cells, and polymorphonuclear leukocytes may be observed, occasionally with myonecrosis.

Meningococcal myocarditis may result in congestive heart failure as well as in pericardial effusion with tamponade. Death may occur suddenly and be associated with involvement of the atrioventricular node.[446]

MYCOPLASMA PNEUMONIAE INFECTION. ECG abnormalities are common during the course of atypical pneumonia, although clinically apparent myocarditis is not. When carditis occurs, it may be serious, and, rarely, fatal.[447] Nonspecific ST segment and T wave abnormalities are the most common manifestations of cardiac involvement; a rare patient may develop complete heart block. The ECG findings usually resolve within 1 to 2 weeks. A cell-mediated autoimmune myocarditis has been postulated as the cause of the changes. Pericarditis may be

FIGURE 48–31. See color plate 29.

a prominent finding, and congestive heart failure is occasionally seen. A protodiastolic gallop and pericardial friction rub may be noted in occasional cases. Complete recovery is the rule in most patients, although occasional patients may have persistent sequelae, including arrhythmias.

PSITTACOSIS. Myocarditis complicating psittacosis is a relatively common occurrence and is characterized by congestive heart failure and acute pericarditis.[448] Pathological changes include fibrinous pericarditis as well as endocarditis and myocarditis. Fever, chest pain, ECG changes, cardiomegaly, systemic emboli, tachycardia, and hypotension may occur. Although most patients recover completely, fatalities have been reported. The systemic infection may be treated effectively with tetracycline, but the effect of the antibiotic on the myocardium is unknown.

SALMONELLOSIS. Symptomatic myocardial involvement during *Salmonella* infections is rare, although ECG abnormalities are often seen, suggesting subclinical myocarditis.[449, 450] Other cardiovascular complications include infected mural thrombi, occasionally resulting in pulmonary and systemic emboli, and mycotic aneurysms. Myocardial abscesses may rupture, producing fatal cardiac tamponade. Myocarditis with congestive heart failure occurs most commonly in children who are severely ill with salmonellosis, and it is associated with a high mortality. When myocarditis occurs, it often develops rapidly, with evidence of biventricular failure, tachycardia, a protodiastolic gallop, an apical systolic murmur of mitral regurgitation, and peripheral edema.

ECG abnormalities include ST segment and T wave changes, prolonged PR or QT intervals, and low QRS voltage.[450]

STREPTOCOCCAL INFECTION. The most commonly detected cardiac finding after beta-hemolytic streptococcal infection is acute rheumatic fever, which is discussed in detail in Chapter 66.

Involvement of the heart by the streptococcus may produce a myocarditis that is distinct from acute rheumatic carditis.[451] It is characterized by an interstitial infiltrate composed of mononuclear cells with occasional polymorphonuclear leukocytes; the infiltrate may be focal or diffuse and may be localized to the subendocardial or perivascular region. There may be small areas of myocardial necrosis. ECG abnormalities, including prolongation of the PR and QT intervals, occur frequently. Although these abnormalities are rarely associated with other clinical manifestations of myocardial involvement, sudden death, conduction disturbances, and arrhythmias may occur.

TUBERCULOSIS. Involvement of the myocardium by *Mycobacterium tuberculosis* (not as a complication of tuberculous pericarditis) is rare, particularly since the introduction of drugs effective against tuberculosis (Fig. 48–31).[452] Most cases of myocardial tuberculosis are clinically silent and are diagnosed only at autopsy. Tuberculous involvement of the myocardium occurs by means of hematogenous or lymphatic spread or directly from contiguous structures; it may lead to arrhythmias, including atrial fibrillation and ventricular tachycardia, complete atrioventricular block, congestive heart failure, left ventricular aneurysms, and sudden death.[452, 453]

WHIPPLE DISEASE

Although overt involvement is rare, intestinal lipodystrophy, or Whipple disease, is not uncommonly associated with cardiac involvement, and periodic acid–Schiff (PAS)-positive macrophages may be found in the myocardium, pericardium, and heart valves of patients with this disorder.[454, 455] Coronary artery lesions, with smooth muscle necrosis, panarteritis, and medial scarring, may be seen. Electron microscopy has demonstrated rod-shaped structures in the myocardium similar to those found in the small intestine, and these represent the causative agent of the disease, *Tropheryma whippelii*, an agent related to the actinomycetes.[454] There may be an associated inflammatory infiltrate and foci of fibrosis. The valvular fibrosis may be severe enough to result in aortic regurgitation and mitral stenosis. Although usually asymptomatic, nonspecific ECG changes are most common; systolic murmurs, pericarditis, complete heart block, and even overt congestive heart failure may occur.[454] The cardiac manifestations of Whipple disease may be overshadowed by the prominent gastrointestinal symptoms that often are present. Antibiotic therapy appears to be effective in treating the basic disease; however, re-

lapses can occur, often more than 2 years after initial diagnosis.

SPIROCHETAL INFECTIONS

LEPTOSPIROSIS (WEIL DISEASE). Most patients with leptospiral infections have mild or subclinical disease and little evidence of heart involvement. Cardiac involvement in severe or fatal leptospirosis is common, however, with 50 to 100 percent of fatal cases demonstrating evidence of myocarditis.[456] Many patients with clinical systemic disease demonstrate atrial fibrillation, first-degree heart block, and transient ST segment and T wave abnormalities, presumably reflecting myocarditis, although significant left ventricular dysfunction is uncommon.[457] Bradycardia despite fever, ventricular premature depolarizations, congestive heart failure, and pericarditis may be seen as well. The pathological findings in the occasional fatal case include petechiae or large loci of hemorrhage (often located in the epicardium), an interstitial myocardial infiltrate (often subendocardial in location), aortitis, and coronary arteritis.

LYME CARDITIS. Lyme disease is caused by a tickborne spirochete (*Borrelia burgdorferi*).[458] It usually begins during the summer months with a characteristic rash (erythema chronicum migrans), followed in weeks to months by neurological, joint, or cardiac involvement; some clinical manifestations may persist for years.[458]

About 10 percent of patients with Lyme disease develop evidence of transient cardiac involvement, the most common manifestation being variable degrees of atrioventricular block[459-461] at the level of the atrioventricular node. Syncope due to complete heart block is frequent with cardiac involvement because often there is an associated depression of ventricular escape rhythms. Ventricular tachycardia occurs uncommonly.[459] Diffuse ST segment and T wave abnormalities and transient, usually asymptomatic, left ventricular dysfunction may be found in some patients, although cardiomegaly or symptoms of congestive heart failure are rare.[460, 462] A positive gallium or indium antimyosin antibody scan may point to suspected cardiac involvement in this disease.[463] The demonstration of spirochetes in myocardial biopsies of some patients with Lyme carditis suggests that the cardiac manifestations are due to a direct toxic effect, although there is speculation that immune-mediated mechanisms may be involved as well.

The value of specific therapy in Lyme carditis remains uncertain, and even without therapy the disease usually is self-limited with complete recovery the rule.[457] Nevertheless, it is thought that treating the early manifestations of the disease may prevent development of late complications.[458] Patients with second-degree or complete heart block should be hospitalized and undergo continuous ECG monitoring. Temporary transvenous pacing may be required for up to a week or longer in patients with high-grade block. Although the efficacy of antibiotics is not established, they are utilized routinely in Lyme carditis. Intravenous antibiotics (ceftriaxone, 2 gm, or penicillin G, 20 million units daily for 14 days) are suggested, although oral antibiotics (doxycycline, 100 mg twice daily, or amoxicillin, 500 mg three times daily for 14 to 21 days) may be used when there is only mild cardiac involvement (first-degree atrioventricular block of less than 40 milliseconds duration).[464] Whether antiinflammatory agents (salicylates, corticosteroids) can ameliorate heart block is not clear.

RELAPSING FEVER. Many infections are currently observed in Ethiopia. During pandemics, mortality may be particularly high, reaching 70 percent, although sporadic cases are often more benign. Cardiac involvement is said to be a common complication and is often implicated as a cause of death, although one report involving 63 children did not find evidence of cardiac involvement.[465] Atrioventricular conduction defects occur frequently and may be responsible for sudden death, although tachyarrhythmias have also been implicated. Numerous petechiae are observed with a diffuse histiocytic interstitial infiltrate, particularly around small arterioles in the left ventricle.

SYPHILIS. Aortitis is the most common manifestation of luetic involvement of the cardiovascular system (see Chap. 40). Aortic regurgitation and coronary ostial narrowing are associated findings. Syphilitic involvement of the myocardium itself in the form of gumma formation is uncommon and usually unsuspected clinically. Involvement of the base of the interventricular septum may result in damage to the conduction system and atrioventicular block. In one case a ruptured left ventricular aneurysm was found as a result of syphilitic endarteritis.[466]

FUNGAL INFECTIONS OF THE HEART

Cardiac fungal infections occur most frequently in patients with malignant disease and/or those receiving chemotherapy, corticosteroids, radiation, or immunosuppressive therapy. Cardiac surgery, intravenous drug abuse, and infection with HIV are also predisposing factors for fungal cardiac involvement.

ACTINOMYCOSIS. Myocarditis is a rare complication of actinomycotic infection, occurring in less than 2 percent of patients; more commonly, it produces pericardial or endocardial disease.[467] However, cardiac involvement is quite serious when it does occur. Involvement of the heart most commonly is the result of direct extension of disease within the thorax. Initially the pericardium is invaded, with eventual obliteration of the pericardial space. The myocardium may be involved by extension of the pericardial process. Myocardial seeding is less common. The myocardial lesion is a suppurative, necrotizing abscess containing the organism, surrounded by granulation tissue. Both right- and left-sided failure are common manifestations.[467] A pericardial rub may be heard, sometimes associated with clinical evidence of a pericardial effusion or constriction.

ASPERGILLOSIS. Myocardial involvement is not uncommon in generalized aspergillosis, and when it occurs it is usually fatal.[468] It is being encountered increasingly in the immunocompromised patient.[469] On pathological examination, myocardial necrosis and infarction caused by thrombosis of vessels that contain fungal mycelia are commonly seen, along with myocardial abscesses and pericardial involvement. The ECG may be normal in the face of significant myocardial damage, but T wave changes may be present. The diagnosis of *Aspergillus* infection is often difficult.[469] Identification of *Aspergillus* through open-lung biopsy, aspiration lung biopsy, transtracheal aspiration, or bronchial brush technique may be successful. Treatment is difficult and usually unsuccessful.

BLASTOMYCOSIS. Involvement of the heart by the fungus is quite uncommon, even in the immunocompromised heart. When involvement occurs, it is most often by direct extension from the pericardium.

CANDIDIASIS. Disseminated candidal infections are common opportunistic infections, particularly in the compromised host. Endocarditis is the most frequent manifestation of cardiac involvement (see Chap. 47), occurring most commonly in cardiac surgical patients or drug addicts, although multiple abscesses of the myocardium may occur as associated or independent findings. Complete heart block may be caused by microabscesses of the conduction system.

COCCIDIOIDOMYCOSIS. Involvement of the heart is rare in patients with generalized coccidioidomycosis. The hearts may be grossly normal, although epicardial lesions with resultant pericarditis are common, and progression to constrictive pericarditis may occur (see Chap. 50). A nonspecific, focal interstitial, and perivascular cellular infiltrate with associated muscle fiber degeneration and interstitial edema is commonly found, although granulomas containing fungi are also seen sometimes.

CRYPTOCOCCOSIS. Cryptococcal infection of the myocardium occurs most commonly in immunocompromised patients with disseminated malignancy or HIV infection. Pathological examination may show cardiac dilatation, with epithelial granulomas, giant cells, and an inflammatory infiltrate.[470] When congestive heart failure occurs, pulmonary congestion and muffled heart sounds may be found on physical examination, and cardiomegaly on the chest roentgenogram. The ECG may show first-degree atrioventricular block and T wave inversions; ventricular arrhythmias have been observed.

HISTOPLASMOSIS. Cardiac involvement in histoplasmosis is rare and usually is related to mediastinal fibrosis, the most serious complication of histoplasmosis.[471] Pericarditis with effusion may occur (see Chap. 50), and superior vena caval obstruction has been observed.[471] Myocardial involvement is uncommon, although atrial arrhythmias and T wave abnormalities have been reported.

MUCORMYCOSIS. Cardiac involvement in the setting of disseminated mucormycosis occurs in about 20 percent of patients and is characterized by fungal invasion of the coronary arteries with resultant areas of myocardial infarction. Valvular and pericardial involvement may be seen as well. Clinical manifestations are nonspecific, and cardiac involvement often is not suspected but may include conges-

tive heart failure, arrhythmias, conduction defects, and endocarditis.[472]

PROTOZOAL MYOCARDITIS

Trypanosomiasis (Chagas Disease)

Chagas disease is caused by the protozoan *Trypanosoma cruzi*. The major cardiovascular manifestation is an extensive myocarditis that typically becomes evident years after the initial infection. The disease is prevalent in Central and South America, particularly in Brazil, Argentina, and Chile, where it is a major public health problem (Fig. 48–32). Upward of 20 million people are thought to be infected with the parasite, and an estimated 100 million are at risk of infection.[473] In rare cases, the disease may be found in nonendemic areas as a consequence of transfusion with contaminated blood products; somewhat more common is emigration of patients with the disease to nonendemic areas.[474]

The natural history of Chagas disease is characterized by three phases: acute, latent, and chronic. During the *acute phase,* the disease is transmitted to humans (usually below the age of 20 years) through the bite of a reduviid bug (subfamily Triatominae), which harbors the parasite in its gastrointestinal tract.[473, 475] This insect acquires the disease from feeding on infected animals, including the armadillo, raccoon, opossum, and skunk as well as domestic dogs and cats. The reduviid bug, popularly known in Argentina as *vinchuca,* meaning "to let oneself drop," lives in the walls and roofs of houses and, during nocturnal feedings, drops from the ceiling onto the sleeping person below. The bug then often bites the person around the eyes, and infection of the human host occurs when the trypanosomes in the animal's feces gain entry through abraded skin or through the conjunctivae.[473] Occasionally, this results in unilateral periorbital edema and swelling of the eyelid, termed the

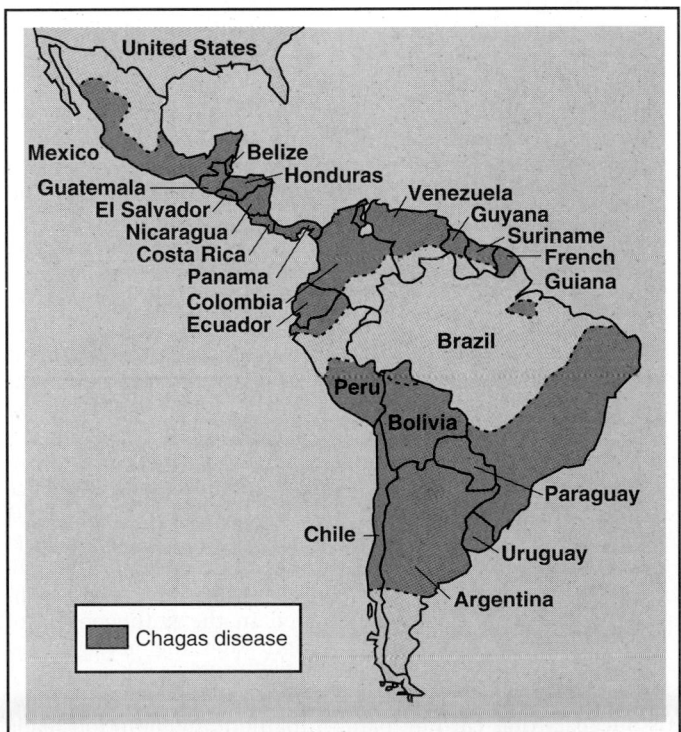

FIGURE 48–32. Distribution of Chagas disease in the Americas. (From Acquatella H: Chagas' disease. *In* Abelmann WH, Braunwald E [eds]: Atlas of Heart Diseases. Vol 2. Cardiomyopathies, Myocarditis, and Pericardial Disease. Philadelphia, Current Medicine, 1995, pp 8.1–8.18.)

Romaña sign, whereas entry through the skin may result in a lesion called a *chagoma.*[473, 475] Transmission may occur through blood transfusions; unfortunately, adequate screening to preclude transfusion-related disease is not possible in many areas due to financial and logistic constraints.[473]

ACUTE TRYPANOSOMIASIS. After inoculation, the protozoa multiply and then migrate widely throughout the body. In less than 10 percent of cases an acute illness occurs; the latter is fatal in about 10 percent of patients.[474, 475] Pathological examination during the acute phase often reveals parasites in the cardiac fibers with a marked cellular infiltrate, particularly around cardiac cells that have ruptured and released the parasites.[475] Involvement may extend into the endocardium, resulting in thrombus formation, and into the epicardium, resulting in pericardial effusion. The pathogenesis of the myocardial lesions of acute Chagas disease appears to relate in large part to immune lysis by antibody and cell-mediated immunity directed against antigens released from *T. cruzi*–infected cells, which become adsorbed onto the surface of infected and noninfected host cells.[473]

Clinical Manifestations. These include fever, muscle pains, sweating, hepatosplenomegaly, myocarditis with congestive heart failure, pericardial effusion, and, occasionally, meningoencephalitis.[473, 475] Most patients recover, and their symptoms resolve over several months. Young children most commonly develop clinical acute disease and generally are more seriously ill than adults.

LATENT AND CHRONIC TRYPANOSOMIASIS. The disease then enters a *latent phase* without clinical symptoms; however, there is evidence of early and progressive subclinical cardiomyopathy. ECG changes often appear at this stage and are a marker for the eventual clinical heart disease and increased mortality to become evident later. At an average of 20 years after the initial (and usually unrecognized) infestation, approximately 30 percent of infected individuals develop findings of *chronic Chagas disease,* the manifestations of which cover a wide spectrum from asymptomatic but seropositive patients through those with ECG abnormalities to those with advanced disease characterized by cardiomegaly, congestive heart failure, arrhythmias, thromboembolic phenomena, atypical chest pain, right bundle branch block, and sudden death.[474] In the advanced stage, cardiac dilatation typically involves all the cardiac chambers, although right-sided enlargement may predominate.[474]

The central paradox in the pathogenesis of this disorder is the poor correlation between the level of parasitemia and the severity of disease.[476] It is not unusual to be unable to detect parasites in patients dying of Chagas disease,[477] although evidence of prior infection may be detected more frequently by the much more sensitive polymerase chain reaction technique.[478] *T. cruzi* antigen is frequently found in biopsy specimens of the heart in chronic Chagas heart disease.[479, 480] An autoimmune etiological mechanism has been proposed, and this may explain the lack of correlation of parasitemia with disease severity.[476, 479, 480] Based on animal models, it appears that self-reactive cytotoxic T lymphocytes develop after the initial infection and produce various cytokines.[476] This results in the lysis of normal host cells, perhaps related to cross-reacting antigens of *T. cruzi* and striated muscle.[474, 481] A variety of antibodies against myocyte sarcoplasmic reticulum, laminin, and other constituents have also been implicated in the pathogenesis of Chagas myocarditis.[479] It is thought that the acute phase results in the release from parasite-modified host cells of self-components that are immunogenic.[474] Another hypothesis suggests that cardiac parasympathetic denervation leads to eventual chronic Chagas disease.[474, 477]

Pathology. Nerves and autonomic ganglia are frequently abnormal, and megaesophagus and megacolon may occur; less commonly, there is dilatation of the stomach, duodenum, ureter, and bronchi. Different strains of *T. cruzi*

may account for the geographical differences in the expression of Chagas disease; megaesophagus and megacolon are common in Brazil but quite uncommon in Central America and Mexico, and megaesophagus is unusual in Venezuela.[473] Lesions of the cardiac nerves are routinely found in patients with chronic Chagas disease, with evidence of cardiac parasympathetic denervation.[473] Pathological cardiac findings include cardiac enlargement, with dilatation and hypertrophy of all cardiac chambers. In more than half the patients, the left (and occasionally right) ventricular apex is thin and bulging, resembling an aneurysm.[477] Thrombus formation is frequent and may fill much of the apex; the right atrium also frequently contains thrombus. It has been suggested that these characteristic apical aneurysms (Fig. 48–33) may be the result of intravascular platelet aggregation leading to focal myocardial necrosis.[479]

The microscopic findings are principally those of extensive fibrosis, particularly of the left ventricle.[474, 482] A chronic cellular infiltrate composed of lymphocytes, plasma cells, and macrophages often is present.[473] Increases in arteriole and capillary diameters have been reported.[482] Preferential involvement of the right bundle branch and the anterior fascicle of the left bundle branch by inflammatory and fibrotic changes explains the frequent occurrence of right bundle branch and left anterior fascicular block.[473] The basement membranes of capillaries, vascular smooth muscle cells, and myocytes are thickened.[479] It is unusual to be able to find parasites in the myofibers of autopsied patients.[477]

Clinical Manifestations. These include anginal chest pain, symptomatic conducting system disease, and sudden death; chronic progressive heart failure, often predominantly right sided, is the rule in advanced cases.[474] Thus, although pulmonary congestion is occasionally noted, the usual findings include fatigue due to diminished cardiac output, peripheral edema, ascites, and hepatic congestion. Tricuspid regurgitation is often present, particularly in patients with severe right-sided heart failure, although mitral regurgitation is frequently present as well. The S_2 is widely split, often with an accentuated pulmonic component, reflecting the combined effects of right bundle branch block and pulmonary hypertension. Autonomic dysfunction is common, with marked abnormalities in the expected reflex changes in heart rate produced by various maneuvers. Deaths result most commonly from pump failure or occur suddenly. Apical aneurysms and left ventricular dilation place patients at high risk for the latter.[483]

Laboratory Findings. The chest roentgenogram often demonstrates severe cardiomegaly, with or without pulmonary venous hypertension. The serum aldolase is usually elevated.[484] ECG abnormalities are the rule late in the course of the disease, particularly in patients who are seroreactive to *T. cruzi* antigen. Right bundle branch block, left anterior hemiblock, atrial fibrillation, and ventricular premature depolarizations are the most common findings in patients with chronic Chagas disease.[473, 485] ST segment and T wave abnormalities also are common, as are Q waves; P wave abnormalities and atrioventricular block are seen less frequently.[473] Early in the disease, the ECG may be normal or nearly so. Administration of the antiarrhythmic agent ajmaline may precipitate the appearance of ECG abnormalities and thus identify patients with as yet clinically silent cardiac involvement.[473] Furthermore, electrophysiological testing of asymptomatic patients, even those with normal ECGs, may demonstrate abnormalities of the conducting system in many.

Ventricular arrhythmias are a prominent feature of chronic Chagas disease.[473, 479, 480] Frequent ventricular premature depolarizations, often with multiple morphologies, are seen frequently, and bouts of ventricular tachycardia may occur. Ventricular arrhythmias are particularly common during and after exercise,[473] occurring in the majority

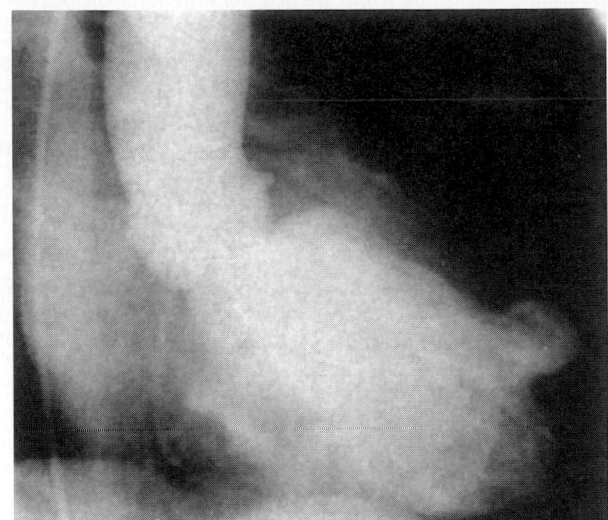
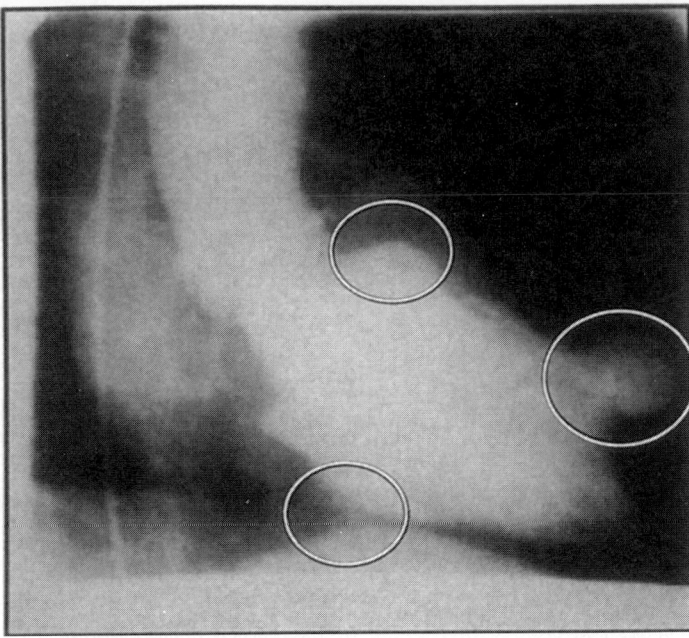

FIGURE 48–33. Left ventriculogram in the right anterior oblique view of a 55-year-old woman with chronic Chagas disease. Multiple left ventricular aneurysms are noted in anterobasal, anterior, and inferior aspects of left ventricle (circled, right). (From Venegoni P, Bhatia HS: Chagas' disease and ventricular arrhythmias. Circulation 96:1363, 1997. Copyright 1997, American Heart Association.)

of patients subjected to stress ECG testing (including some without any clinical evidence of cardiac involvement). Ventricular tachycardia induced by electrophysiological testing is most common in patients with evidence of conduction abnormalities on the ECG, low ejection fraction, and apical left ventricular aneurysm and may predict sudden death.[486, 487] Syncope and sudden death due to ventricular fibrillation are constant threats and may develop even before cardiomegaly or heart failure.[473, 488, 489] Sinus bradycardia may also be seen, even in patients with severe heart failure when a tachycardia would be expected, presumably related to cardiac autonomic dysfunction.[473] Atrial arrhythmias, including atrial fibrillation (often with a slow ventricular response), also may occur.[473] Thromboembolic phenomena are a frequent complication, occurring in more than 50 percent of the patients.[490]

The echocardiographic findings in advanced cases are those of a dilated cardiomyopathy with increased end-diastolic and end-systolic volumes and reduced ejection fraction, often with enlargement of the left atrium and right ventricle.[473] Diastolic filling of the left ventricle is frequently abnormal, even in those without other clinical or echocardiographic evidence of cardiac involvement. In the majority of advanced cases, the echocardiographic appearance is distinctive, with left ventricular posterior wall hypokinesis and relatively preserved interventricular septal motion; an apical aneurysm is often seen on two-dimensional echocardiography. Ten to 15 percent of asymptomatic patients demonstrate apical dyskinesis.

Radionuclide ventriculography may, like echocardiography, demonstrate right or left ventricular wall motion abnormalities in the absence of an overall depression of global ventricular function. Perfusion scanning with thallium-201 may show fixed defects (corresponding to areas of fibrosis) as well as evidence of reversible ischemia.[491] MRI can identify morphological and functional aspects of cardiac involvement; with the use of gadolinium as a contrast medium, it can identify patients with more active myocardial disease.[492]

Left ventricular cineangiography in advanced cases shows a dilated, hypokinetic left ventricle with one large or several apical aneurysms (see Fig. 48–33) containing intra-cavitary thrombus, often with evidence of mitral regurgitation.[473] Coronary angiography is usually normal, although abnormalities of the coronary microcirculation have been suggested as a cause of the clinical manifestations of Chagas disease.

The complement-fixation test (Machado-Guerreiro test) is useful in diagnosis; it has high sensitivity and specificity for the identification of chronic Chagas disease.[473] Also used in diagnosis are the indirect immunofluorescent antibody, the enzyme-linked immunosorbent assay, and the hemagglutination tests.[473] In endemic areas, perhaps the most widely used test is the detection of parasites in the blood of patients with chronic Chagas disease (which occurs in upward of 50 percent of cases) by means of xenodiagnosis.[493] The patient is bitten by reduviid bugs bred in the laboratory; the subsequent identification of parasites in the intestine of the insect is proof of infection in the human host.

MANAGEMENT. The treatment of Chagas disease remains difficult; although slowly progressive at first, once cardiac decompensation develops there is usually a rapid and inexorable progression to death, which is usually due to arrhythmia, although congestive failure and systemic thromboembolism account for additional mortality.[474] Patients at greatest risk of mortality are those with left ventricular enlargement and especially those with impaired left ventricular function.[485, 488] Major efforts are aimed at interrupting transmission of the parasite to humans; such vector control methods have been generally successful.[473] They may prevent not only the initial infection but also reinfection that may play a role in determining the severity of the resulting cardiomyopathy.

Amiodarone appears to be effective in controlling the ventricular arrhythmias frequently seen in Chagas disease, although whether this translates into improved survival remains to be established.[494] ICDs are useful, and the indications are similar to those in patients with life-threatening arrhythmias associated with other causes (see Chap. 23).[495] Anticoagulation may be of some benefit in preventing recurrent thromboembolic episodes.[490] Although antiparasitic agents such as nifurtimox, benzimidazole, and itraconazole are effective in reducing parasitemia and are useful in acute disease, no evidence indicates that they are efficacious in curing the late phases of the disease.[473, 496] A promising avenue of approach appears to be immunoprophylaxis, although a clinically useful vaccine is not yet available. Insertion of an ICD and the latissimus dorsi muscle wrap around the heart (dynamic cardiomyoplasty) have been used sparingly but are not practical options for the vast majority of patients. Similarly, heart transplantation have been performed in a few patients, but the results so far appear to be inferior to those found in other conditions, and episodes of parasitemia and recurrent Chagas disease may be a problem.[497, 498]

AFRICAN TRYPANOSOMIASIS. African sleeping sickness, caused by *Trypanosoma gambiense* or *T. rhodesiense,* may be associated with myocardial abnormalities, although they are usually of less functional significance than in Chagas disease. *T. rhodesiense,* in particular, may lead to cardiac failure,[499] although the central nervous system findings (excessive somnolence) usually dominate the clinical picture.

Pathological examination often reveals pericardial fluid. The heart is not as greatly dilated and hypertrophied as it is in Chagas disease and may appear to be grossly normal. There is often epicardial thickening with a cellular exudate composed of lymphocytes, plasma cells, and histiocytes. The myocardium typically displays a diffuse interstitial infiltrate, often with zones of patchy fibrosis and interstitial edema.

Nonspecific ECG changes, commonly ST segment and T wave abnormalities and prolongation of the QT interval, are observed in at least half of the patients.[499] Unlike Chagas disease, arrhythmias and conduction disturbances are usually not prominent features, and the arterial pressure is usually normal. Some patients have asymptomatic cardiomegaly, although both pulmonary congestion and peripheral edema have been reported.

TOXOPLASMOSIS. *Toxoplasma* infections are caused by an obligate intracellular parasite (*T. gondii*); both congenital and acquired forms may occur. Symptomatic acquired toxoplasmic infections involving the heart are uncommon. They occur most commonly in immunosuppressed patients with malignant diseases and occasionally in patients with the acquired immunodeficiency syndrome and after cardiac or bone marrow transplantation.[500] An inflammatory infiltrate, often with eosinophils and variable degrees of edema and degeneration of the muscle bundles, and pericardial effusion are often present.

Most adult cases are asymptomatic, but *Toxoplasma* infections may produce a severe, fatal disease with multisystemic involvement. Toxoplasmic myocarditis, often with pericarditis, may occur as an isolated disease process or as part of a multisystemic disseminated disease. Manifestations may include arrhythmias (atrial and ventricular), sudden death, atrioventricular block, pericarditis, and heart failure.[501] Large pericardial effusions may be seen on occasion. Diagnosis may be aided by endomyocardial biopsy.[502]

Treatment is with a combination of pyrimethamine and triple sulfonamides, but the response to therapy is variable; treatment appears to have no effect on the cyst form.[500]

MALARIA. Although myocardial changes may be demonstrated during the course of malaria, particularly with *Plasmodium falciparum,* clinical findings to indicate cardiac involvement are rare.[503, 504] The heart generally demonstrates few gross abnormalities. The principal findings are histological. The capillaries are often filled and even distended with an accumulation of parasites, sometimes totally occluding the lumen of the vessels. Thrombosis of the capillaries and ischemic myocardial changes may be seen.[504] Focal myocardial damage may be present, along with an interstitial infiltrate composed of lymphocytes, plasma cells, and macrophages. In rare cases, cardiac failure may contribute to or even cause death.[504] ST segment and T wave changes on the ECG may be the only clinical indications of myocardial involvement.[503]

METAZOAL MYOCARDIAL DISEASE

ECHINOCOCCUS (HYDATID CYST). *Echinococcus* is endemic in many sheep-raising areas of the world, particularly Argentina, Uruguay, New Zealand, Greece, North Africa, and Iceland, but cardiac involvement in hydatid disease is uncommon, occurring in less than 2 percent of cases.[505] The usual host of *Echinococcus granulosus* is the dog, but humans may serve as intermediate hosts (rather than the sheep, the usual intermediate host) if they accidentally ingest ova from contaminated dog feces.

When cardiac involvement is present, the cysts usually are intramyocardial in the interventricular septum or left ventricular free wall (Fig. 48–34); involvement of the right ventricle or atrium may occur.[505] Involvement of the tricuspid valve may be seen on occasion; in most cases, a single cardiac cyst is present.

A myocardial cyst may degenerate and calcify, develop daughter cysts, or rupture. Rupture of the cyst is the most dreaded complication; rupture into the pericardium may result in acute pericarditis, which may progress to chronic constrictive pericarditis.[505] Rupture into the cardiac chambers may result in systemic or pulmonary emboli.[506] Rapidly progressive pulmonary hypertension may occur with rupture of right-sided cysts, with subsequent embolization of hundreds of scolices into the pulmonary circulation. The liberation of hydatid fluid into the circulation may produce profound, fatal circulatory collapse due to an anaphylactic reaction to the protein constituents of the fluid.[505]

Symptoms depend on the location, size, and integrity of the cyst; patients may be asymptomatic or in profound circulatory collapse. It is estimated that only about 10 percent of patients with cardiac hydatid cysts have clinical manifestations.[505] The ECG may reflect the location of the cyst; T wave changes and loss of QRS voltage may occur with left ventricular involvement, whereas atrioventricular conduction defects or right bundle branch block may be seen with involvement of the interventricular septum. Chest pain is usually due to rupture of the cyst into the pericardial space with resultant pericarditis. Large cystic masses may sometimes produce right-sided obstruction.[505]

Diagnosis. Recognition of an echinococcal cyst of the heart is a relatively simple matter if there is evidence of cysts in other organs, particularly the liver and lung. However, a cardiac cyst may be an isolated, solitary finding. The chest roentgenogram frequently shows an abnormal cardiac silhouette or a calcified lobular mass adjacent to the left ventricle.[505] Although CT and MRI may aid in the detection and localization of heart cysts, two-dimensional echocardiography is thought to be the best choice (see Fig. 48–34).[505] Eosinophilia, present in some patients, is a useful adjunctive finding. The Casoni skin test is not very helpful because both false-positive and false-negative results occur. Serological tests, including hemagglutination and complement fixation, may be more useful, but their predictive accuracy is limited.[505]

Management. Until recently, treatment for hydatid disease was limited to surgical excision.[507] Experience suggests that the benzimidazole derivatives mebendazole and albendazole may be somewhat useful in the medical management of this disease.[505, 508] Despite the availability of drug therapy, adjunctive surgical excision is generally recommended, even for asymptomatic patients, because of the significant risk of rupture of the cyst and its attendant serious and sometimes fatal consequences.[505] The surgical results have been generally favorable.

VISCERAL LARVA MIGRANS. People are occasional accidental hosts of the roundworm infestations of dogs due to *Toxocara canis,* but cardiac involvement is rare. Most cases occur in children 1 to 3 years of age.[509] Myocarditis may occur in association with invasion of the myocardium by larvae. The myocardial lesions include granulomas or extensive inflammatory infiltrates (often with eosinophils) with foci of muscle necrosis. Congestive heart failure and death may occur, although asymptomatic cardiac involvement may be seen as well.

SCHISTOSOMIASIS AND RELATED DISEASE. Direct cardiac involvement

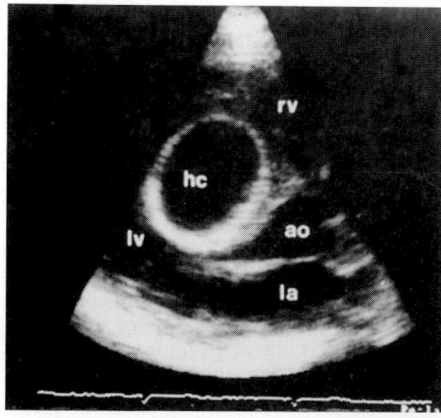
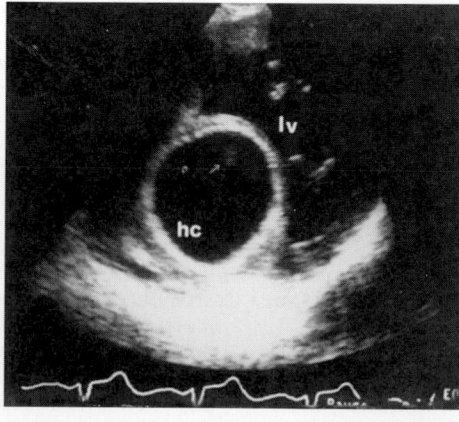

FIGURE 48–34. Involvement of interventricular septum by a hydatid cyst. *Left,* Transthoracic two-dimensional echocardiogram of parasternal long-axis view showing a 3-cm diameter hydatid cyst (hc) in the upper ventricular septum. *Right,* Transesophageal echocardiography showing a hydatid cyst (hc) having a rounded and well-contrasted capsule. la = left atrium; lv = left ventricle; rv = right ventricle; ao = aorta. (From Aupetit J, Ritz B, Ferrini M, et al: Images in cardiovascular medicine: Hydatid cyst of the interventricular septum. Circulation 95:2325, 1997. Copyright 1997, American Heart Association.)

in schistosomiasis, heterophyiasis, and cysticercosis is distinctly unusual. The principal cardiovascular manifestation of schistosomiasis is right-sided heart overload as a consequence of embolization of the ova to the pulmonary vasculature, with attendant pulmonary hypertension.

TRICHINOSIS. Infestation with *Trichinella spiralis* is a common human finding. Mild myocarditis has been said to be a frequent finding, but recent data suggest that clinically detectable cardiac involvement occurs in a minority of patients.[510] Symptomatic involvement is uncommon and may be responsible for the majority of fatalities.[511] Less frequently, death is due to pulmonary embolism secondary to venous thrombosis or to neurologic complications.

Although the parasite may invade the heart, it does not usually encyst there, and it is rare to find larvae or larval fragments in the myocardium. Nonetheless, pathological findings at autopsy may be impressive. The heart may be dilated and flabby, and a pericardial effusion may be present.[510] A prominent focal infiltrate composed of lymphocytes and eosinophils is commonly found, with occasional microthrombi in the intramural arterioles. Areas of muscle degeneration and necrosis are present.

Clinical Manifestations. Myocarditis usually is mild and goes unnoticed, but in occasional cases it is manifested by congestive heart failure and chest pain, usually appearing around the third week of the disease, when the general constitutional symptoms are abating. Physical examination may be normal, or there may be gross cardiomegaly with severe congestive heart failure. Sudden death may occur, usually in the fourth to eighth week of the illness.

ECG abnormalities may be detected in about 10 percent of patients with trichinosis and parallel the time course of clinical cardiac involvement, initially appearing in the second or third week and usually resolving by the seventh week of the illness. The most common ECG abnormalities are repolarization abnormalities and ventricular premature complexes.[510] The ECG changes usually resolve completely.

The diagnosis is usually based on the demonstration of a positive indirect immunofluorescent antibody test in a patient with the clinical features of trichinosis. Eosinophilia, when present, is a supportive finding. The skin test is usually but not invariably positive. Treatment is with anthelmintics and corticosteroids; dramatic improvement in cardiac function has been reported after their use.

Toxic, Chemical, Immune, and Physical Damage to the Heart

A wide variety of substances other than infectious agents may act on the heart and damage the myocardium. In some cases, the damage is acute, transient, and associated with evidence of an inflammatory myocardial infiltrate with myocyte necrosis (e.g., with the arsenicals and lithium); in other cases, a hypersensitivity reaction occurs, without prominent evidence of necrosis (e.g., with sulfonamides). Other agents that damage the myocardium may lead to chronic changes with resulting histological evidence of fibrosis and a clinical picture of a DCM. Furthermore, many offending stimuli may be associated with both acute and chronic phases (e.g., alcohol, doxorubicin). The extent of myocardial damage often is related to the dose and rate of exposure to the toxin.

Numerous chemicals and drugs (both industrial and therapeutic) may lead to cardiac damage and dysfunction. Several physical agents (e.g., radiation and excessive heat) may also result in myocardial damage. Furthermore, myocardial involvement may be evident in a variety of systemic disease, which are described in Part V of this book.

Cocaine

The illicit use of this drug has increased dramatically. It may be associated with a variety of cardiovascular complications, including myocardial ischemia and infarction (unassociated with obstructive coronary artery disease in about one third of cases), accelerated atherosclerosis, arrhythmias and sudden death, electrophysiological effects, coronary vasoconstriction, myocarditis, DCM, rupture of the aorta, cerebrovascular events, increased platelet aggregation, arterial thrombosis, and an apparent predisposition to the development of endocarditis.[512–516] The actual frequency of these complications is in some dispute[517]; the number of adverse events reported in the literature is far less than the casual impression of medical caregivers in inner-city hospitals would suggest. In one study of cocaine abusers who presented to the hospital with chest pain, the frequency of documented myocardial infarction was low.[518] The effects of cocaine on the myocardium itself include transient depression of ventricular function whether the drug is taken acutely or chronically,[519, 520] scattered areas of myocardial necrosis and myocarditis unrelated to coronary artery disease (which in some cases include contraction band necrosis), and fibrosis.[521] In a some cases there has been evidence of dilated cardiomyopathy.[522] Even asymptomatic cocaine abusers may have myocardial depression, albeit clinically silent.[520]

The cardiovascular effects of cocaine likely are related to its principal pharmacological effects: blocking the reuptake of catecholamines in the presynaptic neurons; blocking sodium channels, leading to local anesthetic, membrane-stabilizing effects; and reducing spontaneous sympathetic activity as a result of effects on the brain stem.[521] It has been speculated that the myocardial damage seen with cocaine relates to excess catecholamines damaging myocytes because their reuptake is blocked; this may lead to calcium overload of the cells, or perhaps to local vasoconstriction with subsequent ischemic damage. Coronary vasoconstriction is mediated by action on alpha-adrenergic receptors and is intensified by cigarette smoking and by beta-adrenergic blockade.[523] The increase in myocardial oxygen needs resulting from tachycardia and hypertension, combined with coronary vasoconstriction, can cause myocardial ischemia and is likely responsible for the observation of more than 20-fold increase in the risk of myocardial infarction in the hour after cocaine use.[519] The monocellular infiltrate (myocarditis) that has been found may merely be a reaction to the associated myocyte death, or it could be a hypersensitivity reaction to the cocaine, a metabolite,[524] or a contaminant.

The Coronary Artery Risk Development in Young Adults (CARDIA) study reported that cocaine use was related to being male, single, unemployed, and black, and to higher levels of other substance use.[525] Patients presenting to the emergency department with chest pain are infrequently asked about cocaine use.[524] Although acute myocardial infarction is a real risk in cocaine users, it may be caused by skeletal muscle injury, with elevation of circulating creatine kinase or CK-MB. Therefore, cardiac-specific troponin T or I is especially useful for detecting myocardial necrosis in these patients.[526] Similarly, myocardial perfusion imaging with technetium-99m sestamibi has been found to be useful in excluding infarction in patients with cocaine-associated chest pain.[527]

Treatment of cocaine-induced myocardial ischemia consists of nitrates, alpha-adrenoceptor blockers, calcium antagonists, and thrombolytic therapy (for acute myocardial infarctions). Beta-adrenoceptor blockers probably should be avoided unless hypertension or tachycardia are present, because they have been shown to further reduce coronary blood flow and increase coronary vascular resistance during cocaine use and may predispose to cocaine-mediated cardiac conduction defects.[513, 514, 521] The ACC/AHA Guidelines for the management of unstable angina listed recommend ". . . immediate arteriography, if possible, in patients whose

ST segments remain elevated after nitroglycerin and calcium channel blocker. Thrombolysis if thrombus is detected." Additional recommendations include thrombolytic therapy if ST segments remain elevated despite nitroglycerine and calcium blockers and coronary arteriography is not possible, as well as coronary arteriography, if available, for patients with new ST depression or T-wave changes, who are unresponsive to nitroglycerin and calcium antagonists.[528]

DAUNORUBICIN AND DOXORUBICIN (See Chap. 69)

INTERFERON-ALPHA (see Chap. 69). Interferon-alpha is a leukocyte-derived protein used therapeutically to treat malignancies and HIV infections. Cardiotoxicity, usually consisting of hypotension, tachycardia, and transient arrhythmias, occurs in a minority of patients (perhaps up to 10 percent).[522] Several patients have developed congestive heart failure and the clinical picture of a DCM during interferon-alfa therapy; in at least some patients, the cardiomyopathy resolves rapidly with discontinuation of the drug.[522, 529]

INTERLEUKIN-2 (see Chap. 69). The lymphokine interleukin-2, an antineoplastic agent, has significant cardiovascular toxicity, the most prominent of which is a diffuse capillary leak syndrome with hypotension and tachycardia, although reversible left ventricular dysfunction is seen as well.[529] In about 5 percent of patients, additional cardiotoxicity is seen, consisting of myocardial ischemia, infarction, injury, arrhythmias, and eosinophilic myocarditis.[530]

TRICYCLIC ANTIDEPRESSANTS (see Chap. 70). Although sinus tachycardia, postural hypotension, disturbances in rhythm, abnormalities of atrioventricular conduction, and even sudden death may be seen with the tricyclic antidepressants, particularly when taken as an overdose, important depression of left ventricular function usually does not occur, even in patients with preexisting heart disease.[529] There has been concern when using tricyclic antidepressants in patients with prior myocardial infarction and/or preexisting ventricular arrhythmias, because these agents have a Class I antiarrhythmic effect, prolong the QT interval, and might be proarrhythmic in these settings. The selective serotonin reuptake inhibitors are remarkably free of cardiovascular toxicity and do not appear to depress ventricular function.[529] They may produce side effects by interacting with the metabolism of drugs mediated through the cytochrome-P450 enzyme system.[530]

PHENOTHIAZINES (see Chap. 70). The phenothiazines may be associated with a variety of cardiac disturbances, including ECG changes, atrial and ventricular arrhythmias, and sudden death.[531, 532] Postural hypotension may also be seen. The cardiac effects are largely dose dependent. ECG abnormalities may be observed with as little as 200 mg of thioridazine per day and consist of lengthening of the QT interval and T wave changes. Prolongation of the QT interval may set the stage for the emergence of ventricular arrhythmias, particularly torsades de pointes.[530, 531] Higher doses may lead to frank T wave inversion and increased amplitude of the U wave. Changes in the P wave, QRS complex, and ST segment are usually absent. The ECG abnormalities and arrhythmias resolve with discontinuation of the drug, usually within 48 hours. An occasional patient may require temporary ventricular pacing.

Pathological changes in the hearts of patients who have received phenothiazines and who have died suddenly include the deposition of acid mucopolysaccharide between muscle bundles in periarteriolar regions as well as the conduction system, with myofibrillar degeneration, and endothelial proliferation in the smaller blood vessels, although a direct causal relationship between drug administration and cardiomyopathic changes is only inferential. A variety of explanations have been invoked for the apparent cardiac damage, including direct toxic effects of the phenothiazines on the myocardium, stimulation of higher autonomic centers, and changes in circulating or myocardial levels of catecholamines.

EMETINE. Cardiovascular changes are said to be common with the chronic use of emetine, a drug often employed in the treatment of amebiasis and schistosomiasis as well as the active ingredient in ipecac syrup (used for childhood poisoning).[533] Myocardial lesions may be observed in some patients at autopsy, and similar cardiac damage is noted in experimental animals given emetine. The myocardial lesions consist of myofibrillar degeneration and necrosis, with an interstitial infiltrate of mononuclear cells and histiocytes.

The ECG, which may be abnormal in 50 percent of treated patients, most commonly shows reduced T wave amplitude or inversion. Prolongation of the QT interval and ST segment shifts may also be seen, although abnormalities of the P wave, PR segment, and QRS complex are infrequent. The ECG changes usually resolve within weeks or months after cessation of treatment. Sinus tachycardia and hypotension may also be seen, as well as transient or permanent left ventricular dysfunction.[534] Only rare fatalities have been reported. Dehydroemetine results in ECG abnormalities similar to those of emetine, but they are less prominent and of shorter duration.

METHYSERGIDE. The widespread fibrotic reactions seen with this drug can also involve the heart. Up to 1 percent of patients treated long term may develop typically left-sided valvular lesions, resulting in stenosis and regurgitation.[535]

CHLOROQUINE. This drug has been widely used in the prophylaxis and treatment of a variety of parasitic and other diseases, including collagen and dermatological disorders. ECG changes may be seen with its use, along with conduction disturbances and features of a restrictive cardiomyopathy.[536] In toxic doses, chloroquine may result in depressed cardiac output, bradycardia, arrhythmias, heart block, and death.

ANTIMONY COMPOUNDS. Various antimony compounds, such as stibophen and tartar emetic, have been widely used in the treatment of schistosomiasis; less toxic agents are now becoming available. The antimony compounds are associated with ECG changes in almost all patients. Typical ECG changes include prolongation of the QT interval with flattening or inversion of T waves. ST segment shifts and P wave changes may be seen, although the QRS complex usually demonstrates no abnormality. The majority of patients do not demonstrate cardiac findings, although chest pain, bradycardia, hypotension, ventricular arrhythmias (including paroxysmal ventricular tachycardia and torsades de pointes), congestive heart failure, and sudden death may occur.[537, 538]

LITHIUM (see Chap. 70). Lithium carbonate, used in the treatment of bipolar disorders, is associated with T wave changes in one fourth or more of patients who receive the drug.[539] Clinical evidence of myocardial involvement is usually lacking, although intoxication with lithium may be associated on rare occasions with ventricular arrhythmias, symptomatic sinus node abnormalities, atrioventricular conduction disturbances, congestive heart failure, and in rare cases, death.[539, 540] In fatal lithium toxicity, the heart is said to be dilated, with evidence of myofibrillar degeneration associated with a lymphocytic interstitial infiltrate.

HYDROCARBONS. The fluorinated hydrocarbons, commonly used as aerosol propellants, appear to be cardiac toxins, contrary to their reputation of being inert.[541] In animal models, and occasional humans, the aerosol propellants may cause ventricular tachyarrhythmias, depress myocardial contractility, and lower systemic vascular resistance and arterial pressure.[542] These cardiovascular effects may be involved in the sudden deaths seen in individuals who abuse aerosols for their psychotropic effect.[542]

CATECHOLAMINES. A severe reversible DCM has been observed in conjunction with pheochromocytoma, and the myocardial damage has been attributed to high levels of circulating catecholamines (see Chap. 64).[543, 544] Similar changes have been demonstrated in experimental animals treated with prolonged infusions of l-norepinephrine.[544] Catecholamines also may produce acute myocarditis, with focal myocardial necrosis, inflammation, epicardial hemorrhages, tachycardia, and arrhythmias.[545] Similar findings have been described with excessive use of beta-adrenoceptor agonist inhalants and methylxanthines in the treatment of decompensated pulmonary disease.[546] The cardiomyopathy associated with pheochromocytoma is one of the conditions that should be considered when heart failure suddenly appears without other obvious explanation.[544]

A variety of mechanisms of myocardial damage have been suggested. A direct toxic effect may be involved, or the damage may be secondary to relative tissue hypoxia because of heightened metabolic demands. Alternatively, the damage may result from changes in autonomic tone, enhanced lipid mobility, calcium overload, damaging effects of catecholamine oxidation products (free radicals), or increased sarcolemmal permeability.[545] Catecholamine-induced vasospasm also may play a role.[544]

LEAD. The prominent features in lead poisoning generally center on the gastrointestinal and central nervous systems. However, myocardial involvement may contribute to or be the principal cause of death in some cases.[547] ECG changes, atrioventricular conduction defects, and overt congestive heart failure may occur. The ECG and myocardial changes appear to be reversible with chelation therapy.

CARBON MONOXIDE. Both acute and chronic carbon monoxide toxicity can occur. While central nervous system findings usually dominate the clinical presentation, significant and occasionally fatal cardiac abnormalities have been reported, although some have found no precipitation of arrhythmias following exposure.[548, 549] Because carbon monoxide has a higher affinity for hemoglobin than does oxygen, reduced amounts of oxygen are delivered to the tissues. Thus, the cardiac toxicity may be partially caused by myocardial hypoxia, but a direct toxic effect of the gas on myocardial mitochondria may play an even more important role.[550] The histological features include focal areas of necrosis, most marked in the subendocardium. Focal perivascular infiltrates and punctate hemorrhages are also seen.[550]

Cardiac involvement may appear promptly after exposure, or it may be delayed for up to several days. Palpitations, sinus tachycardia, and various arrhythmias, including ventricular extrasystoles and atrial fibrillation, are common.[551] Bradycardia and atrioventricular block may occur in more severe cases.[551] In patients with ischemic heart disease, angina pectoris and myocardial infarction may be precipitated. ECG ST segment and T wave abnormalities are quite common. Transient right and/or left ventricular wall motion abnormalities may be present.[550] Administration of 100 percent oxygen, bed rest, and surveillance for serious rhythm or conduction abnormalities usually permit rapid recovery.

HYPOCALCEMIA. In rare patients with chronic hypocalcemia (often due to hypoparathyroidism), congestive heart failure may occur (see Chap. 16) and resolve only when the serum calcium level is raised.[552] Rapid transfusion of citrated blood can produce hypocalcemia and reversible myocardial depression, as can ambulatory peritoneal dialysis in patients with chronic renal failure.[553]

HYPOPHOSPHATEMIA. A form of reversible left ventricular dysfunction may be seen with severe hypophosphatemia. Restoration of the serum phosphate level to normal results in hemodynamic recovery.

HYPOMAGNESEMIA. Focal cardiac necrosis is found in experimental magnesium deficiency and may account for the supraventricular and ventricular arrhythmias and ECG changes that are seen clinically. In addition to arrhythmias, coronary spasm and acute myocardial infarction may be seen.[554] A rare case of fatal cardiomyopathy has been reported.[554, 555]

CARNITINE DEFICIENCY. Carnitine, an essential cofactor for the oxidation of fatty acids, produces an HCM or DCM in children who have long-standing carnitine deficiency.[556] Carnitine supplementation can lead to symptomatic and functional improvement; determination of carnitine levels therefore is important in children with unexplained cardiomyopathy. Myocardial carnitine levels may be reduced in the hearts of patients with DCM,[557] but the significance of this observation is not known at present.

SELENIUM DEFICIENCY. Dietary deficiency of the trace element selenium appears to be one of the principal factors responsible for a form of DCM endemic to certain rural areas in China, although the etiological role played by selenium has been questioned.[558] Termed *Keshan disease*, it affects mainly children and young women and apparently is prevented by the prophylactic administration of sodium selenite tablets. A similar cardiomyopathy may be found in westerners subjected to prolonged parenteral hyperalimentation; supplementation with oral selenium may reverse the cardiomyopathy.[559]

SCORPION STING. The venom of the scorpion is mainly neurotoxic, but cardiac findings may be prominent and even fatal, particularly in children.[560] ECG changes and myocardial damage with elevated serum cardiac enzyme levels are common findings. Hearts are normal on gross examination, with prominent microscopic changes usually but not invariably present, particularly in the subendocardial region and papillary muscles. Degeneration and necrosis of muscle fibers are noted, with interstitial edema and a mononuclear infiltrate. The histological features of scorpion sting suggest high levels of circulating catecholamines and are similar to those seen with experimental catecholamine infusion and in pheochromocytoma.[561]

The ECG often initially shows tall, peaked T waves that progress to inversions and ST segment shifts. Q waves may appear, and the QT interval is usually prolonged. Atrial, junctional, and ventricular arrhythmias may occur. Tachycardia, hypertension, anxiety, diaphoresis, and pulmonary edema—findings resembling those of a massive catecholamine effect—are striking in many patients.[561] A smaller number of patients are seen in shock with peripheral vascular collapse. Most deaths are due to pulmonary edema, presumably the result of left ventricular dysfunction.[560] Occasionally, sudden and unexpected deaths occur in a smaller percentage of patients, presumably as a consequence of arrhythmias. Adrenergic blocking agents and the use of specific antivenom appear to be useful in the management of the cardiovascular manifestation of scorpion stings, although a wide variety of agents has been tried.[561]

WASP STINGS. Stings by the vespine wasps may lead to anaphylaxis, with hypotension, circulatory collapse, and cyanosis. Occasional patients may have chest pain and clinical findings compatible with acute myocardial infarction.[562] The mechanism of myocardial damage is unclear; perhaps it merely reflects necrosis from profound hypotension, although a direct toxic effect on the myocardium or an indirect effect on the coronary arteries may be involved.[563]

SNAKE BITE. Cardiac complications are not prominent features of snake bites, and the clinical picture is usually dominated by the neurological, hematological, and vascular damage produced by the snakebite toxin.[564] Myocardial involvement is seen on occasion and may rarely contribute to morbidity and mortality. T wave abnormalities are the most common manifestation of myocardial involvement, although ST segment depression, QRS prolongation, and atrioventricular conduction defects may also be seen.[564, 565] The ECG changes are usually transient, but when persistent they are attributed to direct myocardial damage due to the toxin. Death may occur from circulatory collapse, myocardial depression, or myocardial infarction due to hypotension and coronary artery thrombosis. Coronary artery vasospasm may also be involved.

ARSENIC. Myocardial involvement may be seen in both acute and chronic arsenical poisoning, usually from pesticides; the heart may be dilated, with accumulation of pericardial fluid.[566] Multiple local and confluent areas of subepicardial and subendocardial hemorrhage are characteristic findings. The myocardium is usually abnormal, with evidence of a perivascular mononuclear infiltrate.[566]

Clinically unrecognized interstitial myocarditis is manifested by T wave inversions and ST segment depression, along with prolongation of the QT interval.[566] The ECG changes usually revert to normal within 2 to 4 weeks. The ECG abnormalities appear to resolve more rapidly when BAL (British antilewisite, dimercaprol) is used in therapy.

CYCLOPHOSPHAMIDE (see Chap. 69). High doses of cyclophosphamide have been associated with ECG changes, congestive heart failure, and death from hemorrhagic myocarditis.[529] In the majority of

treated patients, a reversible decrease of QRS voltage and systolic function is seen, often asymptomatic, although more than 20 percent may succumb as a consequence of myopericarditis. The myocardial damage appears to result from direct endothelial damage and resultant fibrin microthrombi in the capillaries.

5-FLUOROURACIL (see Chap. 69). This antineoplastic agent has been associated with cardiotoxicity manifested by chest pain, ECG changes, and arrhythmia.[529] Coronary spasm has been implicated but not proven as the mechanism. There is speculation that 5-fluorouracil may also depress left ventricular dysfunction, but this has not been established with certainty.[529]

HYPERSENSITIVITY

Hypersensitivity to a variety of agents may result in allergic reactions that involve the myocardium. A variety of drugs (most commonly the sulfonamides, hydrochlorothiazide, the penicillins, and methyldopa) or other sensitizers may lead to an allergic myocarditis (Table 48–10), characterized by peripheral eosinophilia and a perivascular infiltration of the myocardium by eosinophils, lymphocytes, and histiocytes; necrosis is seen on occasion.[338] Hypersensitivity myocarditis is rarely recognized clinically and is often first discovered at postmortem examination, although it is occasionally diagnosed on endomyocardial biopsy. Most patients who have hypersensitivity myocarditis are not critically ill, but nevertheless may die suddenly, presumably as a consequence of an arrhythmia. An occasional patient has intense eosinophilic infiltration of the myocardium of no obvious cause, with prominent necrosis evident and findings of hemodynamic collapse; some of these patients may have undiagnosed hypersensitivity myocarditis.[567, 568] Because of the potential for significant deleterious effects, a high index of suspicion for this condition should be maintained. Therapy includes discontinuation of the offending agent and corticosteroids and/or immunosuppression therapy in severe cases.

METHYLDOPA. Although hepatitis is the most frequently encountered serious adverse reaction to methyldopa, sudden and unexpected death has been reported in a number of patients found at necropsy to have had an unsuspected myocarditis.[568, 569] The histological findings have the characteristics of an allergic myocarditis, showing an interstitial inflammatory infiltrate with abundant eosinophils, vasculitis, and focal myocardial necrosis.[568] ECG changes include sinus bradycardia, sinus pauses, and first- and second-degree AV block.

PENICILLIN. Allergic reactions to penicillin are fairly common, but myocardial involvement is rare.[570] Histological findings consist of a perivascular and interstitial infiltrate composed of eosinophils and

▼ **TABLE 48–10. PRINCIPAL DRUGS CAPABLE OF CAUSING HYPERSENSITIVITY MYOCARDITIS**

Antibiotics	**Antiinflammatory**
Amphotericin B	Indomethacin
Ampicillin	Oxyphenbutazone
Chloramphenicol	Phenylbutazone
Penicillin	
Tetracycline	**Diuretics**
Streptomycin	Acetazolamide
	Chlorthalidone
Sulfonamides	Hydrochlorothiazide
Sulfadiazine	Spironolactone
Sulfisoxazole	
	Others
Anticonvulsants	Amitriptyline
Phenindione	Methyldopa
Phenytoin	Sulfonylureas
Carbamazepine	Tetanus toxoid
Antituberculous	
Isoniazid	
Para-aminosalicylic acid	

From Kounis NG, Zavras GM, Soufras GD, Kitrou MP: Hypersensitivity myocarditis. Ann Allergy 62:71, 1989.

mononuclear cells.[568] Both myocardial infarction and pericarditis may occur and account for some of the ECG changes.[570] Transient ECG changes may be the only manifestation of cardiac involvement, with sinus tachycardia, ST segment elevation, and T wave inversion.

SULFONAMIDES. Sulfonamides may result in myocardial damage owing to a hypersensitivity vasculitis as well as a myocarditis.[570] In fatal cases eosinophilic myocarditis, sometimes with granulomas, can be demonstrated.[568] Although usually clinically silent, myocardial involvement may produce severe and even fatal congestive heart failure. ECG changes are usually absent, but nonspecific ST segment and T wave abnormalities may be seen.

TETRACYCLINE. Allergic reactions to antibiotics of the tetracycline class include fever, tachycardia, and first-degree atrioventricular block. Postmortem findings include cardiac dilatation, fibrinoid muscle cell degeneration, and a diffuse interstitial and perivascular infiltrate.[568]

GIANT CELL MYOCARDITIS

Giant cell myocarditis is a rare disease of unknown cause characterized by the presence of multinucleated giant cells in the myocardium. (It is included here because of the possibility that it may be of immune or autoimmune origin.) Also called granulomatous myocarditis, this condition is typically a rapidly fatal disease, often of young to middle-aged adults.[571] Pathological findings are usually impressive. The ventricles are dilated, and mural thrombi may be present. A serpiginous area of myocardial necrosis may be seen involving the right as well as the left ventricle. Multinucleated giant cells are found, particularly at the margins of the areas of myocardial necrosis; a lymphocyte infiltrate is present,[572] with helper or suppressor T cells (Fig. 48–35).[573–575]

FIGURE 48–35. See color plate 29.

ETIOLOGY. Giant cell myocarditis occurs on occasion in association with systemic diseases such as sarcoidosis, systemic lupus erythematosus, drug hypersensitivity, infections (especially syphilis and tuberculosis), thyrotoxicosis and malignant thymoma, but the cause of the disease remains obscure.[338, 576] In many ways the clinical features suggest a viral myocarditis except for the rapid and virulent course. Myocardial infection with coxsackievirus B2 has been reported,[574] and an autoimmune reaction to altered cardiac tissue has been suggested based on the histological findings and the association of giant cell myocarditis with other autoimmune disorders, although there is little direct evidence supporting this view.[571]

CLINICAL MANIFESTATIONS AND TREATMENT. Both sexes are equally affected; the onset typically is rapid, with dyspnea, chest pain, orthopnea, and hypotension. Fever is usually present, with ECG evidence of widespread myocardial involvement. Refractory ventricular arrhythmias, although present in a minority of patients, suggest the diagnosis when present.[571] Overt congestive heart failure and sudden death occur frequently.[571–577] Medical therapy often is unsuccessful, although corticosteroids and immunosuppressive agents appear to have benefited some patients. Because the prognosis in general is poor, an initial attempt at empirical immunosuppressive therapy is warranted.[578, 579] Occasional patients have had long-term survival after medical therapy,[579a] but cardiac transplantation is considered to be the treatment of choice for most patients; there is a risk of fatal recurrent giant cell myocarditis in the transplanted heart.[580]

PHYSICAL AGENTS

RADIATION (see Chap. 69). The use of radiation therapy may result in a variety of cardiac complications, which are usually chronic and which include pericarditis with effusion, tamponade, or constriction; coronary artery fibrosis and myocardial infarction; valvular abnormalities; myocardial fibrosis; and conduction disturbances.[581] Although the heart has been regarded as one of the organs more resistant to the effects of radiation, the clinical significance of radiation-induced heart disease is greater than usually thought.[581] Although radiation probably results in some degree of tissue damage in all patients, clinically significant cardiac involvement occurs in the minority of patients, usually long after the radiation treatment has ended.[582] Radiation-induced cardiac damage is related to the dose of radiation, the mass of heart irradiated, and the dose schedule of the radiation.

The late cardiac damage that may follow irradiation appears to result from a long-lasting injury of the capillary endothelial cells, which leads to cell death, capillary rupture, and microthrombi.[581, 583] Because of this damage to the microvasculature, ischemia results and is followed by myocardial fibrosis. In addition to microvascular damage, the major epicardial coronary arteries may become narrowed, especially at the ostia.[582]

Only an occasional patient manifests acute clinical cardiac abnormality with radiation therapy; typically this consists of acute pericarditis. A mild, transient, asymptomatic depression of left ventricular function may be seen early after radiation therapy. The more common clinical expressions of radiation heart disease occur months or years after the exposure. The pericardium is the most common site of clinical involvement, with findings of chronic pericardial effusion or pericardial constriction (see Chap. 50).[581] Myocardial damage occurs less frequently and is characterized by myocardial fibrosis with or without endocardial fibrosis or fibroelastosis. Left and/or right ventricular dysfunction at rest or with exercise appears to be a common, albeit usually asymptomatic, finding 5 to 20 years after radiation therapy, especially in those in whom the now-outmoded technique of a single anteroposterior port was used.[581] Occasional patients may develop usually asymptomatic left-sided (and rarely right-sided) valvular regurgitation (or on occasion stenosis) that rarely requires valve replacement[582]; often there is a latent period of a decade or more between the radiation exposure and the development of valvular deformity.[583] ECG abnormalities, heart block, and a variety of arrhythmias may be seen months or years after therapeutic radiation, although usually they are of limited clinical significance.[583, 584]

HEAT STROKE

This condition results from failure of the thermoregulatory center following exposure to high ambient temperature. It is manifested principally by hyperpyrexia, renal insufficiency, disseminated intravascular coagulation, and central nervous system dysfunction.[585] However, cardiovascular abnormalities (usually ECG) appear to be common; pulmonary edema, and transient right and/or left ventricular dysfunction may occur, along with hypotension and circulatory collapse. Pathological changes include dilatation of the right side of the heart, particularly the right atrium. Hemorrhages of the subendocardium and the subepicardium are frequently seen at necropsy and often involve the interventricular septum and posterior wall of the left ventricle. Histological findings include degeneration and necrosis of muscle fibers as well as interstitial edema. Factors that have been implicated as possible causes of myocardial damage include direct thermal injury, myocardial hypoxia resulting from circulatory collapse, decreased coronary blood flow, and metabolic abnormalities resulting from widespread injury to other organs.

Sinus tachycardia is invariably present,[585] whereas atrial and ventricular arrhythmias usually are absent. Transient prolongation of the QT interval may be seen, along with ST segment and T wave abnormalities. It may take up to several months for these repolarization abnormalities to resolve. Serum enzyme levels may be elevated and may reflect myocardial damage, at least in part, although comcomitant rhabdomyolysis often is present.

HYPOTHERMIA

Low temperature may also result in myocardial damage. Cardiac dilatation may occur with epicardial petechiae and subendocardial hemorrhages. Microinfarcts are found in the ventricular myocardium, presumably related to abnormalities in the microcirculation. The lesions are not due to the low temperature per se but appear to be the result of the circulatory collapse, hemoconcentration, capillary slugging, and depressed cellular metabolism that accompany hypothermia. Clinical manifestations of hypothermia include sinus bradycardia, conduction disturbances, atrial (and occasionally ventricular) fibrillation, hypotension, a fall in cardiac output, reversible myocardial depression, and a characteristic deflection of the terminal portion of the QRS pattern (Osborn wave).[586] Treatment includes core warming (often utilizing extracorporeal blood warming), cardiopulmonary resuscitation, and management of pulmonary, hematological, and renal complications.[586–588]

REFERENCES

DILATED CARDIOMYOPATHY

1. Sugrue DD, Rodeheffer RJ, Codd MB, et al: The clinical course of idiopathic dilated cardiomyopathy: A population-based study. Ann Intern Med 117:117, 1992.
2. Coughlin SS, Comstock GW, Baughman KL: Descriptive epidemiology of idiopathic dilated cardiomyopathy in Washington County, Maryland, 1975–1991. J Clin Epidemiol 46:1003, 1993.
3. Richardson P, McKenna W, Bristow M, et al: Report of the 1995 World Health Organization/International Society and Federation of Cardiology Task Force on the Definition and Classification of Cardiomyopathies. Circulation 93:841, 1996.
4. Bachinski LL, Roberts R: New theories: Causes of dilated cardiomyopathy. Cardiol Clin 16:603, 1998.
5. Siu SC, Sole MJ: Dilated cardiomyopathy. Curr Opin Cardiol 9:337, 1994.
6. Kasper EK, Agema WR, Hutchins GM, et al: The causes of dilated cardiomyopathy: A clinicopathologic review of 673 consecutive patients. J Am Coll Cardiol 23:586, 1994.
7. Pytlewski G, Georgeson S, Burke J, et al: Endomyocardial biopsy under transesophageal echocardiographic guidance can be safely performed in the critically ill cardiac transplant recipient. Am J Cardiol 73:1019, 1994.
8. Grogan M, Redfield MM, Bailey KR, et al: Long-term outcome of patients with biopsy-proved myocarditis: Comparison with idiopathic dilated cardiomyopathy. J Am Coll Cardiol 26:80, 1995.
9. La Vecchia LL, Bedogni F, Bozzola L, et al: Prediction of recovery after abstinence in alcoholic cardiomyopathy: Role of hemodynamic and morphometric parameters. Clin Cardiol 19:45, 1996.
10. Herskowitz A, Campbell S, Deckers J, et al: Demographic features and prevalence of idiopathic myocarditis in patients undergoing endomyocardial biopsy. Am J Cardiol 71:982, 1993.
11. Martin AB, Webber S, Fricker FJ, et al: Acute myocarditis: Rapid diagnosis by PCR in children. Circulation 90:330, 1994.
12. Kuhl U, Lauer B, Souvatzoglu M, et al: Antimyosin scintigraphy and immunohistological analysis of endomyocardial biopsy in patients with clinically suspected myocarditis—evidence of myocardial cell damage and inflammation in the absence of histologic signs of myocarditis. J Am Coll Cardiol 32:1371, 1998.

Idiopathic Dilated Cardiomyopathy

13. Pelliccia A, Culasso F, Di Paolo FM, et al: Physiologic left ventricular cavity dilatation in elite athletes. Ann Intern Med 130:23, 1999.
14. Dec GW, Fuster V: Medical progress: Idiopathic dilated cardiomyopathy. N Engl J Med 331:1564, 1994.
15. Coughlin SS, Neaton JD, Sengupta A, et al: Predictors of mortality from idiopathic dilated cardiomyopathy in 356,222 men screened for the Multiple Risk Factor Intervention Trial. Am J Epidemiol 139:166, 1994.
16. Adams KF Jr, Zannad F: Clinical definition and epidemiology of advanced heart failure. Am Heart J 135:S204, 1998.
17. Dries DL, Exner DV, Gersh BJ, et al: Racial differences in the outcome of left ventricular dysfunction. N Engl J Med 340:609, 1999.
18. Redfield MM, Gersh BJ, Bailey KR, et al: Natural history of incidentally discovered, asymptomatic idiopathic dilated cardiomyopathy. Am J Cardiol 74:737, 1994.
19. Redfield MM, Gersh BJ, Bailey KR, et al: Natural history of idiopathic dilated cardiomyopathy: Effect of referral bias and secular trend. J Am Coll Cardiol 22:1921, 1993.
20. Manolio TA, Baughman KL, Rodeheffer R, et al: Prevalence and etiology of idiopathic dilated cardiomyopathy (summary of a National Heart, Lung, and Blood Institute workshop). Am J Cardiol 69:1458, 1992.
21. Semigran MJ, Thaik CM, Fifer MA, et al: Exercise capacity and systolic and diastolic ventricular function after recovery from acute dilated cardiomyopathy. J Am Coll Cardiol 24:462, 1994.
22. Fruhwald FM, Dusleag J, Eber B, et al: Long-term outcome and prognostic factors in dilated cardiomyopathy: Preliminary results. Angiology 45:763, 1994.
23. Anguita M, Arizon JM, Bueno G, et al: Clinical and hemodynamic predictors of survival in patients aged < 65 years with severe congestive heart failure secondary to ischemic or nonischemic dilated cardiomyopathy. Am J Cardiol 72:413, 1993.
24. De Maria R, Gavazzi A, Recalcati F, et al: Comparison of clinical findings in idiopathic dilated cardiomyopathy in women versus men. Am J Cardiol 72:580, 1993.
25. Sun JP, James KB, Yang XS, et al: Comparison of mortality rates and progression of left ventricular dysfunction in patients with idiopathic dilated cardiomyopathy and dilated versus nondilated right ventricular cavities. Am J Cardiol 80:1583, 1997.
26. Pelliccia F, d'Amati G, Cianfrocca C, et al: Histomorphometric features predict 1-year outcome of patients with idiopathic dilated cardiomyopathy considered to be at low priority for cardiac transplantation. Am Heart J 128:316, 1994.
27. Brown CA, O'Connell JB: Myocarditis and idiopathic dilated cardiomyopathy. Am J Med 99:309, 1995.
28. Neumann DA: Autoimmunity and idiopathic dilated cardiomyopathy. Mayo Clin Proc 69:193, 1994.
29. Baig MK, Goldman JH, Caforio AL, et al: Familial dilated cardiomyopathy: Cardiac abnormalities are common in asymptomatic relatives and may represent early disease. J Am Coll Cardiol 31:195, 1998.
30. Grunig E, Tasman JA, Kucherer H, et al: Frequency and phenotypes of familial dilated cardiomyopathy. J Am Coll Cardiol 31:186, 1998.
31. McKenna CJ, Codd MB, McCann HA, et al: Idiopathic dilated cardiomyopathy: Familial prevalence and HLA distribution. Heart 77:549, 1997.
32. Bowles KR, Gajarski R, Porter P, et al: Gene mapping of familial autosomal dominant dilated cardiomyopathy to chromosome 10q21-23. J Clin Invest 98:1355, 1996.
33. Durand JB, Bachinski LL, Bieling LC, et al: Localization of a gene responsible for familial dilated cardiomyopathy to chromosome 1q32. Circulation 92:3387, 1995.
34. Li D, Tapscoft T, Gonzalez O, et al: Desmin mutation responsible for idiopathic dilated cardiomyopathy. Circulation 100:461, 1999.
35. Kelly DP, Strauss AW: Inherited cardiomyopathies. N Engl J Med 330:913, 1994.
36. Towbin JA, Hejtmancik JF, Brink P, et al: X-linked dilated cardiomyopathy: Molecular genetic evidence of linkage to the Duchenne muscular dystrophy (dystrophin) gene at the Xp21 locus. Circulation 87:1854, 1993.
37. Leiden JM: The genetics of dilated cardiomyopathy—emerging clues to the puzzle. N Engl J Med 337:1080, 1997.
38. Ortiz-Lopez R, Li H, Su J, et al: Evidence for a dystrophin missense mutation as a cause of X-linked dilated cardiomyopathy. Circulation 95:2434, 1997.
39. Remes AM, Hassinen IE, Ikaheimo MJ, et al: Mitochondrial DNA deletions in dilated cardiomyopathy: A clinical study employing endomyocardial sampling. J Am Coll Cardiol 23:935, 1994.
40. Arbustini E, Diegoli M, Fasani R, et al: Mitochondrial DNA mutations and mitochondrial abnormalities in dilated cardiomyopathy. Am J Pathol 153:1501, 1998.
41. Anan R, Nakagawa M, Miyata M, et al: Cardiac involvement in mitochondrial diseases: A study on 17 patients with documented mitochondrial DNA defects. Circulation 91:955, 1995.
42. Mestroni L: Dilated cardiomyopathy: A genetic approach. Heart 77:185, 1997.
43. Raynolds MV, Bristow MR, Bush EW, et al: Angiotensin-converting enzyme DD genotype in patients with ischaemic or idiopathic dilated cardiomyopathy. Lancet 342:1073, 1993.
44. Bratton SL, Garden AL, Bohan TP, et al: A child with valproic acid–associated carnitine deficiency and carnitine-responsive cardiac dysfunction. J Child Neurol 7:413, 1992.
45. Luppi P, Rudert WA, Zanone MM, et al: Idiopathic dilated cardiomyopathy: A superantigen-driven autoimmune disease. Circulation 98:777, 1998.
46. Keeling PJ, Lukaszyk A, Poloniecki J, et al: A prospective case-control study of antibodies to coxsackie B virus in idiopathic dilated cardiomyopathy. J Am Coll Cardiol 23:593, 1994.
47. Why HJ, Meany BT, Richardson PJ, et al: Clinical and prognostic significance of detection of enteroviral RNA in the myocardium of patients with myocarditis or dilated cardiomyopathy. Circulation 89:2582, 1994.
48. de Leeuw N, Melchers WJ, Balk AH, et al: No evidence for persistent enterovirus infection in patients with end-stage idiopathic dilated cardiomyopathy. J Infect Dis 178:256, 1998.
49. Martino TA, Liu P, Sole MJ: Viral infection and the pathogenesis of dilated cardiomyopathy. Circ Res 74:182, 1994.
50. Pauschinger M, Bowles NE, Fuentes-Garcia FJ, et al: Detection of adenoviral genome in the myocardium of adult patients with idiopathic left ventricular dysfunction. Circulation 99:1348, 1999.
51. Caforio AL, Keeling PJ, Zachara E, et al: Evidence from family studies for autoimmunity in dilated cardiomyopathy. Lancet 344:773, 1994.
52. Limas CJ: Cardiac autoantibodies in dilated cardiomyopathy: A pathogenetic role? Circulation 95:1979, 1997.
53. Pohlner K, Portig I, Pankuweit S, et al: Identification of mitochondrial antigens recognized by antibodies in sera of patients with idiopathic dilated cardiomyopathy by two-dimensional gel electrophoresis and protein sequencing. Am J Cardiol 80:1040, 1997.
54. Limas C, Limas CJ, Boudoulas H, et al: HLA-DQA1 and -DQB1 gene haplotypes in familial cardiomyopathy. Am J Cardiol 74:510, 1994.
55. Fu LX, Magnusson Y, Bergh CH, et al: Localization of a functional autoimmune epitope on the muscarinic acetylcholine receptor-2 in pa-

tients with idiopathic dilated cardiomyopathy. J Clin Invest 91:1964, 1993.

56. Caforio AL, Goldman JH, Baig MK, et al: Cardiac autoantibodies in dilated cardiomyopathy become undetectable with disease progression. Heart 77:62, 1997.

57. Seko Y, Takahashi N, Ishiyama S, et al: Expression of co-stimulatory molecules B7-1, B7-2, and CD40 in the heart of patients with acute myocarditis and dilated cardiomyopathy. Circulation 97:637, 1998.

58. Dorffel WV, Felix SB, Wallukat G, et al: Short-term hemodynamic effects of immunoadsorption in dilated cardiomyopathy. Circulation 95: 1994, 1997.

58a. Felix SB, Staudt A, Dorffel WV, et al: Hemodynamic effects of immunoadsorption and subsequent immunoglobulin substitution in dilated cardiomyopathy: Three-month results from a randomized study. J Am Coll Cardiol 35:1590, 2000.

58b. Muller J, Wallukat G, Dandel M, et al: Immunoglobulin adsorption in patients with idiopathic dilated cardiomyopathy. Circulation 101:385, 2000.

59. Caforio AL: Role of autoimmunity in dilated cardiomyopathy. Br Heart J 72:S30, 1994.

60. Satoh M, Nakamura M, Saitoh H, et al: Tumor necrosis factor-alpha–converting enzyme and tumor necrosis factor-alpha in human dilated cardiomyopathy. Circulation 99:3260, 1999.

61. Bristow MR: Tumor necrosis factor-alpha and cardiomyopathy. Circulation 97:1340, 1998.

62. Bristow MR: Why does the myocardium fail? Insights from basic science. Lancet 352:SI8, 1998.

63. Kanoh M, Takemura G, Misao J, et al: Significance of myocytes with positive DNA in situ nick end-labeling (TUNEL) in hearts with dilated cardiomyopathy: Not apoptosis but DNA repair. Circulation 99:2757, 1999.

64. Herskowitz A, Vlahov D, Willoughby S, et al: Prevalence and incidence of left ventricular dysfunction in patients with human immunodeficiency virus infection. Am J Cardiol 71:955, 1993.

65. Tomita T, Murakami T, Iwase T, et al: Chronic dynamic exercise improves a functional abnormality of the G stimulatory protein in cardiomyopathic BIO 53.58 Syrian hamsters. Circulation 89:836, 1994.

66. Merlet P, Delforge J, Syrota A, et al: Positron emission tomography with 11C CGP-12177 to assess beta-adrenergic receptor concentration in idiopathic dilated cardiomyopathy. Circulation 87:1169, 1993.

67. Bristow MR, Feldman AM: Changes in the receptor-G protein-adenylyl cyclase system in heart failure from various types of heart muscle disease. Basic Res Cardiol 87:15, 1992.

68. Hasenfuss G, Reinecke H, Studer R, et al: Relation between myocardial function and expression of sarcoplasmic reticulum Ca(2+)-ATPase in failing and nonfailing human myocardium. Circ Res 75:434, 1994.

69. Jeck CD, Zimmermann R, Schaper J, et al: Decreased expression of calmodulin mRNA in human end-stage heart failure. J Mol Cell Cardiol 26:99, 1994.

70. Go LO, Moschella MC, Watras J, et al: Differential regulation of two types of intracellular calcium release channels during end-stage heart failure. J Clin Invest 95:888, 1995.

71. Figulla HR, Gietzen F, Zeymer U, et al: Diltiazem improves cardiac function and exercise capacity in patients with idiopathic dilated cardiomyopathy: Results of the Diltiazem in Dilated Cardiomyopathy Trial. Circulation 94:346, 1996.

72. Lanfranchi PA, Braghiroli A, Bosimini E, et al: Prognostic value of nocturnal Cheyne-Stokes respiration in chronic heart failure. Circulation 99:1435, 1999.

73. Singh SN, Fisher SG, Carson PE, et al: Prevalence and significance of nonsustained ventricular tachycardia in patients with premature ventricular contractions and heart failure treated with vasodilator therapy. J Am Coll Cardiol 32:942, 1998.

74. Corey WA, Markel ML, Hoit BD, et al: Regression of a dilated cardiomyopathy after radiofrequency ablation of incessant supraventricular tachycardia. Am Heart J 126:1469, 1993.

75. Katritsis D, Leatham E, Pumphrey C, et al: Low-energy DC catheter ablation of left atrial ectopic tachycardia that had resulted in reversible cardiomyopathy. Pacing Clin Electrophysiol 16:1345, 1993.

76. Luchsinger JA, Steinberg JS: Resolution of cardiomyopathy after ablation of atrial flutter. J Am Coll Cardiol 32:205, 1998.

77. Lazzari JO, Gonzalez J: Reversible high rate atrial fibrillation dilated cardiomyopathy. Heart 77:486, 1997.

78. Pinamonti B, Di Lenarda A, Sinagra G, et al: Restrictive left ventricular filling pattern in dilated cardiomyopathy assessed by Doppler echocardiography: Clinical, echocardiographic and hemodynamic correlations and prognostic implications. J Am Coll Cardiol 22:808, 1993.

79. Vigna C, Russo A, De Rito V, et al: Regional wall motion analysis by dobutamine stess echocardiography to distinguish between ischemic and nonischemic dilated cardiomyopathy. Am Heart J 131:537, 1996.

80. Tauberg SG, Orie JE, Bartlett BE, et al: Usefulness of thallium-201 for distinction of ischemic from idiopathic dilated cardiomyopathy. Am J Cardiol 71:674, 1993.

81. Glamann DB, Lange RA, Corbett JR, et al: Utility of various radionuclide techniques for distinguishing ischemic from nonischemic dilated cardiomyopathy. Arch Intern Med 152:769, 1992.

82. Obrador D, Ballester M, Carrio I, et al: Presence, evolving changes, and prognostic implications of myocardial damage detected in idiopathic and alcoholic dilated cardiomyopathy by 111In monoclonal antimyosin antibodies. Circulation 89:2054, 1994.

83. Inoue T, Sakai Y, Morooka S, et al: Vasodilatory capacity of coronary resistance vessels in dilated cardiomyopathy. Am Heart J 127:376, 1994.

84. Mathier MA, Rose GA, Fifer MA, et al: Coronary endothelial dysfunction in patients with acute-onset idiopathic dilated cardiomyopathy. J Am Coll Cardiol 32:216, 1998.

85. Shannon RP, Komamura K, Shen YT, et al: Impaired regional subendocardial coronary flow reserve in conscious dogs with pacing-induced heart failure. Am J Physiol 265:H801, 1993.

86. Budoff MJ, Shavelle DM, Lamont DH, et al: Usefulness of electron beam computed tomography scanning for distinguishing ischemic from nonischemic cardiomyopathy. J Am Coll Cardiol 32:1173, 1998.

87. Eichhorn EJ, Bristow MR: Medical therapy can improve the biological properties of the chronically failing heart: A new era in the treatment of heart failure. Circulation 94:2285, 1996.

88. Hambrecht R, Fiehn E, Weigl C, et al: Regular physical exercise corrects endothelial dysfunction and improves exercise capacity in patients with chronic heart failure. Circulation 98:2709, 1998.

89. O'Connell JB, Breen TJ, Hosenpud JD: Heart transplantation in dilated heart muscle disease and myocarditis. Eur Heart J 16:137, 1995.

90. Frishman WH: Carvedilol. N Engl J Med 339:1759, 1998.

91. Pitt B, Zannad F, Remme WJ, et al: The effect of spironolactone on morbidity and mortality in patients with severe heart failure. N Engl J Med 341:709, 1999.

92. Cohn JN: Improving outcomes in heart failure. Eur Heart J 19:1124, 1998.

93. Andersson B, Hamm C, Persson S, et al: Improved exercise hemodynamic status in dilated cardiomyopathy after beta-adrenergic blockade treatment. J Am Coll Cardiol 23:1397, 1994.

94. Waagstein F: Efficacy of beta blockers in idiopathic dilated cardiomyopathy and ischemic cardiomyopathy. Am J Cardiol 80:45J, 1997.

95. Eichhorn EJ, Heesch CM, Barnett JH, et al: Effect of metoprolol on myocardial function and energetics in patients with nonischemic dilated cardiomyopathy: A randomized, double-blind, placebo-controlled study. J Am Coll Cardiol 24:1310, 1994.

96. Avezum A, Tsuyuki RT, Pogue J, et al: Beta-blocker therapy for congestive heart failure: A systemic overview and critical appraisal of the published trials. Can J Cardiol 14:1045, 1998.

97. Lechat P, Packer M, Chalon S, et al: Clinical effects of beta-adrenergic blockade in chronic heart failure: A meta-analysis of double-blind, placebo-controlled, randomized trials. Circulation 98:1184, 1998.

97a. Effects of metoprolol CR in patients with ischemic and dilated cardiomyopathy: The randomized evaluation of strategies for left ventricular dysfunction pilot study. Circulation 101:378, 2000.

98. Asseman P, McFadden E, Bauchart JJ, et al: Why do beta-blockers help in idiopathic dilated cardiomyopathy—frequency mismatch? Lancet 344:803, 1994.

99. Sato H, Hori M, Ozaki H, et al: Exercise-induced upward shift of diastolic left ventricular pressure-volume relation in patients with dilated cardiomyopathy: Effects of beta-adrenoceptor blockade. Circulation 88: 2215, 1993.

100. Kim MH, Devlin WH, Das SK, et al: Effects of beta-adrenergic blocking therapy on left ventricular diastolic relaxation properties in patients with dilated cardiomyopathy. Circulation 100:729, 1999.

101. Fazio S, Sabatini D, Capaldo B, et al: A preliminary study of growth hormone in the treatment of dilated cardiomyopathy. N Engl J Med 334:809, 1996.

102. Carson PE: β-Blocker therapy in heart failure: Pathophysiology and clinical results. Curr Probl Cardiol 24:423, 1999.

103. Di Lenarda A, Sabbadini G, Salvatore L, et al: Long-term effects of carvedilol in idiopathic dilated cardiomyopathy with persistent left ventricular dysfunction despite chronic metoprolol. J Am Coll Cardiol 33:1926, 1999.

104. Knight BP, Goyal R, Pelosi F, et al: Outcome of patients with nonischemic dilated cardiomyopathy and unexplained syncope treated with an implantable defibrillator. J Am Coll Cardiol 33:1964, 1999.

105. Cohn JN, Ziesche S, Smith R, et al: Effect of the calcium antagonist felodipine as supplementary vasodilator therapy in patients with chronic heart failure treated with enalapril: V-HEFT III. Circulation 96: 856, 1997.

106. Konstam MA, Remme WJ: Treatment guidelines in heart failure. Prog Cardiovasc Dis 48:65, 1998.

107. Singh SN, Fletcher RD, Fisher SG, et al: Amiodarone in patients with congestive heart failure and asymptomatic ventricular arrhythmia. N Engl J Med 333:77, 1995.

108. Grim W, Hoffmann J, Menz V, et al: Programmed ventricular stimulation for arrhythmia risk prediction in patients with idiopathic dilated cardiomyopathy and nonsustained ventricular tachycardia. J Am Coll Cardiol 32:739, 1998.

109. Gregoratos G, Cheitlin MD, Conill A, et al: ACC/AHA guidelines for implantation of cardiac pacemakers and antiarrhythmia devices: Executive summary—a report of the American College of Cardiology/American Heart Association Task Force on Practice Guidelines (Committee on Pacemaker Implantation). Circulation 97:1325, 1998.

110. Brembilla-Perrot B, Terrier de la Chaise A, Jacquemin L, et al: The signal-averaged electrocardiogram is of limited value in patients with bundle branch block and dilated cardiomyopathy in predicting inducible ventricular tachycardia or death. Am J Cardiol 79:154, 1997.

111. Yi G, Keeling PJ, Goldman JH, et al: Prognostic significance of spectral turbulence analysis of the signal-averaged electrocardiogram in patients

with idiopathic dilated cardiomyopathy. Am J Cardiol 75:494, 1995.

112. Borggrefe M, Chen X, Martinez-Rubio A, et al: The role of implantable cardioverter defibrillators in dilated cardiomyopathy. Am Heart J 127:1145, 1994.

113. Bocker D, Bansch D, Heinecke A, et al: Potential benefit from implantable cardioverter-defibrillator therapy in patients with and without heart failure. Circulation 98:1636, 1998.

114. Ezekowitz M: Antithrombotics for left-ventricular impairment? Lancet 351:1904, 1998.

115. Koniaris LS, Goldhaber SZ: Anticoagulation in dilated cardiomyopathy. J Am Coll Cardiol 31:745, 1998.

116. Cheng JW, Spinler SA: Should all patients with dilated cardiomyopathy receive chronic anticoagulation? Ann Pharmacother 28:604, 1994.

117. Al-Khadra AS, Salem DN, Rand WM, et al: Antiplatelet agents and survival: A cohort analysis from the Studies of Left Ventricular Dysfunction (SOLVD) Trial. J Am Coll Cardiol 31:419, 1998.

118. Garg A, Shiau J, Guyatt G: The ineffectiveness of immunosuppressive therapy in lymphocytic myocarditis: An overview. Ann Intern Med 129:317, 1998.

119. Kass DA, Chen CH, Curry C, et al: Improved left ventricular mechanics from acute DDD pacing in patients with dilated cardiomyopathy and ventricular conduction delay. Circulation 99:1567, 1999.

120. Auricchio A, Stellbrink C, Block M, et al: Effect of pacing chamber and atrioventricular delay on acute systolic function of paced patients with congestive heart failure. Circulation 99:2993, 1999.

120a. Kerwin WF, Botvinick EH, O'Connell JW, et al: Ventricular contraction abnormalities in dilated cardiomyopathy: Effect of biventricular pacing to correct interventricular dyssynchrony. J Am Coll Cardiol 35:1221, 2000.

121. O'Rourke RA: Cardiac pacing: An alternative treatment for selected patients with hypertrophic cardiomyopathy and adjunctive therapy for certain patients with dilated cardiomyopathy. Circulation 100:786, 1999.

122. Bolling SF, Pagani FD, Deeb GM, et al: Intermediate-term outcome of mitral reconstruction in cardiomyopathy. J Thorac Cardiovasc Surg 115:381, 1998.

123. Patel HJ, Polidori DJ, Pilla JJ, et al: Stabilization of chronic remodeling by asynchronous cardiomyoplasty in dilated cardiomyopathy: Effects of a conditioned muscle wrap. Circulation 96:3665, 1997.

124. Popovic Z, Miric M, Gradinac S, et al: Effects of partial left ventriculectomy on left ventricular performance in patients with nonischemic dilated cardiomyopathy. J Am Coll Cardiol 32:1801, 1998.

Alcoholic Cardiomyopathy

125. Fernandez-Sola J, Estruch R, Grau JM, et al: The relation of alcoholic myopathy to cardiomyopathy. Ann Intern Med 120:529, 1994.

126. Preedy VR, Atkinson LM, Richardson PJ, et al: Mechanisms of ethanol-induced cardiac damage. Br Heart J 69:197, 1993.

127. Fernandez-Sola J, Estruch R, Nicolas JM, et al: Comparison of alcoholic cardiomyopathy in women versus men. Am J Cardiol 80:481, 1997.

128. Ballester M, Marti V, Carrio I, et al: Spectrum of alcohol-induced myocardial damage detected by indium-111–labeled monoclonal antimyosin antibodies. J Am Coll Cardiol 29:160, 1997.

129. Jarvis JQ, Hammond E, Meier R, et al: Cobalt cardiomyopathy: A report of two cases from mineral assay laboratories and a review of the literature. J Occup Med 34:620, 1992.

130. Djoenaidi W, Notermans SL, Dunda G: Beriberi cardiomyopathy. Eur J Clin Nutr 46:227, 1992.

131. Teragaki M, Takeuchi K, Takeda T: Clinical and histologic features of alcohol drinkers with congestive heart failure. Am Heart J 125:808, 1993.

132. McKenna CJ, Codd MB, McCann HA, et al: Alcohol consumption and idiopathic dilated cardiomyopathy: A case-control study. Am Heart J 135:833, 1998.

132a. Lazarevic AM, Nakatani S, Neskovic AN, et al: Early changes in left ventricular function in chronic asymptomatic alcoholics: Relation to the duration of heavy drinking. J Am Coll Cardiol 35:1599, 2000.

133. Guillo P, Mansourati J, Maheu B, et al: Long-term prognosis in patients with alcoholic cardiomyopathy and severe heart failure after total abstinence. Am J Cardiol 79:1276, 1997.

134. Seghizzi P, D'Adda F, Borleri D, et al: Cobalt myocardiopathy: A critical review of literature. Sci Total Environ 150:105, 1994.

Arrhythmogenic Right Ventricular Cardiomyopathy

135. Burke AP, Farb A, Tashko G, et al: Arrhythmogenic right ventricular cardiomyopathy and fatty replacement of the right ventricular myocardium: Are they different diseases? Circulation 97:1571, 1998.

136. Mallat Z, Tedgui A, Fontaliran F, et al: Evidence of apoptosis in arrhythmogenic right ventricular dysplasia. N Engl J Med 335:1190, 1996.

137. McKenna WJ, Thiene G, Nava A, et al: Diagnosis of arrhythmogenic right ventricular dysplasia/cardiomyopathy. Task Force of the Working Group Myocardial and Pericardial Disease of the European Society of Cardiology and of the Scientific Council on Cardiomyopathies of the International Society and Federation of Cardiology. Br Heart J 71:215, 1994.

138. Fontaine G, Fontaliran F, Frank R: Arrhythmogenic right ventricular cardiomyopathies: Clinical forms and main differential diagnoses. Circulation 97:1532, 1998.

139. Rampazzo A, Nava A, Miorin M, et al: ARVD4, a new locus for arrhythmogenic right ventricular cardiomyopathy, maps to chromosome 2 long arm. Genomics 45:259, 1997.

140. Marcus FI, Fontaine G: Arrhythmogenic right ventricular dysplasia/cardiomyopathy: A review. Pacing Clin Electrophysiol 18:1298, 1995.

141. Corrado D, Basso C, Thiene G, et al: Spectrum of clinicopathologic manifestations of arrhythmogenic right ventricular cardiomyopathy/dysplasia: A multicenter study. J Am Coll Cardiol 30:1512, 1997.

142. Corrado D, Basso C, Schiavon M, et al: Screening for hypertrophic cardiomyopathy in young athletes. N Engl J Med 339:364, 1998.

143. Nava A, Thiene G, Canciani B, et al: Clinical profile of concealed form of arrhythmogenic right ventricular cardiomyopathy presenting with apparently idiopathic ventricular arrhythmias. Int J Cardiol 35:195, 1992.

144. Pinamonti B, Pagnan L, Bussani R, et al: Right ventricular dysplasia with biventricular involvement. Circulation 98:1943, 1998.

145. Menghetti L, Basso C, Nava A, et al: Spin-echo nuclear magnetic resonance for tissue characterisation in arrhythmogenic right ventricular cardiomyopathy. Heart 76:467, 1996.

146. Schafers M, Lerch H, Wichter T, et al: Cardiac sympathetic innervation in patients with idiopathic right ventricular outflow tract tachycardia. J Am Coll Cardiol 32:181, 1998.

147. Misaki T, Watanabe G, Iwa T, et al: Surgical treatment of arrhythmogenic right ventricular dysplasia: Long-term outcome. Ann Thorac Surg 58:1380, 1994.

148. Ellison KE, Friedman PL, Ganz LI, et al: Entrainment mapping and radiofrequency catheter ablation of ventricular tachycardia in right ventricular dysplasia. J. Am Coll Cardiol 32:724, 1998.

HYPERTROPHIC CARDIOMYOPATHY

149. Morrow AG, Braunwald E: Functional aortic stenosis: A malformation characterized by resistance to left ventricular overflow without anatomic obstruction. Circulation 20:181, 1959.

150. Braunwald E, Morrow AG, Cornell WP, et al: Idiopathic hypertrophic subaortic stenosis: Clinical, hemodynamic and angiographic manifestations. Am J. Med 29:924, 1960.

151. Braunwald E, Lambrew CT, Rockoff SD, et al: Idiopathic hypertrophic subaortic stenosis: I. A description of the disease based upon an analysis of 64 patients. Circulation 30 (Suppl 4):3–119, 1964.

152. Spirito P, Seidman CE, McKenna WJ, et al: The management of hypertrophic cardiomyopathy. N Engl J Med 336:775, 1997.

153. Maron BJ: Hypertrophic cardiomyopathy. Lancet 350:127, 1997.

154. Wigle ED, Rakowski H, Kimball BP, et al: Hypertrophic cardiomyopathy: Clinical spectrum and treatment. Circulation 92:1680, 1995.

155. Louie EK, Edwards LC III: Hypertrophic cardiomyopathy. Prog Cardiovasc Dis 36:275, 1994.

156. Criley JM: Unobstructed thinking (and terminology) is called for in the understanding and management of hypertrophic cardiomyopathy. J Am Coll Cardiol 29:741, 1997.

157. Maron BJ: Hypertrophic cardiomyopathy. Curr Probl Cardiol 18:639, 1993.

158. Maron BJ, Moller JH, Seidman CE, et al: Impact of laboratory molecular diagnosis on contemporary diagnostic criteria for genetically transmitted cardiovascular diseases: Hypertrophic cardiomyopathy, long-QT syndrome, and Marfan-syndrome: A statement for healthcare professionals from the Councils on Clinical Cardiology, Cardiovascular Disease in the Young, and Basic Science, American Heart Association. Circulation 98:1460, 1998.

159. Maron BJ, Pelliccia A, Spirito P: Cardiac disease in young trained athletes: Insights into methods for distinguishing athlete's heart from structural heart disease, with particular emphasis on hypertrophic cardiomyopathy. Circulation 91:1596, 1995.

160. Manolas J, Kyriakidis M, Anastasakis A, et al: Usefulness of noninvasive detection of left ventricular diastolic abnormalities during isometric stress in hypertrophic cardiomyopathy and in athletes. Am J Cardiol 81:306, 1998.

161. Niimura H. Bachinski LL, Sangwatanaroj S, et al: Mutations in the gene for cardiac myosin-binding protein C and late-onset familial hypertrophic cardiomyopathy. N Engl J Med 338:1248, 1998.

162. Yang Q, Sanbe A, Osinska H, et al: A mouse model of myosin binding protein C human familial hypertrophic cardiomyopathy. J Clin Invest 102:1292, 1998.

163. Reddy V, Korcarz C, Weinert L, et al: Apical hypertrophic cardiomyopathy. Circulation 98:2354, 1998.

164. Suzuki J, Watanabe F, Takenaka K, et al: New subtype of apical hypertrophic cardiomyopathy identified with nuclear magnetic resonance imaging as an underlying cause of markedly inverted T waves. J Am Coll Cardiol 22:1175, 1993.

165. Smolders W, Rademakers F, Conraads V, et al: Apical hypertrophic cardiomyopathy. Acta Cardiol 48:369, 1993.

166. McKenna WJ, Coccolo F, Elliott PM: Genes and disease expression in hypertrophic cardiomyopathy. Lancet 352:1162, 1998.

167. Lewis JF, Maron BJ: Clinical and morphologic expression of hypertrophic cardiomyopathy in patients > or = 65 years of age. Am J Cardiol 73:1105, 1994.

168. Wilmshurst PT, Katritsis D: Restrictive and hypertrophic cardiomyopathies in Noonan syndrome: The overlap syndromes. Heart 75:94, 1996.

169. Carvalho JS, Matthews EE, Leonard JV, et al: Cardiomyopathy of glycogen storage disease type III. Heart Vessels 8:155, 1993.

170. Maron BJ, Wolfson JK, Roberts WC: Relation between extent of cardiac muscle cell disorganization and left ventricular wall thickness in hypertrophic cardiomyopathy. Am J Cardiol 70:785, 1992.

171. Clark AL, Coats AJ: Screening for hypertrophic cardiomyopathy. BMJ 306:409, 1993.

172. Mogensen J, Klausen IC, Pedersen AK, et al: Alpha-cardiac actin is a novel disease gene in familial hypertrophic cardiomyopathy. J Clin Invest 103:39R, 1999.

173. Watkins H, Thierfelder L, Hwang DS, et al: Sporadic hypertrophic cardiomyopathy due to de novo myosin mutations. J Clin Invest 90:1666, 1992.

174. Keating M: The devil's in the details: Progress in familial hypertrophic cardiomyopathy. J Clin Invest 93:2, 1994.

175. Jarcho JA, McKenna W, Pare JA, et al: Mapping a gene for familial hypertrophic cardiomyopathy to chromosome 14ql. N Engl J Med 321:1372, 1989.

176. Fananapazir L: Advances in molecular genetics and management of hypertrophic cardiomyopathy. JAMA 281:1746, 1999.

176a. Moolman JA, Reith S, Uhl K, et al: A newly created splice donor site in exon 25 of the MyBP-C gene is responsible for inherited hypertrophic cardiomyopathy with incomplete disease penetrance. Circulation 101:1396, 2000.

177. MacRae CA, Ghaisas N, Kass S, et al: Familial hypertrophic cardiomyopathy with Wolff-Parkinson-White syndrome maps to a locus on chromosome 7q3. J Clin Invest 96:1216, 1995.

178. Watkins H, McKenna WJ, Thierfelder L, et al: Mutations in the genes for cardiac troponin T and alpha-tropomyosin in hypertrophic cardiomyopathy. N Engl J Med 332:1058, 1995.

179. Okamoto S, Ozaki M, Konishi T, et al: A case report of siblings with hypertrophic cardiomyopathy that progressed to dilated cardiomyopathy—case reports. Angiology 44:406, 1993.

180. Solomon SD, Wolff S, Watkins H, et al: Left ventricular hypertrophy and morphology in familial hypertrophic cardiomyopathy associated with mutations of the beta-myosin heavy chain gene. J Am Coll Cardiol 22:498, 1993.

181. Hecht GM, Klues HG, Roberts WC, et al: Coexistence of sudden cardiac death and end-stage heart failure in familial hypertrophic cardiomyopathy. J Am Coll Cardiol 22:489, 1993.

182. Anan R, Shano H, Kisanuki A, et al: Patients with familial hypertrophic cardiomyopathy caused by a PheIIOIle missense mutation in the cardiac troponin T gene have variable cardiac morphologies and a favorable prognosis. Circulation 98:391, 1998.

183. Tardiff JC, Factor SM, Tompkins BD, et al: A truncated cardiac troponin T molecule in transgenic mice suggests multiple cellular mechanisms for familial hypertrophic cardiomyopathy. J Clin Invest 101:2800, 1998.

184. Anan R, Greve G, Thierfelder L, et al: Prognostic implications of novel beta cardiac myosin heavy chain gene mutations that cause familial hypertrophic cardiomyopathy. J Clin Invest 93:280, 1994.

185. Sherrid MV, Chu CK, Delia E, et al: An echocardiographic study of the fluid mechanics of obstruction in hypertrophic cardiomyopathy. J Am Coll Cardiol 22:816, 1993.

186. Betocchi S, Hess OM, Losi MA, et al: Regional left ventricular mechanics in hypertrophic cardiomyopathy. Circulation 88:2206, 1993.

187. Losi MA, Betocchi S, Grimaldi M, et al: Heterogeneity of left ventricular filling dynamics in hypertrophic cardiomyopathy. Am J Cardiol 73:987, 1994.

188. Gwathmey JK, Warren SE, Briggs GM, et al: Diastolic dysfunction in hypertrophic cardiomyopathy: Effect on active force generation during systole. J Clin Invest 87:1023, 1991.

189. Factor SM, Butany J, Sole MJ, et al: Pathologic fibrosis and matrix connective tissue in the subaortic myocardium of patients with hypertrophic cardiomyopathy. J Am Coll Cardiol 17:1343, 1991.

190. Lazzeroni E, Picano E, Morozzi L, et al: Dipyridamole-induced ischemia as a prognostic marker of future adverse cardiac events in adult patients with hypertrophic cardiomyopathy. Circulation 96:4268, 1997.

191. Perrone-Filardi P, Bacharach SL, Dilsizian V, et al: Regional systolic function, myocardial blood flow and glucose uptake at rest in hypertrophic cardiomyopathy. Am J Cardiol 72:199, 1993.

192. Takemura G, Takatsu Y, Fujiwara H: Luminal narrowing of coronary capillaries in human hypertrophic hearts: An ultrastructural morphometrical study using endomyocardial biopsy specimens. Heart 79:78, 1998.

193. Kyriakidis MK, Dernellis JM, Androulakis AE, et al: Changes in phasic coronary blood flow velocity profile and relative coronary flow reserve in patients with hypertrophic obstructive cardiomyopathy. Circulation 96:834, 1997.

194. Kyriakidis M, Triposkiadis F, Dernellis J, et al: Effects of cardiac versus circulatory angiotensin-converting enzyme inhibition on left ventricular diastolic function and coronary blood flow in hypertrophic obstructive cardiomyopathy. Circulation 97:1342, 1998.

195. Yetman AT, McCrindle BW, MacDonald C, et al: Myocardial bridging in children with hypertrophic cardiomyopathy—a risk factor for sudden death. N Engl J Med 339:1201, 1998.

Clinical Manifestations

196. Frank S, Braunwald E: Idiopathic hypertrophic subaortic stenosis: Clinical analysis of 126 patients with emphasis on the natural history. Circulation 37:759, 1968.

197. Chikamori T, Counihan PJ, Doi YL, et al: Mechanisms of exercise limitation in hypertrophic cardiomyopathy. J Am Coll Cardiol 19:507, 1992.

198. Nienaber CA, Hiller S, Spielmann RP, et al: Syncope in hypertrophic cardiomyopathy: Multivariate analysis of prognostic determinants. J Am Coll Cardiol 15:948, 1990.

199. Kar AK, Roy S, Panja M: Aortic regurgitation in hypertrophic cardiomyopathy. J Assoc Physicians India 41:576, 1993.

200. Etchells E, Bell C, Robb K: Does this patient have an abnormal systolic murmur? JAMA 277:564, 1997.

201. Ryan MP, Cleland JG, French JA, et al: The standard electrocardiogram as a screening test for hypertrophic cardiomyopathy. Am J Cardiol 76:689, 1995.

202. Maron BJ, Mathenge R, Casey SA, et al: Clinical profile of hypertrophic cardiomyopathy identified de novo in rural communities. J Am Coll Cardiol 33:1590, 1999.

203. Usui M, Inoue H, Suzuki J, et al: Relationship between distribution of hypertrophy and electrocardiographic changes in hypertrophic cardiomyopathy. Am Heart J 126:177, 1993.

204. Shibata M, Yamakado T, Imanaka-Yoshida K, et al: Familial hypertrophic cardiomyopathy with Wolff-Parkinson-White syndrome progressing to ventricular dilation. Am Heart J 131:1223, 1996.

205. Tamura M, Harada K, Ito T, et al: Abrupt aggravation of atrioventricular block and syncope in hypertrophic cardiomyopathy. Arch Dis Child 73:536, 1995.

206. Maki S, Ikeda H, Muro A, et al: Predictors of sudden cardiac death in hypertrophic cardiomyopathy. Am J Cardiol 82:774, 1998.

207. Stewart JT, McKenna WJ: Management of arrhythmias in hypertrophic cardiomyopathy. Cardiovasc Drugs Ther 8:95, 1994.

208. Fananapazir L, Chang AC, Epstein SE, et al: Prognostic determinants in hypertrophic cardiomyopathy: Prospective evaluation of a therapeutic strategy based on clinical, Holter, hemodynamic, and electrophysiological findings. Circulation 86:730, 1992.

209. Spirito P, Lakatos E, Maron BJ: Degree of left ventricular hypertrophy in patients with hypertrophic cardiomyopathy and chronic atrial fibrillation. Am J Cardiol 69:1217, 1992.

210. Robinson K, Frenneaux MP, Stockins B, et al: Atrial fibrillation in hypertrophic cardiomyopathy: A longitudinal study. J Am Coll Cardiol 15:1279, 1990.

211. Kulakowski P, Counihan PJ, Camm AJ, et al: The value of time and frequency domain, and spectral temporal mapping analysis of the signal-averaged electrocardiogram in identification of patients with hypertrophic cardiomyopathy at increased risk of sudden death. Eur Heart J 14:941, 1993.

212. Counihan PJ, Fei L, Bashir Y, et al: Assessment of heart rate variability in hypertrophic cardiomyopathy: Association with clinical and prognostic features. Circulation 88:1682, 1993.

213. Sneddon JF, Slade A, Seo H, et al: Assessment of the diagnostic value of head-up tilt testing in the evaluation of syncope in hypertrophic cardiomyopathy. Am J Cardiol 73:601, 1994.

214. Klues HG, Roberts WC, Maron BJ: Morphological determinants of echocardiographic patterns of mitral valve systolic anterior motion in obstructive hypertrophic cardiomyopathy. Circulation 87:1570, 1993.

215. Naito J, Masuyama T, Tanouchi J, et al: Analysis of transmural trend of myocardial integrated ultrasound backscatter for differentiation of hypertrophic cardiomyopathy and ventricular hypertrophy due to hypertension. J Am Coll Cardiol 24:517, 1994.

216. Vitale DF, Bonow RO, Calabro R, et al: Myocardial ultrasonic tissue characterization in pediatric and adult patients with hypertrophic cardiomyopathy. Circulation 94:2826, 1996.

217. Klues HG, Proschan MA, Dollar AL, et al: Echocardiographic assessment of mitral valve size in obstructive hypertrophic cardiomyopathy: Anatomic validation from mitral valve specimen. Circulation 88:548, 1993.

218. Grigg LE, Wigle ED, Williams WG, et al: Transesophageal Doppler echocardiography in obstructive hypertrophic cardiomyopathy: Clarification of pathophysiology and importance in intraoperative decision making. J Am Coll Cardiol 20:42, 1992.

219. Schwammenthal E, Nakatani S, He S, et al: Mechanism of mitral regurgitation in hypertrophic cardiomyopathy: Mismatch of posterior to anterior leaflet length and mobility. Circulation 98:856, 1998.

220. Levine RA, Vlahakes GJ, Lefebvre X, et al: Papillary muscle displacement causes systolic anterior motion of the mitral valve: Experimental validation and insights into the mechanism of subaortic obstruction. Circulation 91:1189, 1995.

221. Lin CS, Chen KS, Lin MC, et al: The relationship between systolic anterior motion of the mitral valve and the left ventricular outflow tract Doppler in hypertrophic cardiomyopathy. Am Heart J 122:1671, 1991.

222. Kramer CM, Reichek N, Ferrari VA, et al: Regional heterogeneity of function in hypertrophic cardiomyopathy. Circulation 90:186, 1994.

223. Dong SJ, MacGregor JH, Crawley AP, et al: Left ventricular wall thickness and regional systolic function in patients with hypertrophic cardiomyopathy: A three-dimensional tagged magnetic resonance imaging study. Circulation 90:1200, 1994.

224. Marwick TH, Nakatani S, Haluska B, et al: Provocation of latent left

ventricular outflow tract gradients with amyl nitrite and exercise in hypertrophic cardiomyopathy. Am J Cardiol 75:805, 1995.

225. Cannon RO III, Dilsizian V, O'Gara PT, et al: Myocardial metabolic, hemodynamic, and electrocardiographic significance of reversible thallium-201 abnormalities in hypertrophic cardiomyopathy. Circulation 83:1660, 1991.

226. Dilsizian V, Bonow RO, Epstein SE, et al: Myocardial ischemia detected by thallium scintigraphy is frequently related to cardiac arrest and syncope in young patients with hypertrophic cardiomyopathy. J Am Coll Cardiol 22:796, 1993.

227. Chikamori T, Dickie S, Poloniecki JD, et al: Prognostic significance of radionuclide-assessed diastolic function in hypertrophic cardiomyopathy. Am J Cardiol 65:478, 1990.

Hemodynamics

228. Fananapazir L, McAreavey D: Therapeutic options in patients with obstructive hypertrophic cardiomyopathy and severe drug-refractory symptoms. J Am Coll Cardiol 31:259, 1998.

229. Maron BJ, McIntosh CL, Klues HG, et al: Morphologic basis for obstruction to right ventricular outflow in hypertrophic cardiomyopathy. Am J Cardiol 71:1089, 1993.

230. Kizilbash AM, Heinle SK, Grayburn PA: Spontaneous variability of left ventricular outflow tract gradient in hypertrophic obstructive cardiomyopathy. Circulation 97:461, 1998.

231. Brockenbrough EC, Braunwald E, Morrow AG: A hemodynamic technic for the detection of hypertrophic subaortic stenosis. Circulation 23:189, 1961.

232. Paz R, Jortner R, Tunick PA, et al: The effect of the ingestion of ethanol on obstruction of the left ventricular outflow tract in hypertrophic cardiomyopathy. N Engl J Med 335:938, 1996.

233. Akasaka T, Yoshikawa J, Yoshida K, et al: Phasic coronary flow characteristics in patients with hypertrophic cardiomyopathy: A study by coronary Doppler catheter. J Am Soc Echocardiogr 7:9, 1994.

234. Vassalli G, Seiler C, Hess OM: Risk stratification in hypertrophic cardiomyopathy. Curr Opin Cardiol 9:330, 1994.

235. Maron BJ, Spirito P: Impact of patient selection biases on the perception of hypertrophic cardiomyopathy and its natural history. Am J Cardiol 72:970, 1993.

236. Cannan CR, Reeder GS, Bailey KR, et al: Natural history of hypertrophic cardiomyopathy: A population-based study, 1976 through 1990. Circulation 92:2488, 1995.

237. Cecchi F, Olivotto I, Montereggi A, et al: Hypertrophic cardiomyopathy in Tuscany: Clinical course and outcome in an unselected regional population. J Am Coll Cardiol 26:1529, 1995.

238. Seiler C, Jenni R, Vassalli G, et al: Left ventricular chamber dilatation in hypertrophic cardiomyopathy: Related variables and prognosis in patients with medical and surgical therapy. Br Heart J 74:508, 1995.

239. Maron BJ, Spirito P: Implications of left ventricular remodeling in hypertrophic cardiomyopathy. Am J Cardiol 81:1339, 1998.

240. Watkins H: Sudden death in hypertrophic cardiomyopathy. N Engl J Med 342:422, 2000.

240a. Doevendans PA: Hypertrophic cardiomyopathy: Do we have the algorithm for life and death? Circulation 101:1224, 2000.

241. Yoshida N, Ikeda H, Wada T, et al: Exercise-induced abnormal blood pressure responses are related to subendocardial ischemia in hypertrophic cardiomyopathy. J Am Coll Cardiol 32:1938, 1998.

242. Borggrefe M, Breithardt G: Is the implantable defibrillator indicated in patients with hypertrophic cardiomyopathy and aborted sudden death? J Am Coll Cardiol 31:1086, 1998.

242a. Atiga WL, Fananapazir L, McAreavey D, et al: Temporal repolarization lability in hypertrophic cardiomyopathy caused by beta-myosin heavy-chain gene mutations. Circulation 101:1237, 2000.

243. Almendral JM, Ormaetxe J, Martinez-Alday, JD, et al: Treatment of ventricular arrhythmias in patients with hypertrophic cardiomyopathy. Eur Heart J 14::71, 1993.

244. Olivotto I, Maron BJ, Montereggi A, et al: Prognostic value of systemic blood pressure response during exercise in a community-based patient population with hypertrophic cardiomyopathy. J Am Coll Cardiol 33:2044, 1999.

245. Botvinick EH, Dae MW, Krishnan R, et al: Hypertrophic cardiomyopathy in the young: Another form of ischemic cardiomyopathy? J Am Coll Cardiol 22:805, 1993.

246. Nienaber CA, Gambhir SS, Mody FV, et al: Regional myocardial blood flow and glucose utilization in symptomatic patients with hypertrophic cardiomyopathy. Circulation 87:1580, 1993.

247. Counihan PJ, Frenneaux MP, Webb DJ, et al: Abnormal vascular responses to supine exercise in hypertrophic cardiomyopathy. Circulation 84:686, 1991.

248. Maron BJ, Kogan J, Proschan MA, et al: Circadian variability in the occurrence of sudden cardiac death in patients with hypertrophic cardiomyopathy. J Am Coll Cardiol 23:1405, 1994.

249. Maron BJ, Thompson PD, Puffer JC, et al: Cardiovascular preparticipation screening of competitive athletes: A statement for health professionals from the Sudden Death Committee (Clinical Cardiology) and Congenital Cardiac Defects Committee (Cardiovascular Disease in the Young), American Heart Association. Circulation 94:850, 1996.

250. Maron BJ, Klues HG: Surviving competitive athletics with hypertrophic cardiomyopathy. Am J Cardiol 73:1098, 1994.

251. Maron BJ, Shen WK, Link MS, et al: Efficacy of implantable cardioverterdefibrillators for the prevention of sudden death in patients with hypertrophic cardiomyopathy. N Engl J Med 342:365, 2000.

252. Takagi E, Yamakado T, Nakano T: Prognosis of completely asymptomatic adult patients with hypertrophic cardiomyopathy. J Am Coll Cardiol 33:206, 1999.

253. Gilligan DM, Chan WL, Stewart R, et al: Cardiac responses assessed by echocardiography to changes in preload in hypertrophic cardiomyopathy. Am J Cardiol 73:312, 1994.

Management

254. Gilligan DM, Chan WL, Joshi J, et al: A double-blind, placebo-controlled crossover trial of nadolol and verapamil in mild and moderately symptomatic hypertrophic cardiomyopathy. J Am Coll Cardiol 21:1672, 1993.

255. Wikman-Coffelt J, Stefenelli T, Wu ST, et al: [Ca2+]i transients in the cardiomyopathic hamster heart. Circ Res 68:45, 1991.

256. Gistri R, Cecchi F, Choudhury L, et al: Effect of verapamil on absolute myocardial blood flow in hypertrophic cardiomyopathy. Am J Cardiol 74:363, 1994.

257. Betocchi S, Piscione F, Losi M, et al: Effects of diltiazem on left ventricular systolic and diastolic function in hypertrophic cardiomyopathy. Am J Cardiol 78:451, 1996.

258. Dimitrow PP, Dubiel JS: Effects on left ventricular function of pindolol added to verapamil in hypertrophic cardiomyopathy. Am J Cardiol 71:313, 1993.

259. Fifer MA, O'Gara PT, McGovern BA, et al: Effects of disopyramide on left ventricular diastolic function in hypertrophic cardiomyopathy. Am J Cardiol 74:405, 1994.

260. Matsubara H, Nakatani S, Nagata S, et al: Salutary effect of disopyramide on left ventricular diastolic function in hypertrophic obstructive cardiomyopathy. J Am Coll Cardiol 26:768, 1995.

261. Cecchi F, Olivotto I, Montereggi A, et al: Prognostic value of nonsustained ventricular tachycardia and the potential role of amiodarone treatment in hypertrophic cardiomyopathy: Assessment in an unselected non-referral based patient population. Heart 79:331, 1998.

262. Tendera M, Wycisk A, Schneeweiss A, et al: Effect of sotalol on arrhythmias and exercise tolerance in patients with hypertrophic cardiomyopathy. Cardiology 82:335, 1993.

263. Maron BJ, Cecchi F, McKenna WJ: Risk factors and stratification for sudden cardiac death in patients with hypertrophic cardiomyopathy. Br Heart J 72:S13, 1994.

264. Spirito P, Rapezzi C, Bellone P, et al: Infective endocarditis in hypertrophic cardiomyopathy: Prevalence, incidence, and indications for antibiotic prophylaxis. Circulation 99:2132, 1999.

265. Fananapazir L, Cannon RO III, Tripodi D, et al: Impact of dual-chamber permanent pacing in patients with obstructive hypertrophic cardiomyopathy with symptoms refractory to verapamil and beta-adrenergic blocker therapy. Circulation 85:2149, 1992.

266. Kappenberger L: Pacing for obstructive hypertrophic cardiomyopathy. Br Heart J 73:107, 1995.

267. Maron BJ, Nishimura RA, McKenna WJ, et al: Assessment of permanent dual-chamber pacing as a treatment for drug-refractory symptomatic patients with obstructive hypertrophic cardiomyopathy: A randomized, double-blind, crossover study (M-PATHY). Circulation 99:2927, 1999.

268. Nagueh SF, Lakkis NM, Middleton KJ, et al: Changes in left ventricular diastolic function 6 months after nonsurgical septal reduction therapy for hypertrophic obstructive cardiomyopathy. Circulation 99:344, 1999.

269. Nishimura RA, Trusty JM, Hayes DL, et al: Dual-chamber pacing for hypertrophic cardiomyopathy: A randomized, double-blind, crossover trial. J Am Coll Cardiol 29:435, 1997.

270. Maron BJ: Appraisal of dual-chamber pacing therapy in hypertrophic cardiomyopathy: Too soon for a rush to judgment? J Am Coll Cardiol 27:431, 1996.

271. Linde C, Gadler F, Kappenberger L, et al: Placebo effect of pacemaker implantation in obstructive hypertrophic cardiomyopathy. Am J Cardiol 83:903, 1999.

271a. Erwin JP 3rd, Nishimura RA, Lloyd MA, et al: Dual chamber pacing for patients with hypertrophic obstructive cardiomyopathy: A clinical perspective in 2000. Mayo Clin Proc 75:173, 2000.

272. Cannon RO III, Tripodi D, Dilsizian V, et al: Results of dual-chamber pacing in symptomatic nonobstructive hypertrophic cardiomyopathy. Am J Cardiol 73:571, 1994.

273. Elliott PM, Sharma S, Varnava A, et al: Survival after cardiac arrest or sustained ventricular tachycardia in patients with hypertrophic cardiomyopathy. J Am Coll Cardiol 33:1596, 1999.

274. Primo J, Geelen P, Brugada J, et al: Hypertrophic cardiomyopathy: Role of the implantable cardioverter-defibrillator. J Am Coll Cardiol 31:1081, 1998.

275. Seggewiss H, Gleichmann U, Faber L, et al: Percutaneous transluminal septal myocardial ablation in hypertrophic obstructive cardiomyopathy: Acute results and 3-month follow-up in 25 patients. J Am Coll Cardiol 31:252, 1998.

276. Kim JJ, Lee CW, Park SW, et al: Improvement in exercise capacity and exercise blood pressure response after transcoronary alcohol ablation therapy of septal hypertrophy in hypertrophic cardiomyopathy. Am J Cardiol 83:1220, 1999.

277. Delahaye F, Jegaden O, de Gevigney G, et al: Postoperative and long-

term prognosis of myotomy-myomectomy for obstructive hypertrophic cardiomyopathy: Influence of associated mitral valve replacement. Eur Heart J 14:1229, 1993.

278. Nakatani S, Schwammenthal E, Lever HM, et al: New insights into the reduction of mitral valve systolic anterior motion after ventricular septal myectomy in hypertrophic obstructive cardiomyopathy. Am Heart J 131:294, 1996.

279. Morrow AG, Lambrew CT, Braunwald E: Idiopathic subaortic stenosis: II. Operative treatment and the results of pre- and postoperative hemodynamic evaluations. Circulation 30(Suppl 4):120, 1964.

280. Schulte HD, Bircks WH, Loesse B, et al: Prognosis of patients with hypertrophic obstructive cardiomyopathy after transaortic myectomy: Late results up to twenty-five years. J Thorac Cardiovasc Surg 106:709, 1993.

281. Brunner-La Schonbeck MH, Rocca HP, Vogt PR, et al: Long-term follow-up in hypertrophic obstructive cardiomyopathy after septal myectomy. Ann Thorac Surg 65:1207, 1998.

282. Robbins RC, Stinson EB: Long-term results of left ventricular myotomy and myectomy for obstructive hypertrophic cardiomyopathy. J Thorac Cardiovasc Surg 111:586, 1996.

283. Cannon RO III, Dilsizian V, O'Gara PT, et al: Impact of surgical relief of outflow obstruction on thallium perfusion abnormalities in hypertrophic cardiomyopathy. Circulation 85:1039, 1992.

284. Nishimura RA, Danielson GK: Dual chamber pacing for hypertrophic obstructive cardiomyopathy: Has its time come? Br Heart J 70:301, 1993.

285. McCully RB, Nishimura RA, Tajik AJ, et al: Extent of clinical improvement after surgical treatment of hypertrophic obstructive cardiomyopathy. Circulation 94:467, 1996.

286. Heric B, Lytle BW, Miller DP, et al: Surgical management of hypertrophic obstructive cardiomyopathy: Early and late results. J Thorac Cardiovasc Surg 110:195, 1995.

287. Brown PS Jr, Roberts CS, McIntosh CL, et al: Aortic regurgitation after left ventricular myotomy and myectomy. Ann Thorac Surg 51:585, 1991.

288. Schwammenthal E, Levine RA: Dynamic subaortic obstruction: A disease of the mitral valve suitable for surgical repair? J Am Coll Cardiol 28:203, 1996.

289. Joyce FS, Lever HM, Cosgrove DM III: Treatment of hypertrophic cardiomyopathy by mitral valve repair and septal myectomy. Ann Thorac Surg 57:1025, 1994.

290. Shirani J, Maron BJ, Cannon RO III, et al: Clinicopathologic features of hypertrophic cardiomyopathy managed by cardiac transplantation. Am J Cardiol 72:434, 1993.

RESTRICTIVE AND INFILTRATIVE CARDIOMYOPATHIES

291. Kushwaha SS, Fallon JT, Fuster V: Restrictive cardiomyopathy. N Engl J Med 336:267, 1997.

292. Spyrou N, Foale R: Restrictive cardiomyopathies. Curr Opin Cardiol 9:344, 1994.

293. Benson MD: Hereditary amyloidosis and cardiomyopathy. Am J Med 93:1, 1992.

294. Keren A, Popp RL: Assignment of patients into the classification of cardiomyopathies. Circulation 86:1622, 1992.

295. Garcia MJ, Rodriguez L, Ares M, et al: Differentiation of constrictive pericarditis from restrictive cardiomyopathy: Assessment of left ventricular diastolic velocities in longitudinal axis by Doppler tissue imaging. J Am Coll Cardiol 277:108, 1996.

296. Angelini A, Calzolari V, Thiene G, et al: Morphologic spectrum of primary restrictive cardiomyopathy. Am J Cardiol 80:1046, 1997.

297. Masui T, Finck S, Higgins CB: Constrictive pericarditis and restrictive cardiomyopathy: Evaluation with MR imaging. Radiology 182:369, 1992.

298. Gasperetti CM, Sarembock IJ, Feldman MD: Usefulness of dynamic hand exercise for developing maximal separation of left and right ventricular pressures at end-diastole and usefulness in distinguishing restrictive cardiomyopathy from constrictive pericardial disease. Am J Cardiol 69:1508, 1992.

299. Klein AL, Cohen GI, Pietrolungo JF, et al: Differentiation of constrictive pericarditis from restrictive cardiomyopathy by Doppler transesophageal echocardiographic measurements of respiratory variations in pulmonary venous flow. J Am Coll Cardiol 22:1935, 1993.

299a. Felker GM, Thompson RE, Hare JM, et al: Underlying causes and long-term survival in patients with initially unexplained cardiomyopathy. N Engl J Med 342:1077, 2000.

Amyloidosis

300. Hesse A, Altland K, Linke RP, et al: Cardiac amyloidosis: A review and report of a new transthyretin (prealbumin) variant. Br Heart J 70:111, 1993.

301. Booth DR, Tan SY, Hawkins PN, et al: A novel variant of transthyretin, 59Thr → Lys, associated with autosomal dominant cardiac amyloidosis in an Italian family. Circulation 91:962, 1995.

302. Kyle RA: Amyloidosis. Circulation 91:1269, 1995.

303. Jacobson DR, Pastore RD, Yaghoubian R, et al: Variant-sequence transthyretin (isoleucine 122) in late-onset cardiac amyloidosis in black Americans. N Engl J Med 336:466, 1997.

304. Gertz MA, Kyle RA, Noel P: Primary systemic amyloidosis: A rare complication of immunoglobulin M monoclonal gammopathies and Waldenström's macroglobulinemia. J Clin Oncol 11:914, 1993.

305. Gertz MA, Kyle RA, Thibodeau SN: Familial amyloidosis: A study of 52 North American-born patients examined during a 30-year period. Mayo Clin Proc 67:428, 1992.

306. Dubrey S, Pollak A, Skinner M, et al: Atrial thrombi occurring during sinus rhythm in cardiac amyloidosis: Evidence for atrial electromechanical dissociation. Br Heart J 74:541, 1995.

307. Chamarthi B, Dubrey SW, Cha K, et al: Features and prognosis of exertional syncope in light chain–associated AL cardiac amyloidosis. Am J Cardiol 80:1242, 1997.

308. Reisinger J, Dubrey SW, LaValley M, et al: Electrophysiologic abnormalities in AL (primary) amyloidosis with cardiac involvement. J Am Coll Cardiol 30:1046, 1997.

309. Simons M, Isner JM: Assessment of relative sensitivities of noninvasive tests for cardiac amyloidosis in documented cardiac amyloidosis. Am J Cardiol 69:425, 1992.

310. Tei C, Dujardin KS, Hodge DO, et al: Doppler index combining systolic and diastolic myocardial performance: Clinical value in cardiac amyloidosis. J Am Coll Cardiol 28:658, 1996.

311. Fattori R, Rocchi G, Celletti F, et al: Contribution of magnetic resonance imaging in the differential diagnosis of cardiac amyloidosis and symmetric hypertrophic cardiomyopathy. Am Heart J 136:824, 1998.

312. Tanaka M, Hongo M, Kinoshita O, et al: Iodine-123 metaiodobenzylguanidine scintigraphic assessment of myocardial sympathetic innervation in patients with familial amyloid polyneuropathy. J Am Coll Cardiol 29:168, 1997.

313. Lekakis J, Dimopoulos M, Nanas J, et al: Antimyosin scintigraphy for detection of cardiac amyloidosis. Am J Cardiol 80:963, 1997.

314. Kyle RA, Spittell PC, Gertz MA, et al: The premortem recognition of systemic senile amyloidosis with cardiac involvement. Am J Med 101:395, 1996.

315. Kyle RA, Gertz MA, Greipp PR, et al: A trial of three regimens for primary amyloidosis: Colchicine alone, melphalan and prednisone, and melphalan, prednisone, and colchicine. N Engl J Med 336:1202, 1997.

316. Dubrey S, Mendes L, Skinner M, et al: Resolution of heart failure in patients with AL amyloidosis. Ann Intern Med 125:481, 1996.

317. Pollak A, Falk RH: Left ventricular systolic dysfunction precipitated by verapamil in cardiac amyloidosis. Chest 104:618, 1993.

318. Mathew V, Olson LJ, Gertz MA, et al: Symptomatic conduction system disease in cardiac amyloidosis. Am J Cardiol 80:1491, 1997.

319. Kyle RA: High-dose therapy in multiple myeloma and primary amyloidosis: An overview. Semin Oncol 26:74, 1999.

320. Pelosi F Jr, Capehart J, Roberts WC: Effectiveness of cardiac transplantation for primary (AL) cardiac amyloidosis. Am J Cardiol 79:532, 1997.

Inherited Infiltrative Disorders Causing Restrictive Cardiomyopathy

321. Eng CM, Resnick-Silverman LA, Niehaus DJ, et al: Nature and frequency of mutations in the alpha-galactosidase A gens that cause Fabry disease. Am J Hum Genet 53:1186, 1993.

322. Nakao S, Takenaka T, Maeda M, et al: An atypical variant of Fabry's disease in men with left ventricular hypertrophy. N Engl J Med 333:288, 1995.

323. Pochis WT, Litzow JT, King BG, et al: Electrophysiologic findings in Fabry's disease with a short PR interval. Am J Cardiol 74:203, 1994.

324. Mester SW, Weston MW: Cardiac tamponade in a patient with Gaucher's disease. Clin Cardiol 15:766, 1992.

325. Starzl TE, Demetris AJ, Trucco M, et al: Chimerism after liver transplantation for type IV glycogen storage disease and type 1 Gaucher's disease. N Engl J Med 328:745, 1993.

326. Liu P, Olivieri N: Iron overload cardiomyopathies: New insights into an old disease. Cardiovasc Drugs Ther 8:101, 1994.

327. Porter J, Cary N, Schofield P: Haemochromatosis presenting as congestive cardiac failure. Br Heart J 73:73, 1995.

328. Westra WH, Hruban RH, Baughman KL, et al: Progressive hemochromatotic cardiomyopathy despite reversal of iron deposition after liver transplantation. Am J Clin Pathol 99:39, 1993.

329. Wang TL, Chen WJ, Liau CS, et al: Sick sinus syndrome as the early manifestation of cardiac hemochromatosis. J Electrocardiol 27:91, 1994.

330. Strobel JS, Fuisz AR, Epstein AE, et al: Syncope and inducible ventricular fibrillation in a woman with hemochromatosis. J Interv Card Electrophysiol 3:225, 1999.

331. Cecchetti G, Binda A, Piperno A, et al: Cardiac alterations in 36 consecutive patients with idiopathic haemochromatosis: Polygraphic and echocardiographic evaluation. Eur Heart J 12:224, 1991.

332. Waxman S, Eustace S, Hartnell GG: Myocardial involvement in primary hemochromatosis demonstrated by magnetic resonance imaging. Am Heart J 128:1047, 1994.

333. Politi A, Sticca M, Galli M: Reversal of haemochromatotic cardiomyopathy in beta thalassaemia by chelation therapy. Br Heart J 73:486, 1995.

334. Coleman RA, Winter HS, Wolf B, et al: Glycogen storage disease type III (glycogen debranching enzyme deficiency): Correlation of biochemical defects with myopathy and cardiomyopathy. Ann Intern Med 116:896, 1992.

335. Tse HF, Shek TW, Tai YT, et al: Case report: Lysosomal glycogen storage disease with normal acid maltase: An unusual form of hyper-

trophic cardiomyopathy with rapidly progressive heart failure. Am J Med Sci 312:182, 1996.

Myocardial Sarcoidosis

336. Sharma OP: Myocardial sarcoidosis: A wolf in sheep's clothing. Chest 106:988, 1994.
337. Yazaki Y, Isobe M, Hiramitsu S, et al: Comparison of clinical features and prognosis of cardiac sarcoidosis and idiopathic dilated cardiomyopathy. Am J Cardiol 82:537, 1998.
338. Pisani B, Taylor DO, Mason JW: Inflammatory myocardial diseases and cardiomyopathies. Am J Med 102:459, 1997.
339. Bohle W, Schaefer HE: Predominant myocardial sarcoidosis. Pathol Res Pract 190: 212, 1994.
340. Mitchell DN, du Bois RM, Oldershaw PJ: Cardiac sarcoidosis. BMJ 314: 320, 1997.
341. Angomachalelis N, Hourzamanis A, Salem N, et al: Pericardial effusion concomitant with specific heart muscle disease in systemic sarcoidosis. Postgrad Med J 70:S8, 1994.
342. Le Guludec D, Menad F, Faraggi M, et al: Myocardial sarcoidosis: Clinical value of technetium-99m sestamibi tomoscintigraphy. Chest 106: 1675, 1994.
343. Tawarahara K, Kurata C, Okayama K, et al: Thallium-201 and gallium-67 single photon emission computed tomographic imaging in cardiac sarcoidosis. Am Heart J 124:1383, 1992.
344. Okayama K, Kurata C, Tawarahara K, et al: Diagnostic and prognostic value of myocardial scintigraphy with thallium-201 and gallium-67 in cardiac sarcoidosis. Chest 107:330, 1995.
345. Chandra M, Silverman ME, Oshinski J, et al: Diagnosis of cardiac sarcoidosis aided by MRI. Chest 110:562, 1996.
346. Hirose Y, Ishida Y, Hayashida K, et al: Myocardial involvement in patients with sarcoidosis: An analysis of 75 patients. Clin Nucl Med 19: 522, 1994.
347. Knapp WH, Bentrup A, Ohlmeier H: Indium-111–labelled antimyosin antibody imaging in a patient with cardiac sarcoidosis. Eur J Nucl Med 20:80, 1993.
348. Shammas RL, Movahed A: Successful treatment of myocardial sarcoidosis with steroids. Sarcoidosis 11:37, 1994.
349. Paz HL, McCormick DJ, Kutalek SP, et al: The automated implantable cardiac defibrillator: Prophylaxis in cardiac sarcoidosis. Chest 106:1603, 1994.

Endomyocardial Disease

350. Kutty; VR, Abraham S, Kartha CC: Geographical distribution of endomyocardial fibrosis in south Kerala. Int J Epidemiol 25:1202, 1996.
351. Rashwan MA, Ayman M, Ashour S, et al: Endomyocardial fibrosis in Egypt: An illustrated review. Br Heart J 73:284, 1995.
352. Ribeiro PA, Muthusamy R, Duran CM: Right-sided endomyocardial fibrosis with recurrent pulmonary emboli leading to irreversible pulmonary hypertension. Br Heart J 68:326, 1992.
353. Kartha CC: Endomyocardial fibrosis, a case for the tropical doctor. Cardiovasc Res 30:636, 1995.
354. Weller PF, Bubley GJ: The idiopathic hypereosinophilic syndrome. Blood 83:2759, 1994.
355. Felice PV, Sawicki J, Anto J: Endomyocardial disease and eosinophilia. Angiology 44:869, 1993.
356. Shaper AG: What's new in endomyocardial fibrosis? Lancet 342:255, 1993.
357. Valiathan MS: Endomyocardial fibrosis. Natl Med J India 6:212, 1993.
358. Barbosa MM, Lamounier JA, Oliveira EC, et al: Short report: Endomyocardial fibrosis and cardiomyopathy in an area endemic for schistosomiasis. Am J Trop Med Hyg 58:26, 1998.
359. Andy JJ, Ogunowo PO, Akpan NA, et al: Helminth associated hypereosinophilia and tropical endomyocardial fibrosis (EMF) in Nigeria. Acta Trop 69:127, 1998.
360. Kumari KT, Ravikumar A, Kurup PA: Accumulation of glycosaminoglycans associated with hypomagnesaemia in endomyocardial fibrosis in Kerala: Possible involvement of dietary factors. Indian Heart J 49:49, 1997.
361. Butterfield JH, Gleich GJ: Interferon-alpha treatment of six patients with the idiopathic hypereosinophilic syndrome. Ann Intern Med 121:648, 1994.
362. Parrillo JE: Heart disease and the eosinophil. N Engl J Med 323:1560, 1990.
363. De Cock C, Lemaitre J, Deuvaert FE: Loeffler endocarditis: A clinical presentation as right ventricular tumor. J Heart Valve Dis 7:668, 1998.
364. Rutakingirwa M, Ziegler JL, Newton R, et al: Poverty and eosinophilia are risk factors for endomyocardial fibrosis (EMF) in Uganda. Trop Med Int Health 4:229, 1999.
365. D'Silva SA, Kohli A, Dalvi BV, et al: MRI in right ventricular endomyocardial fibrosis. Am Heart J 123:1390, 1992.
366. Saraclar M, Ozer S, Oztunc F, et al: Echocardiographic findings in endomyocardial fibrosis. Turk J Pediatr 34:47, 1992.
367. Mady C, Barretto AC, Mesquita ET, et al: Maximal functional capacity in patients with endomyocardial fibrosis. Eur Heart J 14:240, 1993.
368. Barretto AC, Mady C, Nussbacher A, et al: Atrial fibrillation in endo-

myocardial fibrosis is a marker of worse prognosis. Int J Cardiol 67:19, 1998.
369. Moraes F, Lapa C, Hazin S, et al: Surgery for endomyocardial fibrosis revisited. Eur J Cardiothorac Surg 15:309, 1999.
370. Schneider U, Jenni R, Turina J, et al: Long-term follow-up of patients with endomyocardial fibrosis: Effects of surgery. Heart 79:362, 1998.
371. Uva MS, Jebara VA, Acar C, et al: Mitral valve repair in patients with endomyocardial fibrosis. Ann Thorac Surg 54:89, 1992.

Carcinoid Heart Disease

372. Pellikka PA, Tajik AJ, Khandheria BK, et al: Carcinoid heart disease: Clinical and echocardiographic spectrum in 74 patients. Circulation 87: 1188, 1993.
373. Waltenberger J, Lundin L, Oberg K, et al: Involvement of transforming growth factor-beta in the formation of fibrotic lesions in carcinoid heart disease. Am J Pathol 142:71, 1993.
374. Kulke MH, Mayer RJ: Carcinoid tumors. N Engl J Med 340:858, 1999.
375. Robiolio PA, Rigolin VH, Wilson JS, et al: Carcinoid heart disease: Correlation of high serotonin levels with valvular abnormalities detected by cardiac catheterization and echocardiography. Circulation 92: 790, 1995.
376. Robiolio PA, Rigolin VH, Harrison JK, et al: Predictors of outcome of tricuspid valve replacement in carcinoid heart disease. Am J Cardiol 75:485, 1995.
377. Connolly HM, Nishimura RA, Smith HC, et al: Outcome of cardiac surgery for carcinoid heart disease. J Am Coll Cardiol 25:410, 1995.
378. Yun D, Heywood JT: Metastatic carcinoid disease presenting solely as high-output heart failure. Ann Intern Med 120:45, 1994.
379. Onate A, Alcibar J, Inguanzo R, et al: Balloon dilation of tricuspid and pulmonary valves in carcinoid heart disease. Tex Heart Inst J 20:115, 1993.
380. Grant SC, Scarffe JH, Levy RD, et al: Failure of balloon dilatation of the pulmonary valve in carcinoid pulmonary stenosis. Br Heart J 67:450, 1992.

MYOCARDITIS

381. Olinde KD, O'Connell JB: Inflammatory heart disease: Pathogenesis, clinical manifestations, and treatment of myocarditis. Annu Rev Med 45:481, 1994.
382. Seko Y, Matsuda H, Kato K, et al: Expression of intercellular adhesion molecule-1 in murine hearts with acute myocarditis caused by coxsackievirus B3. J Clin Invest 91:1327, 1993.
383. Wessely R, Henke A, Zell R, et al: Low-level expression of a mutant coxsackieviral cDNA induces a myocytopathic effect in culture: An approach to the study of enteroviral persistence in cardiac myocytes. Circulation 98:450, 1998.
384. Herskowitz A, Ahmed-Ansari A, Neumann DA, et al: Induction of major histocompatibility complex antigens within the myocardium of patients with active myocarditis: A nonhistologic marker of myocarditis. J Am Coll Cardiol 15:624, 1990.
385. Rose NR, Neumann DA, Herskowitz A: Coxsackievirus myocarditis. Adv Intern Med 37: 411, 1992.
386. Knowlton KU, Badorff C: The immune system in viral myocarditis: Maintaining the balance. Circ Res 85:559, 1999.
387. Brown CS, Bertolet BD: Peripartum cardiomyopathy: A comprehensive review. Am J Obstet Gynecol 178:409, 1998.
388. Hyypia T: Etiological diagnosis of viral heart disease. Scand J Infect Dis 88:25, 1993.
389. Friedrich MG, Strohm O, Schulz-Menger J, et al: Contrast media–enhanced magnetic resonance imaging visualizes myocardial changes in the course of viral myocarditis. Circulation 97:1802, 1998.
390. Ino T, Okubo M, Akimoto K, et al: Corticosteroid therapy for ventricular tachycardia in children with silent lymphocytic myocarditis. J Pediatr 126:304, 1995.
390a. McCarthy RE 3rd, Boehmer JP, Hruban RH, et al: Long-term outcome of fulminant myocarditis as compared with acute (nonfulminant) myocarditis. N Engl J Med 342:690, 2000.
391. Davies MJ, Ward DE: How can myocarditis be diagnosed and should it be treated? Br Heart J 68:346, 1992.
392. Friedman RA, Kearney DL, Moak JP, et al: Persistence of ventricular arrhythmia after resolution of occult myocarditis in children and young adults. J Am Coll Cardiol 24:780, 1994.
393. Dec GW Jr, Waldman H, Southern J, et al: Viral myocarditis mimicking acute myocardial infarction. J Am Coll Cardiol 20:85, 1992.
394. Galiuto L, Enriquez-Sarano M, Reeder GS, et al: Eosinophilic myocarditis manifesting as myocardial infarction: Early diagnosis and successful treatment. Mayo Clin Proc 72:603, 1997.
395. Chida K, Ohkawa S, Esaki Y: Clinicopathologic characteristics of elderly patients with persistent ST segment elevation and inverted T waves: Evidence of insidious or healed myocarditis? J Am Coll Cardiol 25:1641, 1995.
396. Matsuura H, Palacios IF, Dec GW, et al: Intraventricular conduction abnormalities in patients with clinically suspected myocarditis are associated with myocardial necrosis. Am Heart J 127:1290, 1994.
397. Smith SC, Ladenson JH, Mason JW, et al: Elevations of cardiac troponin I associated with myocarditis: Experimental and clinical correlates. Circulation 95:163, 1997.

398. James KB, Lee K, Thomas JD, et al: Left ventricular diastolic dysfunction in lymphocytic myocarditis as assessed by Doppler echocardiography. Am J Cardiol 73:282, 1994.

399. Matsouka H, Hamada M, Honda T, et al: Evaluation of acute myocarditis and pericarditis by Gd-DTPA enhanced magnetic resonance imaging. Eur Heart J 15:283, 1994.

400. Mason JW: Myocarditis. Adv Intern Med 44:293, 1999.

401. Huber SA: Viral myocarditis—a tale of two diseases. Lab Invest 66:1, 1992.

402. Akhtar N, Ni J, Stromberg D, et al: Tracheal aspirate as a substrate for polymerase chain reaction detection of viral genome in childhood pneumonia and myocarditis. Circulation 99:2011, 1999.

403. Frustaci A, Chimenti C, Maseri A: Global biventricular dysfunction in patients with asymptomatic coronary artery disease may be caused by myocarditis. Circulation 99:1295, 1999.

404. Popovic Z, Miric M, Vasiljevic J, et al: Acute hemodynamic effects of metoprolol +/− nitroglycerin in patients with biopsy-proven lymphocytic myocarditis. Am J Cardiol 81:801, 1998.

405. Maisch B, Schonian U, Crombach M, et al: Cytomegalovirus associated inflammatory heart muscle disease. Scand J Infect Dis 88:135, 1993.

406. Mason JW, O'Connell JB, Herskowitz A, et al: A clinical trial of immunosuppressive therapy for myocarditis: The Myocarditis Treatment Trial Investigators. N Engl J Med 333:269, 1995.

407. Drucker NA, Colan SD, Lewis AB, et al: Gamma-globulin treatment of acute myocarditis in the pediatric population. Circulation 89:252, 1994.

408. McNamara DM, Rosenblum WD, Janosko KM, et al: Intravenous immune globulin in the therapy of myocarditis and acute cardiomyopathy. Circulation 95:2476, 1997.

409. Rezkalla SH, Raikar S, Kloner RA: Treatment of viral myocarditis with focus on captopril. Am J Cardiol 77:634, 1996.

410. Yamamoto N, Shibamori M, Ogura M, et al: Effects of intranasal administration of recombinant murine interferon-gamma on murine acute myocarditis caused by encephalomyocarditis virus. Circulation 97:1017, 1998.

411. Nishio R, Matsumori A, Shioi T, et al: Treatment of experimental viral myocarditis with interleukin-10. Circulation 100:1102, 1999.

Viral Myocarditis

412. Nakamura H, Yamamura T, Umemoto S, et al: Autoimmune response in chronic ongoing myocarditis demonstrated by heterotopic cardiac transplantation in mice. Circulation 94:3348, 1996.

413. Hingorani AD: Postinfectious myocarditis. BMJ 304:1676, 1992.

414. Frustaci A, Maseri A: Localized left ventricular aneurysms with normal global function caused by myocarditis. Am J Cardiol 70:1221, 1992.

415. Gowrishankar K, Rajajee S: Varied manifestations of viral myocarditis. Indian J Pediatr 61:75, 1994.

416. Remes J, Helin M, Vaino P, et al: Clinical outcome and left ventricular function 23 years after acute coxsackievirus myopericarditis. Eur Heart J 11:182, 1990.

417. Lowry RW, Adam E, Hu C, et al: What are the implications of cardiac infection with cytomegalovirus before heart transplantation? J Heart Lung Transplant 13:122, 1994.

418. Partanen J, Nieminen MS, Krogerus L, et al: Cytomegalovirus myocarditis in transplanted heart verified by endomyocardial biopsy. Clin Cardiol 14:847, 1991.

419. Schindler JM, Neftel KA: Simultaneous primary infection with HIV and CMV leading to severe pancytopenia, hepatitis, nephritis, perimyocarditis, myositis, and alopecia totalis. Klin Wochenschr 68:237, 1990.

420. Kabra SK, Juneja R, Madhulika, et al: Myocardial dysfunction in children with dengue haemorrhagic fever. Natl Med J India 11:59, 1998.

421. Wali JP, Biswas A, Chandra S, et al: Cardiac involvement in dengue haemorrhagic fever. Int J Cardiol 64:31, 1998.

422. Ursell PC, Habib A, Sharma P, et al: Hepatitis B virus and myocarditis. Hum Pathol 15:481, 1984.

423. Okabe M, Fukuda K, Arakawa K, et al: Chronic variant of myocarditis associated with hepatitis C virus infection. circulation 96:22, 1997.

424. Prati D, Poli F, Farma E, et al: Multicenter study on hepatitis C virus infection in patients with dilated cardiomyopathy. J Med Virol 58:116, 1999.

425. Dalekos GN, Achenbach K, Christodoulou D, et al: Idiopathic dilated cardiomyopathy: Lack of association with hepatitis C virus infection. Heart 80:270, 1998.

426. Hebert MM, Yu C, Towbin JA, et al: Fatal Epstein-Barr virus myocarditis in a child with repetitive myocarditis. Pediatr Pathol Lab Med 15:805, 1995.

427. Craver RD, Sorrells K, Gohd R: Myocarditis with influenza B infection. Pediatr Infect Dis J 16:629, 1997.

428. McGregor D, Henderson S: Myocarditis, rhabdomyolysis and myoglobinuric renal failure complicating influenza in a young adult. NZ Med J 110:237, 1997.

429. Cummins D, Bennett D, Fisher-Hoch SP, et al: Electrocardiographic abnormalities in patients with Lassa fever. J Trop Med Hyg 92:350, 1989.

430. Ozkutlu S, Soylemezoglu O, Calikoglu AS, et al: Fatal mumps myocarditis. Jpn Heart J 30:109, 1989.

430a. Kabakus N, Aydinoglu H, Yekeler H, Arslan IN: Fatal mumps nephritis and myocarditis. J Trop Pediatr 45:358, 1999.

431. Ni J, Bowles NE, Kim YH, et al: Viral infection of the myocardium in endocardial fibroelastosis: Molecular evidence for the role of mumps virus as an etiologic agent. Circulation 95:133, 1997.

432. Hildes JA, Schaberg A, Alcock AUW: Cardiovascular collapse in acute poliomyelitis. Circulation 12:986, 1955.

433. Thomas JA, Raroque S, Scott WA, et al: Successful treatment of severe dysrhythmias in infants with respiratory syncytial virus infections: Two cases and a literature review. Crit Care Med 25:880, 1997.

434. Olesch CA, Bullock AM: Bradyarrhythmia and supraventricular tachycardia in a neonate with RSV. J Paediatr Child Health 34:199, 1998.

435. Frustaci A, Abdulla AK, Caldarulo M, et al: Fatal measles myocarditis. Cardiologia 35: 347, 1990.

436. Degen JA: Visceral pathology in measles. Am J Med Sci 194:104, 1937.

437. Tsintsof A, Delprado WJ, Keogh AM: Varicella zoster myocarditis progressing to cardiomyopathy and cardiac transplantation. Br Heart J 70: 93, 1993.

438. Matthews AW, Griffiths ID: Post-vaccinial pericarditis and myocarditis. Br Heart J 36:1043, 1974.

Rickettsial Myocarditis

439. Chevalier P, Moncada E, Kirkorian G, et al: Q fever−induced EMF. Am Heart J 125:1818, 1993.

439a. Raoult D, Tissot-Dupont H, Foucault C, et al: Q fever 1985−1998. Clinical and epidemiologic features of 1,383 infections. Medicine 79: 109, 2000.

440. Marin-Garcia J, Barrett FF: Myocardial function in Rocky Mountain spotted fever: Echocardiographic assessment. Am J Cardiol 51:341, 1983.

441. Yotsukura M, Aoki N, Fukuzumi N, et al: Review of a case of tsutsugamushi disease showing myocarditis and confirmation of rickettsia by endomyocardial biopsy. Jpn Circ J 55:149, 1991.

Bacterial Myocarditis

442. Jubber AS, Gunawardana DR, Lulu AR: Acute pulmonary edema in Brucella myocarditis and interstitial pneumonitis. Chest 97:1008, 1990.

443. Stevens DL, Troyer BE, Merrick DT, et al: Lethal effects and cardiovascular effects of purified alpha- and theta-toxins from Clostridium perfringens. J Infect Dis 157:272, 1988.

443a. Kadirova R, Kartoglu HU, Strebel PM: Clinical characteristics and management of 676 hospitalized diphtheria cases, Kyrgyz Republic, 1995. J Infect Dis 181(Suppl 1):S110, 2000.

444. Havaldar PV, Patil VD, Siddibhavi BM, et al: Fulminant diptheretic myocarditis. Indian Heart J 41:265, 1989.

445. Armengol S, Domingo C, Mesalles E: Myocarditis: A rare complication during Legionella infection. Int J Cardiol 37:418, 1992.

446. Sandler MA, Pincus PS, Weltman MD, et al: Meningococcaemia complicated by myocarditis: A report of 2 cases. S Afr Med J 75:391, 1989.

447. Agarwala BN, Ruschhaupt DG: Complete heart block from Mycoplasma pneumoniae infection. Pediatr Cardiol 12:233, 1991.

448. Odeh M, Oliven A: Chlamydial infections of the heart. Eur J Clin Microbiol Infect Dis 11:885, 1992.

449. Neuwirth C, François C, Laurent N, et al: Myocarditis due to Salmonella virchow and sudden infant death. Lancet 354:1004, 1999.

450. Wander GS, Khurana SB, Puri S: Salmonella myopericarditis presenting with acute pulmonary oedema. Indian Heart J 44:55, 1992.

451. Maher D, Ostrowski J: Highly virulent Streptococcus pyogenes rheumatic pancarditis and fatal septicaemia with septic shock. J Infect 26: 195, 1993.

452. O'Neill PG, Rokey R, Greenberg S, et al: Resolution of ventricular tachycardia and endocardial tuberculoma following antituberculosis therapy. Chest 100:1467, 1991.

453. Chan AC, Dickens P: Tuberculous myocarditis presenting as sudden cardiac death. Forensic Sci Int 57:45, 1992.

Whipple Disease

454. Silvestry FE, Kim B, Pollack BJ, et al: Cardiac Whipple disease: Identification of Whipple bacillus by electron microscopy of a patient before death. Ann Intern Med 126:214, 1997.

455. Elkins C, Shuman TA, Pirolo JS: Cardiac Whipple's disease without digestive symptoms. Ann Thorac Surg 67:250, 1999.

Spirochetal Infections

456. Singh SS, Vijayachari P, Sinha A, et al: Clinico-epidemiological study of hospitalized cases of severe leptospirosis. Indian J Med Res 109:94, 1999.

457. Rajiv C, Manjuran RJ, Sudhayakumar N, et al: Cardiovascular involvement in leptospirosis. Indian Heart J 48:691, 1996.

458. Sangha O, Phillips CB, Fleischmann KE, et al: Lack of cardiac manifestations among patients with previously treated Lyme disease. Ann Intern Med 128:346, 1998.

459. Haywood GA, O'Connell S, Gray HH: Lyme carditis: A United Kingdom perspective. Br Heart J 70:15, 1993.

460. Asch ES, Bujak DI, Weiss M, et al: Lyme disease: An infectious and postinfectious syndrome. J Rheumatol 21:454, 1994.

461. Ledford DK: Immunologic aspects of vasculitis and cardiovascular disease. JAMA 278:1962, 1997.
462. Rees DH, Keeling PJ, McKenna WJ, et al: No evidence to implicate *Borrelia burgdorferi* in the pathogenesis of dilated cardiomyopathy in the United Kingdom. Br Heart J 71:459, 1994.
463. Stanek G, Klein J, Bittner R, et al: Isolation of *Borrelia burgdorferi* from the myocardium of a patient with long-standing cardiomyopathy. N Engl J Med 322:249, 1990.
464. Rahn DW, Malawista SE: Lyme disease: Recommendations for diagnosis and treatment. Ann Intern Med 14:472, 1991.
465. Mekasha A: Louse-borne relapsing fever in children. J Trop Med Hyg 95:206, 1992.
466. Chino M, Minami T, Nishikawa K: Ruptured ventricular aneurysm in secondary syphilis. Lancet 342:935, 1993.

Fungal Infections of the Heart

467. Bashour TT, Gord C, Baladi N, et al: Intracardiac actinomyocosis. Am Heart J 133:467, 1997.
468. Berarducci L, Ford K, Olenick S, et al: Invasive intracardiac aspergillosis with widespread embolization. J Am Soc Echocardiogr 6:539, 1993.
469. Massin EK, Zeluff BJ, Carrol CL, et al: Cardiac transplantation and aspergillosis. Circulation 90:1552, 1994.
470. Lafont A, Wolff M, Marche C, et al: Overwhelming myocarditis due to *Cryptococcus neoformans* in an AIDS patient. Lancet 2:1145, 1987.
471. Kirchner SG, Hernanz-Schulman M, Stein SM, et al: Imaging of pediatric mediastinal histoplasmosis. Radiographics 11:365, 1991.
472. Jackman JD Jr, Simonsen RL: The clinical manifestations of cardiac mucormycosis. Chest 101:1733, 1992.

Protozoal Myocarditis

473. Hagar JM, Rahimtoola SH: Chagas' heart disease. Curr Probl Cardiol 20:825, 1995.
474. Rossi MA, Bestetti RB: The challenge of chagasic cardiomyopathy: The pathologic roles of autonomic abnormalities, autoimmune mechanisms and microvascular changes, and therapeutic implications. Cardiology 86:1, 1995.
475. Parada II, Carrasco HA, Anez N, et al: Cardiac involvement is a constant finding in acute Chagas' disease: A clinical, parasitological and histopathological study. Int J Cardiol 60:49, 1997.
476. Reis MM, Higuchi M, de la Benvenuti LA, et al: An in situ quantitative immunohistochemical study of cytokines and IL-2R+ in chronic human chagasic myocarditis: Correlation with the presence of myocardial *Trypanosoma cruzi* antigens. Clin Immunol Immunopathol 83:165, 1997.
477. Rossi MA: Comparison of Chagas' heart disease to arrhythmogenic right ventricular cardiomyopathy. Am Heart J 129:626, 1995.
478. Anez N, Carrasco H, Parada H, et al: Myocardial parasite persistence in chronic chagasic patients. Am J Trop Med Hyg 60:726, 1999.
479. Bellotti G, Bocchi EA, de Moraes AV, et al: In vivo detection of *Trypanosoma cruzi* antigens in hearts of patients with chronic Chagas' heart disease. Am Heart J 131:301, 1996.
480. Bestetti RB, Muccillo G: Clinical course of Chagas' heart disease: A comparison with dilated cardiomyopathy. Int J Cardiol 60:187, 1997.
481. Higuchi MD, Ries MM, Aiello VD, et al: Association of an increase in CD8+ T cells with the presence of *Trypanosoma cruzi* antigens in chronic, human, chagasic myocarditis. Am J Trop Med Hyg 56:485, 1997.
482. Higuchi ML, Fukasawa S, De Brito T, et al: Different microcirculatory and interstitial matrix patterns in idiopathic dilated cardiomyopathy and Chagas' disease: A three dimensional confocal microscopy study. Heart 82:279, 1999.
483. Bestetti RB, Dalbo CM, Arruda CA, et al: Predictors of sudden cardiac death for patients with Chagas' disease: A hospital-derived cohort study. Cardiology 87:481, 1996.
484. Carrasco HA, Alarçon M, Olmos L, et al: Biochemical characterization of myocardial damage in chronic Chagas' disease. Clin Cardiol 20:865, 1997.
485. Bestetti RB, Dalbo CM, Freitas QC, et al: Noninvasive predictors of mortality for patients with Chagas' heart disease: A multivariate stepwise logistic regression study. Cardiology 84:261, 1994.
486. Giniger AG, Retyk EO, Laino RA, et al: Ventricular tachycardia in Chagas' disease. Am J Cardiol 70:459, 1992.
487. de Paola AA, Gomes JA, Terzian AB, et al: Ventricular tachycardia during exercise testing as a predictor of sudden death in patients with chronic chagasic cardiomyopathy and ventricular arrhythmias. Br Heart J 74:293, 1995.
488. Carrasco HA, Parada H, Guerrero L, et al: Prognostic implications of clinical, electrocardiographic and hemodynamic findings in chronic Chagas' disease. Int J Cardiol 43:27, 1994.
489. de Paola AA, Gomes JA, Miyamoto MH, et al: Transcoronary chemical ablation of ventricular tachycardia in chronic chagasic myocarditis. J Am Coll Cardiol 20:480, 1992.
490. Braga JC, Labrunie A, Villaca F, et al: Thromboembolism in chronic Chagas' heart disease. Rev Paul Med 113:862, 1995.
491. Marin-Neto JA, Marzullo P, Marcassa C, et al: Myocardial perfusion abnormalities in chronic Chagas' disease as detected by thallium-201 scintigraphy. Am J Cardiol 69:780, 1992.
492. Kalil Filho R, de Albuquerque CP: Magnetic resonance imaging in Chagas' heart disease. Rev Paul Med 113:880, 1995.

493. Ferreira AW, de Avila SD: Laboratory diagnosis of Chagas' heart disease. Rev Paul Med 113:767, 1995.
494. de Paola AA, Gondin AA, Hara V, et al: Medical treatment of cardiac arrhythmias in Chagas' heart disease. Rev Paul Med 113:858, 1995.
495. Muratore C, Rabinovich R, Iglesias R, et al: Implantable cardioverter defibrillators in patients with Chagas' disease: Are they different from patients with coronary disease? Pacing Clin Electrophysiol 20:194, 1997.
496. Apt W, Aguilera X, Arribada A, et al. Treatment of chronic Chagas' disease with itraconazole and allopurinol. Am J Trop Med Hyg 59:133, 1998.
497. Bocchi EA, Bellotti G, Uip D, et al: Long-term follow-up after heart transplantation in Chagas' disease. Transplant Proc 25:1329, 1993.
498. Bocchi EA, Bellotti G, Mocelin AO, et al: Heart transplantation for chronic Chagas' heart disease. Ann Thorac Surg 61:1727, 1996.
499. Tsala Mbala P, Blackett K, Mbonifor CL, et al: Functional and immunologic involvement in human African trypanosomiasis caused by *Trypanosoma gambiense*. Bull Soc Pathol Exot Filiales 81:490, 1988.
500. Hofman P, Drici MD, Gibelin P, et al: Prevalence of *Toxoplasma* myocarditis in patients with the acquired immunodeficiency syndrome. Br Heart J 70:376, 1993.
501. Duffield JS, Jacob AJ, Miller HC: Recurrent, life-threatening atrioventricular dissociation associated with *Toxoplasma* myocarditis. Heart 76:453, 1996.
502. Montoya JG, Jordan R, Lingamneni S, et al: Toxoplasmic myocarditis and polymyositis in patients with acute acquired toxoplasmosis diagnosed during life. Clin Infect Dis 24:676, 1997.
503. Franzen D, Curtius JM, Heitz W, et al: Cardiac involvement during and after malaria. Clin Invest 70:670, 1992.
504. Sharma SN, Mohapatra AK, Machave YV: Chronic falciparum cardiomyopathy. J Assoc Physicians India 35:251, 1987.

Metazoal Myocardial Disease

505. Salih OK, Celik SK, Topcuoglu MS, et al: Surgical treatment of hydatid cysts of the heart: A report of 3 cases and a review of the literature. Can J Surg 41:321, 1998.
506. Benomar A, Yahyaoui M, Birouk N, et al: Middle cerebral artery occlusion due to hydatid cysts of myocardial and intraventricular cavity cardiac origin: Two cases. Stroke 25:886, 1994.
507. Miralles A, Bracamonte L, Pavie A, et al: Cardiac echinococcosis: Surgical treatment and results. J Thorac Cardiovasc Surg 107:184, 1994.
508. Franchi C, Di Vico B, Teggi A: Long-term evaluation of patients with hydatidosis treated with benzimidazole carbamates. Clin Infect Dis 29:304, 1999.
509. Dao AH, Virmani R: Visceral larva migrans involving the myocardium: Report of two cases and review of literature. Pediatr Pathol 6:449, 1986.
510. Lazarevic AM, Neskovic AN, Goronja M, et al: Low incidence of cardiac abnormalities in treated trichinosis: A prospective study of 62 patients from a single-source outbreak. Am J Med 107:18, 1999.
511. Compton SJ, Celum CL, Lee C, et al: Trichinosis with ventilatory failure and persistent myocarditis. Clin Infect Dis 16:500, 1993.

TOXIC, CHEMICAL, IMMUNE, AND PHYSICAL DAMAGE TO THE HEART

512. Eisenberg MJ, Mendelson J, Evans GT Jr, et al: Left ventricular function immediately after intravenous cocaine: A quantitative two-dimensional echocardiographic study. J Am Coll Cardiol 22:1581, 1993.
513. Clarkson CW, Chang C, Stolfi A, et al: Electrophysiological effects of high cocaine concentrations on intact canine heart: Evidence for modulation by both heart rate and autonomic nervous system. Circulation 87:950, 1993.
514. Kimura S, Bassett AL, Xi H, et al: Early afterdepolarizations and triggered activity induced by cocaine: A possible mechanism of cocaine arrhythmogenesis. Circulation 85:2227, 1992.
515. Moliterno DJ, Lange RA, Gerard RD, et al: Influence of intranasal cocaine on plasma constituents associated with endogenous thrombosis and thrombolysis. Am J Med 96:492, 1994.
516. Jennings LK, White MM, Sauer CM, et al: Cocaine-induced platelet defects. Stroke 24:1352, 1993.
517. Lange RA, Willard JE: The cardiovascular effects of cocaine. Heart Dis Stroke 2:136, 1993.
518. Gitter MJ, Goldsmith SR, Dunbar DN, et al: Cocaine and chest pain: Clinical features and outcome of patients hospitalized to rule out myocardial infarction. Ann Intern Med 115:277, 1991.
519. Mittleman MA, Mintzer D, Maclure M, et al: Triggering of myocardial infarction by cocaine. Circulation 99:2737, 1999.
520. Chakko S, Fernandez A, Mellman TA, et al: Cardiac manifestations of cocaine abuse: A cross-sectional study of asymptomatic men with a history of long-term abuse of "crack" cocaine. J Am Coll Cardiol 20:1168, 1992.
521. Kloner RA, Hale S: Unraveling the complex effects of cocaine on the heart. Circulation 87:1046, 1993.
522. Angulo MP, Navajas A, Galdeano JM, et al: Reversible cardiomyopathy secondary to alpha-interferon in an infant. Pediatr Cardiol 20:293, 1999.
523. Pitts WR, Lange RA, Cigarroa JE, Hillis DA: Cocaine-induced myocardial ischemia and infarction: Pathophysiology, recognition, and management. Prog Cardiovasc Dis 40:65, 1997.

524. Hollander JE, Brooks DE, Valentine SM: Assessment of cocaine use in patients with chest pain syndromes. Arch Intern Med 158:62, 1998.

525. Greenlund KJ, Kiefe CI, Gidding SS, et al: Differences in cardiovascular risk factors in black and white young adults: Comparisons among five communities of the CARDIA and the Bogalusa heart studies. Ann Epidemiol 8:22, 1998.

526. McLaurin M, Apple FS, Henry TD, Sharkey SW: Cardiac troponin I and T concentrations in patients with cocaine-associated chest pain. Ann Clin Biochem 33:183, 1996.

527. Kontos MC, Schmidt KL, Nicholson CS, et al: Myocardial perfusion imaging with technetium-99m sestamibi in patients with cocaine-associated chest pain. Ann Emerg Med 33:639, 1999.

528. Braunwald E, Antman EM, Beasley JW, et al: ACC/AHA Guidelines for the management of patients with unstable angina. J Am Coll Cardiol. In press.

529. Feenstra J, Grobbee DE, Remme WJ, et al: Drug-induced heart failure. J Am Coll Cardiol 33:1152, 1999.

530. Goel M, Flaherty L, Lavine S, et al: Reversible cardiomyopathy after high-dose interleukin-2 therapy. J Immunother 11:225, 1992.

531. Le Blaye I, Donatini B, Hall M, et al: Acute overdosage with thioridazine: A review of the available clinical exposure. Vet Hum Toxicol 35: 147, 1993.

532. Schmidt W, Lang K: Life-threatening dysrhythmias in severe thioridazine poisoning treated with physostigmine and transient atrial pacing. Crit. Care Med. 25:1925, 1997.

533. Combs, AB, Acosta, D: Toxic mechanisms of the heart: a review. Toxicol Pathol 18:583, 1990.

534. Ho PC, Dweik R, Cohen MC: Rapidly reversible cardiomyopathy associated with chronic ipecac ingestion. Clin Cardiol 21:780, 1998.

535. Silberstein SD: Methysergide. Cephalalgia 18:421, 1998.

536. Iglesias Cubero G, Rodriguez Reguero JJ, Rojo Ortega JM: Restrictive cardiomyopathy caused by chloroquine. Br Heart J 69:451, 1993.

537. Sundar S, Sinha PR, Agrawal NK, et al: A cluster of cases of severe cardiotoxicity among kala-azar patients treated with a high-osmolarity lot of sodium antimony gluconate. Am J Trop Med Hyg 59:139, 1998.

538. Ortega-Carnicer J, Alcazar R, De la Torre M, et al: Pentavalent antimonial-induced torsades de pointes. J Electrocardiol 30:143, 1997.

539. Groleau G: Lithium toxicity. Emerg Med Clin North Am 12:511, 1994.

540. Terao T, Abe H, Abe K: Irreversible sinus node dysfunction induced by resumption of lithium therapy. Acta Psychiatr Scand 93:407, 1996.

541. Gerhardt RT: Acute halon (bromochlorodifluoromethane) toxicity by accidental and recreational inhalation. Am J Emerg Med 14:675, 1996.

542. Brady WJ Jr, Stremski E, Eljaiek L, et al: Freon inhalational abuse presenting with ventricular fibrillation. Am J Emerg Med 12:533, 1994.

543. Elian D, Harpaz D, Sucher E, et al: Reversible catecholamine-induced cardiomyopathy presenting as acute pulmonary edema in a patient with pheochromocytoma. Cardiology 83:118, 1993.

544. Sardesai SH, Mourant AJ, Sivathandon Y, et al: Phaeochromocytoma and catecholamine induced cardiomyopathy presenting as heart failure. Br Heart J 63:234, 1990.

545. Jiang JP, Downing SE: Catecholamine cardiomyopathy: Review and analysis of pathogenetic mechanisms. Yale J Biol Med 63:581, 1990.

546. Raper R, Fisher M, Bihari D: Profound, reversible, myocardial depression in acute asthma treated with high-dose catecholamines. Crit Care Med 20:710, 1992.

547. Kopp SJ, Barron JT, Tow JP: Cardiovascular actions of lead and relationship to hypertension: A review. Environ Health Perspect 78:91, 1988.

548. Farber JP, Schwartz PJ, Vanoli E, et al: Carbon monoxide and lethal arrhythmias. Res Rep Health Eff Inst 36:1, 1990.

549. Dahms TE, Younis LT, Wiens RD, et al: Effects of carbon monoxide exposure in patients with documented cardiac arrhythmias. J Am Coll Cardiol 21:442, 1993.

550. McMeekin JD, Finegan BA: Reversible myocardial dysfunction following carbon monoxide poisoning. Can J Cardiol 3:118, 1987.

551. Marius-Nunez AL: Myocardial infarction with normal coronary arteries after acute exposure to carbon monoxide. Chest 97:491, 1990.

552. Kudoh C, Tanaka S, Marusaki S, et al: Hypocalcemic cardiomyopathy in a patient with idiopathic hypoparathyroidism. Intern Med 31:561, 1992.

553. Feldman AM, Fivush B, Zahka KG, et al: Congestive cardiomyopathy in patients on continuous ambulatory peritoneal dialysis. Am Kidney Dis 11:76, 1988.

554. Kurnik BR, Marshall J, Katz SM: Hypomagnesemia-induced cardiomyopathy. Magnesium 7:49, 1988.

555. Riggs JE, Klingberg WG, Flink EB, et al: Cardioskeletal mitochondrial myopathy associated with chronic magnesium deficiency. Neurology 42:128, 1992.

556. Paulson DJ: Carnitine deficiency-induced cardiomyopathy. Mol Cell Biochem 180:33, 1998.

557. Ergur AT, Tanzer F, Cetinkaya O: Serum-free carnitine levels in children with heart failure. J Trop Pediatr 45:168, 1999.

558. Huttunen JK: Selenium and cardiovascular diseases—an update. Biomed Environ Sci 10:220, 1997.

559. Levy JB, Jones HW, Gordon AC: Selenium deficiency, reversible cardiomyopathy and short-term intravenous feeding. Postgrad Med J 70:235, 1994.

560. Kumar EB, Soomro RS, al Hamdani A, et al: Scorpion venom cardiomyopathy. Am Heart J 123:725, 1992.

561. Gueron M, Ilia R, Sofer S: Scorpion venom cardiomyopathy. Am Heart J 125:1816, 1993.

562. Ferreira DB, Costa RS, De Oliveira JA, et al: An infarct-like myocardial lesion experimentally induced in Wistar rats with africanized bee venom. J Pathol 177:95, 1995.

563. Wagdi P, Mehan VK, Burgi H, et al: Acute myocardial infarction after wasp stings in a patient with normal coronary arteries. Am Heart J 128: 820, 1994.

564. Lalloo DG, Trevett AJ, Nwokolo N, et al: Electrocardiographic abnormalities in patients bitten by taipans (Oxyuranus scutellatus canni) and other elapid snakes in Papua New Guinea. Trans R Soc Trop Med Hyg 91:53, 1997.

565. Kurnik D, Haviv Y, Kochva E: A snake bite by the burrowing asp, Atractaspis engaddensis. Toxicon 37:223, 1999.

566. Hall JC, Harruff R: Fatal cardiac arrhythmia in a patient with interstitial myocarditis related to chronic arsenic poisoning. South Med J 82:1557, 1989.

Hypersensitivity

567. Getz MA, Subramanian R, Logemann T, et al: Acute necrotizing eosinophilic myocarditis as a manifestation of severe hypersensitivity myocarditis: Antemortem diagnosis and successful treatment. Ann Intern Med 115:201, 1991.

568. Burke AP, Saenger J, Mullick F, et al: Hypersensitivity myocarditis. Arch Pathol Lab Med 115:764, 1991.

569. Webster J, Koch HF: Aspects of tolerability of centrally acting antihypertensive drugs. J Cardiovasc Pharmacol 27 (Suppl 3):S49, 1996.

Giant Cell Myocarditis

570. Garty BZ, Offer I, Livni E, et al: Erythema multiforme and hypersensitivity myocarditis caused by ampicillin. Ann Pharmacother 28:730, 1994.

571. Cooper LT Jr, Berry GJ, Shabetai R: Idiopathic giant-cell myocarditis—natural history and treatment. N Engl J Med 336:1860, 1997.

572. Hyogo M, Kamitani T, Oguni A, et al: Acute necrotizing eosinophilic myocarditis with giant cell infiltration after remission of idiopathic thrombocytopenic purpura. Intern Med 36:894, 1997.

573. Levy NT, Olson LJ, Weyand C, et al: Histologic and cytokine response to immunosuppression in giant-cell myocarditis. Ann Intern Med 128: 648, 1998.

574. Meyer T, Grumbach IM, Kreuzer H, Morguet AJ: Giant cell myocarditis due to coxsackie B2 virus infection. Cardiology 88:296, 1997.

575. Litovsky SH, Burke AP, Virmani R: Giant cell myocarditis: An entity distinct from sarcoidosis characterized by multiphasic myocyte destruction by cytotoxic T cells and histiocytic giant cells. Mod Pathol 9:1126, 1996.

576. Kilgallen CM, Jackson E, Bankoff M, et al: A case of giant cell myocarditis and malignant thymoma: A postmortem diagnosis by needle biopsy. Clin Cardiol 21:48, 1998.

577. Khoury Z, Keren A, Benhorin J, et al: Aborted sudden death in a young patient with isolated granulomatous myocarditis. Eur Heart J 15:397, 1994.

578. Desjardins V, Pelletier G, Leung TK, et al: Successful treatment of severe heart failure caused by idiopathic giant cell myocarditis. Can J Cardiol 8:788, 1992.

579. Nieminen MS, Salminen US, Taskinen E, et al: Treatment of serious heart failure by transplantation in giant cell myocarditis diagnosed by endomyocardial biopsy. J Heart Lung Transplant 13:543, 1994.

579a. Frustaci A, Chimenti C, Pieroni M, Gentiloni N: Giant cell myocarditis responding to immunosuppressive therapy. Chest 117:905, 2000.

580. Laruelle C, Vanhaecke J, van de Werf F, et al: Cardiac transplantation in giant cell myocarditis: A case report. Acta Cardiol 49:279, 1994.

Physical Agents

581. Loyer EM, Delpassand ES: Radiation-induced heart disease: Imaging features. Semin Roentgenol 28:321, 1993.

582. Veeragandham RS, Goldin MD: Surgical management of radiation-induced heart disease. Ann Thorac Surg 65:1014, 1998.

583. Gyenes G, Fornander T, Carlens P, et al: Detection of radiation-induced myocardial damage by technetium-99m sestamibi scintigraphy. Eur J Nucl Med 24:286, 1997.

584. Orzan F, Brusca A, Gaita F, et al: Associated cardiac lesions in patients with radiation-induced complete heart block. Int J Cardiol 39:151, 1993.

585. Dematte JE, O'Mara K, Buescher J, et al: Near-fatal heat stroke during the 1995 heat wave in Chicago. Ann Intern Med 129:173, 1998.

586. Danzl DF, Pozos RS: Accidental hypothermia. N Engl J Med 331:1756, 1994.

587. Walpoth BH, Walpoth-Aslan BN, Mattle HP, et al: Outcome of survivors of accidental deep hypothermia and circulatory arrest treated with extracorporeal blood warming. N Engl J Med 337:1500, 1997.

588. Lazar HL: The treatment of hypothermia. N Engl J Med 337:1545, 1997.

Chapter 49

Primary Tumors of the Heart

WILSON S. COLUCCI · FREDERICK J. SCHOEN

With an incidence of 0.002 to 0.3 percent in autopsy series,[1-7] primary tumors of the heart* are far less common than metastatic tumors to the heart.[8] Benign primary cardiac tumors occur more frequently than malignant ones. The most common cardiac tumor is the myxoma. In a large single-institution series of primary cardiac tumors, comprising 124 cases diagnosed at surgery and autopsy over 40 years (at the University of Minnesota), 42 percent were cardiac myxomas and 16 percent were malignant tumors (sarcomas) (Fig. 49–1).[9] The proportion of myxomas in comparison with other tumors was increased (to 77 percent) when consideration was limited to surgically excised lesions.[9, 10] Before the advent of modern cardiopulmonary bypass surgical techniques, the correct antemortem diagnosis of an intracardiac tumor was largely academic, because effective therapy was not possible. However, now that many cardiac tumors are curable by operation, it is critically important to establish this diagnosis whenever possible. During the past decade, major advances in noninvasive cardiovascular diagnostic techniques—especially echocardiography (see Chap. 7), computed tomography (CT), and magnetic resonance imaging (MRI) (see Chap. 10)—have greatly facilitated this task, and it is now possible safely and readily to screen patients suspected of having a cardiac tumor, in many cases arriving at a definitive diagnosis preoperatively. Nevertheless, a high index of suspicion remains the most important element in diagnosing a cardiac tumor.

CLINICAL PRESENTATION

SYSTEMIC FINDINGS. The cardiac tumor myxoma causes various nonspecific clinical signs and symptoms that often masquerade as many other more common cardiovascular and systemic diseases (Tables 49–1 and 49–2). Cardiac myxoma can produce a broad array of systemic (i.e., noncardiac) findings including fever, cachexia, malaise, arthralgias, Raynaud's phenomenon, rash, clubbing, and episodic bizarre behavior,[11, 12] as well as systemic and pulmonary emboli.[12a] Various laboratory findings have been reported, including hypergammaglobulinemia, elevated erythrocyte sedimentation rate, thrombocytosis, thrombocytopenia, polycythemia, leukocytosis, and anemia. Systemic signs and symptoms frequently resolve when the tumor is removed.

Role of Interleukin-6. The association of constitutional symptoms with cardiac myxoma is likely to be due to the tumor's constitutive synthesis and secretion of interleukin-6 (IL-6),[13-20, 20a] an inflammatory cytokine thought to be a major inducer of the acute phase response, which is associated with fever, leukocytosis, and activation of the complement and clotting cascades.[14] In vitro, IL-6 induces the synthesis of C-reactive protein, serum amyloid A, alpha$_2$-macroglobulin, and fibrinogen by human hepatocytes.[14] High levels of myxoma production of IL-6 may be accompanied by elevated serum concentration in patients who have cardiac myxoma and symptoms characteristic of autoimmune diseases.[18] In some cases, serum IL-6 levels become undetectable and the immunological features resolve on removal of the tumor.[19] Increased titers of antibodies to myocardium[20] and neutrophils[21] have also been found in patients with myxoma and were shown to decline after removal of the tumor. A case of multiple myeloma has been attributed to continuous immunological stimulation by a left atrial myxoma.[22] Because the cardiac findings are nonspecific and may be subtle or absent, it is not unusual for these systemic findings to lead to a diagnosis of collagen-vascular disease, infection, or noncardiac malignant disease.[23-25] Rarely, myxomas may be superinfected by bacteria or fungi.[26-28]

EMBOLIC PHENOMENA. Embolization of tumor fragments or of thrombi from the surface of a tumor is a frequent and often dramatic clinical occurrence.[29-33] Although myxomas are the source of most tumor emboli because of the combination of their friable consistency and intracavitary location (Fig. 49–2), other types of cardiac tumors occasionally may embolize.

The distribution of tumor emboli depends on the location of the tumor and the presence or absence of intracardiac shunts. Left-sided tumors embolize to the systemic circulation, resulting in infarction and hemorrhage of viscera, including the heart,[29] as well as peripheral limb ischemia and vascular aneurysms. The diagnosis of an intracardiac tumor may be made after histological examination of systemic embolic material,[34, 35] and therefore it is of critical importance to make every effort to recover and examine embolic material. In some cases, particularly when petechiae are present, biopsy of skin or muscle[33] can demonstrate intravascular tumor emboli.

Multiple systemic emboli may mimic systemic vasculitis[33] or infective endocarditis, especially when associated with other manifestations of a systemic illness such as fe-

---

*Tumors arising elsewhere in the body and metastasizing to the pericardium and heart are discussed in Chap. 50 (Pericardial Disease) and Chap. 69 (Hematologic-Oncologic Disorders and Heart Disease).

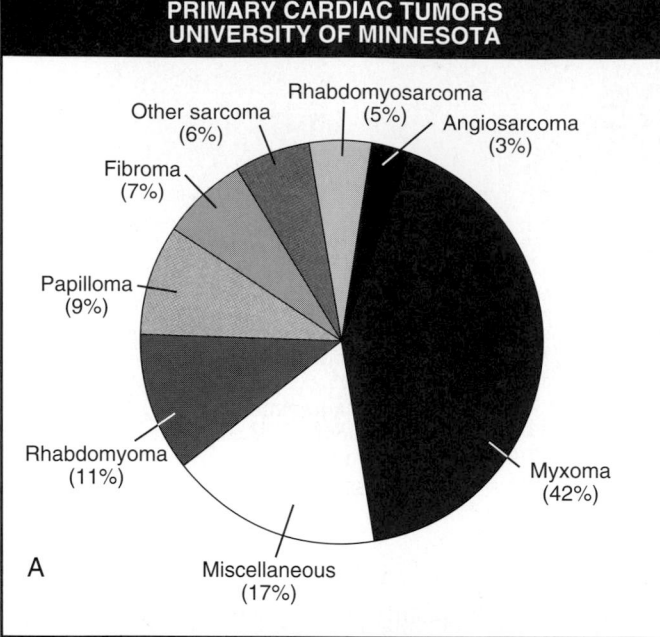

PRIMARY CARDIAC TUMORS
UNIVERSITY OF MINNESOTA

Rhabdomyosarcoma (5%)
Angiosarcoma (3%)
Other sarcoma (6%)
Fibroma (7%)
Papilloma (9%)
Rhabdomyoma (11%)
Miscellaneous (17%)
Myxoma (42%)

A

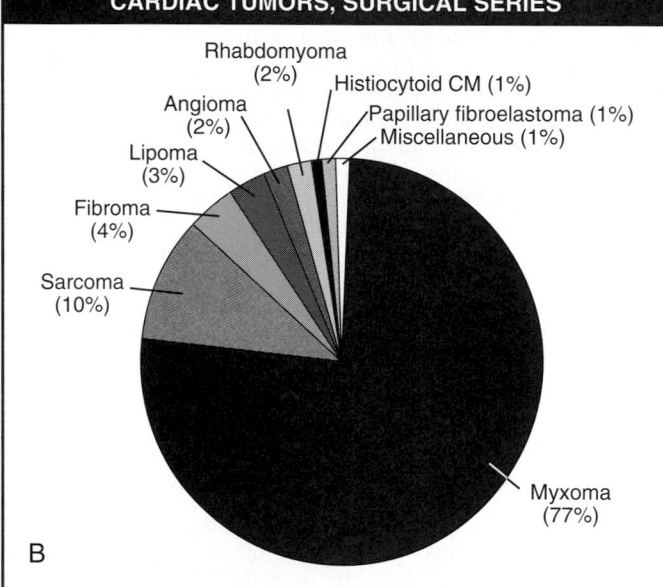

CARDIAC TUMORS, SURGICAL SERIES

Rhabdomyoma (2%)
Histiocytoid CM (1%)
Angioma (2%)
Papillary fibroelastoma (1%)
Miscellaneous (1%)
Lipoma (3%)
Fibroma (4%)
Sarcoma (10%)
Myxoma (77%)

B

FIGURE 49–1. Relative incidence of cardiac tumors. *A,* Incidences of both surgical and autopsy cases are considered. *B,* Relative incidences of only surgical series are considered. When only surgical series are considered, the proportion of myxomas increases. (Adapted from Molina JE, Edwards JE, Ward HB: Primary cardiac tumors: Experience at the University of Minnesota. Thorac Cardiovasc Surg 38:183, 1990.)

ver, weight loss, arthralgias, elevated erythrocyte sedimentation rate, and elevated serum gamma globulins. The finding at angiography of numerous vascular aneurysms secondary to tumor emboli in the cerebral, renal, femoral, and coronary arteries is not infrequent[36] and may lead to the mistaken diagnosis of polyarteritis nodosa.[23] The neurological consequences of embolization include transient ischemic attacks, seizures, syncope, and cerebral, cerebellar, brain stem, spinal cord, or retinal infarction.[37] The neurological event may occasionally be the first or only clinical manifestation of a cardiac tumor. An embolic stroke in a young person without evidence of cerebrovascular disease, particularly in the presence of sinus rhythm, should raise the suspicion of intracardiac myxoma, as well as infective endocarditis and prolapse of the mitral valve.

▼ **TABLE 49–1. SYMPTOMS AND SIGNS OF CARDIAC MYXOMA**

SYMPTOMS	INCIDENCE (%)
Dyspnea on exertion	>75
Paroxysmal dyspnea	~25
Fever	~50
Weight loss	~25
Severe dizziness/syncope	~20
Sudden death	~15
Hemoptysis	~15
SIGNS	**INCIDENCE (%)**
Mitral diastolic murmur	~75
Mitral systolic murmur	~50
Pulmonary hypertension	~70
Right heart failure	~70
Pulmonary emboli	~25
Anemia	>33
Elevated ESR	>33
Third heart sound (tumor plop)	>33
Atrial fibrillation	~15
Elevated globulins	~10
Clubbing	~5
Raynaud's phenomenon	<5

ESR = erythrocyte sedimentation rate.
From Fisher J: Cardiac myxoma. Cardiovasc Rev Rep 9:1195, 1983.

Right-sided cardiac tumors and left-sided cardiac tumors proximal to left-to-right intracardiac shunts may result in pulmonary emboli.[12a, 30, 31] Indeed, serious pulmonary hypertension and secondary cor pulmonale due to chronic recurrent pulmonary emboli from a right atrial myxoma

▼ **TABLE 49–2. CONDITIONS OFTEN CONFUSED WITH ATRIAL MYXOMA**

Left Atrium
Rheumatic mitral valve disease (MS, MR)
Pulmonary hypertension (primary, or secondary to mitral valve disease or LV failure)
Intrinsic lung disease
Cerebrovascular disease (CVA, TIA)
Endocarditis
Rheumatic fever
Myocarditis
Vasculitis (polyarteritis, lupus erythematosus)

Right Atrium
Rheumatic tricuspid valve disease (TS, TR)
Ebstein's anomaly
Atrial septal defect
Pulmonary hypertension
Pulmonary emboli
Constrictive pericarditis
Pleuropericarditis (rub)
Carcinoid heart disease
Cardiomyopathy

Right Ventricle
Pulmonic stenosis
Infundibular stenosis
Pulmonary emboli
Pulmonary hypertension

Left Ventricle
Aortic stenosis
Subaortic stenosis
Cerebrovascular disease
Mural thrombus

MS = mitral stenosis; MR = mitral regurgitation; LV = left ventricular; CVA = cerebrovascular accident; TIA = transient ischemic attack; TS = tricuspid stenosis; TR = tricuspid regurgitation.
From Fisher J: Cardiac myxoma. Cardiovasc Rev Rep 9:1195, 1983.

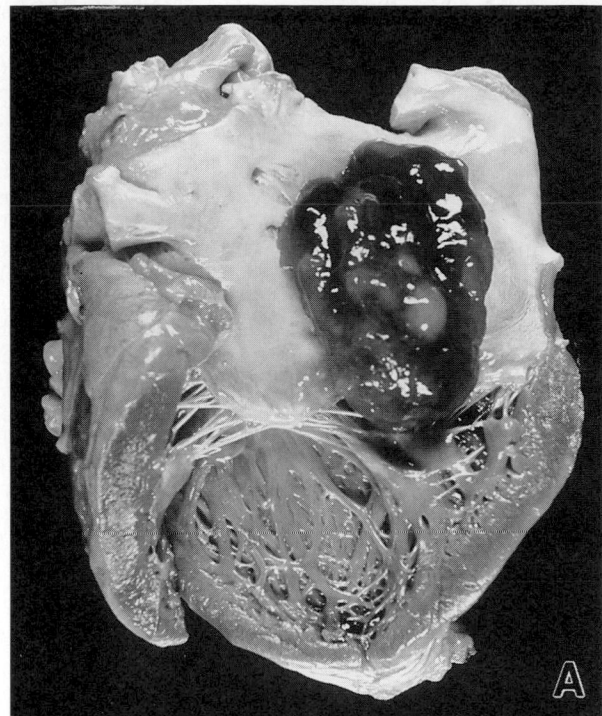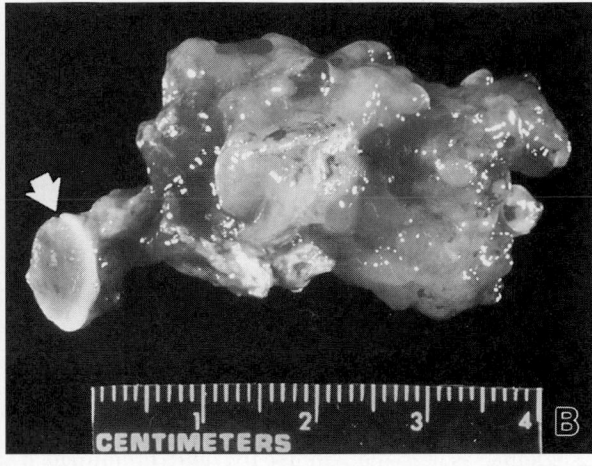

FIGURE 49-2. Photographs of the two most frequent gross appearances of cardiac myxomas. *A,* Polypoid, smooth, round, hemorrhagic left atrial myxoma, noted at autopsy. The tumor mass nearly fills the left atrium and extends into the mitral valve orifice. *B,* irregular gelatinous, friable myxoma mass, surgically removed. The resection margin that surrounds the proximal portion of the stalk is indicated by an arrow. (*A* from Cotran RS, Kumar V, Robbins SL: Robbins' Pathologic Basis of Disease. 5th ed. Philadelphia, WB Saunders, 1994. *B* from Schoen FJ: Interventional and Surgical Cardiovascular Pathology: Clinical Correlations and Basic Principles. Philadelphia, WB Saunders, 1989.)

have been noted.[38] Clinically, the findings may be indistinguishable from pulmonary emboli secondary to venous thromboembolism (see Chap. 52). Although the findings on chest roentgenogram are nonspecific, perfusion lung scanning in such patients may yield results atypical of pulmonary embolism in two respects: (1) The tumor-produced perfusion defects may remain static for long periods, as opposed to typical pulmonary embolic disease in which the defects usually resolve over the course of a few weeks; and (2) flow to one lung may be completely absent while perfusion of the opposite lung is completely normal, a pattern unusual with typical pulmonary emboli.

Cardiac Manifestations

The specific signs and symptoms produced by tumors are more closely related to their precise anatomical location than to their histological types.[39] Thus, it is useful to consider the constellation of findings typical of each location. The presentation of *pericardial tumors* is considered in Chapter 50 and is not discussed here except to point out that primary tumors of the myocardium and endocardium may extend into the pericardial space and produce many of the clinical manifestations of pericardial tumors, including hemorrhagic pericardial effusion and compression of the heart by the effusion or the tumor itself.

MYOCARDIAL TUMORS. When clinically apparent, myocardial tumors most commonly result in disturbances of conduction or rhythm,[40-43] the precise nature of which is determined by the location of the tumor. Thus, tumors in the area of the atrioventricular (AV) node, typically angiomas and mesotheliomas, may produce AV conduction disturbances, including complete heart block, and asystole and can lead to sudden death (see Chap. 26).[40-43] A wide variety of arrhythmias may be produced, including atrial fibril-

lation or flutter, paroxysmal atrial tachycardia with or without block, nodal rhythm, premature ventricular beats, ventricular tachycardia, and ventricular fibrillation (see Chap. 25).[39, 43] Intramural tumors can also produce symptoms by virtue of their size and location. Impairment of ventricular performance may simulate congestive, restrictive, or hypertrophic cardiomyopathy (see Chap. 48). Tumor infiltration of the myocardial wall occasionally causes myocardial rupture.[44]

LEFT ATRIAL TUMORS. Mobile, pedunculated, left atrial tumors may prolapse to various degrees into the mitral valve orifice, resulting in obstruction to AV blood flow and, frequently, mitral regurgitation. The resultant signs and symptoms often mimic those of mitral valve disease[1, 5, 44] (see Table 49-2), especially mitral stenosis (see Chap. 46),[45] and include dyspnea, orthopnea, paroxysmal nocturnal dyspnea, pulmonary edema, cough, hemoptysis, chest pain, peripheral edema, and fatigue. However, weight loss, pallor, syncope, and sudden death—manifestations that are uncommon with mitral valve disease—also occur. It is not unusual for the symptoms to be sudden in onset, intermittent, and related to the patient's body position.[5, 39] Although the majority of symptoms produced by left atrial tumors are nonspecific, the occurrence of paroxysmal symptoms that arise characteristically in a particular body position and are out of proportion to the clinical findings should raise suspicion of a left atrial tumor. The most common primary cardiac tumor presenting in the left atrium is the benign myxoma, which, in the large majority of cases, is solitary.

Physical Examination. The physical examination may disclose signs of pulmonary congestion; an S_4; a loud S_1, which is often widely split; a holosystolic murmur that is loudest at the apex and resembles mitral regurgitation; and a diastolic murmur resulting from obstruction to flow through the mitral orifice produced by the tumor. The loud S_1 that occurs in patients with left atrial myxoma may be due to the late onset of mitral valve closure resulting from prolapse of the tumor through the mitral valve orifice.[46] Consequently, the left ventricular–left atrial pressure cross-over occurs at a higher pressure, as in patients with mitral stenosis or a short PR interval. It has been suggested that the finding of a loud S_1 in the absence of a short PR interval or a mitral diastolic murmur should raise the suspicion of a left atrial tumor.[46] In many cases, an early diastolic sound, termed a *tumor plop,* can be identified. It is thought to be produced as the tumor strikes the endocardial wall or as its excursion is abruptly halted. Although in most cases the tumor plop occurs later than the opening snap of the mitral valve and earlier than the S_3, it is not surprising that this sound is frequently confused with the opening snap or the S_3.

RIGHT ATRIAL TUMORS. Right atrial tumors frequently produce symptoms of right heart failure, including fatigue, peripheral edema, ascites, hepatomegaly, and prominent *a* waves in the jugular vein pulse.[39, 47–50] The average time interval from the symptomatic presentation to the correct diagnosis of right atrial tumor may be years. The development of right-sided heart failure can be rapidly progressive and is often associated with new systolic or diastolic murmurs or both. The murmurs are generally the result of tumor obstruction to tricuspid valve flow or of tricuspid regurgitation caused by tumor interference with valve closure or valve destruction caused directly or indirectly by the tumor.[51] It is not surprising that right atrial tumors have been misdiagnosed as Ebstein's anomaly of the tricuspid valve, constrictive pericarditis, tricuspid stenosis, carcinoid syndrome, superior vena caval syndrome, and cardiomyopathy (see Table 49–2). Pulmonary embolism and pulmonary hypertension occur and may simulate classic thromboembolic disease.[48] Right atrial hypertension may cause right-to-left shunting through a patent foramen ovale, with systemic hypoxia, cyanosis, clubbing, and polycythemia.[50] Whereas myxomas occur much more commonly in the left atrium than in the right atrium, sarcomas occur more commonly in the right atrium.

Physical Examination. The physical examination can reveal peripheral edema, evidence of superior vena cava obstruction, hepatomegaly, and ascites. An early diastolic rumbling murmur, alone or in combination with a holosystolic murmur secondary to tricuspid regurgitation, may demonstrate respiratory or positional variation. Because of the rarity of *isolated* rheumatic tricuspid valvular disease, the lack of other valvular findings should raise the question of a right atrial tumor. A protodiastolic tumor plop has been described and is thought to be similar in etiology to that produced by left atrial tumors.[52] The jugular venous pressure may be elevated, and a prominent *a* wave and steep *y* descent may be present.

RIGHT VENTRICULAR TUMORS. Right ventricular tumors often present with right-sided heart failure as a result of obstruction to right ventricular filling or outflow. Clinical manifestations include peripheral edema, hepatomegaly, ascites, shortness of breath, syncope, and sudden death.

A systolic ejection murmur at the left sternal border is usually found on physical examination. A presystolic murmur and a diastolic rumble[39] have been noted and are thought to be due to obstruction of the tricuspid valve. An S_3 may be audible, and a low-pitched diastolic sound that coincides with the maximal anterior excursion of the tumor has been ascribed either to tumor or to late closure of the pulmonary valve.[53] P_2 is often delayed, and its intensity can be normal, decreased, or increased. Tumor emboli to the pulmonary arteries may result in pulmonary hypertension, and the presence of tumor in the pulmonic valve orifice may lead to pulmonary regurgitation. The jugular veins are frequently distended, with a prominent *a* wave, and may demonstrate Kussmaul's sign (see Chap. 4).

The cardiac findings often lead to a diagnosis of pul-

monic stenosis, restrictive cardiomyopathy, or tricuspid regurgitation. Whereas pulmonic stenosis is often asymptomatic and slowly progressive, the symptoms of right ventricular tumors are often rapidly progressive, and there is no poststenotic dilatation or systolic ejection click.

LEFT VENTRICULAR TUMORS. When left ventricular tumors are predominantly intramural in location, they are often asymptomatic, they can present as conduction disturbances or arrhythmias, or they can interfere with ventricular function. However, when the tumor also has a significant intracavitary component, left ventricular outflow can be obstructed, resulting in syncope and findings consistent with left ventricular failure. Atypical chest pain has also been reported and, in some cases, can reflect obstruction of a coronary artery either directly by tumor involvement or as a result of a tumor embolus to the coronary artery.

Physical Examination. The physical examination reveals a systolic murmur, and both the murmur and the blood pressure may vary with position. Left ventricular tumors may simulate the findings of aortic stenosis, subaortic stenosis, hypertrophic cardiomyopathy, endocardial fibroelastosis, and coronary artery disease.

Benign Versus Malignant Tumors

The types of benign and malignant mesenchymal tumors that can develop in the heart are typical of those occurring in any mass of striated muscle and connective tissue. Although the exact incidence of each specific tumor type cannot be stated, about 75 percent of all cardiac tumors are benign histologically and the remainder are malignant.[1] The majority of benign cardiac tumors are myxomas, followed in frequency by a wide variety of other tumors (Table 49–3). Almost all malignant cardiac tumors are sarcomas, and of these the angiosarcoma and rhabdomyosarcoma are the most common forms (Table 49–4).

Although it is often difficult or impossible to differentiate benign from malignant tumors histologically before operation, certain findings may be helpful. Characteristics suggestive of malignancy include the presence of distant

▼ **TABLE 49–3. RELATIVE INCIDENCE OF BENIGN TUMORS OF THE HEART**

BENIGN TUMOR	% OF GROUP		
	Adults	Children	Infants
Myxoma	46	15	0
Lipoma	21	0	0
Papillary fibroelastoma	16	0	0
Rhabdomyoma	2	46	65
Fibroma	3	15	12
Hemangioma	5	5	4
Teratoma	1	13	18
Mesothelioma of the atrioventricular node	3	4	2
Granular cell tumor	1	0	0
Neurofibroma	1	1	0
Lymphangioma	1	0	0
Hamartoma	0	1	0

Data representing the extensive investigations of the Armed Forces Institute of Pathology as well as the cumulative experience of other researchers. A total of 265, 82, and 49 benign tumors were found in adults (age >16 yr), children (age 1–16 yr), and infants (age <1 yr), respectively. Myxomas were the most common reported benign tumors in adults, whereas rhabdomyomas were the most common benign tumors in both children and infants; benign teratomas also occurred frequently in children and infants.

From Allard MF, Taylor GP, Wilson JE, McManus BM: Primary cardiac tumors. *In* Goldhaber S, Braunwald E (eds): Atlas of Heart Diseases. Philadelphia, Current Medicine, 1995, pp 15.1–15.22.

▼ **TABLE 49–4. RELATIVE INCIDENCE OF PRIMARY MALIGNANT TUMORS OF THE HEART**

TUMOR TYPE	% OF GROUP		
	Adults	Children	Infants
Angiosarcoma	33	0	0
Rhabdomyosarcoma	21	33	66
Mesothelioma	16	0	0
Fibrosarcoma	11	11	33
Malignant lymphoma	6	0	0
Extraskeletal osteosarcoma	4	0	0
Thymoma	3	0	0
Neurogenic sarcoma	3	11	0
Leiomyosarcoma	1	0	0
Liposarcoma	1	0	0
Synovial sarcoma	1	0	0
Malignant teratoma	0	44	0

A total of 117, 9, and 3 malignant tumors were found in adults (age >16 yr), children (age 1–16 yr), and infants (age <1 yr), respectively. Angiosarcomas were the most commonly reported malignant tumors in adults, but rhabdomyosarcomas and mesotheliomas were also relatively common. Malignant teratomas were the most common tumors in children. Rhabdomyosarcomas were the most frequently reported malignant tumors in infants, with fibrosarcomas the second most common.

From Allard MF, Taylor GP, Wilson JE, McManus BM: Primary cardiac tumors. *In* Goldhaber S, Braunwald E (eds): Atlas of Heart Diseases. Philadelphia, Current Medicine, 1995, pp 15.1–15.22.

metastases, local mediastinal invasion, evidence of rapid growth in tumor size, hemorrhagic pericardial effusion, precordial pain, location of the tumor on the right side of the heart or on the atrial free wall, evidence of combined intramural and intracavitary location, and extension into the pulmonary veins. Benign tumors are more likely to occur on the left side of the interatrial septum and to grow slowly. Although benign tumors do not metastasize, distant tumor emboli can mimic peripheral or pulmonary metastases.[54] The preoperative differentiation between benign and malignant tumors can occasionally be made by examination of peripheral tumor emboli recovered by arteriotomy or by biopsy of skin or muscle.[5, 32, 34, 35]

SPECIFIC CARDIAC TUMORS

Benign Tumors

Myxomas

As already pointed out, myxomas are the most common type of primary cardiac tumor, comprising 30 to 50 percent of the total in most pathological series (or higher, when surgically excised tumors are considered).[1–5, 8] The mean age of patients with sporadic myxoma is 56 years, and 70 percent are females. However, myxomas have been described in patients ranging in age from 3 to 83 years and are now not infrequently diagnosed in elderly patients, in whom the symptoms and signs of cardiac tumor may have been attributed to other causes for a substantial time. Approximately 86 percent of myxomas occur in the left atrium, and more than 90 percent are solitary[5, 8] (see Fig. 49–2). In the left atrium, the usual site of attachment is in the area of the fossa ovalis. Myxomas also may occur in the right atrium and, less often, in the right or left ventricle. Several tumors may occur in the same chamber or in a combination of chambers. Although myxomas may occasionally be found on the posterior left atrial wall, tumors presenting in this location should raise the suspicion of malignancy. Myxomas of the mitral and tricuspid valves have been reported.[49, 54]

The clinical signs and symptoms produced by cardiac myxomas include nonspecific manifestations as already discussed, embolization, and mechanical interference with cardiac function (see Table 49–1). Not surprisingly, the symptoms produced by cardiac myxomas may simulate a wide variety of other cardiac and noncardiac conditions (see Table 49–2).

FAMILIAL MYXOMAS. Familial cardiac myxomas constitute approximately 10 percent or less of all myxomas and appear to have an autosomal dominant transmission.[1, 55–57] Some patients with cardiac myxoma have a syndrome, frequently called "syndrome myxoma" or "Carney's syndrome," that also consists of (1) myxomas in other locations (breast or skin), (2) spotty pigmentation (lentigines, pigmented nevi, or both) (Fig. 49–3), and (3) endocrine overactivity (pituitary adenoma, primary pigmented nodular adrenocortical disease, or testicular tumors involving the endocrine components).[58–60; 60a, b] Patients with Carney's syndrome tend to be younger (mean age, 20's), are more likely to have myxomas in locations other than the left atrium, sometimes have bilateral tumors, and are more likely to develop recurrences (Table 49–5).

Although the cause of the syndrome myxoma is unknown, it has been proposed to result from a widespread abnormality resulting in excessive proliferation of certain mesenchymal cells, and excessive glycosaminoglycans production by them, possibly analogous to the neural masses in von Recklinghausen's neurofibromatosis.[61] Patients may have two or more components of this complex, and the first component generally is diagnosed at a relatively young age (mean age, 18 years). Some patients have been said to have the NAME syndrome (*n*evi, *a*trial myxoma, *m*yxoid neurofibroma, *e*phelides)[57, 62] or the LAMB syndrome (*l*entigines, *a*trial *m*yxoma, and *b*lue nevi).[63]

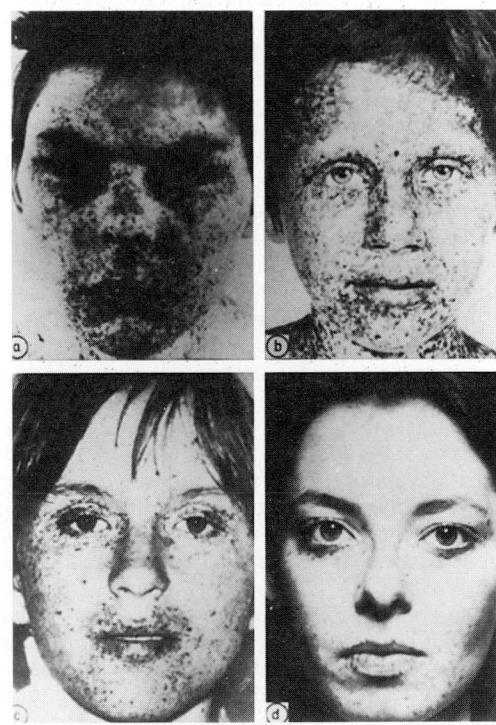

FIGURE 49–3. Four patients with extensive facial freckling, a finding associated with syndrome myxoma. Patients with this syndrome tend to be younger than patients with sporadic myxoma and have a substantially higher incidence of ventricular, multiple, biatrial, recurrent, and familial myxomas of the heart. In addition, these patients, in contrast to patients with sporadic myxoma, may have noncardiac myxomas and endocrine neoplasms. (From Vidaillet HJ Jr, Seward JB, Fyke FE, et al: "Syndrome myxoma": A subset of patients with cardiac myxoma associated with pigmented skin lesions and peripheral and endocrine neoplasms. Br Heart J 57:247, 1987.)

▼ TABLE 49–5. COMPARISON OF THE CLINICAL FEATURES OF SPORADIC MYXOMA AND SYNDROME MYXOMA

FEATURE	SPORADIC	SYNDROME
Age (yr) (range)	56 (39–82)	25 (10–56)
Female/male ratio	2.7 : 1	1.8 : 1
Patients (no.)	70	44
Cardiac myxomas (no.)	72	103
Distributions of myxomas (%)		
Atrial/ventricular	100/0	87/13
Single/multiple	99/1	50/50
Biatrial	0	23
Recurrent	0	18
Familial	0	27
Freckling (%)	0	68
Noncardiac tumors (%)	0	57
Endocrine neoplasm (%)	0	30

From Vidaillet HJ Jr, Seward JB, Fyke FE: "Syndrome myxoma": A subset of patients with cardiac myxoma associated with pigmented skin lesions and peripheral and endocrine neoplasma. Br Heart J 57:247, 1987.

Because cardiac myxomas can be familial, routine echocardiographic screening of first-degree relatives is appropriate, particularly if the patient is young or has many tumors. In one study, screening of families of six patients with familial myxoma yielded four close relatives with cardiac myxoma.[64] Moreover, in patients who have a familial history or other components of the previously described syndrome and who are undergoing resection, a careful search should be made preoperatively for several cardiac myxomas. Postoperatively, these patients should be observed closely for the development of other tumors; this occurs in 12 to 22 percent of such patients.[65] The pathological features of familial myxomas do not differ from those occurring sporadically (discussed later).[66]

PATHOLOGY. Most cardiac myxomas are received by the pathologist as surgically excised specimens that have been removed because of clinical symptoms. Rarely, cardiac myxomas are encountered incidentally at autopsy. The pathological characteristics of myxomas are well described and are independent of location.[1, 54, 67–69]

Gross Pathology. Myxomas are gelatinous (often termed myxoid), smooth, and round, with a glistening surface, or they may be variably friable and either irregular or polypoid (see Fig. 49–3). They are either sessile or pedunculated with a distinct stalk, which may be narrow or broad. In approximately 90 percent of cases arising in the atria, the base of attachment is the atrial septum, usually in the region of the limbus of the fossa ovalis. In approximately 10 percent of cases, the point of origin is the posterior or anterior atrial wall or atrial appendage; valvular myxomas are rare. Cardiac myxomas can be multicentric. Areas of hemorrhage are frequent. The tumors average 4 to 8 cm in diameter but range from less than 1 cm to 15 cm or greater.

Histology. The diagnosis of myxoma is made by the observation of characteristic patterns of cells (often called "lipidic" cells) embedded in a myxoid stroma rich in glycosaminoglycans (Fig. 49–4).[67–69] Myxoma cells have a round, elongated, or polyhedral shape; scant pink cytoplasm; and an ovoid nucleus with an open chromatin pattern. They are occasionally multinuclear. Although they may be present individually, myxoma cells are typically present as cords, rings, or florets, sometimes as many layers surrounding vascular structures. Diagnosis of myxoma requires the presence of characteristic isolated or clustered collections of myxoma cells. Hemorrhages; macrophages; often containing iron pigment; lymphocytes; and plasma cells are variably present. Calcification is present in approximately 10 to 20 percent of cardiac myxomas. Extramedullary hematopoiesis, which comprises glandular structures

lined by mucin-filled goblet cells,[70] and cellular atypia may be present in a minority of cases; these features may simulate malignancy. Because emboli from myxomas usually derive from the most superficial portions, they may have less definitive histological features than the intracardiac lesion from which they originated.

Ultrastructural and Immunohistochemical Findings. Myxoma cells have abundant fine cytoplasmic filaments similar to those of smooth muscle cells.[69] The cells most resemble embryonic mesenchymal cells with multipotential capabilities for cellular differentiation, including vasoformative activity and expression of vascular endothelial growth factor,[69a] and are especially similar to embryonic endocardial cushion tissue.[71] Immunohistochemical studies demonstrate variable positivity for the endothelial cell markers factor VIII–related antigen and Ulex europaeus. More consistent positivity is obtained when myxomas are stained for vimentin, indicative of the mesenchymal derivation of the cells, as well as some neuroendocrine markers and smooth muscle cell antigens. Analysis by immunohistochemistry has not been useful for either diagnostic purposes or elucidation of histogenesis.

Embolization. Although myxomas or other benign cardiac tumors can cause death due to coronary or cerebral embolization,[72] metastatic tumor implantation with wasting is rare. Occasional reports suggest that myxomas may have a malignant counterpart, with local invasion of the interatrial septum, recurrence, or metastasis.[72a] However, some cases of purported malignancy probably represent malignant tumors of other types with extensive areas of myxoid degeneration or of multicentricity that was not appreciated; others may represent inadequate excision or embolization of benign lesions.

Many of the morphological features of organizing mural thrombi resemble those of myxoma, including abundant loose amorphous extracellular matrix, connective tissue cells, and small vascular channels. It is difficult to distinguish between some myxomas and mural thrombi in various stages of organization; indeed, cellular intracardiac thrombi and peripheral thromboemboli occasionally receive an erroneous diagnosis of myxoma. The resemblance to organizing/organized thrombi has been put forth as evidence that myxomas have a thrombotic origin,[73] but most investigators currently find this notion untenable.[67, 71]

Histogenesis. The histogenesis of cardiac myxomas is uncertain, but the weight of evidence favors benign neoplasia, with the tumor probably originating from subendocardial nests of primitive mesenchymal cells that may differentiate into several cell types, including endothelial and lipidic cells. Cytogenetic analyses demonstrating clonal chromosomal abnormalities provide the best support for this concept. Sporadic and familial atrial myxomas have been shown to have heterogeneous clonal telomeric rearrangements and other chromosome abnormalities primarily involving chromosomes 2, 12, and 17; a telomeric association between chromosomes 13 and 15, a rearrangement in 1q32, and loss of the Y chromosome have also been reported.[74–80] Linkage analysis of 11 kindreds affected by Carney's syndrome yielded a chromosomal locus for this disorder mapping to the short arm of chromosome 2 within a 6.4-cM interval (2p16).[74] A gene defect on chromosome 17q (17q2) was associated with Carney's complex in four unrelated families.[76] A most convincing case of clonal structural aberrations was reported by Dijkhuizen and colleagues[80] who found that a cardiac myxoma from a 48-year-old man had normal chromosome number but a complex clonal rearrangement, which included a breakpoint at 12p12, the location of the Ki-ras oncogene. The researchers speculated that Ki-ras might have a role in the origin of cardiac myxoma. Although myocardial hypertrophy and failure as well as endocrine abnormalities such as pituitary and thyroid tumors have been associated with alterations in the hetero-

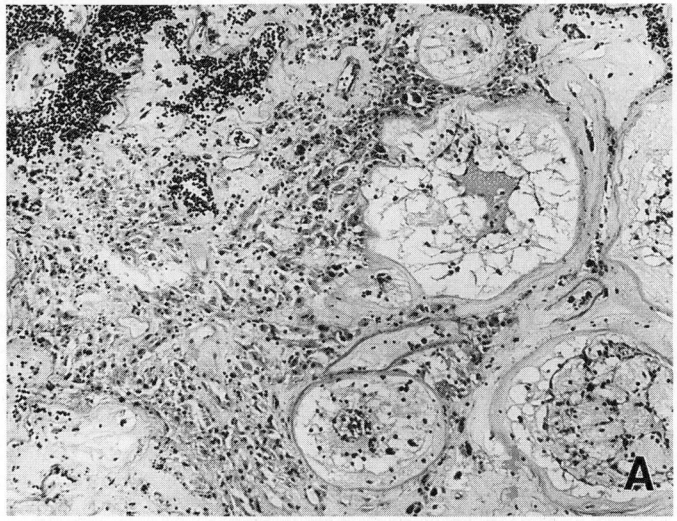

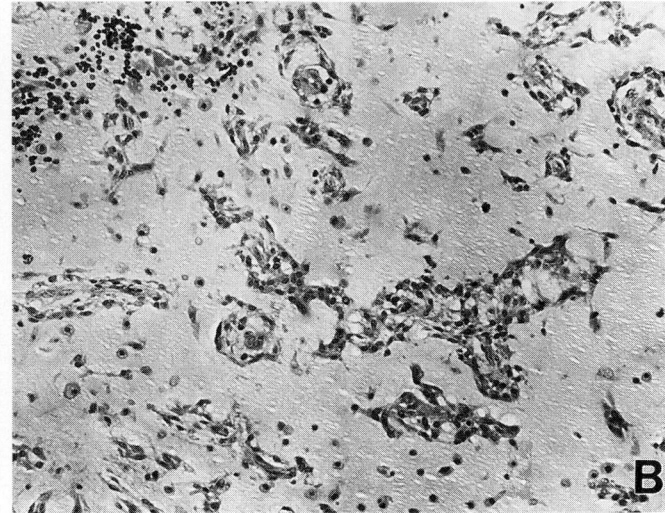

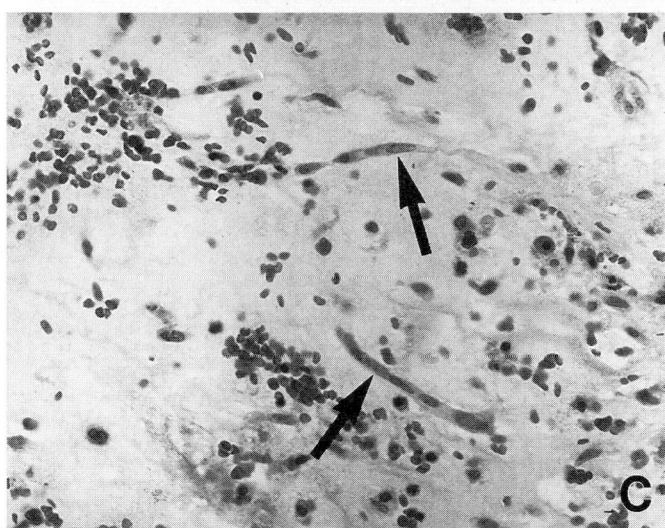

FIGURE 49–4. Characteristic histological features of myxoma. *A,* Low-power view demonstrating individual tumor cells, clusters, and islands scattered throughout the characteristic pale-staining granular extracellular matrix. Hemorrhage is present at upper left. Scattered inflammatory cells are also present. *B,* Medium-power view, demonstrating groups of polygonal myxoma cells. *C,* High-magnification view, showing individual variably rounded to elongated myxoma cells, some arranged in cords (arrows). *A,* 50×; *B,* 175×; *C,* 400×; all stained with hematoxylin and eosin.

trimeric guanosine triphosphate–binding proteins, activating Gsα mutations have not been found in either atrial myxomas or other tumors from patients with Carney's complex.[81] The presence of aneuploidy in some cardiac myxomas provides additional support for the concept of a neoplastic origin.[82]

Before the discussion of nonmyxomatous cardiac tumors is continued later, it should be noted that peculiar microscopic-sized cellular cardiac lesions have been noted incidentally as part of endomyocardial biopsy or surgically removed tissue specimens or at cardiac surgery; these lesions are free floating or loosely attached to a valvular or endocardial mass.[83, 84] Not neoplastic, they have been termed mesothelial monocytic incidental cardiac excrescences (MICE). Histologically, such lesions are composed largely of clusters and ribbons of mesothelial cells and entrapped erythrocytes and leukocytes embedded within a fibrin mesh. Previously considered to be a reactive mesothelial and/or monocytic (histiocytic) hyperplasia, they are now considered to be common artifacts—formed by compaction of mesothelial strips (likely from the pericardium) or other tissue debris and fibrin that are transported via catheters or around an operative site on a cardiotomy suction tip.[85] Such tissue fragments are of importance only in that they should not be confused with metastatic carcinoma.

PAPILLARY TUMORS OF HEART VALVES (PAPILLARY FIBROELASTOMA).

The most common tumors of the cardiac valves, papillary fibroelastomas of the cardiac valves and adjacent endocardium, are not uncommonly found postmortem and may be identified during life by two-dimensional echocardiography.[86, 87] Although many are clinically insignificant, they have the potential to embolize to vital structures[88, 89] or to cause valvular dysfunction, and those on the aortic valve can partially obstruct a coronary arterial orifice.[90] These lesions have a characteristic frondlike appearance resembling a sea anemone. They may be single or numerous; up to 3 or 4 cm in diameter; and occur on any valve or on papillary muscle, chordae tendineae, or endocardium, usually attached by a short pedicle (Fig. 49–5). Most often, the ventricular surface of semilunar valves and the atrial surface of AV valves are affected. The tricuspid valve is most commonly involved in children, and the mitral and aortic valves in adults. Histologically, the tumor is covered by endothelium that surrounds a core of loose connective tissue rich in glycosaminoglycans, collagen, and elastic fibers and containing smooth muscle cells (often as a fine meshwork surrounding a central collagen or dense elastic fiber core).

Pathogenesis. The pathogenesis of these lesions is uncertain, but it appears that they may originate secondary to endocardial trauma and/or the organization of mural thrombi.[73] Papillary tumors are generally distinguished from Lambi's excrescences, which are acellular deposits of thrombus and connective tissue covered by a single layer of endothelium and are found on heart valves at the site of endothelial damage in many adults, particularly along the closure margins of the aortic valve cusps. In contrast, papillary fibroelastomas are unusually found at valvular contact areas.

RHABDOMYOMAS. These are the most common cardiac tumors of infants and children; approximately three-fourths occur in patients younger than 1 year.[91, 92] They occur with equal frequency in the left and right ventricular and septal myocardium; nearly all are multiple. Approximately one-third also involve either one or both atria. In approximately half of affected patients, at least one of the tumors is intracavitary and obstructive. Nonspecific clinical manifestations, including cardiomegaly; right or left ventricular failure or both; and an S_3, S_4, and systolic or diastolic murmurs, may mimic mitral stenosis, mitral atresia, aortic stenosis, subaortic stenosis, or infundibular pulmonic stenosis.

Association with Tuberous Sclerosis. Rhabdomyomas are strongly associated with tuberous sclerosis, a familial syndrome characterized by hamartomas in several organs, epilepsy, mental deficiency, and adenoma sebaceum.[93–95] One study indicated that at least 80 percent

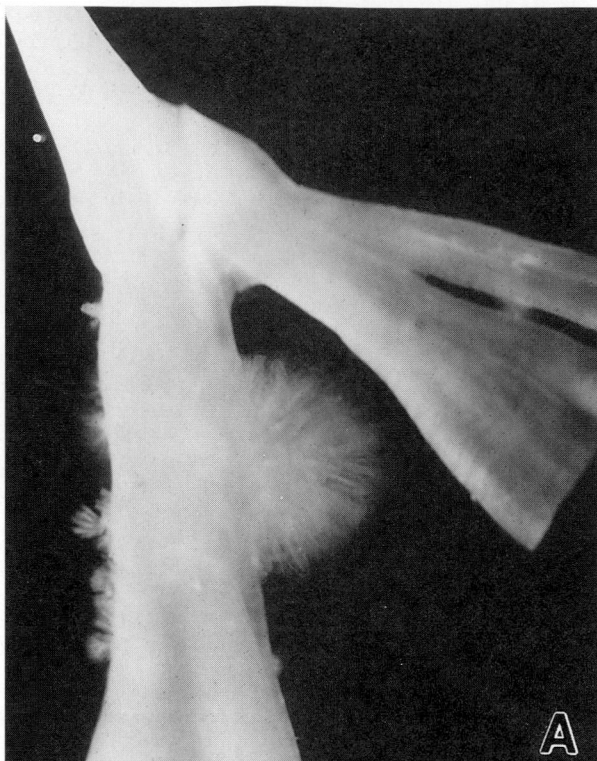 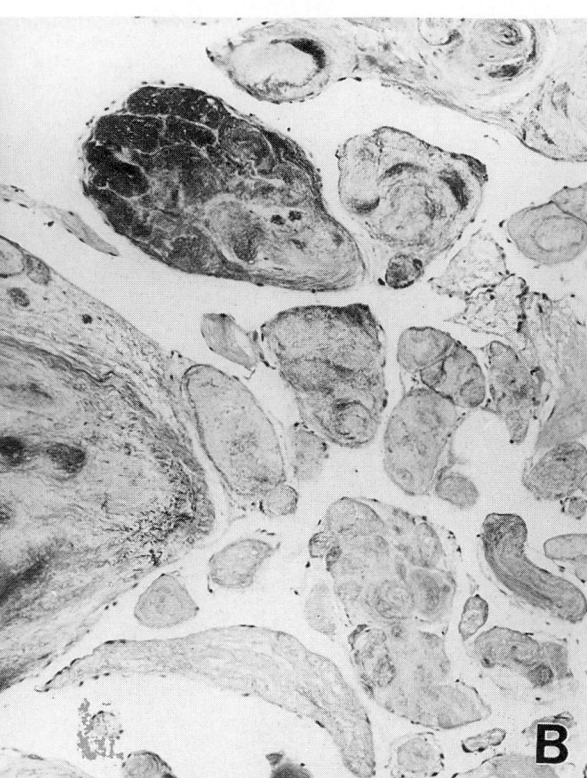

FIGURE 49–5. Papillary fibroelastoma. *A*, Gross photograph demonstrating resemblance of this lesion to a sea anemone, with myriad papillary fronds, arising from the chordae tendineae near the mitral leaflet. In this case, many lesions were present, all associated with the mitral valve apparatus. *B*, Histological appearance of papillary fibroelastoma, demonstrating the numerous papillary fronds consisting of a collagen core surrounded by elastic fibers and loose connective tissue, all covered by endocardial endothelium. 100×; stained with elastica van Gieson stain (elastin black).

of patients with cardiac rhabdomyomas have tuberous sclerosis, and 60 percent of patients less than 18 years old with tuberous sclerosis have cardiac rhabdomyomas.[95] Conversely, approximately 50 percent or more of patients having tuberous sclerosis but no signs or symptoms of cardiac disease have been shown to have echocardiographic findings that are consistent with one or more rhabdomyomas. Rhabdomyomas causing significant intracavity obstruction may result in death within the first 24 hours of life, whereas patients with less severe involvement may either remain asymptomatic or have difficulty during infancy or early childhood.

Pathology. Rhabdomyomas are yellow-gray and range from 1 mm to several centimeters in diameter. They are circumscribed but not encapsulated; microscopically, they are easily distinguished from the surrounding myocardium as clusters of abnormal cells. The microscopic hallmark, termed the *spider cell,* is a large (up to 80-μm diameter) cell containing a central cytoplasmic mass that is suspended by fine fibrillar processes radiating to the periphery, thus giving the appearance of a spider hanging in a net. Such cells are sufficiently characteristic that the tumor may be diagnosed by fine-needle aspiration.[96] The cytoplasm is rich in glycogen and stains positively with periodic acid–Schiff reagent. Electron microscopy demonstrates myofibrils, cytoplasmic and mitochondrial glycogen, and apparent intercellular junctions similar to intercalated discs. Immunohistochemistry reveals diffuse positivity for myoglobin, actin, desmin, and vimentin and the absence of neuroendocrine markers, similar to the staining pattern of the adjacent cardiac muscle. Evidence suggests that rhabdomyomas are actually myocardial hamartomas or malformations rather than true neoplasms. In support of this concept is their multiple occurrence and preponderance in children, especially in those with tuberous sclerosis.

FIBROMAS. Fibromas are benign connective tissue tumors that occur predominantly in children and constitute the second most common type of primary cardiac tumor occurring in the pediatric age group.[97] The majority occur before the age of 10 years, and about 40 percent are diagnosed in infants younger than 1 year. Males and females appear to be equally affected. Derived from fibroblasts and considered low-grade connective tissue tumors, cardiac fibromas resemble and have the same biological behavior as soft tissue fibromatoses at other sites.

Pathology. Almost all cardiac fibromas occur within the ventricular myocardium, most frequently within the anterior free wall of the left ventricle or the interventricular septum and much less often in the posterior left ventricular wall or right ventricle. They typically are gray, firm, circumscribed, and not encapsulated and range in size

from 3 to 10 cm. Grossly, they exhibit a whoried appearance on cut sections. Microscopically, cardiac fibromas consist of elongated fibroblasts admixed with fibrous tissue consisting mostly of collagen. Their cellularity is variable, and mitotic figures are rarely, if ever, seen. Fibrous tissue is intermingled with adjacent myocardial fibers at the margins of the lesion. Calcification and islands of bone formation may be seen microscopically and occasionally radiographically. The *Gorlin syndrome,* the main features of which are multiple nevoid basal cell carcinomas, cysts of the jaw, and skeletal abnormalities, may be associated in some cases with cardiac tumors, either fibromas or fibrous histiocytomas.[98]

Clinical Manifestations. Although fibromas may be incidental findings at postmortem examination, approximately 70 percent at some time cause mechanical interference with intracardiac flow, ventricular contraction abnormalities, or conduction disturbances. Clinical manifestations are protean and include murmurs, atypical chest pain, congestive heart failure and signs of subaortic stenosis, valvular or infundibular pulmonic stenosis with right ventricular hypertrophy, tricuspid stenosis, conduction disturbances, ventricular tachycardia, and sudden death. As in the case of rhabdomyomas, the increased use of echocardiography has rarely resulted in the detection of cardiac fibromas in patients without cardiac signs or symptoms. Surgical excision of cardiac fibromas may be possible.[99, 100]

LIPOMAS AND LIPOMATOUS HYPERTROPHY OF THE ATRIAL SEPTUM. Lipomas occur at all ages and with equal frequency in both sexes. Most range in diameter from 1 to 15 cm, although some have been reported to weigh more than 2 kg. Most tumors are sessile or polypoid and occur in the subendocardium or subpericardium, although about one-fourth are completely intramuscular. Subendocardial tumors with intracavity extension produce symptoms that are characteristic of their location, whereas subepicardial tumors may cause compression of the heart and pericardial effusion. The most common chambers affected are the left ventricle, right atrium, and interatrial septum. Intramural tumors may be asymptomatic or result in arrhythmias, AV or intraventricular conduction disturbances, or mechanical interference. Many tumors are clinically silent, however, and are found only at autopsy or become apparent on a routine chest roentgenogram.

Microscopically, the lesions are usually well encapsulated and composed of typical mature fat cells; they occasionally contain fibrous connective tissue (fibrolipoma), muscular tissue (myolipoma), or vacuolated brown (fetal) fat, resembling a hibernoma.

Whereas lipomas are true neoplasms, a condition termed *lipomatous hypertrophy of the interatrial septum* represents the occurrence of a nonencapsulated hyperplastic accumulation of mature and fetal adipose tissue within the interatrial septum. These lesions range from 1 to 7 cm in dimension, most often protrude into the right atrium, and are more common in obese, elderly, or female patients.[101] Various atrial arrhythmias have been attributed to these lesions, but a cause-and-effect relationship has been difficult to establish.[101] Because this lesion may occasionally be detected by cineangiography, echocardiography, CT, or other diagnostic techniques, the major clinical dilemma is the differential diagnosis and treatment of an intraatrial filling defect.

ANGIOMAS. Composed of benign proliferations of endothelial cells, hemangiomas and lymphangiomas are extremely rare.[102] Anatomically, they may occur in any part of the heart, but usually they are intramural, often in the interventricular septum or AV node, where they may cause complete heart block and sudden death. Cardiac tamponade due to hemopericardium may be the presenting clinical syndrome. More commonly found in the right heart chambers, hemangiomas are red, hemorrhagic, generally sessile or polypoid subendocardial nodules, ranging from 2 to 4 cm in diameter. Histologically, the tumors consist of endothelium-lined spaces that may contain blood, lymph, or thrombi; they are classified according to the predominant type of proliferating vascular channel. Dilated, often thrombosed, subendocardial blood vessels (varices) are frequently mistaken for hemangiomas; they are usually found incidentally.

TERATOMAS. These tumors, which contain elements of all three germ cell layers, occur within the heart less frequently than in the anterior mediastinum.[103] Teratomas are generally observed in children, and when located within the heart, they occur predominantly within the right atrium, right ventricle, or the interatrial or interventricular septum.

CYSTIC TUMOR ("MESOTHELIOMA") OF THE ATRIOVENTRICULAR NODE. Of controversial histogenesis, these small tumors (usually < 15 mm in largest dimension) frequently cause death by complete heart block, ventricular fibrillation,[41] or cardiac tamponade.[104] They occur in patients of virtually any age as poorly circumscribed, often multicystic nodules in the atrial septum, immediately cephalad to the commissure of the septal and anterior leaflets of the tricuspid valve, in the region of the AV node. These lesions are characterized by tubules and cysts lined by flat or cuboidal cells that are devoid of mitotic activity but may have secretory function. Although they are often considered to be derived from mesothelial rests, similar to the adenomatoid tumors of the ovary and testis that they resemble histologically, studies have suggested an endodermal rather than mesothelial origin.[105, 106]

ENDOCRINE TUMORS OF THE HEART. Approximately 2 percent of *paragangliomas* are intrathoracic, and of these, most are located in the posterior mediastinum. However, these tumors can also occur in close association with the left atrial or left ventricular epicardium, where they are thought to have arisen from sympathetic fibers to the heart or from ectopic chromaffin cells. More rarely still, paragangliomas may arise within the interatrial septum. Tumors in any of these locations may secrete catecholamines and therefore can be associated with signs and symptoms characteristic of pheochromocytoma.[107]

Rarely, benign *thyroid tumors* arise within the heart, presumably from ectopic rests of thyroid tissue.[107a] These tumors most often arise from the interventricular septum and present, not infrequently, as obstruction to right ventricular outflow.

Malignant Cardiac Tumors

About one-fourth of all cardiac tumors exhibit malignant histological characteristics and invasive or metastatic behavior. Nearly all of these are sarcomas, thus making these tumors second only to myxomas in overall frequency. Sarcomas may occur at any age but are most common between the third and fifth decades; they are distinctly unusual in infants and children and show no sex preference. In decreasing order of frequency, the sites involved are the right atrium, left atrium, right ventricle, left ventricle, and interventricular septum.

Sarcomas derive from mesenchyme and therefore may display a wide variety of morphological types, including angiosarcoma, rhabdomyosarcoma, fibrosarcoma, osteosarcoma, and others.[108–110]

From a clinical viewpoint, sarcomas characteristically display a rapid downhill course. Death most often occurs from a few weeks to 2 years after the onset of symptoms. These tumors proliferate rapidly and generally cause death through widespread infiltration of the myocardium, obstruction of flow within the heart, or distant metastases. About 75 percent of all patients with cardiac sarcomas have pathological evidence of distant metastases at the time of death.[111, 112] The most frequent sites are the lungs, thoracic lymph nodes, mediastinum, and vertebral column; the liver, kidneys, adrenals, pancreas, bone, spleen, and bowel are less often involved.

The cardiac findings are determined primarily by the location of the tumor and by the extent of intracavitary obstruction. Typical presentations include progressive, unexplained congestive heart failure, particularly of the right side; precordial pain; pericardial effusion; tamponade; arrhythmias; conduction disturbances; obstruction of the venae cavae; and sudden death. Tumors limited to the myocardium without intracavitary extension may produce no cardiac symptoms or may cause arrhythmias and conduction disturbances. Because of the rapid growth potential of sarcomas, they commonly extend into the cardiac chambers, the pericardial space, or both. In about 20 percent of cases, the tumor is sessile or polypoid. When there is extension into the pericardial space, hemorrhagic pericardial effusion is common and tamponade may occur. Because the right side of the heart is most commonly affected, sarcomas frequently cause signs of right-sided heart failure as a result of obstruction of the right atrium, right ventricle, or tricuspid or pulmonic valves. In addition, obstruction of the superior vena cava may result in swelling of the face and upper extremities, whereas obstruction of the inferior vena cava may result in visceral congestion.

ANGIOSARCOMAS. Included within this category are angiosarcomas and Kaposi's sarcomas.[113, 114, 114a, 114b] All 40 patients in one series were adults. In distinction to most other cardiac sarcomas, in which the sex distribution is equal, there appears to be a 2:1 male-to-female ratio among patients with angiosarcomas. These tumors have a striking predilection for the right atrium (Fig. 49–6) and may be infiltrative or polypoid in nature. Microscopically, angiosarcomas are characterized by ill-defined but variable anastomotic vascular channels lined with atypical, often heaped-up, endothelial cells. By electron microscopy, immature endothelial cells, primitive pericytes, and undifferentiated mesenchymal cells may be identified.[115]

RHABDOMYOSARCOMAS. These tumors of striated muscle often diffusely infiltrate the myocardium but may also, on occasion, form a

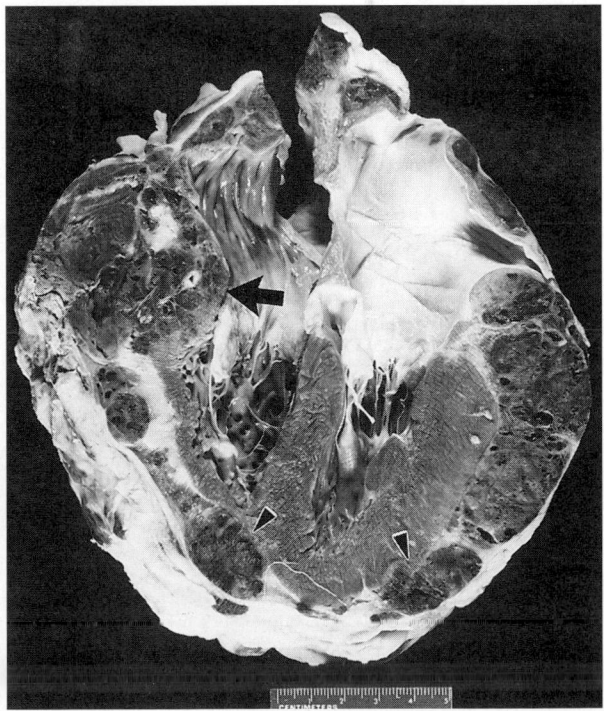

FIGURE 49–6. Massive pericardial angiosarcoma, with deep myocardial invasion at several sites (arrowheads), particularly at the right atrium (arrow). (From Schoen FJ: Interventional and Surgical Cardiovascular Pathology: Clinical Correlations and Basic Principles. Philadelphia, WB Saunders, 1989.)

polypoid extension into the cardiac chambers and therefore have been clinically mistaken for myxoma.[116] Rhabdomyoblasts (cross-striations by light microscopy; thick and thin filaments and Z-band material by electron microscopy) are the histological hallmark of this tumor, and 20 to 30 percent of the tumors have cross-striations.

FIBROSARCOMAS AND MALIGNANT FIBROUS HISTIOCYTOMAS. Fibrosarcomas of the heart have a whitish, soft "fish flesh" consistency characteristic of these tumor types elsewhere in the body.[117] Fibroblastic in differentiation, they are composed of spindle-shaped cells with elongated blunt-ended nuclei and frequent mitoses. They may contain areas of hemorrhage and necrosis and extensively infiltrate the heart, often involving more than one cardiac chamber. A thrombus may form in an obstructed pulmonary vein, in the vena cava, or over the mural surface of the tumor.

LYMPHOMAS. Although cardiac involvement of a systemic lymphoma has been reported in 25 to 36 percent of cases, primary lymphoma involving only the heart or pericardium is much less common.[116, 118] Myocardial infiltration by lymphoma may be nodular or diffuse, and the clinical syndrome of hypertrophic cardiomyopathy has been mimicked. Some of these tumors are predominantly intracavitary.

PULMONARY ARTERY SARCOMAS. Sarcomas of the pulmonary artery trunk, main branches, or pulmonic valves may present as tumor emboli to the lungs or as right ventricular outflow obstruction.[119] These tumors usually present after the fourth decade, show a 2:1 female predominance, and may originate from undifferentiated tissue of the bulbis cordis. Typical symptoms include dyspnea, chest pain, cough, and hemoptysis and may be associated with radiographic findings of a pulmonary hilar mass or cardiomegaly. Right ventricular injection of contrast material helps to delineate the tumor. Although most reported cases were previously diagnosed at autopsy, it is likely that early diagnosis, surgical resection, and possibly chemotherapy may have an impact on survival of future patients with this tumor.[120]

DIAGNOSTIC TECHNIQUES

Although certain clinical manifestations can be suggestive of a cardiac tumor, no clinical finding or set of findings is pathognomonic. Furthermore, the majority of cardiac tumors produce signs and symptoms typical of the common forms of heart disease. The development of modern diagnostic methods has had a major impact on the diagnosis and hence the natural history of cardiac tumors. It is not unusual for cardiac tumors to be diagnosed and cured in patients who are totally asymptomatic or without signs of cardiovascular disease.[121] Although cardiac catheterization made possible the definitive preoperative diagnosis of cardiac tumors, it was not until the advent of echocardiography that it was feasible to evaluate all patients suspected of having this diagnosis. Both M-mode and two-dimensional echocardiography are effective screening techniques. However, two-dimensional echocardiography, and particularly transesophageal imaging (Fig. 49–7), is more sensitive and provides considerably more information about the site of tumor attachment, pattern of tumor movement, and size. In many centers, the information provided by two-dimensional echocardiography (see Chap. 7), CT, or MRI (see Chap. 10) (Fig. 49–8) is considered sufficient to proceed directly to surgery without cardiac catheterization and angiography. However, catheterization and angiography should not be omitted in the absence of a technically adequate two-dimensional echocardiographic study, CT, or MRI that has visualized all four cardiac chambers.

It is imperative that noninvasive evaluation, preferably by two-dimensional echocardiography (or CT or MRI), be performed before cardiac catheterization whenever the diagnosis of cardiac tumor is considered. When left atrial myxoma is suspected, it is safest to visualize the left atrium by injecting the contrast agent into the pulmonary artery and film during the levophase. It is particularly important to avoid the transseptal approach, because this risks dislodgement of fragments of tumor that may be attached in the region of the fossa ovalis. Furthermore, because cardiac tumors may be numerous and present in more than one chamber, all four chambers should be visualized noninvasively before cardiac catheterization whenever possible.

Clinical and Noninvasive Methods

CLINICAL EXAMINATION. When valvular or myocardial disease is suspected on clinical grounds, certain atypical findings can raise the suspicion of cardiac tumor. The intensity of the systolic or diastolic murmur caused by a left atrial myxoma is often exquisitely sensitive to positional change, a finding atypical of valvular heart disease. S_1 may be delayed as a consequence of an elevated left atrial pressure, as in mitral stenosis. It is often intense and widely split, and an early systolic sound may occur, representing tumor movement toward the atrium during systole. In addition, a tumor plop may be present about 100 msec after S_2; it appears to result from the sudden tension of the tumor stalk as it prolapses into the left ventricle during diastole or from the tumor striking the myocardium. The tumor plop *precedes* the end of the rapid filling wave of the apexcardiogram and can thereby be differentiated from an S_3; as noted, it usually occurs later than an opening snap. Systolic time intervals are usually consistent with a reduced stroke

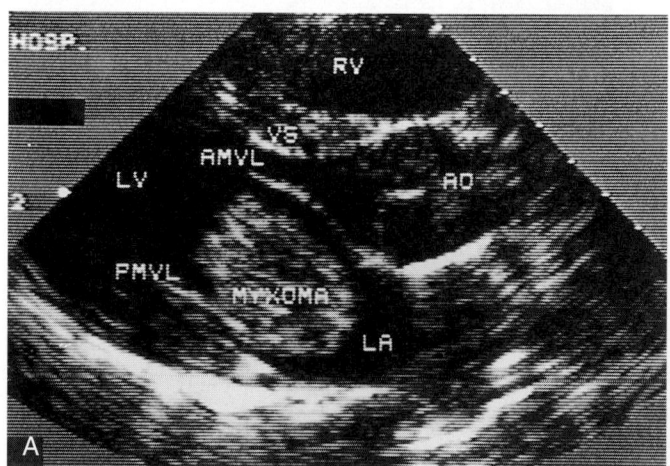
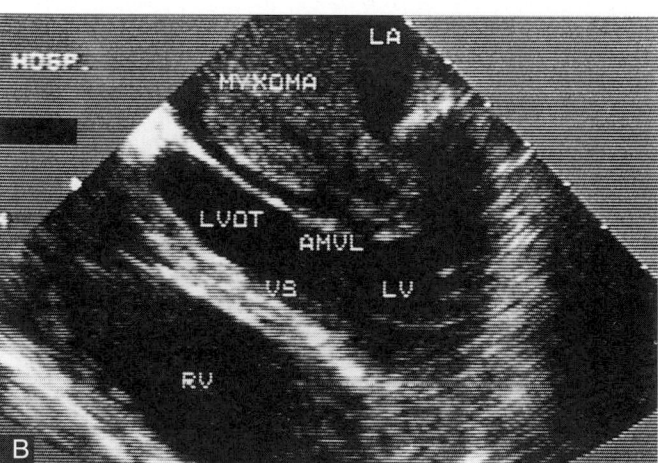

FIGURE 49–7. Transthoracic two-dimensional echocardiogram *(A)* and transesophageal two-dimensional echocardiogram *(B)* showing a left atrial (LA) mass prolapsing into and obstructing the mitral valve orifice. Note the superior resolution of the transesophageal echocardiogram. Although not visible here, the myxoma was attached to the midportion of the atrial septum. (From Allard MF, Taylor GP, Wilson JE, McManus BM: Primary cardiac tumors. *In* Goldhaber SZ, Braunwald E [eds]: Cardiopulmonary Diseases and Cardiac Tumors. Atlas of Heart Diseases. Vol 3. Philadelphia, Current Medicine, 1995, pp 15.1–15.22.)

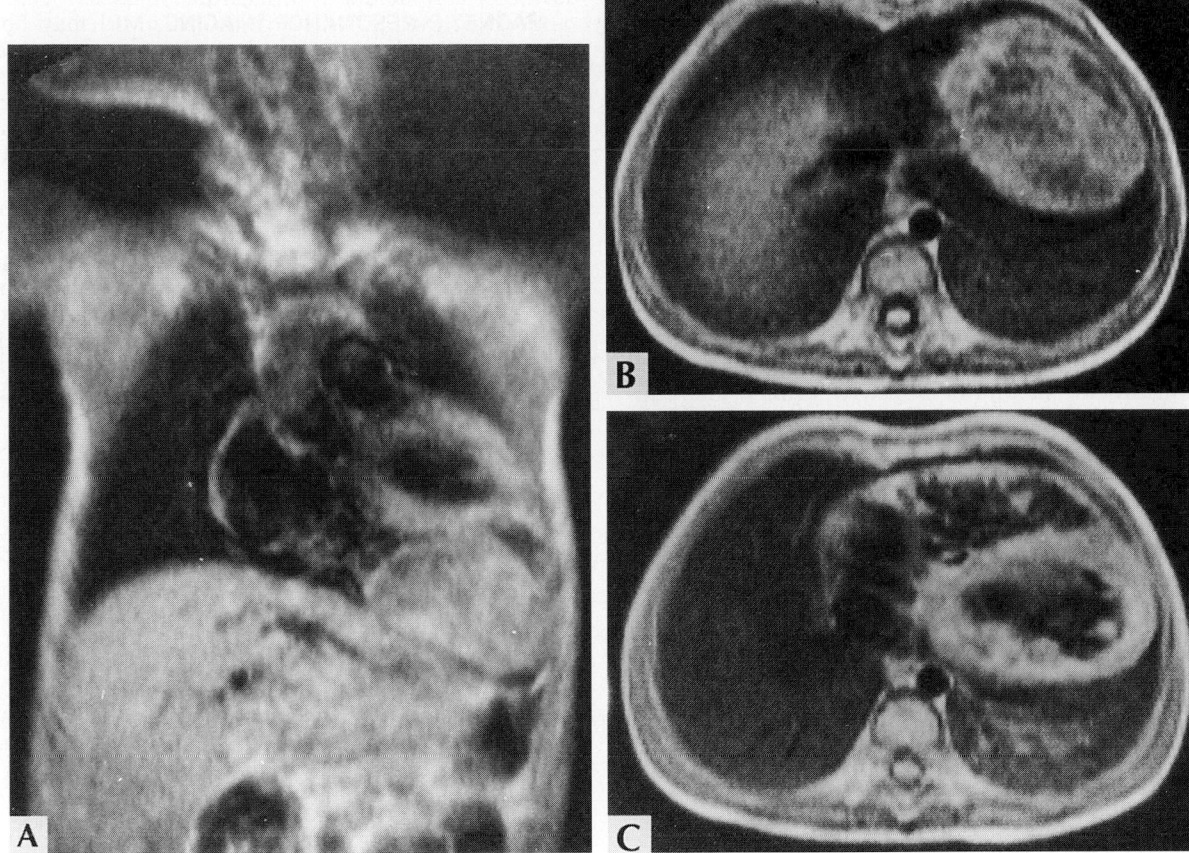

FIGURE 49–8. Magnetic resonance images illustrating a large tumor in the right ventricular apex, impinging on the apical septum. In the coronal view *(A)*, the prominent mass indents the septum. In the axial
views, the tumor shows areas of tissue inhomogeneity *(B)* and indents the ventricular septum *(C)*. (From
Allard MF, Taylor GP, Wilson JE, McManus BM: Primary cardiac tumors. *In* Goldhaber SZ, Braunwald E
[eds]: Cardiopulmonary Diseases and Cardiac Tumors. Atlas of Heart Diseases. Vol 3. Philadelphia, Current
Medicine, 1995, pp 15.1–15.22.)

volume. Apexcardiography often shows a deep notch on
the upstroke, which occurs at the time of extrusion of the
tumor through the mitral valve in early systole.

Right atrial tumors may also result in a widely split S_1
and an early systolic sound. The S_2 may be paradoxically
split as a result of early pulmonic valve closure. A tumor
plop and systolic and diastolic murmurs, which are increased by inspiration, may also occur with right atrial tumors. The jugular venous pulse tracing may reflect obstruction of the tricuspid orifice, demonstrating an accentuated *a*
wave, attenuation of the *x* descent, or an early, broad *v*
wave.

RADIOLOGICAL EXAMINATION

Cardiac tumors may display several findings on plain chest roentgenograms. These include alterations in cardiac contour, changes in overall cardiac size, specific chamber enlargement, alterations in pulmonary vascularity, and intracardiac calcification (see Chap. 8). The
cardiac contour may be normal, may display generalized or specific
chamber enlargement that mimics virtually any type of valvular heart
disease, or may demonstrate a bizarre appearance. Pericardial effusions are rather common and generally indicate invasion of the pericardial space by a malignant tumor. Mediastinal widening, due to hilar
and paramediastinal adenopathy, may indicate spread of a malignant
cardiac tumor. A bumpy, irregular, or fuzzy cardiac border may be
seen when the pericardium is involved. Cardiac enlargement may reflect rapid tumor growth, particularly in the case of sarcomas,
whereas specific chamber enlargement is frequently due to intracavitary obstruction, particularly by pedunculated tumors such as myxomas. Thus, left atrial myxoma may produce the radiological pattern
characteristic of mitral stenosis. A large tumor mass occasionally
displaces the heart and may simulate enlargement of a specific
chamber.

Calcification visible by roentgenographic methods may occur with
several types of cardiac tumor, including rhabdomyomas, fibromas,
hamartomas, teratomas, myxomas, and angiomas. Visualization of intracardiac calcium in an infant or a child is unusual and should immediately raise the question of an intracardiac tumor. Cardiac fluoroscopy and laminography may be helpful in differentiating calcification
of cardiac tumor from that of other structures, such as cardiac valves,
coronary arteries, pericardium, and mural thrombus. Calcified atrial
polypoid tumors may occasionally be seen to prolapse into the ventricle during diastole. Fluoroscopy is also useful in differentiating cardiac tumor from ventricular aneurysm, both of which may result in a
localized protrusion on plain chest roentgenograms. However, on fluoroscopic examination, cardiac tumors do not display the paradoxical
motion during ventricular contraction that is characteristic of ventricular aneurysm.

ECHOCARDIOGRAPHY. Two-dimensional echocardiography provides substantial advantages over conventional
M-mode echocardiography for the diagnosis and preoperative evaluation of intracardiac tumors.[5] In the majority of
cases of cardiac tumors, the information provided by two-
dimensional echocardiography provides adequate information about tumor size, attachment, and mobility to allow
operative resection without preoperative angiography. This
technique is sensitive for detection of small tumors and is
especially useful for detection of left ventricular tumors
and tumors that do not prolapse through the mitral or tricuspid valve orifices (see Figs. 49–7 and 7–115).

Left atrial myxomas have been classified by their echocardiographic appearance as follows: Class I tumors are
small and prolapse through the mitral valve; class II tumors
are small and nonprolapsing; class III tumors are large and
prolapse; and class IV tumors are large and nonprolaps-

ing.[122] The increased sensitivity of two-dimensional echocardiography makes possible the diagnosis of cardiac tumors in neonates and in utero.[123] The improved diagnostic power and widespread use of two-dimensional echocardiography have resulted in an increase in the detection of primary cardiac tumors,[121] in many cases before the onset of clinical signs or symptoms.

Two-dimensional echocardiography may facilitate the differentiation between left atrial thrombus and myxoma, because the former typically produces a layered appearance and is generally situated in the posterior portion of the atrium whereas the latter is often mottled in appearance and rarely occurs in the posterior portion of the atrium. In some atrial myxomas, areas of echolucency may be seen within the tumor mass, corresponding to areas of hemorrhage within the tumor. Because these areas of echolucency are not found in thrombotic or infective lesions, this finding may be of value in the differential diagnosis of an intraatrial mass. Continuous-mode Doppler ultrasonography may be useful for evaluating the hemodynamic consequences of valvular obstruction or incompetence caused by cardiac tumors.[124]

Transesophageal Echocardiography. This approach provides an unimpeded view of both atria and the atrial septum and appears to be superior to transthoracic echocardiography in many patients.[125] The potential advantages of transesophageal echocardiography include improved resolution of the tumor and its attachment (see Figs. 49–7 and 7–115), the ability to detect some masses not visualized by transthoracic echocardiography, and improved visualization of right atrial tumors. In 17 patients suspected of having a cardiac tumor, transthoracic echocardiography yielded four false positives and two false negatives, whereas transesophageal echocardiography resulted in only one false positive and no false negatives.[126] In the same series, transesophageal echocardiography proved to be superior for visualizing anatomical details such as tumor contour, cysts, and calcification and identified a stalk in 10 of 11 tumors subsequently shown to have a stalk at surgery, whereas transthoracic echocardiography identified a stalk in only 5 of the 11 tumors. Transesophageal echocardiography has been used to guide percutaneous biopsy of a right atrial myxoma.[127] Although transesophageal echocardiography does not appear warranted on a routine basis, it should be considered when the transthoracic study is suboptimal or confusing.

RADIONUCLIDE IMAGING. Gated blood pool scanning has been used to identify atrial, ventricular, and intramural tumors.[128] Radionuclide ventriculography generally has a lower rate of resolution than does echocardiography or contrast injection angiography and therefore may be less sensitive for detecting small filling defects. In some cases in which the cardiac tumor was not evident by routine static or dynamic radionuclide imaging, it has been possible to delineate the tumor and its movement during a cardiac cycle by use of a computer-generated composite functional image.[128]

COMPUTED TOMOGRAPHY. CT of the heart has been used to demonstrate cardiac tumors (see Fig. 10–47).[129] Although more experience will be necessary to establish its role, certain advantages are apparent. These include a high degree of tissue discrimination, which may allow definition of the degree of intramural tumor extension; evaluation of the extracardiac structures; and the ability to construct images in any plane. Resolution appears to be improved substantially by gating the computed tomographic acquisition to the cardiac cycle. CT currently appears to be most useful in the evaluation of suspected tumors of the heart to determine the degree of myocardial invasion and the involvement of pericardial and extracardiac structures. Ultrafast CT, a technique that uses electron beam technology, has a short scanning acquisition time that eliminates the motion

artifacts occurring with conventional CT and appears to be useful for assessment of intracardiac masses.[129]

MAGNETIC RESONANCE IMAGING. MRI may be of considerable value in detecting and delineating cardiac tumors and in some cases may depict the size, shape, and surface characteristics of the tumor more clearly than two-dimensional echocardiography.[130] The larger field of view with MRI (see Figs. 49–8, 10–20, and 10–21) provides better definition of tumor prolapse, secondary valve obstruction, and cardiac chamber size than does two-dimensional echocardiography. Contrast enhancement with gadolinium–diethylenetriaminepentaacetic acid and multislice imaging in the transaxial, sagittal, and long axes can provide precise three-dimensional information. MRI can also provide information about tissue composition that can help to differentiate tumors from thrombi.[131]

Angiography

Cardiac catheterization and selective angiocardiography are not necessary in all cases of cardiac tumors, because as already discussed, in many cases adequate preoperative information may be obtained by echocardiography, CT, or MRI. In several circumstances, however, the risk and expense of cardiac catheterization are outweighed by the supplemental information it may provide. These situations include cases in which (1) noninvasive evaluation has not been adequate in fully defining tumor location or attachment; (2) all four cardiac chambers have not been adequately visualized noninvasively; (3) a malignant cardiac tumor is considered likely; or (4) other cardiac lesions may coexist with a cardiac tumor and possibly dictate a different surgical approach. For instance, when a malignant cardiac tumor is suspected, cardiac angiography may provide valuable information about the degree of myocardial, vascular, and/or pericardial invasion. Likewise, in certain cases, such as the presence of pulmonary hypertension or the coexistence of significant valvular or coronary artery lesions, cardiac catheterization and angiography may provide information that significantly affects the surgical approach.[132]

The major angiographic findings in patients with cardiac tumors include (1) compression or displacement of cardiac chambers or large vessels, (2) deformity of cardiac chambers, (3) intracavitary filling defects, (4) marked variations in myocardial thickness, (5) pericardial effusion, and (6) local alterations in wall motion. Displacement of the cardiac chambers or the great vessels without deformation of the internal contour may be observed in both benign and malignant tumors, whereas deformation of a cardiac chamber usually indicates an infiltrating malignant lesion. The most frequent angiographic findings are intracavitary filling defects, which may be either fixed or mobile. Fixed defects may be lobulated or appear as a coarse nodularity of the myocardium that is often difficult to distinguish from a mural thrombus. Such defects may reflect endocardial tumors with broad attachments or intramural tumors with intracavitary extension. Mobile intracavitary defects are usually pedunculated tumors, typically myxomas, although the stalk may be difficult to visualize. Such tumors may prolapse into the AV valve orifice during diastole or, in the case of ventricular tumors, into the left ventricular outflow tract during systole. An atrial ball thrombus may mimic a pedunculated tumor but is more likely to be associated with clot in the atrial appendage.

A localized increase in myocardial wall thickness, especially when accompanied by a pericardial effusion, suggests an infiltrating malignant tumor. It is often difficult to differentiate myocardial thickening from pericardial effusion, but this may be aided by observation of the thickness of the right atrial wall. Because the right atrial wall is seldom infiltrated by tumor, the finding of right atrial thickening to greater than 5 mm suggests a pericardial effusion.[132] In myocardial infiltration, localized areas of disordered wall motion may also be noted by cineangiography. Coronary arteriography may in some cases allow visualization of the vascular supply of the tumor, thus demarcating the extent of tumor invasion, the source of its blood supply, and its relation to the coronary arteries.[133, 134] However, the vascular pattern of cardiac tumors has not proved to be a useful sign of malignancy.

False-negative angiographic results generally occur when the diagnosis is not suspected before catheterization. False-positive results are most often due to thrombus but may also be produced by many entities, such as streaming of nonopaque venous blood, a hematoma in the atrial septum, an aneurysm of the muscular or membranous ventricular septum, Bernheim's syndrome, congenital septal dysplasia, and hydatid cysts of the interventricular septum.

The major risk of angiography is peripheral embolization due to dislodgement of a fragment of tumor or of an associated thrombus. Therefore, thorough evaluation of all cardiac chambers by noninvasive methods before catheterization is recommended for patients suspected of having cardiac tumors so that contrast material can be injected into the chamber proximal (upstream) to the location of the tumor. The transseptal approach to the left atrium is particularly hazardous because of the frequent occurrence of left atrial myxomas in the region of the fossa ovalis.[135]

TREATMENT AND PROGNOSIS

Benign Tumors

Operative excision is the treatment of choice for most benign cardiac tumors and in many cases results in a complete cure.[5, 136-138] Although many tumors are histologically benign, all cardiac tumors are potentially lethal as a result of intracavitary or valvular obstruction, peripheral embolization, and disturbances of rhythm or conduction. Unfortunately, it is not unusual for patients to die or experience a major complication while awaiting operation; therefore, it is mandatory to carry out the operation promptly after the diagnosis has been established.

Although some epicardial tumors may be removed without the aid of extracorporeal circulation, most intramural and intracavitary tumors must be excised under direct vision, requiring use of a heart-lung machine. Closed approaches are not now recommended because of the increased risk of dislodging tumor fragments. In addition, excision cannot be as complete, and adequate inspection of the other cardiac chambers for additional tumors is not possible.

Dislodgement of tumor fragments constitutes a major risk of operation and can result in peripheral emboli or dispersion of micrometastases, which may seed peripherally. To reduce this risk, manipulation of the heart before cardiopulmonary bypass should be minimized. Some surgeons recommend that venous cannulation for cardiopulmonary bypass be performed via the femoral or azygos vein rather than through the right atrium to avoid dislodging an unsuspected right atrial tumor. In addition, the tumor should be removed en bloc when possible and the chamber then irrigated well with saline.

ATRIAL MYXOMAS. Numerous reports document complete cure of left and right atrial myxomas with follow-up periods of 10 to 15 years.[139, 140] In about 1 to 5 percent of cases, a recurrence or second cardiac myxoma has been reported after resection of the initial myxoma.[72a, 141, 142] Possible causes of the second tumor include incomplete excision of the original tumor with regrowth; growth from a second "pretumorous" focus, i.e., metasynchronous; or intracardiac implantation from the original tumor. Because of the first two possibilities, some surgeons have advocated excision of the entire region of the fossa ovalis and repair of the resultant atrial septal defect to remove presumably high concentrations of pretumorous cells thought to be located in that region. In one case, the large size of a myxoma, together with its location on the posterior left atrial wall, necessitated complete removal of the heart, which was followed by autotransplantation, i.e., reimplantation of the patient's excised heart.[143] Laser photocoagulation of a 1-cm area around the stalk attachment site has also been suggested as a way of eradicating pretumorous cells without the need for creating an atrial septal defect.[144] Other surgeons have reported equally successful long-term recurrence-free periods with simple excision of the tumor and a small rim at the base. It now appears that in approximately

7 percent of patients with (1) a familial history of cardiac myxoma, (2) features of the complex of lentigines and other abnormalities, or (3) synchronous tumor appearance (i.e., numerous tumors at the time of presentation), the incidence of a second tumor occurring at some time in the future is in the range of 12 to 22 percent, as compared with approximately 1 percent for patients with sporadic atrial myxoma.[142] It is believed that tumor recurrence in these cases is from a second pretumorous focus of cells. In these high-risk patients, a careful search for additional tumors preoperatively and more extensive resection of the underlying endocardium, atrial septum, or both is recommended. Careful echocardiographic follow-up for detection of metasynchronous tumors is recommended[142] for all patients after resection of a myxoma.

OTHER BENIGN TUMORS. Successful excision has also been reported for ventricular myxomas, as well as most other types of benign cardiac tumor, including rhabdomyoma, hamartoma, fibroma, lipoma, hemangioma, and papillary fibroelastoma.[145-147] The major surgical considerations in excision of ventricular tumors include preservation of adequate ventricular myocardium, maintenance of proper AV valve function, and preservation of as much of the conduction system as possible. Often, however, papillary muscles, chordae tendineae, or the AV conduction system must be sacrificed during the resection of a tumor, thereby necessitating replacement of the AV valve, implantation of a pacemaker, or both.

Malignant Tumors

Operation is not an effective treatment for the great majority of primary malignant tumors of the heart because of the large mass of cardiac tissue involved or the presence of metastases. The major role for surgery in such cases is to establish a diagnosis in order to preclude the possibility of a curable benign tumor. Nevertheless, in some cases, palliation of hemodynamics and/or constitutional symptoms and extension of life can be achieved by aggressive therapy. Survival for 1 to 3 years has been reported after partial resection, chemotherapy, radiation therapy, orthotopic cardiac transplantation, or various combinations of these modalities.[148-152] In some instances, localized recurrences have been eliminated by repeated operations. Some success in palliation of symptoms has been reported after the combination of chemotherapy and radiation therapy[153] and after radiation therapy alone.[152] Lymphosarcoma of the heart frequently responds to chemotherapy, radiation therapy, or both.[154, 155] Unfortunately, many other reports indicate a failure to alter the course of cardiac sarcomas despite various combinations of surgery, chemotherapy, and radiation therapy.

REFERENCES

CLINICAL PRESENTATION

1. Allard MF, Taylor GP, Wilson JE, McManus BM: Primary cardiac tumors. In Goldhaber SZ, Braunwald E (eds): Cardiopulmonary Diseases and Cardiac Tumors: Atlas of Heart Diseases. Vol 3. Philadelphia, Current Medicine, 1995, pp 15.1–15.22.
2. Reynan K: Frequency of primary tumors of the heart. Am J Cardiol 77: 107, 1996.
3. Lam KYL, Dickens P, Chan ACL: Tumors of the heart. Arch Pathol Lab Med 117.1027, 1993.
4. Tazelaar HD, Locke TJ, McGregir CGA: Pathology of surgically excised primary cardiac tumors. Mayo Clin Proc 67:957, 1992.
5. Salcedo EE, Cohen GL, White RD, Davison MB: Cardiac tumors: Diagnosis and treatment. Curr Probl Cardiol 17:73, 1992.
6. Pollia JA, Gogol LJ: Some notes on malignancies of the heart. Am J Cancer 27:329–333, 1996.
7. Burke A, Virmani R: Tumors of the Heart and Great Vessels. Atlas of

Tumor Pathology—3rd series. Armed Forces Institute of Pathology, 1995.

8. Hanson EC: Cardiac tumors: A current perspective. NY State Med 92: 41, 1992.

9. Molina JE, Edwards JE, Ward HB: Primary cardiac tumors: Experience at the University of Minnesota. Thorac Cardiovasc Surg 38:183–191, 1990.

10. Basso C, Valente M, Poletti A, et al: Surgical pathology of primary cardiac and pericardial tumors. Eur J Cardiothorac Surg 12:730–738, 1997.

11. Goodwin JF: Symposium on cardiac tumors: The spectrum of cardiac tumors. Am J Cardiol 21:307, 1968.

12. St. John Sutton MG, Mercier L, Guliani ER, Lie JT: Atrial myxomas: A review of clinical experience in 40 patients. Mayo Clin Proc 55:371, 1980.

12a. Idir M, Oysel N, Guibaud JP, et al: Fragmentation of a right atrial myxoma presenting as a pulmonary embolism. J Am Soc Echocardiogr 13:61–63, 2000.

13. Hirano T, Taga T, Yasukawa K: Human B-cell differentiation factor defined by an anti-peptide antibody and its possible role in autoantibody production. Proc Natl Acad Sci U S A 84:228, 1987.

14. Borden EC, Chin P: Interleukin-6: A cytokine with potential diagnostic and therapeutic roles. J Lab Clin Med 123:824, 1994.

15. Wada A, Kanda T, Hayashi R, et al: Cardiac myxoma metastasized to the brain: Potential role of endogenous interleukin-6. Cardiology 83: 208, 1993.

16. Takahara H, Mori A, Tabata R, et al: Left atrial myxoma with production of interleukin-6. J Jpn Assoc Thorac Surg 40:326, 1992.

17. Seino Y, Ikeda U, Shimada K: Increased expression of interleukin-6 mRNA in cardiac myxomas. Br Heart J 69:565, 1993.

18. Seguin JR, Beigbeder JY, Hvass U, et al: Interleukin-6 production by cardiac myxomas may explain constitutional symptoms. J Thorac Cardiovasc Surg 103:599, 1992.

19. Jourdan M, Bataille R, Sequin J, et al: Constitutive production of interleukin-6 and immunologic features in cardiac myxomas. Arthritis Rheum 33:398, 1990.

20. Curry HLF, Matthews JA, Robinson J: Right atrial myxoma mimicking a rheumatic disorder. Br Med J 1:542, 1967.

20a. Suzuki J, Takayama K, Mitsui F, et al: In situ interleukin-6 transcription in embryonic nonmuscle myosin heavy chain expressing immature mesenchyme cells of cardiac myxoma. Cardiovasc Pathol 9:33–37, 2000.

21. Savige JA, Yeung SP, Davis DJ, et al: Anti-neutrophil cytoplasmic antibodies associated with atrial myxoma. Am J Med 85:755, 1988.

22. Graham SL, Sellers AL: Atrial myxoma with multiple myeloma. Arch Intern Med 139:116, 1979.

23. Leonhardt ETG, Kullenberg KPG: Bilateral atrial myxomas with multiple arterial aneurysms: A syndrome mimicking polyarteritis nodosa. Am J Med 62:792, 1977.

24. Byrd WE, Matthews OP, Hunt RE: Left atrial myxoma presenting as a systemic vasculitis. Arthritis Rheum 23:240, 1980.

25. Feldman AR, Keeling JH: Cutaneous manifestation of atrial myxoma. J Am Acad Dermatol 21:1080, 1989.

26. Quinn TJ, Condini MA, Harris AA: Infected cardiac myxoma. Am J Cardiol 53:381, 1984.

27. Whitman MS, Rovito MA, Klions D, Tunkel AR: Infected atrial myxoma: Case report and review. Clin Infect Dis 18:657, 1994.

28. Revankar SG, Clark RA: Infected cardiac myxoma: Case report and literature review. Medicine 77:337–344, 1998.

29. Hashimoto H, Takahashi H, Fujiwara Y, et al: Acute myocardial infarction due to coronary embolization from left atrial myxoma. Jpn Circ J 57:1016, 1993.

30. De Carli S, Sechi LA, Ciani R, et al: Right atrial myxoma with pulmonary embolism. Cardiology 84:368, 1994.

31. Miyauchi Y, Endo T, Kuroki S, Hayakawa H: Right atrial myxoma presenting with recurrent episodes of pulmonary embolism. Cardiology 81:178, 1992.

32. Eriksen UH, Baandrup U, Jensen BS: Total disruption of left atrial myxoma causing a cerebral attack and a saddle embolus in the iliac bifurcation. Int J Cardiol 35:127, 1992.

33. Boussen K, Moalla M, Blondeau P, et al: Embolization of cardiac myxomas masquerading as polyarteritis nodosa. J Rheumatol 18:283, 1991.

34. Weerasena NA, Groome D, Pollock JG, Pollock JC: Atrial myxoma as the cause of acute lower limb ischemia in a teenager. Scott Med J 34: 440, 1989.

35. Reed RJ, Utz MP, Terezakis N: Embolic and metastatic cardiac myxoma. Am J Dermatopathol 11:157, 1989.

36. Michael AS, Mikhael MA, Christ M: Myxoma of the heart presenting with recurrent episodes of hemorrhagic cerebral infarction: MR findings. J Comput Assist Tomogr 13:123, 1989.

37. Knepper LE, Biller J, Adams HP Jr, Bruno A: Neurologic manifestations of atrial myxoma: A 12-year experience and review. Stroke 19:1435, 1988.

38. Heath D, Mackinnon J: Pulmonary hypertension due to myxoma of the right atrium: With special reference to the behavior of emboli of myxoma in the lung. Am Heart J 68:227, 1964.

39. Harvey WP: Clinical aspects of cardiac tumors. Am J Cardiol 21:328, 1968.

40. Kawano H, Okada R, Kawano Y, et al: Mesothelioma in the atrioventricular node: Case report. Jpn Heart J 35:255, 1994.

41. Balasundaram S, Halees SA, Duran C: Mesothelioma of the atrioventricular node: First successful follow-up after excision. Eur Heart J 13:718, 1992.

42. James TN, Galakhov L: De subitaneis mortibus XXVL: Fatal electrical instability of the heart associated with benign congenital polycystic tumor of the atrioventricular node. Circulation 56:667, 1977.

43. Strauss WE, Asinger RW, Hodges M: Mesothelioma of the AV node: Potential utility of pacing. PACE 11:1296, 1988.

44. Lantz DA, Dougherty TH, Lucca MJ: Primary angiosarcoma of the heart causing cardiac rupture. Am Heart J 118:186, 1989.

45. Mitral stenosis and left atrial myxoma. In Fowler NO (ed): Diagnosis of Heart Disease. New York, Springer-Verlag, 1991, pp 146–159.

46. Gershlick AH, Leech G, Mills PG, Leatham A: The loud first heart sound in left atrial myxoma. Br Heart J 52:403, 1984.

47. Teoh KH, Mulji A, Tomlinson CW, Lobo FV: Right atrial myxoma originating from the eustachian tube. Can J Cardiol 9:441, 1993.

48. Heck HA Jr, Gross CM, Houghton JL: Long-term severe pulmonary hypertension associated with right atrial myxoma. Chest 102:301, 1992.

49. Pessotto R, Santini F, Piccin C, et al: Cardiac myxoma of the tricuspid valve: Description of a case and review of the literature. J Heart Valve Dis 3:344, 1994.

50. Savino JS, Weiss SJ: Right atrial tumor. N Engl J Med 333:1608, 1995.

51. Waxler EB, Kawai N, Kasparian H: Right atrial myxoma: Echocardiographic, phonocardiographic and hemodynamic signs. Am Heart J 82: 251, 1972.

52. Keren A, Chenzbruna A, Schuger L, et al: The etiology of tumor plop in a patient with huge right atrial myxoma. Chest 95:1147, 1989.

53. Hada Y, Wolfe C, Murry CF, Craige E: Right ventricular myxoma: Case report and review of phonocardiographic auscultatory manifestations. Am Heart J 100:871, 1980.

54. Gosse P, Herpin D, Roudant R, et al: Myxoma of the mitral valve diagnosed by echocardiography. Am Heart J 111:803, 1986.

SPECIFIC CARDIAC TUMORS

55. Carney JA, Hruska LS, Beauchamp GD, Gordon H: Dominant inheritance of the complex of myxomas, spotty pigmentation and endocrine overactivity. Mayo Clin Proc 61:165, 1986.

56. Van Galder HM, O'Brien DJ, Staples ED, Alexander JA: Familial cardiac myxoma. Ann Thorac Surg 53:419, 1992.

57. Koopman RJ, Happle R: Autosomal dominant transmission of the NAME syndrome (nevi, atrial myxoma, mucinosis of the skin and endocrine overactivity). Hum Genet 86:300, 1991.

58. Carney JA, Gordon J, Carpenter PC, et al: The complex of myxomas, spotty pigmentation and endocrine overactivity. Medicine 64:270, 1985.

59. Vidaillet HJ Jr, Seward JB, Fyke FE, et al: "Syndrome myxoma": A subset of patients with cardiac myxoma associated with pigmented skin lesions and peripheral and endocrine neoplasms. Br Heart J 57:247, 1987.

60. Bennett WS, Skelton TN, Lehan PH: The complex of myxomas, pigmentation and endocrine overactivity. Am J Cardiol 65:399, 1990.

60a. Cohen C, Turner ML, Stratakis CA: Pigmented lesions of the conjunctiva in Carney's complex. J Am Acad Dermatol 42:145, 2000.

60b. Watson JC, Stratakis CA, Bryant-Greenwood PK, et al: Neurosurgical implications of Carney complex. J Neurosurg 92:413–418, 2000.

61. Carney JA, Behnaz CT: Myxoid fibroadenoma and allied conditions (myxomatosis) of the breast. Am J Surg Pathol 15:713, 1991.

62. Vidaillet HJ Jr, Seward JB, Fyke E, Tajik AJ: NAME syndrome (nevi, atrial myxoma, myxoid neurofibroma, ephelides): A new and unrecognized subset of patients with cardiac myxoma. Minn Med 67:695, 1984.

63. Rhodes AR, Silverman RA, Harrist TJ, Perez-Atayde AR: Mucocutaneous lentigines, cardiomucocutaneous myxoma, and multiple blue nevi: The "LAMB" syndrome. J Am Acad Dermatol 10:72, 1984.

64. Farah MG: Familial cardiac myxoma: A study of relatives of patients with myxoma. Chest 105:65, 1994.

65. McCarthy PM, Peihler JM, Schaff HV, et al: The significance of multiple, recurrent, and "complex" cardiac myxomas. Thorac Cardiovasc Surg 91:389, 1986.

66. Carney JA: Differences between nonfamilial and familial cardiac myxoma. Am J Surg Pathol 9:53, 1985.

67. McAllister HA Jr: Tumors of the heart and pericardium. In Silver MD (ed): Cardiovascular Pathology. 2nd ed. New York, Churchill Livingstone, 1991, p 1297.

68. Burke AP, Virmani R: Cardiac myxoma: A clinicopathologic study. Am J Clin Pathol 100:671, 1993.

69. Ferrans VJ, Roberts WL: Structural features of cardiac myxomas: Histology, histochemistry and electron microscopy. Hum Pathol 4:111, 1973.

69a. Kono T, Koide N, Hama Y, et al: Expression of vascular endothelial growth factor and angiogenesis in cardiac myxoma: a study of fifteen patients. J Thorac Cardiovasc Surg 119:101–107, 2000.

70. Goldman BI, Frydman C, Harpaz N, et al: Glandular cardiac myxomas. Cancer 59:1767, 1987.

71. Lie JT: The identity and histogenesis of cardiac myxomas: A controversy put to rest. Arch Pathol Lab Med 113:724, 1989.

72. Hashimoto H, Takahashi H, Fujiwara Y, et al: Acute myocardial infarction due to coronary embolization from left atrial myxoma. Jpn Circ J 57:1016, 1993.

72a. Terada Y, Wanibuchi Y, Noguchi M, Mitsui T: Metastatic atrial myxoma to the skin at 15 years after surgical resection. Ann Thorac Surg 69:283–284, 2000.

73. Salyer WR, Page DL, Hutchins GM: The development of cardiac myxomas and papillary endocardial lesions from mural thrombus. Am Heart J 89:4, 1975.

74. Stratakis CA, Carney JA, Lin JP, et al: Carney complex, a familial multiple noeplasia and lentiginosis syndrome: Analysis of 11 kindreds and linkage to the short arm of chromosome 2. J Clin Invest 97:699–705, 1996.

75. Basson CT, MacRae CA, Korf B, Merliss A: Genetic heterogeneity of familial atrial myxoma syndromes (Carney complex). Am J Cardiol 79:994–995, 1997.

76. Casey M, Mah C, Merliss AD, et al: Identification of a novel genetic locus for familial cardiac myxomas and Carney complex. Circulation 98:2560–2566, 1998.

77. Dobin S, Speights VO, Donner LR: Addition [1][q32] as the sole clonal chromosomal abnormality in a case of cardiac myxoma. Cancer Genet Cytogenet 96:181–182, 1997.

78. Milunsky J, Huang X-L, Baldwin CT, et al: Evidence for genetic heterogeneity of the Carney complex (familial atrial myxoma syndromes). Cancer Genet Cytogenet 106:173–176, 1998.

79. Richkind KE, Wason D, Vidaillet H: Cardiac myxoma characterization by clonal telomeric association. Genes Chrom Cancer 9:68, 1994.

80. Dijkhuizen T, van den Berg E, Molenaar WM: Cytogenetics of a case of cardiac myxoma. Cancer Genet Cytogenet 73:73, 1992.

81. DeMarco L, Stratakis CA, Boson WL, et al: Sporadic cardiac myxomas and tumors from patients with Carney complex are not associated with activating mutations of the Gsα gene. Hum Genet 98:185–188, 1996.

82. Seidman JD, Berman JJ, Hitchcock CL, et al: DNA analysis of cardiac myxomas: Flow cytometry and image analysis. Hum Pathol 22:494, 1991.

83. Luthringer DJ, Virmani R, Weiss SW, Rosai J: A distinctive cardiovascular lesion resembling histiocytoid (epithelioid) hemangioma. Am J Surg Pathol 14:993, 1990.

84. Veinot JP, Tazelaar HD, Edwards WD, Colby TV: Mesothelial/monocytic incidental cardiac excrescences: Cardiac MICE. Mod Pathol 7:9, 1994.

85. Courtice RW, Stinson WA, Walley VM: Tissue fragments recovered at cardiac surgery masquerading as tumoral proliferations. Am J Surg Pathol 18:167, 1994.

PAPILLARY TUMORS OF HEART VALVES

86. Shahian DW, Labib SB, Chang G: Cardiac papillary fibroelastoma. Ann Thorac Surg 59:538, 1995.

87. LiMandri G, Homma S, Di Tullio MR, et al: Detection of multiple papillary fibroelastomas of the tricuspid valve by transesophageal echocardiography. J Am Soc Echocardiogr 17:315, 1994.

88. Klarich KW, Enriquez-Sarano M, Gura GM, et al: Papillary fibroelastoma: Echocardiographic characteristics for diagnosis and pathologic correlation. J Am Coll Cardiol 30:784–790, 1997.

89. Grinda J-M, Couetil JP, Chauvaud S, et al: Cardiac valve papillary fibroelastoma: Surgical excision for revealed or potential embolization. J Thorac Cardiovasc Surg 117:106–110, 1999.

90. Pomerance A: Papillary "tumours" of the heart valves. J Pathol Bacteriol 87:135, 1981.

91. Fenoglio JJ, McAllister HA, Ferrans VJ: Cardiac rhabdomyoma: A clinicopathologic and electron microscopic study. Am J Cardiol 38:241, 1976.

92. Burke AP, Virmani R: Cardiac rhabdomyoma: A clinicopathologic study. Mod Pathol 4:70, 1991.

93. Bass JL, Breningstall GN, Swaiman KF: Echocardiographic incidence of cardiac rhabdomyoma in tuberous sclerosis. Am J Cardiol 55:137, 1985.

94. Gibbs JL: The heart and tuberous sclerosis: An echocardiographic and electrocardiographic study. Br Heart J 54:596, 1985.

95. Webb DW, Thomas RD, Osborne JP: Cardiac rhabdomyomas and their association with tuberous sclerosis. Arch Dis Child 68:367, 1993.

96. Moriarty AT, Nelson WA, McGahey B: Fine-needle aspiration of rhabdomyosarcoma of the heart. Acta Cytol 34:74, 1990.

97. Van der Hauwaert LG: Cardiac tumours in infancy and childhood. Br Heart J 33:125, 1971.

98. Jones KI, Wolf PL, Jensen P, et al: The Gorlin syndrome: A genetically determined disorder associated with cardiac tumor. Am Heart J 111:1013, 1986.

99. Miralles A, Bracamonte L, Soncul H, et al: Cardiac tumors: Clinical experience and surgical results in 74 patients. Ann Thorac Surg 52:886, 1991.

100. Tazelaar HD, Locke TJ, McGregor CGA: Pathology of surgically excised primary cardiac tumors. Mayo Clin Proc 67:957, 1992.

101. Prior JT: Lipomatous hypertrophy of cardiac interatrial septum. Arch Pathol 78:11, 1964.

102. Chao JC, Reyes CV, Hwang MH: Cardiac hemangioma. South Med J 83:44, 1990.

103. Cox JN, Friedli B, Mechmeche M, et al: Teratoma of the heart. Virchows Arch (A) 402:163, 1983.

104. Meysman M, Noppen M, Demeyer G, Vincken W: Malignant epithelial mesothelioma presenting as cardiac tamponade. Eur Heart J 14:1576, 1993.

105. Monma N, Satodate R, Tashiro A, Segawa I: Origin of so-called mesothelioma of the atrioventricular node. Arch Pathol Lab Med 115:1026, 1991.

106. Burke MAP, Anderson PG, Virmani R, et al: Tumor of the atrioventricular nodal region. Arch Pathol Lab Med 114:1057, 1990.

107. David TE, Lenkei SC, Marquez-Julio A, et al: Pheochromocytoma of the heart. Ann Thorac Surg 41:98, 1986.

107a. Baykut D, Fiegen U, Krian A, Thiel A: Ectopic thyroid tissue in the left ventricular outflow tract. Ann Thorac Surg 69:620–621, 2000.

MALIGNANT CARDIAC TUMORS

108. Putnam JB, Sweeney MS, Colon R, et al: Primary cardiac sarcomas. Ann Thorac Surg 51:906, 1991.

109. Burke AP, Cowan D, Virmani R: Primary sarcoma of the heart. Cancer 69:387, 1992.

110. Thomas CR, Johnson GW, Stoddard MF, Clifford S: Primary malignant cardiac tumors: Update 1992. Med Pediatr Oncol 20:519, 1992.

111. Whorton CM: Primary malignant tumor of the heart. Cancer 2:245, 1949.

112. Burke AP, Virmani R: Osteosarcomas of the heart. Am J Surg Pathol 15:289, 1991.

113. Klima U, Wimmer-Greinecker G, Harringer W, et al: Cardiac angiosarcoma—a diagnostic dilemma. Cardiovasc Surg 1:674, 1993.

114. Herrmann MA, Shankerman RA, Edwards WD, et al: Primary cardiac angiosarcoma: A clinicopathologic study of six cases. J Thorac Cardiovasc Surg 103: 655, 1992.

114a. Dennig K, Lehmann G, Richter T: An angiosarcoma in the left atrium. N Engl J Med 342:443–444, 2000.

114b. Butany J, Yu W: Cardiac angiosarcoma: two cases and a review of the literature. Can J Cardiol 16:197–205, 2000.

115. Keohane ME, Lazzam C, Halperin JL, et al: Angiosarcoma of the left atrium mimicking myxoma: Case report, Hum Pathol 20:599, 1989.

116. Proctor MS, Tracy GP, Von Koch L: Primary cardiac B-cell lymphoma. Am Heart J 118:179, 1989.

117. Basso C, Stefani A, Calabrese F, et al: Primary right atrial fibrosarcoma diagnosed by endocardial biopsy. Am Heart J 131:399, 1996.

118. Kasai K, Kuwao S, Sato Y, et al: Case report of primary cardiac lymphoma: The applications of PCR to the diagnosis of primary cardiac lymphoma. Acta Pathol Jpn 42:667, 1992.

119. Marvasti MA, Obeid AI, Potts JL, Parker FB: Approach in the management of atrial myxoma with long-term folow-up. Ann Thorac Surg 38: 53, 1984.

120. Bleisch N, Kraus F: Polypoid sarcoma of the pulmonary trunk. Cancer 46:314, 1980.

DIAGNOSIS, TREATMENT, PROGNOSIS

121. Lane GE, Kapples EJ, Thompson RC, et al: Quiescent left atrial myxoma. Am Heart J 127:1629, 1994.

122. Charuzi Y, Bolger A, Beeder C, Lew AS: A new echocardiographic classification of left atrial myxoma. Am J Cardiol 55:614, 1985.

123. Dennis MA, Appareti K, Manco-Johnson ML, et al: The echocardiographic diagnosis of multiple fetal cardiac tumors. Ultrasound Med 4: 327, 1985.

124. Panidis IP, Mimtz GS, McAllisterm M: Hemodynamic consequences of the left atrial myxomas as assessed by Doppler ultrasound. Am Heart J 111:927, 1986.

125. Edwards LC, III, Louie EK: Transthoracic and transesophageal echocardiography for the evaluation of cardiac tumors, thrombi, and valvular vegetations. Am J Card Imaging 8:45, 1994.

126. Shyu K-G, Chen J-J, Cheng J-J, et al: Comparison of transthoracic and transesophageal echocardiography in the diagnosis of intracardiac tumors in adults. J Clin Ultrasound 22:381, 1994.

127. Azuma T, Ohira A, Akagi H, et al: Transvenous biopsy of a right atrial tumor under transesophageal echocardiographic guidance. Am Heart J 131:402, 1996.

128. Bough E, Bodem W, Gandsman E, et al: Radionuclide diagnosis of left atrial myxoma with computer-generated functional images. Am J Cardiol 52:1365, 1986.

129. Bleiweis MS, Georgiou D, Brundage BH: Detection of intracardiac masses by ultrafast computed tomography. Am J Card Imaging 8:63, 1994.

130. Fujita N, Caputo GR, Higgins CB: Diagnosis and characterization of intracardiac masses by magnetic imaging. Am J Card Imaging 8:69, 1994.

131. Reddy DB, Jena Col A, Venugopal P: Magnetic resonance imaging (MRI) in evaluation of left atrial masses: An in vitro and in vivo study. J Cardiovasc Surg 35:289, 1994.

132. Fueredi GA, Knetchtges TE, Czarnecki DJ: Coronary angiography in atrial myxoma: Findings in nine cases. Am J Roentgenol 152:737, 1989.

133. Singh RN, Burkholder JA, Magovern GJ: Coronary arteriography as an aid in left atrial myxoma diagnosis. Cardiovasc Intervent Radiol 7:40, 1984.

134. Weyne AE, Heyndrickx GR, Cavelier CC, et al: Cardiac imaging techniques in the diagnosis of angiosarcoma of the heart: Report of two cases. Postgrad Med J 61:271, 1985.

135. Pendyck F, Pierce EC, Baron MG, Lukban SB: Embolization of left atrial myxoma after transseptal cardiac catheterization. Am Cardiol 30:569, 1972.

136. Wiatrowska BA, Walley VM, Masters RG, et al: Surgery for cardiac tumors: The University of Ottawa Heart Institute experience (1980–1991). Can J Cardiol 9:65, 1993.

137. MacGowan SW, Sidhu P, Aherne T, et al: Atrial myxoma: National incidence, diagnosis and surgical management. Ir J Med Sci 162:223, 1993.

138. Aru GM, Falchi S, Cardu G, et al: The role of transesophageal echocardiography in the monitoring of cardiac mass removal: A review of 17 cases. J Card Surg 8:554, 1993.

139. Larsson S, Lepore V, Kennergren C: Atrial myxomas: Results of 25 years' experience and review of the literature. Surgery 105:695, 1989.

140. Bortolotti U, Maraglino G, Rubino M, et al: Surgical excision of intra-cardiac myxomas: A 20-year follow-up. Ann Thorac Surg 49:449, 1990.

141. Waller DA, Ettles DF, Saunders NR, Williams G: Recurrent cardiac myxoma: The surgical implications of two distinct groups of patients. Thorac Cardiovasc Surg 37:226, 1989.

142. McCarthy PM, Piehler JM, Schaff HV, et al: The significance of multiple, recurrent, and "complex" cardiac myxomas. Thorac Cardiovasc Surg 91:389, 1986.

143. Scheld HH, Nestle HW, Kling D, et al: Resection of a heart tumor using autotransplantation. Thorac Cardiovasc Surg 36:40, 1988.

144. Mesnildrey P, Bloch G, Cachera JP, Piwicna A: Atrial myxoma: A new surgical approach using neodynium:yttrium-aluminum-garnet laser photocoagulation. J Thorac Cardiovasc Surg 98:313, 1989.

145. Goldman S, Lortscher R, Pappas G: Surgical treatment for rhabdomyoma of the right atrium causing arrhythmias, J Thorac Cardiovasc Surg 89:802, 1985.

146. Corno A, deSimone G, Catena G, Marcelletti C: Cardiac rhabdomyoma: Surgical treatment in the neonate. Thorac Cardiovasc Surg 37:725, 1984.

147. Orringer MB, Sisson JC, Glazer G, et al: Surgical treatment of cardiac pheochromocytomas. J Thorac Cardiovasc Surg 89:753, 1985.

148. Auflero TX, Pae WE Jr, Clemson BS, et al: Heart transplantation for tumor. Ann Thorac Surg 56:1174, 1993.

149. Yuh DD, Kubo SH, Francis GS, et al: Primary cardiac lymphoma treated with orthotopic heart transplantation: A case report. J Heart Lung Transplant 13:536, 1994.

150. Baay P, Karawande SV, Kushner JP, et al: Successful treatment of a cardiac angiosarcoma with combined modality therapy. J Heart Lung Transplant 13:923, 1994.

151. Crespo MG, Pulpon LA, Pradas G, et al: Hearth transplantation for cardiac angiosarcoma: Should its indication be questioned? J Heart Lung Transplant 82:527, 1993.

152. Baay P Karwande SV, Kushner JP, et al: Successful treatment of a cardiac angiosarcoma with combined modality therapy. J Heart Lung Transplant 13:923, 1994.

153. Hollingworth JH, Sturgill BC: Treatment of primary angiosarcoma of the heart. Am Heart J 78:254, 1969.

154. Terry LN, Kilgerman MM: Pericardial and myocardial involvement by lymphomas and leukemias. The role of radiotherapy. Cancer 25:1003, 1970.

155. Gerfein OB: Lymphosarcoma of the right atrium. Angiographic and hemodynamic documentation of response to chemotherapy. Arch Intern Med 135:325, 1975.

Chapter 50

Pericardial Diseases

DAVID H. SPODICK

PERICARDIAL ANATOMY AND PHYSIOLOGY

Anatomy

Pericardial anatomy is specialized to serve its complex active and passive normal functions (Fig. 50–1).[1, 2] There are two pericardial layers with nerves, lymphatics, and blood vessels. The *serosa* is a sac lined by a monolayer of mesothelial cells attached by loose connective tissue to the heart surfaces and the inner aspect of the fibrosa, lying on the

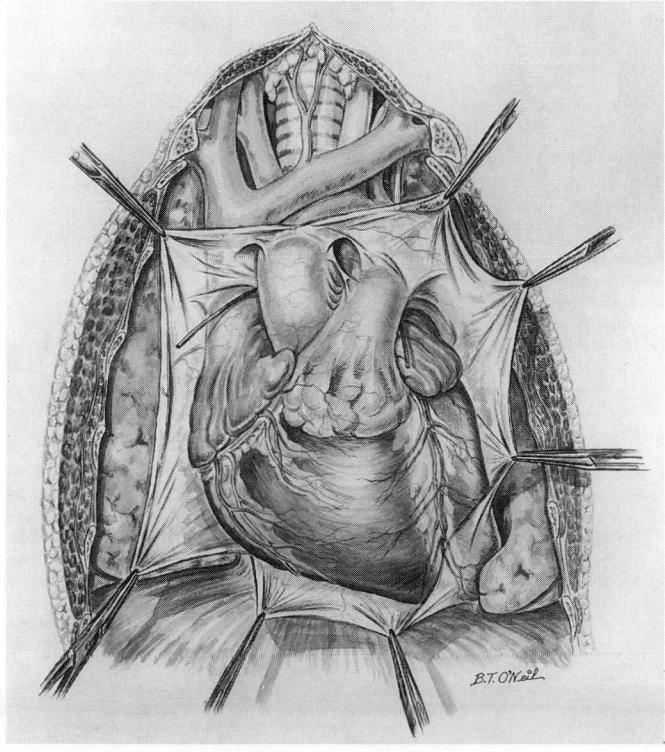

FIGURE 50–1. The opened normal pericardium and heart in situ. The epicardial mesothelium is transparent; the parietal pericardium—mesothelium and fibrosa—is translucent. A curved probe is in the pericardial transverse sinus. (From Spodick DH: Acute Pericarditis. New York, Grune & Stratton, 1959; author's copyright.)

heart like a collapsed rubber glove with finger-like projections over the juxtacardiac great vessels. It contains 15 to 35 ml of serous pericardial fluid, an ultrafiltrate of blood plasma. Externally, it is clasped by the fibrosa and continues upward an average of 6 cm above the aortic root over the aortic arch, where it blends with the deep cervical fascia, and over the venae cavae and pulmonary veins. *Ligaments* attach it to the sternum and the vertebral bodies loosely and to the central tendon of the diaphragm firmly. The serosa directly covering the heart surfaces is the *visceral pericardium* ("the epicardium"; see Fig. 50–1). The fibrosa with the reflections of the serosal sac internally attached to it is the *parietal pericardium* ("the pericardium"). Parietal pericardial thickness varies from 0.8 to 2.5 mm (up to 3.5 mm on magnetic resonance imaging [MRI] and computed tomography [CT]).

PERICARDIAL SINUSES AND RECESSES. The pericardial "cavity" is a nonuniform, mainly potential, space. During life most of the normal fluid is undetectable except in the major sinuses and the atrioventricular (AV) grooves and numerous recesses. In front of the atria and superior venae cavae and behind the proximal ascending aorta and pulmonary artery is a short pericardial passage, the *transverse sinus*, where the serosa encloses the terminal portions of the venae cavae and pulmonary veins, with separate recesses surrounding one third to two thirds of the proximal pulmonary artery. With the pulmonary veins it forms an inverted "U", framing a posterior projection, the *oblique sinus*. CT and MRI disclose numerous smaller recesses not detectable in the open pericardium at surgery and post mortem. The pericardial sinuses and recesses increase the pericardial capacity to accommodate increased fluid (or other contents), contributing to the *pericardial reserve volume*.

THE MESOTHELIUM. Serosal mesothelial cells interdigitate and overlap, maintaining mechanical stability and permitting changes in surface configuration. Projecting *microvilli* presumably reduce friction and facilitate exchange of fluid and ions. *Cytoskeletal filaments* include keratins for structural support and actin. A basal lamina underlies the mesothelium and covers the subepicardial coronary vessels.

THE FIBROSA. The fibrosa, which is composed mainly of *fibrocollagenous tissue*, is wavy in youth, arranged in fascicular bundles and thicker over thinner parts of the heart. The left atrium is tightly clasped by a dense fibrosal mesh. The fibrosa also contains *elastic fibers*.

NERVES, ARTERIES, LYMPHATICS, AND LYMPH NODES. The *phrenic nerves* course upward over the anterior parietal pericardium and supply most of it. (They and their nutrient *pericardiacophrenic artery* must be protected during cardiac and pericardial surgery.) The esophageal plexus supplies vagal fibers. Parietal pericardial lymphatics drain to corresponding anterior and posterior mediastinal nodes while the superficial plexus of the cardiac lymphatics drains the visceral pericardium to the tracheal and bronchial mediastinal nodes.

The internal mammary arteries and small aortic twigs contribute the arterial supply.

SUBEPICARDIAL FAT AND CONNECTIVE TISSUE. Between the heart and the epicardial mesothelium is variable connective tissue and a fat layer that increases with increasing body weight and is disproportionately increased in coronary disease. The fat contains a prostaglandin-like angiogenic factor and important parasympathetic ganglia in a *sinoatrial fat pad.*

Physiology of the Normal Pericardium

PHYSICAL EFFECTS. Purely mechanical pericardial effects belong mainly to the parietal pericardium and are minimal in euvolemic individuals with normal hearts.[3, 4, 4a] The normal parietal pericardium contributes to resting cavitary diastolic pressures and retracts when incised, indicating it is under stress—indeed it exerts a contact stress. Moreover, by exerting stress[5] (magnified by any increase in pericardial fluid pressure) the normal pericardium restricts overall heart filling with a much greater effect on thinner parts like the right ventricle and atrium that probably depend on pericardial constraint for much of their normal pressures and dimensions (after pericardiectomy right ventricular [RV] size increases). The pericardium also limits acute cavitary dilation.

Hypervolemia exaggerates all such effects: when cardiac volume is acutely increased, much of the increased ventricular diastolic pressure is borne by the pericardium, ensuring only minimal change in ventricular diastolic transmural

▼ **TABLE 50–1. ACUTE EFFECTS OF PERICARDIECTOMY/ PERICARDIOTOMY**

GENERAL EFFECTS
Macrophysiological effects are due to absent/reduced constraint of the heart.
  Ventricular interaction:
    Pericardium closed: right ventricle dominates
    Pericardium open: left ventricle dominates
Experimental results depend on protocol:
  Intact conscious closed-chest subjects vs. open-chest anesthetized subjects
  Intact vs. blocked autonomic innervation

SPECIFIC EFFECTS

Decreased
Interactions: ventricular; atrioventricular
Pulmonary volume overload in response to intravascular volume loading:
  Excess intravascular volume redistributed from pulmonary to systemic circulation
RA mean pressure
Systemic vascular resistance during maximal exercise

Increased
Cardiac index and stroke work index due to improved LV systolic performance (Frank-Starling response to increased preload)
LV end-diastolic diameter
LV end-diastolic volume
LV stroke volume
LV transmural pressure
Early LV filling velocity
Early LV filling fraction
LA booster pump function
LA reservoir function
Diastolic discharge frequency of LV mechanoreceptors

Increased Exercise Responses
Maximal O₂ consumption
Maximal cardiac output
Maximal stroke volume
LA pressure
LA stroke volume
LV end-diastolic pressure
  LA = left atrial; LV = left ventricular; RA = right atrial

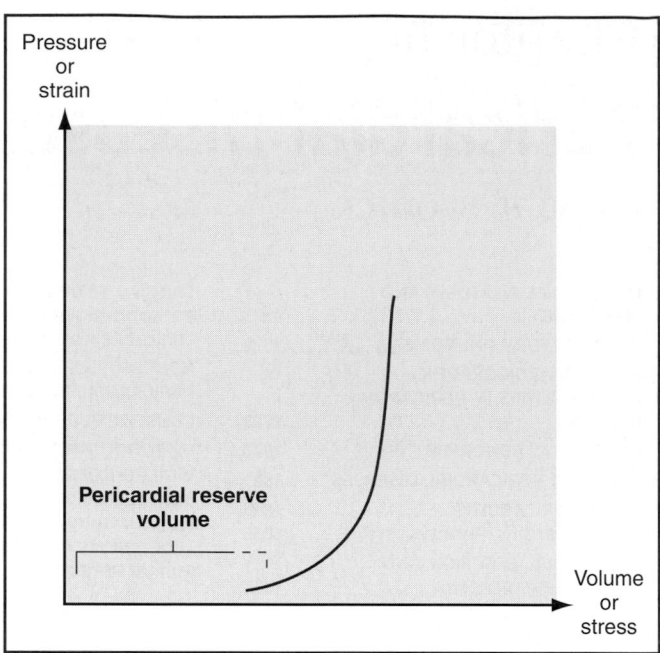

FIGURE 50–2. Schema of stress-strain and pressure-volume curves of the normal pericardium. After the relatively small *pericardial resolve volume* is exhausted by filling of the pericardial sinus and recesses, the curve at first rises gently, with continued filling at some point more acutely; the time scale and exact proportions are variable depending on the *rate of filling* of the intact pericardial sac. (From Spodick DH: The Pericardium: A Comprehensive Textbook. New York, Marcel Dekker, 1997.)

pressures while increasing pericardial constraint. With *euvolemia* the parietal pericardium appears to have minimal direct influence and virtually no effect during *hypovolemia*, probably because decreased preload and reduced heart size free the heart from pericardial constraint. Comparably, nitroglycerin, erect posture, and lower body negative pressure reduce cardiac volume acutely and hence pericardial effects on the myocardium. In contrast, both chronic pericardial effusion and chronic cardiomegaly lead to progressive stretch (time-dependent *stress relaxation* and *creep*) with subsequent hypertrophy of the parietal pericardium increasing its compliance and decreasing its constraining effect on the heart.

Pericardial constraint accounts for most of the resting diastolic right atrial (RA) and RV cavity pressures and contributes substantially to those on the left. Pericardiotomy augments RV filling and stroke volume with improved systolic function by the Frank-Starling relation. The numerous effects of pericardiectomy or pericardiotomy are summarized in Table 50–1.

The parietal pericardium is stiffer than cardiac muscle. Its stiffness is related to regional fiber orientations: more parallel fibers yield more pericardial stiffness.[2] Its mechanical functions mainly relate to (1) its contribution to apparent cardiac stiffness, (2) the effects of a chamber filled with fluid at subatmospheric pressure surrounding the heart, and (3) circulatory "feedback" regulation by pericardial neuroreceptors and mechanoreceptors. On stretching, the parietal pericardium initially "gives," due to extension of its elastic fibers and straightening of its wavy collagen. Thereafter, rapidly increasing resistance to increasing stretch produces characteristic "J"-shaped stress-strain and pressure-volume curves (Fig. 50–2): an initial slow rise in pressure as volume increases—and of strain as stress increases—followed by an angle and a sharp rise. With intact pericardia, ventricular pressure-volume curves are exactly parallel. Acutely increased pericardial fluid or intracardiac volume couple the pericardium to the heart more closely, exaggerating this effect. Removal or opening of the parietal pericardium makes ventricular pressure-volume curves significantly more gentle so that ventricular pressure begins its sharp rise later at a higher cardiac volume and thereafter increases more gradually.

PRESSURE-VOLUME RELATIONSHIPS. Normal intrapericardial pressure (−5 to +5 mm Hg) is nearly always negative and approximates and varies with pleural pressure during respiration. With early increase in pericardial fluid pressure, changes tend to be small, owing to the *pericardial reserve volume*—the volume by which the unstressed pericardium exceeds the cardiac volume. Large increases in right-sided heart pressures, as by volume loading, raise pericardial pressure, but the *myocardial transmural pressure* increase is small and well below the change in pericardial pressure.

THE PERICARDIAL HYDROSTATIC SYSTEM. Normally, pericardial fluid distributes hydrostatic inertial and gravitational (e.g., postural) forces over the cardiac surfaces. This favors approximation of end-diastolic transmural pressure throughout the ventricles and consequently uniform stretch of muscle fibers, tending to balance preload and so permit the Frank-Starling mechanism to operate uniformly. (Note that pericardial contact pressure measured by flat balloons[5] rather than catheters may better represent baseline pericardial constraint of the heart.)

VENTRICULAR INTERDEPENDENCE AND PERICARDIAL CONSTRAINT OF THE HEART. Expressed as ventricular interaction, ventricular interdependence represents the effects of pressure and volume changes in one ventricle on the activities of the other, including filling, contraction, and relaxation. Pericardial contributions to ventricular interaction help to explain reduced ventricular compliance when there is increased pressure in the other ventricle. Although the normal right ventricle is much more compliant than the left, the pericardium constrains both similarly and tends to equalize their compliances (nonpericardial interaction also occurs by means of the circumferential and especially the septal myocardial muscles). *Moreover, either ventricle generates greater isovolumic pressure from any diastolic volume when the pericardium is intact than when it is open or removed.* Diastolic cardiac chamber interactions are greatly magnified by the pericardium, which minimally affects systolic interaction. For example, acutely increased RV size (e.g., cardiocirculatory volume overload or RV infarction) raises intrapericardial pressure significantly, imposing a steeper pressure-volume curve (increased stiffness) on both pericardially constrained ventricles.[6] Interaction operates continuously, although minimally, during normal breathing. Inspiration increases RV filling, which slightly reduces left ventricular (LV) filling, and consequently output, and decreases arterial pressure. Respiratory effects are exaggerated by even small increases in pericardial fluid and markedly in cardiac tamponade; this produces pulsus paradoxus.

TRANSMURAL PRESSURES. Transmural pressures describe the force (related to pressure) balance across a cavity wall. The transmural pressure of the pericardium itself (pericardial pressure minus pleural pressure) approximates zero, although it is usually slightly negative and varies with pleural pressure. *Myocardial transmural pressure* (intracavitary pressure minus intrapericardial pressure) normally is less than 3 mm Hg and depends on pericardial pressure. Transmural pressure at end diastole is a measure of preload (the actual chamber-distending pressure); transmural pressure is thus a true "filling pressure." Therefore, the closed pericardial chamber, normally at slightly subatmospheric pressure, ensures that myocardial transmural pressure stays low relative to even large increases of cavitary diastolic pressures. Myocardial performance is largely determined by end-diastolic fiber length set by end-diastolic chamber volume, which is determined by end-diastolic transmural pressure due to pericardial constraint.

NORMAL RESPIRATORY EFFECTS: RIGHT HEART/LEFT HEART RECIPROCATION (Fig. 50–3). Intrapericardial pressure approximates pleural pressure and varies with its respiratory changes: about −3 mm Hg at end expiration to −6 mm Hg at end inspiration. The normal inspiratory fall in pleural pressure reduces pericardial, RA, RV, wedge, and systemic arterial pressures slightly. However, inspiratory pericardial pressure decreases more than atrial pressures increase, augmenting systemic venous return and right-sided heart filling and, therefore, RV preload and output (pulmonary artery flow velocity increases). Simultaneously, inspiratory aortic flow decreases as aortic transmural pressure increases (which increases impedance to ejection). Moreover, as the increased RV output crosses the lung any inspiratory "pooling" would reduce the gradient for left atrial (LA) filling. The corresponding slight inspiratory decrease in LV transmural pressure and the increased LV afterload (impedance to ejection) reduce LV stroke output. These are directionally identical, with far greater changes in the same measurements during pulsus paradoxus.

PASSIVE PERICARDIAL FUNCTIONS. *Membranous functions* of the pericardium result from its physical presence. It appears to buttress thinner parts of the myocardium, particularly the RA and RV, and to block inflammation from contiguous structures. It reduces friction due to heart movement by means of the pericardial fluid and surfactant phospholipids. *Ligamentous functions* slightly limit cardiac displacement through attachments to adjacent structures.

MICROPHYSIOLOGY OF THE NORMAL PERICARDIUM.[2] Cardiocirculatory feedback regulation by pericardial servomechanisms include (1) *neuroreceptors* in epicardium and fibrosa that detect lung inflation and can alter blood pressure and heart rate through the vagus nerves; (2) *sympathetic efferents* doing the opposite; (3) *mechanoreceptors* sensitive to ventricular stretch, determined by ventricular volume and transmural pressure (myocardial dysfunction is sensed by mechanoreceptors monitoring beat-to-beat changes in cardiac volume, and other mechanoreceptors signal myocardial tension reflexly to match contraction strength with peripheral resistance); and (4) *chemoreceptors* sensitive to substances in the pericardial fluid, which respond to digitalis glycosides and perhaps contribute to their bradycardic effect.

NORMAL PERICARDIAL FLUID.[3] Serous pericardial fluid (normally 15 to 35 ml) is mainly an ultrafiltrate of plasma including some overflow of myocardial interstitial fluid and lymph. Protein concentration is lower than in plasma but with relatively high albumin. Electrolyte concentrations yield an osmolarity less than plasma, consistent with such an ultrafiltrate.

MESOTHELIAL METABOLIC ACTIVITY.[1–3] The mesothelium has cyclooxygenase, prostacyclin synthetase, and lipoxygenase activities; prostaglandin E_1, eicosanoids, and large amounts of prostacyclin (PGI_2) are continually released into the pericardial cavity in response to hypoxia, pericardial stretch, and increased myocardial work and loading conditions. These prostanoids can alter pericardial sympathetic neurotransmission, myocardial work, loading conditions, and myocardial contractility and modulate the caliber and tone of the coronary vessels with multiple effects on cardiac electrophysiology, possibly including reduction of reperfusion-induced arrhythmias. *Prostacyclin also inhibits*

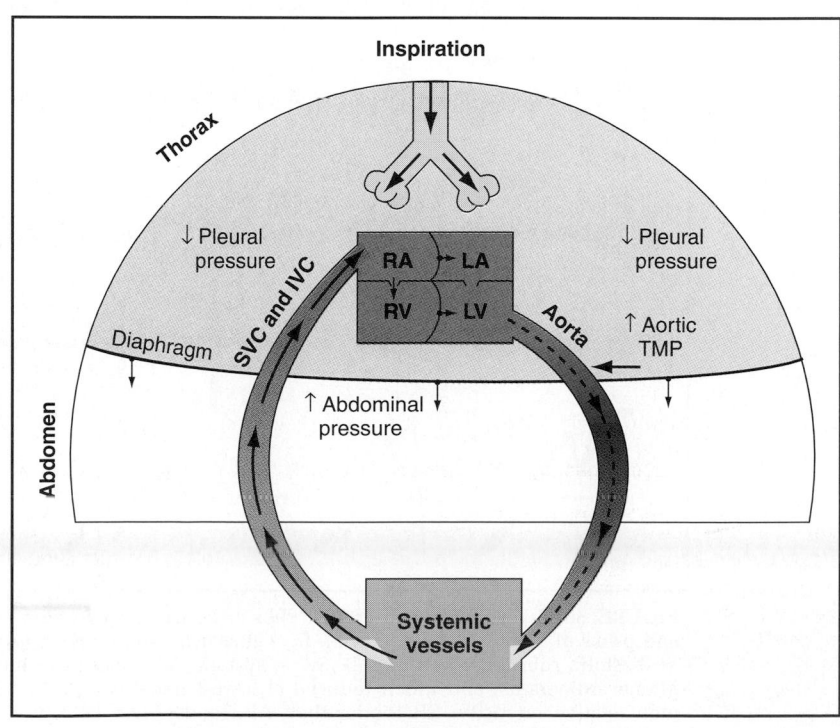

FIGURE 50–3. Inspiratory effects on heart and pericardium (reversed in expiration). Inspiration, by means of diaphragm descent, reduces pleural cavity pressure while increasing abdominal pressure. Venous return to the right side of the heart is sharply increased, with filling at the expense of the left side of the heart (atrial and ventricular septa move to the left). This is accentuated by the fall in aortic transmural pressure, which increases impedance to ejection by the left ventricle. This is the normal response pattern; during compressive pericardial disorders (tamponade, constriction) its degree is increased (pulsus paradoxus). See text. LA = left atrium; LV = left ventricle; RA = right atrium; RV = right ventricle; SVC and IVC = superior and inferior venae cavae.

platelet aggregation and thrombosis in the major coronary vessels as well as clotting during intrapericardial bleeding, whereas fibrinolytic activity by the mesothelium opposes both intrapericardial clotting and adhesion formation. Small amounts of complement (C3, C4, CH_{50}), other immune factors, myocardial cellular enzymes, and related compounds are continually released into the pericardial fluid.[3] During transmural cardiac injury and necrosis, pericardial fluid "washes" the cardiac surfaces, diluting substrates leaked into it that might adversely affect the superficial myocardial sympathetic nerves. A cell-to-cell interaction between pericardial mesothelium and ventricular myocytes in tissue culture may modulate myocyte structure, function, and gene expression, whereas fibroblast growth factor 2 (FGF_2) in pericardial fluid is a major determinant of myocyte growth and functionally significant angiogenesis. Other growth factors modulate activation of macrophages and coronary endothelial cells so that pericardial fluid analyses may give prognostic information with respect to neoangiogenesis and plaque stability. The effects on the heart, its nerves, and the coronary arteries of intrapericardially injected substances permit the pericardial sac to be used for local delivery of therapeutic agents and gene products. This has been accomplished by catheter through the RA appendage and with an instrument specifically designed for access to the normal pericardium (i.e., the perDUCER).[7, 8]

AUSCULTATORY PHENOMENA
(See Chap. 4)

There are five categories of auscultatory phenomena in pericardial disorders: (1) pericardial rubs, (2) abnormal heart sounds, (3) clicks, (4) murmurs, and (5) the effect of pneumohydropericardium.[9, 10]

PERICARDIAL RUB. The pericardial friction sound (rub, "friction rub"; Fig. 50–4), a hallmark of acute pericarditis, occasionally audible in subacute and chronic pericardial disease, is ascribed to friction between inflamed, scarred, or tumor-invaded serosal surfaces *(endopericardial rub)*, including those after sclerotherapy of effusions, or, infrequently, between parietal pericardium and pleura or chest wall *(exopericardial rub)* or both *(endo-exopericardial rub)*. Endopericardial rubs may also be due to destruction of surfactant pericardial phospholipids. The common endoper-

icardial rub, often monotonal, nearly always disappears with resolution of acute inflammation. Exopericardial rubs sometimes result from penetration by severe acute pericarditis but otherwise are due to direct extension, inflammation, or tumor implants from adjacent structures. They may change radically with respiration, have a musical quality, and seem superficial. Like endopericardial rubs, exopericardial rubs also occur after cardiac surgery and with constrictive and nonconstrictive pericardial scarring; most are from adjacent pleuritis—*pleuropericardial rubs*—due to pleural, or both pleural and pericardial, involvement and have both respiratory and cardiac periodicity. *Conus rubs* accompany pulmonary embolism, thyroid "storm" *(Means-Lerman scratches)*, and acute beriberi heart disease; they are ascribed to dilation of the pulmonary conus in a hyperactive heart. In acute pericarditis, rubs usually disappear with accumulation of significant pericardial effusion, but frequently they do not, even during tamponade. Indeed, some rubs, probably exopericardial, "paradoxically" disappear after pericardiocentesis.

Auscultatory Characteristics.[9] Composed of mixed (mainly high) frequency vibrations, most rubs, unlike most murmurs, frequently wax, wane, and transiently disappear. They vary from subtle distant "scrapes" to grating or scratching noises, which may be loud and even palpable. Rubs often give the illusion of "obliterating" or "going through" the heart sounds while seeming superficial. Many change with breathing and body position and do not respect conventional murmur zones of maximum intensity and radiation. Yet, the vast majority of rubs are heard best, or only, along the left mid to lower sternal edge, where palpability is most likely, owing to proximity of the right ventricle to the chest wall. Occasional rubs are sharply localized anywhere along any heart border. Usually loudest in inspiration, particularly with increased pericardial fluid, some rubs have no respiratory predilection; rarely, rubs increase in expiration. Finally, to elicit or accentuate rubs, the examiner should raise all four of the patient's extremi-

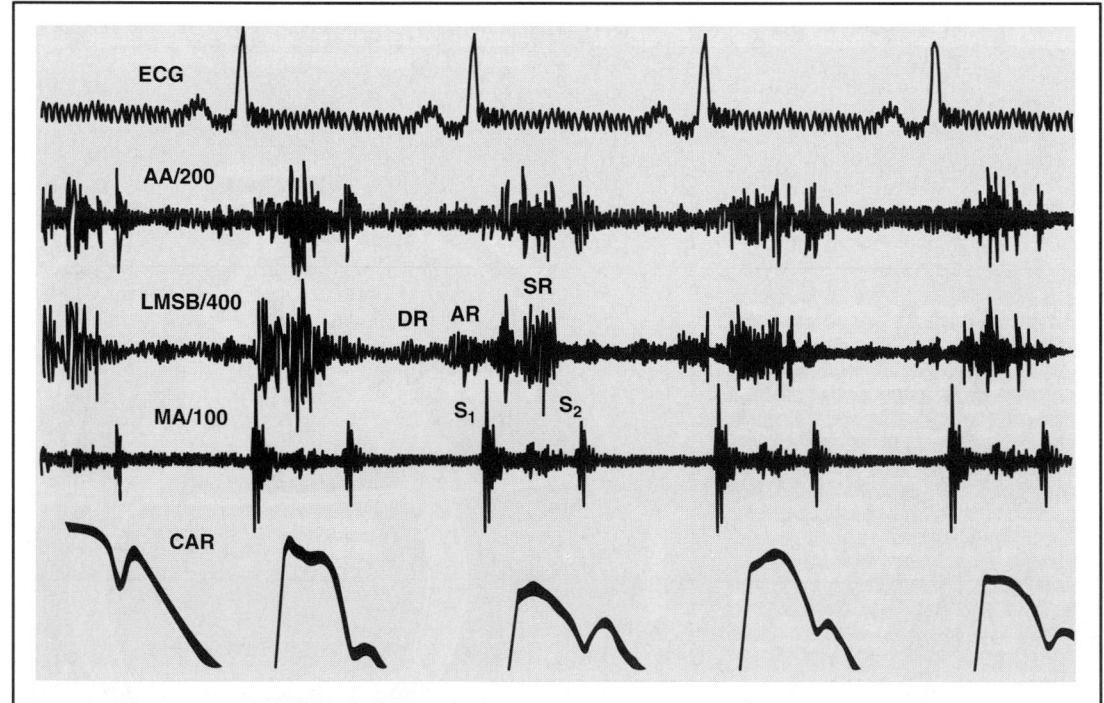

FIGURE 50–4. Triphasic pericardial rub: electrocardiogram *(top)*, multifilter phonocardiograms *(center)*, and peaks of carotid pulse *(bottom)*. S_1 = first heart sound; S_2 = second heart sound. Rub components: DR = diastolic rub; AR = atrial rub; SR = systolic rub. Rub vibrations are mainly high frequency (top two phonocardiograms) and much reduced at lowest frequency (MA/100). This example shows the most common relative intensity: SR louder than AR, louder than DR; only SR remains at lowest filtration. (From Spodick DH: The Pericardium: A Comprehensive Textbook. New York, Marcel Dekker, 1997.)

ties simultaneously to distend the right side of the heart by increased venous return or applying the stethoscope to the precordium while the patient rests on the knee and elbows (Fig. 4–44).

Components. Classically described as biphasic ("to-and-fro"), multiobserver investigations revealed, in patients with heart rates less than 120 beats/min, triphasic rub patterns in well over one half of those in sinus rhythm. The rub occurred with atrial systole *(atrial rub)*, ventricular systole *(systolic rub)*, and early diastole *(early diastolic rub)* (see Fig. 50–4). Only about one third are biphasic (to-and-fro), with some due to absence of atrial systole in rhythm disorders. About 10 percent were monophasic, usually during ventricular systole. At heart rates of more than 100 beats/min the early diastolic and atrial components may fuse *(summation rub)*. Some rubs only appear after exercise; others with one or two components may acquire the remaining components on exercise.

HEART SOUNDS. Pericardial disease can alter heart sounds and their auscultatory appreciation by insulation and particularly by hemodynamic changes.[9] Insulation by pericardial fluid should tend to make heart sounds more distant. Hemodynamic changes common to both tamponade and constriction decrease myocardial compliance and stroke volume, tending to diminish first (S_1) and second (S_2) heart sounds and relatively accentuate the pulmonic component of S_2. Constrictive pericarditis produces its hallmark, the abnormal early diastolic sound[9]—a variant of the third heart sound (S_3; Fig. 50–5)—as well as abnormal splitting of S_2. Effusive constrictive syndromes (simultaneous scar and fluid) produce mixed pictures.

The early diastolic sound of constriction coincides with the abrupt deceleration of excessively rapid early filling[9, 10] and occurs earlier than an abnormal S_3 of myocardial disease and AV valve regurgitation. The early diastolic sound may be the only loud heart sound (sometimes with an intense "knocking" quality) and misinterpreted as S_1, especially during rapid heart rates. At bedside, the S_3 appears after the carotid crest and coincides with the trough of the jugular y descent.[9] A faint or absent S_3 may be revealed by prompt squatting. Patients with heavy calcification can have a particularly loud and sharp early diastolic sound, owing to markedly reduced compliance. Like its timing, early diastolic sound intensity varies directly with the abruptness with which ventricular expansion halts; that is, louder third sounds correlate with high diastolic pressures and steepness of reascent from the typical early diastolic "dip" of ventricular pressure and chest wall displacement curves. In sinus rhythm, a fourth heart sound (S_4) is occasionally present and ascribable to high resistance to active filling. Lack of impairment of atrial systole explains why the S_4 is more common in *elastic constriction* (see p. 1849).

CLICKS. Clicks are high-frequency, discrete vibrations resembling opening snaps of stenosed valves. Classically ascribed to pericardial scarring and articulation of calcifications, this remains speculative, because most clicks are due to intracardiac phenomena related to valves and chordae.[9]

Indeed, pseudoprolapse and true prolapse of mitral and tricuspid leaflets (due to disproportionate shrinkage of ventricular volume in tamponade and constriction) produce clicks.

MURMURS. Murmurs arise from turbulent flow across orifices and tubes. In pericardial disease they are epiphenomena—due to related or unrelated coincident heart disease or when pericardial scarring narrows a valve ring or portion of the heart, aorta, or pulmonary artery.

Murmurs with inflammatory cysts, hematomas, or abscesses are due to compression or actual physical disruption of valves. AV groove compression has produced annular mitral and tricuspid stenosis with murmurs indistinguishable in quality, timing, and respiratory behavior from those of AV valve disease.[10] Selective scarring has also produced systolic murmurs of aortic supravalvular and pulmonic supravalvular and infundibular stenosis. In constrictive pericarditis, unexplained mitral and tricuspid regurgitant murmurs are common. Some murmurs appear only postoperatively; others arise from local inequality within a generalized constricting scar. Coexisting cardiac disease independently produces murmurs that may become modified by constriction.

AUSCULTATORY EFFECTS OF PNEUMOHYDROPERICARDIUM. When air or other gas overlies pericardial fluid, due to trauma, gas-producing organisms, or a fistula from adjacent organs, a metallic tinkle synchronous with systole may be heard if the amount of gas is small. Large amounts produce a churning, splashing, *"mill-wheel sound"* from agitation of the gas-liquid interface by the beating heart.[9]

ELECTROCARDIOGRAPHIC ABNORMALITIES IN PERICARDIAL DISEASE (See Chap. 5)

The pericardium produces no detectable electrical phenomenon, yet pericardial disease can significantly modify the electrocardiogram (ECG).[11] Quasi-specific ST-T wave changes follow spread of pericardial inflammation to the subepicardial myocardium; a superficial myocarditis results.[12] Excess pericardial fluid, fibrin, or dense scar may insulate the heart or short circuit cardiac currents, tending to decrease voltage, although hemodynamic impairment may be as or more important than the size of effusion (unless massive) in reducing voltage. ECG effects of constrictive scarring depend additionally on fibrosis and calcification of the subjacent myocardium; any asymmetry of scarring can mimic disease of a cardiac chamber, valve, or great vessel.

Acute Pericarditis

Acute pericardial inflammation with a superficial shell of myocarditis provokes ST-T abnormalities that, in typical three or four-stage sequence (Table 50–2), are pathognomonic of acute pericarditis.

STAGE 1. This stage alone (Figs. 50–6 and 5–47) is quasi-diagnostic. It mimics "early repolarization" and acute

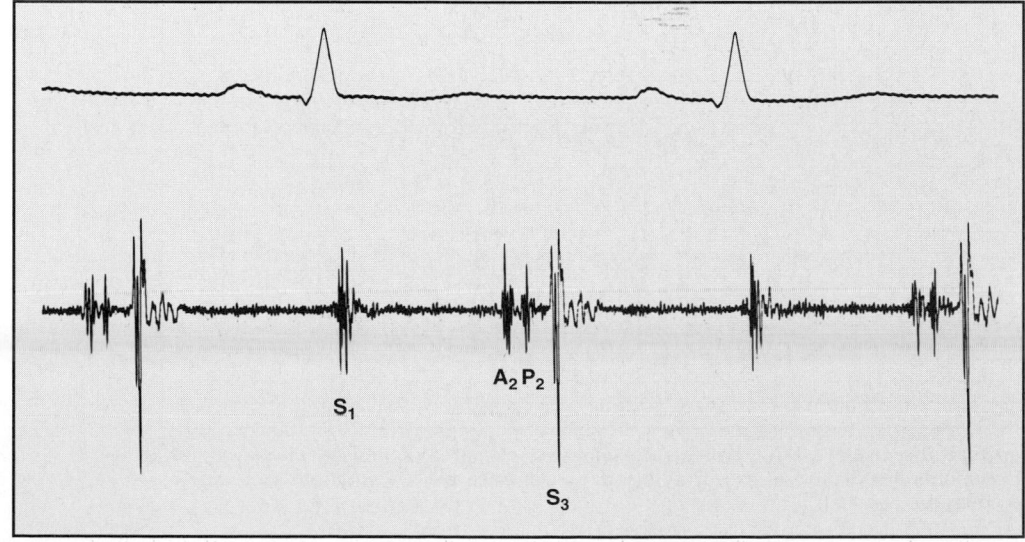

FIGURE 50–5. Constrictive pericarditis: phonocardiogram showing high-amplitude third heart sound (S_3) larger than S_1 and both components (A_2 and P_2) of well-split second heart sound (S_2). (From Spodick DH: The Pericardium: A Comprehensive Textbook. New York, Marcel Dekker, 1997.)

TABLE 50–2. ECG: STAGE I PERICARDITIS VS. "EARLY REPOLARIZATION"

	STAGE 1 PERICARDITIS	"EARLY REPOLARIZATION"
Sex	Either	Virtually all males
Age	Any	Usually younger than 40 years
Prevalence in mental institutions	Sporadic	Relatively common
J-ST evolution	Yes	No
PR segment deviations	Frequent	Occasional
	Ubiquitous	Restricted distribution
	Often conspicuous	Never conspicuous
R-S slurring	Uncommon	Nearly always
T waves		
Amplitude	Normal	Usually tall
Summit	May be blunt	Peaked
J height/T apex V6 (PR segment as baseline)	Usually $\geq 25\%$	Usually $< 25\%$
Tallest precordial R wave	Usually V_5	Usually V_4

Modified from Spodick DH: The Pericardium: A Comprehensive Textbook. New York, Marcel Dekker, 1997.

infarction with anterior and inferior ST segment elevation. Characteristic evolution involves the ST junction (J) and T wave. Unless there is a deeper involvement, there are no QRS complex abnormalities. The entire subepicardial myocardium is involved in generalized pericarditis so that most ECG leads develop simultaneously "in phase" with each other. The mean J-ST vector (axis) is usually directed left and inferiorly ("southeast"), between +30 and +60 degrees in normal hearts. In the thin-walled atrium, myocarditis cannot be superficial and, at least early in acute pericarditis, exaggerates atrial T waves (Ta wave) that appear early, causing PR segment deviations opposite to P wave polarity.

Thus PR segment deviations have a vector (axis) 180 degrees opposite to the P axis—usually at −120 to −150 degrees ("northwest") (see Fig. 50–6). Stage I is virtually pathognomonic of acute pericarditis when it involves virtually all leads. Minimal lead involvement to be considered typical includes I, II, aVL, aVF, and V_3 through V_6.[11] Leads theoretically reflecting "endocardial" events show depressed J points and elevated PR segments. Thus, the ST segment is always depressed in lead aVR, very frequently depressed or isoelectric in V_1, and occasionally depressed in V_2.

STAGE II. This stage is evolutionary; in early stage II, all ST junctions return to the baseline more or less "in phase" with little change in the T wave; PR segments may now be deviated if they had not been in stage I. In late stage II, the T waves progressively flatten and invert mainly in leads that had shown ST segment elevations.

STAGE III. This stage shows generalized T wave inversions in most or all leads. If first recorded in stage III, pericarditis cannot be diagnosed by ECG because stage III is also consistent with diffuse myocardial injury, "biventricular strain," or frank myocarditis. Stage III has become less frequent, presumably due to effective early treatment with antiinflammatory agents.

STAGE IV. In this stage, the ECG returns to its prepericarditis state. Occasionally, stage IV does not occur and there are permanent, generalized or focal T wave inversions and flattenings.

TYPICAL ECG VARIANTS. Typical variants[11] include the following:

1. In stage I, the ST segment may be isoelectric or slightly depressed in lead III with a horizontal or semihorizontal QRS axis; with a vertical axis, the ST segment is isoelectric or slightly depressed in lead aVL and isoelectric in lead I.
2. There may be rapid evolution of stage I to normality, that is, return of the elevated J-ST to the baseline with little or no T wave change.
3. Any stage may be absent.
4. Stage II may persist indefinitely or for long periods, with T wave flattening or inversions indicating a more aggressive process or presaging constrictive evolution.

ATYPICAL ECG VARIANTS. Five atypical variants render the ECG diagnostically nonspecific[11]:

1. There may be no ECG change, either because acute abnormalities are missed (rapid evolution or delayed recording) or be-

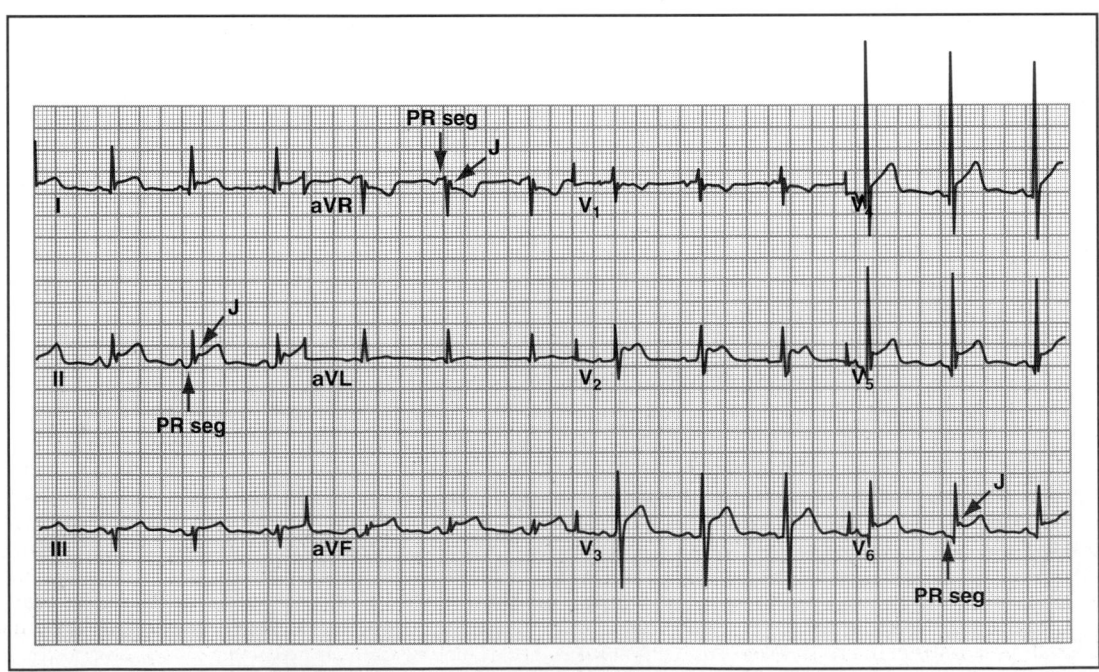

FIGURE 50–6. Acute pericarditis: stage 1 ECG. J points are elevated except aVR and V_1. T waves are essentially normal. PR segments are depressed except aVR and V_1. Absence of PR deviations in a single limb lead (here, aVL) is common. See text.

cause superficial myocarditis is low-grade or absent. Pericarditis of acute myocardial infarction produces only localized pericardial involvement with no general stage I.

2. PR segment deviations alone are not rare; these are very sensitive (with or without ST deviations) but of undetermined specificity.
3. J-ST changes may be restricted to only a few leads, which is misleading because localized cardiac injury is typical of myocardial ischemia. One may suspect this variant because pericarditic changes lack reciprocal ST deviation.
4. T wave inversions before all ST junctions have returned to the baseline, characteristic of myocardial infarction and myopericarditis (in special cases, patients with preexisting T wave abnormalities, especially digitalis effect, may show J-junction deviation while the original T wave abnormalities persist with or without PR segment deviations) and myopericarditis.
5. In stage III there may be T wave inversions only in some leads (usually V_3 or V_4 to V_6).

Nearly half the ECGs in patients with rubs and corresponding clinical syndromes do not present with or evolve a stage I.[11] The majority with typical ECG changes are always recorded on presentation or the first or second day thereafter. Differentiation from myocardial ischemia is crucial because thrombolytic treatment with unrecognized pericarditis can cause hemopericardium.[11] (see Table 50–5 and Chap. 35). Differentiation of stage I from the apparently normal variant of "early repolarization" is summarized in Table 50–2.

RATE AND RHYTHM. Although heart rate is usually rapid (80–130 beats/min), slower rates are noted in patients with autonomic problems—typical of uremic pericarditis. Sinus rhythm is the rule in the absence of heart disease. Indeed, uncomplicated acute pericarditis does not produce significant rhythm disturbances[11] unless there is underlying cardiac disease either preexisting or related through pericardial inflammation, myocardial or pericardial tumor invasion, or associated metabolic abnormality.[11, 12]

PERICARDIAL EFFUSIONS (see pp. 1831, 1838). ECG effects of pericardial effusion are difficult to assess. Low-amplitude ECGs are seen in many, but certainly not all, cases with detectable effusion. Chronic effusions with compression atrophy or scarring of the myocardium may cause permanent low voltage.[11] Yet large effusions without voltage or other ECG abnormalities are not uncommon, especially in patients with voltage-increasing heart disease. ST-T wave abnormalities during pericardial effusion can persist or disappear after paracentesis. They may be related to superficial myocarditis, but in some cases they seem to depend on presence of fluid, possibly due to myocardial compression or ischemia.[11] ST segment displacements are more common with rapid fluid accumulation (as in hemopericardium). P wave voltage reduction usually requires truly massive effusions. Tamponade can reduce voltage even with smaller amounts of fluid, partly due to reduced cardiac volume (Brody effect). Hemolysis of red cells in fluid can produce excess potassium concentrations that affect the ST segment and T wave, including T wave peaking and reversal of previous T wave polarity. Pleural effusions, particularly on the left, may contribute to voltage reduction, whereas generalized fluid retention (as in cirrhosis and heart failure) can reduce ECG voltage without pericardial disease.[11] Note that the presence of *more than minimally increased pericardial fluid raises the energy required for defibrillation and cardioversion.*[13]

CARDIAC TAMPONADE (see p. 1841). Unless massively effusive, chronic pericardial effusion and chronic cardiac tamponade have little ECG effect. In acute tamponade, any ECG stage of acute pericarditis can be found but most often ST (J) segment deviations are absent and T waves are low to inverted. Some patients have nearly normal ECGs. Critical acute hemorrhagic tamponade provokes bradycardia, often of AV junctional origin or with preterminal electromechanical dissociation. QRS-T voltage tends to decrease in tamponade, although the degree of change is unrelated to severity. (Note that preexisting heart disease may account for high or low voltage.) Very few patients have microvoltage, and the P waves usually escape. Whereas purely insulating effects of fluid require large effusions, voltage reduc-

tion in tamponade probably is mainly due to angulation and especially to compression of the heart, which reduces its size. (Occasional tamponade patients develop left-axis deviation, possibly due to ventricular displacement or greater compression of the thin right ventricle.) Some T wave abnormalities may be due to reduced coronary flow in previously diseased coronary arteries, owing to low aortic pressure in tamponade plus epicardial compression of the coronary vessels as well as obliteration of the normal transmural myocardial pressure gradient. Pre-tamponade T wave inversions may be pseudonormalized.[11]

ELECTRICAL ALTERNATION. In the appropriate clinical setting this finding is *almost pathognomonic of tamponade,* occurring in up to one third of cases because of periodic (nearly always 2:1) oscillation of the heart swinging within the effusion.[4] Although typical of large effusions, alternation can occur with as little as 200 ml of pericardial fluid with a thick parietal pericardium. It reflects alternation of the spatial axis of the QRS complex and other waves due to cardiac movements while the ECG electrodes remain in place. T wave alternation is less easily seen, whereas P waves and PR segments rarely visibly alternate. Removal of a small fluid aliquot usually abolishes alternation, just as the same initial decrement usually produces the greatest relative hemodynamic improvement. Alternation is critically related to heart rate: beta-adrenergic blocking agents can slow the rate and make alternation disappear.

EARLY REPOLARIZATION (see Table 50–2). An ECG almost indistinguishable from the J-point deviations of stage I—found mainly in males younger than age 40 and prevalent in mental institutions—may involve most ECG leads and mimic pericarditis. Unlike stage I, this ECG does not acutely evolve and differentiation is sometimes difficult, requiring clinical correlation.[11] In early repolarization, J-point elevations are usually accompanied by a slur, oscillation, or notch at the end of the QRS just before and including the J point and best seen with tall R and T waves (the largest precordial R wave is usually in V_4 rather than V_5). In general, R wave and T wave voltages are large, and a differential test using the PR segment as a baseline is the height of the J point in lead V_6. Pericarditis is likely if the J point is more than 25 percent of the height of the T wave apex.[11]

Constrictive Pericarditis

ECG abnormalities in constrictive pericarditis, although often characteristic, are nonspecific. One "typical" ECG would include mildly low voltage QRS and flattened to inverted T waves in all leads of "epicardial" derivation (Fig. 50–7).[11] (Postoperatively, continued low-voltage predicts reduced survival.) In some patients with chronic and many with acute and subacute constriction, T wave inversions of stage III never improve or regress incompletely. Especially with chronicity, P waves can be wide and bifid (interatrial block), sometimes resembling P-mitrale with P wave axis between + 90 and − 10 degrees; these predict the future occurrence of atrial fibrillation. The P wave in V_1 may indicate LA enlargement (P-terminal force ≥ 4 mV) or RA enlargement (large positive initial component) or both. Yet, many patients have normal ECGs or only nonspecific T wave abnormality. Pleural effusions, ascites, and fluid retention also modify the ECG in constrictive pericarditis. Unlike acute pericarditis, arrhythmias occur in constrictive pericarditis and increase with chronicity (mainly atrial fibrillation and occasionally atrial flutter). Preoperative conversion to sinus rhythm is difficult. Rhythm disturbances are more common with pericardial calcification or an enlarged cardiopericardial silhouette. Arrhythmias always imply cardiac abnormality (see Chap. 25).

QRS ABNORMALITY.[10, 11] In chronic constrictive pericarditis, low voltage and myocardial atrophy are common and probably related. In acute and subacute constrictive pericar-

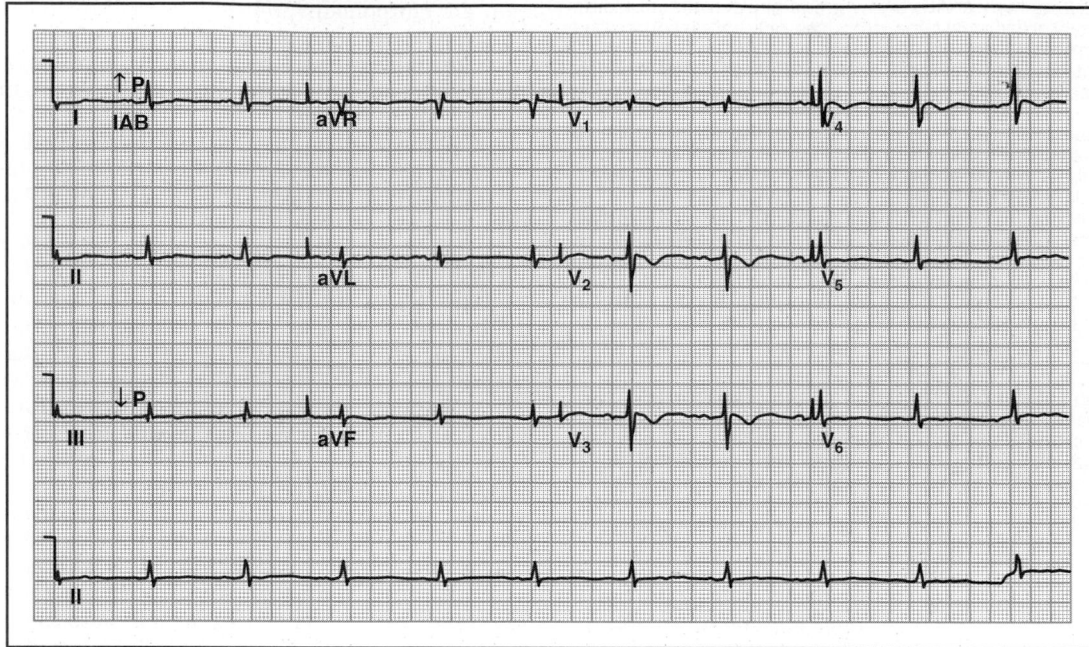

FIGURE 50–7. Constrictive pericarditis (chronic form). Low voltage is evident in ten leads and relatively low voltage occurs in V_2 and V_3, with flat, $-+$, inverted, and frankly inverted T waves. P waves are wide (interatrial block [IAB]) with P axis = 0 degrees: P wave is flat in aVF, inverted in lead III, and upright in lead I (arrows). Wide negative phase of biphasic P wave in V_1 indicates left atrial enlargement (of which IAB is also a strong correlate). (From Spodick DH: The Pericardium: A Comprehensive Textbook. New York, Marcel Dekker, 1997.)

ditis (now the prevalent forms) the QRS axis tends to be normal. In classic chronic constrictive pericarditis, the frontal QRS axis tends to be vertical, in many cases more positive than +60 degrees, and sometimes with right-axis deviation; verticalization increases with chronicity. The vertical tendency may represent disproportionate RV injury and strain or perhaps disuse atrophy of the underloaded left ventricle. Electrical alternation may occur in *effusive-constrictive pericarditis* with dominant parietal pericardial constriction and relatively little effusion. QRS abnormalities typical of RV hypertrophy may evolve in patients with unequal constriction or strategically placed postpericardiectomy scarring affecting the pulmonary artery, the right ventricle, the AV groove, or the mitral valve. Other QRS abnormalities, including abnormal Q waves, reflect myocardial penetration by inflammation, scarring, or focal atrophy. T wave abnormalities are variable. After pericardiectomy, QRS voltage nearly always increases with slow or no evolution in patients with myocardial atrophy. Vertical or right-axis orientation may persist, but there is frequently a limited correction. T wave abnormalities may not change and often temporarily worsen.

CONGENITAL ABNORMALITIES

Most congenital abnormalities of the pericardium are discovered accidentally at cardiac surgery, with routine chest radiography, on fetal echocardiography, or while diagnosing unusual, often unrelated, symptoms.[14] Rarest are *pericardial bands* obstructing the superior vena cava. *Pericardial celomic cysts* are most frequent and usually least important. *Bronchogenic cysts* with congenital partial pericardial defects are important because of potential compression of the heart and vessels.

Congenital Cysts and Diverticula

Cysts occur anywhere on the pericardium (mostly at the right cardiodiaphragmatic angle) and are clinically silent. Usually less than 3 cm in diameter, most are unilocular and smooth and contain clear fluid.[14] Cysts can be associated with chest pain, dyspnea, cough, and significant arrhythmias, probably owing to compression and erosion of adjacent tissues.[15, 16] Rare pedunculated cysts may undergo torsion with chest pain and ischemia-related lesions of the cyst wall. Cysts can become secondarily infected and can complicate related or unrelated pericardial effusion and tamponade. Rapid enlargement is rare, and "spontaneous" resolution is probably due to traumatic rupture.[14] Intrapericardial rupture of large cysts threatens acute tamponade. Indeed, if very large they can mimic pericardial effusion. The principal significance of unilocular and multilocular congenital cysts is simulation of mediastinal tumors (especially when situated away from the diaphragm), loculated pericardial effusions and hematomas, pericardial diverticula, and ventricular pseudoaneurysms.

Diagnosis. This is usually by appropriate imaging and, rarely, thoracoscopy or thoracotomy and aspiration.[14] Cyst fluid, which may contain hyaluronic acid, is yellowish or crystal clear. On imaging, tumors with central necrosis may simulate cysts, whereas unusually shaped and internally bleeding cysts may simulate tumors. Occasionally, a bronchogenic cyst will be "trapped" in or on the pericardium. Benign teratomas, which may undergo malignant change, and lymphangiomas have the same differential diagnosis. Usually CT (especially electron beam), MRI, and, with some difficulty, two- and three-dimensional echocardiography, especially transesophageal (TEE), can be diagnostic.[17] Treatment by TEE-assisted open, or video-assisted thoracoscopic, excision is required for symptomatic, locally compressive, and hemodynamically compromising cysts. Aspiration with or without ablation by a sclerosant (e.g., alcohol) is an option. *Pericardial diverticula* are rarer and resemble cysts except that a comparable developmental abnormality has left a communication with the pericardial cavity.

Absence of the Pericardium

Complete *pericardial agenesis* is rare, often discovered accidentally at cardiac operation or during evaluation of unrelated symptoms, and demonstrable by negative imaging.[17, 18, 18a] Partial loss of any part of the pericardium can occur with or without a defect in the adjacent pleura and very often with some kind of associated congenital cardiac, pulmonary, or skeletal abnormality. Most common is absence of the entire left side of the pericardium. Partial left absence and absent right pericardium are uncommon. Absence of the inferior pericardium with or without diaphragmatic defect or aplasia is rare in adults. Associated diaphragmatic defects may permit intrathoracic, including intrapericardial, herniation of abdominal organs.

Absence of the entire right or (especially) left pericardium permits homolateral cardiac displacement, which is visible on imaging and increased with the patient lying on the side of the defect (particularly the left), which accentuates cardiac mobility. Small increases in preload cause undue ventricular dilation, especially of the right ventricle.

Partial absence of the left pericardium potentially permits herniation and entrapment of parts of the heart like the left atrium, LA appendage, right atrium, right ventricle, and, with apical defects, protrusion through the defects of large parts of both ventricles. Defect edges may compress cardiac chambers, great vessels, and coronary vessels. The phrenic nerves may be displaced to the edges.[19-21]

SYMPTOMS. Acute or chronic symptoms like vague chest pain or dyspnea, including trepopnea, may or may not be related to any pericardial defect, but exacerbation in the left lateral decubitus is typical of left-sided defects.[11, 14, 22] Unusual torsion of the great vessels by unrestrained cardiac mobility may affect filling, ventricular ejection, and coronary flow and has been associated with tricuspic chordal rupture. Ischemic pain and myocardial infarction occur when the edge of a defect critically interrupts a coronary artery.

PHYSICAL FINDINGS.[11] Physical findings usually only support a diagnosis, especially in left-sided absence, and include basal ejection murmurs, wide split S_2, as well as apical midsystolic clicks and systolic murmurs accentuated by inspiration. Extensive left defects produce conspicuous precordial impulses; the apex, frequently in the anterior or midaxillary line, is hypermobile with changes in body position.

ELECTROCARDIOGRAM.[11] Sinus bradycardia is common. Usually, with complete left-sided defects, ECG changes reflect posturally changing anatomical abnormalities and relative volume overload of the right side of the heart. Right-axis deviation and incomplete or complete right bundle branch block are the rule. Leftward displacement of the precordial transition zone is common with poor R wave progression and sometimes QS in leads V_1 to V_3, mimicking anterior infarction: conspicuous single-peaked P waves reflect RA overload.

IMAGING. In extensive or complete left pericardial absence chest radiographs show leftward displacement of the heart and aortic knob with the trachea midline. The pulmonary artery "segment" bulges or fills in to straighten ("mitralize") the left heart border; the right border can be so levodisplaced that the spine is clearly seen. "Air" (projections of lung) between the aorta and pulmonary artery or between the left diaphragm and inferior cardiac border are common. Herniation of the LA appendage is virtually diagnostic of partial left defect but must be distinguished from congenital LA aneurysm. CT and MRI show all the features and are most reliable for absence of pericardial tissue. MRI is more sensitive and can show the typical absence of the preaortic pericardial recess (almost always present in normal hearts) in both partial and complete absence of the left pericardium.[14, 17]

TREATMENT. Treatment, reserved for symptoms (unless herniation threatens) includes partial or complete pericardiectomy, pericardioplasty or extension of the defect to relieve tension on critical structures, and LA appendectomy. Postoperative adhesions help stabilize cardiac position.

ACQUIRED PERICARDIAL DISEASES

Virtually every pathological process, medical and surgical, can involve the pericardium primarily or indirectly.[23, 23a] Thus, freshly diagnosed pericardial disease may or may not be related to other conditions. Classifications in Table 50–3 necessarily overlap; for example, the post-myocardial infarction syndrome belongs both to myocardial/pericardial injury and to the immunopathies.[21] Because of etiopathogenic complexities, protocols for diagnosis and management have been carefully designed and prospectively evaluated.[25]

▼ **TABLE 50–3. ETIOLOGY/PATHOGENESIS OF ACQUIRED DISEASES OF THE PERICARDIUM***

MAJOR CATEGORIES†
  I. Idiopathic pericarditis (syndromes)
  II. Due to living agents—infectious, parasitic
  III. Vasculitis/connective tissue disease
  IV. Immunopathies/hypersensitivity states
  V. Diseases of contiguous structures
  VI. Disorders of metabolism
  VII. Trauma—direct, indirect
  VIII. Neoplasms—primary, metastatic, multicentric
  IX. Of uncertain pathogenesis or in association with various syndromes

  *Considerable overlap (e.g., categories III and IV, V and VIII).
  †See corresponding chapter sections for detailed outlines.
  Modified from Spodick DH: The Pericardium: A Comprehensive Textbook. New York, Marcel Dekker, 1997.

PERICARDIAL RESPONSES TO INFLAMMATION AND IRRITATION. Noxious agents contacting the pericardium set up responses producing clinical disease. For example, microorganisms or antigenic material or immunocytes activated elsewhere can reach the pericardium through the bloodstream, lymphatic vessels, or adjacent organs or by traumatic (including surgical) implantation and set up infective pericarditis. When inflammation is intense, the subjacent myocardium becomes involved, permitting ECG diagnosis; pericardial inflammation is mediated by cytokines, such as tumor necrosis factors and interleukins.[23] Inflamed mesothelium produces increased prostaglandins (inhibition of which may be an effect of antiinflammatory treatment). Intense inflammation involving both myocardium and pericardium produces myopericarditis. Immunopathic mechanisms are increasingly identified in the pathogenesis.[26]

DISEASES OF NEIGHBORING AND CONTIGUOUS STRUCTURES.[23] Diseases of the myocardium, pleura, lungs, diaphragm, esophagus, and mediastinum involve the pericardium by contiguity or by hematogenous or lymphogenous transmission and may or may not become clinically obvious. Sometimes pericarditis is the first clue to disease in a nearby organ. Transmural myocardial infarction virtually always involves the pericardium, but pericardial involvement is diagnosed in fewer than half of patients. Tuberculous pericarditis when not due to hematogenous or lymphogenous implantation can be introduced by adjacent infected mediastinal lymph nodes. Each of the tissues of the pericardium with the exception of the elastic tissue can give rise to primary malignancies and benign tumors, producing irritative (inflammatory) and physical effects that are usually misinterpreted. This is less true for metastatic malignancy. Pericardial fat necrosis is rare, causing nondescript or sharp pain in the left lower chest, often with pleuritic fluctuation suggesting pleuritis or pericarditis. The chest radiograph may show a particularly smudgy pericardial fat pad. Treatment is with antiinflammatory agents or resection.

PERICARDIAL EFFUSION. Pericardial effusion is identified as any excessive pericardial contents due to inflammatory exudation, systemic fluid retention, bleeding, gas (including air), pus, or any combination of these. Pericardial exudation arises mainly if not entirely from the visceral pericardium. Hydropericardium is a transudate and can result after systemic fluid expansion, as in cardiac failure and other conditions with solute and water retention. Hydropericardium is first recognized as enlargement of the cardiac silhouette. There are no recognized clinical consequences except with rare massive hydropericardia that compress lung and other adjacent structures. Inflammatory/irritative effusion is produced from an exudate, which appears when the rate of inflammatory exudation exceeds the resorptive capacity of the serosa, particularly its lymphatics and veins. They may be obstructed by inflammatory disease and compression by the effusion itself.[12, 23] Because large molecules are poorly transported by the pericardium, the tendency to fluid accumulation may be exaggerated by the oncotic effect of protein-rich exudates. Pericardial effusions induce four functional states[12]: (1) slow production of undetected fluid; (2) effusion without cardiac compression; (3) effusion at a rate appropriate to compress the heart significantly but checked by compensatory mechanisms; and (4) cardiac tamponade. In the first two states, either the normal residual capacity of the pericardium is not significantly exceeded or the fibrosa can stretch. Many effusions become stabilized at some level by compensatory mechanisms. *Tamponade is a continuum,* even in patients who never develop corresponding clinical syndromes; florid tamponade is an emergency. Bleeding, thrombosis, neoplastic tissue, and pus modify clinical and imaging aspects.

POLYSEROSITIS.[23] Many conditions causing pericarditis can simultaneously or sequentially inflame other serous sacs. Like pericarditis, polyserositis may appear at any inflammatory state from acute to chronic. Symptoms and signs referable to one or another serosa may dominate the picture. Yet pericardial involvement can be the most distressing because of pericardial pain, emergent tamponade, or the steady deterioration of constriction (e.g., tuberculous serositis); physiologically unimportant pericardial adhesions are common. The vasculitis/connective tissue disease group is most likely to produce true polyserositis (exudates) whereas the acquired immunodeficiency syndrome (AIDS) produces a capillary leak syndrome with noninflammatory transudative effusions much more often than true polyserositis.

HEMOPERICARDIUM. Hemopericardium is always important because of either frank bleeding into the pericardium as in cardiac wounds, erosion of vessels by tumor, an aggressive inflammatory process, or bleeding diatheses, including administration of thrombolytic agents to patients with pericarditis. Detectable bleeding occurs in effusions of almost every etiology. Unless overwhelmed by the rate of bleeding, the fibrinolytic and anticoagulant properties of the pericardial serosa as well as the beating action of the heart (which defibrinates blood) nearly always keeps most or all of the blood liquid and mixed with other pericardial contents. Frank blood and particularly clots, nearly always indicate major bleeding, which must be dealt with at its source. Indeed, clots, recognizable by echocardiography as hyperechoic objects in a pericardial effusion, usually mandate surgical rather than needle drainage. Moreover, any significant amount of blood in the pericardial fluid, especially in the presence of damaged serosa, is the substrate for adhesions and loculations. Malignancy is a major cause of hemopericardium. Subacute and chronic hemopericardium may be "idiopathic" or due to trauma, bleeding disorders, or vascular anomalies. Increasing fluid may be osmotically affected by split proteins (e.g., fibrolysis) and other molecules.

CHYLOPERICARDIUM. This condition results from extravasation of chyle owing to a neoplasm, particularly lymphangiomatous hamartoma or cystic hygroma, or abnormal communication between pericardium and thoracic duct.[27] Many cases follow cardiac and thoracic surgery, suggesting damage to lymphatic channels; many others are idiopathic. Chylopericardium tends to be large and chronic, with an element of tamponade, and is only rarely constrictive.[10] The fluid is milky and alkaline with electrolyte, protein, glucose, and cholesterol levels similar to those of blood serum. Fat studies are typical of chyle and include chylomicrons. In neoplasia, the pericardium can refill so rapidly that reaccumulation of chyle may be visible during operation. No visible communication may be demonstrated between the pericardium and the alimentary tract, especially in nonneoplastic patients. Some communication is indicated in chylopericardium by the following tests: (1) intrapericardial appearance of ingested lipophilic dyes, (2) frequent successful treatment by thoracic duct ligation; (3) lymphangiography demonstrating a relationship between thoracic duct and pericardial cavity; and (4) CT or MRI densities consistent with fat (note that if the patient has not eaten for some time, chylous fluid may become clear). "Primary chylopericardium" denotes an unknown cause.[27] Chylopericardium obligates indefinite assessment for constriction. Although chyle is bactericidal, the effusion can become infected. Enhanced CT with lymphangiography should be diagnostic.[28] Conservative management includes pericardial drainage and a low-fat diet with increased medium-chain triglycerides.[23] More often, low thoracic duct ligation plus a pericardial window or resection is required.

CHOLESTEROL PERICARDITIS. This condition is characterized by high concentrations of cholesterol and other lipids in pericardial fluid and cholesterol crystals in pericardial tissue.[23] Cholesterol effusions tend to be large and subacute or chronic and of multiple etiology. Total pericardial fluid cholesterol approaches or exceeds blood cholesterol (usually normal) with values often more than 500 mg/dl, accompanied by increased total lipids. Cholesterol in most myxedematous effusions lacks crystal formation and usually is in concentrations below the elevated serum level. Cholesterol effusions are turbid, brown, yellow, orange, amber, purple, or coffee color, with a sheen giving a "gold paint" appearance. There may be evidence of recent or remote hemorrhage and leukocytes (mainly lymphocytes).

Specific gravity is nearly always greater than 1.020, whereas electrolyte, total protein, and albumin:globulin ratios approximate those of blood. The pericardium is often thickened by scarring, frequently with variable amounts of fibrin and yellowish nodules, plaques, and papillomatous masses of cholesterol. The epicardium may be visibly inflamed, and constrictive epicarditis is not uncommon. Microscopically, there is often intense fibrosis, with inflammation with many cholesterol clefts and crystals and other lipid crystals. Phagocytes take up considerable lipid and some iron pigment; histocytes have foamy cytoplasm. Crystals and clefts are often surrounded by foreign body giant cells and elements of chronic granulomatous inflammation. Examination under polarized light shows cells containing "Maltese crosses."

Cholesterol effusions occur with pericarditis in tuberculosis, rheumatoid arthritis, and after traumatic hemopericardium, as well as myxedema. In the inflammatory lesions, granulomas are probably a source of the cholesterol as is blood. In "formes frustes" high cholesterol concentration is without crystal formation. Any chronic effusion might result in cholesterol precipitation, particularly with a cholesterol source like blood. Unfortunately, pericardiocentesis frequently results in rapid refilling and sometimes epicardial constriction or unremitting chronic cardiac tamponade.[23, 29] Conservative treatment is drainage, but definitive treatment is pericardial resection and management of any underlying diseases.

LYMPHOPERICARDIUM. This condition is rare and related to local or, more often, generalized lymphangiectasis. Fluid has characteristics of lymph and may contain a predominance of lymphocytes.[23]

PNEUMOPERICARDIUM AND PNEUMOHYDROPERICARDIUM. In adults, pneumopericardium may be "spontaneous" and usually occurs in conjunction with hemopericardium or some type of effusion.[23, 30] It may follow wounds or fistulous communications due to primary disease[31] or instrumentation of adjacent viscera, which can also produce *pyopneumopericardium*. Pericardial infection by gas-producing organisms duplicates the picture. Some cases may be due to malignant destruction of tissue but also to penetrating and nonpenetrating chest and upper abdominal trauma or after single-lung transplantation. Infants and occasional adults on respirators or with severe asthma develop pneumopericardium from alveolar rupture by high-pressure air or oxygen dissecting into the pericardium through weak points in the pericardial reflections over the great vessels.[1] When due to indirect (blunt) trauma, pneumopericardium occurs by three main mechanisms: (1) direct tracheobronchial-pericardial communication; (2) pneumothorax with a pleuropericardial tear; and (3) penetration along pulmonary venous perivascular sheaths from ruptured alveoli to the pericardium. On chest radiography, air-fluid levels indicate pneumohydropericardium. A chest radiograph may show air in the transverse sinus and often subcutaneous emphysema.

TENSION PNEUMOPERICARDIUM.[30] This condition is due to increasing air, gas, or fluid, which produces pneumotamponade, often with marked cyanosis and hypotension. Pneumopericardium and hydropneumopericardium can produce audible clicks and splashes and an "air gap" sign on M-mode echocardiograms.

PERICARDIAL DISORDERS DURING PREGNANCY.[23] There is no evidence that pregnancy affects susceptibility to pericardial disease. However, although tamponade has been observed, the physiological 40 to 50 percent increase in blood volume during pregnancy may moderate its physiological and clinical expression. Many pregnant women normally develop a minimal to moderate clinically silent hydropericardium by the third trimester; this could combine with less than usual exudation by any acute pericarditis to cause cardiac compression. Most pericardial disorders run their accustomed courses during pregnancy and are managed as in nonpregnant patients. Unless contraindicated, treatment with antiinflammatory drugs, antibiotics, and drainage for suppurative pericarditis, drainage of tamponading fluids, and pericardiectomy for constriction, recurrent pericardial effusion, and resistant bacterial pericarditis are indicated.

FETAL PERICARDIAL FLUID. This can be detected by echocardiography after 20 weeks' gestation and is normally 2 mm or less in depth; more fluid should raise questions of hydrops fetalis, Rh disease, hypoalbuminemia, and immunopathy or maternally transmitted mycoplasmal or other infections. However, "idiopathic" pericardial effusion and tamponade may occur in otherwise normal fetuses (necessitating investigation for infection and neoplasia).[32]

PANCREATITIS. Acute and recurrent pericarditis, pericardial effusion, and tamponade associated with pancreatitis may be due to simultaneous infection (presumably viral), immunopathy, or chemical injury by circulating enzymes and rarely by direct pancreatic-mediastinal communication.[23]

BETA-THALASSEMIA. Acute and recurrent "idiopathic" pericarditis with all its consequences and complications occur in up to one half of children with thalassemia major (most often silent or mild), suggesting more than a casual relation. This may represent viral susceptibility or an immunopathy with a possible element of tissue injury by hemosiderin.[33]

FAMILIAL MEDITERRANEAN FEVER.[34] Recurrent pericarditis sometimes accompanies pleuritis and/or peritonitis, making familial Mediterranean fever a polyserositis. Constriction is rare. Treatment is with colchicine.

ACUTE PERICARDITIS

"Dry pericarditis," strictly speaking, indicates pericardial inflammation without effusion, that is, with a fibrinous inflammatory exudate (Fig. 50–8). Because most pericardial irritation evokes at least some fluid clinically, dry pericarditis encompasses cases in which excess pericardial fluid is virtually absent or clinically unimportant.[35, 36] Virtually all etiological forms can present this way (Table 50–4). In some conditions, such as rheumatoid pericarditis, the acute phase is usually missed or discovered by accident, so that the history is that of the etiological illness, except when acute pericarditis is its first sign. Infectious pericarditis may be preceded by local and systemic signs of infection.[36] The classic example is acute viral pericarditis, which is responsible for most cases of "idiopathic" pericarditis and nearly always preceded by a recent respiratory, gastrointestinal, or "flulike" illness. Moreover, symptoms and signs during acute pericarditis may be modified by or coexist with those of an inciting illness. A specific etiological diagnosis (i.e., nonidiopathic) is more easily discovered in "sicker" patients, including those who develop tamponade.[35]

SYMPTOMS. The onset may be abrupt or insidious. Bacterial and viral pericarditis often strike dramatically, whereas the uremic or tuberculous pericarditis often goes unnoticed. Diagnosis can be suggested by symptoms with an abrupt onset, but it may depend on objective manifestations after an insidious onset. Viral pericarditis, for example, can declare itself by crescendoing pain over several hours, whereas uremic or tuberculous pericarditis often presents as fever of unknown origin.

PAIN (Table 50–5). Over the vast range of causes (see Table 50–4), pain is the most common symptom, although it often is absent; thus, rheumatoid pericarditis is nearly always silent whereas acute infectious pericarditis only occasionally lacks pain. Pain can be due to inflammation of the pericardium itself, the phrenic nerves, the adjacent pleura, sympathetic nerves accompanying coronary vessels in the epicardium, or potentiation of the algesic properties of bradykinin by pericardial prostacyclin.[35] Pain can be sharp, "sticking," dull, aching, and pressure-like in individual cases, with intensities varying from 1 to 10. Initially, it tends to be sharp, precordial, and pleuritic and is exacerbated by inspiration, cough, and recumbency; hence, patients sit up for relief. Pain onset, frequently perceived as sudden, particularly when it interrupts sleep, is occasionally related to exertion, which may be coincidental; once established, it worsens with exertion. Characteristic pain relief from sitting up and leaning forward may be related to the biomechanical characteristics of the parietal pericardium. These maneuvers may relieve increased pericardial tissue tension due to inspiration and truncal extension; they also splint the diaphragm.[35] Pain radiation can follow distributions common to angina as well as to the epigastrium, creating problems in differential diagnosis when the pain is not pleuritic or has a pressing quality, and particularly when it radiates to the jaw or one or both shoulders. Shoulder pain must be distinguished from pain in one or both trapezius ridges, usually the left. Trapezius ridge pain

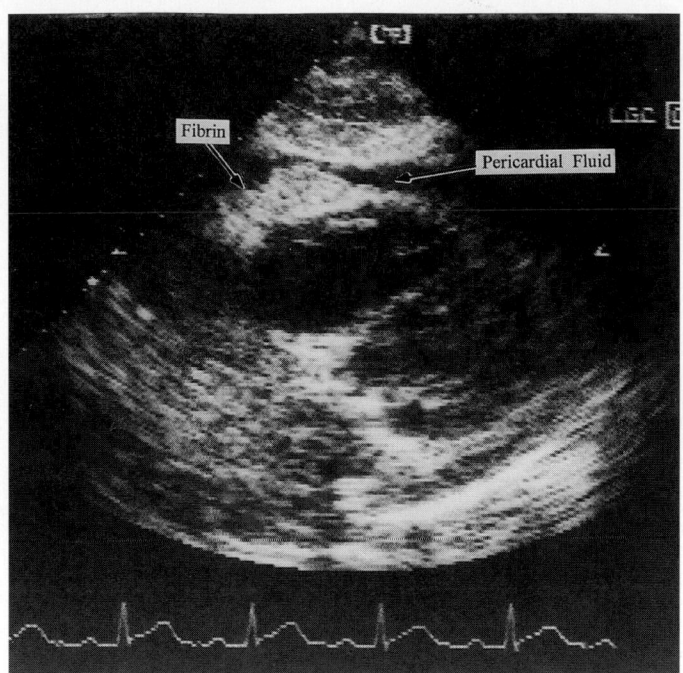

FIGURE 50–8. Fibrinous pericarditis. Large fibrinous exudate on anterior epicardium. Minimal pericardial fluid permits delineation of fibrin.

transmitted through the phrenic nerves is virtually pathognomonic for pericardial irritation.[35] Indeed, some patients perceive pain only in a trapezius ridge. Note that patients must be asked to point to the areas of pain perception because patients and most physicians confuse the trapezius ridge with the shoulder. Pain can also occur in the midposterior thorax or below the left scapula. Palpation of the chest wall may elicit local tenderness revealing costochondritis, Tietze syndrome, or other chest wall syndromes, including rib fractures in patients with traumatic pericarditis.[37] Finally, some patients do not describe "pain" but rather vague precordial distress with or without inspiratory or postural exacerbation. Some patients with myopericarditis (particularly viral) may have skeletal muscle myalgia.

OTHER SYMPTOMS. A nonproductive cough is common, exacerbates pleuritic pain, and may antedate chest symptoms. Productive cough is due to associated illnesses. Hiccup is relatively rare. Odynophagia, rarely the only sign of pericarditis, occurs because of apposition of the esophagus and posterior parietal pericardium; odynophagia and dysphagia also result from pericardial inflammation or effusion due to spread from esophageal inflammation, trauma, or malignancy. Faintness and dizziness are uncommon in the absence of tamponade but can occur when there is considerable pain, tachycardia, or constitutional reaction.

SYSTEMIC REACTION. Fever, usually less than 39°C (102.2°F), is common as a result of pericarditis or accompanying diseases and may herald the clinical onset. Elderly patients lacking mechanisms for cytokine liberation may not be febrile, and some with diseases such as renal failure may be hypothermic. Chills (rigors) are likely to accompany spiking fevers in suppurative pericarditis and some cases of idiopathic (presumably viral) pericarditis. Weakness and depression accompany some cases with marked systemic manifestations. Anxiety is common with very painful or disagreeable precordial sensations, especially in those with preexisting heart disease. Pallor may be a clue to systemic illnesses such as tuberculosis, uremia, neoplasia, and rheumatic carditis. In patients severely ill from antecedent or accompanying disease, symptoms and constitutional reac-

▼ TABLE 50–4. ETIOLOGIES OF ACUTE PERICARDITIS*

I. **Idiopathic Pericarditis**
II. **Pericarditis Due to Living Agents: Infections, Parasitoses**
   A. Bacterial
      1. Suppurative (any organism)
      2. Tuberculous; other mycobacterial
   B. Viral
      1. Coxsackie virus
      2. Influenza virus
      3. Human immunodeficiency virus
      4. Hepatitis B, A, ?C virus
      5. Other
   C. Mycotic (fungal)
   D. Rickettsial
   E. Spirochetal
   F. *Spirillum*
   G. *Mycoplasma pneumoniae*
   H. Infectious mononucleosis
   I. *Leptospira*
   J. *Listeria*
   K. Lymphogranuloma venereum
   L. Psittacosis (Chlamydiaceae)
   M. Parasitic
III. **Pericarditis in the Vasculitis/Connective Tissue Disease Group**
   A. Rheumatoid arthritis
   B. Rheumatic fever
   C. Systemic lupus erythematosus
   D. Drug-induced lupus erythematosus
   E. Scleroderma
   F. Sjögren syndrome
   G. ? Whipple disease (*Tropheryma whippleii* organisms)
   H. Mixed connective tissue disease
   I. Reiter syndrome
   J. Ankylosing spondylitis
   K. Inflammatory bowel diseases
   L. Serum sickness
   M. Wegener granulomatosis
   N. Vasculitis (e.g., temporal/giant cell arteritis)
   O. Polymyositis (dermatomyositis)
   P. Behçet syndrome
   Q. Familial Mediterranean fever
   R. Dermatomyositis
   S. Panmesenchymal reaction of corticosteroid hormone withdrawal
   T. Polyarteritis
   U. Churg-Strauss syndrome
   V. Thrombohemolytic thrombocytopenic purpura
   W. Hypocomplementemic uremic vasculitis syndrome
   X. Leukoclastic vasculitis
   Y. Other
IV. **Pericarditis in Disease of Contiguous Structures**
   A. Myocardial infarction
      1. Acute myocardial infarction
      2. Postmyocardial infarction syndrome
      3. Postpericardiotomy syndrome
      4. Ventricular aneurysm
   B. Dissecting aortic aneurysm
   C. Pleural and pulmonary diseases
      1. Pneumonia
      2. Pulmonary embolism
      3. Pleuritis
V. **Pericarditis in Disorders of Metabolism**
   A. Renal failure
      1. Uremia (chronic/acute renal failure)
      2. "Dialysis" pericarditis
   B. Myxedema
      1. Cholesterol pericarditis
   C. Gout
   D. Scurvy

VI. **Neoplastic Pericarditis**
   A. *Secondary* (metastatic, hematogenous, or by direct extension): carcinoma, sarcoma, lymphoma, leukemia, carcinoid, Sipple syndrome, other
   B. *Primary* mesothelioma, sarcoma, fibroma, lipoma
VII. **Traumatic Pericarditis**
   A. Direct
      1. Pericardial perforation (esp. pneumopericardium)
         a. Penetrating chest injury
         b. Esophageal perforation
         c. Gastric perforation
      2. Cardiac injury: direct trauma
         a. Cardiac surgery (see also V.A3 above) and IX.A below)
         b. During catheterization
            i. Pacemaker insertion
            ii. Catheter ablation for arrhythmias
            iii. Diagnostic
            iv. Percutaneous transluminal coronary angioplasty with coronary dissection
      3. Indirect trauma
         a. Radiation pericarditis
         b. Nonpenetrating chest injury
      4. "Foreign-body" pericarditis
VIII. **Pericarditis of Uncertain Pathogenesis and in Association with Various Syndromes**
   A. Postmyocardial and pericardial injury syndromes (?immune disorders)
   B. Pericardial fat necrosis
   C. Inflammatory bowel disease
      1. Colitis (ulcerative; granulomatous)
      2. Segmental enteritis (Crohn disease)
      3. Whipple disease
      4. Celiac disease
   D. Löffler syndrome
   E. Thalassemia (and other congenital anemias)
   F. "Specific" drug reaction (psicofuranine; ?minoxidil, ? others)
   G. Pancreatitis
   H. Sarcoidosis
   I. Cholesterol pericarditis not associated with myxedema or granulomas
   J. Fat embolism
   K. Bile fistula (to pericardium)
   L. Wissler syndrome
   M. "PIE" syndrome
   N. Stevens-Johnson syndrome
   O. Gaucher disease
   P. Diaphragmatic hernia
   Q. Atrial septal defect
   R. Giant cell aortitis
   S. Takayasu syndrome
   T. Castleman disease (giant lymph node hyperplasia)
   U. Fabry disease
   V. Kawasaki disease
   W. Degos disease
   X. Acute pancreatitis
   Y. Histiocytosis X
   Z. Campylodactyly-pleuritis-pericarditis syndrome
   AA. Farmer's lung
   BB. Yellow nail syndrome
   CC. Myeloid metaplasia
   DD. Afibrinogenemia; hypofibrinogenemia
   EE. Juvenile xanthogranuloma
   FF. Dermatitis herpetiformis
   GG. Hypereosinophilic syndromes
   HH. Other

*Most etiologies can cause both "clinically dry" and effusive pericarditis and constriction.

tion provoked by pericarditis may be submerged in the total picture or suppressed by established treatment.

OBJECTIVE MANIFESTATIONS. The cardinal sign of pericarditis is the pericardial rub (see Fig. 50–4)—three or fewer friction sounds per cardiac cycle[9] (described earlier). Rubs can be transient or intermittent but often last hours to days. Unusually persistent rubs indicate a tendency to chronicity or continuing pericardial irritation as from ma-

	ACUTE PERICARDITIS	ACUTE ISCHEMIA
Onset	More often sudden	Usually gradual, crescendo
Main location	Substernal or left precordial	Same or confined to zones of radiation
Radiation	May be the same as ischemic, also trapezius ridge(s)	Shoulders, arms, neck, jaw, back; not trapezius ridge(s)
Quality	Usually sharp, stabbing; "background" ache or dull and oppressive	Usually "heavy" (pressure sensation) or burning
Inspiration	Worse	No effect unless with infarction pericarditis
Duration	Persistent; may wax and wane	Usually intermittent; <30 min each recurrence, longer for unstable angina
Body movements	Increased	Usually no effect
Posture	Worse on recumbency; improved on sitting, leaning forward	No effect or improvement on sitting
Nitroglycerin	No effect	Usually relief

From Spodick DH: The Pericardium: A Comprehensive Textbook. New York, Marcel Dekker, 1997.

lignant infiltration. Rubs are common in the presence of even large pericardial effusions. Echocardiograms in patients with clinically dry pericarditis may show fibrin with or without a small effusion or with a ragged "sunburst" appearance. ECG abnormalities range from normal to nonspecific to typical stage I ST segment deviations, usually with PR segment deviations (see Fig. 50–6, Table 50–6). Like the pericardial rub, the stage I ECG change is virtually diagnostic of acute pericarditis, always requiring differentiation from certain mimics and particularly when there are typical ECG variants. Occasionally, ECG abnormalities are the only evidence of pericarditis. Finally, any arrhythmias are *not* due to the acute pericarditis itself.[11] Pleural effusions, mainly on the left, are frequent in acute pericarditis. Leukopenia is uncommon and may be due to bone marrow depression by associated disease. Other acute phase reactants,[38] such as the sedimentation rate (ESR) and C-reactive protein (CRP), show mild to marked elevations, the level reflecting the intensity of the process, its inciting disease, or subepicardial myocardial involvement. Serum enzyme elevations derived from myocardium, such as the MB isoenzyme of creatine kinase (CK-MB), aspartate aminotransferase, aldolase, lactate dehydrogenase (LDH), and troponin I, reflect the degree of myocardial involvement by subepicardial myocarditis.[35] Serum myoglobin is usually normal. Patients with the greatest ST segment deviation tend to develop the largest rises, although the correlation is imprecise: some patients do not have significant levels despite ECG changes. Gallium-67 scanning can identify inflammatory and leukemic infiltrations and appears to be superior to scanning with indium-111.[35, 40]

TREATMENT. Treatment aims to relieve symptoms and eliminate etiological agents. Most patients are hospitalized for complete diagnosis and observation for complications, particularly effusion and tamponade. Antiinflammatory and symptomatic treatments resemble those of other conditions producing comparable pain, fever, and malaise and must be individualized. Nonsteroidal antiinflammatory drugs (NSAIDs) are the mainstay, possibly because many inhibit pericardial synthesis of prostaglandin I_2. Any effective NSAID may be used. However, indomethacin should be avoided in adults unless all other options fail, because it reduces coronary flow and has marked side effects. Ibuprofen has an excellent side effect profile and increases coronary flow, with the advantage of the largest dose range of the "classic" NSAIDs.[35, 39] Depending on clinical severity and response, treatment may initially require ibuprofen, 300 to 800 mg every 6 to 8 hours, and can be increased. In many mild cases, particularly of "idiopathic" pericarditis, 1 to 4 days of treatment appears adequate. Finally, all patients should be monitored for side effects; because all NSAIDs affect the gastrointestinal mucosa, it is wise to add misoprostol or other mucosal protectants.[41] Anecdotal evidence is increasing that colchicine added to an NSAID or even as monotherapy is effective for the initial attack and to prevent or treat recurrences.[35] It is well tolerated at 0.6 mg every 12 hours with or without a loading dose but must be monitored for side effects. A well-controlled trial is needed. Corticosteroid therapy should be avoided unless required for a specific illness such as a connective tissue disease or when all else fails, and then it should be used in minimally effective doses and carefully tapered. For pro-

▼ TABLE 50–6. ECG IN ACUTE PERICARDITIS VS. ACUTE ISCHEMIA

	ACUTE PERICARDITIS	ACUTE ISCHEMIA (AP, MI)
J-ST	Diffuse elevation usually concave, without reciprocal depressions	Localized deviation usually convex (with reciprocals in infarct)
PR segment depression	Frequent	Almost never
Abnormal Q waves	None unless with infarction	Common with infarction ("Q wave" infarcts)
T waves	Inverted after J points return to baseline	Inverted while ST segment still elevated (infarct)
Arrhythmia	None (in absence of heart disease)	Frequent
Conduction abnormalities	None (in absence of heart disease)	Frequent

AP = angina pectoris; MI = myocardial infarction.
From Spodick DH: The Pericardium: A Comprehensive Textbook. New York, Marcel Dekker, 1997.

tracted use of prednisone, ibuprofen or another NSAID should be introduced when tapering; after tapering the prednisone, the NSAID should also be tapered. Colchicine appears to improve therapeutic results and facilitate the "weaning" process.[42] Recovered patients should be observed indefinitely for one or more recurrences or later constriction. If patients require anticoagulants (e.g., those with prosthetic cardiac valves), heparin can be used under strict observation while the pericarditis is in progress.

DIFFERENTIAL DIAGNOSIS.[31] Acute pericarditis must be differentiated from syndromes producing similar symptoms and signs (Tables 50–5 to 50–8), bearing in mind that pericarditis may be (1) part of a generalized disease, (2) apparently isolated, or (3) part of a disorder affecting a neighboring organ and (4) occasionally the presenting syndrome of numerous diseases. Pain isolated to or referred to one or both trapezius ridges strongly compels consideration of pericarditis. Central pleuritic chest pain always raises a question of acute pericarditis if pleurisy can be ruled out, but both may occur simultaneously.

When the pain resembles that of cardiac ischemia (see Table 50–8), it may be longer lasting, sharper, and unresponsive to vasodilator therapy. Purely ischemic pain lacks the frequently pleuritic quality of infarction-related forms of pericarditis. Angina produces ECG changes usually with depressed rather than elevated ST segments. Tables 50–5, 50–6, and 50–8 summarize the differentiation of pericarditis from ischemia and infarction. On strictly ECG grounds, up to one third of acute pericarditis cases resemble ischemic heart disease because of atypical ECG evolution (see Chap. 35). Finally, pulmonary embolism can mimic acute pericarditis, particularly if with pleuritic pain (see Chap. 52). The ECG is usually nonspecifically altered and the pleural rub, if any, as well as the pain may not be precordial. Rarely, pulmonary embolism provokes a purely pericardial or pleuropericardial rub, pericardial effusion (usually small), or a pericardial response resembling the post-myocardial infarction syndrome.

Monophasic pericardial rubs, particularly the most common one, the ventricular systolic rub,[9] can mimic murmurs of mitral and especially tricuspid regurgitation and also ventricular septal defect, because all rubs tend to be most intense or occur only at the left mid to lower sternal border where some are palpable.[9] Assisting differential diagnosis are the short-term changeable nature of rubs and their occasionally unpredictable precordial distribution, as well as frequently absent heart disease. A typical stage I ECG is virtually diagnostic, although easily confused with the normal variant "early repolarization." The characteristic widespread ST segment changes are distinguishable from most acute myocardial ischemia and infarctions, which nearly always involve "regional" lead groups with reciprocal ST segment deviations in other leads; reciprocal ST segment depressions virtually never occur in uncomplicated acute pericarditis. Abnormal Q waves do not occur without asso-

ciated or preexisting myocardial disease (see Chaps. 5 and 35).

Myopericarditis/Perimyocarditis

Pericarditis is often accompanied by some degree of myocarditis and vice versa, with one or the other dominating the clinical picture. Most syndromes are primarily myocarditic or pericarditic.

PATHOGENESIS. Systemic disorders with frequent myocarditis, pericarditis, and myopericarditis include immunopathies, the vasculitis/connective tissue disease group, and drug-related pericarditis. Viral and other infections seem most frequent.[43, 44] Cardiotropic viruses can inflame myocardium and pericardium hematogenously, whereas bacterial and other organisms do so through lymphatics or by extension from pericardial infection. In eosinophilic forms, the destructive nature of the eosinophil is evident with high levels of eosinophilic cationic protein.[43] AIDS frequently involves the myocardium, pericardium, or both[45] (see Chap. 68). AIDS myopericarditis results from infection with the human immunodeficiency virus (HIV) and viral co-infection, damage by CD5 and CD8 lymphocytes, and myocardial Kaposi carditis.[45] Immunological mechanisms appear necessary for persistent and recurrent myopericarditis even in the absence of a viral genome.

▼ **TABLE 50–7.** CLINICALLY "DRY" ACUTE PERICARDITIS: PRINCIPAL DIFFERENTIAL DIAGNOSES

MANIFESTATION	TO BE DIFFERENTIATED
Electrocardiogram	
Stage 1	Acute myocardial infarction
	Early repolarization
Stage 2	Ischemia/infarction
Stage 3	Ischemia/infarction/myocarditis
Pain	Myocardial ischemia
	Angina
	Infarction
	Pleuritis
	Pneumonia
	Chest wall pain
	Pulmonary embolus (usually small)
Tachypnea	Pleuropulmonary disease
	Cardiac failure
Pericardial rub	Murmurs
	Pleural rub
	Chest wall sounds
	"Conus rubs"
	Pulmonary embolism
	Acute hyperthyroidism (Means-Lerman "scratch")
	Pacemaker rub (endocardial)

From Spodick DH: The Pericardium: A Comprehensive Textbook. New York, Marcel Dekker, 1997.

▼ **TABLE 50–8.** "CLINICAL FACTORS": ACUTE PERICARDITIS VS. ACUTE ISCHEMIA*

	ACUTE PERICARDITIS	ACUTE ISCHEMIA (AP, MI)
Myocardial enzymes	Normal or elevated	Elevated (infarct)
Pericardial friction	Rub (most cases)	Rub only if with pericarditis
Abnormal S_3	Absent unless preexisting	May be present
Abnormal S_4	Absent unless preexisting	Nearly always present
S_1	Intact	Often dull, mushy after first day
Pulmonary congestion	Absent	May be present
Murmurs	Absent unless preexisting	May be present

*Electrocardiographic differences in Table 50–6.
AP = angina pectoris; MI = myocardial infarction.
From Spodick DH: The Pericardium: A Comprehensive Textbook. New York, Marcel Dekker, 1997.

Almost any acute pericardial or myocardial damage can induce an immunopathy with recurrences (especially enteroviral and cytomegaloviral infections). Viruses provoke antibodies to myolemmal and sarcolemmal membranes (ALMABs and ASABs) and may be pathogenetic because of their cytolytic or cytotoxic properties.[46] The AMLABs and ASABs are part of B-cell–driven immune responses; for example, IgG-type AMLABs are diagnostic of perimyocarditis in tuberculous pericarditis. Drug-induced myopericarditis probably is pathogenetically related through "allergic" or hypersensitivity mechanisms. Finally, disease-specific autoantibodies reflect autoimmune involvement, although they correlate poorly with myocardial biopsy.[46, 47]

Many members of the vasculitis/connective tissue disease group (see Chaps. 48 and 67), classically including acute rheumatic fever, regularly produce myopericarditis.[43] Occasionally, inflammation spreads by contiguity from a primarily pericarditic process to the myocardium or from mediastinitis to the pericardium and myocardium. Pericardial tuberculosis often involves the myocardium, which becomes inflamed and ultimately fibrotic; both active and burned out tuberculosis are evident in tuberculous constriction. In contrast, pure uremic pericarditis may have a brisk inflammatory process in the pericardium and epicardial fat without invading the myocardium.

Evidence of myocardial involvement in pericarditis is summarized in pericarditis (Table 50–9). During myocarditis, pericardial involvement is mainly recognized by a rub or an effusion.[43] The ECG changes of acute pericarditis, as well as QT prolongation, indicate at least superficial myocarditis even when myocardial involvement is subclinical. Reciprocal and regional J (ST) changes (Fig. 50–9) and abnormal Q waves in the absence of infarction represent significant myocarditis disproportionately involving regions of the myocardium. Arrhythmias or conduction disturbances are absent even in severe pericarditis without independent or related disease of the myocardium or valves; myocarditis qualifies as such a related disease.[38]

After even mild idiopathic (presumably viral) pericarditis, transient myocardial functional and wall motion abnormalities can sometimes be detected for months; in more severe cases, global LV or RV dysfunction or eventual dilated cardiomyopathy are strong evidence of a myocarditic component. Occasional patients who, after drainage of pericardial effusion, develop myocardial dilation and acute cardiac failure ("pericardial shock") in the absence of antecedent heart disease almost certainly have had significant myocarditis.[43] Transient cardiac enlargement, usually recognized by imaging in the absence of increased pericardial fluid, and true dyspnea represents myocarditis. In acute pericarditis, when tachycardia persists after fever and pain subside, a myocarditic component is likely. During acute pericarditis, particularly of viral origin, but also with *Mycoplasma, Leptospira,* and *Borrelia* (Lyme disease) infections and skeletal muscle pain (myalgia)

1. *Any* acute ECG QRS complex change, especially if localized or with atypical evolution. Convex ST segment elevation during acute pericarditis. Atrioventricular or interventricular block.
2. Any significant arrhythmia, especially ventricular (in absence of other heart disease)
3. Evidence of myocardial dysfunction (in absence of other heart disease):
   a. Postpericardiocentesis abnormal S_3 (in absence of constrictive pericarditis)
   b. Pulmonary edema
   c. Postpericardiocentesis cardiac failure, especially pulmonary edema
   d. Abnormal imaging and catheterization studies:
      (1) Cardiomegaly
      (2) Abnormal hemodynamics (in absence of constrictive pericarditis)
      (3) Wall motion abnormalities
4. Sinus tachycardia:
   a. Out of proportion to fever, anemia, and/or chest pain
   b. Persistence after resolution of 6 through 10, below
5. Skeletal muscle myalgias, especially during viral pericarditis (suggests a myotropic organism)
6. Pericarditis with transudative effusion fluid
7. Nonpleuritic substernal chest pain with or without radiation (other than to trapezius ridges)
8. Elevated serum levels of cardiac enzymes, especially in presence of elevated serum myoglobin or troponin
9. Positive antimyosin–indium 111 scintigraphy
10. Myocardial production of tumor necrosis factor in absence of septic shock and congestive heart failure
11. Positive ^{99m}technetium pyrophosphate imaging
12. Positive gadolinium (Gd)-67 scintigraphy; Gd-DTPA–enhanced magnetic resonance imaging
13. Positive fibrinogen polymerization test

FIGURE 50–9. Perimyocarditis. *Top,* Acute phase with atypical stage III. T wave inversion in inferolateral distribution with J elevation in many leads in (in typical stage III T wave inversions with J on baselines). *Bottom,* Twenty-two days after onset: J on baseline with T wave inversion in inferolateral ("atypical") distribution consistent with myocarditis.

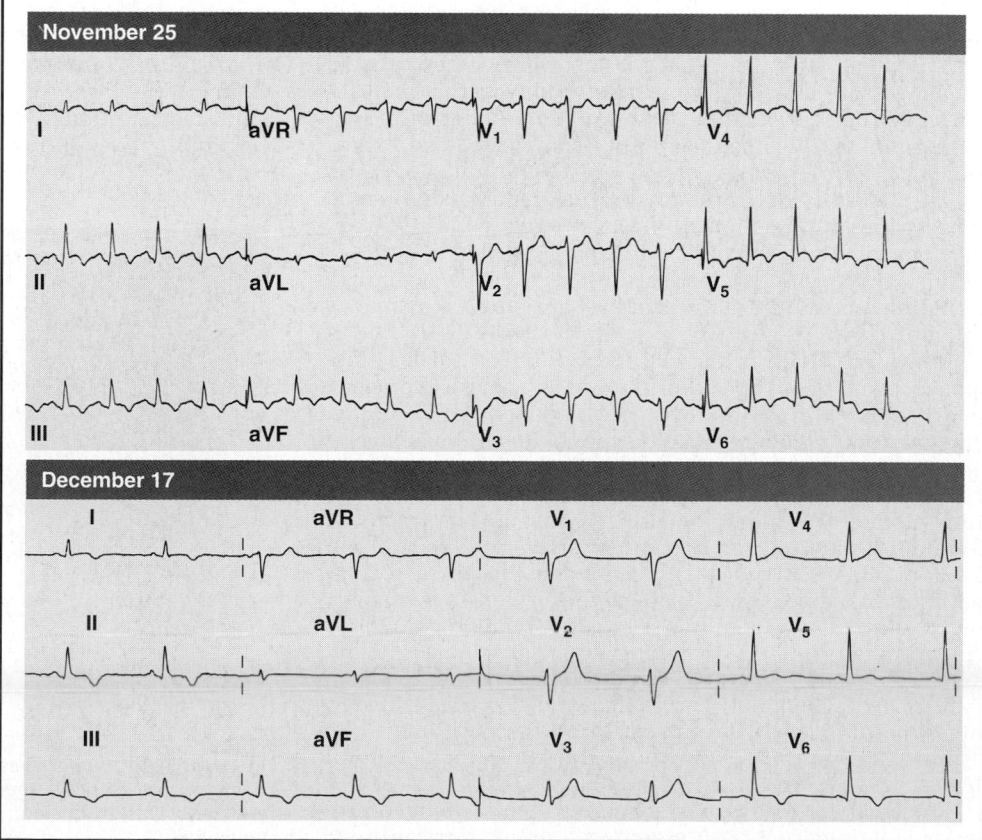

and tenderness, rhabdomyolysis[48] suggests a myotropic organism also involving the myocardium.[43]

Elevations of troponins I and T indicate myocardial damage.[49] Elevated cardiac enzymes with normal myoglobin levels suggest that the pericarditic process has affected only myocardial cell membranes, causing them to leak these substances. This is probably the mildest detectable myopericarditis; elevated serum myoglobin levels may indicate severe (cytoplasmic) damage. Although characteristic ECG changes of acute pericarditis can occur without abnormal enzyme release, in severe cases with significant myopericarditis, CK-MB increases (>10 μg/liter), particularly during ST (J) deviations.[43] Monoclonal antimyosin antibodies labeled with indium-111 are markers of myocarditis,[45] as is detection of proinflammatory cytokine tumor necrosis factor (TNF) in the absence of congestive heart failure and septic shock.

CLINICAL CONSIDERATIONS. Pericarditis with pericardial effusions that are closer to transudates, particularly with severe dyspnea, suggests significant myocardial involvement, whereas exudates indicate at least a strong pericarditic component.[43] Imaging and cardiac catheterization demonstrate transiently or permanently reduced myocardial function, that is, diffuse or localized abnormal ventricular wall motion. MRI shows focal myocardial edema in such zones of segmental or general wall motion abnormality. Finally, auscultation of a new S_3 ("ventricular gallop") is evidence either for myocardial inflammation or some degree of constriction.[43, 50]

Although cardiac enzymes and markers (troponin I and T) are released in most patients with myocarditis and ECG abnormalities, cardiac enzymes may be normal or only slightly increased and enzyme levels can fall while the ST (J) segment is still elevated.[51] Another clue to a myocarditic component during pericarditis is the occasionally convexly elevated J-ST segment, in contrast to the concave ST segment characteristic of acute pericarditis. Occasional patients have mixed forms of pain of both "myocardial" and pleuritic types, with dominance of one kind suggesting the dominant lesion (e.g., squeezing chest pain during apparent pericarditis suggesting significant myocarditis).

Any cardiac asynergy is due to myocardial abnormality and mimics acute infarction. A biopsy specimen obtained by catheter (endomyocardial biopsy) or by thoracoscope (epimyocardial biopsy) can identify myocardial inflammation, preferably if taken from the left ventricle, from which specimens are more often positive. Epimyocardial biopsies are much more productive.[49, 52] An active immune process will yield major histocompatibility complex Class I expression and tissue binding of IgG, IgA, IgM, and C3.[46, 47, 53] Finally, such evidence of myocardial inflammation sometimes persists in patients with constrictive pericarditis and may contribute to postpericardiectomy cardiac dilation and failure. In constrictive pericarditis with active myocarditis,[50] differentiation from restrictive cardiomyopathy may be difficult.

MANAGEMENT. In the absence of myocardial failure, management of myopericarditis is the same as for acute pericarditis.[43] (In both, there are no adequate controlled clinical trials.) Patients may respond to antiinflammatory agents. Corticosteroids should be avoided unless all else fails and the patient is severely ill; near the onset of viral illness, they can stimulate virus replication and paralyze immune responses. Immunosuppressive agents seem useful in autoimmune myocarditis but not conclusively and could be injurious; they appear ineffective for viral (lymphocytic) myocarditis.[54] Interferon may be useful in enteroviral forms. Hyperimmune globulin has been used for cytomegaloviral-associated myopericarditis. Captopril may be of benefit in patients with definite heart failure.[55] Pericardial effusions must be drained with special care because they may "splint" a myocarditic heart, which drainage permits to dilate.

Prognosis for recovery is generally good if the myocarditis is not intense (it is often focal in myopericarditis[56]),

particularly the infective types, although varying degrees of myocardial damage can produce heart failure and, ultimately, dilated or restrictive cardiomyopathy. Rarely, Dressler syndrome (see Chap. 35) ensues.

PERICARDIAL EFFUSION AND HYDROPERICARDIUM

PATHOGENESIS AND CLINICAL CHARACTERISTICS. Pericardial fluid is in dynamic equilibrium with the blood serum, including free exchange of water and electrolytes with surprising pericardial permeability to some large as well as smaller molecules. However, inflamed pericardium may obstruct these exchanges. Most pericardial effusions "weep" from the visceral pericardium.[57] Irritative and inflammatory effusions are associated with local production of substances such as cytokines, tumor necrosis factors, and interleukins.[58] Exudation of proteinaceous material and larger molecules and dissolution of intrapericardial thrombi osmotically attract additional fluid and impede reabsorption. Large effusions usually follow venous and lymphatic obstruction in the epicardium and often occur in the subjacent myocardium (myocardial lymph drainage normally occurs by means of the pericardium and probably contributes to effusions). Surprisingly small fluid increments and even the normal 15 to 35 ml can be identified by imaging.[57] Asymptomatic effusions are typically first suggested by relatively insensitive radiography (Fig. 50–10); a minimum of about 250 ml is needed to fill the pericardial reserve volume (see earlier) sufficiently to detectably increase the cardiopericardial silhouette. Increased pericardial fluid is either hydropericardium (transudate), "true" pericardial effusion (exudate; pyopericardium if purulent), hemopericardium, or mixtures of these, collectively termed "pericardial effusion." Exudates characteristically have more cholesterol, protein, and LDH than transudates, with cholesterol greater than 45 mg/dl, protein concentration more than half the serum level, and LDH greater than 200 U/liter or more than 60 percent of the serum LDH (the serum-effusion albumin gradient may be more valid).[57] However, the exudate-versus-transudate characterization may be indistinct. Moreover, with improving congestive failure, more rapid reabsorption of water than protein and LDH may convert hydropericardium to a pseudoexudate.

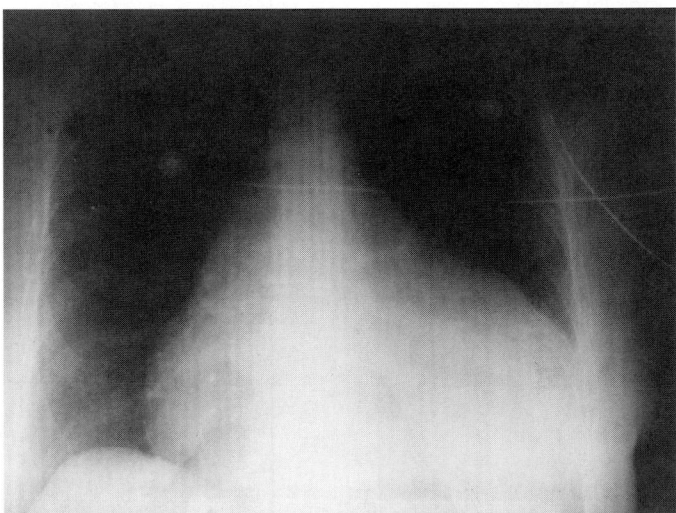

FIGURE 50–10. Large pericardial effusion. Chest radiograph shows a large, featureless bilaterally distended cardiopercardial silhouette and left pleural effusion. Lung fields are clear. (Patient had a low voltage ECG.)

Excess pericardial contents is loosely associated with vague *chest symptoms* such as pressure sensations and aches. Rapid exudation can stretch the pericardium, producing "protopathic" pain. Very large effusions can encroach on neighboring structures, manifest as *dyspnea*, especially on exertion, when compression of lung causes a restrictive pulmonary defect; *dysphagia* from esophageal compression; *cough* from bronchial encroachment; *hiccups* from esophageal compression and involvement of the vagi and phrenic nerves; and *hoarseness* from compression of the recurrent laryngeal nerve.[57]

ETIOLOGY. The causes of exudative pericardial effusion essentially correspond to those of pericardial inflammation and irritation (see Tables 50–3 and 50–4); large exudative effusions are most common with tumors, tuberculous pericarditis, cholesterol pericarditis, myxedema, vasculitis/connective tissue disease, uremic pericarditis, and parasitoses.[59] Unusual conditions include the eosinophilic syndromes, endomyocardial fibrosis, and cardiac transplantation (related to chemotherapy, especially cyclosporin or to rejection). Others occur during bone marrow transplant due to graft-versus-host disease.[57] A small to moderate clinically silent hydropericardium develops by the third trimester in many pregnant women (see Chap. 65). Myopericarditis tends to produce mixed forms, because hydropericardium due to heart failure variably dilutes inflammatory effusions. Drug-related effusions may be difficult to recognize in diseases that can involve the pericardium (e.g., systemic lupus erythematosus [SLE]).

HYDROPERICARDIUM AND CLINICALLY NONCOMPRESSING EFFUSIONS. Hydropericardium, which is usually small, occurs mainly in conditions of fluid retention but less frequently than pleural effusion. It is usually discovered by accident when imaging the chest or heart. "Noncompressing" exudative effusions due to pericardial lesions produce no significant change in blood pressure or cardiac output and no pulsus paradoxus. They may (1) be asymptomatic, (2) present as pericarditic pain or symptoms and signs of the causative condition, or (3) have asymptomatic but significantly increased respiratory fluctuation in ventricular function. Most have symptoms and signs only of "clinically dry" pericarditis. If the effusion is inflammatory, a pericardial rub usually is audible at some time. Slight exaggeration of the normal inspiratory fall in systolic blood pressure suggests "borderline" tamponade.

The *Bamberger-Pins-Ewart sign* is common with very large effusions and is characterized by a dullness and bronchial breathing between the left (rarely the right) scapula and the spine.[57] Otherwise, physical examination is nonspecific and undependable; even with tamponade, heart sounds may not be muffled and precordial percussion is untrustworthy. The ECG is of little or no direct help, although occasionally very large nontamponading effusions induce *electrical alternation* (see Chap. 5) (otherwise associated with critical tamponade). Reduced ECG voltage is nonspecific and undependable; only massive effusions as in severe myxedema produce true microvoltage that may be equally related to myocardial or hemodynamic abnormality.

IMAGING. Radiography can only be suggestive. The shape of the heart shadow on fluoroscopy or static films cannot decisively distinguish true cardiomegaly from pericardial effusion. A "water bottle" silhouette or unusually wide mediastinal shadow (see Fig. 50–10) is suggestive, particularly when the lung fields are not congested. Left pleural effusion is common in both "wet" and "dry" pericarditis, whereas bilateral effusion is more common in congestive heart failure.[57] On a well penetrated lateral film, pericardial fluid is suggested by lucent *pericardial fat lines* within the cardiopericardial shadow. Echocardiography, CT, and MRI define heart size; cardiac function can be determined by echo-Doppler, contrast radiography, nuclear scanning, CT, or MRI.

ECHO-DOPPLER CARDIOGRAPHY (see Chap. 7, Figs. 7–94 to 7–97). Table 50–10 summarizes the results of echo-Doppler investigation of effusions. On the echocardiogram, normal pericardial fluid and small amounts of excess fluid are seen posteriorly, between the LV wall and the parietal pericardium in systole only. With progressive accumulation, posterior fluid appears in both systole and diastole; in larger effusions, fluid appears anterior to the right ventricle. Fluid can be found behind the left atrium (i.e., in the pericardial oblique sinus) but usually with very large often tamponading effusions. *Effusion size* can be estimated by echocardiography: *small:* aggregate echo-free space in systole and diastole less than 10 mm; *moderate:* echo-free space in systole and diastole 10 to 20 mm, at least posteriorly; and *large:* echo-free space or 20 mm or more. As fluid increases, movement of the parietal pericardium decreases. Note that effusion size is a powerful overall predictor of prognosis; large effusions generally mean more serious disease.[57-59] Anterior fluid is frequently absent after cardiac surgery due to anterior adhesions.[60] With only an anterior echo-free space, posterior adhesions might be present, although epicardial fat is usually more likely; occasionally an infiltrative lesion, often malignant, is responsible. Epicardial fat, occasionally simulating posterior and circumcardiac effusions on echocardiography, must be distinguished by CT or MRI (see Chap. 10).

With very large effusions, echocardiography may show cardiac oscillation ("swinging") within the pericardium (see Table 50–10). With some degree of tamponade, often critical, swinging reverses direction on alternate beats instead of on every beat, producing ECG electrical alternation. Large effusions can cause mitral prolapse or pseudoprolapse, as well as midsystolic notching of the aortic or pulmonic valves. TEE is superior to transthoracic echocardiography (TTE), especially for identifying metastases, pericardial thickening, and clots, but it tends to underestimate the volume and distribution of effusions. Three-dimensional echocardiography is promising.[61] Although echocardiography is sufficient in most cases, CT and MRI may be needed if echocardiographic results are equivocal.[57]

MANAGEMENT. Without tamponade (see p. 1841), hemopericardium, or pyopericardium, there are few absolute indications for drainage. Very large nontamponading effusions can be drained to relieve symptoms due to compression of lung and other structures. Pericardial drainage occasionally may be required for diagnosis through examining fluid; pericardial biopsy can be obtained simultaneously. Pericardiocentesis by needle alone can be unrewarding diagnostically, although modern bacteriological and immunocytochemical methods are improving the results (Table 50–11).[59, 62, 63] Adequate fluid with an adequate pericardial biopsy is better and more safely obtained by thoracotomy, subxiphoid incision, or video-assisted thoracoscopic resection and drainage, which also permits efficient and relatively inexpensive removal of thrombi, adhesions, and fibrinous material, minimizing chances for recurrence and cicatrization. Percutaneous balloon pericardiotomy may be used but is best for palliation of malignant tamponade. Loculated effusions may require open surgery or thoracoscopic drainage. The decision for operative intervention depends on (1) urgency of diagnosis and a prognosis requiring aggressive management and (2) probable yield of the diagnostic sample. Thus, persistent illness without an etiological diagnosis warrants obtaining tissue as well as fluid surgically. All patients, especially those with underlying cardiac disease, including myocarditis, should be monitored for postdrainage decompensation.[57]

PERICARDIOCENTESIS. The precise techniques of needle drainage with and without catheter insertion are explained in detail elsewhere.[64] Techniques for nonsurgical drainage for relief of tamponade have been refined over many years, and imaging methods such as echocardiography and CT are now used routinely to locate the effusion and guide needle insertion.[65] Large effusions are more successfully reached; smaller effusions (<5 mm anteriorly) can be missed by the needle, with more frequent complications such as penetration or laceration of cardiac structures. Thick viscous fluids such as pus and partly clotted blood are difficult to aspirate. Patients with severe hemorrhagic disease may tend to bleed. Sites on the chest wall opposite the deepest anterior and inferior fluid collection (determined by imaging) should be used; echocardiographic studies show the apical approach usually to be best.[66] The procedure is best performed in an environment where resuscitation and monitor-

▼ TABLE 50–10. ECHOCARDIOGRAPHIC AND DOPPLER EFFECTS OF PERICARDIAL EFFUSION AND CARDIAC TAMPONADE (VARYING SENSITIVITIES AND SPECIFICITIES)

A. Pericardial effusion
1. Echo-free space:
   a. Posterior to LV (small-to-moderate effusion)
   b. Posterior and anterior (moderate-to-large effusion)
   c. Behind left atrium (large-to-very large effusion and/or anterior adhesion
2. Decreased movement of posterior pericardium-lung interface
3. Brisk RV wall movements unmasked with anterior fluid
4. "Swinging heart" (large effusions, usually tamponade)
   a. RV and LV walls move synchronously
   b. Periodicity 1:1 or 2:1 (one or two swings per cardiac cycle); 2:1 is characteristic of definite tamponade
   c. Pseudoparadoxic motion of LV posterior wall
   d. Mitral/tricuspic pseudoprolapse; occasional true prolapse
   e. Mitral systolic anterior motion
   f. Alternating mitral e-f slope and aortic opening excursion
   g. Aortic valve: midsystolic closure movement
   h. Pulmonic valve: midsystolic notch
5. Hemopericardium: clotted blood identifiable
6. Inspiratory decrease in LV ejection time (with effusion; greater with tamponade)

B. Cardiac tamponade—changes of effusion plus:
1. RV compression
   a. RV diameters decreased, especially outflow tract (≤ 7 mm)
   b. Early diastolic collapse of right ventricle
2. RA free wall indentation (collapse) during late diastole and/or isovolumic contraction lasting at least one third of the cardiac cycle
3. LA free wall indentation (cases with fluid behind left atrium)
4. LV free wall paradoxic motion
5. SVC and IVC congestion (unless volume depletion); IVC >2.2 cm with <50% inspiratory collapse
6. Exaggerated inspiratory effects (especially with pulsus paradoxus with reciprocal right-heart/left-heart effects during inspiration and expiration)

   a. Right ventricle expands
   b. Interventricular septum shifts to left
   c. Left ventricle compressed
   d. Mitral
      (1) d-e amplitude decreased
      (2) e-f slope decreased or rounded
      (3) Open time* decreased; delayed mitral opening
   e. Aortic valve: opening decreased*; premature closure
   f. Echographic stroke volume decreased
7. Notch in RV epicardium during isovolumic contraction
8. Course oscillations of LV posterior wall
9. Pseudohypertrophy: apparent wall thickening due to compression

C. Doppler studies: with any degree of tamponade
1. Major changes on first beats during inspiration and expiration
2. Generally reduced flows/stroke volumes
3. Exaggerated inspiratory augmentation of right-sided and decrease of left-sided flows
4. Respiratory variation in superior and inferior vena caval flow velocities marked in tamponade, less increased with effusion; double-peaked superior vena cava systolic wave. Decreased expiratory diastolic SVC flow.
5. Hepatic vein expiratory effect:
   a. Marked atrial reversal (AR wave)
   b. Marked decrease or reversal of diastolic forward flow
   c. (Occasional) systolic flow reversal
6. (Transesophageal echocardiograms): expiratory increase in pulmonary vein diastolic forward flow
7. Marked inspiratory decrease in LV ejection time; increased RV ejection time
8. Marked inspiratory increase in LV isovolumic relaxation time; decreased RV isovolumic relaxation time
9. Hepatic vein velocity difference between systole and atrial reversal <0 cm/sec

*Often difficult to define during pericardial effusion with tamponade; mitral valve opens late and may open only with atrial systole during inspiration.
SVC and IVC = superior and inferior venae cavae; LA = left atrial; LV = left ventricular; RA = right atrial; RV = right ventricular.
From Spodick DH. The Pericardium: A Comprehensive Textbook. New York, Marcel Dekker, 1997.

ing equipment are available (e.g., the cardiac catheterization laboratory). Cardiac arrhythmias during the procedure will be detected by electrocardiography, but direct monitoring from the needle itself is not an adequate safeguard and may

▼ TABLE 50–11. EXAMINATION OF PERICARDIAL FLUID

BASIC TESTS
1. Hematocrit and cell count
2. Stains: Gram, Ziehl-Nielsen, special
3. Cultures
4. Viral cultures; identification of appropriate immunoglobulins
5. Glucose; protein
6. Cytologic examination
7. Immunocytochemistry

ADDITIONAL TESTS FOR ANTICIPATED DIAGNOSES
1. Lactate dehydrogenase
2. Rheumatoid factor; antinuclear antibody
3. Quantitative complement levels
4. Cholesterol
5. Pathologic examination of cell blocks; cytochemical staining
6. pH
7. Amylase
8. Adenosine deaminase
9. Carcinoembryonic antigen

From Spodick DH: The Pericardium: A Comprehensive Textbook. New York, Marcel Dekker, 1997.

be a handicap.[57, 64, 67] Right-sided heart and arterial catheterization are optimal and may reveal unanticipated effusive-constrictive pericarditis (see Chap 11). Pericardial pressure can be measured through the intrapericardial needle or catheter. An intravenous drip containing isotonic saline or dextrose in water can be used to deliver supporting therapy.

Patients are monitored for cardiac decompensation ("pericardial shock") and for recurrent tamponade due to catheter blockage or reaccumulation of fluid (which is particularly important with bloody fluids or frank hemorrhage because of clotting). Residual clots can later dissolve, producing osmotically active fragments, thus renewing effusion or tamponade.

COMPLICATIONS. The major complications of needle drainage are caused by needle contact with the heart, particularly laceration of a coronary vessel or chamber wall or myocardial perforation. Injuries to coronary veins, the right atrium, and the right ventricle are most dangerous; these are thin walled and likely to bleed briskly, producing hemopericardium. "Simple" perforation of the myocardium, particularly the left ventricle, without laceration is not rare but is well tolerated. Hypotension, probably reflex, can occur at any point, so that atropine should be on hand. Rare penetrations include stomach, colon, and lung. Arrhythmias occur particularly in patients with preexisting heart disease. Direct contact of the needle with the ventricular surface may produce an injury current or ventricular ectopic beats, and contact with the atrial surface may produce atrial ectopic beats.[57]

CARDIAC TAMPONADE

Pathophysiology

INTERACTION BETWEEN THE PERICARDIUM AND ITS CONTENTS. To tamponade the heart, pericardial contents must (1) fill the pericardial reserve volume (see Fig. 50–2), then (2) increase at a rate exceeding the rate of stretch of the parietal pericardium, and (3) exceed the rate at which venous blood volume expands to support the small normal pressure gradient for filling the right side of the heart.[68, 69] Increased pericardial fluid causes loss of normal variations in pericardial contact stress (pressures become uniform over all cardiac chambers), increasing both ventricular and AV interaction. Pericardial volume increases partly by reducing cardiac chamber volumes and ultimately equalizes reduced diastolic compliance in all chambers. The resultant operational defect is restriction of cardiac inflows. (Interaction between the rate of fluid accumulation and parietal pericardial stretch determines pericardial stiffness and consequently the shape of the pericardial pressure-volume curve (Fig. 50–11). With critical tamponade, the heart functions on the steep portion of the pericardial pressure-volume curve so that small fluid increments provoke large pressure increments. With slow fluid accumulation and a yielding pericardium, the initial portion of the pressure-volume curve remains "flat" longer and relatively large fluid volume increases cause relatively little pressure rise (see Fig. 50–11, *right*).

Clinically, cardiac tamponade is defined as the decompensated phase of cardiac compression resulting from increased intrapericardial pressure.[68] Physiologically, tamponade is a continuum,[70] because even small increases in pericardial contents couple the pericardium to the heart, producing significantly increased AV and especially ventricular interaction that exaggerates the normal reciprocal respiratory effects on the right and left sides of the heart.[69]

If unchecked by compensatory mechanisms, rising pericardial contents, such as effusions, blood, pus, gas, and combinations, ultimately produce critical cardiac compression: florid tamponade.

PATHOPHYSIOLOGICAL CONTINUUM OF TAMPONADE. The rate of fluid accumulation determines the clinical response. Intrapericardial hemorrhage, as from wounds, rapidly produces "surgical" tamponade in minutes to hours, whereas a low-intensity inflammatory process can require days to weeks before critical cardiac compression ("medical" tamponade). At any rate of accumulation the system is always subject to sudden breakdown of compensation.

PERICARDIAL STRETCH AND PRESSURE-VOLUME RELATIONS. Pericardial stretch is determined by the rate of increase of its contents and the response of two pericardial "springs": (1) wavy collagen, which tends to be smoothed by expanding pericardial contents, and (2) elastic tissue. Rapid accumulation exhausts these, and the limit of stretch is quickly reached, owing to the pericardium's J-shaped pressure-volume curve (see Fig. 50–11). The ensuing decompensated tamponade tends to be a "last drop" phenomenon, the last bit of fluid putting the pericardium and consequently the cardiac chambers on the steep portion of their pressure-volume curves. Compression of all heart chambers resists cardiac filling, a form of diastolic dysfunction in which at any diastolic volume excessive intracardiac pressure keeps pace with excessive intrapericardial pressure.

Pericardial drainage has a reciprocal effect: the first decrement usually produces the largest hemodynamic improvement by shifting the stretched pericardium back toward the less steep portion of its pressure-volume curve and consequently shifts the parallel myocardial pressure-volume relations.[68, 71]

RIGHT-SIDED HEART AND VENOUS FACTORS. The early point of attack of the rising intrapericardial pressure is on the right atrium and ventricle. The pressures of these thinner chambers equilibrate with rising pericardial pressure before the LA and LV pressures. Normal RA and RV pressures are somewhat lower than in the corresponding left chambers, and the RV wall is much thinner. Thus, rising diastolic pressures paralleling rising pericardial pressure occur first in the right and later in the left sides of the heart.[72] Normally, intrapericardial pressure is lower than RA pressure so that RA (transmural) pressure is normally higher than its cavitary pressure; but with tamponade, rising pericardial pressure progressively reduces, and ultimately makes phasically negative, the transmural pressure of first the right and then the left heart chambers. Cardiac filling is maintained by a parallel rise in systemic and pulmonary venous pressure,[68] the venous beds generating enough pressure to keep both sides of the heart filled.[70] A key factor affecting compensation is the rate of venous volume expansion by fluid transfer from the tissues, from the arterial to the venous side of the cardiovascular system; this requires time and is inoperative in rapid "surgical" tamponade. Finally, diastolic suction probably augments filling.[68]

LEFT-SIDED HEART AND ARTERIAL FACTORS. Pericardial pressure

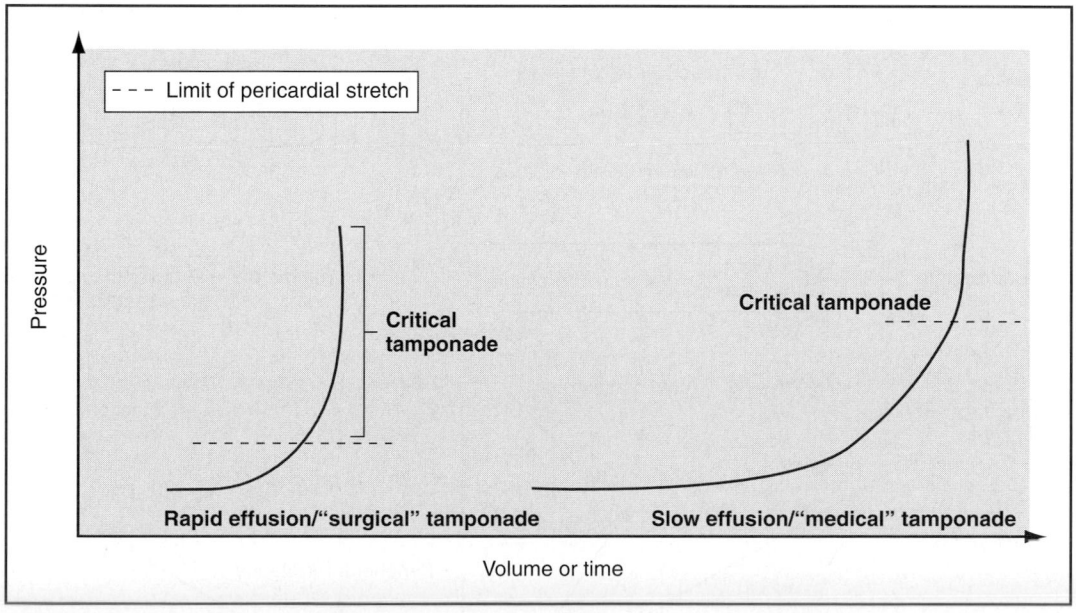

FIGURE 50–11. Cardiac tamponade. Schema of pericardial pressure-volume curves (volume increases over time). At left, rapidly increasing pericardial fluid first fills the pericardial reserve volume (initial flat segment) then rises steeply to exceed the limit of parietal pericardial stretch, causing even steeper rise as smaller fluid increments disproportionately increase the pericardial pressure. At the right, a slower rate of pericardial filling takes longer to exceed pericardial stretch limit because of time available for "give." (From Spodick DH: The Pericardium: A Comprehensive Textbook. New York, Marcel Dekker, 1997.)

equilibrates first with RV diastolic pressure also because pericardial stiffness is inherently greater than RV, but not LV, stiffness. As compensatory mechanisms (Fig. 50–12) are defeated, cardiac filling decreases, pericardial pressure equilibrates with LV diastolic pressure, and cardiac output decreases critically (even the left ventricle ultimately equilibrates due to drastic reduction in volume, producing a very low to phasically negative LV transmural pressure). Eventually, diastolic pressures in both ventricles and the pulmonary artery all equilibrate with mean RA and LA pressures at approximately intrapericardial pressure—the characteristic hemodynamics of "pure" cardiac tamponade.[68-71] During inspiration, left-right heart pressure differences are least or nil and commonly reversed; circulation is assisted by reciprocal flow changes in inspiration and expiration. During pulsus paradoxus the breathing phases have comparable but exaggerated differential effects; with inspiration, pulmonary wedge pressure falls below pericardial pressure. RA pressure also falls but not below pericardial pressure, enhancing inspiratory RV filling.

Transmural Pressure

The true "filling" (distending) cardiac pressures are the *myocardial* transmural pressures: cavity pressure minus intrapericardial pressure. (Cavity pressures are the sum of transmural pressure and pericardial pressures.) Transient reversal of the transmural pressure gradient (negative transmural pressure) causes RV collapse early in diastole (especially the weak RV outflow tract), and the RA, and sometimes LA, collapse in late diastole[73] (Figs. 50–13 and 50–14; see also Figs. 7–95 to 7–97). (The critical negative transmural pressure buckling pressure for the right ventricle is 0.05 to 0.1 mm Hg; for the left ventricle it is 3.0 mm Hg.[74]) The RV inflow tract continues to fill while the outflow tract collapses, suggesting diastolic suction. The thick left ventricle does not collapse *unless* there is loculated high pressure fluid on its free border, RV hypertrophy, pulmonary artery hypertension, or intrapericardial adhesions. The onset of chamber collapses coincides with a 15 to 25 percent decrease in cardiac output[75] while compensatory mechanisms (see Fig. 50–12) still maintain arterial pressure, mainly due to increased peripheral resistance. Thus, at least in euvolemic and hypervolemic patients, RV collapse tends to occur earlier than pulsus paradoxus.

In tamponade, blood mainly enters the heart when blood is leaving it; pericardial volume and pressure vary continuously during the cardiac cycle, reflecting variations in early cardiac chamber volumes, although pericardial fluid continuously compresses the heart. In early diastole, the peak ventricular filling rate is radically reduced along with the filling fraction, emphasizing the importance of atrial contributions.[68, 69] By end-diastole or earlier, the ventricles are filled and maximally expanded within the pericardial sac, raising intrapericardial pressure to its maximum. Although atrial expansion by filling would tend to raise pericardial pressure at end systole, ventricular ejection is complete so the ventricles are at minimal volume, permitting intrapericardial pressure to fall. As the ventricles contract to eject blood and the pericardial "space" is increased, the atrial "floors" are pulled downward and pericardial pressure falls, increasing transmural pres-

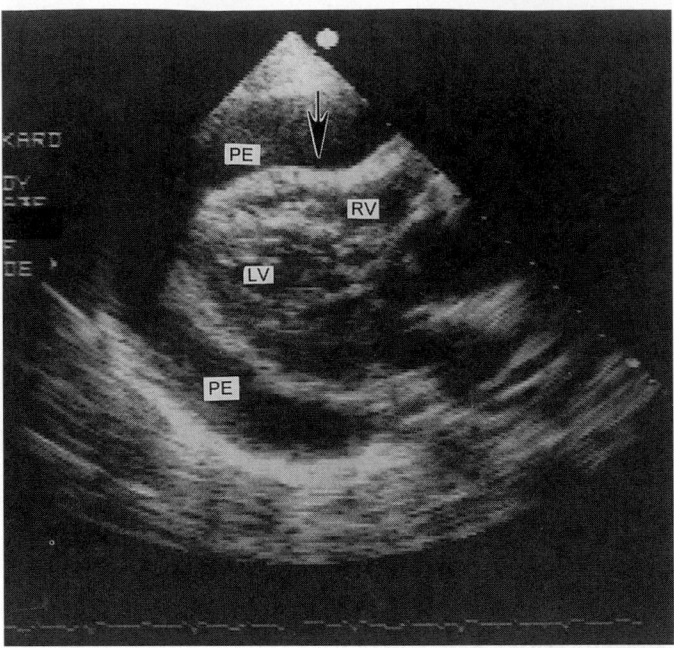

FIGURE 50–13. Large pericardial effusion (PE) with tamponade. Arrow indicates right ventricular (RV) collapse. LV = left ventricle.

sure to enhance atrial filling.[69] Atrial cavitary pressure falls at the same time, producing the *x* descent in atrial pressure curves (Fig. 50–15). Within these dynamics, the ventricles eject reduced stroke volumes but remain underfilled and therefore operate at the low end of their Frank-Starling curves.

High pericardial pressure prevents normally rapid ventricular filling in early diastole. Moreover, the AV valves tend to close early. These factors progressively amputate the *y* descent of the atrial and venous pressure curves, reflecting curtailed and ultimately absent rapid ventricular filling. (Note that the LA *y* descent may be reduced long after elimination of the RA *y* descent.) Atrial reservoir function has increased importance: in severe tamponade the LA may fill only during expiration and the ventricles only during atrial systole.[69] Decreased filling due to premature AV valve closure exacerbates the reduced ventricular preload (shorter fiber length), further contributing to lower stroke volume and decreased ventricular ejection rate. Ultimately, the aortic valve opens only during expiration. During inspira-

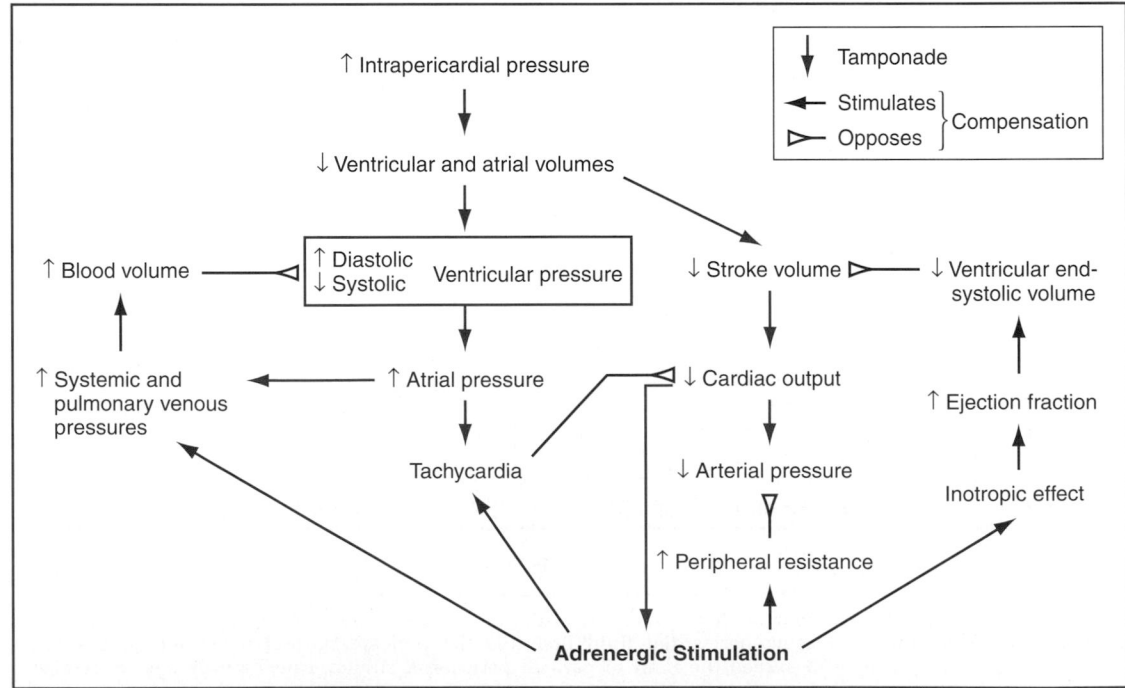

FIGURE 50–12. Cardiac tamponade and compensatory mechanisms. Solid arrowheads = tamponade. (From Spodick DH: The Pericarium: A Comprehensive Textbook. New York, Marcel Dekker, 1997.)

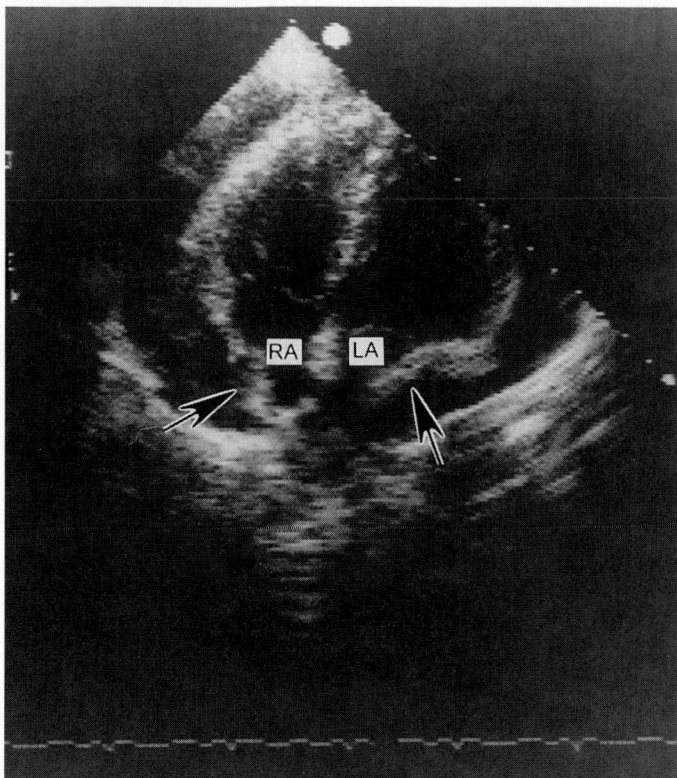

FIGURE 50–14. Large pericardial effusion with tamponade. Biatrial (RA and LA) collapse (arrows).

partly by alpha-adrenergic mechanisms, but thereafter may decline precipitously, owing to falling stroke volume and cardiac output. Good myocardial function permits the ventricles to increase the amount of blood ejected per beat (increased ejection fraction). Diseased or injured left or right ventricles do not maintain compensation as well as normal hearts.[76, 77]

COMPENSATION AND DECOMPENSATION. Compensatory mechanisms (see Fig. 50–12) include time-dependent pericardial stretch and blood volume expansion, tachycardia, increased ejection fraction, and peripheral vasoconstriction due to intense adrenergic stimulation responding to falling cardiac output. Adrenergic stimulation, including increased serum catecholamines, produces (1) alpha-adrenergically increased systemic resistance, which maintains central blood pressure and supports the gradient for coronary flow (increased systemic resistance is not affected by beta blockade but is decreased by alpha blockade, which is potentially decompensating); (2) a beta-adrenergic contribution, which increases heart rate; (3) rising pressure in the right atrium, which also induces tachycardia to defend the minute cardiac output; (4) beta-adrenergic stimulation, which augments diastolic relaxation; and (5) increased inotropy, which minimizes ventricular and systolic volume and improves the ejection fraction. In decompensated tamponade, the blood pressure fall is strongly influenced by an opioid-dependent mechanism, as demonstrated by naloxone-induced blood pressure increase without increasing cardiac output, that is, a large additional increase in systemic resistance.[75]

Owing to arterial and atrial baroreceptor unloading, arterial pressure is augmented by neurohormonal activation, with a limited late contribution by the renin-angiotensin-aldosterone system. Renin, angiotensin II, arginine vasopressin, and aldosterone decrease urine flow and renal sodium and potassium excretion (after mean blood pressure decreases by about 30 percent), followed by increased adrenocorticotropic hormone.[69] A neurogenic antinatriuresis reflexly increases renal sodium and fluid retention, which, teleologically, defends cardiac filling by increased blood volume and venous pressure. Unlike cardiac failure at comparable central pressures, atrial natriuretic factor does not increase because tamponade prevents myocardial stretch. (Teleologically, this is also favorable because atrial natriuretic factor would increase renal sodium and water elimination and is harmful to myocytes, depressing contractility.[77a]) Finally, tamponade can produce a profound arterial respiratory alkalosis.[67] Mixed venous (pulmonary artery) blood pH, Pco_2, and serum bicarbonate are relatively unchanged, but as cardiac output falls critically the difference between arterial and mixed venous Pco_2 increases.

ATYPICAL CARDIAC TAMPONADE. This occurs in four forms: low pressure, occult, right-sided, and hypertensive.[69] In volume-depleted patients, hypovolemia attenuates compensatory increases in venous blood volume and pressure so that cardiac output falls at lower ventricular diastolic pressure: *Low pressure tamponade* may occur at mean diastolic pressures as low as 6 mm Hg with few symptoms at rest and with or without significant systemic hypotension; yet both RV collapse and pulsus paradoxus may be present. Although pulse contours tend to be abnormal, it may be necessary to expand blood volume by an intravenous saline challenge to produce diagnostic pulse morphology. In *occult tamponade*, pericardial pressure equilibrates with RV and often LV diastolic pressure without a compensatory increase in venous pressure. *Right-sided tamponade*, with right diastolic pressures exceeding left, can occur when LV compliance is very low (e.g., LV hypertrophy) or, more commonly, after cardiac surgery, if fluid is loculated over the right side of the heart. In *hypertensive tamponade*, even with significantly low cardiac output there is unusually high (i.e., normal to even hypertensive) systolic arterial pressure, probably due to excessive adrenergic stimulation.[78]

tion, leftward shift of the atrial and ventricular septa[68] further reduce LV chamber compliance and obstruct LV filling. Thus, the ventricular pressure curves show an immediate, shallow to barely visible diastolic rise from a slight lowering just after AV valve opening at the high diastolic levels seen with pressure equilibrium—typically 15 to 30 mm Hg in euvolemic patients (see Fig. 50–15).

CORONARY BLOOD FLOW. This is reduced primarily by increased subepicardial vascular resistance. Yet with normal coronary arteries coronary blood flow remains adequate to support aerobic metabolism because of proportionate reduction in cardiac work; that is, the ventricles are underloaded.[68] Coronary vasodilator reserve, capacitance, and resistance are not critically impaired. Renal and cerebral blood flow during tamponade, though reduced, are partly supported by autoregulation. However, peripheral vascular resistance is high (response to endogenous angiotensin II) with significant hepatic and mesenteric ischemia.

Despite decreased cardiac output, arterial blood pressure is maintained until relatively late in slowly developing ("medical") tamponade,

FIGURE 50–15. Cardiac tamponade; pressure equilibration. Pulmonary artery (PA) diastolic, right atrial (RA) mean, and right ventricular (RV) diastolic pressures are each approximately 15 mm Hg. Respiratory fluctuation of right ventricular systolic pressure is between 23 mm Hg in maximum expiration and 29 mm Hg at peak inspiration. Right atrial pressure has a single conspicuous drop, the *x* descent; there is no *y* descent. Pulmonary artery systolic pressure changes follow the right ventricular systolic pressures at approximately the same levels. (From Spodick DH: The Pericardium: A Comprehensive Textbook. New York, Marcel Dekker, 1997.)

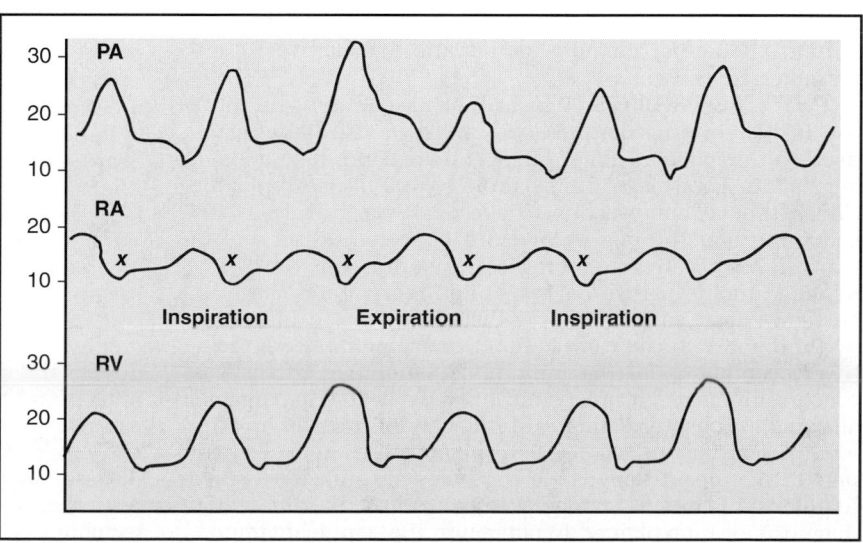

Clinical Features

Pericardial disease of almost any etiology can produce cardiac tamponade, defined as significant compression of the heart by accumulating pericardial contents (liquids, pus, blood, clots, and gas singly or combined).[79] In patients who present with tamponade the great range of pericardial disease requires etiological assessment by probability while anticipating pathogenetic and etiological surprises.[64] Because tamponade is a pathophysiological continuum, patients can have mild to florid tamponade, the latter a form of cardiogenic shock and the former a stage that can progress. Symptoms and signs mirror the rate of physiological impairment. Thus, "medical" and "surgical" tamponade are loose labels conveying relative urgency.[79] "Surgical tamponade," typified by intrapericardial hemorrhage, can quickly overwhelm compensatory mechanisms; with cardiac wounds and intrapericardial rupture of dissecting aortic hematoma as little as 150 ml of blood and clots can be rapidly lethal (see Chap. 51). In contrast, in primarily inflammatory or irritative bloody effusions, slowly escaping blood is prevented from clotting by the pericardium's fibrinolytic activity and defibrination by the "whipping" action of cardiac beating. (Note that almost every form of pericarditis can provoke variably bloody effusion.) In "medical tamponade" fluid exudes at a wide range of rates so that critical cardiac compression may first appear at anywhere from 200 ml to well over a liter. The volume of fluid causing tamponade varies inversely with both parietal pericardial "give" and thickness: disorders that thicken or scar the pericardium such as intense or repeated inflammation can sharply reduce the amount of effusion and bleeding for critical cardiac compression. The clinical onset, ranging from insidious to rapid to sudden, is related to the tempo of physiological impairment. In a patient first discovered to have hundreds of milliliters of fluid, the interplay of exudation rate and pericardial "compliance" permits compensatory responses to keep effusions tolerable longer than in "surgical tamponade."[80]

SYMPTOMS. Patients may have symptoms of an inciting pericardial disease, notably chest discomfort, but in those presenting unconscious, obtunded, or with convulsions there may be no useful history. Tachypnea and dyspnea on exertion progressing to air hunger at rest (occasionally orthopnea) are common, partly related to increased pulmonary interstitial water increasing lung stiffness. Cough and dysphagia are not uncommon and are deceptive as early complaints. Most patients become weak and anorectic and have symptoms ranging from feeling faint to having syncope. Anemia, common in malignancies, exacerbates dyspnea and weakness. Finally, insidiously developing tamponade may present as signs of its complications, such as renal failure, abdominal plethora, or hepatic (shock liver[81]) and mesenteric ischemia.

PHYSICAL FINDINGS. Physical examination is of little use in determining the presence of the pericardial effusion itself, although occasional large effusions produce a Bamberger-Pins-Ewart sign. Tachycardia (>100 beats/min) is the rule, although many patients have heart rates of 90 to 100 beats/min and the rate is lower in hypothyroidism and in many uremic patients. During acute pericarditis with tamponade, uremic pericardial rubs often remain and can even be loud. Heart sounds may be distant, owing to insulation by fluid and reduced cardiac function, sometimes with relative accentuation of the pulmonic component of S_2. The precordium may be quiet and an apex beat not palpable, although, with preexisting cardiomegaly or anterior and apical pericardial adhesions, active pulsations may be palpated. Significant tamponade produces absolute or relative hypotension; indeed, tamponade is part of the differential diagnosis of unexplained hypotension. In "surgical tampon-

ade," shock levels are usual; but in early "medical tamponade," systolic blood pressure is commonly greater than 90 mm Hg. Occasional patients are hypertensive,[78] especially if they have preexisting hypertension; in these patients "normal" blood pressure may be low. (Note that hypertensive blood pressures characterize patients with exaggerated compensatory adrenergic responses and greatly increased peripheral resistance hypertensive tamponade.) Cool extremities, nose, and ears, sometimes with acral cyanosis, are due to vasoconstriction and relative circulatory stasis. Central cyanosis is rare and may be due to a right-to-left shunt, usually through a patent foramen ovale,[82] that disappears after relief of tamponade. Fever is related to etiology, particularly infections. Febrile tamponade may be misdiagnosed as septic shock.

If the patient is not hypovolemic and especially if fluid accumulates sufficiently slowly for expansion of blood volume, jugular venous distention can be anywhere from just visible to striking. Peripheral venous distention can be seen in the forehead, scalp, and ocular fundi. Rapid "surgical tamponade," especially acute hemopericardium, can induce jugular pulsations without distention (i.e., no time for compensatory blood volume expansion). In "medical tamponade," heart rates between 85 and 120 beats/min may yield jugular pulsations slow enough to determine that there is an x descent but absent or greatly attenuated y descent. Indeed, if a venous pressure level can be discerned, this single definitely negative phase can be timed as midsystolic (between S_1 and S_2). These are not outward pulsations; x and y in compressive pericardial disease are "collapses" from a high standing level. Neck veins may also show the normal falling pressure level during inspiration. An inspiratory increase or lack of fall, the so-called Kussmaul sign, belongs to constriction; when verified with tamponade, or after pericardial drainage, it indicates underlying epicardial constriction.

Pulsus Paradoxus (See also Chap. 4)

This is defined as a systolic drop in arterial pressure of 10 mm Hg or more during normal breathing. Most patients with cardiac tamponade have some degree of pulsus paradoxus, often palpable in peripheral arteries (Fig. 50–16). At very low cardiac outputs, however, an arterial catheter may be needed. With a pronounced pulsus paradoxus there may be no Korotkoff sound in inspiration—indeed, the aortic valve may not open in inspiration—with complete inspiratory loss of pulsations in muscular arteries like the radial (the more elastic carotid is less easily evaluated). Pulsus paradoxus may first be appreciated by taking the radial pulse and watching the patient's abdomen during normal breathing. Breathing should not be exaggerated because that can exaggerate the pressure drop. As the abdomen rises, the pulse weakens or disappears.

To quantify the blood pressure difference noninvasively, a cuff is inflated to 15 mm Hg above the apparent highest systolic level and slowly deflated until the first beats are heard and then held at that point during normal respiration (the sequence resembles "bump-bump-bump, silence-silence-silence, bump-bump-bump;" the "bumps"—Korotkoff sounds—are expiratory). Deflation is then continued to where all beats are audible. The difference between the pressures when systolic sounds are first heard and then are continuously heard gives the "size" of the pulsus paradoxus. If a patient is first discovered with pulsus paradoxus, the pericardial variety must be differentiated from other conditions that produce pulsus paradoxus, such as massive pulmonary embolism, profound hemorrhagic shock and other causes of acute hypotension, and obstructive lung disease. In conditions altering tamponade physiology and respiratory mechanisms, pulsus paradoxus may be undetectable.

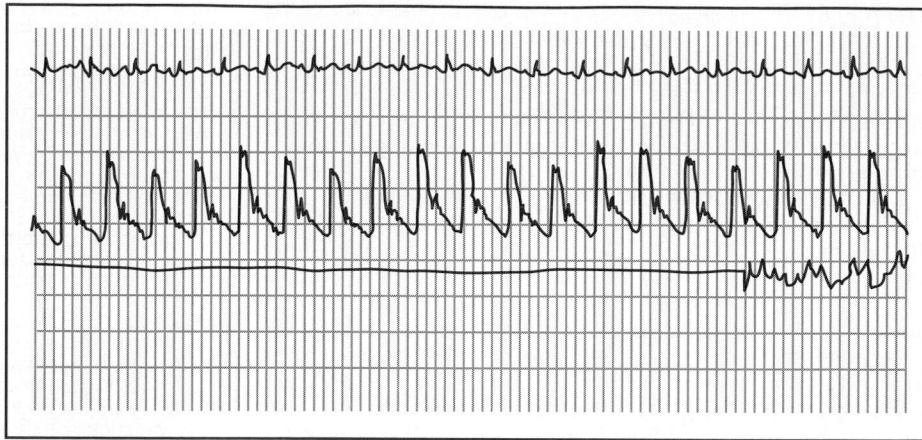

FIGURE 50–16. Pulsus paradoxus during early cardiac tamponade. Brachial artery systolic pressure falls excessively during normal breathing (142 to 124 mm Hg); diastolic pressure is steady at 76 mm Hg. ECG shows marked PR segment depression. (From Spodick DH: The Pericardium: A Comprehensive Textbook. New York, Marcel Dekker, 1997.)

PATHOPHYSIOLOGY. Cyclic cardiocirculatory changes during normal breathing alternately favor right- and left-sided heart filling and ventricular performance, with corresponding pulmonary artery and aortic pressures and flows. Pulsus paradoxus is a pulse (pulsus), not a pressure, change.[83] (There were no blood pressure cuffs or catheters; to Kussmaul it was "paradoxic" since the radial pulse disappeared during inspiration while the apex continued to beat.) Pulsus paradoxus is an exaggeration of the normal inspiratory fall in arterial flow and systolic pressure (see Fig. 50–16) (arbitrarily ≥10 mm Hg). Transmission of pleural pressure variations to the cardiac chambers through the pericardium explains pulsus paradoxus in tamponade whereas their insulation from transmission by scar tends to limit or suppress pulsus paradoxus in constriction. Inspiratory RV volume increase is indispensable for pulsus paradoxus, because when systemic venous return is held constant, tamponade does not cause pulsus paradoxus.[84] Moreover, the right side of the heart is the crux of tamponade dynamics and pulsus can occur in isolated right heart tamponade.[83, 85] Although usually elicited by cuff, pulsus paradoxus is more sensitively revealed by catheter, especially during early tamponade when pericardial pressures are approaching equilibrium with right-sided but not yet with left-sided heart pressures and in low-pressure tamponade. Many such patients have an inspiratory fall in arterial pressure of 10 mm Hg or less that is not quite diagnostic.

Pulsus paradoxus usually signals very large reductions in ventricular volumes and equilibration of mean pericardial and all cardiac diastolic pressures (Fig. 50–17).[83] Breathing now transiently causes the equilibration pressure level to alternate. *Inspiration* decreases pericardial pressure, favoring right-sided heart filling; *expiration* favors left-sided heart filling. Indeed, pulsus occurs as inspiration depresses pulmonary venous pressure below systemic venous pressure so that pulmonary wedge and LA pressures fall below pericardial pressure and the inspiratory decrease in transmitral flow velocity significantly exceeds the normal decrease of 15 percent or less. RA atrial pressure falls, but not below pericardial pressure. Inspiration may also transiently reverse pulmonary venous flow in severe tamponade and thus reduce LA flow.

MECHANISMS

Pulsus paradoxus clearly depends on alternate reciprocal exaggeration of ventricular interaction by the respiratory cycle. The inspiratory systolic pressure fall is also related to the pattern and depth of breathing and hence to the degree of pleural pressure fluctuation. Normally, intrapericardial and pleural pressures vary almost equally during breathing, but in tamponade intrapericardial pressure during inspiration decreases somewhat less than pleural pressures; it increases as the right side of the heart fills, partly because the right side of the heart expands into the pericardial fluid, increasing its already high pressure (see Fig. 50–17). The increased pericardial pressure further compresses the left side of the heart in inspiration, along with a sharp leftward shift of the atrial and ventricular septa, tending to further impede LV filling.[83] The comparable expiratory decreases in right-sided heart filling and cavitary pressures are reflected on echocardiography as maximum RA and RV diastolic collapses during expiration.

Directional respiratory changes in transmural pressures, flow, and filling remain normal and equilibration of approximately 180 degrees out of phase, that is, almost perfectly reciprocal for maximal changes. At the low chamber volumes of tamponade, proportional inspiratory pressure increases are very much greater than normal on the right; corresponding left-side inspiratory pressure decreases are relatively less than on the right, although much greater than normal, dramatically reflected by marked respiratory fluctuation of Doppler transvalvular and intravascular flow velocities. Displacement of the ventricular and atrial septa into the underfilled left ventricle and atrium, enlarging the right side of the heart at the expense of the left is a parallel effect due to inspiratory increase in RV transmural pressure and filling. The septal shifts further impede LV filling, which is also opposed by inspiratory reduction of aortic transmural pressure causing the left ventricle to contract against increased aortic impedance. Aortic flow and systolic pressure decrease promptly, within one beat of the onset of inspiration, immediately after inspiratory merging of pulmonary wedge and intrapericardial pressures. Thus, a large component of the change must be left sided, occurring before any series effect of increased RV output can reach the left atrium.[83] Pulsus paradoxus usually disappears with adequate pericardial drainage.

"NONPERICARDIAL" PULSUS PARADOXUS. Pulsus paradoxus occurs frequently in chronic obstructive airway disease and acute asthma and occasionally in hemorrhagic shock, tension pneumothorax, tracheal compression, RV infarction (possibly due to pericardial constraint), severe pulmonary embolism, restrictive cardiomyopathy, and mediastinal and cardiac compression by mass lesions.

ABSENCE OF PULSUS PARADOXUS. Tamponade without pulsus paradoxus occurs[83]:

1. When LV diastolic pressures and LV stiffness significantly exceed those of the right ventricle; pericardial pressure may effectively equilibrate only with right-sided heart pressures, a form of RV tamponade.
2. When severe aortic regurgitation damps respiratory fluctuations even without LV dysfunction.
3. With atrial septal defect when inspiratory venous return is balanced by shunting to the left atrium.
4. With extreme hypotension in shock, as in severe tamponade, which can make respiration-induced pressure changes unmeasurable.
5. In some cases of acute LV infarction with tamponading effusion.
6. In local (usually postsurgical) cardiac compression.

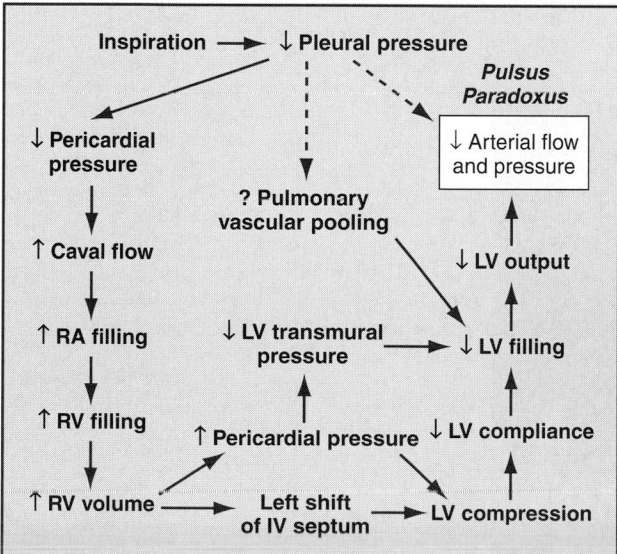

FIGURE 50–17. Physiology of pulsus paradoxus. Complex sequential and simultaneous responses as to inspiratory reduction of pleural pressure produce the inspiratory fall in arterial flow and pressure (see text). (From Spodick DH: The Pericardium: A Comprehensive Textbook. New York, Marcel Dekker, 1997.)

7. With pericardial adhesions, especially over the right side of the heart.

RENAL EFFECTS. Tamponade, like any profound hypotension, induces oliguria because it signals renal sodium and fluid retention. Despite high central circulatory pressures, atrial natriuretic factor cannot increase, owing to the absence of myocardial stretch.

ELECTROCARDIOGRAPHY (see p. 1828 and Chap. 5).[79] The ECG can be normal but most often is nonspecifically altered (mainly ST-T wave abnormalities). It may show acute pericarditis at ECG stages 1, 2, or 3. Electrical alternation of the QRS complex, rarely including the T wave, is quasi-diagnostic. P-QRS or P-QRS-T or P-PR segment-QRS-T alternations (panalternation)[86] are seen only in critical cardiac tamponade. Low voltage is usually due to reduced heart size. Significant vagally mediated bradycardia (overriding normal baroreceptor reflexes) and ultimate electromechanical dissociation (pulseless electric activity) occur in end-stage tamponade, especially in rapid hemopericardium in which critical cardiac compression prevents filling (therefore output) while the ECG is continuously generated.

IMAGING. All imaging methods can demonstrate pericardial effusion. Chest radiographs show an enlarged cardiopericardial silhouette with clear lungs (in the absence of pulmonary disease) (Fig. 50–10, p. 1838). *Echo-Doppler cardiography,* ideally, although not necessarily, TEE, can eliminate the need for invasive hemodynamic measurement by revealing physiological as well as anatomical abnormalities[87, 88](see Table 50–10) (Fig. 50–18; see also Figs. 7–95 to 7–97). Some features are initially blunted in hypervolemic patients.

Echo-Doppler signs are less accurate in patients with pulmonary hypertension and intrapericardial adhesions and of greatly reduced sensitivity after cardiac surgery. If the effusion is large enough, the heart may swing freely in it—the basis of electrical alternation. With large effusions, compression by pericardial fluid permits the entire adult heart to be seen, particularly in the four-chamber scan plane. Cardiac compression may also falsely suggest myocardial hypertrophy (pseudohypertrophy); the left ventricle transiently "remodels."[89]

In the absence of heart disease, systolic function is good, with excellent shortening and ejection fractions, although the ventricles operate at reduced volumes, hence with small stroke outputs. Thus, the heart is underloaded, both "underpreloaded" and "underafterloaded," obviously working hard but prevented by reduced inflow from matching circulatory demand.[79] With hemopericardium, blood and clots are seen, whereas fibrin is common in inflammatory effusions. Collapse of the RV free wall in early diastole (see Fig. 50–13) correlates with obstruction to the atrial *y* descent (i.e., obstruction to rapid filling); it is earliest and most marked in expiration when RV volume is reduced. RA collapse occurs at end diastole and early isovolumic systole; in about 25 percent of cases the left atrium also collapses (see Fig. 50–14). RV diastolic collapse occurs after a 15 to 25

percent drop in cardiac output and before significant decrease in blood pressure in patients who are normovolemic or hypervolemic; it is more specific than RA collapse and more sensitive and specific than pulsus paradoxus in detecting increased intrapericardial pressure, particularly if RV diastolic collapse lasts at least one third of the cardiac cycle. RV diastolic collapse duration is quantitatively related to the pericardial pressure.[73] It may also occur when unilateral or bilateral pleural effusion causes increased pressure in an insignificant pericardial effusion; this is relieved by pleural drainage. Inferior vena cava (IVC) plethora (diameter ≥ 20 mm) and absence of the normal inspiratory IVC collapse (≥50 percent) are seen on subcostal echocardiography. Absence of normal inspiratory IVC collapse implies right-sided heart diastolic pressures of 15 mm Hg or more. Respiratory effects parallel pulsus paradoxus reciprocally, with respiration, as shown by atrial and especially ventricular septal shifts from the right into the left atrium and ventricle in inspiration, reversed in expiration. Although total transvalvular blood volume flows are reduced, flow velocity differences between the right and left sides of the heart are enormously magnified during the breathing cycle. Figure 50–18 shows respiratory variation in transmitral flow. Concurrently, respiratory variations of superior vena cava flow velocities are exaggerated in tamponade. Hepatic vein flow velocities increase during inspiration, with retrograde flow in early expiration.

DIAGNOSIS. Tamponade should be suspected in patients with hypotension and the following findings: elevated systemic venous pressure, falling blood pressure, pulsus paradoxus, tachycardia and dyspnea or tachypnea with clear lungs, chest and abdominal wounds, recent or concurrent evidence of pericarditis, and unexplained "cardiac" enlargement or evidence of pericardial effusion. Moreover, anticoagulant or thrombolytic therapy,[90] certain drugs such as cyclosporine, recent cardiac surgery, blunt chest trauma, malignancies, connective tissue disease, renal failure, and septicemia all precipitate, aggravate, or predispose patients to tamponade. Indwelling instrumentation, particularly of the thin right side of the heart—such as central venous lines, transvenous pacemakers, filtration catheters, and hyperalimentation catheters—can subtly perforate the right atrium or ventricle (see Chap. 11). Some of these provoke hemopericardium; those delivering parenteral fluids can rapidly fill and overload the pericardial cavity.

Certain conditions inhibit or alter the pattern of chamber collapses and respiratory phenomena[79, 91] just as they limit pulsus paradoxus. These include LV hypertrophy and dysfunction, aortic valve disease, pulmonary hypertension, hypertrophy and reduced compliance of the right ventricle, obstruction of heart valves by intrinsic disease or masses, and intrapericardial adhesions. Finally, LV diastolic collapse occurs with loculated, usually postsurgical, effusions over the left ventricle and, rarely, in circumferential tamponade in patients with intrapericardial adhesions, pulmonary artery hypertension, or RV hypertrophy.[91, 92]

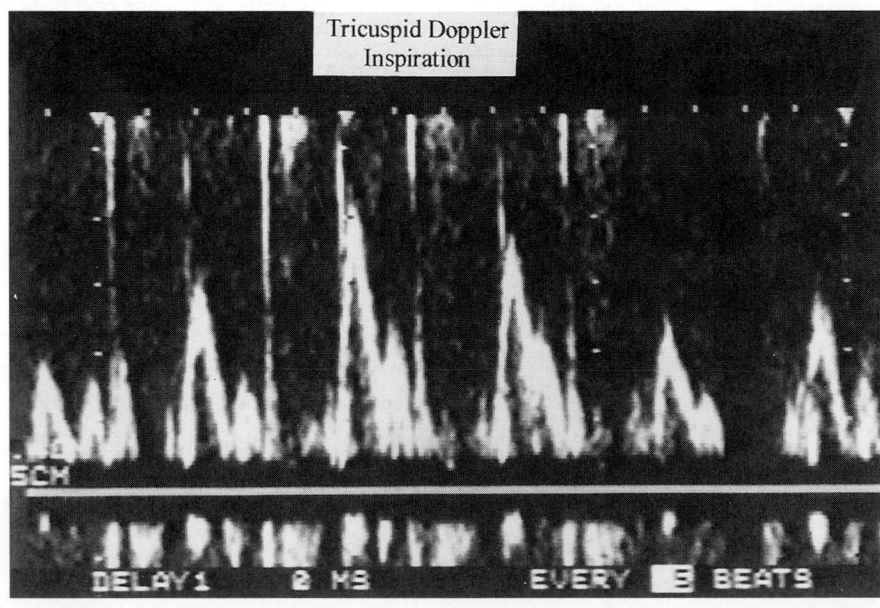

FIGURE 50–18. Cardiac tamponade. Transtricuspid flow velocity "paradoxus." Marked increase in flow velocity occurs with inspiration.

VARIANT FORMS OF CARDIAC TAMPONADE

LOW PRESSURE TAMPONADE.[83] Low pressure tamponade occurs in hypovolemia with severe systemic diseases such as tuberculosis and malignancy as well as in chest trauma with bleeding anywhere. Patients are weak, may seem normotensive, and have dyspnea on exertion, with only mild if any jugular venous distention and no diagnostic pulsus paradoxus. However, they have characteristic respiratory changes in Doppler diastolic inflow signals and isovolumic relaxation time (see Table 50–10). In low-pressure tamponade the low-pressure pericardial effusion equilibrates with RV diastolic pressure only, as in cases of early tamponade, and equilibration occurs first only in inspiration ("inspiratory tracking").

HYPERTENSIVE CARDIAC TAMPONADE. This condition has all the features of cardiac tamponade except that these exceptional patients have high (rarely very high—≥200 mm Hg) blood pressures.[79] Typically, there was antecedent hypertension. Pulsus paradoxus is demonstrable at high pressure. Attempts to reduce the blood pressure may exacerbate the situation and precipitate or greatly exaggerate pulsus paradoxus.[78]

TAMPONADE WITH VENTRICULAR DYSFUNCTION.[89, 90] RV or LV dysfunction can reduce or eliminate pulsus paradoxus. LV dysfunction, especially reduced compliance, notably in hypertensive or severe coronary artery disease, uremia, or aortic valve disease, may be associated with RA and RV collapses at relatively small volumes of excess pericardial fluid. They essentially produce a right-sided heart tamponade at lower intrapericardial pressures than with a normal left ventricle.

PNEUMOTAMPONADE: TENSION PNEUMOPERICARDIUM OR PNEUMOHYDROPERICARDIUM.[79, 93, 94] Increasing air or other gas in the pericardium with or without excess pericardial fluid, blood, pus, or chyle can easily tamponade the heart. Examples include a check-valve mechanism admitting air from lung structures or intrapericardial gas-producing organisms. Diagnostic and therapeutic principles are the same as in liquid tamponade. There is also a tympanitic precordial percussion and frequently the "mill-wheel sound" of the heart splashing in a fluid-gas interface.

REGIONAL CARDIAC TAMPONADE.[79, 95] Loculated effusion over any part of the heart can compress that part. Loculation is usually due to localized pericardial adhesions, especially postsurgically, and induces hemodynamic abnormalities consistent with the compressed chambers or zones. For example, after RV infarction, loculated effusion can cause selective RV tamponade with RV diastolic pressure higher than LV diastolic pressure. Loculated effusions compressing the right atrium (often after surgery) may act similarly and can cause a right-to-left shunt through a patent foramen ovale or atrial septal defect. Occasionally, loculated effusion tamponading the right atrium reproduces all the hemodynamic findings of severe generalized tamponade, including pulsus paradoxus.

EFFUSIVE-CONSTRICTIVE PERICARDITIS. This combination of effusion and constriction with mixed clinical, imaging, and hemodynamic signs can produce tamponade with relatively little fluid when there is a scarred, unyielding parietal pericardium or when a constrictive epicarditis underlies the tamponading fluid.

Cardiac Catheterization

It may be necessary to confirm the diagnosis of tamponade by right heart or complete cardiac catheterization, especially when study of the heart and coronaries becomes desirable. Ideally, catheterization shows high pressures throughout ventricular diastole and near-equilibration (>5 mm Hg) of atrial and ventricular diastolic pressures.[79, 92] Most tamponades equilibrate at 16 to 20 mm Hg (6 to 12 mm Hg in low pressure tamponade). Atrial traces show absent or amputated y descent. Arterial and pericardial catheters disclose exaggerated respiratory pressure fluctuations. Absent coronary disease, compression of the epicardial coronary arteries and veins does not result in anaerobic metabolism as measured by coronary sinus lactate level, demonstrating that the tamponaded (consequently underloaded) myocardium has sufficient blood supply to avoid anoxia, despite the usual tachycardia and strong compensatory adrenergic response. Despite very high central circulatory pressures, tamponade does not cause alveolar pulmonary edema.[79, 96] There may be some interstitial lung edema, but neither alveoli nor septa are affected. Subcostal echocardiography shows that the intrahepatic IVC is plethoric—a more reliable sign than jugular venous distention.[87, 88]

Treatment

Definitive treatment is prompt evacuation of pericardial contents. Only in relatively few patients who had dehydra-

tion and hypovolemia has it been possible to demonstrate effective cardiocirculatory support by medical measures. Volume infusion may also be diagnostically useful only in hypovolemic patients,[97] by revealing the typical hemodynamics of cardiac tamponade, which are otherwise well concealed in some hypovolemic patients (occult tamponade; low-pressure tamponade (see p. 1841).

MEDICAL TREATMENT.[79, 98, 99] Experimental evidence favoring a variety of medical agents is conflicting and investigated in models that do not necessarily apply to human tamponade.[98, 99] Medical treatment may appear temporarily effective (partly because tamponade occasionally remits spontaneously) but usually is ultimately ineffective. It is aimed at supporting compensatory and physiological responses, expanding intravascular volume, increasing or decreasing systemic vascular resistance, and supporting inotropy. The latter is almost predictably useless because most tamponaded hearts without preexisting cardiac disease are under effective endogenous inotropic stimulation with an excellent ejection fraction—but at critically low stroke volume. Supporting filling with various intravenous fluids can help hypovolemic patients but otherwise tends to increase heart volume with a subsequent countervailing increase in pericardial pressure, leaving the patient no better and perhaps worse by decreasing transmural pressure. Agents increasing peripheral resistance to support blood pressure have not been demonstrably effective because tamponade evokes maximal endogenous sympathetic stimulation and perhaps because of untoward cardiac effects. Finally, atropine can be given for depressive vagal reflexes during early and late tamponade.[79]

If drainage equipment is not immediately available, medical measures may be attempted for a transiently favorable effect, perhaps permitting additional pericardial stretch. These include isoproterenol, norepinephrine, dobutamine, and similar agents to support blood pressure and flow. Correction of any metabolic acidosis avoids the myocardial depressant effect of that condition and increases responses to endogenous and exogenous catecholamines. Temporary results may also accrue from vasodilators. Nitroprusside plus blood transfusion improved cardiac output in experimental animals.[98] Hydralazine plus volume infusion appears to raise arterial pressure and cardiac output and improve blood flow to myocardium, central nervous system, and kidney, all locations where slightly improving blood flow has not been critical partly due to autoregulation. Positive-pressure breathing of any kind should be avoided at any stage of tamponade because it will further reduce venous return, RV transmural pressure, and cardiac output. Only after the pericardium is incised or the fluid drained may positive-pressure breathing be used safely.

PERICARDIAL DRAINAGE. Whenever possible, echocardiographically monitored pericardiocentesis or surgical drainage are treatments of choice. Choice of procedure depends on urgency. When death is impending, the quickest method, percutaneous needle paracentesis, can be unavoidable. Yet, with brisk pericardial bleeding, as in wounds, ruptured ventricular aneurysm, or dissecting aortic hematoma, clotting makes needle evacuation impossible. Moreover, bleeding can be slowed by the tamponade pressure so that surgical drainage with suppression of bleeding sources is safer and surer. Drainage should be as complete and prolonged as necessary, whether by catheter or tube or by a window into a neighboring cavity. The choice must be individualized, but a pericardiostomy,[100] with suction drainage for at least 3 to 4 days, is often optimal. Preventing recurrence is important in disorders prone to reaccumulation. Treatment of underlying disease with specific agents may suppress reaccumulation. However, resistant processes such as malignancies and stubborn infections can ultimately require pericardiectomy or obliteration of the pericardial cavity using tetracycline, minocycline, bleomycin (installed with a local anesthetic), or other sclerosants; prolonged tube drainage can stimulate obliterative adhesions and is preferable to use of these painful agents.[79] Traditional percutaneous needle pericardiocentesis[77] is usually effective and relatively safe with inferior fluid accumulation at least l cm deep by echocardiogram. Most effusions can be effectively drained with echocardiographic guidance, which has greatly improved its safety, permitting puncture at any reasonable place on the precordium[101] except over the internal mammary arteries, 2.5 cm on each side of the sternum. An apical or, less often, subxiphoid approach is optimal. Fluoroscopic and even CT guidance are also feasible. Contraindications to thoracotomy, such as pleuropulmonary diseases, which make intolerable even temporary compromise of lung tissue, or extensive pleural adhesions may necessitate prolonged tube drainage or even a pericardioperitoneal shunt performed with special equipment.[79]

SURGICAL DRAINAGE. Subxiphoid surgical incision and thoracoscopic drainage produces little morbidity and can be done in emergencies with only local anesthesia. It permits direct inspection, biopsy of visceral and parietal pericardium, and resection when that is an option. Video-assisted thoracoscopy gives the operator a wide field of view (although a lung, usually the left, must be collapsed). Other chest conditions or failure of thoracoscopic drainage may mandate an open surgical approach.

EFFECTS OF PERICARDIAL DRAINAGE. After pericardiocentesis, cardiac pressure and volume corrections reflect the presence and degree of cardiac compression and are not predictable from the amount of fluid removed. However, because critically tamponaded hearts operate on the steep portion of their pericardial pressure-volume curve (see Fig. 50–11), the initial fluid decrement will produce the greatest improvement in stroke volume. After drainage, RV volume usually increases more than LV volume because the more compliant right ventricle was more compressible. Indeed, the right ventricle occasionally dilates and echocardiography shows abnormal ventricular septal motion characteristic of RV volume overload. Especially if there is myocardial disease, RV dilation may initiate congestive failure. LV dilation can also do this with occasional pulmonary edema ("pericardial shock"). Although pulmonary artery pressure usually falls after drainage, it may rise with a temporary mismatch of ventricular output. Such acute right-sided and particularly left-sided heart failure occurs with ventricles unable to accommodate posttamponade increase in venous return exacerbated by continuing high afterload due to continuing increased peripheral resistance from compensatory adrenergic responses. Hemodynamic and clinical improvements are related to increased stroke volume. Effective drainage is characterized by[79] (1) disappearance of pulsus paradoxus; (2) frequent relief of dyspnea; (3) disappearance of signs of venous engorgement paralleling falling RA pressure; (4) reappearance of *y* descents; (5) loss of vena cava plethora; (6) loss of diastolic pressure equilibration; and (7) prompt loss of electrical alternation. A pericardial catheter (rarely necessary) documents normalization of pericardial pressure.

NONEFFUSIVE SEQUELAE OF PERICARDIAL INFLAMMATION

PERICARDIAL ADHESIONS AND FIBROSIS. Pericarditis can heal without detectable residua or with some scarring of one or both pericardial layers. The plastic fibrinous exudate of acute and subacute pericarditis can be adhesive, but its fate is either fibrinolysis and reabsorption or organization with newly formed collagen fibrils as a matrix for invasion by new blood and lymphatic vessels and later fibrous

or fibrogranulomatous adhesions.[102] A common denominator for intense scarring is bleeding; blood, particularly blood lipids and thrombi, and especially combined with pericardial injury and exudate, is thrombogenic.[102] Cicatrization is probably intensified by locally produced interleukins and tumor necrosis factors found in abnormal pericardial fluids and mesothelial production of a chemical promotant for fibroblasts. The most common cause of intrapericardial adhesions is cardiac surgery.[103]

Local thickenings are not rare on CT in patients with healed myocardial infarctions, rheumatic heart disease, sarcoidosis, and other conditions. More destructive inflammation in severe infectious pericarditis may heal without further consequences but frequently provokes constrictive scarring involving the entire heart, any portion of the heart, or the great vessels, distorting or compressing structures it entraps. Compressive syndromes arise from primarily pericardial lesions, differing from primarily myocardial lesions (e.g., myocardial infarction) that are usually associated with adhesions and fibrosis of little or no dynamic significance. In effusive pericarditis, intrapericardial bands on echocardiography predict significant scarring.[104] Some pericardial adhesions may buttress myocardial wounds or infarcts and contribute mural and microvascular support. Some seal an otherwise fatal myocardial rupture to form a pseudoaneurysm (see Chap. 37).

Clinical Considerations. Adhesions on the outside of the parietal pericardium even when combined with internal adhesions can be due to inflammatory disease of the mediastinum and pleura. Rarely they affect the cardiac silhouette[102] (unusual configurations can be resolved by imaging methods like spin-gated MRI; and CT is optimal for retrosternal adhesions).[105] External adhesions can produce exopericardial rubs and rarely permit systolic tugging on adjacent organs after pleuritis and mediastinitis. On imaging, intrapericardial adhesions modify some effects of tamponade by shifting chamber collapses to unusual locations and restricting swinging.[106] Adhesions are a major problem in the increasing numbers of second and third thoracotomies. Surgical preventive efforts include intrapericardial absorbable polymer patches, plasminogen activator (rt-PA), and hyaluronic acid. Postoperative pericardial closure decreases adhesions but is usually avoided due to unfavorable hemodynamics.[102]

PERICARDIAL CALCIFICATION (PANZERHERZ: "ARMOR HEART"). Dystrophic calcification (rarely ossification) signifies pericardial injury more destructive than conditions healing without calcification.[102] Yet even extensive calcifications may be well tolerated and asymptomatic. However, any degree of calcification may be found in constrictive pericarditis. Local calcification seems related to involvement of areas of least heart movement and of greatest friction between the epicardium and the parietal pericardium: inferiorly the LV apex, the right atrium, the sternal aspect of the right ventricle, and the AV groove. So many cases, especially those with ECG abnormalities, are associated with constriction that constrictive pericarditis should be ruled in or out when pericardial calcification is discovered. Three-dimensional echocardiography, MRI with tagging, and rapid-acquisition spiral or electron-beam CT can simultaneously map calcifications and indicate any hemodynamic impairment.[107, 108] Calcifications increase the technical difficulties of pericardial resection by requiring special instruments, and where calcification invades the myocardium the procedure is particularly difficult and dangerous.

INFLAMMATORY CYSTS.[98] These include pseudocysts as well as encapsulated and loculated pericardial effusions. Pericardial scarring may trap portions of an intrapericardial exudate or hemorrhage, producing a pocket or cystlike structure with or without symptoms and signs requiring drainage or resection. Their capsules are scarred parietal and visceral pericardium with persistent inflammatory activity. Chronic inflammatory cysts must be differentiated from ventricular pseudoaneurysms and true (congenital) pericardial cysts, which tend to be smooth with a predilection for the low right cardiac border, whereas inflammatory pseudocysts, like parasitic cysts, have variable contours and occur anywhere. *Inflammatory diverticula* are related to encapsulated pericardial effusion; they follow exudative pericarditis, especially tuberculous, but acute idiopathic (presumably viral) pericarditis can be a precursor. Unlike inflammatory cysts, only parietal pericardium is primarily involved, and they communicate with the pericardial cavity. Diverticular contents resemble those of inflammatory cysts. Diverticula, for some reason, tend to be right-sided, perhaps because the fibrosa over the right ventricle is particularly thick.

GRANULOMATOUS PERICARDITIS. Granulomas are characterized by simultaneous inflammation and repair, producing subacute and chronic pericardial disease. These are basically nodules or masses composed mainly of vascular fibrous tissue with variable leukocytic infiltration. They can spread throughout the pericardium to form a static, avascular scar, making etiological diagnosis ultimately progressively more difficult. Many granulomas are rich in cholesterol and represent one source of cholesterol pericarditis. There are four main etiological groups of granulomatous pericarditis: (1) of unknown origin; (2) due to systemic diseases such as rheumatoid arthritis (rheumatoid arthritis causes a great number of pericardial adhesions and even pericardial rheumatoid nodules, sometimes with acute or subacute fibrinous pericarditis); (3) infections, particularly tuberculosis and fungi; and (4) foreign-matter reactions, particularly silicosis and asbestosis, which tend to form static scars with uncertain (usually low) constrictive potential.

CONSTRICTIVE PERICARDITIS

CLINICAL CONSIDERATIONS. Constrictive pericarditis "imprisons" the heart.[109, 110] It has important similarities to and differences from cardiac tamponade.[110] Its dominant etiological spectrum has changed (Table 50–12) and its clinical manifestations have changed due to changing tempo of the disease, that is, the aggressiveness of the inciting processes, the point in its development where it becomes significantly compressive or symptomatic and particularly where it becomes diagnosable. With progress in understanding constrictive and restrictive hemodynamics and in testing, diagnosis is only rarely greatly delayed so that most patients are recognized in earlier rather than truly chronic stages. The traditional "*chronic* constrictive pericarditis" is erroneous in most contemporary cases. There remain variably difficult differentiations from restrictive cardiomyopathy, other causes of systemic congestion, particularly RV failure, and hepatic cirrhosis. Sometimes inspection and biopsy of the pericardium and myocardium are required to rule in or out constriction or one of its variants, especially in the presence of systemic diseases that may be related to it. While obliterative adhesions regularly follow cardiac surgery, constrictive scarring is relatively uncommon.[110] Yet, constrictive scarring may follow pericardial resection or pericardiotomy for any condition, including constrictive pericarditis.

PATHOGENESIS. Currently, most cases are of undetermined etiology—"idiopathic." The initial acute pericarditis can be silent or clinically apparent. The essential pathological process is healing with a thick *or thin* scar that restricts cardiac filling usually by total or near-total obliteration of the pericardial "space," although often with lacunae of fluid, pus, or blood. (Loculated fluid and bandlike constriction can compress any portion of the heart including any chamber, valve rings, and great vessels, mimicking disease in those structures.[109, 110]) Traditionally, constriction has been chronic, sometimes with surprising pericardial thickness; recently, thin constricting pericardia are increasingly evident. Early diagnosis and shift of most processes such as tuberculosis to "idiopathic" pericarditis, viral infections, and cardiac surgery[109, 111] cause most contemporary cases to be *subacute* (arbitrarily, 3 to 12 months after the pericardial insult). *Acute* constriction occurs soon after acute pericarditis; healing can cause constricting cicatrization within days after draining tamponade fluid. *Transient constriction* soon after acute pericarditis, usually with effusion, has been observed by echocardiography, inspection of the jugular

▼ **TABLE 50–12. CAUSES OF CONSTRICTIVE PERICARDITIS (WESTERN NATIONS)**

Great Majority: Unknown or uncertain etiology/ "Idiopathic pericarditis"

Relatively Common
Infectious
  Viral or probable viral
  Tuberculous
  Pyogenic
Therapeutic irradiation
Cardiopericardial surgery

Relatively Uncommon (increased incidence in special populations)
Neoplasia
  Metastatic
  Mesothelioma
    Pericardial
    Pleural
Uremia (on dialysis)
Vasculitis/connective tissue disease group
  Especially rheumatoid arthritis, lupus, scleroderma (including CREST syndrome)
Infectious
  Fungal
  Parasitic
Myocardial infarct-related
  Post hemopericardium (from thrombolysis)
  Post-myocardial infarction (Dressler) syndrome
Trauma
  Blunt
  Penetrating
Drugs
  Procainamide (lupus)
  Methysergide
  Practolol
  Hydralazine (lupus)
Hemopericardium/encapsulated hemopericardium in hemorrhagic disorders

Rare
Cholesterol pericarditis
Chylopericardium
Intrapericardial instrumentation
  Automatic implantable cardioverter-defibrillator
  Epicardial pacemaker
Whipple disease
Wegener granulomatosis
Hypereosinophilic syndromes
Cardiac transplant
Hereditary: mulibrey nanism
Sarcoidosis
Asbestosis
Pericardial amyloidosis
Dermatomyositis
Lassa fever
Chemical trauma: sclerotherapy of esophageal varices

veins, venous pulse, and auscultation (transient abnormal S_3) with or without symptoms and resolving in days to weeks.[110] In *chronic* constriction, pericardial tissue usually shows nonspecific fibrosis with few inflammatory cells and frequent myocardial atrophy.

Both subacute and acute constriction show many more inflammatory cells and lighter connective tissue. Depending on etiology there may be giant cells and granulomas.

PATHOPHYSIOLOGY.[109, 110] Constricting pericardial scar, like tamponading fluid, sharply accentuates ventricular pressure-volume relations (see Fig. 50–11) and increases ventricular coupling (ventricular interaction). It *progressively* restricts ventricular filling to earlier diastole until 70 to 80 percent of the reduced filling occurs in the first 25 to 30 percent of diastole[109] (in contrast, tamponade *continuously* restricts filling from the beginning of diastole). Ele-

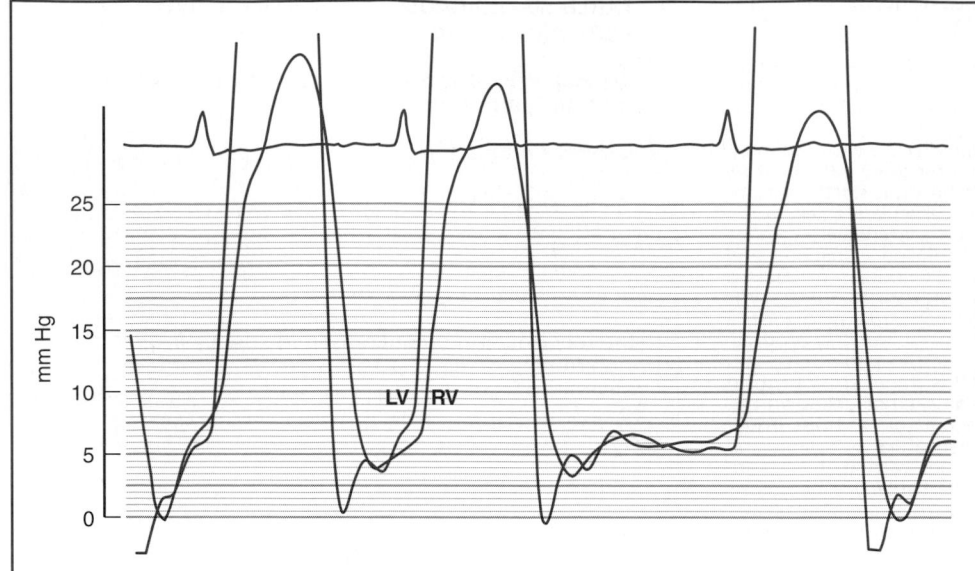

FIGURE 50–19. Constrictive pericarditis. Dip-plateau of left (LV) and right (RV) pressure curves with diastolic equilibrium are best seen in long diastole (patient with atrial fibrillation).

vated atrial pressures reflect elevated ventricular diastolic pressures. Moreover, early diastolic filling is at high velocity, owing to (1) high atrial pressure as the AV valves open and (2) diastolic suction,[112, 113] augmented by elastic recoil (conversion of potential to kinetic energy or "rubber bulb" effect[112]), that is, rebound of the ventricular pericardial scar, which had been contracted like a spring by ventricular systole. Such factors produce the "square root" configuration of ventricular diastolic pressure curves (Fig. 50–19) and other findings (see "Cardiac Catheterization," in Chap. 11).

All cardiac diastolic pressures are nearly equilibrated as in tamponade. Equilibration may be "unbalanced" by vigorous diuretic therapy. Unlike tamponade, venous and atrial pressure waveforms resemble the normal: the y descent is preserved, although deep and usually larger than a more or less deep x descent (Fig. 50–19). (In tamponade the y descent is eliminated or truncated.) Venous flow toward the heart occurs with the x and y descents of venous pressure, with the major acceleration during the y descent rather than as normally during the x descent. There are no systolic abnormalities except with coexisting myocardial lesions, atrophy, or damage, including antecedent or ongoing myocarditis or ischemia. Myocardial atrophy, fibrosis, and calcification are related to chronicity. Ischemia includes intrinsic coronary disease and compression by constricting scar of coronary arteries, veins, or bypass grafts.[114] In uncomplicated constriction, as in tamponade, coronary blood flow is reduced but adequate for aerobic metabolism.

COMPENSATION. Compensation for constriction resembles compensation in cardiac tamponade. Heart rate is the major mechanism defending cardiac output, because stroke volume becomes nearly fixed by filling halted in early diastole. Increased heart rate mainly amputates the diastolic pressure plateau after the abbreviated filling period, so that tachycardia is relatively less detrimental than in conditions without early filling. Humoral, hormonal, and renal responses are similar to those of cardiac failure and tamponade with electrolyte and water retention.[109, 115] Yet, as in tamponade, restricted atrial distensibility prevents significant rise in atrial natriuretic factors. Sodium and water retention and high systemic venous pressure contribute to high hepatic vein pressure, ascites, and edema. The attendant blood volume expansion is more important than the simultaneously elevated systemic vascular resistance in maintaining arterial pressure.[110]

RESPIRATORY EFFECTS. Respiratory responses depend on the effects of pericardial scarring: (1) insulation of the heart from intrathoracic pressure changes and (2) increased ventricular interaction. The heart and pulmonary vessels are intrathoracic. Normally they are simultaneously affected by respiratory pressure changes so that pulmonary venous flow to the left atrium is not significantly changed by breathing. But in classic constriction the heart is totally encased; when inspiration decreases intrathoracic pressure, cardiac pressures remain high. Consequently, pulmonary venous blood cannot easily enter the high pressure left atrium; therefore, total pulmonary venous flow and flow velocity are decreased in inspiration, decreasing LV filling and time to peak filling rate. Respiration does not change superior vena cava pressure or flow velocity. Although the IVC is affected by diaphragmatic movements and abdominal pressure fluctuations, there is diminished (<50 percent) to undetectable respiratory change in IVC diameter.[110, 116] Although inspiration does not

greatly increase RV filling volume, filling *velocities* sharply increase and pulmonary artery flow velocity increases, with much less effect in decreasing aortic pressure. Yet, in some cases, inspiration decreases systolic blood pressure more than 10 mm Hg, particularly if there is an element of tamponade (effusive-constrictive pericarditis) or other cause for pulsus paradoxus, such as pulmonary disease but especially with marked respiratory shifts of the ventricular and atrial septa. Note that both ventricular and atrial septa are free of constriction and respond to pressure differences across them; thus, they often move sharply with respiration.[110]

The *Kussmaul sign,* inspiratory increased venous pressure with jugular venous distention, eliminates the normal inspiratory fall of 3 to 7 mm Hg in mean RA pressure, because the neck veins are extrathoracic and face an impediment to flow into the high pressure right atrium. The right atrium resists inspiratory acceleration of venous blood toward the heart with little or no respiratory variation in RA mean pressure. Other conditions with markedly increased RA and venous pressures that also produce the Kussmaul sign include RV failure, RV myocardial infarct, restrictive cardiomyopathy, chronic cor pulmonale, and acute pulmonary embolism.[110]

Clinical Aspects

CHEST RADIOGRAPH. The cardiopericardial silhouette is usually normal or only modestly enlarged. Its shape depends on the configuration of scar tissue and any remaining fluid.[102, 110] The superior vena cava (SVC) and azygos vein are dilated. Pleural effusions are frequent and usually bilateral. Occasional *constrictive pleuritis* may be missed and discovered by CT, at operation, or post mortem. The only chamber enlargement recognized by chest radiography is LA, particularly with heavy scarring on the left ventricle or the left AV groove (functional mitral stenosis). Pulmonary blood flow often redistributes with upper-zone vascular dilation and decreased lower-zone vessel caliber, particularly with LA enlargement. Kerley B lines may be present, but alveolar edema is rare and implies either unequal chamber constriction or concomitant heart or lung disease.[110] Previously, one third to one half of cases, mainly chronic, had obvious pericardial calcification (Fig. 8–23); diagnostic efficiency has reduced its incidence due to earlier surgery. Calcification is best seen on lateral films (see Chap. 8). With appropriate hemodynamic and clinical findings, calcification strongly favors the diagnosis of constriction but is itself not specific.

CT AND MRI (see Figs. 10–16 and 10–45).[117, 118] Pericardial thickening is best demonstrated by cine and gated MRI and CT with and without contrast medium enhancement. Each technique has high time and spatial resolutions that dependably identify and measure pericardial thickening and geometric changes and are more specific than TTE in differentiating scarring from fluid or tumor. CT and MRI demonstrate the frequently deformed ventricles and atria and enlarged venae cavae that contrast sharply to the aorta, which their diameter normally matches. The atria (particularly the left atrium) may be enlarged and the ventricles narrowed and tubelike. The ventricular septum is frequently sinuous, bowed, or angulated. Pericardial thickness by CT and MRI varies from subtle increase over the normal hairline to 10 to 15 mm (rarely more); any thickening over 3.5 mm helps differentiate constriction from restrictive cardiomyopathy; over 6 mm adds great specificity. However, constricting pericardium may be so thin as not to be recognizable as abnormal by contemporary imaging. CT and MRI permit planning the surgical approach in patients with adequate myocardium by revealing the distribution and varieties of pericardial thickenings and calcifications and any myocardial invasion. Absence of myocardium (especially parts of the LV wall) due to atrophy and fibrosis indicates a poor prognosis, including disastrous postoperative results, particularly irreversible decompensation.[118]

ECHOCARDIOGRAPHY (see Chap. 7).[109, 110, 119, 120] In 40 percent of pericardiectomy patients at the Mayo Clinic, the first clue to constriction came from echocardiography, which reflects constricting anatomical changes, accelerated ventricular filling, and restricted diastolic expansion and filling. Transesophageal and three-dimensional echocardiography display pericardial thickening comparably to CT. TTE is not as reliable. Doppler recording is excellent for dynamic changes. No single echocardiographic or Doppler sign is pathognomonic.

The ventricular and atrial septa, which are pliant compared with the constricted walls, shift leftward with inspiration and rightward with expiration. The ventricular septum often shows paradoxic systolic motion: anterior (type A) or flat (type B). It may be accompanied by reduced to absent diastolic ventricular expansion with a "flat" LV posterior wall almost equally distant from the chest wall signals in early and late diastole. This is characteristic but not specific. Normal or paradoxic septal motion is bracketed by the components of septal "bounce"[109] on two-dimensional echocardiography, which can be further analyzed by M-mode. The "atrial" notch begins in the middle of the P wave and is characterized by rapid posterior or anterior motion, or posterior, then anterior, motion after atrial systole. The ventricular notch is often more abrupt: posterior, posterior-anterior, or, occasionally, an anterior-posterior sequence in early diastole. This "ventricular" septal notch coincides with the early diastolic abnormal S3. The aortic root may show abrupt early diastolic posterior motion. TTE and TEE usually demonstrate enlargement of one or both atria with reduced wall excursion and dimensional change (particularly on the right). Both venae cavae and hepatic veins are dilated with restricted respiratory fluctuations.[109, 110] In the IVC these vary from well under the normal 50 percent of diameter to no change, as in cardiac tamponade and other conditions with 15 mm Hg or more of elevated RA pressure.

ECHO-DOPPLER CARDIOGRAPHY (see Chap. 7).[109, 110, 117, 121] Transmitral and transtricuspid Doppler recordings show rapid forward flow in diastole and reverse flow in later systole (Fig. 7–98). The early-filling and A (late filling) waves are characterized by increased filling velocities and abnormally rapid deceleration from their peaks. Pulmonary venous forward flow velocity is reduced with exaggerated respiratory variation of early diastolic peak velocity and time integral that is even more pronounced than across the mitral valve. Reciprocal respiratory flow changes resemble those in tamponade with decreased left-sided and increased right-sided transvalvular velocities at the very onset (first beat) of inspiration and the reverse at the very onset of expiration. When respiratory variation is blunted or absent due to very high LA pressure, reducing preload by sitting or head-up tilt may unmask it.[122] Doppler tissue imaging shows normal LV expansion velocity and rapid mitral an-

nular velocity. The slope of the color M-mode wave indicates a much more rapid flow from left atrium to left ventricle.

CARDIAC CATHETERIZATION (see Chap. 11). Catheterization is required to quantify pressures and identify concomitant cardiac disease if the sum of other findings only suggests constriction. (Diuretics should be withheld because hypovolemia alters the results.) Moreover, coronary angiography should identify atherosclerosis or any unusual distribution of the coronary arteries and minimize operative accidents. Constrictive hemodynamics are "restrictive" and therefore closely resemble those of restrictive cardiomyopathy, often the principal differential diagnosis. The major finding is near equalization (≤ 5 mm Hg) in all diastolic chamber and venous pressures. Both LV and RV traces have a *dip and plateau*, the *"square root"* configuration (see Fig. 50–19), usually more pronounced in the right ventricle, with the sharp short early diastolic fall toward 0 pressure (dip), rising to a restrictive plateau as the relaxing ventricles spring back with and reach the limit of the tight pericardium. Typically, RV and pulmonary artery systolic pressures are 30 to 45 mm (up to 70 mm) Hg with RV end-diastolic pressure at least one third of RV systolic pressure. Negative atrial waves, like negative venous waves, are preserved, with the y descent usually deeper than the x descent (Fig. 50–20), although they are often equal. In contrast, when x is greater than y effusive constrictive pericarditis is suggested. The nadir of the dip of the ventricular "square root" coincides with the atrial y nadir, ranging from below 0 to well over 20 mm Hg with fluid-filled catheters. High-fidelity catheters show these to be exaggerated; the nadir is usually 4 to 12 mm Hg. *Angiocardiography* shows normal or decreased LV end-systolic and end-diastolic volumes. The SVC is dilated and continuous with a frequently flat RA border. Coronary arteries are usually well within the cardiopericardial silhouette, that is, deep to their normal superficial location, unless the constricting scar is thin. Epicardial coronaries may display less than normal mobility whereas septal coronaries may appear hypermobile.

HISTORY.[109, 110] A history of antecedent pericarditis or pericarditis-inducing disease, drugs, or thoracic irradiation may be clues to diagnosis, but absence of any history of a provocative disorder is common. Constriction (especially chronic) may present deceptively as "congestive failure," pleural effusions, RA thrombosis, and even hepatic coma.

Symptoms and Signs. These reflect the degree of systemic and central venous congestion and fluid retention and may be subtle or overt. Constrictive pericarditis resem-

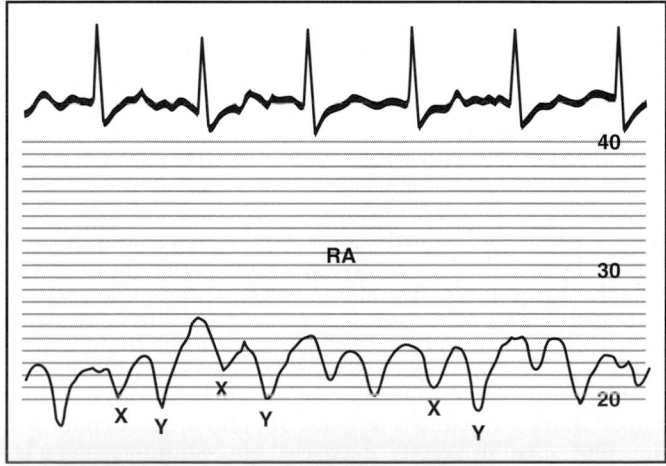

FIGURE 50–20. Constrictive pericarditis. Characteristic right atrial pressure curve has well-formed x and y descents and $y > x$. Mean atrial pressure is approximately 22 mm Hg. Electrocardiogram shows interarterial block. (From Spodick DH: The Pericardium: A Comprehensive Textbook. New York, Marcel Dekker, 1997.)

bles, but is not, "heart failure": the heart has not failed; it has been prevented from "succeeding." Venous congestion resembles right-sided heart failure with appropriate compensatory responses. Patients have pedal edema, ascites, and abdominal discomfort due to splanchnic engorgement. Ascites may be conspicuous, often without peripheral edema. At higher central diastolic pressures (arbitrarily >15 mm Hg), "central" symptoms are more prominent, including dyspnea, easy fatigability, and occasional orthopnea. Cardiac output cannot rise adequately with exercise because of the relatively fixed stroke volume, so that at any pressure level, dyspnea on exertion is characteristic and exacerbated by any pleural effusions, a diaphragm limited by ascites, or increased lung stiffness from interstitial (not alveolar) edema.[110]

PHYSICAL EXAMINATION. Mild tachycardia is the rule, even with light exertion. Chronic or aggressive subacute constriction may be accompanied by atrial fibrillation or other atrial arrhythmias. The blood pressure is normal or relatively low, although occasionally hypertensive. Significant (>10 mm Hg; rarely, 15 mm Hg) pulsus paradoxus occurs if there is effusive-constrictive disease or other extracardiac conditions such as lung disease, or if pliant ventricular and atrial septa have exaggerated respiratory mobility. The Valsalva maneuver produces a square wave response, owing to central vascular congestion.[123] Pedal edema may appear early, or there may be ascites with or without edema. Diminished cardiac output may produce pale, cool extremities with peripheral cyanosis. Jaundice in chronic constriction indicates severe congestive or fibrotic liver impairment. Jugular venous distention is a hallmark, although peripheral venous distention is also easily detected in advanced cases. Neck veins are better seen than in most other conditions because of the high level of venous pressure with sharp x and y descents. These should be sought as collapses from a high standing level. Retinal veins are engorged. Kussmaul sign is common.[110]

Precordial palpation may be "quiet" with no point of maximal impulse or with paradoxical systolic retraction of the chest wall. A sharp early diastolic thrust is common especially in chronic constriction, corresponding to ventricular rapid filling. It coincides with the loud, often palpable, abnormal S_3 (see Fig. 50–5), which sometimes has a "knocking" quality; it is easily mistaken for S_1, especially if the simultaneous diastolic thrust is mistaken for the apex beat.[110] If equivocal or faint, the S_3 is enhanced by squatting, sitting up, or standing or during contrast medium injection. It follows S_2 closely; when it mimics S_1, it follows the carotid pulse peak whereas S_1 precedes it. The jugular x descent occurs approximately with the carotid peak, and the y descent coincides with the S_3 and any diastolic precordial thrust. The liver is often palpable and may have a double pulsation. Ascites is recognized by abdominal protrusion and fluid wave. The spleen may be palpable if portal hypertension ensues.

LABORATORY FINDINGS.[109, 110] The hemogram may be normal or show a normocytic normochromic anemia. Otherwise, especially in less chronic constriction, blood counts reflect etiological agents or processes. Rarely, congestive hypersplenism causes selective cytopenia or pancytopenia. Liver function tests are likely to be abnormal due to hepatic congestion and late cardiac cirrhosis, including increased conjugated and unconjugated bilirubin to the point of cutaneous and conjunctival icterus. Ascitic fluid may be an exudate (typically >2.5 gm/dl protein) or a transudate, (rarely chylous); with chronicity, protein concentration and specific gravity decrease. The serum-ascites albumin gradient tends to exceed 10 gm/dl.

Hypoalbuminemia is common due to liver impairment, protein-losing enteropathy or a proteinuric nephrotic syndrome, each related to chronically high venous pressure and more prominent in children.

ELECTROCARDIOGRAPHY[109] (see also Chap. 5). The ECG is nearly always nonspecifically abnormal, only rarely within normal limits. T waves are almost always low to flat or have general or local inversions; they are usually symmetrical unless digitalis has been given. QRS complex and T wave voltage may be normal or reduced. Interatrial block is common, especially with chronicity, with P waves wider than 100 milliseconds and usually notched. These can resemble P mitrale (which may be present with AV groove constriction). RA enlargement can accompany a large pointed P wave or dominantly positive "±" P in V_1. Local or unequal constriction causes changes due to overload of "upstream" cardiac structures, producing ECGs consistent with RV hypertrophy or "strain" and may show right-axis deviation. In chronic constriction, myocardial atrophy probably contributes to reduced voltage, as do fluid retention and pleural effusions. Myocardial calcification and fibrosis, especially with reduced coronary flow, can produce AV blocks, intraventricular blocks, and even abnormal Q waves. Mixed ECG patterns are particularly common in constriction after cardiac operations because of frequently localized or unequal postoperative scarring and also whatever heart disease required surgery. Finally, constriction can compress even normal coronary arteries sufficiently to produce a positive ECG response to exercise. Subacute and especially chronic constriction is often accompanied by atrial arrhythmias, particularly atrial fibrillation (interatrial block is predictive).

DIFFERENTIAL DIAGNOSIS.[109, 110, 124, 125] Because of variability in scarring and its many mimics, constriction requires an impressive number of tests. Congestive failure due to heart disease is the principal functional diagnosis. Restrictive cardiomyopathy, often due to myocardial fibrosis or amyloidosis, may be difficult because of frequently identical hemodynamics and impairment. Note that restrictive cardiomyopathy patients are poor thoracotomy risks, whereas constricted patients may become unstable when intubated. The basic problem is to distinguish between abnormal chamber stiffness and abnormal muscle stiffness. The principal differential points are the usual thickness of constricting pericardium on imaging and timing of respiratory changes in ventricular systolic pressures; these are discordant in constriction and concordant in restrictive cardiomyopathy. These Doppler flow changes occur within one beat of the onset of inspiration and expiration in constriction but on later beats, if at all, in restrictive cardiomyopathy. The atrial and ventricular septa, free in constriction, are usually restricted in restrictive cardiomyopathy and therefore unlikely to show respiratory mobility. Meticulous Doppler-echocardiography combined if necessary with CT nearly always makes the diagnosis, and Doppler tissue imaging, slope of the color M-mode wave, and mitral annular velocity give clear separation.[126, 127] Occasional cases, particularly those constricted by a thin pericardium will be sufficiently confusing to require myocardial and/or pericardial inspection and biopsy.

Venous obstructive syndromes (e.g., SVC obstruction and nephrotic syndromes), especially with gross edema and ascites, are usually differentiated by imaging, as is abdominal disease with ascites, such as ovarian carcinoma and hepatic cirrhosis. RA tumors, especially myxomas, can mimic constriction by compressing the tricuspid valve; any ventricular involvement adds to the mimicry. In any unclear syndrome, imaging, hemodynamic data, and liver biopsy can be decisive. However, a few patients have simultaneous restrictive cardiomyopathy and constrictive pericarditis, usually due to radiation therapy, and also occurring in transplanted hearts; biopsy may be necessary. Quite suggestive for differentiation are a history of acute pericarditis of almost any etiology, especially purulent, hemorrhagic, or tuberculous. Finally, all segments of the autonomic nervous system are dysfunctional in constriction; in restrictive cardiomyopathy, dysfunction is localized to the sympathetic efferent pathway.[128]

Variants of Constrictive Pericarditis

A variety of cases are not "typical" or "classic," owing to the unpredictable pericardial scarring process, particularly in contemporary patients after cardiac surgery with variants that can resemble other conditions.[110]

UNEQUAL/LOCAL CONSTRICTION. Chambers, valves, and great vessels can be individually or unequally affected by pericardial scarring and calcification, producing murmurs due to locally turbulent blood flow and local ECG and hemodynamic changes. Echocardiography (TEE, TTE, and three-dimensional), MRI, or CT may demonstrate thickened or calcified pericardium. With *LV constriction* the atria, SVC, and IVC are dilated, the right ventricle is normal sized, and the ventricular septum is straight or inclined to the left. With *RV constriction,* the right atrium, IVC, and SVC are dilated and the septum is straight or inclined to the right. *Annular constriction,* mainly in the AV groove, enlarges the atria while the ventricles remain normal or relatively small.

EFFUSIVE-CONSTRICTIVE PERICARDITIS. This form produces symptoms and objective findings due to variable mixtures of effusion or tamponade accompanied by constriction of the visceral pericardium (*constrictive epicarditis*) or constriction with local tamponade of one or more chambers due to loculated effusion. Physical and laboratory findings usually resemble tamponade more than constriction until after the fluid is drained when a constrictive picture emerges.[110] Occasionally, tamponade is suggested by an abnormal S_3, which is ruled out by pure, classic tamponade dynamics (i.e., no rapid filling period). In contrast to pure constriction, significant pulsus paradoxus is frequent. A large dominant x descent ($x > y$) in atrial and venous traces also suggests an element of tamponade. After drainage, pericardial pressure drops to near 0, hemodynamic curves become more typical of constriction, and pulsus paradoxus may disappear. Kussmaul sign in what appears to be dominantly tamponade is a clue to effusive-constrictive pericarditis and may be accentuated after the fluid is drained.

ELASTIC CONSTRICTION. Thick pericardial fluids particularly rich in blood and fibrin may organize and resemble tamponade, owing to continuous elastic compression, usually by clot. The venous and atrial waveforms may show a predominant x descent like tamponade, and there is nearly always no S_3 because there is no early rapid filling; there may be an S_4. Occasionally, malignancies surround the ventricles, producing a similar picture.

LATENT (OCCULT) CONSTRICTION. Patients with dyspnea, fatigue, and mild edema with or without a history of acute pericarditis and no specific cardiac findings may show excessive rises in heart rate and venous pressure with exercise, which may also induce an S_3. Some patients are volume-depleted due to diuretics. Administration of fluids may bring out constrictive dynamics. In this respect the situation is analogous to that in low pressure cardiac tamponade.

TRANSIENT CONSTRICTION. Transient constriction often follows acute pericarditis.

Management

Medical management does not relieve constriction except if with a dynamic inflammatory component responsive to antiinflammatory agents.[109, 110, 129] Any underlying disease should be treated; for specific infection, therapeutic agents should be given before operation and continued afterward. Surgery is definitive and technically easier early before calcification or myocardial abnormalities. Good surgical results follow in patients in better cardiac and systemic condition as well as with less pericardial scarring, calcification, and hepatic congestion. Although AV valve regurgitation (particularly tricuspid) is common in constriction,[110] postoperative regurgitation is a complication.[130]

Currently, most patients respond well. Some have an immediate postoperative diuresis, others a slower recovery over weeks or months. Removal of pericardium should be as extensive as possible (intraoperatively recorded pressure-volume loops clearly reveal the optimal extent[131]), especially the surfaces contacting the ventricles, always taking care to spare both phrenic nerves. A stubbornly adherent epicardial constriction may need to be scored or "meshed," leaving it in place but loosened. Poorer results are seen[131a] with inadequate resection, uncorrected coronary disease, higher New York Heart Association "heart failure" classifications, and older age; after radiation pericarditis; with chronicity, including peripheral organ failure (particularly renal and hepatic[129]; ascites, edema, or both are ominous);

with severe myocardial atrophy and fibrosis; and with significant arrhythmias reflecting myocardial impairment. Preventive therapy (often unsuccessful) depends on adequate treatment of acute pericarditis and drainage of significant collections of blood or pus. *Corticosteroids usually fail to prevent constriction.* Whether colchicine and NSAIDs have a preventive effect is unknown. In specific cases after drainage of bloody fluid, intrapericardial urokinase or streptokinase and, for purulent fluids, streptodornase, may check these substrates for constriction.

INFECTIOUS PERICARDITIS

Infectious agents that reach the pericardium inflame it directly or by various immune responses.[132] While any pericardial infection can be clinically silent, clinical pictures]conform to some degree to the descriptions below, with differences characteristic of particular causes. Acute viral pericarditis is likely to provoke the entire range of subjective and objective acute findings, whereas tuberculous pericarditis can do so but is often overshadowed by systemic disease or complications such as fever or tamponade.

Viral Pericarditis

Viral pericarditis has a wide etiological range, mainly the viruses causing myocarditis, the degree of involvement of either or both tissues depending on host susceptibility, and the particular agent; inflammatory abnormalities are due to immune complexes, direct viral attack, or both.[132–134] Early viral replication in pericardial tissue elicits cellular and humoral immune responses against the virus. If inadequate, there is direct tissue damage or a destructive autoimmune reaction. Viral genomic fragments in pericardial tissue may not replicate, yet they serve as a constant source of antigen to stimulate immune responses. Virus-specific IgM, often with IgG and occasionally IgA, can be found in pericardium and myocardium for years.[132] Most cardiotropic viruses involve the pericardium and myocardium hematogenously, although cardiac and thoracic surgery permit direct implantation. A latent period between a recognized viral infection and the onset of acute pericarditis is compatible with both infective and immunopathic induction of pericarditis.

CLINICAL FEATURES. Most cases of pericarditis of unknown origin, "idiopathic" or "nonspecific," are probably viral; these frequently produce the clinical epitome of acute pericarditis: pain, rub, more or less typical ECG changes, elevated acute-phase reactants (e.g., ESR; CRP), fever, leukocytosis, and variable myocardial enzyme levels. "Variable" ranges from normal to occasionally high levels, reflecting, as does the ECG, variable myocardial inflammation. As with most acute pericarditis, there is a 3:1 to 4:1 male preponderance. Pericarditis may occur during initial viral infection but more often 1 to 3 weeks after an upper respiratory or gastrointestinal syndrome, which is too late to culture the virus.[135] Many patients have pulmonary infiltrates and pleural effusions, often with cough. Any viral pericarditis may be effusive and develop tamponade, although most have little or no effusion.

Clinical illness lasts days to a few weeks, usually resolving within 2 weeks.[132] Complications include unresolved inflammation, particularly recurrent pericarditis due to immunopathy and characterized mainly by pain and often recurrent effusion. One to three recurrences affect up to 50 percent of patients, mainly within 8 months of the initial attack. Typically, recurrences are shorter and milder and usually without ECG changes. They may follow unrelated infection or physical (rarely mental) stress. Pleural effusions, particularly on the left, are common. Acute effusive viral pericarditis, particularly after tamponade, is associated with eventual classic constriction more often than is "dry" pericarditis. Occasionally, especially in children, with a significant element of myocarditis, heart muscle disease may proceed after the pericardial manifestations become clinically silent. Arrhythmias or conduction defects indicate independent heart disease or significant myocarditis (see Chap. 25). Differential diagnoses include acute myocardial infarction, particularly with atypical ECGs. Other conditions include traumatic pericarditis, SLE, and nonviral, especially bacterial, pericarditis. Systemic viral disorders (e.g., hepatitis) should suggest a viral etiology. Infectious mononucleosis usually presents as a severe sore throat, adenopathy, and positive serology; a fourfold increase in neutralizing antibody titer is only supporting evidence.

Newer techniques can identify minute amounts of viral nucleic acid; viral genomes can be demonstrated by the polymerase chain reaction (PCR), which amplifies viral DNA along with in situ hybridization.[133]

Reverse immunoassay (RIA) can demonstrate virus-specific immunoglobulins like IgM, IgG, and IgA. It may not be necessary to use these when the diagnosis seems secure in an otherwise healthy patient, especially since, without tamponade, pericardiocentesis and other invasive procedures add little to management and carry risks.[132]

MANAGEMENT. Effective antiviral agents are not available or even necessary to manage most viral pericarditis. Treatment is for symptoms and complications. Pain, usually pleuritic and limited to the first day or week, is managed by NSAIDs, notably ibuprofen, at doses sufficient to suppress symptoms and fever. Cough can exacerbate pericardial pain and requires antitussive agents. Nontamponading pericardial effusions do not require drainage unless very large. Tamponade requires prompt evacuation of fluid. Usually acute management succeeds. However, virus-specific immunoglobulins are found in many cases of chronic relapsing pericarditis and dilated cardiomyopathy.

Nontuberculous Bacterial (Suppurative) Pericarditis

Acute suppurative pericarditis *(pyopericardium)* simultaneously threatens tamponade and septicemia and is especially serious in children and immunocompromised patients when due to destructive organisms such as staphylococci. Yet, some may be silent, presenting as tamponade or overshadowed by systemic disease and discovered at autopsy. Although many gram-negative organisms such as *Escherichia coli, Salmonella,* other nosocomially acquired infections, and opportunistic organisms have appeared increasingly, the common forms remain streptococcal, pneumococcal, and staphylococcal.[132] Rarely, gas-producing organisms such as *Clostridium* cause pneumopericardium. In adults, pneumopericardium and bacterial pneumopyopericardium are often due to a fistula between the epicardium and a hollow viscus. Invasion from contiguous foci or traumatic implantation include cardiothoracic surgery, mediastinitis, wound infection, myocardial abscess, infective endocarditis, and subdiaphragmatic abscess. Rarely, pericardial invasion spreads along fascial planes from the oral cavity, particularly periodontal and peritonsillar abscesses. Occasionally, infected mediastinal nodes erode the pericardium. Preexisting nonbacterial pericardial effusion as in rheumatoid arthritis, SLE, sarcoid, or uremia can be infected hematogenously.[132] This is probably the pathogenesis of "primary" bacterial pericarditis in which only the pericardium seems to be affected. For example, *Neisseria,* particularly *N. meningitidis* group C, can occur without meningitis, producing "primary" meningococcal pericarditis. Moreover, the *Neisseria* group and other organisms can evoke a sterile, immunopathic effusion, sometimes accompanied by immunopathic or infectious systemic reactions such as arthritis and ophthalmitis.[136] Similarly, *Salmonella* pericarditis, usually due to bacteremia, can occur with or without an enteritic syndrome.

Antimicrobial therapy has decreased the incidence of the common gram-positive infections. Yet there is relative and absolute increase, usually nosocomially acquired, of infections with multiple and gram-negative organisms, especially in immunocompromised patients and after thoracotomy.[132, 133] *Haemophilus influenzae* occurs sporadically in adults, but children are particularly susceptible to it; pericarditis occurs during respiratory illness and even after cellulitis. *H. influenzae* typically provokes a thick, fibrinopurulent exudate similar to cottage cheese or scrambled eggs that can defeat attempts at percutaneous drainage.

CLINICAL FEATURES.[132] Suppurative pericarditis is most often acute and fulminant, arising over several days with rapid development of tamponade or presenting as tamponade. Effusion is the rule; the fluid is a turbid exudate characterized by polymorphonuclear leukocytes, increased LDH, and decreased glucose. There is typically tachycardia, fever, toxicity, chills, and sweating. Chest pain is variable, and a pericardial rub is audible in most patients. Cough is common, especially with pleuropulmonary involvement. In some older patients, infections have a reduced tempo, are often clinically silent, or are overshadowed by systemic disease. Chest radiographs usually show an enlarged cardiopericardial silhouette. With gas-producing organisms there are lucent "bubbles" or an "air"-fluid interface. Leukocytosis with a marked left shift is typical (although limited to absent in debilitated and immunosuppressed patients). Blood and pericardial fluid cultures should disclose organisms. The ECG frequently shows stage I changes, although it may be nonspecifically abnormal if the lesion is discovered late. Imaging will disclose any effusion. Inflammatory infiltration of the pericardium can be identified by scintigraphy with indium-111 or gallium-67 (also responsive to leukemic infiltrations).[137] There may be a tendency to loculation producing pericardial abscesses that may resemble cysts. (Congenital cysts may become infected.) Etiology-specific diagnosis depends on smears, cultures, and more sophisticated searches—e.g., antigen detection, especially when treatment appears to sterilize the fluid. The principal differential diagnoses include tuberculous and viral pericarditis.

PERICARDITIS WITH INFECTIVE ENDOCARDITIS.[132] Pericarditis during endocarditis can be dramatic but is more often found at autopsy. Acute endocarditis may provoke an immunopathic pericardial effusion with immune complex deposition, whereas subacute endocarditis usually causes an infective effusion. Bacterial endocarditis involves the pericardium most often by erosion of a valve-ring abscess or by rupture of an aortic sinus or myocardial abscess. The most common organisms are *Streptococcus viridans* and *Staphylococcus aureus.* Bacteremia can infect both endocardium and pericardium simultaneously. Sterile "sympathetic" (parapericarditic) effusions are not rare,[138] presumably immunopathic. Hemorrhagic effusions follow direct pericardial irritation or bleeding from rupture of a mycotic abscess. Clues to accompanying myocardial and valve-ring invasion include degrees of AV and bundle branch block, each most common with staphylococcal endocarditis.

MANAGEMENT. Systemically administered antibiotics achieve excellent levels in pericardial fluid.[132] Pericardial drainage and exploration, monitored by TEE,[139] are desirable because infections tend to loculate, form adhesions, and constrict. In critical tamponade, simple drainage may first be used for relief, with exploration postponed. Pericardial fluid and tissue should be obtained for gram, acid-fast, and fungal stains, with cultures for aerobes and anaerobes and antimicrobial susceptibility tests.[52] Surgical drainage is preferable over percutaneous drainage, particularly when etiology is uncertain; it permits pericardiectomy when adhesions and loculations predict constriction. With or without definite surgical intervention, urokinase or streptokinase may be used within the pericardium to destroy clots and fibrinous adhesions.[140] Very thick purulent and sanguinopurulent exudates resisting free drainage may require repeated intrapericardial urokinase or streptokinase (to activate the fibrinolytic system) combined with streptodornase (to liquefy viscous nucleoproteins in pus). A clue to loculation and potential constriction is failure to improve after appropriate treatment.[132]

Tuberculous Pericarditis

Pericarditis due to *Mycobacterium tuberculosis* has decreased due to improved public health and effective antimycobacterial treatments. Recently, atypical mycobacteria along with classic tubercle bacilli are increasing in immunocompromised patients, particularly in AIDS due to HIV,[141] lymphocytotrophic, and other viruses. High incidence continues in poorer nations. In the United States its principal importance is differential diagnosis from other syndromes.

PATHOGENESIS.[129] The pericardium may be infected by hematogenous, lymphatic, peribronchial, or contiguous spread of tuberculosis. (Hematogenous dissemination occurs during all primary tuberculosis.) Lymphatic spread is from lung, bronchi, and mediastinal nodes. Contiguous infection involves intrapericardial inoculation from mediastinal nodal, pleural, and, rarely, myocardial tuberculosis.[141a] Some of the material penetrating the pericardium undergoes proteolytic degradation and antigen processing of individual peptides, with immune responses causing much of the morbidity. These include antimyolemmal antibodies,[133] which are very common in tuberculous pericarditis and probably pathogenic. Protein antigens of the bacillus induce delayed hypersensitivity responses stimulating lymphocytes to release lymphokines that activate macrophages and influence granuloma formation. There are four classic pathological stages of tuberculous pericarditis[129]: (1) fibrinous exudation with initial polymorphonuclear leukocytosis, relatively abundant mycobacteria, and beginning granuloma with loose organizations of T cells and macrophages; (2) serous, usually serosanguineous effusions with a mainly lymphocytic exudate with monocytes and foam cells; (3) absorption of effusion with organization of granulomas caseation, and pericardial thickening due to fibrin, collagenosis, and ultimately, fibrosis (mycobacteria become difficult to find); and (4) constrictive scarring: replacement of fibrinous and granulomatous matter by fibrosis, which contracts on the cardiac chambers (constriction can develop despite effective antituberculous therapy). Calcification can occur at any stage, tending to form sheets, plaques, hoops, and bands of calcium salts over any part of the heart. Tuberculous pericarditis may surface as an acute or chronic pericardial effusion and occasionally a variant of cholesterol pericarditis with or without overt tamponade and usually with considerable fibrin, adhesions, and loculations demonstrable by imaging. That noneffusive or minimally effusive acute tuberculous pericarditis often heals without treatment is suggested by the appearance of constriction without a recognizable acute state.

CLINICAL FEATURES.[132] Clinical expression of tuberculous pericarditis depends on the tempo of inflammation, which is typically slow and indolent after an insidious onset and often accidental discovery (especially with large effusions).[142] Occasionally, there is an aggressive course with acute tamponade, often mixed with constrictive components. Children and immunocompromised patients more often present with classic acute pericarditis. Yet most patients have no history of an acute phase and often no history of tuberculosis; evidence of pulmonary tuberculosis is exceptional. However, like tuberculous meningitis, tuberculous pericarditis may erupt during appropriate antimicrobial treatment for tuberculosis elsewhere. When the disease is clinically apparent, patients tend to have lymphocytosis in blood and pericardial fluid with increased proportions of small and l lymphocytes. Tuberculosis may also involve the myocardium, usually without distinctive symptoms unless it is extensive. Eight modes of presentation cover almost any "pericardial" syndrome[132]:

1. Painful acute pericarditis with or without minimal to large effusions and with or without fever, cough, and malaise
2. Silent effusion, often large and chronic
3. Tamponade, usually without other signs except fever
4. Acute constrictive pericarditis (i.e., constriction appearing over

a period of days to a month), usually after drainage of an effusion or disappearance of fluid under therapy
5. Subacute constriction (a course of weeks or months) with varying amounts of fluid (i.e., effusive-constrictive pericarditis)
6. Chronic constrictive pericarditis
7. Pericardial calcifications with or without hemodynamic consequences
8. Fever of unknown origin, usually with constitutional symptoms such as anorexia and weight loss

Tuberculous effusions typically increase slowly with few or no symptoms, leading to tamponade or, after reabsorption or drainage, effusive-constrictive or constrictive pericarditis. Yet tuberculous pericarditis may become recognizable at any stage, more often with tamponade,[143] constriction, or combinations of the two or their complications, as when clinically silent constriction causes hepatic congestion and ascites, simulating cirrhosis ("Pick disease"). Those presenting with constriction may have few constitutional signs and symptoms if the inflammatory process has burned out. Moreover, tuberculous etiology may not be clear because so many forms of pericarditis cause constriction. Few patients have rubs and precordial pain; more often there is nondescript precordial discomfort. Dyspnea, particularly on exertion, may follow cardiac compression or pulmonary restriction due to a very large pericardial effusion with pleural effusion. When presenting as fever of unknown origin, the diagnosis is suggested by an enlarged cardiopericardial silhouette, especially if imaging discloses a more or less chronic pericardial effusion. Finally, tuberculous pericarditis must be ruled in or out when any pericarditis does not rapidly resolve on NSAIDs treatment and in tamponade of obscure origin, particularly in immigrants from Third World countries, elderly patients, and immunocompromised patients, in whom pericardial tuberculosis may be the first manifestation[144] (clinically primary tuberculous pericarditis).

DIAGNOSIS. Identification of *M. tuberculosis* in pericardial fluid or tissue is specific, but negative results do not rule out tuberculous pericarditis.[132, 145] Organisms may be so difficult to find that all fluid drained should be centrifuged and studied by smear, culture, and, if necessary, DNA amplification. Extrapericardial tuberculosis, including lung, pleura, and lymph nodes, indirectly supports the diagnosis, but pericardial tissue should be sampled by subxiphoid incision or pericardioscopy.[52, 132] Yet negative biopsy does not rule out tuberculosis. A positive tuberculin (purified protein derivative [PPD]) skin test can support but not confirm pericardial tuberculosis because it may reflect antecedent extrapericardial tuberculosis, as may positive sputum and gastric aspiration. Negative skin tests imply low risk of tuberculosis but are unhelpful with loss of reactivity in patients with anergy, especially those with severe systemic disease or HIV infection. Early, transiently negative, skin tests may be due to pericardial and pleural sequestration of PPD-reactive T lymphocytes. A "therapeutic test" may be a last diagnostic resort using appropriate antimycobacterial agents for critically ill patients with persistent constitutional signs. Uptake of radionuclides such as gallium-67 and indium-111 indicate pericardial inflammation but are nonspecific because uptake also occurs in purulent and viral pericarditis, leukemic infiltration, and even mesothelioma. High levels (>40 IU/liter) of adenosine deaminase (ADA) activity in pericardial fluid are quasi-specific for tuberculous pericarditis (very high ADA levels appear to predict eventual constriction).[146] Differentiation of neoplastic effusions is virtually absolute, with low levels of ADA accompanying high levels of carcinoembryonic antigen.[132] Complement-fixing antimyolemmal and antimyosin antibodies have been found in most patients with acute tuberculous pericarditis but decrease in late stages and constriction.[52, 133] Mycobacterial antigens have been increasingly detected by enzyme-linked immunosorbent assay (ELISA) with high specificity and sensitivity. Probably optimal is the PCR, which amplifies mycobacterial DNA to "fingerprint" strains of *M. tuberculosis* in pericardial fluid with excellent specificity.[147, 148] It is particularly useful in patients with AIDS/HIV infection who have adenopathy and often atypical mycobacterial infection, especially *M. avium* complex. Moreover, because of 100 percent sensitivity for activity, a negative result excludes *active* tuberculosis. Specificity, virtually 70 percent for active tuberculosis, approaches 90 percent for any tuberculosis infection. False-positive results occur, and blood in pericardial fluid may lead to false-negative results by enzyme inhibition; yet the PCR is superior to bacteriological methods.[147, 148] Cultures should be obtained because of the need for drug susceptibility testing.[132]

MANAGEMENT. Antimycobacterial treatment has greatly decreased mortality in tuberculous pericarditis, although frequently not preventing constriction.[148a] All isolates of *M. tuberculosis* should be tested for antimicrobial susceptibility. Effective multiple drug therapy is mandatory, and severely ill patients benefit from prednisone or other corticosteroid, which will shorten the course, dramatically decrease symptoms and signs in the acute phase, and reduce the death rate.[132, 149] However, corticosteroids reduce constrictive evolution only modestly if at all.[149] Some atypical mycobacteria resist chemotherapy, requiring efforts to find appropriate combinations. Tamponade should be relieved under chemotherapeutic "cover" to prevent extrapericardial spread. Persistent hypotension warrants adrenal function testing because of possible adrenal tuberculosis. Tendencies to nonresolution or worsening (over 6 to 8 weeks), significant pericardial thickening, or signs of constriction mandate pericardiectomy as soon as possible. Indeed, patients with tuberculous pericarditis must be observed indefinitely to detect reactivation, constriction, or reconstriction.[132]

Fungal Pericarditis

In the United States, fungal pericarditis is mainly due to two "geographical" fungi, *Histoplasma* and *Coccidioides*, and to "nongeographical" fungi, *Candida* and *Aspergillus* (*Blastomyces* and *Cryptococcus* are comparatively rare, as is *Pneumocystis carinii*).[132, 150-153] To these are added two "semifungi" (between bacteria and fungi), *Actinomyces* and *Nocardia*. Geographical fungi are locally endemic, whereas nongeographical fungi are largely opportunistic, depending on compromised host defense. All fungi occur preferentially in immunocompromised[153] and severely burned patients, debilitated individuals, infants (especially premature), and those taking corticosteroids that impair antifungal defenses and phagocyte activity. Indeed, apparent cardiac decompensation during fungal infections may be due to tamponade, constriction, or fungal myocarditis.[132] Precise diagnosis is crucial, particularly for the nongeographical fungi, because amphotericin B, a principal antifungal agent, is very toxic. Pericardiectomy is usually crucial for survival.

HISTOPLASMOSIS. This is the most common "naturally" acquired fungal infection. It is frequent in endemic areas of the Ohio and Mississippi River valleys and western Appalachia. Pericarditis usually occurs late after infection elsewhere. Acute fibrinous pericarditis is usually a noninfectious (irritative or immunopathic) complication of infection in adjacent mediastinal lymph nodes that can penetrate the pericardium, causing granulomatous inflammation and occasionally calcification. Pleural effusions are more common with pericarditis than with pulmonary histoplasmosis. *Histoplasma* pericarditis is relatively common in younger, usually immunocompetent patients, whereas disseminated histoplasmosis, like other fungal infections, is more common with immunosuppression. Pericardial involvement can resemble idiopathic pericarditis, resolving within 2 weeks. However, almost half of *Histoplasma*-induced effusions develop hemodynamic compromise. In contrast to other fungal pericarditides, effusion with or without tamponade can be rapid and massive. The fluid is serous, xanthochromic, or hemorrhagic and predominately leukocytic. Pleuropulmonary involvement produces mixed clinical manifestations: it precedes respiratory illness, pleuritic pain, cough, and dyspnea, resembling viral or tuberculous pericarditis.[151] Only occasionally do patients develop constriction or pericardial calcification (rarely, constriction is the presenting feature). If acute pericarditis resolves, relapses occur variably. The diagnosis must be considered in endemic zones. Rising complement fixation titers and the immunodiffusion test are helpful. Moreover, other causes of pericarditis must also be considered in endemic areas even in seropositive patients.[132] With persistent illness, biopsy of lymph nodes, particularly mediastinal nodes, with cultures and methonium silver stains, may be decisive. *Histoplasma* should be identified, because granulomas alone are nonspecific; indeed, tuberculosis may be associated. The principal differential diagnoses are pericarditis due to viruses, tuberculosis, brucellosis, Hodgkin disease, or sarcoid.

Resolution spontaneously or with antiinflammatory agents without antifungal medication indicates almost certainly "immunopathic" or "irritative" pericardial involvement without infection, even if with tamponade. Unless *clearly* recovering, are in no distress, and have a "dry" pericardium on imaging, patients should be hospitalized because of the (infrequent) possibility of tamponade. Antifungal treatment with amphotericin B or ketoconazole is indicated for disseminated histoplasmosis or severe pericardial inflammation.[132] To reduce chest pain, fever, and effusion and suppress the pericardial rub, NSAIDs usually suffice. Tamponade and constriction require decompression. Corticosteroids predispose to dissemination but may be used for severely ill patients. With disseminated histoplasmosis, adrenal function should be assessed because the adrenals may be involved, requiring corticosteroid treatment.

COCCIDIOIDOMYCOSIS. This fungal infection is endemic in the southwest, particularly in the San Joaquin Valley. Spores are inhaled from soil. Pericardial coccidioidomycosis is usually a complication of progressive disseminated infection, although it is rarely "primary" (i.e., confined to the pericardium).[132] Hilar node involvement resembles tuberculosis. Infection causes serofibrinous effusion with a potential for adhesion. The clinical spectrum is wide: from classic acute to chronic adhesive pericarditis and rarely to effusive-constrictive pericarditis. Acute pericardial coccidioidomycosis usually accompanies pneumonia from the same organisms, sometimes with systemic ade-

nopathy, osteomyelitis, or meningitis. The main symptoms may be pneumonitic: cough, dyspnea, fever, and pleuritic pain. Patients are usually chronically ill, debilitated, malnourished, and often immunocompromised. Diagnosis requires histological documentation but is suggested by pericarditis in the endemic zone, especially if with disseminated coccidioidomycosis. Pericarditis may resolve without specific therapy, but anticoccidioidal agents such as fluconazole may be necessary, depending on severity and progress.

"NONGEOGRAPHICAL" FUNGAL INFECTIONS.[132, 150, 152, 153] These related organisms produce similar clinical pictures. Actinomycosis may cause fistulas and sinus tracts to skin and other organs as well as contiguous spread along thoracic and mediastinal tissue planes. Pericarditis tends to be insidious until tamponade or constriction, but acute pericarditis may be followed by chronic effusion with pericardial thickening and adhesions.[154] Acute tamponade may respond to medical and surgical management, only to be followed by rapid constriction. These "semifungi" also cause endocarditis and myocarditis. Although suggested by infection elsewhere, specific diagnosis is by staining and culturing pericardial fluid. Infection is fatal unless treated medically and surgically. *Actinomyces* responds to penicillin and other antibiotics. *Nocardia* responds to sulfonamides, particularly sulfisoxazole. Optimal therapy is combined antimicrobials, surgical drainage, and pericardiectomy as indicated.

PERICARDIAL DISEASE IN AIDS AND AIDS-RELATED COMPLEX (see also Chap. 68).[132, 155, 156] Immunocompromised patients with AIDS and AIDS-related complex respond as do other kinds of immunosuppressed patients, such as those receiving corticosteroids and cytotoxic agents, and include mainly patients on cancer chemotherapy or with serious inflammatory disorders or after organ transplants. AIDS predisposes to infection by multiple organisms, many opportunistic, and to malignancies such as Kaposi sarcoma and non-Hodgkin malignant lymphoma. Complications of AIDS and HIV infection affect the endocardium, myocardium, and pericardium; patients with cardiac involvement have lower T4 cell counts. Pericardial disease, particularly effusion, is relatively frequent but more often discovered by imaging or at autopsy. The most frequent cardiac lesion at autopsy is sterile pericardial effusion.[132] In general, late AIDS-related pericardial effusions imply a grave prognosis, suggesting end-stage HIV disease. Patients with pericarditis often also have myocarditis.

Pericardial involvement in AIDS occurs in six forms[132]:

1. *Silent.* Fibrinous and effusive pericarditis with or without adhesions or apparently sterile pericardial effusion occur as part of a generalized serious effusive process, including ascites and pleural effusion ("capillary leak syndrome"). The specific etiology is often uncertain.
2. *Classic acute pericarditis.* Typically there is pain, rub, and often ECG changes. If effusive, the fluid may be clear, purulent or sanguineous. A search for an infectious etiology is often rewarded. Mycobacteria, fungi, and other opportunistic organisms are frequent.
3. *Cardiac tamponade.* This usually is recurrent with chronicity but it may be the presenting syndrome.
4. *Constrictive pericarditis.*
5. *Neoplasia.* This mainly includes Kaposi sarcoma and aggressive Hodgkin or non-Hodgkin lymphoma.
6. *Myopericarditis.* With definite inflammatory signs there tends to be lymphocytic pericardial infiltration. Sterile hydropericardium may be due to uremia or congestive failure from associated myocarditis or cardiomyopathy. Pericardial effusions of any size are associated with shortened survival.[132] Large effusions may be tuberculous or fungal. Nontuberculous *Mycobacterium* infection occurs late.

At least two forms of *malignancy* are related to AIDS: Kaposi sarcoma and non-Hodgkin malignant lymphoma[157]; Hodgkin and other lymphomas also occur. Kaposi sarcoma involves both visceral and parietal pericardium, with particular predilection for epicardium and subepicardial fat; it produces effusion and occasionally constriction. Although usually disseminated, in AIDS it may appear to be primary in the pericardium with a strong tendency for tamponade.[129] *Malignant lymphoma* is usually multicentric and only rarely primary in the heart, where it typically affects the myocardium more often than the pericardium. Occasionally, an Epstein-Barr viral genome may be discovered.

PARASITIC PERICARDITIS

Pericardial parasitoses appear in endemic areas and in travelers from them in whom mild attacks are often mistaken for idiopathic pericarditis.[132, 158-160] The acute illness typically resembles suppurative bacterial, or occasionally viral, pericarditis. Parasites frequent in the liver such as *Echinococcus* and amebae may also provoke sterile, presumably immunogenic, ("sympathetic") pericardial effusions, which may cause tamponade.[132] Such parasites usually enter the pericardium from perforation through the diaphragm or from secondary lesions in the lung and pleura. Parasitosis elsewhere suggests the diagnosis. In some patients, fluid may be negative for organisms, requiring biopsy. Blood or pericardial fluid *eosinophilia* always suggests parasitic disease.

TOXOPLASMOSIS.[132] Toxoplasmosis (caused by *Toxoplasma gondii*) may be congenital or acquired. Pericarditis is often found at autopsy in patients with more obvious *Toxoplasma* myocarditis. Pericardial affection is mainly chronic, with often a chronic effusion and rarely constriction. Acute pericarditis with or without tamponade is rare and includes fever, rash, and adenopathy; it can resemble SLE. Pericardial involvement may occur during miliary spread, particularly in patients with leukemia and other disorders treated with chemotherapeutic agents or corticosteroids.

ECHINOCOCCOSIS.[159, 160] *Echinococcus granulosus*, an invasive and destructive sporozoan, occurs mainly in sheep-raising countries. It produces hydrated cysts of the myocardium, pericardium, and mediastinum, including great vessels. The pericardium is involved from a ruptured adjacent myocardial cyst or a hepatic cyst penetrating the diaphragm. Chest pain and sharp anaphylactic reactions with eosinophilia are characteristic. Multiple intrapericardial rupture can produce vague to striking symptoms. Pericardial and mediastinal echinococcal cysts also compress the cardiac chambers or great vessels, producing corresponding abnormalities on imaging, which shows well-defined unilocular (occasionally multilocular) cysts with trabeculations due to internal "daughter membranes." Complications include secondary bacterial infection, tamponade, and constriction and even coronary obstruction. Surgical excision (enucleation) may be dangerous due to spillage of active parasites. Evacuation of the cysts and instillation of silver nitrate is usually preferable.

AMEBIASIS.[132] Amebiasis (caused by *Entamoeba histolytica*) occurs mainly in endemic areas and in travelers from them (in whom the syndrome may appear years later). Although patients may also have intestinal amebiasis, liver abscesses, particularly in the left lobe, typically perforate the diaphragm and involve the pericardium. Mortality is high, especially with missed diagnoses. Serofibrinous ("presuppurative") pericarditis with straw-colored or sanguineous fluid can precede gross rupture into the pericardium and is often suspected to be tuberculous. Frank pericardial rupture can be insidious or dramatic with pain, shock, tamponade, and cyanosis. Fluid is brownish; the pus may simulate anchovy paste, an appearance that is quasi-diagnostic. Secondary bacterial infection must be considered in severely ill patients. Occasionally, there is classic acute pericarditis or subacute effusive-constrictive pericarditis with pericardial thickening. Diagnosis is by fluorescent antibody test or amebic enzyme immunoassay supported by a liver scan with technetium-99m.[132] Medical therapy with antiamebic agents such as metronidazole or dehydroemetine is highly successful in hepatic cases, but pericardial involvement requires drainage and, if necessary, resection.

NEMATODAL PERICARDITIS

Filariasis (caused by *Wuchereria bancrofti*), endemic in Africa and India, produces hemorrhagic effusions in which microfilaria are easily found in nocturnal blood smears.[129] Effusions may be clinically silent or massive with rapid or slow tamponade. Cough and constitutional symptoms are common. Persistent pericardial inflammation produces sanguinopurulent pericarditis with chronic lymphocyte inflammatory changes. Survival may produce rapid constriction, even during chemotherapy. Diagnostic clues include other manifestations of filariasis, such as elephantiasis. *Necator americanus* produces eosinophilic pericardial effusion, possibly an "allergic" effect. *Dracunculus* ("guinea worm") has been found in constrictive pericardial scar.

SPIROCHETAL PERICARDITIS

Except for spirochetes transmitted during Lyme carditis[161] and leptospirosis, spirochetal pericarditis is poorly characterized, owing to extreme rarity of discovery in tissue where its presence may be accidental. *Treponema pallidum* is identified only in the rare involvement of the pericardium by localized or miliary syphilitic gummas with a fibrotic reaction or accompanying a hemorrhagic effusion.[132] *Lyme pericarditis* can produce acute pericarditis, pericardial effusion, and myopericarditis. Fatal myopericarditis may ensue with myocardial and conducting tissue involvements. Silver stains of sampled material may demonstrate the spirochetes. However, ELISA can detect IgM and IgG antibodies. Indium-111 antimyosin scintigraphy may be helpful.[162] Leptospirosis[132] (caused by *Leptospira icterohaemorrhagiae*) is mainly a tropical disease and is reported at all ages. Most cases are subclinical. Conjunctival suffusion is a clue. Myocardial and pericardial involvement, often mild, is seen more frequently in patients who are anicteric. Typical acute pericarditis including friction rub and ECG changes may be due either to the organism itself or to an accompanying uremia. Diagnosis is by *Leptospira* agglutination test.

RICKETTSIAL PERICARDITIS

Rickettsiae, particularly *Rickettsia rickettsii*, can produce pericarditis,[132, 163, 164] myocarditis, and vasculitis in endemic areas, including South America, Africa, and the South Central and Atlantic States (Rocky Mountain spotted fever [RMSF]). In Africa tic-transmitted *boutonneuse fever* is due to *Rickettsia conorii*. Q fever, due to *Coxiella burnetii*, is transmitted by sheep and cattle in milk and is found worldwide. It appears to produce more obvious clinical pericarditis than does RMSF and may present as a pericardial effusion. In RMSF, myocarditis and pericarditis can occur with or without vasculitis, the latter being a "toxic" or immunogenic process. Cross-reactive antimy-

olemmal antibodies suggest that apericardial involvement can be immunopathic with pericarditis after extension of myocarditis to the epicardium. Diagnosis is by serological test, including Weil-Felix agglutinins and IgM and IgG antibodies.

CHLAMYDIAL PERICARDITIS

Chlamydiae produce classic acute pericarditis and large effusions.[132] Rare until recently, the Chlamydiaceae, especially *C. trachomatis, C. psittaci*, and *C. pneumoniae*, are increasingly found in immunocompromised patients and patients with malignancies, as well as otherwise healthy hosts. They produce pericarditis, myocarditis, pleuritis, and pneumonitis. Psittacosis follows exposure to psittacine and other birds. (Indeed, pericardial effusion is one of the most common forms in affected birds themselves.) Specific diagnosis is by IgG antibody titers.

PERICARDIAL DISEASE IN METABOLIC DISORDERS

Renal Failure (See Fig. 72–6)

Most *uremic pericarditis* is due to chronic renal failure, which produces all morphological forms of acute pericarditis, effusive and noneffusive, and is usually hemorrhagic, with and without tamponade.[165, 166] *Dialysis pericarditis* accompanies prolonged survival due to effective dialysis, and with it uremic constrictive and effusive constrictive pericarditis have appeared. In acute renal failure, acute uremic pericarditis is usually of less serious significance. Although nitrogen retention is necessary for uremic pericarditis, many patients escape pericarditis so that the pathogenesis is uncertain; "toxic metabolites" are often invoked. Pericardial involvement is unrelated to the etiology of renal failure. Although blood urea nitrogen levels are customarily over 60 mg/dl, there is no strict numerical relationship; and echocardiography reveals excess pericardial fluid in many asymptomatic patients. The incidence of acute pericardial disease in chronic renal failure has plummeted, owing to effective dialysis, hemoperfusion, and renal transplantation (although pericarditis follows transplant in 2 to 3 percent of patients[167]). Small pericardial effusions and noninflammatory hydropericardium due to volume overload and congestive failure (see Chap. 17) are common and usually insignificant.

Cardiac tamponade is the main danger, often precipitated by critically increased bleeding. It may appear as an unexplained fall in blood pressure to a level that varies widely between high, but lower than previously, and shock level. A change in mental status may be the first clue. Fever is variable in the absence of infection and more common in dialysis pericarditis than uremic pericarditis. Chest pain varies from severe to absent. Uremic pericardial rubs tend to be loud, are often palpable, and frequently persist after biochemical abnormalities improve. In uremic pericarditis due to acute and chronic glomerulonephritis and in dialysis pericarditis (especially when precipitated by viral infections), complement-fixing antimyocardial antibodies appear, including antimyolemmal autoantibodies that may be pathogenetic as well as diagnostic.

Uremic pericarditis resembles the spectrum of viral pericarditis and its acute complications, including the characteristics noted earlier. Despite comparable degrees of renal failure, only some, usually younger, patients develop uremic pericarditis, acute myocardial infarction, or hyperparathyroidism.[166, 167] A constant exacerbating factor is the uremic hemorrhagic diathesis from hematological impairments that promote bleeding and abundantly vascular granulation tissue due to uremic inflammation. Pericardial effusions usually predict tamponade in proportion to their size. Uremic exudates contain considerable fibrin and inflammatory cells. All are serosanguineous and, with tamponade, hemorrhagic.[168] Despite destruction of the pericardial mesothelium and gross hemorrhage, pure, that is uninfected, uremic pericarditis is unique: inflammatory cells do not penetrate the myocardium, accounting for the customary absence of typical ECG changes. Indeed, if the ECG is typical of acute pericarditis, intercurrent infection must be suspected. Most often, ECGs are grossly unchanged and reflect associated abnormalities such as LV hypertrophy and "strain," coronary disease, and electrolyte abnormalities. Fluid retention and pleural effusion may reduce ECG voltages with or without pericardial effusion.

DIFFERENTIAL DIAGNOSIS. This may be difficult, especially in mentally confused patients and because nonuremic intercurrent pericarditis of any cause is always possible. For example, when hypertension is not being controlled, dissecting hematoma of the aorta (see Chap. 40) must be considered. Indeed, uremic tamponade may simulate any cardiocirculatory emergency, especially with marked hypotension (often despite fluid overload).[165–168] Conversely, tamponade may be disguised by a relatively or absolutely high pressure level (high pressure tamponade). Confusion of tamponade with florid heart failure may arise from LV hypertrophy, which is frequent in uremics, and myocardial failure, each of which can prevent pulsus paradoxus. Unexplained worsening renal function may be a clue to tamponade. Sepsis of nonrenal origin may coexist and precipitate tamponade; blood cultures may be positive for organisms and pericardial fluid negative. Hepatic congestion due to tamponade may be confused with viral hepatitis. Finally, in uremic patients, frequent autonomic impairment occurs, even during tamponade, so that the *heart rate may be deceptively slow* (60–80 beats/min) despite fever and hypotension.

TREATMENT. This consists of drainage, which should be gradual because of possible "pericardial shock" in patients who may have underlying congestive failure or intercurrent myocarditis that predisposes to postdrainage cardiac dilation. A neurogenic element may also contribute to postdrainage collapse because patients are vagotonic; therefore, during pericardial drainage, patients may need to receive atropine.[166, 169] Intrapericardial hydrocortisone, triamcinolone, or equivalent agents may accelerate improvement by suppressing inflammation. For uremia itself, effective dialysis is mandatory, with careful monitoring of intravascular volume, since with excess pericardial fluid rapid vascular volume reduction can precipitate tamponade.

ACUTE RENAL FAILURE. Patients with hypotension due to shock, sepsis, trauma, or surgery may develop acute renal failure that can be self-limited; but with the blood urea nitrogen of 100 mg/dl or more, uremic pericarditis may appear. This responds to effective treatment of the etiological condition, circulatory support, and acute dialysis. Pericardial involvement is identified by a rub, effusion, or tamponade.

DIALYSIS PERICARDITIS. Adequate dialysis effectively ends uremic pericarditis within a few months. While classic uremic pericarditis is reversed by dialysis, *dialysis pericarditis*, by definition, appears despite otherwise successful dialysis, even in stable patients with good biochemical control.[166] Its pathogenesis is unknown, although it is much less common during peritoneal dialysis than hemodialysis. Immune complex-like material is found in the dialysate, and this "loss" may retard pericarditis.[168, 169] A pathogenetic role for "middle molecules" has been proposed. Several factors are associated with precipitating dialysis pericarditis and effusion, above all inadequate dialysis. Infection, particularly viral, is frequent, with hepatitis and cytomegaloviruses common in dialysis units. Such infections are often systemic, and the pericardial fluid is sterile. Constitutional symptoms, especially fever, are more severe and more common than in uremic pericarditis, and dialysis pericarditis may be preceded by weight gain and hypotension.[166] Effusion with or without hemorrhage is the most important complication and tends to recur. As in classic uremic pericarditis, larger effusions predict tamponade. Survival due to dialysis has allowed uremic constriction to appear.[166]

Treatment is designed to intensify dialysis while avoiding hypotension. Tamponade calls for drainage with maintenance of an intrapericardial catheter for at least 2 or 3 days. While there are no controlled trials, intrapericardial nonabsorbable corticosteroid-like triamcinolone appears to be effective. A trial of peritoneal dialysis for patients who have been on hemodialysis may be therapeutic. For intractable pericardial effusions, pericardial resection is the only effective approach.[166–168]

OTHER RENAL CONDITIONS. Although transplantation is usually successful for renal failure, severe transplant rejection is accompanied by acute pericarditis.[167] Patients with a nephrotic syndrome frequently have pericardial effusions associated with fluid retention (hydropericardium) or actual inflammation. Pericarditis in hepatorenal failure occurs at relatively low blood urea nitrogen levels, does not respond to dialysis, and is almost uniformly fatal.[166]

Hypothyroidism (See also Chap. 64)

Severe hypothyroidism produces large usually clear, high-protein, high-cholesterol, high-specific-gravity pericardial effusions.[165, 166, 170] These are constant in experimental and human myxedema and may precede other signs (especially in primary hypothyroidism). Echocardiography reveals them in 5 to 30 percent. Children with Down syndrome are at special risk for congenital or acquired hypothyroidism, which is often unrecognized because excessive weight, hypotension, and dry skin are classic in Down syndrome and hypothyroidism.[171] With tamponade, dyspnea, fatigue, cardiomegaly, and cyanosis may be attributed to their congenital heart disease.

Many effusions in hypothyroid patients are very large, chronic, asymptomatic, and discovered accidentally by chest radiography.[166] Clinical tamponade[171] is rare because the slow tempo permits pericardial stretch. Three factors may precipitate tamponade: (1) intercurrent acute pericarditis; (2) hemorrhage; and (3) rarely, cholesterol pericarditis with an inflammatory reaction to precipitated cholesterol crystals. Moreover, tamponade can occur with high arterial pressure, presumably due to the increased catecholamines of hypothyroidism.

In severe myxedema, pleural effusion, ascites, and anasarca resemble chronic cardiac failure and constrictive pericarditis.[165] Blood volume is usually increased, whereas in uncomplicated myxedema it tends to be decreased. In some cases, high sedimentation rates suggest an inflammatory component that has been seen on electron microscopy,[166] but the fluid typically has few leukocytes. The ECG may not be altered. However, bradycardia is common, and severely myxedematous patients have distinctly low-voltage to microvoltage QRS.[166] Treatment is thyroid hormone replacement, which is nearly always followed by steady regression of the effusion.[170, 171]

OTHER METABOLIC DISORDERS. Pericarditis has been repeatedly observed during severe crises in patients with *diabetic ketoacidosis* and *adrenal failure* and in some patients with hyperuricemic *gout*.[165, 166] In each case, although bacterial infection, addisonian crisis, or tuberculosis was ruled out, there has not been convincing evidence that pericarditis did not represent an intercurrent inflammation, usually viral, that precipitated that diabetic or adrenal crisis (rarely, tamponade precedes adrenal insufficiency). In Waterhouse-Friderichsen syndrome an accompanying pericarditis is almost certainly meningococcal.[166] In diabetic ketoacidosis, ECGs resembling stage I acute pericarditis have been repeatedly observed both with and without clinical pericarditis.[166] Purely metabolic cholesterol pericarditis occurs in exceptional patients with high serum cholesterol without the usual inciting causes.

NEOPLASTIC PERICARDIAL DISEASE
(See Chaps. 49 and 69)

Three types of neoplastic disease affect the pericardium[172]: (1) primary pericardial tumors, benign or malignant (comparatively rare); (2) secondary malignancies—metastatic and/or from neighboring structures; and (3) nonneoplastic pericardial effusions accompanying malignancy elsewhere. In general, demonstrably malignant effusions imply a prognosis for life of months to a year with breast carcinoma among the "better" prognoses.

SECONDARY MALIGNANCIES: METASTATIC AND INFILTRATIVE

Metastasizing and multicentric malignancies affect the pericardium with or without cardiac involvement, are silent more often and for longer than primary malignancies, and may be the initial sign of malignant disease arising elsewhere.[172–174a] These can present as a pericardial effusion or deceptively when a strong fibrinous reaction mimics acute pericarditis with pain, pericardial rub, fever, and typical or suggestive ECG changes.[172, 173] Usually the ECG is nonspecific even if typical. The J-ST elevations sometimes last for days to weeks, implying persistent pericardial and myocardial injury.[172] In metastatic involvement of the heart by discrete tumors, epicardial lymphatics are nearly always involved. Direct extension occasionally occurs from tumors of the lung, chest wall, or esophagus. Solid tumors may be restricted to the pericardium, invade the myocardium, or appear in both. Lymphomas, Hodgkin disease, leukemias, melanomas, and especially multiple myeloma simultaneously infiltrate the myocardium and pericardium, although each can be isolated to the pericardium. Many of these are associated with local production of cytokines, accounting for associated pericardial inflammation.[175–177] Melanomas, with frequent cardiac involvement often invade the visceral pericardium.[177]

CLINICAL ASPECTS.[172] Secondary neoplasia tends to be insidious and difficult to diagnose unless cancer is recognized elsewhere. Effusions are usually large, especially in patients with hypoalbuminemia, and may be decompensated to tamponade by intrapericardial hemorrhage. Occasional tumors induce constrictive, especially effusive-constrictive pericarditis, with the constriction due to neoplastic tissue, adhesions, or both. Some tumors encase the heart, producing elastic constriction. Occasional tumors involving the pericardium mimic one of the vasculitis-connective disease group. Neoplastic effusions that become suppurative suggest infectious pericarditis, especially in patients immunocompromised due to treatment or to AIDS; the organisms are either common or opportunistic pathogens, especially atypical mycobacteria and fungi.[172]

Pericardial malignancy should be suspected, particularly in patients with malignancy elsewhere[172]: (1) with any large or recurrent effusion; (2) apparently refractory "heart failure" with very high venous pressure; (3) superior vena cava syndrome; or (4) unexplained hepatomegaly. Dyspnea, orthopnea (the most common symptom), unexplained chest pain, and nonproductive cough suggest pericardial involvement. Facial edema and persistent jugular venous distention after drainage of a pericardial effusion may be due to SVC syndrome.

DIAGNOSIS. This may be indicated by chest film, echocardiography, MRI, CT, and radionuclide scanning with indium-111, gallium-67, or technetium.[172, 178] CT and MRI can also reveal tumor contents and texture. For malignant melanoma (over 60 percent with cardiac metastases[177]), MRI is particularly suited because of magnetic scanning. Large effusions or tamponade necessitate studying fluid or tissue, best obtained by video-assisted pericardioscopy, so that samples including *epicardial* biopsy may be obtained safely under direct vision.[52, 179] Cytology, cytometric, and immunohistochemical studies are highly sensitive and specific for most metastatic lesions.[180, 181] False-negative cytology is more common with lymphomas and mesothelioma. Normal mesothelial cells proliferate in response to injury and can show many mitotic figures similar to tumor cells, particularly resembling mesothelioma and adenocarcinoma.[172, 182] Differentiation is by immunohistochemical and ultrastructural methods.[52, 179] Mesothelial cells have keratin and vimentin, whereas carcinoma cells contain carcinoembryonic antigen and LeuM1.[181-183] The ECG is usually abnormal but nonspecific. Malignant effusions usually with tamponade are a common cause of electrical alternation. Fluid obtained by needle or surgical drainage should be studied for cells, including histochemical staining[181-183]; carcinoembryonic antigen and neuron-specific enolase should be sought.[184] Unsatisfactory results require biopsy with the largest possible specimen through the subxiphoid route or by pericardioscopy.

PRIMARY PERICARDIAL NEOPLASM

Benign tumors are found especially in infancy and childhood, whereas *primary malignancies* are discovered mainly in the third and fourth decades.[172] Lipomas and fibromas discovered in mid and later life may grow to giant proportions. Pericardial cysts and particularly hydatid cysts require differential diagnosis, especially if atypically located and if imaging suggests solid tumor.[172] The most important primary malignancies are *mesotheliomas* and *sarcomas* (particularly, *angiosarcoma*), which arise respectively from the pericardial serosa and vasculature and do not metastasize. Pleural mesothelioma can spread to pericardium. They proliferate throughout the pericardium, often invading the myocardium. Mesotheliomas are often related to asbestos or fiberglass exposure, although numerous cases lack either. In general, the signs and symptoms of secondary metastatic and infiltrative malignancies also apply to benign and malignant solid tumors.

CLINICAL FEATURES

Benign tumors usually provoke large effusions even in neonates in whom a cardiorespiratory distress syndrome may appear at or shortly after birth. *Teratomas* are nearly always found in infants with large pericardial effusions; the fluid may be transudate, sanguineous, or, rarely, pyopericardium.[172] Teratomas can compress the right side of the heart and may have detectable calcifications: teeth and bones. Bronchial cysts may resemble teratomas on imaging due to radiopaque contents, but effusions are not common. *Pheochromocytomas* (paragangliomas) and related neurofibromas and neuroblastomas often induce adrenergic hormonal effects, leading to detection by blood and urine tests for catecholamines and localization with iodine-131 metaiodo-benzyl-guanidine. They are hypervascular so that intravenous contrast agents can localize them.[172] *Thymomas* can cause pericardial effusion but may be large enough to be confused with effusion and difficult to identify by imaging if isodense with surrounding structures.[173, 185] Malignant thymomas may present as multisystem disease and autoimmune syndromes as well as cardiac tamponade and SVC obstruction; immunocompromised patients are more susceptible.[172] *Mesotheliomas* may give all the symptoms and signs of metastatic and infiltrate tumors and can mimic idiopathic acute pericarditis with effusion, but with characteristically high levels of hyaluronic acid (hyaluran) in blood and pericardial fluid.[173, 186] They can grow without much exudative reaction to overspread the heart, causing atypical or classic constriction.[173, 181, 182] *Angiosarcomas* grow as blood locules within the pericardial cavity, may or may not deform the cardiopericardial silhouette while enlarging it, and, because of their vascularity, imitate hemopericardium of other origin.[172]

MANAGEMENT

Large refractory and tamponading effusions must be drained. Pericardiocentesis has a high failure rate, except for temporary relief. Percutaneous balloon pericardiotomy[187, 188] or subxiphoid surgical drainage (erroneously termed "window") may be successful in patients with limited survival. Subxiphoid incision permits direct inspection and bi-

opsy; balloon pericardiotomy and pericardiopleural window avoid discomfort and risks of surgery. A pericardioperitoneal shunt may provide prolonged palliation, particularly in children.[172] Extensive pericardial resection is mandatory for persistent recurrence of malignant pericardial constriction; video-assisted pericardio(thoraco)scopic resection is desirable.[172, 173, 179, 189] In patients with very poor prognosis or in whom operation would be hazardous, sclerosing agents have been palliative, although with considerable initial pain.[190] Fortunately, indwelling pericardial drainage tubes act identically, rendering sclerotherapy unnecessary.[172] Yet, there is no convincing evidence that intrapericardial treatment modifies the prognosis for life, which averages 4 months for secondary malignancies except tumors that are unusually sensitive to radiation or systemic chemotherapy.

PERICARDIAL DISEASE IN THE VASCULITIS/ CONNECTIVE TISSUE DISEASE GROUP
(See Chap. 67)

Diseases causing pericarditis, effusion, adhesions, and constriction include most of the vasculitis/connective tissue disease group—a heterogeneous category of disorders that have in common inflammation of blood vessels. Only specific histological lesions in the pericardium confirm the etiology, although characteristic pericardial fluid constituents may be adequate and characteristic clinical behavior often suggests the diagnosis.[191] The primary pathogenic event leading to vasculitis is probably deposition of immune complexes; group members have immunopathic, including autoimmune, features based on immunoglobulin or complement deposition and/or inflammatory cell infiltration in blood vessels and pericardium.[191] Increased or decreased pericardial fluid complement components with normal serum complement levels suggest local complement activation or consumption. With arthritis, synovial tissue and joint fluid abnormalities may resemble those of pericardium and pericardial fluid.[191] Some heterogeneity relates directly or indirectly to exposure to infectious agents (e.g., streptococcal antigen in acute rheumatic fever; hepatitis B antigen in polyarteritis), to unrelated pericardial trauma (e.g., arthritic manifestations with pericarditis in postpericardiotomy and post-myocardial infarction syndromes), or to hypersensitivity, such as "allergic" reactions (e.g., drug-induced lupus) provoking immunopathic responses. Some, such as Wegener granulomatosis[192] and rheumatoid arthritis,[193] feature granulomas. Sarcoidosis, also granulomatous, is less well understood and not strictly a vasculitis.[191] Many patients develop serological evidence, including hypergammaglobulinemia, cryoglobulinemia, hypocomplementemia, circulating immune complexes, and rheumatoid factor, each of which may also be in pericardial fluid. Most of this group affect a preponderance of females, yet males form a disproportionately large part of those with pericardial involvement, reflecting male preponderance in almost every form of pericarditis.[191]

Laboratory studies (e.g., antinuclear antibodies [ANAs]) may support or confirm some diagnoses but alone are not entirely specific.[194, 195] Some malignancies provoke both vasculitis and pericarditis, and some benign and malignant cardiac tumors, including myxoma, may be associated with systemic syndromes resembling those of members of this group.[191]

Rheumatoid Arthritis

Rheumatoid arthritis and its juvenile and adult variants is probably the largest "generator" of pericardial disease. Pericardial involvement is most common in middle-aged white men. Almost half of autopsy patients with rheumatoid arthritis have significant pericardial adhesions, and on echocardiography approximately half have excessive pericardial fluid.[190] Rheumatoid arthritis pericarditis is more common in patients with advanced rheumatoid arthritis with high rheumatoid factor titers.[194] Clinically significant effusions imply a poor prognosis. All morphological forms of pericarditis are associated with rheumatoid arthritis. Acute fibrinous pericarditis, usually subclinical, is demonstrable mainly in patients dying of any reason during arthritis flares. Pericardial effusions, also usually subclinical and small to moderate, can become large, chronic, and even tamponading. Adhesive pericarditis, usually generalized but occasionally localized or with loculated fluid, can provoke all variants of constriction, which tends to occur within 4 to 5 years of the onset of severe rheumatoid arthritis and is comparatively rare with chronicity.[191] Pericardial disease becomes more overt, with severe rheumatoid arthritis particularly in patients with strong serological evidence and only rarely in quiescent disease.[193-196] The most common presentation is a pericardial rub lasting days to years and accidentally discovered in patients without symptoms or with asymptomatic effusion on echocardiography.[190] Recognition of RA pericarditis is confounded not only by its many variants but also by intercurrent diseases, such as viral pericarditis and drug-induced pericarditis (e.g., by phenylbutazone), possible increased susceptibility to other infections and the excellent substrate for bacterial infection afforded by chronic pericardial effusions. Unilateral or bilateral pleural effusions, pleural rubs, and lung lesions (e.g., Caplan syndrome) are common with active disease. Patients with rheumatoid arthritis and systemic congestion ("right-sided heart failure") raise the question of rheumatoid arthritis constriction or tamponade, although common causes of systemic congestion such as true heart failure are more likely.[191]

DIAGNOSIS. Although acute, rheumatoid arthritis pericardial effusions may have more fibrin. Acute and chronic effusions resemble arthritic synovial fluid and rheumatoid pleural effusions.[191, 197] They are mainly serous, often serosanguineous, rarely hemorrhagic, and characterized by low glucose (<45 mg/dl) with a mainly neutrophilic leukocytosis (usually >15,000 cells/mm³), with many cells showing cytoplasmic inclusions that stain for IgM and soluble immune complexes including IgG; complement levels are very low; latex fixation titers for rheumatoid factor are high and relatively specific. Protein is usually more than 5 gm/dl; cholesterol, including crystals, is frequently increased.[191, 196, 197] ECG changes are nonspecific. Cases must be differentiated from tuberculous and bacterial pericarditis, malignancy and, rarely, other causes of cholesterol pericarditis.

MANAGEMENT. Treatment is necessary only for symptomatic pericardial disease. Constriction occurs in rheumatoid arthritis patients despite established antiarthritic treatment with corticosteroids, high-dose aspirin, and other antiinflammatory agents.[191, 198]

ACUTE RHEUMATIC FEVER (See also Chap. 66)

Pericarditis in acute rheumatic fever has declined with decreasing rheumatoid factor in the United States.[191, 198, 199] Mainly a disease of children and adolescents, acute rheumatic fever is associated with antecedent streptococcal infection and has features of immunopathies and other connective tissue diseases. Its pericardial lesions include extensive deposition in the pericardium and in vessels of IgG, IgM, and C3. Most patients have at least discrete fibrotic epicardial milk patches; most of those with chronic valve disease have pericardial adhesions, which frequently are obliterative and which do not appear to constrict. Clinically pericardial involvement is mostly minimal or symptomatic; yet manifest pericardial involvement in acute rheumatic fever usually indicates severe and sometimes fatal pancarditis (almost never without valvulitis[199]), especially if with significant effusion, which may be partly or entirely related to rheumatoid factor myocarditis or heart failure.

Acute pericarditis is a sign of active rheumatic carditis.[192] It usually occurs in the first week after fever and arthritis; chest pain varies from mild to severe; there may be a secondary temperature rise. Disproportionate tachycardia and dyspnea are probably related to myocarditis and pulmonary congestion or edema. The pericardial rub may be intense and last several days. Some degree of effusion is the rule with amber fluid, frequently blood tinged, containing considerable fibrin. Tamponade is rare but must be differentiated from congestive heart failure. Differential diagnosis from other vasculitides is essential, particularly juvenile rheumatoid arthritis in adults who have lymphadenopathy, SLE, and also endocarditis, Lyme disease, and sickle cell crisis. Occasionally, pericarditis is the first sign of acute rheumatic fever. In any child with pericarditis, acute rheumatic fever must be ruled in or out, especially if with a rash and arthralgias, which also occur in viral pericarditis and childhood exanthems.

Without definite carditis, the diagnosis of rheumatic pericarditis is circumstantial and includes (1) fever and arthritis usually preceding pericarditis; (2) relative youth in most cases; and (3) serological positivity for beta-hemolytic streptococci. Nonsteroidal agents may be sufficient treatment. Corticosteroid therapy may be used if nonsteroidal agents fail and may be marginally better.

SYSTEMIC LUPUS ERYTHEMATOSUS

Most patients with SLE develop some form of pericarditis, clinical or subclinical.[191, 194, 200, 201] Pericardial effusion, often large, is common, although tamponade and constriction are comparatively uncommon. SLE pericarditis parallels disease activity[202, 203] and is characterized by epicardial microvasculitis and necrosis and a number of antibodies to nuclear components and phospholipids that form pathogenic antigen-antibody complexes. Immune complexes deposited in the pericardium include IgM, IgG, C3, and, rarely, hematoxylin bodies.[191, 200, 201] SLE causes the entire spectrum and all stages (i.e., acute, subacute, chronic and recurrent) of anatomical and pathophysiological pericardial abnormality. This includes pericarditis; exudative pericardial effusion, which can be serous, serosanguineous, or hemorrhagic; pericardial adhesions; and constrictive pericarditis[191]; any of these may be the first sign.[201] Males are relatively overrepresented, especially among patients who develop constriction.

Pericarditis typically accompanies severe SLE and is often diagnosed during an acute flare that can be painful or painless but virtually always with serological evidence of active disease. Lupus nephropathy is frequent so that uremic pericarditis with effusion may be mistaken for or accompany SLE pericarditis. Increased susceptibility to a range of common and opportunistic bacteria and fungi can be due to the effects of antiinflammatory, immunosuppressive, or cytotoxic treatments and lead to contamination of sterile effusions.[191] Even with infective effusions, blood cultures tend to be negative and some grossly purulent sterile fluids are explained by a very high white blood cell content.

DRUG-INDUCED SLE. This condition is not rare and produces all the pericarditic forms of idiopathic lupus from acute to constrictive but usually spares the kidney.[191] Acute forms clear after discontinuation of offending drugs such as procainamide, isoniazid, hydralazine, methyldopa, or penicillin. Patients with methysergide lupus may develop constriction or, more often, an imitative fibrosing mediastinitis.

MANAGEMENT. Therapy is as for SLE. Tamponade requires drainage, and constriction requires pericardiectomy. However, occasional patients with less than critical tamponade respond to high doses of corticosteroids and even a trial of NSAIDs.

PROGRESSIVE SYSTEMIC SCLEROSIS (SCLERODERMA)

Scleroderma provokes uncontrolled fibroblastic activity leading to abnormal collagen deposition in the microvasculature, skin, synovia, gastrointestinal tract, lungs, heart, kidneys, and pericardium occurring diffusely or in limited systemic scleroderma (CREST syndrome).[191, 204, 205] Although myocardial involvement with failure is common, pericardial scleroderma is the most common cardiac form at autopsy.[191] Echocardiography shows pericardial effusion in almost one half of patients. Although relatively few patients have clinical signs of pericardial scleroderma, these extend from acute fibrinous pericarditis to effusions, which may be chronic recurrent or tamponading, to constriction from relentless fibrosis. Rarely, acute and chronic effusions and even tamponade precede the diagnosis.[191] Scleroderma pericardial effusion, frequently bloody, is an exudate contrasting to exudates in other forms of vasculitis because of the absence of autoantibodies, immune complexes, or complement deposition along with very few white blood cells and a variable protein level.[191, 204] Transudates and pleural effusions are more likely to result from heart failure or uremia. Pericardial scarring in scleroderma is typically slow and associated with gradual obliteration of small vessels. Pericardial involvement occurs with or without myocardial scleroderma, but ECGs, almost always nonspecifically abnormal, reflect myocardial involvement. Consequently, a typical stage I ECG of acute pericarditis should raise the question of intercurrent infection. Because scleroderma is systemic, confounding factors must be considered. Hemodynamics may be affected by pulmonary lesions with pulmonary hypertension, RV hypertrophy, and systemic congestion. Myocardial scleroderma occasionally produces a restrictive cardiomyopathy masquerading as pericardial constriction. As in radiation pericarditis, constrictive pericarditis and restrictive cardiomyopathy may coexist. Renal scleroderma can produce uremic pericarditis. Symptomatic pericardial disease is associated with a poor prognosis.

SJÖGREN SYNDROME

This "sicca syndrome" (dry eyes and dry mouth due to destructive lymphocytic infiltration of exocrine glands) occurs in isolation or in association with connective tissue disorders such as SLE, rheumatoid arthritis, or scleroderma.[191, 206] Pericarditis is of the types associated with the dominant connective tissue disorder, which is usually severe.

POLYMYOSITIS/DERMATOMYOSITIS

These related chronic inflammatory autoimmune diseases of skeletal muscle and skin also affect the heart and pericardium with or without established skeletal muscle involvement.[191, 207] Cardiac and pericardial involvements are usually asymptomatic. Pericarditis, more common in children, is usually discovered incidentally as an effusion on echocardiography, at autopsy, or, occasionally, as fibrinous pericarditis. As in Sjögren syndrome, pericarditis appears to be more frequent in patients with an "overlap syndrome," that is, complicating manifestations of other connective tissue disorders.[191] Effusions, occasionally large, rarely tamponade; constriction is rare. Like SLE, scleroderma can occur with a predominantly myositic syndrome.[207]

PERICARDITIS IN MIXED CONNECTIVE TISSUE DISEASE

Mixed connective tissue disease is a set of "overlap syndromes" with variably combined features of lupus, scleroderma, and dermatomyositis/polymyositis.[191] Pericarditis is the most frequent cardiac finding, particularly at autopsy with pericardial effusions of all sizes.[190] Acute pericarditis or pleuritis can be a presenting feature. Patients have combinations of polyarthritis, Raynaud phenomenon, lymphadenopathy, esophageal dysmotility, skin and muscle involvement, and frequent pulmonary disease with pulmonary artery hypertension; mitral valve prolapse is frequent, often with mitral regurgitation. There are high titers of speckled fluorescent ANA and especially circulating antibodies against nuclear ribonucleoprotein. Echocardiograms frequently show effusion (usually small), and there may be pericardial thickening consistent with postmortem findings of patchy epicardial fibrosis suggesting recurrent episodes. The ECG is nearly always abnormal, frequently showing characteristic ST segment deviations, which is not surprising because of the relative frequency of acute fibrinous pericarditis.[191] Pericardial fluid is serous or serosanguineous but only rarely causes tamponade. Prognosis is surprisingly good in mixed connective tissue disease because pericardial involvement responds to short courses of low-to-moderate dose corticosteroid therapy.

SERONEGATIVE SPONDYLOARTHROPATHIES

This complex group has in common[191] (1) arthritis with a predilection for sacroiliac apophyseal and lumbosacral joints of the spine and the entheses; (2) absence of rheumatoid arthritis serology; (3) male predominance; (4) extraarticular manifestations, including pericarditis, iritis, uveitis, enteric inflammations, myocarditis, and lesions of the aortic root and valve, often with aortic regurgitation; and (5) association with haplotype histocompatibility antigen B27 (HLA-B27). Iritis and cardiopericardial involvement are found primarily in those with B27 positivity, especially syndromes including particularly ankylosing spondylitis, Reiter disease, and the intestinal arthropathies, all associated with dysentery and sometimes urethritis. Dysentery may be related to specific organisms (not necessarily causative). "Psoriatic arthritis" should be included because it can cause constriction. Ankylosing spondylitis is particularly seen in relatively young males with sacroiliitis. Rubs are discovered, and constriction ensues in those with severe acute toxic polyarthritis episodes. Fibrous pericardial adhesions are seen at necropsy. Some patients have had features of Reiter disease. Cardiac involvement is relatively frequent, particularly acute pericarditis with a friction rub[191] and myocarditis[44] with murmurs, gallop rhythms, and conduction abnormalities, all of which may be accompanied by pericardial effusion with increased complement.

The *intestinal arthropathies* include inflammatory bowel disease. In *Crohn disease* and *ulcerative colitis*, acute pericarditis occurs with or without tamponade. *Whipple disease*, a multisystem disorder, has a high proportion of pericardial lesions at necropsy. Serofibrinous pericarditis, sometimes with pleurisy, may accompany seronegative migratory polyarthritis and gastrointestinal symptoms. Pericardial constriction may precede or follow abdominal complaints but is sufficiently rare to suggest intercurrent primary pericarditis.

SYSTEMIC VASCULITIDES

Giant cell arteritis affects medium and larger arteries in any organ including the heart and pericardium.[191, 208] Concomitant pericarditis with or without effusion is of uncertain pathogenesis and possibly is immunopathic. Infections frequently precede giant cell arteritis so that early pericardial syndromes could be mistaken for viral or other infectious pericarditis.[208] Pericarditis and pericardial lesions accompany *temporal (cranial) arteritis* at necropsy and only occasionally clinically, raising the question of intercurrent infection. *Takayasu arteritis* ("pulseless disease"; aortic arch syndrome) is a chronic, idiopathic inflammation of large vessels occurring in relatively young women, with occasional acute pleuritis and pericarditis, sometimes recurrent;

more common is postmortem discovery of pericardial scarring. Tamponade is likely to be due to rupture of a coronary sinus aneurysm. Antiinflammatory, particularly corticosteroid, agents reduce inflammation without effect on ischemia due to arterial lesions.[191]

Polyarteritis (periarteritis nodosa)[209] only occasionally produces acute pericarditis, effusion, or hemopericardium in the absence of uremia. They are more common in patients who are HBsAg positive with associated chronic active hepatitis in some. Patients with coronary arteritis producing myocardial infarcts can develop epistenocardiac pericarditis.

HYPERSENSITIVITY VASCULITIDES

The hypersensitivity vasculitides include *allergic granulomatosis, Churg-Strauss syndrome,* and various *hypereosinophilic syndromes,* all of which have some relation to polyarteritis and produce acute pericarditis, effusion with, or usually without, tamponade and constriction, congestive failure, and acute myocardial infarction.[191, 205, 210, 211] With persistent hypereosinophilia, restrictive cardiomyopathy may result from endocardial involvement. The Churg-Strauss syndrome is a multisystem vasculitis with necrotizing arteritis and eosinophilic infiltrates including extravascular granulomas, particularly in the epicardium. Epicardial and pericardial involvement is relatively frequent, producing all forms of pericarditis and myopericarditis complicated by ischemia due to vasculitis. Characteristically, patients have a history of asthma and allergic rhinitis, which may be transient and episodic. Both blood and pericardial fluid are eosinophilic.

BEHÇET SYNDROME. This is characterized by painful oral and genital ulcers and recurrent hypopyon iritis, sometimes with skin and central nervous system involvement.[191] Arteritis (and venulitis) reveal its relation to the systemic vasculitides. Some patients develop myocarditis, but the *most common cardiac lesion is acute pericarditis.* It is fibrinous or effusive, including pleuropericarditis, each of which may be recurrent but usually self-limited or responding to antiinflammatory agents used for the disease itself. However, Behçet syndrome sometimes provokes thrombosis of major veins, may mimic constriction, and has been associated with chylopericardium and chylothorax.

WEGENER GRANULOMATOSIS. Wegener granulomatosis is characterized by necrotizing local and systemic granulomatous vasculitis of the upper and lower respiratory tract and glomerulonephritis.[191, 212] It overlaps polyarteritis and both giant cell and hypersensitivity arteritides. Diagnosis often requires biopsies of lung or kidney. Serological testing includes antineutrophil, cytoplasmic antibody, and plasma thrombomodulin, which reflects vascular injury. Cardiac involvement occurs in up to 20 percent, including granulomatous myocarditis, endocarditis (including valvulitis), and aortitis; pericarditis occurs in at least half of these, ranging from acute fibrinous to serous or hemorrhagic effusion and occasional tamponade or constriction.

SARCOIDOSIS. Cardiac involvement in sarcoidosis is much more common at necropsy than clinically, because granulomas may be microscopic and not strategically located.[191] Widespread active granulomatous myocarditis and pericarditis, fortunately rare, produce serious and often fatal disease. Pericardial effusions with serous or serosanguineous fluid are relatively common, even during corticosteroid therapy. The majority of pericardial effusions are transudates due to myocardial disease, including heart failure. Constriction has been reported.

SERUM SICKNESS. Serum sickness—with fever, urticaria, lymphadenopathy, myalgia, arthritis, neuritis, vasculitis, and glomulonephritis—can provoke acute pericarditis probably related to pericardial deposition of soluble antigen-antibody complexes when there is an excess of antigen.[191]

MYOCARDIAL INFARCTION–ASSOCIATED PERICARDITIS (See Chap. 35)

Both "early" and "delayed" infarct-associated pericarditis are usually distinct but sometimes without absolute temporal separation, either because one continues into the other or because of the unusually early appearance of pericarditis with characteristics of the delayed form, called *post-myocardial infarction (Dressler) syndrome.*[213, 214] Because the true "early" form is confined to the infarct zone it is known as "infarct pericarditis" or *epistenocardiac pericarditis.*[213] It occurs in almost half of transmural myocardial infarctions but is clinically discovered in many fewer, owing to varying diligence in auscultating a rub, which is usually the only sign. The principal confounding factor in distinguishing epistenocardiac pericarditis from the post-myocardial infarction syndrome is uncertainty as to actual age of any acute infarct; recognition of pericarditis on or near the day of admission usually means epistenocardiac pericarditis, but behavior of the lesion may reveal post-myocardial infarction syndrome.

Infarct Pericarditis

Myocardial infarction-associated pericarditis occurs with anatomically transmural or nearly transmural infarction and is localized to the infarct's "apex" on the epicardium.[213-215] Most ECG changes are localized and nearly always overshadowed by myocardial infarction changes. Thus, generalized stage I ECG changes always raise a question of the post-myocardial infarction syndrome. Acute pericarditis accompanying nontransmural infarct is more likely to be early post-myocardial infarction syndrome. The pericardial exudate is fibrinous; late consequence is a collagenized scar overlying the infarct. Because myocardial infarctions causing detectable epistenocardiac pericarditis are transmural and relatively large, ventricular thrombi, especially apical and RV, are relatively common and probably the reason that systemic embolism is more common in patients who have myocardial infarction pericarditis; with RV infarcts, pulmonary embolism can occur. Moreover, there are more ventricular aneurysms in patients with myocardial infarction pericarditis and more thrombi in them. Such complications reflect the strong tendency for myocardial infarction pericarditis to occur with larger myocardial infarctions and, therefore, associated with higher Killip class and more atrial and ventricular arrhythmias than in patients without pericarditis.[213, 215, 216] Atrial and ventricular arrhythmias are related to heart failure and atrial infarction rather than to pericarditis.[212] Temperature exceeds 37.2°C (99°F) more frequently and lasts longer than without pericarditis.

During the first week of acute myocardial infarction, infarct pericarditis is also a common cause of new chest pain, distinguishable from ischemic pain mainly by its respirophasic and positional ("pleuritic") fluctuations. The importance of larger infarct size with easily discoverable (i.e., rub producing) pericarditis is reflected in late mortality. Despite higher Killip classes, the *in-hospital* prognosis is no different from those without pericarditis. However, *late prognosis* (i.e., 6 months and after) is distinctly worse in those who have myocardial infarction pericarditis.[217, 218]

Patients with infarct pericarditis reflect larger myocardial infarction size by greater (1) myocardial enzyme release, (2) number of ECG leads with elevated ST segments, (3) degree of ST segment elevation, (4) number of leads with infarct Q and QRS abnormality, (5) echocardiographic estimate of myocardial infarction size, (6) aggregate wall motion abnormalities, and (7) radiographic score for extravascular lung water.[213] With infarct pericarditis, anterior and multisite myocardial infarctions are more frequent than with the usually smaller inferior myocardial infarctions. With inferior myocardial infarctions, approximately twice as many patients have pericarditis when there is anterior ST segment depression, which is a sign of a more serious process. Patients have lower ejection fractions that continue to fall up to day 10, whereas without pericarditis depressed ejection fractions tend to rise by 6 to 10 days.[129, 213, 215] With pericarditis there are also more frequent signs of heart failure and increased pulmonary wedge pressure.[216, 217] Early thrombolytic therapy has decreased the incidence of epistenocardiac pericarditis; however, pericarditis appearing despite thrombolysis is a marker of greater damage.[218]

PERICARDIAL EFFUSION.[213, 214, 216, 219, 220] In acute myocardial infarction, pericardial effusions can be irritative (pericarditic) or due to hydropericardium. Effusions tend to develop early, mainly on days 1 to 3, the majority without evidence of pericardial irritation (hydropericardium) and only small to moderate-sized effusions. Larger effusions indicate some degree of heart failure with fluid retention: there is probably increased microvascular permeability associated in some patients with increased extravascular lung water. Increased myocardial interstitial fluid and obstruction of cardiac lymph and venous drainages probably produce the occasional larger irritative effusions that resemble or coincide with hydropericardium.[213] Hydropericardium is more frequent with larger, Q-wave, anterior, and RV myocardial infarctions; they are associated with higher wedge pressures, LV dyssynergy, increased RA pressures, and increased pulmonary alveolar-arterial oxygen difference; reabsorption takes days to weeks.[213-217]

Although tamponade is rare in the absence of bleeding, hydropericardium presages increased mortality because of its association with the foregoing factors.

Anteriorly loculated effusions may cause isolated right-sided heart tamponade by selectively compressing the right ventricle, AV groove, or right atrium; patients develop new hypotension, but pulsus paradoxus usually is absent. The pericardial fluid may contain increased adenosine[219] and beta–fibroblast growth factor.[221] Hemorrhagic pericardial effusion or frankly bloody hemopericardium occurs "spontaneously" or with antithrombotic therapy and, of course, myocardial rupture.[213, 222, 223] Yet any significant pericardial bleeding with myocardial infarction pericarditis is uncommon. However, rapid "cardiac" enlargement, or a loud or persistent pericardial rub or unexplained drop in hemoglobin or hematocrit, with or without tamponade, should be observed for pericardial hemorrhage due to excessive anticoagulation or subacute ventricular rupture. Patients who survive subacute rupture and echocardiography may show echodense material, owing to organizing blood or clots, simulating the texture of intracardiac thrombi but seen between heart and parietal pericardium. Acute ventricular rupture produces rapid tamponade and death, usually with vagally mediated bradycardia culminating in electromechanical dissociation.[213, 224] Because of the frequency of negative taps due to clots and the need to seal the wound, only immediate pericardiotomy and repair offer any faint hope of survival.

PERICARDIAL FRICTION RUB. Most rubs occur within 4 days of onset.[213, 216] A persistent loud or widespread rub may indicate the post-myocardial infarction syndrome or unusually intense myocardial infarction pericarditis requiring intensified observation in patients on antithrombotic therapy. With myocardial infarction pericarditis, most rubs are monophasic, are usually systolic, and can resemble or coexist with murmurs of mitral and tricuspid regurgitation or ventricular septal defect.[213] Disappearance followed by recurrence of rubs may indicate onset of the post-myocardial infarction syndrome. Pericardial rubs with inferior myocardial infarctions are more frequent with RV infarction.

ECG. Infarct pericarditis occurs with transmural (usually Q-wave) myocardial infarction and usually not separately detectable by ECG because it is localized.[11, 213] Failure of evolution of acute ST-T wave changes of myocardial infarction or reversals of ST-T wave evolution in the infarct zone have been associated with infarct pericarditis and impending rupture.[225, 226] Atrial fibrillation is more common after PR segment deviations, a sensitive sign of atrial myopericarditis of unknown specificity and not rare during myocardial infarction pericarditis.[215] Patients with myocardial infarction pericarditis ultimately have more second- and third-degree AV block and more bundle branch and other fascicular blocks, all correlated with larger myocardial infarctions.[213, 216]

THROMBOLYSIS EFFECTS.[213, 218, 224] Effective antithrombotic therapy, administered sufficiently early, usually reperfuses the culprit artery and produces a smaller myocardial infarction, better LV function, and thus less pericardial involvement. Very early thrombolysis decreases the incidence of myocardial infarction pericarditis by at least one half, reduces heart failure among patients with pericarditis, and decreases the incidence of PR segment depression. The rarity of significant pericardial bleeding is remarkable, but thrombolysis has increased the incidence of infarct ruptures and made them earlier. Recanalization of an artery supplying a necrotic myocardial infarction can make the infarct hemorrhagic with bloody pericardial effusion and even tamponade.

DIAGNOSIS. A pericardial rub diagnoses myocardial infarction-associated pericarditis. Pleuritic pain is supporting evidence, whereas pain in one or both trapezius ridges is almost pathognomonic. Stage I ECG changes are uncommon and suggest "early" post-myocardial infarction syndrome,[212] whereas failure to evolve or "resurrection" of previously inverted T waves strongly suggest myocardial infarction pericarditis.[225, 226] Absence of effusion on imaging or a clear pericardial tap exclude subacute ventricular rupture. Dense intrapericardial echoes parallel to the cardiac surfaces suggest subacute rupture.

Conditions to distinguish from myocardial infarction pericarditis (they may coexist) include pulmonary embolism, recurrent ischemia or infarction, acute stress ulcer, mitral and tricuspid regurgitation, ventricular septal rupture, and primary pericarditis without myocardial infarction. "Early" post-myocardial infarction syndrome is distinguished by diffuse ST and PR segment changes and more severe pericarditic symptoms, louder and more persistent rubs, and greater tendency to pericardial effusion and hemorrhage.[213] Primary pericarditis may resemble infarct if the ECG is atypical (see Table 50–5); however, in the absence of myopericarditis, any ST segment elevations are not accompanied by reciprocal changes usual with acute myocardial infarction. Pulmonary embolus, which can also accompany an RV myocardial infarction with pericarditis and mural thrombi,[218] may require lung scan or angiography. Recurrent ischemia should respond to nitrates; pain and ST segment changes of pericarditis will not. Acute mitral and tricuspid regurgitation and ventricular septal defects are distinguishable by murmurs, thrills, and imaging. Their murmurs may resemble rubs, but flows should be demonstrable by Doppler imaging.

Tamponade is rare; yet, particularly in patients on antithrombotic therapy, it must be distinguished from circulatory collapse due to shock and myocardial failure. Injured, low-compliance myocardium may prevent pulsus paradoxus. Diagnosing tamponade thus may require imaging or cardiac catheterization. Even if intrapericardial blood is drained, relieving tamponade, pericardial clots seen on imaging presage recurrence and demand special vigilance.[213] New pleuritic pain favors pericarditis, especially after antithrombotic therapy, which usually prevents pulmonary embolus. With large infarcts, unexplained deterioration should suggest tamponade. If the diagnosis of acute myocardial infarction is mistaken, thrombolysis may produce tamponade from inflamed pericardium[227] or aortic dissection, a mimic of both acute myocardial infarction and acute pericarditis (see Chap. 40).

MANAGEMENT. Myocardial infarction-associated pericarditis is usually mild and responds to aspirin, up to 650 mg every 4 hours for 2 to 5 days. Other nonsteroidal agents risk thinning an infarct (not conclusively demonstrated in humans); ibuprofen, which increases coronary flow is the agent of choice. Corticosteroid therapy may be used for refractory symptoms (usually post-myocardial infarction syndrome) but should be avoided owing to delayed myocardial infarction healing, possible side effects, and dependency. Although more frequent with thrombolysis, hemopericardium remains uncommon in myocardial infarction pericarditis; therefore, heparin and other antithrombotic treatments may not be contraindicated unless there is a widespread or intense pericardial rub[213] (risk of hemopericardium is probably outweighed by benefits of preventing myocardial infarction extension and ventricular thrombi). Yet the problem is compounded by possible "early" post-

myocardial infarction syndrome with diffuse pericarditis and much greater tendency to bleed. Because pericardial bleeding can occur even with clotting indices in the therapeutic range,[222] these must be monitored and the patient watched for tamponade. Finally, any pericardial effusion increases the energy required for defibrillation.[228]

PSEUDOANEURYSM (FALSE VENTRICULAR ANEURYSM)

Pseudoaneurysms represent contained myocardial rupture, most often posterolaterally, limited by the visceral pericardium, with or without adherent parietal pericardium, or by the parietal pericardium alone.[213, 227] They are uncommon and occur with larger infarcts, usually within 5 weeks of onset. They follow ventricular surgery (especially valve replacement), endocarditis, penetrating wounds, and, rarely, tumor infiltration[229] and suppurative pericarditis.[230] Abundant epicardial fat seems to predispose to cardiac rupture[231] but may buttress a pseudoaneurysm.[213] Pseudoaneurysms have a narrow neck communicating with a ventricular cavity; blood flows into the pseudoaneurysm in systole and out in diastole. The neck may be so narrow as to be visible only on color Doppler imaging. Differential diagnosis includes true aneurysm, pericardial cysts, and loculated pericardial effusions.[213]

THE PERICARDIUM AND RIGHT VENTRICULAR MYOCARDIAL INFARCTION

Pericarditis is relatively frequent when inferior myocardial infarction is accompanied by RV myocardial infarction.[213, 229, 232] However, by means of ventricular and AV interaction both the normal and inflamed pericardium constrain the injured right side of the heart, which tends to dilate. RV dilation raises intrapericardial pressure, which decreases LV transmural pressure, thus reducing LV filling, preload, and stroke volume. (Pulmonary embolism can act similarly, with acute right-sided heart dilation imposing acute pericardial constraint.[233]) These represent relative pericardial constriction with constrictive hemodynamics, reduced blood pressure, jugular venous distention, and occasionally an S_3 or Kussmaul sign. Even pulsus paradoxus can appear, related to increased pericardial fluid or septal hyperresponsiveness to the respiratory cycle. These signs may individually depend on the pathophysiological "mix," that is, whether relative constriction due to pericardial tightening or increased intrapericardial pressure dominates. The lungs are usually clear. Thus, the clinical picture usually resembles constriction; with a pericardial rub and pulsus paradoxus it suggests tamponade.[213] Tricuspid regurgitation due to RV myocardial infarction may simulate or obscure a pericardial rub.

POST-MYOCARDIAL INFARCTION SYNDROME (DRESSLER SYNDROME)

This myocardial infarction-associated pericarditis does not require transmural infarction.[213, 234] Most patients have fever, a high sedimentation rate, considerable "pericardial" pain, pleuritis, and sometimes pneumonitis. Its usual onset is from 1 week to several months after clinical onset of myocardial infarction. Some patients have a remote history of pericarditis.[213] Like myocardial infarction pericarditis, the post-myocardial infarction syndrome occurs more often after larger, particularly anterior infarcts, inferior myocardial infarctions with RV infarction, and complicated myocardial infarctions. Post-myocardial infarction syndrome can appear as an extension of epistenocardiac pericarditis, with persistence or recurrence of rub and fever and with considerable malaise in contrast to myocardial infarction pericarditis, which is mild and transient. The usual gap from onset of myocardial infarction symptoms to the post-myocardial infarction syndrome suggests a necessary latent period. (Because approximately 30 percent of Q-wave myocardial infarctions are "silent," following them, post-myocardial infarction syndrome could appear as "idiopathic pericarditis" because post-myocardial infarction syndrome often resembles viral pericarditis.)

The incidence of post-myocardial infarction syndrome remains uncertain, but it is much less than the originally reported 5 percent of acute myocardial infarction.[235] Post-myocardial infarction syndrome occurs with and without antithrombotic treatment but may be more frequent in patients with pericardial bleeding, which can occur during myocardial infarction with or without an antithrombotic regimen.[234]

The post-myocardial infarction syndrome is often considered autoimmune, based on factors in common with other pericardial injury syndromes. These include a latent period, development of antiheart antibodies, and preceding pericardial injury (most cases have had epistenocardiac pericarditis), although it also occurs in nontransmural infarction and, therefore, without direct pericardial injury. Other factors include frequent recurrence; typical prompt response to antiinflammatory agents; frequent associated pleuritis with or without pneumonitis; changes in cellular immunity suggested by altered lymphocyte subsets compared with control patients; and evidence favoring immune complex formation incorporating antibody combined with myocardial antigen, complement pathway activation, and evidence of cellular as well as humoral immunopathic responses.[213]

CLINICAL FEATURES. There may be considerable malaise, marked pleuritic pain, and frequently a rub, pericardial and pleural effusions, and fever up to 40°C (104°F). The ECG occasionally shows ST segment and T wave changes suggesting pericarditis superimposed on evolving myocardial infarction, but it is usually dominated by evolutionary myocardial infarction changes.[213, 234] Telltale PR segment deviations are a strong clue. Pericardial and pleural effusions may be serous or hemorrhagic. Leukocytosis is typically polymorphonuclear (occasionally eosinophilic). The ESR is virtually always high. Recurrence can be single or multiple over weeks or even years. Complications are uncommon but include tamponade relatively early. Late constriction is not surprising because of intrapericardial organization of exudate and blood that can also produce loculated effusions. Rarely, effusions can look purulent because of high neutrophil concentration; taken with the customary fever this mimics purulent pericarditis, but pericardial fluid is sterile.

MANAGEMENT.[213, 234] Patients should be hospitalized and observed for tamponade, differential diagnosis, and adjustments of treatment, including rest and NSAIDs. Recurrences may require a corticosteroid, which should be a last resort with early tapering to discontinuance.

TRAUMATIC PERICARDIAL DISEASE
(See Chap. 51)

Pericardial Reactions to Physical Trauma

The heart and pericardium are only partly protected by the bony thorax.[236-238] A broad range of pericardial injuries evoke responses due to disruption of pericardial tissue and often adjacent and remote tissues. These may be immediate (cellular and vascular inflammation); delayed, including immunopathic (the post-cardiac—pericardial and myocardial—injury syndrome); and due to healing (adhesions, constriction, effusive-constrictive pericarditis). The inflammatory response may be sterile or infected with or without significant effusion. Traumatic tamponade, the most common cause of early death from cardiac wounds, usually is due to bleeding, producing early or late cardiac compression.[236-238] Survival with pericardial adhesions can lead to constrictive or effusive-constrictive pericarditis. Blunt (nonpenetrating) trauma, often more complex than penetrating trauma, occasionally causes cardiac and also pericardial rupture with herniation or entrapment of all or part of the heart. Pericardial laceration is not rare with severe blunt trauma, permitting cardiac displacement.

COMPLICATIONS. Only occasionally does pericardial injury occur in isolation. Concurrent disease or injury of other organs, particularly the heart, modifies the clinical picture, physiological responses, the ECG, and all imaging modalities. These include injuries of the heart, great vessels (especially ascending aorta), conducting system, myocardium, mediastinum, and other chest and abdominal organs. Late pericardial and cardiac sequelae are common, including pericardial effusion, hemopericardium and tamponade, post-cardiac injury syndrome, false aneurysm, congestive failure, and constrictive pericarditis. They require monitoring and long-term follow-up.

Penetrating Trauma

TRAUMATIC AGENTS. Knives, needles, bullets and high-velocity projectiles, intracardiac instrumentation, and cardiac surgery are the most common causes of penetrating trauma.[236, 238, 239] Bullets and shrapnel cause more damage than lacerating and puncturing instruments, the pathways of which may seal over. However, early tamponade is much more common in cardiac stab wounds than bullet wounds. (Nail gun injuries, a new category, require exploration.[240-242]) Any chambers can be involved, but the right ventricle is more common in anterior chest wounds. RA, RV, and great vessel wounds are quickest to tamponade and exsanguinate. The left atrium can be penetrated by posterior chest wounds and has been ruptured by external cardiac massage because of the pericardium's tight clasp of the left atrium. These wounds tend to bleed more slowly than wounds of other chambers and may produce hemothorax rather than hemopericardium or be localized to the adjacent oblique sinus (which may be hemodynamically significant). Anterior esophageal penetration by instruments or swallowed foreign objects such as bones and contaminated surgical instruments is likely to cause suppurative pericarditis. All bullet wounds are potentially infected.[243]

CLINICAL FEATURES. With penetrating trauma the most common causes of immediate death are exsanguination or tamponade and often both. Some patients have rubs, but many do not, or rubs appear with pericardial bleeding and effusion (many patients have serous effusions[244]). ECGs are frequently unhelpful in assessing pericardial damage but may show typical or atypical stage I changes early or late (>24 hours). The principal cause of death—"surgical" tamponade due to hemopericardium or hemopneumopericardium—is difficult to diagnose because of blood loss, vasoconstriction, and frequent hemothorax that are not characteristic of "medical" tamponade. Pulsus paradoxus may be absent or disappear with severe hypotension and shock. There may be tachycardia and abnormal rhythms due to concomitant cardiac injury, or terminal electromechanical dissociation.

TAMPONADE AND HEMOPERICARDIUM. Paradoxically, tamponade can be a correlate of survival.[245] Patients with tamponade reaching emergency departments appear to survive better than nontamponaded patients. The corollary is that untimely release of tamponade without thoracotomy can cause rapid decompensation because clotting of the pericardial hematoma can be hemostatic for cardiac wounds.[246] Thus, especially in unstable patients, thoracotomy in the emergency department or in the operating room is optimal for wound repair. Pericardiocentesis is a temporizing measure for unstable patients while simultaneously preparing for surgery and administering treatment for shock. In stable patients, thoracotomy, subxiphoid pericardial exploration, or video-assisted thoracoscopy are feasible with the option of extending to a full thoracotomy and, if necessary, laparotomy for abdominal wounds (which can also reach the pericardium).

IATROGENIC PERICARDIAL WOUNDS. These are produced by cardiac surgery, percutaneous transluminal coronary angioplasty, stenting and pacing instruments, central venous and pulmonary flotation catheters, arrhythmia ablation, and even needles and catheters for pericardial drainage.[247-250] Pericardial damage during percutaneous transluminal coronary angioplasty can occur with coronary artery dissections, producing local or general pericarditis with or without significant bleeding. Patients may present with new pain, a rub, or tamponade or with hemopericardium. Instruments and pacers may penetrate the right ventricle with or without pericarditic signs or hemopericardium.[246] Central venous catheters tend to penetrate the right atrium and rarely the SVC; fluids administered through them may provoke tamponade or exacerbate tamponade already due to bleeding. *Fetal tamponade* has complicated amniocentesis. Open surgical evacuation is often the optimal management, necessitating rapid transfer to the operating room or thoracotomy in the emergency department.[236]

FOREIGN-BODY AND FOREIGN-SUBSTANCE PERICARDITIS.[236] Smooth-edged foreign bodies less than 1 or 2 cm in diameter may be asymptomatic. Relatively large foreign bodies lying in or near the pericardium, such as metallic fragments, bullets, broken instruments, or needles, are associated with recurrent pericarditis and effusion; they need not penetrate the heart. Asbestos poudrage for coronary disease and cardioverter-defibrillator patches have provoked dense calcification. Silicon-contaminated pacemaker insertion can provoke an exuberant pericardial foreign-body reaction, including giant cells. All can progress to tamponade, adhesions, or constriction. Definitive treatment is removal of the foreign material and any significant adhesions and fluid. Postpericardiotomy syndrome may follow.

SURGICAL PERICARDIAL INFLAMMATION AND EFFUSION.[245, 251, 252] Mild pericarditis and low-grade fever, usually with some bleeding and effusion, are common postoperatively and proportional to the amount of pericardial manipulation, which regularly causes loss of mesothelial cells and provokes fibrinous and leukocyte exudation; significant blood leukocytosis may indicate infection.[245] The ECG tends to reflect this with minor nonspecific or local ST segment changes, yet often with generalized changes that usually do not evolve beyond stage I. Early pericardial effusions are common, tend to appear by the fifth postoperative day, are usually small (<1 cm echo depth), are usually benign, and are frequently associated with a left pleural effusion. Moderate effusions (1–2 cm) are less common, and large effusions (>2 cm) are uncommon. Large and especially increasing early effusions, usually due to bleeding and more common after valve surgery, are harbingers of tamponade. Late effusions (6–60 days after surgery) may also be due to bleeding, especially in patients taking anticoagulants[253] or with a coagulopathy or due to the osmotic ("hydrophilic") effect of slow intrapericardial clot lysis or to immunopathic responses to cardiopericardial trauma.[236]

POSTOPERATIVE TAMPONADE

Nearly all clinically significant effusions are present by the fifth postoperative day. Circumferential and especially localized tamponade remain challenging diagnostic and therapeutic problems.[236] Anticoagulation is associated with tamponade at any time; its principal importance is in the first 3 to 5 days when hemopericardium is most common. Late tamponade, often associated with postpericardiotomy syndrome, is probably inflammatory or immunopathic.[253] Although classic diagnostic signs of tamponade may be present postoperatively, familiar clinical signs such as pulsus paradoxus are often absent. Similarly, echocardiographic and Doppler signs retain their specificity but their sensitivity is greatly reduced.[219] ECG changes are common and of no help whereas the swinging heart and electrical alternation are uncommon (probably due to adhesions). Thus, atypical presentations of tamponade should be anticipated by liberal monitoring of vital signs and catheterization data as well as by echocardiography for chamber collapses and other evidence. TEE is superior to TTE for both tamponade and pericardial thickening.[251, 254]

DIFFERENTIAL DIAGNOSIS. Tamponade must be differentiated from extrapericardial causes of low cardiac output, including[245] (1) ventricular hypokinesis with left, right, or combined ventricular failure; (2) acute LV or RV myocardial infarction; (3) pulmonary embolism; (4) coronary insufficiency; (5) effects of prolonged aortic cross-clamping or inadequate coronary perfusion during cardiopulmonary bypass; (6) severe pulmonary artery hypertension; (7) septic shock; (8) hepatitis (enzyme abnormalities, passive hepatic congestion or injury); or (9) mediastinal hematoma or effusion causing extrapericardial cardiac compression. Apart from elastic constriction[255] by clotted hemopericardium, constrictive pericarditis is not an early consideration but can occur as soon as 2 to 7 weeks (usually much later). Acute cardiac dilatation within a repaired pericardium will have a comparable affect. Each may appear as unexplained dyspnea.[236, 256]

MANAGEMENT.[236] Operative pericarditis and effusions respond quickly to brief therapy with a corticosteroid or NSAID. Coagulation status and platelet levels should be monitored. Early postoperative tamponade is a surgical emergency usually requiring thoracotomy; later tamponade may respond to drainage and observation. Either type can present as sudden deterioration so that clinically and hemodynamically significant effusions of any size should be drained; urokinase or streptokinase can be instilled to aid drainage and inhibit adhesions if further bleeding is ruled out. Coronary bypass grafts are endangered by any blind procedure. Surgical drainage or video-monitored thoracoscopy may be optimal, as determined by particular fluid loculations disclosed by TEE.

Postoperative Pseudoaneurysm.[236, 257] False aneurysms occasionally follow cardiac surgery, especially when a chamber has been vented. These resemble pseudoaneurysms after myocardial infarction.

OTHER.[236, 258, 259] Open-chest *cardiac massage* traumatizes the epicardium, increasing susceptibility to infection, pericardial effusion, tamponade, and ultimate constriction. Removal of *epicardial pacing wires* is usually effected without untoward event, but an epicardial vein or other structure may be traumatized, producing hemopericardium.

CHEMICAL INJURY. More or less sterile chemical injury to pericardium may follow unusual communications of the biliary tract, pancreas, and esophagus, particularly after sclerotherapy of esophageal varices.[260] Pancreatitis may be accompanied by pericardial irritation and effusion even without communication; this is ascribed to hematogenous and lymphogenous transport of pancreatic enzymes to the pericardium.

ELECTRICAL TRAUMA.[236, 261] After lightning strikes, with well-known cardiac consequences, occasional survivors have had pericardial effusion with tamponade or recurrent pericarditis. The latter may be a kind of post-cardiac injury syndrome.

Indirect (Blunt/Nonpenetrating) Pericardial Trauma

Indirect injuries to pericardium, heart, and lung are often more complex than those from penetrating trauma.[236] Blunt trauma to the chest and abdomen follows nonpenetrating thoracic impacts, compression (crush), blast, and traumatic deceleration, producing an injury spectrum from contusion to rupture of the heart, the pericardium, or both.[262] Closed-chest cardiac massage even without rib fractures can also traumatize the heart and pericardium.[259] Any cardiac damage, including exacerbation of antecedent heart or pericardial disease, may complicate a range of pericardial injury, including acute, "clinically dry" pericarditis, or hemopericardium with or without tamponade, pneumopericardium, early and late constriction, and recurrent pericarditis.[236] Indirect forces can displace numerous viscera and may cause the heart and great vessels to acutely "trap" more blood than usual, with directional stresses capable of rupturing the pericardium and other structures. A common cause is deceleration forces, characteristic of transportation-associated accidents, acting in any plane or tangentially. Death usually follows cardiac rupture with acute hemopericardium or pericardial rupture and acute extrusion (herniation; luxation) of some or all of the heart. In general, the more serious the cardiac injury, the more serious the pericardial injury. This may occur in the absence of significant external marks. Isolated parietal pericardial rupture with or without cardiac contusion from blunt injury or after cardiac resuscitation is not rare at autopsy. Fibrinous pericarditis often with some hemorrhage is common. Subacute or late constriction may follow hemopericardium or purulent pericarditis from days to years after injury.

PERICARDIAL LACERATION.[236, 262] Parietal pericardial tears are frequent, especially after falls and other deceleration injuries. Lacerations are rarely isolated or clinically silent; characteristically, cardiac injury accompanies the laceration. The most serious consequence is cardiac herniation: extrusion of all or part of the heart in any direction but usually into the left pleural cavity, frequently with mediastinal and tracheal shift. Herniation is characteristically sudden and nearly always a surgical emergency. (After 72 hours, herniation tends to be restrained by adhesions.) Rupture and laceration of the parietal pericardium occur mainly at either its diaphragmatic or pleural abutments or both.

CLINICAL CONSIDERATIONS.[236, 262a–264] Symptoms occurring after blunt trauma can be nonspecific or multiple, with and without dyspnea or anterior chest or abdominal pain, and may be overshadowed by injuries elsewhere. In hemorrhaging and other hypovolemic trauma patients, an initial favorable response to fluid administration may obscure and delay recognition and treatment of tamponade. All significant or potentially significant chest injuries require careful monitoring for progression or sudden cardiocirculatory deterioration. Nonpenetrating trauma can produce all of the cardiocirculatory physical findings of penetrating trauma and surgical injuries. A pericardial rub, easily missed, may be the only physical sign. Hypotension is the rule, and pulsus paradoxus must be diligently sought but is often deceptively absent. Free air in the pericardium rises to the upper sac. Cardiac contusions may be identified by indium-111 antimyosin scintigraphy. The ECG commonly shows only ST-T wave changes, which occasionally suggest, but only rarely are typical of, acute pericarditis. With cardiac displacement, the QRS axis may shift and occasionally become unusual; there may be altered precordial R wave progression.

IMAGING.[236, 263a] Chest radiographs, preferably with the patient upright, demonstrate any rib and sternal fractures, gas collections, atelectasis, tracheal shift, and displacement of a herniated heart. There may be intrapericardial migration of abdominal organs with unilateral (usually left) diaphragmatic elevation and unusual supradiaphragmatic densities, lucencies, and organ shadows. Rarely, patients do not develop symptoms for months, years, or ever. Echocardiography, optimally TEE, is indispensable and so sensitive that a negative high-quality study significantly decreases the likelihood of complications and sequelae. It will disclose pericardial effusion and fibrinous exudate, RV dilation, ventricular (especially RV) thrombi, and traumatic true and false aneurysms.[263] CT or MRI can discriminate hemopericardium by its density and disclose other cardiac and vascular injuries, angulations, and dilations as well as acute hepatic lymphedema due to cardiac or inferior vena cava compression.[236] Video-assisted thoracoscopy is most specific for selecting appropriate sites and extent of thoracotomy incision.[262a]

MANAGEMENT. Repositioning the patient may permit restitution of a herniated heart's position. Definitive treatment is repair of wounds especially of the heart and vessels and repositioning of displaced organs. The pericardium may have to be sutured, patched, or resected; and some pericardial lacerations may be enlarged to reposition the heart, especially if it dilates.[264]

Post-Cardiac Injury Syndrome; Postpericardiotomy Syndrome

The post-cardiac injury syndrome develops days to months after cardiac and pericardial injury.[236, 253] It so strongly resembles the post-myocardial infarction syndrome that they both appear to be variants of a common immunopathic process. The post-cardiac injury syndrome differs from the post-myocardial infarction syndrome because it acutely provokes a much greater antiheart antibody (AHA) (antiactin and antimyosin) response, probably related to more extensive tissue trauma and more concentrated release of antigenic material.[236] Because even surgery limited to the pericardium can cause the post-cardiac injury syndrome, it is commonly denoted "postpericardiotomy syndrome."

PATHOGENESIS. Myocardial injury releases cellular constituents, possibly autoantigens provoking an autoimmune antibody reaction by AHAs; complement is activated, C3 and C4 levels fall, and leukocytes are mobilized. In the postpericardiotomy syndrome, AHAs appear to be pathogenic in the presence of a dormant or concurrent viral infection that "permits" them to act.[236] (Some trigger is necessary because AHAs alone may not be pathogenic.) A quantitative effect of AHAs is seen in the proportionality between occurrence of the postpericardiotomy syndrome and extent of surgery; correction of congenital defects and of the Wolff-Parkinson-White syndrome have the highest relative incidences. (Postpericardiotomy syndrome after strictly pericardial surgery may challenge the immunopathic hypothesis because no antipericardial antibodies have been identified.) Evidence that post-cardiac injury syndrome/postpericardiotomy is immunopathic includes the following: preceding latent period; frequent recurrences; stimulation of AHAs and complement activation; prompt response to corticosteroids; and clinical characteristics of fever, pulmonary infiltrates, frequent pleuritis (rarely the only sign),[245] and systemic inflammatory symptoms and signs. The "complete" post-cardiac injury syndrome/postpericardiotomy syndrome correlates well with higher titers of AHAs and is rare in patients younger than age 2, possibly owing to hyporeactivity or carryover protection from the mother's immune defenses. The incidence decreases at advanced ages, possibly related to an immune system that has had more extensive encounters with a variety of microorganisms and/or is senescent and therefore hyporeactive. The extent of myocardial damage is not absolutely correlated with provocation of the post-cardiac injury syndrome/postpericardiotomy syndrome.

CLINICAL ASPECTS.[236, 253] The post-cardiac injury syndrome and postpericardiotomy syndrome differ from the usually self-limited postoperative or posttraumatic pericarditis in that more patients develop a form of post-cardiac injury syndrome than clinically significant postsurgical pericarditis. The postinjury latent period usually lasts a week to 6 months, with symptoms and signs more severe, disabling, and prolonged (days to weeks per attack) than uncomplicated posttraumatic pericarditis, although few develop tamponade or constriction. Pericardial fluid tends to be serosanguineous. Recurrences are characteristic, mainly within 6 months of the index attack. Among patients without congenital heart disease, the post-cardiac injury syndrome/postpericardiotomy is more frequent in those with a history of either pericarditis or corticosteroid therapy (especially for rheumatoid arthritis), after aortic valve replacement, and in those with B-negative blood. Most patients have tachycardia, malaise, pleuritic pain, new pericardial and sometimes pleural rubs or both, and mild lymphocytosis or granulocytosis; all patients have low-grade fever, which may simulate a continuation of postoperative or postinjury fever.[236] Most postsurgical pericardial rubs should disappear within a week. The post-cardiac injury syndrome/postpericardiotomy syndrome is considered "complete" if fever, pericarditis, and laboratory evidence of inflammation are present and "incomplete" with only two of these.

DIAGNOSIS.[236, 253] In general, post-cardiac injury syndrome/postpericardotomy syndrome must be considered in patients who after 6 days after surgery or trauma develop fever above 37.8°C (100°F) for over 8 hours with significant pleuritic anterior chest pain and a pericardial rub or two of these, usually with an ESR greater than 40 mm/hr and leukocytosis greater than 11,000 cells/mm³. The echocardiogram usually shows a small to moderate pericardial effusion. Chest radiographs show left or bilateral pleural effusion in most patients and right pleural effusion in a few. The cardiopericardial silhouette may be enlarged, and a few patients have pulmonary infiltrates. The ECG usually reflects myocardial abnormalities. Principal differential diagnoses of post-cardiac injury syndrome/postpericardiotomy syndrome include (1) other causes of postoperative fever including infections and pneumonitis, (2) pulmonary embolism, and (3) myocardial infarction. Perhaps half the patients have ECG changes consistent with acute pericarditis. If new changes are inconsistent with infarct or pericarditis, radionuclide scanning or comparable studies may be useful.

MANAGEMENT.[236, 253] The post-cardiac injury syndrome/postpericardiotomy syndrome usually responds within 48 hours to therapy with aspirin or another NSAID, which should be maintained for 10 days. Corticosteroid therapy is reserved for patients with unresponsive severe symptoms. The unusual tamponading effusion must be drained. Recurrences are often worse than the index attack and should be managed similarly, adding colchicine as tolerated if NSAIDs alone appear ineffective. Pericardiectomy is reserved for intractable effusions that may increase (despite even corticosteroid therapy) and for constriction.

PERICARDIAL SEQUELAE. Pericardial adhesions are generally proportional to the extent of epicardial and pericardial injury and any residual blood after drainage.[245] Loculated effusion or hemorrhage may become manifest early or months postoperatively. Continued inflammatory activity can induce constrictive pericarditis, usually after months to years. Recurrent pericarditis, probably autoimmune, with or without effusion, may follow any pericardial injury, including radiation pericarditis and even pericardial resection. Pseudoaneurysm is rare.

Aortic Dissection and Intramural Hemorrhage

(See Chap. 40)

Aortic dissection, DeBakey types I and II, and aortic intramural hemorrhage often rupture into the pericardium.[213, 265-267] They are almost indistinguishable clinically; this discussion applies to both. Rupture is the most frequent cause of death due to aortic dissection, usually through tamponade with intrapericardial clotting preventing nonsurgical drainage. There is always over 100 ml of blood and usually 400 to 1500 ml.[235, 266] Subacute and chronic bleeding is tolerated with smaller leaks and mitigation by medical treatment of aortic dissecting and shearing forces.[268] A protracted course may allow dilution by pericardial effusion, owing to pericardial irritation and the osmotic affects of intrapericardial hemolysis.

CLINICAL FEATURES.[213, 266, 267] The ECG is seldom normal and may show preexisting LV hypertrophy, acute ischemia, or myocardial infarction. Pericardial irritation by blood that first dissects under the epicardium can provoke a rub and occasionally compress coronary arteries, causing myocardial ischemia and infarction. Occasionally, the ECG resembles stage I acute pericarditis. Occlusion of renal arteries combined with hypotension can produce acute uremic pericarditis. Indeed, dissecting hematoma may first present hours to many days before frank rupture as "acute pericarditis" and without pain typical of dissection,[213, 267] suggesting idiopathic pericarditis, which is much more common. In such relatively slow dissections, misleading ST segment elevations can also be due to release of potassium from intrapericardial hemolysis. In older patients with a history of hypertension, acute pericarditis should always be considered part of another syndrome. In younger patients, in whom idiopathic pericarditis is generally more common, signs of Marfan syndrome[267] or other inherited connective tissues disease or aortic coarctation should be sought. Both aortic regurgitation and dissecting aneurysm are more common in patients with bicuspid aortic valves, congenital aortic stenosis, and coarctation with rib notching on the chest film.

Precise diagnosis as in all acute conditions should be as rapid as practical because of the narrow "windows" for aortic rupture and myocardial salvage. Echocardiography, preferably omniplane TEE (as sensitive as CT and MRI) is optimal to detect pericardial effusion, aortic regurgitation, a false lumen, and an aortic intimal flap. If echocardiography is negative or indecisive, CT, especially helical CT, or spin-echo MRI, which is time consuming and logistically difficult, will usually define aortic mural hemorrhages and intimal flaps.[269] They are safer and more sensitive than aortography (which occasionally becomes necessary[270]). All imaging techniques show pericardial effusions due to aortic dissection usually to be anterior.

MANAGEMENT. The most efficient management when dissection is likely is to do diagnostic procedures in the operating room. Percutaneous pericardial drainage often gives only temporary or no relief, with increase in blood pressure disrupting sealing clots and accelerating intrapericardial leakage, causing frank hemopericardium, shock, electromechanical dissociation, and death. Definitive treatment is surgical relief of tamponade and repair of the aorta. Rarely, aortic dissection involving the pericardium heals spontaneously. Constrictive pericarditis has resulted as early as 7 months later.

PULMONARY THROMBOEMBOLISM AND PULMONARY HYPERTENSION

Pericardial involvement after pulmonary infarction is uncommon. It can be (1) apparently due to contiguity; (2) a complication of antithrombotic therapy for pulmonary embolism; (3) a simultaneous event in pulmonary embolism after trauma including cardiac or other surgery; and (4) rarely, an apparent immunopathy with a pericardial component closely mimicking the post-myocardial infarction syndrome.[271, 272] Infarction of pulmonary segments adjacent to the pericardium can produce pleuropericardial rubs. These are strictly exopericardial and even classic rubs, which rarely may be the first sign of a pulmonary embolus,[213] with or without pleuritic pain. After blunt or penetrating chest trauma or cardiac surgery the mixed picture may be difficult to unravel. Massive pulmonary embolism, such as primary pulmonary hypertension,[271] has been attended by hydropericardium presumably due to right-sided heart failure; such cases may have a conus rub due to acute cor pulmonale without pericarditis. Finally, since pulmonary embolism can be asymptomatic, signs of acute "idiopathic" pericarditis or effusion should alert physicians to search for it in patients who have risk factors for embolism. In general, disorders dilating the right side of the heart increase pericardial constraint of the entire heart, mimicking constriction, and with hydropericardium suggest tamponade, especially with left-sided chamber collapses,[272] which can also be associated with purely pleural effusions.[273]

POST-PULMONARY INFARCTION SYNDROME.[274] Rarely after pulmonary embolism, acute pericarditis with or without effusion appears as a syndrome closely resembling post-myocardial infarction syndrome with strictly pericardial rubs, fever, leukocytosis, elevated ESR, frequent pericardial and pleural effusions, and, rarely, tamponade. Like the post-myocardial infarction syndrome and other immunopathies this syndrome responds to antiinflammatory treatment, particularly rapidly to a corticosteroid. NSAIDs should be tried first.

PERICARDIAL INVOLVEMENT IN GASTROINTESTINAL DISORDERS

ESOPHAGEAL DISEASE.[245] The esophagus overlies the pericardium covering parts of the left atrium and ventricle. Esophageal disorders can involve the pericardium, often catastrophically, frequently with little or no warning, and almost always confusingly because of what appears to be isolated pericardial or cardiac disease or combined esophageal and cardiopericardial signs and symptoms. Most patients who are "candidates" for pericardial involvement include those who have had esophageal surgery and other trauma, gastroesophageal reflux, Barrett esophagus, hiatal hernia, and esophageal strictures. The pericardium is directly involved by fistulas from processes penetrating the esophageal wall such as inflamed esophageal diverticula. These include inflammation (e.g., esophagitis and peptic, bacterial, viral, and fungal ulcers), neoplasms, perforating foreign bodies, corrosive ingestants, and "spontaneous" esophageal rupture. Esophagopericardial fistulas also develop from inflamed surgical and anastomotic suture lines in the esophagus and in patients with colonic interposition for esophageal lesions, resulting in a "thoracic colon"-to-pericardial fistula.

CLINICAL FEATURES. Symptoms and signs depend on the structures involved, including the pericardium itself. Patients may have acute pericarditis, pericardial effusion, pneumopericardium, pneumohydropericardium, or pneumopyopericardium with or without tamponade; any may be the presenting syndrome, including purulent pericarditis, preceding discovery of the fistula. Effusions are usually small and often loculated by adhesions from chronic inflammation. Esophagopericardial fistulas also follow chemical and physical trauma of the esophagus as well as malignancies, including esophageal, pulmonary, or rarely metastatic, and their radiation therapy. Usually there is a history of chronic peptic esophagitis, esophagogastric surgery, or malignancy. Pain can be retrosternal, in the left chest, or in the shoulders or interscapular. Most patients have fever, many have rubs, and patients with acute cases have shock, dyspnea, and cyanosis, any of which can be the initial symptom. A clue is discovery of a pneumohydropericardium or pneumopyopericardium with a "splashing mill wheel" sound. Whereas polymicrobial pericarditis[276, 277] is common, blood cultures may not be positive.

DRUG- AND TOXIN-RELATED PERICARDIAL DISEASE

Certain medications, toxic substances, and some irritants contacting the pericardium can induce acute or subacute pericarditis and effusion, tamponade, adhesions, fibrosis, or constriction (Table 50-13).[278] Anticoagulants and thrombolytic agents may cause an inflamed pericardium to bleed with tamponade or eventual adhesions and constriction, but this is not a specific "pericardiotoxic" effect. Drug and toxin responses are mostly acute pericarditis, inflammatory effusion, or, less commonly, hydropericardium. The importance of these relatively uncommon "pericardiopathies" is their diagnosis and its corollary: excluding other pericardial diseases. Most agents in Table 50-13 are used to treat specific diseases, many of which themselves can cause pericarditis or effusions. In general, acute reactions to these agents resolve when exposure ceases, but some can go on to constriction or recurrent pericarditis. Disorders for which many are given include malignancies, infections, and renal failure, each of which can cause pericarditis. Moreover, distinguishing drug- or toxin-induced pericarditis from idiopathic pericarditis is crucial so that exposure to a pericarditis-inducing agent must be considered in the differential diagnosis of idiopathic pericarditis. For every new case of pericarditis, a thorough history includes exposure to any drugs or noxious agents. Mechanisms include lupus reactions,[279] idiosyncrasy,[280] "serum sick-

▼ **TABLE 50–13. DRUG- AND TOXIN-RELATED PERICARDIAL DISEASE**

A. Drug-induced lupus erythematosus
    Procainamide
    Tocainide
    Hydralazine
    Methyldopa
    Mesalazine
    Reserpine
    Isoniazid
    Hydantoins (phenytoin, dantrolene)
    ? Quinidine

B. Hypersensitivity reaction (often with eosinophilia)
    Penicillins (ampicillin, procaine penicillin)
    Cromolyn sodium
    ? Praziquantel

C. "Idiosyncratic" or hypersensitivity

Methysergide	p-Aminosalicylic acid	5-Fluorouracil
Minoxidil (?also lupus)	Thiazides	Vaccines
Practolol	Streptomycin	Smallpox
Bromocriptine	Thiouracils	Yellow fever
Psicofuranine	Sulfa drugs	Granulocyte-macrophage
Polymer fume inhalation	Cyclophosphamide	colony-stimulating
Cytarabine	Cyclosporine	factor
Phenylbutazone	Amiodarone	
Amiodarone	Mesalazine (Rowasa)	
Streptokinase		

D. Anthracycline derivatives
    Doxorubicin
    Daunorubicin

E. Serum sickness
    Foreign antisera (e.g., antitetanus)
    Blood products

F. Venom
    Scorpion fish sting

G. Foreign-substance reactions (direct pericardial application)
    Talc (magnesium silicate)
    Silicones
    Tetracycline and other sclerosants
    Asbestos

H. Secondary pericardial bleeding/hemopericardium
    Anticoagulants
    Thrombolytic agents

ness,"[281] foreign substance reactions, and immunopathy[282] (see Table 50–13).

IDIOPATHIC PERICARDITIS: PERICARDITIS OF UNKNOWN ETIOLOGY (NONSPECIFIC PERICARDITIS)

No disease is sui genres (i.e., truly idiopathic); rather, etiology is not demonstrable at the contemporary state of knowledge. "Idiopathic" now means "of unknown etiology," usually a syndrome resembling viral pericarditis.[283] Idiopathic pericarditis, that is, any attack resolving without diagnosis, is the most common form of acute pericarditis. However, many diseases can present first as a pericardial disorder. Examples include the vasculitis/connective tissue disease group in which a pericarditic initial presentation is not recognized, particularly lupus; unrecognized myocardial infarction first becoming symptomatic as myocardial infarction pericarditis or even post-myocardial infarction syndrome; aortic dissection; primary and metastatic malignancies; pulmonary embolism; some forms of acute tuberculous pericarditis; Lyme disease; traumatic pericarditis appearing late after trauma, including radiation pericarditis; the seronegative spondyloarthropathies and intestinal inflammatory diseases; acute pancreatitis first presenting as pericardial effusion. Rare diseases exemplify the extreme etiological range, for example, "yellow-nail syndrome," eosinophilic fasciitis (with pericarditis preceding eosinophilia), and celiac disease with dermatitis herpetiformis[284] (here recurrent pericarditis responds to a gluten-free diet). Whereas undiagnosed acute pericarditis with or without effusion often is safely attributed to viral infection, the remarkable range must be considered. Recurrent "idiopathic" pericarditis tends to follow a pattern seen in viral pericarditis. With a missed, (but nonviral) pathogenesis, the causal disease surfaces after the index pericarditis or during a recurrence.[283] In all large prospective studies of patients with acute pericarditis, the largest single group, often the majority, is "idiopathic," often because there have not been comprehensive searches for evidence of viral infection or systemic diseases such as lupus. Treatment is as usual for acute, clinically dry pericarditis and for effusion and tamponade as needed. Eventual identification of any specific pathogenesis requires adequate follow-up and specific treatment.

RECURRENT AND INCESSANT PERICARDITIS

Perhaps 15 to 20 percent of patients do not recover permanently after an initial attack of acute pericarditis. Although exact incidences and natural histories are uncertain, most patients have had acute idiopathic, presumably or manifestly viral, pericarditis; in them, recurrent pericarditis, or continuously active incessant pericarditis, that is, mainly recurrent or incessant pericardial pain, appear to be immunopathic processses.[285] "Incessant" designates pericarditis (or identical pain) in patients who continuously need treatment to suppress symptoms. This can be extended to those who are free of symptoms for periods of less than 6 weeks, an arbitrary figure because of the usual failure of pericardiectomy to end these painful chronic syndrome. Postoperatively, nearly all patients have a brief, unexplained symptom-free 1- to 6-week period (a few patients either appear to be cured completely or for months to years before symptoms return).[285] It is possible that meticulous removal of nearly all the pericardium (pedestals must be left for the phrenic nerves) may yield improved results, but very long follow-up is needed. Anecdotal evidence suggests better results in the less common cases with recurrent pain who also have recurrent effusions.

INCESSANT PERICARDITIS. This condition involves continuous activity surfacing when antiinflammatory, usually corticosteroid, therapy is reduced or discontinued. Most such patients may be said to be "steroid hooked,"[285] a term of art, more dramatic than "steroid dependent," to reflect their desperation. In a minority, repeated or chronic exposure to the inciting agent or process is clearly responsible for recurrences, such as viral and bacterial reinfection (or reactivation of dormant organisms)[283-285] and, more commonly, systemic disorders, notably the vasculitis/connective tissue disease group, especially lupus. Certain pathogenetic possibilities may apply to recurrent and incessant pericarditis: (1) inadequate antiinflammatory treatment of the index or subsequent attack; (2) corticosteroid treatment given early during active viral multiplication that promotes and prolongs viral infection; (3) poorly understood cyclic immune or autoimmune responses to specific or nonspecific agents and processes such as respiratory infections or fatigue; and (4) viral RNA sequences in pericardial tissue acting as constant sources of antigen, although not themselves capable of replication.

RECURRENT IDIOPATHIC PERICARDITIS. "Idiopathic pericarditis" is usually of viral origin because its recurrences are virtually the same syndrome as recurrences after demonstrably viral pericarditis.[262] Recurrent idiopathic pericarditis is perhaps the greatest therapeutic challenge among all pericardial disorders and encompasses both intermittent and incessant forms. Recurrent idiopathic pericarditis and sterile recurrences after viral pericarditis are uncommon without a background of initial or continuing corticosteroid treatment. Characteristically, the incessant form has a threshold level of prednisone below which relapse is certain. Significant effusion is uncommon, and tamponade is rare during recurrences. Constriction appears not to occur in those without effusions.[285] Most recurrent pericarditis seems to represent individual pericardial reactivity to a variety of poorly understood pathogenetic processes and their corticosteroid suppression.

PERICARDIAL IMMUNOPATHY. Strong evidence that most recurrent pericarditis is immunopathic includes[8] (1) latent period after the index attack lasting days to years but usually months; (2) AHAs in some cases, probably those with significant myopericarditis in the index attack; (3) similarity to illnesses such as the post-myocardial infarction and postpericardiotomy syndromes (related to no. 2); (4) frequent allergic personal and/or family history; (5) rapid response to corticosteroid therapy and relapses with decreasing dose or discontinuance; (6) acute recurrent pericarditis during allergic disorders such as reactions to drugs and in celiac disease and dermatitis herpetiformis to foods with gluten; (7) acute recurrent pericarditis in classic serum sickness, including reactions to immunizations (e.g., for smallpox, yellow fever, hepatitis); (8) recurrent pericarditis in diseases of demonstrably autoimmune pathogenesis such as lupus; (9) occasional occurrence with other serositis, mainly pleuritis and rarely peritonitis; (10) frequent arthralgias especially in the post-myocardial infarction and postpericardiotomy syndromes as well as arthritis in the vasculitides; and (11) occasional eosinophilia.

CLINICAL ASPECTS. Recurrences vary from one to dozens over periods of weeks to decades. In no individual cases are patterns of recurrence precisely predictable except during corticosteroid weaning with an established threshold level for recurrence. Some patients can predict a relapse, and symptoms are usually stereotyped for each patient. All have pain resembling pain of the index attack often with strong pleuritic components, which is best described as "annoying" and "disabling" making life unpleasant. Objective manifestations are much less uniform and, while frequently detectable in the first recurrence, often become less common.[285] If significant effusion does not accompany the first recurrence, it is less likely subsequently. Exceptional patients have increasing severity in recurrences during which tamponade may first appear.

Recurrent idiopathic pericarditis is frequently of remote viral origin. Enterovirus-specific IgM responses have been found in many patients with chronic relapsing pericarditis, whereas comparable patients after acute enterovirus, mainly coxsackievirus B, infections elsewhere have only transient evidence of viral infection. Yet, among patients with acute pericarditis the level of IgM antibody was significantly higher in those who later experienced relapse. Host genetic factors are suggested by significantly higher levels of HLA-A2 haplotypes in those who were IgM positive (although extracardiac sites of viral persistence could not be excluded).[285] Thus, many patients with recurrent pericarditis experience persistent viral antigenic stimulation. Recurrences frequently follow new exposure to or infection by viral illnesses. It is not clear why constrictive pericarditis can follow a single attack of viral pericarditis while recurrent pericarditis after repeated comparable "idiopathic" attacks appears not to constrict.

NONIDIOPATHIC RECURRENT PERICARDITIS. Although rare, it is axiomatic that reexposure of susceptible patients to bacterial, particularly tuberculous, and other infections can result in recurrent pericarditis[285-287] and constriction can ensue. Hemopericardium, particularly with pericardial injury, can be associated with recurrent pericarditis.[285] The post-cardiac injury syndromes are especially prone to recurrence. The most important systemic disorders are the vasculitis/connective tissue disease group, especially lupus. In young patients with beta-thalassemia, the frequency of recurrent pericarditis remains unexplained. Recurrent pericarditis with inflammatory bowel disease is on a fairly firm immunopathic basis, as is that accompanying dermatitis herpetiformis, with immune complex deposition as a common basis of recurrent pericarditis.[285] The recurrent polyserositis of familial Mediterranean fever involves the pericardium less often than other serosae and only rarely constricts. Recurrences are in the group with hypersensitivity and manifest "allergy" usually after exposures to ingestants, inhalants, and injectants.

MANAGEMENT. For a confirmed etiology there may be specific therapy. For most patients with recurrent "idiopathic" pericarditis, treatment has been difficult. Patients with the incessant form are corticosteroid dependent. Patients with the intermittent form require treatment only for relapses. Thus the most important preventive consideration is to avoid corticosteroid therapy if possible and to wean patients judiciously from a corticosteroid, relying on aspirin or other NSAIDs, particularly ibuprofen. Immunosuppressive and cytotoxic drugs used in oncology and organ transplantation[288] have not proved effective for recurrent pericarditis. Any effective NSAID may be tried at the lowest adequate dose. Observation is required for gastrointestinal and other side effects, including renal damage partic-

ularly in older patients. The largest challenge, requiring high NSAID doses, its to wean "steroid hooked" patients. Without appropriately designed controlled trials, absolute recommendations cannot be given. "Experience" is a potentially useful alternative. It appears that escalating doses of ibuprofen while slowly reducing prednisone gives good results. Treatment must be individually fine tuned. A "standard decrement" of 1 mg of prednisone permits individualized determination of the intervals between dose reductions (e.g. 1 week to 2 months) while introducing colchicine[289] and increasing ibuprofen doses beginning with 800 mg every 8 hours, if the patient can tolerate it under careful observation and gastrointestinal mucosal protection.

Recurrent Pericardial Effusion. If large or with any degree of tamponade, these should be drained by catheter for several days, while maintaining drug therapy.[285] Failure indicates pericardiectomy.

Exercise Restriction. Personal experience suggests that exercise contributes to exacerbations and recurrences and that restriction of exercise can be a decisive component of treatment in these difficult cases. Absence of appropriately designed controlled trials limits the objectivity of exercise restriction. It is uncertain exactly how to "prescribe" this, but it seems worthwhile.

Radiation Pericardial Disease

Radiation therapy, particularly for Hodgkin disease and other lymphomas and malignancies of the breast, lung or thyroid, involves the pericardium variably, depending on radiation dose, duration of treatment, volume of heart in the field, and radiation source.[236, 290, 291] Incidence increases with survival and follow-up time. (Improved radiation dosing delivery and subcarinal shielding have decreased pericardial involvement.) Peak incidence remains 5 to 9 months after radiation therapy. Prognosis is generally favorable for the pericardial lesion. But, because most significant pericardial involvement is delayed, irradiated patients remain indefinitely susceptible.

PATHOGENESIS. Of all cardiac structures the pericardium is most susceptible to radiation injury, with pericardial syndromes sometimes complicated by injury of the myocardium, coronary arteries, or valves. Although direct radiation injury can be demonstrated, most patients escape significant involvement, raising questions of triggering latent antigens or viral infections, particularly in the delayed forms. Effusions may be serous, sanguineous, or serosanguineous with high concentrations of protein and lymphocytes resembling malignant effusion.[245] Late thickening is more conspicuous in the parietal pericardium with or without occult or obvious constriction. Microvascular ischemia and collagenization of fibrinous exudates contributes to pericardial fibrosis. Radiation involving more than 50 percent of heart volume and delivering over 2500 rads, or 40 to 60 Gy, increases risk with increasing dose and volume of heart irradiation.

CLINICAL ASPECTS.[236, 290] Involvement extends from immediate to variably delayed acute, subacute, and especially chronic syndromes. Acute pericarditis, with or without tamponade, is uncommon, but pericardial rubs are frequent during or within weeks of therapy. Oddly, acute syndromes do not correlate with late disease. Echocardiography shows some effusion in all patients with clinical findings. Subacute disease may appear over months, including effusion, constriction, or effusive-constrictive pericarditis. More common are chronic effusion or constriction, even after years of latency, so that other disease must be considered separately or as a precipitant, raising the question of whether radiation injury makes the pericardium more susceptible to infections. Occult constrictive pericarditis (see p. 1853) is relatively common and identified by catheter monitoring of an intravenous saline challenge.

DIAGNOSIS. Although CT and MRI are more sensitive and specific, TEE is excellent to define the anatomical lesions.[236] Occult constriction may be overlooked in patients with nonspecific complaints (exertional dyspnea, edema, chest pains), which may be attributed to their primary illness. However, radiation therapy is the major cause of combined pericardial constriction and restrictive cardiomyopathy, with the latter a notorious cause of a poor result from pericardiectomy (see p. 1853).

TREATMENT. Mild acute pericarditis and noncompressing effusion do not require specific therapy. Usually, there is no reason to discontinue radiation. Prednisone may be needed for intractable pain but does not prevent constriction. Overt constriction necessitates pericardiectomy, always considering the patient's prognosis and quality of life. Radiation constriction presents technical challenges to the surgeon, and severe involvement of the pulmonary vessels and heart may make it unsuccessful.

Chronic Pericardial Effusion and Chronic Cardiac Tamponade

Chronic pericardial effusion represents excessive pericardial fluid remaining, arbitrarily, for at least 3 months.[292, 293] The vast majority are "idiopathic," presumably autoimmune, or follow viral or other burnt out infections and are large to massive. Chronicity with slow fluid formation permits greater relaxation of the parietal pericardium so that chronic effusions present for 6 months to many years can reach 3 or 4 liters, particularly if of inflammatory origin. Few patients give a history of acute pericarditis.

ETIOLOGY. Pyogenic bacteria have been found in chronic pericardial exudates. Tuberculosis and actinomycosis and other fungi can cause chronic effusions including pericardial cold abscesses.[292] Although pericardial trauma can cause acute tamponade or constriction, it may be followed by chronic hemopericardium[294] and also is occasionally associated with some neoplasms, including primary pericardial sarcoma and Kaposi sarcoma, and various hemorrhagic diseases.[293, 294] The main connective tissue and related disorders associated with chronic effusions include lupus, rheumatic heart disease, scleroderma, polyarteritis, and especially rheumatoid arthritis.[295] *Lymphopericardium* is uncommon and follows lymphatic obstruction, lymphangioma, or rarely communication of thoracic duct and pericardium (usually after cardiothoracic surgery; also implicated in *chylopericardium*). Chronic effusive *cholesterol pericarditis* has multiple causes. *Endomyocardial fibrosis* may be accompanied by and present as a large hydropericardium. Congenital heart lesions, especially atrial septal defect, and *atrial thrombi* rarely are associated with massive chronic effusion. *Irradiation* for thoracic and cervical tumors can produce large, slowly absorbed or nonabsorbed effusions. Metabolic causes include *myxedema* and *uremia*. Hematological disorders associated with chronic pericardial effusion include *polycythemia* and severe, mainly "congenital" anemias—notably *thalassemia* and *pernicious anemia;* rarely, *heterotopic myelopoiesis* in the pericardium provokes a large effusion.[292]

PATHOLOGICAL CHARACTERISTICS. Structural abnormalities and fluid characteristics largely depend on causative disorders. Pericardial tissue usually shows no acute changes and may be strictly fibrotic with adhesions and loculations, sometimes with cyst formation. Specific histological changes are uncommon even in cases related to known diseases.[296] Yet subacute inflammation and fibrinous pericarditis is occasionally superimposed on chronic changes.[292] The fluid, especially in idiopathic chronic effusion, is usually clear and straw colored with mainly exudative characteristics. However, transudate and exudate borderlines may be indistinct. Inflammatory fluids are more often under pressure, producing chronic tamponade with or without associated constriction. Pericardial calcification is occasional and usually confined to the visceral pericardium. Constriction[292, 296, 297] is not rare with chronic effusions of inflammatory origin. Such effusions may contribute independently to cardiac compression depending on an unyielding scarred parietal pericardium. Moreover, constrictive epicarditis is a principal cause of constriction with chronic effusion (i.e., *chronic effusive-constrictive pericar-*

ditis). Yet many large chronic effusions, even with pericardial calcification, do not develop significant constriction or tamponade. Constriction sometimes develops rapidly after drainage of long-standing effusions, possibly by exciting previously low-grade inflammation.[292]

PATHOPHYSIOLOGY.[292, 298] Chronic effusions may have four effects[292]: (1) slow production of small amounts of undetected fluid; (2) demonstrable effusion without symptoms or signs of cardiac compression; (3) smaller or larger effusions compressing the heart but stabilized by compensatory mechanisms; and (4) recurrent or progressive chronic cardiac tamponade. The physiological borderline between a stabilized compressing effusion and progressive tamponade is indistinct; tamponade, acute or chronic, is not "all or none." (In some patients with congestive failure and hydropericardium, drainage decreases both pericardial pressure and cardiac pressures, indicating mild cardiac compression.) If pericardial pressure is elevated but less than RA pressure, drainage reduces only the pericardial pressure. In either case, mean atrial pressures and ventricular diastolic pressures significantly differ from pericardial pressure—in contrast to overt tamponade.[292]

PHYSICAL EFFECTS.[292] Large effusions may encroach on contiguous structures, causing restrictive pulmonary impairment, dyspnea on exertion, hoarseness, hiccough and dysphagia, and a Bamberger-Pins-Ewart sign.

Chronic Cardiac Tamponade

Chronic tamponade resembles chronic constrictive pericarditis. Diminution of cardiac output is comparable.[292-298] Compensatory mechanisms resemble acute tamponade, but circulating blood volume is more expanded. Many patients tolerate even massive chronic effusions amazingly well with minimal or no symptoms and signs, at least at rest.[292, 293] Others reach a stage of relentlessly increasing cardiac compression or one of prolonged debility with complications due to chronically diminished cardiac output and congested viscera.

CLINICAL MANIFESTATIONS. Most symptoms and signs are ascribable to the large pericardial mass, any chronic cardiac compression, and residual pericardial inflammation, modified by any cardiac disease.[272] Chronicity makes symptoms "late" or nil; and such quiet chronic effusions, particularly if "idiopathic," are often accidentally discovered.[292] Symptoms and signs can resemble those of acute effusions or tamponade. However, many patients have vague chest discomfort and chronic fatigue, anorexia, and weight loss.

COURSE.[292-296] The course varies according to pathogenetic factors; bland versus actively inflammatory effusion; pure chronic tamponade; or effusive-constrictive pericarditis. With tamponade, patients tend to develop atrial fibrillation as well as myocardial atrophy (with chronicity); liver congestion,[296] which can ultimately induce "cardiac cirrhosis"; the nephrotic syndrome; or protein-losing enteropathy. Complications may also be precipitated by systemic or respiratory infections.

DIAGNOSIS.[292-298] Identifying pericardial fluid and tamponade by clinical and graphic methods is the same as for acute effusion and tamponade. The ECG is of little value. Low voltage is probably related to myocardial atrophy, fluid retention, and any pleural as well as pericardial effusion.[292] Etiological diagnosis is not possible in most "idiopathic" cases. Pericardial fluid and tissue obtained surgically, by biopsy or necropsy, may yield evidence from appropriate bacteriological, immunological, and histological techniques; and histologically "nonspecific" tissue may yield evidence of prior infection such as traces of tuberculous or viral RNA sequences.

MANAGEMENT.[296, 297] Treatment of chronic effusion is individualized considering presence or absence of (1) cardiac compression, (2) a detectable causative disorder, (3) inflammatory manifestations, and (4) symptoms due to encroachment on adjacent structures. In general, inflammatory effusions tend to require surgical intervention sooner or later particularly if with chronic tamponade; noninflammatory effusions usually respond to treatment of associated disease. Aspiration of pleural effusions and ascites can contribute to symptomatic relief as well as preoperative management. Search for a cause is mandatory, particularly for specific therapeutic targets such as tuberculosis, toxoplasmosis, or myxedema. Management in general is the same as for acute pericardial effusion and tamponade and includes fluid and biopsy for diagnosis and biopsy and drainage for relief. However, drainage without resection is seldom adequate, particularly in idiopathic cases where refilling is common. Signs of persistent inflammation call for antiinflammatory therapy, particularly nonsteroidal agents. Nonabsorbable corticosteroids may be given intrapericardially. In patients for whom complete pericardial resection is not contemplated, chronic systemic congestion calls for sodium restriction and diuretics. Pericardiocentesis should be slow and intermittent to avoid cardiac overloading in patients with poor myocardial function[299]; expanded blood volume and any myocardial atrophy make overloading more likely than in acute tamponade. After paracentesis, incomplete or tardy improvement in the absence of refilling may be due to myocardial impairment; total failure to improve suggests constrictive epicarditis. While pericardiectomy remains a procedure of choice with or without tamponade, it may be postponed in occasional patients with sustained relief from paracentesis or restricted surgical drainage and appropriate medical measures. However, the tendency of inflammatory chronic effusions to eventually constrict and the morbidity from recurrences favor pericardiectomy.[292, 293] Pleuropericardial fenestration is feasible in patients in whom full thoracotomy or thoracoscopic resection are considered unwarranted, principally because of the patient's general condition. Balloon pericardiostomy has been successful. However, fenestration has important disadvantages, including (1) frequent resealing of the stoma, (2) impossibility of complete dependent drainage, (3) potential constrictive scarring due to irritation by the procedure, (4) inadequate inspection of the epicardium, and (5) incomplete removal of adhesive or inflamed and infected tissue.[292]

R E F E R E N C E S

PERICARDIAL ANATOMY AND PHYSIOLOGY

1. Spodick DH: Pericardial macro- and microanatomy: A synopsis. *In* Spodick DH: The Pericardium: A Comprehensive Textbook. New York, Marcel Dekker, 1997, pp 7–14.
2. Spodick DH: Macro- and micro-physiology and anatomy of the pericardium. Am Heart J 124:1046–1051, 1992.
3. Spodick DH: Physiology of the normal pericardium: Functions of the pericardium. *In* Spodick DH: The Pericardium: A Comprehensive Textbook. New York, Marcel Dekker, 1997, pp 15–26.
4. Hammond HK, White FC, Bhargava V, Shabetai R: Heart size and maximal cardiac output are limited by the pericardium. Am J Physiol 263: H1675–H1681, 1992.
4a. Spodick DH: Intrapericardial therapeutics and diagnostics (editorial). Am J Cardiol 85:1012–1014, 2000.
5. Tyberg JV, Smith ER: Ventricular diastole and the role of the pericardium. Hertz 15:354–361, 1990.
6. Santamore WP, Dell'Italia LJ: Ventricular interdependence: Significant left ventricular contributions to right ventricular systolic function. Prog Cardiovasc Dis 40:289–308, 1998.
7. Seferovic P, Ristic A, Maksimovic R, et al: Initial clinical experience with perDUCER device: Promising new tool in the diagnosis and treatment of the pericardial disease. Clin Cardiol 22(Suppl I):I30–I35, 1999.
8. Spodick DH: Microphysiology of the pericardium in relation to intrapericardial therapeutics and diagnostics. Clin Cardiol 22(Suppl I):I2–I3, 1999.

AUSCULTATORY PHENOMENA

9. Spodick DH: Auscultatory phenomena in pericardial disease. *In* Spodick DH: The Pericardium: A Comprehensive Textbook. New York, Marcel Dekker, 1997, pp 27–39.

10. Myers RBH, Spodick DH: Constrictive pericarditis: Clinical and pathophysiologic characteristics. Am Heart J 138:219–232, 1999.

ELECTROCARDIOGRAPHIC ABNORMALITIES

11. Spodick DH: Electrocardiographic abnormalities in pericardial disease. *In* Spodick DH: The Pericardium: A Comprehensive Textbook. New York, Marcel Dekker, 1997, pp 40–64.
12. Spodick DH: Mechanisms of acute pericardial and myocardial injury in pericardial disease. Chest 13:855–856, 1998.
13. Thaker RK, Souza JJ, Troup PJ, et al: Pericardial effusion increases defibrillation energy requirement. PACE 16:1227, 1993.

CONGENITAL ABNORMALITIES

14. Spodick DH: Congenital abnormalities of the pericardium. *In* Spodick DH: The Pericardium: A Comprehensive Textbook. New York, Marcel Dekker, 1997, pp 65–75.
15. Barva GL, Magliani L, Bertoli D, et al: Complicated pericardial cyst: Atypical anatomy and clinical course. Clin Cardiol 21:862–864, 1998.
16. Chopra PS, Duke DJ, Pellett JR, Rahko PS: Pericardial cyst with partial erosion of the right ventricular wall. Ann Thorac Surg 51:840–841, 1991.
17. Hsu T-L, Ho S-J, Wang S-P, et al: Enhanced delineation of pericardial diseases by three-dimensional echocardiography. J Am Coll Cardiol 29: 23a–24a, 1997.
18. Van Son JAM, Danielson GK, Schaff HV, et al: Congenital partial and complete absence of the pericardium. Mayo Clin Proc 68:743–747, 1993.
18a. Gatzoulis MA, Munk MD, Merchant N, et al: Isolated congenital absence of the pericardium: Clinical presentation, diagnosis, and management. Ann Thorac Surg 69:1209–1215, 2000.
19. Oki T, Tabata T, Yamada H, et al: Cross sectional echocardiographic demonstration of the mechanisms of abnormal interventricular septal motion in congenital total absence of the left pericardium. Heart 77: 247–251, 1997.
20. Marani SD, Brunazzi MC, Cotogni A, et al: Congenital absence of the left pericardium: Nuclear magnetic resonance and other imaging techniques. Am J Noninvas Cardiol 6:304–312, 1992.
21. Grassner I, Judmaier W, Fink C: Diagnosis of congenital pericardial defects, including a pathognomic sign for dangerous apical ventricular herniation, on magnetic resonance imaging. Br Heart J 74:60–66, 1995.
22. Rusk RA, Kenny A: Congenital pericardial defect presenting as chest pain. Heart 81:327–328, 1999.

ACQUIRED PERICARDIAL DISEASES

23. Spodick DH: Acquired pericardial disease: Pathogenesis and overview: *In* Spodick DH: The Pericardium: A Comprehensive Textbook. New York, Marcel Dekker, 1997, pp 76–93.
23a. Mehta SM, Myers JL: Congenital Heart Surgery Nomenclature and Database Project: Diseases of the pericardium. Ann Thorac Surg 69(4, Suppl):S191–S196, 2000.
24. Spodick DH: Post-myocardial infarction syndrome (Dressler's syndrome). ACC Curr J Rev 4:35–37, 1995.
25. Permanyer-Miralda G: Indications for pericardiectomy in the absence of constriction. In Soler-Soler J et al (eds): Pericardial Disease. Amsterdam, Kluwer Academic Publishers, 1990, pp 167–181.
26. Maisch B: Pericardial diseases, with the focus on etiology, pathogenesis, pathophysiology, new diagnostic imaging methods, and treatment. Curr Opin Cardiol 9:379–388, 1994.
27. Svedjeholm R, Jansson K, Olin C: Primary idiopathic chylopericardium—a case report and review of the literature. Eur J Cardiothorac Surg 11:387–390, 1997.
28. Yamazaki T, Maruoka S, Takahashi S, Sakamoto K: Lymphoscintigraphy of isolated chylopericardium. Clin Nucl Med 21:575, 1996.
29. Ford EJ, Bear PA, Adams RW: Cholesterol pericarditis causing cardiac tamponade. Am Heart J 122:877–879, 1991.
30. Gorecki PJ, Andrei VE, Schein M: Tension pneumopericardium in chest trauma. J Trauma 46:954–956, 1999.
31. Chapman PR, Boals JR: Pneumopericardium caused by giant gastric ulcer. AJR 171:1669–1670, 1998.
32. Tollens T, Casselman F, Devlieger H, et al: Fetal cardiac tamponade due to an intrapericardial teratoma. Ann Thorac Surg 66:59–60, 1998.
33. Harker LA: Hematologic and oncologic disorders. *In* Rapaport E (ed): Cardiology and Coexisting Disease. New York, Churchill Livingstone, 1994, pp 197–230.
34. Kees S, Langevitz P, Zemer D, et al: Attacks of pericarditis as a manifestation of familial Mediterranean fever (FMF). Q J Med 90:643–647, 1997.

ACUTE PERICARDITIS

35. Spodick DH: Acute, clinically noneffusive ("dry") pericarditis. *In* Spodick DH: The Pericardium: A Comprehensive Textbook. New York, Marcel Dekker, 1997, pp 94–113.
36. Zayas R, Anguita M, Torres F, et al: Incidence of specific etiology and

role of methods for specific etiologic diagnosis of primary acute pericarditis. Am J Cardiol 75:378–382, 1995.

37. Wise CM, Semble EL, Dalton CB: Musculoskeletal chest wall syndromes in patients with noncardiac chest pain: A study of 100 patients. Arch Phys Med Rehabil 73:147–149, 1992.

38. Ilan Y, Oren R, Ben-Chetrit E: Acute pericarditis: Etiology, treatment and prognosis: A study of 115 patients. Jpn Heart J 32:315–321, 1991.

39. Maisch B: Pericardial diseases, with focus on etiology, pathogenesis, pathophysiology, new diagnostic imaging methods, and treatment. Curr Opin Cardiol 9:379–388, 1994.

40. Matsouka H, Hamada M, Honda T, et al: Evaluation of acute myocarditis and pericarditis by Gd-DTPA enhanced magnetic resonance imaging. Eur Heart J 15:283–284, 1994.

41. Koch M, Dezi A, Ferrario F, Capurso L: Prevention of nonsteroidal anti-inflammatory drug-induced gastrointestinal mucosal injury. Arch Intern Med 156:2321–2332, 1996.

42. Adler Y, Finkelstein Y, Guindo J, et al: Colchicine treatment for recurrent pericarditis: A decade of experience. Circulation 97:2183–2185, 1998.

43. Spodick DH: Myopericarditis/perimyocarditis. In Spodick DH: The Pericardium: A Comprehensive Textbook. New York, Marcel Dekker, 1997, pp 114–126.

44. Brodison A, Swann JW: Myocarditis: A review. J Infect 37:99–103, 1998.

45. Barbaro G, Di Lorenzo G, Grisorio B, Barbarini G: Cardiac involvement in the acquired immunodeficiency syndrome: A multicenter clinical-pathologic study. J Heart Dis 1:9, 1999.

46. Maisch B, Herzum M, Hufnagel G, et al: Immunosuppressive treatment for myocarditis and dilated cardiomyopathy. Eur Heart J 16(Suppl O):153–161, 1995.

47. Maisch B, Outzen H, Roth D, et al: Prognostic determinants in conventionally treated myocarditis and perimyocarditis—focus on antimyolemmal antibodies. Eur Heart J 12(Suppl D):81–87, 1991.

48. King DL: Rhabdomyolysis with pericardial tamponade. Ann Emerg Med 23:583–585, 1994.

49. Lauer B, Niederau C, Kuhl U, et al: Cardiac troponin T in patients with clinically suspected myocarditis. J Am Coll Cardiol 30:1354–1359, 1997.

50. Goldstein JA: Differentiation of constrictive pericarditis and restrictive cardiomyopathy. ACC Ed Highlights 10:14–22, 1998.

51. Bergler-Klein J, Sochor H, Stanek G, et al: Indium 111-monoclonal antimyosin antibody and magnetic resonance imaging in the diagnosis of acute Lyme myopericarditis. Arch Intern Med 153:2696–2700, 1993.

52. Maisch B, Bethge C, Drude L, et al: Pericardioscopy and epicardial biopsy—new diagnostic tools in pericardial and perimyocardial disease. Eur Heart J 15(Suppl C):68–73, 1994.

53. Maisch B, Herzum M, Hufnagel G, Bittinger A: Connective or double viral infections in peri(myocarditis). Circulation 96:I697, 1947.

54. Garg A, Shiau J, Guyatt G: The ineffectiveness of immunosuppressive therapy in lymphocytic myocarditis: An overview. Ann Intern Med 128:317–322, 1998.

55. Rezkalla S, Koner RA, Khatib G, Khatib R: Beneficial effects of captopril in coxsackievirus B$_3$ murine myocarditis. Circulation 81:1039–1046, 1990.

56. Gravanis MB, Sternby NH: Incidence of myocarditis: A 10-year autopsy study from Malmo, Sweden. Arch Pathol Lab Med 115:390–392, 1992.

PERICARDIAL EFFUSION

57. Spodick DH: Pericardial effusion and hydropericardium without tamponade. In Spodick DH: The Pericardium: A Comprehensive Textbook. New York, Marcel Dekker, 1997, pp 126–152.

58. Riemann D, Wollert HG, Menschikowski J, et al: Immunophenotype of lymphocytes in pericardial fluid from patients with different forms of heart disease. Int Arch Allergy Immunol 104:48–56, 1994.

59. Merce J, Sagrista-Sauleda J, Permanyer-Miraldo G, Soler-Soler J: Should pericardial drainage be performed routinely in patients who have a large pericardial effusion without tamponade? Am J Med 105:106–109, 1998.

60. D'Cruz I, Rehem AU, Hancock HL: Quantitative echocardiographic assessment in pericardial disease. Echocardiography 14:207–213, 1997.

61. Vazquez de Prada JA, Jiang L, Handschumacher MD, et al: Quantifications of pericardial effusions by three-dimensional echocardiography. J Am Coll Cardiol 24:254–259, 1994.

62. Malmou-Mitsi VD, Zioga AP, Agnantis J: Diagnostic accuracy of pericardial fluid cytology: An analysis of 53 specimens from 44 consecutive patients. Diagn Cytopathol 15:197–204, 1996.

63. Myers DG, Meyers RE, Prendergast TW: The usefulness of diagnostic tests on pericardial fluid. Chest 111:1213–1221, 1997.

64. Spodick DH: Critical care of pericardial disease. In Rippe JM, Irwin RS, Alpert JS, Fink MP: Intensive Care Medicine. 2nd ed. Boston, Little, Brown, 1991, pp 282–295.

65. Callahan JA, Seward JB: Pericardiocentesis guided by two-dimensional echocardiography. J Am Coll Cardiol 14:497–504, 1997.

66. Tsang TSM, Freeman WK, Sinak LJ, Seward JB: Echocardiographically guided pericardiocentesis: Evolution and state-of-the-art technique. Mayo Clin Proc 73:647–652, 1998.

67. Spodick DH: Diagnostic interpretation of pericardial fluids. Chest 111:1156–1157, 1997.

CARDIAC TAMPONADE

68. Spodick DH: Pathophysiology of cardiac tamponade. Chest 113:1372–1378, 1998.

69. Spodick DH: Physiology of cardiac tamponade. In Spodick DH: The Pericardium: A Comprehensive Textbook. New York, Marcel Dekker, 1997, pp 180–190.

70. Reddy PS, Curtiss EI, Uretsky BF: Spectrum of hemodynamic changes in cardiac tamponade. Am J Cardiol 66:1487–1491, 1990.

71. Beloucif S, Takata M, Shimada M, Robotham JL: Influence of pericardial constraint on atrioventricular interactions. Am J Physiol 263(Heart Circ Physiol 32):H125–H134, 1992.

72. Spodick DH: The technique of pericardiocentesis. J Crit Illness 10:807–812, 1995.

73. Reydel B, Spodick DH: Frequency and significance of chamber collapses during cardiac tamponade. Am Heart J 119:1160–1163, 1990.

74. Di Segni E, Feinberg MS, Sheinowitz M, et al: Left ventricular pseudo-hypertrophy in cardiac tamponade: An echocardiographic study in a canine model. J Am Coll Cardiol 21:1286–1294, 1993.

75. Klopfenstein HS, Mathias DW: Influence of naloxone on response to acute cardiac tamponade in conscious dogs. Am J Physiol 259:H512–H517, 1990.

76. Angel J, Domingo E, Anivarro I, et al: Severity of hemodynamic impairment depending on the pattern of cardiac tamponade. Chest 102:128S, 1992.

77. Hoit BD, Fowler NO: Influence of acute right ventricular dysfunction on cardiac tamponade. J Am Coll Cardiol 18:1787–1793, 1991.

77a. Tamima M, Bartunek J, Weinberg EO, et al: Atrial natriuretic peptide has different effects on contractility and intracellular pH in normal and hypertrophied myocytes from pressure-overloaded hearts. Circulation 98:2760–2764, 1998.

78. Ramsaran EK, Benotti JR, Spodick DH: Exacerbated tamponade: Deterioration of cardiac function by lowering excessive arterial pressure in hypertensive cardiac tamponade. Cardiology 86:77–79, 1995.

79. Spodick DH: Cardiac tamponade: Clinical characteristics, diagnosis and management. In Spodick DH: The Pericardium: A Comprehensive Textbook. New York, Marcel Dekker, 1997, pp 153–179.

80. Spodick DH: Acute pericarditis, pericardial effusion, and cardiac tamponade. Bull Saudi Heart Assoc 2:67–76, 1990.

81. Delgado C, Barturen F: Atrial tamponade causing acute ischemic hepatic injury after cardiac surgery. Clin Cardiol 22:242–244, 1990.

82. Thompson RC, Finck SJ, Leventhal JP, Safford RE: Right-to-left shunt across a patent foramen ovale caused by cardiac tamponade: Diagnosis by transesophageal echocardiography. Mayo Clin Proc 66:391–394, 1991.

83. Spodick DH: Pulsus paradoxus. In Spodick DH: The Pericardium: A Comprehensive Textbook. New York, Marcel Dekker, 1997, pp 191–199.

84. Shabetai R: The effects of pericardial effusion on respiratory variations in hemodynamics and ventricular function. J Am Coll Cardiol 17:249–250, 1991.

85. Bhagwat AR, Hoit BD: Respiratory variation of carotid artery flow in cardiac tamponade. Am Heart J 132:1068–1070, 1996.

86. Spodick DH: Truly total electric alternation of the heart. Clin Cardiol 21:427–428, 1998.

87. Merce J, Sagrista-Sauleda J, Permanyer-Miralda G, et al: Correlation between clinical and Doppler echocardiographic findings in patients with moderate and large pericardial effusion: Implications for the diagnosis of cardiac tamponade. Am Heart J 138:759–764, 1999.

88. Mateos M, Carbello J, Garcia H, et al: Relationship between echocardiographic and hemodynamic signs of pericardial tamponade. Echocardiography 15:S43, 1998.

89. Feinberg MS, Popescu BA, Polpescu AC, et al: Transient left ventricular remodelling as a measure of left ventricular compression in patients with cardiac tamponade. Eur Heart J 20(Abstr suppl): 626, 1999.

90. Renkin J, Carler M, De Man P, et al: Cardiogenic shock developing within 48 hours after thrombolysis for acute anterior myocardial infarction may be related to hemorrhagic cardiac tamponade without rupture. J Am Coll Cardiol 29:14A, 1997.

91. D'Cruz KA, Calderon E, Kuri K, Shearin S: Left ventricular diastolic compression in acquired immunodeficiency syndrome with large, non-loculated pericardial effusion. Am Heart J 133:383–384, 1997.

92. D'Cruz IA, Rouse C, Pitts J: Tamponade with focal intrapericardial adhesions: Echocardiographic diagnosis. J Noninvas Cardiol 2:34–36, 1997.

93. Djaiani G, Major E: Pneumopericardium: An unusual cause for cardiac arrest. Anesthesia 53:580–588, 1998.

94. Gorecki PJ, Andrei VE, Schein M: Tension pneumopericardium in chest trauma. J Trauma 46:954–956, 1999.

95. Torelli J, Marwick TH, Salcedo EE: Left atrial tamponade: Diagnosis by transesophageal echocardiography. J Am Soc Echocardiogr 4:413–414, 1991.

96. Spodick DH: Normal and abnormal physiology and diseases of the pericardium. Curr Opin Cardiol 8:496–501, 1993.

97. Angel J, Anivarro I, Domingo E, Soler-Soler J: Cardiac tamponade: Risk and benefit of fluid challenge performed while waiting for pericardiocentesis. Circulation 96:I30, 1997.

98. Spodick DH: Medical treatment of cardiac tamponade. In Caturelli G (ed): Cura intensiva Cardiologica 1991. Rome, TIPAR Poligrafica, 1991, pp 265–268.

99. Spodick DH: Progress in investigation of effusion and tamponade, immunosupression, and constriction in pericarditis and pericardial diseases. Curr Opin Cardiol 7:476–481, 1992.

100. Seferovic PM, Ristic AD, Petrovic P, et al: Percutaneous balloon pericardiotomy with a small size trefoil balloon: A viable treatment option for neoplastic pericardial effusion. Eur Heart J 19:521, 1998.

101. Tsang TSM, Barnes ME, Hayes SN, et al: Clinical and echocardiographic characteristics of significant pericardial effusions following cardiothoracic surgery and outcomes of echo-guided pericardiocentesis for management. Chest 116:322–331, 1999.

102. Spodick DH: Noneffusive sequelae of pericardial inflammation. In Spodick DH: The Pericardium: A Comprehensive Textbook. New York, Marcel Dekker, 1997, pp 200–213.

103. Nkere UU, Whawell SA, Sarraf CE, et al: Perioperative histologic and ultrastructural changes in the pericardium and adhesions. Ann Thorac Surg 58:437–444, 1994.

104. Alio-bosch J, Candell-Riera J, Monge-Rangel L, Soler-Soler J: Intrapericardial echocardiographic images and cardiac constriction. Am Heart J 121:207–208, 1991.

105. Hinds SW, Reisner SA, Ammico AF, Meltzer RS: Diagnosis of pericardial abnormalities by 2D-echo: A pathology-echocardiography correlation in 85 patients. Am Heart J 123:143–150, 1992.

106. D'Cruz IA, Jarrett J, Gross CM, Rogers W: Modification of the echocardiographic features of tamponade by intrapericardial adhesions. Am J Noninvas Cardiol 6:69–74, 1992.

107. Duvernoy O, Malm T, Thuomas KA, et al: CT and MR evaluation of pericardial and retrosternal adhesions after cardiac surgery. J Comput Assist Tomogr 15:555–560, 1991.

108. Spodick DH, Southern JF: A 55-year old man with recurrent pericarditis and pleural effusions after aortic valve replacement: Case Records of the Massachusetts General Hospital, case 32-1992. N Engl J Med 326:1550–1557, 1992.

CONSTRICTIVE PERICARDITIS

109. Myers RBH, Spodick DH: Constrictive percarditis: Clinical and pathophysiologic characteristics. Am Heart J 138:219–232, 1999.

110. Spodick DH: Constrictive pericarditis. In Spodick DH: The Pericardium: A Comprehensive Textbook. New York, Marcel Dekker, 1997, pp 214–259.

111. Lieng LH, Oh JK, Seward JB, et al: Clinical profile of constrictive pericarditis in the modern era: A survey of 135 cases. J Am Coll Cardiol 27:32a–33a, 1996.

112. Bell SP, Fabian J, Watkins MW, LeWinter MM: Decrease in forces responsible for diastolic suction during acute coronary occlusion. Circulation 96:2348–2352, 1997.

113. RuscONI C, Ghizzoni G, Sabatini T, et al: Delayed left ventricular early filling with aging: Loss of restoring forces? J Cardiovasc Diag Proc 14:47–51, 1997.

114. Akasaka T, Yoshida K, Yamamuro A, et al: Phasic coronary flow characteristics in patients with constrictive pericarditis: Comparison with restrictive cardiomyopathy. Circulation 96:1874–1881, 1997.

115. Anand IS, Phil D, Ferrari R, et al: Pathogenesis of edema in constrictive pericarditis. Circulation 83:1880–1887, 1991.

116. Barshar M, Shala A, D'Cruz IA, et al: Echocardiography of the inferior vena cava, superior vena cava, and coronary sinus in right heart failure. Echocardiography 15:787–792, 1998.

117. Oren RM, Grover-Mckay M, Stanford W, Wiess RM: Accurate preoperative diagnosis of percardial constriction using cine computed tomography. J Am Coll Cardiol 22:832–838, 1993.

118. Rienmuller R, Gurgan M, Erdmann E, et al: CT and MR evaluation of pericardial constriction. J Thorac Imag 8:108–121, 1993.

119. D'Cruz I, Rehman AU, Hancock HL: Quantitative echocardiographic assessment in pericardial disease. Echocardiography 14:207–213, 1997.

120. Thamilarasan M, Schvartzman PR, White RD, Klein AL: The accuracy of transesophageal echocardiography in the assessment of pericardial thickness in patients with constrictive pericarditis: A comparison with magnetic resonance imaging. Circulation 100:I294, 1999.

121. Boonyaratavej S, Oh JK, Tajik AJ, et al: Comparison of mitral inflow and superior vena cava Doppler velocities in chronic obstructive pulmonary disease and constrictive pericarditis. J Am Coll Cardiol 32:2043–2048, 1998.

122. Oh JK, Tajik AJ, Appleton CP, et al: Preload reduction to unmask the characteristic Doppler features of constrictive pericarditis: A new observation. Circulation 95:796–799, 1997.

123. Gola A, Leuzzi S, Valle F, et al: Right to left ventricular interaction might trigger Valsalva-induced syncope. Circulation 90:I316, 1994.

124. Garcia MJ, Rodriguez L, Ares M, et al: Differentiation of constrictive pericarditis from restrictive cardiomyopathy. Assessment of left ventricular diastolic velocities in longitudinal axis by Doppler tissue imaging. J Am Coll Cardiol 27:108–114, 1996.

125. Spodick DH: Constrictive pericarditis versus restrictive cardiomyopathy: Difficult differential diagnosis. J Heart Dis 1:112, 1999.

126. Cohen GI, Pietrolungo JF, Thomas JD, Klien AL: A practical guide to assessment of ventricular diastolic function using Doppler echocardiography. J Am Coll Cardiol 27:17530–17560, 1996.

127. Garcia MJ, Thomas JD: Tissue Doppler to assess diastolic left ventricular function. Echocardiography 16:501–508, 1999.

128. Singh M, Juneja R, Bali HK, Varma JS: Autonomic functions in restrictive cardiomyopathy and constrictive pericarditis: A comparison. Am Heart J 136:443–448, 1998.

129. Tirilomis T, Univerdorben S, von der Emde J: Pericardectomy for chronic constrictive pericarditis: Risks and outcome. Eur J Cardiothorac Surg 8:487–492, 1994.

130. Buckingham RE, Furnary AP, Weaver MT, et al: Mitral insufficiency after percardiectomy for constrictive pericarditis. Ann Thorac Surg 58:1171–1174, 1994.

131. Kuroda H, Sakaguchi M, Takano T, et al: Intraoperative monitoring of pressure-volume loops of the left ventricle in pericardectomy for constrictive pericarditis. J Thorac Cardiovasc Surg 112:198–199, 1996.

131a. Ling LH, Oh JK, Schaff HV, et al: Constrictive pericarditis in the modern era: Evolving clinical spectrum and impact on outcome after pericardiectomy. Circulation 100:1380–1386, 1999.

INFECTIOUS PERICARDITIS

132. Spodick DH: Infectious pericarditis. In Spodick DH: The Pericardium: A Comprehensive Textbook. New York, Marcel Dekker, 1997, pp 260–290.

133. Maisch B, Outzen H, Roth D, et al: Prognostic determinants in conventionally treated myocarditis and perimyocarditis—focus on antimyolemmal antibodies. Eur Heart J 12:81–87, 1991.

134. Maisch B, Herzum M, Hufnagel G, Bittinger A: Consecutive or double viral infections in peri (myocarditis). Circulation 96:I697, 1997.

135. Fujioka S, Koide H, Kitaura Y, et al: Molecular detection and differentiation of enteroviruses in endomyocardial biopsies and pericardial effusions from dilated cardiomyopathy and myocarditis. Am Heart J 131:760–765, 1996.

136. Finkelstein Y, Adler Y, Nussinovitch M, et al: A new classification for pericarditis associated with meningococcal infection. Eur J Pediatr 156:585–588, 1997.

137. Coupland DB, Terriff B, Fung AY, Sartori C: The "hot halo" sign: Pyogenic pericarditis on In-111 leukocyte scintigraphy. Clin Nucl Med 17:579–580, 1992.

138. Meyers DG, Meyers RE, Prendergast TW: The usefulness of dianostic tests on pericardial fluid. Chest 111:1213–1221, 1997.

139. Golub RJ, McNulty CM, McClellan JR, et al: Usefulness of transesophageal-Doppler echocardiography in the surgical drainage of a loculated purulent pericardial effusion. Am Heart J 126:724–727, 1993.

140. Mann Segal DD, Shanahan EA, Jones B, Ramasamy D: Purulent pericarditis: Rediscovery of an old remedy. J Thorac Cardiovasc Surg 111:487–488, 1996.

141. Fowler NO: Turberculous pericarditis. JAMA 266:99–103, 1991.

141a. Afzal A, Keohane M, Keeley E, et al: Myocarditis and pericarditis with tamponade associated with disseminated tuberculosis. Can J Cardiol 16:519–521, 2000.

142. Kishk YT, Allam MH, Abdel-Wahab AM: Subclinical pericarditis in 289 patients with pulmonary tuberculosis; further indirect evidence by analysis of 53 patients with pericardial disease. J Am Coll Cardiol 31:220–230, 1998.

143. Suwan PK, Potjalongsilp S: Predictors of constrictive pericarditis after tuberculous pericarditis. Br Heart J 73:187–189, 1995.

144. Ng TTC, Strang JIC, Wilkins EGL: Serodiagnosis of pericardial tuberculosis. Q J Med 88:317–320, 1995.

145. Mueller XM, Tevaearai HT, Hurni M, et al: Etiologic diagnosis of pericardial disease: The value of routine tests during surgical procedures. J Am Coll Surg 184:645–649, 1997.

146. Dogan R, Demircin M, Sarigul A, et al: Diagnostic value of adenosine deaminase activity in pericardial fluids. J Cardiovasc Surg 40:501, 1999.

147. Shah S, Miller A, Mastellone A, et al: Rapid diagnosis of tuberculosis in various biopsy and body fluid specimens by the AMPLICOR Mycobacterium tuberculosis polymerase chain reaction test. Chest 113:1190–1194, 1998.

148. Rana BS, Jones RA, Simpson IA: Recurrent pericardial effusion: The value of polymerase chain reaction in the diagnosis of tuberculosis. Heart 82:246–247, 1999.

148a. Mayosi BM, Volmink JA, Commerford PJ: Interventions for treating tuberculous pericarditis. Cochrane Database Syst Rev (2):CD000526, 2000.

149. Chen WT, Chen CC, Yu FC, et al: Clinical response of tuberculous pericarditis to medical treatment: A retrospective survey. Chin Med J 58:7–11, 1996.

150. Cishek MB, Yost B, Schaefer S: Cardiac aspergillosis presenting as myocardial infarction. Clin Cardiol 19:824–827, 1996.

151. Wheat J: Histoplasmosis: Experience during outbreaks in Indianapolis and review of the literature. Medicine 76:339–354, 1997.

152. Rabinovici R, Szewczyk D, Ovadia P, et al: Candida pericarditis: Clinical profile and treatment. Ann Thorac Surg 63:1200–1204, 1997.

153. Canver CC, Patel AK, Kosolcharoen P, Voytovich MC: Fungal purulent constrictive pericarditis in a heart transplant patient. Ann Thorac Surg 65:1792–1794, 1998.

154. Beier KH, Rusnak RA: Unusual presentation of cervicothoracic actinomycosis complicated by pericardial effusion: A case report. J Emerg Med 15:303–307, 1997.

155. Gouny P, Lancelin C, Girard PM, et al: Percardial effusion and AIDS: Benefits of surgical drainage. Eur J Cardiothorac Surg 13:165–169, 1998.

156. Chyu KY, Birnbaum Y, Naqvi T, et al: Echocardiographic detection of Kaposi's sarcoma causing cardiac tamponade in a patient with acquired immunodeficiency syndrome. Clin Cardiol 21:131–133, 1998.

157. Cesarman E, Chang Y, Moore PS, et al: Kaposi's sarcoma–associated herpesvirus-like DNA sequences in AIDS-related body-cavity–based lymphomas. N Engl J Med 332:1186–1191, 1995.

158. Lazarevic AM, Neskovic AN, Goronja M, et al: Low incidence of cardiac abnormalities in treated trichinosis: A prospective study of 62 patients from a single-source outbreak. Am J Med 107:18–23, 1999.

159. Bashour TT, Alali RK, Mason DT, Saalouke M; Echinococcosis of the heart: Clinical and echocardiographic features in 19 patients. Am Heart J 132:1028–1030, 1996.

160. Birincioglu CL, Bardakci H, Kucuker SA, et al: A clinical dilemma: Cardiac and pericardiac echinococcosis. Ann Thorac Surg 68:1290–1294, 1999.

161. Bruyn GA, de Koning J, Reijsoo FJ, et al: Lyme pericarditis leading to tamponade. Br J Rheumatol 33:862–866, 1994.

162. Bergler-Klein J, Sochor H, Stanek G, et al: Indium 111-monoclonal antimyosin antibody and magnetic resonance imaging in the diagnosis of acute Lyme myopericarditis. Arch Intern Med 153:2696–2700, 1993.

163. Valero F, de Groote P, Millaire A, et al: Pericardial effusion as the initial feature of Q fever. Am Heart J 130:1308–1309, 1995.

164. Nilsson K, Lindquist O, Pahlson C: Association of Rickettsia helvetica with chronic perimyocarditis in sudden cardiac death. Lancet 354:1169–1173, 1999.

PERICARDIAL DISEASE IN METABOLIC DISORDERS

165. Spodick DH: Pericarditis in systemic disease. Cardiol Clin 8:709–716, 1990.

166. Spodick DH: Pericardial disease in metabolic disorders. In Spodick DH: The Pericardium: A Comprehensive Textbook. New York, Marcel Dekker, 1997, pp 291–300.

167. Sever MS, Steinmuller DR, Hayes JM, et al: Pericarditis following renal transplantation. Transplantation 51:1229, 1991.

168. Preston RA, Chakko S, Materson BJ: End-stage renal disease. In Rapaport E (ed): Cardiology and Co-existing Disease. New York, Churchill Livingstone, 1994, pp 175–194.

169. Duvernoy O, Borowiec J, Helmius G, Erikson U: Complications of percutaneous pericardiocentesis under fluoroscopic guidance. Acta Radiol 33:309–314, 1992.

170. Kabadi UM, Kumer SP: Pericardial effusion in primary hypothyroidism. Am Heart J 120:1393, 1990.

171. Bereket A, Yang TF, Dey S, et al: Cardiac decompensation due to massive pericardial effusion: A manifestation of hypothyroidism in children with Down's syndrome. Clin Pediatr 12:749–755, 1994.

NEOPLASTIC PERICARDIAL DISEASE

172. Spodick DH: Neoplastic percardial disease. In Spodick DH: The Pericardium: A Comprehensive Textbook. New York, Marcel Dekker, 1997, pp 301–313.

173. Chow WH, Chow TC, Chiu SW: Pericardial metastasis and effusion as the initial manifestation of malignant thymoma: Identification by cross-sectional echocardiography. Int J Cardiol 37:258–260, 1992.

174. Garrigue S, Robert F, Roudaut R, Bonnet J: Assessment of non-invasive new imaging techniques in the diagnosis of heart liposarcoma. Eur Heart J 16:39–141, 1995.

174a. Warren WH: Malignancies involving the pericardium (In Process Citation). Semin Thorac Cardiovas Surg 12:119–129, 2000.

175. Maisch B: Immunology of cardiac tumors. Thorac Cardiovasc Surg 38:157–163, 1990.

176. Maisch B, Schonian U, Paul R, Gemsa D: Immunologic parameters in patients with neoplastic pericardial effusions. Eur Heart J 16:300, 1995 (abstract).

177. Petropoulakis PN, Steriotis JD, Melanidis JG, Asimakopoulos PJ: Metastatic malignant melanoma as an intracavitary obstructive mass in the right heart. Eur J Cardiothorac Surg 14:256–263, 1998.

178. Mousseaux E, Hernigou A, Azencot M, et al: Evaluation by electron beam computed tomography of intracardiac masses suspected by transesophageal echocardiography. Heart 76:256–263, 1996.

179. Seferovic PM, Ristic AD, Petrovic P, et al: Diagnostic value of pericardial biopsy: Improvement with aggressive sampling enabled by pericardioscopy. Eur Heart J 20(Suppl):625, 1999 (abstract).

180. Bardales RH, Stanley MW, Schaefer RF, et al: Secondary pericardial malignancies: A critical appraisal of the role of cytology, pericardial biopsy, and DNA ploidy analysis. Am J Pathol 106:29–34, 1996.

181. Malamou-Mitsi VD, Zioga AP, Agnantis NJ: Diagnostic accuracy of pericardial fluid cytology: An analysis of 53 specimens from 44 consecutive patients. Diagn Cytopathol 15:197–204, 1996.

182. Henderson DW, Shilkin KB, Whitaker D: Reactive mesothelial hyperplasia vs mesothelioma, including mesothelioma in situ. Am J Clin Pathol 110:397–404, 1995.

183. Thomason R, Schlegel W, Lucca M, et al: Primary malignant mesothelioma of the pericardium: Case report and literature review. Texas Heart Inst J 21:170–174, 1994.

184. Szturmowicz M, Tomkowski W, Fijalkowska A, Filipecki S: The role of carcinoembryonic antigen (CEA) and neuron-specific enolase (NSE) evaluation in pericardial fluid for the recognition of malignant pericarditis. Int J Biol Markers 12(3):96–101, 1997.

185. Wang LS, Huang MH, Lin TS, et al: Malignant thymoma. Cancer 70:443–450, 1992.

186. Knudson W: Tumor-associated hyaluronan: Providing an extracellular matrix that facilitates invasion. Am J Pathol 148:1721–1726, 1996.

187. Palaciosis IG, Tuzcu EM, Ziskind AA, et al: Percutaneous balloon pericardial window for patients with malignant pericardial effusion and tamponade. Cathet Cardiovasc Diagn 22:244–249, 1991.

188. Seferovic PM, Ristic AD, Petrovic P, et al: Triangular, small size percutaneous balloon pericardiotomy: A new treatment option for neoplastic pericardial effusion. J Am Coll Cardiol 31:250c–251c, 1998.

189. Hazelrigg SR, Mack MJ, Landreneau RJ, et al: Thoracoscopic pericardiectomy for effusive pericardial disease. Ann Thorac Surg 56:792–795, 1993.

190. Markiewicz W, Lashevsky I, Rinkevich D, et al: The acute effect of minocycline on the pericardium: Experimental and clinical findings. Chest 113:861–866, 1998.

PERICARDIAL DISEASE IN THE VASCULITIS/CONNECTIVE TISSUE DISEASES

191. Spodick DH: Pericardial disease in the vasculitis-connective tissue disease group. In Spodick DH: The Pericardium: A Comprehensive Textbook. New York, Marcel Dekker, 1997, pp 314–333.

192. Pierfederick A, Muratori M, Castelli G, Baldini A: Pericarditis: A rare beginning for a rare disease. J Cardiovasc Diagn Proc 14:96, 1997.

193. Hara KS, Ballard DJ, Ilstrup DM, et al: Rheumatoid pericarditis: Clinical features and survival. Medicine 69:81–97, 1990.

194. Gulati S, Kumar L: Cardiac tamponade as an initial manifestation of systemic lupus erythematosus in early childhood. Ann Rheum Dis 51:279–280, 1992.

195. Livneh A, Drenth JPH, Klasen IS, et al: Familial Mediterranean fever and hyperimmunoglobulinemia D syndrome: Two diseases with distinct clinical, serologic, and genetic features. J Rheumatol 24:1558–1563, 1997.

196. Turesson C, Lacobsson L, Bergstrom U: Extra-articular rheumatoid arthritis: Prevalence and mortality. Rheumatology 38:668–674, 1999.

197. Meyers DG, Meyers RE, Prendergast TW: The usefulness of diagnostic tests on pericardial fluid. Chest 111:1213–1221, 1997.

198. Ling LH, Oh JK, Schaff HV, et al: Constrictive pericarditis in the modern era: Evolving clinical spectrum and impact on outcome after pericardiectomy. Circulation 100:1380–1386, 1999.

199. Narula J, Chandrasekhar Y, Rahimtoola S: Diagnosis of active rheumatic carditis: The echoes of change. Circulation 100:1576–1581, 1999.

200. Moder KG, Miller TD, Tazelaar HD: Cardiac involvement in systemic lupus erythematosus. Mayo Clin Proc 74:275–284, 1999.

201. Kahl LE: The spectrum of pericardial tamponade in systemic lupus erythematosus: Report of ten patients. Arthritis Rheum 35:1343–1349, 1992.

202. Barletta G, Del Bene R, Brugnolo F, Emmi L: Cardiac involvement in systemic lupus erythematosus: An echocardiographic score of illness activity. J Am Coll Cardiol 31:9C, 1998.

203. Leung WH, Wong KL, Lau CP, et al: Cardiac abnormalities in systemic lupus erythematosus: A prospective M-mode, cross-sectional and Doppler echocardiographic study. Int J Cardiol 27:367–375, 1990.

204. Hata N, Kunimi T, Matsuda H, heta al: Cardiac disorders associated with progressive systemic sclerosis. J Cardiol 32:397–402, 1998.

205. Sattar MA, Guindi RT, Vajcik J: Pericardial tamponade and limited cutaneous systemic sclerosis (CREST syndrome). Br J Rheumatol 29:306–307, 1990.

206. Gyongyosi M, Pokorny G, Jambrik Z, et al: Cardiac manifestations in primary Sjögren's syndrome. Ann Rheum Dis 55:450–454, 1996.

207. Tami LF, Bhasin S: Polymorphism of the cardiac manifestations in dermatomyositis. Clin Cardiol 16:260–264, 1993.

208. Preston J, Warner M: Pericardial effusion as a manifestation of giant cell arteritis. Am J Med 91:439–40, 1991.

209. Hu PJ, Shih IM, Hutchins GM, Hellmann DB: Polyarteritis nodosa of the pericardium: Antemortem diagnosis in a pericardiectomy specimen. J Rheumatol 24:2042–2044, 1997.

210. Guillevin L, Cohen P, Gayraud M, et al: Churg-Strauss syndrome: Clinical study and long-term follow-up of 96 patients. Medicine 78:26–37, 1999.

211. Arima M, Kanoh T: Eosinophilic myocarditis associated with dense deposits of eosinophil cationic protein (ECP) in endomyocardium with high serum ECP. Heart 81:669–675, 1999.

212. Hoffman GS, Kerr GS, Leavitt RY, et al: Wegener granulomatosis: An analysis of 158 patients. 116:488–498, 1992.

MYOCARDIAL INFARCTION-ASSOCIATED PERICARDITIS

213. Spodick DH: Pericardial involvement in diseases of the heart and other contiguous structures. In Spodick DH: The Pericardium: A Comprehensive Textbook. New York, Marcel Dekker, 1997, pp 334–367.

214. Sugiura T, Takehana K, Hatada K, et al: Pericardial effusion after primary percutaneous transluminal coronary angioplasty in first Q-wave acute myocardial infarction. Am J Cardiol 81:1090–1093, 1998.

215. Nagahama Y, Sugiura T, Takehana K, et al: The role of infarction-associated pericarditis on the occurrence of atrial fibrillation. Eur Heart J 19:287–292, 1998.

216. Sugiura T, Takehana K, Abe Y, et al: Frequency of pericardial friction rub ("pericarditis") after percutaneous transluminal coronary angioplasty in Q-wave myocardial infarction. Am J Cardiol 79:362–364, 1997.

217. Spodick DH: Pericardial complications of acute myocardial infarction. In Francis GS, Alper JS (eds): Modern Coronary Care. 2nd ed. Boston, Little, Brown, 1995, pp 331–339.

218. Correale E, Maggioni AP, Romano S, et al: Comparison of frequency, diagnostic and prognostic significance of pericardial involvement in acute myocardial infarction treated with and without thrombolytics. Am J Cardiol 71:1377–1381, 1993.

219. Alam M, Gunda M, Khaja F, et al: Pericardial effusion after acute myocardial infarction. J Heart Dis 1:619, 1999.

220. Gregor P, Widimsky P: Pericardial effusion as a consequence of acute myocardial infarction. Echocardiography 16:317–320, 1999.

221. Jugdutt BI: Right ventricular infarction: Contribution of echocardiography to diagnosis and management. Echocardiography 16:297–304, 1999.

222. Becker RC, Hochman JS, Cannon CP, et al: Fatal cardiac rupture among patients treated with thrombolytic agents and adjunctive thrombin antagonists. J Am Coll Cardiol 33:479–487, 1999.

223. Figueras J, Cortadellas J, Calvo F, Soler-Soler J: Relevance of delayed hospital admission on development of cardiac rupture during acute myocardial infarction: Study in 225 patients with free wall, septal or papillary muscle rupture. J Am Coll Cardiol 32:135–139, 1998.

224. Figueras J, Curos A, Cortadellas J, Soler-Soler J: Reliability of electromechanical dissociation in the diagnosis of left ventricular free wall rupture in acute myocardial infarction. Am Heart J 131:861–864, 1996.

225. Oliva PB, Hammill SC, Edwards WD: Electrocardiographic diagnosis of postinfarction regional pericarditis: Ancillary observations regarding the effect of reperfusion on the rapidity and amplitude of T wave inversion after acute myocardial infarction. Circulation 88:896–904, 1993.

226. Oliva PB, Hammill SC, Talano JV: T wave changes consistent with epicardial involvement in acute myocardial infarction: Observations in patients with a postinfarction pericardial effusion without clinically recognized postinfarction pericarditis. J Am Coll Cardiol 24:1073–1077, 1994.

227. Khoury NE, Borzak S, Gokli A, et al: "Inadvertent" thrombolytic administration in patients without myocardial infarction: Clinical features and outcome. Ann Emerg Med 28:289–293, 1996.

228. Thakur RK, Souza JJ, Troup PJ, et al: Pericardial effusion increases defibrillation energy requirement. PACE 16:1127, 1993.

229. Lee PJ, Spencer KT: Pseudoaneurysm of the left ventricular free wall caused by tumor. J Am Soc Echocardiogr 12:876–878, 1999.

230. de Boer HD, Elzenga NJ, de Boer WJ, Meuzelaar JJ: Pseudoaneurysm of the left ventricle after isolated pericarditis and Staphylococcus aureus septicemia. Eur J Cardiothorac Surg 15:97–99, 1999.

231. Pluenneke A, Stoler RC, Roberts WC: Chest pain. BUMC Proc 12:305–308, 1999.

232. Goldstein JA: Right heart ischemia: Pathophysiology, natural history, and clinical management. Prog Cardiovasc Dis 40:325–341, 1998.

233. Tyberg JV, Smith ER: Ventricular diastole and the role of the pericardium. Herz 15:354–361, 1990.

234. Spodick DH: Post-myocardial infarction syndrome (Dressler's syndrome). ACC Curr J Rev 4:35–37, 1995.

235. Shahar A, Hod H, Barabash GM, et al: Disappearance of a syndrome: Dressler's syndrome in the era of thrombolysis. Cardiology 85:255–258, 1994.

TRAUMATIC PERICARDIAL DISEASE

236. Spodick DH: Traumatic pericardial disease: Accidental, criminal, surgical and biological trauma. In Spodick DH: The Pericardium: A Comprehensive Textbook. New York, Marcel Dekker, 1997, pp 368–410.

237. Hollerman JJ, Fackler ML, Coldwell DM, Ben-Menachem Y: Gunshot wounds: I. Bullets, ballistics, and mechanisms of injury. AJR 155:685–690, 1990.

238. Asensio JA, Berne JD, Demetriades D, et al: One hundred five penetrating cardiac injuries: A 2-year prospective evaluation. J Trauma 44:1073–1082, 1998.

239. Asensio JA, Berne JD, Demetriades D, et al: Penetrating cardiac injuries: A prospective study of variables predicting outcomes. J Am Coll Surg 186:24–34, 1998.

240. Meyer DM, Jesson ME, Grayburn PA: Use of echocardiography to detect occult cardiac injury after penetrating thorac trauma: A prospective study. J Trauma 39:902–909, 1995.

241. Vosswinkel JA, Bilfinger TV: Cardiac nail gun injuries: Lessons learned. J Trauma 47:558–590, 1999.

242. Spodick DH, Moran JJ: Acute traumatic pericarditis: Failed suicide with classic electrocardiogram. Clin Cardiol 22:544, 1999.

243. Fackler ML: Civilian gunshot wounds and ballistics: Dispelling the myths. Emerg Med Clin North Am 16:17–28, 1998.

244. Narins CR, Cunningham MJ, Delehanty JM, et al: Nonhemorrhagic cardiac tamponade after penetrating chest trauma. Am Heart J 132:197–198, 1996.

245. Sabers CJ, Levy NT, Bowen JM: 33-year-old man with chest pain and fever. Mayo Clin Proc 74:181–184, 1999.

246. Nagy KK, Lohmann C, Kim DO, Barrett J: Role of echocardiography in the diagnosis of occult penetrating cardiac injury. J Trauma 38:859–862, 1995.

247. Abramson DC, Giannoti AG: Perforation of the right ventricle with a coronary sinus catheter during preparation for minimally invasive cardiac surgery. Anesthesiology 89:519–521, 1998.

248. Alfonso F, Segovia J, Alswies A: Coronary rupture during stent implantation. Circulation 98:2094, 1998.

249. Jacques B, Gras D, Leclercq C, et al: Péricardité aigue à rechutes inudité par une électrode atriale vissée: À propos de 3 observations. Arch Mal Coeur 89:1389–1395, 1996.

250. Krauss D, Schmidt GA: Cardiac tamponade and contralateral hemothorax after subclavian vein catheterization. Chest 99:517–518, 1991.

251. D'Cruz IA, Overton DH, Pai GM: Pericardial complications of cardiac surgery: Emphasis on the diagnostic role of echocardiography. J Card Surg 7:257–268, 1992.

252. Tomic S, Jovovic L, Zlatanovic M, et al: Echocardiographic evaluation of pericardial effusion after different open heart surgical procedures. Echocardiography 15:543, 1998.

253. Khan AH: The postcardiac injury syndromes. Clin Cardiol 15:67–72, 1992.

254. Jadhav P, Asirvatham S, Craven P, et al: Unusual presentation of late regional cardiac tamponade after aortic surgery. Am J Cardiac Imag 10:204–206, 1996.

255. Konstantakos AK, Gilkeson RC, Brozovich FV, Lee JH: Massive pericardial hematoma simulating constrictive pericarditis: A complication of radiofrequency catheter ablation. J Thorac Cardiovasc Surg 115:726–727, 1998.

256. Dardas P, Tsikaderis D, Ioannides E, et al: Constrictive pericarditis after coronary artery bypass surgery as a cause of unexplained dyspnea: A report of five cases. Clin Cardiol 21:691–694, 1998.

257. Sakai K, Nakamura K, Ishizuka N, et al: Echocardiographic findings and clinical features of left ventricular pseudoaneurysm after mitral valve replacement. Am Heart J 124:975, 1992.

258. Papsin BC, Gorenstein LA, Goldberg M: Delayed myocardial laceration after intrapericardial pneumonectomy. Ann Thorac Surg 55:756–757, 1993.

259. Bitkover Cy, Al-Khalili F, Ribeiro A, Liska J: Surviving resuscitation: Successful repair of cardiac rupture. Ann Thorac Surg 61:710–711, 1996.

260. Lons T, Trinchet JC: La sclerose endoscopique des varices oesophagiennes: Incidents et complications. Gastroenterol Clin Biol 16:50–63, 1992.

261. Arya KR, Taori GK, Kahanna SS: Electrocardiographic manifestations following electric injury. Int J Cardiol 57:100–101, 1996.

262. Buckman RF, Buckman PD: Vertical deceleration trauma: Principles of management. Surg Clin North Am 71:331–340, 1991.

262a. Mineo TC, Ambrogi V, Cristino B, et al: Changing indications for thoracotomy in blunt chest trauma after the advent of videothoracoscopy. J Trauma 42:1088–1091, 1999.

263. Chirillo F, Totis O, Cavarzerani A, et al: Usefulness of transthoracic and transesophageal echocardiography in recognition and management of cardiovascular injuries after blunt chest trauma. Heart 75:301–306, 1996.

264. Feghali NT, Prisant LM: Blunt myocardial injury. Chest 108:1673–1677, 1995.

OTHER PERICARDIAL DISEASES

265. Harris KM, Braverman AC, Gutierrez FR, et al: Transesophageal echocardiographic and clinical features of aortic intramural hematoma. J Thorac Cardiovasc Surg 114:619–626, 1997.

266. Nienaber CA, von Kodolitsch Y, Petersen B, et al: Intramural hemorrhage of the thoracic aorta: Diagnostic and therapeutic implications. Circulation 92:1465–1472, 1995.

267. Pacifico L, Spodick DH: ILEAD—ischemia of the lower extremities due to aortic dissection: The isolated presentation. Clin Cardiol 22:353–356, 1999.

268. Marcus RH, Chuna KG, Hosephson M, et al: Vagolytic therapy in acute cardiac tamponade associated with aortic dissection. Am Heart J 121:926–929, 1991.

269. Nienaber CA, von Kodolitsch Y, Nicolas V, et al: The diagnosis of thoracic aortic dissection by noninvasive imaging procedures. N Engl J Med 328:1–9, 1993.

270. Svensson LG, Labib SB, Eisenhaur AC, Butterly JR: Intimal tear without hematoma: An important variant of aortic dissection that can elude current imaging techniques. Circulation 99:1331–1336, 1999.

271. Hinderliter AL, Willis PW IV, Long W, et al: Frequency and prognostic significance of pericardial effusion in primary pulmonary hypertension. Am J Cardiol 84:481–484, 1999.

272. Anthony P, Chandraratna N, Chan K, et al: Large pleural effusions produce echocardiographic and clinical signs of cardiac tamponade. Circulation 94:I445, 1996.

273. Kisanuki A, Shono H, Kiyonaga K, et al: Two-dimensional echocardiographic demonstration of left ventricular diastolic collapse due to compression by pleural effusion. Am Heart J 122:1173–1175, 1991.

274. Jerjes-Sanchez C, Ramirez-Rivera A, Ibarra-Perez C: The Dressler syndrome after pulmonary embolism. Am J Cardiol 78:343–345, 1996.

275. Miller WL, Osborn MJ, Sinak LJ, Westbrook BM: Pyopneumopericardium attributed to an esophagopericardial fistula: Report of a survivor and review of the literature. Mayo Clin Proc 66:1041–1045, 1991.

276. Hung MJ, Wang CH, Lie DW, Cherng WJ: Spontaneous echo contrast in purulent pericardial effusion due to non-gas-forming organisms. Echocardiography 15:489–494, 1998.

277. Manetta F, Moores DWO, Bennett EV, Edwards NM: Intrapericardial herniation of the stomach after use of the right gastroepiploic artery for coronary artery bypass grafting. J Thorac Cardiovasc Surg 115:479–480, 1998.

278. Spodick DH: Drug- and toxin-related pericardial disease. *In* Spodick DH: The Pericardium: A Comprehensive Textbook. New York, Marcel Dekker, 1997, pp 411–416.

279. Farver DK: Minocycline-induced lupus. Ann Pharmacother 31:1160–1163, 1997.

280. Allen A: The cardiotoxicity of chemotherapeutic drugs. Semin Oncol 19:529–542, 1992.

281. Bensaid J, Denis F: Péricardité aigue bénigne après vaccination contre l'hépatite B. Presse Med 22:269, 1993.

282. Rothenberg ME: Eosinophilia. N Engl J Med 338:1592–1600, 1998.

283. Spodick DH: Idiopathic pericarditis: Pericarditis of unknown origin. *In* Spodick DH: The Pericardium: A Comprehensive Textbook. New York, Marcel Dekker, 1997, pp 417–421.

284. Afrasiabi R, Sirop PA, Albini SM, et al: Recurrent pericarditis and dermatitis herpetiformis: Evidence for immune complex deposition in the pericardium. Chest 97:1006–1007, 1990.

285. Spodick DH: Recurrent and incessant pericarditis. *In* Spodick DH: The Pericardium: A Comprehensive Textbook. New York, Marcel Dekker, 1997, pp 422–432.

286. Farraj RS, McCully RB, Oh JK, Smith TF: *Mycoplasma*-associated pericarditis. Mayo Clin Proc 72:33–36, 1997.

287. Rana BS, Jones RA, Simpson IA: Recurrent pericardial effusion: The value of polymerase chain reaction in the diagnosis of tuberculosis. Heart 82:246–247, 1999.

288. Garg A, Shiau J, Guyatt G: The ineffectiveness of immunosuppressive therapy in lymphocytic myocarditis: An overview. Ann Intern Med 128:317–322, 1998.

289. Adler Y, Finkelstein Y, Guido J, et al: Colchicine treatment for recurrent pericarditis: A decade of experience. Circulation 97:2183–2185, 1998.

290. Arsenian MA: Cardiovascular sequelae of therapeutic thoracic radiation. Prog Cardiovasc Dis 24:299–311, 1991.

291. Karram T, Rinkevitch D, Markiewicz W: Poor outcome in radiation-induced constrictive pericarditis. Int J Radiat Oncol Biol Phys 25:329–331, 1993.

292. Spodick DH: Chronic pericardial effusion and chronic cardiac tamponade. *In* Spodick DH: The Pericardium: A Comprehensive Textbook. New York, Marcel Dekker, 1997, pp 443–452.

293. Merce J, Sagrista-Sauleda J, Permanyer-Miralda G, Soler-Soler J: Should pericardial drainage be performed routinely in patients who have a large pericardial effusion with tamponade? Am J Med 105:106–109, 1998.

294. D'Cruz IA, Overton DH, Pai GM: Pericardial complications of cardiac surgery: Emphasis on the diagnostic role of echocardiography. J Cardiac Surg 7:257–268, 1992.

295. Hara KS, Ballard DJ, Ilstrup DM, et al: Rheumatoid pericarditis: Clinical features and survival. Medicine 69:81–91, 1990.

296. Soler-Soler J: Massive chronic idiopathic pericardial effusion. *In* Soler-Soler J (ed): Pericardial Disease. Dordrecht, The Netherlands, Kluwer Academic Publishers, 1990, pp 153–165.

297. Nugue O, Millaire A, Porte H, et al: Pericardioscopy in the etiologic diagnosis of pericardial effusion in 141 consecutive patients. Circulation 94:1635–1641, 1996.

298. Merce J, Sagrista-Sauleda J, Permanyer-Miralda G, et al: Correlation between clinical and Doppler echocardiographic findings in patients with moderate and large pericardial effusion: Implications for the diagnosis of cardiac tamponade. Am Heart J 138:759–764, 1999.

299. Downey RJ, Bessler M, Weissman C: Acute pulmonary edema following pericardiocentesis for chronic cardiac tamponade secondary to trauma. Crit Care Med 19:1323–1325, 1991.

Chapter 51
Traumatic Heart Disease

KENNETH L. MATTOX • ANTHONY L. ESTRERA
MATTHEW J. WALL, JR.

The earliest reports of traumatic injury to the heart discouraged operative repair, asserting high mortality and the hopelessness of cardiorrhaphy.[1] This pessimism persisted until the first cardiorrhaphy was performed by Rehn[2] in 1898. Rehn subsequently compiled his series of 124 cases over the next 10 years, with a survival of 40 percent.[3] The first cardiac repair for injury in the United States was performed by Hill[4] in 1902 on a kitchen table. In 1959, Isaacs[5] reported a remarkable survival of 89 percent for stab wounds and 43 percent for gunshot wounds to the heart among 60 patients. Enthusiasm for the surgical intervention in traumatic heart disease grew from these reported successes.

Most of the early reports involving traumatic heart disease involved penetrating injuries. Crynes and Hunter[6] reported the first blunt cardiac injury in 1939. In 1955, Des Forges and associates[7] reported the first successful repair for blunt cardiac injury.

Incidence

In the United States, trauma is the fourth leading cause of death, and it is the leading cause of death in those younger than 40 years of age. Thoracic trauma is responsible for 25 percent of the annual 50,000 deaths from vehicular accidents. As high as one fourth of these deaths are due to traumatic cardiac injury.[8] The actual incidence of cardiac injury from all of the diverse etiologies and classifications (including the confusing "cardiac contusion") is unknown. It has been estimated that cardiac injury may account for 10 percent of deaths from gunshot wounds.[9] Penetrating cardiac trauma is a highly lethal injury, with relatively few such patients reaching the hospital. In a series of penetrating cardiac injuries in South Africa where both those reaching the hospital and those being taken directly to the morgue were included, only 6 percent of 1,198 patients reached the hospital with any signs of life.[10] With improvements in organized emergency medical transport systems, up to 45 percent of those who sustain significant traumatic heart injury may reach the emergency department.[11]

Blunt cardiac injuries have been reported less frequently than penetrating injuries. In a population-based study, which included autopsied patients, the incidence of blunt cardiac injury is 0.1 percent.[12] In hospital-based studies, 10 to 70 percent of motor vehicle fatalities may have been the result of blunt cardiac rupture.[13, 14]

ETIOLOGY AND PATTERNS OF CARDIAC TRAUMA

Categorization of traumatic heart disease is based on mechanism of injury (i.e., penetrating, nonpenetrating [blunt], iatrogenic, metabolic, and other) (Table 51–1).

PENETRATING CARDIAC TRAUMA. Penetrating trauma is the most common cause of significant cardiac injury seen in the hospital setting, with the predominant injury being from guns and knives. Penetrating cardiac trauma is secondary to stab wounds in 35 to 96 percent of patients (depending on the instrument used in interpersonal violence in a geographical location), whereas gunshot wounds account for a reported 39 to 66 percent.[15-17] Both of these etiologies vary according to the year of the report and location in the world. One might also postulate that economic factors influence the availability of a penetrating wounding agent. Other mechanisms such as shotguns, ice picks, and fence impalement have also been reported.

The location of injury to the heart often correlates with the location of injury on the chest wall. Because of their anterior location, the anatomical chambers at greatest risk for injury are the right and left ventricles. In a review of 711 patients with penetrating cardiac trauma, 54 percent sustained stab wounds and 42 percent had gunshot wounds. The right ventricle was injured in 40 percent of the cases, the left ventricle in 40 percent, the right atrium in 24 percent, and the left atrium in 3 percent. One third of

▼ TABLE 51–1. ETIOLOGY OF TRAUMATIC HEART DISEASES

I. **Penetrating**
   A. Stab wounds—knives, swords, ice picks, fence posts, wire, sporting
   B. Gunshot wounds—low-high caliber, handgun, rifles, nail guns, lawnmower projectiles
   C. Shotgun wounds—close range, distant
II. **Nonpenetrating (Blunt)**
   A. Motor vehicle accident
      1. Seat belt
      2. Air bag
   B. Vehicular-pedestrian accident
   C. Falls from height
   D. Crushing—industrial accident
   E. Blasts—explosives, grenades
   F. Assault (aggravated)
   G. Sternal or rib fractures
   H. Recreational—sporting events (bull goring), baseball
III. **Iatrogenic**
   A. Catheter induced
   B. Pericardiocentesis induced
IV. **Metabolic**
   A. Traumatic response to injury
   B. "Stunning"
   C. Systemic inflammatory response syndrome (SIRS)
V. **Others**
   A. Burn
   B. Electrical
   C. Factitious—needles, foreign bodies
   D. Embolic—missiles

cardiac injuries involve multiple cardiac structures.[17] Significant intracardiac injuries involved the coronary arteries (39), valvular apparatus (mitral) (2), intracardiac fistulas (i.e., ventricular septal defects [VSD]) (14), and unusual injuries (10). Only 2 percent of patients surviving their initial injury and undergoing an operation required reoperation for a residual defect.[17]

BLUNT CARDIAC TRAUMA. Nonpenetrating or blunt cardiac trauma has replaced the term "cardiac contusion" and ranges from minor bruises of the myocardium to cardiac rupture.[18, 18a] It can be caused by direct energy to the heart or compression of the heart between the sternum and the vertebral column, even including "cardiac contusion" and cardiac rupture during external cardiac massage during cardiopulmonary resuscitation (CPR). Within this spectrum, blunt cardiac injuries may present as free septal rupture, free wall rupture, coronary artery thrombosis, cardiac failure, complex arrhythmia, simple arrhythmia, and/or rupture of chordae tendineae or papillary muscles.[19, 20] The incidence may be as high as three fourths of the patients with severe bodily trauma. Etiologies include motor vehicle accidents, vehicular-pedestrian accidents, falls, crush injuries, blasts, assaults, CPR, and recreational events. Such injury is often associated with sternal or rib fractures. In one report a fatal cardiac dysrhythmia occurred when the sternum was struck by a baseball,[21] which may be a form of commotio cordis.[22]

Cardiac rupture carries a significant mortality. The biomechanics of cardiac rupture include[23]:

- Direct transmission of increased intrathoracic pressure to the chambers of the heart
- Hydraulic effect from a large force applied to the abdominal or extremity veins causing force to be transmitted to the right atrium, resulting in rupture
- Decelerating force, explaining atriocaval tears, between fixed and mobile areas
- Myocardial contusion, necrosis, and delayed rupture
- Penetration from broken rib or fractured sternum

Blunt rupture of the cardiac septum occurs most frequently in late diastole or early systole near the apex of the heart.[19] Multiple ruptures and disruption of the conduction system have been reported.[24] In an autopsy series of 546 patients reported by Parmley and colleagues, blunt cardiac trauma with ventricular rupture most often involved the left ventricle, followed by the right ventricle, and, least often, the left atrium. Thirty cases of VSD were reported, with the most common tear involving both the membranous and muscular portions of the septum. Injury to only the membranous portion of the septum was the least common blunt VSD. Parmley and colleagues also reported that traumatic rupture of the thoracic aorta was associated with lethal cardiac rupture in 22 percent of the cases.[12]

Blunt pericardial rupture results from pericardial tears secondary to increased intraabdominal pressure or lateral decelerative forces. The location of the tears occurs on the left side parallel to the phrenic nerve (64 percent), the diaphragmatic surface of the pericardium (18 percent), the right of the pleuropericardium (9 percent), and the mediastinum (9 percent).[19] Cardiac herniation with cardiac dysfunction can occur with these tears. The heart can be displaced into either pleural cavity or even the peritoneum. In the instance of right pericardial rupture the heart can become torsed and the pericardial cavity is surprisingly found to be "empty" of a heart at a resuscitative left anterolateral thoracotomy. With a left-sided cardiac herniation through a pericardial tear, a distending heart prevents the heart from returning into the pericardium, and the term "incarcerated heart" has been applied. Venous filling is impaired and unless the cardiac herniation is reduced, hypotension and cardiac arrest can occur.

IATROGENIC CARDIAC INJURY. Iatrogenic cardiac injury can occur with central venous line insertion, cardiac catheterization procedures, and pericardiocentesis.

Cardiac injuries caused by central venous lines usually occur with placement from either the left subclavian or the left internal jugular vein.[25] Perforation causing tamponade has also been reported with a right internal jugular introducer sheath for transjugular intrahepatic portocaval shunts.[26] Vigorous insertion of left-sided central lines, especially during dilatation of the line tract, can lead to cardiac perforations. Even appropriate technique carries a discrete rate of iatrogenic injury secondary to central venous catheterization. Common sites of cardiac injury include the superior caval-atrial junction and the superior vena cava–inominate junction. These small perforations often lead to a compensated cardiac tamponade. Drainage by pericardiocentesis is often unsuccessful, and evacuation by the subxiphoid pericardial window or full median sternotomy is required. Once access to the pericardial space is gained, the site of injury has often sealed and may be difficult to find.

Complications from coronary catheterization, including perforation of the coronary arteries, cardiac perforation, and aortic dissection can be catastrophic and require emergency surgical intervention. The incidence of coronary perforation with balloon angioplasty is estimated to be 0.1 to 0.2 percent, but with advanced interventional techniques (e.g., rotablation, directional atherectomy, coronary artery stenting, and laser ablation) the incidence may be as high as 3 percent.[27]

Other potential iatrogenic causes of cardiac injury include external and internal cardiac massage, right ventricular injury during pericardiocentesis, and intracardiac injections.[28]

METABOLIC CARDIAC INJURY. Metabolic cardiac injury (MCI) refers to cardiac dysfunction in response to traumatic injury and may be associated with injuries caused by burns, electrical injury, sepsis, the systemic inflammatory response syndrome, and multisystem trauma.[29-32] The exact mechanism responsible for this dysfunction is unclear, but responses to trauma induce a "mediator storm," and it is this release of cytokines that may have a direct effect on the myocardium. Endotoxin, tumor necrosis factor-alpha, tumor necrosis factor-beta, interleukin-1, interleukin-6, interleukin-10, catecholamines (epinephrine, norepinephrine), cell-adhesion molecules, and nitric oxide are all possible responsible mediators.[33-35]

Metabolic cardiac injury may clinically present as conduction disturbances or decreased contractility leading to decreased output. Myocardial depression can occur in response to the "mediator storm" and alter calcium utilization and depression of the myocyte responsiveness to beta-adrenergic stimulation.[36-39] Horton and coworkers[36] have shown that myocytes have altered calcium utilization in patients with injuries from burns. Ungureanu-Longrois and coworkers[34] reported that the activation of constitutive nitric oxide synthase appears to modulate cardiac responsiveness to cholinergic and adrenergic stimulation and that production of inducible nitric oxide synthase causes depression of myocyte contractile responsiveness to beta-adrenergic agonists. The myocardial depressive effects appear to be reversible.[32]

Treatment of MCI has been supportive with correction of the initiating insults, but some have attempted to address the involved mediators using intravenous milrinone, corticosteroids, arginine, granulocyte-macrophage colony-stimulating factor, and glutamate.[40-43] Use of an intraaortic counterpulsation balloon pump can be considered to treat such myocardial depression, but controlled series do not exist to test this hypothesis.

BURNS. Cardiac complications in the early post-burn period are a major cause of death. The initial cardiovascular effect of burn injury is attributable to the profound reduction in cardiac output that may occur within minutes of the injury. The overall cardiac response has been described as an *ebb* and *flow* pattern, with the initial *ebb* phase lasting between 1 and 3 days and marked by hypovolemia and myocardial depression and the *flow* phase characterized by a prolonged period of increased metabolic demand with increased cardiac output and peripheral blood flow. The reduction in cardiac output observed in the initial period of burn injury is the result of a dramatic and rapid decrease in intravascular volume due to a "capillary leak" and of a direct myocardial depression. Hypovolemia results from the capillary leak caused by endothelial injury and may be mediated by platelet-activating factor, complement, cytokines, arachidonic acid, or oxygen free radicals. Myocardial depression manifested by a decrease in myocardial contractility and abnormalities in ventricular compliance becomes apparent with total body surface area burn of 20 to 25 percent. Myocardial-depressant factor, tumor necrosis factor, vasopressin, oxygen free radicals, and interleukins may be responsible for the depression.[44]

ELECTRICAL INJURY. Cardiac complications are the most common cause of death after electrical injury. An estimated 1100 to 1300 deaths occur annually in the United States from electrical injury (including lightning strikes). The cardiac complications after electrical injury include immediate cardiac arrest, acute myocardial necrosis with or without ventricular failure, pseudoinfarction, myocardial ischemia, dysrhythmias, conduction abnormalities, acute hypertension with peripheral vasospasm, and asymptomatic, nonspecific abnormalities evident on an electrocardiogram (ECG). Damage from electrical injury is due to the direct effects on the excitable tissues, heat generated from the current, and the accompanying associated injuries (e.g., falls, explosions, or fires).[45]

OTHERS. Intrapericardial and intracardiac foreign bodies can cause complications of acute suppurative pericarditis, chronic constrictive pericarditis, foreign body reaction, and hemopericardium.[46] Intrapericardial foreign bodies that have been reported in the literature to result in complications include bullets, hand grenades, shrapnel, knitting needles, and hypodermic needles. Some of these are factitiously inserted by a patient, usually with a psychiatric diagnosis. A report by LeMaire and colleagues[46] advocated removal of intrapericardial foreign bodies that are greater than 1 cm in size, those that are contaminated, and/or those that produce symptoms.

INTRACARDIAC MISSILES. Intracardiac missiles are foreign bodies that are either embedded in the myocardium, retained in the trabeculations of the endocardial surface, free in a cardiac chamber, or in the pericardium. These are the result of direct penetrating thoracic injury or injury to a peripheral vascular structure with embolization to the heart. Location and other conditions determine the type of complications that can occur and the treatment required. Observation might be considered when the missile is (1) right sided, (2) embedded completely in the wall, (3) contained within a fibrous covering, (4) not contaminated, and (5) producing no symptoms. Right-sided missiles can embolize to the lung, at which point they can be removed, or in rare cases they embolize "paradoxically" through a patent foramen ovale or atrial septal defect.[47] Left-sided missiles can present as systemic embolization shortly after the initial injury. Diagnosis is determined with radiographs in two projections, fluoroscopy, echocardiography, or angiography. Treatment of retained missiles is individualized. Removal is recommended for missiles that are left sided, larger than 1 to 2 cm, rough in shape, or produce symptoms.[47] Although direct approach, either with or without cardiopulmonary bypass, has been advocated in the past, a large percentage of right-sided foreign bodies can now be removed by interventional radiologists.

PENETRATING CARDIAC TRAUMA. Wounds involving the precordial "box," which is the anatomical area that includes the epigastrium and precordium within 3 cm of the sternum, carry a high incidence of cardiac injury. Stab wounds present a more predictable path of injury than gunshot wounds. Cardiac injury may present with a clinical spectrum from full arrest with no vital signs to a patient who is asymptomatic with normal vital signs. Up to 80 percent of stab wounds eventually present with tamponade. The weapon injures the pericardium and heart, but as the weapon is removed the pericardium seals and may not allow blood to escape. Rapid bleeding into the pericardium favors clotting rather than defibrination.[48] As pericardial fluid accumulates, a decrease in ventricular filling occurs, leading to a decrease in stroke volume. A compensatory rise in catecholamines leads to tachycardia and increased right-sided heart filling pressures. The limits of distensibility are reached, and the septum shifts toward the left side, further compromising left ventricular function. If this cycle persists, this may lead to worsening of the ventricular function and irreversible shock. As little as 60 to 100 ml of blood in the pericardial sac can produce the clinical picture of tamponade.[48]

The rate of accumulation is dependent on the location of the wound. Owing to a thicker wall, right ventricular wounds seal themselves more readily than right atrial wounds. Injuries to the coronary arteries present with rapid onset of tamponade combined with cardiac ischemia. With injuries to the left ventricle, the decompensated state can worsen, leading to cardiac arrest. Injuries to the right side of the heart can compensate, and rapid deterioration may not occur; this subset of patients may benefit from early diagnosis and immediate intervention.

The classic finding of Beck triad (muffled heart sounds, hypotension, and distended neck veins) may be seen in only 10 percent of patients. Pulsus paradoxus (a substantial fall in systolic blood pressure during inspiration) and Kussmaul sign (increase in jugular venous distention on inspiration) may be present but are not reliable[49] (see Chap. 50). A very valuable and reproducible sign of pericardial tamponade is a narrowing of the pulse pressure. An elevation of the central venous pressure often accompanies rapid and cyclic hyperresuscitation with crystalloid solutions, but in such instances there is a widening of the pulse pressure. Elevation of the central venous pressure and narrowing of the pulse pressure represents a pericardial tamponade syndrome until proven otherwise.

In contrast to stab wounds, gunshot wounds to the heart are more frequently associated with hemorrhage than with tamponade. Twenty percent of gunshot wounds to the heart present as tamponade. With firearms, the kinetic energy is greater and the wounds to the heart and pericardium are frequently larger. Thus, these patients present in arrest more often due to hemorrhage.[49]

NONPENETRATING CARDIAC TRAUMA. As in penetrating cardiac trauma, clinically severe blunt cardiac trauma (e.g., cardiac rupture) presents as either tamponade or as hemorrhage, depending on the status of the pericardium. If the pericardium is intact, tamponade develops; if it is not intact, extrapericardial bleeding occurs and hypovolemic shock ensues. Tamponade may be combined with hypovolemia, thus complicating the clinical presentation.

Blunt cardiac injury can be divided into clinically significant and clinically insignificant injuries. Clinically significant injuries include cardiac rupture (ventricular or atrial), septal rupture, valvular dysfunction, and coronary thrombosis. These injuries present as tamponade, hemorrhage, or severe cardiac dysfunction. Septal rupture and valvular dysfunction (leaflet tear, papillary muscle, or chordal rupture) may initially present without symptoms but later present as the delayed sequelae of heart failure.[48]

Blunt cardiac injury may also present as dysrhythmias, most commonly premature ventricular contractions, the precise mechanism of which is unknown. Ventricular tachycardia can occur and degenerate into ventricular fibrillation. Supraventricular tachyarrhythmias can also occur. These commonly occur within the first 24 to 48 hours.

Small isolated tears in the pericardium may lead to cardiac herniation. This is a rare complication of pericardial rupture and depends on the size of the pericardial tear. If large enough, cardiac herniation can occur, leading to acute cardiac dysfunction. [48]

EVALUATION

Evaluation of the patient with suspected traumatic heart injury is divided among those patients who are clinically stable and those who are in extremis.

INITIAL ASSESSMENT. The diagnosis of traumatic heart injury requires a high index of suspicion (Fig. 51–1). On initial presentation to the emergency center, airway, breathing, and circulation (ABCs) under Advanced Trauma Life Support (ATLS) protocol are evaluated and established.[50] Two large-bore intravenous catheters are inserted, and blood is typed and cross matched. The patient undergoes a Focused Assessment for the Sonographic examination of the Trauma victim (FAST) and is examined for Beck triad of muffled heart sounds, hypotension, and distended neck veins, as well as for pulsus paradoxus and Kussmaul sign. These findings suggest cardiac injury but may be present in only 10 percent of patients with cardiac tamponade. If the FAST demonstrates pericardial fluid in the patient who is unstable (systemic blood pressure <90 mm Hg), immediate transfer to the operating room for definitive repair or damage control is required.

Patients in extremis require immediate surgical intervention and often require emergent thoracotomy for resuscitation. The clear indications for emergency department thoracotomy include the following[51]:

1. Salvageable postinjury cardiac arrest (e.g., patients who have witnessed cardiac arrest with high likelihood of intrathoracic injury, especially penetrating cardiac wounds)

2. Severe postinjury hypotension (i.e., systolic blood pressure <60 mm Hg) due to cardiac tamponade, air embolism, or thoracic hemorrhage

If after resuscitative thoracotomy vital signs are regained, the patient proceeds to the operating room for definitive repair. The patient with confirmed pericardial fluid by FAST with normal vital signs (systemic blood pressure >90 mm Hg) may undergo a thorough evaluation to identify associated injuries. If other injuries are excluded, then open exploration may be required to exclude cardiac injury. In the absence of known causes of pericardial fluid (e.g., malignant pericardial effusion), a missed cardiac injury may lead to delayed bleeding, deterioration, or death.

Chest radiograph is nonspecific, but it can identify hemothorax or pneumothorax and demonstrate an enlarged

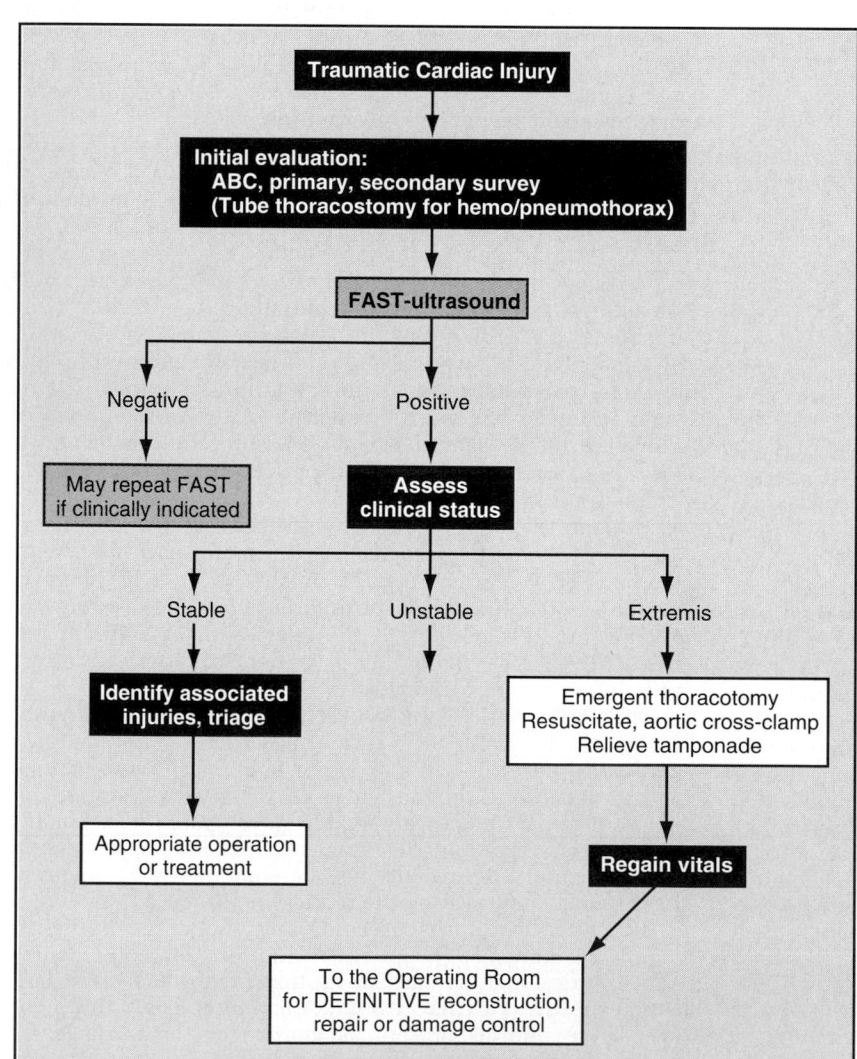

FIGURE 51–1. Algorithm for the initial assessment of traumatic cardiac injury.

cardiac silhouette suggesting pericardial fluid. Other possibly indicated examinations include ultrasonography, central venous pressure measurements, subxiphoid pericardial window, thoracoscopy, laparoscopy, and pericardiocentesis.

ULTRASONOGRAPHY. Surgeons are increasingly performing ultrasonography for thoracic trauma. This increase has paralleled the use of ultrasonography for blunt abdominal trauma. The FAST evaluates four anatomical windows for presence of intraabdominal or pericardial fluid[52] (Fig. 51–2). Ultrasonography in this setting is not intended to reach the precision of studies performed in the radiology suite but is merely intended to determine the presence of abnormal fluid collections, which aid in surgical decision making.[53] Ultrasonography is safe, portable, and expeditious and can be repeated as indicated.[53] If performed by a trained surgeon, the FAST examination has a sensitivity of nearly 100 percent and specificity of 97.3 percent.[54]

To evaluate more subtle findings of blunt cardiac injury in the stable patient, transthoracic (TTE) or transesophageal echocardiography (TEE) may be used. TEE is useful in identifying and characterizing valvular abnormalities and septal defects.

SUBXIPHOID PERICARDIAL WINDOW. Subxiphoid pericardial window has been performed both in the emergency department and in the operating room with the patient under either general or local anesthesia. A subxiphoid vertical incision is made and a small hole made in the pericardium, looking for blood. In a prospective study, Meyer and coworkers[55] compared the subxiphoid pericardial window with echocardiography in penetrating heart injury and reported that the sensitivity and specificity of subxiphoid pericardial window was 100 percent and 92 percent, respectively, compared with 56 percent and 93 percent with echocardiography. They suggested that the difference in the sensitivity may have been due to the presence of hemothorax, which may confuse the pericardial and pleural space, or due to the fact that the blood had drained into the pleura.[55]

The disadvantage of subxiphoid pericardial window is that it is an invasive procedure; and if a major injury is found, a second thoracic incision is required for definitive repair. Although there has been significant controversy in

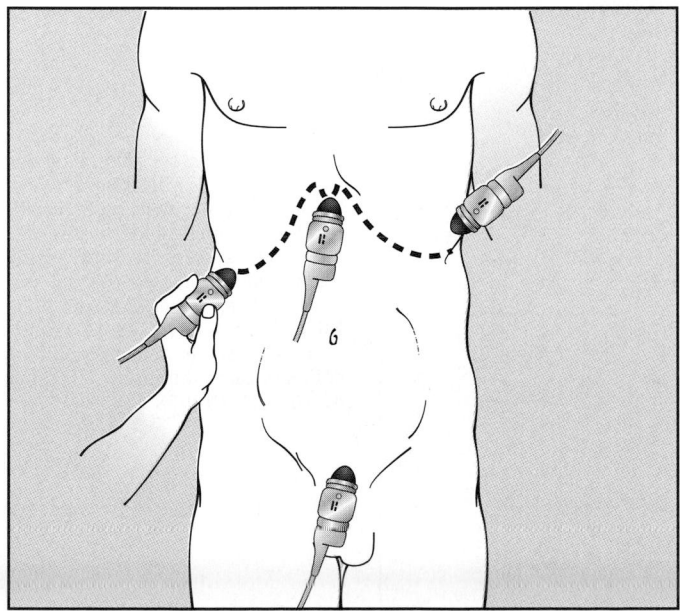

FIGURE 51–2. Focused Assessment for the Sonographic examination of the Trauma victim (FAST). (From Rozycki GS, Feliciano DV, Schmidt JA, et al: The role of surgeon performed ultrasound in patients with possible cardiac wounds. Ann Surg 223:737–746, 1996.)

the indication for subxiphoid pericardial window, recent enthusiasm for ultrasound evaluation has almost eliminated the role of subxiphoid pericardial window in the evaluation of cardiac trauma.

PERICARDIOCENTESIS (See Chap. 50). Pericardiocentesis has had significant historic support, especially at a time when the majority of penetrating cardiac wounds were produced by ice picks and the (surviving) patients arrived several hours and/or days after injury. In such instances there was a natural triage of the more severe cardiac injuries and the intrapericardial blood had become defibrinated and was easy to remove. Currently, many trauma surgeons discourage pericardiocentesis for acute trauma. In general, pericardiocentesis has historically been used as a diagnostic or therapeutic maneuver to drain nonclotted pericardial fluid. In the setting of trauma, cardiac tamponade is acute and due to hemorrhage. Clot forms quickly and is not amenable to needle drainage. Recurrence of tamponade and subsequent increase in mortality, as well as a significant incidence of false-negative results and potential for iatrogenic injury, makes pericardiocentesis a far less than optimal diagnostic tool.[28]

Indications for its use may apply in the iatrogenic injury caused by cardiac catheterization, at which time immediate decompression of the tamponade may be life saving, or in the trauma setting when a surgeon may not be available.

EVALUATION OF BLUNT CARDIAC INJURY

ECG. In blunt cardiac injury, conduction disturbances are common, and, thus, a screening 12-lead ECG may be helpful for evaluation. The most common rhythm disturbance is sinus tachycardia. Other possible disturbances include the following: T wave and ST segment changes (as seen with myocardial bruising), sinus bradycardia, first-degree atrioventricular block, right bundle branch block, right bundle branch block with hemiblock, third-degree block, atrial fibrillation, premature ventricular contractions, ventricular tachycardia, and ventricular fibrillation.[56]

Cardiac Enzymes. Much has previously been written about the use of cardiac enzyme determinations in evaluating blunt cardiac injury. However, no correlation between serum assays (e.g., creatine phosphokinase myocardial band, cardiac troponin T, or cardiac troponin I) and identification and prognosis of injury has been demonstrated with blunt cardiac injury.[57, 58] Therefore, cardiac enzyme assays should not be obtained unless evaluating concomitant coronary artery disease.[56]

TREATMENT

PREHOSPITAL AND EMERGENCY DEPARTMENT. Only a small subset of patients with significant cardiac injury ever reaches the emergency department, and expeditious transport to a designated trauma facility is essential to survival. Transport times of less than 5 minutes and successful endotracheal intubation are positive factors for survival.

DEFINITIVE TREATMENT. Definitive treatment involves surgical exposure through a thoracotomy (Fig. 51–3A) or median sternotomy (see Fig. 51–3B). The mainstay of treatment is relief of tamponade and correction of aberrant physiology. This involves correction of the acidosis and hypothermia and reestablishment of effective coronary perfusion (i.e., resuscitation of the heart).

Cardiorrhaphy should be performed by experienced surgeons (Fig. 51–4). Poor technique may result in enlargement of the lacerations or injury to the coronary arteries. If one is uncomfortable with the suturing technique, digital pressure may be applied until a more experienced surgeon arrives. Other techniques that have been described include the use of a Foley balloon catheter and a skin stapler[17] (Fig. 51–5).

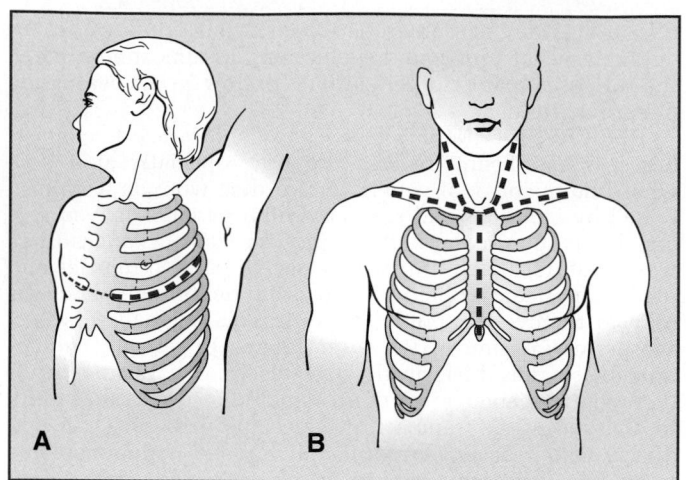

FIGURE 51–3. Incisions for cardiac injury. *A,* Left anterior thoracotomy (extension across the sternum if required). *B,* Median sternotomy (extension to the neck can be performed for exposure of the great vessels).

Exposure to the heart is gained by a left anterolateral thoracotomy, which allows access to the pericardium and heart and exposure for aortic cross-clamping if necessary. This incision may be extended across the sternum to gain access to the right side of the chest and for better exposure of the right atrium or right ventricle. This usually requires ligation of both internal thoracic arteries. Manual access to the right hemithorax from the left side of the chest is achieved through the anterior mediastinum by blunt dissection. This maneuver allows rapid evaluation of the right side of the chest for major injuries without transecting the sternum. Once the left pleural space is entered, the lung is retracted to expose the descending thoracic aorta for cross-clamping of the pericardium for exposure. It is helpful to note how much blood is present in the left side of the chest, which indicates hemorrhage versus tamponade. The pericardial sac anterior to the phrenopericardial vessels and phrenic nerve is opened, injuries are rapidly identified, and repair is performed.

In selected cases, particularly stab wounds to the precordium, the median sternotomy may be used. This incision allows excellent exposure to the anterior structures of the heart, but difficulty with access to the posterior mediastinal structures and descending thoracic aorta for cross-clamping may be encountered.

Mechanical support is not often used in the acute setting.[17]

BLUNT CARDIAC INJURY. Much debate and discussion has occurred over the clinical relevance of "cardiac contusion." Most trauma surgeons conclude this diagnosis should be eliminated because it does not affect how one treats these injuries.[18] Thus, a normotensive patient with a normal initial ECG and suspected blunt cardiac injury is managed with emergency department or "chest pain" observation units with no expected clinical significance. Patients with an abnormal ECG are admitted for monitoring and treated accordingly. Patients who present in cardiogenic shock are evaluated for a structural injury, which is then repaired.

Results

Factors that determine survival in traumatic cardiac injury are mechanism of injury, location of the injury, associated injuries, coronary artery involvement, presence of tamponade, length of prehospital transport, requirement of resuscitative thoracotomy, and experience of the trauma team. The

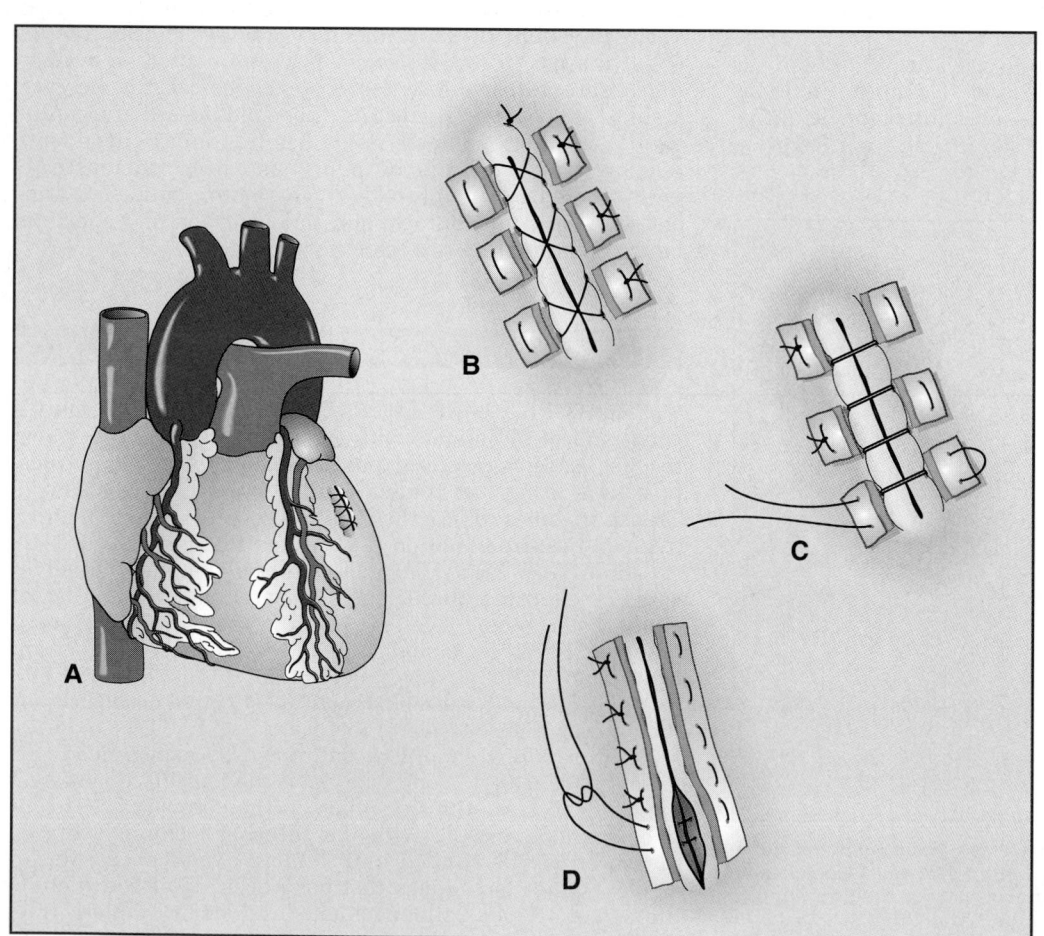

FIGURE 51–4. Technique of suture repair. Cardiorrhaphy *(A).* Should reinforcement be required, interrupted pledgeted sutures *(B),* pledgeted sutures around previously placed staples *(C),* or felt strips *(D)* can be used. (From Wall MJ Jr, Mattox KL, Chen CD, Baldwin JC: Acute management of complex cardiac injuries. J Trauma 42:905–912, 1997.)

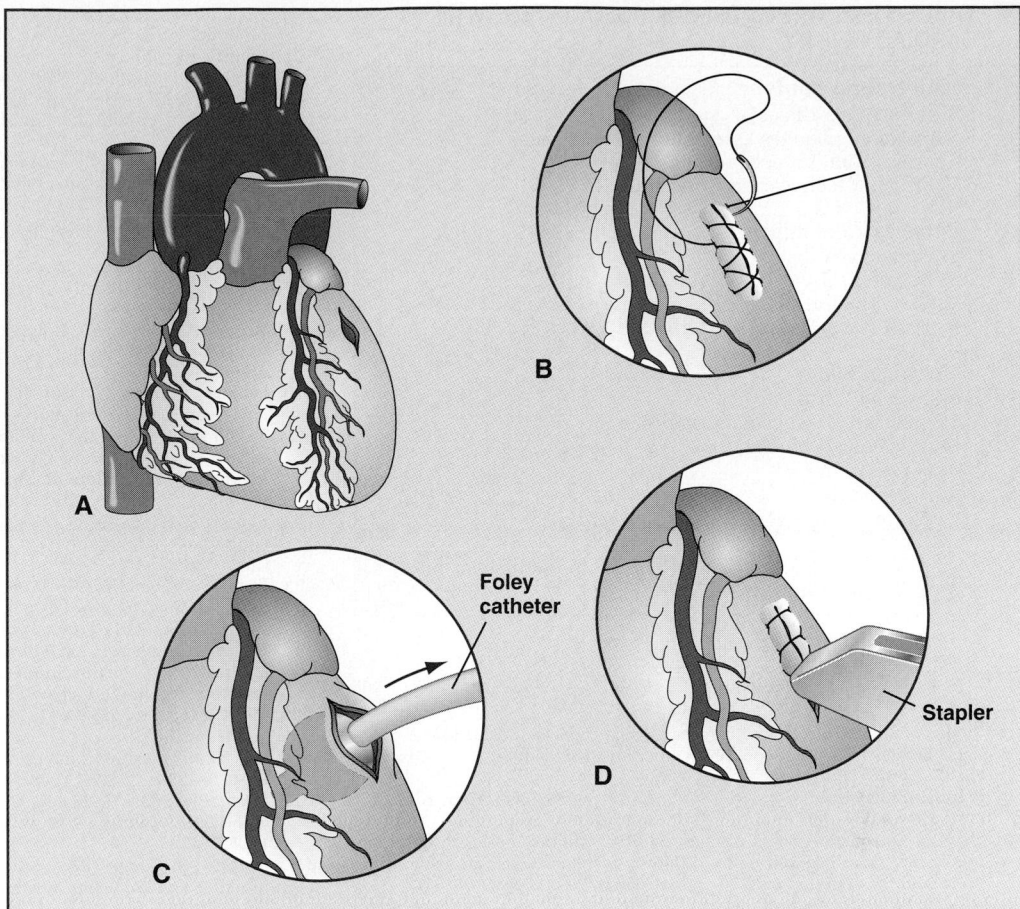

FIGURE 51–5. Temporary techniques to control bleeding. *A,* Stab wound to left ventricle. *B,* Initial management with interrupted or continuous 4-0 polypropylene sutures tied beneath the surgeon's finger. Additional techniques for complex injuries for temporary control include use of Foley balloon catheter *(C)* or skin stapler *(D).* (From Wall MJ Jr, Mattox KL, Chen CD, Baldwin JC: Acute management of complex cardiac injuries. J Trauma 42:905–912, 1997.)

overall hospital survival for penetrating heart injuries ranges from 30 to 90 percent.[17, 59]

The survival from a stab wound is 70 to 80 percent, whereas survival from a gunshot wound is between 30 and 40 percent.[49] Cardiac rupture has a worse prognosis than penetrating injuries to the heart. Calhoun and colleagues[14] reported a 70 percent survival in 10 patients, but most series report a survival of approximately 20 percent.[19]

Complications

Primary injury–related cardiac complications include coronary artery injury, valvular apparatus injury (annulus, papillary muscles, and chordae tendineae), intracardiac fistulas, arrhythmias, and delayed tamponade. These delayed sequelae have been reported to have a broad range (4–56 percent), depending on the definition of complication.[60]

Coronary artery injury is a rare complication, occurring in 5 to 9 percent of cardiac injuries, with a 69 percent mortality.[12, 17] This mortality is due to the associated cardiac injury and other associated injuries and the state of physiologic compromise when the patient arrives. A coronary artery injury is most often controlled by simple ligation, but bypass grafting using saphenous vein may be required for proximal left anterior descending injuries (with utilization of total cardiopulmonary bypass).[17] With a resurrection of the old concept of coronary artery bypass grafting without cardiopulmonary bypass ("off-pump" bypass), this technique may theoretically be used for these injuries in the highly unlikely event that the patient is hemodynamically stable.

Valvular apparatus dysfunction is rare (0.2–9 percent) and may occur with both blunt and penetrating trauma.[12, 17] Most frequently, the aortic valve, followed by the mitral and tricuspid valves, is injured.[12] Often these injuries are identified after the initial cardiorrhaphy and resuscitation has been performed. Timing of repair depends on the patient's condition. If severe cardiac dysfunction exists at the time of the initial operation, immediate valve repair or replacement may be required; otherwise, delayed repair is advised.

Intracardiac fistulas include VSDs, atrial septal defects, and atrioventricular fistulas, with an incidence of 1.9 percent among cardiac injuries.[17] Management depends on symptoms and degree of cardiac dysfunction, with only a minority of these patients requiring repair.[28] These injuries are often identified after primary repair is accomplished and can be repaired after recovery from the original and associated injuries. Cardiac catheterization should be accomplished before repair so that specific anatomic sites of injury and incision planning can be accomplished.

Arrhythmias may occur due to blunt injury, ischemia, or electrolyte abnormalities and are addressed according to the injury (Table 51–2) (see Chap. 25).

Delayed pericardial tamponade is very rare. It has been reported to occur as early as 1 hour after initial operation and as long as 76 days from the injury.[28]

Follow-Up

Secondary sequelae in survivors of cardiac trauma include valvular abnormalities and intracardiac fistulas.[61] These abnormalities may be identified intraoperatively by gross palpation of a thrill[17] or with the use of TEE. TEE, however, may not be feasible in the acutely injured patient. Early postoperative clinical examination and ECG findings are unreliable.[17] Thus, echocardiography is recommended during the initial hospitalization to identify occult injury and establish a baseline study. Because the incidence of late sequelae may be as high as 56 percent, follow-up echocardiography 3 to 4 weeks after injury has been recommended.[61]

▼ TABLE 51-2. ARRHYTHMIAS ASSOCIATED WITH CARDIAC INJURY

Penetrating Injury
Sinus tachycardia
ST segment changes associated with ischemia
Supraventricular tachycardia
Ventricular tachycardia/fibrillation

Blunt Cardiac Injury
Sinus tachycardia
ST segment, T wave abnormalities
Atrioventricular blocks, bradycardia
Ventricular tachycardia/fibrillation

Electrical Injury
Sinus tachycardia
ST segment, T wave abnormalities
Bundle branch blocks
Axis deviation
Prolonged QT
Paroxysmal supraventricular tachycardia
Atrial fibrillation
Ventricular tachycardia, fibrillation (alternating current)
Asystole (lightning strike)

REFERENCES

1. Richardson RG: Billroth and cardiac surgery. Lancet 1:1323, 1963.
2. Rehn L: Ueber penetrirende herzwuden and herzbeutels. Arch Klin Chir 55:315, 1897.
3. Rehn L: Zur chirurgie des herzens und des herzbeutels. Arch Klin Chir 83:723, 1907.
4. Hill LL: A report of a case of successful suturing of the heart, and table of 37 other cases of suturing by different operators with various terminations, and the conclusions drawn. Med Rec 62:846, 1902.
5. Isaacs JP: Sixty penetrating wounds of the heart: Clinical and experimental observations. Surgery 45:696, 1959.
6. Crynes SF, Hunter WC: Traumatic rupture of the pericardium. Arch Intern Med 64:719–746, 1939.
7. Des Forges O, Ridder WP, Lenoci RJ: Successful suture of ruptured myocardium after nonpenetrating injury. N Engl J Med 252:567–569, 1955.
8. Sherman MM, Saini YK, Yarnoz MD, et al: Management of penetrating heart wounds. Am J Surg 135:553, 1978.
9. Ivatury RR: Injury to the heart. In Feliciano DV, Moore EE, Mattox KL (eds): Trauma. 3rd ed. Stamford, CT, Appleton & Lange, 1996.
10. Campbell NC, Thomsen SR, Murkart DJ, et al: Review of 1198 cases of penetrating cardiac trauma. Br J Surg 84:1737, 1997.
11. Foy HM, Arreola-Risa C, Boyle E, et al: Penetrating cardiac injuries: Analysis of combined trauma center and medical examiners experience. Twelfth annual AAST. Halifax, Nova Scotia, Canada, 1995.
12. Parmley LF, Manion WC, Mattingly TW: Nonpenetrating traumatic injury of the heart. Circulation 18:371–396, 1958.
13. Bright EF, Beck CF: Nonpenetrating wounds of the heart: A clinical and experimental study. Am Heart J 10:293–321, 1935.
14. Calhoun JH, Hoffman TH, Trinkle JK, et al: Management of blunt rupture of the heart. J Trauma 26:495–502, 1986.

ETIOLOGY AND PATTERNS OF CARDIAC TRAUMA

15. Hartman PR, Trinkle JK: Injury to the heart. In Moore EE, Mattox KL, Feliciano DV (eds): Trauma. 2nd ed. Norwalk, CT, Appleton & Lange, 1991, pp 373–391.
16. Asensio JA, Berne JD, Demetriades D, et al: One hundred five penetrating cardiac injuries: A 2-year prospective evaluation. J Trauma 44:1073–1082, 1998.
17. Wall MJ Jr, Mattox KL, Chen CD, Baldwin JC: Acute management of complex cardiac injuries. J Trauma 42:905–912, 1997.
18. Mattox KL, Flint LM, Carrico CJ, et al: Editorial: Blunt cardiac injury. J Trauma 33:649–650, 1992.
18a. Kao CL, Chang JP, Chang CH: Acute mediastinal tamponade secondary to blunt sternal fracture. J Trauma 48:157–158, 2000.
19. Funda G, Brathwaite CEM, Rodriguez A, et al: Blunt traumatic rupture of the heart and pericardium: A 10-year experience (1979–1986). J Trauma 31:167–173, 1991.
20. Lin JC, Ott RA: Acute traumatic mitral valve insufficiency. J Trauma 47:165–168, 1999.
21. Amerongen RV, Rosen M, Winnik G, Horwitz J: Ventricular fibrillation following blunt chest trauma from a baseball. Pediatr Emerg Care 13:107, 1997.
22. Maron BJ, Link MS, Wang PJ, et al: Clinical profile of commotio cordis:

An underappreciated cause of sudden death in young during sports and other activities. J Cardiovasc Electrophysiol 10:114–120, 1999.
23. Ivatury RR: Injury to the heart. In Mattox KL, Feliciano DV, Moore EE (eds): Trauma, 4th ed. New York, McGraw-Hill, 1999, pp 545–558.
24. Schaffer RB, Berdat PA, Seiler C, Carrel TP: Isolated rupture of the ventricular septum after blunt chest trauma. Ann Thorac Surg 67:853–854, 1999.
25. Baumgartner FJ, Rayhanabad J, Bongard FS, et al: Central venous injuries of the subclavian-jugular and innominate-caval confluences. Tex Heart Inst J 26:177–181, 1999.
26. Fitt G, Thomson K, Hennessy O: Delayed fatal cardiac perforation by an indwelling long introducer sheath following transjugular intrahepatic portocaval stents. Cardiovasc Intervent Radiol 16:109–110, 1993.
27. Medizinische Klinik IV: Perforation und Ruptur koronaryarterien. Herz 23:311–318, 1998.
28. Ivatury RR, Simon RJ, Rohman M: Cardiac complications. In Mattox KL (ed): Complications of Trauma. New York, Churchill Livingstone, 1994, pp 409–428.
29. Huang YS, Yang ZC, Tan BG, et al: Pathogenesis of early cardiac myocyte damage after sear burns. J Trauma 46:428–432, 1999.
30. Taylor KM: SIRS—the systemic inflammatory response syndrome after cardiac operations. Ann Thorac Surg 61:1607, 1996.
31. Kirkpatrick AW, Chun R, Brown R, Simons RK: Hypothermia and the trauma patient. Can J Surg 42:333–343, 1999.
32. Sharkey SW, Shear W, Hodges M, Herzog CA: Reversible myocardial contraction abnormalities in patients with an acute non-cardiac illness. Chest 114:98–105, 1998.
33. Kumar A, Thota V, Dee L, et al: TNF-alpha and IL-1 are regulators for depression of in vitro myocardial cell contractility induced by serum from humans with septic shock. J Exp Med 183:949–958, 1996.
34. Ungureanu-Longrois D, Balligand JL, Kelly RA, Smith TW: Myocardial contractile dysfunction in the systemic inflammatory response syndrome: Role of cytokine-inducible nitric oxide synthase in cardiac myocytes. J Mol Cell Cardiol 27:155–167, 1995.
35. Meldrum DR, Shenkar R, Sheridan BC, et al: Hemorrhage activates myocardial Nfkappa and increases TNF-alpha in the heart. J Mol Cell Cardiol 29:2849–2854, 1997.
36. Horton JW, Lin C, Maass D: Burn trauma and tumor necrosis factor alpha alter calcium handling by cardiomyocytes. Shock 10:270–277, 1998.
37. Horton JW, Garcia NM, White DJ, Keffer J: Postburn cardiac contractile function and biochemical markers of postburn cardiac injury. J Am Coll Surg 181:289–298, 1995.
38. White M, Wiechmann RJ, Roden RL, et al: Cardiac beta-adrenergic neuroeffector systems in acute myocardial dysfunction related to brain injury. Circulation 92:2183–2189, 1995.
39. Horton JW, White J, Maass D, Sanders B: Arginine in burn injury improves cardiac performance and prevents bacterial translocation. J Appl Physiol 84:695–702, 1998.
40. Heinz G, Geppert A, Delle Karth G, et al: IV milrinone for cardiac output increase and maintenance: Comparison in nonhyperdynamic SIRS/sepsis and congestive heart failure. Intensive Care Med 25:620–624, 1999.
41. Svedjeholm R, Huljebrant I, Hakanson E, Vanhanen I: Glutamate and high dose glucose-insulin-potassium (GIK) in the treatment of cardiac failure after cardiac operations. Ann Thorac Surg 59:S23–S30, 1995.
42. Flohe S, Borgermann J, Dominquez FE, et al: Influence of granulocyte-macrophage colony-stimulating factor (GM-CSF) on whole blood endotoxin responsiveness following trauma, cardiopulmonary bypass, and severe sepsis. Shock 12:17–24, 1999.
43. Giroir BP, Horton JW, White DJ, et al: Inhibition of tumor necrosis factor prevents myocardial dysfunction during burn shock. Am J Physiol 267:H118–H124, 1994.
44. Carleton SC: Cardiac problems associated with burns. Cardiol Clin 13:257, 1995.
45. Carleton SC: Cardiac problems associated with electrical injury. Cardiol Clin 13:263, 1995.
46. LeMaire SA, Wall MJ Jr, Mattox KL: Needle embolus causing cardiac puncture and chronic constrictive pericarditis. Ann Thorac Surg 65:1786–1787, 1998.
47. Symbas PN, Symbas PJ: Missiles in the cardiovascular system. Surg Clin N Am 7:343–349, 1997.

CLINICAL PRESENTATION, PATHOPHYSIOLOGY, AND EVALUATION

48. Ivatury RR: The injured heart. In Mattox KL, Moore EE, Feliciano DV (eds): Trauma. 4th ed. Stamford, CT, Appleton & Lange, 1999.
49. Brown J, Grover FL: Trauma to the heart. Chest Surg Clin North Am 7:325, 1997.
50. American College of Surgeons, Committee on Trauma: Advanced Trauma Life Support. Chicago, American College of Surgeons, 1997.
51. Read RA, Moore EE, Moore JB: Emergency department thoracotomy. In Feliciano DV, Moore EE, Mattox KL (eds): Trauma. 3rd ed. Stamford, CT, Appleton & Lange, 1999.
52. Rozycki GS, Feliciano DV, Schmidt JA, et al: The role of surgeon performed ultrasound in patients with possible cardiac wounds. Ann Surg 223:737–746, 1996.
53. Mattox KL, Wall MJ Jr: Newer diagnostic measures and emergency management. Chest Surg Clin North Am 7:214, 1997.

54. Rozycki GS, Schmidt JA, Oschner MG, et al: The role of surgeon-performed ultrasound in patients with possible penetrating wounds: A prospective multicenter study. J Trauma 45:190, 1998.

55. Meyer DM, Jessen ME, Grayburn PA: Use of echocardiography to detect occult cardiac injury after penetrating thoracic trauma: A prospective study. J Trauma 39:902, 1995.

56. Feliciano DV, Rozycki GS: Advances in the diagnosis and treatment of thoracic trauma. Surg Clin North Am 79:1417–1429, 1999.

57. Adams JE III, Davila-Roman VG, Bessey PQ, et al: Improved detection of cardiac contusion with cardiac troponin I. Am Heart J 131:308–312, 1996.

58. Ferjani M, Droc G, Dreux S, et al: Circulating cardiac troponin T in myocardial contusion. Chest 111:427–433, 1997.

TREATMENT

59. Attar S, Suter CM, Hankins JR, et al: Penetrating cardiac injuries. Ann Thorac Surg 51:711, 1991.

60. Mattox KL, Limacher MC, Feliciano DV, et al: Cardiac evaluation following heart injury. J Trauma 25:758–765, 1985.

61. Demetriades D, Charalambides D, Sareli P, et al: Late sequela of penetrating cardiac injuries. Br J Surg 77:813, 1990.

Chapter 52

Pulmonary Embolism

SAMUEL Z. GOLDHABER

Pulmonary embolism (PE) and deep venous thrombosis (DVT) account for hundreds of thousands of hospitalizations annually in the United States and afflict millions of individuals worldwide. The future holds great promise as advances in molecular biology, diagnostic imaging, and therapy with low-molecular-weight heparin (LMWH) revolutionize our approach to venous thromboembolism. Nevertheless, despite progress in early detection and treatment, the rates of mortality (Fig. 52–1) and recurrent PE remain high.[1] As the population ages, venous thromboembolism will become more prevalent because the incidence of PE increases with age.[1]

Cardiovascular specialists must keep PE in mind when they evaluate patients with unexplained chest discomfort, shortness of breath, and lightheadedness because these symptoms constitute the cardinal clinical presentations for PE. They should implement streamlined diagnostic algorithms and use risk stratification to recommend the most appropriate therapeutic approach. Finally, cardiologists must provide expertise in the treatment of hemodynamically compromised patients with PE as well as those with right ventricular failure who maintain a stable blood pressure and heart rate.

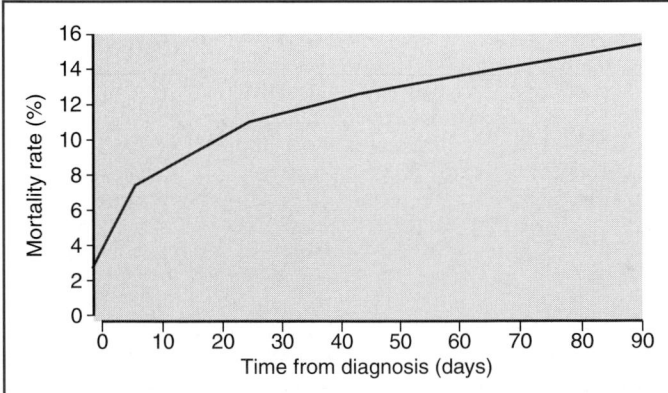

FIGURE 52–1. Overall cumulative mortality due to PE in the International Cooperative Pulmonary Embolism Registry (ICOPER) of 2454 patients was 11.4 percent at 2 weeks and 17.4 percent at 3 months. After exclusion of patients in whom PE was first discovered at autopsy, the mortality rate was 15.3 percent. (From Goldhaber SZ, Visani L, De Rosa M, for ICOPER: Acute pulmonary embolism: Clinical outcomes in the International Cooperative Pulmonary Embolism Registry (ICOPER). Lancet 353:1386, 1999.

PATHOPHYSIOLOGY

Hypercoagulable States

In 1856, Rudolf Virchow postulated that a triad of factors leads to intravascular coagulation: (1) local trauma to the vessel wall, (2) hypercoagulability, and (3) stasis. Classically, the pathogenesis of PE was dichotomized as due to either unusual "inherited" (primary) or commonly "acquired" (secondary) risk factors. Now, however, it appears likely that many patients who develop PE are genetically predisposed (Tables 52–1 and 52–2) but often require a precipitating environmental stress (Table 52–3) to elicit overt thrombosis.[2]

▼ **TABLE 52–1. PRINCIPAL HYPERCOAGULABLE STATES ASSOCIATED WITH VENOUS THROMBOSIS**

HYPERCOAGULABLE STATE	CITATION	COMMENTS
Mutation in factor V gene	Bertina et al[3] Ridker et al[5]	Replaces arginine 506 with glutamine, rendering factor V resistant to inactivation by activated protein C
Resistance to activated protein C	Zöller et al[11]	Molecular background for resistance to activated protein C was found to be heterogeneous
Prothrombin gene mutation	Poort et al[9]	G20210A point mutation increases prothrombin levels
Mutation in protein C gene	Allaart et al[12]	Associated with protein C deficiency
Protein S deficiency	Gladson et al[13]	Protein S a cofactor for protein C
Antithrombin III deficiency	Bucciarelli et al[14]	Autosomal dominant inheritance; has a higher risk for venous thrombosis than the other genetic defects
Hyperhomocysteinemia	den Heijer et al[15] Langman et al[15a] Ridker et al[16]	Doubles or triples risk[15, 15a]; potentiates risk from underlying factor V Leiden[16]
Antiphospholipid antibodies	Greaves[17]	Encompasses anticardiolipin antibodies and lupus anticoagulant; associated with venous and arterial thrombosis

TABLE 52–2A. FREQUENCY OF CLASSIC COAGULATION PROTEIN DEFICIENCIES AMONG PATIENTS WITH VENOUS THROMBOSIS

ABNORMAL	GLADSON ET AL[13] (N = 141)(%)	HEIJBOER ET AL[18] (N = 277)(%)	MALM ET AL[19] (N = 439)(%)
Protein C	4	3	2
Protein S	5	2	2
Antithrombin III	3	1	1
Plasminogen	2	1	0.5

TABLE 52–2B. FREQUENCY OF ACTIVATED PROTEIN C RESISTANCE AMONG PATIENTS WITH VENOUS THROMBOSIS

ABNORMALITY	SVENSSON AND DAHLBÄCK[20] (N = 104)(%)	KOSTER ET AL[21] (N = 301)(%)
Activated protein C resistance	33	21

PRIMARY HYPERCOAGULABLE STATES (see also Chap. 62). The identification of a poor anticoagulant response to activated protein C (aPC) is the most exciting and far-reaching development ever to occur in the field of prothrombotic markers. Normally, a specified amount of aPC can be added to plasma and prolongation of the activated partial thromboplastin time (PTT) can be observed. However, patients with "aPC resistance" have inadequate PTT prolongation. In contrast to classical coagulation protein deficiencies, which are rare (Table 52–2A), aPC resistance occurs frequently among patients with venous thrombosis (Table 52–2B).

The phenotype of aPC resistance is associated with a single point mutation, designated factor V Leiden, in the factor V gene.[3] This mutation results from a single nucleotide substitution of adenine for guanine 1691 that replaces the amino acid arginine with glutamine at position 506. This change eliminates the protein C cleavage site in factor V.[4]

The allelic frequency of this mutation is about 3 percent in healthy male physicians in the United States. In the Physicians' Health Study, no statistically significant differences were found between the incidence of the mutation among previously healthy men who subsequently developed myocardial infarction or stroke compared with men who remained free of cardiovascular disease. However, the incidence of the factor V mutation was three times higher among men who developed DVT.[5]

In a case-control study of premenopausal women who developed DVT, the risk of thrombosis among users of oral

TABLE 52–3. ACQUIRED CONDITIONS THAT MAY PRECIPITATE VENOUS THROMBOSIS

Surgery/immobilization/trauma
Obesity
Increasing age
Cigarette smoking
Systemic arterial hypertension
Oral contraceptives/pregnancy/postpartum
Cancer (sometimes occult adenocarcinoma) and cancer chemotherapy
Stroke/spinal cord injury
Indwelling central venous catheter

contraceptives was increased fourfold. However, the risk of thrombosis among carriers of the factor V Leiden mutation was eightfold that of noncarriers. Among patients with both oral contraceptive use and the mutation, the risk of thrombosis was increased more than 30-fold.[6] The factor V Leiden mutation is also a risk factor for recurrent pregnancy loss[7] and in the Physicians' Health Study is associated with a fourfold increased risk of *recurrent* PE or DVT after completion of a course of anticoagulation.[8]

However, in a cohort of patients with venous thromboembolism in Rome and Milan, the risk of recurrent thrombosis after discontinuing anticoagulation was similar among carriers of factor V Leiden and patients without this mutation.[8a] Furthermore, the prevalence of the factor V Leiden mutation appears to be twice as high in patients with DVT compared with patients with PE. Some investigators speculate that the mutation confers an increased stability and adherence of thrombus to the vein wall, thereby decreasing the frequency of embolization to the lungs.[8b]

A single-point mutation in the 3' untranslated region of the prothrombin gene (G-to-A transition at nucleotide position 20210) is associated with increased levels of prothrombin.[9] In the Physicians' Health Study, the prevalence of the prothrombin gene mutation among control subjects was 3.9 percent, and this G20210A mutation doubled the risk of venous thrombosis.[10] Women with both factor V Leiden and the G20210A prothrombin-gene mutation have a disproportionately high risk of DVT or PE.[10a] Recently, high levels of coagulation factor XI have been described as doubling the risk of venous thrombosis.[10b]

Although molecular medicine can help elucidate pathogenesis, a careful family history is still the most rapid and cost-effective method of identifying a predisposition to venous thrombosis. Investigation with blood tests (see Table 52–1) to detect a hypercoagulable state can be misleading. For example, consumption coagulopathy due to venous thrombosis may be misdiagnosed as deficiency of antithrombin III, protein C, or protein S. Heparin administration can depress antithrombin III levels, and use of warfarin ordinarily causes a mild deficiency of protein C or S. Both oral contraceptives and pregnancy depress protein S levels.

ACQUIRED CONDITIONS THAT MAY PRECIPITATE VENOUS THROMBOSIS. Conditions that increase venous stasis or cause endothelial damage (see Table 52–3) are likely to predispose toward venous thrombosis, especially among patients who already have subclinical hypercoagulable states. Even minor events such as travel and minor surgery increase the venous thromboembolism risk.[21a]

The stasis and immobilization associated with postoperative venous thrombosis may increase after hospital discharge, because many patients who are forced to ambulate during hospitalization may become confined to bed on returning home. PE is increasingly likely to occur *after* hospital discharge because of the contemporary emphasis on minimizing the length of stay after surgery. Among 45,000 total hip and total knee replacement operations in a State of California data base, the diagnosis of venous thromboembolism was made after hospital discharge in 76 percent and 47 percent of the total hip and total knee replacement operations, respectively. The median interval until diagnosis was 17 days for total hip and 7 days for total knee replacements.[22]

Coronary artery bypass grafting has been associated with a 4 percent risk of PE[23] and a 20 percent risk of venous thrombosis of the deep leg veins.[24] After *major trauma*, the DVT rate was 58 percent in a prospective study in which contrast venograms were obtained.[25] Among immobilized *patients in a medical intensive care unit*, the rate of venous thrombosis detected with ultrasonography was 33 percent.[26]

Marked obesity in women was a strong risk factor for PE in both the Framingham Heart Study[27] and the Nurses' Health Study.[28] Other environmental risk factors for PE in the Nurses' Health Study were *cigarette smoking* and systemic arterial *hypertension*.[28]

With respect to *oral contraceptives*, decreasing the estrogen content has diminished the risk of venous thromboembolism. However, third-generation oral contraceptives with the new progestogens, desogestrel and gestodene, are problematic, with an approximate doubling in thrombotic risk even though they are less androgenic, have less effect on carbohydrate and lipid metabolism, and may have stronger suppression of ovarian activity than second-generation oral contraceptives.[29] They appear to cause an acquired resistance to aPC.[30]

Even the low dose of estrogen prescribed for *postmenopausal hormone replacement* doubles the risk of PE.[31] The risk is increased for *raloxifene*, a selective estrogen receptor modulator,[32] as well as for the more commonly used conjugated equine estrogens.

PE is the leading cause of maternal mortality during *pregnancy*. Antenatal DVT is usually left sided, involves the iliofemoral system, and occurs about twice as frequently as postpartum DVT. Increasing age and cesarean section are major risk factors for venous thromboembolism.[33] Conversely, women with serious obstetrical complications have an increased incidence of genetic mutations predisposing them to venous thrombosis.[34]

Cancer promotes the synthesis and secretion of procoagulants and is a risk factor for PE; conversely, venous thromboembolism may be the initial manifestation of an otherwise occult cancer. In a Danish registry, there was a threefold increase in cancer diagnoses during the initial 6 months after DVT or PE became evident. The cancers were often widely metastatic at the time of discovery, and the most frequent cancers were pancreatic, ovarian, primary hepatic, and brain.[35]

Patients receiving chemotherapy for metastatic breast cancer are at risk of developing venous thromboembolic disease. In a randomized controlled trial of very low-dose warfarin versus placebo, 4 percent of the placebo group developed venous thrombosis during the average 6-month follow-up period.[36]

Leg DVT is a common complication of *acute ischemic stroke*, particularly in the paralyzed limb. Even when patients receive 5000 units twice daily of unfractionated heparin for prophylaxis, the venous thrombosis rate is as high as 31 percent.[37] With *spinal cord injury*, there is also a high rate of venous thrombosis.[38]

Thrombotic complications due to indwelling central venous catheters are common and are often associated with catheter sepsis.[39] Indwelling vascular catheters can become engulfed in a thrombin or fibrin sheath that serves as a nidus for subsequent infection.

RELATIONSHIP BETWEEN DEEP VENOUS THROMBOSIS AND PULMONARY EMBOLISM. Most PE result from thrombi that originate in the pelvic or deep veins of the leg; occasionally, thrombi in the axillary or subclavian veins embolize to the pulmonary arteries. In a treatment trial of proximal leg DVT, Moser and colleagues found that nearly 40 percent of patients had asymptomatic PE, based on concomitantly obtained ventilation-perfusion scans.[40] There is also an appreciable risk of asymptomatic PE due to upper-extremity thrombosis.[41] However, many patients with PE do not have detectable DVT.[42]

When venous thrombi detach from their sites of formation, they flow through the venous system toward the pulmonary arterial circulation. If an embolus is extremely large, it may lodge at the bifurcation of the pulmonary artery, forming a saddle embolus (Fig. 52–2 *top*). More commonly, a major pulmonary vessel is occluded (Fig. 52–2 *bottom*).

RIGHT VENTRICULAR DYSFUNCTION. The extent of pulmonary vascular obstruction is probably the most important factor determining whether right ventricular dysfunction ensues. As obstruction increases, pulmonary artery pressures rise. Moreover, the release of vasoconstricting compounds (e.g., serotonin), reflex pulmonary artery vasoconstriction, and hypoxemia may further increase pulmonary vascular resistance and result in pulmonary hypertension.[43]

VENTRICULAR INTERDEPENDENCY. The sudden rise in pulmonary artery pressure reflects an abrupt increase in right ventricular afterload, with consequent elevation of right ventricular wall tension followed by right ventricular dilatation and dysfunction (Fig. 52–3).[44] As the right ventricle dilates, the interventricular septum shifts toward the left ventricle, with resultant underfilling of this chamber due to

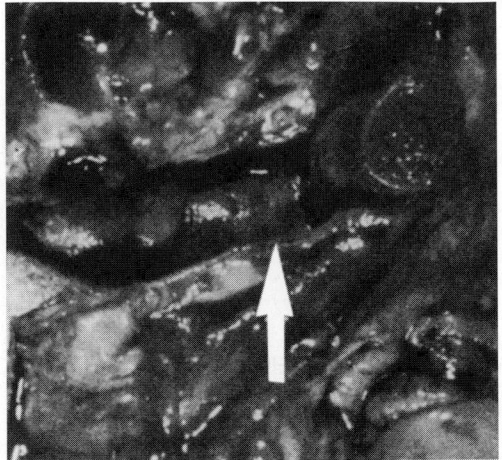

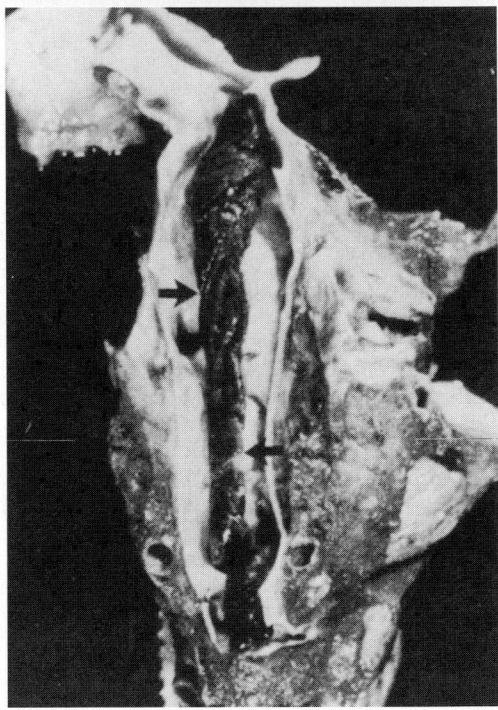

FIGURE 52–2. *Top,* Saddle embolus (arrow) at the bifurcation of the pulmonary artery. *Bottom,* Pulmonary embolus in left lower lobe pulmonary artery, with minimal attachment to the wall of the vessel. The embolus was dark red, typical of venous thrombi, and had indentations believed to represent impressions of the venous valves (arrows). (From Godleski JJ: Pathology of deep venous thrombosis and pulmonary embolism. *In* Goldhaber SZ [ed]: Pulmonary Embolism and Deep Venous Thrombosis. Philadelphia, WB Saunders, 1985, p 17.)

pericardial constraint.[45] In addition, right ventricular contractile dysfunction may decrease right ventricular cardiac output and further reduce left ventricular preload. As the right ventricle distends, coronary venous pressure increases and left ventricular diastolic distensibility decreases.[46]

The reduction in left ventricular preload may also lead to interventricular septal shift toward the left ventricle. With underfilling of the left ventricle, both systemic cardiac output and pressure decrease, potentially compromising coronary perfusion and producing myocardial ischemia, with release of troponin.[47] Elevated right ventricular wall tension following massive PE reduces right coronary flow and increases right ventricular myocardial oxygen demand, which may result in ischemia and possibly cardiogenic shock. Perpetuation of this cycle can lead to right ventricular infarction, circulatory collapse, and death.

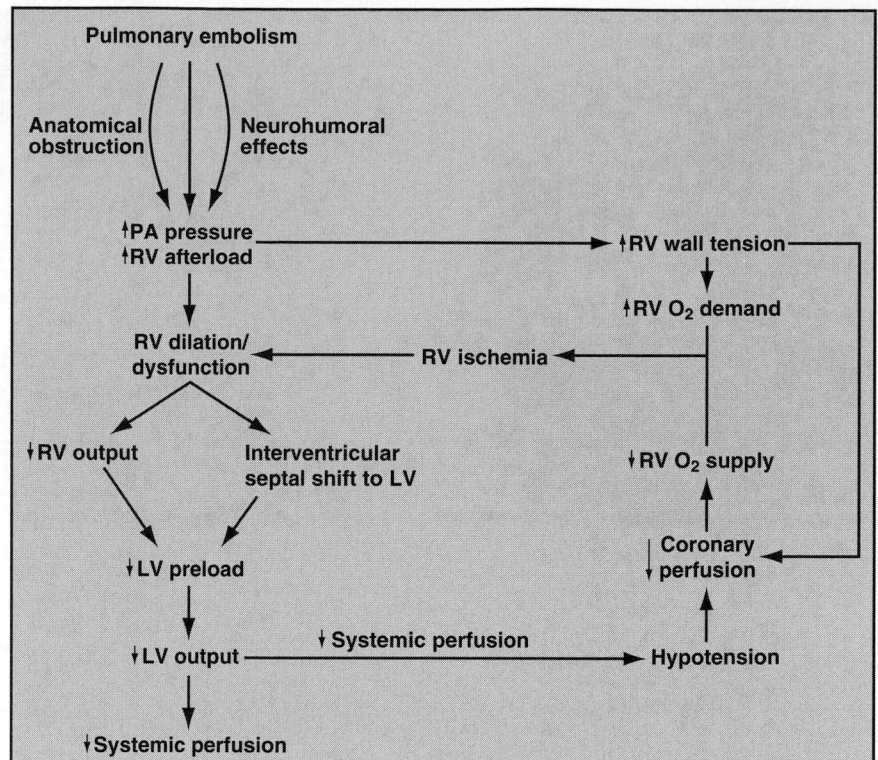

FIGURE 52–3. Pathophysiology of right ventricular dysfunction. PA = pulmonary artery; RV = right ventricle; LV = left ventricle.

SUMMARY OF PATHOPHYSIOLOGY. PE can have the following pathophysiological effects: (1) increased pulmonary vascular resistance due to vascular obstruction, neurohumoral agents, or pulmonary artery baroreceptors; (2) impaired gas exchange due to increased alveolar dead space from vascular obstruction and hypoxemia from alveolar hypoventilation, low ventilation-perfusion units, and right-to-left shunting, as well as impaired carbon monoxide transfer due to loss of gas-exchange surface; (3) alveolar hyperventilation due to reflex stimulation of irritant receptors; (4) increased airway resistance due to bronchoconstriction; and (5) decreased pulmonary compliance due to lung edema, lung hemorrhage, and loss of surfactant.[43]

DIAGNOSIS

Diagnosis of PE is more difficult than treatment or prevention. For patients with PE, the most dangerous period is that preceding the establishment of the correct diagnosis. Fortunately, reliable noninvasive diagnostic approaches have become increasingly available—particularly venous ultrasound, plasma D-dimer enzyme-linked immunosorbent assay (ELISA) chest computed tomography (CT) scanning, and echocardiography. The contemporary diagnostic strategy integrates clinical findings with various diagnostic techniques.[47a]

Clinical Presentation

Clinical suspicion of PE is of paramount importance in guiding diagnostic testing. Dyspnea is the most frequent symptom, and tachypnea is the most frequent sign of PE (Table 52–4). In general, severe dyspnea, syncope, or cyanosis portends a major life-threatening PE. However, pleuritic pain often signifies that the embolism is small and located in the distal pulmonary arterial system, near the pleural lining.

PE should be suspected in hypotensive patients when (1) there is evidence of venous thrombosis or predisposing factors for it and (2) there is clinical evidence of acute cor pulmonale (acute right ventricular failure) such as distended neck veins, an S_3 gallop, a right ventricular heave, tachycardia, or tachypnea, especially if (3) there are echocardiographic findings of right ventricular dilatation and hypokinesis or electrocardiographic (ECG) evidence of acute cor pulmonale manifested by a new S_1-Q_3-T_3 pattern, new incomplete right bundle branch block, or right ventricular ischemia.

DIFFERENTIAL DIAGNOSIS. The differential diagnosis of PE is broad and covers a spectrum from life-threatening disease such as acute myocardial infarction to innocuous anxiety states (Table 52–5). Some patients have concomitant PE and other illnesses. Therefore, for example, if pneumonia or heart failure does not respond to appropriate therapy, the possibility of coexisting PE should be considered.

Distinguishing between PE and primary pulmonary hypertension (see Chap. 53) deserves special vigilance (Table 52–6). Surprisingly, some patients have a hybrid condition that is similar to primary pulmonary hypertension but that includes thrombi. Among these patients, large central pulmonary artery thrombi can develop.[47b] It is often impossible

▼ **TABLE 52–4.** MOST COMMON SYMPTOMS AND SIGNS AMONG THE 2454 PATIENTS IN THE INTERNATIONAL COOPERATIVE PULMONARY EMBOLISM REGISTRY (ICOPER)

SYMPTOM OR SIGN	PERCENT
Dyspnea	82
Respiratory rate >20/min	60
Heart rate >100 beats/min	40
Chest pain	49
Cough	20
Syncope	14
Hemoptysis	7

Adapted from Goldhaber SZ, Visani L, De Rosa M, for ICOPER: Acute pulmonary embolism: Clinical outcomes in the International Cooperative Pulmonary Embolism Registry (ICOPER). Lancet 353:1386, 1999.

▼ TABLE 52–5. DIFFERENTIAL DIAGNOSIS OF PULMONARY EMBOLISM

Myocardial infarction
Pneumonia
Congestive heart failure ("left-sided")
Cardiomyopathy (global)
Primary pulmonary hypertension
Asthma
Pericarditis
Intrathoracic cancer
Rib fracture
Pneumothorax
Costochondritis
"Musculoskeletal pain"
Anxiety

to determine whether these thrombi formed in situ or whether they embolized to the pulmonary arteries from a separate site.

Clinical Syndromes of Pulmonary Embolism

Classification of PE into various syndromes (Table 52–7) is useful for prognostication and for deciding on subsequent clinical management.[48]

MASSIVE PULMONARY EMBOLISM. Patients with massive PE are at risk for cardiogenic shock. They have thrombosis often affecting at least half of the pulmonary arterial system. Clot is almost always present bilaterally. Dyspnea is usually the cardinal symptom, and systemic arterial hypotension requiring pressor support is the predominant sign.

MODERATE TO LARGE PULMONARY EMBOLISM. These patients have right ventricular hypokinesis on echocardiography but normal systemic arterial pressure. Usually, lung scanning indicates that more than 30 percent of the lung is not perfused. These patients have various degrees of right ventricular hemodynamic instability that is masked by normal systemic arterial pressure. They may be at risk for recurrent (and possibly fatal) PE, even with adequate anticoagulation.[49] Therefore, especially if right ventricular dysfunction persists, one should consider using thrombolytics or embolectomy.

▼ TABLE 52–6. PRIMARY PULMONARY HYPERTENSION (PPH) VS. RECURRENT PULMONARY EMBOLISM (PE)

SIMILARITIES	
Symptoms	Fatigue, dyspnea on exertion—most common; chest pain, syncope, hemoptysis, cyanosis—also common
Clinical course	Progressive dyspnea, right-heart failure
Hemodynamics	Elevated right-heart pressures, normal pulmonary capillary wedge pressure
Histology	Thrombotic lesions usually present
Treatment	Includes anticoagulation

DIFFERENCES		
Variable	**PPH**	**Recurrent PE**
Age (years)	20–40	>50
Female/male ratio	4:1	1:1
Clinical course	Continued deterioration	Deterioration, with intermittent stabilization
Perfusion lung scan	No segmental perfusion defects	Segmental or larger perfusion defects
Pulmonary artery systolic pressure	>60 mm Hg	<60 mm Hg
Pulmonary angiogram	"Pruning"	Intraluminal filling defects
Confounding problems with angiogram	Thrombi may occur on or distal to PPH lesions	"Pruning" can also suggest PE
Diagnostic alternatives	Lung biopsy	Pulmonary angioscopy
Therapy	Anticoagulation; high-dose nifedipine or diltiazem; long-term continuous intravenous prostacyclin	Anticoagulation; inferior vena caval interruption; thromboendarterectomy

Adapted from Goldhaber SZ: Strategies for diagnosis. In Goldhaber SZ (ed): Pulmonary Embolism and Deep Vein Thrombosis. Philadelphia, WB Saunders, 1985, p 89.

SMALL TO MODERATE PULMONARY EMBOLISM. This syndrome is characterized by both normal systemic arterial pressure and normal right ventricular function. Patients usually have a good prognosis if anticoagulation or an infe-

▼ TABLE 52–7. SIX SYNDROMES OF ACUTE PULMONARY EMBOLISM

SYNDROME	PRESENTATION	RIGHT VENTRICULAR DYSFUNCTION	THERAPY
Massive	Breathlessness, syncope, and cyanosis with persistent systemic arterial hypotension; typically >50 percent obstruction of pulmonary vasculature	Present	Heparin plus thrombolytic therapy or mechanical intervention
Moderate to large	Normal systemic arterial blood pressure; typically >30 percent perfusion defect on lung scan	Present	Heparin plus or minus thrombolytic therapy or mechanical intervention*
Small to moderate	Normal arterial blood pressure	Absent	Heparin
Pulmonary infarction	Pleuritic chest pain, hemoptysis, pleural rub, or evidence of lung consolidation; typically small peripheral emboli	Rare	Heparin and nonsteroidal antiinflammatory drugs
Paradoxical embolism	Sudden systemic embolic event such as stroke	Rare	Anticoagulation ± closure of right-to-left cardiac shunt
Nonthrombotic embolism	Most commonly air, fat, tumor fragments, or amniotic fluid	Rare	Supportive

* Therapy depends on degree of impairment of right ventricular function and presence or absence of contraindications to thrombolysis or heparin.
Adapted from Goldhaber SZ: Treatment of acute pulmonary embolism. In Goldhaber SZ (ed): Cardiopulmonary Diseases and Cardiac Tumors. In Braunwald E (series ed): Atlas of Heart Diseases. Vol 3. Philadelphia, Current Medicine, 1995, pp 7.1–7.12.

PULMONARY INFARCTION. This syndrome is characterized by unremitting chest pain, occasionally accompanied by hemoptysis. The embolus usually lodges in the peripheral pulmonary arterial tree, near the pleura and close to the diaphragm.[50] Tissue infarction usually occurs 3 to 7 days after embolism. The syndrome at that time often includes fever, leukocytosis, and chest radiological evidence of infarction.

PARADOXICAL EMBOLISM. This syndrome often presents with a sudden, devastating stroke and concomitant PE. Patients often have abnormally elevated pulmonary arterial pressure with a patent foramen ovale evident on echocardiography.[51] Among patients suspected of having paradoxical embolism, occult leg vein thrombosis is frequently present and often is confined to the calves.[52]

NONTHROMBOTIC PULMONARY EMBOLISM. Sources of embolism other than thrombus are less commonly detected than thrombotic PE. Fat embolism syndrome is most often observed after blunt trauma complicated by long-bone fractures.[53] Among patients with cancer, tumor embolism is more difficult to diagnose clinically than thrombotic PE because presenting symptoms and signs are similar in both conditions.[54] Gas embolism,[54a] particularly air embolus, can occur during placement or removal of a central venous catheter.[55] It has also been described as resulting from presumed inadvertent pressure placed on a partially empty plastic intravenous infusion bag.[56]

Intravenous drug abusers tend inadvertently to inject various substances that contaminate their drug supply. Materials commonly found at autopsy include hair, talc, and cotton. These patients are also susceptible to septic PE, which may be accompanied by endocarditis of the tricuspid or pulmonic valves.

Nonimaging Diagnostic Methods

PLASMA D-DIMER ELISA. This is the most promising blood test for pulmonary embolism screening. An abnormally elevated level of *ELISA-determined plasma D-dimer* has more than 90 percent sensitivity for identifying patients with PE proven by lung scan[57] or by angiogram.[58] This test relies on the principle that most patients with PE have ongoing endogenous fibrinolysis that is not effective enough to prevent PE but that does break down some of the fibrin clot to D-dimers. These D-dimers can be assayed by monoclonal antibodies in commercially available kits.

Although elevated plasma concentrations of D-dimers are sensitive for the presence of PE, they are not specific. Levels are elevated in patients for at least 1 week postoperatively and are also increased in patients with myocardial infarction, sepsis, cancer, or almost any other systemic illness.[58a] Therefore the plasma D-dimer ELISA is best used in patients who have suspected PE but no coexisting acute systemic illness.

In the past, plasma D-dimer ELISA was a cumbersome test, especially for emergency use. It was designed, like many ELISAs, to be run in batches; furthermore, skilled technologists were needed to run daily controls and to process the samples. A rapid, individual, and quantitative automated D-dimer ELISA has been validated[59] and approved for use in clinical laboratories. The analytical procedure is straightforward, and turnaround time should be less than 1 hour. This advance in technology promises to expedite the screening of patients with suspected PE.

ARTERIAL BLOOD GASES. Among patients who were suspected of having PE and who underwent angiography in the Prospective Investigation of Pulmonary Embolism Diagnosis (PIOPED) (see p. 1893), determination of the PaO_2 did not discriminate between those with and without PE. There

▼ **TABLE 52–8. ELECTROCARDIOGRAPHIC FINDINGS IN PULMONARY EMBOLISM**

Incomplete or complete right bundle branch block
S in lead I and $aV_L > 1.5$ mm
Transition zone shift to V_5
Qs in leads III and aV_F but not in lead II
QRS axis > 90 degrees or indeterminate axis
Low limb lead voltage
T wave inversion in leads III and aV_F or in leads V_1-V_4

Modified from Sreeram N, Cheriex EC, Smeets JLRM, et al: Value of the 12-lead electrocardiogram at hospital admission in the diagnosis of pulmonary embolism. Am J Cardiol 73:298, 1994.

was no difference between the average PaO_2 (70 mm Hg) among patients with PE compared with those without PE (72 mm Hg) at angiography. Importantly, among patients with angiographically proven PE who had no prior cardiopulmonary disease, the PaO_2 was more than or equal to 80 mm Hg in 26 percent.[60] Furthermore, normal values of the alveolar–arterial oxygen gradient did not preclude the diagnosis of acute PE.[61] Therefore, arterial blood gas determinations should not be part of the diagnostic strategy when investigating suspected PE.

ELECTROCARDIOGRAM. An ECG is useful not only to help preclude acute myocardial infarction but also for rapidly identifying some patients with large PE, who may have ECG manifestations of right-heart strain. In a series of 49 consecutive patients with subsequently proven PE, at least three of seven ECG features suggestive of right ventricular overload (Table 52–8) were identified on 76 percent of ECGs obtained at hospital admission.[62]

IMPEDANCE PLETHYSMOGRAPHY. This is a very indirect approach to DVT diagnosis; it measures changes in electrical resistance caused by obstruction to venous outflow. Impedance plethysmography (IPG) should not be used routinely to detect DVT. In a study of consecutive patients with suspected DVT who underwent both IPG and contrast venography, IPG failed to identify 35 percent of patients with proximal leg DVT.[63]

Imaging Methods

CHEST ROENTGENOGRAPHY. The chest radiograph is usually the first imaging study obtained in patients with suspected PE. Although more than half of patients with PE have an abnormal chest film examination, a near-normal radiograph in the setting of severe respiratory compromise is highly suggestive of massive PE. Classical chest film abnormalities are uncommon but include focal oligemia (Westermark's sign) (Fig. 52–4), indicating massive central embolic occlusion.[64] A peripheral wedge-shaped density above the diaphragm (Hampton's hump) (Fig. 52–5) usually indicates pulmonary infarction.[65] In PIOPED, patients with PE and either a prominent central pulmonary artery or cardiomegaly had higher pulmonary arterial mean pressures than did patients with atelectasis, a pulmonary parenchymal abnormality, or pleural effusion.[66]

One should always search for subtle abnormalities such as distention of the descending right pulmonary artery. The vessel often tapers rapidly after the enlarged portion. The chest radiograph can also help to identify patients with diseases that can mimic PE, such as lobar pneumonia or pneumothorax. Patients with these latter illnesses can also have concomitant PE.[67]

VENOUS ULTRASONOGRAPHY. The primary diagnostic criterion to establish the presence of DVT by ultrasonography is the loss of vein compressibility (Fig. 52–6). Normally, the vein collapses completely when gentle pressure is applied to the skin overlying it. Upper extremity DVT may be more difficult to diagnose because the clavicle can

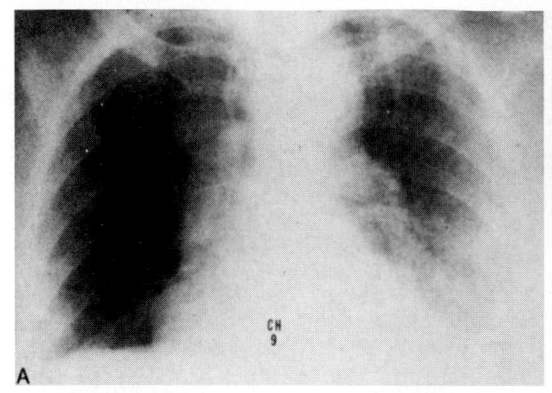
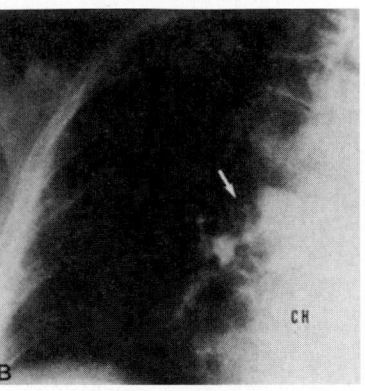

FIGURE 52–4. A, Chest film of a patient with clinical signs of pulmonary embolism; marked oligemia (Westermark's sign) is seen in the entire right lobe. B, Arteriogram from the same patient shows massive saddle embolus in the right main pulmonary artery (arrow). (Courtesy of Dr. Jack L. Westcott, The New York Hospital and Cornell University Medical College.)

hinder attempts to compress the subclavian vein. With acute DVT of either the upper extremity or leg, there is associated passive dilation of the vein.[68]

As many as half of patients with PE have no imaging evidence of DVT.[42] Therefore, if clinical suspicion of PE is high, patients without evidence of DVT should still be investigated for PE. For detection of DVT, ultrasound examination is more accurate than IPG.[69]

Ultrasonography is usually reliable in diagnosing proximal leg DVT in *symptomatic outpatients*.[70] The presence of newly detected DVT may sometimes be a useful surrogate for PE. At selected centers with special expertise, ultrasonography may also be dependable for evaluating suspected symptomatic infrapopliteal DVT.[71] Serial ultrasound measurement of thrombus mass after an episode of acute DVT may allow subsequent correct identification of recurrent DVT.[72] Unfortunately, ultrasonography may yield disappointing results when screening *asymptomatic patients* with possible DVT after orthopedic surgery[73] or after craniotomy.[74]

NUCLEAR VENOGRAPHY. In 1998, the Food and Drug Administration (FDA) approved technetium-99m-apcitide (AcuTect; Diatide, Inc; Londonderry, NH) for the diagnosis of acute leg DVT. A complex of the synthetic peptide apcitide and the radionuclide technetium binds preferentially to the glycoprotein IIb/IIIa receptors found on activated platelets. This diagnostic modality may be complementary to ultrasonography and provide information on pelvic vein thrombosis (not ordinarily imaged by ultrasound), acute DVT superimposed on chronic DVT (not well differentiated by ultrasound), and acute DVT when the ultrasound examination is technically limited owing to body habitus or am-

biguous findings. However, broad clinical experience with this technique has not yet been realized.

CONTRAST PHLEBOGRAPHY. Although contrast phlebography has traditionally been considered the gold standard for DVT diagnosis,[75] venograms are now being obtained with less frequency because of the widespread availability, convenience, and generally excellent results with ultrasonography. Venography is costly and invasive and occasionally results in contrast allergy or contrast-induced phlebitis. Furthermore, there is considerable disagreement in the interpretation of contrast venograms among experienced readers.[76] Patients with massive leg DVT often have nondiagnostic venograms because the contrast agent simply cannot reach the totally obstructed deep leg veins. Consequently, we reserve contrast phlebography for situations in which the ultrasound findings are equivocal or, alternatively, when the ultrasound examination result is normal despite a high clinical suspicion for DVT.

LUNG SCANNING. Although lung scanning remains the principal diagnostic imaging test when PE is suspected, there is increasing dissatisfaction with this approach because the majority of scans do not provide definitive results. Perfusion scintigraphy uses radiolabeled aggregates of albumin or microspheres that are trapped in the pulmonary capillary bed. Six standard views are obtained with a gamma camera. Patients with large PE may have many defects on the perfusion scan. If ventilation scanning is performed on a patient who has PE but no intrinsic lung disease, a normal ventilation study result is expected, yielding a ventilation-perfusion mismatch (Fig. 52–7) and a lung scan interpreted as "high probability for PE."

The utility of the ventilation scan has undergone intense

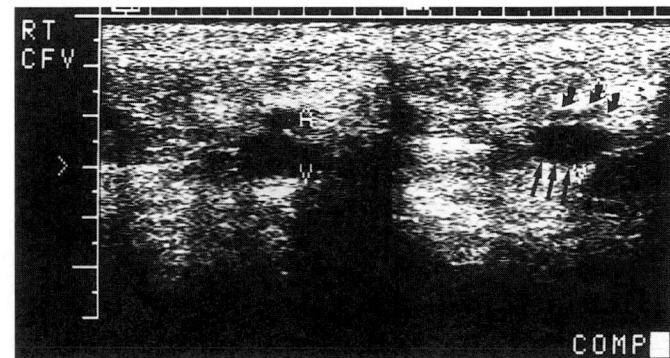

FIGURE 52–5. Posteroanterior chest film of a patient with pulmonary embolism shows a "Hampton's hump" in the right lower lung field, a homogeneous, wedge-shaped density in the peripheral field, convex to the hilum. (Courtesy of Dr. Jack L. Westcott, The New York Hospital and Cornell University Medical College.)

FIGURE 52–6. Right common femoral vein (RT CFV) thrombosis (transverse view) diagnosed by compression ultrasonography. The left half of the image is the baseline ultrasound examination demonstrating the artery (A) superior to the vein (V). During the examination, the artery can be seen to pulsate and appears to wink at the examiner. The vein is typically larger than the artery but normally is not severalfold larger. With compression (COMP) in the right half of the image, the artery is deformed (curved upper arrows), but the vein fails to compress (straight lower arrows).

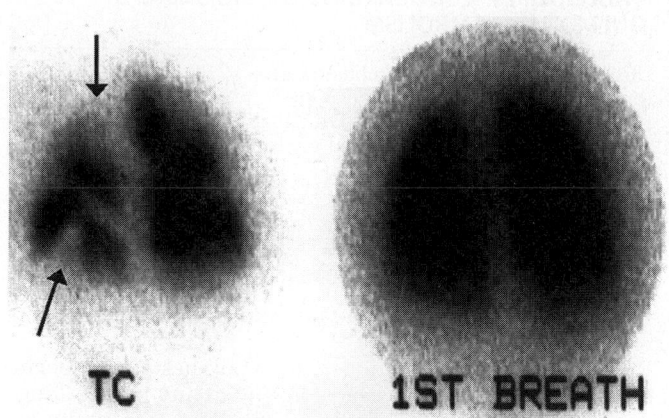

FIGURE 52–7. A 41-year-old woman presented with sudden onset of shortness of breath and retrosternal chest discomfort. Her heart rate was 168 beats/min, respiratory rate 32/min, oxygen saturation 86 percent, and blood pressure 112/70 mm Hg. She underwent a ventilation (*right panel*)-perfusion (*left panel*) lung scan with xenon-133 gas (26 mCi) and technetium-99m macroaggregated albumin (3.2 mCi) in the left posterior oblique position. Numerous scattered segmental (arrows) and subsegmental perfusion defects with near normal ventilation were found. This ventilation-perfusion mismatch was interpreted as high probability for pulmonary embolism.

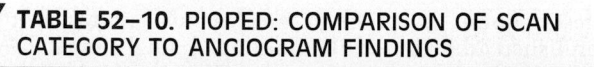

▼ **TABLE 52–10. PIOPED: COMPARISON OF SCAN CATEGORY TO ANGIOGRAM FINDINGS**

| | PULMONARY EMBOLISM | | | NO ANGIO-GRAM | TOTAL N |
	Present	Absent	Uncertain		
Scan category					
High	102	14	1	7	124
Intermediate	105	217	9	33	364
Low	39	199	12	62	312
Near-normal/ normal	5	50	2	74	131
Total	251	480	24	176	931

PIOPED = Prospective Investigation of Pulmonary Embolism Diagnosis.

From the PIOPED Investigators: Value of the ventilation/perfusion scan in acute pulmonary embolism. JAMA 263:2756, 1990.

scrutiny.[76a] In the PIOPED, the ventilation scan was of questionable incremental benefit in establishing or precluding the diagnosis of PE.[77] The European Cardiology Society's Working Group on Thrombosis and Platelets plans to declare that a ventilation scan is no more useful than a chest radiograph for interpretation of perfusion lung scans.

PE is very unlikely in patients with normal and near-normal scans.[78] High-probability scans usually indicate acute PE, but fewer than half of patients with PE have a high-probability scan (Table 52–9). Scans that fall between these extremes of the spectrum should be called intermediate probability.[79] Many patients with low-probability scans but high clinical suspicion for PE do, in fact, have PE at angiography (Table 52–10). Therefore the term *low-probability* scan is a potentially lethal misnomer.[80]

CHEST COMPUTED TOMOGRAPHY. Chest CT is being used with increasing frequency as the initial imaging test in patients with suspected PE (Fig. 52–8). Chest CT is beginning to supplant lung scans because the chest CT result usually is not equivocal. Thrombus is either present or absent, without any "intermediate" or "indeterminate" probability of PE. For patients with intrinsic lung disease and abnormal chest radiograph results, CT scan has the added benefit of potentially suggesting an alternative or concomitant pulmonary disease to explain the clinical presentation.

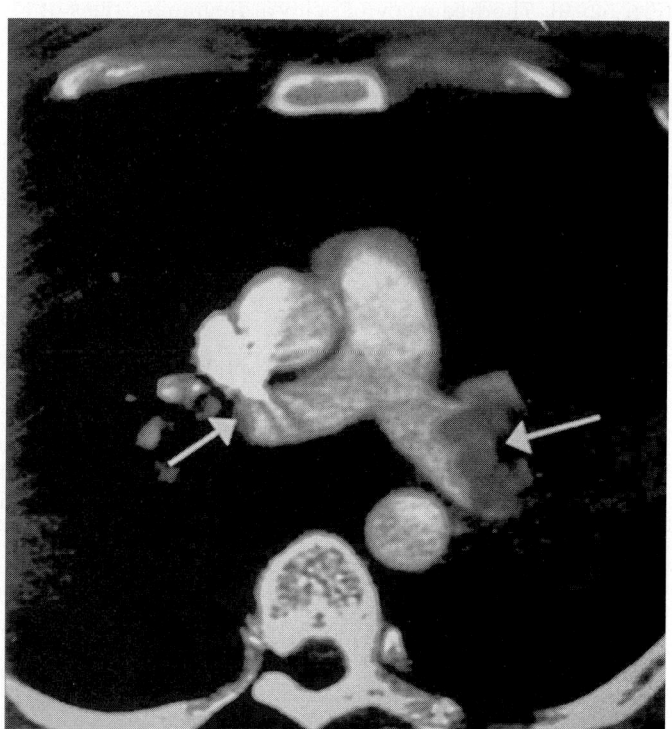

FIGURE 52–8. A 62-year-old physician suffered a massive pulmonary embolism 2 weeks after prostatectomy. Spiral chest CT with contrast provided a definitive diagnosis, with a large thrombus burden apparent in the right and left main pulmonary arteries (arrows).

▼ **TABLE 52–9. PIOPED: PULMONARY EMBOLISM STATUS**

| | CLINICAL PROBABILITY (%) | | | |
	80–100 No. PE/PTs (%)	20–79 No. PE/PTs (%)	0–19 No. PE/PTs (%)	All Probabilities No. PE/PTs (%)
Scan category				
High	28/29 (96)	70/ 80 (88)	5/ 0 (56)	103/118 (87)
Intermediate	27/41 (66)	66/236 (28)	11/ 68 (16)	104/345 (30)
Low	6/15 (40)	30/191 (16)	4/ 90 (4)	40/296 (14)
Near-normal/normal	0/ 5 (0)	4/ 62 (6)	1/ 61 (2)	5/128 (4)
Total	61/90 (68)	170/569 (30)	21/228 (9)	252/887 (28)

PIOPED = Prospective Investigation of Pulmonary Embolism Diagnosis; PE = pulmonary embolism; PTs = patients.

80–100, 20–79, 0–19 represent the clinical probabilities of PE.

No. PE/PTS (%) represents the number and percentage of patients in each subgroup with PE.

From the PIOPED Investigators: Value of the ventilation/perfusion scan in acute pulmonary embolism. JAMA 263:2757, 1990.

The test requires injection of intravenous contrast but is accomplished quickly, while holding a single breath. Although excellent for central large PE, the examination is not reliable for precluding clinically important smaller PE in peripheral pulmonary arteries.[81, 81a]

MAGNETIC RESONANCE IMAGING. Gadolinium-enhanced magnetic resonance (MR) angiography appears comparable to conventional contrast pulmonary angiography in preliminary studies.[82] Unlike standard angiography, MR does not require ionizing radiation or injection of iodinated contrast agent. MR can be performed safely in patients with poor renal function. The test itself imposes virtually no risk to the patient. Finally, MR pulmonary angiography can include assessment of ventricular function; therefore, MR testing can diagnose PE and image right and left ventricular size and pattern of contraction.

ECHOCARDIOGRAPHY (see Chap. 7). Echocardiography is insensitive for the diagnosis of PE but is a rapid, practical, and sensitive technique for detection of right ventricular overload among patients with established and large PE (Fig. 52–9). The frequency of echocardiographic signs of PE (Table 52–11) depends on the population being studied. For those patients in whom transthoracic imaging is unsatisfactory, transesophageal echocardiography can be carried out.[83]

Echocardiographic detection of right ventricular dysfunction at the time of presentation with PE is useful for risk stratification and prognostication. Among patients with major PE, echocardiographic evidence of a patent foramen

▼ TABLE 52–11. ECHOCARDIOGRAPHIC SIGNS OF PULMONARY EMBOLISM

Direct visualization of thrombus (rare)
Right ventricular dilatation
Right ventricular hypokinesis (with sparing of the apex)
Abnormal interventricular septal motion
Tricuspid valve regurgitation
Pulmonary artery dilatation
Lack of decreased inspiratory collapse of inferior vena cava

ovale signifies a high risk of death and paradoxical arterial thromboembolism.[84]

Right ventricular dilatation and hypokinesis may occur in chronic pulmonary hypertension due to any cause. Long-term elevation of right ventricular afterload is usually accompanied by right ventricular hypertrophy. In patients with chronic pulmonary hypertension, the velocity of the tricuspid regurgitant jet may be elevated to a greater level than in patients with acute PE and no underlying cardiopulmonary disease. Right ventricular infarction, cardiomyopathy, and right ventricular dysplasia may also result in right ventricular hypokinesis and dilatation on the echocardiogram. In these conditions, however, the velocity of tricuspid regurgitation is usually less than in acute PE.

It appears that right ventricular contractile dysfunction following PE has a distinct regional pattern in which wall excursion is hypokinetic from the base through the free

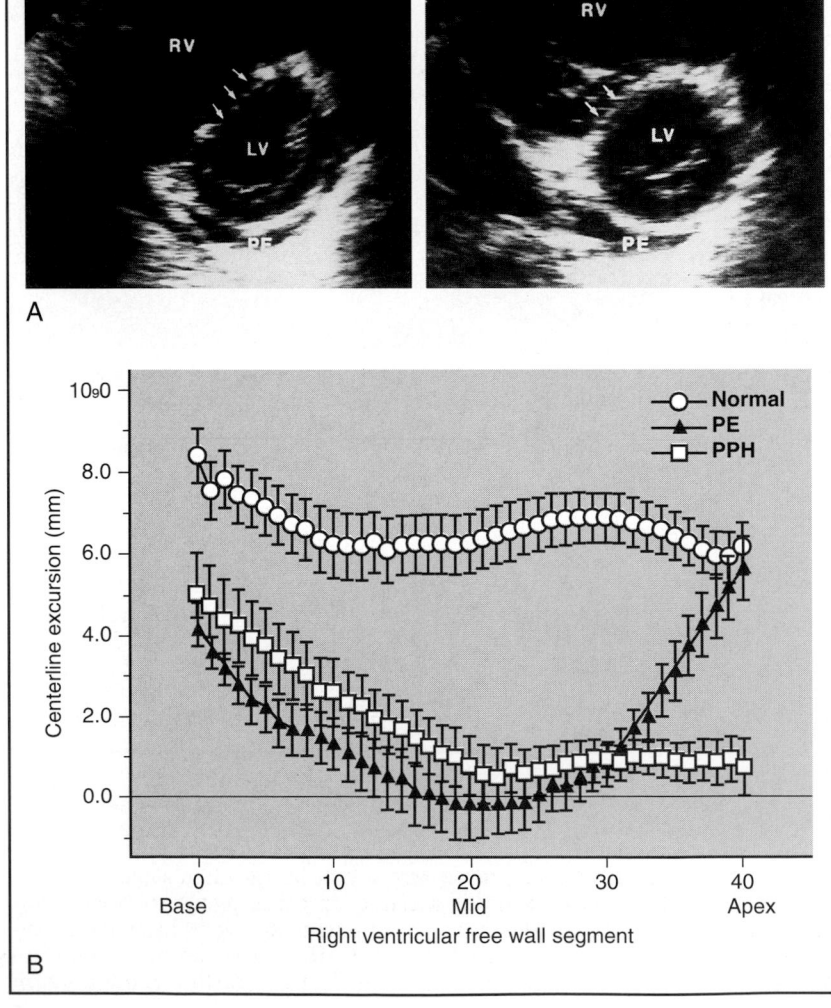

FIGURE 52–9. *A,* Parasternal short-axis views of the right ventricle (RV) and left ventricle (LV) in diastole (*left*) and systole (*right*). Diastolic and systolic bowing of the interventricular septum (arrows) into the LV is compatible with RV volume and pressure overload, respectively. The RV is appreciably dilated and markedly hypokinetic, with little change in apparent RV area from diastole to systole. PE = small pericardial effusion. (From Come PC: Echocardiographic evaluation of pulmonary embolism and its response to therapeutic interventions. Chest 101:151S, 1992.)

B, Segmental RV free wall excursion (mean ± SEM) by centerline analysis in patients with acute pulmonary embolism (PE) or primary pulmonary hypertension (PPH) and in normal persons. The acute increase in afterload in PE results in regional RV dysfunction predominantly affecting the mid free wall as it assumes a more spherical shape to equalize wall stress. The RV apex is spared (McConnell's sign). In contrast, the chronic pressure overload of PPH results in more diffuse RV dysfunction, with limited shape change of the hypertrophied RV. (From McConnell MV, Rayan ME, Solomon SD, et al: Echocardiographic diagnosis of acute pulmonary embolism: A distinct pattern of abnormal right ventricular wall motion. Am J Cardiol 78:469, 1996.)

wall but remains almost normal at the right ventricular apex (McConnell's sign) (Fig. 52–9*B*) This pattern of right ventricular contractile dysfunction differs from the global dysfunction observed in primary pulmonary hypertension.[85] A possible explanation is that in PE, the left ventricle may tether the right ventricular apex, thereby preserving near-normal wall motion in this region.

PULMONARY ANGIOGRAPHY. Standard contrast pulmonary angiography has been considered the gold standard for accurate in vivo diagnosis or exclusion of PE. With appropriate techniques and experience, it can be performed expeditiously and safely in most patients. Angiography is most useful when a diagnostic dilemma persists despite the use of noninvasive tests. This situation is most common when the diagnostic test results are negative or ambiguous in the presence of high clinical suspicion for PE. Pulmonary angiography is obviously also required when interventions are planned such as suction catheter embolectomy, mechanical clot fragmentation, or catheter-directed thrombolysis (discussed later).

PREPARATION OF THE PATIENT. A history of allergy to contrast medium should be sought. If present, high-dose corticosteroids should be administered. Heparin can be discontinued immediately before the procedure, unless the clinical suspicion for PE is very high. Patients should avoid heavy meals for at least 4 hours before angiography.

THE ANGIOGRAPHIC PROCEDURE. The perfusion lung scan serves as a road map to the angiographer, who performs selective angiography rather than injecting into the main pulmonary artery. Obtaining accurate and high-quality recordings of right-heart pressures and waveforms is of paramount importance. If the pressure tracing "dampens" or "wedges" in the proximal pulmonary artery, anatomically massive PE should be suspected before injection of contrast agent. If the pulmonary artery systolic pressure exceeds approximately 50 mm Hg, the differential diagnosis should include chronic PE or acute superimposed on chronic PE.

Our preferred approach is via the femoral vein, although brachial or internal jugular approaches are alternatives. The best means of identifying the correct level for puncture in the groin is with fluoroscopy; the skin incision site should be at the level of the upper region of the femoral neck. We prefer a single wall puncture to avoid the possibility of passing first through the femoral artery before entering the femoral vein. Once access has been obtained, a guidewire is inserted through the needle, and the needle is exchanged for either a pigtail catheter or a sheath with a side arm. To advance through the cardiac chambers and measure right heart pressures, we use either (1) a pigtail catheter with a tip deflector wire or (2) a Swan-Ganz catheter followed by exchange over a guidewire for a pigtail catheter. The pigtail catheter permits a high contrast injection rate with considerable safety.

To carry out a complete diagnostic procedure, at least two views of each lung should be obtained. One view on each side should be the *ipsilateral posterior oblique* (approximately 45 degrees), and the other view can be either an *anteroposterior* view or the *ipsilateral anterior oblique* (approximately 45 degrees). Low-osmolar contrast medium is used because it does not cause the severe coughing that occurs with high-osmolar contrast medium and it gives a greater margin of safety among patients with elevated right-sided heart pressures. The contrast medium is injected usually at a rate of 20 to 25 ml/sec for 2 seconds. If the right-sided heart pressures are elevated, the rate of injection can be decreased, depending on the severity of the elevation. If the right ventricular end-diastolic pressure exceeds 20 mm Hg, consider superselective arteriography with a decreased rate and volume of contrast into the lobe that is most likely to yield a positive result.

We now perform all of our filming for pulmonary arteriography using digital acquisition. The filming rate is 7.5 frames/sec for 1 second before injection (to obtain mask images for digital subtraction), followed by 7.5 frames/sec for the first 3 seconds after the beginning of the injection. However, with digital subtraction, one should view the images in the unsubtracted mode, because subtraction may lead to artifacts that can simulate pulmonary emboli. After the initial rapid filming rate, the filming rate can be decreased to 1 to 2 frames/sec for approximately 5 seconds. If the foregoing views are nondiagnostic, selective magnification angiography (also acquired digitally) of any areas in question can be obtained. If these views do not lead to a diagnostic resolution, balloon occlusion arteriography may be performed.

INTERPRETING THE ANGIOGRAM. A definitive diagnosis of PE depends on visualization in two projections of an intraluminal filling defect in a pulmonary arterial branch or cutoff of a branch with the visualized "tail" of the embolus. Secondary signs of PE reflect decreased perfusion and consist of abrupt occlusion (cutoff) of vessels, oligemia or avascularity of a segment, a prolonged arterial phase with slow filling and emptying of veins, and tortuous, tapering peripheral vessels.[86]

Not all pulmonary artery filling defects or occlusions are due to acute PE. In chronic PE, arteries may appear pouched, and thrombus appears organized with a concave edge. Bandlike defects called *webs* may be present, in addition to intimal irregularities and abrupt narrowing or occlusion of lobar vessels.[87] Other causes of intraluminal filling defects include pulmonary Takayasu's arteritis (see Chap. 40), angiosarcoma, and sarcoidosis.[67]

Overall Strategy: An Integrated Diagnostic Approach

A wide array of diagnostic tests is available for the investigation of suspected PE. Familiarity with each test's strengths and weaknesses (Table 52–12) as well as knowledge of the availability and reliability of specific tests at one's hospital will facilitate a concise and streamlined work-up.

At Brigham and Women's Hospital, we are initiating an interdisciplinary protocol for patients who present to the emergency department with suspected PE (Fig. 52–10). The initial assessment includes the history, physical examination, and ECG, with special attention to the patient's clinical milieu and risk factors for venous thromboembolism. Next we obtain a chest radiograph and a rapid plasma D-dimer ELISA. If both are nondiagnostic, then PE is exceedingly unlikely, and we consider the diagnosis excluded at that point. If either result is abnormal, the diagnostic work-up continues. Most patients then undergo lung scanning, despite its limitations. If the chest radiograph appears abnormal, however, the likelihood of a diagnostic lung scan is low, and we usually perform chest CT with contrast in our emergency department scanner in lieu of lung scanning. For those patients in whom the diagnosis is not clarified with lung scanning or chest CT, the next step is venous ultrasonography. If the result is normal and our clinical suspicion remains high, we usually proceed with contrast pulmonary angiography. We do not consider a low-probability lung scan and a nondiagnostic venous ultrasonogram of the leg to be sufficient to preclude PE in the presence of high clinical suspicion.[88]

Using a similar protocol, investigators collaborating in Geneva and Montreal evaluated 918 consecutive patients suspected of having PE or DVT. After 3 months of follow-up, only 2 percent developed clinical evidence of PE. Pulmonary angiography or contrast venography of the legs was required in only 6 percent of the entire cohort.[89]

MANAGEMENT

Rapid and accurate risk stratification is of paramount importance. Patients with PE present with a wide spectrum of illness, and appropriate care can range from prevention of recurrent PE (with anticoagulation alone or insertion of an IVC filter) to clot dissolution or removal with thrombolysis or embolectomy. Anticoagulation with LMWH is being used with increasing frequency as a bridge to full and therapeutic levels of warfarin.

Adjunctive measures include provision of supplemental oxygen and adequate pain relief, usually most effective with nonsteroidal antiinflammatory medications. Patients who appear toxic and hypoxic should be considered for prompt temporary mechanical ventilation. Those with impending hypotension or poor organ perfusion require rapid institution of an inotrope.

Dobutamine—a beta-adrenergic agonist with positive inotropic and pulmonary vasodilating effects (see Chapter 18) should be considered a first-line agent to treat right-sided heart failure and cardiogenic shock.[89a] In general, volume loading these patients is ill advised because ventricular interdependence can lead to even further reductions in

▼ **TABLE 52–12.** ADVANTAGES AND DISADVANTAGES OF DIAGNOSTIC TESTS FOR SUSPECTED PULMONARY EMBOLISM

DIAGNOSTIC TEST	ADVANTAGES	DISADVANTAGES
Plasma D-dimer ELISA	A normal result makes PE exceedingly unlikely	Level is elevated in many systemic illnesses that mimic PE; unless a rapid assay is available, the turnaround time will be long
(ECG)	Universally available; may indicate acute cor pulmonale	Acute cor pulmonale on ECG is not specific for PE; not a sensitive test
Impedance plethysmography	Portable, inexpensive, easy to use	Inaccurate, with failure to detect major nonobstructive proximal DVT
Chest radiograph	Usually has minor abnormalities but occasionally pathognomonic; may suggest alternative diagnoses; may guide work-up toward chest CT rather than lung scan	Not specific
Venous ultrasonography	Excellent for detecting symptomatic proximal DVT; surrogate for PE	Cannot image iliac vein thrombosis; imaging of calf is operator dependent; DVT may have embolized completely, resulting in a normal result
Nuclear venography	Image pelvic and calf veins; differentiate acute versus chronic DVT	Limited experience with this test
Contrast venography	Used to be gold standard; excellent for calf veins	Can cause chemical phlebitis; uncomfortable; costly; may fail to diagnose massive DVT because veins are filled with thrombus and cannot be opacified
Lung scanning	Standard initial imaging test for PE; high-probability scans are reliable for detecting PE; normal/near-normal scans are reliable for precluding PE	Most scans are neither high probability nor normal/near-normal; ventilation scans are falling out of favor; most test results are equivocal
Chest CT	Excellent for PE in the proximal pulmonary arterial tree	Insensitive for important but distal PE
MRI	Excellent for anatomy and cardiac function	In preliminary use; not widely available; experience very limited
Echocardiography	Excellent for identifying right ventricular dilatation and dysfunction that is not obvious clinically, thus providing an early warning of potentially adverse outcome	Not specific; many patients with PE have normal echocardiograms; the test cannot reliably differentiate causes of right ventricular dysfunction
Pulmonary angiography	Considered the gold standard for diagnosis	Invasive, costly, uncomfortable

ELISA = enzyme-linked immunosorbent assay; PE = pulmonary embolism; ECG = electrocardiogram; DVT = deep vein thrombosis; CT = computed tomography; MRI = magnetic resonance imaging.

left ventricular output. For patients with pulmonary hypertension and a patent foramen ovale, inhaled nitric oxide may reverse right-to-left shunting and improve oxygenation.[90]

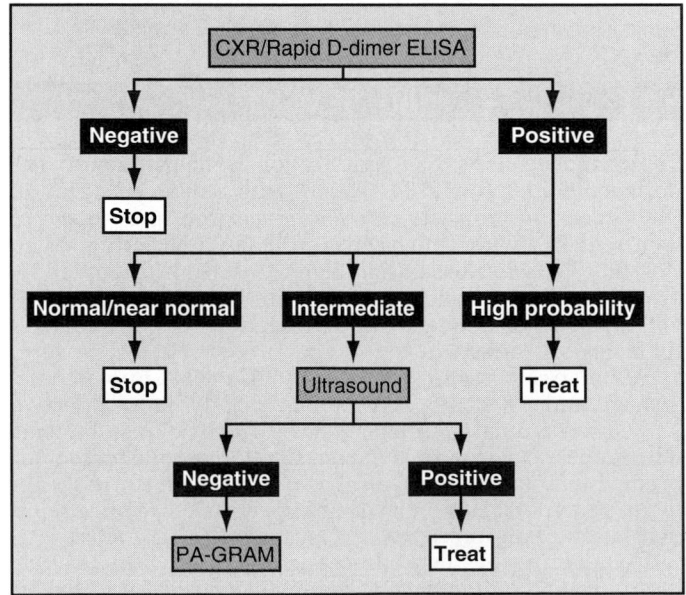

FIGURE 52–10. Pulmonary embolism diagnosis strategy: Overall integrated diagnostic approach. CXR = chest radiograph; ELISA = enzyme-linked immunosorbent assay; PA-GRAM = pulmonary arteriogram.

Prevention of Pulmonary Embolism and Deep Venous Thromboembolism

Heparin

UNFRACTIONATED HEPARIN (see also Chap. 62). Standard, unfractionated heparin is a highly sulfated glycosaminoglycan that is partially purified from either porcine intestinal mucosa or bovine lung. Its molecular weight ranges from 3000 to 30,000 and averages 15,000. Heparin acts primarily by binding to antithrombin III (AT III), an enzyme that inhibits the coagulation factors thrombin (factor IIa), Xa, IXa, XIa, and XIIa. Heparin subsequently promotes a conformational change in AT III that accelerates its activity approximately 100- to 1000-fold.[91] This prevents additional thrombus formation and permits endogenous fibrinolytic mechanisms to lyse clot that has already formed. However, heparin does *not* directly dissolve thrombus that already exists. The efficacy of heparin is limited because clot-bound thrombin is protected from heparin-antithrombin III inhibition.[92] Furthermore, heparin resistance can occur because unfractionated heparin binds to plasma proteins.[93]

LOW-MOLECULAR-WEIGHT HEPARINS (LMWHs). *LMWHs* are fragments of unfractionated heparin that exhibit less binding to plasma proteins and endothelial cells than unfractionated heparin. Therefore, LMWHs have greater bioavailability, more predictable dose response, and longer half-life than unfractionated heparin.[94]

The introduction of LMWHs for treatment of venous thromboembolism is revolutionizing the management of DVT and PE, especially for the majority of patients who are hemodynamically stable. Many large randomized trials of patients with acute DVT have compared subcutaneously administered LMWH with continuous intravenous unfractionated heparin as a bridge to full and therapeutic anticoagulation.[95-97] LMWH was at least as effective and safe as continuous intravenous unfractionated heparin.

A metaanalysis of randomized trials comparing 3674 patients with acute DVT receiving LMWH versus unfractionated heparin[98] demonstrated that LMWH reduced the mortality rate over 3 to 6 months of follow-up by 29 percent. The major bleeding complication rate was reduced by 43 percent. These data were used in a cost-effectiveness analysis that showed that LMWH is highly cost effective compared with unfractionated heparin for DVT management.[99]

The excellent bioavailability and subcutaneous administration of LMWH permit a strategy of weight-based LMWH dosing (without laboratory tests for dose adjustment in most instances) coupled with the possibility of outpatient therapy or an abbreviated hospitalization. With a concerted effort, it appears that the majority of ambulatory patients who present with DVT can be treated as outpatients,[100] as long as an infrastructure has been established to ensure close and meticulous follow-up.[101]

On December 31, 1998, the FDA approved outpatient treatment of DVT *without PE* using enoxaparin 1 mg/kg every 12 hours for a minimum of 5 days. Warfarin is usually begun on the first evening of therapy, and enoxaparin is continued until a stable and therapeutic INR of 2.0 to 3.0 is achieved. The dose of enoxaparin must be decreased in patients with renal insufficiency because LMWH is primarily renally excreted.

The FDA approved the same enoxaparin dosing regimen for inpatient treatment of DVT *with or without PE*. An alternative dosing regimen was also approved for the same indication: 1.5 mg/kg/24 hr of enoxaparin. However, there is less clinical experience with this dosing regimen.[102] Importantly, no trial of patients with symptomatic PE has attempted outpatient or abbreviated hospitalization with LMWH.[103]

MONITORING HEPARIN. An activated PTT that is at least 1½ times greater than the control value should provide a minimum therapeutic level of unfractionated heparin. However, there are many different PTT reagent kits and virtually no standardization of PTT levels.[104] Therefore, an individual hospital's target PTT range for anticoagulation with unfractionated heparin should correspond to a plasma anti-Xa level of approximately 0.4 to 1.0 units/ml. At Brigham and Women's Hospital, we assay the anti-Xa level with a HEPRN pack (Du Pont) in the automated clinical analyzer used for other chemistry tests. This is a chromogenic assay based on the inhibition of factor X_a by heparin-activated antithrombin III.

The plasma anti-Xa level is particularly useful in three situations: (1) monitoring heparin anticoagulation among patients with baseline elevated PTTs due to a lupus anticoagulant or anticardiolipin antibodies, (2) monitoring heparin among DVT and PE patients who require large daily doses of heparin,[105] and (3) monitoring LMWH, which blunts the elevation in the PTT and in the activated clotting time that occurs with unfractionated heparin.

When LMWH is given for prophylaxis, it is administered in a fixed dose, with no or at most slight adjustments based on weight. However, when LMWH is given to achieve full and therapeutic levels of anticoagulation, the dose is based on weight. Ordinarily, no blood tests are needed to monitor LMWH. However, titration of LMWH is warranted for patients with massive obesity or for patients with renal insufficiency. In both circumstances, the dose of LMWH that is administered needs to be adjusted downward from the calculated weight-based dose.

In general, anticoagulation for prophylaxis can be achieved with an anti–factor Xa level of 0.2 to 0.4 units/ml. Full anticoagulation for therapy can be attained with an anti–factor Xa level of 0.4 to 1.0 units/ml. The level peaks approximately 3 hours after subcutaneous injection,[105] and an anti–factor Xa level is optimally obtained during the plateau phase, 4 to 6 hours after injection.[106]

For patients in whom warfarin therapy has failed or who cannot take warfarin (e.g., pregnant women), we treat with LMWH injected subcutaneously and usually teach self-administration.

INITIATING HEPARIN THERAPY. Heparin is the cornerstone of treatment for acute PE. Before heparin therapy is begun, risk factors for bleeding should be considered, such as a prior history of bleeding with anticoagulation, thrombocytopenia, vitamin K deficiency, increasing age, underlying diseases, and concomitant drug therapy. The

most frequently overlooked portion of the physical examination is a rectal examination for occult blood.

There is a transition toward the use of LMWH for patients who present with acute symptomatic PE, even though this approach is not FDA approved. The conventional treatment strategy uses unfractionated heparin, with an initial bolus of 5000 to 10,000 units, followed by a continuous intravenous infusion based on weight. Most patients require at least 30,000 units/24 hr. There are many nomograms, such as Raschke's,[107] to assist in adjusting the dose of continuous intravenous unfractionated heparin, with guidelines provided by the patient's weight and PTT. An automated heparin-delivery system has been described; it controls the PTT based on a computer-generated algorithm and relies on automated venous blood sampling.[108]

Unless a severe bleeding problem such as active gastrointestinal bleeding is detected, heparin can be started before lung scanning or pulmonary angiography. In cases of severe bleeding, heparin therapy should be withheld, and nonpharmacological treatment (secondary prevention) with insertion of an IVC filter should be considered if the diagnosis of PE is confirmed.

COMPLICATIONS. The most important adverse effect of heparin is hemorrhage. Major bleeding during anticoagulation may unmask a previously silent lesion, such as bladder or colon cancer. For most cases of moderate bleeding, cessation of heparin will suffice, and the PTT usually returns to normal within 6 hours because the half-life of unfractionated heparin is only 60 to 90 minutes.

Resumption of heparin at a lower dose or implementing alternative therapy depends on the severity of the bleeding, the risk of recurrent thromboembolism, and the extent to which bleeding may have resulted from excessive anticoagulation. Risk factors for major in-hospital bleeding among anticoagulated patients include the presence of comorbid conditions, age greater than 60 years, the intensity of anticoagulation, concurrent medications, or liver dysfunction that worsens during treatment.[109]

In the event of life-threatening or intracranial hemorrhage, protamine sulfate can be administered at the time heparin is discontinued. Protamine, a strongly basic protein, immediately reverses anticoagulant activity by forming a stable complex with the acidic heparin. For life-threatening hemorrhage, the usual dose is approximately 1 mg/100 units of heparin, administered slowly (e.g., 50 mg over 10 to 30 minutes). Protamine sulfate may cause allergic reactions, particularly in diabetic patients who have had prior exposure to protamine after using neutral protamine Hagedorn (NPH) insulin.[91]

HEPARIN-INDUCED THROMBOCYTOPENIA. This complication is caused by IgG antibodies that recognize complexes of heparin and platelet factor 4, leading to platelet activation via platelet Fc gamma IIa receptors. Formation of procoagulant, platelet-derived microparticles generates thrombin and makes patients especially vulnerable to venous thromboembolism.[110] These clots are often large and bilateral, and they get worse if heparin is continued.

The diagnosis should be suspected if patients develop DVT or PE while receiving heparin, especially if the platelet count decreases to less than 100,000/mm³ or if it decreases by more than 50 percent of baseline. The peak incidence is 4 to 14 days after initiating heparin. Heparin-induced thrombocytopenia occurs much more commonly with unfractionated heparin than with LMWH.[111] However, LMWH usually cross-reacts with unfractionated heparin after heparin-induced thrombocytopenia occurs and therefore should not be used for treatment.

Patients with heparin-induced thrombocytopenia are especially susceptible to venous limb gangrene if warfarin is given before several days of effective antithrombotic therapy[112] such as danaparoid,[113] which reduces thrombin generation, or lepirudin,[114] which inhibits thrombin. Lepirudin currently is the only FDA-approved therapy for heparin-induced thrombocytopenia. The weight-adjusted dose must be reduced in the presence of renal insufficiency, and there is no specific antidote if bleeding occurs. Another direct thrombin inhibitor, argatroban, effectively treats heparin-induced thrombocytopenia.[115] Argatroban does not require dose adjustments with renal dysfunction, and FDA approval is imminent.[115a]

HEPARIN-INDUCED OSTEOPENIA. Patients receiving prolonged heparin therapy may develop osteopenia, osteoporosis, or pathological bone fractures. In most cases, asymptomatic osteopenia is the most severe adverse effect on bone metabolism. This finding is most readily assessed with bone densitometry.[116] Among women who have discontinued heparin after pregnancy, the osteopenia usually resolves within a year.[117] For reasons not well understood, LMWH may cause less osteopenia than does unfractionated heparin.[118]

SPINAL AND EPIDURAL HEMATOMA. Over a 5-year period, the FDA received reports of 43 patients in the United States who suffered spinal or epidural hematoma after receiving LMWH. Emergency decompressive laminectomy was performed in 28, and permanent paraplegia occurred in 16.[119] Consequently, most patients receiving LMWH during pregnancy are switched to unfractionated heparin for several weeks before their due date. Alternatively, LMWH is withheld for at least 24 hours before a scheduled induction of delivery.

HEPARIN-ASSOCIATED TRANSAMINITIS AND HYPERKALEMIA. Heparin-associated elevations in transaminase levels occur commonly, have no relation to whether the heparin is of bovine or porcine origin, and are rarely associated with clinical toxicity.[120, 121] Heparin causes aldosterone depression by an unknown mechanism within 4 to 8 days after initiation of therapy. In patients with a normally functioning renin-angiotensin-aldosterone axis, this is probably of no clinical significance, although serum sodium levels may drop slightly. However, it may cause clinically important hyperkalemia in certain patients, such as those with diabetes or renal failure.[122]

Warfarin Sodium (See also Chap. 62)

Warfarin is a vitamin K antagonist that prevents gamma carboxylation activation of coagulation factors II, VII, IX, and X. The full anticoagulant effect of warfarin may not be apparent for 5 days, even if the prothrombin time, used to monitor warfarin's effect, becomes elevated more rapidly. Elevation in the prothrombin time may initially reflect depletion of coagulation factor VII, which has a half-life of about 6 hours, whereas factor II has a half-life of about 5 days.

OVERLAP WITH HEPARIN. When warfarin therapy is initiated during an active thrombotic state, the levels of protein C and S decline, thus creating a thrombogenic potential. By overlapping heparin and warfarin for 5 days, the procoagulant effect of unopposed warfarin can be counteracted. In a Dutch study, patients with DVT were randomized to oral anticoagulation alone versus heparin plus oral anticoagulation. The recurrent DVT rate was three times higher in the group that received oral anticoagulation alone.[123] This study demonstrates that warfarin should be given with heparin coverage and overlap to patients with an active thrombotic state.

MONITORING WARFARIN. The prothrombin time, used to adjust the dose of warfarin, should be reported according to the International Normalized Ratio (INR), not the prothrombin time ratio or the prothrombin time expressed in seconds. Fewer bleeding complications occur when the INR is used to monitor warfarin dosing rather than the prothrombin time ratio.[124]

INTENSITY AND DURATION OF THERAPY. It is our practice to treat with 5 to 7 days of heparin and to initiate warfarin administration on the first hospital day after documenting a PTT within the therapeutic range[125] or several hours after subcutaneous injection of a therapeutic dose of LMWH. The recurrence rate after completion of anticoagulation is halved by using 6 months of oral anticoagulation rather than 6 weeks.[126] One small study suggests using an indefinite duration of anticoagulation after a first episode of idiopathic venous thromboembolism.[127] However, this approach is not generally accepted. Ongoing trials are investigating the optimal duration and intensity of antiocoagulation among patients at highest risk, those who suffer DVT or PE without recent surgery or antecedent trauma.[128]

There is disagreement about whether patients with venous thromboembolism and factor V Leiden are at increased risk of recurrence after anticoagulation has been discontinued.[8, 8a] The ongoing NIH-sponsored clinical trial, PREVENT, is addressing this issue.[128]

In otherwise healthy patients, I usually initiate warfarin therapy with 5 mg and achieve the target INR in about 5 days.[129] Among systemically ill patients, however, vitamin K deficiency[130] may lead to marked overanticoagulation just after a single modest dose of warfarin. I tend to treat first-time DVT of the calf[131] or upper extremities[132] for 3 months, and proximal DVT or PE for 6 months. The target INR for first-time DVT is 2.0 to 3.0, but I tend to treat PE

more intensively, with a target INR of at least 3.0. Whenever possible, patients who have DVT or PE and who also have the antiphospholipid-antibody syndrome should be maintained with a target INR of at least 3.0.[133]

COMPLICATIONS. The major toxic effect of warfarin is bleeding. The risk of bleeding increases as the INR increases. Risk factors for hemorrhage include severe hepatic or renal disease, alcoholism, drug interactions (including acetaminophen[134]), trauma, malignant disease, and known previous bleeding sites in the gastrointestinal tract. The incidence of rehospitalization for bleeding after hospitalization for DVT is greatest during the first 30 days after discharge. Women and nonwhite patients appear to be at especially increased risk for anticoagulant-related bleeding.[134a]

About 1 to 2 percent of patients will have an extremely low warfarin requirement of 1.5 mg or less in the absence of liver dysfunction, drug interaction, or concomitant disease. A subset is born with CYP2CP variant alleles that are associated with impaired hydroxylation of S-warfarin. If not recognized when warfarin is initiated, these individuals are at a potentially high risk of bleeding complications.[135]

Major life-threatening bleeding requires immediate treatment with enough cryoprecipitate or fresh frozen plasma (FFP) (usually 2 units) to normalize the INR and achieve immediate hemostasis. To treat less serious bleeding, vitamin K has traditionally been administered parenterally; a dose of 10 mg subcutaneously or intramuscularly usually reverses the effects of warfarin in 6 to 12 hours. However, this approach makes patients relatively refractory to warfarin for up to 2 weeks, so that reinstitution of warfarin becomes more difficult. A novel and alternative approach is to administer a single dose of vitamin K. In a cohort of patients who were not bleeding and who had an INR greater than 5.0, a single average dose of 10 mg of vitamin K sufficed to lower the INR to the targeted therapeutic range, without disrupting the subsequent daily dosing of warfarin.[136]

Minor bleeding with a prolonged INR may merely require interruption of warfarin therapy, without administration of FFP, until the INR has returned to the therapeutic range. If bleeding occurs when the INR is within the therapeutic range, occult malignant disease should be suspected and ruled out. Evaluation of cases of minor bleeding and an INR above the therapeutic range is less productive.

Warfarin-induced skin necrosis[137] is a rare but important complication that may be related to warfarin-induced reduction of protein C. The "purple toes syndrome" is another rare complication of warfarin therapy that appears to be caused by cholesterol microembolization.[137] In this syndrome, crystals are released from ulcerated atherosclerotic plaques. It appears that warfarin may worsen cholesterol microembolic disease by interfering with the healing of ulcerated atherosclerotic plaques.

During pregnancy, heparin should generally be used instead of warfarin because warfarin is associated with a markedly higher rate of congenital anomalies. The fetus is particularly susceptible to warfarin embryopathy during the 6th through 12th weeks of gestation. The main features are saddle nose, nasal hypoplasia, frontal bossing, short stature, stippled epiphyses, optic atrophy, cataracts, mental retardation, and flexure contractures. Intracranial bleeding may also lead to secondary central nervous system deformities.[138] Women can take warfarin post partum and breast feed safely, but reliable contraception is essential because warfarin is teratogenic.[139] The level of warfarin in breast milk is so low (25 ng/ml)[140] that it cannot be detected in the baby's plasma.[140]

In the office setting, I routinely assess warfarin dosing with a "point-of-care" device that provides the INR result in 2 minutes by use of a drop of whole blood obtained from a fingertip puncture. Substantial time savings have resulted, and patients leave the office with greater peace of mind and with a more accurate understanding of their warfarin dosing regimen. Appropriately selected patients can self-manage their warfarin dosing at home with a point-of-care device. In a randomized trial comparing self-management with conventional management, the self-managed patients more frequently achieved their target INRs and reported an improved quality of life compared with the conventionally managed group.[141]

ASPIRIN (see also Chap. 62). Aspirin exerts its antithrombotic ef-

▼ TABLE 52–13. INDICATIONS FOR INFERIOR VENA CAVAL FILTERS

Anticoagulation Contraindicated and PE Documented
Active bleeding that might cause exsanguination (e.g., gastrointestinal)
Feared bleeding that might be catastrophic (e.g., postoperative craniotomy)
Ongoing complications of anticoagulation (e.g., heparin-associated thrombocytopenia)
Planned intensive cancer chemotherapy (with anticipated pancytopenia or thrombocytopenia)

Anticoagulation Failure Despite Documentation of Adequate Therapy (e.g., Recurrent PE)

Prophylaxis in High-Risk Patients
Extensive or progressive venous thrombosis
In conjunction with catheter-based or surgical pulmonary embolectomy
Severe pulmonary hypertension or cor pulmonale

PE = pulmonary embolism.

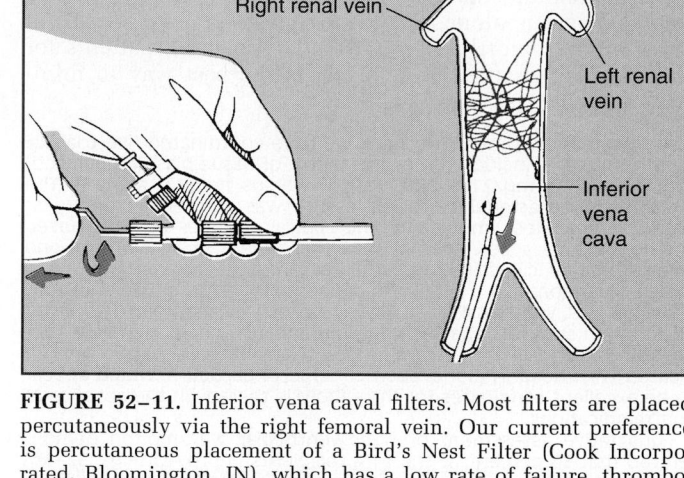

FIGURE 52–11. Inferior vena caval filters. Most filters are placed percutaneously via the right femoral vein. Our current preference is percutaneous placement of a Bird's Nest Filter (Cook Incorporated, Bloomington, IN), which has a low rate of failure, thrombogenicity, and occlusion. The smallness of its sheath may help minimize the risk of bleeding during and after the procedure. To insert the Bird's Nest Filter, the right-angled handle of the wire guide pusher is rotated counterclockwise for 10 to 15 turns to disengage it from the filter. Then the wire guide pusher is removed first, followed by the empty filter catheter. The introducing sheath is left in place so that a postprocedure venacavogram can be obtained. (From Goldhaber SZ: Treatment of venous thrombosis. *In* Goldhaber SZ [ed]: Cardiopulmonary Diseases and Cardiac Tumors. *In* Braunwald E [series ed]: Atlas of Heart Diseases. Vol 3. Philadelphia, Current Medicine, 1995, pp 12.1–12.14.)

fect by eliminating platelet prostaglandin synthesis, thereby blocking thromboxane A_2 formation and causing a moderate decrease in platelet function and a mild hemostatic defect.[142] Consequently, aspirin has at least a modest role in prevention of venous thrombosis.[143] I prescribe low-dose aspirin, usually 81 mg daily, for some patients who have finished their full course of warfarin. This strategy averts an abrupt transition from full anticoagulation to no anticoagulation.

Secondary Prevention: Inferior Vena Caval Interruption

The major indications for placement of an IVC filter are listed in Table 52–13. An IVC filter prevents PE, not DVT.[144] Therefore, when a filter is inserted, anticoagulation should also be used, whenever possible, to prevent further thrombosis.[145]

Most IVC filters are placed below the renal veins. For suprarenal vein placement, the largest experience is with the Greenfield filter. At Brigham and Women's Hospital, we primarily use the bird's nest filter for infrarenal placement (Fig. 52–11).

Primary Treatment

Thrombolysis

Thrombolytic therapy is a useful adjunct to heparin in patients who have PE and who are hemodynamically unsta-

ble.[146] The definition of "hemodynamically unstable" is controversial and varies from systemic arterial hypotension to normal systemic arterial pressure with moderate or severe right ventricular dysfunction. Rapid improvement of right ventricular function and pulmonary perfusion, accomplished with thrombolytic therapy followed by heparin, may lead to a lower rate of death and recurrent PE.[49] Thrombolysis may (1) prevent the downhill spiral of right-sided heart failure by physical dissolution of anatomically obstructing pulmonary arterial thrombus (Fig. 52–12); (2) prevent the continued release of serotonin and other neurohumoral factors that might otherwise lead to worsening pulmonary hypertension; and (3) dissolve much of the source of the thrombus in the pelvic or deep leg veins, thereby decreasing the likelihood of recurrent large PE.

The potential benefits of immediately reversing right heart failure and preventing recurrent PE must be balanced by the risk of hemorrhage. Contraindications to thrombo-

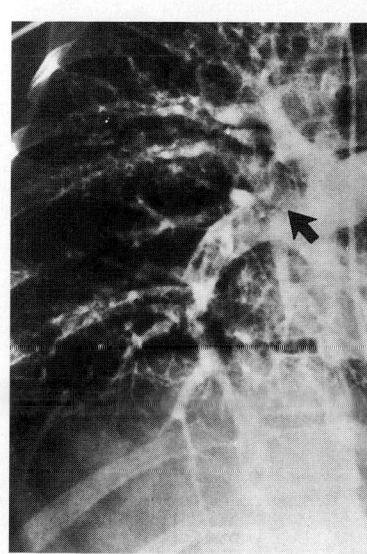
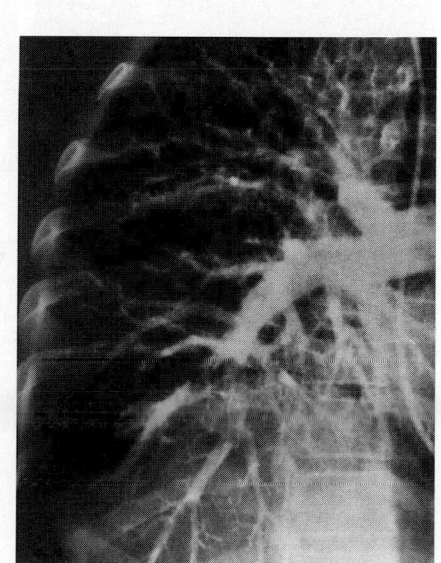

FIGURE 52–12. *Left,* A large embolus in the right pulmonary artery (arrow). *Right,* After a 2-hour infusion of tissue plasminogen activator through a peripheral vein, resolution is pronounced, with only a small amount of residual thrombus in segmental branches. (From Goldhaber SZ, Vaughan DE, Markis JE, et al: Acute pulmonary embolism treated with tissue plasminogen activator. Lancet 2:886, 1986.)

lysis, such as intracranial disease, recent surgery, or trauma, preclude its use in some patients who can safely receive heparin alone. There is a 1 to 2 percent risk of intracranial hemorrhage.[147] Carefully screening patients for contraindications to thrombolysis is the best way to minimize bleeding risk (see Chap. 62).

At Brigham and Women's Hospital, we have coordinated five trials of PE thrombolysis, including the largest trial of tissue plasminogen activator (t-PA, 100 mg/2 hr) plus heparin versus heparin alone.[148] The initial systemic arterial systolic pressure was at least 90 mm Hg in every patient. Most importantly, no clinical episodes of PE recurred among patients receiving t-PA, but there were five (two fatal and three nonfatal) clinically suspected recurrent PEs within 14 days in patients randomized to heparin alone ($p = 0.06$). All five initially showed right ventricular hypokinesis on echocardiogram. This latter observation suggests that echocardiography may help identify a subgroup of patients with PE at high risk of adverse clinical outcomes if treated with heparin alone. Such patients in particular would appear to be excellent candidates for thrombolytic therapy in the absence of contraindications.

Qualitative assessment of right ventricular wall motion demonstrated that 39 percent of the t-PA recipients improved (Figs. 52–13A and B) and 2.4 percent worsened, compared with 17 percent improvement and 17 percent worsening among those who received heparin alone ($p < 0.005$). Quantitative assessment showed that t-PA recipients had a significant decrease in right ventricular end-diastolic area during the 24 hours after randomization compared with none among those allocated to heparin alone ($p < 0.01$). Recipients of t-PA also had an absolute improvement in pulmonary perfusion of 14.6 percent at 24 hours (Fig. 52–13C and D), compared with 1.5 percent improvement among heparin alone recipients ($p < 0.0001$).

Unlike patients with myocardial infarction–thrombolysis, patients with PE have a wide "window" for effective use of thrombolysis. Specifically, patients who receive thrombolysis up to 14 days after new symptoms or signs maintain an effective response,[149] probably because of the bronchial collateral circulation. Therefore, patients suspected of having PE should be considered as potentially eligible for thrombolysis if they have had any new symptoms or signs within the 2 weeks before presentation. Although t-PA 100 mg/2 hr is the only contemporary FDA-approved dosing regimen for PE thrombolysis,[150] other regimens also appear promising, including 1,500,000 units of streptokinase/2 hr[151] and double-bolus reteplase (r-PA) (10-unit bolus followed 30 minutes later by a second 10-unit bolus).[152]

DVT THROMBOLYSIS

Most patients with DVT have contraindications to thrombolysis.[153] Totally occlusive venous thrombosis usually does not lyse if the agent is administered through a peripheral vein.[154] For patients with iliofemoral venous thrombosis, catheter-directed thrombolysis[155] or thrombolysis plus venous angioplasty[156] may be successful.

VENOUS INSUFFICIENCY. Many patients with PE are plagued with chronic lower leg swelling and calf discomfort that can become problematic years after an episode of venous thromboembolism. This is known as *venous insufficiency* or *postthrombotic syndrome*. In most situations, the pathophysiology is damage of venous valves from antecedent DVT. Under extreme circumstances, venous ulceration can occur, particularly in the medial malleolus. The condition is usually manageable with below-knee vascular compression stockings. However, the frequency of venous insufficiency can be halved by preventive use of sized-to-fit compression stockings of 20 to 40 mm Hg.[156a]

Embolectomy

The results of embolectomy can be optimized if patients are referred for this procedure before the onset of cardiogenic shock.[156b] Greenfield's embolectomy device is a classical catheter-based method of extracting pulmonary arterial thrombus (Fig. 52–14).[157] It consists of a 10F steerable catheter with a suction cup attached at the tip. Because of the cup's large size, a surgical venotomy is used, usually to access the right internal jugular vein. A steerable handle controls progression of the catheter through the right cardiac chambers and the pulmonary arterial branches.

Alternative catheterization methods[158] include mechanical fragmentation of thrombus with a standard pulmonary

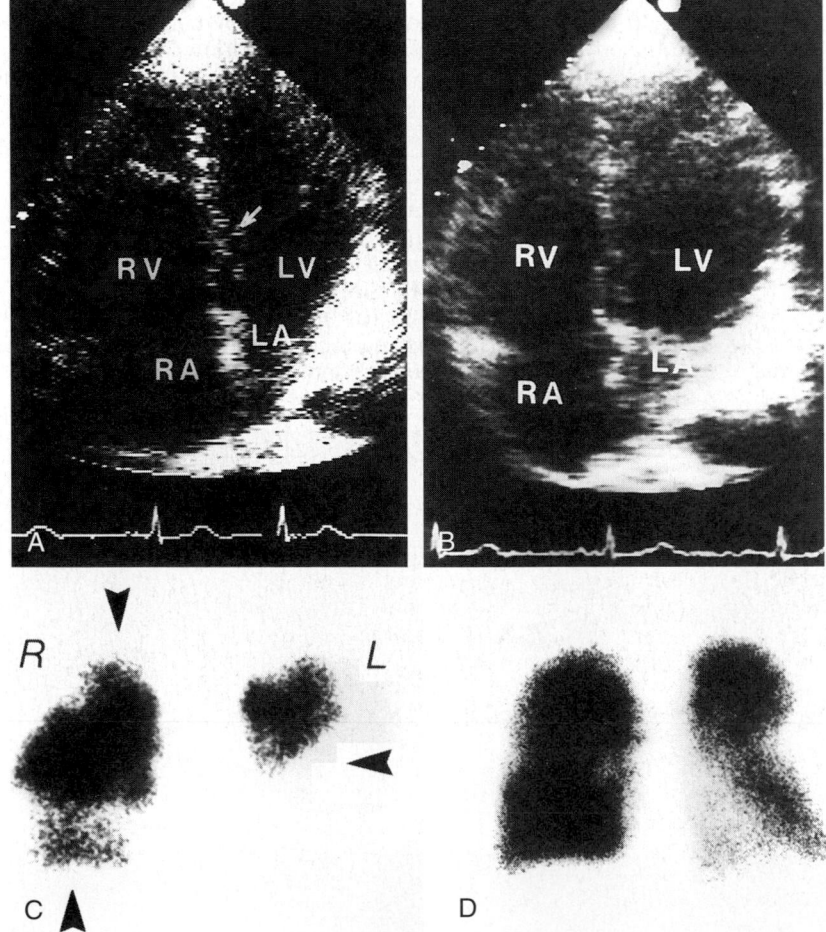

FIGURE 52–13. Echocardiograms (four-chamber view) and perfusion lung scans (anterior view) in a previously healthy 53-year-old man treated with tissue plasminogen activator (t-PA) for pulmonary embolism. *A,* Enlargement of the right ventricle (RV) before treatment. The RV end-diastolic area was 42.9 cm², and the interventricular septum (arrow) was displaced toward the left ventricle (LV). There was moderately severe RV hypokinesis. *B,* Three hours after initiation of t-PA therapy, the size of the RV normalized (with a planimetered area of 25.7 cm²) and the interventricular septum resumed its normal configuration. RV wall motion normalized. *C,* The pretherapy lung scan (*left*) shows absence of perfusion in the right middle lobe (lower arrowhead) and in most of the right upper lobe, particularly the apical segment of the right upper lobe (upper arrowhead). The left lung shows absence of perfusion in the lingula and anterior segment of the left upper lobe (horizontal arrowhead) and irregular perfusion in the apical-posterior segment of the left upper lobe. *D,* The posttherapy scan (*right*) shows marked improvement in perfusion. (From Goldhaber SZ: Treatment of acute pulmonary embolism. *In* Goldhaber SZ [ed]: Cardiopulmonary Diseases and Cardiac Tumors. *In* Braunwald E [series ed]: Atlas of Heart Diseases. Vol 3. Philadelphia, Current Medicine, 1995, pp 3.1–3.25.)

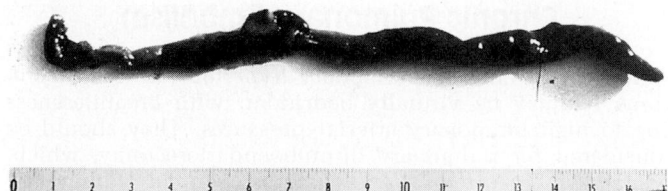

FIGURE 52–14. Philippe Reynaud, M.D., at the Laennec Hospital in Paris, used a Greenfield embolectomy catheter to remove this 17-cm thrombus from a severely compromised patient with PE. Rapid hemodynamic improvement ensued. (From Meyer G, Tamiser D, Reynaud P, Sors H: Acute pulmonary embolectomy. *In* Goldhaber SZ [ed]: Cardiopulmonary Diseases and Cardiac Tumors. *In* Braunwald E [series ed]: Atlas of Heart Diseases. Vol 3. Philadelphia, Current Medicine, 1995, pp 7.1–7.12.)

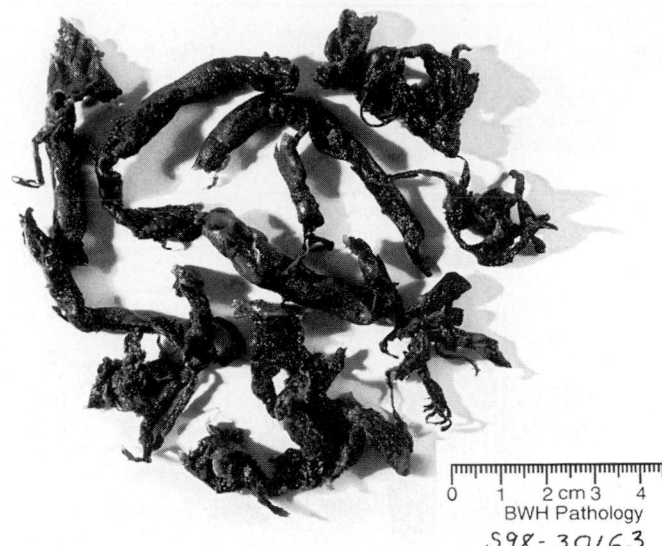

FIGURE 52–16. A 52-year-old woman was on the medical service to treat multiple sclerosis when she became short of breath and collapsed. Her echocardiogram showed a dilated right ventricle and collapsed left ventricle. Shortly thereafter, she suffered cardiac arrest and was immediately taken to the operating room with the presumptive diagnosis of pulmonary embolism. She was placed on cardiopulmonary bypass, and massive amounts of thrombus (*shown above*) were removed from her pulmonary arteries. She subsequently recovered uneventfully.

artery catheter, clot pulverization with a rotating basket catheter, percutaneous rheolytic thrombectomy,[159] and pigtail rotational catheter embolectomy.[160] This 5F Teflon catheter has a distal tip that is divided into four 15-mm bends. The high-speed mechanical rotation of the catheter (about 100,000 rpm) causes centrifugal force to open the distal bends and form a soft flexible helical spiral that can disintegrate thrombus into microscopic particles within seconds.[159] Another approach is simultaneous mechanical clot fragmentation and pharmacological thrombolysis (Fig. 52–15*A* and *B*).[161] Finally, balloon angioplasty has also been used to improve pulmonary arterial flow among patients with PE.[162]

If catheter-based strategies fail, emergency surgical embolectomy with cardiopulmonary bypass can be undertaken (Fig. 52–16).[163] A nonrandomized comparison of t-PA

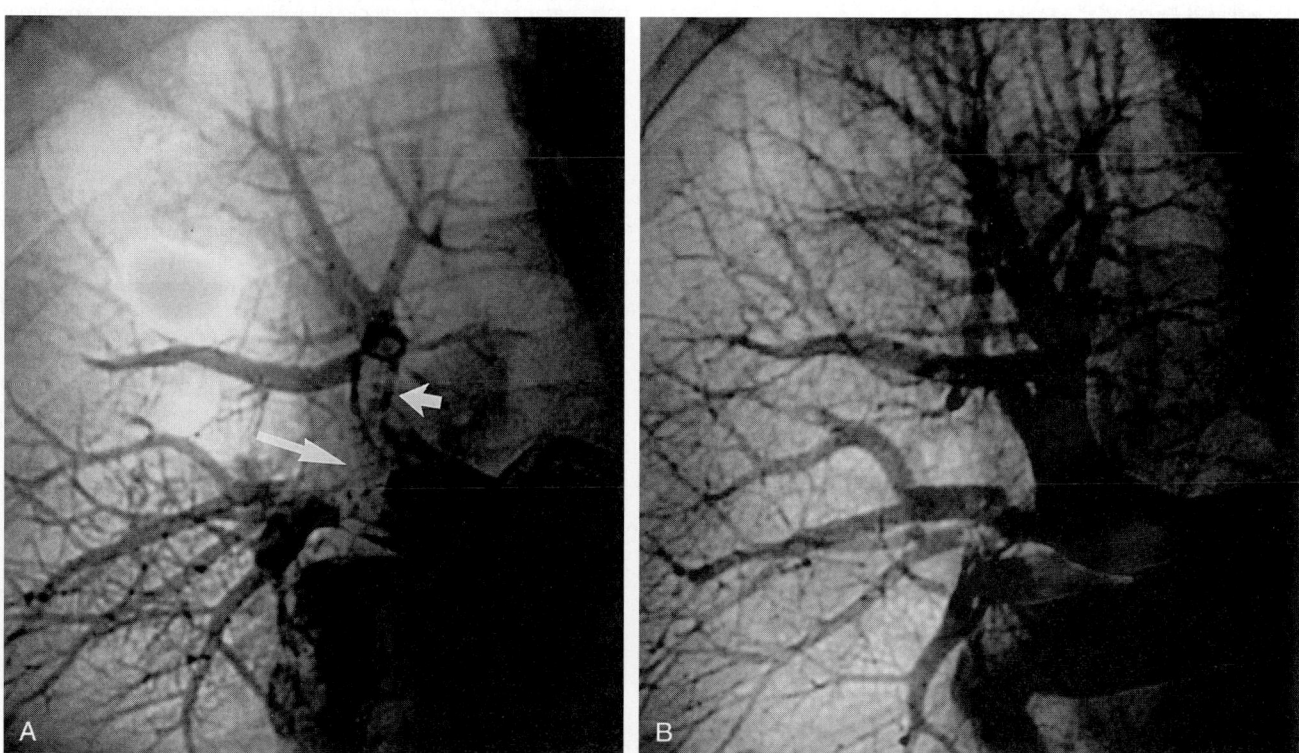

FIGURE 52–15. A 77-year-old woman had right-sided heart failure despite 3 days of full-dose heparin. Therefore, she underwent right heart catheterization and pulmonary angiography. Her pulmonary arterial pressure was 55/30 mm Hg. Seen on her baseline angiogram (*A*) were large right middle and right upper lobe pulmonary emboli (arrows). Because of relative contraindications to full-dose thrombolysis (systemic arterial hypertension and mild dementia), she underwent combined suction catheter embolectomy and catheter-directed thrombolysis with a bolus pulse spray of 8 mg of tissue plasminogen activator followed by an overnight infusion of 1 mg/hr. Her follow-up angiogram (*B*) shows marked improvement and reperfusion.

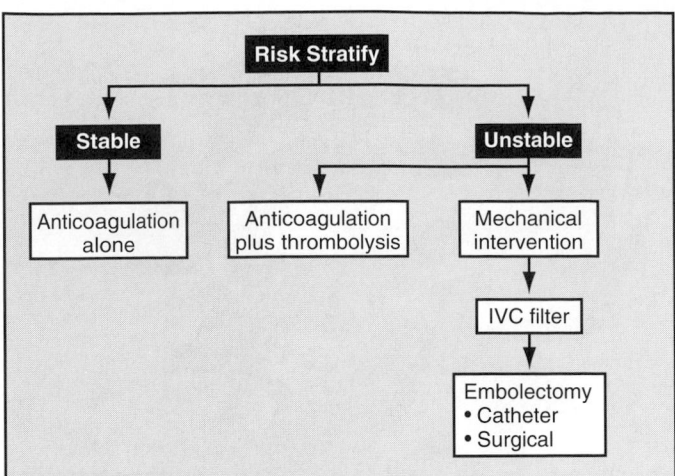

FIGURE 52–17. Proposed strategy for treatment of pulmonary embolism in which risk stratification, often with echocardiography, is undertaken to determine clinical and hemodynamic stability. This evaluation helps to determine prognosis as well as appropriateness of aggressive intervention with thrombolysis or mechanical measures to remove thrombus. IVC = inferior vena caval.

thrombolysis versus surgical embolectomy indicated that both approaches can be life saving in the majority of patients with massive PE.[164] For patients with PE causing hemodynamic instability, pulmonary embolectomy in the catheterization laboratory or operating room should be considered when there are contraindications to thrombolysis or when thrombolysis has failed.[165]

Management Approach for Acute Pulmonary Embolism

Therapy for PE should be tailored according to the anatomical extent of the embolus, the presence of underlying cardiopulmonary disease, and the detection of right-sided-heart dysfunction.[166, 167] The echocardiogram is becoming increasingly important for determination of hemodynamic stability, risk stratification, and prognostication (Fig. 52–17). Primary therapy is being used with increasing frequency for patients with moderate or severe right ventricular dilatation and hypokinesis on echocardiogram, even in the presence of normal systemic arterial pressure. Secondary prevention of recurrent PE is directed toward all patients and appears to suffice in those with small to moderate PE in the absence of major right ventricular dysfunction. Before hospital discharge, obtaining a follow-up perfusion lung scan is useful to establish a new baseline, in case the patient subsequently complains of symptoms suggesting recurrent PE.

EMOTIONAL SUPPORT. Although PE can be as emotionally devastating as myocardial infarction, the psychological burden for patients with PE may be greater. The lay public is not familiar with PE, particularly in terms of the possibility of genetic predisposition, long-term disability, and recurrence of disease. By discussing the implications of PE with patients and their families, the emotional burden may be assuaged. We initiated a Pulmonary Embolism Support Group, co-led by a nurse-physician team, and have been gratified by the experience. Although these sessions have an educational component,[168] the major emphasis is on discussing the anxieties and living difficulties that occur in the aftermath of PE.

Chronic Pulmonary Embolism

Patients with chronic pulmonary hypertension due to previous PE may be virtually bedridden with breathlessness due to high pulmonary arterial pressures. They should be considered for pulmonary thromboendarterectomy, which, if successful, can reduce and at times even cure pulmonary hypertension. The operation involves a median sternotomy, institution of cardiopulmonary bypass, and deep hypothermia with circulatory arrest periods. Incisions are made in both pulmonary arteries into the lower-lobe branches. Pulmonary thromboendarterectomy is always bilateral, with removal of organized thrombus from all involved vessels.

At the University of California at San Diego, more than 1000 patients debilitated by chronic pulmonary hypertension due to PE have undergone pulmonary thromboendarterectomy with good results and at an acceptable risk (Fig. 52–18). The two major causes of mortality are (1) inability to remove sufficient thrombotic material at operation, resulting in persistent postoperative pulmonary hypertension and right ventricular dysfunction; and (2) severe reperfusion lung injury.[169]

Prevention

PE is difficult to diagnose, expensive to treat, and occasionally lethal despite therapy. Therefore, preventive measures are paramount.[170] Various mechanical measures and pharmacological agents can be used. The most recent innovation has been FDA approval of two different LMWHs, one (enoxaparin) for use in patients undergoing total hip or knee replacement or general surgery and another (dalteparin) for patients undergoing total hip replacement or general surgery.

American[171] and European[172] consensus conferences have provided detailed guidelines for prevention of venous thromboembolism. The concept of prophylaxis has gained wide acceptance. This is, at least in part, because of the medicolegal liability of physicians who omit prophylaxis among their hospitalized patients with risk factors for venous thrombosis.[173] Furthermore, a policy of prophylaxis is cost-effective. It is estimated that for every 1,000,000 patients undergoing operation who receive prophylaxis against DVT and PE, approximately $60,000,000 can be saved in direct health care costs.[174]

MECHANICAL MEASURES

GRADUATED COMPRESSION STOCKINGS. These provide continuous stimulation of blood flow and prevent dilation of the venous system

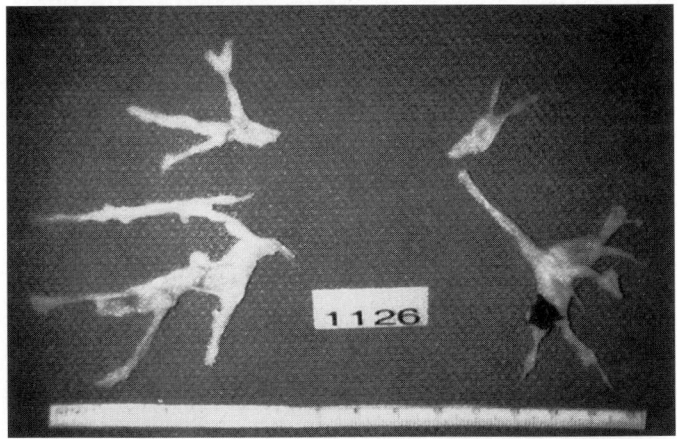

FIGURE 52–18. A 30-year-old man with chronic pulmonary embolism complained of exercise intolerance. His echocardiogram showed mild to moderate right ventricular dysfunction and enlargement. Lung scan, chest CT scan, and pulmonary angiogram showed numerous thrombi. He underwent pulmonary thromboendarterectomy after insertion of a prophylactic inferior vena caval filter. At surgery, a moderate amount of thromboembolic material (*shown above*) was removed from both lungs. His pulmonary artery pressure decreased from a baseline of 35/10 mm Hg to 18/9 mm Hg before the pulmonary artery catheter was removed. He has enjoyed an excellent and uncomplicated recovery. (Courtesy of Dr. Kim M. Kerr.)

in the legs. Graduated compression stockings (GCS) exert more compression at the ankles (usually 18 mm Hg) than at the popliteal fossa or upper thigh (usually 8 mm Hg). In an overview of 12 trials in moderate-risk surgery, GCS reduced the DVT rate by two-thirds.[175] Thus, GCS should be considered first-line prophylaxis for most hospitalized patients and should suffice for prophylaxis among low-risk patients.

INTERMITTENT PNEUMATIC COMPRESSION. Intermittent pneumatic compression (IPC) devices expel blood from the leg veins and thus prevent venous stasis. The mechanical force of compression appears to enhance systemic fibrinolytic activity.[176] IPC is particularly worthwhile among patients who have an absolute contraindication to anticoagulation. In addition, for patients receiving postoperative warfarin prophylaxis, IPC devices have special utility because they are immediately useful, whereas warfarin requires 4 to 5 days of administration before it is entirely effective as an anticoagulant. IPC devices are, in general, used properly in intensive care units. In one survey, however, they were either not applied or applied improperly in the majority of patients after transfer from an intensive care to a regular general surgery unit.[177]

INFERIOR VENA CAVAL INTERRUPTION. (see p. 1899). The most invasive mechanical prophylaxis measure that can be implemented is IVC filter placement. Use of an IVC filter might be appropriate for patients with recently diagnosed PE or DVT who must undergo major surgery that places them at high risk for suffering perioperative PE. The filter prevents PE but not DVT.[144]

PHARMACOLOGICAL AGENTS

UNFRACTIONATED HEPARIN. "Minidose heparin" has traditionally been used to prevent perioperative venous thromboembolism. Unfractionated heparin is administered two or three times daily in a dose of 5000 units subcutaneously. The first injection is usually given 2 hours before the skin incision. An overview of 78 randomized controlled trials with 15,598 patients found a 40 percent reduction in nonfatal PE and a 64 percent reduction in fatal PE.[176] In more recent pharmacological prophylaxis trials, at times, prophylaxis has been deferred until the early postoperative period. Any loss of efficacy resulting from deferring prophylaxis until shortly after surgery is unlikely to be marked.[178]

LOW-MOLECULAR-WEIGHT-HEPARIN. LMWH has a more predictable dose response, more dose-independent mechanisms of clearance, and a longer plasma half-life than unfractionated heparin. LMWHs can achieve higher plasma heparin levels with less bleeding than equivalent doses of unfractionated heparin. Because of its favorable profile (see p. 1896), an increasing number of orthopedic and general surgical patients are receiving once-daily fixed-dose prophylaxis with LMWH rather than injections of minidose unfractionated heparin two or three times daily.

DANAPAROID. Danaparoid is a heparinoid glycosaminoglycuronan that inhibits factors Xa and IIa (thrombin) in a ratio greater than 20.[178a] The active components are heparan sulfate (~ 84 percent), dermatan sulfate (~ 12 percent), and chondroitin sulfate (~ 4 percent). The average molecular weight is about 5500. The only FDA-approved indication is prophylaxis in patients undergoing total hip replacement (in a dose of 750 units administered subcutaneously twice daily).[179] However, it is often used for "off-label" treatment of heparin-induced thrombocytopenia,[180] even though there is about a 10 to 15 percent rate of cross reactivity between unfractionated heparin and danaparoid. Danaparoid can be administered subcutaneously, unlike the only FDA-approved treatment for heparin-induced thrombocytopenia, lepirudin, which can be administered only intravenously.

ASPIRIN. Although aspirin provides modest pharmacological prophylaxis against perioperative venous thromboembolism,[143] it is too weak an agent to be considered the standard of care for prevention of PE or DVT.

PROPHYLAXIS STRATEGIES FOR SPECIFIC CONDITIONS

Fortunately, numerous prophylaxis options are available for preventing PE and DVT in most patients (Table 52-14). The specific prophylaxis modality that is chosen is not nearly as important as upholding a standard that virtually all hospitalized patients receive some preventive measure appropriate to their level of risk.

ORTHOPEDIC SURGERY. Both adjusted-dose warfarin (target INR 2.0 to 3.0) and fixed-dose LMWH effectively prevent most episodes of venous thromboembolism that occur after total hip replacement,[181] total knee replacement, or hip fracture surgery. In one trial, desirudin appeared even more effective than LMWH in preventing venous thromboembolism after total hip replacement[182]; however, it is not commercially available.

To determine whether low-dose aspirin could prevent PE in patients with hip fracture, a megatrial of 13,356 patients was undertaken. They were assigned to 160 mg of enteric-coated aspirin once daily or its placebo in a randomized controlled design. At 5 weeks, 81 patients in the placebo group suffered PE (43 fatal and 38 nonfatal), compared with 46 in the aspirin group (18 fatal and 28 nonfatal), for an overall 43 percent risk reduction (*p* = 0.002) without any increase in major bleeding.[183]

Foot-compression pumps have become popular as a mechanical prophylaxis method, particularly in patients undergoing orthopedic

▼ TABLE 52-14. PREVENTION OF VENOUS THROMBOEMBOLISM

INDICATION	POTENTIAL PROPHYLAXIS REGIMEN
Orthopedic surgery	Enoxaparin 30 mg twice daily
	Enoxaparin 40 mg once daily*
	Dalteparin 5000 units once daily*
	Danaparoid 750 units twice daily*
	Warfarin (target INR = 2.0–3.0)
	GCS plus IPC
General surgery	Enoxaparin 40 mg daily
	Dalteparin 2500 or 5000 units once daily
	GCS plus IPC
Pregnancy	Enoxaparin 40 mg daily
	Dalteparin 5000 units daily
Medical patients	Enoxaparin 40 mg daily
	GCS plus IPC

* Approved only for total hip replacement prophylaxis.
GCS = graduated compression stockings; IPC = intermittent pneumatic compression boots; INR = International Normalized Ratio.

surgery. However, the effectiveness of these pumps in preventing PE and DVT has not been extensively studied. In one trial of patients receiving foot-pump prophylaxis for total knee replacement, 54 percent had postoperative DVT.[184] Thus, these devices cannot be recommended at this time.

Two important concepts have recently emerged. First, DVT occurs with surprisingly high frequency after knee arthroscopy, affecting 18 percent of patients in one series.[185] Second, patients remain at high risk of venous thromboembolism after hospital discharge following total hip or knee replacement.[186] The median time for diagnosis of venous thromboembolism was 17 days postoperatively for total hip replacement and 7 days postoperatively for total knee replacement in a series of approximately 45,000 patients undergoing surgery in California. The FDA has approved prophylaxis for 3 weeks after hospital discharge with enoxaparin 40 mg once daily for patients undergoing total hip replacement.

CARDIAC SURGERY. In a trial of 2786 patients undergoing open-heart surgery, prophylaxis was randomized to pneumatic compression devices plus minidose heparin versus minidose heparin alone. The frequency of PE was 1.5 percent in the combined prophylaxis group versus 4 percent in the group given minidose heparin alone.[187]

MEDICAL PATIENTS. Medical patients have not been nearly as well studied as surgical patients in terms of prevention of venous thromboembolism. In the MEDENOX Trial of 1102 hospitalized medical patients, prophylaxis with enoxaparin 40 mg once daily reduced by two-thirds the frequency of DVT as assessed by bilateral contrast venography between days 6 and 14.[188]

REFERENCES

1. Goldhaber SZ, Visani L, De Rosa M, for ICOPER: Acute pulmonary embolism: Clinical outcomes in the International Cooperative Pulmonary Embolism Registry (ICOPER). Lancet 353:1386, 1999.

HYPERCOAGULABILITY

2. Rosendaal FR: Venous thrombosis: A multicausal disease. Lancet 353: 1167, 1999.
3. Bertina RM, Koeleman BPC, Koster T, et al: Mutation in blood coagulation factor V associated with resistance to activated protein C. Nature 369:64, 1994.
4. Hajjar KA: Factor V Leiden—an unselfish gene? N Engl J Med 331: 1585, 1994.
5. Ridker PM, Hennekens CH, Lindpaintner K, et al: Mutation in the gene coding for coagulation factor V and risks of future myocardial infarction, stroke, and venous thrombosis in apparently healthy men. N Engl J Med 332:912, 1995.
6. Vandenbroucke JP, Koster T, Briët E, et al: Increased risk of venous thrombosis in oral-contraceptive users who are carriers of factor V Leiden mutation. Lancet 344:1453, 1994.
7. Ridker PM, Miletich JP, Buring JE, et al: Factor V Leiden as a risk factor for recurrent pregnancy loss. Ann Intern Med 128:1000, 1008.
8. Ridker PM, Miletich JP, Stampfer MJ, et al: Factor V Leiden and risks of recurrent idiopathic venous thromboembolism. Circulation 92:2800, 1995.
8a. De Stephano V, Martinelli I, Mannucci PM, et al: The risk of recurrent deep venous thrombosis among heterozygous carriers of both factor V Leiden and the G20210A prothrombin mutation. N Engl J Med 341:801, 1999.

8b. Turkstra F, Karemaker R, Kuijer PMM, et al: Is the prevalence of the factor V Leiden mutation in patients with pulmonary embolism and deep venous thrombosis really different? Thromb Haemost 81:345, 1999.

9. Poort SR, Rosendaal FR, Reitsma PH, Bertina RM: A common genetic variation in the 3'-untranslated region of the prothrombin gene is associated with elevated plasma prothrombin levels and an increase in venous thrombosis. Blood 88:3698, 1996.

10. Ridker PM, Hennekens CH, Miletich JP: G20210A mutation in prothrombin gene and risk of myocardial infarction, stroke, and venous thrombosis in a large cohort of US men. Circulation 99:999, 1999.

10a. Gerhardt A, Scharf RE, Beckmann MW, et al: Prothrombin and factor V mutations in women with a history of thrombosis during pregnancy and the puerperium. N Engl J Med 342:374, 2000.

10b. Meijers JCM, Tekelenburg WL, Bouma BN, et al: High levels of coagulation factor XI as a risk factor for venous thrombosis. N Engl J Med 342:696, 2000.

11. Zöller B, Dahlbäck B: Linkage between inherited resistance to activated protein C and factor V gene mutation in venous thrombosis. Lancet 343:1536, 1994.

12. Allaart CF, Poort SR, Rosendaal FR, et al: Increased risk of venous thrombosis in carriers of hereditary protein C deficiency defect. Lancet 341:134, 1993.

13. Gladson CL, Scharrer I, Hach V, et al: The frequency of type heterozygous protein S and protein C deficiency in 141 unrelated young patients with venous thrombosis. Thromb Haemost 59:18, 1988.

14. Bucciarelli P, Rosendaal FR, Tripodi A, et al: Risk of venous thromboembolism and clinical manifestations in carriers of antithrombin, protein C, protein S deficiency, or activated protein C resistance: A multicenter collaborative family study. Arterioscler Thromb Vasc Biol 19:1026, 1999.

15. den Heijer M, Rosendaal FR, Blom HJ, et al: Hyperhomocysteinemia and venous thrombosis: a meta-analysis. Thromb Haemost 80:874, 1998.

15a. Langman LJ, Ray JG, Evrovski J, et al: Hyperhomocyst(e)inemia and the increased risk of venous thromboembolism: More evidence from a case-control study. Arch Intern Med 160:961, 2000.

16. Ridker PM, Hennekens CH, Selhub J, et al: Interrelation of hyperhomocyst(e)inemia, Factor V Leiden, and risk of future venous thromboembolism. Circulation 95:1777, 1997.

17. Greaves M: Antiphospholipid antibodies and thrombosis. Lancet 353:1348, 1999.

18. Heijboer H, Brandjes DPM, Büller HR, et al: Deficiencies of coagulation-inhibiting and fibrinolytic proteins in outpatients with deep-vein thrombosis. N Engl J Med 323:1512, 1990.

19. Malm J, Laurell M, Nilsson IM, Dahlbäck B: Thromboembolic disease—critical evaluation of laboratory investigation. Thromb Haemost 68:7, 1992.

20. Svensson PJ, Dahlbäck B: Resistance to activated protein C as a basis for venous thrombosis. N Engl J Med 330:517, 1994.

21. Koster T, Rosendaal FR, de Ronde H, et al: Venous thrombosis due to poor anticoagulant response to activated protein C: Leiden thrombophilia study. Lancet 342:1503, 1993.

21a. Eekhoff EMW, Rosendaal FR, Vandenbroucke JP: Minor events and the risk of deep venous thrombosis. Thromb Haemost 83:408, 2000.

22. White RH, Romano PS, Zhou H, et al: Incidence and time course of thromboembolic outcomes following total hip or knee arthroplasty. Arch Intern Med 158:1525, 1998.

23. Josa M, Siouffi SY, Silverman AB, et al: Pulmonary embolism after cardiac surgery. J Am Coll Cardiol 21:990, 1993.

24. Goldhaber SZ, Hirsch DR, MacDougall RC, et al: Prevention of venous thrombosis after coronary artery bypass surgery: A randomized trial comparing two mechanical prophylaxis strategies. Am J Cardiol 76:993, 1995.

25. Geerts WH, Code KI, Jay RM, et al: A prospective study of venous thromboembolism after major trauma. N Engl J Med 331:1601, 1994.

26. Hirsch DR, Ingenito EP, Goldhaber SZ: Prevalence of deep venous thrombosis among patients in medical intensive care. JAMA 274:335, 1995.

27. Goldhaber SZ, Savage DD, Garrison RJ, et al: Risk factors for pulmonary embolism: The Framingham study. Am J Med 74:1023, 1983.

28. Goldhaber SZ, Grodstein F, Stampfer MJ, et al: A prospective study of risk factors for pulmonary embolism in women. JAMA 277:642, 1997.

29. Chasen-Taber L, Stampfer MJ: Epidemiology of oral contraceptives and cardiovascular disease. Ann Intern Med 128:467, 1998.

30. Rosing J, Tans G, Nicolaes GAF, et al: Oral contraceptives and venous thrombosis: Different sensitivities to activated protein C in women using second and third generation oral contraceptives. Br J Haematol 97:233, 1997.

31. Grady D, Sawaya G: Postmenopausal hormone therapy increases risk of deep vein thrombosis and pulmonary embolism. Am J Med 105:41, 1998.

32. Cummings SR, Eckert S, Krueger KA, et al: The effect of raloxifene on risk of breast cancer in postmenopausal women. Results from the MORE randomized trial. JAMA 281:2189, 1999.

33. Greer IA: Thrombosis in pregnancy: Maternal and fetal issues. Lancet 353:1258, 1999.

34. Kupferminc MJ, Eldor A, Steinman N, et al: Increased frequency of genetic thrombophilia in women with complications of pregnancy. N Engl J Med 340:9, 1999.

35. Sørensen HT, Mellemkjaer L, Steffensen FH, et al: The risk of a diagno-

sis of cancer after primary deep venous thrombosis or pulmonary embolism. N Engl J Med 338:1169, 1998.

36. Levine M, Hirsch J, Gent M, et al: Double-blind randomised trial of very-low-dose warfarin for prevention of thromboembolism in stage IV breast cancer. Lancet 343:886, 1994.

37. Turpie AGG, Gent M, Côte R, et al: A low-molecular-weight heparinoid compared with unfractionated heparin in the prevention of deep vein thrombosis in patients with acute ischemic stroke: A randomized, double-blind study. Ann Intern Med 117:353, 1992.

38. Green D, Hull RD, Mammen EF, et al: Deep vein thrombosis in spinal cord injury. Summary and recommendations. Chest 102:633S, 1992.

39. Raad II, Luna M, Khalil SAM, et al: The relationship between the thrombotic and infectious complications of central venous catheters. JAMA 271:1014, 1994.

40. Moser KM, Fedullo PF, LitteJohn JK, Crawford R: Frequent asymptomatic pulmonary embolism in patients with deep venous thrombosis. JAMA 271:223, 1994.

41. Prandoni P, Polistena P, Bernardi E, et al: Upper extremity deep vein thrombosis. Risk factors, diagnosis, and complications. Arch Intern Med 157:57, 1997.

42. Turkstra F, Kuijer PMM, van Beek EJR, et al: Diagnostic utility of ultrasonography of leg veins in patients suspected of having pulmonary embolism. Ann Intern Med 126:775, 1997.

PATHOPHYSIOLOGY

43. Elliott CG: Pulmonary physiology during pulmonary embolism. Chest 101:163S, 1992.

44. Lualdi JC, Goldhaber SZ: Right ventricular dysfunction after acute pulmonary embolism: Pathophysiologic factors, detection, and therapeutic implications. Am Heart J 130:1276, 1995.

45. Belenkie L, Dani R, Smith ER, Tyberg JV: The importance of pericardial constraint in experimental pulmonary embolism and volume loading. Am Heart J 123:733, 1992.

46. Watanabe J, Levine MJ, Bellotto F, et al: Effects of coronary venous pressure on left ventricular diastolic distensibility. Circ Res 67:923, 1990.

47. Post F, Voigtlaender T, Mertens D, et al: Troponin I as a severity marker for pulmonary embolism [abstract]. Circulation 98:I-273, 1998.

47a. Perrier A, Miron MJ, Desmarais S, et al: Using clinical evaluation and lung scan to rule out suspected pulmonary embolism: Is it a valid option in patients with normal results of lower-limb venous compression ultrasonography? Arch Intern Med 160:512, 2000.

47b. Moser KM, Fedullo PF, Finkbeiner WE, Golden J: Do patients with primary pulmonary hypertension develop extensive central thrombi? Circulation 91:741, 1995.

48. Goldhaber SZ: Treatment of acute pulmonary embolism. In Goldhaber SZ (ed): Cardiopulmonary diseases and cardiac tumors. In Braunwald E (series ed): Atlas of Heart Diseases. Vol 3. Philadelphia, Current Medicine 1995, p 3.1.

49. Wolfe MW, Lee RT, Feldstein ML, et al: Prognostic significance of right ventricular hypokinesis and perfusion lung scan defects in pulmonary embolism. Am Heart J 127:1371, 1994.

50. Wagenvoort CA: Pathology of pulmonary thromboembolism. Chest 107:10S, 1995.

51. Kasper W, Geibel A, Tiede N, and Just H: Patent foramen ovale in patients with haemodynamically significant pulmonary embolism. Lancet 340:561, 1992.

52. Stöllberger C, Slany J, Schuster I, et al: The prevalence of deep venous thrombosis in patients with suspected paradoxical embolism. Ann Intern Med 119:461, 1993.

53. Fabian TC: Unraveling the fat embolism syndrome. N Engl J Med 329:961, 1993.

54. Goldhaber SZ, Dricker E, Buring JE, et al: Clinical suspicion of autopsy-proven thrombotic and tumor pulmonary embolism in cancer patients. Am Heart J 114:1432, 1987.

54a. Muth CM, Shank ES: Gas embolism. N Engl J Med 342:476, 2000.

55. Phifer TJ, Bridges M, Conrad SA: The residual central venous catheter track—an occult source of lethal air embolism: Case report. J Trauma 31:1558, 1991.

56. Rothenberg F, Schumacher JR, Rosenthal RL: Near-fatal pulmonary air embolus from presumed inadvertent pressure placed on a partially empty plastic intravenous infusion bag. Am J Cardiol 73:1035, 1994.

DIAGNOSIS

57. Bounameaux H, de Moerloose P, Perrier A, Reber G: Plasma measurement of D-dimer as diagnostic aid in suspected venous thromboembolism: An overview. Thromb Haemost 71:1, 1994.

58. Goldhaber SZ, Simons GR, Elliott CG, et al: Quantitative plasma D-dimer levels among patients undergoing pulmonary angiography for suspected pulmonary embolism. JAMA 270:2819, 1993.

58a. Goldhaber SZ: The perils of D-dimer in the medical intensive care unit. Crit Care Med 28:583, 2000.

59. de Moerloose P, Desmarais S, Bounameaux H, et al: Contribution of a new, rapid, and quantitative automated D-dimer ELISA to exclude pulmonary embolism. Thromb Haemost 75:11, 1996.

60. Stein PD, Terrin ML, Hales CA, et al: Clinical, laboratory, roentgenographic, and electrocardiographic findings in patients with acute pul-

monary embolism and no pre-existing cardiac or pulmonary disease. Chest 100:598, 1991.

61. Stein PD, Goldhaber SZ, Henry JW: Alveolar-arterial oxygen gradient in the assessment of acute pulmonary embolism. Chest 107:139, 1995.

62. Sreeram N, Cheriex EC, Smeets JLRM, et al: Value of the 12-lead electrocardiogram at hospital admission in the diagnosis of pulmonary embolism. Am J Cardiol 73:298, 1994.

63. Ginsberg J, Wells PS, Hirsh J, et al: Reevaluation of the sensitivity of impedence plethysmography for the detection of proximal deep vein thrombosis. Arch Intern Med 154:1930, 1994.

64. Westermark N: On the roentgen diagnosis of lung embolism. Acta Radiol 19:357, 1938.

65. Hampton AO, Castleman B: Correlation of postmortem chest teleroentgenograms with autopsy findings with special reference to pulmonary embolism and infarction. AJR 43:305, 1940.

66. Stein PD, Athanasoulis C, Greenspan RH, Henry JW: Relation of plain chest radiographic findings to pulmonary arterial pressure and arterial blood oxygen levels in patients with acute pulmonary embolism. Am J Cardiol 69:394, 1992.

67. Skibo L, Goldhaber SZ: Diagnosis of acute pulmonary embolism. *In* Braunwald E, Goldhaber SZ (eds): Atlas of Heart Diseases. Vol 3. Cardiopulmonary Diseases and Cardiac Tumors. Philadelphia, Current Medicine, 1995, p 2.1.

68. Polak JF: Diagnosis of venous thrombosis. *In* Goldhaber SZ (ed): Cardiopulmonary Diseases and Cardiac Tumors. Vol 3. *In* Braunwald E (series ed). Atlas of Heart Diseases, Philadelphia, Current Medicine, 1995, pp 11.1–11.17.

69. Heijboer H, Büller HR, Lensing AWA, et al: A comparison of real-time compression ultrasonography with impedance plethysmography for the diagnosis of deep-vein thrombosis in symptomatic outpatients. N Engl J Med 329:1365, 1993.

70. Lensing AWA, Prandoni P, Brandjes D, et al: Detection of deep-vein thrombosis by real-time B-mode ultrasonography. N Engl J Med 320:342, 1989.

71. Simons GR, Skibo LK, Polak JF, et al: Utility of leg ultrasonography in suspected symptomatic isolated calf deep venous thrombosis. Am J Med 99:43, 1995.

72. Prandoni P, Cogo A, Bernardi E, et al: A simple ultrasound approach for detection of recurrent proximal-vein thrombosis. Circulation 88:1730, 1993.

73. Wells PS, Lensing AWA, Davidson BL, et al: Accuracy of ultrasound for the diagnosis of deep venous thrombosis in asymptomatic patients after orthopedic surgery: A meta-analysis. Ann Intern Med 122:47, 1995.

74. Jongbloets LMM, Lensing AWA, Koopman MMW, et al: Limitations of compression ultrasound for the detection of symptomless postoperative deep vein thrombosis. Lancet 343:1142, 1994.

75. Rabinov K, Paulin S: Roentgen diagnosis of venous thrombosis in the leg. Arch Surg 104:134, 1972.

76. Couson F, Bounameaux C, Didier D, et al: Influence of variability of interpretation of contrast venography for screening of postoperative deep venous thrombosis on the results of a thromboprophylactic study. Thromb Haemost 70:573, 1993.

76a. de Groot MR, Turkstra F, van Marwijk Kooy M, et al: Value of chest X-ray combined with perfusion scan versus ventilation/perfusion scan in acute pulmonary embolism. Thromb Haemost 83:412, 2000.

77. Stein PD, Terrin ML, Gottschalk A, et al: Value of ventilation/perfusion scans versus perfusion scans alone in acute pulmonary embolism. Am J Cardiol 69:1239, 1992.

78. The PIOPED Investigators: Value of the ventilation/perfusion scan in acute pulmonary embolism: Results of the Prospective Investigation of Pulmonary Embolism Diagnosis (PIOPED). JAMA 263:2753, 1990.

79. Gottschalk A, Sostman HD, Coleman RE, et al: Ventilation-perfusion scintigraphy in the PIOPED study. Part II. Evaluation of the scintigraphic criteria and interpretations. J Nucl Med 34:1119, 1993.

80. Bone RC: The low-probability lung scan: A potentially lethal reading. Arch Intern Med 153:2621, 1993.

81. Drucker EA, Rivitz SM, Shepard JO, et al: Acute pulmonary embolism: Assessment of helical CT for diagnosis. Radiology 209:235, 1998.

81a. Rathbun SW, Raskob GE, Whitsett TL: Sensitivity and specificity of helical computed tomography in the diagnosis of pulmonary embolism: A systematic review. Ann Intern Med 132:227, 2000.

82. Meaney JFM, Weg JG, Chenevert TL, et al: Diagnosis of pulmonary embolism with magnetic resonance angiography. N Engl J Med 336:1422, 1997.

83. Jardin F, Dubourg O, Bourdarias J-P: Echocardiographic pattern of acute cor pulmonale. Chest 111:209, 1997.

84. Konstantinides S, Geibel A, Kasper W, et al: Patent foramen ovale is an important predictor of adverse outcome in patients with major pulmonary embolism. Circulation 97:1946, 1998.

85. McConnell MV, Solomon SD, Rayan ME, et al: Regional right ventricular dysfunction detected by echocardiography in acute pulmonary embolism. Am J Cardiol 78:469, 1996.

86. Wolfe MW, Skibo LK, Goldhaber SZ: Pulmonary embolic disease: Diagnosis, pathophysiologic aspects, and treatment with thrombolytic therapy. Curr Probl Cardiol 18:585, 1993.

87. Auger WR, Fedullo PF, Moser KM, et al: Chronic major-vessel thromboembolic pulmonary artery obstruction: Appearance at angiography. Radiology 182:393, 1992.

88. Meyerovitz MF, Mannting F, Polak JF, Goldhaber SZ: Frequency of pulmonary embolism in patients with low-probability lung scan and negative lower extremity venous ultrasound. Chest 115:980, 1999.

89. Perrier A, Desmarais S, Miron, M-J, et al: Non-invasive diagnosis of venous thromboembolism in outpatients. Lancet 353:190, 1999.

MANAGEMENT

89a. Layish DT, Tapson VF: Pharmacologic hemodynamic support in massive pulmonary embolism. Chest 111:218, 1997.

90. Estagnasié P, Le Bourdellès G, Mier L, et al: Use of inhaled nitric oxide to reverse flow through a patent foramen ovale during pulmonary embolism. Ann Intern Med 120:757, 1994.

91. Kondo NI, Maddi R, Ewenstein BM, Goldhaber SZ: Anticoagulation and hemostasis in cardiac surgical patients. J Cardiovasc Surg 9:443, 1994.

92. Weitz JI, Hudoba M, Massel D, et al: Clot-bound thrombin is protected from inhibition by heparin–antithrombin III but is susceptible to inactivation by antithrombin III–independent inhibitors. J Clin Invest 86:385, 1990.

93. Young E, Prins M, Levine MN, Hirsh J: Heparin binding to plasma proteins, an important mechanism for heparin resistance. Thromb Haemost 67:639, 1992.

94. Weitz JI: Low-molecular-weight heparins. N Engl J Med 337:688, 1997.

95. Koopman MMW, Prandoni P, Piovella F, et al: Treatment of venous thrombosis with intravenous unfractionated heparin administered in the hospital as compared with subcutaneous low-molecular-weight heparin administered at home. N Engl J Med 334:682, 1996.

96. Levine M, Gent M, Hirsh J, et al: A comparison of low-molecular-weight heparin administered primarily at home with unfractionated heparin administered in the hospital for proximal deep-vein thrombosis. N Engl J Med 334:677, 1996.

97. The Columbus Investigators: Low-molecular-weight heparin in the treatment of patients with venous thromboembolism. N Engl J Med 337:657, 1997.

98. Gould MK, Dembitzer AD, Doyle RL, et al: Low-molecular-weight heparins compared with unfractionated heparin for treatment of acute deep venous thrombosis. Ann Intern Med 130:800, 1999.

99. Gould MK, Dembitzer AD, Sanders GD, Garber AM: Low-molecular-weight heparins compared with unfractionated heparin for treatment of acute deep venous thrombosis. Ann Intern Med 130:789, 1999.

100. Harrison L, McGinnis J, Crowther M, et al: Assessment of outpatient treatment of deep-vein thrombosis with low-molecular-weight heparin. Arch Intern Med 158:2001, 1998.

101. Baron RM, Goldhaber SZ: Deep venous thrombosis: Outpatient management is now FDA approved. J Thromb Thrombol 7:113, 1999.

102. Abildgaard U, Eldor BLA, Elias D, et al: Multicenter clinical trial comparing once daily subcutaneous enoxaparin and intravenous heparin in the treatment of acute DVT. Ann Intern Med, in press.

103. Simonneau G, Sors H, Charbonnier B, et al: A comparison of low-molecular-weight heparin with unfractionated heparin for acute pulmonary embolism. N Engl J Med 337:663, 1997.

104. Brill-Edwards P, Ginsberg JS, Johnston M, Hirsh J: Establishing a therapeutic range for heparin therapy. Ann Intern Med 119:104, 1993.

105. Cornelli U, Fareed J: Human pharmacokinetics of low-molecular-weight heparins. Semin Thromb Hemost 25(Suppl 3):57, 1999.

106. Agnelli G, Iorio A, Renga C, et al: Prolonged antithrombin activity of low-molecular-weight heparins. Clinical implications for the treatment of thromboembolic diseases. Circulation 92:2819, 1995.

107. Raschke RA, Reilly BR, Guidry JR, et al: The weight-based heparin dosing nomogram compared with a "standard care" nomogram. A randomized controlled trial. Ann Intern Med 119:874, 1993.

108. Cannon CP, Dingemanse J, Kleinbloesem CH, et al: Automated heparin-delivery system to control activated partial thromboplastin time. Evaluation in normal volunteers. Circulation 99:751, 1999.

109. Landefeld CS, Beyth RJ: Anticoagulant-related bleeding: Clinical epidemiology, prediction, and prevention. Am J Med 95:315, 1993.

110. Warkentin TE: Heparin-induced thrombocytopenia: A ten-year retrospective. Annu Rev Med 50:129, 1999.

111. Warkentin TE, Levine MN, Hirsh J, et al: Heparin-induced thrombocytopenia in patients treated with low-molecular-weight heparin or unfractionated heparin. N Engl J Med 332:1330, 1995.

112. Warkentin TE, Elavathil LJ, Hayward CPM, et al: The pathogenesis of venous limb gangrene associated with heparin induced thrombocytopenia. Ann Intern Med 127:804, 1997.

113. Magnani HN: Heparin induced thrombocytopenia (HIT): An overview of 230 patients treated with Orgaran (Org 10172). Thromb Haemost 70:554, 1993.

114. Greinacher A, Janssens U, Berg G, et al: Lepirudin (recombinant hirudin) for parenteral anticoagulation in patients with heparin-induced thrombocytopenia. Circulation 100:587, 1999.

115. Suzuki S, Sakamoto S, Koide M, et al: Effective anticoagulation by argatroban during coronary stent implantation in a patient with heparin-induced thrombocytopenia. Thromb Res 88:499, 1997.

115a. Lewis BE, Wallis DE, Matthai W, for the ARG-911 Study Investigators: Argatroban provides effective and safe anticoagulation in patients with heparin-induced thrombocytopenia: A prospective, historical controlled study. J Am Coll Cardiol 35:266A (abstract), 2000.

116. Douketis JD, Ginsberg JS, Burrows RF, et al: The effects of long-term heparin therapy during pregnancy on bone density. A prospective matched cohort study. Thromb Haemost 75:254, 1996.

117. Dahlman T, Lindvall N, Hellgren M: Osteopenia in pregnancy during long-term heparin treatment: A radiological study post partum. Br J Obstet Gynaecol 97:221, 1990.

118. Nelson-Piercy C, Letsky EA, de Swiet M: Low molecular weight heparin for obstetric thromboprophylaxis. Experience of 69 pregnancies in 61 women at high risk. Am J Obstet Gynecol 176:1062, 1997.

119. Wysowski DK, Talarico L, Bacsanyi J, et al: Spinal and epidural hematoma and low-molecular weight heparin. N Engl J Med 338:1774, 1998.

120. Dukes GE, Sanders SW, Russo J, et al: Transaminase elevations in patients receiving bovine or porcine heparin. Ann Intern Med 100:646, 1984.

121. Goldhaber SZ, Meyerovitz MF, Green D, et al: Randomized controlled trial of tissue plasminogen activator in proximal deep venous thrombosis. Am J Med 88:235, 1990.

122. Oster JR, Singer I, Fishman LM: Heparin-induced aldosterone suppression and hyperkalemia. Am J Med 98:575, 1995.

123. Brandjes DPM, Heijboer H, Büller HR, et al: Acenocoumarol and heparin compared with acenocoumarol alone in the initial treatment of proximal-vein thrombosis. N Engl J Med 327:1485, 1992.

124. Andrews TC, Peterson DW, Doeppenschmidt D, et al: Complications of warfarin therapy monitored by the international normalized ratio versus the prothrombin time ratio. Clin Cardiol 18:80, 1995.

125. Pearson SD, Lee TH, McCabe-Hassan S, et al: A critical pathway to treat proximal lower extremity deep vein thrombosis. Am J Med 100:283, 1996.

126. Schulman S, Rhedin A-S, Lindmarker P, et al: A comparison of 6 weeks with 6 months of oral anticoagulant therapy after a first episode of venous thromboembolism. N Engl J Med 332:1661, 1995.

127. Kearon C, Gent M, Hirsh J, et al: A comparison of three months of anticoagulation with extended anticoagulation for a first episode of idiopathic venous thromboembolism. N Engl J Med 340:901, 1999.

128. Ridker PM: Long term, low dose warfarin among venous thrombosis patients with and without factor V Leiden mutation: Rationale and design for the Prevention of Recurrent Venous Thromboembolism (PREVENT) trial. Vasc Med 3:67, 1998.

129. Harrison L, Johnston M, Massicotte MP, et al: Comparison of 5-mg and 10-mg loading doses in initiation of warfarin therapy. Ann Intern Med 126:133, 1997.

130. Shearer MJ: Vitamin K. Lancet 345:229, 1995.

131. Lagerstedt CI, Olsson C-G, Fagher BO, et al: Need for long-term anticoagulant treatment in symptomatic calf-vein thrombosis. Lancet 2:515, 1985.

132. Prandoni P, Polistena P, Bernardi E, et al: Upper-extremity deep vein thrombosis: Risk factors, diagnosis, and complications. Arch Intern Med 157:57, 1997.

133. Khamashta MA, Cuadrado MJ, Mujic F, et al: The management of thrombosis in the antiphospholipid antibody syndrome. N Engl J Med 332:993, 1995.

134. Hylek EM, Heiman H, Skates SJ, et al: Acetaminophen and other risk factors for excessive warfarin anticoagulation. JAMA 279:657, 1998.

134a. White RH, Beyth RJ, Zhon H, Romano PS: Major bleeding after hospitalization for deep-venous thrombosis. Am J Med 107:414, 1999.

135. Aithal GP, Day CP, Kesteven PJL, Daly AK: Association of polymorphisms in the cytochrome P450 CYP2C9 with warfarin dose requirement and risk of bleeding complications. Lancet 353:717, 1999.

136. Weintzien TH, O'Reilly RA, Kearns PJ: Prospective evaluation of anticoagulant reversal with oral vitamin K_1 while continuing warfarin therapy unchanged. Chest 114:1546, 1998.

137. Sallah S, Thomas DP, Roberts HR: Warfarin and heparin-induced skin necrosis and purple toe syndrome: Infrequent complications of anticoagulant treatment. Thromb Haemost 78:785, 1997.

138. Wellesley D, Moore I, Heard M, Keeton B: Two cases of warfarin embryopathy: A re-emergence of this condition? Br J Obstet Gynecol 105:805, 1998.

139. Toglia M, Weg JG: Venous thromboembolism during pregnancy. N Engl J Med 335:108, 1996.

140. Orme MLE, Lewis PJ, de Swiet M, et al: May mothers given warfarin breast-feed their infants? BMJ 1:1564, 1977.

141. Sawicki PT: A structured teaching and self-management program for patients receiving oral anticoagulation. JAMA 281:145, 1999.

142. Roth GJ, Calverley DC: Aspirin, platelets, and thrombosis: Theory and practice. Blood 83:885, 1994.

143. Antiplatelet Trialists' Collaboration: Collaborative overview of randomised trials of antiplatelet therapy—III: Reduction in venous thrombosis and pulmonary embolism by antiplatelet prophylaxis among surgical and medical patients. BMJ 308:235, 1994.

144. Decousus H, Leizorovicz A, Parent F, et al: A clinical trial of vena caval filters in the prevention of pulmonary embolism in patients with proximal deep-vein thrombosis. N Engl J Med 338:409, 1998.

145. Becker DM, Philbrick JT, Selby JB: Inferior vena cava filters: Indications, safety, effectiveness. Arch Intern Med 152:1985, 1992.

146. Arcasoy SM, Kreit JW: Thrombolytic therapy of pulmonary embolism. A comprehensive review of current evidence. Chest 115:1695, 1999.

147. Kanter DS, Mikkola KM, Patel SR, et al: Thrombolytic therapy for pulmonary embolism. Frequency of intracranial hemorrhage and associated risk factors. Chest 111:1241, 1997.

148. Goldhaber SZ, Haire WD, Feldstein ML, et al: Alteplase versus heparin in acute pulmonary embolism: Randomised trial assessing right-ventricular function and pulmonary perfusion. Lancet 341:507, 1993.

149. Daniels LB, Parker JA, Patel SR, et al: Relation of duration of symptoms with response to thrombolytic therapy in pulmonary embolism. Am J Cardiol 80:184, 1997.

150. Goldhaber SZ: Contemporary pulmonary embolism thrombolysis. Chest 107:45S, 1995.

151. Meneveau N, Schiele F, Metz D, et al: Comparative efficacy of a two-hour regimen of streptokinase versus alteplase in acute massive pulmonary embolism: Immediate clinical and hemodynamic outcome and one-year follow-up. J Am Coll Cardiol 31:1057, 1998.

152. Tebbe U, Graf A, Kamke W, et al: Hemodynamic effects of double bolus reteplase versus alteplase infusion in massive pulmonary embolism. Am Heart J 138:39, 1999.

153. Markel A, Manzo RA, Strandness DE Jr: The potential role of thrombolytic therapy in venous thrombosis. Arch Intern Med 152:1265, 1992.

154. Meyerovitz MF, Polak JF, Goldhaber SZ: Short-term response to thrombolytic therapy in deep venous thrombosis: Predictive value of venographic appearance. Radiology 184:345, 1992.

155. Comerota AJ, Aldridge SC, Cohen G, et al: A strategy of aggressive regional therapy for acute iliofemoral venous thrombosis with contemporary venous thrombectomy or catheter-directed thrombolysis. J Vasc Surg 20:244, 1994.

156. Marache P, Asseman P, Jabinet JL, et al: Percutaneous transluminal venous angioplasty in occlusive iliac vein thrombosis resistant to thrombolysis. Am Heart J 125:362, 1993.

156a. Brandjes DPM, Büller HR, Heijboer H, et al: Randomised trial of effect of compression stockings in patients with symptomatic proximal-vein thrombosis. Lancet 349:759, 1997.

156b. Brodmann M, Stark G, Pabst E, et al: Pulmonary embolism and intracardiac thrombi—individual therapeutic procedures. Vasc Med 5:27, 2000.

157. Greenfield LJ, Proctor MC, Williams DM, Wakefield TW: Long-term experience with transvenous catheter pulmonary embolectomy. J Vasc Surg 18:450, 1993.

158. Sharafuddin MJA, Hicks ME: Current status of percutaneous mechanical thrombectomy. Part II. Devices and mechanisms of action. J Vasc Interv Radiol 9:15, 1998.

159. Koning R, Cribier A, Gerber L, et al: A new treatment for severe pulmonary embolism. Percutaneous rheolytic thrombectomy. Circulation 96:2498, 1997.

160. Schmitz-Rode T, Janssens U, Schild HH, et al: Fragmentation of massive pulmonary embolism using a pigtail rotation catheter. Chest 114:1427, 1998.

161. Fava M, Loyola S, Flores P, Huete I: Mechanical fragmentation and pharmacologic thrombolysis in massive pulmonary embolism. J Vasc Interv Radiol 8:261, 1997.

162. Voorburg JAI, Cats VM, Buis B, Bruschke AVG: Balloon angioplasty in the treatment of pulmonary hypertension caused by pulmonary embolism. Chest 94:1249, 1988.

163. Ullmann M, Hemmer W, Hannekum A: The urgent pulmonary embolectomy: Mechanical resuscitation in the operating theatre determines the outcome. Thorac Cardiovasc Surg 47:5, 1999.

164. Gulba DC, Schmid C, Borst H-G: Medical compared with surgical treatment for massive pulmonary embolism. Lancet 343:565, 1994.

165. Meyer G, Tamisier D, Reynaud P, Sors H: Acute pulmonary embolectomy. In Goldhaber SZ (ed): Cardiopulmonary diseases and cardiac tumors. In Braunwald E (series ed): Atlas of Heart Diseases. Vol 3. Philadelphia, Current Medicine, 1995, p 6.1.

166. Konstantinides S, Tiede N, Geibel A, et al: Comparison of alteplase versus heparin for resolution of major pulmonary embolism. Am J Cardiol 82:966, 1998.

167. Ribeiro A, Lindmarker P, Johnsson H, et al: Pulmonary embolism: One year follow-up with echocardiography Doppler and five-year survival analysis. Circulation 99:1325, 1999.

168. Walrath K, Berkovitz P, Morrison R, Goldhaber SZ (eds): Frequently asked questions of the Pulmonary Embolism Support Group, Brigham and Women's Hospital: 30 September 1998. http://web.mit.edu/karen/www/faq.html

169. Fedullo PF, Auger WR, Channick RN, et al: A multidisciplinary approach to chronic thromboembolic pulmonary hypertension. In Braunwald E, Goldhaber SZ (eds): Atlas of Heart Diseases. Vol 3. Cardiopulmonary Diseases and Cardiac Tumors. Philadelphia, Current Medicine, 1995, p 7.1.

PREVENTION

170. Goldhaber SZ (ed): Prevention of Venous Thromboembolism. New York, Marcel Dekker, 1993, 607 pp.

171. Clagett GP, Anderson FA, Geerts W, et al: Prevention of venous thromboembolism. Chest 114:531S, 1998.

172. Prevention of venous thromboembolism. International Consensus Statement (guidelines according to scientific evidence). Int Angiol 16:3, 1997.

173. Goldhaber SZ: Malpractice claims relation to PE and DVT. Forum. Cambridge, MA. Risk Management Foundation of the Harvard Medical Institutions, Inc., 1994.

174. Landefeld CS, Hanus P: Economic burden of venous thromboembolism. In Goldhaber SZ (ed): Prevention of Venous Thromboembolism. New York, Marcel Dekker, 1993, p 69.

175. Wells PS, Lensing AWA, Hirsh J: Graduated compression stockings in

the prevention of postoperative venous thromboembolism. Arch Intern Med 154:67, 1994.

176. Comerota AJ, Chouhan V, Harada RN, et al: The fibrinolytic effects of intermittent pneumatic compression. Mechanism of enhanced fibrinolysis. Ann Surg 226:306, 1997.

177. Comerota AJ, Katz ML, White JV: Why does prophylaxis with external pneumatic compression for deep vein thrombosis fail? Am J Surg 164:265, 1992.

178. Collins R, Scrimgeour A, Yusuf S, Peto R: Reduction in fatal pulmonary embolism and venous thrombosis by perioperative administration of subcutaneous heparin: Overview of results of randomized trials in general, orthopedic, and urologic surgery. N Engl J Med 318:1162, 1988.

178a. di Carlo V, Agnelli G, Prandoni P, et al, for the "DOS" (Dermatan sulphate in Oncologic Surgery) Study Group: Dermatan sulphate for the prevention of postoperative venous thromboembolism in patients with cancer. Thromb Haemost 82:30, 1999.

179. Gent M, Hirsh J, Ginsberg JS, et al: Low-molecular-weight heparinoid Orgaran is more effective than aspirin in the prevention of venous thromboembolism after surgery for hip fracture. Circulation 93:80, 1996.

180. Magnani HN: Heparin-induced thrombocytopenia (HIT): An overview of 230 patients treated with Orgaran (ORG 10172). Thromb Haemost 70:554, 1993.

181. Colwell CW, Collis DK, Paulson R, et al: Comparison of enoxaparin and warfarin for the prevention of venous thromboembolic disease after total hip arthroplasty. Evaluation during hospitalization and three months after discharge. J Bone Joint Surg 81-A:932, 1999.

182. Eriksson BI, Wille-Jørgensen P, Kälebo P, et al: A comparison of recombinant hirudin with a low-molecular-weight heparin to prevent thromboembolic complications after total hip replacement. N Engl J Med 337:1329, 1997.

183. Pulmonary Embolism Prevention (PEP) Trial Collaborative Group: Prevention of pulmonary embolism and deep vein thrombosis with low dose aspirin: Pulmonary embolism prevention (PEP) trial. Lancet 355:1295, 2000.

184. Blanchard J, Meuwly J-Y, Leyvraz P-F, et al: Prevention of deep-vein thrombosis after total knee replacement. Randomized comparison between a low molecular-weight heparin (Nadroparin) and mechanical prophylaxis with a foot pump system. J Bone Joint Surg Br 81:654, 1999.

185. Demers C, Marcoux S, Ginsberg JS, et al: Incidence of venographically proved deep vein thrombosis after knee arthroscopy. Arch Intern Med 158:47, 1998.

186. White RH, Romano PS, Zhou H, et al: Incidence and time course of thromboembolic outcomes following total hip or knee arthroplasty. Arch Intern Med 158:1525, 1998.

187. Ramos R, Salem BI, De Pawlikowski MP, et al: The efficacy of pneumatic compression stockings in the prevention of pulmonary embolism after cardiac surgery. Chest 109:82, 1996.

188. Samama MM, Cohen AT, Darmon J-Y, et al: A comparison of enoxaparin with placebo for the prevention of venous thromboembolism in acutely ill medical patients. N Engl J Med 341:793, 1999.

Chapter 53

Pulmonary Hypertension

STUART RICH

▼ Normal Pulmonary Circulation

During the passage of red blood cells through the lungs, hemoglobin is normally oxygenated to nearly full capacity and the blood is cleansed of much particulate matter and bacteria. The lungs, in addition to functioning as a blood oxygenator and filter, play a dominant role in achieving acid-base balance by excreting carbon dioxide, thereby helping maintain optimal blood pH.[1]

PULMONARY BLOOD FLOW, PRESSURE, AND RESISTANCE

PULMONARY CIRCULATION IN THE NORMAL ADULT. The lung has a unique double arterial blood supply from the pulmonary and bronchial arteries, as well as double venous drainage into the pulmonary and azygos veins.[2] The right and left pulmonary arteries carry the entire output of the right ventricle and follow a course adjacent to the airways. Inside the lung each pulmonary artery accompanies the appropriate-generation bronchus and divides with it down to the level of the respiratory bronchiole. Additional supernumerary branches originate without relation to bronchial divisions and directly penetrate into the lung parenchyma. The diameter of the arteries decreases more rapidly than that of the airways they accompany, so in the lung periphery the diameters of the arteries are smaller than those of the adjacent airways. Within the respiratory units the pulmonary arteries and arterioles are centrally located and give rise to precapillary arterioles from which a network of capillaries radiate into the alveolar walls. The alveolar capillaries collect at the periphery of the acini and then drain into venules located within the interlobular and interlobar septa.

The pulmonary arteries are classified as elastic or muscular based on the structure of the tunica media. The elastic arteries are conducting vessels, highly distensible at low transmural pressure. As the arteries decrease in size, the number of elastic laminae decreases and smooth muscle increases. Eventually, in vessels between 1000 and 500 μm, elastic tissue is lost from the media and the arteries become muscular. The intima of the pulmonary arteries consists of a single layer of endothelial cells and their basement membrane. The adventitia is composed of dense connective tissue in direct continuity with the peribronchial connective tissue sheath. The muscular arteries are 500 μm in diameter or less and are characterized by a muscular media bounded by internal and external elastic laminae. In normal adults,

the lumen is wide and the media is thin and represents less than 10 percent of the arterial cross-sectional area. Arterioles are precapillary arteries smaller than 100 μm in outer diameter and composed solely of a thin intima and single elastic lamina. The alveolar capillaries are lined with a continuous layer of endothelium resting on a continuous basement membrane and focally connected to scattered pericytes located beneath the basement membrane.

The bronchial arteries ramify into a capillary network drained by bronchial veins, some of which empty into the pulmonary veins, whereas the remainder empty into the systemic venous bed. The bronchial circulation therefore constitutes a physiological "right-to-left" shunt. The function of the bronchial circulation is to provide nutrition to the airways. Normally, blood flow through this system is quite low and amounts to approximately 1 percent of the cardiac output[3]; the resulting desaturation of left atrial blood is usually trivial. However, in some forms of pulmonary disease, e.g., severe bronchiectasis, and in the presence of many congenital cardiovascular malformations that cause cyanosis, blood flow through the bronchial circulation can increase significantly, account for nearly 30 percent of left ventricular output,[4] and produce a significant right-to-left shunt. In pulmonary disease, significant right-to-left shunting through the bronchial circulation may also result in arterial desaturation. In cyanotic congenital heart disease, bronchial blood is not fully oxygenated; it may participate in gas exchange and improve systemic oxygenation.

Normal pulmonary artery pressure in a person living at sea level has a peak systolic value of 18 to 25 mm Hg, an end-diastolic value of 6 to 10 mm Hg, and a mean value ranging from 12 to 16 mm Hg* (see Chap. 11). Definite pulmonary hypertension is present when pulmonary artery systolic and mean pressures exceed 30 and 20 mm Hg, respectively. Normal mean pulmonary venous pressure is 6 to 10 mm Hg; therefore, the normal arteriovenous pressure difference, which moves the entire cardiac output across the pulmonary vascular bed, ranges from 2 to 10 mm Hg. This small pressure gradient is all the more remarkable when one considers that to move the same amount of blood per minute through the systemic vascular bed, a pressure

---

*All pressures discussed here are in reference to atmospheric pressure at the level of the heart. True transmural pressures are more physiologically meaningful, especially when pulmonary parenchymal disease is present, but are rarely measured.

differential of approximately 90 mm Hg (systemic arterial mean pressure minus right atrial mean pressure) is required.

Pulmonary Vascular Resistance. Thus, the normal pulmonary vascular bed offers less than one-tenth the *resistance* to flow offered by the systemic bed. *Vascular resistance* is generally quantified, by analogy to Ohm's law, as the ratio of pressure drop (ΔP in millimeters Hg) to mean flow (Q in liters per minute). The ratio is commonly multiplied by 79.9 (or 80 for simplification) to express the results in dynes-seconds $\cdot$ centimeters^{-5}. This conversion to metric units may be avoided, i.e., resistance may be expressed in millimeters Hg per liter per minute, which is sometimes referred to as hybrid units, PRU (peripheral resistance units), or Wood units (after the English cardiologist Paul Wood). The calculated pulmonary vascular resistance in normal adults[5] is 67 ± 23 (SD) dyne sec $\cdot$ cm^{-5}, or 1 Wood unit.

Vascular resistance reflects a composite of variables that includes, but is not limited to, the cross-sectional area of small muscular arteries and arterioles. Other determinants are blood viscosity, the total mass of lung tissue (i.e., resistance is higher in infants and children than in adults), proximal vascular obstruction (e.g., pulmonary coarctation, pulmonary embolism, peripheral pulmonic stenosis), and extramural compression of vessels (perivascular edema).

The reduction in resistance in a distensible vascular bed that occurs with increased flow has been offered as the explanation for the absence of pulmonary hypertension in many patients with large left-to-right intracardiac shunts, particularly atrial septal defects.

REGIONAL PERFUSION. A large degree of heterogeneity in regional pulmonary perfusion is characteristic of the pulmonary circulation and can be explained by a fractal branching network.[6] The pulmonary vascular tree can be conceptualized as having a fixed structure that is the primary determinant of overall perfusion and a variable component that can be influenced by passive and active regional factors such as recruitment and/or distention from changing driving or hydrostatic pressures. Active factors such as vasomotion and response to shear stress or hypoxic vasoconstriction influence regional perfusion, which is constantly changing.

PULMONARY CIRCULATION WITH EXERCISE. With moderate exercise, a large increase in pulmonary blood flow is normally accompanied by only a small increase in pulmonary artery pressure. It is important to note that exercise results in an increase in left atrial pressure that is progressive with exercise intensity and accounts for the majority of the increase in pulmonary arterial pressure that is observed.[7] This marked effect of downstream pressure on upstream pressure is unique to the lung circulation inasmuch as systemic arterial pressure during exercise is largely independent of right atrial pressure. Because of the high vascular compliance in the normal lung microcirculation, an increase in left atrial pressure that results from the increased flow will act to distend the small vessels, thereby accounting for the dramatic fall in pulmonary vascular resistance during exercise. Microcirculatory distention increases the surface area for diffusion and slows passage of red cells through the lung, which facilitates oxygen transfer.

FETAL AND NEONATAL CIRCULATION (see also Chap. 43). In the fetus, oxygenated blood enters the heart from the inferior vena cava and streams across the foramen ovale to the left atrium, left ventricle, ascending aorta, and cranial vessels. Desaturated blood returns from the superior vena cava and passes through the tricuspid valve into the right ventricle and pulmonary artery. Because the resistance of the pulmonary vascular bed in the collapsed fetal lung is extremely high, only 10 to 30 percent of the total right ventricular output passes through the lungs, the remainder being shunted across the ductus arteriosus to the descending aorta and then back to the placenta. An abrupt change in the pulmonary circulation occurs at birth. With the first breath, expansion of the lungs and the abrupt rise in PO_2 of blood lead to a release of pulmonary arteriolar vasoconstriction and stretching and dilatation of muscular pulmonary arteries and arterioles, with a marked drop in vascular resistance.[8] This decreased resistance facilitates a large increase in pulmonary blood flow and raises left atrial volume and pressure. The latter closes the flap valve of the foramen ovale, and interatrial right-to-left shunting ordinarily ceases within the first hour of life. Normally, the ductus arteriosus closes over the next 10 hours as a result of contraction of the thick smooth muscle bundles within its wall in response to rising arterial oxygen tension and a change in the prostaglandin milieu. Following the initial dramatic fall in pulmonary vascular resistance at birth, a continuous decline occurs over the first few months of life that is associated with thinning of the media of muscular pulmonary arteries and arterioles until the normal adult pattern is achieved[9] (Fig. 53–1).

AGING AND THE PULMONARY CIRCULATION. Pulmonary artery pressure and pulmonary vascular resistance increase with advanced age, similar to increases that occur in systemic vascular resistance.[10-12] Reduced compliance of the pulmonary vascular bed secondary to intimal fibrosis or increased wall thickness in the muscular pulmonary arteries is a possible cause. It is also possible that some of the changes in the pulmonary arteries relate to reduced compliance of left ventricular filling that is passively reflected back on the pulmonary vascular bed.[11] The prevalence of mild pulmonary hypertension (mean pulmonary artery pressure $\geq$20 mm Hg) may be as high as 13 percent in persons up to 45 years old and 28 percent in those up to 75 years old.[13]

RESPONSE TO HYPOXIA, DRUGS, AND NEURAL AND ENVIRONMENTAL FACTORS

HYPOXIA. Acute *hypoxia* elicits pulmonary vasoconstriction[14] as a self-regulatory mechanism for adjusting capillary perfusion to alveolar ventilation. Hypoxia in humans (PO_2 $\leq$55 mm Hg) is associated with rapid onset of vasoconstriction.[15] Potassium, calcium, and probably chloride channels play important roles in determining pulmonary vascular tone.[16] Ionic control over membrane potential and cytosolic calcium regulates the degree of vasoconstriction and influences proliferation of smooth muscle cells. It seems likely that hypoxia inhibits outward potassium currents, thereby resulting in depolarization of the pulmonary vascular smooth muscle cell membrane, which allows calcium entry into voltage-dependent calcium channels, followed by contraction. Hypoxic pulmonary vasoconstriction is widely variable among healthy people. It also varies markedly with the age of an individual and among different mammalian species. (For further discussion, see Chapter 54.)

NEURAL REGULATION. The media and adventitia of the large elastic pulmonary arteries and the large pulmonary veins are supplied by nerve fibers that influence the distensibility of these capacitance vessels.[3] Although *neural regulation* of pulmonary vascular resistance can be demonstrated[17] and may be particularly important in fetal life, its importance in a normal human adult is less certain.

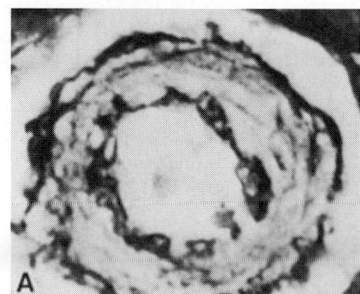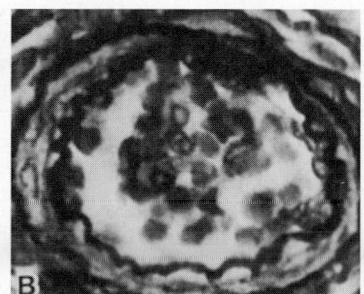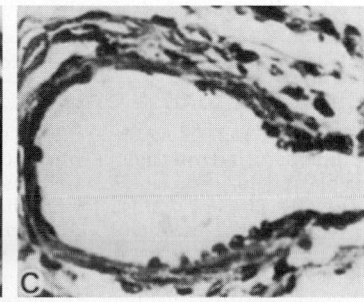

FIGURE 53–1. Changes in pulmonary arteries after birth. Comparison of relative medial thicknesses at birth (*A*), at 2 months of age (*B*), and at 7 months of age (*C*). Elastic–van Gieson stain; magnification $\times$360; reduced 17 percent. (From Petersen RC, Edwards WD: Pulmonary vascular disease in 57 necropsy cases of total anomalous pulmonary venous connections. Histopathology 7:47, 1983.)

ADRENERGIC RECEPTORS. The pulmonary vasculature expresses both alpha and beta adrenoreceptors, both of which help regulate pulmonary vascular tone by producing vasoconstriction or vasodilatation, respectively.[18] Alpha$_1$ adrenoreceptors in the pulmonary arteries have increased affinity and responsiveness to their agonists when compared with other vessels.[19] The downstream signaling events in alpha$_1$-adrenergic stimulation are an increase in ionic calcium levels and activation of protein kinase, which mediate vascular contractile and proliferative responses. The increased sensitivity of alpha$_1$ adrenoreceptors to norepinephrine in the pulmonary arteries may greatly facilitate local regulation of vascular tone in response to acute changes in oxygen concentrations, thereby adjusting regional perfusion. Stimulation of alpha$_1$ adrenoreceptors increases intracellular free calcium levels by at least two mechanisms: (1) coupling to specific G proteins on the cell membrane and (2) blockade of potassium ion channels.[20, 21] Excessive stimulation of alpha$_1$-adrenergic receptors produces smooth muscle contraction, proliferation, and growth. Factors that produce an increase in alpha$_1$ adrenoreceptor gene synthesis, density, and activity greatly enhance pulmonary artery smooth muscle contractile and proliferative responses. Such factors include norepinephrine, appetite suppressants, and cocaine.[22, 23] It also is plausible that an estrogen-induced increase in the number and affinity of vascular alpha$_1$ adrenoreceptors in women is the explanation for the female preponderance noted in conditions associated with pulmonary hypertension[24] (Fig. 53–2).

DRUGS. The alpha-adrenergic blocking agent phentolamine, as well as tolazoline (Priscoline), which also exhibits alpha-adrenergic blocking action, can lower pulmonary vascular resistance. *Beta-adrenergic stimulation* with isoproterenol has been repeatedly shown to cause pulmonary *vasodilatation*. In contrast, beta-adrenergic blockade does not produce any change in pulmonary vascular resistance, which suggests that tonic activation of beta receptors is not necessary for maintenance of the normal low pulmonary vascular resistance. *Acetylcholine* is also a potent relaxant of pulmonary arteries and arterioles and transiently lowers pulmonary vascular resistance in patients with elevated pulmonary vascular resistance with a major reversible component.

PROSTAGLANDINS. Lung tissue is particularly active in the synthesis, metabolism, and release of a number of *prostaglandins*, some of which may play a role in the regulation of pulmonary vascular resistance. Prostaglandins I$_2$ (PGI$_2$) and E (PGE$_2$) are active pulmonary vasodilators, whereas PGF$_2$ alpha and PGA$_2$ are pulmonary vasoconstrictors.[25] Counterregulatory actions have been ascribed to prostacyclin (PGI$_2$) and thromboxane within the pulmonary circulation. Pulmonary endothelial cells have an abundance of prostacyclin synthase, whereas platelets are replete with thromboxane synthase.[26, 27] Both convert the cyclic endoperoxide precursors PGG$_2$ and PGH$_2$ into specific bioactive eicosanoids. Prostacyclin is a powerful vasodilator that also inhibits platelet aggregation through activation of adenylate cyclase. Its metabolic half-life in the bloodstream is less than one circulation time, with its metabolite 6-keto-prostaglandin F$_1$ alpha having little biological activity.[28]

A variety of drugs with diverse mechanisms of action are reported to encourage prostacyclin production and include calcium channel blockers, angiotensin-converting enzyme (ACE) inhibitors, diuretics, and nitrates.[26] Physiologically, prostacyclin is a local hormone rather than a circulating one. Release of prostacyclin by endothelial cells causes relaxation of the underlying vascular smooth muscle and prevents platelet aggregation within the bloodstream. Thromboxane is synthesized in platelets and macrophages.[27] It also has a short half-life. Thromboxane is a potent agonist for platelet aggregation and vasoconstriction, and it may function as a growth factor for smooth muscles by acting via protein kinase C–linked pathways.[29] Because the biological actions of prostacyclin are the opposite those of throm-

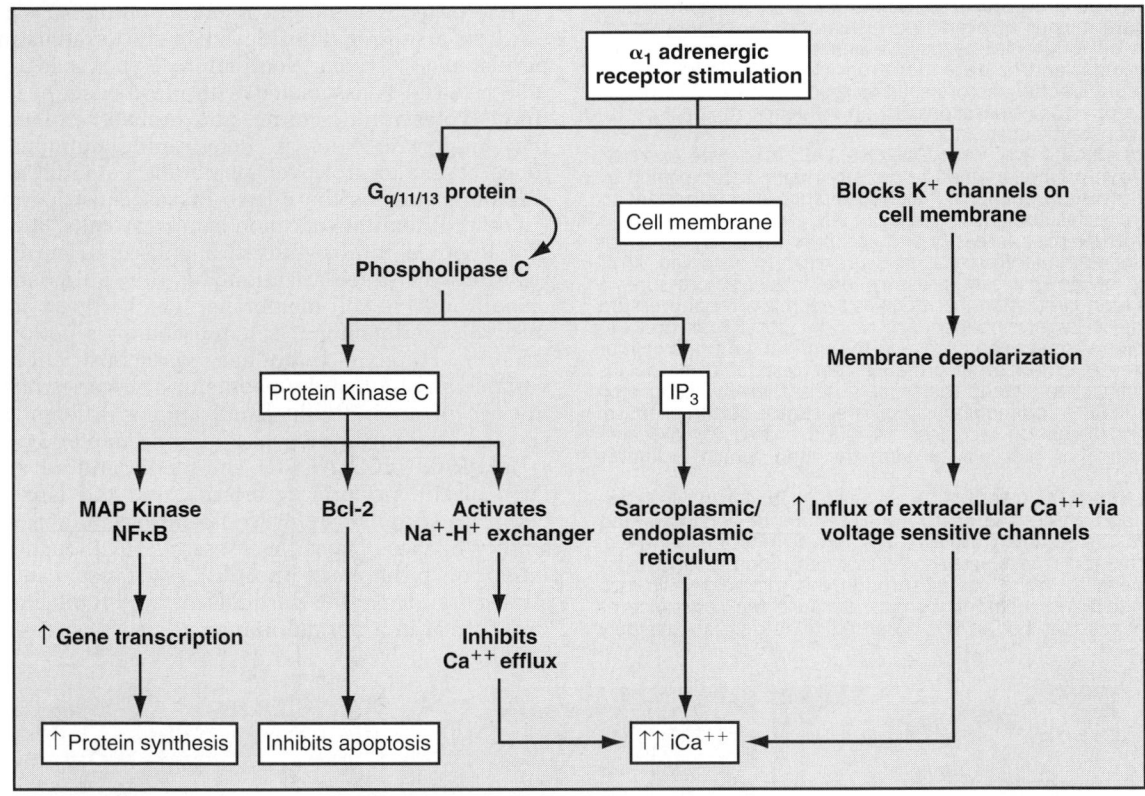

FIGURE 53–2. Signaling pathways of alpha$_1$-adrenergic receptors in smooth muscle cells that lead to pulmonary hypertension. Alpha$_1$-adrenergic receptors activate phospholipase C to produce inositol 1,4,5-triphosphate (IP$_3$), which mobilizes calcium from intracellular stores. Activation of protein kinase C also activates transcription factors such as mitogen-activated protein kinase (MAP kinase) and nuclear factor kappa-B (NFκB), which induce DNA synthesis and cell proliferation. By increasing levels of oncoprotein (Bcl-2) to inhibit apoptosis, the survival of vascular smooth muscle cells is promoted. Alpha$_1$-adrenergic receptors also couple to K$^+$ channels, which leads to entry of calcium from extracellular sources through voltage-sensitive channels. An increase in intracellular calcium is the major signal transduction mechanism responsible for producing smooth muscle contraction via the calcium calmodulin pathway, and protein kinase C activation is the major signal transduction pathway involved in the proliferation of pulmonary vascular smooth muscle cells. (From Salvi SS: α-1 Adrenergic hypothesis for pulmonary hypertension. Chest 115:1708–1719, 1999.)

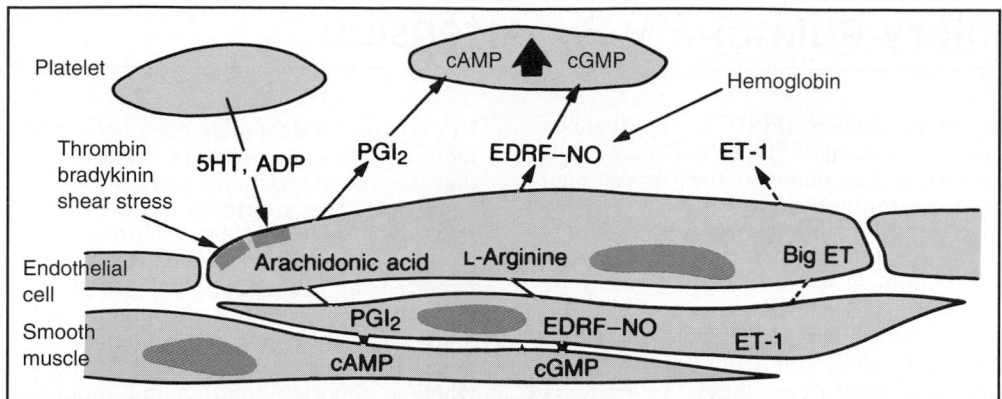

FIGURE 53–3. Generation of prostacyclin (PGI₂), endothelial-derived relaxing factor–nitric oxide (EDRF-NO), and endothelin-1 (ET-1) in endothelial cells. Stimulation of receptors on the cells by serotonin (5HT [5-hydroxytryptomine]) or adenosine diphosphate (ADP) released from platelets or by thrombin, bradykinin, or shear stress leads to the release of vasoactive mediators. PGI₂ relaxes vascular smooth muscle and inhibits aggregation of platelets by increasing levels of cyclic adenosine monophosphate (cAMP). EDRF-NO relaxes vascular smooth muscle and inhibits platelet aggregation and adhesion by increasing levels of cyclic guanosine monophosphate (cGMP). The simultaneous increase in cAMP and cGMP inhibits platelet aggregation. (From Vane JR, Anggard EE, Bolting RM: Regulatory functions of the vascular endothelium. N Engl J Med 323:27, 1990. Copyright © 1990 Massachusetts Medical Society. All rights reserved.)

boxane, the balance between these two peptides appears to control the local environment within the vascular bed.

NITRIC OXIDE. The biological action of nitric oxide (NO) is quite similar to that of prostacyclin in that it relaxes vascular smooth muscle. It differs, however, in that its effects are mediated by changing levels of cyclic guanosine monophosphate (GMP).[30] Endothelial NO synthase is found in the vascular endothelium of the normal pulmonary vasculature, where it is responsible for generating NO to govern vascular tone. Release of NO occurs in response to a multitude of physiological stimuli, which include thrombin, bradykinin, and shear stress.[31] Besides its direct hemodynamic effects, NO inhibits platelet activation and confers an important antithrombotic property on the endothelial surface. NO also inhibits the growth of vascular smooth muscle cells and is probably involved in vascular remodeling in response to injury.[30] NO is also important in the signal transduction of angiogenesis inasmuch as vascular endothelial growth factor receptor activation results in increased NO production[32] (Fig. 53–3).

OTHER VASOACTIVE SUBSTANCES. *Endothelin* is a potent vasoconstrictor peptide that also plays an important role in the regulation of pulmonary vascular tone. Because of its long half-life, subtle disturbances in production or release can lead to sustained vasoconstriction.[33] Several studies have demonstrated an interaction between NO

and endothelin-1 (ET-1) in the vascular endothelium.[34] Expression of endothelin is inversely related to that of NO synthase, thus suggesting an opposite regulatory pathway for these two factors. Two types of ET-1 receptor are known: ETA is expressed mainly on smooth muscle cells and ETB is expressed on endothelial cells.[34] The former mediates vasoconstriction, while the latter mediates vasorelaxation through release of nitric oxide (Fig. 53–4).

Serotonin is an important constituent of platelet dense granules and is released upon activation.[35] Normal endothelial cells respond to serotonin by enhancing the release of NO, thereby leading to vascular smooth muscle relaxation and vasodilatation. In the setting of endothelial dysfunction, serotonin is unable to stimulate NO release and increases vascular smooth muscle tone, thereby leading to vasoconstriction.[36] In addition, serotonin can act as a growth factor and contribute to medial hypertrophy and promote vascular remodeling.[37]

Angiotensin II is generated in the lung by means of enzymatic conversion of angiotensin I, a potent pulmonary vasoconstrictor. Angiotensin II stimulates cell proliferation, extracellular matrix proteins synthesis, and smooth muscle cell migration. Elevated plasma renin and angiotensin II levels have been found during acute hypoxia and hypercapnia in CO₂-retaining patients with chronic obstructive lung disease.[38]

FIGURE 53–4. Regulation of the effects of endothelin (ET). ET may be active in the final stage of transduction of a number of pulmonary smooth muscle contractile and mitogenic factors. Nitric oxide (NO) and prostacyclin (PGI₂), together with atrial natriuretic peptide (ANP), inhibit expression of ET-1. ETA receptors are involved in contraction and in mitogenic effects on smooth muscle cells and fibroblasts. The small resistance arteries in humans appear to have contraction-inducing ETB receptors as well. TGF-β–transforming growth factor-beta. (From Higgenbottam TW, Laude EA: Endothelial dysfunction providing the basis for the treatment of pulmonary hypertension. Chest 114(Suppl):72–79, 1998.)

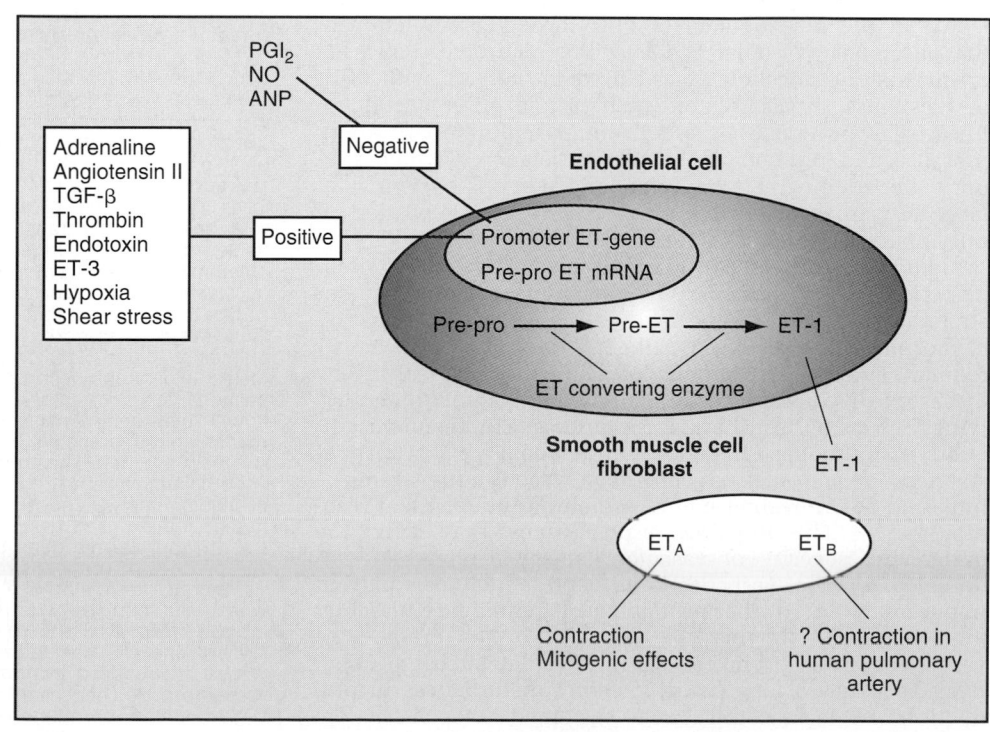

▼ Primary Pulmonary Hypertension

Primary pulmonary hypertension (PPH) is the diagnosis given to patients with pulmonary hypertension of unexplained etiology. Although the name of the disease stems from its distinction from pulmonary hypertension secondary to known cardiac or pulmonary causes, PPH should not be considered as only pulmonary hypertension for which no cause is found. The clinical features, usual age of onset, progression of the disease, and autopsy findings make PPH a distinct clinical entity and distinguish it from many forms of secondary pulmonary hypertension even though its diagnosis requires careful exclusion of secondary causes.[39] The actual incidence of PPH appears to be approximately two cases per million population, thus qualifying it as an orphan disease.[40, 40a]

ETIOLOGY

The precise cause of PPH is unknown, but it probably represents the clinical expression of pulmonary arterial hypertension as the final common pathway from multiple biological abnormalities within the pulmonary circulation. As understanding of vascular biology is improving, many studies point to abnormalities in pulmonary endothelial cell function as causing or contributing to the development of pulmonary hypertension in humans.[41] It is now understood that the endothelial cell regulates pulmonary smooth muscle cell tone.[26] It should be pointed out that even though endothelial cells may appear normal histologically, they may be quite abnormal with respect to function. Dysfunction of the counterregulatory systems within the pulmonary vascular bed seems to be common in pulmonary hypertension. The normal pulmonary vascular endothelial cell maintains the vascular smooth muscle in a state of relaxation.[26] The finding of increased pulmonary vascular reactivity and vasoconstriction in patients with PPH suggests that a marked vasoconstrictive tendency underlies the development of PPH in predisposed individuals,[42] possibly as a result of loss of endothelial cell integrity.[41] The autonomic nervous system has been considered a contributory factor in the development of PPH through stimulation of the pulmonary vascular bed by either neuronally released or circulating catecholamines. In some patients with PPH, the response to vasodilators such as tolazoline, acetylcholine, or isoproterenol is a reduction in pulmonary artery pressure and pulmonary vascular resistance,[43] which supports the notion that the autonomic nervous system is at least in part maintaining a role in constant elevation of pulmonary vascular resistance.

Reduced expression of NO synthase in the endothelium of patients with pulmonary hypertension has been demonstrated and correlates inversely with the extent and severity of morphological lesions.[45] Although it is unsettled whether reduced NO synthase production is a cause or result of the disease, it is consistent with endothelial dysfunction underlying PPH as part of the disease process. Studies of vasodilators in pulmonary hypertension demonstrate that responsiveness to endothelium-dependent vasodilating agents is impaired before response to endothelium-independent vasodilators.[44, 46] This impaired responsiveness may reflect the underlying severity of vascular damage. Conversely, endothelin, a potent vasoconstrictor peptide, may also play an important role in the regulation of pulmonary vascular tone.[34] Its secretion may be enhanced in the presence of vasoconstriction or in the setting of platelet aggregation. Because it has a long half-life, subtle disturbances in production or release could lead to sustained vasoconstriction.

ET_A receptor antagonists have been reported to reduce pulmonary artery pressure in experimental animals.[47] Given that the major resistance vessels in the pulmonary vascular bed are at the arteriolar level, diffuse arteriolar vasoconstriction could easily cause chronically sustained elevations in pulmonary vascular resistance and result in pulmonary hypertension. Elevations in endothelin levels within the pulmonary vasculature of patients with primary and secondary forms of pulmonary hypertension have been documented.[48] This finding would suggest that regardless of whether abnormal endothelial function is the underlying cause of PPH, progression of the disease is invariably accompanied by worsening of endothelial function, which itself can promote disease progression.

A striking feature of the pulmonary vasculature in patients with PPH is intimal proliferation, and in some vessels it causes virtually complete vascular occlusion[49, 50] (Fig. 53–5). Several growth factors have been implicated in the development of this type of vascular pathology, including basic fibroblast growth factor from the endothelium[51] and platelet-derived growth factor[52] and transforming growth factor-beta[53] from platelets. Enhanced growth factor release, activation, and intracellular signaling may lead to smooth muscle cell proliferation and migration, as well as extracellular matrix synthesis. Even advanced lesions show evidence of in situ activity of ongoing synthesis of connective tissue proteins such as elastin, collagen, and fibronectin.[54, 55]

An equally important etiologic feature of PPH is the widespread development of in situ thrombosis of the small pulmonary arteries with resultant vascular obstruction.[49, 50, 56, 57, 57a] Although it was once believed that recurrent, systemic venous microembolism could be an underlying mechanism in PPH, this theory has been essentially rejected for lack of both animal and human data to support it as a clinical entity. Animal studies suggest that more than 22 million thromboemboli in the pulmonary arterioles would be required to raise the mean pulmonary artery pressure 5 mm Hg, yet no source of these emboli has ever been found in patients dying of PPH.[56] Various defects in coagulation; including abnormal platelet function and defective fibrinolysis, have been demonstrated in patients with PPH.[57, 58] In situ thrombosis of the pulmonary vascular bed has been proposed as a causative or contributing feature of pulmonary hypertension.[56, 59] Abnormalities in platelet activation and function and biochemical features of a procoagulant environment within the pulmonary vasculature support a role of thrombosis in disease initiation in some patients.[57, 58, 60, 61] Interactions between growth factors, platelets, and the vessel wall suggest that thrombosis may play a fundamental role in many of the pathobiological processes described in PPH and in disease progression.[62] A prothrombotic state can arise as a consequence of fibrinolysis, enhanced coagulation, or increased platelet activation. Platelet activation not only promotes thrombosis but also leads to the release of granules that contain mitogenic agents and vasoconstrictive substances.[63]

Several studies suggest that local hemodynamics can influence pulmonary vascular remodeling.[64] A classic example is the pulmonary hypertension that occurs in congenital systemic-to-pulmonary shunts. It is believed that endothelial cells can release mediators that induce vascular smooth muscle cell growth in response to changes in pulmonary blood flow or pressure. Experimental data suggest that medial hypertrophy can be converted to a neointimal pattern when pulmonary vascular injury is coupled with increased pulmonary blood flow.[65] These neointimal lesions are composed of smooth muscle cells that are immunoreactive to anti–alpha smooth muscle actin antibody. It is now accepted that hemodynamic shear stress acts through the endothelium to regulate vessel tone and in the chronic restructuring of blood vessels.[64] Endothelial denudation also results in platelet adherence to exposed tissue collagen, with release of platelet-derived smooth muscle mitogens that also have vasoconstrictor properties. This process in turn leads to an inflammatory response and thrombosis, thereby narrowing the lumen of pulmonary vessels. In a person who is susceptible—whether on a genetic or an acquired basis—intense vasoconstriction may lead to fibrinoid necrosis of the arteriolar wall and the development of plexiform lesions. Ultimately, the vessels are reduced in number, and the residua of these destroyed vessels can be seen histologically as "ghost vessels." Destruction of large numbers of pulmonary arterioles reduces the cross-sectional

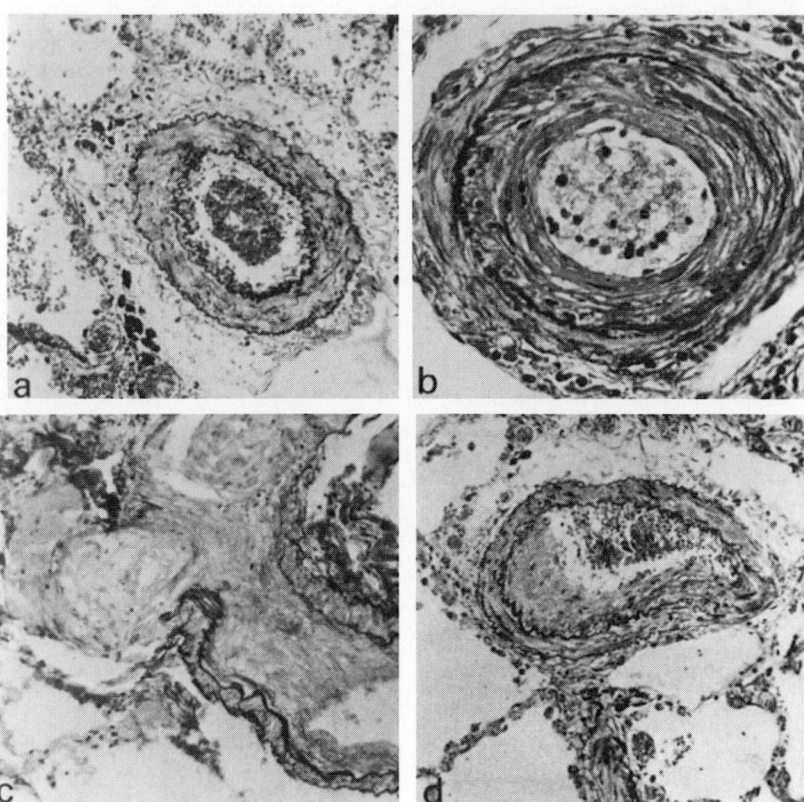

FIGURE 53–5. Photomicrographs of pulmonary arterial histological lesions seen in clinically unexplained pulmonary hypertension. All slides were stained with Verhoeff–van Gieson stain. *A*, Medial hypertrophy (×100). *B*, Concentric laminal intimal fibrosis—seen most often in association with plexiform lesions (×200). *C*, Plexiform lesion demonstrating obstruction in the arterial lumen, aneurysmal dilatation, and proliferation of anastomosing vascular channels (×200). *D*, Eccentric intimal fibrosis—often seen in association with organized microthrombi but also present in many patients with plexiform lesions (×100). (From Palevsky HI, Schloo BL, Pietria CC, et al: Primary pulmonary hypertension. Vascular structure, morphometry and responsiveness to vasodilator agents. Circulation 80: 1207, 1989.)

area of the pulmonary vascular bed, thereby producing a permanent increase in pulmonary vascular resistance and fixed pulmonary hypertension. The latter in turn damages other blood vessels and initiates a vicious circle, with progressively rising pulmonary arterial pressure (Fig. 53–6).

Vascular remodeling is becoming recognized as an important component in the pathogenesis of pulmonary hypertension.[64] An essential role of ACE in the pathogenesis of pulmonary hypertension is strongly suggested by the presence of increased ACE immunoreactivity at sites of increased matrix gene expression in human hypertensive pulmonary arteries.[66] Further supporting a role for ACE in pulmonary vascular remodeling are observations that ACE protein and mRNA expression are focally increased in rat pulmonary arteries with medial hypertrophy from chronic hypoxia.[67]

Increased activity of elastolytic enzymes appears to be important in the pathophysiology of pulmonary vascular disease.[68] High elastin turnover and neosynthesis of elastin have been attributed to degradation of elastin from the increased activity of serine elastase. A cause-and-effect relationship between elastase and pulmonary vascular disease was demonstrated when elastase inhibitors were shown to be effective in attenuating the development and retarding the progression of pulmonary hypertension in monocrotaline-injected and hypoxic rats.[69] Progression of pulmonary hypertension may involve a series of switches in smooth muscle cell phenotype and proliferation to account for the medial hypertrophy and smooth muscle cell migration resulting in neointimal formation. Structural and functional alterations in the endothelial cell could result in loss of barrier function and allow leakage into the subendothelium of a serum factor normally excluded from this region. Enzymes released from precursor or mature smooth muscle cells could activate growth factors normally stored in the extracellular matrix, such as basic fibroblast growth factor and transforming growth factor-beta, which are known to induce smooth muscle cell hypertrophy and proliferation and increase connective tissue protein synthesis. In muscular arteries, release of growth factors would result in hypertrophy of the vessel wall[69] (Fig. 53–7).

Potassium channels are found throughout the pulmonary vascular bed.[35] They consist of voltage-dependent potassium channels and calcium-dependent potassium channels (see also Chap. 22). The role of these channels has been studied primarily in the presence of acute hypoxia in animals. It is believed that potassium channels modulate adult pulmonary vascular tone. It is probable that calcium channels also serve a regulatory role in modulating vascular tone, particularly the L-type calcium channel. Inhibition of the voltage-regulated potassium channel by hypoxia or drugs can produce vasoconstriction and has been described in pulmonary artery smooth muscle cells harvested from patients with PPH.[70] It has been suggested that defects in the potassium channel of pulmonary resistance smooth muscle cells are involved in the initiation or progression of pulmonary hyper-

tension. A genetic defect related to potassium channels in the lungs of patients with PPH that leads to vasoconstriction may be one mechanism for the development of PPH in some patients[70] (Fig. 53–8).

The dysfunctional pulmonary hypertensive endothelial cell phenotype is characterized by uncontrolled proliferation, increased production of vasoconstrictor mediators such as endothelin, expression of 5-lipoxygenase, and decreased synthesis of prostacyclin. In normal lungs, larger proximal pulmonary arteries express more prostacyclin synthase than do smaller arteries.[71] In patients with PPH, expression of prostacyclin synthase is reduced in pulmonary arteries ranging from 1 mm to less than 100 μm in diameter, which suggests that the reduction in prostacyclin synthesis in otherwise morphologically normal to minimally remodeled vessels may play a role in the early stages of pathogenesis. Alternatively, endothelial cells of pulmonary small arteries may become dysfunctional as the disease progresses and pulmonary artery pressure progressively rises. The decrease in prostacyclin production by pulmonary endothelial cells could predispose the lung vessels to additional vasoconstriction and/or in situ thrombosis from enhanced platelet adhesion. Loss of expression of prostacyclin synthase is one of the phenotypic alterations present in pulmonary endothelial cells in severe pulmonary hypertension.[71]

Serotonin may play a role in pulmonary hypertension. Elevations in serotonin levels have been correlated with the pulmonary vascular pressure gradient in patients with acute respiratory distress syndrome.[72] Children with congenital heart disease and pulmonary hypertension have increased turnover of serotonin.[73] PPH has been reported in a patient with familial platelet storage pool disease, which represents a defect in serotonin handling and release.[74]

One series reported increased serotonin in patients with pulmonary hypertension associated with the use of fenfluramine and with collagen-vascular disease.[75] Of interest is that after six of these patients underwent heart/lung transplantation, they had persistently elevated concentrations of plasma serotonin and decreased platelet serotonin concentrations, thus suggesting that the abnormality in platelet serotonin handling was a primary process in the evolution of their pulmonary hypertension.

Genetics

An important emerging concept in the development of PPH is that the disease develops in patients with an underlying genetic predisposition following exposure to specific stimuli, which serve as triggers. Predisposition to the development of pulmonary hypertension has been noted by the marked heterogeneity in responses of the pulmonary vascu-

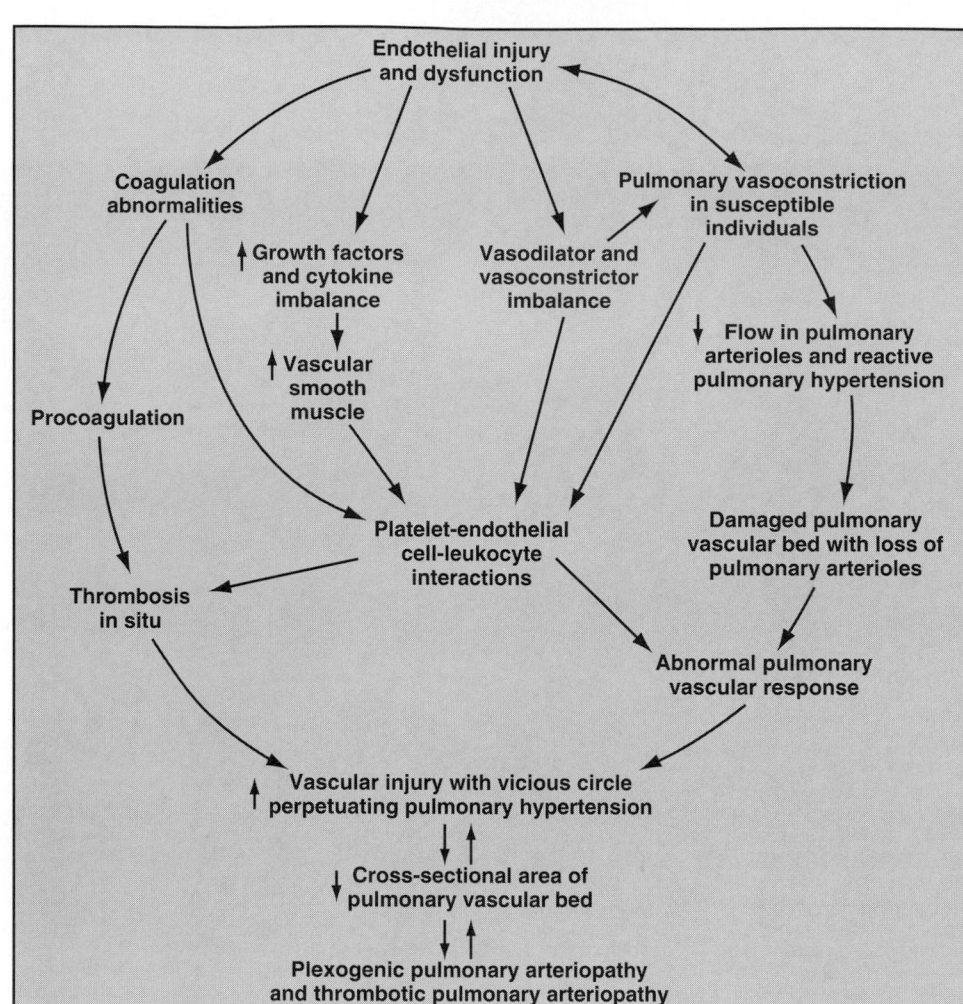

FIGURE 53-6. Possible pathogenesis of primary pulmonary hypertension (PPH). Endothelial injury or dysfunction sets off a cascade of cellular events that lead to the abnormal pulmonary vascular response seen in PPH and subsequently to a perpetuating vicious circle promoting plexogenic and thrombotic pulmonary arteriopathy. (From Rubin L J: ACCP Consensus Statement: Primary pulmonary hypertension. Chest 104:236, 1993.)

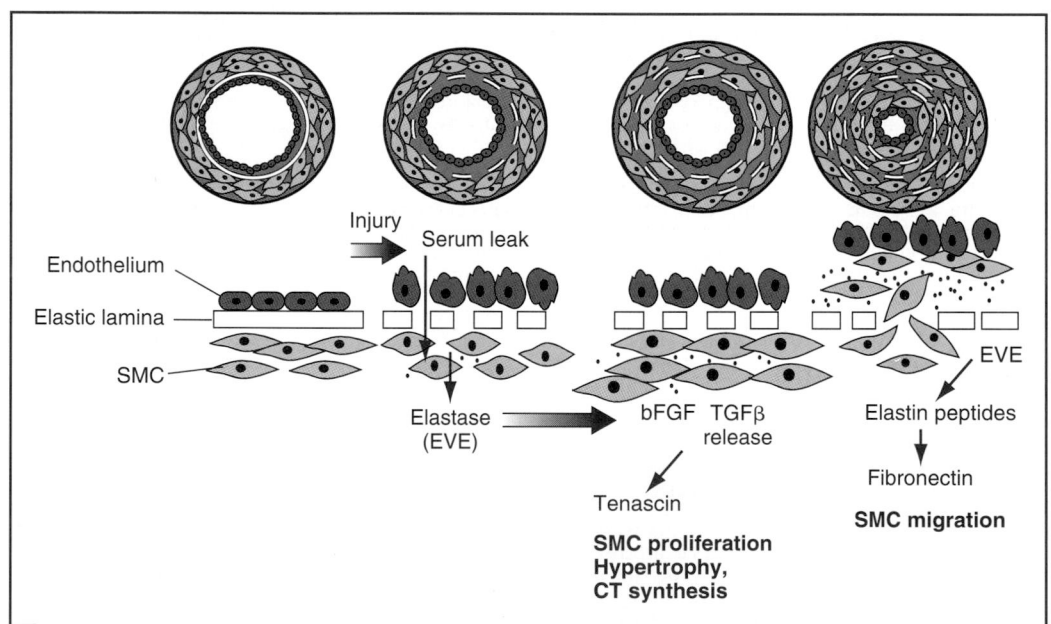

FIGURE 53-7. Schema of the pathophysiology of pulmonary hypertension related to elastase activity. Alterations in the endothelium that result in loss of its barrier function may allow leakage of a serum factor that stimulates smooth muscle cell (SMC) production and release of endogenous vascular elastase (EVE). EVE will degrade elastin and proteoglycans, which serve as storage sites for growth factors such as transforming growth factor-beta (TGFβ) and basic fibroblast growth factor (bFGF). Subsequent stimulation of production of the matrix glycoprotein tenascin leads to an increase in SMC hypertrophy and the synthesis of connective tissue (CT) proteins. The elastin peptides also stimulate production of the matrix glycoprotein fibronectin, which changes SMC from a contractile to a migratory phenotype. (From Rabinovitch M: Pulmonary hypertension: Updating a mysterious disease. Caradiovasc Res 34:268-272, 1997. Copyright 1997, with permission from Elsevier Science.)

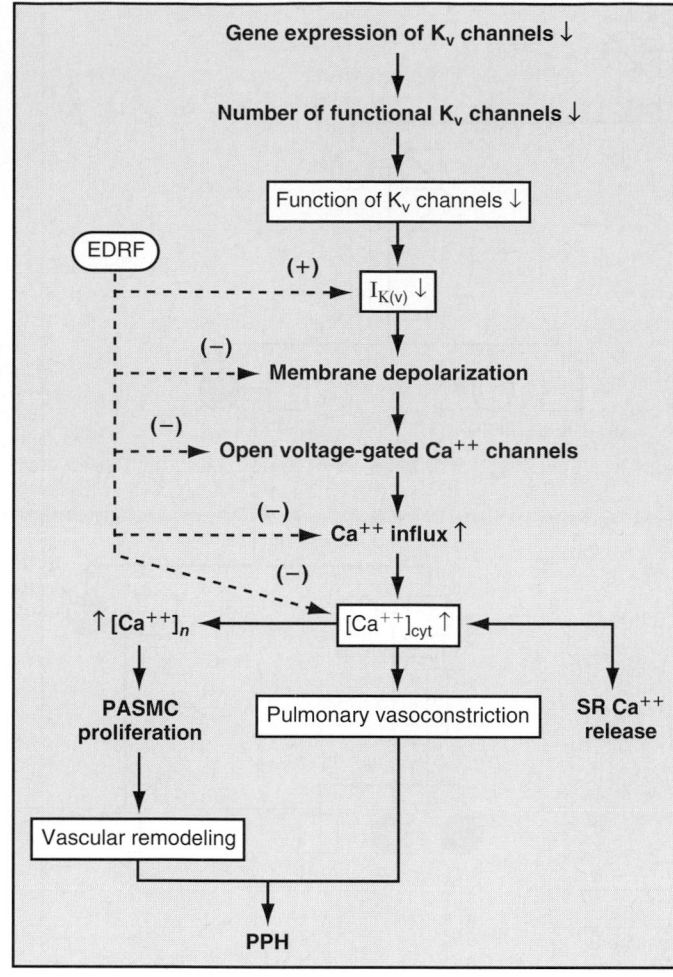

FIGURE 53–8. One proposed cellular mechanism responsible for the development of primary pulmonary hypertension initiated by abnormal gene transcription and expression of voltage-regulated potassium (K_v) channels. Increased calcium influx would raise cytosolic calcium ($[Ca^{2+}]_{cyt}$) and serve to trigger pulmonary vasoconstriction and stimulate cell proliferation with subsequent pulmonary vascular remodeling. Endothelium-derived relaxing factors (EDRFs) also participate in regulating potassium and calcium channels in pulmonary artery smooth muscle cells (PASMCs). (From Yuan JX, Aldinger AM, Juhaszova M, et al: Dysfunctional voltage-gated K^+ channels in pulmonary artery smooth muscle cells of patients with primary pulmonary hypertension. Circulation 98: 1400–1406, 1998.)

lature in a variety of disease states. Examples include the considerable variability among individuals to vasoconstrictive stimuli such as hypoxia or acidosis, which can produce marked pulmonary hypertension in one person and be essentially without effect in another. The pulmonary arterial pressure response to hypoxia is particularly great in individuals with blood group A.[14] This variability in responsiveness of the pulmonary vascular bed undoubtedly accounts for the fact that pulmonary edema develops in only a minority of individuals on exposure to high altitude. Also, the severity of pulmonary hypertension and the level of pulmonary vascular resistance vary considerably among individuals with congenital heart disease and comparably sized ventricular septal defects. Presumably, a genetic basis underlies these differences in pulmonary vascular reactivity, just as there appears to be a genetic basis for the increased reactivity of the systemic vascular bed in essential systemic hypertension.

FAMILIAL PPH. PPH has been diagnosed in families worldwide. The prevalence of familial PPH is uncertain, but it occurs in at least 6 percent of cases and the inci-

dence is probably higher.[76] Many unique features are associated with the transmission and development of PPH in families.[77] The age of onset is variable and penetrance is incomplete. Many individuals in families with PPH inherit the gene and have progeny in whom PPH never develops. The observation that fewer males are born in PPH families than in the population at large suggests that the PPH gene might influence fertilization or cause male fetal wastage.

Patients with familial PPH have a similar female-to-male ratio, age of onset, and natural history of the disease as those with sporadic PPH. Documentation of familial PPH can be difficult since remote common ancestry occurs in patients with apparently sporadic PPH and skip generations caused either by incomplete penetrance or by variable expression can mimic sporadic disease. Because the clinical and pathological features of familial and sporadic PPH are virtually identical, it seems likely that the same genes may be involved in both forms of the disease. It also seems likely that the disease will not be due to an abnormal gene product resulting from a mutation but rather due to abnormal production or regulation of a normal gene product.

Vertical transmission has been demonstrated in as many as five generations in one family and is probably indicative of a single dominant gene that is believed to be autosomal for PPH.[78] Genetic anticipation has been described in familial PPH since the early reports. Trinucleotide repeat expansion, originally described in several neurological disorders, remains the only known biological explanation for genetic anticipation in PPH and raises the possibility that the pathogenesis of familial PPH might have a neurological basis (Fig. 53–9).

The locus of a gene linked to familial PPH has been identified on chromosome 2q31,–33,[78a] and analysis of the genome containing the gene has been reduced to less than 7 million base pairs.[79] PPH-1 is the Human Genome Organization–approved designation DGB:1381541. The low penetrance of this gene confers only about a 10 to 20 percent likelihood of development of the disease.

Risk Factors in the Development of PPH

Although pulmonary hypertension can be the clear result of a disease process affecting the pulmonary parenchyma or vessels directly, a number of conditions have been identified that appear to be associated with the development of primary or unexplained pulmonary hypertension. Risk factors for PPH include drugs, chemical products, and other diseases. Expression of PPH may depend on other clinical features, such as the patient's gender or age at the time of disease expression.[80] The clinical features of PPH in patients with known risk factors are generally determined by the severity of the PPH and whatever influence the risk factor has on the overall medical condition. For example, the association of PPH and cirrhosis would have the combined clinical features of PPH and liver disease.

PORTAL HYPERTENSION

Pulmonary abnormalities have been commonly associated with the development of hepatic cirrhosis and portal hypertension[81] and include hypoxemia and intrapulmonary shunting, portal-pulmonary shunting, impaired hypoxic pulmonary vasoconstriction, and pulmonary hypertension.[82–84] Studies show that the liver plays an important role in regulating pulmonary vascular tone. Although the relative risk associated with the development of pulmonary hypertension in patients with portal hypertension is unknown, a large postmortem study from the Johns Hopkins Hospital showed that the prevalence of unexplained or pulmonary hypertension in patients with cirrhosis was 5.6 times higher than that of PPH alone. A modest increase in pulmonary artery pressure is not unusual in patients with cirrhosis and portal hypertension.[83] The increase in pulmonary artery pressure is usually passive and relates to the increase in cardiac output and/or blood volume and is associated with near-normal pulmonary vascular resistance. Published studies indicate a strong association between portal hypertension and pulmonary hypertension regardless of

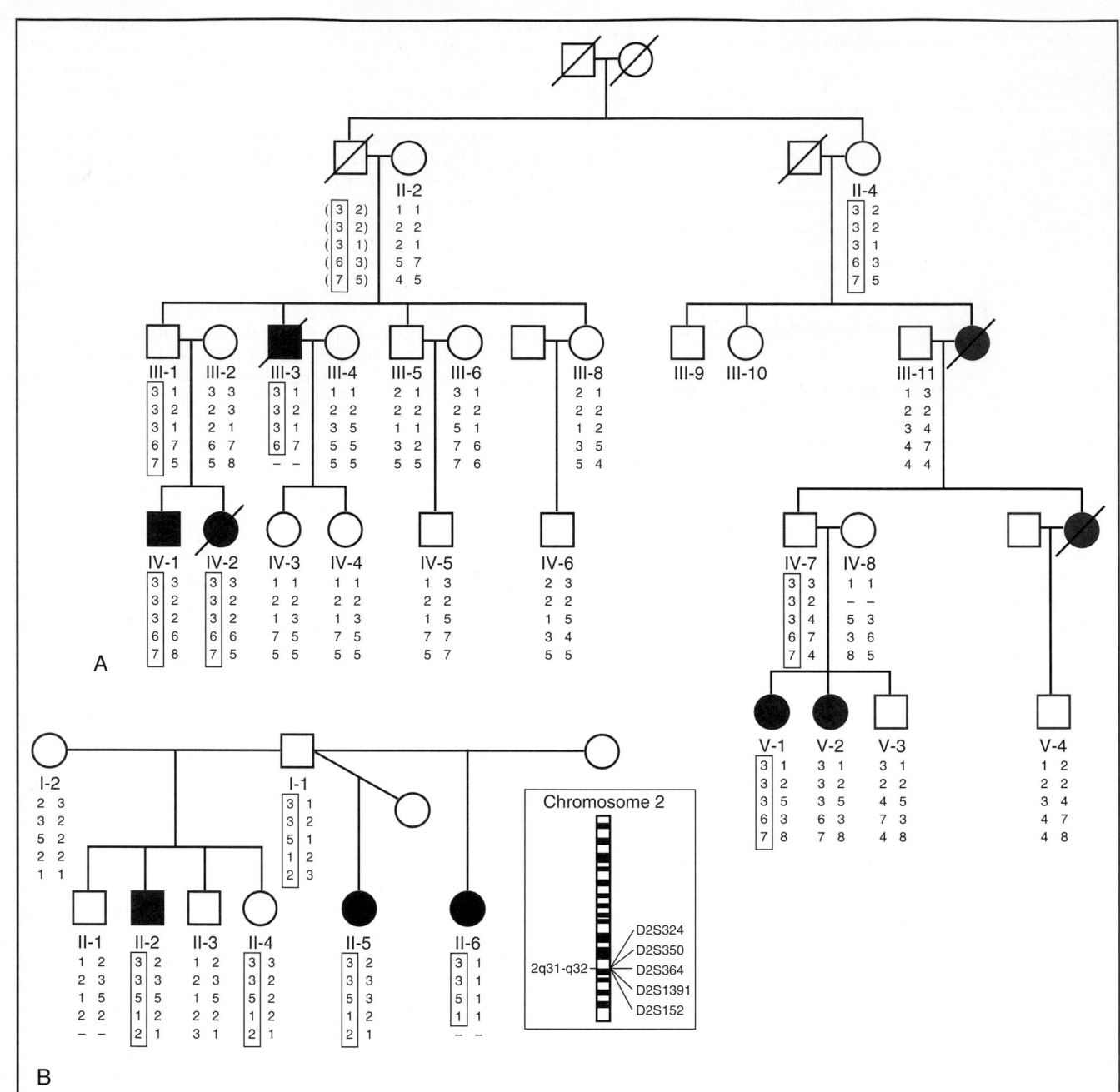

FIGURE 53–9. The pedigrees of two families (*A* and *B*) with familial primary pulmonary hypertension (PPH). Shaded symbols represent affected individuals. Genotyped individuals are indicated by the respective pedigree designations. The PPH-1 region on chromosome 2 (2q31-q32) contains a number of candidate genes. (From Morse JH, Jones AC, Barst RJ, et al: Mapping of familial primary pulmonary hypertension locus (PPH-1) to chromosome 2q31-32. Circulation 95:2603–2606, 1997.)

whether liver disease is present.[84–86] Although the mechanisms are uncertain, several possibilities are consistent. Portal hypertension itself induces numerous modifications in the vascular medium that may trigger a cascade of intracellular signals and/or cause activation or repression of various genes in endothelial and smooth muscle cells.

Pulmonary hypertension may develop in susceptible patients with portal hypertension in response to an increase in vascular wall shear stress caused simply by the increased pulmonary blood flow through the lungs. The presence of a portosystemic shunt may also allow substances normally cleared by the liver to gain access to the pulmonary circulation. Increased levels of several vasoactive mediators, cytokines, and growth factors have been demonstrated in patients with portal hypertension, including serotonin and interleukin-1.[86] Other angiogenic factors such as hepatocyte growth factor or vascular endothelial growth factor may be involved in pulmonary artery remodeling.[87, 88]

Patients in whom PPH develops in association with cirrhosis appear to be similar to patients without cirrhosis with the sole exception that they tend to have higher cardiac output and consequently lower calculated systemic and pulmonary vascular resistance, which is characteristic of the cirrhotic state.[83] Treatment of portal pulmonary hypertension generally follows the guidelines developed for treating patients with PPH. Although severe pulmonary hypertension is considered a contraindication to liver transplantation because of the risk of irreversible right-sided heart failure, successful liver transplantation has been reported in patients with mild pulmonary hypertension.[89, 90] Whether the pulmonary circulation will eventually return to normal posttransplantation remains uncertain.

ANOREXIGENS

Several anorexigens have been demonstrated to cause pulmonary hypertension in humans. The first observation was made in 1967, when an epidemic of PPH was associated with the use of aminorex in Europe coincident with its introduction in the general population.[91] The mechanism by which aminorex causes pulmonary hypertension remains uncertain, but it has similarities to both adrenaline and ephedrine in its chemical structure. The clinical features of pulmonary hypertension were identical to those attributed to PPH.

In 1981 a cause-and-effect relationship between the ingestion of fenfluramine, another appetite suppressant, and the development of pulmonary hypertension was established in a patient in whom PPH developed but reversed upon drug withdrawal and then redeveloped upon rechallenge.[92] The magnitude of the association between the use of appetite suppressants and the development of PPH was clearly defined in the International Primary Pulmonary Hypertension Study (IPPHS), a case-control study conducted in Europe in 1992–1994.[40] In addition to the association between the use of appetite suppressants and the development of pulmonary hypertension, the IPPHS described a dramatic increase in the risk of development of pulmonary hypertension with increased duration of use. The study resulted in severe restriction of the use of appetite suppressants in Europe, only to see their use popularized in the United States. Ultimately, the marked increase in the number of cases of PPH and cardiac valvulopathy ascribed to the use of fenfluramine drugs in the United States led to their withdrawal in 1997. Unfortunately, in the majority of patients the development of pulmonary hypertension has been progressive despite withdrawal of the appetite suppressants.[93, 94, 94a] Although the drugs mainly identified in the IPPHS were the fenfluramines, amphetamine-like anorexigens were also implicated.

The mechanism by which the fenfluramines and aminorex produce pulmonary hypertension has been investigated. Experimental studies have demonstrated that these drugs can cause pulmonary vasoconstriction by inhibiting voltage-gated potassium channels in the smooth muscle cells of resistance-level pulmonary arteries.[95] Although the degree of pulmonary vasoconstriction noted was small, it increased dramatically when NO synthase was inhibited. One recent study compared NO production in patients with PPH and patients with pulmonary hypertension associated with the use of anorexigens.[96] It appears that the latter group had a deficiency in basal NO production when compared with patients with PPH, which suggests that NO may be a compensatory product of the pulmonary arterial endothelium that increases in pulmonary hypertension to counteract the effects of chronic vasoconstriction.

Because of the consistent association with anorexigens and unexplained pulmonary hypertension, clinicians should be exceedingly careful in the use of these drugs in the future, especially in patients who may have increased susceptibility to the development of pulmonary hypertension (Fig. 53–10).

HIV INFECTION

Although well documented, it remains unclear how human immunodeficiency virus (HIV) infection results in an increased incidence of PPH in HIV-infected patients.[97, 98] A direct pathogenic role of HIV seems unlikely inasmuch as no viral constituents have been detected in the vascular endothelium of these patients.[99] On the other hand, reports of pulmonary arteriopathy with intimal proliferation in monkeys experimentally infected with the simian immunodeficiency virus and in a murine model of acquired immunodeficiency syndrome suggest a pathogenetic link between infection with an immunodeficiency virus and the development of PPH, possibly mediated by release of inflammatory mediators or by autoimmune mechanisms.[100] A large case-control study of HIV-associated PPH was recently conducted in the Swiss HIV Cohort Study.[101] The cumulative incidence was 0.6 percent within the entire HIV-infected population. PPH was diagnosed in all stages of HIV infection and without an obvious relationship to immune deficiency. The clinical and hemodynamic features of these patients were similar to those of patients with PPH. Of great interest, however, is that antiretroviral treatment seemed to exert a beneficial effect on the course of hemodynamic progression of the disease.

SYSTEMIC HYPERTENSION

Systemic hypertension is two to three times more common in patients with PPH than in an age-matched population.[40] The underlying mechanisms related to the development of essential hypertension are quite diverse, but the possibility exists that in some patients the mechanism that increases systemic vascular resistance similarly affects the pulmonary vascular bed.[102] It has been suggested that neurohumoral factors may play a role[103] or that the pulmonary vasculature is hypercontractile and overreacts to sympathetic stimulation.[104] Given that essential hypertension is extremely common in the general population, other confounding factors probably contribute to the development of pulmonary hypertension in affected individuals.

INCREASED PULMONARY BLOOD FLOW

For many years it has been observed that PPH can develop in adulthood in patients with atrial septal defect.[105] However, the incidence of this combination is extremely low, thus raising the possibility that they are two completely unrelated events. It is possible that chronically increased pulmonary blood flow may have effects on pulmonary endothelium through some type of mechanical means that would cause perturbations in the integrity of the vascular wall and lead to the development of pulmonary vascular disease. Increased pulmonary blood flow from hyperthyroidism and beriberi have been reported to be associated with the development of unexplained pulmonary hypertension, which suggests that high pulmonary blood flow,[106] rather than mere coincidence, is the basis for the development of pulmo-

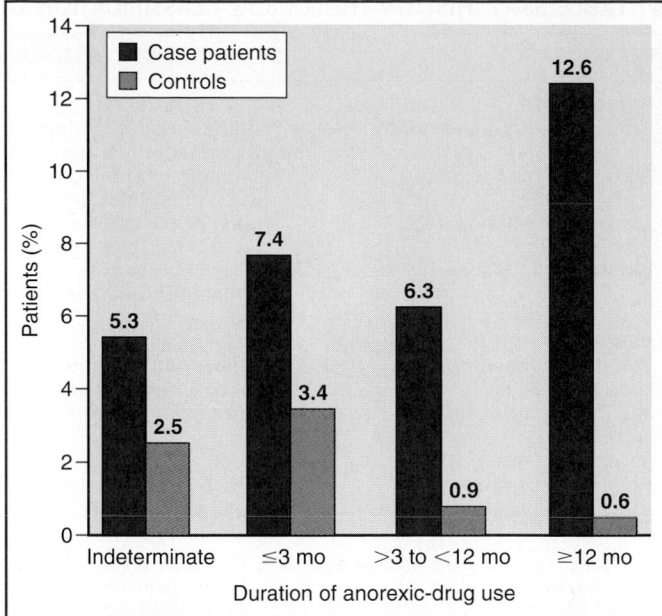

FIGURE 53–10. Relationship between duration of exposure to anorectic drugs and the development of primary pulmonary hypertension (PPH). The odds ratio of PPH developing increases with increased duration of use. The number of controls taking anorectic drugs in whom PPH does not develop diminishes over time, which raises the possibility that a marked increase in duration of exposure could eventually convert all the controls into cases. (From Abenhaim L, Moride Y, Brenot F, et al: Appetite suppressant drugs and the risk of primary pulmonary hypertension. N Engl J Med 335:609–616, 1996. Copyright © 1996 Massachusetts Medical Society. All rights reserved.)

nary hypertension in patients with pretricuspid shunts such as atrial septal defect or anomalous pulmonary venous drainage.

PATHOLOGICAL FINDINGS

Morphological abnormalities in each cell line have been described in PPH.[3, 49, 50] The endothelium in particular displays marked heterogeneity in the pulmonary vascular bed. Although endothelial dysfunction has been clearly described in PPH, discordance between phenotype and function is commonly noted.[107] It is not known at what stage during the evolution of PPH that endothelial cell proliferation occurs. It has been proposed, however, that a somatic mutation rather than nonselective cell proliferation in response to injury may account for the growth advantage of endothelial cells in PPH.[108] Heterogeneity in the smooth muscle and fibroblast populations also contributes to discordance between phenotype and function. Interconversion between cell types (fibroblast to smooth muscle cell or endothelium to smooth muscle cell) in addition to neovascularization may occur.

In the large muscular and elastic arteries, smooth muscle cell hypertrophy and increased connective tissue and extracellular matrix are found.[68, 69] In the subendothelial layer, increased thickness may be the result of recruitment and/or proliferation of smooth muscle–like cells. It is possible that precursor smooth muscle cells are in a continuous layer in the subendothelial layer along the entire pulmonary artery. These cells are similar to the pericytes that are responsible for the appearance of muscle in normally nonmuscular arteries and that contribute to intimal thickening in larger arteries. Alterations in the extracellular matrix secondary to proteolytic enzymes also play a role in the pathology of

▼ **TABLE 53–1. HISTOPATHOLOGICAL CLASSIFICATION OF HYPERTENSIVE PULMONARY VASCULAR DISEASE**

CLASSIFICATION	CHARACTERISTIC HISTOPATHOLOGICAL FEATURES
ARTERIOPATHY	
Isolated medial hypertrophy*	Medial hypertrophy: increase of medial muscle in muscular arteries, muscularization of nonmuscularized arterioles; no appreciable intimal or luminal obstructive lesions. No plexiform lesions
Plexogenic pulmonary arteriopathy	Plexiform and dilatation lesions. Medial hypertrophy; eccentric or concentric-laminar and nonlaminar intimal thickening; fibrinoid necrosis, arteritis, and thrombotic lesions
Thrombotic pulmonary arteriopathy	Thrombi (fresh, organizing, or organized and colander lesions). Eccentric and concentric nonlaminar intimal thickening, varying degrees of medial hypertrophy. No plexiform lesions
Isolated pulmonary arteritis	Active or healed arteritis. Limited to pulmonary arteries; varying degrees of medial hypertrophy, intimal fibrosis, and thrombotic lesions. No plexiform lesions. No systemic arteritis
VENOPATHY	
Pulmonary venoocclusive disease	Eccentric intimal fibrosis and recanalized thrombi within pulmonary veins and venules; arterialized veins, capillary congestion, alveolar edema and siderophages, dilated lymphatics, pleural and septal edema, and arterial medial hypertrophy; intimal thickening and thrombotic lesions
MICROANGIOPATHY	
Pulmonary capillary hemangiomatosis	Infiltrating thin-walled blood vessels throughout pulmonary parenchyma, pleura, bronchi, and walls of pulmonary veins and arteries. Medial hypertrophy and intimal thickening of muscular pulmonary arteries and arterioles

* Medial hypertrophy includes muscularization of arterioles.
Reprinted from Pietra GG: Pathology of primary pulmonary hypertension. *In* Rubin LJ, Rich S (eds): Primary Pulmonary Hypertension. New York, Marcel Dekker, 1997, pp 19–61 by courtesy of Marcel Dekker, Inc.

PPH. Matrix-degrading enzymes can release mitogenically active growth factors that stimulate smooth muscle cell proliferation. In addition, elastase and matrix metalloproteinases contribute to upregulation of proliferation. Degradation of elastin has also been shown to stimulate upregulation of the glycoprotein fibronectin, which in turn stimulates smooth muscle cell migration.[68]

The most common vascular changes in PPH can best be characterized as a *hypertensive pulmonary arteriopathy,* which is present in 85 percent of cases (Table 53–1). These changes involve medial hypertrophy of the arteries and arterioles, often in conjunction with other vascular changes. Isolated medial hypertrophy is uncommon, and when present it has been assumed to represent an early stage of the disease. Plexogenic pulmonary arteriopathy is the most common pattern of hypertensive arteriopathy seen in patients with PPH.[3, 50] It is characterized by medial hypertrophy along with intimal proliferation and other complex lesions. The intimal proliferation may be concentric laminar intimal fibrosis, eccentric intimal fibrosis, or concentric nonlaminar intimal fibrosis. The frequency of these findings differs from case to case and within regions of the same lung in the same patient. In addition, plexiform and dilatation lesions, as well as a necrotizing arteritis, may be seen throughout the lungs. The fundamental nature of the plexiform lesion remains a mystery.[109] It is possible that it represents endothelial cells that are involved prominently in angiogenesis, perhaps akin to a neoplastic process. Morphologically, they represent a mass of disorganized vessels with proliferating endothelial cells, smooth muscle cells, myofibroblasts, and macrophages. Several studies have demonstrated the involvement of growth factors that have been implicated in angiogenesis.[110] Whether the plexiform lesion represents impaired proliferation or angiogenesis remains unclear. These lesions, however, are not pathognomonic for PPH but representative of a chronic, severe pulmonary hypertensive state.

The other major pattern of vascular changes in PPH is that of a *thrombotic pulmonary arteriopathy.*[111] Typical features include medial hypertrophy of the arteries and arterioles with both eccentric and concentric nonlaminar intimal fibrosis. The presence of colander lesions, which represent recanalized thrombi, is also typical. These lesions are believed to arise as a result of primary in situ thrombosis of the small vascular arteries and not from recurrent pulmonary embolism.

On rare occasion, a diffuse pulmonary arteritis with secondary thrombosis has been reported in patients with PPH, predominantly in children.[112] Although the association has not been reported in patients with underlying collagen-vascular disease, it may reflect the vascular response to a specific, but not clearly identified risk factor.

PULMONARY VENOOCCLUSIVE DISEASE

Pulmonary venoocclusive disease is a rare form of PPH observed in approximately 5 percent of cases.[49, 50] The histopathological diagnosis is based on the presence of obstructive eccentric fibrous intimal pads within the pulmonary veins and venules. Arterialization of the pulmonary veins is often present and associated with alveolar capillary congestion. Other changes of chronic pulmonary hypertension such as medial hypertrophy and muscularization of the arterioles with eccentric intimal fibrosis may also be seen. The pulmonary venous obstruction explains the increased pulmonary capillary wedge pressure described in patients in the late stages of the disease and the increase in basilar bronchovascular markings described on the chest radiograph. These clinical findings, along with a perfusion lung scan showing diffuse, patchy nonsegmental abnormalities, is highly suggestive of the diagnosis on a clinical basis.[113–115]

PULMONARY CAPILLARY HEMANGIOMATOSIS

This extremely rare condition is characterized by proliferation of the thin-walled microvessels that infiltrate the peribronchial and perivascular interstitium and lung parenchyma.[116] On occasion, it may be confused with pulmonary venoocclusive disease. The lesions are often patchy and the proliferating vessels may form small nodules within the alveolar interstitial space. These thin-walled vessels are prone to bleeding and may be manifested clinically as overt hemoptysis in affected patients. The perfusion lung scan in these patients may show "hot spots" reflective of local areas within the lung that have increased vascularity. These areas are typically seen at the lung periphery and can be confirmed by pulmonary angiography.[117] The natural history of this form of PPH is not yet defined.[118, 119]

CLINICAL FEATURES

NATURAL HISTORY AND SYMPTOMATOLOGY. The most extensive study on the natural history of PPH was reported from the National Institutes of Health (NIH) Registry on Primary Pulmonary Hypertension from 1981 to 1987.[76] The study included the long-term follow-up of 194 patients in whom PPH was diagnosed by established clinical and hemodynamic criteria. Sixty-three percent of the patients were female, and the mean age was 36 ± 15 years (range, 1 to 81 years) at the time of diagnosis. The mean interval from the onset of symptoms to diagnosis was 2 years, and the most common initial symptoms were dyspnea (80 percent), fatigue (19 percent), syncope or near syncope (13 percent), and Raynaud phenomenon (10 percent). No ethnic differentiation was observed, with 12.3 percent being black and 2.3 percent being Hispanic.

Syncope is a characteristic symptom of PPH and is assumed to be due to a fixed cardiac output. A recent study on the systolic function and interactions of the left and right ventricles in patients with PPH revealed an increased right ventricular end-diastolic volume and reduced right ventricular ejection fraction, with a greater stroke volume than in the left ventricle.[120] The mechanism for maintaining cardiac output with exercise was primarily through an increased heart rate inasmuch as stroke volume actually decreased. The right ventricular ejection fraction decreased with exercise, thus suggesting exercise-induced right ventricular failure. This result is expected because pulmonary artery pressure increases with exercise in PPH. The left ventricular ejection fraction is maintained, however, but left ventricular end-diastolic volume decreases and left ventricular end-systolic volume becomes extremely small, which suggests that the left ventricle is shortening to its maximum extent. The fact that left ventricular end-diastolic and end-systolic volumes decreased whereas right ventricular end-systolic and end-diastolic volumes remained unchanged supports the concept that underfilling and not external compression accounts for the small left ventricular chamber size observed in PPH. Syncope occurs because of exercise-induced right ventricular failure whereby the heart rate becomes the only mechanism available to increase cardiac output, which has limited effectiveness.

On *physical examination,* an increased pulmonic component of the second heart sound was the most common finding (93 percent), with tricuspid regurgitation noted in 40 percent and peripheral edema in 32 percent. In 90 percent of patients the chest radiograph revealed enlargement of the main pulmonary arteries, and the electrocardiogram revealed right ventricular hypertrophy in 87 percent. The clinical profiles of these patients were remarkably similar to those in a previously reported retrospective study of 120 patients from the Mayo Clinic.[57] In the Mayo Clinic series, 75 percent of the patients were women with a mean age of 34 years (range, 3 to 64 years) and a mean interval from onset of symptoms to diagnosis of 1.9 years.

The NIH Registry also revealed that restrictive changes in pulmonary function testing and reduced diffusing capacity for carbon monoxide were very common, with forced vital capacity approximately 80 percent of predicted and diffusing capacity 70 percent of predicted. These changes, however, do not correspond to any measure of severity of the pulmonary hypertension. An additional, virtually universal finding was mild to moderate hypoxemia (mean PO_2 of 72 ± 16 mm Hg), which is attributed to the effect of low mixed venous oxygen from low cardiac output amplified by the underlying ventilation-perfusion inequality.

The hemodynamic findings also suggested that the severity of the disease could be related to a rising right atrial pressure and falling cardiac index, both of which reflect underlying right ventricular dysfunction. The fact that the mean pulmonary artery pressure was similar in patients whose duration of symptoms was less than 1 year and those who were symptomatic for more than 3 years suggests that pulmonary artery pressure rises to fairly high levels early in the course of the disease.

Univariate analysis from the NIH Registry pointed to the mean right atrial pressure, mean pulmonary artery pressure, and cardiac index, as well as the diffusing capacity from carbon monoxide, as significantly related to mortality.[121] In addition, the New York Heart Association classification has also been shown to relate very strongly to survival. Based on estimates obtained from the proportional hazards model, a regression equation was developed that describes the relationship between these three hemodynamic variables and subsequent mortality.

$$P(t) = [(t)]A(x, y, z)$$
$$H(t) = 0.88 - 0.14t + 0.01t^2$$
$$A(x, y, z) = e^{(0.007325x) + (0.0526y) - (0.3275x)}$$

where $P(t)$ = percent survival at t years, t = number of years, x = mean pulmonary artery pressure, y = mean right atrial pressure, and z = cardiac index. This equation has since been validated in two subsequent studies,[122, 123] which suggests that baseline hemodynamic characteristics are very predictive of outcome.

The most common cause of death in patients with PPH in the NIH Registry was progressive right-sided heart failure (47 percent). Sudden cardiac death (both witnessed and unwitnessed) occurred in 26 percent. Of interest is that sudden cardiac death was limited to patients who were New York Heart Association Class IV, thus suggesting that it is a manifestation of end-stage disease rather than a phenomenon that occurs early or unpredictably in the clinical course of the disease. The remainder of the patients died of some other medical complication such as pneumonia or bleeding, which suggests that patients with PPH do not tolerate coexistent medical conditions well. In the NIH Registry experience, no deaths or sustained morbidity was associated with the diagnostic evaluation done at baseline assessment. It should be pointed out, however, that these were university centers with established experience in the management of patients with PPH.

MECHANISMS OF RIGHT VENTRICULAR FAILURE. It is presumed that right ventricular dysfunction in patients with chronic pulmonary hypertension is a result of chronic pressure overload and associated volume overload with the development of tricuspid regurgitation. However, animal studies suggest that right ventricular ischemia may also be a feature and potentially a very common one.[124] The mechanism of right ventricular failure in pulmonary hypertension is complex. The chronic pressure overload that induces right ventricular hypertrophy and reduced contractility has been shown to cause a reduction in coronary blood flow to the right ventricular myocardium, which can produce right ventricular ischemia, both acutely and chronically. Such right ventricular dysfunction appears to be a result of a reduction in right ventricular coronary artery driving pressure. In an interesting animal study by Vlahakes and colleagues[124] acute right ventricular failure secondary to right ventricular hypertension was overcome by increasing central aortic pressure, which resulted in an increase in right ventricular coronary driving pressure. Murray and Vatner[125] reported that a moderate increase in aortic pressure was accompanied by a large increase in right ventricular myocardial perfusion only when the autonomic nervous system was blocked with an alpha blocker. Because the symptom of angina associated with PPH is characteristic of myocardial ischemia, it probably represents ongoing ischemia caused by this phenomenon.

On occasion, patients with pulmonary hypertension may have a reduced left ventricular ejection fraction and even regional wall motion abnormalities of the left ventricle. In the past, these findings had been attributed to mechanisms related to interventricular dependence, which suggests that in some way a dysfunctional right ventricle can lead to a dysfunctional left ventricle.[126] Clearly, the shared interventricular septum can affect the function of both ventricles. More recently, extrinsic compression of the left main coronary artery by the pulmonary artery in patients with chronic pulmonary hypertension has been described and may be associated with classic angina-like symptoms.[127, 128] It is advisable to look for extrinsic compression of the left main coronary artery with coronary angiography in patients with longstanding pulmonary hypertension who have abnormal left ventricular function.

The clinical course of patients with PPH can be highly variable. However, with the onset of overt right ventricular failure manifested by worsening symptoms and systemic venous congestion, patient survival is generally limited to approximately 6 months. Understanding the clinical course of patients with PPH is important, especially when considering major interventional therapy such as organ transplantation.

PHYSICAL EXAMINATION. Findings are consistent with pulmonary hypertension and right ventricular pressure overload: a large *a* wave in the jugular venous pulse; a low-volume carotid arterial pulse with a normal upstroke; a left parasternal (right ventricular) heave; a systolic pulsation produced by a dilated, tense pulmonary artery in the second left interspace; an ejection click and flow murmur in the same area; a closely split second heart sound with a loud pulmonic component; and a fourth heart sound of right ventricular origin. Late in the course, signs of right ventricular failure (hepatomegaly, peripheral edema, and ascites) may be present. Patients with severe pulmonary hypertension may also have prominent *v* waves in the jugular venous pulse as a result of tricuspid regurgitation, a third heart sound of right ventricular origin, a high-pitched early diastolic murmur of pulmonic regurgitation, and a holosystolic murmur of tricuspid regurgitation. Cyanosis is a late finding in PPH and may be worsened by a patent foramen ovale with right-to-left shunting. Other causes of cyanosis include a markedly reduced cardiac output with systemic vasoconstriction and ventilation-perfusion mismatches in the lung. Uncommonly, the left laryngeal nerve becomes paralyzed as a consequence of compression by a dilated pulmonary artery (Ortner syndrome).

LABORATORY FINDINGS

HEMATOLOGICAL AND CHEMICAL STUDIES. Results of these studies are usually normal in patients with PPH. If chronic arterial oxygen desaturation is noted, polycythemia may be present. A number of investigators have reported hypercoagulable states, abnormal platelet function, defects in fibrinolysis, and other abnormalities of coagulation in patients with PPH.[58, 59] Abnormal liver function tests results can indicate right ventricular failure with resultant systemic venous hypertension.

ELECTROCARDIOGRAPHY. The electrocardiogram in PPH usually exhibits right atrial and right ventricular enlargement. A direct correlation between the amplitude of the R wave in V_1, the R/S ratio in V_1, and the level of pulmonary arterial pressure has been reported.

ROENTGENOGRAPHY. Radiographic examination of the chest in patients with PPH shows enlargement of the main pulmonary artery and its major branches, with marked tapering of peripheral arteries. The right ventricle and atrium may also be enlarged. Fluoroscopic examination may disclose exaggerated pulsations of secondary pulmonary arterial branches reflecting an elevation in pulmonary arterial pulse pressure. However, in contrast to the plethoric peripheral lung fields in patients with left-to-right shunts, oligemia is noted in these lung regions in patients with PPH. It has been suggested that survival in PPH correlates inversely with the size of the main pulmonary artery—a reasonable suggestion because the latter correlates with the height of pulmonary arterial pressure. The diameter of the pulmonary artery may be determined from computed tomographic (CT) scans and used to estimate pulmonary artery pressures.[129]

PULMONARY FUNCTION TESTS. Pulmonary function tests typically show mild restriction with a reduced diffusion capacity for carbon monoxide (DLco) and hypoxemia with hypocapnea. Some patients have increased residual volume and reduced maximum voluntary ventilation.

ECHOCARDIOGRAPHY. Echocardiography usually demonstrates enlargement of the right atrium and ventricle, normal or small left ventricular dimensions, and a thickened interventricular septum. The septal/posterior left ventricular wall ratio may be abnormally increased, as in hypertrophic obstructive cardiomyopathy, but other echocardiographic signs characteristic of that condition are not observed. Systolic prolapse of the mitral valve is frequently present, as well as abnormal septal motion of the ventricular septum, as a result of chronic right ventricular pressure overload and reduced left ventricular filling.[130] Doppler echocardiographic evidence of right ventricular systolic hypertension may be obtained by measuring the velocity of the tricuspid regurgitant jet and using the Bernoulli formula (see Chap. 7). Doppler techniques have demonstrated left ventricular diastolic dysfunction with marked dependence on atrial contraction for ventricular filling.[130]

LUNG SCINTIGRAPHY. A perfusion lung scan is an essential component in making the correct diagnosis of PPH. It may reveal a relatively normal perfusion pattern or diffuse, patchy perfusion abnormalities.[131] The severity of the perfusion abnormality in lung scans does not parallel the hemodynamics inasmuch as serial lung scans performed over time in patients with PPH do not show progressive changes consistent with the patients' worsening clinical state. A perfusion lung scan should help distinguish patients with PPH from those who have pulmonary hypertension secondary to chronic pulmonary thromboembolism (Fig. 53–11). The risk associated with lung scans in PPH has been grossly overstated. The early literature reported three patients with pulmonary hypertension who died following lung scans, but it is not clear that the deaths were caused by the procedure. In the NIH Registry on PPH, not one morbid clinical event was associated with the performance of lung scans in any of the patients with pulmonary hypertension.[76]

PULMONARY ANGIOGRAPHY. Pulmonary angiography is essential to establish the correct diagnosis in a patient with presumed PPH in whom a perfusion lung scan suggests segmental or lobar defects. Typically, pulmonary angiography demonstrates large central pulmonary arteries with marked peripheral tapering. Postmortem arteriograms demonstrate the absence of "background haze" secondary to the loss of small, nonmuscular pulmonary arterioles. Although pulmonary angiography carries an increased risk in patients with PPH, it can be performed safely if adequate precautions are taken. The NIH Registry contains no deaths or serious morbidity associated with pulmonary angiography.

Maintenance of adequate oxygenation by the administration of supplemental oxygen and the avoidance of vasovagal reactions (and rapid treatment of those that occur with intravenous atropine) should reduce the associated risk in this patient group. Placement of an arterial line for continuous arterial pressure monitoring is advised, and nonionic contrast agents appear to be better tolerated. Injections are preferably limited to the individual lungs or specific lobes to reduce

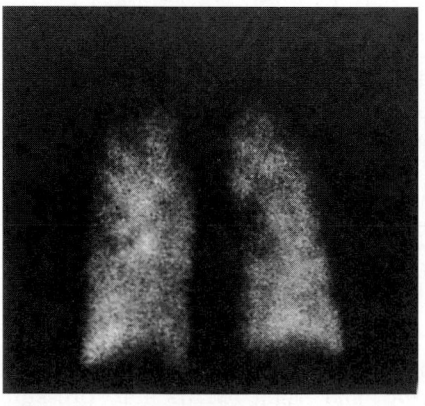
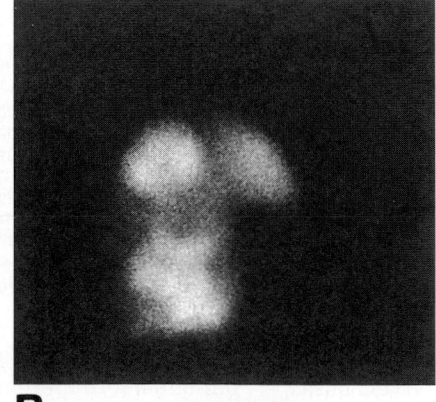

A PPH **B** PTE

FIGURE 53–11. Perfusion lung scans in patients with pulmonary hypertension. *A*, Patient with primary pulmonary hypertension (PPH). *B*, Patient with pulmonary thromboembolism causing pulmonary hypertension (PTE). Both perfusion scans are abnormal. The scan on the patient with PPH shows a mottled distribution in a nonsegmental, nonanatomical manner. The scan on the patient with PTE reveals lobar, segmental, and subsegmental defects highly suggestive of an anatomical obstruction to pulmonary blood flow.

CONDITION	TEST APPLIED	FINDING
Congenital heart disease	Step-up in O_2 saturation in right heart Step-down in O_2 saturation in left heart Cardiac angiography	Left-to-right shunt and location of shunt Right-to-left shunt and location of shunt Anatomical definition
Peripheral pulmonary artery stenoses	Intrapulmonary arterial pressure Pulmonary angiogram	Intrapulmonary arterial pressure gradients Pulmonary arterial branch stenoses
Proximal pulmonary arterial occlusion by clot or tumor*	Selective or main pulmonary angiography	Intravascular filling defect or narrowing, webs, poststenotic dilatation
Mitral stenosis Cor triatriatum Supravalvular mitral ring	Simultaneous wedge and left ventricular pressure recording	An elevated wedge pressure and mean mitral valve diastolic pressure gradient >3 mm Hg at rest, both of which increase with exercise
Mitral regurgitation	Simultaneous wedge and left ventricular pressure recording Left ventriculogram	Large systolic pressure wave in wedge tracing. Regurgitation of contrast from left ventricular angiogram into the left atrium
Left ventricular diastolic dysfunction	Left ventricular pressure	LVEDP >15 mm Hg
Restrictive cardiomyopathy	Right ventricular pressure	LVEDP response to intravenous fluid challenge: normalization of LVEDP with marked reduction in pulmonary artery pressure with intravenous nitroprusside

* Ventilation = perfusion lung scans precede catheterization.
LVEDP = left ventricular end-diastolic pressure.
Modified from Reeves JT, Groves BM: Approach to the patient with pulmonary hypertension. *In* Weir EK, Reeves JT: Pulmonary Hypertension. Mt Kisco, NY, Futura, 1984, p 20.

the contrast load. Pulmonary wedge angiography using a segmental angiographic technique with hand injection of small amounts of angiographic contrast through the terminal lumen of a balloon flotation catheter while the balloon is inflated is not a substitute for pulmonary angiography.

COMPUTED TOMOGRAPHY OF THE CHEST. Chest radiographs, as well as chest CT scans, have been used to determine the presence and severity of pulmonary hypertension based on the diameter of the main pulmonary arteries.[129, 132] This information may be useful when performing chest CT to investigate the lung parenchyma in patients with pulmonary hypertension who are undergoing diagnostic evaluation. In addition, high-resolution chest CT scans have been used successfully in diagnosing chronic thromboembolic pulmonary hypertension.[132] In addition to visualization of thrombi in the pulmonary vasculature with contrast enhancement, a mosaic pattern of variable attenuation compatible with irregular pulmonary perfusion can be determined in the unenhanced CT scan. Marked variation in the size of segmental vessels is also a specific feature of chronic thromboembolic disease. In some institutions, high-resolution CT scanning has replaced lung scintigraphy as a test to make this diagnosis.

EXERCISE TESTING. The use of a symptom-limited exercise test can be very helpful in the evaluation of patients with pulmonary hypertension. Besides allowing objective assessment of the severity of symptoms, exercise testing has been shown to also be predictive of survival. Two types of exercise testing have recently become popularized. The Naughton protocol uses a treadmill with increases in work of 1-MET increments at 2-minute stages to allow patients with very limited exercise tolerance to perform. In the 6-minute walk test, patients are instructed to walk down a 100-ft corridor and cover as much ground as possible within the 6 minutes. The total distance walked is determined by a tester. The application of exercise testing has been particularly helpful in evaluating the efficacy of drug therapy.[133]

CARDIAC CATHETERIZATION. The diagnosis of PPH cannot be confirmed without cardiac catheterization (Table 53–2). Besides allowing the exclusion of other causes, it also establishes the severity of disease and allows an assessment of prognosis. By definition, patients with PPH should have a low or normal pulmonary capillary wedge pressure. Although it has often been stated that one may be unable to obtain an accurate wedge pressure in these patients, such is rarely the case in experienced hands.[76] However, when an increased wedge pressure is obtained, it must be correlated with left ventricular end-diastolic pressure and not attributed to a "falsely elevated" reading.[134] It has been shown that left ventricular diastolic compliance becomes significantly impaired in PPH and parallels the severity of the

disease; thus, pulmonary capillary wedge pressure tends to rise slightly in the late stages of PPH, although it rarely exceeds 16 mm Hg. Measurements of all right-sided pressures are properly made at expiration to avoid incorporating negative intrathoracic pressures.

It can be extremely difficult to pass a catheter into the pulmonary artery in patients with pulmonary hypertension because of the tricuspid regurgitation, dilated right atrium and ventricle, and low cardiac output. Flow-directed thermodilution balloon catheters, which are the proper devices to use, also lack stiffness and can be difficult to place. A specific flow-directed thermodilution balloon catheter has been developed for patients with pulmonary hypertension (American Edwards Laboratories, Irvine, CA); it has an extra port for the placement of a 0.32-inch guidewire to provide better stiffness to the catheter. The risk associated with cardiac catheterization in patients with PPH is extremely low in experienced hands, but deaths have been reported.[76]

DIAGNOSIS (Table 53–3)

It is essential that diagnostic efforts be pursued vigorously in patients with severe pulmonary hypertension to ensure that no patient with secondary pulmonary hypertension is erroneously classified as having PPH. Patients with PPH may tolerate diagnostic procedures poorly. These individuals can experience sudden cardiovascular collapse and even death during or shortly after the induction of general anesthesia for surgical procedures and during cardiac catheterization and angiography.

The *differential diagnosis* of PPH includes a number of well-defined causes of secondary pulmonary hypertension (Table 53–4). Exclusion of mitral stenosis, congenital cardiac defects (including cor triatriatum, pulmonary thromboembolism, and pulmonary venous obstruction by means of catheterization and angiography is imperative. "Silent" mitral stenosis, i.e., without the characteristic diastolic murmur, can be excluded by means of echocardiographic visualization of the motion of the mitral valve and the absence

▼ TABLE 53–3. DIAGNOSTIC STUDIES USEFUL FOR ELUCIDATING CAUSES OF PULMONARY HYPERTENSION

POTENTIAL CAUSE OF PULMONARY HYPERTENSION	DIAGNOSTIC STUDIES
Pulmonary thromboembolic disease	Ventilation/perfusion scans, computed tomography of chest, pulmonary angiography
Pulmonary venous thrombosis or obstruction	Chest x-ray, angiography, computed tomography, magnetic resonance imaging
Congenital intracardiac shunts	Transesophageal echocardiography with contrast
Increased left atrial pressure secondary to mitral or aortic valve disease, left ventricular dysfunction, or systemic hypertension	Pulmonary artery wedge pressure or left atrial pressure (via patent foramen ovale) (>15 mm Hg and LVEDP)
Pulmonary airway disease (e.g., chronic bronchitis and emphysema)	Respiratory function tests (FVC/FEV, chest x-ray)
Hypoxic pulmonary hypertension associated with (1) impaired ventilation, either central (CNS) or peripheral (chest wall problems or upper airway obstruction) and (2) residence at high altitude	Sleep apnea studies and respiratory function tests
Interstitial lung disease, pneumoconioses, and fibrosis (e.g., silicosis, rheumatoid disease, and sarcoidosis)	Chest x-ray, spirometry and carbon monoxide diffusion, high-resolution chest computed tomography
Collagen-vascular disease (e.g., SLE, polyarteritis nodosa, scleroderma)	Serological and immunogenetic studies; skin, muscle, or other tissue biopsy; esophageal motility studies
Parasitic disease (schistosomiasis or filariasis)	Rectal biopsy, complement fixation, skin tests, blood smears
Cirrhosis with portal hypertension	Liver function tests, ultrasonography, computed tomography
Peripheral pulmonary artery stenosis (including Takayasu disease and fibrosing mediastinitis)	Selective pulmonary angiography or pressure gradient at catheterization
Sickle cell disease	Erythrocyte morphology, hemoglobin electrophoresis

CNS = central nervous system; FEV_1 = forced expiratory volume in 1 second; FVC = forced vital capacity; SLE = systemic lupus erythematosus.

Modified from Weir EK: Diagnosis and management of primary pulmonary hypertension. *In* Weir EK, Reeves JT: Pulmonary Hypertension. Mt Kisco, NY, Futura, 1984, p 141.

of a transvalvular pressure gradient (see Chap. 46). *Congenital cardiac defects* with Eisenmengers syndrome can usually be ruled out if significant left-to-right or right-to-left shunts are absent, although occasional patients with equal pulmonary and systemic vascular resistance may have no detectable shunt at rest. Transesophageal echocardiography can reliably detect congenital cardiac defects and distinguish an atrial septal defect from a patent foramen ovale.[135] *Cor triatriatum* (see Chaps. 43 and 44) is recognized by appropriate hemodynamic studies and angiographic visualization of the left atrial membrane. This entity has a characteristic left atrial echocardiogram with normal mitral valve motion. Cardiac catheterization reveals a hemodynamic pattern similar in some ways to mitral stenosis, i.e., a diastolic pressure gradient between the left ventricle and the pulmonary capillary bed. *Pulmonary embolism* (see Chap. 52) can be excluded by pulmonary angiography, and *sickle cell disease with in situ pulmonary vascular thrombosis* (see Chap. 69) can be evaluated by hemoglobin electrophoresis. The presence of severe *pulmonary parenchymal disease* can be recognized by the characteristic physical findings, chest radiograph, pulmonary function tests, and high-resolution chest CT. *Collagen-vascular disease* is suggested by the involvement of other organ systems or the presence of abnormal immunological phenomena such as antinuclear antibodies and LE cells (see Chap. 67).

▼ TABLE 53–4. DIAGNOSTIC CLASSIFICATION OF PULMONARY HYPERTENSION

Pulmonary arterial hypertension
  Primary
    Sporadic
    Familial
  Secondary
    Collagen-vascular disease
    Congenital systemic-to-pulmonary shunts
    Portal hypertension
    HIV infection
    Drugs/toxins
      Anorexigens
      Other
    Persistent pulmonary hypertension of the newborn
    Other
Pulmonary venous hypertension
  Left-sided atrial or ventricular heart disease
  Left-sided valvular heart disease
  Extrinsic compression of central pulmonary veins
    Fibrosing mediastinitis
    Adenopathy/tumors
  Pulmonary venoocclusive disease
  Other
Pulmonary hypertension associated with disorders of the respiratory system and/or hypoxemia
  Chronic obstructive pulmonary disease

Interstitial lung disease
Sleep-disordered breathing
Alveolar hypoventilation disorders
Chronic exposure to high altitude
Neonatal lung disease
Alveolar-capillary dysplasia
Other
Pulmonary hypertension from chronic thrombotic and/or embolic disease
Thromboembolic obstruction of proximal pulmonary arteries
Obstruction of distal pulmonary arteries
  Pulmonary embolism (thrombus, tumor, ova and/or parasites, foreign material)
  In situ thrombosis
  Sickle cell disease
Pulmonary hypertension caused by disorders directly affecting the pulmonary vasculature
Inflammatory
  Schistosomiasis
  Sarcoidosis
  Other
Pulmonary capillary hemangiomatosis

From Rich S (ed): Primary Pulmonary Hypertension: Executive Summary from the World Symposium—Primary Pulmonary Hypertension 1998. Available from the World Health Organization via the Internet (http://www.who.int/ncd/cvd/pph.html).

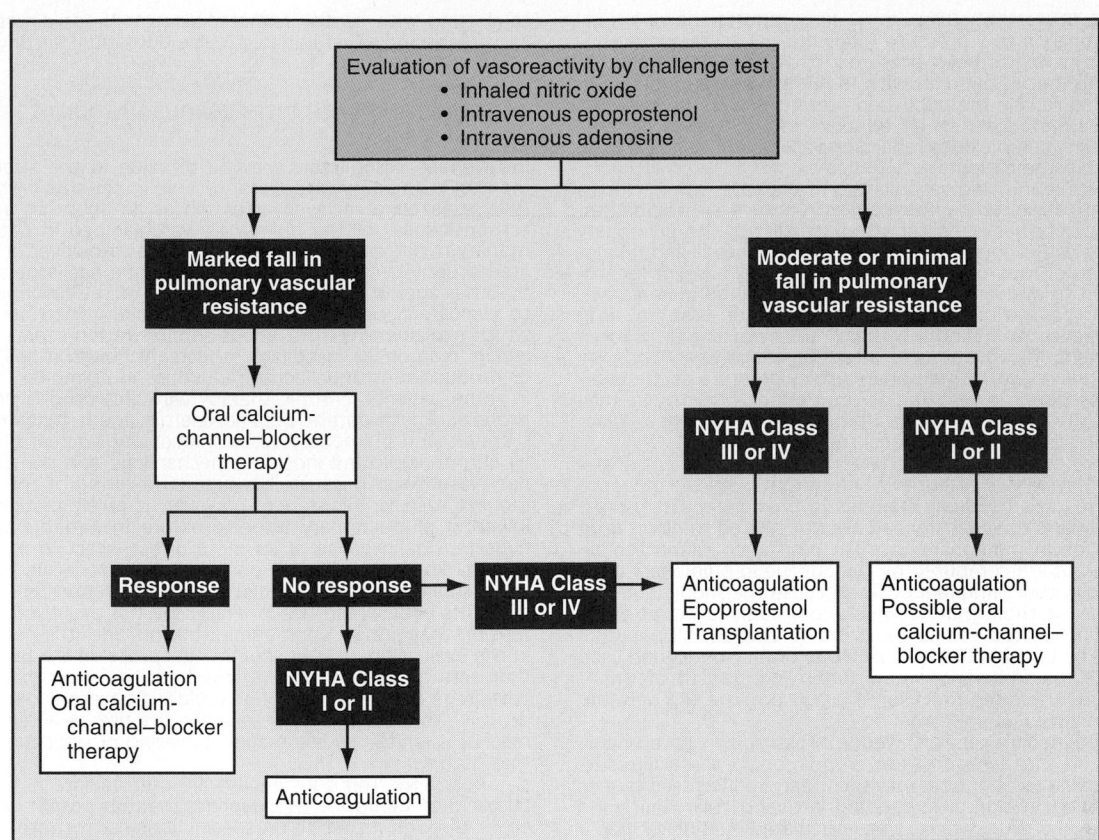

FIGURE 53–12. An algorithm for the management of primary pulmonary hypertension. NYHA = New York Heart Association. (From Rubin IJ: Primary pulmonary hypertension. N Engl J Med 336:111–117, 1997. Copyright © 1997 Massachusetts Medical Society. All rights reserved.)

TREATMENT (Fig. 53–12)

LIFE STYLE CHANGES. The diagnosis of PPH does not necessarily imply total disability for the patient. However, physical activity can be associated with elevated pulmonary artery pressure inasmuch as marked hemodynamic changes have been documented to occur early in the onset of increased physical activity.[136] For that reason, graded exercise activities, such as bike riding or swimming, in which patients can gradually increase their workload and easily limit the extent of their work, are thought to be safer than isometric activities. Isometric activities such as lifting weights or stair climbing can be associated with syncopal events and should be limited or avoided.

The subject of pregnancy should also be discussed with women of childbearing age. The physiological changes that occur in pregnancy can potentially activate the disease and result in death of the mother and/or the child. Besides the increased circulating blood volume and oxygen consumption that will increase right ventricular work, circulating procoagulant factors and the risk of pulmonary embolism from deep vein thrombosis and amniotic fluid are serious concerns. Syncope and cardiac arrest have also been reported to occur during active labor and delivery, and a syndrome of postpartum circulatory collapse has been described.[137] For these reasons, surgical sterilization should be given strong consideration by women with PPH or their husbands.

DIGOXIN. Animal studies performed on the utility of digoxin in right ventricular systolic overload show that prior administration helps prevent the reduction in contractility of the right ventricle. Recently, it has been shown that digoxin can exert a favorable hemodynamic effect when given acutely to patients with right ventricular failure from pulmonary hypertension.[138] An increase in resting cardiac output of approximately 10 percent was noted, which is similar to observations made in patients with left ventricular systolic failure. In addition, it was also observed that digoxin causes a significant reduction in circulating norepinephrine, which was markedly increased. Digitalis toxicity in patients with pulmonary hypertension and normal renal function is uncommon. Consequently, digoxin appears to be a potentially useful medication for patients who have right ventricular failure, either with isolated pulmonary hypertension or in combination with left ventricular systolic failure.

DIURETIC THERAPY. Diuretics appear to be of marked benefit in symptom relief of patients with PPH. Their traditional role has been limited to patients manifesting right ventricular failure and systemic venous congestion. However, patients with advanced PPH can have increased left ventricular filling pressures that contribute to the symptoms of dyspnea and orthopnea, which can be relieved with diuretics. Diuretics may also serve to reduce right ventricular wall stress in patients with concomitant tricuspid regurgitation and volume overload. The fear that diuretics will induce systemic hypotension is unfounded because the main factor limiting cardiac output is pulmonary vascular resistance and not pulmonary blood volume. Patients with severe venous congestion may require high doses of loop diuretics or the use of combined diuretics. In these instances, electrolytes need to be carefully watched to avoid hyponatremia and hypokalemia.

SUPPLEMENTAL OXYGEN THERAPY. Hypoxic pulmonary vasoconstriction can contribute to pulmonary vascular disease in patients with alveolar hypoxia from parenchymal lung disease. Supplemental low-flow oxygen alleviates arterial hypoxemia and attenuates the pulmonary hypertension in these disorders; in contrast, most patients with PPH do not exhibit resting hypoxemia and derive little benefit from supplemental oxygen therapy. Patients who experience arterial oxygen desaturation with activity, however, may benefit from ambulatory supplemental oxygen because increased oxygen extraction develops in the face of fixed oxygen delivery. Patients with severe right-sided heart failure and resting hypoxemia resulting from markedly increased oxygen extraction at rest should be treated with continuous oxygen therapy to maintain their arterial oxygen saturation above 90 percent.[139] Patients with hypoxemia caused by a right-to-left shunt via a patent foramen ovale do not improve their level of oxygenation to an appreciable degree with supplemental oxygen.

VASODILATOR TREATMENT. Because of early reports showing a reduction in pulmonary artery pressure following the acute administration of vasodilators, it has been presumed that vasodilators are the mainstay of treatment in patients with PPH. This presumption, however, is not supported by the published literature over the past two decades. Vasodilators appear to be effective in a subset of patients with PPH, but many complexities regarding vasodilator administration make their use in these patients very difficult.

The first principle in using vasodilators in patients with PPH is to establish accurate baseline hemodynamics. Because substantial hemodynamic variability has been reported to exist in the pulmonary vascular bed and will produce changes in cardiac output and pulmonary artery pressure from moment to moment, serial baseline recordings are required to evaluate the magnitude of change in hemodynamics that may be attributed to variability rather than to drug effect.[140] The practice of attributing "peak" effect of the drug to an administered agent introduces bias into the assessment. Thus, by choosing the highest level of pulmonary artery pressure as the baseline and the subsequent lowest one as drug effect, one may be misled to attribute a favorable influence from a medication when in fact no effect or even an adverse one is occurring.

It must also be emphasized that hemodynamic assessment of the entire circulatory system is essential when determining the influence of drugs in these patients. Small changes in pulmonary artery pressure are probably due to variability and are not related to direct drug influence. Changes in pulmonary vascular resistance cannot be directly measured but are computed by the change in pulmonary pressure and cardiac output simultaneously. Because thermodilution cardiac output, the method that is most commonly used in these patients, can be associated with large errors in reproducibility, particular care should be taken in the methodology of thermodilution used in these patients. In addition, when an underlying right-to-left shunt exists or severe tricuspid regurgitation is a concern, the Fick determination of cardiac output is preferred.

Changes in pulmonary capillary wedge pressure can have important influences on the determination of pulmonary vascular resistance. A rising capillary wedge pressure secondary to increased cardiac output may be the first sign of impending left ventricular failure and an adverse effect of a drug, whereas the calculated pulmonary vascular resistance may become lower and suggest a beneficial effect. Right atrial pressure also reflects the filling characteristics of the right ventricle. A right atrial pressure increase in the face of rising cardiac output suggests right ventricular diastolic dysfunction.[141] The resting heart rate is a physiological parameter of marked importance in patients with congestive heart failure, and treatments that cause an increased heart rate are likely to yield deleterious long-term results. Finally, the systemic arterial oxygen content should be evaluated in patients with PPH. Effective vasodilator drugs can result in vasodilatation of blood vessels supplying poorly ventilated areas of the lung and worsen hypoxemia. This effect is particularly noticeable in patients with underlying chronic lung disease. For all these reasons it has been advocated that vasodilators be initiated only in the hospital setting with central catheter placement for direct hemodynamic recordings and never initiated in the outpatient setting.[139, 142]

ACUTE TESTING WITH INTRAVENOUS VASODILATORS
(Table 53–5)

Intravenous vasodilators may be of value in the short-term assessment of pulmonary vasodilator reserve in patients with PPH.[139] Historically, tolazoline received attention as an agent to acutely test the responsiveness of the pulmonary vascular bed in patients with pulmonary hypertension from several causes. However, it is poorly tolerated acutely because of its side effects and has largely been replaced by other agents. Acetylcholine was one of the first medications used to evaluate patients with PPH. It is rapidly inactivated by the lung, which explains why intravenous administration seems to produce selective pulmonary vasodilator effects. Although it has been reported to produce substantial acute reductions in pulmonary artery pressure in some patients, chronic therapy with this drug is not feasible. Isoproterenol is a potent beta-adrenergic agent that affects both the systemic and pulmonary vascular beds and increases cardiac output by chronotropic and inotropic mechanisms. It is considered a pulmonary vasodilator because it results in lowering of the calculated pulmonary vascular resistance. However, it rarely results in substantial lowering of pulmonary artery pressure in patients with pulmonary hypertension because of its more direct effect in increasing cardiac output. Phentolamine is a potent alpha-adrenergic blocker that has been shown to cause pulmonary vasodilatation in animals and humans. Its widespread use is limited by the profound systemic hypotension that occurs upon administration, and it is not generally used in the evaluation of PPH. Sodium nitroprusside is a potent vasodilator that acts on arterial and venous beds. Its short half-life is also an advantage because the effects rapidly dissipate when infusion of the drug is stopped. Like phentolamine, its use as a test of vasodilator reserve is limited by the marked lowering of systemic blood pressure that occurs.

ADENOSINE. This substance is an intermediate product in the metabolism of adenosine triphosphate that has potent vasodilator properties through its action on specific vascular receptors. In addition to pulmonary vasodilatation, it can also produce systemic and coronary vasodilatation. It is believed to stimulate the endothelial cell and vascular smooth muscle receptors of the A_2 type, which induce vascular smooth muscle relaxation by increasing cyclic adenosine monophosphate.[143] In patients with PPH, adenosine has been shown to be an extremely potent vasodilator and predictive of the subsequent effects of intravenous prostacyclin and oral calcium channel blockers.[144, 145] Adenosine has an extremely short half-life (less than 5 seconds), which provides a safety net by its rapid dissolution should any adverse side effects occur. It is administered intravenously in doses of 50 ng/kg/min and titrated upward every 2 minutes until uncomfortable symptoms develop (such as chest tightness or dyspnea). It should be noted that adenosine is given as an infusion and not as an

▼ **TABLE 53–5.** HEMODYNAMIC ASSESSMENT OF VASODILATORS IN PULMONARY HYPERTENSION

PARAMETER MEASURED	DESIRED ACUTE CHANGES	COMMENTS
Mean pulmonary artery pressure	>25% fall; ideally mean PAP below 30 mm Hg	Must not be any associated significant fall in systemic blood pressure
Pulmonary vascular resistance	>33% fall; ideally, PVR below 6 units	Should be associated with a fall in PA pressure *and* an increase in cardiac output. An increase in cardiac output alone may lead to future RV failure
Right atrial pressure	No change or fall	An increase in RA pressure signals impending RV failure
Pulmonary capillary wedge pressure	No change	An increase in wedge pressure suggests pulmonary venoocclusive disease or coexisting LV dysfunction
Systemic blood pressure	Minimal fall; mean arterial pressure should remain above 90 mm Hg	A significant hypotensive response makes chronic vasodilator therapy contraindicated
Cardiac output	Increase	The increase should be related to increased stroke volume and not solely due to increased heart rate
Heart rate	No significant change	A chronic increased heart rate will result in RV failure. Watch for bradycardia if high doses of diltiazem are used
Systemic arterial oxygen saturation	Increase if reduced on room air, little change if normal	A fall in systemic arterial oxygen saturation suggests lung disease or right-to-left shunting and prohibits chronic use
Pulmonary artery (mixed venous) oxygen saturation	Increase	Should reflect the increase in cardiac output and improved tissue oxygenation

LV = left ventricular; RA = right atrial; RV = right ventricular.
Reprinted from Rubin LJ, Rich S: Medical management. *In* Rubin LJ, Rich S (eds): Primary Pulmonary Hypertension. New York, Marcel Dekker, 1997, pp 271–286 by courtesy of Marcel Dekker, Inc.

intravenous bolus as is used to treat supraventricular tachyarrhythmias.

PROSTACYCLIN. This substance (epoprostenol sodium, or PGI$_2$) is a metabolite of arachidonic acid that is synthesized and released from vascular endothelium and smooth muscle. Its vasodilatory effects are thought to be mediated by activation of specific membrane PGI$_2$ receptors that are also coupled to the adenylate cyclase system.[28] Other effects include inhibition of platelet activation and aggregation, as well as leukocyte adhesion to the endothelium.[146] Prostacyclin has been used as an acute test of vasodilator reserve in patients with PPH. Like adenosine, its short half-life allows use of the drug to be discontinued if any acute adverse effects result. Also similar to adenosine, it is administered incrementally, at 2 ng/kg/min and increased every 15 to 30 minutes until systemic effects such as headache, flushing, or nausea occur, which limits the acute dose titration. Favorable acute effects from prostacyclin appear to be predictive of a favorable response to oral calcium channel blockers.[147]

Adenosine and prostacyclin possess potent inotropic properties, in addition to their ability to vasodilate the pulmonary vascular bed. When using these drugs for the acute testing of patients, one needs to pay particular attention to changes in cardiac output that occur in association with the changes in pulmonary arterial pressure. An increase in cardiac output with no change in pulmonary arterial pressure will result in a reduction in calculated pulmonary vascular resistance and may be erroneously interpreted as a vasodilator response. Instead, one should look at the magnitude of change of each individual parameter to determine the effects that the drug is having on the pulmonary circulation, as well as the type of response that it elicits.

NITRIC OXIDE. This substance, whose activity is identical to that of endothelium-derived relaxing factor, is produced from L-arginine by NO synthase.[148] NO diffuses to vascular smooth muscle and mediates vasodilatation by stimulating soluble guanylate cyclase to produce cyclic GMP. Because it binds very rapidly to hemoglobin with high affinity and is thereby inactivated, inhalation of NO gas results in selective pulmonary vascular effects without influencing the systemic circulation. Inhalation of NO by patients with PPH has been shown to produce a reduction in pulmonary vascular resistance acutely, similar to that achieved with intravenous adenosine, and to also predict the effectiveness of calcium channel blockers.[149, 150] NO has also been shown to be effective in patients with pulmonary hypertension secondary to congenital heart disease and the adult respiratory distress syndrome.[151] Although NO seems to have similar acute effects on pulmonary arterial pressure that are predictive of the chronic response to oral vasodilator agents, it differs importantly from adenosine and prostacyclin in that it has little effect on cardiac output.

Chronic Treatment

CALCIUM CHANNEL BLOCKERS. Of the vasodilators tested in patients with PPH, calcium channel blockers appear to have the widest usage. Early studies using conventional doses failed to demonstrate a chronic sustained benefit. Moreover, calcium channel blockers have properties that could worsen the underlying pulmonary hypertension, including negative inotropic effects on right ventricular function (Fig. 53–13) and reflex sympathetic stimulation, which may increase the resting heart rate.[141] It has been reported that patients with PPH who are challenged with very high doses of calcium channel blockers may manifest a dramatic reduction in pulmonary artery pressure and pulmonary vas-

cular resistance, which upon serial catheterization has been maintained for over 5 years.[122] Importantly, the patient's quality of life is restored with improved functional class, and survival (94 percent rate at 5 years) is improved when compared with nonresponders and historical control subjects (36 percent rate) (Fig. 53–14A). This experience suggests that some patients with PPH have the ability to have their pulmonary hypertension reversed and their quality of life and survival enhanced. It is unknown whether the response to calcium channel blockers identifies two subsets of patients with PPH, different stages of PPH, or a combination of both. However, it is essential to point out that patients who do not exhibit a dramatic hemodynamic response to calcium channel blockers do not appear to benefit from their long-term administration. Unfortunately, it is becoming common practice for physicians to prescribe calcium channel blockers at conventional doses to all patients with pulmonary hypertension, often without hemodynamic guidance. This unfortunate practice may result in quicker deterioration in these patients and should be strongly discouraged.

CHRONIC PROSTACYCLIN INFUSION THERAPY. Continuous-infusion prostacyclin therapy has now been shown in prospective randomized trials to improve quality of life and symptoms related to PPH, exercise tolerance, hemodynamics, and survival.[133, 152–155] (Fig. 53–14B). The initial enthusiasm for prostacyclin was based on the demonstration of pulmonary vasodilator effects when administered to experimental animals with acute pulmonary vasoconstriction and when subsequently administered to patients with PPH. The long-term effects of prostacyclin in PPH include its vasodilator and antithrombotic effects, but its effects may also be importantly related to its ability to restore the integrity of the pulmonary vascular endothelium. A recent study revealed that significant reductions in pulmonary vascular resistance that go beyond acute vasodilation were the rule in the patients treated with intravenous prostacyclin for 1 year.[155] On average, patients had a reduction in pulmonary vascular resistance of greater than 50 percent which occurred even if no acute hemodynamic effects were noted (Fig. 53–15).

Prostacyclin is generally administered through a central venous catheter that is surgically implanted and delivered by an ambulatory infusion system. The delivery system is complex and requires patients to learn the techniques of sterile drug preparation, operation of the pump, and care of the intravenous catheter. Most of the serious complications that have occurred with prostacyclin therapy have been attributable to the delivery system and include catheter-related infections and thrombosis and temporary interruption of the infusion because of pump malfunction. Anecdotal reports of rebound pulmonary hypertension occurring in patients in whom the infusion was interrupted suggest

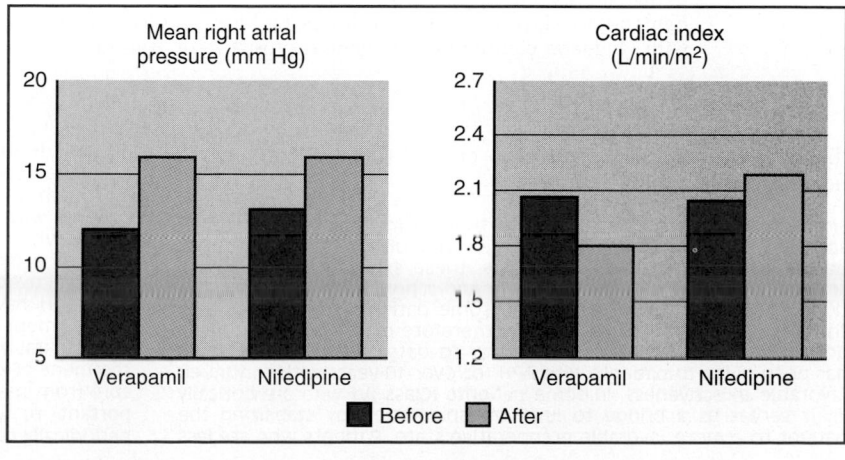

FIGURE 53–13. Adverse effects of calcium channel blockers in pulmonary hypertension. The hemodynamic effects of verapamil and nifedipine in patients with pulmonary hypertension are shown. An increase in right atrial pressure in association with no significant change in cardiac index as produced by nifedipine suggests that right ventricular dysfunction is occurring. The increased right atrial pressure associated with a fall in cardiac index, as produced by verapamil, suggests that negative inotropic effects are producing overt right ventricular failure. (Adapted from Packer M, Medina N, Yushak M: Adverse hemodynamic and clinical effects of calcium channel blockade in pulmonary hypertension secondary to obliterative pulmonary vascular disease. Am Coll Cardiol 4:890, 1994.)

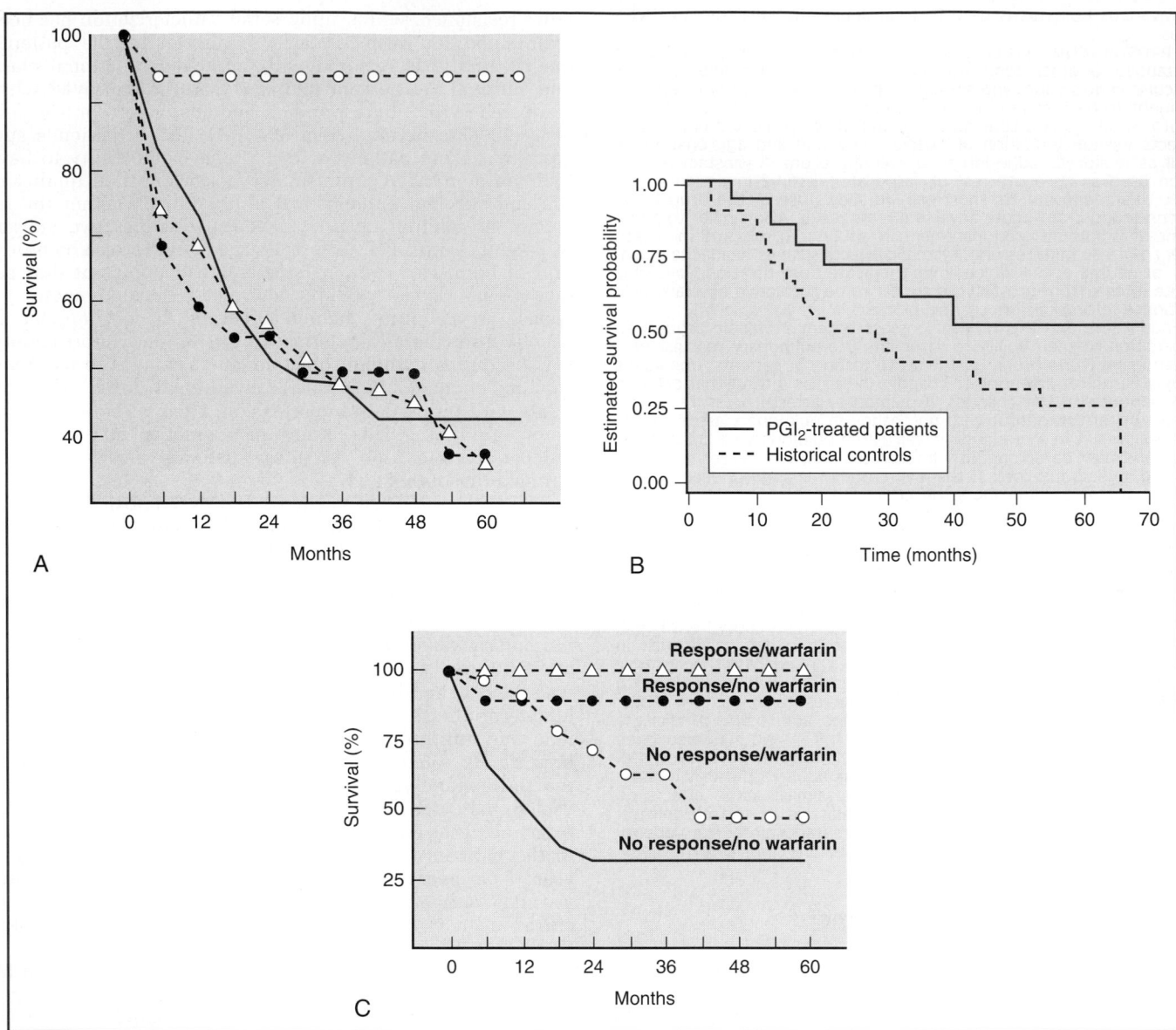

FIGURE 53–14. *A,* Effect of high doses of calcium channel blockers on survival over 5 years in patients with primary pulmonary hypertension (PPH). Patients who responded to the high-dose regimen (open circles) had a 95 percent 5-year survival rate, as opposed to the nonresponders (solid line), who had a 36 percent 5-year survival rate. Rates were similar in patients studied in the National Institutes of Health (NIH) Registry on PPH (triangles), as well as patients from the University of Illinois only (solid circles). *B,* Effect of intravenous prostacyclin (PGI₂) on survival in patients with PPH. The survival of patients given a chronic infusion of prostacyclin and monitored for 5.5 years is compared with that of functional Class III and IV patients from the NIH Registry (historical controls). *C,* Effects of anticoagulation on survival in patients with PPH who did not respond to calcium channel blockers. Patients who received warfarin (open circles) had a marked survival advantage over those who received no warfarin. (*A* and *C* from Rich S, Kaufmann E, Levy PS: The effects of high doses of calcium channel blockers on survival of primary pulmonary hypertension. N Engl J Med 327:76, 1992. Copyright © 1992 Massachusetts Medical Society. All rights reserved. *B* from Barst RJ, Rubin LJ, McGoon MD et al: Survival of primary pulmonary hypertension with long-term continuous intravenous prostacyclin. Ann Intern Med 121:409, 1994.)

that great care must be taken to ensure that the infusion is never stopped.

Side effects related to prostacyclin therapy include flushing, headache, nausea, diarrhea, and a unique type of jaw discomfort that occurs with eating. In most patients, these symptoms are minimal and well tolerated. Chronic foot pain and a poorly defined gastropathy with prolonged use develop in some patients. Tachyphylaxis to the drug develops at low doses and therefore may require a periodic dose increase to maintain its efficacy. To date, chronic prostacyclin has been given to patients with PPH for over 10 years with continued favorable effectiveness. In some patients (Class IV) who are critically ill, it serves as a bridge to lung transplantation by stabilizing the patient to a more favorable preoperative state. Patients who are less

critically ill may do so well with prostacyclin therapy that they may delay the need to consider transplantation, perhaps indefinitely.

A high-cardiac output state has been reported in a large series of patients with PPH receiving chronic prostacyclin therapy and is consistent with the drug having positive inotropic effects.[156] Whether the effect is a direct one on the myocardium or indirect via neurohormonal activation has not been determined. Although most patients with PPH have reduced cardiac output on initial examination, the development of a chronic high-output state could have long-term detrimental effects on underlying cardiac function. The follow-up assessment of patients receiving intravenous prostacyclin is quite variable from medical center to medical center, but it does appear important to determine the cardiac output response to therapy periodically to optimize dosing.[157]

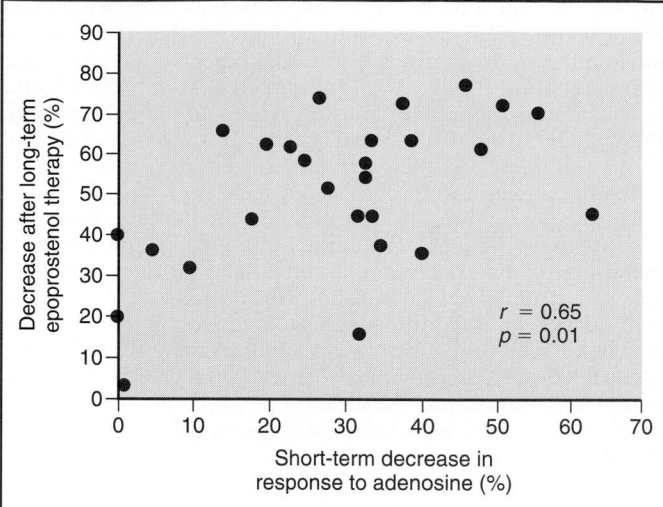

FIGURE 53-15. Long-term reduction in pulmonary vascular resistance (PVR) with chronic therapy with epoprostenol (prostacyclin) for primary pulmonary hypertension (PPH) in relation to the short-term reduction after the administration of adenosine. Although patients with the greatest short-term reduction in PVR had the greatest long-term reduction, patients who had little or no reduction acutely still had a significant reduction in PVR with long-term therapy. This finding suggests that mechanisms other than acute vasodilatation are responsible for the long-term benefit of intravenous prostacyclin therapy in PPH and supports the notion that reversal of pulmonary vascular remodeling is occurring. (From McLaughlin VV, Genthner DE, Panella MM, et al: Reduction in pulmonary vascular resistance with long-term epoprostenol (prostacyclin) therapy in primary pulmonary hypertension. N Engl J Med 338:273–277, 1998. Copyright © 1998 Massachusetts Medical Society. All rights reserved.)

ANTICOAGULANTS. Oral anticoagulant therapy is widely recommended for patients with PPH, although its clinical efficacy as a therapy is difficult to prove. A retrospective review of patients with PPH monitored over a 15-year period at the Mayo Clinic suggested that patients who received warfarin had improved survival over those who did not.[57] The influence of warfarin therapy has been investigated in patients with PPH who failed to respond to high doses of calcium channel blockers.[119] Significant improvement in survival was observed in patients who received anticoagulation, with a 1-year survival rate of 91 percent and 3-year survival rate of 47 percent as compared with 1- and 3-year rates of 62 and 31 percent, respectively, in patients who did not receive anticoagulants (Fig. 53–14C). The current recommendation is to use warfarin in relatively low doses, as has been recommended for prophylaxis of venous thromboembolism, with the international normalized ratio maintained at 2.0 to 2.5 times control.[156] Given its inhibitory effects on smooth muscle proliferation, heparin might be a suitable anticoagulant in PPH, although its use is more difficult. With the recent advent of low-molecular-weight heparins requiring once-a-day administration without the need for adjusting the dose to its antithrombotic effect, treatment with these agents is becoming a more viable alternative. They may be particularly useful in patients who are believed to be at increased risk for pulmonary thromboembolism.

ATRIAL SEPTOSTOMY

The rationale for the creation of an atrial septostomy in PPH is based on experimental and clinical observations suggesting that an intra-atrial defect allowing right-to-left shunting in the setting of severe pulmonary hypertension might be of benefit. Although over 60 patients have undergone this procedure worldwide, it should still be considered investigational.[159–162] Nonetheless, atrial septostomy may represent a real alternative for selected patients with severe PPH. Indications for the procedure include recurrent syncope and/or right

ventricular failure despite maximum medical therapy, as a bridge to transplantation if deterioration occurs in the face of maximum medical therapy, or when no other option exists.[162] Because the disease process in PPH appears to be unaffected by the procedure, the long-term effects of atrial septostomy must be considered palliative.

The procedure-related mortality with atrial septostomy in patients with PPH is high, and thus it should be attempted only in institutions with an established track record in the treatment of advanced pulmonary hypertension and experience in performing atrial septostomy with low morbidity.[161] It should not be performed in a patient with impending death and severe right ventricular failure or a patient receiving maximum cardiorespiratory support. Predictors of procedure-related failure or death have been identified and include a mean right atrial pressure of greater than 20 mm Hg, a pulmonary vascular resistance index of greater than 55 units · m² or a predicted 1-year survival rate of less than 40 percent.

The mechanisms responsible for the beneficial effects of atrial septostomy remain unclear. Possibilities include increased oxygen delivery at rest and/or with exercise, reduced right ventricular end-diastolic pressure or wall stress, improvement in right ventricular function by the Frank Starling mechanism, or relief of ischemia.

HEART-LUNG AND LUNG TRANSPLANTATION. (see also Chap. 20). Heart-lung transplantation has been performed successfully in patients with PPH since 1981.[163] Because these patients have pulmonary vascular disease and severe right ventricular dysfunction, it was originally believed that heart-lung transplantation was the only transplantation option. Widespread application of heart-lung transplantation, however, has been limited by the number of centers with expertise to perform the procedure, the scarcity of suitable donor organs, and the very long waiting times required for

▼ **TABLE 53-6. GENERAL GUIDELINES FOR SELECTION OF LUNG TRANSPLANT RECIPIENTS**

INDICATIONS

Advanced obstructive, fibrotic, or pulmonary vascular disease with a high risk of death within 2 to 3 yr

Lack of success or availability of alternative therapies

Severe functional limitation but preserved ability to walk

Age 55 yr or less for candidates for heart-lung transplantation, age 60 yr or less for candidates for bilateral lung transplantation, and age 65 yr or less for candidates for single-lung transplantation

ABSOLUTE CONTRAINDICATIONS

Severe extrapulmonary organ dysfunction, including renal insufficiency with a creatinine clearance below 50 ml/min, hepatic dysfunction with coagulopathy or portal hypertension, and left ventricular dysfunction or severe coronary artery disease (consider heart-lung transplantation)

Acute, critical illness

Active cancer or recent history of cancer with substantial likelihood of recurrence (except for basal cell and squamous cell carcinoma of the skin)

Active extrapulmonary infection (including infection with HIV, hepatitis B, hepatitis C)

Severe psychiatric illness, noncompliance with therapy, and drug or alcohol dependence

Active or recent (preceding 3 to 6 mo) cigarette smoking

Severe malnutrition (<70% of ideal body weight) or marked obesity (>130% of ideal body weight)

Inability to walk, with poor rehabilitation potential

RELATIVE CONTRAINDICATIONS

Chronic medical conditions that are poorly controlled or associated with target organ damage

Daily requirement for more than 20 mg of prednisone (or equivalent)

Mechanical ventilation (excluding noninvasive ventilation)

Extensive pleural thickening from prior thoracic surgery or infection

Active collagen-vascular disease

Preoperative colonization of the airways with pan-resistant bacteria (in patients with cystic fibrosis)

From Arcasoy SM, Kotloff RB: Lung transplantation. N Engl J Med 340:1081–1091, 1999. Copyright © 1999 Massachusetts Medical Society. All rights reserved.

patients with end-stage right-sided heart failure. More recently, bilateral or double-lung transplantation and single-lung transplantation have been performed successfully in patients with PPH.[164] Hemodynamic studies have shown an immediate reduction in pulmonary artery pressure and pulmonary vascular resistance associated with improvement in right ventricular function.[165]

The ages of recipients of heart-lung and lung transplantation for pulmonary hypertension have ranged from 2 months to 61 years.[166] Operative mortality ranges between 16 and 29 percent and is somewhat higher for recipients of a single-lung transplant. The 1-year survival rate is between 70 and 75 percent, the 2-year survival rate is between 55 and 60 percent, and the 5-year survival rate is between 40 and 45 percent. Transplantation should be reserved for patients with pulmonary hypertension who have progressed in spite of optimal medical management.[167] (Table 53–6).

Patients should be referred for evaluation for transplantation at the appropriate time.[168] The course of the disease and the waiting time must be taken into account, as well as other factors such as the anticipated waiting time before transplantation in the region and the expected survival after transplantation. It is generally accepted that patients should be considered for transplantation when they are New York Heart Association Functional Class III or IV in spite of medical therapy or when treatment with prostacyclin is failing or causing intolerable side effects.

The major long-term complications in patients who survive the operation are the high incidence of bronchiolitis obliterans in the transplanted lungs, acute organ rejection, and opportunistic infection.[169] Although several studies have documented significant improvement in quality of life after heart-lung and lung transplantation for pulmonary hypertension, cost-effectiveness has not yet been addressed. In many patients, prostacyclin may prove to be an ideal bridge to keep patients alive and stable until organs become available.[170]

▼ Secondary Pulmonary Hypertension

Although PPH is relatively rare, with an estimated incidence of 1 to 2 per million in the population, severe pulmonary arterial hypertension associated with other conditions is more common[171-177] (Table 53–7). The most common etiology is associated with collagen-vascular disease states, primarily scleroderma, including the CREST syndrome (calcinosis cutis, Raynaud phenomenon, esophageal dysfunction, sclerodactyly, and telangiectasia), and mixed connective tissue disease.[172] Pulmonary arterial hypertension is also relatively common in patients with congenital heart defects, especially those with ventricular septal defects or a patent ductus arteriosus.[174] Other major etiologies include cirrhosis with portal hypertension and HIV infection.[97, 177] In some instances, increased resistance to pulmonary blood flow downstream leads to what has been referred to as "passive" pulmonary hypertension because in many cases, elevation in pulmonary artery pressure but no significant elevation in pulmonary vascular resistance is observed. Reactive pulmonary hypertension often coexists in these states, with pulmonary artery pressure and pulmonary vascular resistance elevated to levels higher than can be accounted for purely by increased downstream resistance to blood flow. In some instances, relieving the downstream obstruction results in normalization of pulmonary artery pressure and pulmonary vascular resistance, whereas in other instances it may not. Failure of normalization has been believed to be related to chronicity of the reactive pulmonary hypertension leading to irreversible vascular changes, although this hypothesis has never been proved. When reactive pulmonary hypertension occurs, it often results in right ventricular failure, which can predominate in the patient's clinical symptomatology and lead to marked deterioration in functional class and death.

PULMONARY HYPERTENSION ASSOCIATED WITH COLLAGEN-VASCULAR DISEASES (see also Chap. 67)

Scleroderma, either from progressive systemic sclerosis or the CREST syndrome, is the most common etiology of pulmonary hypertension in collagen-vascular disease states.[171, 172] Scleroderma is associated with pulmonary hypertension in as many as one-third of patients, and CREST syndrome in as many as 50 percent.[172, 178] The high incidence suggests that periodic screening with echocardiography in these patients may be a reasonable practice. Although pulmonary hypertension may occur as a result of entrapment and obstruction of the pulmonary microvasculature by interstitial inflammation or fibrosis, patients initially seen with severe pulmonary hypertension usually do not have evidence of interstitial lung disease and have a pulmonary vasculature with histological features that resemble those of PPH.[179] Patients with systemic lupus erythematosus may also have pulmonary hypertension, although less common than in scleroderma. On occasion, pulmonary hypertension may precede the clinical diagnosis of lupus by several years. Mixed connective tissue disease is a less common form of collagen-vascular disease, but pulmonary hypertension may occur in as many as two-thirds of these patients. Pulmonary hypertension has also been described in patients with polymyositis, dermatomyositis, and rheumatoid arthritis.

Because collagen-vascular diseases may have an insidious onset and slowly progressive course, early recognition of the symptoms of pulmonary hypertension may be difficult. Although easy fatigability may be a feature of the collagen-vascular disease, it may also be an initial symptom of pulmonary hypertension. Dyspnea is still the most common initial symptom and should not be attributed to advancing age. Syncope, presyncope, or peripheral edema represents advanced pulmonary hypertension and right-sided heart failure. Physical findings of an elevated jugular venous pressure and an increased pulmonic component of the second heart sound along with a right ventricular fourth heart sound are typical features of pulmonary hypertension and warrant an evaluation for pulmonary hypertension. A murmur of tricuspid regurgitation generally reflects more advanced disease. Arterial hypoxemia is characteristic and should also prompt an evaluation of possible pulmonary hypertension in these patients.

The prognosis of patients with collagen-vascular disease in whom pulmonary hypertension develops is very poor.[179] Conventional therapy with digitalis, diuretics, and supplemental oxygen is used, and

▼ TABLE 53–7. ADVANCED PULMONARY HYPERTENSION BY DISEASE CATEGORY

DISEASE	PREVALENCE	PERCENTAGE OF PATIENTS WITH PH	ESTIMATED NUMBER IN NORTH AMERICA AND EUROPE
Systemic sclerosis	190/million	33	37,620
Congenital heart defects (ASD/VSD/PDA)	300/million	15–20	31,500
Cirrhosis	1600/million	0.6	5760
HIV related	2500/million	0.5	7500
Primary PH	7/million	100	4200

ASD = atrial septal defect; PDA = patent ductus arteriosus; PH = pulmonary hypertension; VSD = ventricular septal defect.

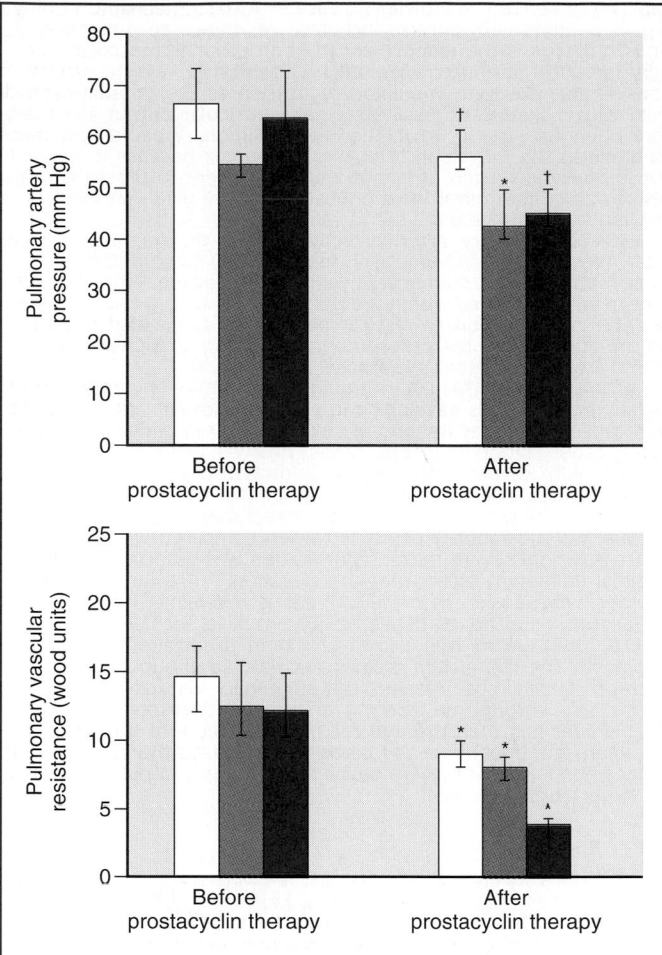

FIGURE 53–16. Mean pulmonary artery pressure (*top*) and pulmonary vascular resistance (*bottom*) before and after prostacyclin therapy in patients with secondary pulmonary hypertension. White bars indicate patients with congenital heart disease, striped bars indicate patients with collagen-vascular disease, and black bars indicate patients with portopulmonary hypertension. *$p < 0.01$. †$p < 0.05$ versus baseline. For all groups combined, mean pulmonary artery pressure fell 23% and pulmonary vascular resistance 50% after chronic (1 year) therapy. (From McLaughlin VV, Genthner DE, Panella MM, et al: Compassionate use of prostacyclin in the management of secondary pulmonary hypertension: A case series. Ann Intern Med 130:740–743, 1999.)

anticoagulation has been recommended to provide a survival benefit similar to the practice in PPH. Although the use of oral vasodilators has been disappointing, intravenous prostacyclin therapy has demonstrated therapeutic efficacy manifested by improved exercise tolerance, hemodynamics, and sense of well-being.[180, 181] Prostacyclin should be considered as a therapeutic intervention as early as possible in patients with pulmonary hypertension secondary to collagen-vascular disease. In patients with associated Raynaud phenomenon, it may provide relief of digital ischemia (Fig. 53–16).

INCREASED RESISTANCE TO PULMONARY VENOUS DRAINAGE

PATHOPHYSIOLOGY. Increased resistance to pulmonary venous drainage is a mechanism common to several conditions of diverse cause in which pulmonary arterial hypertension occurs. Altered resistance to pulmonary venous drainage may be the result of diseases affecting the left ventricle or pericardium, mitral or aortic valvular disease, or rare entities such as cor triatriatum, left atrial myxoma, or pulmonary venoocclusive disease (see below).

The magnitude of pulmonary hypertension depends, in part, on the performance of the right ventricle. In response to an acute stress such as pulmonary embolism, the normal right ventricle of an adult living at sea level can achieve systolic pulmonary pressures of 45 to 50 mm Hg, above which right ventricular failure supervenes. Systolic pressures of 80 to 100 mm Hg can be generated only by a hypertrophied right ventricle that is normally perfused. If right ventricular infarction or ischemia has occurred or if the right and left ventricles are both affected by a myopathic process, right ventricular failure occurs at lower pulmonary vascular pressure and severe pulmonary hypertension may not develop despite an increase in pulmonary vascular resistance.

In the presence of a healthy, nonischemic right ventricle, an increase in left atrial pressure from subnormal levels up to 7 mm Hg results in a fall in both pulmonary vascular resistance and the pressure gradient across the lungs. These reductions may reflect distention of a population of compliant small vessels, recruitment of additional vascular channels, or both. With further increases in left atrial pressure, pulmonary arterial pressure rises along with pulmonary venous pressure; i.e., at a constant pulmonary blood flow, the pressure gradient between the pulmonary artery and veins and pulmonary vascular resistance remains constant. Finally, when pulmonary venous pressure approaches or exceeds 25 mm Hg on a chronic basis, a disproportionate elevation in pulmonary artery pressure occurs; i.e., the pressure gradient between the pulmonary artery and veins rises while pulmonary blood flow remains constant or falls, which is indicative of an elevation in pulmonary vascular resistance that is due, in part, to pulmonary vasoconstriction. The latter occurs to a variable extent in response to passive elevations in pulmonary venous pressure and probably reflects the reactivity of the pulmonary vasculature, which may be variable between and within species.

Considerable variability in pulmonary arterial vasoconstriction is listed in response to pulmonary venous hypertension. Marked reactive pulmonary hypertension with pulmonary artery systolic pressures in excess of 80 mm Hg occurs in somewhat less than one-third of patients with pulmonary venous pressures elevated chronically in excess of 25 mm Hg. The fact that severe reactive pulmonary hypertension develops in less than one-third of patients with severe mitral stenosis also argues in favor of a spectrum of pulmonary vascular reactivity to chronic increases in pulmonary venous pressure.

The mechanism involved in elevating pulmonary vascular resistance is unclear. A neural component may be present; also, an elevation in pulmonary venous pressure may narrow or close airways, which may diminish ventilation and lead to hypoxia and, in turn, elevate pulmonary artery pressure. Finally, interstitial pulmonary edema secondary to pulmonary venous hypertension may encroach on the vascular lumen and contribute to the pulmonary arterial hypertension.

PATHOLOGY. Structural changes in the pulmonary vascular bed develop in association with chronic pulmonary venous hypertension, irrespective of its etiology. At the ultrastructural level, these changes include swelling of pulmonary capillary endothelial cells, thickening of their basal lamina, and wide separation of groups of connective tissue fibrils, indicative of interstitial edema. With persistence of the edema, reticular and elastic fibrils proliferate and the alveolar capillaries become embedded in dense connective tissue. The permeability of interendothelial junctions depends on pulmonary capillary pressure, with leakage of large molecules (40,000 to 60,000 daltons) occurring at capillary pressures in excess of approximately 30 mm Hg.

Light microscopic examination of the lungs of patients with pulmonary venous hypertension shows distention of pulmonary capillaries, thickening and rupture of the basement membranes of endothelial cells, and transudation of erythrocytes through these ruptured membranes into the alveolar spaces, which contain fragments of disintegrating erythrocytes. Pulmonary hemosiderosis is commonly observed and may progress to extensive fibrosis. In the late stages of pulmonary venous hypertension, areas of hemorrhage may be scattered throughout the lungs, edema fluid and coagulum may collect in the alveolar spaces, and widespread organization and fibrosis of pulmonary alveoli may be present. Occasionally, particularly in patients with chronic pulmonary venous hypertension caused by mitral valve disease, the alveolar spaces become ossified. Pulmonary lymphatics may become markedly distended and give the appearance of lymphangiectasis, particularly when pulmonary venous pressure chronically exceeds 30 mm Hg. Structural alterations in the small pulmonary arteries, arterioles, and venules include medial hypertrophy, intimal fibrosis, and rarely, necrotizing arteritis. However, plexiform lesions are not seen. The latter characterize the "irreversible" forms of pulmonary arterial hypertension.

PULMONARY HYPERTENSION SECONDARY TO ELEVATION IN LEFT VENTRICULAR DIASTOLIC PRESSURE

LEFT VENTRICULAR DIASTOLIC FAILURE. This condition may result from hypertension: aortic stenosis; ischemic heart disease; hypertrophic, restrictive, and congestive cardiomyopathies; and constrictive pericarditis. Chronic increases in mean left ventricular filling pressure exceeding 25 mm Hg are uncommon, and the resulting pulmonary arterial hypertension is usually moderate unless reactive pulmonary hypertension also occurs.

Increased pulmonary artery pressure in patients with left ventricular dysfunction is a marker of poor prognosis. Pulmonary hypertension is associated with more frequent episodes of congestive heart failure and excess mortality after heart transplantation.[182] Pulmonary hypertension may result from an increase in left atrial pressure and pulmonary vascular resistance and possibly from the loss of endothelium-dependent vasodilatation of the pulmonary arterial bed. The severity of pulmonary hypertension in patients with left ventricular dysfunction is widely variable and independent of the degree of left ventricular dysfunction or associated functional mitral regurgitation. Many patients will improve considerably if effective medical therapy can be identified that will lower left ventricular end-diastolic pressure.[183] Identifying the basis for the increase in this pressure is essential.

PULMONARY HYPERTENSION SECONDARY TO LEFT ATRIAL HYPERTENSION

Mitral Valve Disease (see also Chap. 46).

MITRAL STENOSIS. This valvular lesion represents an important cause of pulmonary hypertension. Although the pulmonary hypertension associated with mitral stenosis is initially a result of an increase in resistance to pulmonary venous drainage and backward transmission of the elevated left atrial pressure, many patients subsequently exhibit marked pulmonary vasoconstriction and anatomical changes in vessels, so the pulmonary hypertension is "reactive" as well as "passive." The elevation in pulmonary vascular resistance and the associated pulmonary hypertension may come to dominate the clinical picture in mitral stenosis. Thus, patients with mitral stenosis often have what might be considered to be a more proximal obstruction at the level of the pulmonary arterioles and small muscular arteries, with resultant pulmonary hypertension equal to or exceeding systemic arterial pressure during exertion and sometimes even at rest. The clinical picture in such patients is characterized by right ventricular failure with distended neck veins, hepatomegaly, and ascites. These patients exhibit marked fatigue, occasionally a more serious complaint than dyspnea. The murmur of mitral stenosis may be soft or even inaudible, and the opening snap of the stenotic mitral valve may be indistinguishable from a loud pulmonic component of S₂ as a result of narrowing of the S_2 opening snap interval. Pulmonary congestion and edema may not be prominent clinically. Cardiac output is usually markedly reduced. This constellation of findings may obscure the underlying diagnosis of mitral stenosis and suggest instead either PPH or pulmonary hypertension secondary to some other disorder.

Diagnostic Studies. The echocardiogram shows left atrial enlargement and thickened mitral valve leaflets whose mobility is markedly reduced. At cardiac catheterization, the pulmonary arterial hypertension is associated with substantial elevations in pulmonary wedge pressure, and a sizable (> 10 mm Hg) pressure gradient is generally noted between pulmonary capillary wedge and left ventricular diastolic pressure. These findings are of key importance in distinguishing mitral stenosis from pulmonary arterial hypertension, a condition in which left atrial size and the wedge pressure are normal and in which no diastolic pressure gradient can be found between the wedge and left ventricular pressure.

Protection Against Pulmonary Edema. At least three mechanisms that tend to protect against pulmonary edema formation are operative in patients with mitral stenosis and chronic elevations in pulmonary venous pressure in excess of 25 mm Hg (see Chap. 17). First, lymphatic drainage of the pulmonary interstitium increases abruptly when pulmonary venous pressure is increased to 25 mm Hg. Acute increases in pulmonary lymph flow of up to 8 times the resting level occur when pulmonary venous pressure is raised to 30 mm Hg for a 10-minute interval, and the increased lymphatic flow persists at high levels for 30 to 60 minutes after pulmonary venous pressure has returned to normal. In models of *chronic* pulmonary venous pressure elevation, increases in pulmonary lymph flow of up to 28 times normal have been observed.

Diminished permeability of the capillary-alveolar barrier is a second protective mechanism that might be operative in patients with *chronic* pulmonary venous hypertension in excess of 25 mm Hg. There is morphological evidence of thickening of the layer between the capillary lumen and the alveolar space.[184] A third mechanism operating in patients with chronic increased resistance to pulmonary venous drainage is the reactive constriction of small muscular pulmonary arteries and arterioles. This constriction, which results in considerable elevation in pulmonary artery pressure, is usually associated with a significant decline in right ventricular output and therefore pulmonary blood flow). The lower pulmonary blood flow tends to diminish the formation of pulmonary edema because it results in substantially lower left atrial and pulmonary venous pressure at any given size of the mitral valve orifice or for any given impairment in left ventricular function.

Effects of Surgery. After corrective surgery on the mitral valve or after mitral balloon valvuloplasty (see Chap. 46), both pulmonary vascular resistance and pulmonary hypertension decline,[185] the major extent of which is noted within the first postoperative week. The extent of reversal of pulmonary vascular obstruction has varied depending on the adequacy of the procedure in producing an increase in mitral orifice area and whether mitral valve restenosis.[186]

MITRAL REGURGITATION. Although pulmonary hypertension is widely recognized as developing in patients with left atrial hypertension caused by mitral stenosis, it can also occur in patients with pure mitral regurgitation.[187] In one series, nearly half of a cohort of 41 patients with severe mitral regurgitation had pulmonary artery systolic pressures in excess of 50 mm Hg. In this subgroup of patients, pulmonary vascular resistance was three times normal and cardiac output was substantially depressed when compared with that in patients in whom severe mitral regurgitation was associated with only minimal pulmonary artery pressure elevation.[187] Presumably, the pulmonary hypertension in these patients is reversible, just as it is in mitral stenosis, although data on this point have not been reported.

COR TRIATRIATUM (see also Chap. 43). In this malformation, partitioning of the left atrium creates two left atrial subchambers. The posterior subchamber receives the pulmonary venous inflow, which then drains through an opening in the partition into the anterior subchamber and then through the mitral orifice into the left ventricle. When the opening in the partition separating the two left atrial subchambers is small, severe pulmonary venous and pulmonary arterial hypertension result.

INCREASED RESISTANCE TO FLOW THROUGH THE PULMONARY VASCULAR BED

Pulmonary Parenchymal Disease

This important cause of pulmonary hypertension is discussed in Chapter 54.

Eisenmenger Syndrome

(see also Chaps. 43 and 44)

Decreased cross-sectional area of the pulmonary arteriolar bed with irreversible pulmonary hypertension characterizes the so-called Eisenmenger syndrome. This term was used by Wood[188] to refer to patients with congenital cardiac lesions and severe pulmonary hypertension in whom reversal of a left-to-right shunt has occurred. Left-to-right shunts are usually due to congenital cardiovascular malformations (e.g., atrial and ventricular septal defects, patent ductus arteriosus).

PATHOPHYSIOLOGY. Pulmonary hypertension in congenital heart disease may occur simply because of increased pulmonary blood flow. When chronic, the increased pulmonary flow is often associated with a passive reduction in pulmonary resistance and little elevation in pulmonary vascular pressure. In a normal adult with pulmonary blood flow (PBF) of 5 liters/min, pulmonary vascular resistance (PVR) of 60 dyne-sec·cm⁻⁵, and mean left atrial pressure (LA) of 6 mm Hg, the pulmonary artery mean pressure (PA) may be calculated from the expression

$$PVR = \frac{(PA - LA)80}{PBF} = \frac{(PA - 6)80}{5} = 60 \text{ dyne-sec} \cdot cm^{-5}$$

$$PA = \frac{60 \times 5}{80} + 6 = 10 \text{ mm Hg}$$

If PBF is doubled, a reduction in pulmonary vascular resistance to 30 dyne-sec·cm⁻⁵ maintains pulmonary artery mean pressure at a normal level of 10 mm Hg. However, if PBF is increased fourfold to sixfold, the reserve capacity of the pulmonary vascular bed is exceeded, and pulmonary artery pressure rises. Thus, if the pulmonary vascular resistance is 30 dyne-sec·cm^{-5}, a PBF of 30 liters/min is associated with a mean pulmonary artery pressure that is only minimally elevated at 17 mm Hg, although the high right ventricular stroke volumes associated with the augmentation in PBF result in considerably higher values (40 to 45 mm Hg) for pulmonary artery and right ventricular systolic pressure. If no underlying arteriolar vascular disease exists, abolition of the shunt by corrective surgery restores PBF and pulmonary artery pressure to normal.

If a congenital cardiovascular defect causes pulmonary hypertension from the time of birth, the small, muscular arteries of the fetal lung may undergo delayed or only partial involution, with subsequent persistently high levels of pulmonary vascular resistance. This is especially true in lesions in which a left-to-right shunt enters the right ventricle or pulmonary artery directly (i.e., a posttricuspid valve shunt, such as ventricular septal defect or patent ductus arteriosus); these patients experience a higher incidence of severe and irreversible pulmonary vascular damage than do those in whom the shunt is proximal to the tricuspid valve (pretricuspid shunts, as in atrial septal defect and partial anomalous pulmonary venous drainage). In the latter category, pulmonary hypertension may result from a large pretricuspid left-to-right shunt, which enhances the risk of pulmonary vascular damage.

PATHOLOGY. The extent of reversibility of pulmonary vascular obstructive disease in the presence of congenital heart disease varies. From an anatomical point of view, reversible conditions are those in which the decreased pulmonary arteriolar cross-sectional area is the result of medial hypertrophy and vasoconstriction; irreversibility is associated with the presence of necrotizing arteritis and plexiform lesions in these small vessels. The classification by Heath and Edwards[3] of six grades of structural change is widely used to assess the potential reversibility of pulmonary vascular disease and is summarized as follows: *Grade I* is characterized by hypertrophy of the media of small muscular pulmonary arteries and arterioles. In *grade II,* intimal cellular proliferation is added to the medial hypertrophy. *Grade III* is characterized by advanced medial thickening with hypertrophy and hyperplasia, together with progressive intimal proliferation and concentric fibrosis that result in obliteration of many arterioles and small arteries. In *grade IV,* dilatation and so-called plexiform lesions of the muscular pulmonary arteries and arterioles are observed. The latter consist of a plexiform network of capillary-like channels within a dilated segment of a muscular pulmonary artery. The channels are separated by proliferating endothelial cells that often contain thrombi; indeed, the network of capillary channels may constitute recanalization of a thrombus. *Grade V* changes include complex plexiform, angiomatous, and cavernous lesions and hyalinization of intimal fibrosis. Finally, *grade VI* is characterized by the presence of necrotizing arteritis.

The Heath-Edwards classification implies that the morphological alterations are sequential, with grade I being the earliest stage and grade VI being the "end stage" of pulmonary vascular obliterative disease. That such an orderly progression may not in fact occur is suggested by the findings of Wagenvoort, which indicate that plexiform lesions develop gradually in areas affected by necrotizing arteritis. Fibrinoid necrosis of a small segment of a pulmonary arterial branch has been suggested to lead to medial destruction and subsequent aneurysmal dilatation of the vessel, as well as the formation of a fibrin clot in the lumen, often with an admixture of platelets. Organization of the fibrin clot by strands of intimal cells leads to formation of the plexus; the small capillary-like channels within the plexus provide continuity to the distal portion of the artery, which undergoes poststenotic dilatation. With time, the inflammatory component of the process subsides, fibrin disappears, and the strands of intimal cells become fibrotic. Wagenvoort's view is supported by animal experiments in which end-to-end systemic-pulmonary anastomoses resulted in arteritis and fibrinoid necrosis before the appearance of plexiform lesions. Thus, although Heath-Edwards grades I, II,

and III may represent chronological progression, evidence exists that grade VI (necrotizing arteritis) changes appear next, followed by grades IV and V as end-stage alterations.

CLINICAL CONSIDERATIONS. *Eisenmenger syndrome* is applied to any anomalous circulatory communication that leads to obliterative pulmonary vascular disease, including pretricuspid and posttricuspid shunts. Health-Edwards grade IV to VI changes are usual in these patients; occasionally, lesser anatomical changes predominate and may be reversible after successful corrective surgery. The long-term prognosis of patients with the Eisenmenger syndrome is substantially better than that of patients with other conditions associated with pulmonary hypertension.[189] Patients with the Eisenmenger syndrome have an 80 percent survival rate at 10 years, a 77 percent survival rate at 15 years, and a 42 percent survival rate at 25 years.[190, 191] Survival is typically related to mean right atrial pressure and pulmonary vascular resistance.

When pulmonary vascular resistance has increased so that it equals or exceeds systemic resistance and the anatomical changes of the pulmonary vessels are predominantly those of grades IV to VI, surgical closure of the anomalous circulatory communication will be associated with a prohibitive immediate risk and, if the patient survives, will usually fail to relieve pulmonary hypertension. Surgery may in fact hasten death in most survivors who had either balanced shunts or predominant right-to-left shunts because closure of the right-to-left communication merely increases the load on an already overburdened right ventricle. Structural changes in the pulmonary vascular bed are evident in pulmonary arteriograms, which reveal dilated central pulmonary arteries and narrowing of the peripheral branches. These changes can be evaluated by means of quantitative analysis of the pulmonary wedge angiogram.[192]

Intravenous prostacyclin therapy is highly effective and has been shown to improve exercise tolerance, quality of life, and hemodynamics in patients with congenital heart disease irrespective of the severity or duration of the condition[181, 193] (see Fig. 53-16). It is effective in patients who have had previous surgical repair of their defect and in those who have not. No increased incidence of systemic side effects has been noted in patients who have a persistent right-to-left shunt. Long-term prostacyclin therapy may slow the progression of Eisenmenger syndrome and render some patients eligible for partial surgical repair consisting of atrial septostomy.[193] In patients who have bidirectional shunts, the use of prostacyclin may be a therapeutic strategy to enable a patient who is considered inoperable to become eligible for surgery at a later date.

Other Conditions Associated with Decreased Cross-Sectional Area of the Pulmonary Vascular Bed

PERSISTENT FETAL CIRCULATION IN THE NEWBORN (see also Chap. 43). This condition has been reported as a cause of severe pulmonary hypertension.[194, 194a] Affected infants exhibit cyanosis, tachypnea, acidemia, normal pulmonary parenchymal markings on chest radiography, and anatomically normal hearts. Cyanosis is the result of right-to-left shunting across the foramen ovale and through a patent ductus arteriosus. The condition may be due to persistence of extremely muscular small pulmonary arteries, a diminution in the absolute number of these resistance vessels, or a combination of the two.[195]

PULMONARY THROMBOEMBOLISM. This important cause of pulmonary hypertension is discussed in Chapter 52.

NORMAL PULMONARY CIRCULATION

1. Comroe JH: The main functions of the pulmonary circulation. Circulation 33:146, 1966.
2. Pietra GG: The pathology of primary pulmonary hypertension. *In* Rubin LJ, Rich S (eds): Primary Pulmonary Hypertension. New York, Marcel Dekker, 1997, pp 19–61.
3. Wagenvoort CA, Wagenvoort N: Pathology of Pulmonary Hypertension. 2nd ed. New York, John Wiley & Sons, 1977.
4. Fritts HW, Harris P, Chidsey CA, et al: Estimation of flow rate through bronchial-pulmonary vascular anastomoses with use of T-1824 dye. Circulation 23:390, 1961.
5. Barratt-Boyes BG, Wood EH: Cardiac output and related measurements and pressure values in the right heart and associated vessels, together with an analysis of the hemodynamic response to the inhalation of high oxygen mixtures in healthy subjects. J Lab Clin Med 51:72, 1958.
6. Glenny RW: Blood flow distribution in the lung. Chest 114 (Suppl):8–16, 1998.
7. Reeves JT, Taylor AE: Pulmonary hemodynamics and fluid exchange in the lungs during exercise. *In* Rowell LB, Shepherd JT (eds): Handbook of Physiology. New York, Oxford University Press, 1996, pp 585–613.
8. Rudolph AM: The changes in the circulation after birth. Their importance in congenital heart disease. Circulation 41:343, 1970.
9. Bergofsky EH: Mechanisms underlying vasomotor regulation of regional pulmonary blood flow in normal and disease states. Am J Med 57:378, 1974.
10. Davidson WR, Fee EC: Influence of aging on pulmonary hemodynamics in a population free of coronary artery disease. Am J Cardiol 65:1454, 1990.
11. Ghali JK, Liao Y, Cooper RS, et al: Changes in pulmonary hemodynamics with aging in a predominantly hypertensive population. Am J Cardiol 70:367, 1992.
12. Cacciapuoti F, D'Avino M, Lama D, et al: Hemodynamic change in pulmonary circulation induced by effort in the elderly. Am J Cardiol 7:1481, 1993.
13. Rich S, Chomka E, Hasara L, et al: The prevalence of pulmonary hypertension in the United States. Chest 96:236, 1989.
14. Fishman AP: Hypoxia on the pulmonary circulation: How and where it acts. Circ Res 38:221, 1976.
15. Fishman AP: The enigma of hypoxic pulmonary vasoconstriction. *In* Fishman AP (ed): The Pulmonary Circulation: Normal and Abnormal. Philadelphia, University of Pennsylvania Press, 1990, pp 109–129.
16. Weir EK, Reeve HL, Peterson DA, et al: Pulmonary vasoconstriction, oxygen sensing, and the role of ion channels. Chest 114(Suppl):17–22, 1998.
17. Enson Y, Giuntini C, Lewis ML, et al: The influence of hydrogen ion concentration and hypoxia on the pulmonary circulation. J Clin Invest 43:1146, 1964.
18. Salvi SS: α_1-Adrenergic hypothesis for pulmonary hypertension. Chest 115:1708–1719, 1999.
18a. Bevan RD: Influence of adrenergic innervation on vascular growth and mature characteristics. Am Rev Respir Dis 140(Suppl):147–148, 1989.
19. Bevan JA, Oriowo MA, Bevan RD: Physiological variation in α-adrenoreceptor–mediated arterial sensitivity: Relation to agonist affinity. Science 234:196–197, 1986.
20. Minneman KP: α_1-Adrenergic receptor subtypes, inositol phosphates and sources of cell Ca^{2+}. Pharmacol Rev 40:87–119, 1988.
21. Takizawa T, Hara Y, Saito T, et al. α_1-Adrenoreceptor stimulation partially inhibits ATP sensitive K^+ current in guinea pig ventricular cells: Attenuation of the action potential shortening induced by hypoxia and K^+ channel openers. J Cardiovasc Pharmacol 28:799–808, 1996.
22. Weir EK, Reeve HL, Huang JMC, et al: Anorexic agents aminorex, fenfluramine and dexfenfluramine inhibit potassium current in rat pulmonary vascular smooth muscle and cause pulmonary vasoconstriction. Circulation 94:2216–2220, 1996.
23. Schaiberger PH, Kennedy TC, Miller FC, et al: Pulmonary hypertension associated with the long term inhalation of "crank" methamphetamine. Chest 104:614–616, 1993.
24. Bento AC, de Moraes S: Effects of estrogen pretreatment of the spare α_1-adrenoreceptors and the slow and fast components of the contractile response of the isolated female rat aorta. Gen Pharmacol 23:565–570, 1992.
25. Kadowitz PJ, Hyman AL: Differential effects of prostaglandins A_1 and A_2 on pulmonary vascular resistance in the dog. Proc Soc Exp Biol Med 149:282, 1975.
26. Vane JR, Anggard EE, Botting RM: Regulatory functions of the vascular endothelium. N Engl J Med 323:27, 1990.
27. Israels SJ, Cheang T, Roberston G, et al: Impaired signal transduction in neonatal platelets. Pediatr Res 45:687–691, 1999.
28. Moncada S: Prostacyclin, from discovery to clinical application. J Pharmacol 16:71, 1985.
29. Murtha YM, Allen BM, Orr JA: The role of protein kinase C in thromboxane A(2)–induced pulmonary artery vasoconstriction. J Biomed Sci 6:293–295, 1999.
30. Cooper CJ, Landzberg MJ, Anderson TJ: Role of nitric oxide in the local regulation of pulmonary vascular resistance in humans. Circulation 93:266–271, 1996.
31. Cooper CJ, Jevnikar FW, Walsh T, et al: The influence of basal nitric oxide activity on pulmonary vascular resistance in patients with congestive heart failure. Am J Cardiol 82:609–614, 1998.
32. Bouloumie A, Schini-Kerth VB, Busse R: Vascular endothelial growth factor up-regulates nitric oxide synthase expression in endothelial cells. Cardiovasc Res 41:773–780, 1999.
33. Giaid A, Yanagisawa M, Langleben D: Expression of endothelin-1 in the lungs of patients with pulmonary hypertension. N Engl J Med 328:1732–1739, 1993.
34. Giaid A: Nitric oxide and endothelin-1 in pulmonary hypertension. Chest 114(Suppl):208–212, 1998.
35. Weir EK, Reeve HL, Johnson G, et al: A role for potassium channels in smooth muscle cells and platelets in the etiology of primary pulmonary hypertension. Chest 114(Suppl):200–204, 1998.
36. Vanhoutte PM: Endothelial dysfunction and atherosclerosis. Eur Heart J 18:E19–E29, 1997.
37. Fanburg BL, Lee SL: A new role for an old molecule: Serotonin as a mitogen. Am J Physiol 272:L795–L806, 1997.
38. Abraham WT, Raynolds MV, Gottschall B, et al: Importance of angiotensin-converting enzyme in pulmonary hypertension. Cardiology 86(Suppl):9–15, 1995.

PRIMARY PULMONARY HYPERTENSION

39. Rubin LJ: ACCP consensus statement. Primary pulmonary hypertension. Chest 104:236, 1993.
40. Abenhaim L, Moride Y, Brenot F, et al: Appetite-suppressant drugs and the risk of primary pulmonary hypertension. N Engl J Med 335:609–616, 1996.
40a. Lilienfeld DE, Rubin LJ: Mortality from primary pulmonary hypertension in the United States, 1979–1996. Chest 117:796, 2000.
41. Higenbottam TW, Laude EA: Endothelial dysfunction providing the basis for the treatment of pulmonary hypertension. Chest 114(Suppl):72–79, 1998.
42. Wood P: Pulmonary hypertension with special reference to the vasoconstrictive factor. Br Heart J 20:557, 1958.
43. Palevsky HI, Schloo BL, Pietra GG, et al: Primary pulmonary hypertension: Vascular structure, morphometry, and responsiveness to vasodilator agents. Circulation 80:1207–1221, 1989.
44. Uren NG, Ludman PE, Crake T, et al: Response of the pulmonary circulation to acetylcholine, calcitonin, gene-related peptide, substance P_1 and oral nicardipine in patients with primary pulmonary hypertension. J Am Coll Cardiol 19:835, 1992.
45. Giaid A, Saleh D: Reduced expression of endothelial nitric oxide synthase in the lungs of patients with pulmonary hypertension. N Engl J Med 333:214–221, 1995.
46. Celermajer DS, Cullen S, Deanfiled JE: Impairment of endothelium-dependent pulmonary artery relaxation in children with congenital heart disease and abnormal pulmonary hemodynamics. Circulation 87:440, 1993.
47. Okada M, Yamashita C, Okada M, et al: Endothelin receptor antagonists in a beagle model of pulmonary hypertension: Contribution of possible potential therapy. J Am Coll Cardiol 25:1213, 1995.
48. Stewart DJ, Levy RD, Cernacek P, et al: Increased plasma endothelin-1 in pulmonary hypertension: Marker or mediator of disease? Ann Intern Med 114:464, 1991.
49. Pietra GG, Edwards WD, Kay JM, et al: Histopathology of primary pulmonary hypertension. A qualitative and quantitative study of pulmonary blood vessels from 58 patients in the National Heart, Lung, and Blood Institute, Primary Pulmonary Hypertension Registry. Circulation 80:1198, 1989.
50. Edwards WD, Edwards JE: Clinical primary pulmonary hypertension—three pathological types. Circulation 56:884, 1977.
51. Lindner V, Lappi DA, Baird A, et al: Role of basic fibroblast growth factor in vascular lesion formation. Circ Res 63:106–113, 1991.
52. Pierce GF, Mastoe TA, Lingelbach J, et al: Platelet-derived growth factor β and transforming growth factor-β enhance tissue repair activities by unique mechanisms. J Cell Biol 109:429, 1989.
53. Botney MD, Bahadori L, Gold LI: Vascular remodeling in primary pulmonary hypertension. Potential role for transforming growth factor-β. Am J Pathol 144:286, 1994.
54. Bodreau N, Rabinovitch M: Developmentally regulated changes in extracellular matrix in endothelial and smooth muscle cells in the ductus arteriosus may be related to intimal proliferation. Lab Invest 64:187, 1991.
55. Botney MD, Liptay MJ, Kaiser LR, et al: Active collagen synthesis by pulmonary arteries in human primary pulmonary hypertension. Am J Pathol 143:121, 1993.
56. Rich S, Brundage BH: Pulmonary hypertension: A cellular basis for understanding the pathophysiology and treatment. J Am Coll Cardiol 14:545, 1989.
57. Hassell KL: Altered hemostasis in pulmonary hypertension. Blood Coagul Fibrinolysis 9:107–117, 1998.
57a. Wolf M: Thrombotic risk factors in pulmonary hypertension. Eur Resp J 15:395, 2000.
58. Welsh CH, Hassell KL, Badesch DB, et al: Coagulation and fibrinolytic profiles in patients with severe pulmonary hypertension. Chest 110:710–717, 1996.
59. Fuster V, Steele PM, Edwards WD, et al: Primary pulmonary hyperten-

sion: Natural history and the importance of thrombosis. Circulation 70: 580, 1984.
60. Morse JH, Barst RJ, Fotino M, et al: Primary pulmonary hypertension, tissue plasminogen activator antibodies, and HLA-DQ7. Am J Respir Crit Care Med 155:274–278, 1997.
61. Loscalzo J: Endothelial dysfunction in pulmonary hypertension. N Engl J Med 327:117–119, 1992.
62. Ware JA, Helstad DD: Platelet-endothelium interactions. N Engl J Med 328:628, 1993.
63. Nakonechnicov S, Gabbasov Z, Chazova I, et al: Platelet aggregation in patients with pulmonary hypertension. Blood Coagul Fibrinolysis 7: 225–227, 1996.
64. Botney MD: Role of hemodynamics in pulmonary vascular remodeling, implications for primary pulmonary hypertension. Am J Respir Crit Care Med 159:361–364, 1999.
65. Okada K, Bernstein ML, Zhang W, et al: Angiotensin-converting enzyme inhibition delays pulmonary vascular neointimal formation. Am J Respir Crit Care Med 158:939–950, 1998.
66. Schuster DP, Crouch EC, Parks WC, et al: Angiotensin converting enzyme expression in primary pulmonary hypertension. Am J Respir Crit Care Med 154:1087–1091, 1998.
67. Morrell NW, Atochina EN, Morris KG, et al: Angiotensin converting enzyme expression is increased in small pulmonary arteries of rats with hypoxia-induced pulmonary hypertension. J Clin Invest 96:1823–1833, 1995.
68. Rabinovitch M: Insights into the pathogenesis of primary pulmonary hypertension from animal models. In Rubin LJ, Rich S (ed): Primary Pulmonary Hypertension. New York, Marcel Dekker, 1997, pp 63–82.
69. Rabinovitch M: Elastase and the pathobiology of unexplained pulmonary hypertension. Chest 114(Suppl):213–224, 1998.
70. Yuan JX, Aldinger AM, Juhaszova M, et al: Dysfunctional voltage-gated K+ channels in pulmonary artery smooth muscle cells of patients with primary pulmonary hypertension. Circulation 98:1400–1406, 1998.
71. Tuder RM, Cool CD, Geraci MW, et al: Prostacyclin synthase expression is decreased in lungs from patients with severe pulmonary hypertension. Am J Respir Crit Care Med 159:1925–1932, 1999.
72. Sibbald W, Peters S, Lindsay RM: Serotonin and pulmonary hypertension in septic ARDS. Crit Care Med 8:490–494, 1980.
73. Breuer J, Georgaraki A, Sieverding L, et al: Increased turnover of serotonin in children with pulmonary hypertension secondary to congenital heart disease. Pediatr Cardiol 17:214–219, 1996.
74. Herve P, Drouet L, Dosquet C, et al: Primary pulmonary hypertension in a patient with a familial platelet storage pool disease: Role of serotonin. Am J Med 89:117–120, 1990.
75. Herve P, Launay JM, Scrobohaci ML, et al: Increased plasma serotonin in primary pulmonary hypertension. Am J Med 99:249–254, 1995.
76. Rich S, Dantzker DR, Ayres SM, et al: Primary pulmonary hypertension: A national prospective study. Ann Intern Med 107:216–223, 1987.
77. Loyd JE, Newman JH: Familial primary pulmonary hypertension. In Rubin LJ, Rich S (ed). Primary Pulmonary Hypertension. New York, Marcel Dekker, 1997, pp 151–162.
78. Barst R, Loyd JE: Genetics and immunogenetic aspects of primary pulmonary hypertension. Chest 114(Suppl):231–236, 1998.
78a. Deng Z: Fine mapping of PPHI, a gene for familial primary pulmonary hypertension, to a 3-cM region on chromosome 2q33. Am J Resp Crit Care Med 161:1055, 2000.
79. Morse JH, Jones AC, Barst RJ, et al: Mapping of familial primary pulmonary hypertension locus (PPH1) to chromosome 2q31–q32. Circulation 95:2603–2606, 1997.
80. Moride Y, Abenhaim L, Xu J: Epidemiology of primary pulmonary hypertension. In Rubin LJ, Rich S (ed): Primary Pulmonary Hypertension. New York, Marcel Dekker, 1997, pp 163–178.
81. Lange PA, Stoller JK: The hepatopulmonary syndrome. Ann Intern Med 122:521–529, 1995.
82. Hopkins WE, Waggoner AD, Barzilai B: Frequency and significance of intrapulmonary right-to-left shunting in end-stage hepatic disease. Am J Cardiol 70:516, 1992.
83. Groves BM, Brundage BH, Elliott CG, et al: Pulmonary hypertension associated with hepatic cirrhosis. In Fishman AP (ed): The Pulmonary Circulation: Normal and Abnormal. Philadelphia, University of Pennsylvania Press, 1990, pp 359–369.
84. Robalino BD, Moodie DS: Association between primary pulmonary hypertension and portal hypertension: Analysis of its pathophysiology and clinical, laboratory and hemodynamic manifestations. J Am Coll Cardiol 17:492, 1991.
85. Kuo PC, Plotkin JS, Johnson LB, et al: Distinctive clinical features of portopulmonary hypertension. Chest 112:980–986, 1997.
86. Hervé P, Lebrec D, Brenot F, et al: Pulmonary vascular disorders in portal hypertension. Eur Respir J 11:1153–1166, 1998.
87. Goto M, Takei Y, Kuwano S, et al: Tumor necrosis factor and endotoxin in the pathogenesis of liver and pulmonary injuries after orthotopic liver transplantation in the rat. Hepatology 16:487, 1992.
88. Voelkel NF, Tuder RM: Cellular and molecular mechanisms in the pathogenesis of severe pulmonary hypertension. Eur Respir J 8:2129–2138, 1995.
89. Kuo P: Pulmonary hypertension: Considerations in the liver transplant candidate. Transpl Int 9:141–150, 1996.
90. Schott R, Chaouat A, Launoy A, et al: Improvement of pulmonary hypertension after liver transplantation. Chest 115:1748–1749, 1999.
91. Gurtner HP: Pulmonary hypertension, "plexogenic pulmonary arteriopa-

thy" and the appetite depressant drug aminorex: Post or propter? Bull Physiopathol Respir (Nancy) 15:897, 1979.
92. Douglas JG, Monro JF, Kitchin AH, et al: Pulmonary hypertension and fenfluramine. BMJ 283:881, 1981.
93. Brenot F, Herve P, Pettipretz P, et al: Primary pulmonary hypertension and fenfluramine use. Br Heart J 70:537, 1993.
94. Simonneau G, Fartoukh M, Sitbon O, et al: Primary pulmonary hypertension associated with the use of fenfluramine derivatives. Chest 114(Suppl):195–199, 1998.
94a. Rich S, Rubin L, Walker AM, et al: Anorexigens and pulmonary hypertension in the United States: Results from the surveillance of North American pulmonary hypertension. Chest 117:870, 2000.
95. Weir EK, Reeve HL, Huang JM, et al: Anorexic agents aminorex, fenfluramine, and dexfenfluramine inhibit potassium current in rat pulmonary vascular smooth muscle and cause pulmonary vasoconstriction. Circulation 94:2216–2220, 1996.
96. Archer SL, Djaballah K, Humbert M, et al: Nitric oxide deficiency in fenfluramine- and dexfenfluramine-induced pulmonary hypertension. Am J Respir Crit Care Med 158:1061–1067, 1998.
97. Speich R, Jenni R, Opravil M, et al: Primary pulmonary hypertension in HIV infection. Chest 100:1268–1271, 1991.
98. Pettipretz P, Brenot F, Azarian R, et al: Pulmonary hypertension in patients with human immunodeficiency virus infection. Circulation 89:2772, 1994.
99. Mette SA, Palevsky HI, Pietra GG, et al: Primary pulmonary hypertension in association with human immunodeficiency virus infection. Am Rev Respir Dis 145:1196, 1992.
100. Humbert M, Monti G, Fartoukh M, et al: Platelet-derived growth factor expression in primary pulmonary hypertension: Comparison of HIV seropositive and HIV seronegative patients. Eur Respir J 11:554–559, 1998.
101. Opravil M, Pechère M, Speich R, et al: HIV-associated primary pulmonary hypertension: A case control study. Am J Respir Crit Care Med 155:990–995, 1997.
102. Alpert MA, Bauer JH, Parker BM, et al: Pulmonary hypertension in systemic hypertension. South Med J 78:784, 1995.
103. Guazzi MD, DeCasare N, Fiorentini C, et al: Pulmonary vascular supersensitivity to catecholamines in systemic high blood pressure. J Am Coll Cardiol 8:1137, 1986.
104. Moruzzi P, Sganzerla P, Guazzi MD: Pulmonary vasoconstriction overreactivity in borderline systemic hypertension. Cardiovasc Res 23:666, 1989.
105. Yamaki S, Horiuchi T, Miura M, et al: Pulmonary vascular disease in secundum atrial septal defect with pulmonary hypertension. Chest 89:694, 1986.
106. Okura H, Takatsu Y: High-output heart failure as a cause of pulmonary hypertension. Intern Med 33:363, 1994.
107. Voelkel NF, Tuder RM, Weir EK: Pathophysiology of primary pulmonary hypertension: From physiology to molecular mechanisms. In Rubin LJ, Rich S (ed): Primary Pulmonary Hypertension. New York, Marcel Dekker, 1997, pp 83–129.
108. Lee S, Shroyer KR, Markham NE, et al: Monoclonal endothelial cell proliferation is present in primary but not secondary pulmonary hypertension. J Clin Invest 101:927–934, 1998.
109. Tuder RM: Plexiform lesions in primary pulmonary hypertension may represent an abnormal form of angiogenesis. Semin Respir Crit Care Med 15:207–214, 1994.
110. Tuder RM, Groves B, Badesch DB, et al: Exuberant endothelial cell growth and elements of inflammation are present in plexiform lesions of pulmonary hypertension. Am J Pathol 144:275–285, 1994.
111. Wagenvoort CA, Mulder GH: Thrombotic lesions in primary plexogenic arteriopathy. Chest 103:844–849, 1993.
112. Clausen KP, Geer JC: Hypertensive pulmonary arteritis. Am J Dis Child 118:718, 1969.
113. Rich S: Primary pulmonary hypertension. Prog Cardiovasc Dis 31:205, 1988.
114. Swensen SJ, Tashjian JH, Myers JL, et al: Pulmonary venoocclusive disease: CT findings in eight patients. AJR Am J Roentgenol 167:937–940, 1996.
115. Valdes L, Gonzalez-Juanatey JR, Alvarez D, et al: Diagnosis of pulmonary veno-occlusive disease: New criteria for biopsy. Respir Med 92:979–983, 1998.
116. Magee F, Wright JL, Kay MJ, et al: Pulmonary capillary hemangiomatosis. Am Rev Respir Dis 132:922, 1985.
117. Dufour B, Maitre S, Humbert M, et al: High-resolution CT of the chest in four patients with pulmonary capillary hemangiomatosis or pulmonary venoocclusive disease. AJR Am J Roentgenol 171:1321–1324, 1998.
118. Eltorky MA, Headley AS, Winer-Muram H, et al: Pulmonary capillary hemangiomatosis: A clinicopathologic review. Ann Thorac Surg 57:772–776, 1994.
119. Faber CN, Yousem SA, Daubor JH, et al: Pulmonary capillary hemangiomatosis. A report of three cases and a review of the literature. Am Rev Respir Dis 140:808–813, 1989.
120. Nootens M, Wolfkiel CJ, Chomka EV, et al: Understanding right and left ventricular systolic function and interactions at rest and with exercise in primary pulmonary hypertension. Am J Cardiol 73:379, 1995.
121. D'Alonzo GE, Barst RJ, Ayres SM, et al: Survival in patients with primary pulmonary hypertension: Results from a national prospective registry. Ann Intern Med 115:343, 1991.

122. Rich S, Kaufmann E, Levy PS: The effect of high doses of calcium-channel blockers on survival in primary pulmonary hypertension. N Engl J Med 327:76, 1992.

123. Sandoval J, Bauerle O, Palomar A, et al: Survival in primary pulmonary hypertension. Validation of a prognostic equation. Circulation 89:1733, 1994.

124. Vlahakes GJ, Turley K, Hoffman JIE: The pathophysiology of failure in acute right ventricular hypertension: Hemodynamic and biochemical correlations. Circulation 63:87, 1981.

125. Murray PA, Vatner SF: Carotid sinus baroreceptor control of right coronary circulation in normal, hypertrophied, and failing right ventricles of conscious dogs. Circ Res 49:1339, 1981.

126. Nagaya N, Satoh T, Ishida Y, et al: Impaired left ventricular myocardial metabolism in patients with pulmonary hypertension detected by radionuclide imaging. Nucl Med Commun 18:1171–1177, 1997.

127. Patrat J, Jondeau G, Dubourg O, et al: Left main coronary artery compression during primary pulmonary hypertension. Chest 112:842–843, 1997.

128. Kawut SM, Silvestry FE, Ferrari VA, et al: Extrinsic compression of the left main coronary artery by the pulmonary artery in patients with long-standing pulmonary hypertension. Am J Cardiol 83:984–986, 1999.

129. Tan RT, Kuzo R, Goodman LR, et al: Utility of CT scan evaluation for predicting pulmonary hypertension in patients with parenchymal lung disease. Chest 113:1250–1256, 1998.

130. Louie EK, Rich S, Brundage BH: Doppler echocardiographic assessment of impaired left ventricular filling with right ventricular pressure overload due to primary pulmonary hypertension. J Am Coll Cardiol 8:1298, 1986.

131. Rich S, Pietra GG, Kieras K, et al: Primary pulmonary hypertension. Radiographic and scintigraphic patterns of histologic subtypes. Ann Intern Med 105:499, 1986.

132. Bergin CJ, Rios G, King MA, et al: Accuracy of high-resolution CT in identifying chronic pulmonary thromboembolic disease. AJR Am J Roentgenol 166:1371–1377, 1996.

133. Barst RJ, Rubin LJ, McGoon MD, et al: Survival in primary pulmonary hypertension with long-term continuous intravenous prostacyclin. Ann Intern Med 121:409, 1994.

134. Vizza CD, Lynch JP, Ochoa LL, et al: Right and left ventricular dysfunction in patients with severe pulmonary disease. Chest 113:576–583, 1998.

135. Nootens MT, Berarducci LA, Kaufmann E, et al: The prevalence and significance of a patent foramen ovale in pulmonary hypertension. Chest 104:1673, 1993.

136. Janiki JS, Weber KT, Likoff MJ, et al: The pressure-flow response of the pulmonary circulation in patients with heart failure and pulmonary vascular disease. Circulation 72:1270, 1985.

137. Weiss BM, Zemp L, Seifert B, et al: Outcome of pulmonary vascular disease in pregnancy: A systematic overview from 1978 through 1996. J Am Coll Cardiol 31:1650–1657, 1998.

138. Rich S, Seidlitz M, Dodin E, et al: The short-term effects of digoxin in patients with right ventricular dysfunction from pulmonary hypertension. Chest 114:787–792, 1998.

139. Rubin LJ, Rich S: Medical management. In Rubin LJ, Rich S (eds): Primary Pulmonary Hypertension. New York, Marcel Dekker, 1997, pp 271–286.

140. Rich S, D'Alonzo GE, Dantzker DR, et al: Magnitude and implications of spontaneous hemodynamic variability in primary pulmonary hypertension. Am J Cardiol 55:159, 1985.

141. Packer M, Medine N, Yushak M: Adverse hemodynamic and clinical effects of calcium channel blockade in pulmonary hypertension secondary to obliterative pulmonary vascular disease. J Am Coll Cardiol 4:890, 1984.

142. Rich S, Kaufmann L: High dose titration of calcium channel blocking agents for primary pulmonary hypertension: Guidelines for short-term drug testing. J Am Coll Cardiol 18:1323, 1991.

143. McCormack DG, Clarke B, Barnes PJ: Characterization of adenosine receptors in human pulmonary arteries. Am J Physiol 256:H41, 1989.

144. Schrader B, Inbar S, Kaufmann L, et al: Comparison of the effects of adenosine and nifedipine in pulmonary hypertension. J Am Coll Cardiol 19:1060, 1992.

145. Nootens M, Schrader B, Kaufmann E, et al: Comparative acute effects of adenosine and prostacyclin in primary pulmonary hypertension. Chest 107:54, 1995.

146. Dusting GJ, MacDonald PS: Prostacyclin and vascular function: Implications for hypertension and atherosclerosis. Pharmacol Ther 48:323, 1990.

147. Raffy O, Azarian R, Brenot F, et al: Clinical significance of the pulmonary vasodilator response during short-term infusion of prostacyclin in primary pulmonary hypertension. Circulation 93:484, 1996.

148. Mehta S, Stewart DJ, Langleben D, et al: Short-term pulmonary vasodilatation with L-arginine in pulmonary hypertension. Circulation 92:1539, 1995.

149. Pepke-Zaba J, Higgenbottam W, Tuan Ding Xuan A, et al: Inhaled nitric oxide as a cause of selective pulmonary vasodilation in pulmonary hypertension. Lancet 338:1173, 1991.

150. Ricciardi MJ, Knight BP, Martinez FJ, et al: Inhaled nitric oxide in primary pulmonary hypertension, a safe and effective agent for predicting response to nifedipine. J Am Coll Cardiol 32:1068–1073, 1998.

151. Roberts JD, Lang P, Bigatello LM, et al: Inhaled nitric oxide in congenital heart disease. Circulation 87:447, 1993.

152. Barst RJ, Rubin LJ, Long WA, et al: A comparison of continuous intravenous epoprostenol (prostacyclin) with conventional therapy for primary pulmonary hypertension. N Engl J Med 334:296–301, 1996.

153. Barst RJ, Maislin G, Fishman AP: Vasodilator therapy for primary pulmonary hypertension in children. Circulation 99:1197–1208, 1999.

154. Shapiro SM, Oudiz RJ, Cao T, et al: Primary pulmonary hypertension: Improved long-term effects and survival with continuous intravenous epoprostenol infusion. J Am Coll Cardiol 30:343–349, 1997.

155. McLaughlin VV, Genthner DE, Panella MM, et al: Reduction in pulmonary vascular resistance with long-term epoprostenol (prostacyclin) therapy in primary pulmonary hypertension. N Engl J Med 338:273–277, 1998.

156. Badesch DB, Tapson VF, McGoon MD, et al: Continuous intravenous epoprostenol for pulmonary hypertension due to the scleroderma spectrum of disease. A randomized, controlled trial. Ann Intern Med 132:425–434, 2000.

157. Robbins IM, Christman BW, Newman JH, et al: A survey of diagnostic practices and the use of epoprostenol in patients with primary pulmonary hypertension. Chest 114:1269–1275, 1998.

158. Frank H, Mlczoch J, Huber K, et al: The effect of anticoagulant therapy in primary and anorectic drug–induced pulmonary hypertension. Chest 112:714–721, 1997.

159. Rich S, Lam W: Atrial septostomy as palliative therapy for refractory primary pulmonary hypertension. Am J Cardiol 51:1560, 1983.

160. Kirstein D, Levy PS, Hsui DT, et al: Blade balloon atrial septostomy in patients with severe primary pulmonary hypertension. Circulation 91:2028, 1995.

161. Rich S, Dodin E, McLaughlin VV: Usefulness of atrial septostomy as a treatment for primary pulmonary hypertension and guidelines for its application. Am J Cardiol 80:369–371, 1997.

162. Sandoval J, Gaspar J, Pulido T, et al: Graded balloon dilation atrial septostomy in severe primary pulmonary hypertension. J Am Coll Cardiol 32:297–304, 1998.

163. Arcasoy SM, Kotloff RM: Lung transplantation. N Engl J Med 340:1081–1091, 1999.

164. Trulock EP: Lung transplantation. Am J Respir Crit Care Med 155:789–818, 1997.

165. Pasque MK, Trulock EP, Kaiser LR, et al: Single-lung transplantation for pulmonary hypertension: Three-month hemodynamic follow-up. Circulation 84:2275, 1991.

166. Maurer JR, Frost AE, Estenne M, et al: International guidelines for the selection of lung transplant. Transplantation 66:951–956, 1998.

167. Rich S, McLaughlin VV: Lung transplantation for pulmonary hypertension: Patient selection and maintenance therapy while awaiting transplantation. Semin Thorac Cardiovasc Surg 10:135–138, 1998.

168. Nootens M, Freels S, Kaufmann E, et al: Timing of single lung transplantation for primary pulmonary hypertension. J Heart Lung Transplant 13:276–281, 1994.

169. Sundaresan S: The impact of bronchiolitis obliterans on late morbidity and mortality after single and bilateral lung transplantation for pulmonary hypertension. Semin Thorac Cardiovasc Surg 10:152–159, 1998.

170. Conte JV, Gaine SP, Orens JB, et al: The influence of continuous intravenous prostacyclin therapy for primary pulmonary hypertension on the timing and outcome of transplantation. J Heart Lung Transplant 17:679–685, 1998.

SECONDARY PULMONARY HYPERTENSION

171. Maricq HR: Geographic clustering of scleroderma. Br J Rheumatol 29:241–243, 1990.

172. Mitchell H, Bolster MB, LeRoy EC: Scleroderma and related conditions. Med Clin North Am 81:129–149, 1997.

173. Ferencz C: On the birth prevalence of congenital heart disease. J Am Coll Cardiol 16:1701–1702, 1990.

174. Collins-Nakia RL, Rabinovitch M: Pulmonary vascular obstructive disease. Cardiol Clin 11:675–687, 1993.

175. Everhart JE (ed): Digestive Diseases in the United States: Epidemiology and Impact. Bethesda, MD, National Institutes of Health, 1994.

176. Kuo PC, Johnson LB, Plotkin JS, et al: Continuous intravenous infusion of epoprostenol for the treatment of portopulmonary hypertension. Transplantation 63:604–606, 1997.

177. Karon JM, Rosenberg PS, McQuillan G, et al: Prevalence of HIV infection in the United States, 1984 to 1992. JAMA 276:126–131, 1996.

178. Rich S (ed): Primary Pulmonary Hypertension. World Symposium—Primary Pulmonary Hypertension 1998. Available from the World Health Organization via the Internet (http://www.who.int/ncd/cvd/pph.html).

179. Palevsky HI, Gurughagavatula I: Pulmonary hypertension in collagen vascular disease. Compr Ther 25:133–143, 1999.

180. Badesch DB: Clinical trials in pulmonary hypertension. Annu Rev Med 48:399–408, 1997.

181. McLaughlin VV, Genthner DE, Panella MM, et al: Compassionate use of continuous prostacyclin in the management of secondary pulmonary hypertension: A case series. Ann Intern Med 130:740–743, 1999.

182. Sun JP, James KB, Yang XS, et al: Comparison of mortality rates and progression of left ventricular dysfunction in patients with idiopathic dilated cardiomyopathy and dilated versus nondilated right ventricular cavities. Am J Cardiol 80:1583–1587, 1997.

183. Haywood GA, Sneddon JF, Bashir Y, et al: Adenosine infusion for the reversal of pulmonary vasoconstriction in biventricular failure: A good test but a poor therapy. Circulation 86:896–902, 1992.

184. Carabello BA, Grossman W: Calculation of stenotic valve orifice area. *In* Grossman W, Giam DS (eds): Cardiac Catheterization, Angiography, and Intervention. 4th ed. Philadelphia, Lea & Febiger, 1991.

185. Braunwald E, Braunwald NS, Ross J, et al: Effects of mitral valve replacement on pulmonary vascular dynamics of patients with pulmonary hypertension. N Engl J Med 273:509, 1965.

186. Levine MJ, Weinstein JS, Diver DJ, et al: Progressive improvement in pulmonary vascular resistance following percutaneous mitral valvuloplasty. Circulation 79:1061, 1989.

187. Alexopoulos D, Lazzam C, Borrica S, et al: Isolated chronic mitral regurgitation with preserved systolic left ventricular function and severe pulmonary hypertension. J Am Coll Cardiol 14:319, 1989.

188. Wood P: The Eisenmenger syndrome, or pulmonary hypertension with reversed central shunt. BMJ 2:755, 1958.

189. Clabby ML, Canter CE, Moller JH, et al: Hemodynamic data and survival in children with pulmonary hypertension. J Am Coll Cardiol 30:554–560, 1997.

190. Hopkins WE, Ochoa LL, Richardson GW, et al: Comparison of the hemodynamics and survival of adults with severe primary pulmonary hypertension or Eisenmenger syndrome. J Heart Lung Transplant 15:100–105, 1996.

191. Vongpatanasin W, Brickner ME, Hillis LD, et al: The Eisenmenger syndrome in adults. Ann Intern Med 128:745–755, 1998.

192. Rabinovitch M, Keane JF, Fellows KE, et al: Quantitative analysis of the pulmonary wedge angiogram in congenital heart defects. Circulation 63:152, 1981.

193. Rosenzweig EB, Kerstein D, Barst RJ: Long-term prostacyclin for pulmonary hypertension with associated congenital heart defects. Circulation 99:1858–1865, 1999.

194. Steinhorn RH: Persistent pulmonary hypertension of the newborn. Acta Anaesthesiol Scand Suppl 111:135–140, 1997.

194a. Walsh-Sukys MC, Tyson JE, Wright LL, et al: Persistent pulmonary hypertension of the newborn in the era before nitric oxide: Practice variation and outcomes. Pediatrics 105:14, 2000.

195. Winberg P: In search of the keys to the neonatal pulmonary vascular bed. Acta Paediatr 87:357–359, 1998.

Chapter 54

Cor Pulmonale

VALLERIE V. McLAUGHLIN • STUART RICH

Cor pulmonale is defined as right ventricular hypertrophy and dilatation secondary to pulmonary hypertension caused by diseases of the lung parenchyma and/or pulmonary vasculature, unrelated to the left side of the heart. Chronic cor pulmonale traditionally implies pulmonary hypertension related to either obstructive or restrictive lung disease, whereas acute cor pulmonale usually refers to the development of acute pulmonary hypertension from massive pulmonary embolism. The basic anatomy and physiology of the pulmonary circulation is reviewed in Chapter 53. In this chapter the focus is on chronic pulmonary hypertension primarily related to disorders of the respiratory system and/or hypoxemia, chronic thromboembolic disease, and disorders directly affecting the pulmonary vasculature (see Table 53–4, p. 1922). The pathogenic mechanisms that can lead to pulmonary arterial hypertension and cor pulmonale are shown in Table 54–1.

THE EFFECTS OF ALVEOLAR GAS TENSION ON THE PULMONARY CIRCULATION

HYPOXIA (see also p. 1909). The hypoxic pulmonary vasoconstrictor response is an important adaptive mechanism in human physiology.[1] Alveolar hypoxia results in local vasoconstriction so that blood flow is shunted away from hypoxic regions toward better-ventilated areas of the lung, improving the ventilation-perfusion matching within the lung.[2] Although the acute effects of this response are undoubtedly beneficial, chronic hypoxemia can result in sustained elevation of pulmonary artery pressure, vascular remodeling, and the development of cor pulmonale.

Hypoxic pulmonary vasoconstriction can be observed in isolated pulmonary vascular smooth muscle cells.[3] The mechanism of hypoxic pulmonary vasoconstriction involves the inhibition of potassium currents and pulmonary vascular smooth muscle membrane depolarization as a result of changes in the membrane sulfhydryl redox status. Potassium, calcium, and chloride channels all play important roles in determining pulmonary vascular tone and are altered by changes in local oxygen tension in the pulmonary circulation.

Increased calcium (Ca^{2+}) entry into the vascular smooth muscle cells appears to mediate hypoxic pulmonary vasoconstriction.[4] The concentration of Ca^{2+} in the vicinity of the contractile machinery represents a balance between inflow and outflow across the cell membrane and intracellular release and uptake. Within the cell, Ca^{2+} can be mobilized from the sarcoplasmic reticulum and mitochondrial membrane, or the inner aspect of the cell membrane.[5] Although most of the evidence favors an influx of Ca^{2+} from extracellular fluid, the relative contribution of differential mobilization from intracellular stores is unsettled. The mechanism responsible for intracellular mobilization of Ca^{2+} is also unclear.[6, 7]

Mechanisms of Hypoxic Vasoconstriction. The mechanism of acute hypoxic pulmonary vasoconstriction is multifactorial, but the vascular endothelium plays a central role as a mediator of hypoxia-induced pulmonary vasoconstriction. Balanced release of nitric oxide[8] and endothelin[9] by endothelial cells is a key factor in the regulation of tone in the pulmonary circulation. A reduction in nitric oxide production has been demonstrated in the chronically hypoxic piglet[10] and rat,[11] whereas prolonged inhalation of nitric oxide attenuates hypoxic pulmonary vasoconstriction[12] and pulmonary vascular remodeling[13] in rats. Conversely, plasma levels of endothelin-1 are increased in association with hypoxemia in humans.[14] It is believed that endothelin-1 induces a decrease in the calcium-activated potassium current, contributing to hypoxia-induced pulmonary hypertension.[15] Endothelin receptor antagonists have been demonstrated to reduce hypoxic pulmonary vasoconstriction in animals.[16–21]

Pulmonary vascular remodeling in response to hypoxia is also mediated by a number of growth factors. Platelet-derived growth factor-A (PDGF-A) and PDGF-B are elevated in hypoxic rats,[22] and vascular endothelial growth factor (VEGF), which is an endothelial cell–specific mitogen, is upregulated during exposure to chronic hypoxia.[23–25] VEGF is likely involved in pulmonary vascular injury and endothelial cell proliferation in the setting of chronic hypoxic pulmonary vascular remodeling because of its permeability, angiogenesis, proinflammatory properties,[26] and specificity for endothelial cells (Fig. 54–1).

The roles of angiotensin-converting enzyme (ACE) and angiotensin II in the pulmonary circulation are becoming more established. Local increases in right ventricular ACE activity and expression likely play an important role in the pathogenesis of right ventricular hypertrophy secondary to hypoxic pulmonary hypertension. In chronically hypoxic rats the development of pulmonary hypertension and right ventricular hypertrophy is associated with a significant increase in membrane-bound right ventricular ACE activity.[27] ACE inhibitors attenuate the development of pulmonary hypertension in rats exposed to chronic hypoxia,[28, 29] and acute hypoxic pulmonary vasoconstriction is attenuated by type 1 angiotensin II receptor blockade.[30] Treatment of chronically hypoxic rats with ACE inhibitors also reduces right ventricular hypertrophy and fibrosis.[31]

Hypoxia inducible factor-1 (HIF-1)[32] represents a vital link between oxygen sensing, gene transcription, and the

▼ TABLE 54–1. POTENTIAL PATHOGENETIC MECHANISMS LEADING TO PULMONARY ARTERIAL HYPERTENSION AND COR PULMONALE

MECHANISMS	EXAMPLE
Primary	
Anatomical decrease in cross-sectional area (vessel destruction; encroachment on lumen by hypertrophy) of the pulmonary resistance vessels	Interstitial fibrosis and granuloma
Vasoconstriction of pulmonary resistance vessels	Hypoxia and acidosis
Contributory	
Large increments in pulmonary blood flow	Exercise
Increased pressures on the left side of the heart and pulmonary veins	Left ventricular failure or pulmonary venoocclusive disease
Increased viscosity of the blood	Secondary polycythemia or chronic hypoxia
Unproved	
Compression of pulmonary resistance vessels by raised alveolar pressures in their vicinity	Asthmatic bronchitis
Bronchial arterial-pulmonary arterial anastomoses	Expanded bronchial circulation

From Fishman AP: Pulmonary hypertension and cor pulmonale. *In* Fishman AP: Pulmonary Diseases and Disorders. 2nd ed. New York, McGraw-Hill, 1988, p 1001.

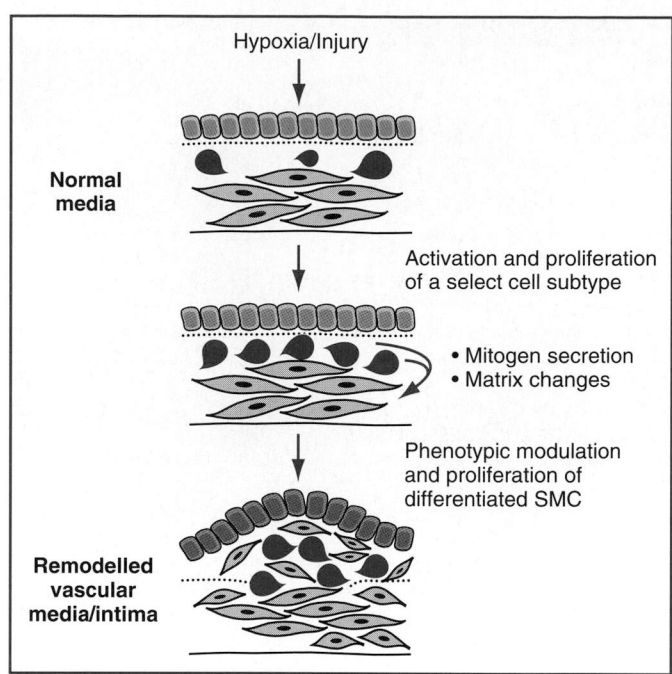

FIGURE 54–1. This diagram demonstrates the existence of phenotypically unique cell subpopulations in the normal vascular media and their contribution to injury-induced vascular remodeling. In response to vascular injury, select cell subpopulations may be activated to migrate, proliferate, and/or change their production of specific matrix proteins. In addition, these cells may also produce autocrine or paracrine growth factors. The selectively activated cell population thus not only expands but also induces changes in other smooth muscle cell subpopulations in the vessel wall. Thus, the final vascular lesion observed in response to physiological stimuli is the collective product of many cell types and several cellular processes. (From Stenmark KR, Frid MG: Smooth muscle cell heterogeneity: Role of specific smooth muscle cell subpopulations in pulmonary vascular disease. Chest 114:82S–90S, 1998.)

physiological adaptation to chronic hypoxia in vivo. One of the classic adaptations to chronic hypoxia is an increased rate of erythropoiesis that is mediated by the glycoprotein growth hormone erythropoietin. HIF-1 has been identified as a nuclear factor that is induced by hypoxia and bound to a site in the erythropoietin response element. HIF-1 expression is tightly regulated by cellular oxygen tension.

Changes in alveolar oxygenation affect the oxygenation of small pulmonary arteries and arterioles by direct gaseous diffusion from the alveoli, respiratory bronchioles, and alveolar ducts in the pulmonary arterioles, even though the latter are "upstream" in relation to the alveoli. This fact, taken together with evidence for a reduction in pulmonary arterial blood volume during hypoxia,[33] supports the view that the small pulmonary arteries and arterioles are the main sites of vasoconstriction and increased resistance in the pulmonary circulation during hypoxia.[33, 34] Although alveolar oxygen tension is a major physiological determinant of pulmonary arteriolar tone, a reduction in the oxygen tension in the mixed venous blood flowing through the small pulmonary arteries and arterioles may also contribute to pulmonary arterial vasoconstriction.[35]

Acidosis significantly increases pulmonary vascular resistance and acts synergistically with hypoxia.[36] In contrast, an increase in arterial P_{CO_2} seems to exert no direct effect but rather operates by way of the induced increase in hydrogen-ion concentration. Hypoxia and acidemia frequently coexist; and their interaction, which is clinically important, follows a predictable pattern.

ALTITUDE. Life at high altitudes is associated with pulmonary hypertension of variable severity, reflecting the range of reactivities of different persons due to the pulmonary vasoconstrictive effect of hypoxia.[37] Altitude decreases the inspired partial pressure of oxygen (P_{IO_2}) because of a decrease in barometric pressure. At sea level, P_{IO_2} is on average 150 mm Hg. At high altitudes (3000 to 5500 m) P_{IO_2} decreases to 80 to 100 mm Hg, and at extreme altitudes, 5500 to 8840 m, P_{IO_2} decreases to 40 to 80 mm Hg. Corresponding alveolar P_{O_2} (P_{AO_2}) and arterial P_{O_2} (P_{aO_2}) depend on the hypoxic ventilatory response and associated respiratory alkalosis. Mild pulmonary hypertension in adult natives at high altitude occurs at rest and may increase substantially with exercise. It is not immediately reversed by breathing of oxygen, does not seem to limit exercise capacity, and is rarely the cause of right ventricular failure.[38, 39] Severe pulmonary hypertension may occur with high altitude pulmonary edema, with infantile or adult forms of subacute mountain sickness, and with chronic mountain sickness. Subacute and chronic mountain sickness may be associated with right-sided heart failure. Subjects susceptible to high-altitude pulmonary edema often present with a slight increase in pulmonary vascular resistance at rest and exercise at sea level and with an enhanced pulmonary vascular reactivity to hypoxia. Transient right ventricular dysfunction has also been described with strenuous exercise at high altitude. In one study, 5 of 14 runners who completed an ultra-marathon at high altitude developed marked right ventricular dilation and hypokinesis, paradoxical septal motion, and pulmonary hypertension.[40] These echocardiographic abnormalities had all normalized at 1-day follow-up.

ASSESSMENT OF PATIENTS WITH COR PULMONALE SECONDARY TO LUNG DISEASE

CLINICAL EXAMINATION. The clinical examination is a relatively insensitive means of detecting pulmonary hyper-

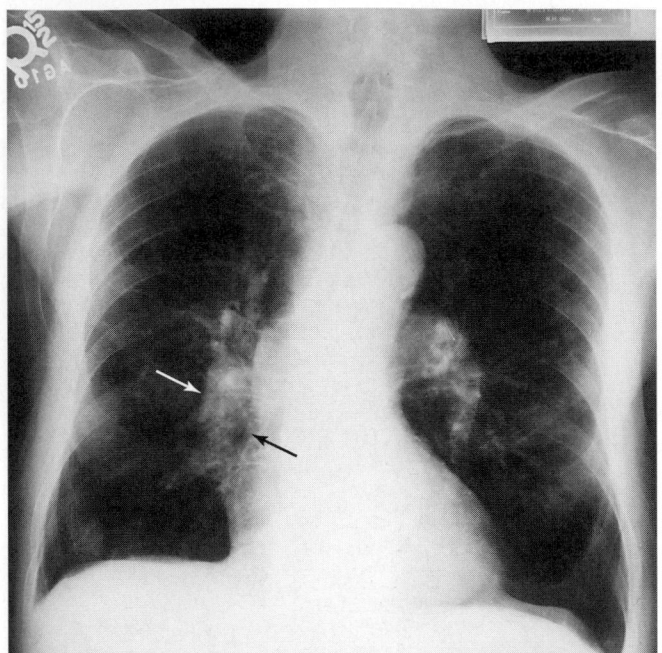

FIGURE 54-2. Upright chest radiograph in the posteroanterior (PA) projection in a man with severe COPD and pulmonary artery hypertension (mean pulmonary artery pressure = 47 mm Hg). The arrows indicate the widest dimensions of the enlarged right descending pulmonary artery. Note also the enlarged main pulmonary artery in the central left hemithorax. An enlarged right descending pulmonary artery (>16 mm Hg) and an enlarged main pulmonary artery on the PA projection are indicative of pulmonary artery hypertension in patients with COPD.

▼ **TABLE 54-2. FREQUENTLY USED ECG CRITERIA FOR RIGHT VENTRICULAR HYPERTROPHY**

Right-axis deviation > 110°
R/S ratio in V_1 > 1
R wave in V_1 ≥ 7 mm
S wave in V_1 < 2 mm
qR pattern in V_1
R wave in V_1 + S wave in V_5 or V_6 > 10.5 mm
R/S ratio in V_5 or V_6 ≤ 1
Onset of intrinsicoid deflection in V_1 = 0.035–0.055 second
rSR[1] in V_1 with R[1] ≥ 10 mm

Adapted from Chou T-C: Right ventricular hypertrophy. *In:* Electrocardiography in Clinical Practice. Philadelphia, WB Saunders 1991, pp 53–68.

tension or right ventricular dysfunction in patients with chronic obstructive pulmonary disease (COPD), because clinical signs are often obscured by hyperinflation of the chest. The jugular venous pressure may also be difficult to assess in patients with COPD because of large swings in intrathoracic pressure. A systolic left parasternal heave indicates right ventricular hypertrophy, whereas the murmur of tricuspid regurgitation suggests right ventricular dilatation, but these are not always present and may be modified by hyperinflation. Accentuation of the pulmonic component of the second heart sound indicating pulmonary hypertension is a specific but insensitive finding in patients with COPD. Peripheral edema can be due to other causes (such as hypoalbuminemia) and does not always occur in patients with pulmonary hypertension. A progressive decrease in exercise tolerance in the absence of worsening pulmonary function should suggest a cardiovascular cause and prompt a thorough evaluation.

CHEST RADIOGRAPH (Fig. 54-2). The presence of pulmonary arterial hypertension in patients with COPD has been shown to be related to the width of the right descending pulmonary artery. A right descending pulmonary artery ranging from greater than 16 mm Hg in its widest dimension[41] to greater than 20 mm Hg has been reported to identify patients with pulmonary arterial hypertension.[42] In addition, a high value for the cardiothoracic ratio was 95 percent sensitive and 100 percent specific for the presence of pulmonary hypertension in patients with COPD.[42] Although measurements on plain chest radiography may be useful as an initial screening test for the presence of pulmonary arterial hypertension, they cannot be used to predict the level of pulmonary arterial pressure in individual patients. Dilatation of the right ventricle gives the heart a globular appearance, but right ventricular hypertrophy or dilatation is not easily discernible on a plain chest radiograph. Encroachment of the retrosternal air space on the

lateral film may be a helpful sign to confirm that the enlarged silhouette is a result of right ventricular dilatation.

ELECTROCARDIOGRAPHY. The detection of right ventricular hypertrophy by the electrocardiogram (ECG) is highly specific but has a low sensitivity (see Chap. 5). Frequently used criteria for the diagnosis of right ventricular hypertrophy are outlined in Table 54-2. However, these ECG abnormalities are usually less pronounced in COPD than other forms of pulmonary hypertension because of the relatively modest degree of pulmonary hypertension that occurs and because of the effects of hyperinflation (Fig. 54-3). Butler and coworkers have introduced three criteria for right ventricular hypertrophy: (1) P wave amplitude <0.25 mV in II, III, aVF, and V_1 or V_2; (2) R wave amplitude ≥0.2 mV in I; and (3) A + R − PL ≥ 0.7 mV (A = R or R′ in V_1 or V_2; R = S in I or V_6; PL = S in V_2).[43] These three criteria achieve 66 percent sensitivity in a group with right ventricular hypertrophy caused by mitral stenosis and 95 percent specificity in normal controls. When these criteria were evaluated in a population with cor pulmonale, their sensitivity was found to be even higher at 89 percent.[44]

ECHOCARDIOGRAPHY. Although echocardiography is an invaluable tool in the evaluation of most forms of pulmonary hypertension (see Chap. 7), its utility is more limited in COPD because hyperinflation of the lungs and marked respiratory variations in intrathoracic pressures often result in suboptimal images. Delayed opening of the pulmonic valve, midsystolic closure, and an increase in the ratio of right ventricular preejection time to total ejection time have been described in patients with pulmonary hypertension.[45] Measurement of the velocity of blood flow in the main pulmonary artery can be used to estimate the pulmonary artery pressure.[46] The interval between the onset of right ventricular ejection and peak velocity, known as the time to peak velocity, correlates fairly well with the mean pulmonary artery pressure in patients with COPD (r = 0.7).[47] However, an adequate recording of the flow velocity from the pulmonary valve may be difficult to obtain. The addition of Doppler echocardiography has improved the assessment of right ventricular systolic ejection flow as an estimate of pulmonary artery systolic pressure[48] by adding the mean right atrial pressure to the peak systolic gradient between the right atrium and right ventricle. It is also possible to estimate the pulmonary end-diastolic pressure noninvasively by summing the mean right atrial pressure and the end-diastolic gradient between the pulmonary artery and the right ventricular outflow track using the pulmonary regurgitation jet. Because obtaining the estimates of peak tricuspid regurgitation velocities in patients with COPD can be difficult at times, saline contrast medium enhancement should be used to improve the accuracy of the measurements.[49]

Two-dimensional echocardiography can be used to assess right ventricular dimensions and wall thickening and right ventricular volume overload in patients with COPD. Detection of right ventricular hypertrophy by echocardiog-

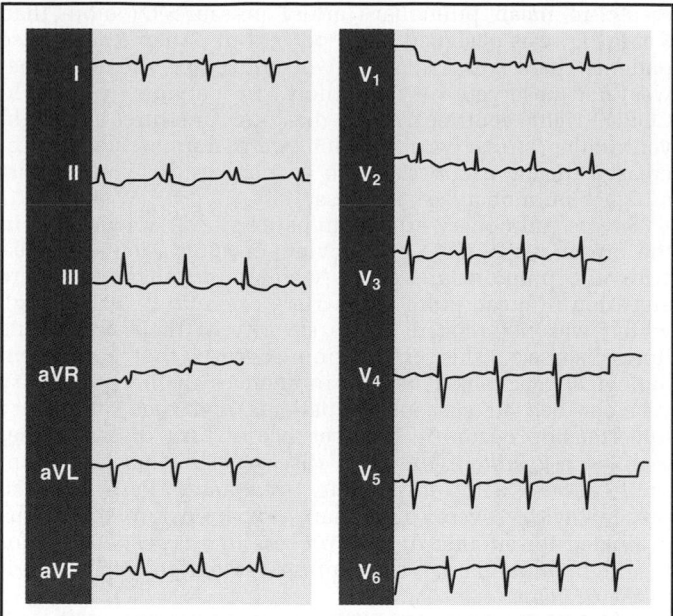

FIGURE 54–3. Electrocardiogram in a patient with emphysema and diffuse lung disease; there is right-axis deviation, "P pulmonale," a qR pattern in V_1 and an rS pattern in V_6. (From McGowan FX, Wagner GS: The electrocardiogram in chronic lung disease. *In* Rubin LJ [ed]: Pulmonary Heart Disease. Boston, Martinus Nijhoff, 1984, p 117.)

raphy is limited by the ability to differentiate the right ventricular wall from its surrounding structures. Moreover, correlations between the thickness of the right ventricular wall and the right ventricular mass are poor, even when measured at autopsy.[50] Measurement of the right ventricular diastolic diameter by echocardiography may be useful in detecting right ventricular enlargement. Right ventricular dysfunction is difficult to quantitate echocardiographically, but the position and curvature of the intraventricular septum gives an indication of right ventricular afterload. The utility of transesophageal echocardiography in the evaluation of pulmonary hypertension has yet to be fully explored, but this technique will usually provide satisfactory imaging of the right-sided heart structures in patients whose transthoracic images are of poor quality.

RADIONUCLIDE VENTRICULOGRAPHY (See also Chap. 9). Radionuclide ventriculography can provide useful information regarding right ventricular function, provided that adequate separation of the cardiac chambers can be accomplished. Because radioactive counts are proportional to volume, variations in the geometric configuration of the ventricles are less important. Although pulmonary artery pressure can not be estimated with this technique, there is an inverse relationship between pulmonary artery pressure and right ventricular ejection fraction in COPD.[51] In most patients with pulmonary vascular disease caused by COPD, the right ventricular ejection fraction is preserved at rest but fails to increase appropriately during exercise.[51] Contractility appears to be maintained until late in the course of the disease, and the abnormal right ventricular response during exercise is most likely due to increased afterload. Patients in whom the right ventricular ejection fraction is reduced usually have more severe pulmonary hypertension or overt signs of right-sided heart failure.

COMPUTED TOMOGRAPHY (See also Chap. 10). CT determined pulmonary arterial cross-sectional diameter correlates well with mean pulmonary artery pressure.[52] A high-resolution CT scan of the chest is also the most accurate noninvasive means of detecting emphysema in vivo.[53] The principal manifestation of emphysema is a hyperlucent re-

gion of lung tissue with no or only a very thin visible wall. Because CT has 10 times the density resolution of conventional radiography, it more readily distinguishes the emphysematous spaces from surrounding lung tissue. Other findings on high-resolution CT include ground-glass opacity, bullae, bronchial wall thickening, mucous plugging of bronchi and bronchioles, overinflation, air trapping (manifest as a lack of expected increase in lung capacity on exhalation scans), central arterial dilatation reflecting pulmonary arterial hypertension, and modest mediastinal lymphadenopathy. CT may demonstrate emphysema in patients with little or no abnormality on pulmonary function tests. Because the aggregate cross-sectional area is so large, the respiratory bronchioles contribute only a small portion of the total resistance to air flow, which causes poor sensitivity of pulmonary function tests.

MAGNETIC RESONANCE IMAGING (See also Chap. 10). MRI is becoming the reference standard for measuring ventricular dimensions because it produces the best images of the right ventricle. This technique is noninvasive and does not impose a radiation burden on the patient, but it is expensive and available only in specialized centers. Studies in patients with COPD have demonstrated a correlation between the right ventricular free-wall volume and both pulmonary artery pressure (r = 0.72, $p > 0.01$) and pulmonary vascular resistance (r = 0.65, $p > 0.01$).[54] Interestingly, the right ventricular free-wall volume as an estimate of wall mass correlates with the $PaCO_2$ but not with the PaO_2.[54] MRI can be used to diagnose right ventricular hypertrophy in patients with COPD and to study the effect of therapeutic interventions. It can also be used to quantify regional right ventricular function to determine the impact of chronic pulmonary hypertension on right ventricular performance.[55]

PULMONARY HYPERTENSION ASSOCIATED WITH RESPIRATORY DISORDERS

Chronic Obstructive Pulmonary Disease

Chronic obstructive pulmonary disease is the fourth leading cause of death in the United States, affecting over 14 million people.[56] The incidence, morbidity, and mortality from COPD is rising and varies widely among countries. In fact, the mortality attributed to COPD in the United States rose by 32 percent during the past decade.[56] This may be related to differences in exposure to risk factors as well as to large variations in individual susceptibility. COPD is a heterogeneous group of diseases that share a common feature: the airways are narrowed, which causes the inability to exhale completely. Although there are numerous disorders that fall under the heading of COPD, the two largest components are emphysema and chronic bronchitis. The American Thoracic Society defines COPD as a disorder characterized by abnormal tests of expiratory flow that do not change markedly either spontaneously over short periods of time or after administration of a bronchodilator.[57] Although clear-cut distinctions can often be made, there is considerable overlap as to the dominant abnormality in the individual patient in whom features of both may be manifest. *Chronic bronchitis* is a condition associated with excessive tracheal bronchial mucous production sufficient to cause cough with expectoration for at least 3 months of the year for more than 2 consecutive years. *Emphysema* is defined as the permanent, abnormal distention of the air spaces distal to the terminal bronchial with destruction of the alveolar septa. In lungs from patients with COPD studied at postmortem, the major site of air flow obstruction has been shown to be in the small airways.

Cigarette smoking is the most commonly identified correlate with COPD and accounts for 80 to 90 percent of the risk of developing COPD.[58] It has been estimated that 15 percent of one-pack-per-day smokers and 25 percent of two-pack-per-day smokers will eventually develop COPD during their lifetime.[58, 59] Why the proportion is so small is not known, but underlying host factors may play a role. Other potential environmental causes include air pollution, occupational exposures, and infection. Individuals who are homozygous for alpha$_1$-antitrypsin deficiency develop severe emphysema in the third and fourth decades of life. Dusty occupational environments are well-established risks but probably not major factors in North America.

PATHOPHYSIOLOGY OF PULMONARY HYPERTENSION. Most commonly, pulmonary hypertension in COPD is due to multiple factors, which include pulmonary vasoconstriction caused by alveolar hypoxia, acidemia, and hypercarbia; the mechanical effects of the high lung volume on pulmonary vessels; the loss of small vessels in the vascular bed in regions of the emphysema and lung destruction; and the increased cardiac output and blood viscosity from polycythemia secondary to hypoxia. Of these causes, hypoxia is undoubtedly the most important and is associated with pathological changes that occur characteristically in the peripheral pulmonary arterial bed.[60] The small pulmonary arteries develop accumulations of vascular smooth muscle cells in their intima that are laid down longitudinally along the length of the vessels. Intimal thickening appears to be an early event that occurs in association with progressive air flow limitation.[61] Medial hypertrophy in the muscular pulmonary arteries, and less commonly fibrinoid necrosis in these vessels, has also been reported in patients with COPD with chronic pulmonary arterial hypertension. Thus, structural change, rather than hypoxic vasoconstriction, is required for the development of sustained pulmonary hypertension in patients with COPD.[62]

Changes in airway resistance may augment pulmonary vascular resistance in patients with COPD by affecting the alveolar pressure. The normal linear relationship between pressure and flow in the pulmonary circulation changes when alveolar pressure is increased. The effect of airway resistance on pulmonary artery pressure may be particularly important when ventilation increases (such as in acute exacerbation of COPD). In patients with COPD, even the small increases in flow that occur during mild exercise may increase pulmonary artery pressure significantly. Alveolar hypoxia is a potent arterial constrictor in the pulmonary circulation, which reduces perfusion with respect to ventilation in an attempt to restore PaO$_2$. In patients with COPD there is a positive correlation between the PaCO$_2$ and the pulmonary artery pressure. Polycythemia, which may develop in response to chronic hypoxemia, increases the blood viscosity, which may also contribute to the severity of pulmonary arterial hypertension. Pulmonary arterial thrombosis may also occur in patients with COPD and may be a result of peripheral airway inflammation.

HEMODYNAMIC CHANGES. The elevation in pulmonary artery pressure tends to be rather mild in patients with COPD. Naeije studied 74 patients with severe, but clinically stable COPD. All presented with episodes of acute and chronic respiratory failure in the past, and almost half presented with peripheral edema.[63] They all had severe air flow limitations (FEV$_1$ 25.7 $\pm$ 1 percent of predicted) and hypoxemia (PaO$_2$ mean 43 mm Hg, range 23 to 67 mm Hg), and the majority were also hypercapnic (PaCO$_2$ mean 51 mm Hg, range 33 to 68 mm Hg). However, the pulmonary artery pressure was only modestly raised to a mean of 35 mm Hg in this group. Although the pulmonary artery pressure may be normal or only slightly elevated when measured at rest in patients with COPD, it may increase to abnormal levels during exercise.[64]

The progression of pulmonary hypertension seems to be related to hypoxemia. In 93 patients with COPD observed for 5 years, hemodynamic worsening, defined as an in-crease in mean pulmonary artery pressure by more than 5 mm Hg, was observed in 29 percent of patients.[65] In these patients there was a marked worsening of hypoxemia that was not observed in the others. In patients with mild COPD, right ventricular end-diastolic pressure and right ventricular stroke work, which were normal at rest, increased during exercise due to an increase in work against a higher pulmonary artery pressure.[66]

Severe pulmonary arterial hypertension is uncommon in the presence of COPD. In a review of 500 patients referred with cor pulmonale, only 6 were found to have severe elevation in mean pulmonary artery pressure (>50 mm Hg), which was not related to the severity of their underlying lung disease.[67] This observation suggests that a different biological mechanism results in changes in the pulmonary vascular bed in susceptible patients and that pulmonary hypertension occurs in the presence of lung disease rather than as a *result* of the lung disease. This has important implications with respect to treatment. Patients who present with severe pulmonary hypertension should be evaluated for another disease process that is responsible for the high pulmonary arterial pressures before attributing it to the COPD.

PROGNOSIS AND PREDICTORS OF SURVIVAL. Although pulmonary arterial hypertension progresses slowly in patients with COPD, its presence confers a poor prognosis. Weitzenblum and coworkers showed a 72 percent 4-year survival rate in those with normal pulmonary artery pressure compared with a 49 percent survival rate in those with an elevated pulmonary artery pressure (mean > 20 mm Hg).[68] Burrows and colleagues studied 50 patients with chronic airway obstruction over 7 years and showed that the pulmonary vascular resistance was the hemodynamic parameter that correlated best with mortality.[69] In this study, none of the patients whose pulmonary vascular resistance exceeded 7 Wood Units survived for more than 3 years. France and colleagues, in a study of 115 patients with COPD, found that a number of variables correlated significantly with mortality, including PaO$_2$, PaCO$_2$, FEV$_1$, and the presence of peripheral edema.[70] Others have reported that patients with COPD who develop peripheral edema have a 5-year survival rate of only 27 to 33 percent.[71]

A 10-year follow-up study conducted on a cohort of 870 patients with severe COPD concluded that (1) patients with COPD have a high mortality rate from acute respiratory failure, cor pulmonale, and lung cancer; (2) patients' age at the time of diagnosis influences the death hazard; (3) patients who need long-term oxygen treatment have a higher death hazard than those who do not; (4) the higher the FEV$_1$ or PaO$_2$ at the time of diagnosis, the lower the death hazard; (5) patients who need and use long-term oxygen treatment have a lower death hazard compared with those who need it but do not use it properly; and (6) patients with a partial reversible airway obstruction who regularly attend the clinic for planned checkups have a lower death hazard compared with those who have the same characteristics but do not show adherence to the care program.[72] In another study, among a cohort of 270 patients with COPD, the median survival was 3.1 years. Death was predicted by the following variables: age, ECG signs of right ventricular hypertrophy, chronic renal failure, ECG signs of myocardial infarction or ischemia, and FEV$_1$ less than 590 ml.[73] Among 166 patients treated with long-term oxygen therapy, the overall survival rates were 78.3 percent and 67.1 percent at 2 and 3 years, respectively. A multivariate analysis showed an independent predictive power for right ventricular systolic pressure, age, and FEV$_1$.[74] Once endotracheal intubation is necessary, the prognosis is usually poor and the survival after 1 year is usually lower than 40 percent.[75] Pulmonary embolism is a common cause of death, with the frequency estimated to be approximately 11 percent.[76]

Among patients with COPD in the intensive care unit, pulmonary embolism was the most frequent cause of death at 40.6 percent.

Treatment

Management goals in COPD are to ameliorate air flow obstruction and improve symptoms, to avoid secondary complications, to maintain functional capacity, and to improve the quality of life. Recent advances in smoking cessation strategies and surgical techniques (lung volume reduction surgery and lung transplantation) and renewed interest in noninvasive positive-pressure ventilation have expanded treatment options to meet the patient's needs. In addition to the specific therapies discussed here, all patients should receive a yearly influenza vaccination and the 23-valent pneumococcal vaccination at least once in their lifetime. For patients who do not receive influenza vaccine and are at risk for influenza type A infection, amantadine, 200 mg/d, or rimantadine, 100 mg twice per day, should be prescribed until the risk of infection has subsided.

SMOKING CESSATION. The importance of smoking cessation cannot be overemphasized. The annual rate of decline of FEV_1 in smokers is approximately 80 ml per year, in contrast to 25 to 30 ml per year in nonsmokers. The Lung Health Study reported that patients who stopped smoking had a small improvement in FEV_1 (57 ml) after 1 year.[77] Thereafter, the rate of decline in lung function is similar to age-matched nonsmokers. The short-term success rates with smoking cessation are variable (18–77 percent), but success is more likely if the patient abstains from smoking within the first 2 weeks of entry into a program. The use of nicotine replacement therapy should always include a structured behavioral modification program to increase the likelihood of success. Pharmacological methods to reduce addictive behavior have not been found to be effective in controlled clinical trials.[78] Recently, the novel antidepressant bupropion (Zyban), which enhances noradrenergic activity, was reported to have a successful smoking cessation rate of 44 percent, compared with 19 percent in the placebo group.[79]

PULMONARY REHABILITATION. Patients with advanced COPD often lead a sedentary lifestyle because of breathlessness during mild to moderate exercise. The lack of exercise leads to deconditioning and worsening dyspnea, even with low levels of activity. The overall goal of a pulmonary rehabilitation program is to maintain the individual's maximal level of independence and functioning in the community. Pulmonary rehabilitation can improve exercise endurance and decrease the sense of breathlessness. Several studies have demonstrated that pulmonary rehabilitation can improve exercise capacity, subjective symptoms, and quality of life.

Because of hyperinflation, deconditioning, and malnutrition, patients with advanced air flow obstruction have weakened ventilatory muscles. Moreover, because of the increased work of breathing, the inspiratory muscles are prone to fatigue. Fortunately, the respiratory muscles can be trained to improve their strength and endurance. Strength training can be achieved by high-intensity, low-frequency stimuli such as inspiring against a closed glottis or shutter valve. Endurance training may also improve inspiratory muscle strength.

OXYGEN. Hypoxemia is a common finding in patients with advanced COPD and is easily corrected with low-flow supplemental O_2. In key clinical trials sponsored by the National Institutes of Health (NIH, Nocturnal Oxygen Therapy Trial [NOTT] Group, 1980) and the British Medical Research Council (1981) long-term oxygen therapy clearly improved the survival of hypoxemic patients with COPD (Fig. 54–4).[80, 81] The British study compared the effect of treatment with oxygen for approximately 15 hours per day with the effects of no oxygen therapy, whereas the NIH

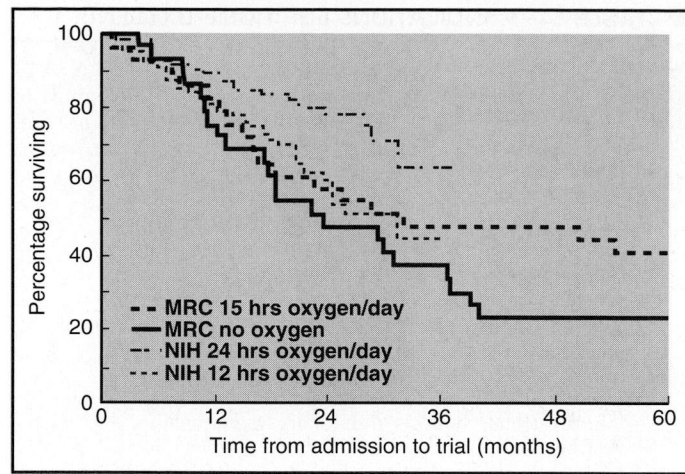

FIGURE 54–4. Survival curves in the MRC (British) and NIH (US) long-term oxygen therapy trials in patients with severe hypoxemia and cor pulmonale. (From Flenley DC, Muir AL: Cardiovascular effects of oxygen therapy for pulmonary arterial hypertension. Clin Chest Med 4:297, 1983.)

study compared nocturnal oxygen therapy (about 12 hours per day) to "continuous" oxygen therapy (at least 19 hours per day). In each study, the mean baseline PaO_2 when the patients were breathing ambient air was 51 mm Hg; the mean FEV_1 was 0.7 to 0.8 liter.

Oxygen therapy was beneficial in both studies (see Fig. 54–4). In the British study, 19 of 42 (45 percent) oxygen-treated patients died within 5 years, whereas 30 of 45 (67 percent) untreated patients died. In the NIH study, the mortality rate after a year was 20.6 percent in the group receiving nocturnal oxygen and 11.9 percent in the group receiving continuous oxygen therapy; and after 2 years, mortality was 40.8 percent and 22.4 percent, respectively. The relative risk of death for nocturnal oxygen therapy compared with continuous oxygen was 1.94. Oxygen therapy is therefore effective, and continuous therapy is more effective than nocturnal therapy only.

HEMODYNAMIC EFFECTS OF OXYGEN. How oxygen therapy improves survival is unknown. Two major hypotheses have been proposed: (1) oxygen relieves pulmonary vasoconstriction, decreasing pulmonary vascular resistance and thus enabling the right ventricle to increase stroke volume, and (2) oxygen therapy improves arterial oxygen content, providing enhanced oxygen delivery to the heart, brain, and other vital organs. These two hypotheses are not mutually exclusive, and each one has supporting evidence. Oxygen therapy clearly alleviates the progressive pulmonary hypertension of untreated COPD. Patients who exhibit a significant decrease in pulmonary artery pressure (>5 mm Hg) after acute oxygen therapy (28 percent oxygen for 1 day) have better survival than patients who do not respond acutely when both groups of patients are subsequently treated with long-term continuous oxygen therapy.[82] Enhanced right ventricular performance during short-term oxygen therapy may also be the direct result of improved tissue (e.g., myocardial) oxygenation rather than decreased pulmonary vascular resistance.[83]

RECOMMENDATIONS. Criteria for chronic home O_2 therapy are shown in Table 54–3. Long-term oxygen therapy is warranted if the resting PaO_2 remains less than 55 mm Hg after a 3-week stabilization period on maximal medical therapy (e.g., bronchodilators, antimicrobial agents, diuretics). Patients with a PaO_2 above 55 mm Hg should be considered for oxygen therapy if they are polycythemic or have clinical evidence (e.g., ECG, physical examination) of pulmonary hypertension.[84] Hypoxemia should be documented after the stabilization period to avoid the cost of long-term

▼ TABLE 54–3. INDICATIONS FOR HOME OXYGEN

Absolute
$PaO_2 \leq 55$ mm Hg or $SaO_2 \leq 88\%$
PaO_2 55–59 mm Hg or $SaO_2 = 89\%$ in the presence of any of the following
  Dependent edema suggesting congestive heart failure
  P pulmonale on the ECG (P wave <3 mm in standard leads II, III, or aVF)
  Erythrocytosis (hematocrit >56%)

Specific Situations
During exercise
  $PaO_2 < 55$ mm Hg or O_2 saturation <88% with low level of exertion
During sleep
  $PaO_2 < 55$ mm Hg or O_2 saturation <88% with associated complications, such as pulmonary hypertension, excessive daytime sleepiness, and cardiac arrhythmias

Adapted from ATS Statement: Comprehensive outpatient management of COPD. Am J Respir Crit Care Med 152(Suppl):S84–S96, 1995.

oxygen therapy in patients who do not require it. In the NOTT study,[81] 45 percent of hypoxemic patients initially selected for study improved enough during 3 to 4 weeks of observation and treatment to suspend plans for long-term oxygen therapy. An even longer observation period of 2 or 3 months may be necessary to exclude patients who eventually achieve acceptable PaO_2 values on medical therapy alone. For sedentary patients already on supplemental O_2, the resting O_2 requirement may be increased by 1 liter/min during mild activities. Oxygen has been shown to delay the onset of fatigue in exercising muscles, thus improving ventilatory endurance and exercise capacity.[85] In addition, it also decreases dyspnea and minute ventilation for a given workload.[86] Nocturnal oxygen therapy may be important in patients with sleep desaturation. Daily activities, such as walking, washing, and eating, are associated with transient oxygen desaturation in patients with moderate to severe COPD, even in the absence of resting hypoxemia.[87] Ambulatory oxygen therapy in patients with COPD and exercise hypoxemia may improve exercise capacity and breathlessness.[88]

Carbon dioxide retention may occur with supplemental O_2, especially with higher O_2 concentrations, and is thought to be due to blunting of hypoxemia driven central respiratory drive. This observation may lead some physicians to withhold O_2 therapy. It is now believed that the main mechanism for CO_2 retention in these patients is worsening ventilation-perfusion inequality due to O_2-induced pulmonary vasodilatation in areas of the lung with poorer ventilation. Ambier and colleagues show that central respiratory drive is normal or slightly increased in patients who develop hypercapnia while on O_2 therapy.[89] If CO_2 retention is associated with systemic acidosis (pH 7.25 or less) and the patient requires high O_2 flow to maintain satisfactory PaO_2, mechanical ventilation should be considered.

ANTICHOLINERGICS. Anticholinergics are the bronchodilators of choice in the management of COPD and appear to be more effective than beta$_2$ agonists.[90] Anticholinergic drugs, typified by atropine, cause bronchodilatation by blocking cholinergic mediated increases in bronchomotor tone. In addition, they also block the afferent limb of the vagally mediated bronchoconstriction induced by nonspecific airway irritants such as cigarette smoke, dust, and fumes. Ipratropium bromide can achieve similar, if not greater, degrees of bronchodilatation than beta agonists and has fewer side effects. It has been suggested that ipratropium bromide should be the initial agent in the chronic therapy for COPD.[91] Combination therapy with anticholinergic and beta$_2$ agonists has been shown to be more effective than either drug alone.[92] Unlike beta agonists, anticho-

linergic drugs have a slower onset of action and a longer half-life. The usual dose of ipratropium bromide is two puffs every 4 to 6 hours. An investigational agent, ipatropium bromide, gives prolonged bronchodilatation lasting over 24 hours and has the advantage of improved compliance with once-daily dosing.[93]

BETA-ADRENERGIC AGONISTS. These are important drugs in the management of chronic air flow obstruction. In contrast to asthma, however, a lesser degree of bronchodilatation is seen in COPD. The absence of a significant bronchodilator response on a single spirometry (post-bronchodilator increase in FEV$_1$ by greater than 15 percent) does not preclude the delayed effectiveness of beta agonists. As many as 70 percent of patients who show no initial response to a beta agonist will show greater than 15 percent improvement in FEV$_1$ on subsequent spirometry.[91] The increases in vital capacity are usually higher than those observed for FEV$_1$, and they are often associated with symptomatic improvement.[94] Recent studies have shown that the long-acting inhaled beta$_2$ agonists salmeterol and formoterol are beneficial in patients with COPD, resulting in improved lung function and symptom control.[95, 96] The side effects of properly used inhaled beta agonists are minimal and limited to skeletal muscle tremors and tachycardia. Although there is no evidence that the regular use of a beta agonist increases mortality in patients as alluded to in asthma, it is generally recommended that a beta agonist should be used on an "as needed" basis. In patients with severe COPD, regularly dosed beta agonists may improve symptoms.[97]

THEOPHYLLINE. The use of theophylline in COPD has been tempered by its frequent side effects, variable hepatic metabolism, and studies showing little symptomatic benefit. However, theophylline is an effective bronchodilator in COPD and will cause a small improvement in results of pulmonary function tests.[98, 99] Long-term use has been associated with an overall 10 to 20 percent increase in the FEV$_1$ from baseline, and an improvement in minute ventilation and gas exchange has also been observed.[98, 100] In addition to improving FEV$_1$, theophylline reduces dyspnea,[98, 101] improves exercise performance,[102] and is associated with a subjective sense of well-being in patients with severe COPD, even if the reduction in dyspnea is not accompanied by a change in functional indices such as FEV$_1$ or arterial blood gases.[101]

CORTICOSTEROIDS. Because there is continued neutrophilic inflammation in COPD, it was thought that inhaled corticosteroids might prevent the progression of disease. However, there is little evidence that inhaled corticosteroids are of benefit to a large percentage of patients.[103] The few patients (approximately 10 percent) who have some response to corticosteroids have asthma. A large study (the European Respiratory Society Study on Chronic Obstructive Pulmonary Disease [EUROSCOP]) in patients with mild COPD showed no overall effect of an inhaled corticosteroid (budesonide, 400 μg twice daily) on the annual rate of decline in lung function, although some subgroups appear to benefit.[104] A recent trial of even higher doses of inhaled budesonide, 1600 μg/d, versus placebo showed no physiological or functional benefit in patients with advanced COPD after 6 months.[105] A 3-year placebo-controlled, parallel group, randomized, double-blinded trial of inhaled budesonide demonstrated no clinical benefit in COPD patients.[106]

The effects of oral corticosteroids are similarly disappointing. Only 10 to 20 percent of COPD patients with judicious use of oral corticosteroids will show improvement in pulmonary symptoms and FEV$_1$ by 20 to 25 percent,[107] as well as decreasing the number of acute exacerbations[108] and airway responsiveness. Clinical criteria that may be useful in predicting corticosteroid responders from nonresponders includes a significant bronchodilator response to a beta agonist, presence of eosinophils in the sputum or blood, and a history of atopy.

DIGITALIS. The effects of digitalis in cor pulmonale are complex. The cardiac glycosides increase the contractility of the RV myocardium, but they also can produce pulmonary vasoconstriction. Furthermore, Sylvester and associates[109] showed that, in dogs, digitalis can reduce venous return, which may adversely affect cardiac output. Intravenous digoxin may also improve diaphragm strength and blood flow in patients with COPD with acute respiratory failure.[110]

Digitalis therapy is indicated in patients with cor pulmonale and coexistent left ventricular failure. In patients with severe COPD and biventricular failure, an improvement in right ventricular ejection fraction has been observed with digoxin,[111] but not in patients with a reduced right ventricular ejection fraction and normal left ventricular function.[112] Recently, it was demonstrated that short-term intravenous digoxin improved cardiac output and reduced circulating norepinephrine[113] in patients with right ventricular dysfunction due to primary pulmonary hypertension. Digitalis therapy may cause an increased incidence of adverse side effects (e.g., cardiac arrhythmias) in patients with obstructive lung disease, presumably in part owing to the effect of hypoxia.

VASODILATORS. No agent other than oxygen has been shown convincingly to vasodilate the pulmonary circulation in patients with COPD. Nonselective beta-adrenergic antagonists may reduce systemic arterial oxygen saturation from intrapulmonary shunting associated with an increase in dyspnea in these patients. Hydralazine and calcium channel blockers have been shown to have essentially no effect on pulmonary hemodynamic measurements in patients with COPD. Currently, there is no role for oral vasodilators in the management of COPD.

NITRIC OXIDE. Inhaled nitric oxide (NO) has been used as a selective pulmonary vasodilator due to its short duration of action and inactivation in the systemic circulation,[114] but it is difficult to use over a prolonged period. A recent study demonstrated that the combined inhalation of NO and O_2 was associated with reductions of the mean pulmonary artery pressure and pulmonary vascular resistance and a remarkable improvement in arterial oxygen saturation.[115] Other studies have suggested that inhaled NO worsens oxygenation in the setting of COPD, potentially by overriding hypoxic pulmonary vasoconstriction.[116, 117] The role of NO in the therapy for COPD has yet to be defined.

ACE INHIBITORS. Angiotensin II is a potent pulmonary and airway constrictor acting through angiotensin II receptors. The role of ACE inhibitors and angiotensin II receptor antagonists is still emerging. In one trial, enalapril reduced pulmonary hypertension and improved renal blood flow in 30 patients with COPD.[118] The angiotensin receptor blocker losartan also reduces pulmonary artery pressure in patients with COPD[119] and therefore may be useful in preventing the progression of pulmonary hypertension and cor pulmonale in patients with severe COPD. Further investigation needs to be completed before making generalized recommendations regarding these agents in patients with COPD.

NONINVASIVE VENTILATION. Noninvasive positive-pressure ventilation (NPPV) has been reported to improve gas exchange, sleep efficiency, quality of life, and functional status in patients with restrictive lung disease and chronic respiratory failure. Its usefulness in patients with COPD is not as well established. The initial interest in using intermittent noninvasive ventilation for patients with severe COPD arose from physiological studies on respiratory muscle function. Hyperinflation in patients with COPD was found to place the respiratory muscles at a mechanical disadvantage. The flattened diaphragms had shortened sarcomere lengths, diminished maximal force, increased muscle tension, and compromised blood supply. Based on these

considerations, investigators hypothesized that noninvasive ventilation would be of value to patients with severe COPD because it would rest the chronically fatigued muscles. Periods of intermittent rest would permit recovery of muscle function, increasing muscle strength, reducing the tendency to fatigue, and improving pulmonary function and gas exchange.

An alternative hypothesis was generated based on sleep studies in COPD. Patients with severe COPD have a high prevalence of sleep-disordered breathing, including not only obstructive sleep apnea but also episodes of hypoventilation associated with oxygen desaturations.[120] Large retrospective analyses have examined outcomes of patients treated with NPPV for periods ranging up to 5 years.[121, 122] Patients with COPD were less likely to continue NPPV treatment than patients with neuromuscular disorders or chest wall deformities, but the average duration of continuation was still 2 to 3 years. Although the survival of patients with COPD treated with long-term NPPV appears to be comparable to that of patients treated with tracheostomies or long-term oxygen therapy, the retrospective and uncontrolled nature of these trials greatly limits any conclusions that can be drawn.

A recent consensus conference suggested that patients with severe CO_2 retention, particularly those with nocturnal oxygen desaturation, appear most likely to respond favorably to NPPV.[123] The statement specifically recommends consideration of NPPV for those patients with COPD and symptoms such as fatigue, dyspnea, and morning headache despite optimal medical management and one of the following physiological criteria: $PaCO_2$ greater than or equal to 55 mm Hg; $PaCO_2$ of 50 to 54 mm Hg and nocturnal desaturation (oxygen saturation < 88 percent for 5 continuous minutes while receiving 2 L/min or more of nasal O_2); or $PaCO_2$ of 50 to 54 mm Hg and hospitalization (two or more times in a 12-month period) related to recurrent episodes of hypercapnic respiratory failure.

LUNG VOLUME REDUCTION SURGERY. Volume reduction surgery, which was originally described by Brantigan, has been advocated in selected patients with advanced emphysema. The surgical technique involves removing 20 to 30 percent of the volume of each lung by means of sternotomy, sequential thoracotomy, or thoracoscopy to reduce the severe hyperinflation commonly seen in patients with severe COPD. The physiological improvement after excision of large bullae in patients with severe emphysema is easy to understand. The compressed normal lung parenchyma expands after bullaectomy, resulting in improved lung function and exercise capacity. In patients with diffuse emphysema, the exact mechanism of these physiological improvements is less clear. The proposed benefits of surgery include the following: restoration of elastic recoil on small airways leading to decreased airway resistance; restoration of normal outward chest recoil; improved ventilation-perfusion matching; and a reduction in end-expiratory lung volume, thereby returning the diaphragm to a more favorable length-tension precontraction length for optimal pressure generation. There are, however, very strict criteria for lung volume reduction surgery (Table 54–4). Although the medical selection criteria are less stringent for lung volume reduction surgery than for lung transplantation, the disease-specific criteria are more restrictive. The residual volume to total lung capacity ratio is the single most important determinant of improvement in pulmonary function after lung volume reduction surgery.[124]

Patients with COPD who are thought to respond best to surgery have the following characteristics: heterogeneous bullous changes within the lung as detected by CT and ventilation-perfusion scan; presence of severe hyperinflation; reduced diaphragmatic excursion; and absence of hypercapnia and pulmonary hypertension. Long-term follow-up data are still not available, and it is not clear how long

▼ **TABLE 54-4. CRITERIA FOR LUNG VOLUME REDUCTION SURGERY**

No age restriction
Marked disability after completing pulmonary rehabilitation (see text)
No tobacco use for at least 4 months
Imaging must show heterogeneous disease (homogeneous disease has more stringent criteria)
Pulmonary function tests (all after bronchodilator administration; lung volumes measured by plethysmography)
    Forced expiratory volume in 1 second (FEV$_1$) ≤ 45%; if age >70 years, an FEV$_1$ ≥ 15% predicted)
    Total lung capacity ≥ 110%
    Residual volume ≥ 150%
    Diffusing capacity of the lung for carbon monoxide ≤ 70%
    Absence of bronchodilator response (FEV$_1$) change ≤ 30% and 300 ml
PaCO$_2$ < 60 mm Hg
PaO$_2$ > 45 mm Hg on room air
Mean pulmonary artery pressure ≤ 35 mm Hg or peak systolic pressure ≤ 45 mm Hg

    Adapted from Dasgupta A, Maurer J: Late-stage emphysema: When medical therapy fails. Cleve Clin J Med 66:415–425, 1999.

▼ **TABLE 54-5. CRITERIA FOR LUNG TRANSPLANTATION FOR COPD**

Ambulatory with rehabilitation potential
80–120% of ideal body weight
Approximate maximum age (years)
    65 (single-lung recipients)
    60 (double-lung recipients)
    55 (heart-lung recipients)
Severely ill despite optimal medical therapy
    NYHA Class III
    FEV$_1$ < 20% of predicted
    Rapid decline in FEV$_1$
    Hypoxia
    Hypercapnia
Minimal corticosteroid use (≤15–20 mg qd)
Creatinine clearance >50 mg ml/min
Contraindications
    Recent or current malignancy
    Significant disease affecting other organ systems
    Extrapulmonary infections
    Substance abuse (including cigarettes) for more than 6 months
    Ventilator dependence

    Adapted from Dasgupta A, Maurer J: Late-stage emphysema: When medical therapy fails. Cleve Clin J Med 66:415–425, 1999.

the improvement in lung function seen after lung volume reduction will persist. Maximal improvement in lung function indices are seen at 6 months after surgery; and although improvements are maintained at 1 year, there may be a trend toward falling indices compared with the 6-month values.[125] Lung volume reduction is palliative to a procedure that does not halt but only slows the rate of functional decline for COPD. The disease will still progress, and symptoms will likely worsen.

LUNG TRANSPLANTATION. COPD is the most common indication for lung transplantation worldwide. In 1995, approximately 60 percent of single lung and 30 percent of bilateral lung transplants were performed on patients with COPD.[126] Lung transplantation is a viable treatment option in patients with advanced pulmonary parenchymal or pulmonary vascular disease who have exhausted medical management. Both the number of patients waiting for lung transplantation and the waiting period have increased. Because of the scarcity of organ donors, the waiting time is now approximately 18 to 24 months in the United States. Patient selection and timing of referral for lung transplantation should take into account this waiting period. Selection criteria are outlined in Table 54–5, although they may differ among lung transplant centers. Currently, both single-lung transplantation and bilateral lung transplantation result in significant improvement in postoperative lung function, exercise capacity, and quality of life.[127] The choice of the procedure needs to be individualized. In general, single-lung transplantation is used for emphysema because of the scarcity of organ donors, lower perioperative morbidity and mortality, and comparable improvement in exercise capacity compared with bilateral lung transplantation.[128] However, postoperative spirometry, single breath diffusing capacity, and arterial oxygen tension are all significantly higher in bilateral lung transplantation compared with single-lung transplantation, which may benefit young patients with emphysema because the higher pulmonary reserve will offset any decline in lung function due to infection or rejection. In most centers, bilateral lung transplantation is reserved for patients with suppurative lung disease or pulmonary vascular disease. The 1-year and 5-year survival for single and bilateral lung transplantation for emphysema is approximately 80 percent and 40 percent, respectively.

Complications associated with lung transplantation recipients are due to infections (i.e., bacterial, viral, or fungal), chronic rejection (bronchiolitis obliterans), and noninfectious complications due to prolonged immunosuppression. Chronic rejection, manifest clinically as progressive deterioration in lung function and pathologically as bronchiolitis obliterans, can occur in 40 percent of lung transplant recipients and is now the most common cause of death among long-term survivors.[129]

Interstitial Lung Disease

Interstitial lung diseases represent a variety of conditions that involve the alveolar walls, perialveolar tissue, and other contiguous supporting structures. Cor pulmonale occurs in a variety of interstitial lung diseases and is often associated with obliteration of the pulmonary vascular bed by lung destruction and fibrosis. The mechanism for pulmonary hypertension may be related to hypoxemia or a loss of effective pulmonary vasculature from lung destruction and/or by indirectly triggering a pulmonary vasculopathy. Interstitial lung disease may be due to environmental inhalant exposures, such as to asbestos, drugs, and chemotherapeutic agents, to radiation, and to recurring aspiration pneumonias. A large number of patients have interstitial lung disease of unknown etiology, the most common being idiopathic pulmonary fibrosis (IPF) and interstitial lung disease associated with collagen vascular diseases.

IDIOPATHIC PULMONARY FIBROSIS. IPF can be associated with pulmonary hypertension, which is difficult to manage because the current medical therapy for IPF is only minimally effective. Most patients are older than 50 years of age and usually report an insidious onset of progressive dyspnea and cough from months to years. The physical findings are typified by inspiratory crackles on chest examination and clubbing of the fingers. The chest radiograph may show bilateral peripheral-based opacities and honeycombing predominantly involving the lower lung zones. Pulmonary function tests show reduced lung volumes with restrictive physiology and a diminished diffusing capacity for carbon monoxide. IPF is a diagnosis of exclusion, and other forms of diffuse parenchymal lung disease need to be ruled out. A definitive diagnosis of IPF requires an open-lung biopsy.[130] Other lung diseases that need to be distinguished include bronchiolitis obliterans with organizing pneumonia, nonspecific interstitial pneumonia, desquamative interstitial pneumonia, acute interstitial pneumonia, lymphocytic interstitial pneumonia, respiratory bronchioli-

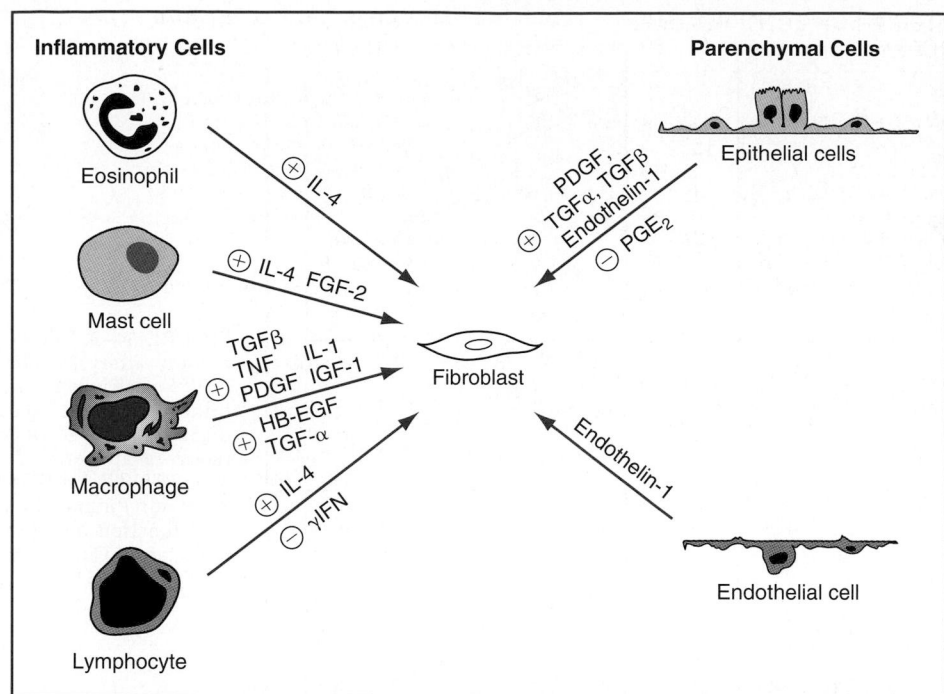

FIGURE 54–5. Pathogenesis of pulmonary fibrosis. There are numerous pathways that can lead to pulmonary fibrosis, and none is mutually exclusive. This scheme poses a problem in that specific targeted therapy would likely be ineffective because of the redundancy of pathways toward fibrosis. However, it is likely that only a few of these pathways are critical in human idiopathic pulmonary fibrosis. Studies with keratinocyte growth factor (KGF) in rats and gene deletion studies in mice indicate that a single growth factor or receptor might be highly effective. Therapy need not be directed at the whole inflammatory response as is the current rationale for corticosteroids and cytotoxic agents. IL-4 = interleukin-4; FGF-2 = fibroblast growth factor-2, basic FGF; TGF-β = transforming growth factor-beta; TNF = tumor necrosis factor; PDGF = platelet-derived growth factor; IL-1 = interleukin-1; IGF-1 = insulin-like growth factor-1; HB-EGF = heparin binding epidermal-like growth factor; IFN = interferon gamma; PGE$_2$ = prostaglandin E$_2$. (From Mason RJ, Schwarz MI, Hunninghake GW, Musson FA: Pharmacological therapy for idiopathic pulmonary fibrosis. Am J Respir Crit Care Med 160:1171–1177, 1999.)

tis–associated interstitial lung disease, and chronic hypersensitivity pneumonitis.

The pathogenesis of pulmonary fibrosis has not been well defined because there are numerous pathways that can lead to pulmonary fibrosis that are not mutually exclusive.[131] Although it is believed that inflammatory cells acting directly on fibroblasts in the lung through a variety of inflammatory mediators play a key role, the interaction of the inflammatory cascade with parenchymal lung cells is also important (Fig. 54–5).

Initial symptoms include dyspnea, effort intolerance, and dry cough without obvious cause. A "ground glass" appearance on high-resolution chest CT is equated histologically with a cellular reaction.[132] A "reticular nodular" appearance denotes more advanced, less cellular fibrotic areas. However, the high-resolution chest CT is normal in approximately 12 percent of biopsy specimen–proven cases of interstitial lung disease.[133]

The major targets of therapy have focused on the inflammatory cells, and this has led to the use of antiinflammatory agents.[134, 135] However, corticosteroids and cytotoxic drugs are only occasionally effective in IPF. Pulmonary hypertension is a complication of pulmonary fibrosis that may warrant more aggressive therapy. Pulmonary hypertension can become the limiting factor in the dyspnea and exercise limitation of patients with IPF and contributes to its mortality. The therapy for pulmonary hypertension should be directed at the underlying disease process and not toward lowering pulmonary artery pressure. Oxygen is indicated in the presence of hypoxemia. Worsening gas exchange and heart failure can be induced by the use of vasodilators, which appear to have no role in disease management. In such patients, therapy with digitalis and diuretics would be appropriate.

ADULT CYSTIC FIBROSIS. Cystic fibrosis (CF) is the most common lethal genetic disease in whites and occurs in approximately 1 of every 2000 live births. As the disease progresses, patients develop disabling lung disease and eventually respiratory failure, pulmonary hypertension, and cor pulmonale. The pathophysiology of pulmonary hypertension and cor pulmonale in CF is believed to be related to progressive destruction of the lung parenchyma and the pulmonary vasculature and to pulmonary vasoconstriction secondary to hypoxemia.[136] The development of cor pulmonale in patients with CF carries a grave prognosis. The mean survival time from the onset of cor pulmonale has been reported to be as short as 8 months. Typically, the patients have severe hypoxemia, which may be a result of and a causative factor of the pulmonary hypertension (Fig. 54–6).

One recent study evaluated patients with CF and cor pulmonale in depth.[137] Right ventricular hypertrophy appears to be a precursor of right ventricular failure and an indicator of the onset of pulmonary hypertension. The severity of the pulmonary hypertension appeared to correlate significantly with declining pulmonary function, as well as with the degree of oxygen desaturation on exercise. In this study, patients who developed pulmonary hypertension had a much worse prognosis (average survival 15 months) compared with those without pulmonary hypertension (average survival 33 months). Once lung function is severely limited (FEV$_1$ < 40 percent predicted), the prevalence of pulmonary hypertension may be as high as 40 percent. Because hypoxemia is universally found, supplemental oxy-

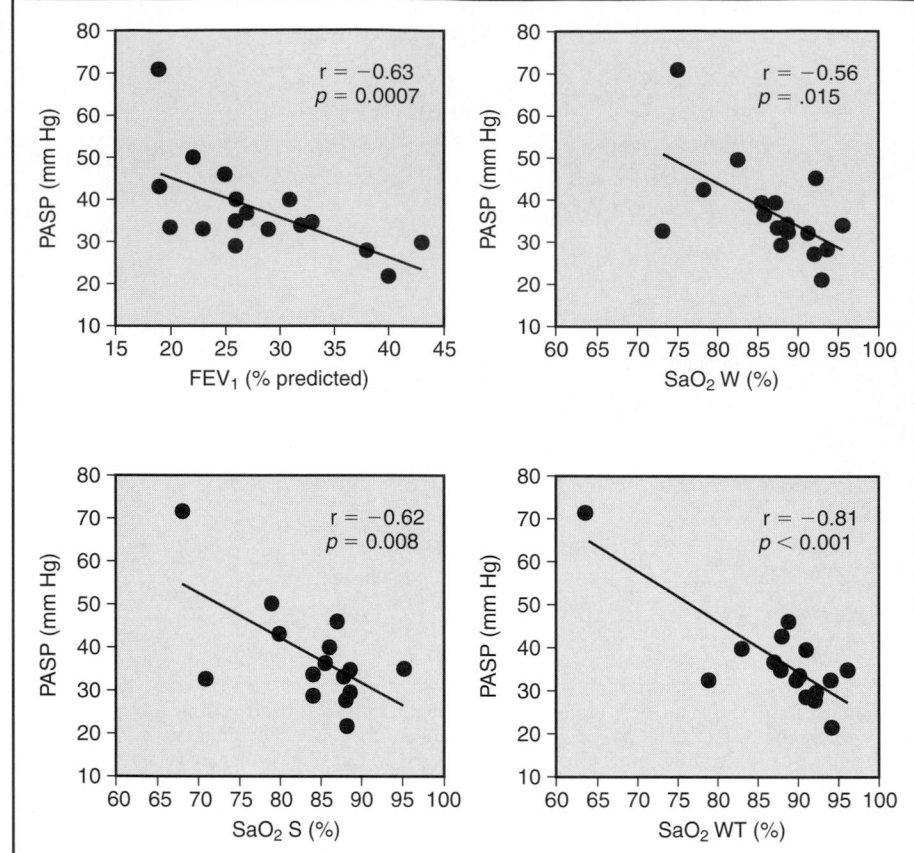

FIGURE 54–6. The correlation between pulmonary artery systolic pressure (PASP) and FEV_1, mean oxygen saturation during wakefulness (SaO_2W), mean oxygen saturation during sleep (SaO_2S), and mean oxygen saturation at the end of a 6-minute walk test (SaO_2WT). (From Fraser KL, Tullis E, Sasson Z, et al: Pulmonary hypertension and cardiac function in adult cystic fibrosis: Role of hypoxemia. Chest 115:1321–1328, 1999.)

gen is considered to be the mainstay of treatment in this group.

Sleep-Disordered Breathing

Sleep apnea, defined as repeated episodes of obstructive apnea and hypopnea during sleep together with daytime sleepiness or altered cardiopulmonary function, is common. Epidemiological studies estimate that the condition affects 2 to 4 percent of middle-aged adults.[138] Only a small proportion of the cases in this group of adults have been diagnosed, which is believed to be related to insufficient awareness of sleep apnea among physicians and the public at large.

The incidence of pulmonary hypertension in the setting of obstructive sleep apnea without clinically significant lung disease ranges from 17 to 41 percent, with most studies suggesting an incidence of 20 percent.[139, 140] Pulmonary hypertension is rarely observed in the absence of daytime hypoxemia, and the severity of nocturnal events (i.e., apnea and hypopnea) does not appear to be the determining factor of pulmonary hypertension (Fig. 54–7). Some studies have demonstrated that a reduced FEV_1 also contributes to pulmonary hypertension in these patients.[141] In most cases, the pulmonary hypertension is mild, similar to COPD.

Patients with sleep apnea also have an increased risk of diurnal hypertension, nocturnal dysrhythmias, right and left ventricular failure, myocardial infarction, and stroke.[142] Symptoms such as sleepiness, fatigue, irritability, and personality change have been attributed to nocturnal desaturation and the chronic sleep deprivation caused by sleep fragmentation. Sleep fragmentation may be the most important predictor of daytime sleepiness. Patient characteristics associated with sleep apnea include male sex, age older than 40 years, habitual snoring, nocturnal gasping, choking, or resuscitative snoring, observed apnea, and a history of sys-

temic hypertension.[143] Symptoms of daytime somnolence, unrefreshed sleep, morning headaches, cognitive impairment, depression, nocturnal esophageal reflux, and nocturia are commonly reported but do not distinguish sleep apnea from other common nonpulmonary, sleep disorders. A sleep study should be performed to confirm the presence of upper airway closure during sleep and to access the patient's level of risk.

Therapeutic strategies for patients with sleep apnea may be grouped into three general categories: behavioral, medical, and surgical. The goals of treatment are to establish normal nocturnal oxygenation and ventilation, abolish snoring, and eliminate disruption of sleep due to upper airway closure. Avoiding factors that increase the severity of upper airway obstruction such as sleep deprivation, the use of alcohol, sedatives, hypnotic agents, and increased weight should be discussed with the patient. In obese patients, weight loss can significantly reduce the severity of the apnea.[144] However, the most important advancement in the medical treatment is positive airway pressure. Positive airway pressure delivered through a mask is the initial treatment of choice in clinically important sleep apnea. Continuous positive pressure is applied to the upper airway with the nasal mask, nasal prongs, or mask that covers both the nose and mouth. The level of positive pressure required to sustain patency of the upper airway during sleep should be determined in the sleep laboratory. Supplemental oxygen can also be used in conjunction with positive airway pressure and assist in maintaining saturation above 90 percent.[145] Patients treated with continuous positive airway pressure delivered nasally have repeatedly demonstrated improvement in neuropsychiatric function and a lessening of daytime sleepiness.[146] Nocturnal desaturation, ventilatory related arousals, nocturnal dysrhythmias, pulmonary hypertension, and right-sided heart failure have also been effectively treated. Retrospective studies suggest that patients

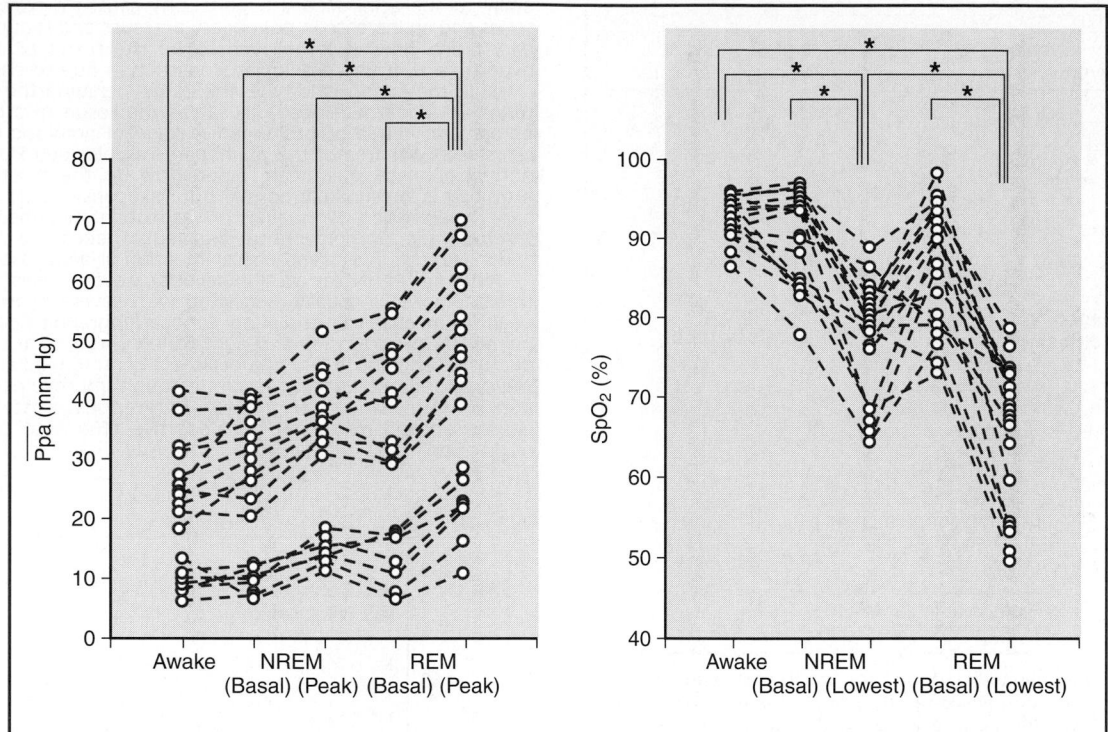

FIGURE 54–7. Mean pulmonary artery pressure (P_{pa}) and oxygen saturation by pulse oximetry (SpO_2) is shown during wakefulness in each sleep stage in patients with obstructive sleep apnea. Mean pulmonary artery pressure appears to be highest during rapid-eye-movement sleep, at a time that oxygen saturation is lowest. During wakefulness, when oxygen saturation is higher, the mean pulmonary artery pressures are considerably lower. (From Niijma M, Kimura H, Edo H, et al: Manifestation of pulmonary hypertension during REM sleep in obstructive sleep apnea syndrome. Am J Respir Crit Care Med 159:1766–1772, 1999.)

treated with nasally delivered continuous positive pressure or tracheostomy have improved survival.[147] Side effects reported by patients usually involve discomfort or irritation related to the nasal mask.

Surgical treatment includes tracheostomy and palatal surgery. For those with severe apnea who cannot tolerate positive airway pressure, tracheostomy can provide dramatic improvement and be life saving, although additional medical and psychosocial morbidity may be associated with this treatment. The most commonly performed palatal surgery, uvulopalatopharyngoplasty, is curative in less than 50 percent of patients. Of 25 patients observed for 4 to 8 years, about half of the patients were clinically and objectively improved over the long term.[148]

The approach to the patient with severe pulmonary hypertension associated with sleep apnea is controversial. Although it is unlikely a result of hypoxemia alone, it is recommended that these patients have documented effective therapy for at least 3 months, before treating the pulmonary arterial hypertension as a separate entity. In this subset, prostacyclin may prove helpful.

Alveolar Hypoventilation Disorders

CHEST WALL DISORDERS. Thoracovertebral deformities that can result in restrictive pulmonary syndromes and chronic alveolar hypoventilation include idiopathic kypho scoliosis, spinal tuberculosis, congenital spinal developmental abnormalities, spinal cord injury and other childhood myelopathies, ankylosing spondylitis, or other congenital and acquired muscular skeletal conditions, such as pectus excavatum. Kyphoscoliosis is a relatively common disorder of the spine in its articulations. When severe,

it can have a profound impact on pulmonary function, characterized by a severe restrictive pattern on pulmonary function testing (Fig. 54–8). In addition, there can be associated inspiratory muscle weakness that appears related to the increased elastic load from reduced lung and chest wall compliance. Scoliosis that appears before the age of 5 years has the worst respiratory prognosis. An angulation of greater than 100 degrees is considered very severe and is strongly associated with chronic alveolar hypoventilation.[149] Pulmonary compliance is often reduced by 50 percent or more as a result of lung underdevelopment and chronic lung hypoinflation. Patients can also have both central and obstructive apneas and hypopneas.

Pulmonary hypertension and chronic cor pulmonale frequently occur in patients with thoracovertebral deformities. Pulmonary hypertension is related to the reduction of the vascular bed because of hypoventilation and hypoxia. Symptoms are commonly slowly progressive. Hypoxemia may be seen from ventilation-perfusion mismatch or underlying atelectasis. When severe, the hypoxemia can also lead to cor pulmonale. In patients with advanced disease, intermittent positive-pressure breathing and noninvasive ventilation have been used successfully, as well as supplemental oxygen in patients who are hypoxemic.[150]

NEUROMUSCULAR DISEASE. The development of right-sided heart failure is an unusual manifestation of respiratory failure solely due to respiratory muscle weakness. It usually develops in response to the hypoxic and hypercapnic stimuli in patients with chronic forms of these disorders. Weakness of the respiratory muscles can be caused by either generalized muscle diseases, such as myopathic infiltrating diseases or muscular dystrophy (see Chap. 71), or more commonly by such neurological disorders as a cord lesion at or below the third cervical vertebrae, amyotrophic

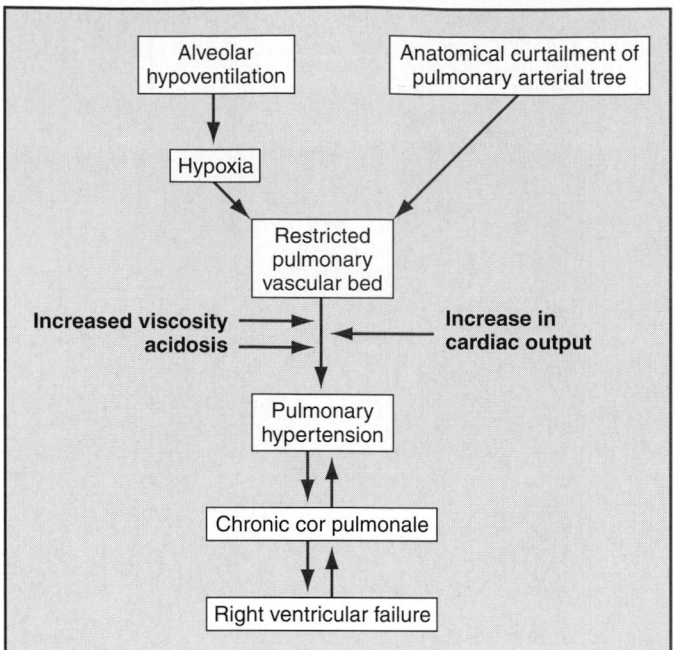

FIGURE 54-8. Pathogenesis of pulmonary hypertension and cor pulmonale in kyphoscoliosis and disorders of ventilatory control. (From Fishman AP: Pulmonary hypertension and cor pulmonale. *In* Fishman AP [ed]: Pulmonary Diseases and Disorders. 2nd ed. New York, McGraw-Hill Book Co, 1988, p 1033.)

lateral sclerosis, myasthenia gravis, poliomyelitis, and Guillain-Barré syndrome. The diagnosis of respiratory muscle weakness is confirmed by the finding of a restrictive ventilatory defect and a marked impairment of maximal respiratory pressures. Nocturnal ventilatory support, with either positive or negative pressure, has become established as effective therapy in appropriate cases, and its beneficial effects are well recognized.[151]

DIAPHRAGMATIC PARALYSIS. Bilateral diaphragmatic paralysis is an uncommon and rarely recognized cause of cor pulmonale. Diaphragmatic paralysis is a result of phrenic nerve injury, which can be traumatic or secondary to an underlying motor neuron disease. It may occur after cardiac surgery, as a manifestation of Lyme disease,[152] after radiation therapy,[153] or as a manifestation of other neurological disorders. When an affected patient is upright, ventilation may be normal or almost so, but when the patient is supine, gas exchange deteriorates. The diagnosis may be suspected in a patient with supine breathlessness, a disturbed sleep pattern, paradoxical motion of the abdomen on inspiration, and a low vital capacity in the upright position.

Patients with nontraumatic bilateral diaphragmatic paralysis may go unrecognized until they present either with respiratory failure or cor pulmonale. The diagnosis can be suspected when the vital capacity is reduced greater than 40 percent of predicted and paradoxic motion of the hemidiaphragms is noted on fluoroscopy.[154] Patients can also have unilateral paralysis of the diaphragm, which is more common but associated with less symptoms and physiological abnormalities. The treatment should always be directed toward correcting the underlying chronic neuromuscular disease, if present, and addressing nocturnal hypoventilation with noninvasive ventilatory techniques. Intermittent positive airway pressure is an effective therapy.[155]

PERSISTENT PULMONARY HYPERTENSION OF THE NEWBORN

Three forms of persistent pulmonary hypertension of the newborn (PPHN) have been described. In the hypertrophic type, the muscular tissue of the pulmonary arteries is hypertrophied and extends periph-erally to the acini. Medial hypertrophy causes narrowing of the arteries and an increase in pulmonary pressure and reduction in pulmonary blood flow. It is believed to be the result of sustained fetal hypertension from chronic vasoconstriction due to chronic fetal distress. In the hypoplastic type, the lungs including the pulmonary arteries are underdeveloped, usually as the result of a congenital diaphragmatic hernia or prolonged leakage of amniotic fluid.[156, 157] The cross-sectional area of the pulmonary vascular bed is inadequate for normal neonatal pulmonary blood flow. In the reactive type, lung histology is presumably normal but vasoconstriction causes pulmonary hypertension. High levels of vasoconstrictive mediators such as thromboxane, norepinephrine, and leukotrienes may be responsible and may result in a streptococcal infection or acute asphyxia at birth.

Although PPHN can vary in severity, severe cases are usually life threatening. It is usually associated with severe hypoxemia and the need for mechanical ventilation. Echocardiographic findings of severe pulmonary hypertension and right-to-left shunting at the level of the ductus arteriosus or foramen ovale are common. Inhaled nitric oxide has provided encouraging results through improvement in oxygenation in these patients (Fig. 54-9). Intravenous prostacyclin has also been used and may even have additive effects to that of inhaled nitric oxide.[158]

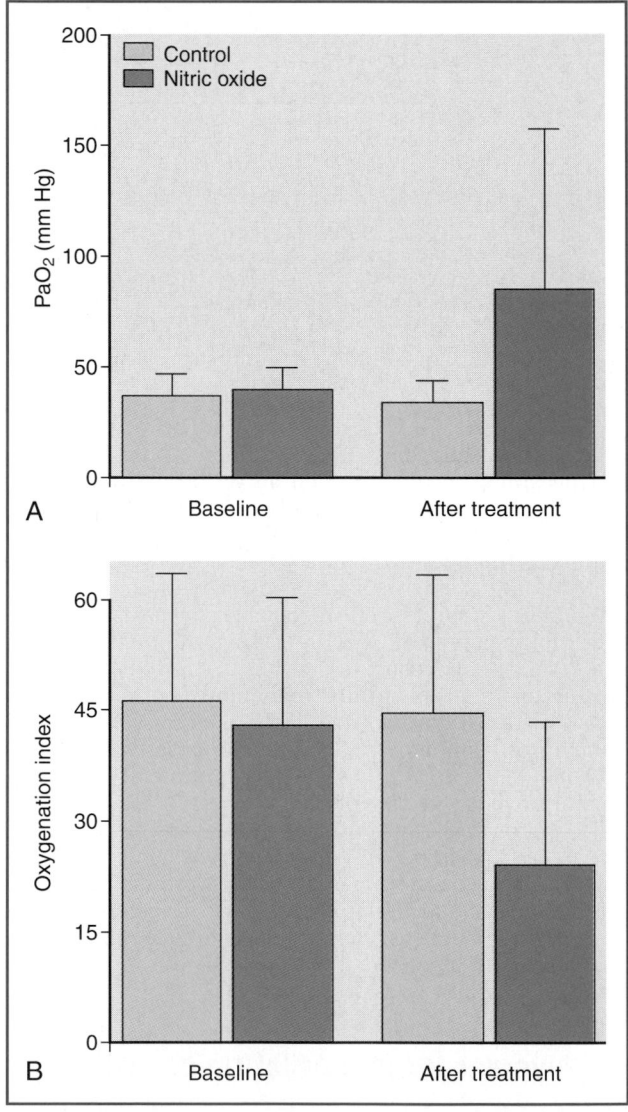

FIGURE 54-9. The short-term effect of inhaled nitric oxide on systemic oxygenation in infants with severe hypoxemia and persistent pulmonary hypertension of the newborn. As compared with conventional treatment with oxygen and mechanical ventilation without nitric oxide (open bars), nitric oxide therapy (solid bars) rapidly increased postductal PaO_2 from baseline (panel A) and decreased the oxygenation index (a value calculated as $100 \times FiO_2 \times$ mean airway pressure and postductal PaO_2). (From Roberts JD Jr, Fineman JR, Morin FC III, et al: Inhaled nitric oxide and persistent pulmonary hypertension of the newborn. N Engl J Med 336:605-610, 1997.)

ALVEOLAR CAPILLARY DYSPLASIA. Alveolar capillary dysplasia is a very rare cause for PPHN and is characterized by a developmental abnormality in the pulmonary vasculature. The antemortem diagnosis can only be made with open-lung biopsy. Despite aggressive treatment with nitric oxide, prostacyclin, and even extracorporeal membrane oxygenation, survival in the setting of alveolar capillary dysplasia is rare.[159]

PULMONARY HYPERTENSION DUE TO CHRONIC THROMBOEMBOLIC DISEASE

Thromboembolic Obstruction of the Proximal Pulmonary Arteries (see also Chap. 62)

Pulmonary thromboembolism, as a single event or as repeated events, rarely leads to the development of chronic pulmonary hypertension.[160] However, in a subset of patients (believed to be less than 0.1 percent of all patients suffering from pulmonary embolism), the outcome is unusual.[161] Rather than having inherent fibrinolytic resolution of the thromboembolism with restoration of vascular patency, the thromboemboli in these patients fails to resolve adequately. They undergo organization and incomplete recanalization and become incorporated into the vascular wall. Commonly, they are in the subsegmental, segmental, and lobar vessels, although it is believed that chronic thromboembolism tends to propagate retrograde, leading to slowly progressive vascular obstruction.[160] It appears that the vast majority of these patients have suffered one major thromboembolic event rather than multiple recurrences.

The slowly progressive nature of the course of chronic thromboembolic pulmonary hypertension (CTEPH) allows right ventricular hypertrophy to ensue and compensate for the increased pulmonary vascular resistance. However, owing to either progressive thrombosis or vascular changes in the "uninvolved" vascular bed,[161] the pulmonary hypertension becomes progressive and the patient manifests the clinical symptoms of dyspnea, fatigue, hypoxemia, and right-sided heart failure.

DIAGNOSIS. The physical examination of a patient with CTEPH is typical of any patient with pulmonary hypertension, with the exception of the following features. These patients tend to have lower cardiac outputs than patients with PPH, which is often reflected by the carotid arterial pulse volume. In addition, on occasion, bruits may be heard over areas of the lung that represent vessels with partial occlusions, but they must be carefully looked for. It is important to make the diagnostic distinction between patients with CTEPH and those with other forms of pulmonary hypertension because the treatment is so different. For the former group, a potentially curative therapy through thromboendarterectomy is available, whereas for the latter group effective pharmacological regimens are now evolving. The symptoms and physical findings of CTEPH are nonspecific and similar to those patients with primary pulmonary hypertension.

The perfusion lung scan is usually adequate to identify patients with this entity and is an important reason why lung scans are recommended for all patients who present with pulmonary hypertension. However, the lung scan typically underestimates the severity of the central pulmonary arterial obstruction.[162] Therefore, patients who present with one or more mismatched segmental or larger defect should undergo pulmonary angiography. Pulmonary angiography can be performed safely in these patients if careful attention is given to the hemodynamic state. Nonionic contrast medium has been demonstrated to cause no major hemodynamic effects even in patients with severe chronic thromboembolic pulmonary hypertension[163] and is preferred. Hypotension and/or bradycardia should be immediately treated with atropine.

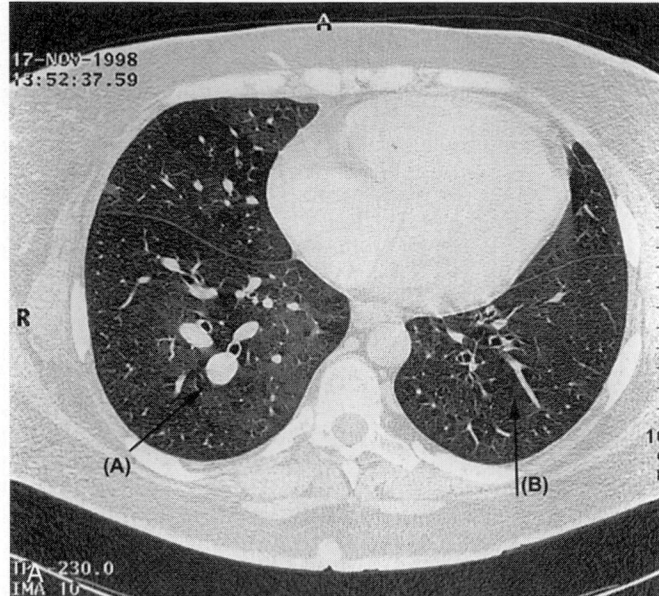

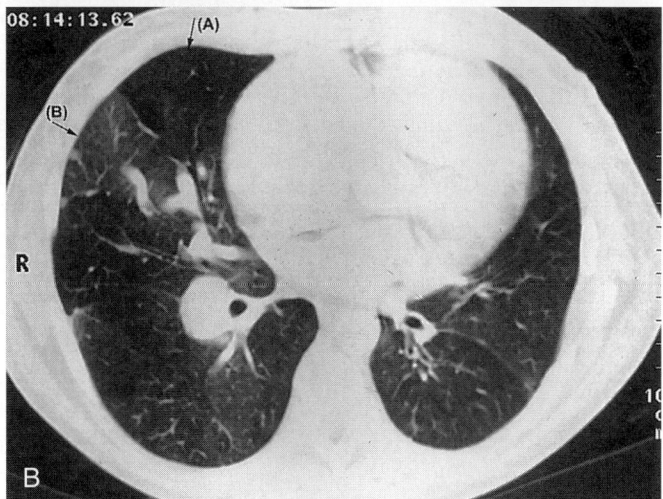

FIGURE 54–10. Chest CT scans in a patient with chronic thromboembolic pulmonary hypertension. In *A*, a helical scan with contrast medium enhancement of the pulmonary vasculature shows a marked disparity in vessel size between the involved vessels (A), which are enlarged from thrombus, and the uninvolved vessels (B). In *B*, a non–contrast medium–enhanced high-resolution scan illustrates a marked mosaic pattern manifest by differences in density of regions of the lung parenchyma reflecting the perfused areas (B) and the nonperfused areas (A), also consistent with underlying thromboembolic disease.

CT can be a great aid in diagnosing CTEPH (Fig. 54–10). Using high-resolution nonenhanced CT, areas of increased attenuation that do not obscure the vessels and that have a ground-glass appearance have been characterized as a mosaic pattern corresponding to hypoperfusion of the lung. Although this pattern is consistent with CTEPH, it may also be seen in cystic fibrosis, bronchiectasis, and the lungs of lung transplant recipients. It is virtually never seen in PPH.[164] Marked variation in the size of the segmental vessels is more specific for CTEPH and is believed to represent involvement of the segmental vessels due to thromboemboli. It has been reported that these findings might also be mimicked in patients with fibrosing mediastinitis.

On cardiac catheterization, patients with CTEPH tend to have higher right atrial pressures and lower cardiac outputs than comparable patients with PPH for the same level of pulmonary artery pressure. Because this is a disease that generally is progressive, the hemodynamic indication for surgical intervention would be an elevation of pulmonary artery pressure and pulmonary vascular resistance for a period of more than 3 months.

TREATMENT. Patients suitable to undergo pulmonary thromboendarterectomy must have thrombi that are accessible to surgical removal and demonstrate a significant increase in the pulmonary vascular resistance.[161] The operative mortality is fairly high, approximately 12 percent in experienced centers.[165] The postoperative management of these patients can be extremely challenging. Patients in whom a large volume of central thrombus is removed, associated with back-bleeding from the distal vascular segments and an immediate fall in the pulmonary artery pressure, usually have an extremely good postoperative course and long-term follow-up. Patients in whom small amounts of thrombus can be removed, in whom the thrombus becomes fragmented at the time of thromboendarterectomy, or in whom there is no distal back-bleeding from the segment where the thrombus was removed usually have a difficult postoperative course. In addition, a lack of significant fall in pulmonary artery pressure and an increase in cardiac output portends a difficult postoperative recovery.

These patients may need mechanical ventilation and inotropic support for days to weeks during periods of slow recovery. Much of their mortality appears to be related to severe right ventricular dysfunction, which actually becomes initially worsened during the surgical procedure. Reperfusion injury, which is manifest by profound hypoxemia and pulmonary infiltrates corresponding to the segments where thrombus was removed, has been reported and can be extensive. The only effective management of this complication is sustained assisted ventilation and oxygen supplementation. Attempts to reverse this with corticosteroids or other agents have not been successful.

Those survivors who have a good result, with a significant reduction in postoperative pulmonary vascular resistance at 48 hours, can expect to realize an improvement in functional class and exercise tolerance.[166, 167] Life-long anticoagulation with a goal international normalized ratio of 2.5 to 3.5 is indicated postoperatively. Right ventricular dysfunction of any magnitude is not considered a contraindication to surgery, because right ventricular function has been noted to improve once the obstruction of the pulmonary blood flow is removed. Certain hypercoagulable states such as lupus anticoagulant may be associated with CTEPH.[168] Some of these patients have also been successfully treated with pulmonary thromboendarterectomy.[169]

Sickle Cell Disease

Cardiovascular system abnormalities are prominent as part of the clinical spectrum of sickle cell disease. Evidence of right ventricular dysfunction, presumably resulting from pulmonary hypertension, is a poorly characterized complication. The incidence of pulmonary hypertension in the setting of sickle cell disease in one series of 60 consecutive patients undergoing echocardiography was 20 percent.[170] The mortality was also significantly greater in patients with pulmonary hypertension than those without (42 percent vs. 8 percent, $p = 0.03$). One must always consider left ventricular dysfunction as a cause of pulmonary hypertension in sickle cell disease because the elevation of pulmonary artery pressure is most often associated with elevation of the pulmonary capillary wedge pressure.[171] Patients with sickle cell disease may also have an increased risk of thromboembolism, and pulmonary thromboendarterectomy may be indicated in certain situations.[172] Sickle cell disease can also affect the lungs by causing embolization of bone marrow elements. Generally, the smaller pulmonary arteries, arterioles, and capillaries are affected. It can be associated with pulmonary infarction or local perivascular fibrosis.

SCHISTOSOMIASIS

Although schistosomiasis is extremely rare in North America, hundreds of millions of people are affected worldwide, particularly in developing countries. The development of pulmonary hypertension almost always occurs in the setting of hepatosplenic disease and portal hypertension.[173] Clinical features appear when ova embolize to the lungs, where they induce formation of delayed hypersensitivity granulomas. In addition, deposition of fibrous tissue causes narrowing, thickening, and occlusion of the pulmonary arterioles. Histologically, focal changes related directly to the presence of schistosome ova may be located either within the alveolar tissue or within the pulmonary arteries, and plexiform or angiomatoid lesions may be found. Fibrosis surrounds most focal lesions.[174] The clinical symptoms and radiographic findings in these patients who develop pulmonary hypertension are not distinctive. In developing countries this condition can be confused with primary pulmonary hypertension.

The diagnosis of schistosomiasis-induced cor pulmonale is confirmed by finding the parasite ova in the urine or stools of persons with symptoms. However, the insidious onset of pulmonary vascular disease years after infection makes finding these parasite ova difficult. Active infections are treated with praziquantel, which kills the adult worms and stops further destruction of tissue by ova deposition.[175] Reversal of pathological lesions in the lungs after therapy has not been documented.

SARCOIDOSIS

Sarcoidosis is a multisystemic granulomatous disease of unknown origin characterized by an enhanced cellular immune response at the sites of involvement.[176] Although any organ can be involved, it most commonly affects the lungs and intrathoracic lymph nodes.[177] The clinical presentation and natural history of sarcoidosis varies greatly, but the lung is involved in over 90 percent of the patients. The most common presenting symptoms are cough and shortness of breath, which is of a progressive nature.[178] As the disease progresses in the lung parenchyma, extensive interstitial fibrosis is the result. In addition, obstructive airway disease, fibrocystic disease, bronchiectasis, endobronchial granulomas, and lobar atelectasis are common consequences of lung involvement.

Cardiac involvement from sarcoidosis appears to be more common than previously thought and may be present in up to one third of the cases (see Chap. 48).[179] Consequently, patients presenting with dyspnea should have a thorough cardiac evaluation for the possibility of cardiac involvement. Noncaseating granulomas may infiltrate the myocardium and leave fibrotic scars; and if enough of the myocardium is involved, the patients will develop clinical features of a restrictive cardiomyopathy. Patients with cardiac involvement from sarcoidosis may also present with varying degrees of heart block, arrhythmias, and/or clinical features of biventricular diastolic heart failure. Sudden death can be a common manifestation of cardiac sarcoid, and it is one of the most feared sequelae. The prognosis of patients with cardiac involvement from sarcoidosis is variable but can be quite poor. Usually a trial of corticosteroids is given in the hope that it will alter the natural history of the disease.

An echocardiogram will often demonstrate either diffuse or regional wall motion abnormalities in patients with cardiac involvement. It is not uncommon, however, to find the features of pulmonary hypertension. Pulmonary hypertension detected by echo-Doppler techniques may be the result of restrictive cardiomyopathy from sarcoid and needs to be clearly distinguished from patients with pulmonary hypertension from direct pulmonary vascular involvement, because their clinical management will differ dramatically.

Cor pulmonale is most commonly the result of chronic severe *fibrocystic* sarcoidosis.[180] Patients have chronic progressive dyspnea with effort, a chest radiograph demonstrating severe diffuse interstitial fibrotic lung disease, and pulmonary function tests that reflect severe restrictive physiology and hypoxemia. In these cases the resulting cor pulmonale is usually mild to moderate and typical of patients presenting with restrictive lung disease of any etiology. The treatment is generally focused on reversing any acute exacerbations of their lung disease and supplemental oxygen when indicated. Some patients with sarcoidosis, however, have mild to moderate restrictive lung disease with severe pulmonary hypertension, presumed from granulomatous vasculitis of the pulmonary vessels. It is critically important in the cardiopulmonary evaluation of the patient presenting with underlying sarcoidosis and dyspnea to distinguish whether the symptoms are from chronic interstitial lung disease, restrictive cardiomyopathy, or pulmonary vascular disease.[181] Although the traditional treatment of these patients has been unsatisfactory, it has recently been demonstrated that some patients have a very favorable response to intravenous prostacyclin therapy.[182] Although interstitial lung involvement from the sarcoidosis can result in mild pulmonary hypertension, a subset of patients present with severe pulmonary hypertension believed to be due to direct pulmonary vascular involvement. It appears that, as with other secondary causes, these patients are predisposed to the development of pulmonary vascular disease that is triggered in some way by the sarcoid disease process. Although the use of intravenous prostacyclin chronically may reverse the right-sided heart failure and dramatically improve their pulmonary hemodynamics, it will have no impact on any underlying fibrotic lung disease and/or hypoxemia, which still may render the patients symptomatic and dyspneic.

PULMONARY CAPILLARY HEMANGIOMATOSIS

Pulmonary capillary hemangiomatosis (PCH) was first described in 1978 as a very rare cause of pulmonary hypertension.[183] Because of the few reports in the medical literature it is hard to characterize this abnormality. The typical chest radiographic appearance is a diffuse bilateral reticular nodular pattern associated with enlarged central pulmonary arteries.[184] Ventilation-perfusion scans are often abnormal and may show matched or unmatched defects. The most characteristic finding on high-resolution CT is diffuse bilateral thickening of the interlobular septa and small centrilobular poorly circumscribed nodular opacities.[185] Diffuse ground-glass opacities have also been described. Histological findings often include irregular small nodular foci of thin-walled capillary sized vessels, which diffusely invade the lung parenchyma, the bronchiolar walls, and the adventitia of large vessels. These nodular lesions are often associated with alveolar hemorrhage. Changes of hypertensive arteriopathy manifest by intimal fibrosis and medial hypertrophy are also common. Most patients appear to be young adults and present with dyspnea and/or hemoptysis. It is very difficult to distinguish PCH from PPH clinically. A hereditary form with probable autosomal recessive transmission has been reported.

The clinical course of these patients is usually one of progressive deterioration leading to severe pulmonary hypertension, right-sided heart failure, and death. Intravenous prostacyclin has been used, but it has been reported with the association of the development of severe pulmonary edema.[186] The only definitive treatment for these patients is bilateral lung transplantation.

R E F E R E N C E S

EFFECTS OF HYPOXIA ON THE PULMONARY CIRCULATION

1. Cutaia M, Rounds S: Hypoxic pulmonary vasoconstriction: Physiologic significant, mechanism and clinic relevance. Chest 97:706–718, 1990.
2. Grover RF, Wagner WW, McMurtry IF, et al: Pulmonary circulation. In Shepherd JT, Abboud FM (eds): Handbook of Physiology, Section 2, The Cardiovascular System, Vol III, Peripheral Circulation and Organ Blood Flow, Part I. Baltimore, MD, Williams & Wilkins, 1983, pp 103–137.
3. Kourembana S, Morita T, Christou H, et al: Hypoxic responses of vascular cells. Chest 114:25S–28S, 1998.
4. McMurtry IF: Bay K 8644, a Ca^{++} channel facilitator, potentiates hypoxic vasoconstriction in isolated rat lungs. Fed Proc 44:2389, 1985.
5. McMurtry IF: Humeral control. In Bergofsky E (ed): Abnormal Pulmonary Circulation. New York, Churchill Livingstone, 1986, pp 83–126.
6. Rabinovitch M, Gamble W, Nadas AS, et al: Rat pulmonary circulation after chronic hypoxia: Hemodynamic and structural features. Am J Physiol 236:H818, 1979.
7. Rabinovitch M, Gamble WJ, Miettinen OS, et al: Age and sex influence on pulmonary hypertension of chronic hypoxia and on recovery. Am J Physiol 240:H62, 1981.
8. Griffith TM, Edwards DH, Davis RL, et al: EDRF coordinates the behavior of vascular resistance vessels. Nature 329:442, 1987.
9. Stewart DJ, Levy RD, Cernacek RP, et al: Increased plasma endothelin-1 in pulmonary hypertension: Marker or mediator of disease? Ann Intern Med 114:464, 1991.
10. Fike CD, Kaplowitz MR, Thomas CJ, et al: Chronic hypoxia decreases nitric oxide production and endothelial nitric oxide synthase in newborn pig lungs. Am J Physiol 274:l517–1526, 1998.
11. Adnot S, Raffestin B, Eddahibi S, et al: Loss of endothelium-dependent relaxant activity in the pulmonary circulation of rats exposed to chronic hypoxia. J Clin Invest 87:155–162, 1991.
12. Liu S, Crawley DE, Barnes PJ, et al: Endothelium-derived relaxing factor inhibits hypoxic pulmonary vasoconstriction in rats. Am Rev Respir Dis 143:32–37, 1991.
13. Horstman DJ, Frank DU, Rich GF: Prolonged inhaled NO attenuates hypoxic, but not monocrotaline-induced, pulmonary vascular remodeling in rats. Anesth Analg 86:74–81, 1998.
14. Cargill RI, Kiely DG, Clark RA, et al: Hypoxaemia and release of endothelin-1. Thorax 50:1308–1310, 1995.
15. Peng W, Michael JR, Hoidal JR, et al: ET-1 modulates KCa-channel activity and arterial tension in normoxic and hypoxic human pulmonary vasculature. Am J Physiol 275:1729–1739, 1998.
16. Chen SJ, Chen YF, Opegenorth TJ, et al: The orally active nonpeptide endothelin A-receptor antagonist A-127722 prevents and reverses hy-

poxia-induced pulmonary hypertension and pulmonary vascular remodeling in Sprague-Dawley rats. J Cardiovasc Pharmacol 29:713–725, 1997.
17. Holm P, Liska J, Clozel M, et al: The endothelin antagonist bosentan: Hemodynamic effects during normoxia and hypoxic pulmonary hypertension in pigs. J Thorac Cardiovasc Surg 112:890–897, 1996.
18. Bialeck RA, Stinson-Fisher C, Murdoch W, et al: A novel orally active endothelin-A receptor antagonist, ZD1611, prevents chronic hypoxia-induced pulmonary hypertension in the rat. Chest 114:91S, 1998.
19. Willette RN, Ohlstein EH, Mitchell MP, et al: Nonpeptide endothelin receptor antagonists: VIII. Attentuation of acute hypoxia-induced pulmonary hypertension in the dog. J Pharmacol Exp Ther 280:695–701, 1997.
20. Haleen S, Schroeder R, Walker D, et al: Efficacy of CI-1020, an endothelin-A receptor antagonist, in hypoxic pulmonary hypertension. J Cardiovasc Pharmacol 31:s331–s335, 1998.
21. Holm P, Liska J, Franco-Cereceda A: The ETA receptor antagonist, BMS-182874, reduces acute hypoxic pulmonary hypertension in pigs in vivo. Cardiovasc Res 37:765–771, 1998.
22. Katayose D, Ohe M, Yamauchi K, et al: Increased expression of PDGF A- and B-chain genes in rat lungs with hypoxic pulmonary hypertension. Am Physiol Soc 1040:l100–l106, 1993.
23. Christou H, Yoshida A, Arthur V, et al: Increased vascular endothelial growth factor production in the lungs of rats with hypoxia-induced pulmonary hypertension. Am J Respir Cell Mol Biol 18:768–776, 1998.
24. Partovian C, Adnot S, Eddahibi S, et al: Heart and lung VEGF mRNA expression in rats with monocrotaline- or hypoxia-induced pulmonary hypertension. Am J Physiol 275:h1948–h1956, 1998.
25. Tuder RM, Flook BE, Voelkel NF: Increased gene expression for VEGF and the VEGF receptors KDR/Flk and Flt in lungs exposed to acute or to chronic hypoxia. J Clin Invest 95:1798–1807, 1995.
26. Clauss M, Gerlach M, Gerlach H, et al: Vascular permeability factor: A tumor-derived polypeptide that induces endothelial cell and monocyte procoagulant activity and promotes monocyte migration. J Exp Med 172:1535–1545, 1990.
27. Morrell NW, Danilov SM, Satyan KB, et al: Right ventricular angiotensin converting enzyme activity and expression is increased during hypoxic pulmonary hypertension. Cardiovasc Res 34:393–403, 1997.
28. Clozel JP, Saunier C, Hartemann D, et al: Effects of cilazapril, a novel angiotensin converting enzyme inhibitor, on the structure of pulmonary arteries of rats exposed to chronic hypoxia. J Cardiovasc Pharmacol 17:36–40, 1991.
29. Nong Z, Stassen JM, Moons L, et al: Inhibition of tissue angiotensin-converting enzyme with quinapril reduces hypoxic pulmonary hypertension and pulmonary vascular remodeling. Circulation 94:1941–1947, 1996.
30. Kiely DG, Cargill RI, Lipworth BJ: Acute hypoxic pulmonary vasoconstriction in man is attenuated by type I angiotensin II receptor blockade. Cardiovasc Res 30:875–880, 1995.
31. Pelouch V, Kolar F, Ost'adal B, et al: Regression of chronic hypoxia-induced pulmonary hypertension, right ventricular hypertrophy, and fibrosis: Effect of enalapril. Cardiovasc Drugs Ther 11:177–185, 1997.
32. Semenza GL, Agani F, Iyer N, et al: Hypoxia-inducible factor: From molecular biology to cardiopulmonary physiology. Chest 114:40s–45s, 1998.
33. Glazier JB, Murray JF: Sites of pulmonary vasomotor reactivity in the dog during alveolar hypoxia and serotonin and histamine infusion. J Clin Invest 50:2550, 1971.
34. Bergofsky EH: Mechanisms underlying vasomotor regulation of regional pulmonary blood flow in normal and disease states. Am J Med 57:378, 1974.
35. Hauge A: Hypoxia and pulmonary vascular resistance: The relative effects of pulmonary arterial and alveolar PO_2. Acta Physiol Scand 76:121, 1969.
36. Enson Y, Guintini C, Lewis ML, et al: The influence of hydrogen ion concentration and hypoxia on the pulmonary circulation. J Clin Invest 43:1146, 1964.
37. Moret P, Covarrubias E, Coudert J, et al: Cardiocirculatory adaptation to chronic hypoxia. Acta Cardiol 27:596, 1972.
38. Heath D, Williams DR: High-Altitude Medicine and Pathology. London, Butterworths, 1989.
39. Ward MP, Milledge JS, West JB: High Altitude Medicine and Physiology, 2nd ed. London, Chapman & Hall Medical, 1995.
40. D'avila-Roman VG, Guest TM, Tuteur PG, et al: Transient right but not left ventricular dysfunction after strenuous exercise at high altitude. J Am Coll Cardiol 30:468–473, 1997.
41. Matthay RA, Schwarz MI, Ellis JH, et al: Pulmonary artery hypertension in chronic obstructive pulmonary disease: Chest radiographic assessment. Invest Radiol 16:95–100, 1981.
42. Chetty KG, Brown SE, Light RW: Identification of pulmonary hypertension in chronic obstructive pulmonary disease from routine chest radiographs. Am Rev Respir Dis 126:338–341, 1982.
43. Butler PM, Leggett SI, Howe CM, et al: Identification of electrocardiographic criteria for diagnosis of right ventricular hypertrophy due to mitral stenosis. Am J Cardiol 57:639, 1986.
44. Behar JV, Howe CM, Wagner NB, et al: Performance of new criteria for right ventricular hypertrophy and myocardial infarction in patients with pulmonary hypertension due to cor pulmonale and mitral stenosis. J Electrocardiol 24:231–237, 1991.

45. Matthay RA, Berger HJ: Noninvasive assessment of right and left ventricular function in acute and chronic respiratory failure. Crit Care Med 11:329–338, 1983.

46. Schiller NB, Sahn DJ: Pulmonary pressure measurement by Doppler and two-dimensional echocardiography in adult and paediatric populations. In Wei EK, Archer SL, Reeves JT (eds): The Diagnosis and Treatment of Pulmonary Hypertension. New York, Futura, 1992, pp 41–59.

47. Migueres M, Escamilla R, Coca F, et al: Pulsed Doppler echocardiography in the diagnosis of pulmonary hypertension and COPD. Chest 98: 280–285, 1990.

48. Masuyama T, Kodama K, Kitabatake A, et al: Continuous wave Doppler echocardiographic detection of pulmonary regurgitation and its application to non-invasive estimation of pulmonary arterial pressure. Circulation 484–492, 1986.

49. Himelman RB, Stulbarg M, Kircher B, et al: Noninvasive evaluation of pulmonary artery pressure during exercise by saline-enhanced Doppler echocardiography in chronic pulmonary disease. Circulation 79:863–871, 1989.

50. Murphy ML: The pathology of the right heart in chronic hypertrophy and failure. In Fisk RL (ed): The Right Heart. Philadelphia, FA Davis, 1987, pp 159–169.

51. Matthay RA, Berger HJ: Cardiovascular-pulmonary interaction in chronic obstructive pulmonary disease with special reference to the pathogenesis and management of cor pulmonale. Med Clin North Am 74:571–618, 1990.

52. Foster WL Jr, Pratt PC, Roggli VL, et al: Centrilobular emphysema: CT-pathologic correlation. Radiology 159:27, 1986.

53. Gurney JW, Jones KK, Robbins RA, et al: Regional distribution of emphysema: Correlation of high-resolution CT with pulmonary function tests in unselected smokers. Radiology 183:457, 1992.

54. Turnball LW, Ridgway JP, Biernacki W, et al: Assessment of the right ventricle by magnetic resonance imaging in chronic obstructive lung disease. Thorax 45:597–601, 1990.

55. Fayad ZA, Ferrari VA, Kraitchman DL, et al: Right ventricular regional function using MR tagging: Normal versus chronic pulmonary hypertension. Magn Reson Med 39:116–123, 1998.

PULMONARY HYPERTENSION WITH RESPIRATORY DISORDERS

56. American Thoracic Society: Statement standards for the diagnosis and care of patients with chronic obstructive pulmonary disease. Am J Resp Crit Care Med 152:s78–s83, 1995.

57. American Thoracic Society: Standards for the diagnosis and care of patients with chronic obstructive pulmonary disease (COPD) and asthma. Am Rev Respir Dis 136:225–244, 1987.

58. US Surgeon General: The Health Consequences of Smoking: Chronic Obstructive Lung Disease. DHHS publication no. 84-50205. Washington, DC, US Department of Health and Human Services, 1984.

59. Sherrill DL, Lebowitz MD, Burrows B: Epidemiology of chronic obstructive pulmonary disease. Clin Chest Med 11:375–388, 1990.

60. Lamb D: Pathology of COPD. In Brewis R, Gibson GJ, Geddes DM (eds): Respiratory Medicine. London, Bailliere Tindall, 1990, pp 497–507.

61. Magee F, Wright JL, Wiggs BR, et al: Pulmonary vascular structure and function in chronic obstructive pulmonary disease. Thorax 43:183–189, 1988.

62. Harris P, Heath D: The pulmonary vasculature in emphysema. In Harris P, Heath D (eds): The human pulmonary circulation. Edinburgh, Churchill Livingstone, 1986, pp 507–521.

63. Naeije R: Should pulmonary hypertension be treated in chronic obstructive pulmonary disease? In Weir EK, Archer SL, Reeves JT (eds): The Diagnosis and Treatment of Pulmonary Hypertension. New York: Futura Publishing, 1992, pp 209–239.

64. Mahler DA, Brent BN, Loke J, et al: Right ventricular performance and central circulatory hemodynamics during upright exercise in patients with chronic obstructive pulmonary disease. Am Rev Respir Dis 130: 722–729, 1984.

65. Weitzenblum E, Sautegeau A, Ehrhart M, et al: Long-term course of pulmonary arterial pressure in chronic obstructive pulmonary disease. Am Rev Respir Dis 130:993–998, 1984.

66. Khaja F, Parker JO: Right and left ventricular performance in chronic obstructive lung disease. Am Heart J 82:319–327, 1971.

67. Stevens D, Sharma K, Rich S, et al: Severe pulmonary hypertension associated with COPD. Am J Respir Crit Care Med 159:A155, 1999.

68. Weitzenblum E, Hirth C, Ducolone A, et al: Prognostic value of pulmonary artery pressure in chronic obstructive pulmonary disease. Thorax 36:752–758, 1981.

69. Burrows B, Fletcher CM, Heard BE, et al: Clinical types of chronic obstructive lung disease in London and in Chicago: A study of 100 patients. Am Rev Respir Dis 90:14–27, 1964.

70. France AJ, Prescott RJ, Biernacki W, et al: Does right ventricular function predict survival in patients with chronic obstructive pulmonary disease? Thorax 43:621–626, 1988.

71. Hodgkin JE: Prognosis in chronic obstructive pulmonary disease. Clin Chest Med 11:555–569, 1990.

72. Piccioni P, Caria E, Bignamini E, et al: Predictors of survival in a group of patients with chronic airflow obstruction. J Clin Epidemiol 51:547–55, 1998.

73. Antonelli I, Fuso L, De Rosa M, et al: Co-morbidity contributes to predict mortality of patients with chronic obstructive pulmonary disease. Eur Respir J 10:2794–800, 1997.

74. Dallari R, Barozzi G, Pinelli G, et al: Predictors of survival in subjects with chronic obstructive pulmonary disease treated with long-term oxygen therapy. Respiration 61:8–13, 1994.

75. Braghiroli A, Zaccaria S, Ioli F, et al: Pulmonary failure as a cause of death in COPD. Monaldi Arch Chest Dis 52:170–175, 1997.

76. Filipecki S, Kober J, Kaminski D, et al: Pulmonary thromboembolism. Monaldi Arch Chest Dis 52:492–493, 1997.

77. Anthonisen NR, Connett JE, Kiley JP, et al: Effects of smoking intervention and the use of an inhaled anticholinergic bronchodilator on the rate of decline of FEV_1: The Lung Health Study. JAMA 272:1497–1505, 1994.

78. Schneider NG, Olmstead RE, Steinberg C, et al: Efficacy of buspirone in smoking cessation: A placebo-controlled trial. Clin Pharmacol Ther 60: 568–575, 1996.

79. Hurt RD, Sachs DPL, Glover ED, et al: A comparison of sustained-released bupropion and placebo for smoking cessation. N Engl J Med 337:1195–202, 1997.

80. Medical Research Council Working Party: Long term domicillary oxygen therapy in chronic hypoxic cor pulmonale complicating chronic bronchitis and emphysema: A clinical trial. Lancet 1:681, 1981.

81. Nocturnal Oxygen Therapy Trial Group: Continuous or nocturnal oxygen therapy in hypoxemic chronic obstructive lung disease. Ann Intern Med 93:931, 1980.

82. Ashutosh K, Mead G, Dunsky M: Early effects of oxygen administration and prognosis in chronic obstructive pulmonary disease and cor pulmonale. Am Rev Respir Dis 127:399–404, 1983.

83. Morrison DA, Henry R, Goldman S: Preliminary study of the effects of low flow oxygen on oxygen delivery and right ventricular function in chronic lung disease. Am Rev Respir Dis 133:390, 1986.

84. Wiedemann HP, Matthay R: The management of acute and chronic cor pulmonale. In Scharf SM, Cassidy SS (eds): Heart-Lung Interactions in Health and Disease. New York, Marcel Dekker, 1989, pp 915–981.

85. Dewan NA, Bell CW: Effect of low flow and high flow oxygen delivery on exercise tolerance and sensation of dyspnea. Chest 105:1061–1065, 1994.

86. Meduri GU, Abou-Shala N, Fox RC, et al: Noninvasive face mask mechanical ventilation in patients with acute hypercapnic respiratory failure. Chest 100:445–454, 1991.

87. Soguel-Schenkel N, Burdet L, deMuralt B, et al: Oxygen saturation during daily activities in chronic obstructive pulmonary disease. Eur Respir J 9:2584–2589, 1996.

88. Wedzicha JA: Ambulatory oxygen in chronic obstructive pulmonary disease. Monaldi Arch Chest Dis 51:243–245, 1996.

89. Ambier M, Murciano D, Fournier M, et al: Central respiratory drive in acute respiratory failure of patients with chronic obstructive pulmonary disease. Am J Rev Respir Dis 122:191–199, 1980.

90. Rennard SI, Serby CW, Ghafouri M, et al: Extended therapy with ipratropium is associated with improved lung function in patients with COPD: A retrospective analysis of data from seven clinical trials. Chest 110:62–70, 1996.

91. Ferguson GT, Cherniack RM: Current concepts: Management of chronic obstructive pulmonary disease. N Engl J Med 328:1017–10222, 1993.

92. Combivent Inhalation Aerosol Study Group. In chronic obstructive pulmonary disease, a combination of ipratropium and albuterol is more effective than either agent alone. Chest 105:1411–1419, 1994.

93. Littner M, Auerbach D, Campbell S, et al: The bronchodilator effects of tiotropium bromide in stable COPD. Am J Respir Crit Care Med 155: A282, 1997.

94. Bellamy D, Hutchison DCS: The effects of salbutamol aerosol on lung function in patients with pulmonary emphysema. Br J Dis Chest 75: 190–196, 1981.

95. Boyd G, Morice AH, Pounsford JC, et al: An evaluation of salmeterol in the treatment of chronic obstructive pulmonary disease (COPD). Eur Respir J 10:815–21, 1997.

96. Cazzola M, Matera MG, Santangelo G, et al: Salmeterol and formoterol in partially reversible severe chronic obstructive pulmonary disease: A dose-response study. Respir Med 89:357–62, 1995.

97. Ziment I: The β-agonist controversy: Impact in COPD. Chest 107:198s–205s, 1995.

98. Murciano D, Auclair MH, Pariente R, et al: A randomized, controlled trial of theophylline in patients with severe chronic obstructive pulmonary disease. N Engl J Med 320:1521–1525, 1989.

99. Thomas P, Pugsley JA, Steward JH: Theophylline and salbutamol improve pulmonary function in patients with irreversible chronic obstruction pulmonary disease. Chest 101:160–165, 1992.

100. Alexander MR, Dull WL, Kasik JE: Treatment of chronic obstructive pulmonary disease with orally administered theophylline: A double-blind, controlled study. JAMA 244:2286–2290, 1980.

101. Mahler DA, Matthay RA, et al: Sustained-release theophylline reduces dyspnea in nonreversible obstructive airway disease. Am Rev Respir Dis 131:22–25, 1985.

102. Fink G, Kaye C, Sulkes J, et al: Effect of theophylline on exercise performance in patients with severe chronic obstructive pulmonary disease. Thorax 49:332–334, 1994.

103. McEvoy CE, Niewoehner DE: Adverse effects of corticosteroid therapy for COPD: A critical review. Chest 111:1609–1619, 1997.

104. Pauwels RA, Lofdahl C, Pride NB, et al: European Respiratory Society

study on chronic obstructive pulmonary disease (EUROSCOP): Hypothesis and design. Eur Respir J 5:1254–1261, 1992.

105. Bourbeau J, Rouleau MY, Boucher S: Randomised controlled trial of inhaled corticosteroids in patients with chronic obstructive pulmonary disease. Thorax 53:477–482, 1998.

106. Vestbo J, Sorensen T, Lange P, et al: Long-term effect of inhaled budesonide in mild and moderate chronic obstructive pulmonary disease: A randomised controlled trial. Lancet 353:1819–1823, 1999.

107. Kerstjens HAM, Brand PLP, Hughes MD, et al: A comparison of bronchodilator therapy with and without inhaled corticosteroid therapy for obstructive airways disease. N Engl J Med 327:1413–1419, 1992.

108. Ziment I: Pharmacologic therapy of obstructive airway disease. Clin Chest Med 11:461–486, 1996.

109. Sylvester JT, Goldberg HS, Permutt S: The role of the vasculature in the regulation of cardiac output. Clin Chest Med 4:222–236, 1983.

110. Aubier M, Murciano D, Viires N, et al: Effects of digoxin on diaphragmatic strength generations in patients with chronic obstructive pulmonary disease during acute respiratory failure. Am Rev Respir 135:544, 1987.

111. Mathur PN, Powles ACP, Pugsley SO, et al: Effect of long-term administration of digoxin on exercise performance in chronic air flow obstruction. Eur J Respir Dis 66:273, 1985.

112. Brown SE, Pakron FJ, Milne N, et al: Effects of digoxin on exercise capacity and right ventricular function during exercise in chronic airflow obstruction. Chest 85:187, 1984.

113. Rich S, Seidlitz M, Dodin E, et al: The short-term effects of digoxin in patients with right ventricular dysfunction from pulmonary hypertension. Chest 114:787–792, 1998.

114. Pepke JZ, Higenbotam TW, Xuan ATD, et al: Inhaled nitric oxide as a cause of selective pulmonary vasodilation in pulmonary hypertension. Lancet 338:1173–1174, 1991.

115. Yoshida M, Taguchi O, Gabazza EC, et al: Combined inhalation of nitric oxide and oxygen in chronic obstructive pulmonary disease. Am J Respir Crit Care Med 155:526–529, 1997.

116. Katayama Y, Higenbottam TW, DiazdeAtauri MJ, et al: Inhaled nitric oxide and arterial oxygen tension in patients with chronic obstructive pulmonary disease and severe pulmonary hypertension. Thorax 52:120–124, 1997.

117. Barbera JA, Roger N, Roca J, et al: Worsening of pulmonary gas exchange with nitric oxide inhalation in chronic obstructive pulmonary disease. Lancet 347:436–440, 1996.

118. Mahajan SK, Sharma VK, Thakral S: Effect of enalapril on renal profile and right ventricular dimensions in chronic cor pulmonale. J Assoc Physicians India 44:323–324, 1996.

119. Kiely DG, Cargill RI, Wheeldon NM, et al: Haemodynamic and endocrine effects of type 1 angiotensin II receptor blockade in patients with hypoxaemic cor pulmonale. Cardiovasc Res 33:201–208, 1997.

120. Fleetham J, West P, Mezon B, et al: Sleep, arousals and oxygen desaturation in chronic obstructive pulmonary disease. Am Rev Respir Dis 126:429–433, 1982.

121. Leger P, Bedicam JM, Cornette A, et al: Nasal intermittent positive pressure: Long-term follow-up in patients with severe chronic respiratory insufficiency. Chest 105:100–105, 1994.

122. Simonds AK, Elliott MW: Outcome of domiciliary nasal intermittent positive pressure ventilation in restrictive and obstructive disorders. Thorax 50:604–609, 1995.

123. Walter J, O'Donohue J, Gay P, et al: Clinical indications for noninvasive positive pressure ventilation in chronic respiratory failure due to restrictive lung disease, COPD, and nocturnal hyperventilation—a consensus conference report. In McIntyre N (ed): National Association for Medical Direction of Respiratory Care. Washington, DC, Chest, 1998, pp 521–534.

124. Fessler HE, Permutt S: Lung volume reduction surgery and airflow limitation. Am J Respir Crit Care Med 157:715–722, 1998.

125. Sciurba FC: Early and long-term functional outcomes following lung volume reduction surgery. Clin Chest Med 18:259–276, 1997.

126. Lynch JP, Martinez F: Lung transplantation: Who's a candidate? (part 1). J Respir Dis 17:304–311, 1996.

127. Lynch JP, Trulock EP: Lung transplantation in chronic airflow limitations. Med Clin North Am 80:657–670, 1996.

128. Low DE, Trulock EP, Kaiser LR, et al: Morbidity, mortality, and early results of single versus bilateral lung transplantation for emphysema. J Thorac Cardiovasc Surg 103:1119–1126, 1992.

129. Patterson GA: Lung transplantation for chronic obstructive pulmonary disease. Clin Chest Med 11:547–554, 1990.

130. Katzenstein AA, Myers JL: Idiopathic pulmonary fibrosis: Clinical relevance of pathologic classification. Am J Respir Crit Care Med 157:1301–1315, 1998.

131. Cherniack RM, Crystal RG, Kalica AR: NHLBI Workshop summary: Current concepts in idiopathic pulmonary fibrosis: A road map for the future. Am Rev Respir Dis 143:680–683, 1991.

132. Remy-Jardin M, Giraud F, Remy J, et al: Importance of ground-glass attenuation in chronic diffuse infiltrative lung disease: Pathologic-CT correlation. Radiology 189:693–698, 1993.

133. Orens JB, Kazerooni EA, Martinez FJ, et al: The sensitivity of high-resolution CT in detecting idiopathic pulmonary fibrosis proved by open lung biopsy: A prospective study. Chest 108:109–115, 1995.

134. Ryu JH, Colby TV, Hartman TE: Idiopathic pulmonary fibrosis: Current concepts. Mayo Clin Proc 73:1085–1101, 1998.

135. Hunninghake G, Kalica AR: Approaches to the treatment of pulmonary fibrosis. Am J Respir Crit Care Med 151:915–918, 1995.

136. Coffey MJ, FitzGerald MX, McNicholas WT: Comparison of oxygen saturation during sleep and exercise in patients with cystic fibrosis. Chest 100:659–662, 1991.

137. Fraser KL, Tullis DE, Sasson Z, et al: Pulmonary hypertension and cardiac function in adult cystic fibrosis: Role of hypoxemia. Chest 115:1321–1328, 1999.

138. Young T, Palta M, Dempsey J, et al: The occurrence of sleep-disordered breathing among middle-aged adults. N Engl J Med 328:1230–1235, 1993.

139. Sanner BM, Doberauer C, Konermann M, et al: Pulmonary hypertension in patients with obstructive sleep apnea syndrome. Arch Intern Med 157:2483–2487, 1997.

140. Kessler R, Chaouat A, Weitzenblum E, et al: Pulmonary hypertension in the obstructive sleep apnea syndrome: Prevalence, causes and therapeutic consequences. Eur Respir J 9:787–794, 1996.

141. Krieger J, Sforza E, Apprill M, et al: Pulmonary hypertension, hypoxemia and hypercapnia in obstructive sleep apnea patients. Chest 96:729–737, 1989.

142. Yamashiro Y, Kryger MH: Why should sleep apnea be diagnosed and treated? Clin Pulm Med 1:250–259, 1994.

143. Flemons WW, Whitelaw WA, Brant R, et al: Likelihood ratios for a sleep apnea clinical prediction rule. Am J Respir Crit Care Med 150:1279–1285, 1994.

144. Smith PL, Gold AR, Meyers DA, et al: Weight loss in mildly to moderately obese patients with obstructive sleep apnea. Ann Intern Med 103:850–855, 1985.

145. Sampol G, Sagales MT, Roca A, et al: Nasal continuous positive airway pressure with supplemental oxygen in coexistent sleep apnoea-hypopnoea syndrome and severe chronic obstructive pulmonary disease. Eur Respir J 9:111–116, 1996.

146. Derderian SS, Bridenbaugh RH, Rajagopal KR: Neuropsychologic symptoms in obstructive sleep apnea improve after treatment with nasal continuous positive airway pressure. Chest 94:1023–1027, 1988.

147. He J, Kryger MH, Zorick FJ, et al: Mortality and apnea index in obstructive sleep apnea: Experience in 385 male patients. Chest 94:9–14, 1988.

148. Janson C, Gislason T, Bengtsson H, et al: Long-term follow-up of patients with obstructive sleep apnea treated with uvulopalatopharyngoplasty. Arch Otolaryngol Head Neck Surg 123:257–262, 1997.

149. Leger P: Long-term noninvasive ventilation for patients with thoracic cage abnormalities. Respir Care Clin North Am 2:241–52, 1996.

150. Simonda AK: Nasal intermittent positive pressure ventilation in neuromuscular and chest wall disease. Monaldi Arch Chest Dis 48:156–168, 1993.

151. Robert D, Gerard M, Leger P, et al: Domiciliary ventilation by tracheostomy for chronic respiratory failure. Rev Fr Mal Respir 11:923–936, 1983.

152. Faul JL, Ruoss S, Doyle RL, et al: Diaphragmatic paralysis due to Lyme disease. Eur Respir J 13:700–702, 1999.

153. DeVito EL, Quadrelli SA, Montiel GC, et al: Bilateral diaphragmatic paralysis after mediastinal radiotherapy. Respiration 63:187–190, 1996.

154. Gierada DS, Slone RM, Fleishman MJ: Imaging evaluation of the diaphragm. Chest Surg Clin North Am 8:237–280, 1998.

155. Lin MC, Liaw MY, Huang CC, et al: Bilateral diaphramatic paralysis—a rare cause of acute respiratory failure manage with nasal mask bilevel positive airway pressure (BiPAP) ventilation. Eur Respir J 10:1922–1924, 1997.

156. Hulsmann AR, van den Anker JN: Evolution and natural history of chronic lung disease of prematurity. Monaldi Arch Chest Dis 52:272–277, 1997.

157. Langer JC: Congenital diaphragmatic hernia. Chest Surg Clin North Am 8:295–314, 1998.

158. Roberts, JD Jr, Fineman JR, Morin FC III, et al: Inhaled nitric oxide and persistent pulmonary hypertension of the newborn. N Engl J Med 336:605–10, 1997.

159. Steinhorn RH, Cox PN, Fineman JR, et al: Inhaled nitric oxide enhances oxygenation but not survival in infants with alveolar capillary dysplasia. J Pediatr 130:417–422, 1997.

PULMONARY HYPERTENSION DUE TO CHRONIC THROMBOEMBOLIC DISEASE

160. Rich S, Levitsky S, Brundage BH: Pulmonary hypertension from chronic pulmonary thromboembolism. Ann Intern Med 108:425, 1988.

161. Moser KM, Daily PO, Peterson K, et al: Thromboembolic pulmonary hypertension. Ann Intern Med 107:560, 1987.

162. Ryan KL, Fedullo PF, Davis GB, et al: Perfusion scan findings understate the severity of angiographic and hemodynamic compromise in chronic thromboembolic pulmonary hypertension. Chest 93:1180–1185, 1988.

163. Pitton MB, Duber C, Mayer E, et al: Hemodynamic effects of nonionic contrast bolus injection and oxygen inhalation during pulmonary angiography in patients with chronic major-vessel thromboembolic pulmonary hypertension. Circulation 94:2485–2491, 1996.

164. King MA, Ysrael M, Bergin CJ: Chronic thromboembolic pulmonary hypertension: CT findings. AJR 170:955–960, 1998.

165. Daily PO, Dembitsky WP, Iversen S, et al: Risk factors for pulmonary thromboendarterectomy. J Thorac Cardiovasc Surg 99:670–678, 1990.

166. Archibald CJ, Auger WR, Fedullo PF, et al: Long-term outcome after pulmonary thromboendarterectomy. Am J Respir Crit Care Med 160:523–528, 1999.

167. Mayer E, Dahm M, Hake U, et al: Mid-term results of pulmonary thromboendarterectomy for chronic thromboembolic pulmonary hypertension. Ann Thorac Surg 61:1788–1792, 1996.

168. Martinuzzo ME, Pombo G, Forastiero RR, et al: Lupus anticoagulant, high levels of anticardiolipin, and anti-beta$_2$-glycoprotein I antibodies are associated with chronic thromboembolic pulmonary hypertension. J Rheumatol 25:1313–1319, 1998.

169. Sandoval J, Amigo MC, Barragan R, et al: Primary antiphospholipid syndrome presenting as chronic thromboembolic pulmonary hypertension: Treatment with thromboendarterectomy. J Rheumatol 23:772–775, 1996.

170. Sutton LL, Castro O, Cross DJ, et al: Pulmonary hypertension in sickle cell disease. Am J Cardiol 74:626–628, 1994.

171. Norris SL, Johnson C, Haywood LJ: Left ventricular filling pressure in sickle cell anemia. J Assoc Acad Minor Phys 3:20–23, 1992.

172. Yung GL, Channick RN, Fedullo PF, et al: Successful pulmonary thromboendarterectomy in two patients with sickle cell disease. Am J Respir Crit Care Med 157:1690–1693, 1998.

173. Morris W, Knauer CM: Cardiopulmonary manifestations of schistosomiasis. Semin Respir Infect 12(2):159–170, 1997.

174. Bethlem EP, Schettino G deP, Carvalho CR: Pulmonary schistosomiasis. Curr Opin Pulm Med 3(5):361–365, 1997.

175. Barbosa MM, Lamounier JA, Oliverira EC, et al: Pulmonary hypertension in schistosomiasis mansoni. Trans R Soc Trop Med Hyg 90:663–665, 1996.

176. Tozman EC: Sarcoidosis: Clinical manifestations, epidemiology, therapy, and pathophysiology. Curr Opin Rheumatol 3:155–159, 1991.

177. Sheffield EA: Pathology of sarcoidosis. Clin Chest Med 18:741–754, 1997.

178. Nagai S, Shigematsu M, Hamada K, Izumi T: Clinical courses and prognoses of pulmonary sarcoidosis. Curr Opin Pulm Med 5:293–298, 1999.

179. Veinot JP, Johnston B: Cardiac sarcoidosis—an occult cause of sudden death: A case report and literature. J Forensic Sci 43:715–717, 1998.

180. Lynch JP III, Kazerooni EA, Gay SE: Pulmonary sarcoidosis. Clin Chest Med 18:755–785, 1997.

181. Mañá J, Badrinas F: Prognosis of sarcoidosis: An unresolved issue. Sarcoidosis 9:15–20, 1993.

182. McLaughlin VV, Genthner DE, Panella MM, et al: Compassionate use of continuous prostacyclin in the management of secondary pulmonary hypertension: A case series. Ann Intern Med 130:740–743, 1999.

183. Masur Y, Remberger K, Hoefer M: Pulmonary capillary hemangiomatosis as a rare cause of pulmonary hypertension. Pathol Res Pract 2:290–295, 1993.

184. Lippert JL, White CS, Cameron EW, et al: Pulmonary capillary hemangiomatosis: Radiographic appearance. J Thorac Imaging 13:49–51, 1998.

185. Dufour B, Mâitre S, Humbert M, et al: High-resolution CT of the chest in four patients with pulmonary capillary hemangiomatosis or pulmonary venoocclusive disease. AJR Am J Roentgenol 171:1321–1324, 1998.

186. Humbert M, Mâitre S, Capron F, et al: Pulmonary edema complicating continuous intravenous prostacyclin in pulmonary capillary hemangiomatosis. Am J Respir Crit Care Med 157:1681–1685, 1998.

MOLECULAR BIOLOGY AND GENETICS

Chapter 55

Principles of Cardiovascular Molecular Biology and Genetics

JEFFREY M. LEIDEN

During the first half of the 20th century revolutionary studies of human and animal physiology led to an elegant understanding of the anatomical, electrical, and mechanical properties of the cardiovascular system. As we enter the new millennium, we are in the midst of a second and equally exciting revolution in cardiovascular medicine—one that involves the application of recent advances in molecular and cellular biology to understanding both normal cardiovascular function and the pathophysiological bases of human cardiovascular disease.

Applications of modern molecular and cellular biology already permeate both cardiovascular diagnostics and therapeutics. During the past 10 years a rapidly expanding list of genes that are involved in the etiology of cardiovascular diseases, including hypertrophic and dilated cardiomyopathies, hypertension, and atherosclerosis, have been identified. Recombinant proteins and antibodies made from cloned genes such as tissue plasminogen activator (t-PA) and glycoprotein IIb/IIIa monoclonal antibodies are currently used to treat or prevent acute coronary thrombosis. Novel gene therapies are being tested for the treatment of ischemic cardiomyopathies and vascular proliferative syndromes such as restenosis after balloon angioplasty or arterial stenting.

Although significant, these advances represent just the beginning of a new era of molecular medicine that promises to fundamentally change the way we practice cardiovascular medicine over the coming decades. In 2000, the sequences of all of the genes in the human genome were reported. This enormous accomplishment will provide a wealth of new information about basic cardiovascular biology as well as large numbers of new diagnostic tools and potential drug targets. Given this rapidly expanding mass of molecular information, it is clear that the practicing cardiologist will soon need to understand as much about the basic principles of molecular biology and human genetics as he or she currently knows about coronary anatomy or cardiac hemodynamics.

In this chapter an overview is provided of the basic terminology, principles, and techniques of molecular and cellular biology. The reader is referred to several excellent texts and in-depth reviews for more detailed information about these topics.[1-5]

ANATOMY OF THE MAMMALIAN CELL

The mammalian cell is a highly dynamic, compartmentalized, and specialized structure that has evolved to carry out a number of functions that are important for survival, replication, and the proper functioning of individual organs and the organism as a whole (Fig. 55–1) (see also Chap. 14).[6, 7]

All human cells share a number of common structures and properties. The outer cell membrane (plasma membrane) is composed of a lipid bilayer studded with extracellular receptors. This membrane provides protection from the extracellular environment while simultaneously enabling the cell to respond to extracellular signals such as hormones, drugs, toxins, or other cells that bind to or otherwise perturb membrane-associated receptors. Mitochondria are specialized subcellular organelles present in all human cells that generate energy in the form of adenosine triphosphate from the oxidation of carbon-containing compounds such as sugars or fats.

The genomic deoxyribonucleic acid (DNA) organized into chromosomes is contained within the membrane-encapsulated cell nucleus. The chromosomes are collections of genes that store the genetic information needed to synthesize all of the component proteins that constitute the **1955**

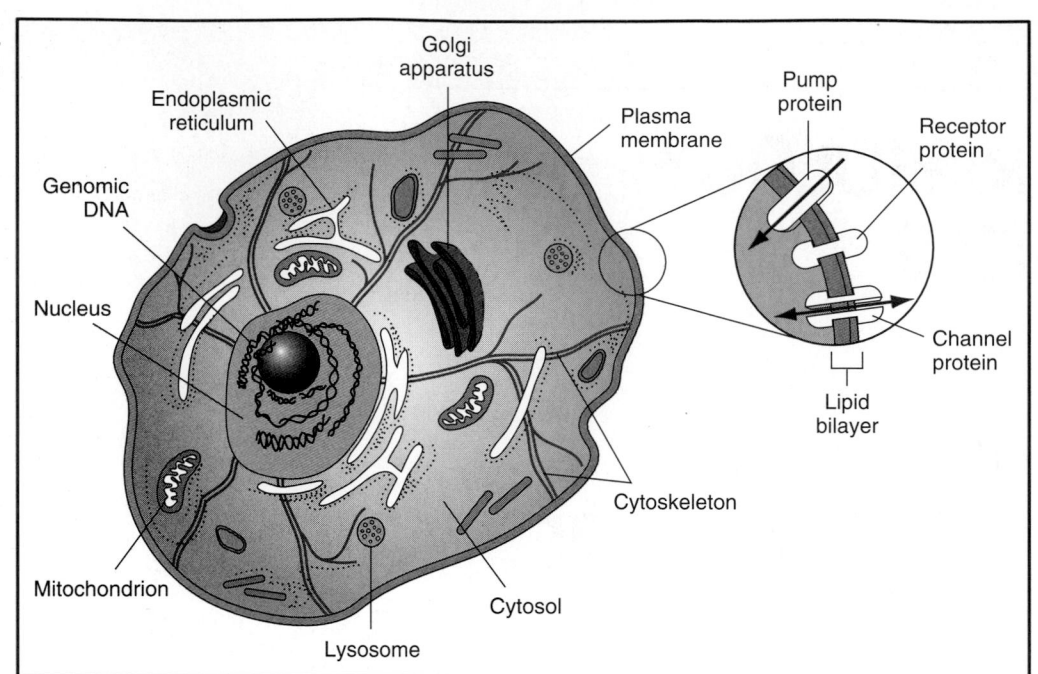

FIGURE 55–1. Anatomy of the mammalian cell. Schematic illustration of an idealized mammalian cell demonstrating structures that are common to most cell types. Note that lineage-specific cell structures, such as sarcomeres, are not included in this illustration. See Figure 14–1 for the latter.

cell and its organelles. As described in more detail later, this DNA is copied or transcribed into ribonucleic acid (RNA) in the nucleus. This RNA is then transported to the cytoplasm (i.e., the nonnuclear portion of the cell), where it is used as a template to direct the synthesis of proteins on specialized synthetic organelles called ribosomes. Newly synthesized proteins are sorted into the cytoplasmic compartment, inserted into membranes, or incorporated into specialized granules for secretion from the cell. These proteins play diverse roles in the physiology of the cell, including functioning as major structural elements; serving as enzymes that catalyze biochemical reactions; and functioning as cell surface receptors that sense and send extracellular signals and as hormones, growth factors, cytokines, or other secreted molecules that help integrate the function of multiple cells and organs within the organism.

In addition to these common structures and organelles, many cells express cell lineage–specific proteins and structures that enable them to carry out their specialized functions within the organism. Thus, for example, striated cardiac muscle cells express a set of contractile proteins assembled into sarcomeres that allow their rhythmic contraction whereas neurons express lineage-specific neurotransmitters and receptors that allow them to interpret and respond to diverse environmental stimuli.

GENETIC MACHINERY AND FLOW OF INFORMATION IN THE CELL

DNA

Despite its remarkably simple structure and limited four-letter alphabet, deoxyribonucleic acid represents one of the most sophisticated and foolproof information storage systems ever discovered.[7, 8] Given its elegant simplicity, it is not surprising that the basic structure and information storage rules of DNA have been highly conserved during evolution from the most simple viruses and bacteria to humans.

DNA is composed of two long strands of polynucleotides wound around each other in a clockwise double helix (Fig. 55–2A). Each strand can contain an unbroken array of millions of nucleotides. The backbone of each strand of the

DNA helix is composed of a linked array of identical deoxyribose phosphate groups, with the phosphate group forming a 5'-3' phosphodiester bond between the fifth carbon of one pentose ring and the third carbon of the adjacent ring. Each deoxyribose sugar on each strand is attached to one of four nucleic acid bases: two purines, adenine and guanine (A and G), and two pyrimidines, cytosine and thymine (C and T). These nucleic acids project at right angles toward the center of the DNA helix and pair with each other according to a very specific set of rules: an A from one strand can only pair with a T from the opposite strand, whereas a C from one strand can only pair with a G from the opposite strand. This nucleic acid pairing, which is stabilized by hydrogen bonding between the two complementary nucleic acids, serves to hold the two strands of the helix together. Of equal importance, the two strands of the helix, which have opposite polarities (one is oriented in the 5' to 3' direction, whereas the other is oriented in a 3' to 5' direction), are complementary copies of each other. Therefore, the sequence of one strand of the helix can be used to easily predict or program the sequence of the opposite strand. This important property of complementarity allows the enzymatic machinery of the nucleus to copy faithfully one strand of DNA into a daughter strand during cell replication and also allows the DNA sequence of a gene to be easily copied into RNA that can be used to program the synthesis of cellular proteins (Fig. 55–2B) (see later).

Chromosomes and Genes

Within the nucleus, the DNA is compacted by being wound around specialized structures called nucleosomes and organized into packages called chromosomes.[9–11] The human genome contains approximately 3×10^9 pairs of nucleotides (called base pairs) organized into 23 pairs of chromosomes.[12–14] One member of each pair of chromosomes is inherited from each parent. Remarkably, almost all of the cells in the human body contain a copy of the entire human genome or all of the instructions necessary to specify the entire organism (erythrocytes and platelets are notable exceptions).

Within a single chromosome, the DNA is organized into individual packets of information called genes[12–14] (Fig. 55–

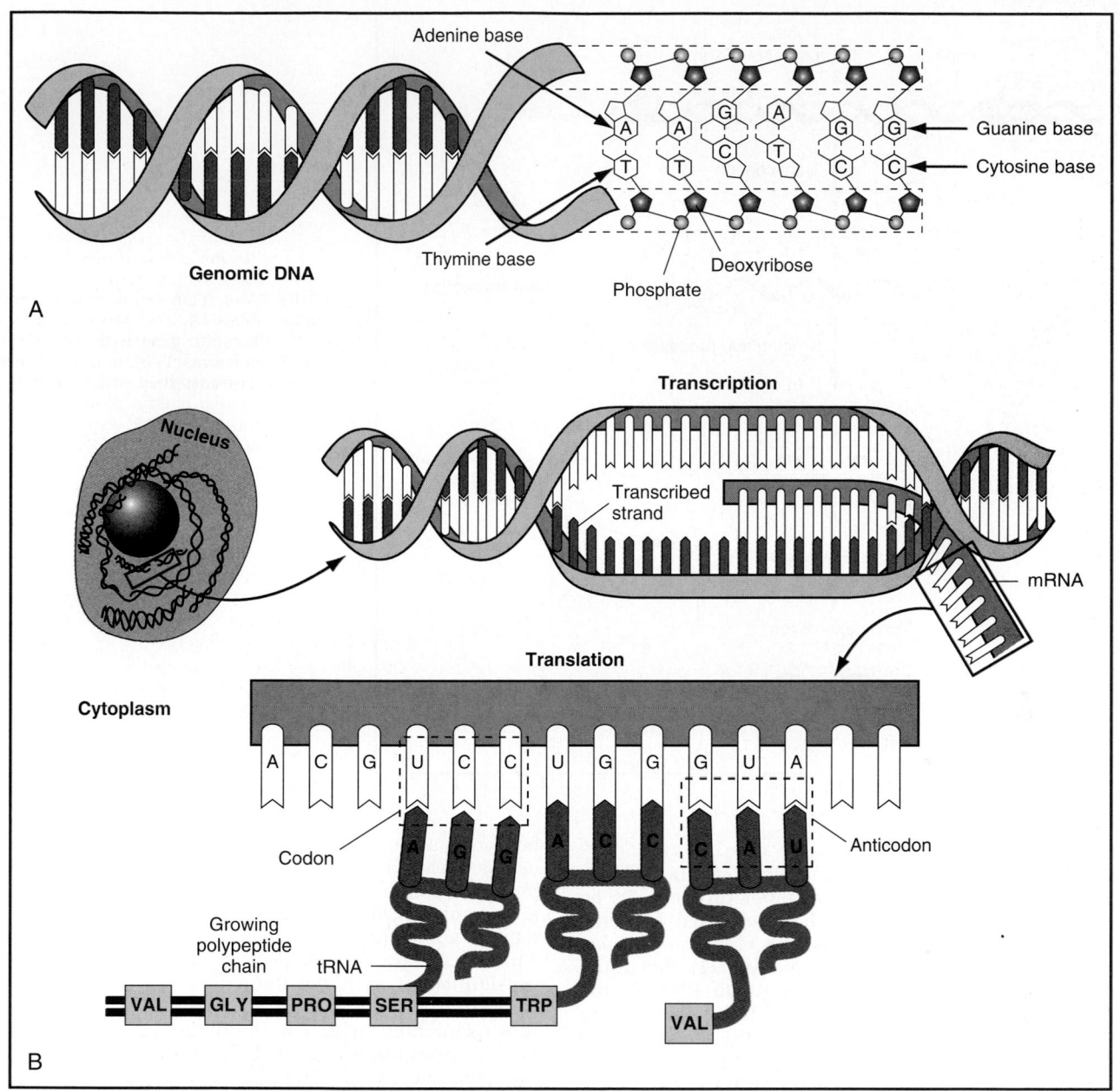

FIGURE 55–2. Flow of genetic information within a eukaryotic cell. *A,* Schematic illustration of the structure of eukaryotic DNA. The double helix at the right edge of the illustration is unfolded to allow visualization of the deoxyribose-phosphate backbone of each strand as well as base pairing between complementary nucleotide bases. *B,* Schematic illustration of transcription and translation of a eukaryotic gene. *Top right,* Genomic DNA being transcribed into messenger ribonucleic acid (mRNA) in the nucleus. *Bottom right,* mRNA being translated into a polypeptide in the cytoplasm. Transfer RNAs (tRNAs) loaded with amino acids are shown binding to the mRNA on a ribosome.

3). Each gene is composed of a unique sequence of nucleotides that comprises the information needed to encode one protein. The capacity of a unique sequence of bases within a gene to encode a unique protein is somewhat analogous to the letters of the alphabet that when assembled in different combinations uniquely define the meaning of individual sentences. The human genome contains an estimated 80,000 to 150,000 distinct genes.[14] The protein coding information contained within a single gene is not continuous but instead is encoded in multiple discontinuous packets called exons.[15] Between these exons are variable-sized stretches of DNA called introns. The function of these introns, which can be thought of as "junk" DNA and which are interspersed in the genes of all eukaryotic cells, remains unclear. However, it has been suggested that they may have facilitated the creation of new genes during evolution by

enabling the duplication, shuffling, and divergence of functional domains of different genes.[15]

In addition to its coding sequence (i.e., the sequence that determines the structure of its encoded protein), each gene also contains regulatory DNA sequences that control its spatial and temporal patterns of expression within different cell types and in response to different extracellular signals. These regulatory sequences, called promoters, enhancers, and silencers, are recognized and bound by a set of specialized nuclear proteins called transcription factors that can promote or inhibit the copying of a gene into an RNA template that can then program the synthesis of its encoded protein.[16–23] Promoters are typically located immediately upstream (or 5′) of the coding region of the gene. Enhancers on the other hand can be located upstream (5′), downstream (3′), or even within the introns of a gene.

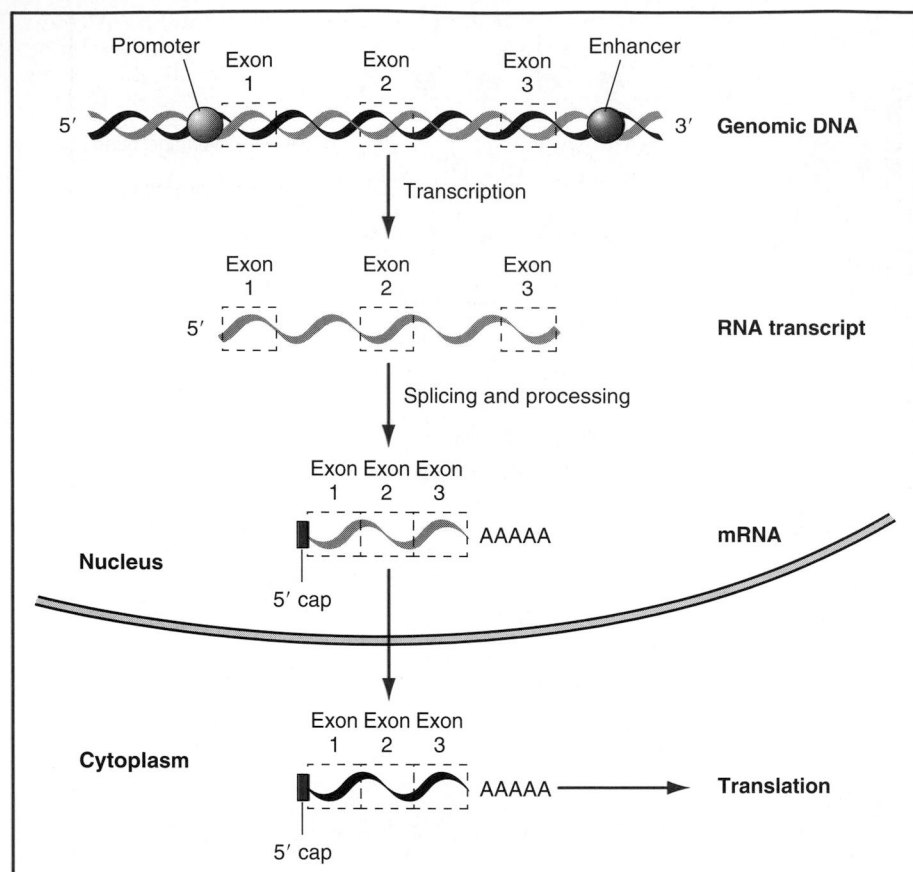

FIGURE 55–3. Transcription and processing of eukaryotic RNA. *Top,* Structure of a prototypical eukaryotic gene with a 5′ promoter, three exons (exons 1–3), and a 3′ enhancer. This gene is transcribed into a primary RNA transcript, which is then processed by splicing and addition of a 5′ cap and 3′ polyA tail. The resulting mature mRNA molecule is exported to the cytoplasm where it is translated into protein on a ribosome.

From Genes to Proteins

TRANSCRIPTION. The genes themselves can be thought of as the code stored in a basic computer program. To be functional, these genes must first be interpreted or translated into the proteins that they specify. This is a complex and highly regulated process that involves (1) the initial copying of the DNA copy of the gene into RNA in the nucleus, (2) processing and transport of this RNA copy to the cytoplasmic compartment (i.e., across the nuclear membrane), (3) translation of the RNA into its encoded protein on ribosomes, and, in some cases, (4) posttranslational modifications of the proteins themselves (see Figs. 55–2 and 55–3). In the first of these steps the antisense strand (3′-5′ strand) of the gene is copied base by base into a single-stranded complementary RNA molecule by cellular RNA polymerases.[19] Like DNA, RNA is a polynucleotide strand composed of a backbone of ribose sugars linked to one of four nucleic acid bases (A, G, C, and U [uracil], instead of T [thymidine]). Thus the sequence of the RNA copy of the antisense strand is identical to the sense strand of the DNA (except that *U*s replace the *T*s). Because this RNA copy contains both the exons (protein coding blocks) and introns (interspersed junk DNA) it must be processed (spliced) to remove all intron sequences and precisely join the exons into a single messenger RNA (mRNA) containing a contiguous region of sequence encoding its cognate protein.[24] Both ends of this single-stranded mRNA are then modified (a cap is added to the 5′ end of the mRNA while the 3′ end has a string of adenine bases added to produce a polyA tail), and the RNA is exported from the nucleus into the cytoplasm, where it is bound by ribosomes in preparation for translation into protein.[25–27]

THE GENETIC CODE. Because DNA and RNA are linear arrays of nucleotides, whereas proteins are linear arrays of amino acids, there must be a code by which the linear sequence of the four nucleotides of the RNA molecule can be translated into the linear sequence of amino acids of its encoded protein. This "genetic code" turns out to be remarkably simple and has been conserved in most (but not all) organisms from viruses to humans.[28, 29] Every three contiguous nucleotides or triplets in the RNA specify a single amino acid (Fig. 55–4). Because there are four nucleotide possibilities at each position, there are 4 × 4 × 4 or 64 different triplet possibilities. One of the triplets, AUG, specifies methionine, which is the amino acid that starts each protein; three other triplets, UAA, UGA, and UAG, program the ribosome to end translation and are therefore called stop codons. The remaining 60 triplets or codons specify one of the 20 amino acids. Because there are 60 codons and only 20 amino acids some amino acids can be specified by two or more different triplets (e.g., cysteine = UGU or UGC). Thus, it is possible to read the sequence of the protein encoded by a gene by simply reading its triplets in order (e.g., ATG TCC TGG TCC = Met Ser Trp Ser).

TRANSLATION. The conversion of the single-stranded mRNA into protein on the ribosome requires special adapter molecules called transfer RNAs (tRNAs) (see Fig. 55–3). One portion of these tRNAs is complementary to the triplet corresponding to the single amino acid it adds to the growing protein chain (e.g., the tRNA for methionine contains a triplet RNA sequence, UAC, that can base pair with the triplet AUG that encodes methionine in the mRNA). A second portion of the tRNA molecule can bind specifically to that amino acid. By docking on the triplet in the mRNA by base pairing, the tRNA brings the correct amino acid into proximity with the growing protein chain, allowing the ribosome to specifically couple it to the carboxy terminus of the nascent polypeptide. The ribosome and tRNAs can therefore be thought of as a reading machine that scans the sequence of the mRNA and converts it into a protein.

EVOLUTIONARY CONSERVATION. The remarkable evolutionary conservation of the structures of DNA, RNA, and

1st nucleotide	2nd nucleotide				3rd nucleotide
	U	**A**	**C**	**G**	
U	Phe	Tyr	Ser	Cys	U
	Leu	STOP	Ser	STOP	A
	Phe	Tyr	Ser	Cys	C
	Leu	STOP	Ser	Trp	G
A	Ile	Asn	Thr	Ser	U
	Ile	Lys	Thr	Arg	A
	Ile	Asn	Thr	Ser	C
	Met	Lys	Thr	Arg	G
C	Leu	His	Pro	Arg	U
	Leu	Gln	Pro	Arg	A
	Leu	His	Pro	Arg	C
	Leu	Gln	Pro	Arg	G
G	Val	Asp	Ala	Gly	U
	Val	Glu	Ala	Gly	A
	Val	Asp	Ala	Gly	C
	Val	Glu	Ala	Gly	G

FIGURE 55–4. The genetic code. The amino acids corresponding to each nucleotide triplet in the mRNA are shown. Note that there are three stop codons (UAG, UAA, and UGA) and a single start codon (AUG).

proteins as well as the genetic code and much of the machinery for RNA and protein production has profound implications for molecular geneticists. It means, for example, that human genes can be transferred into bacteria, yeast, or insect cells where they will be faithfully replicated and copied into RNA and protein. This property constitutes the basis of the recombinant DNA technology used to produce many therapeutic proteins such as t-PA. Similarly, human genes can be spliced into viruses that can be used to infect human cells to transfer genes for therapeutic purposes. Finally, many of the genes involved in human cardiovascular development and function have been highly conserved in mice, fish, and even flies. Thus, these simple organisms can serve as powerful model systems for studying human cardiovascular development and function and for testing novel genetic or pharmacological therapies for human cardiovascular diseases.

Regulation of Gene Expression

Only a small fraction of the genes within the human genome is expressed in any given cell at any given time. These genes can be divided into several subsets based on their patterns of expression. One subset of genes is constitutively expressed in most, if not all, cells. The products of these so-called housekeeping genes are necessary for basic functions of cell survival, replication, and energy generation. A second subset of genes is expressed in a lineage-restricted fashion, for example, only in a cardiomyocyte or an endothelial cell. In fact, it is the precise regulation of expression of this subset of lineage-specific genes that determines the unique identity and function of a particular cell type. A final subset of genes is expressed only in response to a specific environmental stimulus. Given the necessity for these complex and dynamic patterns of differential gene expression, human cells have evolved sophisticated molecular mechanisms to regulate lineage-specific gene expression and to allow rapid and precise changes of gene expression in response to various organismal and environmental signals.

The expression of a specific gene can be regulated at many levels including transcription of the gene into RNA,[16–23] processing and transport of the mRNA into the cytoplasm,[24–27] stability of the cytoplasmic mRNA,[30] translation of the mRNA into protein,[31, 32] posttranslational modification of the protein,[33–37] subcellular localization of the protein,[38] and protein stability.[37] Although each of these mechanisms plays important roles in regulating some genes, two of these, the regulation of gene transcription and protein phosphorylation (and dephosphorylation), appear to represent the major mechanisms used by the cell to control the expression and activity of proteins. Indeed, in many cases these two mechanisms have been linked into distinct signaling pathways that allow cells to respond to developmental, environmental, and organismal signals with complex and precisely orchestrated changes in gene expression. An example of one such signaling pathway is shown in Figure 55–5. In this example, stimulation of a G protein–coupled beta-adrenergic receptor in the plasma membrane by beta-adrenergic agonists such as norepinephrine results in the activation of the enzyme adenylyl cyclase and in the increased production of cyclic adenosine monophosphate (cAMP) in the cytoplasm.[39] This increase in cAMP in turn activates the protein serine kinase, protein kinase A, which migrates to the nucleus where it phosphorylates the transcription factor CREB on a single serine residue (Ser133).[40]

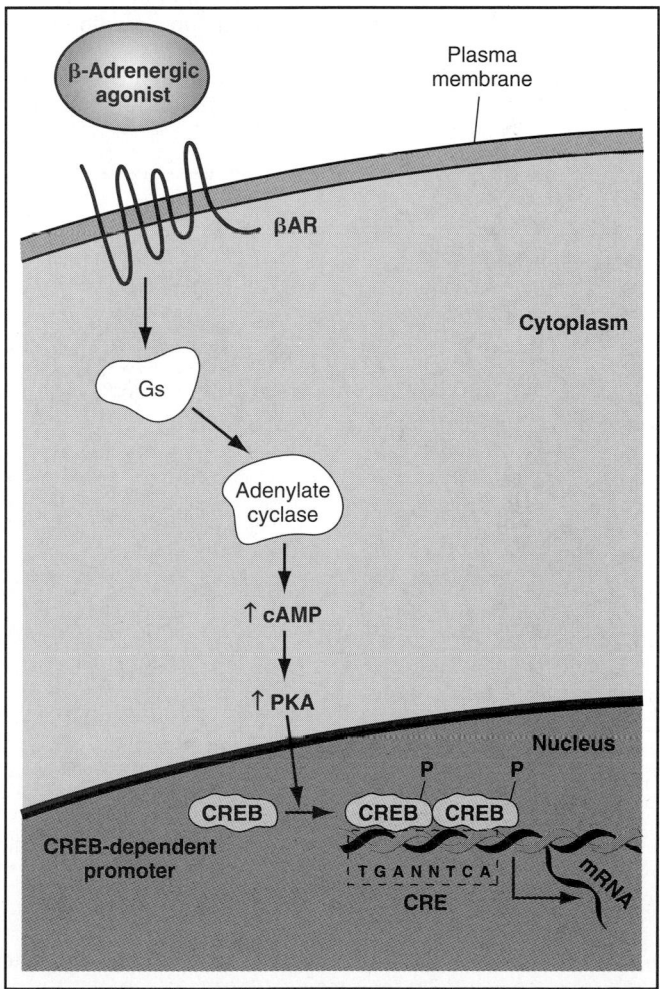

FIGURE 55–5. Schematic illustration of a beta-adrenergic signaling pathway. Binding of a beta-adrenergic agonist to the transmembrane beta-adrenergic receptor (βAR) results in the release of the active G protein, G$_S$. G$_S$ activates adenylate cyclase, which causes increased production of cyclic adenosine monophosphate (cAMP). cAMP in turn activates protein kinase A (PKA), which migrates to the nucleus where it phosphorylates the CREB transcription factor on serine 133. The phosphorylated transcription factor CREB binds as a homodimer to a cAMP response element (CRE)-binding site (TGANNTCA) and activates transcription of a CREB-responsive gene. (See also Figures 14–15 to 14–17.)

Phosphorylated CREB then binds to its specific recognition sequence (TGANNTCA), which is present in the promoters of a set of cAMP–responsive genes, and activates their transcription and expression.[41] Similar types of signaling pathways have evolved to regulate gene expression in response to hormones, cytokines, hypoxia, cell-cell signals, and mechanical stretch.[33, 34]

GENETIC BASES OF HUMAN CARDIOVASCULAR DISEASE

Mutations are alterations in the structures of individual genes that result in corresponding structural changes in the proteins they encode (see also Chap. 56). Because many individual proteins play critical roles in the development and function of the cardiovascular system, such mutations leading to quantitative and qualitative defects in protein function can result in a wide variety of human cardiovascular diseases. Indeed, the preponderance of evidence suggests that genetic mutations often in combination with environmental factors are responsible for the majority of human cardiovascular diseases, including both classical congenital disorders of the heart and vasculature as well as "acquired diseases" such as hypertension, cardiomyopathies, and atherosclerosis.

Different types of mutations affect their encoded proteins in very different ways (Fig. 55–6). "Missense mutations"

result from the substitution of one or more nucleotides in such a way as to change the primary sequence of the encoded protein (e.g., mutation of TTT to TTG causes a single amino acid change of phenylalanine to leucine). Such missense mutations do not typically alter the level of protein expressed but can alter the function of the protein by altering its structure. In contrast, "nonsense mutations" (e.g., TAT to TAA) introduce a premature stop codon into a gene, resulting in a truncated protein product that can display alterations in function or can be unstable. Insertions or deletions of nucleotides can add or subtract amino acids from the resulting proteins if they result in the addition or deletion of triplets of amino acids (i.e., if they occur in multiples of three) or alternatively can result in "frameshifts" in which the codons of the gene are read in the wrong reading frame. Such frameshift mutations typically cause abnormal protein structures that often terminate prematurely, owing to the introduction of out-of-frame termination codons. Mutations in both exons and introns can cause splicing errors that result in alterations in protein structure and/or frameshifts. Finally, mutations in the promoters or enhancers of genes can lead to alterations (either increases or decreases) in the levels of expression of a given protein or, alternatively, can change the temporal or spatial patterns of expression of that protein. In addition to single gene mutations, rearrangements of genes on the same or different chromosomes can also result in human disease. For example, the "in frame" fusion of two different genes by chromosomal rearrangement can result in a fusion protein

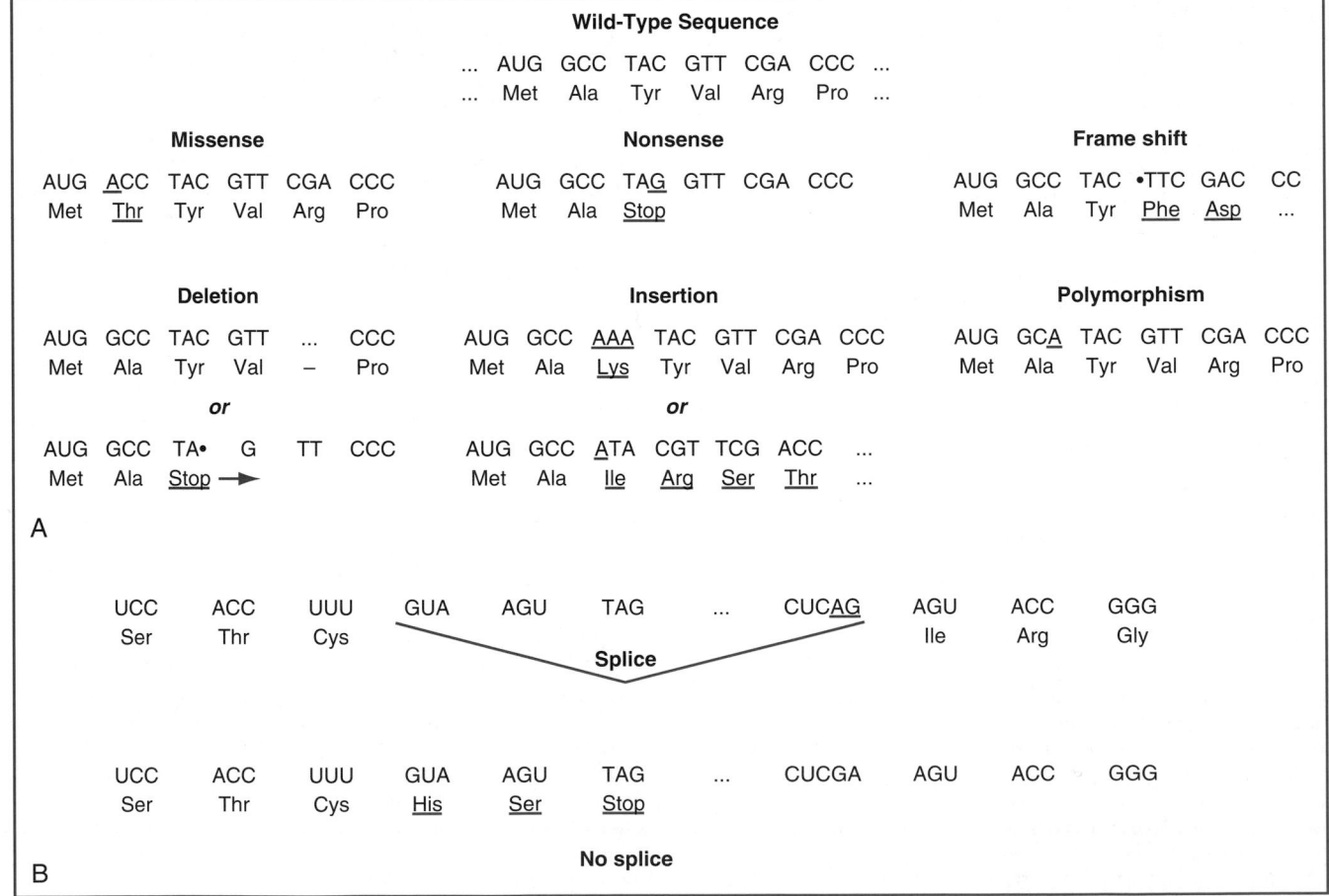

FIGURE 55–6. Different types of mutations alter the structure and expression of human genes. *A*, An example of a wild-type gene sequence is shown in the top panel. The bottom panel shows examples of different types of nucleotide mutations and the resulting alterations in the amino acid sequences of the corresponding protein. Mutations are underlined; deletions are noted by a dot. Polymorphism is a nucleotide substitution that does not alter the primary amino acid structure of the resulting protein. *B*, Splice mutations: an example of a mutation in the 3′ splice acceptor sequence that disrupts splicing, resulting in read-through into the intron and premature termination of the protein.

with a novel and sometimes deleterious function. Similarly, fusion of the promoter of one gene to the coding sequence of a second can lead to an abnormal spatial and temporal pattern of expression of the second gene and protein.

These different types of mutations also lead to different types of diseases (see also Chap. 56). For example, the functional inactivation, deletion, or premature termination of a single gene often results in a "loss of function" of its encoded protein that is manifest as an autosomal recessive trait. That is, only homozygous patients who inherit two copies of the mutated gene (and therefore have a severe deficiency in the amount of protein expressed) manifest the disease. In contrast, heterozygous "carriers" express 50 percent of the normal level of the protein and therefore are usually (but not always) asymptomatic. In contrast, some mutations result in the production of a dominant negative protein that inhibits the function of the normal protein expressed by the other copy of the gene in the patient's cells. Such mutations are often inherited in a dominant fashion; that is, one mutant copy of the gene (allele) is sufficient to produce disease. Similarly, some mutations can result in a gain of function, that is, in constitutive activation or superactivation of the function of the encoded protein. Once again, such mutations are often inherited in an autosomal dominant fashion. Finally, mutations of genes on the X chromosome are often inherited in an X-linked fashion. That is, the disease is only manifest in boys (who have a single X chromosome and therefore are functionally homozygous for the mutation) and is usually inherited from an unaffected mother.

Examples of Genetically Determined Cardiovascular Diseases

Familial Hypertrophic Cardiomyopathy: Genetic Diseases of the Sarcomere (See also Chap. 48)

Familial hypertrophic cardiomyopathy (FHC) is an autosomal dominant inherited disorder with a prevalence of approximately 1 per 500 live births that is characterized by progressive left ventricular hypertrophy, diastolic dysfunction, arrhythmias, and often heart failure and premature death.[42] This disease unfortunately often presents as sudden death in young adults. FHC is genetically heterogeneous; that is, linkage studies in humans demonstrated that the disease maps to a number of different chromosomal loci in different families.[43]

A major breakthrough in cardiovascular genetics occurred when Christine and Jon Seidman and their coworkers identified mutations in the beta-myosin heavy chain (β-MHC) in some families with FHC.[44] The majority of these were missense mutations, that is, they produced a full-length protein with single amino acid substitutions (e.g., in one common β-MHC mutation, the arginine 403 was mutated to a glutamine). In these cases it is likely that the mutant protein serves as a dominant negative inhibitor of sarcomere function—that is, the mutant protein oligomerizes with the normal protein expressed from the wild-type allele and in some way impairs the normal protein's contractile function. This overall impairment in function then stimulates a hypertrophic response (through unknown signaling pathways) that leads to increased diastolic pressures and ultimately to congestive heart failure and arrhythmias.[43] This type of dominant negative phenotype explains how one mutant copy of the gene produces the human disease and is consistent with the dominant pattern of inheritance seen in this disorder.

Subsequently, several groups have identified mutations in other sarcomeric protein genes as the cause of FHC in other families. These include the troponin T gene,[45] the alpha-tropomyosin gene,[45] and the myosin-binding protein C gene.[46] Thus, a picture is now emerging in which many different disruptions of the sarcomeric proteins can lead to cardiac hypertrophy and heart failure.[43, 47] It will be of great interest to understand the molecular pathways by which the cardiomyocyte senses defects in contractile function in patients with FHC and then initiates the hypertrophic program because similar pathways may underlie pathological hypertrophy in patients with acquired hypertrophic cardiomyopathies such as those associated with hypertension and valvular heart disease.

One of the most interesting stories to emerge from the genetic analyses of FHC patients was the notion that one could begin to predict clinical outcomes based on the nature of the mutation causing the disease. Thus, for example, patients with the arginine 403 to glutamine mutation tended to display markedly increased mortality rates, whereas patients with a valine 606 to methionine mutation had normal life expectancies.[48, 48a] This type of genetic prognostication will likely play an increasingly important role in risk stratification in pa-

tients with inherited cardiovascular disorders (see Fig. 48–11). By use of genetic engineering, mutant myosins can be expressed in vivo, permitting functional analysis of the isolated mutant proteins by biophysical techniques in vitro.[48b]

Congenital Long QT Syndrome: A Disease of Cardiomyocyte Ion Channels (See also Chap. 25)

The congenital long QT syndromes are autosomal dominant inherited disorders characterized by repolarization abnormalities (manifest by prolonged QT intervals on an electrocardiogram) and torsades de pointes.[49] Like patients with FHC, long QT syndrome patients often present with syncope and sudden death. Our understanding of both the genetic and pathophysiological bases of this disease were significantly enhanced by Keating and coworkers, who first demonstrated linkage of the disease to three chromosomal loci (LQT1, LQT2, and LQT3) and then cloned the genes responsible at each locus.[50–53] Interestingly, in each case the defective gene encoded a cardiac ion channel: LQT1 is caused by mutations in the KVLQT1 cardiac K channel gene,[53] LQT2 by mutations in the HERG (Human Ether a-go-go Related gene) K channel gene,[51] and LQT3 by mutations in the SCN5A sodium channel gene on chromosome 3p21-24.[52] In the case of the SCN5A gene, in-frame intragenic deletions were shown to disrupt the inactivation of the channel, resulting in enhanced activity during repolarization. Thus, this was essentially a gain of function mutation also consistent with its dominant pattern of inheritance.[54] As in FHC, it appears that mutations in multiple genes involved in regulating the cardiac action potential can give rise to the long QT syndrome.

In addition to inherited long QT syndrome there are a number of environmental long QT syndromes, such as those associated with cardiac ischemia, hypokalemia, type I antiarrhythmic drugs, and certain drug interactions. It is tempting to speculate that polymorphisms (silent mutations or variations) in the same ion channel genes that cause congenital long QT syndrome might confer susceptibility or resistance to these environmental insults. In this regard it will be of interest to sequence these ion channel genes in patients who are very sensitive (or resistant) to hypokalemia or drug-induced QT prolongation.

BASIC TECHNIQUES OF MOLECULAR BIOLOGY

Cloning and Recombinant DNA

Because every human cell contains 3×10^9 base pairs or 80,000 to 150,000 human genes, it is difficult if not impossible to study the structure and function of a single human gene in the context of an intact human cell. To circumvent this problem, molecular biologists have developed simple and elegant techniques for isolating, sequencing, and mutating single genes and copying them millions of times either in simple organisms like bacteria or in the test tube in vitro.[55] Indeed, such gene cloning techniques in many ways represent the foundation of modern molecular biology. As described earlier, the power of gene cloning derives from the fact that bacterial, yeast, and mammalian cells use common mechanisms for copying and expressing DNA. Thus, human genes can be inserted into bacteria, yeast, fruit flies, or mice, where in most cases they are faithfully replicated and expressed into their cognate proteins.

RESTRICTION ENDONUCLEASES. Restriction endonucleases are bacterial proteins that recognize and cleave or cut specific palindromic sequences in DNA.[56] For example, the EcoRI restriction endonuclease from the bacteria *Escherichia coli* recognizes the sequence GAATTC, which occurs approximately every 3000 to 4000 base pairs in human DNA. After recognition of its cognate sequence EcoRI cleaves the two strands of the double helix asymmetrically after the GA to produce overhanging single-stranded sticky ends of ATTC (Fig. 55–7). Three properties of such restriction endonucleases make them extremely useful tools for molecular biologists. First, because the sequence of any gene is unique and generally identical among all members of the species, such endonucleases can be used to reproducibly cleave a given gene at a specific location, thereby resulting in predictably sized cleavage products containing that gene. Second, because there are hundreds of distinct restriction endonucleases each with its own unique recognition sequence, any gene can be reproducibly cut into pieces of almost any size (and the sizes of these fragments

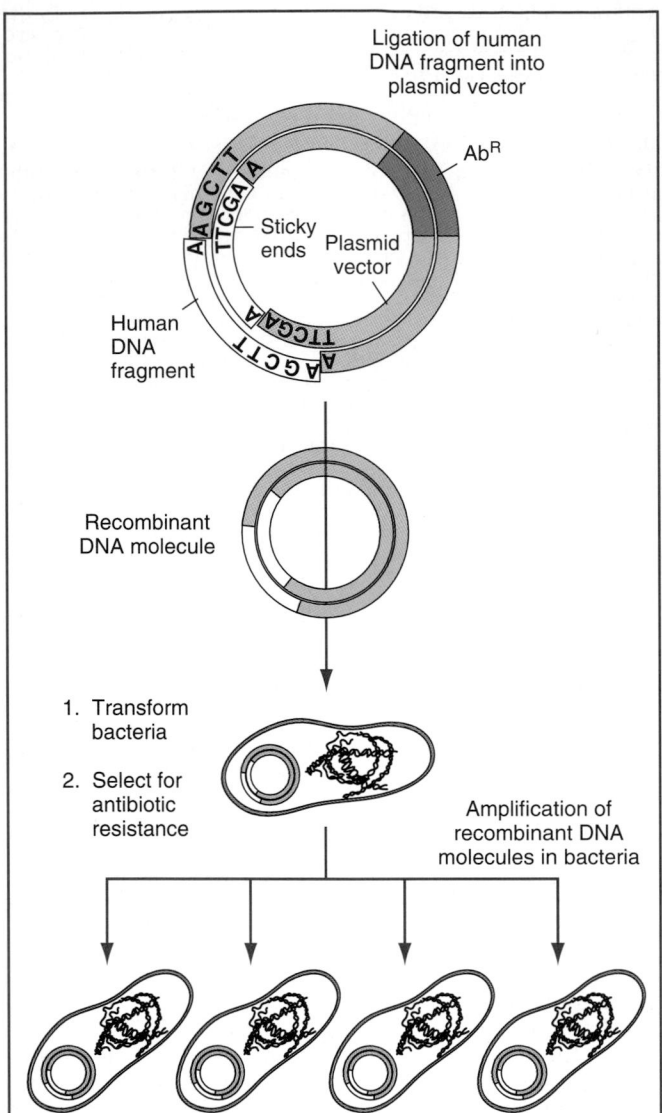

Ligation of human
DNA fragment into
plasmid vector

Ab^R

Sticky
ends Plasmid
vector

Human
DNA
fragment

Recombinant
DNA molecule

1. Transform
   bacteria

2. Select for
   antibiotic
   resistance

Amplification of
recombinant DNA
molecules in bacteria

FIGURE 55–7. Recombinant DNA technology can be used to amplify a human gene. Shown is ligation of a human DNA fragment digested with the restriction endonuclease HindIII into a HindIII-digested bacterial plasmid vector. Hybridization of complementary sticky ends on the two HindIII-digested DNAs allows precise ligation of the two fragments. Ab^R = an antibiotic resistance gene used to select bacteria transformed with the recombinant plasmid. The recombinant plasmid is used to transform bacteria. Bacteria containing the plasmid are selected by growth in antibiotic, resulting in the exponential amplification of the recombinant DNA molecule.

gene cut with that same enzyme ligated into the plasmid DNA to produce a plasmid copy of the human gene (see Fig. 55–7). The resulting plasmid can then be introduced into bacteria. Growth of such genetically modified bacteria in the presence of the appropriate antibiotic yields an essentially pure culture of bacteria, each of which contains between 10 and 500 copies of the single cloned human gene. Because the doubling time of bacteria is on the order of 20 minutes, inoculation of a 1-liter culture of bacterial broth with a single bacterial cell containing 500 copies of a human gene at 6 P.M. results in a culture containing 10^{11} copies of that same gene the next morning. The bacterium serves as a logarithmic gene-duplicating machine with a short replication time—the ideal tool for copying genes.

RECOMBINANT PROTEINS. In addition to their ability to copy genes rapidly and accurately, bacteria can also be used to express the human proteins encoded by cloned genes. By pasting the cloned human gene into a bacterial plasmid containing bacterial transcriptional regulatory sequences, the bacteria can be programmed to make large amounts of the human protein.[58] As long as the protein folds correctly and does not need to be posttranslationally modified by human enzymes (e.g., by adding sugar moieties or phosphate residues), such recombinant proteins made in bacteria will function normally both in vitro and after infusion into patients. In other cases, yeast or mammalian cells can be programmed to synthesize large amounts of recombinant proteins for human therapy.[59, 60]

Example of a Genetically Engineered Protein Used in Therapy: Production of Tissue Plasminogen Activator Using Recombinant DNA Technology

The use of thrombolytic agents has revolutionized the care of patients with acute myocardial infarction (see Chap. 35).[61, 62] Thrombolytic proteins are produced naturally by a wide range of organisms from bacteria to humans. One of the most potent agents, t-PA, was first isolated and purified in substantial amounts from human melanoma cells. However, such cells did not produce sufficient quantities of the active protein for widespread human therapy. Accordingly, there was great interest in using recombinant DNA technologies to engineer the production of large quantities of biologically active and pure t-PA. Although some human proteins such as growth hormone can be produced in their active form from bacteria like *E. coli*, bacteria often cannot properly fold or modify complex human proteins. This proved to be the case with t-PA. After cloning of the gene from melanoma cells[63] (using synthetic oligonucleotides based on the sequence of the purified protein as probes to pick the proper clones), the t-PA complementary DNA (cDNA) was cloned into a restriction endonuclease–digested plasmid containing a drug resistance gene *DHFR)*, and a eukaryotic promoter.[64] After amplification in bacteria this plasmid was transfected into Chinese hamster ovary cells, and clones expressing t-PA were selected by growth in HAT media, which only allowed the survival of cells with large numbers of copies of the *DHFR*-bearing plasmid. These clones of transfected cells were then grown in large numbers in cell fermentors, and the recombinant t-PA that was secreted from the cells was collected and purified from the tissue culture medium.

Nucleic Acid Hybridization

Because the two strands of the DNA helix are complementary to each other, they tend to specifically find and anneal to each other if mixed together under appropriate temperature and salt conditions. Such annealing is stabilized by hydrogen bonding between the complementary base pairs present on each strand of the helix. The annealing of complementary DNA strands is called hybridization and is the basis of many of the techniques used to identify specific genes in large mixtures of genetic material (see blotting techniques and array technologies, later). Hybridization is also employed to specifically join together two pieces of DNA containing complementary single-stranded ends such as occurs after cleavage with a single restriction enzyme and to anneal synthetic single-stranded oligonucleotides to genes during amplification by the polymerase chain reaction (PCR).

can be predicted in advance from the known sequence of the DNA). Finally, the existence of complementary sticky ends on fragments cut by a single restriction endonuclease allows molecular biologists to join together or "ligate" any two fragments of DNA that have been cleaved by that endonuclease. Thus, for example, a human gene fragment digested with EcoRI can be easily ligated to a bacterial gene cut by the same endonuclease. Similarly, a human gene can be ligated into an adenovirus vector after cleavage of both pieces of DNA with a single restriction endonuclease.

GENE CLONING. Plasmids are small circular pieces of DNA that replicate autonomously to high copy number in bacteria.[57] Such plasmids often contain genes encoding antibiotic resistance in bacteria, allowing the selection of bacteria containing them by growth in antibiotic-containing medium. This type of drug resistance plasmid can be cleaved once with a restriction enzyme and a single human

The Polymerase Chain Reaction

As described earlier, bacterial cloning represents an elegant biological solution to the problem of the clonal amplification of genes. An even more rapid technique has been described that allows the clonal amplification of any specific fragment of DNA in less than 2 to 3 hours in a test tube[65-69] (Fig. 55–8). In the PCR a mixture of double-stranded DNA from as little as a single cell is mixed with synthetic oligo-

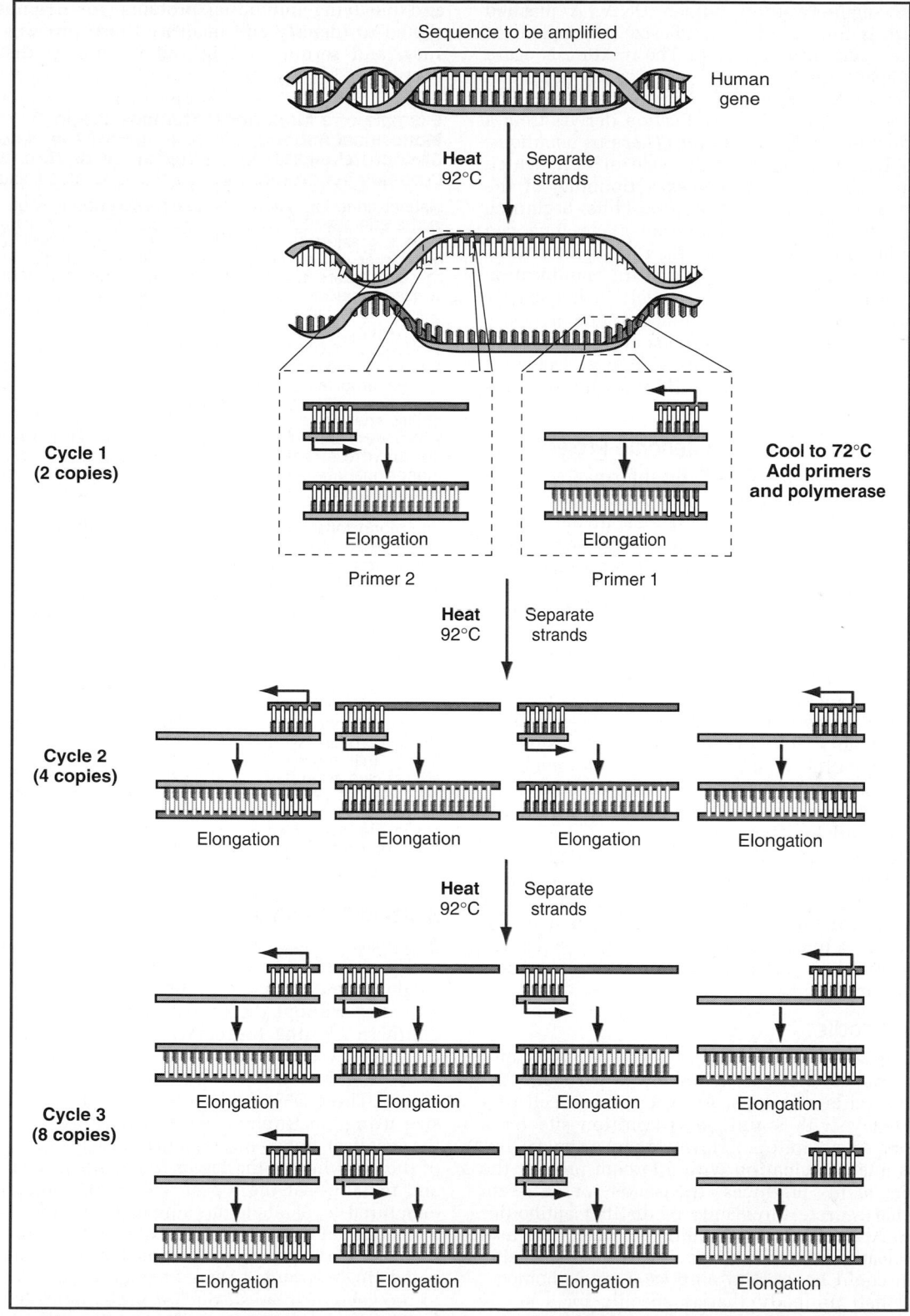

FIGURE 55–8. Gene amplification by the polymerase chain reaction (PCR). Synthetic oligonucleotide primers corresponding to the 5′ and 3′ ends of the DNA sequence to be amplified are chemically synthesized. The double-stranded DNA is melted by heating to 92°C, and primers are annealed by cooling the DNA solution to 72°C. A thermostable DNA polymerase then amplifies each strand of the target sequence, producing two copies of the gene segment. This process is repeated to produce an exponential amplification of the target sequence.

nucleotide primers (small pieces of DNA that are complementary to the ends of the sequence to be amplified). The mixture is heated to melt apart or separate the two strands of human DNA and then cooled to allow the complementary oligonucleotide primers to hybridize or specifically anneal to their complementary sequences, flanking the gene of interest on the single-stranded human DNA. A purified DNA polymerase is then used to synthesize a complementary copy of the fragment of interest. The mixture is again heated to melt apart the complementary strands of human DNA, and the process is repeated. The special heat-stable DNA polymerase used for PCR amplification derives from a bacterium adapted to live in hot water (*Thermus aquaticus*, hence "Taq" polymerase). Each such cycle of PCR, which takes only 3 minutes or so, produces a doubling of the quantity of the gene fragment of interest. Thus, beginning with the DNA from a single cell, in 30 cycles one can produce 2^{30} copies of any gene, more than enough to clone, sequence, or manipulate in vitro. The entire amplification is carried out in a sealed test tube or well in a specially designed machine that can be programmed to automatically heat and cool the sample. This ingenious and simple technology has revolutionized our ability to copy, sequence, mutate, and clone genes beginning with only tiny amounts of a DNA sample.

DNA Sequencing and the Human Genome Project

The human genome contains all of the information necessary for the development and function of the organism. Of equal importance, variations and mutations in the human genome are important determinants of disease susceptibility. Thus, obtaining the sequence of the human genome has been one of the major goals of molecular biology and medicine during the past 20 years. During the 1970s several groups described techniques for sequencing short stretches (several hundred base pairs) of cloned human DNA.[69, 70] The problem was then how to scale up this technology to accomplish the sequencing of the 3×10^9 base pairs contained in each human cell. This scale up has been accomplished in a remarkably short time, particularly considering that a single sequencing reaction still typically generates less than 1000 base pairs of readable DNA sequence. During the past several years the complete sequences of bacteria, yeast, worms, and flies have been determined.[71-74] The sequencing of the entire human genome was completed in 2000. Now that this sequence is in hand, the challenge will become how to organize, search, and manage this vast amount of new information and how to begin to understand the variabilities in sequence between human populations and individuals and how such genetic variability translates into phenotypic variation.

Monoclonal Antibodies

Antibodies recognize and bind to epitopes, specific shapes of molecules such as those assumed by a particular sequence of amino acids or sugars. A single plasma cell produces one antibody with a unique recognition site for a single protein or sugar epitope. However, in a typical immune response after vaccination with a foreign protein, the mammalian organism produces thousands of different plasma cells that secrete thousands of distinct antibodies into the serum. Although such polyclonal antisera are useful, it would clearly be desirable to identify a renewable cell source that could be used to produce a single homogeneous (monoclonal) antibody that is specific for a single epitope on a functionally important human protein. Unfortunately, it is not possible to clone and grow normal plasma cells in tissue culture for long periods of time.

The problem of monoclonal antibody production was solved by Kohler and Milstein,[75] who discovered that they could fuse a normal antibody-producing plasma cell to an immortalized myeloma cell to produce a continuously growing fusion cell that would in many cases continue to produce and secrete large amounts of the plasma cell's antibody. This technique has subsequently been used by many investigators to produce immortalized plasma cells that produce antibodies to proteins of the cardiovascular system. Such monoclonal antibodies are useful for identifying and purifying individual proteins, for diagnostic tests designed to identify and quantify those proteins in cells, tissues, and serum, and in some cases as therapeutic reagents.[17, 76-78]

Example of a Monoclonal Antibody Use in Therapy: Monoclonal Antibody Directed Against the Platelet Glycoprotein IIb/IIIa in the Treatment of Thrombotic Coronary Syndromes (See also Chaps. 35, 36, 38, and 62)

Platelet adhesion, aggregation, and secretion play an important role in the etiology of myocardial infarctions and strokes. Thus, there has been a great deal of interest in developing novel therapeutic reagents that can be used to inhibit platelet function in patients with these disorders. The platelet-specific glycoprotein (GP) IIb/IIIa is a cell surface molecule composed of a 136-kDa A chain and a 100-kDa B chain.[79] GP IIb/IIIa is a member of the integrin family of cellular adhesion receptors. Binding of GPIIb/IIIa to ArgGlyAsp (or RGD) peptide sequences in fibrinogen results in platelet cross-linking, adhesion, spreading, and secretion, and subsequent thrombus propagation.[79]

The importance of the GP IIb/IIIa molecule was demonstrated using RGD (or KGD) containing peptide inhibitors and monoclonal antibodies specific for the fibrinogen binding site of GPIIb/IIIa, both of which were shown to potently inhibit platelet aggregation and function in vitro.[80] These findings led directly to the idea of using such monoclonal antibodies as antiplatelet reagents in patients suffering from unstable coronary syndromes and those undergoing percutaneous revascularization. To avoid immune responses, a high-affinity murine monoclonal antibody directed against the human GP IIb/IIIa molecule (that also recognized the $\alpha_V\beta_3$ vitronectin receptor) was "humanized" using recombinant DNA techniques to render the murine monoclonal antibody less immunogenic and to produce it in large quantities in the supernatants of cultured myeloma cells.

The resulting purified monoclonal antibody abciximab (or ReoPro) was then tested for efficacy in clinical trials in patients undergoing percutaneous coronary revascularization by either balloon angioplasty or stenting.[81-84] These studies have shown a consistent 50 to 60 percent reduction in acute ischemic complications (death, myocardial infarction, and emergency revascularization) in the treated patients. Abciximab appears to be even more efficacious in patients with unstable coronary syndromes undergoing percutaneous revascularization.[85] Small molecule or peptidic GP IIb/IIIa antagonists have similar effects (see also Chaps. 38 and 62). The success of these clinical trials not only has provided us with important new therapeutic reagents for patients undergoing percutaneous revascularization but also has raised the level of enthusiasm concerning the development of additional monoclonal antibody drugs for patients with cardiovascular diseases.

Blotting Techniques

A typical human cell contains thousands of genes, mRNAs and proteins. Blotting techniques allow the identification of single genes, RNAs, or proteins based on their size and sequence without the need to purify individual molecules. Southern blotting begins with the cleavage of human genomic DNA with one or more restriction enzymes, thereby producing a mixture of thousands of DNA fragments of all sizes.[86] These DNA fragments are subsequently separated by size using electrophoresis in an agarose gel. In such a gel the smallest fragments migrate most quickly to the bottom of the gel whereas the larger fragments migrate more slowly and remain near the top of the gel. The fragments are then denatured (separated into single strands) and transferred to a sheet of filter paper to produce a replica of the gel. This filter is then exposed to a radioactive DNA probe (a radiolabeled single-stranded DNA fragment) that is complementary to the gene of interest. Such a probe hybridizes specifically to its complementary gene fragment on the filter and sticks to the filter during washing to remove unbound radioactivity. Because a given gene will only be contained in one or at most a few fragments whose size is based on the occurrence of restriction enzyme sites in and around the gene, the probe will only anneal to a few bands on the filter. Autoradiography of the hybridized and washed filter will allow visualization of these bands and determination of their sizes.

Northern blotting is used to detect specific mRNAs and is based on principles similar to Southern blotting[55] (Fig. 55–9). The mRNA corresponding to each gene displays a characteristic size or sizes. Therefore, a mixture of cellular RNAs of different sizes is separated by electrophoresis on agarose-containing gels, transferred to a filter, and hybridized to a radiolabeled DNA probe complementary to the mRNA of interest. After hybridization the radiolabeled bands are visualized by autoradiography.

Western blotting is an electrophoretic technique used to identify specific proteins. Once again it is based on the principle that different proteins display characteristic sizes and can be recognized specifically by antibodies. A mixture of proteins is separated by size by electrophoresis through a polyacrylamide gel and transferred to a filter. This filter is then incubated with an antibody that is specific for the protein of interest coupled to a radioactive isotope or an enzymatic marker. Specific bands corresponding to the protein of interest are then visualized by autoradiography or colorimetric or photometric reactions.[55]

In addition to allowing the identification of genes, RNAs, and proteins, these blotting techniques allow quantitation of the levels of specific biomolecules in different cell types, in cells from patients with disease, and in response to different developmental or environmental stimuli.

Gene Array Technologies

Blotting techniques allow quantitation and comparison of the levels of expression of a single gene between various cell samples. However, in many cases it would be desirable to compare the expression profiles of hundreds or even thousands of genes in two cell types or tissue samples. For example, it would be fascinating to understand the patterns of expression of all of the genes in the human genome in cardiomyocytes from failing as compared with normal hearts or in vascular smooth muscle cells immediately before and after mechanical injury such as balloon inflation. This type of gene profiling study has become increasingly powerful as the number of sequenced human genes increased over the past several years. Gene array technologies developed during the past 5 years allow the highly accurate and simultaneous quantitation of levels of mRNA expression from thousands of genes.[87–91] Although these technologies differ in their experimental details, they are all based on arraying cDNAs or oligonucleotides corresponding to known gene sequences on a grid of some sort (from a piece of filter paper to a glass slide or a silicon chip) and then hybridizing radiolabled or fluorescent cDNAs (DNA copies of RNA) from different cell samples to the grid. Computer software is then used to analyze the intensity of hybridization to the individual spots on the grid, and statistical analysis can be used to estimate the likelihood of significant changes in the levels of gene expression between the samples.

GENETICALLY MODIFIED MICE AS A MODEL SYSTEM OF HUMAN CARDIOVASCULAR DISEASE

One of the most surprising findings to emerge from molecular genetic studies of the cardiovascular system is the remarkable evolutionary conservation of the molecular pathways that control cardiovascular development and function. It is now clear that similar genes and signaling pathways regulate the development of the heart and vasculature in mice and humans.[2] In some cases these same pathways

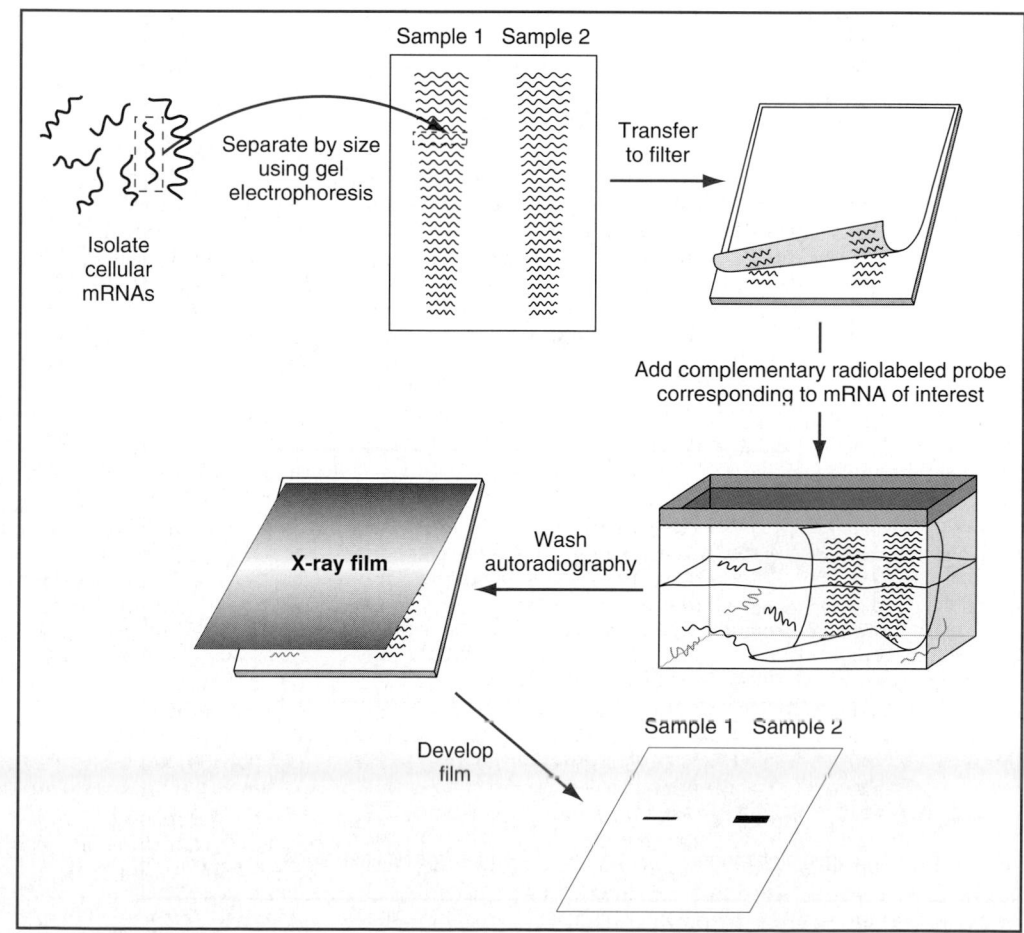

FIGURE 55–9. Northern blot analysis. Cellular mRNAs of different sizes are separated by agarose gel electrophoresis and transferred to a filter membrane. The membrane is incubated in a solution containing a single-stranded radiolabeled DNA probe complementary to the mRNA of interest. This radiolabeled probe hybridizes only to the single band containing the complementary mRNA. Nonspecific binding of the probe is removed by washing the filter, and the band is visualized by exposure of the filter to x-ray film. As shown in the figure, the intensities of the resulting autoradiographic bands correspond to the abundances of the mRNA in the original samples. Hence, the technique can be used to quantitate the levels of gene expression in two different tissue samples.

have even been conserved in reptiles and insects. Thus, we can gain important insights into human cardiovascular biology and disease by studying these processes at the molecular level in lower organisms. In many ways, mice represent an ideal model system for studies of human cardiovascular biology and disease. The mouse is a small animal with a short gestation period (21 days). A great deal is known about murine embryology and genetics. The mouse genome is being sequenced as a part of the genome initiative. Therefore, it will soon be possible to compare the structures of all of the mouse and human genes. Perhaps most importantly, elegant techniques for gene insertion, inactivation, and modification have been devised that allow genetic manipulation of the mouse almost ad libitum.

Transgenic Mice

Overexpression of a wild-type or mutant gene in a mouse represents a powerful tool for understanding both the function of that gene in normal mouse development and, in some cases, its role in specific disease states. The production of a transgenic mouse involves (1) the cloning of the gene of interest, (2) fusion of that gene to transcriptional regulatory sequences that program its expression either in all tissues of the mouse or in specific tissues, (3) injection of the purified transgene into the male pronucleus of a fertilized one-cell mouse embryo, and (4) reimplantation of the injected embryo into a foster mother[35, 92, 93] (Fig. 55–10). In many cases the injected transgene is randomly integrated into a chromosome of the fertilized embryo, resulting in a founder mouse that not only will express the injected transgene but also will pass that transgene on to 50 percent of its progeny. By comparing the phenotype of the transgenic animals with that of their nontransgenic (but otherwise genetically identical) siblings, one can draw firm conclusions about the effects of transgene overexpression on development and function at the cellular, tissue, and organismal levels. Although the production of transgenic animals was originally a technically difficult procedure that could only be carried out in a few specialized research laboratories,[94] it is now possible to produce routinely multiple transgenic founders in less than a month after a single day of embryo injections with the appropriate transgene DNA construct. Thus, the production of transgenic mice has become a standard procedure carried out in many laboratories throughout the world. Moreover, similar techniques have recently been used to produce transgenic rats, rabbits, and pigs.

Promoters have recently been characterized that program transgene expression exclusively in cardiomyocytes, endothelial cells, and vascular smooth muscle cells.[35, 95] Thus, it is now possible to restrict transgene expression to specific cell types in the cardiovascular system. In addition to producing gain-of-function animals by overexpression of the wild-type or even a superactivated mutant gene, it is also possible to use transgenic techniques to eliminate the function of a single gene by overexpressing a dominant negative mutant of that gene whose encoded protein interferes with the function of the wild-type protein.[96, 97] Recently, it has also become possible to produce transgenic mice in which expression of the transgene is turned on or off by adminis-

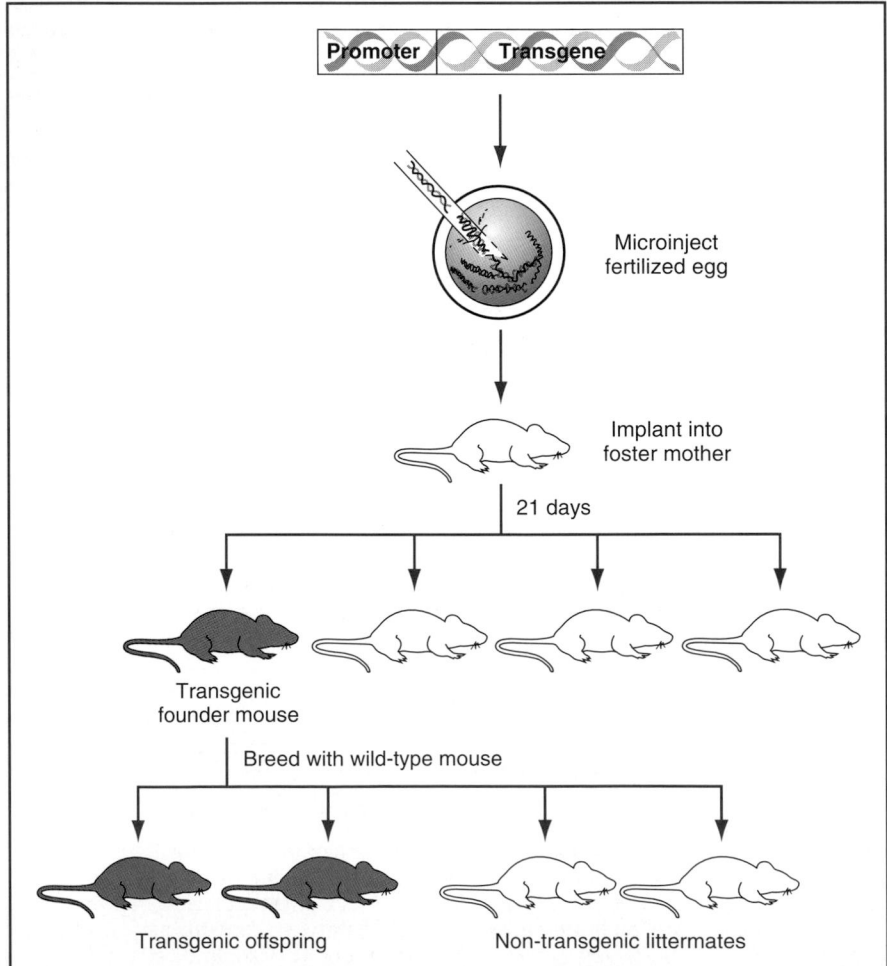

FIGURE 55–10. Production of transgenic mice. The transgene of interest is coupled by recombinant DNA technology to a transcriptional regulatory sequence that directs its expression either in all cells or in specific tissue types of the mouse. This transgene construct is microinjected into the pronucleus of a fertilized mouse egg, which is then implanted into the uterus of a foster mother. Twenty-one days later, this mother gives birth to a litter containing one or more transgenic founder mice that have integrated the transgene cassette into their genomic DNA. Breeding of these founders to wild-type mice results in transmission of the transgene to 50 percent of the resulting offspring. Transgenic mice are shown in black. Nontransgenic mice are shown in white.

tration of a simple drug like tetracycline.[98] Such mice allow precisely timed transgene expression as well as a comparison in the same animal of the phenotypes of transgene-positive and transgene-negative states.

Example of the Use of Genetically Altered Mice to Investigate Cardiovascular Pathophysiology: Transgenic Mice Reveal the Role of Beta-adrenergic Receptor Downregulation in Congestive Heart Failure
(See also Chap. 16)

Chronic overstimulation of beta-adrenergic receptors as is seen in patients with congestive heart failure leads to the downregulation of beta-adrenergic receptor (βAR) signaling in cardiomyocytes.[99] Recent studies have demonstrated that this downregulation results from phosphorylation of the βAR by beta-adrenergic receptor kinase (βARK) and subsequent receptor internalization and uncoupling.[100] Receptor uncoupling, in turn, leads to decreased contractility and an exacerbation of heart failure. Thus, prevention of receptor phosphorylation and internalization might be beneficial in patients with congestive heart failure.[101, 101a]

During the past 5 years, several mouse models of dilated cardiomyopathy and heart failure have been described.[97, 102–105] To ask if the prevention of βAR uncoupling could ameliorate the progression of congestive heart failure in these models, Lefkowitz and colleagues produced transgenic mice that overexpressed a truncated form of βARK (called βARKct).[101] βARKct was known to function as a dominant negative inhibitor of βARK, that is, it prevented βARK from phosphorylating the βAR and therefore prevented βAR internalization. To be certain that the effects of the βARKct transgene were due to its activity in cardiomyocytes, Lefkowitz and colleagues linked the βARKct transgene to the cardiomyocyte-specific alpha-myosin heavy chain (α-MHC) promoter using standard recombinant DNA techniques. After injection of the βARKct transgene into fertilized mouse embryos, Lefkowitz and colleagues produced several lines of transgenic mice that expressed high levels of βARKct only in cardiomyocytes. These βARKct transgenic mice demonstrated increased basal heart rates and contractility as well as enhanced responses to βAR stimulation.[101] To test the effects of βARK inhibition on the progression of heart failure, the βARKct transgenic mice were bred with MLP knockout (KO) mice[102] that develop dilated cardiomyopathy and heart failure. Remarkably, the βARKct transgene prevented the development of congestive heart failure in the MLP KO mice, demonstrating directly that βAR downregulation plays a key role in both the development and progression of heart failure in the MLP KO mice.[106] This exciting genetic experiment confirmed the important role of βARK in this model of heart failure and suggested that drugs that inhibit βARK activity may be useful new therapeutic reagents in patients with congestive heart failure.

Targeted Gene Inactivation ("Knockout") Technologies

Gene knockouts represent a complementary approach to transgenesis for studying the role of a specific gene in mouse development and physiology[107–114] (Fig. 55–11). Unlike transgenic experiments that typically result in overexpression of the transgene product (and hence produce a gain-of-function mouse), gene knockouts eliminate the expression of one or more genes to produce a loss-of-function mutant animal. The classical knockout approach involves transfection of a pluripotent mouse embryonic stem (ES) cell with a targeting construct or copy of the gene of interest containing a deletion or nonsense mutation.[108] Homologous recombination between the targeting construct and one copy of the endogenous gene produces an ES cell with a heterozygous deletion of the gene of interest. This mutant ES cell is then injected into a fertilized mouse blastocyst, which in turn is implanted into a foster mother. The resulting mouse is a chimera in which all tissues (including the gonads) are derived in part from the mutant ES cells and in part from the wild type cells of the injected blastocysts. This chimeric animal is then bred to a wild-type animal. Fertilization of a wild-type egg with a mutant sperm from

the chimera produces a heterozygous KO animal in which one copy of the gene of interest in all cells is mutant and the other copy is wild type. Such heterozygous animals can be bred to produce homozygous knockouts that lack active copies of the gene of interest in all cells. The phenotype of such gene KO animals reveals the essential function(s) of that gene in both normal development and physiology. Unlike transgenesis, gene knockouts are difficult, time consuming, and expensive to produce. It typically takes a skilled investigator 6 to 12 months to produce a single KO mouse strain.

Example of Targeted Gene Deletion to Produce a Disease Model: Apolipoprotein E–Deficient Mice: A Murine Model of Atherosclerosis

Unlike humans, mice are remarkably resistant to atherosclerosis, even when maintained on a high-cholesterol diet.[115] This fact has limited our ability to use mouse models to study the pathogenesis and treatment of atherosclerotic vascular disease. It has been hypothesized that the resistance of mice to atherosclerosis may be due in part to the fact that most of the cholesterol in mouse serum is present in the high-density lipoprotein (IHDL), as opposed to the low-density lipoprotein (LDL) fraction.[115, 116] To alter the lipoprotein pattern in mice and directly test the function of apolipoprotein E (apoE) in cholesterol metabolism, two groups independently used gene targeting to inactivate the apoE gene in mice.[117, 118] Due to delayed clearance of very low density lipoprotein (VLDL) particles lacking apoE, the mutant mice displayed marked elevations in VLDL-like particles and reciprocal decreases in HDL cholesterol (see also Chap. 31). Interestingly, these disorders in lipid metabolism were associated with the development of extensive atherosclerosis when these mice were maintained on a diet similar to those consumed in westernized countries.

These results not only proved the important role of apoE in determining sensitivity to atherosclerosis, but also provided a new animal model of the disease, which could be used to study both pathogenesis and treatment. For example, recent studies have demonstrated that the development of late atherosclerotic lesions in the apoE-deficient mice can be significantly reduced by breeding them to mice deficient in CD154 (or CD40 ligand)[119] or by administration of antibodies against CD154,[120, 120a] a proinflammatory receptor present on T cells, macrophages, vascular smooth muscle cells, and endothelial cells. These findings directly implicated the CD40/CD40L interaction in the progression of atherosclerosis in this model and suggested that strategies to block this pathway may represent novel approaches for the treatment of atherosclerosis.

Newer Gene-Targeting Approaches

Because many genes are required for the early development of multiple cell types and tissues, classical gene knockout approaches can often result in early embryonic lethal phenotypes that are difficult to analyze and understand. Thus, it would be desirable to be able to delete genes in a tissue-specific fashion and/or to inactivate them at different times in development. Moreover, in some cases it is of interest to produce specific mutations of genes rather than to eliminate their expression completely. Recently developed technologies have begun to address these issues.[110–114]

The same types of homologous recombination methods that are used to knockout genes by deletion can be used to introduce specific mutations into wild-type genes. The only major difference in technique is that such "knock-ins" use a targeting construct containing a mutant gene rather than a gene deletion. Moreover, it is possible using homologous recombination to introduce a distinct or unrelated gene into a foreign genetic locus and to thereby regulate the new gene under the control of the promoter of the targeted locus.

Gene deletion can also be carried out in a tissue-specific manner by using an elegant bacterial phage recombination system called Cre-lox.[112, 121] The P1 bacteriophage encodes an enzyme called Cre that catalyzes recombination of DNA between two specific sequences (called loxP sites) that signal recombination.[121] This system can be used in mice by

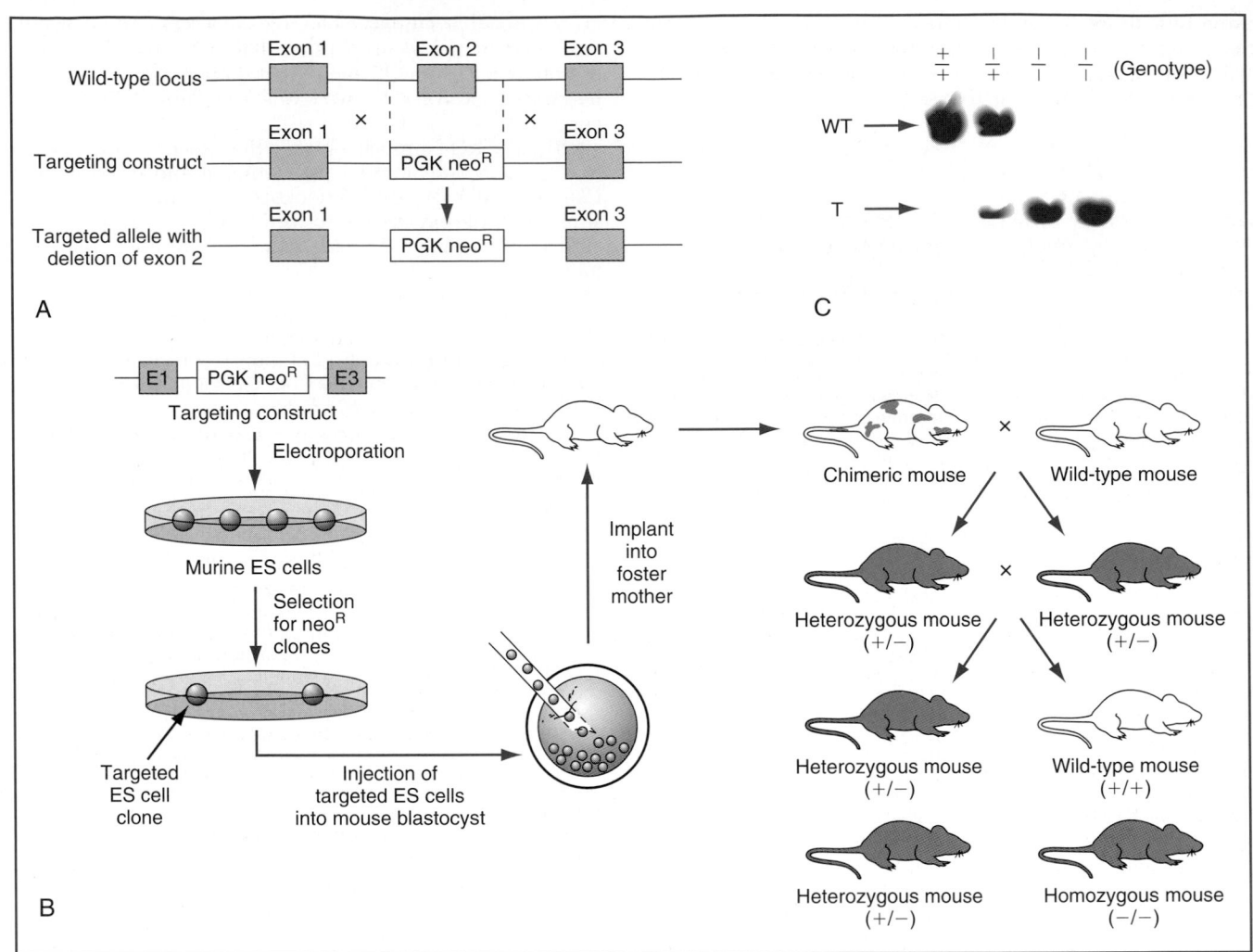

FIGURE 55–11. Gene targeting in mice. *A,* A schematic illustration of a wild-type prototypical eukaryotic gene with three exons *(top),* a targeting construct in which exon 2 has been replaced with a neomycin resistance gene (neo^R) under the control of the phosphoglycerate kinase (PGK) promoter *(middle),* and a targeted allele in which the wild-type gene has been replaced with the targeting construct by homologous recombination *(bottom). B,* Production of gene-targeted mice. The targeting construct produced in *A* is introduced into murine embryonic stem (ES) cells by electroporation. Cells containing the targeted allele produced by homologous recombination are identified by Southern blot analysis and injected into a fertilized mouse blastocyst. Injected blastocysts are implanted into a foster mother, that gives birth 21 days later to chimeric mice in which all of the tissues are derived in part from the targeted ES cells and in part from wild-type cells within the blastocysts. Breeding of the chimeric mouse to a wild-type mouse results in germline transmission of the targeted allele, producing heterozygous mice that contain one targeted and one wild-type allele. Interbreeding of two heterozygous mice produces a litter composed of one-fourth wild-type (+/+) mice, one-fourth homozygous targeted (−/−) mice, and one-half heterozygous (+/−) mice. *C,* Southern blot analysis of a cross between two heterozygous gene-targeted mice. The wild-type (WT) and targeted (T) alleles can be distinguished by their different sizes on Southern blot. The genotypes of resulting mice can be deduced from the patterns of the wild-type and targeted alleles. Wild-type (+/+) mice contain two copies of the wild-type allele. Heterozygous (+/−) mice contain a single copy of the wild-type allele and a single copy of the targeted allele. Homozygous deficient mice (−/−) contain two copies of the targeted allele.

producing a targeting construct in which the gene of interest is flanked by loxP sites (a so-called floxed allele).[112, 121] Mice homozygous for the floxed allele can then be bred with transgenic mice that express the Cre recombinase in a tissue-specific manner. Such mice will then delete the gene of interest only in the tissue expressing the Cre recombinase. By placing the Cre transgene under the control of a tetracycline-responsive promoter it is also possible to program gene deletion only after tetracycline feeding.

By using combinations of transgenesis, gene knockout, and new gene targeting approaches it is now possible to produce gain-of-function and loss-of-function mice in a temporally and spatially regulated fashion. In addition to identifying the function of individual genes at the organis-

mal level, such studies often produce new animal models of human cardiovascular disease that are useful for studies of molecular pathogenesis and therapy. For example, such approaches have already produced mouse models of hypertrophic[122, 123] and dilated cardiomyopathy,[96, 97, 102–105] familial hypercholesterolemia,[124] and congenital cardiac disorders. The completion of the human genome project, announced in June of 2000,[124a, 124b] will lead to the identification of large numbers of variations in gene sequence (polymorphisms), some of which will be associated with specific human diseases. Homologous recombination-mediated knock-ins of these mutations into mice will become an important tool for validating the role of these polymorphisms in the etiology of these diseases.

Advances in Mouse Physiology

To harness the full power of mouse genetics, it is important to be able to perform accurate physiological studies of the cardiovascular system in genetically modified animals. Until recently, the ability to analyze the mouse cardiovascular system was severely limited by both the small size of the heart and vessels in the mouse and by the resting murine heart rate of greater than 500 beats/min. During the last several years, a number of groups have solved this problem by developing miniaturized instrumentation and microsurgical techniques.[3, 96, 125] Using these approaches it is now possible to obtain a wide variety of physiological measurements in anesthetized and intubated closed-chested animals. Such parameters include aortic blood pressures, real-time left ventricular pressure tracings, dP/dt_{max} and dP/dt_{min}, and arterial blood gases and pH both at baseline and after the infusion of pressors such as dobutamine or isoproterenol. In addition, by using high-frequency transducers and customized software it is possible to obtain high-resolution M mode and two-dimensional echocardiograms from mice. These images can be used to determine end-systolic and end-diastolic left ventricular dimensions, left ventricular wall thickness and mass, shortening fraction, and wall stress rate–corrected velocity of fiber shortening (Vefc) relationships. It is also possible to produce myocardial infarctions by coronary artery ligation with or without reperfusion injury and to induce left ventricular hypertrophy by aortic banding or chronic infusion of angiotensin II. Finally, it is now possible to obtain 24-hour electrocardiographic recordings on conscious mice using implanted transducers and to perform limited electrophysiological studies to detect inducible cardiac arrhythmias in these animals.[126] Taken together, these advances make it possible to use the mouse as an accurate and convenient model system for studies of cardiovascular physiology and pathology and, when combined with the genetic manipulations described earlier, suggest that the mouse will become an increasingly useful system for studies of the genetic bases of human cardiovascular disease.

GENE- AND CELL-BASED THERAPIES FOR HUMAN CARDIOVASCULAR DISEASE

Somatic Gene Therapy for Cardiovascular Disease

Somatic gene therapy can be defined as the ability to introduce genetic material into non-germline cells to produce a therapeutic effect at the level of the intact organism. The recent rapid increase in the number of cloned and characterized human genes when coupled with an improved understanding of the genetic pathways involved in normal and pathological cell function has increased the potential usefulness of somatic gene therapy approaches for the treatment of a wide variety of human cardiovascular diseases.[127–130] Indeed, human gene therapy trials have recently been initiated for the treatment of patients with chronic myocardial ischemia[131] and vein graft stenoses.[132]

Gene therapy strategies can be divided into two categories based on the location of cell transduction. Ex vivo approaches are those in which cells or tissues are removed from an animal or patient, transduced with the therapeutic gene in vitro, and then retransplanted into the recipient host. In contrast, in vivo gene therapies involve the transduction of the appropriate cell type in vivo without the need for cell isolation or transplantation. During the past 5 years there has been a paradigm shift in our thinking about gene therapy approaches for human disease. Initial studies focused on the correction of inherited genetic disorders such as familial hypercholesterolemia or muscular dystrophy and often employed ex vivo methods. More recently, it has become clear that gene therapies may also be quite useful for the treatment of acquired disorders such as cardiac ischemia or restenosis and that particularly in the cardiovascular system it is often preferable to develop and employ in vivo gene transduction strategies.[127–130]

Like any successful therapeutic strategy, gene therapies must be tailored to the patient and the patient's disease. Relevant considerations in this design process include an understanding of the cell type that must be transduced and the efficiency of transduction that is needed to correct or prevent the disease. Different disorders require different stabilities of transgene expression. Thus, for example the treatment of an inherited metabolic disorder such as familial hypercholesterolemia requires long-term stable transgene expression (or alternatively the ability to readminister the transgene on a regular basis), whereas the treatment of restenosis likely only requires transient expression of an appropriate transgene. Moreover, some gene therapies such as those designed to treat diabetes mellitus with transgene-encoded insulin clearly require regulated transgene expression whereas others such as the treatment of hemophilia with transgenes encoding coagulation factors XIII or IX simply require constitutive transgene expression. Finally, as with any new therapy it is important to carefully consider the potential risks of any gene therapy, including the effects of overexpression or ectopic transgene expression, the possibility of germline transmission of the transgene, risks associated with the vector used to introduce transgenes into cells (this is particularly true of viral vectors), the chance of mutagenesis of the host genome, and the potential for stimulating host inflammatory and immune responses to the vector or the transgene itself.

Most cardiovascular gene therapy approaches require at least three separate but related components: (1) an appropriate therapeutic transgene, (2) a vector for introducing that transgene into the relevant cell type such as a cardiomyocyte or a vascular smooth muscle cell, and (3) a device (e.g., a catheter or stent) for efficient delivery of the vector to the appropriate location in the cardiovascular system (e.g., to a localized segment of the vasculature or myocardium).

Vectors for Cardiovascular Gene Therapy

To date, five different vector systems have been tested or show promise for cardiovascular gene therapy (Fig. 55–12): (1) "naked" plasmid DNA,[133] (2) synthetic oligonucleotides,[134] (3) replication defective adenoviruses,[135–137] (4) replication defective adeno-associated viruses,[138] and (5) retroviruses/lentiviruses.[135–137] Each of these vectors displays unique advantages and disadvantages, which define their usefulness for the treatment of different cardiovascular diseases (Table 55–1).

"NAKED" DNA. Naked plasmid DNA vectors (i.e., purified plasmids containing only a transgene and an appropriate transcriptional regulatory element) (see Fig. 55–12) are taken up and expressed by small numbers of cardiomyocytes after direct intramyocardial injection.[133, 139] The advantages of such vectors include the simplicity of their production and administration, the stability of their expression (at least 19 months in rodents),[140] and their inability to transduce most other cell types in vivo after intramyocardial injection. However, these advantages are offset by the extremely low efficiency of cardiomyocyte transduction (less than 0.01 percent of the cells in the area of injection),[133, 139, 140] the requirement for direct injection into the myocardium, and their inability to appreciably transduce endothelial cells and smooth muscle cells in the vasculature. Thus, such vectors will likely only be useful for gene therapy strategies that require local expression of transgenes in very small numbers of cardiomyocytes after direct intramyocardial injection. An example of such an approach

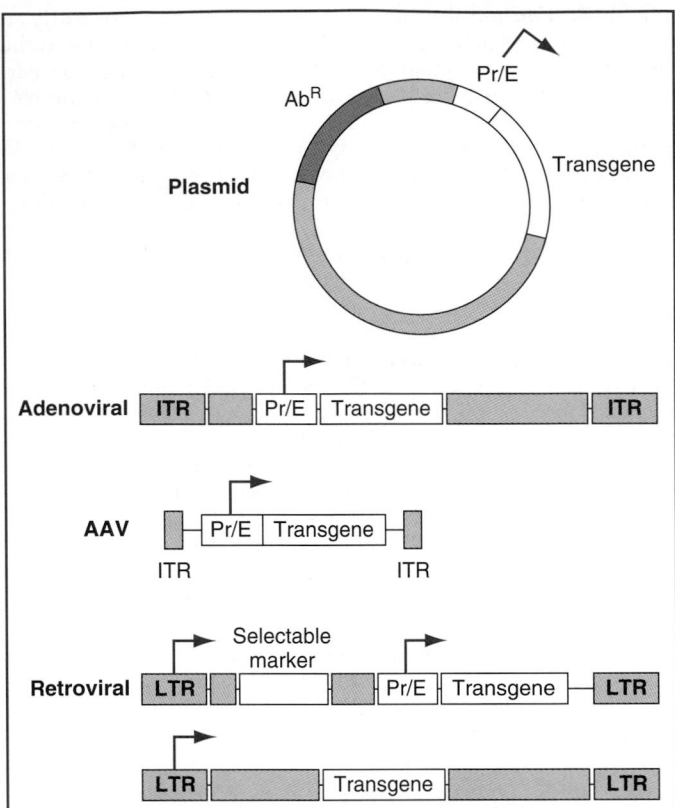

FIGURE 55–12. Commonly used gene therapy vectors. The structures of retroviral, adenoviral, adeno-associated viral (AAV), and plasmid gene therapy vectors are shown. Viral and bacterial sequences are crosshatched. Transgene, promoter/enhancer, and selectable marker sequences are shown as unshaded boxes. LTR = long terminal repeat from the retroviral genome; Pr/E = an eukaryotic promoter/enhancer; ITR = inverted terminal repeat from either the adenoviral or AAV genomes; Ab^R = an antibiotic resistance gene for selection of plasmid-containing bacteria. Arrows show the direction of transcription of transgenes and selectable markers.

in which plasmid vectors are currently being tested in humans is the localized expression of vascular endothelial growth factor (VEGF) to induce angiogenesis after direct injection into regions of ischemic myocardium.[131]

OLIGONUCLEOTIDES. Synthetic oligonucleotides are short (10 to 50 base pair) pieces of chemically synthesized single- or double-stranded DNA that can be used to inhibit the expression of one or more genes after their introduction into cells. The mechanism of action of these oligonucleotides is complex and not fully understood. However, in some cases the single-stranded antisense oligonucleotides (i.e., oligonucleotides whose sequence is complementary to the coding sequence of an mRNA molecule) appear to base pair through hybridization with their complementary mRNAs and thereby to promote their degradation.[74] Double-stranded oligonucleotides corresponding in sequence to the recognition site of a specific transcription factor can serve as decoys that bind and sequester their cognate transcription factor, thereby inhibiting its ability to activate its normal set of target genes.[141] The advantages of such oligonucleotides for gene therapy include their ease of production and their relative safety. Disadvantages include significant batch-to-batch variability in activity, the fact that they are generally limited to turning target genes off as opposed to augmenting the expression of therapeutic transgenes, their nonspecific activities in cells, and their short half-lives (on the order of hours to days) in vivo. In addition, the ability of oligonucleotides to transduce cells in vivo is quite limited, necessitating the use of lipid-viral conjugates to enhance transduction.[142] Thus, such oligonucleotide-mediated

approaches of gene therapy will likely be useful only for transiently turning off the expression of specific genes in localized areas of the cardiovascular system. Indeed, such approaches have been successful in inhibiting vascular smooth muscle cell proliferation and intimal thickening in animal models of balloon angioplasty.[134, 142, 143]

ADENOVIRUS. Adenoviruses are double-stranded DNA viruses that can be used to efficiently transduce a wide variety of tissues and cell types in vivo.[144] These viruses can be genetically engineered to render them replication-defective (i.e., to render them capable of infecting a normal human cell once but incapable of generating infectious progeny and spreading the infection beyond the initial site of administration) and to allow them to program high-level transgene expression in vivo (see Fig. 55–12). The advantages of adenovirus vectors include their very high efficiency of transduction of resting cells (including cardiomyocytes, vascular smooth muscle cells, endothelial cells, and hepatocytes) in vivo, the relative ease of producing large amounts of virus, the ability to deliver the vectors through a catheter, and their relative safety.[145] These vectors have not been associated with persistent infection or malignancy, and they generally do not integrate into the host genome, minimizing the risk of insertional mutagenesis. Unfortunately, these advantages are offset by the fact that adenovirus vectors generally produce potent inflammatory and immune responses both to themselves and to the transgenes that they express.[146–149] These responses produce local tissue damage and usually eliminate virus-transduced cells, thereby limiting the duration of transgene expression to 2 to 3 weeks.[135, 146–149] Moreover, adenovirus vectors generate neutralizing antibodies that prevent readministration of the virus,[148] and in some cases these vectors can break tolerance to self proteins that are related to the transgene protein, thereby producing autoimmunity and/or precluding future gene therapies involving the same transgene.[149] Thus, in their present form these vectors will likely only be useful for gene therapy approaches requiring high-level and efficient but transient transgene expression in vivo. Examples include their use in gene therapy strategies designed to inhibit restenosis and to program myocardial angiogenesis after injection into the myocardium.

Despite the apparent limitations on the use of current-generation adenovirus vectors, recent studies have suggested that in some cases it may be possible to obtain long-term transgene expression in vivo with first-generation adenoviruses (e.g., in the case of expression of a self transgene after injection into skeletal muscle and in the case of adenovirus perfusion of the donor heart before transplantation).[138, 149] Moreover, newer versions of adenovirus vectors in which all of the viral genes have been deleted (so-called helper dependent or gutted adenoviruses) also appear to yield stable transgene expression in vivo.[150–152] Thus, future developments may result in adenovirus vectors that are useful for a wider range of cardiovascular gene therapies.

ADENO-ASSOCIATED VIRUS. Adeno-associated viruses (AAVs) are single-stranded DNA viruses that are nonpathogenic in humans.[153] By replacing all of the viral genes in these vectors with a transgene and promoter cassette it is possible to produce replication-defective AAV vectors that are quite useful for cardiovascular gene therapy[153] (see Fig. 55–12). Like adenoviruses, AAV vectors efficiently infect many resting cell types in vivo, including cardiomyocytes and hepatocytes.[138, 154] Their efficiency of transduction of vascular endothelial and smooth muscle cells remains less clear.[155, 156] Unlike adenoviruses, AAV vectors do not cause significant inflammatory or immune responses. Thus, these vectors can be used to program transgene expression in vivo that is stable for at least 1 year.[157, 158] Cardiomyocytes can be efficiently transduced after either intramyocardial injection or coronary artery perfusion.[138] Moreover, these

VECTOR/TRANSGENE	ADVANTAGES	DISADVANTAGES
Retroviruses	• Stably integrate into host genome • Easily manipulated viral genome • No viral gene products; relatively nonimmunogenic • Highly efficient transduction of many cell types	• Low titers • Capacity for insertional mutagenesis • In vivo instability • Transcriptional shut off in vivo • Require cell proliferation for infection
Adenoviruses	• Maintained as an episome • Highly efficient transduction of replicating and nonreplicating cells • Stable in vivo in absence of immune response • High-level transgene expression in vivo • Relatively nonpathogenic • High titers	• Evoke potent host inflammatory and immune responses that eliminate transgene expression and preclude repeated administration • Difficult to target to specific cell types • Relatively difficult to manipulate viral genome
Adeno-associated virus	• Infects replicating and nonreplicating cells • Potential for site-specific integration • Relatively nonimmunogenic • High titers • Nonpathogenic in humans	• Can accept only small transgenes • Difficult to produce in large quantities • Does not appear to stably transduce all cell types in vivo • Potential for insertional mutagenesis
Plasmid DNA	• Easy to manipulate and produce in large quantities • Nonpathogenic • Relatively nonimmunogenic • Does not require an infectious vector • Maintained as an episome • Can program long-term gene expression in postmitotic cells in vivo	• Very low transduction efficiency
Synthetic oligonucleotides	• Easy to synthesize in large quantities • Relatively high transduction efficiencies if delivered with viral liposomes	• Can only reduce or ablate gene expression • Large number of nonspecific and nonreproducible biological effects • Cannot target specific cell types • Relatively short half-life in vivo
Ribozymes	• Can specifically and effectively target mRNAs	• Can only reduce or ablate gene expression • Difficult to deliver to cells in vivo • Stability in vivo unclear

vectors appear to be quite safe, because they do not produce human disease even in their wild-type form.[153] Limitations of AAV vectors include the difficulty to date in producing large amounts of high-titer vector, the limitation on the size of the transgene that they can accommodate (less than 4.5 kb), and their potential for integration into the host genome.[153] These vectors will quite likely be very useful for gene therapy approaches that require efficient and stable transgene expression in the heart, including the treatment of myocardial ischemia, heart failure, and cardiac arrhythmias.

OTHER VIRAL VECTORS. Retroviruses and lentiviruses are single-stranded RNA viruses that integrate into the host genome after infection[159–162] (see Fig. 55–12). Retroviruses are unlikely to be useful for most cardiovascular gene therapies because they require cell proliferation for efficient infection.[162] Most cardiovascular cell types do not proliferate in vivo. In contrast, lentiviruses based on human or animal immunodeficiency viruses are capable of efficiently transducing many nonproliferating cell types in vivo.[160–163] Like AAV vectors, lentiviral vectors can have most of their viral genes removed and do not appear to trigger inflammatory and immune responses.[163] These vectors can program stable transgene expression in neurons in vivo.[160] Their usefulness in the heart and vasculature has not yet been fully evaluated. Potential disadvantages of these vectors include difficulties producing high-titered virus stocks and the risk of recombination with human immunodeficiency virus or endogenous retroviruses to produce replication-competent pathogenic viruses.

Recent Advances in Vector Development

During the past several years a number of advances have been made that have improved both vector efficacy and safety. These include the use of cell-type specific transcriptional regulatory sequences to produce vectors that express their transgenes in a tissue-specific manner[164] (e.g., smooth muscle cell-specific vectors) and structural modifications of vector coat proteins that enhance their infection of specific cell types.[165] In addition, several systems have been described that allow the regulation of transgene expression in response to exogenously administered drugs.[166, 167] Finally, there has been a great deal of interest in developing systems that will allow the repair of mutant genes in cells in vivo or in vitro. One such system has recently been described that uses chemically synthesized RNA/DNA oligonucleotides called chimeroplasts to direct the cell-mediated repair of single base mutations.[168] The usefulness of this and related gene repair systems for the treatment of inherited cardiovascular diseases will require additional investigation.

Devices for Gene Delivery

The development of devices that can be used for gene delivery has not advanced as quickly as vector development. The design specifications for such gene delivery devices include the ability to efficiently deliver a gene therapy vector to a localized area of the cardiovascular system with minimal invasiveness and no adverse effects on vector viability or efficiency.[169] A variety of catheters have been tested for local vascular gene delivery. These include double-balloon catheters,[128] hydrogel catheters,[170] and porous and microporous balloon catheters.[171, 172] Each of these catheters has been plagued with specific problems, including inefficient or nonuniform transgene delivery, leak of vector into the systemic circulation, and vascular injury due to balloon inflation and/or jetting of vector solution. Similarly, catheters have been described for direct intramyocardial injection. However, to date such devices produce local tissue damage and can result in significant leak of vector into the left ventricular cavity. Importantly, many of these devices have not yet been carefully tested for compatibility with the different vector systems described earlier. Indeed, recent studies have suggested that many of these catheters efficiently and rapidly inactivate adenovirus vectors.[172a] Areas that require more investigation include the use of gene- or vector-coated stents for gene delivery to the vasculature, production of delivery systems that will facilitate intracoronary perfusion with gene therapy vectors, and iontophoresis to enhance the efficiency of localized gene delivery to the heart and vasculature.

Cell-Based Therapies

A variety of cardiovascular cell types including vascular endothelial cells, vascular smooth muscle cells, and embryonic cardiomyocytes can be cultured in the laboratory in vitro. This finding has suggested the possibility of using either wild-type or genetically modified cardiovascular cell transplantation to treat a variety of cardiovascular disorders. Cultured endothelial cells have been used to seed synthetic grafts in an attempt to reduce graft thrombosis.[173, 174] Similarly, endothelial cells genetically modified to produce tissue plasminogen activator have been suggested as a therapy to reduce the thrombotic potential of grafts and native injured coronary arteries.[175]

Cardiomyocytes are terminally differentiated cells that do not retain the capacity to proliferate. Therefore, the heart lacks the capacity for regeneration after ischemic, toxic, or infectious injury. Accordingly, there has been a great deal of recent interest in developing gene- or cell-based therapies for myocardial repair and regeneration.[176] Potential gene-based approaches to this problem include the use of transgenes to stimulate cardiomyocyte proliferation or to program the differentiation of cardiac fibroblasts into cardiomyocytes. Unfortunately, genes with these activities have not yet been discovered. Alternative cell-based approaches would include the injection of either cultured cardiomyocytes or skeletal myocytes into the damaged myocardium. Recent studies have demonstrated that skeletal myocytes injected into the myocardium form a stable graft that may improve global hemodynamics after myocardial injury in rodents.[177–179] However, to date there is no evidence that such grafts form the electrical or functional junctions with the endogenous myocardium that would be required to initiate synchronous contraction of the graft. In contrast, studies from a number of groups have demonstrated stable engraftment of embryonic cardiomyocytes injected into the myocardium with formation of intercalated discs and gap junction between the injected cells and the endogenous cardiomyocytes.[180–182] These findings suggest that such engrafted cells might be capable of forming beating grafts. However, the efficiency of engraftment of such embryonic cardiomyocytes has been low (less than 0.1 percent). Moreover, it will be important to identify a nonembryonic renewable source of such transplantable cardiomyocytes. In this regard it is of interest that recent studies have suggested that such cells can be derived from embryonic stem cells in vitro as well as from adult bone marrow.[181–183] Indeed, adult bone marrow appears to contain pluripotent mesenchymal stem cells with the capacity to differentiate into a variety of cell types, including skeletal and cardiac muscle, hematopoietic cells, cartilage, and fat.[184] Such cells have been reported to repopulate damaged skeletal muscle after intravenous injection.[185] It will be of interest to determine if these cells can similarly repopulate the damaged myocardium after systemic administration.

Example of the Use of Gene Therapy for Cardiovascular Disease: Gene Therapy Approaches for Vascular Proliferative Disorders

Vascular smooth muscle cell (VSMC) migration, proliferation, and extracellular matrix deposition are thought to play important roles in vascular proliferative syndromes such as restenosis after balloon angioplasty or stenting.[186, 187] Despite numerous clinical trials with new drugs and devices, restenosis rates of 20 to 40 percent are still seen with most, if not all, percutaneous coronary revascularization procedures.[188] Thus, there has been interest in developing gene therapy approaches that could be used to treat the vascular proliferative syndromes. Such approaches would require (1) a vector that could efficiently transduce VSMCs at the site of revascularization after delivery through a catheter, (2) an appropriate cytotoxic or cytostatic gene that could either kill or inhibit the proliferation of VSMCs after vessel injury, and (3) a device that could be used to deliver this vector to a localized area of the vasculature.

During the past several years a number of successful gene therapy approaches to this problem have been developed. Nabel and coworkers demonstrated that adenovirus-mediated gene transfer of the herpes simplex virus thymidine kinase (HSV-tk) gene followed by systemic ganciclovir therapy killed proliferating VSMCs and inhibited restenosis by more than 50 percent in a pig model of iliofemoral balloon injury.[130, 189] Using a cytostatic approach, Leiden and coworkers demonstrated that adenovirus-mediated gene transfer of a constitutively active retinoblastoma (Rb) transgene (that inhibits the G1–S transition) or the cyclin-dependent kinase (CDK) inhibitor p21 that prevents Rb phosphorylation prevents smooth muscle cell proliferation and inhibits intimal thickening by 40 to 60 percent in both the rat carotid and porcine iliofemoral models of balloon injury.[189, 190]

Dzau and coworkers demonstrated that double-stranded decoy oligonucleotides containing an E2F binding site (E2F is a transcription factor that is released and activated upon Rb phosphorylation and is needed to drive cells through the G1–S transition) also inhibit restenosis in the rat carotid artery model of balloon injury by more than 70 percent.[143] These investigators have recently gone on to use these same decoy oligonucleotides in a phase I clinical trial of peripheral vein grafting and have reported a statistically significant reduction in graft occlusion after treatment with the E2F decoys.[132] Taken together, these studies suggest that both viral and oligonucleotide-mediated gene therapies may be useful adjuncts to percutaneous and surgical revascularization approaches in patients with atherosclerotic vascular disease.

FUTURE DIRECTIONS OF MOLECULAR CARDIOVASCULAR MEDICINE

Advances in molecular and cellular cardiology have already had a profound impact on cardiovascular biology and medicine. These advances, however, represent only the beginning of a set of revolutionary discoveries that will fundamentally change our understanding of normal cardiovascular function and thereby enhance our ability to diagnose and treat cardiovascular disease. It is impossible to predict the future of this scientific revolution. However, several implications are clear.

The determination of the sequence of all of the genes in the human genome along with the characterization of the role of specific genetic variations in cardiovascular diseases will provide a powerful new set of genetic diagnostic tools. Within 10 years, genetic analyses of a simple blood sample from a child will allow the accurate prediction of the susceptibility of that child to a wide variety of diseases from hypertension, atherosclerosis, and diabetes to cancer and neuropsychiatric disorders. This type of genetic susceptibility testing will fundamentally change the practice of medicine. Rather than treating patients only after they develop symptoms of cardiovascular disease it will be possible to identify those patients at high risk in childhood and intervene to reduce risk factors before disease develops. In addition, it will be possible to predict accurately the response of an individual patient to different drugs. Thus, susceptibility testing will allow the development of a new genetically based preventive medicine.

From the standpoint of basic investigation, the cloned genes and their encoded proteins can be structurally analyzed by nuclear magnetic resonance and crystallographic techniques. The resultant structures will produce important clues about the function of these proteins and will also provide that basis for the rational development of drugs designed to augment or inhibit those functions. Biochemical technologies to unravel protein-protein interactions (for example, one known as the yeast two-hybrid system) will be used to place the newly cloned genes (and proteins) into their intracellular pathways. Such approaches will help to define critical domains in molecules that should help to identify new targets for the development of drug- and gene-based therapies. Finally, newly cloned genes emerging from the genome project will be used in transgenic, knockout, and knock-in strategies in mice to determine, more precisely, their functions, to discover the effects of mutations, and to produce new animal models of human diseases for studies of pathogenesis and new therapies ("functional genomics").

From a therapeutic standpoint, the newly cloned genes will be used to design new in vitro or cell-based strategies that can be used by pharmaceutical companies to screen large libraries of compounds for new drugs. Of equal importance, these genes will form the basis for the development of novel genetic therapies for cardiovascular disease.

Like any powerful new technology, molecular genetics will also raise important ethical questions. Which genetic traits are appropriate for modification? What is the role of germ-line gene therapies that modify the genome in a genetically transmissible fashion? How is the confidentiality of genetic susceptibility data about individual patients guaranteed? And how do we handle information about susceptibility to a disease for which we lack an effective treatment? These questions and many others will be actively debated by physicians, patients, ethicists, and politicians for years to come. Despite these thorny problems, the potential for benefit from molecular genetics significantly outweighs the potential for harm. It is safe to predict that the era of molecular medicine will revolutionize the ability to diagnose and treat patients with cardiovascular diseases.

REFERENCES

1. Chien KR, Braunwald E: Molecular Basis of Cardiovascular Disease: A Companion to Braunwald's Heart Disease. Philadelphia, WB Saunders, 1999.
2. Harvey RP, Rosenthal N: Heart Development. San Diego, Academic Press, 1999.
3. James JF, Hewett TE, Robbins J: Cardiac physiology in transgenic mice. Circ Res 82:407–415, 1998.
4. Schaper W, Winkler B: Of mice and men—the future of cardiovascular research in the molecular era. Cardiovasc Res 39:3–7, 1998.
5. Haber E: Scientific American Molecular Cardiovascular Medicine. New York, Scientific American, 1995.
6. Walker CA, Spinale FG: The structure and function of the cardiac myocyte: A review of fundamental concepts. J Thorac Cardiovasc Surg 118:375–382, 1999.

GENETIC MACHINERY AND FLOW OF INFORMATION IN THE CELL

7. Pienta KJ, Getzenberg RH, Coffey DS: Cell structure and DNA organization. Crit Rev Eukaryot Gene Expr 1:355–85, 1991.
8. Dickerson RE: DNA structure from A to Z. Methods Enzymol 211:67–111, 1992.
9. Ramakrishnan V: Histone structure and the organisation of the nucleosome. Annu Rev Biophys Biomol Struct 26:83–112, 1997.
10. Kornberg RD, Lorch Y: Twenty–five years of the nucleosome, fundamental particle of the eukaryote chromosome. Cell 98:285–294, 1999.
11. Gardiner K: Human genome organization. Curr Opin Genet Dev 5:315–322, 1995.
12. Collins FS: Sequencing the human genome. Hosp Pract (Off Ed) 32:35–43, 46–49, 53–54, 1997.

13. Schuler GD, Boguski MS, Stewart EA, et al: A gene map of the human genome. Science 274:540–546, 1996.
14. Craig IW: Organization of the human genome. J Inherit Metab Dis 17:391–402, 1994.
15. Long M, de Souza SJ, Gilbert W: Evolution of the intron-exon structure of eukaryotic genes. Curr Opin Genet Dev 5:774–778, 1995.
16. Bucher P: [Description of eukaryotic promoters in the EPD database]. Mol Biol (Mosk) 31:616–625, 1997.
17. Weiner LM: An overview of monoclonal antibody therapy of cancer. Semin Oncol 26:41–50, 1999.
18. Novina CD, Roy AL: Core promoters and transcriptional control. Trends Genet 12:351–355, 1996.
19. Fassler JS, Gussin GN: Promoters and basal transcription machinery in eubacteria and eukaryotes: Concepts, definitions, and analogies. Methods Enzymol 273:3–29, 1996.
20. Kadonaga JT: Eukaryotic transcription: An interlaced network of transcription factors and chromatin-modifying machines. Cell 92:307–313, 1998.
21. Patikoglou G, Burley SK: Eukaryotic transcription factor-DNA complexes. Annu Rev Biophys Biomol Struct 26:289–325, 1997.
22. Hanna-Rose W, Hansen U: Active repression mechanisms of eukaryotic transcription repressors. Trends Genet 12:229–234, 1996.
23. Ayer DE: Histone deacetylases: Transcriptional repression with SINers and NuRDs. Trends Cell Biol 9:193–198, 1999.
24. Newman A: RNA splicing. Curr Biol 8:r903–r905, 1998.
25. Lamond AI: Nuclear RNA processing. Curr Opin Cell Biol 3:493–501, 1991.
26. Lewis JD, Izaurralde E: The role of the cap structure in RNA processing and nuclear export. Eur J Biochem 247:461–469, 1997.
27. Herbert A, Rich A: RNA processing and the evolution of eukaryotes. Nat Genet 21:265–269, 1999.
28. Rosenthal N: DNA and the genetic code. N Engl J Med 331:39–41, 1994.
29. Jukes TH: The genetic code—function and evolution. Cell Mol Biol Res 39:685–688, 1993.
30. Ross J: Control of messenger RNA stability in higher eukaryotes. Trends Genet 12:171–175, 1996.
31. Sachs AB, Buratowski S: Common themes in translational and transcriptional regulation. Trends Biochem Sci 22:189–192, 1997.
32. Hentze MW: Translational regulation: Versatile mechanisms for metabolic and developmental control. Curr Opin Cell Biol 7:393–398, 1995.
33. Graves JD, Krebs EG: Protein phosphorylation and signal transduction. Pharmacol Ther 82:111–121, 1999.
34. Patarca R: Protein phosphorylation and dephosphorylation in physiologic and oncologic processes. Crit Rev Oncol 7:343–432, 1996.
35. Hunter JJ, Zhu H, Lee KJ, et al: Targeting gene expression to specific cardiovascular cell types in transgenic mice. Hypertension 22:608–617, 1993.
36. Struhl K: Histone acetylation and transcriptional regulatory mechanisms. Genes Dev 12:599–606, 1998.
37. Ciechanover A: The ubiquitin-proteasome pathway: On protein death and cell life. EMBO J 17:7151–7160, 1998.
38. Eisenhaber F, Bork P: Wanted: Subcellular localization of proteins based on sequence. Trends Cell Biol 8:169–170, 1998.
39. Rockman HA, Koch WJ, Lefkowitz RJ: Cardiac function in genetically engineered mice with altered adrenergic receptor signaling. Am J Physiol 272:h1553–h1559, 1997.
40. Gonzalez GA, Montminy MR: Cyclic AMP stimulates somatostatin gene transcription by phosphorylation of CREB at serine 133. Cell 59:675–680, 1989.
41. Yamamoto KK, Gonzalez GA, Biggs WH, Montminy MR: Phosphorylation–induced binding and transcriptional efficacy of nuclear factor CREB. Nature 334:494–498, 1988.

GENETIC BASES OF HUMAN CARDIOVASCULAR DISEASE

42. Bonne G, Carrier L, Richard P, et al: Familial hypertrophic cardiomyopathy: From mutations to functional defects. Circ Res 83:580–593, 1998.
43. Seidman CE, Seidman JG: Molecular genetic studies of familial hypertrophic cardiomyopathy. Basic Res Cardiol 93:13–16, 1998.
44. Geisterfer-Lowrance AA, Kass S, Tanigawa G, et al: A molecular basis for familial hypertrophic cardiomyopathy: A beta cardiac myosin heavy chain gene missense mutation. Cell 62:999–1006, 1990.
45. Thierfelder L, Watkins H, MacRae C, et al: Alpha–tropomyosin and cardiac troponin T mutations cause familial hypertrophic cardiomyopathy: A disease of the sarcomere. Cell 77:701–712, 1994.
46. Watkins H, Conner D, Thierfelder L, et al: Mutations in the cardiac myosin binding protein-C gene on chromosome 11 cause familial hypertrophic cardiomyopathy. Nat Genet 11:434–437, 1995.
47. Fung DC, Yu B, Littlejohn T, Trent RJ: An online locus-specific mutation database for familial hypertrophic cardiomyopathy. Hum Mutat 14:326–332, 1999.
48. Watkins H, Rosenzweig A, Hwang DS, et al: Characteristics and prognostic implications of myosin missense mutations in familial hypertrophic cardiomyopathy. N Engl J Med 326:1108–1114, 1992.
48a. Marian AJ: Pathogenesis of diverse clinical and pathological phenotypes in hypertrophic cardiomyopathy. Lancet 355:58–60, 2000.
48b. Tyska MJ, Hayes E, Giewat M, et al: Single-molecule mechanics of

R403Q cardiac myosin isolated from the mouse model of familial hypertrophic cardiomyopathy. Circ Res 86:737–744, 2000.

49. el-Sherif N, Turitto G: The long QT syndrome and torsade de pointes. Pacing Clin Electrophysiol 22:91–110, 1999.

50. Curran M, Atkinson D, Timothy K, et al: Locus heterogeneity of autosomal dominant long QT syndrome. J Clin Invest 92:799–803, 1993.

51. Curran ME, Splawski I, Timothy KW, et al: A molecular basis for cardiac arrhythmia: HERG mutations cause long QT syndrome. Cell 80:795–803, 1995.

52. Wang Q, Shen J, Splawski I, et al: SCN5A mutations associated with an inherited cardiac arrhythmia, long QT syndrome. Cell 80:805–811, 1995.

53. Splawski I, Tristani-Firouzi M, Lehmann MH, et al: Mutations in the hminK gene cause long QT syndrome and suppress IKs function. Nat Genet 17:338–340, 1997.

54. Dumaine R, Wang Q, Keating MT, et al: Multiple mechanisms of Na+ channel—linked long-QT syndrome. Circ Res 78:916–924, 1996.

BASIC TECHNIQUES OF MOLECULAR BIOLOGY

55. Sambrook J, Fritsch EF, Maniatis T: Molecular Cloning: A Laboratory Manual. 2nd ed. Cold Spring Harbor, NY, Cold Spring Harbor Laboratory, 1989, p 3v.

56. Kessler C, Manta V: Specificity of restriction endonucleases and DNA modification methyltransferases a review (edition 3). Gene 92:1–248, 1990.

57. Cohen SN, Chang AC: Replication and expression of constructed plasmid chimeras in transformed *Escherichia coli*—a review. Basic Life Sci 5A:35–344, 1975.

58. Buckel P: Recombinant proteins for therapy. Trends Pharmacol Sci 17:450–456, 1996.

59. Sudbery PE: The expression of recombinant proteins in yeasts. Curr Opin Biotechnol 7:517–524, 1996.

60. Koths K: Recombinant proteins for medical use: The attractions and challenges. Curr Opin Biotechnol 6:681–687, 1995.

61. Goldhaber SZ: Thrombolytic therapy. Adv Intern Med 44:311–325, 1999.

62. Collen D: Thrombolytic therapy. Thromb Haemost 78:742–746, 1997.

63. Pennica D, Holmes WE, Kohr WJ, et al: Cloning and expression of human tissue-type plasminogen activator cDNA in *E. coli*. Nature 301:214–221, 1983.

64. Kaufman RJ, Wasley LC, Spiliotes AJ, et al: Coamplification and coexpression of human tissue-type plasminogen activator and murine dihydrofolate reductase sequences in Chinese hamster ovary cells. Mol Cell Biol 5:1750–1759, 1985.

65. White TJ: The future of PCR technology: Diversification of technologies and applications. Trends Biotechnol 14:478–483, 1996.

66. Landegren U: The challengers to PCR: A proliferation of chain reactions. Curr Opin Biotechnol 7:95–97, 1996.

67. Baumforth KR, Nelson PN, Digby JE, et al: Demystified...the polymerase chain reaction. Mol Pathol 52:1–10, 1999.

68. Vosberg HP: The polymerase chain reaction: An improved method for the analysis of nucleic acids. Hum Genet 83:1–15, 1989.

69. Sanger F, Nicklen S, Coulson AR: DNA sequencing with chain-terminating inhibitors. Proc Natl Acad Sci U S A 74:5463–5467, 1977.

70. Maxam AM, Gilbert W: A new method for sequencing DNA. Proc Natl Acad Sci U S A 74:560–564, 1977.

71. Cole ST, Brosch R, Parkhill J, et al: Deciphering the biology of *Mycobacterium tuberculosis* from the complete genome sequence. Nature 393:537–544, 1998.

72. Blattner FR, Plunkett G III, Bloch CA, et al: The complete genome sequence of *Escherichia coli* K-12. Science 277:1453–1474, 1997.

73. Philippsen P, Kleine K, Pohlmann R, et al: The nucleotide sequence of *Saccharomyces cerevisiae* chromosome XIV and its evolutionary implications. Nature 387:93–98, 1997.

74. Stein CA, Cheng YC: Antisense oligonucleotides as therapeutic agents—is the bullet really magical? Science 261:1004–1012, 1993.

75. Kohler G, Milstein C: Continuous cultures of fused cells secreting antibody of predefined specificity. Nature 256:495–497, 1975.

76. Laurino JP, Shi Q, Ge J: Monoclonal antibodies, antigens and molecular diagnostics: A practical overview. Ann Clin Lab Sci 29:158–166, 1999.

77. Farah RA, Clinchy B, Herrera L, Vitetta ES: The development of monoclonal antibodies for the therapy of cancer. Crit Rev Eukaryot Gene Expr 8:321–356, 1998.

78. Ball HJ, Finlay D: Diagnostic application of monoclonal antibody (MAb)-based sandwich ELISAs. Methods Mol Biol 104:127–132, 1998.

79. Phillips DR, Charo IF, Parise LV, Fitzgerald LA: The platelet membrane glycoprotein IIb–IIIa complex. Blood 71:831–843, 1988.

80. Coller BS: Blockade of platelet GPIIb/IIIa receptors as an antithrombotic strategy. Circulation 92:2373–2380, 1995.

81. EPIC: Use of a monoclonal antibody directed against the platelet glycoprotein IIb/IIIa receptor in high-risk coronary angioplasty. The EPIC Investigation. N Engl J Med 330:956–961, 1994.

82. EPILOG: Platelet glycoprotein IIb/IIIa receptor blockade and low-dose heparin during percutaneous coronary revascularization. The EPILOG Investigators. N Engl J Med 336:1689–1696, 1997.

83. Brener SJ, Barr LA, Burchenal JE, et al: Randomized, placebo-controlled trial of platelet glycoprotein IIb/IIIa blockade with primary angioplasty for acute myocardial infarction. ReoPro and Primary PTCA Organization and Randomized Trial (RAPPORT) Investigators. Circulation 98:734–741, 1998.

84. Lincoff AM: Trials of platelet glycoprotein IIb/IIIa receptor antagonists during percutaneous coronary revascularization. Am J Cardiol 82:36p–42p, 1998.

85. Lincoff AM, Califf RM, Anderson KM, et al: Evidence for prevention of death and myocardial infarction with platelet membrane glycoprotein IIb/IIIa receptor blockade by abciximab (c7E3 Fab) among patients with unstable angina undergoing percutaneous coronary revascularization. EPIC Investigators: Evaluation of 7E3 in Preventing Ischemic Complications. J Am Coll Cardiol 30:149–156, 1997.

86. Southern EM: Measurement of DNA length by gel electrophoresis. Anal Biochem 100:319–323, 1979.

87. Johnston M: Gene chips: Array of hope for understanding gene regulation. Curr Biol 8:r171–r174, 1998.

88. Lipshutz RJ, Fodor SP, Gingeras TR, Lockhart DJ: High density synthetic oligonucleotide arrays. Nat Genet 21:20–24, 1999.

89. Huang S: Gene expression profiling, genetic networks, and cellular states: An integrating concept for tumorigenesis and drug discovery. J Mol Med 77:469–480, 1999.

90. Granjeaud S, Bertucci F, Jordan BR: Expression profiling: DNA arrays in many guises. Bioessays 21:781–790, 1999.

91. Duggan DJ, Bittner M, Chen Y, et al: Expression profiling using cDNA microarrays. Nat Genet 21:10–14, 1999.

GENETICALLY MODIFIED MICE AS A MODEL SYSTEM OF HUMAN CARDIOVASCULAR DISEASE

92. Field LJ: Transgenic mice in cardiovascular research. Annu Rev Physiol 55:97–114, 1993.

93. Palmiter RD, Brinster RL: Transgenic mice. Cell 41:343–345, 1985.

94. Palmiter RD: Transgenic mice—the early days. Int J Dev Biol 42:847–854, 1998.

95. Subramaniam A, Jones WK, Gulick J, et al: Tissue-specific regulation of the alpha-myosin heavy chain gene promoter in transgenic mice. J Biol Chem 266:24613–24620, 1991.

96. Fentzke RC, Korcarz CE, Shroff SG, et al: Evaluation of ventricular and arterial hemodynamics in anesthetized closed-chest mice. J Am Soc Echocardiogr 10:915–925, 1997.

97. Fentzke RC, Korcarz CE, Lang RM, et al: Dilated cardiomyopathy in transgenic mice expressing a dominant-negative CREB transcription factor in the heart. J Clin Invest 101:2415–2426, 1998.

98. Kistner A, Gossen M, Zimmermann F, et al: Doxycycline-mediated quantitative and tissue-specific control of gene expression in transgenic mice. Proc Natl Acad Sci U S A 93:10933–10938, 1996.

99. Bristow MR, Hershberger RE, Port JD, et al: Beta-adrenergic pathways in nonfailing and failing human ventricular myocardium. Circulation 82:i12–125, 1990.

100. Pitcher J, Lohse MJ, Codina J, et al: Desensitization of the isolated beta 2-adrenergic receptor by beta-adrenergic receptor kinase, cAMP-dependent protein kinase, and protein kinase C occurs via distinct molecular mechanisms. Biochemistry 31:3193–3197, 1992.

101. Koch WJ, Rockman HA, Samama P, et al: Cardiac function in mice overexpressing the beta-adrenergic receptor kinase or a beta ARK inhibitor. Science 268:1350–1353, 1995.

101a. Lefkowitz RJ, Rockman HA, Koch WJ: Catecholamines, cardiac beta-adrenergic receptors, and heart failure. Circulation 101:1634–1637, 2000.

102. Arber S, Hunter JJ, Ross J Jr, et al: Mlp-deficient mice exhibit a disruption of cardiac cytoarchitectural organization, dilated cardiomyopathy, and heart failure. Cell 88:393–403, 1997.

103. Kubota T, McTiernan CF, Frye CS, et al: Dilated cardiomyopathy in transgenic mice with cardiac-specific overexpression of tumor necrosis factor-alpha. Circ Res 81:627–635, 1997.

104. McConnell BK, Jones KA, Fatkin D, et al: Dilated cardiomyopathy in homozygous myosin-binding protein-C mutant mice. J Clin Invest 104:1235–1244, 1999.

105. Emanueli C, Maestri R, Corradi D, et al: Dilated and failing cardiomyopathy in bradykinin B(2) receptor knockout mice. Circulation 100:2359–2365, 1999.

106. Rockman HA, Chien KR, Choi DJ, et al: Expression of a beta-adrenergic receptor kinase 1 inhibitor prevents the development of myocardial failure in gene-targeted mice. Proc Natl Acad Sci U S A 95:7000–7005, 1998.

107. Muller U: Ten years of gene targeting: Targeted mouse mutants, from vector design to phenotype analysis. Mech Dev 82:3–21, 1999.

108. Capecchi MR: The new mouse genetics: Altering the genome by gene targeting. Trends Genet 5:70–6, 1989.

109. Soriano P: Gene targeting in ES cells. Annu Rev Neurosci 18:1–18, 1995.

110. Smithies O, Maeda N: Gene targeting approaches to complex genetic diseases: Atherosclerosis and essential hypertension. Proc Natl Acad Sci U S A 92:5266–5272, 1995.

111. Lewis J, Yang B, Detloff P, Smithies O: Gene modification via "plug and socket" gene targeting. J Clin Invest 97:3–5, 1996.

112. Sauer B: Inducible gene targeting in mice using the Cre/lox system. Methods 14:381–392, 1998.

113. Kuhn R, Schwenk F: Advances in gene targeting methods. Curr Opin Immunol 9:183–188, 1997.

114. Rajewsky K, Gu H, Kuhn R, et al: Conditional gene targeting. J Clin Invest 98:600–603, 1996.
115. Smith JD: Mouse models of atherosclerosis. Lab Anim Sci 48:573–579, 1998.
116. Breslow JL: Mouse models of atherosclerosis. Science 272:685–688, 1996.
117. Zhang SH, Reddick RL, Piedrahita JA, Maeda N: Spontaneous hypercholesterolemia and arterial lesions in mice lacking apolipoprotein E. Science 258:468–471, 1992.
118. Plump AS, Smith JD, Hayek T, et al: Severe hypercholesterolemia and atherosclerosis in apolipoprotein E–deficient mice created by homologous recombination in ES cells. Cell 71:343–353, 1992.
119. Lutgens E, Gorelik L, Daemen MJ, et al: Requirement for CD154 in the progression of atherosclerosis. Nat Med 5:1313–1316, 1999.
120. Mach F, Schonbeck U, Sukhova GK, et al: Reduction of atherosclerosis in mice by inhibition of CD40 signalling. Nature 394:200–203, 1998.
120a. Schonbeck U, Mach F, Libby P: Molecules in focus: CD154 (CD40 ligand). Review. Int J Biochem Cell Biol 32:687–693, 2000.
121. Hadjantonakis AK, Pirity M, Nagy A: Cre recombinase mediated alterations of the mouse genome using embryonic stem cells. Methods Mol Biol 97:101–122, 1999.
122. Tardiff JC, Factor SM, Tompkins BD, et al: A truncated cardiac troponin T molecule in transgenic mice suggests multiple cellular mechanisms for familial hypertrophic cardiomyopathy. J Clin Invest 101:2800–2811, 1998.
123. Geisterfer-Lowrance AA, Christe M, Conner DA, et al: A mouse model of familial hypertrophic cardiomyopathy. Science 272:731–734, 1996.
124. Ishibashi S, Brown MS, Goldstein JL, et al: Hypercholesterolemia in low density lipoprotein receptor knockout mice and its reversal by adenovirus-mediated gene delivery. J Clin Invest 92:883–893, 1993.
124a. Marshall E: Rival genome sequencers celebrate a milestone together. Science 288:2294–2295, 2000.
124b. Pennisi E: Finally, the book of life and instructions for navigating it. Science 288:2304–2307, 2000.
125. Chien KR: Cardiac muscle diseases in genetically engineered mice: Evolution of molecular physiology. Am J Physiol 269:h755–h766, 1995.
126. Berul CI, Aronovitz MJ, Wang PJ, Mendelsohn ME: In vivo cardiac electrophysiology studies in the mouse. Circulation 94:2641–2648, 1996.

GENE- AND CELL-BASED THERAPIES FOR HUMAN CARDIOVASCULAR DISEASE

127. French BA: Gene therapy and cardiovascular disease. Curr Opin Cardiol 13:205–213, 1998.
128. Nabel EG: Gene therapy for vascular diseases. Atherosclerosis 118(Suppl):S51–S56, 1995.
129. Losordo DW, Vale PR, Isner JM: Gene therapy for myocardial angiogenesis. Am Heart J 138:132–141, 1999.
130. Chang MW, Leiden JM: Gene therapy for vascular proliferative disorders. Semin Interv Cardiol 1:185–193, 1996.
131. Isner JM, Pieczek A, Schainfeld R, et al: Clinical evidence of angiogenesis after arterial gene transfer of phVEGF165 in patient with ischaemic limb. Lancet 348:370–374, 1996.
132. Mann MJ, Whittemore AD, Donaldson MC, et al: Ex-vivo gene therapy of human vascular bypass grafts with E2F decoy: The PREVENT single-centre, randomised, controlled trial. Lancet 354:1493–1498, 1999.
133. Lin H, Parmacek MS, Morle G, et al: Expression of recombinant genes in myocardium in vivo after direct injection of DNA. Circulation 82:2217–2221, 1990.
134. Morishita R, Gibbons GH, Ellison KE, et al: Antisense oligonucleotides directed at cell cycle regulatory genes as strategy for restenosis therapy. Trans Assoc Am Physicians 106:54–61, 1993.
135. Barr E, Carroll J, Kalynych AM, et al: Efficient catheter-mediated gene transfer into the heart using replication-defective adenovirus. Gene Ther 1:51–58, 1994.
136. Ohno T, Gordon D, San H, et al: Gene therapy for vascular smooth muscle cell proliferation after arterial injury. Science 265:781–784, 1994.
137. Schneider MD, French BA: The advent of adenovirus: Gene therapy for cardiovascular disease. Circulation 88:1937–1942, 1993.
138. Svensson EC, Marshall DJ, Woodard K, et al: Efficient and stable transduction of cardiomyocytes after intramyocardial injection or intracoronary perfusion with recombinant adeno-associated virus vectors. Circulation 99:201–205, 1999.
139. Kitsis RN, Buttrick PM, McNally EM, et al: Hormonal modulation of a gene injected into rat heart in vivo. Proc Natl Acad Sci U S A 88:4138–4142, 1991.
140. Acsadi G, Jiao SS, Jani A, et al: Direct gene transfer and expression into rat heart in vivo. New Biol 3:71–81, 1991.
141. Bielinska A, Shivdasani RA, Zhang LQ, Nabel GJ: Regulation of gene expression with double-stranded phosphorothioate oligonucleotides. Science 250:997–1000, 1990.
142. Dzau VJ, Mann MJ, Morishita R, Kaneda Y: Fusigenic viral liposome for gene therapy in cardiovascular diseases. Proc Natl Acad Sci U S A 93:11421–11425, 1996.
143. Morishita R, Gibbons GH, Horiuchi M, et al: A gene therapy strategy using a transcription factor decoy of the E2F binding site inhibits smooth muscle proliferation in vivo. Proc Natl Acad Sci U S A 92:5855–5859, 1995.
144. Kozarsky KF, Wilson JM: Gene therapy: Adenovirus vectors. Curr Opin Genet Dev 3:499–503, 1993.
145. Svensson EC, Tripathy SK, Leiden JM: Muscle-based gene therapy: Realistic possibilities for the future. Mol Med Today 2:166–172, 1996.
146. Yang Y, Nunes FA, Berencsi K, et al: Cellular immunity to viral antigens limits E1-deleted adenoviruses for gene therapy. Proc Natl Acad Sci U S A 91:4407–4411, 1994.
147. Yang Y, Ertl HC, Wilson JM: MHC class I–restricted cytotoxic T lymphocytes to viral antigens destroy hepatocytes in mice infected with E1-deleted recombinant adenoviruses. Immunity 1:433–442, 1994.
148. Yang Y, Li Q, Ertl HC, Wilson JM: Cellular and humoral immune responses to viral antigens create barriers to lung-directed gene therapy with recombinant adenoviruses. J Virol 69:2004–2015, 1995.
149. Tripathy SK, Black HB, Goldwasser E, Leiden JM: Immune responses to transgene-encoded proteins limit the stability of gene expression after injection of replication-defective adenovirus vectors. Nat Med 2:545–550, 1996.
150. Morsy MA, Gu M, Motzel S, et al: An adenoviral vector deleted for all viral coding sequences results in enhanced safety and extended expression of a leptin transgene. Proc Natl Acad Sci U S A 95:7866–7871, 1998.
151. Morsy MA, Caskey CT: Expanded-capacity adenoviral vectors—the helper-dependent vectors. Mol Med Today 5:18–24, 1999.
152. Morral N, O'Neal W, Rice K, et al: Administration of helper-dependent adenoviral vectors and sequential delivery of different vector serotype for long-term liver-directed gene transfer in baboons. Proc Natl Acad Sci U S A 96:12816–12821, 1999.
153. Rabinowitz JE, Samulski J: Adeno-associated virus expression systems for gene transfer. Curr Opin Biotechnol 9:470–475, 1998.
154. Patijn GA, Kay MA: Hepatic gene therapy using adeno-associated virus vectors. Semin Liver Dis 19:61–69, 1999.
155. Rolling F, Nong Z, Pisvin S, Collen D: Adeno-associated virus-mediated gene transfer into rat carotid arteries. Gene Ther 4:757–761, 1997.
156. Lynch CM, Hara PS, Leonard JC, et al: Adeno-associated virus vectors for vascular gene delivery. Circ Res 80:497–505, 1997.
157. Snyder RO, Spratt SK, Lagarde C, et al: Efficient and stable adeno-associated virus-mediated transduction in the skeletal muscle of adult immunocompetent mice. Hum Gene Ther 8:1891–900, 1997.
158. Kessler PD, Podsakoff GM, Chen X, et al: Gene delivery to skeletal muscle results in sustained expression and systemic delivery of a therapeutic protein. Proc Natl Acad Sci U S A 93:14082–14087, 1996.
159. Klimatcheva E, Rosenblatt JD, Planelles V: Lentiviral vectors and gene therapy. Front Biosci 4:d481–d496, 1999.
160. Naldini L, Blomer U, Gallay P, et al: In vivo gene delivery and stable transduction of nondividing cells by a lentiviral vector. Science 272:263–267, 1996.
161. Naviaux RK, Verma IM: Retroviral vectors for persistent expression in vivo. Curr Opin Biotechnol 3:540–547, 1992.
162. Vile RG, Tuszynski A, Castleden S: Retroviral vectors: From laboratory tools to molecular medicine. Mol Biotechnol 5:139–158, 1996.
163. Miyoshi H, Blomer U, Takahashi M, et al: Development of a self-inactivating lentivirus vector. J Virol 72:8150–8157, 1998.
164. Kim S, Lin H, Barr E, et al: Transcriptional targeting of replication-defective adenovirus transgene expression to smooth muscle cells in vivo. J Clin Invest 100:1006–1014, 1997.
165. Kasahara N, Dozy AM, Kan YW: Tissue-specific targeting of retroviral vectors through ligand-receptor interactions. Science 266:1373–1376, 1994.
166. Bohl D, Naffakh N, Heard JM: Long-term control of erythropoietin secretion by doxycycline in mice transplanted with engineered primary myoblasts. Nat Med 3:299–305, 1997.
167. Ye X, Rivera VM, Zoltick P, et al: Regulated delivery of therapeutic proteins after in vivo somatic cell gene transfer. Science 283:88–91, 1999.
168. Cole-Strauss A, Yoon K, Xiang Y, et al: Correction of the mutation responsible for sickle cell anemia by an RNA-DNA oligonucleotide. Science 273:1386–1389, 1996.
169. March KL: Methods of local gene delivery to vascular tissues. Semin Interv Cardiol 1:215–223, 1996.
170. McKay RG: Hydrogel-coated balloon catheter. Semin Interv Cardiol 1:45–46, 1996.
171. Lambert CR, Bikkina M, Sparks KD: Microporous infusion catheter. Semin Interv Cardiol 1:30–1, 1996.
172. Wolinsky H, Lin CS: Use of the perforated balloon catheter to infuse marker substances into diseased coronary artery walls after experimental postmortem angioplasty. J Am Coll Cardiol 17:174b–178b, 1991.
172a. Marshall DJ, Palasis M, Lepore JJ, Leiden JM: Biocompatibility of cardiovascular gene delivery catheters with adenovirus vectors: An important determinant of the efficiency of cardiovascular gene transfer. Mol Ther 1:423–429, 2000.
173. Wilson JM, Birinyi LK, Salomon RN, et al: Implantation of vascular grafts lined with genetically modified endothelial cells. Science 244:1344–1346, 1989.
174. Nabel EG, Plautz G, Boyce FM, et al: Recombinant gene expression in vivo within endothelial cells of the arterial wall. Science 244:1342–1344, 1989.
175. Dichek DA, Anderson J, Kelly AB, et al: Enhanced in vivo antithrombotic effects of endothelial cells expressing recombinant plasminogen

activators transduced with retroviral vectors. Circulation 93:301–309, 1996.

176. Kessler PD, Byrne BJ: Myoblast cell grafting into heart muscle: Cellular biology and potential applications. Annu Rev Physiol 61:219–242, 1999.

177. Koh GY, Klug MG, Soonpaa MH, Field LJ: Differentiation and long-term survival of C2C12 myoblast grafts in heart. J Clin Invest 92:1548–1554, 1993.

178. Taylor DA, Atkins BZ, Hungspreugs P, et al: Regenerating functional myocardium: Improved performance after skeletal myoblast transplantation. Nat Med 4:929–933, 1998.

179. Murry CE, Wiseman RW, Schwartz SM, Hauschka SD: Skeletal myoblast transplantation for repair of myocardial necrosis. J Clin Invest 98: 2512–2523, 1996.

180. Soonpaa MH, Koh GY, Klug MG, Field LJ: Formation of nascent intercalated disks between grafted fetal cardiomyocytes and host myocardium. Science 264:98–101, 1994.

181. Klug MG, Soonpaa MH, Koh GY, Field LJ: Genetically selected cardiomyocytes from differentiating embronic stem cells form stable intracardiac grafts. J Clin Invest 98:216–224, 1996.

182. Leor J, Patterson M, Quinones MJ, et al: Transplantation of fetal myocardial tissue into the infarcted myocardium of rat: A potential method for repair of infarcted myocardium? Circulation 94(Suppl II:II332–II336, 1996.

183. Makino S, Fukuda K, Miyoshi S, et al: Cardiomyocytes can be generated from marrow stromal cells in vitro. J Clin Invest 103:697–705, 1999.

184. Prockop DJ: Marrow stromal cells as stem cells for nonhematopoietic tissues. Science 276:71–74, 1997.

185. Gussoni E, Soneoka Y, Strickland CD, et al: Dystrophin expression in the mdx mouse restored by stem cell transplantation. Nature 401:390–394, 1999.

186. Libby P, Tanaka H: The molecular bases of restenosis. Prog Cardiovasc Dis 40:97–106, 1997.

187. Schwartz RS: The vessel wall reaction in restenosis. Semin Interv Cardiol 2:83–88, 1997.

188. Casterella PJ, Teirstein PS: Prevention of coronary restenosis. Cardiol Rev 7:219–231, 1999.

189. Chang MW, Barr E, Seltzer J, et al: Cytostatic gene therapy for vascular proliferative disorders with a constitutively active form of the retinoblastoma gene product. Science 267:518–522, 1995.

190. Chang MW, Barr E, Lu M-M, et al: Adenovirus-mediated overexpression of the cyclin/cyclin-dependent kinase inhibitor, p21, inhibits vascular smooth muscle cell proliferation and neointima formation in the rat carotid artery model of balloon angioplasty. J Clin Invest 96:2260–2268, 1995.

Chapter 56

Genetics and Cardiovascular Disease

REED E. PYERITZ

GENETIC FACTORS IN DISEASE

Genes contribute to both the cause and the pathogenesis of virtually any abnormality of human physiology and behavior, including, of course, disorders of the heart and vascular system (see Chap. 55). This statement carries two messages in addition to the obvious one. First, the pathology associated with even the most "environmental" of causes, such as trauma, malnutrition, and drug abuse, can be defined only in terms of the human body's response to the insult. How the stress of the initial insult is expressed (the *phenotype*) and how the patient suffers and perhaps recovers depend, to various and yet often poorly defined degrees, on the patient's *genotype*. This idea seems self-evident and verges on the trite, but it is frequently neglected. Some environmental insults, such as massive trauma or poisoning, are lethal to all, regardless of genotype. Nonetheless, as developments in fields such as *pharmacogenetics* and *ecogenetics* are defining genetic susceptibilities to human disease better and more simply, physicians must become increasingly attuned to the importance of the genotype.[1]

Second, the introductory statement emphasizes that genetic factors have roles in *both* cause and process; etiology and pathogenesis, although related, are conceptually distinct.[2] For example, the cause of sickle cell anemia is clearly a single mutant gene, whereas whether a patient homozygous for this mutation expresses all, some, or none of the manifestations of the disease depends on many other genetic and nongenetic factors. Conversely, the cause of pneumococcal pneumonia is equally evident, but the severity and resolution of the disease depend on the patient's immune competence (which in turn depends on genetic and nongenetic factors) as much as on treatment with an antibiotic.

The genotype, therefore, can be detrimental in at least two distinct ways. First, mutant genes can so upset embryology or physiology that a clinical abnormality occurs. Whereas the phenotype of any particular mutation depends on a host of factors, including which homeostatic systems are available to modulate the action of the defect, the genotype has the principal role in causing the disease. It is this class of mutations that are usually referred to as genetic diseases. Second, a mutation can facilitate the action of an extrinsic cause in producing disease. Inherited susceptibilities are part of the pathogenesis of disease and are one reason for taking a patient's family history. Until recently, clinicians could do little to pursue tantalizing facts, such as several relatives' suffering myocardial infarction before age 50. The long-touted prospect of detecting a patient's inherited susceptibilities and intervening before irreversible clinical sequelae occur is becoming reality.

Disorders Due to Microscopic Alterations in Chromosomes

Estimates of the total number of human genes range between 50,000 and 100,000. Two copies (termed *alleles*) of each gene are arrayed along 23 pairs of *chromosomes*. Twenty-two of the chromosomes are called *autosomes* (numbered 1 through 22), and the 23rd pair are the *sex chromosomes,* X and Y. Females have two X chromosomes and males have an X and a Y chromosome. Both autosomal alleles are potentially active in specifying RNA copies of their DNA sequences; whether a gene is active depends on the cell type, the developmental stage of the organism, and the regulatory molecules that interact with promoter and enhancer nucleotide sequences that control transcription of the gene. In cells with two X chromosomes (i.e., in all females, in Klinefelter syndrome in which two Xs and one Y occur, and in other rare conditions), only one X is entirely active after early embryogenesis.

Human chromosomes can be examined by culturing cells capable of mitosis; T lymphocytes obtained from venous blood are the usual source, but fibroblasts, cells from chorionic villi, amniocytes, and leukocyte precursors present in bone marrow are also used clinically. Chromosomes are distinguished from one another by their size, **1977** shape (determined by the position of a constriction called the *centromere,* which functions as the attachment of the mitotic apparatus), and characteristic banding pattern as revealed by any of several staining techniques. The chromosomes are photographed, cut out, and arranged in pairs, from 1 through 22 and the sex chromosomes, in a display called the *karyotype.* This display and its interpretation are the end results of a clinical study of a patient's chromosomes. The chromosome constitution of a cell is designated by first specifying the number of chromosomes present (46 being normal in diploid cells), then specifying the sex chromosomes, and finally describing any abnormalities. For example, a normal male is designated 46,XY, and a female with an extra chromosome 21 is designated 46,XX,+21.

ANEUPLOIDY. Chromosome aberrations, especially too many or too few chromosomes (*aneuploidy*), are extremely common in human embryos; more than one-half of all conceptuses are spontaneously aborted in early pregnancy, and at least one-half of them are aneuploid. Among live-born infants, about 0.5 percent have a chromosome aberration.

Gain or loss of chromosomes generally happens by nondisjunction, or the failure of a homologous pair of chromosomes to separate. Absence of one chromosome is termed *monosomy;* all autosomal monosomies are embryonic lethals, as is presence of only a Y sex chromosome. Presence of three chromosomes is *trisomy,* and presence of an entire extra set of chromosomes (for a total of 69) is *triploidy.* The most common autosomal aneuploidy, trisomy 21 associated with Down syndrome, and aneuploidy for sex chromosomes all are compatible with survival into adulthood.

CHROMOSOME REARRANGEMENTS. A chromosome can break and rejoin within itself, potentially giving rise to an *inversion* of genetic material. Often no apparent phenotypic effect is seen in people with an inversion, but because inversions may disrupt chromosome pairing during meiosis, their offspring may have more profound aberrations.

DELETIONS AND DUPLICATIONS. Just as their names imply, these aberrations are losses or gains of chromosomal material. Many clinical syndromes have been associated with aberrations of specific chromosome regions.[3, 4] The smallest deletion detectable by light microscopy is associated with loss of considerable DNA, on the order of one million base pairs, so more than one gene is potentially disrupted or lost.

A number of conditions, each initially thought to be due to a mutation in a single locus, are associated with small interstitial chromosome aberrations affecting a cluster of genes (Table 56–1). So rather than pleiotropic manifestations of one mutation, these conditions are likely to be due to the effects of several, and perhaps many, mutations and are therefore called *contiguous gene syndromes.*[5] Such defects are potentially heritable, and the occurrence of the disorder in a family behaves as a mendelian dominant.

Disorders Due to Changes in Single Nuclear Genes (See also Chap. 55)

Mutations of genes located on the 22 pairs of autosomes and the two sex chromosomes produce phenotypes inher-

ited according to the two principal tenets of Mendel: alleles segregate and nonalleles assort. The first statement refers to gametes receiving only one of the two alleles at a given locus as a result of meiosis. The second statement describes the results of recombination, the meiotic process of rearranging DNA between the two chromosomes of the pair (*homologous chromosomes*); if two loci are widely spaced along a chromosome, their chances of being separated by recombination are 50-50, and they are said to be *unlinked.*

The Human Genome Project, begun in 1990, has set goals to map all expressed genes, to create a physical map of overlapping pieces of DNA composing the entire genome, and, finally, to sequence all 3 to 3.5 billion nucleotides in the haploid complement of human DNA.[6] The project is well ahead of schedule, and a "rough draft" of the entire sequence became available in 2000. The beginnings and ends of more than 100,000 expressed sequences, most representing genes, have been identified out of a total of perhaps 125,000 genes. More than 10,000 individual loci have been identified on the basis of the phenotype that mutations in single genes produce. The presumption of single-gene defects is based in most instances on the pattern of inheritance in families; segregation of the phenotype according to mendelian principles is the central piece of evidence. For an increasing number of loci, however, molecular genetic techniques have mapped the phenotype to a narrow chromosome region, to a single gene, or even revealed the actual alteration in nucleotide sequence (see also Chap. 55)[7] (Table 56–2). The range of known mendelian variation in humans and information about gene mapping and molecular defects are routinely catalogued and available on-line.[8]

Of the more than 10,000 loci that have been clearly identified on the basis of either an abnormal phenotype or a normal product, 9.1 percent involve the heart.[8] Many others involve other parts of the cardiovascular system. Thousands of loci have been mapped to a restricted region of the genome. Many of these loci cause specific mendelian disorders, and the genetic map of these loci represents the "morbid anatomy of the human genome." Many of the cardiovascular and hemostatic disorders that were mapped by the end of 1999 are shown in Figure 56–1.

DOMINANCE AND RECESSIVENESS. These related concepts are characteristics of the phenotype, *not of the gene.* A phenotype is dominant when the patient is *heterozygous* for a mutation, i.e., when one copy of the mutant allele and one copy of the normal allele are present; this holds for genes on both autosomes and the X chromosome. A phenotype is recessive when the patient has two mutant alleles at the locus causing the condition. If the mutant alleles are identical, the patient is *homozygous* at that locus, a situation usually present either when the allele is identical by descent through both parents (i.e., the parents had a common ancestor and are *consanguin-*

▼ TABLE 56–1. CONTIGUOUS GENE SYNDROMES

	REGION	LOCUS	CARDIOVASCULAR ABNORMALITIES
Syndromes with Cardiovascular Involvement			
Arteriohepatic dysplasia	AHD	del 20p11.23–p12.2	Peripheral pulmonic stenosis/hypoplasia
Cat-eye syndrome	CES	dup22q11	Total anomalous pulmonary venous return
DiGeorge sequence	DGS	del 22q11	Truncus arteriosus, right aortic arch, TOF, PDA
Miller-Dieker syndrome	MDS	del 17p13	PDA ± complex anomalies
Prader-Willi syndrome	PWS/AS	del 15q12	Cor pulmonale (secondary to obesity and central apnea)
WAGR syndrome		del 11p13	Hypertension (secondary to Wilms tumor)
Syndromes Without Frequent Cardiovascular Involvement			
Angelman syndrome		del 15q12*	
Smith-Magenis syndrome		del 17p11.2	

TOF = tetralogy of Fallot; PDA = patent ductus arteriosus; WAGR = Wilms tumor, aniridia, genitourinary, and retardation.

* The deletion is often indistinguishable at the cytogenetic level from that of the Prader-Willi syndrome; genetic imprinting of locus *UBE3A* is thought to account in part for the phenotypic differences. In Prader-Willi Syndrome, the deleted chromosome is always the chromosome 15 inherited from the father, whereas in Angelman syndrome, the deletion affects the maternal chromosome 15.

▼ **TABLE 56–2. MENDELIAN CONDITIONS THAT INVOLVE THE CARDIOVASCULAR SYSTEM WITH KNOWN GENETIC DEFECTS OR GENE MAPPING OF THE PHENOTYPE**

PHENOTYPE	GENE SYMBOL	OMIM NO.*	GENE MAP Locus
Cardiomyopathies			
Adhalinopathy, primary	SGCA	600119	17q12–q21.33
Arrhythmogenic RV dysplasia-1	ARVD1	107970	14q23–q24
Arrhythmogenic RV dysplasia-2	ARVD2	600996	1q42–q43
Arrhythmogenic RV dysplasia-3	ARVD3	602086	14q12–q22
Arrhythmogenic RV dysplasia-4	ARVD4	602087	2q32.1–q32.3
Arrhythmogenic RV dysplasia-5	ARVD5		3p23
Arrhythmogenic RV dysplasia-6	ARVD6		10p12–p14
Becker and Duchenne muscular dystrophies	DMD	310200	Xp21.2
Emery-Dreifuss muscular dystrophy	EMD	310300	Xp28
Emery-Dreifuss muscular dystrophy	LMNA	150330	1q21.2–q21.3
Endocardial fibroelastosis-2	TAZ	302060	Xq28
FDC	ACTC	102540	15q14
FDC-1A	CMD1A	115200	1p11–q11
FDC-1B	CMD1B	600884	9q13
FDC-1C	CMD1C	601493	10q21–q23
FDC-1E	CMD1E	601154	3p25–p22
FDC-1F	CMD1F	602067	6q23
FDC-1G	CMD1G	604145	2q31
FDC-1H	CMD1H		2q14–q22
FDC-2	CMD1D	601494	1q32
FDC, X linked	DMD	310220	Xp21.2
FDC-3A	TAZ	302060	Xq28
FHC-1	MYH7	160760	14q12
FHC-2	TNNT2	191045	1q32
FHC-3	TPM1	191010	15q22.1
FHC-4	MYBPC3	600958	11p11.2
FHC	TNNI3	191044	19q13.4
FHC with WPW	CMH6	600858	7q3
FHC, mid-LV type	MYL2	160781	12q23–q24.3
FHC, mid-LV type	MYL3	160790	3p
Friedreich ataxia	FRDA	229300	9q13
Muscular dystrophy, Duchenne-like	SGCA	600119	17q12–q21.33
Myotonic dystrophy	DMPK	160900	19q13.2–q13.3
Myotonic dystrophy 2	DM2	602668	3q
Noncompaction of LV	TAZ	302060	Xq28
Developmental Disorders			
Alagille syndrome	JAG1	601920	20p12
Atrial septal defect, secundum	ASD1	108800	6p21.3
Atrial septal defect with AV conduction defects	CSX	600584	5q34
AV canal defect-1	AVSD	600309	1p31–p21
Bannayan-Zonana syndrome	PTEN	6011728	10q23.3
Cardiac valve dysplasia-1	CVD1	314400	Xq28
Cat-eye syndrome	CECR	115470	22q11
Conotruncal cardiac defects	CTHM	217095	22q11
DiGeorge syndrome and velocardiofacial syndrome	DGCR	188400	22q11
Down syndrome	DCR	190685	21q22.3
Ellis–van Creveld syndrome	EVC	225500	4p16
Goldenhar syndrome	GHS	141400	7p
Heterotaxy, X-linked visceral	ZIC3	306955	Xq26.2
Holt-Oram syndrome	TBX5	601620	12q24.1
Keutel syndrome	MGP	154870	12p13.1–p12.3
Left-right axis malformation	TGFB4	601877	1q42.1
Noonan syndrome	NS1	163950	12q24
Total anomalous pulmonary venous return	TAPVR1	106700	4p13–q12
Turner syndrome	RPS4X	312760	Xq13.1
Werner syndrome	WRN	277700	8p12–p11.2
Williams syndrome	ELN	130160	7q11.2
Wolf-Hirschhorn syndrome	WHCR	194190	4p16.3
Disorders of Blood Pressure			
Bartter syndrome	SLC12A1	600839	15q15–q21.1
Bartter syndrome with deafness	BSND	602522	1p31
Bartter syndrome, type 2	KCNJ1	600359	11q24
Bartter syndrome, type 3	CLCNKB	602023	1p36
Dysautonomia, familial	DYS	223900	9q31–q33
Hypertension, essential	SAH	145505	16p13.11
Hypertension, essential	PNMT	171190	17q21–q22
Hypertension, essential	AGTR1	106165	3q21–q25

Continued on following page

▼ TABLE 56–2. MENDELIAN CONDITIONS THAT INVOLVE THE CARDIOVASCULAR SYSTEM WITH KNOWN GENETIC DEFECTS OR GENE MAPPING OF THE PHENOTYPE *Continued*

PHENOTYPE	GENE SYMBOL	OMIM NO.*	GENE MAP Locus
Hypertension, essential	GNB3	139130	12p13
Hypertension, essential	AGT	106150	1q42–q43
Hypertension, low renin	HSD11B2	218030	16q22
Hypertension, salt resistant	NPR3	108962	5p14–p12
Hypertension, with brachydactyly	HTNB	112410	12p12.2–p11.2
Liddle syndrome	SCNN1B	600760	16p13–p12
Liddle syndrome	SCNN1G	600761	16p13–p12
Mineralocorticoid excess	HSD11B2	218030	16p22
Orthostatic hypotensive disorder	OHDS	143850	18q
Pheochromocytoma	PCHC	171300	1p
Polycystic kidney disease, adult 1	PKD1	601313	16p13.3–p13.12
Polycystic kidney disease, adult 2	PKD2	173910	4q21–q23
Preeclampsia, susceptibility to	NOS3	163729	7q36
Preeclampsia, susceptibility to	AGT	106150	1q42–q43
Preeclampsia/eclampsia	PEE	189800	4q25–q34
Pulmonary hypertension, familial	PPH1	178600	2q31–q32

Disorders of Coagulation and Thrombosis

PHENOTYPE	GENE SYMBOL	OMIM NO.*	GENE MAP Locus
Antithrombin III deficiency	AT3	107300	1q23–q25
Antithrombin Pittsburgh defect	PI	107400	14q32.1
Coumarin resistance	CYP2A6	122720	19q13.2
Defective thromboxane A2 receptor	TBXA2R	188070	19p13.3
Dysfibrinogenemia, α type	FGA	134820	4q28
Dysfibrinogenemia, β type	FGB	134830	4q28
Dysfibrinogenemia, χ type	FGG	134850	4q28
Dysprothrombinemia	F2	176930	11p11–q12
Factor H deficiency	HF1	134370	1q32
Factor V deficiency	F5	227400	1q23
Factor VII deficiency	F7	227500	13q34
Factor X deficiency	F10	227600	13q34
Factor XI deficiency	F11	264900	4q35
Factor XII deficiency	F12	234000	5q33-qter
Factor XIIIA deficiency	F13A1	134570	6p25–p24
Factor XIIIB deficiency	F13B	134580	1q31–q32.1
Glanzmann thrombasthenia, type A	ITGA2B	273800	17q21.32
Glanzmann thrombasthenia, type B	ITGB3	173470	17q21.32
GNAQ deficiency	GNAQ	600998	9q21
Hemophilia A	F8C	306700	Xq28
Hemophilia B	F9	306900	Xq27.1–q27.2
PAI1 deficiency	PAI1	173360	7q21.3–q22
Plasmin inhibitor deficiency	PLI	262850	17pter-p12
Plasminogen activator deficiency	PLAT	173370	8p12
Plasminogen deficiency	PLG	173350	6q26
Platelet α/δ storage pool deficiency	SELP	173610	1q23–q25
Platelet disorder, familial with myeloid malignancy	FPDMM	601399	21q22.1–q22.2
Platelet glycoprotein IV deficiency	CD36	173510	7q11.2
Platelet-activating factor acetylhydrolase deficiency	PAFAH	601690	6p21.2–p12
Protein C inhibitor deficiency	PCI	601841	14q32.1
Protein S deficiency	PROS1	176880	3p11.1–q11.2
Thrombocythemia, essential	THPO	600044	3q26.3–q27
Thrombocytopenia, neonatal	ITGA2B	273800	17q21.32
Thrombocytopenia, Paris-Trousseau	TCPT	188025	11q23
Thrombocytopenia, X-linked	WAS	301000	Xp11.23–p11.22
Thrombophilia	HRG	142640	3q27
Thrombophilia	PAI1	173360	7q21.3–q22
Thrombophilia	HCF2	142360	22q11
Thrombophilia	THBD	188040	20p11.2
Thrombophilia	PLG	173350	6q26
Thromboxane synthase deficiency	TBXAS1	274180	7q34
Vitamin K–dependent coagulation defect	GGCX	137167	2p12
von Willebrand disease	VWF	193400	12p13.3
Warfarin sensitivity	CYP2C9	601130	10q24

Disorders of Lipid Metabolism

PHENOTYPE	GENE SYMBOL	OMIM NO.*	GENE MAP Locus
Abetalipoproteinemia	MTP	157147	4q22–q24
Abetalipoproteinemia	APOB	107730	2p24
ApoA-I and apoC-III deficiency	APOA1	107680	11q23
ApoA-II deficiency	APOA2	107670	1q21–q23
ApoB-100 ligand defect	APOB	107730	2p24
Cerebrotendinous xanthomatosis	CYP27A1	213700	2q33-qter
Combined familial hyperlipidemia	LPL	238600	8p22

▼ TABLE 56–2. MENDELIAN CONDITIONS THAT INVOLVE THE CARDIOVASCULAR SYSTEM WITH KNOWN GENETIC DEFECTS OR GENE MAPPING OF THE PHENOTYPE *Continued*

1981

Ch 56

PHENOTYPE	GENE SYMBOL	OMIM NO.*	GENE MAP LOCUS
HMG-CoA synthetase-2 deficiency	HMGCS2	600234	1p13–p12
Hypercholesterolemia, familial	LDLR	143890	19p13.2–p13.1
Hypercholesterolemia, familial 3	FH3	603776	1p34.1–p32
Hypertriglyceridemia	APOC3	107720	11q23
Hypertriglyceridemia	APOA1	107680	11q23
Hypoalphalipoproteinemia	APOA1	107680	11q23
Hypobetalipoproteinemia	APOB	107730	2p24
Sitosterolemia	STSL	210250	2p21
Tangier disease	HDLDT1	205400	9q31
Wolman disease	LIPA	278000	10q24–q25
Metabolic Disorders with Primary Effects			
Carnitine acetyltransferase deficiency	CRAT	600184	9q34.1
Carnitine deficiency, systemic	SLC22A5	603377	5q33.1
Metabolic Disorders with Secondary Effects			
Amyloidosis	APOA1	107680	11q23
Amyloidosis, cerebroarterial	APP	104760	21q21.3–q22.05
Cerebral amyloid angiopathy	CST3	105150	20p11.2
Cerebrovascular disease, occlusive	AACT	107280	14q32.1
Coronary spasm, susceptibility to	NOS3	163729	7q36
Fabry disease	GLA	301500	Xq22
Gaucher disease with calcification	GBA	230800	1q21
Glycogen storage disease II (Pompe)	GAA	232300	17q25.2–q25.3
Hemochromatosis	HFE	235200	6p21.3
Homocystinuria	CBS	236200	21q22.3
Homocystinuria, MTHFR deficiency	MTHFR	236250	1p36.3
Menkes syndrome	ATP7A	300011	Xq12–q13
Mucopolysaccharidosis I	IDUA	252800	4p16.3
Mucopolysaccharidosis II	IDS	309900	Xq28
Mucopolysaccharidosis IVA	GALNS	253000	16q24.3
Mucopolysaccharidosis IVB	GLB1	230500	3p21.33
Mucopolysaccharidosis VI	ARSB	253200	5q11–q13
Mulibrey nanism	MUL	253250	17q22–q23
Pseudoxanthoma elasticum	PXE	264800	16p13.1
Neoplastic Disorders			
Carney (NAME) complex	CNC	160980	2p16
Paraganglioma, familial nonchromaffin 1	PGL1	16800	12q23
Paraganglioma, familial nonchromaffin 2	PGL2	601650	11q13.1
von Hippel–Lindau syndrome	VHL	193300	3p26–p25
Primary Disorders of Rhythm and Conduction			
Heart block, progressive familial-1	HB1	113900	19q13.2–q13.3
Jervell and Lange-Nielsen syndrome	KCNQ1	192500	11p15.5
Jervell and Lange-Nielsen syndrome	KCNE1	176261	21q22.1–q22.2
Long QT syndrome-1	KCNQ1	192500	11p15.5
Long QT syndrome-2	KCNH2	152427	7q35–q36
Long QT syndrome-3 and ventricular fibrillation, idiopathic	SCN5A	600163	3p24–p21
Long QT syndrome-4	LQT4	600919	4q25–q27
Long QT syndrome-5	KCNE2	603796	21q22.1
Ventricular tachycardia, idiopathic	GNAI2	139360	3p21
Primary Disorders of Vasculature			
Aneurysm, familial and Ehlers-Danlos, Vascular type	COL3A1	120180	2q31
Cerebral arteriopathy with subcortical infarcts and leukoencephalopathy	NOTCH3	600276	19p13.2–p13.1
Cerebral cavernous malformations-1	CCM1	116860	7q11.2–q21
Cerebral cavernous malformations-2	CCM2	603284	7p15–p13
Cerebral cavernous malformations-3	CCM3	603285	3q25.2–q27
Fibromuscular dysplasia of arteries	COL3A1	120180	2q31
Hemangioma, capillary infantile	HC1	602089	5q31–q33
Hemiplegic migraine, familial	CACNA1A	601011	19p13
Hemiplegic migraine, familial 2	MHP2	602481	1q21–q23
Hemiplegic migraine, familial, susceptibility to	MFTS	300125	Xq
Hereditary hemorrhagic telangiectasia-1	ENG	131195	9q34.1
Hereditary hemorrhagic telangiectasia-2	ACVRL1	601284	12q11–q14
Lymphedema, hereditary	FLT4	136352	5q35.3

Continued on following page

▼ TABLE 56–2. MENDELIAN CONDITIONS THAT INVOLVE THE CARDIOVASCULAR SYSTEM WITH KNOWN GENETIC DEFECTS OR GENE MAPPING OF THE PHENOTYPE *Continued*

PHENOTYPE	GENE SYMBOL	OMIM NO.*	GENE MAP Locus
Marfan syndrome	FBN1	134797	15q21.1
Moyamoya disease	MYMY	252350	3p26–p24.2
Supravalvular aortic stenosis	ELN	130160	7q11.2
Venous malformations, multiple	TEK	600221	9p21

Disorders may have been mapped by the phenotype, by the gene, or both; (?) after a disorder indicates the mapping data are still in limbo. The annotations p and q refer to band patterns in chromosomes detected cytochemically that mark specific regions.

* Refers to the entry for the locus in http://www.ncbi.nlm.nih.gov/htbin-post/Omim.

AV = atrioventricular; FDC = familial dilated cardiomyopathy; FHC = familial hypertrophic cardiomyopathy; LV = left ventricle; RV = right ventricle.

eous) or when the mutant allele is common in the population (e.g., the most prevalent mutation for cystic fibrosis and the mutation for sickle cell anemia). Biochemical and molecular genetic assessment of mutant alleles has shown that the majority of recessive phenotypes are due to two distinct mutant alleles, a situation termed a *genetic compound*, indicative of the widespread heterogeneity in mutations at each locus. Males have but one X chromosome, and each locus is therefore *hemizygous*; a mutant locus is always expressed in the phenotype of a male. Dominance and recessiveness for X-linked traits refer to expression in heterozygous and homozygous women, respectively.

Whether a disorder is called dominant or recessive depends on how carefully the phenotype is assessed and how it is defined. For example, familial hypercholesterolemia is a relatively common hereditary disorder due to defects in the receptor for low-density lipoprotein (see LDL, see also Chap. 31). The vast majority of patients are heterozygous for a mutant allele at the *LDLR* locus on chromosome 19, and the disease is inherited as a mendelian dominant trait. However, if a man and a woman, each heterozygous for an *LDLR* mutation, produce a child, that child has a 25 percent risk of inheriting both of the mutant alleles and thereby is either homozygous or a genetic compound for *LDLR*. Such a child has a much more severe form of familial hypercholesterolemia that is inherited as a mendelian recessive trait. Similarly, homozygosity for the sickle hemoglobin mutation at the β-globin locus on chromosome 11 produces the familiar autosomal recessive disease sickle cell anemia. However, heterozygosity for the same mutation rarely produces disease but produces sickling of erythrocytes if they are examined under conditions of low oxygen tension; this phenotype is transmitted as a dominant trait.

AUTOSOMAL RECESSIVE INHERITANCE. Nearly all deficiencies of enzymatic activity—the classic inborn errors of metabolism first defined by Archibald Garrod in 1903—cause recessive phenotypes. Most homeostatic systems, which include all metabolic pathways, have sufficient flexibility to function well if one of the enzymatic steps functions at half-normal efficiency, as would occur in heterozygosity for a mutant allele at a structural gene for an enzyme. However, homeostasis cannot cope if two mutant alleles cause a reduction in enzymatic activity to a few percent or less of normal activity. The characteristics of autosomal recessive inheritance, features common to such phenotypes, and a typical pedigree are shown in Figure 56–2.

AUTOSOMAL DOMINANT INHERITANCE. Only a few enzyme deficiencies, but many disorders of development and structure, are inherited as dominant traits. The reasons for this are several. One possibility is that developmental homeostasis has a limited repertoire of responses to stress, and when a structural or regulatory macromolecule is reduced to only one-half normal amount, the system cannot cope. Another possibility, illustrated by mutations in procollagen molecules, pertains to gene products that must interact before becoming functional; an aberrant protein combined with a normal one would be a defective multimer, and the effect of being heterozygous for a mutation would be magnified—a *dominant-negative effect*[2, 9] The characteristics of autosomal dominant inheritance, features common to many such phenotypes, and a typical pedigree are shown in Figure 56–3.

Most human dominant traits are *incomplete*, in that the heterozygote is less severely affected than the homozygote. Defects of *LDLR* are illustrative, in which the heterozygote has classic type IIa hyperlipidemia whereas the homozygote has a quantitatively worse form of the same disease. It may well be that homozygosity for most alleles that cause dominant disorders is incompatible with life.

X-LINKED INHERITANCE. The characteristics of X-linked inheritance, features common to such phenotypes, and a typical pedigree are shown in Figure 56–4. Whereas virtually all diseases due to mutations on the X chromosome are more severe in hemizygous males, women heterozygous for the same mutations often show some manifestations, albeit less severe and of later age of onset. For example, most women carriers of α-galactosidase A deficiency (Fabry disease) even-

tually develop cerebrovascular disease or renal failure due to accumulation of sphingolipid.

MITOCHONDRIAL INHERITANCE. Energy generation through oxidative phosphorylation occurs in mitochondria in the cytoplasm of most cell types. Numerous mitochondria, each containing a single chromosome, exist in each cell. Some of the enzymes of oxidative phosphorylation are encoded by genes on the nuclear chromosomes and the proteins transported into the mitochondrion; the rest of the proteins are encoded by genes on the mitochondrial chromosome. Thus, genetic defects of oxidative phosphorylation can be due to mutations of genes on the autosomes or the X chromosome, and the resulting diseases behave as mendelian recessive traits, or mutations of genes on the mitochondrial chromosome, in which case the resulting diseases do not behave as mendelian traits.[10, 11] The differences are explicable by the events of conception. The spermatocyte contributes virtually no mitochondria to the zygote, and the entire complement of mitochondria that will ever be present in the fetus is derived from the mitochondria already present in the cytoplasm of the oocyte. Thus, phenotypes due to mutations of the mitochondrial chromosome show *maternal inheritance*, the characteristics of which are shown in Figure 56–5.

Principles of Clinical Genetics

PLEIOTROPY. Most mutant alleles have effects on more than one organ system, and a mendelian phenotype frequently displays numerous, often diverse manifestations. For example, Marfan syndrome (see p. 2000) is defined by abnormalities in the eye, skeleton, skin, heart, and aorta, and until the recognition of a defect in extracellular microfibrils, the findings could not be linked either etiologically or pathogenetically.[12]

VARIABILITY. The effects of the same mutant allele on phenotype can be different among people heterozygous (for dominant traits), homozygous (for autosomal recessive traits), or hemizygous (for X-linked traits) for the allele. Variability can be described in terms of the frequency of a particular pleiotropic manifestation among patients with the mutation; the severity of the phenotype; and the age of onset of manifestations. If a person has the mutant allele(s) but shows no phenotypic effect, the trait is called *nonpenetrant*. To an important degree, whether or not a clinical phenotype is called nonpenetrant depends on the sensitivity of the techniques used for detection. For example, two decades ago, based on bedside examination, cardiovascular abnormalities were thought to affect about half of people with Marfan syndrome; echocardiography now reveals aortic dilatation in more than 90 percent. The term *incomplete penetrance* should not be used with reference to individuals but to mean a prevalence of the phenotype is less than 100 percent of people known to carry the mutation(s). The Holt-Oram syndrome (see Chap. 43) is an instructive example. In this autosomal dominant syndrome of reduction anomalies of the upper limb and congenital heart defect, patients in the same family can have only arm anomalies, only a heart defect, or both. Moreover, the severity of the reduction defect varies widely, from a proximally

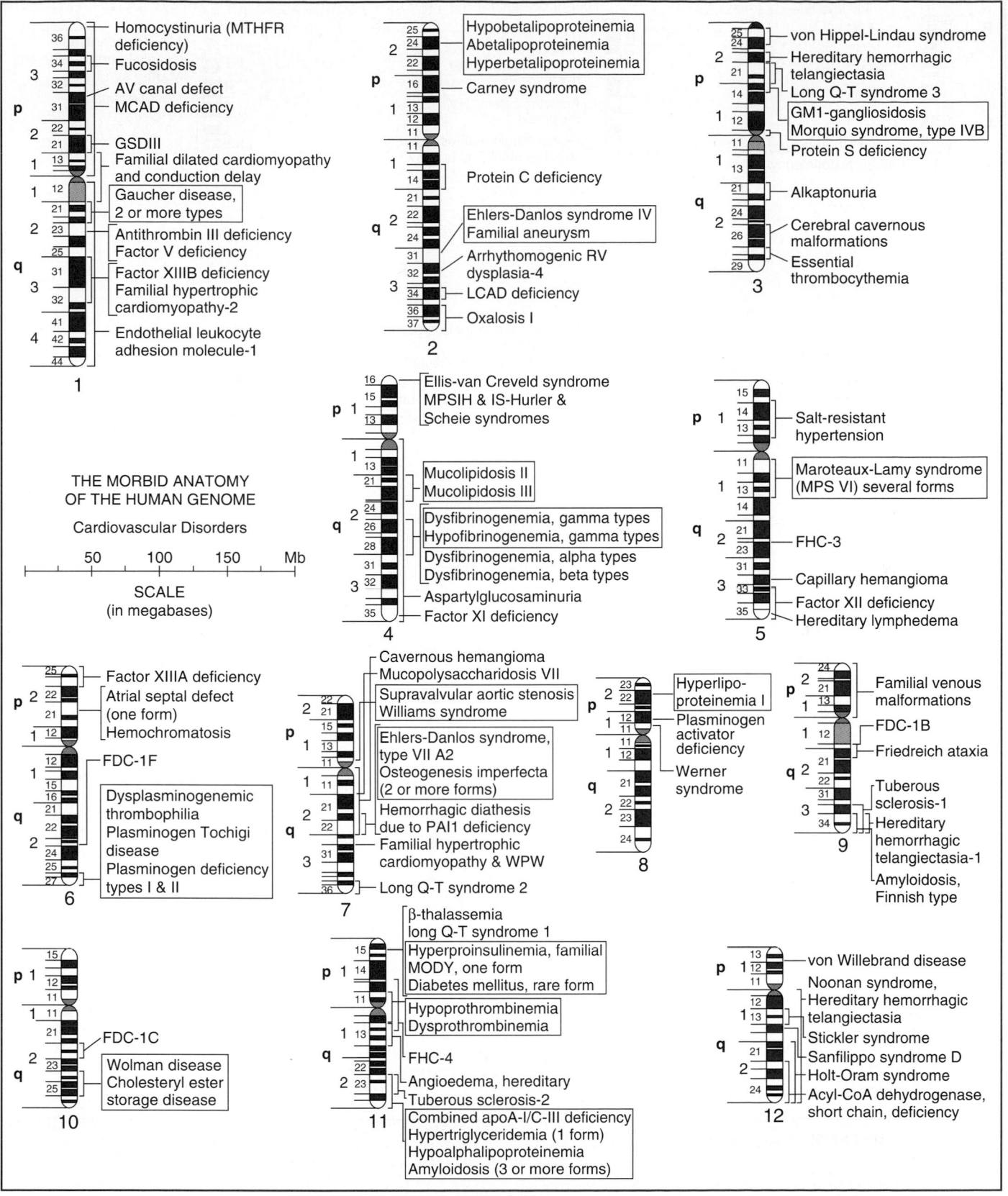

THE MORBID ANATOMY
OF THE HUMAN GENOME

Cardiovascular Disorders

SCALE
(in megabases)

FIGURE 56–1. Chromosomal location of human genes associated with some disorders of the cardiovascular system. These genes affect the structure, function, and metabolism of the heart and blood vessels and hemostasis and have been identified by the deleterious effects of mutations. Numerous additional genes that encode structural proteins important to the cardiovascular system have been identified but not yet associated with disease. In the figure, brackets next to the chromosome show the regional localization of the gene causing a particular disorder. Brackets next to two or more disorders indicate that all of the genes causing the disorders map to the same region. Disorders surrounded by boxes are caused by different mutations at the same gene.

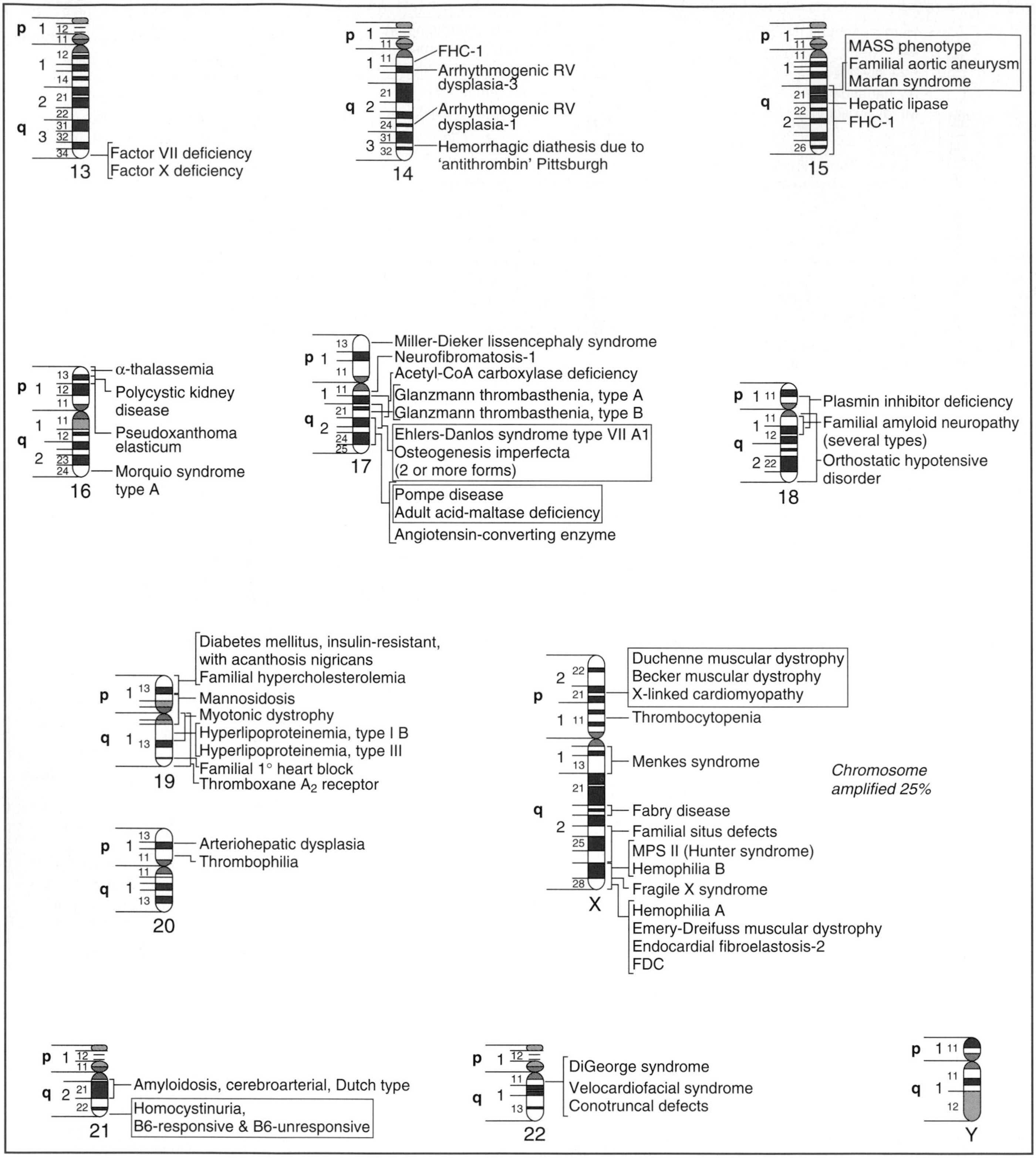

Chromosome 13:
- Factor VII deficiency
- Factor X deficiency

Chromosome 14:
- FHC-1
- Arrhythmogenic RV dysplasia-3
- Arrhythmogenic RV dysplasia-1
- Hemorrhagic diathesis due to 'antithrombin' Pittsburgh

Chromosome 15:
- MASS phenotype
- Familial aortic aneurysm
- Marfan syndrome
- Hepatic lipase
- FHC-1

Chromosome 16:
- α-thalassemia
- Polycystic kidney disease
- Pseudoxanthoma elasticum
- Morquio syndrome type A

Chromosome 17:
- Miller-Dieker lissencephaly syndrome
- Neurofibromatosis-1
- Acetyl-CoA carboxylase deficiency
- Glanzmann thrombasthenia, type A
- Glanzmann thrombasthenia, type B
- Ehlers-Danlos syndrome type VII A1
- Osteogenesis imperfecta (2 or more forms)
- Pompe disease
- Adult acid-maltase deficiency
- Angiotensin-converting enzyme

Chromosome 18:
- Plasmin inhibitor deficiency
- Familial amyloid neuropathy (several types)
- Orthostatic hypotensive disorder

Chromosome 19:
- Diabetes mellitus, insulin-resistant, with acanthosis nigricans
- Familial hypercholesterolemia
- Mannosidosis
- Myotonic dystrophy
- Hyperlipoproteinemia, type I B
- Hyperlipoproteinemia, type III
- Familial 1° heart block
- Thromboxane A$_2$ receptor

Chromosome 20:
- Arteriohepatic dysplasia
- Thrombophilia

Chromosome X:
- Duchenne muscular dystrophy
- Becker muscular dystrophy
- X-linked cardiomyopathy
- Thrombocytopenia
- Menkes syndrome
- Fabry disease
- Familial situs defects
- MPS II (Hunter syndrome)
- Hemophilia B
- Fragile X syndrome
- Hemophilia A
- Emery-Dreifuss muscular dystrophy
- Endocardial fibroelastosis-2
- FDC

Chromosome amplified 25%

Chromosome 21:
- Amyloidosis, cerebroarterial, Dutch type
- Homocystinuria, B6-responsive & B6-unresponsive

Chromosome 22:
- DiGeorge syndrome
- Velocardiofacial syndrome
- Conotruncal defects

Chromosome Y

FIGURE 56–1 *Continued*

placed thumb to near total absence of the arm. The cardiac feature is incompletely penetrant because only about 50 percent of patients have it, but in any individual with the Holt-Oram allele, the heart is either structurally normal or not.

Numerous genetic and environmental factors can affect expression of a gene (Table 56–3), and it is often impossible to determine which of these factors are most important in a specific patient or particular disease. However, the pervasiveness of variable expression emphasizes that phe-notypes determined by single genes are to some extent really "multifactorial."

GENETIC HETEROGENEITY. Similar or even identical phenotypes can be due to fundamentally distinct mutations, a phenomenon termed *genetic heterogeneity*. For example, Marfan syndrome and homocystinuria were long thought to be the same disorder, despite what now appear in retro-spect to be obvious differences in inheritance pattern and intelligence.[13] As in the case of these two disorders, the causes may lie in two different genes whose products are

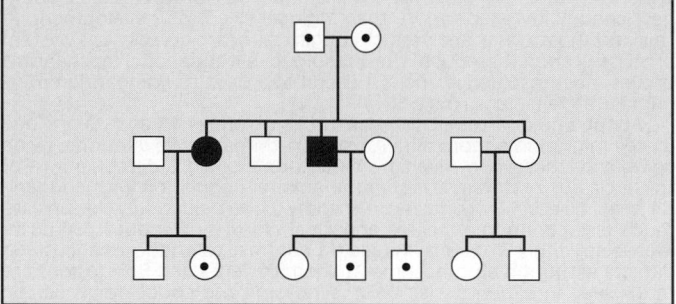

FIGURE 56-2. *Characteristics of autosomal recessive inheritance:*
A single generation is affected.
Both sexes are affected equally frequently.
Each parent is heterozygous (a carrier).
Each offspring of two carriers has a 25 percent chance of being affected, a 50 percent chance of being a carrier, and a 25 percent chance of inheriting neither mutant allele.
Two-thirds of clinically normal offspring are carriers.
The rarer the phenotype, the greater is the likelihood of consanguinity.
Characteristics of autosomal recessive phenotypes:
Often due to enzyme deficiencies.
Often more severe than dominant disorders.
Often early age of onset.

functionally distinct. Osteogenesis imperfecta exemplifies a disorder in which mutations in two genes, $\alpha1(I)$ and $\alpha2(I)$ procollagen, can each produce the same phenotype because the two proteins interact to form type I collagen.[14] Genetic heterogeneity is pervasive at the intragenic level of analysis; except for sickle cell anemia, hemochromatosis, and achondroplasia, virtually all single-gene disorders are due to a wide variety of mutations at a given locus.

Nonpathological Variation in the Cardiovascular System

CARDIAC STRUCTURE AND PHYSIOLOGY. All aspects of the ontogeny of the cardiovascular system are dictated by the genome. If, as seems most credible, few genes have a large effect and many have small contributions, any specific aspect of "normal" cardiovascular phenotype—size, shape, function—exhibits multifactorial inheritance. In other words, to the extent that any given phenotype can be quanti-

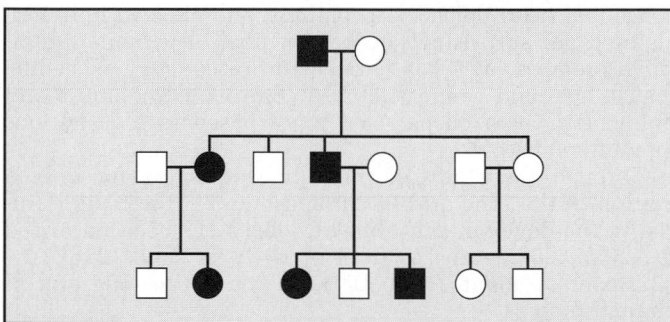

FIGURE 56-3. *Characteristics of autosomal dominant inheritance:*
Several generations are affected.
Both sexes are affected equally frequently.
In familial cases, only one parent need be affected.
Male-to-male transmission occurs.
Offspring of an affected parent has a 50 percent chance of being affected.
The frequency of sporadic cases is higher, the more severe the condition.
Paternal age has an effect in sporadic cases.
Characteristics of autosomal dominant phenotypes:
Often associated with malformations.
Often pleiotropic.
Usually variable.
Often age dependent.

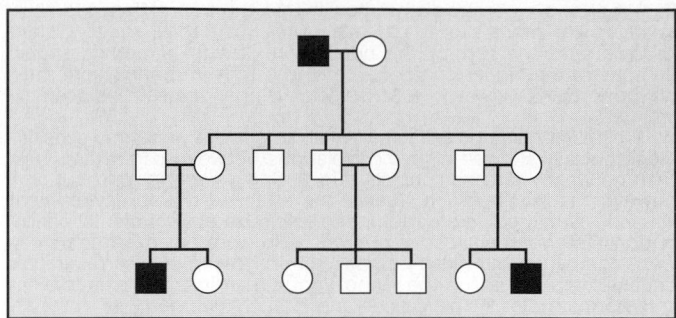

FIGURE 56-4. *Characteristics of X-linked inheritance:*
No male-to-male transmission.
All daughters of affected males are carriers.
Sons of a carrier mother have a 50 percent chance of being affected; daughters have a 50 percent chance of being carriers.
Some mothers of an affected male are not heterozygotes in all cells of their body, but they may have more affected sons if germinal mosaicism is present.
Characteristics of X-linked phenotypes:
More severe in males.
Heterozygous females may be unaffected.
Variable, especially in females.

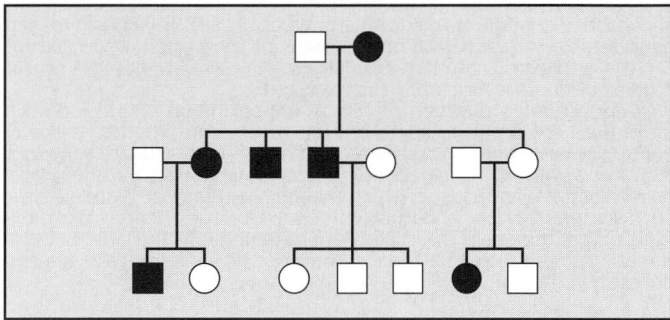

FIGURE 56-5. *Characteristics of disorders due to a mutation of the mitochondrial chromosome:*
Both sexes are equally frequently and severely affected.
Transmission is only through women; offspring of affected men are unaffected.
All offspring of an affected woman may be affected.
Variability of expression can be extreme in a family, including apparent nonpenetrance.
Phenotypes may be age dependent.

▼ **TABLE 56-3. CAUSES OF VARIABILITY OF GENE EXPRESSION**

Genetic background
Age dependence
Sex influence
Sex limitation
Modifying loci: hypostasis and epistasis
Gene alteration
Somatic mutation
Somatic amplification
Transpositions and rearrangements
Mutations
Physiological rearrangements
Variation in X inactivation*
Endogenous complementation*
Maternal factors
Effects of mitochondrial genome
Intrauterine environment
Imprinting
Exogenous and ecological factors
Ecology—temperature, diet
Teratogens
Medical intervention
Chance
* Pertains to female heterozygotes for X-linked disorders.

fied, it shows a normal distribution within the population, and near-relatives are more similar to each other than they are to distant relatives and the rest of the population. The twin method should demonstrate a higher concordance of the trait in monozygotic than dizygotic twins. However, surprisingly few phenotypes have been examined.

Preliminary data on left ventricular dimensions measured echocardiographically showed higher correlations between parent and child than between matched controls, suggesting a genetic contribution[15]; however, as in many such studies, the effect of shared environment was not estimated. In an attempt to minimize environmental contributions, left ventricular sizes of twins who were not exercise trained were compared; the mean intrapair differences in echocardiographic dimensions were less in the monozygotic than in the dizygotic twins and nontwin sibs.[16] The caliber and branch geometry of coronary arteries show familial resemblance, and both parameters are much more similar in monozygotic twins than in other relatives.[17] Further support for the importance of genetic factors in normal development derives from studies that demonstrate ethnic differences in structure. For example, the thickness of the intima and the media of coronary arteries of children who died of noncardiovascular causes varied significantly with the ethnicity of the child.[18]

Measures of cardiac electrophysiology show familial resemblance. Studies of both nuclear families[19, 19a] and twins[20, 21] suggest a genetic contribution to resting heart rate, conduction times, and repolarization time. Genetic control of normal cardiovascular function has been especially difficult to study because of the multitude of environmental (training, diet), stochastic (age), and clinical (subtle, unrecognized pathology) issues that confound comparisons of relatives and controls. Thus far, no strong genetic contribution to an individual's response to physical conditioning has emerged.[16]

VASCULAR SYSTEM. All members of certain inbred animal strains show little variation in arterial anatomy, especially branch angles, and considerable variation with other strains of the same species. Except for the studies of coronary arterial anatomy already noted,[17] similar studies of humans have not been reported.

One intriguing question of clinical importance is whether certain individuals are predisposed to arterial spasm and whether this susceptibility has a genetic basis. An examination of hereditary pathological and polymorphic variation in factors elaborated by endothelial cells, platelets, and leukocytes to maintain patency of blood vessels, such as prostacyclin, endothelium-derived relaxing factor (nitric oxide), or endothelin-1, may prove enlightening.[22-25] Similarly, is there genetic contribution to arterial stiffness or its variation with age and conditioning?

CARDIOVASCULAR DISORDERS ASSOCIATED WITH CHROMOSOME ABERRATIONS

Chromosome aberrations occur in 0.5 percent of the population at birth and are common findings in tumors.[26] Visible alterations of the amount of chromosomal material cause primarily structural defects of the cardiovascular system that are evident in the newborn. The frequency of chromosome aberrations among live-born children with congenital heart defects has been found to range from 5 to 13 percent.[27, 28] Upward of 40 percent of all fetuses with heart defects detected by ultrasonography at 18 to 20 weeks' gestation have chromosome aberrations; most are spontaneously aborted. Most forms of aneuploidy and most duplications and deletions of more than a chromosome band are associated with defects of the cardiovascular system[29] (see Tables 56–1 and 56–3). Exceptions are 47,XXX, 47,XYY, and 47,XXY (Klinefelter syndrome), in which the incidence of congenital heart disease is probably not elevated over the population baseline.

ANEUPLOIDY. How the abnormal phenotypes caused by autosomal aneuploidy develop remains controversial. One view holds that disturbance of the dosage of the genes present on the specific aneuploid chromosome segments is the central issue. The other view is that any aneuploid state disturbs developmental homeostasis in a nonspecific manner. The former theory predicts some distinctiveness of phenotype among the trisomy syndromes that occur in live-born children, whereas the latter predicts shared manifestations. At a coarse level, the clinical pictures are similar, with grave problems of the craniofacies, central nervous system, genitalia, distal limbs, and heart usually present. But when a more refined examination of the phenotypes is obtained, considerable distinctiveness emerges.

The three most common autosomal trisomies—13, 18, and 21—can be readily distinguished at the bedside. In all three, membranous ventricular and atrial septal defects are common. However, the detailed accounting of cardiovascular lesions among large numbers of patients with these trisomies reveals important differences that suggest aneuploidy exerts more than a global effect on development. In this and most other analyses of congenital heart defects, the system of classification based on the presumed pathogenetic mechanisms proves most instructive and is a useful approach to comparing different causative factors (Table 56–4).

About one-quarter of the defects in trisomies 13 and 18 are due to cell migration abnormalities, and two-thirds are flow lesions; when combined, these two mechanisms account for considerably more of these classes of defects than in the general population with congenital heart disease. By contrast, in trisomy 21, left-sided flow lesions are much less common, whereas abnormal closure of endocardial cushions is strikingly frequent. Indeed, in contrast to endocardial cushion defects without a chromosome 21 anomaly, left-sided flow lesions are rarely seen in patients with Down syndrome and endocardial cushion defects.[27, 30] Furthermore, the high incidence of endocardial cushion defects and low incidence of conotruncal and distal aortic anomalies have suggested a distinct pathogenetic mechanism in trisomy 21, potentially involving cell adhesiveness and the extracellular matrix.

TRISOMY 21—DOWN SYNDROME. This most common phenotype due to a human chromosome aberration occurs about once in every 600 births.[31] Most patients have trisomy 21, and the risk of this aberration is exponentially related to maternal age; the risk is lowest for young women and rises steeply after age 35, reaching 4 percent for women older than 45. A small minority (3 percent) of Down syndrome results from an extra copy of all or part of the long arm of chromosome 21 translocated to another chromosome. This situation is relatively more common in mothers younger than 30 years. The phenotypes of the two forms of Down syndrome do not differ. The phenotype tends to be less severe if the trisomy is mosaic (3 percent of Down syndrome) as a result of a mitotic nondisjunctional error in the embryo.

The most common causes of morbidity and mortality in patients with Down syndrome are congenital heart defects (present in 40 to 50 percent of cases),[32] hematological malignant disease, and duodenal atresia. If patients either escape or survive these problems, survival into the fifth decade and beyond is likely but is complicated by progressive dementia of the Alzheimer type. Premature aging may also affect the vasculature, although definitive studies are lacking.

The most characteristic cardiac anomaly in Down syndrome is a defect of closure of the endocardial cushions (see Chap. 43). Complicating the clinical problems in such patients and those with simple septal defects is a seeming predisposition to pulmonary hypertension in the presence of elevated pulmonary blood flow.[33] About one-third of congenital heart defects are complex, and affected individuals tend not surprisingly to be the most ill patients. Mitral valve prolapse (MVP) is found with a frequency exceeding that in age- and gender-matched controls.[34] The aortic and pulmonary valve cusps seem predisposed to fenestrations in adulthood.

Through the study of individuals trisomic for only a portion of the long arm of chromosome 21, the region crucial to the development of heart defects has been narrowed to 1.5 to 2.0 megabases (mb) of DNA in bands 21q22.2–q22.3 out of about 35 mb DNA on the entire long arm of chromosome 21.[35]

Medical treatment of patients with Down syndrome has undergone evolution to more aggressive measures in recent years. Objections and hesitations on medical, societal, and ethical grounds to operative repair of heart defects in Down syndrome have been mollified substantially.[31, 36] More follow-up data are becoming available, and early and late postoperative survival in patients with Down syndrome appears to be comparable to that in other patients with similar defects.[36]

TRISOMY 18. *Edwards syndrome* is the second most common autosomal trisomy. Most cases are due to meiotic disjunction, and there is a strong relationship to maternal age. Routine prenatal diagnostic testing of women older than 34 years would detect all aneuploid fetuses in them, but this would represent only one-third of all auto-

CHROMOSOME ABERRATION	EPONYM	CARDIOVASCULAR MANIFESTATIONS
Triploidy		
69,XXX (or XXY or XYY)		>50% have CHD: ASD and VSD
Aneuploidy		
+13	Patau	~80% have CHD; 75% of CHD is complex: PDA, VSD, ASD, PS, AS, dextrocardia, CoA
+18	Edwards	~90% have CHD: most CHD is complex: VSD, PDA, ASD, bicuspid PV and AV, CoA
+21	Down	~40% have CHD: ECD, TOF; MVP in ~20%; AR
+8 mosaicism		~25% have CHD, most of little clinical consequence: VSD, PDA, CoA, PS
+9 mosaicism		~70% have CHD, usually complex: VSD, PDA, PLSVC
45,X	Turner	~10% have clinically important CHD: 50% of these have CoA; mild CoA is likely much more common; also AS, ARD, VSD, ASD, dextrocardia
47,XXX		CHD not increased
47,XXY	Klinefelter	CHD possibly slightly increased; ? mild conduction changes; venous thromboembolic disease
47,XYY		CHD not increased; ? mild conduction changes
Deletions		
4p−	Wolf-Hirschhorn	~50% have CHD, usually complex: VSD, ASD, PDA, PS
5p−	Cri du chat	~20% have CHD, usually single: VSD, PDA, ASD, PS
7q−		~20% have CHD, various, often complex
13q−		CHD common, often severe, but depend on region deleted
18p−		CHD uncommon
18q−		~25% have CHD, usually single, of little consequence: VSD, PDA, ASD, PS
ring 18		~20% have CHD: CoA, PA hypoplasia, HLH, PLSVC
Duplications		
4p trisomy		~10% have CHD, usually single: no defect predominates
9p trisomy		<10% have CHD: VSD, ASD, AS, PS
10 p trisomy		~30% have CHD, usually single: no defect predominates
10q24−qter trisomy		~50% have CHD, usually complex: ECD, VSD, TOF
22pter−q11 trisomy or tetrasomy	Cat eye	~50% have CHD, usually complex: TAPVR, VSD, TOF
Other Aberrations		
Marker Xq27.3	Fragile X syndrome	~50% have aortic root dilatation, MVP, or both

CHD = congenital heart defect(s); ASD = atrial septal defect; VSD = ventricular septal defect; PDA = patent ductus arteriosus; PS = valvular pulmonic stenosis; AS = aortic stenosis; CoA = coarctation of aorta; PV = pulmonic valve; AV = aortic valve; ECD = endocardial cushion defect; TOF = tetralogy of Fallot; MVP = mitral valve prolapse; AR = aortic regurgitation; PLSVC = persistence of left superior vena cava; ARD = aortic root dilatation; PA = pulmonary artery; HLH = hypoplastic left heart; TAPVR = total anomalous pulmonary venous return.

somal trisomies; in the United States, less than one-half of all women of this advanced age undergo definitive testing. Prenatal detection of trisomies followed by termination of pregnancy is currently having a small but measurable impact on decreasing the incidence of *Down*, *Edwards*, and *Patau* syndromes.

Although the severity of the phenotype rarely enables survival beyond a few months, 10 percent of patients live to 1 year, and a few survive to adulthood, perhaps because of undetected mosaicism for a chromosomally normal cell line. However, central nervous system function is far less than that in Down syndrome and leads to complex medical management and supportive care for long-term survivors.[37]

Cardiovascular defects occur in at least 90 percent of cases and contribute to death. Complex lesions, usually involving septal defects, dysplastic valves that are rarely hemodynamically important, patent ductus arteriosus (PDA), and persistence of the left superior vena cava are common.[38, 39] Right ventricular enlargement is common and may indicate not only shunting from left to right but pulmonary hypertension due to anomalies of the pulmonary vasculature.[38] As in Down syndrome, transposition of the great arteries is virtually unknown in trisomy 18.[39] Rarely should invasive diagnostic procedures or aggressive supportive measures be undertaken in Edwards syndrome.

TRISOMY 13. *Patau syndrome* occurs in about 0.01 percent of live births and in progressively higher frequencies in stillbirths and spontaneous abortions. The external phenotype is usually severe but occasionally not as characteristic as other trisomies; survival beyond a few weeks is rare, and the causes of death involve several organ systems, especially the heart. Cardiovascular anomalies are a bit less frequent than in trisomy 18 and have a slightly different spectrum.[31, 38] Septal defects are the most common isolated lesions; dextrocardia and bicuspid semilunar valves occur in association with other anomalies.

Patients who survive beyond 1 month often are mosaic for a chromosomally normal cell line; thus, prognosis is fraught with uncer-

tainty until detailed analysis is completed. Whether invasive cardiological studies are performed or aggressive management is undertaken can be determined by the severity of involvement of other organ systems, especially the brain, pending cytogenetic investigation.

TURNER SYNDROME. About one in every 2500 females lacks an X chromosome and has a 45,X karyotype, which is by far the most common cause of Turner syndrome. The frequency of a nonmosaic 45,X karyotype is much higher in spontaneous abortuses than in liveborns, and probably less than 2 percent of such conceptuses come to term. The clinical phenotype is variable and often mild; the diagnosis is often not suspected until a child's short stature is evaluated or a woman complains of amenorrhea. Many cases are mosaic for cell lines with 46,XX or 46,XY constitutions. Various structural aberrations involving the X chromosome can cause partial or complete Turner's syndrome.

Among patients with the 45,X karyotype, reported frequencies of congenital cardiovascular defects vary from 20 to 50 percent, depending on how patients were ascertained.[40] Fifty to 70 percent of those with cardiovascular defects have clinically important aortic coarctation, usually of the postductal form.[41] As noninvasive imaging studies of asymptomatic patients became routine, the frequency of coarctation may increase. Various other cardiac malformations may occur, either singly or combined with coarctation. However, there is strong support for left-sided flow abnormalities as a major pathogenetic mechanism. Bicuspid aortic valve and dilatation of the ascending aorta (with a risk of dissection and histopathology showing elastic fiber disruption) occur even in the absence of coarctation,[42] and hypoplastic left heart has been reported.[43] Partial anomalous pulmonary venous drainage without an atrial septal defect is fairly common and should be suspected when right ventricular overload is detected on echocardiography.[44]

Postmortem examination of midtrimester abortuses with 45,X showed a higher incidence of left-sided flow lesions than found at birth, suggesting an association between the pathogenesis of the cardiovascular anomalies and the uniform presence of lymphatic obstruction at the base of the heart.[41]

Blood pressure elevation is common, even without coarctation or after its repair; a high frequency of renal anomalies is one likely cause but not the sole explanation for the prevalence of hypertension.

In about two-thirds of cases, the retained X chromosome derives from the oocyte (maternal X). Because entire chromosomes or regions of a chromosome may be differentially regulated (imprinted)[45] by passage through oogenesis versus spermatogenesis, could some of the variability in phenotype among patients with Turner syndrome be due to the origin of the retained X or the origin of the lost X? In a study of 63 patients, 10 had severe cardiovascular features, and 9 of them had retained the maternal X.[46] This is an idea worthy of further investigation. Women with mosaic karyotypes are less likely to have cardiovascular defects. Some studies also suggest a "critical region" of the X chromosome, which, when deleted, results in most of the features of Turner's syndrome.[47]

CONGENITAL HEART DISEASE
(See Chaps. 43 and 44)

In the past few decades, the reported incidence of structural heart defects in newborns has increased from 5 to 7 per 1000 live births, probably as the result of increased diagnostic sensitivity (especially cross-sectional and Doppler echocardiography and magnetic resonance imaging).[48-52] Supporting this explanation is the lack of change over the same period in the incidence of critical defects diagnosed neonatally at 3.1 to 3.5 per 1000.[48, 53] This enhanced resolving power of noninvasive methods should prove particularly useful in the study of familial structural defects, because apparently unaffected relatives can be evaluated for subclinical evidence of anomalies. Few investigations to date have capitalized on this approach.[54, 55]

As is evident from the previous section, gross aberrations of chromosomes produce an extensive and varied array of structural heart disease, an observation as true for spontaneous abortuses as for live-born children.[56] Unfortunately, cytogenetic aberrations have provided few clues about etiology and pathogenesis of congenital malformations.[57, 58] Better understanding comes from investigating the other two mechanisms by which genes cause congenital heart defects—multifactorial processes and mutations of single genes. In addition to the mendelian syndromes discussed later, evidence for the involvement of genes of large effect derives from studies of incidence of congenital heart disease in populations with a high rate of inbreeding. The increased occurrence of defects in offspring of consanguineous matings suggests that mutations in one or more genes, when homozygous, strongly predispose to abnormal cardiovascular development.[59]

MULTIFACTORIAL PROCESSES. The empirical risks of recurrence of congenital heart defects have increased in recent years,[60, 61] in keeping with the overall higher incidence noted earlier. However, this conclusion has been criticized because the studies focused on the offspring of women probands, in whom the recurrence risk appears higher than in men with congenital heart defects.[62] In addition to this unexplained maternal influence, other factors may be at work. For example, improved detection of subtle lesions, more faithful reporting of patients, and the assiduousness of epidemiologists may have shown a systematic variation. More patients with cardiovascular problems now survive[61-64] to bear children because of improved medical and surgical care; their offspring might be at increased risk because of the severity of the parents' problems, but some evidence refutes this idea.[65]

The familial aggregation of congenital heart defects supports many of the predictions of the threshold liability model of multifactorial inheritance.[53, 66, 67] In most studies, whether focused on populations or families, defects were classified by their pathology; for example, all ventricular

septal defects were considered as one group. There has been bias in reporting families in which one type of defect aggregates, which has led to many reports of "familial atrial septal defect," "familial cardiomyopathy," and so on, without regard to the fact that not all septal defects or cardiopathies have the same structure on careful scrutiny, let alone the same cause.[68, 69]

A major advance has been the movement to examine familial aggregation of defects based on presumed pathogenesis.[52, 70] The scheme developed by Clark[71] and since modified and expanded[72] (Table 56–5), has become widely used. Under this approach, some anatomically distinct lesions are related by common pathogenesis; if the pathogenetic mechanism has substantial genetic control, then the occurrence of distinct defects in the same family would still be consistent with a genetic model. Alternatively, defects unrelated by pathogenesis would require a different interpretation. This model rationalizes examination of apparently unaffected relatives, which increases the chances of detecting subtle manifestations of defective development of cardiovascular structures.

ERRORS IN MESENCHYMAL TISSUE MIGRATION. Included in this category are a wide range of anomalies of the outflow tract, some due to failure of fusion and others due to failure of septation. Relatives of probands with interruption of the aortic arch type B or truncus arteriosus, both uncommon conotruncal malformations, had 2.5 percent and 6.6 percent incidences, respectively, of congenital heart defects.[73] Both recurrence rates were higher than expected. The frequency of congenital malformations was much lower in relatives of patients with other forms of interrupted aortic arch. Moreover, relatives of probands with truncus arteriosus and other defects had a recurrence rate of 13 percent, the majority in the spectrum of conotruncal lesions. Here is an instance in which refined empirical risk data should improve the accuracy of genetic counseling.

Categorizing anatomical defects by presumed pathogenesis emphasizes that all ventricular septal defects are not alike. However, even within an embryologically circumscribed category, the situation is complex. Many perimembranous ventricular septal defects can be considered errors in mesenchymal tissue migration. Evidence exists for the effects of major genes (e.g., as yet unidentified ones in the 22q11 region[74] and *Jagged1*, the gene that when mutated also causes Alagille syndrome[75] and for multifactorial effects.[76]

Conotruncal Development. Considerable progress has been made during the past few years in identifying a region of chromosome 22 that has a major role in development of the conotruncus, the branchial arches, and the face. Interest was first stimulated by detection of small deletions involving 22q11 in patients with *DiGeorge sequence.*[77] This condition includes developmental anomalies of the fourth branchial arch and derivatives of the third and fourth pharyngeal pouches. Hypoplasia of the thymus and parathyroids causes immune deficiency and hypocalcemia. The cardiac defects range from tetralogy of Fallot to ventricular septal defect, truncus arteriosus, interrupted aorta type B, and right aortic arch and are often lethal. Deletion of 22q11 accounts for about 90 percent of instances of DiGeorge sequence.

▼ **TABLE 56–5. CLASSIFICATION OF CONGENITAL HEART DEFECTS BASED ON PATHOGENETIC MECHANISMS**

PATHOGENETIC MECHANISM	EXAMPLES OF DEFECTS
Embryonic blood flow defects	
Left-sided lesions	HLH; bicuspid aortic valve; IAA type A; CoA; PDA
Right-sided lesions	Secundum ASD; PS
Mesenchymal tissue migration defects	TOF; D-TGA
Extracellular matrix defects	ECD
Abnormal cellular death	Ebstein anomaly; muscular VSD
Defects of looping and situs	L-TGA
Abnormalities of targeted growth	TAPVR

HLH = hypoplastic left heart; IAA = interrupted aortic arch; CoA = coarctation of aorta; PDA = patent ductus arteriosus; ASD = atrial septal defect; PS = valvular pulmonic stenosis; TOF = tetralogy of Fallot; TGA = transposition of great arteries; ECD = endocardial cushion defect; VSD = ventricular septal defect; TAPVR = total anomalous pulmonary venous return.

Subsequently, patients with *velocardiofacial syndrome* (VCF, also called Shprintzen syndrome) and what has been called in Japan the *conotruncal anomaly face syndrome* were found to have deletions in the same region, albeit generally smaller ones than in DiGeorge syndrome.[78] Because the deletion is often too small to be detected by routine cytogenetics, fluorescent in situ hybridization (FISH) with a DNA probe for the region is the assay of choice. The VCF syndrome is unlike DiGeorge syndrome and includes an abnormal but characteristic facies, cleft palate, pharyngeal insufficiency, and conotruncal cardiac defects.

This same region of chromosome 22 has been examined in patients with familial occurrence of various congenital cardiac defects and in patients with nonfamilial occurrence, nonsyndromic conotruncal defects, and an important fraction of patients in both categories have submicroscopic deletions of 22q11.[74, 79] Thus, a gene or genes in this region account for much of the recurrence risk of defects due to mesenchymal tissue migration abnormalities. Further, accurate counseling about recurrence risks for this broad range of defects necessitates FISH or molecular analysis for the presence of a deletion in the proband and, if present, in both parents. Deletion of 22q11 occurs in about 13 per 100,000 live births and is, after trisomy 21, the second most common genetic cause of congenital heart disease.[80]

Investigation of a strain of Keeshond dogs prone to conotruncal defects has shown that a single gene can be responsible for pathogenetically related defects of widely varying severity.[81]

FLOW DEFECTS. Left-sided flow lesions comprise a spectrum that includes hypoplastic left heart, congenital aortic stenosis, bicuspid aortic valve, interrupted aortic arch type A, and aortic coarctation. Various components of this spectrum can be present in the same patient. Data from the Baltimore-Washington Infant Study,[52] a population-based case-control study of congenital cardiovascular malformations, were used to show that in first-degree relatives of probands with isolated hypoplastic left heart, the incidence of bicuspid aortic valve was 12 percent; most of the cases were asymptomatic and unrecognized before they were detected by echocardiography as part of this investigation.[59] In an exceptional family, four instances of aortic coarctation occurred in four generations.[82]

The association of coarctation of the aorta, bicuspid aortic valve, and dilatation of the ascending aorta, which may occur as part of *Turner syndrome*, is well known in the general population.[83] Several intriguing questions about the genetics and pathogenesis of this association need to be addressed. To what extent is the ascending aorta intrinsically abnormal and hence predisposed to dilate, and to what extent is the dilatation simply a result of abnormal turbulence created by a bicuspid aortic valve? The fact that some patients with this association also have subtle evidence of a systemic connective tissue abnormality, reminiscent of Marfan syndrome, supports the former hypothesis. It will be of interest to extend the study of left-sided flow lesions to include probands with coarctation or congenital aortic stenosis and to evaluate close relatives with techniques capable of detecting the entire range of flow defects.

EXTRACELLULAR MATRIX ABNORMALITIES. Enough is known about the biochemistry and cell biology of cardiac embryology to state with some confidence that the extracellular matrix ("connective tissue") has an important role. The endocardial cushions have received the most attention as an area where defects in the extracellular matrix might produce malformations.[71] The high frequency of endocardial cushion defects and atrioventricular septal defects in Down syndrome has been noted (see p. 1986). Of interest is the finding of increased adhesiveness of fibroblasts from patients with trisomy 21, a phenomenon that could reflect interaction with the extracellular matrix.[84] The distinctiveness of endocardial cushion defects in patients with normal chromosomes and in those with trisomy 21 has been suggested because of differences in associated cardiovascular malformations.[68] However, of six families in which the proband had an endocardial cushion defect, three had recurrence of the same type of defect in a relative, including two with trisomy 21.[85]

SITUS AND LOOPING DEFECTS. This is an area fraught with difficulties of nomenclature, diagnosis, and heterogeneity of both etiology and pathogenesis. In analysis of clinical data, the most informative approach, but clearly arduous because of the large amount of data required, would be to categorize probands and their relatives by the type of situs (solitus, inversus, dextroversion, and levoversion: see Chap. 43) and each of those by presence or absence of other cardiac and visceral defects. This has not been done on epidemiological cohorts, and in family studies relatives have rarely been subjected to evaluations sufficient to characterize their phenotypes in detail. These variable phenotypes are grouped in a category, *heterotaxy*, that accounts for 3 to 4 percent of all congenital heart defects.

Several mendelian phenotypes point to single genes that have a major effect on determining laterality. In the autosomal recessive *Kartagener syndrome*, a randomization of lateralization of the heart (situs solitus and situs inversus are equally likely in homozygotes)[86] coexists with a defect in ciliary motility, which leads to sinusitis, bronchiectasis, and sperm immotility.[87]

Heterotaxy with splenic and other cardiac defects, particularly of the position of the great vessels, can be inherited as an autosomal recessive, as an autosomal dominant,[88] and as an X-linked recessive.[89] Some of the families with these apparently single-gene disorders have concordance of phenotype, but many do not, suggesting that in

some cases various types of situs defects, polysplenia, and asplenia are different manifestations of the same mutation.[90, 91]

In recent years, investigation of molecular embryology has shed increasing light on cardiovascular development and maldevelopment.[92] The determination of laterality and defects involving heterotaxy have been especially revealing, in both mice and humans.[93, 94] In mice, the *inv* locus has long been associated with left/right asymmetry, and the gene was recently cloned.[95] In humans, mutations of two genes thus far, one encoding the activin receptor type IIB[96] and one encoding the connexin43 gap junction protein,[97] both have been associated with defects of laterality.

Few data define the recurrence risks of defects in the *cell death* (e.g., Ebstein anomaly) and *abnormal targeted growth* (e.g., anomalous pulmonary venous return) categories. Data from the Baltimore-Washington Infant Study do not show an increased risk of any cardiovascular defect in the relatives of a proband with a defect in either of these categories.[52]

DISORDERS OF UNCLEAR CAUSE. A number of disorders include an important likelihood of malformation of the cardiovascular system but are of unclear cause (Table 56-6). Familial recurrence is low enough to be *incompatible* with multifactorial inheritance. Several of these disorders deserve comment.

Certain congenital cardiac defects and other malformations occur together more frequently than expected by chance; this *association* of defects suggests a common cause, pathogenesis, or both, but the following disorders and those in Table 56-7 remain enigmatic on most of these counts. Designation as a *sequence* implies that some evidence exists for a common developmental problem to account for the features.

CHARGE Association (see Table 56-6). Patients with this condition by definition have congenital heart defects.[98, 99] The spectrum of cardiovascular malformations suggests not so much a common pathogenetic scheme as a common time of abnormal development. During gestational days 32 to 45, cardiac septation, fusion of the endocardial cushions and membranous ventricular septum, and formation of the outflow tracts and valves occur. An environmental insult or a breakdown in developmental homeostasis during this period could result in the malformation spectrum of this disorder. The defects in other systems could also arise during this embryological window and would be consistent with either environmental or intrinsic factors.

VACTERL Association (see Table 56-6). This condition has expanded over the years to include *v*ertebral, *v*entricular septal, *a*nal, *c*ardiac *t*racheoesophageal, *r*enal, and *l*imb defects. Omitted from the mnemonic is the single umbilical artery often present.[100] Cardiac defects are present in about one-half of patients with more than two components of this association but usually are not life threatening. VACTERL association occasionally occurs in relatives.[101] Although infants with this condition often fail to thrive initially, the long-term prognosis for health and mental function is good, so aggressive management of the multiple malformations is warranted. It is important to separate as soon as possible those patients who have the features of trisomy 18 or 13q chromosome aberrations, as prognosis in these cases is distinctly unfavorable.

Mendelian Disorders

Some congenital cardiovascular defects segregate in occasional families as predicted of a mendelian phenotype. Strong bias favors reporting such occurrences, and equally strong is a temptation to conclude that, at least in some cases, the defect is caused by mutation in a single gene. However, rarely and by chance alone, a multifactorial trait recurs in a family in a pattern mimicking mendelian segregation. This potential confusion and the resultant uncertainty in counseling patients and families pertains equally well to disturbances of conduction and rhythm, to various cardiomyopathies, to vascular anomalies, and to hypertension, all discussed subsequently. The true cause of the cardiovascular diseases in such families may not become clarified until each is investigated in detail, in concert with efforts to map and sequence the entire human genome.

The subject of this section can therefore be parsed into three broad classes of conditions: congenital cardiac defects that occasionally seem to be inherited as mendelian traits (Table 56-7), pleiotropic mendelian syndromes that always or frequently affect the structure of the cardiovascular system (Table 56-8), and mendelian syndromes that occasionally affect the cardiovascular system (Table 56-9).

PATENT DUCTUS ARTERIOSUS. Most instances of PDA are sporadic occurrences, and a strong association with pre-

▼ **TABLE 56–6.** DISORDERS OF UNCERTAIN CAUSE AND INHERITANCE THAT ARE ASSOCIATED WITH A HIGH INCIDENCE OF CARDIOVASCULAR ABNORMALITIES

DISORDER AND PHENOTYPE	OMIM NO.*	CARDIOVASCULAR ABNORMALITIES†
Aase syndrome (congenital anemia, triphalangeal thumbs)	205600	VSD
Bilateral left-sidedness sequence (polysplenia syndrome)	208530	ASD
Bilateral right-sidedness sequence (asplenia syndrome; Ivemark syndrome)	208530	Situs inversus, ECD, VSD
CHARGE association (*c*oloboma, *h*eart anomaly, choanal *a*tresia, *r*etardation, *g*enital, and *e*ar anomalies)	214800	TOF, PDA, ECD, VSD
Cornelia de Lange syndrome (short stature, retardation, synophrys, hypertrichosis, micromelia, genital anomalies)	122470	~20% have CHD: VSD, PDA, ASD, PLSVC, TOF
DiGeorge sequence‡ (abnormalities of derivatives of 3rd and 4th pharyngeal pouches and 4th branchial arch: hypoplastic thymus with cellular immune deficiency, hyoplastic parathyroids with hypocalcemia)	188400	CHD in ~100%: aortic arch anomalies (especially IAA type B and right-sided aortic arch); PDA, TOF
Goldenhar syndrome (abnormalities of derivatives of 1st and 2nd branchial arch: hemifacial microsomia, microtia, vertebral anomalies)	141400, 164210, 257700	~50% have CHD: VSD, TOF, PDA, CoA, right-sided aortic arch, PLSVC
Klippel-Feil sequence (short neck, limited rotation of the head, cervical anomalies)	118100, 148900, 214300	Variable estimates (5–70%) of CHD: VSD, dextrocardia
"Kabuki make-up" syndrome (dwarfism, peculiar facies, scoliosis, mental retardation)	147920	30% have CHD: ASD, VSD, TOF, CoA, PDA
Pallister-Hall syndrome (hypothalamic hamartoblastoma, hypopituitarism, imperforate anus, postaxial polydactyly)	146510	ECD
Poland sequence (unilateral absence of sternocostal pectoralis major, ipsilateral synbrachydactyly)	173800	~10% have dextrocardia or dextroversion
Rubinstein-Taybi syndrome (short stature, retardation, microcephaly, characteristic facies, broad thumbs)	268600	~20% have CHD: ECD, ASD, TOF, PDA, VSD
VATER association (*v*ertebral defects, *a*nal atresia, *t*racheo-*e*sophageal fistula, *r*adial dysplasia, *r*enal anomaly)	192350	VSD

VSD = ventricular septal defect; ASD = atrial septal defect; TOF = tetralogy of Fallot; PDA = patent ductus arteriosus; ECD = endocardial cushion defect; CHD = congenital heart defect(s); PLSVC = persistence of left superior vena cava; IAA = interrupted aortic arch; CoA = coarctation of aorta; VSD = ventricular septal defect.

* None of these disorders is evidently due to a mutation in a single gene; however, most are listed in Online Mendelian Inheritance in Man (www.ncbi.nlm.nih.gov/omim)[8] and the OMIM no. is provided as a ready source to the literature.

† Cardiovascular defects listed in approximate order of decreasing frequency.

‡ 90% of cases associated with del(22q11); likely a contiguous gene deletion defect.

▼ **TABLE 56–7.** CONGENITAL HEART DEFECTS OCCASIONALLY SHOWING FAMILIAL AGGREGATION CONSISTENT WITH MENDELIAN INHERITANCE

DEFECT	OMIM NO.*	DEFECT	OMIM NO.
Aneurysm, intracranial berry	105800	Hypoplastic left heart	140500, 241550
Aneurysm, abdominal aortic	100070	Hypoplastic right heart	277200
Angioma	106050, 106070, 206570	Lymphedema, congenital	153000, 153100, 153400, 214900, 247440
ASD, ostium primum	209400		
ASD, ostium secundum	108800, 108900, 178650	Mitral valve prolapse	157700
Bicuspid aortic valve	109730	Patent ductus arteriosus	169100
		Pulmonary venous return, anomalous	106700
Conotruncal defect	231060	Pulmonic stenosis	126190, 178650, 193520, 265500, 265600, 270460
Dextrocardia	244400, 304750		
Ebstein anomaly	224700	Subaortic stenosis	271950, 271960
Endocardial fibroelastosis	226000, 227280, 305300		
Hemangioma	106070, 140800, 140900, 234800	Tetralogy of Fallot	187500
Hemangioma, cavernous	116860, 140850	Ventricle, single	234750

ASD = atrial septal defect.

* Data from Online Mendelian Inheritance in Man (www.ncbi.nlm.nih.gov/omim).

▼ **TABLE 56–8. MENDELIAN DISORDERS WITH CONGENITAL DEFECTS OF CARDIOVASCULAR STRUCTURE AS FREQUENT MANIFESTATIONS**

DESCRIPTIVE NAME	EPONYM	OMIM NO.*	CARDIOVASCULAR ABNORMALITIES
Adult polycystic kidney disease		173900	MVP, dilated aortic root, intracranial berry aneurysm
Arteriohepatic dysplasia	Alagille syndrome	118450	PPS
Cataract and cardiomyopathy		212350	HCM
Chondroectodermal dysplasia	Ellis–van Creveld syndrome	225500	ASD (ostium primum), common atrium
Deafness, mitral regurgitation, and short stature	Forney syndrome	157800	MR
Familial collagenoma syndrome		115250	DCM
Heart-hand syndrome	Holt-Oram syndrome	142900	ASD (ostium secundum), VSD, MVP, HLH
Keratosis palmoplantaris	Mal de Meleda	248300	DCM, dysrhythmia
Malignant hyperthermia and skeletal defects	King syndrome	145600	Malignant hyperthermia → cardiac arrest
	Noonan syndrome	163950	PS, HCM
Pulmonic stenosis and deafness		178651	PS
	Smith-Lemli-Opitz syndrome	270400	PDA, ASD, VSD, TOF, ECD, CoA
Velocardiofacial syndrome	Shprintzen syndrome	192430	TOF, tortuous retinal vasculature

MVP = mitral valve prolapse; PPS = peripheral pulmonic stenosis; HCM = hypertrophic cardiomyopathy; ASD = atrial septal defect; MR = mitral regurgitation; DCM = dilated cardiomyopathy; VSD = ventricular septal defect; HLH = hypoplastic left heart; PS = valvular pulmonic stenosis; PDA = patent ductus arteriosus; TOF = tetralogy of Fallot; ECD = endocardial cushion defect; CoA = coarctation of aorta.

* Data from Online Mendelian Inheritance in Man (www.ncbi.nlm.nih.gov/omim).

maturity and all of its antecedents is noted. However, in a number of families that have been described, PDA occurs as an autosomal dominant trait.[102] In some pedigrees, mild facial dysmorphism segregates with PDA; because the facial features differ among families, the number of syndromes remains unclear.[103, 104]

FAMILIAL ATRIAL SEPTAL DEFECT. Two mendelian forms of atrial septal defect exist as autosomal dominant traits. One has no associated problems and has been described in few pedigrees.[105]

The second, more common condition is associated with atrioventricular conduction delay.[106, 107] The defect is of the secundum type, and relatives do not seem to be at increased risk of other cardiac malformations. The severity of heart block rarely progresses to third degree. The electrocardiographic abnormality in a patient with apparently sporadic atrial septal defect should prompt a detailed family history and evaluation of close relatives. Attention should be directed to the upper limbs, particularly the thumbs, to rule out the Holt-Oram syndrome; radiographic examination of the upper limbs of the proband is helpful on this account.

In patients with atrial septal defect due to aneuploidy (a syndrome with extracardiac features), when one of the autosomal dominant forms is excluded, the recurrence risk of secundum atrial septal defect is about 3 percent, a value that conforms closely to the multifactorial threshold model.

Several pleiotropic mendelian conditions have defects of the atrial septum as frequent manifestations.

HOLT-ORAM SYNDROME. This autosomal dominant condition, first elaborated in 1960, shows marked variability within a pedigree.[108] The cardinal manifestations are dysplasia of the upper limbs and atrial septal defect. In heterozygotes for the mutation, arm deformity ranges from undetectable through distally placed thumbs and hypoplastic thenar eminences, triphalangeal thumbs, anomalies of the carpus, and radial aplasia, to phocomelia and hypoplasia of the clavicles and shoulders. Upper-extremity deformity is usually bilateral but may be asymmetrical in severity, with the left side more affected. Similarly, the atrial involvement ranges from none to a large secundum defect with early, severe hemodynamic compromise. Other cardiac malformations have been reported, with ventricular septal defects and PDA the most frequent.[109] The skeletal and cardiac manifestations are not correlated in individuals, and how a parent is affected is not a reliable predictor of effects on offspring.[110] Prenatal diagnosis by ultrasonography was reported in a fetus with severe limb abnormalities; a large septal defect could presumably be detected as well. Other manifestations include dermatoglyphic abnormalities, pectus excavatum, hypoplastic peripheral arteries, and cardiac conduction disturbance, the last usually involving the atrioventricular node and present in patients with septal defects. Although the Holt-Oram syndrome bears some resem-

▼ **TABLE 56–9. MENDELIAN DISORDERS WITH CARDIOVASCULAR ABNORMALITIES AS OCCASIONAL MANIFESTATIONS**

SYNDROME	EPONYM	OMIM NO.*	CARDIOVASCULAR ABNORMALITIES
Acrocephalosyndactyly type I	Apert syndrome	101200	PS, PPS, VSD, EFE
Acrocephalopolysyndactyly type II	Carpenter syndrome	201000	PDA, VSD, PS, TGA
Hereditary angioedema		106100	Coronary arteritis
Imperforate anus with hand, foot, and ear anomalies	Townes-Brocks syndrome	107480	Sporadic cases have CHD: VSD, ASD
Mandibulofacial dysostosis	Treacher Collins syndrome	154500, 248390	10% have CHD; variable
Neuronal ceroid lipofuscinosis	Batten disease	204200	HCM
Orofacial digital syndrome type II	Mohr syndrome	252100	Variable
Short rib–polydactyly syndrome	Saldino-Noonan syndrome	263530	TGA, ECD, hypoplastic right heart
Thrombocytopenia—absent radius syndrome		274000	TOF

PS = valvular pulmonic stenosis; PPS = peripheral pulmonic stenosis; VSD = ventricular septal defect; EFE = endocardial fibroelastosis; PDA = patent ductus arteriosus; TGA = transposition of great arteries; CHD = congenital heart defect(s); ASD = atrial septal defect; HCM = hypertrophic cardiomyopathy; ECD = endocardial cushion defect; TOF = tetralogy of Fallot.

* Data from Online Mendelian Inheritance in Man (www.ncbi.nlm.nih.gov/omim).

blance to the VACTERL association, the clear mendelian nature and lack of more extensive organ system involvement of the former indicate that the two conditions do not represent a pathogenetic spectrum.

The diagnosis of Holt-Oram syndrome is most likely to be missed in a patient with an unknown or unremarkable family history, a secundum septal defect, and minimal or no thumb anomaly. In any "sporadic" case of an atrial septal defect, the patient and the parents should be carefully examined for limb malformations and the family history studied in detail. Detection of a subtle limb defect alters the recurrence risk in offspring of the proband from the empirical risk of an isolated septal defect of 3 percent to the 50 percent of an autosomal dominant trait.

Mutations in the *TBX5* gene, which is a transcriptional regulator, cause one form of Holt-Oram syndrome.[111] Different mutations have more or less effect on limb and cardiac development, which accounts for much of the interfamilial variability. Not all families with Holt-Oram syndrome are linked to this locus at 12q2, so at least one additional gene can cause this spectrum of defects.[112, 113]

ELLIS–VAN CREVELD SYNDROME (Fig. 56–6). This rare autosomal recessive chondrodysplasia is found among the old order Amish because of a founder effect and consanguinity. Short stature, metaphyseal dysplasia, dysplastic nails and teeth, and postaxial polydactyly are the pleiotropic manifestations in addition to congenital heart disease.[114] The last is present in more than one-half of homozygotes, and most of the defects affect the atrial septum. The majority are defects of endocardial cushion closure, including ostium primum defects of widely varying size up to a single atrium. This disorder has long been thought to be due to a yet unknown defect in the extracellular matrix, which would fit with the high frequency of endocardial cushion lesions. However, defects thought due to abnormal embryonic flow (coarctation, hypoplastic left heart, and patent ductus arteriosus) occur in about 20 percent of cases. The gene maps to 4p16 in patients of all ethnic derivations.[115] A gene of unknown function within this locus has been called

EVC, with the finding of pathological mutations in a number of patients.[115a] Ellis–van Creveld syndrome can be diagnosed prenatally by detection of polydactyly by ultrasonography.

FAMILIAL ATRIOVENTRICULAR CANAL DEFECTS. This spectrum of defects occasionally occurs in an autosomal dominant pattern in families and is unassociated with features in other systems. Because the cardiac defect is suggestive of that in Down syndrome, linkage to chromosome 21 markers was pursued, to no avail. In a large kindred that showed variable expression of nonsyndromic atrioventricular canal defects, analysis of shared markers among those clearly affected identified a region on chromosome 1 (1p31–p21) that must harbor a gene that effects susceptibility to failure of closure of the endocardial cushions.[116]

VENTRICULAR SEPTAL DEFECT. This malformation does not seem to be inherited as an isolated mendelian malformation, and no syndromes include it as a common, isolated manifestation.

SUPRAVALVULAR AORTIC STENOSIS. This congenital lesion, which may be asymptomatic and detected long after birth because of an ejection murmur, occurs in at least three settings. It can be a sporadic anomaly, a component of Williams syndrome, or an autosomal dominant trait associated with peripheral pulmonic stenoses and a diffuse arteriopathy.

Williams syndrome is usually sporadic but, in more instances than previously recognized, is a highly variable autosomal dominant condition. The full spectrum includes infantile hypercalcemia, abnormal (elfin) facies (see Fig. 43–35), mental deficiency, short stature, numerous peripheral pulmonic stenoses, and supravalvular aortic stenosis.[117–119] Although patients usually survive the problems of infancy and show catch-up growth, progressive problems of joint contractures, genitourinary and gastrointestinal dysfunction, hypertension, and psychosocial adjustment define the long-term prognosis.[120–122]

Supravalvular aortic stenosis (SVAS) is due to heterozygosity for a mutation in tropoelastin (discussed later). Because elastic fibers are

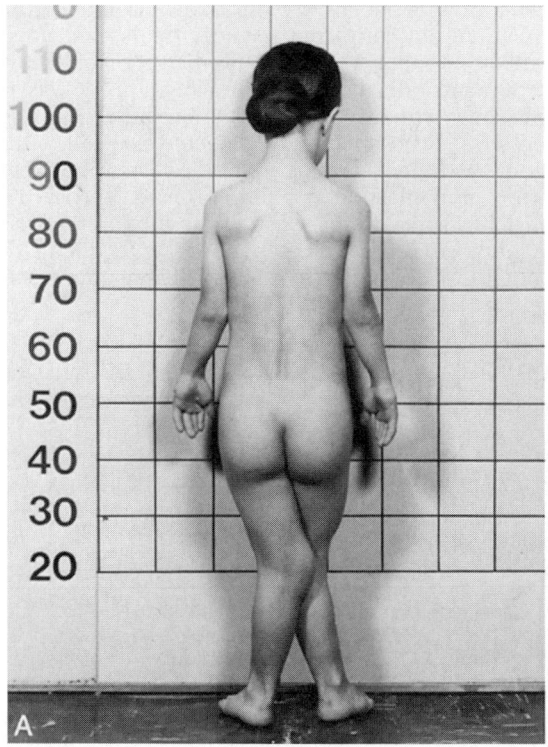
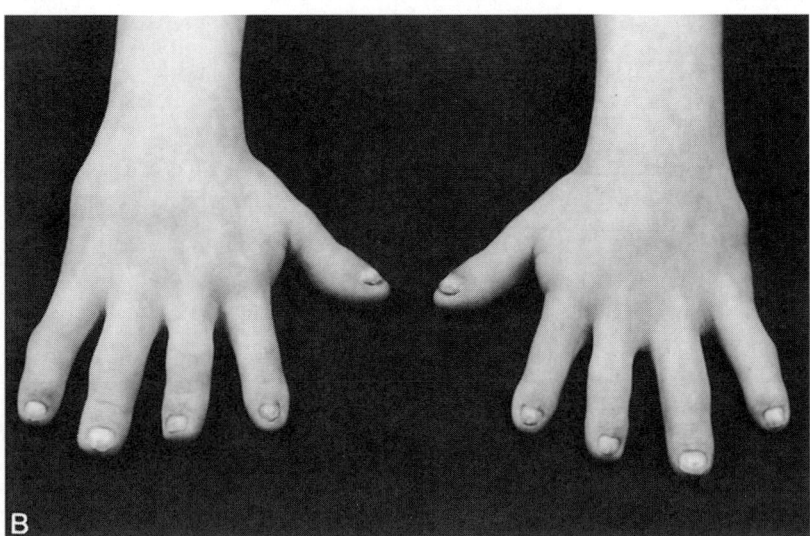

FIGURE 56–6. Ellis–van Creveld syndrome in a young woman. *A,* Note short stature, joint contractures at the elbows, and marked genu valgum. *B,* The fingers are short and the nails dysplastic. Note the protuberances along the ulnar edges of the hands where sixth digits were amputated.

intrinsic to the media of elastic and muscular arteries, a diffuse, progressive arteriopathy develops, with thickening of the wall and reduction of the lumen. The natural history of the arterial disease is just emerging as patients with Williams syndrome live longer and are monitored prospectively.[123] A predisposition to cerebrovascular disease seems certain.[124, 125]

Virtually all patients with Williams syndrome who have been tested have a deletion of the long arm of chromosome 7.[126, 127] Those with SVAS have a deletion that involves the tropoelastin locus. The crucial gene(s) involved in the rest of the Williams phenotype lie telomeric to the tropoelastin locus; considerable effort is currently being directed at identifying these gene(s) that have a role in development of the face, in calcium metabolism, and in development of personality and cognitive capability.

Autosomal dominant SVAS is an entity distinct from Williams syndrome,[128-130] although some patients have subtle defects in personality and intelligence. Peripheral pulmonary artery stenoses may be present but rarely cause hemodynamic problems. The aortic lesion requires surgery in less than half of patients.

MITRAL VALVE PROLAPSE. (see Chap. 46). This trait is of heterogeneous cause and pathogenesis; although it has been called the most common abnormality of human heart valves.[131] MVP is equally clearly not always an abnormality.[132, 133] Here only the heritable forms of MVP are discussed. These can be classified into three groups. The first is a familial form with minimal extracardiac involvement. The second is an autosomal dominant condition that is clinically variable and at one end of its spectrum merges with Marfan syndrome; it could just as well be discussed as a heritable disorder of connective tissue. The third category is composed of the various mendelian syndromes that include MVP as a pleiotropic manifestation. In all of these categories, prolapse of the tricuspid valve is a frequent accompaniment.

The first category, which some have called MVP syndrome or familial MVP,[134] includes a condition that is centered on the mitral valve. The development of actual prolapse shows the age- and gender-dependent behavior characteristic of the idiopathic form.[134, 135] Formal genetic studies in most families confirm *autosomal dominance with variable expression*. This category has been partitioned into those patients with billowing of the mitral leaflets and those with excessive systolic mitral annular expansion; because this phenotype breeds relatively true, two distinct autosomal dominant forms may exist.[136] The cause(s) of these entities is unknown. Moreover, when and how the phenotype of this condition can be distinguished from the sporadic cases of MVP and the cases with obvious evidence of a systemic disorder of connective tissue are unclear. The only consistent extracardiac manifestations are excessive arm span in women and relatively low body weight and systolic pressure.[137, 138] Susceptibility to myxomatous degeneration of all cardiac valves can be inherited as an X-linked trait that maps to Xq28.[139]

Many clinical geneticists and cardiologists have referred patients with a suspicion of Marfan syndrome (see p. 1983) or Ehlers-Danlos syndrome (see p. 1986). Some of these patients do not meet minimal diagnostic criteria for a recognized connective tissue disorder[140, 141] but clearly have extracardiac features consistent with a defect of the extracellular matrix described later. MVP is commonly but not always present; when it is and when evidence of a systemic abnormality of connective tissue is lacking, the patient should be considered to have the condition described in the preceding paragraph, what some call primary MVP.[142] The clinical spectrum of the patients with syndromic MVP includes abnormal striae atrophicae, excessive arm span and leg length, joint hypermobility, pectus excavatum, scoliosis, reduction in thoracic kyphosis ("straight back"), myopia, and mild aortic root dilatation.[143] Aortic dilatation beyond 3 SD above the mean for body surface area, aortic dissection, ectopia lentis, or a family history of any of these three features *removes* a patient from this category. For the remainder of patients, the acronym MASS phenotype, for *m*itral *v*alve, *a*orta, *s*kin, and *s*keletal, describes what cer-

tainly is a heterogeneous grouping of patients and families. The aorta is mentioned specifically because of the appropriate concern that progressive dilatation and dissection will occur; in fact, neither has been the case, although prospective evaluation has been unsystematic. Many of the associations between MVP and deformity of the thoracic cage and spontaneous pneumothorax are explained by the MASS phenotype.[144]

Finally, as described later, MVP frequently accompanies Marfan syndrome, several of the Ehlers-Danlos syndromes, and cutis laxa and occurs more often than expected in osteogenesis imperfecta, Larsen syndrome, pseudoxanthoma elasticum, and other mendelian syndromes (Table 56–10). In addition, occasional families with otherwise unclassified heritable disorders of connective tissue have prominent involvement of the mitral apparatus, with myxomatous deterioration, calcification, or both.[145]

NOONAN SYNDROME. Among the pleiotropic mendelian syndromes that have frequent cardiovascular involvement, Noonan syndrome is important because of its relatively high prevalence and clinical variability. This autosomal dominant condition has been called the male Turner syndrome in the past because of the short stature, cubitus valgus, neck webbing, congenital lymphedema, and congenital heart defects that coexist in the 45,X Turner syndrome. However, Noonan syndrome is distinct, not simply because both men and women are affected. Patients with Noonan syndrome often have an unusual deformity of the sternum, mental dullness, hypertelorism, ptosis, and cryptorchidism.[146] The cardiovascular defects, although widely varied, do not include an increased incidence of coarctation of the aorta. Because of the dysmorphism of the facies and the cardiac involvement, Noonan syndrome is often classified, along with William, leopard, King, and Watson syndromes, as a cardiofacial syndrome.

The entire phenotype of Noonan syndrome is highly variable, and affected persons can escape clinical problems (or accurate diagnosis) even if they have obvious manifestations.[147] Similarly, a wide range of cardiovascular involvement can occur. *Valvular pulmonic stenosis* was the first defect identified, and Noonan syndrome should always be considered in a patient with this lesion.[148] The valve cusps are thickened and dysplastic, even in the absence of hemodynamic compromise. Obstruction to right-sided flow can also occur in patients with Noonan syndrome because of pulmonary artery hypoplasia or infundibular subvalvular changes. The latter finding reflects a generalized predisposition to hypertrophic cardiomyopathy, often asymmetrical, that can affect either ventricle.[149] *Atrial septal defect* occurs in about one-third of patients, usually in association with pulmonic stenosis.

▼ **TABLE 56–10. CARDIOVASCULAR DEFECTS ASSOCIATED WITH PRENATAL EXPOSURE TO TERATOGENS**

TERATOGEN	CARDIOVASCULAR ABNORMALITIES*
Ethanol	~50% have CHD: VSD (~50% close spontaneously), TOF, ASD, ECD, absence of a pulmonary artery
Hydantoin	~10% have CHD: VSD, ASD, PS
Lithium	<3% have Ebstein anomaly
Phenylalanine	~20% have CHD: TOF
Retinoic acid	>50% have CHD: TGA, TOF, VSD, IAA
Rubella	>50% have CHD: PDA with or without ASD, VSD, PPS, IAA
Trimethadione	~50% have CHD: complex combinations most frequent (involving VSD, ASD, PDA, AS, PS), VSD, TOF
Valproic acid	>50% have CHD: left- and right-sided flow lesions: CoA, HLH, ASD, VSD, pulmonary atresia
Vitamin D	Supravalvular aortic stenosis is the cardinal manifestation; PPS
Warfarin	~10% have CHD: PDA, PS; rarely, intracranial hemorrhage.

CHD = congenital heart defect(s); VSD = ventricular septal defect; TOF = tetralogy of Fallot; ASD = atrial septal defect; ECD = endocardial cushion defect; PS = valvular pulmonic stenosis; TGA = transposition of great arteries; IAA = interrupted aortic arch; PPS = peripheral pulmonic stenosis; PDA = patent ductus arteriosus; AS = aortic stenosis; CoA = coarctation of aorta; HLH = hypoplastic left heart.

* Among patients with the full clinical spectrum associated with each teratogen; cardiovascular defects listed in decreasing order of prevalence.

Ventricular septal defects and patent ductus arteriosus each occur in about 10 percent. Congenital anomalies of coronary arteries are occasionally and unexpectedly found during evaluation of more obvious defects. The electrocardiogram often shows left anterior hemiblock and a deep precordial S wave, a pattern not common in pulmonic stenosis of other causes.

Lymphatic dysplasia, especially of the lower limbs, is common but causes clinical difficulties in less than 20 percent.[146] Although evidence of lymphedema often disappears during childhood, chylothorax and a protein-losing enteropathy represent the severe end of the spectrum.[150]

Noonan syndrome shares features with other cardiofacial syndromes, and in sporadic cases (which account for 50 percent of Noonan syndrome) diagnosis can be difficult. All are *autosomal dominant,* so genetic counseling is somewhat easier. Affected males have reduced reproductive capabilities because of testicular abnormalities. Susceptibility to malignant hyperthermia can be detected by family history, elevated skeletal muscle creatine kinase levels, or muscle biopsy. Despite the relatively high frequency of Noonan syndrome, estimated to be as great as 1 per 1000, neither its cause nor its pathogenesis is clear. One gene has been mapped to 12q24.2–q 24.31, but interlocus genetic heterogeneity is likely.[151, 152] Intriguing issues that may shed light on these uncertainties are the overlap in phenotype with type I neurofibromatosis[153, 154] (the gene for which is on chromosome 17), and the frequent coexistence of Noonan syndrome and deficiency of coagulation factor XI.[155]

Teratogenic Effects

A teratogen is any agent that adversely affects embryonic or fetal development, such as infectious vectors, radiation, drugs, and other chemicals (see Table 56–10).[156] Teratogenic effects on the cardiovascular system are considered in this chapter for several reasons: First, the phenotypes are often reminiscent of those due to chromosomal aberrations and single-gene mutations. Second, clinical geneticists and dysmorphologists are involved in diagnosing, managing, and investigating both teratogenic and genetic syndromes. Finally, how the organism responds to an encounter with a potential teratogen is largely determined by its genome. The entire field of ecogenetics and part of pharmacogenetics are concerned with these issues.

The abilities to resist disruption of normal human embryogenesis and development involve systems quite distinct from physiological homeostasis and related only in part with developmental homeostasis. Genetic susceptibilities to teratogens can be illustrated by diverse mechanisms: reduced or inaccurate repair of radiation-induced DNA damage; enhanced receptiveness to viral entry or replication; immune deficiencies that prevent inactivation of infectious vectors or maintenance of immunity; slow inactivation of a compound that exerts a direct deleterious effect; or rapid conversion of an inoffensive drug to a teratogenic metabolite. These types of hereditary variation may be determined by single genes, with susceptibility inherited as a mendelian trait, or by many genes, each of small effect. Either situation can account for the well-known fact that only a fraction of pregnancies exposed to a given agent are affected adversely. Variation in dose and timing of exposure also confound interpretation of epidemiological and family data. It is not surprising, then, that the actual appearance of the abnormal phenotype is not amenable to traditional pedigree analysis. Rather, examination of the biochemical susceptibilities have proved, and will continue to prove, more enlightening.

Some teratogens, such as *warfarin,* have a clear action that explains how the pleiotropic manifestations emerge. The action of other teratogens, such as alcohol, is obscure. Finally, in some teratogenic syndromes, such as that in offspring of women with diabetes mellitus, the actual offensive agent is unclear, and numerous pathogenetic mechanisms seems to pertain.[157, 158] Regardless of cause and pathogenetic mechanism, the phenotypes of many teratogens often share manifestations, especially prenatal growth retardation, abnormalities of the craniofacies, and mental retar-

dation.[159] The following syndromes have prominent consequences on the cardiovascular system.

FETAL ALCOHOL SYNDROME. Ethanol is the most common teratogen to which the human embryo and fetus are exposed. The period of greatest vulnerability is the first trimester, and the risks are clearly related to the amount of alcohol consumed; the risk of the fetal alcohol syndrome's occurring in an offspring of a chronic alcoholic woman is 30 to 50 percent. The features are highly variable and include growth retardation, mild to moderate mental retardation, hyperactivity, short palpebral fissures, a smooth philtrum with a thin upper lip, and small distal phalanges.[160, 161] Congenital heart defects occur in more than one-half of children with the full spectrum of the phenotype; ventricular septal defects are most common and often insignificant, but atrial septal defects, tetralogy of Fallot, and aortic coarctation can occur.

FETAL HYDANTOIN SYNDROME. Virtually all antiseizure medications can affect the fetus. Hydantoin was the first to be identified as a teratogen. The risk to the fetus depends in part on the genotype of the fetus; defects in arene oxidase predispose to the full syndrome.[162, 163] The features include prenatal and postnatal growth retardation, mild mental retardation, a broad face with a short nose, short distal phalanges with small nails, and hip dislocation. Cardiovascular defects, which are an inconstant part of the syndrome, include septal defects, right- and left-sided flow defects, and a single umbilical artery.

RETINOIC ACID EMBRYOPATHY. Isotretinoin was not recognized as a teratogen until after it was licensed for the treatment of acne. The vulnerable period extends from the first week through the fourth month of gestation. Isotretinoin increases the risks of miscarriage and stillbirth. The phenotype includes anomalies of the craniofacies and gross neuroanatomical disruption. Cardiovascular defects are common and emphasize various conotruncal malformations.[164] Liveborn infants often succumb to the cardiac and brain anomalies. Although the mechanism of action is not certain, vitamin A derivatives such as retinoic acid function as *morphogens* during embryogenesis, serving as signals for cell migration. The fact that the cardiovascular defects are primarily those of rotation and folding suggests disruption of a normal developmental homeostatic system.

WARFARIN EMBRYOPATHY. Coumarin-related vitamin K antagonists are usually prescribed for various cardiovascular problems to women of childbearing age and can cause diverse cardiovascular and other organ damage to the fetus. Coumarin interferes with embryogenesis directly when administered during gestational weeks 6 through 9. The most pronounced effects are on cartilage because of inhibition of enzymes of extracellular matrix metabolism. Congenital cardiac defects are perhaps increased in frequency but fit no specific pathogenetic mechanism.[165] The second pattern of coumarin effects involves exposure during the second and third trimesters and includes spontaneous abortion, stillbirth, and various central nervous system defects. The last are not due simply to intracranial hemorrhage as was once assumed.[165]

What predisposes to the adverse fetal effects of coumarin remains to be discovered. First, more than 75 percent of women who take coumarin derivatives throughout pregnancy have normal offspring; reassuring most women while identifying those at risk for adverse effects has obvious advantages. Second, placing all pregnant women on a regimen of heparin is not an acceptable solution, because heparin can cause stillbirth or premature fetal loss in about 20 percent of exposures, is not as effective as coumarin in some indications for anticoagulation, and is more trouble to administer and regulate.

MATERNAL PHENYLKETONURIA. The inborn error of metabolism phenylketonuria (PKU), produces severe mental retardation unless the phenylalanine content of the diet is markedly reduced soon after birth.[166] Deficiency of phenylalanine hydroxylase in the fetus produces no harm because fetal blood levels of phenylalanine are regulated by the heterozygous mother's enzyme. Because neonatal screening for this disease is now routine in all states, virtually all patients receive treatment and grow to adulthood with average intelligence. Many patients discontinue the rigorous dietary therapy during adolescence when the elevated phenylalanine levels have far less deleterious effects. The embryopathy occurs when a woman with homozygous deficiency for phenylalanine hydroxylase becomes pregnant and her fetus is exposed to high levels of the amino acid, which overwhelm its ability to metabolize. The result is highly predictable if the mother does not restart dietary restriction of phenylalanine for the entire gestation: moderate to severe mental retardation, prenatal and postnatal growth retardation, microcephaly, and various cardiovascular defects in 15 to 20 percent.[167] This condition can largely be prevented by effective counseling of female patients with PKU.

FETAL RUBELLA EFFECTS (see Chapter 29). About 50 percent of fetuses become infected with the rubella virus when the mother is infected during the first trimester. An infected fetus not only suffers varied and severe interference with development and organogenesis but acquires a chronic viral illness that can persist for years. The most common features of the embryopathy are mental deficiency, deafness, cataract, and cardiovascular defects. PDA is common, as are septal defects. Peripheral pulmonary stenosis and fibromuscular proliferation of medium and small arteries often improve postnatally.

CARDIOMYOPATHIES (See also Chap. 48)

Each of the three clinical categories of primary cardiomyopathy—hypertrophic, dilated, and restrictive—can be caused by mutations in single genes as judged by mendelian inheritance of a consistent phenotype in numerous families. Many other mendelian and mitochondrial disorders also cause cardiomyopathies as a secondary consequence of their basic metabolic disturbance.

Hypertrophic Cardiomyopathy

In the more than four decades since the recognition of hypertrophic cardiomyopathy as a clinical entity, many aspects of its natural history, pathology, and management have been substantially clarified.[168, 169] The phenotype is most clearly defined anatomically and histologically and consists of myocardial hypertrophy without secondary cause; cellular and myofiber disarray; myocardial fibrosis; and mediointimal proliferation of small coronary arteries. None of these features is pathognomonic; for example, myofiber disorganization is present in the normal human heart during embryogenesis and in congenital heart defects that place strain on the right-sided circulation.

About half of probands with idiopathic hypertrophic cardiomyopathy of any segment of the left ventricle have affected first-degree relatives, and in those families the phenotype is inherited as an autosomal dominant, familial hypertrophic cardiomyopathy (FHC). There is wide variability of expression within a family, in part because of age dependence of the trait.[168] Later generations of relatives in adolescence and childhood may not have developed echocardiographic evidence of hypertrophy. Hence, pedigree screening by phenotype for clinical, counseling, or investigative purposes should not be considered complete until the following criteria are satisfied: Two-dimensional echocardiography is used to ensure that segmental hypertrophy is detected; a person at risk has normal echocardiographic findings and no evidence of electrocardiographic abnormality or important dysrhythmia after about age 20; and a person of any age has left ventricular hypertrophy without any other explanation, such as hypertension or aortic stenosis.

FHC is a disease of the sarcomere, with primary defects of thick and thin filaments now defined. Mutations of at least six and perhaps more loci cause FHC (see Table 56–2). The first gene identified was the cardiac β-myosin heavy chain gene (*MYH7*). Depending on the population studied, about 50 percent of all FHC mutations occur in *MYH7,* and many mutations have been described.[169, 170] Patients with neither parent affected may also have *MYH7* mutations, suggesting that the genetic alteration occured in the egg or sperm of a parent.[171] The likelihood of germline mosaicism is strongly suggested by two sibs with FHC and the same mutation in *MHY7,* even though neither parent shows the mutation in leukocyte DNA[171a] Mutations that alter charge of the beta-myosin heavy chain generally carry a worse prognosis in terms of age of detection, electrocardiographic abnormalities, and sudden death.[172–174] Thus, defining the specific gene involved, followed by the specific mutation, has likely clinical importance.[175] However, because of the substantial technical challenges and expense of identifying the specific mutation in any given patient with FHC, genetic testing is not yet routine.[176] How the mutant protein interacts with other components of the sarcomere of both cardiac and skeletal muscle to produce the phenotype is another area of active research, as is the generation and characterization of animal models of FHC.[177]

Although intergenic and intragenic heterogeneity account for much of the interfamilial variability in the FHC phenotype, considerable variation remains among relatives who share the same mutation. Both environmental and genetic factors have impacts. A possible example of the latter is the angiotensin I–converting enzyme (ACE) genotype, with different polymorphic variants of ACE associated with more or less hypertrophy.[178]

The importance of presymptomatic and even prehypertrophy diagnosis through mutation analysis in families will become more important as improved methods of therapy evolve.[178a]

Dilated Cardiomyopathy

The prevalence of idiopathic dilated cardiomyopathy is about double that of the hypertrophic form, or about 2 to 8 per 100,000.[179–181] Although numerous occurrences of familial dilated cardiomyopathy (FDC) are reported, few investigations have been conducted of an unselected series of probands for clinical and subclinical evidence of cardiac disease.[182] Thus, it is unclear what fraction of patients with idiopathic dilated cardiomyopathy have a mendelian disease, how many have a new mutation for a mendelian disease, and how many have phenocopies of nongenetic causes. Estimates of a positive family history, which could suggest a mendelian condition or a shared environmental cause, range from 7 to 30 percent.[168, 169, 182]

Because of the risk of severe dysrhythmia in dilated cardiomyopathy, early detection of individuals with the disorder can be life saving. Two-dimensional echocardiography is a sensitive method for detecting affected relatives with subclinical disease. Individuals who have equivocal left ventricular enlargement or dysfunction can have ambulatory electrocardiographic monitoring and, if the diagnosis is still uncertain, can have serial examinations. Certainly every patient with idiopathic dilated cardiomyopathy should have a detailed family history; about 20 percent reveal an affected relative.[182] If any close relative has a history consistent with cardiomyopathy, dysrhythmia, or sudden death at a relatively young age, counseling about the risk of a familial disease and the potential benefits of pedigree screening should be offered.

The majority of instances of FDC fit autosomal dominant inheritance, but X-linked, autosomal recessive, and mitochondrial forms exist.[168, 183–185] Clinical variability characterizes virtually all pedigrees; variation in severity, clinical phenotype, and age of onset is typical.

In late 1999, the causes of most of the autosomal dominant forms of FDC were unknown. Mutation of the cardiac actin gene (*ACTC*) causes one uncommon form of FDC.[186] In some families with autosomal dominant disease, a mild proximal skeletal myopathy of type I fibers coexists with cardiac involvement.[187]

In one family, cardiomyopathy developed only in association with pregnancy.[188] Although peripartum cardiomyopathy is a well-recognized, usually sporadic disorder, its occurrence in five women in two generations suggests a hereditary predisposition.

Histological examination of myocardium generally shows nonspecific hypertrophy and fibrosis. By electron microscopy, however, mitochondria are distinctly abnormal, a finding not seen in congestive heart failure due to other causes.[189] Although various mutations of the mitochondrial chromosome can cause dilated cardiomyopathy, including of childhood onset, the inheritance pattern in most cases does not suggest maternal transmission.[185]

Some pedigrees show convincing evidence of X linkage of dilated cardiomyopathy. At least three loci have been identified. In *Barth syndrome,* cardiac involvement is associated with skeletal myopathy, proportionate short stature, and neutropenia. The cause is mutation of the (*TAZ*) gene at Xq28.[189, 190] Mutations of this gene can also cause isolated FDC and noncompaction of the left ventricle.[168, 191]

Many males with *Duchenne* and some with *Becker muscular dystrophy* develop myocardial dysfunction (see Chap. 71).[192] In the Becker form, right ventricular involvement may be unassociated with left ventricular dysfunction.[193] Deletion of exon 49 of the dystrophin gene predisposes to cardiomyopathy. This pleiotropic feature in a disease that presents as a skeletal myopathy prompted evaluation of the dystrophin locus in pedigrees with apparently isolated cardiomyopathy. Mutations in the 5' end of the dystrophin gene have been found to account for some instances of X-linked dilated cardiomyopathy.[194, 195] Why some dystrophin mutations are selectively expressed in cardiac muscle (and other in brain) is unclear.

Emery-Dreifuss muscular dystrophy (see Chap. 71) is distinguishable clinically from the Duchenne and Becker forms by absence of pseudohypertrophy of skeletal muscle, early involvement of the arms with elbow contractures, and early onset of cardiac conduction abnormalities and atrial dysrhythmia.[192, 196] Autosomal dominant and X-linked recessive forms occur. In the latter, female heterozygotes are also commonly affected, albeit more mildly than males.[197] The disease was mapped to the distal region of Xq28, and a previously unknown gene, called emerin, was found to be mutated.[198] Hearts show replacement of myocardium, especially in the atria, with fat and fibrosis. Even though the conduction system is not primarily affected histologically, sudden death is common in both hemizygous men and heterozygous women; thus, carrier detection can be life saving.

The dominant form of Emery-Dreifuss muscular dystrophy is caused by mutations in the lamin A/C gene.[199] Both emerin and lamin A/C are expressed in the nuclear membrane of skeletal and heart muscle.

An autosomal recessive form of limb-girdle muscular dystrophy with dilated cardiomyopathy has been found to be due to mutations in the gene encoding β sarcoglycan.[200] In a number of families with severe, adult-onset autosomal dominant skeletal myopathy, cardiac conduction defects, and cardiomyopathy have been due to mutations in the gene encoding the intermediate filament protein, desmin.[200a]

Restrictive Cardiomyopathy

The pathogenesis of the majority of cases of restrictive cardiomyopathy involves infiltration or replacement of the myocardium or both. The causes are varied and can be nongenetic or genetic; the latter are mostly metabolic diseases with secondary effects on the heart and are summarized in Table 56–9; some are reviewed subsequently. One form of restrictive cardiomyopathy that has primary genetic forms among many other causes is endocardial fibroelastosis. Other mutations produce restriction through pericardial constriction. Isolated pedigrees of primary myocardial fibrosis without secondary cause and leading to restrictive hemodynamics are not classifiable.[201, 202]

ENDOCARDIAL FIBROELASTOSIS (see Chap. 48). This abnormality is characterized by thickening of the endocardium, which leads to decreased compliance and impaired diastolic function. Primary forms, discussed here, are unassociated with other cardiac anomalies (see Table 56–9). In infants there is often an indolent course of failure to thrive, tachypnea, and tachycardia, until a precipitant such as an upper respiratory infection leads to rapid cardiac decompensation. Treatment of children with primary endocardial

fibroelastosis is ineffective; cardiac transplantation now offers some hope. Autopsy shows enlargement of the left ventricle and perhaps other chambers, no abnormality of lung vessels, and collapse of the left lower lobe. Histopathological study reveals extensive deposition of extracellular matrix, primarily collagen and elastic fibers, in the endocardium.

X-linked recessive inheritance is the most firmly established of the single-gene causes. Some pedigrees show mainly small, contracted cardiac chambers, whereas others have chamber dilatation; both are compatible with the functional pathophysiology described by the term "restrictive." Males are affected earlier and more severely by both forms, and death in infancy is not unusual.[203] The condition must be distinguished from X-linked dilated cardiomyopathy and Barth syndrome (see also earlier on this page).[189] Morphological abnormalities of mitochondria occur on ultrastructural studies of heart and leukocytes. Insufficient longitudinal experience is recorded to know whether females heterozygous for this mutation develop a dilated or restrictive cardiomyopathy later in life.

Several pedigrees suggestive of autosomal recessive inheritance of primary endocardial fibroelastosis were reported before the routine availability of laboratory methods to diagnose metabolic derangements, especially defects in fatty acid catabolism.[204] The occurrence of hydrocephalus, endocardial fibroelastosis, and neonatal cataracts may be due to a single gene mutation but could represent sequelae of a viral infection.[205] Endocardial fibroelastosis can be a prominent finding at autopsy in patients with autosomal dominant dilated cardiomyopathy[206], whether the endocardial changes are primary, representing yet another mendelian form of this disorder, or whether they are secondary is unclear.

Restrictive cardiomyopathy often occurs with both hemodynamic evidence of impaired diastolic filling and wall thickening; any of the conditions causing pseudohypertrophy of the myocardium can eventually exhibit restrictive pathophysiology. Hemochromatosis and the amyloidoses, both hereditary and acquired forms, are especially likely to present in this manner. Connective tissue replaces myocytes or infiltrates the interstitium in a number of conditions. Fibrosis of the myocardium may cause pseudohypertrophy, but the clinical consequences are more those of restriction. Restrictive pathophysiology often accompanies fibrosis of the myocardium, at least in the early stages. Replacement of myocytes or infiltration of the interstitium by collagen and proteoglycan occurs in various conditions, such as muscular dystrophies and disorders that predispose to ischemia due to coronary artery occlusion, such as diabetes mellitus, hemoglobinopathies associated with sickling, Fabry disease, and the mucopolysaccharidoses. Severe fibrosis may produce considerable thickening of the myocardium, or pseudohypertrophy. Finally, a number of hereditary conditions are associated with endocardial fibroelastosis (Table 56–11).

CONSTRICTIVE PERICARDITIS (see also Chap. 50). Two rare autosomal recessive disorders include fibrous thickening of the pericardium as a manifestation. In both, signs and symptoms of constrictive pericarditis develop insidiously, and treatment by pericardiotomy is life saving. One condition was first described in Finland and given the name *MULIBREY* nanism, a combination of a mnemonic from *muscle, liver, brain,* and *eye* and an archaic word for dwarfism (nanism). Growth failure from an early age is common, and growth does not improve once pericardial constriction is abated. Subsequently, more than a dozen patients, generally with consanguineous parents, have been reported from around the world.[207] The disease locus has been mapped to 17q.[208]

The *arthropathy-camptodactyly syndrome* previously had been reported because of the skeletal and rheumatological manifestations before pericardial effusion and fibrous thickening of the pericardium were recognized as manifestations.[209] The disease locus was mapped in consanguineous kindreds by homozygosity by descent to 1q25–q31, and mutations occur in the gene, *CACP*, that encodes a secreted proteoglycan.[210, 211]

▼ **TABLE 56-11. DISORDERS ASSOCIATED WITH RESTRICTIVE CARDIOMYOPATHY**

	OMIM NO.*
Primary Endocardial Fibroelastosis	
Familial endocardial fibroelastosis	226000, 305300
Faciocardiorenal syndrome	227280
Secondary Endocardial Fibroelastosis	
As a Relatively Common Manifestation	
Maternal lupus erythematosus	
Pseudoxanthoma elasticum	177850, 264800
Systemic carnitine deficiency	212140
Trisomy 18	
As a Relatively Infrequent Manifestation	
Cornelia de Lange syndrome	122470
Rubinstein-Taybi syndrome	268600
Secondary Infiltrative Cardiomyopathy	
Familial amyloidoses I and III	176300
Fabry disease	301500
Gaucher disease type I	230800
Glycogen storage disorder II	232300
Glycogen storage disorder III	232400
Hemochromatosis	235200
Mucopolysaccharidosis IH	252800
Mucopolysaccharidosis II	309900

* Data from Online Mendelian Inheritance in Man (www.ncbi.nlm.nih.gov/omim).

Cardiomyopathies Secondary to Other Causes

INBORN ERRORS OF METABOLISM. These can affect the left ventricle by various mechanisms (Table 56–12) and produce diverse anatomical, histological, and functional disturbances. The most common anatomical result is an apparent hypertrophic cardiomyopathy, which is actually *pseudohypertrophic* because the thickened walls are not due to myocardial cell hypertrophy but to cellular or interstitial infiltration by metabolites. Abnormalities of both systolic and diastolic function result, outflow obstruction may occur, and in some cases the hemodynamic characteristics resemble a restrictive cardiomyopathy. The offending metabolite may be an incompletely degraded macromolecule such as glycogen (*glycogen storage disorder II* [Pompe disease] and *glycogen storage disorder III*), proteoglycan and glycosaminoglycan (*mucopolysaccharidoses I, III, IV, VI, and VII*), sphingolipid (*Fabry disease, Tay-Sachs disease, Farber disease, Refsum disease, and Gaucher disease*), glycoprotein (*fucosidosis and mannosidosis*), and amyloid (*familial amyloidoses I and III*) or a small molecule such as iron in *hemochromatosis*. Some of these disorders are discussed later. True myocardial hypertrophy occurs as a part of mendelian syndromes, such as *Noonan syndrome, von Recklinghausen neurofibromatosis*,[212] and *leopard syndrome*,[213, 214] and monogenic errors of metabolism, notably those producing *hyperthyroidism* and *pheochromocytoma*. Any of the mendelian disorders that cause hypertension may, over time, produce true myocardial hypertrophy.

Dilated cardiomyopathy often results from inborn errors of energy production, especially fatty acid metabolism. Various disorders associated with *carnitine deficiency, mitochondrial* and *peroxisomal dysfunction*, and *muscle dysfunction* can present with symptoms of congestive heart failure or dysrhythmia.

PRIMARY DISORDERS OF RHYTHM AND CONDUCTION

Virtually every dysrhythmia and conduction abnormality has been reported to occur in relatives.[215, 216] For example, *familial disturbance of conduction* occurs, without evident cause, at the sinus node,[217, 218] atrioventricular node,[219, 220] and bundle branches.[221, 222] However, understanding the genetics of cardiac electrophysiology has been hampered by several characteristics of this extensive literature: Most families have been small, so that mode of inheritance, or even whether the inheritance is mendelian, is uncertain; many of the families show a mixture of different defects, partly because the disease is progressive[223, 224]; and some specific conduction defects are associated with hereditary myocardial diseases, such as familial cardiomyopathy,[168, 225] atrial cardiomyopathy,[226] and familial amyloidosis.[227] As noted earlier, there seems to be genetic control of normal electrical conduction, so it would not be surprising to find mutations in single genes that produced clinically important disturbance.

Several important causes of complete heart block, although not mendelian, nonetheless involve genetic factors. The association between rheumatic diseases and heart block was clearly established when the offspring of mothers with acquired disorders of connective tissue, especially lupus erythematosus, were found to have complete heart block.[228-230] Many examples of "autosomal recessive" congenital heart block represent this familial but nonmendelian etiology. The risk is not related to severity of the maternal disease but is highest in children of women with antibodies to ribonucleoprotein (anti-Ro[SS-A])[231] and at least one allele for HLA-DR3.[232] Thus, it may be the maternal genotype that determines susceptibility to inflammation of the fetal heart at vulnerable periods, such as gestational weeks 3 to 4, when the atrioventricular node is forming. Also, genetic susceptibility to inflammation of the atrioventricular node of patients themselves is suggested by the relatively high association of HLA-B27 in adults requiring permanent pacemakers[233]; not all of these patients have overt evidence of HLA-B27–associated rheumatic diseases.

Familial dysrhythmia is also not uncommon.[215] Nodal rhythm,[234] ventricular irritability,[235] and tachydysrhythmia associated with accessory atrioventricular pathways[236, 237] have been reported in families. Familial atrial fibrillation has been genetically mapped to 10q22–q24.[238] In one family, three generations were affected by a syndrome of ventricular extrasystoles and tachydysrhythmias with recurrent syncope, hypoplasia of the distal toes, and hypoplasia of the mandible (Robin sequence).[239]

ARRHYTHMOGENIC RIGHT VENTRICULAR DYSPLASIA. Hereditary cardiomyopathies are another cause of familial dysrhythmia, and a notable example is arrhythmogenic right ventricular dysplasia (ARVD), an autosomal dominant condition with variable expression[240, 241] (see also Chap. 25). Although ARVD is uncommon, the familial form shows clusters of high incidence (0.4 percent) in some regions of Italy and is an underappreciated cause of life-threatening dysrhythmia.[242] The right ventricle is involved primarily in most cases, with thinning and replacement of myocardium by fat and fibrosis.[243, 243a] Dysrhythmia, usually ventricular but occasionally supraventricular, may precede signs of right ventricular dysfunction. About one-third of cases are familial, generally in an autosomal dominant pattern. At least six loci can cause ARVD (see Table 56–2).[244, 244a] Whether the pathogenesis is homogeneous or not and whether true dysplasia, degeneration (due to a metabolic defect or muscular dystrophy), or inflammation has the leading role are unclear.

LONG QT SYNDROME (see Chap. 26). Familial syncope and sudden death have long been associated with ventricular dysrhythmia, but a distinct syndrome was not recognized until Ward[245] and Romano,[246] working independently three decades ago, reported the characteristic prolonged QT interval. Subsequent investigations of numerous families have clearly established that the defect in repolarization is inherited as an *autosomal dominant*. Although a long QT_c is consistently present, other abnormalities of conduction also occur, although they may not be evident on the resting electrocardiogram.[247] Long QT syndrome is generally unassociated with systemic abnormalities, but three patients with a negative family history for long QT had syndactyly of multiple fingers and toes.[248]

► TABLE 56–12. MENDELIAN ERRORS OF METABOLISM WITH MANIFESTATIONS IN THE CARDIOVASCULAR SYSTEM

DISORDER	EPONYM OR COMMON NAME	OMIM NO.*	PATHOGENESIS	CARDIOVASCULAR INVOLVEMENT	BIOCHEMICAL DEFECT	GENE LOCUS†	ANIMAL MODEL‡
Aminoacidopathies							
Alkaptonuria	Ochronosis	203500	Deposition of homogentisic acid in connective tissue	AS; atherosclerosis			
Cystinosis, nephropathic type		219800	Lysosomal storage	Hypertension from renal failure, vascular wall thickening	?	?	Syrian hamster
Homocystinuria		236200	Unknown	Early CAD: venous thrombosis; pulmonary embolism	Cystathionine-β-synthase	CBS	
Oxalosis I	Hyperoxaluria	259900	Vascular and tissue accumulation of oxalate	Conduction defect; vascular occlusions; Raynaud's phenomenon	Peroxisomal alanine: glyoxylate aminotransferase	AGT	
Defects in Fatty Acid Metabolism							
Carnitine transport defect	Primary carnitine deficiency	212140	Lipid myopathy; defective energy generation	DCM: ECF	?	?	
MCAD deficiency		201450	Lipid myopathy; defective energy generation	DCM	Medium-chain acyl-CoA dehydrogenase	ACADM	
LCAD deficiency		201460	Lipid myopathy; defective energy generation	DCM	Long-chain acyl-CoA dehydrogenase	ACADL	
Glycogen Storage Disorders							
GSD I	Pompe	252300	Lysosomal storage	Pseudohypertrophic CM; short PR interval; ECF	α-1,4-glucosidase	GAA	Canine and bovine
GSD II	Adult acid maltase deficiency	232300	Lysosomal storage	Primarily skeletal muscle; respiratory insufficiency; cor pulmonale	α-1,4-glucosidase		
GSD III	Forbes; debrancher deficiency	232400	Intracellular glycogen accumulation fibrosis	Pseudohypertrophic CM	Amylo-1,6-glucosidase		
Phosphorylase kinase deficiency	GSD of the heart			DCM	Phosphorylase kinase		
Glycoproteinoses							
Fucosidosis, severe		230000	Lysosomal storage	Myocardial thickening	α-Fucosidase	FUCA1	
Fucosidosis, mild		230000	Lysosomal storage	Angiokeratoma	α-Fucosidase	FUCA1	
Mannosidosis		248500	Lysosomal storage	Myocardial thickening; valvular thickening; conduction disturbance	α-Mannosidase	MANB	
Aspartylglycosaminuria		208400	Lysosomal storage	Valvular thickening	Aspartylglycosylamine amino hydrolase	AGA	
Mucolipidoses							
ML II	I-cell	252500	Lysosomal storage	Same as MPS IH	Acetylglucosamine-1-phosphotransferase	GNPTA	
ML III	Pseudo-Hurler polydystrophy	252500	Lysosomal storage	Valvular thickening and dysfunction, esp. AS, AR	Acetylglucosamine-1-phosphotransferase	GNPTA	
Mucopolysaccharidoses (MPS)							
MPS IH	Hurler	252800	Lysosomal storage	Early CAD: PH and OAD → CP; valvular dysfunction, esp. MR, AR; pseudohypertrophic CM	α-L-Iduronidase	IDUA	Canine and feline
MPS IS	Scheie	252800	Lysosomal storage	Valvular dysfunction, esp. AS	α-L-Iduronidase	IDUA	
MPS IH/S	Hurler-Scheie	252800	Lysosomal storage	Same as MPS IH	α-L-Iduronidase	IDUA	
MPS II	Hunter	209900	Lysosomal storage	Same as MPS IH; less severe in mild MPS II variant	Sulfoiduronate sulfatase	IDS	
MPS III A	Sanfilippo A	252900	Lysosomal storage	Valvular thickening and occasional dysfunction	Heparin sulfate sulfatase	SGSH	
MPS III B	Sanfilippo B	252920	Lysosomal storage	Valvular thickening and occasional dysfunction	N-Acetyl-α-D-glucosaminidase	NAGLU	
MPS III C	Sanfilippo C	252930	Lysosomal storage	Valvular thickening and occasional dysfunction	Acetyl-CoA; α-glucosaminidase N-acetyltransferase	MPS3C	

Disorder	Eponym	OMIM[*]	Biochemical mechanism	Cardiac features	Enzyme/Protein	Gene[†]	Animal model[‡]
MPS III D	Sanfilippo D		Lysosomal storage	Valvular thickening and occasional dysfunction	N-Acetylglucosamine-6-sulfatase	GNS	
MPS IV A	Morquio A	253000	Lysosomal storage	Valvular dysfunction, esp. AR	Galactosamine-6-sulfatase	GALNS	
MPS IV B	Morquio B	253010	Lysosomal storage	Milder than MPS IV A	β-Galactosidase	GLB1	
MPS VI	Maroteaux-Lamy	253200	Lysosomal storage	Same as MPS IH	Arylsulfatase B	ARSB	Feline
MPS VII	Sly	253220	Lysosomal storage	Valvular thickening	β-Glucuronidase	GUSB	Mouse and canine
Sphingolipidoses							
α-Galactosidase A deficiency	Fabry	301500	Cellular accumulation of trihexosyl ceramide, esp. endothelium	Early CAD, valvular thickening and dysfunction; pseudohypertrophic CM; short PR interval; arteriolar occlusion; angiokeratoma	α-Galactosidase A	GLA	
Ceramidase deficiency	Farber	228000	Histiocytic infiltration	Nodular thickening of valves	Ceramidase	?	
Glucocerebrosidase deficiency	Gaucher, adult form	230800	Cellular accumulation of glucocerebroside	PH → CP; interstitial infiltration of myocytes by Gaucher cells; constrictive pericarditis	β-Glucocerebroside	GBA	
Miscellaneous Disorders							
Acid lipase deficiency	Wolman	278000	↑ Cholesterol; foam cell infiltration	Atherosclerosis	Lysosomal acid lipase	LIPA	
Acid lipase deficiency	Cholesterol ester storage disease	278000	↑ Cholesterol; foam cell infiltration	Atherosclerosis; PH	Lysosomal acid lipase	LIPA	
Geleophysic dysplasia		231050	Lysosomal storage	Valvular dysfunction	?	?	
Hereditary angioedema		106100	Complement and kinin activation	Angioedema	C1 esterase inhibitor ?	CINH	

CAD = coronary artery disease; DCM = dilated cardiomyopathy; ECF = endocardial fibroelastosis; CM = cardiomyopathy; AS = aortic stenosis; AR = aortic regurgitation; PH = pulmonary hypertension; OAD = obstructive airway disease; CP = cor pulmonale; MR = mitral regurgitation; GSD = glycogen storage disease.

* Data from Online Mendelian Inheritance in Man (www.ncbi.nlm.nih.gov/omim).
† Gene symbol; for chromosomal locus see Table 56–2.
‡ Naturally occurring mutants; does not include transgenic and knockout rodent models.

Long QT syndrome is genetically heterogeneous, and mutations of at least 5 loci can produce similar disorders (see Table 56–2). Each gene identified encodes a protein involved with a cation channel.[249] Most mutations in individuals with an autosomal dominant form of long QT occur in potassium channel, rather than sodium channel gene.[250] Long QT syndrome should be suspected as a cause of sudden death, especially in young people without other evident cardiovascular risk factors, and especially when the death is associated with exercise or fright.[251] A positive family history of sudden death would obviously heighten the suspicion of long QT, but in many families penetrance is reduced.[252] Use of genotype to determine unequivocally who is heterozygous for the mutation has permitted assessment of both penetrance and the reliability of electrocardiographic criteria for diagnosis.[253] Not unexpectedly, the criterion of a corrected QT interval greater than 0.44 second is good, but it is less than 90 percent sensitive and specific. Treatment with beta-adrenergic blockade or an automatic implanted defibrillator is effective. Individuals heterozygous for the mutant gene should be identified through a detailed family history, clinical assessment, and, if necessary, DNA testing, and counseled appropriately. In some instances, the nature of the mutation has prognostic implications and can be used to guide the aggressiveness of therapy.[254, 255] However, given the extensive intergenic and intragenic heterogeneity, molecular testing, especially of a person with no family history, is not warranted, given the current technology.[176]

The association of familial syncope, sudden death, and congenital deafness was codified by Jervell and Lange-Nielsen in 1957,[256] although as with most eponymous syndromes, reports of affected individuals occurred previously. As would be expected for a rare autosomal recessive condition, the parents of affected children are more likely than average to be consanguineous. The frequency of a long QT_c among deaf children is about 1 per 100, so routine electrocardiographic screening of anyone with congenital deafness is warranted. Fright and rage clearly precipitate syncope and sudden death.

Patients with this disorder are homozygous or compound heterozygotes for mutations of several of the same cation-channel genes that cause dominant long QT syndrome.[257]

DISORDERS OF CONNECTIVE TISSUE

The two broad classes of disorders of connective tissue are those due to mutations in single genes that determine or somehow affect components of the extracellular matrix and those due to extrinsic factors affecting the extracellular matrix, such as rheumatoid arthritis and systemic lupus erythematosus. The former category includes many disorders that affect the cardiovascular system. Susceptibility to so-called acquired disorders of connective tissue is, in part, determined by genes, and this specific aspect is reviewed.

Mendelian Disorders of the Extracellular Matrix

Close to 200 distinct phenotypes now compose this category, which was first defined less than four decades ago with fewer than 10 disorders.[258] Several reviews and textbooks describe the phenotypes, genetics, and causes of many of the conditions (Table 56–13).[14, 259–262]

Marfan Syndrome

This *autosomal dominant* disorder is relatively frequent (~1 per 10,000), occurs in all races and ethnic groups, and is often not diagnosed during life.[262] In light of the classical

▼ TABLE 56–13. CARDIOVASCULAR MANIFESTATIONS OF HERITABLE DISORDERS OF CONNECTIVE TISSUE

DISORDER	OMIM NO.*	CARDIOVASCULAR MANIFESTATIONS
Cutis laxa	219100	PS, PPS, CP
	123700	MVP
Ehlers-Danlos I	130000	MVP
II	130010	MVP
III	130020	MVP
IV	130050	Arterial rupture, MVP
VI	225400	MVP
VIII	130080	MVP
X	225310	MVP, aortic root dilatation
Osteogenesis imperfecta I	166200	MVP, mild aortic root dilatation
II	166210	CP, arterial calcification
III	259420	MVP
IV	166220	Aortic root dilatation
Marfan syndrome	154700	MVP, aortic root dilatation, aortic dissection
MASS phenotype	157700	MVP, mild aortic root dilatation
Pseudoxanthoma elasticum	177850	Arteriolar sclerosis, claudication, myocardial infarction, endocardial fibroelastosis

PS = valvular pulmonic stenosis; PPS = peripheral pulmonic stenosis; CP = cor pulmonale; MVP = mitral valve prolapse.
* Data from Online Mendelian Inheritance in Man (www.ncbi.nlm.nih.gov/omim).

phenotype, failure to diagnose Marfan syndrome may seem surprising; however, marked clinical variability, age dependence of all of the manifestations, and a high (~30 percent) rate of new mutation all conspire to make detection of mildly affected, young, sporadic patients challenging.[262a] Even with the discovery of the genetic and biochemical bases of the condition, the diagnosis of Marfan syndrome outside of families with the classical phenotype remains entirely clinical. Current criteria (Table 56–14) depend on the manifestations in the cardinal organ systems—the eye, the skeleton, the heart, and the aorta—and other systems, as well as the family history[141, 176] (Fig. 56–7). The presence of manifestations more specific for Marfan syndrome, such as aortic dilatation, aortic dissection in a nonhypertensive young person, ectopia lentis, and dural ectasia, clearly is more important diagnostically than features common in other connective tissue disorders and in the general population, such as scoliosis, joint hypermobility, myopia, and MVP.

The most common cardiovascular features are MVP and dilatation of the sinuses of Valsalva.[263, 264] Associated clinical problems of mitral regurgitation, aortic regurgitation, and aortic dissection account, if untreated, for most of the early mortality that results in an average age of death in the fourth and fifth decades of life.[265] Children tend to be more severely affected by mitral valve disease,[266, 267] whereas aortic problems are progressive and more likely in adolescence and beyond.

MITRAL VALVE INVOLVEMENT. MVP (see also Chap. 46) is age dependent and more common in women with Marfan syndrome. The incidence reaches 60 to 80 percent when patients are studied by two-dimensional echocardiography,[142] and the valve leaflets generally have an elongated and redundant appearance. Progression of severity, as judged by appearance or worsening of mitral regurgitation by clinical and echocardiographic criteria, occurs in at least one-quarter of patients,[268] a much higher rate than in MVP found in the general population.[133] The mitral annulus di-

▼ TABLE 56–14. DIAGNOSTIC CRITERIA FOR MARFAN SYNDROME PHENOTYPIC MANIFESTATIONS*

Skeleton
Joint hypermobility, tall stature, pectus excavatum, reduced thoracic kyphosis, scoliosis, arachnodactyly, dolichostenomelia, pectus carinatum, erosion of the lumbosacral vertebrae from dural ectasia†

Eye
Myopia, retinal detachment, elongated globe, ectopia lentis†

Cardiovascular
Mitral valve prolapse, endocarditis, dysrhythmia, dilated mitral annulus, mitral regurgitation, tricuspid valve prolapse, aortic regurgitation, aortic dissection†, dilatation of the aortic root†

Pulmonary
Apical blebs, spontaneous pneumothorax

Skin and Integument
Inguinal hernias, incisional hernias, striae atrophicae

Central Nervous System
Attention deficit disorder, hyperactivity, verbal-performance discrepancy, dural ectasia†, anterior pelvic meningocele†

If the family history is positive for a close relative clearly affected by Marfan syndrome, to make the diagnosis in the patient, a major criterion should be present as well as findings in one other system.
If the family history is negative or unknown, to make the diagnosis, the patient should have one major criterion and manifestations in two other systems.

* Manifestations are listed within each organ system in increasing specificity for Marfan syndrome, although none is completely specific; those indicated by † are the most specific and constitute major criteria.[141]

lates and contributes to the regurgitation, as do stretching and occasional rupture of chordae. About 10 percent of patients with marked prolapse have calcification of the mitral annulus. Standard treatment for chronic mitral regurgitation is indicated, but coexistent aortic root dilatation usu-

ally requires that increasing inotropy be avoided. When mitral regurgitation becomes severe enough to warrant surgical intervention, two considerations must be added to the balance: (1) Repair of the mitral apparatus is often successful and durable in Marfan syndrome.[269, 270] Repair is less easily accomplished when the cusps are extremely redundant, there is marked chordal damage, or the annulus is heavily calcified. (2) The aorta may be enlarged enough to permit concomitant repair. In Marfan syndrome, as in virtually all of the heritable disorders of connective tissue, there is an increased susceptibility to dehiscence of prosthetic mitral valves, regardless of the care taken in placing them.

AORTIC ROOT INVOLVEMENT (See also Chap. 40). The sinuses of Valsalva are often dilated at birth, and the rate of progression varies widely among patients in general and also among relatives (Fig. 56–8). Thus, predicting long-term risks of developing aortic regurgitation (which clearly is positively associated with aortic root diameter[271]), suffering aortic dissection (which is less clearly associated with diameter), or requiring aortic surgery is fraught with uncertainty. Transthoracic echocardiography is sufficient for detecting and monitoring changes in diameter, because in the absence of dissection, dilatation is limited to the proximal ascending aorta, and the rate of change is slow, measured in millimeters per year. Rare exceptions of principal dilatation of the thoracic aorta can be monitored with transesophageal echocardiography or magnetic resonance imaging. Patients with dilatation less than 1.5 times the mean diameter predicted for their body size[272] can be observed annually; as the diameter increases, more frequent evaluation is necessary. Aortic regurgitation often appears in adults at a diameter of 50 mm but may be absent at diameters of more than 60 mm.[271, 272] The risk of dissection increases with the size of the aorta and fortunately occurs infrequently below a diameter of 55 mm in the adult. Many physicians have adopted the criterion of a 50 to 55 mm maximal aortic root dimension for performing elective surgery in adult patients with Marfan syndrome, regardless of the severity of the aortic regurgitation,[270] although patients with a family history of aortic dissection should have surgery at the lower end of this range. The perioperative results of both elective and emergency repair of the aortic

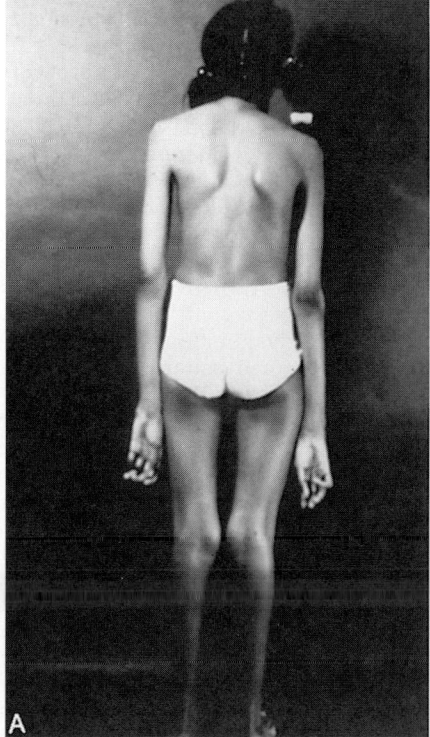
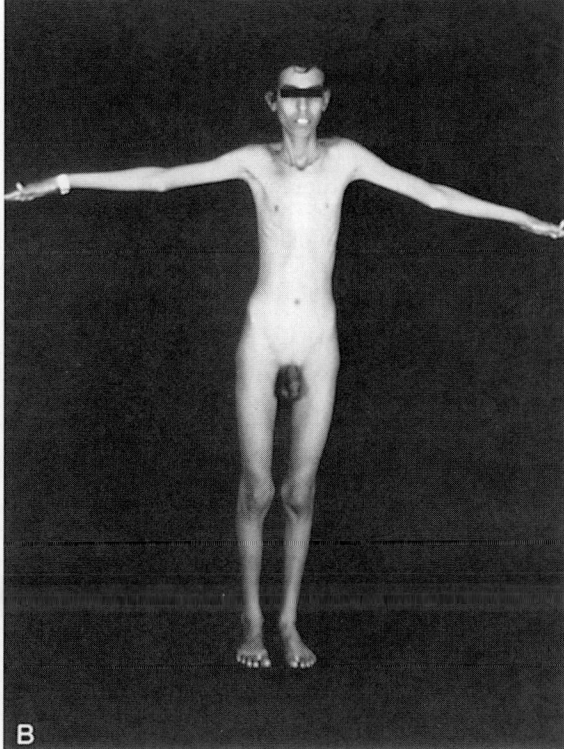

FIGURE 56–7. External phenotype of a patient with Marfan syndrome, showing long extremities and digits, tall stature, and pectus carinatum.

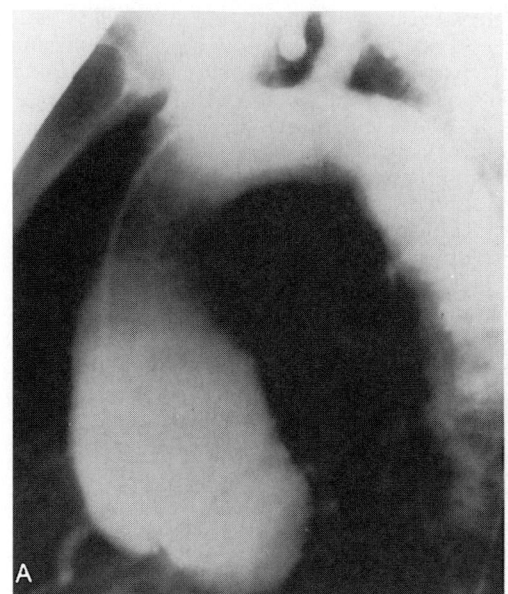 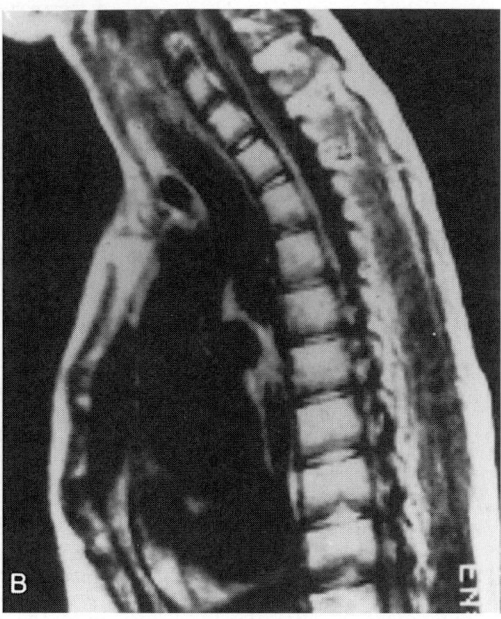

FIGURE 56-8. Dilatation of the aortic root in Marfan syndrome. *A,* Lateral angiogram of the ascending aorta showing dilatation of the sinuses of Valsalva and proximal ascending aorta and relatively normal caliber of the ascending aorta. *B,* Lateral magnetic resonance imaging of the same patient.

root have been excellent and a marked improvement from the pre–composite graft era that ended in the mid 1970s. Long-term results of operation are limited by the problems of endocarditis and anticoagulation, common to all prosthetic valves, but in the absence of chronic aortic dissection appear favorable for patients with Marfan syndrome.[270, 273, 274, 275]

Several approaches to repairing the dilated or dissected aortic root while preserving the native aortic valve have been developed.[276] Both short- and now long-term follow-up of patients with Marfan syndrome who have undergone this repair have been quite favorable.[270, 276a] The operation must be performed before the root is widely dilated and the valve commisures and cusps markedly stretched. This approach is increasingly being taken in all patients when the maximal root dimension reaches 50 mm, and it is an especially suitable procedure for women of childbearing age who want to consider pregnancy, as well as for all others in whom anticoagulation is contraindicated.

THORACIC ABNORMALITIES. Severe *pectus excavatum* may complicate cardiovascular surgery by hampering exposure of the heart by median sternotomy. For elective cardiovascular surgery, repair of the sternal deformity some months in advance permits sufficient healing of the costochondral junctions that a stable and functionally and cosmetically improved thoracic cage will facilitate further surgery and postoperative recovery.[277] Simultaneous repair of cardiac and sternal defects, although possible, is a long procedure, and intraoperative bleeding from bone can be considerable because of the anticoagulation associated with cardiopulmonary bypass.

AORTIC DISSECTION (see also Chap. 40). This complication usually begins just above the coronary ostia (type A in the Stanford scheme) and extends the entire length of the aorta (type I in DeBakey scheme). About 10 percent of dissections begin distal to the left subclavian (type B or III), but rarely is dissection limited to the abdominal aorta. Angiography, magnetic resonance imaging, and transesophageal echocardiography all have a role in the diagnosis of acute dissection in Marfan syndrome, with the capabilities and experience of the medical center and the stability of the patient important determinants of the approach. Because many acute dissections of the ascending aorta in Marfan syndrome have a stuttering course that culminates in death due to rupture or hemopericardium, rapid transfer to a facility prepared to perform immediate repair is essential.

Not all acute dissections in Marfan syndrome involve severe, tearing chest pain that radiates to the back; indeed, some extensive dissections have been occult. This experience reinforces the need for a high index of suspicion by physicians whenever a tall, nearsighted young person with a thoracic cage deformity arrives at an emergency department with vague complaints of lightheadedness, chest or abdominal discomfort, or a murmur of aortic regurgitation. Similarly, patients known to have Marfan syndrome and their close relatives need to be educated about the signs and symptoms of aortic dissection. In general, the management of acute and chronic dissection in Marfan syndrome follows standard practice, with several departures. First, all dissections of the ascending aorta should be repaired promptly, preferably with a composite graft. Second, regular evaluation with magnetic resonance imaging is important, as the diameter of any region of dissected aorta is likely to expand over time.[278, 279] Third, reduction of systolic blood pressure and administration of negative-inotropic doses of beta-adrenergic blockers should be even more strictly adhered to than in dissections without a connective tissue abnormality. In most instances, any region of the aorta should be repaired when complications of further dissection, branch vessel occlusion, or dilatation beyond about 50 mm occur. A staged approach to total replacement of the Marfan aorta is now both feasible and successful.[280]

DYSRHYTHMIAS. Some patients develop serious ventricular or supraventricular dysrhythmia. The latter often accompanies chronic mitral regurgitation, but the former may be of high grade and difficult to suppress when only MVP is present. Some patients have the syndrome of autonomic dysfunction, atypical chest pain, and palpitations seen in some patients with MVP unassociated with a flagrant connective tissue abnormality.

MANAGEMENT. Routine cardiological management of Marfan syndrome is multifaceted: regular clinical and echocardiographic examinations; routine endocarditis prophylaxis for dental and other procedures; restriction of activity from heavy weightlifting, contact sports, and any exertion at maximal capacity; and long-term beta-adrenergic blockade form the basic approach, with individual variation often appropriate. Support for the role of beta blockade comes from several prospective studies that show a reduction in the rate of aortic dilatation and the risk of aortic dissection in patients treated with negatively inotropic doses of propranolol or atenolol.[281, 282] However, short-term administration of propranolol to patients with large sinus of

Valsalva aneurysms, although reducing heart rate and peak systolic pressure, did not improve the impedance characteristics recorded in the ascending aorta. However, in the presence of studies that emphasize the importance of central pulse pressure to aortic dilation,[284] use of beta blockade seems warranted.[283]

A woman with Marfan syndrome has two concerns about pregnancy (see also Chap. 65). The first is the 50:50 risk that any child will inherit the condition; prenatal diagnosis can currently be attempted in selected situations. The second is the risk of dissection that the hemodynamic stresses of pregnancy place on the aorta. Several dozen case reports attest to the heightened incidence of dissection during the third trimester, parturition, and the first month post partum.[285, 286] However, in the majority of instances, serious aortic dilatation was present. Prospective evaluation of 21 women through 45 pregnancies confirmed our earlier recommendation that the cardiovascular risks are relatively low if the aortic diameter does not exceed 40 mm and cardiac function is not compromised[286], a view shared by others.[287]

ETIOLOGY. Marfan syndrome is caused by mutations in the gene that encodes fibrillin-1 (*FBN1*), the major constituent of microfibrils, components of the extracellular matrix that are widely dispersed and perform numerous functions.[262, 288, 289]

Microfibrils and tropoelastin form elastic fibers. Fragmentation and disorganization of elastic fibers in the aortic media have long been a histological marker (inappropriately called cystic medial necrosis) of Marfan syndrome,[263] although similar microscopic pathology occurs in familial aortic aneurysms and aging aortas of the normal population. A defect in microfibrils explains all of the pleiotropic manifestations of Marfan syndrome.[262, 290]

More than 100 distinct mutations in *FBN1*, the gene that encodes fibrillin-1, have been found in different families, and only a few have occurred, by chance, in unrelated patients.[290, 291] Because *FBN1* is such a large gene (~ 9000 nucleotides in the mRNA), finding a mutation is still not a simple matter.[176, 292] Once the mutation is identified, diagnosis in that family is straightforward. In families with several alive and cooperative affected members, linkage analysis can be used for presymptomatic and prenatal diagnosis. The use of molecular testing is confounded, however, by the discovery that autosomal dominant ectopia lentis, familial tall stature, MASS phenotype, and familial aortic aneurysm all are phenotypes found to be due to mutations in *FBN1* and are exactly the conditions clinicians are interested in excluding in their patients of questionable diagnosis.[290]

Mutations in *FBN1* have distinct effects on microfibril formation: Some affect synthesis, others secretion, and others incorporation of fibrillin-1 monomers into the extracellular matrix.[293, 294]

MITRAL VALVE PROLAPSE AND THE MASS PHENOTYPE. This heterogeneous group of conditions, described earlier (see p. 1993) likely contains large numbers of patients and families who have a defect of the extracellular matrix underlying the phenotypes. Some but not all have mutations in *FBN1*.[262, 290]

Ehlers-Danlos Syndrome

This group of heterogeneous conditions is linked by variable involvement of the skin and the joints, with hyperelasticity and fragility of the former occurring with hypermobility of the latter[261, 295] (Fig. 56–9). Mitral valve prolapse is clearly increased in frequency in most of the clinical types,[296] but aortic root dilatation is an uncommon finding.

The most serious cardiovascular problems occur in the *vascular form of Ehlers-Danlos syndrome* with spontaneous rupture of large- and medium-caliber arteries.[296a] Various defects of type III collagen are the cause of the phenotype in virtually all patients studied.[297] Analysis of collagen production by cultured skin fibroblasts should be

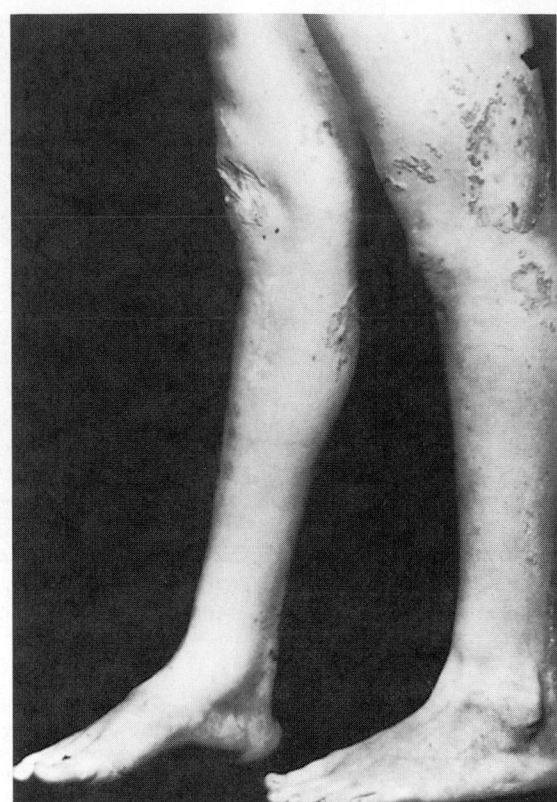

FIGURE 56–9. Legs of a patient with Ehlers-Danlos syndrome type IV who died of rupture of the subclavian artery. Note the mild joint hypermobility and the striking dermal abnormalities—elastosis perforans serpiginosa and thin, atrophic scars over areas of recurrent trauma.

used to confirm the diagnosis.[14] True aneurysms rarely form; rather, a rupture without dissection usually occurs as a catastrophic event. Most prone are the abdominal aorta and its branches, the great vessels of the aortic arch, and the large arteries of the limbs. False aneurysms and fistulas[298] may be one result in those patients who do not die of the initial rupture. Vascular surgery is difficult, as the normal-appearing vessels around the rent fail to hold sutures. As a consequence, elective surgery to repair vascular anomalies, such as false aneurysms, that are causing no immediate problem is contraindicated in most cases. The vascular form of Ehlers-Danlos syndrome is often sporadic but, when familial, is usually autosomal dominant.[298a] Prenatal diagnosis is possible by examining collagen production in amniocytes. However, pregnancy is particularly hazardous to women with this condition because of vascular rupture, although some mutations may not be as dangerous.[297, 299]

Pseudoxanthoma Elasticum (PXE)

This is a clinically variable and genetically heterogeneous disorder of unknown cause. Histopathological examination of affected tissues shows fragmentation and calcification of elastic fibers. The skin, the eyes, the gastrointestinal system, and the cardiovascular system are the organs most severely affected.[261, 300] The skin shows highly characteristic raised yellowish papules (pseudoxanthoma) overlying areas of flexural stress, such as the neck, cubital and popliteal fossae, and groin (Fig. 56–10). Breaks in the elastic lamella, Bruch membrane of the choroid, produce the funduscopic finding of angioid streaks. Gastrointestinal hemorrhage is common and potentially fatal; mucosal arterioles bleed, and because the calcified elastic fibers prevent effective vessel retraction, hemostasis is difficult. Selective arterial embolization was life saving in one instance.[301] The heart is affected in a number of ways. Endocardial fibroelastosis is common, but because primarily the atria are involved, a restrictive cardiomyopathy is uncommon. One patient with marked endocardial fibroelastosis was helped by resection of calcified elastic bands within the left ventricle.[306] Mitral valve prolapse may be increased in frequency[302, 303] but is rarely a clinical problem. Coronary artery disease with myocardial ischemia and infarction is a common cause of early death.[304, 305]

Elastic and muscular arteries, including the coronaries, develop a type of arteriosclerosis similar to Mönckeberg; progressive luminal narrowing occurs and can produce complete occlusion. This is initially most evident at the radial and ulnar arteries, where absence of pulses

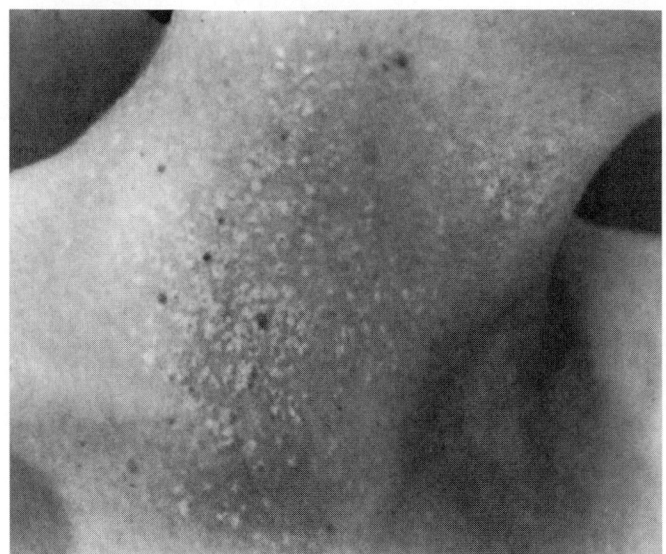

FIGURE 56–10. Skin of a young man with pseudoxanthoma elasticum. The neck is a typical location to notice the raised, yellowish papules from which the name of the condition derives.

and a positive Allen test result are noted early in the course.[304] Because narrowing progresses slowly, collaterals form, and peripheral ischemia is a late complication. Because the arterial stenoses tend to be diffuse, bypassing them often involves extensive surgery. Because of a positive association between phenotypic severity and dietary calcium intake, patients can be advised to restrict consumption of dairy products and to avoid calcium supplements.[307] Hypertension and all risk factors for atherosclerosis should be aggressively controlled.

Through linkage analysis, both the recessive and dominant forms of PXE have been mapped to the same region of chromosome 16.[308]

Genetic Susceptibility to Acquired Disorders of Connective Tissue

Genetic factors are clearly implicated in the susceptibility to many of the rheumatic disorders and to specific complications of specific conditions.[233] The cardiovascular manifestations of these disorders are particularly interesting in this regard. For example, study of HLA-DR antigen frequencies suggests that immune-response factors are involved in the pathogenesis of chronic rheumatic heart disease in blacks.[309]

INBORN ERRORS OF METABOLISM THAT AFFECT THE CARDIOVASCULAR SYSTEM

Hundreds of biochemical defects that affect human metabolism have direct or secondary impact on the cardiovascular system (see Table 56–12). Several examples are reviewed, selected for their relevance to clinical practice or their instructive lessons about pathophysiology.

Aminoacidopathies

Inborn errors of amino acid metabolism result in the accumulation of precursors and a deficit of end products, either or both of which can be detrimental.

Alkaptonuria

An intermediate of tyrosine catabolism polymerizes to homogentisic acid, which readily accumulates in the extracellular matrix.[310] Over many years, connective tissue of cartilage, heart valves, and arteries becomes increasingly abnormal. Aortic stenosis and arteriosclerosis are the cardiological sequelae.

Homocystinuria

This condition is caused by a deficiency of cystathionine beta-synthase; the pathogenesis of the pleiotropic manifestations is largely unknown.[13, 311, 312] Perhaps the amino acid sulfhydryl groups bind to collagen, fibrillin, and other macromolecules and interfere with cross-linking. The clinical features, once confused with Marfan syndrome, include tall stature, skeletal deformity, ectopia lentis, mental retardation, psychiatric disturbances, and a predilection for venous and arterial thromboses. Those patients with mutations that render the enzyme activity able to be increased by pharmacological doses of pyridoxine are less severely affected; early treatment can prevent most aspects of the phenotype.[313, 313a] Patients unresponsive to pyridoxine can be helped by a low-protein diet to reduce intake of methionine and by oral betaine, a co-factor essential for remethylation of homocysteine.

Myocardial infarction, pulmonary embolism, and stroke are the most common causes of death. The pathogenesis of the vascular complications was once thought to involve abnormal platelet function, but platelet survival in untreated patients is normal.[314] Growing evidence supports a susceptibility of heterozygotes, who have none of the external phenotype of the disease, to atherosclerosis.[315–317] Various actions of homocysteine on endothelial receptors, stimulation of smooth muscle growth, and production of extracellular matrix components are being explored for clinical relevance.[318, 319] Current therapeutic approaches are focused on maintaining physiological levels of the co-factors involved in metabolism of sulfurated amino acids—folate and vitamins B_6 and B_{12}.[320]

Disorders of Fatty Acid Metabolism

Although most organs can metabolize fatty acids when faced with hypoglycemia, only the heart depends on fatty acids as the primary source of energy generation. Thus, it is not surprising that virtually all genetic defects in fatty acid metabolism, including generalized defects in mitochondria and peroxisomes, are associated with myocardial dysfunction. Other substrates—glucose, lactate, and oxaloacetate—also generate energy in myocardial cells by entry into mitochondria and the tricarboxylic acid (Krebs) cycle. Thus, defects in conversion of pyruvate to acetyl coenzyme A and in any point along the tricarboxylic acid cycle and the respiratory chain have a major impact on myocardial energy generation. Quite likely, some sporadic and familial instances of idiopathic cardiomyopathy may represent undiagnosed or undefined metabolic disorders.

CARNITINE DEFICIENCIES. Carnitine is a required co-factor for entry of long-chain fatty acids into mitochondria and is both synthesized endogenously and available from dietary sources.[321] Deficiency of carnitine effectively blocks metabolism of long-chain fatty acids throughout the body and hepatic metabolism of ketones. Because of their relative dependence on fatty acids, muscle cells, including myocytes, suffer out of proportion to other tissue when carnitine levels are low for any reason. Cytoplasmic inclusions of lipid are characteristic findings in myocytes and hepatocytes.

Several mendelian defects produce primary or secondary carnitine deficiency. An autosomal recessive defect in carnitine palmitoyltransferase I leads to increased plasma carnitine and a skeletal muscle myopathy with little effect on the heart.[321] So-called systemic carnitine deficiency can have various causes: primary deficiency of intake, synthesis, or function, and secondary deficiency, the majority now known to be a result of defects in fatty acid metabolism. The latter group of conditions usually does not respond to pharmacological doses of carnitine.[321, 323]

Primary carnitine deficiency usually presents in infancy with hypoglycemia, coma, and congestive heart failure due to dilated cardiomyopathy. In the few cases reported, problems largely resolve with carnitine treatment; they can be prevented from recurring by oral supplementation with L-carnitine.[323, 324] Primary systemic carnitine deficiency is due to a defect in carnitine transport, which leads to excessive urinary loss and which affects muscle but not liver.[322] Thus, muscle cells still may be relatively deficient in carnitine, despite supplementation, and long-term prognosis is uncertain.

DEFECTS OF BETA-OXIDATION. At least 20 steps are involved when a molecule of free fatty acid leaves the plasma, enters beta-oxidation in the mitochondrion, and generates electrons and acetyl-CoA.[321] At each turn of the oxidation spiral, two carbons are removed from the fatty acid, and the enzymes involved in this step are specific for substrates of only certain chain length: long-chain, medium-chain, and short-chain acetyl-CoA dehydrogenases, or LCAD, MCAD, and SCAD. Thus far, patients with defects in nine of the steps have been characterized.

Patients homozygous for these generally autosomal recessive disorders develop episodic hypoketotic hypoglycemia, usually associated with fasting or intercurrent illness. Deficiency of MCAD is the most common cause and occurs in about 1 of every 7000 newborns in the United States. Hypoglycemic crises can rapidly progress to coma and death, and 50 to 60 percent of affected infants die in the first 2 years of life.[325] Because infants between episodes or before a fatal crisis appear normal, MCAD deficiency accounts for a proportion of so-called sudden infant deaths.[326] Histopathological examination shows microvesicular accumulation of fat in cardiac and skeletal muscle. One mutation in MCAD (A985G) accounts for a large percentage of all alleles that predispose to this lethal disorder, and various approaches to newborn screening are being investigated.

MITOCHONDRIAL MYOPATHIES. All of the enzymes of fatty acid oxidation are encoded by genes located on nuclear chromosomes, but the components of the electron transport chain are encoded by both nuclear and mitochondrial genes. Several syndromes involving various types of myopathies have been shown to be due to mutations in the mitochondrial chromosome.[10, 11] The *Kearns-Sayre* syndrome includes pigmentary degeneration of the retina, ophthalmoplegia, and cardiomyopathy as its most prominent manifestations; all of the affected tissues rely nearly exclusively on oxidative phosphorylation for energy generation.

The *MELAS* syndrome (*m*yopathy, *e*ncephalopathy, *l*actic *a*cidosis, and *s*trokelike episodes) is due to mutations in mitochondrial transfer RNA genes.[328, 329] In addition to the features that define the acronym, hypertrophic cardiomyopathy and diffuse coronary angiopathy are common. Various other mtDNA mutations are associated with hypertrophic or dilated cardiomyopathy.[185, 330]

Variations in both the actual mutations and the fraction of abnormal mitochondria in the cells of the different organs (heteroplasmy) account for many of the clinical differences in phenotype, severity, and age of onset among patients with this disorder. Inheritance is maternal for patients with mitochondrial mutations; apparent autosomal recessive and dominant inheritance may indicate that mutations of nuclear genes can impair electron transport similarly to mitochondrial mutations. Some patients have been treated with moderate success over the short term with coenzyme Q[331] and with cardiac transplantation in one case.[332]

Glycogenoses

Three of the glycogen storage disorders affect cardiac muscle.

GLYCOGEN STORAGE DISEASE II. This autosomal recessive condition is due to deficiency of the lysosomal enzyme α-1,4-glucosidase and results in the lysosomal accumulation of glycogen in most tissues. Several allelic variants occur.[333] The condition with infantile onset is called *Pompe disease,* and cardiac involvement is profound.[334] Infants with Pompe disease appear well initially but soon fail to thrive and develop hypotonia, tachypnea, and tachycardia; the disease progresses during the first year to irreversible congestive heart failure and death due to pneumonia or cardiopulmonary failure. Auscultation typically reveals no murmurs until late in the course when obstruction develops, and hypoglycemia does not appear because the nonlysosomal pathway of glycogen catabolism is intact. The diagnosis is suggested by massive cardiomegaly on examination and chest radiography and by characteristic echocardiographic abnormalities of a short PR interval and markedly increased QRS voltage.[335] Echocardiography shows tremendously thickened (pseudohypertrophic) ventricles, and Doppler interrogation or catheterization may reveal subaortic and subpulmonic pressure gradients characteristic of obstructive cardiomyopathy.

Reduced diastolic function of a restrictive cardiomyopathy develops eventually, and endocardial fibroelastosis is common.[335, 336] With these findings, the diagnosis of Pompe disease is virtually certain, but it can be confirmed by analysis of α-1,4-glucosidase activity in cultured fibroblasts. Prenatal diagnosis is possible by enzymatic assay of amniocytes. Treatment is supportive, but cardiac transplantation could correct the cardiac problem; unfortunately, involvement of other organs, including the lungs, liver, and skele-

tal muscle, might eventually prove just as serious as the cardiomyopathy. Bone marrow transplantation might be a solution if performed early in the course. An animal model of α-1,4-glucosidase deficiency exists in cattle and develops cardiac pathology typical of human Pompe disease.[337]

Cardiomyopathy may develop in the juvenile-onset form of α-1,4-glucosidase deficiency,[338] but it is not invariable because of allelic heterogeneity. In one sibship without cardiac involvement, three brothers had extensive hepatic, skeletal muscle, and arterial smooth muscle accumulation of glycogen, and each died of rupture of a basilar artery aneurysm.[339] The adult-onset form usually presents with insidious onset of respiratory insufficiency, and clinically important cardiac disease is rare.[340]

GLYCOGEN STORAGE DISEASE III. The striking clinical variability in phenotype associated with deficiency of α-1,4-glucosidase is due in large part to the extensive array of mutations that occur at the *GAA* locus.[341] This autosomal recessive deficiency of amylo-1,6-glucosidase results in infantile- and juvenile-onset syndromes of muscle weakness, wasting, and hepatomegaly. Clinical cardiac disease is not common, although both cytoplasmic (nonlysosomal) and intermyofibril glycogen is routinely present in the heart and causes pseudohypertrophy and increased voltage on electrocardiography. The diagnosis has been established by enzymatic assay of an endomyocardial biopsy specimen.[342-344]

GLYCOGEN STORAGE DISEASE IV. This is caused by deficiency of α-1,4-glucan: α-1,4-glucan 6-glycosyl transferase. It usually causes a fatal disorder of early childhood characterized by hepatic failure; although extensive deposition of polysaccharide occurs in the heart, death intervenes before cardiac symptoms appear. In the most severe form, the fetus has hydrops and generalized muscle degeneration.[345] As with all of the glycogen storage diseases, extensive allelic heterogeneity results in milder forms of the classic disorders. Patients with diagnosis later in adolescence tend to have more severe cardiomyopathy.[346, 347] Liver transplantation has been life saving in some cases and has, somewhat surprisingly, resulted in a reduction of glycogen deposits in the heart and skeletal muscles.[348, 349]

CARDIAC PHOSPHORYLASE KINASE DEFICIENCY. Few cases of this enzyme deficiency have been reported: deposition of glycogen is confined to the heart, which may be massively thickened and enlarged, and leads to early death.[350, 351]

GLYCOPROTEINOSES. This group of disorders results in the lysosomal accumulation of various compounds that cannot be catabolized further because of the specific enzyme deficiency (see Table 56–12). Some have prominent cardiac pathology, generally of pseudohypertrophy and valvular thickening, which present with congestive failure, valvular dysfunction, conduction defects, or dysrhythmia.[352]

Hematological Disorders (See Chap. 69)

HEMOCHROMATOSIS. This autosomal recessive disorder of unknown cause results in iron deposition in many tissues, including the myocardium. The manifestations include diabetes mellitus, skin hyperpigmentation, hypogonadism, hepatic failure with cirrhosis, hepatoma, and congestive heart failure; severity is less, and age of onset later in women because of the autophlebotomy provided by menstruation.[353] The cause of the most common form of hereditary hemochromatosis is a gene, *HFE,* that is closely linked to the major histocompatibility locus on chromosome 6. One specific mutation accounts for a large proportion of the mutant alleles among whites.[354] Fully 10 percent of the population is heterozygous for a hemochromatosis mutation, suggesting that at an incidence of 2 to 3 per 1000, this disease is underdiagnosed. This frequency has given rise to interest in population screening by molecular genetic techniques, but for now traditional clinical laboratory approaches are appropriate.[355] Diagnosis depends on finding increased serum iron, ferritin, and, especially, transferrin saturation in the absence of any obvious cause of excessive iron intake.[356]

Cardiac involvement often appears first as dysrhythmia or congestive heart failure. Dysrhythmia, conduction abnormalities, and low QRS voltage are typical electrocardiographic findings; cardiomegaly is seen on chest radiography, and a dilated cardiomyopathy with reduced systolic function can be documented on echocardiography.[357, 358] Occasional patients have a restrictive pattern on cardiac catheterization.[359]

Treatment by repeated phlebotomy is most effective if begun before organ damage is irreversible. If a patient with congestive heart failure has not yet developed serious compromise in other organs, cardiac transplantation may be contemplated, as may combined heart-liver replacement.

HEMOGLOBINOPATHIES (See also Chap. 69). *Sickle cell disease* and other hemoglobinopathies associated with sickling can produce ischemia and infarction in numerous organs by occlusion of small vessels[360]; however, the heart is relatively resistant.[361] Nonetheless, the combination of chronic hypoxemia and anemia produces a sustained high-output state that leads to congestive heart failure in many adults. The cardiovascular system can also be compromized by systemic hypertension due to renal infarction, pulmonary embolism and infarction (the chest pain of which often causes concern about myocardial ischemia), pulmonary hypertension,[362] stroke,[360] and hemosiderosis from chronic transfusions.

In addition to a hyperdynamic congestive failure, iron overload is the principal risk to the myocardium in other causes of decreased erythrocyte production *(thalassemias)* and increased erythrocyte consumption *(hemolytic anemias)* requiring repeated transfusions. Treatment with daily injections of deferoxamine can, if begun early, prevent the development of severe cardiac and hepatic disease.[363] Development of an oral iron chelator would greatly improve compliance and efficacy. Various approaches to management of sickle cell disease, including hydroxyurea, show promise.[364] Combined heart-liver transplantation has been used in a case of end-stage organ failure with homozygous beta-thalassemia.[365]

Mucopolysaccharidoses and Disorders of Targeting Lysosomal Enzymes

Many of the specific disorders in these two groups share phenotypical manifestations and are caused by various defects in the ability of lysosomes to catabolize proteoglycan and glycosaminoglycan. Short stature, progressive coarsening of facial features, a skeletal dysplasia termed dysostosis multiplex, corneal clouding, and protean effects on the cardiovascular system are common[366-370] (Fig. 56-11). Only MPS IS (Schele syndrome), the mild form of MPS IH (mild Hunter syndrome), MPS IV (Morquio syndrome), and MPS VI (Maroteaux-Lamy syndrome) have minimal or no mental impairment.

CARDIOVASCULAR MANIFESTATIONS. The cardiovascular complications (see Table 56-12), which are all progressive and usually insidious, arise from engorgement of cells and tissues with macromolecular storage material.[371] First, the ventricular walls become pseudohypertrophic, and systolic function gradually deteriorates. The electrocardiogram shows reduced QRS voltages; rarely is any conduction disturbance present. Second, coronary arteries narrow because of intimal and medial thickening.[372] Myocardial infarction is common in MPS IH and the severe form of MPS II, although the patients are usually too retarded to complain of classical symptoms, and the diagnosis is made post mortem.[373] Third, valve leaflets thicken and cause progressive dysfunction that is oddly specific for individual disorders. For example, aortic stenosis is common in MPS IS, and mitral regurgitation is frequently found in MPS IH and MPS IV. Finally, narrowing of the upper and middle airways causes obstructive apnea, chronic hypoxemia and hypercarbia, pulmonary hypertension, and eventually cor pulmonale.[374, 375]

MANAGEMENT. Treatment of children with those conditions that caused mental retardation has in the past been supportive. Increasing experience with bone marrow transplantation in many of the conditions shows that in the survivors of the transplant, somatic accumulation of mucopolysaccharide can be reduced, with clinical improvement in cardiopulmonary function.[366, 376, 377] However, improvement of central nervous system function has been marginal or absent. Nonetheless, bone marrow transplantation may have a role, especially in MPS IV and MPS VI, in which cardiopulmonary compromise can greatly shorten otherwise productive lives. Attempts at cardiovascular surgery, indeed of any procedure requiring general anesthesia, are fraught with risks of difficult intubation, hyperextension of the neck with cervical cord damage (the odontoid process is often hypoplastic), and prolonged efforts to wean from mechanical ventilation.[374]

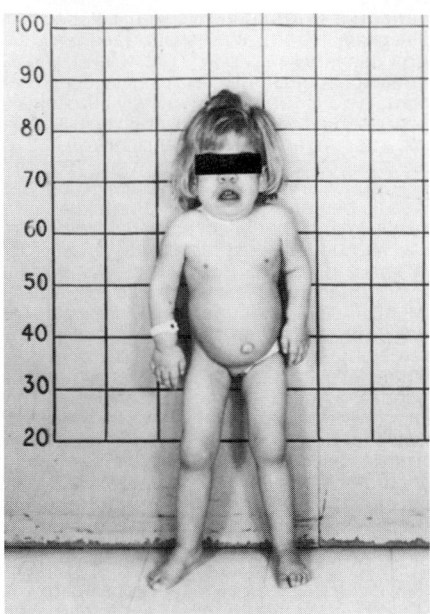

FIGURE 56-11. Hurler syndrome in a 4-year-old girl. Note short stature and coarse facial features.

Sphingolipidoses

FABRY DISEASE. This X-linked condition deserves comment because the diagnosis is often not made until adulthood, when serious end-organ damage has occurred.[378] As a result of deficiency of α-galactosidase A, ceramide trihexoside and other glycosphingolipids accumulate in lysosomes of many cells and organs, especially endothelial cells, glomerular and tubular cells of the kidneys, and the heart. Microangiopathy causes the characteristic skin lesion, angiokeratoma, and may contribute, along with primary nerve involvement, to acroparesthesias and painful crises. Proteinuria and hypertension precede renal failure, which has often led to death in males and often leads by the fourth decade to the need for long-term dialysis or renal transplantation. A successful kidney allograft does not correct the systemic metabolic defect,[379] and the disease usually progresses in other organs.[380] Infusion of purified human α-galactosidase A shows promise of reducing tissue storage of glycosphingolipid.[380a]

CARDIAC MANIFESTATIONS. Structural and functional cardiac involvement is qualitatively similar to that in the mucopolysaccharidoses. Thickening of the myocardium is pseudohypertrophy due to deposition of glycosphingolipid in lysosomes; the diagnosis has been made by endocardial biopsy during the evaluation of unexplained ventricular hypertrophy or frank obstructive cardiomyopathy.[381-384] Chronic hypertension can exaggerate left ventricular dysfunction, as can ischemia and infarction due to diffuse luminal narrowing of the coronary arteries. Echocardiography is useful for serial documentation of myocardial function.[385] Although valvular thickening and MVP are common, hemodynamically important mitral regurgitation is not.[386] The pulmonary vasculature becomes narrowed and right-sided pressures rise, but cor pulmonale is rarely a problem. The electrocardiogram often shows a shortened PR interval, increased left ventricular voltages, and dysrhythmia. Medium-sized arteries throughout the body develop luminal narrowing, with cerebrovascular disease the most common cause of death after renal failure.

Heterozygous females generally show some clinical manifestations, especially in the eyes, and at much later ages than hemizygous males develop renal, cerebrovascular, and cardiac disease.[378, 385-387] Prenatal diagnosis is possible, and a detailed family history and genetic counseling are essential whenever the disease is found. Various mutations occur in the gene for α-galactosidase A and account for much of the clinical variability.[382, 384, 388]

Familial Amyloidoses (See also Chap. 48)

Various disorders, defined initially by clinical phenotype and due to progressive accumulation of amyloid in organs and tissues, are beginning to be categorized by the underlying biochemical and genetic defects.[389] The several conditions termed familial amyloidosis with polyneuropathy and originally classified as separate autosomal dominant disorders are now known to be due to different mutations in the same gene encoding transthyretin, a thyroxine- and retinol-binding protein also called prealbumin. Although polyneuropathy dominates the early course during young adulthood, renal failure and restrictive cardiomyopathy supervene later and cause death in most cases. The age of onset, severity, and predilection for kidney and cardiac involvement are determined by the type of mutation, with males affected earlier and more severely.[390–392]

Liver transplatation can prevent progression of the disease and potentially reverse some tissue accumulation[393]; when the myocardium is severely infiltrated, combined liver-heart transplant offers the only hope.

NEUROMUSCULAR DISORDERS (See Chap. 71)

CARDIAC TUMORS (See also Chap. 49)

The three most common tumors that originate in the heart are myxomas, fibromas, and rhabdomyomas. All occur as part of hereditary syndromes and as sporadic events. The new occurrence of any of these tumors, especially in a child, may represent the first manifestation of a systemic condition, so a detailed general examination and family history are always indicated.[394–397] For example, 51 to 86 percent of cardiac rhabdomyomas occur because of tuberous sclerosis.[398, 398a] Tumors due to hereditary disorders tend to be multiple and to recur after resection. An example is the NAME syndrome (for *n*evi, *a*trial myxoma, *m*yxoid neurofibromata, and *e*phelides; the acronym ignores the numerous endocrine tumors) also called Carney complex, in which many myxoma can occur throughout the myocardium.[399–404]

INHERITED DISORDERS OF THE CIRCULATION

Hereditary Hemorrhagic Telangiectasia

This autosomal dominant condition, often called Osler-Rendu-Weber disease, is more common than appreciated. Because of marked intrafamilial and interfamilial variability, the condition may remain undiagnosed in affected patients for years despite mild manifestations.[405, 406, 406a] Mucocutaneous telangiectases, 0.5 to 3 mm in diameter, occur on the tongue, lips, and fingertips most commonly. Small and moderate-sized arteriovenous fistulas occur in the nose, leading to recurrent epistaxis, in the gastrointestinal system, where they cause recurrent bleeding and occult anemia, and in the lungs, resulting in hypoxemia, hemoptysis, polycythemia, clubbing, paradoxical embolization through the right-to-left shunt, and a hyperdynamic circulation. Less common sites of vascular malformations are the brain,[407, 408] liver,[409] and the kidneys.[410] Diffuse ectasia of the coronary arteries was noted in one patient.[411] and hemorrhagic pericarditis with tamponade in another.[412] Bleeding is facilitated, even in the presence of normal platelet function and clotting function, because of the lack of resistance channels in the telangiectatic lesions.[413]

Patients with hereditary hemorrhagic telangiectasia (HHT) and their close relatives should be screened for pulmonary arteriovenous malformations through auscultation, arterial blood gas analysis, and chest radiography. A low PaO$_2$ should prompt consideration of angiography and therapeutic balloon occlusion of the feeding arteries of any sizable malformation to prevent systemic embolization, especially to the brain.[414] In a few patients, epistaxis and gastrointestinal blood loss have been reduced by antifibrinolytic therapy with danazol or aminocaproic acid.[415–417]

Controlled trials of various approaches to chronic management, taking into account clinical and genetic variables, are sorely needed.

At least three genes are capable of causing HHT, and two have been mapped, to 9q33–q34 and to 3p22. The former locus encodes a transforming growth factor-beta–binding protein called endoglin, and various mutations segregate with HHT in different families.[418] The other locus encodes an activin receptor–like kinase 1 gene,[419] which is a member of the serine-threonine kinase receptor family, expressed in endothelial cells. This suggests that defects in this gene might affect development or repair of vessels. Yet a third locus is likely.[420] Thus, by mutation detection or linkage analysis, presymptomatic and prenatal diagnosis is available to a large number of patients with a potentially life-threatening disorder.

Von Hippel–Lindau Syndrome

The features of this autosomal dominant condition involve malformations and abnormal growth of small blood vessels. Retinal angioma, hemangioblastoma of the cerebellum, and hemangioma of the spinal cord occur in association with renal cell carcinoma, pancreatic and epididymal cystadenomas, and pheochromocytoma.[421, 422] Secondary hypertension due to renal disease and pheochromocytoma, which is often bilateral, occurs and predisposes to subarachnoid hemorrhage. The cause is a tumor suppressor gene, *VHL*, at 3p26–p25.[423] Patients inherit a germline mutation (and there is great diversity among families in the actual mutations)[424] that is present in all cells. When a somatic mutation in the normal allele occurs in a susceptible cell, such as in the renal parenchyma or adrenal medulla, the cell becomes functionally homozygous for a lack of the gene product, and the cascade toward neoplasia is initiated.[425] How this gene product stimulates or permits angiomatous malformations is unclear.

Disorders Primarily Affecting Arteries

Mendelian disorders are associated with a diverse array of arterial pathology, and some were described or catalogued earlier in this chapter. This section deals with two categories of disorders caused by a single mutant gene: pleiotropic syndromes better known for affecting organ systems other than the vasculature, and primary abnormalities of arteries.

ADULT POLYCYSTIC KIDNEY DISEASE (APKD). This relatively common autosomal dominant disease affects 0.5 million people and accounts for 8 to 10 percent of all long-term hemodialysis in the United States. Development of renal cysts is age dependent, and presymptomatic detection of heterozygotes, even by ultrasonography, can be uncertain into adulthood.[426, 427] About one-half of patients are hypertensive, one-half have hepatic cysts, one-half eventually develop severe renal failure, and an unknown (but probably high) fraction have colonic diverticula. Elevated plasma renin levels contribute to hypertension long before renal failure occurs.[428] The cardiovascular manifestations include MVP in one-quarter, mild dilatation of the aortic root, occasional thoracic and abdominal aneurysms, and a predisposition to regurgitation of the aortic, mitral, and tricuspid valves.[429–431] The association of diverticula, organ cysts, and cardiovascular lesions reminiscent of but milder than Marfan syndrome suggests some involvement of the extracellular matrix.

The most serious vascular problem is typical berry aneurysms of the cerebral circulation, which occur in about 10 percent of heterozygotes but may remain asymptomatic throughout life. Hypertension predisposes to subarachnoid hemorrhage. How to screen for and treat intracranial aneurysms in patients without neurological symptoms remains controversial. Cerebral angiography carries higher risks in patients with APKD because of dissection and heightened vascular reactivity. Magnetic resonance imaging detects most saccular aneurysms down to 2 to 3 mm in diameter. Whether to attempt prophylactic repair when a small aneurysm is detected has not been investigated systematically. Without question, aggressive blood pressure control is indicated in any patient with APKD.

At least three genes cause APKD. The greatest portion of cases are due to mutations in a gene called *PBP* at the *PKD1* locus (16p13.3).[432a]

In most of the rest of families, the disease maps to the *PKD2* locus in the region 4q23–q23. Families affected by mutations in *PKD2* tend to develop renal failure later and have a milder course.[433] In both *PKD1* and *PKD2*, the multiorgan cysts develop when a somatic mutation occurs in the normal allele at the respective mutant locus, analogous to the two-hit model so familiar with tumorigenesis.[434, 435] A French Canadian family with disease typical of *PKD1* is unlinked to either locus, indicating that a *PKD3* gene exists.[436]

ARTERIOHEPATIC DYSPLASIA. An autosomal dominant disorder of marked variability, *Alagille syndrome* causes neonatal jaundice due to aplasia of intrahepatic bile ducts and congestive heart failure in the most severely affected infants but may be asymptomatic in heterozygous relatives.[437, 438] The cardiovascular findings include peripheral pulmonic and systemic arterial stenoses in the majority, occasionally associated with septal defects or PDA. A diffuse vasculopathy is present in some patients.[439] Renal disease may produce hypertension. The locus was initially mapped by studying chromosomes and finding in some patients that part or all of band 20p12 was missing (an interstitial deletion). The *Jagged1* gene, which mapped to this exact region, was then identified as the cause.[440, 441]

ARTERIAL ANEURYSM, ECTASIA, OR DISSECTION (see also Chaps. 30, 40, and 41). Pedigrees abound in which dilatation of the aortic root, aneurysm of the abdominal aorta, aortic dissection without dilatation, or a combination of these problems occurs in an autosomal dominant pattern without evidence of a recognized heritable disorder of connective tissue.[442–444] Because of the variable presentation and natural history of the aortic disease, presymptomatic detection of presumed heterozygotes is uncertain, as is reassurance of relatives at risk who are of childbearing age and would prefer not to pass this condition to offspring.

The association of dissection of the ascending aorta with bicuspid aortic valve and aortic coarctation is well known, although the cause and pathogenesis remain unclear. In such cases, the aortic wall shows abnormalities of elastic fibers.[445] A person with a congenitally bicuspid aortic valve or aortic coarctation should be screened for dilatation of the aortic root, and first-degree relatives should be screened for both lesions. This recommendation is based, in part, on bicuspid aortic valve being a congenital heart defect of the left-sided flow category, with a relatively high recurrence risk.

In two families with autosomal dominant transmission of arterial aneurysms and mild increased skin fragility and bruisability, different mutations in the gene encoding type III procollagen occurred.[446, 447] Thus, depending on the mutation, deficiency of type III collagen can cause the vascular form of Ehlers-Danlos syndrome (see p. 2003) or a form of the much subtler but just as deadly syndrome, familial arterial rupture. For these families in which the mutations have been defined, reliable presymptomatic and prenatal diagnoses are at hand. However, suggestions that mutations in type III collagen would account for the majority of aortic aneurysms, including abdominal aneurysms in the elderly, have proved unfounded.[448]

A predisposition to cervical arterial dissection in young people was found to be associated with diffuse lentiginosis in several families, with a suggestion of autosomal recessive inheritance.[449] An association is also noted between cervical dissection and intracranial hemorrhage, which is increased when congenital cardiovascular defects are present, especially bicuspid aortic valve or aortic coarctation.[450, 451]

Formal genetic analysis of 91 families ascertained through a proband with *abdominal aortic aneurysm* suggests that an autosomal recessive predisposition exists for late-onset aneurysms.[452] This study and others[453] provide a rationale for offering ultrasound screening to sibs of patients with abdominal aortic dilatation.

FAMILIAL ARTERIAL TORTUOSITY. This is a rare, possibly autosomal recessive condition of unknown cause. Diffuse ectasia of all systemic arteries occurs with, paradoxically, peripheral pulmonic stenoses.[454]

FAMILIAL INTRACRANIAL HEMORRHAGE. In addition to APKD, three syndromes predispose to subarachnoid or cerebral hemorrhage. *Berry aneurysms* without pleiotropic manifestations in other organs are a rare but well-documented autosomal dominant trait.[455] How aggressively near relatives should be screened for intracranial aneurysms remains controversial because of the relatively low risk of hemorrhage compared with the morbidity and mortality of current surgical techniques for repairing defects.[456, 457, 457a] A defect in type III collagen was suggested by linkage analysis, but sequence analysis of the gene in 55 unrelated patients found no mutations.[458]

The *cerebral arterial type of familial amyloidosis* (type VI) is an autosomal dominant condition due to a defect in the proteinase inhibitor cystatin O.[459] This disease is rare outside of Iceland and Holland. The walls of cerebral arteries are thickened by a material resembling amyloid, and the vessels become tortuous and fragile. Recurrent cerebral hemorrhage is common in the fifth and sixth decades of life.[460]

Familial hemangiomas have been reported infrequently to occur as an autosomal dominant condition.[461] The brain and retina are the principal sites of vascular malformation, although in some pedigrees, cutaneous lesions occur. The intracranial hemangioma can be large and present with varied neurological symptoms, including hemorrhage. A more benign familial disorder of primarily isolated cutaneous hemangiomas also exists.[462]

FAMILIAL ARTERIAL OCCLUSIVE DISEASES.[463] *Fibromuscular dysplasia* of the renal and other arteries occurs in *von Recklinghausen neurofibromatosis* and, along with pheochromocytoma, can be a cause of hypertension.[464, 465] Severe deficiency of α_1-antiprotease is another cause of fibromuscular dysplasia.[466] The arterial lesion can occur by itself in families and produce stroke, myocardial infarction, intermittent claudication, and hypertension at young ages, as early as childhood.[467] Inheritance is most consistent with autosomal dominance.[468]

Familial hypoplasia of the carotid arteries,[469] *familial arteriopathy* caused by concentric thickening of systemic and pulmonic arteries,[470] familial moyamoya disease (which has been mapped to 3p24.2–p26),[471] and generalized *arterial calcification of infancy*[472] all are rare, possibly mendelian, syndromes of unknown cause.

Cerebral autosomal dominant arteriopathy with subcortical infarcts and leukoencephalopathy (CADASIL) is due to mutations in the *NOTCH3* gene.[472a] Characteristic inclusions occur in vascular smooth muscle cells, and the deep, perforating cerebral arterioles develop occlusions that produce insidious onset of symptoms and transient ischemic attacks.

FAMILIAL HEMIPLEGIC MIGRAINE. The migraine syndrome is commonly familial and occurs in many generations. A severe form, associated with recurrent hemiplegia, is inherited as an autosomal dominant trait and is due to mutations in a sodium channel gene.[473, 474] However, some families with hemiplegic migraine and others with simple migraine are unlinked to this locus.[475, 476] In the same region of 19p is a locus causing autosomal dominant cerebral arteriopathy with subcortical infarcts.[477] Whether the two conditions are related through allelism is unclear.

FAMILIAL PULMONARY HYPERTENSION (see also Chap. 53). Primary pulmonary hypertension (PPH) is occasionally familial.[478–480] Inheritance is most consistent with an autosomal dominant predisposition with sex influence favoring expression in females. A locus for PPH occurs in the region 2q31–q32 and the defect in some way leads to monoclonal proliferation of endothelial cells.[481–483] Molecular defects favoring recurrent microemboli to the pulmonary circulation afford another area to explore.

Pulmonary hypertension can occur in *neurofibromatosis* due to pulmonary fibrosis.[484]

Disorders Primarily Affecting Veins

VARICOSE VEINS. Although a familial susceptibility to varicosities of the lower extremities clearly exists and favors women in a ratio of 2:1, mendelian inheritance has not been confirmed. *Marfan syndrome*, various *Ehlers-Danlos syndromes*, and an autosomal recessive condition featuring distichiasis (a double row of eyelashes)[485] predispose to varicose veins.

ATRETIC VEINS. Some patients with the *Klippel-Trénaunay-Weber syndrome* of cutaneous hemangioma and hemihypertrophy have atresia of the deep venous system.[486] The concomitant superficial varicosities should not be stripped, lest the remaining venous drainage of the lower extremity be removed. This is a confusing syndrome that overlaps with several others; mendelian inheritance is uncertain. Renal arterial aneurysm and hemangioma occurred in one patient.[487]

CAVERNOUS ANGIOMAS. Cavernous angiomas represent at least 15 percent of vascular malformations of the central nervous system, and familial occurrence is common.[488] These are not arteriovenous malformations but primarily a tortuous collection of veins. Seizure is the most common presenting feature, followed by headache, stroke, and progressive neurological deficit. Magnetic resonance (T_2-weighted) imaging is the procedure of choice because it is sensitive, and arteriography is not likely to detect the venous malformation. In some families, hepatic angiomas are an important feature.[489] The cause of one form has been identified as a gene, *KRIT1*, of unclear function.[490–492]

ARTERIOVENOUS MALFORMATIONS. The most common mendelian cause of arteriovenous malformations (AVM) is the various forms of hereditary hemorrhagic telangiectasia. However, AVM, especially of the brain, are relatively common findings,[493] and other genetic susceptibilities may exist.

Disorders Primarily Affecting Lymphatics

Several forms of *hereditary lymphedema* exist, with the best studied inherited as autosomal dominants. An early-onset form bears the eponym *Nonne-Milroy lymphedema* and can cause a protein-losing enteropathy and pleural effusion. *Meige lymphedema* does not appear until about the time of puberty and is most severe in the legs, although one family with late-onset edema had involvement of the arms and face.[494] Considerable intrafamilial variability in age of onset is noted, however, and whether two or more distinct conditions exist remains unclear. Mutations in one of the receptors for vascular endothelial growth factor, *FLT4,* have been found in some families.[495, 496]

GENETIC FACTORS PREDISPOSING TO ATHEROSCLEROSIS (see also Chap. 31)

Various genetic factors, in addition to the well-studied errors of lipid metabolism, clearly predispose to atherosclerosis. Few genes outside of those involved in lipid metabolism have such an overwhelming impact as to be identifiable from the family history. However, genes that predispose to hypertension and diabetes mellitus; control arterial diameter, reactivity, and branching angles; affect platelet adhesiveness, thrombosis, and fibrinolysis; and regulate endothelial and smooth muscle function all can be considered candidate genes for study in families predisposed to atherosclerosis.[497-499] Screening numerous genes for common mutations and polymorphisms that convey risk information will be increasing possible.[501, 502]

ABNORMAL REGULATION OF BLOOD PRESSURE (see also Chap. 28)

Blood pressure is a quantifiable trait that shows continuous variation within the population. Although many genes and environmental factors undoubtedly affect a person's blood pressure, familial transmission of some arbitrarily defined disease "hypertension" follows neither mendelian nor multifactorial inheritance.[503-505] Various cybernetic systems operate to maintain the blood pressure within tolerable limits. When this physiological homeostasis goes awry or its limits are too lax, pathological and clinical consequences occur.[509] For example, sensitivity of the baroreflex was impaired in patients who had untreated essential hypertension and a positive family history of hypertension compared with hypertensive patients with no family history and to nonhypertensive controls.[506] The complexities of such systems are considerable, and two approaches have been taken in recent years to focus the analysis.[505, 507-509] One involves a candidate-gene approach in humans, based on loci known to be involved in physiological pathways, and the second involves naturally occurring and experimentally created strains of animals.

STUDIES OF HUMANS. All of the classical approaches to detecting genetic influences in diseases—twin studies, familial aggregation, adoption—confirm that genes have a role, but less than 5 percent of patients with hypertension have a defined genetic cause.

Occasional families show striking mendelian segregation of hypertension without being associated with one of the identifiable syndromes listed in Table 56–13. One example, in which early, severe hypertension is inherited as an autosomal dominant trait, is *Liddle syndrome.*[510, 511] Because of hypokalemia, aldosteronism was suspected, but both aldosterone and renin levels were low. Attention then focused on sodium resorption in the distal nephron and its regulation. Mutations discovered in the beta subunit of the epithelial sodium channel render the channel insensitive to the usual regulators.

Another example of successful application of the candidate gene approach is investigation of *glucocorticoid-remediable aldosteronism.*[512] The phenotype was mapped to chromosome 8q21, a region already known to contain two candidate genes, aldosterone synthase and 11β-hydroxylase. By honing in on these loci, mutations creating a chimeric gene by unequal recombination were found to be the cause.[513] As a result of the fusion, aldosterone synthase comes under regulation of adrenocorticotropic hormone. The actual frequency of such mutational events is considerably higher than suspected in the population, and the molecular means are now available to assess the epidemiology of what will likely be a common cause of early hypertension.

Angiotensinogen, the gene for which is in the region 1q42–q43, is a logical candidate gene to investigate because of the central role of its product in blood pressure regulation. Several polymorphic variants involving single amino acid substitutions occur; at positions 174 and 235, either methionine (M) or threonine (T) can exist. The special effects of these polymorphisms on activity, if any, are unclear, but persons homozygous for the 235T allele have plasma angiotensinogen levels 20 percent higher than those with the 235M alleles. Some but not all studies have found an association between the 174M and 235T alleles and hypertension.[514-516] The importance of these polymorphisms seems to depend on the ethnic background.[517]

The ACE gene, at 17q23, contains a common insertion/deletion polymorphism, termed I and D, respectively, that permits both association and linkage studies. The three possible genotypes are DD, ID, and II, and the plasma level of ACE is highest, for unclear reasons, in persons who are DD and lowest in those who are II. The DD genotype has been associated with predisposition to coronary artery disease and to myocardial infarction, which may account for a relative decrease of hypertensive patients with the DD genotype at older ages.[518, 519]

Pregnancy is a clear risk factor for hypertension. A susceptibility locus for preeclampsia has been identified.[520, 521]

The opposite of hypertension, inappropriate control of pressure on the low side, also has numerous genetic bases (Table 56–15).[504, 522, 523]

STUDIES IN ANIMALS. The stroke-prone spontaneously hypertensive (SHRSP) rat is an example of an animal model for a human disease that arose in nature. The phenotype of the rat is clearly polygenic and is thus particularly relevant to much of essential hypertension in humans. Using polymorphic markers spread throughout the rat genome, it has been possible to conduct linkage analyses of hundreds of markers with hypertension when SHRSP animals were crossed with a nonhypertensive strain. Two loci have been identified, and one lies close to where ACE maps.[524] This general approach, called quantitative trait mapping or linkage (QTL), is increasingly being applied to various phenotypes in animals and humans. Determining the actual gene involved in the animal model should then suggest that the homologous locus in the human is a candidate for participation in normal and abnormal regulation of the trait.

A second approach in animals involves transgenic or knockout techniques to create and breed a new, specific genotype. In simplest terms, a given gene can be eliminated, can be mutated in a specific way, can be moved to a different strain (genetic background), or can be overexpressed (See also Chap. 55). For example, eliminating function of the gene that encodes atrial natriuretic peptide in the mouse resulted in moderate elevation of blood pressure when sodium intake was low or somewhat high. Mice heterozygous for the mutation had normal blood pressure on these salt loads but became abnormally hypertensive when fed a high-salt diet.[525, 526]

A number of mendelian conditions, most of which are rare, cause major deviations of blood pressure from an appropriate physiological range (see Table 56–15). These disorders are likely to be underdiagnosed.

▼ **TABLE 56–15. MENDELIAN DISORDERS ASSOCIATED WITH ABNORMAL BLOOD PRESSURE**

DISORDER	OMIM NO.*	PATHOGENESIS
Primarily elevated blood pressure		
Adrenal hyperplasia IV	202010	11-β-hydroxylase deficiency $\rightarrow$ ↑ 11-deoxycorticosterone
Adrenal hyperplasia V	202110	17-α-hydroxylase deficiency $\rightarrow$ ↑ 11-deoxycorticosterone
Aldosteronism	103900	↑ Aldosterone
Alport syndrome	104200	Renal failure
	301050	
Amyloidosis, familial visceral (amyloidosis VIII)	105200	Nephropathy
Arterial calcification of infancy	208000	Arteriosclerosis
Arterial fibromuscular dysplasia	135580	Renal artery stenosis $\rightarrow$ ↑ renin
Arteriohepatic dysplasia	118450	Renal dysplasia; renal arterial stenosis
Bartter syndrome	241200	Secondary to hyperaldosteronism
Fabry disease	301500	Renal failure; renal arterial stenosis; arteriolar stenosis $\rightarrow$ ↑ peripheral resistance
Liddle syndrome	177200	Defective epithelial sodium channel $\rightarrow$ ↓ k^+ ↓ aldosterone, ↓ renin, ↓ angiotensin
Multiple endocrine neoplasia I	131100	Adrenocortical adenoma $\rightarrow$ ↑ Cushing syndrome
Multiple endocrine neoplasia II	171400	Pheochromocytoma $\rightarrow$ ↑ catecholamines
Nail-patella syndrome	161200	Nephropathy
Neurofibromatosis type I	162200	Pheochromocytoma $\rightarrow$ ↑ catecholamines; and renal arterial fibromuscular dysplasia
Paraganglioma	168000	↑ Catecholamines
		Pheochromocytoma $\rightarrow$ ↑ catecholamines
Pheochromocytoma, familial	171300	↑ Catecholamines
Polycystic kidney disease, adult	173900,	↑ Renin; renal failure
	173910	
Porphyria, acute intermittent	176000	?, but only during acute attacks
Pseudohypoaldosteronism, type I	264350	Aldosterone receptor deficiency
Pseudohypoaldosteronism, type II	145260	Defective renal secretion of potassium
Pseudoxanthoma elasticum	177850,	Arteriosclerosis
	264800	
Riley-Day syndrome	223900	Dysautonomia
von Hippel–Lindau syndrome	193300	Pheochromocytoma $\rightarrow$ ↑ catecholamines
Wilms tumor	194070,	
	194071,	
	194090	?
Primarily low blood pressure†		
Dopamine β-hydroxylase deficiency	223360	↑ Synthesis of epinephrine
Fabry disease	301500	↓ Peripheral vascular tone
Hyperbradykininism	143850	↑ Bradykinin
Pelizaeus-Merzbacher, late-onset	169500	?
Peripheral motor neuropathy and dysautonomia	252320	?
Pheochromocytoma, familial	171300	↑ Catecholamines (epinephrine)
Shy-Drager syndrome	146500	Primary autonomic insufficiency

* Data from Online Mendelian Inheritance in Man (www.ncbi.nlm.nih.gov/omim).

†Does not include hypovolemia, obstruction of blood flow, and cardiogeneic causes of hypotension, each of which subsumes numerous hereditary disorders as primary causes.

REFERENCES

GENETIC FACTORS IN DISEASE

1. Childs B: Genetic Medicine: A Logic of Disease. Baltimore, Johns Hopkins University Press, 1999.
2. Murphy EA, Pyeritz RE. Pathogenetics. In Rimoin DL, Connor JM, Pyeritz RE (eds): Principles and Practice of Medical Genetics. 3rd ed. New York, Churchill Livingstone, 1997, pp 359–370.
3. Gardner RJ, Sutherland GR: Chromosome Abnormalities and Genetic Counseling. New York, Oxford University Press, 1989.
4. Borgaonkar D: Chromosomal Variation in Man. 8th ed. New York, John Wiley & Sons, 1997.
5. Ledbetter DH, Ballabio A: Molecular cytogenetics of continuous gene syndromes: Mechanisms and consequences of gene dosage imbalance. In Scriver CR, Beaudet AL, Sly WA, Valle D (eds): The Metabolic and Molecular Bases of Inherited Disease. New York, McGraw-Hill, 1995, p 811.
6. Collins FS: Shattuck Lecture—Medical and societal consequences of the Human Genome Project. N Engl J Med 341: 28–37, 1999.
7. Pyeritz RE: Genetic approaches to cardiovascular disease. In Chien KR, Breslow JL, Leiden JM, et al (eds): Molecular Basis of Cardiovascular Disease. Philadelphia, WB Saunders, 1999, pp 19–36.
8. Online Mendelian Inheritance in Man. www.ncbi.nlm.nih.gov/omim
9. Pyeritz RE: Marfan syndrome and related disorders of connective tissue. Annu Rev Med (in press).
10. Wallace DC, Brown MD, Lott MT: Mitochondrial genetics. In Rimoin DL, Connor JM, Pyeritz RE (eds): Principles and Practice of Medical Genetics. 3rd ed. New York, Churchill Livingstone, 1997, pp 277–332.

11. Johns DR: The other human genome: Mitochondrial DNA and disease. Nat Med 2:1065–1068, 1996.
12. Pyeritz RE: Pleiotropy revisited: Molecular explanations of a classic concept. Am J Med Genet 34:124, 1989.
13. Pyeritz RE: Homocystinuria. In Beighton P (ed): McKusick's Heritable Disorders of Connective Tissue. 5th ed. St. Louis, CV Mosby, 1993, p 137.
14. Byers PH: Disorders of collagen biosynthesis and structure. In Scriver CR, Beaudet AL, Sly WA, Valle D (eds): The Metabolic and Molecular Bases of Inherited Disease. New York, McGraw-Hill, 1995. p 4029.
15. Diano R, Bouchard C, Dumesnil J, et al: Parent-child resemblance in left ventricular echocardiographic measurements. Can J Appl Sport Sci 5:4, 1980.
16. Adams TD, Yanowitz FG, Fisher AG, et al: Heritability of cardiac size: An echocardiographic and electrocardiographic study of monozygotic and dizygotic twins. Circulation 71:39, 1985.
17. Herrington DM, Pearson TA: Clinical and angiographic similarities in twins with coronary artery disease. Am J Cardiol 59:366, 1987.
18. Vlodaver Z, Kahn HA, Neufeld HN: The coronary arteries in early life in three different ethnic groups. Circulation 39:541, 1969.
19. Moller P, Heiberg A: Atrioventricular conduction time—a heritable trait? II. Family studies. Clin Genet 18:454, 1980.
19a. Friedlander Y, Lapidos T, Sinnreich R, Kark JD: Genetic and environmental sources of QT interval variability in Israeli families: The kibbutz settlements family study. Clin Genet 56:200–209, 1999.
20. Moller P, Heiberg A, Berg K: The atrioventricular conduction time—a heritable trait? III. Twin studies. Clin Genet 21:181, 1982.
21. Hawlik RJ, Garrison RJ, Fabsitz R, et al: Variability of heart rate, P-R, QRS and QT durations in twins. J Electrocardiol 13:45, 1980.
22. Dinerman JL, Mehta JL: Endothelial, platelet and leukocyte interactions

in ischemic heart disease: Insights into potential mechanisms and their clinical relevance. J Am Coll Cardiol 16:207, 1990.

23. Wang XL, Mahaney MC, Sim AS, et at: Genetic contribution of the endothelial constitutive nitric oxide synthase gene to plasma nitric oxide levels. Arterioscler Thromb Vasc Biol 17:3147–3153, 1997.

24. Rudic RD, Sessa WC: Human Genetics '99: The cardiovascular system: Nitric oxide in endothelial dysfunction and vascular remodeling: Clinical correlates and experimental links. Am J Hum Genet 64:673–377, 1999.

25. Zannad F, Visvikis S, Gueguen R, et al: Genetics strongly determines the wall thickness of the left and right carotid arteries. Hum Genet 103:183–188, 1998.

CARDIOVASCULAR DISORDERS ASSOCIATED WITH CHROMOSOME ABERRATIONS

26. Popescu NC, Zimonjic DB: Molecular cytogenetic characterization of cancer cell alterations. Cancer Genet Cytogene 93:10–21, 1997.

27. Ferencz C, Neill CA, Boughman JA, et al: Congenital cardiovascular malformations associated with chromosome abnormalities: An epidemiologic study. J Pediatr 114:79, 1989.

28. Berg KA, Clark EB, Astemborski JA, et al: Prenatal detection of cardiovascular malformations by echocardiography: An indication for cytogenetic evaluation. Am J Obstet Gynecol 159:477, 1988.

29. van Karnebeek CDM, Hennekam RCM: Associations between chromosomal anomalies and congenital heart defects: A database search. Am J Med Genet 84:158–166, 1999.

30. De Biase L, Di Ciommo V, Ballerini L, et al: Prevalence of left-sided obstructive lesions in patients with atrioventricular canal without Down syndrome. J Thorac Cardiovasc Surg 91:467, 1986.

31. Tolmie JL: Down syndrome and other autosomal trisomies. In Rimoin DL, Connor JM, Pyeritz RE (eds): Principles and Practice of Medical Genetics. 3rd ed. New York, Churchill Livingstone, 1997, pp 925–972.

32. Freeman SB, Taft LF, Dooley KJ, et al: Population-based study of congenital heart defects in Down syndrome. Am J Med Genet 80:213–217, 1998.

33. Clapp S, Perry BL, Farooki ZQ, et al: Down's syndrome, complete atrioventricular canal, and pulmonary vascular obstructive disease. J Thorac Cardiovasc Surg 100:115, 1990.

34. Goldhaber SZ, Rubin IL, Brown W, et al: Valvular heart disease (aortic regurgitation and mitral valve prolapse) among institutionalized adults with Down's syndrome. Am J Cardiol 57:278, 1986.

35. Korenberg J, Bradley C, Disteche C: Down syndrome: Molecular mapping of congenital heart disease and duodenal stenosis. Am J Hum Genet 50:294–302, 1992.

36. Schneider DS, Zahka KG, Clark EB, et al: Patterns of cardiac care in infants with Down syndrome. Am J Dis Child 143:363, 1989.

37. Van Dyck DC, Allen M: Clinical management considerations in long-term survivors with trisomy 18. Pediatrics 58:893, 1976.

38. Musewe NN, Alexander DJ, Teshima I, et al: Echocardiographic evaluation of the spectrum of cardiac anomalies associated with trisomy 13 and trisomy 18. J Am Coll Cardiol 15:673, 1990.

39. Van Praagh S, Truman T, Firpo A, et al: Cardiac malformations in trisomy-18: A study of 41 postmortem cases. J Am Coll Cardiol 13:1586, 1989.

40. Saenger P: Turner's syndrome. N Engl J Med 335:1749–1754, 1996.

41. Lacro RV, Lyons Jones K, Benirschke K: Coarctation of the aorta in Turner syndrome: A pathologic study of fetuses with nuchal cystic hygromas, hydrops fetalis and female genitalia. Pediatrics 81:445, 1988.

42. Allen DB, Hendricks SA, Levy JM: Aortic dilation in Turner syndrome. J Pediatr 109:302, 1986.

43. Natowicz M, Kelley RI: Association of Turner syndrome with hypoplastic left-heart syndrome. Am J Dis Child 141:218, 1987.

44. Moore JW, Kirby WC, Rogers WM, et al: Partial anomalous pulmonary venous drainage associated with 45,X Turner's syndrome. Pediatrics 86:273, 1990.

45. Sapienza C, Hall JG: Genetic imprinting in human disease. In Scriver CR, Beaudet AL, Sly WA, Valle D (eds): The Metabolic and Molecular Bases of Inherited Disease. New York, McGraw-Hill, 1995, p 437.

46. Jacobs P, Dalton P, James R, et al: Turner syndrome: A cytogenetic and molecular study. Ann Hum Genet 61:471–483, 1997.

47. Zinn AR, Tonk VS, Chen Z, et al: Evidence for a Turner syndrome locus or loci at Xp11.2-p22.1. Am J Hum Genet 63:1757–1766, 1998.

CONGENITAL HEART DISEASE

48. Fixler DE, Pastor P, Chamberlin M, et al: Trends in congenital heart disease in Dallas County births: 1971–1984. Circulation 81:137, 1990.

49. Helmcke F, de Souza A, Nanda NC, et al: Two-dimensional and color Doppler assessment of ventricular septal defect of congenital origin. Am J Cardiol 63:1112, 1989.

50. Hanna EJ, Nevin NC, Nelson J: Genetic study of congenital heart defects in Northern Ireland (1974–1978). J Med Genet 31:858, 1994.

51. Simpson IA, Sahn DJ, Valdes-Cruz LM, et al: Color Doppler flow mapping in patients with coarctation of the aorta: New observations and improved evaluation with color flow diameter and proximal acceleration as predictors of severity. Circulation 77:736, 1988.

52. Ferencz C, Loffredo CA, Correa-Villaseñor A, Wilson P: Genetic and Environmental Risk Factors of Major Cardiovascular Malformations: The Baltimore-Washington Infant Study 1981–1989. Armonk, NY, Futura, 1997.

53. Lin AE, Herring AH, Scharenberg K, et al: Cardiovascular malformations: Changes in prevalence and birth status, 1972–1990. Am J Med Genet 84:102–110, 1999.

54. Brenner JL, Berg KA, Schneider DS, et al: Cardiac malformations in relatives of infants with hypoplastic left-heart syndrome. Am J Dis Child 143:1492, 1989.

55. Pyeritz RE, Murphy EA: The genetics of congenital heart disease: Perspectives and prospects. J Am Coll Cardiol 13:1458, 1989.

56. Ursell PC, Byrne JM, Strombino BA: Significance of cardiac defects in the developing fetus: A study of spontaneous abortuses. Circulation 72:1232, 1985.

57. Devriendt K, Matthijs G, Dael RV, et al: Delineation of the critical deletion region for congenital heart defects on chromosome 8p23.1. Am J Hum Genet 64:1119–1126, 1999.

58. Clayton-Smith J, Donnai D: Human malformations. In Rimoin DL, Connor JM, Pyeritz RE (eds): Principles and Practice of Medical Genetics. 3rd ed. New York, Churchill Livingstone, 1997, pp 383–394.

59. Sadiq M, Stümper O, Wright JGC, et al: Influence of ethnic origin on the pattern of congenital heart defects in the first year of life. Br Heart J 73:173, 1995.

60. Whittemore R, Hobbins JC, Engle MA: Pregnancy and its outcome in women with and without surgical treatment of congenital heart disease. In Engle MA, Perloff JK (eds): Congenital Heart Disease After Surgery. New York, Yorke Medical Books, 1983, p 362.

61. Rose VR, Gold JM, Lindsay G, et al: A possible increase in the incidence of congenital heart defects among the offspring of affected parents. J Am Coll Cardiol 6:376, 1985.

62. Nora JJ, Berg K, Nora AH: Cardiovascular disease—genetics, epidemiology and prevention. Am J Hum Genet 50:450, 1992.

63. Boughman JA: Familial risks of congenital heart defects [letter]. Am J Med Genet 29:233, 1988.

64. Murphy JG, Gersh BJ, McGoon MG, et al: Long-term outcome after surgical repair of isolated atrial septal defect: Follow-up at 27 to 32 years. N Engl J Med 323:1645, 1990.

65. Gold RJM, Rose V, Yau Y: Severity and recurrence risk of congenital heart defects exemplified by atrial septal defect secundum. Clin Genet 32:148, 1987.

66. Sanchez-Cascos A: The recurrence risk in congenital heart disease. Eur J Cardiol 7:197, 1978.

67. Lathrop GM, Terwilliger JD, Weeks DE: Multifactorial inheritance and genetic analysis of multifactorial disease. In Rimoin DL, Connor JM, Pyeritz RE (eds): Principles and Practice of Medical Genetics. 3rd ed. New York, Churchill Livingstone, 1997, pp 333–346.

68. Digilio MC, Marino B, Toscanno A, et al: Atrioventricular canal defect without Down syndrome: A heterogeneous malformation. Am J Med Genet 85:140–146, 1999.

69. Marino B, Digilio MC: Inlet ventricular septal defect is not a partial atrioventricular septal defect. Am J Med Genet 87:195, 1999.

70. Corone P, Bonaiti C, Feingold J, et al: Familial congenital heart disease: How are the various types related? Am J Cardiol 51:942, 1983.

71. Clark EB: Mechanisms in the pathogenesis of congenital cardiac malformations. In Pierpont MEM, Moller JH (eds): Genetics of Cardiovascular Disease. Boston, Martinus Nihjoff, 1986, p 3.

72. Maestri NE, Beaty TH, Liang K-Y, et al: Assessing familial aggregation of congenital cardiovascular malformations in case-control studies: Genet Epidemiol 5:343, 1988.

73. Pierpont MEM, Gobel JW, Moller JH, et al: Cardiac malformations in relatives of children with truncus arteriosus or interruption of the aortic arch. Am J Cardiol 61:423, 1988.

74. Goldmuntz E, Clark BJ, Mitchell LE, et al: Frequency of 22q11 deletions in patients with conotruncal defects. J Am Coll Cardiol 32:492–498, 1998.

75. Krantz ID, Smith R, Colliton RP, et al: Jagged1 mutationsin patients ascertained with isolated congenital heart defects. Am J Med Genet 84:56–60, 1999.

76. Ewing CK, Loffredo CA, Beaty TH: Paternal risk factors for isolated membranous ventricular septal defects. Am J Med Genet 71:42–46, 1997.

77. Desmaze C, Prieur M, Amblard F, et al: Physical mapping by FISH of the DiGeorge critical region (DGCR): Involvement of the region in familial cases. Am J Hum Genet 53:1239, 1993.

78. Matsuoka R, Takao A, Kimura M, et al: Confirmation that the conotruncal anomaly face syndrome is associated with a deletion within 22q11.2. Am J Med Genet 53:285, 1994.

79. Funke B, Puech A, Saint-Jore B, et al: Isolation and characterization of a human gene containing a nuclear localization signal from the critical region for velo-cardiofacial syndrome on 22q11. Genomics 53:146–154, 1998.

80. Goodship J, Cross I, LiLing J, Wren C: A populations study of chromosome 22q11 deletions in infancy. Arch Dis Child 79:348–351, 1998.

81. Patterson DF, Pexieder T, Schnarr WR, et al: A single major-gene defect underlying cardiac conotruncal malformations interferes with myocardial growth during embryonic development: Studies in the CTD line of Keeshond dogs. Am J Hum Genet 52:388, 1993.

82. Beekman RH, Robinow M: Coarctation of the aorta inherited as an autosomal dominant trait. Am J Cardiol 56:818, 1985.

83. Lindsay J Jr: Coarctation of the aorta, bicuspid aortic valve and abnormal ascending aortic wall. Am J Cardiol 61:182, 1988.

84. Wright TC, Orkin RW, Destrempes M, et al: Increased adhesiveness of Down syndrome fetal fibroblasts in vitro. Proc Natl Acad Sci U S A 81: 2426, 1984.

85. Ferencz C, Boughman JA, Neill CA, et al: Congenital cardiovascular malformations: Questions on inheritance. J Am Coll Cardiol 14:756, 1989.

86. Moreno A, Murphy EA: Inheritance of Kartagener syndrome. Am J Med Genet 8:305, 1981.

87. Afzelius BA, Mossberg B: Immotile-cilia syndrome (primary ciliary dyskinesia), including Kartagener syndrome. In Scriver CR, Beaudet AL, Sly WA, Valle D (eds): The Metabolic and Molecular Bases of Inherited Disease. New York, McGraw-Hill, 1995, p 3943.

88. Alonso S, Pierpont ME, Radtke W: Geterotaxia syndrome and autosomal dominant inheritance. Am J Med Genet 56:12, 1995.

89. Casey B, Devoto M, Jones KL, et al: Mapping a gene for familial situs abnormalities to human chromosome Xq24-q27.1. Nature Genet 5:403, 1993.

90. Anderson C, Devine WA, Anderson RH, et al: Abnormalities of the spleen in relation to congenital malformation of the heart: A survey of necropsy findings in children. Br Heart J 63:122, 1990.

91. Phoon CK, Neill CA: Asplenia syndrome: Insight into embryology through an analysis of cardiac and extracardiac anomalies. Am J Cardiol 73:581, 1994.

92. Olson EN, Srivastava D: Molecular pathways controlling heart development. Science 272:671–676, 1996.

93. Casey B: Two rights make a wrong: Human left-right malformations. Hum Mol Genet 7:1565–1571, 1998.

94. Towbin JA, Casey B, Belmont J: Human Genetics '99: The cardiovascular system: The molecular basis of vascular disorders. Am J Hum Genet 64:678–684, 1999.

95. Mochizuki T, Saijoh U, Tsuchiya K, et al: Cloning of inv, a gene that controls left/right asymmetry and kidney development. Nature Genet 395:177–181, 1998.

96. Kosaki R, Gebbia M, Kosaki K, et al: Left-right axis malformations associated with mutations in ACVR2B, the gene for human activin receptor type IIB. Am J Med Genet 82:70–76, 1999.

97. Britz-Cunningham SH, Shah MM, Zuppan CW, et al: Mutations of the Connexin43 gap-junction gene in patients with heart malformations and defects of laterality. N Engl J Med 332:1323–1329, 1995.

98. Cyran SE, Martinez R, Daniels S, et al: Spectrum of congenital heart disease in CHARGE association. J Pediatr 110:576, 1987.

99. Oley CA, Baraitser M, Grant DB: A reappraisal of the CHARGE association. J Med Genet 25:147, 1988.

100. Weaver DD, Mapstone CL, Yu P: The VATER association: Analysis of 46 patients. Am J Dis Child 140:225, 1986.

101. Nezarati MM, McLeod DR: VACTERL manifestations in two generations of a family. Am J Med Genet 82:40–42, 1999.

102. Woods CG, Sheffield LJ: Further family with autosomal dominant patent ductus arteriosus. J Med Genet 31:659, 1994.

103. Davidson HR: A large family with patent ductus arteriosus and unusual face. J Med Genet 30:503, 1992.

104. Slavotinek A, Clayton-Smith J, Super M: Familial patent ductus arteriosus: A further case of CHAR syndrome. Am J Med Genet 71:229–232, 1997.

105. Lynch HT, Bachenberg K, Harris RE, et al: Hereditary atrial septal defect: Update of a large kindred. Am J Dis Child 132:600, 1978.

106. Basson CT, Solomon SD, Weissman B, et al: Genetic heterogeneity of heart-hand syndromes. Circulation 91:1326–1329, 1995.

107. Schott J-J, Benson DW, Basson CT, et al: Congenital heart disease caused by mutations in the transcription factor NKX2-5. Science 281: 108–111, 1998.

108. Gall JC, Stern AM, Cohen MM, et al: Holt-Oram syndrome: Clinical and genetic study of a large family. Am J Hum Genet 18:187, 1966.

109. Sletten LJ, Pierpont MEM: Variation in severity of cardiac diseases in Holt-Oram syndrome. Am J Med Genet 65:128–132, 1996.

110. Basson CT, Cowley GS, Solomon SD, et al: The clinical and genetic spectrum of the Holt-Oram syndrome (heart-hand syndrome). N Engl J Med 330:885, 1994.

111. Basson CT, Huang T, Lin RC, et al: Different TBX5 interactions in heart and limb defined by Holt-Oram syndrome mutations. Proc Natl Acad Sci U S A 96:2919–2924, 1999.

112. Terrett JA, Newbury-Ecob R, Cross GS, et al: Holt-Oram syndrome is a genetically heterogeneous disease with one locus mapping to human chromosome 12q. Nature Genet 6:401, 1994.

113. Fryns JP, Bonnet D, De Smet L: Holt-Oram syndrome with associated postaxial and central polysyndactyly: Further evidence for genetic heterogeneity in the Holt-Oram syndrome. Genet Counsel 7:323–324, 1996.

114. McKusick VA, Egeland JA, Eldridge R, et al: Dwarfism in the Amish: I. The Ellis-van Creveld syndrome. Bull Johns Hopkins Hosp 115:306, 1964.

115. Polymeropoulos MH, Ide SE, Wright M, et al: The gene for Ellis-van Creveld syndrome is located on chromosome 4p16. Genomics 35:1–5, 1996.

115a. Ruiz-Perez VL, Ide SE, Strom TM, et al: Mutations in a new gene in Ellis-van Creveld syndrome and Weyers acrodental dysostosis. Nature Genet 24:283–286, 2000.

116. Sheffield VC, Pierpont ME, Nishimura D, et al: Identification of a complex congenital heart defect susceptibility locus by using DNA pooling and shared segment analysis. Hum Mol Genet 6:117–121, 1997.

117. Preus M: The Williams syndrome: Objective definition and diagnosis. Clin Genet 25:422, 1984.

118. Maisuls H, Alday LE, Thuer O: Cardiovascular findings in the Williams-Beuren syndrome. Am Heart J 114:897, 1987.

119. Hallidie-Smith KA, Karas S: Cardiac anomalies in Williams-Beuren syndrome. Arch Dis Child 63:809, 1988.

120. Morris CA, Demsey SA, Leonard CO, et al: Natural history of Williams syndrome: Physical characteristics. J Pediatr 113:318, 1988.

121. Morris CA, Leonard CO, Dilts C, et al: Adults with Williams syndrome. Am J Med Genet 6 (Suppl):102–107, 1990.

122. Broder K, Reinhardt E, Ahern J, et al: Elevated ambulatory blood pressure in 20 subjects with Williams syndrome. Am J Med Genet 83:356–360, 1999.

123. Wessel A, Pankau R, Kececioglu D, et al: Three decades of follow-up of aortic and pulmonary vascular lesions in the Williams-Beuren syndrome. Am J Med Genet 52:297, 1994.

124. Ardinger RH Jr, Goertz KK, Mattioli LF: Cerebrovascular stenoses with cerebral infarction in a child with Williams syndrome. Am J Med Genet 51:200, 1994.

125. van Son JAM, Edwards WD, Danielson GK: Pathology of coronary arteries, myocardium, and great arteries in supravalvular aortic stenosis: Report of five cases with implications for surgical treatment. J Thorac Cardiovasc Surg 108:21, 1994.

126. Tassabehji M, Metcalfe K, Karmiloff-Smith A, et al: Williams syndrome: Use of chromosomal microdeletions as a tool to dissect cognitive and physical phenotypes. Am J Hum Genet 64:118–125, 1999.

127. Francke U: Williams-Beuren syndrome: Genes and mechanisms. Hum Mol Genet 8:1947–1954, 1999.

128. Chiarella F, Bricarelli FD, Lupi G: Familial supravalvular aortic stenosis: A genetic study. J Med Genet 26:86, 1989.

129. Ensing GJ, Schmidt MA, Hagler DJ, et al: Spectrum of findings in a family with nonsyndromic autosomal dominant supravalvular aortic stenosis: A Doppler echocardiographic study. J Am Coll Cardiol 13:413, 1989.

130. Schmidt MA, Ensing GJ, Michels VV, et al: Autosomal dominant supravalvular aortic stenosis: Large three-generation family. Am J Med Genet 32:384, 1989.

131. Devereux RB, Kramer-Fox R, Shear MK, et al: Diagnosis and classification of severity of mitral valve prolapse: Methodologic, biologic, and prognostic considerations. Am Heart J 113:1265, 1987.

132. Nishimura RA, McGoon MD: Perspectives on mitral-valve prolapse. N Engl J Med 341:48–50, 1999.

133. Freed LA, Levy D, Levine RA, et al: Prevalence and clinical outcome of mitral-valve prolapse. N Engl J Med 341:1–7, 1999.

134. Devereux RB, Kramer-Fox R: Inheritance and phenotypic features of mitral valve prolapse. In Boudoulas H, Wooley CF (eds): Mitral Valve Prolapse and the Mitral Valve Prolapse Syndrome. Mt. Kisco, NY, Futura, 1988, p 109.

135. Strahan NV, Murphy EA, Fortuin NJ, et al: Inheritance of the mitral valve prolapse syndrome. Discussion of a three-dimensional penetrance model. Am J Med 74:967, 1983.

136. Pini R, Greppi B, Kramer-Fox R, et al: Mitral valve dimensions and motion and familial transmission of mitral valve prolapse with and without mitral leaflet billowing. J Am Coll Cardiol 12:1423, 1988.

137. Hickey AJ, Narunsky L, Wilcken DEL: Bodily habitus and mitral valve prolapse. Aust N Z J Med 15:326, 1985.

138. Devereux RB, Brown WT, Lutas EM, et al: Association of mitral valve prolapse with low body weight and low blood pressure. Lancet 2:792, 1982.

139. Kyndt F, Schott JJ, Trochu JN, et al: Mapping of X-linked myxomatous valvular dystrophy to chromosome Xq28. Am J Hum Genet 62:627–632, 1998.

140. Beighton P, de Paepe A, Danks D, et al: International nosology of heritable disorders of connective tissue, Berlin, 1986. Am J Med Genet 29:581, 1988.

141. DePaepe A, Deitz HC, Devereux RB, et al: Revised diagnostic criteria for the Marfan syndrome. Am J Med Genet 62:417–426, 1996.

142. Roman MJ, Devereux RB, Kramer-Fox R, et al: Comparison of cardiovascular and skeletal features of primary mitral valve prolapse and the Marfan syndrome. Am J Cardiol 3:317, 1989.

143. Glesby MJ, Pyeritz RE: Association of mitral valve prolapse and systemic abnormalities of connective tissue: A phenotypic continuum. JAMA 262:523, 1989.

144. Shamberger RC, Welch KJ, Sanders SP: Mitral valve prolapse associated with pectus excavatum. J Pediatr 111:404, 1987.

145. Rogan K, Sears-Rogan P, Vermani R, et al: Familial myxomatous valvular disease. Am J Cardiol 63:1149, 1989.

146. Mendez HMM, Opitz JM: Noonan syndrome: A review. Am J Med Genet 21:493, 1985.

147. Allanson JE, Hall JG, Hughes HE, et al: Noonan syndrome: The changing phenotype. Am J Med Genet 21:507, 1985.

148. Noonan JA, Ehmke DA: Associated noncardiac malformations in children with congenital heart disease. J Pediatr 63:468, 1963.

149. Battisle CE, Feldt RH, Lie JT: Congestive cardiomyopathy in Noonan's syndrome. Mayo Clin Proc 52:661, 1977.

150. Miller M, Motulsky AG: Noonan syndrome in an adult family presenting with chronic lymphedema. Am J Med 65:379, 1978.

151. Brady AF, Jamieson CR, van der Burgt I, et al: Further delineation of the critical region for Noonan sysndrome on the long arm of chromosome 12. Eur J Hum Genet 5:336–337, 1997.

152. Legius E, Schollen E, Matthijs G, Fryns J-P: Fine mapping of Noonan/cardiofacio-cutaneous syndrome in a large family. Eur J Hum Genet 6: 32–37, 1998.

153. Quattrin T, McPherson E, Putnam T: Vertical transmission of the neurofibromatosis/Noonan syndrome. Am J Med Genet 26:645, 1987.

154. van der Burgt I, Berends E, Lommen E, et al: Clinical and molecular studies in a large Dutch family with Noonan syndrome. Am J Med Genet 53:187, 1994.

155. Kitchens CS, Alexander JA: Partial deficiency of coagulation factor XI as a newly recognized feature of Noonan syndrome. J Pediatr 102:224, 1983.

156. Hanson JW: Human teratology. In Rimoin DL, Connor JM, Pyeritz RE (eds): Principles and Practice of Medical Genetics. 3rd ed. New York, Churchill Livingstone, 1997, pp. 697–724.

157. Khoury MJ, Becerra JE, Cordero JF, et al: Clinical-epidemiologic assessment of patterns of birth defects associated with human teratogens: Application to diabetic embryopathy. Pediatrics 83:658, 1989.

158. Beckman DA. Brent RL: Mechanisms of teratogenesis. Annu Rev Pharmacol Toxicol 24:483, 1984.

159. Shepard TH: Catalog of Teratogenic Agents. 9th ed. Baltimore, Johns Hopkins Press, 1998.

160. Jones KL: Fetal alcohol syndrome. Pediatr Rev 8:122, 1986.

161. Bagheri MM, Burd L, Martsolf JT, Klug MG: Fetal alcohol syndrome. J Perinat Med 26:263–269, 1998.

162. Finnell RH, Chernoff GF: Genetic background. The elusive component in the fetal hydantoin syndrome. Am J Med Genet 19:459, 1984.

163. Strickler SM, Dansky LV, Miller MA, et al: Genetic predisposition to phenytoin-induced birth defects. Lancet 2:746, 1985.

164. Lammer EJ: Retinoic acid embryopathy. N Engl J Med 313:837, 1985.

165. Hall JG, Pauli RM, Wilson KM: Maternal and fetal sequelae of anticoagulation during pregnancy. Am J Med 68:122, 1980.

166. Scriver CR, Kaufman S, Eisensmith RC, et al: The hyperphenylalaninemias. In Scriver CR, Beaudet AL, Sly WA, Valle D (eds): The Metabolic and Molecular Bases of Inherited Disease. New York, McGraw-Hill, 1995, p 1015.

167. Lenke RR, Levy HL: Maternal phenylketonuria and hyperphenylalaninemia. N Engl J Med 303:1202, 1980.

CARDIOMYOPATHIES

168. Vosberg H-P, McKenna WJ. Cardiomyopathies. In Rimoin DL, Connor JM, Pyeritz RE (eds): Principles and Practice of Medical Genetics. 3rd ed. New York, Churchill Livingstone, 1997, pp. 843–878.

169. Seidman CE, Seidman JG: Molecular genetics of inherited cardiomyopathies. In Chien KR, Breslow JL, Leiden JM, et al: (eds). Molecular Basis of Cardiovascular Disease. Philadelphia, WB Saunders, 1999, pp 251–263.

170. Fung DCY, Yu B, Littlejohn T, et al: An online locus-specific mutation database for familial hypertrophic cardiomyopathy. Hum Mutat 14:326–332, 1999.

171. Watkins H, Thierfelder L, Hwang DS, et al: Sporadic hypertrophic cardiomyopathy due to de novo myosin mutations. J Clin Invest 90:1666, 1992.

171a. Forissier J-F, Richard P, Briault S, et al: First description of germline mosaicism in familial hypertrophic cardiomyopathy. J Med Genet 37: 132–134, 2000.

172. Jeschke B, Uhl K, Weist B, et al: A high risk phenotype of hypertrophic cardiomyopathy associated with a compound genotype of two mulated β-myosin heavy chain genes. Hum Mutat 102:299–304, 1998.

173. Tesson F, Richard P, Charron P, et al: Genotype-phenotype analysis in four families with mutations in β-myosin heavy chain gene responsible for familial hypertrophic cardiomyopathy. Hum Mutat 12:385–392, 1998.

174. Richard P, Isnard R, Carrier L, et al: Double heterozygosity for mutations in the β-myosin heavy chain and in the cardiac myosin binding protein C genes in a family with hypertrophic cardiomyopathy. J Med Genet 36:542–545, 1999.

175. Yu B, French JA, Jeremy RW, et al: Counseling issues in familial hypertrophic cardiomyopathy. J Med Genet 35:183–188, 1998.

176. Maron BJ, Moller JH, Seidman CE, et al: Impact of laboratory molecular diagnosis on contemporary diagnostic criteria for genetically transmitted cardiovascular diseases: Hypertrophic cardiomyopathy, long-QT syndrome, and Marfan syndrome. Circulation 98:1460–1471, 1998.

177. Cuda G. Fannapazir L, Zhu WS, et al: Skeletal muscle expression and abnormal function of β-myosin in hypertrophic cardiomyopathy. J Clin Invest 91:2861, 1993.

178. Lechin M, Quinones MA, Omran A, et al: Angiotensin I converting enzyme genotypes and left ventricular hypertrophy in patients with hypertrophic cardiomyopathy. Circulation 92:1808, 1995.

178a. Maron BJ, Shen W-K, Link MS, et al: Efficacy of implantable cardioverter-defibrillators for the prevention of sudden death in patients with hypertrophic cardiomyopathy. N Engl J Med 342:365–373, 2000.

179. Codd MB, Sugrue DD, Gersh BJ, et al: Epidemiology of idiopathic dilated and hypertrophic cardiomyopathy: A population-based study in Olmsted County, Minnesota, 1975–1984. Circulation 80:564, 1989.

180. Dec GW, Fuster V: Idiopathic dilated cardiomyopathy. N Engl J Med 331:1564, 1994.

181. Manolio TA, Baughman KL, Rodeheffer R, et al: Prevalence and etiology of idiopathic dilated cardiomyopathy. Am J Cardiol 69:1458, 1992.

182. Michels VV, Moll PP, Miller FA, et al: The frequency of familial dilated cardiomyopathy in a series of patients with idiopathic dilated cardiomyopathy. N Engl J Med 326:77, 1992.

183. Maeda M, Holder E, Lowes B, et al: Dilated cardiomyopathy associated with deficiency of the cytoskeletal protein metavinculin. Circulation 95: 17–20, 1997.

184. Jung M, Poepping I, Perrot A, et al: Investigation of a family with autosomal dominant dilated cardiomyopathy defines a novel locus on chromosome 2q14-q22. Am J Hum Genet 65:1068–1077, 1997.

185. Vilarinho L, Santorelli FM, Rosas MJ, et al: The mitochondrial A3243G mutation presenting as severe cardiomyopathy. J Med Genet 34:607–609, 1997.

186. Mayosi BM, Khogali SS, Zhang B, et al: Cardiac and skeletal actin gene mutations are not a common cause of dilated cardiomypathy. J Med Genet 36:796–797, 1999.

187. Caforio ALP, Rossi B, Risaliti R: Type 1 fiber abnormalities in skeletal muscle of patients with hypertrophic and dilated cardiomyopathy: Evidence of subclinical myogenic myopathy. J Am Coll Cardiol 14:1464, 1989.

188. Voss EG, Reddy CVR, Detremo R, et al: Familial dilated cardiomyopathy. Am J Cardiol 54:456, 1984.

189. Barth PG, Scholte JA, Berden JA, et al: An X-linked mitochondrial disease affecting cardiac muscle, skeletal muscle and neutrophil leukocytes. J Neurol Sci 62:327, 1983.

190. Bione S, D'Adamo P, Maestrini E, et al: A novel X-linked gene, G4.5. is responsible for Barth syndrome. Nat Genet 12:385–389, 1996.

191. Digilio MC, Marino B, Bevilacqua M, et al: Genetic heterogeneity of isolated noncompaction of the left ventricular myocardium. Am J Med Genet 85:90–91, 1999.

192. Emery AEH: Duchenne and other X-linked muscular dystrophies. In Rimoin DL, Connor JM, Pyeritz RE (eds): Principles and Practice of Medical Genetics. 3rd ed. New York, Churchill Livingstone, 1997, pp 2337–2354.

193. Melacini P, Fanin M, Danieli GA, et al: Cardiac involvement in Becker muscular dystrophy. J Am Coll Cardiol 22:1927, 1993.

194. Muntoni F, Cau M, Ganau A, et al: Deletion of the dystrophin muscle-promoter region associated with X-linked dilated cardiomyopathy. N Engl J Med 329:921, 1993.

195. Towbin JA, Hejtmancik JF, Brink P, et al: X-linked dilated cardiomyopathy: Molecular genetic evidence of linkage to the Duchenne muscular dystrophy (dystrophin) gene at the Xp21 locus. Circulation 87:1854, 1993.

196. Bushby KMD: Autosomally inherited muscular dystrophies. In Rimoin DL, Connor JM, Pyeritz RE (eds): Principles and Practice of Medical Genetics. 3rd ed. New York, Churchill Livingstone, 1997, pp 2355–2366.

197. Fishbein MC, Siegel RJ, Thompson CE, et al: Sudden death of a carrier of X-linked Emery-Dreifuss muscular dystrophy. Ann Intern Med 119: 900, 1993.

198. Bione S, Maestrini E, Rivella S, et al: Identification of a novel X-linked gene responsible for Emery-Dreifuss muscular dystrophy. Nat Genet 8: 323, 1994.

199. Morris GE, Manilal S: Heart to heart: From nuclear proteins to Emery-Dreifuss muscular dystrophy. Hum Mol Genet 8:1847–1851, 1999.

200. Barresi R, Di Blasi C, Negri T, et al: Disruption of heart sarcoglycan complex and severe cardiomyopathy caused by β sarcoglycan mutations. J Med Genet 37:102–107, 2000.

200a. Dalakas MC, Park K-Y, Semino-Mora C, et al: Desmin myopathy, a skeletal myopathy with cardiomyopathy caused by mutations in the desmin gene. N Engl J Med 342:770–780, 2000.

201. Aroney C, Bett N, Radford D: Familial restrictive cardiomyopathy. Aust N Z J Med 18:877, 1988.

202. Fitzpatrick AP, Shapiro LM, Richards AF, et al: Familial restrictive cardiomyopathy with atrioventricular block and skeletal myopathy. Br Heart J 63:114, 1990.

203. Hodgson S, Child A, Dyson M: Endocardial fibroelastosis: Possible X-linked inheritance. J Med Genet 24:210, 1987.

204. Opitz JM: Genetic aspects of endocardial fibroelastosis. Am J Med Genet 11:92, 1982.

205. Devi AS, Eisenfeld L, Uphoff D, et al: New syndrome of hydrocephalus, endocardial fibroelastosis, and cataracts (HEC) syndrome. Am J Med Genet 56:62, 1995.

206. Ross RS, Bulkley BH, Hutchins GM, et al: Idiopathic familial myocardiopathy in three generations: A clinical and pathologic study. Am Heart J 96:170, 1978.

207. Voorhees ML, Hussan GS, Blackman MS: Growth failure with pericardial constriction: The syndrome of mulibrey nanism. Am J Dis Child 130:1146, 1976.

208. Avela K, Lipsanen-Nyman M, Perheentupa J, et al: Assignment of the mulibrey nanism gene to 17q by linkage and linkage-disequilibrium analysis. Am J Hum Genet 60:896–902, 1997.

209. Martinez-Lavin M, Buendia A, Delgado E, et al: A familial syndrome of pericarditis, arthritis and camptodactyly. N Engl J Med 309:224, 1983.

210. Bahabri SA, Suwairi WM, Laxer RM, et al: The camptodactyly-arthropathy-coxa vara-pericarditis syndrome: Clinical features and genetic mapping to human chromosome 1. Arthritis Rheum 41:730–735, 1998.

211. Marcelino J, Carpten JD, Suwairi WM, et al: CACP, encoding a secreted proteoglycan, is mutated in camptodactyly-arthropathy-coxa vara-pericarditis syndrome. Nat Genet 23:319–322, 1999.

212. Fitzpatrick AP, Emanuel RW: Familial neurofibromatosis and hypertrophic cardiomyopathy. Br Heart J 60:247, 1988.

213. Sommer A, Contras SB, Craenen JM, et al: A family study of the LEOPARD syndrome. Am J Dis Child 121:520, 1971.

214. Coppin BD, Temple IK: Multiple lentigines syndrome (LEOPARD) syndrome or progressive cardiomyopathic lentiginosis. J Med Genet 24: 582–586, 1997.

PRIMARY DISORDERS OF RHYTHM AND CONDUCTION

215. Marks ML, Keating MT: Familial dysrhythmias. *In* Rimoin DL, Connor JM, Pyeritz RE (eds): Principles and Practice of Medical Genetics. 3rd ed. New York, Churchill Livingstone, 1997, pp. 879–898.

216. Priori SG, Barhanin J, Hauer RNW, et al: Genetic and molecular basis of cardiac arrhythmias: Impact on clinical management Part I and II. Circulation 99:518–528, 1999.

217. Gambetta M, Weese J, Ginsburg M. et al: Sick sinus syndrome in a patient with familial PR prolongation. Chest 64:520, 1973.

218. Surawicz B, Hariman RJ: Follow-up of the family with congenital absence of sinus rhythm. Am J Cardiol 61:467, 1988.

219. Balderston SM, Shaffer EM, Sondheimer HM, et al: Hereditary atrioventricular conduction defect in a child. Pediatr Cardiol 10:37, 1989.

220. Wolkowicz J, Burgess JH: Complete heart block in an Inuit family. Can J Cardiol 4:352, 1988.

221. Stephan E: Hereditary bundle branch system defect: Survey of a family with four affected generations. Am Heart J 95:89, 1978.

222. Lorber A, Maisuls E, Naschitz J: Hereditary right axis deviation: Electrocardiographic pattern of pseudo left posterior hemiblock and incomplete right bundle branch block. Int J Cardiol 20:399, 1988

223. Van Der Merwe P-L, Weymar HW, Torrington M, et al: Progressive familial heart block (type I): A follow up study after 10 years. S Afr Med J 73:275, 1988.

224. Torrington M, Weymar HW, van der Merwe PL, et al: Progressive familial heart block: Pt I. Extent of the disease. S Afr Med J 70:354, 1986.

225. Kothari SS, Agrawal SM, Kirshnaswami S: Familial complete heart block in hypertrophic cardiomyopathy. Int J Cardiol 20:294, 1988.

226. Stables RH, Bailey C, Ormerod OJM: Idiopathic familial atrial cardiomyopathy with diffuse conduction block, Q J Med 264:325, 1989.

227. Olofsson B-V, Eriksson P, Eriksson A: The sick sinus syndrome in familial amyloidosis with polyneuropathy. Int J Cardiol 4:71, 1983.

228. Winkler RB, Nora AH, Nora JJ: Familial congenital complete heart block and maternal systemic lupus erythematosus. Circulation 56:1103, 1977.

229. McCue CM, Mantakas ME, Tingelstad JB, et al: Congenital heart block in newborns of mothers with connective tissue disease. Circulation 56: 82, 1977.

230. Chameides L, Truex RC, Vetter V, et al: Association of maternal systemic lupus erythematosus with congenital complete heart block. N Engl J Med 297:1204, 1977.

231. Scott JS, Maddison PJ, Taylor PV, et al: Connective-tissue disease, antibodies to ribonucleoprotein, and congenital heart block. N Engl J Med 309:209, 1983.

232. Lockshin MD, Gibofsky A, Peebles CL, et al: Neonatal lupus erythematosus with heart block: Familial study of a patient with anti-SS-A and SS-B antibodies. Arthritis Rheum 26:210, 1983.

233. Bergfeldt L: HLA-B27-Associated cardiac disease. Ann Intern Med 127: 621–629, 1997.

234. Bacos JM, Eagan JT, Orgain ES: Congenital familial nodal rhythm. Circulation 22:887, 1960.

235. Chen Q, Kirsch GE, Zhang D, et al: Genetic basis and molecular mechanism for idiopathic ventricular fibrillation. Nature 392:293–296, 1998.

236. Chia BL, Yew FC, Chay SO, et al: Familial Wolff-Parkinson-White syndrome. J Electrocardiol 15:195, 1982.

237. Vidaillet HJ, Pressley JC, Henke E, et al: Familial occurrence of accessory atrioventricular pathways: Preexcitation syndrome. N Engl J Med 317:65, 1987.

238. Brugada R, Tapscott T, Czernuszewicz GZ, et al: Identification of a genetic locus for familial atrial fibrillation. N Engl J Med 336:905–911, 1997.

239. Stoll C, Kieny JR, Dott B, et al: Ventricular extrasystoles with syncopal episodes, perodactyly, and Robin sequence in three generations: A new inherited MCA syndrome? Am J Med Genet 42:480, 1992.

240. Laurent M, Descases C, Biron Y, et al: Familial form of arrhythmogenic right ventricular dysplasia. Br Heart J 113:827, 1987.

241. Ruder MA, Winston SA, Davis JC, et al: Arrhythmogenic right ventricular dysplasia in a family. Am J Cardiol 56:799, 1985.

242. Wiesfeld ACP, Crijns JGM, Van Dijk RB, et al: Potential role for endomyocardial biopsy in the clinical characterization of patients with idiopathic ventricular fibrillation. Am Heart J 127:1421, 1993.

243. McKenna WJ, Thiene G, Nava A, et al: Diagnosis of arrhythmogenic right ventricular dysplasia/cardiomyopathy. Br Heart J 72:215, 1994.

243a. Watzinger N, Lercher P, Kern R, et al: Biventricular dysplasia. Circulation 101:1479–1482, 2000.

244. Severini GM, Krajinovic M, Pinamonti B, et al: A new locus for arrhythmogenic right ventricular dysplasia on the long arm of chromosome 14. Genomics 31:193–200, 1996.

244a. Li D, Ahmad F, Gardner MJ, et al: The locus of a novel gene responsible for arrhythmogenic right-ventricular dysplasia characterized by early onset and high penetrance maps to chromosome 10p12-p14. Am J Hum Genet 66:148–156, 2000.

245. Ward OC: A new familial cardiac syndrome in children. J Ir Med Assoc 54:103, 1964.

246. Romano C: Congenital cardiac arrhythmia. Lancet 1:658, 1965.

247. Greenspon AJ, Kidwell GA, Barrasse LD, et al: Hereditary long QT syndrome associated with cardiac conduction system disease. PACE 12: 479, 1989.

248. Marks ML, Whisler SL, Clericuzio C, et al: A new form of long QT syndrome associated with syndactyly. J Am Coll Cardiol 25:59, 1995.

249. Vincent GM: The molecular genetics of the long QT syndrome: Genes causing fainting and sudden death. Annu Rev Med 49:263–274. 1998.

250. Wattanasirichaigoon D, Vesely MR, Duggal P, et al: Sodium channel abnormalities are infrequent in patients with long QT syndrome: Identification of two novel *SCN5A* mutations. Am J Med Genet 86:470–476, 1999.

251. Ackerman MJ, Tester DJ, Porter CJ, et al: Molecular diagnosis of the inherited long-QT syndrome in a woman who died after near-drowning. N Engl J Med 341:121–125, 1999.

252. Priori SG, Napolitano C, Schwartz PJ: Low penetrance in the long-QT syndrome. Circulation 99:529–533, 1999.

253. Vincent GM, Timothy KW, Leppert M, et al: The spectrum of symptoms and QT intervals in carriers of the gene for the long-QT syndrome. N Engl J Med 327:846, 1992.

254. Zareba W, Moss AJ, Schwartz PJ, et al: Influence of the genotype on the clinical course of the long-QT syndrome. N Engl J Med 339:690–695, 1998.

255. Priori SG, Barhanin J, Hauer RNW, et al: Genetic and molecular basis of cardiac arrhythmias: Impact on clinical management. Part III. Circulation 99:674–681, 1999.

256. Jervell A, Lange-Nielsen F: Congenital deaf-mutism, functional heart disease with prolongation of Q-T interval and sudden death. Am Heart J 54:59, 1957.

257. Splawski I, Timothy KW, Vincent GM, et al: Molecular basis of the long-QT syndrome associated with deafness. N Engl J Med 336:1562–1567, 1997.

DISORDERS OF CONNECTIVE TISSUE

258. McKusick VA: Heritable Disorders of Connective Tissue. St. Louis, CV Mosby, 1956.

259. Royce PM, Steinmann B (eds): Connective Tissue and Its Heritable Disorders: Molecular, Genetic and Medical Aspects. New York, Wiley-Liss, 1993.

260. Pyeritz RE: Heritable disorders of connective tissue. *In* Pierpont ME, Moller JH (eds): The Genetics of Cardiovascular Disease. Boston, Martinus Nijhoff, 1987, p 265.

261. Beighton P (ed): McKusick's Heritable Disorders of Connective Tissue. 5th ed. St. Louis, CV Mosby, 1993.

262. Pyeritz RE: Disorders of fibrillins and microfibrilogenesis: Marfan syndrome, MASS phenotype, contractural arachnodactyly and related conditions. *In* Rimoin DL, Connor JM, Pyeritz RE (eds): Principles and Practice of Medical Genetics. 3rd ed. New York, Churchill Livingstone, 1997, pp 1027–1066.

262a. Pyeritz RE: The Marfan syndrome. Ann Rev Med 51:481–510, 2000.

263. McKusick VA: The cardiovascular aspects of Marfan's syndrome: A heritable disorder of connective tissue. Circulation 11:321, 1955.

264. Marsalese DL, Moodie DS, Vacante M, et al: Marfan's syndrome: Natural history and long-term follow-up of cardiovascular involvement. J Am Coll Cardiol 14:422, 1989.

265. Murdoch JL, Walker BA, Halpern BL, et al: Life expectancy and causes of death in the Marfan syndrome. N Engl J Med 286:804, 1972.

266. Sisk HE, Zahka KG, Pyeritz RE: The Marfan syndrome in early childhood: Analysis of 15 patients diagnosed less than 4 years of age. Am J Cardiol 52:353, 1983.

267. Morse RP, Rockenmacher S, Pyeritz RE, et al: Diagnosis and management of Marfan syndrome in infants. Pediatrics 86:888, 1990.

268. Pyeritz RE, Wappel MA: Mitral valve dysfunction in the Marfan syndrome. Am J Med 74:797, 1983.

269. Gillinov AM, Hulyalkar A, Cameron DE, et al: Mitral valve operation in patients with the Marfan syndrome. J Thorac Cardiovasc Surg 107:724, 1994.

270. Gott VL, Greene PS, Alejo DE, et al: Surgery for ascending aortic disease in Marfan patients: A multi-center study. N Engl J Med 340:1307–1313, 1999.

271. Lima SD, Lima JAC, Pyeritz RE, et al: Relationship of mitral valve prolapse to left ventricular size in Marfan's syndrome. Am J Cardiol 55: 739, 1985.

272. Roman MJ, Rosen SE, Kramer-Fox R, et al: Prognostic significance of the pattern of aortic root dilation in the Marfan syndrome. J Am Coll Cardiol 22:1470, 1993.

273. Crawford ES: Marfan's syndrome: Broad spectral surgical treatment: Cardiovascular manifestations. Ann Surg 198:487, 1983.

274. Svensson LG, Crawford ES, Coselli JS, et al: Impact of cardiovascular operation on survival in the Marfan patient. Circulation 80:233, 1988.

275. Silverman DI, Burton KJ, Gray J, et al: Life expectancy in the Marfan syndrome. Am J Cardiol 75:157, 1995.

276. David TE: Aortic valve repair in patients with Marfan syndrome and ascending aorta aneurysms due to degenerative disease. J Card Surg 9(Suppl):182–187, 1994.

276a. Birks EJ, Webb C, Child A, et al: Early and long-term results of a valve-sparing operation for Marfan syndrome. Circulation 100(suppl II): 29–35, 1999.

277. Arn PH, Scherer LR, Haller JA Jr, et al: Outcome of pectus excavatum

in patients with Marfan syndrome and in the general population. J Pediatr 115:954, 1989.

278. Schaefer S, Peshock RM, Malloy CR, et al: Nuclear magnetic resonance imaging in Marfan's syndrome. J Am Coll Cardiol 9:70, 1987.

279. Soulen RL, Fishman E, Pyeritz RE, et al: Evaluation of the Marfan syndrome: MR imaging versus CT. Radiology 165:697, 1987.

280. Crawford ES, Crawford JL, Stowe CL, et al: Total aortic replacement for chronic aortic dissection occurring in patients with and without Marfan's syndrome. Ann Surg 199:358, 1984.

281. Shores J, Borger KR, Murphy EA, et al: Chronic β-adrenergic blockade protects the aorta in the Marfan syndrome: A prospective, randomized trial of propranolol. N Engl J Med 330:1335, 1994.

282. Salim MA, Alpert BS, Ward JC, et al: Effect of beta-adrenergic blockade on aortic root rate of dilation in the Marfan syndrome. Am J Cardiol 74: 629, 1994.

283. Yin FCP, Brin KP, Ting C-T, et al: Arterial hemodynamics in the Marfan syndrome. Circulation 79:854, 1989.

284. Jondeau G, Boutouyrie P, Lacolley P, et al: Central pulse pressure is a major determinant of ascending aorta dilatation in Marfan syndrome. Circulation 99:2677–2681, 1999.

285. Pyeritz RE: Maternal and fetal complications of pregnancy in the Marfan syndrome. Am J Med 71:784, 1981.

286. Rossiter JP, Morales AJ, Repke JT, et al: A prospective longitudinal evaluation of pregnancy in the Marfan syndrome. Am J Obstet Gynecol 173:1599, 1995.

287. Lipscomb KJ, Clayton-Smith J, Clarke B, et al: Outcome of pregnancy in women with Marfan's syndrome. Br J Obstet Gynaecol 104:210–216, 1997.

288. Hollister DW, Godfrey M, Sakai LY, et al: Marfan syndrome: Immunohistologic abnormalities of the elastin-associated microfibrillar fiber system. N Engl J Med 323:152, 1990.

289. Sakai LY, Keene DR, Engvall E: Fibrillin, a new 350-kD glycoprotein, is a component of extracellular microfibrils. J Cell Biol 103:2499, 1986.

290. Pyeritz RE, Dietz HC: The Marfan syndrome and other fibrillinopathies. In Royce PM, Steinmann B (eds): Connective Tissue and Its Heritable Disorders: Molecular, Genetic and Medical Aspects. 2nd ed. New York, Wiley-Liss (in press).

291. Collod-Beroud G, Beroud C, Ades L: Marfan Database (3rd ed): New mutations and new routines for the software. Nucl Acids Res 26:229–233, 1998.

292. Yuan B, Thomas JP, von Kodolitsch Y, Pyeritz RE: Comparison of heteroduplex analysis, direct sequencing and enzyme mismatch cleavage for detecting mutations in a large gene, FBN1. Hum Mutat 14:440–446, 1999.

293. Milewicz DMcG, Pyeritz RE, Crawford ES, et al: Marfan syndrome: Defective synthesis, secretion and extracellular matrix formation of fibrillin by cultured dermal fibroblasts. J Clin Invest 89:79, 1992.

294. Aoyama T, Francke U, Dietz H, et al: Quantitative differences in biosynthesis and extracellular deposition of fibrillin in cultured fibroblasts distinguish five groups of Marfan syndrome patients and suggest distinct pathogenic mechanisms. J Clin Invest 94:130, 1994.

295. Beighton P, De Paepe A, Steinmann B, et al: Ehlers-Danlos syndromes: Revised nosology, Villefranche, 1997. Am J Med Genet 77:31–37, 1998.

296. Leier CV, Call TD, Fulkerson PK, et al: The spectrum of cardiac defects in the Ehlers-Danlos syndrome, types I and III. Ann Intern Med 92:171, 1980.

296a. Pyeritz RE: Ehlers-Danlos syndrome. N Engl J Med 342:730–732, 2000.

297. Gilchrist D, Schwarze U, Shields K, et al: Large kindred with Ehlers-Danlos syndrome type IV due to a point mutation (G571S) in the COL3A1 gene of type III procollagen: Low risk of pregnancy complications and unexpected longevity in some affected relatives. Am J Med Genet 82:305–311, 1999.

298. Fox R, Pope FM, Narcisi P, et al: Spontaneous carotid cavernous fistula in Ehlers-Danlos syndrome. J Neurol Neurosurg Psychiatry 51:984, 1988.

298a. Pepin M, Schwarze U, Superti-Furga A, Byers PH: Clinical and genetic features of Ehlers-Danlos syndrome type IV, the vascular type. N Engl J Med 342:673–680, 2000.

299. Rudd NL, Nimrod C, Holbrook KA, et al: Pregnancy complications in type IV Ehlers-Danlos syndrome. Lancet 1:50, 1983.

300. Pope FM: Pseudoxanthoma elasticum, cutis laxa, and other disorders of elastic tissue. In Rimoin DL, Connor JM, Pyeritz RE (eds): Principles and Practice of Medical Genetics. 3rd ed. New York, Churchill Livingstone, 1997, pp 1083–1120.

301. Cunningham JR, Lippman SM, Renie WA, et al: Pseudoxanthoma elasticum: Treatment of gastrointestinal hemorrhage by arterial embolization and observations of autosomal dominant inheritance. Johns Hopkins Med J 147:168, 1980.

302. Lebwohl MG, Distefano D, Prioleau PG, et al: Pseudoxanthoma elasticum and mitral-valve prolapse. N Engl J Med 307:228, 1982.

303. Pyeritz RE, Weiss JL, Renic WA, et al: Pseudoxanthoma elasticum and mitral-valve prolapse. N Engl J Med 307:1451, 1982.

304. Goodman RM, Smith EW, Paton D, et al: Pseudoxanthoma elasticum: A clinical and histopathological study. Medicine 42:297, 1963.

305. Lebwohl M, Halperin J, Phelps RG: Occult pseudoxanthoma elasticum in patients with premature cardiovascular disease. N Engl J Med 329: 1237, 1993.

306. Challenor VF, Conway N, Monro JL: The surgical treatment of restrictive cardiomyopathy in pseudoxanthoma elasticum. Br Heart J 59:266, 1988.

307. Renie WA, Pyeritz RE, Combs J, et al: Pseudoxanthoma elasticum: High calcium intake in early life correlates with severity. Am J Med Genet 19:235, 1984.

308. Struk B, Neldner KH, Rao VS, et al: Mapping of both autosomal recessive and dominant variants of pseudoxanthoma elasticum to chromosome 16p13.1. Hum Mol Genet 6:1823, 1997.

309. Maharaj B, Hammond MG, Appadoo B, et al: HLA-A, B, DR, and DQ antigens in black patients with severe chronic rheumatic heart disease. Circulation 76:259, 1987.

INBORN ERRORS OF METABOLISM THAT AFFECT THE CARDIOVASCULAR SYSTEM

310. La Du BN: Alkaptonuria: In Scriver CR, Beaudet AL, Sly WA, Valle D (eds): The Metabolic and Molecular Bases of Inherited Disease. New York, McGraw-Hill, 1995, p 1371.

311. Mudd SH, Levy HL, Skovby F: Disorders of transsulfuration. In Scriver CR, Beaudet AL, Sly WA, Valle D (eds): The Metabolic and Molecular Bases of Inherited Disease. New York, McGraw-Hill, 1995, p 1279.

312. Kraus JP, Janosik M, Kozich V, et al: Cystathionine β-synthase mutations in homocystinuria. Hum Mutat 13:362–375, 1999.

313. Mudd SH, Skovby F, Levy HL, et al: The natural history of homocystinuria due to cystathionine beta-synthase deficiency. Am J Hum Genet 37: 1, 1985.

313a. Wilcken DEL, Wilcken B: The natural history of vascular disease in homocystinuria and the effects of treatment. J Inher Metab Dis 20:295–300, 1997.

314. Hill-Zobel RL, Pyeritz RE, Scheffel U, et al: Kinetics and biodistribution of 122In-labeled platelets in homocystinuria. N Engl J Med 307:781, 1982.

315. Selhub J, Jacques PF, Bostom AG, et al: Association between plasma homocysteine concentrations and extracranial carotid-artery stenosis. N Engl J Med 332:286, 1995.

316. Kang S-S, Passen EL, Ruggie N, et al: Thermolabile defect of methylenetetrahydrofolate reductase in coronary artery disease. Circulation 88: 1463, 1993.

317. Eikelboom JW, Lonn E, Genest J Jr, et al: Homocyst(e)ine and cardiovascular disease: A critical review of the epidemiologic evidence. Ann Intern Med 131:363–375, 1999.

318. Hajjar KA: Homocysteine-induced modulation of tissue plasminogen activator binding to its endothelial cell membrane receptor. J Clin Invest 91:2873, 1993.

319. Majors A, Ehrhart LA, Pezacka EH: Homocysteine as a risk factor for vascular disease. Enhanced collagen production and accumulation by smooth muscle cells. Arterioscler Thromb Vasc Biol 17:2074–2081, 1997.

320. Stampfer MJ, Manilow MR: Can lowering homocysteine levels reduce cardiovascular risk? N Engl J Med 332:328, 1995.

321. Roe CR, Coates PM: Mitochondrial fatty acid oxidation disorders. In Scriver CR, Beaudet AL, Sly WA, Valle D (eds): The Metabolic and Molecular Bases of Inherited Disease. New York, McGraw-Hill, 1995, p 1501.

322. Treem WR, Stanley CA, Finegold DN, et al: Primary carnitine deficiency due to a failure of carnitine transport in kidney, muscle, and fibroblasts. N Engl J Med 319:1331, 1988.

323. Waber LJ, Valle D, Neill C, et al: Carnitine deficiency presenting as familial cardiomyopathy: A treatable defect in carnitine transport. J Pediatr 101:700, 1982.

324. Tripp ME, Katcher ML, Peters HA, et al: Systemic carnitine deficiency presenting as familial endocardial fibroelastosis. N Engl J Med 305:385, 1981.

325. Goodman SI: Organic acid metabolism. In Rimoin DL, Connor JM, Pyeritz RE (eds): Principles and Practice of Medical Genetics. 3rd ed. New York, Churchill Livingstone, 1997, pp 1977–1990.

326. Brackett JC, Sims HF, Steiner RD, et al: A novel mutation in medium chain Acyl-CoA dehydrogenase causes sudden neonatal death. J Clin Invest 94:1477, 1994.

327. de Vries HG, Niezen-Koning K, Kliphuis JW, et al: Prevalence of carriers of the most common medium-chain acyl-CoA dehydrogenase (MCAD) deficiency mutation (G985A) in The Netherlands. Hum Genet 98:1–2, 1996.

328. Anan R, Nakagawa M, Miyata M, et al: Cardiac involvement in mitochondrial diseases. A study of 17 patients with documented mitochondrial DNA defects. Circulation 91:955, 1995.

329. Merante F, Tein L, Benson L, et al: Maternally inherited hypertrophic cardiomyopathy due to a novel T-to-C transition at nucleotide 9997 in the mitochondrial tRNAglycine gene. Am J Hum Genet 55:437, 1994.

330. Van Hove JLK, Shanske S, Ciacci F, et al: Mitochondrial myopathy with anemia, cardiomyopathy and lactic acidosis: A distinct late onset mitochondrial disorder. Am J Med Genet 51:115, 1994.

331. Ogashara S, Engel AG, Frens D, et al: Muscle coenzyme Q deficiency in familial mitochondrial encephalomyopathy. Proc Natl Acad Sci U S A 86:2379, 1989.

332. Channer KS, Channer JL, Campbell MJ, et al: Cardiomyopathy in the Kearns-Sayre syndrome. Br Heart J 59:486, 1988.

333. Chen Y-T, Burchell A: Glycogen storage diseases. In Scriver CR, Beaudet AL, Sly WA, Valle D (eds): The Metabolic and Molecular Bases of Inherited Disease. New York, McGraw-Hill, 1995, p 935.

334. Ehlers KH, Hagstrom JWC, Lukas DS, et al: Glycogen-storage disease of the myocardium with obstruction to left ventricular outflow. Circulation 25:96, 1962.

335. Bharati S, Serratto M, Du Brow I, et al: The conduction system in Pompe's disease. Pediatr Cardiol 2:25, 1982.

336. Bonnici F, Shapiro R, Joffe HS, et al: Angiocardiographic and enzyme studies in a patient with type II glycogenosis. S Afr Med J 58:860, 1980.

337. Robinson WF, Howell JM, Dorling PR: Cardiomyopathy is generalised glycogenosis type II in cattle. Cardiovasc Res 17:238, 1982.

338. Suzuki Y, Tsuji A, Omura K, et al: Km mutant of acid alpha-glucosidase in a case of cardiomyopathy without signs of skeletal muscle involvement. Clin Genet 33:376, 1988.

339. Makos MM, McComb RD, Hart MN, et al: Alpha-glucosidase deficiency and basilar artery aneurysm: Report of a sibship. Ann Neurol 22:629, 1987.

340. Kretzschmar HA, Wagner H, Hubner G, et al: Aneurysm and vacuolar degeneration of cerebral arteries in late-onset acid maltase deficiency. J Neurol Sci 98:169, 1990.

341. Martiniuk F, Mehler M, Tzall S, et al: Extensive genetic heterogeneity in patients with acid alpha glucosidase deficiency as detected by abnormalities of DNA and mRNA. Am J Hum Genet 47:73, 1990.

342. Olson LJ, Reeder GS, Noller KL, et al: Cardiac involvement in glycogen storage disease III. Morphological and biochemical characterization with endomyocardial biopsy. Am J Cardiol 53:980, 1984.

343. Coleman RA, Winter HS, Wolf B, et al: Glycogen debranching enzyme deficiency: Long-term study of serum enzyme activities and clinical features. J Inherit Metab Dis 15:869, 1992.

344. Talente GM, Coleman RA, Alter C, et al: Glycogen storage diseases in adults. Ann Intern Med 120:218, 1994.

345. Cox PM, Brueton LA, Murphy KW, et al: Early-onset fetal hydrops and muscle degeneration in siblings due to a novel variant of type IV glycogenosis. Am J Med Genet 86:187–193, 1999.

346. Servidei S, Metlay LA, Chodosh J, et al: Fatal infantile cardiopathy caused by phosphorylase b kinase deficiency. J Pediatr 113:82, 1988.

347. Schroder JM, May R, Shin YS: Juvenile hereditary polyglucosan body disease with complete branching enzyme deficiency (type IV glycogenosis). Acta Neuropathol 85:419, 1993.

348. Howell RR: Continuing lessons from glycogen storage diseases [editorial]. N Engl J Med 324:55, 1991.

349. Selby R, Starzl TE, Yunis E, et al: Liver transplantation for type IV glycogen storage disease. N Engl J Med 324:39, 1991.

350. Eishi Y, Takemura T, Sone R, et al: Glycogen storage disease confined to the heart with deficient activity of cardiac phosphorylase kinase: A new type of glycogen storage disease. Hum Pathol 16:193, 1987.

351. Elleder M, Shin YS, Zuntova A, et al: Fatal infantile hypertrophic cardiomyopathy secondary to deficiency of heart specific phosphorylase b kinase. Virchows Arch A 423:303, 1993.

352. Leroy JG: Oligosaccharidoses. In Rimoin DL, Connor JM, Pyeritz RE (eds): Principles and Practice of Medical Genetics. 3rd ed. New York, Churchill Livingstone, 1997, pp 2081–2104.

353. Bothwell TH, Charlton RW, Motulsky AG: Hemochromatosis. In Scriver CR, Beaudet AL, Sly WA, Valle D (eds): The Metabolic and Molecular Bases of Inherited Disease. New York, McGraw-Hill, 1995, p 2237.

354. Olynyk JK, Cullen DJ, Aquilia S, et al: A population-based study of the clinical expression of the hemochromatosis gene. N Engl J Med 341:718–724, 1999.

355. Burke W, Thomson E, Khoury MJ, et al: Hereditary hemochromatosis: Gene discovery and its implications for population-based screening. JAMA 280:172–178, 1998.

356. Edwards CQ: Early detection of hereditary hemochromatosis. Ann Intern Med 101:707, 1984.

357. Olson LJ, Baldus WP, Tajik AJ, Echocardiographic features of idiopathic hemochromatosis. Am J Cardiol 60:885, 1987.

358. Porter J, Cary N, Schofield P: Haemochromatosis presenting as congestive cardiac failure. Br Heart J 73:73, 1995.

359. Cutler DJ, Isner JM, Bracey AW, et al: Hemochromatosis heart disease: An unemphasized cause of potentially reversible restrictive cardiomyopathy. Am J Med 69:923, 1980.

360. Adams RJ: Sickle cell disease and stroke. J Child Neurol 10:75–76, 1995.

361. Weatherall DJ, Clegg JB, Higgs DR, et al: The hemoglobinopathies. In Scriver CR, Beaudet AL, Sly WA, Valley D (eds): The Metabolic and Molecular Bases of Inherited Disease. New York, McGraw-Hill, 1995, p 3417.

362. Sutton LL, Castro O, Cross DJ, et al: Pulmonary hypertension in sickle cell disease. Am J Cardiol 74:626, 1994.

363. Brittenham GM, Griffith PM, Nienhuis AW, et al: Efficacy of deferoxamine in preventing complications of iron overload in patients with thalassemia major. N Engl J Med 331:567, 1994.

364. Steinberg MH: Management of sickle cell disease. N Engl J Med 340:1021–1030, 1999.

365. Olivieri NF, Liu PP, Sher GD, et al: Combination liver and heart transplantation for end-stage iron-induced organ failure in an adult with homozygous beta-thalassemia. N Engl J Med 330:1125, 1994.

366. Spranger J: Mucopolysaccharidoses. In Rimoin DL, Connor JM, Pyeritz RE (eds): Principles and Practice of Medical Genetics. 3rd ed. New York, Churchill Livingstone, 1997, pp 2071–2080.

367. Johnson GL, Vine DL, Cottrill CM, et al: Echocardiographic mitral valve deformity in the mucopolysaccharidoses. Pediatrics 67:401, 1981.

368. Gross DM, Williams JC, Caprioli C, et al: Echocardiographic abnormalities in the mucopolysaccharide storage diseases. Am J Cardiol 61:170, 1988.

369. John RM, Hunter D, Swanton RH: Echocardiographic abnormalities in type IV mucopolysaccharidosis. Arch Dis Child 65:746, 1990.

370. Pyeritz RE: Storage disorders. In Pierpont ME, Moller JH (eds): The Genetics of Cardiovascular Disease. Boston, Martinus Nijhoff Publishing, 1987, p 215.

371. Nelson J, Shields MD, Mulholland HC: Cardiovascular studies in the mucopolysaccharidoses. J Med Genet 27:94, 1990.

372. Brosius FC III, Roberts WC: Coronary artery disease in the Hurler syndrome: Qualitative and quantitative analysis of the extent of coronary narrowing at necropsy in six children. Am J Cardiol 47:649, 1981.

373. Renteria VG, Ferrans VJ, Roberts WC: The heart in the Hurler syndrome: Gross, histologic and ultrastructural observations in five necropsy cases. Am J Cardiol 38:487, 1976.

374. Semenza GL, Pyeritz RE: Respiratory complications of the mucopolysaccharide storage disorders. Medicine 67:209, 1988.

375. Young ID, Harper PS: Long-term complications in Hunter's syndrome. Clin Genet 16:125, 1979.

376. Armitage JO: Bone marrow transplantation. N Engl J Med 330:827, 1994.

377. Whitley CB, Belani KG, Chang P-N, et al: Long-term outcome of Hurler syndrome following bone marrow transplantation. Am J Med Genet 46:209, 1993.

378. Rutledge SL, Percy AK: Gangliosidoses and related lipid storage diseases. In Rimoin DL, Connor JM, Pyeritz RE (eds): Principles and Practice of Medical Genetics. 3rd ed. New York, Churchill Livingstone, 1997, pp 2105–2130.

379. Spence MW, MacKinnon KE, Burgess JK, et al: Failure to correct the metabolic defect by renal allotransplantation in Fabry's disease. Ann Intern Med 84:13, 1976.

380. Kramer W, Thormann J, Mueller K, et al: Progressive cardiac involvement by Fabry's disease despite successful renal allotransplantation. Int J Cardiol 7:72, 1985.

380a. Schiffmann R, Murray GJ, Treco D, et al: Infusion of α-galactosidase A reduces tissue globotriaosylceramide storage in patients with Fabry disease. Proc Natl Acad Sci U S A 97:365–370, 2000.

381. Colucci WS, Lorell BH, Schoen FJ, et al: Hypertrophic obstructive cardiomyopathy due to Fabry's disease. N Engl J Med 307:926, 1982.

382. von Scheidt W, Eng CM, Fitzmaurice TF, et al: An atypical variant of Fabry's disease with manifestations confined to the myocardium. N Engl J Med 324:395, 1991.

383. Hillsley RE, Hernandez E, Steenbergen C, et al: Inherited restrictive cardiomyopathy in a 74-year-old woman: A case of Fabry's disease. Am Heart J 129:199–202, 1995.

384. Nakao S, Takenaka T, Maeda M, et al: An atypical variant of Fabry's disease in men with left ventricular hypertrophy. N Engl J Med 333:288–293, 1995.

385. Goldman ME, Cantor R, Schwartz MF, et al: Echocardiographic abnormalities and disease severity in Fabry's disease. J Am Coll Cardiol 7:1157, 1986.

386. Sakuraba H, Yanagawa Y, Igarashi T, et al: Cardiovascular manifestations in Fabry's disease: A high incidence of mitral valve prolapse in hemizygotes and heterozygotes. Clin Genet 29:276, 1986.

387. Mutoh T, Senda Y, Sugimura K, et al: Severe orthostatic hypotension in a female carrier of Fabry's disease. Arch Neurol 34:468, 1988.

388. Bernstein HS, Bishop DF, Astrin KH, et al: Fabry disease: Six gene rearrangements and an exonic point mutation in the alpha-galactosidase gene. J Clin Invest 83:1390, 1989.

389. Thomas PK, Harding AE. Hereditary motor and sensory neuropathies. In Rimoin DL, Connor JM, Pyeritz RE (eds): Principles and Practice of Medical Genetics. 3rd ed. New York, Churchill Livingstone, 1997, pp 2249–2268.

390. Backman C, Olofsson BO: Echocardioraphic features in familial amyloidosis with polyneuropathy. Acta Med Scand 214:273, 1983.

391. Eriksson A, Eriksson P, Olofsson B-O, et al: The cardiac atrioventricular conduction system in familial amyloidosis with polyneuropathy: A clinico-pathologic study of six cases from Northern Sweden. Acta Pathol Microbiol Immunol Scand 91:343, 1983.

392. Booth DR, Tan SY, Hawkins PN, et al: A novel variant of transthyretin, 59[Thr-Lys], associated with autosomal dominant cardiac amyloidosis in an Italian family. Circulation 91:962, 1995.

393. Skinner M, Lewis WD, Jones LA, et al: Liver transplantation as a treatment for familial amyloidotic polyneuropathy. Ann Intern Med 120:133, 1994.

394. Vidaillet HJ Jr: Cardiac tumors associated with hereditary syndromes. Am J Cardiol 61:1355, 1988.

395. Burke AP, Rosado-de-Christenson M, Templeton PA, et al: Cardiac fibroma: Clinicopathologic correlates and surgical treatment. J Thorac Cardiovasc Surg 108:862, 1994.

396. Roach ES, DiMario FJ, Kandt RS, Northrup H: Tuberous sclerosis complex consensus conference: Recommendations for diagnostic evaluation. J Child Neurol 14:401–407, 1999.

397. Sperling D, Smith M: Novel 23-base-pair duplication mutation in TSC1 exon 15 in an infant presenting with cardiac rhabdomyomas. Am J Med Genet 84:346–349, 1999.

398. Harding CO, Pagon RA: Incidence of tuberous sclerosis in patients with cardiac rhabdomyoma. Am J Med Genet 37:443, 1990.

398a. Astrinidis A, Khare L, Carsillo T, et al: Mutational analysis of the tuberous sclerosis gene TSC2 in patients with pulmonary lymphangioleiomyomatosis. J Med Genet 37:55–57, 2000.

399. Liebler GA, Magovern GJ, Park SB, et al: Familial myxomas in four siblings. J Thorac Cardiovasc Surg 71:605, 1976.

400. Carney JA, Gordon H, Carpenter PC, et al: The complex of myxomas, spotty pigmentation, and endocrine overactivity. Medicine 64:270, 1985.

401. Handley J, Carson D, Sloan J, et al: Multiple lentigines, myxoid tumours and endocrine overactivity: Four cases of Carney's complex. Br J Dermatol 126:367, 1992.

402. Goldstein MM, Casey M, Carney JA, et al: Molecular genetic diagnosis of the familial myxoma syndrome (Carney complex). Am J Med Genet 86:62–65, 1999.

INHERITED DISORDERS OF THE CIRCULATION

403. Basson CT, MacRae CA, Korf B, Merliss A: Genetic heterogeneity of familial atrial myxoma syndromes (Carney complex). Am J Cardiol 79: 994–995, 1997.

404. Stratakis CA, Carney JA, Lin J-P, et al: Carney complex, a familial multiple neoplasia and lentiginosis syndrome: Analysis of 11 kindreds and linkage to the short arm of chromosome 2. J Clin Invest 97:699–705, 1996.

405. Peery WH: Clinical spectrum of hereditary hemorrhagic telangiectasia (Osler-Weber-Rendu disease). Am J Med 82:989, 1987.

406. Haitjema T, Disch F, Overtoom TTC, Westermann CJJ: Screening family members of patients with hereditary hemorrhagic telangiectasia. Am J Med 99:519–524, 1995.

406a. Shovlin CL, Guttmacher AE, Buscarini E, et al: Diagnostic criteria for hereditary hemorrhagic telangiectasia (Rendu-Osler-Weber syndrome). Am J Med Genet 91:66–67, 2000.

407. Guillén B, Guizar J, de la Cruz J, et al: Hereditary hemorrhagic telangiectasia: Report of 15 affected cases in a Mexican family. Clin Genet 39: 214, 1991.

408. Fulbright RK, Chaloupka JC, Putman CM, et al: MR of hereditary hemorrhagic telangiectasia: Prevalence and spectrum of cerebrovascular malformations. Am J Neuroradiol 19:477–484, 1998.

409. Nikolopoulos N, Xynos E, Vassilakis JS: Familial occurrence of hyperdynamic circulation status due to intrahepatic fistulae in hereditary hemorrhagic telangiectasia. Hepatogastroenterology 35:167, 1988.

410. Cooke DAP: Renal arteriovenous malformation demonstrated angiographically in hereditary haemorrhagic telangiectasia (Rendu-Osler-Weber disease). J R Soc Med 79:744, 1986.

411. Kurnik PB, Heymann WR: Coronary artery ectasia associated with hereditary hemorrhagic telangiectasia. Arch Intern Med 149:2357, 1989.

412. Kopel L, Lage SG: Cardiac tamponade in hereditary hemorrhagic telangiectasia. Am J Med 105:252–253, 1998.

413. Braverman IM, Keh A, Jacobson BS: Ultrastructure and three-dimensional organization of the telangiectases of hereditary hemorrhagic telangiectasia. J Invest Dermatol 95:422, 1990.

414. Lee DW, White RI Jr, Egglin TK, et al: Embolotherapy of large pulmonary arteriovenous malformations: Long-term results. Ann Thorac Surg 64:930–940, 1997.

415. Haq AU, Glass J, Netchvolodoff CV, et al: Hereditary hemorrhagic telangiectasia and danazol. Ann Intern Med 109:171, 1988.

416. Saba HI, Morelli GA, Logrono LA: Treatment of bleeding in hereditary hemorrhagic telangiectasia with aminocaproic acid. N Engl J Med 330: 1789, 1994.

417. Phillips MD: Stopping bleeding in hereditary telangiectasia. N Engl J Med 331:1822, 1994.

418. McAllister KA, Grogg KMM, Johnson DW, et al: Endoglin, a TGF-β binding protein of endothelial cells, is the gene for hereditary haemorrhagic telangiectasia type 1. Nat Genet 8:345, 1994.

419. Johnson DW, Berg JN, Baldwin MA, et al: Mutations in the activin receptor-like kinase 1 gene in hereditary haemorrhagic telangiectasia type 2. Nat Genet 13:189–195, 1996.

420. Piantanida M, Buscarini E, Dellavecchia C, et al: Hereditary haemorrhagic telangiectasia with extensive liver involvement is not caused by either HHT1 or HHT2. J Med Genet 33:441–443, 1996.

421. Jennings AM, Smith R, Cole DR, et al: Von Hippel-Lindau disease in a large British family: Clinicopathological features and recommendations for screening and follow-up. Q J Med 66:233, 1988.

422. Lamiell JM, Salazar FG, Hsia YE: Von Hippel-Lindau disease affecting 43 members of a single kindred. Medicine 68:1, 1989.

423. Latif F, Troy K, Gnarra J, et al: Identification of the von Hippel-Landau disease tumor suppressor gene. Science 260:1317, 1993.

424. Zbar B, Kishida T, Chen F, et al: Germline mutations in the Von Hippel-Lindau disease (VHL) gene in families from North America, Europe, and Japan. Hum Mutat 8:348–357, 1996.

425. Prowse AH, Webster AR, Richards FM, et al: Somatic inactivation of the VHL gene in Von Hippel-Lindau disease tumors. Am J Hum Genet 60:765–771, 1997.

426. Parfrey PS, Bear JC, Morgan J, et al: The diagnosis and prognosis of autosomal dominant polycystic kidney disease. N Engl J Med 323:1085, 1990.

427. Gabow PA: Autosomal dominant polycystic kidney disease. N Engl J Med 329:332, 1993.

428. Chapman AB, Johnson A, Gabow PA, et al: The renin-angiotensin aldosterone system and autosomal dominant polycystic kidney disease. N Engl J Med 323:1091, 1990.

429. Leier CV, Baker PB, Kilman JW, et al: Cardiovascular abnormalities associated with adult polycystic kidney disease. Ann Intern Med 100: 683, 1984.

430. Hossack KF, Leddy CL, Johnson AM, et al: Echocardiographic findings in autosomal dominant polycystic kidney disease. N Engl J Med 319: 907, 1988.

431. Chapman JR, Hilson AJW: Polycystic kidneys and abdominal aortic aneurysms. Lancet 1:646, 1980.

432. Chapman AB, Rubinstein D, Hughes R, et al: Intracranial aneurysms in autosomal dominant polycystic kidney disease. N Engl J Med 327:916, 1992.

432a. Watnick T, Phakdeekitcharoen B, Johnson A, et al: Mutation detection of PKD1 identifies a novel mutation common to three families with aneurysms and/or very-early-onset disease. Am J Hum Genet 65:1561–1571, 1999.

433. Hateboer N, van Dijk MA, Bogdanova N, et al: Comparison of phenotypes of polycystic kidney disease types 1 and 2. Lancet 353:103–107, 1999.

434. Koptides M, Hadjimichael C. Koupepidou P, et al: Germinal and somatic mutations in the PKD2 gene of renal cysts in autosomal dominant polycystic kidney disease. Hum Mol Genet 8:509–513, 1999.

435. Qian F, Watnick TJ, Onuchic LF, et al: The molecular basis of focal cyst formation in human autosomal dominant polycystic kidney disease type I. Cell 87:979–987, 1996.

436. Daoust MC, Reynold DM, Bichet DG, et al: Evidence for a third genetic locus for autosomal dominant polycystic kidney disease. Genomics 25: 733, 1995.

437. Shulman SA, Hyams JS, Gunta R, et al: Arteriohepatic dysplasia (Alagille syndrome): Extreme variability among affected family members. Am J Med Genet 19:325, 1984.

438. Dhorne-Pollet S, Deleuze J-F, Hadchouel M, et al: Segregation analysis of Alagille syndrome. J Med Genet 31:453, 1994.

439. Woolfenden AR, Albers GW, Steinberg GK, et al: Moyamoya syndrome in children with Alagille syndrome: Additional evidence of a vasculopathy. Pediatrics 103:505–508, 1999.

440. Yuan Z-R, Kohsak T, Ikegaya T, et al: Mutational analysis of the Jagged 1 gene in Alagille syndrome families. Hum Mol Genet 7:1363–1369, 1998.

441. Li L, Krantz ID, Deng Y, et al: Alagille syndrome is caused by mutations in human Jagged1, which encodes a ligand for Notch1. Nat Genet 16:243–251, 1997.

442. Nicod P, Bloor C, Godfrey M, et al: Familial aortic dissecting aneurysms. J Am Coll Cardiol 13:811, 1989.

443. Biddinger A, Rocklin M, Coselli J, Milewicz DM: Familial thoracic aortic dilatations and dissections: A case control study. J Vasc Surg 25: 506–511, 1997.

444. Milewicz DM, Chen H, Park E-S, et al: Reduced penetrance and variable expressivity of familial thoracic aortic aneurysms/dissections. Am J Cardiol 82:474–479, 1998.

445. Roberts CS, Roberts WC: Dissection of the aorta associated with congenital malformation of the aortic valve. J Am Coll Cardiol 17:712, 1994.

446. Kontusaari S, Tromp G, Kuivaniemi H, et al: Inheritance of RNA splicing mutation (G^{+1} IVS$_{20}$) in the type III procollagen gene (COL3AI) in a family having aortic aneurysms and easy bruisability: Phenotypic overlap between familial arterial aneurysms and Ehlers-Danlos syndrome type IV. Am J Hum Genet 47:112, 1990.

447. Kontusaari S, Tromp G, Kuivaniemi H, et al: A mutation in the gene for type III procollagen (COL3AI) in a family with aortic aneurysms. J Clin Invest 86:1465, 1990.

448. Tromp G, Wu Y, Prockop DJ, et al: Sequencing of cDNA from 50 unrelated patients reveals that mutations in the triple-helical domain of type III procollagen are an infrequent cause of aortic aneurysms. J Clin Invest 91:2539, 1993.

449. Schievink WI, Michaels VV, Mokri B, et al: A familial syndrome of arterial dissections with lentiginosis. N Engl J Med 332:576, 1995.

450. Majamaa K, Portimojarvi H, Sotaniemi KA, et al: Familial aggregation of cervical artery dissection and cerebral aneurysm. Stroke 25:1704, 1994.

451. Schievink WI, Mokri B, Piepgras DG, et al: Intracranial aneurysms and cervicocephalic arterial dissections associated with congenital heart disease. J Neurosurg 39:685–690, 1996.

452. Majumder PP, St. Jean PL, Ferrell RE, et al: On the inheritance of abdominal aortic aneurysm. Am J Hum Genet 48:164, 1991.

453. Fitzgerald P, Ramsbottom D, Burke P, et al: Abdominal aortic aneurysm in the Irish population. Br J Surg 82:483–486, 1995.

454. Pletcher BA, Fox JE, Boxer RA, et al: Four sibs with arterial tortuosity. Am J Med Genet 66:121–128, 1996.

455. Halal F, Mohr G, Toussi T, et al: Intracranial aneurysms: A report of a large pedigree. Am J Med Genet 15:89, 1983.

456. Caplan LR: Should intracranial aneurysms be treated before they rupture? N Engl J Med 339:1774–1775, 1998.

457. Magnetic Resonance Angiography Study Group: Risks and benefits of screening for intracranial aneurysms in first-degree relatives of patients with sporadic subarachnoid hemorrhage. N Engl J Med 241:1344–1350, 1999.

457a. Gaist D, Væth M, Tsiropoulos I, et al: Risk of subarachnoid haemorrhage in first degree relatives of patients with subarachnoid haemorrhage: Follow up study based on national registries in Denmark. BMJ 320:141–145, 2000.

458. Kuivaniemi H, Prockop DJ, Wu Y, et al: Exclusion of mutations in the gene for type III collagen (COL3A1) as a common cause of intracranial

aneurysms or cervical artery dissections: Results from sequence analysis of the coding sequences of type III collagen from 55 unrelated patients. Neurology 43:2652, 1993.

459. Abrahamson M: Human cysteine proteinase inhibitors: Isolation, physiological importance, inhibitory mechanism, gene structure and relation to hereditary cerebral hemorrhage. Scand J Clin Lab Invest 48:21, 1988.

460. Wattendorf AR, Bots GTAM, Went LN, et al: Familial cerebral amyloid angiopathy presenting as recurrent cerebral haemorrhage. J Neurol Sci 55:121, 1982.

461. Pasyk KA, Argenta LC, Erickson RP: Familial vascular malformations: Report of 25 members of one family. Clin Genet 26:221, 1984.

462. Walter JW, Blei F, Anderson JL, et al: Genetic mapping of a novel familial form of infantile hemangioma. Am J Med Genet 82:77–83, 1999.

463. Iadecola C: Genetics of cerebrovascular disease. N Engl J Med 339:216, 1998.

464. Stanley JC: Arterial fibrodysplasia. Arch Surg 110:561, 1975.

465. Kousseff BG, Gilbert-Barness EF: Vascular neurofibromatosis and infantile gangrene. Am J Med Genet 34:221, 1989.

466. Schievink WI, Björnsson J, Parisi JE, et al: Arterial fibromuscular dysplasia associated with severe α_1-antitrypsin deficiency. Mayo Clin Proc 69:1040, 1994.

467. Petit H, Bouchez B, Destee A, et al: Familial form of fibromuscular dysplasia of the internal carotid artery. J Neuroradiol 10:15, 1983.

468. Rushton AR: The genetics of fibromuscular dysplasia. Arch Intern Med 140:233, 1980.

469. Austin JG, Stear JC: Familial hypoplasia of both internal carotid arteries. Arch Neurol 24:1, 1971.

470. McDonald AH, Gerlis LM, Somerville J: Familial arteriopathy with associated pulmonary and systemic arterial stenoses. Br Heart J 31:375, 1969.

471. Ikeda H, Sasaki T, Yoshimoto T, et al: Mapping of a familial Moyamoya disease gene to chromosome 3p24.2-p26. Am J Hum Genet 64:533–537, 1999.

472. Van Dyck M, Proesmans W, VanHollebeke E, et al: Idiopathic infantile arterial calcification with cardiac, renal and central nervous system involvement. Eur J Pediatr 148:374, 1989.

472a. De Lange RPJ, Bolt J, Reid E, et al: Screening British CADASIL families for mutations in the NOTCH3 gene. J Med Genet 37:224–225, 2000.

473. Ophoff RA, Terwindt GM, Vergouwe MN, et al: Familial hemiplegic migraine and episodic ataxia type-2 are caused by mutations in the Ca^{2+} channel gene CACNL1A4. Cell 87:543–552, 1996.

474. Ducros A, Denier C, Joutel A, et al: Recurrence of the T666M calcium channel CACNA1A gene mutation in familial hemiplegic migraine with progressive cerebellar ataxia. Am J Hum Genet 64:89–98, 1999.

475. Joutel A, Ducros A, Vahedi K, et al: Genetic heterogeneity of familial hemiplegic migraine. Am J Hum Genet 55:1166, 1994.

476. Hovatta I, Kallela M, Färkkilä M, et al: Familial migraine: Exclusion of the susceptibility gene from the reported locus of familial hemiplegic migraine on 19p. Genomics 23:707, 1994.

477. Tournier-Lasserve E, Joutel A, Melki I, et al: Cerebral autosomal dominant arteriopathy with subcortical infarcts and leukoencephalopathy maps to chromosone 19q12. Nat Genet 3:256, 1993.

478. Melmon KL, Braunwald E: Familial pulmonary hypertension. N Engl J Med 269:770, 1963.

479. Kingdon HS, Cohen LS, Roberts WC, et al: Familial occurrence of primary pulmonary hypertension. Arch Intern Med 118:422, 1966.

480. Loyd JE, Primm RK, Newman JH: Familial primary pulmonary hypertension: Clinical patterns. Am Rev Respir Dis 129:194, 1984.

481. Nichols WC, Koller DL, Slovis B, et al: Localization of the gene for familial primary pulmonary hypertension to chromosome 2q31-32. Nat Genet 15:277–280, 1997.

482. Morse JH, Jones AC, Barst RJ, et al: Mapping of familial primary pulmonary hypertension locus (PPH1) to chromosome 2q31-q32. Circulation 95:2603–2606, 1997.

483. Lee S-D, Shroyer KR, Markham NE, et al: Monoclonal endothelial cell proliferation is present in primary but not secondary pulmonary hypertension. J Clin Invest 101:927–934, 1998.

484. Porterfield JK, Pyeritz RE, Traill TA: Pulmonary hypertension and interstitial fibrosis in von Recklinghausen neurofibromatosis. Am J Med Genet 25:531, 1986.

485. Goldstein S, Qazi QH, Fitzgerald J, et al: Distichiasis, congenital heart defects and mixed peripheral vascular anomalies. Am J Med Genet 20:283, 1985.

486. Lindenauer SM: The Klippel-Trenaunay-Weber syndrome: Varicosity, hypertrophy and hemangioma with no arteriovenous fistula. Ann Surg 162:303, 1965.

487. Campistol JM, Agusti C, Torras A, et al: Renal hemangioma and renal artery aneurysm in the Klippel-Trenaunay syndrome. J Urol 140:134, 1988.

488. Dellemijn PLI, Vanneste JAL: Cavernous angiomatosis of the central nervous system: Usefulness of screening the family. Acta Neurol Scand 88:259, 1993.

489. Drigo P, Mammi I, Battistella PA, et al: Familial cerebral, hepatic, and retinal cavernous angiomas: A new syndrome. Childs Nerv Syst 10:205, 1994.

490. Craig HD, Gunel M, Cepeda O, et al: Multilocus linkage identifies two new loci for a Mendelian form of stroke, cerebral cavernous malformation, at 7p15-13 and 3q25.2–27. Hum Mol Genet 7:1851–1858, 1998.

491. Gunel M, Awad IA, Finberg K, et al: A founder mutation as a cause of cerebral cavernous malformation in Hispanic Americans. N Engl J Med 334:946–951, 1996.

492. Laberge-le Couteulx S, Jung HH, Labauge P, et al: Truncating mutations in CCM1, encoding KRIT1, cause hereditary cavernous angiomas. Nat Genet 23:189–193, 1999.

493. Duong DH, Hartmann A, Isaacson S, et al: Arteriovenous malformations of the brain in adults. N Engl J Med 340:1812–1818, 340.

494. Herbert FA, Bowen PA: Hereditary late-onset lymphedema with pleural effusion and laryngeal edema. Arch Intern Med 143:913, 1983.

495. Ferrell RE, Levinson KL, Esman JH, et al: Hereditary lymphedema: Evidence for linkage and genetic heterogeneity. Hum Mol Genet 7:2073–2078, 1998.

496. Evans AL, Brice G, Sotirova V, et al: Mapping of primary congenital lymphedema to the 5q35.3 region. Am J Hum Genet 64:547–555, 1999.

497. Cambien F, Poirier O, Lecerf L, et al: Deletion polymorphism in the gene for angiotensin-converting enzyme is a potent risk factor for myocardial infarction. Nature 359:641, 1992.

498. Fowkes FGR, Connor, JM, Smith FB, et al: Fibrinogen genotype and risk for peripheral atherosclerosis. Lancet 339:693, 1992.

499. Ishigami T, Umemura S, Iwamoto T, et al: Molecular variant of angiotensinogen gene is associated with coronary atherosclerosis. Circulation 91:951, 1995.

500. von Kodolitsch Y, Pyeritz RE, Rogan PK: Splice site mutations in atherosclerosis candidate genes: Relating individual information to phenotype. Circulation 100:693–699, 1999.

501. Hacia JG, Collins FS: Mutational anaysis using oligonucleotide microarrays. J Med Genet 36:730–736, 1999.

502. Elston RC: Linkage and association. Genet Epidemiol 15:565–576, 1998.

503. Burke W, Motulsky AG: Hypertension. In King RA, Rotter JI, Motulsky AG (eds): The Genetic Basis of Common Diseases. New York, Oxford University Press, 1992, p 170.

504. Murphy EA, Pyeritz RD: Homeostasis: VII. A conspectus. Am J Med Genet 24:735, 1986.

505. Corvol P, Soubrier F, Jeunemaitre X: Molecular genetics of hypertension. In Rimoin DL, Connor JM, Pyeritz RE (eds): Principles and Practice of Medical Genetics. 3rd ed. New York, Churchill Livingstone, 1997, pp 899–908.

506. Parmer RJ, Cervenka JH, Stone RA: Baroflex sensitivity and heredity in essential hypertension. Circulation 85:497, 1992.

507. Lindpainter K: Genes, hypertension and cardiac hypertrophy. N Engl J Med 330:1678, 1994.

508. Lifton RP: Molecular genetics of human blood pressure variation. Science 272:676–680, 1996.

509. Halushka MK, Fan JB, Bentley K, et al: Patterns of single-nucleotide polymorphisms in candidate genes for blood-pressure homeostasis. Nat Genet 22:239–247, 1999.

510. Shimkets RA, Warnock DG, Bositis CM, et al: Liddle's syndrome: Heritable human hypertension caused by mutations in the β subunit of the epithelial sodium channel. Cell 79:407, 1994.

511. Gordon RG, Klemm SA, Tunny TJ, et al: Primary aldosteronism: Hypertension with a genetic basis. Lancet 340:159, 1992.

512. Gordon RD: Heterogeneous hypertension. Nat Genet 11:6, 1995.

513. Lifton RP, Dluhy RG, Powers M, et al: A chimeric 11β-hydroxylase/aldosterone synthase gene causes glucocorticoid-remediable aldosteronism and human hypertension. Nature 355:262, 1992.

514. Hata A, Namikawa C, Sasaki M, et al: Angiotensinogen as a risk factor for essential hypertension in Japan. J Clin Invest 93:1285, 1994.

515. Jeunemaitre X, Soubrier F, Kotelevtsev YV, et al: Molecular basis of human hypertension: Role of angiotensinogen. Cell 71:169, 1992.

516. Caulfield M, Lavendar P, Farral M, et al: Linkage of the angiotensinogen gene to essential hypertension. N Engl J Med 33:1629, 1994.

517. Niu T, Xu X, Rogus J, et al: Angiotensinogen gene and hypertension in Chinese. J Clin Invest 101:188–194, 1998.

518. Barley J, Carter N, Crews D, et al: Angiotensin 1 converting enzyme (ACE) polymorphism in different groups and its association with hypertension, plasma renin activity and aldosterone. J Med Genet 31:172, 1994.

519. Morris BJ, Zee RYL, Schrader AP: Different frequencies of angiotensin-converting enzyme genotypes in older hypertensive individuals. J Clin Invest 94:1085, 1994.

520. Arngrimsson R, Hayward C, Nadaud S, et al: Evidence for a familial pregnancy-induced hypertension locus in the eNOS-gene region. Am J Hum Genet 61:354–362, 1997.

521. Arngrimsson R, Siguroardottir S, Frigge ML, et al: A genome-wide scan reveals a maternal susceptibility locus for pre-eclampsia on chromosome 2p13. Hum Mol Genet 8:1799–1805, 1999.

522. DeStefano AL, Baldwin CT, Burzstyn M, et al: Autosomal dominant orthostatic hypotensive disorder maps to chromosome 18q. Am J Hum Genet 63:1425–1430, 1998.

523. Schwartz F, Baldwin CT, Baima J, Gavras H: Mitochondrial DNA mutations in patients with orthostatic hypotension. Am J Med Genet 86:145–150, 1999.

524. Jacob HJ, Lindpainter K, Lincoln SE, et al: Genetic mapping of a gene causing hypertension in the stroke-prone spontaneously hypertensive rat. Cell 67:213, 1991.

525. John SWM, Krege JH, Oliver PM, et al: Genetic decreases in atrial natriuretic peptide and salt-sensitive hypertension. Science 267:679, 1995.

526. Cohen LS, Friedman JM, Jefferson JW, et al: A reevaluation of risk of in utero exposure to lithium. JAMA 271:146, 1994.

PART VII

CARDIOVASCULAR DISEASE IN SPECIAL POPULATIONS

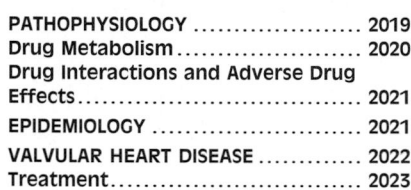

Chapter 57

Cardiovascular Disease in the Elderly

MELVIN D. CHEITLIN • DOUGLAS P. ZIPES

PATHOPHYSIOLOGY

The age at which patients become "elderly" is difficult to define because aging is a continuum, with blurred boundaries between middle and old age. Ideally, the term "elderly" should be marked by distinct changes in physiology, but the rate of physiological aging varies and may not advance in lock step with chronological changes, so that one can be physiologically young but chronologically old, and vice versa. In some reports the elderly are defined by eligibility for Medicare benefits (65 years). In others, age cutoffs of 70 or even 75 years are used.

Aging is characterized by a gradual loss of function in many organ systems, unrelated to a pathological condition. Certainly, in many old individuals comorbid diseases complicate the aging process; but independent of associated diseases, aging produces major cardiovascular changes, including decreased elasticity and compliance of the aorta and great arteries.[1] These alterations result in a higher systolic arterial pressure and an increased impedance to left ventricular (LV) ejection, and subsequent mild LV hypertrophy and interstitial fibrosis.[2] A decrease in the rate of myocardial relaxation also occurs. As a result, the LV becomes stiffer and takes longer to relax and fill in diastole, thus increasing the importance of a properly timed atrial contraction in contributing to a normal LV end-diastolic volume (Fig. 57–1) and forming the basis for diastolic dysfunction and congestive heart failure (CHF).[3] There is also a 50 to 75 percent loss of pacemaker cells in the sinus node, accompanied by a decrease in intrinsic and maximum sinus rate. The number of atrioventricular (AV) nodal cells seems to be preserved, although an increase in AV nodal delay (PR interval) is common. Increased fibrosis of the fibrous skeleton of the AV annuli occur, along with fibrosis and loss of specialized cells in the His bundle and bundle branches that can result in heart block. Heart valves thicken, and calcification results at the base of the aortic valve and mitral annulus.[4] Aging causes a decreased sensitivity of the heart to beta-adrenergic agonists and a diminished reactivity to chemoreceptors and baroreceptors.[5] There is no decrease in myocardial contractility solely as a result of aging, but diseases that do result in decreased contractility, such as hypertension (HTN) and coronary artery disease (CAD), are common in this age group.

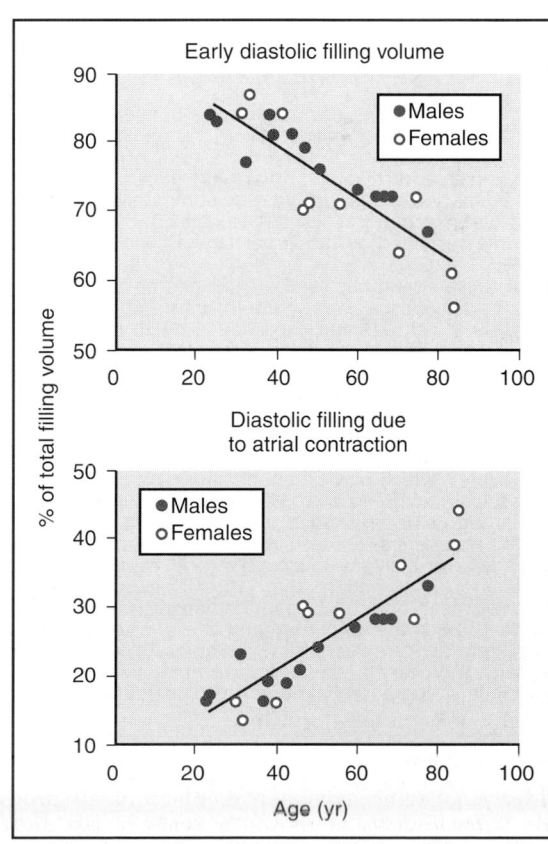

FIGURE 57–1. Effect of age on early diastolic filling and on atrial contribution to diastolic filling by echo-Doppler in healthy Baltimore Longitudinal Study on Aging (BLSA) participants. (From Geokas MC, Lakatta EG, Makinodon T, et al: The aging process. Ann Intern Med 113:455–466, 1990.)

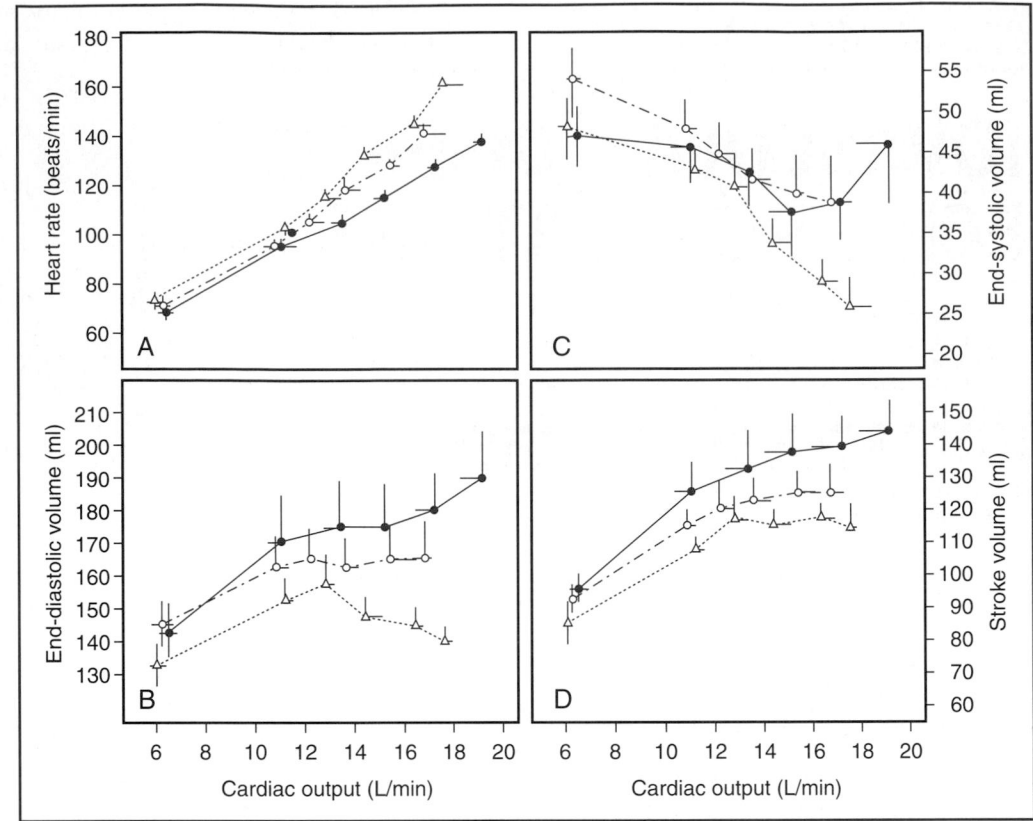

FIGURE 57–2. Exercise-related changes in heart rate *(A)*, end-diastolic volume *(B)*, end-systolic volume *(C)*, and stroke volume *(D)* in young (ages 25–44 years) *(triangles)*, middle-aged (ages 45–64 years) *(open circles)*, and elderly (ages 65–80 years) *(closed circles)* healthy men, according to increasing cardiac output with exercise. All groups had similar increase in cardiac output up to a workload of 150 watts. Note that the elderly increase cardiac output by increasing end-diastolic volume and stroke volume with exercise. (From Gerstenblith G, Renlund DG, Lakatta EG: Cardiovascular response to exercise in younger and older men. Fed Proc 46:1834–1839, 1987.)

Cardiac output remains normal at rest, but with a slower heart rate there is an increased reliance on the Frank-Starling mechanism to increase stroke volume and keep the cardiac output normal.[6] With exercise, a decrease in the ability to achieve maximum heart rate and oxygen consumption is seen in older as compared with younger patients. However, ejection fraction (EF) is kept normal by the increased stroke volume sustained by the larger LV diastolic volume seen with exercise[6] (Fig. 57–2).

Many of these alterations can be explained at cellular and subcellular levels. Cardiac fibrosis, reduction in the number of cardiac myocytes, increase in cell size and capacitance by 20 to 80 percent, and decreased responsiveness to beta-adrenergic receptor stimulation are typical changes found in older animal hearts. Interestingly, some of the same structural alterations parallel those that occur during development of myocardial hypertrophy. Aging hearts recapitulate the fetal phenotype in many aspects. Aging increases the magnitude of the L-type calcium current (ICa-L) in parallel with enlargement of cardiac myocytes, which may be important to help preserve contractile function (see Chaps. 14 and 15). The increase in ICa-L is balanced by the enlarged cell size in aged myocytes so that, despite the increase in the numbers of ICa-L channels, the overall density becomes normalized by the increase in cell size and capacitance. However, ICa-L inactivation is slowed so that larger calcium influx can occur with each heartbeat.[7] Altered calcium homeostasis predisposes to calcium overload. Both the amplitude and the density of the transient outward current (Ito) are decreased with aging.[8] These changes in Ito, together with the delay in ICa-L inactivation, may largely account for prolongation in action potential duration as hearts age.

Drug Metabolism

The elderly consume a large percentage of all drugs prescribed. Three fourths of those 75 years of age and older receive drugs of some kind. Elderly outpatients in the community take 2 or 3 medications per day, and institutionalized geriatric patients take 3 to 8 or as many as 15 per day.[9] The pharmacokinetics of drugs have been evaluated mostly in the 65- to 75-year age group, and this information is extrapolated to old and very old patients of ages 80 to 85, because few studies in this age group have been done. Aging affects both the pharmacodynamics and pharmacokinetics of drugs (see Chap. 23).

PHARMACOKINETICS

ABSORPTION. Although drugs can be given intravenously, subcutaneously, or intramuscularly, most cardiovascular drugs are given orally and are absorbed by passive diffusion through the intestinal mucosa rather than by active transport. Aging decreases gastric acidity, slows intestinal motility, and decreases by 30 percent the mucosal area for absorption in, and decreases the blood flow to, the small intestine; yet none of these seems to affect cardiovascular drug absorption significantly.

DISTRIBUTION. With aging, there is a decrease in lean body mass, and therefore a decrease in the volume of total body water. Diuretics, by decreasing the extracellular fluid, further decrease the volume of distribution and reduce the loading dose of the drug needed to achieve therapeutic levels.

With illness comes a decrease in serum albumin level, counterbalanced partly by an increase in alpha-acid glycoprotein.[10] Although these changes may not be of major importance to a drug's effect, diseases that result in the loss of all plasma proteins such as renal failure can have a major effect. Furthermore, highly protein-bound drugs that compete for binding sites on the albumin can displace other drugs, increasing the free-drug plasma concentration and increasing the effect of the drug. This explains why warfarin, which is 98 percent protein bound, has so many drug-drug interactions.

ELIMINATION. The major sites of drug elimination are through the kidney and metabolism by liver enzymes. Hepatic metabolism biotransforms the drug to a biologically inactive or a hydrophilic polar compound, cleared by the kidney. There are two phases of liver metabolism: Phase I reactions are discrete oxidative pathways of cytochrome P450 (CYP) occurring in the endoplasmic reticulum, whereas phase II reactions, those of conjugation, including glucuronidation, sulfation, and acetylation, occur in the cytosome. Aging results in a decrease in liver mass, and often also in the activity of the most important CYP enzymes involved in drug metabolism. Phase II conjugative reactions do not decrease with age.[11] Obviously, liver disease can affect the capacity of the liver to metabolize drugs.

Biotransformation can be influenced by drugs that either inhibit or cause induction of the CYP syndrome. Common drugs such as cimetidine, macrolide antibiotics, and quinidine inhibit the system, and drugs such as phenytoin and glucocorticoids induce the enzymes. For drugs metabolized by this CYP system, inhibition causes an increase in the plasma concentration and half-life, whereas induction causes a decrease.

Aging results in a decrease in the number of renal glomeruli and tubules, as well as in renal blood flow and glomerular filtration rate (GFR).[12] With a decrease in GFR, the dose of renally excreted drugs must be reduced parallel to this decline in GFR. Digoxin is an excellent example of a renally excreted drug.

Another important renal effect of aging involve angiotensin-converting enzyme (ACE) inhibitors and non-steroidal anti-inflammatory agents (NSAIDs). ACE inhibitors reduce conversion to angiotensin II and increase levels of bradykinin; aldosterone excretion is also decreased. This serves to decrease the constriction of the glomerular efferent arterioles and can result in decreasing renal function and even renal failure in the presence of renal artery stenosis. The decrease in aldosterone secretion with ACE inhibitors can increase serum potassium levels and result in hyperkalemia. These effects are exaggerated in the elderly patient.

NSAIDs inhibit the synthesis of prostaglandins, which are responsible in part for regulating renal blood flow. In elderly patients with a low GFR, CHF, or liver disease, NSAIDs can further reduce renal function, causing hyperkalemia or frank renal failure from tubular necrosis or interstitial nephritis.[13] In the elderly patient using ACE inhibitors or NSAIDs, reduced doses of these drugs, with careful monitoring of renal function and serum electrolytes, are required.

PHARMACODYNAMICS. Aging is associated with a decrease in cardiovascular responsiveness to beta$_1$-adrenergic stimulation, probably related to a decrease in adrenergic receptors[5] and in baroreceptor sensitivity. In the elderly patient, this accounts for less bradycardia with beta blockers than is seen in younger patients. The decrease in baroreceptor and beta$_1$-adrenergic responsiveness can result in a lack of compensatory tachycardia and exaggerated hypotension with the use of vasodilators and nitrates in elderly patients. Sensitivity to various calcium channel blockers appears to be increased in elderly patients, with a greater decrease in heart rate and blood pressure (BP) to the same serum concentration of verapamil or diltiazem than seen in the younger patient.[14]

Drug Interactions and Adverse Drug Effects

Age brings an increased incidence of adverse drug effects, occurring in one fourth of older patients and accounting for 3 to 10 percent of all hospital admissions for elderly patients.[15] Elderly patients often take multiple drugs; the number of medications taken is the most important risk factor for adverse drug reactions.[16] This polypharmacy results in noncompliance, because the elderly often confuse the drug schedule, especially for drugs given more than once a day. Another reason for noncompliance is the high cost of drugs, which may result in patients electing not to have prescriptions filled. Polypharmacy also results in adverse drug reactions from drug-drug interactions, owing to the interference of the pharmacokinetics of one drug on another. Another common reason for drug-drug interaction is competition between two highly protein-bound drugs for receptor sites, with displacement of one drug and a resultant increase in free drug in the plasma and drug effectiveness.

Other factors predicting poor compliance include a complicated drug regimen, multiple drugs, noncomprehension of instructions, mental impairment, visual or hearing disabilities, and no helper or relative at home. Legible instructions in the patient's language on easily opened bottles, certain memory aids, and the aid of visiting nurses can all improve compliance.

Drugs with similar effect can produce an additive pharmacological action (e.g., excessive bradycardia from a combination of verapamil and digoxin). Cardiovascular drugs that cause the most drug interactions are digoxin, warfarin, lidocaine, quinidine, and amiodarone.[17]

Basic principles of therapeutics in the elderly are as follows:

1. Know all the drugs the patient is taking.
2. Regularly review the drug regimen; insist that the patient bring all medicines to the next visit.
3. Take a careful drug history because of multiple drugs from multiple sources, including self-medication with over-the-counter drugs.
4. Know the pharmacokinetics and side effects of the drugs.
5. Start the drugs in the elderly at a low dose and increase in small increments and larger intervals than in younger patients until the desired effect is obtained.
6. Use the simplest drug regimen possible.
7. Adjust the dose by the patient's response.
8. Educate patient, family, and friends about the medicines, what they are for, and how to take them; also tell them about the major side effects. Be alert to drug-induced illness; in the elderly, this can be subtle or mistaken for symptoms due to the patient's disease. Drug-related effects can present as somnolence, confusion and even delirium, nausea, frequent falls, or urinary incontinence.
9. Expect noncompliance, and tell the patient what to do if the dose is missed or in cases of confusion about whether or not the drug was taken.

EPIDEMIOLOGY

Average life expectancy has risen from 47 years in the United States in 1890 to 72 years for men and 79 years for women by the end of the 20th century. At present, a person reaching the age of 65 has an average life expectancy of 18 more years; at age 85, this is 7 years.[18] The average maximum length of life, however, is 85 to 90 years and has not changed much.[19]

The population 65 years and older has grown from 20 million in 1970 to 35 million in 2000, and it is estimated that there will be 69 million by the year 2030 (20 percent of the U.S. population, up from 13 percent in 1997). By 2030, the fastest-growing segment of that elderly population will be those aged 85 and older,[18] growing from 2 million in 1970 to 4.5 million in 2000, and 8 million (estimated) by 2030.[18] The number of persons in the world who are 60 years old or older is estimated to be nearly 600 million in 1999 and is projected to be about 2 billion by 2050. At that time, the elderly population will exceed that of children from birth to 14 years of age for the first time in human history. At present, one in every 10 people is 60 years or older. By 2050, this is projected to become 1 in every 5. The percentage is growing fastest in the developed regions of the world. The older population itself is aging: currently, the oldest old (80 years or older) comprise 11 percent of the population 60 and older; by 2050, they are projected to comprise 19 percent. The number of those 100 years and older is projected to increase from 145,000 in 1999 to 2.2 million by 2050.[19] The aging pyramid, instead of becoming smaller in number as the age groups increase, will become more of a trapezoid, especially as the "baby boomers" become the elderly population.

In this older population cardiovascular disease plays a significant role and is the most common cause of morbidity and mortality.[20] Heart failure (HF) is the most common diagnostic-related group in the Medicare population 65 years old and older. In the Framingham Heart Study, 44 percent of men and 28 percent of women aged 75 to 84 had cardiovascular disease; in the 85 to 94 age group, the prevalence was 48 percent in men and 43 percent in women.[21] CAD and HTN (especially isolated systolic HTN) increase as the population ages. In the United States, in people older than 65, HTN is present in about half the patients (Fig. 57-3).[22]

The overall cost of treating cardiac disease in people older than the age of 65 years was estimated at $58 billion in 1995.[18] Hospital and nursing home care is the largest proportion of this cost. A recent study in 80- to 98-year olds found that most would rather extend their lives in

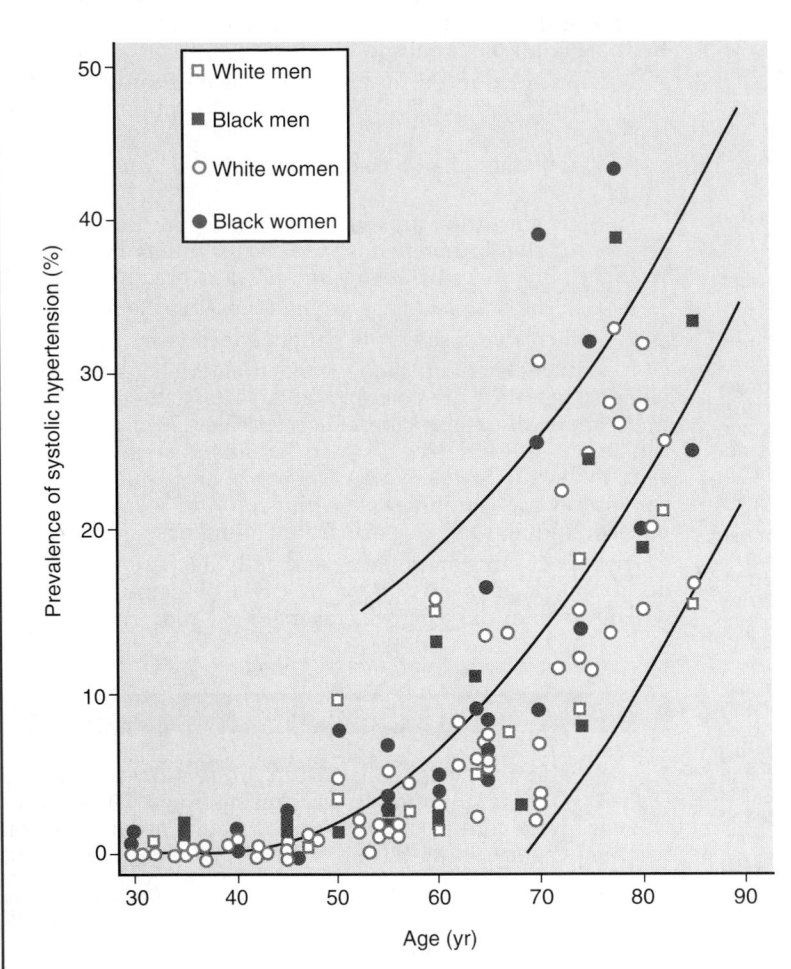

FIGURE 57-3. Prevalence of isolated systolic hypertension by the midpoint of the age classes reported in various studies. As shown by the unweighted regression line, the prevalence of systolic hypertension increases curvilinearly with age. The 95 percent confidence interval for the prediction of individual points is presented for the age range of 50 to 90 years. (From Staessen J, Amery A, Fagard R: Isolated systolic hypertension in the elderly. J Hypertens 8:393–405, 1990.)

their present state of compromised health than live shorter lives in excellent health.[23]

VALVULAR HEART DISEASE
(see also Chap. 46)

Although any valve lesion can be seen in the elderly population, the most common valve diseases are calcific aortic stenosis (AS) and mitral regurgitation (MR) due to myxomatous mitral valve. MR due to ischemia, or previous myocardial infarction, resulting in a failure of the papillary muscle/LV complex to allow proper coaptation of the mitral leaflets, is also a common cause, along with LV failure for any reason. Mild to moderate MR usually occurs in patients with calcification of the mitral annulus. Ruptured chordae, endocarditis, trauma, and aortic dissection are other causes of aortic regurgitation (AR) and MR.

Aortic valve sclerosis, as a result of stiffening and calcification of the aortic annulus and base of the semilunar cusps, causes an early-peaking systolic ejection murmur that is short and grade III-VI or less in loudness. It does not represent significant obstruction. No physical findings of obstruction are present, nor is LV hypertrophy, but it is associated with other manifestations of atherosclerotic disease, especially CAD,[24] and indeed it may result from the atherosclerotic process. It can be found in about 30 percent of the elderly, whereas significant AS is seen in 2 to 3 percent.[24] The cause of AS in the older age group is calcific or degenerative, almost always on a normally tricuspid semilunar valve. Calcification is at the base and body of the

semilunar cusps, and the commissures are not fused. Rheumatic heart disease is much less common, as is congenital AS. Patients with a bicuspid aortic valve are seen in the elderly age group, but most who develop calcification and severe obstruction do so between the ages of 40 and 60.[25] In the elderly AR can be due to rheumatic heart disease, but more often it is due to myxomatous changes and prolapse of the aortic cusp, aneurysmal aortic root dilation, infective endocarditis (possibly on a bicuspid aortic valve), or dissecting aorta.

Primary valve disease in the elderly rarely causes tricuspid and pulmonic valve regurgitation, which is usually secondary to pulmonary HTN and dilatation of the right ventricle. Pulmonary HTN can be due to LV diseases such as ischemia or cardiomyopathy, mitral stenosis, or intrinsic pulmonary disease. Primary tricuspid regurgitation due to infective endocarditis almost always occurs in intravenous drug users, who are rare in this age group. Primary tricuspid valve regurgitation (TR) can rarely be seen in elderly patients after trauma. Infrequently, an elderly patient is found with Ebstein disease and TR, or pulmonic valve regurgitation after tetralogy of Fallot repair with a patch-enlarged pulmonary outflow tract and annulus.

DIAGNOSIS. The diagnosis of significant valve disease can be difficult in the elderly population; echocardiographic-Doppler imaging can be of great help (see Chap. 7). The loudness of an aortic stenotic murmur depends on the generated LV systolic pressure as well as on the stroke volume and the loudness of MR murmur on the regurgitant volume. If the cardiac output is low, the murmur of AS or MR may be soft or even absent. The loudness of the murmur also depends on the nearness of the site of origin of the murmur to the chest wall. Accompanying clues to severity can also be absent or confusing in the elderly. For instance, an S_4 gallop or the presence of LV hypertrophy in a young person with AS is a sign strongly suggesting hemodynamic severity of the AS. In the older patient, an S_4 is often present without AS, as is LV hypertrophy, especially in those patients who have had a long history of systolic HTN. In the elderly, the carotid upstroke can feel normal in severe AS because of the stiff aorta.

The severity of AR can be difficult to judge by physical examination in the elderly because of the frequent occurrence of a wide pulse pressure due to a stiff atherosclerotic aorta rather than to severe AR. Acute AR masks many of the peripheral signs of severe AR, because the LV filling pressure is high and the forward effective stroke volume is low, thus decreasing the rise of the systolic aortic pressure, increasing the diastolic pressure, and narrowing the pulse pressure. If the AR is very severe, the diastolic regurgitant gradient between the aorta and LV is small, and with tachycardia there may be little or no diastolic murmur. The collapsing quality of the carotid pulse and Duroziez sign, that is, the systolic and diastolic bruit heard on compression of the femoral artery by the bell of the stethoscope, remain as signs of severe AR.

Treatment

A problem with selecting therapy for the elderly is that, until recently, they have been excluded from most controlled trials, and information about treatment comes mostly from registries and observational studies. Medical therapy for elderly patients with valve disease is generally similar to that for younger patients.[26] In elderly patients, even with mild mitral valve disease, atrial fibrillation (AF) is common, and represents a markedly increased threat of systemic embolization and stroke. Anticoagulation, unless absolutely contraindicated, is essential.

VALVE SURGERY. Deciding to send an elderly patient with significant valvular stenosis or regurgitation to surgery can be difficult and must be individualized because of the diversity of problems found in this age group. Generally, the patient younger than 75 has a similar morbidity and mortality to a younger patient with a similar problem. As the patient enters the late 60s and early 70s, a higher prevalence of comorbidity exists, with increased coronary, cerebrovascular, renal, hepatic, and pulmonary disease that add to surgical morbidity and mortality.[27] After age 75 to 80, surgical morbidity and mortality are increased, even beyond the impact of comorbidities, because age per se becomes an increasing risk factor for valvular surgery. In patients older than 75, the risk of neurological problems and stroke with cardiopulmonary bypass surgery increases.[28] The elderly have more problems than younger patients with mechanical valve replacement, mostly because of the increased complications from anticoagulation.[29]

The goals of valve surgery in the elderly are somewhat different from those in younger patients. In the older patient the major goal becomes relief of symptoms, with improvement in activity and quality of life rather than prolongation of life.

Aortic Stenosis. After the occurrence of symptoms of HF, exertional syncope, angina, or myocardial infarction without obstructive CAD, mortality in patients with severe AS increases rapidly, so that the mean survival is 3 years for symptomatic patients, shorter with HF symptoms, and somewhat longer with angina. In all probability, survival is even less in the elderly. Also, the incidence of sudden death increases in the symptomatic patient with AS, accounting for one fifth to one fourth of all deaths (see Chap. 46). Surgery should be recommended once symptoms begin, depending on the overall status of the patient and the number and severity of comorbidities. Only in the presence of a decreasing EF, or possibly with increasing runs of nonsustained ventricular tachycardia, should a patient not complaining of symptoms be offered surgery.[26]

Patients with AR who undergo aortic valve replacement do not fare as well as patients with AS, especially if they are in New York Heart Association (NYHA) Class III or IV or have a decreased LV EF.[30] Long-term morbidity and mortality are increased in patients with moderate to severe AR if they have symptoms, an EF less than 50 to 55 percent, comorbidities, or an increased LV end-systolic diameter by echocardiography (>25 mm/m^2).[26, 31] Surgery is, therefore, indicated in these patients.

Aortic Valve Replacement. In younger patients who have pliable valves and AS due to commissural fusion, successful commissurotomy, either surgically or by balloon valvotomy, is possible, with good results lasting 15 to 30 years.[32] In elderly patients with AS of whatever cause, the aortic valve is always severely calcified, and valvotomy, either by surgery or balloon, has a limited, short-lived success. With severe AR, valve replacement is the rule, except for ascending aortic aneurysm or AR with aortic dissection, in which ascending aortic grafting with valve resuspension can be done with long-term success.[33]

In most series of patients older than 70 years, perioperative mortality varies from 2.4 to 12.4 percent, depending on comorbid conditions, increasing patient age, the presence of other cardiac lesions or concomitant operations such as mitral valve repair or replacement, or coronary artery bypass graft (CABG).[34]

As experience has increased, perioperative mortality has fallen to 6 to 10 percent for aortic replacement and CABG[35] and 4 to 7 percent with isolated aortic replacement. Factors that predict perioperative mortality in patients older than 75 years are NYHA functional therapeutic Class IV, decreased LV EF, chronic HF, the presence of comorbid diseases such as pulmonary or renal disease or diabetes, and concomitant procedures such as mitral valve surgery, coronary artery surgery, or surgery performed as an urgent procedure. Other independent predictors of hospital mortality include cardiomegaly, serum creatinine level greater than 150 mmol, and operation as an emergency procedure. Predictors of late mortality are comorbid diseases such as severe renal, pulmonary, or coronary disease and poor LV function.[30, 36] Patients with coexisting minimal-to-moderate AS or AR who have cardiac surgery for other than aortic valve disease (e.g., coronary surgery or mitral valve replacement) generally experience very slow progression of the aortic valve disease. Consequently, there is no indication to replace the aortic valve at that time.[37] However, the higher the aortic valve gradient and the heavier the aortic valve calcification, the more likely the AS will progress, and therefore the more reasonable it becomes to replace the aortic valve at the time of the primary surgery.

As many as 40 percent of patients with AS in the elderly age group have at least one significantly obstructed coronary artery.[38] The presence of atheromas in the descending aorta by transesophageal echocardiography is a good predictor of CAD.[39] Although stress echocardiography has been recommended to detect CAD in patients with AS,[40] stress testing is generally unnecessary, because in this age group coronary arteriography is justified preoperatively to assess the status of the coronary arteries[26] (see Chaps. 6 and 7). Aortic valve débridement can result in relief of severe calcific AS; however, it has been abandoned by most surgeons because there is a rapid restenosis and, with some techniques, a high incidence of increased AR (see Chap. 46). Occasionally it can be beneficial.[41]

A biological tissue valve, rather than a mechanical valve, is most often placed in this elderly age group because of their shorter life expectancy, because biological valves are less subject to tissue failure in elderly patients,[27, 42] and because of the dangers of anticoagulants in the elderly.[29] For most tissue valves, even in younger patients, there is no significant failure for 5 to 10 years, long enough to last the natural life of the elderly patient.[42] With aortic valve replacement, operative mortality is slightly increased with age and more markedly increased with comorbidity and severity of disease; however, the results of surgery are excellent, with a definite increase in quality of life.

Mitral Valve Repair/Replacement. With MR, because of multiple causes and especially CAD causing severe MR, the results of valve replacement are not as good as with AS; 5-year survival after both coronary surgery and mitral valve replacement is only about 50 percent.[43] With mitral valve replacement, the major risk factor for mortality is the presence of CAD.[44] Patients do well after repair of MR, with perioperative mortality of 4 percent and 25 months late mortality of 6 percent.[45] Thus, the elderly undergoing mitral valve surgery do not do as well as those having aortic valve replacement or younger patients and fare better with mitral valve repair than with replacement.

Balloon Valvotomy. For calcific AS, balloon valvotomy increases aortic valve area, but rapid restenosis follows. Because balloon valvotomy is not an alternative to valve replacement, its use is restricted to very old, extremely symptomatic patients who are poor candidates for surgery, where the procedure might improve cardiac output and peripheral organ perfusion, and relieve afterload on the LV enough to allow surgical valve replacement at a later time. It can also be useful in those patients who are not candidates for surgery because of comorbid problems and who are repeatedly hospitalized for HF. Balloon valvotomy can keep these patients out of the hospital for a variable period of time, and improve quality of life.[46] Balloon valvotomy for MS has become the procedure of choice when the valve is not heavily calcified and MR is absent or minimal. The results of balloon valvotomy are equivalent to those of open commissurotomy, and both are better than closed commissurotomy.[47] Mitral valve calcification, frequent in the elderly, reduces the success rate and increases mortality and complications.[48]

CORONARY ARTERY DISEASE
(see also Chaps. 35 through 37)

PREVALENCE AND INCIDENCE. As the population ages, the prevalence and annual incidence of the development of overt CAD increases substantially with age, as does the total number of people with clinical CAD (Fig. 57–4). The severity and diffuse distribution of the coronary obstruction also increases, presumably as a result of prolonged exposure to atherosclerotic risk factors. There is a striking gender difference, with men developing CAD at a younger age than women (37 percent in men aged 65 to 74 vs. 22 percent in women of the same age range). The prevalence of CAD in the Framingham cohort aged 75 to 84 years was 44 percent in men and 28 percent in women. In the 85- to 94-year age range, the prevalence of CAD was 48 percent in men and 43 percent in women.[49] The lifetime risk of developing CAD at age 40 is 49 percent for men and 32 percent for women, decreasing to 35 percent for men and 24 per-

cent for women at age 70, or 1 in 3 for men and 1 in 4 for women.[50]

MORTALITY. Almost 85 percent of people who die of CAD are age 65 or older. According to data from the Health Care Financing Administration, in 1995, $98 billion ($3,769 to $11,110 per discharge) was paid by Medicare to Medicare beneficiaries for CAD. Of 2.3 million Americans discharged from hospitals with a first-listed diagnosis of CAD in 1996, 57 percent were 65 years of age or older.[51] CAD mortality is about twice as high in men as in women and higher in blacks than in whites. After age 70, mortality in white men is higher than in black men. In women, mortality in blacks exceeds that in whites until age 85.[52] Although mortality from CAD has been declining since 1970, the decline is greater in white men and women than in blacks (average annual percentage change 3 to 4 percent vs. 2 to 3 percent), more robust than in the age groups up to 85 but still 1 to 2 percent in even the oldest age groups.[52] After adjustment for major risk factors, with each decade of advancing age, a twofold to threefold increase in coronary vascular mortality persists.

RISK FACTORS
(See Chaps. 31, 32, and 39)

The impact of many risk factors for CAD, such as HTN, diabetes, and LV hypertrophy, increases with age. Although the benefits of risk-factor reduction in the elderly for some risk factors is incomplete, excellent evidence exists that control of BP, for example, reduces cardiovascular events even in the older age group.

HYPERTENSION (see Chaps. 28 & 29). Because HTN is so common in the older population, and the number and type of effective drugs so numerous, this is one of the most controllable of the risk factors. Fifty-seven percent of men and 61 percent of women aged 65 to 74 and 64 percent of men and 77 percent of women aged 75 and older have HTN, as defined by at least one ambulatory BP reading of 140 mm Hg systolic or 90 mm Hg diastolic or higher.[18] Both systolic and diastolic elevation of BP is associated with an increased risk of CAD in men and women. People older than 65 years with systolic pressure greater than 180 mm Hg have a threefold to fourfold increase in risk of CAD compared with people with a systolic pressure of less than 120 mm Hg. A diastolic pressure greater than 105 mm Hg increased the risk two to three times compared with a diastolic pressure of less than 75 mm Hg.[53]

Isolated systolic HTN (systolic pressure greater than 140 mm Hg with a diastolic pressure less than 90 mm Hg)[54] is very frequent in the elderly and is partially related to the loss of elasticity and compliance of the aorta and arterial branches. The risk of stroke, CHF, renal disease, renal insufficiency, and probably coronary artery events decreases with a decrease in the degree of systolic HTN, as shown in the Systolic Hypertension in the Elderly Program (SHEP trial) (see Chap. 29). Treatment of HTN in the elderly population reduces the risk of cardiovascular events, especially stroke and CHF, and probably decreases the incidence of myocardial infarction.[55]

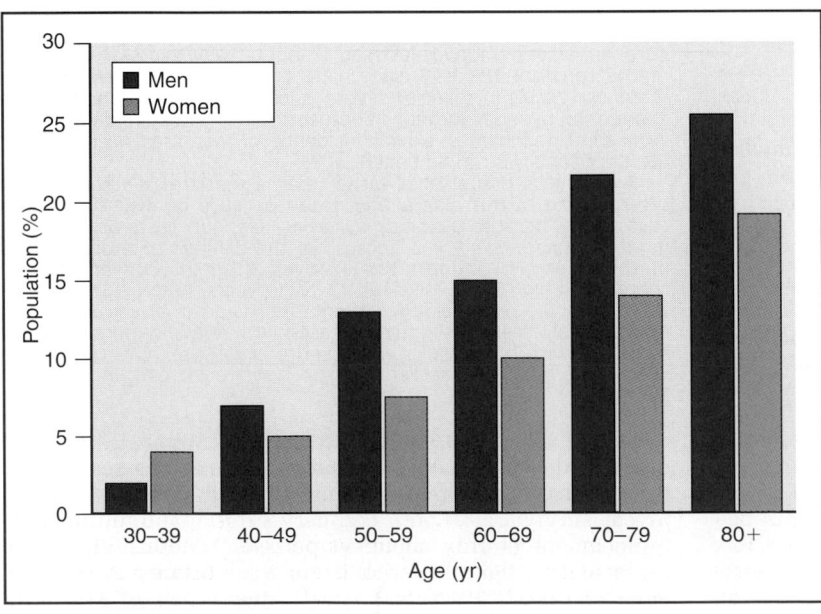

FIGURE 57–4. Prevalence of coronary heart disease by age and sex. (NHAHES III, US 1988–1991.) (From Kannel WB, Wilson WF, Larson MG, et al: Coronary risk factors and coronary prevention in octogenarians. *In* Wenger NK [ed]: Cardiovascular Disease in the Octogenarian and Beyond. 1st ed. London, Martin Dunitz, 1999, p. 143.)

SMOKING (see Chaps. 31, 32, and 39). Cigarette smoking declines in prevalence with advancing age to about 15 percent of men and 11.5 percent of women age 65 and older.[56] Although smoking is a powerful risk factor in the younger patient, it is unclear if smoking exerts the same risk in the older population[57] and whether smoking cessation in elderly patients decreases the incidence of coronary events. In the Coronary Artery Surgery Study (CASS) registry, patients older than age 70, all of whom had CAD, who continued to smoke, had three times the risk of death or myocardial infarction during a 60-year follow-up period compared with those who stopped smoking. In the British Physicians' Study[58] and the U.S. Nurses' Health Study,[59] smoking was an independent risk factor for coronary events in both younger and older age groups. However, the Framingham Heart Study showed that in individuals older than age 65 the incidence of lung cancer is accelerated, but there was no correlation between the incidence of smoking and CAD.[60] The explanation for the latter may be that, although there is increased risk of CAD from smoking, there is increased mortality from other smoking-related diseases in this age group. It is also possible that those susceptible to CAD from smoking died at a younger age, and among the persons who survive to age 65, fewer patients are susceptible to CAD from smoking.

HYPERLIPIDEMIA (see Chap. 31). Serum cholesterol concentration increases progressively until age 50 in men and age 65 in women and then begins to decline. High-density lipoprotein value is higher in both men and women and stays constant with aging.[61] Among people 65 to 74 years of age, 22 percent of men and 41 percent of women have a total serum cholesterol value of greater than 240 mg/dl; for those older than 75 years, 20 percent of men and 38 percent of women have cholesterol levels greater than 240 mg/dl.[18] Although the association between the risk factor of an elevated serum cholesterol level and the development of CAD is less striking in the elderly, the ratio of total to high-density lipoprotein cholesterol remains a strong predictor of CAD in the elderly.[62] Elevated triglycerides have been independently associated with an increased risk of CAD in elderly women but not men.[63] Treatment with HMG-CoA reductase drugs can reduce the incidence of acute cardiac events in patients up to 75 years of age; older patients have not been studied.[64]

DIABETES MELLITUS (see Chap. 63). In 1996, there were 503,000 Americans discharged from the hospital with a first-listed diagnosis of diabetes mellitus. Of these, 39 percent were older than 65 years of age. The prevalence of physician-diagnosed diabetes in patients aged 60 and older is 12 to 13 percent for men and women. The vast majority of patients older than age 70 have non–insulin-dependent (type II) diabetes. Its presence doubles the risk of CAD and, when combined with hyperlipidemia, increases the risk 15-fold.[65]

PHYSICAL INACTIVITY. Approximately one third of men and women aged 65 to 74, and 38 percent of men and 51 percent of women aged older than 75 years, report no leisure-time physical activity. Frequent exercise raises high-density lipoprotein cholesterol, controls obesity, and lowers systolic and diastolic BP even in patients 60 to 80 years old and reduces insulin resistance.[66] Even moderate amounts of exercise have been shown to protect against CAD events in middle-aged and older men in the Framingham Heart Study.[67]

Other risk factors for CAD, such as lipoprotein (a) and other apolipoproteins, are still being investigated. A high homocystine level is not uncommon in elderly men and is strongly associated with increased prevalence of coronary heart disease and cerebrovascular disease.[68] After an acute myocardial infarction (AMI), patients with depression who are socially isolated have an increased recurrence rate and mortality[69] (see Chaps. 39 and 70). This social isolation is more common in the elderly.

Clinical Presentation

Elderly patients have more multivessel disease and lower EF than do younger patients.[70] Although angina pectoris is a common first presentation of CAD in the elderly, angina may not occur until the CAD is well advanced because of often markedly decreased activity. For this reason, acute ischemic syndromes are common initial presentations of CAD.[70] Also, many symptoms of discomfort that would alert a younger person are explained away in the elderly patient as a consequence of "getting old."

When angina occurs, the precipitating factors and the description, with radiation and its relief by rest, are similar to that in younger patients. However, with advancing age, a frequent presenting symptom is increasing fatigability and shortness of breath during activity because of the ischemic effects on systolic and diastolic myocardial function. In patients with documented CAD, anginal pain without dyspnea is reported in 25 to 43 percent of persons older than age 65, dyspnea without chest discomfort in 8 to 25 percent, and both dyspnea and angina in almost 50 percent.[71] Others have reported the initial manifestation of CAD in the

elderly to be angina in 80 percent.[72] As many as 30 percent have silent ischemia.

With increasing age, the gender composition of patients with AMI changes from 80 percent men younger than 55 to about 50 percent men aged 75 to 84 and only one third men aged older than 83.[73] Sudden pulmonary edema is a common presentation of AMI in the elderly, but chest pain is still the most common, as it is in younger patients. Neurological symptoms as a presentation of AMI, such as syncope, stroke, or confusion, are more likely seen in the elderly, as is painless AMI. Non-Q-wave myocardial infarctions are more common in the elderly. Physical examination, especially during the ischemic episode, can be very helpful. Unlike younger patients, an S_4 gallop rhythm is very common in elderly patients with and without CAD; however, the appearance or increase in the loudness of an S_4 or S_3 gallop or MR murmur during the chest discomfort or dyspnea and its disappearance with relief of the chest discomfort or dyspnea are strong evidence in favor of a transient decrease in diastolic ventricular function, the most common cause of which is CAD. For the same reason, an electrocardiogram (ECG) taken during the time of the discomfort that shows definite ST segment elevation or depression, or marked T wave inversion, which reverses after the discomfort abates, is excellent evidence of severe CAD. Because LV hypertrophy is common in elderly patients, ST segment/T wave changes can be present chronically on a resting ECG and are of limited help in diagnosing myocardial ischemia unless the ST segment/T wave changes are transient and associated with chest discomfort.

SILENT ISCHEMIA. The presence of significant CAD without symptoms increases with age. Because only about 20 percent of people older than 80 have clinically evident CAD[74] and over 50 percent have significant CAD at autopsy,[75] a large number of elderly people must have significant CAD without symptoms. About one third of asymptomatic hypertensive elderly patients have a myocardial infarction discovered incidentally on ECG. An equal number have silent ischemia. The reason for increased silent ischemia in the elderly patient is not known, but it may be related to mental status changes impairing perception or recall of ischemic pain, to the development of collaterals that reduce the severity of the myocardial ischemia, to autonomic dysfunction, or to increased sensitivity to endogenous endomorphins.[76] Although the presence of silent ischemia may not predict a worse prognosis for the patient with CAD than its absence, most people with silent ischemia have a positive exercise test result and so probably have more extensive CAD.

Diagnosis

The diagnosis of CAD in the elderly can be suspected by finding a history of typical angina or atypical symptoms related to exertion, and by a careful physical examination, as indicated earlier. Stress testing is done to establish the diagnosis and to determine risk stratification and prognosis (see Chap. 6). The high prevalence and increased severity of CAD in the elderly, by Bayesian principles, increases the sensitivity of stress testing but makes it harder to exclude significant disease because of more false-negative test results.[77]

The criteria for a positive exercise test result in the elderly do not differ significantly from those in the younger patient.[77] As in younger patients, the test is less likely to be positive with single-vessel disease but is 80 to 85 percent sensitive in identifying patients with three-vessel or left main CAD. In patients older than 60 to 65 years, the sensitivity for diagnosing the presence of significant CAD varies from 62 to 84 percent, and the specificity from 56 to 93 percent, depending on the population studied. The ability to walk through the second stage of Bruce protocol (>6 minutes) predicts low risk.[77]

The increased number of false-positive test results seen in the elderly is probably attributable to an abnormal resting ECG, the presence of LV hypertrophy from HTN or valve disease, or intraventricular conduction defects. Prognosis depends on the amount of ischemic and nonfunctioning myocardium, reflecting the effect of severity and extent of CAD on LV function. For risk stratification, attention should be paid to the chronotropic and inotropic responses to exercise, exercise-induced arrhythmias, and the duration of exercise. Arrhythmias are common in the elderly, especially at high workloads, but are not necessarily an adverse feature unless they occur with other signs of ischemia.[77] Inability to increase the heart rate to 85 percent of age-predicted maximum, or a hypotensive response to exercise, are poor prognostic factors, similar to those seen in younger patients.

PROGNOSTIC VALUE OF STRESS TESTING. Stress testing offers challenges to the elderly. Many have orthopedic or neurological problems that prevent active walking on a treadmill. Many are physically deconditioned and may have an abnormal resting ECG, making criteria of ST segment shifts for positivity less reliable. In a study of patients older than 65 years observed for 2 years, those with ST segment depression during stress testing had a 17 percent cardiac death rate, whereas the incidence was only 2 percent in those without ST segment depression.[78] In patients older than 70 years who had exercise stress testing 3 weeks after an AMI and were observed for a mean of 4.5 years, of those who failed to increase double product from rest to exercise by more than 1500, and also developed ventricular arrhythmias with exercise, only 25 percent were still alive at the end of the follow-up time, whereas in the absence of either response, 77 percent were still alive.[78a] Patients after AMI who are unable to increase systolic BP with exercise greater than 30 mm Hg have a 1-year mortality of 15 percent compared with 2 percent for those who did increase their BP.[78b] Using the Duke treadmill score combining ST segment depression, chest pain, and exercise duration is useful to predict significant (>75 percent) stenosis and severe three-vessel or left main disease.[77]

When the patient can exercise, but the resting ECG is abnormal or has a feature that makes it impossible to diagnose ischemia (left bundle branch block, pacemaker, or marked ST segment changes), then myocardial perfusion study at rest and after exercise, using tracers such as thallium-201, technetium-99m sestamibi or technetium-99m tetrofosmin single-photon emission computed tomographic imaging (see Chap. 9), or stress echocardiography (see Chap. 7) can be used to detect areas of scarring or ischemia. When exercise cannot be done, pharmacological tests using dipyridamole or adenosine to vasodilate coronary arterioles and increase coronary blood flow maximally to areas without stenotic arteries, or dobutamine to increase myocardial oxygen demand and create ischemia, can be used. Dobutamine stress testing is safe in the elderly. These techniques are more sensitive than exercise testing in identifying single- and two-vessel disease, and, like exercise testing, are also useful for risk stratification. With the use of thallium-201 perfusion tests on 120 patients older than 70 years with known or suspected CAD, three variables were associated with a cardiac event: (1) a maximum ST segment depression of ≥2 mm (27 percent with vs. 6 percent without), (2) peak exercise beyond stage 1 of the Bruce protocol (18 percent event rate in those who could not go beyond this stage vs. 6 percent in those who could), and (3) the presence of either a fixed or a reversible thallium defect (18 percent event rate with vs. 2 percent without). The combination of inability to attain peak exercise beyond stage 1 and the presence of any thallium defect were the most powerful predictors, with a relative risk of 5.3 at 1 year.[79]

Acute Myocardial Infarction

(see also Chap. 35)

In the elderly, AMI results in an increase in mortality compared with younger patients. Eighty percent of all deaths due to AMI occur in those 65 years of age and older.[74] In a population-based study over a 20-year period between 1975 and 1995, patients aged 55 to 64 were 2.2 times more likely to die of AMI during hospitalization than were patients younger than 55, whereas patients aged 65 to 74, 75 to 84, and older than 85 years were at 4.2, 7.8, and 10.2 times greater risk of dying.[73] In the Global Utilization of Streptokinase and TPA for Occluded Coronary Arteries (GUSTO)-I study of 41,021 patients, in-hospital mortality from AMI younger than age 65 was 3 percent as opposed to 9.5 percent at age 65 to 74, 19.6 percent at age 75 to 85, and 30.3 percent in those older than 85 (Fig. 57–5).[80] Age alone can result in changes that increase mortality from AMI due to increasing diastolic dysfunction, altered baroreceptor and beta-adrenergic receptor responsiveness, and age-related decreases in renal and pulmonary function, all of which make the patient vulnerable to increased complications. Older patients have an increased comorbidity with pulmonary, renal, and hepatic disease. A more adverse baseline status in AMI prevails with higher NYHA functional class, prior history of CHF, prior myocardial infarction, angina, HTN or diabetes mellitus, low EF, and cardiovascular disease; and more of the elderly are women.[81] Complications of myocardial infarction are also more frequent in the elderly, includ-

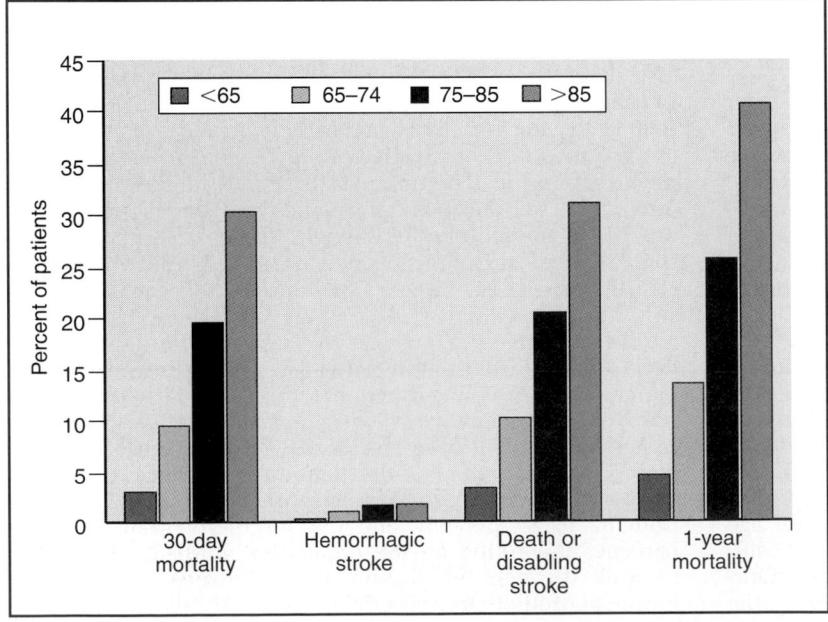

FIGURE 57–5. Effects of age on mortality and stroke, GUSTO-1 trial. Of 41,021 patients, 24,708 were younger than 65 years, 11,201 were 65 to 74 years, 4625 were 75 to 85 years, and 412 were older than 85 years. All patients had ST segment elevation and were treated with thrombolytic agents. Postdischarge 1-year mortality remained high in the oldest groups (6.1 percent and 10.3 percent, respectively) and continued to be low (1.5 percent) in the younger than 65 group. (From White HD, Barbash GI, Califf RM, et al for the GUSTO-1 Investigators: Age and outcome with contemporary thrombolytic therapy: Results from the GUSTO-1 Trial. Circulation 94: 1826–1833, 1996.)

ing CHF, atrial arrhythmias, cardiogenic shock, and cardiac rupture.[82]

Management

Management of AMI

MEDICAL TREATMENT. Treatment of patients with angina, acute ischemic syndromes, and AMI is similar to that in younger patients (see Chaps. 35 and 36). For angina and acute ischemic syndromes, aspirin, nitrates, beta-blockers, calcium-channel blockers, ACE inhibitors, and anticoagulants such as heparin have all been found to be as effective in elderly as in younger patients.[83] In the older population, attention should be paid to impaired baroreceptor reflexes, decreased beta-adrenergic responsiveness, and stiff aorta. With ACE inhibitors or nitrates, especially short-acting nitroglycerin with venodilatation, postural hypotension can result in falls and injury. Combinations of digoxin, amiodarone, and calcium channel blockers can also produce profound bradycardia more easily in the elderly. These drugs should be initiated cautiously, beginning with lower doses than in younger patients and carefully watching for toxicity.[84]

In a study of 10,018 patients older than 65, after an AMI with no absolute contraindication to aspirin use, aspirin was associated with a 22 percent reduction in 30-day mortality.[85] Beta blockers are the antiischemic drugs of choice in elderly patients with stable angina,[86] and all appear to be equally effective in controlling angina.[87] Many studies demonstrate the effectiveness of beta blockers in reducing mortality after AMI, including in patients older than age 65.[88] Beta blockers are often not given to patients with chronic obstructive pulmonary disease, type I diabetes mellitus, a low LV EF, or a history of HF, even though they have been shown to reduce mortality in these groups also. Despite evidence of effectiveness, aspirin and beta blockers are underprescribed in the elderly, and patients with the highest risk for in-hospital death appear to be least likely to receive beta blockers. ACE inhibitors have also been shown to reduce mortality, and to prevent LV remodeling and the onset of CHF in patients after a large AMI[89] (see Chaps. 35 and 39). Calcium channel blockers are equally effective, as are beta blockers, in controlling anginal pain.[87] Because of the tendency of rapid-acting calcium channel blockers to cause vasodilation, a drop in BP, and increased sympathetic tone, short-acting calcium channel blockers should be avoided. The use of slow-release, or new-generation long-acting, dihydropyridines are the calcium antagonists of choice.[87] After an AMI, however, calcium channel blockers have not been shown to decrease mortality; and in certain patients there is evidence that they are harmful, especially in those with decreased ventricular function, CHF, or bradyarrhythmias.[84] It is a consensus of the American College of Cardiology/American Heart Association AMI group that calcium channel blockers are used too often in patients with AMI and that beta blockers are the more appropriate choice.[84, 90]

Heparin is recommended in acute ischemic syndromes and has been shown to decrease the development of AMI and/or mortality in patients given aspirin compared with those given aspirin alone.[91] Most studies have not investigated patients older than age 75, where the incidence of intracranial bleeding is higher than in younger patients. No trial has specifically investigated fractionated or low-molecular-weight heparin, with varying molecular weights that bind specifically to antithrombin III in patients 75 years of age and older.[91] Two major trials of the platelet glycoprotein IIb-IIIa inhibitors have been reported, with reduction in combined endpoints of myocardial infarction and death, but the number of patients older than 65 was small and no specific comments can be made.[91]

FIBRINOLYTIC THERAPY. There is evidence that the older population with AMI benefits from fibrinolytic drugs with reduced mortality and preserved LV function. Pooled results from five major thrombolytic trials showed an absolute reduction in mortality of 3.5 percent in patients older than age 65 compared with 2.2 percent in the younger population.[92] There was also an absolute excess of strokes and other bleeding complications of less than 1 percent. Elderly patients take longer to reach the hospital after the onset of chest pain and are less likely to receive thrombolysis.[93, 94] Depending on the study, 10 to 50 percent of the elderly are excluded from thrombolytic therapy solely on the basis of age.[95] Observational studies indicate that older patients are at slightly greater risk of hemorrhagic stroke after fibrinolysis than younger patients.[96] In the elderly, especially those older than age 75, the incidence of serious bleeding, especially intracranial bleeding, must be balanced against any possible benefit derived from the use of fibrinolytics during an AMI.

THROMBOLYSIS VERSUS PRIMARY ANGIOPLASTY. Several trials have shown no advantage to early angioplasty compared with medical management in patients with non–ST segment elevation myocardial infarction, except for those with ongoing ischemia.[91] However, none of these has addressed the elderly specifically. In patients with ST segment elevation AMI, percutaneous transluminal coronary angiography (PTCA) can restore antegrade flow in the infarct-related occluded artery, with Thrombolysis in Myocardial Infarction (TIMI) grade 3 flow in 90 percent of patients.[84] In a post-hoc analysis of high-risk patients (those older than age 75 with anterior myocardial infarction or tachycardia on presentation), mortality was only 2 percent in those with primary angioplasty, and 10 percent in those receiving thrombolysis ($p < 0.01$).[97] The difference was in part related to an excessive incidence of cerebrovascular hemorrhage with death in the thrombolytic group. The cardiac-related deaths were similar in the two groups.

Management of CAD

PERCUTANEOUS CORONARY INTERVENTION (PCI). Coronary arteriography is more likely to be performed in elderly patients who are symptomatic and have CAD than in younger patients.[98] Elderly patients with high-risk CAD or angina not responding to medical management are being sent for PCI in increasing numbers because it is a less invasive procedure than coronary bypass surgery.[99] Although patients in general do very well, some studies document increasing procedural morbidity and mortality with advancing age, particularly past 80 years.

Multivessel PCI is successful in patients aged 65 and older, with an overall angioplasty success rate of 96 percent. Complete revascularization was accomplished in 52 percent, and 3.2 percent had a myocardial infarction or other major in-hospital complications. Independent predictors of mortality were EF less than 40 percent ($p < 0.001$), three-vessel disease ($p < 0.01$), female gender ($p < 0.02$), and PTCA from 1985 or earlier.[100] In one study, the octogenarian was more likely to be a woman and have multivessel disease, with high-grade stenoses and more complex lesions than the younger patient.[101] Procedural mortality rose fivefold in those older than 80 years compared with those younger than 60 years. The rate of postprocedural myocardial infarction was also one and one-half times higher in the elderly than in the younger patients. Angiographic success was equal to that in younger patients, and the rate of in-hospital bypass surgery after intervention was less than that in younger patients.[101]

CORONARY ARTERY BYPASS SURGERY. There are no randomized studies comparing surgery to medical management in patients older than 65 years. Although there is limited information from randomized studies of coronary surgery compared with angioplasty that have included elderly patients,[102] and many reports of elderly patients from the same institution who had either CABG or angioplasty,[103] the conclusions from such studies are limited. With medical advances in the treatment of CAD, and with more patients with lesser degrees of CAD receiving angioplasty, coronary surgery is being done more often than in the past on older patients with more complicated CAD. As age increases, the proportion of men to women undergoing CABG increases, as does the prevalence of severe angina and CHF. The severity of the distribution of coronary stenoses also increases with age, as well as the incidence of complications, including neurological events, wound infections, and death, increasing in every decade after age 40. In most surgical series, morbidity and mortality are greater in the elderly, particularly in those older than 75 years.[104] Perioperative mortality in the elderly patient varies in different studies, from less than 2 percent to 10 percent.[102, 104] Morbidity and mortality depend on the presence of comorbidity, the EF, and the diffuseness of the CAD but are generally higher in the elderly.[104] The elderly patient also has a higher incidence of complications such as stroke, renal failure, prolonged ventilation, and postoperative cardiac arrest.[104, 105] Carotid artery disease is also more common in the elderly.

In the Bypass Angioplasty Revascularization Investigation (BARI) trial, 709 patients aged 65 to 80 with multivessel CAD were randomized to bypass surgery or angioplasty.[102] Mortality at 30 days was 0.7 percent for PTCA and 1.1 percent for CABG. For patients both older and younger than 65, it was 1.7 percent. CABG resulted in greater angina relief and fewer repeat procedures in both younger and older patients. In older patients compared with younger patients, stroke was more common after CABG than after PTCA (1.7 vs. 0.2 percent), and HF and pulmonary edema were more common after PTCA (4.0 vs. 1.3 percent). The 5-year survival rate was 91.5 percent after CABG and 89.5 percent after PTCA in the younger patients and 85.7 percent after CABG and 81.4 percent after PTCA in the older. Stents[106] and minimally invasive or "off-pump" coronary artery surgery[107] offer advantages in the elderly for low risk revascularization. There is evidence of substantial improvement in health-related quality of life after PTCA in the elderly similar to that seen in the younger patients.[107a]

CARDIAC REHABILITATION (see Chap. 39). Fewer than half of eligible patients, and most elderly patients after a myocardial infarction or CABG do not participate in rehabilitation programs.[108] Because exercise capacity is reduced in the elderly after a cardiac event, exercise rehabilitation is especially important in this age group. Women and older patients are less likely to participate, as are those with lesser degrees of education and employment.[109]

Psychological depression is common after AMI and coronary surgery, especially in the elderly.[69, 110] Education and reinforcement that this reaction is a normal response to a major cardiovascular event, and mostly transient, can be very helpful. Erectile dysfunction is especially common after coronary surgery or AMI and should be inquired about. The energy used during sexual activity is usually less than 5 METs.[111] Most patients can return to normal sexual activity within 3 to 4 weeks after an acute event. If erectile dysfunction is a problem, encouragement to resume sexual activity gradually should be given; and drugs such as sildenafil, or intracavernosal or intraurethral prostacyclin, can be very effective. The patient should be cautioned about the need to avoid taking nitrates within 24 hours of taking sildenafil.[111]

Exercise prescriptions designed for the individual show substantial evidence for benefit of exercise in the elderly, with an increase in exercise tolerance and capacity, obesity indices, lipid profile, overall levels of physical fitness, and quality of life.[112] The greatest reduction in mortality with exercise training may occur in elderly men.[113] The benefits of cardiac rehabilitation have been shown to occur equally well in elderly women.[114] Rehabilitation programs for the elderly are safe. Data from 57,000 patients with over 2 million exercise hours identified only 21 cardiac events, including three fatal and eight nonfatal myocardial infarctions, during exercise training, or one cardiac event per 100,000, one AMI per 300,000, and one death per 1 million exercise hours.[115, 116]

HEART FAILURE

Heart failure is the leading first-listed diagnosis among hospitalized older adults[117] (Fig. 57–6). Among an estimated 4 million U.S. residents with HF, 70 percent were older than 60 years. The National Hospital Discharge Survey estimated 871,000 hospital admissions annually with a first-listed diagnosis of HF from 1985 to 1995; the numbers of hospitalizations for any diagnosis of HF increase to 2.6 million, or 53 percent, over the 10-year period in question. About 78 percent of men and 85 percent of women hospitalized with HF were older than 65 years.

The etiology of HF in the elderly is the same as that in the younger populations. In the Framingham Heart Study, the prevalence of HF increased from 0.8 percent in the 50- to 59-year age group to 9.1 percent in the population 80 years and older.[118] Also in the Framingham study, the annual incidence of HF in men increased from 0.2 percent in the 45- to 54-year age group to 1.4 percent in the 75- to 84-year age group to 5.4 percent in the 85- to 94-year age group.[118] Whereas the majority of patients with HF younger than 65 years are men, of those over that age 60 percent are women, and the proportion increases with age.[119] Furthermore, there was a 27 percent increase in the incidence of initial hospitalization for HF in those 65 years and older from 1986 to 1993.[120]

The mortality from HF is very high in the elderly, particularly with advanced HF, and may be 10 to 15 percent at 1 month and as high as 30 percent or more at 1 year. Mortality rate increases exponentially after age 65 in both men and women.[120a] HF is not only an important reason for

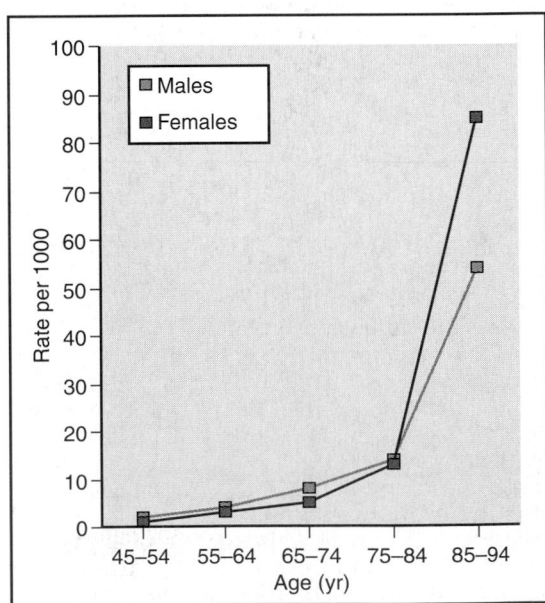

FIGURE 57–6. Incidence of heart failure by age and sex: 30-year follow-up from the Framingham Heart Study. (From Kannel WB, Belanger AJ: Epidemiology of heart failure. Am Heart J 121:951–957, 1991.)

hospitalization but also is second only to HTN as a reason for outpatient physician visits, accounting for 12 million office visits per year in the United States.[121] HF in the older population consumes the most resources, with an estimated annual expenditure of $40 billion.[121]

PATHOPHYSIOLOGY (see Chap. 16). With aging, LV hypertrophy occurs as a result of increased afterload, a slowing of LV muscle relaxation, and stiffening of the LV, all of which lead to diastolic dysfunction as a prominent feature of HF. With a stiff LV, atrial contraction becomes most important in delivering a normal LV diastolic volume and keeping stroke volume normal (see Fig. 57–1). Therefore, AF often precipitates, or markedly increases, symptoms of HF in the elderly population.[122] In fact, with advancing age, the proportion of people with LV failure but normal systolic function approaches 50 percent or more.[123] Diastolic dysfunction as a pathophysiological function of HF occurs more often in women than in men and also more often with hypertensive cardiovascular disease and diabetes.

DIAGNOSIS. The diagnosis of HF can be difficult in the older individual. Symptoms of dyspnea on exertion or easy fatigability are often taken as signs of "getting older" or deconditioning or can result from other diseases, especially pulmonary disease, thyroid abnormality, anemia, or depression. Edema of the lower extremity is not unusual in older patients, because the skin turgor decreases and the patient is increasingly sedentary, with legs dependent much of the time. Edema-related liver and renal disease is also not uncommon. Symptoms of increasing orthopnea or development of nocturnal cough, shortness of breath, or paroxysmal nocturnal dyspnea should alert the clinician to the possibility of the diagnosis of HF.

Physical examination is particularly helpful with the findings of rales, tachycardia, and an S_3 gallop rhythm; with right-sided HF, an elevated jugular venous pressure or positive hepatojugular reflux can be seen, as well as a right-sided S_3 gallop rhythm. Chest radiography showing cardiomegaly, pulmonary congestion, or vascular redistribution confirms the diagnosis.

Echocardiography is especially helpful in identifying the presence of a dilated, hypokinetic LV. With pure diastolic dysfunction as a cause of HF, the patient often has LV hypertrophy, although LV systolic function may appear to be normal, with normal or near-normal EF. An S_4 gallop rhythm and echo-Doppler signs of delayed LV filling and diastolic dysfunction are frequently present. Clinical signs and symptoms of HF in the presence of a normal EF makes the diagnosis of pure diastolic dysfunction.

Management

(see also Chaps. 18, 19, and 21)

The management of HF in the elderly follows the same principles as those in younger patients[124] (see Chaps. 18 and 21). The goals of therapy are also the same, including a decrease or elimination of symptoms, reduction in rehospitalization, and improvement in quality of life. Prolongation of life is desirable but of lower priority in the aged person with HF. Treatment requires consideration of the etiology of the heart disease, the factors that can precipitate HF, and the medical management. For instance, the patient with HF due to AS requires aortic valve replacement; HF due to ischemic but viable myocardium requires revascularization. Managing problems that precipitate HF in patients with underlying heart disease can be important in their medical management. For example, in the patient with diastolic dysfunction who develops HF along with AF, conversion to normal sinus rhythm or, less desirable, control of ventricular rate is the most important treatment.[125]

Noncompliance with medical therapy, excessive salt intake and volume overload in the patient with renal failure, and infection are all causes of exacerbation of HF requiring rehospitalization. These factors contribute to 30 to 50 percent of recurrent episodes of HF in the elderly[126] and are the major reasons why between one third and one half of all patients hospitalized with HF are readmitted within 3 to 6 months of initial discharge.[126]

An effective way of managing elderly patients with HF is through a multidisciplinary approach and follow-up of patients at home through telephone calls, home visits by nursing personnel, and other patient contacts between office visits. Such an approach decreased the 90-day readmission rate by 32 percent in a group of 137 patients 80 to 96 years of age,[127] with improved quality-of-life scores and decreased overall cost. This multidisciplinary approach involves ongoing patient education, dietary consultation, medication review, daily weighings, and help with psychosocial problems and results in better compliance with medication[128] and overall cost reduction due to decreased rehospitalization.[129]

Although medications for HF are the same as those for the younger population, care must be taken not to cause hypovolemia, with marked reduction in stroke volume. Also, electrolyte levels should be monitored closely, especially in those patients taking digoxin and ACE inhibitors, because of the danger of renal dysfunction, hypokalemia, and hyperkalemia. A danger of hypovolemia is precipitation of falls in elderly patients, with subsequent hip fracture.[130] Another problem in elderly patients is that many are receiving NSAIDs, which can increase the risk of HF in elderly patients taking diuretics.[131]

DRUG THERAPY

ACE inhibitors, underprescribed in the elderly, are as effective in improving quality of life and reducing mortality as in younger patients.[132] Digoxin is useful in patients with HF who are in AF and/or are symptomatic on diuretics and ACE inhibitors.[133] However, in the elderly, lean body mass is decreased and renal function frequently is impaired; digoxin dosage is therefore lower than in the younger patient, and the danger of toxicity is greater. The Digitalis Investigation Group (DIG) reported that there was no decrease in overall mortality, but there was a decrease in hospitalization and mortality due to HF in patients receiving digoxin. Older age was an independent risk factor for all-cause mortality and rehospitalization, as well as for HF rehospitalizations and deaths.[134]

Angiotensin II type 1 receptor antagonists are probably as effective as ACE inhibitors, but they are still being evaluated in the elderly, although side effects are probably less often noted.[135] Candesartan was effective in improving exercise tolerance, as well as symptoms and signs of HF.[136] In patients unable to take ACE inhibitors or angiotensin II type 1 receptor blockers, hydralazine and isosorbide have been shown to reduce mortality in patients with HF (see Chap. 18).

Beta blockers, if started in the usual dosage in patients with HF, will worsen the patient's clinical status; however, beta blockers started in small doses with titration upward have been shown to be very effective in improving quality of life of patients with HF, as well as increasing EF and exercise tolerance.[137] In the U.S. carvedilol study, patients with chronic HF and EF less than 35 percent were randomized to carvedilol versus placebo. Mortality was 65 percent lower in the carvedilol group in a 6.5-month follow-up.[138] Patients older than 60 years had results similar to younger patients. In this study, few patients were older than age 75 years. After AMI, beta blockers have been shown to decrease late mortality in the elderly population.[139]

In general, first-generation calcium channel blockers have been associated with adverse effects in patients with HF and as a result are usually contraindicated. If calcium channel blockers are indicated for ischemia, then those with little negative inotropic effect, such as amlodipine or felodipine, should be used.

DIASTOLIC DYSFUNCTION

The treatment of diastolic dysfunction in the elderly has not been well studied. If the symptoms are predominantly pulmonary congestion, then treatment with diuretics and/or long-acting nitrates will lower the filling pressure and decrease shortness of breath. However, overdiuresis can markedly drop the stroke volume and cause hypotension and prerenal azotemia. Beta blockers, by slowing the heart rate and increasing the diastolic filling period, can lower the filling pressure and improve LV compliance by decreasing LV hypertrophy. Similar benefits can result from ACE inhibitors and calcium channel blockers, and all of these drugs have been used in patients with HF and EF greater than 40 percent. Verapamil has been shown to improve symptoms in exercise capacity and diastolic function in older patients with HF and EF less than 45 percent.[140] Whether results with spironolactone will be similar in patients older than age 75 years is unknown but likely (see Chap. 18).

HYPERTENSION
(see also Chaps. 28 and 29)

Both essential and secondary HTN, especially with renoarterial disease, are found in the elderly (see Fig. 57–3). Isolated systolic HTN, as defined by a systolic BP greater than 140 mm Hg and a diastolic BP reading less than 90 mm Hg, is especially prominent in the elderly as a result of the decrease in arterial compliance and concomitant LV systolic stiffening.[3] The diagnosis of HTN should be made only after the BP is found to be elevated on three separate occasions. In the elderly, there are several problems in obtaining a correct BP using the BP cuff.[141] With noncompliant arteries, changes in stroke volume can result in wide variations in systolic BP. The patient should therefore be allowed to rest for 3 minutes before BP is taken.[141] Each time, BP should be taken two or three times and the results averaged. The "white coat" effect can be seen in 15 to 20 percent of all hypertensives, and it is especially common in the elderly.[142] Systolic BPs can vary as much as 20 to 40 mm Hg. For this reason, home or ambulatory BP recordings can be helpful in ascertaining the patient's usual BP.[143]

Another problem, termed "pseudohypertension," is caused by a brachial artery that is calcified and sclerotic and therefore not easily compressed by the BP cuff. The diagnosis of pseudohypertension can be made for certain only by comparing cuff systolic BPs to intraarterial pressures. Recently, doubt has been cast on the validity and usefulness of "Osler's maneuver," that of continuing to palpate a radial pulse with the BP cuff above auscultated systolic BP.[144] Falsely low systolic BPs can also occur because of the "auscultatory gap" in 20 percent of the elderly.[145] Here, Korotkoff sounds may be heard at 180 mm Hg, disappear, and then reappear at 130 mm Hg. If the BP cuff is not inflated to more than 180 mm Hg, the systolic BP will be incorrectly read as 130 mm Hg. This auscultatory phenomenon, the cause of which is unknown, is associated with age, female gender, increased arterial stiffness, and increased prevalence of carotid atherosclerotic plaques.[145] Pseudohypotension occurs when the BP is measured in an arm with an atherosclerotic obstruction proximal to the brachial artery. It can be suspected when there is a 30 mm Hg difference in BPs between the arms. A unilateral supraclavicular bruit is often heard. BP should always be taken initially in both arms and followed in the arm with the higher pressure.

HYPOTENSION. Orthostatic hypotension, defined as a drop of more than 20 mm Hg in pressure on going from a supine or sitting to a standing position for 1 to 3 minutes, was present in the Systolic Hypertension in the Elderly Program (SHEP) study before therapy in one of every six elderly patients with HTN.[146] Orthostatic HTN is more likely to occur in an elderly person because of the noncompliant vessels and is especially likely to occur with hypovolemia due to diuretics or drugs interfering with vasoconstriction, such as alpha-adrenergic blockade given for HTN or benign prostatic hypertrophy.

Postprandial hypotension is especially common in elderly patients, occurring 30 to 120 minutes after a meal and causing drops in BP of more than 20 mm Hg. It is associated with lightheadedness, syncope, and falls and may be caused by vasodilation associated with excessive insulin response to a glucose load.[147] Decisions regarding BP control or change in therapy for HTN should take into account how long after the last meal the BP is taken.

EPIDEMIOLOGY

HTN is more common in blacks than in whites: About 45 percent of white, but 60 percent of black, men and women have HTN at ages 65 to 74.[148] In a study from a university geriatrics practice of 459 men and 1360 women, mean age 80 ± 8 years (range 59 to 101 years), HTN was present in 58 percent.[149] Because of its prevalence in the elderly, isolated systolic HTN was thought to be a natural consequence of aging. To the extent that there are changes in the arterial wall with aging that lead to less compliant vessels, a rise in systolic BP is a consequence of aging. That isolated systolic HTN is not a normal consequence of aging is reflected in the fact that epidemiological studies show a rise in systolic BP with age occurring only infrequently in most nonindustrialized societies. In a study in which participants at ages 50 to 89 were surveyed as to leisure activity (classified into light, moderate, heavy, and no physical activity), BP decreased with increasing levels of activity.[150] It appears, therefore, that there are environmental and life-style influences on the late rise in systolic BP with aging.

HTN remains the most common cause of HF, both with systolic and diastolic dysfunction. It is a strong risk factor for the development of CAD in both men and women. The Framingham Heart Study found that people 65 to 94 years of age with systolic BPs greater than 180 mm Hg had a threefold to fourfold increase in the risk of CAD compared with those whose systolic BP was less than 120 mm Hg.[53] A diastolic BP greater than 105 mm Hg caused a twofold to threefold higher rise in CAD than in those with a diastolic BP less than 75 mm Hg. Mortality is increased in elderly patients with HTN, mainly owing to HF and CAD.[53] In addition to mortality, the complications of HTN can be especially devastating: almost two thirds of those older than age 60 with untreated HTN will have a cerebrovascular accident, HF, myocardial infarction, or aortic dissection within 5 years.[151] Similar morbidity and mortality have been shown to occur in patients with isolated systolic HTN as in those with systolic and diastolic HTN.[152]

Although there is no doubt that lowering BP will reduce mortality, in old patients aged 80 to 85, there is paradoxical evidence of higher mortality with lower than with higher systolic or diastolic BP.[153] In one study of 561 people, including 82 percent of women aged older than 85, the 5-year mortality was lower in hypertensive (41 percent) than normotensive (72 percent) patients. It was highest in those with the lowest systolic BP (< 120 mm Hg) or diastolic BP (< 70 mm Hg) and was lowest in those with systolic BP greater than 160 mm Hg or diastolic BP greater than 90 mm Hg.[153] Another study found that patients with a mean age older than 75 with the lowest diastolic BP (< 75 mm Hg) had the highest cardiovascular disease and all-cause mortality, whereas the highest diastolic BPs predicted higher survival.[154] The higher mortality in patients with the lowest diastolic BP suggests the possibility of decreased coronary perfusion pressure and subendocardial ischemia. This paradox of increased mortality in very old patients with a lower systolic BP and diastolic BP has been termed the "J curve,"[155] which is probably related to the effects of cardiac, respiratory, and neoplastic disease in those with low BP versus good myocardial function in those with HTN. Therefore, one cannot conclude that patients older than 75 to 80 years will not benefit from BP reduction. The SHEP study found no evidence of a J curve in treated patients with isolated systolic HTN.[156] However, a recent population-based cohort study[157] reported a risk of myocardial infarction in elderly patients with treatment of diastolic BP to less than 90 mm Hg, after adjusting for all other coronary risk factors.

Treatment
(see also Chap. 29)

The recommendations for the treatment of HTN in the elderly do not differ from those for younger patients.[54, 158] Lowering even isolated systolic HTN decreases cardiovascular and total mortality, as well as hypertensive complications of HF, renal failure, and stroke.[55, 156] The goal of treatment of HTN in elderly patients should be a lowering of systolic BP to less than 140 mm Hg without creating postural hypotension or symptoms of organ hypoperfusion, such as elevated blood urea nitrogen or renal insufficiency.[158] If this is not possible, lowering systolic BP by 20 mm Hg is considered an acceptable response and has been associated with useful reduction in clinical cardiovascular events.[64] Benefits occur regardless of the class of antihypertensive drugs used.

The Swedish Trial in Old Patients with Hypertension (STOP-H) randomized 1627 patients with systolic/diastolic HTN, aged 70 to 84, to placebo versus atenolol, metoprolol, pindolol, or hydrochlorothiazide and amiloride. In a 25-month follow-up, a 28 percent decrease in fatal myocardial infarction, a 67 percent decrease in sudden death, and a 47 percent decrease in stroke resulted.[159] A meta-analysis of

1670 patients aged 80 or more, from randomized controlled trials of antihypertensive drugs, suggested that treatment prevented 34 percent of strokes and decreased the incidence of major cardiovascular events by 22 percent and HF by 39 percent. However, there was no treatment benefit for cardiovascular or total deaths. This suggests, in patients older than age 80, that there is benefit in reducing nonfatal cardiovascular events but not total mortality.[160]

Because of the expense and potential benefit in patients with CAD, diuretics and beta blockers are often the first choice in antihypertensive treatment in the elderly. In the patient with HF, ACE inhibitors should be used together with other drugs to decrease BP. Nitrates have recently been advocated in patients with isolated systolic HTN because they have an effect on arterial distensibility, reducing systolic BP without affecting mean BP or diastolic BP.[161] This has the theoretical benefit of not decreasing myocardial perfusion and would benefit those patients with HTN and concurrent CAD and cerebrovascular disease.

Nonpharmacological therapy, consisting of increased exercise, salt restriction, weight loss, and limited alcohol intake can be useful for patients with mildly elevated BP.[54, 158] There are few studies in elderly hypertensives of the effectiveness of this approach in decreasing BP and no evidence (unlike in pharmacological therapy) that it would decrease complications of HTN and mortality. The elderly have increased sensitivity to salt, so that salt loading increases BP and salt restriction reduces it.[162] In a meta-analysis of 11 randomized controlled trials, 5 included patients older than 60 years of age and 6 included patients with a mean age of 60. When all trials were pooled, a chronic high sodium chloride intake significantly increased systolic BP and diastolic BP by 6 and 3.5 mm Hg, respectively, and there was a significant association between salt intake and systolic BP. A high sodium chloride diet in elderly patients with essential HTN is associated with a higher systolic BP and diastolic BP, and the effect is more pronounced in the older patient.[163] In 300,000 elderly nursing home patients (mean age, 83 years), HTN was diagnosed in 27 percent. About one fourth had six or more comorbid conditions. Seventy percent of these patients were receiving antihypertensive drugs, with calcium channel blockers the most common (26 percent), followed by diuretics (25 percent), ACE inhibitors (22 percent), and beta blockers (8 percent). The oldest subjects (>85 years) and those with marked physical or cognitive impairment were less likely to receive treatment.[164]

CARDIOMYOPATHY
(see also Chap. 48)

Both dilated (DCM) (congestive) and hypertrophic (HCM) cardiomyopathy occur in the elderly. Most DCMs are of unknown etiology, just as they are in younger patients.

Amyloid Cardiomyopathy

Amyloid DCM is noted primarily in older people. Although small deposits of amyloidosis (senile amyloidosis) are often seen at autopsy, they are of no clinical significance in people younger than 85 years. Reactive amyloidosis, seen in chronic rheumatoid arthritis or bronchiectasis, usually does not involve the heart. In amyloid heart disease the amyloid, an abnormal fibrillar protein, is deposited intercellularly and in the walls of small coronary arteries[165] (see Chap. 48).

The amyloid can involve only certain organs, or it can be a generalized disorder. The heart and tongue, with and without skeletal involvement, and the autonomic nervous system, are frequently involved. Amyloid infiltration of the heart causes thickening of the ventricles, which become less compliant to diastolic filling, resulting in the picture of restrictive cardiomyopathy. Senile amyloidosis, in the past thought to be a consequence of aging without clinical significance, is now known to contribute to HF in patients older than 85.[166] Of 142 men and 90 women with primary immunoglobulin light-chain amyloidosis, the median age at diagnosis was 59 years, with a range of 29 to 85 years, and was unusual in those younger than 40 (3.0 percent) and in nonwhites (6.5 percent). Macroglossia was seen in 27 percent. Patients most often demonstrated features of multisystem

dysfunction, and cardiac amyloidosis was seen in isolation in only 3.9 percent. With cardiac involvement, the median survival was 1 year from diagnosis; and with the onset of HF, it was 9 months. Cardiac amyloidosis should be suspected in elderly patients with HF and a hypertrophied LV, possibly with "sparkling" myocardial characteristics and normal chamber sizes on echocardiography (see Chap. 7), low ECG voltage (see Chap. 5), and evidence of multisystemic disease.[167] An abnormal echocardiogram and signal-averaged ECG predict both all-cause and sudden cardiac death mortality, whereas an abnormal signal-averaged ECG independently predicts SD in those patients with an abnormal echocardiogram.[168]

Hypertrophic Cardiomyopathy

Hypertrophic cardiomyopathy is another important disease that is being diagnosed increasingly in the elderly patient.[169] HCM in elderly patients has been found in 4 percent of an unselected population of 379 elderly patients (mean age = 83 years) in a long-term health care facility.[170] In an echocardiographic survey of 15,137 people in a 33-month period, 44 patients with HCM (0.29 percent) were found, aged 16 to 87 years (mean age 57), 14 of whom were older than 60 years. Eighty-three percent had few or no symptoms; in 8 patients, symptoms began at age 70 or older. Resting systolic gradients were found in 38 percent of the patients. It is clear that HCM can remain clinically silent and undetected for many years, often to an advanced age.[171]

Compared with younger patients, the elderly with HCM have more mild HTN and fewer have a history of syncope. Echocardiography shows that the elderly have relatively mild LV wall thickening, generally confined to the basilar septum.[172] Another study showed that elderly patients with HCM had more concentric hypertrophy than younger ones. Microscopically, there is less marked septal myocyte disarray and intramural coronary artery thickening and less sudden cardiac death (see Chaps. 26 and 48) in older patients with HCM than in younger patients.[173]

In the symptomatic patient, beta blockers and calcium channel blockers are still the first line of treatment. Controlled trials with synchronous AV pacing have yielded mixed results, although most find a moderate to marked decrease in systolic LV outflow tract gradient. Some note a decrease in symptoms, increased quality of life measures, and increased exercise capacity[174]; but others find no subjective or objective benefits.[175]

When medical management fails, surgical septal myomectomy has proven successful over the years, with an early mortality from isolated myomectomy of 3.6 percent. During the past 10 years, mortality was only 1.9 percent.[176] In 346 patients followed up to 26 years after surgery, the annual mortality was 0.6 percent compared historically to an annual mortality in unoperated patients that varied from 1.7 to 4 percent. The surgical patients also had long-lasting improvement in symptoms, exercise capacity, and quality-of-life indices.

Alcohol-induced transcoronary ablation of septal hypertrophy has been reported, with low mortality and significant improvement manifested by reduction in septal thickness, LV outflow tract gradient, and improvement in NYHA functional class and exercise capacity. There is also a significant improvement in LV passive filling volume,[177] a decrease in LV filling pressures at rest, and during exercise.[178] High-grade AV block can result.[178]

In those patients surviving a cardiac arrest or who have ventricular tachycardia (see Chap. 25), or those judged to be at high risk for a life-threatening cardiac arrhythmia, an implanted cardioverter-defibrillator (see Chaps. 24 and 26) has proven to be very effective.[179]

Supraventricular Arrhythmias

The frequency of both supraventricular and ventricular arrhythmias increases with age. Premature atrial complexes (PACs) are extremely frequent in elderly people. Isolated PACs can be seen in resting ECGs of 5 to 10 percent of normal people older than age 60. With 24-hour ambulatory ECGs, the majority of patients older than age 65 have PACs, and even short runs of supraventricular tachycardia (SVT) of mostly three to five beats.[180] In mostly healthy subjects 65 years of age and older in the Cardiovascular Health Study, short runs of paroxysmal SVT (PSVT) were seen in about 50 percent of subjects, nearly doubling in prevalence from the late 60s age group to the 80s.[180] Both isolated PACs and short runs of PSVT have no prognostic significance for CAD in elderly patients over a 10-year follow-up period in the Baltimore Longitudinal Study of Aging Project.[181]

In general, patients with PACs or short runs of asymptomatic PSVT need no treatment except reassurance. If the patient is unpleasantly symptomatic, type IA or IC antiarrhythmic drugs are effective but should not be given to patients with underlying heart disease. Amiodarone or sotalol can be tried. PSVT, either AV nodal reentry, atrial tachycardia, or SVT associated with a bypass tract, is treated just as in younger patients. Adenosine can be used effectively and safely in elderly patients.[182] Although beta blockers, calcium channel blockers, and type IC antiarrhythmic drugs are effective for patients with repeated prolonged episodes of some SVTs, radiofrequency catheter ablation is done with success rates similar to that seen in younger patients.[183]

ATRIAL FIBRILLATION. This is the most common chronic arrhythmia and increases with age. It is seen in 3 to 4 percent of subjects 60 to 65 years of age, a prevalence 10 times as high as that in the general population. The incidence doubles for each decade after age 60,[184] reaching 8.8 percent of the population older than 80 years.[185] About one third of patients with AF have paroxysmal episodes on 24-hour ambulatory ECG, and two thirds have chronic AF.[184] The prevalence of AF in men and women without cardiovascular disease in the Cardiovascular Health Study was 1.6 percent, rising to 4.6 percent in patients with subclinical, and to 9.1 percent in those with overt, cardiovascular disease.[186] Age-adjusted prevalence of AF increases strikingly in men with a prior myocardial infarction (4.9 to 17.4 percent).[187] AF most often occurs with underlying heart disease such as HTN, CAD, mitral valve disease, and HF. The presence of any cardiovascular disease increases the risk of AF by twofold to fivefold.[188] In elderly patients, thyrotoxicosis can manifest mainly by the onset of AF with a rapid ventricular response, so-called apathetic thyrotoxicosis.[189]

Symptoms and morbidity occur in older patients with AF. The rapid ventricular response can cause unpleasant palpitations; but also, with loss of atrial contraction, the booster-pump function of atrial systole is lost and stroke volume decreases (see Fig. 57–1). If the rate is very rapid, BP may drop significantly. In the elderly, because of the less compliant LV, loss of atrial contraction is especially important. Uncontrolled rapid ventricular response can lead to HF or "tachycardia-mediated cardiomyopathy." In elderly patients with sick sinus syndrome, paroxysmal AF can result in syncope when the arrhythmia terminates and there is a long pause before sinus node function returns or if the subsequent rhythm is marked bradycardia (see Chaps. 23 and 25). A most important problem associated with AF is that of thromboembolism, because of stasis of blood flow, especially in the atrial appendage, with thrombus formation and possible thromboembolism. In the Framingham Heart Study, the incidence of stroke in patients with AF rose from 1.5 percent in the 50- to 59-year age group to 23.5 percent in those older than age 80.[190]

A small number of older patients with AF have neither HTN nor any other cardiovascular disease and represent cases of so-called "lone" AF. The Framingham study found lone AF in 17 percent of men and 6 percent of women, with a mean age of 71 and 68 years, respectively. Follow-up for new cardiovascular events over a mean of 16 years revealed similar rates of CAD and HF as in control patients without AF, but a fourfold increase in the rate of stroke.[191] Patients younger than 60 years with lone AF do not have an increased risk of embolic stroke,[192] but increasing age increases the risk.[193] Risk factors that increase the incidence of thromboembolism and stroke during AF include diabetes, HF, advanced age, smoking, recent myocardial infarction, HTN, and enlarged left atrial diameter greater than 40 mm.[185] Patients older than age 75 years with diabetes, HTN, or prior transient ischemic attack/stroke have an annual stroke incidence of 8 to 12 percent.[192]

Warfarin reduces the incidence of stroke in patients with nonvalvular AF (see Chap. 25), but the risk of bleeding, particularly intracerebral hemorrhage, is higher, especially in patients older than 75.[194] Nevertheless, in elderly patients it appears safe to use adjusted-dose warfarin with a low risk of major hemorrhage, if the international normalized ratio (INR) is maintained in the 2 to 3 range.[195, 196] Therefore, it is recommended that all elderly patients with AF without contraindications (active ulcer, recent surgery, bleeding diathesis, dementia, frequent falls or trauma) be anticoagulated to an INR between 2 and 3, with avoidance of higher INRs. In those who cannot take warfarin, an antiplatelet drug such as aspirin, 325 mg/d, although clearly not as effective as warfarin, is recommended.[197] Patients younger than 65 with lone AF can be treated with aspirin, or without antithrombotic therapy. In those older than age 75, therapeutic benefit must be balanced against the risk of intracerebral bleeding, but anticoagulation with INR between 2 and 3 is recommended with risk factors present that increase the chance of stroke. In others, aspirin should be considered.

In elderly patients with AF, an attempt to convert to sinus rhythm, preferably by direct-current cardioversion after 3 to 4 weeks of anticoagulation, can be made. Maintenance of sinus rhythm is most successful if the AF is not long standing (i.e., less than a year) and with minimal left atrial enlargement.[198] If this is not possible, or if the patient reverts to AF despite antiarrhythmic drug therapy, control of ventricular response is necessary with beta blockers, calcium channel blockers, or digoxin. If drugs fail to slow the ventricular rate, modification of AV nodal conduction by radiofrequency catheter ablation is successful. Radiofrequency ablation can also be used to eliminate rapidly discharging foci causing AF (see Chap. 25).

Atrial flutter responds to low-energy direct-current cardioversion, which is the procedure of choice when the ventricular response is rapid. It can be an unstable rhythm, reverting to sinus rhythm or AF. If atrial flutter persists, RF catheter ablation can eliminate further episodes (see Chap. 25). Although the incidence of thromboembolism is lower than with AF, anticoagulation is generally indicated for patients with atrial flutter, as in patients with AF.[199]

Ventricular Arrhythmias

Premature ventricular complexes (PVCs), like PACs, increase in prevalence and frequency with age and include simple and complex PVCs, ventricular couplets, and short bursts of ventricular tachycardia.[180, 184, 200] With exercise, PVCs increase in prevalence from 11 percent in the third decade to 57 percent in the ninth.[200] The prognostic significance of isolated or even complex PVCs depends on the presence or absence of underlying cardiovascular disease.[201]

The treatment of PVCs, even complex PVCs, is not indicated in asymptomatic patients who have no underlying cardiac disease. In symptomatic patients, beta blockers are often the initial drug of choice. Treatment of nonsustained and sustained ventricular tachyarrhythmias in the elderly in general is no different than in younger patients (see Chap. 25).[202]

Conduction Defects

The changes in the sinus and AV nodes due to aging, along with the decreased sensitivity to adrenergic stimulation, create an increased incidence of sick sinus syndrome, as well as AV and bundle branch conduction disease. Individuals older than 80 years without cardiovascular disease are reported not to have sinus bradycardia less than 43 beats/min or pauses of more than 2 seconds.[180] Consequently, sinus bradycardia less than 40 beats/min or sinus pauses of more than 2 seconds may be manifestations of sick sinus syndrome. However, pacemaker implantation is not indicated in asymptomatic patients with these findings. In contrast, in the patient with syncope or presyncope or taking medications that aggravate the sick sinus syndrome, a pacemaker is indicated.

With aging, the incidence of AV and bundle branch block is increased, possibly as a result of increasing fibrosis and calcification of the fibrous skeleton of the heart.[201] Types 1 and 2 degree AV block can be benign unless associated with digitalis toxicity or symptoms and are usually the result of enhanced vagal tone. The presence of Mobitz type II and third-degree AV block is unusual, even in older patients,[201] and is always associated with advanced conduction system disease, requiring pacemaker implantation[203] (see Chaps. 23 through 25). In paced patients 65 to 79 years of age with isolated AV block, the survival rate was similar to matched individuals without AV block, whereas in those older than 80 years, the survival rate was lower than in matched controls.[204]

The QRS axis shifts leftward with age, becoming −30 degrees in 20 percent by age 90, perhaps due to increased LV mass or interstitial fibrosis of the anterior fascicular radiation. Right bundle branch block is found in 3 percent of healthy people older than 85 years, and in 8 to 10 percent of those with heart disease.[201, 205] The presence of left bundle branch block correlates strongly with age and may be a marker of slowly progressive degenerative disease affecting the myocardium. In 855 men older than 50 years observed for 30 years, 1 percent of those aged 50 and 17 percent at age 80 developed bundle branch block. No relationship between bundle branch block and ischemic heart disease or mortality was found. Men who developed bundle branch block had a larger-volume heart at age 50 and developed diabetes and HF during follow-up more often than control subjects.[206] In the Framingham Heart Study, 2 percent of subjects older than age 70 developed a nonspecific intraventricular conduction defect exceeding 120 milliseconds, which was associated with the presence of organic heart disease.[207] The presence of bundle branch block should lead to a search for underlying cardiac disease, but unless it progresses to advanced heart block it needs no therapy.

R E F E R E N C E S

PATHOPHYSIOLOGY

1. Vaitkevicius PV, Fleg JL, Engel JH, et al: Effects of age and aerobic capacity on arterial stiffness in healthy adults. Circulation 88:1456–1462, 1993.
2. Chen CH, Nakayama M, Nevo E, et al: Coupled systolic-ventricular and vascular stiffening with age: Implications for pressure regulation and cardiac reserve in the elderly. J Am Coll Cardiol 32:1221–1227, 1998.
3. Gardin JM, Arnold AM, Bild DE, et al: Left ventricular diastolic filling in the elderly: The cardiovascular health study. Am J Cardiol 82:345–351, 1998.
4. Shirani J, Yousefi J, Roberts WC: Major cardiac findings at necropsy in 366 American octogenarians. Am J Cardiol 75:151–156, 1995.
5. Davies CH, Ferrara N, Harding SE: Beta-adrenoceptor function changes with age of subject in myocytes from non-failing human ventricle. Cardiovasc Res 31:152–156, 1996.
6. Lakatta EG: Cardiovascular regulatory mechanisms in advanced age. Physiol Rev 73:413–467, 1993.
7. Zhou YY, Lakatta EG, Xiao RP: Age-associated alterations in calcium current and its modulation in cardiac myocytes. Drugs Aging 13:159–171, 1998.
8. Cerbai E, Barbieri M, Li Q, Mugelli A: Ionic basis of action potential prolongation of hypertrophied cardiac myocytes isolated from hypertensive rats of different ages. Cardiovasc Res 28:1180–1187, 1994.
9. Johnson RE, Vollmer WM: Comparing sources of drug data about the elderly. J Am Geriatr Soc 39:1079–1084, 1991.
10. Veering BT, Burm AG, Souverijn JH, J et al: The effect of age on serum concentrations of albumin and alpha 1-acid glycoprotein. Br J Clin Pharmacol 29:201–206, 1990.
11. Tateishi T, Fujimura A, Shiga T, et al: Influence of aging on the oxidative and conjugative metabolism of propranolol. Int J Clin Pharmacol Res 15:95–101, 1995.
12. Lindeman RD: Changes in renal function with aging: Implications for treatment. Drugs Aging 2:423–431, 1992.
13. Lamy PP: Renal effects of nonsteroidal antiinflammatory drugs: Heightened risk to the elderly? J Am Geriatr Soc 34:361–367, 1986.
14. Schwartz JB: Aging alters verapamil elimination and dynamics: Single dose and steady-state responses. J Pharmacol Exp Ther 255:364–373, 1990.
15. Chrischilles EA, Segar ET, Wallace RB: Self-reported adverse drug reactions and related resource use: A study of community-dwelling persons 65 years of age and older. Ann Intern Med 117:634–640, 1992.
16. Chutka DS, Evans JM, Fleming KC, Mikkelson KG: Symposium on geriatrics: I. Drug prescribing for elderly patients. Mayo Clin Proc 70:685–693, 1995.
17. Podrazik PM, Schwartz JB: Principles of cardiovascular pharmacology at advanced age. In Wenger NK (ed): Cardiovascular Disease in the Octogenarian and Beyond. London: Martin Dunitz, 1999, p 127.
18. U.S. National Center for Health Statistics: Health, United States 1999; with Health and Aging Chartbook. Hyattsville, MD, The Center, 1999.
19. United Nations, Population Division, Department of Economic and Social Affairs, April 18, 2000. Web site: www.undp.org/popn/wdtrends/a99/99note.htm
20. Roberts WC, Shirani J: Comparison of cardiac findings at necropsy in octogenarians, nonagenarians, and centenarians. Am J Cardiol 82:627–631, 1998.
21. Cupples LA, D'Agostino RJ: The Framingham Study: An Epidemiologic Investigation of Cardiovascular Disease. Section 23. Some Risk Factors Related to the Annual Incidence of Cardiovascular Disease and Death, Using Pooled Repeated Biennial Measurements: Framingham Heart Study, 30-Year Follow-Up. Springfield, VA, US Department of Commerce, 1987.
22. Wei JY: Advanced aging and the cardiovascular system. In Wenger NK (ed): Cardiovascular Disease in the Octogenarian and Beyond. London, Martin Dunitz, 1999, p 9.
23. Tsevat J, Dawson NV, Wu AW, et al: Health values of hospitalized patients 80 years or older. HELP Investigators. Hospitalized Elderly Longitudinal Project. JAMA 279:371–375, 1998.
24. Otto CM, Lind BK, Kitzman DW, et al: Association of aortic-valve sclerosis with cardiovascular mortality and morbidity in the elderly. N Engl J Med 341:142–147, 1999.
25. Braverman AC: Bicuspid aortic valve and associated aortic wall abnormalities. Curr Opin Cardiol 11:501–503, 1996.
26. Bonow RO, Carabello B, de Leon AC, et al: ACC/AHA Guidelines for the Management of Patients With Valvular Heart Disease. Executive Summary: A report of the American College of Cardiology/American Heart Association Task Force on Practice Guidelines (Committee on Management of Patients With Valvular Heart Disease). J Heart Valve Dis 7:672–707, 1998.
27. Cohen G, David TE, Ivanov J, et al: The impact of age, coronary artery disease, and cardiac comorbidity on late survival after bioprosthetic aortic valve replacement. J Thorac Cardiovasc Surg 117:273–284, 1999.
28. Hogue CW Jr, Murphy SF, Schechtman KB, Davila-Roman VG: Risk factors for early or delayed stroke after cardiac surgery. Circulation 100:642–647, 1999.
29. Arom KV, Emery RW, Nicoloff DM, Petersen RJ: Anticoagulant related complications in elderly patients with St. Jude mechanical valve prostheses. J Heart Valve Dis 5:505–510, 1996.
30. Verheul HA, van den Brink RB, Bouma BJ, et al: Analysis of risk factors for excess mortality after aortic valve replacement. J Am Coll Cardiol 26:1280–1286, 1995.
31. Dujardin KS, Enriquez-Sarano M, Schaff HV, et al: Mortality and morbidity of aortic regurgitation in clinical practice: A long-term follow-up study. Circulation 99:1851–1857, 1999.
32. Kirklin JW, Barratt-Boyes BG: Congenital aortic stenosis. In Kirklin JW, Barratt-Boyes BG (eds): Cardiac Surgery: Morphology, Diagnostic Criteria, Natural History, Techniques, Results and Indications. 2nd ed. New York, Churchill Livingstone, 1993, p 1195.

33. David TE, Armstrong S, Ivanov J, Webb GD: Aortic valve sparing operations: An update. Ann Thorac Surg 67:1840–1842, 1999.
34. Gilbert T, Orr W, Banning AP: Surgery for aortic stenosis in severely symptomatic patients older than 80 years: Experience in a single UK centre. Heart 82:138–142, 1999.
35. Zaidi AM, Fitzpatrick AP, Keenan DJ, et al: Good outcomes from cardiac surgery in the over 70s. Heart 82:134–137, 1999.
36. Kolh P, Lahaye L, Gerard P, Limet R: Aortic valve replacement in the octogenarians: Perioperative outcome and clinical follow-up. Eur J Cardiothorac Surg 16:68–73, 1999.
37. Vaturi M, Porter A, Adler Y, et al: The natural history of aortic valve disease after mitral valve surgery. J Am Coll Cardiol 33:2003–2008, 1999.
38. Bessou JP, Bouchart F, Angha S, et al: Aortic valvular replacement in octogenarians: Short-term and mid-term results in 140 patients. Cardiovasc Surg 7:355–362, 1999.
39. Tribouilloy C, Peltier M, Rey JL, et al: Use of transesophageal echocardiography to predict significant coronary artery disease in aortic stenosis. Chest 113:671–675, 1998.
40. Lin SS, Roger VL, Pascoe R, et al: Dobutamine stress Doppler hemodynamics in patients with aortic stenosis: Feasibility, safety, and surgical correlations. Am Heart J 136:1010–1016, 1998.
41. Weinschelbaum E, Stutzbach P, Oliva M, et al: Manual debridement of the aortic valve in elderly patients with degenerative aortic stenosis. J Thorac Cardiovasc Surg 117:1157–1165, 1999.
42. Grunkemeier GL, Bodnar E: Comparison of structural valve failure among different "models" of homograft valves. J Heart Valve Dis 3:556–560, 1994.
43. Herlitz J, Brandrup-Wognsen G, Caidahl K, et al: Mortality and morbidity among patients who undergo combined valve and coronary artery bypass surgery: Early and late results. Eur J Cardiothorac Surg 12:836–846, 1997.
44. Akins CW, Daggett WM, Vlahakes GJ, et al: Cardiac operations in patients 80 years old and older. Ann Thorac Surg 64:606–614, 1997.
45. Bolling SF, Deeb GM, Bach DS: Mitral valve reconstruction in elderly, ischemic patients. Chest 109:35–40, 1996.
46. Cheitlin MD: Severe aortic stenosis in the sick octogenarian: A clear indicator for balloon valvuloplasty as the initial procedure. Circulation 80:1906–1908, 1989.
47. Ben Farhat M, Ayari M, Maatouk F, et al: Percutaneous balloon versus surgical closed and open mitral commissurotomy: Seven-year follow-up results of a randomized trial. Circulation 97:245–250, 1998.
48. Meneveau N, Schiele F, Seronde MF, et al: Predictors of event-free survival after percutaneous mitral commissurotomy. Heart 80:359–364, 1998.

CORONARY ARTERY DISEASE

49. Kannel WB, Vokonas PS: Demographics of the prevalence, incidence, and management of coronary heart disease in the elderly and in women. Ann Epidemiol 2:5–14, 1992.
50. Lloyd-Jones DM, Larson MG, Beiser A, Levy D: Lifetime risk of developing coronary heart disease. Lancet 353:89–92, 1999.
51. American Heart Association: Coronary heart disease and angina pectoris. December 8, 1999. Web site: www.amhrt.org/statistics/04corny.html
52. U.S. Department of Health and Human Services, Public Health Service, Centers for Disease Control and Prevention: Morbidity and Mortality: Chartbook on Cardiovascular Lung and Blood Diseases. Bethesda, MD, The Department, 1996.
53. Kannel WB: Blood pressure as a cardiovascular risk factor: Prevention and treatment. JAMA 275:1571–1576, 1996.
54. The sixth report of the Joint National Committee on prevention, detection, evaluation, and treatment of high blood pressure. Arch Intern Med 157:2413–2446, 1997.
55. Prevention of stroke by antihypertensive drug treatment in older persons with isolated systolic hypertension. Final results of the Systolic Hypertension in the Elderly Program (SHEP). SHEP Cooperative Research Group. JAMA 265:3255–3264, 1991.
56. American Heart Association: Older Americans and cardiovascular diseases. Biostatistical fact sheet. April 20, 2000. Web site: www.americanheart.org/biostats/biool.htm
57. LaCroix AZ, Lang J, Scherr P, et al: Smoking and mortality among older men and women in three communities. N Engl J Med 324:1619–1625, 1991.
58. Doll R, Peto R, Wheatley K, et al: Mortality in relation to smoking: 40 years' observations on male British doctors. BMJ 309:901–911, 1994.
59. Kawachi I, Colditz GA, Stampfer MJ, et al: Smoking cessation in relation to total mortality rates in women: A prospective cohort study. Ann Intern Med 119:992–1000, 1993.
60. Castelli WP, Wilson PW, Levy D, Anderson K: Cardiovascular risk factors in the elderly. Am J Cardiol 63:12H–19H, 1989.
61. Johnson CL, Rifkind BM, Sempos CT, et al: Declining serum total cholesterol levels among US adults. The National Health and Nutrition Examination Surveys JAMA 269:3002–3008, 1993.
62. Kannel WB, Wilson PW: An update on coronary risk factors. Med Clin North Am 79:951–971, 1995.
63. LaRosa JC: Triglycerides and coronary risk in women and the elderly. Arch Intern Med 157:961–968, 1997.
64. Prevention of cardiovascular events and death with pravastatin in patients with coronary heart disease and a broad range of initial cholesterol levels. The Long-Term Intervention with Pravastatin in Ischaemic Disease (LIPID) Study Group. N Engl J Med 339:1349–1357, 1998.
65. Assmann G, Schulte H: Diabetes mellitus and hypertension in the elderly: Concomitant hyperlipidemia and coronary heart disease risk. Am J Cardiol 63:33H–37H, 1989.
66. Williams PT: Coronary heart disease risk factors of vigorously active sexagenarians and septuagenarians. J Am Geriatr Soc 46:134–142, 1998.
67. Kannel WB, Sorlie P: Some health benefits of physical activity. The Framingham Study. Arch Intern Med 139:857–861, 1979.
68. Stehouwer CD, Weijenberg MP, van den Berg M, et al: Serum homocysteine and risk of coronary heart disease and cerebrovascular disease in elderly men: A 10-year follow-up. Arterioscler Thromb Vasc Biol 18:1895–1901, 1998.
69. Frasure-Smith N, Lesperance F, Talajic M: Depression and 18-month prognosis after myocardial infarction. Circulation 91:999–1005, 1995.
70. Reynen K, Bachmann K: Coronary arteriography in elderly patients: Risk, therapeutic consequences and long-term follow-up. Coron Artery Dis 8:657–666, 1997.
71. Coodley EL: Coronary artery disease in the elderly. Postgrad Med 87:223–228, 1990.
72. O'Rourke RA, Chatterjee K, Wei JY: Cardiovascular disease in the elderly: Coronary heart disease. J Am Coll Cardiol 10:52A–56A, 1987.
73. Goldberg RJ, McCormick D, Gurwitz JH, et al: Age-related trends in short- and long-term survival after acute myocardial infarction: A 20-year population-based perspective (1975–1995). Am J Cardiol 82:1311–1317, 1998.
74. Wenger NK: Cardiovascular disease in the elderly. Curr Probl Cardiol 17:609–690, 1992.
75. Elveback L, Lie JT: Continued high incidence of coronary artery disease at autopsy in Olmsted County, Minnesota, 1950 to 1979. Circulation 70:345–349, 1984.
76. Ambepitiya G, Roberts M, Ranjadayalan K, Tallis R: Silent exertional myocardial ischemia in the elderly: A quantitative analysis of anginal perceptual threshold and the influence of autonomic function. J Am Geriatr Soc 42:732–737, 1994.
77. Gibbons RJ, Balady GJ, Beasley JW, et al: ACC/AHA Guidelines for Exercise Testing: A report of the American College of Cardiology/American Heart Association Task Force on Practice Guidelines (Committee on Exercise Testing). J Am Coll Cardiol 30:260–311, 1997.
78. Glover DR, Robinson CS, Murray RG. Diagnostic testing in 104 patients over 65 years of age. Eur Heart J 1984:5(SupplE):59–61.
78a. Saunamaki KI: Early post-myocardial infarction exercise testing in subjects 70 years or more of age: Functional and prognostic evaluation. Eur Heart J 5(SupplE) 93–96, 1984.
78b. Fioretti P, Deckers JW, Brower RW, et al. Predischarge stress test after myocardial infarction in old age: results and prognostic valve. Eur Heart J 1984:5(SupplE):101–104.
79. Hilton TC, Shaw LJ, Chaitman BR, et al: Prognostic significance of exercise thallium-201 testing in patients aged greater than or equal to 70 years with known or suspected coronary artery disease. Am J Cardiol 69:45–50, 1992.
80. White HD, Barbash GI, Califf RM, et al: Age and outcome with contemporary thrombolytic therapy: Results from the GUSTO-I trial. Global Utilization of Streptokinase and TPA for Occluded coronary arteries trial. Circulation 94:1826–1833, 1996.
81. Paul SD, O'Gara PT, Mahjoub ZA, et al: Geriatric patients with acute myocardial infarction: Cardiac risk factor profiles, presentation, thrombolysis, coronary interventions, and prognosis. Am Heart J 131:710–715, 1996.
82. Rask-Madsen C, Jensen G, Kober L, et al: Age-related mortality, clinical heart failure, and ventricular fibrillation in 4259 Danish patients after acute myocardial infarction. Eur Heart J 18:1426–1431, 1997.
83. Smith JCJ: Drug treatment after acute myocardial infarction: Is treatment the same for the elderly as in the young patient? Am J Geriatr Cardiol 7:60, 1998.
84. Ryan TJ, Antman EM, Brooks NH, et al: 1999 update: ACC/AHA guidelines for the management of patients with acute myocardial infarction: A report of the American College of Cardiology/American Heart Association Task Force on Practice Guidelines (Committee on Management of Acute Myocardial Infarction). J Am Coll Cardiol 34:890–911, 1999.
85. Krumholz HM, Radford MJ, Ellerbeck EF, et al: Aspirin in the treatment of acute myocardial infarction in elderly Medicare beneficiaries: Patterns of use and outcomes. Circulation 92:2841–2847, 1995.
86. Messerli FH, Grossman E, Goldbourt U: Are beta-blockers efficacious as first-line therapy for hypertension in the elderly? A systematic review. JAMA 279:1903–1907, 1998.
87. Gibbons RJ, Chatterjee K, Daley J, et al: ACC/AHA/ACP-ASIM guidelines for the management of patients with chronic stable angina: A report of the American College of Cardiology/American Heart Association Task Force on Practice Guidelines (Committee on Management of Patients With Chronic Stable Angina). J. Am Coll Cardiol 33:2092–2197, 1999.
88. Krumholz HM, Radford MJ, Wang Y, et al: National use and effectiveness of beta-blockers for the treatment of elderly patients after acute myocardial infarction: National Cooperative Cardiovascular Project. JAMA 280:623–629, 1998.
89. Schroeder AP, Sorensen K, Nielsen JC, et al: Clinical assessment of indication for ACE-inhibitor treatment early after acute myocardial infarction. Scand Cardiovasc J 33:137–142, 1999.

90. Rogers WJ, Bowlby LJ, Chandra NC, et al: Treatment of myocardial infarction in the United States (1990 to 1993). Observations from the National Registry of Myocardial Infarction. Circulation 90:2103–2114, 1994.

91. Braunwald E, Antman EM, Beasley JW, et al: ACC/AHA guidelines for the management of patients with unstable angina: A report of the American College of Cardiology/American Heart Association Task Force on Practice Guidelines (Committee on Management of Patients with Unstable Angina). J Am Coll Cardiol, in press.

92. Rich MW: Therapy for acute myocardial infarction. Clin Geriatr Med 12:141–168, 1996.

93. Barakat K, Wilkinson P, Deaner A, et al: How should age affect management of acute myocardial infarction? A prospective cohort study. Lancet 353:955–959, 1999.

94. McLaughlin TJ, Gurwitz JH, Willison DJ, et al: Delayed thombolytic treatment of older patients with acute myocardial infarction. J Am Geriatr Soc 47:1222–1228, 1999.

95. Krumholz HM, Murillo JE, Chen J, et al: Thrombolytic therapy for eligible elderly patients with acute myocardial infarction. JAMA 277:1683–1688, 1997.

96. Woods KL, Ketley D: Utilisation of thrombolytic therapy in older patients with myocardial infarction. Drugs Aging 13:435–441, 1998.

97. Grines CL, Browne KF, Marco J, et al: A comparison of immediate angioplasty with thrombolytic therapy for acute myocardial infarction. The Primary Angioplasty in Myocardial Infarction Study Group. N Engl J Med 328:673–679, 1993.

98. Elder AT, Shaw TR, Turnbull CM, Starkey IR: Elderly and younger patients selected to undergo coronary angiography. BMJ 303:950–953, 1991.

99. Thompson RC, Holmes DR Jr, Grill DE, et al: Changing outcome of angioplasty in the elderly. J Am Coll Cardiol 27:8–14, 1996.

100. Bedotto JB, Rutherford BD, McConahay DR, et al: Results of multivessel percutaneous transluminal coronary angioplasty in persons aged 65 years and older. Am J Cardiol 67:1051–1055, 1991.

101. Wennberg DE, Makenka DJ, Sengupta A, et al: Percutaneous transluminal coronary angioplasty in the elderly: Epidemiology, clinical risk factors, and in-hospital outcomes. The Northern New England Cardiovascular Disease Study Group. Am Heart J 137:639–645, 1999.

102. Mullany CJ, Mock MB, Brooks MM, et al: Effect of age in the Bypass Angioplasty Revascularization Investigation (BARI) randomized trial. Ann Thorac Surg 67:396–403, 1999.

103. Sollano JA, Rose EA, Williams DL, et al: Cost-effectiveness of coronary artery bypass surgery in octogenarians. Ann Surg 228:297–306, 1998.

104. Craver JM, Puskas JD, Weintraub WW, et al: 601 octogenarians undergoing cardiac surgery: Outcome and comparison with younger age groups. Ann Thorac Surg 67:1104–1110, 1999.

105. Almassi GH, Sommers T, Moritz TE, et al: Stroke in cardiac surgical patients: Determinants and outcome. Ann Thorac Surg 68:391–397, 1999.

106. De Gregorio J, Kobayashi Y, Albiero R, et al: Coronary artery stenting in the elderly: Short-term outcome and long-term angiographic and clinical follow-up. J Am Coll Cardiol 32:577–583, 1998.

107. Tasdemir O, Vural KM, Karagoz H, Bayazit K: Coronary artery bypass grafting on the beating heart without the use of extracorporeal circulation: Review of 2052 cases. J Thorac Cardiovasc Surg 116:68–73, 1998.

107a. Seto TB, Talra DA, Berezin R, et al. Percutaneous coronary revascularization in elderly patients: Impact on functional status and quality of life. Ann Intern Med 132:955–958, 2000.

108. Evenson KR, Rosamond WD, Luepker RV: Predictors of outpatient cardiac rehabilitation utilization: The Minnesota Heart Surgery Registry. J Cardiopulm Rehabil 18:192–198, 1998.

109. Lavie CJ, Milani RV, Cassidy MM, et al: Benefits of cardiac rehabilitation and exercise training in older persons. Am J Geriatr Cardiol 4:42, 1995.

110. Milani RV, Lavie CJ: Prevalence and effects of cardiac rehabilitation on depression in the elderly with coronary heart disease. Am J Cardiol 81:1233–1236, 1998.

111. Cheitlin MD, Hutter AM Jr, Brindis RG, et al: Use of sildenafil (Viagra) in patients with cardiovascular disease. Technology and Practice Executive Committee Circulation 99:168–177, 1999.

112. Lavie CJ, Milani RV: Effects of cardiac rehabilitation programs on exercise capacity, coronary risk factors, behavioral characteristics, and quality of life in a large elderly cohort. Am J Cardiol 76:177–179, 1995.

113. Kannel WB, Belanger A, D'Agostino R, Israel I: Physical activity and physical demand on the job and risk of cardiovascular disease and death: The Framingham Study. Am Heart J 112:820–825, 1986.

114. Lavie CJ, Milani RV: Cardiac rehabilitation in the aged patient. *In* Wenger NK, (ed): Cardiovascular Disease in the Octogenarian and Beyond. London, Martin Dunitz; 1999, p 227.

115. Van Camp SP, Peterson RA: Cardiovascular complications of outpatient cardiac rehabilitation programs. JAMA 250:1100–1103, 1986.

116. Schmitz C, Weiz A, Reichart B: Is cardiac surgery justified in patients in the ninth decade of life? J Cardiac Surg 13:113, 1998.

HEART FAILURE

117. Haldeman GA, Croft JB, Giles WH, Rashidee A: Hospitalization of patients with heart failure: National Hospital Discharge Survey, 1985 to 1995. Am Heart J 137:352–360, 1999.

118. Kannel WB, Belanger AJ: Epidemiology of heart failure. Am Heart J 121:951–957, 1991.

119. Ho KK, Pinsky JL, Kannel WB, Levy D: The epidemiology of heart failure: The Framingham Study. J Am Coll Cardiol 22:6A–13A, 1993.

120. Croft JB, Giles WH, Pollard RA, et al: National trends in the initial hospitalization for heart failure. J Am Geriatr Soc 45:270–275, 1997.

120a. Gillum RF: Epidemiology of heart failure in the United States [Editorial]. Am Heart J 126:1042–1047, 1993.

121. O'Connell JB, Bristow MR: Economic impact of heart failure in the United States: Time for a different approach. J Heart Lung Transpl 13 (Suppl):S107, 1994.

122. Rich MW: Epidemiology, pathophysiology, and etiology of congestive heart failure in older adults. J Am Geriatr Soc 45:968–974, 1997.

123. Davie AP, Francis CM, Caruana L, et al: The prevalence of left ventricular diastolic filling abnormalities in patients with suspected heart failure. Eur Heart J 18:981–984, 1997.

124. Fishkind D, Paris BE, Aronow WS: Use of digoxin, diuretics, beta blockers, angiotensin-converting enzyme inhibitors, and calcium channel blockers in older patients in an academic hospital-based geriatrics practice. J Am Geriatr Soc 45:809–812, 1997.

125. Van den Berg MP, Tuinenburg AE, Crijns HJ, et al: Heart failure and atrial fibrillation: Current concepts and controversies. Heart 77:309–313, 1997.

126. Krumholz HM, Parent EM, Tu N, et al: Readmission after hospitalization for congestive heart failure among Medicare beneficiaries. Arch Intern Med 157:99–104, 1997.

127. Rich MW, Beckham V, Wittenberg C, et al: A multidisciplinary intervention to prevent the readmission of elderly patients with congestive heart failure. N Engl J Med 333:1190–1195, 1995.

128. Rich MW, Gray DB, Beckham V, et al: Effect of a multidisciplinary intervention on medication compliance in elderly patients with congestive heart failure. Am J Med 101:270–276, 1996.

129. Stewart S, Vandenbroek AJ, Pearson S, Horowitz JD: Prolonged beneficial effects of a home-based intervention on unplanned readmissions and mortality among patients with congestive heart failure. Arch Intern Med 159:257–261, 1999.

130. Gales BJ, Menard SM: Relationship between the administration of selected medications and falls in hospitalized elderly patients. Ann Pharmacother 29:354–358, 1995.

131. Heerdink ER, Leufkens HG, Herings RM, et al: NSAIDs associated with increased risk of congestive heart failure in elderly patients taking diuretics. Arch Intern Med 158:1108–1112, 1998.

132. Garg R, Yusuf S: Overview of randomized trials of angiotensin-converting enzyme inhibitors on mortality and morbidity in patients with heart failure. Collaborative Group on ACE Inhibitor Trials JAMA 273:1450–1456, 1995.

133. Aronow WS: Therapy of congestive heart failure in elderly persons. Compr Ther 23:639–647, 1997.

134. The effect of digoxin on mortality and morbidity in patients with heart failure. The Digitalis Investigation Group. N Engl J Med 336:525–533, 1997.

135. Burrell LM, Johnston CI: Angiotensin II receptor antagonists: Potential in elderly patients with cardiovascular disease. Drugs Aging 10:421–434, 1997.

136. Riegger GA, Bouzo H, Petr P, et al: Improvement in exercise tolerance and symptoms of congestive heart failure during treatment with candesartan cilexetil. Symptom, Tolerability, Response to Exercise Trial of Candesartan Cilexetil in Heart Failure (STRETCH) Investigators. Circulation 100:2224–2230, 1999.

137. Doughty RN, Rodgers A, Sharpe N, MacMahon S: Effects of beta-blocker therapy on mortality in patients with heart failure: A systematic overview of randomized controlled trials. Eur Heart J 18:560–565, 1997.

138. Packer M, Bristow MR, Cohn JN, et al: The effect of carvedilol on morbidity and mortality in patients with chronic heart failure. U.S. Carvedilol Heart Failure Study Group. N Engl J Med 334:1349–1355, 1996.

139. Gottlieb SS, McCarter RJ, Vogel RA: Effect of beta-blockade on mortality among high-risk and low-risk patients after myocardial infarction. N Engl J Med 339:489–497, 1998.

140. Setaro JF, Zaret BL, Schulman DS, et al: Usefulness of verapamil for congestive heart failure associated with abnormal left ventricular diastolic filling and normal left ventricular systolic performance. Am J Cardiol, 66:981–986, 1990.

HYPERTENSION

141. Parati G, Frattola A, Di Rienzo M, et al: Broadband spectral analysis of blood pressure and heart rate variability in very elderly subjects. Hypertension 30:803–808, 1997.

142. Pickering TG: The ninth Sir George Pickering memorial lecture. Ambulatory monitoring and the definition of hypertension [Editorial]. J Hypertens 10:401–409, 1992.

143. Appel LJ, Stason WB: Ambulatory blood pressure monitoring and blood pressure self-measurement in the diagnosis and management of hypertension. Ann Intern Med 18:867–882, 1993.

144. Belmin J, Visintin JM, Salvatore R, et al: Osler's maneuver: Absence of usefulness for the detection of pseudohypertension in an elderly population. Am J Med 98:42–49, 1995.

145. Cavallini MC, Roman MJ, Blank SG, et al: Association of the ausculta-

tory gap with vascular disease in hypertensive patients. Ann Intern Med 124:877–883, 1996.

146. Applegate WB, Davis BR, Black HR, et al: Prevalence of postural hypotension at baseline in the Systolic Hypertension in the Elderly Program (SHEP) cohort. J Am Geriatr Soc 39:1057–1064, 1991.

147. Masuo K, Mikami H, Ogihara T, Tuck MI: Mechanisms mediating postprandial blood pressure reduction in young and elderly subjects. Am J Hypertens 9:536–544, 1996.

148. Statement on hypertension in the elderly. The Working Group on Hypertension in the Elderly. JAMA 256:70–74, 1986.

149. Mendelson G, Ness J, Aronow WS: Drug treatment of hypertension in older persons in an academic hospital-based geriatrics practice. J Am Geriatr Soc 47:597–599, 1999.

150. Reaven PD, Barrett-Connor E, Edelstein S: Relation between leisure-time physical activity and blood pressure in older women. Circulation 83:559–565, 1991.

151. Veterans Administration Cooperative Study on Antihypertensive Agents: Double blind control study of antihypertensive agents: III. Chlorothiazide alone and in combination with other agents; preliminary results. Arch Intern Med 110:230, 1962.

152. Himmelmann A, Hedner T, Hansson L, et al: Isolated systolic hypertension: An important cardiovascular risk factor. Blood Press 7:197–207, 1998.

153. Mattila K, Haavisto M, Rajala S, Heikinheimo R: Blood pressure and five year survival in the very old. BMJ (Clin Res Ed) 296:887–889, 1988.

154. Langer RD, Ganiats TG, Barrett-Connor E: Factors associated with paradoxical survival at higher blood pressures in the very old Am J Epidemiol 134:29–38, 1991.

155. Kaplan NM: The appropriate goals of antihypertensive therapy: Neither too much nor too little. Ann Intern Med 116:686–690, 1992.

156. Implications of the systolic hypertension in the elderly program. The Systolic Hypertension in the Elderly Program Cooperative Research Group. Hypertension 21:335–343, 1993.

157. Merlo J, Ranstam J, Liedholm H, et al: Incidence of myocardial infarction in elderly men being treated with antihypertensive drugs: Population based cohort study. BMJ 313:457–461, 1996.

158. 1999 World Health Organization–International Society of Hypertension: Guidelines for the management of hypertension. Guidelines Subcommittee. J Hypertens 17:151–183, 1999.

159. Dahlof B, Lindholm LH, Hansson L, et al: Morbidity and mortality in the Swedish Trial in Old Patients with Hypertension (STOP-Hypertension). Lancet 338:1281–1285, 1991.

160. Gueyffier F, Bulpitt C, Boissel JP, et al: Antihypertensive drugs in very old people: A subgroup meta-analysis of randomised controlled trials. INDANA Group [Comment]. Lancet 353:793–796, 1999.

161. Van Bortel LM: Influence of aging on arterial compliance. J Hum Hypertens 12:583, 1998.

162. Shimamoto H, Shimamoto Y: Time course of hemodynamic responses to sodium in elderly hypertensive patients. Hypertension 16:387–397, 1990.

163. Alam S, Johnson AG: A meta-analysis of randomised controlled trials (RCT) among healthy normotensive and essential hypertensive elderly patients to determine the effect of high salt (NaCl) diet of blood pressure. J Hum Hypertens 13:367–374, 1999.

164. Gambassi G, Lapane K, Sgadari A, et al: Prevalence, clinical correlates, and treatment of hypertension in elderly nursing home residents. SAGE (Systematic Assessment of Geriatric Drug Use via Epidemiology) study group. Arch Intern Med 158:2377–2385, 1998.

CARDIOMYOPATHY

165. Gertz MA, Kyle RA: Primary systemic amyloidosis—a diagnostic primer. Mayo Clin Proc 64:1505–1519, 1989.

166. Kyle RA, Spittell PC, Gertz MA, et al: The premortem recognition of systemic senile amyloidosis with cardiac involvement. Am J Med 101:395–400, 1996.

167. Dubrey SW, Cha K, Anderson J, et al: The clinical features of immunoglobulin light-chain (AL) amyloidosis with heart involvement. QJ Med 91:141–157, 1998.

168. Dubrey SW, Bilazarian S, LaValley M, et al: Signal-averaged electrocardiography in patients with AL (primary) amyloidosis. Am Heart J 134:994–1001, 1997.

169. Fay WP, Taliercio CP, Ilstrup DM, et al: Natural history of hypertrophic cardiomyopathy in the elderly. J Am Coll Cardiol 16:821–826, 1990.

170. Aronow WS, Kronzon I: Prevalence of hypertrophic cardiomyopathy and its association with mitral anular calcium in elderly patients. Chest 94:1295–1296, 1988.

171. Maron BJ, Mathenge R, Casey SA, et al: Clinical profile of hypertrophic cardiomyopathy identified de novo in rural communities. J Am Coll Cardiol 33:1590–1595, 1999.

172. Lai ZY, Shih CM, Chang NC, Wang TC: Clinical and morphologic features of hypertrophic cardiomyopathy in elderly patients 85 years or older. Jpn Heart J 40:155, 1999.

173. Litovsky SH, Rose AG: Clinicopathologic heterogeneity in hypertrophic cardiomyopathy with regard to age, asymmetric septal hypertrophy, and concentric hypertrophy beyond the pediatric age group. Arch Pathol Lab Med 122:434–441, 1998.

174. Gadler F, Linde C, Daubert C, et al: Significant improvement of quality of life following atrioventricular synchronous pacing in patients with hypertrophic obstructive cardiomyopathy: Data from 1 year of follow-up. Pacing In Cardiomyopathy (PIC) study group. Eur Heart J 20:1044–1050, 1999.

175. Maron BJ, Nishimura RA, McKenna WJ, et al: Assessment of permanent dual-chamber pacing as a treatment for drug-refractory symptomatic patients with obstructive hypertrophic cardiomyopathy: A randomized, double-blind, crossover study (M-PATHY). Circulation 99:2927–2933, 1999.

176. Schulte HD, Borisov K, Gams E, et al: Management of symptomatic hypertrophic obstructive cardiomyopathy—long-term results after surgical therapy. Thorac Cardiovasc Surg 47:213–218, 1999.

177. Nagueh SF, Lakkis NM, Middleton KJ, et al: Doppler estimation of left ventricular filling pressures in patients with hypertrophic cardiomyopathy. Circulation 99:254–261, 1999.

178. Gietzen FH, Leuner CJ, Raute-Kreinsen U, et al: Acute and long-term results after transcoronary ablation of septal hypertrophy (TASH). Catheter interventional treatment for hypertrophic obstructive cardiomyopathy. Eur Heart J 20:1342–1354, 1999.

179. Maron BJ, Shen WK, Link MS, et al: Efficacy of implantable cardioverter-defibrillators for the prevention of sudden death in patients with hypertrophic cardiomyopathy. N Engl J Med 342:365–373, 2000.

ARRHYTHMIAS

180. Kantelip JP, Sage E, Duchene-Marullaz P: Findings on ambulatory electrocardiographic monitoring in subjects older than 80 years. Am J Cardiol 57:398–401, 1986.

181. Fleg JL, Kennedy HI: Long-term prognostic significance of ambulatory electrocardiographic findings in apparently healthy subjects greater than or equal to 60 years of age. Am J Cardiol 70:748–751, 1992.

182. Camaiti A, Del Rosso A, Morettini A, et al: Efficacy and safety of adenosine in diagnosis and treatment of regular tachycardia in the elderly. Coron Artery Dis 9:591–596, 1998.

183. Zado ES, Callans DJ, Gottlieb CD, et al: Efficacy and safety of catheter ablation in octogenarians. J Am Coll Cardiol 35:458–462, 2000.

184. Manolio TA, Furberg CD, Rautaharju PM, et al: Cardiac arrhythmias on 24-h ambulatory electrocardiography in older women and men: The Cardiovascular Health Study. J Am Coll Cardiol 23:916–925, 1994.

185. Ryder KM, Benjamin EJ: Epidemiology and significance of atrial fibrillation. Am J Cardiol 84(Suppl):131R–138R, 1999.

186. Furberg CD, Psaty BM, Manolio TA, et al: Prevalence of atrial fibrillation in elderly subjects (the Cardiovascular Health Study). Am J Cardiol 74:236–241, 1994.

187. Wolf PA, Benjamin EJ, Belanber AJ, et al: Secular trends in the prevalence of atrial fibrillation: The Framingham Study. Am Heart J 131:790, 1996.

188. Alpert JS, Mackstaller LL: Atrial fibrillation in the very old: Incidence, mechanism and therapy. In Wenger NK (ed): Cardiovascular Disease in the Octogenarian and Beyond. London, Martin Dunitz, 1999, p 305.

189. Kahaly GJ, Nieswandt J, Mohr-Kahaly S: Cardiac risks of hyperthyroidism in the elderly. Thyroid 8:1165–1169, 1998.

190. Wolf PA, Abbott RD, Kannel WB: Atrial fibrillation as an independent risk factor for stroke: The Framingham Study. Stroke 22:983–988, 1991.

191. Brand FN, Abbott RD, Kannel WB, Wolf PA: Characteristic and prognosis of lone atrial fibrillation: 30-year follow-up in the Framingham Study. JAMA 254:3449–3453, 1985.

192. Atrial Fibrillation Investigators: Risk factors for stroke and efficacy of antithrombotic therapy in atrial fibrillation: Analysis of pooled data from five randomized controlled trials. Arch Intern Med 154:1449–1457, 1994.

193. Kopecky SL, Gersh BJ, McGoon MD, et al: Lone atrial fibrillation in elderly persons: A marker for cardiovascular risk. Arch Intern Med 159:1118–1122, 1999.

194. Aronow WS, Ahn C, Kronzon I, Gutstein H: Incidence of new thromboembolic stroke in persons 62 years and older with chronic atrial fibrillation treated with warfarin versus aspirin. J Am Geriatr Soc 47:366–368, 1999.

195. Gullov AL, Koefoed BG, Petersen P: Bleeding during warfarin and aspirin therapy in patients with atrial fibrillation: The AFASAK 2 study. Atrial Fibrillation Aspirin and Anticoagulation. Arch Intern Med 159:1322–1328, 1999.

196. Brass LM, Krumholz HM, Scinto JD, et al: Warfarin use following ischemic stroke among Medicare patients with atrial fibrillation. Arch Intern Med 158:2093–2100, 1998.

197. Laupacis A, Albers G, Dalen J, et al: Antithrombotic therapy in atrial fibrillation. Chest 108:352S–359S, 1995.

198. Pritchett EL: Management of atrial fibrillation. N Engl J Med 326:1264–1271, 1992.

199. Lanzarotti CJ, Olshansky B: Thromboembolism in chronic atrial flutter: Is the risk underestimated? J Am Coll Cardiol 30:1506–1511, 1997.

200. Fleg JL: Electrocardiographic findings in older persons without clinical heart disease. In Tresch DD, Aronow WS (eds): Cardiovascular Disease in the Elderly Patient. New York, Dekker, 1994, p 43.

201. Aronow WS: Correlation of arrhythmias and conduction defects on the resting electrocardiogram with new cardiac events in 1,153 elderly patients. Am J Noninvas Cardiol 5:88, 1991.

202. Panotopoulos PT, Axtell K, Anderson AJ, et al: Efficacy of the implantable cardioverter-defibrillator in the elderly. J Am Coll Cardiol 29:556–560, 1997.

203. Gregoratos G, Cheitlin MD, Conill A, et al: ACC/AHA guidelines for implantation of cardiac pacemakers and antiarrhythmia devices: A report of the American College of Cardiology/American Heart Association Task Force on Practice Guidelines (Committee on Pacemaker Implantation). J Am Coll Cardiol 31:1175–1209, 1998.

204. Shen WK, Hammill SC, Hayes DL, et al: Long-term survival after pacemaker implantation for heart block in patients > or = 65 years. Am J Cardiol 74:560–564, 1994.

205. Rajala SA, Geiger UK, Haavisto MV, et al: Electrocardiogram, clinical findings and chest x-ray in persons aged 85 years or older. Am J Cardiol 55:1175–1178, 1985.

206. Eriksson P, Hansson PO, Eriksson H, Dellborg M: Bundle-branch block in a general male population: The study of men born 1913. Circulation 98:2494–2500, 1998.

207. Kreger BE, Anderson KM, Kannel WB: Prevalence of intraventricular block in the general population: The Framingham Study. Am Heart J 117:903–910, 1989.

Chapter 58

Coronary Artery Disease in Women

PAMELA S. DOUGLAS

Approximately one third of all deaths in women are attributed to coronary artery disease (CAD), making it the most common cause of death in women as well as in men (Fig. 58–1). The proportion rises to over half of all deaths if all forms of cardiovascular disease are included, and CAD is increasingly important as longevity is enhanced and the population ages.[1, 2] Yet, in contrast to the dramatic decrease in cardiovascular mortality achieved for men in the past 20 years, there has been little improvement for women.

An enormous amount of scientific investigation is directed at understanding the causes and cures of CAD. Recognizing the influences of gender on basic biology may provide important keys to cardiovascular pathophysiology that may eventually benefit both sexes. In the clinical arena, CAD is increasingly thought of as a preventable disease as medicine acquires the knowledge and tools to reduce its incidence and modify its consequences. However, the benefits have not been as readily extended to women. This chapter addresses the similarities and differences in CAD risk factors, symptoms, diagnosis, and treatment between men and women. Knowledge of these and their incorporation into clinical practice will improve care for women and reduce the large health risk and burden of CAD.

RISK FACTORS FOR CAD IN WOMEN AND THEIR MODIFICATION

Perhaps the most important risk factor for CAD in women is the misperception that coronary artery disease is not a woman's disease—that it is somehow more benign or less important in women than in men.[3] This misconception, shared by both patients and providers, is gradually being corrected but still has important influences on all aspects of prevention, diagnosis, and treatment. If CAD is not believed to pose a significant risk, it is unlikely that patients will implement difficult life-style changes to prevent it or seek emergency care on development of symptoms. This underestimation of risk extends to offspring of women with CAD, who, despite a significant burden of modifiable risk factors, perceive their risk of CAD as being below average.[4] Similarly, providers have been shown to underestimate the likelihood of CAD presence, leading to neglect of formal risk assessment and failure to aggressively treat CAD once it has been detected. In addition, a woman's presentation style alters physicians' estimates of the likelihood of CAD, so that an actress whose demeanor was more business-like was judged to have a much higher probability of disease than one who behaved histrionically, despite identical histories and test results.[5] To reduce CAD mortality in women, it is critical that patients, providers, and the public recognize the importance of CAD and its prevention and treatment.

Factors associated with higher cardiac risk in men, including age, family history, smoking, hypertension, lipoproteins, and diabetes mellitus (see Chap. 31), are also associated with increased cardiac risk in women[6–10]; however, they may have a different relative importance. Moreover, additional factors such as hormonal status are equally powerful predictors of CAD in women. These differences have been formally incorporated into a variety of gender-specific risk assessment algorithms published by the American Heart Association (AHA) and others.[1, 7, 11] Furthermore, the

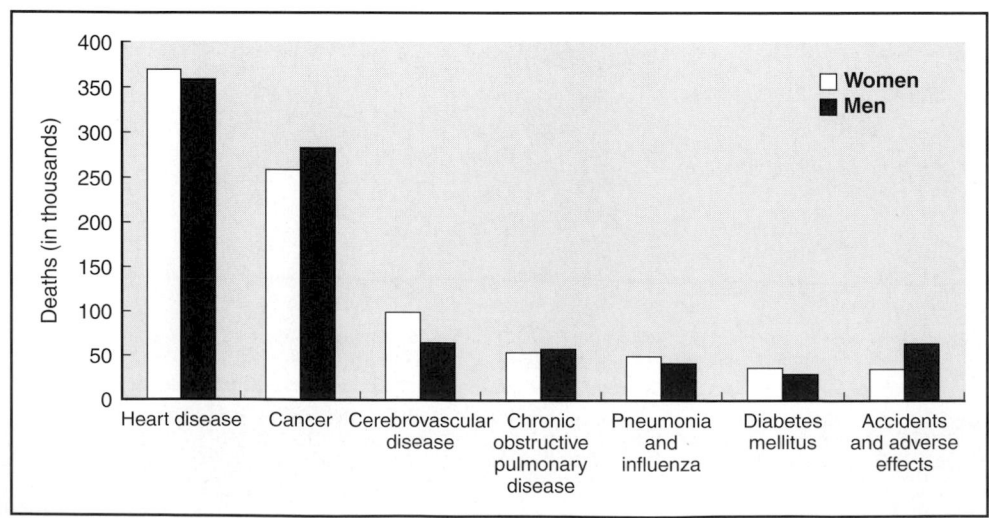

FIGURE 58–1. Number of deaths due to the seven leading causes of death in women and men in the United States in 1997, ranked in order for women. (Data from National Vital Statistics Report 47[June 30], 1999.)

approach to management of CAD risk differs somewhat in women. In recognition of this, the AHA and American College of Cardiology have published comprehensive guidelines for primary and secondary prevention of CAD in women.[7]

LIPIDS (see also Chaps. 31–33): Elevated total cholesterol and low-density lipoprotein (LDL) levels are only weakly associated with CAD in women and only in women 65 years old or younger.[8–13] Instead, high-density lipoprotein (HDL) cholesterol is closely and inversely associated with CAD risk.[10, 14] Triglycerides are an independent predictor of CAD, particularly in older women.[10, 15, 16] Lipoprotein(a), a composite of LDL, apolipoprotein B-100, and apolipoprotein(a), is also associated with higher cardiac risk in women.[17, 17a]

Treatment of dyslipidemia is generally accomplished by the same life-style changes and medications in men and women, although dietary interventions may be less effective in women.[18] Although clinical trials have generally not included women in sufficient numbers for independent prospective analysis, several recent studies employing aggressive, multifactorial treatment for lipid lowering have documented an equal or greater effect in women, for both primary and secondary prevention,[19–21] and after bypass surgery (see Chap. 33).[22] Women, as well as men, display angiographic regression of coronary atherosclerosis and reduction in coronary events and death, even with normal baseline cholesterol levels.

In general, recommended dietary and pharmacological lipid-lowering strategies are similar in men and women and should be as aggressively employed. However, hormone replacement therapy may be a preferred primary therapy for postmenopausal women with low HDL[8, 23] (Table 58–1). Effects of estrogen may be additive to or even supplant those of conventional lipid-lowering medications,[24, 25] because they include other beneficial effects in addition to lipid lowering, such as coronary vasodilation and antioxidant properties (see later).[26, 27] However, estrogen increases triglycerides in 20 to 25 percent of women, particularly those with elevated baseline levels,[28] who may therefore be less likely to benefit from hormone replacement therapy. An elevated baseline level therefore mandates careful monitoring of lipid levels after institution of hormonal therapy and consideration of transdermal rather than oral administration. Newer regimens include selective estrogen receptor modulators (SERMs), soy compounds such as isoflavenoids, and phytoestrogens, all proven to have beneficial effects on serum lipids in women,[29–31] but their place in the therapeutic armamentarium has not been established by large-scale randomized clinical trials.

Current recommendations for initiation of treatment and therapeutic goals (National Cholesterol Education Program [NCEP]-II) are similar in men and women and are based on LDL levels.[23] Despite the fact that HDL is a more powerful determinant of CAD risk in women, the NCEP-II guidelines do not include HDL except as a modifying factor, and then at a fairly low level for women. Similarly, triglycerides are not considered as a primary indication for treatment. Strong arguments have been made to alter these recommendations in favor of more aggressive therapy for indications other than LDL-lowering in women, particularly because it is not clear how well NCEP-II guidelines address the needs of women or the very elderly, who are predominantly female. The strikingly positive results achieved in recent statin trials suggest that these agents should be included in most lipid-lowering regimens designed for primary or secondary prevention of CAD for women.

DIABETES (see also Chap. 63). Diabetes is a risk factor for the presence and severity of coronary artery disease in both men and women but carries a greater incremental risk in women, completely eliminating the "female advantage."[6, 9, 11, 32] The AHA awards twice the weight to diabetes in women in calculating CAD risk,[11] similar to that of a systolic blood pressure of 173 mm Hg or above or a cholesterol level of 316 mg/dl or above. Even more than in men, diabetes dramatically increases the mortality of myocardial infarction in women.[9, 33]

Non-insulin-dependent diabetes is associated with obesity, abdominal and upper body fat distribution, hypertension, and insulin resistance, all of which have been associated with higher coronary artery disease risk.[32] This complex of abnormalities may be causally related to high circulating insulin levels. More so than in men, obesity and body fat distribution appear to be independent coronary artery disease risk factors in women.[6, 32] Diabetes is also linked with the presence of hyperlipidemia (elevated triglycerides, reduced HDL), especially in women,[32] although the lipoprotein response to adequate diabetic treatment is variable.[34] Finally, diabetes is associated with a variety of platelet abnormalities and endothelial dysfunction, additional contributors to CAD.[35] Regardless of mechanism, recent data from the Diabetes Control and Complications Trial suggest that intensive diabetes therapy reduces cardiovascular complications in young (younger than age 40) men and women.[36]

HYPERTENSION (see also Chaps. 28 and 29). The prevalence of hypertension in women greatly increases with age so that nearly 80 percent of women older than age 75 are hypertensive.[37] Hypertension carries an independent coronary artery disease risk for both men and women and substantially enhances the risks associated with hyperlipidemia, smoking, obesity, and diabetes. Antihypertensive treatment reduces both overall mortality and cardiac morbidity as well as the incidence of stroke; these effects are most striking in the elderly.[37, 38]

▼ **TABLE 58–1. EFFECT OF HORMONE REPLACEMENT THERAPY ON LIPOPROTEIN LEVELS (% INCREASE OR DECREASE)**

	PLACEBO	E ALONE	E + PA (CYCLIC)	E + PA (CONTINUOUS)	E + PA (CYCLIC)
TC	−11	−20	−36	−36	−20
LDL	−11	−37	−46	−43	−38
HDL	−3	+14	+4	+3	+11
Triglycerides	−4	+15	+14	+13	+15
LP(a)	0	−17	−26	−20	−22

E = conjugated equine estrogen 0.625 mg daily; E + PA (cyclic) = conjugated equine estrogen 0.625 mg daily plus medroxyprogesterone acetate, 10 mg/d for 12 days each month; E + PA (continuous) = E + PA 2.5 mg/d; E + P (cyclic) = E + micronized progesterone, 200 mg/d for 12 days each month.

Adapted from The Postmenopausal Estrogen/Progestin Interventions (PEPI) Trial: Effects of estrogen or estrogen/progestin regimens on heart disease risk factors in postmenopausal women. JAMA 273:199, 1995. Copyright 1995, American Medical Association. Additional data from Espeland MA, Marcovina SM, Miller V, et al: Effect of postmenopausal hormone therapy on lipoprotein(a) concentration. Circulation 97:979, 1998.

SMOKING. Smoking is a strong independent risk factor for coronary artery disease in both men and women; although smoking rates in the United States are falling overall, they are currently increasing among young women.[39] This risk is present even with minimal exposure (<5 cigarettes/day) and is not improved by use of low-yield cigarettes. Smoking risk is strikingly synergistic with that of oral contraceptive use, especially in women older than age 35, and leads to an earlier menopause, another coronary artery disease risk unique to women.[40] Cessation of smoking appears to gradually eliminate the excess risk in women,[41] although women more often smoke to lose or maintain body weight and find it harder to quit than do men.

HEMOSTASIS. Elevated fibrinogen levels appear to be an independent cardiac risk factor in men and women, although women have not been as well studied.[42] The mechanism(s) by which fibrinogen enhances risk are poorly understood, although high fibrinogen levels have been associated with other CAD risk factors, including hypertension, diabetes, smoking, obesity, hyperlipidemia, and menopause, and lower levels have been associated with exercise, hormone replacement therapy, and high HDL.[43] Gender differences in platelet function and hemostasis are virtually unexplored. Factor V Leiden mutation may be a marker for atherothrombotic risk in postmenopausal women taking estrogen replacement or, conversely, may identify those who can take such medication without such side effects.[44]

EXERCISE. A sedentary life style is associated with CAD in both men and women, although the data for women are sparse.[45] The reported beneficial effects of exercise on CAD risk profile are less marked in women compared with men, with lesser increases in HDL and less weight loss resulting from similar exercise training.[18] In prospective observational studies, a lower fitness level has been associated with a 4.7-fold increased risk for all-cause mortality in women,[46] and higher activity levels have been associated with decreased relative risks for CAD (0.44) and stroke (0.51), independent of other vascular risk factors.[47] Recent data from the Nurses' Health Study defines the amount of exercise needed to prevent CAD, with a convincing dose-response relationship between the intensity of exercise and the reduction in risk.[48] Two aspects of this study were particularly important: brisk walking conferred the same benefit as vigorous exercise, and sedentary women who became active late in life reaped similar benefits as those who remained active throughout.

PSYCHOSOCIAL FACTORS (see also Chap. 70). The interaction of psychosocial and biobehavioral factors and heart disease is complex but perhaps has been more extensively studied in women than in men.[49, 50] Several of the cardiovascular risk factors discussed earlier are related to behavior (obesity, smoking, exercise) and are optimally treated with its modification. Perceived stress and its balance with situational control have been found to affect CAD risk in women as well as in men. Acute and chronic stress are thought to "trigger" myocardial infarction in both sexes by contributing to plaque rupture.[51] Social networks and support influence CAD outcome both independently and through the likelihood of compliance with therapeutic strategies (e.g., cardiac rehabilitation). The lack of social support has been associated with a worse outcome in both men and women, but its impact may be greater in women and women are more likely to survive their partners and live alone. Depression appears to be an independent risk factor for poor outcome after cardiac events or surgery in women, and cardiovascular outcome can be improved by specific therapy.[52]

INFLAMMATION (see also Chap. 31). Inflammation is increasingly recognized as a risk factor for CAD in women. In the Women's Health Study, C-reactive protein was as powerful an independent predictor as any other single fac-

tor.[52a, 52b] Women with the highest quartile of C-RP had a fivefold to sevenfold increased risk of cardiac and vascular events over a 3-year follow-up period. Other markers with lower, but still significant, risk include serum amyloid A, soluble intercellular adhesion molecule-1, and interleuken 6.

HORMONES: RISKS AND BENEFITS OF ESTROGEN

The ovary produces both estrogenic and androgenic hormones until menopause, when production decreases gradually over several years but does not fully cease. The risk of CAD in women rises thereafter, equaling that in men by age 75. Women who have an early menopause and/or bilateral oophorectomy experience a higher risk of CAD. Menopause, or estrogen deprivation, is associated with detrimental changes in cardiovascular risk factors, including an increase in LDL cholesterol, a small decrease in HDL, and an increased total ratio of cholesterol to HDL.[53, 54] Furthermore, menopause decreases aortic root elasticity and blunts nocturnal reductions in blood pressure, in association with the more subtle changes of concentric left ventricular remodeling and reduced contractility.[55, 56] Natural menopause seems to have little immediate effect on blood pressure, glucose tolerance, insulin levels, body weight, or physical activity other than that of advancing age.[54]

ORAL CONTRACEPTIVES. Current low-dose oral contraceptives generally contain a synthetic estrogen, such as ethinyl estradiol, and a synthetic progestin, and pose only a very negligible cardiovascular risk for most patients.[53, 57, 58] The risk of arterial and venous thrombosis is low but is magnified by advancing age and especially by smoking. The risk of myocardial infarction is not increased by oral contraceptives unless the patient is older than age 35 and/or smokes cigarettes, and it appears to be entirely caused by thromboembolism rather than by coronary atherosclerosis, because the angiographic coronary plaque burden is actually lower in oral contraceptive users than in age-matched nonusers with myocardial infarction.

Because most regimens employ a combination of hormones, the effect of any given oral contraceptive on circulating lipoproteins represents the sum of estrogenic effects (higher HDL and triglycerides, lower LDL) and progestogenic effects (higher LDL, lower HDL). Newer agents such as norethindrone, gestodene, desogestrel, and norgestimate have beneficial effects on lipoprotein levels but may increase thromboembolic complications.[58]

ESTROGEN AND CARDIAC RISK FACTOR MODIFICATION. Observations of the low risk of CAD in premenopausal women led to the hypothesis that estrogen is protective and led to clinical trials of estrogen therapy in men in the 1950s and 1960s. These studies used high-dose conjugated estrogens (up to 10 mg/day) and generally resulted in poor drug tolerance, little in the way of favorable risk factor modification, and an excess of thrombophlebitis, cholecystitis, and embolic events without evidence of cardioprotection. Large, randomized trials in women have only begun recently; results from many trials will not be available for several years. Currently, our knowledge of the value of hormonal replacement therapy in women is based on its prospectively demonstrated beneficial effects on cardiac risk factors, observational evidence of primary and secondary protection, and the negative results of the one secondary prevention trial published to date (Heart and Estrogen/Progestin Replacement Study [HERS]).[59]

In postmenopausal women, exogenous estrogen results in higher HDL (especially HDL_2) and apolipoprotein A1, and lower LDL, apolipoprotein B-100, and Lp(a),[17a, 53, 60–62] (see Table 58–1). Importantly, the Postmenopausal Estrogen/Progestin Interventions (PEPI) trial showed that the addition of a progestin to estrogen did not interfere with the LDL cholesterol-lowering effect of the latter but reduced endometrial hyperplasia. The use of micronized progestin was associated with an increase in HDL cholesterol.[60] Triglycerides and LDL are often increased in a dose-dependent manner; and although these increases are highly variable in magnitude, they may limit the use of estrogen in some patients. Transdermal estrogens appear to have lesser effects on all lipoproteins, suggesting that first-pass liver metabolism is important in mediating these effects. This mode of drug delivery may be preferred in women with marked triglyceride elevations at baseline or in response to the oral route.[63] Indeed, the alterations in lipoprotein metabolism result largely from estrogen receptor–mediated actions on apolipoprotein gene expression in the liver.

Actions of Estrogen

Estrogen was once thought to mediate all of its beneficial effects through alterations in lipid metabolism; however, this mechanism accounts for only one fourth to one third of its actions. The other, multiple beneficial effects provide additional "biological plausibility" for the observed reduction in CAD among premenopausal women or postmenopausal women taking hormone replacement therapy.[64, 65] Estrogen mediates most of its effects through specific receptors (at least two types, alpha and beta, have been described) that function as transcription factors altering gene expression when they are activated. Estrogen receptors are found throughout the vasculature as well as in reproductive tissues, bone, liver, and brain. Estrogen decreases the atherogenic oxidation of LDL both in vivo and in vitro and decreases the incorporation of lipids into the vessel wall, both protective mechanisms for estrogen replacement.[66, 67] Data from the Atherosclerosis Risk in Communities (ARIC) study suggest that estrogen's effect is largely physiological and not structural or anatomical.[61, 68] In support of this, estrogen is a direct vasodilator, with effects on nitric oxide release and calcium and potassium ion channels. Estrogen acutely decreases the paradoxical coronary vasoconstriction response to acetylcholine[69] and potentiates the endothelium-dependent vasodilation of conductance and resistance coronary beds and forearm vessels in women.[70] This effect may account for its symptomatic benefit in women with Syndrome X.[71]

Estrogen also regulates expression of a variety of vascular-related genes important in CAD. These include prostacyclin, endothelin-1, collagen, matrix metalloproteinase 2, E-selectin, vascular adhesion molecule, and vascular endothelial growth factor. A similar array of actions is noted on nonvascular genes, also deemed to be important in CAD, including growth and development genes (TGF-beta, epidermal growth factor, platelet-derived growth factor, flt-4 tyrosine), coagulation- and fibrinolysis-related genes (tissue factor, fibrinogen, protein S, coagulation factors VII and XII, PAI-1, tPA, and antithrombin III) and signaling-related genes. Together, these actions suggest a powerful role for estrogen in regulating vascular tone, the response to injury and repair, atherosclerosis, and coagulation. Clinical studies confirm estrogen's association with many of these systems. These effects include a decrease in thrombotic potential,[60, 72] enhanced fibrinolysis,[73] and lowered serum angiotensin-converting enzyme activity.[74] Reports of an idiosyncratic elevation in blood pressure and improved insulin sensitivity have not been confirmed by more recent clinical studies.[60, 61] At present, which of the many beneficial effects of estrogen are most important for the prevention of CAD has not been determined. An active area of research, this knowledge is critical to future development of clinical tools for the prevention and treatment of CAD in both men and women.

CAD Prevention with Estrogen

More than 30 epidemiological studies have examined the utility of estrogen in the primary prevention of CAD, and the vast majority report a significant benefit.[53, 75–81] The largest of these studies, the Nurses' Health Study, reported a relative risk of 0.56 for myocardial infarction or death in women currently using estrogen and 0.83 in ever-users, after adjustment for age and risk factors.[81] Meta-analyses[75, 77, 80] have determined composite relative risks of 0.50 to 0.65 for both the development of and death from CAD in estrogen users.

Other documented benefits of estrogen therapy include the alleviation of menopausal symptoms, including vasomotor instability, prevention of urogenital atrophy and urinary tract infections, prevention of osteoporosis and fatal hip fracture (relative risk for death is 0.75 for users of estrogen), and prevention of colon cancer (relative risk 0.80).[53, 75, 79] A possible protective effect against stroke has been noted in several studies[82] but is not significant in others, including the large Nurses' Health Study (relative risk 0.97 for current users) and another recent meta-analysis.[75] It is possible that the relatively young cohorts examined may have influenced these findings (median age for stroke in women is 83 years). Estrogen replacement may also have beneficial effects on cognitive function, particularly in symptomatic women.[83]

The beneficial effect of reproductive hormones also extends to selective estrogen receptor modulators (SERMs). Tamoxifen, a first-generation estrogen agonist/antagonist with selective tissue effects, has been shown to have salutary effects on circulating lipoproteins[84] and to reduce the number of hospital admissions resulting from CAD and deaths due to myocardial infarction and vascular causes.[85] Raloxifene, a second-generation SERM, also has a beneficial effect on cardiac risk factors[29, 86] and does not cause breast or uterine hyperplasia, although its clinical cardiovascular benefit is unproven. In rabbits, it is a nitric oxide-dependent coronary vasodilator acting through estrogen receptor binding.[87] Studies in monkeys fed an atherogenic diet showed that, whereas raloxifene reduced LDL, it did not prevent plaque formation, as conjugated estrogens did.[88] The data regarding phytoestrogens and soy products (isoflavenoids) are even less clear. However, some women may prefer these agents, because they are seen as dietary supplements rather than pharmacological interventions, and the U.S. Food and Drug Administration has approved labeling of soy products as possessing efficacy in lipid lowering. These are very active areas of investigation and drug development, and many new prescription and over-the-counter compounds will be introduced in the near future, including those suitable for use in men. Ultimately, recommendations regarding their use await performance of randomized trials with clinical (and not surrogate) endpoints and demonstration of relative merit to conventional estrogen replacement therapy.

A smaller number of studies have evaluated the utility of estrogen in the secondary prevention of coronary artery disease. Women who were current or ever-users of estrogen had less severe angiographic coronary artery disease than never-users, even after correction for age, cholesterol, smoking, diabetes, and hypertension.[89] Long-term survival in women with a similar extent of angiographically documented coronary disease or after coronary artery bypass grafting is greater in women taking estrogen,[90, 91] and restenosis is reduced after angioplasty.

Although these observations are compelling, completion of the first randomized prospective trial of hormone replacement therapy, HERS, has caused a dramatic rethinking of the potential benefit.[59] Contrary to expectations, there were no reductions in nonfatal myocardial infarction, coronary death, and overall mortality during 4.1 years of follow-up in 3763 postmenopausal women with CAD (Fig. 58–2). Instead, there was an excess of thrombotic events, particularly in years 1 and 2. As an alternative to abandonment of the hypothesis that estrogen is protective, investigators have cited the possible mitigating effects of concomitant progestin. However, the hormone replacement therapy regimen used (0.625 mg conjugated equine estrogens plus 2.5 mg medroxyprogesterone daily) did have beneficial lipid effects, raising HDL 10 percent and lowering LDL 11 percent, but also caused more thromboembolic events and

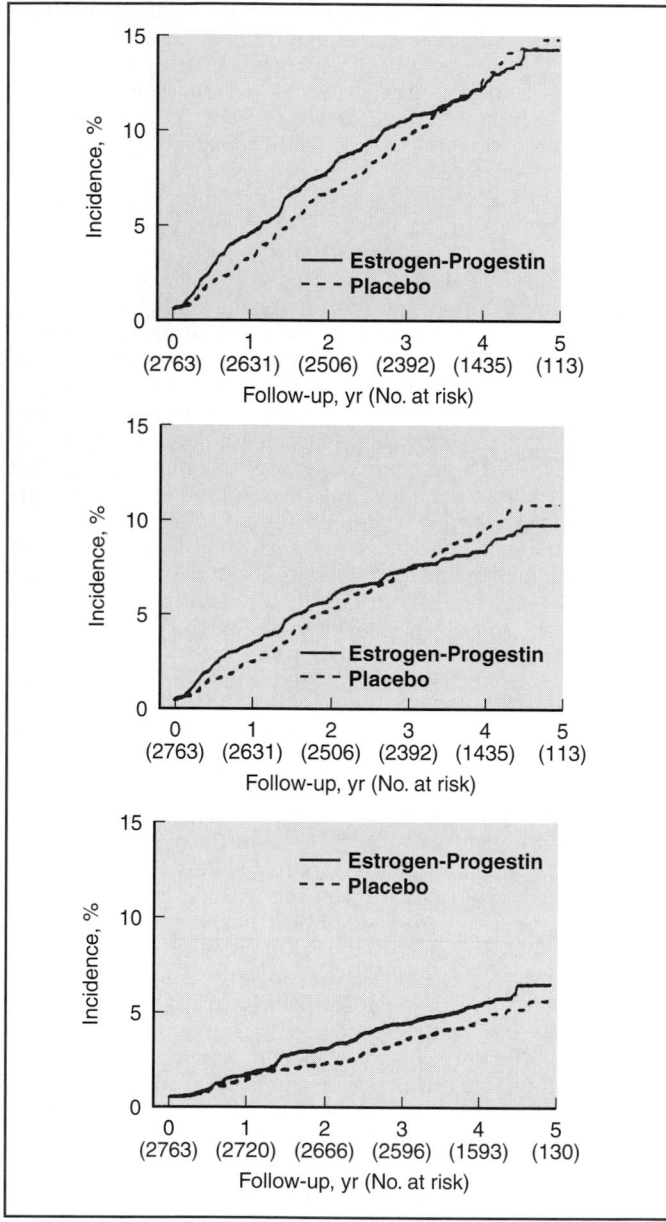

FIGURE 58–2. Coronary artery disease (CAD) events *(left)*, nonfatal myocardial infarction *(center)*, and CAD deaths *(right)* in the Heart and Estrogen/Progestin Replacement Study (HERS): Kaplan-Meier estimates of the cumulative incidence of events. The number of women observed at each year of follow-up and still free of an event are provided in parentheses. Log rank *p* values are 0.91 for primary CAD events, 0.46 for nonfatal myocardial infarction, and 0.23 for CAD death. (From Hulley S, Grady D, Bush T, et al: Randomized trial of estrogen plus progestin for secondary prevention of coronary heart disease in postmenopausal women. JAMA 280:609, 1998. Copyright 1998, American Medical Association.)

gallbladder disease. Another possible explanation is attrition of women with an early increased risk, such as for thromboembolism.[92] This hypothesis is supported by close examination of the time trends that reveal excess CAD events early and fewer later in the follow-up period. Further, there are questions regarding the statistical power of the HERS population and follow-up.[92a] A final hypothesis, that estrogen may increase vascular inflammation, is supported by several recent studies showing increased C-reactive protein among estrogen users,[93, 94] which may override antiinflammatory effects of lowered E-selectin in some individuals and is associated with increased cardiovascular risk.[52a]

In the light of these data it is hard to recommend initiation of estrogen replacement therapy for secondary prevention of CAD, yet patients currently on therapy should probably continue. Many questions remain.[92, 92a, 95] Some have suggested that use of a lower dose or different hormone regimen or the addition of aspirin would modify the early thromboembolic side effects. It is also unclear how these results should be applied to decisions regarding use of estrogen replacement therapy for primary prevention. Trial participants are currently being followed for longer term results, and other studies are in progress.

In addition to the questions HERS raises about efficacy, and the methodological limitations in other available studies, there are significant risks associated with estrogen use and logistic problems with its prescription. Chief among the risks of estrogen use is endometrial cancer, for which unopposed estrogen therapy carries a fivefold to eightfold increased risk, associated with an estimated threefold increased risk of death.[75, 78] Women without a uterus obviously do not share this risk, and it has been proposed that the addition of a progestin nullifies it. A potential detrimental effect on the cardioprotective action of estrogen of adding progestins has been anticipated because of their androgenic effect on circulating lipids; however, recent studies suggest that this factor may have negligible effects or may even be beneficial.[60, 80]

BREAST CANCER. Estrogen may increase breast cancer risk, with meta-analyses showing little increased risk for short-term therapy, whereas a higher relative risk, up to 1.5, has been associated with long-term use (over 10 years) in the Nurses' Health Study.[75, 96, 97] This a strong psychological, if not biological, deterrent to estrogen replacement, especially in women with a personal or family history of breast cancer and a low likelihood of developing (i.e., no risk factors for) CAD. Women with established CAD or with risk factors and no family history of breast cancer would remain good candidates for estrogen replacement, and SERMs, which may actually reduce breast cancer risk,[98] could be preferred agents in others. The effects of the addition of progestins to estrogen on the incidence of breast cancer are unknown, but they appear to be minimal.[97]

WEIGHING RISKS AND BENEFITS OF ESTROGEN. Three recent meta-analyses of estrogen replacement reviewed all available data on its effects on endometrial and breast cancers, hip fracture, stroke, and coronary artery disease.[75–77, 80] Combining these data with other information regarding the incidence and mortality of these diseases, detailed estimates of the gain/loss in life expectancy or assessment of summed risk weights with hormone therapy were derived. In these analyses, for most women, estrogen replacement enhanced longevity somewhat and SERMs added little benefit. However, simple life expectancy calculations may not address some women's concerns adequately.[99]

Other considerations in the decision to use estrogen replacement include the drug's side effects, such as vaginal bleeding, the need for careful monitoring for breast and uterine cancers and endometrial hyperplasia, and the costs of therapy and of monitoring.[75–77] The risk of thrombophlebitis is unclear at the doses currently employed,[100] but it is likely elevated[59]; it is unclear if aspirin use offsets this risk or if testing for prothrombotic tendencies, such as factor V Leiden mutation, can be used to exclude women at higher risk.[44] Finally, compliance with estrogen replacement therapy taken to relieve menopause symptoms is poor; there is no reason to think that this will improve in asymptomatic women taking estrogen for the prevention of future disease.[95]

A full evaluation of the risks and benefits of estrogen replacement cannot be made without considering the methodological flaws inherent in all available data and those crucial areas in which information is lacking. For primary prevention, the reliance on observational studies in the absence of randomized trials raises issues of selection bias, especially because women using estrogen are more likely to see their physicians frequently, to adopt healthy behaviors such as exercise, prudent diet, and smoking cessation, and to be of higher socioeconomic status.[101] For any woman, patient preference after careful counseling should be a dominant factor. Published patient algorithms are helpful in this regard.[76, 99, 102]

The most commonly used estrogen is conjugated equine estrogens at a daily dose of 0.625 mg. There is no evidence that cardioprotection is enhanced or even preserved at a higher dose, and side effects are often worse; indeed there is evidence that a dose of 0.3 mg is equally cardioprotective.[102a] Similarly, the optimal formulation, dosage, and regimen for progestins are unclear. The optimal timing of estrogen replacement is also unknown. Some workers suggest starting the drug at menopause and continuing indefinitely for women at high risk. The usefulness of beginning therapy at a more advanced age (e.g., with the first manifestation of CAD) is unknown, particularly in light of the HERS study.

ESTROGEN REPLACEMENT THERAPY GUIDELINES. The American College of Physicians and others have published guidelines for counseling postmenopausal women about primary preventive hormone therapy that are well grounded in available knowledge.[76, 102] These guidelines suggest that, based on available data, estrogen replacement is likely of value in women with a high risk of developing osteoporosis or CAD. This proposal represents an enormous potential change in cardiovascular therapeutics and practice, as yet unsupported by data from randomized controlled trials, such as the Women's Health Initiative, which will not become available until 2005. It is important to recognize that whereas salutary effects of estrogen replacement on lipids have been demonstrated in prospective randomized trials, clinical benefits in primary prevention thus far are limited to observational studies and secondary prevention was not beneficial in the single large study completed to date.[59] It may be that untested, newer agents such as the SERMs or phytoestrogens[102b] may ultimately be preferred treatment. Ongoing randomized trials of primary and secondary prevention will prove whether the use of estrogen replacement in postmenopausal women is a viable strategy.

EVALUATION OF CHEST PAIN IN WOMEN

Clinical Syndromes and Natural History

It has long been assumed that the clinical expression of CAD is similar in men and women, yet available information suggests that gender differences in presentation and disease manifestations exist and should be considered in the evaluation of the patient with chest pain. Several studies document that women are more likely than men to present with angina and less likely to present with a concrete event such as myocardial infarction as either the first

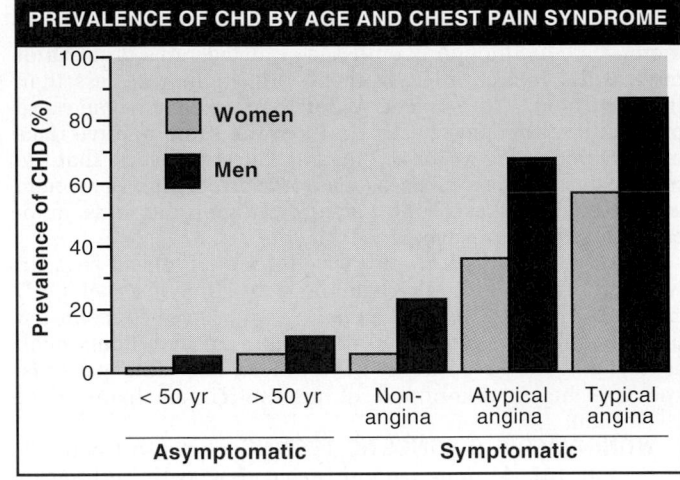

FIGURE 58–3. Prevalence of angiographically documented coronary heart disease (CHD) in men and women according to age and chest pain syndrome. (Modified from DeSanctis RW: Clinical manifestations of coronary artery disease: Chest pain in women. *In* Wenger NK, Speroff L, Packard B [eds]: Cardiovascular Health and Disease in Women. Greenwich, CT, Le Jacq Communications, 1993, p 68.)

or subsequent manifestations of CAD.[3] Furthermore, women are on average 5 to 10 years older at the time of presentation. Perhaps even more than in men, the prevalence of angiographic coronary disease varies dramatically according to the nature of the chest pain, the patient's age, and the presence and type of coronary risk factors[103–105] (Fig. 58–3). This underlines the importance of good history taking and careful cardiovascular risk factor assessment in the evaluation of women with chest pain.[106]

A variety of factors influence the evaluation of chest pain in women, including patient and physician perception of disease risk (see earlier). Compared with men, women with chronic stable angina are older and more likely to have hypertension, diabetes, and congestive heart failure but are less likely to have had a prior myocardial infarction or revascularization.[107] Although equally likely to have effort angina, such women are more likely to experience pain at rest, during sleep, or with mental stress. Similarly, women undergoing a myocardial infarction are more likely to have nausea and jaw, back, or neck pain, or palpitations, and are less likely to report diaphoresis than men.[108, 109] These differences make the evaluation of a new symptom or disability more complex and make essential a gender-based approach to education of both lay and health personnel in the presentation of acute ischemic syndromes.

The reasons for these differences in symptoms are unclear. Women with acute myocardial infarction have similar angiographic findings, suggesting that the mechanism of infarction does not vary by gender.[110] However, women do have higher prevalences than men do of vasospastic angina and of microvascular angina,[104, 105] both of which are associated with atypical chest pain patterns, are often treated differently, and have a more favorable prognosis than epicardial coronary disease. Recent data suggest that such chest pain syndromes are related to myocardial ischemia with altered phosphocreatine metabolism documented by PET scan.[110a] Even in the presence of angiographically documented disease, gender differences in plaque components (more cellular and fibrous tissue in women), endothelial function (estrogen-induced coronary vasodilation), and hemostasis (higher fibrinogen and factor VII levels in women) may influence the pathophysiology and, therefore, the clinical manifestations of coronary disease.[43, 111] Finally, women more commonly have noncoronary chest pain syndromes, further complicating their clinical assessment.

Women with chest pain are less likely to experience a subsequent myocardial infarction or coronary death than men.[3, 112, 113] Although overall age-adjusted rates of death or myocardial infarction in women with angina are less than those in men,[112] of subjects older than age 65, women and men with exertional chest pain have the same relative risks of CAD death (2.7 vs. 2.4).[114] Other data suggesting that the prognosis of coronary disease is not more benign in women include the similar (if not worse) early mortality after myocardial infarction in women.[115]

Thus, determination of the etiology of chest pain in women can be difficult, hampered by the onset of CAD later in life, a setting of greater frailty and concomitant disease, the more common appearance of symptoms such as rest angina in patients with otherwise stable patterns, and the higher likelihood of alternative mechanisms of chest pain.

NONINVASIVE DIAGNOSTIC TESTING (see also Chaps. 6, 7, 9, and 13). Although noninvasive diagnostic testing for CAD does not fully resolve the difficulties inherent in evaluating chest pain in women, careful test selection and interpretation can provide valuable information regarding the presence and severity of CAD in women. The general principles underlying noninvasive diagnostic testing do not differ in men and women.[116] The simplest diagnostic test, the resting electrocardiogram, reveals a higher prevalence of repolarization (ST-T wave) abnormalities in women with suspected coronary disease than in men (32 vs. 23 percent).[103]

Treadmill exercise testing carries a higher false-positive rate in women (38 to 67 percent) than in men (7 to 44 percent) in the same studies, in part because of a lower pretest likelihood of disease.[104] However, women have a low false-negative rate (12 to 22 percent) that compares favorably to that in men (12 to 40 percent) and suggests that routine testing reliably *excludes* the presence of CAD in women with negative tests. The exercise electrocardiogram also provides useful prognostic information in women.[117, 118] Variables contributing to test accuracy are resting ST-T wave abnormalities, peak exercise heart rate, number of diseased vessels, typical angina, age, gender, drug use (digitalis, diazepam), hyperventilation, conduction abnormalities, left ventricular hypertrophy, mitral valve prolapse, vasospasm, and hormonal influences. Although less common in women, false-negative studies may be contributed to by gender-specific characteristics, including reduced exercise tolerance and the higher prevalence of single-vessel disease in women.

The addition of imaging to electrocardiographic stress testing markedly improves its accuracy in women, as noted by recent meta-analyses[119, 120] and reviews[121] (Fig. 58–4; Table 58–2). Planar thallium scans during treadmill exercise testing suggest moderate increases in sensitivity and specificity in women.[118, 119, 121] The use of single-photon emission computed tomography (SPECT) may not improve accuracy in women as it does in men.[122] Much of the inaccuracy of thallium scanning in women has been attributed to breast attenuation, which is reduced by use of higher-energy isotopes such as technetium-99m-sestamibi and by newer algorithms for attenuation correction (see Chap. 9).[123] Coupling exercise testing with echocardiographic visualization of wall motion (i.e., exercise echocardiography) also improves diagnostic accuracy in women,[119, 121, 124] even more so than in men.[120] Similarly, the use of pharmacological stress agents (e.g., adenosine, dipyridamole, dobutamine) in women coupled with either echocardiographic or nuclear imaging shows substantial improvements in test performance over electrocardiographic results alone.[121]

Because few direct comparisons between exercise echocardiography and exercise-thallium or sestamibi testing have been reported, the objective basis for selecting one

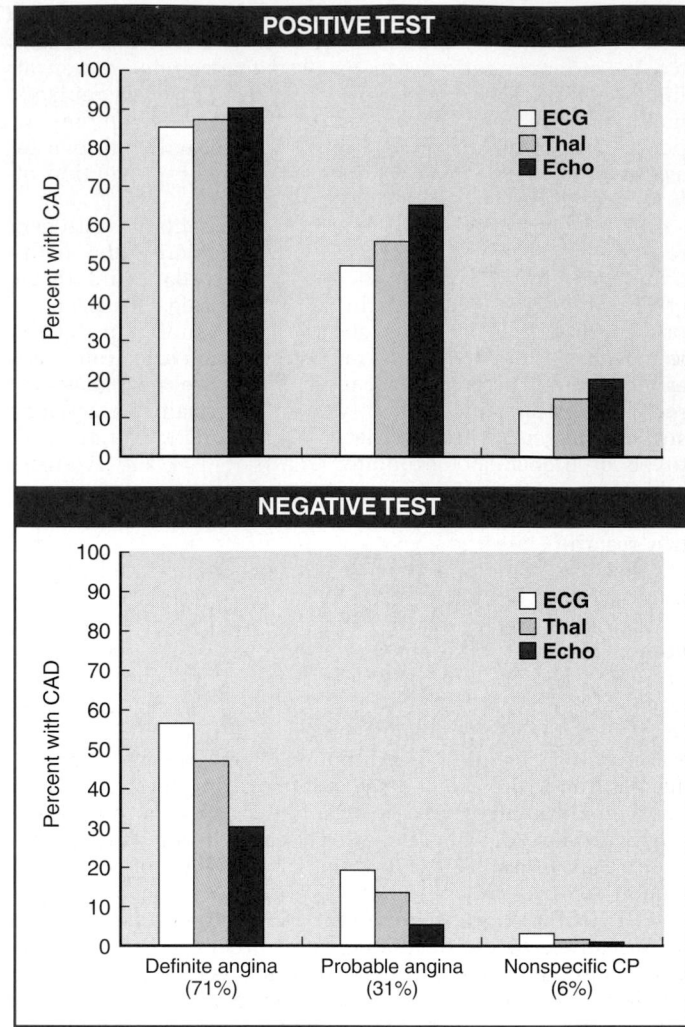

FIGURE 58–4. Posttest likelihood of coronary artery disease (CAD) in a 55-year-old woman, depending on test results (positive, top; negative, bottom), type of chest pain (CP), and pretest probability of disease (in parentheses) as described in CASS (Edmond M, Mock MB, Davis KB, et al: Long-term survival of medically treated patients in the coronary artery surgery study [CASS] registry. Circulation 90:2645, 1994) and type of stress test performed (exercise electrocardiogram [ECG], thallium perfusion [Thal], echocardiographic imaging [Echo]). (Data from Kwok Y, Kim C, Grady D, et al: Meta-analysis of exercise testing to detect coronary artery disease in women. Am J Cardiol 83:660, 1999.)

modality over another must rely on meta-analysis and cost-effectiveness modeling. Recent meta-analyses[119, 120] have shown exercise echocardiography to have similar sensitivity and superior specificity to nuclear perfusion studies, with the accuracy of exercise ECG and exercise nuclear studies showing gender dependence, whereas that of exercise echocardiography is similar in men and women. Several formal cost-effectiveness models show stress echocardiography to dominate over nuclear techniques,[124–126] suggesting that diagnostic testing strategies employing exercise echocardiography as the first test might be superior.

CORONARY ANGIOGRAPHY. Few studies have examined gender differences in invasive diagnostic testing. Women are more likely than men to experience vascular and renal complications from diagnostic angiography, possibly due to more advanced age, higher prevalence of diabetes, and smaller body size; the incidence of myocardial infarction, stroke, and death is similar.[127]

GENDER BIAS. A 1987 study reporting that men with positive nuclear exercise tests were 6.3 times more likely to

▼ TABLE 58–2. WEIGHTED MEAN TEST CHARACTERISTICS FOR EXERCISE STRESS
TESTING IN THE DIAGNOSIS OF CORONARY ARTERY DISEASE IN WOMEN

2045

Ch 58

EXERCISE TEST	NO. WOMEN	SENSITIVITY	SPECIFICITY	LIKELIHOOD RATIO (+)	LIKELIHOOD RATIO (−)
ECG	3721	61%	70%	2.25	0.55
Thallium	842	78%	64%	2.87	0.36
Echo	296	86%	79%	4.29	0.18

Modified from Kwok Y, Kim C, Grady D, et al: Meta-analysis of exercise testing to detect coronary artery disease in women. Am J Cardiol 83:660, 1999.

be referred to cardiac catheterization than women[128] gave rise to concerns that female patients were receiving inadequate or inappropriate care, a conclusion that has been supported by several subsequent studies. Coronary angiography is performed 28 to 45 percent more often and revascularization 15 to 27 percent more often in men than in women with a diagnosis of CAD.[129] Although awareness of gender differences is growing, these discrepancies still exist, such that both gender and race influence management of chest pain.[130]

It is clear that less aggressive treatment strategies in women do not represent optimal care even for patient groups with differences in disease prevalence, nor do they accurately reflect the difficulties in diagnosing coronary disease in women. Although women undergoing diagnostic stress testing[131] were equally likely to have a positive stress electrocardiogram (29 percent in women vs. 30 percent in men) or stress thallium examination (23 vs. 27 percent), they were less commonly referred for additional noninvasive testing (4 vs. 20 percent) or catheterization (34 vs. 45 percent). However, subsequent event rates were higher in women, whether they had a normal initial test (1.6 percent/yr death or myocardial infarction vs. 0.8 per cent in men) or an abnormal one (14.3 vs. 6.0 percent/yr). Both male and female patients who did undergo revascularization had no events, whereas women who were not revascularized had a worse prognosis than similarly untreated men. These data demonstrate not only a gender-based difference in clinical practice but a worse patient outcome in women treated less aggressively.

MANAGEMENT OF CHRONIC CAD IN WOMEN

MEDICAL THERAPY. Because fewer studies have examined the medical treatment of chronic CAD in women, there is less evidence as to whether women respond similarly to men to conventional therapy. A recent review of gender differences in the efficacy of CAD treatment found evidence for similar benefit of antiplatelet therapy, beta blockade, nitroglycerin, thrombolytics, and angiotensin-converting enzyme inhibitors[132] (Fig. 58–5). Calcium channel blockade was not effective in either men or women. Although early data regarding aspirin were conflicting, newer observational studies suggest benefit but still await confirmation by a randomized clinical trial. The Nurses' Health Study showed that women older than 50 taking one to six aspirin per week had a 32 percent lower likelihood of myocardial infarction,[133] a borderline significant reduction that did not apply to younger women or higher doses. Another observational study in women with CAD revealed reduced adjusted relative risk for cardiovascular (relative risk 0.61) and all-cause (0.66) mortality. Diabetic, elderly, and symptomatic women benefited most, as did women with prior myocardial infarctions.[134] Aspirin and other antiplatelet agents also reduced vascular events in women.[135]

Interestingly, glycoprotein IIb-IIIa inhibitors provide additional benefit over aspirin in unstable coronary syndromes in women but not in men.[136] This finding suggests that, in women, platelets may play a more important role or may require more aggressive inhibition.

Cross-sectional studies reveal that women with CAD are more likely than men to be receiving nitrates, calcium channel blockers, sedatives, diuretics, and other antihypertensive agents but are equally or less likely to have been prescribed aspirin and beta blockers.[107, 131] Although this has improved somewhat, treatment levels are not yet equal, especially in older patients. The impact, if any, of these differences on the prognosis of coronary disease is unknown. Although the Coronary Artery Surgery Study (CASS) shows that women treated medically had better 12-year survival with angiographically documented zero-, one- or two-vessel disease than did men with similar anatomy,[137] other studies suggest that undertreatment of women is related to a worse outcome.[138]

REVASCULARIZATION. Many studies have addressed the relative effectiveness of revascularization procedures (angioplasty and coronary artery bypass grafting [CABG]) in men and women. Unfortunately, comparisons of the results of medical management and percutaneous and operative revascularization are few. Instead, these studies have focused on gender differences in the population under study, making difficult the application of these data to the optimal care of individual patients. Virtually all data for both angioplasty and CABG have been derived from post hoc subgroup analyses of studies designed to address other issues.

Percutaneous Coronary Intervention (PCI) (see also Chap. 38). Virtually all PCI studies note a greater prevalence of comorbidities in women, including advanced age, hypertension, congestive heart failure, diabetes, severe concomitant noncardiac disease, and hypercholesterolemia.[138–146] The severity of angina is also greater in women, the condition being more likely to be unstable or to be of Canadian Class III or IV severity.[139, 141–143]

The likelihood of *angiographic success* of the application of balloon angioplasty or of new devices is similar in men and women in current series,[141–143] with lower success rates in women reported only in the older studies. In contrast, in most balloon angioplasty series, women experience higher complication and mortality rates, including groin complications, acute closure, and death, but not myocardial infarction or emergency coronary artery bypass grafting[140] (Table 58–3). Indeed, the proportional risk of death from procedural complications is greater in women.[145, 146] The difference in outcome has been variously attributed to women's older age, smaller body size, greater severity of angina, more fragile vessels, and greater burden of comorbidity.[143, 147] More recent preliminary data from the National Heart Lung and Blood Institute (NHLBI) Dynamic Registry (1997–1998) and Northern New England Data Bases (1990–1993 and 1994–1996) suggest that the gender gap is narrowing, particularly with the growing use of new devices.[145, 148, 149]

The late outcome of PCI appears to be similar in men and women, with women more likely to experience an-

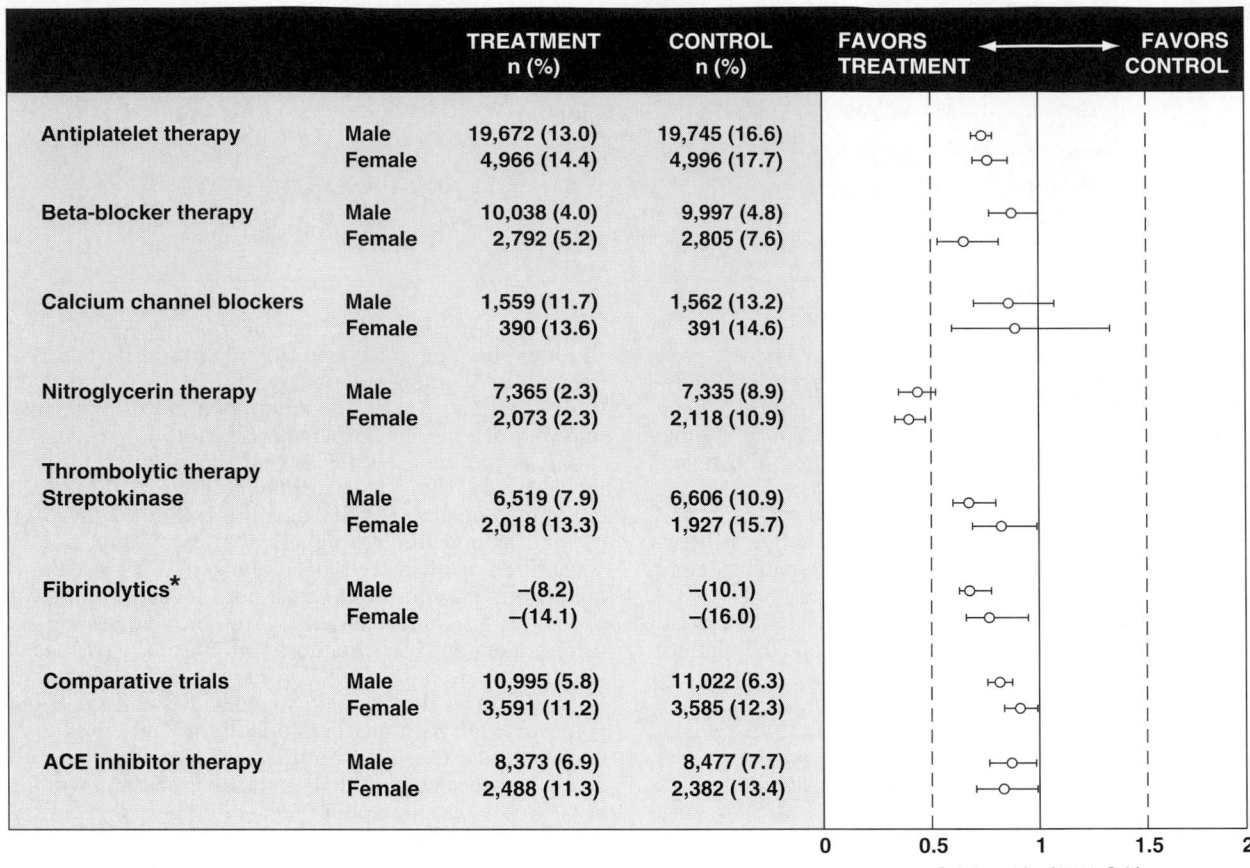

		TREATMENT n (%)	CONTROL n (%)	FAVORS TREATMENT ← → FAVORS CONTROL
Antiplatelet therapy	Male	19,672 (13.0)	19,745 (16.6)	
	Female	4,966 (14.4)	4,996 (17.7)	
Beta-blocker therapy	Male	10,038 (4.0)	9,997 (4.8)	
	Female	2,792 (5.2)	2,805 (7.6)	
Calcium channel blockers	Male	1,559 (11.7)	1,562 (13.2)	
	Female	390 (13.6)	391 (14.6)	
Nitroglycerin therapy	Male	7,365 (2.3)	7,335 (8.9)	
	Female	2,073 (2.3)	2,118 (10.9)	
Thrombolytic therapy Streptokinase	Male	6,519 (7.9)	6,606 (10.9)	
	Female	2,018 (13.3)	1,927 (15.7)	
Fibrinolytics*	Male	–(8.2)	–(10.1)	
	Female	–(14.1)	–(16.0)	
Comparative trials	Male	10,995 (5.8)	11,022 (6.3)	
	Female	3,591 (11.2)	3,585 (12.3)	
ACE inhibitor therapy	Male	8,373 (6.9)	8,477 (7.7)	
	Female	2,488 (11.3)	2,382 (13.4)	

0   0.5   1   1.5   2
Odds ratio (95% C.I.)

FIGURE 58–5. Proportional effects of treatment strategies on morbidity and mortality in women versus men from randomized controlled trials. Antiplatelet trials evaluated aspirin, dipyridamole, ticlopidine, sulfinpyrazone, or suloctidil versus active or placebo control in vascular disease (not coronary artery disease); beta blocker trials assessed atenolol, metoprolol, or propranolol versus control; calcium channel blocker studies evaluated diltiazem or verapamil versus control; the nitroglycerin trial assessed transdermal glyceryl trinitrate versus control; fibrinolytic trials tested streptokinase, anistreplase, urokinase, or alteplase versus control; comparative thrombolytic trials assessed streptokinase versus alteplase; and angiotensin-converting enzyme (ACE) inhibitor trials assessed captopril, lisinopril, or enalapril versus control. Unless otherwise specified, summary frequencies and odds ratios with 95 percent confidence intervals (C.I.) are presented. Asterisk indicates multivariable-adjusted odds ratio, percentages of patients only. (Modified from Fetters JK, Peterson ED, Shaw LJ, et al: Sex-specific differences in coronary artery disease risk factors, evaluation, and treatment: Have they been adequately evaluated? Am Heart J 131:804, 1996.)

gina and men more likely to experience cardiac events (myocardial infarction, revascularization or death).[140–143, 146, 147] Two observational studies have suggested that estrogen use in postmenopausal women reduces restenosis,[150, 151] perhaps through acceleration of endothelial repair.

Coronary Artery Bypass Grafting (see also Chap. 37). Gender differences in outcome after CABG are well established and remain present even in the mid 1990s.[152–154] As with angioplasty, virtually every study has shown women to have more comorbidities and less favorable patient characteristics preoperatively. Women are also more likely than men to undergo urgent or emergent surgery. Women and men undergoing CABG are equally symptomatic, but women are more likely to have preserved ventricular function and less likely to have multivessel or three-vessel disease.

The mortality of women is higher than of men, with risk ratios of 1.4 to 4.4. This is particularly true for low- and medium-risk patients, with no difference in highest-risk patients, suggesting that other factors predominate.[154] In addition, women are less likely to receive internal mammary grafts or undergo complete revascularization and are more likely to experience the complications of heart failure, perioperative infarction, and hemorrhage.[152, 153]

The causes of this higher mortality appear to be multiple, including technical factors such as smaller body size

and coronary diameter, advanced age, comorbidities such as diabetes and hypertension, and clinical factors such as the urgency of the procedure. Disease-related factors such as the extent and severity of angiographic stenoses and left ventricular dysfunction are also important in determining outcome, yet these factors tend to be more favorable in women. As with angioplasty, patient-related factors and comorbidities seem increasingly important to outcome, with more recent studies reporting continuing gender differences in outcome.[154] The impact of new techniques such as minimally invasive bypass surgery and grafting performed without circulatory arrest is unknown, but it may be greater in the frailer, older female population.

Women have a lower likelihood of being free of angina than do men and experience greater physical disability and less return to work. Rates of long-term survival, infarction, and reoperation are similar.

ACUTE CORONARY SYNDROMES
(see also Chaps. 35 and 36)

Women have a different clinical presentation and hospital course after acute coronary syndromes and acute myocardial infarction and respond differently to both medical and

STUDY, YEAR, REFERENCE	SERIES	ANGIOGRAPHIC SUCCESS (%)		COMPLICATIONS (%)		MORTALITY (%)	
		Women	Men	Women	Men	Women	Men
Cowley, et al., 1985[139]	NHLBI 1978–1982	56.6	56.6	27.2	19.4	1.7	0.3
Kelsey, et al., 1993[140]	NHLBI 1985–1986	89	89	29	20	2.6	0.3
Arnold, et al., 1994[141]	Cleveland Clinic 1980–1988	93.6	93.3	9	7	1.1	0.3
Weintraub, et al., 1994[142]	Emory 1980–1991	90.8	89.7			0.7	0.1
Bell, et al., 1993[143]	Mayo Clinic 1979–1987	83	82			1.0	1.2
	Mayo Clinic 1988–1990	87	90			2.9	1.4
Welty, et al., 1994[144]	Deaconess 1981–1989	89.6	91.2			0.6	0.9
Malenka, et al., 1999[145]	Northern New England 1990–1993					0.6	2.2
Keelan, et al., 1997[146]	Mayo Clinic 1981–1993 (unstable angina)	87.9	87.2	8.3	7.8	4.1	3.2
O'Connor, et al., 1999[147]	Northern New England 1994–1996					1.3	0.96

procedural therapies. Gender differences in acute myocardial infarction have been reviewed.[155]

CLINICAL SYNDROMES. Women suffering from an acute coronary syndrome or myocardial infarction are likely to be older and more likely to have a history of hypertension, diabetes, unstable angina, hyperlipidemia, and congestive heart failure, and they are less likely to be smokers than their male counterparts.[155–171] Women are also more likely to experience neck and shoulder pain, abdominal pain, nausea, vomiting, fatigue, and dyspnea in addition to chest pain.[163–164] It is unclear if they are more likely to have silent infarctions.[3] Perhaps due in part to these more atypical symptoms, women seek medical attention more slowly[166] and even after hospital arrival may experience greater delays in receiving care.[157, 159, 163]

Women admitted to a hospital for acute coronary syndromes are more likely to have experienced a prior non-transmural infarction.[161] Women with infarction have more serious presentations, with greater prevalences of tachycardia, rales, heart block, and a higher Killip class on initial presentation.[157, 159, 161, 164, 166] Nevertheless, women are less likely to receive thrombolysis (even after controlling for eligibility)[156, 163, 164, 166, 167] and receive it later than do men.[159, 162] Women are also less likely to be admitted to a coronary care unit[166, 168] or to be hospitalized in an institution in which catheterization is available.[161] Most[161, 163, 165, 168] but not all[169, 170] studies find that women with acute infarction are less likely to undergo diagnostic catheterization during their hospital stay, even after controlling for age and a variety of clinical characteristics. Some studies have reported equal or near-equal rates of angioplasty and bypass surgery among catheterized patients,[159, 160, 165, 169] suggesting that differences in treatment disappear once disease is documented angiographically.[169, 171] However, this is not true in all series.[163, 164]

Women have higher rates of in-hospital complications from infarction, including bleeding, stroke, shock, myocardial rupture, and recurrent chest pain, than do men, although most of these differences disappear on correction for controlling for age and comorbidities.[159, 160, 172] Women with acute infarction are more likely to be treated with nitrates, digoxin, and diuretics than are men and are less likely to receive thrombolytics, antiarrhythmics, antiplatelet agents, and beta blockers.[158, 162, 166] Even after discharge, women are less likely to be scheduled for exercise tests or referred for cardiac rehabilitation, and recovery from infarction appears delayed with slower return to work and full resumption of all activities, with more sleep disturbance and psychiatric and psychosomatic complaints experienced.[173]

MORTALITY. Mortality in non-Q-wave myocardial infarction appears to be similar to that in men, whereas women with unstable angina are less likely to have angiographic CAD or reinfarction and death.[174, 175] In acute myocardial infarction, early or in-hospital mortality in women is greater than in men, and adjustment for age and/or clinical characteristics serves to reduce this difference but not to eliminate it fully. This is particularly true in younger women (Fig. 58–6).[115, 156, 176, 177] Analysis of a very large scale, population-based data set (as opposed to post hoc analysis of thrombolytic trial study populations[178]) indicated that gender differences in mortality decrease with age.[177] In part, this gap may be due to a higher rate of prehospital sudden death in men,[164] but this cannot explain the twofold greater mortality in women younger than 50 years of age compared with similarly aged men. Mortality 1 to 3 years after hospital discharge is similar in men and women, when adjustments are made for age and other baseline characteristics.[115, 179]

TREATMENT. The reduction in mortality from thrombolysis in men and women with acute myocardial infarction is likely similar.[110, 163, 176, 179] The efficacy of thrombolysis also appears similar in men and women with similar rates of intracoronary thrombosis on pretreatment angiography[110] and of thrombolytic-induced, infarct-related artery patency and left ventricular function.[157, 160] However, complication rates, particularly hemorrhagic stroke and recurrent myocardial infarction, appear to be higher in women.[159, 160, 180, 181] Primary angioplasty is equally, if not more effective in women, as demonstrated by the Primary Angioplasty in Myocardial Infarction (PAMI) trial, in part due to the reduction in hemorrhagic stroke.[182, 183]

Medical treatment after hospital discharge appears to carry somewhat different benefits for men and women. Aspirin likely prevents reinfarction in women[134]; calcium channel blockers are not of benefit. Two studies suggest

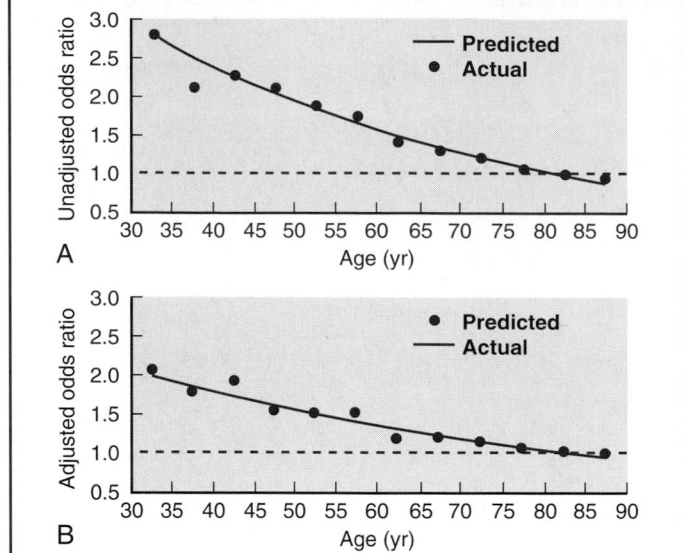

FIGURE 58–6. Odds ratios for death during hospitalization for myocardial infarction in women as compared with men, according to age. *A,* The unadjusted odds ratios were derived from the model that included sex, age, the interaction between sex and age, and the year of discharge. *B,* The adjusted odds ratios were derived from the model that also included race, insurance status, medical history, severity of clinical abnormalities at admission, type of management in the first 24 hours after admission, and time to presentation. (From Vaccarino V, Parsons L, Every NR, et al: Sex-based differences in early mortality after myocardial infarction. N Engl J Med 341:220, 1999. Copyright 1999, Massachusetts Medical Society.)

that men may experience more benefit than women when treated with angiotensin-converting enzyme inhibitors postinfarction.[184, 185] In contrast, beta blockade clearly provides a substantial improvement in postinfarction survival in women that is equal to, if not greater than, that seen in men.[186–188] Unfortunately, women are less likely to be discharged on beta blockers.[158, 162, 166]

CONCLUSIONS

Although gender differences in the epidemiology of CAD have long been appreciated, we have only recently begun to critically examine and analyze differences in heart disease between men and women. Application of this new knowledge to patient care requires education of both patients and providers, yet it is essential for optimal medical practice. Although the diagnostic and therapeutic management of CAD are based on principles common to men and women, differences exist in risk factors, hormonal influences, clinical presentation, diagnostic evaluation, treatment, and outcomes of interventions for coronary artery disease. Similar differences exist in heart failure.[189] The astute practitioner will be able to incorporate knowledge of these differences into the care of each individual.

In the past 5 years, knowledge of gender-based cardiovascular pathophysiology and therapeutics has dramatically increased and will continue to grow as the many studies in progress close the gaps in our understanding of CAD in women. In particular, hormones and hormone replacement therapy, central to women's care, remain a large and unresolved area awaiting further elucidation of the basic biology and its translation into clinical care.

REFERENCES

RISK FACTORS

1. Mosca L, Manson JE, Sutherland SE, et al: Cardiovascular disease in women: A statement for healthcare professionals from the AHA. Circulation 96:2468, 1997.
2. Roger VL, Jacobsen SJ, Weston SA, et al: Trends in heart disease deaths in Olmsted County, Minnesota, 1979–1994. Mayo Clin Proc 74:651, 1999.
3. Lerner DJ, Kannel WB: Patterns of coronary heart disease morbidity and mortality in the sexes: 26-year follow-up of the Framingham population. Am Heart J 111:383, 1986.
4. Allen JK, Blumenthal RS: Risk factors in the offspring of women with premature coronary heart disease. Am Heart J 135:428, 1998.
5. Birdwell BG, Herbers JE, Kroenke K: Evaluating chest pain. Arch Intern Med 153:1991, 1993.
6. Rich-Edwards JW, Manson JE, Hennekens CH, et al: The primary prevention of coronary heart disease in women. N Engl J Med 332:1758, 1995.
7. Mosca L, Grundy SM, Judelson D, et al: Guide to preventive cardiology for women. Circulation 99:2480, 1999.
8. Detection, Evaluation, and Treatment of High Blood Cholesterol in Adults (Adult Treatment Panel II). Circulation 89:1329, 1994.
9. Jousilahti P, Vartiainen E, Tuomilehto J, Puska P: Sex, age, cardiovascular risk factors, and coronary heart disease: A prospective follow-up study of 14,786 middle-aged men and women in Finland. Circulation 99:1165, 1999.
10. Denke MA: Primary prevention of coronary heart disease in postmenopausal women. Am J Med 107(2A):48S, 1999.
11. Grundy SM, Pasternak R, Greenland P, et al: Assessment of cardiovascular risk by use of multiple risk-factor assessment equations: A statement for healthcare professionals from the American Heart Association and the American College of Cardiology. Circulation 100:1481, 1999.

Lipoproteins

12. LaRosa JC: Lipoproteins and lipid disorders. *In* Douglas PS (ed): Cardiovascular Health and Disease in Women. Philadelphia, WB Saunders, 1993, p 175.
13. Eaker ED, Castelli WP: Coronary heart disease and its risk factors among women in the Framingham Study. *In* Eaker ED, Packer B, Wenger N, et al (eds): Coronary Heart Disease in Women. New York, Haymarket Doyma, 1987, p 122.
14. Miller VT: Lipids, lipoproteins, women and cardiovascular disease. Atherosclerosis 108:S73, 1994.
15. Criqui MH, Heiss G, Cohn R, et al: Plasma triglyceride level and mortality from coronary heart disease. N Engl J Med 328:1220, 1993.
16. LaRosa JC: Triglycerides and coronary risk in women and the elderly. Arch Intern Med 157:961, 1997.
17. Bostom AG, Gagnon DR, Cupples A, et al: A prospective investigation of elevated lipoprotein a detected by electrophoresis and cardiovascular disease in women: The Framingham Heart Study. Circulation 90:1688, 1994.
17a. Shlipak MG, Simon JA, Vittinghoff E, et al: Estrogen and progestin, lipoprotein(a), and the risk of recurrent coronary heart disease events after menopause. JAMA 283:1845–1852, 2000.
18. Bush TL, Fried LP, Barrett-Connor E: Cholesterol, lipoproteins, and coronary heart disease in women. Clin Chem 34:B60, 1988.
19. Scandinavian Simvastatin Survival Study Group (4S): Randomized trial of cholesterol lowering in 4444 patients with coronary heart disease: The Scandinavian Simvastatin survival study. Lancet 344:1383, 1389, 1994.
20. Lewis SJ, Sacks FM, Mitchell JS, et al: Effect of pravastatin on cardiovascular events in women after myocardial infarction: The cholesterol and recurrent events (CARE) trial. J Am Coll Cardiol 32:140, 1998.
21. Downs JR, Clearfield M, Weis S, et al: Primary prevention of acute coronary events with lovastatin in men and women with average cholesterol levels. JAMA 279:1615, 1998.
22. The Post-Coronary Bypass Graft Trial Investigators: The effect of aggressive lowering of low-density lipoprotein cholesterol levels and low-dose anticoagulation on obstructive changes in saphenous-vein coronary-artery bypass grafts. N Engl J Med 336:153, 1997.
23. Summary of the Second Report of the National Cholesterol Education Program (NCEP) Expert Panel on Detection, Evaluation, and Treatment of High Blood Cholesterol in Adults (Adult Treatment Panel II): Expert Panel on Detection, Evaluation and Treatment of High Blood Cholesterol in Adults. JAMA 269:3015, 1993.
24. Darling GM, Johns JA, McCloud PI, Davis SR: Estrogen and progestin compared with simvastatin for hypercholesterolemia in postmenopausal women. N Engl J Med 337:595, 1997.
25. Davidson MH, Testolin LM, Maki KC, et al: A comparison of estrogen replacement, pravastatin, and combined treatment for the management of hypercholesterolemia in postmenopausal women. Arch Intern Med 157:1186, 1997.
26. Koh KK, Cardillo C, Bui MN, et al: Vascular effects of estrogen and cholesterol-lowering therapies in hypercholesterolemic postmenopausal women. Circulation 99:354, 1999.
27. Herrington DM, Werbel BL, Riley WA, et al: Individual and combined effects of estrogen/progestin therapy and lovastatin on lipids and flow-

mediated vasodilation of postmenopausal women with coronary artery disease. J Am Coll Cardiol 33:2030, 1999.

28. Walsh BW, Schiff I, Rosner B, et al: Effects of postmenopausal estrogen replacement on the concentrations and metabolism of plasma lipoproteins. N Engl J Med 325:1196, 1991.

29. Walsh BW, Kuller LH, Wild RA, et al: Effects of raloxifene on serum lipids and coagulation factors in healthy postmenopausal women. JAMA 279:1445, 1998.

30. Potter SM, Baum JA, Teng H, et al: Soy protein and isoflavones: Their effects on blood lipids and bone density in postmenopausal women. Am J Clin Nutr 68:1375S, 1998.

31. Wagner JD, Cefalu WT, Anthony MS, et al: Dietary soy protein and estrogen replacement therapy improve cardiovascular risk factors and decrease aortic cholesteryl ester content in ovariectomized cynomolgus monkeys. Metabolism 46:698, 1997.

Diabetes

32. Spelsberg A, Ridker PM, Manson JE: Carbohydrate metabolism, obesity, and diabetes. In Douglas PS (ed): Cardiovascular Health and Disease in Women. Philadelphia, WB Saunders, 1993, p 191.

33. Zuanetti G, Latini R, Maggioni AP, et al: Influence of diabetes on mortality in acute myocardial infarction: Data from the GISSI-2 study. J Am Coll Cardiol 22:1788, 1993.

34. Diabetes Control and Complications Trial Research Group: The effect of intensive treatment of diabetes on the development and progression of long-term complications in insulin-dependent diabetes mellitus. N Engl J Med 329:977, 1993.

35. Sowers JR: Diabetes mellitus and cardiovascular disease in women. Arch Intern Med 158:617, 1998.

36. Diabetes Control and Complications Trial Research Group: Effect of intensive diabetes management on macrovascular events and risk factors in the diabetes control and complications trial. Am J Cardiol 75:894, 1995.

Hypertension

37. Bittner V, Oparil S: Hypertension. In Douglas PS (ed): Cardiovascular Health and Disease in Women. Philadelphia, WB Saunders, 1993, p 63.

38. Hayes SN, Taler SJ: Hypertension in women: Current understanding of gender differences. Mayo Clin Proc 73:157, 1998.

Smoking

39. Fried LP, Becker DM: Smoking and cardiovascular disease. In Douglas PS (ed): Cardiovascular Health and Disease in Women. Philadelphia, WB Saunders, 1993, p 217.

40. Shapiro S, Sloane D, Rosenberg L, et al: Oral contraceptive use in relation to myocardial infarction. Lancet 1:743, 1979.

41. Hermanson B, Omenn GS, Kronmal RA, et al: Beneficial six-year outcome of smoking cessation in older men and women with coronary artery disease: Results from the CASS registry. N Engl J Med 319:1365, 1988.

Hemostasis

42. Eriksson M, Egberg N, Wamala S, et al: Relationship between plasma fibrinogen and coronary heart disease in women. Arterioscler Thromb Vasc Biol 19:67, 1999.

43. Weksler BB: Hemostasis and thrombosis. In Douglas PS (ed): Cardiovascular Health and Disease in Women. Philadelphia, WB Saunders, 1993, p 231.

44. Glueck CJ, Wang P, Fontaine RN, et al: Effect of exogenous estrogen on atherothrombotic vascular disease risk related to the presence or absence of Factor V Leiden mutation (resistance to activated protein C). Am J Cardiol 84:549, 1999.

Exercise

45. O'Toole ML: Exercise and physical activity. In Douglas PS (ed): Cardiovascular Health and Disease in Women. Philadelphia, WB Saunders, 1993, p 253.

46. Blair SN, Kohl HW, Paffenbarger RS, et al: Physical fitness and all-cause mortality: A prospective study of healthy men and women. JAMA 262:2395, 1989.

47. Manson JE, Stampfer MJ, Willet WC, et al: Physical activity and incidence of coronary heart disease and stroke in women. Circulation 91:927, 1995.

48. Manson JE, Hu FB, Rich-Edwards JW, et al: A prospective study of walking as compared with vigorous exercise in the prevention of coronary heart disease in women. N Engl J Med 341:650, 1999.

Psychosocial

49. Haynes SG, Czajkowski SM: Psychosocial and environmental correlates of heart disease. In Douglas PS (ed): Cardiovascular Health and Disease in Women. Philadelphia, WB Saunders, 1993, p 269.

50. Brezinka V, Kittel F: Psychosocial factors of coronary heart disease in women. Soc Sci Med 42:1351, 1996.

51. Muller JE, Abela GS, Nesto RW, Tofter GH: Triggers, acute risk factors and vulnerable plaques: The lexicon of a new frontier. J Am Coll Cardiol 23:809, 1994.

52. Milani RV, Lavie CJ, Cassidy MM: Effects of cardiac rehabilitation and exercise training programs on depression in patients after major coronary events. Am Heart J 132:726, 1996.

52a. Ridker PM, Hennekens CH, Buring JE, Rifai NC: C-reactive protein and other markers of inflammation in the prediction of cardiovascular disease in women. N Engl J Med 342:836–843, 2000.

52b. Ridker PM, Buring JE, Shih J, et al: Prospective study of C-reactive protein and the risk of future cardiovascular events among apparently healthy women. Circulation 98:731–733, 1998.

HORMONES

53. Lobo RA: Hormones, hormone replacement therapy, and heart disease. In Douglas PS (ed): Cardiovascular Health and Disease in Women. Philadelphia, WB Saunders, 1993, p 153.

54. Matthews KA, Meilahn E, Kuller LH, et al: Menopause and risk factors for coronary heart disease. N Engl J Med 321:641, 1989.

55. Karpanou EA, Vyssoulis GP, Papakyriakou SA, et al: Effects of menopause on aortic root function in hypertensive women. J Am Coll Cardiol 28:1562, 1996.

56. Schillaci G, Verdecchia P, Borgioni C, et al: Early cardiac changes after menopause. Hypertension 32:764, 1998.

57. Chasan-Taber L, Stampfer MJ: Epidemiology of oral contraceptives and cardiovascular disease. Ann Intern Med 128:467, 1998.

58. Dunn N, Thorogood M, Faragher B, et al: Oral contraceptives and myocardial infarction: Results of the MICA case-control study. BMJ 318:1579, 1999.

59. Hulley S, Grady D, Bush T, et al: Randomized trial of estrogen plus progestin for secondary prevention of coronary heart disease in postmenopausal women. JAMA 280:605, 1998.

60. The Writing Group for the PEPI Trial: Effects of estrogen or estrogen/progestin regimens on heart disease risk factors in postmenopausal women. The Postmenopausal Estrogen/Progestin Interventions (PEPI) Trial. JAMA 273:199, 1995. Final results: http://www.epibiostat.ucsf.edu/HERS/

61. Nabulsi AA, Folsom AR, White A, et al: Association of hormone replacement therapy with various cardiovascular risk factors in postmenopausal women. The Atherosclerosis Risk in Communities Study Investigators. N Engl J Med 328:1069, 1993.

62. Espeland MA, Marcovina SM, Miller V, et al: Effect of postmenopausal hormone therapy on lipoprotein(a) concentration. Circulation 97:979, 1998.

63. Crook D, Cust MP, Gangar KF, et al: Comparison of transdermal and oral estrogen-progestin replacement therapy: Effects on serum lipids and lipoproteins. Am J Obstet Gynecol 166:950, 1992.

64. Gerhard M, Ganz M: How do we explain the clinical benefits of estrogen? Circulation 92:5, 1995.

65. Mendelsohn ME, Karas RH: The protective effects of estrogen on the cardiovascular system. N Engl J Med 340:1801, 1999.

66. Sack MN, Rader DJ, Cannon RO III: Oestrogen and inhibition of oxidation of low-density lipoproteins in postmenopausal women. Lancet 343:269, 1994.

67. Keaney JF Jr, Shwaery GT, Xu A, et al: 17-Beta-estradiol preserves endothelial vasodilator function and limits low-density lipoprotein oxidation in hypercholesterolemic swine. Circulation 89:2251, 1994.

68. Nabulsi AA, Folsom AR, Szklo M, et al: No association of menopause and hormone replacement therapy with carotid artery intima-media thickness. Circulation 94:1857, 1996.

69. Reis SE, Gloth ST, Blumenthal RS, et al: Ethinyl estradiol acutely attenuates abnormal coronary vasomotor responses to acetylcholine in postmenopausal women. Circulation 89:52, 1994.

70. Lieberman EH, Gerhard MD, Uehata A, et al: Estrogen improves endothelium-dependent, flow-mediated vasodilation in postmenopausal women. Ann Intern Med 121:936, 1994.

71. Rosano GMC, Peters NS, Lefroy D, et al: 17-Beta-estradiol therapy lessens angina in postmenopausal women with Syndrome X. J Am Coll Cardiol 28:1500, 1996.

72. Gebara OC, Mittleman MA, Sutherland P, et al: Association between increased estrogen status and increased fibrinolytic potential in the Framingham Offspring Study. Circulation 91:1952, 1995.

73. Koh KK, Mincemoyer R, Bui MN, et al: Effects of hormone-replacement therapy on fibrinolysis in postmenopausal women. N Engl J Med 336:683, 1997.

74. Proudler AJ, Ahmed AIH, Crook D, et al: Hormone replacement therapy and serum angiotensin-converting-enzyme activity in postmenopausal women. Lancet 346:89, 1995.

75. Grady D, Rubin SM, Petitti DB, et al: Hormone therapy to prevent disease and prolong life in postmenopausal women. Ann Intern Med 117:1016, 1992.

76. Col NF, Eckman MH, Karas RH, et al: Patient-specific decisions about hormone replacement therapy in postmenopausal women. JAMA 277:1140, 1997.

77. Col NF, Pauker SG, Goldberg RJ, et al: Individualizing therapy to prevent long-term consequences of estrogen deficiency in postmenopausal women. Arch Intern Med 159:1458, 1999.

78. Grady D, Gebretsadik T, Kerlikowske K, et al: Hormone replacement therapy and endometrial cancer risk: A meta-analysis. Obstet Gynecol 85:304, 1995.

79. Grodstein F, Newcomb PA, Stampfer MJ: Postmenopausal hormone therapy and the risk of colorectal cancer: A review and meta-analysis. Am J Med 106:574, 1999.

80. Stampfer MJ, Colditz GA: Estrogen replacement therapy and coronary heart disease: A quantitative assessment of the epidemiologic evidence. Prev Med 20:47, 1991.

81. Stampfer MJ, Colditz GA, Willett WC, et al: Postmenopausal estrogen therapy and cardiovascular disease: Ten-year follow-up from the Nurses' Health Study. N Engl J Med 325:756, 1991.

82. Finucane FF, Madans JH, Bush TL, et al: Decreased risk of stroke among postmenopausal hormone users: Results from a national cohort. Arch Intern Med 153:73, 1993.

83. Yaffe K, Sawaya G, Lieberburg I, Grady D: Estrogen therapy in postmenopausal women: Effects on cognitive function and dementia. JAMA 279:688, 1998.

84. Love RR, Newcomb PA, Wiebe DA, et al: Effects of tamoxifen therapy on lipid and lipoprotein levels in postmenopausal patients with node-negative breast cancer. J Natl Cancer Inst 82:1327, 1990.

85. Rutqvist LE, Mattsson A: Cardiac and thromboembolic morbidity among postmenopausal women with early-stage breast cancer in a randomized trial of adjuvant tamoxifen: The Stockholm Breast Cancer Study Group. J Natl Cancer Inst 85:1398, 1993.

86. Khovidhunkit W, Shoback DM: Clinical effects of raloxifene hydrochloride in women. Ann Intern Med 130:431, 1999.

87. Figtree GA, Lu Y, Webb CM, Collins P: Raloxifene acutely relaxes rabbit coronary arteries in vitro by an estrogen receptor–dependent and nitric oxide–dependent mechanism. Circulation 100:1095, 1999.

88. Clarkson TB, Anthony MS, Jerome CP: Lack of effect of raloxifene on coronary artery atherosclerosis of postmenopausal monkeys. J Clin Endocrinol Metab 83:721, 1998.

89. Sullivan JM, Vander Zwaag R, Lemp GF, et al: Postmenopausal estrogen use and coronary atherosclerosis. Ann Intern Med 108:358, 1988.

90. Sullivan JM, Vander Zwaag R, Hughes JP, et al: Estrogen replacement and coronary artery disease: Effect on survival in postmenopausal women. Arch Intern Med 150:2557, 1990.

91. Sullivan JM, El-Zeky F, Vander Zwaag R, Ramanathan KK: Estrogen replacement therapy after coronary artery bypass surgery: Effect on survival. Circulation 345:669, 1995.

92. Herrington DM: The HERS trial results: Paradigms lost? Ann Intern Med 131:463, 1999.

92a. Blumenthal RS, Zacur HA, Reis SE, Post WS: Beyond the null hypothesis—Do the HERS results disprove the estrogen/coronary heart disease hypothesis? Am J Cardiol 85:1015–1017, 2000.

93. Ridker PM, Hennekens CN, Rifai N, et al: Hormone replacement therapy and increased plasma concentration of C-reactive protein. Circulation 100:713, 1999.

94. Cushman M, Legault C, Barrett-Connor E, et al: Effect of postmenopausal hormones on inflammation-sensitive proteins: The postmenopausal estrogen/progestin interventions (PEPI) study. Circulation 100:717, 1999.

95. Petitti DB: Hormone replacement therapy and heart disease prevention: Experimentation trumps observation. JAMA 280:650, 1998.

96. Henrich JB: The postmenopausal estrogen/breast cancer controversy. JAMA 268:1900, 1992.

97. Colditz GA, Hankinson SE, Hunter DJ, et al: The use of estrogens and progestins and the risk of breast cancer in postmenopausal women. N Engl J Med 332:1589, 1995.

98. Cummings SR, Eckert S, Krueger KA, et al: The effect of raloxifene on risk of breast cancer in post-menopausal women: Results from the MORE (Multiple Outcomes of Raloxifene Evaluation) trial. JAMA 281:2189, 1999.

99. Connelly MT, Ferrari N, Hagen N, Inui TS: Patient-identified needs for hormone replacement therapy counseling: A qualitative study. Ann Intern Med 131:265, 1999.

100. Devor M, Barrett-Connor E, Renvall M, et al: Estrogen replacement therapy and the risk of venous thrombosis. Am J Med 92:275, 1992.

101. Posthuma WFM, Westendorp RGJ, Vandenbroucke JP: Cardioprotective effect of hormone replacement therapy in postmenopausal women: Is the evidence biased? BMJ 308:1268, 1994.

102. American College of Physicians: Guidelines for counseling postmenopausal women about preventive hormone therapy. Ann Intern Med 117:1038, 1992.

102a. Grodstein F, Stampfer MJ, Manson JE, et al: Postmenopausal estrogen and progestin use and the risk of cardiovascular disease. N Engl J Med 332:1589, 1996.

102b. Lissin LW, Cooke JP: Phytoestrogens and cardiovascular health. J Am Coll Cardiol 35:1403–1410, 2000.

EVALUATION OF CHEST PAIN IN WOMEN

103. Weiner DA, Ryan TJ, McCabe CH, et al: Correlations among history of angina, ST-segment response and prevalence of coronary artery disease in the coronary artery surgery study (CASS). N Engl J Med 301:230, 1979.

104. DeSanctis RW: Clinical manifestations of coronary artery disease: Chest pain in women. In Wenger NK, Speroff L, Packard B (eds): Cardiovascular Health and Disease in Women. Greenwich, CT, Le Jacq Communications, 1993, p 67.

105. Sullivan AK, Holdright DR, Wright CA, et al: Chest pain in women: Clinical, investigative, and prognostic features. BMJ 308:883, 1994.

106. Douglas PS, Ginsburg GS: The evaluation of chest pain in women. N Engl J Med 334:1311, 1996.

107. Pepine CJ, Abrams J, Marks RG, et al: Characteristics of a contemporary population with angina pectoris. Am J Cardiol 74:226, 1994.

108. Milner K, Funk M, Richards S, et al: Gender differences in symptom presentation associated with coronary heart disease. Am J Cardiol 84:396, 1999.

109. Peterson ED, Alexander KP: Learning to suspect the unexpected: Evaluating women with cardiac syndromes. Am Heart J 136:186, 1998.

110. Woodfield SL, Lundergan CF, Reiner JS, et al: Gender and acute myocardial infarction: Is there a different response to thrombolysis? J Am Coll Cardiol 29:35, 1997.

110a. Buchtal SD, den Hollander JA, Merz CNB, et al: Abnormal myocardial phosphorus-31 nuclear magnetic resonance spectroscopy in women with chest pain but normal coronary angiograms. N Engl J Med 342:829–835, 2000.

111. Mautner SL, Lin F, Mautner GC, Roberts WC: Comparison in women versus men of composition of atherosclerotic plaques in native coronary arteries and in saphenous veins used as aortocoronary conduits. J Am Coll Cardiol 21:1312, 1992.

112. Murabito JM, Evans JC, Larson MG, Levy D: Prognosis after the onset of coronary heart disease: An investigation of differences in outcome between the sexes according to initial coronary disease presentation. Circulation 88:2548, 1993.

113. Orencia A, Bailey K, Yawn BP, Kottke TE: Effect of gender on long-term outcome of angina pectoris and myocardial infarction/sudden unexpected death. JAMA 270:2392, 1993.

114. LaCroix AZ, Guralnik JM, Curb JD, et al: Chest pain and coronary heart disease mortality among older men and women in three communities. Circulation 81:437, 1990.

115. Vaccarino V, Krumholz HM, Berkman LF, Horwitz RI: Sex differences in mortality after myocardial infarction. Circulation 91:1861, 1995.

116. Lualdi JC, Douglas PS: Considerations in the selection of noninvasive testing for the diagnosis of coronary artery disease. Cardiol Rev 6:278, 1998.

117. Weiner DA, Ryan TJ, Parsons L, et al: Long-term prognostic value of exercise testing in men and women from the coronary artery surgery study (CASS) registry. Am J Cardiol 75:865, 1995.

118. Alexander KP, Shaw LJ, Delong ER, et al: Value of exercise treadmill testing in women. J Am Coll Cardiol 32:1657, 1998.

119. Kwok Y, Kim C, Grady D, et al: Meta-analysis of exercise testing to detect coronary artery disease in women. Am J Cardiol 83:660, 1999.

120. Fleischmann KE, Hunink MGM, Kuntz KM, Douglas PS: Exercise echocardiography or exercise SPECT imaging? A meta-analysis of diagnostic test performance. JAMA 280:913, 1998.

121. Tong AT, Douglas PS: Stress echocardiography in women. Cardiol Clin 17:573, 1999.

122. Fintel DJ, Links JM, Brinker JA, et al: Improved diagnostic performance of exercise thallium-201 single photon emission computed tomography over planar imaging in the diagnosis of coronary artery disease: A receiver operating characteristic analysis. J Am Coll Cardiol 13:600, 1989.

123. Taillefer R, DePuey EG, Udelson JE, et al: Comparative diagnostic accuracy of Tl-201 and Tc-99m sestamibi SPECT imaging (perfusion and ECG-gated SPECT) in detecting coronary artery disease in women. J Am Coll Cardiol 29:69, 1997.

124. Marwick TH, Anderson T, Williams MJ, et al: Exercise echocardiography is an accurate and cost-efficient technique for detection of coronary artery disease in women. J Am Coll Cardiol 26:335, 1995.

125. Kuntz KM, Fleischmann KE, Hunink MGM, Douglas PS: Cost-effectiveness of diagnostic strategies for patients with chest pain. Ann Intern Med 130:709, 1999.

126. Kim C, Kwok YS, Saha S, Redberg RF: Diagnosis of suspected coronary artery disease in women: A cost-effectiveness analysis. Am Heart J 137:1019, 1999.

127. Steen MK, Jacobs AK, Freney D, et al: Gender related differences in complications during coronary angiography. Circulation 86(Suppl I):254, 1992.

Gender Bias

128. Tobin JN, Wassertheil-Smoller S, Wexler JP, et al: Sex bias in considering coronary bypass surgery. Ann Intern Med 107:19, 1987.

129. Ayanian JZ, Epstein AM: Differences in the use of procedures between women and men hospitalized for coronary heart disease. N Engl J Med 325:221, 1991.

130. Schulman KA, Berlin JA, Harless W, et al: The effect of race and sex on physicians' recommendations for cardiac catheterization. N Engl J Med 340:618, 1999.

131. Shaw LJ, Miller DD, Romeis JC, et al: Gender differences in the noninvasive evaluation and management of patients with suspected coronary artery disease. Ann Intern Med 120:559, 1991.

MANAGEMENT OF CAD

132. Fetters JK, Peterson ED, Shaw LJ, et al: Sex-specific differences in coronary artery disease risk factors, evaluation, and treatment: Have they been adequately evaluated? Am Heart J 131:796, 1996.

133. Manson JE, Stampfer MJ, Colditz GA, et al: A prospective study of aspirin use and primary prevention of cardiovascular disease in women. JAMA 266:521, 1991.

134. Harpaz D, Benderly M, Goldbourt U, et al: Effect of aspirin on mortality in women with symptomatic or silent myocardial ischemia. Am J Cardiol 78:1215, 1996.

135. Antiplatelet Trialists' Collaboration: Collaborative overview of randomi-

sed trials of antiplatelet therapy: II. Maintenance of vascular graft or arterial patency by antiplatelet therapy. BMJ 308:159, 1994.

136. Goldschmidt-Clermont PJ, Schulman SP, Bray PF, et al: Refining the treatment of women with unstable angina: A randomized, double-blind, comparative safety and efficacy evaluation of Integrelin versus aspirin in the management of unstable angina. Clin Cardiol 19:869, 1996.

137. Edmond M, Mock MB, Davis KB, et al: Long-term survival of medically treated patients in the coronary artery surgery study (CASS) registry. Circulation 90:2645, 1994.

138. Schwartz LM, Fisher ES, Tosteson NA, et al: Treatment and health outcomes of women and men in a cohort with coronary artery disease. Arch Intern Med 157:1545, 1997.

139. Cowley MJ, Mullin SM, Kelsey SF, et al: Sex differences in early and long-term results of coronary angioplasty in the NHLBI PTCA registry. Circulation 71:90, 1985.

140. Kelsey SF, James M, Holubkov AL, et al: Results of percutaneous transluminal coronary angioplasty in women: 1985–1986 NHLBI coronary angioplasty registry. Circulation 87:720, 1993.

141. Arnold AM, Mick MJ, Piedmonte MR, Simpfendorfer C: Gender differences for coronary angioplasty. Am J Cardiol 74:18, 1994.

142. Weintraub WS, Wenger NK, Kosinski AS, et al: Percutaneous transluminal coronary angioplasty in women compared with men. J Am Coll Cardiol 24:81, 1994.

143. Bell MR, Holmes DR, Berger PB, et al: The changing in-hospital mortality of women undergoing percutaneous transluminal coronary angioplasty. JAMA 269:2091, 1993.

144. Welty FK, Mittleman MA, Healy RW, et al: Similar results of percutaneous transluminal coronary angioplasty for women and men with postmyocardial infarction ischemia. J Am Coll Cardiol 23:35, 1994.

145. Malenka DJ, O'Rourke D, Miller MA, et al: Cause of in-hospital death in 12,232 consecutive patients undergoing percutaneous transluminal coronary angioplasty. Am Heart J 137:632, 1999.

146. Keelan ET, Nunez BD, Grill DE, et al: Comparison of immediate and long-term outcome of coronary angioplasty performed for unstable angina and rest pain in men and women. Mayo Clin Proc 72:5, 1997.

147. O'Connor GT, Malenka DJ, Quinton H, et al: Multivariate prediction of in-hospital mortality after percutaneous coronary interventions in 1994–1996. J Am Coll Cardiol 34:681, 1999.

148. Greenberg MA, Mueller HS: Why the excess mortality in women after PTCA? Circulation 87:1030, 1993.

149. Jacobs AK, Yeh W, Kelsey SF, et al: Gender differences in patients undergoing contemporary percutaneous coronary intervention: The 1997–1998 NHLBI Dynamic Registry. Circulation 98:I-198, 1998.

150. O'Brien JE, Peterson ED, Keeler GP, et al: Relation between estrogen replacement therapy and restenosis after percutaneous coronary interventions. J Am Coll Cardiol 28:1111, 1996.

151. O'Keefe JH Jr, Kim SC, Hall RR, et al: Estrogen replacement therapy after coronary angioplasty in women. J Am Coll Cardiol 29:1, 1997.

Coronary Artery Bypass Grafting

152. King KB, Clark PC, Hicks GL: Patterns of referral and recovery in women and men undergoing coronary artery bypass grafting. Am J Cardiol 69:179, 1992.

153. O'Connor GT, Morton JR, Diehl MJ, et al, for the Northern New England Cardiovascular Disease Study Group: Differences between men and women in hospital mortality associated with coronary artery bypass graft surgery. Circulation 88:2104, 1993.

154. Edwards FH, Carey JS, Grover FL, et al: Impact of gender on coronary bypass operative mortality. Ann Thorac Surg 66:125, 1998.

ACUTE CORONARY SYNDROMES

155. Collins LJ, Douglas PS: Acute coronary syndromes. In Charney P (ed): Coronary Artery Disease in Women: Prevention, Diagnosis and Management. Philadelphia, American College of Physicians, 1999, p 401.

156. Maynard C, Litwin PE, Martin JS, Weaver WD: Gender differences in the treatment and outcome of acute myocardial infarction: Results from the Myocardial Infarction Triage and Intervention Registry. Arch Intern Med 152:972, 1992.

157. Jenkins JS, Flaker GC, Nolte B, et al: Causes of higher in-hospital mortality in women than in men after acute myocardial infarction. Am J Cardiol 73:319, 1994.

158. Wilkinson P, Laji K, Ranjadayalan K, et al: Acute myocardial infarction in women: Survival analysis in first six months. BMJ 309:566, 1994.

159. White HD, Barbash GI, Modan M, et al: After correcting for worse baseline characteristics, women treated with thrombolytic therapy for acute myocardial infarction have the same mortality and morbidity as men except for a higher incidence of hemorrhagic stroke. The Investigators of the International Tissue Plasminogen Activator/Streptokinase Mortality Study. Circulation 88:2097, 1993.

160. Lincoff AM, Califf RM, Ellis SG, et al: Thrombolytic therapy for women with myocardial infarction: Is there a gender gap? Thrombolysis and angioplasty in myocardial infarction study group. J Am Coll Cardiol 22:1780, 1993.

161. Kostis JB, Wilson AC, O'Dowd KO, et al: Sex differences in the management and long-term outcome of acute myocardial infarction: A statewide study. Circulation 90:1715, 1994.

162. Chandra NC, Ziegelstein RC, Rogers WJ, et al: Observations of the treatment of women in the United States with myocardial infarction. Arch Intern Med 158:981, 1998.

163. Weaver WD, White HD, Wilcox RG, et al: Comparisons of characteristics and outcomes among women and men with acute myocardial infarction treated with thrombolytic therapy. JAMA 275:777, 1996.

164. Tunstall-Pedoe H, Morrison C, Woodward M, et al: Sex differences in myocardial infarction and coronary deaths in the Scottish MONICA population of Glasgow 1985 to 1991: Presentation, diagnosis, treatment, and 28-day case fatality of 3,991 events in men and 1,551 events in women. Circulation 93:1981, 1996.

165. Maynard C, Weaver WD: Treatment of women with acute MI: New findings from the MITI registry. J Myocardial Ischemia 4:27, 1992.

166. Clarke KW, Gray D, Keating NA, Hampton JR: Do women with acute myocardial infarction receive the same treatment as men? BMJ 309:563, 1994.

167. Yarzebski J, Col N, Pagley P, et al: Gender differences and factors associated with the receipt of thrombolytic therapy in patients with acute myocardial infarction: A community-wide perspective. Am Heart J 131:43, 1996.

168. Adams JN, Jamieson M, Rawles JM, et al: Women and myocardial infarction: Agism rather than sexism? Br Heart J 73:87, 1995.

169. Krumholz HM, Douglas PS, Lauer MS, Pasternak RC: Selection of patients for coronary angiography and coronary revascularization early after myocardial infarction: Is there evidence for a gender bias? Ann Intern Med 116:785, 1992.

170. Funk M, Griffey KA: Relation of gender to the use of cardiac procedures in acute myocardial infarction. Am J Cardiol 74:1170, 1994.

171. Healy B: The Yentl syndrome. N Engl J Med 325:274, 1991.

172. Greenland P, Reicher-Reiss H, Goldbourt U, Behar S: In-hospital and 1-year mortality in 1,524 women after myocardial infarction: Comparison with 4,315 men. Circulation 83:484, 1991.

173. Hamilton GA: Recovery from acute myocardial infarction in women. Cardiology 77(Suppl 2):58, 1990.

174. Hochman JS, McCabe CH, Stone PH, et al: Outcome and profile of women and men presenting with acute coronary syndromes: A report from TIMI IIIB. TIMI investigators. Thrombolysis in myocardial infarction. J Am Coll Cardiol 30:141, 1997.

175. Hochman JS, Tamis JE, Thompson TD, et al: Sex, clinical presentation, and outcome in patients with acute coronary syndromes. N Engl J Med 341:226, 1999

176. Lee KL, Woodlief LH, Topol EJ, et al: Predictors of 30-day mortality in the era of reperfusion for acute myocardial infarction: Results from an international trial of 41,021 patients. Circulation 91:1659, 1995.

177. Vaccarino V, Parsons L, Every NR, et al: Sex-based differences in early mortality after myocardial infarction. N Engl J Med 341:217, 1999.

178. Malacrida R, Genoni M, Maggioni AP, et al: A comparison of the early outcome of acute myocardial infarction in women and men. N Engl J Med 338:8, 1998.

179. Moen EK, Asher CR, Miller DP, et al: Long-term follow-up of gender-specific outcomes after thrombolytic therapy for acute myocardial infarction from the GUSTO-I trial. J Womens Health 6:285, 1997.

180. Maggioni AP, Franzosi MG, Santoro E, et al, and the Gruppo Italiano per lo studio della sopravvivenza nell'infarto miocardico II (GISSI-2), and the International Study Group: The risk of stroke in patients with acute myocardial infarction after thrombolytic and antithrombotic treatment. N Engl J Med 327:1, 1992.

181. Becker RC, Terrin M, Ross R, et al, and the Thrombolysis in Myocardial Infarction Investigators: Comparison of clinical outcomes for women and men after acute myocardial infarction. Ann Intern Med 120:638, 1994.

182. Grines CL, Browne KF, Marco J, et al, for the Primary Angioplasty in Myocardial Infarction Study Group: A comparison of immediate angioplasty with thrombolytic therapy for acute myocardial infarction. N Engl J Med 328:673, 1993.

183. Stone GW, Grines CL, Browne KF, et al: A comparison of in-hospital outcome in men versus women treated by either thrombolytic therapy or primary coronary angioplasty for acute myocardial infarction. Am J Cardiol 75:987, 1995.

184. Pfeffer MA, Braunwald E, Moye LA, et al, on behalf of the SAVE investigators: Effect of captopril on mortality and morbidity in patients with left ventricular dysfunction after myocardial infarction: Results of the survival and ventricular enlargement trial. N Engl J Med 327:669, 1992.

185. ISIS-4 (Fourth International Study of Infarct Survival) Collaborative Group: A randomised factorial trial assessing early oral captopril, oral mononitrate, and intravenous magnesium sulphate in 58,050 patients with suspected acute myocardial infarction. Lancet 345:669, 1995.

186. Rodda BE: The Timolol Myocardial Infarction Study: An evaluation of selected variables. Circulation 67:I-101, I-106, 1983.

187. ISIS-1 Collaborative Group: Randomised trial of intravenous atenolol among 16,027 cases of suspected acute myocardial infarction. Lancet 2:57, 1986.

188. Yusuf S, Peto R, Lewis J, et al: Beta-blockade during and after myocardial infarction: An overview of the randomized trials. Progr Cardiovasc Dis 27:335, 1985.

189. Petrie MC, Dawson NF, Murdoch DR, et al: Failure of women's hearts. Circulation 99:2334, 1999.

Chapter 59

Cardiovascular Disease in Athletes

BARRY J. MARON

During the past several years, the medical community and the lay public have become increasingly interested in and concerned about the causes of sudden and unexpected deaths in young trained athletes.[1] Such catastrophes are always unexpected events and, though relatively uncommon,[2, 3] nevertheless achieve high visibility and have a particularly tragic and devastating impact on the community.[4] As a consequence, the cardiovascular diseases[4-15] and circumstances[16, 17, 17a] responsible for sudden death in athletes participating in sporting activities have been the subject of several reports, and a large measure of clarification has resulted.

CAUSES OF SUDDEN DEATH

Several autopsy-based studies have documented the cardiovascular diseases responsible for sudden death in young competitive athletes or youthful asymptomatic individuals with active sports-related life styles.[2, 5-9] Of note, these structural abnormalities should not be confused with the normal physiological adaptations in cardiac dimensions evident in many trained athletes and consisting of increased left ventricular mass with end-distolic cavity enlargement or occasionally increased wall thickness.[18-20] It is also important to be cautious in assigning frequency estimates for various cardiovascular diseases as causes of sudden death in athletes; patient selection biases unavoidably influence the acquisition of such data in the absence of a systematic national registry.

Young Athletes

It has been convincingly demonstrated that the vast majority of sudden deaths in young athletes (age < 35 years) are due to various congenital cardiovascular diseases (>20) (see Figs. 59-1 to 59-4.)[2, 4-9] Indeed, virtually any disease capable of causing sudden death in young individuals may also do so in young athletes. It should be emphasized that all of these diseases are uncommon within the general population and do not occur with the same frequency as causes of sudden death in young athletes; indeed, most of the diseases are responsible for just 5 percent or less of all athletic field deaths.[4, 5]

HYPERTROPHIC CARDIOMYOPATHY (HCM) (see Chap. 48). The majority of studies show HCM to be the single most common cause of sudden death in young athletes, accounting for about one-third of these catastrophes.[5] HCM is a primary and familial cardiac malformation characterized by asymmetrical left ventricular hypertrophy and nondilated ventricular cavities[21-24] (Fig. 59-2), with heterogeneous expression and diverse clinical course. Disease-causing mutations in nine genes encoding proteins of the sarcomere (and >100 mutations) have been reported.[23, 24]

HCM is a relatively common genetically transmitted disease, occurring in about 0.2 percent (1 in 500) of the general population.[25]

Not uncommonly, HCM is responsible for sudden cardiac death in young and asymptomatic individuals and frequently occurs during moderate or severe exertion.[21, 22] Indeed, the stress of intense training and competition (and associated alterations in blood volume, hydration, and electrolytes) undoubtedly increases that risk to some degree.[26] In HCM, particularly strenuous physical activity may act as a trigger mechanism for generating potentially lethal ventricular tachyarrhythmias, given the underlying electrophysiologically unstable myocardial substrate composed of replacement fibrosis (which is probably the consequence of

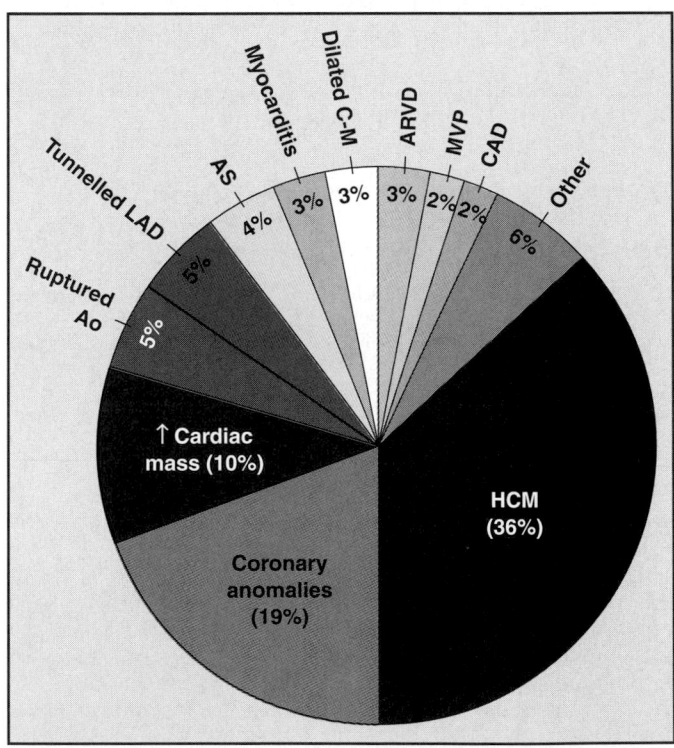

FIGURE 59-1. Causes of sudden cardiac death in young competitive athletes (median age, 17 years) based on systematic tracking of 158 athletes in the United States, primarily 1985-1995. In an additional 2 percent of the patients, no evidence of cardiovascular disease sufficient to explain death was identified at necropsy. ↑ (increased) cardiac mass = hearts with increased weight and some morphological features consistent with (but not diagnostic of) hypertrophic cardiomyopathy. (From Maron BJ, Thompson PD, Puffer JC, et al: Cardiovascular preparticipation screening of competitive athletes. Circulation 94:850–856, 1996. Adapted and reproduced with permission of the American Heart Association.)

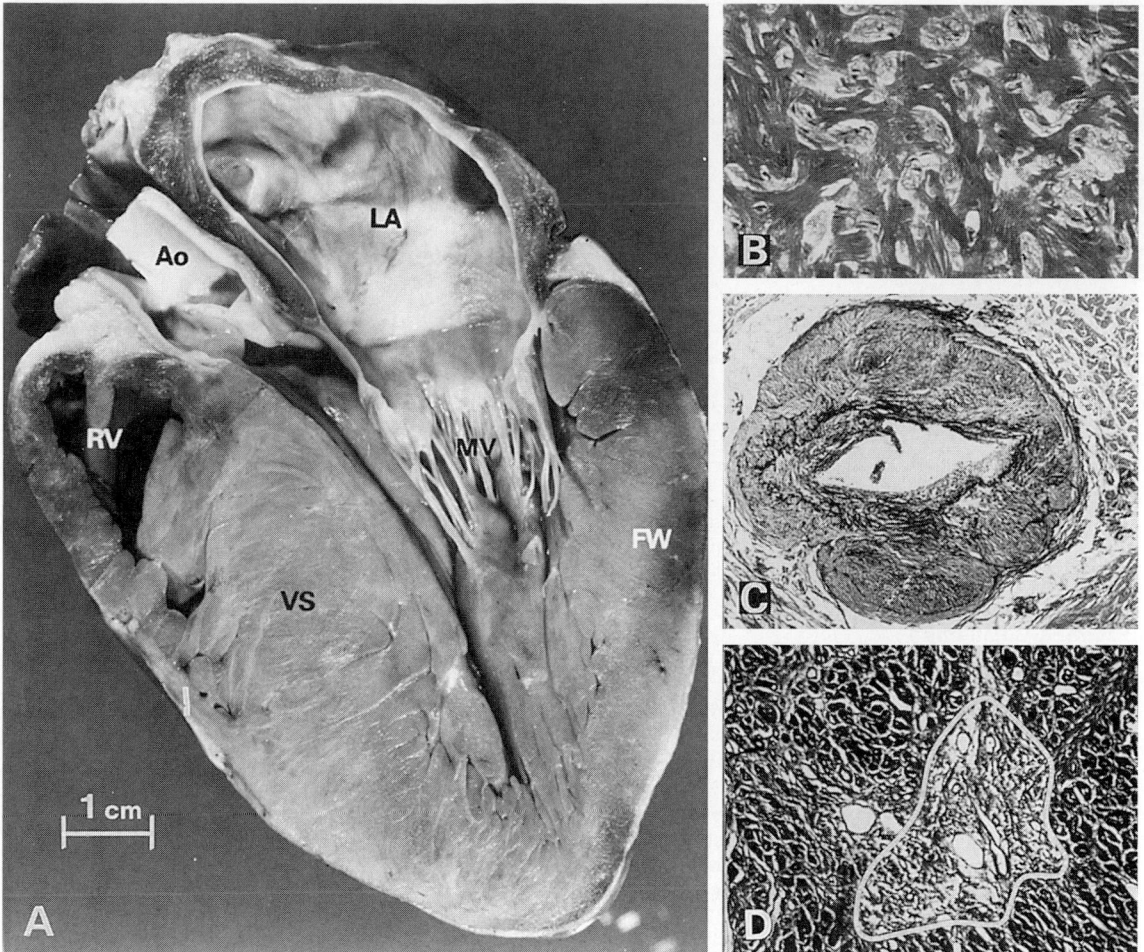

FIGURE 59–2. Morphological components of the disease process in hypertrophic cardiomyopathy (HCM), the most common cause of sudden death in young competitive athletes. *A,* Gross heart specimen sectioned in a cross-sectional plane similar to that of the echocardiographic (parasternal) long axis; left ventricular wall thickening shows an asymmetrical pattern and is confined primarily to the ventricular septum (VS), which bulges prominently into the left ventricular outflow tract. The left ventricular cavity appears reduced in size. FW = left ventricular free wall. *B–D,* Histological features characteristic of left ventricular myocardium in HCM. *B,* Markedly disordered architecture with adjacent hypertrophied cardiac muscle cells arranged at perpendicular and oblique angles. *C,* An intramural coronary artery with thickened wall, due primarily to medial hypertrophy, and with apparently narrowed lumen. *D,* Replacement fibrosis in an area of ventricular myocardium adjacent to an abnormal intramural coronary artery, and probably a consequence of ischemia. Ao = aorta; LA = left atrium; RV = right ventricle. (From Maron J: Hypertrophic cardiomyopathy. Lancet 350:127–133, 1997.)

ischemia) and disorganized cardiac muscle cells (see Fig. 59–2).

Disease variables that appear to identify those individuals at greatly increased risk include prior aborted cardiac arrest or sustained ventricular tachycardia, family history of sudden or other premature HCM-related death (or high-risk genotype), multiple-repetitive nonsustained ventricular tachycardia on ambulatory Holter electrocardiographic (ECG) recording, recurrent syncope particularly when exertional and in the young, massive degrees of left ventricular hypertrophy, and possibly hypotensive blood pressure response to exercise.[22] Patients who have HCM and who are judged to be at high risk for sudden death may be considered for primary prevention of sudden death with prophylactic cardioverter-defibrillator implants.[27]

Although HCM may be suspected during preparticipation sports evaluations by the prior occurrence of exertional syncope, a family history of HCM or premature cardiac death, or the presence of a heart murmur, these features are relatively uncommon among all individuals affected by the disease.[22] Consequently, screening procedures limited to customary history and physical examination cannot be expected to identify HCM reliably and consistently.[28]

In some young athletes, segmental ventricular septal thickening (13 to 15 mm) consistent with a relatively mild morphological expression of HCM may be difficult to distinguish from the physiological and benign form of left ventricular hypertrophy that represents an adaptation to athletic training (i.e., "athlete's heart").[28a, 28b] Athletes within this morphological "gray zone" present an important and not uncommon clinical problem in which the differential diagnosis between HCM and athlete's heart can often be resolved by noninvasive testing[29] (Fig. 59–3). This distinction may have particularly important implications, given that young athletes with an unequivocal diagnosis of HCM are discouraged from participation in most competitive sports to minimize risk (with the possible exception of those sports considered to be of low intensity).[30] Conversely, improper diagnosis of cardiac disease in an athlete may lead to unnecessary withdrawal from athletics, thereby depriving that individual of the varied benefits of sports.

In addition, hearts encountered at autopsy not infrequently have increased mass (and left ventricular wall thickness) and nondilated ventricular cavities suggestive of HCM, but with other objective morphological findings not sufficiently striking to permit a definitive diagnosis.[5] It is

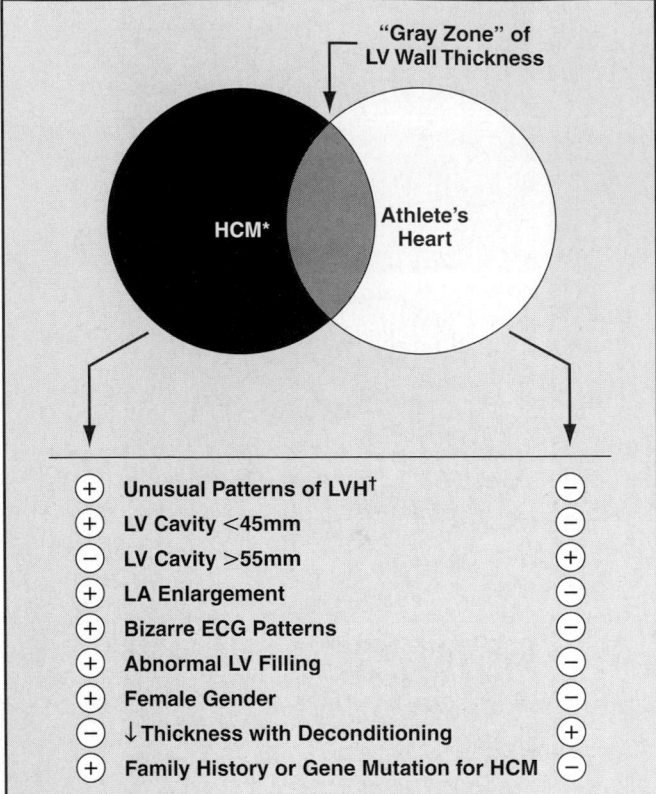

"Gray Zone" of LV Wall Thickness

HCM*

Athlete's Heart

(+) Unusual Patterns of LVH†	(−)
(+) LV Cavity <45mm	(−)
(−) LV Cavity >55mm	(+)
(+) LA Enlargement	(−)
(+) Bizarre ECG Patterns	(−)
(+) Abnormal LV Filling	(−)
(+) Female Gender	(−)
(−) ↓ Thickness with Deconditioning	(+)
(+) Family History or Gene Mutation for HCM	(−)

FIGURE 59–3. Chart depicting the criteria used to distinguish hypertrophic cardiomyopathy (HCM) from athlete's heart when the left ventricular (LV) wall thickness is within the shaded gray zone of overlap (13 to 15 mm), consistent with both diagnoses. *Assumed to be the nonobstructive form of HCM in this discussion, because the presence of substantial mitral valve systolic anterior motion would confirm, per se, the diagnosis of HCM in an athlete. †May involve various abnormalities, including heterogeneous distribution of left ventricular hypertrophy (LVH) in which asymmetry is prominent, and adjacent regions may be of greatly different thicknesses, with sharp transitions evident between segments. Also, patterns in which the anterior ventricular septum is spared from the hypertrophic process and the region of predominant thickening may be in the posterior portion of the septum or anterolateral or posterior free wall. ↓ = decreased; LA = left atrial. (From Maron BJ, Pelliccia A, Spirito P: Cardiac disease in young trained athletes: Insights into methods for distinguishing athlete's heart from structural heart disease with particular emphasis on hypertrophic cardiomyopathy. Circulation 91:1596–1601, 1995. Reproduced with permission of the American Heart Association.)

uncertain whether some of these cases represent mild morphological expressions of HCM or, conceivably, unusual examples of marked physiological left ventricular hypertrophy associated with deleterious consequences.

CONGENITAL CORONARY ARTERY MALFORMATIONS (see Chaps. 43 and 44). Second in importance and frequency to HCM are the congenital coronary artery anomalies of wrong aortic sinus origin (occurring in about 20 percent).[5] The most common of these lesions causing sudden death in athletes appears to be anomalous origin of the left main coronary artery from the right (anterior) sinus of Valsalva,[31-33] although the mirror-image malformation, anomalous right coronary artery from the left aortic sinus, has also been incriminated in these catastrophes[33] (Fig. 59–4). Such malformations are difficult to recognize during life because they are usually unassociated with symptoms (e.g., exertional syncope or chest pain) or alterations in the 12-lead or exercise ECG; therefore, diagnosis requires a high index of suspicion.[31] Indeed, occurrence of one or more episodes of exertional syncope in a young athlete

FIGURE 59–4. See color plate 30.

necessitates definitive exclusion of a coronary anomaly. It may also be possible to identify (or raise a strong suspicion of) anomalous coronaries of wrong sinus origin using transthoracic or transesophageal echocardiography,[4, 34] which can then lead to anatomical confirmation with coronary arteriography. However, congenital coronary artery malformations cannot be reliably identified by standard preparticipation athletic screening.

These coronary malformations should result in exclusion from intense competitive sports to reduce the risk of a cardiac event.[26] Also, wrong sinus anomalies are amenable to surgical correction with bypass grafting, which is the most common approach to restore distal coronary flow.[4, 31-33]

Myocardial ischemia (see Chap. 34) in young individuals with coronary artery anomalies involving wrong sinus origin probably occurs in infrequent bursts, cumulative with time, ultimately resulting in patchy myocardial necrosis and fibrosis; this process could predispose to lethal ventricular tachyarrhythmias by creating an electrically unstable myocardial substrate. Potential mechanisms that have been advanced include (1) acute angled takeoff and kinking or flaplike closure at the origin of the coronary artery and (2) compression of the anomalous artery between the aorta and pulmonary trunk during exercise. Furthermore, the proximal portion of the artery may be intramural (i.e., within the aortic tunica media), which could further aggravate coronary obstruction, particularly with aortic expansion during exercise.

Other unusual causes of exercise-related sudden deaths in young athletes include hypoplasia of the right coronary and left circumflex arteries, left anterior descending or right coronary artery origin from the pulmonary trunk, virtual absence of the left coronary artery, and spontaneous coronary arterial intussusception and coronary artery dissection.[5, 8, 9]

CORONARY ARTERY DISEASE (see Chaps. 35 to 37). Atherosclerotic coronary artery disease may be responsible for sudden death during physical exertion in youthful athletes[2, 5-9] and can be associated with acute plaque rupture[35] (Fig. 59–5). Indeed, Corrado and colleagues[36] have emphasized the occurrence of premature atherosclerotic coronary disease as a prominent cause of sudden death in young persons (including some competitive athletes) in the Veneto region of northeastern Italy. The coronary disease is usually confined to the left anterior descending coronary artery and is due to obstructive fibrous and smooth muscle cell plaques in the absence of acute thrombus. In one study of sports-related sudden deaths, not limited to competitive athletes, atherosclerotic coronary artery disease (as well as HCM) was the leading cause of sudden death.[6]

MYOCARDITIS (see Chap. 48). Although myocarditis is an acknowledged cause of sudden death in young athletes, with or without prior symptoms, definitive diagnosis may be difficult clinically (and at autopsy), particularly in the healed phase.[30] Indeed, the importance of myocarditis as a cause of sudden death in the young may have been previously exaggerated owing to overinterpretation of histological data[37] or the lack of standardized morphological criteria[30]; others have suggested that this diagnosis is now probably underestimated.[4] In a large autopsy-based series of 134 competitive athletes, only 6 percent showed areas of myocardium with acute inflammatory changes, consistent with acute myocarditis,[5] or areas of idiopathic myocardial scarring possibly representing healed myocarditis. The inflammatory process of myocarditis (see Fig. 59–5) is usually triggered by several viral agents, often enterovirus but

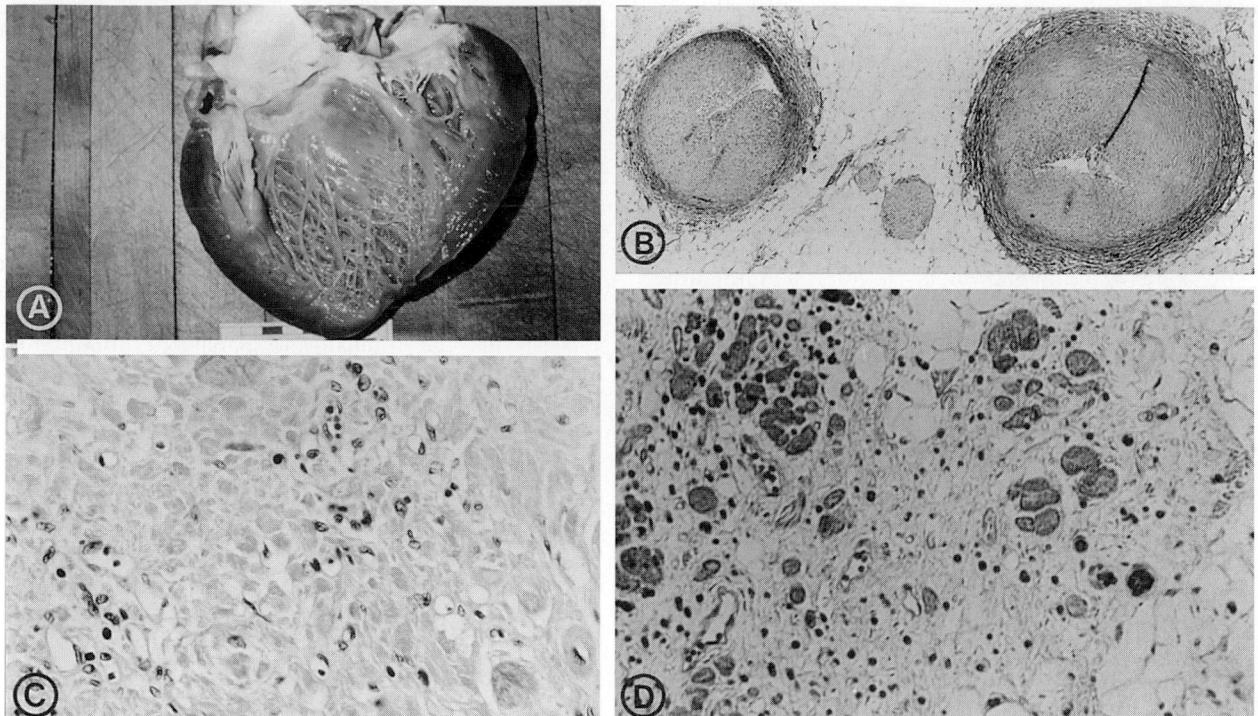

FIGURE 59–5. Cardiac morphological findings at autopsy in four competitive athletes who died suddenly. A, Gross specimen from an athlete with greatly enlarged ventricular cavities, consistent with dilated cardiomyopathy. B, Histological section of the left anterior descending coronary artery (*left*) and diagonal branch (*right*) showing severe (>95 percent) cross-sectional luminal narrowing by atherosclerotic plaque. C, Foci of inflammatory cells consistent with myocarditis. D, Histological section of the right ventricular wall showing islands of myocytes within a matrix of fatty and fibrous replacement characteristic of arrhythmogenic right ventricular cardiomyopathy. (Adapted from Maron BJ, Shirani J, Poliac LC, et al: Sudden death in young competitive athletes: Clinical, demographic, and pathological profiles. JAMA 276:199–204, 1996. Reproduced with permission of the American Medical Association.)

also adenovirus.[38] Chronic cocaine use may provoke a similar clinical and pathological profile.[39]

Myocarditis does not necessarily require permanent withdrawal from competitive athletics. Athletes should, however, undergo a prudent convalescent period of about 6 months after the onset of clinical manifestations and should be allowed to resume competition when ventricular function and cardiac dimensions have returned to normal and clinically relevant arrhythmias are absent on ambulatory monitoring and stress testing.[30]

INTRAMURAL CORONARY ARTERY (see Chaps. 34 and 37). It is unresolved whether the presence of short segments of the left anterior descending coronary artery (1 to 3 cm), tunneled and completely surrounded by left ventricular myocardium (i.e., myocardial "bridges"), constitutes a potentially lethal anatomical variant responsible for sudden unexpected death in otherwise healthy young individuals during exertion.[40] Some regard muscle bridges to have the potential for producing critical systolic arterial narrowing (and residual diastolic compression), resulting in myocardial ischemia and, in one report, increased risk for cardiac arrest in young patients with HCM.[41] Short-acting beta blockers may alleviate anginal symptoms and ischemia by increasing luminal diameter of tunneled coronary segments and normalizing flow velocities, thereby suggesting that myocardial bridges may have pathophysiological significance.[42] Nevertheless, coronary blood flow occurs predominantly during diastole, and necropsy studies have frequently documented tunneled coronary arteries in patients who had not died suddenly.

AORTIC RUPTURE (AND MARFAN SYNDROME) (see Chaps. 40 and 56). Young athletes uncommonly die suddenly as a result of rupture of the aorta,[2, 5, 8, 9] including some with the physical stigmata of Marfan syndrome, in whom disruption of the aortic media with decreased numbers of elastic fibers is usually evident at autopsy (i.e., cystic medial necrosis). Certain individuals with Marfan syndrome may successfully participate in strenuous competitive sports for many years without experiencing a catastrophic event, presumably before the time aortic dilatation becomes marked and predisposition for dissection or rupture increases critically. Indeed, the presence of aortic dilatation is the primary determinant of whether athletes with Marfan syndrome should be judged medically ineligible for competition.[26]

VALVULAR HEART DISEASE (see Chap. 46). Aortic valvular stenosis has proved to be an uncommon cause of sudden death in young athletes,[2, 5, 6, 8, 9] although older hospital-based studies suggested that this lesion much more frequently caused sudden unexpected death in children and young asymptomatic adults.[37] This is probably because aortic stenosis is likely to be identified early in life (including during preparticipation screening), by virtue of the characteristically loud heart murmur, thereby leading to disqualification from competitive sports.[28] Despite its frequency within the general population (probably <3 percent),[43] mitral valve prolapse appears to be a very uncommon cause of morbidity or sudden death in young competitive athletes.[30, 43, 44]

CARDIAC CONDUCTION SYSTEM ABNORMALITIES (see Chap. 25). A spectrum of congenital or acquired abnormalities confined to the cardiac conduction system (in the absence of other structural cardiac abnormalities) has occasionally been regarded as the cause of sudden death in competitive athletes and other young people, presumably by producing heart block and bradyarrhythmias.[45, 46] These

FIGURE 59–6. See color plate 30.

include malformations of the atrioventricular conduction tissue, such as accessory atrioventricular pathways, or morphologically abnormal small intramural arteries to the sino-atrial node or atrioventricular nodes with thickened vessel walls and narrowed lumen. Such vascular abnormalities have been incriminated as determinants of sudden death and myocardial ischemia by virtue of tissue degeneration, scarring, and hemorrhage in the surrounding conducting tissue.

ARRHYTHMOGENIC RIGHT VENTRICULAR CARDIOMYOPATHY (ARVC) (see Chaps. 25 and 48). ARVC is an unusual, often familial condition that may be associated with important ventricular or supraventricular arrhythmias and has been cited as a cause of sudden death in young individuals, including athletes.[47-49] ARVC is characterized morphologically by cell death in the right ventricular wall, in which myocytes are replaced by fibrous or adipose tissue, often associated with myocarditis and evidence of programmed cell death (Fig. 59–6; see Chap. 48). This disease process may be segmental or may diffusely involve the right ventricle. In several autopsy studies of sudden death of young athletes, ARVC is uncommon (i.e., <5 percent).[4-6, 9] An exception is reports from the Veneto region of Italy, where ARVC is the single most common cause of sudden death in competitive athletes (and HCM is uncommon),[7] because of either a unique genetic substrate or the long-standing Italian national screening program for competitive athletes,[50] which has probably identified and disqualified far greater numbers of athletes with HCM than ARVC.[51]

APPARENTLY NORMAL HEARTS. Occasionally, no evidence of structural cardiovascular disease is demonstrable in athletes dying suddenly even after careful examination of the heart. In such instances (about 2 percent of athletic field deaths),[4, 5] it may not be possible to preclude with certainty noncardiac factors, such as substance abuse (see Chap. 70).[39] It is also possible that such deaths are due to either occult conduction system disease,[45, 46] clinically unidentified Wolff-Parkinson-White syndrome, rare conditions in which structural cardiac abnormalities are characteristically lacking at necropsy such as idiopathic ventricular fibrillation[52] and long QT syndrome,[53] or unrecognized segmental ARVC (see Chap. 25).[47, 49]

Older Athletes

Older athletes (age >35 years) may also harbor occult cardiac disease and die suddenly and unexpectedly while participating in intense (often competitive) athletic activities. Unlike in youthful athletes, in older conditioned athletes, the cause of death is usually atherosclerotic coronary artery disease (see Chaps. 35 to 37). The remaining deaths in older athletes are due to diseases unrelated to atherosclerosis, such as HCM or valvular heart disease.[30, 54]

Older trained athletes who have died suddenly of coronary heart disease, reported in several necropsy-based investigations,[10, 11, 13-15] compose a heterogeneous athletic population including runners training for competitive long-distance races and recreational joggers, as well as participants in sports such as rugby, squash, and golf. Most of these deaths occur during or just after physical activity. In contrast to young competitive athletes, most older athletes who have died of coronary heart disease had either known risk factors, cardiovascular symptoms, or prior myocardial infarction, with severe coronary artery involvement (atherosclerotic narrowing of two or three major extramural coronary arteries) and myocardial scarring.

Prevalence and Significance

In young athletes, the frequency of sudden unexpected death that occurs during competitive sports and is due to cardiovascular disease appears to be low, occurring in about 1:200,000 individual student-athletes per academic high school year[3] and in 1:70,000 during a 3-year career. In comparison, older athletes have somewhat higher rates of exercise-related sudden death, reported to be 1:15,000 to 1:50,000 per year, usually in apparently healthy male athletes,[12] joggers,[11] and marathon racers.[15] Such estimates may suggest that the intense and persistent public interest in these tragic events in young individuals is perhaps disproportionate to their overall numerical significance. However, the emotional and social impact of athletic field catastrophes remains high because competitive athletes, to much of the lay public and physician community, intuitively represent the healthiest element of society.[1, 4]

Demographics

Based primarily on data assembled from broad-based United States populations,[2-6, 9] a profile of young competitive athletes who die suddenly has emerged. Athletes had participated in a large number and variety of sports, the most frequent being basketball and football (about 70 percent[5]), probably reflecting the relatively high participation level in these team sports as well as their intensity. In European studies, the most common sport associated with sudden death is soccer.[47, 51] The vast majority of athletic field deaths occurred in males (about 90 percent), largely of high school age (about 60 percent[5]); however, others achieved collegiate or even professional levels of competition.

The vast majority of athletes who incur sudden death are free of cardiovascular symptoms during their lives, with their underlying cardiovascular disease completely unsuspected. Sudden collapse has been associated with exercise in 90 percent of athletes, predominantly in the late afternoon and early evening hours, corresponding to the peak periods of competition and training (particularly for organized team sports).[5] These observations substantiate that, in the presence of certain structural cardiovascular diseases, physical activity represents a trigger and an important precipitating factor for sudden death on the athletic field.

Although the majority of reported sudden deaths in competitive athletes have been in white males, one study showed a substantial proportion (about 40 percent) to be in African Americans.[55] The substantial occurrence of HCM-related sudden death in young black male athletes contrasts sharply with the infrequent identification of black patients with HCM in hospital-based populations and may be explained by disproportionate access to subspecialty medical care, which makes it less likely for African American patients to achieve a cardiovascular diagnosis such as HCM.

Screening and Preparticipation Detection of Cardiovascular Abnormalities

Detection of preexisting cardiovascular abnormalities with the potential for significant morbidity or sudden death is an important objective of the widespread practice of preparticipation screening for high school– and college-aged athletes.[56] Athletic screening in the United States has customarily been performed in the context of a personal and family history and physical examination.[4, 28, 56, 56a] However, the utility of these routine evaluations for both U.S. high school– and college-aged student-athletes is limited by the complex nature of the responsible cardiovascular abnormalities and the infrequency with which they occur within the general population, as well as apparent inadequacies in the preparticipation cardiovascular screening process.[56a] For example, the approved history and physical examination questionnaires (which serve as guides to examiners) may be suboptimal for 25 percent or more of high school– and college-aged athletes.[56, 56a] Indeed, one retrospective study reported that potentially lethal cardiovascular abnormalities were suspected by preparticipation history and physical examination in only 3 percent of high school and collegiate athletes who ultimately died suddenly of these diseases (including only 2 percent of the HCM victims examined).[5]

Citing medical and ethical considerations, an American Heart Association consensus panel[28] recommended preparticipation cardiovascular screening, as well as a more systematic approach to implementation, to enhance the likelihood of suspecting or identifying important cardiovascular abnormalities. These recommendations included a personal and family history and physical examination targeted to detect those lesions known to predispose to sudden cardiac death.

Although the addition of noninvasive testing (e.g., echocardiography or ECG) to the screening process would undoubtedly enhance detection of many of the responsible lesions (particularly HCM),[51] this would be an unrealistic aspiration on a national scale in the United States owing to the prohibitive cost and other practical obstacles. It should be emphasized that no available screening design (even with diagnostic testing) is capable of detecting all important lesions and affected athletes, and medical clearance for participation in sports does not necessarily connote the absence of cardiovascular disease.

Eligibility Considerations for Athletes with Known Cardiovascular Disease

When a cardiovascular abnormality is identified in a competitive athlete, the following considerations arise: (1) the magnitude of risk for sudden cardiac death (or disease progression) associated with continued participation in competitive sports and (2) criteria for discerning whether individual athletes should be withdrawn from sports competition. In this regard, the 26th Bethesda Conference[26] affords prospective consensus panel recommendations for athletic eligibility and disqualification, taking into account the severity of relevant cardiovascular abnormalities as well as the intensity of sports training and competition. These recommendations are predicated on the assumption that intense physical exertion in the context of competitive sports may act as a trigger in certain predisposed athletes with underlying structural heart disease. Although that risk cannot be quantified with precision, temporary or permanent withdrawal of selected athletes with cardiovascular disease from participation in certain competitive sports is regarded as a prudent strategy for diminishing the likelihood of sudden death.[5, 26, 30] The Bethesda Conference report[26] provides clear benchmarks for the expected standard of care that may be used to resolve future medicolegal disputes and has been cited by a U.S. Appellate Court as consensus expert guidelines that team physicians should rely on in formulating appropriate decisions regarding the eligibility of competitive athletes with cardiovascular disease.[57]

Cardiac Risks of Sports Unrelated to Structural Cardiovascular Disease

Although uncommon, virtually instantaneous cardiac arrest may result from a relatively modest and nonpenetrating blunt blow to the chest, in the *absence* of underlying cardiovascular disease or resultant structural injury to the chest wall or heart itself (i.e., commotio cordis) (see Chap. 51).[16, 17, 17a] Such occurrences are produced either by a pro-

jectile (most commonly a baseball, softball, or hockey puck) or by bodily contact with another athlete. The blow to the chest is not perceived as unusual for the sporting event, nor of sufficient magnitude to result in a catastrophe. A common scenario is that of a young baseball player at bat struck in the chest by a pitched ball thrown from a standard distance. Of note, many of these catastrophes have occurred in purely recreational situations at home or on the playground, with the fatal injuries often inflicted by family members.

There appear to be three determinants of a commotio cordis event: (1) chest impact located directly over the heart, usually of relatively low energy[16, 17a]; (2) precise timing of the blow to a narrow 15-msec segment of the cardiac cycle vulnerable to potentially lethal ventricular arrhythmias, just before the T wave peak,[17] apparently also involving activation of the potassium–ATP channel (K_{ATP})[58]; and (3) a narrow, compliant chest wall, typical of young children.[16]

Certain measures aimed at prevention of commotio cordis events have been considered. Softer than standard (safety) baseballs reduced the risk for ventricular fibrillation in an experimental model of this syndrome, suggesting that sudden death prevention may be achieved through modification of athletic equipment.[17, 17a] Wider use of padding designed to cover the precordium would theoretically protect against the occurrence of commotio cordis in youngsters competing in sports such as baseball, ice hockey, karate, lacrosse, and football. However, the infrequency of commotio cordis events represents an obstacle to documenting the effectiveness of any protective intervention.

Commotio cordis events are not uniformly fatal; about 10 percent of the reported victims are known to have survived, usually because of reasonably prompt cardiopulmonary resuscitation and defibrillation.[4] With enhanced public awareness of this syndrome, emergency measures are likely to be implemented more rapidly on the athletic field, possibly avoiding many future catastrophes.

REFERENCES

1. Maron BJ: Sudden death in young athletes: Lessons from the Hank Gathers affair. N Engl J Med 329:55–57, 1993.
2. Liberthson RR: Sudden death from cardiac causes in children and young adults. N Engl J Med 334:1039–1044, 1996.
3. Maron BJ, Gohman TE, Aeppli D: Prevalence of sudden cardiac death during competitive sports activities in Minnesota high school athletes. J Am Coll Cardiol 32:1881–1884, 1998.
4. Maron BJ: Cardiovascular risks to young persons on the athletic field. Ann Intern Med 129:379–386, 1998.

CAUSES OF SUDDEN DEATH

5. Maron BJ, Shirani J, Poliac LC, et al: Sudden death in young competitive athletes: Clinical, demographic and pathological profiles. JAMA 276: 199–204, 1996.
6. Burke AP, Farb A, Virmani R, et al: Sports-related and non–sports-related sudden cardiac death in young athletes. Am Heart J 121:568–575, 1991.
7. Corrado D, Thiene G, Nava A, et al: Sudden death in young competitive athletes: Clinicopathologic correlations in 22 cases. Am J Med 39:588–596, 1990.
8. Maron BJ, Roberts WC, McAllister HA, et al: Sudden death in young athletes. Circulation 62:218–229, 1980.
9. Van Camp SP, Bloor CM, Mueller FO, et al: Nontraumatic sports death in high school and college athletes. Med Sci Sports Exer 27:641–647, 1995.
10. Virmani R, Robinowitz M, McAllister HA: Nontraumatic death in joggers. A series of 30 patients at autopsy. Am J Med 72:871–874, 1982.
11. Thompson PD, Funk EJ, Carleton RA, et al: Incidence of death during jogging in Rhode Island from 1975 through 1980. JAMA 247:2535–2538, 1982.
12. Siscovick DS, Weiss NS, Fletcher RH, et al: The incidence of primary cardiac arrest during vigorous exercise. N Engl J Med 311:874–877, 1984.
13. Northcote RJ, Evans ADB, Ballantyne D: Sudden death in squash players. Lancet 21:148–151, 1984.

14. Waller BF, Roberts WC: Sudden death while running in conditioned runners aged 40 years or over. Am J Cardiol 45:1292–1300, 1980.

15. Maron BJ, Poliac LC, Roberts WO: Risk for sudden cardiac death associated with marathon running. J Am Coll Cardiol 28:428–431, 1996.

16. Maron BJ, Poliac LC, Kaplan JA, et al: Blunt impact to the chest leading to sudden death from cardiac arrest during sports activities. N Engl J Med 33:337–342, 1995.

17. Link MS, Wang PJ, Pandian NG, et al: An experimental model of sudden death due to low-energy chest-wall impact (commotio cordis). N Engl J Med 338:1805–1811, 1998.

17a. Maron BJ, Links MS, Wang PJ, et al: Clinical profile of commotio cordis: An under-appreciated cause of sudden death in the young during sports and other activities. J Cardiovasc Electrophysiol 10:114–120, 1999.

18. Pelliccia A, Maron BJ, Spataro A, et al: The upper limit of physiologic cardiac hypertrophy in highly trained elite athletes. N Engl J Med 324:295–301, 1991.

19. Pelliccia A, Culasso F, Di Paolo F, et al: Physiologic left ventricular cavity dilatation in elite athletes. Ann Intern Med 130:23–31, 1999.

20. Pelliccia A, Maron BJ, Culasso F: Athlete's heart in women: Echocardiographic characterization of highly trained elite female athletes. JAMA 276:211–215, 1996.

21. Wigle ED, Sasson Z, Henderson MA, et al: Hypertrophic cardiomyopathy. The importance of the site and extent of hypertrophy. A review. Prog Cardiovasc Dis 28:1–83, 1985.

22. Maron BJ: Hypertrophic cardiomyopathy. Lancet 350:127–133, 1997.

23. Schwartz K, Carrier L, Guicheney P, et al: Molecular basis of familial cardiomyopathies. Circulation 91:523–540, 1995.

24. Maron BJ, Moller JH, Seidman CE, et al: Impact of laboratory molecular diagnosis on contemporary diagnostic criteria for genetically transmitted cardiovascular diseases: Hypertrophic cardiomyopathy, long-QT syndrome, and Marfan syndrome. Circulation 98:1460–1471, 1998.

25. Maron BJ, Gardin JM, Flack JM, et al: Assessment of the prevalence of hypertrophic cardiomyopathy in a general population of young adults: Echocardiographic analysis of 4111 subjects in the CARDIA study. Circulation 92:785–789, 1995.

26. Maron BJ, Mitchell JH: 26th Bethesda Conference. Recommendations for determining eligibility for competition in athletes with cardiovascular abnormalities. J Am Coll Cardiol 24:845–899, 1994.

27. Maron BJ, Shen W-K, Link MS, et al: Efficacy of implantable cardioverter-defibrillators for the prevention of sudden death in patients with hypertrophic cardiomyopathy. N Engl J Med 342:365–373, 2000.

28. Maron BJ, Thompson PD, Puffer JC, et al: Cardiovascular preparticipation screening of competitive athletes. Circulation 94:850–856, 1996.

28a. Stolt A, Karjalainen J, Heinonen OJ, Kujala UM: Left ventricular mass, geometry and filling in elite female and male endurance athletes. Scand J Med Sci Sports 10(1):28–32, 2000.

28b. Zandrino F, Molinari G, Smeraldi A, et al: Magnetic resonance imaging of athlete's heart: myocardial mass, left ventricular function, and cross-sectional area of the coronary arteries. Eur Radiol 10:319–325, 2000.

29. Maron BJ, Pelliccia A, Spirito P: Cardiac disease in young trained athletes: Insights into methods for distinguishing athlete's heart from structural heart disease with particular emphasis on hypertrophic cardiomyopathy. Circulation 91:1596–1601, 1995.

30. Maron BJ, Isner JM, McKenna WJ: 26th Bethesda Conference: Recommendations for determining eligibility for competition in athletes with cardiovascular abnormalities. Task Force 3: Hypertrophic cardiomyopathy, myocarditis, and other myopericardial diseases, and mitral valve prolapse. In Maron BJ, Mitchell JH (eds): 26th Bethesda Conference: Recommendations for determining eligibility for competition in athletes with cardiovascular abnormalities. J Am Coll Cardiol 24:880–885, 1994.

31. Cheitlin MD, De Castro CM, McAllister HA: Sudden death as a complication of anomalous left coronary origin from the anterior sinus of Valsalva, a not-so-minor congenital anomaly. Circulation 50:780–787, 1974.

32. Taylor AJ, Rogan KM, Virmani R: Sudden cardiac death associated with isolated congenital coronary artery anomalies. J Am Coll Cardiol 20:640–647, 1992.

33. Roberts WC, Kragel AH: Anomalous origin of either the right or left main coronary artery from the aorta with subsequent coursing of the anomalously arising artery between aorta and pulmonary trunk. Am J Cardiol 62:1263–1267, 1988.

34. Alam M, Brymer J, Smith S: Transesophageal echocardiographic diagnosis of anomalous left coronary artery from the right aortic sinus. Chest 103:1617–1618, 1993.

35. Burke AP, Farb A, Malcom GT, et al: Plaque rupture and sudden death related to exertion in men with coronary artery disease. JAMA 281:921–926, 1999.

36. Corrado D, Basso C, Poletti A, et al: Sudden death in the young. Is acute coronary thrombosis the major precipitating factor? Circulation 90:2315–2323, 1994.

37. Lambert EC, Menon VA, Wagner HR, et al: Sudden unexpected death from cardiovascular disease in children. A cooperative international study. Am J Cardiol 34:89–96, 1974.

38. Pauschinger M, Bowles NE, Fuentes-Garcia FJ, et al: Detection of adenoviral genome in the myocardium of adult patients with idiopathic left ventricular dysfunction. Circulation 99:1348–1354, 1999.

39. Isner JM, Estes NAM III, Thompson PD, et al: Acute cardiac events temporally related to cocaine abuse. N Engl J Med 315:1438–1443, 1986.

40. Morales AR, Romanelli R, Boucek RJ: The mural left anterior descending coronary artery, strenuous exercise and sudden death. Circulation 62:230–237, 1980.

41. Yetman AJ, McCrindle BW, MacDonald C, et al: Myocardial bridging in children with hypertrophic cardiomyopathy—a risk factor for sudden death. N Engl J Med 339:1201–1209, 1998.

42. Schwarz ER, Klues HG, vom Dahl J: Functional, angiographic and intracoronary Doppler flow characteristics in symptomatic patients with myocardial bridging: Effect of short-term intravenous beta-blocker medication. J Am Coll Cardiol 27:1637–1645, 1996.

43. Freed LA, Levy D, Levine RA, et al: Prevalence and clinical outcome of mitral valve prolapse. N Engl J Med 341:1–7, 1999.

44. Dollar AL, Roberts WC: Morphologic comparison of patients with mitral valve prolapse who died suddenly with patients who died from severe valvular dysfunction or other conditions. J Am Coll Cardiol 17:921–931, 1991.

45. Bharti S, Lev M: Congenital abnormalities of the conduction system in sudden death in young adults. J Am Coll Cardiol 8:1096–1104, 1986.

46. Burke AP, Subramanian R, Smialek J, et al: Nonatherosclerotic narrowing of the atrioventricular node artery and sudden death. J Am Coll Cardiol 21:117–122, 1993.

47. Thiene G, Nava A, Corrado D, et al: Right ventricular cardiomyopathy and sudden death in young people. N Engl J Med 318:129–133, 1988.

48. Marcus FI, Fontaine GH, Guiraudon G, et al: Right ventricular dysplasia: A report of 24 adult cases. Circulation 65:384–398, 1982.

49. Corrado D, Basso C, Thiene G, et al: Spectrum of clinicopathologic manifestations of arrhythmogenic right ventricular cardiomyopathy/dysplasia: A multicenter study. J Am Coll Cardiol 30:1512–1520, 1997.

50. Pelliccia A, Maron BJ: Preparticipation cardiovascular evaluation of the competitive athlete: Perspectives from the 30 year Italian experience. Am J Cardiol 75:827–828, 1995.

51. Corrado D, Basso C, Schiavon M, et al: Screening for hypertrophic cardiomyopathy in young athletes. N Engl J Med 339:364–369, 1998.

52. Survivors of out-of-hospital cardiac arrest with apparently normal heart. Need for definition and standardized clinical evaluation. Circulation 95:265–272, 1997.

53. Vincent GM, Timothy KW, Leppert M, et al: The spectrum of symptoms and QT intervals in carriers of the gene for the long-QT syndrome. N Engl J Med 327:846–852, 1992.

54. Noakes TD, Rose AG, Opie LH: Hypertrophic cardiomyopathy associated with sudden death during marathon racing. Br Heart J 41:624–627, 1979.

55. Maron BJ, Poliac LC, Mathenge R: Hypertrophic cardiomyopathy as an important cause of sudden cardiac death on the athletic field in African-American athletes (abstract). J Am Coll Cardiol 29 (Suppl A):462A, 1997.

PROFILE AND DEMOGRAPHICS

56. Glover DW, Maron BJ: Profile of preparticipation cardiovascular screening for high school athletes. JAMA 279:1817–1819, 1998.

56a. Pfister GC, Puffer JC, Maron BJ: Preparticipation cardiovascular screening for US collegiate student-athletes. JAMA 283:1597–1599, 2000.

57. Maron BJ, Mitten MJ, Quandt EK, et al: Competitive athletes with cardiovascular disease—the case of Nicholas Knapp. N Engl J Med 339;1632–1635, 1998.

58. Link MS, Wang PJ, VanderBrink BA, et al: Selective activation of the K_{ATP}^+ channel is a mechanism by which sudden death is produced by low energy chest wall impact (commotio cordis). Circulation 100:413–418, 1999.

Chapter 60

Medical Management of the Patient Undergoing Cardiac Surgery

DAVID H. ADAMS · ELLIOTT M. ANTMAN

Several advances have occurred in cardiac surgery that make operative repair of a variety of cardiac lesions a viable therapeutic alternative for an increasing number of patients with cardiovascular disease. These advances include improvements in tools for assessment of perioperative risk, surgical and anesthesia techniques for myocardial revascularization, valve repair and replacement, and repair of complex congenital cardiac defects, as well as new approaches to management of patients with left ventricular dysfunction and cardiac arrhythmias.[1-3] Advances relating to minimally invasive cardiac surgical procedures have added additional options in the comprehensive care of patients with surgical cardiovascular disease.[4-9] Perioperative medical and surgical supportive measures have progressed, including the proliferation of intraoperative transesophageal echocardiography,[9a] ventricular assist devices, pharmacological supportive strategies, and comprehensive blood conservation programs. Evidence suggests that translation of these improvements into routine surgical practice and institution of regular quality control surveillance measures have led to a reduction in risk-adjusted operative mortality for coronary artery bypass grafting (CABG) to less than 2 percent for the general population and 3 to 4 percent for the Medicare population.[10-12] However, the profile of patients referred for surgery has also changed and is characterized by greater proportions of patients with advanced age, depressed left ventricular function, multiple comorbidities, prior revascularization operations, and failed acute interventional procedures, which has led to higher mortality rates in tertiary care referral centers that are called upon to operate on such patients with greater frequency.[13-19b]

This chapter summarizes the information required by the cardiologist, whose important responsibilities include collaboration with the surgical team for both preoperative and postoperative care, especially care of the medical complications that may develop.

PREOPERATIVE EVALUATION

GENERAL MEDICAL CONDITION. Except for life-threatening conditions (e.g., proximal aortic dissection,[20] cardiogenic shock caused by ruptured papillary muscle in acute myocardial infarction, penetrating wound of the heart), it behooves the consulting cardiologist to assess the overall medical condition of the patient and advise the surgical team if postponement of the operation seems warranted[21-29] (Table 60–1). Particular attention should be paid to the patient's potential for development of one or more of the following complications: (1) bleeding during cardiopulmonary bypass while heparinized or while anticoagulated after

▼ TABLE 60–1. PREOPERATIVE LABORATORY EVALUATION OF PATIENTS UNDERGOING CARDIAC SURGERY

PREOPERATIVE LABORATORY TEST	ABNORMAL FINDING	COMMENT
Complete blood count	1. Anemia, especially Hct <35%	1. Anticipate that hemodilution will occur on cardiopulmonary bypass and blood loss will occur intraoperatively. In stable patients, preoperative iron supplementation (weeks) or erythropoietin therapy (days) should be considered. Patients with unstable angina, congestive heart failure, aortic stenosis, and left main coronary artery disease should be advised against autologous donation of blood in the preoperative period.
	2. WBC >10,000	2. Search for possible infection
Coagulation screen	1. Prolonged bleeding time 2. Elevated PT and/or PTT 3. Thrombocytopenia	All these laboratory abnormalities suggest that the patient is at risk for bleeding postoperatively and may have excessive chest tube drainage. Corrective measures (e.g., vitamin K, fresh frozen plasma, platelet transfusions) should be considered preoperatively, and surgery may need to be postponed. Hematological consultation may be required if an inherited defect in coagulation (e.g., von Willebrand factor deficiency) is suspected

Table continued on following page

PREOPERATIVE LABORATORY TEST	ABNORMAL FINDING	COMMENT
Chemistry profile	1. Elevated BUN/creatinine	1. Abnormal renal function that may worsen in the perioperative period (caused by nonpulsatile flow on cardiopulmonary bypass and potential low flow postoperatively); may necessitate temporary or even permanent hemodialysis
	2. Potassium <4.0 mEq/liter and/or magnesium <2.0 mEq/liter	2. Electrolyte deficits may place the patient at risk of arrhythmias perioperatively and should be corrected before induction of anesthesia
	3. Abnormal liver function tests	3. Patient may clear anesthetic agents as well as other cardioactive drugs more slowly. Low albumin level may indicate a state of relative malnutrition that may need to be corrected with nutritional support perioperatively
Stool Hematest	Positive for occult blood	Because heparinization will take place while on the cardiopulmonary bypass apparatus, the patient may be at risk for GI bleeding perioperatively. The source of GI heme loss should be investigated preoperatively if clinical circumstances permit. The potential for bleeding in the future may influence the choice of prosthetic valve inserted.
Pulmonary function	Reduced VC or prolonged FEV_1	Anticipate longer than usual process of weaning from ventilator postoperatively if FEV_1 <65% of VC or FEV_1 <1.5–2.0 liters. Obtain baseline arterial blood gas analysis on room air to help guide respiratory management postoperatively
Thyroid function	These tests are not ordered routinely but should be performed in cases of suspected hypothyroidism or hyperthyroidism, known thyroid dysfunction during replacement therapy, and atrial fibrillation in patients who have not undergone evaluation of thyroid function	Hypothyroid patients require prolonged period of ventilatory support postoperatively because of slower clearance of anesthetic agents Hyperthyroid patients have a hypermetabolic state that places them at increased risk of myocardial ischemia, vasomotor instability, and poorly controlled ventricular rate in atrial fibrillation
Echocardiography	1. Decreased LV ejection fraction	1. Patients with decreased LV function are at higher perioperative risk for surgery. Selected patients should undergo viability assessment
	2. Decreased RV function	2. RV dysfunction increases perioperative risk and identification may lead to preoperative assessment of reversibility of pulmonary hypertension
	3. Aortic stenosis	3. Mild to moderate aortic stenosis (gradient <25 mm Hg) may be treated by prophylactic valve replacement in selected low-risk patients
	4. Aortic insufficiency	4. Ventricular dimension will help guide decisions to perform valve replacement in addition to revascularization in patients with combined aortic regurgitation and coronary disease.
	5. Mitral insufficiency	5. Moderate or severe mitral regurgitation may warrant valve exploration in patients undergoing coronary revascularization
	6. LV aneurysm	6. May alert surgeons to the need of aneurysmectomy in selected patients
	7. Ventricular septal defect	7. Identification will suggest the need for early surgical intervention
Cardiac catheterization	1. Elevated LV end-diastolic pressure and pulmonary capillary wedge pressure	1. May remain elevated in the early postoperative period and indicate a need for careful attention to maintenance of adequate preload postoperatively
	2. Elevated right atrial pressure	2. May reflect tricuspid regurgitation or RV dysfunction from prior infarction. Such patients require vigorous volume expansion postoperatively to maintain adequate cardiac output.
	3. Elevated pulmonary artery pressure (and pulmonary vascular resistance)	3. Fixed pulmonary vascular resistance should be suspected when the pulmonary artery diastolic pressure exceeds the mean pulmonary capillary wedge pressure. Vigorous oxygenation and pharmacological support with a pulmonary vasodilator (isoproterenol, prostaglandin E_1) are important in such cases. Patients with a pulmonary artery diastolic pressure equal to the pulmonary capillary wedge pressure usually have more rapid resolution of pulmonary hypertension postoperatively
	4. LV mural thrombus	4. Increased risk of stroke perioperatively
	5. Status of internal mammary arteries	5. Highly desirable arterial conduits for planned revascularization surgery.[40, 41] Particular care required during reoperation if patent internal mammary artery bypass is in place from previous surgery
	6. Status of saphenous vein grafts	6. "Pseudoextravasation" of dye outside the lumen in a patent graft with slow flow probably represents thrombus-filled atherosclerotic aneurysm of the graft

BUN = blood urea nitrogen; FEV_1 = volume of air expired at 1 second; GI = gastrointestinal; Hct = hematocrit; LV = left ventricular; PT = prothrombin time; PTT = partial thromboplastin time; RV = right ventricular; VC = vital capacity; WBC = white blood cell count.

insertion of a mechanical heart valve prosthesis [30]; (2) deterioration in renal function; (3) arrhythmias secondary to electrolyte imbalance; (4) sepsis from incompletely treated pulmonary, urinary tract, or dental infection or dermatological infection over the sternum or saphenous vein harvest site; (5) need for prolonged ventilatory support postoperatively because of underlying pulmonary disease and preoperative malnutrition; and (6) exacerbation of a neurological deficit because of carotid artery disease or prior stroke.[22] When perioperative intraaortic balloon pump support may be needed, the status of the iliofemoral circulation should be assessed bilaterally. Of note, the risk of limb ischemia may be reduced by the use of sheathless, small-caliber balloon pump catheters.[31] Despite the increased risk of perioperative morbidity and mortality, recent data indicate that patients with combined coronary artery disease and peripheral vascular disease have a greater likelihood of long-term survival and freedom from myocardial infarction with CABG surgery versus medical therapy, particularly in the presence of two- and three-vessel coronary artery disease.[32]

The *protein-calorie malnutrition* associated with cardiac cachexia has been shown to compromise cardiac function and is associated with a greater risk of respiratory failure, sepsis, and prolonged hospitalization. If the clinical situation allows, patients in whom cardiac cachexia is diagnosed should receive a few weeks of preoperative nutritional support before undergoing elective cardiac surgery. The general principles of nutritional support in cardiac surgical patients are outlined in Figure 60–1.

RISK FACTORS FOR CARDIAC MORBIDITY AND MORTALITY. Risk factors for morbidity and mortality after coronary revascularization surgery have been analyzed extensively.[33–36b] A commonly used, simple clinical severity scoring system is shown in Table 60–2. Although patients with low-risk scores may be considered candidates for "fast-track" cost-saving measures such as admission on the day of surgery or early extubation postoperatively, those with higher-risk scores are likely to experience increased morbidity, required longer intensive care unit (ICU) stays and more consultations by specialists, and consume a greater proportion of medical resources. Furthermore, clinical severity scoring is helpful in identifying patients at high risk for operative mortality (score >10). By assembling and reviewing the data necessary for accurate assessment of a patient's operative risk, cardiologists can help with the appropriate clinical triage of patients, contain hospital costs, and facilitate consultations with other medical specialists (e.g., dialysis team) as needed. Patients at increased risk of mediastinal infection include the elderly and those suffering from diabetes mellitus, malnutrition, severe pulmonary disease that is likely to lead to prolonged postoperative ventilatory support, and macromastia in women.[37–39]

VENTRICULAR DYSFUNCTION. An especially important aspect of the preoperative evaluation of a cardiac surgical patient involves estimating the extent of underlying ventricular dysfunction. Evidence exists that unrevascularized viable myocardium after myocardial infarction serves as a substrate for recurrent ischemic events.[39–43] Also, patients with severe multivessel disease and akinetic myocardial zones who suffer from chronic congestive heart failure as a result of hibernating myocardium (see Chap. 37) experience improved ventricular function after CABG.[39] Contemporary techniques that should be used for assessing myocardial viability in dysfunctional regions include imaging procedures that correlate perfusion with cell membrane integrity (thallium reperfusion), metabolic activity (positron-emission tomography), or contractile reserve (stress echocardiography).[39–40a] Clinicians should rely on imaging modalities with which they are most familiar and that are available at their institution.

Careful consideration should be given to the possibility of *right ventricular dysfunction* (see Table 60–1), which

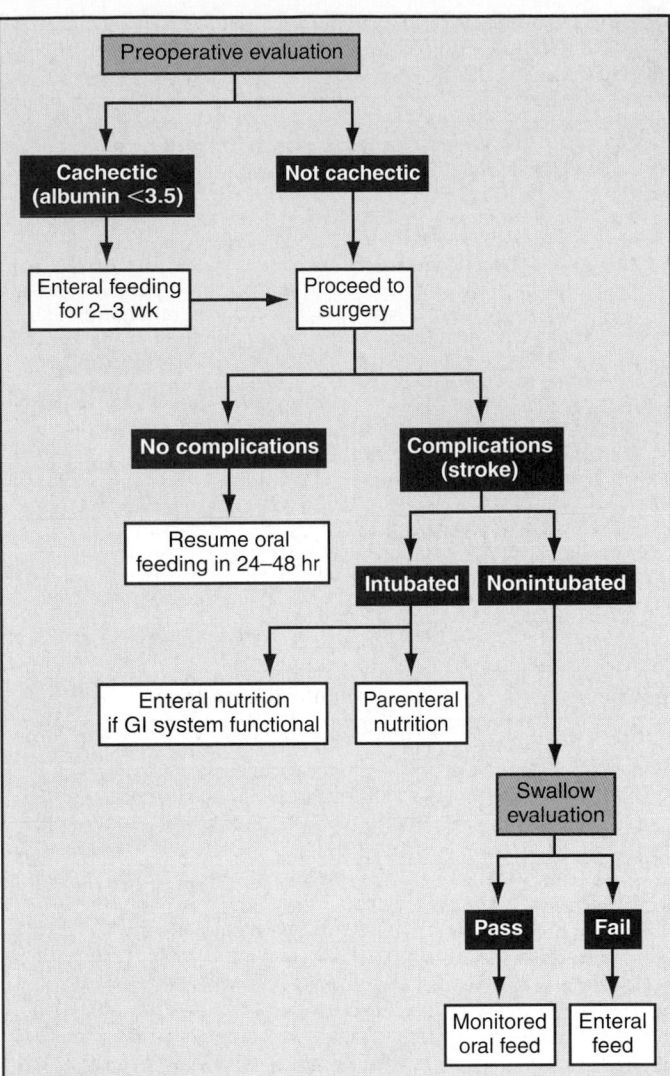

FIGURE 60–1. The nutritional status of cardiac patients has a significant impact on their postoperative outcome. Patients who are cachectic before elective cardiac surgery should be nutritionally bolstered for 2 to 3 weeks prior to surgery. Postoperative patients are in a hypermetabolic state and require increased nutrition to meet metabolic demands and facilitate wound healing. Oral diet is resumed 24 hours after uncomplicated surgery, and the diet is advanced as rapidly as tolerated. For patients who have perioperative complications such as stroke, a swallow evaluation is needed to assess the patient's ability to protect the airway during meals. If the patient fails the swallow evaluation or if the patient is intubated, nutritional requirements are met by early enteral feeding except in cases of gastrointestinal dysfunction. Oral feeding tubes are useful in the short term, while prolonged nutritional support is best handled by placement of an enteral tube.

should be suspected in patients with preoperatively elevated pulmonary artery systolic pressure (>60 mm Hg), a history of inferoposterior left ventricular infarction (which may be associated with right ventricular infarction), and longstanding tricuspid regurgitation. Patients with right ventricular dysfunction should receive an inotropic agent with vasodilating actions such as milrinone (5 μg/kg/min) or dobutamine (5 μg/kg/min) in addition to supplemental oxygen perioperatively in an attempt to lower pulmonary vascular resistance and improve right ventricular systolic performance. Intravenous nitrate infusions, in the perioperative period have also been shown to reduce pulmonary hypertension and ameliorate right ventricular failure. Inhaled agents, including aerosolized prostacyclin and nitric oxide, have also been shown to effectively lower pulmo-

▼ TABLE 60–2. PREOPERATIVE RISK FACTORS FOR ADVERSE OUTCOMES IN PATIENTS UNDERGOING CABG SURGERY: A CLINICAL SEVERITY SCORING SYSTEM AND EVENT CURVES (NORTHERN NEW ENGLAND CARDIOVASCULAR DISEASE STUDY GROUP)

PREOPERATIVE ESTIMATION OF RISK OF MORTALITY, CEREBROVASCULAR ACCIDENT, AND MEDIASTINITIS

For use *only* in isolated CABG surgery

Directions: Locate outcome of interest, e.g., mortality. Use the score in that column for each relevant preoperative variable, and then sum these scores to get the total score. Take the total score and look up the approximate preoperative risk in the table below

PATIENT OR DISEASE CHARACTERISTICS	MORTALITY SCORE	CVA SCORE	MEDIASTINITIS SCORE
Age 60–69	2	3.5	
Age 70–79	3	5	
Age ≥80	5	6	
Female sex	1.5		
EF <40%	1.5	1.5	2
Urgent surgery	2	1.5	1.5
Emergency surgery	5	2	3.5
Prior CABG	5	1.5	
PVD	2	2	
Diabetes			1.5
Dialysis or creatinine ≥2	4	2	2.5
COPD	1.5		3.5
Obesity (BMI 31–36)			2.5
Severe obesity (BMI ≥37)			3.5
Total score			

PERIOPERATIVE RISK

TOTAL SCORE	MORTALITY (%)	CVA (%)	MEDIASTINITIS (%)
0	0.4	0.3	0.4
1	0.5	0.4	0.5
2	0.7	0.7	0.6
3	0.9	0.9	0.7
4	1.3	1.1	1.1
5	1.7	1.5	1.5
6	2.2	1.9	1.9
7	3.3	2.8	3.0
8	3.9	3.5	3.5
9	6.1	4.5	5.8
10	7.7	≥6.5	≥6.5
11	10.6		
12	13.7		
13	17.7		
14	≥28.3		

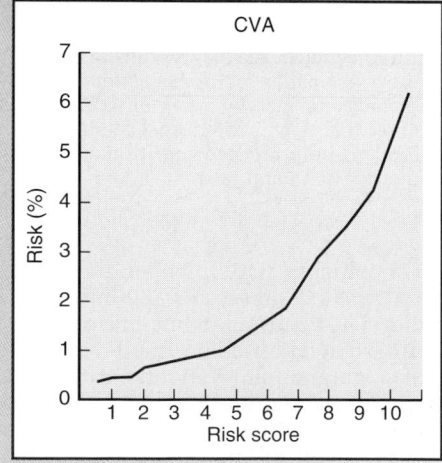

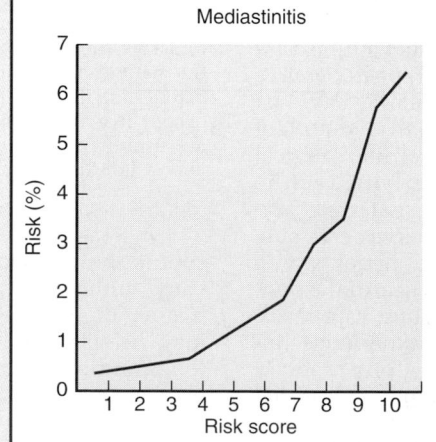

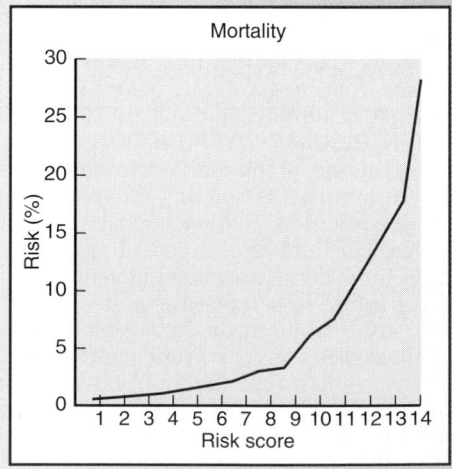

nary vascular resistance and improve perioperative right ventricular performance.[44]

Patients with mitral regurgitation and severe heart failure should undergo preoperative afterload reduction with such agents as oral angiotensin-converting enzyme (ACE) inhibitors and intravenous sodium nitroprusside to a systolic pressure of about 90 to 100 mm Hg. Potential contraindications to such preoperative afterload reduction include

▼ **TABLE 60-2.** PREOPERATIVE RISK FACTORS FOR ADVERSE OUTCOMES IN PATIENTS UNDERGOING CABG SURGERY: A CLINICAL SEVERITY SCORING SYSTEM AND EVENT CURVES (NORTHERN NEW ENGLAND CARDIOVASCULAR DISEASE STUDY GROUP) *Continued*

2063

Ch 60

DEFINITIONS

EF <40% (left ventricular ejection fraction): The patient's current EF is less than 40%

Urgent: Medical factors require patient to stay in hospital to have operation before discharge. The risk of immediate morbidity and death is believed to be low

Emergency: Patient's cardiac disease dictates that surgery be performed within hours to avoid unnecessary morbidity or death.

PVD (peripheral vascular disease): Cerebrovascular disease including prior CVA, prior TIA, prior carotid surgery, carotid stenosis by history or radiographic studies, or carotid bruit. Lower extremity disease including claudication, amputation, prior lower extremity bypass, absent pedal pulses, or lower extremity ulcers

Diabetes: Currently treated with oral medications or insulin.

Dialysis or creatinine ≥2: Peritoneal dialysis– or hemodialysis-dependent renal failure or creatinine ≥2 mg/dl

COPD (chronic obstructive pulmonary disease): Treated with bronchodilators or steroids

Obesity: Find the approximate height and weight in the table below to classify the person as obese or severely obese. Obesity: BMI 31–36. Severe obesity: BMI ≥37.

Example: A patient 5'7" and weighing 200 lb is classified as obese. If the patient weighed 236 lbs or more, that patient would be classified as severely obese

HEIGHT (FEET AND INCHES)	WEIGHT (LB)		HEIGHT (FEET AND INCHES)	WEIGHT (LB)	
	Obesity: BMI 31–36	Severe Obesity: BMI ≥37		Obesity: BMI 31–36	Severe Obesity: BMI ≥37
5'0"	158–184	≥189	5'8"	203–236	≥244
5'1"	164–190	≥195	5'9"	209–243	≥250
5'2"	169–196	≥202	5'10"	215–250	≥258
5'3"	175–203	≥208	5'11"	222–258	≥265
5'4"	180–209	≥215	6'0"	228–265	≥272
5'5"	186–217	≥222	6'1"	235–273	≥280
5'6"	191–222	≥228	6'2"	241–280	≥287
5'7"	198–229	≥236	6'3"	248–288	≥296

BMI = body mass index; CABG = coronary artery bypass surgery; CVA = cardiovascular accident; TIA = transient ischemic attack.

From Eagle KA, Guyton RA, Davidoff R, et al.: ACC/AHA guidelines for coronary artery bypass surgery. J Am Coll Cardiol 34:1262–1347, 1999. Reprinted with permission from the American College of Cardiology.

concomitant severe aortic stenosis and hemodynamically significant cerebral or renal vascular disease. In these patients, early intervention with intraaortic balloon counterpulsation may be useful. Intraaortic balloon support is also commonly used in the setting of severe decompensation from acute mitral regurgitation secondary to conditions such as papillary muscle rupture. Infarct-related ventricular septal defect is another hemodynamically significant lesion that may require pharmacological and intraaortic balloon support in the perioperative period.

RISK OF MYOCARDIAL ISCHEMIA. Acute thrombolytic and interventional catheterization treatment regimens for acute myocardial infarction may not successfully restore coronary perfusion because of inadequate thrombolysis, reocclusion of the infarct-related artery following initially successful thrombolysis, or dissection/acute thrombosis of the target vessel during angioplasty.[45, 46] Identification of patients for referral for emergency bypass surgery and decisions regarding the timing of such surgery remain a challenging clinical problem, particularly in view of the high perioperative mortality rate for patients who require surgery within 24 to 48 hours of thrombolysis.[46, 47]

Potential indications for emergency bypass surgery following failed attempts at reperfusion in acute myocardial infarction include significant left main stenosis and inability to maintain patency of the infarct-related artery, severe multivessel coronary artery disease with anatomy unsuitable for angioplasty and ischemic dysfunction of the noninfarct zones, and inability to maintain patency of an infarct-related artery that places a large amount of myocardium in jeopardy (proximal left anterior descending) in patients with an infarct of less than 6 hours' duration.[45, 46] Although some clinical reports suggest that patients in cardiogenic shock who undergo urgent revascularization have improved survival in comparison to those who are not revascularized, these series suffer from potential selection bias, and definitive recommendations regarding the management of patients with cardiogenic shock and acute myocardial infarction must await the results of ongoing randomized trials.[45]

Patients who are referred for emergency revascularization surgery should be supported by an intraaortic balloon pump and, if technically feasible, an intracoronary perfusion catheter. Other methods for mechanical assistance of the failing circulation are described in Chap-

ter 19. Because patients who undergo emergency bypass surgery within 6 to 12 hours of administration of a thrombolytic agent are at greater risk for intraoperative and postoperative hemorrhage, they should receive a hemostatic agent such as aprotinin (2 million kallikrein-inhibiting units [KIU] over a 20-minute period, followed by a continuous infusion of 500,000 KIU/hr).[48]

Patients with other manifestations of an acute coronary syndrome such as active unstable angina may also be in tenuous hemodynamic balance as they proceed to the operating room, particularly if significant left main coronary artery stenosis or severe three-vessel coronary artery disease associated with left ventricular dysfunction and/or mitral regurgitation is present. Delays while awaiting surgery and the time between the induction of anesthesia and the institution of cardiopulmonary bypass are high-risk periods during which a vicious spiral of myocardial ischemia and low-output syndrome can rapidly develop. Such patients should be protected by an intraaortic balloon pump inserted preoperatively and infusion of nitroglycerin.

ANESTHESIA FOR CARDIAC SURGERY. The details of the practice of cardiac anesthesia are beyond the scope of this chapter and are available in other sources.[49] High-dose synthetic narcotics that do not cause vasodilatation, such as fentanyl and sufentanil, have replaced morphine in many centers. Early extubation protocols are now followed in most cardiac units for patients with low or moderate risk. Advantages of early extubation include a decrease in respiratory complications, ventilatory support, and length of stay in the ICU. To achieve early extubation within 6 hours of surgery, anesthetic techniques have included combinations of inhalational anesthetics, such as enflurane and isoflurane, together with low to moderate amounts of intravenous opioids, such as fentanyl and sufentanil, along with the intravenous anesthetic propofol. The newer, inhaled anesthetics that have replaced nitrous oxide still have the potential to cause vasodilatation. Patients with critical aortic stenosis, critical mitral stenosis, and large right-to-left shunts may experience a dramatic reduction in cardiac output as ventricular stroke volume falls with a reduction in preload. Preoperative volume expansion and even administration of vasopressor agents may be necessary to avoid this problem.

Although supraventricular arrhythmias after cardiac surgery are seldom life threatening, they frequently provoke disturbing symptoms, may jeopardize hemodynamic stability, and are associated with an increased incidence of postoperative stroke, increased length of stay in the ICU, and increased hospital costs.[50–52]

In the past it was a common preoperative practice in many institutions to administer digitalis prophylactically to all patients undergoing cardiac surgery, not only for inotropic support but also for "control" of the ventricular rate if atrial fibrillation (AF) occurred postoperatively.[52] There is little reason to believe that digoxin prevents the development of AF; indeed, clinical trails do not clearly substantiate either a lower incidence of AF or a slower ventricular rate in AF in patients treated prophylactically with digoxin.[53] Futhermore, hypoxia, hypokalemia, elevated catecholamine levels, and reduced clearance of digoxin are common postoperatively, and these conditions may predispose the patient to digoxin toxicity.

ATRIAL FIBRILLATION

Because of the hazards of postoperative AF, considerable effort has been devoted to identifying preoperative factors associated with an increased risk of postoperative arrhythmia.[52] Such factors include advanced age and male gender. It has been proposed that a prolonged P wave duration recorded on a signal-averaged electrocardiogram (ECG) and greater than 70 percent narrowing of the lumen of the right coronary artery are associated with an increased risk of postoperative AF.[54, 55] However, for a substantial number of patients with postoperative AF, no apparent preoperative risk factor can be identified. Cox has presented clinical data suggesting that about one-third of patients undergoing cardiac operations are vulnerable to postoperative AF because of mild nonuniformity in the distribution of their trial refractory periods.[56] Intraoperative atrial ischemia associated with rapid rewarming of the atria during prolonged periods of cold cardioplegic arrest may increase the dispersion of refractoriness in the atria of such patients and thereby increase the risk of postoperative AF.

Because of difficulties in reliably identifying patients at risk for AF preoperatively, it is common clinical practice to provide prophylactic therapy to the majority of patients undergoing CABG surgery. Beta-adrenoceptor blocking agents are most suitable for prophylaxis against AF.[52, 53] In the *absence* of an ejection fraction less than 30 percent, severe bronchospastic lung disease, or bradyarrythmias, we advocate the use of prophylactic beta blockers in patients undergoing CABG. Conclusive data regarding the use of prophylactic antiarrhythmic therapy to prevent postoperative AF are lacking, although prophylactic amiodarone in selected patients has appeared promising in several clinical trials.[57, 58]

BRADYARRHYTHMIAS AND ATRIOVENTRICULAR AND INTRAVENTRICULAR BLOCK.
Patients with high-grade (third-degree or type II second-degree) atrioventricular block and hemodynamic compromise (systolic pressure <90 mm Hg) are at high risk during general anesthesia unless a temporary transvenous pacemaker wire is inserted preoperatively.

In patients in whom a permanent pacemaker has been implanted, its specifications (model, mode, and settings) and, if possible, a statement regarding the pacemaker dependency of the patient should be noted in the medical record (see Chap. 24). The possibility of postoperative malfunction in the permanent pacing system because of the effects of anesthesia, electrocautery, and surgical manipulation of the leads (e.g., during atrial cannulation) should be anticipated.[59] Clinicians should have the appropriate pacemaker programming equipment available postoperatively because many problems (secondary to electromagnetic interference from the electrocautery apparatus) can be quickly resolved by interrogation of the generator and reprogramming in the recovery area.

The risk of permanent, complete heart block postoperatively is increased with multiple valve replacements, particularly in patients who have had previous valve surgery. However, implantation of a permanent epicardial pacing lead is rarely needed at the time of surgery because of the ease of implantation of a transvenous endocardial system postoperatively. An exception would be patients who are undergoing tricuspid valve replacement with a mechanical prosthesis, especially if they are simultaneously undergoing an aortic or mitral valve operation. Because of the contraindication to passing a transvenous lead through the mechanical tricuspid prosthesis, the surgical team should be alerted to the need for placement of permanent epicardial leads intraoperatively.

Patients with previously implanted cardioverter-defibrillator devices should have their unit disabled prior to surgery to minimize the risk of inappropriate shocks from sensing of electrocautery signals intraoperatively. Until the device is reactivated in the postoperative period, equipment for rapid external defibrillation should be available.

Perioperative Drug Therapy

With the exception of oral anticoagulation with warfarin, most medications can and should be continued up to the time of surgery. Clinical trials of patients receiving saphenous vein bypass grafts demonstrated the importance of initiating antiplatelet therapy in the perioperative period.[60] Because of the increased risk of postoperative bleeding, some surgical groups discontinue aspirin use for several days preoperatively in elective cases. Many cardiologists are concerned about the risk of "breakthrough" episodes of ischemia if aspirin therapy is discontinued preoperatively and prefer to continue it up to the time of surgery and rely on preoperative donations of autologous red cells, cell saver techniques, autotransfusion of shed blood intraoperatively and postoperatively, and drugs such as aprotinin to minimize the need for and potential hazards of homologous blood transfusion. If aspirin is witheld preoperatively, it should be restarted within 24 to 48 hours after surgery to reduce the risk of vein graft occlusion.[60] Warfarin therapy should be stopped 2 to 3 days preoperatively and, if necessary, treatment with heparin or low-molecular-weight dextran initiated.

Although definitive data are not available, it is our usual practice to continue both aspirin and clopidogrel up to the time of surgery in patients who have undergone implantation of a stent in the coronary circulation within the preceeding 2 weeks in order to minimize the risk of stent thrombosis preoperatively. For patients who have had a stent implanted more than 2 weeks prior to surgery, we discontinue clopidogrel administration but continue aspirin up to the time of surgery. For patients receiving long-term clopidogrel as secondary prevention for vascular disease, we discontinue use of the drug 5 to 7 days preoperatively.

To minimize the risk of intraoperative bleeding, if patients are undergoing interventional catheterization procedures and have normal renal function and if cardiac surgery is likely to take place within the ensuing 24 to 48 hours, we prefer to use a short-acting intravenous glycoprotein IIb/IIIa inhibitor such as eptifibatide or tirofiban rather than a long-acting agent such as abciximab. Treatment with the short-acting agent is usually discontinued 6 to 12 hours preoperatively to permit platelet function to return toward normal. We prefer to use abciximab in patients with renal dysfunction since the small, short-acting inhibitors are cleared predominantly through renal elimination. When abciximab is used, we discontinue the infusion at least 12 hours prior to surgery.

For patients who have received an intravenous glycoprotein IIb/IIIa inhibitor and must proceed urgently to cardiac surgery, the antiplatelet effects of abciximab may be reversed by platelet transfusions.[60a] In contrast, the high excess of free drug versus bound drug in the case of eptifibatide or tirofiban limits the ability of platelet transfusions to restore normal platelet function. In cases in which urgent removal of epifibatide or tirofiban from the circulation is desired, hemodialysis may be necessary.

Calcium antagonists previously prescribed for control of ischemic heart disease should be continued up to the time of surgery to reduce the chance of myocardial ischemia from withdrawal of the drug. In the case of diltiazem and verapamil, the dose may need to be reduced because these agents may provoke bradycardia and a low-output syndrome postoperatively, especially if a beta blocker or amiodarone is given concurrently or the patient is elderly. Profound atropine- and isoproterenol-resistant bradyarrhythmias may occur postoperatively in patients treated with these calcium antagonists, particularly when the patient has not yet recovered from the hypothermia that is imposed intraoperatively; temporary dual-chamber pacing support should be available to manage such patients.

CONTINUATION OF ANTIARRHYTHMICS. With the exception of amiodarone, antiarrhythmic drugs that have been prescribed for hemodynamically compromising or life-threatening ventricular tachyarrhythmias should be continued up to the time of surgery because of the risk of "breakthrough" of a potentially lethal ventricular arrhythmia in the preoperative period.

Patients with a documented history of resuscitation from sudden cardiac death who are receiving amiodarone should continue to receive this drug up to the time of surgery. However, in cases in which amiodarone was prescribed for a less overtly life-threatening arrhythmia (e.g., AF), the maintenance dosage has been greater than 200 mg/d, and the patient has a history of lung disease, we recommend at least a 3-month period of abstinence from the drug before subjecting the patient to elective cardiopulmonary bypass.

IMPLANTABLE CARDIOVERTER-DEFIBRILLATORS. Prophylactic implantation of cardioverter-defibrillators at the time of CABG in patients at high risk for ventricular arrhythmias (ejection fraction ≤ 35 percent, abnormal signal-averaged ECG) does not improve survival.[5]

INTRAOPERATIVE MANAGEMENT

Despite increased risks, particularly related to age and advanced disease, cardiac surgery patients today enjoy markedly improved outcomes when compared with patients operated on 10 years ago. Important intraoperative surgical advances that have contributed to this improval outcome include epiaortic echocardiographic scanning in patients with ascending aortic atherosclerosis, transesophageal echocardiography, retrograde blood cardioplegia, retrograde cerebral perfusion in patients requiring circulatory arrest, and performance of all vascular anastomoses with a single aortic cross-clamp under cardioplegic arrest. Emphasis on modern strategies to ensure blood conservation and minimize hemostatic complications has significantly decreased or eliminated homologous blood exposure for most patients undergoing cardiac surgery (Fig. 60–2).

Until recently, nearly all cardiac surgical procedures were performed via a standard median sternotomy with the use of cardiopulmonary bypass and cardiac arrest to provide a bloodless, motionless field (Fig. 60–3). Cardiac surgeons have recently explored less invasive approaches to coronary and valvular heart disease. The impetus for this change has been to decrease overall surgical trauma associated with full sternotomy and cardiopulmonary bypass without compromising the efficacy and safety of procedures. In valvular heart disease, cardiopulmonary bypass is essential, and therefore the focus has been on reducing trauma through a variety of less invasive incisions (Fig. 60–4). In coronary surgery, smaller incisions have also been used with or without cardiopulmonary bypass, particulary to perform single-vessel bypass to the left anterior descending artery. Recent technical advances in myocardial stabilization (Fig. 60–5) have now focused attention on off-pump multivessel coronary bypass through a full sternotomy.[60b] This approach is particularly appealing in selected high-risk patients, including those with ascending aortic atherosclerosis, renal dysfunction, and severe pulmonary disease. Wider adoption of less invasive cardiac surgical techniques can be anticipated if ongoing clinical trials demonstrate short-term patient benefit and medium- and long-term results comparable to those obtained with standard techniques.[60c]

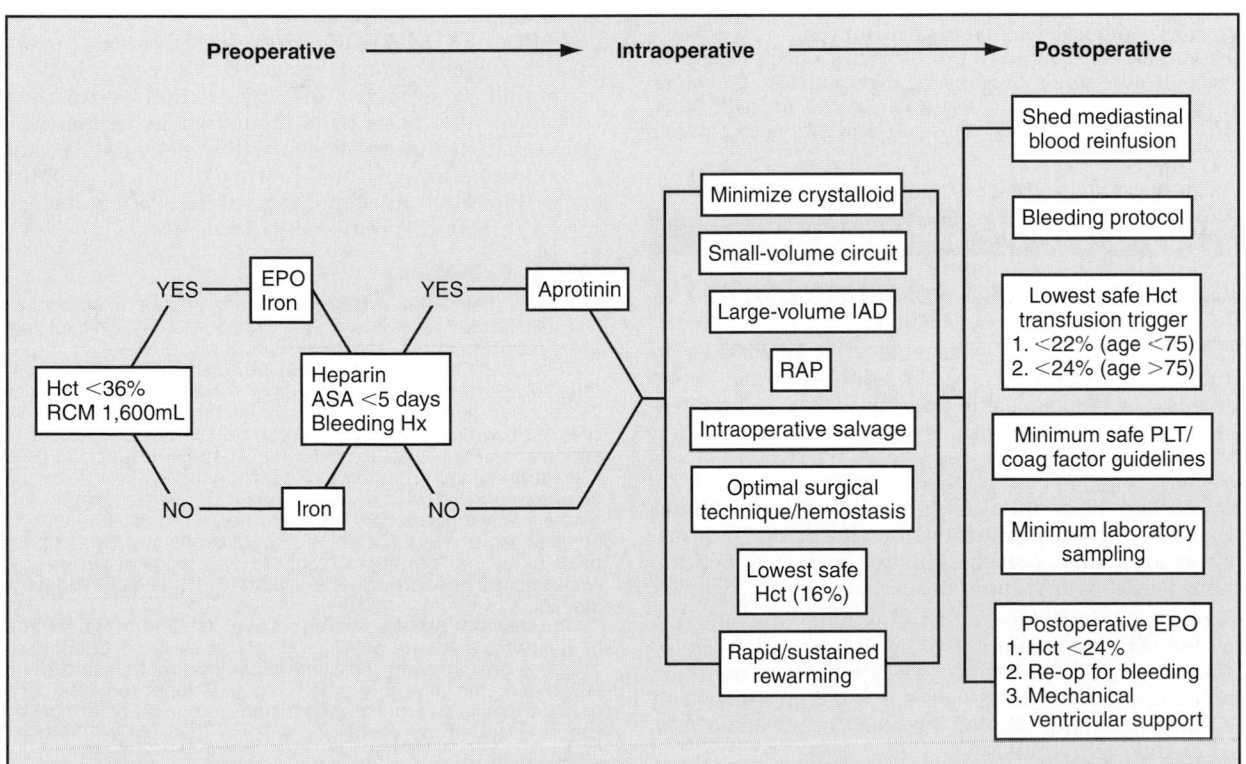

FIGURE 60–2. Multimodality algorithm designed to optimize blood conservation in cardiac surgical patients. Preoperative, intraoperative, and postoperative strategies are all important to eliminate the requirement for homologous blood transfusion. ASA = aspirin; coag = coagulation; EPO = erythropoietin; Hct = hematocrit; Hx = history; IAD = intraoperative autologous donation; PLT = platelet; RAP = retrograde autologous priming; RCM = red cell mass. (From Rosengart TK: Open heart surgery without transfusion in high-risk patients. Am J Cardiol 83:31B–37B, 1999.)

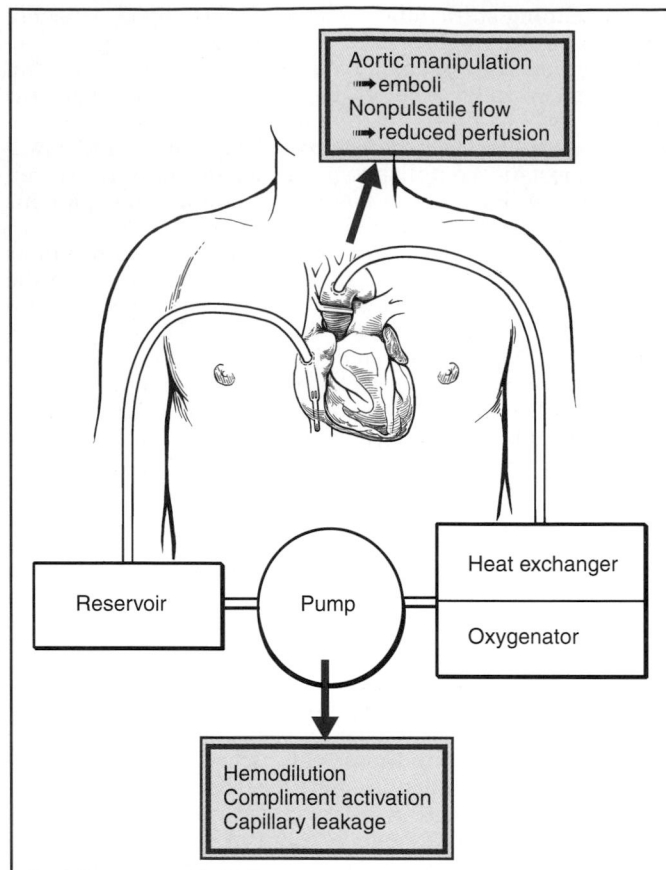

FIGURE 60–3. Schematic diagram of a typical cardiopulmonary bypass circuit. Venous blood is drained by a cannula from the right atrium into a reservoir and then pumped through an oxygenator and heat exchanger and returned via an aortic cannula to the ascending aorta. Although cardiopulmonary bypass is extremely safe in the current era, morbidity may occur in selected patients. Cerebral emboli may result from aortic manipulation. End-organ perfusion may be reduced as a result of loss of pulsatile flow. Finally, the bypass circuit may cause hemodilution and trigger systemic activation.

POSTOPERATIVE MANAGEMENT

Fluid, Electrolyte, and Acid-Base Balance

Extracorporeal circulation is associated with an increase in extracellular fluid and total exchangeable sodium, along with a decrease in exchangeable potassium. The cumulative experience in many centers has led to the following basic principles of management:

1. For the first 48 hours after surgery, free water is limited to about 1000 ml/d and intravenous fluids are administered in the form of 5 percent glucose in water. Sodium replacement varies with volume needs.

2. Serum potassium levels can fluctuate dramatically; therefore, frequent measurement of serum potassium is indicated, especially in diabetics. We attempt to maintain serum potassium in the range of 4.5 ± 0.5 mEq/liter and magnesium at 2.0 mEq/liter or greater to minimize the chance of cardiac arrhythmias.

3. Serum glucose levels are frequently elevated (250 to 400 mg/dl), as a result of glucose-containing intravenous solutions and surgically induced increases in cortisol and catecholamine levels. In nondiabetic patients, insulin therapy is not usually required, whereas it is routinely used in insulin-requiring diabetic patients to avoid uncontrolled hyperglycemia.

4. Mild metabolic acidosis or metabolic alkalosis may be present for the first 24 hours postoperatively, particularly during rewarming. These acid-base abnormalities usually do not require correction in the absence of preoperative renal dysfunction or development of acute renal failure postoperatively.[61] Significant metabolic acidosis (pH <7.35) should be avoided during the rewarming phase, particularly if patients are dependent on an inotropic agent. Hyperventilation (PCO_2 <35 mm Hg) and treatment with sodium bicarbonate should be instituted.

5. Serum total calcium, phosphorus, and magnesium levels are frequently depressed for about 24 to 48 hours in normally convalescing patients, partly because of the effects of hemodilution. These electrolyte abnormalities are usually self-correcting, and replacement therapy is not generally required. A possible exception is hypomagnesemia, which may predispose to the development of cardiac arrhythmias.[52]

Respiratory Management

EFFECTS OF ANESTHESIA, STERNOTOMY, AND CARDIOPULMONARY BYPASS ON PULMONARY FUNCTION. Four broad areas should be considered, as outlined in Table 60–3.[62, 63] most all patients experience alveolar dysfunction after open-heart surgery because of right-to-left intrapulmonary shunting of blood from various intrinsic alveolar abnormalities (e.g., atelectasis, edema, infection) and pulmonary vascular events (e.g., extravasation of fluid, inhibition of hypoxia-induced vasoconstriction). Central respiratory drive and respiratory muscle function are depressed postoperatively because of a combination of pharmacological effects and mechanical derangements of thoracic function. Patients with preexisting pulmonary disease may experience more profound depression of respiratory function necessitating vigorous pulmonary toilette.

EARLY EXTUBATION. Historically, most postoperative cardiac surgery patients received between 6 and 18 hours of ventilatory support (Table 60–4). Early extubation protocols have now been widely adopted in cardiac ICUs, and stable patients are extubated within 4 hours. Advantages of early extubation include improved patient mobility with early transition to step-down units. Patient selection for early extubation is outlined in Table 60–4.

SPECIAL PROBLEMS

Failure to meet early extubation criteria may result from a variety of factors. Careful assessment will usually identify one or more etiologies resulting in respiratory dysfunction.

INCREASED ALVEOLAR-ARTERIAL GRADIENT. An increased alveolar-arterial gradient postoperatively is a serious problem that demands thorough evaluation. The ventilator settings should be checked and a chest radiograph obtained to ascertain the position of the tip of the endotracheal tube (to exclude, for example, intubation of the right main stem bronchus) and to rule out pneumothorax, lobar atelectasis or pneumonia, or a large pleural effusion. Hemodynamic monitoring by means of a pulmonary artery catheter can cause pulmonary hemorrhage from overinflation of the balloon, and bronchoscopy may need to be performed to diagnose and manage the problem (e.g., occlusion of the bronchus draining the bleeding segment of the lung).

PULMONARY EDEMA (see also Chap. 17). The most common cause of pulmonary edema postoperatively is elevated pulmonary venous pressure arising from left ventricular dysfunction and/or a valvular lesion (e.g., mitral regurgitation). Such patients require aggressive diuresis, as well as vasodilator/inotropic and possibly intraaortic balloon support. Mechanical ventilation with positive end-expiratory pressure (PEEP) is used until the patient's ventricular function improves. Repeat surgery may be needed if pulmonary edema persists despite attempts to control severe mitral regurgitation medically.

In a minority of patients, pulmonary edema after cardiac surgery is due to the adult respiratory distress syndrome. In its most extreme form, this disorder is associated with a generalized whole-body *post-pump syndrome* characterized by increased capillary permeability, interstitial edema, fever, leukocytosis, renal dysfunction, and hemodynamic collapse.

UNDERLYING CHRONIC LUNG DISEASE. General surgical preparation

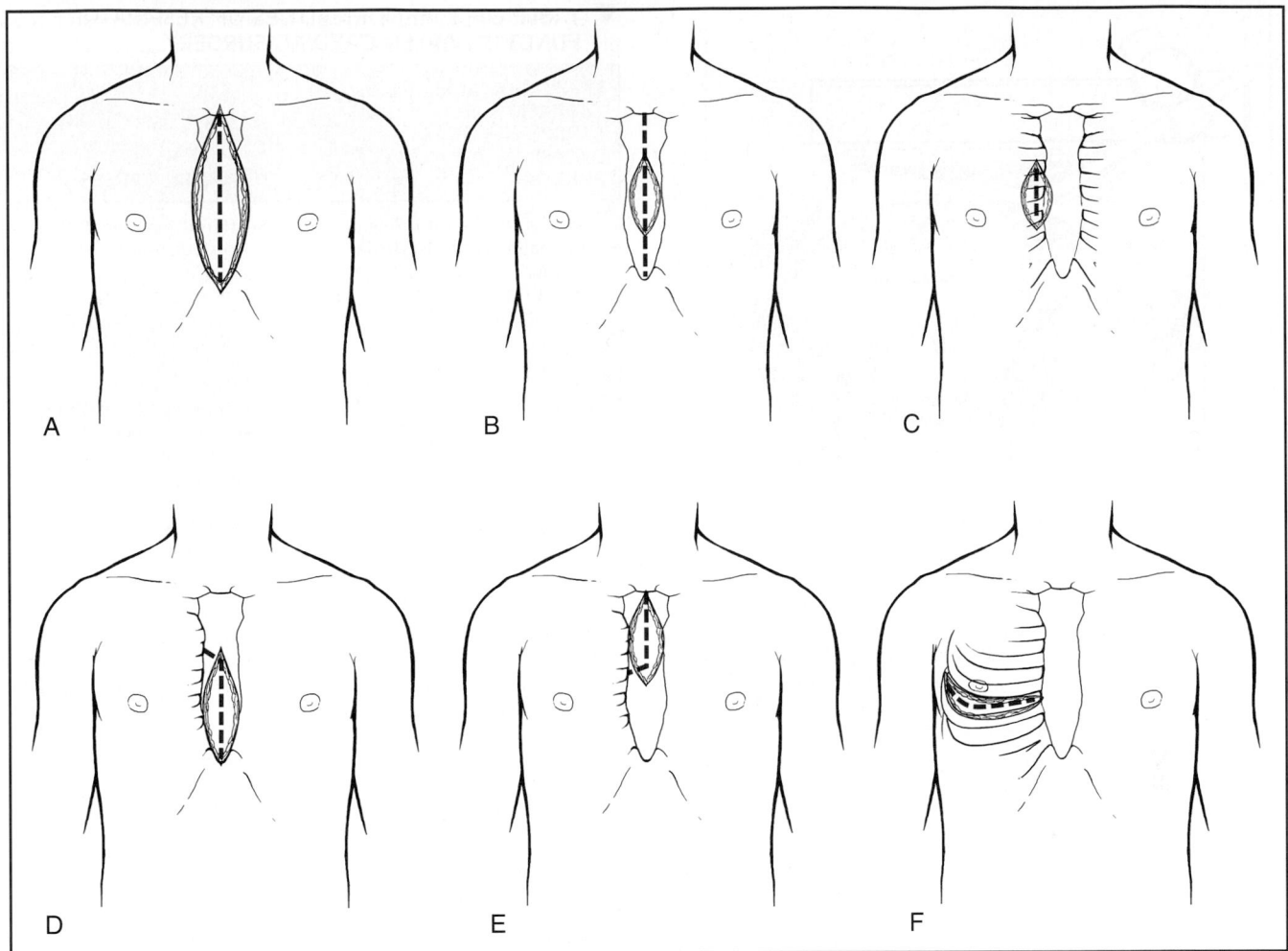

FIGURE 60–4. Schematic representation of traditional incision and sternotomy (*A*) compared with a variety of less invasive incisions (dotted lines represent chest wall incisions). Limited skin incision/full sternotomy (*B*) is gaining in popularity because of improved cosmetics and reduced trauma from the limited chest wall retraction. Although once popular, the parasternal approach (*C*) is used less frequently because of the residual chest wall defect. Partial lower or upper sternotomy (*D* and *E*) has been used predominantly in valve procedures. Right anterior thoracotomy (*F*) is a useful approach, particularly in mitral valve reoperations. Left anterior thoracotomy has been described for coronary bypass procedures.

of patients with obstructive lung disease, including antibiotics, bronchodilators, and cessation of cigarette smoking, may help minimize the risk of respiratory failure from postoperative atelectasis and pneumonia.[62, 63] Inhaled bronchodilators should be continued postoperatively. Refractory patients may require a short course of corticosteroids (e.g., methylprednisolone 0.5 mg/kg every 6 hours for 3 days) to be weaned from the ventilator.[62] Previous enthusiasm for intravenous methylxanthines has waned because of evidence of limited efficacy and the risk of agitation, arrhythmias, and grand mal seizures.[64] Intravenous theophylline should therefore be reserved for extremely refractory cases and administered in a dose of 0.4 mg/kg/hr with careful monitoring of plasma levels to maintain them in the range of 10 to 15 μg/ml.

We have successfully operated on patients with severe respiratory compromise, including those with a forced expiratory volume in 1 second (FEV$_1$) of less than 0.8 liters who require home oxygen therapy. All patients with severe pulmonary dysfunction are considered for early extubation. It is important to maintain the arterial carbon dioxide tension close to the patient's baseline level to ensure an adequate respiratory drive.

DIAPHRAGMATIC FAILURE. Diaphragmatic dysfunction after cardiac surgical procedures usually occurs as a result of injury to the phrenic nerve(s). An elevated hemidiaphragm may be seen on postoperative radiographs in 25 percent of patients who undergo myocardial preservation including topical ice slush and harvesting of an internal mammary artery.[65] A simple bedside test of diaphragmatic function is to ask the patient to protrude the umbilicus, a movement that requires diaphragmatic functional integrity. Of note, an elevated hemidiaphragm is not usually associated with increased postoperative morbidity or mortality.

Recovery of the hemidiaphragm to normal position occurs in 80 percent of patients at 1 year and nearly all patients by 2 years postoperatively. Clinically important diaphragmatic dysfunction caused by unilateral or bilateral phrenic nerve injury develops in less than 1 percent of patients after cardiac surgery.

Evidence of diaphragmatic failure includes an inability to wean the patient from the ventilator, vital capacity less than 500 cc, and paradoxical movement of the diaphragm on fluoroscopy (abnormal "sniff" test)[62] or ultrasonography.

PROLONGED VENTILATORY INSUFFICIENCY. Patients who fail to be weaned from the ventilator within 48 hours require special attention. Because of the risk of stress-induced gastritis, H$_2$ receptor blockers (e.g., ranitidine 50 mg intravenously every 8 to 12 hours) or a mucosal cytoprotective agent (sucralfate 1 gm orally two to four times per day) is administered. Nutritional support is critical to provide metabolic needs and prevent the catabolism of respiratory muscles (see Fig. 60–1). Pressure support ventilation strategies are particularly useful for patients in need of prolonged ventilation. Barotrauma is minimized and patient comfort improved while permitting incremental weaning in small steps.

High-compliance, low-pressure cuff (<20 mm Hg) endotracheal tubes have reduced the risk of mechanical complications (e.g., tracheal stenosis) and permit patients to remain intubated for several weeks. Nonetheless, we believe that patients requiring prolonged ventilatory support beyond 10 to 14 days will generally benefit from a decision to

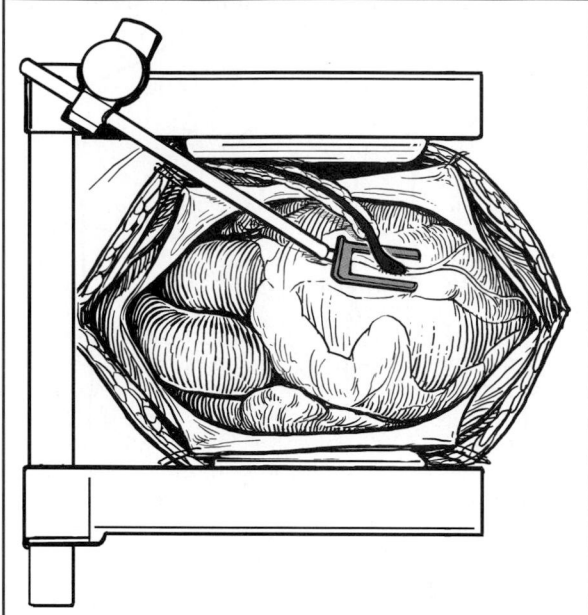

FIGURE 60–5. Off-pump coronary bypass surgery on the beating heart has been facilitated by the development of platform stabilization systems to provide isolated immobilization during the performance of distal anastomoses. The left anterior descending artery is most amenable to platform stabilization as opposed to the posterolateral circulation.

proceed with early tracheostomy.[65a] Tracheostomy provides improved patient comfort and greater pulmonary toilet and enhances weaning by minimizing pulmonary dead space. Percutaneous tracheostomy offers the advantage of bedside insertion with minimal surgical trauma and is particularly useful in patients with reasonable ventilatory mechanics but heavy secretions.

▼ **TABLE 60–3.** ABNORMALITIES OF RESPIRATORY FUNCTION AFTER CARDIAC SURGERY

EFFECTS OF ANESTHESIA, THORACIC SURGERY, AND CARDIOPULMONARY BYPASS ON PULMONARY FUNCTION	POTENTIAL CAUSES
Alveolar dysfunction (e.g., widened alveolar-arterial oxygen gradient because of right-to-left intrapulmonary shunting)	Scattered regions of atelectasis with preserved perfusion
	Pulmonary edema (e.g., cardiogenic, noncardiogenic "postpump" alveolar capillary leak)
	Infection
	Inhibition of hypoxic pulmonary vasoconstriction by anesthetic agents
	Exacerbation of ventilation/perfusion mismatch by vasodilating agents used postoperatively (e.g., nitroprusside)
Decreased central respiratory drive	General anesthetics
	Narcotic analgesics
	Cerebral insult in perioperative period
Decreased respiratory muscle function	Thoracic pain (incision, chest tubes)
	Persistent effects of muscle relaxants
	Age
	Obesity
	Depressed cardiac function
	Primary diaphragmatic dysfunction (e.g., phrenic nerve injury)
Exacerbation of underlying chronic pulmonary disease	Increase in airway resistance
	Increased secretions and worsening bronchitis
	Pneumonia

▼ **TABLE 60–4.** CARDIAC SURGERY EARLY EXTUBATION PROTOCOL

Definition	Extubation within 4 hr after surgery
Patient selection	
Inclusion criteria	All patients ≤80 yr old, LV ejection fraction >25%
Exclusion criteria	High inotropic requirement, postoperative bleeding or ischemia
Anesthetic management	
Intraoperative	Low-dose synthetic narcotics and inhalation agents
Postoperative	Muscle relaxant reversal
	Propofol 0.1 ml/kg/hr
	Minimize narcotic use
Ventilatory management	
Postoperative	SIMV mode
	Check ABGs and decrease ventilatory support every 20 min
	Always keep between pH 7.35 and 7.45
	Always keep PO_2 >75 mm Hg
Extubation guidelines	
Oxygenation	PO_2 >75 mm Hg at an FIO_2 ≤0.50
Respiratory drive	PCO_2 <45 mm Hg and pH >7.35
	Spontaneously breathing
Mechanics	Respiratory rate <25 breaths/min
	Negative inspiratory pressure >20 cm H_2O
	Tidal volume >8 cc/kg
	Vital capacity >10 cc/kg
Airway protection	Alert with gag reflex
	Absence of heavy secretions
Cardiovascular	Cardiac index >2.0 liters/min/m²
	MAP >80 and <120 mm Hg

ABG = arterial blood gas; LV = left ventricular; MAP = mean arterial pressure; SIMV = synchronized intermittent mandatory ventilation.

Hypertension

Postoperative hypertension has been defined variably in the literature,[66] but we consider it to be present if systolic pressure exceeds 140 mm Hg.[67] The incidence of postoperative hypertension ranges from 40 to 60 percent. It occurs more commonly in patients with a preoperative history of hypertension, prior maintenance therapy with a beta blocker, and well-preserved left ventricular function.[68] Postoperative hypertension is especially frequent after CABG and surgical relief of left ventricular outflow tract obstruction (e.g., aortic valve replacement, correction of coarctation of the aorta).

The mechanism of postoperative hypertension probably varies from patient to patient but usually includes (1) a "rebound" effect from withdrawal of beta blockade administered preoperatively; (2) excessive sympathetic nervous system activity with elevated levels of circulating catecholamines (especially norepinephrine)[69]; (3) pressor reflexes originating in the heart, great vessels, or coronary arteries[70]; and (4) a drop in aortic pressure proximal to the site of the corrected coarctation with resultant stimulation of aortic and carotid baroreceptors by apparent "hypotension." The renin-angiotensin system is stimulated and peripheral resistance is increased. Sudden exposure of vascular beds downstream from the coarctation to "undamped" aortic pressure has also been reported to cause mesenteric arteritis.

The adverse consequences of elevated systemic pressure include an increased risk of postoperative bleeding, suture line disruption, and aortic dissection[61]; elevated left ventricular afterload and a consequent reduction in left ventricular output; and injury to aortocoronary bypass grafts and postoperative stroke.

MANAGEMENT. Although a variety of agents may be used for treating acute postoperative hypertension, we prefer those that are rapidly acting and titratable and have a short half-life. Nitroglycerin is our first-choice agent, beginning at a dose of 25 μg/min and titrating up to a dose of 300 μg/min. Sodium nitroprusside (0.5 to 2 μg/kg/min) may be required in hypertension refractory to nitroglycerin therapy. Because of its prominent vasodilatory effects, sodium nitroprusside should be administered with caution for the first 3 to 4 hours after surgery since volume shifts may occur during the rewarming phase. The ultrashort-acting beta blocker esmolol (50 to 250 μg/kg/min) may be useful in patients with a hyperdynamic circulation. It is initially preferred over longer-acting beta blockers when evaluating patient tolerance to beta blockade (e.g., moderately severe left ventricular dysfunction). The need for transition to oral antihypertensive therapy is assessed on an individual basis; chronic treatment is usually required in patients with a preoperative history of hypertension.

Perioperative Myocardial Infarction

(See also Chap. 35)

Despite modern intraoperative myocardial protection and improvements in surgical technique, some degree of ischemia occurs nearly uniformly during CABG. Only a minority of patients (5 to 15 percent of patients undergoing CABG), however, actually experience a *perioperative myocardial infarction*, even in tertiary care centers currently operating on higher-risk patients, including those with failed interventional procedures.[71-73] Potential causes of myocardial ischemia and infarction in the perioperative period include incomplete revascularization; diffuse atherosclerotic disease of the distal coronary arteries; spasm, embolism, or thrombosis of the native coronary vessels or bypass grafts[74, 75]; technical problems with graft anastomoses; inadequate myocardial preservation intraoperatively; increased myocardial oxygen needs, as in left ventricular hypertrophy; and hemodynamic derangements in the postoperative period (e.g., hypotension, hypertension, tachycardia). Although initially one might suspect that perioperative myocardial infarction results from occlusion of bypass grafts placed to circumvent diseased coronary arteries, autopsy studies have shown that bypass grafts are usually patent in patients dying of a perioperative myocardial infarction.[76] This observation lends support to the concept that poor myocardial protection or a mismatch between myocardial oxygen supply and demand postoperatively accounts for much of the infarction noted.

DIAGNOSIS. The diagnosis of a myocardial infarction after cardiac surgery is more difficult than at other times because of the nonspecific ST-T wave abnormalities on ECG and nearly universal elevation of creatine kinase (CK) levels postoperatively. A number of diagnostic findings (Table 60-5) must be carefully interpreted and then integrated as shown in the algorithm displayed in Table 60-6.

A 12-lead ECG should be obtained immediately on the patient's arrival in the ICU after surgery and no less frequently than once every 24 hours for the first few postoperative days. Measurements of total CK and CK-MB should be made every 8 hours for the first 24 to 36 hours if perioperative myocardial infarction is suspected.

TROPONIN. Experience with newer, more sensitive serum markers of cardiac injury, such as troponin I and troponin T, is limited.[77, 78] However, initial reports suggest that cardiac-specific troponin I and

▼ **TABLE 60-5. DIAGNOSIS OF MYOCARDIAL INFARCTION AFTER CARDIAC SURGERY**

DIAGNOSTIC FINDING	COMMENT
Symptoms	
Early (<24 hr postop)	Not reliable because of residual effects of anesthesia and postoperative analgesics
Late (>24 hr postop)	Potentially reliable but may be confused with incisional pain and pleuritic pain from chest tubes, pericarditis
Electrocardiogram	
New, persistent Q waves	Most reliable diagnostic finding, but only if the Q waves persist on serial ECGs over several days
Evolutionary ST-T changes	Supportive data favoring the diagnosis of MI only if a typical evolutionary pattern is observed. Because of the effects of cardiopulmonary bypass, hypothermia, postoperative pericarditis, mediastinal chest tubes, and medications (e.g., digitalis), a variety of nonspecific ST-T wave abnormalities may be seen and should not be relied on for diagnosing perioperative MI
Myocardial-specific enzymes	
Total CK	Elevated total CK levels postoperatively may arise from multiple sources, including skeletal muscle in the thorax and calf, as well as myocardium
CK-MB	Myocardial-specific CK may be released from ischemia occurring during cardiopulmonary bypass, as well as myocardial and aortic incisions made intraoperatively (e.g., right atrium for cannulation of the cavae). Because of the nearly universal release of CK-MB, a diagnosis of MI should not be made unless CK-MB is significantly elevated (e.g., >30 units/liter)
Echocardiogram	A regional wall motion abnormality is a helpful finding, particularly if it can be shown to be a new finding by comparison with a preoperative study. Paradoxical motion of the high anterior portion of the interventricular septum is a common finding postoperatively in the absence of MI and should not be taken as the sole evidence of new perioperative myocardial necrosis

CK = creatine kinase; MI = myocardial infarction.

▼ TABLE 60–6. ALGORITHM FOR DIAGNOSIS OF PERIOPERATIVE MYOCARDIAL INFARCTION AFTER CARDIAC SURGERY

NEW Qs ON ECG	CK-MB >30 IU/LITER	NEW RWMA ON ECHO*	DIAGNOSIS	COMMENT
Yes	Yes	Yes	Definite MI	
Yes	Yes	No	Probable MI	New zone of necrosis not evident on ECHO. The persistence of new Q waves and abnormally elevated CK-MB suggests that Q waves are not a "benign" postoperative finding
Yes	No	Yes	Definite MI	CK-MB peak probably missed because of infrequent sampling
Yes	No	No	Possible MI	New Q waves may be false-positive finding
No	Yes	Yes	Probable MI	Non–Q-wave MI
No	Yes	No	MI unlikely	Small non–Q-wave MI cannot be entirely excluded
No	No	Yes	MI unlikely	Removal of "restraining" effect of pericardium may result in new RWMAs, especially in high anterior septal area
No	No	No	No MI	Although small patchy areas of necrosis may be seen histologically, these abnormalities are probably not of clinical significance

* Perioperative echocardiography is not *required* for the diagnosis of a perioperative MI but can provide useful supportive data or aid in the diagnosis in unclear cases, especially if obtained acutely.

ECHO = echocardiography; MI = myocardial infarction; RWMA = regional wall motion abnormality.

troponin T are elevated postoperatively in virtually all patients who undergo CABG surgery. Patients who experience a perioperative myocardial infarction release greater quanitities of troponin such that serum measurements may remain 10- to 20-fold higher than the upper limit of the reference interval for at least 4 to 5 days postoperatively. Even in patients not experiencing perioperative myocardial infarctions by conventional diagnostic criteria, the relative increase in proteins such as cardiac troponin I over preoperative baseline values is greater than that of CK-MB, which suggests that troponin measurements can detect small amounts of myocardial tissue damage that are not detected by CK-MB.

ELECTROCARDIOGRAPHY. The ECG is the most reliable tool for diagnosing a perioperative myocardial infarction. New and persistent Q waves accompanied by new, persistent, and evolutionary ST-T wave abnormalities are the most helpful criteria. Pathological Q waves resulting from perioperative myocardial infarction may appear with an earlier time course (i.e., immediately on arrival from the operating room) than in a nonrevascularized patient.

ECHOCARDIOGRAPHY. Bedside echocardiograms (transthoracic and if necessary transesophageal) play an important role in establishing the diagnosis of a perioperative myocardial infarction by detecting new regional wall motion abnormalities in cases in which the ECG or serum marker measurements are unclear. It is especially helpful to compare new echocardiograms with the preoperative studies that are almost always available.

RISKS AND CONSEQUENCES OF PERIOPERATIVE INFARCTION. Variables that have been found to correlate with the development of perioperative myocardial infarction in patients undergoing CABG include emergency surgery, aortic cross-clamp time greater than 100 minutes, a recent myocardial infarction (within the prior week), and a history of previous revascularization (either percutaneous transluminal coronary angioplasty or CABG surgery).[73]

Patients with a perioperative myocardial infarction have increased hospital mortality (about 10 to 15 percent) when compared with patients undergoing CABG who have not sustained a perioperative myocardial infarction (about 1 percent).[73, 79]

Characteristics of patients who are especially at risk of increased short-term mortality after a perioperative myocardial infarction include age older than 65 years, unstable angina preoperatively, a myocardial infarction within 1 week before surgery, left ventricular aneurysm, intraventricular conduction disturbance (e.g., left bundle branch block), and the need for reoperation for bleeding. About two-thirds of the postoperative mortality is due to pump failure and one-third is due to malignant ventricular tachyarrhythmias.[79] Perioperative myocardial infarction also adversely affects the long-term prognosis, particularly if associated with inadequate revascularization and depressed left ventricular function.[80]

MANAGEMENT OF MYOCARDIAL ISCHEMIA AFTER CABG. Patients with evidence of myocardial ischemia after coronary bypass surgery require an integrated assessment of clinical findings and laboratory tests on an individualized basis to define the appropriate management strategy. At the center of the decision pathway are the 12-lead ECG and hemodynamic observations (Fig. 60–6). Patients with ST elevations and a low cardiac index require intraaortic balloon pump support. Two-dimensional echocardiography is useful to detect new wall motion abnormalities that may necessitate coronary angiography and a percutaneous revascularization procedure in selected patients.

Low-Output Syndrome and Shock States

RECOGNITION. Sometimes, diagnosis of low-output syndrome and a shock state after cardiac surgery is difficult. Because cold extremities and mottled skin may result from hypothermia postoperatively, these observations lack sufficient specificity. Although reduced systolic pressure is the most striking manifestation of this disorder, low-output syndrome may be present even if the arterial systolic pressure exceeds 100 mm Hg because increased systemic vascular resistance (>1500 dyne-sec $\cdot$ cm^{-2}) may be supporting the peripheral perfusion pressure. It is important to recognize this syndrome because of the strong relationship between cardiac index in the early postoperative period and the probability of cardiac death after surgery. Common clinical features of the low-output syndrome and shock states after cardiac surgery include cold extremities, mottled skin, reduced systolic pressure (<90 mm Hg), decreased urine output (<30 ml/hr), low cardiac index (<2.0 liter/min/m²), low mixed venous oxygen saturation (<50 percent), and acidosis.

One should make careful hemodynamic measurements and integrate them with bedside echocardiographic recordings to confirm the diagnosis of low-output syndrome and attempt to segregate the findings into one of the patterns (*reduced preload, cardiogenic shock,* or *sepsis*) in Table 60–7. Although the hemodynamic findings among these patterns overlap and the coexistence of multiple disorders (e.g., bradycardia and hypovolemia) may blur the distinction between patterns, they offer a clinically useful approach to the evaluation of a patient with low-output syndrome. In addition to the specific treatment measures discussed below, a number of general measures are applicable to all patients who are in a shock-like condition after cardiac surgery, including prompt correction of any electrolyte and acid-base disturbances, transfusion to a hematocrit

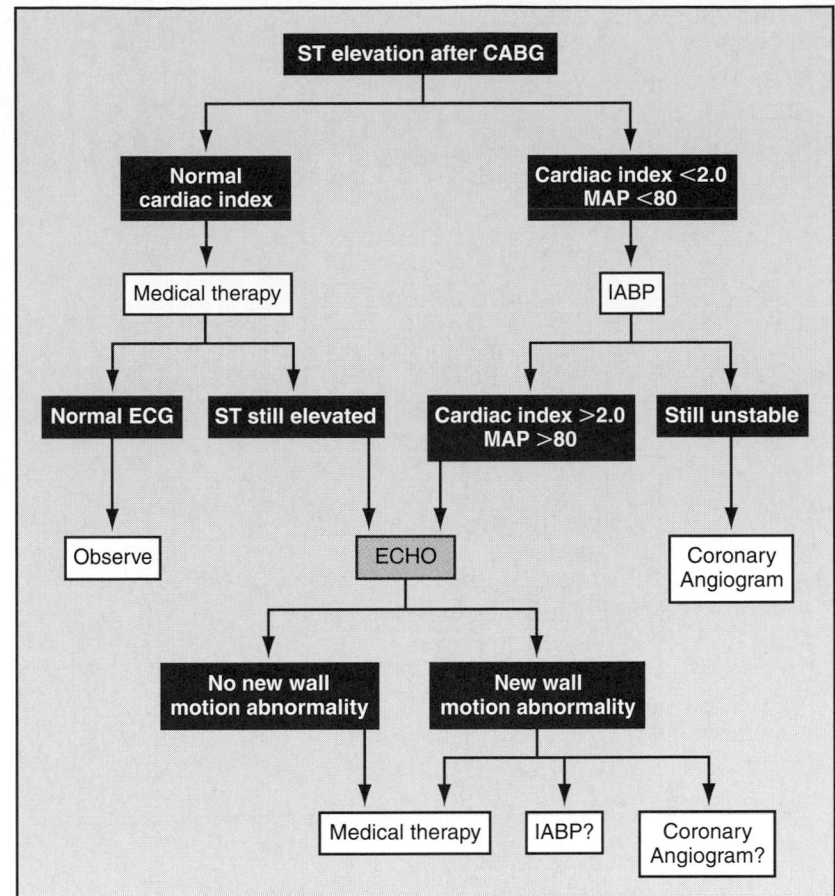

FIGURE 60–6. Myocardial ischemia after coronary bypass grafting is frequently observed. Hemodynamic assessment and ensurance of adequate coronary and systemic perfusion dictate early management strategies. Echocardiographic evaluation helps further tailor postoperative care. CABG = coronary artery bypass graft surgery; ECG = electrocardiogram; ECHO = echocardiography; IABP = intraaortic balloon pumping; MAP = mean arterial pressure.

over 30 percent for improved oxygen-carrying capacity of the blood, and a "low threshold" for mechanical ventilatory support to minimize the work of breathing and thereby reduce total-body oxygen needs.

REDUCED PRELOAD

Hypovolemia. Low ventricular filling pressure, normal systemic vascular resistance, and a reduced cardiac index, coupled with echocardiographic demonstration of small ventricular volume with preserved systolic function, are indicative of *hypovolemia.* Possible causes include bleeding, excessive diuresis, the "leaky capillary state" associated with the postpump syndrome, and less frequently, inadequate vascular volume because of insufficient return of fluids at the conclusion of cardiopulmonary bypass. Rarely, adrenal cortical insufficiency as a result of perioperative hemorrhage into the adrenals has been reported as a cause of hypovolemic hypotension after cardiac surgery.

Therapeutic maneuvers include the administration of intravenous fluids (normal saline solution, lactated Ringer solution), transfusion with packed red blood cells if the hemoglobin is less than 8 gm/dl, and administration of colloid-type volume expanders. It is also important to discontinue any vasodilators or antihypertensives that may have been prescribed during a period when the patient was hypertensive. While waiting for the above measures to take effect, the patient may require transient infusion of a vasoconstrictor (usually phenylephrine [Neo-Synephrine]) or an inotropic pressor (usually dopamine or epinephrine).

Vasodilatation. Inhibition of sympathetic tone by the effects of anesthetic agents may cause peripheral vasodilatation. In combination with the increased venous capacitance that may occur during rewarming, a low-output syndrome may develop as a result of markedly reduced systemic vascular resistance (<1000 dyne-sec $\cdot$ cm^{-5}). This situation is best treated by infusion of a vasoconstrictor such as norepi-

nephrine in a dose of 1 to 10 μg/min until the systemic vascular resistance returns to a normal level.

CARDIOGENIC SHOCK. When right ventricular and left ventricular filling pressures are in the normal range and systemic vascular resistance is not reduced, a frequent cause of a cardiac index less than 2 liters/min/m^2 is *bradycardia.* Because the cardiac index is the product of stroke volume and heart rate, this abnormality is easily corrected by atrial or atrioventricular pacing at 85 to 100 beats/min.

Left Ventricular Failure. The pattern of predominant *left ventricular failure* in the early postoperative state is characterized by a disproportionately elevated pulmonary capillary wedge pressure in comparison to right atrial pressure, a low cardiac index, and normal or elevated systemic vascular resistance. Echocardiography usually reveals a dilated, poorly contractile left ventricle, often exhibiting multiple regional wall motion abnormalities.

DIAGNOSIS. The differential diagnosis of left ventricular failure after cardiac surgery includes the following conditions (which may coexist in the same patient): preoperative left ventricular dysfunction, inadequate surgical correction of the cardiac lesion (e.g., residual left ventricular outflow tract obstruction after repair of idiopathic hypertrophic subaortic stenosis, residual ventricular septal defect), complication of a surgical procedure (e.g., prosthetic valve leak or thrombosis, depression of stroke volume after correction of mitral regurgitation caused by elevation of afterload), dysrhythmia, depressant effect of a pharmacological agent (e.g., antiarrhythmic drug), acid-base or electrolyte disturbance, or myocardial ischemia and/or infarction. Bedside echocardiography can usually help identify mechanical disorders such as prosthetic valve dysfunction and dysrhythmias, and metabolic abnormalities and toxic drug levels can be readily recognized by ECG and laboratory measurements.[81]

Management. The objectives of hemodynamic management of patients with *left ventricular failure* postoperatively are to correct hypotension if present, increase forward left ventricular output, and return left and right ventricular fill-

▶ **TABLE 60–7. HEMODYNAMIC DISTURBANCES FOLLOWING CARDIAC SURGERY**

	REDUCED PRELOAD		Bradycardia (Inappropriately Slow HR Postoperatively)	CARDIOGENIC SHOCK			SEPSIS
	Hypovolemia	Vasodilatation		LV Failure	RV Failure	Cardiac Tamponade	
Hemodynamics							
RA	<8	<8	≦10	≧10	>10	>15	<10
PCW	<15	<15	>15	>20	≦15*	>15	<15
CI	<2.0	<2.0	<2.0	<2.0	<2.0	<2.0	≧2.0
SVR	>1200	<1000	>1200	>1000	>1000	>1000	<1000
Other			HR <60		PCW >15 if LV failure is present	RA = PCW = PAd (within 5 mm Hg) unless "asymmetrical" tamponade occurs because of pericardial clots	Narrow A-V O₂ difference
Echocardiogram	Small ventricular chambers with vigorous systolic contraction unless LV dysfunction was present preoperatively	Small ventricular chambers with normal systolic contraction unless LV dysfunction was present preoperatively	Normal-sized ventricular chambers with vigorous systolic contraction, albeit at a slow rate	Dilated LV with reduced systolic performance; regional wall motion abnormalities may reflect old or new myocardial ischemia and/or infarction	Dilated RA and RV with reduced RV systolic contraction. TR often present on Doppler study. LV contractile performance is variable	Small cardiac chambers with diastolic collapse of RA and RV. Systolic contraction of RV and LV usually normal unless dysfunction was present preoperatively or coexistent LV or RV failure has occurred postoperatively	Small ventricular chambers with normal or slightly depressed contractile function (myocardial depressant factor)
Management	IV fluids Transfusion if Hgb <10 Inotropes	Vasopressors	Cardiac pacing	Search for correctible lesion, offending agent, or laboratory abnormality Inotropes Vasopressors and vasodilators Mechanical assistance	Supplemental O₂ Pulmonary vasodilators Inotropes Mechanical assistance	Reexploration Supportive measures: IV fluids, inotropes	IV fluids Antibiotics Vasopressors Inotropes

CI = cardiac index; Hgb = hemoglobin; HR = heart rate; IV = intravenous; LV = left ventricular; PAd = pulmonary artery diastolic; PCW = pulmonary capillary wedge; RA = right atrial; RV = right ventricular; SVR = systemic vascular resistance; TR = tricuspid regurgitation.

ing pressures to the normal range. These parameters are intimately related, and treatment may require careful titration of several intravenous agents for pharmacological support of the failing circulation. Boluses of calcium chloride (0.5 to 1.0 gm) increase myocardial contractility, but the effect is modest and short-lived. A continuous infusion of dopamine (5 to 10 μg/kg/min) or epinepherine (1 to 4 μg/kg/min) is preferable if the primary goal is to increase systemic arterial pressure and cardiac output. Dobutamine (2 to 5 μg/kg/min), amrinone (bolus of 0.75 mg/kg and infusion of 5 to 10 μg/kg/min), or milrinone (bolus of 50 μg/kg/min and infusion of 0.375 to 0.75 μg/kg/min) also augment cardiac output and should be selected if a reduction in ventricular filling pressure is desired; systemic arterial pressure is usually unchanged or may even drop slightly because of the peripheral vasodilatory effects of these drugs.[61, 82, 83] A commonly used combination is dopamine (2 μg/kg/min) to achieve greater renal perfusion in conjunction with dobutamine (2 to 5 μg/kg/min) for augmentation of cardiac output. If the mean arterial pressure is equal to or greater than 90 mm Hg, vasodilator therapy with nitroglycerin increases forward cardiac output and lowers pulmonary capillary wedge pressure further. When hypotension is profound (e.g., systolic pressure <70 mm Hg), norepinephrine or epinepherine 1 to 10 μg/min may be necessary to prevent coronary hypoperfusion.[61, 82]

We prefer to use an intraaortic balloon pump (see Chap. 19) for mechanical support of the circulation along with pharmacotherapy early in the course of management of postoperative left ventricular failure that does not respond to the initial pharmacological maneuvers already discussed. This protocol has the advantages of avoiding a continuous upward titration of the dose of sympathomimetic inotropic agents and vasoconstrictors associated with downregulation of beta-adrenoceptors and diminished perfusion of the renal, mesenteric, and coronary vascular beds. Also, intraaortic balloon counterpulsation does not increase myocardial oxygen demand. The intraaortic balloon pump is particularly helpful if significant mitral regurgitation is present but may be contraindicated in the presence of severe aortic regurgitation and if an abdominal aortic aneurysm is present. Delayed sternal closure is another important adjunct in the management of cardiogenic shock following surgery (see Fig. 60–7). If the patient fails to improve despite a combination of intraaortic balloon pumping, open-chest management, and pharmacotherapy, a ventricular assist device may be inserted for temporary support or as a "bridge" to cardiac transplantation until a donor is located.[84, 85] Serial evaluations of left ventricular function over time and under different loading conditions and supportive measures are best obtained with transesophageal echocardiograms.[86]

RIGHT VENTRICULAR FAILURE. The pattern of predominant *right ventricular failure* is characterized by a disproportionate elevation in right atrial pressure in comparison to pulmonary capillary wedge pressure. In severe cases of postoperative right ventricular failure, right atrial pressure may exceed 20 mm Hg while pulmonary capillary wedge pressure remains equal to or less than 15 mm Hg. When left ventricular failure is present simultaneously, the difference between right atrial and pulmonary capillary wedge pressure lessens and differentiation from cardiac tamponade becomes difficult. Bedside echocardiography is useful for making a proper diagnosis (see Table 60–7).

Postoperatively, predominant right ventricular failure may be seen as a result of one or more of the following conditions: elevated pulmonary vascular resistance (persistently elevated from preoperative elevations in pulmonary artery pressure; postoperative hypoxia, pulmonary embolus, or pneumothorax), primary right ventricular ischemia/infarction,[87] or a mechanical lesion (tricuspid regurgitation, residual shunt flow, right ventriculotomy).

Massive pulmonary embolism is a rare occurrence after cardiac surgery (see Chap. 52). The diagnosis should be suspected when sudden deterioration in oxygenation occurs in association with confusion, systemic hypotension, tachycardia, ECG abnormalities (unexplained right axis deviation, right bundle branch block, a right ventricular strain pattern), and elevation of right atrial pressure. Angiographic confirmation of the diagnosis is not usually necessary. Ex-

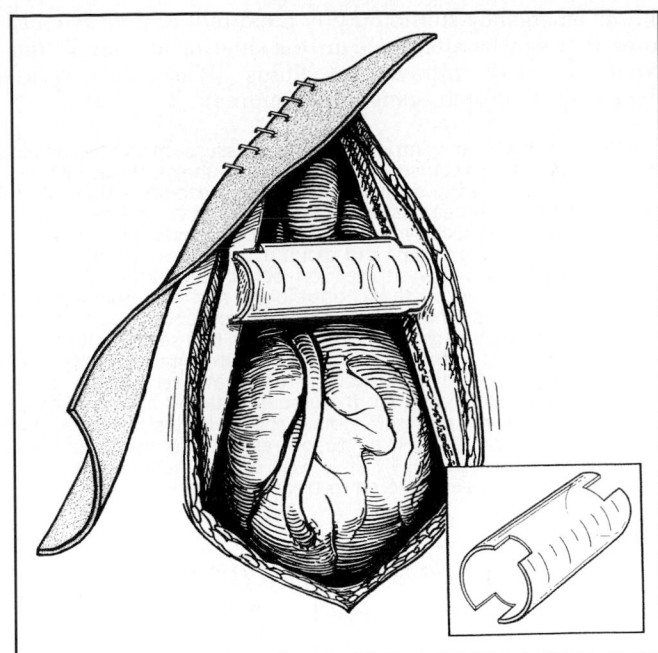

FIGURE 60–7. Patients in a low output state may not tolerate immediate sternal closure, particularly in the setting of significant mediastinal and myocardial edema associated with prolonged cardiopulmonary bypass. A modified barrel syringe is inserted between the sternal tables and the wound is then covered with an Esmarch dressing. After resolution of edema and recovery of myocardial function, the patient is returned to the operating room for a standard sternal closure.

peditious noninvasive confirmation by echocardiography is advisable in patients in whom the diagnosis remains uncertain.

MANAGEMENT. Hemodynamic management of predominant right ventricular failure should focus on improvement in right ventricular output to allow adequate filling of the left ventricle. Supplemental oxygen and hyperventilation to decrease Pco_2 levels help lower pulmonary artery pressure. Bradycardia (>60 beats/min) is corrected by atrial or atrioventricular pacing, isoproterenol (1 to 2 μg/min in an average adult) increases right ventricular contractility and also causes pulmonary vasodilatation. Pulmonary hypertension may also be reduced by prostaglandin E_1[88] and intravenous nitroglycerin.

Cardiac Tamponade (see Chap. 50). Postoperative echocardiography has shown that virtually all patients have pericardial effusion after cardiac surgery and that many such effusions are asymmetrical and loculated.[89] Even with mediastinal drains in place, it is possible for cardiac tamponade to develop postoperatively; recognition of this condition requires a high index of suspicion and assessment of hemodynamics at the bedside.[90]

Recognition. Important clinical features of tamponade, such as diminished heart sounds and pulsus paradoxus, may be obscured by mechanical ventilation. Asymmetrical, loculated accumulation of blood and clots in the mediastinum and pericardial space may cause isolated tamponade of one or two cardiac chambers and produce unusual elevations in diastolic pressure (e.g., right atrial tamponade with elevation of central venous pressure without an increase in right ventricular end-diastolic pressure or pulmonary capillary wedge pressure).[91] Beside two-dimensional transthoracic and transesophageal echocardiography is usually helpful for diagnosing pericardial effusions and assessing the hemodynamic significance of fluid collections.[92] Diastolic collapse of the right atrium and right ventricle is an indication of a hemodynamically significant external compressive force and should prompt urgent treatment.

Treatment. Although pericardiocentesis may be helpful in nonsurgical tamponade, it is unlikely to be successful in evacuating the organized pericardial and mediastinal material that develops after cardiac surgery; subxiphoid drainage and/or emergency sternotomy is preferred. Supportive measures that can be attempted in the interim include volume expansion with intravenous fluids (Plasmanate, whole blood) and inotropic agents (dobutamine).

SEPTIC SHOCK. Low ventricular filling pressure, markedly reduced systemic vascular resistance, and a normal or unexpectedly high cardiac index in the setting of hypotension and a shocklike state should raise suspicion of the early stages of *sepsis*. With progression of septic shock, a capillary leak syndrome develops (hypovolemia) and myocardial depression may occur and result in a somewhat reduced contractile pattern of the ventricles on echocardiography. Combined therapy with intravenous fluids, antibiotics, and inotropic agents is required to interrupt the vicious cycle of hypotension, acidosis, and diminished coronary perfusion. Most patients in a septic state during the first several days after cardiac surgery are infected with a skin organism (e.g., indwelling catheters) or from seeding the bloodstream from a pulmonary or urinary source. Broad antibiotic coverage (e.g., vancomycin plus ceftazidine) should be instituted. Because the offending organism is likely to be resistant to the prophylactic antibiotic given preoperatively, it is wise to not include it as one of the empirical antibiotics selected to treat sepsis.

Perioperative Arrhythmias

(See also Chap. 25)

EVALUATION AND TREATMENT. There appear to be two peaks in the incidence of arrhythmias perioperatively: The first occurs in the operating room (most commonly during induction of anesthesia, weaning from cardiopulmonary bypass, rewarming), and the second occurs in the ICU between the second and fifth postoperative days. The electrophysiological mechanisms underlying perioperative arrhythmias are incompletely understood, but they can probably be ascribed to a combination of the effects of circulating catecholamines, alterations in autonomic nervous system tone, transient electrolyte imbalance, myocardial ischemia or infarction, and mechanical irritation of the heart.

APPROACH TO THE PATIENT. Several factors may predispose to the development of arrhythmias, including ventilatory dysfunction, fever, electrolyte imbalance (hypokalemia, hypomagnesemia, hypocalcemia), anemia, myocardial ischemia or infarction, low cardiac output and reflex increase in sympathetic tone, hypertension, pericardial inflammation, and toxic effects of cardioactive medications (e.g., digitalis toxicity, bradycardia induced by diltiazem).[52, 93] *Every effort should be made to look for and eliminate any of the factors that may be provoking the arrhythmia.*

Although antiarrhythmic drug therapy and direct-current cardioversion are traditional methods for treating postoperative arrhythmias, cardiac pacing techniques have a number of advantages, including more rapid onset and offset of action, avoidance of potential drug toxicity (especially proarrhythmia), elimination of the need for anesthesia (required for cardioversion), reduced anxiety for the patient, greater safety in patients receiving digitalis, and perhaps most important, the ability to repeat the pacing protocol if the arrhythmia should recur, a not infrequent event. In addition to terminating arrhythmias, cardiac pacing can be used to suppress arrhythmias in many patients by atrial, atrioventricular sequential, or ventricular stimulation at a critical rate (e.g., 85 to 100 beats/min).

Surface Electrocardiogram.
The value of a 12-lead ECG and simultaneously recorded multiple standard ECG lead rhythm strips cannot be overemphasized if one is attempting to analyze a wide complex tachycardia. Unfortunately, a number of the criteria for differentiating supraventricular tachycardia with aberrant conduction from ventricular tachycardia (VT) (see Chap. 25) may not be applicable to postoperative patients because of previous or newly acquired infarction patterns, transient conduction defects (seen in 5 to 15 percent of patients in the early recovery period), and nonspecific repolarization patterns.

Epicardial Electrodes.
It is desirable to place two wires on the free wall of the right atrium and the right ventricle to allow for bipolar atrial recording and pacing or dual-chamber pacing. The advantages of bipolar pacing include a smaller stimulus artifact, the ability to record a bipolar atrial electrogram during ventricular pacing, and a reduced

likelihood of precipitating undesired atrial arrhythmias if an atrial wire is used as the indifferent electrode during unipolar ventricular pacing. Schematic diagrams showing the typical intrathoracic positioning of the atrial and ventricular wires are shown in Figure 60-8.

Supraventricular Arrhythmias

ATRIAL PREMATURE DEPOLARIZATIONS. The hemodynamic consequences of atrial premature depolarizations are almost always minor, and one should resist the urge to suppress them with antiarrhythmic drugs. Instead, they should be considered a signal that the patient is possibly hypoxic or that an electrolyte imbalance is present and a warning that the patient is at risk for more serious arrhythmia such as AF or atrial flutter. In the absence of such correctable abnormalities, one may want to administer a beta blocker to inhibit the effects of circulating catecholamines and also to slow the ventricular rate if AF should develop.

ATRIAL FLUTTER. Control of the ventricular rate in atrial flutter is more difficult than in AF because of the limited number of ventricular responses to atrial activation (usually 2:1, 4:1, but rarely an odd-numbered multiple). Atrial flutter may be difficult to terminate with antiarrhythmic agents. Cardioversion with an energy of 25 to 50 watt-seconds delivered as a single discharge can be expected to terminate atrial flutter in more than 90 percent of patients.

Atrial flutter can also be terminated by rapid atrial pacing with the temporary epicardial atrial wires placed at the time of surgery (Fig. 60-9). The likelihood of success is increased if one uses sufficiently rapid rates of pacing (up to 140 percent of the spontaneous atrial rate), a sufficient duration of pacing (10 to 30 seconds) with adequate strength (5 to 20 mA), and pretreatment of the patient with procainamide.[94] To achieve the high drive rates required, a special stimulator is used.

ATRIAL FIBRILLATION. Despite the fact that AF is an extremely common arrhythmia following cardiac surgery, the optimal management strategy has not been established. Even after prophylactic therapy with beta-adrenoceptor blockers, transient symptomatic AF occurs in at least 25 to 30 percent of patients after CABG and in 50 percent of patients following valvular surgery; AF appears with greatest incidence on the second or third postoperative day.[52]

Management. Unless hemodynamic collapse is present, in which case direct-current cardioversion should be performed, the initial treatment of choice in a postoperative patient is to slow the ventricular rate. Provided that the patient's ventricular function is adequate, acute intravenous administration of beta blockers (e.g., metoprolol 5 mg every 5 minutes for up to three doses), verapamil (5-mg bolus every 5 to 10 minutes for three or four doses), or diltiazem (0.25- to 0.35-mg/kg bolus over a period of 2 minutes) is a more desirable option. Esmolol, an ultrashort-acting cardioselective beta blocker, when administered intravenously in a dose of 50 to 250 $\mu g/kg/min$, provides the option of rapid onset; in the event of hemodynamic deterioration, the effects of the drug are usually dissipated within 15 to 30 minutes after discontinuation of the infusion. In addition, the probability of conversion to sinus rhythm with esmolol appears to be better than with other agents such as verapamil.[95]

ANTICOAGULANTS. Epidemiological observations suggest that the development of postoperative AF is associated with a marked increase in the risk of stroke (odds ratio 3.0) and prolonged hospitalization.[50-52] No consensus has been reached regarding anticoagulation recommendations in patients with postoperative AF. The risk of hemorrhage in the early postoperative period must be weighed against the risk of systemic thromboembolism.[96] When AF develops beyond the second postoperative day, we generally advocate adherence to the guidelines established for nonsurgical patients and initiate anticoagulation (intravenous heparin followed by oral warfarin) in patients who have been in the arrhythmia for more than 48 hours, especially if the patient has a history of systemic embolism or if mitral valve disease or cardiomyopathy is present.[97]

Beyond control of the ventricular rate acutely, the two treatment strategies for management of postoperative AF are similar to those

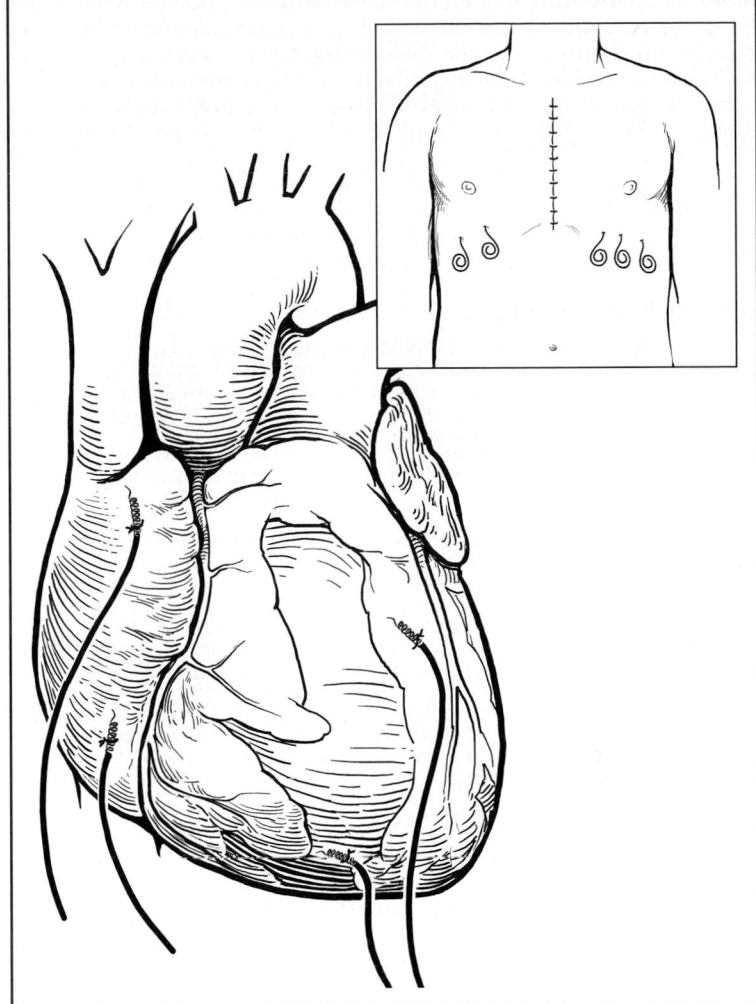

FIGURE 60–8. Epicardial electrodes in patients undergoing cardiac surgery. The precise number and location of pacing wires may vary among institutions and also by the complexity of the operation (e.g., no atrial wires for routine coronary artery bypass surgery but both atrial and ventricular wires for valve surgery). In the example shown, the two atrial wires exit to the patient's right while the ventricular wires are the first two leads exiting to the patient's left; the subcutaneous ground wire is the one closest to the left anterior axillary line.

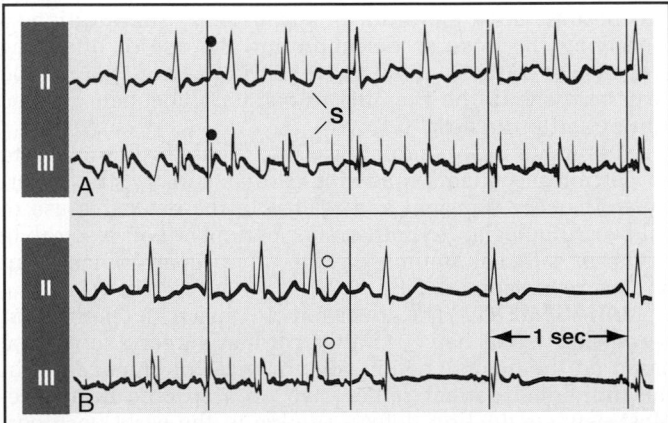

FIGURE 60–9. Recording of electrocardiographic leads II and III in a patient with atrial flutter. Panels *A* and *B* are not continuous tracings. The dots in *A* mark the onset of rapid atrial pacing at 350 beats/min with a pacing stimulator capable of high drive rates. The morphology of the atrial complexes changes dramatically such that by the end of the trace in *A,* the atrial complexes are positive in leads II and III. Panel *B* shows the termination of 30 seconds of atrial pacing at 350 beats/min. The circles represent the last paced atrial beat. With abrupt termination of the rapid atrial pacing, sinus rhythm appears. S = stimulus artifact. Time lines are at 1-second intervals. (From Waldo AL, MacLean WAH: Diagnosis and Treatment of Cardiac Arrhythmias Following Cardiac Surgery. Mt Kisco, NY, Futura, 1980.)

for nonsurgical patients: chronic anticoagulation while administering rate-controlling agents versus restoration of sinus rhythm and attempts at suppression of recurrence of AF. Because large-scale clinical trial data are not available to guide decision-making in this area, therapeutic approaches must be individualized.[96] Ibutilide, a class III antiarrhythmic agent, has been shown to be effective in the acute conversion of post-CABG AF when administered intravenously, albeit with a small risk (<2 percent) of torsades de pointes.[98] Procainamide is frequently used for the treatment of AF after open-heart surgery, although present evidence indicates that it has limited effectiveness in suppressing recurrence of AF.[99] Furthermore, any treatment decision formulated during hospitalization should be readdressed at the first postoperative visit (typically 4 to 6 weeks) to determine whether it is still a desirable course of action once the inflammation and metabolic alterations of the postoperative state have dissipated.

Patients with depressed left ventricular function or striking ventricular hypertrophy who experience troublesome dyspnea and/or hypotension when in AF postoperatively are suitable candidates for a trial of restoration of sinus rhythm.

Permanent suppressive antiarrhythmic therapy is often necessary in patients with rheumatic heart disease and a preoperative history of AF despite successful aortic or mitral valve surgery even if sinus rhythm is present during the early postoperative period.

PAROXYSMAL SUPRAVENTRICULAR TACHYCARDIA. The reentrant forms of paroxysmal supraventricular tachycardia (PSVT)—atrioventricular nodal reentry tachycardia and atrioventricular reentry tachycardia—occur less frequently in postoperative patients than does AF or atrial flutter but, fortunately, retain their responsiveness to vagal maneuvers and pharmacotherapy designed to inhibit atrioventricular nodal conduction. The antiarrhythmic agent adenosine, an endogenous nucleoside, has a number of features that make it the drug of choice for treating PSVT in postoperative patients.[100] A rapid (2 seconds) intravenous bolus of 6 mg terminates about 60 percent of episodes of PSVT within 20 seconds; a subsequent bolus of 12 mg administered 1 to 2 minutes later terminates PSVT in virtually all patients who failed to respond to the lower dose. Because adenosine is rapidly transported into the cell or degraded enzymatically to inosine, the physiological effects of adenosine are dissipated in less than 5 minutes. Untoward reactions such as flushing, chest pain, or dyspnea, although common, are mild and short-lived.

PSVT may also be diagnosed by atrial recordings and terminated by burst atrial pacing or randomly delivered ventricular or atrial premature depolarizations that invade the reentrant circuit and interrupt the arrhythmia.

Ventricular Arrhythmias

VENTRICULAR PREMATURE DEPOLARIZATIONS. Isolated ventricular premature depolarizations (VPDs) commonly occur after cardiac surgery. An increase in the density of VPDs may be seen in patients with a preoperative history of VPDs, or they may appear de novo in patients with no history of ventricular arrhythmias. Although a fall in arterial pressure may be associated with isolated VPDs, this decreased pressure is usually extremely brief and of no significant hemodynamic consequence to the patient unless prolonged periods of bigeminy occur.

Management. We advocate a conservative approach focusing on prompt detection and correction of provocative factors, liberal use of beta blockers in patients with an ejection fraction greater than 30 percent, overdrive atrial or atrioventricular sequential pacing between 85 and 100 beats/min, and restriction of suppressive antiarrhythmic therapy to patients with a preoperative history of serious ventricular tachyarrhythmias.[52] If the decision is made to suppress VPDs in a patient without a history of symptomatic ventricular arrhythmias, the treatment period should be brief (6 to 24 hours) and the patient should not be automatically converted to treatment with an oral antiarrhythmic drug regimen without careful reconsideration of the indications for treatment.

VENTRICULAR TACHYCARDIA. Many of the same arguments cited above for isolated VPDs can be applied to paroxysms of nonsustained VT. No definitive guidelines are available, but we believe that symptomatic episodes of nonsustained VT in the absence of correctable factors and attempts at overdrive atrial or atrioventricular sequential pacing are indications for antiarrhythmic therapy, especially if the episodes are associated with hemodynamic compromise. *Sustained VT* is a serious emergency that should be handled in an orderly approach. If the clinical situation permits, a 12-lead ECG should be obtained for future reference and confirmation of the diagnosis; simultaneous recording of surface ECG leads with electrograms from the epicardial wires may be helpful in establishing the mechanism of a wide complex tachycardia.

Attempts at acute conversion of the tachycardia include the following maneuvers in the sequence listed: thumpversion, burst ventricular pacing, and boluses of antiarrhythmic agents (lidocaine 100 mg, procainamide up to 500 to 1000 mg over a period of 20 minutes, amiodarone 75 to 150 mg infused over a 10-minute period, or bretylium 500 to 1000 mg over a period of 5 to 10 minutes). In urgent circumstances, synchronized direct-current cardioversion with a low-energy shock (25 to 50 watt-seconds) may be used. Unsynchronized shocks of 100 to 200 watt-seconds should be administered if the tachycardia rate is greater than 160 beats/min and/or has a sinusoidal waveform on ECG. After conversion, a search for correctable disorders should be undertaken, and if none is found, a continuous infusion of lidocaine (2 mg/min), procainamide (2 mg/min), amiodarone (1.0 mg/min for 6 hours followed by a maintenance infusion of 0.5 mg/min), or bretylium (1 to 2 mg/min) is started.

VENTRICULAR FIBRILLATION. As in nonsurgical patients, ventricular fibrillation (VF) must be promptly treated with an unsynchronized direct-current shock. VF can often be reverted with shocks of 200 watt-seconds, provided that the intervention is performed promptly. It should be possible to defibrillate postoperative patients in the ICU expeditiously; therefore, the higher energies (360 to 400 watt-seconds)

used in the "field" are probably unnecessary—at least initially. Because of the small number of patients experiencing unexpected sustained, hemodynamically compromising VT or VF, epidemiological data on provocative factors and the prognosis of these arrhythmias are difficult to evaluate.[52, 101, 102] Unexplained VT or VF occurring within 24 hours after CABG surgery is associated with very high in-hospital mortality, probably resulting from perioperative ischemia, infarction, and/or pump failure.[101] Episodes of VT or VF occurring more than 24 hours after bypass surgery have a slightly less ominous prognosis and may be due to reperfusion of previously ischemic zones, early postoperative occlusion of coronary bypass grafts, or transmembrane shift of electrolytes during the process of recovery.[103, 104]

Risk stratification of patients experiencing VT or VF postoperatively should include assessment of left ventricular function, coronary arteriography if ischemia/infarction is suspected, and consideration of an electrophysiological study to establish the most appropriate course of therapy.[105] Because of the numerous metabolic fluxes taking place in the early postoperative period, electrophysiological study should, if possible, be postponed until at least 5 to 7 days following surgery.[52] Serious consideration should be given to use of an implantable cardioverter-defibrillator in patients without an identifiable reversible cause of their arrhythmia, particularly those with a depressed ejection fraction.

ATRIOVENTRICULAR JUNCTIONAL RHYTHMS. Nonparoxysmal atrioventricular junctional rhythms (rate >45 beats/min) can be seen after mitral or aortic valve surgery. Trauma and tissue swelling from surgical débridement and suture placement are believed to be the provocative mechanisms. Such rhythms are typically transient (≤48 hours) and easily treated with atrial or atrioventricular sequential pacing at a rate above that of the intrinsic junctional mechanism.[106]

Bradyarrhythmias

Sinus bradycardia or sinus arrest with emergence of a slow atrioventricular junction escape rhythm may be seen postoperatively when one or more of the following factors are present: advanced age, hypothermia, drug effects (diltiazem, beta blocker, digitalis, procainamide), preoperative sinus node dysfunction, intraoperative trauma to the sinus node, and postoperative elevation in vagal tone.[107] In addition to modifying the dose or discontinuing the use of offending drugs (such as those noted above), atrial pacing at 85 to 100 beats/min should be initiated to maintain adequate cardiac output and urine flow.

Although a new conduction defect may develop in up to 45 percent of patients following cardiac surgery, the majority are usually transient and related to the extensive use of cold cardioplegia, hypothermia, perioperative electrolyte shifts, or surgical trauma during valve repair/replacement or closure of septal defects.[108, 109]

MANAGEMENT. The decision to insert a permanent pacemaker (see Chap. 24) after cardiac surgery should be based on the hemodynamic consequences of bradycardia in the individual patient rather than on a specific heart rate. Most new conduction defects resolve in the early postoperative period, but some persist for as long as 2 weeks. Few data are available to guide the decision about timing of implantation of a permanent pacemaker. We are willing to monitor a younger patient (<65 years) following CABG surgery with a temporary pacing system postoperatively to see whether a conduction defect resolves. However, we have a low threshold for implanting a permanent pacemaker following aortic or mitral valve surgery or if antiarrhythmic therapy or beta-blocker treatment is contemplated because these pharmacological measures might "stress" a diseased conduction system. We advocate early insertion of a permanent pacemaker in elderly patients with symptomatic bradycardia because the recuperative process is facilitated, the period of relative immobilization and ECG monitoring is minimized, and hospital stay is shortened.[110] Finally, we are more aggressive about implantation of permanent pacemakers in patients with persistent advanced atrioventricular block than in to patients with isolated sinus bradycardia.

CARDIOVERSION. Direct-current cardioversion should be used in postsurgical patients with the following additional considerations. The recent cardiotomy with resultant pericardial and mediastinal inflammation, the presence of chest tubes and/or pleural effusions, and elevated catecholamine levels after surgery may all contribute to higher energy requirements for reversion of arrhythmias such as AF than are commonly required in patients who have not recently undergone cardiac surgery. To achieve the maximum transcardiac spread of current after median sternotomy, the anterior paddle should be placed to the *right* of the sternum between the third and sixth intercostal space, and the other paddle should be positioned in the fourth to sixth intercostal space as far in the left axilla as possible or in a posterior location under the tip of the left scapula. Firm pressure is applied to the paddles to maintain contact with the chest wall as the discharge buttons are depressed.

Hemostatic Disturbances (See Chap. 62)

Multifactorial derangement of the hemostatic system develops in all patients who undergo cardiopulmonary bypass. These abnormalities are caused by exposure of the blood to artificial surfaces, hemodilution, and the effects of heparin[111-115] (Table 60-8). Platelet dysfunction is the most significant hemostatic abnormality that occurs after cardiopulmonary bypass, although diminution of coagulation factor levels may assume greater significance in patients with preoperative deficiencies in hemostasis. Administration of the following drugs before surgery may predispose the patient to excessive bleeding: aspirin and other antiplatelet agents, nonsteroidal antiinflammatory agents, thrombolytic agents,[113] certain antibiotics (carbenicillin, ticarcillin, moxalactam, cefamandole, third-generation cephalosporins), dextran, amrinone, quinidine, cytotoxic agents, gold, phenylbutazone, and fish oils.[113]

MANAGEMENT. The most obvious evidence of bleeding in a postoperative cardiac surgical patient is by means of chest tube drainage. "Acceptable" rates of bleeding are usually less than 100 ml/hr. In our institution, guidelines for returning to the operating room because of excessive bleeding include more than 500 ml/hr for 1 hour, more than 300 ml/hr for 3 hours, and 200 to 300 ml/hr for 5 hours.

These guidelines may be tempered by correctable extenuating circumstances, such as uncontrolled hypertension postoperatively, failure to achieve normothermia, or an abnormal coagulation status that is being corrected. Emergency medical maneuvers that can be attempted after sending coagulation studies to the laboratory include the use of PEEP up to 10 cm H_2O for mediastinal tamponade, empirical "correction" of putative platelet dysfunction with desmopressin acetate (DDAVP, a synthetic analog of arginine vasopressin that increases plasma levels of von Willebrand factor) 0.3 μg/kg infused over a period of 15 to 30 minutes, and empirical administration of a small dose of protamine sulfate 25 to 50 mg because heparin may be liberated from the patient's fat stores as rewarming occurs.[116]

Once the coagulation profile returns, additional therapy in the form of platelet transfusions for a platelet count less than 100,000/mm³ and fresh frozen plasma to correct an elevated prothrombin time can be prescribed. Aprotinin therapy (2 × 10⁵ KIU loading bolus followed by infusion of 0.5 × 10⁵ KIU/hr for 4 hours) is helpful in cases of excessive postoperative bleeding by virtue of its ability to inhibit fibrinolysis and replenish platelet glycoprotein Ib receptors and von Willebrand factor activity.[117, 117a] When monitoring bleeding from a chest tube, it is important to be alert to sudden cessation of hemorrhage, which may indicate that the chest tubes have clotted and the fluid is now draining into the mediastinum or the pleural spaces. Serial chest radiographs may be helpful while observing a patient during a bleeding episode. With correct medical management, less than 5 percent of patients need to return to the operating room for control of bleeding, preferably within 3 to 4 hours of the original surgery, before hemodynamic destabilization occurs and large volumes of blood products are administered.

ANTITHROMBOTIC THERAPY IN CARDIAC SURGICAL PATIENTS. A wide spectrum of patients recovering from cardiac surgery may require either short- or long-term antithrombotic therapy[118] (Table 60-9). Furthermore the intensity of therapy will be dictated by the estimated risk of thromboembolism. Variables that may have an impact on the risk of thromboembolism include insertion of a prosthetic valve (mechanical more than bioprosthetic), valve location (mitral more than aortic), the presence of AF, size of the left atrium, history of thromboembolism, left atrial thrombi visualized at surgery, and ventricular wall motion abnormalities associated with mural thrombi.

▼ TABLE 60-8. HEMOSTATIC DISTURBANCES FOLLOWING CARDIOPULMONARY BYPASS

ABNORMALITY	CAUSE

Exposure of blood to artificial surfaces
1. Platelet dysfunction
  A. Prolonged bleeding time
  B. Decreased adhesiveness
	1. Depletion of platelet alpha granules, reduced response to wounds, and increased plasma levels of platelet factor 4 and beta-thromboglobulin[111]

2. Inflammatory response	2. Activation of the complement, coagulation, fibrinolytic, and kallikrein cascades; activation of neutrophils with degranulation and protease enzyme release; oxygen free radical production; and synthesis of cytokines (tumor necrosis factor, interleukin-1, interleukin-6, interleukin-8)
Hemodilution 1. Thrombocytopenia	1. Priming of extracorporeal bypass circuit with crystalloid solutions. Heparin-mediated immune thrombocytopenia may occur in about 5% of patients*
2. Coagulation factor depletion	2. Most coagulation factor levels are reduced by hemodilution by about 50%; factor V is reduced to 20-30% of normal and factor VIII is relatively unaffected. Factor levels usually return to normal within 12 hr after completion of cardiopulmonary bypass. Although plasminogen and fibrinogen levels are decreased by about 50%, fibrin degradation products usually do not appear in the plasma during bypass[113]
Heparinization	Thrombus formation is inhibited and excessive bleeding is avoided intraoperatively by maintaining the activated clotting time between 400 and 480 sec

* Note: reversal of heparin effects is accomplished with protamine sulfate. Vascular collapse has been reported in some patients during protamine treatment. To avoid the problem of heparin-induced thrombocytopenia and because heparin may not effectively inhibit all the thrombin generated during cardiopulmonary bypass ("heparin rebound"), novel antithrombins are being evaluated as alternatives to heparin during surgery.[114, 115]

▼ **TABLE 60–9.** ANTICOAGULATION GUIDELINES FOR ANTITHROMBOTIC THERAPY IN CARDIAC SURGERY PATIENTS

SURGERY	ANTICOAGULANT	INR*
Mitral mechanical valve	Warfarin	2.5–3.5
Aortic mechanical valve	Warfarin	2.0–3.0
Tricuspid mechanical valve	Warfarin	2.5–3.0
Atrial fibrillation	Warfarin	2.0–2.5
Mitral tissue valve	Warfarin	2.0–3.0 for 6 wk
Mitral valve repair	Warfarin	2.0–2.0 for 6 wk
Tricuspid tissue valve	Warfarin	2.0–3.0 for 6 wk
Tricuspid repair	Warfarin	2.0–3.0 for 6 wk
LV thrombus	Warfarin	2.0–3.0 for 6 mo
LV aneurysm repair	Warfarin	2.0–3.0 for 6 wk
Aortic tissue valve	Aspirin (80 mg/d)	
Coronary artery bypass	ASA 325 mg/d, 81 mg/d if taking Coumadin	

* The target international normalized ratio is the midpoint of the range.
ASA = acetylsalicylic acid (aspirin); LV = left ventricular.

Infection

FEVER. Despite its nonspecific nature, fever is the most common initial clinical sign of a postoperative infection.[119] It should be emphasized, however, that patients who experience a normal course of convalescence continue to show an elevated temperature for up to 6 days postoperatively.[120] In the absence of infection, such early fevers are believed to be caused by alterations in blood components after cardiopulmonary bypass. In addition to infectious causes, fevers that occur beyond 6 days may be due to drug reactions, phlebitis at the site of intravenous lines, atelectasis, pulmonary emboli, or the postpericardiotomy syndrome.

WOUND AND INCISION

Leg. Infections of the leg wound are typically manifested by fever, induration, pain, erythema, local warmth, and drainage from the suture line. The usual infectious agents include *Staphylococcus*, *Strepto*-

coccus, and aerobic gram-negative bacilli. Wound aspiration and Gram stain should be used to guide antibiotic treatment. More advanced cases require wound débridement and open drainage. Techniques of minimally invasive saphenous vein harvesting now make it possible to avoid a long leg incision, which decreases the risk of postoperative leg infection[120a] (Fig. 60–10).

Recurrent bacterial cellulitis in the leg used for saphenous vein harvest may be a recalcitrant problem that appears months to years after surgery. Antibiotic courses directed against staphylococcal and streptococcal species for each individual occurrence may be insufficient, and a long-term course of antibiotic therapy may be needed. It is important to search for evidence of superficial fungal infections in the affected leg because persistent tinea pedis infection has been reported to cause recurrent lower extremity cellulitis.[121] If a fungal infection is identified, treatment with topical miconazole or clotrimazole should be given in addition to antibacterial therapy.

Mediastinitis. Mediastinitis and sternal osteomyelitis are among the most serious complications of median sternotomy.[37, 122] If one excludes operations that occur after thoracic trauma, it is estimated that mediastinitis occurs in about 2 percent of patients who undergo median sternotomy.

Most cases of mediastinitis occur within 2 weeks after sternotomy. Important diagnostic features of patients in whom mediastinitis

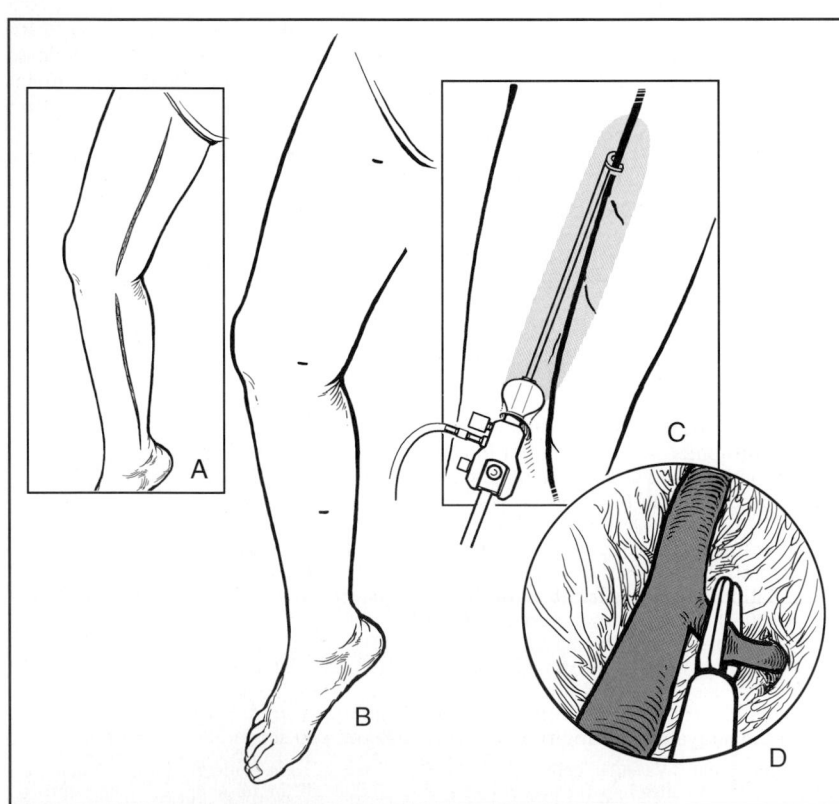

FIGURE 60–10. Minimally invasive approaches to saphenous vein harvesting have significantly reduced incisional morbidity. Traditional harvesting requires long leg incisions (*A*), as compared with the less invasive videoscopic harvesting (*B*). A dissection cannula is introduced through a small incision (*C*), and branches are later divided (*D*) under videoscopic guidance.

develops early after cardiac surgery include persistent fever in excess of 101°F beyond the fourth postoperative day, a systemic toxic condition, leukocytosis, bacteremia, and a purulent discharge from the sternal wound. Recognition of mediastinitis requires a high index of suspicion and a vigorous, repetitive search for evidence of sternal wound drainage in patients who are persistently febrile late into the first week after surgery and who have no other obvious focus of infection, such as pneumonia or urinary tract infection.[123] The diagnosis can be confirmed by needle aspiration from the subxiphoid approach followed by Gram's stain and culture.

Risk Factors and Diagnosis. Risk factors for the development of mediastinitis include prolonged cardiopulmonary bypass time, excessive postoperative bleeding with reexploration for control of hemorrhage, and diminished cardiac output in the postoperative period. The incidence of mediastinitis is increased when both internal mammary arteries are mobilized bilaterally for use as bypass conduits.[124] Therefore, many surgeons prefer to use only the left internal mammary artery, particularly in elderly diabetic patients, who may already be predisposed to delayed sternal wound healing.

The spectrum of microorganisms that cause mediastinitis includes *Staphylococcus* (*aureus* and *epidermidis*) in about 50 percent of patients and a variety of gram-negative bacilli in about 40 percent of cases.[123–125] Mixed infections and fungal infections are rare. The organism isolated frequently is resistant to the prophylactic antibiotic used preoperatively, especially if the isolate includes a gram-negative bacillus or a beta-lactamase–producing *S. aureus*.

DIAGNOSIS OF STERNAL WOUND INFECTION. Definitive diagnosis requires exploration of the wound and culture of suspicious areas. In the past, closed (débridement, reclosure, and antibiotic irrigation) and open (débridement, packing, closure by secondary intent) approaches were commonly used. To facilitate functional recovery, we now favor early plastic surgical flap techniques to allow for immediate primary closure with vascularized tissue.[126, 127] Regardless of the sternal closure strategy used, bacterial-specific intravenous antibiotics are typically administered for 6 weeks.

INFECTIVE ENDOCARDITIS (see Chap. 47)

It has been convincingly shown that perioperative antibiotic prophylaxis is of benefit in patients undergoing cardiac surgery.[128] Although the antibiotic regimen varies, in part related to local differences in microbiological flora and personal preference, it is directed against gram-positive cocci (the most frequent causative pathogens in infections after cardiac surgery) and usually contains a cephalosporin. The regimen used in our institution consists of 1 gm of cefazolin intravenously 30 minutes before the skin incision and then repeated at 8-hour intervals for 48 hours after surgery.

PROSTHETIC VALVE ENDOCARDITIS (see Chaps. 46 and 47). Prosthetic valve endocarditis is a rare, but extremely serious complication of cardiac surgery, frequently arising from nosocomial bacteremias.[129, 130] It is estimated to occur in only 2 to 4 percent of patients; about half of the cases are classified as "early" (<60 days from the date of surgery) and half as "late" (>60 days from the date of surgery).[129–131] Pooled data from several series indicate that the organism responsible for early prosthetic valve endocarditis includes a *Staphylococcus* species in about 50 percent of cases.[131] The remainder of early cases of prosthetic valve endocarditis are caused by gram-negative bacilli, diphtheroids, and fungi.

Management. Features of prosthetic valve endocarditis that have been associated with increased mortality include invasive infection (i.e., extension into the myocardium), congestive heart failure resulting from dysfunction of the prosthesis, and the presence of antibiotic resistant, virulent microorganisms or a fungal organism.[131] Appropriate antibiotic therapy for prosthetic valve endocarditis is discussed in Chapter 47.

VIRAL. Viral infections that occur after cardiac surgery are almost exclusively the result of infectious complications of transfusion therapy and, with the exception of human immunodeficiency virus, primarily result in hepatitis. The incidence of viral infections after cardiac operations is decreasing as a result of a reduction in the number of transfusions of blood bank products (e.g., cell saver techniques and preoperative autologous blood donations) and improved screening techniques in contemporary blood bank practice. Cytomegalovirus infection is a febrile syndrome that typically occurs 1 month postoperatively. It is characterized by high-spiking fevers, abnormalities in liver function test results, and arthralgias. A self-limited illness, it is best treated with antipyretics and supportive fluid therapy.

FUNGAL. Fungal infections that involve the heart are rare. They are typically seen in cases of fungemia and are usually fatal. Although the problem of fungemia is well described in immunocompromised hosts (e.g., heart transplant recipient), in an autopsy study of 60 patients

with fungal infections of the heart, 25 percent of cases occurred in association with conventional valvular surgery.[132] About half of fungal infections of the heart are confined to the endocardium, and half involve both the endocardium and the myocardium. Extracardiac involvement is common, with spread of infection to the lungs, cerebrospinal fluid, urine, and skin. The most commonly encountered organisms, in descending order of frequency, are *Candida*, *Aspergillus*, and *Cryptococcus* species. Patients who appear to be at particular risk of fungal involvement of the heart are those who have received corticosteroids and long courses of antibiotic treatment postoperatively.

Peripheral Vascular Complications

Most adults who undergo cardiac surgery—especially coronary revascularization—have atherosclerosis of the peripheral vasculature (e.g., ileofemoral system) and may experience lower extremity ischemia after surgery because of low flow in the perioperative period with in situ thrombosis, embolism from the heart or aorta, or vascular compromise from an intraaortic balloon pump catheter. Management consists of anticoagulation and removal of indwelling catheters, if clinically feasible. Thrombectomy and even revascularization surgery of the lower extremities (e.g., femorofemoral, femoropopliteal, or axillofemoral bypass) may be required to salvage threatened limbs.

Asymptomatic deep venous thrombosis of the calf can develop before hospital discharge in about one-third to one-half of patients who receive saphenous vein bypass grafts. Occasionally, these thrombi propagate to the proximal leg veins; only rarely do they cause massive pulmonary embolism.[30, 133] The best strategy is rigorous perioperative prophylaxis against venous thromboembolism in all such patients. Low-molecular-weight heparin (e.g., enoxaparin 30 to 40 mg subcutaneously every 12 hours) appears to be efficacious.

Other Complications

PERICARDITIS (see Chap. 50). Postoperative tamponade is discussed on p. 55. Pericardial friction rubs are frequently audible in the early postoperative period and are probably the result of mechanical irritation from the mediastinal chest tubes. They usually disappear by the second or third postoperative day and are asymptomatic because of the narcotic analgesics prescribed at that stage of recovery. Although pericardial rubs develop in some patients toward the end of the first postoperative week, they are usually benign, do not indicate a need for prolongation of hospitalization, and do not require treatment. A separate clinical syndrome that appears late in the first postoperative month is the *postpericardiotomy syndrome*.[134] The relationship between postpericardiotomy syndrome and chronic constrictive pericarditis is not firmly established, but a number of patients with *postoperative constrictive pericarditis* have a history of postpericardiotomy syndrome.

RENAL FAILURE (see Chap. 72). All patients who undergo cardiac surgery experience a reduction in renal blood flow and the glomerular filtration rate (GFR) as a consequence of both anesthesia and cardiopulmonary bypass. Risk factors for the development of persistent renal failure after cardiac surgery include a preoperative history of renal dysfunction or left ventricular dysfunction, prolonged bypass time (>180 minutes), prolonged aortic cross-clamping (>60 minutes), perioperative hypotension, advanced age (>70 years), and the development of medical complications postoperatively.[135]

Most cases of acute renal failure after cardiac surgery result from renal ischemia that lowers the GFR directly (prerenal disease) or, if severe or prolonged, can induce acute tubular necrosis. Possible additional contributory factors include sepsis, nephrotoxic drugs, radiocontrast material injection, cholesterol plaque embolization in the renal circulation, increased urine free hemoglobin levels from hemolysis while undergoing cardiopulmonary bypass, and the effects of ACE inhibitors on glomerular capillary pressure.[136] The detrimental effects of ACE inhibitors are most likely to occur when renal perfusion pressure is low because of renal artery stenosis or systemic hypotension caused by cardiac failure.

Urine output is variable in patients with postoperative acute renal failure. Anuria is uncommon and, if present, should raise the suspicion of urinary tract obstruction (e.g., occluded Foley catheter). More commonly, patients are either oliguric (<400 mg/d) or nonoliguric. Oliguric acute renal failure occurs less frequently than nonoliguric renal failure, usually reflects more severe renal injury, and is associated with a greater probability of requiring dialysis during the acute phase.[136]

Differentiation Between Prerenal Azotemia and Acute Tubular Necrosis. Important diagnostic studies in all patients with acute renal failure include urinalysis and estimation of pulmonary capillary wedge pressure and cardiac output by means of pulmonary artery catheterization. Prerenal azotemia should be suspected if the urine sodium level is less than 20 mEq/liter, the fractional excretion of sodium is less than 1 percent, and urine osmolality is greater than 500 mOsm/liter. Acute tubular necrosis should be suspected if the urine sodium level is greater than 40 mEq/liter, fractional excretion of sodium is greater than 2 percent, and urine osmolality is less than 350 mOsm/liter.[136]

Treatment. Essential elements of therapy for both prerenal azotemia and acute tubular necrosis include optimization of intravascular fluid volume and cardiac output. The latter is best accomplished with vasodilators and inotropic agents rather than vasopressors to avoid further reductions in renal blood flow. Experimental studies suggest that several modalities may protect against the development of progressive renal failure in models of acute renal ischemic injury (e.g., renal artery clamping that simulates the effects of suprarenal aortic cross-clamping while undergoing cardiopulmonary bypass). Mannitol (which washes out obstructing casts), a loop diuretic (which decreases energy requirements in the thick ascending limb of the loop of Henle, thereby decreasing ischemic injury), and the combination of dopamine and atrial natriuretic peptide (but neither alone) have all been effective.[137]

It is prudent to undertake a trial of furosemide and mannitol (only if the patient can tolerate the volume load of the latter) within the first 12 to 24 hours after the development of oliguria. The aim of such therapy is to increase urine output. Because of the renal vasodilating effects of dopamine (2 to 3 μg/kg/min), patients with both oliguric and nonoliguric renal failure may experience an increase in urine output.[138]

If oliguria persists beyond 12 hours, a number of supportive measures must be initiated, including careful attention to electrolyte balance, specifically avoiding hyperkalemia; avoidance of excessive free water administration, which might lead to hyponatremia; correction of acidosis (adding bicarbonate to daily fluids); and adjustment of medication dosages for delayed excretion if the drug is cleared by renal mechanisms. Analysis should be carried out for pericarditis, refractory hyperkalemia, uremic encephalopathy, or colitis. Continuous arteriovenous hemofiltration can be used to remove excess fluid.[136]

Cardiac Surgery in Patients with Chronic Renal Failure. Patients with chronic renal failure who undergo surgery have an increased risk of exacerbation of renal dysfunction perioperatively. Deterioration in renal function may require temporary or even permanent hemodialysis, and these eventualities should be addressed with the patient and the cardiac surgical team preoperatively. Surgery can be safely performed in patients who are already maintained by hemodialysis, but careful coordination of the surgical and dialysis schedules is essential to minimize postoperative problems with fluid and electrolyte management.

GASTROINTESTINAL COMPLICATIONS. Serious gastrointestinal complications after cardiac surgery[139, 140] are rare (occurring in about 1 percent of patients) and can usually be handled by a conservative approach. Only about 0.5 percent of patients who undergo cardiac surgery require a general surgical operation for a gastrointestinal complication.[140, 141] Patients with circulatory compromise and those who require intraaortic balloon pump support are more likely to have gastrointestinal complications. Despite their relative rarity, gastrointestinal complications are associated with significant mortality (approaching 40 percent in some series), thus highlighting the need for careful monitoring and repeated physical examination in high-risk patients.[139, 140] Most complications occur within 7 days of surgery.

NEUROLOGICAL COMPLICATIONS. Neurological complications after cardiac surgery are quite common, particularly in the elderly, if one is attentive to the subtle cognitive (short-term memory loss, lack of concentration) and psychological (depression, increased sense of dependency) changes seen early after surgery.[22, 142, 142a] A positive and supportive attitude on the part of the staff and enlistment of the aid of family members help minimize these problems. Although many patients return to their postoperative state by 4 to 6 weeks after surgery, about 10 percent continue to show deterioration in neuropsychological functioning over the next 6 months, especially if they are older than 65.[22, 142] More serious neurological complications such as stroke occur in 1 to 5 percent of patients but may be seen in as many as 10 percent of patients older than 65.[22]

Symptomatic visual defects may be seen after cardiac surgery and result from retinal emboli, occipital lobe infarction, or anterior ischemic optic neuropathy. Risk factors for cerebrovascular accident (CVA) or transient ischemic attack (TIA) after cardiac surgery include preoperative carotid bruit, previous CVA or TIA, postoperative AF, prolonged cardiopulmonary bypass (>2 hours), and preoperative left ventricular mural thrombus.[22, 143]

Neuropathies in the upper extremities have been reported after cardiac operations. A pattern of injury involving predominantly the ulnar nerve and medial antebrachial cutaneous nerve suggests that the lesion involves brachial plexus compression or a traction injury.[144] The average duration of symptoms after such an injury is 2 months,

but some patients show a slower time course of improvement extending over 6 to 12 months.

REHABILITATION AND PREPARATION FOR DISCHARGE (see Chap. 39)

A coordinated, multidisciplinary cardiac exercise program is essential to overcome the physical deconditioning and psychosocial upheaval associated with cardiac surgery. Emphasis should be placed on early mobilization and progressively more patient self-care, including initiation of these measures in the ICU during the first 24 hours postoperatively. After transfer out of the ICU, the patient should be encouraged to engage in low-density (2 to 3 METS) isotonic activities such as walking and range-of-motion exercises.[145] The nursing staff should monitor the patient's progress while being alert to any undue acceleration in heart rate (>120 beats/min) or hemodynamically compromising arrhythmias.

Patients should also participate in an education program focusing on instructions regarding postoperative medications and initiation of secondary measures targeted at preventing graft occlusion and progression of atherosclerosis.[60, 146, 147] Because of the overwhelming evidence indicating that platelet inhibition is critical to prevention of graft occlusion, all patients undergoing bypass surgery should receive long-term therapy with aspirin unless contraindicated. Ticlopidine may be useful in aspirin-intolerant patients, but there is no evidence of significant benefit from the routine use of either dipyridamole or sulfinpyrazone. Fast-track discharge protocols are now standard, and uncomplicated patients are typically discharged on the fifth postoperative day.[148]

REFERENCES

1. Eagle KA, Guyton RA, Davidoff R, et al: ACC/AHA guidelines for coronary artery bypass graft surgery. J Am Coll Cardiol 34:1262–1347, 1999.
2. Bech-Hanssen O, Caidahl K, Wall B, et al: Influence of aortic valve replacement, prosthesis type, and size on functional outcome and ventricular mass in patients with aortic stenosis. J Thorac Cardiovasc Surg 118:57–65, 1999.
3. Di Carli MF, Maddahi J, Rokhsar S, et al: Long-term survival of patients with coronary artery disease and left ventricular dysfunction: Implications for the role of myocardial viability assessment in management decisions. J Thorac Cardiovasc Surg 116:997–1004, 1998.
4. Trachiotis GD, Weintraub WS, Johnston TS, et al: Coronary artery bypass grafting in patients with advanced left ventricular dysfunction. Ann Thorac Surg 66:1632–1639, 1998.
5. Bigger JT Jr: Prophylactic use of implanted cardiac defibrillators in patients at high risk for ventricular arrhythmias after coronary-artery bypass graft surgery. Coronary Artery Bypass Graft (CABG) Patch Trial Investigators. N Engl J Med 337:1569–1575, 1997.
6. Aklog L, Adams DH, Couper GS, et al: Techniques and results of direct-access minimally invasive mitral valve surgery: A paradigm for the future. J Thorac Cardiovasc Surg 116:705–715, 1998.
7. Machler HE, Bergmann P, Anelli-Monti M, et al: Minimally invasive versus conventional aortic valve operations: A prospective study in 120 patients. Ann Thorac Surg 67:1001–1005, 1999.
8. Magovern JA, Benckart DH, Landreneau RJ, et al: Morbidity, cost, and six-month outcome of minimally invasive direct coronary artery bypass grafting. Ann Thorac Surg 66:1224–1229, 1998.
9. Allen KB, Griffith GL, Heimansohn DA, et al: Endoscopic versus traditional saphenous vein harvesting: A prospective, randomized trial. Ann Thorac Surg 66:26–32, 1998.
9a. Byrne JG, Aklog L, Adams DH: Assessment and management of functional or ischaemic mitral regurgitation. Lancet 335:1743–1744, 2000.
10. Katz NM, Gersh BJ, Cox JL: Changing practice of coronary bypass surgery and its impact on early risk and long-term survival. Curr Opin Cardiol 13:465–475, 1998.
11. Aldea GS, Gaudiani JM, Shapira OM, et al: Effect of gender on postoperative outcomes and hospital stays after coronary artery bypass grafting. Ann Thorac Surg 67:1097–1103, 1999.
12. Mullany CJ, Mock MB, Brooks MM, et al: Effect of age in the Bypass Angioplasty Revascularization Investigation (BARI) randomized trial. Ann Thorac Surg 67:396–403, 1999.
13. Blanche C, Khan SS, Chaux A, et al: Cardiac reoperations in octogenarians: Analysis of outcomes. Ann Thorac Surg 67:93–98, 1999.

14. Adams DH, Chen RH, Kadner A, et al: Impact of small prosthetic valve size on operative mortality in the elderly after aortic valve replacement for aortic stenosis: Does gender matter? J Thorac Cardiovasc Surg 118: 815–822, 1999.

15. Jamieson WR, Edwards FH, Schwartz M, et al: Risk stratification for cardiac valve replacement. National Cardiac Surgery Database. Database Committee of The Society of Thoracic Surgeons. Ann Thorac Surg 67: 943–951, 1999.

16. Lazar HL, Jacobs AK, Aldea GS, et al: Factors influencing mortality after emergency coronary artery bypass grafting for failed percutaneous transluminal coronary angioplasty. Ann Thorac Surg 64:1747–1752, 1997.

17. Gott JP, Thourani VH, Wright CE, et al: Risk neutralization in cardiac operations: Detection and treatment of associated carotid disease. Ann Thorac Surg 68:850–857, 1999.

18. Duarte IG, Murphy CO, Kosinski AS, et al: Late survival after valve operation in patients with left ventricular dysfunction. Ann Thorac Surg 64:1089–1095, 1997.

19. Couper GS, Dekkers RJ, Adams DH: The logistics and cost-effectiveness of circulatory support: Advantages of the ABIOMED BVS 5000. Ann Thorac Surg 68:646–649, 1999.

19a. Erickson LC, Torchiana DF, Schneider EC, et al: The relationship between managed care insurance and use of lower-mortality hospitals for CABG surgery. JAMA 283:1976–1982, 2000.

19b. Alexander KP, Anstrom KJ, Muhlbaier LH, et al: Outcomes of cardiac surgery in patients age ≥ 80 years: Results from the National Cardiovascular Network. J Am Coll Cardiol 35:731–738, 2000.

PREOPERATIVE EVALUATION

20. Rizzo R, Aranki S, Aklog L, et al: Rapid noninvasive diagnosis and surgical repair of acute ascending aortic dissection. J Thorac Cardiovasc Surg 108:567, 1994.

21. Akins CW: Combined carotid endarterectomy and coronary revascularization operation. Ann Thorac Surg 66:1483–1484, 1998.

22. Hornick P, Smith P, Taylor K: Cerebral complications after coronary bypass grafting. Curr Opin Cardiol 9:670, 1994.

23. Moore W, Barnett H, Beebe H, et al: Guidelines for carotid endarterectomy: A multidisciplinary consensus statement from the ad hoc committee, American Heart Association. Circulation 91:566, 1995.

24. Allie DE, Lirtzman M, Malik AP, et al: Rapid-staged strategy for concomitant critical carotid and left main coronary disease with left ventricular dysfunction: IABP use. Ann Thorac Surg 66:1230–1235, 1998.

25. Aranki SF, Adams DH, Rizzo RJ, et al: Determinants of early mortality and late survival in mitral valve endocarditis. Circulation 92 (Suppl 2): 143–149, 1995.

26. Lytle BW, McElroy D, McCarthy P, et al: Influence of arterial coronary bypass grafts on the mortality in coronary reoperations. J Thorac Cardiovasc Surg 107:675, 1994.

27. Edwards F, Clark R, Schwartz M: Impact of internal mammary artery conduits on operative mortality in coronary revascularization. Ann Thorac Surg 57:27, 1994.

28. Uva MS, Braunberger E, Fisher M, et al: Does bilateral internal thoracic artery grafting increase surgical risk in diabetic patients? Ann Thorac Surg 66:2051–2055, 1998.

29. Engoren M, Buderer NF, Zacharias A, Habib RH: Variables predicting reintubation after cardiac surgical procedures. Ann Thorac Surg 67: 661–665, 1999.

30. Kondo NI, Maddi R, Ewenstein BM, Goldhaber SZ: Anticoagulation and hemostasis in cardiac surgical patients. J Card Surg 9:443, 1994.

31. Tatar H. Cicek S, Demirkilic U, et al: Vascular complications of intraaortic balloon pumping: Unsheathed versus sheathed insertion. Ann Thorac Surg 55:1518, 1993.

32. Rihal C, Eagle K, Mickel M, et al: Surgical therapy for coronary artery disease among patients with combined coronary artery and peripheral vascular disease. Circulation 91:46, 1995.

33. Higgins T, Estafanous F, LIoyd F, et al: Stratification of morbidity and mortality outcome by preoperative risk factors in coronary artery bypass patients: A clinical severity score. JAMA 207:2344, 1992.

34. Edwards FH, Carey JS, Grover FL, et al: Impact of gender on coronary bypass operative mortality. Ann Thorac Surg 66:125–131, 1998.

35. Ferraris VA, Ferraris SP: Risk factors for postoperative morbidity. J Thorac Cardiovasc Surg 111:731–741, 1996.

36. Tu JV, Jaglal SB, Naylor CD, Steering Committee of the Provincial Adult Cardiac Care Network of Ontario: Multicenter validation of a risk index for mortality, intensive care unit stay, and overall hospital length of stay after cardiac surgery. Circulation 91:677, 1995.

36a. Brooks MM, Jones RH, Bach RG, et al: Predictors of mortality and mortality from cardiac causes in the Bypass Angioplasty Revascularization Investigation (BARI) randomized trial and registry. Circulation 101: 2082–2089, 2000.

36b. Vogt A, Grube E, Glunz HG, et al: Determinants of mortality after cardiac surgery: Results of the Registry of the Arbeitsgemeinschaft Leitender Kardiologischer Krankenhausarzte (ALKK) on 10 525 patients. Eur Heart J 21:28–32, 2000.

37. Borger MA, Rao V, Weisel RD, et al: Deep sternal wound infection: Risk factors and outcomes. Ann Thorac Surg 65:1050–1056, 1998.

38. He GW, Ryan WH, Acuff TE, et al: Risk factors for operative mortality and sternal wound infection in bilateral internal mammary artery grafting. J Thorac Cardiovasc Surg 107:196, 1994.

39. Palazzo R, Barner HB: Surgery for ischemic heart disease. Curr Opin Cardiol 9:216, 1994.

40. Vanoverschelde, J-LJ, Gerber DL, D'Hondt AM, et al: Preoperative selection of patients with severely impaired left ventricular function for coronary revascularization: Role of low-dose dobutamine echocardiography and exercise-redistribution-reinjection thallium SPECT. Circulation 92:37, 1995.

40a. Pasquet A, Lauer MS, Williams MJ, et al: Prediction of global left ventricular function after bypass surgery in patients with severe left ventricular dysfunction. Impact of preoperative myocardial function, perfusion, and metabolism. Eur Heart J 21:125–136, 2000.

41. Lee K, Marwick T, Cook S, et al: Prognosis of patients with left ventricular dysfunction, with and without viable myocardium after myocardial infarction: Relative efficacy of medical theraphy and revascularization. Circulation 90:2687, 1994.

42. Salati M, Lemma M, Di Mattia DG, et al: Myocardial revascularization in patients with ischemic cardiomyopathy: Functional observations. Ann Thorac Surg 64:1728–1734, 1997.

43. Lomboy C, Schulman D, Grill H, et al: Rest-redistribution thallium-201 scintigraphy to determine myocardial viability early after myocardial infarction. J Am Coll Cardiol 25:210, 1995.

44. Fullerton DA, Jones SD, Jaggers J, et al: Effective control of pulmonary vascular resistance with inhaled nitric oxide after cardiac operation. J Thorac Cardiovasc Surg 111:753–762, 1996.

45. Alvarez JM: Emergency coronary bypass grafting for failed percutaneous coronary artery stenting: Increased costs and platelet transfusion requirements after the use of abciximab. J Thorac Cardiovasc Surg 115: 472–473, 1998.

46. Tardiff BE, Califf RM, Morris D, et al: Coronary revascularization surgery after myocardial infarction: Impact of bypass surgery on survival after thrombolysis. GUSTO Investigators. Global Utilization of Streptokinase and Tissue Plasminogen Activator for Occluded Coronary Arteries. J Am Coll Cardiol 29:240–249, 1997.

47. Braxton JH, Hammond GL, Letsou GV, et al: Optimal timing of coronary artery bypass graft surgery after acute myocardial infarction. Circulation 92:66, 1995.

48. Misfeld M, Dubbert S, Eleftheriadis S, et al: Fibrinolysis-adjusted perioperative low-dose aprotin reduces blood loss in bypass operations. Ann Thorac Surg 66:792–799, 1998.

49. Kirklin J, Barratt-Boyes B: Anesthesia for cardiovascular surgery. In Kirklin J, Barratt-Boyes B (eds): Cardiac Surgery. New York, Churchill Livingstone, 1993, p 167.

50. Creswell L, Schuessler R, Rosenbloom M, Cox J: Hazards of postoperative atrial arrhythmias. Ann Thorac Surg 56:539, 1993.

51. Aranki S, Shaw D, Adams D, et al: Predictors of atrial fibrillation following coronary artery surgery: Current trends and impact on hospital resources. Circulation 94:390–397, 1996.

52. Lauer M, Eagle K: Arrhythmias following cardiac surgery. In Podrid P, Kowey P (eds): Cardiac Arrhythmia. Mechanisms, Diagnosis, and Management. Baltimore, Williams & Wilkins, 1995, p 1206.

53. Andrews TC, Relmold SC, Berlin JA, Ahlman EM: Prevention of supraventricular arrhythmias after coronary artery bypass surgery: A meta-analysis of randomized control trials. Circulation 84(Suppl 3):236, 1991.

54. Steinberg J, Zelenkofske S, Wong S, et al: Value of the P wave signal-averaged ECG for predicting atrial fibrillation after cardiac surgery. Circulation 88:2618, 1993.

55. Mendes L, Connelly G, McKenney P, et al: Right coronary artery stenosis: An independent predictor of atrial fibrillation after coronary artery bypass surgery. J Am Coll Cardiol 25:198, 1995.

56. Cox J: A perspective on postoperative atrial fibrillation in cardiac operations. Ann Thorac Surg 56:405, 1993.

57. Redle JD, Khurana S, Marzan R, et al: Prophylactic oral amiodarone compared with placebo for prevention of atrial fibrillation after coronary artery bypass surgery. Am Heart J 138:144–150, 1999.

58. Daoud EG, Strickberger SA, Man KC, et al: Preoperative amiodarone as prophylaxis against atrial fibrillation after heart surgery. N Engl J Med 337:1785–1791, 1997.

59. Lamas G, Rebecca G, Braunwald N, Antman E: Pacemaker malfunction after nitrous oxide anesthesia. Am J Cardiol 56:995, 1985.

60. Pearson T, Rapaport E, Criqui M, et al: Optimal risk factor management in the patient after coronary revascularization: A statement for healthcare professionals from an American Heart Association writing group. Circulation 90:3125, 1994.

60a. Lemmer JH Jr, Metzdorff MT, Krause AH Jr, et al: Emergency coronary artery bypass graft surgery in abciximab-treated patients. Ann Thorac Surg 66:90–95, 2000.

60b. Cartier R, Brann S, Dagenais F, et al: Systematic off-pump coronary artery revascularization in multivessel disease: Experience of three hundred cases. J Thorac Cardiovasc Surg 119:221–229, 2000.

60c. Berger PB, Alderman EL, Nadel A, Schaff HV: Frequency of early occlusion and stenosis in a left internal mammary artery to left anterior descending artery bypass graft after surgery through a median sternotomy on conventional bypass: Benchmark for minimally invasive direct coronary artery bypass. Circulation 100:2353–2358, 1999.

POSTOPERATIVE MANAGEMENT

61. Kirklin J, Barratt-Boyes B: Postoperative care. In Kirklin J, Barratt-Boyes B (eds): Cardiac Surgery. New York, Churchill Livingstone, 1993, p 195.

62. Lippmann M, Goldberg S, Walkenstein M: Pulmonary complications of open heart surgery. *In* Kotler M, Alfieri A (eds): Cardiac and Noncardiac Complications of Open Heart Surgery: Prevention, Diagnosis, and Treatment. Mt Kisco, NY, Futura, 1992, p 239.

63. Walden S, Meyer P: Pulmonary management. *In* Baumgartner W, Owens S, Cameron D, Reitz B (eds): The Johns Hopkins Manual of Cardiac Surgical Care. St Louis, CV Mosby, 1994, p 161.

64. Lam A, Newhouse M: Management of asthma and chronic airflow limitation. Chest 98:44, 1990.

65. Katz MG, Katz R, Schachner A, Cohen AJ: Phrenic nerve injury after coronary artery bypass grafting: Will it go away? Ann Thorac Surg 65:32–35, 1998.

65a. Stamenkovic SA, Morgan IS, Pontefract DR, Campanella C: Is early tracheostomy safe in cardiac patients with median sternotomy incisions? Ann Thorac Surg 69:1152–1154, 2000.

66. Weiss SJ, Longnecker DE: Perioperative hypertension: An overview. Coron Artery Dis 4:401, 1993.

67. Gray RJ, Bateman TM, Czer LS, et al: Use of esmolol in hypertension after cardiac surgery. Am J Cardiol 56:56, 1985.

68. Cooper TJ, Clutton BTH, Jones SN, et al: Factors relating to the development of hypertension after cardiopulmonary bypass. Br Heart J 54:91, 1985.

69. O'Dwyer JP, Yorukoglu D, Harris MN: The use of esmolol to attenuate the haemodynamic response when extubating patients following cardiac surgery—a double-blind controlled study. Eur Heart J 14:701, 1993.

70. James T, Hageman G, Urthaler F. Anatomic and physiologic considerations of a cardiogenic hypertensive reflex. Am J Cardiol 44:852, 1979.

71. Hamm CW, Reimers J, Ischinger T, et al: A randomized study of coronary angioplasty compared with bypass surgery in patients with symptomatic multivessel coronary disease: German Angioplasty Bypass Surgery Investigation (GABI). N Engl J Med 331:1037, 1994.

72. King SE, Lembo NJ, Weintraub WS, et al: A randomized trial comparing coronary angioplasty with coronary bypass surgery: Emory Angioplasty Versus Surgery Trial (EAST). N Engl J Med 331:1044, 1994.

73. Greaves S, Rutherford J, Aranki S, et al: Current incidence and determinants of perioperative myocardial infarction in coronary artery surgery. Am Heart J 132:572–573, 1996.

74. Lemmer JH Jr, Kirsh MM: Coronary artery spasm following coronary artery surgery. Ann Thorac Surg 46:108, 1988.

75. Obarski TP, Loop FD, Cosgrove DM, et al: Frequency of acute myocardial infarction in valve repairs versus valve replacement for pure mitral regurgitation. Am J Cardiol 65:887, 1990.

76. Bulkley BH, Hutchins GM: Myocardial consequences of coronary artery bypass graft surgery: The paradox of necrosis in areas of revascularization. Circulation 56:906, 1977.

77. Katus H, Schoeppenthau M, Tanzeem A, et al: Non-invasive assessment of perioperative myocardial cell damage by circulating cardiac troponin T. Br Heart J 65:259, 1991.

78. Mair J, Larue C, Mair P, et al: Use of cardiac troponin I to diagnose perioperative myocardial infarction in coronary artery bypass grafting. Clin Chem 40:2066, 1994.

79. Bateman T, Matloff J, Gray R: Myocardial infarction during coronary artery bypass surgery—benign event or prognostic omen? Int J Cardiol 6:259, 1984.

80. Force T, Hibberd P, Weeks G, et al: Perioperative myocardial infarction after coronary artery bypass surgery. Circulation 82:903, 1990.

81. Joffe II, Jacobs LE, Lampert C, et al: Role of echocardiography in perioperative management of patients undergoing open heart surgery. Am Heart J 131:162, 1995.

82. Baumgartner W, Owens S, Cameron D, Reitz B: The Johns Hopkins Manual of Cardiac Surgical Care. St Louis, CV Mosby, 1994, p 546.

83. Feneck RO: Intravenous milrinone following cardiac surgery: I. Effects of bolus infusion followed by variable dose maintenance infusion: The European Milrinone Multicentre Trial Group. J Cardiothorac Vasc Anesth 6:554, 1992.

84. Lee WA, Gillinov AM, Cameron DE, et al: Centrifugal ventricular assist device for support of the failing heart after cardiac surgery. Crit Care Med 21:1186, 1993.

85. Oz M, Rose E, Levin H: Selection criteria for placement of left ventricular assist devices. Am Heart J 129:173, 1995.

86. Reichert CL, Koolen JJ, Visser CA: Transesophageal echocardiographic evaluation of left ventricular function during intraaortic balloon pump counterpulsation. J Am Soc Echocardiogr 6:490, 1993.

87. Reichert CL, Visser CA, Van den Brink RB, et al: Prognostic value of biventricular function in hypotensive patients after cardiac surgery as assessed by transesophageal echocardiography. J Cardiothorac Vasc Anesth 6:429, 1992.

88. Mikawa K, Maekawa N, Goto R, et al: Use of prostaglandin F_1 to treat perianaesthetic pulmonary hypertension associated with mitral valve disease. J Int Med Res 21:161, 1992.

89. Pepi M, Muratori M, Barbier P, et al: Pericardial effusion after cardiac surgery: Incidence, site, size, and haemodynamic consequences. Br Heart J 72:327, 1994.

90. Chuttani K, Tischler MD, Pandian NG, et al: Diagnosis of cardiac tamponade after cardiac surgery: Relative value of clinical, echocardiographic, and hemodynamic signs. Am Heart J 127:913, 1994.

91. Russo AM, O'Connor WH, Waxman HL: Atypical presentations and echocardiographic findings in patients with cardiac tamponade occurring early and late after cardiac surgery. Chest 104:71, 1993.

92. Schoebrechia B, Herregods MC, Van de Werf F, De Geest H: Usefulness of transesophageal echocardiography in patients with hemodynamic deterioration late after cardiac surgery. Chest 104:1631, 1993.

93. Moore SL, Wilkoff BL: Rhythm disturbances after cardiac surgery. Semin Thorac Cardiovasc Surg 3:24, 1991.

94. Olshansky B, Okumura K, Hess PG, et al: Use of procainamide with rapid atrial pacing for successful conversion of atrial flutter to sinus rhythm. J Am Coll Cardiol 11:359, 1988.

95. Platia EV, Fitzpatrick P, Wallis D, et al: Esmolol vs verapamil for the treatment of recent-onset atrial fibrillation/flutter. J Am Coll Cardiol 11:170, 1988.

96. Eckman MH, Levin HJ, Pauker SG. Making decisions about antithrombotic therapy in heart disease: Decision analytic and cost-effectiveness issues. Chest 106(Suppl):457, 1995.

97. Laupacis A, Albers GW, Dalen JE, et al: Antithrombotic therapy in atrial fibrillation. Chest 108(Suppl):352, 1995.

98. VanderLugt JT, Mattioni T, Denker S, et al: Efficacy and safety of ibutilide fumarate for the conversion of atrial arrhythmias after cardiac surgery. Circulation 100:369–375, 1999.

99. Raitt MH, Dolack GL, Kino K, et al: Procainamide has limited effectiveness for the treatment of atrial fibrillation after open heart surgery. Circulation 90(Supp 1):376, 1994.

100. Ganz L, Friedman P: Medical progress: Supraventricular tachycardia. N Engl J Med 332:162, 1995.

101. Gottipaty V, Kocovic D, Kinchla N, et al: Timing and impact on survival of in-hospital cardiac arrest after coronary artery bypass graft surgery. Circulation 88(Suppl 1):166, 1993.

102. Carlson M, Biblo L, Waldo A: Post open heart surgery ventricular arrhythmias. Cardiovasc Clin 22.241, 1992.

103. Holman W, Spruell R, Vicente W, Pacifico A: Electrophysiological mechanisms for postcardioplegia reperfusion ventricular fibrillation. Circulation 90(Suppl 2):293, 1994.

104. Willems S, Weiss C, Meinertz T: Tachyarrhythmias following coronary artery bypass graft surgery: Epidemiology, mechanisms, and current therapeutic strategies. Thorac Cardiovasc Surg 45:232–237, 1997.

105. Costeas XF, Schoenfeld MH: Usefulness of electrophysiologic studies for new-onset sustained ventricular tachyarrhythmias shortly after coronary artery bypass grafting. Am J Cardiol 72:1291, 1993.

106. Scott WA: Temporary DDD pacing after surgically induced heart block. Am J Cardiol 71:1123, 1993.

107. Hippeläinen M, Mustonen P, Manninen H, Rehnberg S: Predictors of conduction disturbances after coronary bypass grafting. Ann Thorac Surg 57:1284, 1994.

108. Tuzcu EM, Emre A, Goormastic M, et al: Incidence and prognostic significance of intraventricular conduction abnormalities after coronary bypass surgery. J Am Coll Cardiol 16:607, 1990.

109. Emlein G, Huang S, Pires L, et al: Prolonged bradyarrhythmias after isolated coronary artery bypass graft surgery. Am Heart J 126:1084, 1993.

110. Tsai T, Matloff J: Cardiac surgery in the elderly. *In* Matloff RGAJ (ed): Medical Management of the Cardiac Surgical Patient. Baltimore, Williams & Wilkins, 1990. p 27.

111. Kestin AS, Valeri CR, Khuri SF, et al: The platelet function defect of cardiopulmonary bypass. Blood 82:107, 1993.

112. Morse DS, Adams DH, Magnani B: Platelet and neutrophil activation during cardiac surgical procedures: Impact of cardiopulmonary bypass. Ann Thorac Surg 65:691–695, 1998.

113. Kajani M, Waxman H: Hematologic problems after open heart surgery. *In* Kotler M, Alfieri A (eds): Cardiac and Noncardiac Complications of Open Heart Surgery: Prevention, Diagnosis, and Treatment. Mt Kisco, NY, Futura, 1992, p 219.

114. Brister SJ, Ofosu FA, Buchanan MR: Thrombin generation during cardiac surgery: Is heparin the ideal anticoagulant? Thromb Haemost 70:259, 1993.

115. Mossad E, Estafanous F: Blood use in cardiac surgery and the limitations of hemodilution. Curr Opin Cardiol 10:584, 1995.

116. Baumgartner W, Owens S: Hemorrhage and tamponade. *In* Baumgartner W, Owens S, Cameron D, Reitz B (eds).: The Johns Hopkins Manual of Cardiac Surgical Care. St Louis, CV Mosby, 1994, p 183.

117. Royston D: Aprotinin in patients having coronary artery bypass graft surgery. Curr Opin Cardiol 10:591, 1995.

117a. Levi M, Cromheecke ME, de Jonge E, et al: Pharmacological strategies to decrease excessive blood loss in cardiac surgery: A meta-analysis of clinically relevant endpoints. Lancet 354:1940–1947, 2000.

118. Stein PD, Alpert JS, Copeland JG III, et al: Antithrombotic therapy in patients with mechanical and biological prosthetic heart valves. Chest 108(Suppl):371–379, 1995.

119. Verkkala V, Valtonen V, Jarvinen A, Tolppanen E: Fever, leukocytosis and C-reactive protein after open-heart surgery and their value in the diagnosis of postoperative infections. Thorac Cardiovasc Surg 35:78, 1987.

120. Livelli F, Johnson R, McEnany M, et al: Unexplained in-hospital fever following cardiac surgery: Natural history, relationship to postpericardiotomy syndrome, and a prospective study of therapy with indomethacin versus placebo. Circulation 57:968, 1978.

120a. Carpino PA, Khabbaz KR, Bojar RM, et al: Clinical benefits of endoscopic vein harvesting in patients with risk factors for saphenectomy wound infections undergoing coronary artery bypass grafting. J Thorac Cardiovasc Surg 119:69–76, 2000.

121. Greenberg J, DeSanctis RW, Mills RMJ: Vein-donor-leg cellulitis after coronary artery bypass surgery. Ann Intern Med 97:565, 1982.

122. The Parisian Mediastinitis Study Group: Risk factors for deep sternal wound infection after sternotomy: A prospective, multicenter study. J Thorac Cardiovasc Surg 111:1200–1207, 1996.

123. Greenblatt J, Fischer R: Complications of cardiac surgery: Infections. *In* Kotler M, Alfieri A (eds): Cardiac and Noncardiac Complications of Open Heart Surgery: Prevention, Diagnosis, and Treatment. Mt Kisco, NY, Futura, 1992, p 145.

124. He GW, Ryan WH, Acuff TE, et al: Risk factors for operative mortality and sternal wound infection in bilateral internal mammary artery grafting. J Thorac Cardiovasc Surg 107:196–202, 1994.

125. Milano CA, Georgiade G, Muhlbaier LH, et al: Comparison of omental and pectoralis flaps for poststernotomy mediastinitis. Ann Thorac Surg 67:377–381, 1999.

126. Ringelman PR, Vander Kolk CA, Cameron D, et al: Long-term results of flap reconstruction in median sternotomy wound infections. Plast Reconstr Surg 93:1208–1216, 1994.

127. Rand RP, Cochran RP, Aziz S, et al: Prospective trial of catheter irrigation and muscle flaps for sternal wound infection. Ann Thorac Surg 65:1046–1049, 1998.

128. Hall J, Christiansen K, Carter M, et al: Antibiotic prophylaxis in cardiac operations. Ann Thorac Surg 56:916, 1993.

129. Threlkeld M, Cobbs C: Infectious disorders of prosthetic valves and intravascular devices. *In* Mandell G, Douglas R, Bennett J (eds): Principles and Practice of Infectious Diseases. New York, Churchill-Livingstone, 1990, p 706.

130. Fang G, Keys T, Gentry I, et al: Prosthetic valve endocarditis resulting from nosocomial bacteremia: A prospective multicenter study. Ann Intern Med 119:500, 1993.

131. Niwaya K, Knott-Craig CJ, Santangelo K, et al: Advantage of autograft and homograft valve replacement for complex aortic valve endocarditis. Ann Thorac Surg 67:1603–1608, 1999.

132. Atkinson JB, Connor DH, Robinowitz M, et al: Cardiac fungal infections: Review of autopsy findings in 60 patients. Hum Pathol 15:935, 1984.

133. Gillinov AM, Davis EA, Alberg AJ, et al: Pulmonary embolism in the cardiac surgical patient. Ann Thorac Surg 53:988, 1992.

134. Khan AH: The postcardiac injury syndromes. Clin Cardiol 15:67, 1992.

135. Kellerman PS: Perioperative care of the renal patient. Arch Intern Med 154:1674, 1994.

136. Kobrin S, Tobias S: Renal complications of open heart surgery. *In* Kotler M, Alfieri A (eds): Cardiac and Noncardiac Complications of Open Heart Surgery: Prevention, Diagnosis, and Treatment. Mt Kisco, NY, Futura, 1992, p 311.

137. Rose B: Acute renal failure—prerenal disease versus acute tubular necrosis. *In* Rose B (ed): Pathophysiology of Renal Disease. New York, McGraw-Hill, 1987, p 63.

138. Casale A, Ulrich S: Complications in other organ systems. *In* Baumgartner W, Owen S, Cameron D, Reitz B (eds): The Johns Hopkins Manual of Cardiac Surgical Care. St Louis, CV Mosby, 1994, p 271.

139. Egleston CV, Wood AE, Gorey TF, McGovern EM: Gastrointestinal complications after cardiac surgery. Ann R Coll Surg Engl 75:52, 1993.

140. Tsiotos GG, Mullany CJ, Zietlow S, Van Heerden JA: Abdominal complications following cardiac surgery. Am J Surg 167:553, 1994.

141. Taggart DP, Browne SM, Halligan PW, Wade DT: Is cardiopulmonary bypass still the cause of cognitive dysfunction after cardiac operations? J Thorac Cardiovasc Surg 118:414–420, 1999.

142. Kallis P, Unsworth-White J, Munsch C, et al: Disability and distress following cardiac surgery in patients over 70 years of age. Eur J Cardiothorac Surg 7:306, 1993.

142a. Puskas JD, Winston AD, Wright CE, et al: Stroke after coronary artery operation: Incidence, correlates, outcome, and cost. Ann Thorac Surg 69:1053–1056, 2000.

143. Kuroda Y, Uchimoto R, Kaieda R, et al: Central nervous system complications after cardiac surgery: A comparison between coronary artery bypass grafting and valve surgery. Anesth Analg 76:222, 1993.

144. Seyfer AE, Grammer NY, Bogumill GP, et al: Upper extremity neuropathies after cardiac surgery. J Hand Surg [Am] 10:16, 1985.

REHABILITATION AND PREPARATION FOR DISCHARGE

145. Fletcher G, Balady G, Froelicher V, et al: Exercise standards: A statement for healthcare professionals from the American Heart Association. Circulation 91:580, 1995.

146. van der Meer J, Hillege H, Koostra G, et al: Prevention of one-year vein-graft occlusion after aortocoronary-bypass surgery: A comparison of low-dose aspirin, low-dose aspirin plus dipyridamole, and oral anticoagulants. Lancet 342:257, 1993.

147. Daida H, Yokoi H, Miyano H, et al: Relation of saphenous vein graft obstruction to serum cholesterol levels. J Am Coll Cardiol 25:193, 1995.

148. Walji S, Peterson RJ, Neis P, et al: Ultra-fast track hospital discharge using conventional cardiac surgical techniques. Ann Thorac Surg 67:363–370, 1999.

Chapter 61

General Anesthesia and Noncardiac Surgery in Patients with Heart Disease

LEE GOLDMAN • JOSHUA ADLER

The cardiovascular system of patients undergoing general anesthesia and noncardiac surgical procedures is subject to numerous stresses owing to depression of myocardial contractility and respiration as well as fluctuations in temperature, arterial pressure, ventricular filling pressures, blood volume, and activity of the autonomic nervous system. Complications of anesthesia and operation, such as hemorrhage, infection, fever, pulmonary embolism, and myocardial infarction, impose additional burdens on the cardiovascular system. Patients who have cardiac disease and who are compensated preoperatively may be unable to meet these increased demands during the perioperative period, in which case arrhythmias, myocardial ischemia, and/or heart failure may develop.[1-3] As a consequence, a substantial proportion of all deaths in most series of noncardiac operations results from cardiovascular complications.

Because both the frequency and the seriousness of cardiovascular complications of general anesthesia and operation are considerably increased in patients with known cardiovascular disease, the magnitude of these risks must be appreciated to decide on the advisability of noncardiac surgery in cardiac patients. In addition, both the life expectancy and the quality of life of patients must be taken into account. For instance, a noncardiac surgical procedure with a high risk, directed to correct a disorder that is not life threatening, may be difficult to justify if the patient's cardiac condition precludes a survival period sufficient to allow the patient to reap the benefits of the operation. Obviously, the dangers and disability of the disease for which an operation is being proposed must also be balanced against the risk of the operation itself.

ANESTHESIA

Changes in cardiovascular function during general anesthesia are due to many factors, including direct effects of the anesthetic agent(s) and indirect effects mediated primarily through the autonomic nervous system. In addition, if respiration is inadequately maintained, the resulting hypoxemia, hypercarbia, and acidosis may further depress myocardial contractility and increase cardiac irritability. The interplay of these several variables may produce changes in arterial and central venous pressures, cardiac output, and rate and rhythm. To minimize the risk of operation in patients with a compromised cardiovascular system, it is essential to minimize these changes.[3]

The choice of the anesthetic approach and the specific anesthetic agents to be used should be made by a qualified anesthesiologist, commonly after careful evaluation of the patient's medical and cardiac condition and often after consultation with the surgeon and the internist or cardiologist. Different anesthesiologists may prefer different anesthetic techniques, and the anesthesiological literature clearly indicates that there is little, if any, correlation between the anesthetic route or agents and the likelihood of major clinical complications. Thus, the skill and experience of the anesthesiologist, including the ability to monitor hemodynamics and respond quickly, are far more important than the specific agent or technique that is used. Although the cardiological consultant should not expect to dictate the anesthetic approach, the quality of the consultation will be improved if the consultant appreciates the clinical pharmacology of the anesthetic agent.

General Anesthesia

The induction of general anesthesia is usually accomplished with intravenous anesthetics. The common agents used for the induction of anesthesia, barbiturates and benzodiazepines, lower systemic arterial pressure by about 20 to 30 percent in healthy patients but sometimes by a greater amount in hypertensive patients.[3] Barbiturates reduce blood pressure through depression of myocardial contractility and sympathetic tone. Benzodiazepines act primarily by venodilation and have a more modest effect on blood pressure. Ketamine, a phencyclidine derivative, stimulates the sympathetic nervous system and thus does not lower blood pressure but can increase myocardial oxygen demand. It is most often used in severely hypovolemic patients. During laryngoscopy and tracheal intubation, blood pressure can increase by 20 to 30 mm Hg.[3] Such increases can be avoided by adequate topical anesthesia because the hypertension appears to be caused by the laryngoscopy rather than by the passage of a tube into the trachea. Maintenance of general anesthesia can be achieved with inhalational or intravenous agents. In most cases, a combination of agents is used, so-called balanced anesthesia.

INHALATION AGENTS. These agents enter the bloodstream by way of the alveoli and are excreted across the alveoli essentially unchanged. The predominant hemodynamic effects of the commonly used inhalational agents (halothane, enflurane, and isoflurane) are depression of myocardial contractility and reduction in arterial blood pressure.[4] Nitrous oxide also decreases myocardial contractility but does not result in significant hypotension because of reflex vasoconstriction. Although the physiological and pharmacological properties of the inhalational agents differ slightly, no single agent has been shown to be appreciably safer in patients with cardiac disease.[5-7]

INTRAVENOUS ANESTHETICS. Narcotics are the principal intravenous agents used for maintenance of general anesthesia. Most narcotics cause some degree of hypotension through venodilation, with little effect on myocardial contractility. The short-acting agents fentanyl, sufentanyl, and alfentanyl are less likely to cause hypotension than morphine.[4] Propofol is an attractive agent because of its very rapid onset and, particularly, offset of action. It may, however, cause moderate to severe hypotension principally due to venodilation. It is often used as a sedative agent in intensive care settings as well as a general anesthetic agent.

MUSCLE RELAXANTS. Drugs used for muscle relaxation also may have cardiovascular effects. *Succinylcholine* can cause bradycardia, which can be reversed or prevented by administration of atropine. In patients anesthetized with halothane, *pancuronium* and *gallamine* cause an increase in heart rate, arterial pressure, and cardiac output, whereas *tubocurarine* and *metocurine* result in a fall in mean arterial pressure with mild elevations in heart rate and little, if any, change in cardiac output. *Vecuronium* has essentially no cardiovascular side effects.

Spinal and Epidural Anesthesia

Spinal and epidural anesthesia cause sympathetic denervation, which produces peripheral arteriodilation and venodilation. Systemic vascular resistance may be reduced by 10 to 15 percent. Venodilation may cause a marked reduction in right ventricular preload as a consequence of sympathetic denervation. Under these circumstances, right ventricular preload depends critically on the effects of gravity on the patient's position, as well as on the total blood volume.

In four randomized trials comparing general anesthesia with either spinal/epidural anesthesia or combined general plus spinal/epidural anesthesia, no differences in cardiac outcomes have been found.[8-11] Furthermore, in an informal meta-analysis combining the data from these trials, still no difference was noted.[12] The choice of anesthetic technique should ultimately be left to the anesthesiologist.

REGIONAL AND LOCAL ANESTHESIA. Cardiovascular effects from peripheral nerve blocks with local anesthetic agents are uncommon but can occasionally result from absorption of local anesthetic agents into the bloodstream. A major concern with local or regional anesthesia is whether the technique provides adequate anesthesia and analgesia for the planned procedure; the cardiological consultant should not underestimate the cardiovascular consequences of inadequate anesthesia.

Intraoperative Hemodynamics and Arrhythmias

During the operative procedure, it is not uncommon for systolic blood pressure to fall into the range of 95 to 105 mm Hg. Such blood pressure reductions are often brief and may respond to a lightening of the anesthesia, to a brisk fluid challenge, or to the use of intravenous sympathomimetic agents. Such blood pressure reductions are equally likely with general versus spinal/epidural anesthesia.[13] Any severe reduction in arterial pressure in patients with ischemic heart disease can reduce coronary flow and precipitate myocardial ischemia. In general, transient reductions in blood pressure are not associated with major cardiac complications. Marked or sustained reductions in blood pressure, such as a 33 percent reduction below the

preoperative blood pressure lasting more than 10 minutes, have been associated with increased cardiac complication rates.[14, 15]

Positive-pressure ventilation during general anesthesia reduces the return of blood to the right side of the heart and tends to reduce ventricular preload. Fluid that is administered during positive-pressure ventilation does not increase preload to the extent that it would in patients who are ventilating spontaneously. When the positive-pressure ventilation of general anesthesia ceases, ventricular preload increases, often abruptly, and hypertension or pulmonary congestion may result. Analogous physiological changes can occur with the cessation of spinal or epidural anesthesia because the venodilation caused by these agents also reduces right ventricular preload.

Transient bradycardias, such as sinus bradycardia and junctional rhythm, can occur during periods of vagal stimulation. These bradyarrhythmias commonly respond to a lightening of the anesthesia or to the administration of atropine or beta$_1$-adrenoceptor agonists such as isoproterenol or epinephrine. Tachyarrhythmias can result from hypovolemia or vasodilation as well as from sensitization of the myocardium to catecholamines that are circulating and/or released by sympathetic nerve endings in the heart.[16] Tachycardia is poorly tolerated by patients with mitral stenosis (see Chap. 46) and can cause myocardial ischemia in patients with coronary artery disease. Therapy with specific antiarrhythmic medications is usually indicated only when the arrhythmia causes circulatory compromise and does not respond to changes in the depth of anesthesia or to attention to problems such as hypoxemia, hypovolemia, hypotension, or potentially precipitating surgical manipulation.

Mild hypothermia frequently occurs during the intraoperative period. For most patients, there are few if any consequences from a transient decline in body temperature. In a study of patients undergoing vascular surgery, however, intraoperative hypothermia was associated with an increased risk of myocardial ischemia.[17] Furthermore, in a randomized trial comparing routine thermal care with supplemental warming during the intraoperative and early postoperative period in patients undergoing vascular surgery, postoperative cardiac morbidity was reduced in the warmed group.[18]

MONITORING. In patients who have severe underlying heart disease and who are undergoing noncardiac surgery, it is mandatory to monitor cardiac function during anesthesia,[19] including cardiac rate and rhythm and directly recorded arterial blood pressure. A radial artery line permits not only monitoring of intraarterial pressure but also frequent sampling for determination of blood gas values. In the presence of peripheral vasoconstriction, indirect (cuff) blood pressure measurements may greatly underestimate true arterial pressure.

Multiple lead monitoring of cardiac rhythm and ST segments has become the standard of care in high-risk patients with coronary artery disease. Although intraoperative ischemia is less predictive of adverse cardiac outcomes than either preoperative or postoperative ischemia, prolonged episodes of intraoperative ischemia are associated with adverse cardiac events.[20]

The use of pulmonary artery (PA) catheters to measure pulmonary artery capillary wedge pressure and cardiac output is controversial. Many small studies have shown no reduction in adverse cardiac outcomes with the use of an intraoperative PA catheter in unselected high-risk patients undergoing vascular surgery.[21, 22] Nevertheless, in certain situations, a PA catheter may be helpful, such as in patients with severe left ventricular dysfunction, in patients who have severe aortic stenosis or unstable angina and who are undergoing high-risk surgery, and to monitor intracardiac fluid status closely.[23, 24] The decision to use an intraoperative PA catheter should be left to the anesthesiologist, but it is appropriate for the cardiological consultant to recommend consideration of its use in very high-risk patients.

THE OPERATION

Just as consultant cardiologists must understand the pharmacological effects of anesthesia, they must also recognize the physiological effects of surgery, including the direct consequences of the operation and the expected responses to postoperative recuperation.

NATURE OF THE OPERATION. A key element in perioperative risk assessment is an estimation of the baseline risk. This is the average risk of a particular procedure at a particular institution. This baseline risk may then be modified by the clinical characteristics of an individual patient. Among noncardiac surgical procedures, the highest cardiovascular complication rates are commonly associated with abdominal aortic aneurysm surgery,[25] which causes substantial myocardial stress because of aortic cross-clamping and major shifts in fluid and electrolytes. The risk of cardiac complications is also higher in other major abdominal and thoracic procedures than in procedures on the extremities, in large part because of the more difficult postoperative course.[26] Patients who undergo operation for aortic aneurysm, carotid arterial disease, or peripheral vascular disease often have substantial coronary artery disease as well, and the extent of the latter may be underestimated because of the limitations caused by the peripheral arterial disease. At the other end of the spectrum, ophthalmalogical surgery, upper endoscopy, and transurethral prostate resection can be safely performed even in patients with heart disease.[27, 28] The estimated risk of myocardial infarction or cardiac death due to various surgical procedures is shown in Table 61-1.

DURATION. The risk of cardiovascular mortality and morbidity is generally correlated with the duration of anesthesia, but this is principally because the longest operations are more often on the aorta or in the abdomen or chest than on the extremities. The risk of major cardiovascular complications does not appear to correlate with the duration of surgery after controlling for the type of surgery, unless the operation is prolonged because of intraoperative complications.

EMERGENCY OPERATION. When an operation is carried out under emergency conditions, it is associated with greatly increased mortality in patients with cardiovascular disease. The risk of postoperative cardiac complications, including postoperative myocardial infarction or cardiac death, is increased anywhere from 2.5- to 4-fold in emergency compared with elective surgery.[13, 25, 29, 30] Part of this increased risk is because patients undergoing emergency operations may often have poorly controlled or unappreciated general medical problems, such as fluid and electrolyte imbalance or hepatic dysfunction.[13, 25] However, emergency surgery appears to be an important correlate of postoperative complications, even after controlling for the underlying medical disease.[25, 29, 30]

ESTIMATION OF RISK. A few patients have such compelling reasons for operation (e.g., leaking abdominal aortic aneurysm or perforated viscus) that estimation of operative risk is an academic exercise, because failure to operate almost certainly will result in the patient's death. The timing or even the performance of an operation is often elective, however, and under these circumstances estimation of operative risk is an important aspect of the medical consultant's role.

One convenient method to estimate surgical risk is to use multifactorial indices. The original index of Goldman and colleagues[29] and its modification[31] weighted several clinical factors based on their relative significance as predictors of adverse cardiac outcomes (Table 61-2). Both indices have been validated in prospective series of general surgical patients[25] and in other studies.[32-35] Because these indices were developed on general surgical patients, they tend to underestimate risk in patients undergoing vascular surgery and in patients with stable coronary artery disease.[36] Moreover, these indices were based on data from the 1970s and early 1980s; most patients undergoing surgery in 1999 had a low risk score, thus limiting the indices' ability to discriminate among patients.[31, 32]

A revised cardiac risk index has been developed using data from the 1990s.[37] In this study, Lee and colleagues identified six independent and relatively equally important predictors of postoperative adverse cardiac outcomes (see Table 61-2). In this simple index, the number of predictors correlated with the risk of cardiac morbidity and mortality. When compared with the older indices and with the American Society of Anesthesiologists (ASA) class, the revised index was found to be superior.[37] Moreover, the revised index appears to predict risk accurately in vascular surgery,

▼ TABLE 61-1. RISK OF MYOCARDIAL INFARCTION OR CARDIAC DEATH FOR NONCARDIAC PROCEDURES*

High risk (often >5%)	Aortic surgery
	Peripheral vascular surgery
	Emergent major operations, particularly in the elderly
	Anticipated prolonged surgical procedures associated with larger fluid shifts or blood loss
Intermediate risk (1–5%)	Intrathoracic and intraperitoneal surgery
	Carotid endarterectomy
	Head and neck surgery
	Orthopedic surgery
	Open prostate surgery
Low risk (generally <1%)	Endoscopic procedures
	Cataract surgery
	Superficial procedures and biopsies
	Transurethral prostate surgery

*Adapted from ACC/AHA Task Force Report: Guidelines for perioperative cardiovascular evaluation for noncardiac surgery. J Am Coll Cardiol 93:1278, 1996.

with the exception of abdominal aortic aneurysm surgery. The optimal use of cardiac risk indices may be to modify a baseline risk such as that shown in Table 61-1 rather than to predict an absolute risk of complications.[38, 39] Furthermore, indices should generally serve as an adjunct to a thorough evaluation of specific cardiac conditions.

INFLUENCE OF SPECIFIC CARDIOVASCULAR DISORDERS

Ischemic Heart Disease

Assessment of Risk

CLINICAL. Ischemic heart disease is a major determinant of perioperative morbidity and mortality. The incidence of perioperative myocardial infarction is increased 5- to 50-fold in patients who have previously suffered infarcts compared with patients who do not have a clinical history of coronary disease.

During the 1970s, several studies reported about a 30 percent risk of reinfarction or cardiac death when patients were operated on within 3 months of the previous myocardial infarction, about a 15 percent risk when the operation was performed 3 to 6 months after a prior infarction, and about a 5 percent risk when the operation was performed more than 6 months after the infarction.[13] Complication rates were subsequently reduced during the 1980s.[36, 40, 41] For example, Rao and colleagues[40] reported only a 6 percent reinfarction rate within 3 months after preoperative myocardial infarction and only a 2 percent reinfarction rate between 3 and 6 months after a myocardial infarction, and they then confirmed these low risks in a subsequent report.[41] The reduction in cardiac morbidity and mortality has been attributed to the use of perioperative monitoring and careful regulation of hemodynamic status, cardiac rhythm, oxygenation, electrolytes, and hematocrit.

Obviously, truly life-saving procedures must be performed almost regardless of the cardiac risk, and purely elective surgery should commonly be delayed for 6 months after infarction, when the cardiovascular risks will have returned to a stable, long-term baseline risk. The more difficult issue is in patients in whom the operation is not truly emergent but is also not purely elective—for example, a patient with severe symptomatic peripheral vascular dis-

RISK FACTOR	POINTS	INTERPRETATION
Goldman et al*		
Age >70 yr	5	
MI in previous 6 mo	10	Class I 0–5 points } low risk
S$_3$ gallop or jugular venous distention	11	
Important aortic stenosis	3	Class II 6–12 points } intermediate risk
Rhythm other than sinus or PACs on last preoperative ECG	7	
>5 PVCs/min documented at any time before operation	7	Class III 13–25 points } high risk
		Class IV >26 points
PO$_2$ <60 or PCO$_2$ >50 mm Hg; K < 3.0 or HCO$_3$ <20 mEq/L; BUN >50 or Cr >3.0 mg/dl; abnormal AST, signs of chronic liver disease, or bedridden from noncardiac causes	3	
Intraperitoneal, intrathoracic, or aortic operation	3	
Emergency operation	4	
Detsky et al†		
MI in previous 6 mo	10	
MI >6 mo previously	5	
Canadian Cardiovascular Society Angina		
Class III	10	
Class IV	20	
Unstable angina in previous 6 mo	10	<15 points = low risk
Alveolar pulmonary edema		
Within 1 wk	10	
Ever	5	>15 points = high risk
Suspected critical aortic stenosis	20	
Rhythm other than sinus or sinus plus PACs on last preoperative ECG	5	
>5 PVCs/min at any time before surgery	5	
Poor general medical status	5	
Age >70 yr	5	
Emergency operation	10	
Lee et al‡		
Intrathoracic, intraperitoneal, or infrainguinal vascular surgery	1	
History of ischemic heart disease	1	0–1 point = low risk
History of congestive heart failure	1	2 points = intermediate risk
Insulin treatment for diabetes mellitus	1	3 or more points = high risk
Serum creatinine level >2.0 mg/dl	1	
History of cerebrovascular disease	1	

PAC = premature atrial complexes; ECG = electrocardiogram; PVC = premature ventricular complexes; BUN = blood urea nitrogen; Cr = creatinine; AST = aspartate aminotransferase; K = potassium; HCO$_3$ = bicarbonate.

* Adapted from Goldman L, Caldera DL, Nussbaum SR, et al: Multifactorial index of cardiac risk in noncardiac surgical procedures. N Engl J Med 297: 845, 1977.

† Adapted from Detsky AS, Abrams HB, McLaughlin JR, et al: Predicting cardiac complications in patients undergoing noncardiac surgery. J Gen Intern Med 1:211, 1986.

‡ Adapted from Lee TH, Marcantonio ER, Mangione CM, et al: Derivation and prospective validation of a simple index for prediction of cardiac risk of major noncardiac surgery. Circulation 100:1043, 1999.

ease or a patient with a potentially resectable malignant tumor. In such situations, one would like to delay operation sufficiently long for cardiac risk to be reduced but not wait a full 6 months. Because full healing of a myocardial infarction usually takes about 4 to 6 weeks, one rational approach is to evaluate the patient with post-myocardial infarction prognostic studies, such as a submaximal exercise tolerance test, and to use the patient's clinical and cardiological conditions as the guide for surgery sometime between 4 weeks and 3 months after the infarction.

A recent preoperative myocardial infarction increases a patient's relative risk of reinfarction with operation, but the absolute risk depends on various factors in addition to the timing of the infarction. Patients who have good exercise tolerance and left ventricular function after infarction and who can resume normal activity levels within 4 to 6 weeks after infarction should be able to undergo operation with relatively small absolute risks, even if their relative risk might be slightly lower if one could wait the full 6 months. By comparison, risks are likely to be substantially higher in patients who have postinfarction angina or who have evidence of ischemia on exercise electrocardiography, thallium scintigraphy, or dobutamine stress echocardiography.

When a patient with angina pectoris is evaluated, the patient's current (preoperative) exercise tolerance should be ascertained and an assessment made about whether the anginal pattern is stable or unstable (see Chap. 36). In patients who can carry objects such as two grocery bags or a young child up a flight of stairs without stopping and without appreciable symptoms, most surgical procedures are generally well tolerated.[42] Physicians should avoid relying on the *frequency* of angina because patients who voluntarily reduce their activity level may also greatly reduce their symptoms. This phenomenon is especially true in patients whose surgical conditions, such as orthopedic disorders or peripheral vascular disease, limit ambulation.

NONINVASIVE TESTING FOR ISCHEMIA. *Exercise treadmill testing* is an objective means for assessing exercise tolerance and is especially beneficial if the history is unreliable. Unfortunately, the limited sensitivity and specificity of standard electrocardiographic exercise tolerance testing limit the use of this test for diagnosing coronary artery disease (see Chap. 6). In studies of patients undergoing vascular surgery, postoperative cardiac complications were significantly less common in patients who exercised to higher heart rates and cardiac workloads.[27] The prognostic value of limited exercise tolerance has also been reported in persons older than 65[35, 43] in whom the inability to perform 2 minutes of bicycle exercise in a supine position and to raise the heart rate above 99 beats/min was an independent important predictor of cardiac complications in noncardiac surgery. Of note was that poor exercise capacity was an independent predictor of cardiac complications but that electrocardiographic changes with exercise were not.

In patients who are unable to exercise because of noncardiac disability (e.g., intermittent claudication or orthopedic abnormalities), dipyridamole thallium imaging, ambulatory ischemia monitoring, or stress echocardiography can be used to assess perioperative risk. Dipyridamole thallium imaging (see Chap. 9) has been successful in identifying high-risk patients among selected subgroups of patients who are referred for the test before undergoing vascular surgery, and it is especially appealing for patients who have abnormal resting electrocardiograms or are taking medications such as digoxin that make electrocardiographic monitoring unreliable for the detection of ischemia.

Among 1410 patients in the five largest series of such patients,[44–48] a reversible defect on thallium scintigraphy had a sensitivity of 85 percent for predicting postoperative cardiac complications and a specificity of 60 percent; the relative risk of cardiac complications in a patient with a reversible defect was 9.0. When dipyridamole thallium scintigraphy was used in *unselected* consecutive patients having abdominal aneurysm or major vascular surgery, it was *not* proved useful for predicting perioperative myocardial infarction, myocardial ischemia, or cardiac death.[49, 50] In the largest single series of 451 *consecutive* unselected patients, the presence of a reversible thallium defect had a sensitivity of just 36 percent, a specificity of 65 percent, and a relative risk of 1.0 (i.e., it was of no value whatsoever) for predicting major perioperative cardiac events.

Ambulatory electrocardiographic (Holter) recording can identify up to 90 percent of patients who will develop major postoperative ischemic complications.[51] Patients with asymptomatic preoperative ischemia or asymptomatic postoperative ischemia have as high as a 30 percent risk of developing a clinical event, including myocardial infarction, unstable angina, ischemic pulmonary edema, or cardiac death.[20, 51, 52] In contrast, asymptomatic intraoperative ischemia is less predictive.[20, 53] Asymptomatic postoperative ischemia, which is found in a substantial minority of patients with or at risk for atherosclerotic disease,[54, 55] commonly precedes a clinical event by an hour or more[52, 56]; longer episodes of postoperative ischemia are associated with a higher risk of a major clinical event.[56] Patients with perioperative ischemia also have more late cardiac events well after surgery.[53, 57] The requirement for a near-normal resting electrocardiogram and a 24-hour testing period generally makes this test less practical than either dipyridamole thallium scintigraphy or stress echocardiography.

Although some investigators have used radionuclide ventriculography to predict risk,[58] in other studies data from resting and/or exercise radionuclide ventriculography did not add important independent information for predicting overall perioperative cardiac risk.[35, 49, 59, 60] Similarly, routine transthoracic echocardiography adds little for the prediction of postoperative complications.[61]

Stress echocardiography after exercise or agents such as dipyridamole or dobutamine can be used to identify patients at markedly increased risk on the basis of the provocation of left ventricular wall motion abnormalities with stress.[62–69] Poldermans and colleagues studied 300 consecutive unselected patients undergoing major vascular surgery with dobutamine stress echocardiography. Of 72 patients with a stress-induced new regional wall motion abnormality, 17 suffered a perioperative myocardial infarction or cardiac death. None of the 228 patients without a stress-induced wall motion abnormality suffered a cardiac complication.[65] Stress echocardiography appears to be at least as good as dipyridamole thallium scintigraphy or ambulatory ischemia monitoring for predicting complications.

Many studies have evaluated the extent to which specific clinical variables can be used to select patients for preoperative noninvasive ischemia testing. In patients undergoing vascular surgery, Eagle and colleagues found that age greater than 70 years, a history of ventricular arrythmias requiring treatment, angina, diabetes mellitus, and abnormal Q waves on the electrocardiogram were independent predictors of cardiac complications.[44] Patients with none of these variables were at low risk for complications, and those with three or more were at high risk regardless of the results of dipyridamole thallium scintigraphy. In the group with one or two of these variables, dipyridamole thallium scintigraphy accurately identified patients as either high or low risk. In a similar study, L'Italien and colleagues added a history of congestive heart failure as an independent predictor of adverse cardiac outcomes and found coronary revascularization within 5 years to have a protective effect.[70] Thallium scintigraphy added useful predictive information only to the group of patients found to be at intermediate risk on the basis of assessment using clinical variables.

Fewer data are available on dobutamine stress echocardiography. However, in patients with low-risk clinical variables, it appears that dobutamine echocardiography does not add appreciably to the clinical risk assessment. Unlike thallium scintigraphy, however, a normal dobutamine stress echocardiogram result in a patient with high-risk clinical variables may predict a low risk of perioperative complications.[65] Hypotension during dobutamine echocardiography predicts perioperative cardiac events.[65a] In conclusion, most data support the use of noninvasive ischemia testing in preoperative evaluation of patients found to be at intermediate risk on clinical assessment.

PRIOR CORONARY REVASCULARIZATION. Patients who have undergone successful coronary revascularization can undergo major noncardiac surgical procedures with a low mortality rate,[71] except perhaps in the first 30 days postoperatively.[71a] An analysis of patients in the Coronary Artery Surgery Study registry[71] showed that total operative mortality was 2.4 percent in 458 patients who had significant coronary artery disease and underwent noncardiac operations without prior coronary artery bypass grafting (CABG). By comparison, operative mortality was 0.9 percent among 399 patients who had had a CABG procedure performed before noncardiac surgery. The mortality was higher in patients who had more severe left ventricular dysfunction or dyspnea on exertion and in patients who used nitrates, were older, and had diabetes. The risk of myocardial infarction, however, was not significantly different between the patients with and without preoperative CABG, and the cardiac death rates were only 0.4 percent and 1.3 percent, respectively, in the two groups. Subsequent studies have confirmed that prior CABG, particularly if within 5 years of subsequent noncardiac surgery, is associated with a decreased risk of perioperative cardiac death.[70]

Fewer data are available to evaluate the effects of preoperative percutaneous transluminal coronary angioplasty (PTCA). In three different series of high-risk patients who underwent PTCA before vascular surgery, the mortality with noncardiac surgery was less than 3 percent.[72–74]

APPROACH TO RISK ASSESSMENT. A practical approach to patients with known ischemic heart disease or with specified high-risk characteristics[44] should use information from the history as well as diagnostic tests.[38, 39, 75–77] If the history reliably indicates that the patient has Canadian Cardiovascular Society class I or class II angina, the patient is able to raise the double product (the heart rate multiplied by the systolic blood pressure) above the range to be expected with general anesthesia and surgery and hence

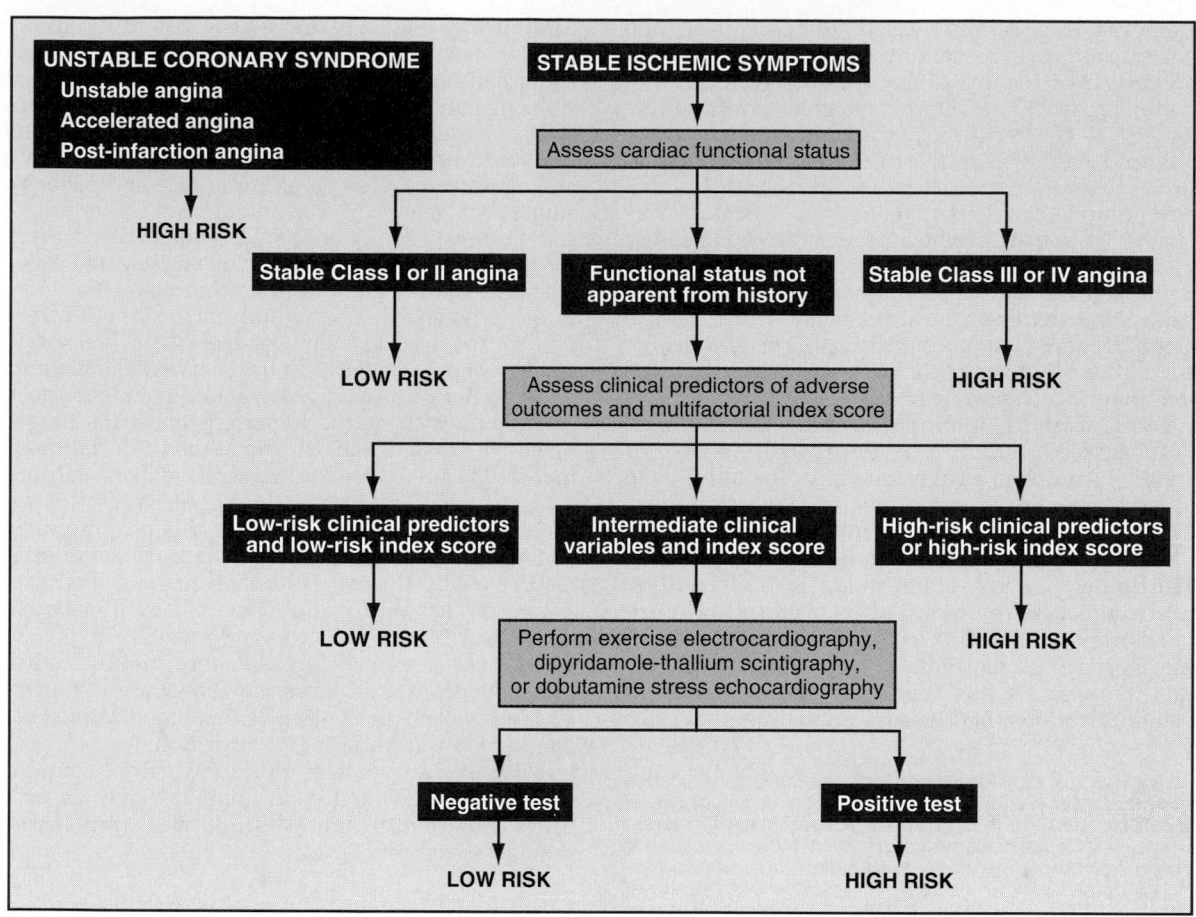

FIGURE 61–1. Risk assessment in patients with ischemic heart disease.

should be able to withstand the stress of the procedure.[71] If the history is unreliable, exercise testing to assess physical function[35, 44] will aid in risk assessment. If the patient is unable to exercise because of noncardiac conditions, dipyridamole thallium imaging or stress echocardiography should be considered, particularly for patients believed to be at intermediate risk on clinical assessment. An approach to risk assessment in patients with ischemic heart disease is shown in Figure 61–1.

Patients who have angina or who have had a myocardial infarction but who can exercise to class I or II level or have normal dipyridamole thallium imaging or stress echocardiography results can undergo most operations with acceptable risk, roughly a 4 to 5 percent risk of myocardial infarction and a 1 percent mortality. Patients who cannot perform class I or II activities or who have positive dipyridamole thallium or stress echocardiography results are likely to have a 5 to 25 percent risk of myocardial infarction and a 5 to 25 percent mortality. For any patient with an appropriate indication for noninvasive ischemia testing or coronary angiography independent of planned noncardiac surgery, such testing should generally precede surgery, particularly if the results may lead to a coronary revascularization procedure.

RISK REDUCTION STRATEGIES. Medications. All baseline preoperative cardiac medications should be continued up to and including the day of surgery and resumed promptly once the patient is eating. In three small studies, the institution of prophylactic beta-blocking agents immediately before surgery was associated with decreased intraoperative ischemia and, in one of these studies, a decreased risk of postoperative myocardial infarction.[78–80] A randomized controlled trial of prophylactic atenolol in patients with known coronary artery disease or at high risk for it demonstrated a significant reduction in both 6-month and

12-month mortality but no reduction in perioperative mortality or cardiac morbidity.[81] In a more recent study of prophylactic beta-adrenergic blockade, 112 high-risk patients were randomized to either preoperative bisoprolol or placebo before undergoing major vascular surgery. Oral bisoprolol, at a dose of 5 mg or 10 mg daily, was begun at least 7 days before surgery and continued until the 30th postoperative day. The combined incidence of perioperative cardiac death or nonfatal myocardial infarction was 34 percent in the placebo group compared with 3.4 percent in the bisoprolol group.[82] This difference was highly statistically significant. There is now sufficient evidence to recommend the routine use of prophylactic bisoprolol or atenolol in high-risk patients who are undergoing major surgery and are not already taking beta-blocking agents.[82a]

Nitrates have been shown in multiple studies to reduce intraoperative ischemia but have never demonstrated a reduction in adverse cardiac outcomes.[83] Prophylactic nitrates, most commonly intravenous nitroglycerin, should therefore be considered only for high-risk patients. Few data are available on the use of prophylactic calcium channel blocking agents during the perioperative period; thus, no firm recommendations can be made.

The alpha-adrenergic blockers may also be useful to reduce perioperative risk. Clonidine has been shown to reduce perioperative ischemia but has not demonstrated a reduction in cardiac morbidity.[84, 85] A newer agent, mivazerol, also appears to reduce ischemia and in a single study was associated with a decreased risk of myocardial infarction in patients undergoing vascular surgery.[86, 87] At the present time, however, beta-blocking agents are the preferred method to reduce risk in patients with ischemic heart disease.

Preoperative Cardiac Optimization. In patients found to be at high risk because of poor cardiac functional status or a positive result of a noninvasive ischemia test, one approach is to optimize the cardiac medications and then reevaluate cardiac status in a few weeks. Although not proved in clinical trials, an improvement in cardiac functional status or in the results of ischemia testing may be associated with a reduction in the risk of cardiac complications.

Intensive preoperative hemodynamic optimization has been advocated by some to reduce perioperative morbidity in high-risk patients. Three randomized controlled trials have demonstrated a reduction in perioperative morbidity,[23,88,89] and a fourth shows no difference,[90] with the use of immediate preoperative optimization of hemodynamic parameters. In these studies, patients were admitted to an intensive care setting where a PA catheter was placed. Intravenous fluid infusions, inotropic agents, and afterload-reducing agents were used to achieve goal values for the pulmonary capillary wedge pressure (usually 8 to 15 mm Hg) and oxygen delivery (usually 600 ml/min/m²). Although goal values were achieved for most patients, the reduction in complication risk was independent of achieving the goal values. On the other hand, in other studies, when hemodynamics were optimized in medical and postoperative patients in an intensive care unit, there was no reduction in mortality or morbidity.[91, 92] Preoperative hemodynamic optimization of this type can be considered for high-risk patients undergoing high-risk operations.

CORONARY REVASCULARIZATION. In patients who have an indication for coronary angiography and/or revascularization independent of planned noncardiac surgery, it is advisable to perform the cardiac procedures first. This is particularly important in high-risk patients. The use of prophylactic coronary revascularization, however, is controversial. No randomized controlled trials have evaluated the use of prophylactic coronary revascularization before noncardiac surgery. Two decision analyses attempted to define the precise role of prophylactic revascularization.[93, 94] Both concluded that routine revascularization is not warranted and that the subgroups most likely to benefit remain undefined. Patients found to be at low risk have roughly a 1 percent cardiac mortality with noncardiac surgery.[95] The mortality from CABG or PTCA ranges from 0.5 to 2 percent.[96] Therefore, prophylactic revascularization is not likely to reduce *total* mortality in low-risk patients.

In high-risk patients, prophylactic revascularization may be a reasonable strategy because such patients face a 5 to 25 percent mortality with noncardiac surgery.[44] Furthermore, if one considers potential long-term mortality reduction, prophylactic revascularization seems reasonable in certain groups. For example, high-risk patients undergoing vascular surgery, particularly those with diabetes mellitus, have significantly reduced long-term survival largely because of premature cardiac death and thus may be the most likely to benefit from prophylactic revascularization[97], particularly surgical revascularization.[97a]

The risk of thrombosis is significant in patients soon after percutaneous coronary stent placement, particularly if anticoagulation is stopped too soon. Thus, noncardiac surgery should not immediately follow a stent procedure.

PREOPERATIVE TRANSFUSION. No large randomized clinical trials have determined the optimal hemoglobin level before surgery or the appropriate threshold for transfusion. Most data suggest that perioperative morbidity and mortality increase as the preoperative hemoglobin level decreases.[98, 99] This relationship appears to be more pronounced in patients with cardiovascular disease.[98] At preoperative hemoglobin levels below 9.0 g/dl, the risk of mortality appears to increase sharply. Thus, in patients with cardiac disease, particularly ischemic heart disease, it is reasonable to consider preoperative blood transfusion when the hemoglobin level is less than 9 gm/dl. In general, however, the risks and benefits of transfusion should be individualized on the basis of the patient's comorbidities and the anticipated surgical blood loss. It is important to consider that the combined risk of transmission of human immunodeficiency virus, hepatitis C, or hepatitis B through transfusion of one unit of allogeneic blood is estimated to be 1 in 34,000.[100]

Hypertension (see Chap. 28)

Several studies have documented that patients with hypertension have higher risks of suffering major cardiac complications during or shortly after noncardiac operation than do patients who have always been normotensive. However, most of this increased risk is because of the ischemic heart disease, left ventricular dysfunction, renal failure, or other abnormalities that often occur in patients with hypertension. In patients with mild to moderate hypertension, diastolic pressures less than 110 mm Hg, and systolic blood pressure less than 200 mm Hg, and no evidence of serious end-organ damage, general anesthesia and major noncardiac surgery are generally well tolerated.[15] Hypertensive patients are, however, at higher risk for labile blood pressures and for hypertensive episodes during surgery and especially just after extubation. Thus, it is neither mandatory nor desirable to delay noncardiac operation for the weeks or months that may be required to achieve ideal blood pressure control in stable patients who have mild to moderate hypertension but who have no hypertensive end-organ damage.

Patients with severe hypertension in the immediate preoperative period are at increased risk for perioperative myocardial infarction and congestive heart failure.[15] In such patients, blood pressure should be controlled before surgery. Commonly used agents for this purpose include intravenous sodium nitroprusside and labetalol because they may be easily titrated. Although uncontrolled early studies suggested that the continuation of any hypertensive agents might increase the risk of perioperative hypotension, substantial subsequent data from more careful studies indicate that patients whose hypertension is well controlled do at least as well, if not better, if their medications are, in fact, continued up to the time of operation.[15]

Thiazide and other diuretics cause some degree of chronic volume depletion, and patients receiving these drugs may require more fluid administration early during the operative procedure.

Valvular Heart Disease (see Chap. 46)

Patients who have valvular heart disease and who are undergoing anesthesia and noncardiac operation are subject to many potential hazards: heart failure, infection, tachycardia, and embolization. As might be expected, patients with no or only mild limitation of activity (i.e., those in Class I or II) tolerate operation well and probably require little more than careful perioperative care and prophylaxis for infective endocarditis. Those with more serious impairment of cardiac reserve (i.e., those in Class III or IV) tolerate major noncardiac operations poorly, and their prognosis for surviving major surgery is distinctly worse.[13, 26]

Patients with symptomatic critical aortic stenosis[29] are at increased risk for sudden death or acute pulmonary edema during the perioperative period, if demands on cardiac output are suddenly increased or if atrial fibrillation and a rapid ventricular rate are precipitated by anesthesia or operation.

The risk associated with severe aortic stenosis may be most prominent when the valvular disease is not known to the surgical or anesthesia team before surgery.[101] It is therefore crucial to make the diagnosis of severe aortic stenosis before surgery to allow for appropriate preoperative and intraoperative treatment. In general, patients with symptomatic severe aortic stenosis should undergo corrective valve surgery or, when appropriate, valvuloplasty, before noncardiac surgery.[102, 103] On the other hand, in two series of patients with severe aortic stenosis, defined as an aortic valve area less than 1.0 cm², and normal left ventricular function who underwent major noncardiac surgery, only 2 of 36 patients died during the perioperative period.[101, 104] This suggests that when preoperative correction of the valvular lesion is not feasible, surgery may be performed with an acceptable risk. In such cases, appropriate anesthetic care may involve invasive hemodynamic monitoring and anesthetic agents or techniques that minimize reductions in preload.

In patients with mitral stenosis, control of heart rate and, particularly, avoidance of atrial fibrillation with a rapid ventricular response are important to prevent perioperative congestive heart failure.[27] In patients with severe mitral stenosis, corrective valve surgery or valvuloplasty should precede noncardiac surgery.

Perioperative cardiac morbidity in patients with aortic or mitral regurgitation appears to be largely related to the associated congestive heart failure. Therefore, preoperative control of heart failure is crucial. This should include the use of diuretic agents and afterload-reducing agents.

HYPERTROPHIC CARDIOMYOPATHY (see Chap. 48). Patients with hypertrophic cardiomyopathy are intolerant of hypovolemia, which may lead to both a reduction in the elevated preload necessary to maintain cardiac output and an increase in the obstruction to left ventricular outflow. Similarly, decreases in afterload may also increase dynamic outflow obstruction. With careful perioperative, intraoperative, and postoperative care, however, the risk of major cardiac complications in such patients is small. In the two largest series of noncardiac operations in patients with hypertrophic cardiomyopathy, no deaths and only two myocardial infarctions ensued after a total of 133 operations. Reversible cardiac complications were common, however. Arrhythmias occured in more than 20 percent of patients, congestive heart failure in 16 percent, and hypotension requiring vasopressor therapy in 14 percent.[105, 106] It has previously been suggested that spinal anesthesia may be relatively contraindicated in patients with hypertrophic obstructive cardiomyopathy because of its tendency to reduce systemic vascular resistance and increase venous pooling and thereby increase the severity of obstruction to outflow.[105] However, Haering and colleagues[106] did not find spinal anesthesia to be associated with an increase in cardiac complications. Hemodynamic monitoring is not routinely required but may be helpful when these patients undergo major aortic, abdominal, or thoracic procedures.

PROSTHETIC HEART VALVES. Most patients with mechanical prosthetic heart valves receive anticoagulants on a long-term basis to prevent thromboembolic complications (see Chap. 46). If these medications are continued through the period of noncardiac operation, hematoma formation and persistent postoperative bleeding can ensue. Anticoagulants can be temporarily discontinued during the perioperative period with minimal risk of thrombosis. In one study,[107] no thromboembolic complications occurred in 159 patients who had prosthetic valves and were undergoing 180 noncardiac operations when warfarin was discontinued an average of 2.9 days preoperatively and resumed 2.7 days postoperatively.[107] Using a similar approach, Katholi and associates did not observe thromboembolic complications in 25 noncardiac operations on patients with prosthetic aortic valves[108]; however, two such complications occurred in the 10 patients with mitral valve prostheses when anticoagulants were discontinued for noncardiac operations, although these patients had Kay-Shiley caged-disc valves, which are associated with a somewhat higher risk of thromboembolic complications. Using a decision analytical approach, Kearon and Hirsh concluded that perioperative heparinization with either intravenous standard heparin or subcutaneous low-molecular-weight heparin in patients with mechanical heart valves leads to a substantial increase in major bleeding risk and only a modest reduction in thromboembolic risk.[109] They recommended discontinuation of warfarin 4 days before surgery and resumption as soon as possible after surgery. Because it takes 4 days on average for the International Normalized Ratio (INR) to drop below 1.5 in patients with a baseline INR of 2.0 to 3.0, the number of days with normal anticoagulation is usually only 2 or 3 using this approach.[109] In certain patients, the risk of perioperative thromboembolism may be particularly high, such as in those with a caged-disc valve or those who have had a recent embolic event. In such patients, perioperative heparinization may be justified. Warfarin should be discontinued 4 days before surgery and heparin (intravenous standard heparin or subcutaneous low-molecular-weight heparin) begun once the INR has dropped below 1.5. Heparin is then stopped 6 hours before surgery and resumed at least 12 hours after surgery if considered safe by the surgeon. Analyses indicate that these various anticoagulation regimens are cost-effective, provided that they do not result in lengthening the hospitalization.[110] Even 1 day of additional hospitalization is relatively costly, and the daily risk of thromboembolic complications is low. Thus, perioperative anticoagulation management should focus on regimens that provide reasonable protection from thromboembolic disease but that permit patients to be discharged when the surgical condition itself permits.[110]

Endocarditis Prophylaxis (see Chap. 47)

Numerous surgical procedures are associated with the development of transient bacteremia with organisms that may cause endocarditis.[111] However, the risk of developing endocarditis after surgery is low,[111, 112] and a reduction in risk with the use of prophylactic antibiotics has not been demonstrated in controlled clinical trials. Nevertheless, because the risks associated with prophylactic antibiotics are low and the potential morbidity of endocarditis is high, antibiotic prophylaxis is recommended for patients with moderate- or high-risk structural cardiac lesions undergoing procedures with a high risk of bacteremia.

Congenital Heart Disease (see Chap. 44)

Depending on the nature of the malformation, patients with congenital heart disease may be subject to one or more potentially serious complications, such as infection, bleeding, hypoxemia, hypotension, and paradoxical embolization during general anesthesia and operation. As is the case for patients with valvular heart disease, patients who have congenital heart disease and who are to undergo a surgical procedure require prophylaxis to prevent infective endocarditis.

Patients with cyanotic congenital heart disease tolerate systemic hypotension poorly because this increases the right-to-left shunt and the severity of hypoxemia. In one large series, induction was commonly accomplished using ketamine or fentanyl to avoid hypotension, and anesthesia was maintained with morphine and nitrous oxide or with large doses of fentanyl with or without nitrous oxide. With use of careful anesthetic techniques, the risk of major anesthetic complications is extremely low even in very ill and cyanotic patients.[113] However, spinal anesthesia, which causes peripheral arterial vasodilation and reduces venous return, can have deleterious hemodynamic effects in patients with cyanotic congenital heart disease. Infusion of a vasoconstrictor such as phenylephrine may occasionally be required to raise systemic vascular resistance and thereby decrease the magnitude of the right-to-left shunt. Because patients with right-to-left shunts are subject to the risk of paradoxical emboli, including air emboli, meticulous techniques with regard to intravenous solutions and injections are mandatory to prevent such complications.

Congestive Heart Failure

(see Chaps. 17 and 18)

Congestive heart failure is a major determinant of perioperative risk, irrespective of the nature of the underlying cardiac disorder. Mortality with noncardiac surgery increases with worsening cardiac class[13, 42] and with the presence of pulmonary congestion,[13, 25] especially when a third heart sound is noted.[29] The perioperative mortality rate appears to depend more on a patient's condition at the time of operation than on the most severe depression of cardiovascular status the patient has ever experienced. Patients with well-controlled congestive heart failure have an increased risk of developing postoperative pulmonary edema but little excess mortality.[49] When heart failure is not well controlled, as evidenced by the presence of an S_3 gallop, rales on lung examination, or pulmonary edema on chest radiograph, the risk of death may be as high as 15 percent.[13] It is therefore advisable to control heart failure preoperatively with the use of diuretics and afterload-reducing agents. In such patients, it is important to avoid overdiuresis in the immediate preoperative period because the risk of severe intraoperative hypotension is increased in intravascularly volume-depleted patients. It is therefore desirable, if possible, to stabilize a patient's condition by treating heart failure for approximately 1 week rather than for only 1 or 2 days before the contemplated operation. Perioperative cardiogenic pulmonary edema develops in about 2 percent of patients who are older than 40 years and are undergoing major noncardiac surgery without prior congestive heart failure, in about 6 percent of patients whose heart failure is well controlled, and in about 16 percent of patients whose heart failure persists on physical examination or chest radiograph before surgery.[13]

Digitalis is one of the most common causes of iatrogenic complications in hospitalized patients, and it may be associated with a higher risk of intraoperative bradyarrhythmias.[13] Therefore, preoperative digitalization is *not* recommended except in patients whose congestive heart failure is sufficiently severe that they would normally meet the criteria for long-term digitalization.

Arrhythmias (see Chap. 25)

Arrhythmias may be a manifestation of the severity of underlying left ventricular dysfunction and of coronary artery disease and hence are frequently markers for the likelihood of perioperative cardiac complications. Because patients who have ventricular premature complexes but no evidence of underlying heart disease on detailed examination have an apparently normal cardiac prognosis, ventricular premature complexes in the *absence* of underlying heart disease should not be considered a risk factor for cardiac complications with noncardiac surgery.

Although it would be ideal for arrhythmias to be well controlled preoperatively, the risks associated with arrhythmias appear to be related more to the underlying cardiac disease than to the arrhythmias per se. Furthermore, the frequency of preoperative ventricular premature complexes or nonsustained ventricular tachycardia in patients with known structural heart disease does not appear to correlate with adverse cardiac outcomes.[114] Therefore, no current evidence shows that asymptomatic ventricular premature complexes or episodes of nonsustained ventricular tachycardia require aggressive preoperative control or prophylactic intraoperative suppression. Similarly, in patients with well-controlled atrial fibrillation, cardioversion need not be carried out specifically because of planned noncardiac surgery if such a management option would not otherwise be appropriate. Careful rhythm monitoring during surgery and in the immediate postoperative period would be prudent.

Patients who are most at risk for the development of postoperative supraventricular tachyarrhythmias include elderly patients undergoing pulmonary surgery, patients with subcritical valvular stenoses, and patients with prior histories of supraventricular tachyarrhythmias. Although previous data suggested that digitalis may reduce the risk of development of postoperative supraventricular tachycardia and decrease the ventricular rate when it does occur,[13] the use of prophylactic digitalis has not been formally studied. Given the effectiveness of beta-adrenergic blocking agents, calcium channel antagonists, and adenosine for the treatment of supraventricular arrhythmias, it may be most prudent simply to treat the arrhythmia when it occurs rather than use prophylactic digitalis.

Several studies have shown that pretreatment with amiodarone or sotalol reduces the incidence of postoperative atrial fibrillation after CABG or cardiac valve surgery.[115–118] In a randomized controlled trial of 85 patients, the use of prophylactic sotalol begun 24 to 48 hours before cardiac surgery and continued for 4 days was associated with a 12 percent incidence of postoperative atrial fibrillation, compared with 38 percent in the placebo group.[118] Similarly, intravenous amiodarone administered immediately after cardiac surgery was associated with a 35 percent incidence of atrial fibrillation, compared with 47 percent for placebo.[115] Such results are promising and justify consideration of prophylactic therapy in patients at risk for developing atrial fibrillation after cardiac surgery. It is not known whether prophylactic therapy with amiodarone or sotalol is effective for noncardiac surgery; therefore, it is not currently recommended for routine use.

CONDUCTION DEFECTS. Patients with *complete heart block* must respond to the demands for an increased cardiac output by augmenting stroke volume, but this compensatory response is prevented in many patients by a concurrent impairment of cardiac contractility. In addition, most anesthetic agents depress myocardial contractility and/or produce peripheral vasodilatation. Furthermore, anesthesia can cause further depression of the automaticity, and therefore the ventricular rate, of patients with heart block. Thus, patients with untreated complete heart block may be unable to meet the increased demands placed on the cardiovascular system by anesthesia and operation, and a permanent or temporary pacemaker should be inserted before the use of general anesthesia, even in asymptomatic patients (see Chaps. 24 and 25).

Another problem is presented by patients with *chronic bifascicular block* (see Chap. 25). A significant fraction of patients developing this abnormality in the course of an acute myocardial infarction progress to complete heart block, often accompanied by sudden severe hemodynamic compromise. Progression from bifascicular to complete heart block has not been documented during the perioperative period in patients without a previous history of third-degree heart block. Prophylactic pacemaker placement for such patients or for patients with first-degree atrioventricular (AV) block or type I second-degree AV block (Wenckebach) is not recommended, although a pacemaker should always be available in the operating room for emergency placement.[27] However, in patients who have bifascicular block and type II second-degree AV block and who have a history of unexplained syncope or transient third-degree AV block, the risk of development of complete heart block is much higher, and a temporary pacemaker should be inserted preoperatively.

In general, a prophylactic *temporary pacemaker* should be inserted before noncardiac operations only if the patient meets the indications for permanent pacemaker insertion and the operation should not be delayed for the time required for a permanent pacemaker insertion, or if the operative course is likely to be complicated by transient bacteremia. In such situations, a temporary pacemaker should be placed initially, and the permanent pacemaker can be inserted after the operation.

PATIENTS WITH A PERMANENT PACEMAKER OR DEFIBRILLATOR (see Chap. 24). When a patient with a permanent pacemaker or defibrillator in situ is about to undergo operation, the device should be carefully evaluated to ensure that it is functioning properly preoperatively. Demand pacemakers and defibrillators are sensitive to electromagnetic interference, such as that produced by the electrocautery, which may result in failure to pace or provoke defibrillator discharge. The danger of this potentially hazardous interaction can be reduced by placing the indifferent plate of the cautery unit as far as possible from the lead and pacemaker pulse generator, and the electrocautery should be used in brief bursts rather than continuously. Also, a magnet should be available in the operating room to convert the pacemaker from the demand to the fixed-rate mode. Defibrillators should have sensing inactivated preoperatively to prevent the device from sensing electrocautery as ventricular fibrillation and delivering a shock. Because the cautery may also interfere with the electrocardiographic monitor and render results temporarily uninterpretable, arterial pressure should be monitored directly when the cautery is being used.

GENERAL MEDICAL PROBLEMS. Patients with heart disease and with a general medical status complicated by diabetes, renal insufficiency, hepatic abnormalities, hypoxemia, or electrolyte abnormalities have a higher risk of cardiac complications, presumably because these nonmedical conditions exacerbate the stress placed on the heart by the operation.[13, 25, 29] Morbidity is also higher in markedly obese patients[118a] because obesity is often associated with abnormal cardiorespiratory function, metabolic function, and hemostasis. Every effort should be made to correct any of these noncardiac problems before operation, and the potential long-term benefits of surgery must also be interpreted in light of the patient's general prognosis.

POSTOPERATIVE COMPLICATIONS

MYOCARDIAL INFARCTION. Transient intraoperative ischemia does not appear to be a major correlate of postoperative ischemic events in patients undergoing noncardiac surgery,[20, 53] but most clinical postoperative ischemic events are preceded by asymptomatic episodes of postoperative ischemia that can be detected by ambulatory ischemic monitoring.[20, 52–54, 56] Although series from before 1980 showed a peak in the risk of myocardial infarction on about the third postoperative day, more recent series show that a combination of frequent electrocardiograms and cardiac enzymes detects many non-Q-wave infarctions in the first 24 hours postoperatively.[34, 51, 119–121] Although care must be taken in interpreting cardiac enzymes in the perioperative period,[120] it may be that supply-demand imbalances cause an early peak in non-Q-wave postoperative infarctions, whereas the hypercoagulable postoperative state leads to a later (3 to 5 days postoperatively) peak in Q wave infarctions. For both types of infarction, postoperative stresses include general surgical complications, hypoxia and other pulmonary complications, fluid and electrolyte abnormalities, and the stresses of modern postoperative ambulation protocols. Substantial data indicate that prophylactic anticoagulation with low-dose heparin reduces the risk of postoperative venous thromboembolic complications,[122] and such therapy is routinely indicated in most cardiac patients who undergo noncardiac operations. In fact, such anticoagulation regimens may permit a more gradual postoperative ambulation protocol in cardiac patients and hence possibly lower the incidence of postoperative myocardial infarction.

The diagnosis of postoperative myocardial infarction can be difficult. Roughly 50 percent of patients who have postoperative myocardial infarctions are pain free.[13, 95] Other signs such as hypotension, hypertension, arrhythmias, or altered mental status may often be the only clue to the presence of myocardial ischemia or infarction. In patients with signs or symptoms of myocardial ischemia or infarction, measurement of serum cardiac enzyme levels may be helpful. Elevated troponin I levels (>1.0 ng/ml) may be somewhat more specific for myocardial ischemia or infarctions than are elevations in CK-MB isoenzymes.[121, 123]

HYPERTENSION. Postoperative hypertension is most likely to occur soon after the cessation of positive-pressure ventilation or in the recovery room, and it is more common after carotid endarterectomy and major abdominal vascular procedures.[15]

Common precipitants include fluid overload after cessation of positive-pressure ventilation, hypoxemia, anxiety, and pain. The principal therapeutic approaches should therefore concentrate on ensuring adequate oxygenation, pain control, and fluid control. In general, supplemental oxygen, morphine, and diuretics are the mainstays of the treatment of postoperative hypertension. Nitroprusside and labetalol (see Chap. 29) are the preferred medications for more severe hypertension. Intravenous hydralazine in small doses is effective for treating postoperative hypertension, but it has the potential of precipitating supraventricular tachyarrhythmias.

CONGESTIVE HEART FAILURE. Although postoperative heart failure can be precipitated by myocardial infarction or ischemia, a substantial proportion of the cases are directly caused by excess fluid administration. Heart failure tends to occur soon after cessation of positive-pressure ventilation and again at about 24 to 48 hours after operation, when the fluid that was given in the perioperative period is mobi-

lized from the extravascular sites. Diuretics, often given intravenously and occasionally supplemented with afterload-reducing agents, are usually sufficient therapy for postoperative congestive heart failure.

POSTOPERATIVE ARRHYTHMIAS. Arrhythmias are common after operation and are often a manifestation of a noncardiac complication, such as bleeding, infection, or an acid-base or electrolyte imbalance occurring in a patient with heart disease. Management of such arrhythmias often requires recognition and correction of extracardiac factors.

A new postoperative supraventricular tachyarrhythmia should prompt a search for remediable medical problems. Direct antiarrhythmic therapy is often unnecessary and is usually secondary in importance to correction of the underlying cause of the arrhythmia.

Sinus tachycardia is the most common rhythm disturbance in postoperative patients. Many noncardiac etiological factors have been identified, including pain, hypovolemia, hypervolemia, fever, anemia, hypoxemia, pulmonary emboli, anxiety, infection, hypotension, and electrolyte abnormalities (especially hypokalemia). These noncardiac factors are much more common causes of sinus tachycardia in postoperative cardiac patients than is either myocardial infarction or heart failure. Sinus tachycardia not caused by congestive heart failure does not slow with cardiac glycosides.

Atrial fibrillation is also a common postoperative arrhythmia. Atrial dilatation, which lowers the threshold for development of this arrhythmia, can result from heart failure, mitral valve disease, and/or hypervolemia. Noncardiac precipitants include pneumonia, atelectasis, and pulmonary emboli. Initially, postoperative patients with atrial fibrillation should be treated with a beta-blocking agent, calcium channel antagonist, or digitalis. Cardioversion is usually delayed until the precipitating factors have been eliminated, because patients who undergo cardioversion before clearing of the atelectasis or pneumonia frequently have reversion to atrial fibrillation, whereas patients whose pulmonary problem or congestive heart failure is adequately treated often have spontaneous reversion to sinus rhythm.

In the case of coronary artery or cardiac valve surgery, postoperative atrial fibrillation is very common, occurring in up to 40 percent of patients,[124] and is associated with thromboembolic complications and prolonged hospital stays. Unlike the noncardiac surgery setting, most cases of postoperative atrial fibrillation do not appear to be associated with reversible noncardiac conditions. Therefore, early cardioversion can be beneficial. In one study, intravenous ibutilide was shown to be effective and safe for the treatment of postoperative atrial fibrillation following cardiac surgery.[125] It is not known whether ibutilide is as useful in the noncardiac surgery setting; however, these data suggest that when urgent cardioversion is indicated after noncardiac surgery, ibutilide should be considered.

Atrial flutter is often poorly tolerated because of the rapid ventricular rate and the difficult pharmacological management. Cardioversion is the treatment of choice.

IMPLICATIONS OF POSTOPERATIVE COMPLICATIONS FOR LONG-TERM MANAGEMENT. When a patient develops a perioperative myocardial infarction, the evaluation and the recuperative process generally should be analogous to when a myocardial infarction occurs in other patients (see Chap. 35). Because postoperative congestive heart failure is commonly precipitated by iatrogenic fluid overload, the patient commonly does not need long-term therapy for congestive heart failure. Similarly, perioperative arrhythmias are often precipitated by specific stimuli, and patients with a postoperative arrhythmia should not automatically be consigned to long-term antiarrhythmic therapy. In patients who develop either postoperative congestive heart failure or arrhythmias, it is often appropriate to discontinue new cardiac therapies several days before discharge and to observe patients to see whether long-term therapy is indicated.

THE ROLE OF THE MEDICAL CONSULTANT

The physician called on to evaluate the status of a patient with suspected or overt cardiac disease before elective or emergency noncardiac surgery first must determine whether cardiovascular disease is present and, if it is, must identify those factors that can increase the risk of operation. It may be necessary to invest considerable time and effort to prepare patients for operation. In addition, patients must be carefully monitored after operation to detect and manage the cardiac problems that frequently complicate the postoperative period.

PREPARATION OF PATIENTS FOR ANESTHESIA AND OPERATION. Careful preparation of cardiac patients for operation may diminish the frequency and seriousness of intraoperative and postoperative complications. The medical consultant should, after appropriate discussion with the surgeon, be prepared to urge postponement or cancellation of an elective operation or to insist on sufficient time to institute any measures that are necessary to minimize risk. The consultant should attempt to be brief and to the point and to provide a limited number of explicit, relevant suggestions. The cardiological consultant should work closely with the anesthesiologist and the surgeon so that their talents may be combined to maximize the likelihood of a favorable outcome.

REFERENCES

ANESTHESIA

1. Breslow MJ, Miller CF, Rogers M (eds): Perioperative Management. St. Louis, CV Mosby, 1990.
2. Mangano DT (ed): Perioperative Cardiac Assessment. Philadelphia, JB Lippincott, 1990.
3. Longnecker DE, Tinker JH, Morgan GE (eds): Principles and Practice of of Anesthesiology, 2nd ed. St. Louis, Mosby-Year Book, 1998.
4. Fleisher LA: Anesthetic management and perioperative surveillance. Prog Cardiovasc Dis 40:441, 1998.
5. Slogoff S, Keats AS, Dear WE. et al: Steal-prone coronary anatomy and myocardial ischemia associated with four primary anesthetic agents in humans. Anesth Analg 72:23, 1991.
6. Slogoff S, Keats AS: Randomized trial of primary anesthetic agents on outcome of coronary artery bypass operations. Anesthesiology 70:179, 1989.
7. Forrest JB, Cahalan MK, Redher K, et al: Multicenter study of general anesthesia. II. Results. Anesthesiology 72:262, 1990.
8. Bode RH Jr, Lewis KP, Zarich SW, et al: Cardiac outcome after peripheral vascular surgery: Comparison of general and regional anesthesia. Anesthesiology 84:3, 1996.
9. Cook PT, Davies MJ, Cronin KD, et al: A prospective randomised trial comparing spinal anaesthesia using hyperbaric cinchocaine with general anaesthesia for lower limb vascularity surgery. Anaesth Intens Care 14:373, 1986.
10. Christopherson R, Beattie C, Frank SM, et al: Perioperative morbidity in patients randomized to epidural or general anesthesia for lower extremity vascular surgery. Perioperative Ischemia Randomized Trial Study Group. Anesthesiology 79:422, 1993.
11. Damask MC, Weissman C, Todd G: General versus epidural anesthesia for femoral-popliteal bypass surgery. J Clin Anesth 2:71, 1990.
12. Go AS, Browner WS: Cardiac outcomes after regional or general anesthesia, do we have the answer. Anesthesiology 84:1, 1996.
13. Goldman L, Caldera DL, Southwick FS, et al: Cardiac risk factors and complications in non-cardiac surgery. Medicine 57:357, 1978.
14. Charlson ME, MacKenzie CR, Gold JP, et al: The preoperative and intraoperative hemodynamic predictors of postoperative myocardial infarction or ischemia in patients undergoing noncardiac surgery. Ann Surg 210:637, 1989.
15. Goldman L, Caldera DL: Risks of general anesthesia and elective surgery in the hypertensive patient. Anesthesiology 50:285, 1979.
16. Ellis J, Drijvers G, Pedlow S, et al: Premedication with oral and transdermal clonidine provides safe and efficacious postoperative sympatholysis. Anesth Analg 79:1133, 1994.
17. Frank SM, Beattie C, Christopherson R, et al: Unintentional hypothermia is associated with postoperative myocardial ischemia. Anesthesiology 78:468, 1993.

18. Frank SM, Fleisher LA, Breslow MJ, et al: Perioperative maintenance of normothermia reduces the incidence of morbid cardiac events. JAMA 277:1127, 1997.
19. Eisenberg MJ, London MJ, Leung JM, et al: Monitoring for myocardial ischemia during noncardiac surgery. A technology assessment of transesophageal echocardiography and 12-lead electrocardiography. JAMA 268:210, 1992.
20. Mangano DT, Browner WS, Hollenberg M, et al: Association of perioperative myocardial ischemia with cardiac morbidity and mortality in men undergoing noncardiac surgery. N Engl J Med 323:1781, 1990.
21. Isaacson IJ, Lowdon JD, Berry AJ, et al: The value of pulmonary artery and central venous monitoring in patients undergoing abdominal aortic reconstructive surgery: A comparative study of two selected, randomized groups. J Vasc Surg 12:754, 1990.
22. Joyce WP, Provan JL, Amelis FM, et al: The role of haemodynamic monitoring in abdominal aortic surgery: A prospective randomized study. Eur J Vasc Surg 4:633, 1990.
23. Berlauk JF, Abrams JH, Gilmour IJ, et al: Preoperative optimization of cardiovascular hemodynamics improves outcome in peripheral vascular surgery. A prospective, randomized clinical trial. Ann Surg 214:289, 1991.
24. American Society of Anesthesiologists Task Force on Pulmonary Artery Catheterization: Practice guidelines for pulmonary artery catheterization. Anesthesiology 78:380, 1993.
25. Larsen SF, Olesen KH, Jacobsen E, et al: Prediction of cardiac risk in non-cardiac surgery. Eur Heart J 8:179, 1987.
26. Forrest JB, Rehder K, Cahalan MK, Goldsmith CH: Multicenter study of general anesthesia. III. Predictors of severe perioperative adverse outcomes. Anesthesiology 76:3, 1992.
27. Eagle KA, Brundage BH, Chaitman BR, et al: Guidelines for perioperative cardiovascular evaluation for noncardiac surgery. A report of the American College of Cardiology/American Heart Association Task Force on Practice Guidelines. Circulation 93:1278, 1996.
28. Lee JG, Krucoff MW, Brazer SR: Periprocedure myocardial ischemia in patients with severe symptomatic coronary artery disease undergoing endoscopy: Prevalence and risk factors. Am J Med 99:270, 1995.
29. Goldman L, Caldera DL, Nussbaum RR, et al: Multifactorial index of cardiac risk in noncardiac surgical procedures. N Engl J Med 297:845, 1977.
30. Shah KB, Kleinman BS, Rao TLK, et al: Angina and other risk factors in patients with cardiac diseases undergoing noncardiac operations. Anesth Analg 70:240, 1990.
31. Detsky AS, Abrams HB, McLaughlin JR, et al: Predicting cardiac complications in patients undergoing non-cardiac surgery. J Gen Intern Med 1:211, 1986.
32. Prause G, Ratzenhofer-Comenda B, Pierer G, et al: Can ASA grade or Goldman's cardiac index predict perioperative mortality? Anaesthesia 52:203, 1997.
33. Prause G, Offner A, Ratzenhofer-Comenda B, et al: Comparison of two preoperative indices to predict perioperative mortality in non-cardiac surgery. Eur J Cardiothorac Surg 11:670, 1996.
34. Charlson ME, MacKenzie CR, Ales KL, et al: Surveillance for postoperative myocardial infarction after noncardiac operations. Surg Gynecol Obstet 167:407, 1988.
35. Gerson MC, Hurst JM, Hertzberg VS, et al: Cardiac prognosis in noncardiac geriatric surgery. Ann Intern Med 103:832, 1985.
36. Jeffrey CC, Kunsman J, Cullen DJ, Brewster DC: A prospective evaluation of cardiac risk index. Anesthesiology 58:462, 1983.
37. Lee TH, Marcantonio ER, Mangione CM, et al: Derivation and prospective validation of a simple index for prediction of cardiac risk of major noncardiac surgery. Circulation 100:1043, 1999.
38. Goldman L: Cardiac risk in noncardiac sursery: An update. Anesth Analg 80:810, 1995.
39. Mangano DT, Goldman L: Preoperative assessment of the patient with known or suspected coronary disease. N Engl J Med 333:1750, 1995.

INFLUENCE OF SPECIFIC CARDIOVASCULAR DISORDERS

40. Rao TLK, Jacobs KH, El-Etr AA: Reinfarction following anesthesia in patients with myocardial infarction. Anesthesiology 59:499, 1983.
41. Shah KB, Kleinman BS, Sami H, et al: Reevaluation of perioperative myocardial infarction in patients undergoing noncardiac operations. Anesth Analg 71:231, 1990.
42. McPhail N, Menkis A, Shariatmadar A, et al: Statistical prediction of cardiac risk in patients who undergo vascular surgery. Can J Surg 28:404, 1985.
43. Gerson MC, Hurst JM, Hertzberg VS, et al: Prediction of cardiac and pulmonary complications related to elective abdominal and noncardiac thoracic surgery in geriatric patients. Am J Med 88:101, 1990.
44. Eagle KA, Coley CM, Newell JB, et al: Combining clinical and thallium data optimizes preoperative assessment of cardiac risk before major vascular surgery. Ann Intern Med 110:859, 1989.
45. Brown KA, Rowen M: Extent of jeopardized viable myocardium determined by myocardial perfusion imaging best predicts perioperative cardiac events in patients undergoing noncardiac surgery. J Am Coll Cardiol 21:325, 1993.
46. Hendel RC, Whitfield SS, Villegas BJ, et al: Prediction of late cardiac events by dipyridamole thallium imaging in patients undergoing elective vascular surgery. Am J Cardiol 70:1243, 1992.

47. Lette J, Waters D, Cerino M, et al: Preoperative coronary artery disease risk stratification based on dipyridamole imaging and a simple three-step, three-segment model for patients undergoing noncardiac vascular surgery or major general surgery. Am J Cardiol 69:1553, 1992.

48. Bry JDL, Belkin M, O'Donnell TF Jr, et al: An assessment of the positive predictive value and cost-effectiveness of dipyridamole myocardial scintigraphy in patients undergoing vascular surgery. J Vasc Surg 19:112, 1994.

49. Baron JF, Mundler O, Bertrand M, et al: Dipyridamole-thallium scintigraphy and gated radionuclide angiography to assess cardiac risk before abdominal aortic surgery. N Engl J Med 330:663, 1994.

50. Mangano DT, London MJ, Tubau JF, et al: Dipyridamole thalium-201 scintigraphy as a preoperative screening test. A re-examination of its predictive potential. Circulation 84:493, 1991.

51. Raby KE, Goldman L, Creager MA, et al: Correlation between preoperative ischemia and major cardiac events after peripheral vascular surgery. N Engl J Med 321:1296, 1989.

52. Pasternack PF, Grossi EA, Baumann FG, et al: Silent myocardial ischemia monitoring predicts late as well as perioperative cardiac events in patients undergoing vascular surgery. J Vasc Surg 15:171, 1992.

53. Raby KE, Barry J, Creager MA, et al: Detection and significance of intraoperative and postoperative myocardial ischemia in peripheral vascular surgery. JAMA 268:222, 1992.

54. Mangano DT, Hollenberg M, Fegert G, et al: Perioperative myocardial ischemia in patients undergoing noncardiac surgery—I. Incidence and severity during the 4 day perioperative period. J Am Coll Cardiol 17:843, 1991.

55. Mangano DT, Wong MG, London MJ, et al: Perioperative myocardial ischemia in patients undergoing noncadiac surgery—II. Incidence and severity during the first week after surgery. J Am Coll Cardiol 17:851, 1991.

56. Landesberg G, Luria MH, Cotev S, et al: Importance of long-duration postoperative ST-segment depression in cardiac morbidity after vascular surgery. Lancet 341:715, 1993.

57. Mangano DT, Browner WS, Hollenberg M, et al, for the *McSPI* Research Group: Long-term cardiac prognosis following noncardiac surgery. JAMA 268:233, 1992.

58. Pasternack PF, Imparato AM, Riles TS, et al: The value of the radionuclide angiogram in the prediction of perioperative myocardial infarction in patients undergoing lower extremity revascularization procedures. Circulation 72(Suppl 2):13, 1985.

59. Franco CD, Goldsmith J, Veith FJ, et al: Resting gated pool ejection fraction: A poor predictor of perioperative myocardial infarction in patients undergoing vascular surgery for infrainguinal bypass grafting. J Vasc Surg 10:656, 1989.

60. McCann RL, Wolfe WG: Resection of abdominal aortic aneurysm in patients with low ejection fractions. J Vasc Surg 10:240, 1989.

61. Halm EA, Browner WS, Tubau JF, et al, for the *McSPI* Research Group: Echocardiography for preoperative assessment of cardiac risk in noncardiac surgery. J Gen Intern Med 9:31, 1994.

62. Tischler MD, Lee TH, Hirsch AT, et al: Prediction of major cardiac events after peripheral vascular surgery using dipyridamole echocardiography. Am J Cardiol 68:593, 1991.

63. Langan AM, Youkey JR, Franklin DP, et al: Dobutamine stress echocardiography for cardiac risk assessment before aortic surgery. J Vasc Surg 18:905, 1993.

64. Poldermans D, Fioretti PM, Forster T, et al: Dobutamine stress echocardiography for assessment of perioperative cardiac risk in patients undergoing major vascular surgery. Circulation 87:1506, 1993.

65. Poldermans D, Arnese M, Fioretti PM, et al: Improved cardiac risk stratification in major vascular surgery with dobutamine-atropine stress echocardiography. J Am Coll Cardiol 26:648, 1995.

65a. Day SM, Younger JG, Karavite D, et al: Usefulness of hypotension during dobutamine echocardiography in predicting perioperative cardiac events. Am J Cardiol 85:478, 2000.

66. Davila-Roman VG, Waggoner AD, Sicard GA, et al: Dobutamine stress echocardiography predicts surgical outcome in patients with an aortic aneurysm and peripheral vascular disease. J Am Coll Cardiol 21:957, 1993.

67. Lane RT, Sawada SG, Seger DS, et al: Dobutamine stress echocardiography for assessment of cardiac risk before noncardiac surgery. Am J Cardiol 68:976, 1991.

68. Laika SG, Sawada SG, Dalsing MC, et al: Dobutamme stress echocardiography as a predictor of cardiac events associated with aortic surgery. J Vasc Surg 15:831, 1992.

69. Eichelberger JP, Schwarz KQ, Black ER, et al: Predictive value of dobutamine echocardiography just before noncardiac vascular surgery. Am J Cardiol 72:602, 1993.

70. L'Italien GJ, Paul SD, Hendel RC, et al: Development and validation of a bayesian model for perioperative cardiac risk assessment in a cohort ot 1081 vascular surgery candidates. J Am Coll Cardiol 27:779, 1996.

71. Foster ED, Davis KB, Carpenter JA, et al: Risk of noncardiac operation in patients with defined coronary disease. The Coronary Artery Surgery Study (CASS) registry experience. Ann Thorac Surg 41:42, 1986.

71a. Kaluza GL, Joseph J, Lee JR, et al: Catastrophic outcomes of noncardiac surgery soon after coronary stenting. J Am Coll Cardiol 35:1288, 2000.

72. Elmore JR, Hallett JW Jr, Gibbons RJ, et al: Myocardial ravascularization before abdominal aortic aneurysmorrhaphy: Effect of coronary angioplasty. Mayo Clin Proc 68:637, 1993.

73. Huber KC, Ebans MA, Bresnahan JF, et al: Outcome of noncardiac operations in patients with severe coronary artery disease successfully treated preoperatively with coronary angioplasty. Mayo Clin Proc 67:15, 1992.

74. Allen JR, Helling TS, Hartzler GO: Operative procedures not involving the heart after percutaneous transluminal coronary angioplasty. Surg Gynecol Obstet 173:285, 1991.

75. Fleisher LA, Barash PG: Preoperative cardiac evaluation for noncardiac surgery: A functional approach. Anesth Analg 74:586, 1992.

76. Granieri R, Macpherson DS: Perioperative care of the vascular surgery patient. The perspective of the internist. J Gen Intern Med 7:102, 1992.

77. Wong T, Detsky AS: Preoperative cardiac risk assessment for patients having peripheral vascular surgery. Ann Intern Med 115:743, 1992.

78. Pasternack PF, Imparato AM, Baumann FG, et al: The hemodynamics of beta-blockade in patients undergoing abdominal aortic aneurysm repair. Circulation 76(Suppl III):III-1, 1987.

79. Stone JG, Foex P, Sear JW, et al: Myocardial ischemia in untreated hypertensive patients: Effect of a small oral dose of a beta-adrenergic blocking agent. Anesthesiology 68:495, 1988.

80. Pasternack PF, Grossi EA, Baumann FG, et al: Beta blockade to decrease silent myocardial ischemia during peripheral vascular surgery. Am J Surg 158:113, 1989.

81. Mangano DT, Layug EL, Wallace AW, Tateo I: Effect of atenolol on mortality and cardiovascular morbidity after noncardiac surgery. N Engl J Med 335:1713, 1996.

82. Poldermans D, Boersma E, Bax JJ, et al: The effect of bisoprolol on perioperative mortality and myocardial infarction in high-risk patients undergoing vascular surgery. N Engl J Med 341:1789, 1999.

82a. Warltier DC, Pagel PS, Kersten JR: Approaches to prevention of perioperative myocardial ischemia. Anesthesiology 92:253, 2000.

83. Coriat P, Daloz M, Bousseau D, et al: Prevention of intraoperative myocardial ischemia during noncardiac surgery with intravenous nitroglycerine. Anesthesiology 61:193, 1984.

84. Ellis J, Drijvers G, Pedlow S, et al: Premedication with oral and transdermal clondine provides safe and efficacious postoperative sympatholysis. Anesth Analg 79:1133, 1994.

85. Dorman BH, Zucker JR, Verrier ED, et al: Clonidine improves perioperative myocardial ischemia, reduces anesthetic requirements, and alters hemodynamic parameters in patients undergoing coronary artery bypass surgery. J Cardiothorac Vasc Anesth 7:386, 1993.

86. McSPI-Europe Research Group: Perioperative sympatholysis. Anesthesiology 86:346, 1997.

87. Oliver M, Goldman L, Julian DG, Holme I, for the Mivazerol Trial Investigators Research Group: Effect of mivazerol on perioperative cardiac complications during non-cardiac surgery in patients with coronary heart disease: The European mivazerol trial (EMIT). Anesthesiology 91:951, 1999.

88. Boyd O, Grounds RM, Bennett ED: A randomized clinical trial of the effect of deliberate perioperative increase of oxygen delivery on mortality in high-risk surgical patients. JAMA 270:2699, 1993.

89. Wilson J, Woods I, Fawcett J, et al: Reducing the risk of major elective surgery: Randomised controlled trial of preoperative optimisation of oxygen delivery. BMJ 318:1099, 1998.

90. Ziegler DW, Wright JG, Choban PS, Flancbaum L: A prospective randomized trial of preoperative optimization of cardiac function in patients undergoing elective peripheral vascular surgery. Surgery 122:584, 1997.

91. Shoemaker WC, Kram HB, Appel PL, et al: Prospective trial of supranormal values of survivors as therapeutic goals in high risk surgical patients. Chest 94:1187, 1988.

92. Yu M, Levy MM, Smith P, et al: Effect of maximizing oxygen delivery on morbidity and mortality rates in critically ill patients: A prospective, randomized, controlled study. Crit Care Med 21:830, 1993.

93. Fleisher LA, Skolnick ED, Holroyd KJ, et al: Coronary artery revascularization before abdominal aortic aneurysm surgery: A decision analytic approach. Anesth Analg 79:661, 1994.

94. Mason JJ, Owens DK, Harris RA, et al: The role of coronary angiography and coronary revascularization before noncardiac vascular surgery. JAMA 273:1919, 1995.

95. Ashton CM, Petersen NJ, Wray NP, et al: The incidence of perioperative myocardial infarction in men undergoing noncardiac surgery. Ann Intern Med 118:504, 1993.

96. Hartz AJ, Kuhn EM, Pryor DB, et al: Mortality after coronary angioplasty and coronary artery bypass surgery (the national Medicare experience). Am J Cardiol 70:179, 1992.

97. Cohen MC, Curran PJ, L'Italien GJ, et al: Long-term prognostic value of preoperative dipyridamole thallium imaging and clinical indexes in patients with diabetes mellitus undergoing peripheral vascular surgery. Am J Cardiol 83:1038, 1999.

97a. Detre KM, Lombardero MS, Mori Brooks M, et al: The effect of previous coronary artery bypass surgery on the prognosis of patients with diabetes who have acute myocardial infarction. N Engl J Med 342:989, 2000.

98. Carson JL, Duff A, Poses RM, et al: Effect of anaemia and cardiovascular disease on surgical mortality and morbidity. Lancet 348:1055, 1996.

99. Nelson AH, Fleisher LA, Rosenbaum SH: Relationship between postoperative anemia and cardiac morbidity in high-risk vascular patients in the intensive care unit. Crit Care Med 21:860, 1993.

100. Wahr JA: Myocardial ischaemia in anaemic patients. Br J Anaesth 81 (Suppl 1):10, 1998.

101. Torsher LC, Shub C, Rettke SR, Brown DL: Risk of patients with severe aortic stenosis undergoing noncardiac surgery. Am J Cardiol 81:448, 1998.

102. Hayes SN, Holmes DR Jr, Nishimura RA, Reeder GS: Palliative percutaneous aortic balloon valvuloplasty before noncardiac operations and invasive diagnostic procedures. Mayo Clin Proc 64:753, 1989.

103. Roth RB, Palacios IF, Block PC: Percutaneous aortic balloon valvuloplasty: Its role in the management of patients with aortic stenosis requiring major noncardiac surgery. J Am Coll Cardiol 13:1039, 1989.

104. O'Keefe JH, Shub C, Rettke SR: Risk of noncardiac surgical procedures in patients with aortic stenosis. Mayo Clin Proc 64:400, 1989.

105. Thompson RC, Liberthson RR, Lowenstein E: Perioperative anesthetic risk of noncardiac surgery in hypertrophic obstructive cardiomyopathy. JAMA 254:2419, 1985.

106. Haering JM, Comunale ME, Parker RA, et al: Cardiac risk of noncardiac surgery in patients with asymmetric septal hypertrophy. Anesthesiology 85:254, 1996.

107. Tinker JH, Tarhan S: Discontinuing anticoagulant therapy in surgical patients with cardiac valve prostheses. JAMA 239:738, 1978.

108. Katholi RE, Nolan SP, McGuire IB: Living with prosthetic heart valve. Subsequent noncardiac operations and the risk of thromboembolism or hemorrhage. Am Heart J 92:162, 1976.

109. Kearon C, Hirsh J: Management of anticoagulation before and after elective surgery. N Engl J Med 336:1506, 1997.

110. Eckman MH, Beshansky JR, Durand-Zaleski L, et al: Anticoagulation for noncardiac procedures in patients with prosthetic heart valves. JAMA 263:1513, 1990.

111. Durack DT: Prevention of infective endocarditis. N Engl J Med 332:38, 1995.

112. Dajani AS, Taubert KA, Wilson W, et al: Prevention of bacterial endocarditis. Recommendations by the American Heart Association. JAMA 277:1794, 1997.

113. Ammash NM, Connolly HM, Abel MD, Warnes CA: Noncardiac surgery in Eisenmenger syndrome. J Am Coll Cardiol 33:222, 1999.

114. Mahla E, Rotman B, Rehak P, et al: Perioperative ventricular dysrhythmias in patients with structural heart disease undergoing noncardiac surgery. Anesth Analg 86:16, 1998.

115. Guarnieri T, Nolan S, Gottlieb SO, et al: Intravenous amiodarone for the prevention of atrial fibrillation after open heart surgery: The amodarone reduction in coronary heart (ARCH) trial. J Am Coll Cardiol 34:343, 1999.

116. Redle JD, Khurana S, Marzan R, et al: Prophylactic oral amiodarone compared with placebo for prevention of atrial fibrillation after coronary artery bypass surgery. Am Heart J 138:144, 1999.

117. Daoud EG, Strickberger SA, Man KC, et al: Preoperative amiodarone as prophylaxis against atrial fibrillation after heart surgery. N Engl J Med 337:1785, 1997.

118. Gomes JA, Ip J, Santoni-Rugiu F, et al: Oral d,l sotalol reduces the incidence of postoperative atrial fibrillation in coronary artery bypass surgery patients: A randomized double-blind placebo-controlled study. J Am Coll Cardiol 34:334, 1999.

118a. Thomas EJ, Goldman L, Mangione CM, et al: Body mass index as a correlate of postoperative complications and resource utilizations. Am J Med 102:277, 1997.

POSTOPERATIVE COMPLICATIONS

119. Charlson ME, MacKenzie CR, Ales KL, et al: The post-operative electrocardiogram and creatine kinase: Implications for diagnosis of myocardial infarction after non-cardiac surgery. J Clin Epidemiol 42:25, 1989.

120. Rettke SR, Shub C, Naessens JM, et al: Significance of mildly elevated creatine kinase (myocardial band) activity after elective abdominal aortic aneurysmectomy. J Cardiothorac Vasc Anesth 5:425, 1991.

121. Adams JE III, Scicard GA, Allen BT, et al: Diagnosis of perioperative myocardial infarction with measurement of cardiac troponin I. N Engl J Med 330:670, 1994.

122. Bick RL, Haas SK: International consensus recommendations. Summary statement and additional suggested guidelines. European consensus conference, November 1991. American College of Chest Physicians consensus statement of 1995. International consensus statement, 1997. Med Clin North Am 82:613, 1998.

123. Lee TH, Thomas EJ, Ludwig LE, et al: Troponin T as a marker for myocardial ischemia in patients undergoing noncardiac surgery. Am J Cardiol 77:1031, 1996.

124. Pires LA, Wagshal AB, Lancey R, et al: Arrhythmias and conduction disturbances after coronary artery bypass graft surgery: Epidemiology, management and prognosis. Am Heart J 129:799, 1995.

125. Vanderlugt JT, Mattioni T, Denker S, et al: Efficacy and safety of ibutilide fumarate for the conversion of atrial arrhythmias after cardiac surgery. Circulation 100:369, 1999.

GUIDELINES

SUMMARY OF GUIDELINES FOR REDUCING CARDIAC RISK WITH NONCARDIAC SURGERY

Thomas M. Lee

Guidelines on the assessment and management of perioperative risk of coronary artery disease in noncardiac surgery were published by the American College of Physicians (ACP) in 1997[1] and an American College of Cardiology/American Heart Association (ACC/AHA) task force in 1996.[2] These guidelines preceded research demonstrating the beneficial impact of beta blockers on high-risk patients undergoing noncardiac surgery,[3, 4] as well as the publication of the Revised Cardiac Risk Index.[5]

Both the ACP and the ACC/AHA guidelines emphasize the importance of using clinical data to stratify patients according to their risk of major cardiac complications. The ACP guidelines recommend use of a modification[6] of the Cardiac Risk Index of Goldman and colleagues.[7] Compared with this modification and other algorithms available when these guidelines were developed, the revised cardiac risk index[5] is more accurate and identifies a larger percentage of patients as having intermediate or high risk. Thus, this new index may be incorporated into future guidelines.

Low-risk patients may proceed directly to surgery, whereas special risk-reducing strategies (e.g., coronary angiography and revascularization) may be appropriate for very high-risk patients (Table 61–G–1). Among patients undergoing vascular surgery, both guidelines also recommend focusing use of noninvasive testing for further risk stratification on those with intermediate clinical risk. The ACP guidelines differ from the ACC/AHA guidelines by recommending against noninvasive testing in nonvascular patients with an intermediate risk determined by clinical evaluation.

These recommendations may be influenced in future revisions by randomized trial data demonstrating marked reductions in perioperative risk associated with treatment with bisoprolol in a population of patients who had abnormal results of stress echocardiography examinations and who underwent major vascular surgery.[3] These findings raise the possibility that an appropriate strategy may be to use beta blockers for intermediate- and high-risk patients rather than use noninvasive testing or coronary angiography to identify patients for revascularization. No prospective data show that testing or revascularization strategies can improve overall outcomes for patients undergoing noncardiac surgery.

Issue	Class I	Class II	Class III
Recommendations for preoperative noninvasive evaluation of left ventricular function	Patients with current or poorly controlled CHF	Patients with prior CHF and patients with dyspnea of unknown cause	As a routine test of left ventricular function in patients without prior CHF
Perioperative therapy with beta blockers*	Beta blockers required in the recent past to control symptoms of angina or patients with symptomatic arrhythmias or hypertension	Preoperative assessment identifies untreated hypertension, known coronary disease, or major factors for coronary disease	Contraindication to beta blockade
Recommendations for intraoperative nitroglycerin	High-risk patients previously on nitroglycerin who have active signs of myocardial ischemia without hypotension	As a prophylactic agent for high-risk patients to prevent myocardial ischemia and cardiac morbidity, particularly in those who have required nitrate therapy to control angina	Patients with signs of hypovolemia or hypotension
Intraoperative use of pulmonary artery catheters	Patients at risk for major hemodynamic disturbances that are most easily detected by a pulmonary artery catheter who are undergoing a procedure that is likely to cause these hemodynamic changes in a setting with experience in interpreting the results (e.g., suprarenal aortic aneurysm repair in a patient with angina)	Either the patient's condition or the surgical procedure (but not both) places the patient at risk for hemodynamic disturbances (e.g., total hip replacement in a patient with chronic renal insufficiency)	No risk of hemodynamic disturbances

* Recommendations precede prospective randomized trials demonstrating beneficial impact of beta blockade on outcomes.[3, 4]
CHF = congestive heart failure; Class I = Appropriate indication; Class II = equivocal indication; Class III = contraindicated. For definitions, see p. 1714.
From Guidelines for perioperative evaluation for noncardiac surgery: Report of the American College of Cardiology/American Heart Association Task Force on Practice Guidelines. Circulation 93:1278–1317, 1996.

References

1. American College of Physicians: Guidelines for assessing and managing the perioperative risk from coronary artery disease associated with major noncardiac surgery. Ann Intern Med 127:309–312, 1997.
2. Guidelines for perioperative cardiovascular evaluation for noncardiac surgery: Report of the American College of Cardiology/American Heart Association Task Force on Practice Guidelines. Circulation 93:1278–1317, 1996.
3. Poldermans D, Boersma E, Bax JJ, et al: The effect of bisoprolol on perioperative cardiac death and myocardial infarction in high-risk patients undergoing vascular surgery. N Engl J Med 341:1789, 1999.
4. Mangano DT, Layug EL, Wallace A, Tateo I, for the Multicenter Study of Perioperative Ischemia Research Group. Effect of atenolol on mortality and cardiovascular morbidity after noncardiac surgery. N Engl J Med 335:1713–1720, 1996.
5. Lee TH, Marcantonio EM, Mangione CM, et al: Derivation and prospective validation of a simple index for prediction of cardiac risk of major noncardiac surgery. Circulation 100:1043–1049, 1999.
6. Detsky AS, Abrams HB, McLaughlin JR, et al: Predicting cardiac complications in patients undergoing noncardiac surgery. J Gen Intern Med 1:211–219, 1986.
7. Goldman L, Caldera DL, Nussbaum SR, et al: Multifactorial index of cardiac risk in noncardiac surgical procedures. N Engl J Med 297:845–850, 1977.

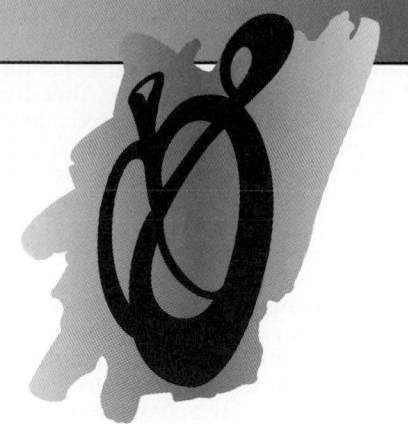

▼ PART VIII

CARDIOVASCULAR DISEASE AND DISORDERS OF OTHER ORGAN SYSTEMS

Chapter 62

Hemostasis, Thrombosis, Fibrinolysis, and Cardiovascular Disease

ANDREW I. SCHAFER • NADIR M. ALI
GLENN N. LEVINE

BASIC MECHANISMS OF HEMOSTASIS AND THROMBOSIS

The human hemostatic system has evolved as a remarkably orchestrated scheme of linked activities designed to preserve the integrity of blood circulation. Hemostasis is regulated to promote blood fluidity under normal circumstances. It is also prepared to clot blood with speed and precision at sites of vascular damage to arrest blood flow and prevent exsanguination whenever and wherever the integrity of the circulation is disrupted. Finally, hemostasis has the capability to restore blood flow and perfusion upon subsequent healing of a damaged vessel. The major components of the hemostatic system include (1) the vessel wall itself, (2) plasma proteins (the coagulation and fibrinolytic factors), and (3) platelets (and probably other formed elements of blood, such as monocytes and red cells). These constituents function virtually inseparably (Fig. 62–1). Although they are discussed in this chapter individually, it is important to recognize the interdependence of the actions of the vessel wall, plasma clotting factors, and platelets.

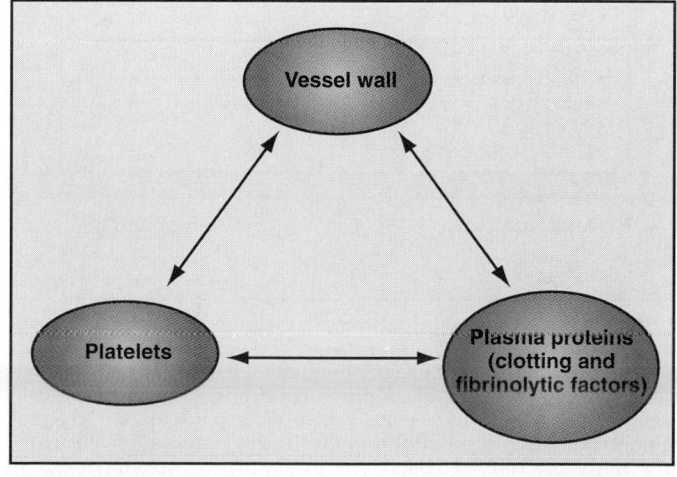

FIGURE 62–1. Interactions between the major components of the hemostatic system: the vessel wall, plasma proteins (clotting and fibrinolytic factors), and platelets.

Vascular Endothelium

A monolayer of endothelial cells lines the intimal surface of the entire circulatory tree, thereby representing the only stationary cell type that components of blood ever come in contact with under normal circumstances. The endothelial surface of the adult human is enormous: It is composed of about 1 to 6 $\times$ 10[13] cells, weighs approximately 1 kg, and covers a surface area equivalent to about six tennis courts.[1, 2] Yet, as recently as the first half of the 20th century, endothelial cells were viewed simply as barriers of blood flow, acting "merely in a negative manner," "similarly to a layer of paraffin or oil."[3] Today, we recognize that endothelium is a dynamic organ with complex metabolic capabilities, including the ability to control vascular permeability, the flow of biologically active molecules and nutrients, cell-cell and cell-matrix interactions within the vessel wall, blood flow and vascular tone, interactions of blood cells, the inflammatory response, and angiogenesis.

Endothelium is also an ideal regulator of hemostasis.[4, 5] It is endowed with a remarkable repertoire of activities that permit it to rapidly transform from a potent antithrombotic to a prothrombotic surface wherever the need arises. Indeed, attempts to reproduce these properties in clinical settings such as cardiovascular prostheses, extracorporeal circuits, and bypass grafts by pharmacological or even gene transfer methods have proven suboptimal, leading to more recent approaches to tissue engineering of vessels.[6]

Normal, quiescent endothelium constitutively displays a potent antithrombotic (thromboresistant) surface to blood (Fig. 62–2). It expresses anticoagulant, profibrinolytic, and platelet inhibitory properties. Whenever endothelium is activated or perturbed, however, it is rapidly transformed to a prothrombotic surface that actually promotes coagulation, inhibits fibrinolysis, and activates platelets. These are not entirely uniform phenomena, however. Throughout the cir-

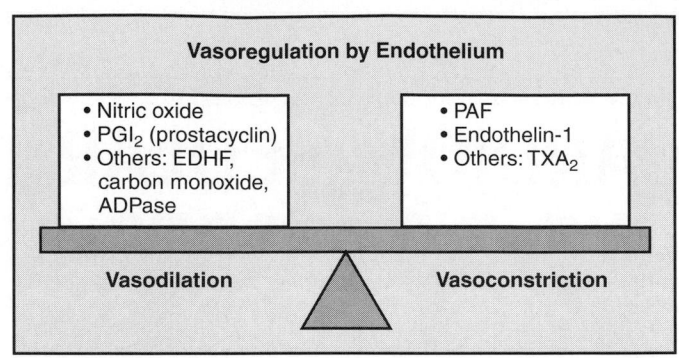

FIGURE 62–3. Regulation of vascular tone by the balance of endothelium-derived vasodilators and vasoconstrictors. ADPase = adenosine diphosphatase; EDHF = endothelium-derived hyperpolarizing factor; PAF = platelet-activating factor; TXA$_2$ = thromboxane A$_2$.

culatory tree, even within a single organ, there is marked heterogeneity in the phenotype of endothelial cells.[7–11] With respect to hemostasis, for example, endothelial cells from different tissues are heterogeneous in their expression of von Willebrand factor, plasminogen activators, and tissue factor.[1, 12, 13] This endothelial heterogeneity is determined by both genetic and environmental factors. Exposure to different microenvironmental stimuli, including variable hemodynamic forces and cellular and humoral mediators, contributes significantly to the heterogeneity of endothelial phenotypes that develops throughout the circulation.[14]

The specific antithrombotic and prothrombotic properties of endothelial cells that are shown in Figure 62–2 are described in more detail in the following sections. The hemostatic conversion of the vessel wall is triggered by mechanical damage or by perturbation and activation of the vascular cells by agents such as cytokines, endotoxin, hypoxia, and hemodynamic forces.

Similarly, as illustrated in Figure 62–3, a delicate balance exists in the capability of endothelial cells to modulate vascular tone. An important physiological vasodilator released by endothelial cells is nitric oxide (NO), a simple diatomic gas synthesized from the terminal guanidino nitrogen atoms of L-arginine by the action of a group of enzymes known as nitric oxide synthases (NOSs).[15–18] The major isoform of NOS present in endothelial cells, eNOS, is constitutively active and is further activated by stimuli that increase intracellular calcium, including several receptor-dependent agonists (e.g., thrombin) and hemodynamic forces (shear stress and cyclic stretch).[19] NO acts as a potent vasodilator as well as an inhibitor of platelet adhesion and platelet aggregation by stimulating soluble guanylate cyclase and thereby elevating intracellular levels of cyclic guanosine monophosphate in vascular smooth muscle cells and platelets. Prostaglandin I$_2$ (PGI$_2$, prostacyclin) is a major endothelium-derived oxygenation product of arachidonic acid, synthesized by the sequential actions of cyclooxygenase (COX) and prostacyclin synthase.[4, 20, 21] Prostacyclin, like NO, is both a vasodilator and inhibitor of platelet aggregation (but not adhesion), exerting these actions by stimulating adenylate cyclase and thereby elevating intracellular cyclic adenosine monophosphate (AMP) in target vascular smooth muscle and platelets. Endothelium-derived hyperpolarizing factor (EDHF)[21–23] and carbon monoxide (CO), a byproduct of heme metabolism to biliverdin by heme oxygenases,[24] are also direct vasodilators elaborated by endothelial cells. Endothelial ecto-adenosine diphosphatase (ADPase), recently identified as CD39,[25] is a membrane-associated platelet inhibitor but may also indirectly promote vasodilation by generating adenosine.[5] These vasodilator properties of endothelium are counterbalanced by endothelium-derived vasoconstrictors, including plate-

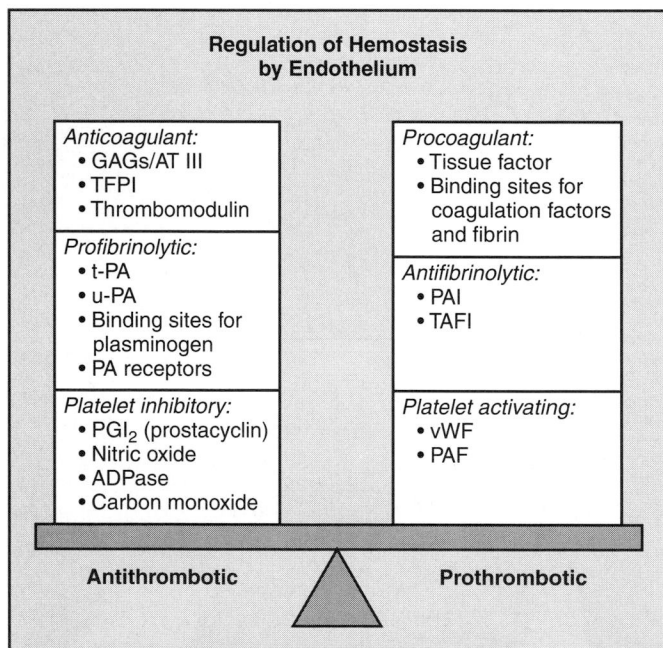

FIGURE 62–2. Balance of antithrombotic and prothrombotic properties of vascular endothelium. In general, antithrombotic properties dominate in quiescent endothelium under normal physiological conditions. In contrast, prothrombotic properties are expressed whenever endothelium is perturbed or activated. GAGs = glycosaminoglycans; AT III = antithrombin III; TFPI = tissue factor pathway inhibitor; t-PA = tissue-type plasminogen activator; u-PA = urokinase-type plasminogen activator; PAI = plasminogen activator inhibitor; TAFI = thrombin-activatable fibrinolysis inhibitor; vWF = von Willebrand factor; PAF = platelet-activating factor.

let-activating factor,[26, 27] endothelin-1,[28–30] and thromboxane A₂ (TXA₂).[31]

In many cases, endothelium-derived vasodilators are also platelet inhibitors and, conversely, endothelium-derived vasoconstrictors can also be platelet activators. The net effect of vasodilation and inhibition of platelet function is to promote blood fluidity, whereas the net effect of vasoconstriction and platelet activation is to promote hemostasis. Thus, as indicated in Figures 62–2 and 62–3, blood fluidity and hemostasis can be exquisitely regulated by the balance of antithrombotic/prothrombotic and vasodilatory/vasoconstrictor properties of endothelial cells, which are often coordinately modulated by their relative states of quiescence and activation.[5]

Coagulation

Plasma coagulation proteins ("clotting factors") normally circulate in plasma in their biologically inactive zymogen (or proenzyme) forms. When the thromboresistant nature of the vascular system is altered, by either mechanical injury or inflammatory and other systemic stimuli, (e.g., coronary plaque rupture in patients who develop unstable angina), the coagulation system is activated. If the physiological antithrombotic defenses can be overwhelmed, the result will be the formation of hemostatic thrombi composed of platelets and fibrin. In cases where activation of the coagulation system is triggered by focal vascular injury, the occlusive hemostatic thrombus will be precisely localized at and limited to the site of damage.

The sequence of coagulation protein reactions that culminate in the formation of fibrin was originally described as a "waterfall" or a "cascade" (Fig. 62–4). The coagulation cascade is a highly coordinated and regulated series of linked enzymatic reactions that involves the sequential activation of plasma zymogens to serine proteases. Each protease then catalyzes the subsequent zymogen-protease transition by cleavage of peptide bonds. This creates a biochemical amplifier in which a small initiating stimulus rapidly generates high levels of the end product fibrin.[32–34] Our understanding of the coagulation cascade has been refined with the recognition that it actually involves a series of linked enzymatic multiprotein complexes, each consisting of a serine protease, one or more cofactor proteins, divalent cations, and a cellular surface (e.g., platelet membranes) on which these components can be assembled.[34]

Two pathways of blood coagulation have been recognized: the so-called intrinsic or contact activation pathway and the so-called extrinsic or tissue factor pathway. These two pathways of activation of the coagulation cascade converge to form a "common" pathway, which leads to the generation of the pivotal coagulation enzyme thrombin. As illustrated in Figure 62–4, thrombin not only catalyzes the conversion of fibrinogen to fibrin but also serves an important role in sustaining the cascade by feedback activation of coagulation factors at several strategic sites.

INTRINSIC PATHWAY. This pathway of coagulation is triggered by the autoactivation of factor XII to its active serine protease form (factor XIIa) on "negatively charged" surfaces, optimally in the presence of two other contact activation proteins, prekallikrein and high-molecular-weight kininogen.[35] The physiological negatively charged surface for contact activation of factor XII and the intrinsic pathway of coagulation is really the cell membrane, which serves as a foundation for the assembly and activation of these proteins.[36] Factor XIIa converts the zymogen factor XI to its corresponding serine protease, factor XIa. Factor XIa, in turn, then serves as an activator of factor IX to IXa. The final step in the intrinsic pathway is the activation of the plasma zymogen factor X to factor Xa by factor IXa, a reaction that requires the activated form of the plasma cofactor, factor VIIIa. Factor VIIIa is generated by thrombin-induced limited proteolysis of factor VIII.

In vivo, however, coagulation is probably not initiated primarily by this intrinsic pathway. The most compelling support of this is the

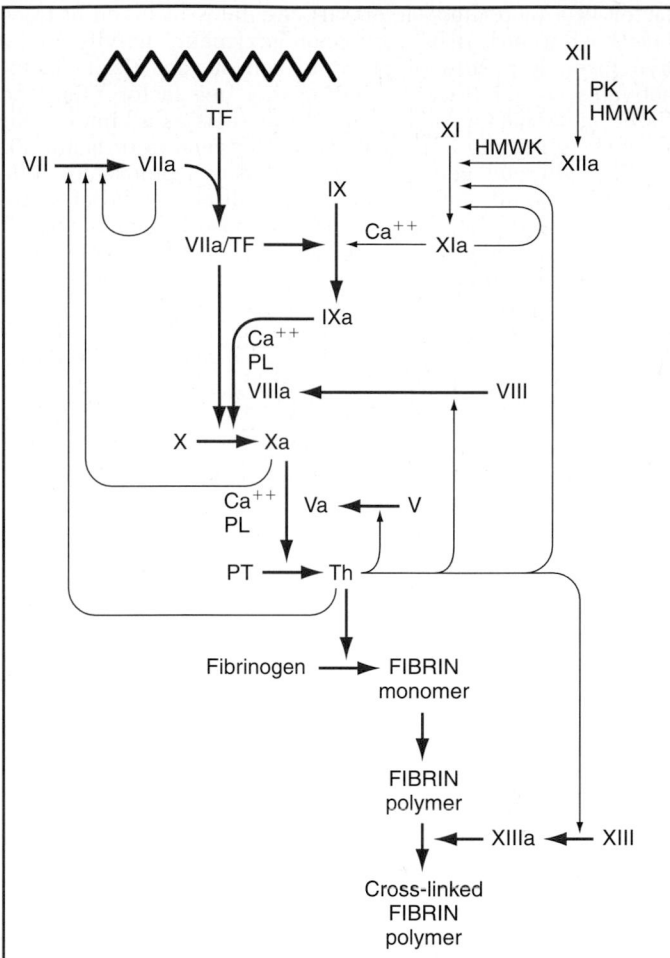

FIGURE 62–4. The coagulation cascade. This scheme emphasizes recent understanding of the importance of the tissue factor pathway in initiating clotting in vivo, the interactions between pathways, and the pivotal role of thrombin in sustaining the cascade by feedback activation of coagulation factors. TF = tissue factor; PK = prekallikrein; HMWK = high-molecular-weight kininogen; PL = phospholipid; PT = prothrombin; Th = thrombin. (Modified from Schafer AI: The primary and secondary hypercoagulable states. *In* Schafer AI [ed]: Molecular Mechanisms of Hypercoagulable States. Austin, TX, Landes Bioscience, 1997, pp 1–48.)

clinical observation that individuals with inherited deficiencies of any of the contact activation factors (factor XII, prekallikrein, high-molecular-weight kininogen) do not have a bleeding tendency. Thus, it has been argued that this system has little to do with the initiation of hemostasis.[36] In fact, these proteins may play important roles in other physiological systems, such as vasoregulation and as antithrombotic and profibrinolytic agents.[37] In contrast, individuals with deficiencies of factors XI, IX, or VIII do have clinical bleeding tendencies; and, therefore, these proteins in the intrinsic pathway do appear to play important roles in hemostasis. The participation of factor XI in hemostasis is therefore probably not dependent on its activation by factor XIIa but rather on its positive feedback activation by thrombin. Thus, this positive feedback loop (see Fig. 62–4) would permit factor XIa to function in the propagation and amplification, rather than in the initiation, of the coagulation cascade.

EXTRINSIC PATHWAY. Coagulation in vivo is probably initiated predominantly through the extrinsic pathway. The immediate trigger is the injury-induced expression of the integral membrane glycoprotein tissue factor[38–40] on the surfaces of activated endothelial cells and circulating blood cells (particularly leukocytes), cells that normally do not express tissue factor activity on their surfaces.[41] Alternatively, vascular damage can expose blood to tissue factor that is constitutively expressed on the surfaces of subendothelial cellular components of the vessel wall, such as smooth muscle cells and fibroblasts. The serine protease factor VIIa (activated factor VII) circulates in blood at trace levels[42] but possesses very poor enzymatic activity in its free form. Exposure of blood to cell surface tissue factor activates coagulation by binding this free factor VIIa. The tissue factor/factor VIIa complex then acts as a bimolecular enzyme to rapidly autocatalyze the conversion of factor VII to VIIa, thereby generating more tissue factor/factor VIIa complexes and amplifying this initial hemostatic response.[43] Factor Xa and thrombin can also induce factor VII activation (see Fig. 62–4); in fact, these two enzymes may be kinetically preferred over the tissue factor/factor VIIa complex as physiological activators of factor VII.[44] The final reaction in the extrinsic pathway is the activation of factor X to factor Xa. This can be catalyzed directly by the tissue factor/factor VIIa bimolecular enzyme complex. Alternatively, the complex can indirectly activate factor X by initially converting factor IX to factor IXa (providing communication between the extrinsic and intrinsic pathways of coagulation), which then activates factor X. This indirect route of factor X activation is probably the one that is favored kinetically.

COMMON PATHWAY. Factor Xa, which can be formed through the actions of either the tissue factor/factor VIIa complex or factor IXa (with factor VIIIa as a cofactor), initiates the common pathway of coagulation by converting the inactive plasma zymogen prothrombin to thrombin, the pivotal protease of the coagulation system. The essential cofactor for this reaction is factor Va, a plasma protein that shares about 30 percent sequence identity to the other plasma coagulation cofactor, factor VIIIa. Like the homologous factor VIIIa, factor Va is produced by thrombin-induced limited proteolysis of factor V. As noted earlier and further described later, thrombin is a multifunctional enzyme, but its major role in the common pathway is to convert soluble plasma fibrinogen to an insoluble fibrin matrix.[45] Fibrin polymerization involves an orderly process of intermolecular associations.[46] Thrombin also activates factor

XIII (fibrin-stabilizing factor) to factor XIIIa, a transglutaminase that covalently cross-links and thereby stabilizes the fibrin clot.[46, 47]

The coagulation cascade that culminates in fibrin formation would occur extremely inefficiently and slowly in fluid phase plasma. However, the assembly of these clotting factors on activated cell membrane surfaces greatly accelerates their reaction rates and also serves to localize blood clotting to sites of vascular injury.[32, 34, 38] In addition, proteases in the coagulation factor complexes assembled on cell surfaces are sequestered from inactivation by their physiological antithrombotic regulators described later, further enhancing the efficiency of membrane-dependent reactions. The critical cell membrane components on which these coagulation reactions proceed are acidic phospholipids. These phospholipid species are not normally exposed on resting cell membrane surfaces. However, when platelets, monocytes, and endothelial cells are activated by vascular injury or inflammatory stimuli, the procoagulant head groups of the membrane anionic phospholipids become translocated to the surfaces of these cells, making them available to support and promote the plasma coagulation reactions.[48, 49]

PROTHROMBINASE COMPLEXES. Major membrane phospholipid-associated enzyme complexes in the coagulation cascade include the "Xase" (or tenase) and "prothrombinase" complexes (Fig. 62–5). Each complex consists of a serine protease enzyme, its zymogen substrate, and its cofactor assembled in association with each other on the membrane surface. The "extrinsic Xase" complex consists of the tissue factor/factor VIIa enzyme complex and its zymogen substrates, factor IX and factor X. The "intrinsic Xase" complex consists of factor IXa as the enzyme, factor X as its substrate, and factor VIIIa as the cofactor. The "prothrombinase complex" consists of factor Xa as the enzyme, prothrombin (factor II) as its substrate, and factor Va as the cofactor. Factor IXa generated by the "extrinsic Xase" complex becomes the enzyme of the "intrinsic Xase" com-

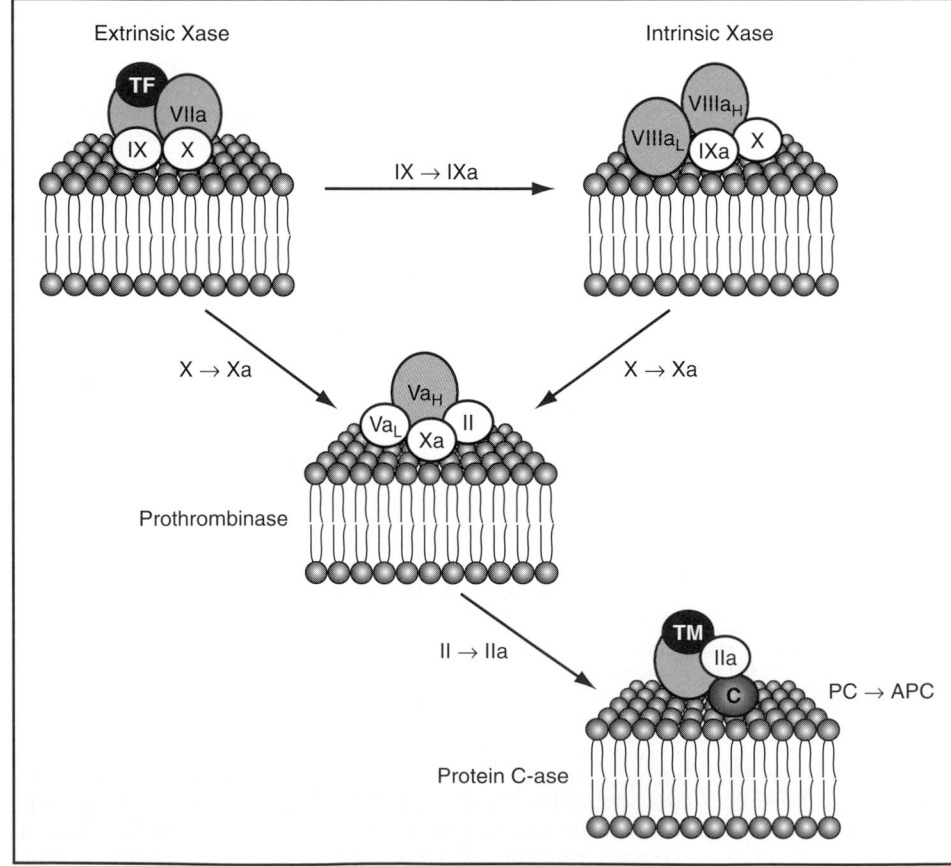

FIGURE 62–5. Schematic representation of the phospholipid membrane-associated enzyme complexes of coagulation. Each vitamin K–dependent serine protease (factors VIIa, IXa, and Xa and α-thrombin [IIa]) is shown in association with its cofactor protein (tissue factor [TF], factors VIIIa and Va, and thrombomodulin [TM]) and zymogen substrate(s) (factors IX and X, prothrombin [II] and protein C [C]) on the membrane surface. The cofactor proteins, factor VIIIa and factor Va, are characterized by a two-domain structure and consist of heavy (H) and light (L) chains that are bridged together by Ca^{2+} ions. Both domains are required for cofactor-membrane association and cofactor-protease binding. (Modified from Jenny NS, Mann KG: Coagulation cascade: An overview. *In* Loscalzo J, Schafer AI [eds]: Thrombosis and Hemorrhage. 2nd ed. Baltimore, Williams & Wilkins, 1998, pp 3–27.)

plex. Factor Xa generated by either the "extrinsic Xase" or the "intrinsic Xase" complex becomes the enzyme of the "prothrombinase" complex. These successive reaction complexes of coagulation most likely occur by diffusion of products along the same cell membrane surface.[34]

The final enzyme product, thrombin, is detached from cell membranes and out into the blood to serve its multiple purposes. A major terminating reaction, also shown in Figure 62–5, involves membrane assembly of the "protein Case" complex in which free thrombin (factor IIa) binds to the integral membrane protein, thrombomodulin, which serves as the site for activation of protein C, a major antithrombotic protein discussed later in the chapter.

Anticoagulant (Antithrombotic) Mechanisms

Several physiological antithrombotic mechanisms act in concert to prevent clotting under normal circumstances. Optimal activity of each of the anticoagulant systems depends on the integrity of vascular endothelium. Thus, these physiological mechanisms operate to preserve blood fluidity in the intact circulation and also to limit blood clotting to specific focal sites of vascular injury.[50]

Endothelial PGI$_2$, nitric oxide, ADPase, and carbon monoxide are physiological platelet inhibitory mediators (see Fig. 62–2). Other anticoagulant systems are designed to limit fibrin accumulation. Several of these mechanisms, including antithrombin, the protein C/protein S/thrombomodulin system and tissue factor pathway inhibitor (TFPI), act at different sites in the coagulation cascade to dampen fibrin accumulation. Fibrin that forms despite these anticoagulant defenses is then degraded by the fibrinolytic system. The sites of action of the major physiological antithrombotic pathways are shown in Figure 62–6.

ANTITHROMBIN. Antithrombin (or antithrombin III) is the major plasma protease inhibitor of thrombin and the other clotting factors in the intrinsic and common pathways of coagulation. It is a single-chain glycoprotein that is synthesized primarily in the liver and belongs to the serine protease inhibitor ("serpin") family of proteins.[51, 52] Antithrombin neutralizes thrombin and other activated coagulation factors by forming a complex between the active site of the enzyme and the reactive center (Arg393 and Ser394) of antithrombin. The rate of formation of these inactivating complexes increases by a factor of several thousand in the presence of heparin. This is the major anticoagulant mechanism of action of heparin (see later). Heparin and heparan sulfate proteoglycans are actually present as endogenous components of the vessel wall. Thus, antithrombin inactivation of thrombin and other activated clotting factors probably occurs physiologically on vascular surfaces, where heparins are present to catalyze these reactions, rather than in fluid phase plasma. Inherited quantitative or qualitative deficiencies of antithrombin lead to a lifelong predisposition to venous thromboembolism.[11, 32, 50, 53]

PROTEIN C/PROTEIN S/THROMBOMODULIN. Protein C is another plasma glycoprotein synthesized by the liver, which becomes an anticoagulant when it is activated by thrombin through cleavage of an Arg169-Leu170 bond in its heavy chain.[54, 55] The thrombin-induced activation of protein C occurs physiologically on thrombomodulin, a transmembrane proteoglycan binding site for thrombin on endothelial cell surfaces.[56, 57] Thrombomodulin thus serves an antithrombotic function both by binding and thereby removing thrombin from the circulation and also by promoting generation by thrombus of anticoagulantly active protein C. Activated protein C acts as an anticoagulant by cleaving multiple bonds and thereby destroying the membrane-bound activated forms of coagulation factors V (Va)

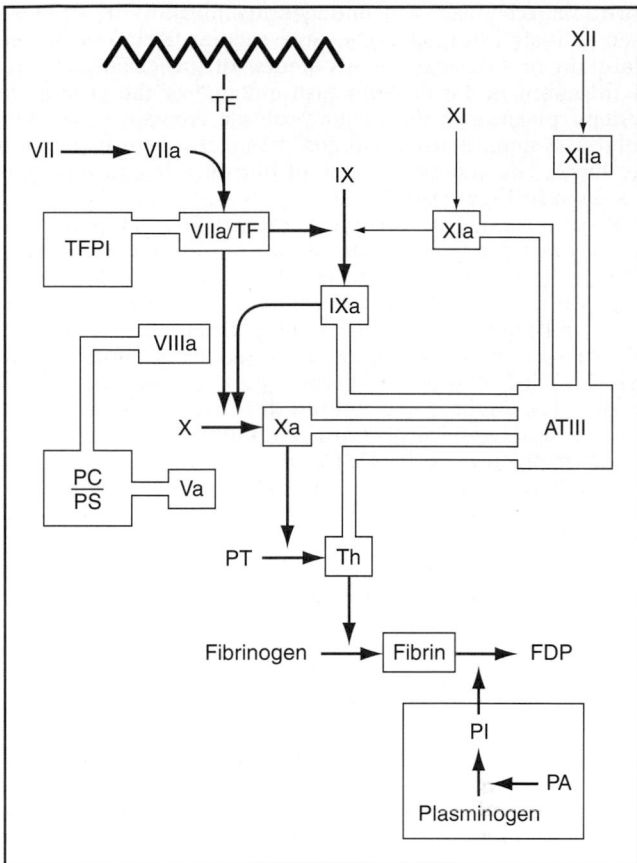

FIGURE 62–6. Sites of action of the four major physiological antithrombotic pathways: antithrombin (AT); protein C/protein S (PC/PS); tissue factor pathway inhibitor (TFPI); and the fibrinolytic system, consisting of plasminogen, plasminogen activator (PA), and plasmin (Pl). (From Schafer AI: The primary and secondary hypercoagulable states. *In* Schafer AI [ed]: Molecular Mechanisms of Hypercoagulable States. Austin, TX, Landes Bioscience, 1997, pp 1–48.)

and VIII (VIIIa). This reaction is accelerated by a cofactor, protein S. Like protein C, protein S is a glycoprotein that undergoes vitamin K–dependent posttranslational carboxylations to form gamma-carboxyglutamic acid ("Gla") residues that allow it to bind to negatively charged phospholipid surfaces. Protein S acts as a cofactor by increasing the affinity of activated protein C for phospholipids in the formation of the membrane-bound protein Case complex (see Fig. 62–5). Quantitative or qualitative deficiencies of protein C or protein S, or resistance to the action of activated protein C by a specific mutation at its target cleavage site in factor Va (factor V Leiden), lead to hypercoagulable states.[11, 32, 50, 53]

TISSUE FACTOR PATHWAY INHIBITOR. TFPI is a plasma protease inhibitor that regulates the tissue factor–induced extrinsic pathway of coagulation.[58] Unlike other coagulation inhibitors, which are members of the serpin family, TFPI is a multivalent Kunitz-type serine protease inhibitor. This structure permits TFPI to exert dual inhibitory actions against both tissue factor/factor VIIa (mediated by its Kunitz-1 domain binding to factor VIIa), as shown in Figure 62–6, as well as factor Xa (mediated by its Kunitz-2 binding to factor Xa). Circulating plasma TFPI is bound to lipoproteins. TFPI can also be released by heparin from endothelial cells, where it is bound to glycosaminoglycans, and from platelets.

THE FIBRINOLYTIC SYSTEM. Any thrombin that escapes the inhibitory effects of the physiological anticoagulant systems described earlier is available to convert fibrinogen to fibrin. In response, the endogenous fibrinolytic system is then activated to dispose of intravascular fibrin and thereby maintain or reestablish the patency of the circulation. Just as thrombin is the key protease enzyme of the coagulation system, plasmin is the major protease enzyme of the fibrinolytic system, acting to digest fibrin to fibrin degradation products. The general scheme of fibrinolysis and its control is shown in Figure 62–7.

Plasminogen, the inactive zymogen form of plasmin, is synthesized primarily in the liver and circulates in plasma in high (micromolar) concentrations. It is a single-chain glycoprotein, which has significant sequence homology with apolipoprotein (a). Elevated plasma levels of lipoprotein (a) are associated with atherosclerotic cardiovascular risk.[59] Indeed, one possible atherogenic mechanism for lipoprotein (a) might be to inhibit fibrinolysis by competing with plasminogen for plasmin generation.

Plasminogen Activators. These cleave the Arg560-Val561 bond of plasminogen to generate the active enzyme plasmin, a two-chain molecule that derives its heavy chain (or A chain) from the amino-terminal region and its light chain (or B chain) from the carboxy-terminal region of plasminogen. The enzyme-active site of plasmin is localized in the B chain, whereas the A chain contains lysine-binding sites. The lysine-binding sites of plasmin (and plasminogen) permit it to bind to fibrin, so that physiological fibrinolysis is "fibrin specific." Plasmin is a serine protease the actions of which are not limited to fibrinolysis; plasmin also plays important roles in tissue remodeling, wound healing, angiogenesis, and cell migration.[60]

The major physiological plasminogen activators that convert plasminogen to plasmin are tissue-type plasminogen activator (t-PA) and urokinase-type plasminogen activator (u-PA). Both are serine proteases that are released by endothelial cells into plasma in trace concentrations. Plasmin can convert t-PA from its single-chain form to a two-chain molecule, in which the heavy and light chains are disulfide bonded. Both the single-chain and two-chain forms of t-PA are catalytically active to convert plasminogen to plasmin. In contrast, single-chain u-PA (scu-PA) has little enzyme activity and must be converted to its disulfide bonded, two-chain active form by hydrolysis of a Lys158-Ile159 bond. t-PA and u-PA are released from endothelial cells by a variety of humoral factors (e.g., growth factors, hormones, and cytokines), as well as hemodynamic forces, but many of these stimuli also induce the release of plasminogen activator inhibitors.

Both plasminogen (through its lysine-binding sites) and t-PA possess specific affinity for fibrin and thereby bind selectively to clots. In the absence of fibrin, t-PA activates

plasminogen to plasmin relatively slowly. Fibrin provides a surface for the sequential binding of t-PA and plasminogen. The assembly of a ternary complex, consisting of fibrin, plasminogen, and t-PA, promotes the localized interaction between plasminogen and t-PA and thereby greatly accelerates the rate of plasminogen activation to plasmin. Moreover, partial degradation of fibrin by plasmin exposes new plasminogen and t-PA binding sites in carboxy-terminus lysine residues of fibrin fragments to enhance further these reactions. Thus, early fibrin digestion by plasmin further accelerates fibrinolysis, thereby amplifying the process. This creates a highly efficient mechanism to generate plasmin focally on the fibrin clot, which then becomes plasmin's substrate for digestion to fibrin degradation products. Thus, the fibrin surface itself is an important regulator of its own degradation by providing binding sites for fibrinolytic proteins.

In addition to its interactions with fibrin, components of the fibrinolytic system are also efficiently assembled on cell surfaces, similar to the coagulation system, to localize and kinetically optimize the generation of plasmin.[61, 62] Specific binding sites for plasminogen and t-PA are present on the surfaces of endothelial cells, identified with annexin II, and other cell surfaces[63] to catalyze plasminogen activation. The presence of u-PA receptors (u-PAR) has also been identified on endothelial cells and other cell types.

The capacity of endothelial cells to synthesize and release plasminogen activators and then to bind these and other components of the fibrinolytic system provides a powerful paracrine mechanism to concentrate and activate fibrinolysis in proximity to intravascular thrombi contiguous to sites of endothelial damage. At the same time, receptors for the fibrinolytic proteins are also present on the surfaces of other cell types, including platelets and leukocytes that accumulate within thrombi.[64]

Plasmin cleaves fibrin at different rates at different sites of the fibrin molecule. This orderly process leads to the generation of characteristic fibrin fragments during the process of fibrinolysis. At the end of this sequential proteolysis, the D and E domains of fibrin are liberated. The sites of plasmin cleavage of fibrin are the same as those in fibrinogen. However, when plasmin acts on covalently cross-linked fibrin, D-dimers are released; hence, D-dimers can be measured in plasma as a relatively specific test of fibrin (rather than fibrinogen) degradation. Fibrin(ogen) degradation products may have potent anticoagulant and antiplatelet actions, thereby further contributing to the net antithrombotic effects of fibrinolysis.

Fibrinolytic Inhibitors. As shown in Figure 62–7, physiological regulation of fibrinolysis occurs primarily at two levels: (1) Plasminogen activator inhibitors (PAIs), specifically PAI-1 and PAI-2, inhibit the physiological plasminogen activators, and (2) alpha$_2$-antiplasmin inhibits plasmin. PAI-1 is the primary inhibitor of t-PA and u-PA in plasma.[65, 66] This serine protease inhibitor is a single-chain glycoprotein derived from endothelial cells and other cell types. PAI-1 inhibits t-PA by the formation of a complex between the active site of t-PA and the "bait" residues (Arg346-Met347) of PAI-1.[67]

PAI-2, which also belongs to the serpin superfamily, was originally identified in trophoblastic epithelium and hence is referred to as placental-type PAI.[68] Particularly elevated plasma levels of PAI-2 are found in pregnant women. Alpha$_2$-antiplasmin is a single-chain glycoprotein serpin that is synthesized predominantly by the liver. It is the main inhibitor of plasmin in human plasma, forming a 1:1 stoichiometric complex with plasmin that inactivates the enzyme.[67] Alpha$_2$-macroglobulin also inhibits plasmin, but at a much slower rate than alpha$_2$-antiplasmin; therefore, alpha$_2$-macroglobulin is of questionable importance in the physiological regulation of fibrinolysis.

Platelets

Platelets are cytoplasmic fragments that are released into blood from bone marrow megakaryocytes and circulate with an average life span of 7 to 10 days.[69] These terminal cell fragments are anucleate and therefore possess minimal capacity to synthesize new protein.

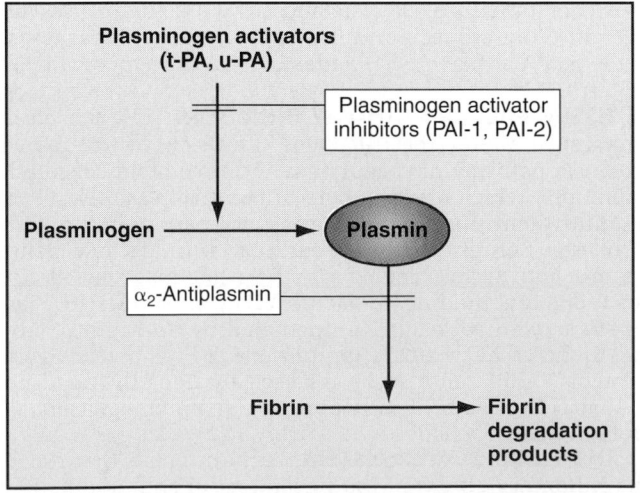

FIGURE 62–7. Scheme of the fibrinolytic system and its control.

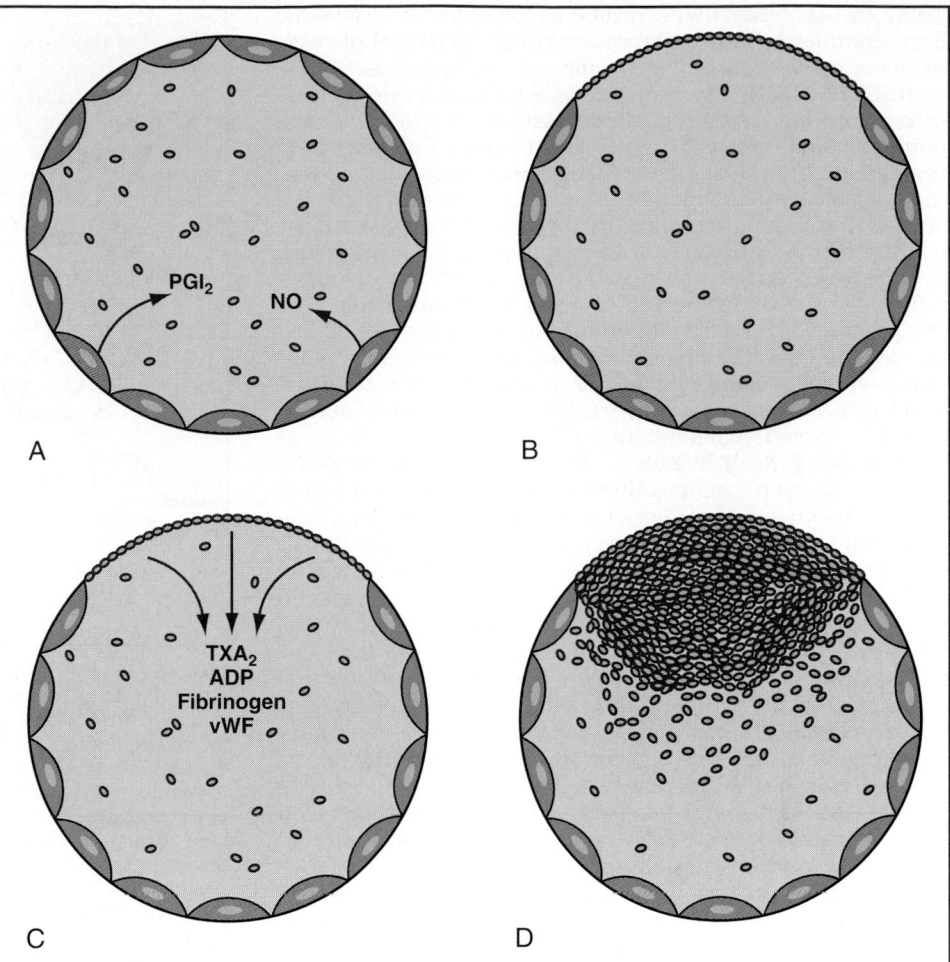

FIGURE 62–8. Sequence of events in platelet activation. *A,* Under normal conditions, a monolayer of endothelial cells lines the intimal surface of the circulatory tree, releasing platelet-inhibitory mediators such as PGI_2 (prostacyclin) and nitric oxide (NO). *B,* At a site of vascular injury, endothelium is lost and platelets undergo "adhesion" (platelet-vessel wall interactions) to subendothelial structures that are now exposed (e.g., collagen). *C,* Adherent platelets are activated, and release granule constituents (e.g., ADP, fibrinogen, von Willebrand factor) and thromboxane A_2 (TXA_2). *D,* Substances released from activated platelets recruit additional platelets from the circulation to the site of injury and mediate the process of platelet "aggregation" (platelet-platelet interactions), resulting in the formation of an occlusive platelet plug.

The antithrombotic properties of intact vascular endothelium include potent platelet inhibitors (see Fig. 62–2 and Fig. 62–8A). These inhibitors include PGI_2, NO, and CO, which are labile molecules that are released by endothelial cells and act locally as autocoids, and ADPase, an ectonucleotidase of endothelial membranes that breaks down platelet-activating ADP.

ADHESION. On vascular intimal injury, the antiplatelet properties of endothelium are diminished locally, while previously cryptic, thrombogenic subendothelial substances (e.g., collagen) become exposed to flowing blood. Circulating platelets recognize sites of vascular disruption and undergo the process of adhesion to the site of injury (see Fig. 62–8B). Adhesion results in the formation of a monolayer of platelets that are attached to the denuded vascular intimal surface. Platelet adhesion (i.e., platelet-vessel wall interaction) is mediated primarily by von Willebrand factor (vWF), a multimeric protein consisting of a wide spectrum of polymerized subunits that create a mature protein with a molecular mass that ranges from about 550 to more than 10,000 kDa, one of the largest soluble proteins in plasma.[70, 71] vWF is synthesized by both endothelial cells and megakaryocytes, where it is stored in Weibel-Palade bodies and alpha granules, respectively, before its regulated secretion. Released vWF is present in both plasma and in the extracellular matrix of the subendothelial vessel wall, to which the platelets are anchored. The large vWF multimers serve as the primary "molecular glue" to attach platelets to a damaged vessel wall with sufficient strength to withstand the high levels of shear stress that would tend to detach them with the flow of blood. The receptor for vWF on the platelet surface is localized in membrane glycoprotein (Gp) Ib, part of the platelet membrane Gp Ib/IX-V complex.[72, 73]

Higher levels of shear stress on the arterial side of the circulation promote the interaction between vWF and platelet membrane Gp Ib, probably through subtle shear-induced changes in the vWF molecule and/or its platelet receptor.[74] Platelet adhesion is also facilitated by direct binding to subendothelial collagen by means of specific platelet membrane collagen receptors.[75–77]

ACTIVATION. Adherent platelets then become activated[78] (Fig. 62–8C). The platelet activation process results from the combined actions of several agonists that bind to their respective membrane receptors on adherent platelets and transmit platelet-activating intracellular signals. These platelet stimuli include humoral mediators in plasma (e.g., epinephrine, thrombin), mediators released from activated cells (e.g., ADP, serotonin), and vessel wall extracellular matrix constituents that come in contact with adherent platelets (e.g., collagen, vWF). Several of these stimuli can synergistically activate platelets[79, 80] and may also act in concert with shear forces to which platelets are simultaneously exposed.[81] Activated platelets undergo the release reaction, during which they secrete prepackaged constituents of their cytoplasmic granules: ADP, adenosine triphosphate, and serotonin from the dense granules; soluble adhesive proteins (fibrinogen, vWF, thrombospondin, fibronectin); growth factors (including platelet-derived growth factor, transforming growth factor-alpha and transforming growth factor-beta); and procoagulants (platelet factor 4, factor V) from the alpha granules.[82] Simultaneously, activated platelets synthesize *de novo* and release the potent platelet activator and vasoconstrictor TXA_2. TXA_2 is the major cyclooxygenase product of arachidonic acid metabolism in platelets. As described later in the section on antiplatelet agents, aspirin inhibits cyclooxygenase and thereby blocks TXA_2 synthesis in platelets.

TXA_2 acts in concert with several of the substances released from granules to induce the activation of additional platelets in the microenvironment of the developing thrombus.[83, 84]

AGGREGATION. The products of the platelet release reaction, including secreted granule constituents and TXA_2, mediate the final phase of platelet activation, the process of aggregation (see Fig. 62–8D). During platelet aggregation (platelet-platelet interaction) additional platelets are recruited from the circulation to the site of vascular injury, leading to the formation of an occlusive platelet thrombus. As discussed earlier, the platelet plug is anchored and stabilized by the fibrin mesh that develops simultaneously as the product of the coagulation cascade. At lower shear levels (e.g., in the venous circulation), the "molecular glue" that mediates aggregation is fibrinogen, which can be derived either from plasma or from the alpha-granule releasate of activated platelets. At higher shear levels (e.g., in arteries), vWF itself, which is also the ligand that mediates platelet adhesion, can substitute for fibrinogen as the ligand of aggregation.[74] Fibrinogen or vWF binds to specific platelet membrane receptors that are located in the Gp IIb/IIIa integrin complex.[85, 86] Integrins are widely distributed on the surfaces of adherent eukaryotic cells. All receptors in the integrin superfamily contain an alpha and a beta subunit. Individual integrins can often bind to more than one ligand; thus, platelet Gp IIb/IIIa can recognize both fibrinogen and vWF, as well as some other adhesive proteins.

The Gp IIb/IIIa complex is the most abundant receptor on the platelet surface. Its alpha subunit (Gp IIb) is expressed specifically on platelets, but its $beta_3$ subunit (Gp IIIa) is shared by other integrins, including receptors on vascular cells. The heterodimeric, ligand-binding Gp IIb/IIIa complexes are not normally exposed in their active forms on the surfaces of quiescent circulating platelets. However, platelet activation converts Gp IIb/IIIa into competent receptors by means of specific signal transduction pathways,[86, 87] enabling Gp IIb/IIIa to bind to fibrinogen and vWF. The binding of these adhesive proteins requires that they contain the specific tripeptide sequence Arg-Gly-Asp (RGD). Recognition of fibrinogen and other ligands by the active Gp IIb/IIIa complex involves the RGD tripeptide sequence (located at positions 95–97 and 572–574 of each of the two A-alpha chains of fibrinogen). When two activated platelets with functional Gp IIb/IIIa receptors each bind the same fibrinogen molecule, a fibrinogen bridge is created between the two platelets (Fig. 62–9). Because the surface of each platelet has about 50,000 Gp IIb/IIIa fibrinogen binding sites, numerous activated platelets recruited to the site of vascular injury can rapidly form an occlusive aggregate by means of a dense network of intercellular fibrinogen bridges.[88] In addition to its RGD sequences, the gamma chains of fibrinogen also contain a 12-amino acid residue (dodecapeptide HHLGGAKQAGDV) that also has the ability to bind to the platelet Gp IIb/IIIa receptor. These events of ligand binding to activated platelet membrane Gp IIb/IIIa receptors, which mediate the process of platelet aggregation, have served as targets for antiplatelet therapy with Gp IIb/IIIa antagonists.

Central Role of Thrombin

Thrombin plays a pivotal role in coordinating, integrating, and regulating hemostasis. Depending on the circumstances, it can either promote or prevent blood clotting. This multifaceted effect of thrombin has been referred to as the "thrombin paradox."[89] The balance of prothrombotic and antithrombotic activities of thrombin is determined by at least two variables: (1) the concentration of free thrombin in blood and (2) the presence or absence of endothelial cells at thrombin's site of action.

When free thrombin is available in blood at high concentrations, particularly at a site of vascular injury where

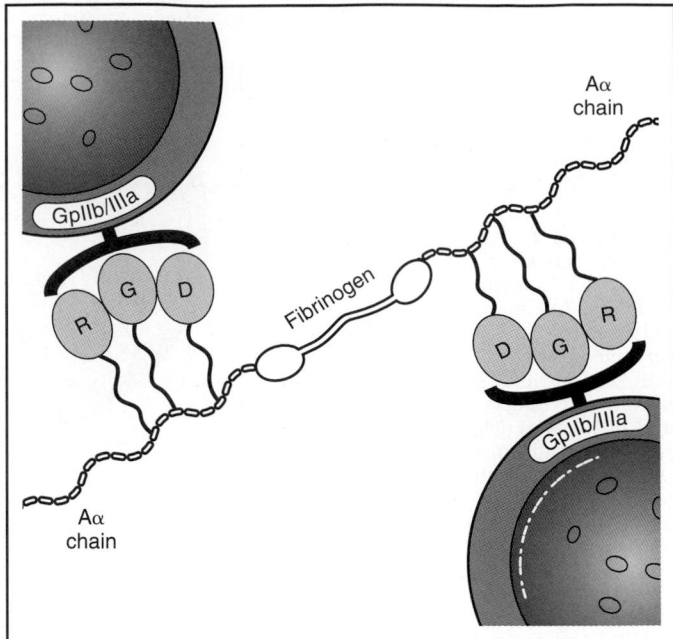

FIGURE 62–9. Linkage of two activated platelets by fibrinogen, which binds to its receptors in the platelet Gp IIb/IIIa complex by means of tripeptide RGD (arginine-glycine-aspartic acid) sequences located on the α chains of dimeric fibrinogen. The high density of Gp IIb/IIIa complexes on the surfaces of activated platelets permits the rapid formation of a network of fibrinogen bridges, leading to platelet aggregation at the site of vascular injury. (In regions of high shear stress, such as in diseased coronary arteries, von Willebrand factor may replace fibrinogen as the primary aggregating ligand. Like fibrinogen, the von Willebrand factor molecule has RGD sequences that mediate this process.) The result of platelet aggregation is the formation of an occlusive platelet thrombus. (From Schafer AI: Antiplatelet therapy with glycoprotein IIb/IIIa receptor inhibitors and other novel agents. Tex Heart Inst J 24:90–96, 1997.)

the antithrombotic influence of endothelium is lost, thrombin is a potent inducer of clotting (Fig. 62–10). This enzyme catalyzes several coagulation factor activation reactions that lead to fibrin formation, factor XIII activation to promote fibrin cross-linking, and activation and aggregation of platelets. In fact, under these procoagulant conditions, reciprocal, interdependent, and mutually self-amplifying interaction occurs between thrombin generation and platelet activation. Membranes of activated platelets facilitate thrombin generation by providing a surface for the assembly of coagulation factors and cofactors (Fig. 62–11 and described earlier). Conversely, thrombin is a potent activator of platelets, stimulating the availability of additional activated platelet surface for further thrombin generation. Thus, this reciprocal interaction between thrombin and platelets promotes and amplifies the formation of a tightly focused hemostatic plug composed of platelets and fibrin.

At lower concentrations of thrombin and in the presence of intact endothelium, the antithrombotic effects of thrombin predominate (see Fig. 62–10). Low levels of thrombin stimulate increased levels of the endogenous circulating anticoagulant, activated protein C.[90] Accordingly, as shown in Figure 62–12, a J curve describes the relationship between the thrombotic potential of blood and free thrombin concentration.[89] Furthermore, in the presence of normal endothelial cells in the intact circulation (see Fig. 62–10), endothelial thrombomodulin removes free thrombin from blood and low concentrations of thrombin stimulate t-PA release and the release of antiplatelet PGI_2 and NO from endothelial cells. Thus, thrombin plays a central role in modulating the state of blood coagulability, depending on its free concentration in blood and the presence or absence of intact endothelial cells at its site of action.

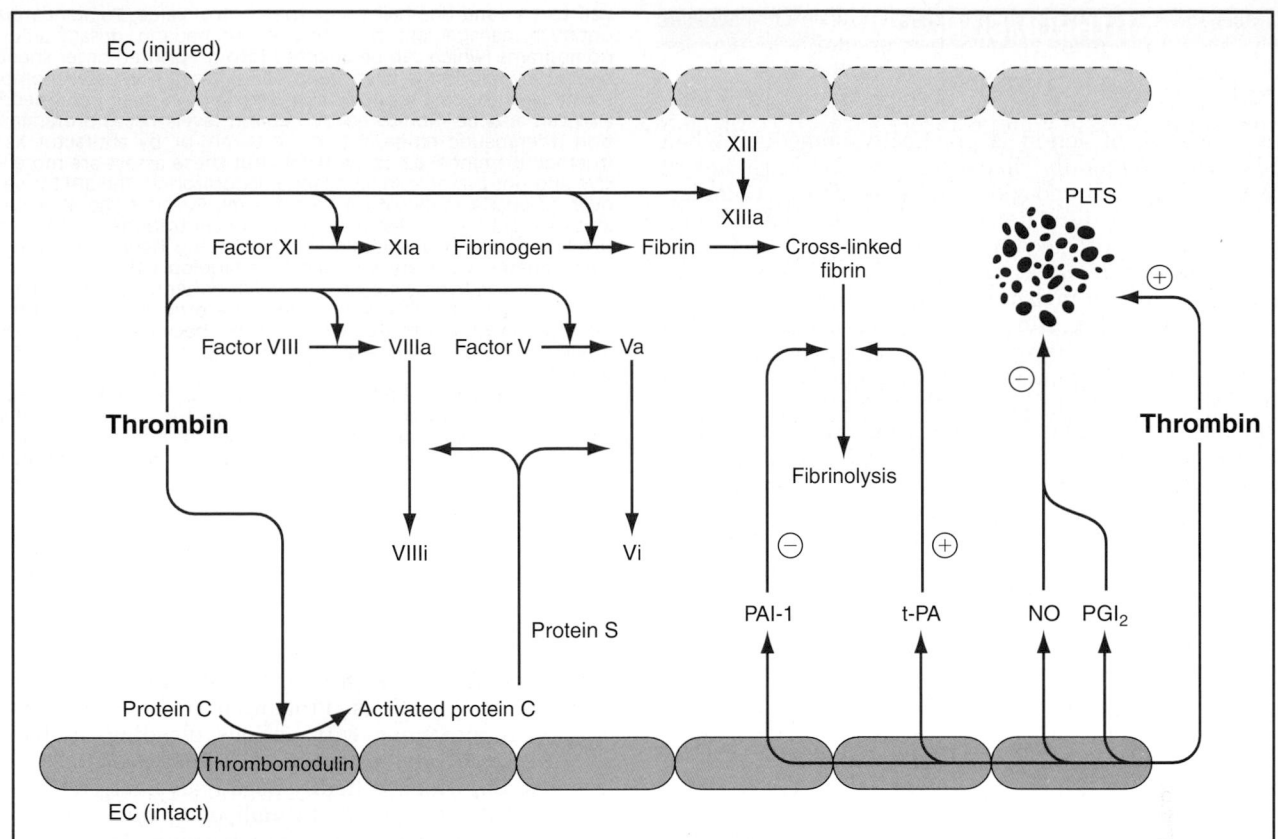

FIGURE 62–10. Central role of thrombin in modulating the state of blood coagulability, depending on the presence or absence of intact endothelial cells (EC) at its site of action. In the presence of intact EC *(lower part of figure),* free thrombin is removed from the circulation by EC thrombomodulin and the antithrombotic effects of thrombin predominate: activation of protein C, release of tissue-type plasminogen activator (t-PA), and release of platelet-inhibitory nitric oxide (NO) and prostaglandin I₂ (PGI₂) by intact EC. In the absence of intact EC *(upper part of figure),* free thrombin is available in blood at higher concentrations and its prothrombotic effects predominate: activation of coagulation factors, fibrin formation and cross-linking, and activation of platelets (PLTS). PAI-1 = plasminogen activator inhibitor-1.

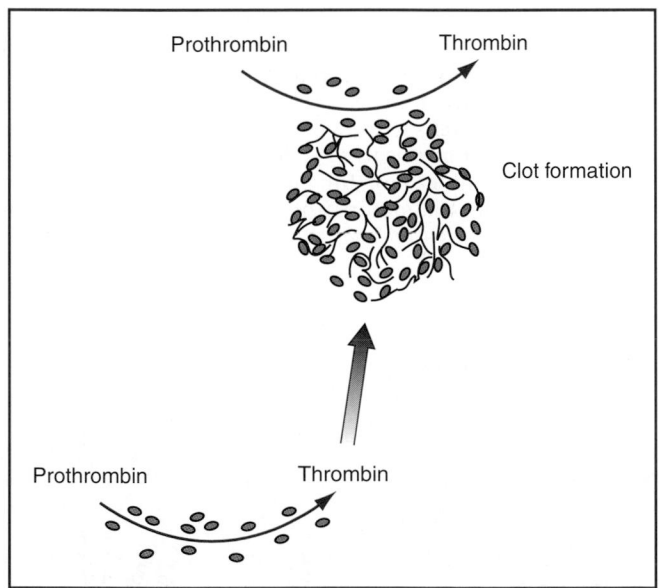

FIGURE 62–11. Reciprocal interaction between thrombin generation and platelet activation. Membranes of activated platelets facilitate thrombin generation by providing a surface for assembly of coagulation factors. Conversely, thrombin is a potent activator of platelets, thus acting to promote and amplify activation of the coagulation system. This reciprocal interaction results in the accelerated and tightly focused formation of a hemostatic plug composed of platelets and fibrin. (From Schafer AI: The primary and secondary hypercoagulable states. *In* Schafer AI [ed]: Molecular Mechanisms of Hypercoagulable States. Austin, TX, Landes Bioscience, 1997, pp 1–48.)

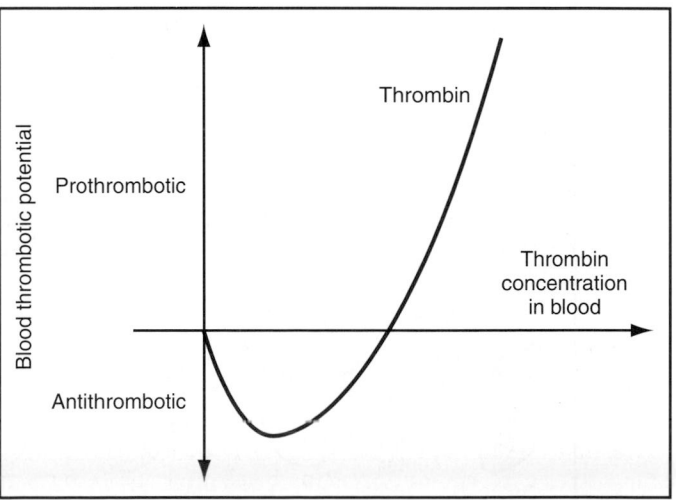

FIGURE 62–12. The thrombin paradox. At low concentrations of thrombin, protein C is activated and elevated activated protein C exhibits antithrombotic activity. At increasingly higher levels of thrombin, the procoagulant properties of thrombin become dominant and prothrombotic potential is markedly increased. (Adapted from Griffin JH: The thrombin paradox. Nature 378:337–338, 1995.)

Heparin

Because its onset of action is practically immediate when administered parenterally, heparin is the anticoagulant of choice when rapid anticoagulation is required.[91] Commercial preparations of unfractionated heparin consist of a heterogenous mixture of glycosaminoglycans, with molecular weights ranging from 3000 to 30,000.[91, 92] However, only about one third of the molecules in these products are anticoagulantly active. Heparin exerts its anticoagulant effect by interacting with antithrombin III (AT), as shown in Figure 62–13. A specific pentasaccharide sequence in heparin accounts for its ability to bind with high affinity to lysine sites on AT. In the absence of heparin, AT binds to and neutralizes thrombin and other activated clotting factors (see earlier) slowly; however, heparin-bound AT undergoes a conformational change that dramatically accelerates its ability to bind to and neutralize these factors. In these reactions, arginine reactive centers in AT bind to the enzyme active center serines of thrombin and other serine protease coagulation factors, thereby inhibiting their activities. Heparin then dissociates from these complexes and can be reused to bind to other AT molecules. Heparin thus acts as a true catalyst in accelerating the neutralization of thrombin and other activated clotting factors by AT.[93] Fibrin-bound thrombin is relatively protected from inactivation by the heparin/AT complex.

Heparin is poorly absorbed from the gastrointestinal tract and therefore must be administered parenterally. The complex pharmacokinetics of unfractionated heparin are due to its nonspecific binding to many plasma proteins (including some acute-phase reactants) and to vascular and blood cells. Provided that the doses used are adequate, the efficacy and safety of heparin are comparable when administered by continuous intravenous infusion or by subcutaneous injection.[94] Intermittent intravenous injections of heparin are associated with more bleeding complications than is continuous intravenous infusion.

HEPARIN MONITORING. Because of unfractionated heparin's often unpredictable pharmacokinetics and its narrow therapeutic range, therapy with this agent requires laboratory monitoring for proper dosing.[95] This is conventionally performed with the activated partial thromboplastin time (aPTT), a test that is sensitive to the inhibitory effects of heparin on thrombin, factor Xa, and factor IXa. For the treatment of deep venous thrombosis or pulmonary embolism, heparin is usually initiated with an intravenous bolus of 5000 U, followed by continuous intravenous infusion of 30,000 to 35,000 U/24 hours that is subsequently adjusted to maintain the aPTT at one and one-half to two and one-half times the control value. To standardize and optimize management with intravenous heparin, dosage-adjustment nomograms (which can be adapted into preprinted order sheets) and computer algorithms have been used. Weight-adjusted nomograms for heparin treatment of unstable angina have been published.[96] Heparin can also be monitored by heparin levels using protamine titration (therapeutic range: 0.2 to 0.4 U/ml), or by antifactor Xa levels (therapeutic range: 0.3 to 0.6 U/ml), but these assays are more expensive and not available in all hospital laboratories. The aPTT is sensitive over a heparin range of 0.1 to 1.0 U/ml. Because the aPTT becomes immeasurably prolonged at heparin concentrations of more than 1.0 U/ml, this test is unsuitable for monitoring heparin dosage during percutaneous coronary interventions (angioplasty and stenting) and during cardiac bypass surgery, in which patients require higher levels of anticoagulation with heparin. In these procedures, heparin can be monitored by the activated clotting time, because this test provides a graded response to heparin concentrations in the range of 1 to 5 U/ml.[91]

Low-dose subcutaneous unfractionated heparin has also been used to prevent (rather than treat) venous thromboembolism in high risk patients. Doses of 5000 U every 8 or 12 hours generally do not prolong the aPTT and therefore do not require monitoring in this setting.

COMPLICATIONS. The major complication of heparin is bleeding. Factors that predispose to increased bleeding risk include advanced age, serious concurrent illness, heavy consumption of alcohol, concomitant use of aspirin, and renal failure.[92] Due to its relatively short half-life, simple discontinuation of heparin is usually adequate to control bleeding complications. Protamine sulfate can be used in emergency situations with serious bleeding. Protamine, a strongly basic protein, practically instantaneously neutralizes heparin, which is highly negatively charged.

Two distinct types of thrombocytopenia are associated with heparin therapy. The more common form, which may occur in up to 15 percent of patients receiving therapeutic doses of heparin, is a benign and self-limited side effect. This dose-dependent, non–immune-mediated type of thrombocytopenia rarely causes severe reductions in the platelet count or clinical complications and usually does not require discontinuation of heparin. In contrast, the rarer, immune form of heparin-induced thrombocytopenia (HIT) can, paradoxically, cause serious, limb- and life-threatening arterial as well as venous thrombosis. The mechanism in these cases is the interaction of antibody (usually IgG) with a complex of heparin and platelet factor 4 (PF4) on the surfaces of platelets from which PF4 is released upon activation.[97, 98] This complex results in the activation of platelets through their FcγIIa receptors and their intravascular aggregation, which may cause apparently paradoxical thrombosis in the presence of thrombocytopenia. In HIT, the platelet count decreases, often precipitously, characteristically 5 to 10 days after starting heparin.

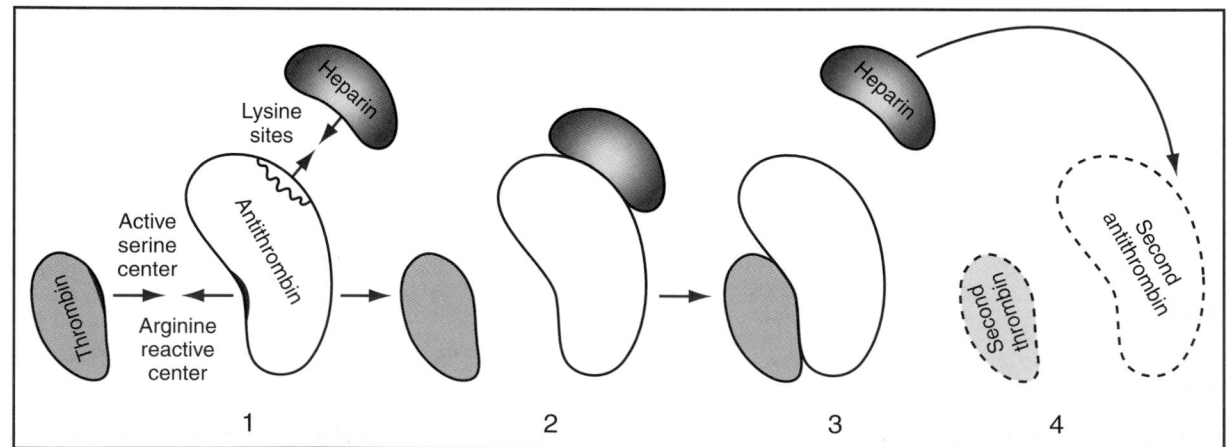

FIGURE 62–13. Mechanism of heparin action. (Modified from Rosenberg RD: Hemorrhagic disorders: I. Protein interactions in the clotting mechanism. *In* Beck WS [ed]: Hematology. 5th ed. Cambridge, MIT Press, 1991, pp 507–542.)

The decline in platelet count in HIT is usually moderate, with a typical nadir of 50,000 to 60,000/mm³. However, HIT can cause severe thrombocytopenia even in the absence of thrombosis; and, conversely, heparin-induced thrombosis can actually occur with a normal platelet count. Immune-mediated HIT is not heparin dose dependent and can develop with low-dose heparin or even with heparin flushes or the use of heparin-bonded catheters. There is no single, definitive laboratory test to ascertain the diagnosis of HIT. Laboratory testing for HIT can involve functional assays in which the heparin-induced activation of platelets in vitro is tested by aggregation, serotonin release, or platelet activation markers.[98] Alternatively, enzyme immunoassays of antibody-heparin-PF4 complexes can be used to test for HIT.[99]

When HIT is suspected, any source or route of heparin being administered to the patient must be discontinued immediately. Because many such patients need continued anticoagulation for the underlying problem that required heparin, alternative treatment may include danaparoid, a mixture of low-molecular-weight anticoagulant glycosaminoglycans with relatively weak cross-reactivity with HIT sera,[100] or a direct thrombin inhibitor such as hirudin[101] or argatroban, a small-molecule synthetic antithrombin.[102] Low-molecular-weight heparins (LMWH) should not be substituted for heparin because they have stronger cross-reactivity with HIT sera.[98, 103]

Other side effects of heparin include cumulative dose-dependent osteoporosis, skin necrosis, alopecia, hypersensitivity reactions, and hypoaldosteronism.[92] Heparin is the anticoagulant of choice during pregnancy; unlike warfarin, it does not cross the placenta and is not teratogenic.

Low-Molecular-Weight Heparins

Low-molecular-weight heparins are manufactured from standard, unfractionated heparin by chemical or enzymatic depolymerization that yields fragments about one-third the size of unfractionated heparin.[104–106] An important mechanism of action of LMWH that presumably provides them with therapeutic and safety advantages over unfractionated heparin is their ability to inhibit and neutralize factor Xa relatively selectively. Inhibition of thrombin requires that heparin bind to both AT and thrombin, thereby forming a ternary complex (Fig. 62–14).[104] Ternary complex formation requires that heparin contain at least 18 saccharide residues, including the high-affinity pentasaccharide sequence that binds to AT. In contrast, inhibition of factor Xa requires that heparin bind only to AT; hence, only the pentasaccharide sequence of heparin is needed for this simpler reaction. Most heparin chains in LMWH preparations have less than 18 saccharide units and therefore are of insufficient length to bind to both AT and thrombin. However, the shorter heparin fragments in LMWH are able to catalyze the inhibition of factor Xa by AT, provided that they contain the essential pentasaccharide sequence. Thus, the effects of LMWH in the coagulation cascade are restricted to relatively selective inactivation of factor Xa, while standard (unfractionated) heparin has equivalent inhibitory activity against factor Xa and thrombin.

LMWH has been considered theoretically superior to standard heparin in several additional ways.[106, 106a] First, unlike unfractionated heparin, it can inhibit platelet-bound factor Xa and therefore should be a more effective anticoagulant. Second, LMWH binds less readily to plasma proteins (including acute phase reactants) and vascular and blood cells, and LMWH is more resistant to neutralization by platelet factor 4; this produces a longer plasma half-life, more predictable bioavailability, and more favorable pharmacokinetics than standard heparin. Third, LMWH has less pronounced effects on platelet function and vascular integrity, properties that presumably contribute to its lower risk of bleeding complications than standard heparin. The longer plasma half-life and more predictable anticoagulant response of LMWH preparations allow their administration as fixed-dose, once-daily or twice-daily subcutaneous injections, without need for laboratory monitoring. The convenience of use of LMWH has been extended to outpatient management of patients with uncomplicated acute venous thromboembolism, a situation that previously required continuous intravenous heparin infusion in the hospital.[105] Although several LMWH preparations have been approved for use in North America and Europe, they are prepared by different depolymerization methods and have somewhat different molecular compositions, pharmacological properties, and anticoagulant profiles.[107] Therefore, caution should be exercised in the interchangeability of these LMWH products.

Many (though not all) studies have shown that LMWH

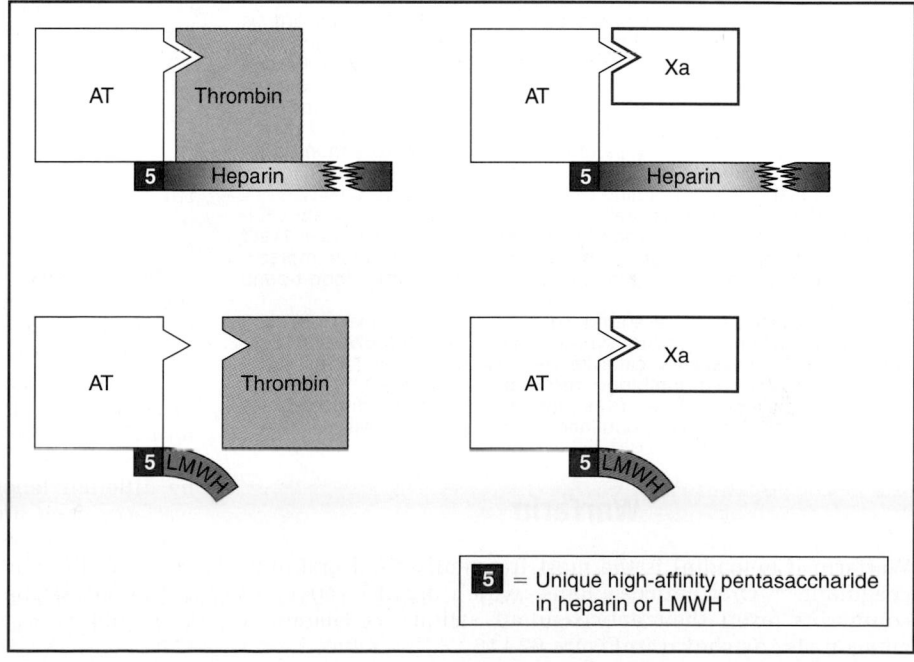

FIGURE 62–14. Mechanisms of inhibitory action of unfractionated heparin (heparin) and low-molecular-weight heparin (LMWH) on thrombin and factor Xa. Both unfractionated heparin and LMWH bind to antithrombin (AT) through a high-affinity pentasaccharide sequence (5) that both types of heparin contain. Inhibition of thrombin (left side of figure) requires formation of a ternary complex of heparin with both antithrombin (AT) and thrombin. Unfractionated heparins have sufficient length (≥ 18 saccharide residues, including the pentasaccharide sequence) to accomplish this, but LMWHs do not. In contrast, inhibition of factor Xa (right side of figure) requires that heparin bind only to AT, which unfractionated heparin and LMWH can catalyze equally effectively through their common pentasaccharide sequences. Thus, LMWH (but not unfractionated heparin) inactivates factor Xa selectively relative to thrombin.

5 = Unique high-affinity pentasaccharide in heparin or LMWH

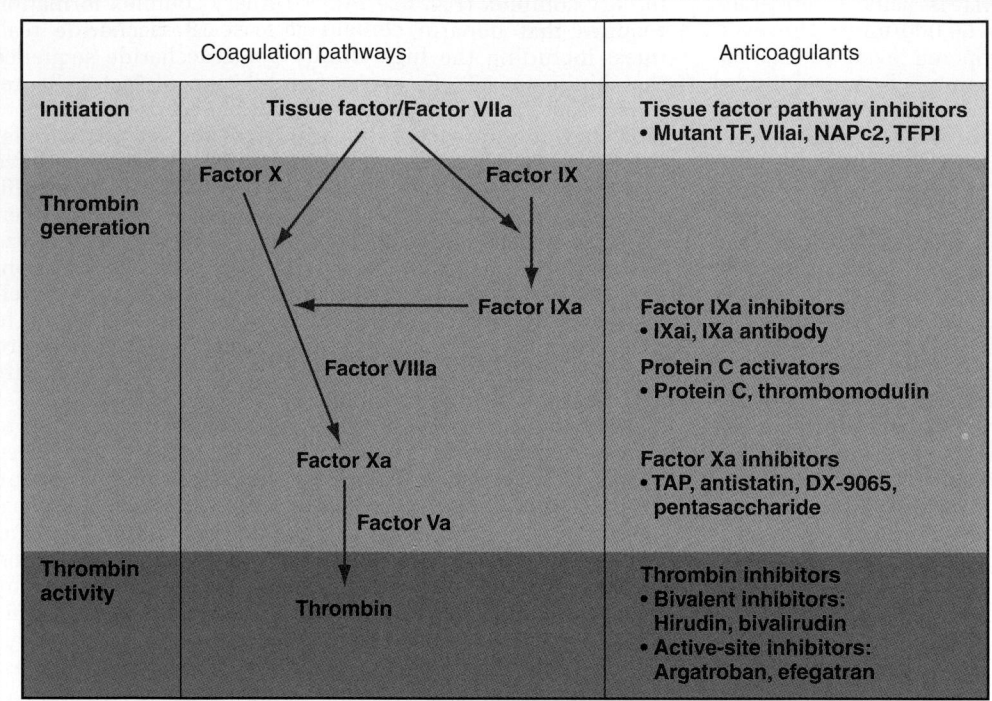

Coagulation pathways		Anticoagulants
Initiation	**Tissue factor/Factor VIIa**	**Tissue factor pathway inhibitors** • Mutant TF, VIIai, NAPc2, TFPI
Thrombin generation	**Factor X** **Factor IX**	
	Factor IXa	**Factor IXa inhibitors** • IXai, IXa antibody
	Factor VIIIa	**Protein C activators** • Protein C, thrombomodulin
	Factor Xa	**Factor Xa inhibitors** • TAP, antistatin, DX-9065, pentasaccharide
	Factor Va	
Thrombin activity	**Thrombin**	**Thrombin inhibitors** • Bivalent inhibitors: Hirudin, bivalirudin • Active-site inhibitors: Argatroban, efegatran

FIGURE 62–15. Activation and inhibitors of coagulation. New anticoagulants act by inhibiting the tissue factor pathway (initiation), thrombin generation, and thrombin activity. (Modified from Hirsh J, Weitz JI: New antithrombotic agents. Lancet 353:1431–1436, 1999.)

are associated with a lower incidence of major bleeding complications than standard, unfractionated heparin. Furthermore, the frequency of immune-mediated HIT is much lower with LMWH.[108] Osteoporosis also occurs less often with long-term administration of LMWH than with standard heparin.[109]

OTHER GLYCOSAMINOGLYCAN-DERIVED DRUGS (NEW HEPARINS)

Heparan sulfate, dermatan sulfate, and proteoglycans are endogenous heparin-like molecules with antithrombotic activity.[110] Several of these endogenous glycosaminoglycans have been developed as clinical anticoagulants.[111, 112]

Danaparoid (Orgaran, formerly ORG 10172) is a mixture of low-molecular-weight anticoagulant glycosaminoglycans, predominantly heparan sulfate (84 percent) and dermatan sulfate (12 percent).[98, 113] It preferentially inhibits factor Xa and has a lesser degree of antithrombin activity. Bioavailability of danaparoid is essentially 100 percent by subcutaneous dosing, and twice-daily administration is required when using this route. Rapid full anticoagulation is better achieved by an initial intravenous bolus.[114] Danaparoid is a weak anticoagulant as measured by the prothrombin time (PT) and aPTT tests. Therefore, laboratory monitoring of danaparoid can only be performed using anti–factor Xa levels. However, in view of the predictable dose-dependent anticoagulant response to danaparoid, laboratory monitoring is not required in most patients. Because danaparoid is excreted largely unchanged into the urine, dose reduction and laboratory monitoring are required in patients with renal failure. A disadvantage of danaparoid is the inability of protamine sulfate to neutralize its activity.

Dermatan sulfate, a naturally occurring glycosaminoglycan, catalyzes the inactivation of thrombin by heparin cofactor II. Like direct thrombin inhibitors (see later), and unlike standard and low-molecular-weight heparins, dermatan sulfate can inactivate fibrin-bound thrombin.[115]

Pentasaccharide, representing the high-affinity heparin binding site for antithrombin, and its synthetic analogs (SR90107A/ORG31540, SANORG 32701) selectively catalyze the inactivation of factor Xa by antithrombin without inhibiting thrombin (Fig. 62–15).[116] Definitive clinical trials will be required to demonstrate the superiority of these and other heparin mimetics obtained by chemical synthesis.[117]

Warfarin

Warfarin (Coumadin) is the most frequently used oral anticoagulant.[118] Oral anticoagulants, which are derivatives of coumarins, exert their anticoagulant actions as vitamin K antagonists. As shown in Figure 62–16,[119] the reduced form of vitamin K, vitamin KH_2, is normally required as a cofactor for the gamma-carboxylation of glutamic acid residues in coagulation factors II (prothrombin), VII, IX, and X. This posttranslational modification of these clotting factors is necessary for them to function physiologically in the coagulation cascade by allowing them to bind to and form calcium-dependent complexes on cellular phospholipid surfaces. Oral anticoagulants block the reductase enzymes that are required to recycle vitamin K epoxide to vitamin KH_2 after the gamma-carboxylation reaction, thereby depleting the active vitamin K cofactor.

Warfarin is rapidly and almost completely absorbed from the gastrointestinal tract and circulates bound to albumin with a mean plasma half-life of approximately 40 hours.[104, 120] Numerous drugs alter the anticoagulant response to warfarin by pharmacokinetic or pharmacodynamic interactions. Drugs such as phenylbutazone, erythromycin, fluconazole, cimetidine, amiodarone, clofibrate, isoniazid, and propranolol increase warfarin levels, whereas drugs such as cholestyramine, barbiturates, rifampin, and sucralfate decrease warfarin levels. Dietary variations in vitamin K likewise alter warfarin's anticoagulant effects; high vitamin K intake in the diet (including nutritional supplements and vitamin preparations) reduces the anticoagulant response to warfarin. Conversely, liver disease, malabsorption, and hypermetabolic states enhance the anticoagulant effect of warfarin.

MONITORING. Oral anticoagulant therapy requires laboratory monitoring with the PT test. Commercially available thromboplastin reagents that are used in the PT assay vary considerably in their clotting ability. This problem previously created major variability in the PT values reported by different laboratories. To standardize PT reporting, the international normalized ratio (INR) is now used. The INR corrects for differences in the thromboplastin reagents used by different laboratories. The optimal therapeutic range of warfarin dose for the prevention of venous thromboembolism and for the prevention of systemic embolism from atrial fibrillation and tissue heart valves targets an INR of 2.0 to 3.0. Higher intensity anticoagulation (INR 2.5 to 3.5) is required in patients with mechanical prosthetic heart valves.

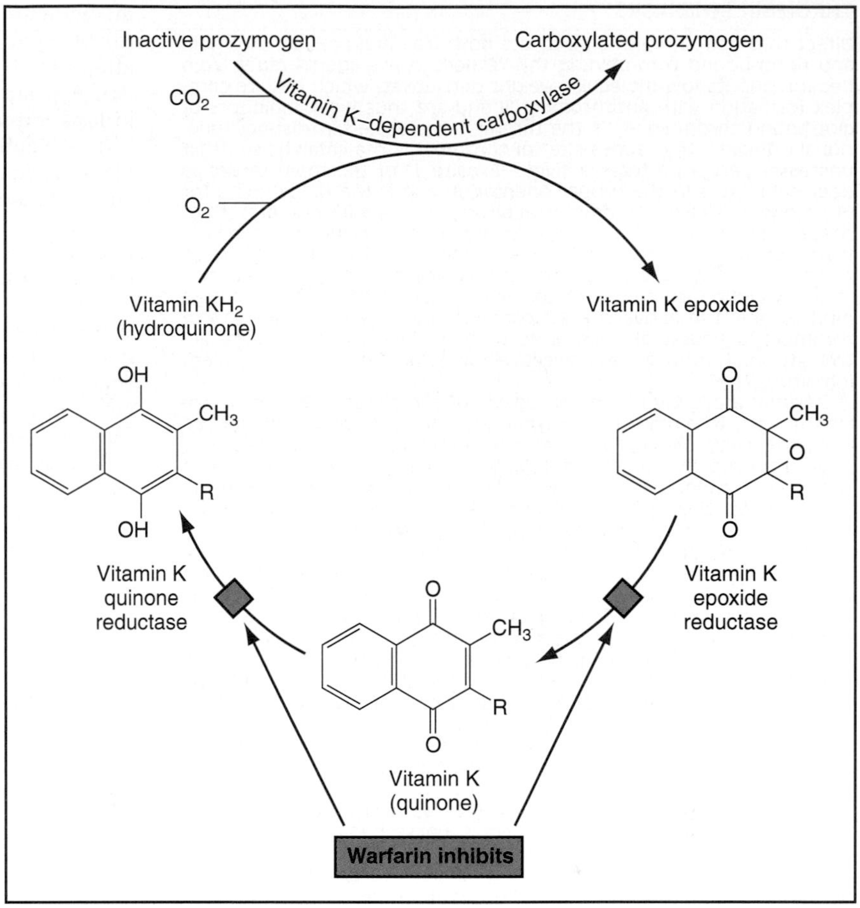

FIGURE 62–16. Vitamin K cycle and its inhibition by warfarin. Warfarin inhibits vitamin K epoxide reductase and vitamin K quinone reductase and so blocks the conversion of vitamin K epoxide to vitamin KH_2. Vitamin KH_2 is a cofactor for the carboxylation of inactive proenzymes (factors II, VII, IX, and X) to their active forms. (From Furie B, Furie BC: Molecular basis of vitamin K–dependent gamma-carboxylation. Blood 75:1753–1762, 1990.)

"Loading doses" of warfarin should not be employed in initiating oral anticoagulation. Although warfarin has a rapid onset of action, its optimal antithrombotic effect requires several days. The activity of all four of the vitamin K–dependent clotting factors must be inhibited to achieve clinically effective anticoagulation. The effects of warfarin require depletion of circulating clotting factors that are already gamma-carboxylated and hence biologically active when warfarin is started. The vitamin K–dependent clotting factors have different half-lives, with factor VII having the shortest. Therefore, the initial increase in the INR is predominantly due to a decrease in functional factor VII. A large "loading dose" of warfarin (i.e., 10 mg or more per day) will thus create a selective, severe factor VII deficiency state, with its attendant bleeding risk, while still failing to provide antithrombotic effect. In addition, a precipitous reduction in the plasma level of protein C, a vitamin K–dependent anticoagulant (rather than clotting) factor, which has the shortest half-life of all vitamin K–dependent proteins, can lead to a transient paradoxical hypercoagulable state during the first 36 hours of warfarin therapy (see later).[121, 122] Therefore, the initial dose of warfarin should approximate the chronic maintenance dose that is anticipated, generally in the range of 4 to 6 mg/d in most adults.[120]

COMPLICATIONS. Skin necrosis is a very rare complication that occurs within the first few days of starting warfarin therapy and tends to occur in patients with underlying inherited protein C or protein S deficiency. As noted earlier, it is likely to be related to the initial precipitous decrease in protein C levels (especially in individuals who may already have a congenitally low level of protein C). This leads to a transient prothrombotic imbalance, particularly with the use of large loading doses of warfarin. Warfarin should be avoided in pregnancy because of its potential to cause embryopathy and peripartum neonatal and maternal bleeding complications.

As with heparin, bleeding complications are the most frequent adverse effects of warfarin. For an individual patient, the cumulative risk of bleeding complications is directly related to the intensity and duration of anticoagulant therapy.[123] Major bleeding on warfarin occurs at a rate of 5 to 7 percent per year.[124] As noted earlier, the INR can vary despite a stable, chronic dose of warfarin as a function of changes in other medications or diet. When the INR exceeds the therapeutic range, discontinuing or reducing the dose of warfarin is usually sufficient; stopping warfarin generally normalizes the INR within about 3 days. If more rapid reversal of warfarin effect is required because of extreme elevations of the INR or clinical bleeding, vitamin K can be administered orally or parenterally. However, particularly when vitamin K is given at higher doses, a transient resistance to re-anticoagulation with warfarin may be encountered subsequently. Emergency reversal of warfarin effect can be rapidly achieved by infusion of fresh frozen plasma (usually starting with 2 to 4 units). Algorithms for the management of elevated INR with or without bleeding have been proposed.[120, 125]

Thrombin Inhibitors and Other Specific Coagulation Inhibitors

New anticoagulants have been developed that specifically target inactivation of thrombin, factor Xa, factor IXa, and the factor VIIa/tissue factor complex, as well as inactivation of factors VIIIa and Va by enhancement of the protein C anticoagulant pathway.[116] The sites of action of these anticoagulants are shown in Figure 62–15. Except for the direct thrombin inhibitors, most of these agents have yet to be evaluated in phase 3 trials.

Direct thrombin inhibitors inactivate both free (fluid-phase) thrombin and fibrin-bound thrombin. In this respect, these agents differ from heparin and its low-molecular-weight derivatives, which require complex formation with antithrombin III and are thus weak inhibitors of clot-bound thrombin.[126–128] The thrombin molecule has distinct functional domains. The "active site" of thrombin is the catalytic site that possesses serine protease activity. "Exosite 1" of thrombin serves to dock substrates in the proper orientation and is the binding site for fibrin(ogen).[129] Direct thrombin inhibitors interact with one or both of these sites. Hirudin and bivalirudin are more specific for thrombin than active-site inhibitors because they are bivalent, binding to thrombin at both the active site and exosite 1. In contrast, low-molecular-weight thrombin inhibitors such as argatroban and efegatran bind to only the active site of thrombin. Because the active site of thrombin is structurally similar to other serine proteases, these active-site inhibitors are less selective for thrombin than the bivalent inhibitors.[116, 128]

Hirudin (desirudin) is the prototype of the direct thrombin inhibitors. It is a 65-amino acid polypeptide that was originally isolated from the saliva of *Hirudo medicinalis*, the medicinal leech. Hirudin is now produced by recombinant DNA technology. It binds tightly to thrombin, forming a slowly reversible, 1:1 stoichiometric complex. In this complex, the amino-terminal of hirudin binds to the active site and its carboxy-terminal binds to exosite 1 of thrombin.

Bivalirudin (formerly Hirulog) is a synthetic 20-amino acid polypeptide. It is composed of a peptide sequence (D-Phe-Pro-Arg-Pro) that is directed at the active site of thrombin, linked to a dodecapeptide analog of the exosite 1–binding carboxy-terminal of hirudin.[130] Thus, like hirudin, bivalirudin interacts bivalently with both the active site and exosite 1 of thrombin, forming a 1:1 stoichiometric complex. However, once bound, thrombin cleaves the Arg-Pro bond and thereby removes the active site binding part of bivalirudin, leaving only a low-affinity, weaker inhibitory interaction with thrombin. Consequently, the potent thrombin inhibitory effect of bivalirudin is short lived, conferring on it a potential safety advantage.

Hirudin, bivalirudin, and other direct thrombin inhibitors have theoretical advantages over heparin. First, as noted earlier, they can inactivate clot-bound thrombin. Second, unlike heparin, they do not bind to plasma proteins. Therefore, they have the pharmacokinetic advantage of a more predictable anticoagulant response. This should permit their administration without laboratory monitoring. However, the narrow therapeutic window for hirudin makes its monitoring necessary and may prove to be a significant limitation. In clinical trials of hirudin, used in conjunction with thrombolytic therapy in patients with acute myocardial infarction, concentrations of hirudin were selected that produced a prolongation of the aPTT similar to that achieved with heparin. The excessive bleeding observed with hirudin in these trials suggests that hirudin causes more bleeding than heparin when these agents are used in doses that prolong the aPTT to the same extent,[131] and it points out the potential pitfalls of extrapolating from the experience of heparin when choosing a laboratory test to monitor a new antithrombotic agent.[126] The better benefit-to-risk profile of bivalirudin appears to permit its administration in weight-adjusted doses without laboratory monitoring.[130]

Several low-molecular-weight direct thrombin inhibitors have been developed. These less-specific agents target only the active site of thrombin. Argatroban is the prototype of the noncovalent class of these active site inhibitors, which also includes napsagatran, inogatran, and melagatran. Efegatran and boroarginine derivatives are reversible-covalent active site inhibitors of thrombin. They serve as pseudosubstrates for thrombin, which are cleaved by thrombin to form a covalent enzyme-inhibitor adduct.[130]

OTHER SPECIFIC COAGULATION INHIBITORS

Inhibitors of factor Xa (see Fig. 62–15)[128, 132] include tick anticoagulant peptide (TAP) and antistatin. Both are potent and specific factor Xa inhibitors that are available in recombinant forms. DX-9065[133] is a synthetic, low-molecular-weight, reversible factor Xa inhibitor that has oral bioavailability. Experimental agents that are inhibitors of factor IXa include a monoclonal antibody and an active site-blocked factor IXa.[134] Specific inhibitors of the tissue factor pathway under study include a soluble mutant form of tissue factor that has decreased cofactor function for factor VIIa–induced activation of factor X[135]; active-site–blocked factor VIIa (VIIai), which competes with factor VII for tissue factor binding; NAPc2, a small, nematode-derived anticoagulant protein that binds to factor X and inhibits factor VIIa within the factor VII/tissue factor complex[136]; and recombinant TFPI.[137] Protein C activators that have been studied as therapeutic anticoagulants include plasma and recombinant forms of protein C and recombinant soluble thrombomodulin.[116]

Thrombolytic (Fibrinolytic) Drugs

The fibrinolytic system has been described previously and is illustrated in Figure 62–7 (see p. 2104). The common mechanism of action of currently available thrombolytic (fibrinolytic) agents, including streptokinase, urokinase, alteplase (recombinant tissue-type plasminogen activator [rt-PA]), and anistreplase (anisoylated plasminogen streptokinase activator complex [APSAC]), involves the conversion of the inactive plasma zymogen, plasminogen, to the active fibrinolytic enzyme, plasmin.[138] Plasmin has relatively weak substrate specificity and can degrade not only fibrin but any protein that has an arginyl-lysyl bond available for enzymatic attack, including fibrinogen. Because indiscriminate plasmin lysis of both fibrin and fibrinogen can produce a systemic state of fibrin(ogen)olysis (or "systemic lytic state"), which might cause a serious systemic bleeding tendency, attempts have been made to develop thrombolytic agents that generate plasmin preferentially at the fibrin surface in a preformed thrombus ("fibrin specific agents"). Plasmin associated with fibrin is protected from rapid inhibition by alpha$_2$-antiplasmin (see earlier) and can thereby effectively degrade the fibrin of a clot.[139] Thus, the biochemical strategy was to develop fibrinolytic agents that bind to fibrin and thereby produce only fibrin-bound plasmin from fibrin-bound plasminogen.

Streptokinase and urokinase induce a systemic lytic state, with extensive systemic activation of the fibrinolytic system, deplete alpha$_2$-antiplasmin, and degrade circulating fibrinogen. In contrast, the physiological plasminogen activators t-PA and scu-PA, as well as staphylokinase, activate plasminogen preferentially at the fibrin surface.[140] The promise of a marked reduction in the risk of hemorrhage with "second generation" fibrin-specific agents has not been fulfilled in large clinical trials, however. This may be due to the inability of plasmin to discriminate between fibrin in pathological thrombi, which is the desired target, and fibrin in physiological hemostatic plugs, the lysis of which will induce bleeding.

Streptokinase

Streptokinase is isolated from hemolytic streptococci and is produced from bacterial cultures. The mechanism of activation of plasminogen by streptokinase is unique among plasminogen activators in that streptokinase itself possesses no enzymatic activity.[141] Streptokinase forms a complex with plasminogen, and it is the streptokinase-plasminogen complex that actually possesses enzymatic activity toward plasminogen. The streptokinase-plasminogen complexes are thereby converted to streptokinase-plasmin complexes, and the enzyme active sites in the streptokinase-plasmin complexes are the same as those in plasmin. The streptokinase-plasmin(ogen) complexes activate circulating and fibrin-bound plasminogen relatively indiscriminately, producing a systemic lytic state.

Because of its bacterial source, streptokinase is antigenic. Most individuals have preexisting antibodies resulting from previous streptococcal infection. The administration of streptokinase stimulates the rapid formation of high titers of neutralizing antistreptokinase antibodies, which are sufficient to neutralize standard doses of streptokinase. Although antibody titers may return to near-baseline levels as early as 2 years after a single dose,[142] once streptokinase has been used then subsequent thrombolytic treatment should be with an immunologically unrelated agent because of the uncertain efficacy of repeated treatment.[140] Streptokinase causes transient hypotension in many patients and significant allergic reactions in some, including a serum sickness-type syndrome, fever, rash, and bronchospasm.[143]

Anisoylated Plasminogen/Streptokinase Activator Complex

Although the streptokinase/plasmin complex possesses high plasmin-generating efficiency, it is rapidly inactivated in plasma by protease inhibitors. This limitation led to the synthesis of anisoylated plasminogen-streptokinase activator complex (APSAC; anistreplase), in which streptokinase is noncovalently associated with plasminogen and the enzyme active site of plasminogen is protected by the covalent addition of a *p*-anisoyl group. APSAC retains the fibrin-binding properties of the streptokinase-plasminogen complex, but it is enzymatically inert. Therefore, when injected intravenously, APSAC circulates to the site of fibrin deposition. APSAC cannot be inactivated by plasma alpha$_2$-antiplasmin because its enzyme active site is inaccessible. Deacylation of fibrin-bound APSAC then uncovers the catalytic center, which converts plasminogen to plasmin. APSAC thereby permits fibrin-targeted thrombolysis.

Compared with streptokinase, APSAC has greater stability in plasma (fibrinolytic half-life of 12 to 18 minutes vs. 40 to 60 minutes), and can be administered rapidly as a single intravenous bolus without hypotension. Like streptokinase, the bacterial origin of APSAC causes immunological complications. Some individuals with preexisting antistreptococcal antibodies demonstrate a blunted fibrinolytic response to APSAC, and high titers of neutralizing antibodies following a single treatment persist for months.[144] As with streptokinase, APSAC can also cause allergic reactions in a small percentage of patients.

Urokinase

Urokinase, or two-chain urokinase-type plasminogen activator (tcu-PA), is a trypsin-like serine protease composed of two polypeptide chains with molecular masses of 20 and 34 kDa, respectively, linked by a disulfide bridge. Urokinase is produced from cultures of human fetal kidney cells. It directly activates plasminogen to plasmin, leading to relatively nonspecific degradation of fibrin, fibrinogen and other plasma proteins, depletion of circulating alpha$_2$-antiplasmin, and a systemic lytic state. Urokinase is not antigenic and does not cause allergic reactions.[138]

Single-Chain Urokinase-Type Plasminogen Activator

Single-chain urokinase-type plasminogen activator (scu-PA; prourokinase) is a naturally occurring 54 kDa protein that is the zymogenic precursor of urokinase; scu-PA is converted to proteolytically active urokinase (two-chain u-PA) by means of limited hydrolysis by plasmin and kallikrein. In plasma, scu-PA is mostly inactive. Although scu-PA does not directly bind to fibrin, it induces plasminogen activation in the presence of fibrin, leading to relative fibrin-specific plasminogen activation. Urokinase-type plasminogen activator receptors (u-PAR) on endothelial cells and leukocytes may also modulate scu-PA fibrinolytic activity. Plasmin generation is enhanced by binding of scu-PA to u-PAR.[141, 145]

Tissue-Type Plasminogen Activator

Tissue-type plasminogen activator (t-PA) is a naturally occurring molecule released from vascular endothelial cells. For therapeutic thrombolysis, it is produced commercially by recombinant DNA technology (rt-PA; alteplase) and, as a "second-generation" agent, it is relatively fibrin specific.

t-PA is a single-chain serine protease composed of 527 amino acids with a molecular mass of 68 kDa. It activates plasminogen directly and follows Michaelis-Menten kinetics.[141] The efficiency of plasminogen activation by t-PA is significantly enhanced in the presence of fibrin. The basis for the relative fibrin specificity of t-PA action is described previously in the section on the fibrinolytic system. Briefly, fibrin provides a surface for the sequential binding of enzyme (t-PA) and substrate (plasminogen). The assembly of this ternary complex thereby promotes the activation of plasminogen to plasmin that is efficiently localized to the

fibrin clot; fibrin then becomes the substrate for lysis by the plasmin that is generated on its surface.

t-PA is converted by plasmin to a disulfide-linked two-chain form by hydrolysis of the Arg 275—Ile276 bond; alteplase consists mainly of the single-chain form of t-PA. Both the single-chain and two-chain forms of t-PA are cleared from plasma according to a two-compartment model, with initial half-lives of 3 to 6 minutes and terminal half-lives of 40 to 50 minutes. The currently preferred dosage regimen of fibrin-selective alteplase for coronary thrombolysis consists of weight-adjusted, accelerated ("front-loaded") administration. The front-loaded administration of alteplase achieves a mean steady-state plasma concentration during the initial 30 minutes that is 45 percent higher than that achieved with standard infusion, although it does not alter the plasma half-life.[141, 146]

VARIANTS, CHIMERAS, AND CONJUGATES OF PLASMINOGEN ACTIVATORS

These thrombolytic agents have been engineered to favorably alter the pharmacokinetic and functional properties of currently used drugs. They are designed to have prolonged half-lives, improved enzymatic efficiency, enhanced local concentrations in the clot by altered binding to fibrin and stimulation by fibrin, and resistance to plasma protease inhibitors.[140, 141, 147] Several of these agents have begun to undergo clinical trial.[148]

Reteplase (r-PA) is a single-chain nonglycosylated deletion variant of t-PA, containing only the kringle-2 and serine protease domains. This deletion mutant has a prolonged half-life and, therefore, can be administered by bolus injection.[149] A mutant of rt-PA, TNK-rt-PA, contains amino acid substitutions at three sites: threonine (T) at position 103 is replaced by asparagine; asparagine (N) at position 117 is replaced by glutamine; and four amino acids, lysine (K), histidine, arginine, and arginine, are replaced by alanine-alanine-alanine-alanine at positions 296 through 299. TNK-rt-PA is characterized by a prolonged half-life, improved fibrin specificity, and increased resistance to inhibition by PAI-1.[150] Another third-generation agent that is a modification of wild-type t-PA is lanoteplase (n-PA), which has an even longer half-life than TNK-rt-PA and can be administered by single-bolus, weight-adjusted injection.[151] Prolonged half-lives have also been obtained by substitution or deletion of one or more selected amino acids in the finger or epidermal growth factor domains of t-PA.[140, 147] One of these t-PA variants is E6010, in which Cys is replaced by Ser at position 84; it possesses a half-life of 23 minutes or more after a single intravenous bolus. The t-PA of saliva from the vampire bat *Desmodus rotundus* (bat-PA) has potent and relatively fibrin-specific thrombolytic properties.[152, 153] Different molecular forms of bat-PA have been purified, characterized, cloned, and expressed.

Antibody targeting of thrombolytic agents is a potentially powerful approach to localizing the actions of these drugs to specific components of different types of thrombi (e.g., directed at platelet antigens in arterial thrombi, or thrombin in recently formed thrombi). This can be achieved by conjugating plasminogen activators with monoclonal antibodies that are specific, for example, for fibrin but do not cross react with fibrinogen.[154] These bifunctional molecules are engineered to contain both a highly specific antigen-binding site that concentrates the drug at the clot and an effector site that promotes thrombolysis.

STAPHYLOKINASE

Staphylokinase[155–157] is isolated from *Staphylococcus* species. Like streptokinase, it forms a 1:1 stoichiometric complex with plasminogen. Unlike the streptokinase-plasminogen complex, however, the staphylokinase-plasminogen complex is enzymatically inactive; it must be converted to staphylokinase-plasmin to become a potent plasminogen activator. Also unlike streptokinase-plasmin(ogen), the staphylokinase-plasmin complex is rapidly neutralized in the circulation by alpha$_2$-antiplasmin. After inhibition by alpha$_2$-antiplasmin, staphylokinase is released from the complex and is recycled to bind other plasminogen molecules. The relative fibrin selectivity of staphylokinase resides in the ability of fibrin to largely (> 100-fold) protect it from inhibition by alpha$_2$-antiplasmin. As a bacterial plasminogen activator, staphylokinase is an antigenic thrombolytic agent that induces antibody formation and resistance to repeated administration.

Antiplatelet Agents

The sequence of events involved in the process of platelet activation is described in detail in the previous section on platelets and is summarized in Figures 62–8 (p. 2105) and 62–17. Inhibition of platelet function can be targeted at any

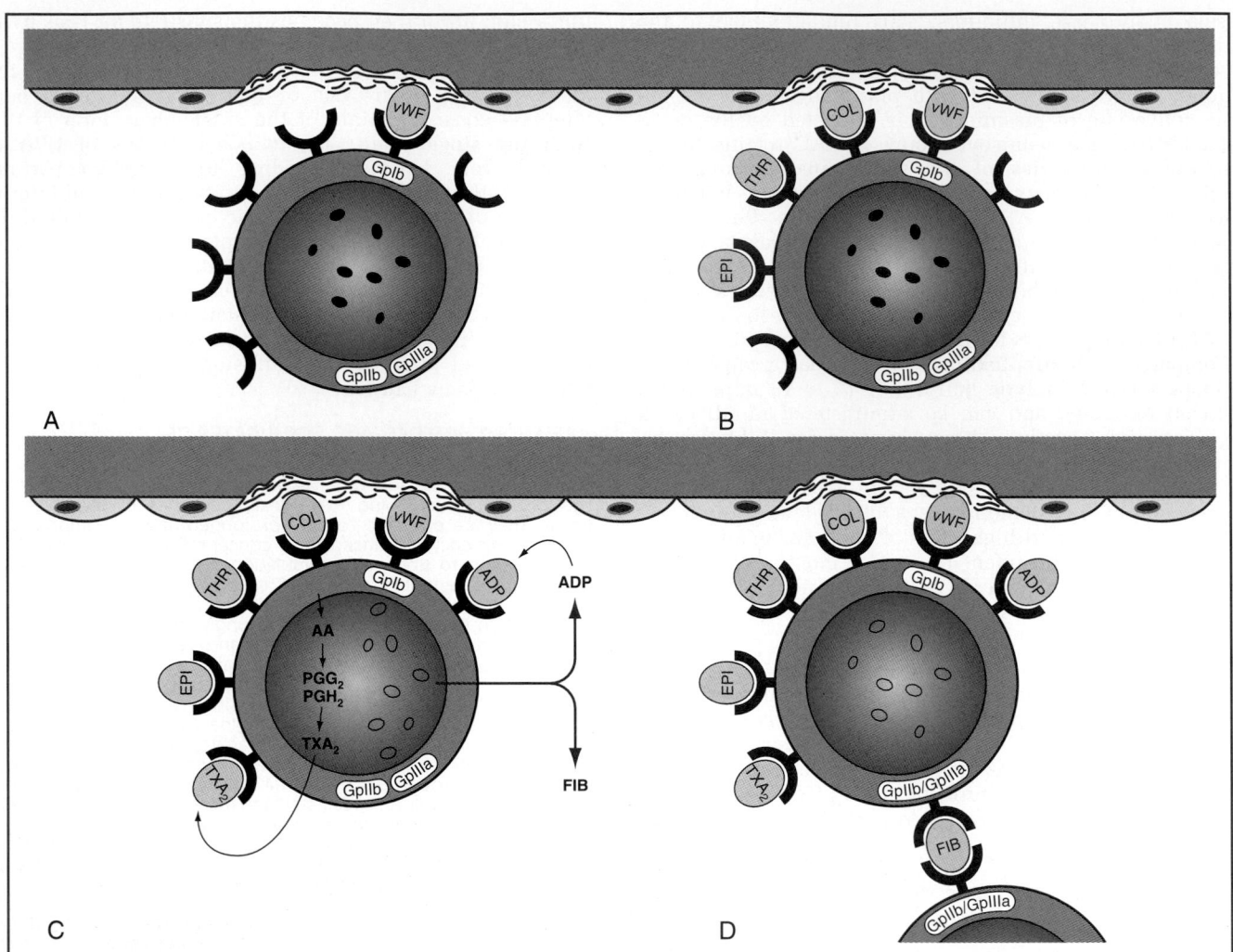

FIGURE 62–17. Sequence of events in platelet activation, with potential targets for antiplatelet therapy. *A,* Platelet adhesion to the injured vascular intimal surface is mediated by von Willebrand factor (vWF) binding to its receptor on platelet membrane Gp Ib. *B,* Adherent platelets are also anchored to the damaged vessel wall by binding of subendothelial collagen (COL) to its platelet surface COL receptors. Other platelet stimuli in blood, including thrombin (THR) and epinephrine (EPI), bind to their respective receptors. *C,* In response to these different stimuli, adherent platelets are activated and release thromboxane A_2 (TXA$_2$) and adenosine diphosphate (ADP), which bind to their own respective platelet receptors and amplify the activation process. AA = arachidonic acid; PGG$_2$ and PGH$_2$ = labile prostaglandin endoperoxides. *D,* Platelet aggregation is mediated by fibrinogen (FIB) binding to its receptors on adjoining platelets, forming fibrinogen bridges. The FIB receptor is formed by the complexing of Gp IIb/IIIa in the membrane of activated platelets. (Modified from Schafer AI: Antiplatelet therapy with glycoprotein IIb/IIIa receptor inhibitors and other novel agents. Tex Heart Inst J 24:90–96, 1997.)

one of these activation steps. Platelet blockade would be expected to be most effective if it is directed at either the initial (adhesion) (see Fig. 62–17*A*) or final (aggregation) (see Fig. 62–17*D*) points in the sequence. Antiplatelet agents targeted at any one of the intermediate events should be less potent, because platelet adhesion is followed by the binding of several specific agonists to their respective receptors and the activation of several simultaneous intracellular pathways (e.g., ADP release, TXA$_2$ synthesis) that act in concert to induce the final step of platelet aggregation. Therefore, pharmacological interruption of only one of these intermediate steps (e.g., with aspirin, antithrombins, ticlopidine, clopidogrel) may permit platelet activation through alternative, uninhibited pathways. Agents that block the interaction of vWF with its platelet membrane Gp Ib receptor should inhibit adhesion (see Fig. 62–17*A*) as well as the subsequent downstream cascade of platelet activation events, including secretion of mitogens into the vessel wall and platelet aggregation.[158] Therapeutic approaches to inhibit adhesion could involve anti-vWF or anti-Gp Ib

monoclonal antibodies or agents that interfere with vWF-platelet Gp-Ib binding. These strategies have yet to be translated to clinical practice, however. In contrast, considerable clinical evidence has now validated various powerful therapeutic strategies to block the final step of platelet aggregation that is mediated by the interaction of fibrinogen (or vWF) with its platelet Gp IIb/IIIa receptors (see Fig. 62–17*D*).

Aspirin

Aspirin (acetylsalicylic acid), which has been used medicinally since antiquity and has been demonstrated to have antithrombotic efficacy for almost 50 years, has stood the test of time as an effective, inexpensive, and relatively safe drug for the prevention of various thrombotic and vascular disorders, particularly in the arterial circulation where platelets are the predominant participants in the thrombotic process.[159, 159a] Until recently, aspirin has been essentially the only available, clinically effective antiplatelet drug. However, there are several clinical settings in which aspirin

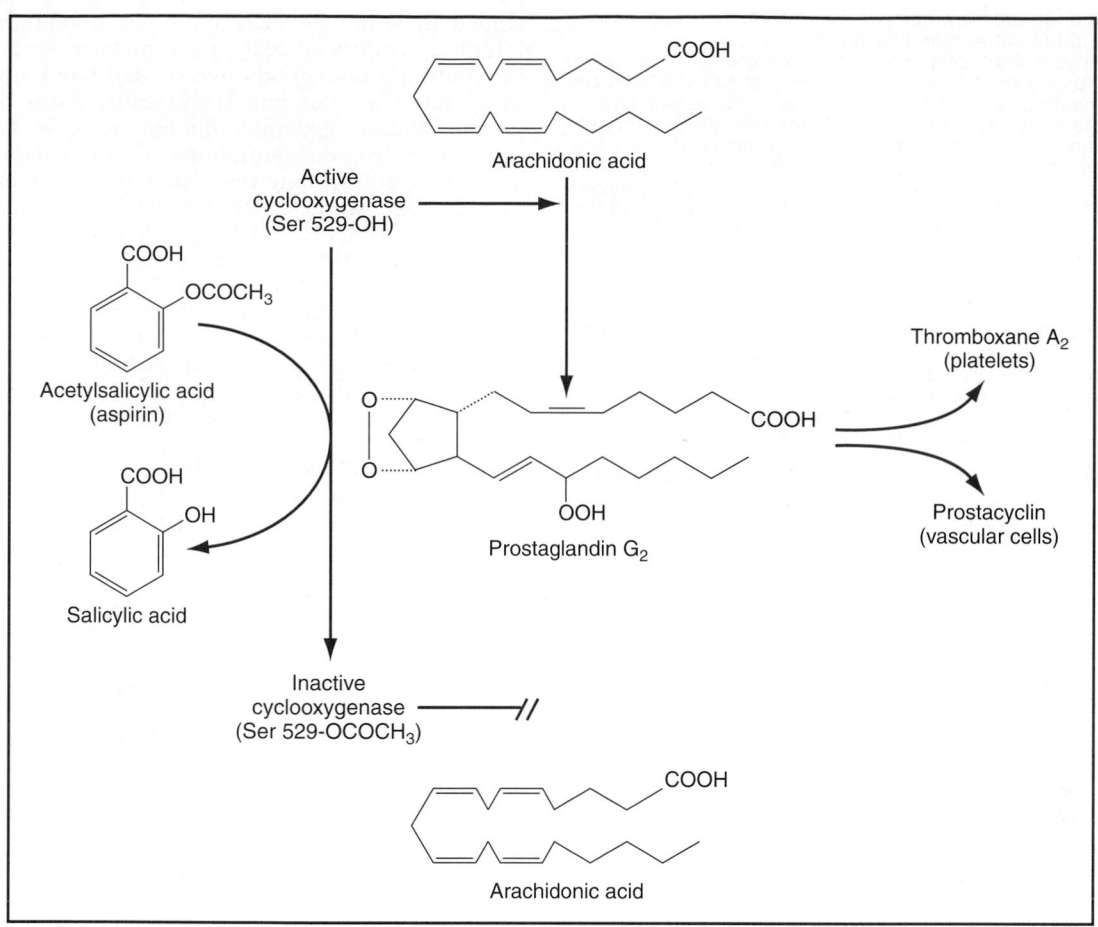

FIGURE 62–18. Aspirin (acetylsalicylic acid) inhibition of cyclooxygenase (prostaglandin-G/H synthase). Aspirin acetylates serine at position 529 of cyclooxygenase, rendering the enzyme inactive. Acetylated cyclooxygenase does not function to catalyze the oxygenation of arachidonic acid to prostaglandin G_2. Aspirin thereby blocks the formation of thromboxane A_2 (in platelets) and prostacyclin (in vascular cells). (From Loscalzo J, Schafer AI: Anticoagulants, antiplatelet agents, and fibrinolytics. *In* Loscalzo J, Creager MA, Dzau MV [eds]: Vascular Medicine: A Textbook of Vascular Biology and Diseases. Philadelphia: Lippincott Williams & Wilkins, 1996.)

fails to provide full (or even partial) antithrombotic benefit.[160]

Aspirin is readily absorbed from the stomach and upper small intestine and is then hydrolyzed to release free acetyl groups. As shown in Figure 62–18, this moiety acetylate serine residues at position 529 of cyclooxygenase (COX; prostaglandin G/H synthase), which leads to irreversible inactivation of the enzyme.[161, 162] Inactive, acetylated COX is unable to function to catalyze the oxygenation of arachidonic acid to prostaglandin G_2. Aspirin thereby blocks the formation of TXA_2, a potent mediator of platelet aggregation and vasoconstrictor. Because anucleate platelets are essentially unable to synthesize new, unacetylated COX, aspirin blocks the function of platelets exposed to it for their remaining lifetime (normally 7 to 10 days) in the circulation. This accounts for the lengthy therapeutic effect of aspirin despite its plasma half-life of only 20 minutes.

The inhibitory effects of aspirin on platelet TXA_2 production and ex vivo aggregation are rapid, with maximal effects achieved within 15 to 30 minutes of oral administration of a dose as low as 81 mg.[163] A single oral dose of 100 mg of aspirin almost completely suppresses platelet TXA_2 synthesis in both normal individuals and in patients with cardiovascular disease. Daily administration of only 30 to 50 mg of aspirin exerts a cumulative effect and likewise results in almost complete inhibition of platelet TXA_2 production within 7 to 10 days.[159] These aspirin effects on platelet TXA_2 formation generally correlate well with inhibition of ex vivo platelet aggregability and prolongation of the skin bleeding time. Although platelet function remains

impaired for 4 to 7 days after a single dose of aspirin, reflecting the life span of irreversibly inhibited platelets, the prolonged bleeding time generally returns to normal within 24 to 48 hours of aspirin ingestion: This discrepancy is due to the release from bone marrow into the circulation of a sufficient cohort of uninhibited platelets after the elimination of aspirin from blood to restore normal in vivo hemostasis (bleeding time) even before complete normalization of ex vivo platelet function.

Aspirin also inhibits COX in vascular endothelial cells, leading to suppression of platelet inhibitory and vasodilatory endothelium-derived PGI_2; this would be expected to offset the antiplatelet effects of aspirin. Attempts to design "platelet selective" aspirin regimens have not translated to clinical feasibility. Nevertheless, there is ample evidence that the antithrombotic effects of aspirin predominate in vivo, possibly due to mechanisms in addition to platelet TXA_2 inhibition.[161]

NON-ASPIRIN NONSTEROIDAL ANTIINFLAMMATORY DRUGS (NSAIDS)

Non-aspirin NSAIDs likewise inhibit COX. Unlike aspirin, however, these other NSAIDs are reversible inhibitors of the enzyme; and, therefore, their durations of TXA_2 and platelet inhibitory action are dependent on the clearance of the drugs from the circulation.[164] Thus, there is considerable variability in the extent and duration of the effects of various NSAIDs on ex vivo platelet aggregation and bleeding time prolongation.[164] Non-aspirin NSAIDs reversibly inhibit COX by preventing its arachidonic acid substrate from gaining access to the active site of the enzyme.[165] Interaction of NSAIDs with COX may prevent acetylation of the enzyme by aspirin. This suggests that the concomitant administration of non-aspirin NSAIDs may actually antagonize the effects of aspirin on COX by competitive interaction, and consequently blunt aspirin's antiplatelet efficacy.[166]

The constitutive isoform of COX, COX-1, is the one that is present in platelets and produces TXA_2. Aspirin and the traditional NSAIDs are nonselective inhibitors of both COX-1 and COX-2. The newer COX-2-specific inhibitors are designed to maximize the antiinflammatory effects that are mediated by the COX-2 isoform, while minimizing the common side effects (e.g., bleeding) that are attributed to the COX-1 isoform. Therefore, the antiplatelet potency of the new COX-2 inhibitors is several orders of magnitude lower than that of aspirin and the standard NSAIDs[167, 168] and generally cannot be assumed to afford antithrombotic protection.[169]

OTHER THROMBOXANE INHIBITORS

Figure 62–17C illustrates other opportunities to interrupt platelet TXA_2 synthesis and/or action in addition to COX blockade. The reduced incidence of atherosclerotic cardiovascular disease in Greenland Eskimos has been attributed, at least in part, to their diets rich in fish oils containing omega-3 polyunsaturated fatty acids. A major omega-3 fatty acid in fish oils is eicosapentaenoic acid (EPA), which incorporates into cell membrane phospholipids and competes with arachidonic acid as substrate for COX. The product of EPA oxygenation is TXA_3, an eicosanoid that is devoid of the potent platelet activating and vasoconstrictor actions of arachidonic acid–derived TXA_2. Large and often unpalatable doses (> 10 gm EPA daily) of medicinal fish oils are required to simulate changes in platelet membrane fatty acid content attained with Eskimo diets and thereby produce antiplatelet actions.[158] Thromboxane synthase inhibitors (e.g., dazoxiben) and TXA_2 receptors antagonists, as well as dual thromboxane synthase/TXA_2 receptor inhibitors (e.g. ridogrel), have been developed but have generally not been found to be superior to aspirin in limited clinical trials.[158, 170]

Ticlopidine and Clopidogrel

Ticlopidine (Ticlid) and clopidogrel (Plavix) are structurally related thienopyridine derivatives. They produce their antiplatelet effects by inhibiting the ADP-dependent pathway of platelet activation.[171] After oral administration, both drugs apparently require modification to active forms. They exert a permanent effect on a platelet protein(s),[162] which is the ADP receptor itself or a platelet membrane component closely related to the ADP receptor. As ADP receptor blockers, these drugs inhibit ADP-induced platelet aggregation (see Fig. 62–17C).

Presumably because they must be converted to an active form in vivo, ticlopidine and clopidogrel have a relatively slow onset of antiplatelet action, which may make them less than optimal agents in clinical settings where rapid effect is desired (e.g., unstable angina). Full platelet inhibitory effect is achieved only 3 to 5 days after oral administration of ticlopidine, and the bleeding time does not become maximally prolonged until 5 to 6 days after starting treatment. Regimens involving bolus administration of these thienopyridines may accelerate their antiplatelet effects. The effect of ticlopidine on platelets persists for 4 to 8 days after discontinuation of the drug, reflecting the circulating lifetime of platelets and consistent with an irreversible antiplatelet effect.

Severe neutropenia, which is usually reversible with discontinuation of the drug, has been noted in up to 1 percent of patients on ticlopidine. The risk of this adverse effect is much lower (about 0.1 percent) with clopidogrel. (See also Chapter 67.) In addition, thrombotic thrombocytopenic purpura (TTP), a serious and sometimes fatal disorder, is a rare complication of therapy with ticlopidine. TTP typically occurs within 2 to 8 weeks of initiation of ticlopidine[172] and has been noted in 0.02 percent of patients receiving ticlopidine after coronary stenting.[173, 173a] More recently, TTP has also been reported after the initiation of clopidogrel therapy, often within the first two weeks of treatment.[173a] Other side effects, including gastrointestinal symptoms, pruritus, urticaria, and bleeding, also appear to occur less often with clopidogrel than with ticlopidine.[171]

Dipyridamole

The mechanism of antiplatelet action of dipyridamole is unclear. Although this drug has been previously demonstrated to stimulate PGI_2 synthesis, potentiate the platelet inhibitory effects of PGI_2, raise platelet cyclic AMP levels by inhibiting phosphodiesterase, and block uptake of adenosine into vascular and blood cells, these potential antiplatelet actions generally do not occur at therapeutically achievable drug concentrations.[158] Unlike aspirin, dipyridamole does not prolong the bleeding time or inhibit ex vivo platelet aggregation at therapeutic doses. Although numerous clinical trials have failed to demonstrate antithrombotic efficacy of dipyridamole when it is used alone in any clinical setting, it may enhance the effect of warfarin in preventing systemic embolization from mechanical heart valve prostheses and add to the beneficial effect of aspirin in preventing the progression of peripheral occlusive arterial disease or, when used in a sustained release preparation, in the secondary prevention of ischemic stroke.[174]

Glycoprotein IIb/IIIa Antagonists

Regardless of the stimulus for their activation, the aggregation of platelets is finally regulated through their membrane binding sites for fibrinogen in the Gp IIb/IIIa receptor complex (see Fig. 62–17D). This provides the rationale for pharmacological intervention directed against the platelet Gp IIb/IIIa complex.[175, 176] The role of the platelet Gp IIb/IIIa complex in platelet activation is discussed in more detail earlier in the section on platelets. Because Gp IIb/IIIa antagonists do not block TXA_2 production by activated platelets,[177] concomitant use of aspirin may enhance their antithrombotic efficacy.

Platelet Gp IIb/IIIa antagonists generally belong to one of the following classes: (1) monoclonal antibody against Gp IIb/IIIa; (2) peptide (peptidomimetic) antagonists, many of which contain the RGD sequence that can compete with fibrinogen for its Gp IIb/IIIa binding site; and (3) nonpeptide (nonpeptide-mimetic) antagonists of Gp IIb/IIIa. Three drugs currently available for coronary intervention or acute coronary syndromes represent the prototypes for these groups: Abciximab (c7E3 Fab, ReoPro) is a monoclonal antibody, eptifibatide (Integrilin) is a peptide antagonist, and tirofiban (Aggrastat) is a nonpeptide mimetic. These agents are approved for intravenous administration, but numerous oral Gp IIb/IIIa antagonists are currently under development and in phase II trials for chronic antiplatelet therapy.[175, 178, 179] Although the mechanism of action of these agents (i.e., inhibition of ligand binding to the receptor) is similar, it should not be assumed that they react at the same site within the receptor or that the consequences of their binding to Gp IIb/IIIa are identical.[179] Monoclonal antibody has a relatively extended duration of antiplatelet action, whereas the peptides and nonpeptide mimetics have a shorter elimination half-life.

Abciximab is the Fab fragment of a monoclonal antibody to Gp IIb/IIIa that has been humanized (mouse/human chimera) to reduce immunogenicity.[180] Abciximab is not specific to platelet Gp IIb/IIIa: It cross reacts with the related integrin, $alpha_v$-$beta_3$, the vitronectin receptor that is present on vascular cells. This cross reactivity was originally considered to be of potential therapeutic benefit in the prevention of coronary restenosis and inhibition of thrombin generation.[181, 182] Abciximab is presently administered as an intravenous bolus followed by infusion for 12 to 24 hours for coronary interventions.[175] Because abciximab is derived from an antibody, concern has been raised about repeat administration. However, initial data indicate that readministration is safe and efficacious and that the same indications for first-time use can apply to subsequent readministration.[183]

Eptifibatide is a synthetic cyclic heptapeptide that contains a modified lysine-glycine-aspartic acid (KGD), rather than RGD, sequence that recognizes the binding site of platelet Gp IIb/IIIa[184] (see Fig. 62–9). The rationale for eptifibatide is that the substitution of a single lysine (K) for arginine (R) makes this agent specific for the platelet Gp IIb/IIIa integrin. Whether this is an advantageous or disadvantageous property (see earlier) has yet to be definitely determined. Eptifibatide is administered by bolus intravenous injection followed by infusion for up to 72 hours in acute coronary syndromes.[175] Patients who undergo coronary interventions are usually continued on eptifibatide infusion for 18 to 24 hours after intervention. Eptifibatide is not immunogenic and is safe for repeated administration.[185]

Tirofiban (Aggrastat) is a nonpeptide mimetic. In contrast to the RGD (or KGD) peptidomimetics, which inhibit platelet aggregation by binding competitively to the RGD recognition site of Gp IIb/IIIa, the nonpeptides mimic the geometric, stereotactic, and charge characteristics of the RGD sequence.[88]

The clinical development of oral Gp IIb/IIIa antagonists has proven to be challenging.[88a] A major problem has been the question of optimal inhibition and monitoring of platelet function. Although 80 percent Gp IIb/IIIa blockade has been found to be effective and relatively safe with brief intravenous administration of the currently available agents in a controlled hospital environment, appropriate dosing of oral agents for chronic therapy remains problematic. Interindividual variability of response to chronic inhibition may be caused by genetic polymorphism of the Gp IIb/IIIa complex. Rapid, simple laboratory monitoring of Gp IIb/IIIa antagonist therapy will be required,[186, 187] and "therapeutic range" of inhibition of platelet function may have to be established for long-term administration. Chronic oral Gp IIb/IIIa blockade with certain agents may also be complicated by a paradoxical prothrombotic effect due to partial agonist effects at certain doses.[188]

COMPLICATIONS. Bleeding complications with currently approved intravenous platelet Gp IIb/IIIa antagonists have primarily involved vascular access puncture sites in patients undergoing percutaneous intervention. Reduction and weight-adjustment in adjunctive heparin dosing in patients undergoing coronary interventions have reduced the incidence of these bleeding problems. No increase in intracerebral hemorrhage has been observed with the Gp IIb/IIIa antagonists. Therefore, the need for platelet transfusion to treat life-threatening bleeding is extremely rare, particularly with the short-acting agents eptifibatide and tirofiban.[175] Severe thrombocytopenia (platelet count $<20,000/\mu l$) occurs in 0.1 to 0.5 percent of patients treated with the intravenous agents, and the incidence appears to be slightly higher with abciximab.[175, 179] There may be more than one mechanism for thrombocytopenia: A precipitous decrease in platelet count may occur within 1 to 2 hours of initial exposure, or there may be a significant decline several days after initiation of therapy.

ANTITHROMBOTIC AND THROMBOLYTIC THERAPY IN CARDIOVASCULAR DISEASE

Primary Prevention of Ischemic Heart Disease

Three major trials have now evaluated the potential benefits of aspirin and/or warfarin in the primary prevention of ischemic heart disease. Two trials, the United States Physicians' Health Study[189] and the British Doctors' Trial,[190] compared aspirin therapy with placebo. The ultimate design of the Thrombosis Prevention Trial was a 2 × 2 factorial design comparing warfarin with placebo and comparing aspirin with placebo.[191]

ASPIRIN. In the Physicians Health Study, over 22,000 healthy male physicians were treated with either aspirin (325 mg every other day) or placebo for 5 years. Although treatment with aspirin reduced the risk of a first myocardial

infarction by 44 percent, the absolute risks of myocardial infarction in both aspirin and placebo groups were low (0.2 percent/year and 0.4 percent/year, respectively). This reduction in myocardial infarction risk was manifest only in those 50 years of age or older, and hemorrhagic stroke and gastrointestinal bleeding tended to occur more frequently in those treated with aspirin. There was no difference in the incidence of cardiovascular mortality, the primary study endpoint.

In the British Doctors' Trial,[190] 5139 male physicians were randomized to take either aspirin (500 mg daily in most cases) or to avoid aspirin. After 6 years of therapy, there was no difference in the rates of myocardial infarction or cardiovascular death. Disabling strokes were more common in those treated with aspirin. When the Physicians' Health Study and the British Doctors' Trial are considered together, aspirin therapy resulted in a 32 percent reduction in nonfatal myocardial infarction and a 13 percent reduction in any vascular event, although there was no difference in total cardiovascular death and there was a trend toward increased risk of nonfatal stroke.[192]

In one arm of the Thrombosis Prevention Trial,[191] approximately 4000 men aged 45 to 69 years at high risk for the development of ischemic heart disease were randomized to either aspirin (75 mg daily of controlled-release formulation) or placebo. Aspirin therapy reduced the incidence of nonfatal myocardial infarction by 32 percent, corresponding to an absolute reduction of 2.3 events/1000 person-years. There was no reduction in fatal myocardial infarction. Overall stroke rates were similar, although there tended to be more hemorrhagic strokes in those treated with aspirin.

The previous three trials enrolled only men, and as of yet there are no randomized data examining aspirin therapy in women for primary prevention. The results of three prospective observational studies and one case-control study of aspirin in women have yielded conflicting results.[193] Two studies showed a reduced incidence of myocardial infarction, one showed no effect on ischemic heart disease, and one showed no effect on acute myocardial infarction but an increased risk of overall ischemic heart disease. The ongoing Women's Health Study, in which 40,000 women are randomized to either aspirin (100 mg every other day) or placebo, should yield important information on the role of aspirin for primary prevention of ischemic cardiac events in women.

WARFARIN. In the other arm of the Thrombosis Prevention Trial design, patients were treated with either warfarin (target INR 1.5) or placebo. Warfarin therapy reduced the incidence of nonfatal myocardial infarction by 10 percent, fatal myocardial infarction by 39 percent, and the combined endpoint of ischemic cardiac events by 21 percent. There tended to be more hemorrhagic and all-cause strokes, as well as a greater incidence of aortic aneurysm rupture, in those treated with warfarin. The all-cause mortality rate was reduced by warfarin therapy by a statistically significant 17 percent.

In patients who received both warfarin and aspirin therapy, nonfatal and fatal myocardial infarctions were reduced 35 percent and 29 percent, respectively, when compared with placebo therapy. This reduction was, however, accompanied by an increase in hemorrhagic and fatal strokes. Of note, approximately half of all patients in the Thrombosis Prevention Trial had withdrawn from treatment by the time the study was completed. Figure 62–19 displays the results of the Thrombosis Prevention Trial for the four treatment groups (placebo, aspirin alone, warfarin alone, aspirin plus warfarin).

RECOMMENDATIONS. Although aspirin therapy does appear to reduce the incidence of nonfatal myocardial infarction in men, the absolute reduction is extremely modest (two to five events per 1000 subjects per year), has only been shown to be of benefit in those at least 45 to 50 years old, and may be accompanied by a small increased risk of hemorrhagic stroke. Therefore, it is difficult to recommend the widespread use of aspirin for the primary prevention of myocardial infarction. Aspirin therapy may have some modest benefit in selected higher risk patients older than 45 to 50 years. The utility of aspirin in the primary prevention of myocardial infarction in women is at present unresolved, and recommendations regarding its use must await the results of the Women's Health Initiative.

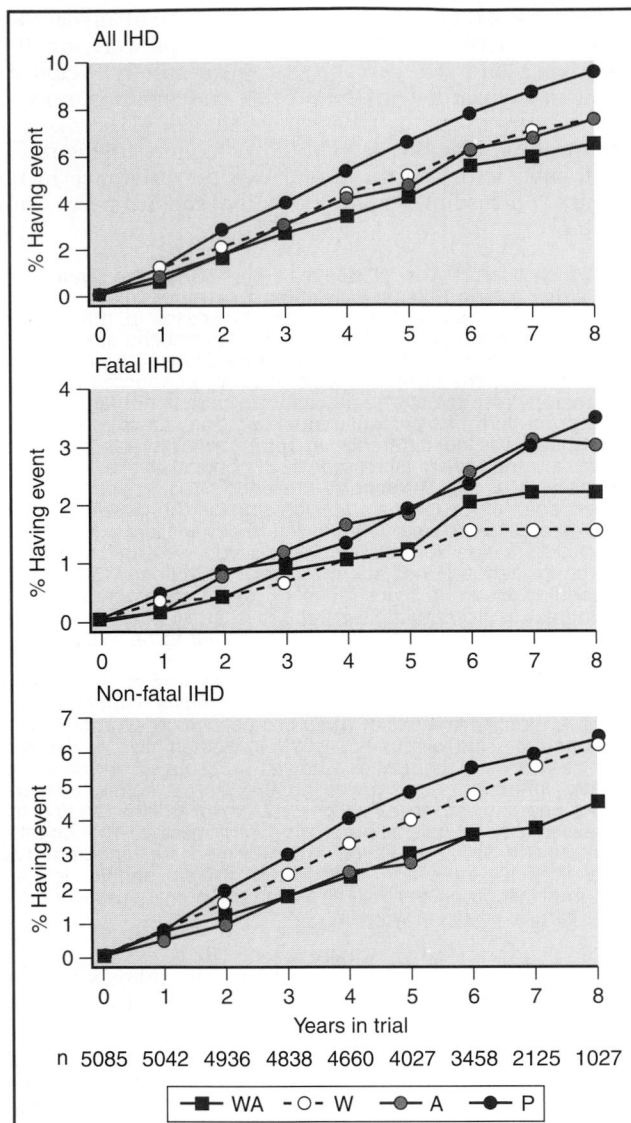

FIGURE 62–19. Cumulative proportion of men in the four treatment groups (WA = warfarin + aspirin; W = warfarin; A = aspirin; P = placebo) with fatal or nonfatal myocardial infarction (All IHD), fatal myocardial infarction (Fatal IHD), or nonfatal myocardial infarction (Nonfatal IHD). (From Medical Research Council's General Practice Research Framework: Thrombosis prevention trial: Randomized trial of low-intensity oral anticoagulation with warfarin and low-dose aspirin in the primary prevention of ischemic heart disease in men at increased risk. Lancet 351:238, 1998.)

Warfarin therapy in high-risk male subjects does lead to a reduction in the risk of myocardial infarction and overall mortality. However, as with aspirin therapy, the absolute reductions are modest (three ischemic cardiac events and one death per 1000 men per year) and this benefit appears to be accompanied by a small risk of serious adverse events. Combination warfarin and aspirin therapy may lead to the greatest reduction in ischemic cardiac events, but it may also be accompanied by an increased risk of hemorrhagic and fatal stroke. Furthermore, as suggested by the results of the Thrombosis Prevention Trial, many patients will discontinue treatment over time, owing to bleeding or other factors. The modest benefits in absolute terms of warfarin or combination therapy must therefore be balanced by physicians and patients against the small but real risks of bleeding and the inconveniences of anticoagulation monitoring.

Secondary Prevention of Ischemic Heart Disease (See also Chap. 37)

ANTIPLATELET AGENTS FOR SECONDARY PREVENTION. The fissuring of atherosclerotic plaque with subsequent platelet deposition and activation of the coagulation cascade are key events in the pathogenesis of acute coronary syndromes. Thus, antiplatelet agents and anticoagulants are useful therapeutic strategies for prevention of vascular events in patients with stable or unstable angina as well as post-myocardial infarction.[194–200]

The 1994 Antiplatelet Trialists' Collaboration is a meta-analysis of the effect of prolonged antiplatelet therapy on prevention of vascular events including myocardial infarction, stroke, and cardiovascular death.[201] This overview included over 70,000 high-risk patients with known atherosclerotic disease. Among these categories, about 20,000 patients were post-myocardial infarction, 10,000 were post stroke or transient ischemic attack (TIA), 4000 had unstable angina, and 16,000 were in the other vascular disease categories (e.g., stable angina, percutaneous transluminal coronary angioplasty). The absolute reduction of vascular events for every 1000 patients treated was 40 events in patients with myocardial infarction treated for 2 years, 40 events in patients with previous strokes treated for 3 years, 50 events in patients with unstable angina treated for 6 months, and 20 events in patients belonging to the other vascular disease categories treated for 1 year (Fig. 62–20). This benefit was separately statistically significant in middle-aged and older patients, men and women, hypertensive and normotensive patients, and diabetic and nondiabetic patients. Doses of aspirin in the range of 75 to 325 mg/d were as effective as higher doses of aspirin or other antiplatelet regimens in this meta-analysis. The reader is directed to a review of individual randomized trials of antiplatelet therapy for secondary prevention of vascular events in patients post-myocardial infarction.[202]

Since publication of the 1994 Antiplatelet Trialists' Collaboration overview, the Clopidogrel versus Aspirin in Patients at Risk of Ischemic Events (CAPRIE) trial has addressed secondary prevention in patients with vascular disease.[203] This trial enrolled 19,185 patients with atherosclerotic vascular disease manifested as either recent ischemic stroke, recent myocardial infarction, or symptomatic peripheral arterial disease to a regimen of clopidogrel (75 mg once daily) or aspirin (325 mg once daily). The study had initially planned to enroll 15,000 patients with 5000 patients in each of the major subgroups of vascular disease. However, the sample size had to be increased partly because of a lower than expected incidence of the composite endpoints in the active control or aspirin group. The primary endpoint of reduction in vascular events defined as ischemic stroke, myocardial infarction, or cardiovascular death occurred in 5.32 percent of patients assigned to clopidogrel and 5.83 percent of patients assigned to aspirin after a mean follow-up of 1.91 years ($p = 0.043$, relative risk reduction of 8.7 percent). Although the overall endpoint was slightly in favor of clopidogrel, the subgroup of patients enrolled with previous myocardial infarction did not have a reduction in the composite endpoint, which occurred in 5.03 percent of patients on clopidogrel and 4.84 percent of patients on aspirin. There were no major differences in adverse effects between the two agents. The incidence of neutropenia was only 0.1 percent, unlike in previous large trials with ticlopidine, a congener of clopidogrel. However, the rather modest benefit of clopidogrel for prevention of vascular events when compared with aspirin presently makes its major indication for patients who are intolerant to or have true aspirin allergy. The mechanism for inhibition of platelet aggregation is different for the two agents, with clopidogrel working through the ADP pathway and aspirin working through the thromboxane pathway. Thus, combination therapy may have the potential for synergistic clinical benefit. This strategy is being explored in ongoing clinical trials.

ANTICOAGULANTS FOR SECONDARY PREVENTION. The value of long-term oral anticoagulation with warfarin in survivors of acute myocardial infarction remains unresolved after more than five decades of clinical research. The early trials such as the Working Party on Anticoagulant Therapy in Coronary Thrombosis (MRC) and the Veterans Administration Cooperative long-term therapy study (VA Coop) performed in the 1950s to 1970s suggested relative reduction in mortality of 10 to 30 percent as well as significant reduction in reinfarction, venous thrombosis, and embolic events.[204, 205] This efficacy was at the cost of an increase in both total and serious bleeding complications (an absolute increase in total bleeding events by 8 to 15 percent over 5 years). These trials were the basis for long-term

Category of trial	No. of trials with data	MI, Stroke, or Vascular Death		O-E	Variance	Odds ratio and confidence interval (antiplatelet: control)	% Odds reduction (SD)
		Antiplatelet	Adjusted controls				
Prior MI	11	1331/987 (13.5%)	1693/9914 (17.1%)	−158.5	561.6		25% (4)
Acute MI	9	992/9388 (10.6%)	1348/9385 (14.4%)	−177.9	−510.3		29% (4)
Prior stroke/TIA	18	1076/5837 (18.4%)	1301/5870 (22.2%)	−98.5	386.5		22% (4)
Other high risk	104	784/11434 (6.9%)	1058/11542 (9.2%)	−134.0	−352.5		32% (4)
All high risk (four main categories)	142	4183/36536 (11.4%)	5400/36711 (14.7%)	−568.8	1810.9		27% (2)
All low risk (primary prevention)	3	652/14608 (4.46%)	708/14604 (4.85%)	−28.5	273.5		10% (6)
All trials (high or low risk)	145	4835/51144 (9.5%)	6108/51315 (11.9%)	−597.3	2084.4		25% (2)

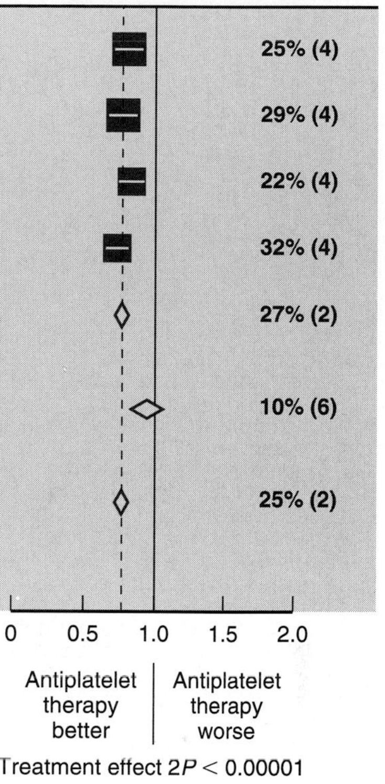

0   0.5   1.0   1.5   2.0

Antiplatelet therapy better | Antiplatelet therapy worse

Treatment effect 2P < 0.00001

FIGURE 62–20. Prevention of death, myocardial infarction (MI), and stroke by prolonged antiplatelet therapy. SD = standard deviation; TIA = transient ischemic attack. (From Antiplatelet Triallists' Collaboration. Collaborative overview of randomised trials of antiplatelet therapy—1: Prevention of death, myocardial infarction, and stroke by prolonged antiplatelet therapy in various categories of patients. BMJ 308:81–106, 1994.)

anticoagulant therapy after myocardial infarction as standard of care (Fig. 62–21 and Table 62–1). The decline in the use of oral anticoagulants in the late 1970s and 1980s was related to the results of the German-Austrian Aspirin (GAMIS) and the Enquête de Prévention Secondaire de L'Infarctus du Myocarde (EPSIM) trials, suggesting that benefits of a magnitude similar to those derived from oral anticoagulants can be realized by chronic treatment with aspirin.[194, 206]

The GAMIS trial randomized 946 patients who had survived a myocardial infarction for 30 to 42 days to aspirin (1.5 gm/d), phenprocoumon, or placebo. Total mortality after 2 years of follow-up was lower but not statistically significant in the aspirin group (8.5 percent) than in the placebo (10.3 percent) and phenprocoumon (12.1 percent) groups. Similar reductions in cardiovascular death and myocardial infarction were observed in the aspirin group compared with either oral anticoagulation or placebo groups but failed to reach statistical significance. The EPSIM trial enrolled 1303 patients to a treatment of either aspirin or oral anticoagulants for secondary prevention after myocardial infarction. After a mean follow-up of 29 months there was identical mortality between the two groups. The incidences of total and severe bleeding were increased in the anticoagulant arm, with rates of 16 percent versus 5 percent and 3 percent versus 1 percent, respectively. The aspirin group was associated with a higher incidence of gastritis and peptic ulceration. These two trials shifted the pendulum in favor of aspirin for secondary prevention of vascular events in survivors of myocardial infarction at least in North America.

The Warfarin-Aspirin Reinfarction Study (WARIS) trial revived the debate of the benefits of long-term oral anticoagulation after myocardial infarction.[207] The trial randomized 1214 patients to a regimen of warfarin (target INR of 2.8 to 4.8) versus placebo for an average treatment period of 37 months. The total mortality based on intention-to-treat was reduced from 20 to 15 percent, a relative risk reduction of 24 percent with warfarin therapy. When the analysis was

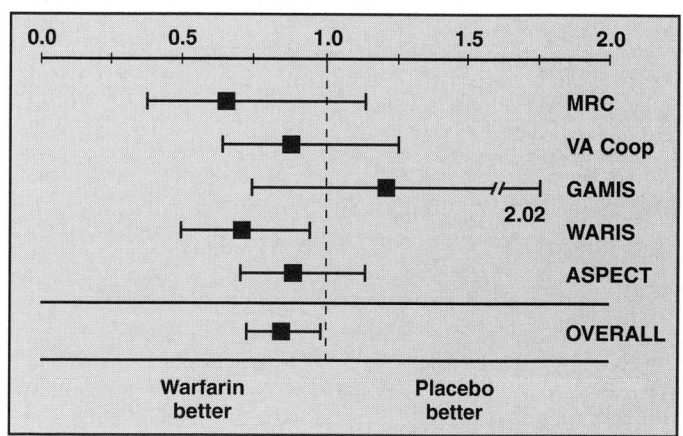

FIGURE 62–21. Long-term therapy with warfarin (Coumadin) in survivors of MI. The figure shows the odds ratio with 95 percent confidence interval for mortality comparing warfarin versus placebo in the major randomized trials spanning over four decades. Pooling of data from all trials shows a significant but modest overall treatment benefit. (From Loscalzo J, Schafer AI [eds]: Thrombosis and Hemorrhage. 2nd ed. Baltimore, Williams & Wilkins, 1998, p 1320.)

▼ TABLE 62–1. LONG-TERM COUMADIN THERAPY IN SURVIVORS OF MYOCARDIAL INFARCTION (MI): RESULTS OF MAJOR RANDOMIZED TRIALS

STUDY	YEAR	NO. RANDOMIZED	TARGET INR	WEEKS AFTER MI*	YR OF FOLLOW-UP	INR IN TARGET RANGE (%)
MRC[204]	1955–60	383	2.0–2.5	4–6	4	60
VA Coop[205]	1957–60	739	2.0–2.5	3	5	82
GAMIS[194]	1970–77	626	2.5–5.0	4–7	2	62–75
WARIS[207]	1983–86	1214	2.8–4.8	4	5	75
ASPECT[208]	1986–91	3404	2.8–4.8	2	3	74

*Enrollment time = weeks after MI.
INR = International normalized ratio.
From Loscalzo J, Schafer AI (eds): Thrombosis and Hemorrhage. 2nd ed. Baltimore, Williams & Wilkins, 1998, p 1320.

based on patients actually receiving treatment, striking reductions in mortality (35 percent), reinfarction (43 percent), and cerebrovascular accident (61 percent) were observed. The magnitude of survival benefit afforded by warfarin in this trial was larger than that possible with the use of aspirin alone after myocardial infarction. The investigators attributed the lower mortality to the greater degree of anticoagulation achieved (higher target INRs) and to maintaining a higher proportion of patients in the therapeutic range compared with earlier trials of oral anticoagulation.

The Anticoagulation in the Secondary Prevention of Events in Coronary Thrombosis (ASPECT) trial was initiated before the publication of the WARIS trial.[208] The results of this trial were thus crucial to confirm the magnitude of benefits of oral anticoagulants suggested by the WARIS trial. The ASPECT trial randomized 3404 hospital survivors of myocardial infarction to anticoagulant (target INR 2.8 to 4.8) or placebo treatment within 6 weeks of discharge. During a mean follow-up of 37 months, total mortality was reduced by 10 percent, a difference that was not statistically significant. However, significant reductions of recurrent myocardial infarction by 53 percent, cerebrovascular events by 40 percent, and all vascular events by 35 percent were observed. This efficacy on secondary endpoints was at the cost of 3.87-fold increase in bleeding events with anticoagulation.

Because aspirin and oral anticoagulants mediate their antithrombotic effect through different pathways, the potential for additive or synergistic clinical benefit when the two agents are combined was explored in the Coumadin Aspirin Reinfarction Study (CARS) and in the Combination Hemotherapy and Mortality Prevention (CHAMP) trial.[209, 210] The CARS trial was designed to evaluate whether a combination of low-dose warfarin and low-dose aspirin would reduce vascular events compared with aspirin monotherapy without excessive bleeding risk in patients with previous myocardial infarction. The trial randomized 8803 patients to daily therapy with (1) aspirin (160 mg), (2) warfarin (3 mg) with aspirin (80 mg), or (3) warfarin (1 mg) with aspirin (80 mg). The design reflects the observational data that high doses of aspirin in combination with standard anticoagulation (target INR of 2.5 to 4.5) predisposes patients to an unacceptably high rate of bleeding complications, predominantly gastrointestinal. There were no significant reductions in the incidence of vascular events defined as reinfarction, nonfatal ischemic stroke, or cardiovascular death at 1 year between the groups (8.6 percent, 8.4 percent, and 8.8 percent, respectively). This lack of difference in benefit was associated with a significant increase in spontaneous bleeding complications in the 3 mg warfarin plus 80 mg aspirin group (1.4 vs. 0.7 percent, $p = 0.014$). The CARS trial provides compelling evidence that a combination of low fixed-dose warfarin with 80 mg of aspirin does not provide clinical benefit beyond that achievable with 160-mg aspirin monotherapy. The results of the CHAMP trial also have not demonstrated any benefit of the combination of warfarin and aspirin in comparison with aspirin alone. In summary, the meta-analysis of both antiplatelet and oral anticoagulant trials as well as the more recent combination hemotherapy study demonstrate reductions in all-cause mortality and recurrent myocardial infarctions and cerebrovascular accidents with these agents.

RECOMMENDATIONS. All survivors of myocardial infarction should be treated with aspirin, 160 to 325 mg daily The magnitude of benefit in most survivors of myocardial infarction with oral anticoagulant alone or in combination with aspirin over and above aspirin monotherapy does not appear large enough to justify the increased rate of nonfatal major hemorrhage and the greater cost and complexity associated with their use. However, patients who develop atrial fibrillation, congestive heart failure, mobile mural thrombus, or systemic/pulmonary embolism after myocardial infarction may benefit from oral anticoagulant therapy.

Acute Coronary Syndromes and ST Segment Elevation Myocardial Infarction

Antiplatelet, anticoagulant, and fibrinolytic therapy have become a mainstay of the modern management of acute myocardial infarction. These important therapies are discussed in the chapter on acute myocardial infarction (see Chap. 35).

Prevention of Cardiac Chamber and Prosthetic Valvular Thromboembolism

PREVENTION OF LEFT VENTRICULAR THROMBOEMBOLISM AFTER MYOCARDIAL INFARCTION (See also Chap. 35). The underlying substrate for ventricular mural thrombus formation is multifactorial and probably related to a combination of regional myocardial akinesis/dyskinesis, abnormal endocardial surface, aberrant blood flow dynamics associated with low cardiac output, and concomitant atrial fibrillation. The early short-term anticoagulation studies such as the MRC, Bronx Municipal Hospital study, and VA Cooperative study in aggregate demonstrated an absolute reduction in mortality (4.2 percent) and thromboembolism (7.9 percent) with early heparinization soon after the diagnosis of acute myocardial infarction followed by oral anticoagulation.[202, 212–214] However, changing practices of the care of patients with acute myocardial infarction, such as the advent of coronary care units, thrombolytic therapy, aspirin use, and early mobilization of patients, have challenged the applicability of these early trials to contemporary practice.

The earlier observations that anterior myocardial infarctions are associated with a higher incidence of mural thrombi have been validated by the predischarge echocardiographic observations of the 8326-patient Gruppo Italiano per lo Studio della Sopravivenza nell'Infarto Miocardico-3 (GISSI-3) trial.[215] Although the overall incidence of thrombi in patients at low to medium risk for left ventricular (LV) thrombus formation (patients with severe pump failure and Killip class IV were excluded) was 5.1 percent, the incidence in patients with anterior myocardial infarction was 11.5 percent compared with 2.3 percent for patients with myocardial infarction at other sites ($p < 0.0001$). In addition, patients with LV ejection fraction (LVEF) less than 40 percent had a higher incidence of ventricular thrombi (10.5 percent) compared with those with an EF greater than 40 percent (4 percent).

In a serial echocardiographic study of 99 consecutive patients with anterior wall infarction, Mooe and coworkers observed a 44 percent incidence of LV thrombi during hospitalization and a 30 percent incidence at discharge.[216] Repeat echocardiogram at 1 month, 3 months, and 12 months after hospital discharge showed that the thrombi had resolved in 81 percent, 84 percent, and 90 percent of the patients, respectively. Oral anticoagulants were used in 24 percent of patients and did not enhance the resolution of thrombi at 1 month. Patients with LV thrombi during the hospital stay had more extensive myocardial dysfunction and significantly higher mortality during the follow-up period of over 3 years than those without thrombi (23 vs. 7 percent, $p < 0.01$).

In an observational analysis of 2231 patients post-myocardial infarction enrolled in the Survival and Ventricular Enlargement (SAVE) trial the rate of stroke was 1.5 percent per year of follow-up.[217] The independent risk factors for cerebral thromboembolic event included a lower EF (for every decrease of 5 percentage points in the EF there was an 18 percent increase in the risk of stroke), older age, and the absence of aspirin or anticoagulant therapy (administered on a non-randomized basis). There was an 81 percent reduction in risk of stroke with anticoagulation in this trial. (This was not a specified endpoint of this trial of angiotensin-converting enzyme inhibitor administration on mortality post-myocardial infarction.) This reduction was of greater magnitude than the reduction in stroke observed in either the ASPECT (39 percent) or the WARIS (55 percent) trials. The use of aspirin was associated with a 56 percent risk reduction for cerebrovascular accidents in the SAVE trial. The limitations of this study include the lack of data on the intensity of anticoagulation and the fact that therapy with aspirin and anticoagulant agents was not randomly assigned.

Randomized trials of high-dose subcutaneous heparin versus placebo during the hospital stay in patients with acute myocardial infarction have shown that this therapy is effective at reducing the formation of LV thrombi by 50 to 66 percent.[218-220] However, these trials had an adequate sample size only to evaluate the surrogate endpoint of resolution of LV thrombi with active treatment and should not be taken as evidence of benefit in preventing thromboembolic or vascular events.

RECOMMENDATIONS. Oral anticoagulation with warfarin should be used in patients with large anterior myocardial infarction for 3 to 6 months at a target INR of 2 to 3. Although it is prudent to use oral anticoagulant in patients with protruding or mobile LV thrombi, the routine administration in all patients after acute myocardial infarction must await further clarification.[220]

DILATED CARDIOMYOPATHY (See also Chap. 48). Patients with LV systolic dysfunction due to either ischemic or nonischemic dilated cardiomyopathy are at risk of developing both arterial and venous thromboembolic events.[221] The presence of regional wall motion abnormality, of poor contractility creating areas of relative stasis, of concomitant atrial fibrillation, and of chronic hypercoagulable state are factors that predispose to thromboembolism in these patients.[222] The incidence of thromboembolic events has ranged from 37 to 50 percent in older autopsy studies.[223] However, when clinically apparent events are evaluated, the incidence has been much lower. Fuster and coworkers observed 3.5 clinically apparent embolic events per 100 patient-years in a retrospective analysis of 104 patients with nonischemic dilated cardiomyopathy.[224] In a prospective follow-up of 264 patients with dilated cardiomyopathy, Katz and coworkers observed that the incidence of stroke was 1.7 per 100 patient-years.[225] In a more recent retrospective analysis by Natterson and coworkers of 224 patients awaiting cardiac transplantation, an arterial embolization rate of 3.2 per 100 patient-years was observed.[226]

The observational analysis of the factors predisposing to mortality and cerebral thromboembolism in the large prospective heart failure trials evaluating the use of angiotensin converting enzyme inhibitors (V-HEFT, SOLVD, and SAVE) has been published.[217, 227-229] Although these trials are not directly comparable to those of patients with dilated cardiomyopathy, the factors predisposing to thromboembolic events for patients with chronically depressed LV systolic function are relevant. These studies, which are elaborated here, have the following limitations: (1) The oral anticoagulant or antiplatelet regimens were not randomly allocated, (2) the intensity or the duration of anticoagulation is unknown, and (3) the number of patients on aspirin alone or warfarin alone is not available from the data base.

The observational analysis of the Veterans Affairs Vasodilator-Heart Failure Trials (V-HEFT I and II) included 642 men with heart failure who were followed for an average of 2.28 years (V-HEFT I) and 804 men were followed for an average of 2.56 years (V-HEFT II).[229] The incidence of all thromboembolic events in V-HEFT I was 2.7 per 100 patient-years, and in V-HEFT II was 2.1 per 100 patient-years; and it was not reduced in patients treated with warfarin.

Patients with lower peak oxygen consumption (MVO_2) and lower EF had a higher risk of thromboembolic events, but only the difference in MVO_2 was significant. The use of oral anticoagulants was associated with a small but statistically insignificant increase in thromboembolic events in this analysis. There was no significant difference in the rate of thromboembolism between patients with ischemic and non-ischemic cardiomyopathy in this trial.

The retrospective analysis of Studies of Left Ventricular Dysfunction (SOLVD) was limited to the 6378 patients who were in sinus rhythm because of the confounding influence of atrial fibrillation on thromboembolic events.[228] The annual incidence of thromboembolic events was higher in women (2.4 percent) than in men (1.8 percent). Multivariate analysis revealed a 53 percent increased risk of thromboembolism for every 10 percent reduction in EF in women ($p = 0.02$), but no increased risk was observed in men. The use of anticoagulants alone or the combination of anticoagulants plus antiplatelet agents was not associated with significant risk reduction on the incidence of thromboembolism in either men or women. However, aspirin monotherapy resulted in 23 percent risk reduction in men ($p = 0.06$) and 53 percent risk reduction in women ($p = 0.03$).

A separate analysis focusing on warfarin anticoagulation and mortality in the 6797 patients enrolled in the SOLVD prevention and treatment trials has also been reported.[227] This cohort was divided into 861 patients on warfarin and 5652 patients on no oral anticoagulants. The patients on warfarin were sicker, as evidenced by lower mean EF, higher prevalence of atrial fibrillation, and cerebrovascular disease. When all-cause mortality was evaluated without adjusting for differences in baseline characteristics, there was no benefit of warfarin. However, after adjusting for baseline differences, warfarin use was a highly significant predictor of favorable outcome with a hazard ratio of 0.76 (95 percent confidence interval 0.65 to 0.89, $p = 0.0006$). A similar analysis after adjusting for differences in baseline characteristics has not been reported for the V-HEFT. These differences in baseline variables may explain the higher thromboembolic event rate (although not statistically significant) in patients on anticoagulants in the V-HEFT study. The reduction in the relative risk of stroke with anticoagulation (81 percent) and antiplatelet agents (56 percent) in the SAVE trial has been elaborated in the section on prevention of LV thrombi post-myocardial infarction.[217]

RECOMMENDATIONS. A placebo-controlled randomized trial of long-term anticoagulation in patients with dilated cardiomyopathy has not yet been performed. Thus, the routine use of oral anticoagulants cannot be universally recommended, especially in view of the observed benefits of aspirin monotherapy from CARS and several nonrandomized trials.[209, 220] Oral anticoagulation should thus be individualized to patients with high-risk characteristics such as large, protruding, or mobile ventricular thrombi and in patients with concomitant atrial fibrillation.

Prosthetic Heart Valves (See also Chap. 46)

Risks associated with implantation of prosthetic heart valves include thromboembolism, particularly stroke, and valve thrombosis. Although patients with bioprosthetic valves are at risk for thromboembolic events primarily during the first 90 days after surgery, those with mechanical valves remain at significant risk indefinitely.[230, 231] In one analysis, the incidence of major embolism in the absence of antithrombotic therapy was calculated to be 4 per 100 patient-years.[232] Factors that are associated with an increased risk of thromboembolism include the presence of older "first generation" mechanical valves (e.g., Starr-Edwards "ball and cage" valve), valves in the mitral position, the presence of more than one prosthetic valve, prior embolism, atrial fibrillation, enlarged left atrium, low LVEF, and advanced age.[232-236]

ANTIPLATELET THERAPY ALONE. There have been no randomized placebo-controlled trials assessing antiplatelet therapy alone as an antithrombotic regimen in patients with mechanical heart valves. Nonrandomized studies of aspirin, dipyridamole, or both in patients with mechanical heart valves have shown only modest or no significant protective effect.[232, 237] In one open prospective randomized trial of patients with mitral or aortic Starr-Edwards valves, combination antiplatelet therapy (aspirin plus dipyridamole or aspirin plus pentoxifylline) was associated with a higher incidence of thromboembolism when compared with treatment with warfarin.[238] Based on the previous reports, antiplatelet therapy alone is not considered to provide adequate antithrombotic protection in patients with mechanical prostheses.[239]

There have likewise been no randomized nor placebo-controlled trials of antiplatelet therapy alone in patients with bioprosthetic valves. One series of 185 patients with bioprosthetic valves in the mitral or mitral and aortic positions who were in sinus rhythm reported no thromboembolic events with a mean follow-up of 32 months in patients treated with aspirin (500 mg every other day to 1 gm/d).[240]

WARFARIN THERAPY. Studies of patients with bileaflet mechanical valves (such as the commonly used St. Jude valve) have shown that oral anticoagulation to achieve lower INRs is not associated with a clinically significant increase in thromboembolic complications compared with those with higher INRs. In one prospective study, subset analysis of patients in sinus rhythm with nonenlarged left atria showed little difference in thromboembolic events when INR values of 1.8 to 2.7 were compared with those of 2.5 to 3.2.[241] In a large series of patients from the Netherlands, patients with bileaflet valves had no more complications at INRs of 2.0 to 2.9 than INRs of 3.0 to 3.9 or 4.0 to 4.9, although those with tilting disc or caged ball or disc valves had less overall adverse outcomes at higher INRs. In the AREVA study, patients at low risk for embolic events randomized to anticoagulation at an INR of 2.0 to 3.0 had similar thromboembolic events and less hemorrhagic events than those randomized to anticoagulation at an INR of 3.0 to 4.5.[242]

Patients treated with bioprosthetic valves, especially in the mitral position, are at significant risk of thromboembolism during the first 90 days after surgery; and this risk is decreased with anticoagulation therapy.[230] In one study of patients who received bioprosthetic valves, those randomized to anticoagulation with an INR of 2.0 to 2.25 had thromboembolic rates comparable to those treated with a target INR of 2.5 to 4.0.[243]

These and other studies have led to lower recommended INR ranges for the prevention of thromboembolic events in patients with mechanical valves (particularly those with St. Jude valves) and with bioprosthetic valves.[231, 239, 244, 245]

WARFARIN PLUS ANTIPLATELET THERAPY. Several trials have evaluated the utility of combined warfarin and antiplatelet therapy compared with warfarin therapy alone. Turpie and colleagues randomized a group of patients consisting of those with either mechanical heart valves or high-risk characteristics and bioprosthetic valves to treatment with warfarin (target INR 3.0 to 4.5) and either aspirin (100 mg daily) or placebo. Major systemic embolism of vascular death occurred at a rate of 1.9 percent/year in those treated with aspirin and 8.5 percent/year in those treated with placebo. All-cause death occurred in 2.8 percent and 7.4 percent of patients, respectively. Although bleeding was more common in the combined therapy group, most of the increased incidence of bleeding was due to minor bleeding.[246] A meta-analysis of five randomized trials comparing warfarin therapy alone with warfarin therapy combined with antiplatelet therapy (aspirin or dipyridamole) found that combination therapy reduced embolism by 67 percent and overall mortality by 40 percent. Although the risk of bleeding was increased with combination therapy, the benefits of combination therapy appeared to outweigh this increased bleeding risk.[247]

In a trial comparing the combination of lower-intensity anticoagulation with warfarin (INR 2.5 to 3.5) and aspirin (100 mg/d) with higher-intensity anticoagulation alone (INR 3.5 to 4.5), the incidence of thromboembolic events was similar; bleeding tended to be more common in patients treated with higher-intensity anticoagulation therapy.[248] Altman and coworkers found no difference in systemic embolization or vascular death in patients treated with combination therapy between those who received relatively low-dose aspirin (100 mg/d) and those treated with high-dose aspirin (650 mg/d).[249] Thus, combination warfarin and antiplatelet therapy in many patients appears to reduce the risk of thromboembolic events without unacceptably increasing bleeding complications. Antiplatelet therapy with as low as 100 mg/d of aspirin in this setting appears adequate.

RECOMMENDATIONS. Recommendations regarding antithrombotic therapy in patients with prosthetic heart valves have been published from a consensus conference of the American College of Chest Physicians (ACCP)[239] and others[231, 244, 245] based on the above and other data. The following summarizes in simplified form the latest (as of this writing) ACCP guidelines.

All patients with mechanical prosthetic heart valves should be treated with oral anticoagulants. The intensity of anticoagulation recommended in specific situations can be thought of as a three-tier system, based on the presence or absence of certain factors associated with increased risk of thromboembolism and on the just discussed studies. For patients with a bileaflet valve (e.g., "St. Jude") in the aortic position, without other factors that have been correlated with increased risk of thromboembolism (enlarged left atrium, atrial fibrillation, low LVEF), treatment should be with warfarin with a target INR of 2.5 (range 2.0 to 3.0). For patients with a bileaflet or tilting disc valve in the aortic position with atrial fibrillation or with bileaflet or tilting disc valve in the mitral position, treatment should be with either (1) warfarin alone with a target INR of 3.0 (range 2.5 to 3.5) or with (2) warfarin with a target INR of 2.5 (range 2.0 to 3.0) plus aspirin (80 to 100 mg/d). For patients with caged ball (e.g., "Starr Edwards") or caged disc valves or those with any mechanical valves and other factors associated with increased risk of thromboembolism, combined therapy with warfarin with a target INR of 3.0 (range 2.5–3.5) and aspirin (80–100 mg/d) is recommended.

Patients with bioprosthetic heart valves should be treated with warfarin with a target INR of 2.5 (range 2.0–3.0) for 3 months. After this period, those not at risk of systemic embolism from other factors (e.g., atrial fibrillation) can be treated with aspirin (162 mg/d).

Percutaneous Coronary Interventions

Antiplatelet and anticoagulant therapy has made modern percutaneous arterial interventions practical.[250] The strategies for using these therapies in patients undergoing coronary interventions are discussed in detail in Chapter 38. A summary of the key findings follows.

ANTIPLATELET AGENTS IN PERCUTANEOUS CORONARY INTERVENTIONS. In the era of balloon angioplasty alone, before the advent of stents, the utility of aspirin for prevention of periprocedural myocardial infarction and/or recurrent ischemia requiring urgent revascularization was established. The quest to reduce further ischemic complications of percutaneous coronary intervention in the 1990s was aided by the introduction of potent new antiplatelet agents such as the Gp IIb/IIIa receptor inhibitors.[251–256] The Gp IIb/IIIa receptor antagonists have been evaluated in five major prospective, randomized, double-blind, placebo-controlled trials in patients undergoing balloon angio-

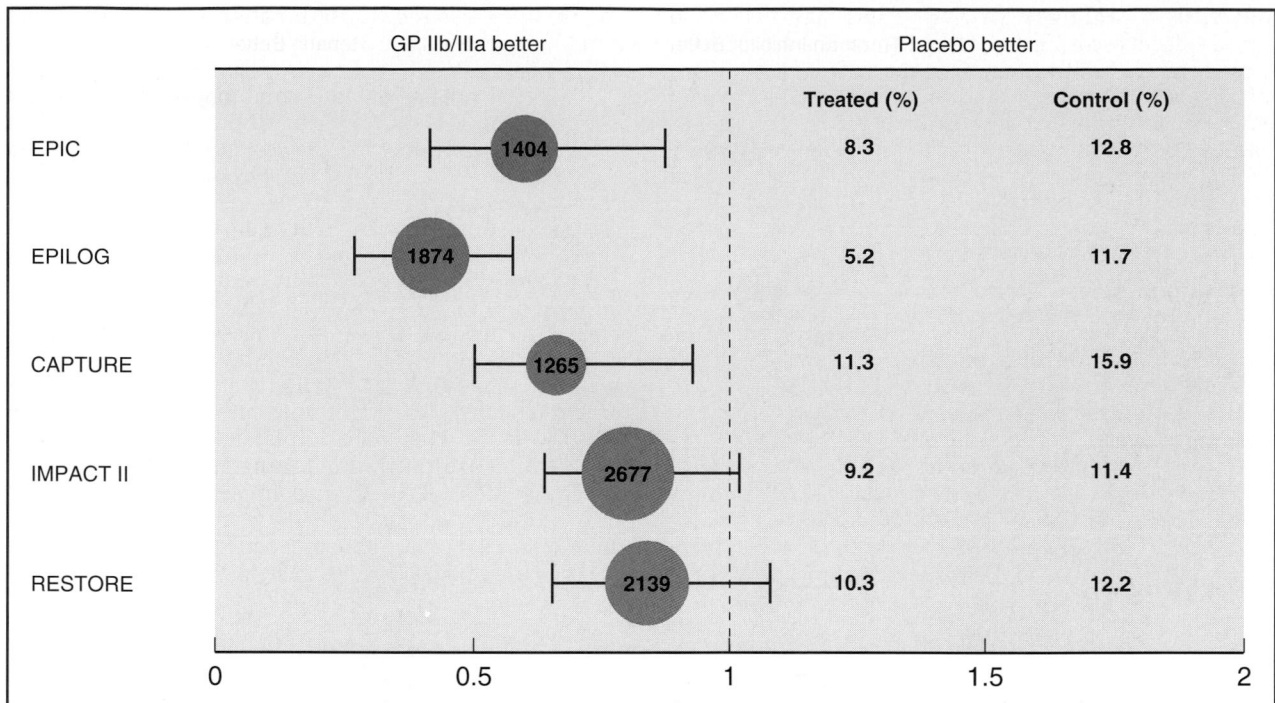

FIGURE 62–22. The reduction in acute ischemic complications after percutaneous transluminary coronary angioplasty defined as death, myocardial infarction, or urgent target vessel revascularization (triple composite) in trials of GP IIb/IIIa inhibitors versus placebo at 30 days. The odds ratio with 95 percent confidence intervals for each trial is shown. The odds ratio circle for each trial is relatively proportional to its sample size, which is also shown as a number. The embedded table shows the event rate in the treated and control groups. (Adapted from Lincoff AM, Tcheng JE, Califf RM, et al: Sustained suppression of ischemic complications of coronary intervention by platelet GP IIb/IIIa blockade with abciximab: One-year outcome in the EPILOG trial. Evaluation in PTCA to Improve Long-term Outcome with abciximab GP IIb/IIIa blockade. Circulation 99:1951–1958, 1999. Copyright 1999, American Heart Association.)

plasty.[251-253, 257] Although there are some differences between studies, the overall direction has been one of marked reduction in ischemic complications of balloon angioplasty with the use of these agents (Fig. 62–22).

The success of these early Gp IIb/IIIa inhibitor trials, along with the potential drawbacks of monoclonal Fab fragments such as immunogenicity, a finite incidence of thrombocytopenia (≈5 percent), and the extended duration of antiplatelet effect, created an impetus to evaluate other Gp IIb/IIIa receptor antagonists.[258-261] Two phase III clinical trials using cyclic RGD peptides (eptifibatide) or nonpeptide RGD mimetics (tirofiban) that compete for ligand binding to the Gp IIb/IIIa receptor have been reported. Their results show a similar reduction in triple composite endpoint in the first 24 to 72 hours after percutaneous transluminal coronary angioplasty. However, clinical efficacy with these shorter-acting agents was not sustained at 30 days and 6 months.[252, 253]

ANTICOAGULANTS IN PERCUTANEOUS CORONARY INTERVENTIONS. Coronary interventions before the Gp IIb/IIIa inhibitor era were often performed by using approximately 150 U/kg of heparin (with a 10,000- to 15,000-unit initial bolus), targeted to an activated clotting time (ACT) between 300 and 350 seconds.[262, 263] The rationale for this level of anticoagulation during angioplasty was the observation of an inverse relationship between ACT and the risk of ischemic complications. Periprocedural ischemic events increase the synthesis of heparin-binding proteins and potentiate the local release of platelet factor 4 (PF4) by platelets.[264] This leads to heparin resistance and/or inactivation with consequent reduction in ACT and aPTT values. These shortcomings of heparin along with the biochemical advantages afforded by the direct thrombin inhibitors hirudin and its congener bivalirudin provided an impetus to test these agents for prevention of ischemic complications and restenosis after angioplasty.[265] After encouraging preliminary

studies, two large prospective randomized trials evaluated the two direct thrombin inhibitors in patients undergoing percutaneous coronary intervention (Fig. 62–23).[266, 267] The failure of the direct thrombin inhibitor to substantially alter the long-term outcome in patients undergoing percutaneous coronary intervention or in acute coronary syndromes may be multifactorial, possibly related to continued thrombin generation during, as well as rebound increase in thrombin activity upon cessation of, infusion.[268]

ANTITHROMBOTIC THERAPY AFTER DEPLOYMENT OF CORONARY STENTS. Coronary stenting has outpaced balloon angioplasty as the most frequently performed percutaneous revascularization procedure.[250] The early experience with coronary stenting was associated with a 5 to 20 percent incidence of stent thrombosis that frequently resulted in clinical events such as death, myocardial infarction, or urgent target lesion revascularization.[269-271] The tendency for ischemic complications after stenting occurred despite intense anticoagulation during the procedure with high-dose heparin, dextran, and postprocedure warfarin administration to an INR of 3.0 to 4.5.[271] The need to optimize oral anticoagulation during heparin infusion as well as bleeding complications as a result of intense anticoagulation led to prolonged hospitalizations. The introduction of thienopyridine ADP antagonists (ticlopidine and clopidogrel) and the optimization of stent deployment techniques have eliminated the need to treat patients with warfarin after coronary stenting. Trials have now shown the superiority of the combination antiplatelet regimen of aspirin and ticlopidine over aspirin alone, or aspirin plus oral anticoagulation with warfarin, not only in patients with optimal stent deployment but also in patients who are at high risk of stent thrombosis[272-276] (Fig. 62–24).

Although ticlopidine has proven to be effective in preventing stent thrombosis in multiple trials, the enthusiasm

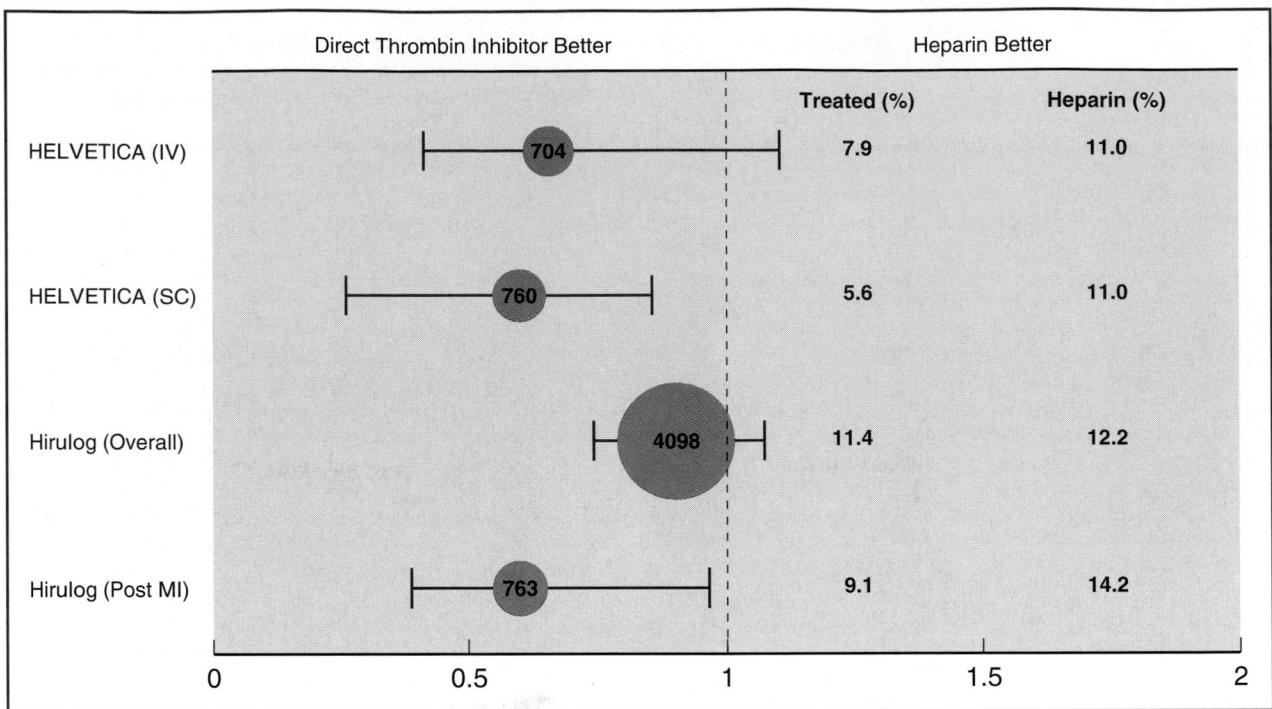

FIGURE 62–23. The reduction in acute ischemic complications after PTCA defined as death in the hospital, myocardial infarction (MI), abrupt vessel closure, or rapid clinical deterioration of cardiac origin in the HELVETICA and Hirulog in Angioplasty trials. The odds ratio with 95 percent confidence intervals for each trial is shown. The odds ratio of the intravenous (IV) and subcutaneous (SC) arms of HELVETICA, the overall group as well as the postinfarction angina subgroup in the Hirulog in Angioplasty trial, are shown. The odds ratio circle for each trial is relatively proportional to its sample size, which is also shown as a number. The embedded table shows the event rate in the treated and control groups.

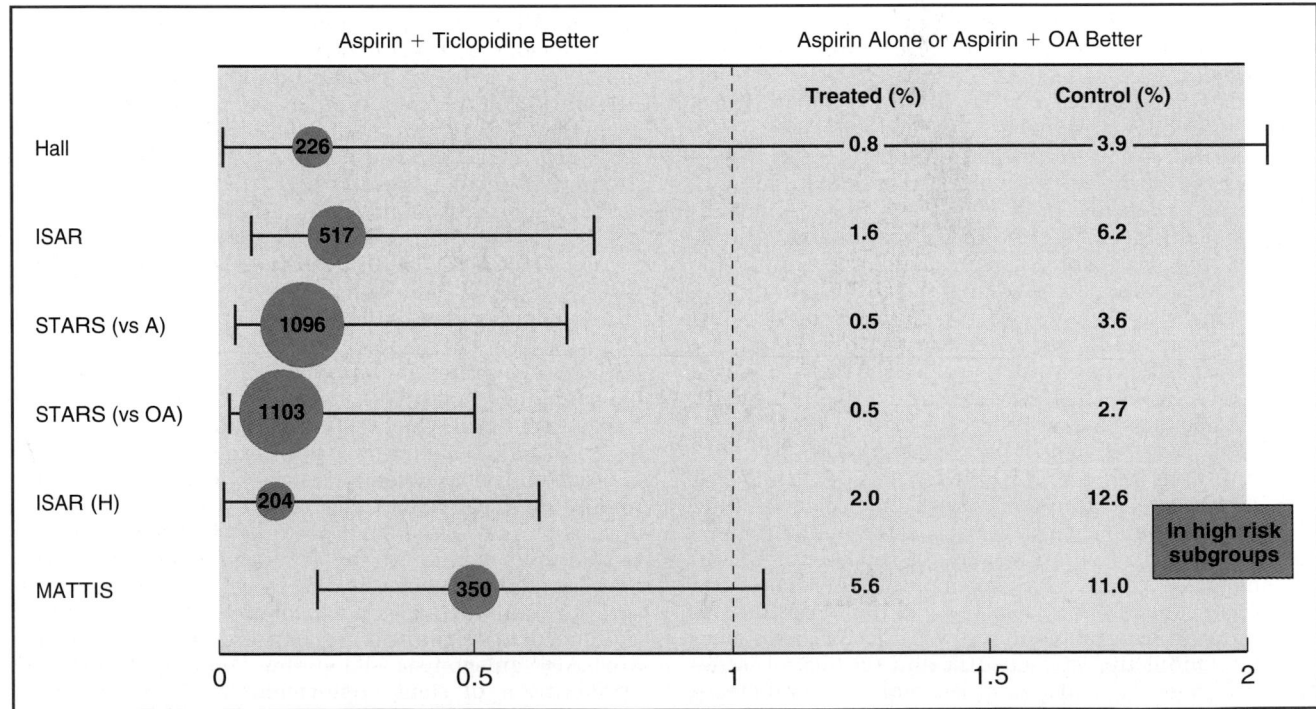

FIGURE 62–24. The reduction in clinical sequelae of stent thrombosis defined as death, myocardial infarction, revascularization of the target lesion, or angiographically evident thrombosis within 30 days in the stent trials. The odds ratio with 95 percent confidence intervals for each trial is shown. The event rate in the control groups is either for aspirin treatment alone (STARS vs. A and Hall and coworkers) or aspirin plus oral anticoagulation with warfarin (STARS vs. OA, ISAR, ISAR H [denoting high-risk group] and MATTIS). The ISAR (H) and the MATTIS trial enrolled patients who were at high risk of stent thrombosis. The odds ratio circle for each trial is relatively proportional to its sample size, which is also shown as a number. The embedded table shows the event rate in the treated and control groups.

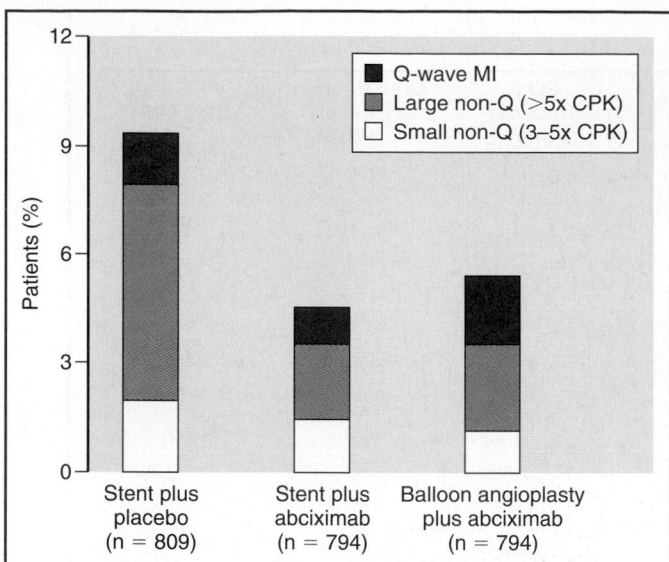

FIGURE 62–25. The incidence and type of each myocardial infarction for each treatment group in the EPISTENT trial. The predominant effect of abciximab was in the reduction of large non-Q wave myocardial infarction which comprised 86 percent of the benefit. (From EPISTENT Investigators: Randomised placebo-controlled and balloon-angioplasty-controlled trial to assess safety of coronary stenting with use of platelet glycoprotein-IIb/IIIa blockade. Evaluation of Platelet IIb/IIIa Inhibitor for Stenting. Lancet 352:87–92, 1998.)

for this agent was tempered by a small but finite incidence of hematological side effects such as neutropenia and thrombotic thrombocytopenic purpura.[277–288] This provided the impetus to evaluate clopidogrel, a congener of ticlopidine.[289] The preliminary results of the CLASSICS (Clopidogrel plus ASA vs. Ticlopidine plus ASA in patients with stents) study suggest that clopidogrel provides comparable efficacy and fewer side effects than ticlopidine.[211] Recently, TTP has been described in association with clopidogrel as well as with ticlopidine, albeit at lower frequency.[173a]

ROLE OF GP IIB/IIIA INHIBITORS IN CORONARY STENTING. The EPISTENT trial was designed to evaluate the synergism between optimization of luminal rheology with coronary stenting and potent platelet blockade with Gp IIb/IIIa inhibitors.[254] In this trial, 2399 patients were randomized to a strategy of balloon angioplasty with abciximab, stent deployment with abciximab, and stent deployment with routine anticoagulation with weight-based heparin (100 U/kg). There was a dramatic reduction in the triple composite endpoint of death, myocardial infarction, and urgent target vessel revascularization at 30 days in the two abciximab groups (6.9 and 5.3 percent) compared with stent deployment on the background of routine heparin therapy (10.8, $p < 0.007$, and 0.001, respectively). The predominant effect of abciximab was in the reduction of large non-Q wave myocardial infarction that comprised 86 percent of the benefit (Fig. 62–25). The best outcome was in the stent plus abciximab group, indicating that there is synergism between optimization of luminal rheology and potent platelet inhibition. Preliminary data regarding the durability of benefit for the combined abciximab/stent strategy versus stenting alone for reduction of death rates (0.8 percent vs. 2.4 percent) at 1 year are now available. The ESPRIT study is evaluating the potential benefit of treatment with eptifibatide in patients primarily without traditional high-risk clinical or angiographic features who are undergoing coronary stent implantation. Results of this study should be forthcoming.

ANTITHROMBOTIC THERAPY FOR PREVENTION OF CORONARY RESTENOSIS. The paradigm that coronary restenosis is predominantly a result of mural thrombosis that provides a scaffold for the subsequent migration and proliferation of neointimal smooth muscle cells has recently been challenged by serial intravascular ultrasound studies in patients undergoing percutaneous transluminal coronary angioplasty.[290] These observations have highlighted the importance of both acute vessel recoil and late vascular remodeling as the major factors contributing to luminal narrowing after this procedure.[291] Thus, it is not surprising that a decade of animal and clinical studies with both conventional antiplatelet agents and antithrombins has yielded negative results for the prevention of coronary restenosis.[250]

RECOMMENDATIONS. All patients undergoing percutaneous coronary intervention should be pretreated with aspirin (160–325 mg/d) in the absence of specific contraindications such as true aspirin allergy. Whereas Gp IIb/IIIa inhibitors should be considered in most patients undergoing percutaneous coronary intervention, their use is strongly recommended for patients at high risk of ischemic complications such as intracoronary thrombus, post-myocardial infarction, and unfavorable lesion morphology. Combination antiplatelet therapy with aspirin and a thienopyridine (ticlopidine or clopidogrel) should be used in all patients undergoing intracoronary stenting for 2 to 4 weeks after stent implantation (and aspirin alone should then be continued indefinitely).

Antithrombotic Therapy after Coronary Artery Bypass Surgery (See also Chap. 37)

The disease process in the vein grafts is initiated at the time of explantation from the leg and progresses through an early thrombotic phase in the first month after surgery, followed by intimal hyperplasia over the next 12 months, which creates a substrate for accelerated atherosclerosis.[292–296] Saphenous vein graft occlusion in the first month is therefore a result of thrombotic occlusion and is reported to occur in 3 to 12 percent of grafts. The predisposition to thrombosis is initiated at the time of harvesting when high pressure distention is required to overcome venous spasm.[297–300] This results in prominent endothelial cell loss and medial damage, with consequent deposition of fibrin, platelets, and neutrophils on the denuded luminal surface. In addition, the disruption of endothelial integrity results in reduction of tissue plasminogen activator production, impairment of thrombomodulin mediated inhibition of the coagulation cascade, and exposure of tissue factor.[301] The thrombotic tendency in the first several weeks after aortocoronary bypass led to the use of antiplatelet agents in an effort to prevent graft occlusion (Fig. 62–26).[292, 293, 296, 302–305]

Landmark clinical trials conducted in the 1980s by Chesebro and coworkers as well as Goldman and coworkers have shown that (1) aspirin (100 to 975 mg daily) when initiated either before, on the day of, or 1 day after bypass surgery is effective at reducing thrombotic graft occlusion; (2) the combination of dipyridamole and aspirin is no more effective than aspirin alone; (3) initiation of aspirin before bypass surgery is associated with an increase in perioperative bleeding events without an increase in graft patency when compared with aspirin therapy started within the first 24 hours after surgery; (4) aspirin therapy after the first 48 hours is not effective in preventing graft occlusion; and (5) there are no benefits on vein bypass graft patency of aspirin therapy for longer than 1 year.[306]

For patients who are intolerant of or allergic to aspirin, ticlopidine started within the first 2 days after grafting is a viable alternative based on the study by Limet and coworkers.[302] There are no studies of combination therapy with aspirin and ticlopidine or clopidogrel, which is a potentially useful regimen because these agents mediate their

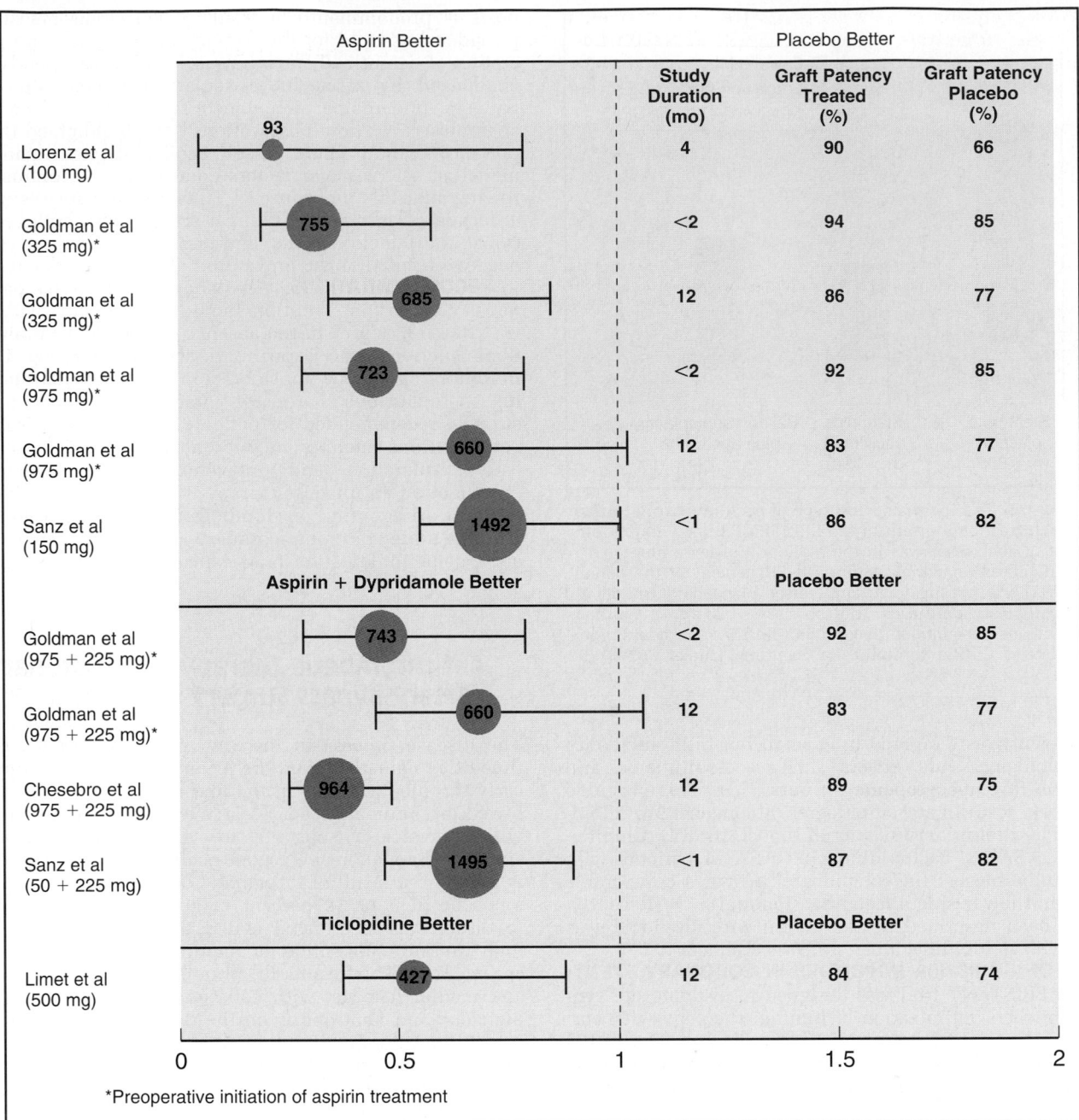

FIGURE 62–26. The effect of antithrombotic therapy with aspirin alone (100–975 mg), aspirin plus dipyridamole, or ticlopidine compared with placebo on saphenous vein graft patency in different trials is depicted as odds ratio with 95 percent confidence intervals for each trial. The odds ratio circle for each trial is relatively proportional to number of vein grafts evaluated, which is also shown as a number. The embedded table shows the duration of follow-up and the rate of graft patency in the treated versus the control groups.

antiplatelet effect by different pathways. On the basis of the efficacy of combined therapy with aspirin plus ticlopidine or aspirin plus clopidogrel in reducing subacute stent thrombosis, it is reasonable to evaluate the potential synergy of these regimens for prevention of vein graft thrombosis.[289, 307]

The use of oral anticoagulants initiated before or immediately after surgery provides no additional improvement in graft patency when compared with aspirin therapy.[308–310] In addition, bleeding complications occurred more frequently in the oral anticoagulant group.[308, 309] The Post CABG study evaluated whether aggressive lowering of low-density lipoprotein cholesterol levels or low-dose anticoagulation would delay the progression of atherosclerosis in vein grafts.[311] The study enrolled 1351 patients 1 to 11 years

after bypass surgery with at least one patent vein graft in a 2 × 2 factorial design to aggressive or moderate treatment to lower low-density lipoprotein cholesterol and to treatment with warfarin or placebo. The warfarin group achieved a mean INR of only 1.4. The primary outcome in this trial was angiographic progression of disease that was lowered by aggressive lipid-lowering therapy. However, warfarin was not superior to placebo in influencing rates of disease progression (34 vs. 32 percent; $p = 0.48$) or graft occlusion. These angiographic outcomes were accompanied by no differences in the rates of myocardial infarction (5.0 vs. 5.0 percent) or the need for revascularization (7.8 vs. 7.9 percent) between the warfarin-treated and placebo-treated patients.

The improved understanding of the pathogenesis of early

thrombotic occlusion of vein grafts has led to experimental studies using innovative strategies.[294, 312, 313] The saphenous vein grafts are ideal targets for gene therapy because the explanted veins are available for ex vivo transfer of exogenous genetic material before grafting. The replication-defective adenoviral vectors have been successfully used to transfer genes in experimental porcine vein graft models.[314] In addition, cultured human saphenous veins have been successfully transfected with an adenoviral vector encoding bovine endothelial NOS, yielding a marked increase in venous endothelial NO production.[313] This strategy, if clinically feasible, has the potential to provide a potent local antithrombotic milieu in the early vulnerable period of thrombosis after graft implantation. The administration of platelet selective NO donors and the modulation of tissue factor with anti–tissue factor antibody are some of the other approaches undergoing investigation in experimental animal models.[312, 315]

RECOMMENDATIONS. Early antiplatelet therapy with aspirin should be used in all patients after coronary artery bypass surgery to prevent vein graft occlusion. Preoperative aspirin may increase intraoperative bleeding and is not more beneficial than aspirin started within the first 24 to 48 hours after surgery. Therefore, for elective surgery and if the clinical situation permits, aspirin should be withheld until after the operation. Aspirin at doses of 100 to 325 mg/d should be started immediately after surgery. A delay in the initiation of aspirin beyond 48 hours is associated with reduced efficacy. The addition of dipyridamole to aspirin has not been shown to enhance vein graft patency.

The appropriate duration of antiplatelet therapy after surgery is controversial. Studies suggest that aspirin therapy for at least 1 year reduces vein graft occlusion. Although studies do not show an improvement in vein graft patency with antiplatelet therapy beyond the first year, the beneficial effects of aspirin for secondary prevention of coronary artery disease argue that it be continued indefinitely in these patients. For patients allergic to aspirin, ticlopidine, 250 mg twice daily, beginning 48 hours after surgery has been reported to be effective and may be considered as an alternative.

R E F E R E N C E S

BASIC MECHANISMS OF HEMOSTASIS AND THROMBOSIS

1. Cines DB, Pollak ES, Buck CA, et al: Endothelial cells in physiology and in the pathophysiology of vascular disorders. Blood 91:3527–3561, 1998.
2. Henderson AH: Endothelium in control. Br Heart J 65:116–125, 1991.
3. Schafer AI: Preface. In Schafer AI (ed): Molecular Mechanisms of Hypercoagulable States. Austin, Landes Bioscience, 1997.
4. Wu KK, Thiagarajan P: Role of endothelium in thrombosis and hemostasis. Annu Rev Med 47:315–331, 1996.
5. Schafer AI: Vascular endothelium: In defense of blood fluidity. J Clin Invest 99:1143–1144, 1997.
6. Niklason LE, Gao J, Abbott WM, et al: Functional arteries grown in vitro. Science 284:489–493, 1999.
7. Risau W: Differentiation of endothelium. FASEB J 9:926–933, 1995.
8. Garlanda C, Dejana E: Heterogeneity of endothelial cells: Specific markers. Arterioscler Thromb Vasc Biol 17:1193–1202, 1997.
9. Schnittler HJ: Structural and functional aspects of intercellular junctions in vascular endothelium. Basic Res Cardiol 93(Suppl 3):30–39, 1998.
10. Thorin E, Shreeve SM: Heterogeneity of vascular endothelial cells in normal and disease states. Pharmacol Ther 78:155–166, 1998.
11. Rosenberg RD, Aird WC: Vascular-bed-specific hemostasis and hypercoagulable states. N Engl J Med 340:1555–1564, 1999.
12. Drake TA, Cheng J, Chang A, et al: Expression of tissue factor, thrombomodulin, and E-selectin in baboons with lethal Eschericia coli sepsis. Am J Pathol 142:1458, 1993.
13. Levin EG, Osborn KG: The expression of endothelial cell tissue plasminogen activator in vivo: A function defined by vessel size and anatomic location. J Cell Sci 11:139, 1997.
14. Augustin HG, Kozian DH, Johnson RC: Differentiation of endothelial cells: Analysis of the constitutive and activated cell phenotypes. Bioessays 16:901, 1994.
15. Moncada S, Higgs A: The L-arginine-nitric oxide pathway. N Engl J Med 329:2002–2012, 1993.
16. Dinerman JL, Lowenstein CJ, Snyder SH: Molecular mechanisms of nitric oxide regulation: Potential relevance to cardiovascular disease. Circ Res 73:217–222, 1993.
17. Cook JP, Dzau VJ: Nitric oxide synthase: Role in the genesis of vascular disease. Annu Rev Med 48:489–509, 1997.
18. Xu WM, Liu LZ: Nitric oxide: From a mysterious labile factor to the molecule of the Nobel Prize: Recent progress in nitric oxide research. Cell Res 8:251–258, 1998.
19. Venema RC, Sayegh HS, Armal JF, et al: Role of the enzyme calmodulin-binding domain in membrane association and phospholipid inhibition of endothelial nitric oxide synthase. J Biol Chem 270:14705, 1995.
20. Vane JR, Botting RM: Pharmacodynamic profile of prostacyclin. Am J Cardiol 75:3a–10a, 1995.
21. Vanhoutte PM, Mombouli JV: Vascular endothelium: Vasoactive mediators. Prog Cardiovasc Dis 39:229–238, 1996.
22. Cohen RA, Vanhoutte PM: Endothelium-dependent hyperpolarization: Beyond nitric oxide and cyclic GMP. Circulation 92:3337–3349, 1995.
23. Garland CJ, Plane F, Kemp BK, et al: Endothelium-dependent hyperpolarization: A role in the control of vascular tone. Trends Biol Sci 16:23, 1995.
24. Durante W, Schafer AI: Carbon monoxide and vascular cell function. Int J Mol Med 2:255–263, 1998.
25. Marcus AJ, Broekman MJ, Drosopoulos JHF, et al: The endothelial cell ecto-ADPase responsible for inhibition of platelet function is CD39. J Clin Invest 99:1351–1360, 1997.
26. Zimmerman GA, Elstad MR, Lorant DE, et al: Platelet-activating factor (PAF): Signaling and adhesion in cell-cell interactions. Adv Exp Med Biol 416:297–304, 1996.
27. Feuerstein G, Rabinovici R, Leor J, et al: Platelet-activating factor and cardiac diseases: Therapeutic potential for PAF inhibitors. J Lipid Mediat Cell Signal 15:255–284, 1997.
28. La M, Reid JJ: Endothelin-1 and the regulation of vascular tone. Clin Exp Pharmacol Physiol 22:315–323, 1995.
29. Ferro CJ, Webb DJ: The clinical potential of endothelin receptor antagonists in cardiovascular medicine. Drugs 51:12–27, 1996.
30. Schiffrin EL, Touyz RM: Vascular biology of endothelin. J Cardiovasc Pharmacol 32(Suppl 3):s2–s13, 1998.
31. Luscher TF, Tanner FC, Tschudi MR, et al: Endothelial dysfunction in coronary artery disease. Annu Rev Med 44:395–418, 1993.
32. Schafer AI: The primary and secondary hypercoagulable states. In Schafer AI (ed): Molecular Mechanisms of Hypercoagulable States. Austin, Landes Bioscience, 1997, pp 1–48.
33. Rock G, Wells P: New concepts in coagulation. Crit Rev Clin Lab Sci 34:475–501, 1997.
34. Jenny NS, Mann KG: Coagulation cascade: An overview. In Loscalzo J, Schafer AI (eds): Thrombosis and Hemorrhage. 2nd ed. Baltimore, Williams & Wilkins, 1998, pp 3–27.
35. Wachtfogel YT, DeLa Cadena RA, Colman RW: Structural biology, cellular interactions and pathophysiology of the contact system. Thromb Res 72:1–21, 1993.
36. Schmaier AH: Contact activation: A revision. Thromb Haemost 78:101–107, 1997.
37. Schmaier AH: Contact activation. In Loscalzo J, Schafer AI (eds): Thrombosis and Hemorrhage. 2nd ed. Baltimore, Williams & Wilkins, 1998, pp 105–127.
38. Broze GJ Jr: Tissue factor pathway inhibitor and the revised theory of coagulation. Annu Rev Med 46:103–112, 1995.
39. Toomey JR, Kratzer KE, Lasky NM, et al: Targeted disruption of the murine tissue factor gene results in embryonic lethality. Blood 88:1583–1587, 1996.
40. Osterud B: Tissue factor: A complex biological role. Thromb Haemost 78:755–758, 1997.
41. Lorenzet R, Napoleone E, Celi A, et al: Cell-cell interaction and tissue factor expression. Blood Coag Fibrinolysis Suppl 1:s49–s59, 1998.
42. Morrissey JH, Macik BG, Neuenschwander PF, et al: Quantitation of activated factor VII levels in plasma using a tissue factor mutant selectively deficient in promoting factor VII activation. Blood 81:734–744, 1993.
43. Edgington TS, Dickinson CD, Ruf W: The structural basis of function of the TF VIIa complex in the cellular initiation of coagulation. Thromb Haemost 78:401–405l, 1997.
44. Butenas S, Mann KG: Kinetics of human factor VII activation. Biochemistry 35:1904–1910, 1996.
45. Mosesson MW: Fibrinogen and fibrin polymerization: Appraisal of the binding events that accompany fibrin generation and fibrin clot assembly. Blood Coagul Fibrinolysis 8:257–267, 1997.
46. Mosesson MW: Fibrinogen structure and fibrin clot assembly. Semin Thromb Hemost 24:169–174, 1998.
47. Anwar R, Gallivan L, Edmonds SD, et al: Genotype/phenotype correlations for coagulation factor XIII: Specific normal polymorphisms are associated with high or low factor XIII specific activity. Blood 93:897–905, 1999.
48. Zwaal RF, Comfurius P, Bevers EM: Lipid–protein interactions in blood coagulation. Biochim Biophys Acta 1376:433–453, 1998.
49. Dachary-Prigent J, Toti F, Satta N, et al: Physiopathological significance of catalytic phospholipids in the generation of thrombin. Semin Thromb Hemost 22:157–164, 1996.

50. Schafer AI: Hypercoagulable states: Molecular genetics to clinical practice. Lancet 344:1739–1742, 1994.

51. van Boven HH, Lane DA: Antithrombin and its inherited deficiency states. Semin Hematol 34:188–204, 1997.

52. Lane DA, Bayston TA: Molecular basis of antithrombin action and deficiency. In Schafer AI (ed): Molecular Mechanisms of Hypercoagulable States. Austin, Landes Bioscience, 1997, pp 49–77.

53. De Stefano V, Finazzi G, Mannucci PM: Inherited thombophilia: Pathogenesis, clinical syndromes and management. Blood 87:3531–3544, 1996.

54. Dahlbäck B: The protein C anticoagulant system: Inherited defects as basis for venous thrombosis. Thromb Res 77:1–42, 1995.

55. Simmonds RE, Lane DA: Regulation of coagulation. In Loscalzo J, Schafer AI (eds): Thrombosis and Hemorrhage. 2nd ed. Baltimore, Williams & Wilkins, 1998, pp 45–76.

56. Esmon CT: Molecular events that control the protein C anticoagulant pathway. Thromb Haemost 70:29–35, 1993.

57. Sadler JE: Thrombomodulin structure and function. Thromb Haemost 78:392–395, 1997.

58. Broze GJ Jr: The tissue factor pathway of coagulation. In Loscalzo J, Schafer AI (eds): Thrombosis and Hemorrhage. 2nd ed. Baltimore, Williams & Wilkins, 1998, pp 77–104.

59. Dobroski DR, Rabbani LE, Loscalzo J: The relationship between thrombosis and atherosclerosis. In Loscalzo J, Schafer AI (eds): Thrombosis and Hemorrhage. 2nd ed. Baltimore, Williams & Wilkins, 1998, pp 837–861.

60. Mignatti P, Rifkin DB: Plasminogen activators and matrix metalloproteinases in angiogenesis. Enzyme Protein 49:117–137, 1996.

61. Hajjar KA: Changing concepts in fibrinolysis. Curr Opin Hematol 2: 345–350, 1995.

62. Lijnen HR, Collen D: Endothelium in hemostasis and thrombosis. Prog Cardiovasc Dis 39:343–350, 1997.

63. Hajjar KA, Jacovina AT, Chacko J: An endothelial cell receptor for plasminogen/tissue plasminogen activator: I. Identity with annexin II. J Biol Chem 269:21191–21197, 1994.

64. Plow EF, Ugarova T, Miles TA: Interaction of the fibrinolytic system with the vessel wall. In Loscalzo J, Schafer AI (eds): Thrombosis and Hemorrhage. 2nd ed. Baltimore, Williams & Wilkins, 1998, pp 373–385.

65. Eitzman DT, Ginsberg D: Of mice and men: The function of plasminogen activator inhibitors (PAIs) in vivo. Adv Exp Med Biol 425:131–141, 1997.

66. Vaughn DE: Plasminogen activator inhibitor-1: A common denominator in cardiovascular disease. J Invest Med 46:370–376, 1998.

67. Vaughn DE, Declerk PJ: Fibrinolysis and its regulation. In Loscalzo J, Schafer AI (eds): Thrombosis and Hemorrhage. 2nd ed. Baltimore, Williams & Wilkins, 1998, pp 155–170.

68. Astedt B, Lindoff C, Lecander I: Significance of the plasminogen activator inhibitor of placental type (PAI-2) in pregnancy. Semin Thromb Hemost 24:431–435, 1998.

Platelets

69. Kaushansky K: Thrombopoietin. N Engl J Med 339:746–754, 1998.

70. Ruggeri ZM: von Willebrand factor. J Clin Invest 100(Suppl 11):S41–46, 1997.

71. Sadler JE: Biochemistry and genetics of von Willebrand factor. Annu Rev Biochem 67:395–424, 1998.

72. Lopez JA, Dong JF: Structure and function of the glycoprotein Ib-IX-V complex. Curr Opin Hematol 4:323–329, 1997.

73. Ware J: Molecular analyses of the platelet glycoprotein Ib-IX-V receptor. Throm Haemost 79:466–478, 1998.

74. Kroll MH, Hellums JD, McIntire LV, et al: Platelets and shear stress. Blood 88:1525–1541, 1996.

75. Savage B, Almus-Jacobs F, Ruggeri ZM: Specific synergy of multiple substrate-receptor interactions in platelet thrombus formation under flow. Cell 94:657–666, 1998.

76. Nakamura T, Kambayashi J, Okuma M: Activation of the GP IIb–IIIa complex induced by platelet adhesion to collagen is mediated by both alpha$_2$-beta$_1$ integrin and Gp VI. J Biol Chem 274:11897–11903, 1999.

77. Di Paloa J, Federici AB, Mannucci PM, et al: Low platelet alpha$_2$beta$_1$ levels in type I von Willebrand disease correlate with impaired platelet function in a high shear stress system. Blood 93:3578–3582, 1993.

78. Blockmans D, Deckmyn H, Vermylen J: Platelet activation. Blood Rev 9: 143–156, 1995.

79. Mustonen P, Lassila R: Epinephrine augments platelet recruitment to immobilized collagen in flowing blood—evidence for a von Willebrand factor-mediated mechanism. Thromb Haemost 75:175–181, 1996.

80. Vanags DM, Lloyd JV, Rodgers SE, et al: ADP, adrenaline and serotonin stimulate inositol 1,4,5-triphosphate production in human platelets. Eur J Pharmacol 358:93–100, 1998.

81. Wagner CT, Kroll MH, Chow TW, et al: Epinephrine and shear stress synergistically induce platelet aggregation via a mechanism that partially bypasses VWF-GP IB interactions. Biorheology 33:209–229, 1996.

82. Harrison P, Cramer EM: Platelet alpha-granules. Blood Rev 7:52–62, 1993.

83. Armstrong RA: Platelet prostanoid receptors. Pharmacol Ther 72:171–191, 1996.

84. Thomas DW, Mannon RB, Mannon PJ, et al: Coagulation defects and altered hemodynamic responses in mice lacking receptors for thromboxane A$_2$. J Clin Invest 102:1994–2001, 1998.

85. Lefkovits J, Plow EF, Topol EJ: Platelet glycoprotein IIb/IIIa receptors in cardiovascular medicine. N Engl J Med 332:1553–1559, 1995.

86. Peerschke EIB, Lopez JA: Platelet membranes and receptors. In Loscalzo J, Schafer AI (eds): Thrombosis and Hemorrhage. 2nd ed. Baltimore, Williams & Wilkins, 1998, pp. 229–260.

87. Nurden AT, Poujol C, Nurden P: Different activation states of Gp IIb/IIIa complexes in platelets. Blood Coagul Fibrinolysis 10(Suppl 1):S67–S70, 1991.

88. Schafer AI: Antiplatelet therapy with glycoprotein IIb/IIIa receptor inhibitors and other novel agents. Tex Heart Inst J 24:90–96, 1997.

88a. Verstraete M: Synthetic inhibitors of platelet glycoprotein IIb/IIIa in clinical development. Circulation 101:E76–80, 2000.

89. Griffin JH: The thrombin paradox. Nature 378:337–338, 1995.

ANTITHROMBOTIC DRUGS

90. Hanson SR, Griffin JH, Harker LA, et al: Antithrombotic effects of thrombin-induced activation of endogenous protein C in primates. J Clin Invest 92:2003–2012, 1993.

91. Hirsh J, Warkentin TE, Raschke R, et al: Heparin and low-molecular-weight heparin. Chest 114:489s–510s, 1998.

92. Hirsh J: Heparin. N Engl J Med 324:1565–1574, 1991.

93. Rosenberg RD: Hemorrhagic disorders: I. Protein interactions in the clotting mechanism. In Beck WS (ed): Hematology. 5th ed. Cambridge, MIT Press, 1991, pp 507–542.

94. Hommes DW, Bura A, Mazzolai L, et al: Subcutaneous heparin compared with continuous intravenous heparin administration in the initial treatment of deep vein thrombosis: A meta-analysis. Ann Intern Med 116:279–284, 1992.

95. Kher A, Al Dieri R, Hemker HC, et al: Laboratory assessment of antithrombotic therapy: What tests and if so why? Hemostasis 27:211–218, 1997.

96. Braunwald E, Jones RH, Mark DB, et al: Diagnosing and managing unstable angina: Agency for Health Care Policy and Research. Circulation 90:613–622, 1994.

97. Aster RH: Heparine induced thrombocytopenia and thrombosis. N Engl J Med 332:1374–1376, 1995.

98. Warkentin TE: Heparin-induced thrombocytopenia: A ten-year retrospective. Annu Rev Med 50:129–147, 1999.

99. Newman PM, Swanson RL, Chong BH: Heparin-induced thrombocytopenia: IgG binding to PF4-heparin complexes in the fluid phase and cross-reactivity with low molecular weight heparin and heparinoid. Thromb Haemost 80:292–297, 1998.

100. Magnani HN: Organan (danaparoid sodium) use in the syndrome of heparin-induced thrombocytopenia. Platelets 8:74–81, 1997.

101. Greinacher A, Volpel H, Janssens U, et al: Recombinant hirudin (lepirudin) provides safe and effective anticoagulation in patients with heparin-induced thrombocytopenia: A prospective study. Circulation 99:73–80, 1999.

102. Lewis BE, Walenga JM, Wallis DE: Anticoagulation with Novastan (argatroban) in patients with heparin-induced thrombocytopenia and thrombosis syndrome. Semin Thromb Hemost 23:197–202, 1997.

103. Warkentin TE: Heparin-induced thrombocytopenia: Pathogenesis, frequency, avoidance, and management. Drug Saf 17:325–241, 1997.

104. Kearon C, Hirsh J: Anticoagulation in venous thromboembolism. In Smith TW (ed): Cardiovascular Therapeutics. Philadelphia, WB Saunders, 1996, pp 442–455.

105. Schafer AI: Low-molecular-weight heparin—an opportunity for home treatment of venous thrombosis. N Engl J Med 334:724–725, 1996.

106. Schafer AI: Low-molecular-weight heparin for venous thromboembolism. Hosp Pract 31:99–101, 1997.

106a. Kaul S, Shah PK: Low molecular weight heparin in acute coronary syndrome: Evidence for superior or equivalent efficacy compared with unfractionated heparin? J Am Coll Cardiol 35:1699–1712, 2000.

107. Fareed J, Jeske W, Hoppensteadt D, et al: Low-molecular-weight heparins: Pharmacologic profile and product differentiation. Am J Cardiol 82:3l–10l, 1998.

108. Warkentin TE, Levine MN, Hirsh J, et al. Heparin-induced thrombocytopenia in patients treated with low-molecular-weight heparin or unfractionated heparin. N Engl J Med 332:1330–1335, 1995.

109. Monreal M, Lafoz E, Olive A, et al: Comparison of subcutaneous unfractionated heparin with a low molecular weight heparin (fragmin) in patients with venous thromboembolism and contradictions to coumarin. Thromb Haemost 71:7–11, 1994.

110. Freedman JE, Scharfstein JS, Gold HK, et al: New antithrombotic strategies. In Loscalzo J, Schafer AI (eds): Thrombosis and Hemorrhage, 2nd ed. Baltimore, Williams & Wilkins, 199., pp 1259–1277.

111. Nurmohamed MT, ten Cate H, ten Cate JW: Low molecular weight heparin(oid)s: Clinical investigation and practical recommendations. Drugs 53:736–751, 1997.

112. Bates SM, Weitz JI: The new heparins. Coron Artery Dis 9:65–74, 1998.

113. Wilde MI, Markham A: Danaparoid. Drugs 54:903–924, 1997.

114. Laposata M, Green D, Van Cott EM, et al: College of American Pathologists Conference XXXI on laboratory monitoring of anticoagulant therapy. The clinical use and laboratory monitoring of low-molecular-weight heparin, danaparoid, hirudin and related compounds, and argatroban. Arch Pathol Lab Med 122:799–807, 1998.

115. Bendayan P, Coccalon H, Dupuoy D, et al: Dermatan sulfate is a more potent inhibitor of clot-bound thrombin than unfractionated and low molecular weight heparins. Thromb Haemostas 1: 576–580, 1977.
116. Hirsh J, Weitz JI: New antithrombotic agents. Lancet 353:1431–1436, 1999.
117. Petitou M, Herault JP, Bernat A, et al: Synthesis of thrombin-inhibiting heparin mimetics without side effects. Nature 398:417–422, 1999.

Warfarin

118. Keller C, Matzdorff AC, Kemkes-Matthes B: Pharmacology of warfarin and clinical implications. Semin Thromb Hemost 25:13–16, 1999.
119. Furie B, Furie BC: Molecular basis of vitamin K-dependent gamma-carboxylation. Blood 75:1753–1762, 1990.
120. Horton JD, Bushwick BM: Warfarin therapy: Evolving strategies in anticoagulation. Am Fam Physician 59:635–646, 1999.
121. Hirsh J, Dalen JE, Deykin D, et al: Oral anticoagulants: Mechanism of action, clinical effectiveness, and optimal therapeutic range. Chest 108(Suppl 4): 231s–234s, 1995.
122. Harrison L, Johnston M, Massicotte MP, et al: Comparison of 5-mg and 10-mg loading doses in initiation of warfarin therapy. Ann Intern Med 126:133–136, 1997.
123. Levine MN, Raskob G, Landefeld S, et al: Hemorrhagic complications of anticoagulant treatment. Chest 108(Suppl):276s–290s, 1995.
124. Schafer AI: Venous thrombosis as a chronic disease. N Engl J Med 340: 955–956, 1999.
125. Jeske W, Messmore HL Jr, Fared J: Pharmacology of heparin and oral anticoagulants. In Loscalzo J, Schafer AI (eds): Thrombosis and Hemorrhage. 2nd ed. Baltimore, Williams & Wilkins, 1998, pp 1193–1213.
126. Hall RD, Pineo GF, Raskob GE: Hirudin versus heparin and low-molecular-weight heparin: And the winner is. . . J Lab Clin Med 132:171–174, 1998.
127. Fenton JW II, Ofosu FA, Brezniak DR, et al: Thrombin and antithrombotics. Semin Thromb Hemost 24:87–91, 1998.
128. Hauptmann J, Stürzebecher J: Synthetic inhibitors of thrombin and factor Xa: From bench to bedside. Thromb Res 93:203–241, 1999.
129. Stubbs MT, Bode W: A player of many parts: The spotlight on thrombin's structure. Thromb Res 69:1–58, 1993.
130. Bates SM, Weitz JI: Direct thrombin inhibitors for treatment of arterial thrombosis: Potential differences between bivalirudin and hirudin. Am J Cardiol 82(8b):12p–18p, 1998.
131. Klement P, Liao P, Hirsh J, et al: Hirudin causes more bleeding than heparin in a rabbit ear bleeding model. J Lab Clin Med 132:180–185, 1998.
132. Eisenberg PR, Siegel JE, Abendschein DR, et al: Importance of factor Xa in determining the procoagulant activity of whole-blood clots. J Clin Invest 91:1877–1883, 1993.
133. Herbert JM, Bernat A, Dol F, et al: DX-9056A, a novel, synthetic, selective and overly active inhibitor of factor Xa: In vitro and in vivo studies. J Pharmacol Exp Ther 276:1030–1038, 1996.
134. Spanier TB, Oz MC, Mianov OP, et al: Heparinless cardiopulmonary bypass with active-site blocked factor IXa: A preliminary study on the dog. J Thorac Cardiovasc Surg 115:1179–1188, 1998.
135. Kelley RF, Refino CJ, O'Connell MP, et al: A soluble tissue factor mutant is a selective anticoagulant and antithrombotic agent. Blood 89: 3219–3227, 1997.
136. Stanssens P, Bergum PW, Gansemans Y, et al: Anticoagulant repertoire of the hookworm Ancylostoma caninum. Proc Natl Acad Sci U S A 93: 2149–2154, 1996.
137. Broze GJ Jr: The role of tissue factor pathway inhibitor in a revised coagulation cascade. Semin Hematol 29:159–169, 1992.

Thrombolytic (Fibrinolytic) Drugs

138. Bell WR Jr: Evaluation of thrombolytic agents. Drugs 54(Suppl 3):11–16, 1997.
139. Collen D, Lijnen HR: Basic and clinical aspects of fibrinolysis and thrombolysis. Blood 78:3114–3124, 1991.
140. Collen D: Thrombolytic therapy. Thromb Haemost 78:742–746, 1997.
141. Leopold JA, Keaney JF Jr, Loscalzo J: Pharmacology of thrombolytic agents. In Loscalzo J, Schafer AI (eds): Thrombosis and Hemorrhage. 2nd ed. Baltimore, Williams & Wilkins, 1998, pp 1215–1258.
142. McGrath K, Hogan C, Hunt D, et al: Neutralising antibodies after streptokinase treatment for myocardial infarction: A persisting puzzle. Br Heart J 74:122–123, 1995.
143. Lee HS, Yule S, McKenzie A, et al: Hypersensitivity reactions to streptokinase in patients with high pre-treatment antistreptokinase antibody and neutralisation titres. Eur Heart J 14:1640–1643, 1993.
144. Lee HS, Cross S, Davidson R, et al: Raised levels of antistreptokinase antibody and neutralization in titres from 4 to 54 months after administration of streptokinase and antistreplase. Eur Heart J 14:84–89, 1993.
145. Schwartz BS, Espana F: Two distinct urokinase-serpin interactions regulate the initiation of cell surface-associated plasminogen activation. J Biol Chem 274:15278–15283, 1999.
146. Tanswell P, Tebbe U, Neuhaus KL, et al: Pharmacokinetics and fibrin specificity of alteplase during accelerated infusions in acute myocardial infarction. J Am Coll Cardiol 19:1071–1075, 1992.
147. Madison EL: Probing structure-function relationships of tissue-type plasminogen activator by site-specific mutagenesis. Fibrinolysis 8:221–236, 1994.

148. Ross AM: New plasminogen activators: A clinical review. Clin Cardiol 22:165–171, 1999.
149. Noble S, McTavish D: Reteplase: A review of its pharmacological properties and clinical efficacy in the management of acute myocardial infarction. Drugs 52:589–605, 1996.
150. Keyt BA, Paoni NF, Refino CJ, et al: A faster-acting and more potent form of tissue plasminogen activator. Proc Natl Acad Sci U S A 91: 3670–3674, 1994.
151. den Heijer P, Vermeer F, Ambrosioni E, et al: Evaluation of a weight-adjusted single-bolus plasminogen activator in patients with myocardial infarction: A double-blind, randomized angiographic trial of lanoteplase versus alteplase. Circulation 98:2117–2125, 1998.
152. Witt W, Maas B, Baldus B, et al: Coronary thrombolysis with Desmodus salivary plasminogen activator in dogs: Fast and persistent recanalization by intravenous bolus administration. Circulation 90:421–426, 1994.
153. Toschi L, Bringmann P, Petri T, et al: Fibrin selectivity of the isolated protease domains of tissue-type and vampire bat salivary gland plasminogen activators. Eur J Biochem 252:108–112, 1998.
154. Haber E: Antibody targeting: A strategy for improving thrombolytic therapy. In Haber E (ed): Molecular Cardiovascular Medicine. New York, Scientific America, 1995, pp 145–155.
155. Collen D, Lijnen HR: Staphylokinase: A fibrin-specific plasminogen activator with therapeutic potential? Blood 84:680–686, 1994.
156. Collen D: Staphylokinase: A potent, uniquely fibrin-selective thrombolytic agent. Nat Med 4:279–284, 1998.
157. Jespers L, Vanwetswinkel S, Lijnen HR, et al: Structural and functional basis of plasminogen activation of staphylokinase. Thromb Haemost 81: 479–485, 1999.

Antiplatelet Agents

158. Schafer AI: Antiplatelet therapy. Am J Med 101:199–209, 1996.
159. Schafer AI: Aspirin and antiplatelet agents in cardiovascular disease. In Smith TW (ed): Cardiovascular Therapeutics. Philadelphia, WB Saunders, 1996, pp 427–442.
159a. Awtry EH, Loscalzo J: Aspirin. Circulation 101:1206–1218, 2000.
160. Folts JD, Schafer AI, Loscalzo J, et al: A perspective on the potential problems with aspirin as an antithrombotic agent: A comparison of studies in an animal model with clinical trials. J Am Coll Cardiol 33: 295–303, 1999.
161. Patrono C: Aspirin as an antiplatelet drug. N Engl J Med 330:1287–1294, 1994.
162. Calverly DC, Roth GJ: Antiplatelet therapy. Aspirin, ticlopidine/clopidogrel, and anti-integrin agents. Hematol/Oncol Clin North Am 12: 1231–1249, 1998.
163. Dabaghi SF, Kamat SG, Payne J, et al: Effects of low-dose aspirin on in vitro platelet aggregation in the early minutes after ingestion in normal subjects. Am J Cardiol 74:720–723, 1994.
164. Schafer AI: Effects of nonsteroidal anti-inflammatory therapy on platelets. Am J Med 106(5b):25s–36s, 1999.
165. Picot D, Loll PJ, Garavito RM: The x-ray crystal structure of the membrane protein prostaglandin H_2 synthase-1. Nature 367:243–249, 1994.
166. Loll PJ, Picot D, Ekabo D, et al: Synthesis and use of iodinated nonsteroidal anti-inflammatory drug analogs as crystallographic probes of the prostaglandin H_2 synthase cyclooxygenase active site. Biochemistry 35: 7330–7340, 1996.
167. Klein T, Nüsing RM, Pfeilschifter J, et al: Selective inhibition of cyclooxygenase 2. Biochem Pharmacol 48:1605–1610, 1994.
168. Riendeau D, Percival MD, Boyce S, et al: Biochemical and pharmacologic profile of a tetrasubstituted furanone as a highly selective COX-2 inhibitor. Br J Pharmacol 121:105–107, 1997.
169. McAdam B, Catella-Lawson F, Mardini L, et al: Systemic biosynthesis of prostacyclin by cyclooxygenase (COX)-2: The human pharmacology of a selective inhibitor of Cox-2. Proc Natl Acad Sci U S A 96:272–277, 1999.
170. The RAPT Investigators. Randomized trial of ridogrel, a combined thromboxane A_2 synthase inhibitor and thromboxane A_2/prostaglandin endoperoxide receptor antagonist, versus aspirin as adjunct to thrombolysis in patients with acute myocardial infarction. Circulation 89:588–595, 1994.
171. Sharis PJ, Cannon CP, Loscalzo J: The antiplatelet effects of ticlopidine and clopidogrel. Ann Intern Med 129:394–405, 1998.
172. Chen DK, Kim JS, Sutton DM: Thrombotic thrombocytopenic purpura associated with ticlopidine use: A report of 3 cases and review of the literature. Arch Intern Med 159:311–314, 1999.
173. Steinhubl SR, Tan WA, Foody JM, et al: Incidence and clinical course of thrombotic thrombocytopenia purpura due to ticlopidine following coronary stenting. EPISTENT Investigators. Evaluation of platelet IIb/IIIa inhibitor for stenting. JAMA 281:806–810, 1999.
173a. Bennett CL, Connors JM, Carwile JM, et al: Thrombotic thrombocytopenic purpura associated with clopidogrel. N Engl J Med 342:1773–1777, 2000.
174. Diener H, Cuhla L, Forbes C, et al: European Stroke Prevention Study 2: Dipyridamole and acetylsalicylic acid in the secondary prevention of stroke. J Neurol Sci 143:1–13, 1996.
175. Coller BS: Blockade of platelet GpIIb/IIIa receptors as an antithrombotic strategy. Circulation 92:2373–2380, 1995.
176. Vorcheimer DA, Badimon JJ, Fuster V: Platelet glycoprotein IIb/IIIa receptor antagonists in cardiovascular disease. JAMA 281:1407–1414, 1999.

177. Byrne A, Moran N, Maher M, et al: Continued thromboxane A₂ formation despite administration a platelet glycoprotein IIb/IIIa antagonist in patients undergoing coronary angioplasty. Arteriosc Thromb Vasc Biol 17:3224–3229, 1997.

178. Madan M, Berkowitz SD, Tcheng JE: Glycoprotein IIb/IIIa integrin blockade. Circulation 98:2629–2635, 1998.

179. Topol EJ, Byzova TV, Plow EF: Platelet GpIIb-IIIa blockers. Lancet 353:227–231, 1999.

180. Jordan RE, Mascelli MA, Nakada MT, et al: Pharmacology and clinical development of abciximab (c7E3 Fab, ReoPro). In Sasahara AA, Loscalzo J (eds): New Therapeutic Agents in Thrombosis and Thrombolysis. New York, Marcel Dekker, 1997, pp 291–313.

181. Reverter JC, Beguin S, Kessels H, et al: Inhibition of platelet-mediated, tissue factor–induced thrombin generation by the mouse/human chimeric 7E3 antibody: Potential implications for the effect c7E3 Fab treatment on acute thrombosis and "clinical restenosis." J Clin Invest 98:863–874, 1996.

182. Topol EJ, Ferguson JJ, Weisman HF, et al: Long-term protection from myocardial ischemic events in a randomized trial of brief integrin β3 blockade with percutaneous coronary intervention. JAMA 278:479–484, 1997.

183. Tcheng JE, Kereiakes DJ, Braden GA, et al: Readministration of abciximab: Interim report of the ReoPro Readministration Registry. Am Heart J 138:33–38, 1999.

184. Goa KL, Noble S: Eptifibatide: A review of its use in patients with acute coronary syndromes and/or undergoing percutaneous coronary intervention. Drugs 57:439–462, 1999.

185. Lorenz TJ, Macdonald F, Kitt MM: Nonimmunogenieity of eptifibatide, a cyclic heptapeptide inhibitor of platelet glycoprotein IIb–IIIa. Clin Ther 21:128–137, 1999.

186. Coller BS: Monitoring platelet Gp IIb/IIIa antagonist therapy. Circulation 97:5–9, 1998.

187. Smith JW, Steinhubl SR, Lincoff AM, et al: Rapid platelet-function assay: An automated and quantitative cartridge-based method. Circulation 99:620–625, 1999.

188. Peter K, Schwarz M, Ylanne J, et al: Induction of fibrinogen binding and platelet aggregation as a potential intrinsic property of various glycoprotein IIb/IIIa (αIIb β3) inhibitors. Blood 92:3240–3249, 1998.

ANTITHROMBOTIC AND THROMBOLYTIC THERAPY IN CARDIOVASCULAR DISEASE

189. Steering Committee of the Physicians' Health Study Research Group: Final report on the aspirin component of the ongoing Physicians' Health Study. N Engl J Med 321:129–135, 1989.

190. Peto R, Gray R, Collins R, et al: Randomised trial of prophylactic daily aspirin in British male doctors. BMJ 296:313–316, 1988.

191. Medical Research Council's General Practice Research Framework: Thrombosis prevention trial: Randomized trial of low-intensity oral anticoagulation with warfarin and low-dose aspirin in the primary prevention of ischaemic heart disease in men at increased risk. Lancet 351:233–241, 1998.

192. Hennekens CH, Buring JE, Sandercock P, et al: Aspirin and other antiplatelet agents in the secondary and primary prevention of cardiovascular disease. Circulation 80:749–756, 1989.

193. Levine GN, Stein B, Ali MN: Antithrombotic therapy in cardiovascular disease. In Loscalzo J, Schafer AI (eds): Thrombosis and Hemorrhage, pp 1309–1336. Baltimore, Williams & Wilkins, 1998.

194. Breddin K, Loew D, Lechner K, et al: The German-Austrian aspirin trial: A comparison of acetylsalicylic acid, placebo and phenprocoumon in secondary prevention of myocardial infarction. On behalf of the German-Austrian Study Group. Circulation 62:v63–72, 1980.

195. Elwood PC, Cochrane AL, Burr ML, et al: A randomized controlled trial of acetylsalicylic acid in the secondary prevention of mortality from myocardial infarction. BMJ 1:436–440, 1974.

196. Elwood PC, Sweetnam PM: Aspirin and secondary mortality after myocardial infarction. Lancet 2:1313–1315, 1979.

197. The Coronary Drug Project Research Group: Aspirin in coronary heart disease. Circulation 62:v59–v62, 1980.

198. The Persantine-Aspirin Reinfarction Study Research Group: Persantine and aspirin in coronary heart disease. Circulation 62:449–461, 1980.

199. The Aspirin Myocardial Infarction Study Group: The aspirin myocardial infarction study: Final results. Circulation 62:v79–v84, 1980.

200. Klimt CR, Knatterud GL, Stamler J, et al: Persantine-Aspirin Reinfarction Study: II. Secondary coronary prevention with persantine and aspirin. J Am Coll Cardiol 7:251–269, 1986.

201. Antiplatelet Trialists' Collaboration: Collaborative overview of randomised trials of antiplatelet therapy: I. Prevention of death, myocardial infarction, and stroke by prolonged antiplatelet therapy in various categories of patients. BMJ 308:81–106, 1994.

202. Fiore LD, Deykin D: Use of antiplatelet agents and anticoagulants in post-myocardial infarction. Cardiol Clin 12:451–476, 1994.

203. CAPRIE Steering Committee: A randomised, blinded, trial of clopidogrel versus aspirin in patients at risk of ischaemic events (CAPRIE). Lancet 348:1329–1339, 1996.

204. MRC Trial: Working party on anticoagulant therapy in coronary thrombosis to the Medical Research Council: An assessment of long-term anticoagulant administration after cardiac infarction: Second report. BMJ 2:837–843, 1964.

205. Ebert RV: Long-term anticoagulant therapy after myocardial infarction: Final report of the Veterans Administration cooperative study. JAMA 207:2263–2267, 1969.

206. EPSIM Research Group: A controlled comparison of aspirin and oral anticoagulants in prevention of death after myocardial infarction. N Engl J Med 307:701–708, 1982.

207. Smith P, Arnesen H, Holme I: The effect of warfarin on mortality and reinfarction after myocardial infarction. N Engl J Med 323:147–152, 1990.

208. The ASPECT Research Group: Effect of long-term oral anticoagulant treatment on mortality and cardiovascular morbidity after myocardial infarction. Anticoagulants in the Secondary Prevention of Events in Coronary Thrombosis (ASPECT). Lancet 343:499–503, 1994.

209. CARS Investigators: Randomised double-blind trial of fixed low-dose warfarin with aspirin after myocardial infarction. Coumadin Aspirin Reinfarction Study. Lancet 350:389–396, 1997.

210. Cairns JA, Markham BA: Economics and efficacy in choosing oral anticoagulants or aspirin after myocardial infarction. JAMA 273:965–967, 1995.

211. Ferguson JJ: Meeting Highlights: Highlights of the 48th scientific sessions of the American College of Cardiology. Circulation 100:570–575, 1999.

Prevention of Cardiac Chamber and Prosthetic Valvular Thromboembolism

212. Chalmers TC, Matta RJ, Smith HJ, et al: Evidence favoring the use of anticoagulants in the hospital phase of acute myocardial infarction. N Engl J Med 297:1091–1096, 1977.

213. The MRC Study Group: Assessment of short-anticoagulant administration after cardiac infarction. Report of the Working Party on Anticoagulant Therapy in Coronary Thrombosis to the Medical Research Council. BMJ 1:335–342, 1969.

214. Drapkin A, Merskey C: Anticoagulant therapy after acute myocardial infarction: Relation of therapeutic benefit to patient's age, sex, and severity of infarction. JAMA 222:541–548, 1972.

215. Chiarella F, Santoro E, Domenicucci S, et al: Predischarge two-dimensional echocardiographic evaluation of left ventricular thrombosis after acute myocardial infarction in the GISSI-3 study. Am J Cardiol 81:822–827, 1998.

216. Mooe T, Teien D, Karp K, et al: Long-term follow up of patients with anterior myocardial infarction complicated by left ventricular thrombus in the thrombolytic era. Heart 75:252–256, 1996.

217. Loh E, Sutton MS, Wun CC, et al: Ventricular dysfunction and the risk of stroke after myocardial infarction. N Engl J Med 336:251–257, 1997.

218. Turpie AG, Robinson JG, Doyle DJ, et al: Comparison of high-dose with low-dose subcutaneous heparin to prevent left ventricular mural thrombosis in patients with acute transmural anterior myocardial infarction. N Engl J Med 320:352–357, 1989.

219. Randomised controlled trial of subcutaneous calcium-heparin in acute myocardial infarction. The SCATI (Studio sulla Calciparina nell'Angina e nella Trombosi Ventricolare nell'Infarto) Group. Lancet 2:182–186, 1989.

220. Hirsh J, Fuster V: Guide to anticoagulant therapy: II. Oral anticoagulants. Circulation 89:1469–1480, 1994.

221. Koniaris LS, Goldhaber SZ: Anticoagulation in dilated cardiomyopathy. J Am Coll Cardiol 31:745–748, 1998.

222. Yamamoto K, Ikeda U, Furuhashi K, et al: The coagulation system is activated in idiopathic cardiomyopathy. J Am Coll Cardiol 25:1634–1640, 1995.

223. Roberts WC, Siegel RJ, McManus BM: Idiopathic dilated cardiomyopathy: Analysis of 152 necropsy patients. Am J Cardiol 60:1340–1355, 1987.

224. Fuster V, Gersh BJ, Giuliani ER, et al: The natural history of idiopathic dilated cardiomyopathy. Am J Cardiol 47:525–531, 1981.

225. Katz SD, Marantz PR, Biasucci L, et al: Low incidence of stroke in ambulatory patients with heart failure: A prospective study. Am Heart J 126:141–146, 1993.

226. Natterson PD, Stevenson WG, Saxon LA, et al: Risk of arterial embolization in 224 patients awaiting cardiac transplantation. Am Heart J 129:564–570, 1995.

227. Al-Khadra AS, Salem DN, Rand WM, et al: Warfarin anticoagulation and survival: A cohort analysis from the Studies of Left Ventricular Dysfunction. J Am Coll Cardiol 31:749–753, 1998.

228. Dries DL, Rosenberg YD, Waclawiw MA, et al: Ejection fraction and risk of thromboembolic events in patients with systolic dysfunction and sinus rhythm: Evidence for gender differences in the studies of left ventricular dysfunction trials [published erratum appears in J Am Coll Cardiol 32:555, 1998]. J Am Coll Cardiol 29:1074–1080, 1997.

229. Dunkman WB, Johnson GR, Carson PE, et al: Incidence of thromboembolic events in congestive heart failure. The V-HeFT VA Cooperative Studies Group. Circulation 87:vi94–vi101, 1993.

Prosthetic Heart Valves

230. Heras, M, Chesebro JH, Fuster V, et al: High risk of thromboembolic events early after bioprosthetic cardiac valve replacement. J Am Coll Cardiol 25:1111–1119, 1995.

231. Tiede DJ, Nishimura RA, Gastineau DA, et al: Modern management of prosthetic valve anticoagulation. Mayo Clin Proc 73:665–680, 1998.
232. Cannegieter SC, Rosendaal FR, Briet E: Thromboembolic and bleeding complications in patients with mechanical heart valve prostheses. Circulation 89:635–641, 1994.
233. Cannegister SC, Rosendaal FR, Wintzen AR, et al: Optimal oral anticoagulant therapy in patients with mechanical heart valves. N Engl J Med 333:11–17, 1995.
234. Horstkotte D, Scharf RE, Schultheiss HP: Intracardiac thrombosis: Patient-related and device-related factors. J Heart Valve Dis 4:114–120, 1995.
235. Horstkotte D, Schulte HD, Bircks W, et al: Lower intensity anticoagulation therapy results in lower complication rates with the St. Jude medical prosthesis. J Thorac Cardiovasc Surg 107:1136–1145, 1994.
236. Isreal DH, Sharma SK, Fuster V: Antithrombotic therapy in prosthetic heart valve replacement. Am Heart J 127:400, 1994.
237. Israel DH, Fuster V, Ip JH, et al: Intracardiac thrombosis and systemic embolization. In Colman RW, Hirsh J, Marder VJ, Salzman EW (eds): Hemostasis and Thrombosis: Basic Principles and Clinical Practice. Philadelphia, JB Lippincott, 1994, pp 1452–1468.
238. Mok DC, Boey J, Wang R, et al: Warfarin versus dipyridamole-aspirin and pentoxifylline-aspirin for the prevention of prosthetic heart valve thromboembolism: A prospective randomized clinical trial. Circulation 72:1059, 1985.
239. Stein PD, Alpert JS, Dalen JE, et al: Antithrombotic therapy in patients with mechanical and biological prosthetic heart valves. Chest 114:602s–610s, 1998.
240. Nunez L, Aguado GM, Larrea JL, et al: Prevention of thromboembolism using asprin after mitral valve replacement with porcine bioprosthesis. Ann Thorac Surg 37:84–87, 1984.
241. Horstkotte D, Schulte H, Bircks W, et al: Unexpected findings concerning thromboembolic complications and anticoagulation after complete 10 year follow-up of patients with St. Jude medical prosthesis. J Heart Valve Dis 2:291–301, 1993.
242. Acar J, Iung B, Boissel JP, et al: AREVA: Multicenter randomized comparison of low-dose versus standard dose anticoagulation in patients with mechanical prosthetic heart valves. Circulation 94:2107–2112, 1996.
243. Turpie AGG, Gunstensen J, Hirsh J, et al: Randomised comparison of two intensities of oral anticoagulant therapy after tissue heart valve replacement. Lancet 1:1242–1245, 1988.
244. Study Group of the Working Group on Valvular Heart Disease of the European Society of Cardiology: Guidelines for prevention of thromboembolic events in valvular heart disease. Eur Heart J 16:1320–1330, 1995.
245. Hirsh J, Fuster V: AHA medical/scienfific statement: Guide to anticoagulant therapy: II. Oral anticoagulants. Circulation 89:1469–1480, 1994.
246. Turpie AGG, Gent M, Laupacis A, et al: A comparison of aspirin with placebo in patients treated with warfarin after heart-valve replacement. N Engl J Med 329:524–529, 1993.
247. Cappelleri JC, Fiore LD, Brophy MT, et al: Efficacy and safety of combined anticoagulant and antiplatelet therapy versus anticoagulant monotherapy after mechanical heart-valve replacement: A metaanalysis. Am Heart J 130:547–552, 1995.
248. Meschengieser SS, Fondevila CG, Frontroth J, et al:: Low-intensity oral anticoagulation plus low-dose aspirin versus high-intensity oral anticoagulation alone: A randomized trial in patients with mechanical prosthetic heart valves. J Thorac Cardiovasc Surg 113:910–916, 1997.
249. Altman R, Rouvier J, Gurfinkel E, et al: Comparison of high-dose with low-dose aspirin in patients with mechanical heart valve replacement treated with oral anticoagulant. Circulation 94:2113–2116, 1996.

Percutaneous Coronary Interventions

250. Bittl JA: Medical progress—advances in coronary angioplasty. N Engl J Med 335:1290–1302, 1996.
251. EPIC Investigators: Use of a monoclonal antibody directed against the platelet glycoprotein IIb/IIIa receptor in high-risk coronary angioplasty. The EPIC Investigation. N Engl J Med 330:956–961, 1994.
252. RESTORE Investigators: Effects of platelet glycoprotein IIb/IIIa blockade with tirofiban on adverse cardiac events in patients with unstable angina or acute myocardial infarction undergoing coronary angioplasty. Randomized Efficacy Study of Tirofiban for Outcomes and Restenosis. Circulation 96:1445–1453, 1997.
253. IMPACT-II Investigators: Randomised placebo-controlled trial of effect of eptifibatide on complications of percutaneous coronary intervention: IMPACT-II. Integrilin to Minimise Platelet Aggregation and Coronary Thrombosis-II. Lancet 349:1422–1428, 1997.
254. EPISTENT Investigators: Randomised placebo-controlled and balloon-angioplasty–controlled trial to assess safety of coronary stenting with use of platelet glycoprotein-IIb/IIIa blockade. Evaluation of Platelet IIb/IIIa Inhibitor for Stenting. Lancet 352:87–92, 1998.
255. Schwartz L, Bourassa MG, Lesperance J, et al: Aspirin and dipyridamole in the prevention of restenosis after percutaneous transluminal coronary angioplasty. N Engl J Med 318:1714–1719, 1988.
256. Colombo A, Hall P, Nakamura S, et al: Intracoronary stenting without anticoagulation accomplished with intravascular ultrasound guidance. Circulation 91:1676–1688, 1995.
257. CAPTURE Investigators: Randomised placebo-controlled trial of abcixi-mab before and during coronary intervention in refractory unstable angina: The CAPTURE Study. Lancet 349:1429–1435, 1997.
258. Berkowitz SD, Sane DC, Sigmon KN, et al: Occurrence and clinical significance of thrombocytopenia in a population undergoing high-risk percutaneous coronary revascularization: Evaluation of c7E3 for the Prevention of Ischemic Complications (EPIC) Study Group. J Am Coll Cardiol 32:311–319, 1998.
259. Jenkins LA, Lau S, Crawford M, et al: Delayed profound thrombocytopenia after c7E3 Fab (abciximab) therapy. Circulation 97:1214–1215, 1998.
260. Ferrari E, Thiry M, Touati C, et al: Acute profound thrombocytopenia after c7E3 Fab therapy. Circulation 96:3809–3810, 1997.
261. Berkowitz SD, Harrington RA, Rund MM, et al: Acute profound thrombocytopenia after C7E3 Fab (abciximab) therapy. Circulation 95:809–813, 1997.
262. McGarry TFJ, Gottlieb RS, Morganroth J, et al: The relationship of anticoagulation level and complications after successful percutaneous transluminal coronary angioplasty. Am Heart J 123:1445–1451, 1992.
263. Narins CR, Hillegass WBJ, Nelson CL, et al: Relation between activated clotting time during angioplasty and abrupt closure. Circulation 93:667–671, 1996.
264. Eitzman DT, Chi L, Saggin L, et al: Heparin neutralization by platelet-rich thrombi: Role of platelet factor 4. Circulation 89:1523–1529, 1994.
265. Ali MN, Villarreal-Levy G, Schafer AI: The role of thrombin and thrombin inhibitors in coronary angioplasty. Chest 108:1409–1419, 1995.
266. Bittl JA, Strony J, Brinker JA, et al: Treatment with bivalirudin (Hirulog) as compared with heparin during coronary angioplasty for unstable or postinfarction angina. Hirulog Angioplasty Study Investigators. N Engl J Med 333:764–769, 1995.
267. Serruys PW, Herrman JP, Simon R, et al: A comparison of hirudin with heparin in the prevention of restenosis after coronary angioplasty. Helvetica Investigators. N Engl J Med 333:757–763, 1995.
268. Zoldhelyi P, Bichler J, Owen WG, et al: Persistent thrombin generation in humans during specific thrombin inhibition with hirudin. Circulation 90:2671–2678, 1994.
269. Serruys PW, Strauss BH, Beatt KJ, et al: Angiographic follow-up after placement of a self-expanding coronary-artery stent. N Engl J Med 324:13–17, 1991.
270. Schatz RA, Baim DS, Leon M, et al: Clinical experience with the Palmaz-Schatz coronary stent: Initial results of a multicenter study. Circulation 83:148–161, 1991.
271. George BS, Voorhees WD, Roubin GS, et al: Multicenter investigation of coronary stenting to treat acute or threatened closure after percutaneous transluminal coronary angioplasty: Clinical and angiographic outcomes. J Am Coll Cardiol 22:135–143, 1993.
272. Schomig A, Neumann FJ, Kastrati A, et al: A randomized comparison of antiplatelet and anticoagulant therapy after the placement of coronary-artery stents. N Engl J Med 334:1084–1089, 1996.
273. Bertrand ME, Legrand V, Boland J, et al: Randomized multicenter comparison of conventional anticoagulation versus antiplatelet therapy in unplanned and elective coronary stenting: The full anticoagulation versus aspirin and ticlopidine (fantastic) study. Circulation 98:1597–1603, 1998.
274. Schuhlen H, Hadamitzky M, Walter H, et al: Major benefit from antiplatelet therapy for patients at high risk for adverse cardiac events after coronary Palmaz-Schatz stent placement: Analysis of a prospective risk stratification protocol in the Intracoronary Stenting and Antithrombotic Regimen (ISAR) trial. Circulation 95:2015–2021, 1997.
275. Urban P, Macaya C, Rupprecht HJ, et al: Randomized evaluation of anticoagulation versus antiplatelet therapy after coronary stent implantation in high-risk patients: The multicenter aspirin and ticlopidine trial after intracoronary stenting (MATTIS). Circulation 98:2126–2132, 1998.
276. Leon MB, Baim DS, Popma JJ, et al: A clinical trial comparing three antithrombotic-drug regimens after coronary-artery stenting. Stent Anticoagulation Restenosis Study Investigators. N Engl J Med 339:1665–1671, 1998.
277. Ariyoshi K, Shinohara K, Ruirong X: Thrombotic thrombocytopenic purpura caused by ticlopidine, successfully treated by plasmapheresis. Am J Hematol 54:175–176, 1997.
278. Bennett CL, Kiss JE, Weinberg PD, et al: Thrombotic thrombocytopenic purpura after stenting and ticlopidine. Lancet 352:1036–1037, 1998.
279. Bennett CL, Weinberg PD, Rozenberg-Ben-Dror K, et al: Thrombotic thrombocytopenic purpura associated with ticlopidine: A review of 60 cases. Ann Intern Med 128:541–544, 1998.
280. Centurioni R, Candela M, Leoni P, et al: Is ticlopidine really responsible for thrombotic thrombocytopenic purpura (TTP)? Haematologica 78:196–197, 1993.
281. Ellie E, Durrieu C, Besse P, et al: Thrombotic thrombocytopenic purpura associated with ticlopidine [letter]. Stroke 23:922–923, 1992.
282. Jamar S, Vanderheyden M, Janssens L, et al: Thrombotic thrombocytopenic purpura: A rare but potential life-threatening complication following ticlopidine administration. Acta Cardiol 53:285–286, 1998.
283. Kovacs MJ, Soong PY, Chin-Yee IH: Thrombotic thrombocytopenic purpura associated with ticlopidine. Ann Pharmacother 27:1060–1061, 1993.
284. Kupfer Y, Tessler S: Ticlopidine and thrombotic thrombocytopenic purpura. N Engl J Med 337:1245, 1997.
285. Mukamal KJ, Wu B, McPhedran P: Ticlopidine-associated thrombotic thrombocytopenic purpura. Ann Intern Med 129:837, 1998.

286. Muszkat M, Shapira MY, Sviri S, et al: Ticlopidine-induced thrombotic thrombocytopenic purpura. Pharmacotherapy 18:1352–1355, 1998.
287. Page Y, Tardy B, Zeni F, et al: Thrombotic thrombocytopenic purpura related to ticlopidine. Lancet 337:774–776, 1991.
288. Vianelli N, Catani L, Belmonte MM, et al: Ticlopidine in the treatment of thrombotic thrombocytopenic purpura: Report of two cases. Haematologica 75:274–277, 1990.
289. Moussa I, Oetgen M, Roubin G, et al: Effectiveness of clopidogrel and aspirin versus ticlopidine and aspirin in preventing stent thrombosis after coronary stent implantation. Circulation 99:2364–2366, 1999.
290. Schwartz RS, Holmes DR Jr, Topol EJ: The restenosis paradigm revisited: An alternative proposal for cellular mechanisms. J Am Coll Cardiol 20:1284–1293, 1992.
291. Mintz GS, Kent KM, Pichard AD, et al: Intravascular ultrasound insights into mechanisms of stenosis formation and restenosis. Cardiol Clin 15:17–29, 1997.

Antithrombotic Therapy after Coronary Artery Bypass Surgery

292. Goldman S, Copeland J, Moritz T, et al: Improvement in early saphenous vein graft patency after coronary artery bypass surgery with antiplatelet therapy: Results of a Veterans Administration Cooperative Study. Circulation 77:1324–1332, 1988.
293. Goldman S, Copeland J, Moritz T, et al: Saphenous vein graft patency 1 year after coronary artery bypass surgery and effects of antiplatelet therapy: Results of a Veterans Administration Cooperative Study. Circulation 80:1190–1197, 1989.
294. Motwani JG, Topol EJ: Aortocoronary saphenous vein graft disease: Pathogenesis, predisposition, and prevention. Circulation 97:916–931, 1998.
295. Stein PD, Dalen JE, Goldman S, et al: Antithrombotic therapy in patients with saphenous vein and internal mammary artery bypass grafts. Chest 114:658s–665s, 1998.
296. Sanz G, Pajaron A, Alegria E, et al: Prevention of early aortocoronary bypass occlusion by low-dose aspirin and dipyridamole. Grupo Espanol para el Seguimiento del Injerto Coronario (GESIC). Circulation 82:765–773, 1990.
297. Boyle EMJ, Lille ST, Allaire E, et al: Endothelial cell injury in cardiovascular surgery: Atherosclerosis. Ann Thorac Surg 63:885–894, 1997.
298. Sellke FW, Boyle EMJ, Verrier ED: Endothelial cell injury in cardiovascular surgery: The pathophysiology of vasomotor dysfunction. Ann Thorac Surg 62:1222–1228, 1996.
299. Verrier ED, Boyle EMJ: Endothelial cell injury in cardiovascular surgery. Ann Thorac Surg 62:915–922, 1996.
300. Roubos N, Rosenfeldt FL, Richards SM, et al: Improved preservation of saphenous vein grafts by the use of glyceryl trinitrate-verapamil solution during harvesting. Circulation 92:ii31–ii36, 1995.
301. Boyle EMJ, Verrier ED, Spiess BD: Endothelial cell injury in cardiovascular surgery: The procoagulant response. Ann Thorac Surg 62:1549–1557, 1996.
302. Limet R, David JL, Magotteaux P, et al: Prevention of aorta-coronary bypass graft occlusion: Beneficial effect of ticlopidine on early and late patency rates of venous coronary bypass grafts: A double-blind study. J Thorac Cardiovasc Surg 94:773–783, 1987.
303. Chesebro JH, Fuster V, Elveback LR, et al: Effect of dipyridamole and aspirin on late vein-graft patency after coronary bypass operations. N Engl J Med 310:209–214, 1984.
304. Goldman S, Copeland J, Moritz T, et al: Starting aspirin therapy after operation: Effects on early graft patency. Department of Veterans Affairs Cooperative Study Group. Circulation 84:520–526, 1991.
305. Lorenz RL, Schacky CV, Weber M, et al: Improved aortocoronary bypass patency by low-dose aspirin (100 mg daily): Effects on platelet aggregation and thromboxane formation. Lancet 1:1261–1264, 1984.
306. Goldman S, Copeland J, Moritz T, et al: Long-term graft patency (3 years) after coronary artery surgery: Effects of aspirin: Results of a VA cooperative study. Circulation 89:1138–1143, 1994.
307. Leon M, Baim D, Gordon P, et al: Clinical and angiographic results from the Stent Anticoagulant Regimen Study (STARS). Circulation 96(Suppl I):I–685, 1996.
308. van der Meer J, Hillege HL, Kootstra GJ, et al: Prevention of one-year vein-graft occlusion after aortocoronary-bypass surgery: A comparison of low-dose aspirin, low-dose aspirin plus dipyridamole, and oral anticoagulants. The CABADAS Research Group of the Interuniversity Cardiology Institute of The Netherlands. Lancet 342:257–264, 1993.
309. McEnany MT, Salzman EW, Mundth ED, et al: The effect of antithrombotic therapy on patency rates of saphenous vein coronary artery bypass grafts. J Thorac Cardiovasc Surg 83:81–89, 1982.
310. Pantely GA, Goodnight SHJ, Rahimtoola SH, et al: Failure of antiplatelet and anticoagulant therapy to improve patency of grafts after coronary-artery bypass: A controlled, randomized study. N Engl J Med 301:962–966, 1979.
311. The Post Coronary Artery Bypass Graft Trial Investigators: The effect of aggressive lowering of low-density lipoprotein cholesterol levels and low-dose anticoagulation on obstructive changes in saphenous-vein coronary-artery bypass grafts. N Engl J Med 336:153–162, 1997.
312. deBelder A, Salas E, Langford E, et al: S-nitrosoglutathione inhibits coronary artery vein graft platelet activation in vivo. Eur Heart J 17(Suppl):545, 1996.
313. Cable DG, O'Brien T, Schaff HV, et al: Adenoviral transfection of human saphenous veins with eNOS: Gene therapy applied to coronary bypass conduits. Circulation 94(Suppl I):I–295, 1996.
314. Chen SJ, Wilson JM, Muller DW: Adenovirus-mediated gene transfer of soluble vascular cell adhesion molecule to porcine interposition vein grafts. Circulation 89:1922–1928, 1994.
315. Annex BH, Fulton GJ, Channon KM, et al: Local delivery of an anti-tissue factor antibody decreases leukocyte infiltration but fails to limit intimal hyperplasia in experimental vein grafts. Circulation 94(Suppl I):I–4, 1996.

Chapter 63

Diabetes Mellitus and the Cardiovascular System

RICHARD W. NESTO • PETER LIBBY

SCOPE OF THE PROBLEM

In the coming decades, the burden of cardiovascular diseases (CVDs) related to diabetes will increase substantially. Diabetes, formerly thought of as a problem of glucose metabolism, actually produces most of its harm by effects on the cardiovascular system.[1, 2, 2a] Microvascular disease underlies the pathogenesis of diabetic retinopathy, a common cause of blindness. Microvascular disease also causes diabetic renal disease, a major contributor to need for dialysis therapy.

Most diabetics die of CVD, and atherosclerosis accounts for some 80 percent of all diabetic mortality. About three-quarters of the cardiovascular deaths from diabetes result from coronary artery disease (CAD). The remaining quarter results from cerebral or peripheral vascular disease. Atherosclerotic disease causes some three-quarters of all hospitalizations for diabetic complications. Tight control of glycemia consistently reduces the risk of microvascular complications of diabetes in large clinical trials. However, the benefits of glycemic control on the macrovascular complications of diabetes are less firmly established. With the success of currently available hypoglycemic agents in mitigating microvascular disease, a shift toward a preponderance of macrovascular complications may well occur.

The burden of diabetic disease in the population will increase markedly in the coming years. In the United States, the prevalence of diabetes has increased from approximately 2 million cases in the early 1960s to some 15 million in the year 2000. Current estimates project 22 million cases by the year 2025. This increase goes hand in hand with an epidemic of obesity, which affected approximately 18 percent of the U.S. population in 1998.[3] During the 7 years from 1991 to 1998, the body weight of American men increased over 3 percent and that of women almost 5 percent. The significant clustering of atherogenic risk factors, including glucose levels and body weight, links the current epidemic of obesity and diabetes mellitus.[4]

The coming wave of CVD related to diabetes will take a particularly heavy toll in certain minority populations. Hispanics, blacks, Native Americans, and Asian Indians will bear a disproportionate burden of diabetic CVD.[5] The predilection of these ethnic groups to the development of obesity and glucose intolerance on a Western diet may have a genetic basis. The ability to store fat may have conferred a survival advantage in populations subject to famine. This selective pressure could enrich the population in genes that facilitate fat storage, the so-called thrifty gene hypothesis.[6, 7] As discussed below, diabetics with CVD fare worse than their nondiabetic counterparts. Hence, physicians caring for patients with CVD have a compelling need to have a working knowledge of the effects of diabetes mellitus on the heart and blood vessels.

NEW DIAGNOSTIC CRITERIA. In 1997, the American Diabetes Association promulgated new criteria for the diagnosis of diabetes mellitus. These criteria use a single blood glucose determination after an 8-hour fast (fasting plasma glucose [FPG]) as the major diagnostic criterion (Table 63–1). An FPG of less than 110 mg/dl is considered normal. A new diagnostic category known as impaired fasting glucose

▼ TABLE 63–1. CRITERIA FOR THE DIAGNOSIS OF DIABETES MELLITUS

NORMAL	IMPAIRED FASTING GLUCOSE AND IMPAIRED GLUCOSE TOLERANCE	DIABETES MELLITUS
FPG <110 mg/dl	FPG ≥110 mg/dl and <126 mg/dl (IFG)	FPG ≥126 mg/dl
2-hr PG* <140 mg/dl	2-hr PG* ≥140 mg/dl and <200 mg/dl (IGT)	2-hr PG* ≥200 mg/dl
2-hr PG*		Symptoms of DM and random plasma glucose concentration ≥200 mg/dl

*Rather than using the classic glucose tolerance curve with multiple time points sampled, the new criteria use, in parallel with fasting plasma glucose (FPG) measurements, a 2-hour post–glucose load (PG) set of criteria. The plasma sample is obtained 2 hours following an oral administration of 75 gm of anhydrous glucose in aqueous solution.
IFG = impaired fasting glucose; IGT = impaired glucose tolerance.
From The Expert Committee on the Diagnosis and Classification of Diabetes Mellitus: Report of the Expert Committee on the Diagnosis and Classification of Diabetes Mellitus. Diabetes Care 22(Suppl 1):5–19, 1999. Reproduced with permission of The American Diabetes Association, Inc.

encompasses FPGs greater than 110 but less than 126 mg/dl. An FPG greater than 126 mg/dl establishes the diagnosis of diabetes mellitus.

Type II diabetics, previously known as noninsulin-dependent diabetics, represent about 90 percent of the diabetic population. However, those with type I diabetes (previously known as insulin-dependent or juvenile diabetes) also have an independently higher risk of cardiovascular events, and their disease generally develops at a much younger age than in the type II diabetic population.

PATHOPHYSIOLOGY OF THE CARDIOVASCULAR COMPLICATIONS OF DIABETES

A number of metabolic, cellular, and molecular mechanisms underlie diabetic CVD (Table 63–2). A brief discussion of the most important pathophysiological concepts follows:

DYSLIPIDEMIA AND ASSOCIATED METABOLIC ABNORMALITIES (see also Chap. 31). The longest studied, best understood, and most substantiated mechanism for enhanced atherogenesis in type II diabetes is the dyslipidemia and associated cluster of risk factors known as the "metabolic syndrome" (Table 63–3). Increased hepatic production of very low-density lipoproteins (VLDLs) by the liver lies at the center of the pathogenesis of diabetic dyslipidemia (Fig. 63–1). The liver increases its production of VLDL in response to increased delivery of fatty acid from several sources. Uptake of free fatty acids by striated muscle depends on insulin. Under conditions of insulin resistance, striated muscle takes up less free fatty acids, which increases the presentation of free fatty acids to the liver. In addition, central obesity increases the delivery of free fatty acids to the liver. Abdominal obesity, particularly in men, consists primarily of increased visceral adipose tissue that is drained by the portal vein and delivers an excessive load of free fatty acid to the liver, where it furnishes the substrate for increased VLDL synthesis. The accumulation of triglyceride-rich lipoproteins in plasma depends not only on increased production of VLDL by the liver but also on decreased catabolism of triglyceride-rich lipoproteins, including dietary chylomicrons. Lipoprotein lipase activity decreases in uncontrolled type II diabetes. This enzyme

▼ **TABLE 63–2. MECHANISMS OF VASCULAR ABNORMALITIES IN DIABETES MELLITUS**

Hyperglycemia
  Increased diacylglycerol, protein kinase C activation
  Increased sorbitol
Hyperinsulinemia
Oxidative stress
  Reactive oxygen species
  Carbonyl overload
Advanced glycation end products (AGEs)
  Activation of nuclear factor kappa B (NF-κB)
  Overproduction of inflammatory cytokines
Dyslipidemia
  Small dense LDL
  Low HDL
  Hypertriglyceridemia
Procoagulant, antifibrinolytic state
  Elevated fibrinogen
  Increased plasminogen activator inhibitor (PAI)
  Heightened platelet function
Genetic abnormalities
  Peroxisomal proliferation-activating receptor-gamma (PPAR-γ) mutations

HDL = high-density lipoprotein; LDL = low-density lipoprotein.

▼ **TABLE 63–3. COMPONENTS OF THE CARDIOVASCULAR DYSMETABOLIC SYNDROME**

Insulin resistance
Hyperglycemia
Dyslipidemia
Hypercoagulability
Obesity
Hypertension

plays a key role in clearing postprandial lipemia, which largely consists of triglyceride-rich particles.

The increase in triglyceride-rich lipoprotein partially accounts for the low levels of high-density lipoprotein (HDL) characteristic of diabetic dyslipidemia. The high concentration of triglyceride-rich lipoproteins provides an increase in substrate for cholesterol ester transfer protein, which promotes the flux of cholesterol from HDL particles and decreases the level of HDL cholesterol. Part of HDL's protective effect against atherosclerosis may result from its ability to reduce the oxidation of low-density lipoprotein (LDL). In addition to a quantitative decrease in HDL cholesterol levels in uncontrolled diabetes, recent evidence suggests qualitative differences in HDL particles from poorly controlled type II diabetic patients. In particular, HDL isolated from such patients protects LDL from oxidation less effectively than does HDL from nondiabetic subjects.[8]

Curiously, diabetics tend to not have markedly elevated plasma LDL concentrations. However, LDL particles in uncontrolled type II diabetic patients characteristically have qualitative alterations as well. In particular, LDL from such diabetic subjects tends to be smaller and denser than typical LDL particles. These small, dense LDL particles show greater susceptibility to oxidative modification in vitro. Moreover, LDL from poorly controlled type II diabetics has increased susceptibility to oxidation because of decreased antioxidant defense mechanisms in the plasma of diabetics.[9]

Alterations in the traditional variables of the lipoprotein profile go hand in hand with other risk factors in diabetic patients. In addition to the triad of increased triglycerides, decreased HDL, and small dense LDL, insulin-resistant patients tend to have hypertension and obesity, as well as hyperglycemia (see Table 63–3). Abnormalities in coagulation and fibrinolysis in type II diabetes are considered below. The mechanistic link between visceral adiposity and diabetic dyslipidemia has already been discussed. Many life style or hygienic issues contribute to insulin resistance. For example, the visceral adiposity at the root of diabetic dyslipidemia commonly results from excessive caloric intake in the face of limited physical activity.

Genetic Predisposition. Increasing evidence, however, supports the concept that genetic predisposition may contribute to the development of type II diabetes. Recent work has defined a specific mutation that leads to severe insulin resistance, diabetes mellitus, and hypertension. In two kindreds, dominant negative mutations in a transcription factor known as peroxisomal proliferation-activating receptor-gamma (PPAR-gamma) caused this insulin resistance constellation in members of two affected kindreds at a relatively young age.[10] Interestingly, the thiazolidinedione family of insulin-sensitizing agents acts by binding and activating the nuclear receptor/transcription factor PPAR-gamma. While this single-gene mutation probably accounts for the insulin resistance syndrome in a small number of individuals, it illustrates how a genetic abnormality can cause this condition. With completion of the human genome project and study of single-nucleotide polymorphisms increasingly practicable, other genetic predisposing factors for type II diabetes will probably emerge. These factors may well in-

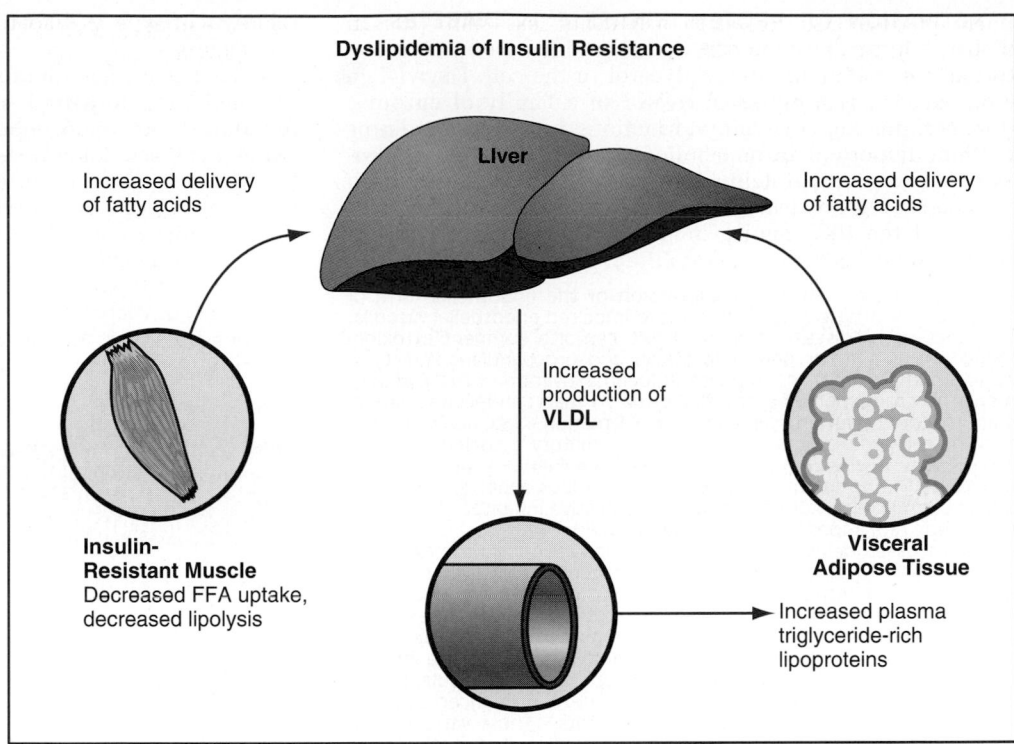

FIGURE 63-1. Pathogenesis of diabetic dyslipidemia. Increased production of very low-density lipoprotein by the liver results from increased delivery of fatty acids because of decreased utilization by muscle and increased delivery of fatty acids from visceral abdominal fat to the liver via the portal circulation. Decreased catabolism of postprandial triglyceride-rich lipoprotein particles because of reduced lipoprotein lipase activity accentuates diabetic dyslipidemia (not shown here; see Fig. 31–4).

In figure:

Dyslipidemia of Insulin Resistance

Liver

Increased delivery of fatty acids

Increased delivery of fatty acids

Increased production of **VLDL**

Insulin-Resistant Muscle
Decreased FFA uptake, decreased lipolysis

Visceral Adipose Tissue

Increased plasma triglyceride-rich lipoproteins

---

volve haplotypes or polygenic conditions, as well as single-gene mutations, as illustrated by the PPAR-gamma mutation.

OXIDATIVE STRESS IN DIABETES MELLITUS. Numerous basic science and clinical studies indicate an increased level of oxidative stress in diabetes.[11] Hyperglycemia leads to increased production of reactive oxygen species by several cell types. The reactive oxygen species can, in turn, augment the formation of reactive carbonyl species. Nonoxidative reactions can also increase the concentrations of reactive carbonyl compounds under hyperglycemic conditions. The reactive carbonyl species can derivatize proteins and lipids. The products of reactions of proteins with reactive oxygen and carbonyl species include the advanced glycation end products (AGEs) discussed below. There is little doubt that products of glycation accumulate in diabetic patients. However, they accumulate in nondiabetic elderly individuals as well.[11] Recent evidence suggests that inundation of the detoxification mechanisms for reactive carbonyl groups may account for the increase in oxidant and carbonyl stress in diabetics.

From a practical standpoint, the issue of whether oxidant stress causes diabetic complications or merely serves as a marker of deranged metabolism is crucial. In several recent clinical trials that included diabetic subjects, the lack of a protective effect of antioxidant compounds suggests the importance of emphasizing measures known to improve cardiovascular outcomes in diabetic subjects, such as lipid management and angiotensin-converting enzyme (ACE) inhibitor administration, while awaiting further information regarding the potential benefits of antioxidant strategies.

ADVANCED GLYCATION END PRODUCTS AND THEIR RECEPTORS. The hyperglycemia characteristic of diabetes leads to nonenzymatic glycation of macromolecules. Use of hemoglobin A_{1c} allows the clinician to gauge the extent of hyperglycemia in a patient by measurement of this glycated form of hemoglobin. In hyperglycemic states, many other proteins and even lipids can become glycated. The chemistry of nonenzymatic glycation involves the formation of a labile covalent link between the aldehyde function on the glucose molecule and amino side chains on sugars and lipids, which results in the formation of an aldimine or Schiff base. The aldimine slowly undergoes a chemical reaction to form a ketoamine by the Amadori rearrangement. The glycated hemoglobin commonly used to monitor diabetic patients is one such Amadori product.

However, more complex chemical reactions can ensue and allow condensation into larger heterocyclic derivatives of sugars linked to macromolecules. These structures, known as AGEs, are fluorescent and actually cause the macromolecule to take on a brown hue. Numerous chemical studies have characterized the structure of AGEs. A great deal of information is emerging regarding the potential significance of AGEs in the pathobiology of the complications of diabetes, notably, the accelerated vascular disease characteristic of this condition.[11–14] Recent studies have shown accumulation of AGE-modified proteins, aside from hemoglobin, in diabetic subjects. The presence of glycated forms of LDL can engender an immune response and otherwise contribute to macrovascular disease.[15] Phospholipids and apolipoproteins can form AGEs.[16] AGE-modified LDL apoprotein and LDL lipid increase in diabetic subjects in comparison to nondiabetics.[16]

Cells contain several receptors for AGEs that mediate their biological effects. Exposure to AGE-modified proteins can elicit the production of inflammatory cytokines from vascular cells, cause impaired endothelial-dependent vasodilator function, and augment the endothelial expression of various leukocyte adhesion molecules implicated in atherogenesis in vivo.[17, 18] One extensively characterized receptor for AGEs is known as the receptor for advanced glycation end products, or RAGE.[19] Recent experiments support a functional role for RAGEs in the development of experimental atherosclerosis. Mice lacking the apolipoprotein E gene are susceptible to atherosclerosis. Administration of an antibody fragment that neutralizes RAGEs attenuated the atherosclerosis in these mutant mice. This beneficial effect on atherosclerotic lesion development did not depend on a change in blood sugar or lipoprotein profile.[20] These data support a role for AGEs in atherogenesis. However, they do not explain why the link between glycemic control and macrovascular disease in diabetes has proved so elusive.

EFFECTS OF THE DIABETIC STATE ON THROMBOSIS AND FIBRINOLYSIS. Type II diabetes and its associated metabolic abnormalities favor an imbalance in the coagulation/fibrinolytic systems that support clot formation and stability.[21] Diabetic patients have increased levels of fibrinogen[22] and plasminogen activator inhibitor type 1 (PAI-1) in the plasma and in lesions.[23, 24] They also appear to have abnormal platelet function.[25] These various abnormalities may contribute to heightened susceptibility to the thrombotic complications of atherosclerosis.

ACTIVATION OF PROTEIN KINASE C IN DIABETES. In diabetes, hyperglycemia can lead to an increased concentration of the metabolite diacylglycerol in the cell. Diacylglycerol, in turn, is a classic activator of a family of enzymes that perform key regulatory functions by phosphorylating proteins important in metabolic control. This family of enzymes, known as protein kinase C (PKC), has some dozen members. A great deal of recent work has implicated activation of the PKC family in the cardiovascular complications of diabetes.[26, 27]

Activation of PKC can inhibit expression of the endothelial form of nitric oxide synthase and thus promote impaired endothelial vasodilator function, as discussed below.[28] PKC can also augment cytokine-induced tissue factor gene expression and procoagulant activity in human endothelial cells.[29] Glucose-induced activation of PKC can augment the production of extracellular matrix macromolecules that accumulate during atherosclerotic lesion formation.[27] PKC activation can also increase the production of proinflammatory cytokines and the proliferation of vascular wall cells.[27] In vivo evidence supports a role of PKC activation in the pathogenesis of various aspects of vascular dysfunction in vivo. Administration of a selective inhibitor of PKC-beta to diabetic rats improves retinal blood flow.[30]

As discussed below, considerable evidence supports the existence of a diabetic form of cardiomyopathy distinct from ischemia. PKC activation may contribute not only to vascular dysfunction but also to cardiomyopathy in diabetes. Indeed, PKC-beta activity increases in the hearts of diabetic rats. Cardiac hypertrophy and fibrosis develop in transgenic mice overexpressing a PKC-beta isoform in the heart.[31] Early thickening of the interventricular septum, left ventricular hypertrophy, and a decrease in left ventricular dP/dt in concert with increased activity of PKC develop in diabetic rats.[32] These various studies provide evidence in vitro and in diabetic animals of a role of the PKC system in diabetic cardiovascular complications. Studies currently in progress will evaluate the relevance of this intriguing laboratory work to the clinical situation.

ABNORMAL VASODILATOR FUNCTION IN DIABETES. The ability to measure vasodilator function in intact humans has furnished a new window into mechanisms of vascular dysfunction. Numerous studies have documented impaired endothelial-dependent vasodilator function in human arteries. Type I diabetics without hypertension or dyslipidemia had impaired endothelial-dependent vasodilator function when compared with age-matched nondiabetic subjects. The diabetic and nondiabetic groups had similar responses to endothelial-independent vasodilators.[33] Type II diabetic patients appear to have defects in both endothelial-dependent vasodilation and smooth muscle function.[34, 35] Experimental studies have indicated that overproduction of oxygen-derived free radicals in response to elevated glucose contributes to endothelial cell dysfunction.[36] Indeed, high doses of the antioxidant vitamin C can improve endothelial-dependent vasodilation in both type II[37] and type I[38] diabetic subjects. Further mechanistic studies have shown a significant correlation between insulin sensitivity and endothelial nitric oxide production.[39] Insulin's well-known vasodilator response depends in part on endothelial nitric oxide production. Type II diabetic subjects do not show improvement in endothelial-dependent vasodilation in comparison to lean nondiabetic controls when infused with insulin in glucose clamp experiments.[40] Acute hyperglycemia impairs endothelial-dependent vasodilation in both microvessels and macrovessels in normal subjects.[41] In type II diabetics, treatment of the dyslipidemia with a fibric acid derivative improves both fasting and postprandial endothelial function.[42] This finding shows that dyslipidemia, as well as hyperglycemia, can contribute to impaired endothelial vasodilator responses in diabetic humans. It further demonstrates the ability of therapy to improve endothelial-dependent vasodilation in humans.

As noted above, firm evidence now supports a link between genetics and the insulin-resistant syndrome. In this regard, first-degree relatives of type II diabetic patients who are normotensive and without overt diabetes show impaired endothelial-dependent vasodilation and insulin resistance, as determined by clamp studies.[43] This impaired endothelial vasodilatory function in the young first-degree relatives of type II diabetics did not depend on traditional risk factors.

Recent work has identified a novel potential mechanism for mediating impaired endothelial-dependent vasodilator function.[43a] An endogenous competitive inhibitor of nitric oxide synthase known as asymmetrical dimethylarginine (ADMA) is augmented in hypercholesterolemics.[44] Accumulation of ADMA may result from inhibition of its catabolism because of a reduction in activity of the enzyme dimethylarginine dimethylaminohydrolase.[45] Recent evidence suggests that dysregulation of this enzyme may raise levels of ADMA in diabetics.[45, 45a] These new findings provide yet another potential molecular pathway of impaired vascular function in diabetes.

EPIDEMIOLOGY OF CARDIOVASCULAR DISEASE IN DIABETES MELLITUS AND IMPAIRED GLUCOSE TOLERANCE

The prevalence of both diabetes and impaired fasting glucose is increasing within the U.S. population (see Fig. 63–1).[46] Approximately 6 percent of the U.S. population has diabetes, and only half of those cases have been diagnosed. Moreover, impaired glucose tolerance occurs twice as frequently as overt diabetes. This disease places a major demand on resources of the health care system. Data from a managed care organization on the 1-year cost of treating more than 85,000 patients with diabetes as compared with age- and sex-matched nondiabetic counterparts confirm the impact of CVD in diabetes.[47] The largest proportion (17 percent) of the excess cost associated with diabetes was attributable to CAD. In contrast, end-stage renal disease accounted for 11 percent of the excess costs of treatment. The general population in the United States has enjoyed impressive declines in the mortality associated with heart disease in the last decades. However, the drop in cardiovascular mortality in diabetic men and women has lagged well behind that of the general population.[48] Two other important factors—aging of the U.S. population overall and the increasing prevalence of diabetes—suggest that the relationship between diabetes and coronary heart disease (CHD) morbidity and mortality will become even more important in the future.

CHD MORBIDITY AND MORTALITY IN TYPE II DIABETES MELLITUS

The clinical association between diabetes, elevated glucose, and CVD has been intensively studied for many years.[49] The excess morbidity and mortality remain even after adjustment for traditional CHD risk factors. In the Framingham Study, 20-year follow-up of individuals aged 45 to 74 years at the initial screening showed a twofold to threefold elevation in the risk of clinically evident atherosclerotic disease in those with diabetes as compared with the nondiabetic cohort.[50] These data also showed loss of the protection against CHD in women with diabetes, who had a rate of CHD mortality as high as that in diabetic men. In the Multiple Risk Factor Intervention Trial (MRFIT), more than 5000 men (out of approximately 350,000 screened) who reported taking medications for diabetes were monitored for an average of 12 years.[51] For every age stratum, ethnic background, and risk factor level, men with diabetes had an absolute risk of CHD death more than three times higher than that in the nondiabetic cohort, even after adjustment for established risk factors. Similar findings were seen in a large cohort of 11,554 white men and 666 black men between the ages of 35 and 64 screened from 1967 to 1973 and monitored prospectively for 22 years.[52] A recent Finnish study showed that diabetics without a prior myocardial infarction had the same risk of a first myocardial infarction as did nondiabetic survivors of myocardial infarction (Fig. 63–2).[53] Data from the Rancho Bernardo Study and the Nurses' Health Study show that women with diabetes experience a disproportionately greater impact from diabetes than do men with diabetes.[54, 55]

CHD MORTALITY IN TYPE I DIABETES MELLITUS

Type II diabetes accounts for more than 90 percent of all cases of diabetes, and most studies of CHD risk have evaluated middle-aged or

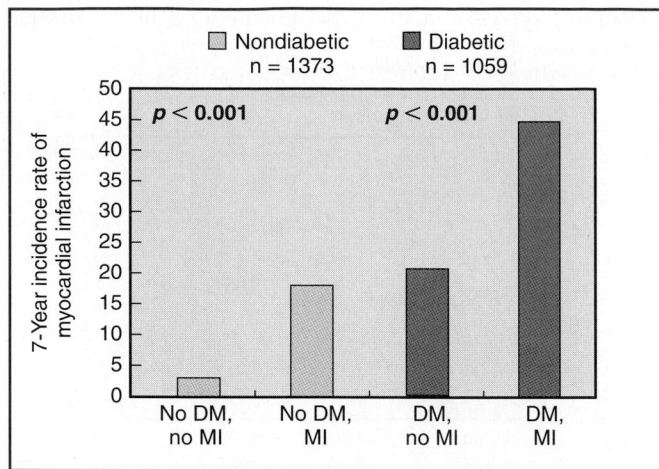

FIGURE 63–2. Marked increase in the risk of coronary artery disease in type II diabetics. These data show a striking increase in the risk of a first or recurrent myocardial infarction in diabetics as compared with nondiabetic subjects in a population-based study in Finland over a 7-year follow-up period. These data also show that a diabetic without a history of previous myocardial infarction has an approximately equal risk for a first myocardial infarction as a nondiabetic subject who has already sustained myocardial infarction. These data support recent recommendations from the American Diabetes Association to treat diabetic subjects as though they already have established coronary artery disease. (From Haffner SM, Lehto S, Ronnemaa T, et al: Mortality from coronary heart disease in subjects with type 2 diabetes and in nondiabetic subjects with and without prior myocardial infarction. N Engl J Med 339:229–234, 1998.)

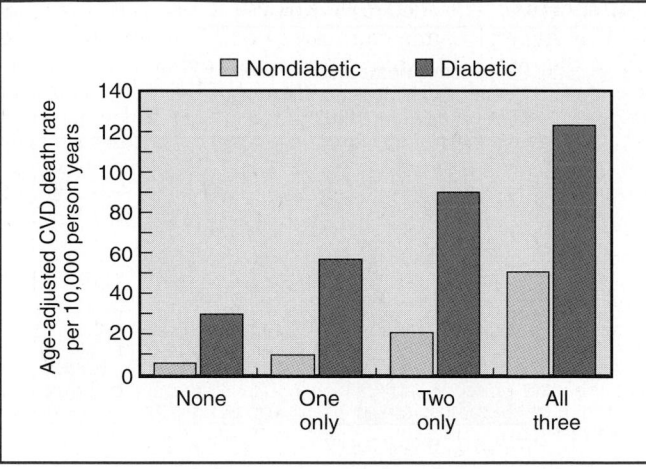

FIGURE 63–3. Age-adjusted cardiovascular disease death rates according to the presence of a number of risk factors for men with and without diabetes at baseline who were screened for the MRFIT. The presence of diabetes confers a steep increase in the cardiovascular death rate at any level of concomitant risk factors. (From Stamler J, Vaccaro O, Neaton JD, et al: Diabetes, other risk factors, and 12-yr cardiovascular mortality for men screened in the Multiple Risk Factor Intervention Trial. Diabetes Care 16:434–444, 1993. Reproduced with permission of the American Diabetes Association, Inc.)

elderly populations consisting of mostly type II diabetics. However, a smaller collection of data also identifies an increased risk of CHD in patients with type I diabetes. In the Framingham Study, 292 patients with type I diabetes monitored for 20 to 40 years had a cumulative CAD mortality that was approximately 4 times that seen in nondiabetics (35 vs. 8 percent by age 55).[56] Regardless of the age of onset, the first deaths related to CAD occurred by the fourth decade of life, and the cumulative mortality rate increased at a similar rate in the subsequent 20 years. The increase in CAD mortality after age 30 appeared particularly striking in patients with renal complications, who had an estimated risk of CAD that was 15 times higher than that in patients without persistent proteinuria. Observational studies in other populations have made similar findings.[57–59] These data identify persistent proteinuria as a strong predictor of the development of CAD in this population. Proteinuria serves as a marker of generalized vascular damage that on a wider scale emerges as a predisposition to cardiovascular disease.

Aggregation of Traditional CHD Risk Factors in Diabetes

The high prevalence of "established" risk factors for CHD in diabetics complicates the epidemiological assessment of CHD in this patient population.[60–62] CHD risk factors such as hypertension, dyslipidemia, and obesity cluster in patients with diabetes.[4] In type II diabetics at time of diagnosis, over 50 percent have hypertension and over 30 percent have hypercholesterolemia. In MRFIT, the "classic" risk factors known to predict CVD mortality in nondiabetics— serum cholesterol (≥ 200 mg/dl), systolic blood pressure (≥ 120 mm Hg), and cigarette smoking—independently predict CVD mortality in diabetic subjects.[51] Most men in either the diabetic or nondiabetic group had one or more of these risk factors, with the majority having two or more. Within each stratum of risk (no risk factors, one only, two only, all three), CVD mortality was substantially higher for men with diabetes (Fig. 63–3). Notably, there was a synergistic effect of diabetes and other risk factors such that the presence of any single risk factor or the combination of any two or all three was associated with a steeper increase in CVD mortality in men with diabetes than in those without it.

The United Kingdom Prospective Diabetes Study (UKPDS) has provided perhaps the most compelling data to support the importance of risk factor aggregation in enhancing the CHD risk profile of patients with newly diagnosed diabetes.[63] This study evaluated a large number of middle-aged subjects with newly detected type II diabetes (n = 3055), in 335 of whom CAD developed during a median follow-up of 8 years. CAD was significantly associated with increased concentrations of LDL cholesterol, decreased concentrations of HDL cholesterol, increased levels of hemoglobin A_{1c} and systolic blood pressure, and a history of smoking as measured at baseline.

Plasma Glucose as an Independent Risk Factor for Atherosclerosis

Although diabetes clusters with the admixture of traditional risk factors for CHD mentioned above, the rate of CHD morbidity and mortality in diabetics exceeds the rate expected from the interaction of these multiple risk factors by approximately 50 percent. Hyperglycemia itself has emerged as a leading candidate responsible for this excess CHD risk in diabetes.

Compelling data in this regard have emerged from prospective observations of patients with type II diabetes in which patients were stratified by fasting glucose levels.[64, 65] In one such study, the average fasting blood glucose level independently related to all-cause ($p = 0.0002$), cardiovascular ($p = 0.0006$), and ischemic heart disease ($p = 0.03$) mortality (Fig. 63–4). No obvious threshold level for this association was noted; rather, the lower the fasting blood glucose level, the better the outcome. Comparable results in the San Antonio Heart Study substantiate a dose-response relationship between hyperglycemia and CVD mortality.[65] In this study, diabetic subjects in the top quartile of FPG had a risk of CVD mortality 4.7 times greater than did diabetic subjects in quartiles 1 and 2 combined ($p = 0.01$). This increase in risk remained after adjustment for other potential risk factors. The graded, continuous pattern linking hyperglycemia and CVD risk in type II diabetes also applies to subjects with type I diabetes. Ten year follow up in the Wisconsin Epidemiological Study of type I diabetics showed that for each 1 percent increase in glycated hemoglobin, the hazard ratio for CHD mortality nearly doubled.[66] Indeed, even in individuals without frank diabetes, evidence points to a continuum of CHD risk that is dependent on glucose levels across the spectrum from normal glucose tolerance through impaired glucose tolerance to diabetes.[67] Data from a cohort study performed in Rancho Bernardo showed that in both men and women, the incidence of myocardial infarction and stroke correlated positively with glucose tolerance status. Other studies in diverse populations have also gen-

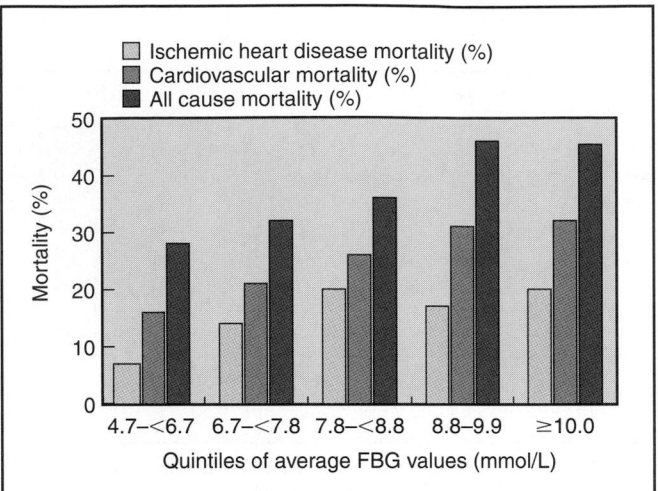

FIGURE 63–4. All-cause mortality, cardiovascular mortality, and ischemic heart disease mortality in patients with type II diabetes by quintiles of average fasting blood glucose. Cardiovascular mortality and all-cause mortality increase throughout the range of fasting plasma glucose levels in a graded fashion. (From Andersson DK, Svardsudd K: Long–term glycemic control relates to mortality in type II diabetes. Diabetes Care 18:1534–1543, 1995. Reproduced with permission of the American Diabetes Association, Inc.)

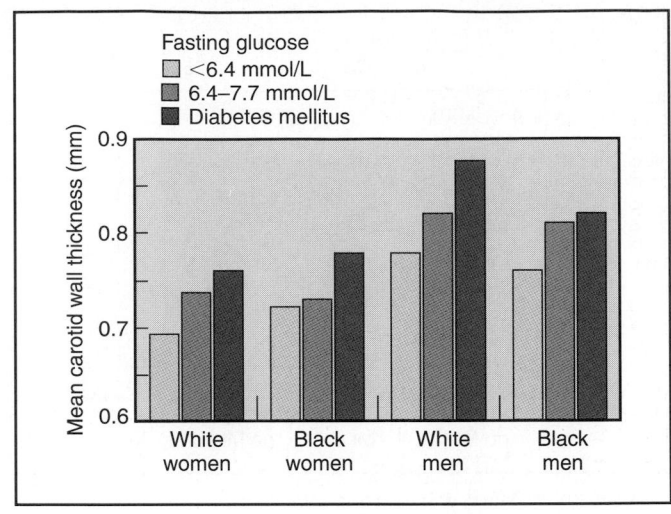

FIGURE 63–5. Sex- and race-specific associations between average carotid artery intima-media thickness (IMT) by fasting glucose status and the presence of diabetes mellitus in participants free of cardiovascular disease at baseline in the Atherosclerosis Risk in Communities (ARIC) Study from 1987 to 1989. The average carotid IMT increases across the entire range of fasting glucose levels. (From Folsom AR, Eckfeldt JH, Weitzman S, et al: Relation of carotid artery wall thickness to diabetes mellitus, fasting glucose and insulin, body size, and physical activity. Atherosclerosis Risk in Communities [ARIC] Study Investigators. Stroke 25:66–73, 1994. By permission of the American Heart Association.)

erally shown a graded relationship between glucose tolerance and the rate of CHD events.[52, 68, 69]

Investigations into the relationship between glucose and CHD risk in the studies noted above focused on CHD or ischemic mortality as the endpoint. Although powerful indicators of the graded, continuous effect of glucose, these studies do not provide any evidence of glucose's effect on the vessel wall itself. Several studies have evaluated intima-media thickness (IMT) of the carotid artery by ultrasound.[70–73] Carotid IMT correlates well with cardiovascular risk factors and the occurrence of CHD.[74] In the Atherosclerosis Risk in Communities (ARIC) Study, carotid wall thickness correlated with fasting glucose tolerance in all gender and race subgroups in a large and diverse sample of 15,800 subjects aged 45 to 64 without symptomatic CVD (Fig. 63–5).[70]

It is still unclear whether CVD risk is distributed across a continuum of glucose values in diabetic subjects or whether a critical value exists above which CVD rates increase. Also, whether evidence of an association is altered by the method of evaluating plasma glucose (postchallenge vs. fasting) requires further investigation. In a study from Japan in a population cohort of men, postchallenge glucose was a better predictor of CVD death than wave fasting glucose levels.[75] In general, the results of studies examining this relationship are difficult to compare because of differences in study design (e.g., longitudinal vs. cross-sectional), endpoints (e.g., CVD event rates vs. changes in carotid IMT), and patient populations.

Insulin Resistance as an Independent Risk Factor

As stated previously, diabetes clusters with other CVD risk factors, among them hypertension, obesity, and dyslipidemia. Almost all subjects with a combination of these metabolic disorders also have insulin resistance.[76] Hyperinsulinemia may provide the crucial link between hyperglycemia and CVD (see Table 63–3).[77] This collective occurrence of multiple metabolic abnormalities in an individual patient has been variously termed syndrome X, the insulin resistance syndrome, and cardiovascular dysmetabolic syndrome. Data from a number of studies indicate that hyperinsulinemia independently predicts CVD risk. For example, in a large (n = 1625) triethnic population consisting of equal numbers of subjects with diabetes, hyperglycemia, and normal glucose tolerance, insulin resistance correlated positively with atherosclerosis as assessed by carotid IMT.[78] Since insulin resistance typically precedes the development of hyperglycemia, these findings may explain, in part, the elevated risk of CHD that is found in individuals with newly diagnosed type II diabetes.

Other data suggest that endogenous insulin itself, rather than insulin resistance, may have direct adverse effects on the cardiovascular system. One case-control study monitored over 2000 nondiabetic men without apparent ischemic heart disease at baseline for 5 years.[79] Individuals who had experienced a CHD event had fasting insulin concentrations at baseline that were 18 percent higher than in controls ($p < 0.001$), an association that remained valid after adjusting for the potentially confounding effects of systolic blood pressure, plasma triglycerides, apolipoprotein B, and LDL and HDL cholesterol.

RISK FACTOR INTERVENTION TO REDUCE CHD IN PATIENTS WITH DIABETES MELLITUS
(see also Chap. 32)

Intensive Glycemic Control

Numerous studies have shown a positive correlation between CHD endpoints and increasing glucose levels in patients with diabetes. In the UKPDS, hemoglobin A_{1c} levels above 6.2 percent were associated with an increased risk of macrovascular disease.[63] For each 1 percent elevation in hemoglobin A_{1c}, CHD risk increased by 11 percent. However, it also appeared that the relative risk of CHD did not increase in association with hemoglobin A_{1c} levels below 7 percent, thus suggesting a threshold. Therefore, several clinical trials have sought to determine whether intensive treatment of blood glucose levels can reduce the risk of CHD associated with diabetes.

In the Diabetes Control and Complications Trial (DCCT), 1441 patients with type I diabetes (mean age of 27 years) and no significant retinopathy at baseline were randomized to intensive glycemic control (external insulin pump or three or more insulin injections per day) or conventional therapy (one to two insulin injections per day).[80] Patients were monitored prospectively for a mean of 6.5 years, with regular assessment of microvascular and macrovascular outcomes. After 5 years, the cumulative incidence of retinopathy was approximately 50 percent less in the intensive-treatment group than in the conventional-treatment group ($p < 0.001$). Intensive therapy also reduced the risk of macrovascular disease (cardiovascular and peripheral vascular disease) by 41 percent, although the difference between groups lacked statistical significance. A second, smaller Veterans Affairs (VA) Study that tested the feasibility of intensive blood glucose control in type II diabetics also showed no significant differences in cardiovascular endpoints between treatment arms.[81] These two trials had a number of important limitations. Both lacked adequate power to detect a difference in macrovascular events between treatment groups given the small number of events in each group. In the DCCT, the low event rate probably resulted from the relative youth of the study population, and in the VA Study, it probably resulted from the small patient population and a short follow-up period.

Larger, adequately powered studies such as UKPDS showed a nonsignificant trend in favor of intensive blood glucose control in terms of reduction of myocardial infarction.[82] This trial randomized 3867 patients with newly diagnosed type II diabetes to intensive therapy (diet plus oral therapy or insulin) or conventional therapy. Patients entered into the study had a low background prevalence of CHD and a low rate of CHD risk factors. Patients were monitored for approximately 10 years. As in the DCCT, microvascular endpoints were improved in the intensive-therapy arm. A trend toward a reduced rate of myocardial infarction was also noted in the group receiving intensive blood glucose control ($p = 0.052$).[82]

Treatment of Hypertension in Diabetics

(see also Chaps. 28 and 29)

Hypertension and diabetes frequently occur together as part of the dysmetabolic syndrome. The addition of hypertension to the clinical picture of diabetes amplifies the already high risk of CVD in these patients. In addition, hypertension significantly contributes to the development of microalbuminuria and retinopathy in diabetes. The role of antihypertensive therapy in reducing cardiovascular morbidity and mortality in patients with diabetes has engendered controversy, as in patients without diabetes. In nondiabetics, older trials of diuretic and beta blocker antihypertensive therapy did not show a reduction in cardiovascular mortality. The deleterious effects of these agents on metabolic indices (triglycerides, HDL, and blood sugar) may have accounted for these findings. Contemporary antihypertensive agents, including calcium channel blockers (CCBs) and ACE inhibitors, do not adversely affect metabolic factors that might counteract the benefits of blood pressure lowering.

Two recent trials compared the effects of CCBs and ACE inhibitors in patients with type II diabetes.[83, 84] They showed a greater reduction in CHD endpoints with an ACE inhibitor than with a dihydropyridine CCB. The results of these two studies suggested that CCBs did not benefit and might even harm diabetic patients at high risk for cardiovascular events. Although the results of these trials imply that ACE inhibitors would be the preferred agents for treating diabetic patients, interpretation of these relatively small studies in which cardiovascular endpoints were not the primary outcome measure requires caution.[85] More rigorously designed studies, such as the UKPDS and the Systolic Hypertension in Europe Trial (Syst-Eur), have not supported the findings of the two smaller trials noted above and have shown beneficial effects for both ACE inhibitors and CCBs in patients with diabetes (Table 63-4).[85a] For example, in the UKPDS,[86] 1148 hypertensive patients with type II diabetes responded equally well to captopril or atenolol in terms of achieving blood pressure control and had similar reductions in the risk of macrovascular disease. Myocardial infarction declined 21 percent in the group randomized to tight blood pressure control ($p = NS$). This group also had a 44 percent reduction in the risk of fatal and nonfatal stroke when compared with the group assigned to less tight blood pressure control. Although the blood pressure achieved in the UKPDS subgroup assigned to tight blood pressure control was good (144/82), data from the Syst-Eur Trial[87, 89] and the Hypertension Optimal Treatment (HOT) Trial[88] indicate that achieving even lower blood pressure goals is associated with low rates of cardiovascular complications during CCB-based therapy. A recent analysis of initially nondiabetic subjects in the Atherosclerosis Risk in Communities (ARIC) Study showed no increased risk of developing diabetes when treated with ACE inhibitors, CCB, or thiazides.[00a] However, there was a 28% increased risk of developing diabetes in those who received beta blockers in this study.

Treatment of Dyslipidemia in Diabetics

(see also Chaps. 31 and 33)

The central role of diabetic dyslipidemia in accelerating atherosclerosis in type II diabetics has major therapeutic implications. While strict glycemic control in and of itself does not appear to consistently reduce macrovascular disease, tight glycemic control can ameliorate features of the lipoprotein profile associated with increased risk. Thus, as in all individuals with or at risk for atherosclerosis, individuals with impaired glucose intolerance or frank diabetes or those with a strong family history of type II diabetes should have intense counseling regarding life style modification. In particular, achieving and maintaining an ideal body weight and performing regular aerobic exercise can improve insulin sensitivity. Even though LDL levels often lie within the average range in type II diabetic subjects, treatment with 3-hydroxy-3-methylglutaryl coenzyme A (HMG CoA) reductase inhibitors reduces coronary risk.[90, 91] Furthermore, treatment with fibric acid derivatives targets in particular the low HDL and high triglycerides characteristic of diabetic dyslipidemia. The results of the recent Veterans Affairs High-Density Lipoprotein Cholesterol Intervention Trial (VA-HIT) suggest that a population of individuals, many of whom have a lipoprotein profile of insulin resistance, show a reduction in coronary events and stroke when treated with a fibric acid derivative.[92] The recent Diabetes Atherosclerosis Intervention Study (DAIS) showed delayed angiographic progression of coronary atherosclerosis in diabetic patients treated with fenofibrate.[92a] The thiazolidinedione agents improve insulin sensitivity by activating PPAR-gamma. Future work should define the role of the thiazolidinediones in preventing the cardiovascular complications of type II diabetes inasmuch as the rationale for a beneficial effect appears strong.

TREATMENT OF ACUTE CORONARY SYNDROMES IN DIABETES MELLITUS

PROGNOSIS. Diabetic patients have higher mortality than nondiabetics do during the acute phase of myocardial infarction, as well as in short- and long-term follow-up. The diabetic population will comprise a greater proportion of patients with myocardial infarction in the future. Numerous mechanisms in diabetic patients conspire to increase the risk of myocardial infarction. This section will review the state of knowledge regarding optimizing treatments for this important population with acute coronary syndromes

FIBRINOLYTIC THERAPY IN DIABETICS (see also Chap. 35). Fibrinolytic therapy has reduced early and late mortality from acute myocardial infarction in patients with and without diabetes. Despite some concern that the elevated levels of PAI-1, fibrinogen, coagulation factors, and reactive platelets commonly encountered in diabetes might reduce the likelihood of successful reperfusion,[93] both the Thrombolysis and Angioplasty in Myocardial Infarction (TAMI) and the Global Utilization of Streptokinase and Tissue Plasminogen Activator for Occluded Coronary Arteries (GUSTO-1) thrombolysis trials demonstrated similar infarct-related artery patency rates in diabetic and nondiabetic subgroups.[94–96] Indeed, diabetic patients experience the same or greater benefit from thrombolysis as nondiabetics do. In the Second International Study of Infarct Survival (ISIS-II), diabetic patients receiving streptokinase had a 31 percent improvement in survival in comparison to placebo, greater than the 23 percent improvement seen in the nondiabetic group. Pooled data from five recent major thrombolysis trials show that 30-day mortality has been substantially reduced to 11 percent in diabetics and 6 percent in nondiabetics—an odds ratio similar to that observed in the earlier literature. Formerly, concern about hemorrhage from diabetic retinopathy made diabetes a contraindication to thrombolysis. However, only 1 of 6011 (0.02 percent) diabetic patients receiving thrombolytic therapy experienced intraocular hemorrhage.[97]

▼ **TABLE 63–4.** LARGE STUDIES EVALUATING ANTIHYPERTENSIVE THERAPY IN PATIENTS WITH DIABETES MELLITUS

SOURCE, YEAR	NO. OF PATIENTS (% WITH DIABETES)	STUDY ENTRY CRITERIA	TYPE OF DRUGS
PLACEBO-CONTROLLED STUDIES			
SHEP,[5] 1996	583 (12.3)	Systolic hypertension defined as 160–219 mm Hg; diastolic, <90 mm Hg	Placebo vs. diuretic-based (chlorthalidone)
Syst-EUR,[6] 1999	492 (10.5)	Systolic hypertension defined as 160–219 mm Hg; double-blind; diastolic, <95 mm Hg	Placebo vs. nitrendipine
HOPE,[7] 2000	3578 (38.5)*	Diabetes and 1 other cardiovascular risk factor or No diabetes and history of cardiovascular disease	Ramipril and vitamin E vs. placebo
TREAT TO BLOOD PRESSURE TARGET STUDIES			
HOT,[8] 1998	1501 (8)	Diastolic hypertension defined as 100–115 mm Hg; randomized into 3 target blood pressure groups of approximately 500	Felodipine-based and angiotensin-converting enzyme inhibitor, β-blocker, or diuretic
UKPDS,[4, 9] 1998	1148 (100)†	Open randomization	Less tight blood pressure control vs. tight control; further randomization to captopril or atenolol
ANGIOTENSIN-CONVERTING ENZYME INHIBITION VS OTHER AGENTS STUDIES			
CAPPP,[10] 1999	572 (5.2)‡	Diastolic hypertension defined as >100 mm Hg	Captopril vs. diuretic or β-blocker
ABCD,[11] 1998	470 (100)	Diabetes and diastolic hypertension defined as ≥90 mm Hg	Nisoldipine vs. enalapril
FACET,[12] 1998	380 (100)	Systolic hypertension defined as >140 mm Hg or diastolic hypertension defined as >90 mm Hg	Amlodipine vs. fosinopril

SHEP = Systolic Hypertension in the Elderly Program; Syst-EUR = Systolic Hypertension in Europe; HOPE = Heart Outcomes Prevention Evaluation; HOT = Hypertension Optimal Treatment; UKPDS = United Kingdom Prospective Diabetes Study; CAPPP = Captopril Prevention Project; ABCD = Appropriate Blood Pressure Control in type II diabetes trial; FACET = Fosinopril versus Amlodipine Cardiovascular Events randomized Trial.
* Of the 3578, 1808 received placebo and 1770 received ramipril.

MECHANISMS OF AGGRAVATION OF OUTCOMES. Mortality after acute myocardial infarction correlates with the severity of left ventricular dysfunction. The nature and time course of left ventricular remodeling are major determinants of this risk. Numerous factors related to diabetes may adversely affect remodeling. Previous silent infarction, diabetic cardiomyopathy, hypertension,[98] and autonomic dysfunction[99] are conditions that either alone or in combination can affect non–infarct zone function and predispose to ventricular remodeling.[85, 100, 101] Endothelial cell dysfunction may result in impaired coronary perfusion and lead to ischemia.[102] Diabetes also retards coronary collateral development.[103]

Metabolic changes in diabetes may also contribute to the worsened prognosis of this group of patients with acute coronary syndromes. Insulin resistance impairs the ability of the heart to metabolize free fatty acids. Ordinarily, ischemia increases levels of the glucose transporter protein GLUT-4 (the predominant insulin-sensitive glucose transporter) in human myocardium, which augments glycolysis and adenosine triphosphate (ATP) production. In diabetes, elevated free fatty acid levels depress GLUT-4 activity and, hence, glucose entry and glycolysis in myocardial cells. This shift in substrate supply results in less efficient ATP production and the generation of oxygen free radicals, both of which impair left ventricular contractile performance.[104]

Autonomic nervous system (ANS) dysfunction in diabetes can also contribute to excess mortality (see below for an extended discussion of a cardiovascular autonomic neuropathy in diabetes). Approximately 50 percent of people with diabetes for 10 or more years have impaired heart rate variability because of parasympathetic denervation, which results in a relative increase in sympathetic tone. Sympathovagal imbalance may alter hemostasis in favor of thrombosis, lower the threshold for coronary plaque disruption, alter the circadian pattern of ischemia, and increase the risk for reinfarction and ventricular arrhythmia.[105–107] Elevated levels of PAI-1, fibrinogen, and coagulation factors (factors VII, IX, X, and XII), combined with hyperaggregable platelets, also contribute to an increased risk for early and late reinfarction in diabetic patients.[93, 108, 109]

Such factors may also account for the twofold higher risk of death conferred by diabetes that was observed in the control treatment arms of trials that evaluated the efficacy of platelet glycoprotein IIb/IIIa inhibitors in unstable angina/non-Q-wave infarction, such as the PURSUIT (Platelet Glycoprotein IIb/IIIa in Unstable Angina: Receptor Suppression Using Integrilin Therapy) Trial or the PRISM PLUS (Platelet Receptor Inhibition in Ischemic Syndrome Management in Patients Limited by Unstable Signs and Symptoms) Study. At 7 and 30 days, diabetics with unstable coronary syndromes experienced a mortality rate similar to that of nondiabetics with Q wave infarction.[110, 111]

Medical Therapy

ASPIRIN

Studies have consistently shown that patients with either type I or type II diabetes have enhanced platelet aggregation in response to a variety of agonists.[112] Platelets from diabetic patients exhibit increased production of thromboxane, a potent vasoconstrictor and platelet agonist.[113] In the Early Treatment of Diabetic Retinopathy Study (ETDRS), patients with type I or type II diabetes randomized to aspirin 650 mg/d had a significantly lowered risk of myocardial infarction without incurring an increase in the risk of vitreous or retinal bleeding, even in patients with retinopathy.[114] In the Bezafibrate Infarction Prevention Study (BIPS), an observational analysis of aspirin use by individuals with a history of CAD, the absolute benefit per 100 patients treated with aspirin in diabetic patients exceeded that in nondiabetic patients (cardiac mortality reduction, 5 vs. 2.1 percent; total mortality, 7.8 vs. 4.1 percent).[115] The American Diabetes Association currently recommends enteric-coated aspirin in a dose of 81 to 325 mg/d (1) as secondary prevention in men and women with diabetes and evidence of macrovascular disease and (2) as primary prevention in persons with type I or II diabetes and additional coronary risk factors.[116]

BETA-ADRENERGIC BLOCKING AGENTS

Despite overwhelming evidence that beta-adrenergic blocking agents (beta blockers) reduce mortality and reinfarction in patients with myocardial infarction, their use in diabetic patients has only recently become accepted. Beta blockers produced an early and late post-

FOLLOW-UP, YEARS	BLOOD PRESSURE EFFECTS	MAIN RESULTS
4.5	Difference between diuretic and placebo group was 9.8 mm Hg systolic and 2.2 mm Hg diastolic	Benefit of drug similar to cohort without diabetes; 34% decrease in cardiovascular events in cohort with diabetes
2§	Difference between nitrendipine and placebo group was 8.6 mm Hg systolic and 3.9 mm Hg diastolic	Drug benefit greater than in cohort without diabetes; decrease in total mortality (55%), cardiovascular mortality (76%), and cardiovascular events (69%) in cohort with diabetes
4.5¶	Difference between ramipril and placebo group was <2 mm Hg systolic and 1 mm Hg diastolic	Angiotensin-converting enzyme inhibitor superior, decrease in primary outcome (24%) and total mortality (25%) in cohort with diabetes
3.8§	Difference among the 3 groups at end point was approximately 4 mm Hg	Benefit only detected in cohort with diabetes; decrease in cardiovascular mortality (67%) and events (51%) in cohort with diabetes with the lowest levels of blood pressure
8.4§	Less tight blood pressure control, 154/87 mm Hg; tight control, 144/82 mm Hg; similar reduction in blood pressure with both drugs	Captopril treatment not superior; decrease in diabetes-related events (24%) and death (32%); decrease in acute myocardial infarction (21%) in tight blood pressure cohort
>6§	Baseline blood pressure greater in captopril group; similar reduction with both drugs	Captopril treatment superior in cohort with diabetes; decrease in primary end point (40%), acute myocardial infarction (65%), and all cardiovascular events (33%) in cohort with diabetes treated with captopril
5¶	Similar reduction in blood pressure with both drugs	Fatal and nonfatal acute myocardial infarction for 25 patients taking nisodipine and 5 cases taking enalapril
<3§	Similar reduction in blood pressure with both drugs	Decrease in cardiovascular events for patients taking fosinopril (14/189 vs. 27/191)

† Of the 1148, 390 had less tight blood pressure control. The 758 who had tight blood pressure control were randomized, and 400 received captopril and 358 received atenolol.
‡ Of the 572, 309 received captopril vs. 263 who received a diuretic or β-blocker.
§ Values are expressed as medians.
¶ Values are expressed as means.
From Cooper ME, Johnston CI: Optimizing treatment of hypertension in patients with diabetes. JAMA 283:3178–3179, 2000.

myocardial infarction survival benefit in comparison to placebo in patients with diabetes that exceeded the degree of benefit seen in their nondiabetic counterparts in several studies.[117] Although these data derive from retrospective subgroup analyses of trials in the prethrombolytic era, they concur with more recent results. The National Cooperative Cardiovascular Project reviewed over 45,000 patients, 26 percent of whom had diabetes. After adjusting for confounding variables, beta blocker use was associated with a lower 1-year mortality rate in diabetic patients without an increase in diabetes-related complications.[118] Furthermore, a recent post hoc analysis of the BIPS Study demonstrated that the use of beta blockers was associated with improved long-term survival in a large group of type II diabetic subjects, 30 percent of whom had never experienced a prior myocardial infarction.[119]

The greater relative benefit of beta blockers in the presence of diabetes may derive from several factors. Beta blockers can help restore sympathovagal balance in diabetic patients with autonomic neuropathy. These drugs may also decrease free fatty acid utilization within the myocardium and hence reduce oxygen need. Beta blockers can, however, mask the warning signs of hypoglycemia by suppressing glycogenolysis, interfere with insulin release, and further impair glucose tolerance in patients with diabetes. In addition, some clinicians have concerns that beta blockers may elevate serum triglycerides, reduce HDL, and increase LDL and thereby potentially counteract some of the widely accepted cardioprotective benefits of these drugs. However, recent data indicate that the currently used beta blockers may not adversely affect the lipid profile.[120] Much of the concern surrounding the use of these drugs in diabetes stems from earlier experience with noncardioselective agents in higher dosage. The risk of hypoglycemia in diabetic hypertensive patients taking cardioselective beta blockers was no different from that of patients taking placebo.[121] Cardioselective agents have less tendency to worsen glycemic control than nonselective agents do, although diabetes may develop in over 20 percent of nondiabetic hypertensive patients given beta blockers.[89a]

ANGIOTENSIN-CONVERTING ENZYME INHIBITORS

ACE inhibitors reduce infarct size, limit ventricular remodeling, improve survival after myocardial infarction, and may be of particular benefit in patients with diabetes.[85] A post hoc analysis of one thrombolytic trial (Grupo Italiano per lo Studio della Sopravivenza nell'Infarto Miocardico-3 [GISSI-3]) revealed that early administration of lisinopril in the setting of acute myocardial infarction reduced 6-week and 6-month mortality comparatively more in diabetic versus nondiabetic patients (30 vs. 5 percent reduction at 6 weeks and 20 vs. 0 percent at 6 months, respectively). Lisinopril administration resulted in 37 lives saved per 1000 treated diabetic patients. Another retrospective analysis, the Trandolapril in Patients with Reduced Left Ventricular Function after AMI (TRACE) Study, compared the effect of oral trandolapril versus placebo in anterior myocardial infarction in patients with and without diabetes.[122] Patients with diabetes experienced a greater relative improvement in survival over 5 years of follow-up than did the nondiabetic cohort. Furthermore, ACE inhibitor treatment reduced by nearly 50 percent the risk of sudden death, reinfarction, and progression of congestive heart failure (CHF) in patients with diabetes, whereas subjects without diabetes experienced only trends in protection against these secondary outcomes.

Many factors may explain the particular benefits of ACE inhibitors in diabetic patients with acute myocardial infarction. These agents can prevent or limit remodeling of the ventricle, particularly when administered early in the course of acute myocardial infarction,[123] reduce recurrent ischemic events,[124] and restore sympathovagal imbalance.[125] ACE inhibitors may also improve endothelial function in diabetes,[126] counteract reduced fibrinolysis by suppression of PAI-1 expression,[127] and decrease insulin resistance.[128] In one recent study (Heart Outcomes Prevention Evaluation [HOPE]), ramipril significantly reduced the rates of myocardial infarction, stroke, and cardiovascular death in diabetic subjects with or without a prior history of CAD or CHF over a 5-year period when compared with placebo.[129] The ACE inhibitor's efficacy in the absence of a clinical history of CHF and hypertension in the majority of patients in the HOPE Study points to the importance of these nonhemodynamic benefits of ACE inhibitors.

GLYCOPROTEIN IIb/IIIa BLOCKERS
(see also Chaps. 36 and 62)

These potent antiplatelet agents have improved outcomes in patients with unstable angina and non-Q-wave infarction. Overall, glycoprotein IIb/IIIa antagonists have equal or better efficacy in diabetic than nondiabetic patients. Adverse effects (mostly bleeding) also appear equivalent in diabetics.

The PRISM PLUS Study compared heparin with heparin plus tirofiban in 362 patients with diabetes and 1208 without diabetes.[111] At 7 days, the cumulative endpoint of death, myocardial infarction, refractory ischemia, or rehospitalization for unstable angina in diabetic patients was reduced from 21.8 percent with heparin alone to 14.8 percent with heparin plus tirofiban. In nondiabetic subjects, the cumulative endpoint was reduced from 16.7 to 12.4 percent when tirofiban was added to heparin. Despite the increased aggregability of platelets in patients with diabetes, no significant difference was observed in the ability of standard dosing of abciximab to achieve 80 percent or greater platelet inhibition during a 12-hour infusion in patients with and without diabetes.[130]

In the EPILOG (Evaluation of PTCA to Improve Long-Term Outcomes by c7E3 Glycoprotein IIb/IIIa Receptor Blockade) Trial, abciximab treatment resulted in fewer acute adverse events after percutaneous transluminal coronary angioplasty (PTCA) in both the diabetic and nondiabetic groups, although longer-term follow-up revealed a higher rate of target vessel revascularization if diabetes were present.[131] In the EPISTENT (Evaluation of Platelet IIb/IIIa Inhibition in Stenting) Trial, however, a highly significant 51 percent decrease (8.1 vs. 16.6 percent; $p = 0.02$) in target vessel revascularization at 6 months was experienced by stented diabetic patients randomized to abciximab versus stented diabetic patients receiving placebo.[132]

INSULIN

Recent studies have evaluated the role of strict glycemic control in diabetic patients during the acute phase of myocardial infarction. The blood glucose level may increase in proportion to infarct size and hemodynamic stress in nondiabetic patients with myocardial infarction as catecholamines, cortisol, and growth hormone are released. These hormones may create "transient" insulin resistance, with serum glucose returning to normal at discharge. In some cases, a very high admission glucose level out of proportion to infarct size indicates previously undiagnosed diabetes. Nevertheless, substantial evidence points to the admission glucose level as an independent predictor of early and late mortality after myocardial infarction in patients with and without diabetes mellitus.[133-136]

The Diabetes and Insulin-Glucose Infusion in Acute Myocardial Infarction (DIGAMI) Study randomized 620 diabetic patients with acute myocardial infarction to either intensive insulin therapy (insulin-glucose infusion for 24 hours, followed by subcutaneous insulin injection for 3 months) or a standard glycemic control strategy.[137] Those receiving the intensive insulin regimen had a lower blood glucose level during the first hour (9.6 vs. 11.7 mmol/liter; $p < 0.01$) and at discharge (8.2 vs. 9.0 mmol/liter; $p < 0.01$) than the control group did. The infusion group had a significant reduction in 1-year mortality when compared with the control group (19 vs. 26 percent; $p < 0.027$). The two groups were similar in baseline characteristics and in other treatments received. After 3.4 years, mortality remained lower in the insulin infusion group than the group receiving conventional care (33 percent in the infusion group and 44 percent in the control group; $p = 0.011$). Predictors of mortality were age, history of CHF, diabetes duration, admission glucose, and admission hemoglobin A_{1c} level.[138] The greatest survival benefit was seen in the subgroup whose diabetes had been managed with diet or oral hypoglycemic drugs before infarction.

Several mechanisms may explain the findings of the DIGAMI Trial. Insulin-glucose infusion may (1) increase the availability of glucose as a substrate for ATP generation in cardiac muscle; (2) reduce lipolysis and decrease the generation of free fatty acids, which can impair myocardial contractility and trigger ventricular arrhythmia; and (3) shift cardiac metabolism from free fatty acid oxidation to glycolysis. In addition, tight glycemic control can reverse hyperglycemia-induced platelet reactivity and reduce the typically elevated PAI-1 activity in patients with diabetes. Part of the benefit derived from the use of insulin in the tight control arm may have resulted from the removal of any potential cardiac risk associated with the use of sulfonylureas (see below).

SULFONYLUREAS

In the 1970s, the University Group Diabetes Program (UGDP), a prospective trial evaluating the efficacy of tolbutamide versus insulin in patients with type II diabetes, reported an increase in cardiovascular mortality and CAD in the group assigned to tolbutamide.[139] A smaller study reported similar results.[140] Despite controversy at the time, the sulfonylurea class of hypoglycemic agents have become widely used as the benefits of improved glycemic control in preventing diabetes-related microvascular complications have become established.

The UKPDS investigated the impact of tight glycemic control with a variety of treatment strategies on the incidence and severity of microvascular and macrovascular complications in newly diagnosed diabetes. A higher incidence of sudden death or myocardial infarction was not seen in patients assigned to sulfonylureas over a 10-year follow-up.[82] A retrospective study recently identified sulfonylurea use as a risk factor for in-hospital mortality among diabetic patients undergoing PTCA for acute myocardial infarction.[141]

Concern over the use of sulfonylureas, particularly in the setting of myocardial injury, stems from their blockade of ATP-sensitive potassium channels (K^+-ATP).[142, 143] In the pancreas, such inhibition results in the secretion of insulin, thus accounting for the hypoglyce-

mic effect of these drugs. In the myocardium, however, blockade of K^+-ATP channels may limit ischemic preconditioning, a cardioprotective mechanism, and attenuate coronary vasodilation.[144-146] In patients undergoing PTCA 90 minutes after receiving either glibenclamide or placebo, intracoronary electrocardiograms (ECGs) were recorded at the end of the first and second balloon inflations. The group pretreated with glibenclamide experienced no difference in the degree of ST segment shift from the first to the second inflation. The placebo group, however, demonstrated less ST segment shift and had less pain with the second balloon inflation, which is an indication of induction of ischemic preconditioning not present in the sulfonylurea-treated patients.[147] Another study using treadmill-induced ischemia showed no abolition of ischemic preconditioning with glibenclamide versus placebo.[148] The number of sulfonylurea drugs has grown since the initial concerns raised by the UGDP Study. Glibenclamide but not glimepiride significantly inhibited the forearm vasodilator response to the activation of K^+-ATP channels by diazoxide, which suggests that different sulfonylureas have different specificities for vascular and/or myocardial K^+-ATP channels.[149] Sulfonylureas may be either proarrhythmic or antiarrhythmic, depending on the presence or absence of ischemia, as a result of the role of the K^+-ATP channel in regulating the duration of the cardiac action potential.[150, 151] The choice of specific sulfonylureas for patients with diabetes on the basis of the presence or absence of coronary disease remains unclear at this time.

Coronary Revascularization
(see also Chaps. 37 and 38)

PERCUTANEOUS TRANSLUMINAL CORONARY ANGIOPLASTY. Large-scale trials have generally not shown a benefit of aggressive revascularization after thrombolytic therapy for acute myocardial infarction. Similar considerations apply to diabetic patients.[152] Although diabetic and nondiabetic patients have similar rates of initial angioplasty success,[153] diabetics have higher restenosis rates after PTCA[154, 155] and worse longer-term outcomes.[156, 157]

Diabetics also have a higher risk of in-hospital mortality, restenosis, and long-term mortality after coronary artery stenting and atherectomy.[155, 158] Although stenting has reduced restenosis rates in both diabetics and nondiabetics overall, smaller lumina in the stented vessels and a significantly higher restenosis rate (55 vs. 20 percent; $p = 0.001$) were seen in diabetics within 4 months of the procedure despite similar baseline and procedural characteristics.[158] The mechanisms underlying the increased restenosis rate in diabetes after coronary intervention is unclear. Serial intravascular ultrasonography has suggested that exaggerated intimal hyperplasia develops in diabetics after intervention.[159] Histological study found increased collagen-rich fibrous tissue in atherectomy specimens from diabetics.[160]

CORONARY ARTERY BYPASS GRAFT SURGERY. Most studies comparing outcomes in diabetic and nondiabetic patients undergoing coronary artery bypass graft surgery (CABG) show an increased risk of postoperative death, 30-day and long-term mortality, and need for subsequent reoperation. Diabetic patients have a worse risk profile, tend to be older, and have more extensive CAD and poorer left ventricular function than nondiabetic patients do.[161] However, their higher long-term mortality is in part independent of these factors and continues to diverge from that in nondiabetic patients during long-term follow-up. This difference probably reflects accelerated disease progression in both the nonbypassed and the bypassed native coronary vessels.

The Bypass Angioplasty Revascularization Investigation (BARI) Trial, which included 641 patients with and 2962 patients without diabetes, evaluated the role of CABG in diabetic patients.[162] Five-year mortality was higher in diabetic patients. After 5 years of follow-up, Q wave myocardial infarction occurred more frequently in diabetic patients (8 vs. 4 percent). CABG significantly reduced the mortality after a myocardial infarction when compared with angioplasty, whereas no such protective effect of surgery was noted in nondiabetic patients experiencing myocardial infarction.

▼ **TABLE 63–5. INDICATIONS FOR CARDIAC TESTING IN DIABETIC PATIENTS**

Testing for CAD is warranted in patients with the following:
Typical or atypical cardiac symptoms
Resting electrocardiogram suggestive of ischemia or infarction
Peripheral or carotid occlusive arterial disease
Sedentary life style, age ≥35 yr, and plans to begin a vigorous exercise program
Two or more of the following risk factors in addition to diabetes
Total cholesterol ≥240 mg/dl, LDL cholesterol ≥160 mg/dl, or HDL cholesterol <35 mg/dl
Blood pressure >140/90 mm Hg
Smoking
Family history of premature CAD
Positive microalbuminuria/macroalbuminuria test

CAD = coronary artery disease; HDL = high-density lipoprotein; LDL = low-density lipoprotein.

Taken from Consensus Development Conference on the Diagnosis of Coronary Heart Disease in People With Diabetes. Diabetes Care 21:1551–1568, 1998.

CABG VERSUS PTCA. In general, randomized trials comparing PTCA with CABG have reported similar outcomes. Diabetes, however, may alter the outcomes of these different revascularization treatments.[163] The BARI Trial, which randomized patients with multivessel disease to CABG or PTCA, found that bypass surgery in treated diabetic patients was associated with a higher survival rate at 5 years than was PTCA (80.6 vs. 65.5 percent; $p = 0.003$).[164] The benefit of CABG accrued primarily in patients receiving internal mammary artery conduits. Cardiac mortality was 2.9 percent when an internal mammary artery graft was used as compared with 18.2 percent when only saphenous vein grafts were used, a mortality similar to that observed with PTCA.[165]

Screening for Coronary Artery Disease

Because diabetics have blunted anginal symptoms and a poor outcome following coronary events, the issue of screening for CAD in patients with diabetes mellitus has particular importance.[166] A recent American College of Cardiology/American Diabetes Association Consensus Development Conference established guidelines for screening diabetic individuals for CAD (Table 63–5).[167] Screening in asymptomatic diabetic individuals will establish a diagnosis of significant CAD in 5 to 15 percent of those without diabetic complications, in 20 to 60 percent of patients with peripheral or carotid arterial disease, and in the majority of those with chronic renal failure.[168] A number of factors specific to diabetic patients may interfere with the sensitivity and specificity of noninvasive diagnostic tests for myocardial ischemia.[168] However, most agree on the need to perform screening in diabetic patients before major noncardiac or vascular surgery or before initiation of an exercise program.[169] These subgroups face definable periods of excess cardiac risk, and discovery of significant CAD can have a major impact on management.

DIABETIC CARDIOMYOPATHY

Over the years, substantial evidence has accumulated that a specific, "true" diabetic cardiomyopathy distinct from ischemic injury does indeed exist.[170–172] The exact prevalence, nature, and cause of cardiac dysfunction directly attributable to diabetes have given rise to considerable debate inasmuch as other factors common in diabetes, such as hypertension, coronary atherosclerosis, and microvascular dysfunction, can independently impair myocardial performance.

EPIDEMIOLOGICAL EVIDENCE. Data from the Framingham Heart Study corroborated early observations suggesting the existence of a diabetic cardiomyopathy. In the Framingham cohort, after adjustment for age, blood pressure, cholesterol level, obesity, and history of CAD, the presence of diabetes quadrupled the risk for CHF in men 35 to 64 years old and doubled it in men 65 years or older. In women 35 to 64 years of age, diabetes entailed an eightfold increase in CHF and a fourfold increase in risk in older women.[173]

More recent epidemiological studies using case-control analyses have confirmed the association between diabetes and idiopathic cardiomyopathy in men[174] and in women[175] and have emphasized a possible interaction between diabetes and a history of hypertension. In men screened for the MRFIT Study who had cardiomyopathy, diabetes was a risk factor for mortality.[176] By combining the original Framingham Study Cohort and the Framingham Offspring Study, gender-specific linear regression analysis probed the contribution of diabetes and glucose intolerance to age-adjusted echocardiographic parameters in more than 4500 men and women. Diabetic individuals, particularly women, had higher heart rates and greater left ventricular wall thickness and cardiac mass than unaffected subjects did.[177]

PATHOLOGY. Early postmortem studies in diabetic subjects revealed myocyte hypertrophy, myofibril depletion with replacement fibrosis, interstitial deposition of periodic acid–Schiff–positive material, and perivascular fibrosis. Coronary arterioles demonstrate increased thickening of basement membranes and microaneurysms in autopsy specimens, as well as in tissue obtained at the time of coronary bypass surgery.[178, 179] More recently, endomyocardial biopsies from patients with diabetes have demonstrated a range of ultrastructural changes, including capillary basement membrane thickening and interstitial fibrosis, that are accentuated by coexisting hypertension.[180] Coexisting hypertension and diabetes accentuate myocardial fibrosis and collagen content.[98]

Noninvasive methods have confirmed fibrosis as a key feature of the heart in diabetic patients without evident cardiac disease. Ultrasound tissue characterization with backscatter analysis has been used to evaluate the myocardium of type I diabetic individuals with normal systolic function but with a variety of diabetes-related complications. When compared with an age-matched population, the diabetic group exhibited cardiac acoustic abnormalities suggesting increased collagen content of the myocardium.[181] Another study compared 26 type I diabetic subjects without hypertension or CAD with an age- and sex-matched control group by using a similar technique to assess myocardial acoustic properties. This study documented increased myocardial echodensity suggestive of increased collagen deposition despite normal septal and posterior wall thickness.[182]

MECHANISMS OF DIABETIC CARDIOMYOPATHY (Table 63–6). AGEs accumulate in tissue exposed to hyperglycemia and may contribute to the vascular complications of diabetes mellitus, as discussed above.[12, 13] Accumulation of AGE-modified extracellular matrix results in inelasticity of the vessel wall and could interfere with myocardial function as well. Serum levels of AGEs correlate with microvascular and renal complications in type I diabetes. In 52 patients with type I diabetes, prolongation of the isovolumic relaxation time as assessed by Doppler echocardiography correlated with serum levels of AGEs after adjustment for age, diabetes duration, renal function, blood pressure, and autonomic function parameters.[183] Experimental studies in diabetic dogs have also shown decreased left ventricular compliance associated with intramyocardial deposition of collagen in the absence of hypertrophy.[184] These data help explain the clinical observation that diabetic patients can have CHF as a result of diastolic dysfunction in the absence of hypertension and/or increased wall thickness.

Abnormalities in myocardial calcium handling may also contribute to abnormal cardiac mechanics in the diabetic heart.[185] Insulin-dependent diabetes impairs sarcoplasmic reticular Ca^{2+} pump activities, which reduces the rate of calcium removal from the cytoplasm in

▼ **TABLE 63–6. POSSIBLE CONTRIBUTORS TO DIABETIC CARDIOMYOPATHY**

Collagen accumulation decreasing myocardial compliance, accumulation of advanced glycosylation end product–modified extracellular matrix proteins leading to diastolic dysfunction[183, 184]

Abnormalities in myocardial calcium handling may also contribute to abnormal cardiac mechanics in the diabetic heart[185–188]

Activation of protein kinase C triggered by increased intracellular diacylglycerol[27]

Cardiac autonomic neuropathy[189]

Genetic abnormalities[190–192]

diastole. Such alterations may contribute to the increased diastolic stiffness that characterizes diabetic cardiomyopathy.[186, 187] Diabetes-related changes in troponin T, the contractile regulatory protein of the thin myofilament, may also contribute to both diastolic and systolic dysfunction.[188] In addition, activation of PKC may contribute to cardiac hypertrophy and failure, as discussed above.[27] In addition, a possible major cause of or contributor to chronic left ventricular dysfunction (cardiomyopathy) may be the direct effects of hyperglycemia and insulin resistance on myocardial cellular metabolism. The unavailability of glucose as an energy substrate and the shift in intracellular metabolism from glycolysis to free fatty acid oxidation can result in inadequate ATP generation and increased production of oxygen free radicals, both of which lead to depressed contractile function.[188a]

A recent study showed that a subset of type I diabetics without overt cardiac disease had abnormal left ventricular function with exercise despite normal contractile indices at rest. This decrement in left ventricular reserve correlated with evidence of reduced sympathetic innervation (see below), thus implicating dysautonomia in the pathogenesis of diabetic cardiac dysfunction.[189]

Genetic abnormalities may predispose to the development of cardiomyopathy in diabetics. Mitochondrial DNA mutations and deletions associated with diabetes mellitus may increase the risk for cardiac disease.[190, 191] A recent cross-sectional analysis evaluated the relationship between the ACE I/D genotypes and left ventricular mass in 289 type II diabetic subjects.[192] Presence of the ACE D/D genotype was independently associated with an increase in left ventricular mass.

CLINICAL FEATURES. In diabetic patients, the range of pathological and cellular abnormalities in the diabetic myocardium discussed above can reduce left ventricular compliance and cause shortness of breath out of proportion to the degree of systolic dysfunction. The natural history of diabetic cardiomyopathy is poorly understood. Many diabetic patients have diastolic dysfunction recognized on clinical grounds, but subsequent systolic dysfunction does not appear to develop. In others, left ventricular systolic dysfunction does intervene to produce a typical "congestive" cardiomyopathy.

Even young, asymptomatic type I diabetics frequently have echocardiographic evidence of diastolic dysfunction.[193, 194] It is more difficult to isolate diabetes-specific abnormalities in left ventricular function in type II diabetics because many of these individuals also have hypertension and/or CAD, which alone or together can cause diastolic and/or systolic dysfunction. However, considerable evidence suggests more decline in both systolic and diastolic function in diabetics than nondiabetics.[195, 196]

As noted above in the Framingham Study (without separation into type I and type II), women with diabetes had increased wall thickness, end-diastolic dimensions, and cardiac mass when compared with their nondiabetic counterparts.[177] Women with glucose intolerance showed similar, but less significant trends in these echocardiographic parameters, thus supporting the concept that changes in cardiac structure and function may occur in the setting of insulin resistance before the onset of hyperglycemia and a diagnosis of diabetes. In addition, the increased relative risk for cardiac death in diabetic women as opposed to diabetic men may result in part from these sex-specific effects on cardiac mass, an important independent predictor of outcome in the Framingham Study. Increased cardiac mass in the normotensive nondiabetic obese population is strongly associated with the degree of insulin resistance measured by the insulin and glucose response to an intra-

venous glucose tolerance test.[197] This relationship was independent of body weight, age, and blood pressure. A hemodynamic study comparing diastolic function in lean and obese nonhypertensive and hypertensive adults without CAD showed that left ventricular chamber stiffness was highest in the obese hypertensive individuals.[198] These subjects had the highest fasting glucose levels (within the normal range), which implicates insulin resistance as an important cofactor for the development of decreased left ventricular compliance even in the absence of diabetes. Elevated plasma insulin levels may induce myocardial hypertrophy by a direct growth-stimulating effect on myocardial cells.[199] Hyperinsulinemia increases salt reabsorption by the kidney. The expanded extracellular fluid compartment and blood volume could also lead to an increase in cardiac mass over time. When combined with hypertension, itself a cause of increased cardiac mass, these factors may result in proportionately more left ventricular hypertrophy than when hypertension is not associated with insulin resistance.

CARDIOVASCULAR AUTONOMIC NERVOUS SYSTEM DYSFUNCTION IN DIABETES MELLITUS

Cardiovascular autonomic neuropathy (CAN) probably contributes to the poor prognosis of CVD in both type I and type II diabetes mellitus. The majority of patients with CAN come to clinical attention with complaints of postural hypotension, resting tachycardia, exercise intolerance, or painless myocardial ischemia or infarction. The risk for CAN depends on the duration of diabetes and the degree of glycemic control and tends to parallel the development of other end-organ diseases related to diabetes such as retinopathy, nephropathy, and vasculopathy. Symptoms and signs of CAN often occur relatively late in the natural history of this complication. Because reliable and quantitative noninvasive methods to assess ANS function have now become available, the diagnosis of CAN may now precede the development of symptoms. Most clinicians regard CAN as a major complication of type I diabetes because the challenge of managing this complication often dominates the care of these patients. CAN tends to be less fully expressed in a patient with type II diabetes, who is typically older and has a wider variety of comorbid conditions.

DIAGNOSIS. A variety of tests can assess parasympathetic and sympathetic function in diabetics. A series of bedside maneuvers can aid in the diagnosis of CAN and differentiate the relative contribution of parasympathetic and sympathetic dysfunction in CAN. These tests use the ECG to measure beat-to-beat heart rate variation during deep breathing, at assumption of an upright posture, and during the Valsalva maneuver.[200] Recently, tests have emerged that can detect the presence of CAN before symptoms develop. A number of methods assess heart rate variability during 24-hour recordings and thereby permit detection of subtle disorders in autonomic balance. Cardiac radionuclide imaging with the norepinephrine analog metaiodobenzylguanidine (MIBG) can directly image the sympathetic nerve activity of the myocardium. Diabetic individuals generally have less myocardial MIBG uptake with more pronounced regional differences from base to apex than do patients without diabetes. In addition, positron-emission tomographic (PET) scanning with the sympathetic neurotransmitter analog ^{11}C-labeled hydyoxyephedrine can evaluate myocardial sympathetic innervation. These noninvasive methods, alone or in combination with the standard bedside examination, can establish the presence and severity of CAN and be used to evaluate the effects of interventions.[201]

PREVALENCE. The prevalence of CAN varies with the method used and the population studied, but CAN appears to be quite common. In a large group of type I and II diabetic subjects, heart rate variability on 24-hour ambulatory ECG showed abnormalities in nearly 50 percent of diabetics, far more than in controls.[202] MIBG scintigraphy in patients with type I diabetes for at least 10 years who had CAD excluded by thallium single-photon emission computed tomography (SPECT) revealed regional adrenergic denervation in 18 of 24 subjects.[203] In newly diagnosed type I diabetic individuals examined by a battery of tests, 8 percent had definite CAN.[200]

PROGNOSIS. Numerous studies have documented increased mortality in diabetic patients with CAN.[204-206] In type I diabetics, 5-year mortality in patients with CAN exceeded the 5-year mortality in those without CAN by fivefold.[205] Another study involving both type I and type II patients examined the relationship between ANS function and retinopathy, nephropathy, glycemic control, and cardiovascular risk factors. CAN conferred excess mortality beyond that attributable to other risk factors.[207] The relationship of ANS dysfunction to outcome in type II diabetic patients is less well characterized. In a Finnish study, 70 men with newly diagnosed type II diabetes and baseline, 5-year, and 10-year assessment of heart rate variability were compared with a control group. Sympathetic ANS dysfunction at the 5-year examination predicted the 10-year cardiovascular mortality.[99]

EFFECTS OF TREATMENT. Institution of strict glycemic control in type I diabetic patients can reverse abnormalities in heart rate variability in diabetic patients with early CAN[208] and reduce the degree of left ventricular sympathetic denervation on PET scanning with labeled hydroxyephedrine.[209] Pancreatic-kidney transplantation in type I patients can result in an improvement in cardiovascular reflexes.[210] Other treatment modalities found to improve autonomic function include the antioxidant alpha-lipoic acid,[211] an ACE inhibitor,[212, 213] and aldose reductase inhibition.[214, 215]

Mechanisms Responsible for Increased Morbidity and Mortality

Numerous mechanisms may underlie the increased cardiovascular morbidity and mortality associated with CAN in diabetes mellitus (Table 63-7).

IMPAIRED ANGINA PERCEPTION. Clinicians have recognized for some time that myocardial ischemia or infarction may be associated with less severe angina in a diabetic versus a nondiabetic patient. CAN may explain the blunted appreciation of cardiac ischemic pain in diabetic patients. Instead of typical angina, patients may have shortness of breath, diaphoresis, gastrointestinal complaints, profound fatigue, or abrupt changes in glycemic control. When compared with nondiabetic patients with exercise-induced ischemia, diabetic individuals are less apt to be limited by angina at the time of ST segment depression than nondiabetics are.[216] In one study that used ambulatory ST segment monitoring to examine diabetic patients with documented

▼ TABLE 63-7. CARDIOVASCULAR AUTONOMIC NEUROPATHY AND INCREASED CARDIOVASCULAR MORBIDITY AND MORTALITY IN DIABETES MELLITUS

EFFECTS OF SYMPATHOVAGAL IMBALANCE
Impairs angina recognition
Silent ischemia and infarction
Alters threshold for ischemia
Increased resting heart rate and blunted chronotropic response to exercise
Impaired coronary vasomotor regulation
Causes abnormal diastolic and systolic function
Factor in cardiac cardiomyopathy
Increases risk for ventricular arrhythmia
In presence or absence of myocardial ischemia
Alters circadian pattern of triggering of acute cardiac events
Loss of nocturnal protection against myocardial infarction
Alters circadian blood pressure regulation
Increased cardiac mass
Risk factor for microalbuminuria and diabetic nephropathy
Adversely affects the natural history of congestive heart failure
Causes hemodynamic instability in the perioperative period

CAD, over 90 percent of ischemic episodes were asymptomatic.[106] Shortness of breath reflecting ischemia-induced heart failure may precede the perception of angina during treadmill testing and correlates with the degree of CAN on cardiovascular reflex testing[217, 218] and MIBG scanning,[219] thus suggesting a direct link between autonomic neuropathy and defective angina recognition. Histological damage to cardiac afferent nerve fibers has been demonstrated in diabetic patients with silent myocardial infarction.[220] The blunted recognition of ischemia because of CAN may delay treatment and worsen the outcome.[96, 221] Blunted perception also makes it difficult to monitor antiischemic treatment or determine whether restenosis has occurred after coronary intervention.

CAN AND MYOCARDIAL INFARCTION TRIGGERING. Diabetic patients with CAN show a homogeneous distribution of myocardial infarction throughout the full 24-hour period,[106] while diabetics without CAN have a circadian pattern of ischemia like that seen in nondiabetic patients, with a typical prominence in the early morning.[105, 222, 223]

CAN AND THE THRESHOLD FOR MYOCARDIAL ISCHEMIA. Myocardial ischemia occurs when there is an imbalance between myocardial oxygen supply and demand, both of which can be affected by CAN. Resting tachycardia caused by parasympathetic denervation, an early manifestation of CAN, increases myocardial oxygen demand and can place diabetic patients with CAD closer to their ischemic threshold. Even transient sympathovagal imbalance can trigger ischemia-mediated sudden death. In a small group of patients with CAD who had sudden cardiac death during Holter monitoring, transient decreases in heart rate variability preceded onset of the ST segment shift and precipitated life-threatening arrhythmias in all eight cases.[224]

EFFECT OF CAN ON CORONARY BLOOD FLOW REGULATION. The status of the ANS can affect coronary blood flow regulation independent of mechanisms mediated by endothelial cell function.[225] Diabetic patients with sympathetic nervous system dysfunction have impaired dilation of coronary resistance vessels in response to cold pressor testing when compared with diabetics without defects in cardiac adrenergic nerve density.[226] In another study, global myocardial blood flow and coronary flow reserve in response to adenosine were subnormal in diabetics with CAN as defined by similar PET criteria.[227] The aspects of CAN described above may well provoke ischemic episodes by upsetting the balance between myocardial supply and demand.

CAN AND SUDDEN CARDIOVASCULAR DEATH IN DIABETICS. It has been recognized for some time that sudden death can occur in the absence of CAD in patients with diabetes mellitus. The association of abnormal cardiovascular reflex testing and sudden cardiac death in early case studies pointed to a direct link between autonomic balance and arrhythmogenesis. The relationship of sudden death (defined as unexpected death within 1 or 24 hours of symptoms) to glucose intolerance was examined in 8006 Japanese-American men after 23 years' follow-up in the Honolulu Heart Program.[228] After adjustment for recognized cardiac risk factors, the relative risks for sudden death within 24 hours in subjects with high normal glucose (151 to 224 mg/dl), asymptomatic high glucose values (>225 mg/dl), and diabetes versus those with lower glucose values (<151 mg/dl) were 1.59, 2.22, and 2.76, respectively ($p < 0.05$).

The recognition that sympathetic imbalance relates to the pathophysiology of sudden death in the familial long QT syndrome has supported CAN as a risk factor for premature cardiac death in individuals with diabetes. Prolongation of the corrected QT interval in diabetic patients correlates with the degree of autonomic neuropathy.[229] Newer methods to assess arrhythmogenic potential have firmly established CAN as a risk factor for sudden death in diabetes. The presence of QT dispersion on the 12-lead ECG reflects dispersion of ventricular refractoriness and increased risk for arrhythmia. When compared with a nondiabetic control group and a diabetic group without CAN, QT dispersion was greatest in diabetic patients with CAN.[230] Diabetic patients with the most advanced cardiovascular sympathetic denervation have the highest mortality rate. This apparent paradox may be explained by recent data demonstrating that diabetic patients with severe autonomic neuropathy can have marked heterogeneity in left ventricular sympathetic neuronal uptake on PET scanning with the neurotransmitter analog ^{11}C-hydroxyephedrine.[231]

PERIOPERATIVE HEMODYNAMIC INSTABILITY. Perioperative hemodynamic instability in the setting of CAN may contribute to the twofold to threefold greater risk of cardiac morbidity and mortality in diabetics undergoing noncardiac surgery. During induction of general anesthesia, heart rate and blood pressure may decline to a greater degree than in patients without diabetes. In rare cases, cardiovascular collapse has occurred after brachial plexus block.[232] Diabetics with autonomic neuropathy require perioperative pharmacological support with pressors to stabilize blood pressure more often than do diabetics without CAN.[233] Despite the preponderance of data linking diabetes and perioperative cardiac risk, no relationship was seen between autonomic function and hemodynamic behavior in a recent study comparing diabetic and nondiabetic patients undergoing CABG surgery.[234]

FUTURE PERSPECTIVES

Cardiovascular complications have emerged over the last decade as the key target to reduce morbidity and mortality in diabetics. The focus in treatment of diabetes is shifting from blood sugar to the blood vessel. Future studies will doubtless more often specify cardiovascular events as major endpoints rather than merely specifying surrogates such as glycemia. Evaluation of the possible cardiovascular protective effects of new classes of agents such as the insulin sensitizers (thiazolidinediones) is under way, for example. The role of fibrates in place of or in addition to statins for the treatment of diabetic dyslipidemia needs careful evaluation. The benefits of initiating treatment of individuals with impaired glucose tolerance to slow the progression to overt diabetes also merits study. Inevitably, this challenging group of patients will become more and more an integral part of the daily practice of cardiology in the years to come.

REFERENCES

SCOPE OF THE PROBLEM

1. Libby P, Rabbani L, Brogi E, et al: The challenge of diabetic vascular disease. *In* Bagdade J (ed): Year Book of Endocrinology. St Louis, Mosby, 1993.
2. Grundy SM, Benjamin IJ, Burke GL, et al: Diabetes and cardiovascular disease: A statement for healthcare professionals from the American Heart Association. Circulation 100:1134–1146, 1999.
2a. Friesinger GC 2nd, Gavin JA 3rd: Diabetes and cardiologists: A call to action. J Am Coll Cardiol 35:1130–1133, 2000.
3. Mokdad AH, Serdula MK, Dietz WH, et al: The spread of the obesity epidemic in the United States, 1991–1998. JAMA 282:1519–1522, 1999.
4. Wilson PW, Kannel WB, Silbershatz H, et al: Clustering of metabolic factors and coronary heart disease. Arch Intern Med 159:1104–1109, 1999.
5. Brancati FL, Kao WHL, Folsom AR, et al: Incident type 2 diabetes mellitus in African American and white adults: The atherosclerosis risk in communities study. JAMA 283:2253–2259, 2000.
6. Carter JS, Pugh JA, Monterrosa A: Non–insulin-dependent diabetes mellitus in minorities in the United States. Ann Intern Med 125:221–232, 1996.

PATHOPHYSIOLOGY OF THE CARDIOVASCULAR COMPLICATIONS OF DIABETES

7. Lindeman RD, Romero LJ, Hundley R, et al: Prevalences of type 2 diabetes, the insulin resistance syndrome, and coronary heart disease in an elderly, biethnic population. Diabetes Care 21:959–966, 1998.

8. Gowri MS, Van der Westhuyzen DR, Bridges SR, et al: Decreased protection by HDL from poorly controlled type 2 diabetic subjects against LDL oxidation may be due to the abnormal composition of HDL. Arterioscler Thromb Vasc Biol 19:2226–2233, 1999.
9. Tsai EC, Hirsch IB, Brunzell JD, et al: Reduced plasma peroxyl radical trapping capacity and increased susceptibility of LDL to oxidation in poorly controlled IDDM. Diabetes 43:1010–1014, 1994.
10. Barroso I, Gurnell M, Crowley VE, et al: Dominant negative mutations in human PPARgamma associated with severe insulin resistance, diabetes mellitus and hypertension. Nature 402:880–883, 1999.
11. Baynes JW, Thorpe SR: Role of oxidative stress in diabetic complications: A new perspective on an old paradigm. Diabetes 48:1–9, 1999.
12. Stitt AW, Bucala R, Vlassara H: Atherogenesis and advanced glycation: Promotion, progression, and prevention. Ann N Y Acad Sci 811:115–127, 1997.
13. Wautier JL, Guillausseau PJ: Diabetes, advanced glycation endproducts and vascular disease. Vasc Med 3:131–137, 1998.
14. Brownlee M: Negative consequences of glycation. Metabolism 49:9–13, 2000.
15. Witztum JL: Role of modified lipoproteins in diabetic macroangiopathy. Diabetes 46(Suppl 2):112–114, 1997.
16. Bucala R, Makita Z, Koschinsky T, et al: Lipid advanced glycosylation: Pathway for lipid oxidation in vivo. Proc Natl Acad Sci U S A 90:6434–6438, 1993.
17. Vlassara H, Fuh H, Makita Z, et al: Exogenous advanced glycosylation end products induce complex vascular dysfunction in normal animals: A model for diabetic and aging complications. Proc Natl Acad Sci U S A 89:12043–12047, 1992.
18. Vlassara H, Fuh H, Donnelly T, et al: Advanced glycation endproducts promote adhesion molecule (VCAM-1, ICAM-1) expression and atheroma formation in normal rabbits. Mol Med 1:447–456, 1995.
19. Schmidt AM, Yan SD, Wautier JL, et al: Activation of receptor for advanced glycation end products: A mechanism for chronic vascular dysfunction in diabetic vasculopathy and atherosclerosis. Circ Res 84:489–497, 1999.
20. Park L, Raman KG, Lee KJ, et al: Suppression of accelerated diabetic atherosclerosis by the soluble receptor for advanced glycation endproducts. Nat Med 4:1025–1031, 1998.
21. Reaven GM, Lithell H, Landsberg L: Hypertension and associated metabolic abnormalities—the role of insulin resistance and the sympathoadrenal system. N Engl J Med 334:374–381, 1996.
22. Imperatore G, Riccardi G, Iovine C, et al: Plasma fibrinogen: A new factor of the metabolic syndrome. A population-based study. Diabetes Care 21:649–654, 1998.
23. Sobel BE, Woodcock-Mitchell J, Schneider DJ, et al: Increased plasminogen activator inhibitor type 1 in coronary artery atherectomy specimens from type 2 diabetic compared with nondiabetic patients: A potential factor predisposing to thrombosis and its persistence. Circulation 97:2213–2221, 1998.
24. Meigs JB, Mittleman MA, Nathan DM, et al: Hyperinsulinemia, hyperglycemia, and impaired hemostasis: The Framingham Offspring Study. JAMA 283:221–228, 2000.
25. Trovati M, Anfossi G: Insulin, insulin resistance and platelet function: Similarities with insulin effects on cultured vascular smooth muscle cells. Diabetologia 41:609–622, 1998.
26. Feener EP, King GL: Vascular dysfunction in diabetes mellitus. Lancet 350(Suppl 1):9–13, 1997.
27. Koya D, King GL: Protein kinase C activation and the development of diabetic complications. Diabetes 47:859–866, 1998.
28. Kuboki K, Jiang ZY, Takahara N, et al: Regulation of endothelial constitutive nitric oxide synthase gene expression in endothelial cells and in vivo: A specific vascular action of insulin. Circulation 101:676–681, 2000.
29. Terry CM, Callahan KS: Protein kinase C regulates cytokine-induced tissue factor transcription and procoagulant activity in human endothelial cells. J Lab Clin Med 127:81–93, 1996.
30. Ishii H, Jirousek MR, Koya D, et al: Amelioration of vascular dysfunctions in diabetic rats by an oral PKC beta inhibitor. Science 272:728–731, 1996.
31. Wakasaki H, Koya D, Schoen FJ, et al: Targeted overexpression of protein kinase C beta2 isoform in myocardium causes cardiomyopathy. Proc Natl Acad Sci U S A 94:9320–9325, 1997.
32. Giles TD, Ouyang J, Kerut EK, et al: Changes in protein kinase C in early cardiomyopathy and in gracilis muscle in the BB/Wor diabetic rat. Am J Physiol 274:H295–H307, 1998.
33. Johnstone MT, Creager SJ, Scales KM, et al: Impaired endothelium-dependent vasodilation in patients with insulin-dependent diabetes mellitus. Circulation 88:2510–2516, 1993.
34. McVeigh GE, Brennan GM, Johnston GD, et al: Impaired endothelium-dependent and independent vasodilation in patients with type 2 (non-insulin-dependent) diabetes mellitus. Diabetologia 35:771–776, 1992.
35. Williams SB, Cusco JA, Roddy MA, et al: Impaired nitric oxide–mediated vasodilation in patients with non–insulin-dependent diabetes mellitus. J Am Coll Cardiol 27:567–574, 1996.
36. Tesfamariam B, Cohen RA: Free radicals mediate endothelial cell dysfunction caused by elevated glucose. Am J Physiol 263:H321–H326, 1992.
37. Ting HH, Timimi FK, Boles KS, et al: Vitamin C improves endothelium-dependent vasodilation in patients with non–insulin-dependent diabetes mellitus. J Clin Invest 97:22–28, 1996.

38. Timimi FK, Ting HH, Haley EA, et al: Vitamin C improves endothelium-dependent vasodilation in patients with insulin-dependent diabetes mellitus. J Am Coll Cardiol 31:552–557, 1998.

39. Petrie JR, Ueda, S, Webb DJ, et al: Endothelial nitric oxide production and insulin sensitivity. A physiological link with implications for pathogenesis of cardiovascular disease. Circulation 93:1331–1333, 1996.

40. Steinberg HO, Chaker H, Leaming R, et al: Obesity/insulin resistance is associated with endothelial dysfunction. Implications for the syndrome of insulin resistance. J Clin Invest 97:2601–2610, 1996.

41. Akbari CM, Saouaf R, Barnhill DF, et al: Endothelium-dependent vasodilatation is impaired in both microcirculation and macrocirculation during acute hyperglycemia. J Vasc Surg 28:687–694, 1998.

42. Evans M, Anderson RA, Graham J, et al: Ciprofibrate therapy improves endothelial function and reduces postprandial lipemia and oxidative stress in type 2 diabetes mellitus. Circulation 101:1773–1779, 2000.

43. Balletshofer BM, Rittig K, Enderle MD, et al: Endothelial dysfunction is detectable in young normotensive first-degree relatives of subjects with type 2 diabetes in association with insulin resistance. Circulation 101:1780–1784, 2000.

43a. Cooke JP: Does ADMA cause endothelial dysfunction? Arterioscler Thromb Vasc Biol, in press.

44. Boger RH, Bode-Boger SM, Szuba A, et al: Asymmetric dimethylarginine (ADMA): A novel risk factor for endothelial dysfunction: Its role in hypercholesterolemia. Circulation 98:1842–1847, 1998.

45. Ito A, Tsao PS, Adimoolam S, et al: Novel mechanism for endothelial dysfunction: Dysregulation of dimethylarginine dimethylaminohydrolase. Circulation 99:3092–3095, 1999.

45a. Fard A, Tuck C, Donis J, et al: Acute elevations of plasma asymmetric dimethylarginine and impaired endothelial function in response to a high-fat meal in patients with Type 2 diabetes. Arterioscler Thromb Vasc Biol, in press.

46. Harris MI: Diabetes in America: Epidemiology and scope of the problem. Diabetes Care 21(Suppl 3):C11–C14, 1998.

47. Selby JV, Ray GT, Zhang D, et al: Excess costs of medical care for patients with diabetes in a managed care population. Diabetes Care 20:1396–1402, 1997.

48. Gu K, Cowie CC, Harris MI: Diabetes and decline in heart disease mortality in US adults. JAMA 281:1291–1297, 1999.

49. Bierman EL: George Lyman Duff Memorial Lecture. Atherogenesis in diabetes. Arterioscler Thromb 12:647–656, 1992.

50. Kannel WB, McGee DL: Diabetes and cardiovascular disease. The Framingham study. JAMA 241:2035–2038, 1979.

51. Stamler J, Vaccaro O, Neaton JD, et al: Diabetes, other risk factors, and 12-yr cardiovascular mortality for men screened in the Multiple Risk Factor Intervention Trial. Diabetes Care 16:434–444, 1993.

52. Lowe LP, Liu K, Greenland P, et al: Diabetes, asymptomatic hyperglycemia, and 22-year mortality in black and white men. The Chicago Heart Association Detection Project in Industry Study. Diabetes Care 20:163–169, 1997.

53. Haffner SM, Lehto S, Ronnemaa T, et al: Mortality from coronary heart disease in subjects with type 2 diabetes and in nondiabetic subjects with and without prior myocardial infarction. N Engl J Med 339:229–234, 1998.

54. Barrett-Connor EL, Cohn BA, Wingard DL, et al: Why is diabetes mellitus a stronger risk factor for fatal ischemic heart disease in women than in men? The Rancho Bernardo Study. JAMA 265:627–631, 1991.

55. Manson JE, Colditz GA, Stampfer MJ, et al: A prospective study of maturity-onset diabetes mellitus and risk of coronary heart disease and stroke in women. Arch Intern Med 151:1141–1147, 1991.

56. Krolewski AS, Warram JH, Rand LI, et al: Epidemiologic approach to the etiology of type I diabetes mellitus and its complications. N Engl J Med 317:1390–1398, 1987.

57. Borch-Johnsen K, Kreiner S: Proteinuria: Value as predictor of cardiovascular mortality in insulin dependent diabetes mellitus. BMJ 294:1651–1654, 1987.

58. Koivisto VA, Stevens LK, Mattock M, et al: Cardiovascular disease and its risk factors in IDDM in Europe. EURODIAB IDDM Complications Study Group. Diabetes Care 19:689–697, 1996.

59. Orchard TJ, Dorman JS, Maser RE, et al: Prevalence of complications in IDDM by sex and duration. Pittsburgh Epidemiology of Diabetes Complications Study II. Diabetes 39:1116–1124, 1990.

60. Nathan DM, Meigs J, Singer DE: The epidemiology of cardiovascular disease in type 2 diabetes mellitus: how sweet it is . . . or is it? Lancet 350(Suppl 1):4–9, 1997.

61. Lehto S, Ronnemaa T, Haffner SM: Dyslipidemia and hyperglycemia predict coronary heart disease events in middle-aged patients with NIDDM. Diabetes 46:1354–1359, 1997.

RISK FACTOR INTERVENTION TO REDUCE CHD IN PATIENTS WITH DIABETES MELLITUS

62. Standl E, Balletshofer B, Dahl B, et al: Predictors of 10-year macrovascular and overall mortality in patients with NIDDM: The Munich General Practitioner Project. Diabetologia 39:1540–1545, 1996.

63. Turner RC: The U.K. Prospective Diabetes Study. A review. Diabetes Care 21(Suppl 3):C35–C38, 1998.

64. Andersson DK, Svardsudd K: Long-term glycemic control relates to mortality in type II diabetes. Diabetes Care 18:1534–1543, 1995.

65. Wei M, Gaskill SP, Haffner SM, et al: Effects of diabetes and level of glycemia on all-cause and cardiovascular mortality. The San Antonio Heart Study. Diabetes Care 21:1167–1172, 1998.

66. Klein R, Klein BE, Moss SE: The Wisconsin Epidemiologic Study of Diabetic Retinopathy. XVI. The relationship of C-peptide to the incidence and progression of diabetic retinopathy. Diabetes 44:796–801, 1995.

67. Wingard DL, Barrett-Connor EL, Scheidt-Nave C, et al: Prevalence of cardiovascular and renal complications in older adults with normal or impaired glucose tolerance or NIDDM. A population-based study. Diabetes Care 16:1022–1025, 1993.

68. Kuusisto J, Mykkanen L, Pyorala K, et al: Non-insulin-dependent diabetes and its metabolic control are important predictors of stroke in elderly subjects. Stroke 25:1157–1164, 1994.

69. Rodriguez BL, Lau N, Burchfiel CM, et al: Glucose intolerance and 23-year risk of coronary heart disease and total mortality: The Honolulu Heart Program. Diabetes Care 22:1262–1265, 1999.

70. Folsom AR, Eckfeldt JH, Weitzman S, et al: Relation of carotid artery wall thickness to diabetes mellitus, fasting glucose and insulin, body size, and physical activity. Atherosclerosis Risk in Communities (ARIC) Study Investigators. Stroke 25:66–73, 1994.

71. Temelkova-Kurktschiev TS, Koehler C, Leonhardt, W, et al: Increased intimal-medial thickness in newly detected type 2 diabetes: Risk factors. Diabetes Care 22:333–338, 1999.

72. Wagenknecht LE, D'Agostino RB Jr, Haffner SM, et al: Impaired glucose tolerance, type 2 diabetes, and carotid wall thickness: The Insulin Resistance Atherosclerosis Study. Diabetes Care 21:1812–1818, 1998.

73. Hanefeld M, Koehler C, Schaper F, et al: Postprandial plasma glucose is an independent risk factor for increased carotid intima-media thickness in non-diabetic individuals. Atherosclerosis 144:229–235, 1999.

74. O'Leary DH, Polak JF, Kronmal RA, et al: Carotid-artery intima and media thickness as a risk factor for myocardial infarction and stroke in older adults. Cardiovascular Health Study Collaborative Research Group. N Engl J Med 340:14–22, 1999.

75. Tominaga M, Eguchi H, Manaka H, et al: Impaired glucose tolerance is a risk factor for cardiovascular disease, but not impaired fasting glucose. The Funagata Diabetes Study. Diabetes Care 22:920–924, 1999.

76. Bonora E, Kiechl S, Willeit J, et al: Prevalence of insulin resistance in metabolic disorders: The Bruneck Study. Diabetes 47:1643–1649, 1998.

77. Deedwania PC: The deadly quartet revisited. Am J Med 105:1S–3S, 1998.

78. Howard G, O'Leary DH, Zaccaro D, et al: Insulin sensitivity and atherosclerosis. The Insulin Resistance Atherosclerosis Study (IRAS) Investigators. Circulation 93:1809–1817, 1996.

79. Despres JP, Lamarche B, Mauriege P, et al: Hyperinsulinemia as an independent risk factor for ischemic heart disease. N Engl J Med 334:952–957, 1996.

80. The effect of intensive treatment of diabetes on the development and progression of long-term complications in insulin-dependent diabetes mellitus. The Diabetes Control and Complications Trial Research Group. N Engl J Med 329:977–986, 1993.

81. Abraira C, Colwell J, Nuttall F, et al: Cardiovascular events and correlates in the Veterans Affairs Diabetes Feasibility Trial. Veterans Affairs Cooperative Study on Glycemic Control and Complications in Type II Diabetes. Arch Intern Med 157:181–188, 1997.

82. Intensive blood-glucose control with sulphonylureas or insulin compared with conventional treatment and risk of complications in patients with type 2 diabetes (UKPDS 33). UK Prospective Diabetes Study (UKPDS) Group. Lancet 352:837–853, 1998.

83. Tatti P, Pahor M, Byington RP, et al: Outcome results of the Fosinopril Versus Amlodipine Cardiovascular Events Randomized Trial (FACET) in patients with hypertension and NIDDM. Diabetes Care 21:597–603, 1998.

84. Estacio RO, Schrier RW: Antihypertensive therapy in type 2 diabetes: Implications of the appropriate blood pressure control in diabetes (ABCD) trial. Am J Cardiol 82:9R–14R, 1998.

85. Nesto RW, Zarich, S: Acute myocardial infarction in diabetes mellitus: Lessons learned from ACE inhibition. Circulation 97:12–15, 1998.

85a. Cooper ME, Johnston CI: Optimizing treatment of hypertension in patients with diabetes. JAMA 283:3177–3179, 2000.

86. Efficacy of atenolol and captopril in reducing risk of macrovascular and microvascular complications in type 2 diabetes: UKPDS 39. UK Prospective Diabetes Study Group. BMJ 317:713–720, 1998.

87. Tuomilehto J, Rastenyte D, Birkenhager WH, et al: Effects of calcium-channel blockade in older patients with diabetes and systolic hypertension. Systolic Hypertension in Europe Trial Investigators. N Engl J Med 340:677–684, 1999.

88. Hansson L, Zanchetti A, Carruthers SG, et al: Effects of intensive blood-pressure lowering and low-dose aspirin in patients with hypertension: Principal results of the Hypertension Optimal Treatment (HOT) randomised trial. HOT Study Group. Lancet 351:1755–1762, 1998.

89. Staessen JA, Fagard R, Thijs L, et al: Randomised double-blind comparison of placebo and active treatment for older patients with isolated systolic hypertension. The Systolic Hypertension in Europe (Syst-Eur) Trial Investigators. Lancet 350:757–764, 1997.

89a. Gress TW, Nieto FJ, Shahar E, et al: Hypertension and hypertensive therapy as risk factors for type 2 diabetes mellitus. Atherosclerosis Risk in Communities Study. N Engl J Med 342:905–912, 2000.

90. Goldberg RB, Mellies MJ, Sacks FM, et al: Cardiovascular events and their reduction with pravastatin in diabetic and glucose-intolerant myo-

cardial infarction survivors with average cholesterol levels: Subgroup analyses in the cholesterol and recurrent events (CARE) trial. The Care Investigators. Circulation 98:2513–2519, 1998.

91. Haffner SM, Alexander CM, Cook TJ, et al: Reduced coronary events in simvastatin-treated patients with coronary heart disease and diabetes or impaired fasting glucose levels: Subgroup analyses in the Scandinavian Simvastatin Survival Study. Arch Intern Med 159:2661–2667, 1999.

TREATMENT OF ACUTE CORONARY SYNDROMES IN DIABETICS

92. Rubins HB, Robins SJ, Collins D, et al: Gemfibrozil for the secondary prevention of coronary heart disease in men with low levels of high-density lipoprotein cholesterol. Veterans Affairs High-Density Lipoprotein Cholesterol Intervention Trial Study Group. N Engl J Med 341:410–418, 1999.

92a. Steiner G: Lipid intervention trials in diabetes. Diabetes Care 23(Suppl2):B49–53, 2000.

93. Gray RP, Yudkin JS, Patterson DL: Enzymatic evidence of impaired reperfusion in diabetic patients after thrombolytic therapy for acute myocardial infarction: A role for plasminogen activator inhibitor? Br Heart J 70:530–536, 1993.

94. Granger CB, Califf RM, Young S, et al: Outcome of patients with diabetes mellitus and acute myocardial infarction treated with thrombolytic agents. The Thrombolysis and Angioplasty in Myocardial Infarction (TAMI) Study Group. J Am Coll Cardiol 21:920–925, 1993.

95. Woodfield SL, Lundergan CF, Reiner JS, et al: Angiographic findings and outcome in diabetic patients treated with thrombolytic therapy for acute myocardial infarction: The GUSTO-I experience. J Am Coll Cardiol 28:1661–1669, 1996.

96. Mak KH, Moliterno DJ, Granger CB, et al: Influence of diabetes mellitus on clinical outcome in the thrombolytic era of acute myocardial infarction. GUSTO-I Investigators. Global Utilization of Streptokinase and Tissue Plasminogen Activator for Occluded Coronary Arteries. J Am Coll Cardiol 30:171–179, 1997.

97. Mahaffey KW, Granger CB, Toth CA, et al: Diabetic retinopathy should not be a contraindication to thrombolytic therapy for acute myocardial infarction: Review of ocular hemorrhage incidence and location in the GUSTO-I trial. Global Utilization of Streptokinase and t-PA for Occluded Coronary Arteries. J Am Coll Cardiol 30:1606–1610, 1997.

98. van Hoeven KH, Factor SM: A comparison of the pathological spectrum of hypertensive, diabetic, and hypertensive-diabetic heart disease. Circulation 82:848–855, 1990.

99. Toyry JP, Niskanen LK, Mantysaari MJ, et al: Occurrence, predictors, and clinical significance of autonomic neuropathy in NIDDM. Ten-year follow-up from the diagnosis. Diabetes 45:308–315, 1996.

100. Jacoby RM, Nesto RW: Acute myocardial infarction in the diabetic patient: Pathophysiology, clinical course and prognosis. J Am Coll Cardiol 20:736–744, 1992.

101. Iwasaka T, Takahashi N, Nakamura S, et al: Residual left ventricular pump function after acute myocardial infarction in NIDDM patients. Diabetes Care 15:1522–1526, 1992.

102. Nahser PJ Jr, Brown RE, Oskarsson H, et al: Maximal coronary flow reserve and metabolic coronary vasodilation in patients with diabetes mellitus. Circulation 91:635–640, 1995.

103. Abaci A, Oguzhan A, Kahraman S, et al: Effect of diabetes mellitus on formation of coronary collateral vessels. Circulation 99:2239–2242, 1999.

104. Depre C, Vanoverschelde JL, Taegtmeyer H: Glucose for the heart. Circulation 99:578–588, 1999.

105. Bernardi L, Ricordi L, Lazzari P, et al: Impaired circadian modulation of sympathovagal activity in diabetes. A possible explanation for altered temporal onset of cardiovascular disease. Circulation 86:1443–1452, 1992.

106. Zarich S, Waxman S, Freeman RT, et al: Effect of autonomic nervous system dysfunction on the circadian pattern of myocardial ischemia in diabetes mellitus. J Am Coll Cardiol 24:956–962, 1994.

107. Muller JE, Tofler GH, Stone PH: Circadian variation and triggers of onset of acute cardiovascular disease. Circulation 79:733–743, 1989.

108. Gray RP, Patterson DL, Yudkin JS: Plasminogen activator inhibitor activity in diabetic and nondiabetic survivors of myocardial infarction. Arterioscler Thromb 13:415–420, 1993.

109. Thompson SG, Kienast J, Pyke SD, et al: Hemostatic factors and the risk of myocardial infarction or sudden death in patients with angina pectoris. European Concerted Action on Thrombosis and Disabilities Angina Pectoris Study Group. N Engl J Med 332:635–641, 1995.

110. Inhibition of platelet glycoprotein IIb/IIIa with eptifibatide in patients with acute coronary syndromes. The PURSUIT Trial Investigators. Platelet Glycoprotein IIb/IIIa in Unstable Angina: Receptor Suppression Using Integrilin Therapy. N Engl J Med 339:436–443, 1998.

111. Inhibition of the platelet glycoprotein IIb/IIIa receptor with tirofiban in unstable angina and non-Q-wave myocardial infarction. Platelet Receptor Inhibition in Ischemic Syndrome Management in Patients Limited by Unstable Signs and Symptoms (PRISM-PLUS) Study Investigators. N Engl J Med 338:1488–1497, 1998.

112. Davi G, Catalano I, Averna M, et al: Thromboxane biosynthesis and platelet function in type II diabetes mellitus. N Engl J Med 322:1769–1774, 1990.

113. Colwell JA: Aspirin therapy in diabetes. Diabetes Care 20:1767–1771, 1997.

114. Aspirin effects on mortality and morbidity in patients with diabetes mellitus. Early Treatment Diabetic Retinopathy Study report 14. ETDRS Investigators. JAMA 268:1292–1300, 1992.

115. Harpaz D, Gottlieb S, Graff E, et al: Effects of aspirin treatment on survival in non–insulin-dependent diabetic patients with coronary artery disease. Israeli Bezafibrate Infarction Prevention Study Group. Am J Med 105:494–499, 1998.

116. Aspirin therapy in diabetes. American Diabetes Association. Diabetes Care 20:1772–1773, 1997.

117. Kjekshus J, Gilpin E, Cali G, et al: Diabetic patients and beta-blockers after acute myocardial infarction. Eur Heart J 11:43–50, 1990.

118. Chen J, Marciniak TA, Radford MJ, et al: Beta–blocker therapy for secondary prevention of myocardial infarction in elderly diabetic patients. Results from the National Cooperative Cardiovascular Project. J Am Coll Cardiol 34:1388–1394, 1999.

119. Jonas M, Reicher-Reiss H, Boyko V, et al: Usefulness of beta-blocker therapy in patients with non–insulin-dependent diabetes mellitus and coronary artery disease. Bezafibrate Infarction Prevention (BIP) Study Group. Am J Cardiol 77:1273–1277, 1996.

120. Lakshman MR, Reda DJ, Materson BJ, et al: Diuretics and beta-blockers do not have adverse effects at 1 year on plasma lipid and lipoprotein profiles in men with hypertension. Department of Veterans Affairs Cooperative Study Group on Antihypertensive Agents. Arch Intern Med 159:551–558, 1999.

121. Shorr RI, Ray WA, Daugherty JR, et al: Antihypertensives and the risk of serious hypoglycemia in older persons using insulin or sulfonylureas. JAMA 278:40–43, 1997.

122. Gustafsson I, Torp-Pedersen C, Kober L, et al: Effect of the angiotensin-converting enzyme inhibitor trandolapril on mortality and morbidity in diabetic patients with left ventricular dysfunction after acute myocardial infarction. Trace Study Group. J Am Coll Cardiol 34:83–89, 1999.

123. Pfeffer MA, Greaves SC, Arnold JM, et al: Early versus delayed angiotensin-converting enzyme inhibition therapy in acute myocardial infarction. The healing and early afterload reducing therapy trial. Circulation 95:2643–2651, 1997.

124. Rutherford JD, Pfeffer MA, Moye LA, et al: Effects of captopril on ischemic events after myocardial infarction. Results of the Survival and Ventricular Enlargement trial. SAVE Investigators. Circulation 90:1731–1738, 1994.

125. Binkley PF, Haas GJ, Starling RC, et al: Sustained augmentation of parasympathetic tone with angiotensin-converting enzyme inhibition in patients with congestive heart failure. J Am Coll Cardiol 21:655–661, 1993.

126. O'Driscoll G, Green D, Maiorana A, et al: Improvement in endothelial function by angiotensin-converting enzyme inhibition in non–insulin-dependent diabetes mellitus. J Am Coll Cardiol 33:1506–1511, 1999.

127. Vaughan DE, Rouleau JL, Ridker PM, et al: Effects of ramipril on plasma fibrinolytic balance in patients with acute anterior myocardial infarction. HEART Study Investigators. Circulation 96:442–447, 1997.

128. Torlone E, Britta M, Rambotti AM, et al: Improved insulin action and glycemic control after long-term angiotensin-converting enzyme inhibition in subjects with arterial hypertension and type II diabetes. Diabetes Care 16:1347–1355, 1993.

129. Yusuf S, Sleight P, Pogue J, et al: Effects of an angiotensin-converting-enzyme inhibitor, ramipril, on cardiovascular events in high-risk patients. The Heart Outcomes Prevention Evaluation Study Investigators. N Engl J Med 342:145–153, 2000.

130. Steinhubl SR, Kottke-Marchant K, Moliterno DJ, et al: Attainment and maintenance of platelet inhibition through standard dosing of abciximab in diabetic and nondiabetic patients undergoing percutaneous coronary intervention. Circulation 100:1977–1982, 1999.

131. Platelet glycoprotein IIb/IIIa receptor blockade and low-dose heparin during percutaneous coronary revascularization. The EPILOG Investigators. N Engl J Med 336:1689–1696, 1997.

132. Lincoff AM, Califf RM, Moliterno DJ, et al: Complementary clinical benefits of coronary-artery stenting and blockade of platelet glycoprotein IIb/IIIa receptors. Evaluation of Platelet IIb/IIIa Inhibition in Stenting Investigators. N Engl J Med 341:319–327, 1999.

133. Bellodi G, Manicardi V, Malavasi V, et al: Hyperglycemia and prognosis of acute myocardial infarction in patients without diabetes mellitus. Am J Cardiol 64:885–888, 1989.

134. Oswald GA, Smith CC, Betteridge DJ, et al: Determinants and importance of stress hyperglycaemia in non-diabetic patients with myocardial infarction. BMJ 293:917–922, 1986.

135. Fava S, Aquilina O, Azzopardi J, et al: The prognostic value of blood glucose in diabetic patients with acute myocardial infarction. Diabet Med 13:80–83, 1996.

136. Capes SE, Hunt D, Malmberg K, et al: Stress hyperglycemia and increased risk of death after myocardial infarction in patients with and without diabetes: A systematic overview. Lancet 355:773–778, 2000.

137. Malmberg K, Ryden L, Efendic S, et al: Randomized trial of insulin-glucose infusion followed by subcutaneous insulin treatment in diabetic patients with acute myocardial infarction (DIGAMI study): Effects on mortality at 1 year. J Am Coll Cardiol 26:57–65, 1995.

138. Malmberg K, Norhammar A, Wedel H, et al: Glycometabolic state at admission: Important risk marker of mortality in conventionally treated patients with diabetes mellitus and acute myocardial infarction: Long-term results from the Diabetes and Insulin-Glucose Infusion in Acute Myocardial Infarction (DIGAMI) study. Circulation 99:2626–2632, 1999.

139. A study of the effects of hypoglycemia agents on vascular complica-

tions in patients with adult-onset diabetes. VI. Supplementary report on nonfatal events in patients treated with tolbutamide. Diabetes 25:1129–1153, 1976.

140. Rytter L, Troelsen S, Beck-Nielsen H: Prevalence and mortality of acute myocardial infarction in patients with diabetes. Diabetes Care 8:230–234, 1985.

141. Garratt KN, Brady PA, Hassinger NL, et al: Sulfonylurea drugs increase early mortality in patients with diabetes mellitus after direct angioplasty for acute myocardial infarction. J Am Coll Cardiol 33:119–124, 1999.

142. Brady PA, Terzic A: The sulfonylurea controversy: More questions from the heart. J Am Coll Cardiol 31:950–956, 1998.

143. Engler RL, Yellon DM: Sulfonylurea KATP blockade in type II diabetes and preconditioning in cardiovascular disease. Time for reconsideration. Circulation 94:2297–2301, 1996.

144. Cleveland JC Jr, Meldrum DR, Cain BS, et al: Oral sulfonylurea hypoglycemic agents prevent ischemic preconditioning in human myocardium. Two paradoxes revisited. Circulation 96:29–32, 1997.

145. Katsuda Y, Egashira K, Ueno H, et al: Glibenclamide, a selective inhibitor of ATP-sensitive K⁺ channels, attenuates metabolic coronary vasodilatation induced by pacing tachycardia in dogs. Circulation 92:511–517, 1995.

146. Davis CA 3rd, Sherman AJ, Yaroshenko Y, et al: Coronary vascular responsiveness to adenosine is impaired additively by blockade of nitric oxide synthesis and a sulfonylurea. J Am Coll Cardiol 31:816–822, 1998.

147. Tomai F, Crea F, Gaspardone A, et al: Ischemic preconditioning during coronary angioplasty is prevented by glibenclamide, a selective ATP-sensitive K⁺ channel blocker. Circulation 90:700–705, 1994.

148. Correa SD, Schaefer S: Blockade of K(ATP) channels with glibenclamide does not abolish preconditioning during demand ischemia. Am J Cardiol 79:75–78, 1997.

149. Bijlstra PJ, Lutterman JA, Russel FG, et al: Interaction of sulphonylurea derivatives with vascular ATP-sensitive potassium channels in humans. Diabetologia 39:1083–1090, 1996.

150. Cole WC, McPherson CD, Sontag D: ATP-regulated K⁺ channels protect the myocardium against ischemia/reperfusion damage. Circ Res 69:571–581, 1991.

151. Kubota I, Yamaki M, Shibata T, et al: Role of ATP-sensitive K⁺ channel on ECG ST segment elevation during a bout of myocardial ischemia. A study on epicardial mapping in dogs. Circulation 88:1845–1851, 1993.

152. Mueller HS, Cohen LS, Braunwald E, et al: Predictors of early morbidity and mortality after thrombolytic therapy of acute myocardial infarction. Analyses of patient subgroups in the Thrombolysis in Myocardial Infarction (TIMI) trial, phase II. Circulation 85:1254–1264, 1992.

153. Baim DS, Diver DJ, Feit F, et al: Coronary angioplasty performed within the Thrombolysis in Myocardial Infarction II study. Circulation 85:93–105, 1992.

154. Van Belle E, Bauters C, Hubert E, et al: Restenosis rates in diabetic patients: A comparison of coronary stenting and balloon angioplasty in native coronary vessels. Circulation 96:1454–1460, 1997.

155. Levine GN, Jacobs AK, Keeler GP, et al: Impact of diabetes mellitus on percutaneous revascularization (CAVEAT-I). CAVEAT-I Investigators. Coronary Angioplasty Versus Excisional Atherectomy Trial. Am J Cardiol 79:748–755, 1997.

156. Stein B, Weintraub WS, Gebhart SP, et al: Influence of diabetes mellitus on early and late outcome after percutaneous transluminal coronary angioplasty. Circulation 91:979–989, 1995.

157. Kip KE, Faxon DP, Detre KM, et al: Coronary angioplasty in diabetic patients. The National Heart, Lung, and Blood Institute Percutaneous Transluminal Coronary Angioplasty Registry. Circulation 94:1818–1825, 1996.

158. Carrozza JP Jr, Kuntz RE, Fishman RF, et al: Restenosis after arterial injury caused by coronary stenting in patients with diabetes mellitus. Ann Intern Med 118:344–349, 1993.

159. Kornowski R, Mintz GS, Kent KM, et al: Increased restenosis in diabetes mellitus after coronary interventions is due to exaggerated intimal hyperplasia. A serial intravascular ultrasound study. Circulation 95:1366–1369, 1997.

160. Moreno PR, Fallon JT, Murcia AM, et al: Tissue characteristics of restenosis after percutaneous transluminal coronary angioplasty in diabetic patients. J Am Coll Cardiol 34:1045–1049, 1999.

161. Cohen Y, Raz I, Merin G, et al: Comparison of factors associated with 30-day mortality after coronary artery bypass grafting in patients with versus without diabetes mellitus. Israeli Coronary Artery Bypass (IS-CAB) Study Consortium. Am J Cardiol 81:7–11, 1998.

162. Detre KM, Lombardero MS, Brooks MM, et al: The effect of previous coronary-artery bypass surgery on the prognosis of patients with diabetes who have acute myocardial infarction. Bypass Angioplasty Revascularization Investigation Investigators. N Engl J Med 342:989–997, 2000.

163. Weintraub WS, Stein B, Kosinski A, et al: Outcome of coronary bypass surgery versus coronary angioplasty in diabetic patients with multivessel coronary artery disease. J Am Coll Cardiol 31:10–19, 1998.

164. Comparison of coronary bypass surgery with angioplasty in patients with multivessel disease. The Bypass Angioplasty Revascularization Investigation (BARI) Investigators. N Engl J Med 335:217–225, 1996.

165. Influence of diabetes on 5-year mortality and morbidity in a randomized trial comparing CABG and PTCA in patients with multivessel disease: The Bypass Angioplasty Revascularization Investigation (BARI). Circulation 96:1761–1769, 1997.

166. Prevalence of unrecognized silent myocardial ischemia and its association with atherosclerotic risk factors in noninsulin-dependent diabetes mellitus. Milan Study on Atherosclerosis and Diabetes (MiSAD) Group. Am J Cardiol 79:134–139, 1997.

167. Consensus development conference on the diagnosis of coronary heart disease in people with diabetes: 10–11 February 1998, Miami, Florida. American Diabetes Association. Diabetes Care 21:1551–1559, 1998.

DIABETIC CARDIOMYOPATHY

168. Nesto RW: Screening for asymptomatic coronary artery disease in diabetes. Diabetes Care 22:1393–1395, 1999.

169. Manske CL, Wilson RF, Wang Y, et al: Atherosclerotic vascular complications in diabetic transplant candidates. Am J Kidney Dis 29:601–607, 1997.

170. Zarich SW, Nesto RW: Diabetic cardiomyopathy. Am Heart J 118:1000–1012, 1989.

171. Fein FS, Sonnenblick EH: Diabetic cardiomyopathy. Prog Cardiovasc Dis 27:255–270, 1985.

172. Fein FS, Sonnenblick EH: Diabetic cardiomyopathy. Cardiovasc Drugs Ther 8:65–73, 1994.

173. Kannel WB, Hjortland M, Castelli WP: Role of diabetes in congestive heart failure: The Framingham study. Am J Cardiol 34:29–34, 1974.

174. Coughlin SS, Pearle DL, Baughman KL, et al: Diabetes mellitus and risk of idiopathic dilated cardiomyopathy. The Washington, DC Dilated Cardiomyopathy Study. Ann Epidemiol 4:67–74, 1994.

175. Coughlin SS, Tefft MC: The epidemiology of idiopathic dilated cardiomyopathy in women: The Washington DC Dilated Cardiomyopathy Study. Epidemiology 5:449–455, 1994.

176. Coughlin SS, Neaton JD, Sengupta A, et al: Predictors of mortality from idiopathic dilated cardiomyopathy in 356,222 men screened for the Multiple Risk Factor Intervention Trial. Am J Epidemiol 139:166–172, 1994.

177. Galderisi M, Anderson KM, Wilson PW, et al: Echocardiographic evidence for the existence of a distinct diabetic cardiomyopathy (the Framingham Heart Study). Am J Cardiol 68:85–89, 1991.

178. Fischer VW, Barner HB, Leskiw ML: Capillary basal laminar thickness in diabetic human myocardium. Diabetes 28:713–719, 1979.

179. Factor SM, Okun EM, Minase T: Capillary microaneurysms in the human diabetic heart. N Engl J Med 302:384–388, 1980.

180. Kawaguchi M, Techigawara M, Ishihata T, et al: A comparison of ultrastructural changes on endomyocardial biopsy specimens obtained from patients with diabetes mellitus with and without hypertension. Heart Vessels 12:267–274, 1997.

181. Perez JE, McGill JB, Santiago JV, et al: Abnormal myocardial acoustic properties in diabetic patients and their correlation with the severity of disease. J Am Coll Cardiol 19:1154–1162, 1992.

182. Di Bello V, Talarico L, Picano E, et al: Increased echodensity of myocardial wall in the diabetic heart: An ultrasound tissue characterization study. J Am Coll Cardiol 25:1408–1415, 1995.

183. Berg TJ, Snorgaard O, Faber J, et al: Serum levels of advanced glycation end products are associated with left ventricular diastolic function in patients with type 1 diabetes. Diabetes Care 22:1186–1190, 1999.

184. Avendano GF, Agarwal RK, Bashey RI, et al: Effects of glucose intolerance on myocardial function and collagen-linked glycation. Diabetes 48:1443–1447, 1999.

185. Schaffer SW, Mozaffari M: Abnormal mechanical function in diabetes: Relation to myocardial calcium handling. Coron Artery Dis 7:109–115, 1996.

186. Allo SN, Lincoln TM, Wilson GL, et al: Non–insulin-dependent diabetes–induced defects in cardiac cellular calcium regulation. Am J Physiol 260:C1165–C1171, 1991.

187. Schaffer SW, Mozaffari MS, Artman M, et al: Basis for myocardial mechanical defects associated with non–insulin-dependent diabetes. Am J Physiol 256:E25–E30, 1989.

188. Akella AB, Sonnenblick EH, Gulati J: Alterations in myocardial contractile proteins in diabetes mellitus. Coron Artery Dis 7:124–132, 1996.

188a. Depre C, Vanoverschelde JL, Taegtmeyer H: Glucose for the heart. Circulation 99:578–588, 1999.

189. Scognamiglio R, Avogaro A, Casara D, et al: Myocardial dysfunction and adrenergic cardiac innervation in patients with insulin-dependent diabetes mellitus. J Am Coll Cardiol 31:404–412, 1998.

190. Takeda N: Mitochondrial DNA mutations in diabetic heart. Diabetes Res Clin Pract 31(Suppl):123–126, 1996.

191. Shiotani H, Ueno H, Inoue S, et al: Diabetes mellitus and cardiomyopathy–association with mutation in the mitochondrial tRNA(Leu)(UUR) gene. Jpn Circ J 62:309–310, 1998.

192. Estacio RO, Jeffers BW, Havranek EP, et al: Deletion polymorphism of the angiotensin converting enzyme gene is associated with an increase in left ventricular mass in men with type 2 diabetes mellitus. Am J Hypertens 12:637–642, 1999.

193. Zarich SW, Arbuckle BE, Cohen LR, et al: Diastolic abnormalities in young asymptomatic diabetic patients assessed by pulsed Doppler echocardiography. J Am Coll Cardiol 12:114–120, 1988.

194. Gotzsche O, Darwish A, Hansen LP, et al: Abnormal left ventricular diastolic function during cold pressor test in uncomplicated insulin-dependent diabetes mellitus. Clin Sci (Colch) 89:461–465, 1995.

195. Mustonen JN, Uusitupa MI, Laakso M, et al: Left ventricular systolic

function in middle-aged patients with diabetes mellitus. Am J Cardiol 73:1202–1208, 1994.

196. Celentano A, Vaccaro O, Tammaro P, et al: Early abnormalities of cardiac function in non–insulin-dependent diabetes mellitus and impaired glucose tolerance. Am J Cardiol 76:1173–1176, 1995.

197. Sasson Z, Rasooly Y, Bhesania T, et al: Insulin resistance is an important determinant of left ventricular mass in the obese. Circulation 88:1431–1436, 1993.

CARDIOVASCULAR AUTONOMIC NERVOUS SYSTEM DYSFUNCTION IN DIABETES MELLITUS

198. Jain A, Avendano G, Dharamsey S, et al: Left ventricular diastolic function in hypertension and role of plasma glucose and insulin. Comparison with diabetic heart. Circulation 93:1396–1402, 1996.

199. Ito H, Hiroe M, Hirata Y, et al: Insulin–like growth factor-I induces hypertrophy with enhanced expression of muscle specific genes in cultured rat cardiomyocytes. Circulation 87:1715–1721, 1993.

200. Ziegler D, Dannehl K, Volksw D, et al: Prevalence of cardiovascular autonomic dysfunction assessed by spectral analysis and standard tests of heart-rate variation in newly diagnosed IDDM patients. Diabetes Care 15:908–911, 1992.

201. Spallone V, Menzinger G: Diagnosis of cardiovascular autonomic neuropathy in diabetes. Diabetes 46(Suppl 2):67–76, 1997.

202. Ewing DJ, Neilson JM, Shapiro CM, et al: Twenty four hour heart rate variability: Effects of posture, sleep, and time of day in healthy controls and comparison with bedside tests of autonomic function in diabetic patients. Br Heart J 65:239–244, 1991.

203. Kreiner G, Wolzt M, Fasching P, et al: Myocardial m-[123I]iodobenzylguanidine scintigraphy for the assessment of adrenergic cardiac innervation in patients with IDDM. Comparison with cardiovascular reflex tests and relationship to left ventricular function. Diabetes 44:543–549, 1995.

204. Sampson MJ, Wilson S, Karagiannis P, et al: Progression of diabetic autonomic neuropathy over a decade in insulin-dependent diabetics. Q J Med 75:635–646, 1990.

205. O'Brien IA, McFadden JP, Corrall RJ: The influence of autonomic neuropathy on mortality in insulin-dependent diabetes. Q J Med 79:495–502, 1991.

206. Orchard TJ, Lloyd CE, Maser RE, Kuller LH: Why does diabetic autonomic neuropathy predict IDDM mortality? An analysis from the Pittsburgh Epidemiology of Diabetes Complications Study. Diabetes Res Clin Pract 34(Suppl):165–171, 1996.

207. Spallone V, Maiello MR, Cicconetti E, et al: Autonomic neuropathy and cardiovascular risk factors in insulin-dependent and non insulin-dependent diabetes. Diabetes Res Clin Pract 34:169–179, 1997.

208. Burger AJ, Weinrauch LA, D'Elia JA, et al: Effect of glycemic control on heart rate variability in type I diabetic patients with cardiac autonomic neuropathy. Am J Cardiol 84:687–691, 1999.

209. Stevens MJ, Raffel DM, Allman KC, et al: Regression and progression of cardiac sympathetic dysinnervation complicating diabetes: An assessment by C-11 hydroxyephedrine and positron emission tomography. Metabolism 48:92–101, 1999.

210. Hathaway DK, Abell T, Cardoso S, et al: Improvement in autonomic and gastric function following pancreas-kidney versus kidney-alone transplantation and the correlation with quality of life. Transplantation 57:816–822, 1994.

211. Ziegler D, Schatz H, Conrad F, et al: Effects of treatment with the antioxidant alpha-lipoic acid on cardiac autonomic neuropathy in NIDDM patients. A 4-month randomized controlled multicenter trial (DEKAN Study). Deutsche Kardiale Autonome Neuropathie. Diabetes Care 20:369–373, 1997.

212. Kontopoulos AG, Athyros VG, Didangelos TP, et al: Effect of chronic quinapril administration on heart rate variability in patients with diabetic autonomic neuropathy. Diabetes Care 20:355–361, 1997.

213. Malik RA: Can diabetic neuropathy be prevented by angiotensin-converting enzyme inhibitors? Ann Med 32:1–5, 2000.

214. Giugliano D, Marfella R, Quatraro A, et al: Tolrestat for mild diabetic neuropathy. A 52-week, randomized, placebo-controlled trial. Ann Intern Med 118:7–11, 1993.

215. Ikeda T, Iwata K, Tanaka Y: Long–term effect of epalrestat on cardiac autonomic neuropathy in subjects with non–insulin dependent diabetes mellitus. Diabetes Res Clin Pract 43:193–198, 1999.

216. Nesto RW, Phillips RT, Kett KG, et al: Angina and exertional myocardial ischemia in diabetic and nondiabetic patients: Assessment by exercise thallium scintigraphy. Ann Intern Med 108:170–175, 1988.

217. Marchant B, Umachandran V, Stevenson R, et al: Silent myocardial ischemia: Role of subclinical neuropathy in patients with and without diabetes. J Am Coll Cardiol 22:1433–1437, 1993.

218. Ambepityia G, Kopelman PG, Ingram D, et al: Exertional myocardial ischemia in diabetes: A quantitative analysis of anginal perceptual threshold and the influence of autonomic function. J Am Coll Cardiol 15:72–77, 1990.

219. Langer A, Freeman MR, Josse RG, et al: Metaiodobenzylguanidine imaging in diabetes mellitus: Assessment of cardiac sympathetic denervation and its relation to autonomic dysfunction and silent myocardial ischemia. J Am Coll Cardiol 25:610–618, 1995.

220. Faerman I, Faccio E, Milei J, et al: Autonomic neuropathy and painless myocardial infarction in diabetic patients. Histologic evidence of their relationship. Diabetes 26:1147–1158, 1977.

221. Indications for fibrinolytic therapy in suspected acute myocardial infarction: Collaborative overview of early mortality and major morbidity results from all randomised trials of more than 1000 patients. Fibrinolytic Therapy Trialists' (FTT) Collaborative Group. Lancet 343:311–322, 1994.

222. Morning peak in the incidence of myocardial infarction: Experience in the ISIS-2 trial. ISIS-2 (Second International Study of Infarct Survival) Collaborative Group. Eur Heart J 13:594–598, 1992.

223. Hjalmarson A, Gilpin EA, Nicod P, et al: Differing circadian patterns of symptom onset in subgroups of patients with acute myocardial infarction. Circulation 80:267–275, 1989.

224. Pozzati A, Pancaldi LG, Di Pasquale G, et al: Transient sympathovagal imbalance triggers "ischemic" sudden death in patients undergoing electrocardiographic Holter monitoring. J Am Coll Cardiol 27:847–852, 1996.

225. Di Carli MF, Tobes MC, Mangner T, et al: Effects of cardiac sympathetic innervation on coronary blood flow. N Engl J Med 336:1208–1215, 1997.

226. Di Carli MF, Bianco-Batlles D, Landa ME, et al: Effects of autonomic neuropathy on coronary blood flow in patients with diabetes mellitus. Circulation 100:813–819, 1999.

227. Stevens MJ, Dayanikli F, Raffel DM, et al: Scintigraphic assessment of regionalized defects in myocardial sympathetic innervation and blood flow regulation in diabetic patients with autonomic neuropathy. J Am Coll Cardiol 31:1575–1584, 1998.

228. Curb JD, Rodriguez BL, Burchfiel CM, et al: Sudden death, impaired glucose tolerance, and diabetes in Japanese American men. Circulation 91:2591–2595, 1995.

229. Kahn JK, Sisson JC, Vinik AI: QT interval prolongation and sudden cardiac death in diabetic autonomic neuropathy. J Clin Endocrinol Metab 64:751–754, 1987.

230. Wei K, Dorian P, Newman D, et al: Association between QT dispersion and autonomic dysfunction in patients with diabetes mellitus. J Am Coll Cardiol 26:859–863, 1995.

231. Stevens MJ, Raffel DM, Allman KC, et al: Cardiac sympathetic dysinnervation in diabetes: Implications for enhanced cardiovascular risk. Circulation 98:961–968, 1998.

232. Lucas LF, Tsueda K: Cardiovascular depression after brachial plexus block in two diabetic patients with renal failure. Anesthesiology 73:1032–1035, 1990.

233. Burgos LG, Ebert TJ, Asiddao C, et al: Increased intraoperative cardiovascular morbidity in diabetics with autonomic neuropathy. Anesthesiology 70:591–597, 1989.

234. Keyl C, Lemberger P, Palitzsch KD, et al: Cardiovascular autonomic dysfunction and hemodynamic response to anesthetic induction in patients with coronary artery disease and diabetes mellitus. Anesth Analg 88:985–991, 1999.

Chapter 64

The Heart in Endocrine Disorders

ELLEN W. SEELY · GORDON H. WILLIAMS

In 1835, Robert Graves described "three cases of violent and long-continued palpitation in females" with thyrotoxicosis.[1] Twenty years later, Thomas Addison reported that patients with disease of the "suprarenal capsules" had a "pulse, small and feeble . . . excessively soft and compressible." As the disease progressed, "the body wastes . . . the pulse becomes smaller and weaker, and . . . the patient at length gradually sinks and expires."[2] Thus, since the mid-19th century, it has been known that deranged hormonal secretion can significantly alter cardiovascular function. The purpose of this chapter is to summarize the more important cardiovascular manifestations of endocrine and nutritional diseases.

ACROMEGALY

The anterior pituitary gland secretes at least seven polypeptide hormones. Four (adrenocorticotropic hormone [ACTH] and related peptides, follicle-stimulating hormone, luteinizing hormone, and thyroid-stimulating hormone [TSH]) primarily produce their biological effect indirectly by altering hormonal secretion from a specific target gland (adrenal cortex, gonad, or thyroid). Thus, the pathophysiological manifestations of a derangement in their secretion are the same as those of their target organs and will be discussed later. No cardiovascular manifestations of altered prolactin secretion are known, but acromegaly (growth hormone [GH] excess) is associated with a number of clinical signs and symptoms related to the cardiovascular system.

ACTIONS OF GROWTH HORMONE. GH is only one of a family of peptides whose overall function is to regulate growth of the organism.[3, 4] Two hormones secreted by the hypothalamus (somatotropin-releasing hormone and somatostatin) regulate the release of GH from the anterior pituitary, with the former stimulating and the latter suppressing its release.[5, 6] A variety of other factors also modify GH release, many of which work through a GH secretagogue receptor.[7] An orally active agonist of this receptor, MK-677, can stimulate GH release in normal and elderly individuals.[8, 9] Whether it can do so in pathophysiological states in which GH is suppressed is uncertain.

After GH is released into the circulation, it binds to a plasma protein that is identical in amino acid composition to the extracellular domain of the GH receptor. The purpose of the binding protein is unclear. It may prolong the plasma half-life of GH and thereby its biological effect. Contrariwise, GH-binding protein can compete with the GH receptor and thereby reduce GH's biological effect. The GH receptor consists of nearly equal extracellular and intracellular domains with two GH-binding sites per receptor.[10] It is a member of the cytokine receptor superfamily and mediates its effects via activation of the JAK (Janus Kinase) family of intracellular tyrosine kinases and the STAT (signal transducer and activator of transcription) family of

transcription factors.[11] GH mediates its effects in two ways: directly and by increasing the production of somatomedins (insulin-like growth factors [IGFs] I and II).[3, 4, 11] GH's predominant effect is on modifying IGF-I's synthesis as suggested by the following: GH-deficient individuals are deficient in IGF-I but not IGF-II, and IGF-I reduces GH release from the pituitary.

In humans, the gene for IGF-I is located on chromosome 12 and that for IGF-II on chromosome 11 near the insulin gene. Expression of mRNA from these genes occurs in many tissues, particularly in the fetus. They are homologs of the proinsulin molecule and exert biological effects that are qualitatively similar to those of insulin.[3, 12] Postpartum, mRNA levels are highest in the liver but are also found in a number of other tissues. IGF is synthesized in the liver in response to GH and, for the most part, is bound to one of six specific binding proteins. Because production of these binding proteins can be regulated by growth factors, they may play a functional role by producing a readily available circulating reservoir of growth factors.[13] While many of the actions attributed to GH are actually produced by IGFs, GH does have direct effects, some of them the opposite those of IGFs. For example, GH antagonizes the action of insulin while the IGFs mimic it. GH's other direct effects include increasing amino acid transport and incorporation in the heart and stimulating outgrowth of vascular smooth muscle cells in culture. However, in this chapter, by convention the term *growth hormone effects* is used, although most of these effects are probably mediated by the IGFs, particularly IGF-I.

Much of our knowledge of GH's action comes from animal and/or in vitro studies with all their limitations, and relatively little information is available in humans because of the scarcity of human GH until recently. Thus, the following description needs to be interpreted with caution until more human data are available. GH's effects influence many metabolic processes, but the net effect is anabolic. Thus, when GH is administered to a GH-deficient individual, positive nitrogen balance with retention of calcium, sodium, potassium, magnesium, and chloride is manifested within days.[3, 4]

GH also induces changes in both fat and carbohydrate metabolism.[3, 4] When administered for a short time, it increases the uptake and utilization of glucose by fat cells, thus increasing lipogenesis. However, when administered over a long period, it promotes lipolysis, thus increasing plasma free fatty acid levels and their oxidation and promoting ketogenesis, particularly in diabetic patients or animals. GH reduces glucose uptake by fat and muscle cells, increases gluconeogenesis, and increases peripheral resistance to insulin; as a consequence, plasma glucose levels rise. Because of this reduced tissue uptake of glucose and the increased blood levels of free fatty acids and ketones, tissues, such as the myocardium, that are able to use these latter compounds as energy substrates do so. In contrast, if IGF-I is administered to patients with noninsulin-dependent diabetes mellitus, glycemic control improves and insulin sensitivity increases.[14]

EFFECT OF GROWTH HORMONE AND SOMATOSTATIN ON THE HEART. Specific receptors for GH and IGF-I in the heart promote cardiac remodeling and inotropism. Activation of these receptors induces the expression of genes for specific contractile proteins and also those responsible for myocyte hypertrophy. GH also increases the force of contraction and shifts the myosin form to the low–adenosine triphosphatase (ATPase) activity V_3 isoform[15] (see Chap. 14). Short-term administration of GH to normal subjects, which produces changes in GH levels similar to those observed in patients with mild acromegaly, increases the heart rate and myocardial contractility, the latter reflected in fractional shortening of the left ventricle and mean circumferential shortening of velocity as determined by echocardiography.[16] GH has no effect on mean arterial blood pressure. In adults with GH deficiency, replacement therapy also modifies cardiac function, but the changes differ from those observed in normal subjects given GH. Left ventricular mass, stroke volume, and cardiac output increase significantly, whereas total peripheral resistance and arterial pressure decrease. However, systolic blood pressure does not change either at rest or during exercise.[17]

Somatostatin has an effect on the heart beyond that induced by its effect on GH secretion. Infusion of somatostatin causes bradycardia and a fall in cardiac output. Furthermore, in some cases of supraventricular arrhythmias, somatostatin administration restores sinus rhythm.[18] Finally, cardiac nerves have been shown to contain somatostatin, which suggests that this hormone may be an important physiological regulator of cardiac conduction.

CLINICAL AND BIOCHEMICAL MANIFESTATIONS. Acromegaly is almost invariably the result of a GH producing chromophobic or eosinophilic pituitary adenoma, although it may rarely be secondary to ectopic production of GH or somatotropin-releasing hormone.[19]

A derangement in carbohydrate metabolism is the most common metabolic consequence of chronic overproduction of GH. Impaired glucose tolerance is found in half the patients, and hyperinsulinemia is present in nearly all; thus, a state of insulin resistance exists. However, clinical diabetes mellitus is present in only 20 to 30 percent of patients, which suggests that only in those who are predisposed and have limited insulin reserve does overt disease actually develop.[3, 19] The insulin-resistant state may also contribute to other features of the disease, e.g., the hypertension. Nearly three-quarters of subjects are overweight. Thus, it might be anticipated that hyperlipidemia would be common in acromegaly. Yet, it is in fact infrequently observed except in patients with clinical diabetes mellitus.[3, 4, 17] Even in these patients it is probably secondary to the decreased secretion of insulin rather than the increased secretion of GH.

Cardiovascular Manifestations

The cardiac manifestations of acromegaly include cardiac enlargement that is greater than would be anticipated for the generalized organomegaly. In addition, the frequency of a number of other cardiovascular disorders is increased in patients with acromegaly: hypertension, premature coronary artery disease, congestive heart failure, and cardiac arrhythmias, particularly frequent ventricular premature beats and intraventricular conduction defects.[16, 20] Indeed, because of the frequent occurrence of congestive heart failure and cardiac arrhythmias in patients who otherwise have no predisposing factors (e.g., no hypertension or arteriosclerosis), it has been suggested that a specific acromegalic cardiomyopathy exists (see below).

CARDIOMEGALY. Nearly all patients with acromegaly have cardiomegaly (Fig. 64–1), particularly after the fifth decade.[16, 20, 21] Echocardiographic assessment suggests that cardiac mass is frequently increased, particularly asymmet-

rical septal hypertrophy, with a sizable minority having left ventricular dilatation and a reduced ejection fraction.[20–22] Although the cardiomegaly may be related to the generalized effect of GH on protein synthesis, some data suggest that other factors may also be important. For example, enlargement of the heart is often greater than that of other organs. Furthermore, no direct relationship can be found between the degree of cardiomegaly and the level of circulating GH.[20, 21] However, the duration of acromegaly correlates with the severity of cardiac hypertrophy. Other factors that may be important in the genesis of cardiomegaly include the hypertension and atherosclerosis that occur with increased frequency in acromegaly. Focal cardiac interstitial fibrosis and myocarditis with a lymphocytic infiltrate have also been reported in the majority of cases.[16] The former is probably due to the effect of GH on collagen synthesis. Additionally, small-vessel disease of the myocardium may occasionally be present. The resultant dysfunction in cardiac contraction secondary to any of these pathological changes could also contribute to the cardiac enlargement. Finally, the cardiomyopathy characteristic of acromegaly may also contribute to the cardiomegaly.

HYPERTENSION. The most common cardiovascular manifestation of acromegaly, hypertension, occurs in 25 to 50 percent of patients in most studies if individuals with hypopituitarism are excluded. However, the frequency of hypertension may be overestimated if hypertension is defined by 24-hour blood pressure monitoring. Minniti and colleagues found that 60 percent of patients with acromegaly reported to be hypertensive by traditional criteria were normotensive by 24-hour ambulatory blood pressure data.[23] Hypertensive acromegalic patients tend to be older and to have had their acromegaly longer than nonhypertensive acromegalic patients. The underlying pathophysiology is uncertain. However, the hypertension is usually mild, uncomplicated, and readily responsive to drugs.[19] Most investigators either have searched for factors other than GH that could cause hypertension or have attempted to determine how GH itself may produce hypertension. In many respects, patients with acromegaly appear to have an expanded plasma volume; the presence of an increase in the glomerular filtration rate, renal plasma flow, extracellular fluid volume, and sodium space and a reduction in plasma renin activity all support this hypothesis.[3, 4, 24] Indeed, the striking increase in plasma volume in active acromegaly is reduced following treatment.

A number of studies have suggested that GH itself may be responsible for the hypertension. Thus, pituitary irradia-

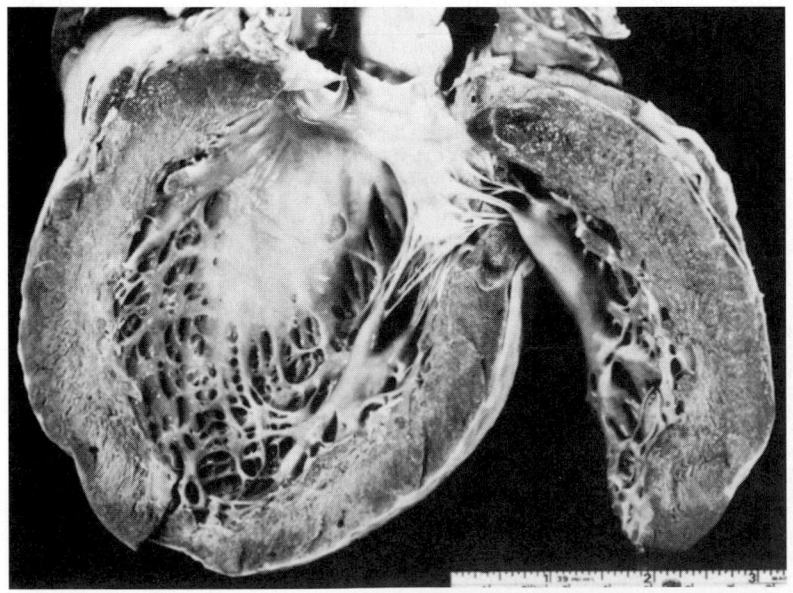

FIGURE 64–1. Opened left ventricle of the heart of an acromegalic patient showing marked dilatation and hypertrophy, with fibrosis in the left septal endocardium. (From Rossi L, Thiene G, Caragaro L, et al: Dysrhythmias and sudden death in acromegalic heart disease. A clinicopathologic study. Chest 72:496, 1977.)

tion or hypophysectomy significantly reduces arterial pressure in hypertensive acromegalic patients, even with full glucocorticoid replacement, unless GH levels are not normalized.[21] Indeed, the apparent volume expansion may relate directly to the elevated GH levels because administration of GH can produce retention of sodium, expansion of extracellular fluid volume, and abnormalities in white blood cell sodium transport. It has been proposed that the pathophysiology of the hypertension in acromegaly may be similar to that in essential hypertension. In both conditions, cardiac output may be initially elevated secondary to expansion of the extracellular fluid volume (see Chap. 28). This response could elevate arterial pressure and ultimately lead to changes in the peripheral vasculature that produce fixed hypertension.

ATHEROSCLEROSIS. In view of the alterations in carbohydrate and lipid metabolism caused by GH (see above), as well as the high incidence of hypertension, it is not surprising that premature atherosclerosis occurs in patients with acromegaly. What is uncertain is its frequency.[19]

Acromegalic Cardiomyopathy

Some patients with acromegaly but no evidence of hypertension or atherosclerosis have significant cardiac dysfunction.[20, 25] They primarily have cardiomegaly, congestive heart failure, and/or cardiac arrhythmias[10, 20, 25–27]; the congestive heart failure is particularly resistant to conventional therapy. It has been suggested that these manifestations of acromegalic cardiomyopathy are related to the higher collagen content per gram of heart than found in normal myocardium. Histological observations show cellular hypertrophy, patchy fibrosis, and myofibrillar degeneration (Fig. 64–2). Sudden death has been associated with inflammatory and degenerative damage to the sinoatrial perinodal nerve plexus and degeneration of the atrioventricular (AV) node.

It is not clear whether acromegalic cardiomyopathy is a specific entity. The evidence favoring this view, although indirect, comes from five types of observations: (1) Nearly 50 percent of acromegalic patients have electrocardio-graphic abnormalities.[26] The most common findings are ST segment depression with or without T wave abnormalities, patterns consistent with left ventricular hypertrophy, intraventricular conduction disturbances—specifically, bundle branch block—and supraventricular or ventricular ectopic rhythms. Indeed, in one controlled study, 48 percent of acromegalic patients had complex ventricular arrhythmias as compared with 12 percent of normal subjects. Although no correlation has been found between the severity of ventricular arrhythmias and GH levels, the frequency of premature ventricular contractions increases with the duration of acromegaly.[26] Although hypertension or signs of atherosclerosis are present in many, 10 to 20 percent of patients with acromegaly and electrocardiographic changes have no evidence of these conditions. (2) Ten to 20 percent of acromegalics have overt congestive heart failure. Perhaps a fourth of such individuals have no known predisposing cause.[27] (3) The majority of patients with acromegaly but without hypertension or atherosclerosis have subclinical evidence of cardiac, particularly diastolic, dysfunction.[20] (4) Approximately half of all patients with acromegaly, including patients without hypertension, have echocardiographic evidence of left and right ventricular hypertrophy.[20, 27–29] These patients have GH levels that are significantly higher than those of patients without left ventricular hypertrophy. Half of the patients with left ventricular hypertrophy exhibit asymmetrical septal hypertrophy, and these patients have a significantly greater percentage of internal dimensional shortening during systole than do either patients with concentric hypertrophy or those without left ventricular hypertrophy. (5) The most compelling evidence for a specific effect of GH hypersecretion inducing cardiac abnormalities comes from the impact of administration of the somatostatin analogs octreotide and lanreotide, which inhibit secretion of GH. In one study, 7 patients with acromegaly, 3 of whom had refractory congestive heart failure, were given octreotide subcutaneously three times daily. Right-heart catheterization performed before and after 3 months of therapy showed an 18 percent increase in stroke volume and a return of the cardiac index to normal. Within 40 days of treatment, the 3 patients with congestive heart

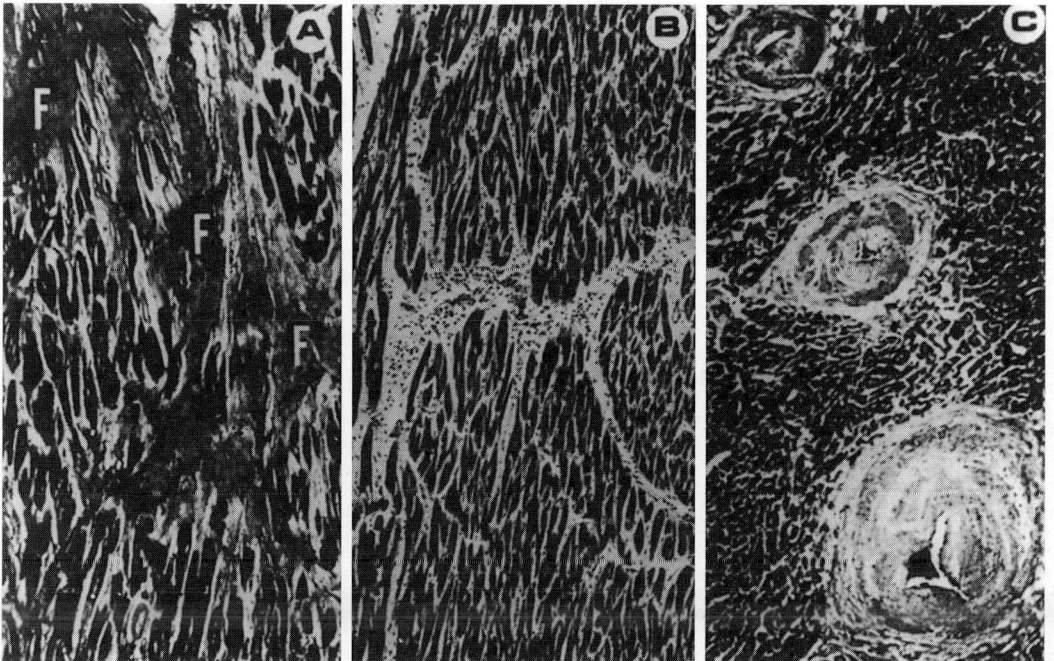

FIGURE 64–2. Histopathological features of acromegalic heart disease. *A,* Nonspecific myocardial hypertrophy and interstitial fibrosis (F). *B,* Myocarditis with predominantly lymphomononuclear cell infiltrate. *C,* Small-vessel disease (proliferative fibrous wall thickening) or intramural coronary artery branches. (From Lie JT: Acromegaly and heart disease. Prim Cardiol 7:53, 1981.)

failure had dramatic clinical improvement that was sustained for up to 3 years.[30] In a second study, within 1 week of initiating octreotide therapy, left ventricular mass was reduced, as assessed by echocardiography.[31] In a third study in 11 normotensive patients with active acromegaly, 6 months of octreotide therapy produced a significant reduction in left ventricular mass index, mean wall thickness, and isovolumic relaxation time, as well as a significant increase in the ratio of early to late peak velocity of right ventricular filling. This improvement in diastolic function was not accompanied by significant differences in systolic function indices.[32] Finally, 1 patient treated for 1 year with octreotide had substantial improvement in the histopathological appearance of myocardial biopsy specimens.[33] However, improvement in left ventricular function does not universally occur following correction of the excess GH production. In some patients who have had longstanding active acromegaly, left ventricular filling abnormalities may be only partly reversible. In these patients, presumably nonreversible interstitial fibrosis prevents correction of the GH-induced cardiomyopathy.[34]

DIAGNOSIS AND TREATMENT

The *diagnosis* of acromegaly is established by documenting the non-suppressibility of serum GH levels following glucose loading.[5, 4] In most laboratories, GH concentrations in normal subjects are less than 2 ng/ml 120 minutes after the oral administration of 100 gm of glucose. IGF-I levels may be more useful than GH levels to diagnose and monitor the course of the disease after treatment because of IGF-I's greater stability and longer serum half-life. It is also important to evaluate the integrity of the other pituitary hormones and, in hypertensive patients, to rule out an associated pheochromocytoma or aldosteronoma. The presence of sinus tachycardia or atrial fibrillation in a patient with acromegaly warrants a careful search for coexisting hyperthyroidism.

Surgery and irradiation remain the mainstays of treatment. The surgical approach is more often transsphenoidal rather than transfrontal; heavy-particle (proton beam) instead of conventional irradiation is often used.[3] Because of the delayed reduction in GH levels with the latter method, progression of cardiovascular disease in acromegalics continues even though GH levels are falling if they are not normal.[21] Secretion of GH can be suppressed in some acromegalics with somatostatin analogs.[30-33] Whether these agents have any effect on tumor growth, however, is unclear.

Acromegalic patients with cardiovascular abnormalities usually respond to conventional therapeutic measures for hypertension, heart failure, and arrhythmias. Two caveats should be taken into consideration: (1) Those with hypertension appear particularly responsive to volume-depleting maneuvers, i.e., diuretics and sodium restriction, perhaps even more so than patients with essential hypertension; (2) on the other hand, some patients with congestive heart failure, primarily those *without* underlying hypertensive heart disease (i.e., those who are considered to have acromegalic cardiomyopathy), appear particularly resistant to therapy.

THYROID DISEASE

Thyroid hormone has a profound effect on a number of metabolic processes in virtually all tissues, with the heart being particularly sensitive to its effects. Therefore, it is not surprising that thyroid dysfunction can produce dramatic cardiovascular effects, often mimicking primary cardiac disease. Thyroid's actions on the heart can be grouped into three broad categories: (1) direct cardiac effects, (2) effects mediated by thyroid hormone's action on the sympathetic nervous system, and (3) effects secondary to hemodynamic changes.

ACTION OF THYROID HORMONE. Two biologically active hormones are secreted by the thyroid: thyroxine (T_4) and triiodothyronine (T_3). Most studies support the hypothesis that T_3 is the final mediator and T_4 is a prohormone, primarily because of the universal presence of T_3 but not T_4 nuclear receptors in tissues responsive to thyroid hormone, specifically the heart.[35-38]

Nuclear-Mediated Effects of Thyroid Hormone. The majority of thyroid hormone's effects are mediated via a change in the expression of responsive genes. This process begins with diffusion of T_4 and T_3 across the plasma membrane because of their lipid solubility. In the cytosol, T_4 is converted into T_3 by the action of 5'-monodelodinase, the concentration of which varies from tissue to tissue in direct relation to the tissue's responsiveness to thyroid hormone. Then, the circulating and newly synthesized T_3 passes through the nuclear membrane to bind to specific thyroid hormone receptors (THRs). The THR is part of the nuclear receptor superfamily of proteins, which also includes proteins that act as receptors for steroids, vitamin D, and retinoic acid.

There are two THR genes—THRα located on chromosome 17 and THRβ located on chromosome 3. The predominant THR form in the heart is alpha$_1$, whereas the predominant receptor form in the pituitary and liver is the beta isoform. Several other isoforms have also been reported, the functions of which are unclear.[39] The THR is located almost exclusively within the nucleus. After interacting with T_3 and other protein transcription factors, the entire complex binds to thyroid response elements (TREs) located on the promoter region on specific genes (for additional details, the reader is referred to a review by Tsai and O'Malley[40]).

Thyroid hormone's effect on the synthesis of specific proteins can be either direct or indirect. Indirect effects include a change in production of an intermediate factor necessary for the function or activity of a more distant targeted protein. Thyroid hormone can have a positive or negative effect on regulating gene transcription. Positive effects have been documented for the following genes: myosin heavy-chain alpha,[41] Ca^{2+}-ATPase,[42] Na^+, K^+-ATPase,[43] beta$_1$-adrenergic receptor,[44] glucose transporter (Glut-4),[45] cardiac troponin,[46, 47] and atrial natriuretic protein.[48] Thyroid hormone also can negatively regulate genes, e.g., myosin heavy-chain beta and the glucose transporter Glut-1, at least neonatally.[45]

Thyroid Extranuclear Actions. Whereas the predominant effects of thyroid hormone are via its effect in regulating gene expression as noted above, thyroid hormone has also been clearly documented to have extranuclear effects. For example, T_3 increases both glucose and calcium uptake by the heart. Although some of these effects could be nuclear-mediated events, some studies suggest that thyroid hormone must also have a membrane effect. Evidence supporting a membrane effect includes rapid onset (for calcium uptake, maximum effect is achieved within 30 seconds), independence from new protein synthesis, and thyroid hormone specificity in that analogs of thyroid hormone that have no biological effect do not produce similar changes.[37, 49, 50]

In summary, thyroid hormone's nuclear and extranuclear effects on the heart lead to changes in the proportion of myosin heavy-chain protein from beta to alpha, thereby increasing myosin V_1 and decreasing myosin V_3 isoenzyme levels and thus leading to an increased velocity of contraction and diastolic relaxation. It also increases transcription of the calcium-ATPase gene. Extranuclear effects include thyroid hormone's direct effect on calcium current and cytosolic calcium changes induced by inotropic factors, including isoproterenol and the external calcium concentration.[51, 52]

As a secondary event, thyroid hormone also increases ATP consumption. However, because less of the chemical energy is used in the contractile process and more is dissipated as heat, myocardial metabolism is less efficient.[35, 51, 52]

RELATIONSHIP BETWEEN THE THYROID AND THE SYMPATHETIC NERVOUS SYSTEM

It has been proposed that some of the effects of thyroid hormone on the heart are indirect and secondary to changes in activity of the sympathetic nervous system (Table 64–1). Many of the cardiovascular effects of hyperthyroidism, i.e., tachycardia, systolic hypertension, increased cardiac output, and myocardial contractility, can be abolished or reduced by blocking the activity of the sympathetic nervous system.[53] Thyroid hormone may alter the relationship between the sympathetic nervous and cardiovascular systems either by increasing the activity of the sympathoadrenal system or by enhancing the response of cardiac tissue to normal sympathetic stimulation. Also, it has been suggested that sympathetic stimuli merely exert a direct additive effect on cardiovascular function above that produced by thyroid hormone. On the other hand, evidence has also been presented that hyperthyroidism reduces the sensitivity of cardiac tissue to sympathetic stimuli.[49]

Thus, the results of experiments on the relationship between the sympathoadrenal system and hyperthyroidism have evoked considerable controversy. Thyroid hormone's effect in three areas has been explored: adrenergic output, adrenergic receptors, and adrenergic transduction mechanisms. Plasma and urine levels of norepinephrine, epinephrine, dopamine, and beta-hydroxylase are either low or normal in hyperthyroidism and either normal or elevated in hypothyroidism. Therefore, the sympathomimetic features of hyperthyroidism cannot be due simply to an overall increase in adrenergic activity but are rather due to a change in the affinity of catecholamines for their receptors or a change in receptor number or to modification of a postreceptor mechanism. In the rat heart, which has been the organ most extensively studied, administration of thyroid hormone causes an increase in both the number of receptors and their affinity for their ligand, while hypothyroidism induces the opposite effect.[49] Thyroid hormone also increases mRNA levels for the beta$_1$-adrenergic receptor.[44, 49]

▼ TABLE 64–1. CLINICAL FEATURES OF HYPERTHYROIDISM

DIRECT THYROID HORMONE EFFECT*	BETA-ADRENERGIC–LIKE EFFECT*
Resting heart rate >90/min (90%)†	Resting heart rate >90/min (90%)
Palpitations (85%)	Palpitations (85%)
Atrial fibrillation (10%)	Exertional dyspnea (80%)
Pedal edema (30%)	Increased pulse pressure (systolic hypertension)
Increased oxygen consumption (basal metabolism)	Active apical impulse
Weight loss	Loud first heart sound and pulmonic component of the second heart sound
Skeletal muscle myopathy	
Increased bone turnover (occasional osteoporosis or hypercalcemia)	Midsystolic murmur, usually basal
Fair skin	Third heart sound (occasional)
Fine brittle hair	Means-Lerman scratch (rare)‡
Brittle nails	Tremor
Oligomenorrhea or amenorrhea	Brisk reflexes
Increased bowel frequency	Increased perspiration
	Heat intolerance
	Insomnia
	Anxiety
	Stare, lid lag§

* Both types of effects contribute to the tachycardia and palpitations.

† Numbers in parentheses are approximate prevalence of the findings compiled from several large series. Goiter is almost always present, although in elderly patients thyroid enlargement may be minimal or absent.

‡ A systolic scratch or click in the 2nd left intercostal space that is probably generated by the pleura and pericardium rubbing together.

§ These effects reflect upper lid retraction. Infiltrative ophthalmyopathy with exophthalmos is found only when Graves disease is the cause of the hyperthyroidism and is not related to the hyperthyroid state per se.

From Kaplan MM: The thyroid and the heart: How do they interact? J Cardiovasc Med 7:893, 1982.

These changes in receptor number and affinity then lead to changes in sensitivity of the myocardium to beta adrenoceptor agonists. For example, stimulation of adenylate cyclase activity by isoproterenol is increased in hyperthyroidism and reduced in hypothyroidism. Changes are also seen in the force of contraction, with increased sensitivity of ventricular muscle to isoproterenol-induced contraction in hyperthyroidism and reduced sensitivity in hypothyroidism.[49] These effects were also observed in vivo in dogs, in which propranolol-induced reductions in heart rate and myocardial contractility were greater in hyperthyroid than euthyroid animals.[54]

Circulating blood elements have also provided additional evidence in support of the concept that thyroid hormone "upregulates" beta adrenoceptors. When patients are used as their own control, both the number of beta adrenoceptors and the sensitivity of adenylate cyclase to isoproterenol stimulation in mononuclear cells are increased by thyroid hormone.[55, 56] Additionally, in circulating reticulocytes of hypothyroid animals, the number of receptors is decreased.[49]

Evidence supporting an effect of thyroid hormone in modifying the transduction mechanisms mediating adrenergic effects is less clear. In cultured developing rat myocardial cells, the addition of T_3 increased the level of $G_{s\alpha}$ protein while reducing $G_{s\alpha}$ and the beta subunits of G proteins. These results suggest that thyroid hormone elevates G protein subunits that activate adenylate cyclase and suppresses those that inhibit it. However, Levine and colleagues could not document an effect of thyroid hormone on $G_{s\alpha}$ subunits in adult rat ventricles, although an apparent inhibitory effect of thyroid hormone on $G_{s\alpha}$ 2 and 3 protein, G_β 1 and 2 protein, polypeptide, and mRNA levels was confirmed.[57] Similar effects have been reported for adipose tissue,[58] which probably explains the reduced lipolytic response to catecholamines in hypothyroidism. Thus, thyroid hormone has a complex interaction with the adrenergic nervous system. Hyperthyroidism increases the number and potentially the affinity of beta-adrenergic receptors and also modifies the intracellular G protein milieu to enhance the transduction potential of agonists binding to the adrenergic receptor.

Effect of Thyroid Hormone on the Heart

Abundant evidence indicates that thyroid hormone may alter cardiac function directly, as noted above. additionally, the increased heart rate and myocardial contractility observed in experimental hyperthyroidism are not completely reversed by either sympathetic or parasympathetic blockade.[54] Finally, T_4 enhances the rate of contraction of cardiac muscle, even in the presence of adrenergic blockade. Right ventricular papillary muscles isolated from cats rendered hyperthyroid exhibited augmented myocardial contractility, as reflected in an upward shift of the myocardial force-velocity curve, along with greatly increased velocity of myocardial fiber shortening, reduced time to peak tension during isometric contraction, and development of augmented peak tension. Single ventricular myocytes isolated from hyperthyroid rats exhibited marked augmentation in twitch velocity and abbreviated contraction and relaxation times. Prior catecholamine depletion by pretreatment with reserpine did not alter this inotropic effect of hyperthyroidism, thus providing further evidence for a direct cardiac effect. This hypothesis has been assessed in intact conscious animals. The results suggest that the major actions of T_4 on the left ventricle are (1) a direct positive inotropic effect and (2) an increase in the size of the ventricular cavity without a change in end-diastolic pressure or length of the sarcomere in diastole, although hypothyroidism does not necessarily impair pump function.[49]

The available data suggest that the direct effect of thyroid hormone on the heart is primarily mediated via a change in protein synthesis, as described above. Specifically, synthesis of myosin heavy chains is changed from the beta to the alpha form, thereby increasing the level of the more mobile myosin isoenzyme (V_1). With the reduction in mRNA levels for beta-myosin heavy chain, the slower V_3 myosin isoform is substantially reduced. Goto and associates demonstrated in the hyperthyroid rabbit heart that an increase in the myosin isoform V_1/V_3 ratio is associated with decreased contractile efficiency and increased energy cost of excitation-contraction coupling.[59] This change produces a less efficient system, thereby leading to more heat production per contractile response. In contrast to thyroid hormone's marked effect on myosin isoenzyme composition in rats and rabbits, in humans there appears to be much less of an effect. The myosin heavy-chain beta form is the isoenzyme overwhelmingly present in human hearts and is little affected by thyroid status. Even the alpha form increases very little when thyroid hormone is given to severely hypothyroid subjects.[60]

Thyroid hormone's effect on cardiac contractility also appears to be mediated in part by changes in intracellular calcium handling. Thyroid hormone increases expression of sodium-calcium-ATPase, which augments transsarcolemmal calcium influx in cultured ventricular cells.[61]

In ferret ventricular muscle, hypothyroidism reduces peak tension and prolongs the duration of contraction in association with changes in cytosolic calcium that are decreased and prolonged in relation to ventricular muscle obtained from euthyroid animals (Fig. 64–3). Hyperthyroidism produces the opposite changes. Thus, alteration in intracellular calcium handling, specifically that related to recycling of calcium by the sarcoplasmic reticulum, may account for the thyroid-induced changes in myocardial contractile function.[62] Finally, the effect of T_4 on myosin isoenzyme appears to be localized primarily to the ventricles, with atrial isoenzymes relatively unaltered by changes in thyroid hormone. Thus, while thyroid hormone itself has a major direct effect on modifying protein synthesis, changes in cardiac workload may also contribute. Studies using heterotrophic cardiac isografts suggest that the changes in myosin enzyme levels may in part be secondary to changes in workload.[63] Again, how much the changes described in rodents apply to humans is uncertain.

Thyroid hormone modifies the electrical activity of the heart by several mechanisms. It increases recruitment of slower inactivating sodium channels.[64] It also modifies the expression and/or composition and thereby the activity of

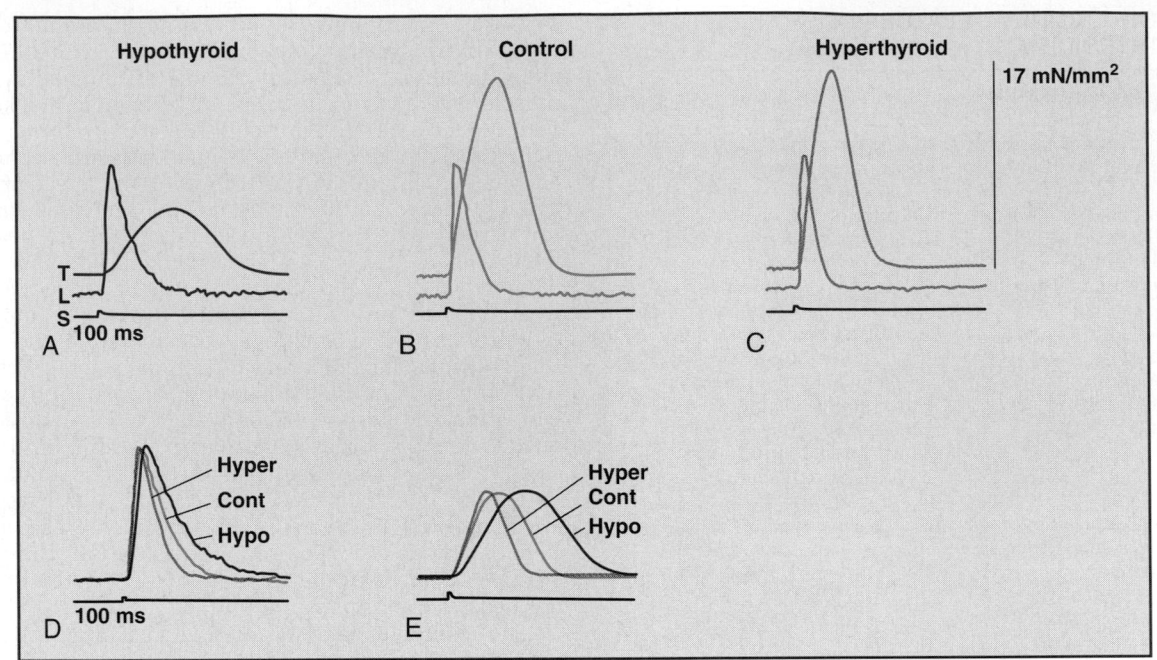

FIGURE 64–3. The thyroid state influences the time course of the isometric contraction and the Ca²⁺ transient. The isometric tension (T) and the aequorin light signal, reflecting intracytoplasmic [Ca]²⁺ (L), were recorded from myocardium obtained from a hypothyroid (*A*), euthyroid (*B*), and hyperthyroid (*C*) ferret at 30°C, 0.33 Hz stimulation. I is expressed in millinewtons per square meter muscle cross-sectional area. The Ca²⁺ transients (aqueorin signals) are scaled to equal amplitudes and superimposed in *D*. In *E*, the tensions have been scaled to equal amplitudes and superimposed. The time from the beginning of the stimulus sweep (S) to the stimulus represents 100 milliseconds. (From MacKinnon R, Gwathmey JK, Allen PD, et al: Modulation by the thyroid state of intracellular calcium and contractility in ferret ventricular muscle. Circ Res 63:1080, 1988. By permission of the American Heart Association.)

one or more potassium channels and several calcium channels.[52, 65–67] These effects probably result from altered gene transcription because of thyroid hormone. In general, these channel effects lead to a reduction in early repolarization in the absence of thyroid hormone and an accelerated decline in the action potential when thyroid hormone is present in excess. The tachycardia observed in hyperthyroidism appears to be due to a combination of an increased rate of diastolic depolarization and a decreased duration of the action potential in the sinoatrial node cells. The propensity for the development of atrial fibrillation may be due to the shortened refractory period of atrial cells.

Hyperthyroidism

Hyperthyroidism is the clinical state resulting from excess production of T₄, T₃ or both. The most common cause is a diffuse toxic goiter (Graves disease). Although the etiology of this condition is still unknown, the hyperproduction of T₄ and T₃ is thought to result from circulating IgG autoantibodies that bind to the thyrotropin receptor on the thyroid gland. The second most common form of hyperthyroidism is nodular toxic goiter, a condition in which localized areas of the gland function excessively and autonomously.[68]

Hyperthyroidism is a relatively common disease that occurs four to eight times more often in women than men, with a peak incidence in the third and fourth decades. Commonly associated signs and symptoms (see Table 64–1) include fatigue, hyperactivity, insomnia, heat intolerance, palpitations, dyspnea, increased appetite with weight loss, nocturia, diarrhea, oligomenorrhea, muscle weakness, tremor, emotional lability, increased heart rate, systolic hypertension, hyperthermia, warm moist skin, lid lag, stare, and brisk reflexes. Serum T₄ levels are increased and serum TSH is suppressed.

CARDIOVASCULAR MANIFESTATIONS. The heart is among the most responsive organs to thyroid hormone. Cardiovascular signs and symptoms are therefore important clinical features of hyperthyroidism.[68, 69] Palpitations, dyspnea, tachycardia, and systolic hypertension are common findings. Diastolic hypertension can also occur. Typically noted are a hyperactive precordium with a loud first heart

sound, an accentuated pulmonic component of the second heart sound, and a third heart sound; occasionally, a systolic ejection click is heard. Midsystolic murmurs along the left sternal border are common, and a systolic scratch, the so-called Means-Lerman scratch, is occasionally heard in the 2nd left intercostal space during expiration. It may represent a pulmonic flow murmur related to cardiac output.

As would be anticipated, the cardiac and stroke volume index, mean systolic ejection rate, velocity and extent of wall shortening (Fig. 64–4), and coronary blood flow are all increased, the systolic ejection period and preejection period are abbreviated, the pulse pressure is widened, and systemic vascular resistance is reduced in hyperthyroidism. The changes in left ventricular performance induced by thyroid hormone appear to be secondary to augmented contractility rather than alterations in loading conditions or a change in heart rate. If the hyperthyroidism is relatively mild, many of the indices of left ventricular function are normal, with exercise needed to bring out abnormalities.[69] It has been suggested that many of the changes in cardiac function are secondary to the increased metabolic demands of peripheral tissue. However, the increase in cardiac output is greater than would be predicted on the basis of the increased total-body oxygen consumption, thus supporting the view that thyroid hormone exerts a direct cardiac stimulant action independent of its effect on general tissue metabolism, as noted above. Furthermore, normalization of the myocardial contractile response to exercise may not occur until several months after normalization of thyroid function. However, it is likely that the overall pathological consequences associated with thyrotoxicosis result from an interaction between the effect of thyroid hormone on the heart and its effect on the peripheral circulation (Fig. 64–5).

Roentgenographic and electrographic changes are common, but nonspecific in hyperthyroidism.[69] Thus, on chest x-ray the left ventricle, aorta, and pulmonary artery are

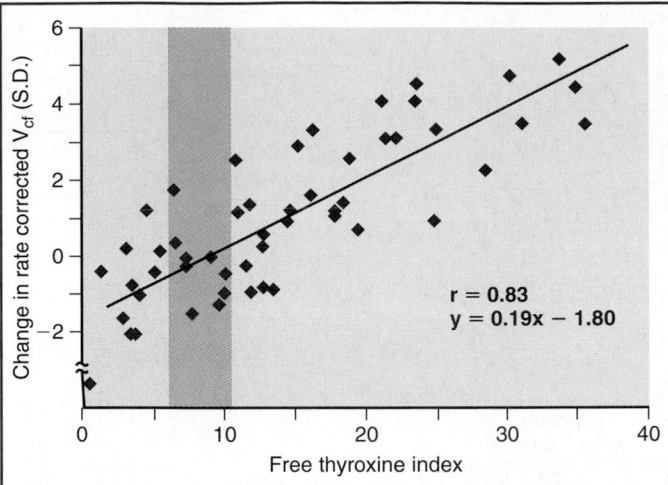

FIGURE 64-4. Rate-corrected velocity of shortening in SD units from the normal mean regression line obtained from 11 patients at varying levels of the free thyroxine index. A strong positive correlation can be seen between the level of thyroid hormone and the change in contractile state. The shaded area represents the normal range for the serum free thyroxine index. (From Feldman T, Borow KM, Sarne DH, et al: Myocardial mechanics in hyperthyroidism: Importance of left ventricular loading conditions, heart rate and contractile state. J Am Coll Cardiol 7:967, 1986. Reprinted with permission from the American College of Cardiology.)

prominent, and in some cases, generalized cardiac enlargement can be noted. In patients with sinus rhythm, the magnitude of the tachycardia in general parallels the severity of the disease. Sinus tachycardia is present in 40 percent of patients with hyperthyroidism and occurs most frequently in the younger age groups and often at night.[70] Ten to 15 percent of patients with hyperthyroidism have persistent atrial fibrillation, which is often heralded by one or more transient episodes of this arrhythmia.[69] Shortening of the AV conduction time and functional refractory period results in an increased frequency at which the AV conduction system transmits rapid atrial impulses. Intraatrial conduction disturbances, manifested by prolongation or notching of the P wave and prolongation of the PR interval in the absence of treatment with digitalis, occur in 15 and 5

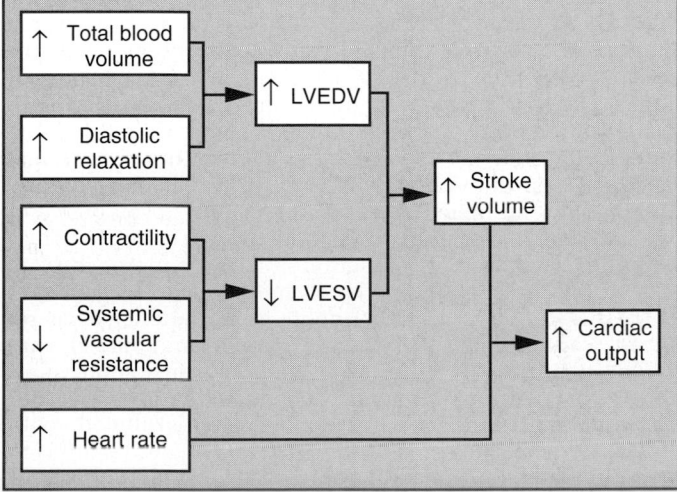

FIGURE 64-5. Cardiovascular effects of hyperthyroidism. Cardiac output is increased as a result of thyroid hormone augmentation of the hemodynamic parameters indicated in the figure. LVEDV = Left ventricular end-diastolic volume; LVESV = left ventricular end-systolic volume. (Modified from Woeber KA: Thyrotoxicosis and the heart. N Engl J Med 327:94, 1992.)

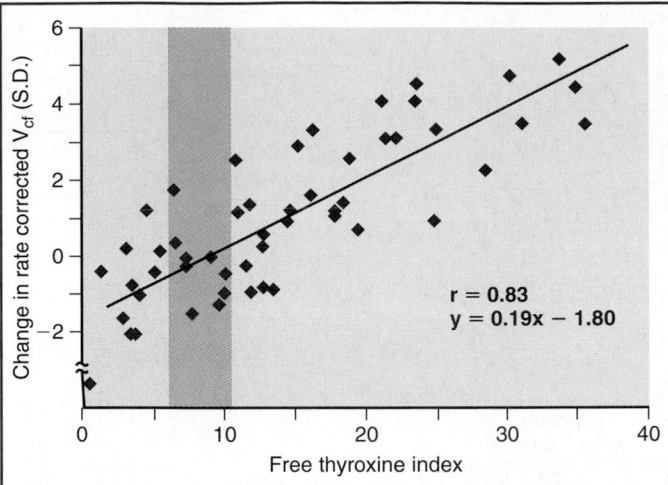percent of patients with hyperthyroidism, respectively. Occasionally, second- or third-degree heart block may result. The cause of the AV conduction disturbance is not clear because animal experiments have shown that the functional refractory period of the AV conduction system and the conduction time were shortened in dogs with hyperthyroidism and prolonged in dogs with hypothyroidism.[71] Intraventricular conduction disturbances, most commonly right bundle branch block, occur in about 15 percent of patients with hyperthyroidism without associated heart disease of other etiology. Paroxysmal supraventricular tachycardia and flutter are rare in hyperthyroidism. Finally, occult thyrotoxicosis may underlie either chronic or paroxysmal isolated atrial fibrillation.[72]

Both angina pectoris and heart failure occur in patients with hyperthyroidism. For many years it was assumed that these conditions were seen only in the presence of underlying cardiovascular disease. More recently, however, five lines of evidence have suggested otherwise: (1) Congestive heart failure has been produced in experimental animals by simply administering T_4. (2) Congestive heart failure may develop in children with thyrotoxicosis and no underlying cardiac disease.[73] (3) Angina has been reported in a hyperthyroid patient with normal coronary arteries, presumably secondary to thyroid-induced coronary artery spasm. (4) The abnormal left ventricular function observed during exercise in hyperthyroid subjects is not reversed by beta blockade but is reversed by treating the hyperthyroidism.[49, 68, 69] (5) Finally, Ebisawa and coauthors reported that the cardiomyopathy in patients with thyrotoxicosis may be irreversible. Four patients with this condition had increased left ventricular end-diastolic volumes and reduced ejection fractions, even 13 to 15 years following treatment of their hyperthyroidism. Myocardial biopsies, performed in two patients, showed no specific light microscopic abnormalities.[74]

Thus, when it is severe and persistent, thyrotoxicosis can overtax even a normal heart, although in most instances the development of clinical manifestations of heart failure and myocardial ischemia in patients with hyperthyroidism signifies the presence of underlying cardiac or coronary vascular disease. The frequency of hyperthyroidism is also increased in patients with familial hypertrophic cardiomyopathy. In one kindred, 3 of 17 members with hypertrophic cardiomyopathy also had hyperthyroidism.[75] Finally, hyperthyroidism is associated with mitral value prolapse in more than a third of cases.[49, 68, 69]

TREATMENT OF CARDIOVASCULAR DISEASE IN HYPERTHYROIDISM. Hyperthyroid patients with cardiovascular disease are particularly resistant to therapy. It has been well documented that both heart failure and arrhythmias are resistant to conventional doses of cardiac glycosides. Although the specific mechanisms underlying these altered responses remain obscure, they may be related to both systemic and local effects.[76] First, serum levels of cardiac glycosides are diminished in hyperthyroidism, not primarily because its metabolism is increased but because its volume of distribution is greater. Second, experimental hyperthyroidism reduces the enhancement in myocardial contractile force and the prolongation in the AV nodal refractory period produced by these agents.[76] Because of this decreased sensitivity to cardiac glycosides, toxicity may develop at a dose that has relatively little therapeutic effect.

DIAGNOSIS AND TREATMENT OF HYPERTHYROIDISM

The mainstay of treatment is beta-adrenergic blocking agents pending initiation of more definite treatment of the hyperthyroidism. Hyperthyroidism in most patients is clinically manifested as described above. The diagnosis is confirmed with a low TSH level, which reflects an elevated level of thyroid hormone in the blood. In elderly patients with apathetic hyperthyroidism, cardiovascular manifestations predominate, specifically, atrial fibrillation and/or congestive heart failure, and therefore evaluation of thyroid function in such patients is particularly important.

Definitive treatment of hyperthyroidism is surgical removal of the gland or irradiation with radioactive iodide. In severely ill patients, particularly those with thyroid storm, significant cardiovascular symptoms, or both, neither of these therapies is appropriate. Thus, medical therapy is directed at reducing both the production and the biological effect of thyroid hormone with thionamides and beta blockers.[76-78] Tachycardia, palpitations, tremor, restlessness, muscle weakness, and heat intolerance are reversed by these agents, which offer the additional benefit of inhibiting the conversion of T_4 to the biologically active T_3 in peripheral tissues.

TREATMENT OF CARDIOVASCULAR MANIFESTATIONS OF HYPERTHYROIDISM.

Prompt treatment of hyperthyroidism can significantly reduce, if not eliminate the associated cardiovascular symptoms. About half of patients with concurrent onset of hyperthyroidism and angina pectoris experience complete remission of this symptom after treatment of hyperthyroidism.[78] Furthermore, in 30 to 40 percent of thyrotoxic patients with atrial fibrillation sustained for 1 week or longer, spontaneous reversion to sinus rhythm occurs when they become euthyroid.[49, 68, 69]

Beta blockers can be administered orally or intravenously, but because these drugs interfere with the effects of sympathetic stimulation on the heart, they must be used with caution in patients with congestive heart failure. However, if the heart failure is in part related to the tachycardia, beta blockade may be beneficial.[77] Beta-blocking drugs also slow the ventricular rate in atrial fibrillation. The most useful agents for correcting the fundamental defect are thionamides such as propylthiouracil,[76] which inhibits thyroid hormone synthesis. Iodine inhibits the release of thyroid hormones from the thyrotoxic gland, and its beneficial effects occur more rapidly than those of thionamides. It is therefore useful for rapid amelioration of the hyperthyroid state in patients with thyroid heart disease. Ipodate may be particularly useful for this purpose. Iodine may also be used along with antithyroid agents to control thyrotoxicosis following ^{131}I treatment until the radioactive iodide has had time to take effect. Most hyperthyroid patients, however, escape from the effects of iodide after 10 to 14 days.

Hypothyroidism

Hypothyroidism results from reduced secretion of both T_4 and T_3, which occurs in most cases as a consequence of destruction of the thyroid gland itself, usually by an inflammatory process. The most common cause in the United States is Hashimoto's thyroiditis. Less commonly, it is secondary to decreased secretion of TSH because of either pituitary or hypothalamic disease. In secondary hypothyroidism, the signs and symptoms associated with deficiency of other pituitary hormones are also usually present. The incidence of hypothyroidism peaks between the ages of 30 and 60 years, and it is twice as common in women as men. The following signs and symptoms are common: cold intolerance, dryness of the skin, weakness, impairment in memory, personality changes, shortness of breath, constipation, hoarseness, menorrhagia and other forms of menstrual dysfunction, and occasionally, heart failure.

CARDIOVASCULAR MANIFESTATIONS

(Fig. 64–6). The heart in overt myxedema is often pale, flabby, and grossly dilated. Histological examination discloses myofibrillar swelling, loss of striations, and interstitial fibrosis. With early detection and treatment of hypothyroidism, the classic findings of cardiac enlargement, cardiac dilatation, significant bradycardia, weak arterial pulses, hypotension, distant heart sounds, low electrocardiographic voltage, nonpitting facial and peripheral edema, and evidence of congestive heart failure, such as ascites, orthopnea, and paroxysmal dyspnea, are now seen only infrequently. However, exertional dyspnea and easy fatigability continue to be common complaints.

Myxedema is associated with increased capillary permeability and subsequent leakage of protein into the interstitial space; these abnormalities result in pericardial effusion, a common clinical finding in overt myxedema that occurs in about one-third of all patients. Rarely, it is complicated

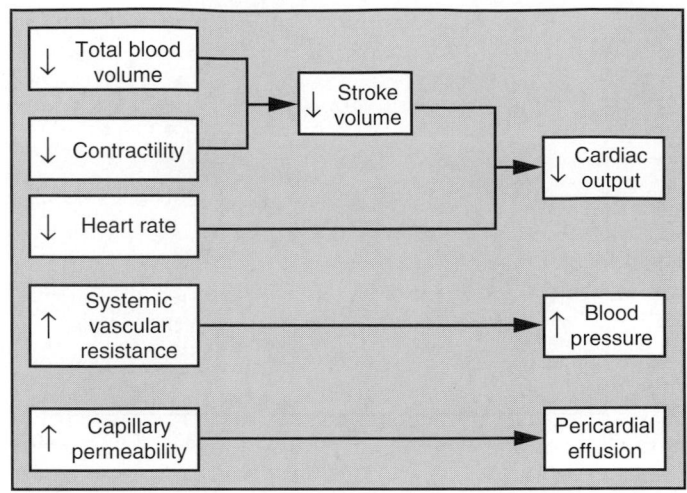

FIGURE 64–6. Cardiovascular effects of hypothyroidism. Cardiac output is decreased because of diminished total blood volume, impaired left ventricular contractility, and bradycardia. Hypertension results from increased systemic vascular resistance. Pericardial effusion results from increased capillary permeability and interstitial protein leak.

by cardiac tamponade.[49, 68] Echocardiography is the most useful method of establishing the diagnosis. The effusions disappear with thyroid replacement therapy. Myxedema-associated cardiogenic shock has also rarely been reported, and it, too, responds to thyroid replacement therapy.[79]

Electrocardiographic changes include sinus bradycardia and prolongation of the QT interval. The P wave amplitude is usually very low. It is possible that hypothyroidism may contribute to reentrant ventricular arrhythmias,[80] which may be due to prolonged action potential duration.[80a] The incidence of AV and intraventricular conduction disturbances is about three times greater in patients with myxedema than in the general population. Incomplete or complete right bundle branch block has been observed, and a primary myocardial abnormality suggestive of cardiomyopathy has been reported.[81] Other electrocardiographic changes are those associated with pericardial effusion.

The frequency of hypertension is increased in patients with hypothyroidism, although not in patients with severe myxedema.[49, 68] In one study of 477 patients, 15 percent of the hypothyroid subjects had a blood pressure greater than 160/95 as compared with 5.5 percent in age-matched euthyroid subjects. Replacement of thyroid hormone resulted in a substantial reduction in blood pressure in the hypertensive patients.[82] In a study of 688 consecutive hypertensive patients, hypothyroidism was found in 25 (3.6 percent). In nearly one-third of this subgroup, treatment of the hypothyroidism lowered the blood pressure to within the normal range.[83] Thus, individuals with mild to moderate hypothyroidism have an increased possibility of the development of hypertension, particularly diastolic hypertension, whereas individuals with severe hypothyroidism are more likely to have normal or slightly low blood pressure.[82, 83]

MYOCARDIAL EFFECTS.

Hypothyroid patients have reduced cardiac output, stroke volume, and blood and plasma volume.[49, 68, 84] Right- and left-heart filling pressures are usually within normal limits unless they are elevated by pericardial effusion. Blood flow is redistributed, with mild reductions in cerebral and renal flow and significant reductions in cutaneous flow. The ventricular isovolumetric relaxation time is prolonged but is normalized during T_4 replacement.[85] The impact of hypothyroidism on cardiac function can occur quickly in patients rendered hypothyroid for assessment of thyroid status in the treatment of thyroid cancer. Two weeks after discontinuing thyroid medication, the left ventricular end-diastolic diameter and peak velocity of early diastolic filling, as well as the heart rate, were reduced. No changes were observed in systolic or diastolic blood pressure.[86]

Cardiac muscle isolated from cats with experimentally produced hypothyroidism exhibited reduced contractility characterized by depression of the myocardial force-velocity curve, a reduction in the rate of tension development, and prolongation of the contractile response.

Congestive heart failure is not common in myxedema, nor does it occur in the absence of other cardiac disease. Presumably, the depressed myocardial contractility is sufficient to sustain the reduced workload placed on the heart in hypothyroidism. However, it may be difficult to distinguish between symptoms of myxedema and heart failure. Dyspnea, edema, effusions, cardiomegaly, and T wave changes occur in both conditions. In left-sided heart failure, pulmonary arterial pressure is usually elevated during exercise, cardiac output fails to rise normally, and the Valsalva response is normal, whereas the opposite occurs in myxedema. Also, the hemodynamic changes in myxedema respond to thyroid hormone administration.

Cardiac catecholamine levels are not reduced in hypothyroidism. Neither the sensitivity of the mechanical performance of the heart to sympathetic nerve stimulation nor the response of cardiac adenylate cyclase to norepinephrine is altered in hypothyroidism. However, the total number of myocardial beta receptors is reduced.[62, 56] Both isoproterenol-stimulated contractility and the accumulation of cyclic adenosine monophosphate are reduced in hearts obtained from hypothyroid rats. In experimental hypothyroidism, calcium in isolated myocardial sarcoplasmic reticulum particles is reduced, which may explain the altered contractile state.[59]

Finally, while the clinical and morphological cardiac features of hypothyroidism resemble those associated with dilated cardiomyopathy few clinical data are available to support a connection between these conditions. Fruhwald and colleagues examined the prevalence of thyroid abnormalities in 61 patients with idiopathic dilated cardiomyopathy. By ultrasonography, 8 percent had morphological abnormalities of the thyroid. Yet none had clinical or biochemical evidence of hyperthyroidism or hypothyroidism. In the 10 patients who were taking amiodarone, the frequency of morphological thyroid abnormalities was similar to the frequency of abnormalities with the rest of the patients.[87]

ATHEROSCLEROSIS. It has been suggested that patients with hypothyroidism have an increased risk of atherosclerosis because of significant changes in lipid metabolism. Hypercholesterolemia and hypertriglyceridemia, which are associated with the development of premature coronary artery disease, are commonly found in patients with hypothyroidism.[88] Treatment of the hypothyroidism corrects the abnormal lipid pattern. For example, Arem and Patsch noted a 22 percent reduction in the mean low-density lipoprotein (LDL) cholesterol concentration after 4 months of thyroid replacement therapy.[89] High-density lipoprotein (HDL) cholesterol levels did not change appreciably. Support for a connection between hypothyroidism and atherosclerosis has come from several sources, including the documentation that the latter occurs with twice the frequency in patients with myxedema than in age- and sex-matched controls and that the development of atherosclerosis in cholesterol-fed animals is enhanced by the presence of hypothyroidism and reduced when thyroid hormone is administered. Yet myocardial infarction and angina pectoris are relatively uncommon in hypothyroidism. This low frequency of cardiac complications from atherosclerosis may simply reflect the decreased metabolic demand on the myocardium in hypothyroidism. However, the known effects of hypothyroidism on serum enzyme concentrations do complicate the assessment of chest pain in patients with myxedema.

Diagnosis is made by documentation of an elevated serum TSH level. Caution must be exercised in treating hypothyroid patients who are elderly and who may have underlying heart disease to avoid precipitating myocardial infarction or severe congestive heart failure; a slow replacement program is indicated in these individuals.

Treatment of congestive heart failure is particularly difficult in patients with myxedema, both because of the effect of thyroid hormone on the heart and because the heart's response to cardiac glycosides is altered. Patients with severe angina pectoris and untreated myxedema pose a difficult clinical dilemma because angina may be exacerbated by thyroid hormone replacement and the usual medical management of angina with beta blockers may induce severe bradycardia. Coronary arteriography often shows severe coronary artery disease in these patients, and an excellent surgical team can perform successful coronary revascularization with minimal thyroid replacement. Full thyroid replacement can then be safely achieved during the postoperative period, without the recurrence of angina.[90]

Amiodarone and the Thyroid

The widespread use of amiodarone for cardiac arrhythmias is now one of the most common causes of thyroid abnormalities in patients with cardiovascular disease[91, 92] (see also Chap. 23). Amiodarone has structural similarity to T_4 and T_3 and is also rich in iodine. Amiodarone decreases the peripheral conversion of T_4 to T_3, which leads to elevated levels of circulating T_4 and lower levels of circulating T_3. Since this inhibition occurs in the pituitary gland as well, a transient increase in TSH is seen early in treatment but usually resolves over the next 3 months.[93, 94] These laboratory test changes are common and not usually associated with any clinical manifestations of thyroid dysfunction.

HYPOTHYROIDISM. Hypothyroidism, the most common clinical manifestation of amiodarone-induced thyroid dysfunction in the United States and United Kingdom, occurs in as many as 13 percent of patients.[91, 92] The mechanism of this dysfunction is not clearly defined but may be related to the effect of the large iodine load on inhibition of thyroid hormone release and synthesis superimposed on underlying autoimmune thyroid disease.[95] It has also been suggested that amiodarone itself may cause autoimmune thyroid dysfunction by altering T-cell function.

Symptoms are the same as those seen in other forms of hypothyroidism, and the diagnosis is confirmed with the demonstration of an elevated TSH level. Some patients will regain normal thyroid function several months after stopping amiodarone therapy, although others will have permanent hypothyroidism. If thyroid function does not return to normal with discontinuation of therapy or if amiodarone administration is continued, thyroid hormone replacement at a dose that normalizes the TSH level will treat the condition.

HYPERTHYROIDISM. Amiodarone-induced hyperthyroidism most commonly occurs in areas of the world with iodine deficiency but can be seen in iodine-replete individuals as well.[91, 92] Patients may demonstrate typical symptoms of hyperthyroidism such as weight loss, heat intolerance, and tremor, but at times the initial symptom may be the onset or recurrence of cardiac arrhythmias. Diagnosis is made by the patient's history, clinical examination, and thyroid function testing, which shows low TSH and elevated T_4. Since low TSH and elevated T_4 levels can also be commonly seen in the early phase of amiodarone therapy without symptoms, measurement of total T_3 may be helpful in distinguishing these conditions. In the early phase of treatment with amiodarone, T_3 levels are decreased, whereas in hyperthyroidism, the T_3 level is increased.[96]

Two mechanisms have been proposed for amiodarone-induced hyperthyroidism. Type I occurs in abnormal thyroid glands and is caused by iodine-induced increased thyroid hormone synthesis in subjects with nodular goiters or latent Graves disease. Type II occurs in what is a normal gland. It is presumably secondary to a thyroid-destructive process caused by iodine or amiodarone per se.[97] In the latter case, amiodarone may induce thyrotropin receptor antibodies, which then cause the hyperthyroid state.[98] Some investigators have suggested that type I (hypervascular state) and type II (hypovascular state) thyrotoxicosis can be distinguished by color flow Doppler sonography. Another sometimes useful distinguishing feature is an increased serum interleukin-6 level in type II but not type I. It has been reported to be important to distinguish these two types since their treatments differ. Patients with type II but not type I sometimes respond very well to glucocorticoids.[99]

Cessation of amiodarone therapy will lead to eventual resolution of the hyperthyroidism, although normalization can sometimes take several months. However, amiodarone therapy often cannot be stopped, in which case other treatment modalities must be instituted. The two primary modalities are thionamides and surgery. Propylthiouracil or methimazole may be successful, but not in all cases. When medical management fails, thyroidectomy may be the procedure of choice to allow continuation of amiodarone therapy. Radioactive iodine therapy is most commonly not an option because of the high iodine content of amiodarone and the resultant increased thyroidal stores leading to very low radioactive iodine uptake by the thyroid.

THYROID MONITORING. Because of the frequency of thyroid dysfunction with amiodarone therapy, routine monitoring of thyroid function tests is recommended. Several algorithms for monitoring have been published. One such algorithm is depicted in Figure 64–7.

DISEASES OF THE ADRENAL CORTEX

Since Addison's description in 1855 of adrenal insufficiency,[2] it has been appreciated that steroids secreted by the adrenal cortex exert a significant effect on the cardiovascular system. For many years, the primary influence was assumed to be mediated by the adrenal steroids' effect in modifying blood pressure. Recently, it has been proposed that these steroids, particularly aldosterone, have a much broader impact on cardiovascular function. Yet diseases of the adrenal cortex are often associated with changes in blood pressure. Adrenal insufficiency is characterized by hypotension, whereas hypertension often accompanies excessive production of adrenal steroids.

Three classes of steroids are secreted by the adrenal cortex: glucocorticoids, e.g., cortisol; mineralocorticoids, e.g., aldosterone; and androgens, e.g., dehydroeplandrosterone. In this section, the physiology and pathophysiology of glucocorticoid and mineralocorticoid secretion are addressed.

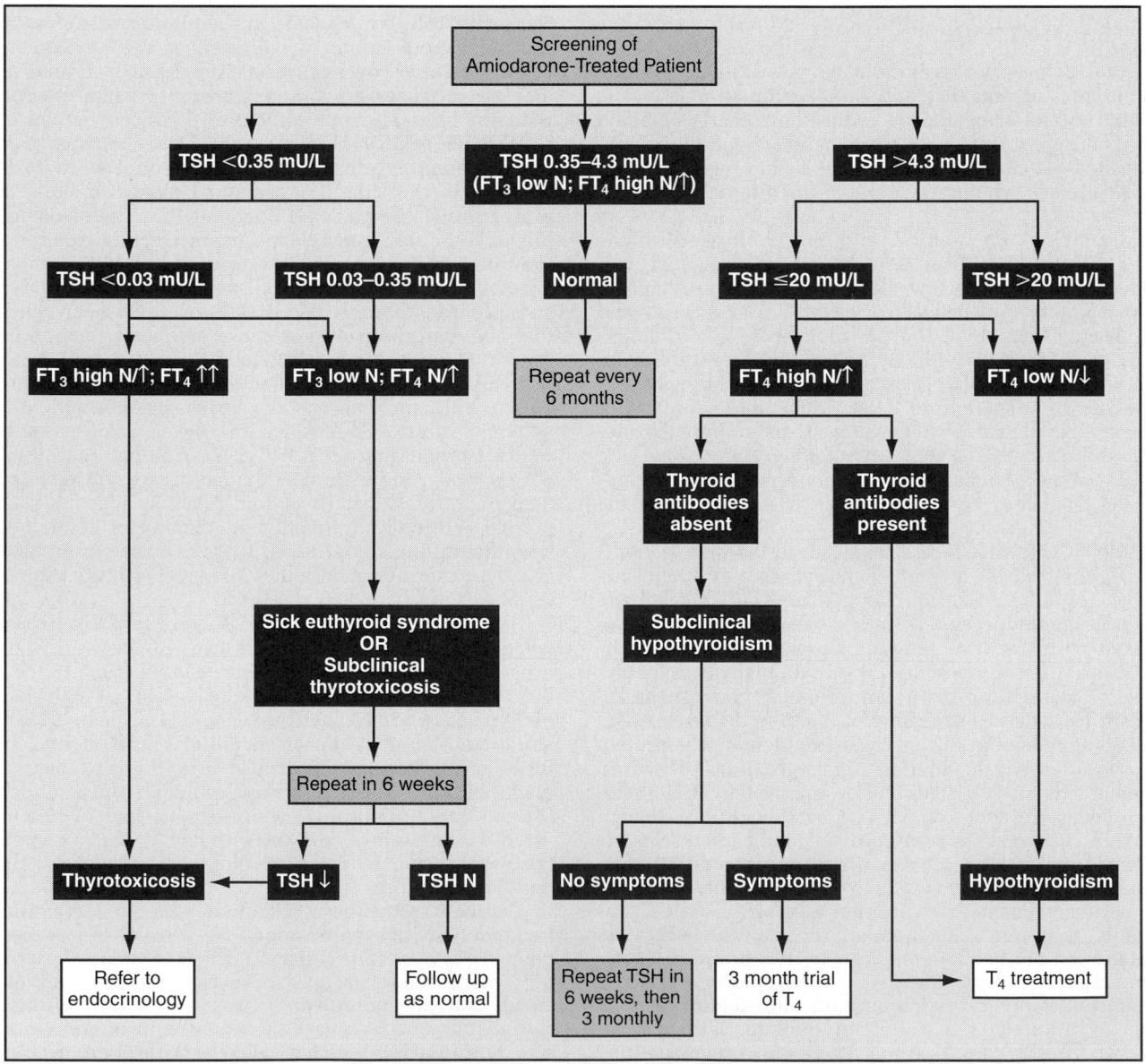

FIGURE 64–7. Algorithm for evaluating thyroid status in patients taking amiodarone. Amiodarone withdrawal may also be appropriate in some cases. TPO = thyroid peroxidase. (Adapted from Newman CM, Price A, Davies DW, et al: Amiodarone and the thyroid: A practical guide to the management of thyroid dysfunction induced by amiodarone therapy. Heart 79:121, 1998.)

HORMONE ACTIONS

CORTISOL. The primary glucocorticoid, cortisol, is synthesized from cholesterol in the inner layers of the adrenal cortex. Its average plasma concentration is 15 μg/dl in the morning, which falls to 5 μg/dl by early evening.[100] The fundamental mechanism of action of the glucocorticoids is similar to that of other steroid hormones. They enter a target tissue by diffusion and combine with a specific high-affinity intracellular receptor protein. The receptor-cortisol complex can then bind to promoters of target genes and regulate their transcription. The major action of glucocorticoids is to promote gluconeogenesis, and in that respect, they have both catabolic and antiinsulin properties.

Glucocorticoids also have antiinflammatory effects. They maintain normal vascular responsiveness to circulating vasoconstrictors such as norepinephrine and have a major effect on both the distribution and excretion of body water.

ALDOSTERONE. The major mineralocorticoid produced by the human adrenal gland is aldosterone. It is also synthesized from cholesterol, but almost exclusively in the outer layer (glomerulosa) of the adrenal cortex. Aldosterone has two important functions: (1) It is a major regulator of extracellular fluid volume by its effect on sodium retention, and (2) It is a major determinant of potassium metabolism. Aldosterone acts predominantly on the distal convoluted tubule and/or collecting duct of the kidney, where it promotes the reabsorption of sodium. Potassium then diffuses into the lumen of the tubules because of the change in electrochemical gradient produced by active reabsorption of the positively charged sodium ion. Hydrogen ion may also be more freely excreted because of this change in the electrochemical gradient. Although aldosterone also acts on salivary and sweat glands and on epithelial cells of the gastrointestinal tract, these actions have little impact on total-body sodium and potassium homeostasis.

Three well-defined mechanisms control aldosterone release.[100, 101]

1. The renin-angiotensin system is the major system for control of extracellular fluid volume by regulating aldosterone secretion. Aldosterone is linked in a negative feedback loop with the renin-angiotensin system. Thus, during periods registered as volume deficiency, release of the enzyme renin from the juxtaglomerular cells of the kidney is increased. Renin then increases the production of angiotensin I from its substrate. Angiotensin I is rapidly converted into the biologically active angiotensin II, which increases aldosterone secretion. Angiotensin II also produces vasoconstriction, thereby raising blood pressure and reducing blood flow to a variety of tissues, especially the kidney.
2. Potassium ion also regulates aldosterone secretion independent of the renin-angiotensin system; an elevated potassium concentration increases aldosterone secretion and vice versa. The adrenal cortex is very sensitive to changes in potassium concentration, with as little as a 0.1-mEq/liter increment producing significant changes in plasma aldosterone levels.
3. ACTH also affects aldosterone secretion profoundly. However, because control of aldosterone release is not appreciably altered in patients who have been on a long-term regimen of steroid therapy, ACTH probably has a smaller role than the other two factors do in maintaining normal aldosterone secretion.

In addition to these major stimuli controlling aldosterone secretion, salt-losing hormones such as atrial natriuretic peptide and dopamine inhibit aldosterone secretion, particularly in response to angiotensin II.[101] Finally, poor dietary intake of both sodium and potassium alters the magnitude of the aldosterone response to acute stimulation, sodium restriction, and potassium loading, both of which enhance the response of the adrenal, perhaps by modifying the local (adrenal) renin-angiotensin system.[100, 101]

ALDOSTERONE: A CARDIOVASCULAR RISK FACTOR.

While diseases of the adrenal cortex primarily affect the cardiovascular system via changes in blood pressure or volume homeostasis, even at physiological levels aldosterone may enhance the risk of cardiovascular damage. This increased risk is mediated, in part, by aldosterone's classic action on epithelial cells (e.g., renal tubular cells) whereby sodium, volume, and potassium homeostasis is modified and in part, by several nonclassic effects on nonepithelial cells (e.g., myocytes and fibroblasts) in which a variety of functions are modified. For example, aldosterone has a direct effect on collagen metabolism in cardiac fibroblasts. In rats treated with a high-salt diet and aldosterone, cardiac fibrosis develops within 6 weeks.[102–105] A clinical correlate of this effect is a reactive perivascular and interstitial cardiac fibrosis in patients with primary aldosteronism that does not seem to be due to pressure overload alone. In the stroke-prone, spontaneously hypertensive rat, administering an angiotensin-converting enzyme (ACE) inhibitor markedly

attenuates the early death rate.[106] Since this manipulation will reduce both angiotensin II and aldosterone levels, either could be involved in mediating this damage. When Rocha and colleagues returned angiotensin II levels to normal with an infusion of angiotensin II, the damage recurred unless the animals were adrenalectomized or the mineralocorticoid receptor blocked biochemically before the infusion began. By this technique, not only the cardiac damage but also the renal and cerebral damage was prevented even in the face of an increased angiotensin II level and persistently elevated blood pressure.[107–109, 109a, 109b] These data strongly support the hypothesis that it is aldosterone and not angiotensin II that is the principal mediator of this damage. Finally, aldosterone also may increase plasminogen activator inhibitor type 1 (PAI-1) expression and secretion and contribute to the inflammatory response accompanying microvascular disease.[109a, 109b]

Support for these experimentally derived data comes from clinical studies. Increased plasma aldosterone levels in patients with essential hypertension are associated with decreased systemic arterial compliance.[110] Plasma aldosterone levels more closely correlate with left ventricular mass than does plasma renin activity.[111] Finally, results of the Randomized Aldosterone Evaluation Study (RALES) provide strong support for a role of aldosterone independent of effects on electrolytes[112] (see also Chap. 18). Over 1600 patients with New York Heart Association (NYHA) Class III or IV heart failure were randomized to treatment with a low-dose mineralocorticoid receptor antagonist (spironolactone) or placebo on top of standard therapy (ACE inhibitors, loop diuretics, and in the majority, digoxin). A highly significant (30 percent) reduction was noted in all-cause mortality in the treatment group. The magnitude of this effect, observed despite concomitant therapy with an ACE inhibitor, is comparable in magnitude to the benefit of an ACE inhibitor alone in this population. The applicability of these findings to other cardiovascular diseases and milder forms of hypertension awaits the results of future studies.

Cushing Syndrome

(see also Chap. 28)

In 1932, Harvey Cushing reported a syndrome characterized by truncal obesity, hypertension, fatigue, weakness, amenorrhea, hirsutism, purple abdominal striae, glucosuria, edema, and osteoporosis.[113] The majority of cases are secondary to bilateral adrenal hyperplasia, with the predominant feature being excess production of glucocorticoids and androgens.[100] Some cases are due to ACTH-producing tumors of either the pituitary gland (Cushing disease) or nonendocrine tissue (ectopic ACTH production). Fifteen to 20 percent of cases are due to primary adrenal neoplasia, either adenoma or carcinoma. Most patients have a typical body habitus: central obesity and slender extremities with proximal muscle weakness. Hypertension is present in 80 to 90 percent of patients, and diabetes occurs in 20 percent, probably in individuals with a predisposition.[100] Evidence of androgen excess may also be present, including hirsutism, amenorrhea, and clitorimegaly.

Laboratory tests disclose evidence of excess production of both glucocorticoids and androgens in the majority of cases. Thus, urinary metabolites of these steroids, 17-ketosteroids and 17-hydroxysteroids, are characteristically increased. Most patients show some evidence of glycosuria or hyperglycemia.

CARDIOVASCULAR MANIFESTATIONS. Before the development of effective therapy for Cushing syndrome, accelerated atherosclerosis was a common finding. Early death usually occurred from myocardial infarction, congestive heart failure, or stroke. Even with more effective treatment, the mortality of patients with Cushing syndrome is still significantly higher than that in the general population, primarily because of an increased risk of cardiovascular disease.[114] Although the pathophysiology of the accelerated atherosclerosis is not clear, the hypertensive process probably contributes. Chronic excess production of cortisol leads to hyperlipidemia and hypercholesterolemia, both of which may promote the development of atherosclerosis.[100]

The pathophysiology of the hypertension in Cushing syndrome has been much debated. Early studies suggested that it was secondary to volume expansion as a result of cortisol's mineralocorticoid properties. Support for this mechanism comes from the demonstration of increased levels of atrial natriuretic hormone in patients with Cushing syndrome, which suggests a volume-expanded state.[115] However, recent studies have not supported this hypothesis. Alternative hypotheses include glucocorticoid potentiation of the response of vascular smooth muscle to vasoconstrictive agents and ACTH- or cortisol-induced increases in renin substrate.[100] The latter thesis suggests that the increased blood pressure is secondary to increased generation of angiotensin II. Support for the potentiation hypothesis comes from a documented increased vascular response to both angiotensin II and catecholamines in patients with Cushing syndrome as compared with normal subjects.[116, 117] A final possibility is increased vasoconstrictor sensitivity to cortisol itself, which has been suggested to occur in essential hypertension, probably by modifying renal vascular resistance.[118, 119] Thus, the pathophysiology of the hypertension may be multifactorial and related to volume expansion, increased production of vasoactive agents, e.g., angiotensin II, and increased sensitivity of vascular smooth muscle to vasoactive agents.

Hemodynamic, electrocardiographic, and roentgenographic studies of patients with Cushing syndrome have revealed no specific abnormalities except those that are in general associated with either hypertension or hypokalemia. PR intervals tend to be shorter than normal. Echocardiograms have shown ventricular hypertrophy with asymmetrical septal thickening. The frequency of these abnormalities is greater than that seen in patients with essential hypertension and equivalent levels of blood pressure.[120]

Rarely, Cushing syndrome and cardiac myxoma occur in the same individual. In addition to having these two conditions, 80 percent of patients have a cutaneous abnormality. In most, it is a pigmented lesion; in some, it is a subcutaneous myxoma. Histologically, the adrenal glands show nodular hyperplasia.[121]

DIAGNOSIS AND TREATMENT. The diagnosis of Cushing syndrome is established by the lack of appropriate suppression of cortisol secretion by dexamethasone. The best screening test is the administration of 1 mg of dexamethasone at bedtime with measurement of plasma cortisol between 7 and 10 the next morning.[100] In normal subjects, cortisol levels are less than 5 μg/dl. Some patients, particularly the obese, may have false-positive responses, but false-negative responses occur only rarely. Definitive diagnosis of Cushing syndrome is made by the administration of 0.5 mg of dexamethasone every 6 hours for 2 days, with measurement of either plasma cortisol levels at the end of the second day (normal, <5 μg/dl) or the 24-hour cortisol excretory rate on the second day of dexamethasone suppression (normal, <10 μg/24 hr).[100]

Therapy for Cushing syndrome is usually directed at the specific cause. Thus, patients with adrenal carcinoma or adenoma or an ACTH-producing pituitary tumor are treated surgically. In some cases, patients with adrenal carcinoma have nonresectable lesions, and therefore surgery is combined with chemotherapy. Treatment of patients with bilateral hyperplasia but no evidence of an ACTH-producing tumor is controversial because the cause is often unknown. In some centers, bilateral adrenalectomy is the treatment of choice, while more commonly, therapy directed at the pituitary (either surgery or irradiation) is used.[100]

Treatment of the *cardiovascular abnormalities* associated with Cushing syndrome is directed at lowering blood pressure and correcting the hypokalemia if present. Caution

should be exercised in treating the hypertension with potassium-losing diuretics because of the tendency for hypokalemia to develop in these patients. Thus, potassium-sparing diuretics or potassium supplements are often required. As in all clinical conditions in which hypokalemia may be present, cardiac glycosides should be used with caution in patients with Cushing syndrome.

The hypertension is often resistant to conventional antihypertensive programs. Fallo and coworkers reported that only 15 percent of their hypertensive patients with Cushing syndrome had control of blood pressure with conventional medications: diuretics, calcium antagonists, and ACE inhibitors either as single agents or in combination. In 12 patients who failed conventional therapy, treatment with ketoconazole, an adrenal enzyme inhibitor, normalized blood pressure in all but 1 subject. In that 1 subject cortisol levels were not decreased. Thus, specific therapy directed at lowering cortisol production appears to be more effective than conventional antihypertensive therapy is in controlling hypertension in patients with Cushing syndrome.[122]

Hyperaldosteronism

(see also Chap. 28)

CLINICAL AND BIOCHEMICAL MANIFESTATIONS. Aldosteronism is a syndrome associated with hypersecretion of aldosterone. Primary aldosteronism signifies that the stimulus for the excess aldosterone production resides within the adrenal. In secondary aldosteronism, the stimulus is of extraadrenal origin.

In patients with primary aldosteronism, which is most commonly due to an aldosterone-producing adrenal adenoma, hypertension, hypokalemia, and metabolic alkalosis are common.[100, 123] Polyuria may exist because of the hypokalemia, and glucose intolerance is increased in frequency. Muscle cramps secondary to the hypokalemia may be present, but little else distinguishes this type from other forms of hypertension. Laboratory studies confirm the presence of hypokalemic alkalosis with a low specific gravity of urine and normal levels of adrenal glucocorticoids. The incidence of primary aldosteronism is between 0.5 and 2 percent of the hypertensive population, and it occurs twice as frequently in females as in males, with the initial manifestation usually occurring between the ages of 30 and 50 years.[100]

CARDIOVASCULAR MANIFESTATIONS. Many of the cardiovascular effects of aldosteronism are nonspecific and are related to aldosterone's effect on atrial pressure and potassium balance. Thus, T wave flattening or U wave prominence on the electrocardiogram and the presence of premature ventricular contractions and other arrhythmias as a result of hypokalemia are observed. Traditionally, it has been assumed that primary aldosteronism is not associated with significant cardiovascular complications. However, recent studies do not support this conclusion.[124–129] Nishimura and colleagues identified cardiovascular complications in 34 percent of their patients, with 16 percent having strokes and 7 percent having renal insufficiency.[128] Halimi and Mimram reported that albuminuria was greater and more frequent in patients with primary aldosteronism than in those with essential hypertension matched for age, gender, and severity and duration of hypertension.[126] Finally, strokes occur in 11 to 16 percent of patients with glucocorticoid-remediable aldosteronism (see below) before the age of 30.[129] Thus, these data support the hypothesis that in hypertensive patients, the presence of hyperaldosteronism represents an independent cardiovascular risk factor.

DIAGNOSIS AND TREATMENT. The diagnosis of primary aldosteronism is made by the presence of diastolic hypertension without edema, hypersecretion of aldosterone that fails to be appropriately suppressed during volume expansion, hyposecretion of renin, and hypokalemia with inappropriate urinary potassium loss during salt loading. The state of the renin-angiotensin system is often used to distinguish primary aldosteronism from other conditions that produce hypertension and hypokalemia. For example, hypertension and hypokalemia may be part of the clinical picture of secondary aldosteronism that accompanies malignant or accelerated hypertension or is associated with renal artery stenosis. Secondary aldosteronism can be readily distinguished from primary aldosteronism by plasma renin activity, which is increased in the former and reduced in the latter. However, the combination of hypertension and low plasma renin activity does not necessarily mean primary aldosteronism. Between 15 and 30 percent of patients with essential hypertension have low renin levels, so-called low-renin essential hypertension.[123] The possibility of excess mineralocorticoid secretion has been extensively evaluated in these patients; however, no definitive evidence for such exists (see Chap. 28).

Another entity that mimics primary aldosteronism is glucocorticoid-remediable aldosteronism (see also Chaps. 28 and 56). This condition is an inherited hypertensive disorder with dysregulation of aldosterone secretion secondary to a gene mutation. The mutation is a fusion gene product between two genes coding for the enzymes responsible for the last step in the biosynthesis of aldosterone and cortisol, i.e., 11-beta-hydroxylase/aldosterone synthase. This chimeric enzyme is expressed in fasciculata cells, thereby leading to ACTH control of aldosterone synthase—a condition that normally does not occur. These patients can be distinguished by either genetic assessment or measurement of unique 18-hydroxycortisol steroids in the urine.[130]

The principal therapy for primary aldosteronism is surgical removal of the aldosterone-producing adenoma. In some cases, removal is not possible because of the excessive risk imposed by the general physical status of the patient, in which case spironolactone, which pharmacologically blocks the effects of aldosterone, is used long-term. This form of therapy may bc of limited benefit in men because compliance is reduced by the undesirable side effects of gynecomastia and impotence, particularly when doses greater than 200 mg/d are required.[100]

In some patients, primary aldosteronism is due not to a solitary adenoma but to bilateral hyperplasia.[123] Although the clinical characteristics of these two conditions are similar, their responses to surgery are different. In both cases, hypokalemia is corrected, but patients with bilateral hyperplasia often do not exhibit a reduction in arterial pressure. Patients with bilateral hyperplasia are best treated with aldosterone receptor antagonists (e.g., spironolactone) and other antihypertensive agents. Thus, preoperative distinction between bilateral hyperplasia and an adrenal adenoma by adrenal venography or adrenal scanning is important.

Adrenal Insufficiency

Clinically, patients with adrenal insufficiency can be divided into four types[100]: (1) the most common, primary insufficiency (Addison disease); (2) secondary insufficiency caused by a lack of ACTH; (3) selective hypoaldosteronism; and (4) enzyme deficiency (congenital adrenal hyperplasia).

Addison disease may occur at any age and affects both genders equally. It is commonly due to a destructive process involving both adrenal glands; this process is sometimes infectious, but most often it is autoimmune.[100] Nearly all patients with primary adrenal insufficiency have weakness, increased skin pigmentation, significant weight loss, anorexia, nausea, vomiting, and hypotension, particularly postural. As the disease progresses, serum levels of sodium, chloride, and bicarbonate are gradually reduced, and potassium levels are increased.

CARDIOVASCULAR MANIFESTATIONS. The most common cardiovascular finding in adrenal insufficiency is arterial hypotension. In severe cases, blood pressure may be in the range of 80/50 mm Hg, with postural accentuation. Indeed, syncope occurs in a significant percentage of patients. In severe cases, heart size and peripheral pulses decrease. The most common electrocardiographic abnormalities are low or inverted T waves, sinus bradycardia, a prolonged

QT_c interval, and low voltage. Conduction defects also occur, with first-degree block present in 20 percent of patients. Changes secondary to the hyperkalemia are not common, and cardiac failure is unusual.[131]

DIAGNOSIS AND TREATMENT. Decreased response of the adrenal cortex to ACTH establishes the diagnosis of Addison disease. The best screening test is the administration of synthetic ACTH (cosyntropin) 0.25 mg intramuscularly or intravenously, with measurement of plasma cortisol levels 30 to 60 minutes later. Cortisol levels double or increase by 10 μg/dl in normal subjects. Definitive evaluation is by prolonged (usually 24-hour) infusion of ACTH with assessment of either plasma cortisol excretion of cortisol or both.[100]

It is possible to differentiate primary adrenal insufficiency from secondary adrenal insufficiency, isolated hypoaldosteronism, or congenital adrenal hyperplasia because one of the adrenal hormonal functions is normal in each of the latter three conditions.

An increasingly common form of hypoaldosteronism is that associated with hyporeninism. Most commonly, this syndrome is observed in older diabetic patients with a mild degree of renal impairment and hypertension; acidosis is also common. Usually, these patients have unexplained hyperkalemia. The cause is unknown but may be secondary to damage to the juxtaglomerular apparatus and/or reduced conversion of a renin precursor into the active enzyme. This clinical syndrome is particularly important in the presence of cardiovascular disease. Furthermore, commonly used drugs (beta blockers and calcium antagonists) can exacerbate this condition by further compromising aldosterone release.[132]

Treatment of adrenal insufficiency is accomplished by replacement of the deficient steroid. In adults with primary or secondary insufficiency, hydrocortisone 20 to 30 mg daily is administered in divided doses, usually two-thirds in the morning and one-third in midafternoon. In patients with associated aldosterone deficiency, 9-alpha-fluorohydrocortisone 0.05 to 0.10 mg daily is given. During periods of significant stress (surgery, infection, or trauma), the glucocorticoid dose should be increased.

PHEOCHROMOCYTOMA
(see also Chap. 28)

Effects of Catecholamines on the Cardiovascular System

The adrenal medulla and sympathetic nervous system are linked morphologically, biochemically, and physiologically and are often referred to as the sympathoadrenal system.[133, 134] In addition to their important effects on the cardiovascular system, cathecholamines also have significant metabolic effects consisting of stimulation of glycogenolysis and gluconeogenesis, that is, increasing the production of glucose from glycogen and amino acid precursors and stimulating lipolysis.

CLINICAL AND BIOCHEMICAL MANIFESTATIONS. A pheochromocytoma is a catecholamine-producing tumor derived from chromaffin cells. Those arising from extraadrenal chromaffin cells are called nonadrenal pheochromocytomas or paraganglionomas. Rarely, these tumors occur in the heart or pericardium.[135, 136] Probably less than 0.1 percent of patients with hypertension have a pheochromocytoma. Although it is an uncommon disease, pheochromocytomas generate a great deal of interest, largely because of the significant morbidity and mortality associated with these tumors, with detection often resulting in cure. Pheochromocytomas are highly vascular tumors; less than 10 percent are malignant as indicated by local invasion or metastasis, but as with other endocrine tumors, malignancy cannot always be determined by microscopic appearance alone.

Although the vast majority of tumors occur sporadically, approximately 5 percent are inherited as an autosomal trait, by which they are often part of a pluriglandular neoplastic syndrome,[133, 134] which in addition to pheochromocytoma may consist of medullary carcinoma of the thyroid, parathyroidadenoma, and retinal or cerebellar hemangioblastomas. Most pheochromocytomas are solitary adrenal tumors, with 10 percent being bilateral and 10 percent nonadrenal. However, in the familial form of pheochromocytoma, nearly half of patients have bilateral adrenal tumors.

CARDIOVASCULAR MANIFESTATIONS. Hypertension is the major cardiovascular manifestation of pheochromocytoma. The features that suggest pheochromocytoma in hypertensive patients are (1) paroxysmal attacks of any kind, (2) headaches, (3) excessive sweating, (4) signs of hypermetabolism, (5) orthostatic hypotension, and (6) unusual blood pressure elevation as a result of trauma or surgery.[133, 134] Many of the features are similar to those of hyperthyroidism. Although paroxysmal attacks are the hallmark of pheochromocytoma, more than half the patients have fixed hypertension and nearly 10 percent are normotensive.

The lability of blood pressure in patients with pheochromocytoma has been suggested to be due not only to episodic discharge of catecholamines but also to a reduction in plasma volume, as well as impaired sympathetic reflexes. A number of observations suggest that chronic volume depletion is present.[137] For example, alpha adrenoceptor blockade or removal of the tumor produces severe hypotension, which is correctable by volume expansion.[133] Cardiac output has been reported to be normal, whereas the heart rate is increased and orthostatic hypotension is accompanied by decreased stroke volume and inadequate adjustments in peripheral resistance indicative of impaired peripheral vascular reflexes.[133] An occasional patient has markedly elevated central aortic pressure and severe systemic hypotension resulting from severe arterial vasoconstriction. Patients with pheochromocytoma may also have acute pulmonary edema.[138] Some patients with pheochromocytoma have hemodynamic features indistinguishable from those of essential hypertension. These results suggest that long-term exposure to high circulating levels of catecholamines may produce a different clinical picture than that observed after acute administration. These differences may be due to desensitization induced by chronic exposure to catecholamines.[137]

The electrocardiogram is abnormal in as many as 75 percent of patients with pheochromocytoma. Changes consist of T wave inversion, left ventricular hypertrophy, sinus tachycardia, and in some cases, other alterations in rhythm, such as frequent supraventricular ectopic beats or paroxysmal supraventricular tachycardia.[139, 140] An occasional patient has a short PR interval and a narrow QRS complex, which suggests that catecholamines are modifying the AV conduction system. When arterial pressure increases markedly, changes suggestive of myocardial damage are present, including transient ST segment elevations, marked diffuse T wave inversions, and depression of ST segments. These changes are usually transient, and the electrocardiographic pattern reverts to normal after removal of the tumor or pharmacological blockade.[134] However, the acute rise in blood pressure does not seem to be related to the development of complex arrhythmias. These hypertensive events are associated with a significant reduction in vagal tone. However, this finding is similar to what is observed in essential hypertension.[139] Some of the electrocardiographic abnormalities are presumably due to hypertensive heart disease or myocardial ischemia. However, a specific catecholamine-induced myocarditis and/or cardiomyopathy has also been suggested.[138, 141, 142] Interestingly, a patient with catecholamine-induced cardiomyopathy was treated with captopril, with resolution of the cardiomyopathy within 2 weeks.[143] In rats with pheochromocytoma, treatment with captopril also markedly attenuated the cardiomyopathy but did not modify contraction of isolated rings of the thoracic aorta in response to either epinephrine or angiotensin II.[144] The mechanism by which captopril produced these beneficial effects is unclear but could be related to inhibiting angiotensin II–induced cardiac fibrosis.[103]

The echocardiogram often shows left ventricular hypertrophy with normal left ventricular systolic function but occasionally mimics hypertrophic obstructive cardiomyopathy.[140] During a hypertensive crisis the electrocardiogram may show systolic anterior involvement of the anterior mitral leaflet, paradoxical septal motion, and proximal excursion of the posterior wall.

Myocarditis. Pathologically, the myocarditis consists of focal necrosis with infiltration of inflammatory cells, perivascular inflammation, and contraction band necrosis[133, 145, 146] (Fig. 64–8), finally resulting in fibrosis. In some studies, 50 percent of patients who died of pheochromocytoma had myocarditis, usually accompanied by left ventricular failure and pulmonary edema. Although coronary atherosclerosis is usually present, medial thickening is the most characteristic lesion of the coronary arteries. When norepinephrine is infused into the rabbit, sustained coro-

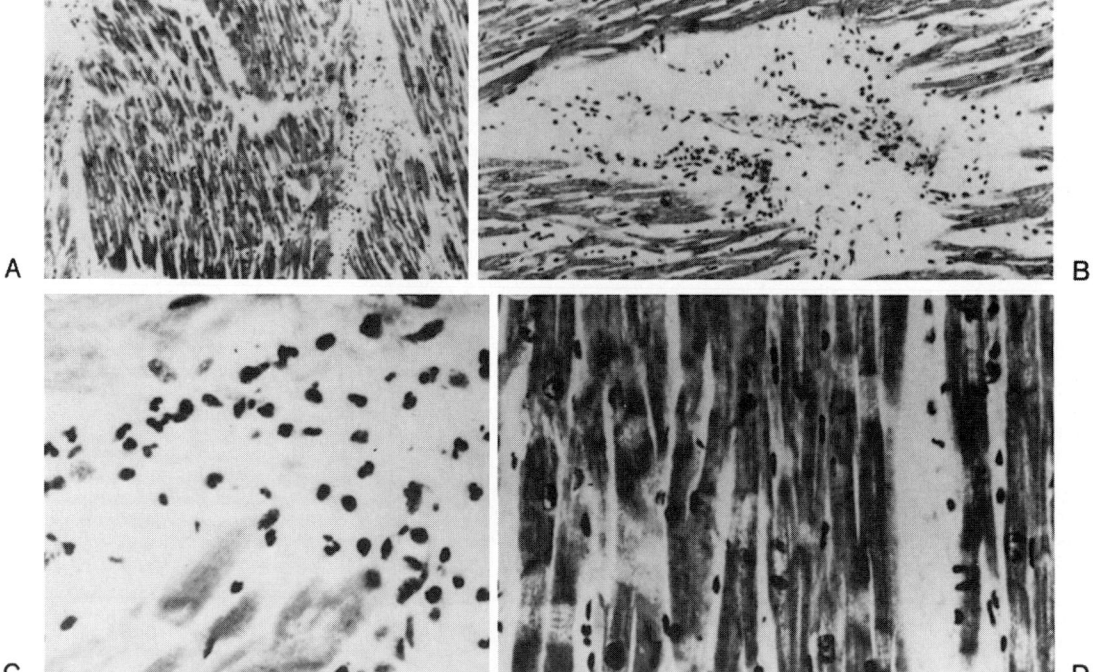

FIGURE 64–8. Left ventricular myocardium with acute myocarditis and contraction band necrosis in a patient with pheochromocytoma dying of catecholamine crisis. *A,* Diffuse infiltration by inflammatory cells through myocardium. *B,* Perivascular inflammation. *C,* Close-up of the inflammatory infiltrate. *D,* Contraction band necrosis of myocytes. Hematoxylin-eosin; original magnification ×20 (*A*), ×45 (*B*), ×540 (*C*), ×330 (*D*). (From McManus, BM, Fleury TA, Roberts WC: Fatal catecholamine crisis in pheochromocytoma: Curable cause of cardiac arrest. Am Heart J 102:930, 1981.)

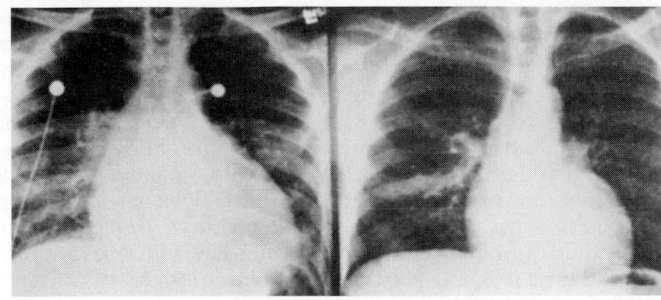

FIGURE 64–9. Pheochromocytoma-induced cardiomyopathy. *Left,* Chest x-ray on admission. Cardiomegaly, right pleural effusion, and signs of congestive heart failure are present. *Right,* One month after removal of the tumor, no signs of congestion and a significant decrease in heart size are noted. (From Velasquez G, D'Souza VJ, Hackshaw BT, et al: Phaeochromocytoma and cardiomyopathy. Br J Radiol 57:89, 1984.)

nary vasoconstriction occurs and within 48 hours leads to histologically documented myocardial damage.[147] Occasionally, patients with pheochromocytoma have manifestations of cardiomyopathy that may be reversed when the tumor is removed (Fig. 64–9). The myositis is not necessarily limited to the myocardium; it may also occur in skeletal muscle.[148]

DIAGNOSIS AND TREATMENT. The diagnosis of pheochromocytoma is established by documenting increased urinary or plasma levels of catecholamines or one of their metabolites.[133] Three tests are commonly used: (1) total catecholamines, (2) vanillylmandelic acid, and (3) metanephrine. The last two are metabolites of catecholamine and were first used to screen for phcochromocytoma because they are present in greater quantities. When reliably performed, these tests are probably equivalent in accuracy. The probability of pheochromocytoma being present in a hypertensive patient with a single normal urine level is less than 5 percent. It is most desirable to measure both the catecholamines and one of the two metabolites, preferably metanephrine, when screening for pheochromocytoma. If the blood pressure fluctuates, it is particularly important to collect the urine at a time when the pressure is elevated. Chromogranin A blood levels are another potential screening test for pheochromocytoma. Chromogranin A is a cosecretory product from neuroendocrine tumors and does not have a known biological effect. Reliability, sensitivity, and precision estimates in comparison to urine hormonal measurements have not yet been reported, however.[149] Specific pharmacological tests to screen for pheochromocytoma are of limited benefit, usually hazardous, and therefore warranted only in unusual circumstances. Clonidine has been proposed as a useful definitive test for pheochromocytoma, although it is necessary only in unusual cases. Catecholamine levels are suppressed in normal subjects via stimulation of central alpha adrenoceptors; after clonidine administration in patients with pheochromocytoma, however, catecholamine levels are not suppressed.[150] Unfortunately, profound and prolonged hypotension has been reported in some patients during the course of this test.

Once the diagnosis of pheochromocytoma is established, specific pharmacological blockade should be initiated.[133] Administration of phenoxybenzamine hydrochloride should be begun, with the initial dosage being 10 mg every 12 hours; the dose is then gradually increased every 2 to 3 days until arterial pressure is restored to normal. Alternatively, prazosin may be used. However, it should be noted that alpha adrenoceptor blockade may induce a decline in arterial pressure accompanied by serious postural hypotension, presumably because of the vasodilation occurring in the presence of hypovolemia. This hypotensive response can be prevented by adequate sodium intake; if the re-

sponse is very striking, infusion of saline may be required. Adequate control of arterial pressure is essential before any arteriographic procedure, before initiating beta adrenoceptor blockade, and before surgery. Calcium antagonists may be useful both in treating the hypertension associated with pheochromocytoma and in reducing catecholamine production.

Beta adrenoceptor blockade is useful in patients with pheochromocytoma who have significant tachycardia, palpitations, and catecholamine-induced arrhythmias. However, beta blockade with a drug affecting $beta_2$ receptors must not be initiated prior to inadequate alpha blockade since severe *hypertension* may occur as a result of unopposed alpha-stimulating activity of the circulating catecholamines.

Definitive treatment is surgical removal of the tumor, usually after localization with computed tomography, arteriography, or scanning with a radioactive iodide derivative of guanethidine as the scanning agent.[151, 152] Scanning may be particularly important in localizing extraadrenal, e.g., thoracic, pheochromocytomas. Precise definition of the anatomical boundaries of this tumor is important preoperatively if surgery is to be successful.[153] In patients with inoperable lesions, long-term use of a combination of alpha and beta adrenoceptor blockers has been helpful. Drugs that inhibit the biosynthesis of catecholamines, such as alphamethyltyrosine, and generalized chemotherapeutic agents have also been used in patients with malignant pheochromocytoma.[154] Although rare, of particular importance to the cardiologist is the presence of a cardiac pheochromocytoma.[135, 136, 153]

PARATHYROID DISEASE

Disordered parathyroid secretion is associated with two cardiovascular disturbances: cardiac arrhythmias and hypertension. Changes in calcium metabolism, as well as a direct effect of parathyroid hormone (PTH) on the cardiovascular system, appear to be responsible.

CLINICAL AND BIOCHEMICAL MANIFESTATIONS. PTH is a single-chain polypeptide of 84 amino acids. Its major biological effect is to increase mobilization of calcium into the extracellular fluid from a variety of tissues; this action is linked in a negative feedback loop with the serum unbound calcium concentration. Thus, an increase in serum calcium concentration reduces PTH release and vice versa.[155] PTH also increases urinary excretion of phosphate, augments bone resorption, and reduces the urinary excretion of calcium.

Primary hyperparathyroidism, the excess production of PTH, is usually secondary to a solitary parathyroid adenoma. Occasionally, generalized parathyroid hyperplasia exists, and infrequently, carcinoma of the parathyroid gland is found. The signs and symptoms of primary hyperparathyroidism are related to the direct effects of PTH on kidney or bone or those associated with the hypercalcemia. Nearly half the patients have signs and symptoms of renal dysfunction, such as polyuria, nocturia, renal stones, and in severe cases, nephrocalcinosis and renal failure.

Cardiac hypertrophy is found with increased frequency in patients with hyperparathyroidism, even in the absence of hypertension. In one study, 5 of 18 patients with hypertrophic cardiomyopathy had raised serum PTH levels but normal serum calcium levels. In contrast, left ventricular hypertrophy did not occur in 6 patients with hypercalcemia alone.[155]

Cardiovascular Manifestations of Parathyroid Diseases

CARDIAC EFFECTS. Although most of the effects of PTH on the heart are probably secondary to a change in extracellular calcium, PTH also has direct effects on the heart that result in an increased beating rate of isolated heart cells and positive inotropic action.[156–160] These effects are probably mediated by PTH binding to specific receptors, which leads to increased entry of calcium into cardiac cells, and by PTH increasing the release of endogenous myocardial norepinephrine. The direct effect of PTH may be deleteri-

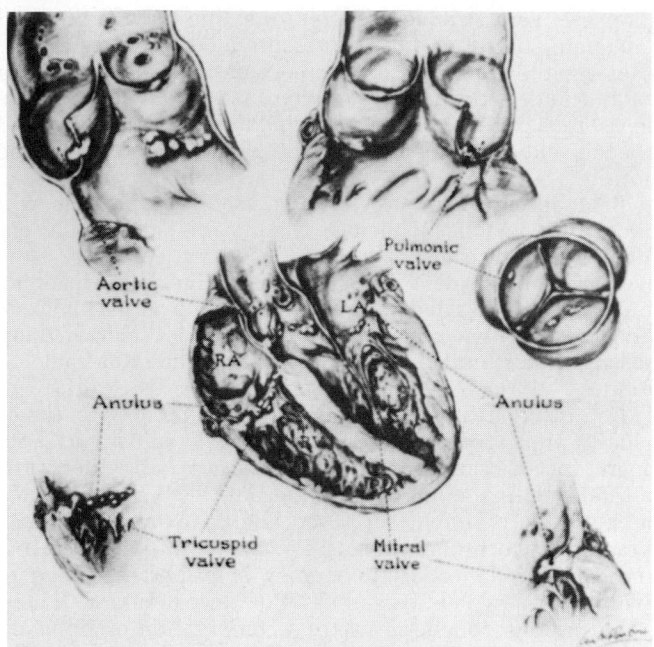

FIGURE 64–10. Heart showing the distribution of calcific deposits in the tricuspid and mitral valve annuli and at the bases of both pulmonic and aortic valve cusps in a 43-year-old woman with hypercalcemia secondary to primary hyperparathyroidism. (From Roberts WC, Waller BF: Effect of chronic hypercalcemia on the heart: An analysis of 18 necropsy patients. Am J Med 71:371, 1981.)

ous because it causes necrosis of rat myocytes and may be directly responsible for the increased accumulation of calcium in dystrophic muscles and for the heart damage found in uremia. On the other hand, hypoparathyroidism may cause a dilated cardiomyopathy, presumably secondary to the hypocalcemia.[161, 162] However, because longstanding hypocalcemia does not necessarily produce left ventricular dysfunction,[163] hypomagnesemia and reduced circulating PTH may also be involved. PTH also has a direct effect on vascular smooth muscle and causes vasodilation.

Chronic hypercalcemia from a variety of causes is associated with increased deposition of calcium in the fibrous skeleton of the heart and valvular cusps, as well as in coronary arteries and myocardial fibers[164] (Fig. 64–10). Chronic hypercalcemia may also be a risk factor for accelerated coronary atherosclerosis.[162]

The plateau of the action potential of cardiac fibers is prolonged by low and shortened by high extracellular calcium concentrations (see Chap. 22). The changes in duration of the action potential are accompanied by corresponding changes in duration of the refractory period, the ST segment, and the QT interval. Thus, the major electrocardiographic change in hypercalcemia is shortening of the QT interval. Less frequently, disorders of intraventricular conduction have been reported with shortening of the PR interval. Complete heart block occurs only rarely.

Hypocalcemia produces the opposite effect on the electrocardiogram: prolongation of the QT interval and nonspecific ST and T wave changes. Normal contractile function of cardiac muscle requires calcium, and heart failure has been reported in patients with chronic hypocalcemia secondary to hypoparathyroidism.[165]

HYPERTENSION. Hypercalcemic patients detected by routine serum calcium screening techniques have higher arterial pressure than do matched normocalcemic subjects.[162] Yet in patients with hyperparathyroidism, the level of serum calcium is similar in those who are normotensive and those who have hypertension, which suggests that hypercalcemia per se is not the dominant cause of the hyper-

tension. Thus, the pathophysiology of the hypertension is uncertain and may be multifactorial.[166–168] Hypercalcemia produces nephrocalcinosis, which may lead to renal failure and hypertension. Thus, reversal of hypertension after successful parathyroid surgery is more likely to occur when renal function is normal. Increased serum calcium also increases myocardial contractility, peripheral resistance, and release of or vascular sensitivity to vasoconstrictor agents such as angiotensin II and norepinephrine. Although hypercalcemia can increase cardiac contractility and arterial pressure acutely, it is unlikely that this action produces a significant alteration in cardiac output or performance on a long-term basis in the absence of PTH. Thus, elevated peripheral resistance is the most likely cause of the hypertension associated with hyperparathyroidism. Although PTH itself is a vasodilator, except subacutely,[166] characteristic changes in other hormones that occur in hyperparathyroidism may contribute to the hypertension. For example, PTH increases 1-alpha-hydroxylation of 25(OH) vitamin D, thereby leading to higher levels of 1,25(OH)$_2$ vitamin D. 1,25(OH)$_2$ vitamin D enhances vascular reactivity,[169] and the higher levels in hyperparathyroidism could contribute to hypertension. Finally, a circulating hypertensive factor produced in the parathyroid gland has been identified and termed "parathyroid hypertensive factor" (PHF).[170, 171] PHF is distinct from PTH and has the ability to increase the intracellular calcium concentration in vascular smooth muscle cells primarily via opening L-type calcium channels.[172] PHF was first found in the parathyroid glands of spontaneously hypertensive rats,[171] but it has since been found in the circulation of essential hypertensives, especially those who are salt sensitive and have low renin levels.[173] Elevated levels have been reported to predict a beneficial response to calcium channel blockers.[174] However, further support for the existence and physiological role of PHF is required.

DIAGNOSIS AND TREATMENT

An elevated or even a normal concentration of PTH in the presence of hypercalcemia establishes the diagnosis of hyperparathyroidism; many patients with this condition manifest hypercalcemia for the first time after starting thiazide therapy for the associated hypertension. Treatment consists of surgical removal of the parathyroid tumor or hyperplastic glands.

Patients with hypertension should have a determination of serum calcium levels before therapy is begun. If thiazide diuretics are used in treatment, serum calcium levels should be determined every 6 months. If thiazide-induced hypercalcemia occurs, serum calcium should be determined for 2 to 3 months after discontinuation of thiazide treatment. Persistence of the hypercalcemia suggests that the patient has primary hyperparathyroidism.[165]

Patients with hypoparathyroidism and hypocalcemia are usually treated with calcium supplementation and vitamin D or one of its metabolites such as calcitriol (1,25-dihydroxyvitamin D).

GONADAL HORMONES AND THE CARDIOVASCULAR SYSTEM

Estrogen
(see also Chap. 58)

The past several years have witnessed an explosion in the investigation of estrogen's effects on the cardiovascular system. It has long been observed that premenopausal women enjoy protection against cardiovascular disease and that this protection is lost at menopause. Based on this observation, it has been hypothesized that it is the loss of estradiol with menopause that is responsible for the loss of cardiovascular protection. It has therefore been postulated that giving postmenopausal women estrogen as hormone replacement therapy would reduce cardiovascular risk. The role of estrogen in cardiovascular protection remains controversial.

Several mechanisms that involve different systems have been proposed to explain the cardiovascular benefit induced by estrogen.[175] Some of these mechanisms include alterations in lipid metabolism and coagulation, as well as direct vascular effects. Oral estrogen increases HDL and lowers LDL cholesterol. This potential benefit appears to account for only 30 percent of the benefit seen. More recently, the effect of estrogen on coagulation has been investigated, and it has been shown that estrogen lowers levels of plasminogen activator inhibitor type I, thereby leading to more fibrinolysis. Estrogen causes vasodilation of both peripheral vessels and coronary arteries. Most of this effect appears to be mediated by the vascular endothelium and release of nitric oxide.

Observational studies have demonstrated a decrease in cardiac risk factors in postmenopausal women taking estrogen. The Rancho Bernado study of 1057 postmenopausal women showed that estrogen users were more likely than nonusers to have lower weight, diastolic blood pressure, fasting insulin, and total cholesterol, with higher HDL cholesterol.[176] A similar benefit in altering cardiovascular risk factors was seen in the Atherosclerosis Risk in Community study of 4958 postmenopausal women.[177]

Furthermore, observational studies have demonstrated a reduction in coronary heart disease in postmenopausal women who use estrogen. The Nurses Health Study of 48,470 postmenopausal women monitored for up to 10 years demonstrated that the use of estrogen was associated with a relative risk of 0.56 for major coronary disease and 0.72 for death from cardiovascular disease.[178]

Despite the mechanistic and epidemiological data supporting a cardiovascular benefit of estrogen, the only published randomized prospective study showed no benefit on coronary heart disease prevention. The Heart and Estrogen/Progestin Replacement Study (HERS) studied 2763 postmenopausal women with a prior history of coronary heart disease in a prospective secondary prevention trial. With an average follow-up of 4 years, no reduction in cardiovascular events was seen in the group of women receiving estrogen (0.625 mg conjugated equine estrogen) given in combination with medroxyprogesterone (2.5 mg).[179] Whether estrogen is beneficial as primary prevention should be answered by the ongoing Women's Health Initiative.[180] In addition, whether other estrogens or combinations with other progestins will provide a benefit remains to be determined.

Selective Estrogen Receptor Modulators

Because concern about an increased risk for breast cancer is a major deterrent to estrogen use, the class of drugs termed selective estrogen receptor modulators (SERMs) has been developed. These drugs do not bind well to the breast or uterine estrogen receptor. The effects that they will have on cardiovascular disease are not known as yet. The first drug of this class in common use was tamoxifen, which has been used primarily in the treatment of breast cancer. Several studies of tamoxifen in the treatment of breast cancer have shown a decrease in either fatal myocardial infarction or hospital admissions for cardiac disease.[181, 182] Caution must be used in viewing these results since the studies were not designed to look at heart disease as a primary endpoint. Tamoxifen has been shown to lower LDL cholesterol as a potential mechanism for its cardiovascular benefit.[183] The only other SERM now approved for use is raloxifene, which is indicated for the prevention and treatment for osteoporosis. Raloxifene lowers LDL cholesterol without increasing HDL cholesterol.[184] Whether raloxifene will have any benefit on cardiovascular morbidity or mortality is currently under investigation.

Oral Contraceptives

The literature on the association between oral contraceptive use and coronary heart disease is controversial. The controversy is due in large part to the decreasing estrogen content in oral contraceptives over the past 40 years, as well as the incorporation of varying progestins with different androgenic potencies. The changing spectrum of oral contraceptive composition also makes it difficult to extend data based on earlier agents to today's preparations. Several studies have shown an increased risk of myocardial infarction in oral contraceptive users.[185] However, prior oral contraceptive use does not confer an increased risk for cardiovascular disease. Studies of the effect of newer contraceptive agents are not available.[186]

BLOOD PRESSURE EFFECTS OF ORAL CONTRACEPTIVES AND HORMONAL REPLACEMENT THERAPY

Oral contraceptive use has been associated with a rise in blood pressure since their widespread use in the 1960s. When blood pressure rises, it usually remains within the normotensive range; rarely, it increases into the hypertensive (> 140/90 mm Hg) range. Even with the earlier-generation oral contraceptives, which used a higher estrogen dose and varied progestins, data were conflicting regarding whether whether blood pressure rises.[187-189] Differences in responses to oral contraceptives may depend on the quantity of estrogen, the type of progestin, and the race and genetic background of the user. Studies of the new generation of oral contraceptives, which contain no greater than 35 μg ethinyl estradiol and less androgenic progestins, are more limited. Available data on desogestrel-containing oral contraceptives include a multicenter trial of more than 1600 women monitored over 23,000 cycles. No significant change in mean blood pressure over a 2-year period of use was observed, and only a 0.3 percent incidence of hypertension was noted.[190] Other studies of this agent have revealed similar results.[191, 192] Although activation of the renin-angiotensin-aldosterone axis occurs in oral contraceptive users, the degree of activation may be greater in those who remain normotensive than those who became hypertensive. Thus, the etiology of oral contraceptive–induced hypertension remains unclear.

The belief that estrogens used for hormone replacement therapy induce hypertension is largely based on the older oral contraceptive literature. In fact, the use of estrogen in many trials is associated with no change in blood pressure. It is likely that estrogens differ in their effect on blood pressure. Estrone and estradiol, natural estrogens, may actually lead to a fall in blood pressure.

ANDROGENS AND THE HEART. Similar to the view that women are protected against cardiovascular disease because of estrogen, it has been assumed that the increased incidence of cardiovascular disease in men is in part related to testosterone levels. However, studies designed to examine this link, although limited in number and size, have instead suggested that testosterone has a neutral or perhaps even beneficial effect on cardiovascular risk in men.

Observational studies have failed to show a positive relationship between testosterone levels and cardiovascular disease in men. Several studies of over 3000 men in different countries have shown no relationship between baseline testosterone levels and the future development of cardiovascular disease in men.[193, 194] Since these studies are cross-sectional, it is possible that the lower testosterone levels are a consequence of the coronary heart disease, not a cause.

Unfortunately, at this time, few intervention studies are available to help determine the cause-and-effect relationship. In a study of 62 men with a history of angina, men were randomized to receive placebo or oral testosterone. Of note, the serum testosterone levels of these men were normal, but significantly lower than controls at baseline. The group that received testosterone had a significant reduction in anginal symptoms and improvement in ST segment changes on electrocardiographic and Holter monitoring.[195] A more recent study evaluated the effect of acute intravenous testosterone on 14 men with a history of angina and angiographically proven coronary artery disease and low serum testosterone levels. In this study, the time to ST segment depression on exercise tolerance tests was prolonged by 20 percent in men receiving testosterone versus placebo.[196]

CARDIOVASCULAR CONSEQUENCES OF OBESITY

The prevalence of obesity is increasing in many developing countries and in the United States. Estimates based on the

National Health and Nutritional Examination Survey III study indicate that as of 1994, 33 percent of the U.S. population was obese,[197] and this percentage is predicted to steadily increase. Obesity is associated with higher levels of blood pressure, dyslipidemia, and type II diabetes mellitus, all contributors to cardiovascular disease. However, in addition, obesity appears to be an independent predictor of coronary artery disease in both men and women.[198, 199] Recent studies indicate that it is not just obesity that is associated with increased cardiovascular disease, but that upper body obesity further increases the risk.[200]

Evidence of circulatory dysfunction in the massively obese, in association with cardiac enlargement during life and at autopsy, was first described by Smith and Willius in 1933.[201] Cardiac changes in obesity may often be related to concomitant hypertension. The elevated leptin levels seen in obesity may be mediators of the hypertensive process.[201a] Left ventricular hypertrophy also may be present in the absence of systemic hypertension.[202] Right ventricular hypertrophy may also be seen, most commonly as a result of obesity-related obstructive sleep apnea and pulmonary hypertension. Much of the cardiovascular risk associated with obesity is probably associated with the concomitant insulin resistance (see Chap. 63).

TREATMENT OF THE CARDIOVASCULAR MANIFESTATIONS OF OBESITY. Although weight reduction would seem to be the most beneficial treatment of cardiovascular disease in obesity, conclusive longitudinal studies are lacking. However, with weight reduction often comes improvement in the hypertension, dyslipidemia, and insulin resistance seen in obesity. Weight reduction is also associated with regression of left ventricular hypertrophy independent of blood pressure changes,[203] as well as shortening of the prolonged QT_c seen in obese patients.[204]

CARDIAC COMPLICATIONS OF WEIGHT LOSS. Rapid weight loss has been associated with cardiac arrhythmias and sudden death.[205] In some cases, these complications are probably secondary to inadequate electrolyte supplementation. In others, they may be related to a reduction in myocardial protein and cardiac atrophy. Although initially associated with a liquid protein diet, sudden death may occur under any circumstance associated with rapid weight loss.[206]

MALNUTRITION

Malnutrition, particularly protein-calorie deficiency, is prevalent in many underdeveloped areas of the world. However, in recent years, it has also become a concern in developed countries in individuals who have chronic diseases, in whom it exists as a result of both anorexia and hypermetabolism, and in otherwise healthy individuals with anorexia nervosa.

CARDIAC CHANGES IN MALNUTRITION. The circulatory status of patients with severe nutritional depletion and electrolyte imbalance is precarious: Cardiac output, systolic pressure, and pulse pressure are abnormally low, and massive, generalized edema may be present; the PR interval may be shortened. Loss of subcutaneous fat may be observed, as well as general wasting and atrophy of most organs, including the heart, which is thin walled, pale, and flabby on gross examination. Histological study reveals atrophy of muscle fibers. Treatment of a dehydrated or severely anemic patient with protein-calorie malnutrition involves correction of hematological, fluid, and electrolyte imbalance. Congestive heart failure can be avoided if care is taken to avoid overloading with sodium, water, or blood.

ANOREXIA NERVOSA. This common psychiatric condition, seen particularly in young women, is associated with significant cardiac morbidity and mortality. Many of the cardiac changes relate to protein-calorie malnutrition, including destruction of cardiac myofibrils.[207] Echocardiographic findings include small ventricular chamber size and mass, even when corrected for weight, reduced cardiac index, and abnormalities in mitral valve function.[208] Hypocalcemia and hypomagnesemia may contribute to arrhythmias, heart failure, and sudden death since bradycardia thought to be secondary to increased vagal tone is common. QT_c prolongation can also be seen and may indicate a predisposition to arrhythmias and sudden death. Predictors of QT_c prolongation are weight, body mass index, and rapidity of weight loss even in the absence of electrolyte disturbances.[209]

REFERENCES

1. Graves RJ: Clinical lectures. London Med Surg J (Part II) 7:516, 1835.
2. Addison T: On the Constitutional and Local Effects of Diseases of the Suprarenal Capsules. London, Highley, 1855.

ACROMEGALY

3. Thorner MO, Vance ML, Laws ER Jr, et al: The anterior pituitary. *In* Wilson JD, Foster DW, Kronenberg HM, et al (eds): Williams Textbook of Endocrinology. 9th ed. Philadelphia, WB Saunders, 1998, p 249.
4. Strob JS, Thomas MJ: Human growth hormone. Pharmacol Rev 46:1, 1994.
5. Hartman ML, Veldhuis JD, Thorner MO: Normal control of growth hormone secretion. Horm Res 40:37, 1993.
6. Wass JAH: Somatostatin. *In* DeGrool LJ, Besser M, Burger HG, et al (eds): Endocrinology. Vol 1. 3rd ed. Philadelphia, WB Saunders, 1995, p 266.
7. Pong SS, Chaung LYP, Dean DC, et al: Identification of a new G-protein–linked receptor for growth hormone secretagogues. Mol Endocrinol 10:57, 1996.
8. Scopinschi G, Vanonderbertgen A, Lhermitebaleriaux M, et al: Effects of a 7-day treatment with a novel, orally active, growth hormone (GH) secretagogue, MK-677, on 24-hour GH profiles, insulin-like growth factor I, and adrenocortical function in normal young men. J Clin Endocrinol Metab 81:2776, 1996.
9. Chapman IM, Bach MA, Van Cauter E, et al: Stimulation of the growth hormone (GH)–insulin-like growth factor I axis by daily oral administration of a GH secretagogue (MK-677) in healthy elderly subjects. J Clin Endocrinol Metab 81:4249, 1996.
10. Menon RK, Stephan DA, Singh M, et al: Cloning of the promoter-regulatory region of the murine growth hormone receptor gene. Identification of a developmentally regulated enhancer element. J Biol Chem 270:8851, 1995.
11. Carter-Su C, Schwartz J, Smit LS: Molecular mechanism of growth hormone action. Annu Rev Physiol 58:187, 1996.
12. Oh Y, Muller H, Neely EK, et al: New concepts in insulin-like growth factor receptor physiology. Growth Regul 3:113, 1993.
13. Jones JI, Clemmons DR: The insulin-like growth factors and their binding proteins: Biologic actions. Endocr Rev 16:3, 1995.
14. Froesch ER, Zenobi PD, Hussain M: Metabolic and therapeutic effects of insulin-like growth factor I. Horm Res 42:66, 1994.
15. Lombardi G, Colao A, Ferone D, et al: Effect of growth hormone on cardiac function. Horm Res 48 (Suppl)4:38, 1997.
16. Sacca L, Cittadini A, Fazio S: Growth hormone and the heart. Endocr Rev 15:55, 1994.
17. Caidahl K, Eden S, Bengtsson BA: Cardiovascular and renal effects of growth hormone. Clin Endocrinol 40:393, 1994.
18. Greco AV, Ghirlanda G, Barona C, et al: Somatostatin in the paroxysmal supraventricular and junctional tachycardia. BMJ 288:28, 1984.
19. Ezzat S, Forster MJ, Berchtold P, et al: Acromegaly. Clinical and biochemical features in 500 patients. Medicine (Baltimore) 73:233, 1994.
20. Fazio S, Cittadini A, Cuocolo A, et al: Impaired cardiac performance is a distinct feature of uncomplicated acromegaly. J Clin Endocrinol Metab 79:441, 1994.
21. Hradec J, Marek J, Kral J, et al: Long-term echocardiography follow-up of acromegalic heart disease. Am J Cardiol 72:204, 1993.
22. Cuocolo A, Nicolai E, Fazio S, et al: Impaired left ventricular diastolic filling in patients with acromegaly: Assessment with radionuclide angiography. J Nucl Med 36:196, 1995.
23. Minniti G, Moroni C, Jaffrain-Rea ML, et al: Prevalence of hypertension in acromegalic patients: Clinical measurement versus 24-hour ambulatory blood pressure monitoring. Clin Endocrinol 48:149, 1998.
24. Kraatz C, Benker G, Weber F, et al: Acromegaly and hypertension: Prevalence and relationship to the renin-angiotensin-aldosterone system. Klin Wochenschr 68:583, 1990.
25. Lopez-Velasco R, Escobar-Morreale HF, Vega B, et al: Cardiac involvement in acromegaly: Specific myocardiopathy or consequence of systemic hypertension? J Clin Endocrinol Metab 82:1047, 1997.
26. Kahaly G, Olshausen KV, Mohr-Kahaly S, et al: Arrhythmia profile in acromegaly. Eur Heart J 13:51, 1992.
27. Aono J, Nobuoka S, Nagashima J, et al: Heart failure in 3 patients with acromegaly: Echocardiographic assessment. Intern Med 37:599, 1998.
28. Ozbey N, Oncul A, Bugra Z, et al: Acromegalic cardiomyopathy: Evaluation of the left ventricular diastolic function in the subclinical stage. J Endocrinol Invest 20:305, 1997.
29. Fazio S, Cittadini A, Sabatini D, et al: Evidence for biventricular involvement in acromegaly: A Doppler echocardiographic study. Eur Heart J 14:26, 1993.
30. Chanson P, Timsit J, Masquet C, et al: Cardiovascular effects of the somatostatin analog octreotide in acromegaly. Ann Intern Med 113:921, 1990.
31. Lim MJ, Barkan AL, Buda AJ: Rapid reduction of left ventricular hypertrophy in acromegaly after suppression of growth hormone hypersecretion. Ann Intern Med 117:719, 1992.
32. Merola B, Cittadini A, Colao A, et al: Chronic treatment with the somatostatin analog octreotide improves cardiac abnormalities in acromegaly. J Clin Endocrinol Metab 77:790, 1993.

33. Nishiki M, Murakami Y, Sohmiya M, et al: Histopathological improvement of acromegalic cardiomyopathy by intermittent subcutaneous infusion of octreotide. Endocr J 44:655, 1997.

34. Rossi E, Zuppi P, Pennestri F, et al: Acromegalic cardiomyopathy. Left ventricular filling and hypertrophy in active and surgically treated disease. Chest 102:1204, 1992.

THYROID DISEASE

35. Dillmann WH: Biochemical basis of thyroid hormone action in the heart. Am J Med 88:626, 1990.

36. Polikar R, Burger AG, Scherrer U, Nicod P: The thyroid and the heart. Circulation 87:1435, 1993.

37. Davis PJ, Davis FB: Acute cellular actions of thyroid hormone and myocardial function. Ann Thorac Surg 56(Suppl):16, 1993.

38. Dillmann WH: Cardiac function in thyroid disease: Clinical features and management considerations. Ann Thorac Surg 56(Suppl):9, 1993.

39. Lazar MA: Thyroid hormone receptors: Multiple forms, multiple possibilities. Endocrinol Rev. 14:184, 1993.

40. Tsai MJ, O'Malley BW: Molecular mechanisms of action of steroid/thyroid receptor superfamily members. Annu Rev Biochem 63:451, 1994.

41. Tsika RW, Bahl JJ, Leinwand LA, Morkin E: Thyroid hormone regulates expression of a transfected human α-myosin heavy chain fusion gene in fetal rat heart cells. Proc Natl Acad Sci U S A 87:379, 1990.

42. Zarain-Herzberg A, Marques J, Sukovich D, Pariasmy M: Thyroid hormone receptor modulates the expression of the rabbit cardiac sarco (endo) plasmic reticulum Ca(2+)-ATPase gene. J Biol Chem 269:1460, 1994.

43. Orlowski J, Lingrell JB: Thyroid and glucocorticoid hormones regulate the expression of multiple Na, K-ATPase genes in cultured neonatal rat cardiac myocyte. J Biol Chem 265:3462, 1990.

44. Bahouth SW: Thyroid hormones transcriptionally regulate the β-1 adrenergic receptor gene in cultured ventricular myocyte. J Biol Chem 266:15863, 1991.

45. Castello A, Rodriguez-Manazaneque JC, Camps M, et al: Perinatal hypothyroidism impairs the normal transition of GLUT4 and GLUT1 glucose transporters from fetal to neonatal levels in heart and brown adipose tissue. Evidence for tissue-specific regulation of GLUT4 expression by thyroid hormone. J Biol Chem 269:5905, 1994.

46. Averyhart-Fullard V, Fraker LD, Murphy AM, Solaro RJ: Differential regulation of slow-skeletal and cardiac troponin I mRNA during development and by thyroid hormone in rat heart. J Mol Cell Cardiol 26:609, 1994.

47. Dieckman LJ, Solaro RJ: Effect of thyroid status on thin-filament Ca^{2+} regulation and expression of troponin I in perinatal and adult rat hearts. Circ Res 67:344, 1990.

48. Fullerton MJ, Stuchbury S, Krozowski ZS, Funder JW: Altered thyroidal status and the in vivo synthesis of atrial natriuretic peptide in the rat heart. Mol Cell Endocrinol 69:227, 1990.

49. Dillmann WH: Thyroid hormones and the heart: Basic mechanistic and clinical issues. Thyroid Today 19:1, 1996.

50. Segal J: Calcium is the first messenger for the action of thyroid hormone at the level of the plasma membrane: First evidence for an acute effect of thyroid hormone on calcium uptake in the heart. Endocrinology 126:2693, 1990.

51. Morgan JP: Thyroid hormone effects on intracellular calcium and inotropic responses of rat ventricular myocardium. Am J Physiol 267:H1112, 1994.

52. Han J, Leem C, So L, et al: Effects of thyroid hormone on the calcium current and isoprenaline-induced background current in rabbit ventricular myocytes. J Mol Cell Cardiol 26:925, 1994.

53. Levey GS, Klein L: Catecholamine-thyroid interactions and the cardiovascular manifestation of hyperthyroidism. Am J Med 88:642, 1990.

54. Rutherford JP, Vatner SF, Braunwald E: Adrenergic control of myocardial contractility in conscious hyperthyroid dogs. Am J Physiol 237:590, 1980.

55. Anderson RGG, Nilsson OR, Kuo JF: β-Adrenoreceptor adenosine 3'-5'-monophosphate system in human leukocytes before and after treatment for hyperthyroidism. J Clin Endocrinol Metab 56:42, 1993.

56. Bahouth SW: Regulation of steady-state levels of beta-adrenergic receptors and G-proteins by thyroid hormones in cultured rat myocardial cells. FASEB J 4:A1779, 1990.

57. Levine MA, Feldman AM, Robishaw JD, et al: Influence of thyroid hormone status on expression of genes encoding G protein subunits in the rat heart. J Biol Chem 265:3553, 3560, 1990.

58. Rapiojko PJ, Watkins DC, Ros M, Malbon CC: Thyroid hormones regulate G-protein beta-subunit mRNA expression in vivo. J Biol Chem 264:16183, 1989.

59. Goto Y, Slinker BK, LeWinter MM: Decreased contractile efficiency and increased nonmechanical energy cost in hyperthyroid rabbit heart: Relation between O$_2$ consumption and systolic pressure-volume area or force-time interval. Circ Res 66:999, 1990.

60. Ladenson PW, Sherman SI, Baughman KL, et al: Reversible alterations in myocardial gene expression in a young man with dilated cardiomyopathy. Proc Natl Acad Sci U S A 89:5251, 1992.

61. Kim D, Smith TW, Marsh JD: Effect of thyroid hormone on slow calcium channel function in cultured chick ventricular cells. J Clin Invest 80:88, 1987.

62. MacKinnon R, Gwathmey JK, Allen PD, et al: Modulation by the state of intracellular calcium and contractility in ferret ventricular muscle. Circ Res 63:1080, 1988.

63. Korecky B, Zak R, Schwartz K, et al: Role of thyroid hormone in regulation of isomyosin composition, contractility, and size of heterotypically isotransplanted rat heart. Circ Res 60:824, 1987.

64. Dudley SC Jr, Baumgarten CM: Bursting of cardiac sodium channels after acute exposure to 3,5,3'-triiodo-L-thyronine. Circ Res 73:301, 1993.

65. Shimoni Y, Severson DL: Thyroid status and potassium currents in rat ventricular myocyte. Am J Physiol 268:H576, 1995.

66. Shimoni Y, Banno H: Thyroxine effects on temperature dependence of ionic currents in single rabbit cardiac myocytes. Am J Physiol 265:H1875, 1993.

67. Gotzsche BH: L-Triiodothyronine acutely increases Ca(2+)-uptake in the isolated, perfuse rat heart. Changes in L-type C(2+)-channels and beta-receptors during short- and long-term hyper- and hypothyroidism. Eur J Endocrinol 130:171, 1994.

68. Larsen, PR, Davies TF, Hay ID: The thyroid gland. In Wilson JD, Foster DW, Kronenberg HM, et al (eds): Williams Textbook of Endocrinology. 9th ed. Philadelphia, WB Saunders, 1998, p 389.

69. Woeber KA: Thyrotoxicosis and the heart. N Engl J Med 327:94, 1992.

70. Olshausen K, Bischoll S, Kahaly G, et al: Cardiac arrhythmias and heart rate in hyperthyroidism. Am J Cardiol 63:930, 1989.

71. Goel BG, Hanson CS, Han J: A-V conduction in hyper- and hypothyroid dogs. Am Heart J 83:504, 1972.

72. Seibers MJ, Drinka PJ, Vergauwen C: Hyperthyroidism as a cause of atrial fibrillation in long-term care. Arch Intern Med 152:2063, 1992.

73. Cavallo A, Joseph CJ, Casta A: Cardiac complications in juvenile hyperthyroidism. Am J Dis Child 138:479, 1984.

74. Ebisawa K, Ikeda U, Maruta M, et al: Irreversible cardiomyopathy due to thyrotoxicosis. Cardiology 84:274, 1994.

75. Wilson R, Gibson TC, Terrien CM, Levy AM: Hyperthyroidism and familial hypertrophic cardiomyopathy. Arch Intern Med 143:378, 1983.

76. Klein I, Becken DV, Levey GS: Treatment of hyperthyroid disease. Ann Intern Med 121:281, 1994.

77. Geffner DL, Hershman JM: β-Adrenergic blockade for the treatment of hyperthyroidism. Am J Med 93:61, 1992.

78. Ladenson PW: Recognition and management of cardiovascular disease related to thyroid dysfunction. Am J Mcd 88:638, 1990.

79. Mackerrow SD, Osborn LA, Levey H, et al: Myxedema-associated cardiogenic shock treated with intravenous thyronine. Ann Intern Med 117:1014, 1992.

80. Kumar A, Bhandari AK, Rahimtoola SH: Torsade de pointes and marked QT prolongation in association with hypothyroidism. Ann Intern Med 106:712, 1987.

80a. Sun ZQ, Ojamaak-Coetzee WA, Artman M, Klein I: Effects of thyroid hormone on action potential and repolarizing currents in rat ventricular myocytes. Am J Physiol 278:E302–E307, 2000.

81. Bernstein R, Midtbo K, Smith G, et al: Incidence of hypertrophic cardiomyopathy in hypothyroidism. Thyroid 5:277, 1995.

82. Saito I, Kunihiko I, Saruta T: Hypothyroidism as a cause of hypertension. Hypertension 5:112, 1983.

83. Streeten DHP, Andersen GH, Howland T, et al: Effects of thyroid function on blood pressure: Recognition of hypothyroid hypertension. Hypertension 11:78, 1988.

84. Wieshammer S, Keck FS, Waitzinger J, et al: Left ventricular function at rest and during exercise in acute hypothyroidism. Br Heart J 60:204, 1988.

85. Vora J, O'Malley BP, Petersen S, et al: Reversible abnormalities of myocardial relaxation in hypothyroidism. J Clin Endocrinol Metab 61:269, 1985.

86. Grossman NG, Wieshammer S, Keck FS, et al: Doppler echocardiographic evaluation of left ventricular diastolic function in acute hypothyroidism. Clin Endocrinol 40:227, 1994.

87. Fruhwald FM, Ramschak-Schwarzer S, Pichler B, et al: Subclinical thyroid disorders in patients with dilated cardiomyopathy. Cardiology 88:156, 1997.

88. Elder J, McLelland A, O'Reilly DS, et al: The relationship between serum cholesterol and serum thyrotropin, thyroxine and tri-iodothyronine concentrations in suspected hypothyroidism. Ann Clin Biochem 36:110, 1990.

89. Arem N, Patsch W: Lipoprotein and apolipoprotein levels in subclinical hypothyroidism. Arch Intern Med 150:2097, 1990.

90. Klemperer JD, Klein I, Gomez M, et al: Thyroid hormone treatment after coronary-artery bypass surgery. N Engl J Med 333:1522, 1995.

91. Newman CM, Price A, Davies DW, et al: Amiodarone and the thyroid: A practical guide to the management of thyroid dysfunction induced by amiodarone therapy. Heart 79:121, 1998.

92. Thorne SA, Barnes I, Cullinan P, et al: Amiodarone-associated thyroid dysfunction: Risk factors in adults with congenital heart disease. Circulation 100:140, 1000.

93. Drvota V, Carlsson B, Haggblad J, et al: Amiodarone is a dose-dependent noncompetitive and competitive inhibitor of T3 binding to thyroid hormone receptor subtype beta 1, whereas disopyramide, lidocaine, propafenone, metoprolol, dl-sotalol, and verapamil have no inhibitory effect. J Cardiovasc Pharmacol 26:222, 1995.

94. Iervasi G, Clerico A, Bonini R, et al: Acute effects of amiodarone administration on thyroid function in patients with cardiac arrhythmia. J Clin Endocrinol Metab 82:275, 1997.

95. Pitsiavas V, Smerdely P, Boyages SC: Amiodarone compared with io-

dine exhibits a potent and persistent inhibitory effect on TSH-stimulated cAMP production in vitro: A possible mechanism to explain amiodarone-induced hypothyroidism. Eur J Endocrinol 140:241, 1999.

96. Harjai KJ, Licata AA: Effects of amiodarone on thyroid function. Ann Intern Med 126:63, 1997.

97. Bartalena L, Brogioni S, Grasso L, et al: Treatment of amiodarone-induced thyrotoxicosis, a difficult challenge: Results of a prospective study. J Clin Endocrinol Metab 81:2930, 1996.

98. Sato K, Yamazaki K, Kanaji Y, et al: Amiodarone-induced thyrotoxicosis associated with thyrotropin receptor antibody. Thyroid 8:1123, 1998.

99. Bogazzi F, Bartalena L, Brogioni S, et al: Color flow Doppler sonography rapidly differentiates type I and type II amiodarone- induced thyrotoxicosis. Thyroid 7:541, 1997.

DISEASES OF THE ADRENAL CORTEX

100. Williams GH, Dluhy RG: Diseases of the adrenal cortex. In Braunwald E, Fauci AS, Kasper DL, et al (eds): Harrison's Principles of Internal Medicine. 15th ed. New York, McGraw-Hill, 2000.

101. Mortensen RM, Williams GH: Aldosterone action: Physiology. In DeGroot LJ, Beaser M, Burger HG, et al (eds): Endocrinology. Vol 1, 4th ed. Philadelphia, WB Saunders, 2000.

102. Brilla CG, Matsubana LS, Weber KT: Antifibrotic effects of spironolactone in preventing myocardial fibrosis in systemic arterial hypertension. An J Cardiol 71:12A 1993.

103. Brilla CG, Zhou G, Matsubana L, Weben KT: Collagen metabolism in cultured rat cardiac fibroblasts: Response to angiotensin II and aldosterone. J Mol Cell Cardiol 26:809, 1994.

104. Fullerton MJ, Funder JW: Aldosterone and cardiac fibrosis: In vitro studies. Cardiovasc Res 28:1863, 1994.

105. Funder JW, Krozowski Z, Myles K, et al: Mineralocorticoid receptors, salt, and hypertension. Recent Prog Horm Res 52:247, 1997.

106. Stier CT Jr, Sim GJ, Mahboubi K, et al: Prevention of stroke and hypertensive renal disease by the angiotensin II receptor antagonist DuP 753 in salt-loaded stroke-prone SHR. In McGregor GA, Server PS (eds): Current Advances in ACE Inhibition. ed 2. London, Churchill Livingstone, 1991, p 252.

107. Rocha R, Chander PN, Khanna K, et al: Mineralocorticoid blockade reduces vascular injury in stroke-prone hypertensive rats. Hypertension 31:451, 1998.

108. Stier CT Jr, Chander PN, Zuckerman A, et al: Vascular protective effect of a selective aldosterone receptor antagonist in stroke-prone spontaneously hypertensive rats. Am J Cardiol in press.

109. Rocha R, Chander PN, Zuckerman A, et al: Role of aldosterone in renal vascular injury in stroke-prone hypertensive rats. Hypertension 33:232, 1999.

109a. Brown NJ, Kim KS, Chen YQ, et al: Synergistic effect of adrenal steroids and angiotension II on plasminogen ac inhibitor-1 production. J Clin Endocrinol Metab 85:336−344, 2000.

109b. Rocha R, Stier CT, Kifor I, et al: Aldosterone: A mediator of myocardial infarction and renal arteriopathy in rats. Endocrinology 2000 (in press).

110. Blacher J, Amah G, Girerd X, et al: Association between increased plasma levels of aldosterone and decreased systemic arterial compliance in subjects with essential hypertension. Am J Hypertens 10:1326, 1997.

111. Schunkert H, Hense H-W, Muscholl M, et al: Associations between circulating components of the renin-angiotensin-aldosterone-system and left ventricular mass. Heart 77:24, 1997.

112. Pitt B, Zannad F, Remme WJ, et al: The effects of spironolactone on morbidity and mortality in patients with severe heart failure. N Engl J Med 341:709, 1999.

113. Cushing H: The basophil adenomas of the pituitary body and their clinical manifestations (pituitary basophilism). Bull Johns Hopkins Hosp 50:137, 1932.

114. Etxabe J, Vazquez JA: Morbidity and mortality in Cushing's disease: An epidemiological approach. Clin Endocrinol 40:479, 1994.

115. Soszynski P, Slowinska-Srzednicka J, Kasperlik-Zaluska A, Zglicaynski S: Endogenous natriuretic factors: Atrial natriuretic hormone and digitalis-like substance in Cushing's syndrome, J. Endocrinol 129:453, 1991.

116. Mantero F, Boscaro M: Glucocorticoid-dependent hypertension. J Steroid Biochem Mol Biol 43:409, 1992.

117. Yasuda, G. Shionoiri H, Umeura S, et al: Exaggerated blood pressure response to angiotensin II in patients with Cushing's syndrome due to adrenocortical adenomas. Eur J Endocrinol 131:582, 1994.

118. Walker BR, Best R, Shackleton CH, et al: Increased vasoconstrictor sensitivity to glucocorticoids in essential hypertension. Hypertension 27:190, 1996.

119. Whitworth JA, Kelly JJ, Brown MA, et al: Glucocorticoids and hypertension in man. Clin Exp Hypertens 19:871, 1997.

120. Sugihara N, Shimizu M, Kita Y, et al: Cardiac characteristics and postoperative courses in Cushing's syndrome. Am J Cardiol 69:1475, 1992.

121. Carney JA, Gordon H, Carpenter PC, et al: The complex of myxomas, spotty pigmentation, and endocrine overactivity. Medicine (Baltimore) 64:270, 1985.

122. Fallo F, Paoletta A, Tona F, et al: Response of hypertension to conventional antihypertensive treatment and/or steroidogenesis inhibitors in Cushing's syndrome. J Intern Med 234:595, 1993.

123. Conlin PR, Dluhy RG, Williams GH: Disorders of the renin-angiotensin-aldosterone system. In Schrier RW (ed): Renal and Electrolyte Disorders. 4th ed. Boston, Little, Brown, 1992, p 405.

124. Pessina AC, Sacchetto A, Rossi GP: Left ventricular anatomy and function in primary aldosteronism and renovascular hypertension. Adv Exp Med Biol 432:63, 1997.

125. Rossi GP, Sacchetto A, Pavan E, et al: Remodeling on the left ventricle in primary aldosteronism due to Conn's adenoma. Circulation 95:1471, 1997.

126. Halimi J-M, Mimram A: Albuminuria in untreated patients with primary aldosteronism or essential hypertension. J Hypertens 13:1801, 1995.

127. Takeda R, Matsubara T, Miyamori I, et al: Vascular complications in patients with aldosterone producing adenoma in Japan. Comparative study with essential hypertension. J Endocrinol Invest 18:370, 1995.

128. Nishimura M, Uzu T, Fuji T, et al: Cardiovascular complications in patients with primary aldosteronism. Am J Kidney Dis 33:261, 1999

129. Litchfield WR, Anderson BF, Weiss RJ, et al: Intracranial aneurysm and hemorrhagic stroke in glucocorticoid remediable aldosteronism. Hypertension 31:445, 1998.

130. Lifton RP, Dluhy RG, Powers M, et al: A chimeric 11 β-hydroxylase/aldosterone synthase gene causes glucocorticoid-remediable aldosteronism in human hypertension. Nature 355:262, 1992.

131. Dorin RI, Kearns PJ: High output circulatory failure in acute adrenal insufficiency. Crit Care Med 16:296, 1988.

132. Lee TH, Salomon DR, Rayment CM, Antman E: Hypotension and sinus arrest with exercise-induced hyperkalemia and combined verapamil/propranolol therapy. Am J Med 80:1203, 1986.

PHEOCHROMOCYTOMA

133. Gifford RW, Manger WM, Bravo EL: Pheochromocytoma. Endocrinol Metab Clin North Am 23:387, 1994.

134. Walther MM, Keiser HR, Linehan WM: Pheochromocytoma: Evaluation, diagnosis, and treatment. World J Urol 17:35, 1999.

135. Jirari A, Charpentier A, Popescu S, et al: A malignant primary cardiac pheochromocytoma. Ann Thorac Surg 68:565, 1999.

136. Dresler C, Cremer J, Logemann F, et al: Intrapericardial pheochromocytoma. Thorac Cardiovasc Surg 46:100, 1998.

137. Bravo E, Fouad-Tarazi F, Rossi G, et al: A reevaluation of the hemodynamics of pheochromocytoma. Hypertension 15:1128, 1990.

138. Gatzoulis KA, Tolis G, Theopistou A, et al: Cardiomyopathy due to a pheochromocytoma: A reversible entity. Acta Cardiol 53:277, 1998.

139. Dabrowska B, Dabrowski A, Pruszczyk P, et al: Heart rate variability before sudden blood pressure elevations or complex cardiac arrhythmias in phaeochromocytoma. J Hum Hypertens 10:43, 1996.

140. Munakata M, Aihara A, Imai Y, et al: Altered sympathetic and vagal modulations of the cardiovascular system in patients with pheochromocytoma: Their relations to orthostatic hypotension. Am J Hypertens 12: 572, 1999.

141. Nanda AS, Feldman A, Liang CS: Acute reversal of pheochromocytoma-induced catecholamine cardiomyopathy. Clin Cardiol 18:421, 1995.

142. Huddle KR, Kalliatakis B, Skoularigis J: Pheochromocytoma associated with clinical and echocardiographic features simulating hypertrophic obstructive cardiomypopathy. Chest 109:1394, 1995.

143. Slathe M, Weiss P, Ritz R: Rapid reversal of heart failure in a patient with phaeochromocytoma and catecholamine-induced cardiomyopathy who was treated with captopril. Br Heart J 68:527, 1992.

144. Hu ZW, Billingham M, Tuck M, Hoffman BB: Captopril improves hypertension and cardiomyopathy in rats with pheochromocytoma. Hypertension 15:210, 1990.

145. McManus BM, Fleury TA, Roberts WC: Fatal catecholamine crisis in pheochromocytoma. Curable form of cardiac arrest. Am Heart 102:930, 1981.

146. Baratella MC, Menti L, Angelini A, et al: An unusual case of myocarditis. Int J Cardiol 65:305, 1998.

147. Simon M, Downing SE: Coronary vasoconstriction and catecholamine cardiomyopathy. Am Heart J 109:297, 1985.

148. Bhatnagar D, Carey P, Pollard A: Focal myositis and elevated creatinine kinase levels in a patient with phaeochromocytoma, Post grad Med 62: 197, 1986.

149. Ferrari L, Seregni E, Martinetti A, et al: Chromogranin A measurement in neuroendocrine tumors. Int J Biol Markers 13:3, 1998.

150. Lenz T, Ross A, Schumm-Draeger P, et al: Clonidine suppression test revisited. Blood Press 7:153, 1998.

151. Roelants V, Goulios C, Beckers C, et al: Iodine-131-MIBG scintigraphy in adults: Interpretation revisited? J Nucl Med 39:1007, 1998.

152. Sisson JC, Shulkin BL: Nuclear medicine imaging of pheochromocytoma and neuroblastoma. Q J Nucl Med 43:217, 1999.

153. Jebara VA, Uva MS, Farge A, et al: Cardiac pheochromocytomas Ann Thorac Surg 53:356, 1992.

154. Steinsapir J, Carr AA, Prisant LM, et al: Metyrosine and pheochromocytoma. Arch Intern Med 157:901, 1997.

155. Brown EM: Physiology of calcium metabolism. In Becker KL (ed): Principles and Practice of Endocrinology and Metabolism. Philadelphia, JB Lippincott, 1990, p 423.

156. Schluter KD, Piper HM: Cardiovascular actions of parathyroid hormone and parathyroid hormone−related peptide. Cardiovasc Res 37:34, 1998.

157. Hara M, Liu YM, Zhen L, et al: Positive chronotropic actions of para-

thyroid hormone and parathyroid hormone–related peptide are associated with increases in the current, I (f), and the slope of the pacemaker potential. Circulation 96:3704, 1997.

158. Schluter KD, Weber M, Piper HM: Parathyroid hormone induces protein kinase C but not adenylate cyclase in adult cardiomyocytes and regulates cyclic AMP levels via protein kinase C–dependent phosphodiesterase activity. Biochem J 310:439, 1995.

159. Ogino K, Burkhoff D, Bilezikian JP: The hemodynamic basis for the cardiac effects of parathyroid hormone (PTH) and PTH-related protein. Endocrinology 136:3024, 1995.

160. Ebisawa K, Kimura K, Nakayama T, et al: Cardiac electrophysiologic effects of parathyroid hormone in the guinea pig. Heart Vessels 10:128, 1995.

161. Suzuki T, Ikeda U, Fujikawa H, et al: Hypocalcemic heart failure: A reversible form of heart muscle disease. Clin Cardiol 21:227, 1998.

162. Stefenelli T, Abela C, Frank H, et al: Cardiac abnormalities in patients with primary hyperparathyroidism: Implications for follow-up. J Clin Endocrinol Metab 82:106, 1997.

163. Vered L, Vered Z, Perez JE, et al: Normal left ventricular performance documented by Doppler echocardiography in patients with long-standing hypocalcemia. Am J Med 86:413, 1989.

164. Roberts WC, Waller BF: Effect of chronic hypercalcemia on the heart: An analysis of 18 necropsy patients. Am J Med 71:371, 1981.

165. Csanady M, Forster T, Julesz J. Reversible impairment of myocardial function in hypoparathyroidism causing hypocalcaemia. Br Heart J 63:58, 1990.

166. Fliser D, Franek E, Fode P, et al: Subacute infusion of physiological doses of parathyroid hormone raises blood pressure in humans. Nephrol Dial Transplant 12:933, 1997.

167. Resnick LM: Calciotropic hormones in salt-sensitive essential hypertension: 1,25-dihydroxyvitamin D and parathyroid hypertensive factor. J Hypertens Suppl 12:3, 1994.

168. Morfis L, Smerdely P, Howes LG: Relationship between serum parathyroid hormone levels in the elderly and 24 h ambulatory blood pressures. J Hypertens 15: 1271, 1997.

PARATHYROID DISEASE

169. Hatton DC, Xue H, DeMerritt JA, McCarron DA: 1,25(OH)$_2$ vitamin D$_3$–induced alterations in vascular reactivity in the spontaneously hypertensive rat. Am J Med Sci 307(Suppl):154, 1994.

170. Benishin CG, Lewanczuk RZ, Pang PK: Purification of parathyroid hypertensive factor from plasma of spontaneously hypertensive rats. Proc Natl Acad Sci USA 88:6372, 1991.

171. Benishin CG, Labeda T, Guo DD, et al: Identification and purification of parathyroid hypertensive factor from organ culture of parathyroid glands from spontaneously hypertensive rats. Am J Hypertens 6:134, 1993.

172. Pang PK, Benishin CG, Shan J, Lewanczuk RZ. PHF: The new parathyroid hypertensive factor. Blood Press 3:148, 1994.

173. Lewanczuk RZ, Benishin CG, Shan J, Pang PK: Clinical aspects of parathyroid hypertensive factor, J Cardiovasc Pharmacol 23(Suppl):23, 1994.

174. Lewanczuk RZ, Resnick LM, Ho MS, et al: Clinical aspects of parathyroid hypertensive factor. J Hypertens Suppl 12:11, 1994.

GONADAL HORMONES AND THE CARDIOVASCULAR SYSTEM

175. Mendelsohn ME, Karas RH: The protective effects of estrogen on the cardiovascular system. N Engl J Med 340:1801–1811, 1999.

176. Barrett-Connor E, Wingard DL, Criqui MH: Postmenopausal estrogen use and heart disease risk factors in the 1980s. JAMA 261:2095–2100, 1989.

177. Nabulsi AA, Folson AR, White A, et al: Association of hormone-replacement therapy with various risk factors in postmenopausal women. The Atherosclerosis Risk in Community Study Investigators. N Engl J Med 328:1069–1075, 1993.

178. Grodstein F, Stampfer MJ, Manson JF, et al: Postmenopausal estrogen and progestin use and risk of cardiovascular disease. N Engl J Med 335:453–461, 1996.

179. Hulley S, Grady D, Bush T, et al: Randomized trial of estrogen plus progestin for secondary prevention of coronary heart disease in postmenopausal women. JAMA 280:605–613, 1998.

180. Women's Health Initiative Study Group: Design of the Women's Health Initiative clinical trial and observational study. Control Clin Trials 19: 61–109, 1998.

181. McDonald CC, Stewart HJ, Scottish Breast Cancer Study Committee: Fatal myocardial infarction in the Scottish adjuvant tamoxifen trial. BMJ 303:435–437, 1991.

182. Rutqvist LE, Mattsson A, Stockholm Breast Cancer Study Group: Cardiac and thromboembolic morbidity among postmenopausal women with early stage breast cancer in a randomized trial of adjuvant tamoxifen. J Natl Cancer Inst 85:1398–1406, 1993.

183. Grey AB, Stapleton JP, Evans MC, Reid IR: The effect of the anti-estrogen tamoxifen on cardiovascular risk factors in normal postmenopausal women. J Clin Endocrinol Metab 80:3191–3195, 1995.

184. Walsh BW, Kuller LH, Wild RA, et al: Effects of raloxifene on serum lipids and coagulation factors in healthy postmenopausal women. JAMA 279:1145–1451, 1998.

185. Webber LS, Hunter SM, Baugh JG, et al: The interaction of cigarette smoking, oral contraceptive use, and cardiovascular risk factor variables in children: The Bogalusa Heart Study. Am J Publ Health 72:266, 1982.

186. Stampfer MJ, Willett WC, Colditz GA, et al: A prospective study of past use of oral contraceptive agents and risk of cardiovascular diseases. N Engl J Med 319, 1313, 1988.

187. Ramcharan S, Pellegrin FA, Hoag EJ: The occurrence and course of hypertensive disease in users and nonusers of oral contraceptive drugs. In Ramacharan S (ed): The Walnut Creek Contraceptive Drug Study: A prospective study of the side effects of oral contraceptives. Vol. 2. U.S. Department of Health, Education and Welfare Publications No. (NIH) 76-563. Washington, DC, U.S. Government Printing Office, 1976, p. 1.

188. Prentice RL: On the ability of blood pressure effects to explain the relation between oral contraceptives and cardiovascular disease. Am J Epidemiol 127:213, 1988.

189. Blumenstein BA, Douglas MB, Hall WD: Blood pressure changes and oral contraceptive use: A study of 2676 black women in the southeastern United States. Am J Epidemiol 112:539, 1980.

190. Rekers H: Multicenter trial of a monophasic oral contraceptive containing ethinyl estradiol and desogestrel. Acta Obstet Gynecol Scand 67:171, 1988.

191. Walling M: A multicenter efficacy and safety study of an oral contraceptive containing 150 μg desogestrel and 30 μg ethinyl estradiol. Contraceptive 46:313, 1992.

192. Shoupe D: Multicenter randomized comparison of two low-dose triphasic combined oral contraceptive containing desogestrel or norethindrone. Obstet Gynecol 83:679, 1994.

193. Yarnell JW, Beswick AD, Sweetman PM, Riad-Fahmy D: Endogenous sex hormones and ischemic heart disease in men, The Caterpilly prospective study. Arterioscler Thromb 13:517–520, 1993.

194. Barrett-Connor E, Khaw KT: Endogenous sex hormones and cardiovascular disease in men. A prospective population-based study. Circulation 78:539–545, 1988.

195. Wu S, Weng X: Therapeutic effects of an androgenic preparation on myocardial ischemia and cardiac function in 62 elderly male coronary heart disease patients. Chin Med J 106:415, 1993.

196. Webb CM, Adamson DL, de Zeigler D, Collins P: Effect of acute testosterone on myocardial ischemia in men with coronary artery disease. Am J Cardiol 83:437–439, 1999.

CARDIOVASCULAR CONSEQUENCES OF OBESITY

197. Kuczmarski RS, Flegal KM, Campbell SM, et al: Increasing prevalence of overweight among US adults. The National Health and Nutritional Survey. JAMA 272:205–211, 1994.

198. Garrison RJ, Castelli WP: Weight and thirty-year mortality of men in the Framingham Study. Ann Intern Med 103:1006–1009, 1985.

199. Manson JE, Willett WC, Stampfer MJ, et al: Body weight and mortality among women. N Engl J Med 333:677–685, 1995.

200. Kaplan NM: The deadly quartet. Upper-body obesity, glucose intolerance, hypertriglyceridemia, and hypertension. Arch Intern Med 149:1514–1520, 1989.

201. Smith HL, Willius RA: Adiposity of the heart. A clinical and pathological study of one hundred and thirty-six obese patients. Ann Intern Med 52:911, 1933.

201a. Aizawa-Abe M, Ogawa Y, Masuki H, et al: Pathophysiological role of leptin in obesity-related hypertension. J Clin Invest 105:1243–1252, 2000.

202. Van Itallie TB: Health implications of overweight and obesity in the United States. Ann Intern Med 103:983–988, 1985.

203. Himeno E, Nishino K, Nakashima Y, et al: Weight reduction regresses left ventricular mass regardless of blood pressure level in obese subjects. Am Heart J 131:313–319, 1996.

204. Mshui ME, Saikawa T, Ito K, et al: QT interval and QT dispersion before and after diet therapy in patients with simple obesity. Proc Soc Exp Biol Med 220:133–138, 1999.

205. Webb JG, Kiess MC, Chan-Yan CC: Malnutrition and the heart. Can Med Assoc J 135:753–758, 1986.

206. Pringle TH, Scoble IN, Murray RG, et al: Prolongation of the QT interval during therapeutic starvation: A substrate for malignant arrhythmias. Int J Obes 7:253–261, 1988.

207. Schocken DD, Holloway JD, Powers PS: Weight loss and the heart. Effects of anorexia nervosa and starvation. Arch Intern Med 149:877–881, 1989.

208. de Simone G, Scalfi L, Galderisi M, et al: Cardiac abnormalities in young women with anorexia nervosa. Br Heart J 71:287–292, 1994.

209. Swenne I, Larsson PT: Heart risk associated with weight loss in anorexia nervosa and eating disorders: Risk factors for QTc interval prolongation and dispersion. Acta Paediatr 88:304–309, 1999.

Chapter 65

Pregnancy and Cardiovascular Disease

URI ELKAYAM

CARDIOVASCULAR PHYSIOLOGY DURING PREGNANCY AND THE PUERPERIUM

PREVALENCE. Although heart disease is limited to only 0.5 to 1.0 percent of pregnant women, it remains an important cause of maternal morbidity and even mortality and has a significant effect on fetal outcome.[1-3] Pregnancy and the peripartum period are associated with important cardio-circulatory changes[4] that can lead to marked clinical deterioration in the woman with heart disease. Hemodynamic changes occurring during pregnancy are summarized in Table 65-1.

BLOOD VOLUME. Blood volume increases substantially during pregnancy, starting as early as the sixth week and rising rapidly until midpregnancy, when the rise continues but at a much slower rate[4] (Fig. 65-1). The degree of maximum volume expansion varies considerably in the individual patient (20 to 100 percent) and averages 50 percent. This increase is reported to correlate with fetal weight, placental mass, weight of the products of conception, and maternal and neonatal weight.[4] A higher increment in blood volume is reported in multigravidas and in women with multiple pregnancies.[3]

Because increase in plasma volume is more rapid than increase in red blood cell mass (see Fig. 65-1), hemoglobin concentration falls during pregnancy gradually until week 30, causing the "physiological anemia of pregnancy" with hematocrit levels that can be as low as 33 to 38 percent, a condition that can be partially corrected with iron therapy.[4] Changes in blood volume during pregnancy are attributable to estrogen-mediated stimulation of the renin-aldosterone system,[5, 6] which results in sodium and water retention. Changes in other hormones, including deoxycorticosterone, prostaglandins, estrogen, prolactin, placental lactogen, growth hormone, adrenocorticotropic hormone, and atrial natriuretic peptides, may also be involved in water retention during pregnancy.[4, 7]

CARDIAC OUTPUT, STROKE VOLUME, AND HEART RATE. Cardiac output during pregnancy is estimated to increase by approximately 50 percent.[4] It begins to rise around the fifth week and increases rapidly until the 24th week, when it plateaus or continues to rise slightly[4, 8, 9] (Fig. 65-2, Table 65-1). During the third trimester, body position can substantially influence cardiac output, which increases in the lateral position and declines in the supine position, owing to caval compression by the gravid uterus and decreased venous return to the heart. The increase in cardiac output early in pregnancy is predominantly due to augmentation in stroke volume, whereas in the third trimester it is largely due to an accelerated heart rate and stroke volume does not change or even declines as a result of caval compression (see Fig. 65-2). Increase in cardiac output seems to be enhanced in subsequent pregnancies.[9]

Heart rate peaks during the third trimester with an average increase of 10 to 20 beats/min[4, 9] (see Fig. 65-2), although on occasion it may be markedly faster. Pregnancy with multiple fetuses is associated with an even higher heart rate.

BLOOD PRESSURE AND SYSTEMIC VASCULAR RESISTANCE. Systemic arterial pressure begins to fall during the first trimester, reaches a nadir in mid pregnancy, and returns toward pregestational levels before term[4, 9] (see Table 65-1). Because diastolic blood pressure decreases substantially more than systolic pressure, the pulse pressure widens.[4] Reduction in blood pressure is caused by a decline in systemic vascular resistance due to reduced vascular tone,[10] probably mediated by (1) gestational hormonal activity, increased levels of circulating prostaglandins, and atrial natriuretic peptides,[4, 11] as well as endothelial nitric oxide[12]; (2) increased heat production by the developing fetus; and (3) the creation of low-resistance circulation in the pregnant uterus.

SUPINE HYPOTENSIVE SYNDROME OF PREGNANCY. The supine hypotensive or the uterocaval syndrome of

▼ **TABLE 65-1. CARDIOCIRCULATORY CHANGES DURING NORMAL PREGNANCY**

PARAMETER	CHANGES AT VARIOUS TIMES (WEEKS)					
	5	12	20	24	32	38
Heart rate	↑	↑↑↑	↑↑↑	↑↑↑	↑↑↑↑	↑↑↑↑
Systolic blood pressure	↔	↓	↓	↔	↑	↑↑
Diastolic blood pressure	↔	↓↓	↓↓	↓	↔	↑↑
Stroke volume	↑	↑↑↑↑	↑↑↑	↑↑↑	↑↑↑	↑↑↑↑
Cardiac output	↑↑↑	↑↑↑↑↑	↑↑↑↑↑	↑↑↑↑↑	↑↑↑↑	↑↑↑↑↑
Systemic vascular resistance	↓↓	↓↓↓↓	↓↓↓↓↓	↓↓↓↓	↓↓↓↓	↓↓↓↓
Left ventricular ejection fraction	↑	↑↑	↑↑	↑↑	↑	↓↓

↑, ≤5%; ↑↑, 6-10%; ↑↑↑, 11-15%; ↑↑↑↑, 16-20%; ↑↑↑↑↑, 21-30%; ↑↑↑↑↑↑, >30%; ↑↑↑↑↑↑↑, >40%.

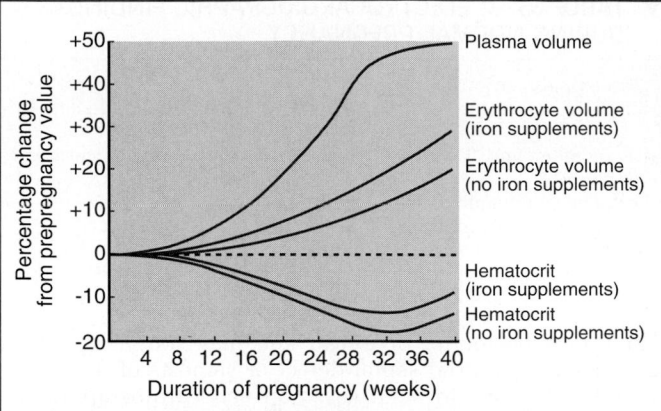

FIGURE 65–1. Changes in plasma volume, erythrocyte volume, and hematocrit during pregnancy. Increase in plasma volume is more rapid than increase in erythrocyte volume, causing the "physiological anemia of pregnancy," which can be partially corrected with iron supplements. (From Pitkin RM: Nutritional support in obstetrics and gynecology. Clin Obstet Gynecol 19:489, 1976.)

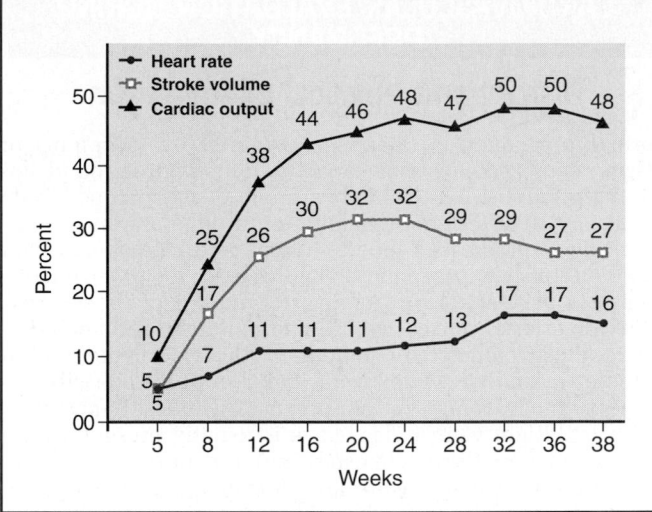

FIGURE 65–2. Percent changes of heart rate, stroke volume, and cardiac output measured in the lateral position throughout pregnancy compared with prepregnancy values. (Modified from Robson SC, Hunter S, Boys RJ, Dunlop W: Serial study of factors influencing changes in cardiac output during human pregnancy. Am J Physiol 256:H1060–H1065, 1989.)

pregnancy occurs with significant decreases in heart rate and blood pressure in up to 11 percent of pregnant women.[4] These hemodynamic changes are associated with weakness, lightheadedness, nausea, dizziness, and even syncope and are explained by acute occlusion of the inferior vena cava by the enlarged uterus (Fig. 65–3). When the supine position is abandoned, these hemodynamic effects and symptoms usually are promptly relieved.

HEMODYNAMIC CHANGES DURING LABOR AND DELIVERY. Hemodynamics are altered substantially during labor and delivery secondary to anxiety, pain, and uterine contractions.[4] Oxygen consumption increases threefold; and cardiac output rises progressively during labor owing to increase in both stroke volume and heart rate, and it is higher in the lateral position. Both systolic and diastolic blood pressures increase markedly during contractions, with greater augmentation during the second stage.[4, 13] Hemodynamic changes during labor and delivery are greatly influenced by the form of anesthesia and analgesia.[4, 13] Reduction of pain and apprehension by local, caudal, and epidural anesthesia may limit hemodynamic changes and rise in oxygen consumption.[4, 13]

HEMODYNAMIC EFFECTS OF CESAREAN SECTION. To avoid the hemodynamic changes associated with vaginal delivery, cesarean section is frequently recommended for women with cardiovascular disease. However, this form of delivery can also be associated with considerable hemodynamic fluctuations related largely to intubation, drugs used for anesthesia and analgesia,[14] larger extent of blood loss, the relief of caval compression, extubation, and postoperative awakening.[3]

HEMODYNAMIC CHANGES POST PARTUM. A temporary increase in venous return may occur immediately after delivery due to relief of caval compression and, in addition, blood shifting from the contracting uterus into the systemic circulation (autotransfusion).[14] This change in effective blood volume occurs despite blood loss during delivery and can result in a substantial rise in ventricular filling pressure, stroke volume, and cardiac output and may lead to clinical deterioration. Both heart rate and cardiac output return to prelabor values by 1 hour after delivery and mean blood pressure and stroke volume by 24 hours after delivery.[4, 13] Hemodynamic adaptation to pregnancy persists post partum and gradually returns to prepregnancy values within 12 to 24 weeks after delivery.[4]

FIGURE 65–3. Venocaval compression of the inferior vena cava and abdominal aorta by the gravid uterus can lead to reduced venous return and thus to decreased cardiac output. (From Lee W, Shah PK, Amin DK, et al: Hemodynamic monitoring of cardiac patients during pregnancy. In Elkayam U, Gleicher N: Cardiac Problems in Pregnancy. 2nd ed. New York, Alan R. Liss, 1990, p 61.)

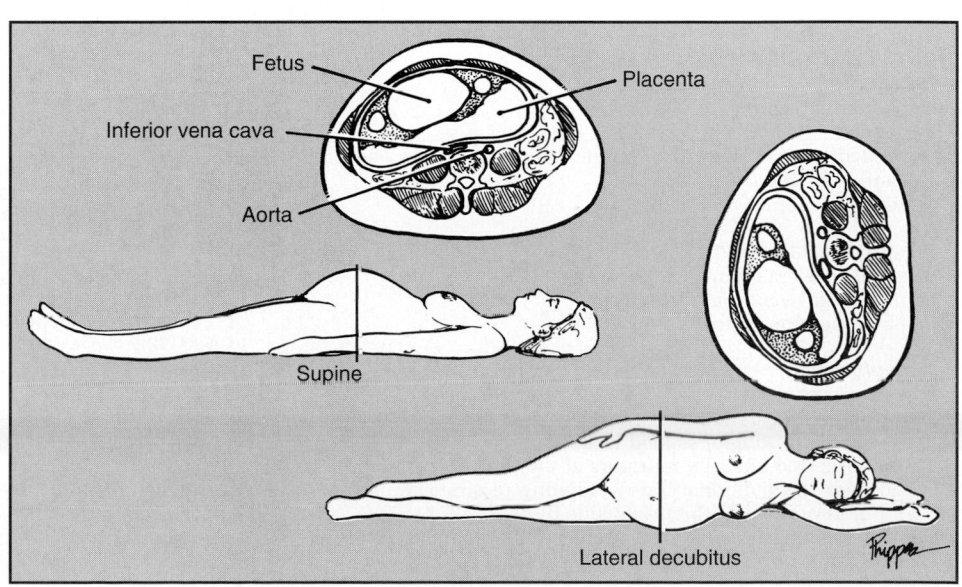

CARDIOVASCULAR EVALUATION DURING PREGNANCY

History and Physical Examination

Normal pregnancy is often accompanied by symptoms of fatigue, decreased exercise capacity, hyperventilation, dyspnea, palpitations, lightheadedness, and even syncope (Table 65–2).[15, 16] In addition, augmentation of jugular venous pulsation due to increased blood volume, and leg edema (often observed in late pregnancy), could lead to an erroneous diagnosis of heart failure or overestimation of its severity. Systemic arterial pulses are full and collapsing and are similar to those palpated in patients with aortic regurgitation or hyperthyroidism. A left ventricular impulse is easily detected in most women in late pregnancy and is hyperactive and brisk. Right ventricular heave is usually present during the second and third trimester, and the pulmonary trunk and pulmonic valve closure are often palpable. This group of findings may result in difficulty in assessing the presence and/or severity of pulmonary hypertension.

CARDIAC AUSCULTATION (see Chap. 4). Especially after the first trimester, auscultation often reveals an increased first heart sound (S_1) with exaggerated splitting that may be misinterpreted as a fourth heart sound (S_4) or as a systolic click.[15] The second heart sound (S_2) is often increased in late pregnancy and may exhibit persistent splitting when the patient is examined in the lateral position. These changes in S_2 may be interpreted as signs of pulmonary hypertension (loud P_2) or atrial septal defect (systolic murmur and splitting of S_2). Auscultation of the third heart sound (S_3) and S_4 is uncommon in normal pregnancy.

Innocent Systolic Murmurs. These can be heard in most pregnant women and are the result of the hyperkinetic circulation of pregnancy. Murmurs are usually midsystolic and soft, are heard best at the lower left sternal edge and over the pulmonic area, and radiate to the suprasternal notch and more to the left than to the right side of the neck.[15] Not uncommonly the benign murmur of preg-

▼ **TABLE 65–2. CARDIAC SYMPTOMS AND FINDINGS DURING NORMAL PREGNANCY**

SYMPTOMS
Decreased exercise capacity
Tiredness
Dyspnea
Orthopnea
Palpitations
Lightheadedness
Syncope
PHYSICAL FINDINGS
Inspection
Hyperventilation
Peripheral edema
Distended neck veins with prominent a and v waves and brisk x and y descents
Capillary pulsation
Precordial Palpation
Brisk, diffuse, and displaced left ventricular impulse
Palpable right ventricular impulse
Palpable pulmonary trunk impulse
Auscultation
Pulmonary basilary rales
Increased first heart sound with exaggerated splitting
Exaggerated splitting of second heart sound
Midsystolic ejection-type murmurs at the lower left sternal edge and over the pulmonary area radiating to suprasternal notch and more to the left than right side of neck
Continuous murmurs (cervical venous hum, mammary souffle)
Diastolic murmurs (rare)

▼ **TABLE 65–3. ELECTROCARDIOGRAPHIC FINDINGS DURING NORMAL PREGNANCY**

QRS axis deviation
Small Q wave and inverted P wave in lead III (abolished by inspiration)
ST segment and T wave changes (ritodrine tocolysis, cesarean section)
Frequent sinus tachycardia
Higher incidence of arrhythmias
Increase R/S ratio in leads V_2 and V_1

nancy may be louder or longer and may sound like those associated with atrial septal defect or stenosis of one of the semilunar valves. In such cases an echocardiographic and Doppler evaluation is warranted to rule out an abnormal cardiac condition. Two benign continuous murmurs that may be heard during gestation are the cervical venous hum and mammary souffle. The venous hum is usually heard maximally over the right supraclavicular fossa but can radiate to the contralateral area and sometimes to the area below the clavicle. The mammary souffle may be either systolic or continuous, is heard over the breast late in gestation or in the lactating woman, and is caused by increased flow in the mammary vessels. Characteristically, the murmur decreases or vanishes when pressure is applied to the stethoscope or when the patient moves to the upright position.[15] Diastolic murmurs may be heard in normal pregnant women due to increased blood flow through the atrioventricular valve.[15] Such a finding, however, is infrequent in the healthy pregnant woman and therefore requires careful diagnostic work-up to rule out organic disease.

Laboratory Examinations

ELECTROCARDIOGRAPHY (see Chap. 5). In normal pregnancy, the QRS axis may shift to either the left or the right, but it usually stays within normal limits[15] (Table 65–3). A small Q wave and an inverted P wave in lead III that vary with respiration as well as a greater r wave amplitude in lead V_2 may be present. A high incidence of ST segment depression mimicking myocardial ischemia but not associated with wall motion abnormalities has been described between induction of anesthesia and the end of surgery in patients undergoing cesarean section.[17, 18] Increased susceptibility to arrhythmias during pregnancy is manifested by the frequent finding of sinus tachycardia and atrial and/or ventricular premature beats.[16] There is an increased incidence of paroxysmal supraventricular tachycardia during normal pregnancy,[19] and several cases of ventricular tachycardia have been reported in healthy women.[20]

CHEST RADIOGRAPHY (see Chap. 8). Although the radiation dose associated with a routine chest radiograph is minimal, because of the potential for adverse biological effects from any amount of radiation the pelvic area should be shielded by protective lead material[21] (Table 65-4).

Changes seen on chest films in normal pregnancy may simulate cardiac disease and should be interpreted with caution.[22] Straightening of the left upper cardiac border because of prominence of the pulmonary conus is often seen. The heart may seem enlarged because of its horizontal positioning secondary to the elevated diaphragm. In addition, an increase in lung markings may simulate a pattern of flow redistribution seen with increased pulmonary venous pressure. Pleural effusion is often found early post partum. It is usually small and resorbs 1 to 2 weeks after delivery.[15]

DOPPLER ECHOCARDIOGRAPHY (see Chap. 7). Gestational use of both maternal and fetal cardiac ultrasound is considered safe.[23, 23a] Transesophageal echocardiography has been increasingly used in pregnancy and seems to be well tolerated by both mother and fetus[24] (Table 65-5).

▼ **TABLE 65–4. CHEST RADIOGRAPHIC FINDINGS DURING NORMAL PREGNANCY**

Straightening of the left upper cardiac border
Horizontal position of the heart
Increased lung marking
Small plural effusion in early postpartum period

▼ TABLE 65–5. DOPPLER AND ECHOCARDIOGRAPHIC FINDINGS DURING NORMAL PREGNANCY

Slightly increased systolic and diastolic left ventricular dimensions (when patient examined in the lateral position)

Unchanged or slightly improved left ventricular systolic function

Moderate increase in size of right atrium, right ventricle, and left atrium

Progressive dilation of pulmonary, tricuspid, and mitral valve annuli

Functional pulmonary, tricuspid, and mitral regurgitation

Small pericardial effusion

Pericardial effusion, usually small or minimal, has been noted in normal pregnant women late in pregnancy.[25] There is a progressive increase in all cardiac chamber dimensions with an approximately 20 percent increase in the size of the right atrium and the right ventricle, 12 percent in left atrial size, and 6 percent in left ventricular size.[26, 27] Post partum these changes gradually return toward baseline but may remain different from prepregnancy values for several months.[9] In addition, there is early and progressive dilatation of mitral, tricuspid, and pulmonary annuli, which is associated with increase in valvular regurgitation.[28]

STRESS TESTING (see Chap. 6). An exercise test using bicycle ergometry or a treadmill can be carried out during pregnancy to help establish the diagnosis of ischemic heart disease and to assess functional capacity and cardiac reserve.[29] The safety of such testing in pregnancy has not been fully established. Because fetal bradycardia has been reported with maximal but not with submaximal exercise,[29, 30] a low-level exercise protocol allowing heart rate increase to 70 percent of maximal predicted heart rate with fetal monitoring is recommended when stress testing is indicated.[15]

RADIATION. Exposure of the embryo to irradiation during the first 10 days post conception would most likely have either no effect or lead to resorption.[31] Irradiation during organ formation (days 10–50) may cause a teratogenic effect, whereas after completion of organogenesis, it may cause intrauterine growth retardation, central nervous system abnormalities, and possible increased incidence of childhood cancer or leukemia. Current recommendations related to intrauterine radiation exposure are

- Less than 5 rads—patient can be reassured of very low likelihood of risk.
- Five to 10 rads—patient should be counseled regarding low risk of problems.
- Ten to 15 rads during first 6 weeks—individual considerations for termination of pregnancy should be made.
- More than 15 rads—termination of pregnancy recommended.

Routine chest radiography is associated with radiation of 20 mrad to the chest. Standard fluoroscopy could deliver 1 to 2 rads/min to the chest and high level fluoroscopy or cine as much as 5 to 10 rads/min. The amount of radiation scattered to the uterus and absorbed by the embryo is less than 5 percent of radiation absorbed by the directly radiated tissue. Direct irradiation to the fetus should be avoided and can be prevented by covering the patient with a lead apron during radiographic procedures. The use of a lead apron, however, is of little help in reducing fetal irradiation due to Compton-scattered photons.[31]

Radiation to the fetus from nuclear medicine procedures is mainly due to distribution of radiopharmaceuticals to the bladder or the placenta or directly across the placental barrier. The expected radiation with thallium-201 or technetium-99m–labeled sestamibi diagnostic procedures is less than 1 rad per examination. Cardiac function studies with technetium-99m–labeled red blood cells is associated with fetal radiation of 1 to 2 rads, peripheral contrast radiographic venography of 0.5 rad or less, and pulmonary scintigraphy with technetium-macroaggregated albumin of 0.05 rad or less.[31]

MAGNETIC RESONANCE IMAGING (see Chap. 10). Although magnetic resonance imaging poses no known risks to the fetus, experience with this technique is limited and its safety has not been fully established.[32] Currently, the U.S. Food and Drug Administration recommends prudence in using magnetic resonance imaging during pregnancy.[32] This technique should therefore be used only when evaluation cannot be delayed until after pregnancy, and if possible after the first trimester.

PULMONARY ARTERY CATHETERIZATION. Hemodynamic monitoring with the aid of a pulmonary artery catheter can be of great help in managing patients at high risk during pregnancy, labor, delivery, and the postpartum period.[33] The ability to insert and position the flotation catheter with pressure monitoring without the need for fluoroscopy makes it particularly attractive for use during pregnancy. Hemodynamic monitoring is recommended throughout labor and delivery for any patient with symptomatic cardiac disease during pregnancy or with the potential for deterioration due to valvular, myocardial, or ischemic heart disease. Because significant circulatory changes that may lead to hemodynamic deterioration occur in the early postpartum period,[4] hemodynamic monitoring should be continued for at least several hours after delivery to ensure stability.

CARDIAC CATHETERIZATION (see Chap. 11). Cardiac catheterization may be indicated in rare instances of cardiac decompensation when sufficient information cannot be obtained by noninvasive techniques, especially if cardiac surgery, coronary angioplasty, or balloon valvuloplasty is being considered. Although this technique provides high-quality images, it is associated with a relatively high dose of radiation. To minimize radiation to the pelvic and abdominal areas, the brachial rather than the femoral approach is preferred, fluoroscopy and cine time should be reduced to the minimum required, and direct irradiation to the fetus should be avoided.

PREGNANCY IN WOMEN WITH CONGENITAL HEART DISEASE (See Chap. 44)

Because of increased survival in children with congenital heart disease, pregnancy has become more common in this patient population.[34, 35] Preconception management should include careful history and assessment of risk for both the mother and the fetus.[35–37]

The patient should be counseled regarding contraceptive alternatives,[38] potential maternal and fetal risks of pregnancy,[39, 40] and, when appropriate, expected long-term maternal morbidity and survival as well as the risk of congenital malformations in the offspring.[41] In addition, guidance concerning anticoagulation and prophylactic antibiotics, if needed, should be provided.[42]

MATERNAL AND FETAL OUTCOME. In general, a good maternal outcome can be expected in most cases with noncyanotic congenital heart disease. Maternal outcome is determined by the nature of the disease, surgical repair, presence and severity of cyanosis, increased pulmonary vascular resistance, maternal functional capacity, myocardial dysfunction, left ventricular obstruction, and history of arrhythmias[42a, 42b] or other prior cardiac events.[40] Unfavorable outcome, including development of congestive heart failure, arrhythmias, and hypertension, is commonly seen in patients with impaired functional status and those with cyanosis.[40–42] Other reported complications include angina, infective endocarditis, and thromboembolic phenomena.

Maternal functional capacity and cyanosis also determine fetal outcome.[43, 44] Fetal wastage was reported in 45 percent of cyanotic mothers compared with 20 percent in acyanotic mothers with congenital heart disease.[44] Low birth weight for gestational age and prematurity are common in cyanotic mothers and correlate with maternal hemoglobin and hematocrit values.[43, 44] Risk of congenital heart disease is increased for the offspring of mothers with congenital heart disease with a reported incidence of 4 to 8 percent.[45, 46] In addition, there are a greater number of noncardiac congenital malformations, as well as mental and physical impairments in children born to mothers with congenital heart disease.

LABOR AND DELIVERY. Elective induction of labor when fetal maturity is confirmed may be used in high-risk patients for better planning of hemodynamic monitoring and availability of expert personnel[34] during labor and delivery. Vaginal delivery is preferred for most patients, and cesarean section is indicated in the stable patients only for obstetric reasons. Oxygen should be given to hypoxemic mothers, and hemodynamic as well as blood gas monitoring is recommended in most patients with impaired functional capacity, cardiac dysfunction, pulmonary hypertension, and cyanotic malformations. Blood volume loss must be anticipated and treated promptly.

ANTIBIOTIC PROPHYLAXIS. Official recommendations by the American Heart Association suggest that antibiotic prophylaxis for an uncomplicated delivery is unnecessary except for cases with a prosthetic heart valve or a surgically constructed systemic-to-pulmonary shunt.[47] Because of difficulties in predicting complicated deliveries and potential devastating consequences of endocarditis,[48] antibiotic prophylaxis for vaginal delivery in all patients with congenital heart disease (except those with an isolated secundum type of atrial septal defect and those 6 months or more after repair of septal defects or surgical ligation and division of patent ductus arteriosus) seems reasonable.

Specific Malformations

ATRIAL SEPTAL DEFECT (see also Chap. 44). Atrial septal defect is usually well tolerated in pregnancy even in patients with large left-to-right shunts. The development of pulmonary hypertension and atrial arrhythmias rarely occurs in the childbearing age. Because endocarditis is rare, antibiotic prophylaxis is not indicated in patients with secundum-type atrial septal defect. Recommendations concerning pregnancy in patients with atrial septal defect should be made on an individual basis, considering accompanying lesions, functional status, and the level of pulmonary vascular resistance.[34]

VENTRICULAR SEPTAL DEFECT (see also Chap. 44). Women with isolated ventricular septal defect usually tolerate pregnancy well, although congestive heart failure and arrhythmias have been reported.[34] The risk posed by pregnancy after closure of an uncomplicated ventricular septal defect should not differ from that in patients without heart disease. The incidence of ventricular septal defect in offspring has been reported to be 4 to 11 percent.[34] Marked reduction in blood pressure during or after delivery as a result of blood loss or anesthesia can lead to shunt reversal in patients with pulmonary hypertension. The use of vasopressors and volume replacement to stabilize blood pressure should prevent further complications.

PATENT DUCTUS ARTERIOSUS (see also Chap. 44). Maternal outcome in patients with patent ductus arteriosus with left-to-right shunt is usually favorable[34, 42]; however, clinical deterioration and congestive heart failure can occur in some patients. There were no maternal deaths among a large number of patients with patent ductus arteriosus.[40, 48] The need for surgical intervention during pregnancy is rare. A fall in systemic vascular resistance during gestation and hypotension early post partum can lead to shunt reversal in women with pulmonary hypertension. Peripartum decrease in systemic blood pressure should be corrected by means of vasopressor agents.

CONGENITAL AORTIC VALVE DISEASE (see also Chap. 44). Most patients with mild aortic stenosis have favorable outcome of pregnancy provided that they receive early diagnosis and appropriate care, including hemodynamic monitoring during labor and delivery and appropriate anesthesia.[3, 34, 49] At the same time, however, moderate and severe aortic stenosis is likely to be associated with symptomatic deterioration during pregnancy and may lead to maternal morbidity and even mortality.[3]

Symptoms usually develop in the second or third trimester and may include exertional dyspnea, chest pain, lightheadedness, and syncope. Increased incidence of cardiac defects has been reported in liveborn infants of mothers with left ventricular outflow obstruction.[43] Because of the risk involved, patients with severe aortic stenosis (aortic valve area <1.0 cm²) should consider undergoing valve replacement before becoming pregnant. Optional management strategies of a pregnant patient with severe aortic stenosis include (1) early abortion followed by valve replacement and repeat pregnancy and (2) continuation of pregnancy and plan for percutaneous balloon valvuloplasty or surgical intervention in patients who show clinical deterioration not controlled by medical therapy.[50, 51]

Both replacement of aortic valve and percutaneous balloon valvuloplasty have been performed successfully in pregnant women with aortic stenosis.[50–53] These procedures, however, are not free of complications. Although valvuloplasty obviates the general anesthesia and cardio-pulmonary bypass required for surgery, it can be associated with prolonged radiation exposure and hemodynamic fluctuations that can lead to immediate and late fetal complications. Surgical replacement of the aortic valve during pregnancy can be associated with increased incidence of maternal complications and fetal loss.[53] These procedures should therefore be considered only in symptomatic patients with severe disease not manageable by medical therapy and should be avoided when possible during the first trimester.

COARCTATION OF THE AORTA (see also Chap. 44). Both maternal and fetal outcome is usually favorable in cases with aortic coarctation.[54–56] At the same time, however, cases of severe hypertension, congestive heart failure, and aortic dissection have been reported.[42, 56] A recent study reported congenital heart disease in 3 percent of newborns born to patients with corrected coarctation.[57] Because a higher incidence of infective endocarditis in the mother and of congenital heart disease in the fetus have been shown in cases with surgically uncorrected compared with corrected coarctation,[43] it seems advisable to correct aortic coarctation before pregnancy.[57]

Measures to reduce the incidence of aortic dissection and rupture of cerebral aneurysms during pregnancy consist of limiting physical activity and controlling blood pressure. Excessive blood pressure reduction, however, may compromise uteroplacental blood flow and should be avoided. Surgical correction of coarctation has been performed successfully during pregnancy[57] and may be indicated in patients with severe, uncontrollable systolic hypertension or heart failure.

PULMONIC STENOSIS (see also Chap. 44). Isolated pulmonic stenosis is usually well tolerated during pregnancy.[3, 34, 34a] When possible, however, severe stenosis should be corrected before conception. In the rare instance of progressive right ventricular failure or symptoms clearly related to the stenotic valve, or in a patient with intracardiac shunt at either the atrial or ventricular level with cyanosis, percutaneous balloon valvotomy should be considered during pregnancy.

TETRALOGY OF FALLOT (see also Chap. 44). Hemodynamic changes associated with pregnancy may become severe and cause clinical deterioration in women with surgically uncorrected or only partially corrected tetralogy of Fallot. Increase in blood volume and venous return to the right atrium raises right ventricular pressure, which combined with a fall in systemic vascular resistance can produce or exacerbate right-to-left shunt and cyanosis. Labor and delivery are particularly important because a fall in blood pressure can also increase right-to-left shunt and the degree of cyanosis. Maternal hematocrit above 60 percent, arterial oxygen saturation below 80 percent, right ventricular hypertension, and syncopal episodes are poor prognostic signs. Pregnancies in women with cyanosis are associated with high rate of spontaneous abortion, premature deliveries, and fetal growth retardation.[43, 44, 45, 58, 59]

Close monitoring of systemic blood pressure and blood gases during labor and delivery is recommended for cyanotic or symptomatic patients. Incidence of cardiac defects reported in born infants ranges between 3 and 17 percent.[40]

Patients who have undergone only palliative procedures or who have significant residual defects after repair, such as residual ventricular septal defect, pulmonic stenosis or regurgitation, and ventricular dysfunction, are still at higher risk during pregnancy. Patients who had undergone shunt procedures to improve cyanosis may develop pulmonary hypertension, which increases the risk of pregnancy. Because maternal and fetal outcomes seem to be markedly improved after surgical repair, this procedure should be performed before conception. Because revision of an incompletely repaired defect is recommended in patients with residual ventricular septal defect when the pulmonary/systemic flow ratio is greater than 1.5:1.0, in those with right ventricular outflow obstruction (right ventricular systolic pressure >60 mm Hg), and in those with right ventricular failure due to pulmonic regurgitation, such revision should be performed before conception in a woman who plans to conceive.

EISENMENGER SYNDROME (see also Chap. 44). This condition continues to be associated with a high risk of maternal morbidity and mortality. A recent review of 55 women who had at least one pregnancy showed maternal mortality of 39 percent.[34] Similarly, a recent analysis of 65 published cases with Eisenmenger syndrome from more than 20 countries showed 43 percent maternal mortality.[60] Cause of maternal death is often unclear; it usually occurs in the first few days after delivery and is preceded by desaturation and hemodynamic deterioration. Eisenmenger syndrome is also associated with a poor fetal outcome, with a high incidence of fetal loss, prematurity, intrauterine growth retardation, and perinatal death.[34, 34a]

Because of the high risk of maternal mortality, patients with Eisenmenger syndrome should be advised against pregnancy and early abortion should be recommended for patients who are already pregnant. Management of a patient who decides to proceed to term must include close follow-up for early detection of clinical deterioration. Because of increased incidence of peripartum thromboembolism, anticoagulant therapy seems indicated in the third trimester of gestation and for 4 weeks post partum. Because premature delivery is common, women with Eisenmenger syndrome should be hospitalized for any sign of premature uterine activity. For this reason and to ensure restriction of activity and close follow-up, early elective hospitalization is recommended. Spontaneous labor is preferred to induction and should lower the chance of prematurity or the need for cesarean section. Blood pressure, electrocardiographic, and blood gas monitoring are essential during labor and delivery to ensure early detection and correction of problems; high concentrations of oxygen may be helpful. Most patients in stable condition will tolerate vaginal delivery; however, an attempt should be made to shorten the second stage of labor by the use of forceps or vacuum extraction. Because of the higher risk of fetal distress during vaginal delivery and potential need for emergency cesarean section, a planned cesarean section is often preferred. Insertion of a Swan-Ganz catheter may be difficult and associated with the development of arrhythmias, and its routine use is not recommended.[61] Inhaled nitric oxide has been used successfully to reduce pulmonary pressure and improve oxygenation during labor and the early postpartum period in two patients with Eisenmenger syndrome.[62, 63] Both patients gave birth to live infants but died 2 and 21 days post partum.

EBSTEIN ANOMALY. Pregnancy in women with noncyanotic Ebstein anomaly is well tolerated. In cyanotic cases pregnancy is associated with increased risk of maternal heart failure, prematurity, and fetal loss.[64, 65] The approach to labor and delivery in symptomatic or cyanotic patients with Ebstein anomaly includes antibiotic prophylaxis, oxygen administration, hemodynamic and blood gas monitoring, and efforts to prevent a drop in systemic blood pressure in response to peripheral vasodilation or blood loss.

COMPLEX CYANOTIC CONGENITAL HEART DISEASE. The more widespread use of palliative and corrective surgical procedures for complex cyanotic congenital cardiac anomalies has allowed more women who are so affected to reach childbearing age.[34] Although successful pregnancies have been reported in patients with partially corrected and uncorrected cyanotic heart disease, including pulmonary and tricuspid atresia,[44, 66] transposition of the great vessels,[64-70] truncus arteriosus,[71] single ventricle,[72-74] double-outlet right ventricle,[75] and double-inlet left ventricle,[76] pregnancy is associated with increased risk in these patients. A report[44] of 96 pregnancies in 44 patients with cyanotic heart disease without Eisenmenger reaction demonstrated cardiovascular complications in 32 percent of the patients. These complications included heart failure, thromboembolic events, supraventricular tachycardia, and peripartum bacterial endocarditis resulting in postpartum maternal death in one patient. In addition, a high incidence of fetal wastage (57 percent), premature deliveries, small-for-gestational-age newborns, and both cardiac and noncardiac congenital malformations have been reported.[34]

Although the incidence of rheumatic heart disease is declining in the United States, the disease continues to be prevalent in many developing countries and may be associated with significant morbidity and even mortality.[3, 77]

ACUTE RHEUMATIC FEVER (see Chap. 66). This disease occurs most often in children, before puberty, and only rarely during pregnancy.[77] The management of acute rheumatic fever during pregnancy is similar to that of nonpregnant patients. Because heart failure is usually due to an incompetence of the mitral or aortic valve, diuretics and vasodilators should be the therapy of choice. Surgical repair of valvular incompetence should be performed in patients not responding to medical therapy. The results of mitral valve repair in patients with acute rheumatic disease, however, are inferior to those seen in patients with other forms of valvular regurgitation. Mild cases of heart failure require only bed rest and treatment of streptococcal pharyngitis and comorbidity, including anemia and nutritional difficulty.[77]

CHRONIC RHEUMATIC VALVULAR DISEASE (see Chap. 46). Patients with chronic rheumatic valvular disease should be managed individually according to the site and severity of the lesion. However, certain general guidelines apply to the care of all patients. These include (1) restriction of physical activity in symptomatic patients to reduce cardiovascular load and prevent hemodynamic and symptomatic worsening and (2) prophylactic antibiotic treatment to prevent streptococcal infection and recurrence. Although antibiotic prophylaxis during labor and delivery has not been uniformly recommended,[47] it is commonly used for vaginal and abdominal deliveries. Hemodynamic monitoring is strongly recommended from the onset of labor to approximately 24 hours post partum in any patient who experiences symptoms of heart failure during pregnancy and for those with severe valvular disease, left ventricular dysfunction, or pulmonary hypertension.

MITRAL STENOSIS (see also Chap. 46). This condition is the most common rheumatic valvular lesion in pregnancy.[77] The majority of patients with moderate to severe mitral stenosis demonstrate a worsening of one or two classes in the New York Heart Association functional status during gestation.[3, 77] Although mitral stenosis is often accompanied by some degree of mitral regurgitation, hemodynamic problems are related predominantly to flow obstruction. The pressure gradient across the narrowed mitral valve may increase greatly secondary to the physiological increase in heart rate and blood volume of pregnancy.[3] Increased left atrial pressure can result in atrial flutter or fibrillation, substantially accelerating the ventricular rate and further elevating left atrial pressure. In addition, decreased serum colloid osmotic pressure during pregnancy and excessive peripartum intravenous fluid administration can both predispose to pulmonary edema. A recent study has demonstrated a high incidence of worsening of functional class and the development of heart failure, which led to the need for hospitalizations and either starting or increasing the dose of cardiac medications in patients with moderate to severe mitral stenosis. In addition, there was a marked increase in the rate of prematurity and fetal growth retardation in these cases. Despite marked increase in maternal morbidity, there was no mortality.[3]

Treatment. The therapeutic approach to patients with significant mitral stenosis should aim to reduce the heart rate and decrease blood volume. Both heart rate and symptoms can be controlled effectively by restricting physical activity and administering beta-adrenergic receptor blockers.[77-79] In patients with atrial fibrillation, digoxin may also be useful for control of ventricular rate. Blood volume can be decreased through restriction of salt intake and the use of oral diuretics; aggressive use of diuretic agents should, however, be avoided to prevent hypovolemia and reduction of uteroplacental perfusion.

Although careful medical therapy allows successful completion of pregnancy in the great majority of women,[77] repair or replacement of the valve during pregnancy may be indicated in some patients with severe symptoms in spite of adequate medical therapy.[80-82] In both mitral valve commissurotomy (open or closed) and replacement, the risk in pregnant patients is comparable to that in nonpregnant patients.[81] In contrast, however, open commissurotomy and valve replacement are likely to result in increased fetal loss.[81, 82] Closed mitral commissurotomy is associated with only minimal risk to the fetus; it is, therefore, preferable to the open technique.[83] However, it should be recommended only in centers where it is performed routinely.

Balloon Valvuloplasty (see also Chap. 46). The use of percutaneous mitral balloon valvuloplasty during pregnancy has been reported in an increasing number of pregnant patients with mitral stenosis.[84-89] In the majority of cases, hemodynamic and symptomatic improvement has been achieved without apparent untoward maternal and fetal effects. At the same time, however, serious complications have occasionally been reported, including initiation of uterine contraction,[86] maternal arrhythmia leading to fetal distress,[87] cardiac tamponade requiring surgical intervention, and systemic embolization.[88] In addition, this procedure is associated with some risk to the fetus secondary to unavoidable ionizing radiation. This information suggests that percutaneous mitral balloon valvuloplasty is an attractive alternative to surgery during pregnancy, but it is limited by the exposure to radiation and possible complications that may result in fetal distress or require surgical intervention during pregnancy. The procedure should be avoided if possible during the first trimester[77] and should be performed by experienced operators with adequate abdominal and pelvic shielding with minimum radiation exposure or under echocardiographic guidance, if possible.

Mitral Valve Repair or Replacement (see also Chap. 46). For all of the aforementioned reasons, mitral valve repair or replacement during pregnancy should be considered only in cases with severe mitral stenosis (mitral valve area < 1.0 cm²) refractory to optimal medical therapy or when close follow-up during pregnancy, labor, and delivery is not possible. When valve replacement is indicated, selection of the type of prosthesis should be based on its hemodynamic profile and durability and the need for anticoagulation.

Vaginal delivery can be permitted in most patients with mitral stenosis. In symptomatic patienvs, those with moderate or severe stenosis (mitral valve area <1.5 cm²), hemodynamic monitoring is recommended during labor and delivery. Initiation of monitoring at onset of labor allows hemodynamic optimization by means of intravenous diuretics, digoxin (in case of atrial fibrillation), beta blockers, or nitroglycerin and prevention of a rise in left atrial pressure during labor and delivery. With delivery and thus relief of venocaval obstruction due to the gravid uterus, there is an immediate increase in venous return, which may lead to a substantial increase in pulmonary artery wedge pressure. For this reason, hemodynamic monitoring should be continued for at least several hours post partum.

Epidural anesthesia is the most appropriate form of analgesia in patients with mitral stenosis for both vaginal and abdominal delivery. This form of anesthesia is often associated with a significant fall in pulmonary arterial and left atrial pressures due to systemic vasodilation. With this approach, the great majority of patients with mitral stenosis, even if it is severe, can be delivered with few complications.

MITRAL REGURGITATION (see also Chap. 46). This condition is usually well tolerated in pregnancy, presumably because of left ventricular unloading secondary to the physiological fall in systemic vascular resistance. In symptomatic patients, drug therapy with diuretics is indicated,

and digoxin may be useful in those with impaired left ventricular systolic function. Because hydralazine has been shown to be safe for use during pregnancy,[90] it may be used for further reduction of left ventricular afterload and prevention of hemodynamic worsening associated with isometric exercise during labor.[91]

AORTIC STENOSIS (see also Chap. 46). Rheumatic aortic stenosis is rare during pregnancy and occurs in conjunction with mitral valve disease in approximately 5 percent of pregnant patients with rheumatic valvular disease.[77] Although most patients with aortic stenosis and valve area greater than 1.0 cm² tolerate pregnancy well, patients with more severe stenosis may demonstrate clinical deterioration with exertional dyspnea, near-syncope, or syncope and pulmonary edema.[3, 92] Development of serious symptoms during pregnancy, especially if resistant to medical therapy, may require termination of pregnancy or repair of the valve either surgically (valve replacement) or by percutaneous balloon valvuloplasty.[81, 93]

AORTIC REGURGITATION (see also Chap. 46). Similar to mitral regurgitation, aortic regurgitation is also well tolerated during pregnancy, probably because of reduced systemic vascular resistance and increased heart rate, which results in shortening of diastole. In symptomatic patients, diuretics, digoxin, and hydralazine for left ventricular afterload reduction can be safely used.

Other Conditions Affecting the Valves, Aorta, and Myocardium

Mitral Valve Prolapse (see also Chap. 46)

The prevalence of mitral valve prolapse in the general population has been recently found to be 2.4 percent and was reported in approximately 1.2 percent of pregnant women. Because of high incidence of systolic functional murmurs and wide splitting of the first heart sound during pregnancy, mitral valve prolapse may be falsely diagnosed and needs to be confirmed by echocardiographic criteria.[94] At the same time, the incidence of prolapse-related auscultatory and echocardiographic findings may decrease during gestation as a result of an increase in left ventricular end-diastolic volume.[95]

For the few patients with mitral valve prolapse with chest pain or cardiac arrhythmias, the emphasis should be on reassurance and attempts to avoid the use of medications during pregnancy. Beta-adrenergic blocking agents are recommended when therapy is indicated. Patients with mitral valve prolapse, especially those with a thickened mitral valve and mitral regurgitation, are at increased risk for infective endocarditis. Although antibiotic prophylaxis for uncomplicated vaginal delivery has not been uniformly recommended, the development of bacteremia during vaginal delivery and cesarean section cannot always be predicted. For this reason, prophylaxis for labor and delivery in patients with mitral valve prolapse accompanied by valve thickening and/or regurgitation seems warranted.

Marfan Syndrome (See also Chap. 40)

Pregnancy in women with Marfan syndrome poses a twofold problem: (1) cardiovascular complications and (2) a high risk of having a child who will inherit the condition.[96, 97] Cardiovascular complications during pregnancy include dilatation of the ascending aorta, which may lead to the development of aortic regurgitation and congestive heart failure, and proximal and distal dissections of the aorta with occasional involvement of the iliac and coronary arteries (see Fig. 65-3). The risk of aortic dissection is significantly higher in patients with a dilated aorta or a history of previous dissection. Patients with Marfan syndrome who have only minor involvement of the cardiovascular system and aortic diameter less than 40 mm usually

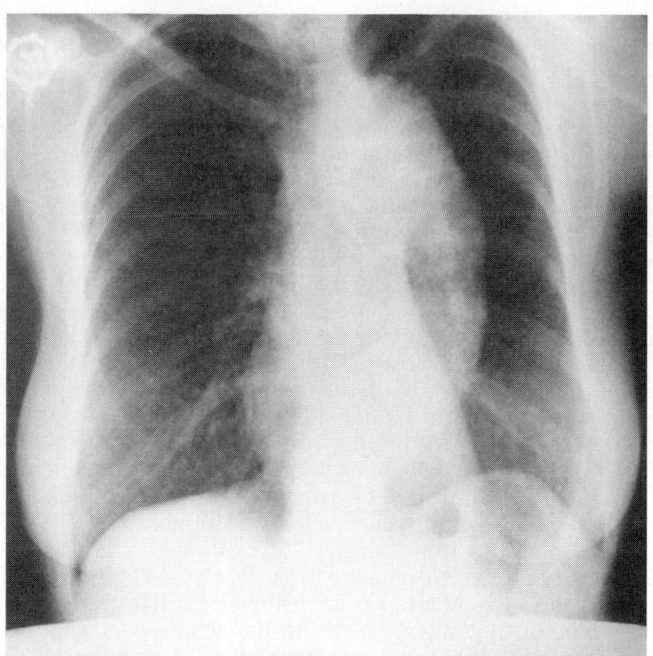

FIGURE 65-4. Chest radiograph demonstrating severe dilatation of the thoracic aorta in a 23-year-old woman with Marfan syndrome who presented with sharp chest pain radiating to the back during her 16th week of gestation. The patient was found to have thoraco-abdominal aortic aneurysm and descending aortic dissection and had an elective abortion at 19 weeks.

tolerate pregnancy well without subsequent worsening of their cardiovascular status attributable to pregnancy.[98] The majority of complications are developed in the later phase of pregnancy. Marfan syndrome may also be responsible for cervical incompetence, abnormal placental site, and postpartum hemorrhagic complications.[99]

The management of pregnancy in women with Marfan syndrome should include preconception counseling to discuss potential maternal and fetal risks.[96] Women with significant cardiac involvement—in particular, dilatation of the aorta and previous history of aortic dissection—are at high risk for complications during gestation and should be advised against conception or, if they are already pregnant, to have an early abortion (Fig. 65-4). In contrast, the risk in patients without cardiac complications and with a normal aortic diameter is significantly lower. Still, a favorable outcome is not guaranteed, and aortic dissection can occur, albeit infrequently, in patients with a normal-sized aorta.[96] Preconception echocardiographic assessment of the aorta and periodic follow-up during pregnancy are highly recommended.[98] Because aneurysms and dissections of the aorta can occasionally involve the descending aorta, the use of transesophageal echocardiography seems preferred to transthoracic examination.[100] During pregnancy, vigorous physical activity should be avoided. Beta blockers, which have been shown to reduce the rate of aortic dilatation and the risk of complications in patients with Marfan syndrome, should be administered.[101] In case of substantial dilatation of the aorta during pregnancy, therapeutic abortion or surgical intervention should be considered.[96] In women with aortic dilatation, aortic dissection, or other cardiac complications, abdominal delivery by cesarean section should be the preferred mode of delivery to minimize hemodynamic changes associated with vaginal delivery.[96, 98]

Cardiomyopathies (See Chap. 48)

HYPERTROPHIC CARDIOMYOPATHY. Reported experience in over 100 pregnancies in patients with hypertrophic cardiomyopathy reveals a favorable outcome in most cases but at the same time a potential for increased morbidity and even mortality.[102, 103] New onset or worsening of congestive heart failure has been reported in approximately 20 percent of cases, and a few patients experienced chest pain, palpitations, dizzy spells, and syncope. Poorly tolerated resistant supraventricular tachycardia with fetal distress[104] has also been reported as well as new-onset atrial fibrillation leading to hemodynamic deterioration and direct-current cardioversion.[105] Few patients had ventricular arrhythmias, which proved fatal in one,[102] and in one patient sudden death occurred at 28 weeks during moderate exertion.[106] Fetal outcome in most cases does not seem to be affected by maternal hypertropic cardiomyopathy. The risk of inheriting the disease may be as high as 50 percent in familial cases and less in sporadic cases.[102]

The therapeutic approach to the pregnant patient with hypertrophic cardiomyopathy depends on the presence of symptoms and left ventricular outflow obstruction. In the symptomatic patient with obstructive hypertrophic cardiomyopathy, an attempt should be made to avoid blood loss and use of drugs that can lead to vasodilation or sympathetic stimulation during labor and delivery. Indications for drug therapy during gestation include arrhythmias and symptoms other than those caused by normal pregnancy. Symptoms associated with elevated left ventricular filling pressure should be treated with beta-adrenergic blocking agents, with diuretics and calcium antagonists added if beta blockers alone are not sufficient.[102] Dual-chamber pacing may be considered before pregnancy in symptomatic patients.[107] Because of the potential arrhythmogenic effect of pregnancy, implantation of an automatic defibrillator before pregnancy should be considered in patients with hypertrophic cardiomyopathy with aborted syncope, or life-threatening arrhythmias.

Vaginal delivery has been shown to be safe in women with hypertrophic cardiomyopathy.[88] In those with symptoms or outflow obstruction, the second stage of labor may be shortened by the use of forceps. The use of prostaglandins to induce uterine contractions may be risky in a patient with obstructive hypertrophic cardiomyopathy, owing to their vasodilatory effect, whereas oxytocin should be well tolerated. Because tocolytic agents with beta-adrenergic receptor activity may aggravate left ventricular outflow tract obstruction, other medications such as magnesium sulfate are preferred. Similarly, spinal and epidural anesthetics should be used with caution in obstructive hypertrophic cardiomyopathy because of their vasodilatory effect, and excessive blood loss should be avoided or replaced promptly with intravenous fluid or blood.[102, 103]

Because the risk for infective endocarditis is increased in hypertrophic cardiomyopathy, especially the obstructive form, and in patients with mitral valve abnormalities, antibiotic prophylaxis should be considered for labor and delivery.

PERIPARTUM CARDIOMYOPATHY. Peripartum cardiomyopathy is a form of dilated cardiomyopathy with left ventricular systolic dysfunction that results in signs and symptoms of heart failure. Symptoms usually occur during the last trimester of gestation, and diagnosis is usually made in the early peripartum period.[108, 108a] Because there is no specific test available for the diagnosis of peripartum cardiomyopathy, it is established by exclusion of other causes of left ventricular dilatation and systolic dysfunction (Table 65-6). The reported incidence of the disease in the United States is approximately 1 in 15,000 with a higher incidence (up to 1 in 1,000) in certain parts of Africa.[108]

Common symptoms and signs are shortness of breath, fatigue, chest pain, palpitations, weight gain, peripheral edema, peripheral or pulmonary embolization, and arrhythmias. Physical examination often reveals an enlarged heart, S_3, and murmurs of mitral and tricuspid regurgitation. The electrocardiogram may show tachycardia, ST-T wave

▼ TABLE 65–6. MODIFIED CRITERIA FOR DIAGNOSIS OF PERIPARTUM CARDIOMYOPATHY

Development of cardiac failure during pregnancy or within 6 months of delivery
Absence of a determinable cause for cardiac failure
Demonstrable impairment in left ventricular systolic function

changes, conduction abnormalities, and arrhythmias. Chest radiography usually shows cardiomegaly, pulmonary venous congestion with interstitial or alveolar edema, and occasionally pleural effusion. Doppler echocardiography commonly shows enlargement of all four cardiac chambers, with marked reduction in left ventricular systolic function. Small-to-moderate pericardial effusion and mitral, tricuspid, and pulmonic regurgitation may be evident. The clinical presentation and hemodynamic changes are indistinguishable from those found in other forms of dilated cardiomyopathy.[109] A few patients with high-output heart failure have been reported.[110]

The incidence of peripartum cardiomyopathy is greater in multiparous women and in those with preeclampsia and twin pregnancies, as well as in women older than 30 years of age.[111] Although the etiology of peripartum cardiomyopathy is still unknown, the unique nature of this syndrome is suggested by its relation to pregnancy, its occurrence at a relatively young age when compared with other forms of dilated cardiomyopathy, the relatively rapid recovery of cardiac size and function in a large number of patients, and the recurrence of left ventricular depression with subsequent pregnancies.[108] Association between myocarditis and peripartum cardiomyopathy was suggested by some investigators who reported a high incidence of myocarditis documented by endomyocardial biopsy.[112] Later reports, however, have indicated a low incidence of myocarditis in patients with peripartum cardiomyopathy that was comparable to that found in an age- and sex-matched nonpregnant, control population with idiopathic dilated cardiomyopathy.[108, 113]

The clinical course of peripartum cardiomyopathy varies, with 50 to 60 percent of patients showing complete or near-complete recovery of clinical status and cardiac function, usually within the first 6 months postpartum[111]; the rest of the patients demonstrate either further clinical deterioration, leading to cardiac transplantation or early death, or persistent left ventricular dysfunction and chronic heart failure.

Management. Acute heart failure should be treated vigorously with oxygen, diuretics, digitalis, and vasodilator agents. The use of hydralazine as an afterload-reducing agent is safe during pregnancy.[90] The use of organic nitrates, dopamine, dobutamine, or milrinone has been reported in pregnancy in a limited number of cases. Nitroprusside has been used successfully during pregnancy, but experiments in animals have shown the potential for fetal toxicity.[90] Angiotensin-converting enzyme inhibitors have a

teratogenic effect, may cause fetal renal dysfunction, and should therefore not be used during pregnancy.[114] Because of the increased incidence of thromboembolic events in peripartum cardiomyopathy, anticoagulant therapy is recommended. Because the disease may be reversible, the temporary use of an intraaortic balloon pump or left ventricular assist device may help stabilize the patient's condition pending improvement.[115, 116] A small retrospective study of intravenous immune globulin showed a favorable effect on recovery of left ventricular dysfunction in patients with peripartum cardiomyopathy.[117] Further evaluation of this therapy seems warranted. The presence of preeclampsia may be associated with greater improvement in left ventricular dysfunction post partum.[111] Because of the high risk of mortality, patients with severe heart failure, who do not recover early, should be considered for cardiac transplantation. Two reports comparing results of cardiac transplantation in age-matched females with peripartum cardiomyopathy and idiopathic cardiomyopathy showed favorable and comparable long-term survival in both groups.[118, 119] Although mortality from peripartum cardiomyopathy was reported to be over 40 percent in early studies,[108] two recent studies reported incidence of death or cardiac transplantation to be in the range of 12 to 18 percent.[111, 112]

Subsequent pregnancies in women with peripartum cardiomyopathy are often associated with relapse, leading to left ventricular dysfunction, symptomatic deterioration, and even to death. Although the likelihood of such relapse is greater in patients with persistently abnormal cardiac function, it has also been reported in women in whom left ventricular function is restored after the first episode.[120] Two recent surveys on the risk of subsequent pregnancy in women with history of peripartum cardiomyopathy reported mortality of 0 to 2 percent in patients with normal left ventricular ejection fraction before the subsequent pregnancy and 8 to 17 percent in patients with depressed left ventricular ejection fraction (Table 65–7).[120, 121] For these reasons, subsequent pregnancies should be discouraged in patients with peripartum cardiomyopathy who have persistent cardiac dysfunction; women with recovered cardiac function cannot be guaranteed an event-free pregnancy, and recurrence of the disease is possible. The risk of mortality in such cases, however, seems to be small.

Hypertension in Pregnancy

(See Chap. 28)

Hypertensive disorders are the most common medical complications of pregnancy and are a major cause of maternal and perinatal morbidity and mortality.[2, 122] In general, hypertension in pregnancy is defined as blood pressure greater than 140 mm Hg systolic and 90 mm Hg diastolic on at least two occasions 6 hours apart.[123] Hypertension complicates 8 to 10 percent of all pregnancies and is an important cause of maternal mortality and morbidity, including abruptio placentae, pulmonary edema, respiratory failure, disseminated intravascular coagulation, cerebral hemor-

▼ TABLE 65–7. MATERNAL AND FETAL OUTCOME IN 67 SUBSEQUENT PREGNANCIES IN 60 PATIENTS WITH A HISTORY OF PERIPARTUM CARDIOMYOPATHY

GROUPS	MATERNAL OUTCOMES			FETAL OUTCOME		
	Normal (%)	Left Ventricular Dysfunction (%)	Death (%)	Live birth (%)	Abortions (%)	Still birth (%)
A	74	23	2	93	5	2
B	37	54	8	83	17	0

Group A—43 pregnancies in 40 patients with history peripartum cardiomyopathy who had recovery of left ventricular function.
Group B—24 pregnancies in 23 patients with history of peripartum cardiomyopathy and persistent left ventricular dysfunction

TABLE 65–8. MODIFIED CLASSIFICATION OF THE AMERICAN COLLEGE OF OBSTETRICIANS AND GYNECOLOGISTS

Pregnancy-Induced Hypertension
Hypertension that develops as a consequence of pregnancy and regresses post partum
Hypertension without proteinuria or pathological edema
Preeclampsia: with proteinuria or pathological edema
  Mild
  Severe
Eclampsia: with proteinuria or pathological edema

Pregnancy-Aggravated Hypertension
Underlying hypertension worsened by:
  Superimposed preeclampsia
  Superimposed eclampsia

Coincidental Hypertension
Chronic hypertension that antecedes pregnancy or persists post partum

rhage, hepatic failure, and acute renal failure.[123] Fetal complications include prematurity, intrauterine growth retardation, stillbirth, and neonatal death. Hypertensive disorders in pregnancy can be divided into three broad categories: chronic hypertension, gestational hypertension,[124] and preeclampsia (Table 65–8).

CHRONIC HYPERTENSION. Chronic hypertension is defined as hypertension that precedes pregnancy, hypertension that occurs before the 20th gestational week, and hypertension that persists beyond the 6th postpartum week.[123] It occurs in 1 to 5 percent of pregnancies and is associated with increased complications (15 percent), such as fetal growth retardation, premature delivery, abruptio placentae, acute renal failure, and hypertensive crisis; most of these complications occur in patients older than age 30 years with a longer duration of hypertension or those who develop superimposed preeclampsia. Drug therapy is recommended for patients with high-risk characteristics. Therapy options for patients with high-risk chronic hypertension are shown in Table 65–9.

GESTATIONAL HYPERTENSION. This is defined as hypertension induced by pregnancy beginning after 20 weeks of gestation and resolving by the sixth postpartum week.[123] Gestational hypertension is further classified as transient hypertension (hypertension without proteinuria) and preeclampsia (hypertension with proteinuria). Transient hypertension usually presents in the late third trimester with

return of blood pressure to normal by the 10th postpartum day. It should be noted that the presence of proteinuria can occur late in the course of preeclampsia and the distinction between transient hypertension and preeclampsia can be difficult and made retrospectively. For this reason, in uncertain situations, preeclampsia should be considered and seizure prophylaxis should be instituted empirically in patients with blood pressure greater than 160/110 mm Hg. Pregnancy outcome is usually favorable, and use of antihypertensive therapy should be reserved for patients with blood pressure greater than 160/110 mm Hg. Recommended drugs include parenteral hydralazine, parenteral labetolol, and oral nifedipine.[124]

PREECLAMPSIA-ECLAMPSIA. Preeclampsia usually occurs after 20 weeks' gestation in the first pregnancy and near term in multiparous women. Preeclampsia can be subclassified into mild and severe.[123] In mild preeclampsia, systolic blood pressure is greater than 140 mm Hg but less than 160 mm Hg, and diastolic blood pressure is greater than 90 mm Hg but less than 110 mm Hg, and mild proteinuria (<5.0 g/24 hr) is the only laboratory abnormality. In severe preeclampsia, blood pressure is greater than 160 mm Hg systolic or more than 110 mm Hg diastolic, proteinuria is greater than 5.0 g/24 hr, platelet count is less than 100.000/ml, and there is evidence for microangiopathic hemolytic anemia or elevated levels of hepatic enzymes. Other symptoms consistent with severe disease are persistent headache, visual disturbance, pulmonary edema, and epigastric pain. Preeclampsia is always associated with increased risk to both mother and fetus and can progress to eclampsia, a life-threatening convulsive phase. Preeclampsia usually regresses within 24 to 48 hours post partum. In the minority of cases, postpartum eclampsia with hypertension, proteinuria, and convulsions occurs within 10 days after delivery.[123]

Patients with stable, mild preeclampsia may be followed until fetal pulmonary maturity is verified or until after 37 weeks of gestation with cervical ripening.[124] There is no evidence for need or benefit of antihypertensive drug therapy in this subgroup of patients. Severe preeclampsia can be rapidly progressive, leading to sudden deterioration of the status of both mother and fetus. Patients with severe preeclampsia who are at or past 34 weeks' gestation should be delivered promptly. Patients with severe preeclampsia who are at 24 to 34 weeks' gestation may receive expectant management that includes admission, bed rest, 24 hours of intravenous magnesium sulfate for seizure prophylaxis, blood pressure control, fetal assessment, and corticosteroids for acceleration of fetal lung maturity. Indicators for deliv-

TABLE 65–9. ANTIHYPERTENSIVE DRUGS IN PREGNANCY

CLASS	DRUG	STARTING DOSE	MAXIMUM DOSE
Drugs for Long-Term Treatment of Hypertension			
Central alpha$_2$-agonist	Methyldopa	250 mg tid	4 g/d
	Clonidine	0.1–0.3 mg bid	1.2 mg/d
Alpha$_1$-adrenergic blocker	Prazosin	1 mg bid	20 mg/d
Calcium channel blocker	Nifedipine	10 mg qid	120 mg/d
Beta-adrenergic blocker	Atenolol	100 mg qd	100 mg/bid
Alpha/beta-adrenergic blocker	Labetalol	100 mg tid	2400 mg/d
Diuretics	Hydrochlorothiazide	25 mg qd	50 mg/d

CLASS	DRUG	DOSE	
Drugs for Acute Treatment of Severe Hypertension			
Arterial dilator	Hydralazine	5–10 mg IV q 15–30 min	
	Diazoxide	30–60 mg IV q 10–15 min	
Calcium channel blocker	Nifedipine	10–20 mg PO q 30 min	
Alpha/beta-adrenergic blocker	Labetalol	20–40–80 mg IV q 10–20 min (up to 300 mg)	
Arterial/venous dilator	Sodium nitroprusside	(50 mg/250 mL saline): 0.5–5.0 μg/kg/min	

ery include eclampsia, resistant, severe hypertension (refractory to maximum doses of three antihypertensive drugs), completion of 34 weeks of gestation, HELLP syndrome (hemolysis, elevated liver enzymes, low platelet count), and fetal testing suggesting a problem is present.[123] Because of potential risks to the mother and fetus, conservative management of severe preeclampsia has been recommended only at tertiary perinatal centers under a very close maternal and fetal monitoring. The primary goal of treatment is to prevent cerebral complications. Recommended goal of therapy is reduction of mean blood pressure below 126 mm Hg but not less than 105 mm Hg and diastolic blood pressure between 90 and 105 mm Hg. Use of intravenous hydralazine is recommended as initial therapy, given intravenously in 5-mg bolus doses at intervals of 20 minutes up to cumulative dose of 20 mg. If not effective or associated with maternal side effect (tachycardia, headache, nausea), labetalol (20 mg intravenously) or nifedipine (10 mg orally) should be given.

PREGNANCY AFTER CARDIAC TRANSPLANTATION
(See Chap. 20)

A recent study conducted to determine the outcome of pregnancy in cardiac allograft recipients identified 47 pregnancies in 35 heart transplant recipients, which resulted in 35 (74 percent) live births.[125] Therapeutic abortion was performed in five cases owing to a short interval between transplantation and conception. Maternal hemodynamic changes during gestation seemed well tolerated, and rejection episodes were rare. At the same time, however, a higher incidence of maternal complications was reported, including chronic hypertension, preeclampsia, worsening kidney failure, premature rupture of membranes, and infections.[126] Although fetal loss does not seem to be increased, an increased incidence of preterm deliveries and fetal growth retardation and cesarean sections were reported. No maternal deaths were reported during pregnancy. The incidence of late death, however, was high compared with age-matched healthy women. None of the newborns was found to have congenital malformations, supporting a lack of teratogenic effect of immunosuppressive agents.[126] This limited information suggests, therefore, that pregnancy in women after cardiac transplantation is not associated with increased maternal mortality; however, it results in increased maternal morbidity, preterm deliveries, and fetal growth retardation. In addition, the patients and their families should be informed regarding risk of shorter life span after delivery in patients after heart transplantation.

CORONARY ARTERY DISEASE (See Chaps. 35–37)

PATHOGENESIS. Although coronary artery disease is encountered during pregnancy with increasing frequency because of increasing maternal age and fertility,[127] it is still rare among women of childbearing age; and the occurrence of peripartum acute myocardial infarction is anecdotal.[128]

Risk factors for coronary artery disease in women younger than the age of 50 years include cigarette smoking, high levels of total plasma cholesterol, low levels of high-density lipoproteins, diabetes mellitus, hypertension, a family history of coronary artery disease, toxemia of pregnancy, and the use of oral contraceptives.[127–130] The combination of heavy smoking or hypertension and concurrent use of oral contraceptives has been shown to be a powerful predictor of acute myocardial infarction.[130]

In the assessment of risk factors for coronary artery disease during pregnancy it should be noted that total cholesterol, low-density lipoprotein cholesterol, and triglyceride levels are significantly increased during pregnancy.[131]

ACUTE MYOCARDIAL INFARCTION (see also Chap. 35). Peripartum acute myocardial infarction has been reported at any stage of pregnancy and at ages between 16 and 45. The highest incidence, however, occurs in the third trimester and in women older than age 33 years. In addition, acute myocardial infarction has been noted to occur more commonly in multigravidas and its location to be more commonly in the anterolateral wall. Most maternal death occurred either at the time of infarction or within 2 weeks.[128] To reduce the risk for acute myocardial infarction, oral contraceptives should be avoided or formulations with lower effective doses of estrogen should be used in cigarette smokers and in women with hypertension.

Although atherosclerotic disease seems to be the primary cause of acute myocardial infarction[128, 132–134] peripartum acute myocardial infarction is often associated with normal coronary angiograms and has been suggested as being due to a decrease in coronary perfusion caused by spasm or in situ thrombosis. Although the presence of spasm has not been documented and its cause is not clear, it has been suggested as a cause of myocardial infarction in some instances with pregnancy-induced hypertension and with the administration of ergot derivatives, bromocriptine,[135] oxytocin, and prostaglandin[136] used to suppress lactation or uterine bleeding and in patients with pheochromocytoma.[137] Coronary arterial dissection mostly in the immediate postpartum period has been commonly associated with peripartum acute myocardial infarction.[128, 135, 138, 139] The dissection involves the left anterior descending artery in approximately 80 percent of cases and the right coronary artery in most other cases. Other potential causes of acute myocardial infarction during pregnancy have been collagen vascular disease, Kawasaki disease, sickle cell anemia, and hemostatic abnormalities.[128, 135, 140]

DIAGNOSIS. The diagnostic approach to ischemic myocardial disease in pregnancy is influenced to some extent by whether a diagnostic procedure could harm the fetus and by normal changes seen during pregnancy that may mimic pathological changes. T wave inversion, Q wave in lead III, and increased R/S ratio in leads V_1 and V_2 are commonly seen in normal pregnancy. ST segment depression, not associated with chest pain or echocardiographic wall motion abnormalities, has been described during elective cesarean section and can mimic myocardial ischemia. Because fetal bradycardia has been reported during maximal exercise in normal women, a submaximal exercise protocol with fetal monitoring is recommended for the evaluation of ischemic myocardial disease during pregnancy.

Radionuclide myocardial perfusion scans and radionuclide ventriculography expose the fetus to some radiation and should be used only when the potential benefits seem to outweigh fetal risk. For similar reasons, cardiac catheterization involving fluoroscopy and cineangiography should be used only when relevant information cannot be obtained by other, noninvasive methods. The diagnosis of myocardial ischemia and infarction has been reported to be delayed during pregnancy because of the low level of suspicion.[128] Concentrations of myoglobin, creatine kinase, and creatine kinase MB were found to be increased twofold 30 minutes after delivery, whereas level of troponin I remained below the cutoff value for discriminating myocardial infarction. For this reason, troponin should be used to diagnose myocardial infarction after delivery.[141]

MANAGEMENT. Both maternal and fetal considerations should influence the therapeutic approach to ischemic heart disease during pregnancy. Morphine sulfate does not cause congenital defects. Because it crosses the placenta, it can cause neonatal respiratory depression when given shortly before delivery.[128] Available reports on the use of thrombolytic therapy during pregnancy do not support a teratogenic effect, and the majority of reported cases resulted in favorable maternal and fetal outcome.[128, 133, 142] This therapy, however, is associated with risk of maternal hemorrhage, especially when given at the time of delivery. Because of their safety in pregnancy, beta blockers appear to be the drugs of choice. The use of organic nitrates and calcium antagonists in patients with acute myocardial ischemia or infarction has been described in a limited number of patients. These drugs should be given cautiously to prevent maternal hypotension and potential fetal distress. Use of high-dose aspirin during pregnancy is debatable, because it has been reported to cause fetal growth retardation and bleeding in the neonate and in the mother.[143] Use of low-dose aspirin, however, is safe during pregnancy.[143, 144]

Coronary reperfusion by means of percutaneous transluminal coronary angioplasty[133, 145, 146] or coronary artery bypass graft surgery[134, 139, 147] has been reported to be successful during pregnancy although experience is still limited. Such procedures should be avoided during the first trimester, if possible, owing to the potential deleterious fetal effects due to ionizing radiation as well as cardiopulmonary bypass.

Risk stratification after acute myocardial infarction during pregnancy should be determined by noninvasive methods. Total cholesterol, low density lipoprotein cholesterol, and triglyceride levels are significantly increased during pregnancy.[131] Coronary angiography should be done only in cases in which coronary angioplasty or bypass surgery seems indicated during pregnancy.

Management of the Pregnancy. Management should focus on reducing cardiovascular stress during pregnancy and the peripartum period. Termination of pregnancy may be required in patients with intractable ischemia or heart failure in the early phase of gestation. During labor, adequate analgesia and supplemental oxygen should be given; and, if desired, cardiac output can be increased by placing the patient in the left lateral decubitus position. Labor in the supine position, however, may decrease venous return and thus reduce right and left ventricular filling pressures. Low forceps can be used to shorten the second stage of labor. Pulmonary artery catheterization with hemodynamic monitoring can help in the early detection and correction of hemodynamic abnormalities during labor and delivery.[148] Although elective cesarean section is not indicated in every case, it should be used in patients with active ischemia or hemodynamic instability despite adequate medical therapy.[149] Continued hemodynamic monitoring is advisable for several hours post partum to detect hemodynamic worsening associated with postpartum hemodynamic changes described earlier.

ARRHYTHMIAS (See Chap. 25)

Pregnancy is associated with an increased incidence of arrhythmias in women both with and without structural heart disease.[16, 150-153] In healthy women, multiple and even frequent atrial and ventricular premature complexes may occur, usually without effect on either the mother or the fetus.[16] There is also a strong suggestion for an increased frequency of paroxysmal supraventricular tachycardia during pregnancy.[152, 153]

ATRIAL FLUTTER AND ATRIAL FIBRILLATION. Atrial flutter and fibrillation are rare during normal pregnancy and are usually associated with rheumatic mitral valve disease.[3] Recent reports have described atrial fibrillation during gestation accompanied by treatment with magnesium sulfate[154] and in a patient with preexcitation.[155] Ventricular tachycardia is a rare occurrence in pregnancy. It has been reported in women without structural disease,[156, 157] but it is usually associated with structural heart disease, drugs,[158-160] electrolyte abnormalities,[161] or eclampsia.[162]

Although palpitations, dizziness, and even syncope are relatively common symptoms in normal pregnancy, these are rarely associated with cardiac arrhythmias.[16] Cardiac arrhythmias, however, when they occur, can be hemodynamically significant even in patients with a normal heart during gestation.[19] Reduction in blood pressure occasionally associated with such arrhythmias can result in fetal bradycardia and the need for immediate treatment with antiarrhythmic drugs, electric cardioversion, or urgent cesarean section. The effect of pregnancy on women with the hereditary long QT syndrome has been reported.[163] The postpartum interval was associated with a significant increase in the risk for cardiac events, including death, aborted cardiac arrest, and syncope. Treatment with beta-adrenergic blockers was independently associated with a decrease in the risk for cardiac events.

Synchronized electrical cardioversion has been performed safely during all stages of pregnancy[157, 164, 165] and can be used in patients with tachyarrhythmias unresponsive to drug therapy that are associated with hemodynamic decompensation. Insertion of an implantable cardioverter-defibrillator has not been reported during pregnancy; however, pregnancies in women with an implantable cardioverter-defibrillator have been reported to be uneventful.[166]

COMPLETE HEART BLOCK. This condition has been described during pregnancy and is usually congenital.[167-169] Patients with complete heart block may remain asymptomatic during pregnancy and have an uncomplicated labor and delivery without treatment.[167] Improvement of atrioventricular nodal conduction during two successive uncomplicated pregnancies in a patient with congenital heart block has been reported.[170] Symptomatic patients with conduction abnormalities, including bifascicular block,[171] second-degree atrioventricular block,[172] and complete heart block,[173] have been treated during pregnancy with either temporary or permanent pacemakers; and numerous pregnancies have been reported in patients after pacemaker implantation. In an attempt to reduce exposure to ionizing radiation, placement of a pacemaker during pregnancy has been done with electrocardiographic and echocardiographic guidance in some cases.[172, 174] Skin irritation and ulceration at the implant site due to enlargement of the breast and abdomen during pregnancy have been reported.

MANAGEMENT OF ARRHYTHMIAS. A complete evaluation is indicated in patients with arrhythmias during pregnancy to rule out a treatable cause such as electrolyte imbalance, thyroid disease, and arrhythmogenic effects of drugs, alcohol, caffeine, and cigarette smoking. An identified cause should be treated and antiarrhythmic drug therapy initiated only if the arrhythmia persists and is symptomatic, hemodynamically important, or life threatening. When drug therapy seems necessary, the smallest therapeutic dose of drugs known to be safe for the fetus should be used (Table 65–10). Therapeutic blood levels and the indication for continuous drug therapy should be reevaluated periodically. Electrophysiological evaluation is usually postponed until the postpartum period but can be performed under echocardiographic guidance if indicated during pregnancy.[174] Because of the unpredictable exposure to ionizing radiation, catheter ablation procedures should be performed, if possible, after delivery.

OTHER CARDIOVASCULAR DISORDERS

Aortic Dissection (See also Chap. 40)

A predisposition to aortic dissection during gestation has been suggested.[175, 176] Over the past 50 years, approximately 200 cases of aortic dissection in association with pregnancy have been reported. The incidence is increased among multiparous women older than age 30 years with coarctation of the aorta and Marfan syndrome. Pregnancy-related aortic dissection may be due to alterations in the structure of the vascular wall[175, 177] and seems to occur most often during the third trimester and peripartum period.

Transesophageal echocardiography provides a powerful and safe tool for establishing the diagnosis of aortic dissection during pregnancy.[178] This method is preferable to computed tomography, which involves radiation exposure, and to magnetic resonance imaging, the safety of which during gestation has not been fully established.[32]

The combination of intravenous nitroprusside and beta-adrenergic blocking agents is currently recommended to control hypertension in nonpregnant patients with aortic dissection. Because nitroprusside can result in fetal toxicity, it should be used only post partum or in patients refractory to other drugs during pregnancy and can be substituted by hydralazine or nitroglycerin.[90] To avoid blood pressure elevation associated with labor and vaginal delivery in women with aortic dissection, cesarean section using epidural anesthesia is recommended.[179, 180]

Takayasu Arteritis (See Chap. 67)

Because Takayasu arteritis often occurs in young women, there is a high likelihood of pregnancy in patients with this condition.[181] Review of the literature revealed information on pregnancies in over 50 women with Takayasu disease.[182] The majority of more recently published cases have reported favorable maternal outcome, although increase in blood pressure during pregnancy and the development of heart failure have been described.[183, 184] Although fetal growth retardation and premature labor and delivery are common,[185-187] favorable fetal outcome has been reported in most cases. Mode of delivery in the majority of cases was vaginal, and forceps were often used to expedite the second stage of labor. Cesarean section delivery has been performed mainly for obstetrical indications or maternal hypertension and vascular disorders. In the great majority of patients, abdominal delivery has been performed under epidural anesthesia with

DRUG	USE IN PREGNANCY	POTENTIAL SIDE EFFECTS	SAFETY	BREASTFEEDING[213]	RISK FACTORS[219]*
Adenosine[19]	Maternal and fetal arrhythmias	No side effects reported in >30 cases treated for maternal arrhythmia; data on use during first trimester, however, are limited to few patients.	Safe	NA	C
Amiodarone[215]	Maternal and fetal arrhythmias	IUGR, prematurity, hypothyroidism	Unsafe	Not recommended	C
Angiotensin-converting enzyme inhibitors[216]	Hypertension	Oligohydramnios, IUGR, prematurity, neonatal hypotension, renal failure, anemia, and death. Skull ossification defect, limb contractures, patent ductus arteriosus	Unsafe	Compatible	D
Beta-adrenergic blocking agents[217]	Hypertension, maternal arrhythmias, myocardial ischemia, mitral stenosis, hypertrophic cardiomyopathy, hyperthyroidism, Marfan syndrome	Fetal bradycardia, low placental weight, prolonged labor, low birth weight, hypoglycemia, respiratory dysfunction	Safe	Compatible; monitoring of infant's heart rate recommended	B
Digoxin[218]	Maternal and fetal arrhythmias, heart failure	Low birth weight, prematurity	Safe	Compatible	C
Disopyramide[215]	Maternal arrhythmias	May induce uterine contraction and delivery	Limited data	Compatible	C
Diuretics[219]	Hypertension, congestive heart failure	Reduced uteroplacental perfusion	Potentially unsafe	Compatible	C–D
Flecainide[215]	Maternal and fetal arrhythmias	Two cases of fetal death after successful maternal treatment for fetal supraventricular tachycardia reported. Neither death could be attributed with certainty to flecainide.	Limited data	Compatible	C
Lidocaine[215]	Local anesthesia, maternal arrhythmias	May cause infants central nervous depression at birth with high dose	Safe	Compatible	C
Mexiletine[215]	Maternal arrhythmias	Fetal bradycardia, IUGR, low Apgar score, and neonatal hypoglycemia have been reported	Limited data	Compatible	C
Nifedipine[90]	Hypertension	Fetal distress due to maternal hypotension reported	Safe	Compatible	C
Organic nitrates[90]	Myocardial infarction and ischemia, hypertension, pulmonary edema, tocolysis	Fetal heart rate deceleration and bradycardia	Limited data	NA	C
Procainamide[215]	Maternal and fetal arrhythmias	None reported	Probably safe	Compatible	C
Propafenone[215]	Maternal and fetal arrhythmias	Fetal death reported after direct intrauterine administration in fetuses with nonimmune fetal hydrops	Limited data	NA	C
Quinidine[215]	Maternal and fetal arrhythmias	Minimal oxytoxic activity, high doses may cause premature labor and abortion. Transient neonatal thrombocytopenia and damage to eighth nerve reported	Safe	Compatible	C
Sodium nitroprusside[90]	Hypertension, aortic dissection	Potential thiocyanate toxicity with high-dose, fetal mortality reported in animals	Potentially unsafe	NA	C
Sotalol[217]	Maternal arrhythmias, hypertension, fetal tachycardia	Fetal bradycardia, IUGR	Limited data	Compatible; significant quantities in breast milk, careful monitoring of infants recommended	B

* Risk factors have been assigned based on level of risk to the fetus[214]:

Category A: Controlled studies in women fail to demonstrate a risk to the fetus in the first trimester (and there is no evidence of a risk in later trimesters), and the possibility of fetal harm appears remote.

Catetory B: Either animal-reproduction studies have not demonstrated a fetal risk but there are no controlled studies in pregnant women or animal-reproduction studies have shown an adverse effect (other than a decrease in fertility) that was not confirmed in controlled studies in women in the first trimester (and there is no evidence of a risk in later trimesters).

Category C: Either studies in animals have revealed adverse effects on the fetus (teratogenic or embryocidal, or other) and there are no controlled studies in women or studies in women and animals are not available. Drugs should be given only if the potential benefit justifies the potential risk to the fetus.

Category D: There is positive evidence of human fetal risk, but the benefits from use in pregnant women may be acceptable despite the risk (e.g., if the drug is needed in a life-threatening situation or for a serious disease for which safer drugs cannot be used or are ineffective).

IUGR = intrauterine growth retardation; NA = no data available.

favorable results. A study of C-reactive protein scores and digital plethysmography showed improvement rather than deterioration of Takayasu arteritis with pregnancy.

Primary Pulmonary Hypertension (See Chap. 53)

Primary pulmonary hypertension is one of the few cardiovascular conditions in which pregnancy can be associated with a high maternal mortality. Review of the literature has revealed maternal mortality of 30 to 40 percent.[188, 189] Clinical deterioration during pregnancy or death cannot be predicted on the basis of the patient's preconceptual clinical status. Symptomatic deterioration usually occurs in the second trimester and is manifested by fatigue, exertional dyspnea, syncope, chest pain, palpitations, nonproductive cough, hemoptysis, and leg edema. Worsening of symptoms during pregnancy led to early hospitalization in many reported cases. Death has occurred a few hours to several days post partum, usually due to sudden death or progressive right ventricular failure. Although the exact cause of death in patients with primary pulmonary hypertension is not clear, right ventricular ischemia and failure, cardiac arrhythmias, and pulmonary embolism are likely mechanisms. In addition to high maternal risk, primary pulmonary hypertension is associated with poor fetal outcome with high incidence of fetal loss, prematurity, and fetal growth retardation.[188]

Because of the potential deleterious effect of pregnancy on both mothers with primary pulmonary hypertension and their fetuses, pregnancy should be avoided in these patients and tubal ligation should be recommended. Because an etiological link between pulmonary hypertension and estrogen-containing oral contraceptives has been suggested, this form of birth control is not recommended for women with primary pulmonary hypertension. Early abortion is indicated in patients with primary pulmonary hypertension who become pregnant. If the patient elects to continue the pregnancy, physical exertion should be restricted to reduce the circulatory load. The incidence of premature deliveries is increased in patients with primary pulmonary hypertension and should be anticipated. Because of the beneficial effect of anticoagulation in patients with primary pulmonary hypertension[190, 191] and the increased incidence of thromboembolism during pregnancy, such therapy is recommended throughout gestation or at least during the third trimester and early postpartum phase. Hemodynamic monitoring and blood gas measurements should be performed continuously during labor and delivery. Oxygen should be provided to prevent hypoxemia, and every effort should be made to prevent or immediately correct blood loss during delivery.[188]

Most patients can tolerate vaginal delivery, and spontaneous labor is preferable to induction. Because of the high rate of early postpartum maternal death, close monitoring is recommended for several days post partum. Successful short-term use of calcium antagonists has been reported in patients with primary pulmonary hypertension during pregnancy.[192] Prostaglandins have also been used to lower pulmonary pressure for a short period during pregnancy.[192] The safety of these drugs, when used chronically, however, is not known.

Cardiac Surgery During Pregnancy

Because heart disease that requires surgery is usually diagnosed and treated before pregnancy, cardiac surgery during gestation is uncommon; and the experience continues to be anecdotal.[193, 194] The effects of anesthesia and the surgical procedure, especially cardiopulmonary bypass, on the uteroplacental circulation and fetal outcome are still not well understood. Recent review of the literature published between 1984 and 1996[194] identified 161 cases of various cardiovascular operations, 137 with and 24 without cardiopulmonary bypass.[195] Surgery during pregnancy resulted in high fetal-neonatal mortality of 30 percent. Week of gestation at time of surgery, surgery with cardiopulmonary bypass, longer duration, and temperature of cardiopulmonary bypass did not influence fetal-neonatal outcome. Operations performed during pregnancy resulted in a moderately high maternal mortality at 6 percent, and surgery performed immediately after delivery was associated with even higher mortality at 12 percent. Hospitalization after the 27th gestational week and emergency surgery were associated with poor maternal outcome. Nine percent maternal mortality was reported in cases that involved valvular surgery and 22 percent in cases of aortic or arterial dissection repairs and pulmonary embolectomies. Maternal risk associated with peripartum cardiovascular surgery seems therefore higher than risk of similar surgery in nonpregnant patients.

Because of high incidence of fetal wastage and moderate increase in maternal risk, surgery should be recommended only for patients who do not respond to medical therapy. To minimize the risk of teratogenicity, surgery should be avoided during the first trimester. Because heart surgery is indicated after failure of medical therapy, many of these patients will be hemodynamically unstable and will require hemodynamic evaluation and optimization before operation and monitoring during surgery. Anesthetic agents should be selected on the basis of their hemodynamic effects and fetal safety. When the patient is at or near term, abdominal delivery by cesarean section can be performed before cardiac surgery, once fetal maturity has been confirmed. Fetal heart monitoring should be performed continuously during surgery by experienced personnel.

Pregnancy in Patients with Prosthetic Heart Valves (See Chap. 46)

VALVE SELECTION. The selection of a prosthetic heart valve for women of childbearing age remains difficult.[195, 196] New-generation mechanical valves offer excellent durability, low risk of reoperation, and superior hemodynamic profile. However, the need for anticoagulation is associated with an increased risk of maternal bleeding and fetal loss. Tissue valves have a high incidence of deterioration in young patients, which is further accelerated during pregnancy,[197-200] with a 30 percent expected rate of valve replacement within 10 years, and an inferior hemodynamic profile, especially with small valve sizes in the aortic position.[201] Although homograft valves and new pericardial valves appear to have better hemodynamics, information regarding pregnancy in women with these valves is limited.[202, 203] Because of their durability and hemodynamic advantage, and, with careful anticoagulation, only a small risk of thromboembolic as well as bleeding complications, second-generation mechanical prostheses seem to be the preferred choice in all women of childbearing age who need valve replacement and who can be closely monitored.

Risks associated with pregnancy in women with prosthetic valves are related mainly to the increased hemodynamic burden and incidence of thromboembolic events as well as to fetal untoward effects caused by cardiovascular drugs and anticoagulation. Experience in more than 1000 pregnancies indicates that most asymptomatic or mildly symptomatic patients before gestation tolerate the hemodynamic burden of pregnancy, although decreased functional capacity and need to start or increase drug therapy are not uncommon.[197-204]

Increased thromboembolic events have been reported, with an incidence as high as 10 to 15 percent. Approximately two thirds of these patients present with valve thrombosis, leading to death in 40 percent of them.[197-200] Thromboembolism, however, has been reported mostly with older-generation mechanical prostheses in the mitral position.[197-200, 204] Heparin has been considered the anticoagulant of choice during pregnancy because of its proven safety for both the patient and the fetus.[205] Oral anticoagu-

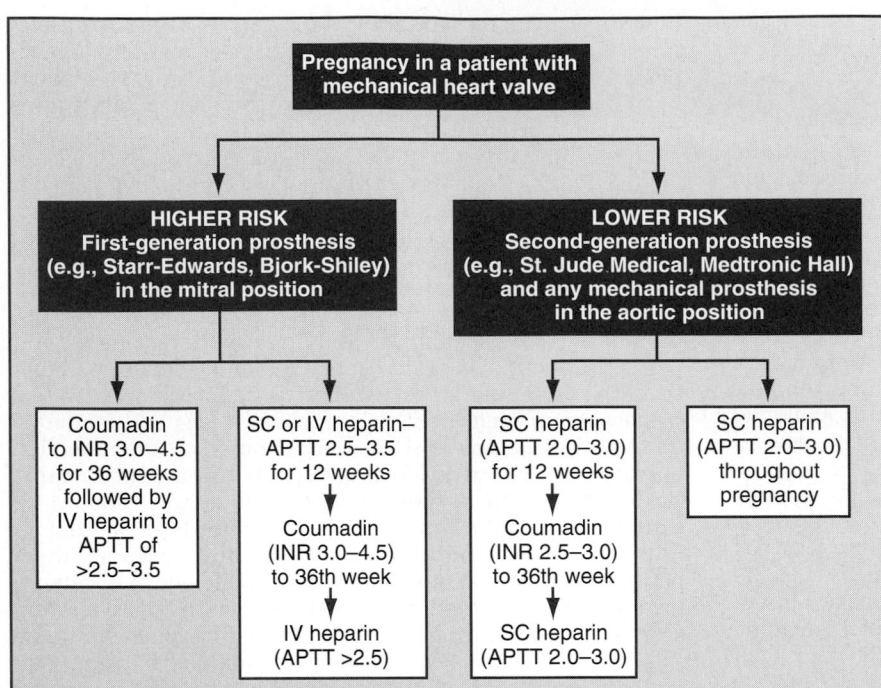

FIGURE 65–5. Suggested algorithm for the management of anticoagulation in patients with mechanical prosthetic heart valves during pregnancy.

lant agents have been considered contraindicated in pregnancy because of their teratogenic effect, increased fetal bleeding complications, and risk of central nervous system damage during gestation. Reports of increased incidence of mechanical valve thrombosis during use of subcutaneous heparin during pregnancy[198, 199, 204] have raised concern regarding the effectiveness of heparin in pregnant women with mechanical heart valves.[206] This has led to recommendations for the use of warfarin as an anticoagulant of choice for the first 35 weeks of pregnancy in patients with a mechanical prosthetic valves.[198, 204, 207, 208] These recommendations have been problematic and have not been adopted by both patients and physicians, especially in the United States.[209, 210] The concern regarding use of warfarin during pregnancy is related to the risk of warfarin-induced embryopathy (depressed nasal bridge, nasal hypoplasia, small nasal bones, hypoplastic alae nasi, telacanthus, upper airway obstruction due to choanal stenosis, and punctate epiphyseal dysplasia of the long bones and the cervical and lumbar vertebral plates) and increased risk of intracranial bleeding.[205] The incidence of warfarin-induced embryopathy is 5 to 9 percent and is dose related.[206, 211] Limited information indicates that in patients with new-generation mechanical prosthetic valves the use of adjusted-dose heparin either throughout pregnancy or during the first trimester and after the 35th to 36th week of gestation is safe.[195]

ANTICOAGULATION (see also Chap. 46). Our recommendations for anticoagulation during pregnancy in patients with mechanical valve prosthesis are shown in Figure 65–5. Thromboembolic prophylaxis of women seems to be best achieved with oral anticoagulation with first-generation prosthetic valves in the mitral position, especially in those patients who can achieve therapeutic anticoagulation with less than 5 mg/d of warfarin (international normalized ratio of 3.0–4.5) for the first 35 weeks. An alternative therapy for patients electing to avoid warfarin in the first gestational trimester is intravenous or subcutaneous heparin with aggressive monitoring and appropriate dose adjustment[206] for the first trimester, followed by warfarin between 13 and 36 weeks and then intravenous or subcutaneous heparin until delivery. High heparin intensity should be used in patients at high risk, aiming at antifactor Xa levels of 0.55 to 0.8 U/ml or an activated partial thromboplastin time of 2.5 to 3.5.

Because of a high incidence of premature labor in patients with prosthetic heart valves,[204, 209] warfarin should be substituted for heparin at the 35th or 36th week to avoid onset of labor during warfarin therapy. The switch from warfarin to heparin should be performed in the hospital. In lower-risk patients, including those with an aortic prosthetic valve and second-generation prosthesis in the mitral position, subcutaneous heparin therapy is advocated throughout pregnancy (activated partial thromboplastin time of 2.0–3.0).[195, 196, 205] Use of warfarin during weeks 13 to 35 or 36 is an alternative regimen in cases in which self-injection of heparin is not desirable by the patient or is associated with side effects. A higher level of anticoagulation seems justified in patients with mechanical prostheses in the mitral position, in patients with more than one mechanical prosthesis, in patients with atrial fibrillation, and/or in patients with a history of systemic embolization. The intensity of anticoagulation should be frequently monitored and immediately corrected if needed. Because a small dose of aspirin is safe during pregnancy[143] and can reduce the incidence of systemic embolization or death when added to oral anticoagulation,[212] 80 mg of aspirin may be added to maximize the antithrombolic effect.

Safe use of low-molecular-weight heparin has been reported in few patients with prosthetic heart valve.[195] Low-molecular-weight heparin provides a better effect, owing to its superior bioavailability and longer half-life, and may reduce the risk of bleeding and osteoporosis. This drug, however, is less readily reversible by protamine sulfate and may be more difficult to handle during labor and delivery. More information is therefore required before low-molecular-weight heparin can be routinely recommended for anticoagulation in a patient with a prosthetic valve during gestation. For more information on cardiovascular drugs, see Table 65–10.[213–219]

REFERENCES

CARDIOVASCULAR PHYSIOLOGY DURING PREGNANCY AND THE PUERPERIUM

1. Tan J, de Sweet M: Prevalence of heart disease diagnosed de novo in pregnancy in a West London population. Br J Obstet Gynaecol 105: 1185–1188, 1998.

2. Berg CJ, Atrash HK, Koonin LM, Tucker M: Pregnancy-related mortality in the United States, 1987–1990. Obstet Gynecol 88:161–167, 1996.

3. Hameed AB, Wani OR, Karaalp IS, et al: Valvular disease in pregnancy: Effects on maternal and fetal outcome. Circulation 100:1–148, 1999.

4. Elkayam U, Gleicher N: Hemodynamic and cardiac function during normal pregnancy and the puerperium. In Elkayam U, Gleicher N (eds): Cardiac Problems in Pregnancy. 3rd ed. New York, Wiley-Liss, 1998, pp 3–20.

5. Thomsen JK, Fogh-Andersen N, Jaszczak P: Atrial natriuretic peptide, blood volume, aldosterone, and sodium excretion during twin pregnancy. Acta Obstet Gynecol Scand 73:14–20, 1994.

6. Brown MA, Gallery ED: Volume homeostasis in normal pregnancy and preeclampsia: Physiology and clinical implications. Baillieres Clin Obstet Gynecol 8:287–310, 1994.

7. Duvekot JJ, Peeters LLH: Renal hemodynamics and volume hemostasis in pregnancy. Obstet Gynecol Survey 49:830–839, 1994.

8. Thomsen JK, Fogh-Andersen N, Jaszczak P: Atrial natriuretic peptide, blood volume, aldosterone, and sodium excretion during twin pregnancy. Acta Obstet Gynecol Scand 73:14–20, 1994.

9. Clapp JF III, Capeless E: Cardiovascular function before, during and after the first and subsequent pregnancies. Am J Cardiol 80:1469–1473, 1997.

10. Poppas A, Shroff SG, Korcarz CE, et al: Serial assessment of the cardiovascular system in normal pregnancy. Circulation 95:2407–2415, 1997.

11. Itoh H, Sagawa N, Mori T, et al: Plasma brain natriuretic peptide level in pregnant women with pregnancy-induced hypertension. Obstet Gynecol 82:71, 1993.

12. Podjarny E, Mandelbaum A, Bernheim J: Does nitric oxide play a role in normal pregnancy and pregnancy-induced hypertension? Nephrol Dial Transplant 9:1527–1540, 1994.

13. Robson SC, Dunlop W, Boys RJ, et al: Cardiac output during labour. BMJ 295:1169, 1987.

14. Lee W, Rokey R, Cotton DB, et al: Maternal hemodynamic effects of uterine contractions by M-mode and pulsed-Doppler echocardiography. Am J Obstet Gynecol 161:974–977, 1989.

CARDIAC EVALUATION DURING PREGNANCY

15. Elkayam U, Gleicher N: Cardiac evaluation during pregnancy. In Elkayam U, Gleicher N (eds): Cardiac Problems in Pregnancy. 3rd ed. New York, Wiley-Liss, 1998, pp 23–32.

16. Shotan A, Ostrzega E, Mehra A, et al: Incidence of arrhythmias in normal pregnancy and relation to palpitations, dizziness and syncope. Am J Cardiol 79:1061–1064, 1997.

17. Kleinman B: Electrocardiographic changes during cesarean section. Anesthesiology 78:997–998, 1993.

18. Zakowski MI, Ramanathan S, Baratta JB, et al: Electrocardiographic changes during cesarean section is cause for concern? Anesth Analg 76: 162–167, 1993.

19. Elkayam U, Goodwin TM: Adenosine therapy for supraventricular tachycardia during pregnancy. Am J Cardiol 75:521–523, 1995.

20. Brodsky M, Doria R, Allen B, et al: New onset ventricular tachycardia during pregnancy. Am Heart J 123:933–941, 1992.

21. Wagner CK, Leser RG, Saldana LR: Exposure of the Pregnant Patient to Diagnostic Radiation: A Guide to Medical Management. Philadelphia, JB Lippincott, 1985, p 52.

22. Fidler JL, Patz EF, Ravin CE: Cardiopulmonary complications of pregnancy: Radiographic findings. AJR Am J Roentgenol 161:937–942, 1993.

23. Bioeffects Committee of the American Institute of Ultrasound in Medicine. J Ultrasound Med Biol 2:R14, 1983.

23a. Allan L: Antenatal diagnosis of heart disease. Heart 83:367, 2000.

24. Stoddard MF, Longaker RA, Vuocol LM, Dawkins PR: Transesophageal echocardiography in the pregnant patient. Am Heart J 124:785, 1992.

25. Abduljabbar HS, Marzouki KM, Zawawi TH, Khan AS: Pericardial effusion in normal pregnant women. Acta Obstet Gynecol Scand 70:291–294, 1991.

26. Robson SC, Hunter S, Boys RJ, Dunlop W: Serial study of factors influencing changes in cardiac output during human pregnancy. Am J Physiol 256:H1060–H1065, 1989.

27. Campos O: Doppler echocardiography during pregnancy: Physical and abnormal findings. Echocardiography 13:135–146, 1996.

28. Campos O, Andrade JL, Bocanegra J, et al: Physiologic multivalvular regurgitation during pregnancy: A longitudinal Doppler echocardiographic study. Int J Cardiol 40:265–272, 1993.

29. Erkkola RU, Pirhonen JP, Kivijarvi AK: Flow velocity waveforms in uterine and umbilical arteries during submaximal bicycle exercise in normal pregnancy. Obstet Gynecol 79:611–615, 1992.

30. Van-Dorn MB, Lotgering FK, Struijk C, et al: Maternal and fetal cardiovascular responses to strenuous bicycle exercise. Am J Obstet Gynecol 166:854–859, 1992.

31. Colletti PM, Lee K: Cardiovascular imaging in the pregnant patient. In Elkayam U, Gleicher N (eds): Cardiac Problems in Pregnancy. 3rd ed. New York, Wiley-Liss, 1998, pp 33–36.

32. Colletti PM, Sylvestre PB: Magnetic resonance imaging in pregnancy. MRI Clin North Am 2:291–307, 1994.

33. American College of Obstetricians and Gynecologists: Invasive hemodynamic monitoring in obstetrics and gynecology. ACOG technical bulletin 175. Int J Gynecol Obstet 42:199–205, 1993.

34. Warnes CA, Elkayam U: Congenital heart disease and pregnancy. In Elkayam U, Gleicher N (eds): Cardiac Problems in Pregnancy. 3rd ed. New York, Wiley-Liss, 1998, pp 39–53.

34a. Weiss BM, Hess OM: Pulmonary vascular disease and pregnancy: Current controversies, management strategies, and perspectives. Eur Heart J 21:104–115, 2000.

35. Oakely C: Pregnancy and congenital heart disease. Heart 78:12–14, 1997.

36. Zuber M, Gautschi N, Oechslin E, et al: Outcome of pregnancy in women with congenital shunt lesions. Heart 81:271–275, 1999.

37. Swan L, Hillis WS, Cameron A: Family planning requirements of adults with congenital heart disease. Heart 78:9–11, 1997.

38. Kjos SL: Fertility control in the cardiac patient. In Elkayam U, Gleicher N (eds): Cardiac Problems in Pregnancy. 3rd ed. New York, Wiley-Liss, 1998, pp 451–456.

39. Mendelson MA: Pregnancy in the women with congenital heart disease. Am J Cardiac Imaging 9:44–52, 1995.

40. Sin SC, Sermer M, Harrison DA, et al: Risk and predictors for pregnancy-related complications in women with heart disease. Circulation 96:2789–2794, 1997.

41. Ardinger RH Jr: Genetic counseling in congenital heart disease. Pediatr Ann 26:99–104, 1997.

42. Perloff JK: Congenital heart disease. In Gleicher N (ed): Principles and Practice of Medical Therapy in Pregnancy. 2nd ed. Norwalk, CT, Appleton & Lange, 1992, p 788.

42a. Copel JA, Liang RI, Demasio K, et al: The clinical significance of the irregular fetal heart rhythm. Am J Obstet Gynecol 182:813–817, 2000.

42b. Lisowski LA, Verheijen PM, Benatar AA, et al: Atrial flutter in the perinatal age group: Diagnosis, management and outcome. J Am Coll Cardiol 35:771–777, 2000.

43. Whittemore R, Hobbins JC, Engle MA: Pregnancy and its outcome in women with and without surgical treatment of congenital heart disease. Am J Cardiol 50:641, 1982.

44. Presbitero P, Somerville J, Stone S, et al: Pregnancy in cyanotic congenital heart disease: Outcome of mother and fetus. Circulation 89:2673–2676, 1994.

45. Whittemore R, Wells JA, Castellsague X: A second-generation study of 427 probands with congenital heart defects and their 837 children. J Am Coll Cardiol 23:1459–1467, 1994.

46. Driscoll DJ, Michels VV, Gersony WM, et al: Occurrence risk for congenital heart disease in relatives of patients with aortic stenosis, pulmonary stenosis, or ventricular septal defect. Circulation 87(Suppl I):I-114–I-120, 1993.

47. Dajani AS, Taubert KA, Wilson W, et al: Prevention of bacterial endocarditis. Recommendations by the American Heart Association. JAMA 277:1794–1801, 1997.

48. Ebrahimi R, Leung CY, Elkayam U, Reid CL: Infective endocarditis. In Elkayam U, Gleicher N (eds): Cardiac Problems in Pregnancy. 3rd ed. New York, Wiley-Liss, 1998, pp 191–198.

49. Lao TT, Sermer M, MaGee L, et al: Congenital aortic stenosis and pregnancy—a reappraisal. Am J Obstet Gynecol 169:540, 1993.

50. Lao TT, Adelman, AG, Sermer M, Colman JM: Balloon valvuloplasty for congenital aortic stenosis in pregnancy. Br J Obstet Gynaecol 100:1141, 1993.

51. Banning AP, Pearson JF, Hall RJC: Role of balloon dilatation of the aortic valve in pregnant patients with severe aortic stenosis. Br Heart J 70:544, 1993.

52. Bhargava B, Agarwal R, Yadav R, et al: Percutaneous balloon aortic valvuloplasty during pregnancy: Use of the Inoue balloon and the physiologic antegrade approach Cathct Cardiovasc Diagn 45:422–425, 1998.

53. Chambers CE, Clark SL: Cardiac surgery during pregnancy. Clin Obstet Gynecol 37:316–323, 1994.

54. Faclouach S, Azzouzi L, Tahiri A, Chararbi PV: Aortic coarctation and pregnancy: A propos of 3 cases followed-up during a period of 10 years. Ann Cardiol Angiol 45:262–265, 1994.

55. Zeira M, Zohar S: Pregnancy and delivery in women with coarctation of the aorta. Harefuah 124:756–758, 1993.

56. Connolly HM, Ammash NM, Warnes CA: Pregnancy in women with coarctation of the aorta (abstract). J Am Coll Cardiol 27 (Suppl A):43A, 1996.

57. Saidi AS, Bezold LI, Altman CA, et al: Outcome of pregnancy following intervention for coarctation of the aorta. Am J Cardiol 82:786–788, 1998.

58. Patton DE, Lee W, Cotton DB, et al: Cyanotic maternal heart disease in pregnancy. Obstet Gynecol Surv 45:594–600, 1990.

59. Larsen-Disney P, Price D, Meredith J: Undiagnosed maternal Fallot tetralogy presenting in pregnancy. Aust NZ J Obstet Gynecol 32:169–171, 1992.

60. Branko WM, Otto H: Preoperative cardiovascular evaluation for noncardiac surgery: Congenital heart disease and heart disease in pregnancy deserve better guidelines. Circulation 95:530–531, 1997.

61. Devitt JH, Noble WH, Byrick RJ: A Swan-Ganz catheter related complication in a patient with Eisenmenger's syndrome. Anesthesiology 57: 335–337, 1982.

62. Goodwin TM, Gherman RB, Hameed A, Elkayam U: Favorable response of Eisenmenger's syndrome to inhaled nitric oxide during pregnancy. Am J Obstet Gynecol 180:64–67, 1999.

63. Lust KM, Boots RJ, Dooris M, Wilson J: Management of labor in Eisenmenger syndrome with inhaled nitric oxide. Am J Obstet Gynecol 181: 419–423, 1999.

64. Donnelly JE, Brown JM, Radford DJ: Pregnancy outcome and Ebstein's anomaly. Br Heart J 66:368–371, 1991.

65. Connolly HM, Warnes CA: Ebstein's anomaly: Outcome of pregnancy. J Am Coll Cardiol 23:1194–1198, 1994.

66. Lao TT, Sermer M, Colman JM: Pregnancy after the Fontan procedure for tricuspid atresia: A case report. J Reprod Med 41:287–290, 1996.

67. Clarkson PM, Wilson NJ, Neutze JM, et al: Outcome of pregnancy after the Mustard operation for transposition of the great arteries with intact ventricular septum. J Am Coll Cardiol 24;190–193, 1994.

68. Lao TT, Sermer M, Colman JM: Pregnancy following surgical correction for transposition of the great arteries. Obstet Gynecol 83:665–668, 1994.

69. Dellinger EH, Haidi HA: Maternal transposition of the great arteries in pregnancy: A case report. J Reprod Med 39:324–326, 1994.

70. Rousselil MP, Irion O, Beguim F, et al: Successful term pregnancy after Mustard operation for transposition of the great arteries. Eur J Obstet Gynecol Reprod Biol 59:111–113, 1995.

71. Perry CP: Childbirth after surgical repair of truncus arteriosus. J Reprod Med 35:65–67, 1990.

72. Fong J, Druzin M, Gimbel AA, Fisher J: Epidural anesthesia for labour and cesarean section in a parturient with a single ventricle and transposition of the great arteries. Can J Anesth 27:680–684, 1990.

73. Summer D, Melville C, Smith CD, et al: Successful pregnancy in a patient with a single ventricle. Eur J Obstet Gynecol Reprod Biol 4: 239–241, 1992.

74. Zavisca FG, Johnson MD, Holubec JT, et al: General anesthesia for cesarean section in a parturient with a single ventricle and pulmonary atresia. J Clin Anesth 5:315–320, 1993.

75. Rowbottom SJ, Gin T, Cheung LD: General anesthesia for caesarean section in a patient with Douceted complex cyanotic heart disease. J Anaesth Intensive Care 22:74–78, 1994.

76. Walsh, Savage R, Hess DB: Successful pregnancy in a patient with double inlet left ventricle treated with septation procedure. South Med J 83:358–359, 1990.

RHEUMATIC HEART DISEASE

77. Essop MR, Sareli P: Rheumatic valvular disease and pregnancy. In Elkayam U, Gleicher N (eds): Cardiac Problems in Pregnancy. 3rd ed. New York, Wiley-Liss, 1998, pp 55–60.

78. Avila WS, Grinberg M, D'ecourt LV, et al: Clinical course of women with mitral valve stenosis during pregnancy and puerperium. Arq Bras Cardiol 58:359, 1992.

79. Al Kasab SM, Sabag T, Al Zaibag M, et al: β-Adrenergic receptor blockade in the management of pregnant women with mitral stenosis. Am J Obstet Gynecol 163:37, 1990.

80. Cohen RG, Castro LJ: Cardiac surgery during pregnancy. In Elkayam U, Gleicher N (eds): Cardiac Problems in Pregnancy. 3rd ed. New York, Wiley-Liss, 1998, pp 277–283.

81. Chambers CE, Clark SL: Cardiac surgery during pregnancy. Clin Obstet Gynecol 37:316–323, 1994.

82. Born D, Massonetto JC, de Almeida PA, et al: Heart surgery with extracorporeal circulation in pregnant women: Analysis of materno-fetal outcome. Arq Bras Cardiol 64:207–211, 1995.

83. De Swiet M, Deverall P: Editorial note: Pregnancy—Still an indication for closed mitral valvotomy. Int J Cardiol 26:323, 1990.

84. Farhat MB, Maatouk F, Betbout F, et al: Percutaneous balloon mitral valvuloplasty in eight pregnant women with severe mitral stenosis. Eur Heart J 13:1658, 1992.

85. Rothlisberger C, Essop MR, Skudicky D, et al: Results of percutaneous balloon mitral valvotomy in young adults. Am J Cardiol 72:73–77, 1993.

86. Lung B, Cormier B, Elias J, et al: Usefulness of percutaneous balloon commissurotomy for mitral stenosis during pregnancy. Am J Cardiol 73: 398, 1994.

87. Glatz JC, Pomerantz RM, Cunningham MJ, Woods JR. Percutaneous balloon valvuloplasty for severe mitral stenosis during pregnancy: A review of therapeutic options. Obstet Gynecol Surv 48:503, 1993.

88. Sharma S, Loya YS, Desai DM, Pinto RJ: Percutaneous mitral valvotomy in 200 patients using Inoue balloon—immediate and early haemodynamic results. Indian Heart J 45:169, 1993.

89. Ribiero PA, Al Zaibag M: Mitral balloon valvotomy in pregnancy (editorial). J Heart Valve Dis 1:206, 1992.

90. Calvin SE: Use of vasodilators during pregnancy. In Elkayam U, Gleicher N (eds): Cardiac Problems in Pregnancy. 3rd ed. New York, Wiley-Liss, 1998, pp 391–398.

91. Roth A, Shotan A, Elkayam U: A randomized comparison between the hemodynamic effects of hydralazine and nitroglycerin alone and in combination at rest and during isometric exercise in patients with chronic mitral regurgitation. Am Heart J 125:155, 1993.

92. Lao TT, Sermer M, MaGee L, et al: Congenital aortic stenosis and pregnancy—a reappraisal. Am J Obstet Gynecol 169:540, 1993.

93. Banning AP, Pearson JF, Hall RJC: Role of balloon dilatation of the aortic valve in pregnant patients with severe aortic stenosis. Br Heart J 70:544, 1993.

94. Freed LA, Levy D, Levine RA, et al: Prevalence and clinical outcome of mitral-valve prolapse. N Engl J Med 341:1–7, 1999.

95. Rayburn WF: Mitral valve prolapse and pregnancy. In Elkayam U, Gleicher N (eds): Cardiac Problems in Pregnancy. 3rd ed. New York, Wiley-Liss, 1998, pp 175–182.

96. Elkayam U, Ostrzega E, Shotan A, Mehra A: Marfan syndrome and pregnancy. In Elkayam U, Gleicher N (eds): Cardiac Problems in Pregnancy. 3rd ed. New York, Wiley-Liss, 1998, pp 211–221.

97. Simpson LL, Athanassions AM, D'Alton ME: Marfan syndrome in pregnancy. Curr Opin Obstet Gynecol 9:337–341, 1997.

98. Rossiter JP, Repke JT, Morales AJ, et al: A prospective longitudinal evaluation of pregnancy in the Marfan's syndrome. Am J Obstet Gynecol 173:1599–1606, 1995.

99. Paternoster DM, Santarossa C, Vettore N, et al: Obstetric complications in Marfan's syndrome. Min Gynecol 50:441–443, 1998.

100. Simpson IA, deBelder MA, Treasure T, et al: Cardiovascular manifestations of Marfan's syndrome: Improved evaluation by transesophageal echocardiography. Br Heart J 69:104, 1993.

101. Shores J, Berger KR, Murphy EA, Pyeritz RE: Progression of aortic dilatation and the benefit of long-term beta adrenergic blockade in Marfan's syndrome. N Engl J Med 330:1335, 1994.

OTHER CONDITIONS AFFECTING THE VALVES, AORTA, OR MYOCARDIUM

102. Elkayam U, Dave R: Hypertrophic cardiomyopathy and pregnancy. In Elkayam U, Gleicher N (eds): Cardiac Problems in Pregnancy. 3rd ed. New York, Wiley-Liss, 1998, pp 211–221.

103. Autore C, Brauneis S, Fabrizio A, et al: Epidural anesthesia for cesarean section in patients with hypertrophic cardiomyopathy: A report of three cases. Anesthesiology 90:1205–1207, 1999.

104. Gras D, Mabo P, Kermarrec A, et al: Radiofrequency ablation of atrioventricular conduction during the 5th month of pregnancy. Arch Mal Coeur Vaiss 85:1873–1877, 1992.

105. Coven G, Zizzi S, Cimino F, et al: Electric cardioversion in pregnant patients with obstructive hypertrophic cardiomyopathy: A clinical case. Min Anestesiol 1994;60:725–728, 1994.

106. Pelliccia F, Cianfrocca C, Gaudig C, Reale A: Sudden death during pregnancy in hypertrophic cardiomyopathy. Eur Heart J 13:421, 1992.

107. Rowe T: Hypertrophic cardiomyopathy in pregnancy: A case study. J Cardiovasc Nurs 8:69, 1994.

108. Lang RM, Lampert MB, Poppas A, et al: Peripartal cardiomyopathy. In Elkayam U, Gleicher N (eds): Cardiac Problems in Pregnancy. 3rd ed. New York, Wiley-Liss, 1998, pp 87–100.

108a. Pearson GD, Veille JC, Rahimtoola S, et al: Peripartum cardiomyopathy: National Heart, Lung, and Blood Institute and Office of Rare Diseases (National Institutes of Health) workshop recommendations and review. JAMA 283:1183–1188, 2000.

109. van Hoevan KH, Kitsis RN, Katz SD, Factor SM: Peripartum versus idiopathic dilated cardiomyopathy in young women—a comparison of clinical, pathological and prognostic features. Int J Cardiol 40:57, 1993.

110. Marin-Neto JA, Maciel BC, Teran Urbanetz LL, et al: High output failure in patients with peripartum cardiomyopathy: A comparative study with dilated cardiomyopathy. Am Heart J 121:134, 1990.

111. Tummala PP, Rao KS, Akhter MW, et al: Peripartum cardiomyopathy: Clinical profile of 100 patients diagnosed in the United States. Circulation 100(18):I-579, 1999.

112. Midei MC, DeMent, SH, Feldman AM, et al: Peripartum myocarditis and cardiomyopathy. Circulation 81:922, 1990.

113. Rizeg MN, Rickembacher PR, Fowler MB, Billingham ME: Incidence of myocarditis in peripartum cardiomyopathy. Am J Cardiol 74:474, 1994.

114. Shotan A, Widerhorn J, Hurst A, Elkayam U: Risks of angiotensin-converting enzyme inhibition during pregnancy: Experimental and clinical evidence, potential mechanisms, and recommendations for use. Am J Med 96:451, 1994.

115. Hoffman AC, Masouye P, Rifat K, Suter PM: Peripartum cardiomyopathy: A case report. Acta Anesthesiol Scand 35:784–785, 1991.

116. Hovsepian PG, Ganzel B, Sohi GS, et al: Peripartum cardiomyopathy treated with a left ventricular assist device as a bridge to cardiac transplantation. South Med J 82:527, 1989.

117. Bozkurt B, Villanueva FS, Halubkov R, et al: Intravenous immune globulin in the therapy of peripartum cardiomyopathy. J Am Coll Cardiol 34:177–180, 1999.

118. Keogh A, McDonald P, Spratt P, et al: Outcome in peripartum cardiomyopathy after heart transplantation. J Heart Lung Transplant 13:202–207, 1994.

119. Peter R, Rickenbacher MD: Long-term outcome after heart transplantation for peripartum cardiomyopathy. Am Heart J 127:1318–1323, 1994.

120. Tummala PP, Akhter MW, Hameed AB, et al: Risk of subsequent pregnancies in women with a history of peripartum cardiomyopathy. Circulation 100(18):I-381, 1999.

121. Ostrzega E, Elkayam U: Risk of subsequent pregnancy in women with a history of peripartum cardiomyopathy: Results of a survey (abstract). Circulation 92 (Suppl I):1-333, 1995.

122. Witlin A, Sibai B: Hypertension. Clin Obstet Gynecol 41:533–544, 1998.

123. Chari RS, Frangieh AY, Sibai BM: Hypertension during pregnancy: Diagnosis, pathophysiology, and management. In Elkayam U, Gleicher N (eds): Cardiac Problems in Pregnancy. 3rd ed. New York, Wiley-Liss, 1998, pp 257–273.

124. Sibai BM: Treatment of hypertension in pregnant women. N Engl J Med 335:257–265, 1996.

125. Branch KR, Wagoner LE, McGrory CH, et al: Risks of subsequent pregnancies on mother and newborn in female heart transplant recipient. J Heart Lung Transplant 17:698–792, 1998.

126. Alami WS, Young JB: Pregnancy after cardiac transplantation. *In* El-kayam U, Gleicher N (eds): Cardiac Problems in Pregnancy. 3rd ed. New York, Wiley-Liss, 1998, pp 327–337.

CORONARY ARTERY DISEASE

127. Rutherford JD: Coronary artery disease in the childbearing age. *In* El-kayam U, Gleicher N (eds): Cardiac Problems in Pregnancy. 3rd ed. New York, Wiley-Liss, 1998, pp 121–130.
128. Roth A, Elkayam U: Acute myocardial infarction and pregnancy. *In* Elkayam U, Gleicher N (eds): Cardiac Problems in Pregnancy. 3rd ed. New York, Wiley-Liss, 1998, pp 131–151.
129. Hannaford P, Ferry S, Hirsch S: Cardiovascular sequelae of toxaemia of pregnancy. Heart 77:154–158, 1997.
130. Acute myocardial infarction and combined oral contraceptives: Results of an international multicenter case-control study. WHO collaborative study of cardiovascular disease and steroid hormone contraception. Lancet 349:1202–1209, 1997.
131. Brizzi P, Tonalo G, Esposito F, et al: Lipoprotein metabolism during normal pregnancy. Am J Obstet Gynecol 181:430–434, 1999.
132. Santos G, Sadaniantz A: Postpartum acute myocardial infarction. Am J Obstet Gynecol 177:1553–1555, 1997.
133. Weber MD, Halligan RE, Schumacher JA: Acute infarction, intracoronary thrombolysis, and primary PTCA in pregnancy. Cathet Cardiovasc Diagn 42:38–43, 1997.
134. Garry D, Leikim E, Fleisher AG, Tejani N: Acute myocardial infarction in pregnancy with subsequent medical and surgical management. Obstet Gynecol 87:802–804, 1996.
135. Badui E, Enciso R: Acute myocardial infarction during pregnancy and puerperium. Rev Angiol 47:739–756, 1996.
136. Chen FG, Koh KF, Chong YS: Cardiac arrest associated with sulprostone: Use during cesarean section. Anaesth Intensive Care 26:298–301, 1998.
137. Hamada S, Hinokio K, Naka O, et al: Myocardial infarction as a complication of pheochromocytoma in a pregnant woman Eur J Obstet Gynecol Reprod Biol 70:197–200, 1996.
138. Athanassiou AM, Turrentine MA: Myocardial infarction and coronary artery dissection during pregnancy associated with type IV Ehlers-Danlos syndrome. Am J Perinatol 13:181–183, 1996.
139. Klutstein MW, Tzivoni D, Bitran D, et al: Treatment of spontaneous coronary artery dissection: Report of three cases. Cathet Cardiovasc Diagn 40:372–376, 1992.
140. Ulm MR, Obwegesser R, Ploeckinger B, et al: A case of myocardial infarction complicating pregnancy—a role for prostacyclin synthesis stimulating plasma factor and lipoprotein. Thromb Res 83:237–242, 1996.
141. Shivvers SA, Wians FH Jr, Keffer JH, Ramin SM: Maternal cardiac troponin I levels during normal labor and delivery. Am J Obstet Gynecol 180:122–127, 1999.
142. Schumacher B, Belfort MA, Card RJ: Successful treatment of acute myocardial infarction during pregnancy within tissue plasminogen activator. Am J Obstet Gynecol 176:716–719, 1997.
143. Ginsberg JS, Hirsch J: Use of antithrombotic agents during pregnancy. Chest 114:524S–531S, 1998.
144. Cartis S, Sibai B, Houth J, et al: Low-dose aspirin to prevent preeclampsia in women at high risk. National Institute of Child Health and Human Development, network of maternal-fetal medicine unit. N Engl J Med 338:701–705, 1998.
145. Ascarelli MH, Grider AR, Hsu HW: Acute myocardial infarction during pregnancy managed with immediate percutaneous transluminal coronary angioplasty. Obstet Gynecol 88:655–657, 1996.
146. Eickman FM: Acute coronary artery angioplasty during pregnancy. Cathet Cardiovasc Diagn 38:369–372, 1996.
147. Silberman S, Fink D, Berko RS, et al: Coronary artery bypass surgery during pregnancy. Eur J Cardiothorac Surg 10:925–926, 1996.
148. Shalev Y, Ben-Hur II, Hagay Z, et al: Successful delivery following myocardial ischemia during the second trimester of pregnancy. Clin Cardiol 16:754, 1993.
149. Hameed AB, Tummala PP, Godwin TM, et al: Unstable angina during pregnancy in two patients with premature coronary atherosclerosis and aortic stenosis secondary to familial hypercholesterolemia. Am J Obstet Gynecol 182:1152–1155, 2000.

ARRHYTHMIAS

150. Brodsky M, Doria R, Allen B, et al: New-onset ventricular tachycardia during pregnancy. Am Heart J 123:933, 1992.
151. Widerhorn JK, Widerhorn AIM, Rahimtoola SH, Elkayam U: WPW syndrome during pregnancy: Increased incidence of supraventricular arrhythmias. Am Heart J 124:796, 1992.
152. Tawam M, Levine J, Mendelson M, et al: Effect of pregnancy on paroxysmal supraventricular tachycardia. Am J Cardiol 72:838, 1993.
153. Lee SH, Chen SA, Wu TJ, et al: Effects of pregnancy on first onset and symptoms of paroxysmal supraventricular tachycardia. Am J Cardiol 76:675–678, 1995.
154. Oettinger M, Pelitz Y: Asymptomatic paroxysmal atrial fibrillation during intravenous magnesium sulfate treatment in preeclampsia. Gynecol Obstet Invest 36:24:1993.

155. Penkala M, Hancock EW: Wide-complex tachycardia in pregnancy. Hosp Pract 28:63–64, 1993.
156. Field LM, Barton FL: The management of anaesthesia for caesarean section in a patient with paroxysmal ventricular tachycardia. Anaesthesia 48:593, 1993.
157. Leung CY, Brodsky MA: Cardiac arrhythmias and pregnancy. *In* El-kayam U, Gleicher N (eds): Cardiac Problems in Pregnancy. 3rd ed. New York, Wiley-Liss, 1998, pp 155–175.
158. Braden GL, Von Oeyen PT, Germain MI, et al: Ritodrin- and terbutaline-induced hypokalemia in preterm labor: Mechanisms and consequences. Kidney Int 51:1867–1875, 1997.
159. Feldman JM: Cardiac arrest after succinylcholine administration in a pregnant patient recovered from Guillain-Barre syndrome. Anesthesiology 72:942, 1990.
160. Swartjes JM, Schutte MF, Bleker OP: Management of eclampsia: Cardiopulmonary arrest resulting from magnesium sulfate overdose. Eur J Obstet Gynaecol Reprod Biol 47:73, 1992.
161. Varon ME, Sherer DM, Abramowicz JS, Akiyama T: Maternal ventricular tachycardia associated with hypomagnesemia. Am J Obstet Gynecol 167:1352, 1992.
162. Naido DP, Bhorat L, Moodley J, et al: Continuous electrocardiographic monitoring in hypertensive crises in pregnancy. Am J Obstet Gynecol 164:530, 1991.
163. Rashba EJ, Zareba W, Moss AJ, et al: Influence of pregnancy on the risk for cardiac events in patients with hereditary long QT syndrome. Circulation 97:451–456, 1998.
164. Doig JC, McComb JM, Reid DC: Incessant atrial tachycardia accelerated by pregnancy. B Heart J 67:266, 1992.
165. Murphy JJ, Hutchon DJ: Incessant atrial tachycardia accelerated by pregnancy (letter). Br Heart J 68:342, 1992.
166. Natale A, Davidson T, Geiger MJ, Newby K: Implantable cardioverter-defibrillators and pregnancy: A safe combination? Circulation 96:2808–2812, 1997.
167. Dalvi BV, Chaudhuri A, Kulkarni HL, Kale PA: Therapeutic guidelines for congenital complete heart block presenting in pregnancy. Obstet Gynecol 79:802, 1992.
168. Lau CP, Lee, CP, Wong CK, et al: Rate responsive pacing with a minute ventilation sensing pacemaker during pregnancy and delivery. PACE 13:158, 1990.
169. Ramsewak S, Persad P, Perkins S, Narayaansingh G: Twin pregnancy in a patient with complete heart block. Clin Exp Obstet Gynecol 19:166, 1992.
170. Holdright DR, Sutton GC: Restoration of sinus rhythm during two consecutive pregnancies in a woman with congenital complete heart block. Br Heart J 64:338, 1990.
171. Emori T, Goto Y, Maeda T, et al: Multiple coronary artery dissections diagnosed in vivo in a pregnant woman. Chest 104:289, 1993.
172. Jordaens LJ, Vandenbogaerde JF, van De Bruaene P, De Buyzere M: Transesophageal echocardiography for insertion of a physiological pacemaker in early pregnancy. PACE 13:955, 1990.
173. Terhaar M, Schakenbach L: Care of the pregnant patient with a pacemaker. J Perinatol Neonatal Nurs 5:1, 1991.
174. Lee MS, Evans SJL, Blumberg S, et al: Echocardiographically guided electrophysiologic testing in pregnancy J Am Soc Echocardiogr 7:182, 1994.

OTHER CARDIOVASCULAR DISORDERS

175. Elkayam U, Hameed A: Vascular dissections and aneurysms during pregnancy. *In* Elkayam U, Gleicher N (eds): Cardiac Problems in Pregnancy. 3rd ed. New York, Wiley-Liss, 1998, p. 201.
176. Nolte JE, Rutherford RB, Nawaz S, et al: Arterial dissections associated with pregnancy. J Vasc Surg 21:515–520, 1995.
177. Anderson RA, Fineron FW: Aortic dissection in pregnancy: Importance of pregnancy-induced changes in the vessel wall and bicuspid aortic valve in pathogenesis. Br J Obstet Gynaecol 101:1085–1088, 1994.
178. Sommer T, Fehske W, Holzknecht N, et al: Aortic dissection: A comparative study of diagnosis with spiral CT, multiplanar transesophageal echocardiography, and MR imaging. Radiology 198:347–352, 1996.
179. Wahlers T, Lass J, Alken A, Borst HG: Repair of acute type A aortic dissection after cesarean section in the thirty-ninth week of pregnancy (letter). J Thorac Cardiovasc Surg 107:314–315, 1994.
180. Jayram A, Carp HM, Davis L, Jacobson SL: Pregnancy complicated by aortic dissection: cesarean delivery during extradural anaesthesia. Br J Anaesth 1995; 75:358–360.
181. Kerr GS: Takayasu's arteritis. Rheum Dis Clin North Am 21:1041–1058, 1995.
182. Elkayam U, Hameed A: Takayasu's arteritis and pregnancy. *In* Elkayam U, Gleicher N (eds): Cardiac Problems in Pregnancy. 3rd ed. New York, Wiley-Liss, 1998, p 237.
183. Crofts SL, Wilson E: Epidural analgesia for labour in Takayasu's arteritis. Br J Obstet Gynaecol 98:408–409, 1991.
184. Winn HN, Setaro JF, Mazor M, et al: Severe Takayasu's arteritis in pregnancy: The role of central hemodynamic monitoring. Am J Obstet Gynecol 159:1135–1136, 1988.
185. Matsumura A, Moriwaki R, Numano F: Pregnancy in Takayasu arteritis from the view of internal medicine. Heart Vessel Suppl 7:120–124, 1992.
186. Bassa A, Desai DK, Moodley J: Takayasu's disease and pregnancy: Three case studies and a review of the literature. S Afr Med J 85:107–112, 1995.

187. Fignon A, Marret H, Alle C, et al: Association of Takayasu's arteritis, pregnancy and Still's disease. J Gynecol Obstet Biol Reprod (Paris) 24: 747–750, 1995.

188. Elkayam U, Dave R, Bokhari SWH: Primary pulmonary hypertension in pregnancy. *In* Elkayam U, Gleicher N (ed): Cardiac Problems in Pregnancy. 3rd ed. New York, Wiley-Liss, 1998, p 183.

189. Weiss BM. Zemp L. Seifert B, Hess OM: Outcome of pulmonary vascular disease in pregnancy: A systematic overview from 1978 through 1996. J Am Col Cardiol 31:1650–1657, 1998.

190. Rubin LJ: Primary pulmonary hypertension. N Engl J Med 336:111–117, 1997.

191. Weiss BM, Hess OM: Pulmonary vascular disease and pregnancy: Current controversies, management strategies, and perspectives. Eur Heart J 21:104–115, 2000

192. Easterling TR, Ralph DD, Schmucker BC: Pulmonary hypertension in pregnancy: Treatment with pulmonary vasodilator. Obstet Gynecol 93: 494–498, 1999.

CARDIAC SURGERY DURING PREGNANCY

193. Parry AJ, Westaby S: Cardiopulmonary by pass during pregnancy. Perfusion Rev 3:8–18, 1994.

194. Weiss BM, von Segesser LK, Alon E, et al: Outcome of cardiovascular surgery and pregnancy: A systematic review of the period 1984–1996. Am J Obstet Gynecol 179:1643–1653, 1998.

195. Elkayam U: Pregnancy through a prosthetic heart valve. J Am Coll Cardiol 33:1642–1645, 1999.

196. Elkayam U, Khan SS: Pregnancy in the patient with artificial heart valve. *In* Elkayam U, Gleicher N, (eds): Cardiac Problems in Pregnancy. 3rd ed. New York, Wiley-Liss, 1998, pp 61–78.

197. Born D, Martinez EE, Almeida PA, et al: Pregnancy in patients with prosthetic heart valves: The effect of anticoagulation on mother, fetus and neonate. Am Heart J 1992; 124:413–417, 1992.

198. Sbarouni E, Oakley CM: Outcome of pregnancy in women with valve prostheses. Br Heart J 71:196–201, 1993.

199. Hanania G, Thomas D, Michel PL, et al: Grossesses chez les porteuses de prostheses valvulaires: Etude cooperative retrospective francaise (155 cas). Arch Mal Coeur 87:429–437, 1994

200. Lee CN, Wu CC, Lin PY, et al: Pregnancy following cardiac prosthetic valve replacement. Obstet Gynecol 83:353–356, 1994

201. Vongpatanasin W, Hills LD, Lange RA: Prosthetic heart valves. N Engl J Med 335:407–416, 1996

202. Denbow CE, Matadiol L, Sivapragasam S, et al: Pregnancy in patients after homograft cardiac valve replacement. Chest 88:540, 1982.

203. Dore A, Somerville J: Pregnancy in patients with pulmonary autograft valve replacement. Em Heart J 18:1659–1662, 1997.

204. Salazar E, Izaguirre R, Verdejo J, et al: Failure of adjusted doses of subcutaneous heparin to prevent thromboembolic phenomena in pregnant patients with mechanical cardiac valve prostheses. J Am College Cardiol 27:1698–1703, 1996.

205. McGehee W: Anticoagulation in pregnancy. *In* Elkayam U, Gleicher N (eds): Cardiac Problems in Pregnancy. 3rd ed. New York, Wiley-Liss, 1998, pp 407–417.

206. Chan WS, Anand S, Ginsberg JS: Anticoagulation of pregnant women with mechanical heart valves: A systemic review of the literature. Arch Intern Med 160:191–196, 2000.

207. Gohlke-Barwolf C, Acar J, Oakely C, et al: Guidelines for prevention of thromboembolic events in valvular heart disease: Study group of the working group on valvular heart disease of the European Society of Cardiology. Eur Heart J 16;1320–1330, 1995.

208. Bonow RO, Carobelo B, DeLeon AC, et al: ACC/AHA Guidelines for the management of patients with valvular heart disease. J Am Coll Cardiol 32:1486–1588, 1998.

209. Elkayam U: Anticoagulation in pregnant women with prosthetic heart valves: a double jeopardy. J Am Coll Cardiol 27:1704–1706, 1990.

210. Evans W, Laifer SA, McNanley TJ, et al: Management of thromboembolic disease associated with pregnancy. J Maternal-Fetal Med 6:21–27, 1997.

211. Vitale N, DeFeo M, Salvatore De Santo L, et al: Dose-dependent fetal complications of warfarin in pregnant women with mechanical heart valves. J Am Coll Cardiol 33:1637–1641, 1999.

212. Cappelen JC, Flore LD, Brophy MT, et al: Efficacy and safety of combined anticoagulant and antiplatelet therapy versus anticoagulant monotherapy after mechanical heart valve replacement: A metaanalysis. Am Heart J 130:547–552, 1995.

213. Committee on Drugs, American Academy of Pediatrics: The transfer of drugs and other chemicals into human milk. Pediatrics 93:137–150, 1994.

214. Briggs GG, Freeman RK, Yaffe SJ: Drugs in Pregnancy and Lactation. Baltimore, Williams & Wilkins, 1994.

215. Shotan A, Hurst AK, Widerhorn J, et al: Antiarrhythmic drugs during pregnancy and lactation. *In* Elkayam U, Gleicher N (eds): Cardiac Problems in Pregnancy. 3rd ed. New York, Wiley-Liss, 1998.

216. Shotan A, Widerhorn J, Hurst A, Elkayam U: Risks of angiotensin-converting enzyme inhibition during pregnancy: Experimental and clinical evidence, potential mechanisms, and recommendations for use. Am J Med 96:451–456, 1994.

217. Hurst AK, Hoffman K, Frishman WH, Elkayam U: The use of beta-adrenergic blocking agents in pregnancy and lactation. *In* Elkayam U, Gleicher N (eds): Cardiac Problems in Pregnancy. 3rd ed. New York, Wiley-Liss, 1998, pp 357–372.

218. Steinberg I, Mitani GM, Harrison EL, Elkayam U: Digitalis glycosides in pregnancy. *In* Elkayam U, Gleicher N (eds): Cardiac Problems in Pregnancy. 3rd ed. New York, Wiley-Liss, 1998, pp 419–433.

219. Cohen E, Garty M: Diuretics in pregnancy. *In* Elkayam U, Gleicher N (eds): Cardiac Problems in Pregnancy. 3rd ed. New York, Wiley-Liss, 1998, pp 351–356.

GUIDELINES

MANAGEMENT OF VALVULAR DISEASE IN PREGNANCY

Thomas H. Lee

Recommendations for management of valvular heart disease in pregnancy are included in the 1998 ACC/AHA guidelines on valvular disease.[1] These guidelines do not recommend routine antibiotic prophylaxis in patients with valvular heart disease undergoing uncomplicated vaginal delivery or cesarean section unless infection is suggested. For high-risk patients, such as those with prosthetic heart valves or prior histories of endocarditis, antibiotics are considered optional.

Complex guidelines are offered on anticoagulation for patients with mechanical prosthetic heart valves (Table 65–G–1). These guidelines reflect high complication rates in pregnant women managed with subcutaneous heparin and support the use of intravenous heparin during the first trimester. After the 36th week of pregnancy, transition from warfarin to heparin is recommended in anticipation of labor. Data on low-molecular-weight heparin in this setting were too sparse for the development of recommendations.

REFERENCES

1. Bonow RO, Carabello B, de Leon AC Jr, et al: ACC/AHA guidelines for the management of patients with valvular heart disease: Executive summary. A report of the American College of Cardiology/American Heart Association Task Force on Practice Guidelines (Committee on Management of Patients With Valvular Heart Disease). Circulation 98:1949–1984, 1998.

2. Gohlke-Barwolf C, Acar J, Oakley C, et al: Guidelines for prevention of thromboembolic events in valvular heart disease: Study Group of the Working Group on Valvular Heart Disease of the European Society of Cardiology. Eur Heart J 16:1320–1330, 1995.

TABLE 65–G–1. GUIDELINES FOR ANTICOAGULATION DURING PREGNANCY IN PATIENTS WITH MECHANICAL PROSTHETIC VALVES

Indication	Class I	Class IIa	Class IIb	Class III
Anticoagulation during pregnancy in patients with mechanical prosthetic valves: weeks 1 through 35	The decision whether to use heparin during the first trimester or to continue oral anticoagulation throughout pregnancy should be made after full discussion with the patient and her partner; if she chooses to change to heparin for the first trimester, she should be made aware that heparin is less safe for her, with a higher risk of both thrombosis and bleeding, and that any risk to the mother also jeopardizes the baby.[2] High-risk women (a history of thromboembolism or an older-generation mechanical prosthesis in the mitral position) who choose *not* to take warfarin during the first trimester should receive continuous unfractionated heparin intravenously in a dose to prolong the midinterval (6 hours after dosing) aPTT to two to three times control. Transition to warfarin can occur thereafter.	In patients receiving warfarin, INR should be maintained between 2.0 and 3.0 with the lowest possible dose of warfarin, and low-dose aspirin should be added.	Women at low risk (no history of thromboembolism, newer low-profile prosthesis) may be managed with adjusted-dose subcutaneous heparin (17,500 to 20,000 U b.i.d.) to prolong the mid-interval (6 hours after dosing) aPTT to two to three times control.	
Anticoagulation during pregnancy in patients with mechanical prosthetic valves: after the 36th week		Warfarin should be stopped no later than week 36 and heparin substituted in anticipation of labor. If labor begins during treatment with warfarin, a cesarean section should be performed. In the absence of significant bleeding, heparin can be resumed 4 to 6 hours after delivery and warfarin begun orally.		

aPTT = activated partial thromboplastin time; INR = international normalized ratio.

Chapter 66

Rheumatic Fever

ADNAN S. DAJANI

Rheumatic fever (RF) is generally classified as a connective tissue disease or collagen-vascular disease. Its anatomical hallmark is damage to collagen fibrils and to the ground substance of connective tissue. The rheumatic process is expressed as an inflammatory reaction that involves many organs, primarily the heart, the joints, and the central nervous system. The clinical manifestations of acute RF follow a group A streptococcal (GAS) infection of the tonsillopharynx after a latent period of approximately 3 weeks. The major importance of acute RF is its ability to cause fibrosis of heart valves, leading to crippling hemodynamics of chronic heart disease.

RF is the most common cause of acquired heart disease in children and young adults worldwide. Although the incidence of RF declined sharply in many developed countries, the disease remains a major problem in many developing countries. The precise reasons for the fluctuations in the incidence of the disease remain only partly understood. Although RF has been studied extensively, the pathogenesis of the disease is not well defined.

Epidemiology

The incidence of RF and prevalence of rheumatic heart disease are markedly variable in different countries.[1, 2] At the beginning of the 20th century, the incidence of RF in the United States exceeded 100 per 100,000 population, ranged between 40 and 65 per 100,000 between 1935 and 1960, and is currently estimated at less than 2 per 100,000. Beginning in 1984, several outbreaks of acute RF were reported from a number of geographically distinct areas in the United States.[2] These focal outbreaks were not associated with a national increase in the incidence of RF.[3] The decline in the incidence of RF in industrialized countries is in sharp contrast to the persistent high incidence of the disease in nonindustrialized countries.

In many developing countries, the incidence of acute RF approaches or exceeds 100 per 100,000.[1] In keeping with the falling incidence of RF in industrialized countries, the prevalence of rheumatic heart disease has declined. Table 66-1 compares the prevalence of rheumatic heart disease in school-age children in different regions of the world.

The decline in incidence of RF and prevalence of rheumatic heart disease has been attributed to several factors. Although the decline preceded the introduction of antimicrobial agents for the treatment of streptococcal pharyngitis, some reports suggest that the use of these agents may have enhanced the rate of this decline.[4] Improved economic standards, better housing conditions, decreased crowding in homes and schools, and access to medical care are often credited, at least in part, for the marked decline in RF.[1] Epidemiological observations in the United States[5] and the United Kingdom[6] show periodic shifts in the appearance and disappearance of specific M types in a particular geographical location. Such shifts may be another explanation for the decline and resurgence of RF in some parts of the world.

Because of the causal relationship between RF and GAS pharyngitis, the epidemiologies of the two illnesses are very similar. Initial attacks of RF occur most commonly between the ages of 6 and 15 years, and RF rarely occurs before the age of 5 years.[7] The risk of RF is increased in populations at high risk for streptococcal pharyngitis, such as military recruits, persons living in crowded conditions, and those in close contact with school-age children. The incidence of RF is equal in male and female patients. The seasonal incidence of RF also parallels that of streptococcal pharyngitis. The peak incidence of RF in Europe and the United States is in spring. Although RF used to be considered a disease of temperate climates, it is now more common in warm tropical climates, particularly in developing countries.

Pathogenesis

The evidence that GAS is the agent causing initial and recurrent attacks of RF is strong but indirect. It is based on clinical, epidemiological, and immunological observations. Factors that contribute to the pathogenesis of RF are related to both the putative causative agent and the host (Table 66-2).

THE ETIOLOGICAL AGENT. An untreated GAS tonsillopharyngitis is the antecedent event that precipitates RF.[8] RF does not follow streptococcal skin infection (impetigo). Proper antimicrobial treatment of streptococcal pharyngitis with eradication of the organism virtually eliminates the risk of RF.[8] In situations conducive to epidemic streptococcal pharyngitis (such as the military population, crowding), as many as 3 percent of untreated acute streptococcal sore throats may be followed by RF.[9] Endemic infections result in much lower attack rates. It has been well documented that about one-third of all cases of acute RF follow mild, almost asymptomatic pharyngitis. The lack of symptomatic pharyngitis was particularly striking in most of the recent outbreaks of acute RF in which the majority of patients (58 percent) had no history of pharyngitis.[2] This is an alarming observation, because primary prevention of acute RF relies on identification and proper treatment of streptococcal pharyngitis.

The major factors that are related to the risk of RF are the magnitude of the immune response to the antecedent streptococcal pharyngitis and persistence of the organism during convalescence.[9] Variations in the rheumatogenicity of GAS strains are a factor influencing the attack rate of RF.[10] The concept that RF is associated with infections due to virulent encapsulated (mucoid) strains capable of inducing strong type-specific immune responses to M protein and other streptococcal antigens[11] has been strengthened by observations made during the outbreaks of acute RF in the

▼ **TABLE 66-1. RHEUMATIC HEART DISEASE IN SCHOOL-AGE CHILDREN**

LOCATION	PREVALENCE PER 1000
United States	0.6
Japan	0.7
Asia (other)	0.4–21.0
Africa	0.3–15.0
South America	1.0–17.0

▼ TABLE 66–2. PATHOGENESIS OF RHEUMATIC FEVER

GROUP A STREPTOCOCCUS

Tonsillopharyngeal infection, no other sites
Intensity of the infection
  Brisk antibody response
  Persistence of the organism
Rheumatogenic strains
  M types 1, 3, 5, 6, 14, 18, 19, 27, and 29
  Distinct structural characteristics of M proteins
    Long terminal antigenic domain
    Epitopes shared with human heart tissue
  Heavily encapsulated, forming mucoid colonies
  Resistance to phagocytosis
  Does not produce opacity factor

SUSCEPTIBLE HOST
Genetic predisposition
  Presence of specific B-cell alloantigen
  High incidence of class II HLA antigens

---

mid-1980's. The streptococci isolated from patients with RF and their sibling contacts during these outbreaks were primarily strains belonging to M types 1, 3, 5, 6, and 18.[12] M proteins of rheumatogenic streptococci show distinct structural characteristics: They share a long terminal antigenic domain[13] and contain epitopes that are shared with human heart tissue, particularly sarcolemmal membrane proteins and cardiac myosin.[14, 15]

THE HOST. Although only a small proportion of individuals with untreated streptococcal pharyngitis may develop RF (3 percent), the incidence of the disease after streptococcal pharyngitis in patients who have had a previous episode of RF is substantially greater (about 50 percent). Numerous epidemiological studies also indicate familial predisposition to the disease. These observations and more recent studies strongly suggest a genetic basis for susceptibility to RF. A specific B-cell alloantigen, identified by monoclonal antibodies, has been described in almost all patients (99 percent) with RF but in only a small number (14 percent) of controls.[16] Furthermore, susceptibility to RF has been linked with HLA-DR 1, 2, 3, and 4 haplotypes in various ethnic groups.[17]

Pathology

The acute phase of RF is characterized by exudative and proliferative inflammatory reactions involving connective or collagen tissue. Although the disease process is diffuse, it affects primarily the heart, joints, brain, and cutaneous and subcutaneous tissues. A generalized vasculitis affecting small blood vessels is commonly noted, but unlike the vasculitis of some other connective tissue disorders, thrombotic lesions are not seen in RF.

The basic structural change in collagen is fibrinoid degeneration. The interstitial connective tissue becomes edematous and eosinophilic, with fraying, fragmentation, and disintegration of collagen fibers. This is associated with infiltration of mononuclear cells including large modified fibrohistiocytic cells (Aschoff's cells). Some of the histiocytes are multinucleated and form Aschoff's giant cells.

The Aschoff's nodule in the proliferative stage is considered pathognomonic of rheumatic carditis. These nodules have been found almost invariably in the autopsies of patients who died of rheumatic carditis; however, more recent observations indicate that Aschoff's nodules are observed in only 30 to 40 percent of biopsy specimens from patients with primary or recurrent episodes of RF.[18] Aschoff's bodies may be seen in any area of the myocardium but not in other affected organs such as joints or brain. They are most often noted in the interventricular septum, the wall of the left ventricle, or the left atrial appendage. Aschoff's nodules persist for many years after a rheumatic attack, even in patients with no evidence of recent or active inflammation.

Inflammation of valvular tissue accounts for the more commonly recognized clinical manifestations of rheumatic carditis. Initial inflammation leads to valvular insufficiency. The histological findings in endocarditis consist of edema and cellular infiltration of the valvular tissue and the chordae tendineae. Hyaline degeneration of the affected valve leads to the formation of verrucae at its edge, preventing total approximation of the leaflets. Fibrosis and calcification of the valve occur if inflammation persists. This process may eventually lead to valvular stenosis.

DIAGNOSIS

No specific clinical, laboratory, or other test establishes the diagnosis of RF.[18a] In 1944, T. Duckett Jones formulated his criteria for the diagnosis of RF[19]; these criteria are still valuable. They have been modified, revised, edited, and updated by the Committee on Rheumatic Fever, Endocarditis, and Kawasaki Disease of the Council on Cardiovascular Disease in the Young (American Heart Association).[20] The most recent guidelines (Table 66–3) emphasize the diagnosis of *initial attacks* of RF. Dividing clinical and laboratory findings into major and minor manifestations is based on the diagnostic importance of a particular finding. If supported by evidence of preceding GAS infection, the presence of two major manifestations or of one major and two minor manifestations indicates a high probability of acute RF.

Major Clinical Manifestations

CARDITIS. Rheumatic carditis is a pancarditis affecting the endocardium, myocardium, and pericardium to various degrees. Clinically, rheumatic carditis is almost always associated with a murmur of valvulitis. The severity of carditis is variable. In its most severe form, death due to cardiac failure may occur. More commonly, carditis is less intense, and the predominant effect is subsequent scarring of the heart valves. Evidence of carditis may be very subtle; signs of valvular involvement may be mild and transient and may be easily missed on auscultation. Baseline studies, including electrocardiographs and echocardiographs, should be obtained in patients in whom RF is suspected. Patients who show no clear evidence of carditis on initial examination should be closely monitored for a few weeks to assess cardiac involvement.

Carditis is often regarded as the most specific manifesta-

▼ TABLE 66–3. GUIDELINES FOR THE DIAGNOSIS
OF INITIAL ATTACKS OF RHEUMATIC FEVER
(JONES CRITERIA, UPDATED 1992)

MAJOR MANIFESTATIONS	MINOR MANIFESTATIONS
Carditis	Clinical findings
Polyarthritis	Arthralgia
Chorea	Fever
Erythema marginatum	Laboratory findings
Subcutaneous nodules	Elevated acute phase reactants
	Erythrocyte sedimentation rate
	C-reactive protein
	Prolonged PR interval

SUPPORTING EVIDENCE OF ANTECEDENT A STREPTOCOCCAL INFECTION
Positive throat culture or rapid streptococcal antigen test
Elevated or rising streptococcal antibody titer

From Dajani AS, Ayoub EM, Bierman FZ, et al: Guidelines for the diagnosis of rheumatic fever: Jones Criteria, updated 1992. JAMA 268: 2069, 1992. Copyright 1992 American Medical Association.

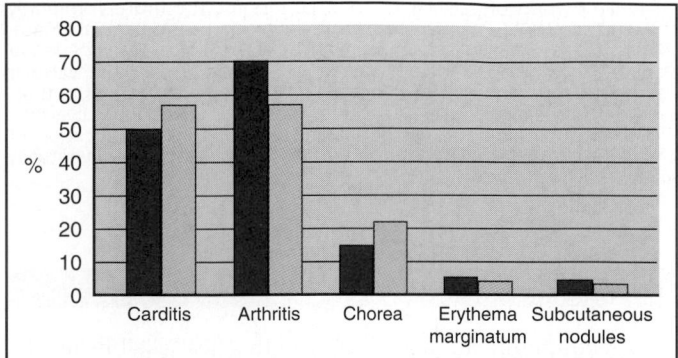

FIGURE 66–1. Relative frequency of major manifestations of rheumatic fever in earlier (dark bars) and more recent (light bars) reports in the 1980s.

tion of RF. It is noted in at least 50 percent of patients with acute RF (Fig. 66–1). Recent outbreaks in the United States suggested that the frequency of carditis was somewhat higher than traditionally reported and may be in part due to more sophisticated diagnostic methods.[2] In one report, carditis was diagnosed in 72 percent of cases by auscultation and in 91 percent of cases by Doppler ultrasonography. The risk of overdiagnosing valvular incompetence by echocardiography should be emphasized, and overreliance on this tool in diagnosing rheumatic carditis should be avoided.

Valvulitis (endocarditis) involving mitral and aortic valves and the chordae of the mitral valve is the most characteristic component of rheumatic carditis. Mitral regurgitation is the hallmark of rheumatic carditis. Aortic regurgitation is less common and usually associated with mitral regurgitation. The pulmonic and tricuspid valves are rarely involved. Residual valvular damage is a major concern in patients with RF and may lead to intractable cardiac failure requiring surgical intervention.

Myocarditis or pericarditis in the *absence* of valvulitis is *not* likely to be due to RF. Tachycardia is an early sign of myocarditis but may also be due to fever or cardiac failure. Transient arrhythmias may occur in patients with myocarditis. Severe myocarditis or valvular regurgitation may lead to cardiac failure. Cardiac enlargement occurs when severe hemodynamic changes result from valvular, myocardial, or pericardial disease. Inflammation of the visceral and parietal surfaces of the pericardium occurs, resulting in pericarditis and the accumulation of pericardial fluid.

ARTHRITIS. Polyarthritis is the most common major manifestation of RF (see Fig. 66–1) but the least specific. It is almost always asymmetric and migratory and involves larger joints (knees, ankles, elbows, and wrists). Swelling, redness, heat, severe pain, limitation of motion, and tenderness to touch are characteristic. The arthritis of RF is benign and does not result in permanent joint deformity. Joint fluid shows findings characteristic of inflammation (not infection). In untreated cases, arthritis usually lasts 2 to 3 weeks. A striking feature of rheumatic arthritis is its dramatic response to salicylates. Indeed, if a patient does not improve substantially after 48 hours of adequate salicylate treatment, the diagnosis of RF should be in doubt.

Some patients may develop arthritis and other multisystem manifestations after acute streptococcal pharyngitis that do not fulfill the Jones criteria for the diagnosis of acute RF. This "syndrome" has been referred to as poststreptococcal reactive arthritis (PSRA). The arthritis of PSRA does not respond dramatically to antiinflammatory agents. Some patients with PSRA may have silent or delayed-onset carditis[21]; therefore, these patients should be carefully observed for several months for the subsequent development of carditis.

CHOREA. Sydenham's chorea, St. Vitus' dance, or chorea minor occurs in about 20 percent of patients with RF (see Fig. 66–1). The rheumatic inflammatory process in the central nervous system specifically involves the basal ganglia and caudate nuclei. Chorea is a *delayed* manifestation of RF, usually appearing 3 months or longer after the onset of the precipitating streptococcal infection. This is in sharp contrast to the latent period of carditis or arthritis, which is usually 3 weeks. As such, chorea is frequently the only manifestation of RF. Furthermore, evidence of a recent GAS infection may be difficult to document, and other supporting historical, clinical, or laboratory findings to fulfill the Jones criteria may be lacking. The diagnosis of RF can be made in a patient with chorea without strictly adhering to the Jones criteria.

Sydenham's chorea is characterized clinically by purposeless and involuntary movements, muscle incoordination and weakness, and emotional lability. The manifestations are more evident when a patient is awake and under stress and may disappear during sleep. All muscles may be involved, but primarily muscles of the face and extremities. Speech may be affected, being explosive and halting. Handwriting deteriorates, and patients become uncoordinated and easily frustrated. The symptoms of Sydenham's chorea must be distinguished from tics, athetosis, conversion reactions, hyperkinesis, and behavior problems. Symptoms usually resolve in 1 to 2 weeks, even without treatment.

ERYTHEMA MARGINATUM. This distinctive rash is a rare manifestation of RF, occurring in less than 5 percent of patients. It is an evanescent, erythematous, macular, nonpruritic rash with pale centers and rounded or serpiginous margins. Lesions vary greatly in size and occur mainly on the trunk and proximal extremities, not on the face. The rash may be induced by application of heat.

SUBCUTANEOUS NODULES. These are firm, painless, freely movable nodules that measure 0.5 to 2 cm. They are rarely seen in patients with RF (about 3 percent); when present, they are most often seen in patients with carditis. They are usually located over extensor surfaces of the joints (particularly elbows, knees, and wrists), in the occipital portion of the scalp, or over spinous processes. The overlying skin is freely movable, shows no discoloration, and is not inflamed.

Minor Manifestations

CLINICAL FINDINGS. Fever and arthralgia are nonspecific, common findings in patients with acute RF. Their diagnostic value is limited because they are encountered commonly in various other diseases. They are used to support the diagnosis of RF when only a single major manifestation is present. Fever is noted during the acute stages of the disease and has no characteristic pattern. Arthralgia is pain in one or more large joints without objective findings on examination and must not be considered a minor manifestation if arthritis is present. Epistaxis and abdominal pain may also occur but are not included as minor diagnostic criteria for RF.

LABORATORY FINDINGS. Elevated acute phase reactants offer objective but nonspecific indications of tissue inflammation. The erythrocyte sedimentation rate (ESR) and C-reactive protein (CRP) level are almost always elevated during the acute stages of the disease in patients with carditis or polyarthritis but are usually normal in patients with chorea. The ESR is useful in monitoring the course of the disease; it usually returns to normal as the rheumatic activity subsides. The ESR may be elevated in patients with anemia and may be suppressed to normal levels in patients with congestive cardiac failure. Unlike the ESR, the CRP level is unaffected by anemia or cardiac failure.

A common finding in patients with acute RF is a prolonged PR interval for age and rate on electrocardiography. This finding alone is not diagnostic of carditis and does not correlate with the ultimate development of chronic rheumatic cardiac disease. Other findings on electrocardiography include tachycardia, atrioventricular block, and QRS–T changes suggestive of myocarditis; these changes are not considered minor manifestations.

Leukocytosis may be observed in the acute stages of RF, but the leukocyte count is variable and not dependable. Anemia is usually mild or moderate and normocytic normochromatic in morphology (anemia of chronic inflammation). Chest roentgenograms are useful in assessing cardiac size; however, normal findings on a chest roentgenogram do not preclude the presence of carditis. Pericarditis, pulmonary edema, and increased pulmonary vascularity are also detected by this examination. Echocardiography may be helpful in detecting endocardial, myocardial, and pericardial involvement. Antimyosin antibody imaging has been reported to be useful in the detection of rheumatic carditis.[21a]

Antecedent Group A Streptococcal Infection

A number of illnesses mimic acute RF, and no laboratory test or tests establish a specific diagnosis of RF. It is therefore important to establish an antecedent streptococcal infection by demonstrating GAS in the tonsillopharynx or an elevated or rising streptococcal antibody titer. *Evidence of an antecedent streptococcal infection is required for confirmation of the initial diagnosis of acute RF.*

At the time of diagnosis of acute RF, only about 11 percent of patients have throat cultures positive for GAS.[2] The paucity of positive cultures is due, in part, to elimination of the organism by host defense mechanisms during the latent period between the onset of the infection and the subsequent development of RF. Several rapid GAS antigen detection tests are commercially available. These tests vary in method. Most have a high degree of specificity but a low sensitivity in a clinical setting. A negative test result does not preclude the presence of GAS in the pharynx. A positive throat culture result or rapid antigen test does not distinguish between a recent infection that can be associated with acute RF and chronic pharyngeal carriage of the organism.

Because the presence of GAS in the pharynx may not represent active infection, elevated or rising antistreptococcal antibody titers provide more reliable evidence of a recent streptococcal infection than does a positive culture or a positive rapid antigen test result. The most commonly used antibody tests are the antistreptolysin O (ASO) and antideoxyribonuclease B (anti-DNase B). The ASO test is usually performed first, and if results are not elevated, the anti-DNase B test is done. Elevated titers for both tests may persist for several weeks or months. ASO titers rise and fall more rapidly than anti-DNase B. A commercially available slide agglutination test measures antibodies to several streptococcal antigens. It is simple to perform, rapid, and widely available; however, the test is not well standardized and not very reproducible and is not recommended as a definitive test for evidence of a preceding GAS infection.

TREATMENT

GENERAL. Whenever possible, patients should be admitted to a hospital for close observation and appropriate work-up. Bed rest is generally considered important because it lessens joint pain. The duration of bed rest may be variable and individually determined. Ambulation may be attempted once fever abates and acute phase reactants return to normal. Patients should be allowed to return to a reasonably active life with normal physical activity. Strenuous physical exercise should be avoided, however, particularly if carditis was present. Although throat cultures are rarely positive for GAS at the time of onset of RF, patients should receive a 10-day course of penicillin therapy. Patients allergic to penicillin should be treated with erythromycin.

If heart failure intervenes, patients should receive diuretics, oxygen, and digitalis and be on a restricted sodium diet. Digitalis preparations should be used cautiously because cardiac toxicity may occur with conventional dosages.

ANTIRHEUMATIC THERAPY. There is no specific treatment for the inflammatory reactions initiated by RF. Supportive therapy is aimed at reducing constitutional symptoms, controlling toxic manifestations, and improving cardiac function.

Patients with mild or no carditis usually respond well to salicylates. Salicylates are particularly effective in relieving joint pain; such pain usually abates within 24 hours of starting salicylates. Indeed, if joint pain persists after salicylate treatment, the diagnosis of RF may be questionable and patients should be reevaluated. Because no specific diagnostic tests for RF exist, antiinflammatory therapy should be withheld until the clinical picture has become sufficiently clear to allow for a diagnosis. Early administration of antiinflammatory agents may suppress clinical manifestations and prevent appropriate diagnosis. For optimal antiinflammatory effect, serum salicylate levels around 20 mg percent are required. Aspirin, at doses of 100 mg/kg/d, given four to five times daily, usually results in adequate serum levels to achieve a clinical response. Optimal salicylate therapy must be individualized, however, to ensure adequate response and avoid toxicity. Tinnitus, nausea, vomiting, and anorexia are common dose-related toxicities associated with salicylism. Side effects may subside after a few days of treatment despite continuation of the medication.

Patients with significant cardiac involvement—particularly those with pericarditis or congestive heart failure—respond more promptly to corticosteroids than to salicylates. Indeed, steroids may be life saving in very ill patients. Patients who do not respond to adequate doses of salicylates may occasionally benefit from a trial course of corticosteroids. Prednisone, 1 to 2 mg/kg/d, is the usual dose.

There is no evidence that salicylate or corticosteroid therapy affects the course of carditis or diminishes the incidence of residual heart disease. Therefore, the duration of therapy with antiinflammatory agents is arbitrarily based on an estimate of the severity of the episode and the promptness of the clinical response.

Mild attacks with little or no cardiac involvement may be treated with salicylates for about 1 month or until there is sufficient clinical and laboratory evidence of inflammatory inactivity. In more severe cases, therapy with corticosteroids may be continued for 2 to 3 months. The medication is then gradually reduced over the next 2 weeks. Even with prolonged therapy, some patients (approximately 5 percent) continue to demonstrate evidence of rheumatic activity for 6 months or more. A "rebound," manifested by reappearance of mild symptoms or of acute phase reactants, may occur in some patients after antiinflammatory medications have been discontinued, usually within 2 weeks. Modest symptoms usually subside without treatment; more severe symptoms may require treatment with salicylates. Some physicians recommend the use of salicylates (aspirin, 75 mg/kg/d) during the period when corticosteroids are being tapered and believe that such an approach may reduce the likelihood of a rebound.

Information about the use of salicylates other than aspirin is very limited. No evidence shows that other nonsteroidal antiinflammatory agents are more effective than aspirin. In patients who cannot tolerate aspirin or who are allergic to it, a trial of other nonsteroidal agents may be warranted. Aspirin preparations that are coated or that contain alkali or buffers may also be tried; however, little evidence shows that such preparations are better tolerated, and some may have undesirable side effects.

PREVENTION

Primary Prevention

Prevention of primary attacks of RF depends on prompt recognition and proper treatment of GAS tonsillopharyngitis. Eradication of GAS from the throat is essential. Although appropriate antimicrobial therapy started up to 9 days after the onset of acute streptococcal pharyngitis is effective in preventing primary attacks of rheumatic fever,[8] early therapy is advisable because it reduces both morbidity and the period of infectivity. In selecting a regimen for the treatment of GAS pharyngitis, various factors should be considered, including bacteriological and clinical efficacy; ease of adherence to the recommended regimen (frequency of daily administration, duration of therapy, palatability); cost; spectrum of activity of the selected agent; and potential side effects.[22]

Penicillin is the antimicrobial agent of choice for the treatment of GAS, except in patients with history of allergy to penicillin.[23, 24] Penicillin has a narrow spectrum of activity, has a longstanding proven efficacy, and is the least expensive regimen. GAS resistant to penicillin has not been documented.[25] Penicillin may be administered intramuscularly or orally (Table 66-4), depending on the patient's likely adherence to an oral regimen.

Intramuscular benzathine penicillin G is preferred, particularly for patients who are unlikely to complete a 10-day course of oral therapy and for patients with a personal or family history of RF or rheumatic heart disease. Benzathine penicillin G injections should be given as a single dose in a large muscle mass. This formulation is painful; injections that contain procaine penicillin in addition to benzathine penicillin G are less painful. Less discomfort is associated with intramuscular benzathine penicillin G if the medication is warmed to room temperature before administration.

The oral antibiotic of choice is penicillin V (phenoxymethyl penicillin). Patients should take oral penicillin regularly for an entire 10-day period, although they are likely to be asymptomatic after the first few days. Although the broader-spectrum amoxicillin is often used for treatment of GAS pharyngitis, it offers no microbiological advantage over penicillin.

Oral erythromycin is acceptable for patients allergic to penicillin. Treatment should also be prescribed for 10 days. Erythromycin estolate (20 to 40 mg/kg/d in two to four divided doses), or erythromycin ethyl succinate (40 mg/kg/d in two to four divided doses) is effective in treating streptococcal pharyngitis; however, efficacy of a twice-daily regimen in adults requires further study. The maximal dose of erythromycin is 1 gm/d. Although strains of GAS resistant to erythromycin are prevalent in some areas of the world and have resulted in treatment failures,[26] they are uncommon in most parts of the United States.[25]

The macrolide azithromycin has similar susceptibility to that of erythromycin against GAS but may cause fewer gastrointestinal side effects. Azithromycin can be administered once daily and produces high tonsillar tissue concentrations. A 5-day course of azithromycin is approved by the Food and Drug Administration as a second-line therapy for the treatment of patients 16 years of age or older with GAS pharyngitis. The recommended dosage is 500 mg as a single dose on the first day followed by 250 mg once daily for 4 days.[27]

A 10-day course of an oral cephalosporin is an acceptable alternative, particularly for penicillin-allergic patients. Narrower-spectrum cephalosporins, such as cefadroxil or

▼ **TABLE 66-4. PREVENTION OF RHEUMATIC FEVER**

AGENT	DOSE	ROUTE	DURATION
Primary Prevention			
Benzathine penicillin G	600,000 units for patients ≤27 kg 1,200,000 units for patients >27 kg	IM	Once
or			
Penicillin V	Children: 250 mg 2–3 times daily Adolescents and adults: 500 mg 2–3 times daily	PO	10 days
For patients allergic to penicillin:			
Erythromycin	40 mg/kg/d 2–4 times daily (maximum 1 gm/d)	PO	10 days
Secondary Prevention			
Benzathine penicillin G	1,200,00 units every 3–4 wk	IM	See Table 66-5
or			
Penicillin V	250 mg b.i.d.	PO	See Table 66-5
or			
Sulfadiazine	0.5 gm once daily for patients ≤27 kg (60 lb) 1.0 gm once daily for patients >27 kg (60 lb)	PO	See Table 66-5
For patients allergic to penicillin and sulfadiazine:			
Erythromycin	250 mg b.i.d.	PO	See Table 66-5

IM = intramuscularly; PO = orally.
Modified from Dajani AS, Taubert K, Ferrieri P, et al: Treatment of streptococcal pharyngitis and prevention of rheumatic fever. Pediatrics 96:758, 1995. Reproduced by permission of Pediatrics.

cephalexin, are probably preferable to the broader-spectrum cephalosporins such as cefaclor, cefuroxime, cefixime, and cefpodoxime. Some penicillin-allergic persons (<15 percent) are also allergic to cephalosporins, and these agents should not be used by patients with immediate (anaphylactic-type) hypersensitivity to penicillin.

Several reports indicate that a 10-day course with an oral cephalosporin is superior to 10 days of oral penicillin in eradicating GAS from the pharynx.[28-31] Reports suggest that a 5-day course with selected oral cephalosporins is comparable to a 10-day course of oral penicillin in eradicating GAS from the pharynx.[32-34]

Certain antimicrobials are not recommended for treatment of streptococcal upper respiratory tract infections.[24] Tetracyclines should not be used because of the high prevalence of resistant strains. Sulfonamides and trimethoprim-sulfamethoxazole will not eradicate GAS in patients with pharyngitis and should not be used to treat active infections. Chloramphenicol is not recommended because of unpredictable efficacy and potential serious toxicity.

Secondary Prevention

Patients who have suffered a previous attack of RF and who develop streptococcal pharyngitis are at high risk for a recurrent attack of RF. A GAS infection need not be symptomatic to trigger a recurrence. Furthermore, RF can recur even when a symptomatic infection is optimally treated. For these reasons, prevention of recurrent RF requires continuous antimicrobial prophylaxis rather than recognition and treatment of acute episodes of streptococcal pharyngitis. Continuous prophylaxis is recommended for patients with a well-documented history of RF (including cases manifested solely by Sydenham's chorea) end those with definite evidence of rheumatic heart disease. Such prophylaxis should be initiated as soon as acute RF or rheumatic heart disease is diagnosed. A full therapeutic course of penicillin (as outlined in Table 66–4) should first be given to patients with acute RF to eradicate residual GAS even if a throat culture is negative at that time. Streptococcal infections occurring in family members of rheumatic patients should be treated promptly.

CONTINUOUS ANTIMICROBIAL PROPHYLAXIS. This provides the most effective protection from RF recurrences. Risk of recurrence depends on several factors. Risk increases with several previous attacks, whereas the risk decreases as the interval since the most recent attack lengthens. The likelihood of acquiring a streptococcal upper respiratory tract infection is an important consideration. Patients with increased exposure to streptococcal infections include children and adolescents; parents of young children; teachers, physicians, nurses, and allied health personnel in contact with children; military recruits; and others in crowded housing. A higher risk of recurrences in economically disadvantaged populations has been demonstrated.

Physicians must consider each individual situation when determining appropriate duration of prophylaxis. Patients who have had rheumatic carditis are at a relatively high risk for recurrences of carditis and are likely to sustain increasingly severe cardiac involvement with each recurrence. Therefore, patients who have had rheumatic carditis should receive long-term antibiotic prophylaxis, perhaps for life. Duration of prophylaxis depends on whether residual valvular disease is present or absent (Table 66–5). Prophylaxis should continue even after valve surgery, including prosthetic valve replacement. Patients who have had RF without carditis are at considerably less risk of cardiac involvement with a recurrence. Therefore, prophylaxis may be discontinued in these individuals after several years.[35] In general, prophylaxis should continue until 5 years have elapsed since the last RF attack or age 21 years, whichever is longer. The decision to discontinue prophylaxis or reinstate it should be made after discussion with the patient of potential risks and benefits and careful consideration of the epidemiological risk factors enumerated earlier.

An injection of 1,200,000 units of long-acting penicillin preparation every 4 weeks is the recommended regimen for secondary prevention in most circumstances in the United States (see Table 66–4). In countries where the incidence of RF is particularly high, in special circumstances, or in certain high-risk individuals, such as patients with residual rheumatic carditis, the administration of benzathine penicillin G every 3 weeks is recommended.[36] Long-acting penicillin is of particular value in patients with a high risk of recurrence of RF. The advantages of benzathine penicillin G must be weighed against inconvenience to patients and pain of injection, which cause some patients to discontinue prophylaxis.

Successful oral prophylaxis depends primarily on patients' adherence to prescribed regimens. Patients need careful and repeated instructions about the importance of continuing prophylaxis. Most failures of prophylaxis occur in nonadherent patients. Even with optimal patient adherence, risk or recurrence is higher in individuals receiving oral prophylaxis compared with those receiving intramuscular benzathine penicillin G.[22] Oral agents are more appropriate for patients at lower risk for rheumatic recurrence. Accordingly, some physicians switch patients to oral prophylaxis when they have reached late adolescence or young adulthood and have remained free of rheumatic attacks for at least 5 years.

Penicillin V is the preferred oral agent (see Table 66–4). There are no published data about the use of other penicillins, macrolides, or cephalosporins for secondary prevention of RF. Although sulfonamides are not effective in eradication of GAS, they do prevent infection. Sulfadiazine and sulfisoxazole appear to be equivalent; the use of sulfisoxazole is acceptable on the basis of extrapolation from data demonstrating that sufladiazine has proven effectiveness in secondary prophylaxis. The recommended dose of sulfisoxazole is the same as that for sulfadiazine. Sulfonamide prophylaxis is contraindicated in late pregnancy because of transplacental passage of the drugs and potential competition with bilirubin for albumin-binding sites. Erythromycin is recommended for patients who are allergic to penicillin and sulfisoxazole.

Infective Endocarditis Prophylaxis

(See also Chap. 47)

Patients with rheumatic valvular heart disease also require additional short-term antibiotic prophylaxis before certain surgical and dental procedures to prevent possible development of infective endocarditis. Patients with prosthetic valves or previous endocarditis are at particularly high risk. *Antibiotic regimens used to prevent recurrences of acute RF are inadequate for prevention of bacterial endocarditis.* The current recommendations of the American Heart Association concerning prevention of bacterial endocarditis should be followed.[37] Because alpha-hemolytic streptococci in the oropharynx may have developed resistance to oral penicillin being used for secondary prevention of RF, the agent selected to prevent endocarditis should not be a penicillin. Patients who have had RF but who do not have evidence of rheumatic heart disease do not need endocarditis prophylaxis.

REFERENCES

General

Narula J, Virmanil R, Reddy KS, Tandon R: Rheumatic Fever. American Registry of Pathology. Washington, DC, Armed Forces Institute of Pathology, 1999.

EPIDEMIOLOGY

1. World Health Organization: Rheumatic fever and rheumatic heart disease. WHO Technical Report Series 764. Geneva, World Health Organization, 1988.
2. Dajani AS. Current status of nonsuppurative complications of group A streptococci. Pediatr Infect Dis J 10:S25, 1991.
3. Taubert KA, Rowley AH, Shulman ST: Seven-year national survey of Kawasaki disease and acute rheumatic fever. Pediatr Infect Dis J 13:704, 1994.
4. Massell BF, Chute CG, Walker AM, et al: Penicillin and the marked decrease in morbidity and mortality from rheumatic fever in the United States. N Engl J Med 318:280, 1988.
5. Schwartz B, Facklam RR, Breiman RF: Changing epidemiology of group A streptococcal infection in the USA. Lancet 336:1167, 1990.

▼ **TABLE 66–5. DURATION OF SECONDARY PROPHYLAXIS IN PATIENTS WITH RHEUMATIC FEVER**

CATEGORY	DURATION
Rheumatic fever with carditis and residual valvular disease	At least 10 yr after last episode and at least until age 40 Sometimes lifelong prophylaxis
Rheumatic fever with carditis but no residual valvular disease	10 yr or well into adulthood, whichever is longer
Rheumatic fever without carditis	5 yr or until age 21, whichever is longer

From Dajani AS, Taubert K, Ferrieri P, et al: Treatment of streptococcal pharyngitis and prevention of rheumatic fever. Pediatrics 96:758, 1995; with permission.

6. Colman G, Tanna A, Efstatiou A, et al: The serotypes of *Streptococcus pyogenes* present in Britain during 1980–1990 and their association with disease. J Med Microbiol 39:165, 1993.
7. Bland EF, Jones TD: Rheumatic fever and rheumatic heart disease: A twenty-year report on 1000 patients followed since childhood. Circulation 4:836, 1951.
8. Denny FW, Wannamaker IW, Brink WR, et al: Prevention of rheumatic fever: Treatment of the preceding streptococcal infection. JAMA 143:151, 1950.
9. Siegel AC, Johnson EE, Stollerman GH: Controlled studies of streptococcal pharyngitis in a pediatric population. I. Factors related to the attack rate of rheumatic fever. N Engl J Med 265:559, 1961.
10. Stollerman GH: Rheumatogenic group A streptococci and the return of rheumatic fever. Adv Intern Med 35:1, 1990.
11. Stollerman GH: Rheumatogenic streptococci and autoimmunity. Clin Immunol Immunopathol 61:131, 1991.
12. Kaplan EL, Johnson DR, Cleary PP: Group A streptococcal serotypes isolated from patients and sibling contacts during the resurgence of rheumatic fever in the United States in the mid-1980s. J Infect Dis 159:101, 1989.
13. Bessen D, Jones KF, Fischetti VA: Evidence for two distinct classes of streptococcal M protein and their relationship to rheumatic fever. J Exp Med 169:269, 1989.
14. Krisher K, Cunningham MW: Myosin: A link between streptococci and heart. Science 227:413, 1985.
15. Dale JB, Beachey EH: Sequence of myosin cross-reactive epitopes of streptococcal M protein. J Exp Med 164:1785, 1986.
16. Khanna AK, Buskirk DR, Williams RC, et al: Presence of non-HLA B cell antigen in rheumatic fever patients and their families as defined by a monoclonal antibody. J Clin Invest 83:1710, 1989.
17. Ayoub EM, Barrett DJ, Maclaren NK, et al: Association of class II human histocompatibility leukocyte antigens with rheumatic fever. J Clin Invest 77:2019, 1986.
18. Narula J, Chopra P, Talwar KK, et al: Does endomyocardial biopsy aid in the diagnosis of active rheumatic carditis? Circulation 88:2198, 1993.
18a. Kim EJ: Index of suspicion. Case #6. Diagnosis: Acute rheumatic fever (ARF). Pediatr Rev 21:26, 2000.

DIAGNOSIS AND TREATMENT

19. Jones TD: Diagnosis of rheumatic fever. JAMA 126:481, 1944.
20. Dajani AS, Ayoub EM, Bierman FZ, et al: Guidelines for the diagnosis of rheumatic fever: Jones criteria, updated 1992. JAMA 268:2069, 1992.
21. Schaffer FM, Agarwal R, Helm J, et al: Poststreptococcal reactive arthritis and silent carditis: A case report and review of the literature. Pediatrics 93:837, 1994.
21a. Narula J: Usefulness of antimyosin antibody imaging for the detection of active rheumatic myocarditis. Am J Cardiol 84:946, 1999.

PREVENTION

22. Dajani AS: Adherence to physicians' instructions as a factor in managing streptococcal pharyngitis. Pediatrics 97:976, 1996.
23. Markowitz M, Gerber MA, Kaplan EL: Treatment of streptococcal pharyngotonsillitis: Reports of penicillin's demise are premature. J Pediatr 123:679, 1993.
24. Dajani AS, Taubert K, Ferrieri P, et al: Treatment of streptococcal pharyngitis and prevention of rheumatic fever. Pediatrics 96:758, 1995.
25. Coonan KM, Kaplan EL: In vitro susceptibility of recent North American group A streptococcal isolates to eleven oral antibiotics. Pediatr Infect Dis J 13:630, 1994.
26. Seppala H, Nissinen A, Jarvinen H, et al: Resistance to erythromycin in group A streptococci. N Engl J Med 326:292, 1992.
27. Hooton TM: A comparison of azithromycin and penicillin V for the treatment of streptococcal pharyngitis. Am J Med 91:23S, 1991.
28. Pichichero ME, Margolis PA: A comparison of cephalosporins and penicillin in the treatment of group A streptococcal pharyngitis: A meta-analysis supporting the concept of microbial copathogenicity. Pediatr Infect Dis J 10:275, 1991.
29. Block SL, Hedrick JA, Tyler RD: Comparative study of the effectiveness of cefixime and penicillin V for the treatment of streptococcal pharyngitis in children and adolescents. Pediatr Infect Dis J 11:919, 1992.
30. Gooch WM, McLinn S, Aronovitz GH, et al: Efficacy of cefuroxime axetil suspension compared with that of penicillin V suspension in children with group A streptococcal pharyngitis. Antimicrob Agents Chemother 37:159, 1993.
31. Dajani AS, Kessler SL, Mendelson R, et al: Cefpodoxime proxetil vs penicillin V in pediatric streptococcal pharyngitis/tonsillitis. Pediatr Infect Dis J 12:275, 1993.
32. Pichichero ME, Gooch WM, Rodriguez W, et al: Effective short-course treatment of acute group A beta-hemolytic streptococcal tonsillopharyngitis; Ten days of penicillin V vs 5 days or 10 days of cefpodoxime therapy in children. Arch Pediatr Adolesc Med 148:1053, 1994.
33. Aujard Y, Boucut I, Brahimi N, et al: Comparative efficacy and safety of four-day cefuroxime axetil and 10-day penicillin treatment of group A beta-hemolytic streptococcal pharyngitis in children. Pediatr Infect Dis J 14: 295, 1995.
34. Dajani AS: Pharyngitis/tonsillitis: European and United States experience with cefpodoxime proxetil. Pediatr Infect Dis J 14:S7, 1995.
35. Berrios X, del Campo E, Guzman B, et al: Discontinuing rheumatic fever prophylaxis in selected adolescents and young adults. Ann Intern Med 118:401, 1993.
36. Lue HC, Wu MH, Wang JK, et al: Long-term outcome of patients with rheumatic fever receiving benzathine penicillin G prophylaxis every three weeks versus every four weeks. J Pediatr 125:812, 1994.
37. Dajani AS, Taubert KA, Wilson W, et al: Prevention of bacterial endocarditis: Recommendations by the American Heart Association. JAMA 277: 1794, 1997.

Chapter 67

Rheumatic Diseases and the Cardiovascular System

BRIAN F. MANDELL • GARY S. HOFFMAN

Systemic rheumatologic conditions are pleomorphic and often involve the cardiovascular system. Patients may present because of musculoskeletal disease, fever of uncertain origin, regional or visceral ischemia, organ failure (e.g., uremia, hypoxemia, dementia, congestive heart failure), or inflammation (e.g., pericarditis, pleurisy). The cardiologist is usually not the initial source of care but becomes involved through the consultative process. However, in certain circumstances, cardiologists or cardiothoracic surgeons may be the first to recognize clinical "outliers" for which systemic autoimmune disease should be part of the differential diagnosis. Several examples include young patients with ischemic heart disease, aortic aneurysms and valvular regurgitation, claudication, or multifocal thrombi or any patient in whom cardiovascular abnormalities occur in the setting of systemic illness. The varied presentations and treatments of rheumatic illnesses and their cardiovascular manifestations are the subjects of this chapter.

Vasculitis

Vasculitis is the common denominator of rheumatic diseases that affect the cardiovascular system, although each of the many forms of systemic vasculitis is uncommon. This fact alone makes it a challenge for the clinician. Additionally, all forms of vasculitis are readily confused with other systemic illnesses for which immunosuppressive therapy may have adverse or lethal consequences. Processes that may be confused with vasculitis include sepsis (particularly bacterial endocarditis), drug toxicities and poisonings (especially with agents that are likely to produce vasospasm, e.g., cocaine, amphetamines), coagulopathies, malignancies, cardiac myxomas, and multifocal emboli from large vessel aneurysms[1] (Table 67–1). The most certain diagnosis of vasculitis lies in the identification of compatible clinical features and pathologic proof of vasculitis. In some instances, vasculitis may present as a characteristic constellation of findings within systemic illness. For example, the presence of upper and lower airway inflammation and red blood cell casts in the urine sediment, with or without renal insufficiency, would suggest Wegener granulomatosis. Hypertension and upper extremity claudication in a young individual, especially if female, should suggest Takayasu arteritis. Unfortunately, many patients with vasculitis do not present with such readily recognizable features. Instead, one may have to rely on combinations of less typical clues. A patient with fever, active urinary sediment, and peripheral neuropathy is likely to have vasculitis, especially if the

previously noted competing diagnoses have already been ruled out. The presence of a purpuric rash, particularly if it is palpable, furthers the probability of this diagnosis, which can be confirmed by a simple skin biopsy. When such features occur in a patient with an already established autoimmune disease (e.g., rheumatoid arthritis, systemic lupus erythematosus, Sjögren syndrome, or relapsing polychondritis), the likelihood of vasculitis being present increases.

The incidence of vasculitis appears to be on the rise, with aging of the population.[1a, 1b, 1c] The considerable social and economic costs of the vasculitides may have been underestimated in the past.[1d] A recent bibliography provides an update on the literature of the vasculitic syndromes.[1e]

PROOF OF DIAGNOSIS. Definitive proof depends on visualizing vasculitic lesions in affected tissue, and the greatest success in achieving a tissue diagnosis comes from biopsy of abnormal or symptomatic sites. In patients with proven vasculitis, the yield from biopsies of clinically normal sites is considerably less than 20 percent. Therefore, a biopsy of apparently normal tissue is not recommended.[2, 3] Biopsies of abnormal organs provide diagnostically useful information in over 65 percent of cases. Yield is less than 100 percent because uniform involvement of vessels in vasculitis is uncommon.

A biopsy may not be practical in an illness with symptoms of visceral ischemia, carotidynia, or findings of unequal pulses or blood pressures. Biopsies of large vessels and diagnostic laparotomy, in the absence of an acute abdomen, are usually impractical. In this setting, angiography may be helpful. Evidence of vascular injury may be apparent from areas of vascular stenosis and/or aneurysm formation that cannot be explained on the basis of atherosclerosis. Angiography is particularly useful for patients with diseases that involve large (Takayasu arteritis, giant cell

▼ **TABLE 67–1. DIAGNOSIS OF VASCULITIS: DISEASES THAT CAN MIMIC PRIMARY SYSTEMIC VASCULITIS**

Sepsis, especially endocarditis
Drug toxicity/poisoning
Coagulopathy
Malignancy
Cardiac myxoma
Multifocal emboli from large vessel aneurysms (cholesterol, mycotic)

(From Hoffman GS: Textbook of Rheumatology, Systemic Vasculitis. Update 28. Philadelphia, WB Saunders, 1998.)

arteritis of the elderly [GIA]) and medium-sized vessels (e.g., polyarteritis nodosa). Serological tests may provide additional information.[3a, 3b]

Once the diagnosis of vasculitis is clearly established and based on the strongest of circumstantial evidence or biopsy proof of vascular inflammatory injury, one must still consider whether such lesions are due to *secondary vasculitis* from bacterial, fungal, and viral infections (e.g., hepatitis B or C and, in immunologically compromised patients, human immunodeficiency virus or cytomegalovirus) or malignancies. Paraneoplastic vasculitis should be considered on the basis of a suspicious history or laboratory finding, or in patients who fail to respond to usually effective aggressive immunosuppressive therapy.

Takayasu Arteritis

Takayasu arteritis (TA), an idiopathic large-vessel vasculitis in young individuals, affects the aorta and its major branches (Fig. 67–1A and B). Histologically, TA is characterized by intense mononuclear leukocyte infiltration and the presence of giant cells (see Fig. 67–1C). Women are affected about 10 times more often than men. Morbidity results from arterial stenosis and organ ischemia, as well as aneurysm formation, especially of the aortic root, where it may produce aortic regurgitation. Hypertensive or primary cardiac, renal, and central nervous system vascular disease account for most deaths. Estimates of mortality range from 3 percent at 8 years[4] to 35 percent at 5 years follow-up.[5]

Symptoms of large-vessel abnormalities or the finding of hypertension, especially in young patients, necessitate careful examination of extremity pulses and blood pressures for asymmetry as well as a search for vascular bruits. Other indications of active disease include increasing extremity or visceral ischemia, malaise, myalgias, arthralgias, night sweats, and fever. Occurrence of such symptoms that take place in the presence of an elevated erythrocyte sedimentation rate suggests active disease. However, a significant number of patients may not have any constitutional or new vascular symptoms, and as many as 50 percent may have normal sedimentation rates and still experience progressive disease.[6–8] The occurrence of active TA in this setting has been documented by the finding of (1) new vascular abnormalities on sequential angiographic studies in patients who were thought to be in remission and (2) inflammatory changes in bypass specimens from patients in whom surgery was performed because of critical flow abnormalities, in the setting of clinically "quiescent" disease.[7–9] Until we are able to judge more accurately the degree of disease activity in TA, outcomes will be compromised. Studies using refinements in magnetic resonance imaging techniques may enable the clinician to detect qualitative abnormalities in the vessel wall that imply inflammatory change.[10] These abnormalities may then be followed sequentially to determine response to therapy.

The cardiac sequelae of TA are far more commonly due to aortic regurgitation and inadequately treated hypertension than arteritis affecting the coronary vessels.[6, 11] When coronary artery vasculitis occurs, it is most frequent in the ostial regions. However, more distal involvement can also occur and both types of lesions may coexist in the same patient. These observations underscore the importance of considering vasculitis in the differential diagnosis of young patients with ischemic syndromes.[12]

TREATMENT. Approximately 60 percent of patients with TA respond to corticosteroid therapy (e.g., prednisone, 1 mg/kg/d), with subsequent resolution of symptoms and stabilization of arteriographically demonstrable abnormalities. However, progressive tapering of corticosteroid therapy has been associated with disease relapse in over 40 percent of patients. Corticosteroid-resistant or relapsing patients may

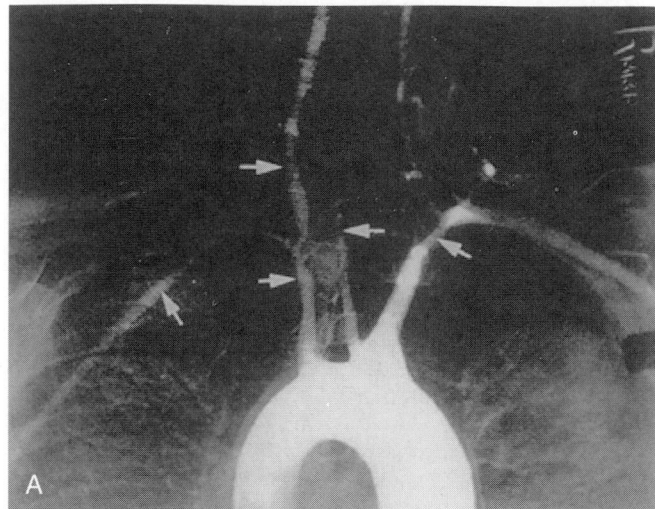

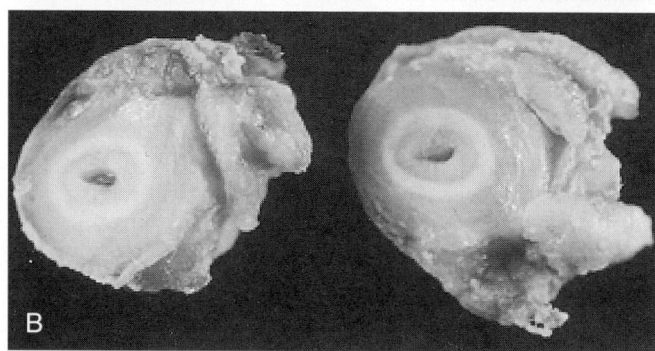

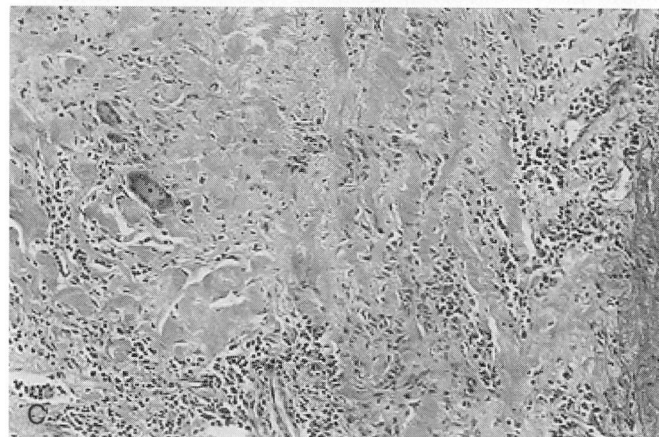

FIGURE 67–1. Takayasu arteritis. *A,* The arrows in this aortic arch angiogram show the characteristic narrowing that occurs in the brachiocephalic, carotid, and subclavian arteries. *B,* Gross photography of the same patient at autopsy shows two cross sections of the right carotid artery with pronounced intimal thickening and minimal residual lumen. *C,* This histologic section illustrates arterial media destruction by mononuclear inflammation with giant cells that takes place in active Takayasu aortitis. (From Schoen FJ, Cotran RS: Blood vessels. *In* Cotran RS, Kuman V, Collins T [eds]: Robbins Pathologic Basis of Disease. 6th ed. Philadelphia, WB Saunders, 1999, pp 493–541.)

respond to the addition of daily therapy with cyclophosphamide (~2 mg/kg) or weekly therapy with methotrexate (~20 mg).[7, 9, 13] About 40 percent of patients who are treated with a cytotoxic agent and a corticosteroid will achieve remission, but over time about half of these patients will also experience relapse, leading to the requirement for chronic immunosuppressive therapy in approximately 25 percent of all patients with TA.

A discussion of pharmacological therapy for TA addresses only one important aspect of care. Other important

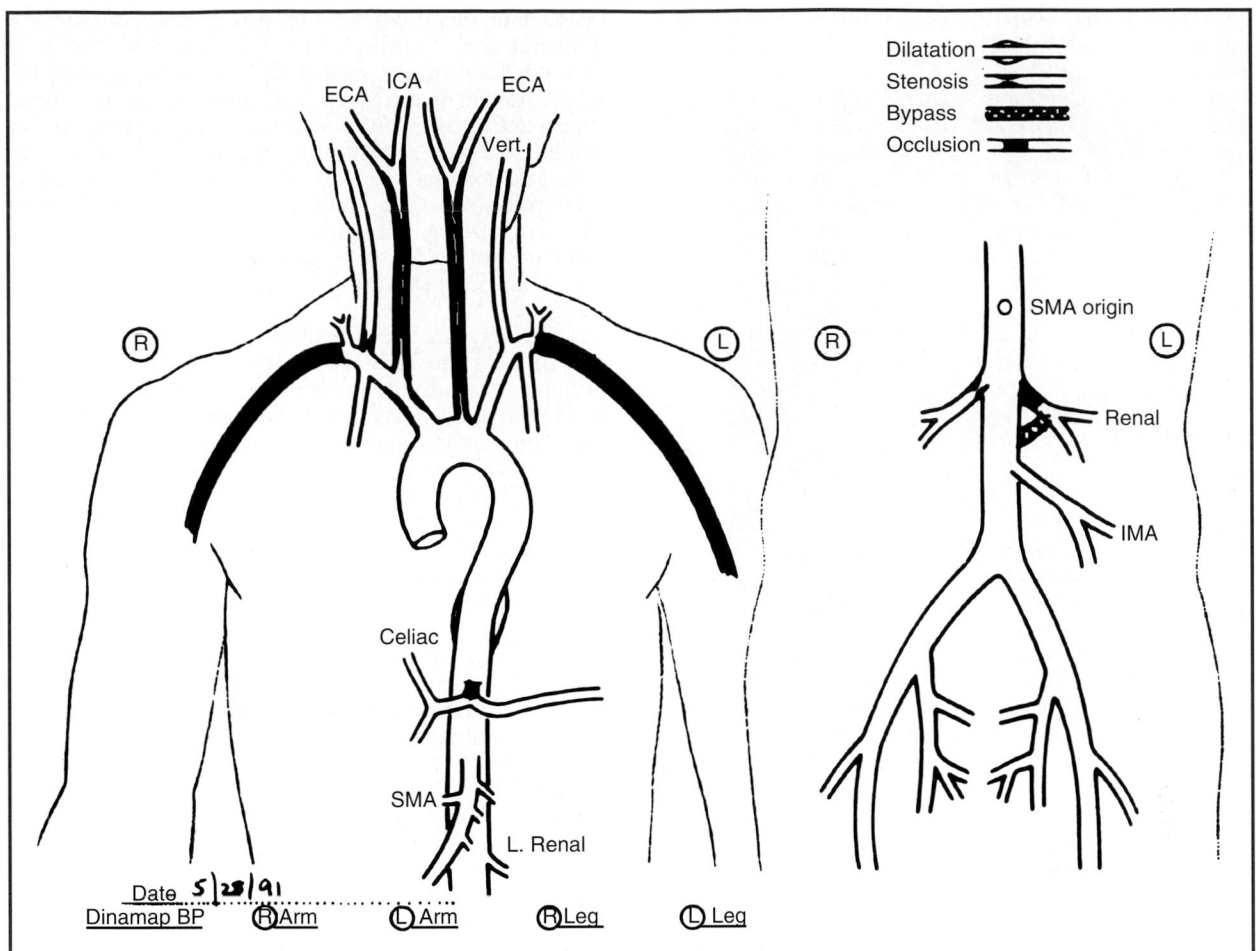

FIGURE 67–2. Takayasu arteritis. Standard Takayasu arteritis diagram used by the Cleveland Clinic Center for Vasculitis Care and Research. In this young man, occlusion of both subclavian arteries has led to leg pressures being the only reliable measure of central aortic pressure. He has also had a left renal artery bypass for a stenotic lesion, which was responsible for severe hypertension. Also note bilateral common carotid stenosis.

issues include treatment of the anatomic effects of vascular lesions. Patients with TA may have signs of clinical deterioration caused by fixed critical stenoses or aneurysms. Hypertension affects 21 to 90 percent of patients.[7, 9, 14–16] In Asia and Mexico, TA is one of the most common causes of hypertension in the adolescent and young adult population. Inadequately treated hypertension may lead to cerebral, cardiac, and renal injury. One of the most common errors in clinical management occurs when the physician does not know whether blood pressure recordings in an extremity are representative of aortic root pressure. Because over 90 percent of patients have stenotic lesions and the most common site of stenosis is the subclavian artery(s), blood pressure in one or both arms may underestimate pressure in the aorta. Elevated aortic root pressure, unrecognized and untreated, enhances the risks of hypertensive complications. This potential pitfall can best be avoided by recording arterial pressures when performing angiography (Fig. 67–2). These observations emphasize the importance of knowing the distribution and severity of all vascular lesions. In the setting of renal insufficiency, the potential contrast agents to cause further renal impairment may limit exploration of the extent of all potential vascular lesions. However, in the absence of contraindications, the entire aorta and its primary branches should be included in vascular imaging studies. Magnetic resonance angiography lacks the ability to measure intravascular pressures. If the clinical examination does not suggest the presence of extremity lesions or show unequal extremity pressures, a magnetic resonance study

may be sufficient to delineate other vascular lesions without resorting to invasive contrast angiography. Whenever feasible, anatomic correction of clinically significant lesions should be considered, especially when renal artery stenosis and hypertension are present.

Aortic root involvement may lead to valvular insufficiency, angina, and congestive heart failure in about 20 percent of patients.[7, 16] Severe or progressive changes may require aortic surgery, with or without valve replacement. Because determining disease activity based solely on clinical and laboratory parameters may be difficult, *all* such surgeries should include histopathological evaluation of vascular specimens.[7–9] It is always preferable to operate on patients with TA when their disease is in apparent remission. Pathology findings from surgical specimens should guide the need for postoperative immunosuppressive treatment.

The care of patients with TA requires a team approach that includes clinicians familiar with the proper use of immunosuppressive therapies, vascular imaging/intervention specialists, and, in the setting of critical stenoses or aneurysms, cardiovascular physicians and surgeons. For most patients, medical and surgical therapies are palliative.

Giant Cell Arteritis of the Elderly

Giant cell arteritis (GCA) and Takayasu arteritis are the principal diseases associated with sterile granulomatous in-

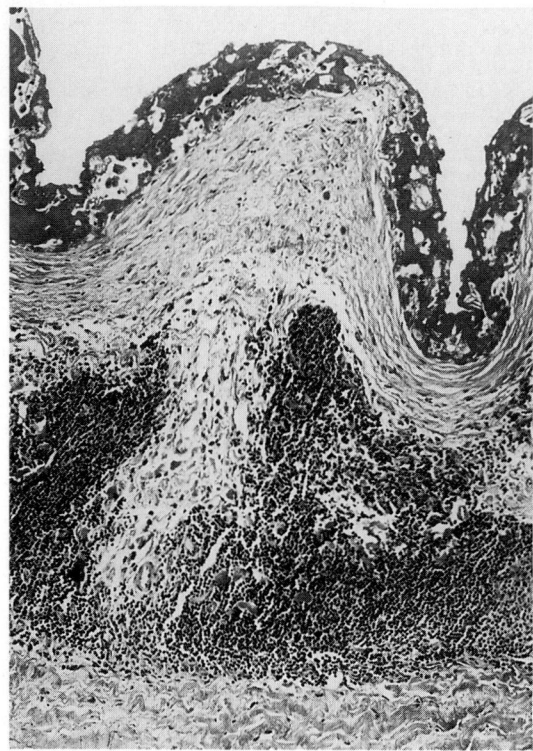

FIGURE 67–3. Temporal (giant cell) arteritis: Active aortitis with perivascular lymphoplasmacytic infiltrate in the adventitia, unorganized periadventitial fibrin and secondary infarcts and patchy scarring involving approximately 50 per cent of the media in giant cell arteritis. (Courtesy of F. J. Schoen.)

flammation of large and medium-sized vessels (Fig. 67–3). GCA affects people 50 years of age and older (mean = 70 years). Although women are more often affected (2–3:1), this gender difference is not as striking as in TA (6–10:1). The demographic characteristics of GCA are the same as for patients with polymyalgia rheumatica and, in fact, 30 to 50 percent of patients with GCA may concurrently present features of polymyalgia rheumatica. The most characteristic features of GCA include new onset of atypical and often severe headaches, scalp and temporal artery tenderness, acute visual loss, and pain in the muscles of mastication (Table 67–2).[17] When such abnormalities occur in conjunction with an elevated erythrocyte sedimentation rate, a clinical diagnosis of GCA can be presumed and treatment initiated even without the benefit of a temporal artery bi-

▼ **TABLE 67–2. GIANT CELL ARTERITIS: CLINICAL PROFILE**

ABNORMALITY	FREQUENCY (%)
Atypical headache	60–90
Tender temporal artery	40–70
Systemic symptoms not attributable to other diseases	20–50
Fever	20–50
Polymyalgia rheumatica	30–50
Acute visual abnormalities	12–40
Transient ischemic attacks or stroke	5–10
Claudication	
"Jaw"	30–70
Extremities	5–15
Aortic aneurysm	15–20
Dramatic response to corticosteroid	~100
Positive temporal artery biopsy	~50+

(From Hoffman GS: Textbook of Rheumatology, Systemic Vasculitis. Update 28. Philadelphia, WB Saunders, 1998.)

opsy. The diagnosis is doubtful if dramatic improvement does not occur within 24 to 72 hours. The specific findings of a positive biopsy would be helpful in guiding treatment when typical features are not present, but the diagnosis is suggested because of vague systemic symptoms, atypical headache in the setting of normal or elevated sedimentation rate, and exclusion of all other reasonable diagnoses have been ruled out. The yield of positive temporal artery biopsies in patients clinically diagnosed with GCA has been estimated to be 50 to 80 percent, depending in part on the size of the biopsy and whether bilateral samples have been obtained.

GCA may produce aortitis in at least 15 percent of cases and involve the primary branches of the aorta in a similar number of individuals.[18–21] Consequently, some patients with GCA may present with features that resemble those of TA. The same considerations and precautions must be applied in GCA among the elderly with large vessel inflammatory diseases in patients with TA (e.g., the need to identify an extremity that provides a reliable blood pressure equivalent to aortic root pressure; follow-up should include careful observation for new bruits, pulse and blood pressure asymmetry, and the possible development of aortic aneurysms). Recent studies have demonstrated that patients with GCA were more than 17 times more likely than age-matched controls to have thoracic aortic aneurysms and about two times more likely than aged-matched controls to have abdominal aortic aneurysms.[19, 20] Fifty-five percent of patients with thoracic aortic aneurysms died as a result of those lesions. Because aneurysms were found either in the course of routine care or at postmortem, these may be conservative estimates. The finding of large vessel disease, including aortic aneurysms, in elderly persons with GCA should not merely be assumed to be secondary to atheromatous disease.

It is not surprising that objective features of cardiac disease would be present in about half of all patients with GCA.[22] However, it appears that myocardial infarction due to GCA is rare[23] or rarely appreciated because histopathological findings in coronary arteries are infrequently sought in patients with a mean age of 70 years.

Corticosteroids continue to be the most effective therapy for GCA. Prednisone (~0.7–1 mg/kg/d) will reduce symptoms within 1 to 2 days and often eliminates symptoms within a week. Tapering of corticosteroids can begin about 1 month after clinical and laboratory parameters (particularly the erythrocyte sedimentation rate) have normalized. Unfortunately, the erythrocyte sedimentation rate does not always normalize even with disease control, so it should not be relied on as the only measure of disease activity. Occasional patients may either not achieve complete remission or not respond to tapered-off corticosteroids. Some authors have recommended cytotoxic or immunosuppressive agents for such individuals, but the utility of these agents has not been proven, as demonstrated in controlled comparative trials.

Idiopathic Aortitis

Aortitis, a recognized feature of TA and GCA, may also occur in uncommon diseases such as Behçet disease and Cogan syndrome and as a complication of Kawasaki disease in children. Occasionally, it is an unanticipated finding in patients undergoing surgery for aortic valve regurgitation, aneurysm resection, or coarctation. Little is known about the frequency and clinical characteristics of idiopathic aortitis.

A recent 20-year review of pathological specimens from consecutive aortic surgeries at the Cleveland Clinic Foundation revealed that 52 of 1204 specimens (4.3 percent) were classified as idiopathic aortitis, a designation that required exclusion of vasculitis associated with postoperative infections, atherosclerosis, or inflammation occurring around surgical materials from prior operations. Sixty-seven percent of patients with idiopathic aortitis were women. In 96 percent of cases, aortitis was present in the thoracic aorta. If one considered only thoracic aortic aneurysms, 12 percent of 386 thoracic specimens had idiopathic inflammatory features. In 96 percent of cases, symptoms of systemic illness had not been present at the time of surgery. In 69 percent of cases, idiopathic aortitis was not related to a current or past history of systemic disease. In 31 percent (16/52), aortitis was associated with a past history of giant cell arteritis, Takayasu arteritis, systemic lupus, Wegener granulomatosis, and a variety of other disorders. Over a mean follow-up period of 42 months, new aneurysms were identified among 6 of 25 patients who were not treated with glucocorticosteroids and none of 11 patients who were treated with glucocorticosteroids. Although the observations on nonrandomized patients could indicate a benefit of such therapy in this setting, marked variation of dose and duration of therapy raises uncertainty about the efficacy of therapy. Because 17 percent of patients subsequently developed new aneurysms, it is prudent for patients with idiopathic aortitis, identified at the time of surgery, to be periodically evaluated for recurrent or persistent disease. If proof of recurrent disease is present, treatment should be pursued, as recommended for Takayasu arteritis and GCA.

The broad spectrum of aortitis includes patients who may have systemic illnesses known to affect large vessels. However, in the setting of a cardiovascular surgery practice, aortitis may first become apparent only after pathological evaluation of excised specimens.

KAWASAKI DISEASE (See also Chap. 45)

Kawasaki disease (KD) is an acute febrile illness that primarily affects children younger than 4 years of age and almost never affects children older than 8 years (mean age in Japan is 12 months, and in the United States it is 2.8 years).[24] The most prominent features are included in the Centers for Disease Control and Prevention case definition guidelines (Table 67–3). KD is usually self-limiting within 4 to 8 weeks; its mortality rate is 2 percent. Deaths usually result from acute thrombosis of coronary artery aneurysms, the result of prior vasculitis. Case studies using noninvasive techniques find coronary artery aneurysms in 20 percent of patients, compared with 60 percent discovered by angiography. Data from postmortem studies have also demonstrated vasculitis of the aorta and celiac, carotid, subclavian, and pulmonary arteries. Rare case reports of gut vasculitis in KD exist.[25, 26] Gastrointestinal morbidity may depend more on small-vessel than large-vessel disease. Treatment with high doses of aspirin (30 mg/kg/d) or intravenous gamma globulin may prevent aneurysms or hasten their regression.

VASCULITIS OF SMALL/MEDIUM-SIZED VESSELS THAT MAY AFFECT THE CARDIOVASCULAR SYSTEM

Hypersensitivity vasculitis, Henoch-Schönlein purpura, Wegener granulomatosis, microscopic polyangiitis, polyarteritis nodosa, and Churg-Strauss syndrome (CSS) may all have cardiac consequences.[26a] Surveys of the literature and the original observations of Churg and Strauss indicate that CSS (asthma, eosinophilia, and vasculitis) may be complicated by congestive heart failure (25–50 percent), acute or constric-

▼ **TABLE 67–3. CDC CASE DEFINITION OF KAWASAKI DISEASE**

Fever ≥ 5 days, without other explanation, plus at least four of the following:
1. Bilateral conjunctival injection
2. Mucous membrane changes: injected or fissured lips; injected pharynx or "strawberry" tongue
3. Extremity abnormality: erythema of palms/soles, edema of hands/feet or generalized or peripheral desquamation
4. Rash
5. Cervical lymphadenopathy
Note: 80% of cases occur in children younger than 4 years old; it is rare in children older than 8 years old.

tive pericarditis (10–30 percent), hypertension (30–75 percent), myocarditis, and, rarely, myocardial infarction. The majority of deaths in CSS relate to cardiovascular disease.[27–30] Cardiac involvement is associated with an increased relative risk of death in CSS, polyarteritis nodosa, and related vasculitides of small and medium-sized vessels.[31, 32] Patients with cardiac involvement almost always have an established diagnosis based on prior recognition of more specific disease manifestations. Treatment of active inflammatory lesions of the heart is the same as would be applied to other sites of vasculitis. Because vasculitis usually involves small vessels, opportunities for invasive therapeutic measures are limited.

Rheumatoid Arthritis

Rheumatoid arthritis (RA) is the most common form of chronic inflammatory polyarthritis. Present in approximately 70 percent of patients, rheumatoid factor does not confirm the diagnosis of RA, and it is frequently present in other diseases, including chronic viral hepatitis and bacterial endocarditis. Systemic complications of RA include pericarditis, pleuritis, systemic necrotizing arteritis, compressive neuropathies, interstitial lung disease, and Sjögren and Felty syndromes.

PERICARDIAL DISEASE (see also Chap. 50). RA affects the pericardium in approximately 50 percent of patients, as indicated by echocardiographic and necropsy studies (see Chap. 50). Chronic, asymptomatic effusive pericardial disease is more common than acute pericarditis.[33–35] Although the frequency of symptomatic pericarditis among outpatients with RA has been estimated as less than 0.5 percent, in a series of 41 selected patients with severe RA, 75 percent had symptoms compatible with acute pericarditis.[33] Patients with rheumatoid pericardial disease are generally older and have long-standing RA. Although it may show characteristic changes in acute pericarditis, the electrocardiogram is usually normal in patients with chronic pericardial disease. Coexistent small pleural effusions are common and may reflect rheumatoid serositis or hemodynamic effects of the pericarditis. Pericardial calcification has been reported,[36] mimicking tuberculous pericarditis. Limited data have been published on the nature of pericardial fluid in RA. Fluid is frequently blood tinged, and leukocyte counts range from scant to more than 30,000/mm³, generally with a neutrophil predominance. The glucose level may be quite low when compared with serum glucose values, similar to markedly depressed glucose levels reported in rheumatoid pleural effusions. The presence of rheumatoid factor in the fluid does not confirm the diagnosis of RA pericarditis. Infection must be excluded. Constrictive pericarditis has been reported, and it must be distinguished from restrictive cardiomyopathy, a rare complication of secondary amyloidosis in patients with long-standing RA. Treatment of clinical pericarditis includes the use of nonsteroidal antiinflammatory drugs, intensified systemic immunosuppressive therapy, pericardial steroid injections, and surgical decompression. A pericardial window may be required if systemic therapy is ineffective or already at an intense level. The pressure of pericardial constriction usually requires surgical treatment. Chest pain due to costochondritis is far more common than pericarditis. The use of aggressive medical therapy early in the course of rheumatoid disease may decrease the frequency of pericardial involvement.

OTHER CARDIOVASCULAR INVOLVEMENT. Patients with RA have a decreased life expectancy, and their leading cause of death is cardiovascular disease.[37] Potential risk factors for coronary artery disease (CAD) in patients with RA include the systemic inflammatory state, the use of corticosteroids, which may accelerate atherosclerosis, and possibly the use of methotrexate, which can elevate levels of circulating homocysteine, although the relative contributions of these factors to acceleration of CAD are not clear.[38, 39] Significant ischemic disease may be clinically silent owing to the relative physical inactivity of patients

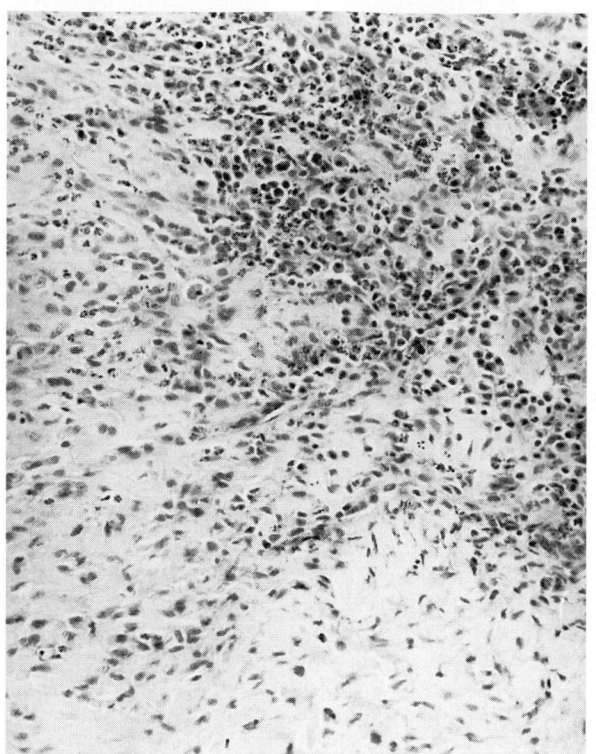

FIGURE 67–4. Aortic valve in a patient with rheumatoid arthritis with florid chronic active inflammation including numerous plasma cells, lymphocytes, and polymorphonuclear leukocytes. (Courtesy of F. J. Schoen.)

with severe rheumatoid disease. Coronary arteritis is a rarely reported complication of RA.[40] Treatment of CAD does not differ from that of patients without RA. Coronary arteritis, occurring along with systemic arteritis, is treated with combination immunosuppressive therapy, including corticosteroids plus cyclophosphamide or other agents.

RA is not usually associated with clinically significant myocarditis or congestive heart failure. Secondary amyloidosis is rare in rheumatoid disease, but it can cause cardiomyopathy and atrioventricular conduction abnormalities. Tachyarrhythmias can occur as a result of rheumatoid pericarditis. Focal myocardial involvement with rheumatoid disease has been well described and may result in conduction system abnormalities. Rheumatoid nodules involving the conduction system have been reported.[41] All levels of conduction block have been described and, once established, do not generally respond to antiinflammatory therapy.

Autopsy studies have indicated frequent involvement of the cardiac valves (Fig. 67–4) and aorta, but these abnormalities are rarely of clinical significance. Slowly progressive granulomatous valvulitis may be difficult, if not impossible, to distinguish from disease unrelated to RA. A rapidly progressive inflammatory aortic valvulitis of the aortic valve, advancing to need for valve replacement over less than 5 years has been described previously.[42] Rheumatoid aortitis, with involvement of the aortic valve, has been reported,[43] but aortitis is not frequently recognized ante mortem. RA does not cause primary pulmonary hypertension, but secondary pulmonary hypertension may result from rheumatoid lung disease.

HLA-B27–Associated Spondyloarthropathies

The rheumatoid factor–negative spondyloarthropathies share several features that distinguish them from rheumatoid arthritis. Unlike rheumatoid arthritis, the entire spine, not just the cervical region, may be involved. Involvement of the sacroiliac joint occurs frequently, and it may be the only musculoskeletal manifestation. Large peripheral joints are commonly involved. Inflammation of the tendon sheaths and bone insertions (enthesitis) occurs frequently. Diffuse tendon sheath involvement may produce "sausage digits." There is an increased frequency of the HLA-B27 gene in these disorders. Although approximately 10 percent of healthy American whites have the HLA-B27 gene, it is present in 90 percent of American whites with ankylosing spondylitis and approximately 60 percent of patients with inflammatory bowel–related spondylitis. These percentages are much lower in African Americans and Asians. Presence of the gene predisposes to anterior uveitis, cardiac conduction disease, and proximal aortitis. Thus, some patients with psoriatic arthritis, enteropathic arthritis, reactive arthritis including Reiter syndrome, and ankylosing spondylitis are predisposed to these complications. Patients may express extraskeletal HLA-B27–related complications without overt rheumatic disease.

Pericarditis, although reported,[44] is not characteristic of these diseases (see also Chap. 50). CAD does not occur at an increased rate, and arteritis is not expected. Diastolic dysfunction has been reported[45] in patients who have the HLA-B27 gene but is rarely of clinical significance. Cardiac conduction disease has been well described in patients with ankylosing spondylitis as well as Reiter syndrome. It has been estimated that up to one third of patients with ankylosing spondylitis develop conduction disease.[46] Initially, the atrioventricular conduction block may be intermittent, but it tends to progress. Conduction disease occurs more commonly in males, and as many as 20 percent of males with permanent pacemakers carry the HLA-B27 gene.[47] Conduction disease may be the only abnormality associated with the HLA-B27 gene. Electrophysiological studies indicate that the level of block is usually at the atrioventricular node, not fascicular.[48, 49] It has been suggested that atrial fibrillation occurs more commonly than expected in patients who carry the HLA-B27 gene.

AORTIC ROOT DISEASE (see also Chap. 40). This condition, with involvement of the aortic valve, has been reported in up to 100 percent of patients in autopsy series and 30 percent in echocardiographic studies. Characteristic findings have included thickening of the aortic root with subsequent dilatation. Aortic cusp nodularity with proximal thickening comprises the "subaortic bump."[50] Transesophageal echocardiography located the subaortic bump in 74 percent of 44 patients with ankylosing spondylitis.[51] In this study, aortic regurgitation developed in 50 percent of patients and 20 percent of patients developed congestive heart failure, underwent valve replacement, suffered a stroke, or died as compared with only 3 percent of age- and sex-matched volunteers. The aortic lesions progressed in 24 percent of patients and resolved in an additional 20 percent of patients over approximately a 2-year follow-up. The severity of aortic root disease was associated with the patients' age and duration of spondylitis. Because dilatation and stiffening of the aortic root contributes to the aortic regurgitation, the regurgitant murmur may be best heard along the right sternal border. Inflammatory aortic disease can occasionally extend to the mitral valve, causing mitral regurgitation.

Systemic Lupus Erythematosus

(See also Chap. 51)

Systemic lupus erythematosus (SLE) is a systemic autoimmune disease characterized by the presence of immune complexes and a constellation of clinical features that may include serositis, arthritis, glomerulonephritis, central nervous system dysfunction, hemolytic anemia, thrombocytopenia, leukopenia, and autoantibodies. Histologically, the arteritis of SLE can include fibrinoid necrosis as well as intense peri-

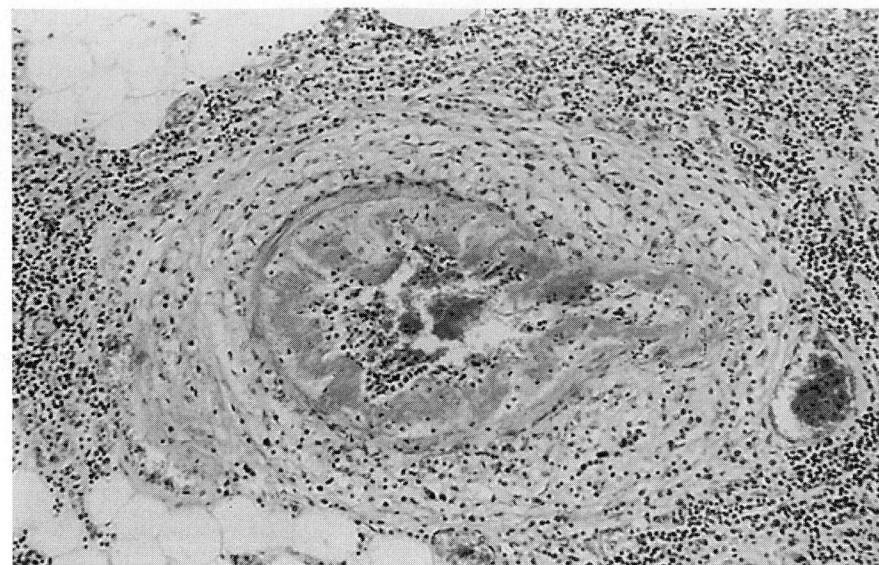

FIGURE 67–5. Systemic lupus erythematosus. Vasculitis with fibrinoid necrosis. (From Schoen FJ, Cotran RS: Blood vessels. *In* Cotran RS, Kuman V, Collins T [eds]: Robbins Pathologic Basis of Disease. 6th ed. Philadelphia, WB Saunders, 1999, pp 493–541.)

vascular cuffing by leukocytes (Fig. 67–5). Antiphospholipid antibodies (APLAs) are present in more than 20 percent of lupus patients. The disease is more common in women, and it can occur at any age. Idiopathic and drug-induced lupus have cardiac manifestations. Drug-induced lupus is well recognized after treatment with various cardiac medications, including procainamide, quinidine, and hydralazine. Over 90 percent of patients with SLE have antinuclear antibodies, although the presence of even high titers of antinuclear antibodies is *not* diagnostic of SLE. Anti–double-stranded DNA is present in 50 to 70 percent of patients with idiopathic SLE and is most common in those with glomerulonephritis.

PERICARDIAL DISEASE (see also Chap. 50). Imaging and autopsy series demonstrate pericardial involvement in more than 60 percent of patients, and clinically significant pericarditis occurs in less than 30 percent,[52] making pericarditis the most common cardiac problem among patients with SLE.[53] Although unexplained chest pain is common in these patients, it is more likely caused by causes other than pericarditis. Pericarditis may occur as the initial manifestation of SLE, but it may also appear at any point during the disease course or as a complication of chronic renal disease. Pericardial fluid, when obtained, has generally demonstrated a high neutrophil predominance,[53] an elevated protein level, and a low or normal glucose level. Complement levels in the fluid tend to be low, but this is not a characteristic unique to SLE. Indeed, the fluid is indistinguishable from that obtained from patients with bacterial pericarditis. Pericardial tamponade may occur at any point in the course of SLE, including the initial presentation.[54] When effusions occur in the setting of chronic renal failure, it is difficult to distinguish uremic from lupus pericarditis. Patients with mild pericarditis without hemodynamic compromise are generally treated with NSAID therapy, unless there is a contraindication to such therapy, such as renal insufficiency. If corticosteroid therapy does not engender a prompt response, large sterile pericardial effusions, particularly those accompanied by fever and/or hemodynamic compromise, are best treated with drainage and consideration of a pericardial window. Pericarditis, as well as tamponade, can occur with drug-induced lupus. Constrictive pericarditis, presumably as a sequela of lupus pericarditis, has been reported. Pericardial thickening has been described in approximately 30 percent of patients with SLE.

CORONARY ARTERY DISEASE. Coronary arteritis that results in ischemic syndromes occurs in patients with SLE. The distinction between CAD and coronary arteritis may require sequential angiographic studies, with documentation of more rapid change in luminal images than is usu-

ally seen with CAD. Despite the young age of many patients with lupus, atherosclerosis remains the most common cause of ischemic cardiac disease. The prevalence of subclinical CAD is quite high, as measured by thallium exercise testing and autopsy studies, and angina or myocardial infarction occurs in less than 20 percent of patients. As patients live longer with their disease, the prevalence of clinical events will increase.

Cardiovascular disease is the most common cause of death in patients with long-standing SLE. There are reports of young patients with SLE who suffer myocardial infarction as the initial manifestation of their CAD. Middle-aged women with lupus are more than 50 times more likely to experience myocardial infarction[55] than other women of similar age. Risk factors include disease duration, period of time treated with corticosteroids, postmenopausal status, and hypercholesterolemia. Additional causes of acute coronary syndromes include thrombosis, often related to the presence of APLAs, and embolism from nonbacterial vegetative endocarditis (Libman-Sacks). The presence of APLAs predisposes to thrombosis in some patients and has been associated with valvular thickening and nonbacterial endocarditis. Antiendothelial antibodies may accelerate atherogenesis. In this regard, APLAs were an independent predictor of CAD in a subset analysis of the Helsinki heart study.[56] Treatment of ischemic disease in patients with SLE is similar to those patients with "routine" atherosclerotic disease. Exceptions include the rare patients with coronary arteritis, who should be treated aggressively with high doses of corticosteroids, and those patients with thrombotic disease related to APLAs. These latter patients should be treated with long-term high-dose anticoagulation. Aspirin is *not* sufficient. Thrombocytopenia is common in patients with APLAs and may complicate therapy.

MYOCARDIAL DISEASE. Myocardial dysfunction in lupus is usually multifactorial and may result from immunologic injury, ischemia, valvular disease, or coexistent problems such as hypertension. Acute myocarditis is infrequent, but it can be the initial presentation of SLE. Patients with peripheral skeletal myositis are reportedly at increased risk for myocarditis.[57] Measurement of cardiotroponin-I may be of value in documenting cardiac involvement, but the MB fraction of CPK may be elevated in the presence of skeletal myositis, even in the absence of myocarditis. Echocardiographic and systolic time interval studies have demonstrated abnormal cardiac function in patients with active SLE. These changes usually reverse with control of disease activity. In the absence of other contributing factors,[58] acute or chronic congestive heart failure due to SLE is not common. Findings on endomyocardial biopsy specimens are not specific, generally revealing patches of myocardial fibrosis, sparse interstitial mononuclear cell infiltrates, and occasional myocyte necrosis.[59] If acute left ventricular failure occurs in patients with active SLE in the absence of CAD or valve disease, a trial of corticosteroid therapy is indicated.

ARRHYTHMIAS. Tachyarrhythmias can occur in patients with SLE secondary to pericarditis or ischemia. Sinus tachycardia may be the earliest manifestation of myocarditis. A gallium scan may be abnormal in lupus myocarditis.[60] Abnormal heart rate variability has been described and may be due to autonomic dysfunction or to occult myocarditis. Abnormal heart rate variability and abnormal myocardial single-photon emission computed tomography have been described, including some patients with normal resting echocardiograms.[61] Unexplained sinus tachycardia that resolves with treatment of SLE can occur in the presence of active SLE even without demonstrable cardiac dysfunction. Occult pulmonary embolism should always be considered as a cause of tachycardia in patients with SLE, especially in the presence of antiphospholipid antibodies.

Infants born to mothers with SLE and other systemic autoimmune diseases have an increased incidence of congenital complete heart block. The pathogenic mechanism is the transmission of maternal anti-Ro and anti-La antibodies in utero, which causes myocardial inflammation and fibrosis of the conduction system.[62, 63] The risk for development of third-degree atrioventricular block in infants born to mothers carrying this antibody is quite low. However, women with systemic autoimmune diseases should be screened for antibody presence before pregnancy. If they are present, the patients should be examined with fetal ultrasound studies throughout pregnancy to detect complete heart block or hydrops. Heart block usually appears after the first trimester of pregnancy; it is almost always irreversible. If recognized early, dexamethasone in utero may be successful in reversing myocarditis.[64] Plasmapheresis and intravenous gamma-globulin therapy may also be tried. It is frequently necessary to place a pacemaker in the infant shortly after delivery.[65]

VALVULAR DISEASE. Valvular involvement in SLE is common. Recognized 50 years ago as noninfectious vegetations (Libman-Sacks endocarditis), transesophageal studies have shown valvular abnormalities in over 50 percent of patients with SLE.[66] Valvular thickening is the most striking finding, followed by vegetations and valvular insufficiency. The vegetations are generally located on the atrial side of the mitral valve and the arterial side of the aortic valve; they are usually immobile. Over time, the lesions may either resolve or worsen, and fibrosis may cause retraction of the valve, causing insufficiency. Less commonly, the vegetations on the valve may occlude the orifice causing stenosis.[67] Valvulitis, with valve fenestrations and rapidly progressing dysfunction, may occur. There are descriptions of mitral and aortic valve replacement in patients with SLE.[68] Valve repair has also been described.[69] Recurrence of valve disease, particularly thrombosis, may affect prosthetic valves. The nonbacterial vegetations rarely embolize and cause stroke syndromes. Several studies have demonstrated an increased prevalence of cardiac valve dysfunction in the presence of APLA, with or without SLE.[70] Because vegetations may occur in APLA-negative patients with SLE,[71] there appear to be multiple mechanisms that affect heart valves in lupus patients. Because of the high prevalence of valvular abnormalities in SLE patients, these patients should receive consideration for antibiotic prophylaxis for endocarditis. However, at present no adequate studies to evaluate this intervention have been performed.

Pulmonary artery hypertension is common in patients with SLE as assessed noninvasively.[72] Clinically significant pulmonary hypertension is less common. Causes for development of pulmonary hypertension include thromboembolic disease due to APLA, intimal proliferation of the pulmonary artery, chronic vasospastic disease associated with peripheral Raynaud disease, and, very rarely, arteritis of the pulmonary vessels. Successful heart-lung transplantation has been reported in a patient with SLE and progressive pulmonary hypertension.[73] Aortitis rarely occurs in patients with SLE.[74]

Antiphospholipid Antibody Syndrome

Antiphospholipid antibody syndrome (APLAS) is defined as the presence of either APLA or a lupus anticoagulant *and* a history of otherwise unexplained recurrent venous or arterial thrombosis, or frequent second- or third-trimester miscarriages. Mild thrombocytopenia and livedo reticularis are also common. APLAs are quite common in patients with SLE, although not all of these patients will exhibit the clinical syndrome. Low to moderate levels of APLA can also be found in association with a number of infectious and other autoimmune diseases, usually without clinical consequence. In the absence of another systemic disease, APLAS is termed *primary*.

Primary APLAS is not associated with pericarditis, myocarditis, or conduction disease. Cardiac manifestations include thrombotic CAD, intracardiac thrombi,[75] and nonbacterial endocarditis.[76] Heart valve abnormalities can be found in approximately 30 percent of patients with primary APLAS. Valvular involvement can include thrombotic masses extending from the valve ring or leaflets, vegetations, or thickening. The mitral valve is affected more frequently than aortic valve; regurgitation is far more common than stenosis. Most valvular involvement is clinically silent. The first manifestation of valvular involvement with APLAS may be a thromboembolic event such as stroke. The incidence of superimposed bacterial endocarditis is not known.

Thrombosis in the setting of APLAs is treated with full-dose anticoagulation with warfarin (Coumadin) using a target international normalized ratio of 3.0. Treatment of clinically significant valvular or intracardiac masses is high-dose anticoagulation with warfarin,[77] with or without the addition of aspirin. Patients likely can also be treated with full therapeutic doses of heparin. Management of heparin dosing, in the setting of a lupus anticoagulant that prolongs the baseline PTT, may require consultation with the coagulation laboratory.[78] The lack of prospective controlled trials with matched patients precludes making any firm recommendations about the long- and short-term utility of adding acetylsalicylic acid to either anticoagulation regimen, although this is often done in patients with recurrent thrombosis despite anticoagulation. Treatment needs to be tailored to the unique clinical circumstances that are present in each patient. There are no data to direct decisions regarding anticoagulation in the setting of APLAS and valvular disease, without thrombosis. Vegetations may resolve with anticoagulation therapy over several months.[79] Patients with APLAS are at risk for myocardial infarction and reocclusion after angioplasty or bypass grafting. Aggressive prophylactic anticoagulation should be employed perioperatively in patients with APLAS and previous thrombosis.[80] Pulmonary hypertension can occur in patients with APLAS secondary to chronic thromboembolic disease. It has also been proposed that APLAs can directly stimulate pulmonary artery intimal proliferation.

Scleroderma

Scleroderma (progressive systemic sclerosis [PSS]/CREST syndrome) and its variants are characterized by the presence of microvascular disease and various patterns of cutaneous and parenchymal fibrosis; antinuclear antibodies are present in more than 90 percent of patients. Generalized scleroderma (PSS) includes proximal cutaneous fibrosis; Raynaud phenomenon, which occurs in 90 percent of patients and is often severe; gastrointestinal dysmotility; pulmonary fibrosis; and cardiac disease. These patients are at risk to develop scleroderma renal crisis.[81] Most of the manifestations of scleroderma are due to fibrosis, not to acute inflammation. Corticosteroids are not the mainstay of treatment.

The more limited CREST variant includes calcinosis, Raynaud phenomenon, esophageal dysmotility, sclerodactyly, and telangiectasia. Patients with CREST syndrome may develop isolated pulmonary hypertension and cardiac conduction disease, but they are not prone to pulmonary fibrosis or renal crisis.

Pericardial involvement is common in scleroderma and includes fibrinous pericarditis in up to 70 percent of patients at autopsy (see also Chap. 50).[82] Small pericardial effusions are demonstrated at echocardiography in 40 percent or less of patients. Acute pericarditis syndromes, including significant effusions, also occur.[83] The presence of moderate or large pericardial effusions is an independent risk factor for mortality.[84] Pericarditis with effusions may require corticosteroid therapy, but there is concern over the risk of inducing scleroderma renal crisis with the use of corticosteroids.

Necropsy and endomyocardial biopsy demonstrate the presence of patchy myocardial fibrosis, occasionally with contraction band necrosis. The latter finding has been attributed to intermittent and intense ischemia produced by microvascular occlusion, perhaps due to vasospasm.[85] Extramural coronary arteries are generally normal. However, approximately 80 percent of PSS and 65 percent of CREST patients have fixed perfusion defects on thallium imaging.[86] Myocardial infarctions have been documented in PSS patients with angiographically normal coronary arteries.[85] Ventricular conduction abnormalities are common and, along with a septal pseudoinfarct pattern, correlate with reduced myocardial function with exercise.[87] Electrical abnormalities can be found throughout the conduction system, and ventricular ectopy is present in more than 60 percent of patients. Patients with scleroderma, especially those with a history of palpitations or syncope, are prone to sudden death, a risk that is further increased in patients with coexistent skeletal myositis.[88] Primary valvular disease is not common. Renal crisis may be associated with variable degree of hypertension, rapidly rising creatinine levels, microangiopathy, and left ventricular failure. Treatment is with angiotensin-converting enzyme inhibitors, not corticosteroids.

Pulmonary hypertension is a major clinical problem that occurs in both limited scleroderma and PSS. In PSS, it may be due to intrinsic pulmonary artery disease or be secondary to interstitial fibrosis.[89] Patients with CREST and PSS should have periodic echocardiograms to screen for asymptomatic pulmonary hypertension,[90] which may respond to vasodilator therapy.[91]

Polymyositis and Dermatomyositis

Polymyositis and dermatomyositis are characterized by inflammation and resultant weakness of proximal greater than distal skeletal muscles; both can be associated with fever and interstitial lung disease. Respiratory muscles may be involved in severe cases. Other visceral organ involvement is uncommon in adults. Dermatomyositis has characteristic skin lesions that include extensor tendon erythema; Gottron papules overlying knuckles, elbows, and knees; edema of the eyelids; and a photosensitive diffuse papular eruption with scale. In a minority of cases, dermatomyositis may be a paraneoplastic syndrome. Both polymyositis and dermato-

myositis are associated with progressive proximal muscle weakness. Acute disease may be associated with intense myalgia as well as weakness.

Although pericarditis is uncommon, it can be seen when polymyositis occurs as part of an overlap syndrome with other autoimmune diseases such as SLE or PSS (see also Chap. 50). Coronary arteritis and ischemic CAD would be rare as part of these syndromes. Localized or generalized myocardial dysfunction is common by echocardiographic assessment but infrequently causes clinical failure.[92] The cardiomyopathy may be corticosteroid responsive. Corticosteroid myopathy generally affects skeletal, but not respiratory or cardiac, muscle.

Polymyositis and dermatomyositis frequently affect the conduction system. In an electrocardiographic study of 77 patients, 23 percent had conduction block,[93] which can occur in the absence of cardiomyopathy and may be progressive. Pulmonary hypertension can occur but is usually secondary to interstitial lung disease.

Sarcoidosis (See also Chap. 48)

Sarcoidosis is a granulomatous inflammatory disease of unknown etiology that primarily affects the lung parenchyma. It can also cause significant adenopathy, arthropathy, myositis, fever, and renal, liver, skin, and cardiac disease.

Pericarditis has been frequently described, and necropsy studies have documented cardiac involvement in 27 percent of patients.[94] This granulomatous, infiltrative disease of the myocardium is often

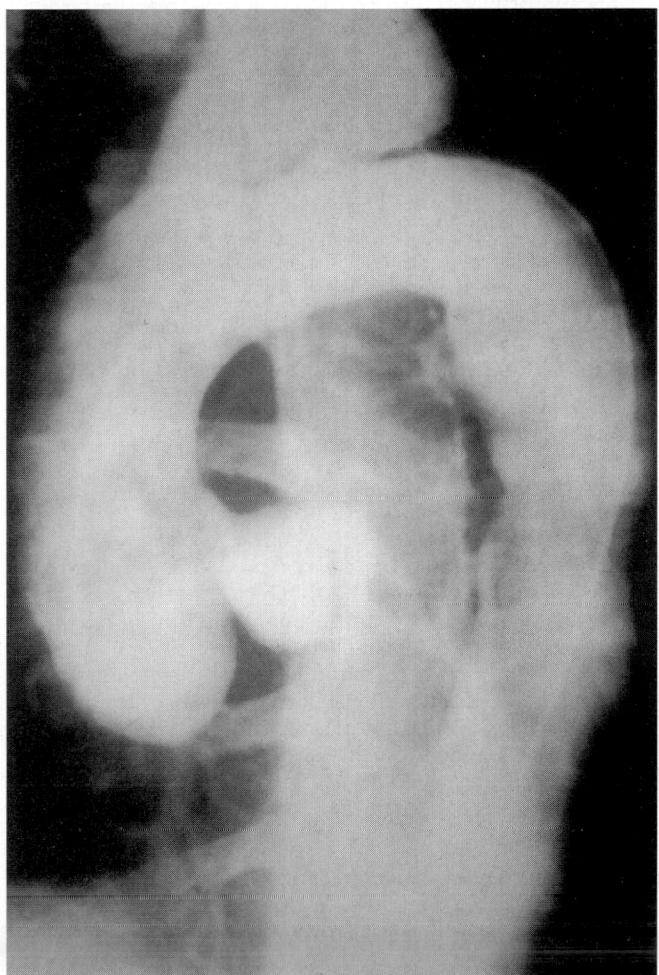

FIGURE 67–6. Sarcoid vasculitis. Aortogram from a 20-year-old African-American male who presented with chronic polyarthritis, uveitis, Bell palsy, and upper extremity claudication. He has had occlusion of both the subclavian and innominate vessels, which led to claudication, and also has aneurysmal dilatation of the entire aorta.

▼ TABLE 67–4. RELATIVE FREQUENCIES OF CARDIAC INVOLVEMENT IN SELECTED SYSTEMIC AUTOIMMUNE DISORDERS

	PERICARDIAL	ISCHEMIC ARTERITIS/THROMB.	MYOPATHY	CONDUCTION	VALVULAR	PULMONARY HYPERTENSION	AORTITIS
RA	++++	+/++++	+	++	+	+	+++
B27	+		+	++++	+++		++++
Spondylo.					(aortic)		
SLE	++++	++/++++	+++	++++*	++++	+++	+
APLA		−/++++			++++	+++	
Scleroderma	++++	−/+	++	++++		++++	
Polymyositis	+		+++	+++			
Sarcoidosis	+++		+	++		+++	++

RA = Rheumatoid arthritis; B27 Spondylo. = HLA-B27–associated spondyloarthropathies; SLE = systemic lupus erythematosus; APLA = antiphospholipid antibody syndrome; ARTERITIS/THROMB. = coronary arteritis/thrombotic or atherosclerosis-related coronary artery disease.
+ = reported; ++ = rare; +++ = well described; ++++ = frequently reported.
* Congenital complete heart block.

asymptomatic, but it can cause arrhythmias, conduction disease, and, rarely, otherwise unexplained congestive heart failure.[95] Granulomatous infiltration may be patchy, and there is a predilection toward involvement of the left ventricle, particularly the upper septal area. This distribution may influence the results of diagnostic right-sided endomyocardial biopsy. Use of gallium imaging may be helpful in determining the need and duration of immunosuppressive therapy.[96] Sarcoid dilated cardiomyopathy may be difficult to distinguish from idiopathic cardiomyopathy or giant cell myocarditis. Conduction disease is more common in patients with sarcoidosis,[97] and thallium perfusion defects tend to preferentially affect the anterior septal and apical regions. Biopsy may help to distinguish sarcoidosis from giant cell myocarditis,[98] but the diagnostic yield of endomyocardial biopsy is low.[99] Sarcoidosis is at least somewhat steroid responsive. Pulmonary artery hypertension can occur in sarcoidosis, generally as a result of pulmonary fibrosis.

Systemic vasculitis is an uncommon complication of sarcoidosis. Its precise frequency remains unknown. Sarcoid vasculitis can affect small- to large-caliber vessels, including the aorta. The latter presentation can be easily confused with Takayasu arteritis (Figure 67–6). African-American patients appear predisposed to the development of large vessel involvement. Although corticosteroid therapy may be palliative for all forms of sarcoid vasculitis, relapses of the disease are common and often preclude withdrawal of treatment. Morbidity from disease and treatment is common. Deaths from sarcoid vasculitis occur in a minority of reported cases.[100]

Summary

The different rheumatic diseases can affect the heart in distinct patterns (Table 67–4). Occasionally, cardiac involvement represents the initial manifestation of a systemic autoimmune disease. The clinical pattern of involvement may provide a clue as to the underlying diagnosis. Cardiologists will encounter patients with these diseases and their cardiac and extracardiac complications and should remain vigilant to recognize these patterns when they occur.

REFERENCES

1. Hoffman GS, Kerr GS: Recognition of systemic vasculitis in the acutely ill patient. In Mandell BF (ed): Management of Critically Ill Patients with Rheumatologic and Immunologic Diseases. New York, Marcel Dekker, 1994, pp 279–308.
1a. Watts RA, Lane SE, Bentham G, Scott DG: Epidemiology of systemic vasculitis: A ten-year study in the United Kingdom. Arthritis Rheum 43:414–419, 2000.
1b. Scott DG, Watt RA: Systemic vasculitis: Epidemiology, classification, and environmental factors. Ann Rheum Dis 59:161–163, 2000.
1c. Stone JJ, Hoffman GS: Vasculitis at the millennium [editorial]. Curr Opin Rheumatol 12:1–2, 2000.
1d. Cotch MF: The socioeconomic impact of vasculitis. Curr Opin Rheumatol 12:20–23, 2000.
1e. Bibliography. Current world literature. Vasculitis syndromes. Rheumatol 12:B1–B13, 2000.
2. Albert DA, Rimon D, Silverstein MD: The diagnosis of polyarteritis nodosa: I. A literature-based decision analysis approach. Arthritis Rheum 31:1117–1127, 1988.
3. Albert DA, Silverstein MD, Paunicka K, et al: The diagnosis of polyarteritis nodosa: II. Empirical verification of a decision analysis model. Arthritis Rheum 31:1128–1134, 1988.
3a. Schultz DR, Diego JM: Antineutrophil cytoplasmic antibodies (ANCA) and systemic vasculitis: Update of assays, immunopathogenesis, controversies, and report of a novel de novo ANCA-associated vasculitis after kidney transplantation. Semin Arthritis Rheum 29:267–285, 2000.
3b. Harper L, Savage CO: Pathogenesis of ANCA-associated systemic vasculitis. J Pathol 190:349–359, 2000.

TAKAYASU ARTERITIS

4. Koide K: Takayasu arteritis in Japan. Heart Vessels 7(S):48–54, 1992.
5. Kerr GS, Hallahan CW, Giordano J, et al: Takayasu's arteritis. Ann Intern Med 120:919–929, 1994.
6. Morales E, Pineda C, Martinez-Lavin M: Takayasu's arteritis in children. J Rheumatol 18:1081–1084, 1991.
7. Hoffman GS: Treatment of resistant Takayasu's arteritis. Rheum Dis Clin North Am 21:73–80, 1995.
8. Lagneau P, Michel JB, Vuong PN: Surgical treatment of Takayasu's disease. Ann Surg 205:157–166, 1987.
9. Hoffman GS: Takayasu's arteritis: Lessons from the American National Institutes of Health experience. Int J Cardiol 54(Suppl):83–86, 1996.
10. Flamm SD, White RD, Hoffman GS: The clinical application of "edema-weighted" magnetic resonance imaging in the assessment of Takayasu's arteritis. Int J Cardiol 66(Suppl):151–159, 1998.
11. Hashimoto Y, Tanaka M, Hata A, et al: Four years followup study in patients with Takayasu arteritis and severe aortic regurgitation: Assessment by echocardiography. Int J Cardiol 54(Suppl):173–176, 1997.
12. Amano J, Suzuki A: Coronary artery involvement in Takayasu's arteritis: Collective review and guidelines for surgical treatment. J Thorac Cardiovasc Surg 102:554–560, 1991.
13. Hoffman GS, Leavitt RY, Kerr GS, et al: Treatment of Takayasu's with methotrexate. Arthritis Rheum 37:578–582, 1994.
14. Sharma BK, Sagar S, Singh AP, Suri S: Takayasu arteritis in India. Heart Vessels 7(Suppl):37–43, 1992.
15. Ito I: Medical treatment of Takayasu arteritis. Heart Vessels 7(Suppl):133–137, 1992.
16. Giordano JM, Hoffman GS, Leavitt RY: Takayasu's disease. In Rutherford RB (ed): Vascular Surgery. 4th ed. Philadelphia, WB Saunders, 1995, pp 245–253.

GIANT CELL ARTERITIS OF THE ELDERLY

17. Rodriguez-Valverde V, Sarabia JM, Gonzalez-Gay MA, et al: Risk factors and predictive models of giant cell arteritis in polymyalgia rheumatica. Am J Med 102:331–336, 1997.
18. Evans J, Hunder GG: The implications of recognizing large-vessel in-

volvement in elderly patients with giant cell arteritis. Curr Opin Rheumatol 9:37–40, 1997.

19. Evans JM, O'Fallon WM, Hunder GG: Increased incidence of aortic aneurysm and dissection in giant cell (temporal) arteritis. Ann Intern Med 122:502–507, 1995.

20. Liu G, Shupak R, Chiu BK: Aortic dissection in giant cell arteritis. Semin Arthritis Rheum 25:160–171, 1995.

21. Greene GM, Lain D, Sherwin RM, et al: Giant cell arteritis of the legs. Am J Med 81:727–733, 1986.

22. Matteson EL, Gold KN, Block DA, Hunder GG: Long term survival of patients with giant cell arteritis in the American College of Rheumatology giant cell arteritis classification criteria cohort. Am J Med 100:193–196, 1996.

23. Lie JT: Aortic and extracranial large vessel giant cell arteritis: A review of 72 cases with histologic documentation. Semin Arthritis Rheum 24:422–431, 1995.

KAWASAKI DISEASE

24. Bell DM, Brink EW, Nitzkin JL, et al: Kawasaki's syndrome: Description of two outbreaks in the United States. N Engl J Med 304:1568–1575, 1981.

25. Murphy DJ Jr, Morrow R, Harberg FJ, Hawkins EP: Small bowel obstruction as a complication of Kawasaki disease. Clin Pediatr 26:193–196, 1987.

26. Fan ST, Lau WY, Wong KK: Ischemic colitis in Kawasaki's disease. J Pediatr Surg 21:964–965, 1986.

26a. Osman A, McCreery CJ: Cardiac vasculitis in Henoch-Schonlein purpura. Circulation 101:E69–E70, 2000.

VASCULITIS OF SMALL/MEDIUM-SIZED VESSELS

27. Churg J, Strauss L: Allergic granulomatosis, allergic angiitis, and periarteritis nodosa. Am J Pathol 27:277–301, 1951.

28. Hoffman GS: From Textbook of Rheumatology, Systemic Vasculitis. Update 28. Philadelphia, WB Saunders, 1998.

29. Lanham JG, Elkon KB, Pusey CD, Hughes GR: Systemic vasculitis with asthma and eosinophilia: A clinical approach to Churg Strauss syndrome. Medicine 63:65–81, 1984.

30. Guillevin L, Lhote F, Gayraud M, et al: Prognostic factors in polyarteritis nodosa and Churg Strauss syndrome. Medicine 75:17–28, 1996.

31. Lanham JG, Churg J: Churg Strauss syndrome. In Churg A, Churg J (eds): Systemic Vasculitides. New York, Igaku-Shoin, 1991, pp 102–120.

32. Fortin PR, Larson MG, Watters AK, et al: Prognostic factors in systemic necrotizing vasculitis of the polyarteritis nodosa group—a review of 45 cases. J Rheumatol 22:78–84, 1995.

RHEUMATOID ARTHRITIS

33. Hara KS, Ballard DJ, Ilstrup DM, et al: Rheumatoid pericarditis: Clinical features and survival. Medicine 69:81–91, 1990.

34. Kelly CA, Bourke JP, Malcome A, Griffiths ID: Chronic pericardial disease in patients with rheumatoid arthritis: A longitudinal study. Q J Med 73:461–470, 1990.

35. McRorie ER, Wright RA, Errington ML, Luqmani RA: Rheumatoid constrictive pericarditis. Br J Rheumatol 36:100–103, 1997.

36. Manui H, Raven P: Calcific constrictive pericarditis due to rheumatoid arthritis. Postgrad Med J 66:57–58, 1990.

37. Myllykangas-Luosujarvi R, Aho K, Kautiainen H, Isomaki H: Cardiovascular mortality in women with rheumatoid arthritis. J Rheumatol 22:1065–1067, 1995.

38. Frederich CA, Rader DJ: Management of lipid disorders. Rheum Dis Clin North Am 25:507–520, 1999.

39. Willberg-Jonsson S, Ohman ML, Rantap Dahlqvist S: Cardiovascular morbidity and mortality in patients with seropositive rheumatoid arthritis in northern Sweden. J Rheumatol 24:445–451, 1997.

40. Swezey RL: Myocardial infarction due to rheumatoid arteritis: An antemortem diagnosis. JAMA 199:855–857, 1967.

41. Nomeir AM, Turner RA, Watts LE: Cardiac involvement in rheumatoid arthritis: Follow-up study. Arthritis Rheum 22:561–564, 1979.

42. Levine AJ, Dimitri WR, Bonser RS: Aortic regurgitation in rheumatoid arthritis necessitating aortic valve replacement. Eur J Cardiothorac Surg 15:213–214, 1999.

43. Gravellese EM, Corson JM, Coblyn JS, et al: Rheumatoid aortitis: A rarely recognized but clinically significant entity. Medicine 68:95–106, 1989.

HLA-B27–ASSOCIATED SPONDYLOARTHROPATHIES

44. Wilkinson M, Bywaters EG: Clinical features and course of ankylosing spondylitis as seen in a follow up of 222 hospital referred cases. Ann Rheum Dis 17:209–228, 1958.

45. Crowley JJ, Donnelly SM, Tobin M, et al: Doppler echocardiographic evidence of left ventricular diastolic dysfunction in ankylosing spondylitis. Am J Cardiol 71:1337–1340, 1993.

46. Bergfeldt L, Edhag O, Vallin H: Cardiac conduction disturbances, an underestimated manifestation in ankylosing spondylitis: A 25-year follow-up study of 68 patients. Acta Med Scand 212:217–223, 1982.

47. Bergfeldt L: HLA-B27–associated rheumatic diseases with severe cardiac bradyarrhythmias: Clinical features and prevalence in 223 men with permanent pacemakers. Am J Med 75:210–215, 1983.

48. Bergfeldt L: HLA-B27–associated cardiac disease. Ann Intern Med 127:621–629, 1997.

49. Bergfeldt L, Vallin H, Edhag L: Complete heart block in HLA B27 associated disease: Electrophysiological and clinical characteristics. Br Heart J 51:184–188, 1984.

50. Bulkley BH, Roberts WC: Ankylosing spondylitis and aortic regurgitation: Description of the characteristic cardiovascular lesion from study of eight patients. Circulation 48:1004–1027, 1973.

51. Roldan CA, Chavez J, Wiest PW, et al: Aortic root disease associated with ankylosing spondylitis. J Am Coll Cardiol 32:1397–1404, 1998.

SYSTEMIC LUPUS ERYTHEMATOSUS

52. Moder KG, Miller TD, Tazelaar HD: Cardiac involvement in systemic lupus erythematosus. Mayo Clin Proc 74:275–284, 1999.

53. Mandell BF: Cardiovascular involvement in systemic lupus erythematosus. Semin Arthritis Rheum 17:126–141, 1987.

54. Kahl LE: The spectrum of pericardial tamponade in systemic lupus erythematosus. Arthritis Rheum 35:1343–1349, 1992.

55. Manzi S, Meilahn EN, Rairie JE, et al: Age-specific incidence rates of myocardial infarction and angina in women with systemic lupus erythematosus: Comparison with the Framingham study. Am J Epidemiol 145:408–415, 1997.

56. Vaarala O, Manttari M, Manninen V, et al: Anti-cardiolipin antibodies and risk for myocardial infarction in a prospective cohort of middle-aged men. Circulation 91:23–27, 1995.

57. Borenstein DG, Fye WB, Arnett FC, Stevens MB: The myocarditis of systemic lupus erythematosus: Association with myositis. Ann Intern Med 89:619–624, 1978.

58. Winslow TM, Ossipov MA, Fazio GP, et al: The left ventricle in systemic lupus erythematosus: Initial observations and a five-year follow-up in a university medical center population. Am Heart J 125:1117–1122, 1993.

59. Bulkley BH, Roberts WC: The heart in systemic lupus erythematosus and the changes induced in it by corticosteroid therapy: A study of 36 necropsy patients. Am J Med 58:243–264, 1975.

60. Jolles PR, Tatum JL: SLE myocarditis. Detection by Ga-67 citrate scintigraphy. Clin Nucl Med 21:284–286, 1996.

61. Lagan R, Schillaci O, Tubani L, et al: Lupus carditis: Evaluation with technetium-99m MIBI myocardial SPECT and heart rate variability. Angiology 50:143–148, 1999.

62. Finkelstein Y, Adler Y, Harel L, et al: Anti-Ro (SSA) and anti-La (SSB) antibodies and complete congenital heart block. Ann Med Interne 148:204–208, 1997.

63. Buyon JP, Winchester R: Congenital complete heart block: A human model of passively acquired autoimmune injury. Arthritis Rheum 33:609–614, 1990.

64. Carreira PE, Gutierrez-larraya F, Gomez-Reino JJ: Successful intrauterine therapy with dexamethasone for fetal myocarditis and heart block in a woman with systemic lupus erythematosus. J Rheumatol 20:1204–1207, 1993.

65. Deloof E, Devlieger H, Van Hoestenberghe R, et al: Management with a staged approach of the premature hydropic fetus due to complete congenital heart block. Eur J Pediatr 156:521–523, 1997.

66. Roldan CA, Shively BK, Crawford MH: An echocardiographic study of valvular heart disease associated with systemic lupus erythematosus. N Engl J Med 335:1424–1430, 1996.

67. Hussain R, Neligan MC: Systemic lupus erythematosus: A rare cause of mitral stenosis. Thorac Cardiovasc Surg 41:125–126, 1993.

68. Morin AM, Boyer A, Nataf P, Gandjbakhch I: Mitral insufficiency caused by systemic lupus erythematosus requiring valve replacement: Three case reports and a review of the literature. Thorac Cardiovasc Surgeon 44:313–316, 1996.

69. Kalangos A, Panos A, Sezerman O: Mitral valve repair in lupus valvulitis: Report of a case and review of the literature. J Heart Valve Dis 4:202–207, 1995.

70. Leung W-H, Wong K-L, Lau C-P, et al: Association between antiphospholipid antibodies and cardiac abnormalities in patients with systemic lupus erythematosus. Am J Med 89:411–419, 1990.

71. Gleason CB, Stoddard MC, Wagner SG, et al: A comparison of cardiac valvular involvement in the primary antiphospholipid syndrome versus anticardiolipin-negative systemic lupus erythematosus. Am Heart J 125:1123–1129, 1993.

72. Winslow TM, Ossipov MA, Fazio GP, et al: Five-year follow-up study of the prevalence and progression of pulmonary hypertension in systemic lupus erythematosus. Am Heart J 129:510–515, 1995.

73. Levy RD, Guerraty AJ, Yacoub MH, Loertscher R: Prolonged survival after heart-lung transplantation in systemic lupus erythematosus. Chest 104:1903–1905, 1993.

74. Peguero A, Rabb H, Morgan M, et al: Lupus aortitis and aneurysm: Case report and review of the literature. J Clin Rheumatol 5:32–36, 1999.

ANTIPHOSPHOLIPID ANTIBODY SYNDROME

75. Asherson TA, Hughes GRV: The expanding spectrum of Libman Sacks endocarditis: The role of antiphospholipid antibodies. Clin Exp Rheumatol 7:226–228, 1989.

76. Hojnik M, George J, Ziporen L, Shoenfeld Y: Heart valve involvement (Libman-Sacks endocarditis) in the antiphospholipid syndrome. Circulation 92:1579–1587, 1996.
77. Khamashta MA, Cuadrado MJ, Mujic F, et al: The management of thrombosis in the anti-phospholipid-antibody syndrome. N Engl J Med 332:993–997, 1995.
78. Bartholomew J: Dosing of heparin in the presence of a lupus anticoagulant. J Clin Rheumatol 4:307–311, 1998.
79. Agirbasli MA, Hansen DE, Byrde BF: Resolution of vegetations with anticoagulation after myocardial infarction in primary antiphospholipid syndrome. Echocardiography 10:877–880, 1997.
80. Ciocca RG, Choi J, Grahm: Antiphospholipid antibodies lead to increased risk of cardiovascular surgery. Am J Surg 170:198–200, 1995.

SCLERODERMA

81. Steen V D: Scleroderma renal crisis. Rheum Dis Clin North Am 22:861–878, 1996.
82. Byers RJ, Marshall DAS, Freemont AJ: Pericardial involvement in systemic sclerosis. Ann Rheum Dis 45:393–394, 1997.
83. Deswal A, Follansbee WP: Cardiac involvement in scleroderma. Rheum Dis Clin North Am 22:841–860, 1996.
84. Clements PJ, Lachenbruch PA, Furst DE, et al: Cardiac score: A semiquantitative measure of cardiac involvement that improves prediction of prognosis in systemic sclerosis. Arthritis Rheum 34:1371–1376, 1991.
85. Bulkley BH Klacsmann PG, Hutchins GM: Angina pectoris, myocardial infarction, and sudden cardiac death with normal coronary arteries: A clinicopathologic study of nine patients with progressive systemic sclerosis. Am Heart J 95:563–568, 1978.
86. Clements PJ, Furst DE: Heart involvement in systemic sclerosis. Clin Dermatol 12:267–275, 1994.
87. Follansbee WP, Curtiss EI, Rahko PS, et al: The electrocardiogram in systemic sclerosis (scleroderma): Study of 102 consecutive cases with functional correlations and review of the literature. Am J Med 79:183–192, 1985.
88. Follansbee WP, Zerbe TR, Medsger TA: Cardiac and skeletal muscle disease in systemic sclerosis (scleroderma): A high risk association. Am Heart J 125:194–203, 1993.

89. Koh ET, Lee P, Gladman DD, Abu-Shakra M: Pulmonary hypertension in systemic sclerosis: An analysis of 17 patients. Br J Rheumatol 35:989–993, 1996.
90. Murata I, Takenaka K, Yoshinoya S, et al: Clinical evaluation of pulmonary hypertension in systemic sclerosis and related disorders: A Doppler echocardiographic study of 135 Japanese patients. Chest 111:36–43, 1997.
91. Menon N, McAlpine L, Peacock AJ, Madhok R: The acute effects of prostacyclin on pulmonary hemodynamics in patients with pulmonary hypertension secondary to systemic sclerosis. Arthritis Rheum 41:466–469, 1998.

POLYMYOSITIS AND DERMATOMYOSITIS

92. Askari D, Heuttner TL: Cardiac abnormalities in polymyositis/dermatomyositis. Semin Arthritis Rheum 127:208–219, 1982.
93. Stern R, Godblold J, Chess Q, Kagen L: ECG abnormalities in polymyositis. Arch Intern Med 144:2185–2188, 1984.

SARCOIDOSIS

94. Silverman KJ, Hutchins GM, Bulkley BH: Cardiac sarcoid: A clinicopathologic study of 84 unselected patients with systemic sarcoidosis. Circulation 58:1204–1211, 1978.
95. Oakley C: Cardiac sarcoidosis. Thorax 44:371–372, 1989.
96. Kurata C, Sakata K, Taguchi T, et al: SPECT imaging with Tl-201 and Ga-67 in myocardial sarcoidosis. Clin Nucl Med 17:408–411, 1990.
97. Yazaki Y, Isobe M, Hiramitsu S, et al: Comparison of clinical features and prognosis of cardiac sarcoidosis and idiopathic dilated cardiomyopathy. Am J Cardiol 82:537–540, 1998.
98. Litovsky SH, Burke AP, Virmani R: Giant cell myocarditis: An entity distinct from sarcoidosis characterized by multiphasic myocyte destruction by cytotoxic T cells and histiocytic giant cells. Mod Pathol 9:1126–1134, 1996.
99. Uemura A, Morimoto SI, Hiramissu S, et al: Histologic diagnostic rate of cardiac sarcoidosis: Evaluation of endomyocardial biopsies. Am Heart J 138:299–302, 1999.
100. Fernandes SRM, Singsen BH, Hoffman GS: Sarcoidosis and systemic vasculitis. Semin Arthritis Rheum 30:33–46, 2000.

Chapter 68

Cardiovascular Abnormalities in HIV-Infected Individuals

STACY D. FISHER · STEVEN E. LIPSHULTZ

Infection with the human immunodeficiency virus (HIV) is one of the leading causes of acquired heart disease and specifically of symptomatic heart failure (Table 68–1). The cardiac complications of HIV infection tend to occur late in the disease and are therefore becoming more prevalent in our society as therapy and longevity improve. Mean annual incidence is estimated at 15.9 cases of cardiac disease per 1000 HIV-infected patients.[1]

The Joint United Nations Program on HIV/AIDS estimated that, worldwide, 33.4 million people were living with HIV infection or acquired immunodeficiency syndrome (AIDS) in 1998.[2] The incidence of new HIV infection in the United States has decreased substantially over the past 5 years. Deaths related to HIV infection decreased 42 percent in 1996–1997 and 20 percent in 1997–1998 because of improved antiretroviral therapies and better identification and treatment of opportunistic infections. By the end of 1998, about 300,000 people in the United States were living with AIDS and the number of long-term survivors was increasing.[3] Early in the epidemic, HIV infections were chiefly found in homosexual males; however, now most new cases occur in injection drug users and heterosexual partners of infected persons. Minority groups are overrepresented.[3]

The range of cardiac abnormalities caused by HIV infection is suggested in one recent autopsy study of 440 patients. Eighty-two had cardiac involvement: the conditions, in order of frequency, were pericardial effusion, lymphocytic interstitial myocarditis, dilated cardiomyopathy (frequently with myocarditis), infective endocarditis, and malignancy (myocardial Kaposi's sarcoma and B-cell immunoblastic lymphoma).[4]

Left Ventricular Systolic Dysfunction

CLINICAL PRESENTATION. In HIV-infected patients, concurrent pulmonary infections, pulmonary hypertension, anemia, portal hypertension, malnutrition, or malignancy may alter or confuse the characteristic signs that define heart failure in other populations. Thus, patients with left ventricular systolic dysfunction may be asymptomatic or may present with New York Heart Association Class III or IV heart failure.

Echocardiography is a useful test to assess left ventricular systolic function in this population and, in addition to left ventricular dysfunction, often reveals either low-to-normal wall thickness or left ventricular hypertrophy and a dilated left ventricular chamber. Electrocardiography (ECG) may reveal nonspecific conduction defects or repolarization changes. In one multicenter trial, 57 percent of asymptomatic HIV-infected individuals had baseline ECG abnormalities, including supraventricular and ventricular ectopic beats.[5] The chest radiograph has low sensitivity and specificity for congestive heart failure in patients with HIV infection.

Encephalopathy is associated with symptomatic heart failure in HIV-infected individuals, suggesting that it may be comorbid with cardiac dysfunction in late-stage HIV infection.[6]

INCIDENCE. One prospective study of asymptomatic HIV-infected adults with initial CD4 counts of more than 400 cells/ml found that 76 of 952 (8 percent) had significant left ventricular dysfunction (diffuse left ventricular hypokinesis with an ejection fraction less than 45 percent and left ventricular end-diastolic volume index greater than 80 ml/m^2) over 60 months follow-up.[1] Almost all had fewer than 400 CD4-positive cells/ml at the time of diagnosis of cardiomyopathy. The mean annual incidence for asymptomatic patients was calculated at 15.9 cases of dilated cardiomyopathy per 1000 patients. Cardiomyopathy was diagnosed 28 ± 10 (mean standard deviation) months after enrollment.[1]

A 4-year observational study of 296 patients with a spectrum of HIV-related disease found 44 (15 percent) with dilated cardiomyopathy (fractional shortening less than 28 percent, with global left ventricular hypokinesis), 13 (4 percent) patients with isolated right ventricular dysfunction (right ventricle larger than left ventricle on standard two-dimensional views), and 12 (4 percent) patients with borderline left ventricular dysfunction (left ventricular end-systolic diameter greater than 58 mm, but fractional shortening greater than 28 percent, or global dysfunction reported by one or two, but not all three observers) (Fig. 68–1).[7] Dilated cardiomyopathy was strongly associated with a CD4 count of less than 100 cells/ml.[7]

Left ventricular dysfunction is a common consequence of HIV infection in children. In a study of 205 vertically (mother to child) HIV-infected children (enrolled at a median age of 22 months and followed with echocardiography every 4 to 6 months and ECG, Holter monitoring, and chest radiography every year), the prevalence of decreased left ventricular function (fractional shortening <28 percent)

2211

TYPE	POSSIBLE ETIOLOGIES AND ASSOCIATIONS	INCIDENCE

Dilated cardiomyopathy	Infectious
	  HIV documented in myocytes
	  Toxoplasma gondii
	  Coxsackievirus group B
	  Epstein-Barr virus
	  Cytomegalovirus
	  Adenovirus
	Autoimmune response to infection
	Drug-related
	  Cocaine
	  Possibly nucleoside analogues
	  Interleukin-2, doxorubicin, interferon
	Metabolic/Endocrine
	  Nutritional deficiency/wasting
	    Selenium, vitamin B_{12}, carnitine
	  Thyroid hormone
	  Growth hormone
	  Adrenal insufficiency
	  Hyperinsulinemia
	Cytokines
	  Tumor necrosis factor-alpha, nitric oxide, tumor
	    growth factor-beta, endothelin-1
	Hypothermia
	Hyperthermia
	Autonomic Insufficiency
	Encephalopathy
	Acquired Immunodeficiency
	  HIV viral load
	  Length of infection
		Estimated 15.9 patients/1000 asymptomatic HIV-infected persons[1]

Pericardial effusion	Bacteria
	  Staphylococcus aureus
	  Streptococcus pneumoniae
	  Proteus mirabilis
	  Nocardia asteroides
	  Staphylococcus epidermidis
	  Pseudomonas aeruginosa
	  Klebsiella pneumoniae
	  Enterococcus species
	  Listeria species
	Mycobacteria
	  Mycobacterium tuberculosis
	  Mycobacterium avium-intracellulare
	  Mycobacterium kansaii
	Viral Pathogens
	  HIV
	  Herpes simplex virus
	  Herpes simplex virus type 2
	  Cytomegalovirus
	Other Pathogens
	  Cryptococcus neoformans
	  Toxoplasma gondii
	  Histoplasma capsulatum
	Malignancy
	  Kaposi's sarcoma
	  Malignant lymphoma
	Capillary leak/wasting/malnutrition
	Hypothyroidism
	Low CD4 count
	Prolonged acquired immunodeficiency
		11%/year[26]
		Spontaneous resolution in up to 42% of affected patients[16, 26]

Infective endocarditis	Autoimmune response to infection
	Bacterial
	  Staphylococcus aureus
	  Salmonella species
	  Streptococcus species
	  Enterococcus
	  Hemophilus parainfluenzae
	  Staphylococcus epidermidis
	  Pseudalleschira boydii
	Fungal/Yeast
	  Aspergillus fumigatus
	  Candida species
	  Cryptococcus neoformans
		Up to 6% incidence[29]

TYPE	POSSIBLE ETIOLOGIES AND ASSOCIATIONS	INCIDENCE
Nonbacterial thrombotic endocarditis (generally tricuspid valve)	Underlying valvular endothelial damage, vitamin C deficiency, valvular injury secondary to catheters or injected impurities (intravenous drug use), disseminated intravascular coagulation, hypercoagulable state, malnutrition, wasting, prolonged acquired immunodeficiency	Rare (<3–5%) incidence[29, 32]

Malignancy (Kaposi's sarcoma, non-Hodgkin's lymphoma, leiomyosarcoma)	Prolonged immunodeficiency, low CD4 count
	Viral Associations
	   Human herpesvirus-8
	   Epstein-Barr virus
		1% incidence (3/440)[33]

Isolated right ventricular and pulmonary disease	Recurrent bronchopulmonary infections, pulmonary arteritis, microvascular pulmonary emboli due to thrombus or drug injection	
Primary pulmonary hypertension	Plexogenic pulmonary arteriopathy Mediator release from endothelium	0.5% incidence[38]

Vasculitis
   Systemic necrotizing
   Hypersensitivity
   Henoch-Schönlein purpura
   Lymphomatoid granulomatosis
   Primary central nervous system angiitis
	Drug therapy (antibiotic and antiretroviral)	Case reports becoming more common

Accelerated atherosclerosis
   Coronary artery disease
   Cerebrovascular disease
	Protease inhibitor therapy, atherogenesis by virus-infected macrophages, chronic inflammation	Up to 8% prevalence by autopsy and case reports[42, 44]

Autonomic dysfunction	Associated nervous system disease Drug therapy side effects Prolonged immunodeficiency Malnutrition	Common in late-stage disease[47]
Arrhythmias	Drug therapy Pentamidine Autonomic dysfunction	Unknown

was 5.7 percent. The 2-year cumulative incidence was 15.3 percent.[8] The cumulative incidence of symptomatic congestive heart failure and/or the use of cardiac medications was 10 percent over 2 years.[8]

Global estimates of HIV-infected people range from 33.4 to 120 million people worldwide between the years 1998 and 2000.[2] If there is a 10 percent incidence of symptomatic congestive heart failure over the 2 years,[8] then there would be 3.34 to 12 million cases of congestive heart failure during a 2-year interval.

PATHOGENESIS. A wide variety of possible etiological agents have been postulated in HIV-related cardiomyopathy (see Table 68–1), including myocardial infection with HIV itself, opportunistic infections, viral infections, autoimmune response to viral infection, cardiotoxicity from therapeutic or illicit drugs, nutritional deficiencies, cytokine overexpression, and many others.[9]

Myocarditis (see Chap. 48). Myocarditis is perhaps the best studied of the possible causes. Dilated cardiomyopathy may be related to a direct action of HIV on the myocardial tissue or to an autoimmune process induced by HIV alone or in conjunction with co-infecting viruses.[1, 9a] *Toxoplasma gondii,* coxsackievirus group B, Epstein-Barr virus, cytomegalovirus, adenovirus, and HIV in myocytes have been found in biopsy specimens.[10] Postmortem biopsy samples of children with HIV revealed histological evidence of myocarditis in 11 of 32 and borderline myocarditis in another 13 cases, possibly relating to the development of cardiomyopathy and to rapid progression of HIV disease.[10a]

Right ventricular biopsy performed on 76 patients within 1 month of the diagnosis of cardiomyopathy revealed evidence of myocarditis in 63, HIV nucleic acid sequences in cardiac myocytes in 58, and active myocarditis in 36.[1] In the 36 patients with active myocarditis, 9 had coexisting viral infections (coxsackievirus group B [n = 6], cytomegalovirus [n = 2], or Epstein-Barr virus [n = 1]).[1]

Autopsy and biopsy results have revealed only scant and patchy inflammatory cell infiltrates in the myocardium.[11] HIV virions appear to infect myocardiocytes in patchy distributions. The infected cells are not surrounded by an inflammatory response, and no clear association has been made between the infection and functional disability. Nevertheless, myocardial biopsy may be clinically helpful, because it may reveal lymphocytic infiltrates suggesting myocarditis or treatable opportunistic infections (by special stains), permitting aggressive therapy for an underlying pathogen.

Notably, HIV-related cardiomyopathy is often not associated with any specific opportunistic infection, and approximately 40 percent of patients have not experienced any opportunistic infection before the onset of cardiac symptoms.[12]

Cytokine Alterations. HIV infection increases the production of tumor necrosis factor-alpha, which alters intracellular calcium homeostasis and increases nitric oxide (NO) production, tumor growth factor-beta, and endothelin-1 upregulation.[12, 13] NO induced in high levels has been shown experimentally to have a negative inotropic effect and to be cytotoxic to myocytes.

In one study, HIV-infected individuals with dilated cardiomyopathy were much more likely to have myocarditis, and had a broader spectrum of viral infections, than did HIV-negative patients with idiopathic dilated cardiomyopathy.[14] Also, levels of tumor necrosis factor-alpha and induced NO synthase were higher in myocytes from the HIV-infected patients with dilated cardiomyopathy (particularly those with viral co-infections) and levels varied inversely with the CD4 count. Barbaro and associates postulate that immunodeficiency may favor the selection of viral variants of increased pathogenicity or enhance the cardiovirulence of viral strains.[14]

Nutritional Deficiencies. Nutritional deficiencies are

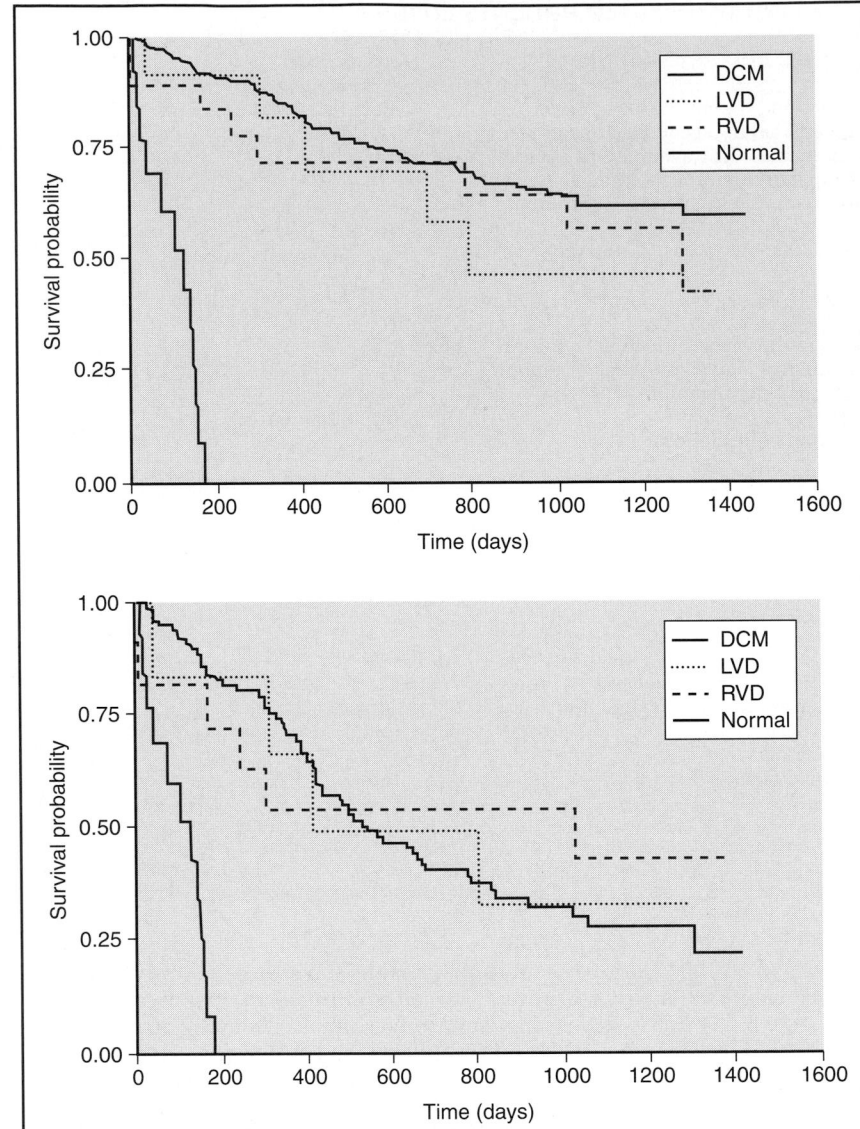

FIGURE 68–1. *Top,* Survival curves for 296 HIV-infected patients with structurally normal hearts, dilated cardiomyopathy (DCM), left ventricular dysfunction (LVD), or right ventricular dysfunction (RVD). *Bottom,* Time to death related to AIDS in 81 patients with CD4+ cell counts less than 20 × 10⁶ cells per liter. (From Currie PF, Jacob AJ, Foreman AR, et al: Heart muscle disease related to HIV infection: Prognostic implications. BMJ 309:1605, 1994.)

common in HIV infection, particularly in late-stage disease. Poor absorption and diarrhea both lead to electrolyte imbalances and deficiencies in elemental nutrients. Deficiencies of trace elements have been associated with cardiomyopathy. For example, selenium deficiency increases the virulence of coxsackievirus to cardiac tissue.[15] Selenium replacement reverses cardiomyopathy and restores left ventricular function in nutritionally deplete patients. Levels of vitamin B₁₂, carnitine, and growth and thyroid hormone may also be altered in HIV disease; all have been associated with left ventricular dysfunction.

Pathogenesis in Children. In children with vertically transmitted HIV infection, two mechanisms of pathogenesis have been described. One is the dilation of the left ventricle with a reduction in thickness-to-end-systolic dimension ratio of the ventricle. The other is concentric hypertrophy of the muscle; with dilation, the thickness-to-end-systolic dimension ratio remains normal or is increased.[6]

COURSE OF DISEASE. Patients with asymptomatic left ventricular dysfunction (fractional shortening less than 28 percent, with global left ventricular hypokinesis) may have transient disease by echocardiographic criteria. In one serial echocardiographic study, three of six patients with abnormal fractional shortening had normal readings after a mean of 9 months. The three with persistently depressed left ventricular function died within 1 year of baseline.[16]

Prognosis. Mortality in HIV-infected patients with car-diomyopathy is increased independent of CD4 count, age, sex, and risk group. The median survival to AIDS-related death was 101 days in patients with left ventricular dysfunction and 472 days in patients with a normal heart, at similar infection stage (see Fig. 68–1).[7] Isolated right ventricular dysfunction or borderline left ventricular dysfunction did not place patients at risk. Compared with idiopathic cardiomyopathy, patients with HIV-related cardiomyopathy had a hazard ratio of 4.0 (95% confidence interval 2.80–5.74) for death over a mean follow-up period of 4.4 years.[16a]

In the P²C² HIV study of children with vertically transmitted HIV infection (median age, 2.1 years), 5-year cumulative survival was 64 percent.[17] Mortality was higher in children with baseline depressed left ventricular fractional shortening or increased left ventricular dimension, thickness, mass, wall stress, heart rate, or blood pressure (Fig. 68–2). Decreased left ventricular fractional shortening and increased wall thickness were also predictive of survival after adjustment for age, height, CD4 count, HIV RNA copy number, clinical center, and encephalopathy.[6, 17] Fractional shortening was abnormal for up to 3 years before death, whereas wall thickness identified a population at risk only 18 to 24 months before death. Thus, in children, fractional shortening may be a useful long-term predictor and wall thickness a useful short-term predictor of mortality.[18]

Rapid-onset congestive heart failure has a grim prognosis

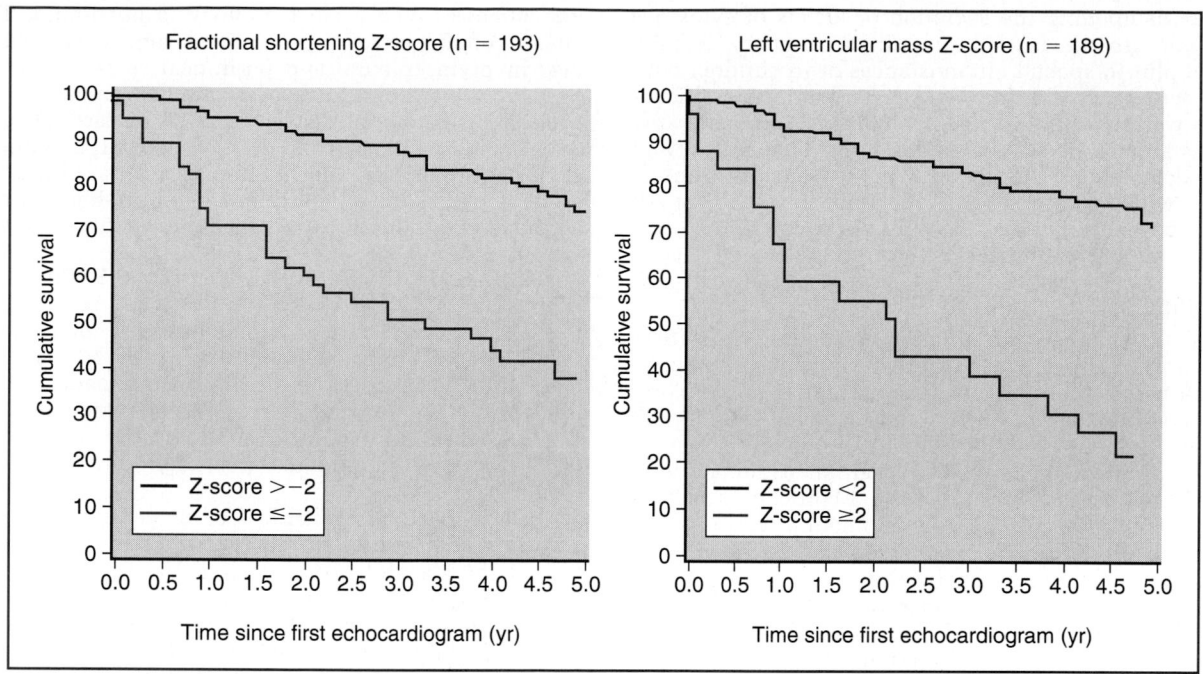

FIGURE 68–2. Kaplan-Meier cumulative survival curves for 193 HIV-infected children according to baseline echocardiographic measurements after prospective follow-up. Patients are stratified by Z scores adjusted for age or body surface area for each measurement. *Left,* Fractional shortening. *Right,* Left ventricular mass. (Based on data from Lipshultz SE, Easley KA, Orav EJ, et al: Cardiac dysfunction and mortality in HIV-infected children: The prospective P²C² HIV multicenter study. Circulation, in press.)

in HIV-infected adults and children, with over half of patients dying of primary cardiac failure within 6 to 12 months of presentation.[6, 12] Chronic-onset heart failure may respond better to medical therapy in this patient population.[12]

Therapy

Therapy for dilated cardiomyopathy associated with HIV infection is generally similar to therapy for nonischemic cardiomyopathy and includes diuretics, digoxin, and angiotensin-converting enzyme inhibitors as tolerated. No studies have investigated the efficacy of specific cardiac therapeutic regimens other than intravenous immunoglobulin.[19, 20]

Opportunistic or other infections should be sought aggressively and treated, with potential to improve or resolve the cardiomyopathy.[21] Right ventricular biopsy may be useful in identifying infectious causes of heart failure to institute targeted therapy.[21] However, right ventricular biopsy is probably underused.

After medical therapy is begun, serial echocardiographic studies should be performed at 4-month intervals.[21] Monitoring recommendations for testing and timing of follow-up are based on studies relating impairment of fractional shortening to a worse prognosis.[21] If function continues to worsen or the clinical course deteriorates, a biopsy should be considered.

Intravenous immunoglobulins have had some success in acute congestive cardiomyopathy and nonspecific myocarditis in HIV-uninfected patients.[20] Immunoglobulin therapy is beneficial in Kawasaki disease, an immunologically mediated illness with cardiac dysfunction resembling that seen with HIV disease.[22, 23] Monthly immunoglobulin infusions in HIV-infected pediatric patients have been associated with minimized left ventricular dysfunction, an increase in left ventricular wall thickness, and a reduction in peak left ventricular wall stress (Fig. 68–3), suggesting that both impaired myocardial growth and left ventricular dysfunction may be immunologically mediated.[18]

The apparent efficacy of immunoglobulin therapy may be the result of immunoglobulins removing cardiac autoan-

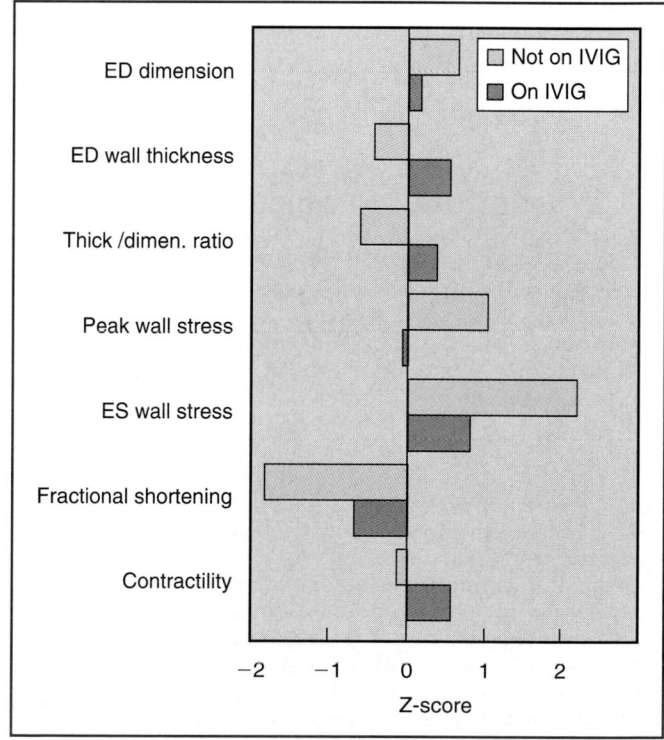

FIGURE 68–3. Mean echocardiographically measured cardiac dimensions in patients taking intravenous immunoglobulin (IVIG) and patients not taking it. All measurements are presented as age- or body surface area–adjusted Z scores. ED = end diastolic; ES = end systolic. (From Lipshultz SE, Orav EJ, Sanders SP, et al: Immunoglobulins and left ventricular structure and function in pediatric HIV infection. Circulation 92:2220, 1995. Copyright 1995, American Heart Association.)

tibodies or dampening the secretion or effects of cytokines and cellular growth factors. Immunomodulatory therapy may be helpful in special circumstances or in children with declining left ventricular function. A randomized, multicenter trial is warranted to evaluate the efficacy of this therapy.

Patients should be evaluated for nutritional status, and any with deficiencies should receive supplements. Supplementation with selenium, carnitine, multivitamins, or all three may be helpful, especially in anorexic patients or in those with wasting or diarrheal syndromes.

Animal Models

Chronic pathogenic simian immunodeficiency virus (SIV) infection in rhesus macaques resulted in significant depression of left ventricular ejection fraction and extensive coronary arteriopathy suggestive of a cell-mediated immune response.[24] Notably, two thirds of chronically infected macaques that died of SIV had myocardial pathology with lymphocytic myocarditis in 9 of 15 and coronary arteriopathy in 9 of 15 (6 alone and 3 in combination with myocarditis). Coronary arteriopathy was associated with evidence of vessel occlusion and recanalization, with associated areas of myocardial necrosis in 4 macaques. Two animals had marantic endocarditis, and 1 had a left ventricular mural thrombus on pathological examination. Macaques with cardiac pathology were emaciated to a greater extent than macaques with SIV and similar periods of infection who did not experience cardiac disease.[24]

Left Ventricular Diastolic Dysfunction

Clinical and echocardiographic findings suggest that diastolic dysfunction is relatively common in long-term survivors of HIV infection. Left ventricular diastolic dysfunction may precede systolic dysfunction.[25] One large multicenter echocardiographic study found that asymptomatic HIV-infected patients had 34.6 percent lower E/A ratio (Doppler-derived parameter of diastolic dysfunction: peak early [E] over peak atrial [A] velocity) and 19.7 percent longer isovolumetric relaxation time than healthy adults.[5]

Pericardial Effusion (see Chap. 50)

CLINICAL PRESENTATION. HIV-infected patients with pericardial effusions generally have a lower CD4 count, marking more advanced disease, than those without effusions.[26] Effusions are generally asymptomatic.

INCIDENCE. Asymptomatic pericardial effusions are common in HIV-infected patients.[16, 26, 27] The 5-year Prospective Evaluation of Cardiac Involvement in AIDS (PRECIA) study found that 16 of 231 patients (59 subjects with asymptomatic HIV, 62 with AIDS-related complex, and 74 with AIDS) developed pericardial effusions.[26] Three subjects had an effusion on enrollment, and 13 developed effusions during follow-up (12 of them had AIDS). Pericardial effusions were small (maximum pericardial space less than 10 mm at end diastole) in 80 percent and asymptomatic in 87 percent of patients with effusion. The incidence of pericardial effusion among those with AIDS was 11 percent per year.[26] The prevalence of effusion in AIDS patients rises over time, reaching a mean in asymptomatic patients of about 22 percent after 25 months of follow-up.[26]

HIV infection should be suspected whenever young patients have pericardial effusion or tamponade. In a retrospective series of cardiac tamponade cases in a city hospital, 13 of 37 patients (35 percent) had HIV infection.[28]

PATHOGENESIS. Pericardial effusion may be related to an opportunistic infection or to malignancy (see Table 68–

1), but most often a clear etiology is not found. The effusion is often part of a generalized serous effusive process also involving pleural and peritoneal surfaces. This "capillary leak" syndrome may be related to enhanced cytokine production in the later stages of HIV disease. Other causes may include uremia from HIV-associated nephropathy or drug nephrotoxicity. Fibrinous pericarditis with or without effusion is also well described, comprising 9 percent of cardiac lesions found in AIDS patients in one autopsy series.[26]

COURSE OF DISEASE AND PROGNOSIS. Effusion markedly increases mortality.[16, 26, 26a] For example, in the PRECIA study, it nearly tripled the risk of death among AIDS patients (Fig. 68–4).[26] Also 2 of 16 patients with effusions developed pericardial tamponade. Pericardial effusion may, however, resolve spontaneously in up to 42 percent of patients.[16, 26] Mortality was still markedly increased in patients who had developed an effusion.[16, 26]

MONITORING AND THERAPY. Screening echocardiography is recommended in HIV-infected individuals, regardless of the stage of disease. All HIV-infected patients with evidence of heart failure, Kaposi's sarcoma, tuberculosis, or other pulmonary infections should have baseline echocardiography, Holter monitoring, and ECG testing.[27] Patients should undergo pericardiocentesis if they have pericardial effusion and clinical signs of tamponade (e.g., elevated jugular venous pressure, dyspnea, hypotension, tachycardia, and pulsus paradoxus) or echocardiographic signs of tamponade (e.g., valvular inflow respiratory variation by continuous wave Doppler, septal bounce, right ventricular diastolic collapse) and a large effusion.

Patients with pericardial effusion without tamponade should be evaluated for treatable opportunistic infections such as tuberculosis and for malignancy. Highly active antiretroviral therapy should be considered if this has not already been instituted. Repeat echocardiography is recommended after 1 month, or sooner if clinical symptoms of tamponade develop in the interim.

Infective Endocarditis (See Chap. 47)

Injection drug users are at greater risk than the general population for infective endocarditis, chiefly of right-sided heart valves. Surprisingly, HIV-infected patients may not

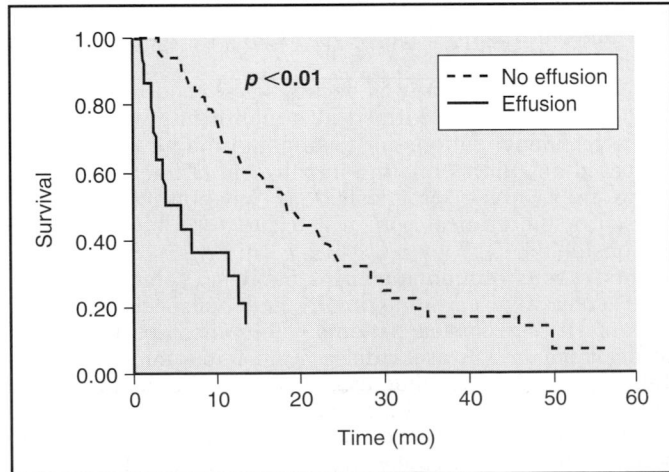

FIGURE 68–4. Survival of patients with and without pericardial effusions at AIDS diagnosis. (From Heidenreich PA, Eisenberg MJ, Kee LL, et al: Pericardial effusion in AIDS: Incidence and survival. Circulation 92:3229, 1995. Copyright 1995, American Heart Association.)

have a higher incidence of endocarditis than people with similar risk behaviors.[29]

Because the autoimmune response to bacterial endocarditis is often largely responsible for valvular destruction associated with endocarditis, variations in the course of the disease in HIV-infected patients may occur. For example, HIV-infected patients have a higher risk of developing *Salmonella* endocarditis than immunocompetent patients because they are more likely to develop *Salmonella* bacteremia during *Salmonella* infection. However, they respond better to antibiotic therapy and may be less likely to sustain valvular damage because of their impaired immune response.[29-31]

Common organisms associated with endocarditis in HIV-infected patients include *Staphylococcus aureus* and *Salmonella* species.[29, 31] Fungal endocarditis with organisms such as *Aspergillus fumigatus*, *Candida* species, and *Cryptococcus neoformans* is more common in intravenous drug users with HIV than in those without it and, again, may be responsive to therapy (see Table 68–1).[29]

Fulminant courses of infective endocarditis with high mortality may occur in patients with late-stage AIDS with poor nutritional status and severely compromised ability to fight infection, but several cases have been successfully treated with antibiotic therapy.[29] Operative indications in HIV-infected patients with endocarditis include hemodynamic instability, failure to sterilize cultures after appropriate intravenous antibiotics, and severe valvular destruction in patients with a reasonable life expectancy after recovery from surgery.

Nonbacterial Thrombotic Endocarditis

Nonbacterial thrombotic endocarditis (or marantic endocarditis) involves large friable sterile vegetations that form on the cardiac valves. These lesions have been associated with disseminated intravascular coagulation and systemic embolization. Lesions are rarely diagnosed ante mortem; among patients who do receive the diagnosis, clinically relevant emboli occur in an estimated 42 percent of cases.[29, 32] In the early HIV epidemic, several case series suggested a high incidence of this uncommon disorder; however, very few cases have since been reported, and almost none have been found in prospective series. Marantic endocarditis should be suspected in any patient with systemic embolization; yet it should be considered rare in AIDS patients.

Treatment of nonbacterial thrombotic endocarditis should focus on reducing the underlying disease state causing coagulation abnormalities and/or valvular endothelial damage. Anticoagulation risk/benefit assessment must be made on an individual basis.

Cardiovascular Malignancy (See Chap. 49)

Malignancy affects many AIDS patients, generally in the later stages of disease. Cardiac malignancy is usually metastatic disease.

Kaposi's sarcoma (angiosarcoma) is associated with human herpesvirus-8 and affects up to 35 percent of AIDS patients, particularly homosexuals, with an incidence inversely related to the CD4 count. Autopsy found that 28 percent of HIV-infected patients with widespread Kaposi's sarcoma had cardiac involvement, and rarely described it as a primary cardiac tumor.[33, 34] An endothelial cell neoplasm with a predilection in the heart for subpericardial fat around the coronary arteries, Kaposi's sarcoma has not been found invading the coronary arteries.[33]

Kaposi's sarcoma involving the heart is generally an incidental finding at autopsy, rarely causing cardiac symptoms. Specific symptoms may be related to pericardial effusion associated with the epicardial location of the tumor. Pericardial fluid in patients with cardiac Kaposi's sarcoma is typically serosanguineous without malignant cells or infection.[33] Kaposi's sarcoma is difficult to treat. Most patients die of opportunistic infections related to the advanced stage of immunodeficiency, rather than from the malignancy.

Primary cardiac malignancy associated with HIV infection is generally due to cardiac lymphoma. Non-Hodgkin lymphomas are 25 to 60 times more common in HIV-infected individuals. They are the first manifestation of AIDS in up to 4 percent of new cases.[35, 36] Primary cardiac lymphoma may present as dyspnea, right-sided heart failure, biventricular failure, chest pain, or arrhythmias.[36] Cardiac lymphoma is associated with rapid progression to cardiac tamponade, symptoms of congestive heart failure, myocardial infarction, tachyarrhythmias, conduction abnormalities, or superior vena cava syndrome.[33] Pericardial fluid typically reveals malignant cells but may be histologically normal. Systemic multiagent chemotherapy with and without concomitant radiation or surgery has been beneficial in some patients, but overall the prognosis is poor.[33, 36]

Leiomyosarcoma, associated with Epstein-Barr virus, is a rare, malignant tumor of smooth muscle origin with an increased incidence in children with AIDS. Leiomyosarcomas are largely noncardiac and often involve the arterial wall.[33] An intracardiac mass in late-stage HIV infection is associated with a uniformly poor prognosis.

Isolated Right Ventricular Disease and Pulmonary Disease (See Chap. 54)

Isolated right ventricular hypertrophy with or without right ventricular dilation is relatively uncommon in HIV-infected individuals and is generally related to pulmonary disease that increases pulmonary vascular resistance. Possible causes include multiple bronchopulmonary infections, pulmonary arteritis from the immunological effects of HIV disease, or microvascular pulmonary emboli caused by thrombus or contaminants in injected drugs.[37]

Primary pulmonary hypertension has been described in a disproportionate number of HIV-infected individuals, primarily in case reports. Primary pulmonary hypertension is estimated to occur in about 0.5 percent of hospitalized AIDS patients.[38] In one series of 6 AIDS patients with pulmonary hypertension associated with right ventricular hypertrophy and failure, clinical findings included dyspnea on exertion, hypoxemia, restrictive lung disease with decreased diffusing lung capacity for carbon monoxide, and right ventricular hypertrophy on ECG.[38]

Plexogenic pulmonary arteriopathy was demonstrated on lung histology from 5 of 12 patients reported as having primary pulmonary hypertension and HIV infection.[39] All of these patients had clear lung fields on examination and chest radiograph and normal perfusion scans.

Pulmonary hypertension is often explained by lung infections, venous thromboembolism, or left ventricular dysfunction. Pulmonary hypertension found on screening echocardiography or right-sided heart catheterization warrants further examination for treatable pulmonary infections.

Primary pulmonary hypertension has been reported in HIV-infected patients without a history of thromboembolic disease, intravenous drug use, or pulmonary infections associated with HIV.[37-40] One autopsy and one biopsy specimen revealed precapillary muscular pulmonary artery and arteriole medial hypertrophy, fibroelastosis, and eccentric intimal fibrosis without direct viral infection of pulmonary artery cells.[40] This suggests mediator release from infected cells elsewhere. Primary pulmonary hypertension has also been found in hemophiliacs receiving lipophilized factor VIII, intravenous drug users, and patients with left ventricular dysfunction, obscuring any relationship with HIV.[37] It may be that HIV causes endothelial damage and mediator-related vasoconstriction of the pulmonary arteries.[16, 38, 40] Therapy includes anticoagulation (based on individual risk/benefit analysis) and vasodilator agents as tolerated.

Vasculitis

Vasculitis is being reported more often in HIV-infected patients.[40a] It should be suspected in patients with fever of unknown origin, unexplained multisystem disease, unexplained arthritis or myositis, glomerulonephritis, peripheral neuropathy (especially mononeuritis multiplex), or unexplained gastrointestinal, cardiac, or central nervous system ischemia. Many types of vasculitis have been described in HIV-infected patients (see Table 68–1).[41] Successful immunomodulatory therapy, chiefly with systemic corticosteroid therapy, has been described.

Accelerated Atherosclerosis

(See Chaps. 30 through 32)

Accelerated atherosclerosis has been observed in young HIV-infected individuals without traditional coronary risk factors.[42–44] Significant coronary lesions were discovered at autopsy in 8 HIV-positive subjects aged 23 to 32 who died unexpectedly.[42] Cytomegalovirus was present in 2, and hepatitis B virus was found in 2. None of the 8 patients had evidence of cocaine use.

Premature cerebrovascular disease is common in AIDS patients. An 8 percent stroke prevalence in AIDS patients was estimated in an autopsy study in the 1980s.[45] Of the patients with stroke, 4 of 13 had evidence of cerebral emboli and 3 of those 4 had a clear cardiac source of embolus.

Protease inhibitor therapy significantly alters lipid metabolism and may be associated with premature atherosclerotic disease. Angiographically proven advanced symptomatic coronary artery disease has been reported in three men younger than age 40 treated with protease inhibitors.[46] Chronic inflammatory states have also been associated with premature atherosclerotic vascular disease.

Autonomic Dysfunction

Early clinical signs of autonomic dysfunction in HIV-infected patients include syncope and presyncope, diminished sweating, diarrhea, bladder dysfunction, and impotence. In one study, heart rate variability, Valsalva ratio, cold pressor testing, and hemodynamic responses to isometric exercise, tilt table testing, and standing showed that autonomic dysfunction occurred in patients with AIDS-related complex and was pronounced in AIDS patients. Patients with HIV-associated nervous system disease had the greatest abnormalities in autonomic function.[47, 47a]

Complications of Therapy for HIV

Potent antiretroviral medications and highly active antiretroviral therapy, which generally combines three or more agents and usually includes a protease inhibitor, have clearly increased the life span and quality of life of HIV-infected patients.[48–51] However, protease inhibitors, particularly when used in combination therapy or in highly active antiretroviral therapy, are associated with lipodystrophy, fat wasting and redistribution, metabolic abnormalities, hyperlipidemia, insulin resistance, and increased atherosclerotic risk profiles.[52–54] HIV-infected patients treated with protease inhibitors have reported substantial decreases in total body fat with peripheral lipodystrophy (fat wasting of the face, limbs, and buttocks) and relative conservation or enhancement of central adiposity (truncal obesity, breast enlargement, and "buffalo hump") compared with patients who have not received protease inhibitors.[54] Lipid alterations associated with protease inhibitors include higher triglyceride, total cholesterol, insulin, lipoprotein(a) and C-peptide levels, and lower high-density lipoprotein levels (all promoting an atherogenic profile).[52–54b] Flow-dependent vasodilation measured in the brachial artery by venous occlusion plethysmography was impaired in HIV-infected patients taking protease inhibitors.[54a]

Lipid abnormalities vary with different protease inhibitors.[53] Ritonavir had the largest adverse effects on lipids, with a mean increase in total cholesterol of 2.0 mmol/liter and a mean increase in triglyceride level of 1.83 mmol/liter. More modest increases of total cholesterol without significant triglyceride increases were found in patients taking indinavir and nelfinavir. Combination with saquinavir did not further elevate the total cholesterol. Protease inhibitor therapy increased lipoprotein(a) by 48 percent in patients with pretreatment elevated values (>20 mg/dL).[53] In some cases, switching protease inhibitors can reverse both elevations in triglyceride levels and abnormal fat deposition. At this time, increased coronary artery disease secondary to protease inhibitor related dyslipidemia has not been shown.[54c, 54d]

Zidovudine (azidothymidine) has been implicated in skeletal muscle myopathies.[55, 56] In culture, zidovudine causes a dose-dependent destruction of human myotubes.[56] Human-cultured cardiac muscle cells treated with zidovudine develop mitochondrial abnormalities.[56] However, cardiac myopathies have not been evident in clinical data. In a combined retrospective and prospective analysis, both HIV-infected and HIV-negative children born to HIV-infected women and exposed to zidovudine in utero were not more likely to have abnormal left ventricular structure and function than children who were not exposed to zidovudine.[56b] Rare patients with left ventricular dysfunction, however, have improved with cessation of zidovudine therapy and normal troponin T levels have been measured in some of these patients.[56a]

A transgenic versus wild-type mouse model demonstrated cardiomyopathy by HIV infection alone that is enhanced by zidovudine therapy. Zidovudine-treated mice had mitochondrial ultrastructural damage in cardiac myocytes.[57]

Intravenous pentamidine, used to treat *Pneumocystis carinii* pneumonia in patients intolerant of trimethoprim/sulfamethoxazole, has been associated with cases of torsades de pointes and refractory ventricular tachycardia.[21, 58, 59] Recommendations for the use of intravenous pentamidine are outlined in Figure 68–5.

Multiple medication reactions and interactions have occurred during the treatment of HIV infection and are a significant cause of cardiac emergencies in HIV-infected patients. Common cardiac drug interactions are outlined in Table 68–2.

Perinatal Transmission and Vertically Transmitted HIV Infection

Most pediatric patients with HIV are infected in the perinatal period, but HIV transmission can be minimized if moth-

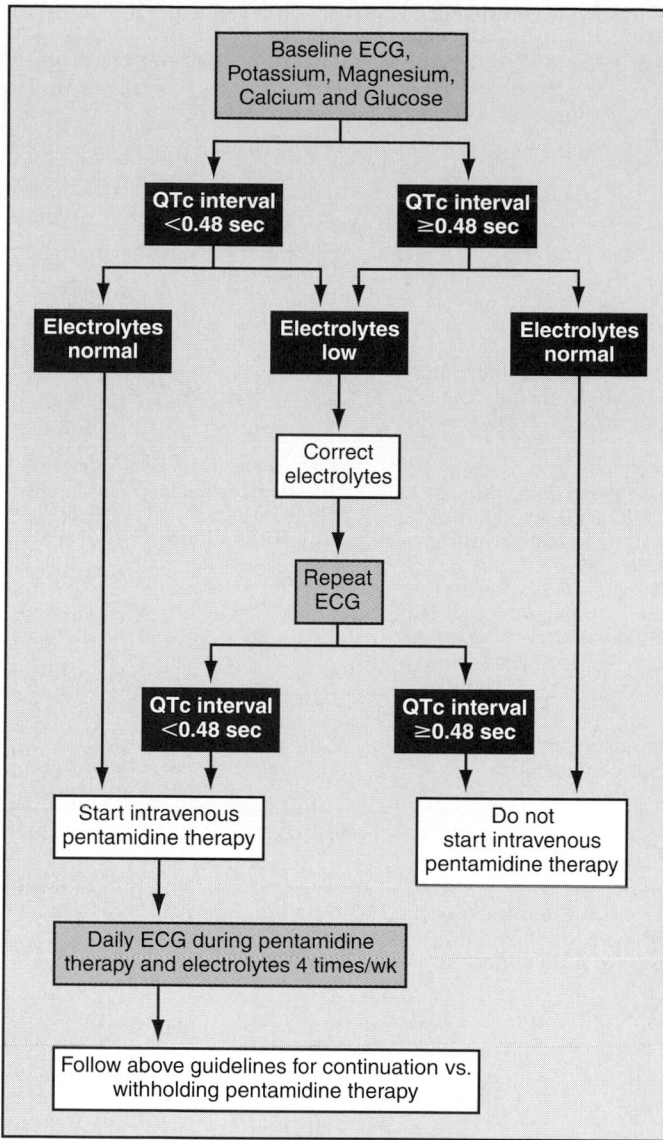

FIGURE 68–5. Recommendations for HIV-infected patients starting intravenous pentamidine treatment. (From Moorthy LN, Lipshultz SE: Cardiovascular monitoring of HIV-infected patients. *In* Lipshultz SE [ed]: Cardiology in AIDS. New York, Chapman & Hall, 1998, p 345. Data based on Eisenhauer MD, Eliasson AH, Taylor AJ, et al: Incidence of cardiac arrhythmias during intravenous pentamidine therapy in HIV-infected patients. Chest 105:389, 1994.)

ers are given courses of zidovudine in the second and third trimesters or short courses before parturition.[60–67]

Rates of congenital cardiovascular malformations in cohorts of HIV-uninfected and HIV-infected children born to HIV-infected mothers ranged from 5.6 to 8.9 percent. These rates were 5 to 10 times higher than reported in population-based epidemiological studies but not higher than in normal populations similarly screened.[68]

In the same cohorts, serial echocardiograms performed at 4- to 6-month intervals found subclinical cardiac abnormalities to be common, persistent, and often progressive.[6, 68a] Some had dilated cardiomyopathy (left ventricular contractility 2 standard deviations or more below the normal mean and left ventricular end-diastolic dimension 2 standard deviations above the mean or more) and inappropriate left ventricular hypertrophy (elevated left ventricular mass in the setting of decreased height and weight). Depressed left ventricular function correlated with immune dysfunction at baseline but not longitudinally, suggesting that the CD4 cell count may not be a useful surrogate marker of HIV-associated left ventricular dysfunction. The development of encephalopathy was highly correlated with a decline in fractional shortening.

In children with vertically transmitted HIV-1 infection, disease may progress rapidly or slowly.[69] Rapid progressors have higher heart rates, higher respiratory rates, and lower fractional shortening on serial examinations than nonrapid progressors and HIV-uninfected children similarly screened. Rapid progressors have higher 5-year cumulative mortality, higher HIV-1 viral loads, and lower CD8+ (cytotoxic) T cell counts than nonrapid progressors.[69] Knowing the patterns of disease allows more aggressive therapy to be initiated earlier in rapid progressors.

Monitoring Recommendations

Routine, systematic cardiac evaluation including a comprehensive history and thorough cardiac examination is essential for the care of HIV-infected adults and children. Asymptomatic cardiac disease may be fatal, and cardiac symptoms are often confounded by secondary effects of HIV-infection; thus, systematic echocardiographic monitoring is warranted.

HIV-infected individuals without cardiac symptoms should undergo annual echocardiography and should have Holter monitoring and ECG every 2 years.[21] Patients with serious noncardiac illness should undergo echocardiography, ECG, and Holter monitoring followed by echocardiography every 8 months and ECG and Holter monitoring every year.[21] Patients with cardiac symptoms should have a formal cardiac assessment including baseline echocardiography, ECG, and Holter monitoring and should begin directed therapy.[21] Recommendations for Holter monitoring are based on studies illustrating the frequency of high-grade arrhythmias and abnormal conduction patterns. Holter monitoring recommendations have not been tested and are a suggestion based on available data.

In patients with left ventricular dysfunction, serum troponin assays are indicated. Serum troponin elevations warrant consideration of cardiac catheterization and endomyocardial biopsy. Myocarditis proven by biopsy warrants considering therapy with intravenous immunoglobulin. Cytomegalovirus inclusions on the biopsy specimen warrant antiviral therapy, and abnormal mitochondria should encourage consideration of a "drug holiday" from zidovudine. Ultrasound examination should be repeated after 2 weeks of therapy to allow a more aggressive approach if left ventricular dysfunction persists or worsens and to encourage continued therapy if improvement has occurred.[21]

Conclusions

The longer HIV-infected patients live and the more advanced their disease, the higher the risk of cardiac complications.[1, 4, 60] An epidemic number of HIV-infected individuals will present with cardiac complications in the next decade as long-term viral infection, co-infections, drug therapy, and immunosuppression take a toll on the heart. The impact that highly active antiretroviral therapy will have on the incidence and prevalence of cardiac complications in HIV-infected patients is unknown. Early screening and therapy of HIV infected patients, regardless of the stage of disease, will identify the potentially fatal complications of HIV disease and therapy and allow them to be treated.

CLASS	DRUGS	CARDIAC DRUG INTERACTIONS	CARDIAC SIDE EFFECTS
Antiretroviral Nucleoside reverse transcriptase inhibitors	Abacavir (Ziagen) Didanosine (ddI, Videx) Lamivudine (3TC, Epivir) Stavudine (d4T, Zerit) Zalcitabine (ddC, Hivid) Zidovudine (AZT, Retrovir)	Dipyridamole	Rare—lactic acidosis Hypotension with abacavir Skeletal muscle myopathy with Zidovudine
Nonnucleoside reverse transcriptase inhibitors	Delavirdine (Rescriptor) Efavirenz (Sustiva) Nevirapine (Viramune)	Calcium channel blockers, warfarin Warfarin Beta blockers, nifedipine, quinidine, steroids, theophylline. May decrease effects of warfarin.	
Protease inhibitors	Amprenavir (Agenerase) Indinavir (Crixivan) Nelfinavir (Viracept) Ritonavir (Norvir) Saquinavir (Invirase, Fortovase)	All are metabolized by cytochrome P-450 and interact with sildenafil, amiodarone, lidocaine, quinadine, warfarin, and "statins." Calcium channel blockers, prednisone, quinine; increases beta blocker levels 1.5–3 ×; warfarin may increase levels three times	Implicated in premature atherosclerosis, dyslipidemia, insulin resistance, fat wasting and redistribution
Antiinfective Antibiotics	Erythromycin	Cytochrome P-450 metabolism and drug interactions	Orthostatic hypotension, ventricular tachycardia, bradycardia, torsades (with drug interactions)
	Trimethoprim-sulfamethoxazole (Bactrim)	Increases warfarin effects	Orthostatic hypotension, anaphylaxis
Antifungal agents	Amphotericin B Ketoconazole Itraconazole (Sporanox)	Digoxin toxicity Cytochrome P-450 metabolism and drug interactions; increases levels of sildenafil, warfarin, "statins," nifedipine, and digoxin	Hypertension, arrhythmia, renal failure, hypokalemia, thrombophlebitis, angioedema
Antiviral agents	Foscarnet Ganciclovir	 Zidovudine	Reversible cardiac failure, electrolyte abnormalities Ventricular tachycardia, hypotension
Antiparasitic	Pentamidine (IV)		Hypotension, arrhythmias (torsades), ventricular tachycardia, hyperglycemia, hypoglycemia, sudden death
Chemotherapy agents	Vincristine Interferon alfa Interleukin-2 Doxorubicin (Adriamycin)	Decreases digoxin level Decreases digoxin level	Arrhythmia, myocardial infarction, cardiomyopathy Orthostatic hypotension (only $1/26$ non-HIV, common in HIV patients), myocardial infarction, cardiomyopathy, ventricular and supraventricular arrhythmias, atrioventricular block Hypotension, arrhythmia, sudden death, myocardial infarction, cardiac failure, capillary leak, thyroid alterations Myocarditis, cardiomyopathy, cardiac failure
Other Systemic corticosteroids		Decreases salicylate levels and increases gastric ulceration in combination with salicylates.	Ventricular hypertrophy, cardiomyopathy, hyperglycemia
Pentoxifylline			Decreased triglyceride levels, arrhythmias, chest pain
Growth hormone			Ventricular hypertrophy, activation of the renal angiotension system (hypertension)
Medroxyprogesterone (Megace)			Edema, thrombophlebitis, hyperglycemia

REFERENCES

1. Barbaro G, Di Lorenzo G, Grisorio B, et al: Incidence of dilated cardiomyopathy and detection of HIV in myocardial cells of HIV-positive patients. N Engl J Med 339:1093, 1998.
2. UNAIDS: Report on the Global HIV/AIDS Epidemic. Geneva, Switzerland, UNAIDS, June 1998. http://www.unaids.org/highband/document/epidemio/wadr98e.pdf; 1998.
3. Centers for Disease Control and Prevention: HIV/AIDS Surveillance Report. MMWR Morbid Mortal Wkly Rep 11:1–43, 1999.
4. Barbaro G, Di Lorenzo G, Grisorio B, et al: Cardiac involvement in the acquired immunodeficiency syndrome: A multicenter clinical-pathological study. AIDS Res 14:1071, 1998.

LEFT VENTRICULAR SYSTOLIC DYSFUNCTION

5. Barbaro G, Barbarini G, Di Lorenzo G: Early impairment of systolic and diastolic function in asymptomatic HIV-positive patients: a multicenter echocardiographic and echo-Doppler study. AIDS Res 12:1559, 1996.
6. Lipshultz SE, Easley KA, Orav EJ, et al: Left ventricular structure and function in children infected with human immunodeficiency virus. The Prospective P²C² HIV Multicenter Study. Circulation 97:1246, 1998.
7. Currie PF, Jacob AJ, Foreman AR, et al: Heart muscle disease related to HIV infection: Prognostic implications. Br Med J 309:1605, 1994.
8. Starc TJ, Lipshultz SE, Kaplan S, et al: Cardiac complications in children with human immunodeficiency virus infection. Pediatrics 104(2): e14, 1999.
9. Mann JM: AIDS—the second decade: A global perspective. J Infect Dis 165:245, 1992.
9a. Shannon RP, Simon MA, Mathier MA, et al: Dilated cardiomyopathy associated with simian AIDS in nonhuman primates. Circulation 101: 185–193, 2000.
10. Acierno LJ: Cardiac complications in acquired immunodeficiency syndrome (AIDS): A review. J Am Coll Cardiol 13:1144, 1989.
10a. Bowles NE, Kearney DL, Ni J, et al: The detection of viral genomes by polymerase chain reaction in the myocardium of pediatric patients with advanced HIV disease. J Am Coll Cardiol 34:857, 1999.
11. Herskowitz A: Cardiomyopathy and other symptomatic heart diseases associated with HIV infection. Curr Opin Cardiol 11:325, 1996.
12. Herskowitz A, Willoughby SB, Vlahov D, et al: Dilated heart muscle disease associated with HIV infection. Eur Heart J 16(Suppl O):50, 1995.
13. Finkel TH, Banda NK: Indirect mechanisms of HIV pathogenesis: How does HIV kill T cells? Curr Opin Immunol 6:605, 1994.
14. Barbaro G, Di Lorenzo G, Soldini M, et al: Intensity of myocardial expression of inducible nitric oxide synthase influences the clinical course of human immunodeficiency virus–associated cardiomyopathy. Circulation 100:933, 1999.
15. Luginbuhl LM, Orav EJ, McIntosh K, et al: Cardiac morbidity and related mortality in children with HIV infection. JAMA 269:2869, 1993.
16. Blanchard DG, Hagenhoff C, Chow LC, et al: Reversibility of cardiac abnormalities in human immunodeficiency virus (HIV)-infected individuals: a serial echocardiographic study. J Am Coll Cardiol 17:1270, 1991.
16a. Felker MG, Thompson RE, Hare JM, et al: Underlying causes and long-term survival in patients with initially unexplained cardiomyopathy. N Engl J Med 342:1077, 2000.
17. Lipshultz SE, Easley KA, Orav EJ, et al: Cardiac dysfunction and mortality in HIV-infected children: The prospective P²C² HIV multicenter study. Circulation, in press.
18. Lipshultz SE, Orav EJ, Sanders SP, et al: Immunoglobulins and left ventricular structure and function in pediatric HIV infection. Circulation 92:2220, 1995.
19. Drucker NA, Colan SD, Lewis AB, et al: Gamma-globulin treatment of acute myocarditis in the pediatric population. Circulation 89:252, 1994.
20. McNamara DM, Rosenblum WD, Janosko KM, et al: Intravenous immune globulin in the therapy of myocarditis and acute cardiomyopathy. Circulation 95:2476, 1997.
21. Moorthy LN, Lipshultz SE: Cardiovascular monitoring of HIV-infected patients. In Lipshultz SE (ed): Cardiology in AIDS. New York, Chapman & Hall, 1998, p 345.
22. Newburger JW, Sanders SP, Burns JC, et al: Left ventricular contractility and function in Kawasaki syndrome. Effect of intravenous gamma-globulin. Circulation 79:1237, 1989.
23. Newburger JW, Takahashi M, Beiser AS, et al: A single intravenous infusion of gamma globulin as compared with four infusions in the treatment of acute Kawasaki syndrome. N Engl J Med 324:1633, 1991.
24. Shannon RP, Simon MA, Mathier MA, et al: Dilated cardiomyopathy associated with Simian AIDS in nonhuman primates. Circulation 101: 185, 2000.
25. Coudray N, de Zuttere D, Force G, et al: Left ventricular diastolic function in asymptomatic and symptomatic human immunodeficiency virus carriers: an echocardiographic study. Eur Heart J 16:61, 1995.

PERICARDIAL EFFUSION

26. Heidenreich PA, Eisenberg MJ, Kee LL, et al: Pericardial effusion in AIDS: Incidence and survival. Circulation 92:3229, 1995.
26a. Rerkpattanapipat P, Wongpraparut N, Jacobs LE, et al: Cardiac manifestations of acquired immunodeficiency syndrome. Arch Intern Med 160: 602, 2000.

27. Silva-Cardoso J, Moura B, Martins L, et al: Pericardial involvement in human immunodeficiency virus infection. Chest 115:418, 1999.
28. Kwan T, Karve MM, Emerole O: Cardiac tamponade in patients infected with HIV. A report from an inner-city hospital. Chest 104:1059, 1993.

INFECTIVE ENDOCARDITIS

29. Currie PF, Sutherland GR, Jacob AJ, et al: A review of endocarditis in acquired immunodeficiency syndrome and human immunodeficiency virus infection. Eur Heart J 16:15, 1995.
30. Bestetti RB, Figueiredo JF, Da Costa JC, et al: Salmonella tricuspid endocarditis in an intravenous drug abuser with human immunodeficiency virus infection. Int J Cardiol 30:361, 1991.
31. Nahass RG, Weinstein MP, Bartels J, et al: Infective endocarditis in intravenous drug users: A comparison of human immunodeficiency virus type 1-negative and -positive patients. J Infect Dis 162:967, 1990.
32. Lopez JA, Ross RS, Fishbein MC, et al: Non-bacterial thrombotic endocarditis: A review. Am Heart J 113:773, 1987.

CARDIOVASCULAR MALIGNANCY

33. Jenson HB, Pollock BH: Cardiac cancers in HIV-infected patients. In Lipshultz SE (ed): Cardiology in AIDS. New York, Chapman & Hall, 1998, p 255.
34. Silver MA, Macher AM, Reichert CM, et al: Cardiac involvement by Kaposi's sarcoma in acquired immune deficiency syndrome (AIDS). Am J Cardiol 53:983, 1984.
35. Beral V, Peterman T, Berkelman R, et al: AIDS-associated non-Hodgkin lymphoma. Lancet 337:805, 1991.
36. Duong M, Dubois C, Buisson M, et al: Non-Hodgkin's lymphoma of the heart in patients infected with human immunodeficiency virus. Clin Cardiol 20:497, 1997.

ISOLATED RIGHT VENTRICULAR DISEASE AND PULMONARY DISEASE

37. Saidi A, Bricker JT: Pulmonary hypertension in patients infected with HIV. In Lipshultz SE (ed): Cardiology in AIDS. New York, Chapman & Hall, 1998, p 187.
38. Himelman RB, Dohrmann M, Goodman P, et al: Severe pulmonary hypertension and cor pulmonale in the acquired immunodeficiency syndrome. Am J Cardiol 64:1396, 1989.
39. Aarons EJ, Nye FJ: Primary pulmonary hypertension and HIV infection. AIDS 5:1276, 1991.
40. Coplan NL, Shimony RY, Ioachim HL, et al: Primary pulmonary hypertension associated with human immunodeficiency viral infection. Am J Med 89:96, 1990.
40a. Chetty R, Batitang S, Nair R: Large artery vasculopathy in HIV-positive patients: another vasculitic enigma. Hum Pathol 31:374–379, 2000.

VASCULITIS AND ACCELERATED ATHEROSCLEROSIS

41. Calabrese LH: Vasculitis and infection with the human immunodeficiency virus. Rheum Dis Clin North Am 17:131, 1991.
42. Tabib A, Greenland T, Mercier I, et al: Coronary lesions in young HIV-positive subjects at necropsy. Lancet 340:730, 1992.
43. Capron L, Kim YU, Laurian C, et al: Atheroembolism in HIV-positive individuals. Lancet 340:1039, 1992.
44. Constans J, Marchand JM, Conri C, et al: Asymptomatic atherosclerosis in HIV-positive patients: A case-control ultrasound study. Ann Intern Med 27:683, 1995.
45. Berger JR, Harris JO, Gregorios J, et al: Cerebrovascular disease in AIDS: A case-control study. AIDS 4:239, 1990.
46. Henry K, Melroe H, Huebsch J, et al: Severe premature coronary artery disease with protease inhibitors. Lancet 351:1328, 1998.

AUTONOMIC DYSFUNCTION

47. Saidi A, Moodie D, Garson A, et al: Electrocardiography and 24-hour electrocardiographic ambulatory recording (Holter monitor) studies in children of mothers infected with human immunodeficiency virus type 1. Pediatr Cardiol 21:189, 2000.
47a. Gluck T, Degenhardt E, Scholmerich J, et al: Autonomic neuropathy in patients with HIV: course, impact of disease stage, and medication. Clin Auton Res 10:17–22, 2000.

COMPLICATIONS OF THERAPY FOR HIV

48. Mocroft A, Vella S, Benfield TL, et al: Changing patterns of mortality across Europe in patients infected with HIV-1. EuroSIDA Study Group. Lancet 352:1725, 1998.
49. Palella FJ Jr, Delaney KM, Moorman AC, et al: Declining morbidity and mortality among patients with advanced human immunodeficiency virus infection—HIV outpatient study investigators. N Engl J Med 338:853, 1998.

50. Vittinghoff E, Scheer S, O'Malley P, et al: Combination antiretroviral therapy and recent declines in AIDS incidence and mortality. J Infect Dis 179:717, 1999.

51. Detels R, Munoz A, McFarlane G, et al: Effectiveness of potent antiretroviral therapy on time to AIDS and death in men with known HIV infection duration. JAMA 280:1497, 1998.

52. SoRelle R: Vascular and lipid syndromes in selected HIV-infected patients. Circulation 9:829, 1998.

53. Periard D, Telenti A, Sudre P, et al: Atherogenic dyslipidemia in HIV-infected individuals treated with protease inhibitors. Circulation 100:700, 1999.

54. Carr A, Samaras K, Burton S, et al: A syndrome of peripheral lipodystrophy, hyperlipidaemia and insulin resistance in patients receiving HIV protease inhibitors. AIDS 12:F51, 1998.

54a. Falutz J, Turcot D: Cardiovascular profile in the HIV/HAART lipodystrophy (HAL) syndrome. J Am Coll Cardiol 35(Suppl A):299, 2000.

54b. Sosman JM, Klein MA, Bellehurneur JL, et al: Endothelial dysfunction is associated with the use of human immunodeficiency virus-1 protease inhibitors. Program and abstracts of the 7th Conference on Retroviruses and Opportunistic Infections. San Francisco, California, Abstract 29, 2000.

54c. Cheminot N, Gariepy J, Chironi G, et al: Diagnosis and determinants of subclinical arterial disease in HIV-1-infected patients on HAART. Program and abstracts of the 7th Conference on Retroviruses and Opportunistic Infections. San Francisco, California, Abstract 31, 2000.

54d. Lenormand-Walckenaer C, Joly V, Matheron S, et al: Detection of myocardial ischemia in protease inhibitor (PI)-treated HIV-infected patients with hyperlipemia. Program and Abstracts of the 7th Conference on Retroviruses and Opportunistic Infections. San Francisco, California, Abstract 35, 2000.

55. Cupler EJ, Danon MJ, Jay C, et al: Early features of zidovudine-associated myopathy: Histopathological findings and clinical correlations. Acta Neuropathol 90:1, 1995.

56. Lamperth L, Dalakas MC, Dagani F, et al: Abnormal skeletal and cardiac muscle mitochondria induced by zidovudine (AZT) in human muscle in vitro and in an animal model. Lab Invest 65:742, 1991.

56a. Dagan T, Sable C, Taylor P, et al: Reversible cardiac dysfunction associated with zidovudine exposure in HIV-infected children. J Am Coll Cardiol 35(Suppl A):513, 2000.

56b. Lipshultz SE, Easley KA, Orav EJ, et al: Is antiretroviral therapy with zidovudine cardiotoxic? The prospective P²C² HIV multicenter study. New Engl J Med. In press, 2000.

57. Lewis W, Grupp IL, Grupp G, et al: Cardiac dysfunction occurs in the HIV-1 transgenic mouse treated with zidovudine. Lab Invest 80:1, 2000.

58. Wharton JM, Demopulos PA, Goldschlager N: Torsades de pointes during administration of pentamidine isethionate. Am J Med 83:571, 1987.

59. Eisenhauer MD, Eliasson AH, Taylor AJ, et al: Incidence of cardiac arrhythmias during intravenous pentamidine therapy in HIV-infected patients. Chest 105:389, 1994.

60. Connor EM, Sperling RS, Gelber R, et al: Reduction of maternal-infant transmission of human immunodeficiency virus type 1 with zidovudine treatment. N Engl J Med 331:1173, 1994.

PERINATAL TRANSMISSION AND VERTICALLY TRANSMITTED HIV INFECTION

61. Lindegren ML, Byers RH, Fleming P, et al: Status of the perinatal HIV epidemic in the United States: Success in perinatal prevention. In Program and abstracts of the XIIth World AIDS Conference, Geneva, Switzerland (abstract 23306), 1998.

62. Stiehm ER, Lambert JS, Mofenson LM, et al: Efficacy of zidovudine and human immunodeficiency virus (HIV) hyperimmune immunoglobulin for reducing perinatal HIV transmission from HIV-infected women with advanced disease: Results of Pediatric AIDS Clinical Trials Group protocol 185. J Infect Dis 179:567, 1999.

63. Mofenson LM: Short-course zidovudine for prevention of perinatal infection. Lancet 353:766, 1999.

64. Shaffer N, Chuachoowong R, Mock PA, et al: Short-course zidovudine for perinatal HIV-1 transmission in Bangkok, Thailand: A randomised controlled trial. Lancet 353:773, 1999.

65. Wiktor SZ, Ekpini E, Karon JM, et al: Short-course oral zidovudine for prevention of mother-to-child transmission of HIV-1 in Abidjan, Cote d'Ivoire: A randomised trial. Lancet 353:781, 1999.

66. Wade NA, Birkhead GS, Warren BL, et al: Abbreviated regimens of zidovudine prophylaxis and perinatal transmission of the human immunodeficiency virus. N Engl J Med 339:1409, 1998.

67. Guay LA, Musoke P, Fleming T, et al: Intrapartum and neonatal single-dose nevirapine compared with zidovudine for prevention of mother-to-child transmission of HIV-1 in Kampala, Uganda: HIVNET 012 randomised trial. Lancet 354:795, 1999.

68. Lai WW, Lipshultz SE, Easley KA, et al: Prevalence of congenital cardiovascular malformations in children of human immunodeficiency virus-infected women: The prospective P2C2 HIV Multicenter Study. J Am Coll Cardiol 32:1749, 1998.

68a. Hornberger LK, Lipschultz SE, Easley KA, et al: Cardiac structure and function in fetuses of human immunodeficiency virus (HIV)-infected mothers: the prospective NHLBI P²C² study. Am Heart J. In Press, 2000.

69. Shearer WT, Lipshultz SE, Easley KA, et al: Alterations in cardiac and pulmonary function in pediatric rapid human immunodeficiency virus type 1 disease progressors. Pediatrics 105:e9, 2000.

Chapter 69

Hematological-Oncological Disorders and Cardiovascular Disease

RICHARD M. STONE • KENNETH R. BRIDGES
PETER LIBBY

A dialogue between cardiologists and hematologist-oncologists is often required in the care of patients with a variety of disorders encompassing both fields. Intrinsic cardiac disease in patients with neoplastic or benign hematological disorders affects the natural history of the underlying condition as well as the therapeutic possibilities. How primary hematological disorders can affect the cardiovascular system is illustrated by hypercoagulability due to cancer, bleeding, and/or anemia from bone marrow failure and also by hyperviscosity in polycythemia. Tumors that invade or involve the heart are not uncommon. These two disciplines also frequently intersect because of the generally negative effect of antineoplastic drugs on cardiac function. Such agents may have direct effects on the myocardium or act indirectly owing to chemotherapy-induced myelosuppression with associated sepsis.

IRON AND THE HEART

Iron metabolism and its derangements,[1] especially those associated with deficiency or excess, may have profound effects on the cardiovascular system. Iron-deficiency anemia has been the primary hematological problem faced by humans throughout history. In many parts of the world it continues to be a major scourge. Iron overload (Table 69–1) has become a problem only with advances in medical care that have prolonged life and with advances in medical technology that have made feasible repeated blood transfusions. Hereditary hemochromatosis, the best characterized genetic cause of iron overload, generally manifests after about the third decade of life. As late as 1890, the median life expectancy in Europe was only 40 years, meaning that most people with hereditary hemochromatosis died of other causes before developing complications of the disorder. The longer life spans that we currently enjoy have brought this condition to the forefront.

Transfusions are of equally recent advent. Medical researchers discovered blood antigens only at the beginning of the 20th century. Routine blood transfusion was not feasible until the 1940s. Before the 1960s when repeated transfusion therapy became widespread in the industrialized world, patients with chronic severe anemias, such as thalassemia major, succumbed largely to cardiac complications of the anemia.

Iron overload has relatively uniform manifestations, irrespective of cause. Cardiac dysfunction is a primary cause of death in people with iron overload. The heart does not accumulate iron disproportionately to the other organs. The key to the heart's central role in the pathology of iron overload lies in the need for the complex array of cells and structures in the heart to function coordinately. Half of the liver for instance can be lost to fibrosis or cirrhosis, and a person can still survive. Obviously, this is not true of the heart.

ETIOLOGY OF IRON OVERLOAD. Hereditary hemochromatosis results from a fractional increase in dietary iron absorption. Tissue iron reaches dangerous levels after 30 or 40 years. The gene responsible for hereditary hemochromatosis, *HFE,* resides on chromosome 6. Discovered in 1996, the gene encodes a protein that is homologous to Class I human leukocyte antigens. The alteration in HFE protein that produces hereditary hemochromatosis in 90 percent of those with the disease involves the mutation of a cysteine to tyrosine at position 282 (C282Y).[2] Individuals who have one copy of the mutant *HFE* gene are carriers who only rarely develop iron overload (usually in association with a second defect). People with two copies of the mutant allele

▼ **TABLE 69–1. CAUSES OF IRON OVERLOAD**

I. Primary Hemochromatosis—genetically transmitted (autosomal recessive)
  A. Men affected more than women
  B. Alcohol increases iron absorption and worsens disease
II. Secondary Hemochromatosis—transfusion related
  A. With intestinal hyperabsorption: thalassemias
  B. Without intestinal hyperabsorption: bone marrow failure states
    1. Aplastic anemia
    2. Pure red cell aplasia
    3. Myelodysplastic syndromes
    4. Agnogenic myeloid metaplasia/myelofibrosis

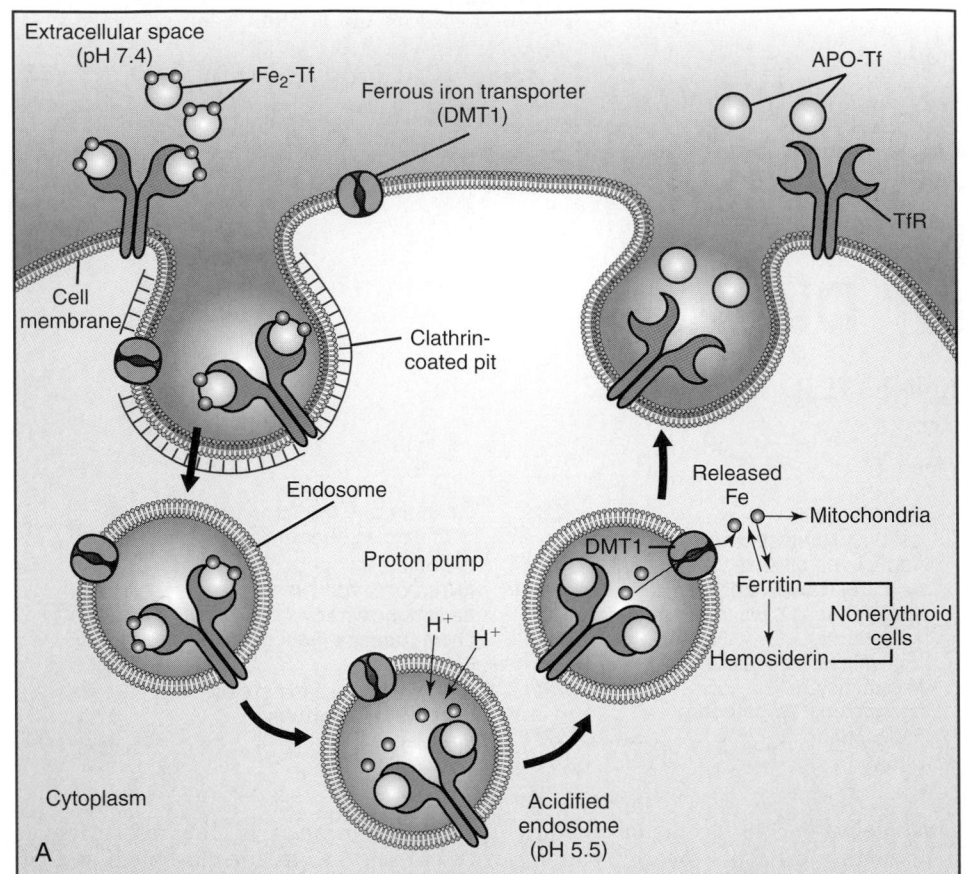

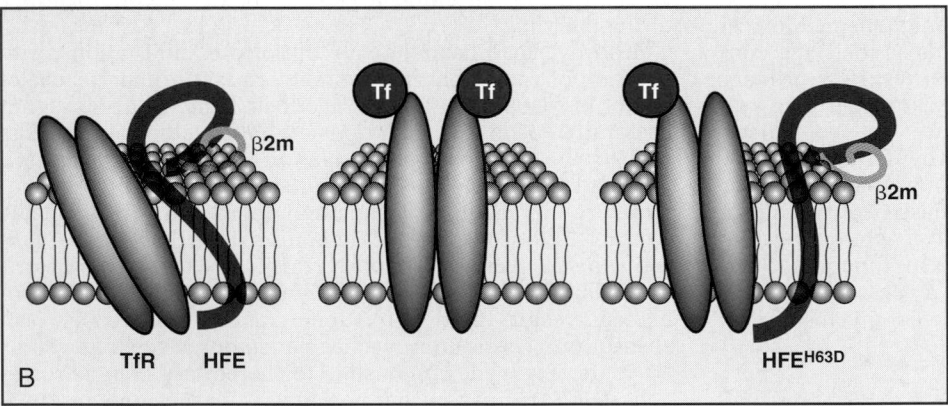

FIGURE 69–1. *A,* The transferrin shuttle pathway. Iron is released from its transferrin-bound state in the circulation intracellularly in endosomes due to proton-pump—mediated acidic pH. The HFE protein, mutated in hemochromatosis, acts as a brake on iron internalization by binding to transferrin receptors. (From Andrews NC: Medical progress: Disorders of iron metabolism. N Engl J Med 341:1985–1986, 1999.) *B,* The transferrin receptor (TFR)–HFE complex. Wild-type HFE protein is associated with beta$_2$-microglobulin and binds to TFR, decreasing transferrin binding *(left).* The C282 mutant HFE protein does not associate with beta$_2$-microglobulin, allowing TFR free to bind transferrin *(center).* The H63D mutant HFE does associate with beta$_2$-microglobin but fails to decrease TFR affinity for transferrin *(right).* (From Andrews NC, Levy JE: Iron is hot: An update on the pathophysiology of hemochromatosis. Blood 92:1845–1851, 1998.)

can develop iron overload, which engenders a vast array of clinical problems.

Only recently have investigators gained insight into the mechanism by which the mutation in *HFE* alters cellular iron metabolism. Iron in the circulation binds to transferrin, the protein that maintains it in a soluble, nontoxic state. The plasma membrane of cells contains transferrin receptors that mediate cellular iron uptake. Transferrin receptors bind iron-transferrin complexes and mediate their internalization through endosomes. Iron is separated from transferrin in the endosome and is shuttled into the interior of the cell (Fig. 69–1A). The iron-free transferrin (apotransferrin) recycles into the circulation and is free to bind and transport additional iron atoms. The HFE protein associates with transferrin receptors in the plasma membrane, thereby reducing transferrin binding to the receptor and slowing the internalization process.[3]

The cysteine 282 to tyrosine mutation C282Y disrupts the folding of the HFE protein. The mutant HFE protein does not associate with the transferrin receptor and does not act as a brake on iron uptake by cells (see Fig. 69–1B).[4] These insights do not fully explain the increase in gastrointestinal iron absorption, which is the root of hereditary hemochromatosis. They do, however, mechanistically connect HFE and iron metabolism. Improved understanding of the complex process of intestinal iron absorption should provide a better pathophysiological explanation for the clinical manifestations of hereditary hemochromatosis.

Hereditary hemochromatosis is remarkably common. Ten to 12 percent of individuals of European background are heterozygous for the condition.[5] The incidence of homozygosity for the condition approaches 1 in 300,[6] making hereditary hemochromatosis one of the most prevalent genetic conditions in the world.[7] Nonetheless, the clinical incidence of the disorder is less than predicted by the genetic frequency calculations. Variable penetrance, perhaps related to secondary genetic or environmental conditions, must influence clinical manifestations. The C282Y mutation appears to be an uncommon cause of iron overload in people of African[8] or Asian origin.[9]

TRANSFUSIONAL IRON OVERLOAD. A unit of blood (250 ml) contains about 225 mg of iron. Iron is an integral component of the heme moiety in hemoglobin and cannot be removed from the blood in that state. Reticuloendothelial cells destroy senescent red cells, primarily in the liver and spleen. The iron from the hemoglobin is not excreted but, rather, is used to make new red cells or placed in storage (primarily in hepatocytes).

Those with severe chronic anemias often require regular transfusions to survive. Patients with thalassemia major, a condition in which the genes encoding hemoglobin produce defective protein and consequently defective red cells, require up to 2 units of blood every 3 weeks to avoid the deadly consequences of their severe anemia.[10] Nearly all of

Fenton reaction:

$$O_2^- + Fe^{+3} \rightarrow O_2 + Fe^{+2}$$
$$Fe^{+2} + H_2O_2 \rightarrow Fe^{+3} + HO\cdot + OH^-$$

Net:
$$O_2^- + H_2O_2 \rightarrow O_2 + HO\cdot + OH^-$$

FIGURE 69–2. Reactive oxygen species derived from intracellular free iron by Fenton chemistry. (Courtesy of N. C. Andrews.)

the iron from the transfused red cells goes into storage and eventually produces severe iron overload. Therefore, the major problem confronting those patients is not anemia but organ damage from iron.[11] Inherited disorders, such as thalassemia major, or acquired conditions, such as myelodysplastic syndrome, can lead to transfusional iron overload. The redistribution of the excess iron to storage sites means that these patients suffer the same consequences as those with hereditary hemochromatosis.

MECHANISMS OF CARDIAC DAMAGE BY IRON OVERLOAD. Iron deposition in the cardiac myocytes is the initial event in iron-mediated cardiac injury. Transferrin receptors on the cell surface mediate this process through the well-characterized transferrin cycle just described. Iron-saturated transferrin attaches to these receptors and releases iron to the interior of the cell. The excess iron is stored in association with the hemosiderin protein.

Iron that is stored in hemosiderin is innocuous.[12] This iron is in equilibrium, however, with a very small pool of so-called free iron in the cell. This pool of iron is so small that its precise size has eluded determination. Better termed loosely bound iron, this material catalyzes the formation of reactive oxygen species through Fenton chemistry (Fig. 69–2). These reactive oxygen species can mediate cell injury.

Among the several reactive oxygen species promoted by iron overload, the most damaging is the hydroxyl radical.[13, 14] This molecule is extremely short-lived and yet highly active in its interaction with biological molecules.[15] Lipid peroxides, protein disulfide bridges, and DNA cross-linking are some of the consequences of iron-mediated generation of reactive oxygen species.[16]

Cardiac cells are particularly sensitive to oxidant-mediated injury because they must perform a number of complex functions, which include contraction and transmission of electrical impulses. With iron loading, cardiac cells in culture begin to fail, including loss of their characteristic pattern of beating. Desferrioxamine, a powerful iron chelator that binds iron in culture and prevents generation of

reactive oxygen species by the Fenton reaction, can restore normal cellular activity.[17]

CLINICAL MANIFESTATIONS OF CARDIAC IRON OVERLOAD (see also Chap. 40). Restrictive cardiomyopathy (Fig. 69–3) is the most common cardiac defect that occurs with iron overload, but other problems have been described, including pericarditis, restrictive cardiomyopathy, and angina without coronary artery disease. A strong correlation exists between the cumulative number of blood transfusions and functional cardiac derangements in patients with thalassemia.[18] Echocardiographic assessment of patients with beta-thalassemia major who receive concurrent chelation therapy with desferrioxamine shows no difference relative to controls in the fractional shortening.[19] A pronounced pattern of integrated backscatter of the interventricular septum and posterior wall is an important echocardiographic finding indicating iron deposition.

The physical examination reveals surprisingly little even in patients with heavy cardiac iron deposition. Once evidence of cardiac failure appears, however, heart function rapidly deteriorates, often resisting medical intervention. Biventricular failure produces pulmonary congestion, peripheral edema, and hepatic engorgement. This potentially lethal cardiac complication has been reversed on occasion by vigorous iron chelation.

Iron deposition in the bundle of His and the Purkinje system impairs signal conduction from the atrial pacemaker to the ventricles. Patients sometimes die suddenly, presumably due to arrhythmias. At one time, patients treated with the chelator desferrioxamine for transfusional iron overload received supplements of ascorbic acid in the range of 15 to 30 mg/kg/d to promote iron mobilization. Reports of sudden death prompted cessation of this practice. At lower doses (2 to 4 mg/kg), ascorbic acid is a safe adjunct to chelation therapy in patients with transfusional iron overload.

Echocardiography in children and radionuclide ventriculography in adults are the most useful noninvasive diagnostic techniques to detect iron-overload–induced cardiomyopathy. The echocardiographic abnormalities correlate roughly with the number of transfusions. Exercise radionuclide ventriculograms are particularly sensitive in the detection of cardiac dysfunction in patients with iron overload.

Treatment of Cardiac Iron Overload

The degree to which aggressive iron chelation therapy can reverse cardiac dysfunction has given rise to vigorous debate. A number of short-term studies suggested that chelation can restore function in patients with significant cardiac compromise.[20] More recently, investigators examined a cohort of patients with beta-thalassemia major who were

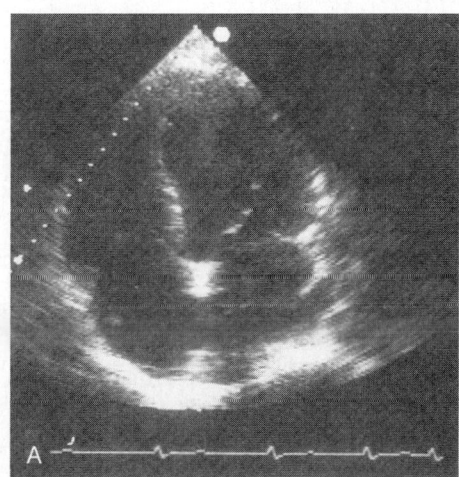
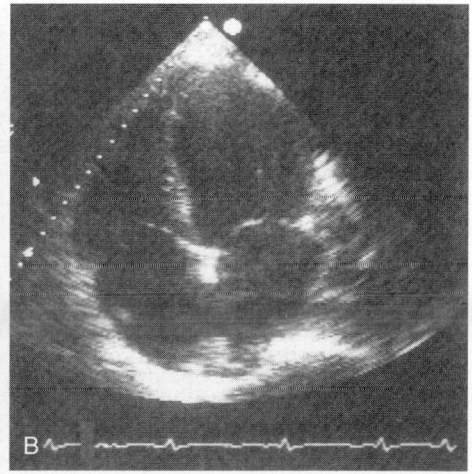

FIGURE 69–3. Consequences of cardiac hemochromatosis. Apical four-chamber views in diastole (A) and in systole (B), demonstrating moderate biventricular enlargement with markedly reduced systolic performance (ejection fraction, 18 percent). In addition, marked biatrial enlargement is noted. (From Passen EL, Rodriguez ER, Neumann A, et al: Cardiac hemochromatosis. Circulation 94:2302–2303, 1996. Copyright 1996, American Heart Association.)

transfused while receiving chelation therapy.[21] In this series only persistent plasma ferritin values of greater than 2500 ng/ml were associated with cardiac-related death. Another group of investigators recently reviewed the outcome of aggressive treatment of patients who had transfusional iron overload with associated cardiac dysfunction.[22] This group of 19 patients suffered from severe congestive heart failure and/or cardiac arrhythmias. The patients received intravenously administered desferrioxamine on a 24-hour per day regimen. For routine iron chelation, most physicians administer the drug over 12- to 16-hour intervals. In addition to the aggressive iron chelation therapy, the investigators administered current conventional cardiac regimens.

The dramatic results revealed an increase in the mean ejection fraction of the patients with congestive heart failure from 30 to 50 percent. Arrhythmias were controlled, and no patient died suddenly. Sudden death occurs commonly in iron-overloaded patients, presumably resulting from malignant arrhythmias. The iron chelation regimens appeared to facilitate management of arrhythmias in this cohort. The plasma ferritin values exceeded 10,000 ng/ml in many of the patients at the onset of treatment. These values declined but never approached normal values (15–400 ng/ml in men).

Bone marrow transplantation now offers a potential cure for some patients with beta-thalassemia major.[23, 24] The correction of the underlying hemolytic anemia creates a clinical situation analogous to hereditary hemochromatosis: patients are iron-overloaded with normal hemoglobin values. Some investigators have taken advantage of this situation to use phlebotomy as a means of removing the iron that has accumulated over years of transfusion therapy, even in patients who continue on an iron-chelation regimen.[25] This strategy removes iron and improves cardiac function in most of these patients.[26]

The lessons from these reports are twofold. First, early iron chelation therapy prevents cardiac dysfunction in patients with transfusional iron overload. Second, congestive cardiomyopathy and arrhythmias in these patients are potentially reversible. Unlike the situation with ischemic cardiomyopathy, the cardiac myocytes have not been destroyed by the pathological events that produced the dysfunction. Iron overload injures myocytes by production of free radicals that interfere with their function. Until irreversible damage leading to cell death occurs, the injury can be halted and reversed by chelators that remove the iron, indirectly blocking production of free radicals. Aggressive intervention with cardiac support and chelation therapy is indicated in patients with iron-mediated cardiac dysfunction.

Iron as a Coronary Risk Factor

An important question concerning iron and the heart is whether body iron stores in the normal range increase susceptibility to myocardial infarction. A number of small anecdotal reports lie on either side of the issue and are uninformative. A study published in 1992 examined the relationship between plasma ferritin levels, a reasonable surrogate measure of body iron stores, and coronary artery disease in a cohort of about 2000 men in Finland.[27] The data indicated that elevated plasma ferritin levels increased the risk of acute myocardial infarction by over twofold. However, a variety of common problems including chronic inflammation and smoking can elevate the serum ferritin level. These investigators attempted to compensate for this factor by using a newer test, the plasma transferrin receptor assay, in a small sample of about 200 men.[28] Results of this smaller study agreed with those that the group reported in 1992.

Investigators from the first National Health and Nutrition Examination Survey Epidemiologic Follow-up Study (NHANES) also addressed the question, using a multivariate Cox proportional-hazards model.[29] Using transferrin saturation as an index of body iron stores, the researchers analyzed data on over 4500 people between the years of 1971 and 1987. They found no statistically significant relationship between transferrin saturation and coronary heart disease. Results of an epidemiological study involving about 2000 men in Iceland agreed with those of the NHANES report.[30] The issue of the role of body iron stores in the "normal" range in coronary artery disease remains open. The variable results in epidemiological studies from different countries suggests that iron plays a small role, if any, in this arena.

ANEMIA AND CARDIAC FUNCTION

The heart and blood comprise a single functional unit with two principal purposes: (1) to deliver oxygen and nutrients to peripheral tissues and (2) to remove metabolic waste products. The Fick principle states that cardiac output is proportional to oxygen consumption and the arteriovenous oxygen difference (Fig. 69–4). The level of hemoglobin in the blood is the primary determinant of arteriovenous oxygen difference. As the hemoglobin content falls (anemia), cardiac output increases to keep pace with tissue oxygen consumption. Cardiac output depends on the functional capacity of the heart. An important question then, is whether anemia *per se* compromises cardiac function.

One group of investigators examined the question by studying systolic and diastolic left ventricular function in patients with chronic severe anemia (hemoglobin levels of less than 7 gm/dl for more than 3 months). The assessments were done by M-mode, two-dimensional, and Doppler echocardiography.[31] In most instances, the anemia was due to iron deficiency, meaning no primary cardiac insult existed. The cardiac output was elevated as expected, owing to a higher stroke volume and heart rate. Left ventricular contractility was higher than normal, and no evidence existed of diastolic dysfunction. The investigators concluded that, in the absence of primary cardiac disease, anemia does not produce congestive heart failure, at least over the time span studied.

More severe anemia can, however, produce left ventricular dysfunction and circulatory congestion. A group of otherwise healthy children with hemoglobin levels of less than 6 gm/dl due to iron deficiency were also assessed by echocardiography.[32] Left ventricular preload was significantly higher, and left ventricular afterload was significantly lower in the patients relative to controls. Cardiac index was also significantly higher in the severely anemic patients. Iron supplementation eliminated the discrepancy. The interpretation of these results requires consideration that iron deficiency of this severity could impair synthesis of important heme-dependent enzymes, such as the cyto-

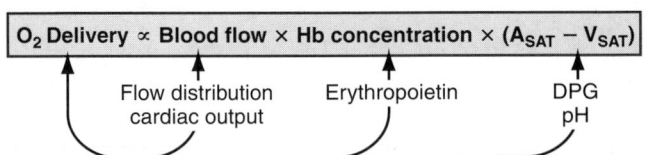

FIGURE 69–4. The Fick principle: Cardiac output is proportional to oxygen consumption and the arteriovenous oxygen difference and the hemoglobin concentration. Compensation for hypoxia may be affected by an increase in cardiac output, an increase in erythropoietin production, or shift to the right in the oxygen dissociation curve due to blood pH-mediated increase in red blood cell 2,3-diphosphoglycerate. (From Bunn HF: Pathophysiology of the anemias. *In* Harrison's Principles of Internal Medicine. 13th ed. New York, McGraw-Hill, 1994, p 1720.)

chromes. Cardiac myocytes depend tremendously on these enzymes required for oxidative metabolism. Therefore, the cardiac dysfunction in these severely anemic patients could result in part from compromised myocardial metabolism. Nutritional deficiency that often accompanies very severe iron deficiency can also contribute to cardiac dysfunction.[33]

One way to avoid possible confounding due to secondary contributions of anemia, as might occur with severe iron deficiency, is to examine cardiac function in patients with genetically determined anemia. Investigators have carefully examined cardiac function in patients with thalassemia major. The presentation of these studies is complicated, because most people with thalassemia major have some degree of iron overload due to repeated transfusion (see earlier). In contrast to thalassemia, people with sickle cell disease usually do not receive chronic transfusions.

Patients with sickle cell disease typically have hemoglobin values in the range of 7 to 9 gm/dl. Cardiomegaly with ventricular dilation develops early in the course of the condition. Early on, patients with sickle cell disease have hyperdynamic hearts with high ejection fractions and a cardiac index that substantially exceed normal values. The heart's ability to maintain this high state of activity declines over time. By early adulthood, many patients begin to exhibit diastolic dysfunction.[34] Volume overload is required to maintain the cardiac index in the face of the low hemoglobin level. Despite the vasoocclusive nature of the disease, definite episodes of typical transmural myocardial infarction are rare. The slow decline in cardiac reserves means that by the fourth or fifth decades these patients begin to have clinically apparent evidence of cardiac dysfunction. Intolerance to the fluid loading used to treat sickle cell vasoocclusive crises is often the harbinger of cardiac involvement in this disease.

HEMATOLOGICAL DISORDERS AND THE CARDIOVASCULAR SYSTEM

Efficient oxygen delivery to cardiac and peripheral tissues requires adequate blood flow, sufficient oxygen-carrying capacity, and a gradient allowing release of oxygen from hemoglobin. In anemia, compensatory responses include increased blood flow owing to increase in cardiac work and a left shift in the oxygen dissociation curve. In contrast, rheological effects of decreased blood flow due to hyperviscosity can be profound, leading to deleterious consequences, including tissue infarction. Hematological/oncological disorders in which hyperviscosity occurs include plasma cell neoplasms (multiple myeloma and Waldenström macroglobulinemia), myeloproliferative disorders (polycythemia vera, essential thrombocytosis, and, in rare cases, chronic myeloid leukemia), lymphoma (if associated with cryoglobulinemia), and acute leukemia (hyperleukocytosis in certain subtypes of acute myeloid leukemia). Patients with a variety of neoplasms, particularly those with mucin-producing adenocarcinomas of the gastrointestinal tract, have an increased risk of thrombotic complications. This so-called hypercoagulable state associated with cancer is not due to increased blood viscosity (see Chap. 62).

Polycythemia

True or absolute polycythemia refers to a condition in which the red cell mass is above normal. Polycythemia must be distinguished from states in which the hematocrit (red cell volume/plasma volume) is increased due to a decrease in plasma volume. An example of a spurious elevation in the hematocrit is Geisboch syndrome, typically seen in middle-aged, overweight hypertensive men.[35] Reducing the red cell mass by phlebotomy or other means does not alter their predisposition to thrombosis, which is likely related to standard atherogenesis rather than to elevated hematocrit.[36] A red cell mass test[37] using chromium-labeled red blood cells is needed to determine if a further work-up for polycythemia is required.

The polycythemias are subclassified into primary disorders and secondary conditions (Table 69–2)[38] in which the increase in red cell mass results from increased production of erythropoietin, the oxygen-tension regulated protein hormone elaborated by the kidney. Erythropoietin production can be increased in any disorder associated with hypoxemia, such as high-altitude chronic lung disease and cyanotic forms of congenital heart disease[39]; impaired release of oxygen by certain hemoglobin variants (e.g., hemoglobin Hallamshire), which cause a shift in the oxygen dissociation curve to the left,[40] also leads to an increase in cell mass. The inappropriate production of erythropoietin or erythropoietin-like protein can be the cause of the erythrocytosis associated with certain tumors, such as cerebellar hemangioblastoma,[41] renal cell carcinoma,[42] and hepatocellular carcinomas.[43] An erythropoietin-independent or autonomously driven increase in the red cell mass is the hallmark of polycythemia vera, one of the myeloproliferative disorders.[37]

Whereas there is an increased incidence of symptoms due to thrombosis or impaired blood flow in patients with polycythemia vera,[37] whether the increased red cell mass wholly accounts for these problems is unclear. Supporting the role of erythrocytosis as the major culprit are (1) the known decrease in oxygen transport with increased blood viscosity based on capillary tube experiments (Fig. 69–5) and (2) the symptomatic relief achieved by patients when the hematocrit is reduced by phlebotomy.[44] On the other hand, patients with secondary erythrocytosis rarely experience the plethora of nonspecific symptoms (e.g., visual disturbances, dizziness, confusion) typ-

▼ **TABLE 69–2. DIFFERENTIAL DIAGNOSIS OF POLYCYTHEMIA**

ERYTHROCYTOSIS ASSOCIATED WITH A NORMAL OR REDUCED RED BLOOD CELL MASS
Acute or chronic hemoconcentration
Spurious polycythemia (stress polycythemia, relative polycythemia, or Gaisböck syndrome)

ERYTHROCYTOSIS ASSOCIATED WITH AN ELEVATED RED BLOOD CELL MASS (ABSOLUTE POLYCYTHEMIA)
Secondary Polycythemia
Increased erythropoietin production (physiologically appropriate)
  High altitude
  Cardiopulmonary disease
  Decreased blood oxygen-carrying capacity due to carboxyhemoglobin
  Impaired oxygen delivery, hemoglobin with increased oxygen affinity or congenital decreased red cell 2, 3-diphosphoglycerate
  Renal artery stenosis
  Familial elevated erythropoietin with appropriate physiological response
Autonomous erythropoietin production
  Tumors
    Hypernephroma
    Cerebellar hemangioblastoma
    Hepatoma
    Uterine fibroids
    Pheochromocytoma
    Adrenal cortical adenoma
    Ovarian carcinoma
  Renal disorders
    Cysts
    Hydronephrosis
    Bartter syndrome
    Transplantation
  Familial polycythemia due to autonomous erythropoietin production

Polycythemia Vera

From Fruchtman SM, Berk PD: Polycythemia vera. *In* Handin RI, Lux SE, Stossel TP (eds): Blood: Principles and Practice of Hematology. Philadelphia, JB Lippincott, 1995.

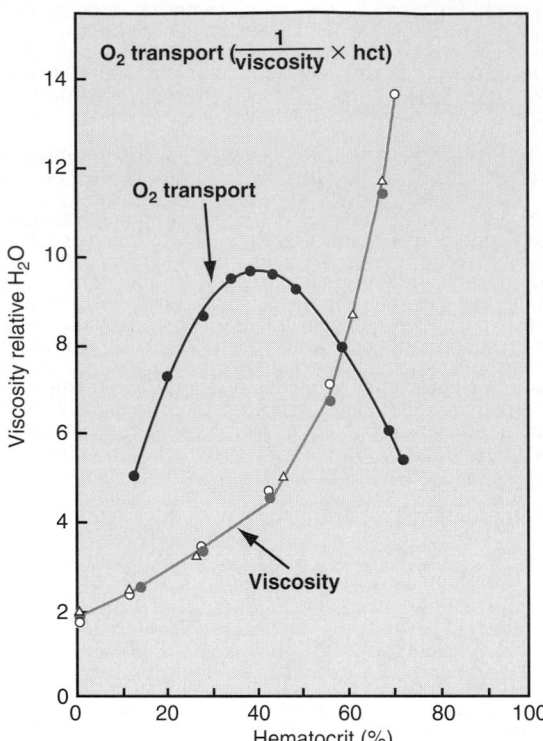

FIGURE 69–5. Capillary tube experiment that documents the relationship between blood viscosity and oxygen transport. Blood that is too viscous due to polycythemia does not carry oxygen efficiently. (From Jandl JH: Blood: Textbook of Hematology. 2nd ed. Boston, Little, Brown, 1996, p 159.)

ical of the patient suffering from polycythemia vera.[37] Second, those with polycythemia vera often have persistent symptoms requiring antineoplastic therapy, which can lead to an amelioration in symptoms when the hematocrit has already been lowered by phlebotomy, perhaps because the platelets in this condition are intrinsically abnormal (e.g., reduced expression of the thrombopoietin receptor c-mpl).[45]

Polycythemia Vera

Polycythemia vera is a clonal chronic myeloproliferative disorder that is characterized by an increase in the red cell mass.[46] Other cell lineages including leukocytes and platelets may also be elevated. Splenomegaly is common. Studies have suggested that the cause of this disorder is an increased sensitivity of hematopoietic progenitor cells to regulatory factors such as erythropoietin.[47, 48] Patients with polycythemia vera usually have serum erythropoietin levels that are quite low even after phlebotomies have lowered the hemoglobin level. A defect in the cell signaling cascade may cause hypersensitivity to erythropoietin, although some have suggested that red blood cell production in this disease is completely independent of erythropoietin.[49] The *SHP1* gene, which encodes an intracellular phosphatase involved in cell signaling pathways, is potentially dysregulated in polycythemia vera.[50] Mutations in the erythropoietin receptor gene have been reported in a handful of families with familial polycythemia vera.[51]

CLINICAL MANIFESTATIONS. Patients with polycythemia vera[52] may present with a variety of nonspecific complaints, including headache, weakness, pruritus (especially after showering), dizziness, sweating, abnormal vision, paresthesias, arthralgias, weight loss, or abdominal pain. On physical examination, patients have a ruddy complexion, organomegaly, and hypertension. Both thrombosis and hemorrhage may occur. Thrombosis occurs in up to 30 to 40 percent of patients with the disorder, including deep venous thrombosis of the lower extremities, pulmonary em-

bolism, and coronary, cerebrovascular, or peripheral occlusions.[53] The splanchnic bed is particularly susceptible to thrombosis in patients with polycythemia vera. Cardiac valvular abnormalities also occur in patients with polycythemia vera (usually mitral valve thickening or nonbacterial vegetations). Hepatic or vena caval thrombosis, the Budd-Chiari syndrome, is a serious and not unusual event in patients with polycythemia vera. Of all patients with Budd-Chiari syndrome, up to 10 percent have polycythemia vera.[54] The risk of thrombosis may be related to excessive homocysteine levels.[55] Neurological abnormalities including transient ischemic attacks, cerebral infarction or hemorrhage, fluctuation in mental status, confusional states, and choreic syndromes also have been described. Dizziness, visual disturbances, scalp tenderness, and headache may occur because of increased blood viscosity and reduced cerebral blood flow caused by the erythrocytosis. Basilar artery insufficiency as well as carotid territory strokes may also occur. Peripheral arterial thrombosis, peripheral vascular disease, and erythromelalgia, characterized by burning pain in the digits and potential ulceration, are further manifestations of the circulatory problems typically seen in those with polycythemia vera. Gastrointestinal and cerebral hemorrhage[56] have been described, particularly after the use of antiplatelet agents.

DIAGNOSIS AND TREATMENT. The polycythemia study group has developed clinical and laboratory criteria for diagnosis[57] that require the presence of an elevated red cell mass and any three of the following criteria: (1) normal arterial oxygen saturation in the presence of erythrocytosis, (2) splenomegaly, (3) thrombocytosis and leukocytosis, (4) bone marrow hypercellularity associated with mature megakaryocytes without myelofibrosis, (5) low serum erythropoietin levels, and (6) abnormal marrow proliferative capacity as manifested by formation of erythroid colonies in the absence of erythropoietin.

Therapy requires individualization; there is no curative therapy other than perhaps bone marrow transplantation[58] in the rare patient with severe clinical manifestations. For most patients it is appropriate to reduce the blood cell count to normal as rapidly as possible with phlebotomy (1 to 2 units every other day as needed).[59] The hematocrit should be maintained in the 42 to 45 percent range. Pruritus, if present may be treated with cyproheptadine or even interferon alfa.[60] Elective surgery should be delayed until the red cell mass is in the normal range, if possible. Aspirin should be used carefully in a patient with polycythemia vera owing to the risk of hemorrhagic complications.[61] Hydroxyurea, an oral antimetabolite chemotherapy agent, may be helpful in cases where the hematocrit cannot be controlled by phlebotomy alone.[62] The alkylating agent busulfan should be avoided, owing to an increased risk of bone marrow fibrosis and leukemogenesis. Use of phlebotomy alone as a treatment strategy is associated with a higher risk of thrombosis.[59] The risk of leukemogenesis from hydroxyurea is low but real,[63] so this agent must be used carefully as a means of reducing the risk of thrombosis.

THROMBOCYTOSIS

An elevated (>450,000/ml) platelet count can result from physiologically appropriate stimuli, such as those occurring after general surgery, splenectomy, pregnancy, or iron deficiency. Such reactive thrombocytoses are not associated with an increased number of thrombotic events, in contrast to primary or essential thrombocytosis, which is one of the myeloproliferative disorders. In essential thrombocytosis there is a tendency toward increased clotting (as well as to hemorrhage due to intrinsic platelet dysfunction), sometimes with disastrous results, especially in younger patients with this condition.[56, 64, 65] Myocardial infarction is actually less common in those with essential thrombocytosis than with polycythemia vera.[57, 65] The use of hydroxyurea to lower the platelet count (and ameliorate the clonal stem cell defects as well) has been associated with reduction in cardiac risk.[66] The effect of anagrelide, which reproducibly lowers the platelet count, on the natural history of essential thrombocytosis is unclear.[67]

LEUKOCYTOSIS

Leukocytosis in patients with acute leukemia may provoke a host of cardiovascular problems during the course of the disease. Sepsis associated with profoundly myelosuppressive and gut-damaging chemotherapy can be associated with severe, albeit reversible, depression of cardiac function.[68] Two important issues relating leukemia to cardiac physiology are discussed later in this chapter: leukemic cell invasion of the myocardium or pericardium and direct toxic effect of antileukemic drugs, particularly anthracyclines. Occasionally, a very elevated white blood cell count may lead to circulatory compromise. Patients with chronic and acute lymphoid leukemia can tolerate extremely high white blood cell counts (more than several hundred thousand per microliter) without evident problems. However, patients with acute myeloid leukemia, particularly those with the acute monocytic or acute myelomonocytic subtype, may experience so-called leukostatic phenomena.[69, 70] Probably due to adhesion molecules expressed on the leukemia cell surface in those acute myeloid leukemia subtypes, aggregates of such neoplastic cells may cause thrombosis and hemorrhages in microcapillaries of the brain,[71] producing encephalopathy or, in the lung, producing pulmonary infiltrates and hypoxemia.[72, 73] In instances of cerebral or pulmonary leukostasis, rapid lowering of the white blood cell count is required. Usually, such reduction can be accomplished by institution of hydroxyurea or definitive antileukemic chemotherapy[74]; occasionally, limited radiation to the brain[74] and/or leukophoresis[75] is required to prevent severe complications. Patients with chronic myeloid leukemia in stable phase who may often have high white blood cell counts, composed of mid-range and mature myeloid cells, occasionally experience leukostatic/thrombotic complications[76] such as priapism or stroke.

HYPERVISCOSITY DUE TO QUANTITATIVE OR QUALITATIVE ABNORMALITIES IN PLASMA PROTEINS

Plasma cell neoplasms are characterized by a clonal proliferation of cells capable of elaborating a single immunoglobulin molecule, either light chains or heavy chains or a structurally complete multimeric protein. The so-called M-component may, depending on its biochemical properties and level, interfere with normal process such as nerve conduction[77] or coagulation[78] owing to effects on clotting factors and/or platelet function. The hyperviscosity syndrome, characterized by circulating immune complexes, is more likely at a given level of IgM excess than in the more common IgG myeloma. Patients with an IgM M-spike and an accumulation of plasmacytoid lymphocytes in the marrow and/or lymph nodes have Waldenström macroglobulinemia[79] syndrome. When suspected on clinical grounds, the hyperviscosity syndrome can be confirmed by actual measurements of serum viscosity.[80] Hyperviscosity, a medical emergency, requires a prompt reduction in the M-component,[81] usually through a combination of plasmapheresis plus tumor burden reduction with chemotherapy. Elaboration of proteins that can aggregate at low temperature (cryoglobulins)[82] can result from a host of infections, as well as inflammatory or neoplastic conditions such as lymphoma, and can impose peripheral circulating problems, as discussed later.

PLASMA CELL NEOPLASMS

Multiple myeloma and other plasma cell tumors are neoplasms of plasma cells or plasmacytoid lymphocytes. These disorders may result from dysregulation of normal growth suppression genes. Overproduction of interleukin-6, which serves as an autocrine growth factor for myeloma cells, may also contribute to the development of this disease.[83]

Clinical manifestations of multiple myeloma include bone pain, renal insufficiency, anemia, hypercalcemia, infection, bleeding, and neurological symptoms. Hyperviscosity, especially in patients with IgG subclass myeloma,[84] has been described. Hyperviscosity may also be associated with bleeding. The diagnosis can be made by measuring serum viscosity[80] and by eyeground examination, which discloses the slow blood flow in the retinal blood vessels. Plasmapheresis[81] is the appropriate treatment. The overabundantly elaborated monoclonal protein can be deposited in tissues such as the kidney and heart, producing secondary amyloidosis. Cardiac amyloidosis may lead to cardiomyopathy, characterized by a speckled appearance on echocardiography.

The diagnosis of myeloma[85] rests on finding one major and one minor criteria or at least three minor criteria. The major criteria include plasmacytoma on tissue biopsy, marrow plasmacytosis greater than 30 percent, monoclonal protein of significant height (IgG greater than 3.5 gm/dl, IgA greater than 2 gm/dl, or light-chain [Bence Jones] protein in the urine greater than 1 gm/24 hr). The minor criteria include marrow plasmacytosis of 10 to 29 percent, monoclonal protein present but less than the levels defined for major criteria, osteolytic bone lesions, or a decrease in uninvolved immunoglobulins.

Waldenström macroglobulinemia[79] is characterized by marrow infiltration with lymphoplasmacytoid cells and high levels of IgM in the blood; lymphadenopathy or splenomegaly, rare in and multiple myeloma, is present in at least 40 percent of those with Waldenström macroglobulinemia. Complications caused by the macroglobulin production such as hyperviscosity, cold hemolytic anemia, peripheral neuropathy, renal disease, and bleeding are often the presenting manifestations. Although serum viscosity is elevated in most patients with Waldenström disease, only 15 to 20 percent have symptoms related to this problem. Congestive heart failure is not unusual, owing to the anemia and expanded plasma volume as well as the increased viscosity.

Patients with asymptomatic multiple myeloma should not be treated until there is clear evidence of disease progression. The aggressive therapeutic approach to multiple myeloma includes up-front high-dose dexamethasone or a vincristine/doxorubicin/dexamethase (VAD) regimen followed by autologous bone marrow transplantation once a reasonable response has been achieved.[86] Patients who are not candidates for high-dose chemotherapy should be treated for at least 12 months with one of the available regimens, including dexamethasone or VAD. Anemia can be corrected in many patients by administration of erythropoietin.[87] Hypercalcemia should be treated. The use of bisphosphonates such as pamidronate to stabilize bone matrix has resulted in a lower incidence of skeletal complications and improved outcome in patients with myeloma.[88] Patients with Waldenström macroglobulinemia are usually managed with combination chemotherapy.[79] Thalidomide, which may work by inhibiting angiogenesis, has efficacy in patients with refractory myeloma.[89]

CRYOGLOBULINS

Cryoglobulins are immunoglobulins that produce high-molecular-weight aggregates at temperatures below 37°C (98.6°F). To detect the presence of these proteins, blood should be drawn through a preheated syringe and stored at body temperature.[82] Hepatitis C virus is a particularly important etiological agent.[90] The chief symptoms are peripheral vasculitis. Skin and joint manifestations are most common, but central nervous system dysfunction, renal failure, and even severe hypertension leading to cardiovascular and cerebrovascular accidents have been described in severe cases.[91] Interferon alfa to treat hepatitis C–associated disease[92] and cytotoxic drugs to treat the vascular disease[93] are potentially useful therapeutic modalities.

CARDIAC MANIFESTATIONS OF NEOPLASTIC DISEASE

Based on autopsy series, tumors affecting the heart are much more likely to have originated from a neoplasm elsewhere than to have primarily occurred in the heart.[94] Primary cardiac tumors are discussed in Chapter 49. Metastatic tumors reach the heart most commonly by hematogenous dissemination, which cause multiple nodules, occasionally so diffuse as to lead to restrictive cardiomyopathy.[95] Direct extension, especially from mesotheliomas,[96] sarcomas,[97, 98] and mediastinal lymphomas[99, 100] (Hodgkin and non-Hodgkin) also occur (Fig. 69–6).

Essentially, any tumor may spread to cardiac structures, including the myocardium, pericardium, and valves. The most common tumors to spread to the heart in descending order of frequency are carcinoma of the lung, breast, malignant melanoma, and leukemia. General autopsy series shows cardiac involvement in 1 to 20 percent of patients with malignant diseases; the frequency ranges as high as 60 percent in those with melanoma.[95]

Clinical manifestations of tumors metastatic to the myocardium are generally nonexistent, in distinction to the effects of tumors invading the pericardium, which may produce life-threatening tamponade. Myocardial invasion can occasionally produce tachyarrhythmias, atrioventricular block, or congestive heart failure.[101, 102] The diagnosis of myocardial metastasis ante mortem may be noted on echocardiographic examination, magnetic resonance imaging, gallium scanning, computed tomography, or positron-emission tomography.[103–105] Such studies may be particularly helpful in cases in which direct extension plays a role.

Pericardial Involvement

(See also Chap. 50)

Hematogenous spread (e.g., breast cancer, melanoma, sarcoma, leukemia)[106–109] or direct extension of a thoracic tumor (e.g., mesothelioma, lymphoma, or lung cancer)[96, 110] can lead to pericardial involvement. Pericardial involve-

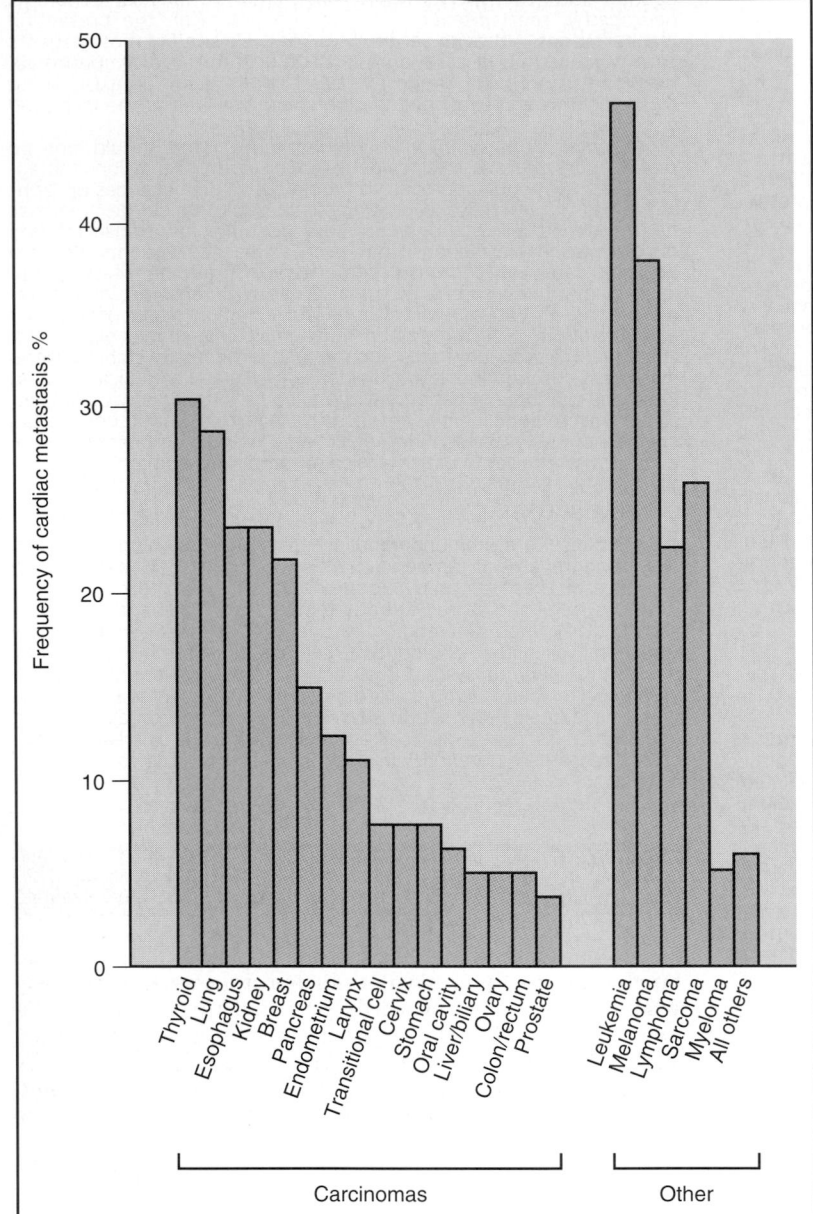

FIGURE 69–6. Frequency of metastatic tumors to the heart and pericardium. (From English JC, et al: Metastatic tumors of the heart. *In* Goldhaber SZ [ed]: Cardiopulmonary Diseases and Cardiac Tumors. *In* Braunwald E [series ed]: Atlas of Heart Diseases. Vol 3. Philadelphia, Current Medicine, 1995, pp 116.1–116.6. Adapted from McAllister HA, Fenoglio JJ: Tumors of the cardiovascular system. *In* Atlas of Tumor Pathology. 2nd ed. Washington, DC, Armed Forces Institute of Pathology, 1978, pp 111–119.)

ment[111] can be classified as either primarily infiltrative, with thickening and adherence to or infiltration of the myocardium, or as effusive, where there is significant reactive expansion of pericardial fluid. Although these two categories are not mutually exclusive, the infiltrative form tends to cause constrictive physiology whereas the effusive form results in pericardial tamponade.

Symptoms of pericardial tamponade include dyspnea and tachycardia due to a failure of cardiac output to meet oxygen demand, especially with exercise; cough and chest pain may also occur, although the key to suspecting the diagnosis is unexplained dyspnea and tachycardia in a cancer patient with normal resting oxygen saturation.

Pulsus paradoxus and paradoxical movement of the jugular venous pulse are important clinical signs of tamponade and should be sought during the physical examination, although their absence does not rule out the syndrome, which may occur only in the setting of relatively advanced pathological findings (see also Chap. 50). Once the diagnosis of pericardial tamponade is suspected, an echocardiogram should be obtained. Although at cardiac catheterization demonstration of equal diastolic pressure on both sides of the heart is the hemodynamic key to diagnosis, echocardiography also provides critical physiological insight. As intrapericardial pressure rises, the relatively thin right ventricular wall will collapse, particularly in diastole.[112] Such diastolic right ventricular wall collapse is quite sensitive for hemodynamically significant tamponade; sometimes an echocardiogram will also actually delineate the metastasis. Computed tomography or magnetic resonance imaging is more suitable in situations in which pericardial infiltration/constriction is the more prominent physiology.

Not every pericardial effusion in a patient with cancer is due to malignant disease. Prior chest radiation therapy[113, 114] for lung cancer or lymphoma can produce pericardial disease as a late complication. Such radiation-induced effusions do not usually cause tamponade, but extreme care must be taken to exclude this eventuality.

The management of cancer patients with tamponade often requires surgical drainage[115] (e.g., creation of a pericardial window) by thoracotomy, subxiphoid pericardiotomy, or video-assisted thoracoscopy,[116] which offers a good balance between invasiveness and effectiveness. In patients with lymphoma who present with minimal tamponade early in the course of the disease, chemotherapy can result in rapid amelioration of symptoms.[117]

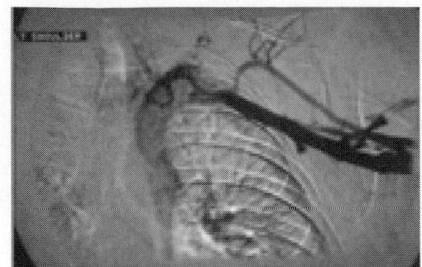

FIGURE 69–7. The radiographic appearance of SVC syndrome. Chest venography. (From Roberts JR, et al: Multimodality treatment of malignant superior vena caval syndrome. Chest 116:835–837, 1999.)

Superior Vena Cava Syndrome

Compression of the easily distensible superior vena cava, with or without associated thrombosis, by a thoracic tumor such as carcinoma of the lung or lymphoma can produce significant clinical consequences. The so-called superior vena cava syndrome[118] often presents as facial swelling, headache, and arm edema. A prominent venous pattern can be observed on inspection of the anterior chest wall. The diagnosis can be established by scintigraphy, angiography, or high-resolution contrast medium–enhanced computed tomography (Fig. 69–7). Although rarely life threatening, the superior vena cava syndrome can lead to considerable morbidity and discomfort. Emergent radiation treatment is the treatment of choice.[119] In patients with responsive tumors such as Hodgkin disease or non-Hodgkin lymphoma, chemotherapy should be initiated as soon as possible. The likelihood of symptomatic relief with antineoplastic therapy depends on the duration of the obstruction and the intrinsic chemosensitivity of the tumor. Local therapies such as stenting, angioplasty, clot removal, or lysis are currently being developed[120–123] (see also Chap. 42). The role of anticoagulation is controversial[124, 125]; some authorities recommend an angiographic evaluation (e.g., magnetic resonance angiogram) to document thrombosis before initiating such therapy.

Arrhythmias

Arrhythmias, typically due to electrolyte imbalance or decreased oxygen-carrying capacity (hypoxia due to pulmonary involvement with tumor or infection; or anemia) are common in patients with cancer. Tumor involvement of cardiac structures may also lead to nonspecific rhythm disturbances, including low voltage, sinus tachycardia, and ST segment and T wave charges. Atrial fibrillation or flutter can occur due to any of the aforementioned issues or to tumor invasion of the atria or of the coronary arteries that supply this chamber. In rare cases, atrioventricular node involvement will occur, leading to complete heart block.[110] Carotid sinus syncope[126] has been associated, in rare cases, with tumorous involvement of cervical lymph nodes.

Ischemic Heart Disease and Malignancy

In addition to the patient with intrinsic arteriosclerotic coronary disease who also happens to have cancer, there is sometimes a relationship between the malignancy and the ischemic heart disease. For example, tumor emboli can occlude[127] or tumor mass can compress the coronary artery.[128] The hypercoagulable state associated with malignancy, especially mucin-secreting adenocarcinoma, can predispose a patient to develop a coronary thrombosis. Radiation therapy promotes arteriosclerosis[129] (see next section).

Myocardial infarction was suspected as the cause of death in 4 percent of 816 patients with solid tumors undergoing autopsy.[95] In most of the nonarteriosclerotic cases

(which account for the majority of such infarctions), extrinsic compression of a coronary artery is the cause of the infarction. Typical angina rarely precedes the coronary event in this setting.

Nonbacterial Thrombotic Endocarditis

(See also Chap. 47)

Although the cardiac valves may be directly involved with metastatic tumor, the most common cause of valvular heart disease in the cancer patient is nonbacterial thrombotic endocarditis (NBTE).[130–133] NBTE generally involves the aortic and mitral valve and occurs in patients with advanced adenocarcinoma of the gastrointestinal tract and lung. Although the precise pathophysiology of NBTE remains uncertain, associated features include tumor-associated immune complexes and the presence of catheters, especially in right-sided valvular lesions. The clinical signs of NBTE may be subtle and resemble those of subacute bacterial endocarditis; more dramatic findings such as stroke[133] or myocardial infarction have been noted. Echocardiography can establish the diagnosis; yet treatment is difficult, in great part owing to the generally advanced stage of cancer in these patients.

INFLAMMATORY MEDIATORS ASSOCIATED WITH CARDIAC DISEASE

The carcinoid syndrome (see also Chaps. 46 and 48) is characterized by the elaboration of serotonin and its metabolites from a neoplastic proliferation of neoendocrine cells derived from ectoderm.[134] Clinical findings may include flushing, hypotension, and/or valvular lesions (Fig. 69–8).[135, 136] The best treatment is reduction of tumor burden by surgery, although cisplatin-based chemotherapy may offer palliation.[134]

In the hypereosinophilic syndrome (see also Chap. 48),[137] a myeloproliferative disorder, eosinophils infiltrate the bone marrow and circulate in high numbers in the peripheral blood. Cardiac involvement may result from the elaboration of mediators of inflammation as well as from direct invasion by the eosinophils.[138] Because corticosteroids can cause lysis of eosinophils, these drugs have been used successfully to treat cardiac complications such as cardiomegaly with a thickened right ventricular wall (leading to restrictive physiology[139]), mural thrombosis, and right-sided valvular dysfunction.[140] Mast cell neoplasms, including systemic mastocytosis, can also lead to valvular heart disease by a mechanism[141] similar to that described in association with hypereosinophilic syndrome. Massive release of vasodilatory substances during anesthesia has led to cardiovascular collapse in patients with mastocytosis.[142]

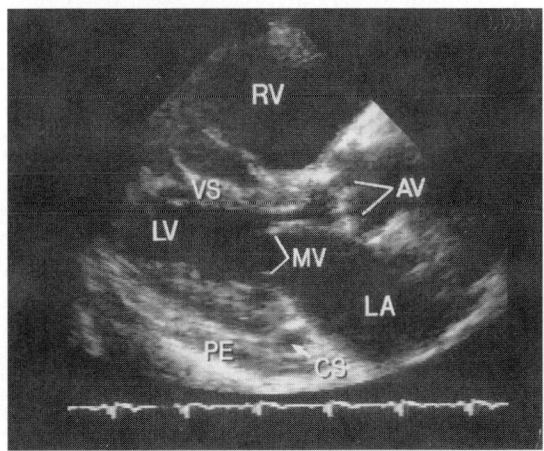

FIGURE 69–8. Carcinoid tumor involving the heart. Echocardiogram demonstrating thickened aortic and mitral valves, a small pericardial effusion and dilated right ventricle. AV = aortic valve; CS = coronary sinus; LA = left atrium; LV = left ventricle; MV = mitral valve; PE = pericardial effusion; RV = right ventricle; VS = ventricular septum. (From Pellikka PA, et al: Carcinoid heart disease: Clinical and echocardiographic spectrum in 74 patients. Circulation 87:1188–1196, 1993. Copyright 1993, American Heart Association.)

As understanding of the pathophysiology of neoplasia grows, it is hoped that molecules that specifically target the genetic lesions accounting for a given neoplasm will allow for a markedly improved therapeutic index (likelihood of benefit compared with toxicity). The successful use of all-trans retinoic acid in acute promyelocytic leukemia, characterized by a translocation of the retinoic acid receptor alpha gene to the promyelocytic leukemia gene, is one such example of relatively specific therapy, albeit in a rare disease.[143] However, for the most part, chemotherapy or irradiation entails significant side effects that always must be weighed against the goals of treatment, be they palliative or curative. Although many antineoplastic approaches are particularly toxic to tissues with a high cell turnover rate, such as the bone marrow, hair, and gastrointestinal tract, the heart is frequently adversely affected. In particular, as patients live longer after the diagnosis and therapy of cancer, late cardiac toxicity can lessen the quality of life.

Radiation Therapy

Therapeutic ionizing radiation to the chest is used to prevent local recurrence of breast cancer, to improve disease control in lung cancer and esophageal cancer, as well as to improve the cure rate with Hodgkin and non-Hodgkin lymphoma of the mediastinum. Essentially, all cardiac structures, including the pericardium, myocardium, and coronary arteries may be affected by such efforts.

MECHANISMS OF RADIATION-INDUCED CARDIAC INJURY. Damage to both normal and neoplastic tissues occurs due to the free electrons, liberated due to the impact of high-energy proton beams, which directly damage DNA or do so indirectly, resulting in the creation of hydroxyl radicals from water.[144] Although the degree of DNA damage induced by radiation is most closely linked with cytotoxicity and therefore generally involves proliferating cells, more long-lived cells can also be affected. Radiation also induces early response genes such as c-*jun*, *fos*, and *EGR1*, cytokines such as tumor necrosis factor, and fibroblast growth factor, which may also contribute to the toxic effect. Moreover, radiation-induced apoptosis, or programmed cell death, may be a key component of tumor radiosensitivity, as well as cardiac toxicity, owing to endothelial cell damage mediated in this fashion.[145]

The subacute radiation injury to the heart noted clinically may result from a combination of microvascular destruction and apoptosis. The microvascular destruction can lead to coronary artery disease, ischemia, progressive cellular loss, and fibrosis. Late tissue injury to the myocardium, valves, and pericardium[146–149] may occur. Cardiotoxicity is common at doses over 45 Gy, indicating increased radiosensitivity compared with the brain, esophagus, or bladder.[144]

Radiation-Induced Pericardial Disease

(See also Chap. 50)
Radiation therapy can produce acute or delayed effects on the pericardium. Especially with radiation techniques employed before the 1990s, almost all patients who received over 40 Gy to the anterior mediastinum would develop pericardial effusion or thickening within 9 months of treatment,[150] but symptoms of pericardial disease can be delayed for up to 10 years.[151, 152] Such symptoms occur in a minority of irradiated patients in whom up to 70 percent may have pathological evidence of radiation-related pericardial disease.[153] Late pericardial fibrosis with development of constrictive pericarditis occurred in 3 of 102 Hodgkin

patients treated with mediastinal reduction in the 1970s.[154] In the case of pericardial effusions that produce tamponade physiology, a pericardectomy with creation of a window can be a critical therapeutic and diagnostic maneuver, because it is also important to rule out recurrence of the neoplasm. Removal of the entire pericardium may be alternatively necessary and may be required in patients with constrictive disease. The actual rate of pericardectomy was reported to be 4 percent at 17 years in one study that followed children and adolescents with Hodgkin disease.[154] However, postpericardectomy mortality is high,[155] presumably because of the problems associated with diffuse damage to the entire heart, such as coronary artery disease, conduction system disturbances (e.g., sinus node disease),[156] and atrioventricular block,[157] and valvular pathology.[153, 158]

Radiation-Induced Myocardial and Ischemic Disease

Although radiation-induced myocardial fibrosis is common,[153] it is more difficult to show that left ventricular dysfunction derives solely from radiation therapy, as opposed to combined modality therapy with anthracycline chemotherapy. Children are certainly at risk for late effects due to chest radiotherapy. The incidence of late electrocardiographic abnormalities in children who received spinal or mediastinal irradiation in childhood is as high as 31 percent; cardiac-limited exercise dysfunction occurs in over 70 percent of children undergoing spinal irradiation, compared with 32 percent who had received flank/mediastinal radiation.[159] However, the most common and arguably the most important late effect is myocardial ischemia/infarction. The distribution of proximal coronary artery narrowing at autopsy[160] may result from the design of radiation ports that tend to primarily encompass the origin of these vessels.

One of the best retrospective series documenting the risk of significant coronary heart disease due to radiation is the Stanford study,[161] which examined the records of 635 individuals younger than the age of 21 treated for Hodgkin disease. Seven of 12 patients who experienced fatal cardiac events had a myocardial infarction (6–22 years post therapy), each of whom received 42 to 45 Gy to the mediastinum between ages 9 and 20 (relative risk was 41.5 percent [95 percent confidence interval was 18.1–82.1 percent]). Chemotherapy did not add risk for myocardial infarction. The actuarial risk of a fatal or nonfatal myocardial infarction was 8 percent at 22 years after therapy. Adults may be at somewhat lower risk, given the case-cohort study of 4665 patients[162] demonstrating an age-adjusted relative risk of death due to myocardial infarction of 2.56 percent after mediastinal irradiation. It has been strongly suggested that patients receiving mediastinal radiation be longitudinally screened for the presence of preclinical cardiac disease.[163]

Given the frequent use of radiation therapy in women with breast cancer after conservative surgery, concerns have been raised about the potentially increased risk of coronary disease in this setting. In 244 patients with stage I or II breast cancer who received breast tangential irradiation (45 Gy with a 16-Gy boost) either before or after doxorubicin-containing chemotherapy regimens, there was no increase in cardiac events in those with either left- or right-sided breast cancer.[164] The trend toward the use of either chemotherapy only or low-dose radiation after chemotherapy for Hodgkin disease will likely result in a markedly decreased incidence of cardiac disease compared with the era when curative intent radiation was primarily employed.[165, 166] Amifostine is a thiol that can salvage the oxygen-derived free radicals that mediate irradiation (and chemotherapy)–induced cytotoxicity and may be selectively taken up by normal, compared with neoplastic, tissues.[167] There are, however, no data at this point supporting the administration of this agent to protect the heart from the damaging effects of radiation.[168]

There is little prospectively collected data concerning the risk of radiation-induced heart disease. Based largely on retrospective series, the following points are clear: (1) accelerated coronary artery narrowing results from chest irradiation and may lead to serious clinical consequences[160, 162, 169, 170]; (2) irradiation during childhood or adolescence carries greater impact than similar therapy given later in life[161, 171, 172]; (3) effects of radiation impairing function of noncardiac site such as the thyroid, gonads, skeleton, and lungs can have important indirect cardiac effects[163]; and (4) improvements in radiation techniques such as more focused high-energy beams, careful field design, modified fractionation, and better shielding are lessening the incidence of this problem.[163]

Chemotherapy-Induced Cardiac Disease

Combination chemotherapy leads to cures in patients with germ cell neoplasms, acute leukemias, and lymphomas and performs a critical adjunctive role, along with local tumor control in many other neoplasms, including breast cancer, lung cancer, and colorectal cancer. Toxicities of such regimens that contain cell-cycle or S-phase specific antineoplastic agents generally most markedly impact tissues such as the gastrointestinal tract and bone marrow, characterized by rapid cell tumor. However, chemotherapy-induced myocardial damage is a considerable problem, particularly in patients who are either cured or experience major palliation. Because long-surviving patients may be at risk for a delayed-onset cardiomyopathy, understanding risk factors for and minimizing the likelihood of development of this problem represents a major direction of research in the fields of both oncology and cardiology. The anthracyclines (doxorubicin, daunorubicin, idarubicin, and epirubicin) and the related anthracenedione mitoxantrone are the chemotherapeutic agents most widely recognized for causing cardiotoxicity; however, many other agents, including those in the biological response modifier class, are associated with cardiovascular pathology (Table 69–3).

PATHOGENESIS OF ANTHRACYCLINE-INDUCED CARDIAC INJURY

Anthracyclines are part of curative therapy for acute leukemias, Hodgkin and non-Hodgkin lymphoma, breast cancer, and sarcomas of the bone. They are employed as palliative therapy in a variety of other neoplasms. These drugs contain an aromatic ring structure that intercalates in-between DNA base pairs; however, the mechanism of cytotoxicity appears to be inhibition of the function of topoisomerase II, an enzyme critical in allowing DNA to undergo efficient repair. Second, these drugs generate free radicals, which can damage cell membranes, in part by lipid peroxidation. The latter effect correlated most closely with cardiac toxicity; members of this class such as amsacrine and mitoxantrone, which produce lower quantities of free radicals, are less likely to cause cardiomyopathy.[173]

Enzymes such as P450 reductase, xanthine oxidase, and mitochondrial NADH oxidase are plentiful in the energy-dependent and mitochondrial-rich cardiac tissue and are responsible for reducing the anthracyclines to their corresponding semiquinone free radicals. However, the heart may have relatively low ability to detoxify the free radicals because of the presence of only small amounts of catalase, which converts hydrogen peroxide to water.[174] Lack of general free

radical scavenging may be less important than the chelation of iron by the anthracyclines. The anthracycline-iron complexes generate tissue-damaging hydroxyl radicals in the immediate vicinity of the target.[173] Consequently, dexrazoxane (Zinacard), a drug that undergoes hydrolysis to a carboxylamine capable of accepting the iron from the anthracycline-iron complex, is the only clinically effective cardioprotectant.[168, 175] General free radical scavengers such as N-acetylcysteine are ineffective.[176]

Downstream effects of the free-radical–mediated damage induced by the anthracyclines include defective calcium binding by the sarcoplasmic reticulum; decreased actin, troponin, and myosin light chain 2 gene expression; and release of vasoactive amines and proinflammatory cytokines, such as tumor necrosis factor and interleukin-2.[177] Moreover, the presence of free radicals may activate certain intracellular signaling pathways,[178, 179] which turn on the apoptotic or programmed cell death machinery.[180] The disturbance in sarcoplasmic structures corresponds to ultrastructural damage to these elements and may cause calcium overload leading to deleterious transient activation of contractile proteins.[181] The findings of myofibrillar loss, mitochondrial swelling cisternal disruption, (Fig. 69–9), and nuclear degeneration are the histopathological consequences of the biochemical changes noted earlier. Second, myocyte loss on the basis of apoptotic cell death has been documented. The degree of pathological changes has been used to establish a grading system to classify the severity of injury.[182] Serial endomyocardial biopsies are seldom used now because of the invasiveness and lack of predictive value of this technique relative to other monitoring strategies.

Clinical Aspects of Anthracycline-Induced Cardiotoxicity

In rare cases, a single dose of anthracycline produces acute or subacute cardiac toxicity. The most common acute toxicities include electrophysiological abnormalities, among them nonspecific ST and T wave abnormalities, decreased QRS voltage, and prolongation of the QT interval.[177] Rhythm disturbances including sinus tachycardia, ventricular and supraventricular arrhythmias, as well as conduction system alterations including atrioventricular block and bundle branch block can occur.[183, 184] Very rare cases of an acute myocarditis-pericarditis syndrome causing sudden death or rapidly progressive heart failure within 2 weeks of administration of the drug have been described.[184]

The common, clinically relevant type and potentially severe anthracycline-induced cardiac toxicity is the chronic cardiomyopathy that results from cumulative exposure to these agents. Although many risk factors, including older age and antecedent heart disease, for the development of anthracycline-induced cardiomyopathy have been described, the most important is cumulative dose of the drug. There is a nonlinear increase in the incidence of cardiomyopathy from 0.15 percent or lower at 400 mg/m² or less cumulative doses, compared with a 7 percent incidence at 550 mg/m² (Fig. 69–10). Although endomyocardial biopsies demonstrate a progressive loss in cardiac myocytes with increasing doses beginning at a low level of total drug ad-

▼ TABLE 69–3. CARDIOTOXICITY ANTINEOPLASTIC AGENTS

DRUG	TOXIC DOSE RANGE*	COMMENTS
Doxorubicin	> 550 mg/m² (total dose)	Congestive heart failure (cumulative toxic effect), arrhythmias
	> 550 mg/m² (total dose)	Cardiac toxicity with additional risk factors
Daunorubicin	> 550 mg/m² (total dose)	Same toxicity as doxorubicin
Mitoxantrone	> 100–140 mg/m² (total dose)	Congestive heart failure, decreases in left ventricular ejection fraction
Cyclophosphamide	> 100–120 mg/kg over 2 days	Congestive heart failure, hemorrhagic myocarditis/pericarditis/necrosis
5-Fluorouracil	Conventional dose	Angina/myocardial infarction
Vincristine	Conventional dose	Myocardial infarction
Vinblastine	Conventional dose	Myocardial infarction
Busulfan	Conventional oral daily dose	Endocardial fibrosis
Mitomycin C	Conventional dose	Myocardial damage similar to radiation-induced injury
Cisplatin	Conventional dose	Acute myocardial ischemia
Amsacrine	Conventional dose	Ventricular arrhythmias
Taxol	Conventional dose	Bradycardia
Interferons	Conventional dose	Exacerbates underlying cardiac disease
Interleukin-2	Conventional dose	Acute myocardial injury, ventricular arrhythmias, hypotension

*Route of administration is intravenous unless otherwise indicated. Conventional dose is the commonly accepted therapeutic range.
From Holland JF: Cancer Medicine. 4th ed. Baltimore, Williams & Wilkins, 1997, p 897.

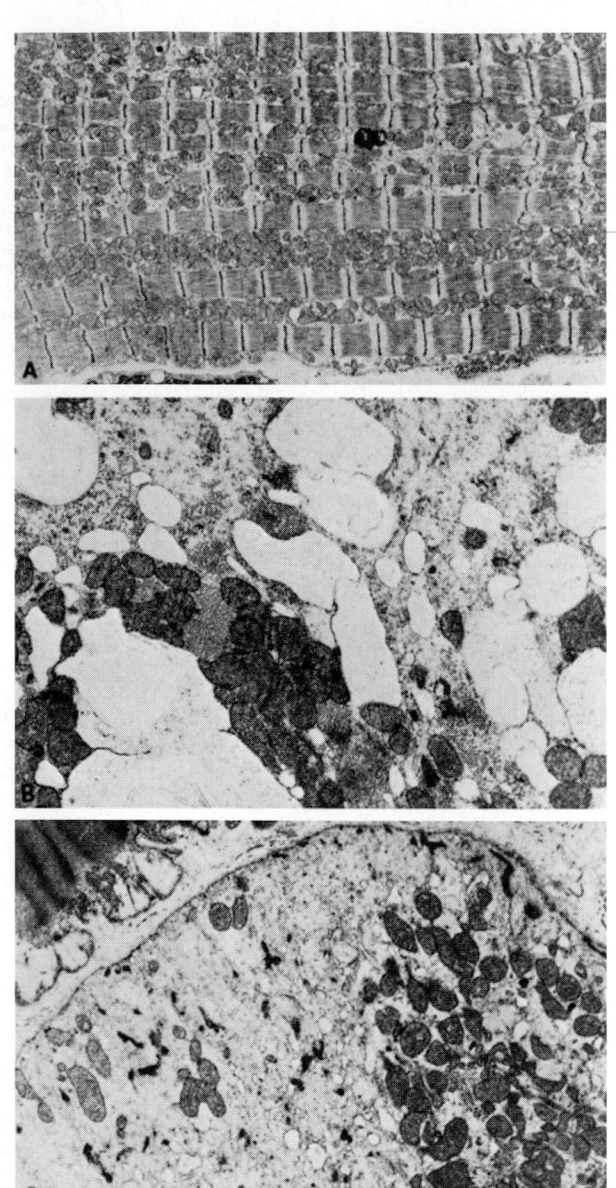

FIGURE 69–9. Ultrastructural features of an anthracycline-induced cardiac toxicity. *A,* Normal. *B,* Vacuolation. *C,* Myofibrillar dropout. *B* and *C* are after doxorubicin therapy. (From Ali MD, Ewer MS: Cancer and the Cardiopulmonary System. New York, Raven Press, 1984, pp 62–63.)

ministered, the clinical expression of the dilated congestive cardiomyopathy generally does not occur until a threshold cumulative dose (which differs for each anthracycline) is reached. Although mortality for anthracycline-induced cardiomyopathy was formerly believed to be as high as 40 percent, recent reports in the current era of afterload reduction suggest a better prognosis. Nonetheless, once heart failure due to long-term exposure to these agents becomes clinically apparent, the disease should be taken very seriously. In a recently published study in which the outcomes of 1230 patients with cardiomyopathies were assessed with a median follow-up of 4.4 years, patients with doxorubicin-associated cardiomyopathy had an inferior survival (hazard ratio 3.46, 95 percent confidence interval 1.67–7.18) compared with patients with idiopathic cardiomyopathy[185] (Fig. 69–11). The timing of the onset of clinical symptoms of congestive heart failure relative to anthracycline exposure can vary substantially. In one small series, heart failure developed at a mean time of 4 weeks (range, 1–17 weeks)

from the last dose of chemotherapy. The course was more severe in those patients who had a higher (>300 mg/m²) dose of doxorubicin.[186]

Standard therapy including inotropic agents, diuresis, and afterload reduction represent the typical medical management of patients with anthracycline-induced cardiomyopathy; some studies have suggested that beta-receptor antagonists might also have a role.[187–189] Selected patients with severe cardiomyopathy who also have a lower likelihood of responding to medical therapy have undergone successful heart transplantation.[190, 191]

Chronic cardiomyopathy resulting in overt congestive heart failure that might require such a drastic intervention as cardiac transplantation is probably less common than the so-called late-onset anthracycline cardiotoxicity, which can cause a more subtle degree of ventricular dysfunction and/ or arrhythmias[177] many years after the anthracyclines have been given.[192] Such delayed-onset effects are a particularly important issue in children who have received moderate to large doses of anthracyclines during therapy for acute lymphoblastic leukemia.[193–195] Because several studies that have observed patients longitudinally after exposure to anthracyclines during childhood have shown that echocardiographic abnormalities progress over time, there is concern about the potentially widened scope of eventual clinical cardiac dysfunction in such patients. For example, a reduction in intraventricular septum and posterior wall diastolic dimensions is more pronounced 7 years after exposure to anthracyclines than in control subjects.[196] The long-term clinical relevance of such findings is unclear. Moreover, whether the low level of elevation in serum cardiac troponin-T levels, indicating some degree of acute injury, which occurs during acute therapy with doxorubicin, has any clinical impact is unclear, although elevations correlated with abnormal echocardiograms 9 months after chemotherapy.[197] Some clinical deterioration of cardiac function can be detected more readily with the specialized technique of automatic border detection compared with conventional echocardiography[198] or with indium-111/antimyosin scintigraphy.[199] Echocardiographic abnormalities are more common in girls and those patients exposed at a young age to a high cumulative dose of doxorubicin.[200] Although the eventual clinical impact of the type of systolic and diastolic dysfunction documented as a late effect in children and adults treated with anthracyclines remains unclear, the onset of laboratory evidence of cardiac abnormality has correlated with congestive symptoms in patients with cardiomyopathies due to other causes.[201]

MONITORING OF PATIENTS RECEIVING ANTHRACYCLINES. The ideal monitoring system for the occurrence of anthracycline-induced cardiotoxicity would be noninvasive, a reliable predictor of eventual clinical dysfunction, and detect disease early enough so that an effective therapeutic strategy could be used. Endomyocardial biopsy, radionuclide angiocardiography, resting echocardiography, and exercise echocardiography have each been used in an effort to predict the development of the so-called early or classic cardiomyopathy. Although endomyocardial biopsy grade can predict the rate of potential clinical progression, sampling errors due to patchy myocardial involvement, invasiveness, and expense have limited the routine use of this technique.[177, 202]

Patients receiving anthracyclines over time are often followed with radionuclide ventriculography, based on an earlier study that suggested that a 15 percent decline in left ventricular ejection fraction (LVEF), or a LVEF of less than 40 percent, occurred in those at high risk for clinical cardiac decompensation.[203] However, concerns have been raised regarding the problem that by the time the LVEF falls a significant amount of myocardium has already been irretrievably lost. Echocardiographic features, such as meas-

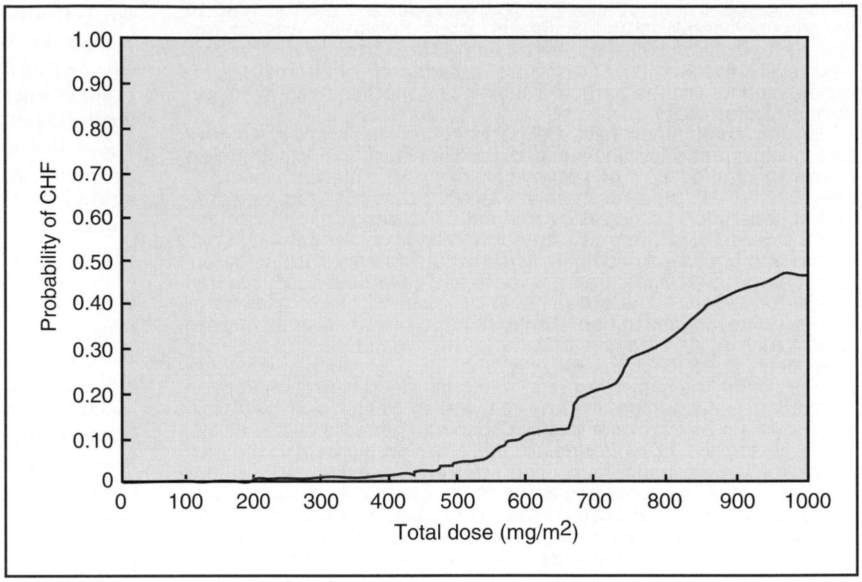

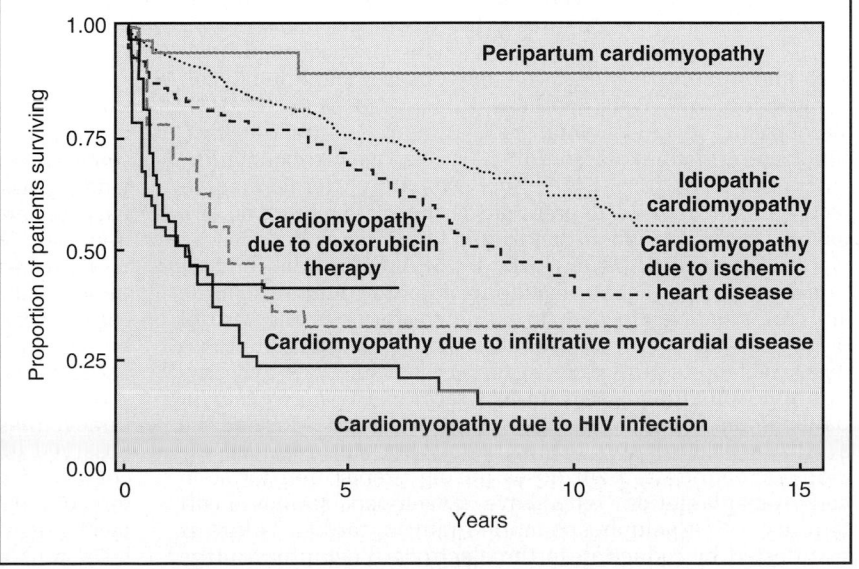

FIGURE 69–10. Anthracycline cardiotoxicity: relationship of dose to the incidence of congestive heart failure. (From Shan K, et al: Anthracycline-induced cardiotoxicity. Ann Intern Med 125:47–58, 1996.)

urement of the rate of relaxation and fractional shortening of diastolic filling, can also serve as a potentially sensitive means of detecting the early onset anthracycline-induced chronic cardiomyopathy.[204]

The value of very sensitive tests of ventricular function to detect so-called late-onset cardiomyopathy has been discussed earlier with regard to findings on echocardiography or radionuclide angiography in children many years after receiving anthracyclines. Dobutamine/exercise echocardiography and exercise radionuclide angiography have each been somewhat predictive of this late-onset cardiac dysfunction in patients with normal resting cardiac function.[177] However, the importance of these relatively subtle abnormalities, generally of diastolic dysfunction, is even more unclear in the case of late-onset cardiomyopathy, compared with that of early detection of the chronic dilated cardiomyopathy, which occurs much earlier relative to the chemotherapy treatment.[205]

PREVENTION OF ANTHRACYCLINE-INDUCED CARDIO-TOXICITY. Strategies for minimizing cardiotoxic effects of anthracyclines include altering the dose and schedule, use of new formulation of anthracyclines (e.g., liposome-encapsulated), calcium channel or beta-adrenergic blocker phar-

macological approaches, and "true" cardioprotection using iron-chelating agents and/or free radical scavengers. Each of these strategies has shown some ability to limit cardiotoxicity. However, ensuring antineoplastic efficacy remains a major issue with regard to most of the putative cardioprotective agents. It has been recognized for more than 20 years that administration of a given dose of doxorubicin in smaller fractions or by continuous infusion schedules would produce less cardiac toxicity without any apparent compromise of antineoplastic activity.[206–209] Examples of changes in dose schedule to produce less cardiotoxicity include weekly dosing of doxorubicin (rather than every 3 weeks) in breast cancer patients, continuous infusion of doxorubicin in patients with multiple myeloma or non-Hodgkin lymphoma (which might also have better activity in drug-resistant cells), or giving the drug over 6 hours.[210]

Liposome-encapsulated anthracyclines may allow administration of a higher total with less cardiotoxicity. Endomyocardial biopsies indicate less marked histopathological changes at a given dose of anthracycline when given by the liposomal route.[211-214] However, it remains of critical importance to ensure that the use of liposome-encapsulated anthracyclines does not reduce antitumor efficacy. A recent provocative study compared docetaxel, a taxane, versus doxorubicin, in patients with metastatic breast cancer who had received previous

FIGURE 69–11. Mortality from various causes of cardiomyopathy. (From Felker GM, et al: Underlying causes and long-term survival in patients with initially unexplained cardiomyopathy. N Engl J Med 342:1077–1084, 2000.)

alkylating-agent chemotherapy.[215] Not only was the median time to progression longer in the docetaxel group but there was no cardiotoxicity in this group, compared with four deaths in the patients who received doxorubicin. Therefore, substitution of alternative efficacious agents for the anthracyclines is yet another strategy for reducing cardiotoxicity.

Several compounds have been tested for their ability to protect against anthracycline-induced cardiomyopathy, including dexrazoxane, amifostine, glutathione, vitamin E, mesna, and ORG 2766.[168, 175, 216, 217] These drugs block toxicity by either reducing free radical generation or increasing free radical scavenging. Dexrazoxane, which has received the most attention, readily penetrates cell membranes and appears to complex with metal cofactors, including iron. Chelation of intracellular iron may decrease doxorubicin-induced free radical formation.[175] The drug should be given within 30 minutes of anthracycline administration. Three randomized, placebo-controlled clinical trials of dexrazoxane in patients with advanced breast cancer have been conducted in which a total of 626 patients were enrolled.[175, 218-220] The mean decrease in left ventricular injection fraction by radionuclide scanning was lower in women treated with dexrazoxane. However, dexrazoxane was not shown to increase overall or disease-free survival. At higher doses, there was an increase in the incidence of myelosuppression, and concern remains that tumor response rates may be decreased.[168] Moreover, it is not known whether the drug can protect against delayed-onset cardiotoxicity. The vagueness of the American Cancer Society Clinical Practice Guidelines reflects the many unanswered questions regarding the use of the agent. In fact, the only setting in which the agent is recommended even for consideration is in patients who have received 300/mg/m² or more of doxorubicin yet who might benefit from further anthracycline.[168]

Other agents with antioxidant effect, such as probucol, coenzyme Q10, and melatonin, may provide cardioprotection without affecting tumor response rates, at least based on animal data.[221-224] These promising early results await additional confirmatory studies. Pilot data with calcium antagonists[225] and beta-adrenergic blockers,[189, 226] such as metoprolol, have also been developed. Finally, a transgenic mouse overexpressing the human complementary DNA for multiple drug resistance, driven by an alpha-cardiac myosin gene, has been developed.[227] The animals are resistant to doxorubicin-mediated myocyte dropout.

Cardiotoxicity of Other Antineoplastic Agents

5-FLUOROURACIL (5-FU). This is a fluorinated pyrimidine that undergoes under intracellular metabolism to deoxy-5-fluorouracil monophosphate, an inhibitor of the enzyme thymidylate synthase (as well as interfering with DNA and RNA metabolism). 5-FU is used to treat several important solid tumors, including colorectal cancer, squamous cell carcinoma of the head and neck, and breast cancer. Although it is not a common cause of cardiotoxicity, patients with prior coronary disease and/or those receiving concurrent radiation therapy are at risk for 5-FU-induced heart disease. Vasoocclusive complications, particularly acute myocardial infarction, may be somewhat more likely in patients receiving 5-FU-based chemotherapy. Clinical manifestations of 5-FU cardiotoxicity, which occurs in less than 2 percent of patients receiving this drug, include typical ischemic electrocardiographic changes, chest pain, nausea, and diaphoresis.[228] 5-FU may cause endothelial cell contraction and lysis, perhaps on a vasospastic basis.[229] Vasospastic-type ischemia, arrhythmias, contractile dysfunction, and frank infarction have also been documented in connection with 5-FU.[230-232] Fortunately, the cardiac effects, including mild depression of contractile function, are usually reversible when the drug is withdrawn.[233-237]

CYCLOPHOSPHAMIDE AND IFOSFAMIDE. The bifunctional alkylating agents cyclophosphamide and ifosfamide are converted in the liver to an active form. In the case of cyclophosphamide, hepatic microsomal mixed function oxidases metabolize the drug to the active moiety, 4-hydroxycyclophosphamide. A severe myocardiopathy may occur in patients receiving high doses of these drugs. Most of the available data comes from patients who have received cyclophosphamide at high doses during preparation for stem cell transplantation who have developed serious heart failure.[238, 239] Cyclophosphamide-induced cardiac failure is manifested by reduction in the electrocardiographic voltage

on systolic function and increase in myocardial mass due to edema, with pathology indicating acute myocyte necrosis, hemorrhagic myopericarditis, and endothelial injury. Preexisting heart disease is a predisposing factor,[240] and mortality approaches 33 percent. Six of 19 women undergoing autologous bone marrow transplantation for breast cancer developed transient clinical and chest radiographic evidence of moderate congestive heart failure during the course of recovery from transplantation, with a median time of onset on day 13 after chemotherapy. The median area under the curve of cyclophosphamide concentration was lower in those patients who developed cardiotoxicity, presumably owing to a high rate of conversion of parent compound to the active metabolite.[239] Ifosfamide can cause a similar syndrome of heart failure.[241]

OTHER AGENTS. Preparative regimens for bone marrow transplantation involving high doses of cyclophosphamide, frequently along with total-body radiation, are not infrequently associated with subacute cardiotoxicity.[242] Life-threatening cardiotoxicity is rare (less than 2 percent) in the posttransplant setting; however, cardiac events seem to be more common in those with a reduced ejection fraction at baseline. Consequently, most transplant protocols eliminate from eligibility patients who have impaired cardiac function at the time of transplant. It is possible that with the advent of so-called miniallogeneic transplant protocols[243] in which the dose of conditioning regimens is decreased in favor of the graft-versus-cancer effect, that such cardiotoxicity will be less common in the future.

Although cisplatin,[244] bleomycin,[245] and *Vinca* alkaloids[246] do not generally cause direct cardiac muscle damage, each of these agents does have potential endothelial and vasospastic[247] effects. As such, it is perhaps not surprising that myocardial infarction has been described. Moreover, because cisplatin causes renal tubular potassium and magnesium wasting, electrocardiographic abnormalities are not uncommon.

The taxanes, relatively new to the clinic, are useful in patients with a host of neoplasms, including breast, lung, and ovarian cancer. Paclitaxel and docetaxel have been associated with the development of brachycardia; it is now recognized that such events are rare (<10 percent), may have been due to the formerly used carrier, and are generally not clinically significant.[248] These agents do not appear to have any long-term cardiac side effects. Minimal added toxicity from the addition of paclitaxel to doxorubicin for the treatment of breast cancer has been noted.[249, 250] Interferon alfa, which is used in hairy cell leukemia, chronic myelogenous leukemia, and Kaposi sarcoma, can occasionally cause a severe congestive cardiomyopathy with myocardial dysfunction, which is generally reversible with discontinuation of the drug.[251, 252]

High-dose interleukin-2, which may have a role in the treatment of selected patients with renal cancer and melanoma, can cause high fevers and myalgias, as well as, in some cases, life-threatening capillary leak syndromes, including tissue edema, hypotension, noncardiogenic pulmonary edema, renal failure, and an occasional myocardial infarction.[252-254]

Trastuzamab (Herceptin) is a humanized monoclonal antibody that targets the human epidermal growth factor receptor (HER-2), which is overexpressed in 30 percent of breast carcinomas. This novel agent is associated with clinical responses in HER-2, overexpressing breast cancer when given alone[255] or with other agents such as taxanes or anthracyclines.[256] However, a cardiomyopathy similar to that observed after doxorubicin therapy has been noted. In the context of the known expression of HER-2 or HER-3 receptors in myocardial tissue, this is of concern. The precise mechanism and incidence, if any, of Herceptin-mediated heart problems requires evaluation.[257]

HEMATOLOGICAL EFFECTS OF CARDIAC MEDICATIONS
(See also Chap. 62)

Reports exist linking virtually every drug with hematological abnormalities. The focus in this section is primarily on the more common and clinically important hematological effects produced by medications currently employed in the clinical practice of cardiovascular medicine. For a broader discussion of hematological effects of cardiac medications currently less used, the reader can consult previous editions of this text. This discussion considers, in turn, thrombocytopenia, granulocytopenia/aplastic anemia, and anemia.

Thrombocytopenia

HEPARIN-INDUCED THROMBOCYTOPENIA (HIT) (see also Chap. 62). Heparin, a commonly used anticoagulant in cardiovascular diseases, frequently causes thrombocytopenia. Two forms of HIT can occur. In type I HIT, thrombocytopenia occurs within days of initiating therapy. Type I HIT causes modest thrombocytopenia with levels seldom below 75,000 cells/μL. This form of HIT probably results from increased aggregation of platelets that have been crosslinked by the highly negatively charged heparin molecule. Type I HIT is common, occurring in several percent of patients receiving heparin therapy. Type I HIT generally improves with time, even with continuation of heparin treatment.

In contrast, type II HIT produces more severe thrombocytopenia with levels often below 50,000 cells/cm³. Type II HIT occurs later after initiation of therapy, typically between 4 days and 2 weeks of treatment. In type II HIT, thrombosis as well as bleeding can occur. The mechanism of type II HIT involves binding of exogenously administered heparin to a platelet surface protein known as platelet factor 4 (PF4). When an IgG antibody that recognizes this PF4/heparin complex binds, the ternary complex associates with platelet receptors for the Fc portion of the immunoglobulin molecule. Ligation of the Fc receptors causes platelet activation and thrombosis. The second form of HIT requires immediate cessation of heparin therapy. Even heparin flushes of peripheral intravenous catheters should be avoided. Low-molecular-weight heparin is associated with a much lower incidence of HIT.[258] Thrombin inhibitors such as hirudin and argatroban may be very useful as replacement for heparin in type HIT, when even low-molecular-weight heparin must be used with caution.[259]

GLYCOPROTEIN (GP) IIb/IIIa ANTAGONISTS (see also Chap. 62). The introduction of IIb/IIIa antagonists represents one of the major advances in cardiology in the past decade. Numerous studies have shown improved outcomes after coronary intervention and the acute coronary syndromes due to administration of these agents.[260] GP IIb/IIIa antagonists currently available for intravenous use include a chimeric antibody (abciximab), small organic molecules (e.g., tirofiban), and a cyclic oligopeptide (eptifibatide). A number of orally active agents exist as well. Each of these drugs can cause thrombocytopenia[261] (Fig. 69-12). Defining clinically significant thrombocytopenia as less than 50,000/μL, the incidence with small molecules is 0.6 to 0.8 percent, with abciximab up to 2 percent.

Administration of these agents requires careful monitoring for thrombocytopenia. A baseline platelet count should be obtained; a basal level of less than 100,000/μL is a relative contraindication to GP IIb/IIIa antagonist use. A platelet count should be obtained 1 to 4 hours after administration of a GP IIb/IIIa antagonist. If the platelet count falls below 50 percent of baseline or less than 100,000/μL,

Agent	No. of patients
Abciximab	6,272
Tirofiban	7,159
Eptifibatide	15,486
Lamifiban	3,758
GP IIb/IIIa + heparin	27,196
GP IIb/IIIa, no heparin	6,038

FIGURE 69-12. A meta-analysis of rates of thrombocytopenia associated with use of intravenous GP IIb/IIIa antagonists. Data shown compile results from 28 clinical trials. The odds ratio (OR) and 95% confidence intervals (CI) for each agent are depicted on the whisker plots. (After Giugliano RP; from Madan M, Berkowitz SD: Understanding thrombocytopenia and antigenicity with glycoprotein IIb-IIIa inhibitors. Am Heart J 138:317-326, 1999.)

the agent should be discontinued. Because the clinical indications for GP IIb/IIIa and heparin therapy are similar, coadministration of these agents occurs commonly. Hence, the differential diagnosis of thrombocytopenia due to GP IIb/IIIa antagonists versus heparin-induced thrombocytopenia is a common clinical dilemma. Clues to the differential diagnosis include the time course of onset of the thrombocytopenia. The decline in platelet count with GP IIb/IIIa antagonists typically occurs during the first day, whereas there is a delay of 3 to 4 days in type I HIT. Laboratory evaluation of heparin/PF4/IgG complexes can also aid the differential diagnosis.

Several mechanisms may account for the thrombocytopenia associated with GP IIb/IIIa antagonist administration.[262] One mechanism is analogous to the "innocent bystander" mechanism often responsible for drug-induced hemolytic anemia. In this situation, an antibody binds to the drug, as well as to the platelets. Complement-induced lysis, or enhanced clearance by the spleen due to opsonization, can reduce platelet number. Another potential mechanism involves an antibody response directed against a conformational epitope on the IIb/IIIa complex itself. When a ligand binds to GP IIb/IIIa, it can induce a shape change that uncovers a new antigenic determinant, or epitope, a ligand-induced binding site. The immune response targets a normally concealed part of the GP IIb/IIIa molecule revealed upon binding of the antagonist.

Another potential mechanism is applicable specifically to the chimeric antibody abciximab.[263] In this situation, a portion of the chimeric antibody that retains mouse sequences in the hinge region of the immunoglobulin molecule can engender an antibody response. This mechanism has been called a human anti-chimeric antibody reaction. Because this mechanism requires generation of a antibody response to the foreign epitope (mouse sequences in the chimeric antibody), its onset would be later than most GP IIb/IIIa antagonist-induced thrombocytopenic episodes. Complement-induced lysis of platelet binding the antibody presumably causes the thrombocytopenia. Readministration of abciximab within 2 weeks can lead to profound thrombocytopenia in approximately 12 percent of patients.[264]

The treatment of thrombocytopenia associated with administration of GP IIb/IIIa antagonists involves stopping the drug. Platelet transfusion may prove necessary if the platelet count drops below 20,000/μL3. Although the mechanisms may differ, all three structurally distinct classes of GP IIb/IIIa antagonists can cause thrombocytopenia. Curiously, a number of recent trials with oral GP IIb/IIIa antagonists have shown not only no benefit in terms of event reduction but also a tendency to increase events.[265] The reason for the unexpected lack of efficacy of the oral GP IIb/IIIa antagonists remains uncertain.

THIENOPYRIDINES AND THROMBOTIC THROMBOCYTOPENIC PURPURA. The introduction of thienopyridine antiplatelet agents has proven a boon in interventional cardiology and for aspirin-allergic patients with atherosclerotic disease. These drugs (ticlopidine and clopidogrel) bind to an adenosine diphosphate receptor on the surface of platelets that mediates platelet activation and propagation of platelet aggregation. Before the use of thienopyridine agents, abrupt thrombosis represented a major limitation to the use of coronary stents. Lengthy hospital stays to achieve therapeutic anticoagulation with warfarin were inconvenient for patients, expensive, fraught with the risk of bleeding with intensive warfarin therapy, and eventually proved less effective than administration of aspirin and thienopyridine after coronary stenting.[266]

Patients with atherosclerosis with indications for aspirin who are unable to take this agent due to allergy have also benefited from thienopyridine therapy.[267] Considerable data establish the utility of agents of this class in reducing unstable coronary events and stroke in patients at risk. However, the possibility of developing thrombotic thrombocytopenic purpura (TTP) requires careful thought when considering use of thienopyridines. First recognized with ticlopidine, and subsequently with clopidogrel, TTP due to thienopyridines presents as the classic findings of thrombocytopenia, microangiopathic hemolytic anemia, central nervous system abnormalities, and renal dysfunction. Because prevention of recurrent strokes is a common indication for this class of drugs, mental status changes due to TTP can present a diagnostic challenge. TTP due to ticlopidine occurs in approximately 1 in 1600 treated patients.[268] The incidence of clopidogrel-induced TTP requires more extensive study but is probably substantially lower.[269]

TTP is life threatening. Death occurs in about a third of patients with ticlopidine-associated TTP. Plasmapheresis should be instituted as soon as the diagnosis is made and appears to strikingly reduce mortality (from 60 percent from patients not undergoing plasmapheresis to 22 percent of those plasmapheresed).[268] The physician should remain vigilant in all patients receiving thienopyridines for early clinical signs of TTP, including rashes or confusion. The finding of schistocytes on a peripheral blood smear supports the diagnosis of TTP. Fortunately, most episodes of TTP due to thienopyridines occur during the first 3 months of therapy, after which point patients require less surveillance.

The precise mechanism of thienopyridine-induced TTP remains elusive. However, it may involve generation of an antibody that inhibits a metalloproteinase important for processing large multimers of von Willebrand factor.[270, 271] Antibody-induced inhibition of this metalloproteinase favors the accumulation of the large von Willebrand factor multimers, which more effectively promote platelet aggregation and cross-linking than lower molecular weight forms.

TTP, although rare, is a serious and frequently lethal complication of thienopyridine therapy. In patients requiring coronary stent placement, the risk/benefit ratio of thienopyridine use, limited to a few weeks, supports the use of these agents to prevent the otherwise common and often disastrous complication of abrupt thrombosis. In candidates for antiplatelet therapy with aspirin allergy, selection of a thienopyridine also likely has a net benefit for the patient. In patients able to tolerate aspirin, individual decisions regarding the use of thienopyridines based on the particular clinical scenario seem warranted.

QUINIDINE. Quinidine, once a mainstay of antiarrhythmic therapy, has lost popularity in recent years. Hematological side effects, including thrombocytopenia, in addition to a potential proarrhythmic effect, has contributed to the decline in quinidine's use in the clinic. The mechanism of quinidine-induced thrombocytopenia probably involves a humoral immune response.[272] Cessation of the drug generally leads to a gradual increase in platelet number over a period of days. Alkalization of the urine can help promote the elimination of quinidine, a weak base. Intravenous immunoglobulin may also mitigate quinidine-induced thrombocytopenia.[273]

OTHER CARDIOVASCULAR MEDICATIONS ASSOCIATED WITH THROMBOCYTOPENIA. Several other cardiac medications cause thrombocytopenia less frequently. However, several of these agents are in very common clinical use, resulting in the number of patients at risk is considerable (Table 69–4). These agents include the thiazide diuretics, furosemide, digoxin, procainamide, and the phosphodiesterase inhibitor inotropic agents, such as amrinone or milrinone.[274] A comprehensive listing of drugs that induce thrombocytopenia can be found on the Internet at http://moon.ouhsc.edu/jgeorge.

Leukopenia/Aplastic Anemia

Granulocytopenia can occur during treatment with a wide variety of cardiovascular drugs.[275] The sulfhydryl group containing angiotensin-converting enzyme inhibitors (the "prils") represents one class of cardiac medications that with increasing use occasionally causes leukopenia. Procainamide (particularly sustained-release procainamide) can cause severe leukopenia.[276, 277] The granulocytopenia improves after cessation of procainamide treatment. Interestingly, the leukopenia can occur independently of the well-known procainamide-induced lupus syndrome.[278] Granulocyte colony-stimulating factor is one therapeutic option for drug-induced thrombocytopenia.[279] Other cardiovascular drugs that can cause agranulocytosis or aplastic

▼ **TABLE 69–4. CURRENTLY USED CARDIAC DRUGS IMPLICATED IN DRUG-INDUCED THROMBOCYTOPENIA***

AGENT	FREQUENCY OF USE	INCIDENCE	BLEEDING	THROMBOSIS	CLINICAL IMPORTANCE
Furosemide	++++	+	+	−	+++
Heparin	++++	+++	+	+++	++++
Thiazides	++++	+	+	−	+
Aspirin	+++	+	+++	−	+
Digoxin/digitoxin	+++	+	++	−	+
Glycoprotein IIb/IIIa blockers	+++	++	++	−	+++
Thienopyridines	+++	+	++	++	++
Quinine/quinidine	++	++	+++	−	++
Alpha-methyldopa	+	++	++	−	+
Amrinone, milrinone	+	++	++	−	+
Procainamide	+	+	++	−	+

*Plus (+) and minus (−) signs indicate subjective impressions of the frequency and importance of selected aspects of drug-induced thrombocytopenia, ranging from very low (−) to very high (++++).

Adapted from Giugliano RP: Drug-induced thrombocytopenia: Is it a serious concern for glycoprotein IIb/IIIa receptor inhibitors? J Thromb Thrombolysis 5:191–202, 1998.

anemia include beta blockers, such as propranolol, dipyridamole, digoxin, and nifedipine.[275] The thienopyridine ticlopidine causes granulocytopenia in about 2.5 percent of recipients. A leukocyte count should be obtained before and at 2-week intervals during the first 3 months. If the drug is omitted during the first 3 months of therapy, a follow-up white blood cell count should be monitored for an additional 2 weeks, because patients are at risk for leukopenia even after stopping ticlopidine. Among the immunosuppressants used in cardiac transplantation recipients, azathioprine can cause a dose-related decrease in white blood cell count. This represents a mechanism-based toxicity related to the drug's primary mode of action as an immunosuppressant.

Anemia

Cardiac medications seem to cause anemia less commonly than thrombocytopenia or leukopenia. Hemolytic anemia due to methyldopa is seen less frequently, because use of this antihypertensive agent has declined. One currently used medication associated with hemolytic anemia is quinidine. Phenytoin, now uncommonly used as an antiarrhythmic agent, and triamterene, a common component of combination diuretic drugs, can cause megaloblastic anemia.

REFERENCES

IRON AND THE HEART

1. Andrews NC: Disorders of iron metabolism. N Engl J Med 341:1986–1995, 1999.
2. Brandhagen DJ, Fairbanks VF, Batts KP, et al: Update on hereditary hemochromatosis and the HFE gene. Mayo Clin Proc 74:917–921, 1999.
3. Feder JN, Penny DM, Irrinki A, et al: The hemochromatosis gene product complexes with the transferrin receptor and lowers its affinity for ligand binding. Proc Natl Acad Sci U S A 95:1472–1477, 1998.
4. Andrews NC, Levy JE: Iron is hot: An update on the pathophysiology of hemochromatosis. Blood 92:1845–1851, 1998.
5. Cardoso EM, Stal P, Hagen K, et al: HFE mutations in patients with hereditary haemochromatosis in Sweden. J Intern Med 243:203–208, 1998.
6. Ryan E, O'Keane C, Crowe J: Hemochromatosis in Ireland and HFE. Blood Cells Mol Dis 24:428–432, 1998.
7. Powell LW, George DK, McDonnell SM, et al: Diagnosis of hemochromatosis. Ann Intern Med 129:925–931, 1998.
8. Monaghan KG, Rybicki BA, Shurafa M, et al: Mutation analysis of the HFE gene associated with hereditary hemochromatosis in African Americans. Am J Hematol 58:213–217, 1998.
9. Merryweather-Clarke AT, Pointon JJ, Shearman JD, et al: Global prevalence of putative haemochromatosis mutations. J Med Genet 34:275–278, 1997.
10. Giardina PJ, Hilgartner MW: Update on thalassemia. Pediatr Rev 13:55–62, 1992.
11. Piomelli S, Loew T: Management of thalassemia major (Cooley's anemia). Hematol Oncol Clin North Am 5:557–569, 1991.
12. Bonkovsky HL: Iron and the liver. Am J Med Sci 301:32–43, 1991.
13. McCord JM: Human disease, free radicals, and the oxidant/antioxidant balance. Clin Biochem 26:351–357, 1993.
14. Farber JL: Mechanisms of cell injury by activated oxygen species. Environ Health Perspect 102(Suppl 10):17–24, 1994.
15. Abdalla DS, Campa A, Monteiro HP: Low density lipoprotein oxidation by stimulated neutrophils and ferritin. Atherosclerosis 97:149–159, 1992.
16. Enright HU, Miller WJ, Hebbel RP: Nucleosomal histone protein protects DNA from iron-mediated damage. Nucl Acids Res 20:3341–3346, 1992.
17. Link G, Konijn AM, Hershko C: Cardioprotective effect of alpha-tocopherol, ascorbate, deferoxamine, and deferiprone: Mitochondrial function in cultured, iron-loaded heart cells. J Lab Clin Med 133:179–188, 1999.
18. Scopinaro F, Banci M, Vania A, et al: Radioisotope assessment of heart damage in hypertransfused thalassaemic patients. Eur J Nucl Med 20:603–608, 1993.
19. Vanotti D, Gennari P, Pisani E, et al: Quantitative ultrasonic analysis of myocardium in patients with thalassemia major and iron overload. Circulation 87:748–754, 1993.
20. Aldouri MA, Wonke B, Hoffbrand AV, et al: High incidence of cardiomyopathy in beta-thalassaemia patients receiving regular transfusion and iron chelation: Reversal by intensified chelation. Acta Haematol 84:113–117, 1990.
21. Olivieri NF, Nathan DG, MacMillan JH, et al: Survival in medically

treated patients with homozygous beta-thalassemia. N Engl J Med 331:574–578, 1994.
22. Davis BA, Porter JB: Long-term outcome of continuous 24-hour deferoxamine infusion via indwelling intravenous catheters in high-risk β-thalassemia. Blood 95:1229–1236, 2000.
23. Lucarelli G, Galimberti M, Polchi P, et al: Marrow transplantation in patients with thalassemia responsive to iron chelation therapy. N Engl J Med 329:840–844, 1993.
24. Giardini C, Angelucci E, Lucarelli G, et al: Bone marrow transplantation for thalassemia. Experience in Pesaro, Italy. Am J Pediatr Hematol Oncol 16:6–10, 1994.
25. Angelucci E, Muretto P, Lucarelli G, et al: Treatment of iron overload in the "ex-thalassemic." Report from the phlebotomy program. Ann NY Acad Sci 850:288–293, 1998.
26. Mariotti E, Angelucci E, Agostini A, et al: Evaluation of cardiac status in iron-loaded thalassaemia patients following bone marrow transplantation: Improvement in cardiac function during reduction in body iron burden. Br J Haematol 103:916–921, 1998.
27. Salonen JT, Nyyssonen K, Korpela H, et al: High stored iron levels are associated with excess risk of myocardial infarction in eastern Finnish men. Circulation 86:803–811, 1992.
28. Tuomainen TP, Punnonen K, Nyyssonen K, et al: Association between body iron stores and the risk of acute myocardial infarction in men. Circulation 97:1461–1466, 1998.
29. Sempos CT, Looker AC, Gillum RF, et al: Body iron stores and the risk of coronary heart disease. N Engl J Med 330:1119–1124, 1994.
30. Magnusson MK, Sigfusson N, Sigvaldason H, et al: Low iron-binding capacity as a risk factor for myocardial infarction. Circulation 89:102–108, 1994.
31. Bahl VK, Malhotra OP, Kumar D, et al: Noninvasive assessment of systolic and diastolic left ventricular function in patients with chronic severe anemia: A combined M-mode, two-dimensional, and Doppler echocardiographic study. Am Heart J 124:1516–1523, 1992.
32. Hayashi R, Ogawa S, Watanabe Z, et al: Cardiovascular function before and after iron therapy by echocardiography in patients with iron deficiency anemia. Pediatr Int 41:13–17, 1999.
33. Kwiatkowski JL, West TB, Heidary N, et al: Severe iron deficiency anemia in young children. J Pediatr 135:514–516, 1999.
34. San M, Demirtascedil M, Burgut R, et al: Left ventricular systolic and diastolic function in patients with sickle cell anemia. Int J Angiol 7:185–187, 1998.
35. Carneskog J, Safai-Kutti S, Suurkula M, et al: The red cell mass, plasma erythropoietin and spleen size in apparent polycythaemia. Eur J Haematol 62:43–48, 1999.
36. Watts EJ, Lewis SM: Spurious polycythaemia—a study of 35 patients. Scand J Haematol 31:241–247, 1983.
37. Messinezy M, Pearson TC: ABC of clinical haematology: Polycythaemia, primary (essential) thrombocythaemia and myelofibrosis. BMJ 314:587–590, 1997.
38. Berlin NI: Diagnosis and classification of the polycythemias. Semin Hematol 12:339–351, 1975.
39. Swan L, Hillis WS: Management of polycythaemia in adults with cyanotic congenital heart disease. Heart 81:451, 1999.
40. Leach M, Greaves M, Porter N, et al: Haemoglobin Hallamshire (beta146 HIS → TYR): A new high oxygen affinity haemoglobin responsible for familial erythrocytosis. Clin Lab Haematol 18:237–239, 1996.
41. Trimble M, Caro J, Talalla A, et al: Secondary erythrocytosis due to a cerebellar hemangioblastoma: Demonstration of erythropoietin mRNA in the tumor. Blood 78:599–601, 1991.
42. Shiramizu M, Katsuoka Y, Grodberg J, et al: Constitutive secretion of erythropoietin by human renal adenocarcinoma cells in vivo and in vitro. Exp Cell Res 215:249–256, 1994.
43. Muta H, Funakoshi A, Baba T, et al: Gene expression of erythropoietin in hepatocellular carcinoma. Intern Med 33:427–431, 1994.
44. Landolfi R, Rocca B, Patrono C: Bleeding and thrombosis in myeloproliferative disorders: Mechanisms and treatment. Crit Rev Oncol Hematol 20:203–222, 1995.
45. Moliterno AR, Hankins WD, Spivak JL: Impaired expression of the thrombopoietin receptor by platelets from patients with polycythemia vera. N Engl J Med 338:572–580, 1998.
46. Gilliland DG, Blanchard KL, Levy J, et al: Clonality in myeloproliferative disorders: Analysis by means of the polymerase chain reaction. Proc Natl Acad Sci U S A 88:6848–6852, 1991.
47. Goyal RK, Longmore GD: Abnormalities of cytokine receptor signalling contributing to diseases of red blood cell production. Ann Med 31:208–216, 1999.
48. Tefferi A: Diagnosing polycythemia vera: A paradigm shift. Mayo Clin Proc 74:159–162, 1999.
49. Correa PN, Eskinazi D, Axelrad AA: Circulating erythroid progenitors in polycythemia vera are hypersensitive to insulin-like growth factor-1 in vitro: Studies in an improved serum-free medium. Blood 83:99–112, 1994.
50. Wickrema A, Chen F, Namin F, et al: Defective expression of the SHP-1 phosphatase in polycythemia vera. Exp Hematol 27:1124–1132, 1999.
51. Arcasoy MO, Harris KW, Forget BG: A human erythropoietin receptor gene mutant causing familial erythrocytosis is associated with deregulation of the rates of Jak2 and Stat5 inactivation. Exp Hematol 27:63–74, 1999.
52. Bilgrami S, Greenberg BR: Polycythemia rubra vera. Semin Oncol 22:307–326, 1995.

53. Rossi C, Randi ML, Zerbinati P, et al: Acute coronary disease in essential thrombocythemia and polycythemia vera. J Intern Med 244:49–53, 1998.
54. Dayal S, Patti HP, Acharya SK: Polycythemia vera: Overt to latent form in a patient with Budd-Chiari syndrome. J Clin Gastroenterol 22:76–77, 1996.
55. Gisslinger H, Rodeghiero F, Ruggeri M, et al: Homocysteine levels in polycythaemia vera and essential thrombocythaemia. Br J Haematol 105:551–555, 1999.
56. Schafer AI: Bleeding and thrombosis in the myeloproliferative disorders. Blood 64:1–12, 1984.
57. Michiels JJ, Juvonen E: Proposal for revised diagnostic criteria of essential thrombocythemia and polycythemia vera by the Thrombocythemia Vera Study Group. Semin Thromb Hemost 23:339–347, 1997.
58. Stobart K, Rogers PC: Allogeneic bone marrow transplantation for an adolescent with polycythemia vera. Bone Marrow Transplant 13:337–339, 1994.
59. Gilbert HS: Historical perspective on the treatment of essential thrombocythemia and polycythemia vera. Semin Hematol 36:19–22, 1999.
60. Barbui T, Finazzi G: Treatment of polycythemia vera. Haematologica 83:143–149, 1998.
61. Willoughby S, Pearson TC: The use of aspirin in polycythaemia vera and primary thrombocythaemia. Blood Rev 12:12–22, 1998.
62. Najean Y, Rain JD: Treatment of polycythemia vera: The use of hydroxyurea and pipobroman in 292 patients under the age of 65 years. Blood. 90:3370–3377, 1997.
63. Cacciola E, Cacciola RR, Guglielmo P, et al: Acute myeloid leukemia occurring in a patient with polycythemia vera in treatment with hydroxyurea. Haematologica 84:755–756, 1999.
64. Barbui T, Finazzi G, Dupuy E, et al: Treatment strategies in essential thrombocythemia: A critical appraisal of various experiences in different centers. Leuk Lymphoma 22(Suppl 1):149–160, 1996.
65. Cortellazzo S, Viero P, Finazzi G, et al: Incidence and risk factors of thrombotic complications in a historical cohort of 100 patients with thrombocythemia. J Clin Oncol 8:556–562, 1990.
66. Michiels JJ, van Genderen PJ, Lindemans J, et al: Erythromelalgic, thrombotic and hemorrhagic manifestations in 50 cases of thrombocythemia. Leuk Lymphoma 22(Suppl 1):47–56, 1996.
67. Tefferi A, Silverstein MN, Petitt RM, et al: Anagrelide as a new platelet-lowering agent in essential thrombocythemia: Mechanism of actin, efficacy, toxicity, current indications. Semin Thromb Hemost 23:379–383, 1997.
68. Raymond RM: When does the heart fail during shock? Circ Shock 30:27–41, 1990.

LEUKEMIA AND THE CIRCULATORY SYSTEM

69. Wurthner JU, Kohler G, Behringer D, et al: Leukostasis followed by hemorrhage complicating the initiation of chemotherapy in patients with acute myeloid leukemia and hyperleukocytosis: A clinicopathologic report of four cases. Cancer 85:368–374, 1999.
70. Creutzig U, Ritter J, Budde M, et al: Early deaths due to hemorrhage and leukostasis in childhood acute myelogenous leukemia: Associations with hyperleukocytosis and acute monocytic leukemia. Cancer 60:3071–3079, 1987.
71. Hug V, Keating M, McCredie K, et al: Clinical course and response to treatment of patients with acute myelogenous leukemia presenting with a high leukocyte count. Cancer 52:773–779, 1983.
72. Lester TJ, Johnson JW, Cuttner J: Pulmonary leukostasis as the single worst prognostic factor in patients with acute myelocytic leukemia and hyperleukocytosis. Am J Med 79:43–48, 1985.
73. Ventura GJ, Hester JP, Smith TL, et al: Acute myeloblastic leukemia with hyperleukocytosis: Risk factors for early mortality in induction. Am J Hematol 27:34–37, 1988.
74. Strauss RA, Gloster ES, McCallister JA, et al: Acute cytoreduction techniques in the early treatment of hyperleukocytosis associated with childhood hematologic malignancies. Med Pediatr Oncol 13:346–351, 1985.
75. Porcu P, Danielson CF, Orazi A, et al: Therapeutic leukapheresis in hyperleukocytic leukaemias: Lack of correlation between degree of cytoreduction and early mortality rate. Br J Haematol 98:433–436, 1997.
76. Vadher BD, Machin SJ, Patterson KG, et al: Life–threatening thrombotic and haemorrhagic problems associated with silent myeloproliferative disorders. Br J Haematol 85:213–216, 1993.

PARAPROTEINEMIA AND HYPERVISCOSITY SYNDROME

77. Meier C: Polyneuropathy in paraproteinaemia. J Neurol 232:204–214, 1985.
78. Farhangi M, Merlini G: The clinical implications of monoclonal immunoglobulins. Semin Oncol 13:366–379, 1986.
79. Dimopoulos MA, Alexanian R: Waldenstrom's macroglobulinemia. Blood 83:1452–1459, 1994.
80. Rosenson RS, Tangney C: Intraindividual variability in plasma viscosity measurements. Thromb Haemost 79:1063–1064, 1998.
81. Siami GA, Siami FS: Plasmapheresis and paraproteinemia: Cryoprotein-induced diseases, monoclonal gammopathy, Waldenström's macroglobulinemia, hyperviscosity syndrome, multiple myeloma, light chain disease, and amyloidosis. Ther Apher 3:8–19, 1999.
82. Della Rossa A, Trevisani G, Bombardieri S: Cryoglobulins and cryoglobulinemia: Diagnostic and therapuetic considerations. Clin Rev Allergy Immunol 16:249–264, 1998.

CANCERS METASTATIC TO THE HEART AND PERICARDIUM

83. Klein B, Zhang XG, Lu ZY, et al: Interleukin-6 in human multiple myeloma. Blood 85:863–872, 1995.
84. Lindsley H, Teller D, Noonan B, et al: Hyperviscosity syndrome in multiple myeloma: A reversible, concentration-dependent aggregation of the myeloma protein. Am J Med 54:682–688, 1973.
85. Durie BG, Salmon SE: A clinical staging system for multiple myeloma: Correlation of measured myeloma cell mass with presenting clinical features, response to treatment, and survival. Cancer 36:842–854, 1975.
86. Attal M, Harousseau JL, Stoppa AM, et al: A prospective, randomized trial of autologous bone marrow transplantation and chemotherapy in multiple myeloma. Intergroupe Français du Myelome. N Engl J Med 335:91–97, 1996.
87. Alexanian R, Dimopoulos M: The treatment of multiple myeloma. N Engl J Med 330:484–489, 1994.
88. Berenson JR, Lichtenstein A, Porter L, et al: Efficacy of pamidronate in reducing skeletal events in patients with advanced multiple myeloma. Myeloma Aredia Study Group. N Engl J Med 334:488–493, 1996.
89. Singhal S, Mehta J, Desikan R, et al: Antitumor activity of thalidomide in refractory multiple myeloma. N Engl J Med 341:1565–1571, 1999.
90. Horcajada JP, Garcia-Bengoechea M, Cilla G, et al: Mixed cryoglobulinaemia in patients with chronic hepatitis C infection: Prevalence, significance and relationship with different viral genotypes. Ann Med 31:352–358, 1999.
91. Dispenzieri A, Gorevic PD: Cryoglobulinemia. Hematol Oncol Clin North Am 13:1315–1349, 1999.
92. McHutchison JG, Gordon SC, Schiff ER, et al: Interferon alfa-2b alone or in combination with ribavirin as initial treatment for chronic hepatitis C. Hepatitis Interventional Therapy Group. N Engl J Med 339:1485–1492, 1998.
93. Lamprecht P, Gause A, Gross WL: Cryoglobulinemic vasculitis. Arthritis Rheum 42:2507–2516, 1999.
94. Lam KY, Dickens P, Chan AC: Tumors of the heart: A 20-year experience with a review of 12,485 consecutive autopsies. Arch Pathol Lab Med 117:1027–1031, 1993.
95. Abraham KP, Reddy V, Gattuso P: Neoplasms metastatic to the heart: Review of 3314 consecutive autopsies. Am J Cardiovasc Pathol 3:195–198, 1990.
96. Meysman M, Noppen M, Demeyer G, et al: Malignant epithelial mesothelioma presenting as cardiac tamponade. Eur Heart J 14:1576–1577, 1993.
97. Ling FT, David TE, Merchant N, et al: Intracardiac extension of intravenous leiomyomatosis in a pregnant woman: A case report and review of the literature. Can J Cardiol 16:73–79, 2000.
98. Seibert KA, Rettenmier CW, Waller BF, et al: Osteogenic sarcoma metastatic to the heart. Am J Med 73:136–141, 1982.
99. Peterson CD, Robinson WA, Kurnick JE: Involvement of the heart and pericardium in the malignant lymphomas. Am J Med Sci 272:161–165, 1976.
100. Goldsbrough DR, Carder PJ: Rapidly progressive cardiac failure due to lymphomatous infiltration of the myocardium. Postgrad Med J 65:688, 1989.
101. English JC, Allard MF, Babul S, et al: Metastatic tumors of the heart. In Goldhaber SZ (ed): Cardiopulmonary Diseases and Cardiac Tumors, Atlas of Heart Diseases. Vol 3. Philadelphia, Current Medicine, 1995.
102. Almange C, Lebrestec T, Louvet M, et al: [Complete atrio-ventricular block caused by a metastatic tumor of the heart.] Semin Hop 54:1419–1424, 1978.
103. Mousseaux E, Meunier P, Azancott S, et al: Cardiac metastatic melanoma investigated by magnetic resonance imaging. Magn Reson Imaging 16:91–95, 1998.
104. Burn PR, Chinn R, King DM: Right atrial metastatic melanoma detected by dynamic contrast enhanced spiral CT. Br J Radiol 72:395–396, 1999.
105. Atra A, Shankar AG, Padhani AR: Metastatic cardiac osteosarcoma—imaging features. Br J Radiol 71:336–339, 1998.
106. Khabele D, Chasen S: Cardiac tamponade as an unusual presentation of advanced breast cancer in pregnancy. J Reprod Med 44:989–991, 1999.
107. de Costa CM, de Camargo B, Gutierrez y Lamelas R, et al: Cardiac tamponade complicating hyperleukocytosis in a child with leukemia. Med Pediatr Oncol 33:120–123, 1999.
108. Gibbs P, Cebon JS, Calafiore P, et al: Cardiac metastases from malignant melanoma. Cancer 85:78–84, 1999.
109. Lopez FF, Mangi A, Mylonakis E, et al: Atrial fibrillation and tumor emboli as manifestations of metastatic leiomyosarcoma to the heart and lung. Heart Lung 29:47–49, 2000.
110. Giudici MC, Sadler RL, Robken JA, et al: Complete atrioventricular block due to large cell lymphoma: Resolution with chemotherapy. Clin Cardiol 19:262–264, 1996.

PERICARDIAL TAMPONADE AND CONSTRICTION IN NEOPLASIA

111. Hancock EW: Neoplastic pericardial disease. Cardiol Clin 8:673–682, 1990.

112. Tsang TS, Oh JK, Seward JB: Diagnosis and management of cardiac tamponade in the era of echocardiography. Clin Cardiol 22:446–452, 1999.

113. Myers RB, Spodick DH: Constrictive pericarditis: Clinical and pathophysiologic characteristics. Am Heart J 138:219–232, 1999.

114. Posner MR, Cohen GI, Skarin AT: The differentiation of malignant from idiopathic and radiation-induced pericarditis. Am J Med 71:407, 1981.

115. Allen KB, Faber LP, Warren WH, et al: Pericardial effusion: Subxiphoid pericardiostomy versus percutaneous catheter drainage. Ann Thorac Surg 67:437–440, 1999.

116. Maisch B, Pankuweit S, Brilla C, et al: Intrapericardial treatment of inflammatory and neoplastic pericarditis guided by pericardioscopy and epicardial biopsy—results from a pilot study. Clin Cardiol 22:I17–I22, 1999.

117. Kirn D, Mauch P, Shaffer K, et al: Large-cell and immunoblastic lymphoma of the mediastinum: Prognostic features and treatment outcome in 57 patients. J Clin Oncol 11:1336–1343, 1993.

118. Sawka AM, Prakash UB: 59–year-old man with epistaxis, headache, and cough. Mayo Clin Proc 75:193–196, 2000.

SUPERIOR VENA CAVA SYNDROME

119. Markman M: Diagnosis and management of superior vena cava syndrome. Cleve Clin J Med 66:59–61, 1999.

120. Thony F, Moro D, Witmeyer P, et al: Endovascular treatment of superior vena cava obstruction in patients with malignancies. Eur Radiol 9:965–971, 1999.

121. Schindler N, Vogelzang RL: Superior vena cava syndrome: Experience with endovascular stents and surgical therapy. Surg Clin North Am 79:683–694, 1999.

122. Hochrein J, Bashore TM, O'Laughlin MP, et al: Percutaneous stenting of superior vena cava syndrome: A case report and review of the literature. Am J Med 104:78–84, 1998.

123. Roberts JR, Bueno R, Sugarbaker DJ: Multimodality treatment of malignant superior vena caval syndrome. Chest 116:835–837, 1999.

124. Ostler PJ, Clarke DP, Watkinson AF, et al: Superior vena cava obstruction: A modern management strategy. Clin Oncol 9:83–89, 1997.

125. Abner A: Approach to the patient who presents with superior vena cava obstruction. Chest 103:394s–397s, 1993.

126. Bauer CA, Redleaf MI, Gartlan MG, et al: Carotid sinus syncope in head and neck cancer. Laryngoscope 104:497–503, 1994.

127. Ackermann DM, Hyma BA, Edwards WD: Malignant neoplastic emboli to the coronary arteries: Report of two cases and review of the literature. Hum Pathol 18:955–959, 1987.

OTHER CARDIOVASCULAR COMPLICATIONS OF NEOPLASIA

128. Weinberg BA, Pinkerton CA, Waller BF: External compression by metastatic squamous cell carcinoma: A rare cause of left main coronary artery narrowing. Clin Cardiol 13:360–366, 1990.

129. Virmani R, Farb A, Carter AJ, et al: Comparative pathology: Radiation-induced coronary artery disease in man and animals. Semin Intervent Cardiol 3:163–172, 1998.

130. Gonzalez Quintela A, Candela MJ, Vidal C, et al: Nonbacterial thrombotic endocarditis in cancer patients. Acta Cardiol 46:1–9, 1991.

131. Ojeda VJ, Frost F, Mastaglia FL: Nonbacterial thrombotic endocarditis associated with malignant disease: A clinicopathological study of 16 cases. Med J Aust 142:629–631, 1985.

132. Blanchard DG, Ross RS, Dittrich HC: Nonbacterial thrombotic endocarditis: Assessment by transesophageal echocardiography. Chest 102:954–956, 1992.

133. Glass JP: The diagnosis and treatment of stroke in a patient with cancer: Nonbacterial thrombotic endocarditis (NBTE): A case report and review. Clin Neurol Neurosurg 95:315–318, 1993.

134. Kulke MH, Mayer RJ: Carcinoid tumors. N Engl J Med 340:858–868, 1999.

135. Jacobsen MB, Nitter-Hauge S, Bryde PE, et al: Cardiac manifestations in mid-gut carcinoid disease. Eur Heart J 16:263–268, 1995.

136. Pellikka PA, Tajik AJ, Khandheria BK, et al: Carcinoid heart disease: Clinical and echocardiographic spectrum in 74 patients. Circulation 87:1188–1196, 1993.

137. Weller PF, Bubley GJ: The idiopathic hypereosinophilic syndrome. Blood 83:2759–2779, 1994.

138. Zientek DM, King DL, Dewan SJ, et al: Hypereosinophilic syndrome with rapid progression of cardiac involvement and early echocardiographic abnormalities. Am Heart J 130:1295–1298, 1995.

139. Spyrou N, Foale R: Restrictive cardiomyopathies. Curr Opin Cardiol 9:344–348, 1994.

140. Hayashi S, Isobe M, Okubo Y, et al: Improvement of eosinophilic heart disease after steroid therapy: Successful demonstration by endomyocardial biopsied specimens. Heart Vessels 14:104–108, 1999.

141. Smith GB, Gusberg RJ, Jordan RH, et al: Histamine levels and cardiovascular responses during splenectomy and splenorenal shunt formation in a patient with systemic mastocytosis. Anaesthesia 42:861–867, 1987.

142. Vaughan ST, Jones GN: Systemic mastocytosis presenting as profound cardiovascular collapse during anaesthesia. Anaesthesia 53:804–807, 1998.

143. Fenaux P, Chastang C, Chevret S, et al: A randomized comparison of all transretinoic acid (ATRA) followed by chemotherapy and ATRA plus chemotherapy and the role of maintenance therapy in newly diagnosed acute promyelocytic leukemia. The European APL Group. Blood 94:1192–1200, 1999.

RADIATION THERAPY AND THE CARDIOVASCULAR SYNDROME

144. Weichselbaum RR, Chen G, Hallahan DE: Biological and physical basis of radiation. In Holland JF, Frei EI, Bast RCJ, et al (eds): Cancer Medicine. Baltimore, Williams & Wilkins, 1997.

145. Haimovitz-Friedman A, Kan CC, Ehleiter D, et al: Ionizing radiation acts on cellular membranes to generate ceramide and initiate apoptosis. J Exp Med 180:525–535, 1994.

146. Om A, Ellahham S, Vetrovec GW: Radiation-induced coronary artery disease. Am Heart J 124:1598–1602, 1992.

147. Carlson RG, Mayfield WR, Normann S, et al: Radiation-associated valvular disease. Chest 99:538–545, 1991.

148. Arsenian MA: Cardiovascular sequelae of therapeutic thoracic radiation. Prog Cardiovasc Dis 33:299–311, 1991.

149. Schultz-Hector S: Radiation–induced heart disease: Review of experimental data on dose response and pathogenesis. Int J Radiat Biol 61:149–160, 1992.

150. Kreuser ED, Voller H, Behles C, et al: Evaluation of late cardiotoxicity with pulsed Doppler echocardiography in patients treated for Hodgkin's disease. Br J Haematol 84:615–622, 1993.

151. Toyofuku M, Okimoto T, Tadehara F, et al: Cardiac disease late after chest radiotherapy for Hodgkin's disease: A case report. Jpn Circ J 63:803–805, 1999.

152. Applefeld MM, Slawson RG, Spicer KM, et al: Long-term cardiovascular evaluation of patients with Hodgkin's disease treated by thoracic mantle radiation therapy. Cancer Treat Rep 66:1003–1013, 1982.

153. Veinot JP, Edwards WD: Pathology of radiation-induced heart disease: A surgical and autopsy study of 27 cases. Hum Pathol 27:766–773, 1996.

154. Zinzani PL, Gherlinzoni F, Piovaccari G, et al: Cardiac injury as late toxicity of mediastinal radiation therapy for Hodgkin's disease patients. Haematologica 81:132–137, 1996.

155. Ni Y, von Segesser LK, Turina M: Futility of pericardiectomy for postirradiation constrictive pericarditis? Ann Thorac Surg 49:445–448, 1990.

156. Pohjola-Sintonen S, Totterman KJ, Kupari M: Sick sinus syndrome as a complication of mediastinal radiation therapy. Cancer 65:2494–2496, 1990.

157. Slama MS, Le Guludec D, Sebag, C, et al: Complete atrioventricular block following mediastinal irradiation: A report of six cases. Pacing Clin Electrophysiol 14:1112–1118, 1991.

158. Lund MB, Ihlen H, Voss BM, et al: Increased risk of heart valve regurgitation after mediastinal radiation for Hodgkin's disease: An echocardiographic study. Heart 75:591–595, 1996.

159. Jakacki RI, Goldwein JW, Larsen RL, et al: Cardiac dysfunction following spinal irradiation during childhood. J Clin Oncol 11:1033–1038, 1993.

160. Brosius FC, Waller BF, Roberts WC: Radiation heart disease: Analysis of 16 young (aged 15 to 33 years) necropsy patients who received over 3,500 rads to the heart. Am J Med 70:519–530, 1981.

161. Hancock SL, Donaldson SS, Hoppe RT: Cardiac disease following treatment of Hodgkin's disease in children and adolescents. J Clin Oncol 11:1208–1215, 1993.

162. Boivin JF, Hutchison GB, Lubin JH, et al: Coronary artery disease mortality in patients treated for Hodgkin's disease. Cancer 69:1241–1247, 1992.

163. Lipshultz SE, Sallan SE: Cardiovascular abnormalities in long-term survivors of childhood malignancy. J Clin Oncol 11:1199–1203, 1993.

164. Hardenbergh PH, Recht A, Gollamudi S, et al: Treatment-related toxicity from a randomized trial of the sequencing of doxorubicin and radiation therapy in patients treated for early stage breast cancer. Int J Radiat Oncol Biol Phys 45:69–72, 1999.

165. Salloum E, Tanoue LT, Wackers FJ, et al: Assessment of cardiac and pulmonary function in adult patients with Hodgkin's disease treated with ABVD or MOPP/ABVD plus adjuvant low-dose mediastinal irradiation. Cancer Invest 17:171–180, 1999.

166. Shulman LN, Mauch PM: Current role of radiotherapy in Hodgkin's and non-Hodgkin's lymphoma. Curr Opin Oncol 7:421–425, 1995.

167. Coleman CN, Bump EA, Kramer RA: Chemical modifiers of cancer treatment. J Clin Oncol 6:709–733, 1988.

168. Hensley ML, Schuchter LM, Lindley C, et al: American Society of Clinical Oncology clinical practice guidelines for the use of chemotherapy and radiotherapy protectants. J Clin Oncol 17:3333–3355, 1999.

169. Joensuu H: Acute myocardial infarction after heart irradiation in young patients with Hodgkin's disease. Chest 95:388–390, 1989.

170. O'Donnell L, O'Neill T, Toner M, et al: Myocardial hypertrophy, fibrosis and infarction following exposure of the heart to radiation for Hodgkin's disease. Postgrad Med J 62:1055–1058, 1986.

171. Green DM, Gingell RL, Pearce J, et al: The effect of mediastinal irradiation on cardiac function of patients treated during childhood and adolescence for Hodgkin's disease. J Clin Oncol 5:239–245, 1987.

172. Piovaccari G, Ferretti RM, Prati F, et al: Cardiac disease after chest

irradiation for Hodgkin's disease: Incidence in 108 patients with long follow-up. Int J Cardiol 49:39–43, 1995.

CARDIAC COMPLICATIONS OF CHEMOTHERAPY

173. Myers C: Anthracyclines and DNA intercalators. *In* Holland JF, Frei E III, Bast RC Jr, et al (eds): Cancer Medicine. Vol 1. Baltimore, Williams & Wilkins, 1997, pp 977–988.
174. Doroshow JH: Doxorubicin-induced cardiac toxicity. N Engl J Med 324:843–845, 1991.
175. Speyer JL, Green MD, Kramer E, et al: Protective effect of the *bis*-piperazinedione ICRF-187 against doxorubicin-induced cardiac toxicity in women with advanced breast cancer. N Engl J Med 319:745–752, 1988.
176. Myers C, Bonow R, Palmeri S, et al: A randomized controlled trial assessing the prevention of doxorubicin cardiomyopathy by *N*-acetylcysteine. Semin Oncol 10:53–55, 1983.
177. Shan K, Lincoff AM, Young JB: Anthracycline-induced cardiotoxicity. Ann Intern Med 125:47–58, 1996.
178. Zhu W, Zou Y, Aikawa R, et al: MAPK superfamily plays an important role in daunomycin-induced apoptosis of cardiac myocytes. Circulation 100:2100–2107, 1999.
179. Aihara Y, Kurabayashi M, Arai M, et al: Molecular cloning of rabbit CARP cDNA and its regulated expression in adriamycin-cardiomyopathy. Biochim Biophys Acta 1447:318–324, 1999.
180. Kumar D, Kirshenbaum L, Li T, et al: Apoptosis in isolated adult cardiomyocytes exposed to adriamycin. Ann NY Acad Sci 874:156–168, 1999.
181. Wang YX, Korth M: Effects of doxorubicin on excitation-contraction coupling in guinea pig ventricular myocardium. Circ Res 76:645–653, 1995.
182. Billingham ME, Bristow MR: Evaluation of anthracycline cardiotoxicity: Predictive ability and functional correlation of endomyocardial biopsy. Cancer Treatment Symposia 3:71–76, 1984.
183. Steinberg JS, Cohen AJ, Wasserman AG, et al: Acute arrhythmogenicity of doxorubicin administration. Cancer 60:1213–1218, 1987.
184. Bristow MR, Billingham ME, Mason JW, et al: Clinical spectrum of anthracycline antibiotic cardiotoxicity. Cancer Treat Rep 62:873–879, 1978.
185. Felker GM, Thompson RE, Hare JM, et al: Underlying causes and long-term survival in patients with initially unexplained cardiomyopathy. N Engl J Med 342:1077–1084, 2000.
186. Moreb JS, Oblon DJ: Outcome of clinical congestive heart failure induced by anthracycline chemotherapy. Cancer 70:2637–2641, 1992.
187. Matsui H, Morishima I, Numaguchi Y, et al: Protective effects of carvedilol against doxorubicin-induced cardiomyopathy in rats. Life Sci 65:1265–1274, 1999.
188. Shaddy RE, Tani LY, Gidding SS, et al: Beta-blocker treatment of dilated cardiomyopathy with congestive heart failure in children: A multi-institutional experience. J Heart Lung Transplant 18:269–274, 1999.
189. Shaddy RE, Olsen SL, Bristow MR, et al: Efficacy and safety of metoprolol in the treatment of doxorubicin-induced cardiomyopathy in pediatric patients. Am Heart J 129:197–199, 1995.
190. Musci M, Loebe M, Grauhan O, et al: Heart transplantation for doxorubicin-induced congestive heart failure in children and adolescents. Transplant Proc 29:578–579, 1997.
191. Levitt G, Bunch K, Rogers CA, et al: Cardiac transplantation in childhood cancer survivors in Great Britain. Eur J Cancer 32a:826–830, 1996.
192. Steinherz LJ, Steinherz PG, Tan CT, et al: Cardiac toxicity 4 to 20 years after completing anthracycline therapy. JAMA 266:1672–1677, 1991.
193. Lipshultz SE, Colan SD, Gelber RD, et al: Late cardiac effects of doxorubicin therapy for acute lymphoblastic leukemia in childhood. N Engl J Med 324:808–815, 1991.
194. Yeung ST, Yoong C, Spink J, et al: Functional myocardial impairment in children treated with anthracyclines for cancer. Lancet 337:816–818, 1991.
195. Steinherz LJ, Steinherz PG, Tan C: Cardiac failure and dysrhythmias 6–19 years after anthracycline therapy: A series of 15 patients. Med Pediatr Oncol 24:352–361, 1995.
196. Leandro J, Dyck J, Poppe D, et al: Cardiac dysfunction late after cardiotoxic therapy for childhood cancer. Am J Cardiol 74:1152–1156, 1994.
197. Lipshultz SE, Rifai N, Sallan SE, et al: Predictive value of cardiac troponin T in pediatric patients at risk for myocardial injury. Circulation 96:2641–2648, 1997.
198. Hashimoto I, Ichida F, Miura M, et al: Automatic border detection identifies subclinical anthracycline cardiotoxicity in children with malignancy. Circulation 99:2367–2370, 1999.
199. Kremer LC, Tiel-van Buul MM, Ubbink MC, et al: Indium-111–antimyosin scintigraphy in the early detection of heart damage after anthracycline therapy in children. J Clin Oncol 17:1208, 1999.
200. Lipshultz SE, Lipsitz SR, Mone SM, et al: Female sex and drug dose as risk factors for late cardiotoxic effects of doxorubicin therapy for childhood cancer. N Engl J Med 332:1738–1743, 1995.
201. Rihal CR, Nishimura RA, Hatle LK, et al: Systolic and diastolic dysfunction in patients with clinical diagnosis of dilated cardiomyopathy: Relation to symptoms and prognosis. Circulation 90:792–798, 1994.
202. Pegelow CH, Popper RW, de Wit SA, et al: Endomyocardial biopsy to monitor anthracycline therapy in children. J Clin Oncol 2:443–446, 1984.
203. Alexander J, Dainiak N, Berger HJ, et al: Serial assessment of doxorubicin cardiotoxicity with quantitative radionuclide angiocardiography. N Engl J Med 300:278–283, 1979.
204. Schmitt K, Tulzer G, Merl M, et al: Early detection of doxorubicin and daunorubicin cardiotoxicity by echocardiography: Diastolic versus systolic parameters. Eur J Pediatr 154:201–204, 1995.
205. Suzuki J, Yanagisawa A, Shigeyama T, et al: Early detection of anthracycline-induced cardiotoxicity by radionuclide angiocardiography. Angiology 50:37–45, 1999.
206. Legha SS, Benjamin RS, Mackay B, et al: Reduction of doxorubicin cardiotoxicity by prolonged continuous intravenous infusion. Ann Intern Med 96:133–139, 1982.
207. Valdivieso M, Burgess MA, Ewer MS, et al: Increased therapeutic index of weekly doxorubicin in the therapy of non–small cell lung cancer: A prospective randomized study. J Clin Oncol 2:207, 1984.
208. Shapira J, Gottfried M, Lishner M, Ravid M: Reduced cardiotoxicity of doxorubicin by a 6-hour infusion regimen: A prospective randomized evaluation. Cancer 65:870, 1990.
209. Anders RJ, Shanes JG, Zeller FP: Lower incidence of doxorubicin-induced cardiomyopathy by once-a-week low-dose administration. Am Heart J 111:755–759, 1986.
210. Speyer J, Wasserheit C: Strategies for reduction of anthracycline cardiac toxicity. Semin Oncol 25:525–537, 1998.
211. Berry G, Billingham M, Alderman E, et al: The use of cardiac biopsy to demonstrate reduced cardiotoxicity in AIDS Kaposi's sarcoma patients treated with pegylated liposomal doxorubicin. Ann Oncol 9:711–716, 1998.
212. Alberts DS, Garcia DJ: Safety aspects of pegylated liposomal doxorubicin in patients with cancer. Drugs 54:30–35, 1997.
213. Fichtner I, Arndt D, Elbe B, et al: Cardiotoxicity of free and liposomally encapsulated rubomycin (daunorubicin) in mice. Oncology 41:363–369, 1984.
214. Treat J, Greenspan A, Forst D, et al: Antitumor activity of liposome-encapsulated doxorubicin in advanced breast cancer: Phase II study. J Natl Cancer Inst 82:1706–1710, 1990.
215. Chan S, Friedrichs K, Noel D, et al: Prospective randomized trial of docetaxel versus doxorubicin in patients with metastatic breast cancer. The 303 Study Group. J Clin Oncol 17:2341–2354, 1999.
216. Links M, Lewis C: Chemoprotectants: A review of their clinical pharmacology and therapeutic efficacy. Drugs 57:293–308, 1999.
217. Konorev EA, Kennedy MC, Kalyanaraman B: Cell-permeable superoxide dismutase and glutathione peroxidase mimetics afford superior protection against doxorubicin-induced cardiotoxicity: The role of reactive oxygen and nitrogen intermediates. Arch Biochem Biophys 368:421–428, 1999.
218. Swain SM, Whaley FS, Gerber MC, et al: Cardioprotection with dexrazoxane for doxorubicin-containing therapy in advanced breast cancer. J Clin Oncol 15:1318–1332, 1997.
219. Swain SM, Whaley FS, Gerber MC, et al: Delayed administration of dexrazoxane provides cardioprotection for patients with advanced breast cancer treated with doxorubicin-containing therapy. J Clin Oncol 15:1333–1340, 1997.
220. Wiseman LR, Spencer CM: Dexrazoxane: A review of its use as a cardioprotective agent in patients receiving anthracycline-based chemotherapy. Drugs 56:385–403, 1998.
221. Iliskovic N, Singal PK: Lipid lowering: An important factor in preventing adriamycin-induced heart failure. Am J Pathol 150:727–734, 1997.
222. Siveski-Iliskovic N, Hill M, Chow DA, et al: Probucol protects against adriamycin cardiomyopathy without interfering with its antitumor effect. Circulation 91:10–15, 1995.
223. Morishima I, Matsui H, Mukawa H, et al: Melatonin, a pineal hormone with antioxidant property, protects against adriamycin cardiomyopathy in rats. Life Sci 63:511–521, 1998.
224. Sugiyama S, Yamada K, Hayakawa M, et al: Approaches that mitigate doxorubicin-induced delayed adverse effects on mitochondrial function in rat hearts; liposome-encapsulated doxorubicin or combination therapy with antioxidant. Biochem Mol Biol Int 36:1001–1007, 1995.
225. Akimoto H, Bruno NA, Slate DL, et al: Effect of verapamil on doxorubicin cardiotoxicity: Altered muscle gene expression in cultured neonatal rat cardiomyocytes. Cancer Res 53:4658–4664, 1993.
226. Liu XK, Engelman RM, Agrawal HR, et al: Preservation of membrane phospholipids by propranolol, pindolol, and metoprolol: A novel mechanism of action of beta-blockers. J Mol Cell Cardiol 23:1091–1100, 1991.
227. Dell'Acqua G, Polishchuck R, Fallon JT, et al: Cardiac resistance to adriamycin in transgenic mice expressing a rat alpha-cardiac myosin heavy chain/human multiple drug resistance 1 fusion gene. Hum Gene Ther 10:1269–1279, 1999.
228. Anand AJ: Fluorouracil cardiotoxicity. Ann Pharmacother 28:374–378, 1994.
229. Cwikiel M, Eskilsson J, Wieslander JB, et al: The appearance of endothelium in small arteries after treatment with 5-fluorouracil: An electron microscopic study of late effects in rabbits. Scanning Microsc 10:805–818, 1996.
230. Frishman WH, Sung HM, Yee HC, et al: Cardiovascular toxicity with cancer chemotherapy. Curr Probl Cardiol 21:225–286, 1996.
231. Ensley JF, Patel B, Kloner R, et al: The clinical syndrome of 5-fluorouracil cardiotoxicity. Invest New Drugs 7:101–109, 1989.

232. Robben NC, Pippas AW, Moore JO: The syndrome of 5-fluorouracil cardiotoxicity: An elusive cardiopathy. Cancer 71:493–509, 1993.

233. Meyer CC, Calis KA, Burke LB, et al: Symptomatic cardiotoxicity associated with 5-fluorouracil. Pharmacotherapy 17:729–736, 1997.

234. Becker K, Erckenbrecht JF, Haussinger D, et al: Cardiotoxicity of the antiproliferative compound fluorouracil. Drugs 57: 475–484, 1999.

235. Aziz SA, Tramboo NA, Mohi-ud-Din K, et al: Supraventricular arrhythmia: A complication of 5-fluorouracil therapy. Clin Oncol 10:377–378, 1998.

236. Keefe DL, Roistacher N, Pierri MK: Clinical cardiotoxicity of 5-fluorouracil. J Clin Pharmacol 33:1060–1070, 1993.

237. Grandi AM, Pinotti G, Morandi E, et al: Noninvasive evaluation of cardiotoxicity of 5-fluorouracil and low doses of folinic acid: A one-year follow-up study. Ann Oncol 8:705–708, 1997.

238. Goldberg MA, Antin JH, Guinan EC, et al: Cyclophosphamide cardiotoxicity: An analysis of dosing as a risk factor. Blood 68:1114–1118, 1986.

239. Ayash LJ, Wright JE, Tretyakov O, et al: Cyclophosphamide pharmacokinetics: Correlation with cardiac toxicity and tumor response. J Clin Oncol 10:995–1000, 1992.

240. Braverman AC, Antin JH, Plappert MT, et al: Cyclophosphamide cardiotoxicity in bone marrow transplantation: A prospective evaluation of new dosing regimens. J Clin Oncol 9:1215–1223, 1991.

241. Quezado ZM, Wilson WH, Cunnion RE, et al: High–dose ifosfamide is associated with severe, reversible cardiac dysfunction. Ann Intern Med 118:31–36, 1993.

242. Herenstein B, Stefanic M, Schmeiser T, et al: Cardiac toxicity of bone marrow transplantation: Predictive value of cardiologic evaluation before transplant. J Clin Oncol 12:998–1004, 1998.

243. Champlin R, Khouri I, Kornblau S, et al: Reinventing bone marrow transplantation: Reducing toxicity using nonmyeloablative, preparative regimens and induction of graft-versus-malignancy. Curr Opin Oncol 11:87–95, 1999.

244. Icli F, Karaoguz H, Dincol D, et al: Severe vascular toxicity associated with cisplatin-based chemotherapy. Cancer 72:587–593, 1993.

245. Burkhardt A, Holtje WJ, Gebbers JO: Vascular lesions following perfusion with bleomycin: Electron-microscopic observations. Virchows Arch [A] Pathol Anat Histol 372:227–236, 1976.

246. Aisner J, Van Echo DA, Whitacre M, et al: A phase I trial of continuous infusion VP16-213 (etoposide). Cancer Chemother Pharmacol 7:157–160, 1982.

247. Fukuda M, Oka M, Itoh N, et al: Vasospastic angina likely related to cisplatin-containing chemotherapy and thoracic irradiation for lung cancer. Intern Med 38:436–438, 1999.

248. Hochster H, Wasserheit C, Speyer J: Cardiotoxicity and cardioprotection during chemotherapy. Curr Opin Oncol 7:304–309, 1995.

249. Hudis C, Riccio L, Seidman A, et al: Lack of increased cardiac toxicity with sequential doxorubicin and paclitaxel. Cancer Invest 16:67–71, 1998.

250. Sparano JA: Doxorubicin/taxane combinations: Cardiac toxicity and pharmacokinetics. Semin Oncol 26:14–19, 1999.

251. Deyton LR, Walker RE, Kovacs JA, et al: Reversible cardiac dysfunction associated with interferon alfa therapy in AIDS patients with Kaposi's sarcoma. N Engl J Med 321:1246–1249, 1989.

252. Schechter D, Nagler A, Ackerstein A, et al: Recombinant interleukin-2 and interferon alpha immunotherapy following autologous bone marrow transplantation: A case report of cardiovascular toxicity with serial echocardiographic evaluation. Cardiology 80:168–171, 1992.

253. Osanto S, Cluitmans FH, Franks CR, et al: Myocardial injury after interleukin-2 therapy. Lancet 2:48–49, 1988.

254. Nora R, Abrams JS, Tait NS, et al: Myocardial toxic effects during recombinant interleukin-2 therapy. J Natl Cancer Inst 81:59–63, 1989.

255. Baselga J, Tripathy D, Mendelsohn J, et al: Phase II study of weekly intravenous trastuzumab (Herceptin) in patients with HER2/neu-overexpressing metastatic breast cancer. Semin Oncol 26:78–83, 1999.

256. Shak S: Overview of the trastuzumab (Herceptin) anti-HER2 monoclonal antibody clinical program in HER2-overexpressing metastatic breast cancer. Herceptin Multinational Investigator Study Group. Semin Oncol 26:71–77, 1999.

257. Ewer MS, Gibbs HR, Swafford J, et al: Cardiotoxicity in patients receiving transtuzumab (Herceptin): Primary toxicity, synergistic or sequential stress, or surveillance artifact? Semin Oncol 26:96–101, 1999.

HEMATOLOGIC EFFECTS OF CARDIAC MEDICATIONS

258. Mammen EF: Low molecular weight heparins and heparin-induced thrombocytopenia. Clin Appl Thromb Hemost 5(Suppl 1):S72–S75, 1999.

259. Januzzi JL Jr, Jang IK: Heparin induced thrombocytopenia: Diagnosis and contemporary antithrombin management. J Thromb Thrombolysis 7:259–264, 1999.

260. Vorchheimer DA, Badimon JJ, Fuster V: Platelet glycoprotein IIb/IIIa receptor antagonists in cardiovascular disease. JAMA 281:1407–1414, 1999.

261. Llevadot J, Coulter SA, Giugliano RP: A practical approach to the diagnosis and management of thrombocytopenia associated with glycoprotein IIb/IIIa receptor inhibitors. J Thromb Thrombolysis 9:175–180, 2000.

262. Giugliano RP: Drug-induced thrombocytopenia: Is it a serious concern for glycoprotein IIb/IIIa receptor inhibitors? J Thromb Thrombolysis 5: 191–202, 1998.

263. Madan M, Berkowitz SD: Understanding thrombocytopenia and antigenicity with glycoprotein IIb–IIIa inhibitors. Am Heart J 138:317–326, 1999.

264. Tcheng JE: Perspectives on the future of platelet glycoprotein IIb/IIIa blockade therapy. Texas Heart Inst J 25:49–56, 1998.

265. O'Neill WW, Serruys P, Knudtson M, et al: Long-term treatment with a platelet glycoprotein-receptor antagonist after percutaneous coronary revascularization. N Engl J Med 342:1316–1324, 2000.

266. Schomig A, Neumann FJ, Kastrati A, et al: A randomized comparison of antiplatelet and anticoagulant therapy after the placement of coronary-artery stents. N Engl J Med 334:1084–1089, 1996.

267. Caprie SC: A randomized, blinded trial of clopidogel versus aspirin in patients at risk of ischemic events (CAPRIE). Lancet 348:1329–1339, 1996.

268. Bennett CL, Davidson CJ, Raisch DW, et al: Thrombotic thrombocytopenic purpura associated with ticlopidine in the setting of coronary artery stents and stroke prevention. Arch Intern Med 159:2524–2528, 1999.

269. Bennett CL, Connors JM, Carwile JM, et al: Trombotic thrombocytopenic purpura associated with colpidogrel. N Engl J Med 342:1773–1777, 2000.

270. Furlan M, Robles R, Galbusera M, et al: von Willebrand factor–cleaving protease in thrombotic thrombocytopenic purpura and the hemolytic-uremic syndrome. N Engl J Med 339:1578–1584, 1998.

271. Tsai HM, Lian EC: Antibodies to von Willebrand factor–cleaving protease in acute thrombotic thrombocytopenic purpura. N Engl J Med 339: 1585–1594, 1998.

272. Chong BH, Berndt MC, Koutts J, et al: Quinidine-induced thrombocytopenia and leukopenia: Demonstration and characterization of distinct antiplatelet and antileukocyte antibodies. Blood 62:1218–1223, 1983.

273. Ray JB, Brereton WF, Nullet FR: Intravenous immune globulin for the treatment of presumed quinidine-induced thrombocytopenia. DICP 24: 693–695, 1990.

274. Kikura M, Lee MK, Safon RA, et al: The effects of milrinone on platelets in patients undergoing cardiac surgery. Anesth Analg 81:44–48, 1995.

275. Kelly JP, Kaufman DW, Shapiro S: Risks of agranulocytosis and aplastic anemia in relation to the use of cardiovascular drugs. The International Agranulocytosis and Aplastic Anemia Study. Clin Pharmacol Ther 49: 330–341, 1991.

276. Hoyt RE: Severe neutropenia due to sustained-release procainamide. South Med J 80:1196–1197, 1987.

277. Ellrodt AG, Murata GH, Riedinger MS, et al: Severe neutropenia associated with sustained-release procainamide. Ann Intern Med 100:197–201, 1984.

278. Abe H, Suzuka H, Tasaki H, et al: Sustained-release procainamide-induced reversible granulocytopenia after myocardial infarction. Jpn Heart J 36:483–487, 1995.

279. Winfred RI, Nanda S, Horvath G, et al: Captopril-induced toxic epidermal necrolysis and agranulocytosis successfully treated with granulocyte colony-stimulating factor. South Med J 92:918–920, 1999.

Chapter 70

Psychiatric and Behavioral Aspects of Cardiovascular Disease

ARTHUR J. BARSKY

Daily life offers ample empirical evidence of an intimate relationship between the psyche and the heart. Intense emotions such as anxiety, anger, elation, and sexual arousal are accompanied by predictable increases in heart rate and blood pressure. Our everyday speech is filled with cardiac metaphors; the heart "races" with excitement, "pounds" in eager anticipation, "stands still" in dread, "aches" with grief. Many cultures have regarded the heart as the seat of emotion, the origin of love, the source of courage, or the abode of the soul. Generous people have "big hearts," and stingy people are "heartless." When you first met your first love, your heart "skipped a beat," and you were "broken hearted" when you parted ways soon thereafter. We attend funerals with a "heavy heart" and offer our "heartfelt" condolences. The interaction of heart and psyche is bidirectional. Emotions and stressful experiences affect the heart directly through the autonomic nervous system and indirectly through neuroendocrine pathways. Conversely, cardiac activity and function can reach conscious awareness and may be experienced as symptoms.

PSYCHIATRIC AND BEHAVIORAL ASPECTS OF CORONARY HEART DISEASE

Type A Behavior Pattern and Hostility

Clinicians dating back to Sir William Osler have observed that a surprising number of coronary heart disease (CHD) patients seem to be compulsive, driven overachievers who are unable to relax and quick to feel angry and frustrated when things do not proceed as planned. Such observations were reified in the 1960s by Friedman and Rosenman, who advanced the concept of Type A behavior, which was actually a cluster of psychological traits and behavioral patterns. Type A individuals struggled to obtain numerous objectives, as rapidly as possible, from an environment that continually seemed to oppose their efforts. Type A behavior is suffused with ambition, time urgency, and anger and hostility. Type A persons are excessively competitive and aggressive, with an extreme desire for achievement and rec-

ognition—impatient people leading fast-paced lives in continual and strenuous pursuit of a goal. This was contrasted to Type B individuals who are relaxed, unhurried, and less aggressive and who do not get as upset when thwarted. Large-scale, prospective studies in the 1970s and 1980s (including the Western Collaborative Group Study) conducted on initially healthy individuals showed that those with Type A behavior pattern, versus Type B individuals, had a significantly elevated rate of developing CHD (two times higher) and myocardial infarction (five times higher) at 5- to 8½-year follow-up and had more extensive CHD at the time of angiography.[1] Some additional longitudinal studies replicated these findings, but a substantial number, including the Multiple Risk Factor Intervention Trial (MRFIT), failed to support this association. In particular, several studies did not find that Type A behavior pattern predicted the subsequent incidence of cardiac events among patients with already established CHD. This suggested that perhaps the association between Type A and the development of CHD might be stronger than the association between Type A and the progression of disease.

These contradictory findings led to a search for more specific features or components of Type A behavior that might be more closely associated with CHD. A body of work emerged suggesting that anger and/or suppressed anger are the pathogenic components of Type A personality,[2] and laboratory studies provided evidence of pathophysiological changes that were associated with anger and hostility. Hostility is thought of as an underlying, enduring personality trait that encompasses a cynical, suspicious, and denigrating attitude toward others. This attitude then results in more frequent, intense, or longer-lasting episodes of anger when the individual is provoked, challenged, or otherwise stressed. Anger, hostility, antagonistic interactions, cynicism, and mistrust have been associated in long-term, prospective studies with the incidence of CHD, coronary events, and total mortality; and this literature suggests that such anger and hostility are independent risk factors for the development of CHD.[2, 3] In a 7-year, follow-up study of 1305 men, for instance, the relative risk for men with the greatest levels of anger was 2.66 for cardiac events (cardiac death, nonfatal myocardial infarction, and angina) as compared with men with the lowest levels of anger.[4] In the Western Electric study, the baseline hostility scores of 1877 middle-aged men were predictive of CHD events over a 10-year period.[5] Most recently, in a sample of 2890 middle-aged men observed for more than 8 years, suppressed anger was a significant predictor of a major cardiac event (relative odds = 1.70; 95 percent confidence interval [CI] = 1.26 to 2.29), and this relationship persisted after controlling for physiological, psychosocial, and behavioral risk factors.[6] Several cross-sectional angiographic studies also report an association between the degree of hostility and the extent of CHD.

Other studies, however, have not found an association between anger and CHD, and the evidence linking irritability, anger, and hostility to CHD prognosis and mortality is less conclusive than its association with the incidence of CHD. It has been reported in a 3-year, follow-up study that anger was significantly associated with CHD mortality in men with already established heart disease and with the incidence of restenosis after angioplasty,[7] but in general it appears that hostility and anger may predispose more to the initial cardiac event than they adversely influence the course of already established coronary artery disease. It is unclear to what degree hostility's effect may be mediated through its influence on other risk factors, such as lack of social supports, smoking, diet, and alcohol use. Possible associations between anger and race, socioeconomic status, and gender also represent potential confounds. In sum, although more research is necessary to establish the specifics of the relationship, it appears that anger and hostility do play a role in the development of CHD.

Depression and Anxiety

DEPRESSION. Recent work has begun to focus on the influence of depression and, to a lesser degree, anxiety on the onset, course, and outcome of CHD. A substantial body of prospective research indicates that major depression and subthreshold depressive symptoms, in both healthy individuals and in patients with CHD, confer an increased risk for subsequent cardiac events. Depression is prevalent in patients with CHD. Clinically significant depressive symptoms are found in 40 to 65 percent of patients after a myocardial infarction, and the prevalence of major depressive disorder is 20 to 25 percent in such patients.[8, 9] In one study, 31.5 percent of post-myocardial infarction patients experienced major depression in the hospital or within 1 year after discharge.[10] The prevalence of depression is also elevated in patients with stable CHD who have not had a recent myocardial infarction or other cardiac event (as high as 20 percent in some studies) and in patients who have undergone coronary artery bypass surgery.[11] Although most subjects in these studies have been male, there is evidence that the risk of depression in women with CHD is twice as high as that of men. Studies also reveal that depression is consistently underdiagnosed by cardiologists and primary care physicians in these patients.

Depression is of course important in and of itself because of the very considerable suffering it imposes. But in addition, depression exacerbates, prolongs, and amplifies cardiac symptoms. CHD patients with depression have more severe cardiac symptoms than nondepressed CHD patients, even after controlling for the severity of cardiac disease. Thus, depressed patients have greater levels of angina during exercise treadmill testing, terminate the treadmill test sooner, and have more persistent angina after myocardial infarction. In addition, depression engenders disability and role impairment, adversely affects compliance with medical therapy, and is detrimental to cardiac rehabilitation. In a 1-year, prospective study of patients who had undergone catheterization for documented CHD, physical

functioning and interference with activities were better predicted by baseline depression and anxiety than by the number of stenosed vessels, even after controlling for medical comorbidity and treatment.[12] Although major depression is most powerful in this regard, less severe forms of depression that do not meet diagnostic criteria for major depressive disorder also produce significant functional impairment, after controlling for individual differences in cardiac and medical comorbidity.

Depression also exerts a negative prognostic influence on the course and outcome of CHD. In patients with documented CHD, depression predicts future cardiac events and is associated with significantly elevated rates of cardiac mortality.[8, 13, 14] Major depressive disorder at the time of cardiac catheterization is a significant predictor of subsequent myocardial infarction, angioplasty, coronary artery bypass grafting, and death in patients with evidence of CHD, and this effect is independent of CHD severity, left ventricular ejection fraction, and smoking.[13] After myocardial infarction, depression increases the risk of future coronary events, including reinfarction, cardiac arrest, and death, after taking the severity of CHD into account.[8, 14, 15] In an important longitudinal study of 222 patients, baseline depression was a significant predictor of cardiac mortality 6 and 18 months after myocardial infarction, and this association persisted after taking into account the effects of baseline left ventricular dysfunction, Killip class, previous myocardial infarction, and frequency of premature ventricular contractions.[8, 14] For longer periods, from 6 to 27 years, the relative risk of myocardial infarction or cardiac mortality associated with depression has been reported to be between 1.5 and 6, after controlling for severity of cardiac disease.[14, 16, 17]

The degree of risk associated with depression is as great as that associated with traditional risk factors (e.g., cholesterol, smoking, hypertension) and is largely independent of them. This risk is elevated for women as well as men and not limited to diagnosable, major depressive disorder but also includes depressive symptoms. That is, there is a continuous, linear relationship between the number of depressive symptoms and the risk of subsequent cardiac events. An interaction effect may exist, in which the co-occurrence of both depression and ventricular arrhythmias exerts a particularly poor prognostic influence.[14] Interestingly, optimism seems to have a positive influence on prognosis; optimism at the time of coronary artery bypass surgery is associated with a lower rate of rehospitalization for cardiac events over the subsequent 6 months, after controlling for sociodemographic differences and disease severity.[18]

Depression also appears to be a risk factor for the development of CHD, although the evidence here is less extensive and somewhat less conclusive, especially since depression tends to co-occur with other risk factors for CHD. Some prospective studies report a modest association between depression and the incidence of CHD, but others fail to find a correlation. In longitudinal studies of initially healthy, community residents without a history of CHD, depression has been associated with a relative risk between 1.5 and 2 for the subsequent development of CHD, myocardial infarction, and cardiac death over periods from 6 to 40 years, and this risk is largely independent of the more traditional risk factors.[16, 17, 19-21] For example, in a prospective study of 2832 healthy adults, depressed mood was a significant predictor of subsequent fatal and nonfatal CHD.[16] Similar prospective findings have been reported in men and women over a 27-year period and in men over 40 years. Other work, however, has failed to confirm these findings: depression was not associated with an increased risk of CHD over a 15-year period in a study of 2573 adults,[22] nor was it associated with an increased risk of myocardial infarction in a 5-year follow-up of elderly individuals with hypertension.[23]

In sum, the evidence at this point indicates that depression confers an increased cardiovascular risk on healthy individuals and on individuals with already established CHD. Both major depressive disorder and elevated levels of depressive symptoms are significant in this regard. The degree of risk associated with major depression is comparable to that associated with other, established risk factors and is largely independent of them.

This relationship between depression and CHD may be mediated by several different behavioral and physiological mechanisms. Depression may operate through its influence on behavior: Depressed individuals may take poorer care of themselves, pay less attention to diet, drink more alcohol, smoke more, have less motivation and energy to exercise regularly, and be less likely to seek medical care and adhere to the medical regimen. There is, however, only limited empirical evidence bearing on this hypothesis. In addition, depression hinders recovery and causes poorer psychosocial adjustment to, and coping with, disease. Depressed post-myocardial infarction patients are more likely to experience social readjustment problems in the year after myocardial infarction than nondepressed post-myocardial infarction patients, are slower to return to work, and report more associated stress. Depression has an additional adverse consequence: It is associated with poorer adherence to the medical regimen[24] and to cardiac risk factor modification and rehabilitation programs, and depressed patients are more likely to drop out of exercise programs.

At least three separate pathophysiological mechanisms may link depression to CHD.[25, 26] First, depression results in autonomic arousal with hypothalamic-adrenocortical and sympathoadrenal hyperactivity. Depressed patients show hyperactivity of the hypothalamic-pituitary-adrenocortical axis and hypercortisolemia, and corticosteroids have atherogenic effects, including the induction of high blood pressure and increases in cholesterol and free fatty acids. In addition, there is hypersecretion of norepinephrine in depression, and such sympathoadrenal activation can contribute to cardiovascular disease through the direct effects of catecholamines on cardiac function, blood vessels, and platelets. Second, depressed patients exhibit diminished heart rate variability, and this has been found specifically in depressed cardiac patients as well.[27] This is believed to result from a relative increase in sympathetic tone and/or a relative decrease in parasympathetic tone, and it places depressed cardiac patients at greater risk for fatal arrhythmias. Third, depression may be accompanied by changes in platelet aggregability. Serotonin, which plays a role in depression, influences thrombogenesis and enhances platelet activation and responsiveness to other thrombogenic agents.

ANXIETY. In addition to depression, chronic anxiety and anxiety disorders such as panic disorder and phobias appear to exert a negative influence on the heart, and several studies suggest a relationship between anxiety disorder and increased cardiac morbidity and mortality. Anxiety has been found to predict CHD mortality and sudden cardiac death in a large, population-based, prospective study, after adjusting for a range of potential confounding variables.[28] In another study, anxiety was an independent predictor of cardiac events after myocardial infarction, after the influence of depression was taken into account.[29] There is also suggestive evidence for anxiety as a risk factor predisposing one to the development of CHD. Thus, initially healthy men who reported phobic anxiety were found to have a strikingly increased likelihood of subsequent death due to CHD, even after taking other CHD risk factors into account.[30] Possible mechanisms explaining this association include a decrease in vagal activity and consequently in heart rate variability in intensely anxious patients, microvascular angina, or idiopathic cardiomyopathy.

Psychosocial Factors

A number of psychosocial, cultural, and environmental factors increase the risk of CHD, either independently or in combination. These include social isolation and lack of social support, life stresses such as job strain, and sociodemographic characteristics. It is important to remember that these psychosocial risk factors tend to be associated with each other and therefore to co-occur within the same individuals. For example, job strain and socioeconomic position may be inversely correlated, and depression may be positively associated with social isolation. These psychosocial factors also tend to be associated with life-style behaviors that are unhealthy. For example, life stress may be correlated with smoking and increased alcohol consumption and body weight, and people with fewer social supports are less likely to stop smoking or to adhere to the medical regimen. This co-occurrence or clustering of psychosocial factors within the same individual is important because they may have a synergistic and not merely an additive effect in elevating risk. This interaction effect also makes studying the role of these variables more difficult.

SOCIAL ISOLATION, LACK OF SOCIAL SUPPORT, AND SOCIAL DISRUPTION. The literature on social support and cardiac disease emerged from population-based, cross-sectional surveys revealing that measures of social integration (such as being married, having regular contact with friends, and belonging to organizations) were associated with lower levels of CHD. Subsequent work substantiated this, revealing that social isolation and low social support (living alone, having few friends or family members, and not belonging to organizations, clubs, or churches) are associated with an increased incidence of CHD and a poorer outcome after the first diagnosis of CHD. Thus, those who live alone, are unmarried, or are without a confidante have a higher rate of recurrent myocardial infarction, fatal myocardial infarction, and all-cause cardiac mortality than those who are more socially integrated. Among patients with documented CHD, being unmarried and without a confidante confers a significantly worse 5-year prognosis, even after medical risk factors have been taken into account.[31] Berkman and associates found that elderly men and women who reported less emotional support from others before they sustained a myocardial infarction were almost three times more likely to die in the 6 months after it, after controlling for severity of infarction, comorbidity, coronary artery disease, and socioeconomic status.[32] This effect may be particularly robust in men.

However, many studies of social support and survival after myocardial infarction are retrospective or do not adequately assess and control for comorbid disease. There is suggestive evidence of an interaction effect between low social support and Type A behavior pattern such that low social support is a negative cardiac influence in Type A individuals but not in Type B individuals. Interestingly, animal studies also suggest social support has a protective role against atherogenesis. Thus the fondling by research personnel of laboratory rabbits placed on an atherogenic diet retards the development of coronary artery disease.[33] Crowding and social disruption of animal colonies on the one hand and isolation of individual laboratory animals on the other[34] both result in significantly increased rates of atherogenesis, and this effect is not due to increases in serum lipids.

Acculturation also influences the development of CHD. A classic epidemiological survey compared Japanese men living in Japan, Hawaii, and California. Traditional Japanese culture and lifestyle declined across the three groups, and this was accompanied by an increased incidence of CHD.[35] Similar findings emerged when comparing Japanese-Americans living in California who retained the traditional Japanese culture to varying degrees.[36] Animal work is also provocative in this regard. Dominant male monkeys fed an atherogenic diet develop coronary atherosclerosis at an accelerated rate when repeatedly moved from one social group to another rather than when left in a single, stable group.

Several mechanisms of action have been proposed to explain the relationship between social integration and CHD. First, concerned and supportive others may encourage healthy behaviors and adherence to the medical regimen and provide a motivation for altering unhealthy, behavioral risk factors. Conversely, loneliness may foster unhealthy behaviors such as smoking and drinking. Second, social support may attenuate and buffer the individual's emotional and/or physiological response to environmental stress. This may occur by virtue of the emotional benefits of comfort, encouragement, and consolation, as well as through practical assistance that mitigates the impact of stressful life events, for example, lending money, assisting with errands, and providing transportation.

LIFE STRESS AND JOB STRAIN. There has long been interest in the relationship between life stress and the development and progression of CHD. In animal studies ranging from mice to primates, stressful experimental paradigms that increase aggression and fear, and that decrease social affiliation and disturb stable social hierarchies, are associated with atherosclerosis. Thus, monkeys moved repeatedly from one stable monkey society to another developed more CHD than control monkeys.[37] In humans, two different forms of stress have received particular attention: major life events that tax one's abilities to adapt (such as getting divorced, moving, encountering financial difficulties, or being involved in a lawsuit) and more minor, recurrent irritants and daily frustrations. Some studies of individuals undergoing major, stressful life events have found an association with the incidence of myocardial infarction, the development of CHD, or cardiac mortality, whereas other prospective studies have not found a statistically significant association. At this point, the evidence remains inconclusive.

When turning to daily life stress, job strain and other forms of work-related stress have received considerable attention. Job strain is defined as the combination of high job demands with little autonomy or control over one's working conditions, routine, or schedule. Job strain has been associated with an increased risk of CHD in previously healthy people,[38] but its impact on the prognosis of already developed CHD is less clear. Cross-sectional studies in both the United States and Europe disclose that both male and female workers high in job strain have a higher prevalence of CHD and a higher incidence of myocardial infarction than do those with low job strain.[39] Longitudinal studies also provide some support for this hypothesis. In a large, 1-year prospective study, both men and women in higher-strain jobs had significantly higher rates of myocardial infarction.[40] Johnson and associates[41] conducted a longitudinal study of 12,517 Swedish men over a 14-year period and found that low levels of control over one's work conditions were an independent risk factor for cardiovascular disease mortality. After adjusting the data for the influences of age, smoking, exercise, and social class, workers with low levels of control over their jobs had a relative risk of 1.83 (95 percent CI = 1.19 to 2.82) for cardiovascular mortality. Workers with both low control over their work and low levels of social support had a relative risk of 2.62 (95 percent CI = 1.27 to 5.61) for cardiovascular mortality.

SOCIODEMOGRAPHIC CHARACTERISTICS. Health status in general is correlated with socioeconomic position, and persons of lower position have higher rates of CHD and a poorer prognosis after myocardial infarction. Lower socioeconomic status (whether assessed by education, occupation, or income) prospectively predisposes healthy people to an increased risk of CHD and CHD patients to a poorer prognosis. The decline in cardiovascular disease mortality over the past 30 years in the United States has been more pronounced among those of higher socioeconomic status, and the reasons for this are not clear. Because beneficial health habits (including not smoking and weight control) tend to be associated with socioeconomic status, they may play a role. Poorer nutrition and difficulty obtaining medical care may contribute. In addition, exposure to stressful life events, greater job strain, lack of social support, and diminished sense of self-control may also contribute to the relationship between socioeconomic status and CHD. Finally, hostility and depression may be inversely correlated with social position. There are also complex racial and ethnic differences in cardiovascular disease that remain poorly understood. Because race and ethnicity tend to be confounded with differences in socioeconomic position, it has been difficult to isolate their effects on the incidence, prevalence, course, and outcome of CHD.

Acute Mental Stress

Sudden, acute mental stress has negative cardiovascular consequences. Cardiovascular mortality rises in the month immediately after the death of a loved one,[42] and the incidence of cardiac events also rises immediately after natural disasters and among civilians subjected to military attack. The direct cardiovascular effects of sudden, acute mental stress have been observed during daily life with continuous, ambulatory monitoring and with laboratory paradigms that induce stress experimentally. These laboratory paradigms involve performing tasks that are aversive, challenging, or demanding, such as public speaking or accomplishing difficult intellectual tasks under time pressure or in frustrating circumstances. Such stressors reliably increase heart rate, blood pressure, and myocardial oxygen demands. The effect of acute mental stress on the heart already damaged by preexisting CHD has been studied extensively. Recent work has employed relatively sensitive measures of myocardial ischemia, including regional myocardial perfusion (measured with positron emission tomography) and wall motion abnormalities (assessed with radionuclide ventriculography and echocardiography). Such stress can precipitate myocardial ischemia in 30 to 60 percent of CHD patients.[43]

Mental stress–induced ischemia occurs at lower heart rates and at a lower level of myocardial work than does exercise-induced ischemia, suggesting that decreases in myocardial perfusion may play a role in mental stress–induced ischemia. In a representative study, 59 percent of CHD patients (and 8 percent of controls) exhibited myocardial ischemia during periods of experimentally induced stress using radionuclide ventriculography to detect wall motion abnormalities indicative of ischemia.[44] One third of the CHD patients had a decrease of at least 5 percent in ejection fraction. Clinical characteristics, such as extent of CHD, did not differentiate between those who did and did not develop ischemia when stressed.[44] Such mental stress–induced ischemia is more likely to be "silent" or asymptomatic than is the ischemia induced by exercise. In the study just referred to, 83 percent of mental stress–induced ischemic episodes were asymptomatic.[44]

When patients with preexisting CHD are monitored during daily life, mental challenges, in the absence of strenuous physical exertion, are frequently accompanied by transient myocardial ischemia. Such ischemia has been observed, for example, while driving and during public speaking. Whereas most ischemic episodes during daily life do not appear to be precipitated by psychological or mental stress, a sizable minority (perhaps as many as one fourth) are.[45, 46] Methodological difficulties however, make it difficult to establish the relative frequency of such psychological stressor—induced episodes.

CHD patients who exhibit mental stress—induced ischemia during daily life or in the laboratory setting appear to be at increased risk of subsequent fatal and nonfatal cardiac events.[47, 48] This relationship persists after other risk factors (including age, left ventricular function, and prior myocardial infarction) have been taken into account.[47] Acute stress may promote ischemic heart disease in a number of ways. First, stress increases myocardial oxygen demands as a result of its hemodynamic effects. There may also be a decrease in coronary blood flow secondary to vasospasm, especially in more severely diseased vessels.[49] Stress also activates the sympathoadrenal medullary and pituitary-adrenocortical systems, with increases in circulating cortisol and catecholamines, which activate platelets and promote platelet aggregation and which increase cholesterol and decrease high-density lipoproteins. The net result of all these effects is to increase cardiac demand while at the same time decreasing coronary blood supply and to promote plaque rupture and increase thrombus formation.

Sudden Emotion

The work on anger, depression, and anxiety discussed earlier deals with the long-term consequences and sequelae of enduring, persistent emotions. There is also a body of work on the immediate and acute effects of sudden, intense, negative emotion on the cardiovascular system. Because much of this work focuses on its role in triggering arrhythmias and sudden cardiac death, it will be reviewed in the next section. It is important to note here, however, that mental activities leading to intense anger and, to a lesser degree, to anxiety are also potent triggers of myocardial ischemia.[50, 51] Thus, there is a twofold increase in the risk of myocardial infarction in the 2 hours after an episode of intense anger.[52] Because these intense, negative emotional states involve sympathetic arousal, they may act by triggering coronary vasospasm, rupture of atherosclerotic plaques, and increased platelet aggregation. Anger and hostility in particular have been associated with increased platelet adhesion.[53] Hostility is also associated with decreased parasympathetic arousal during ambulatory monitoring.[54] When anger is experimentally induced, patients scoring higher on hostility scales exhibit greater sympathetic nervous system—mediated cardiovascular responses than those who are less hostile.[55]

ARRHYTHMIAS AND SUDDEN CARDIAC DEATH

Increasing evidence links mentally stressful and emotionally powerful events with lethal arrhythmias and sudden cardiac death (SCD). Intense emotions such as anxiety and anger, and the events that arouse them, have been associated with both benign and lethal arrhythmias, including ventricular premature contractions, ventricular tachycardia, and ventricular fibrillation. This effect is most evident in hearts that are already diseased, ischemic, or electrically unstable. There are at least three lines of investigation into the arrhythmogenic potential of stress, emotion, and psychiatric distress: epidemiologic surveys examining the role of life stress or psychiatric distress in predisposing to the subsequent development of lethal arrhythmias or SCD; psychophysiological experiments and anecdotal case reports of sudden, intense emotion or acute stress as immediate precipitants of arrhythmias or SCD; and investigations of the central nervous system's influence over cardiac rate and rhythm.

It has long been suspected that acutely stressful events and sudden, intense emotion can on occasion precipitate fatal arrhythmias and SCD. In 1971, Engel, using reliable, historical anecdotes, compiled a series of cases in which individuals were observed to die suddenly at the peak of intensely stressful and overwhelmingly emotional or traumatic experiences.[56] Reich and colleagues[57] subsequently conducted a careful, retrospective, psychiatric interview of patients hospitalized after a documented episode of ventricular tachycardia or ventricular fibrillation. They found that 21 percent had a major emotional disturbance or psychological trigger in the preceding 24 hours.[57] These included interpersonal conflicts, bereavement, public humiliation, marital separation, and business losses. Other studies produced comparable findings: one fourth to one half of SCD victims were thought to have died within minutes to hours after major psychological stress and acute emotional arousal.[58, 59] Although studies like these tend to suffer from problems of retrospective bias and selective recall, inadequate or absent control groups, and sampling bias, when taken together they nonetheless suggest that acute stress (perhaps in conjunction with other factors such as preexisting ischemic heart disease) can precipitate lethal arrhythmias and contribute to sudden cardiac death in a sizable fraction of cases.

Another line of research has examined the link between emotionally provocative daily stresses and arrhythmias. In healthy subjects, increases in ventricular ectopy occur during driving, public speaking, and stressful interviews. Among cardiac patients undergoing ambulatory monitoring, daily life stresses (but not major life change events) are statistically associated with ectopy. Lown[60, 61] and others have shown that experimentally induced psychological stress lowers the ventricular vulnerable period and the threshold for ventricular fibrillation and increases the frequency of ventricular ectopic beats in patients with preexisting ventricular arrhythmias. The acute, arrhythmogenic effect of stress-induced, sympathetic arousal has been demonstrated in patients with the long QT syndrome. Thus it is clear that stressful experiences and events can produce rhythm changes in both normal subjects and CHD patients. The clinical importance of this remains to be established, but the combination of severe, acute mental distress and a myocardium made vulnerable by virtue of preexisting disease can result in lethal arrhythmias and SCD.

Stressful events and the emotional distress that they evoke also have a less immediate and more prolonged effect in predisposing the individual to lethal arrhythmias and SCD over the long term. Thus, a number of studies report increases in life stress in the months preceding SCD. One prospective study of post-myocardial infarction patients found that a measure of life stress predicted sudden cardiac death in the following 3 years. However, for the most part this research is based on retrospective recall by a spouse or other informant and is subject to systematic reporting bias. In addition, many of these studies lack suitable control groups and/or employ problematic measures of life stress.[62]

EPIDEMIOLOGICAL SURVEYS. These suggest that some psychiatric disorders may also predispose to SCD. Anxiety disorders in particular appear to confer an increased risk of cardiac events, cardiac mortality, and SCD.[26, 63, 64] However, these studies are limited in number and generalizability. In one study, psychiatric distress during hospitalization for myocardial infarction predicted ventricular arrhythmias during ambulatory monitoring in the year after the infarct,[61] although a subsequent study by the same investigators failed to confirm these findings.[65] In retrospective work, female SCD victims with no prior history of cardiovascular disease were more likely to have had a psychiatric history than demographically matched, healthy controls.[66] Depression was the most common psychiatric diagnosis in these studies, and hopelessness may be the most toxic element of depression in this regard.[26] However a number of possible confounds make this work difficult to interpret, and on balance the evidence at this time must be considered equivocal.

Sociocultural and sociodemographic factors may also play a role in SCD. The inverse relationship found between socioeconomic status and cardiac mortality in general is especially robust for SCD, although this may be confounded by an association between socioeconomic status and access to emergency medical care. Other work has disclosed that cardiac mortality is significantly higher immediately after, as compared with immediately before, an important religious holiday. There are also well-recognized, culture-specific syndromes in which sudden death follows ritualized events that have a powerful, culture-specific significance (such as "voodoo death").

The link between stress and arrhythmias has been explored in experimental animal work. When dogs are subject to aversive restraint and electric shock, there is a 49 to 66 percent decrease in the repetitive extrasystole threshold.[67] If a coronary artery occlusion is first produced experimentally, then the same stressful paradigm induces spontaneous ventricular fibrillation.[68] Similarly, when pigs with a coronary artery occlusion are placed in a stressful environment, there is a high incidence of spontaneous ventricular fibrillation.[69] Conditioning and adaptation to the stress reduce its arrhythmogenic effect.

NEURAL CONTROL OF RHYTHM. A number of pathways mediate neural control of heart rate and rhythm. First, activation of the hypothalamic-adrenomedullary axis, with a resulting increase in circulating catecholamines, increases myocardial irritability and decreases the threshold for inducing ventricular fibrillation. Second, direct sympathetic innervation of the heart exerts a proarrhythmic effect, increasing ventricular ectopy and lowering the threshold for inducing ventricular arrhythmias, especially in the heart with preexisting ischemic damage or electrical instability. This effect is moderated by an antiarrhythmic, protective effect exerted by the parasympathetic system through the vagus nerve. Animal work has revealed evidence of cortical and brain stem control of cardiac rhythm. Pathways run from the frontal cortex and hypothalamus to the brain stem nuclei controlling cardiovascular function. Stimulation of the lateral and posterior hypothalamus lowers the ventricular fibrillation threshold, and blockade of these corticofrontal pathways can raise the threshold. In humans, electrocardiographic (ECG) changes in rhythm and/or repolarization are seen in many patients suffering cerebrovascular accidents involving the cortex.[70]

Finally, extreme stress and acute psychological trauma can result in myocardial necrosis. In animal models, large quantities of catecholamines, either exogenously administered or stress induced, can result in myofibrillar degeneration and myocardial necrosis. Pathological examination reveals widespread calcification, the result of peroxidation of myocardial lipid membranes and blockage of the calcium channel pump. This same lesion has also been reported in humans who died suddenly at the peak of extreme psychic stress and trauma.[71]

PSYCHIATRIC AND BEHAVIORAL ASPECTS OF HYPERTENSION AND CONGESTIVE HEART FAILURE

Hypertension (see also Chap. 28)

Stress, conditioned learning, and autonomic arousal can all elevate blood pressure. Stimulation of brain sites with con-

nections to the sympathetic nervous system elevates blood pressure, and many of these sites are in turn connected with higher centers involved in the perception of the environment. But the transient elevations of blood pressure that humans manifest in stressful and provocative situations may be unrelated to the persistent, sustained elevation that constitutes the disease of hypertension.

STRESS AND BLOOD PRESSURE. Stressful environments and situations that are challenging or aversive transiently increase the blood pressure of both normotensive and hypertensive individuals. This has been demonstrated in field studies using ambulatory monitoring of blood pressure during daily life and in laboratory studies assessing blood pressure reactivity to a discrete stimulus or specific experimental stressor. Some individuals exhibit greater reactivity than others, consistently responding to psychological stressors with greater increases in blood pressure and heart rate, more vasoconstriction and catecholamine secretion, and a more prolonged recovery phase. These individual differences in cardiovascular reactivity emerge early in life and appear to be stable and enduring over time. Such physiological hyperreactivity has long been thought to predispose to the eventual development of hypertension and atherosclerosis, but the hypothesis remains unproven and the evidence is still inconclusive. Patients with clinically diagnosed hypertension have been reported to show greater blood pressure responses to behavioral challenge than normotensive individuals,[72] and some prospective studies suggest that greater cardiovascular reactivity to stress is associated with subsequent, higher systolic and diastolic blood pressure.[73, 74] But the use of laboratory challenges is problematic, and it is not clear that transient blood pressure increases in response to such stressors are precursors of pathological, sustained hypertension.[75] A number of studies have examined whether normotensive individuals with a family history of hypertension show greater cardiovascular reactivity to experimental mental stressors than normotensive individuals without such a family history. The results of this work remain inconclusive and equivocal.[76]

In surveys examining the relationship between naturally occurring stress and blood pressure, major life stress has been associated with the onset or worsening of essential hypertension. Job strain in particular has been associated with an elevated prevalence and incidence of hypertension in men (although this is less clear in women), and the blood pressures of people in more stressful occupations tend to be higher than those in less stressful jobs. However, it appears that such chronic stress requires the simultaneous presence of other etiological factors (e.g., genetic endowment, dietary factors, or renal disease) to cause sustained hypertension. This situation may be analogous to that emerging from animal work. In animals predisposed to hypertension by genetic endowment or salt ingestion, repeated exposure to stress can lead to sustained hypertension.[77] But sustained hypertension does not appear to result in healthy animals without such predisposing factors.

PSYCHOLOGICAL INFLUENCES. Anger and anxiety are accompanied by increases in peripheral vascular resistance and blood pressure. Anger has been thought to predispose to the development of essential hypertension, but this is controversial, particularly because much of the relevant research is either retrospective or cross-sectional.[78] Hostile individuals respond to provocation, conflict, and disagreement with larger increases in blood pressure than do people who are less hostile.[79] There have been reports of higher levels of anger and suppressed anger among hypertensive patients, but the direction, significance, and certainty of this association remains unclear. In a prospective study, increases in trait anger in women did predict increases in blood pressure over a 3-year period, after controlling for biological and genetic variables.[80] However, it does not appear that the prevalence of essential hypertension is elevated in hostile, Type A individuals. Studies of minority populations tend to disclose a closer link between anger and hypertension than do studies of nonminorities.

Recent work has focused on the more-difficult-to-measure construct of repressed or *suppressed* emotion (particularly anger), and there are reports of an association between emotional inhibition and essential hypertension. A meta-analysis concluded that there does appear to be an association between *suppressed* anger and resting blood pressure.[81] In one prospective study, men who suppressed their feelings when faced with an interpersonal conflict were more likely to be hypertensive at follow-up.[82] But, in general, this literature is still inconclusive, in part because of the difficulty in distinguishing transient angry states from anger as a stable, enduring personality trait.

Other studies have examined the role of anxiety. There is some evidence that chronically anxious persons develop greater increases in systolic blood pressure over the ensuing years[80, 83] and may also be at increased risk of developing essential hypertension.[80, 84] It has been suggested that psychological stressors tend to produce more anger in males and more anxiety in females.[79] Both of these affective states are accompanied by arousal of the sympathetic nervous system, and this suggests that chronically increased sympathetic tone is a final common pathway to elevated blood pressure.[80] Finally, the possible etiological role of depression has also been investigated. The prevalence of hypertension is reported to be higher in depressed community residents, depressed medical patients, and depressed psychiatric patients than in nondepressed comparison groups.

Based on this work, therapies such as relaxation training and meditative techniques, blood pressure and heart rate biofeedback, and psychotherapy incorporating relaxation training have all been employed to treat hypertension. Relaxation techniques and meditation apparently decrease blood pressure by lowering total peripheral resistance and vasoconstrictive tone.[85] One potential weakness of such therapies is that the treatment effect may decay upon discontinuation of active treatment. Some studies, however, have found that the beneficial effects of relaxation training (combined with pharmacotherapy) were still evident at long-term follow-up after the behavioral treatment ended.[86] In one study, relaxation training lowered blood pressure while the exercises were being practiced, but ambulatory blood pressure readings during daily life did not decline.[87] In sum, although these behavioral techniques are not very effective when used alone, they may provide some incremental benefit when added to the conventional antihypertensive regimen.[78] They may lead to modest reductions in blood pressure or enable the physician to employ lower doses of antihypertensive medication.[78] The latter outcome is of more than trivial significance because nonadherence to the antihypertensive medication regimen is very common and constitutes a major impediment to effective treatment.

SOCIOCULTURAL FACTORS. Epidemiological and animal studies suggest a relationship between high blood pressure and sociocultural conditions. Essential hypertension tends to be less prevalent in societies with stronger cultural traditions and more widely held value systems and in those that are safer and more stable, than in societies with more disintegration, higher crime rates, and less stable social orders. In societies undergoing transition, conflict, or disintegration, blood pressures tend to rise over time, but many factors (e.g., changes in diet) may be contributing.[88] Individuals in more crowded and stressful living and working environments tend to show increased levels of catecholamines, increased cardiovascular reactivity, and higher average blood pressures. Animal studies seem to corroborate these findings: Mice subjected to crowding and ex-

posed to threat from cats develop sustained high blood pressure.[89]

Congestive Heart Failure (see also Chap. 17)

The psychiatric and behavioral aspects of congestive heart failure (CHF) have only recently been subjected to scrutiny. It appears that the sorts of psychosocial factors that influence the course and outcome of CHD may also influence CHF. Stress and emotional distress have been linked to the onset or exacerbation of CHF, perhaps by increasing heart rate and blood pressure and/or by provoking myocardial ischemia in patients with preexisting, severe CHD. Emotional factors have been reported to precede admission in 49 percent of hospitalizations for CHF.[90] It has been suggested that left ventricular function is impaired during psychological stress,[91] and stress-induced heart failure has been described. In a study of patients with idiopathic cardiomyopathy, experimental psychological stress (mental arithmetic) was shown to induce changes in left ventricular diastolic function.[92]

Depression has received particular attention in CHF populations because it is chronic and debilitating, and because of its increased prevalence in the elderly. Freedland and coworkers[93] found that 17 percent of elderly patients hospitalized with CHF had current, major depression, and Havranek and colleagues[94] found a significantly higher prevalence of depressive symptoms in outpatients with CHF than in outpatients with hypertension. Others, however, have not found an elevated rate of depression in CHF. This research is complicated by difficulty in differentiating CHF from depressive disorders. The anorexia, fatigue, weakness, and insomnia (resulting from orthopnea and paroxysmal nocturnal dyspnea) accompanying CHF can be confused with the symptoms of depression, and the cardiac cachexia of end-stage CHF may also suggest severe depression. When CHF is severe enough to cause cerebral ischemia, then cognitive dysfunction, confusion, and delirium with psychotic symptoms may result. This may at times be difficult to distinguish from anxiety disorder and panic.

Social support appears to be an important moderator of the clinical course of CHF. Elderly women hospitalized with CHF who have no sources of emotional support have a more than threefold increase in the risk of cardiovascular events in the ensuing year than comparable patients with emotional support.[95] Elderly men without emotional support were not at increased risk. This work also underscored the importance of social ties, because patients without social ties had a more than twofold increase in cardiovascular events, even after taking emotional support into account.[95]

CARDIAC SYMPTOMS: CHEST PAIN AND PALPITATIONS (see also Chap. 3)

Chest Pain

Chest pain, the classic symptom of CHD, is a nonspecific, insensitive, and unreliable indicator of ischemia. Pain does not bear a fixed, one-to-one relationship to demonstrable pathology; many patients with chest pain have no heart disease, and ischemia and infarction are often asymptomatic. Approximately one fourth of myocardial infarctions are "silent," and 70 to 80 percent of out-of-hospital, ischemic episodes in CHD patients are asymptomatic. Conversely, no cardiac cause is found for the vast majority of complaints of chest pain. Even in patients with documented CHD, two thirds of chest pain episodes occur in the absence of ST segment depression indicative of ischemia.[51]

In one study of primary care patients presenting with chest pain that led to a diagnostic work-up, a definite medical cause could be established in only 5 of 80 patients, at a cost of $4354 per diagnosis.[96] Even among patients undergoing coronary angiography for chest pain, 10 to 30 percent have minimal or no angiographic evidence of CHD.

The absence of demonstrable heart disease, however, does not mean that the patient's chest pain is either inconsequential or self-limited. Follow-up studies of chest pain patients with negative angiography and/or negative exercise stress testing reveal persistent distress and disability. Although rates of myocardial infarction and of cardiac morbidity and mortality remain low in these populations, these patients continue to exhibit elevated levels of symptoms, disability, and medical care utilization. At least half of these patients continue to report recurrent chest pain, the persistent belief that they have serious heart disease, and impaired functioning (at work, socially, and in daily activities) comparable to that of patients with myocardial infarction and angina.[97, 98]

Psychological, psychiatric, and behavioral factors mediate the relationship between CHD on the one hand and the resulting symptoms and disability on the other. Emotional distress is correlated with reports of chest pain in both CHD patients and in those free of cardiac disease.[12] Generalized psychological distress and body awareness is higher in patients with chest pain and normal coronary arteries than in those with CHD.[99] Mood and daily activities may account for as much of the variability in ambulatory patients' reports of chest pain as does ST depression indicative of ischemia.[51] The level of disability in patients with medically unexplained chest pain is strongly associated with the presence of psychiatric morbidity.[98]

Several psychological factors tend to differentiate chest pain patients with and without demonstrable cardiac disease. When those with normal angiography or normal stress tests are compared with those with positive tests, the former group is younger, more likely to be female, and has more psychological distress and a higher prevalence of diagnosable psychiatric disorder.[100, 101] Patients with medically unexplained chest pain have a higher than expected prevalence of depressive and anxiety disorder.[100] When compared with chest pain patients with positive findings on angiography, they have elevated rates of panic disorder (35 to 50 percent vs. 5 percent) and of major depressive disorder (approximately 35 to 40 percent vs. 5 to 8 percent). Of course, cardiac and psychiatric disorders are not mutually exclusive and not infrequently co-occur. Thus, 5 to 23 percent of patients with angiographic evidence of CHD also have panic disorder. These cases of psychiatric and cardiac comorbidity pose especially difficult diagnostic dilemmas, and it is in them that panic disorder is most likely to be overlooked. The chest pain seen in panic disorder is more likely to be atypical in clinical character and to be accompanied by palpitations, dizziness, paresthesias, and multiple other somatic symptoms.

Palpitations

Palpitations are among the most common symptoms encountered in medical practice, reported by 16 percent of patients in a large survey of a primary care clinic.[102] Yet this subjective sensation corresponds very poorly to demonstrable abnormalities of cardiac rate or rhythm: Most palpitations are not accompanied by arrhythmias, and most arrhythmias are not perceived and reported as palpitations. When patients complaining of palpitations undergo 24-hour, ambulatory ECG monitoring, 39 to 85 percent manifest a rhythm disturbance (the vast majority being benign and clinically insignificant). Approximately three fourths

of these patients with arrhythmias report at least one palpitation during 24 hours of monitoring, but in less than 15 percent of them do their symptoms coincide in time with the arrhythmia. Thus, accurate symptom reports occur in less than 10 percent of all patients being monitored.

Because palpitations are rarely accompanied by a clinically significant arrhythmia, it is not surprising that a high proportion of such patients either have a psychiatric cause for their symptom or no etiology can be established. In a careful survey of 190 patients presenting with palpitations, 31 percent were judged to have a psychiatric basis for their presenting symptom and no etiology could be established in an additional 16 percent.[103] The most common psychiatric cause of palpitations is panic disorder, which is found in more than a fourth of ambulatory medical patients complaining of palpitations. In one study, 31 percent of 229 such patients had panic disorder or panic attacks, and in another study, 28 percent of patients referred for 24-hour ambulatory ECG monitoring for palpitations met criteria for lifetime panic disorder and 19 percent met criteria for current panic disorder.[104] In the latter study, a high prevalence of depressive disorder was also reported.

Palpitations that have no demonstrable cardiac basis are nonetheless a persistent and disturbing problem for many patients. In a naturalistic, 1-year follow-up study, 75 percent of palpitation patients were found to have experienced recurrent symptoms, 19 percent reported impairment of their work performance, and 37 percent reported impairment in their role functioning at home.[103] In another study, 84 percent of palpitation patients remained symptomatic 6 months after initially presenting, and they had an elevated rate of medical utilization during the follow-up interval.[105]

Panic attacks and arrhythmias may be difficult to distinguish clinically. Both may present with palpitations, shortness of breath, and lightheadedness, and both not infrequently occur in the young and in those who are otherwise healthy. Frank syncope, however, is unusual in panic disorder and if there have been multiple episodes, panic attacks are more stereotyped and more consistent from episode to episode. Recurrent panic attacks tend to lead to agoraphobia, in which the patient first becomes apprehensive about, and then avoids, situations such as being left alone, trapped in large crowds, and journeying far from home. Conversely, to make matters more difficult, the sympathetic arousal that may accompany an arrhythmia (and other acute cardiac events such as pulmonary emboli, acute valvular dysfunction, and myocardial ischemia as well) may be experienced and reported by the patient as acute anxiety or panic rather than as a cardiac event.

Delay and Denial of Cardiac Symptoms

Myocardial infarction patients commonly ignore, rationalize, or explicitly deny their symptoms, so that the average interval between the onset of symptoms and arrival in an emergency department is between 3 and 9 hours, depending on the study.[106] Delay before seeking medical attention for acute myocardial infarction is a serious problem, in part because a high proportion of myocardial infarction deaths occur soon after the event and in part because the newer therapies to preserve myocardial tissue (e.g., intravenous thrombolysis) require early intervention (see Chap. 36). Delay is greater in women and in the elderly[107, 108] and (paradoxically) in those with a history of previous myocardial infarction.[107] From a practical standpoint, a crucial determinant of the length of delay is the interval before the myocardial infarction sufferer informs someone else of his or her symptoms; once the patient informs another person of his or her distress, help is usually rapidly obtained.

Acute Care of the Hospitalized Patient

The onset or sudden progression of cardiac disease is a frightening and powerful emotional experience. Pain and physical discomfort, the specter of sudden death or invalidism, and the knowledge that one has a chronic and potentially lethal disease are all profoundly distressing. The initial reaction is almost always one of anxiety. Fears of premature, sudden death loom, and worries about physical, sexual, social, and occupational incapacity materialize and plague patients. They may become terrified of any physical activity or strong emotion, fearing that these can immediately trigger sudden death. As time passes and chronicity sets in, anxiety may be replaced with despondency and a heightened sense of physical vulnerability and of one's mortality. The individual may come to feel damaged or diminished. Patients may feel that their job performance and future livelihood have been irrevocably compromised, that they are old and decrepit, and that they face a restricted and empty future. They may feel guilty and blame themselves for falling ill, ascribing their plight to their failure to exercise enough, diet sufficiently, or maintain other "healthy" habits. All of this may lead to a clinically significant, depressive episode.

Several psychiatric and behavioral problems commonly arise in patients hospitalized for an acute cardiac event. In addition to the illness itself, the experience of hospitalization (and in particular admission to the coronary care or intensive care unit) can be frightening and stressful. Patients suddenly find themselves in an unfamiliar, alien, and terrifying world, surrounded by fearsome machines with blinking lights and beeping alarms, subjected to painful procedures and tests about which they know little and understand less, while their lives seemingly hang in the balance from moment to moment. The daily routine and the food are alien, and patients feel cut off from family, friends, neighbors, and all that is familiar. Sustained sleep is next to impossible, and many are afraid to fall asleep, believing that the heart is in greater jeopardy during sleep. Their worst fears may seem to come true when they witness a cardiac arrest, or even the death, of another patient.

Hospitalized patients should be kept well informed about what is transpiring, what is being done medically for them, and why. They should be told what to expect before procedures are carried out; the functions of equipment should be explained; and the effects and (especially) side effects of medications should be described in advance. The patient should be reassured that anxiety is a normal and entirely appropriate reaction. Anxiolytics are often prescribed because anxiety is not only uncomfortable but its concomitant sympathetic arousal can be medically dangerous. Benzodiazepines are most commonly used for this purpose and should be prescribed on a regular, round-the-clock (rather than as needed) basis. In the elderly and in those with compromised liver function, the shorter-acting benzodiazepines (e.g., oxazepam or lorazepam) are preferred, because they are cleared primarily by the kidneys. The pharmacology of anxiolytics is discussed in the following section.

DELIRIUM. This condition is not infrequent in hospitalized cardiac patients, especially after cardiac surgery. Delirium is characterized by an altered level of consciousness and a fluctuating state of confusion. The delirious patient is disoriented to time and place, has impaired memory and attention, develops delusional ideas, and experiences perceptual disturbances such as illusions or hallucinations. The sleep-wake cycle is disrupted, and the level of consciousness and arousal is disturbed, so that the patient may be either stuporous or obtunded, or hyperalert, restless, and agitated. The onset of delirium may be insidious (e.g., insomnia, mild nocturnal confusion, and restlessness) and go unnoticed by the staff, or it may be dramatic and abrupt. The patient begins to misinterpret sensory information (for instance mistaking a shadow for someone lurking in a corner of his or her room) and becomes suspicious and increasingly frightened. As confusion, fear, and excitement mount, frank paranoia sets in and the patient may become agitated, disruptive, belligerent, and out of control. This is a psychiatric emergency, because in their confusion and frenzy, delirious patients may harm themselves accidentally, fall, or pull out therapeutic life lines, catheters, and implanted devices. The incidence of delirium after cardiac surgery is as high as 30 percent in some studies,[109] typically following a lucid interval of 3 to 5 days after surgery. The risk factors for postcardiotomy delirium are advanced age (older than age 70 years); more extensive aortic atherosclerosis (large atheromas may be liberated by surgical manipulation of the aorta); a prior history of neurological disease, particularly preexisting cerebrovascular disease; a history of pulmonary disease, with the concomitant risks of poorer cerebral oxygenation and more hypoxia; and surgery that is more extensive and of longer duration.[110]

Treatment of Delirium. This rests on rapid identification and correction of the underlying cause of the delirium, medication for behavioral control if necessary, and supportive measures to provide comfort and safety. The etiological search is paramount. This means checking for cerebral hypoperfusion or hypoxia, acid-base disturbance, inadequate hydration, fluid and electrolyte imbalance, renal or hepatic failure, endocrine dysfunction, infection, and nutritional deficiency. Medications must be carefully reviewed because anticholinergics, narcotics, sedative-hypnotics, and H_2 blockers are common causes of delirium. Common offenders include cimetidine, digoxin, aminophylline, anticonvulsants, and all sedatives and hypnotics. Alcohol or drug withdrawal is a frequent cause, and the history must be searched carefully with this possibility in mind.

If the patient is agitated, combative, or confused enough to require behavioral control, high-potency antipsychotic drugs can be administered. Haloperidol has been widely used for this purpose and is safe and effective in critically ill patients, whether given orally or parenterally (including intravenously in emergency situations).[111, 112] Mild, delirious agitation is treated with 0.5 to 2 mg of haloperidol and moderate delirium with 5 to 10 mg; and the severely delirious patient can be given 10 or more mg of haloperidol. If the agitation persists unabated after 20 to 30 minutes, twice the original dose may be readministered. It has a minimal effect on heart rate, blood pressure, and respiration, and extrapyramidal effects are rare when it is administered intravenously. Parenteral droperidol is sometimes used. If excitement, hyperarousal, and motor agitation are especially prominent, the antipsychotic may be supplemented with a short-acting benzodiazepine such as lorazepam. Antipsychotic agents are discussed in the following section.

Supportive measures should be undertaken to calm, orient, and comfort the delirious patient. He or she should be reoriented frequently by the staff, and a clock and calendar should be prominently displayed to aid in this process. It is helpful to preserve as much of a day-night cycle as is feasible considering the hospital routine and to limit awakenings by staff during the night as much as possible. Family visitation should be encouraged because it is helpful in reassuring and calming the patient and in reducing paranoia. Familiar objects, such as family photographs, should be prominently displayed and plainly visible. Staff need to continually reintroduce themselves, educate the patient about what they are doing, and repeatedly explain the situation. Physical restraint should be employed whenever necessary to prevent self-harm or harm to the staff.

Convalescence and Recovery

In the weeks after hospital discharge, depression is common, although it varies widely in severity. It is often self-limited, gradually diminishing as the patient resumes his or her old activities and as the specter of the acute episode and the hospitalization recede into the past. Frank discussion of the patient's concerns and educational information about common myths and fears are helpful. Lingering anxiety may have led patients to avoid activities or situations that they fear will provoke symptoms, cardiac events, or even sudden death. Early, progressive mobilization is the best antidote to anxiety and depression. The patient may be shocked and dismayed at the degree of exhaustion produced by even mild exertion, and although this easy fatigability is actually the result of deconditioning, it is mistakenly interpreted as evidence of permanent cardiac damage. As a result, exercise may be assiduously avoided, which only exacerbates the problem.

Patients are often apprehensive about returning to work because of the stress is engenders. Many believe that strong emotions can be lethal and try to protect themselves by assiduously avoiding all situations or activities that arouse strong feelings, such as sexual activity or watching sports on television. Sexual activity in particular is diminished, and sexual dysfunction is common in both women and men with cardiac disease.[113] Such concerns should be elicited by the physician and then discussed frankly and openly. Recommendations should be as specific as possible about which activities are prescribed and proscribed; simply saying "use your judgment" or "do it in moderation" is not helpful.[114] Group meetings of cardiac patients (such as post-myocardial infarction groups) to share common concerns, provide support, obtain educational information, and guide the progressive resumption of activities can be helpful in recuperation.

If depression lasts more than several weeks and is profound enough to meet diagnostic criteria for major depressive disorder, as happens in one third of patients in the year after myocardial infarction,[10] aggressive therapy is indicated. If left untreated, depression imposes a serious psychosocial burden, medical rehabilitation and recovery are impeded, and the depression itself is likely to become chronic. More than three fourths of post-myocardial infarction patients with major depressive disorder remain depressed 6 to 12 months later.[115, 116] It is thought that successful treatment (psychopharmacological and/or psychosocial) of depression in post-myocardial infarction patients will reduce subsequent cardiac morbidity and mortality, and large-scale, multiinstitutional intervention trials (e.g., Sertraline Antidepressant Heart Attack Randomized Trial [SADHART], Enhancing Recovery in Coronary Heart Disease [ENRICHD]) are now underway to test this hypothesis. The pharmacotherapy of depression is discussed in the following section.

Over the long term, some cardiac patients adopt a persistent coping style that is maladaptive and dysfunctional.[114] They may ignore the episode and deny their illness entirely, maintaining that nothing serious has happened at all. They may refuse to acknowledge any limitations or adhere to a therapeutic regimen, and generally overdo things. Alternatively, they may capitulate completely to their illness and retreat into unwarranted invalidism, becoming "cardiac cripples" who are preoccupied with their health, terrified by every benign twinge or cramp, and living a life of psychological invalidism and disability. Each of these profoundly maladaptive coping patterns deserves psychiatric attention.

Primary prevention programs attempt to modify behavioral risk factors in individuals who have not yet manifested significant disease, with the aim of preventing cardiac events from occurring or of delaying their onset. Secondary prevention programs focus on similar factors in patients who already have clinical evidence of disease, with the aim of retarding its progression. These psychosocial, educational, and behavioral programs may include many different components. Most programs assist patients to modify lifestyle behavioral risk factors, including smoking cessation, curtailing alcohol abuse, lowering saturated fat intake, and controlling weight. Almost all emphasize a formal program of graduated, progressive, aerobic exercise. Many programs include educational counseling about CHD, its risk factors and its treatment. Many also attempt to modify hostility or Type A behavior with cognitive/behavioral therapy.

Rehabilitation programs for patients who have sustained a cardiac event often aim to promote psychosocial adjustment and may include psychotherapy (see Chap. 39). Most programs include stress management and relaxation training, in which patients are taught to identify social and environmental stressors, improve their use of social supports, and develop new skills for managing stressful situations and the disturbing effects that they evoke. Relaxation training generally combines elements of progressive muscle relaxation, diaphragmatic breathing, and focused attention. Patients are taught these techniques and are then encouraged to practice them regularly.

It is difficult to summarize the effectiveness of these heterogeneous psychotherapeutic, psychosocial, and behavioral programs because they vary so widely in quality, content, design, and intensity. Many intervention trials are flawed by small sample size, high dropout rates, insufficient long-term follow-up, and inadequate comparison or control groups. In addition, as standard cardiac care improves so substantially, it becomes more difficult to demonstrate the incremental benefit of these programs in terms of hard cardiac endpoints.[117] Trials reporting positive benefits have generally not been replicated. Nonetheless, it generally appears that when added to standard medical care, many of these programs are more effective than usual care alone in reducing psychiatric distress and morbidity, and in improving quality of life, disability status, and role functioning, and probably in reducing cardiac morbidity and mortality as well.[118-122]

A careful meta-analysis of 23 randomized, controlled intervention trials involving over 2000 patients, disclosed that when added to standard cardiac care, psychosocial interventions resulted in significant reductions in systolic blood pressure, heart rate, and serum cholesterol, and significantly lower rates of cardiac mortality and cardiac morbidity. These benefits were most evident in the 2 years after the intervention and became less evident thereafter.[118] Two meta-analyses of psychoeducational therapies found favorable effects on cardiac mortality, systolic blood pressure, and on exercise and diet.[123, 124] Finally a recent, thorough meta-analysis of 37 programs with varying components of psychoeducation and stress management found that they resulted in a 34 percent reduction in cardiac mortality and a 29 percent reduction in recurrent myocardial infarction, as well as significant effects on blood pressure and weight.[125]

PSYCHOSOCIAL INTERVENTIONS. There is a growing interest in supportive, psychosocial interventions designed particularly to improve social support and lessen social isolation, often in combination with counseling or other treatment for depression and anxiety. In one study of 435 post-myocardial infarction patients randomized to a nursing-based psychosocial intervention or to medical care as usual, 1-year cardiac mortality was half as high in the intervention group[126] and the incidence of recurrent myocardial infarction was significantly lower at 7-year follow-up.[127] On the other hand, three large, randomized trials of multimodal, case management interventions conducted by nurses or health visitors[128-130] failed to demonstrate a clear reduction in depression or psychological dysphoria. Two of these studies found no effect on cardiac disease outcomes,[128, 129] and one study showed a marginally significant, negative impact of the intervention on cardiac outcomes in women.[130]

RELAXATION TRAINING. Stress management techniques and relaxation therapy have been found to improve cardiac outcomes in some studies. Various combinations of these techniques have been shown to decrease the incidence and frequency of anginal episodes,[131] fatal and nonfatal cardiac events,[126] and disability and role impairment[132] and to improve quality of life. Relaxation training alone has been found to decrease fatal and nonfatal myocardial infarction[133] and to improve cardiac function.[134] In one large-scale study, a 4-month program of stress management was compared with exercise training and usual care in patients with documented CHD. At follow-up an average of 3 years later, the former group had a lower incidence of cardiac events and fewer ischemic episodes.[135] On the contrary, other studies disclose either a very limited and transient benefit (i.e., seen only in the first month after the intervention) or no benefit at all in terms of anginal frequency, cardiac events, or reduction in blood pressure.[129, 136] Jones and West, for example, randomized over 2000 patients with a recent myocardial infarction to a psychosocial treatment or to care as usual and found no significant differences between the groups in cardiac mortality after 1 year.[128] In summarizing this outcome literature, it appears that these psychosocial and stress reduction programs, when they are focused, well designed, and added to standard cardiac care, do decrease psychiatric distress and improve health-related quality of life and role functioning. They probably also decrease cardiac morbidity and/or mortality, but this has not yet been definitively established.

PSYCHOLOGICAL TREATMENT OF HOSTILITY AND TYPE A BEHAVIOR. Several intervention trials have specifically assessed psychological treatments to modify hostility and Type A behavior. These treatment programs are manualized and protocol driven. They aim to enhance the awareness and effective management of anger and other negative feelings and thoughts and to improve problem solving and communications skills. A meta-analysis of 18 such controlled trials concluded that treatment had a moderately large effect size in modifying anger, hostility, impatience, and time urgency.[137] The authors also found a marginally significant effect on cardiac events and mortality in the year after treatment. In a recent, controlled, randomized trial of an eight-session workshop to reduce hostility, the intervention was found to significantly decrease hostility at 2-month follow-up.[140] In the Recurrent Coronary Prevention Project (RCPP), the addition of

Type A behavior counseling to a standard psychosocial rehabilitation program of 862 post-myocardial infarction patients produced a significant reduction in Type A behavior and a 44 percent reduction in nonfatal myocardial infarction and cardiac death at 3-year follow-up.[138] The effect on nonfatal myocardial infarction persisted 4½ years after the intervention.[139]

Graduated, aerobic exercise training is another keystone of many cardiac rehabilitation programs. Such training improves exercise capacity and lowers blood pressure and body weight, as well as improving subjective, health-related quality of life. It is less clear, however whether these risk factor reductions in turn lead to significant differences in cardiac outcomes.[120] This may be because a sizable fraction of patients do not continue to adhere to the exercise regimen over long periods of time after the program ends.

PSYCHOPHARMACOLOGY IN THE CARDIAC PATIENT

Cardiovascular Aspects of Psychotropic Agents

Antidepressants (Table 70–1)

SEROTONIN REUPTAKE INHIBITORS (SRIs). The SRIs have superseded the tricyclic antidepressants (TCAs) as the first-line agents for treating the cardiac patient with major depressive disorder. Their efficacy is comparable to that of

▼ **TABLE 70–1. ANTIDEPRESSANTS**

AGENT	STARTING DOSE	MAXIMUM DOSE	SIDE EFFECTS	CARDIOVASCULAR EFFECTS	
Serotonin Reuptake Inhibitors					
Sertraline	12.5–25 mg/d	200 mg/d	Sexual dysfunction Nausea, diarrhea Headache		Benign bradycardia
Fluoxetine	5–10 mg/d	80 mg/d	Anxiety, agitation, insomnia Somnolence, sedation		
Paroxetine	10 mg/d	50 mg/d	Tremor		
Tricyclics					
Amitriptyline	10–25 mg h.s.	300 mg/d	Sedation, somnolence	Dry mouth Blurry vision	Increase QT, PR, QRS intervals Decrease T wave amplitude
Imipramine	10–25 mg h.s.	300 mg/d		Constipation Urinary retention	Tachycardia Arrhythmias
Nortriptyline	10 mg/d	150 mg/d	Anxiety, insomnia	Postural hypotension Weight gain	Postural hypotension
Desipramine	25 mg/d	300 mg/d			
Psychostimulants					
Methylphenidate	2.5 mg b.i.d.	20 mg b.i.d.	Anxiety, agitation Insomnia Anorexia Paranoia		Tachycardia (mild) Hypertension (mild)
Other Agents					
Bupropion	75 mg/d	150 mg t.i.d.	Anorexia, nausea Anxiety, agitation Insomnia Seizures		
Venlafaxine	12.5 mg b.i.d.	125 mg t.i.d.	Nausea Headache Sexual dysfunction Anxiety, insomnia Somnolence Dizziness		Hypertension (dose related)
Trazadone	25 mg/d	600 mg/d	Sedation Nausea Headache Priapism (rare)		Postural hypotension Arrhythmias (rare)
Mirtazapine	15 mg q.h.s.	45 mg q.h.s.	Sedation, somnolence Weight gain Dry mouth, anticholinergic effects Dizziness Agranulocytosis (rare)		

the older TCAs, they are better tolerated and safer in overdose, and they have less pharmacological action on the heart. The serotonergic antidepressants have little anticholinergic, antihistaminic, or noradrenergic activity. However, because they have become available only relatively recently, there has been less systematic study of their efficacy and safety in CHD populations and in the elderly, and few randomized, controlled trials in these populations have been completed. Although more extensive investigation is still necessary, the data thus far suggest that the SRIs have minimal cardiovascular effects and a large margin of safety in treating patients with even very severe heart disease.[141]

In healthy patients, the SRIs have no adverse effects on cardiac contractility or conduction and there is no evidence of cardiotoxicity in overdose. In cardiac populations, they do not appear to cause significant electrocardiographic or blood pressure changes, although they can slow heart rate. Only very rarely do they produce a clinically significant degree of sinus bradycardia. The SRIs have the potential to interact with a number of medications used to treat cardiac disease. They inhibit hepatic cytochrome P450 isoenzymes,[142] a series of isoenzymes involved in the oxidative metabolism of many drugs. These include lipophilic beta blockers (e.g., metoprolol and propranolol), calcium channel blockers, type IC antiarrhythmics, angiotensin-converting enzyme inhibitors, anticonvulsants, antihistamines, benzodiazepines, TCAs, codeine, and warfarin. The SRIs therefore can raise the blood levels of these other agents when co-administered. However, although these interactions can be demonstrated in vitro, their significance in clinical practice is still unclear. Caution should be exercised when giving SRIs to patients on these medications, and in particular the prothrombin time of patients receiving both warfarin and an SRI should be monitored closely. Because the SRIs are highly protein bound, they may displace other protein-bound drugs when co-administered, thereby increasing their bioavailability. This interaction can occur with warfarin and digitoxin, but it does not appear to be clinically significant in magnitude.

TRICYCLIC ANTIDEPRESSANTS (TCAs). TCAs were previously the mainstay of antidepressant pharmacotherapy and remain effective agents that are still widely employed. However, their multiple cardiovascular side effects and their potential lethality in overdose are disadvantages in patients with cardiac disease. TCAs act on adrenergic neurons in the central nervous system, and in the periphery have anticholinergic properties, have quinidine-like effects, and produce alpha-adrenergic receptor blockade. They affect heart rate, rhythm, conduction, contractility, and blood pressure. Accordingly, these agents are not generally used in the presence of rhythm or conduction disturbances, severe congestive heart failure, or within 4 to 6 weeks of a myocardial infarction. A guiding principle when using them in the elderly and those with cardiac disease is to initiate treatment with low doses and to titrate the dosage upward slowly and carefully. Among the TCAs, the tertiary amines (e.g., imipramine and amitriptyline) are associated with more side effects, and the secondary amines (e.g., nortriptyline) have a preferable side-effect profile in cardiac patients.[143]

The TCAs are type IA antiarrhythmic agents (see Chap. 23) and accordingly depress cardiac conduction, decrease ventricular irritability, and suppress ectopic activity. They slow atrial and ventricular depolarization; increase the QT, PR, and QRS intervals; and decrease T wave amplitude. In the absence of preexisting conduction abnormalities, this action is unlikely to be clinically significant at therapeutic doses. However, second-degree heart block, sick sinus syndrome, bundle branch block, a prolonged QT interval, and the concurrent administration of antiarrhythmic agents are all considered contraindications to their use. In contrast to this antiarrhythmic effect, the TCAs can on occasion be

arrhythmogenic. This is probably due to their prolongation of the QT interval and/or an increase in myocardial norepinephrine resulting from their peripheral inhibition of norepinephrine reuptake. Although the most common arrhythmias are atrial or ventricular premature beats, these may give way to more malignant ventricular arrhythmias. These toxic, proarrhythmic effects are seen primarily in overdose, and at therapeutic levels they are rare and more likely in those with preexisting CHD, a prolonged QT interval, electrical instability, or a recent myocardial infarction.[144] At toxic levels, in overdose, any type of arrhythmia may be seen. These may last for 3 to 4 days after the ingestion. The TCAs also elevate heart rate 5 to 20 beats per minute, as a result of their anticholinergic blockade. Although this does not pose a problem in relatively healthy patients, it may be a consideration in those with heart disease.

TCAs produce postural hypotension in up to 20 percent of patients. In the elderly, in whom orthostatic hypotension can produce cerebral hypoperfusion and lead to falls and fractures, this side effect can be crucial. In these patients, blood pressure should be checked immediately after standing up when treatment is initiated and after increments in dosage. Elderly patients should be advised to stand up slowly after lying or sitting for prolonged periods. The magnitude of this effect is related to the magnitude of pretreatment orthostatic hypotension,[145] and it is more likely to be clinically significant in patients with CHF, impaired left ventricular function, volume depletion, or in patients who are taking antihypertensive medications.[146] Orthostatic hypotension is less likely to be a problem with nortriptyline than with amitriptyline or imipramine. Caution is indicated when treating patients with poor ejection fractions because in animal studies, TCAs exert a depressant effect on myocardial contractility. However, in humans this effect is evident only at toxic doses and only rarely aggravates CHF.[147]

TCAs are generally not prescribed within 4 to 6 weeks after an uncomplicated, acute myocardial infarction. However, the decision of whether or when to initiate treatment with these agents after a myocardial infarction must be made on an individual basis, weighing the particular indications and contraindications (CHF, arrhythmias, and conduction abnormalities) on a case-by-case basis.

OTHER ANTIDEPRESSANTS. Psychostimulants such as *methylphenidate* and *dextroamphetamine* are used to treat depression in medically compromised and elderly patients.[148] These agents tend to be used when depression is life threatening and immediate treatment response is crucial (because they have a rapid onset of action) and in depressions with very prominent anergia and apathy. Although there is considerable clinical support for their use, there are few rigorously controlled trials demonstrating their sustained efficacy over time. Serious cardiovascular side effects such as tachycardia, hypertension, and arrhythmias are relatively rare, but caution must be exercised when administering these medications to patients with significant hypertension, tachycardia, or ventricular ectopy, and blood pressure and heart rate should be monitored.

Bupropion, a nontricyclic antidepressant that acts on both the dopamine and norepinephrine systems, causes less hypotension than the TCAs; does not affect cardiac rate, conduction, or contractility; and is safely used in patients with cardiac disease.[149] It does not exacerbate ventricular arrhythmias or conduction block in patients with these conditions.[149] An increased incidence of seizures is seen at higher doses, and bupropion may occasionally elevate blood pressure.

Venlafaxine affects the reuptake of both serotonin and norepinephrine. It appears to have very few cardiovascular actions and no effect on the electrocardiogram.[150] At higher doses, however, venlafaxine has been associated with elevation in blood pressure.[151] Unlike the SRIs, it does not inhibit P450 cytochrome isoenzymes and may therefore be useful in patients on cardiac medications.

Trazodone, a triazolopyridine antidepressant, is often used in low doses as a hypnotic. Cardiovascular complications from trazodone are very rare. It has few, if any, antiarrhythmic properties, although it has very rarely been associated with heart block and ventricular arrhythmias.[152] Because of its weak alpha-adrenergic blockade, it may also produce orthostatic hypotension.

Mirtazapine is a tetracyclic antidepressant with a complex mechanism of action. It has not been studied in patients with cardiovascular disease, but in noncardiac populations it does not affect blood pressure significantly and does not affect cardiac conduction.[153] It has no anticholinergic activity, but it may increase heart rate slightly.[153]

Neuroleptics (Table 70-2)

Neuroleptic or antipsychotic drugs are used in the treatment of schizophrenia, organic psychoses, and mood disorders with psychotic features. They are also widely used in geriatric patients for agitation, confusion, excitement, and behavioral dyscontrol. In general, neuroleptic drugs affect cardiac conduction and rhythm and produce hypotension. They have alpha-adrenergic blocking and quinidine-like properties, along with anticholinergic activity. They can produce prolongation of the PR and QT intervals, ST segment depression, T wave changes, ventricular arrhythmias, and heart block. Although the quinidine-like effects of the neuroleptics are usually negligible, they can become significant in patients already taking type I antiarrhythmics or in those with hypokalemia or with clinically significant conduction delays.[154] When administering a low-potency neuroleptic along with an antiarrhythmic, the ECG should be monitored for conduction delays. The lower-potency neuroleptics produce more orthostatic hypotension (by means of alpha-adrenergic blockade) and tachycardia (by means of anticholinergic action), and this is of particular concern in the elderly and in the acute myocardial infarction patient.[155] Orthostasis is more likely to be a problem when these agents are combined with antihypertensives.

The higher-potency neuroleptic agents, such as haloperidol and the piperazine phenothiazines, produce less of these effects and are therefore preferred in the presence of significant cardiac disease (especially conduction problems) and after cardiac surgery.[111] Haloperidol in particular has been frequently used with safety and efficacy in severely ill cardiac patients. Oral haloperidol does not significantly affect the ECG, and intravenous haloperidol is used in acute emergencies such as agitated deliria. Intravenous administration can on rare occasions cause torsades de pointes, and the QT interval should therefore be monitored during aggressive, intravenous haloperidol therapy.[156]

Experience with the newer, "atypical" antipsychotics in cardiac patients is much more limited but suggests a generally similar profile. Clozapine can cause tachycardia and orthostatic hypotension and has significant anticholinergic activity (along with a risk of myelosuppression and agranulocytosis). There are recent reports of an infrequent association of clozapine with ECG changes, arrhythmias, myocarditis, and congestive heart failure.[157, 157a] Olanzapine produces mild orthostatic hypotension but has little effect on the electrocardiogram. Sertindole prolongs the QT interval and may therefore pose a problem in cardiac patients. Risperidone produces hypotension and has a quinidine-like effect, prolonging the QT interval, although this may occur only in overdose.

Mood Stabilizers (Table 70-3)

LITHIUM. Lithium exerts minimal cardiotoxicity at therapeutic doses in most patients and can be used safely in cardiac disease if initiated at a low dose, increased gradually, and monitored carefully. Benign, reversible T wave changes (including inversion and flattening) are common with lithium administration and are not clinically significant. Clinically significant cardiovascular side effects of lithium are very rare; they may include sinus node dysfunction and increases in ventricular irritability. The major toxic effects of lithium are neural (confusion, sedation), and the primary concern in cardiac patients is lithium toxicity resulting from decreased renal clearance or hypovolemia. This is of concern in patients with congestive heart failure, and it is exacerbated by their restricted sodium intake and the use of diuretics. Sodium depletion decreases renal clearance of lithium. In the kidney, lithium is filtered out at

▼ **TABLE 70-2. NEUROLEPTIC (ANTIPSYCHOTIC) AGENTS**

AGENT	STARTING DOSE	MAXIMUM DOSE	SIDE EFFECTS	CARDIOVASCULAR EFFECTS
Haloperidol	0.5 mg/d	>10 mg q.i.d.	Akathisia Dystonia Parkinsonism Tardive dyskinesia Neuroleptic malignant syndrome Rash Anticholinergic effects	Tachycardia Increase QT interval Torsades de pointes
Clozapine	12.5 mg q.h.s. or b.i.d.	200–300 mg t.i.d.	Dizziness Somnolence Weight gain Hypersalivation Seizures Agranulocytosis Anticholinergic effects	Tachycardia Postural hypotension
Olanzapine	5 mg/d	20 mg/d	Sedation Constipation Weight gain Seizures Akathisia Extrapyramidal symptoms	Postural hypotension (mild)
Risperidone	0.25–0.5 mg/d	>6 mg/d	Somnolence Fatigue Nausea, diarrhea Weight gain Sexual dysfunction Nasal congestion Extrapyramidal symptoms	Hypotension QT interval prolongation Tachycardia

▼ TABLE 70–3. MOOD STABILIZERS

AGENT	STARTING DOSE	MAXIMUM DOSE	SIDE EFFECTS	CARDIOVASCULAR EFFECTS
Lithium	300 mg b.i.d.	2100 mg/d (titrate against serum concentration)	Drowsiness, sedation Confusion Nausea, diarrhea Metallic taste Polyuria/polydipsia Tremor Hypothyroidism	T wave inversion or flattening Sinus node dysfunction Ventricular irritability
Carbamazepine	100 mg b.i.d.	1600 mg/d	Dizziness Drowsiness, sedation Ataxia Diplopia, blurred vision Rash Nausea Leukopenia Hyponatremia	Depressed cardiac conduction
Valproate	250 mg b.i.d.–t.i.d.	3500 mg/d–4500 mg/d	Nausea, vomiting, anorexia Sedation Confusion Weight gain Tremor	

the glomerulus and then reabsorbed in the proximal tubules. Sodium depletion, such as with diuretics, causes an increased proximal reabsorption of sodium, and lithium is reabsorbed more efficiently at the same time. A given lithium dose thus results in a higher blood lithium level. Lithium may still be administered to the patient on diuretics, but lithium levels must be monitored and lithium dosage may need to be reduced as much as 25 to 50 percent. The elderly also require lower lithium doses because of a decline in the glomerular filtration rate. On rare occasion, lithium may worsen arrhythmias in patients with sinus node dysfunction.[158]

ANTICONVULSANTS. These drugs are increasingly prescribed to stabilize the mood of patients with bipolar disorder (manic-depressive illness). Their use in cardiac patients has not yet been systematically studied. It is known that carbamazepine has quinidine-like effects and can aggravate heart block,[159] and it may also exacerbate CHF.[160] Carbamazepine can also produce hyponatremia, and this effect is potentiated by other factors that cause hyponatremia, such as diuretics and CHF.[161] Valproate, although not yet studied widely in cardiac populations, does not appear to have adverse cardiac effects. It can, however, lower the platelet count, decrease fibrinogen levels, and increase the prothrombin time.

Benzodiazepines (Table 70–4)

Benzodiazepines have anxiolytic, sedative, anticonvulsant, and muscle relaxant properties. Anxiety disorders, especially panic disorder and generalized anxiety disorder, are prevalent in patients with cardiac disease. Panic disorder is treated either with a benzodiazepine with antipanic efficacy (such as clonazepam, lorazepam, or alprazolam) or an antidepressant. Generalized anxiety disorder can also be treated with benzodiazepines, buspirone, or SRIs. Hospitalized cardiac patients are acutely anxious, and because anxiety itself can threaten cardiac status, benzodiazepines are widely and almost routinely used in coronary care units. They can decrease respiratory drive in patients with chronic obstructive pulmonary disease and chronic hypercapnia but are free of cardiac side effects and can safely be used in seriously ill cardiac patients, even in the period immediately after myocardial infarction.

Benzodiazepines with longer half-lives (e.g., diazepam, flurazepam, chlordiazepoxide) accumulate in the body with repeated administration. A steady state is reached very slowly, and clearance of the drug after discontinuation is prolonged. Intramuscular absorption of these agents, other than lorazepam and midazolam, is erratic and unpredictable. The most prominent side effects are sedation, fatigue, memory complaints, and psychomotor impairment. In hospitalized patients and in the elderly, these effects can result in oversedation or delirium. Patients with preexisting cognitive impairment or organic brain syndromes often react to benzodiazepines with further confusion, increased memory loss, behavioral disinhibition, and belligerence. Ambulatory patients should be cautioned about driving and participating in activities requiring a high degree of alertness.

▼ TABLE 70–4. BENZODIAZEPINES

AGENT	STARTING DOSE	MAXIMUM DOSE	SIDE EFFECTS	CARDIOVASCULAR EFFECTS
Short-Acting Benzodiazepines				
Oxazepam	10 mg b.i.d.	120 mg/d		
			Sedation, drowsiness	
Lorazepam	0.5 mg b.i.d.	10 mg/d	Slowed psychomotor function	
			Exacerbation of underlying cognitive impairment	
Long-Acting Benzodiazepines			Ataxia/falls in elderly	
Diazepam	1–2 mg q.d.	60 mg/d	Respiratory depression	
Chlordiazepoxide	5 mg q.d.	100 mg/d	Tolerance/addiction	
Clonazepam	0.25 mg/d	6 mg/d	Amnesia	
Alprazolam	0.25 mg b.i.d.	8 mg/d		

Psychiatric Side Effects of Cardiovascular Drugs

ANTIHYPERTENSIVES. Many antihypertensive agents have central nervous system side effects.[162] Depression is not uncommon with methyldopa, clonidine, reserpine, and guanethidine. Therefore, calcium channel blockers and angiotensin-converting enzyme inhibitors may be preferable in the hypertensive patient with a history of depression. Abrupt discontinuation of antihypertensive agents can cause anxiety, agitation, and vivid dreams.[163] Clonidine and methyldopa are relatively common causes of insomnia.

BETA-ADRENERGIC RECEPTOR ANTAGONISTS. There is a long-standing clinical impression that beta blockers can cause depression. Although there are reports that patients maintained on these agents have an elevated rate of concurrent antidepressant pharmacotherapy,[164] other studies have failed to find an association between beta blocker use and depression.[165] Some of the confusion may stem from the fact that these agents cause sedation, lethargy, fatigue, and impotence, side effects that overlap with, and may be confused with, depression. Depression may be more likely in those with a past history or family history of depression, with the more lipophilic agents (e.g., propranolol, metoprolol),[162] and when using higher doses. Beta blockers are also occasionally the cause of vivid dreams and nightmares, hallucinations, and other psychotic symptoms. These tend to occur more often in the elderly.

CALCIUM CHANNEL BLOCKERS. In general, calcium channel blockers do not have prominent psychiatric side effects. There are isolated case reports of depression associated with their administration, but this has not yet been demonstrated conclusively.

ANGIOTENSIN-CONVERTING ENZYME INHIBITORS. These agents appear to have relatively few central nervous system side effects, although they may, on rare occasion, induce depression.

ANTIARRHYTHMICS. Lidocaine is a relatively common cause of anxiety, confusion, disorientation, hallucinations, and central nervous system excitement. Confusion, hallucinations, and delirium have also been reported with high doses of quinidine. Procainamide may cause depression, hallucinations, and other psychotic symptoms.

DIGITALIS. Anxiety, depression, visual illusions (e.g., yellow halos), and confusion may be the first signs of digitalis toxicity, but psychiatric symptoms may emerge at therapeutic serum levels as well.[166]

DIURETICS. Diuretics can induce cognitive mental status changes as a result of their producing electrolyte imbalances (e.g., hyponatremia) or hypovolemia, and a secondary mood disorder may also occur, often characterized by anorexia, lethargy, and weakness.

Interactions of Psychotropic and Cardiac Drugs (Table 70–5)

Because many cardiac and psychotropic agents lower blood pressure, additive hypotensive effects are not uncommon, as for example between the TCAs and antihypertensives. Many psychotropic agents slow conduction and prolong the PR, QRS, and QT intervals, and synergistic effects can occur when they are used in conjunction with antiarrhythmic medications, resulting in heart block or the long QT syndrome. There are several interactions between the TCAs and cardiac medications. The TCAs interfere with neuronal reuptake of clonidine and guanethidine and thus antagonize their antihypertensive action. They may potentiate the antihypertensive action of prazosin. And the dry mouth induced by TCAs may hinder the absorption of sublingual nitrates.

Serotonin reuptake inhibitors (e.g., fluoxetine, sertraline,

▼ **TABLE 70–5. INTERACTIONS OF PSYCHOTROPIC AND CARDIAC DRUGS**

MEDICATION	EFFECT ON CARDIAC AGENT
Interactions Involving Tricyclic Antidepressants	
Type IA antiarrhythmics	Potentiate delay in cardiac conduction; heart block
Antihypertensives: guanethidine, clonidine, reserpine	Antagonize antihypertensive effect; potentiate orthostatic hypotension
Sublingual nitrates	Oral absorption hindered by dry mouth
Alpha-adrenergic blocking agents	Potentiate antihypertensive effect
Interactions Involving Serotonergic Antidepressants	
Lipophilic beta blockers Calcium channel blockers Type IC antiarrhythmics Angiotensin-converting enzyme inhibitors Warfarin	Increase blood levels due to decreased hepatic degradation
Digitoxin Warfarin	Increase bioavailability due to displacement from protein-binding sites
MEDICATION	EFFECT ON PSYCHOTROPIC AGENT
Interactions Involving Lithium	
Diuretics that cause sodium loss	Increase blood lithium levels
Calcium channel blockers	Enhance lithium toxicity; bradycardia
Angiotensin-converting enzyme inhibitors	Enhance lithium toxicity
Methyldopa	Enhance lithium toxicity
MEDICATION	EFFECT ON PSYCHOTROPIC OR CARDIAC AGENT
Interactions Involving Carbamazepine	
Calcium channel blockers	Enhance carbamazepine toxicity
Antiarrhythmics	Potentiate delay in cardiac conduction

paroxetine, and fluvoxamine) are bound to plasma proteins and can displace other protein-bound drugs, thereby increasing the level of active drug and resulting in possible toxicity. This is particularly salient with warfarin and digitoxin, although the clinical significance of these interactions is not yet clear.[160] As noted earlier, diuretics may raise lithium levels into the toxic range. This can generally be dealt with by reducing the lithium dose, although during acute diuresis the proper adjustment of lithium is difficult because of the massive shifts in sodium and fluid balance.[160]

There are reports of idiosyncratic toxic reactions and of bradycardia when lithium is co-administered with the calcium channel blockers verapamil and diltiazem, and of lithium toxicity precipitated by the use of angiotensin-converting enzyme inhibitors. Methyldopa seems to have a number of interactions with psychotropic agents, including possible toxicity when combined with lithium. The metabolic degradation of carbamazepine may be inhibited by calcium channel blockers, thereby increasing the risk of carbamazepine toxicity.[167] Carbamazepine and antiarrhythmics may have additive effects in slowing cardiac conduction.

REFERENCES

PSYCHIATRIC ASPECTS OF CORONARY HEART DISEASE

1. Rosenman RH, Brand RJ, Jenkins CD, et al: Coronary heart disease in the Western Collaborative Group Study: Final follow-up experience of 8½ years. JAMA 233:872–877, 1975.

2. Miller TQ, Smith TW, Turner CW, et al: A meta-analytic review of research on hostility and physical health. Psychol Bull 119:322–348, 1996.

3. Barefoot JC, Larsen L, von der Leith L, Schroll M: Hostility, incidence of acute myocardial infarction and mortality in a sample of older Danish men and women. Am J Epidemiol 142:477–484, 1995.

4. Kawachi I, Sparrow D, Spiro A, et al: A prospective study of anger and coronary heart disease: The Normative Aging Study. Circulation 94:2090–2095, 1996.

5. Shekelle RB, Gale M, Ostfield A, et al: Hostility, risk of coronary heart disease, and mortality. Psychosom Med 45:109–114, 1983.

6. Gallacher JE, Yarnell JW, Sweetnam PM, et al: Anger and incident heart disease in the Caerphilly study. Psychosom Med 61:446–454, 1999.

7. Goodman M, Quigley J, Moran G, et al: Hostility predicts restenisis after percutaneous transluminal coronary angioplasty. Mayo Clin Proc 71:729–734, 1996.

8. Frasure-Smith N, Lespérance F, Talajic M: Depression following myocardial infarction: Impact on 6-month survival. JAMA 270:1819–1825, 1993.

9. Carney RM, Rich MW, Tevelde A, et al: Major depressive disorder in coronary artery disease. Am J Cardiol 60:1273–1275, 1987.

10. Lespérance F, Frasure-Smith N, Talajic M: Major depression before and after myocardial infarction: Its nature and consequences. Psychosom Med 58:99–110, 1996.

11. McKhann GM, Borowicz LM, Goldsborough MA, et al: Depression and cognitive decline following coronary artery bypass grafting. Lancet 349:1282–1284, 1996.

12. Sullivan MD, LaCroix AZ, Baum C, et al: Functional status in coronary artery disease: A one-year prospective study of the role of anxiety and depression. Am J Med 103:348–356, 1997.

13. Carney RM, Rich MW, Freedland KE, Saini J: Major depressive disorder predicts cardiac events in patients with coronary artery disease. Psychosom Med 50:627–633, 1988.

14. Frasure-Smith N, Lespérance F, Talajic M: Depression and 18-month prognosis after myocardial infarction. Circulation 91:999–1005, 1995.

15. Frasure-Smith N: In-hospital symptoms of psychological stress as predictors of long-term outcome after acute myocardial infarction in men. Am J Cardiol 67:121–127, 1991.

16. Anda R, Williamson D, Jones D, et al: Depressed affect, hopelessness, and the risk of ischemic heart disease in a cohort of U.S. adults. Epidemiology 4:285–294, 1993.

17. Barefoot JC, Schroll M: Symptoms of depression, acute myocardial infarction, and total mortality in a community sample. Circulation 93:1976–1980, 1996.

18. Scheier MF, Matthews KA, Owens JF, et al: Optimism and rehospitalization after coronary artery bypass surgery. Arch Intern Med 159:829–835, 1999.

19. Aromaa A, Raitasalo R, Reunanen A, et al: Depression and cardiovascular diseases. Acta Psychiatr Scand 377(Suppl):77–82, 1994.

20. Ford DE, Mead LA, Chang PP, et al: Depression is a risk factor for coronary artery disease in men. Arch Intern Med 158:1422–1426, 1998.

21. Hippisley-Cox J, Fielding K, Pringle M: Depression as a risk factor for ischemic heart disease in men: Population based case-control study. BMJ 316:1714–1719, 1998.

22. Vogt T, Pope C, Mullooly J, Hollis J: Mental health status as a predictor of morbidity and mortality. Am J Public Health 84:227–231, 1994.

23. Wassertheil-Smoller S, Applegate WB, Berge K, et al: Change in depression as a precursor of cardiovascular events. SHEP Cooperative Research Group (Systolic Hypertension in the Elderly). Arch Intern Med 56:553–561, 1996.

24. Carney RM, Freedland KE, Eisen S, Mulcahy R: Major depression and medication adherence in elderly patients with coronary artery disease. Health Psychol 14:88–90, 1995.

25. Musselman DL, Evans DL, Wemeroff CB: The relationship of depression to cardiovascular disease: Epidemiology, biology, and treatment. Arch Gen Psychiatry 55:580–592, 1998.

26. Rozanski A, Blumenthal JA, Kaplan J: Impact of psychological factors on the pathogenesis of cardiovascular disease and implications for therapy. Circulation 99:2192–2217, 1999.

27. Carney RM, Saunders RD, Freedland KE, et al: Association of depression with reduced heart rate variability in coronary artery disease. Am J Cardiol 76:562–564, 1995.

28. Kawachi I, Sparrow D, Vokonas PS, Weiss ST: Symptoms of anxiety and risk of coronary heart disease: The Normative Aging Study. Circulation 90:2225–2229, 1994.

29. Frasure-Smith N, Lespérance F, Talajic M: The impact of negative emotions on prognosis following myocardial infarction: Is is more than depression? Health Psychol 14:388–398, 1995.

30. Kawachi I, Colditz GA, Ascherio A, et al: Prospective study of phobic anxiety and risk of coronary heart disease in men. Circulation 89:1992–1997, 1994.

31. Williams RB, Barefoot JC, Califf RM, et al: Prognostic importance of social and economic resources among medically treated patients with angiographically documented coronary artery disease. JAMA 267:520–524, 1992.

32. Berkman LF, Leo-Summers L, Horwitz RI: Emotional support and survival following myocardial infarction: Findings from a prospective, population-based study of the elderly. Ann Intern Med 117:1003–1009, 1992.

33. Nerem RM, Levesque MJ, Cornhill JF: Social environment as a factor in diet-induced atherosclerosis. Science 208:1475–1476, 1980.

34. Shively CA, Clarkson TB, Kaplan JR: Social deprivation and coronary atherosclerosis in female cynomolgus monkeys. Atherosclerosis 77:69–76, 1989.

35. Robertson TL, Kato H, Rhoads GG, et al: Epidemiologic studies of coronary heart disease and stroke in Japanese men living in Japan, Hawaii, and California: Incidence of myocardial infarction and death from coronary heart disease. Am J Cardiol 39:239–243, 1977.

36. Marmot MG, Syme SL: Acculturation and coronary heart disease in Japanese-Americans. Am J Epidemiol 104:225–247, 1976.

37. Kaplan JR, Manuck SB, Clarkson TB, et al: Social stress and atherosclerosis in normocholesterolemic monkeys. Science 220:733–735, 1983.

38. Bosma H, Peter R, Siegrist J, Marmot M: Two alternative job stress models and the risk of coronary heart disease. Am J Public Health 88:68–74, 1998.

39. Karasek RA, Theorell TG, Schwartz J, et al: Job, psychological factors, and coronary heart disease: Swedish prospective findings and U.S. prevalence findings using a new occupational inference method. Adv Cardiol 29:62–87, 1982.

40. Alfredsson L, Spetz CL, Theorell T: Type of occupation and near-future hospitalization for myocardial infarction and some other diagnoses. Int J Epidemiol 14:378–388, 1985.

41. Johnson JV, Stewart W, Hall EM, et al: Long-term psychosocial work environment and cardiovascular mortality among Swedish males. Am J Public Health 86:324–331, 1996.

42. Kaprio J, Koskenvuo M, Rita H: Mortality after bereavement: A prospective study of 95,647 persons. Am J Public Health 77:283–287, 1987.

43. Krantz DS, Kop WJ, Santiago HT, Gottdiener JS: Mental stress as a trigger of myocardial ischemia and infarction. Cardiol Clin 14:271–287, 1996.

44. Rozanski A, Bairey CN, Krantz DS: Mental stress and the induction of silent myocardial ischemia in patients with coronary artery disease. N Engl J Med 318:1005–1012, 1988.

45. Barry J, Selwyn AP, Nabel EG, et al: Frequency of ST-segment depression produced by mental stress in stable angina pectoris from coronary artery disease. Am J Cardiol 61:989–993, 1988.

46. Campbell S, Barry J, Rebecca GS, et al: Active transient myocardial ischemia during daily life in asymptomatic patients with positive exercise tests and coronary artery disease. Am J Cardiol 57:1010–1016, 1986.

47. Jiang W, Babyak M, Krantz DS, et al: Mental stress-induced myocardial ischemia and cardiac events. JAMA 21:1651–1656, 1996.

48. Jain D, Burg M, Soufer P, et al: Prognostic implications of mental stress-induced silent left ventricular dysfunction in patients with stable angina pectoris. Am J Cardiol 76:31–35, 1995.

49. Yeung AC, Vekshtein NI, Krantz DS, et al: The effect of atherosclerosis on the vasomotor response of coronary arteries to mental stress. New Engl J Med 325:1551–1556, 1991.

50. Gabbay FH, Krantz DS, Kop WJ, et al: Triggers of myocardial ischemia during daily life in patients with coronary artery disease: Physical and mental activities, anger, and smoking. J Am Coll Cardiol 27:585–592, 1996.

51. Krantz DS, Hedges SM, Gabbay FH, et al: Triggers of angina and ST-segment depression in ambulatory patients with coronary artery disease: Evidence for uncoupling of angina and ischemia. Am Heart J 128:703–712, 1994.

52. Mittelman MA, Maclure M, Sherwood JB, et al: Triggering of acute myocardial infarction onset by episodes of anger: Determinants of myocardial infarction onset study investigators. Circulation 92:1720–1725, 1995.

53. Markowitz JH: Hostility is associated with increased platelet activity in coronary heart disease. Psychosom Med 60:586–591, 1998.

54. Sloan RP, Shapiro PA, Bigger JT Jr, et al: Cardiovascular autonomic control and hostility in healthy subjects. Am J Cardiol 74:298–300, 1994.

55. Suarez EC, Kuhn CM, Schanberg SM, et al: Neuroendocrine, cardiovascular, and emotional responses of hostile men: The role of interpersonal challenge. Psychosom Med 60:78–88, 1998.

ARRHYTHMIAS AND SUDDEN DEATH

56. Engel GL: Sudden and rapid death during psychological stress: Folklore or folk wisdom? Ann Intern Med 74:771–782, 1971.

57. Reich P, DeSilva RA, Lown B, Murawski BJ: Acute psychological disturbance preceding life-threatening ventricular arrhythmias. JAMA 246:233–235, 1981.

58. Myers A, Dewan HA: Circumstances attending 100 sudden deaths from coronary artery disease with coroner's necropsies. Br Heart J 7:1133–1143, 1975.

59. Rissanen V, Romo M, Siltanen P: Premonitory symptoms and stress factors preceding sudden death from ischemic heart disease. Acta Med Scand 204:000–000, 1978.

60. Lown B, DeSilva RA: Roles of psychological stress and autonomic nervous system changes in provocation of ventricular premature complexes. Am J Cardiol 41:979–985, 1978.

61. Follick MJ, Gorkin L, Capone RJ, et al: Psychological stress as a predictor of ventricular arrhythmias in a post-myocardial infarction population. Am Heart J 116:32–36, 1988.

62. Kamarck T, Jennings JR: Biobehavioral factors in sudden cardiac death. Psychol Bull 109:42–75, 1991.

63. Coryell W, Noyes R, Clancy J: Excess mortality in panic disorder. Arch Gen Psychiatry 39:701–703, 1982.
64. Haines AP, Imeson JD, Meade TW: Phobic anxiety and ischemic heart disease. BMJ 295:297–299, 1987.
65. Follick MJ, Ahern DK, Gorkin L, et al: Relation of psychosocial and stress reactivity variables to ventricular arrhythmias in the Cardiac Arrhythmia Pilot Study (CAPS). Am J Cardiol 66:63–67, 1990.
66. Talbott E, Kuller LH, Perper J, Murphy PA: Sudden unexpected death in women: Biologic and psychosocial origins. Am J Epidemiol 114:671–682, 1981.
67. Matta RJ, Lawler JE, Lown B: Ventricular electrical instability in the conscious dog: Effects of psychologic stress and beta-adrenergic blockade. Am J Cardiol 34:594–598, 1976.
68. Corbalan R, Verrier R, Lown B: Psychological stress and ventricular arrhythmias during myocardial infarction in the conscious dog. Am J Cardiol 34:692–696, 1974.
69. Skinner JE, Lie JT, Entman ML: Modification of ventricular fibrillation latency following coronary artery occlusion in the conscious pig. Circulation 51:656–666, 1975.
70. Samuels MA: Electrocardiographic manifestations of neurologic disease. Semin Neurol 4:453–461, 1984.
71. Cebelin M, Hirsch CS: Human stress cardiomyopathy. Hum Pathol 11:123–132, 1980.

BEHAVIORAL ASPECTS OF HYPERTENSION AND HEART FAILURE

72. Fredrikson M, Matthews KA: Cardiovascular responses to behavioral stress and hypertension: A meta-analytic review. Ann Behav Med 12:30–39, 1990.
73. Light KC, Dolan CA, Davis MR, et al: Cardiovascular responses to an active coping challenge as predictors of blood pressure patterns 10 to 15 years later. Psychosom Med 54:217–230, 1992.
74. Matthews KA, Woodall KL, Allen MT: Cardiovascular reactivity to stress predicts future blood pressure status. Hypertension 22:479–485, 1993.
75. Pickering TG: Challenge response predictors. Am J Hypertens 4:611S–614S, 1991.
76. Muldoon MF, Terrell DF, Bunker CH, Manuck SB: Family history studies in hypertension research: Review of the literature. Am J Hypertens 6:76–88, 1993.
77. Henry JP, Stephens PM: The social environment and essential hypertension in mice: Possible role of the innervation of the adrenal cortex. In Stress, Health, and the Social Environment. New York, Springer-Verlag, 1977.
78. Niaura R, Goldstein MG: Psychological factors affecting physical conditions: Cardiovascular disease literature review: II. Psychosomatics 33:146–155, 1992.
79. Smith TW, Gallo LG: Hostility and cardiovascular reactivity during marital interaction. Psychosom Med 61:436–445, 1999.
80. Markowitz JH, Matthews KA, Wing RR, et al: Psychological, biological, and health behavior predictors of blood pressure changes in middle-aged women. J Hypertension 9:399–406, 1991.
81. Suls J, Wan CK, Costa PT: Relationship of trait anger to resting blood pressure: A meta-analysis. Health Psychol 14:444–456, 1995.
82. Kahn HA, Medalie JH, Neufeld HN, et al: The incidence of hypertension and associated factors: The Israeli ischemic heart disease study. Am Heart J 84:171–182, 1972.
83. Pernini C, Muller FB, Buhler FR: Suppressed aggression accelerated early development of essential hypertension. J Hypertension 9:499–503, 1991.
84. Jonas BS, Franks P, Ingram DD: Are symptoms of anxiety and depression risk factors for hypertension? Longitudinal evidence from the National Health and Nutrition Survey I Epidemiologic Follow-up Study. Arch Fam Med 6:43–49, 1997.
85. Barnes VA, Treiber FA, Turner JR, et al: Acute effects of transcendental meditation on hemodynamic functioning in middle aged adults. Psychosom Med 61:525–531, 1999.
86. Agras WS, Southam MA, Taylor CB, et al: Long-term persistence of relaxation-induced blood pressure lowering during the working day. J Consult Clin Psychol 51:792–794, 1983.
87. Jacob RG, Shapiro AP, Reeves RA, et al: Comparison of relaxation therapy for hypertension with placebo, diuretics and beta-blockers. Arch Intern Med 146:2335–2340, 1986.
88. Salmond CE, Joseph JG, Prior IAM, et al: Longitudinal analyses of the relationship between blood pressure and migration: The Tokelan Island Migrant Study. Am J Epidemiol 122:291–301, 1985.
89. Henry JP, Meehan JP, Stephens PM: The use of psychosocial stimuli to induce prolonged systolic hypertension in mice. Psychosom Med 29:408–432, 1967.
90. Perlman LV, Ferguson S, Bergum K, et al: Precipitation of congestive heart failure: Social and emotional factors. Ann Intern Med 75:1–7, 1971.
91. Feenstra J, Grobee DE, Jonkman FAM, et al: Prevention of relapse in patients with congestive heart failure: The role of precipitating factors. Heart 80:432–436, 1998.
92. Giannuzzi P, Shabetai R, Imparato A, et al: Effects of mental exercise in patients with dilated cardiomyopathy and congestive heart failure: An echocardiographic Doppler study. Circulation 83(Suppl 4):155–165, 1991.
93. Freedland KE, Carney RM, Rich MW, et al: Depression in elderly patients with congestive heart failure. Int J Geriatr Psychiatry 24:59–71, 1991.
94. Murberg TA, Bru E, Aarsland T, Svebak S: Functional status and depression among men and women with congestive heart failure. Int J Psychiatr Med 28:273–291, 1998.
95. Krumholtz HM, Butler J, Miller J, et al. Prognostic impact of emotional support for elderly patients hospitalized with heart failure. Circulation 97:958–964, 1998.

CHEST PAIN AND PALPITATIONS

96. Kroenke K, Mangelsdorff AD: Common symptoms in ambulatory care: Incidence, evaluation, therapy, and outcome. Am J Med 86:262–266, 1989.
97. Potts SG, Bass CM: Psychosocial outcome and use of medical resources in patients with chest pain and normal or near-normal coronary arteries: A long-term follow-up study. Q J Med 86:583–593, 1993.
98. Isner JM, Salem DN, Banas JS, Levine HJ: Long-term clinical course of patients with normal coronary arteriography: Follow-up study of 121 patients with normal or nearly normal coronary arteriograms. Am Heart J 102:645–653, 1981.
99. Costa PT, Zonderman AB, Engel BT, et al: The relation of chest pain symptoms to angiographic findings of coronary artery stenosis and neuroticism. Psychosom Med 47:285–293, 1985.
100. Katon W, Hall ML, Russo J, et al: Chest pain: Relationship of psychiatric illness to coronary arteriographic results. Am J Med 84:1–9, 1988.
101. Channer KS, James MA, Papouchado M, Rees JR: Anxiety and depression in patients with chest pain referred for exercise testing. Lancet 2:820–822, 1985.
102. Kroenke K, Arrington ME, Mangelsdorff AD: The prevalence of symptoms in medical outpatients and the adequacy of therapy. Arch Intern Med 150:1685–1690, 1990.
103. Weber BE, Kapoor WN: Evaluation and outcomes of patients with palpitations. Am J Med 100:138–148, 1996.
104. Barsky AJ, Cleary PD, Sarnie MK, Ruskin JN: Panic disorder, palpitations, and the awareness of cardiac activity. J Nerv Ment Dis 182:63–71, 1994.
105. Barsky AJ, Cleary PD, Coeytaux RR, Ruskin JN: The clinical course of palpitations in medical outpatients. Arch Intern Med 155:1782–1788, 1995.
106. Kenyon LW, Ketterer MW, Gheorghiade M, Goldstein S: Psychological factors related to prehospital delay during acute myocardial infarction. Circulation 84:1969–1976, 1991.
107. Meischke H, Larsen MP, Eisenberg MS: Gender differences in reported symptoms for acute myocardial infarction: Impact of prehospital delay time interval. Am J Emerg Med 16:363–366, 1998.
108. Leizorovicz A, Haugh MC, Mercier C, et al: Prehospital and hospital time delays in thrombolytic treatment in patients with suspected myocardial infarction. Eur Heart J 18:248–253, 1997.

PSYCHIATRIC CARE OF THE HOSPITALIZED PATIENT

109. Smith LW, Dimsdale JE: Postcardiotomy delirium: Conclusions after 25 years? Am J Psychiatry 146:452–458, 1989.
110. Roach GW, Kanchuger M, Mangano CM, et al: Adverse cerebral outcomes after coronary bypass surgery. N Engl J Med 335:1857–1863, 1996.
111. Tesar GE, Murray GB, Cassem NH: Use of high-dose intravenous haloperidol in the treatment of agitated cardiac patients. J Clin Psychopharmacol 5:344–347, 1985.
112. Goldstein MG, Haltzman SD: Intensive care. In Stoudemire A, Fogel BS (eds): Psychiatric Care of the Medical Patient. New York, Oxford University Press, 1993, pp 241–265.
113. McLane M, Krop H, Mehta J: Psychosexual adjustment and counseling after myocardial infarction. Ann Intern Med 92:514–519, 1980.
114. Cassem NH: Psychiatric problems in patients with acute myocardial infarction. In Karliner JS, Gregoratos G (eds): Coronary Care. London, Churchill Livingstone, 1981, pp 829–846.
115. Stern MJ, Pascale L, Ackerman A: Life adjustment post myocardial infarction: Determining predictive variables. Arch Intern Med 137:1680–1685, 1977.
116. Ladwig KH, Roll G, Breithardt G, et al: Post-infarction depression and incomplete recovery 6 months after acute myocardial infarction. Lancet 343:20–23, 1994.
117. Frasure-Smith N, Lespérance F: Psychosocial risks and cardiovascular disease: Report for the 1998 Canadian Cardiovascular Society Consensus Conference. Can J Cardiol 15(suppl G):93G–97G, 1999.
118. Linden W, Stossel C, Maurice J: Psychosocial interventions for patients with coronary artery disease—a meta-analysis. Arch Intern Med 156:745–752, 1996.
119. Oldridge NB, Guyat G, Jones N, et al: Effects on quality of life with comprehensive rehabilitation after acute myocardial infarction. Am J Cardiol 67:1084–1089, 1991.
120. Oldridge NB, Guyat G, Fischer ME: Cardiac rehabilitation after myocardial infarction: Combined experience of randomized clinical trials. JAMA 260:945–950, 1988.
121. Langosch W: Psychological effects of training in coronary patients: A critical review of the literature. Circulation 80:234–244, 1988.

122. Blumenthal JA, Emery CF: Rehabilitation of patients following myocardial infarction. J Consult Clin Psychol 56:374–381, 1988.

123. Ketterer MW: Secondary prevention of ischemic heart disease. Psychosomatics 34:478–484, 1993.

124. Mullen PD, Mains DA, Velez R: A meta-analysis of controlled trials of cardiac patient education. Patient Ed Counsel 19:143–162, 1992.

125. Dusseldorp E, van Elderen T, Maes S, et al: A meta-analysis of psychoeducational programs for coronary heart disease patients. Health Psychol 18:506–519, 1999.

126. Frasure-Smith N, Prince R: The ischemic heart disease life stress monitoring program: Impact on mortality. Psychosom Med 47:431–445, 1985.

127. Frasure-Smith N, Prince R: Long-term follow-up of the Ischemic Heart Disease Life Stress Monitoring Program. Psychosom Med 51:485–513, 1989.

128. Jones DA, West RR: Psychological rehabilitation after myocardial infarction: Multicentre, randomised, controlled trial. BMJ 313:1517–1521, 1996.

129. Taylor CB, Miller NH, Smith PM, DeBusk RF: The effect of a home-based, case-managed, multifactorial risk-reduction program on reducing psychological distress in patients with cardiovascular disease. J Cardiopulm Rehabil 17:157–162, 1997.

130. Frasure-Smith N, Lespérance F, Prince RH, et al: Randomized trial of home-based psychosocial nursing intervention for patients recovering from myocardial infarction. Lancet 350:473–479, 1997.

131. Bundy C, Carroll D, Wallace L, Nagle R: Psychosocial treatment of stable angina pectoris. Psychol Health 10:69–74, 1994.

132. Lewin B, Cay EL, Todd I, et al: The angina management rehabilitation program: A rehabilitation treatment. Br J Cardiol 221–226, 1995.

133. Langosch W, Seer P, Grodner G, et al: Behavior therapy with coronary heart disease patients: Results of a comparative study. J Psychosom Res 26:475–484, 1982.

134. van Dixhoorn J, Duivenvoorden HJ, Staal HA, Pool J: Physical training and relaxation therapy in cardiac rehabilitation assessed through a composite criterion for training outcome. Am Heart J 118:545–552, 1989.

135. Blumenthal JA, Jiang W, Babyak MA, et al: Stress management and exercise training in cardiac patients with myocardial ischemia: Effects on prognosis and evaluation of mechanisms. Arch Intern Med 157:2213–2223, 1997.

136. Payne TJ, Johnson CA, Penzien DB, et al: Chest pain self-management training for patients with coronary artery disease. J Psychosom Res 38:409–418, 1994.

137. Nunes EV, Frank KA, Kornfeld D: Psychologic treatment for the Type A behavior pattern and for coronary heart disease: A meta analysis of the literature. Psychosom Med 48:159–173, 1987.

138. Friedman M, Thoresen CE, Gill JJ, et al: Alteration of Type A behavior and reduction in cardiac recurrences in postmyocardial infarction patients. Am Heart J 108:237–248, 1984.

139. Friedman M, Thoresen CE, Gill JJ, et al: Alteration of Type A behavior and its effects on cardiac recurrences in post myocardial infarction patients: Summary of results of the Recurrent Coronary Prevention Project. Am Heart J 112:653–665, 1986.

140. Gidron Y, Davidson K, Bata I: The short-term effects of a hostility-reduction intervention in CHD patients. Health Psychol 18:416–420, 1999.

PSYCHOPHARMACOLOGY

141. Roose SP, Glassman AH, Attia E, et al: Cardiovascular effects of fluoxetine in depressed patients with heart disease. Am J Psychiatry 155:650–655, 1998.

142. Harvey AT, Preskorn SH: Cytochrome P450 enzymes: Interpretation of their interactions with selective serotonin reuptake inhibitors: I. J Clin Psychopharmacol 16:273–285, 1996.

143. Nelson JC, Kennedy JS, Pollock BG, et al: Treatment of major depression with nortriptyline and paroxetine in patients with ischemic heart disease. Am J Psychiatry 156:1024–1028, 1999.

144. Glassman AH, Roose SP, Bigger JT Jr: The safety of tricyclic antidepressants in cardiac patients: Risk-benefit reconsidered. JAMA 269:2673–2675, 1993.

145. Neshkes RE, Gerner R, Jarvik LF, et al: Orthostatic effect of imipramine and doxepin in depressed geriatric outpatients. J Clin Psychopharmacol 5:102–106, 1985.

146. Stoudemire A, Moran MG, Fogel BS: Psychotropic drug use in the medically ill: I. Psychosomatics 31:377–391, 1990.

147. Glassman AH, Preud'homme XA: Review of the cardiovascular effects of heterocyclic antidepressants. J Clin Psychiatry 54(Suppl):16–22, 1993.

148. Masond PS, Tesar GE: Use of stimulants in the medically ill. Psychiatr Clin North Am 19:515–547, 1996.

149. Roose SP, Dalack GW, Glassman AH, et al: Cardiovascular effects of bupropion in depressed patients with heart disease. Am J Psychiatry 148:512–516, 1991.

150. Beliles K, Stoudemire A: Psychopharmacologic treatment of depression in the medically ill. Psychosomatics 39:S2–S19, 1998.

151. Feighner JP: Cardiovascular safety in depressed patients: Focus on venlafaxine. J Clin Psychopharmacol 56:574–579, 1995.

152. Spar JE: Plasma trazodone concentrations in elderly depressed inpatients: Cardiac effects and short-term efficacy. J Clin Psychopharmacol 7:406–409, 1987.

153. Nelson JC: Safety and tolerability of the new antidepressants. J Clin Psychiatry 58(Suppl):26–31, 1997.

154. Stoudemire A, Moran MG, Fogel BS: Psychotropic drug use in the medically ill: II. Psychosomatics 32:34–46, 1991.

155. Stoudemire A, Moran MF: Psychopharmacology in the medically ill patient. In Schatzberg AF, Nemeroff CB (eds): Textbook of Psychopharmacology. Washington, DC, American Psychiatric Press, 1998, pp 931–959.

156. Hunt N, Stern TA: The association between intravenous haloperidol and torsades de pointes. Psychosomatics 36:541–549, 1995.

157. Lieberman JA: Maximizing clozapine therapy: Managing side-effects. J Clin Psychiatry 59(Suppl 3):38–43, 1998.

157a. Kilian JG, Kerr K, Lawrence C, Celermajer DS: Myocarditis and cardiomyopathy associated with clozapine. Lancet 354:1841–1845, 1999.

158. Stekler TL: Lithium- and carbamazepine-associated sinus node dysfunction: Nine-year experience in a psychiatric hopsital. J Clin Psychopharmacol 14:336–339, 1994.

159. Benassi E, Bo GP, Cociot L, et al: Carbamazepine and cardiac conduction disturbances. Ann Neurol 22:280–281, 1999.

160. Levenson JL: Cardiovascular disease. In Stoudemire A, Fogel BS (eds): Psychiatric Care of the Medical Patient. New York, Oxford University Press, 1993, pp 539–563.

161. Lohr MB: Hyponatremia during carbamazepine therapy. Clin Pharmacol Ther 37:693–696, 1985.

162. Gengo FM, Gabos C: Central nervous systems considerations in the use of beta-blockers, angiotension-converting enzyme inhibitors and thiazide diuretics in managing essential hypertension. Am J Cardiol 116:305–310, 1988.

163. Houston MC, Hodge R: Beta-adrenergic blocker withdrawal syndromes in hypertension and other cardiovascular diseases. Am Heart J 116:515–522, 1988.

164. Thiessen BQ, Wallace SM, Blackburn JL: Increased prescribing of antidepressants subsequent to beta-blocker therapy. Arch Intern Med 150:2286–2290, 1990.

165. Schleifer SJ, Slater WR, Macari-Hinson MM, et al: Digitalis and beta-blocking agents: Effects on depression following myocardial infarction. Am Heart J 121:1397–1402, 1991.

166. Eisendrath SJ, Sweeney MA: Toxic neuropsychiatric effects of digoxin at therapeutic serum concentrations. Am J Psychiatry 144:506–507, 1987.

167. Ketter TA, Post RM, Worthington K: Principles of clinically important drug interactions with carbamazepine: II. J Clin Psychopharmacol 11:306–313, 1991.

Chapter 71

Neurological Disorders and Cardiovascular Disease

WILLIAM J. GROH · DOUGLAS P. ZIPES

Cardiovascular disease that occurs secondary to an underlying neurological disorder is related either to direct involvement of the heart or due to induced neurohormonal abnormalities that act on the heart. In several neurological disorders, the cardiovascular manifestations can be responsible for a greater risk of morbidity and mortality than the neurological manifestations. This chapter reviews those neurological disorders associated with important cardiovascular sequelae.

THE MUSCULAR DYSTROPHIES

The muscular dystrophies are a diffuse group of heritable disorders in which direct involvement of cardiac muscle is present to a variable degree. The muscular dystrophies can be classified into:

- 1. Duchenne and Becker muscular dystrophies
- 2. Myotonic muscular dystrophy
- 3. Emery-Dreifuss muscular dystrophy
- 4. Limb girdle muscular dystrophy
- 5. Facioscapulohumeral muscular dystrophy

Duchenne and Becker Muscular Dystrophies

GENETICS

Both Duchenne and Becker muscular dystrophies are X-linked recessive disorders in which the genetic locus has been identified as an abnormality in the dystrophin gene.[1, 2] This gene is the largest identified in humans to date.[3, 4] Dystrophin messenger RNA is expressed predominantly in skeletal, cardiac, and smooth muscle with lower levels in brain. The dystrophin protein complexes with muscle cytoskeleton, possibly functioning to link contractile proteins to the cell membrane.[5] Its absence can lead to membrane fragility, resulting in myofibril necrosis and eventual loss of muscle fibers with fibrotic replacement. In Duchenne muscular dystrophy, dystrophin is nearly absent; whereas in Becker muscular dystrophy, dystrophin is present but reduced in size or amount.[6, 7] This leads to the characteristic rapidly progressive skeletal muscle disease in Duchenne muscular dystrophy and the more benign course in Becker muscular dystrophy. The heart as a muscle is also involved. Indeed, studies have recognized a distinct clinical syndrome of X-linked dilated cardiomyopathy producing a progressive and severe cardiomyopathy with minimal skeletal muscle weakness that involves a dystrophin mutation.[8, 9] Involvement of the heart with sparing of skeletal muscle occurs secondary to selective abnormalities in certain dystrophin isotype transcripts, allowing functional dystrophin expression in all tissue but cardiac muscle.[10]

CLINICAL PRESENTATION. Duchenne muscular dystrophy is the most common inherited neuromuscular disorder, with an incidence of 30 per 100,000 live male births. Patients with disease become symptomatic before age 5, presenting with skeletal muscle weakness that progresses such that the boy becomes wheelchair-bound before the age of 13 years (Fig. 71–1). Death occurs commonly by age 20 to 25 years primarily from respiratory failure or cardiac arrest. Becker muscular dystrophy is less common (3 per 100,000 live male births), has a more variable presentation of skeletal muscle weakness (Fig. 71–2), and has a better prognosis, with most patients surviving to age 40 to 50 years.

CARDIOVASCULAR MANIFESTATIONS. Virtually all patients with Duchenne muscular dystrophy develop a cardiomyopathy, but clinical recognition may be masked by severe skeletal muscle weakness. Preclinical cardiac involvement is present in one fourth by age 6, with the onset of clinically apparent cardiomyopathy after age 10 being common.[11] Predilection for involvement in the posterobasal and posterolateral left ventricle has been observed (Fig. 71–3). This has been hypothesized to be related to the increased axial stress that cardiac myocytes encounter in the posterior wall and thus a more important role for dystrophin in limiting sarcolemma damage.[12] As with the skeletal muscle weakness, cardiac involvement in Becker muscular dystrophy is more variable, ranging from none or subclinical to severe cardiomyopathy requiring transplant.[13, 14] Cardiac involvement in Becker muscular dystrophy is independent of the severity of skeletal muscle involvement, with some investigators observing increased likelihood of cardiovascular disease in older individuals.[14, 15] More than one half of patients with subclinical or benign skeletal muscle disease were noted to have cardiac involvement when carefully evaluated.[16] In follow-up studies, progression in the severity of cardiac involvement is common.[15] Cardiomyopathy can initially only involve the right ventricle.[16]

The cardiovascular examination in Duchenne muscular dystrophy may be altered by thoracic deformities and a high diaphragm. A reduction in the anteroposterior chest dimension is commonly responsible for a systolic impulse displaced to the left sternal border, a grade 1–3/6 short midsystolic murmur in the second left interspace, and a loud pulmonary component of the second heart sound. In both Duchenne and Becker muscular dystrophy, mitral regurgitation is commonly observed. This is believed related to posterior papillary muscle dysfunction in Duchenne muscular dystrophy and to mitral annular dilatation in Becker muscular dystrophy.[17]

Electrocardiography. In patients with Duchenne mus-

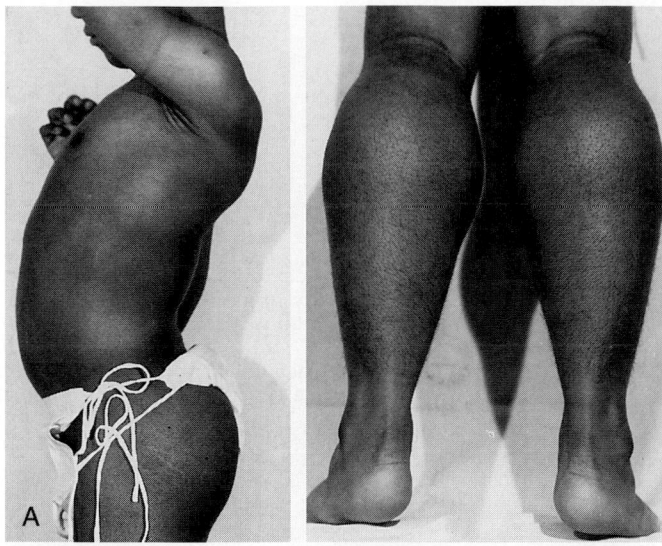

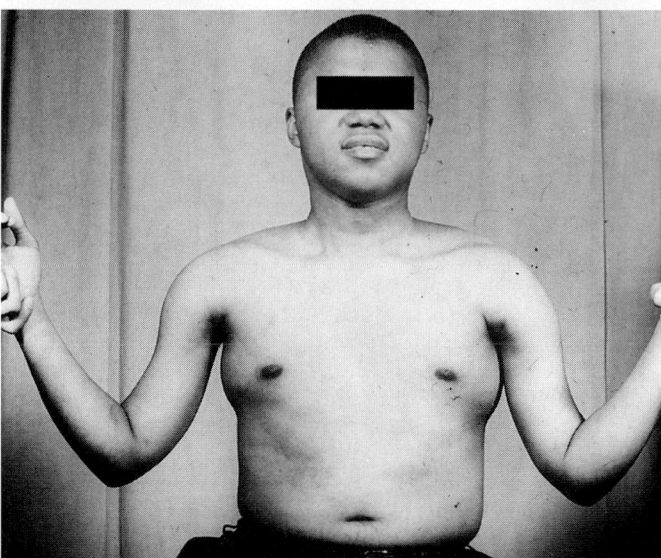

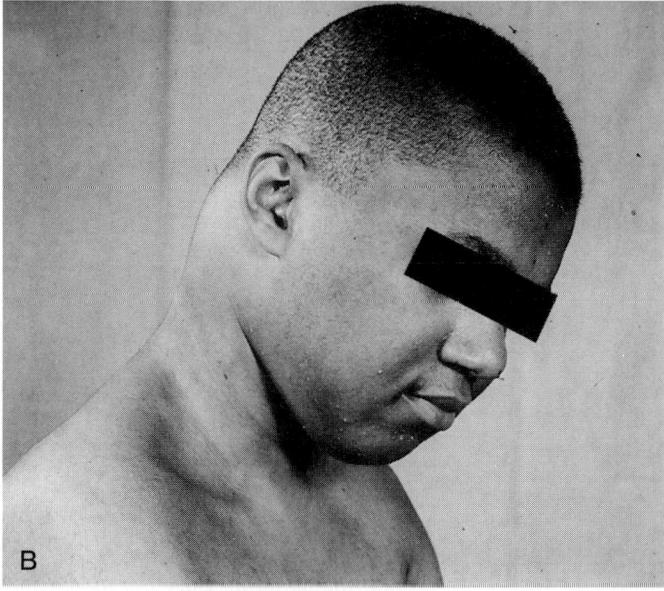

FIGURE 71–1. *A,* Classic X-linked muscular dystrophy. *Left,* Exaggerated lumbar lordosis. *Right,* Calf pseudohypertrophy and shortening of the Achilles tendons. *B,* Seventeen-year-old boy with Duchenne muscular dystrophy. There is striking enlargement (hypertrophy/pseudohypertrophy) of the deltoid and pectoralis major muscles (upper panel) and of the trapezius (lower panel). There was also striking enlargement of both calves (not shown). (*A* and *B* courtesy of Joseph K. Perloff, M.D.)

cular dystrophy the electrocardiogram (ECG) is abnormal in 90 percent, demonstrating a distinctive pattern of tall R waves and an increased R/S amplitude in V_1 and deep narrow Q waves in the left precordial leads related to the characteristic posterolateral left ventricular involvement (Fig. 71–4). In patients with Becker muscular dystrophy ECG abnormalities are present in up to 75 percent.[14, 15] The ECG abnormalities observed include tall R waves and an increased R/S amplitude in V_1, similar to that seen in Duchenne muscular dystrophy, but may also show frequent incomplete right bundle branch block. This may be related to early involvement of the right ventricle. In patients with congestive heart failure, left bundle branch block is common (Fig. 71–5).[15]

In both Duchenne and Becker muscular dystrophies, elevated serum creatinine kinase activity is observed, over 10-fold and 5-fold normal values, respectively.[18]

Arrhythmias. In Duchenne muscular dystrophy, arrhythmias secondary to disturbances in both rhythm and conduction are observed. Persistent or labile sinus tachycardia is the most recognized abnormality.[19] The pathogenesis of this tachycardia is unknown but does not appear related to abnormal autonomic function.[20] Atrial arrhythmias including atrial fibrillation and atrial flutter occur commonly as a preterminal rhythm.[21] Abnormalities in atrioventricular (AV) conduction have been observed. Up to 10 percent of individuals have PR intervals of less than 120 milliseconds, with an additional 10 percent having prolonged PR intervals.[22] Ventricular arrhythmias occur on monitoring in 30 percent (primarily ventricular premature complexes). More complex ventricular arrhythmias have been reported as well. These are more commonly present in individuals with severe muscle disease.[19, 23] Sudden death occurs in Duchenne muscular dystrophy, primarily in patients with severe skeletal muscle weakness. Whether this is an arrhythmic death is not clear.

Arrhythmic manifestations in Becker muscular dystrophy tend to correspond to the degree of the associated dilated cardiomyopathy but are not well characterized.[24] Distal conduction system disease with complete heart block and bundle branch reentry ventricular tachycardia have been observed.[25, 26]

Female carriers of Duchenne muscular dystrophy are at increased risk of dilated cardiomyopathy.[27, 28, 28a]

TREATMENT AND PROGNOSIS. Duchenne muscular dystrophy is a progressive disorder with respiratory or cardiac death common by age 20 to 25. A primary cardiac etiology for death occurs in about one fourth of patients with an equal distribution of death from progressive heart failure and sudden death.[19, 21] Intravenous verapamil used for preterminal atrial arrhythmias can lead to acute respiratory failure.[29] A report of the use of an implantable cardioverter-defibrillator for recurrent drug refractory ventricular tachycardia resulted in a periprocedural respiratory death.[30]

In Becker muscular dystrophy or female carriers of Duchenne muscular dystrophy, it is not known whether therapy to decrease myocardial wall stress is beneficial in preventing or delaying progression to cardiac failure. Once heart failure is established, conventional therapy is indicated. Orthotopic cardiac transplantation has been reported.[31]

Myotonic Muscular Dystrophy

GENETICS

Adult myotonic muscular dystrophy (dystrophica myotonia, Steinert disease) is a heredofamilial disease (autosomal dominant) characterized by reflex and percussion myotonia, weakness, and atrophy of distal skeletal muscles as well as systemic manifestations of early balding, gonadal atrophy, cataracts, mental retardation, and cardiac involvement (Fig. 71–6).[32] The genetic abnormality responsible for this diffuse systemic disease is an amplified and unstable trinucleotide (cytosine-thymine-guanine [CTG]) repeat found on the long arm of chromosome 19. This repeat sequence is located in the 3′ untrans-

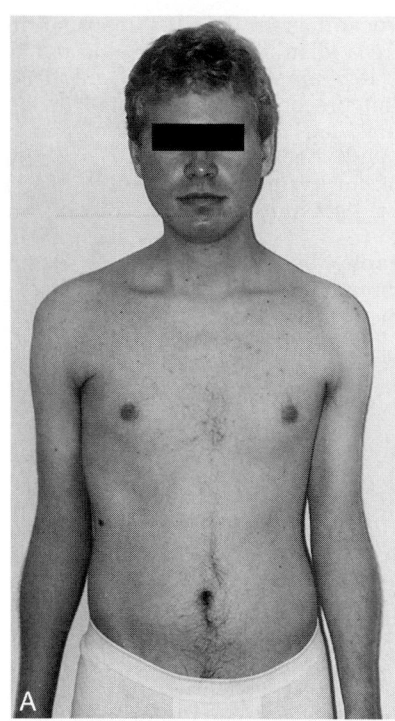
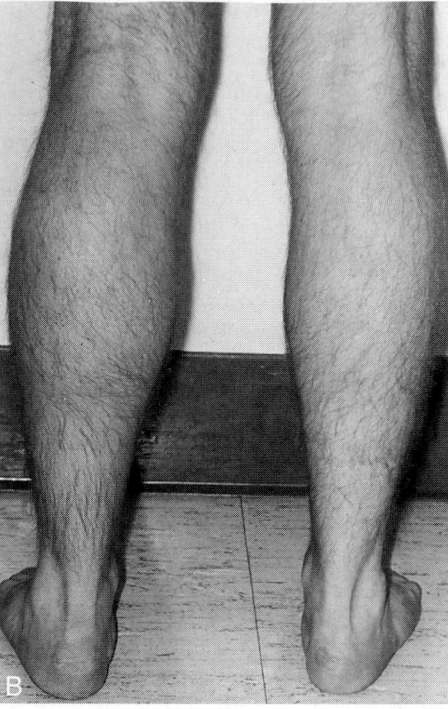

FIGURE 71–2. Late onset, slowly progressive Becker muscular dystrophy in a 22-year-old man. A, There is dystrophy of the shoulder girdle, arms, and pelvic girdle (last not shown). B, Asymmetric calf pseudohypertrophy is greater on the left than on the right. Dystrophy of proximal leg muscles is not shown. (A and B courtesy of Joseph K. Perloff, M.D.)

lated region of a gene encoding a protein homologous to serine/threonine protein kinases, identified as myotonic protein kinase (Mt-PK or DMPK).[33–35] In individuals without myotonic dystrophy, between 5 and 37 copies of this CTG repeat are present. In individuals with myotonic dystrophy, 50 to several thousand CTG repeats are observed. A direct correlation exists between an increasing number of CTG repeats and earlier age at onset and increasing severity of neuromuscular involvement.[36–38] Whether increasing CTG expansion correlates with increasing cardiac involvement is debated.[39–42]

MECHANISM. The mechanism by which the amplified CTG repeat flanking Mt-PK leads to the characteristic involvement in myotonic dystrophy is not clear but likely involves alterations in tissue phosphorylation related to reduction in Mt-PK activity and possibly a resultant change in ion channel structure or function.[43, 44] Studies using transgenic mice deficient in Mt-PK have shown divergent results regarding the replication of the skeletal muscle disease.[45, 46] Cardiac conduction disease was observed in the transgenic mouse model, similar to what is seen in the human disease, although without characteristic degenerative pathology.[47] Other mechanisms for the cardiac

involvement have been hypothesized, including a potential relationship to a second gene adjacent to Mt-PK known to be responsible for progressive familial heart block, impaired glucose utilization possibly related to abnormal protein kinase function, and abnormal coronary reserve.[48–50]

CLINICAL PRESENTATION. Myotonic dystrophy is the most common inherited neuromuscular disorder in patients presenting as adults. The global incidence has been estimated to be 1 in 8000, although it is higher in certain populations, such as French Canadians, and lower to nonexistent in other populations, such as African blacks.[32] The age at onset of symptoms and diagnosis averages 20 to 25 years. Common early manifestations are weakness in the muscles of the face, neck, and distal extremities. On examination, myotonia (delayed muscle relaxation) can be dem-

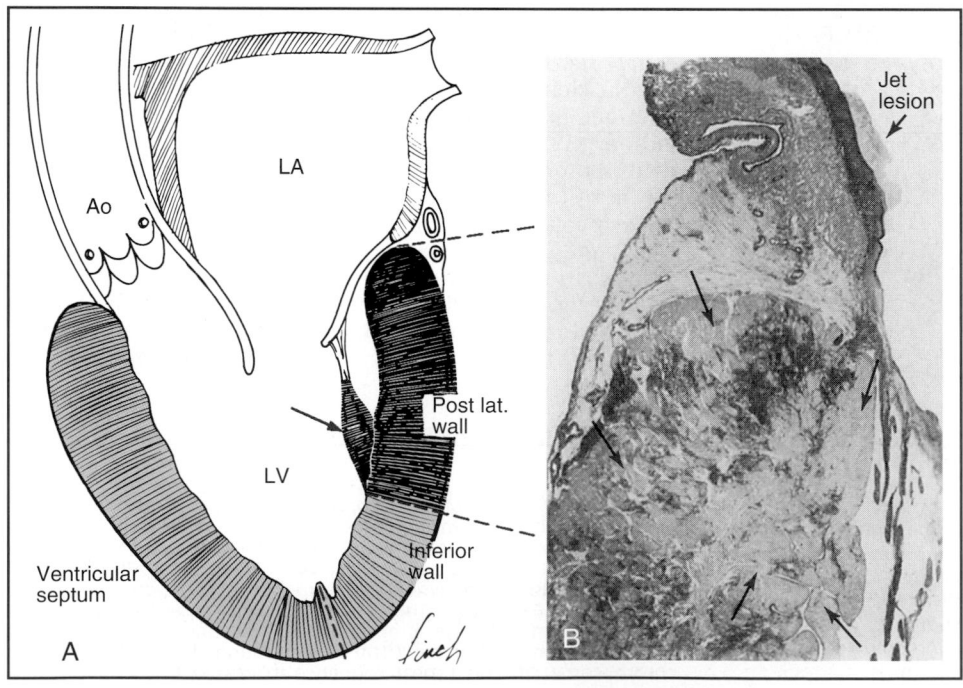

FIGURE 71–3. A, Schematic illustration showing the typical posterobasal myocardial involvement with lateral extension in classic Duchenne muscular dystrophy. The posterolateral papillary muscle is involved (arrow). LA = left atrium; LV = left ventricle; Ao = aorta. B, Necropsy section showing posterobasal involvement (arrows) of the left ventricle (LV) in a boy with classic Duchenne muscular dystrophy. The posterolateral papillary muscle was involved, resulting in mitral regurgitation and the jet lesion shown at upper right. (A and B courtesy of Joseph K. Perloff, M.D.)

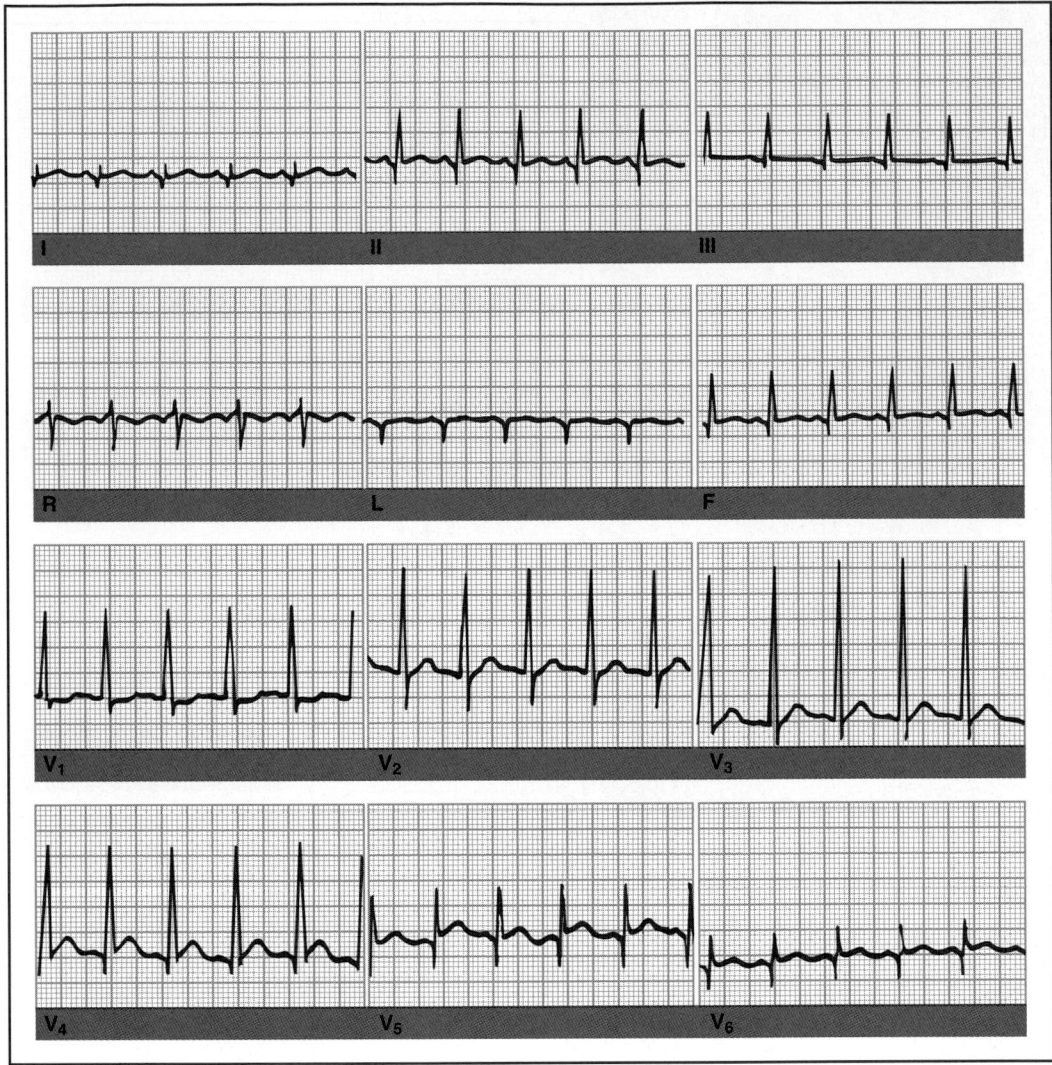

FIGURE 71-4. Electrocardiogram from a 12-year-old boy with classic Duchenne muscular dystrophy. Sinus tachycardia is observed. The QRS complex is typical of Duchenne dystrophy, showing tall R waves in lead V_1 and deep, narrow Q waves in leads I, aVL, and V_4 to V_6. (Courtesy of Charles Fisch, M.D., Indiana University School of Medicine, Indianapolis, IN.)

onstrated in the grip, thenar muscle group, and tongue (Fig. 71–7). Diagnosis when the individual is asymptomatic is possible using electromyography and genetic testing. Symptomatic myotonic dystrophy tends to present at an earlier age and with increasing severity in successive generations. This property is called anticipation and is related to the increasing amplification of CTG repeat length in successive generations.[38, 51] In general, cardiac symptoms occur after the onset of skeletal muscle weakness but can be the initial manifestation of the disease.

CARDIOVASCULAR MANIFESTATIONS. Cardiac pathology is commonly seen in myotonic dystrophy and primarily involves degeneration (fibrosis and fatty infiltration) of the specialized conduction tissue, including the sinus node, AV node, and His-Purkinje system. Degenerative changes are observed in working atrial and ventricular tissue but only rarely progress to symptomatic cardiomyopathy (Fig. 71–8).[52, 53] It is not surprising, based on this preferential degeneration of conduction tissue, that the primary cardiac manifestations of myotonic dystrophy are arrhythmias.

Electrocardiography and Arrhythmias. The majority of adult patients with myotonic dystrophy have ECG abnormalities. In several large series, atrial fibrillation or atrial flutter was observed in 6 to 11 percent, first-degree AV block was found in 20 to 60 percent, right bundle branch block in 2 to 11 percent, and left bundle branch block in 5

to 13 percent. Q waves not associated with a known myocardial infarction are common. ECG abnormalities often progress over time (Fig. 71–9).

Mitral valve prolapse is often observed on echocardiography and is believed to be related to papillary muscle dysfunction. The heart may be involved before myocardial degenerative changes in a manner similar to the myotonia in skeletal muscle. This has been hypothesized to be manifest by echocardiographic evidence of delayed early diastolic relaxation of the left ventricle.[54]

At electrophysiological study, the most common abnormality found is a prolonged His-ventricular (H-V) interval. This was observed in 56 to 90 percent of selected patients and in follow-up studies does appear to progress.[42, 55] Other findings at electrophysiological study include prolongation in the atrial-His (A-H) interval and inducible atrial arrhythmias, primarily atrial fibrillation. In patients without previously known ventricular tachycardia, the likelihood of inducing a sustained ventricular tachycardia is low.

Conduction system disease can progress to symptomatic AV block and necessitate pacemaker implantation. Current prevalence of permanent cardiac pacing in patients with myotonic dystrophy varies between 3 and 22 percent (or higher).[42, 56] Patient selection and indication for pacing is not clear or consistent in these series. Slowed conduction in the ventricles is present, as evidenced by a significant

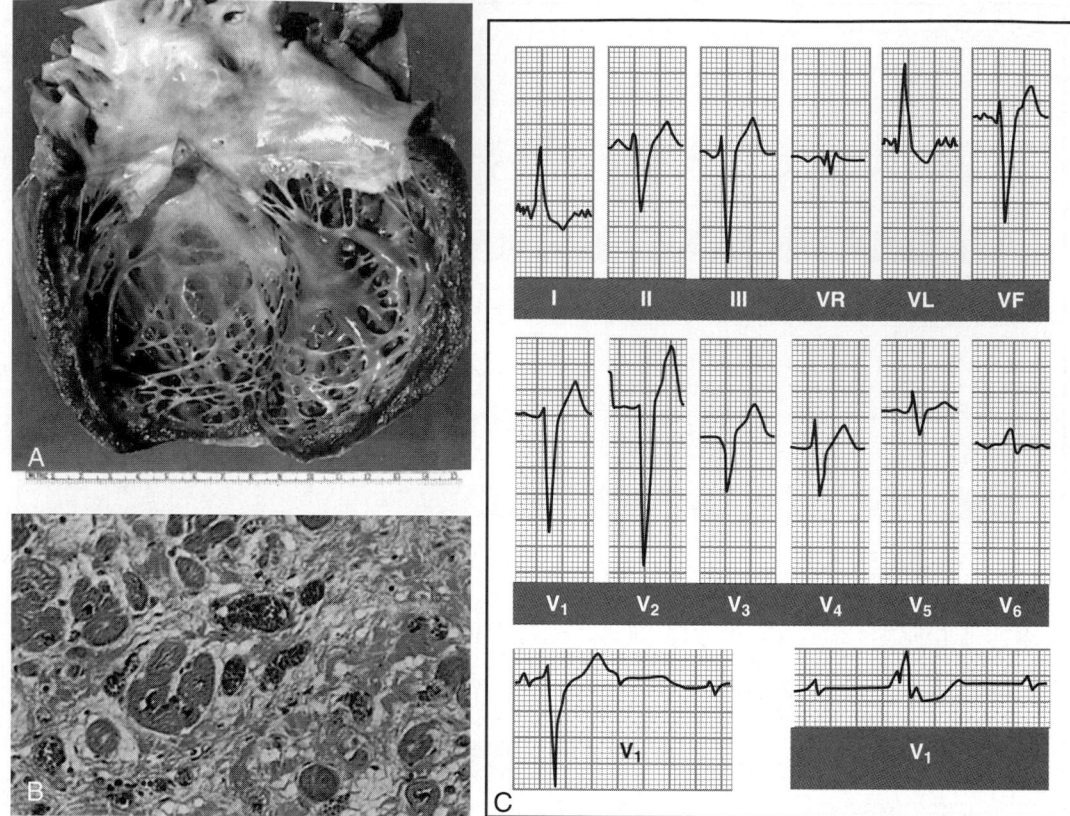

FIGURE 71–5. Gross and microscopic cardiac pathological specimens and the electrocardiogram from a 45-year-old man with late-onset, slowly progressive Becker muscular dystrophy. *A,* Dilated, flabby left ventricle with focal endocardial thickening. *B,* Microscopic section from the left ventricle shows marked confluent scarring with variations in fiber size; there was no significant coronary artery disease. *C,* Electrocardiogram recorded at age 40 years. The 12-lead tracing shows left-axis deviation, a QRS of 0.14 second, small Q waves in leads I and aVL, and loss of R waves in leads V_2 and V_3. The lower tracings, taken 4 years later (a year before death), show complete heart block with a variable QRS configuration. (From Perloff JK, et al: The cardiomyopathy of progressive muscular dystrophy. Circulation 33:625, 1966. Copyright 1966, The American Heart Association.)

incidence of late potentials on signal-averaged ECGs.[57, 57a] Atrial arrhythmias, primarily atrial fibrillation and atrial flutter, are common in myotonic dystrophy, being seen in approximately 10 percent of a general population, and are more common in those patients with more severe neuromuscular disease.[58–61] Ventricular tachycardia can occur in patients with myotonic dystrophy.[62–65] In at least two reports and a series of six patients, the ventricular tachycardia observed was related to reentry in the diseased distal conduction system, as characterized by bundle branch reentry and interfascicular reentry tachycardia (see Chap. 25).[62, 65] Therapy with right bundle branch and/or fascicular radiofrequency ablation resulted in absence of further inducible ventricular tachycardia.[62, 65]

Sudden Death. The incidence of sudden death in patients with myotonic dystrophy is substantial and believed to be primarily caused by arrhythmias. In a registry of 180 myotonic dystrophy patients from the Netherlands collected from 1950 to 1997, 29 percent of all deaths were classified as sudden, presumably secondary to arrhythmias.[66] This was secondary only to pneumonia (31 percent) as a cause of death. In a 10-year study of mortality in a cohort of 367 patients from Quebec, 75 (20 percent) patients died.[67] In these 75 deaths, 31 percent were characterized as secondary to cardiovascular causes, with 11 percent sudden. The mechanisms leading to sudden death in myotonic dystrophy are not clear. Both bradyarrhythmias and ventricular tachyarrhythmias may be responsible. Bradyarrhythmias can cause sudden death in that distal conduction disease producing AV block may result in a lack of an appropriate automatic escape rhythm and asystole or bradycardia-mediated ventricular fibrillation. Sudden death can occur in myotonic dystrophy despite previous permanent cardiac pacing, implicating the role of ventricular tachyarrhythmias.

TREATMENT. Cardiac management in individuals with myotonic dystrophy is not well established. In patients in whom a dilated cardiomyopathy does develop, standard

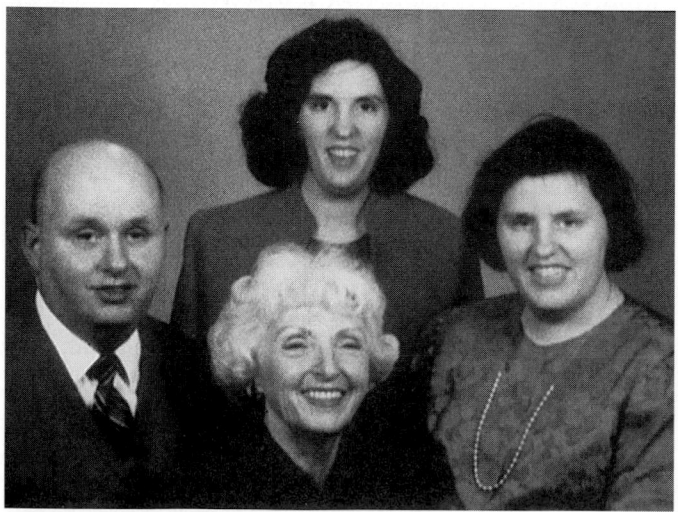

FIGURE 71–6. Myotonic muscular dystrophy in three siblings. Note the unaffected mother (front). Demonstrated is premature balding (left) and characteristic thin facies (rear).

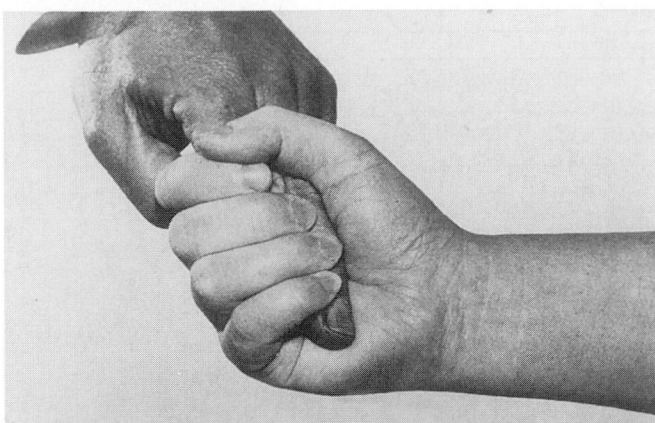

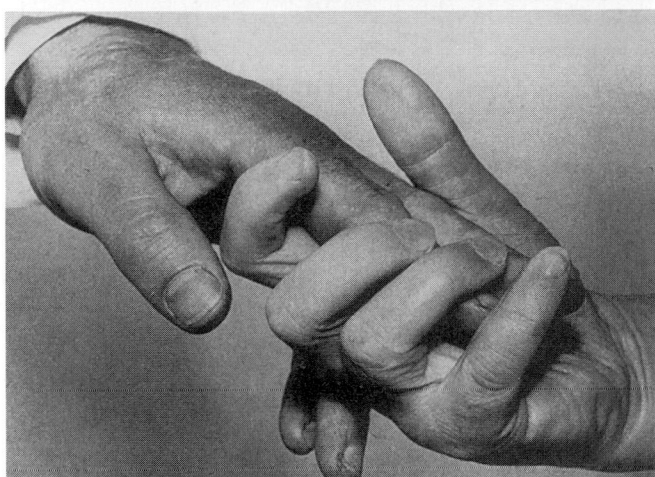

FIGURE 71-7. Grip myotonia in myotonic muscular dystrophy. Inability to release (bottom) after exerting grip (top). (Reproduced by permission from Harper PS, et al: Myotonic dystrophy. In Engel AG, Franzini-Armstrong C [eds]: Myology: Basic and Clinical. 2nd ed. vol. II. New York, McGraw-Hill, 1994, p 1195.)

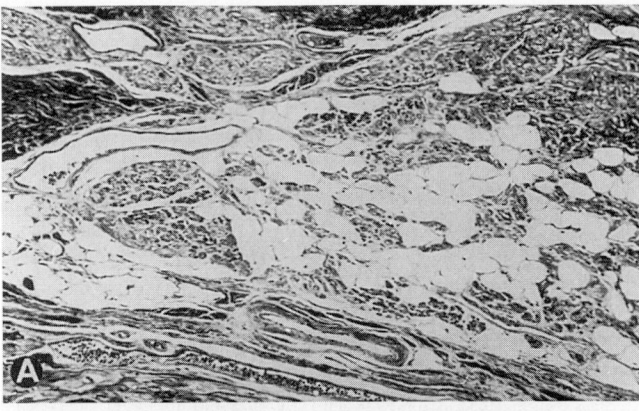

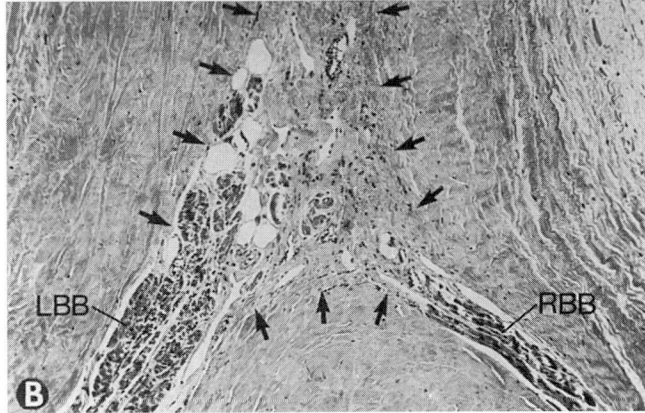

FIGURE 71-8. Histopathology of the atrioventricular bundle in myotonic dystrophy. *A*, Fatty infiltration in a 57-year-old man (Masson trichrome stain, ×90). *B*, Focal replacement fibrosis and atrophy in a 48-year-old woman. Arrows demarcate expected size and shape of the branching atrioventricular bundle (Hematoxylin and eosin stain, ×90). LBB = left bundle branch, RBB = right bundle branch. (From Nguyen HH, et al: Pathology of the cardiac conduction system in myotonic dystrophy: A study of 12 cases. J Am Coll Cardiol 11:662, 1988. Copyright 1988, American College of Cardiology.)

therapy including angiotensin-converting enzyme (ACE) inhibitors and beta-blocking agents has improved symptoms.[68] Patients presenting with symptoms indicative of arrhythmic disease such as syncope and palpitations should undergo an extensive evaluation, including electrophysiological study, to determine an etiology. A low threshold for permanent pacing is warranted. In individuals who are asymptomatic from a cardiac standpoint the degree of appropriate screening is not well established. Most authors recommend ECGs yearly and consideration for 24-hour ambulatory monitoring. Whether significant or progressive ECG abnormalities require intervention (prophylactic pacing, invasive electrophysiological evaluation) is uncertain. In one series, in which 45 individuals with myotonic dystrophy were followed for a mean of 4.6 years, ECG evidence of conduction abnormalities increased from 38 to 62 percent.[60] In this study, baseline or progression of ECG abnormalities did not correlate with the need for pacemaker insertion (5 individuals) or sudden death (1 individual). More recently, a series of 53 patients observed for a mean time period of 6.3 years determined that a PR interval of 240 milliseconds or greater was useful in predicting cardiac events (atrial fibrillation, complete heart block, syncope, and sudden death).[69] The appropriate therapy for this higher risk group was not discussed. Trials encompassing more patients using a multicenter approach have been recommended.[56] Some groups have advocated invasive electrophysiological evaluation and prophylactic permanent pacing in a high proportion of myotonic dystrophy patients.[42] Certain families may be more prone to arrhythmic manifestations of myotonic dystrophy and should be considered for

more careful evaluation.[70] Anesthesia in individuals with myotonic dystrophy can increase the risk of AV conduction block and other arrhythmias, and therefore these individuals should be carefully monitored and prophylactic temporary pacing considered.

In patients presenting with wide complex tachycardia, invasive electrophysiological testing with careful evaluation for bundle branch reentry tachycardia should be done. The use of class I antiarrhythmic agents in suppressing ventricular tachycardia in myotonic dystrophy has had limited efficacy. Sotalol may be more effective.[63] Whether implantable cardioverter-defibrillators are appropriate or useful has not been described.

PROGNOSIS. The course of neuromuscular abnormalities in myotonic dystrophy is highly variable. Death from progressive weakness and respiratory difficulty can occur in advanced muscular disease. Other individuals may be only minimally limited by weakness to ages of 60 to 70 years.[32] Sudden death may significantly reduce survival in patients with myotonic dystrophy, including those minimally symptomatic from a neuromuscular status. What evaluation and interventions are appropriate, and the degree of effectiveness to decrease the risk of sudden death, are unclear.

Emery-Dreifuss Muscular Dystrophy

GENETICS

Emery-Dreifuss muscular dystrophy is a rare familial disorder in which skeletal muscle symptoms are often mild but with cardiac involvement common and life threatening.[71, 72] The disease is primarily inherited in an X-linked recessive fashion, but there is heterogeneity in

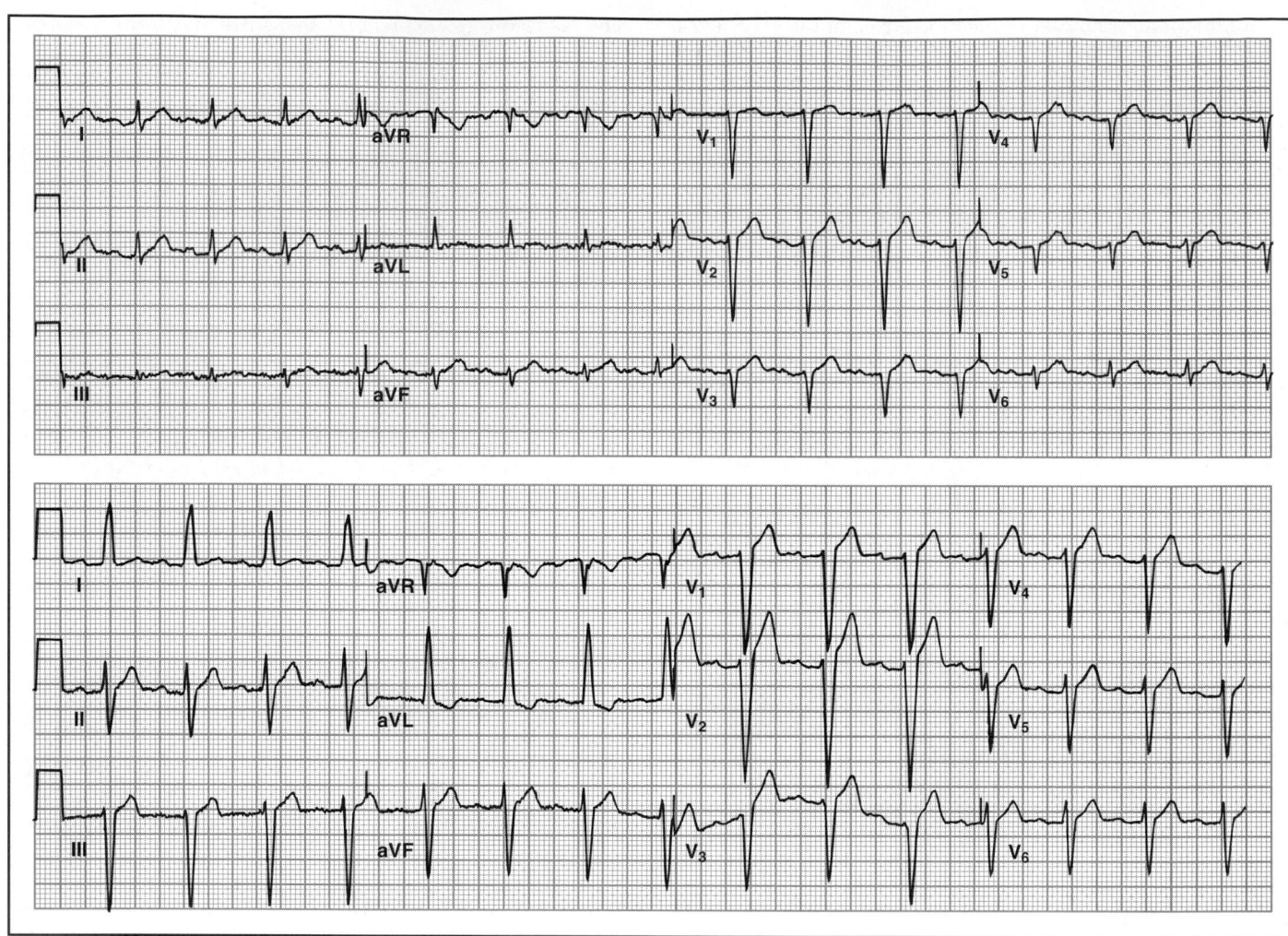

FIGURE 71–9. Electrocardiograms obtained 1 year apart in a 36-year-old man with myotonic dystrophy (top older). Note the abnormal Q waves in the precordial leads. An increasing PR interval and QRS duration are observed consistent with increasing severity of conduction disease.

that families have been reported that fit an autosomal dominant and recessive inheritance pattern.

A gene responsible for the X-linked recessive Emery-Dreifuss muscular dystrophy was identified in 1994.[73] The candidate gene found on chromosome Xq28, *STA*, encodes a nuclear membrane protein called emerin.[74–76] The lack of emerin in skeletal and cardiac muscle is responsible for the disease phenotype. Recently, the autosomal dominant Emery-Dreifuss muscular dystrophy was linked to chromosome 1 with a candidate gene encoding proteins of the nuclear lamina.[77]

CLINICAL PRESENTATION. Emery-Dreifuss muscular dystrophy is characterized by a triad of (1) early contractures of the elbow, Achilles tendon, and posterior cervical muscles; (2) slowly progressing muscle weakness and atrophy; and (3) cardiac involvement.[71, 72]

The disorder has been labeled "benign X-linked muscular dystrophy" to differentiate the slowly progressive muscular weakness from that of Duchenne muscular dystrophy. A definitive diagnosis can be made in Emery-Dreifuss muscular dystrophy and in carriers using antiemerin antibodies.[78, 79]

CARDIOVASCULAR MANIFESTATIONS. Arrhythmias are the primary manifestation of cardiac disease in Emery-Dreifuss muscular dystrophy.[79a] Abnormalities in impulse generation and conduction are exceedingly frequent. ECGs are generally abnormal by age 20 to 30 years, commonly showing first-degree AV block. The atria appear to be involved earlier than the ventricles, with atrial fibrillation and atrial flutter or, more classically, permanent atrial standstill and junctional bradycardia, observed. Abnormalities in impulse generation or conduction are present in virtually all indi-

viduals by age 35 to 40 years, and permanent ventricular pacing is often required. Sudden death (presumed cardiac) before age 50 is exceedingly common and is reported to occur in as high as 40 percent of individuals.[80] This may be diminished with prophylactic permanent pacing.

Arrhythmia. Ventricular tachyarrhythmias including sustained ventricular tachycardia and ventricular fibrillation have been reported. Invasive electrophysiological study data are limited in this rare condition. Mild prolongation of the H-V interval, atrial, AV nodal, and ventricular refractory periods has been observed.[81] Female carriers of Emery-Dreifuss muscular dystrophy do not develop skeletal muscle disease but do develop late cardiac disease, including conduction abnormalities; and sudden death can occur.[82] The characteristic arrhythmic involvement in Emery-Dreifuss muscular dystrophy may be related to the unique localization of emerin in desmosomes and fascia adherens of the intercalated discs.[83] If emerin functions in maintaining cell-to-cell adhesion, then its absence may impair conduction.

Localization of emerin in intercalated discs has not been observed by all investigators.[84] Although arrhythmic disease is the most common presentation of cardiac involvement in Emery-Dreifuss muscular dystrophy, a dilated cardiomyopathy can develop. This may be more common in patients in whom survival has been improved with permanent pacemaker implantation.[85] Both autopsy and endomyocardial biopsy have shown abnormal cardiac fibrosis.[85, 86]

TREATMENT AND PROGNOSIS. Affected males should be carefully monitored for development of ECG abnormalities of conduction. Ambulatory electrocardiography may reveal arrhythmic abnormalities during sleep that are not apparent during short-term ECG recording.[86] AV block can occur with anesthesia.[87] Permanent ventricular pacing is recommended once conduction disease is evident and can be life saving. After ventricular pacing, other cardiac manifestations can occur, including ventricular tachyarrhythmias and/or ventricular dysfunction. Female carriers do develop conduction disease, and ECG monitoring on a routine basis is appropriate. Whether prophylactic ventricular pacing is indicated in this group is not clear.

Cardiac disease including sudden death remains responsible for significant mortality in Emery-Dreifuss muscular dystrophy despite early pacing. Whether other therapy (implantable cardioverter-defibrillators) would diminish this mortality has not been tested.

Limb Girdle Muscular Dystrophy

GENETICS

Limb girdle muscular dystrophy constitutes a group of disorders with a limb/pelvic girdle distribution of weakness but with otherwise heterogeneous inheritance and clinical features.[88] Classically, the disorder is inherited in an autosomal recessive fashion, although autosomal dominant and sporadic genetic inheritance has been observed. Positional cloning has improved an understanding of the genetics of limb girdle muscular dystrophy. Abnormalities have been identified in a number of genes most commonly expressed as dystrophin-associated proteins.[89]

CLINICAL PRESENTATION. The onset of muscle weakness is variable but usually occurs before age 30 years. Patients commonly present with complaints of difficulty with walking or running secondary to pelvic girdle involvement. As the disease progresses, involvement of the shoulder muscles and then more distal muscles occurs, with sparing of facial involvement. Slow progression to severe disability and/or death is common.

CARDIOVASCULAR MANIFESTATIONS. Historically, cardiac involvement in limb girdle muscular dystrophy has been considered to be rare. However, as more has been understood about the genetic constitution and heterogeneity of this group of disorders, a greater realization of the potential for cardiac involvement is emerging.

An autosomal recessive or sporadic limb girdle muscular dystrophy caused by a deficiency in the sarcoglycan complex associated with dystrophin may be associated with a dilated cardiomyopathy.[90-92] ECGs from several patients showed abnormalities such as increased R wave in V_1, consistent with the pattern of dystrophin-related cardiomyopa-

thy, as seen in Duchenne muscular dystrophy. Cardiac abnormalities seen with ECG or echocardiographic evaluation have been detected in up to 80 percent, but with a much smaller proportion of patients being symptomatic.[92, 93]

A recently recognized autosomal dominant limb girdle muscular dystrophy with a high incidence of cardiac arrhythmic involvement has been linked to chromosome 1q11-21.[94] In these families, affected members develop high-degree AV block by age 35 to 45 years. Sudden death believed to be cardiac was reported in eight individuals at a median age of 50 years, including those in whom permanent pacing was previously instituted. A dilated cardiomyopathy was diagnosed in two individuals. In one individual, postmortem examination revealed extensive cardiac fibrosis, including replacement of the specialized conduction tissue. Others have reported families with limb girdle muscular dystrophy in whom AV block, cardiomyopathy, and sudden death were the primary manifestations.[95, 96]

TREATMENT AND PROGNOSIS. Because of the heterogeneous nature of limb girdle muscular dystrophy, specific recommendations for routine cardiac evaluation are difficult to make. In families in whom cardiac disease has been shown to be associated with their neuromuscular disorder, cardiac evaluation for arrhythmic disease and ventricular dysfunction should be considered. In individual families, prophylactic permanent pacing can be indicated.[95]

Facioscapulohumeral Muscular Dystrophy

GENETICS

Facioscapulohumeral muscular dystrophy is an autosomal dominant disorder in which the genetic locus has been mapped to chromosome 4q35.[97] Genetic heterogeneity has been reported.[98] Neither the definitive gene nor the gene product responsible for facioscapulohumeral muscular dystrophy has been identified.[99]

CLINICAL PRESENTATION. Muscle weakness tends to follow a slowly progressive but variable course presenting with facial muscle weakness and progressing to involve the shoulders, foot extensors, and pelvis (Fig. 71–10).[100]

CARDIOVASCULAR MANIFESTATIONS. Cardiac involvement in facioscapulohumeral muscular dystrophy has been reported but does not constitute a significant problem in prevalence or severity as it does in many of the other muscular dystrophies. In one series of 31 patients evaluated by physical examination, chest radiograph, ECG, and echocardiogram, no evidence of cardiac abnormalities was found.[101] Other series have reported a propensity toward

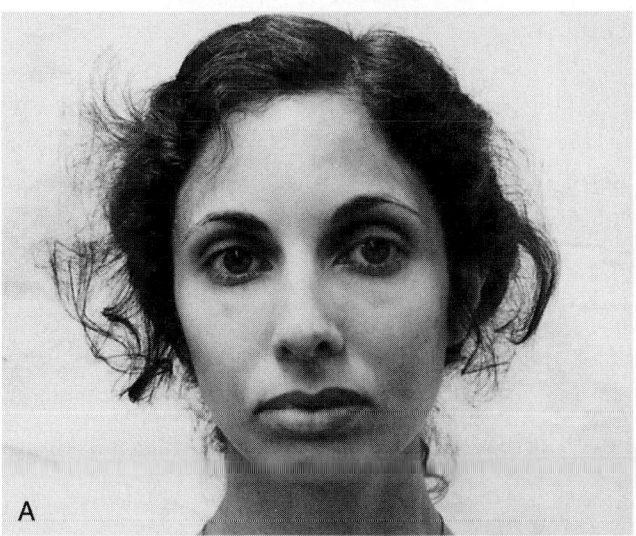
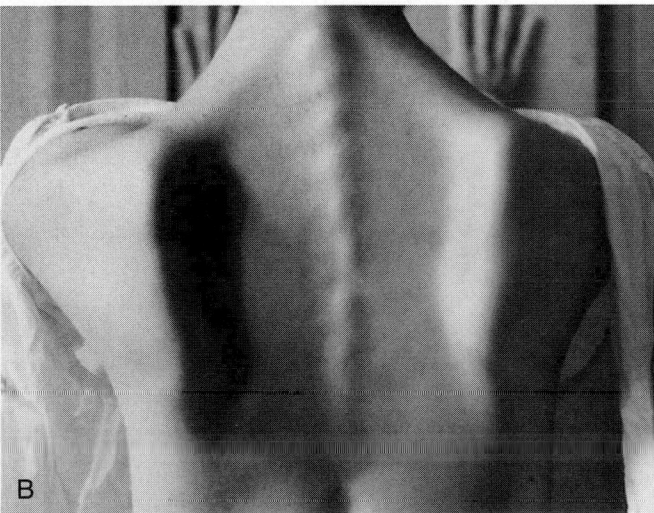

A   B

FIGURE 71–10. Facioscapulohumeral muscular dystrophy in a 32-year-old woman. *A*, The face is in repose (myopathic) with dimpling of the corners of the mouth. *B*, Typical winging of the scapulae. (*A* and *B* courtesy of Joseph K. Perloff, M.D.)

arrhythmias.[102, 103] In 30 patients (mean age, 35 years), ECGs were abnormal in 26, primarily with atrial abnormality or minor conduction disease. Ten patients underwent invasive electrophysiological study with findings of abnormal sinus node function in 3, prolonged H-V interval in 1, and inducible sustained or unsustained episodes of atrial fibrillation or atrial flutter with single atrial extrastimuli in 8. In 100 patients with facioscapulohumeral muscular dystrophy genetically linked to chromosome 4q35, 5 percent were found to have arrhythmic disease in the absence of cardiovascular risk factors.[103] Three patients were symptomatic, with one requiring pacemaker implantation for AV block. Clinical correlation and follow-up was not available in either of these studies. Early reports of permanent atrial paralysis in facioscapulohumeral muscular dystrophy are likely cases of Emery-Dreifuss muscular dystrophy.

TREATMENT AND PROGNOSIS. Because significant clinical cardiac involvement is rare in facioscapulohumeral muscular dystrophy, specific monitoring or treatment recommendations are not well defined. One group has recommended yearly ECGs.[103]

FRIEDREICH ATAXIA

GENETICS

Friedreich ataxia is a progressive spinocerebellar degenerative disease characterized clinically by ataxia of the limbs and trunk, dysarthria, loss of deep tendon reflexes, sensory abnormalities, skeletal deformities, and cardiac involvement. It is inherited in an autosomal recessive fashion with linkage to chromosome 9.[104] The gene responsible has been identified and has been found to encode a 210-amino acid protein, frataxin.[105] Frataxin is a mitochondrial protein important in iron homeostasis and respiratory function.[106, 107] Abnormalities in frataxin leads to mitochondrial dysfunction, poor cellular response to oxidative stress, and apoptosis.[108, 109]

Messenger RNA for frataxin is highly expressed in the heart. The mutations identified have been primarily an amplified and unstable trinucleotide (guanine-adenine-adenine [GAA]) repeat found in the first intron. Increasing size of this expansion has been found to correlate with the age at onset and severity of neurological symptoms and the degree of left ventricular hypertrophy by echocardiography.[110–112]

CLINICAL PRESENTATION. The estimated prevalence of Friedreich ataxia is 1 in 50,000. Neurological symptoms usually manifest around puberty and almost always before age 25. Progressive loss of neuromuscular function, with the individual wheelchair-bound 10 to 20 years after symptom onset, is the norm. Neurological symptoms precede cardiac symptoms in most but not all cases.

CARDIOVASCULAR MANIFESTATIONS. Friedreich ataxia is frequently associated with a concentric hypertrophic cardiomyopathy (Fig. 71–11).[112] Asymmetric septal hypertrophy is also observed. A left ventricular outflow gradient has been reported in some cases. Presentation with a dilated cardiomyopathy is more rare but can occur (Fig. 71–12). Whether the dilated cardiomyopathy occurs as a progressive transition from the hypertrophic cardiomyopathy or is a distinct entity is not known. A recent study would support the former.[113] The prevalence of hypertrophy varies between studies but does increase in likelihood with younger age at diagnosis and with increasing GAA trinucleotide repeat length.[112, 114] As high as 95 percent of neurologically symptomatic patients have cardiac abnormalities on ECG and echocardiographic evaluation. Findings are consistent with ventricular hypertrophy. On ECGs, left ventricular hypertrophy is not always present despite echocardiographic evidence.[114a] Widespread T wave inversion is common (Fig. 71–13).

Arrhythmias. These can occur but are less common then what might be expected considering the high incidence of cardiac muscle involvement and hypertrophy. Atrial arrhythmias including atrial fibrillation and atrial flutter are associated with the dilated cardiomyopathy.[115] Clinically relevant disorders of impulse formation or conduction have not been reported despite histopathological evidence of conduction system involvement.[115] Ventricular tachycardia in the setting of dilated cardiomyopathy has been observed.[116] However, ventricular tachyarrhythmias are not associated with the hypertrophic cardiomyopathy. Sudden death can occur, but the mechanism of this death has not been well characterized.

Endomyocardial Biopsy. This procedure has demonstrated myocyte hypertrophy and interstitial fibrosis.[117] His-

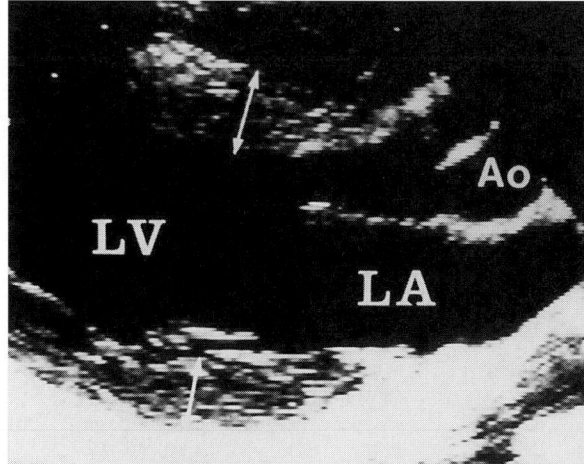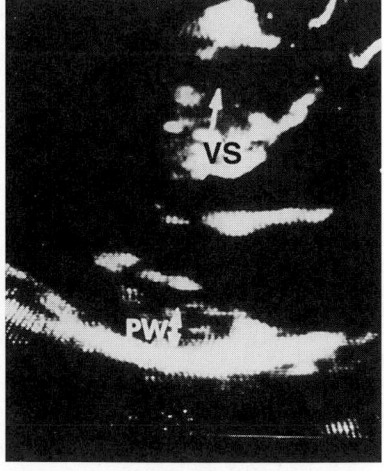

FIGURE 71–11. *A,* Two-dimensional echocardiogram (parasternal long axis diastolic frames) from a 14-year-old girl with Friedreich ataxia and concentric hypertrophy (arrows) of the left ventricle (LV). *B,* Two-dimensional echocardiogram (parasternal long axis) from a 17-year-old boy with Friedreich ataxia and hypertrophic cardiomyopathy characterized by disproportionate thickness (arrows) of the ventricular septum (VS) compared with the posterior wall (PW). Ao = aorta; LA = left atrium. (From Perloff JK: Cardiac manifestations of neuromuscular disease. *In* Abelmann WH [ed]: Cardiomyopathies, Myocarditis, and Pericardial Disease. vol. 2. *In* Braunwald E [series ed]: Atlas of Heart Diseases. Philadelphia, Current Medicine, 1995, pp 6.1–6.19.)

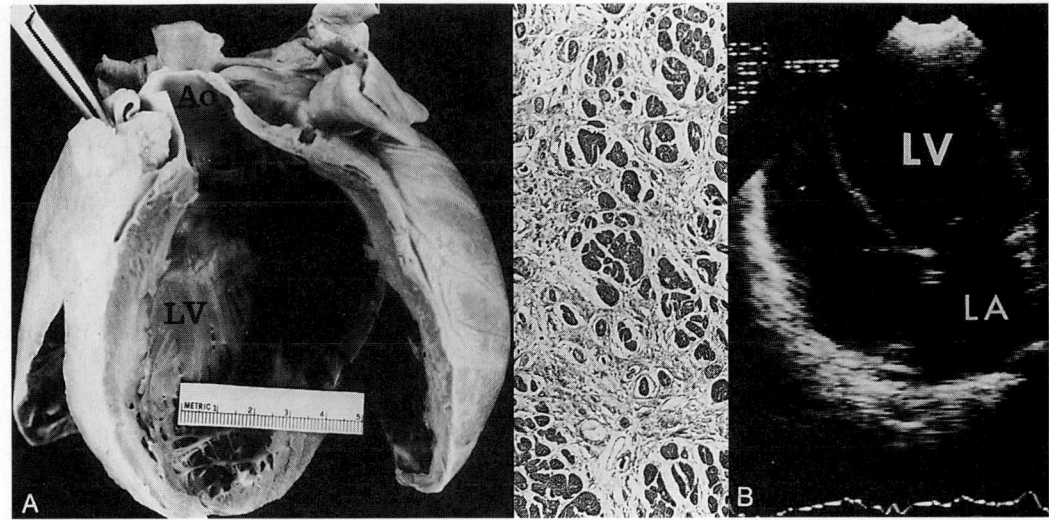

FIGURE 71–12. *A,* Gross and histological specimens from a 17-year-old boy with Friedreich ataxia whose echocardiogram progressed from normal at age 13 years to a minimally dilated, hypocontractile left ventricle 3 to 4 years later. The gross specimen shows a mildly dilated left ventricle (LV) with normal wall thickness; the walls were flabby. The microscopic section from the left ventricular free wall shows marked connective tissue replacement. Although specifically sought, small-vessel coronary artery disease was not identified. *B,* Two-dimensional echocardiogram (apical window) showing the mildly dilated, thin-walled left ventricle (LV). LA = left atrium. (From Child JS, et al: Cardiac involvement in Friedreich ataxia. J Am Coll Cardiol 7:1370, 1986. Copyright 1986, American College of Cardiology.)

topathological examination, at the time of autopsy, revealed myocyte hypertrophy and degeneration, interstitial fibrosis, active muscle necrosis, bizarre pleomorphic nuclei, and periodic acid-Schiff–positive deposition in both large and small coronary arteries. Degeneration and fibrosis in cardiac nerves and ganglia and the conduction system have also been observed.[115, 117] Myocardial fiber disarray, as observed in genetic hypertrophic cardiomyopathy, is rare.[115] Deposition of calcium salts and iron have been reported. How

these cardiac pathological findings relate to abnormalities in the protein frataxin is unknown.

TREATMENT AND PROGNOSIS. No specific therapy for the neurological or cardiac disease is available. Progressive neurological dysfunction is common, with death from respiratory failure or infection occurring in the fourth or fifth decades. Cardiac death can occur, primarily in those developing a dilated cardiomyopathy. These patients tend to do poorly, with rapid progression to end-stage congestive heart failure.

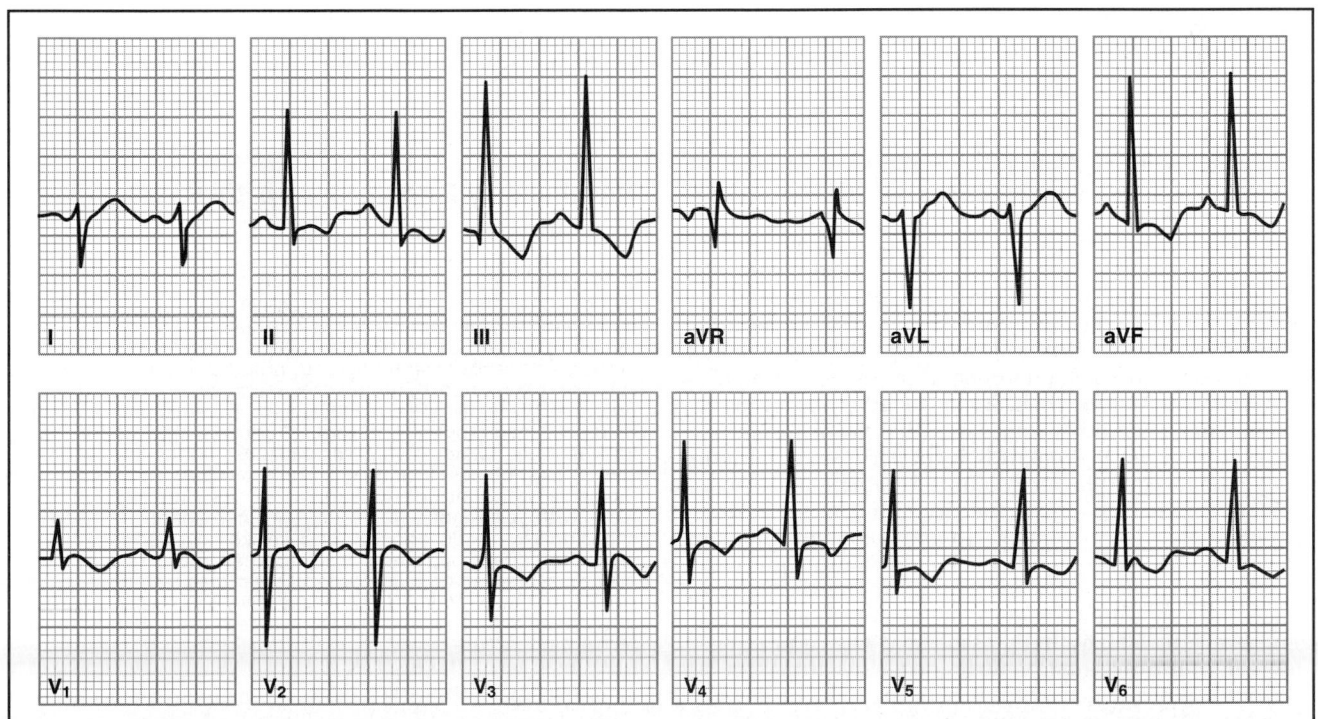

FIGURE 71–13. Electrocardiogram from a 34-year-old man with Friedreich ataxia. Widespread ST and T changes are observed. (Courtesy of Charles Fisch, M.D., Indiana University School of Medicine, Indianapolis, IN.)

The Periodic Paralyses

GENETICS

The primary periodic paralyses are rare, nondystrophic, autosomal dominant disorders that result from abnormalities in ion channel genes. They can be classified into hypokalemic and hyperkalemic (potassium-sensitive) periodic paralysis with several subclassifications in each. Hypokalemic periodic paralysis is characterized by episodic attacks of weakness in association with decreased serum potassium levels. Penetrance is complete in males and approximately 50 percent in females.[118] Hypokalemic periodic paralysis has been mapped to chromosome 1q31-32 with subsequent identification of mutations in the alpha₁ subunit of the dihydropyridine-sensitive calcium channel.[119, 120] The disease may be genetically heterogeneous, as observed with the identification of a family with hypokalemic periodic paralysis and a mutation in the skeletal muscle sodium channel (SCN4A).[118]

Hyperkalemic periodic paralysis also manifests as episodic weakness but with symptoms worsening with potassium supplementation. Complete penetrance is observed. Potassium levels are usually high but may be normal during an attack. Hyperkalemic periodic paralysis is due primarily to mutations in the alpha subunit of SCN4A found on chromosome 17.[121] Multiple different mutations in this gene have been reported and result in a potassium-sensitive failure of inactivation in the sodium channel.[122] Hyperkalemic periodic paralysis is genetically heterogeneous. Andersen syndrome, a potassium-sensitive periodic paralysis associated with characteristic dysmorphic features and ventricular arrhythmias, is not secondary to SCN4A mutations or known long QT syndrome genetic loci (Fig. 71–14).[123] The genetic abnormality in this disease remains unknown.

CLINICAL PRESENTATION. Episodic weakness is usually the presenting symptom in both of the periodic paralyses. Attacks of weakness tend to be more severe and of longer duration with hypokalemic periodic paralysis than with hyperkalemic periodic paralysis. In both diseases, cold and rest after exercise can trigger an attack. Ingestion of carbohydrates can trigger an attack in hypokalemic periodic paralysis but may ameliorate an attack in hyperkalemic periodic paralysis.[124]

CARDIOVASCULAR MANIFESTATIONS. Patients with the periodic paralyses are at an increased risk of ventricular tachycardias with occurrence more common with hyperkalemic periodic paralysis. In both, bidirectional ventricular tachycardia has been observed independent of digitalis intoxication.[123, 125] The bidirectional ventricular tachycardia occurs independent of attacks of muscle weakness, generally does not correlate with serum potassium levels, and can convert to sinus rhythm with exercise. Ventricular ectopy is common, often seen interspersed with bidirectional ventricular tachycardia (see Chap. 25).

Prolonged QT interval can be observed. In some reports, this is episodic and associated with weakness, hypokalemia, or antiarrhythmic therapy. In other cases, a prolonged QT interval can be constant. Andersen syndrome is more commonly associated with a prolonged QT interval and ventricular tachycardia. Sudden death has been reported.

TREATMENT AND PROGNOSIS. The episodes of weakness commonly respond to measures that work to normalize potassium levels.[124] Weakness in hyperkalemic periodic paralysis can respond to mexiletine. Treatment of electrolytes usually does not improve arrhythmias or, if it does, only transiently. Improvement in symptomatic nonsustained ventricular tachycardia associated with a prolonged QT interval has been reported with beta-blocker therapy. Class 1A antiarrhythmic agents can worsen muscle weakness and exacerbate arrhythmia associated with a prolonged QT interval.[125] Bidirectional ventricular tachycardia, not associated with a prolonged QT interval, may not respond to beta-blocker therapy. Imipramine has been observed to decrease the episodes of bidirectional ventricular tachycardia.[125] Whether other antiarrhythmic therapies have a role in the treatment of the periodic paralyses is unknown.

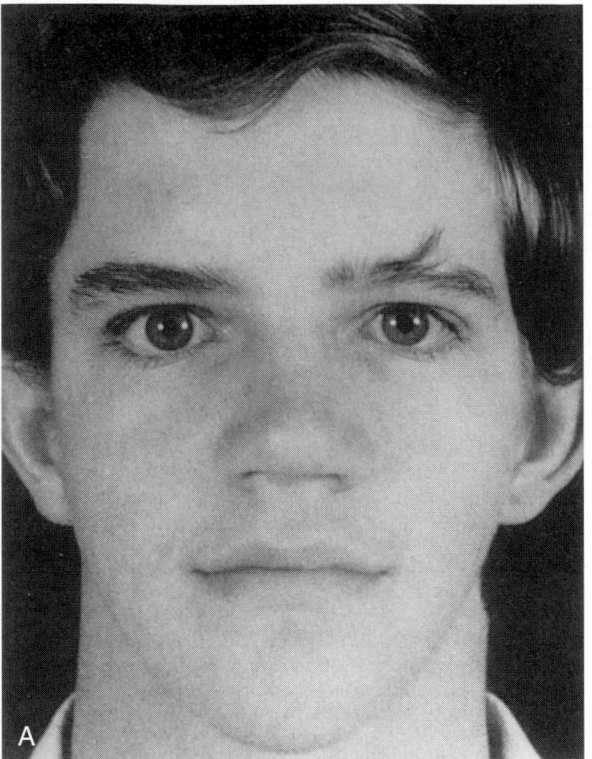

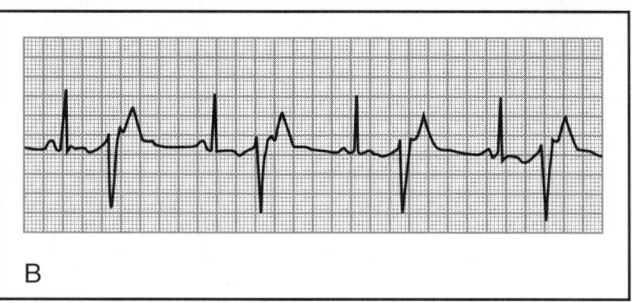

FIGURE 71–14. Andersen syndrome in a 22-year-old man. Characteristic low-set ears and hypoplastic mandible. *B,* Electrocardiographic recording revealing ventricular bigeminy. (From Tawil R, et al: Andersen syndrome: Potassium-sensitive periodic paralysis, ventricular ectopy, and dysmorphic features. Ann Neurol 35:326, 1994. Copyright 1994, American Neurological Association.)

Mitochondrial Encephalomyopathies

GENETICS

The mitochondrial encephalomyopathies are a heterogeneous group of disorders resulting from mutations in mitochondrial DNA.[126] The number of distinct disorders is extensive. Mitochondrial DNA is inherited maternally, and the majority of these disorders are thus transmitted from mother to children of both sexes. Some of the disorders occur sporadically or are inherited in an autosomal fashion. It is not surprising, based on the important metabolic function of mitochondria, that these disorders manifest with systemic pathology involving metabolic, neurological, and cardiac function. Mitochondrial encephalomyopathies, which have cardiac manifestations, present as several clinical phenotypes, including chronic progressive external ophthalmoplegia, which includes the Kearns-Sayre syndrome; myoclonus epilepsy with red ragged fibers [MERRF]; mitochondrial myopathy, encephalopathy, lactic acidosis, and strokelike episodes [MELAS]; and Leber hereditary optic neuropathy. Other, more rare mitochondrial disorders present primarily with cardiac manifestations, often a dilated cardiomyopathy.[127] Chronic progressive external ophthalmoplegia is primarily a sporadic disease, whereas the others listed are maternally inherited.

CLINICAL PRESENTATION. *Kearns-Sayre syndrome* is characterized by the clinical triad of progressive external ophthalmoplegia, pigmentary retinopathy, and AV block (Fig. 71–15). Diabetes, deafness, and ataxia can also be associated. Clinical features of MERRF include myoclonus,

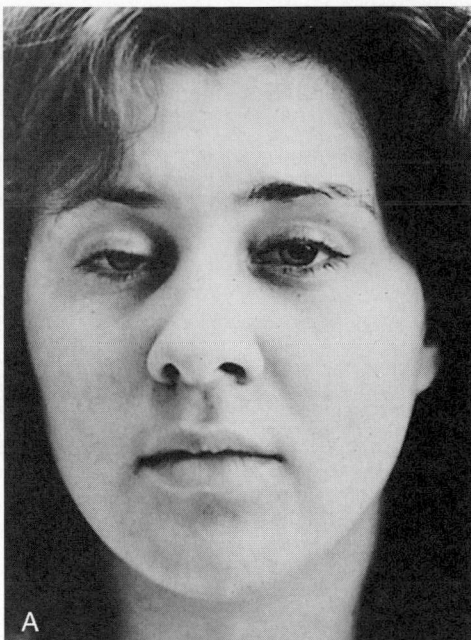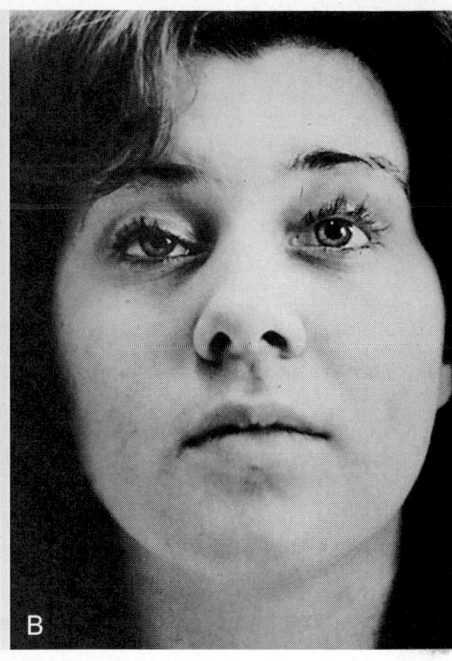

FIGURE 71–15. An 18-year-old girl with Kearns-Sayre syndrome and bilateral asymmetrical ptosis. Within 24 months, her electrocardiogram changed from normal to bifascicular block (complete right bundle branch block and left anterior fascicular block). *A,* Asymmetrical ptosis when the patient looks straight ahead. *B,* Ptosis of the right lid persists when the patient looks up. She also had typical pigmentary retinopathy. (*A* and *B* courtesy of Joseph K. Perloff, M.D.)

seizures, ataxia, dementia, and skeletal muscle weakness. MELAS is the most common of the maternally inherited mitochondrial disorders and is characterized by encephalopathy, subacute strokelike events, migraine-like headaches, recurrent emesis, extremity weakness, and short stature. *Leber hereditary optic neuropathy* manifests as a severe, subacute, painless loss of central vision, predominantly affecting young men.

CARDIOVASCULAR MANIFESTATIONS. In chronic progressive external ophthalmoplegia, primarily in the *Kearns-Sayre syndrome,* cardiac involvement manifests as conduction abnormalities.[128, 129] A dilated cardiomyopathy has also been reported.[130] In the Kearns-Sayre syndrome, AV block is exceedingly common, usually presenting after eye involvement becomes manifest. In one series reporting 5 cases and reviewing 30 additional cases, Stokes-Adams syncope occurred in 29 percent, 34 percent had permanent pacemakers implanted, and in 7 patients (20 percent) AV block was believed to contribute to death.[128] The H-V interval is prolonged, consistent with distal conduction disease.[131]

Leber hereditary optic neuropathy can be associated with a short PR interval and preexcitation syndromes in a significant proportion.[132] In a review of 55 patients from eight pedigrees, 16 were noted to have a PR interval less than 120 milliseconds, with 5 manifesting preexcitation. Supraventricular tachycardia has been reported.

In MERRF and MELAS, cardiac involvement manifesting as hypertrophic cardiomyopathy (symmetrical or asymmetrical) has been observed.[129, 133] These patients can develop chest pain with ECG abnormalities and myocardial perfusion defects.[134] Progression (or questionably a second entity) to dilated cardiomyopathy can occur with heart failure and death.

Preexcitation has been described with MELAS.[129]

Several mitochondrial DNA mutations can be associated with dilated cardiomyopathy in the absence of other clinical abnormalities.[126]

TREATMENT AND PROGNOSIS. In *Kearns-Sayre syndrome,* the prophylactic implantation of a pacemaker has been advocated when distal conduction disease is evident. Pacing appears to improve survival.[128, 129] The degree of distal conduction disease that warrants prophylactic pacing is not clear. In *Leber hereditary optic neuropathy,* a baseline ECG may be prudent. In the other mitochondrial disorders, an understanding of the potential for cardiac involvement is necessary. Whether specific evaluation in these disorders without symptoms is necessary is uncertain.

Spinal Muscular Atrophy

GENETICS

Spinal muscular atrophies are a group of lower motor neuron disorders presenting as progressive, symmetrical muscle weakness. In most cases, an autosomal recessive pattern of inheritance is observed but there is genetic heterogeneity.[135] By means of linkage analysis, the spinal muscular atrophies were mapped to chromosome 5q11.2-q13.3.[136] Mutations in a particular gene, *SMN* (survival of motor neuron), are responsible for this disorder.[137] Severity of the disease is correlated with the degree of reduction of the protein product of this gene.[138]

CLINICAL PRESENTATION. Spinal muscular atrophies are divided into three clinical groups characterized by the age at onset, degree of muscular weakness, and survival.[139] Type I (Werdnig-Hoffmann disease) and type II have early childhood onset with severe limitation of life span. Spinal muscular atrophy type III (Kugelberg-Welander disease) is characterized by childhood or adolescent onset of atrophy and weakness in proximal muscles with slow progression.

CARDIOVASCULAR MANIFESTATIONS. Cardiac involvement in spinal muscular atrophies include coexisting complex congenital heart disease, cardiomyopathy, and arrhythmias. Congenital heart disease has been associated with type I and III spinal muscular atrophies.[140] The most common abnormality is atrial septal defect, with other abnormalities reported. In spinal muscular atrophy type III, a dilated cardiomyopathy may occur with endomyocardial biopsy specimens demonstrating fibrosis.[141] Progression leading to a fatal outcome has been reported. Arrhythmic abnormalities including atrial standstill, atrial fibrillation, atrial flutter, and AV block may be the most common cardiac manifestation in these diseases.[141] Permanent pacing for atrial standstill and AV block has been reported.

TREATMENT AND PROGNOSIS. The skeletal muscle involvement in spinal muscular atrophy type I and II limit life span so significantly that treatment of associated cardiac abnormalities is often not indicated. In spinal muscular atrophy type III, awareness of the potential of associated cardiac abnormalities is necessary. Permanent pacing may be required.

Guillain-Barré Syndrome

CLINICAL PRESENTATION. The Guillain-Barré syndrome is an acute inflammatory demyelinating neuropathy characterized by peripheral, cranial, and autonomic nerve dysfunction.[142] It is the most common acquired demyelinating neuropathy, with an annual incidence of 1.7 per 100,000 population. The syndrome usually occurs 3 days to 3 weeks after a viral respiratory illness, a gastrointestinal infection, an immunization, or surgery. This disorder usually presents as symmetrical limb weakness that can progress to involve cranial and respiratory muscles. Approximately one third of individuals require assisted ventilation.

CARDIOVASCULAR MANIFESTATIONS. Cardiac involvement in Guillain-Barré syndrome is related to accompanying autonomic nervous system dysfunction that manifests as hypertension, orthostatic hypotension, resting sinus tachycardia, loss of heart rate variability, ST segment abnormalities, and both bradyarrhythmias and tachyarrhythmias.[143, 144] Significant autonomic nervous system dysfunction occurs primarily in severe cases of Guillain-Barré syndrome. Microneurographic recordings have shown increased sympathetic outflow during an acute phase of the disease that normalized with recovery.[145]

Life-threatening arrhythmias are common in severe cases of Guillain-Barré syndrome, primarily those requiring assisted ventilation. In a prospective study of 100 patients, serious arrhythmias occurred in 11 of 33 patients requiring ventilation.[143] This included asystole in 6, bradycardia of less than 30 beats/min in 1, rapid atrial fibrillation in 2, and ventricular tachycardia/fibrillation in 2. Thirteen deaths occurred, with four due to arrhythmias. All individuals with serious arrhythmias had signs of autonomic dysfunction. In this series and in other reports, asystole was commonly associated with tracheal suction.[143]

TREATMENT AND PROGNOSIS. In addition to supportive care, early plasmapheresis and intravenous immunoglobulin can improve recovery.[142] In patients requiring ventilation, cardiac rhythm monitoring is mandatory. If serious bradycardia or asystole is observed, temporary or permanent pacing can improve survival. Atropine or isoproterenol during tracheal suction can be of benefit. The mortality rate in individuals hospitalized with Guillain-Barré syndrome is as high as 20 percent. In individuals who recover from Guillain-Barré syndrome, autonomic function also recovers, and no long-term arrhythmia risk has been observed.

Myasthenia Gravis

CLINICAL PRESENTATION. Myasthenia gravis is a disorder of neuromuscular transmission resulting from production of antibody targeted against the nicotinic acetylcholine receptor.[146] The primary symptom, fluctuating weakness, usually begins with the eye and facial muscles and later can involve the large muscles of the limbs. Patients can present at any age, most commonly at a younger age in women and an older age in men. Myasthenia gravis is usually associated with hyperplasia or a benign or malignant tumor (thymoma) of the thymus gland. The prevalence in the United States is 1 per 33,000.

CARDIOVASCULAR MANIFESTATIONS. A myocarditis can be associated with myasthenia gravis, especially that occurring with thymoma.[147] A cardiac muscle antibody may be responsible.[148] Whereas cardiac pathological changes at autopsy are believed to be common, signs and symptoms of cardiac disease have been historically considered to be more rarely observed and nonspecific. This lack of symptomatic involvement may not always be true. In one series of 108 myasthenia gravis patients, 17 (16 percent) had evidence of cardiac

abnormalities not explained by another etiology.[147] In 11 (10 percent) of these patients, clinical cardiac manifestations primarily arrhythmic occurred. These included atrial fibrillation, AV block, asystole, and unexplained sudden death. Cardiac abnormalities were more common in thymoma patients (50 percent) than among non-thymoma patients (12 percent). Autopsy findings were consistent with myocarditis.

TREATMENT AND PROGNOSIS. Myasthenia gravis is treated with anticholinesterase and immunosuppressive agents. Thymectomy is often indicated. Anticholinesterase agents may slow heart rate and lead to hypotension.[149] No specific therapy has been discussed for the cardiac involvement. Whether immunosuppressive agents or thymectomy improves cardiac disease is unknown. Use of quinidine and propranolol in patients with myasthenia gravis may precipitate an acute exacerbation of weakness.[147, 150]

ACUTE CEREBROVASCULAR DISEASE

CARDIOVASCULAR MANIFESTATIONS. Acute cerebrovascular diseases, including subarachnoid hemorrhage, other stroke syndromes, and head injury, can be associated with severe cardiac manifestations.[151] The mechanism by which this occurs appears to be related to abnormal autonomic nervous system function, primarily a markedly increased sympathetic and parasympathetic output. Hypothalamic stimulation can reproduce the ECG changes observed in acute cerebrovascular disease. ECG changes associated with hypothalamic stimulation or blood in the subarachnoid space can be prevented or diminished with spinal cord transection, stellate ganglion blockade, vagolytics, and adrenergic blockers.

Electrocardiography. Abnormalities on ECGs are observed in as high as 80 to 90 percent of individuals with subarachnoid hemorrhage.[151, 152] Abnormalities including ST segment elevation and depression, T wave inversion, and pathological Q waves are observed.[151, 153] Peaked inverted T waves and a prolonged QT interval may occur in 25 to 40 percent of patients (Fig. 71-16). Hypokalemia is

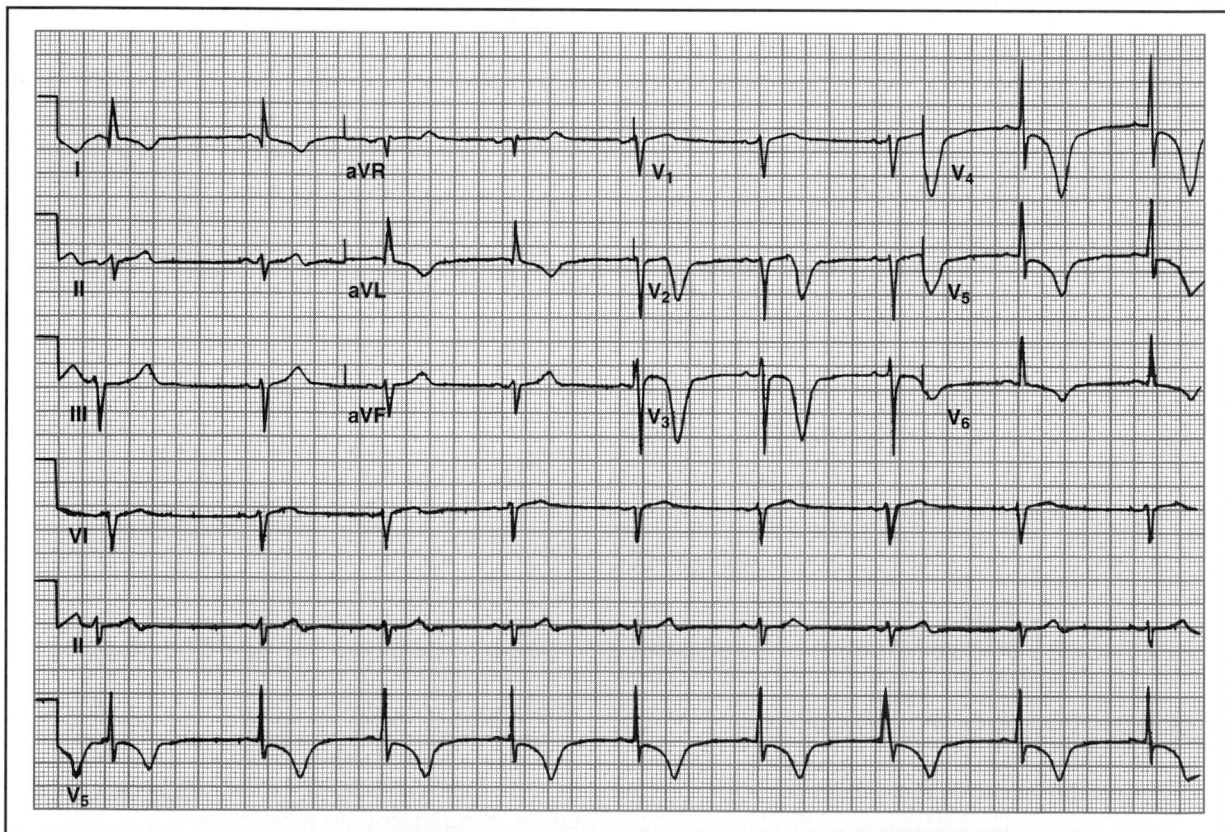

FIGURE 71–16. Electrocardiogram from a patient with cerebral hemorrhage. Deep and symmetrical T wave inversions are observed. (Courtesy of Charles Fisch, M.D., Indiana University School of Medicine, Indianapolis, IN.)

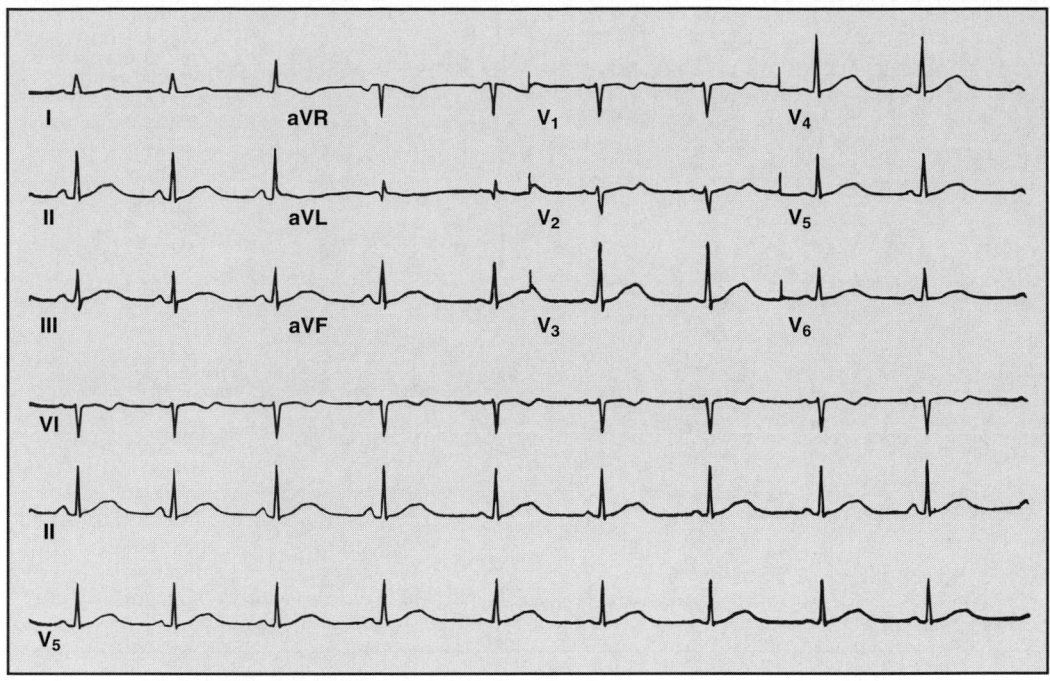

A

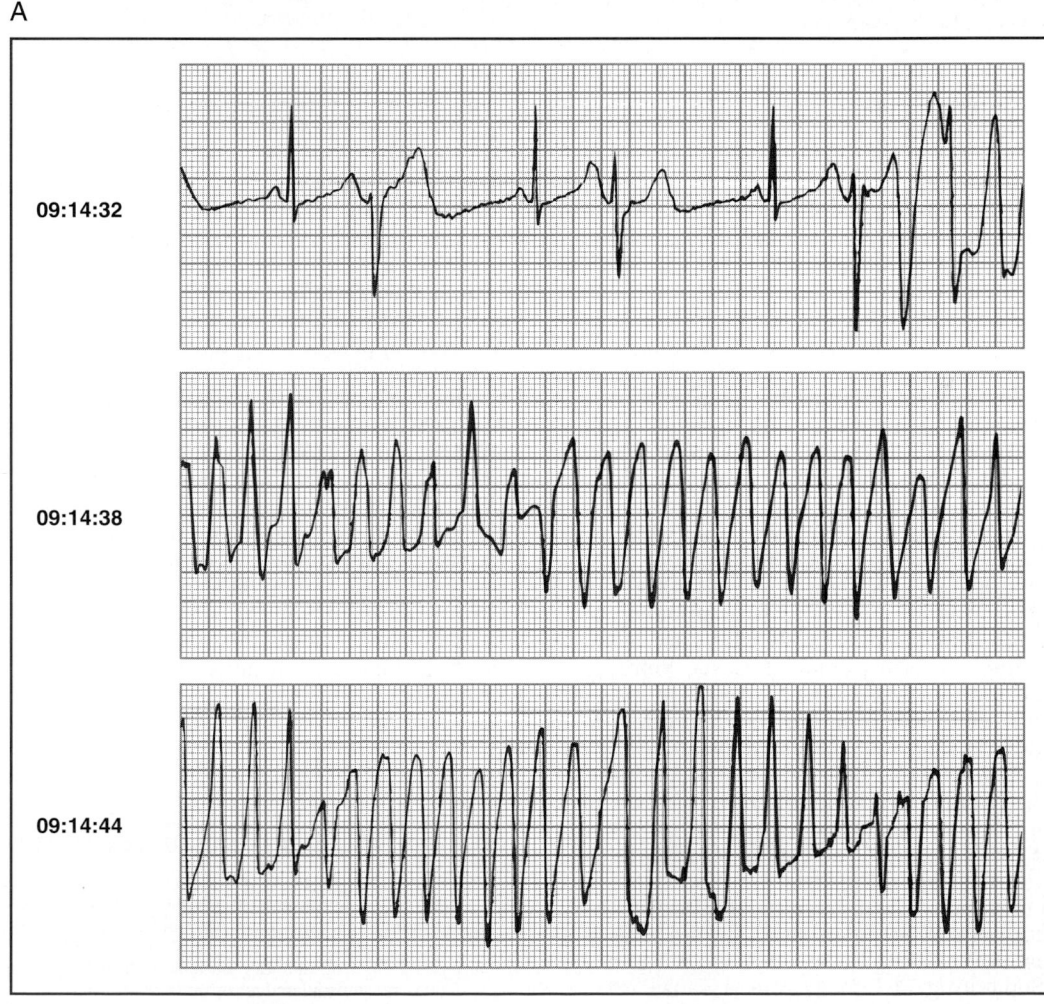

B

FIGURE 71-17. A 49 year old patient with cerebral hemorrhage. *A,* Electrocardiogram recorded within 3 hours of admission and 4 hours after onset of symptoms. QT interval prolongation is observed. *B,* Electrocardiographic monitoring at 6 hours after admission. Ventricular bigeminy precedes the onset of polymorphic ventricular tachycardia. Cardioversion was required. The patient was subsequently treated with a beta-adrenergic blocker without further ventricular tachycardia. *C,* Electrocardiogram done 2 weeks after admission. QT interval has normalized.

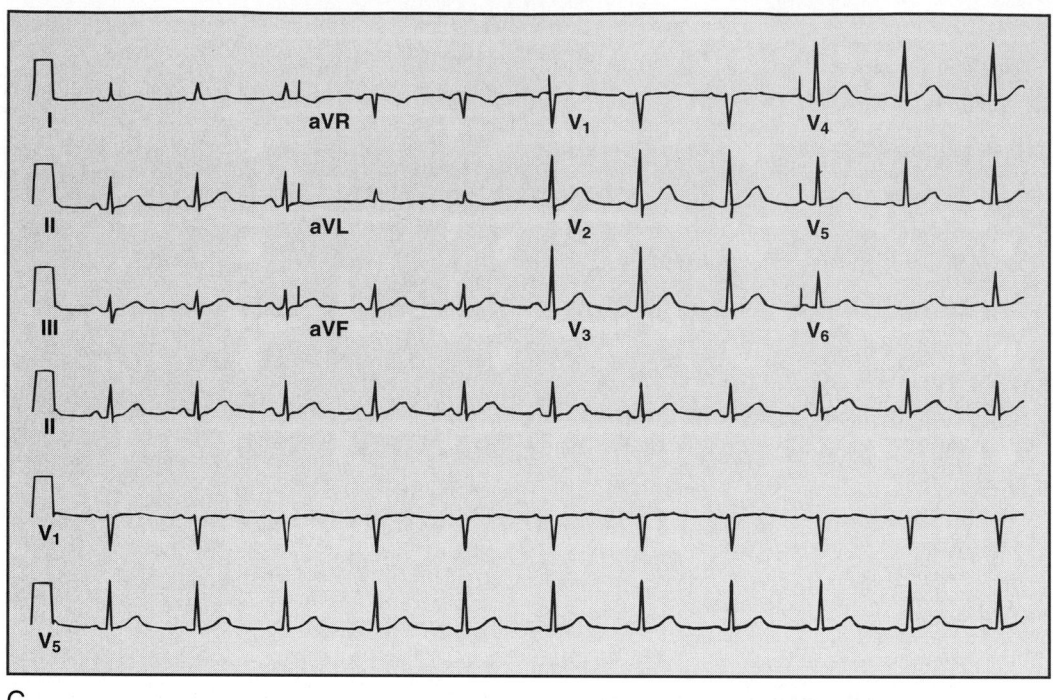

C

FIGURE 71–17 *Continued*

observed in up to 50 percent of patients with subarachnoid hemorrhage, and this increases the likelihood of QT interval prolongation.[154]

Other stroke syndromes are often associated with abnormal ECGs, but whether these are related to the stroke syndrome or to underlying intrinsic cardiac disease is often difficult to discern.[151] A prolonged QT interval is more common in subarachnoid hemorrhage than other stroke syndromes. Closed-head trauma can cause similar ECG abnormalities as subarachnoid hemorrhage, including a prolonged QT interval. Myocardial damage with liberation of myocardial enzymes and subendocardial hemorrhage or fibrosis at autopsy can occur in the setting of acute cerebrovascular disease. Like the ECG changes, these abnormalities are believed related to local myocardial catecholamine excess.

Neurogenic pulmonary edema may accompany the acute neurological insult.[155, 156] This edema can have both a cardiogenic component, related to systemic hypertension, and a noncardiogenic (pulmonary capillary leak) component.

Arrhythmia. Life-threatening arrhythmias can occur in the setting of acute cerebrovascular disease. Ventricular tachycardia or fibrillation has been observed in patients with subarachnoid hemorrhage and head trauma.[154, 157] A torsades de pointes type of ventricular tachycardia can occur (Fig. 71–17). Often this is observed in the setting of a prolonged QT interval and hypokalemia. Stroke syndromes, other than subarachnoid hemorrhage, appear to be only rarely associated with serious ventricular tachycardias.[151] Atrial tachyarrhythmias including atrial fibrillation and regular supraventricular tachycardia have been observed.[151, 152, 154] Atrial fibrillation is most common in individuals presenting with what is believed to be an acute thromboembolic stroke.[151] Separating an effect from a cause may be difficult. Bradyarrhythmias including sinoatrial block, sinus arrest, and AV block occur in up to 10 percent of individuals with subarachnoid hemorrhage.[154] Bradyarrhythmias are less common in other stroke syndromes.

TREATMENT AND PROGNOSIS. Beta-adrenergic blockers appear effective in decreasing myocardial damage and in controlling both supraventricular and ventricular tachyarrhythmias associated with subarachnoid hemorrhage and

head trauma.[158] Beta-adrenergic blockers can increase the likelihood of bradyarrhythmias.[154] Life-threatening arrhythmias appear to occur in the first day after the neurological event.[154] Continuous ECG monitoring during this period is indicated. Careful monitoring of potassium levels especially in patients with subarachnoid hemorrhage is warranted. Refractory ventricular tachyarrhythmias can be controlled effectively with stellate ganglion blockade.[159]

ECG abnormalities reflect adverse intracranial factors but do not appear to portend a poor cardiovascular outcome.[153, 160, 160a]

Head injury (blunt trauma or gunshot wound) and cerebrovascular accident are the leading causes of brain death in individuals being considered as heart donors. These donors may manifest ECG abnormalities, hemodynamic instability, and myocardial dysfunction related primarily to adrenergic storm and not to intrinsic cardiac disease. Experimental studies on whether contractile performance recovers with transplantation are still controversial.[161–163] Optimization of volume status and inotropic support with careful echocardiographic evaluation and possibly left-sided heart catheterization may allow the use of some donor hearts that would have otherwise been rejected.

REFERENCES

DUCHENNE AND BECKER MUSCULAR DYSTROPHY

1. Kunkel LM: Analysis of deletions in DNA from patients with Becker and Duchenne muscular dystrophy. Nature 322:73–77, 1986.
2. Hoffman EP, Kunkel LM: Dystrophin abnormalities in Duchenne/Becker muscular dystrophy. Neuron 2:1019–1029, 1989.
3. Koenig M, Hoffman EP, Bertelson CJ, et al: Complete cloning of the Duchenne muscular dystrophy (DMD) cDNA and preliminary genomic organization of the DMD gene in normal and affected individuals. Cell 50:509–517, 1987.
4. Hoffman EP, Brown RH Jr, Kunkel LM: Dystrophin: The protein product of the Duchenne muscular dystrophy locus. Cell 51:919–928, 1987.
5. Klietsch R, Ervasti JM, Arnold W, et al. Dystrophin-glycoprotein complex and laminin colocalize to the sarcolemma and transverse tubules of cardiac muscle. Circ Res 72:349–360, 1993.
6. Ibraghimov-Beskrovnaya O, Ervasti JM, Leveille CJ, et al: Primary structure of dystrophin-associated glycoproteins linking dystrophin to the extracellular matrix. Nature 355:696–702, 1992.

7. Matsumura K, Nonaka I, Tome FM, et al: Mild deficiency of dystrophin-associated proteins in Becker muscular dystrophy patients having in-frame deletions in the rod domain of dystrophin. Am J Hum Genet 53:409–416, 1993.

8. Muntoni F, Cau M, Ganau A, et al: Brief report: Deletion of the dystrophin muscle-promoter region associated with X-linked dilated cardiomyopathy. N Engl J Med 329:921–925, 1993.

9. Ortiz-Lopez R, Li H, Su J, et al: Evidence for a dystrophin missense mutation as a cause of X-linked dilated cardiomyopathy. Circulation 95:2434–2440, 1997.

10. Muntoni F, Wilson L, Marrosu G, et al: A mutation in the dystrophin gene selectively affecting dystrophin expression in the heart. J Clin Invest 96:693–699, 1995.

11. Nigro G, Comi LI, Politano L, et al: The incidence and evolution of cardiomyopathy in Duchenne muscular dystrophy. Int J Cardiol 26:271–277, 1990.

12. Cziner DG, Levin RI: The cardiomyopathy of Duchenne's muscular dystrophy and the function of dystrophin. Med Hypoth 40:169–173, 1993.

13. Steare SE, Dubowitz V, Benatar A Subclinical cardiomyopathy in Becker muscular dystrophy. Br Heart J 68:304–308, 1992.

14. Melacini P, Fanin M, Danieli GA, et al: Cardiac involvement in Becker muscular dystrophy. J Am Coll Cardiol 22:1927–1934, 1993.

15. Hoogerwaard EM, de Voogt WG, Wilde AA, et al: Evolution of cardiac abnormalities in Becker muscular dystrophy over a 13-year period. J Neurol 244:657–663, 1997.

16. Melacini P, Fanin M, Danieli GA, et al: Myocardial involvement is very frequent among patients affected with subclinical Becker's muscular dystrophy. Circulation 94:3168–3175, 1996.

17. Saito M, Kawai H, Akaike M, et al: Cardiac dysfunction with Becker muscular dystrophy. Am Heart J 132:642–647, 1996.

18. Bakker E, Van Ommen GB: Duchenne and Becker muscular dystrophy. In Emery AE (ed): Neuromuscular Disorders: Clinical and Molecular Genetics. Chichester, John Wiley & Sons, 1998, p 61.

19. Yanagisawa A, Miyagawa M, Yotsukura M, et al: The prevalence and prognostic significance of arrhythmias in Duchenne type muscular dystrophy. Am Heart J 124:1244–1250, 1992.

20. Miller G, D'Orsogna L, O'Shea JP: Autonomic function and the sinus tachycardia of Duchenne muscular dystrophy. Brain Dev 11:247–250, 1989.

21. Perloff JK: Cardiac rhythm and conduction in Duchenne's muscular dystrophy: A prospective study of 20 patients. J Am Coll Cardiol 3:1263–1268, 1984.

22. Sanyal SK, Johnson WW: Cardiac conduction abnormalities in children with Duchenne's progressive muscular dystrophy: Electrocardiographic features and morphologic correlates. Circulation 66:853–863, 1982.

23. Chenard AA, Becane HM, Tertrain F, et al: Ventricular arrhythmia in Duchenne muscular dystrophy: Prevalence, significance and prognosis. Neuromuscul Disord 3:201–206, 1993.

24. Nigro G, Comi LI, Politano L, et al: Evaluation of the cardiomyopathy in Becker muscular dystrophy. Muscle Nerve 18:283–291, 1995.

25. Quinlivan R, Ball J, Dunckley M, et al: Becker muscular dystrophy presenting with complete heart block in the sixth decade. J Neurol 242:398–400, 1995.

26. Negri SM, Cowan MD: Becker muscular dystrophy with bundle branch reentry ventricular tachycardia. J Cardiovasc Electrophysiol 9:652–654, 1998.

27. Politano L, Nigro V, Nigro G, et al: Development of cardiomyopathy in female carriers of Duchenne and Becker muscular dystrophies. JAMA 275:1335–1338, 1996.

28. Hoogerwaard EM, Bakker E, Ippel PF, et al: Signs and symptoms of Duchenne muscular dystrophy and Becker muscular dystrophy among carriers in The Netherlands: A cohort study. Lancet 353:2116–2119, 1999.

28a. Ogata H, Nakagawa H, Hamabe K, et al: A female carrier of Duchenne muscular dystrophy complicated with cardiomyopathy. Intern Med 39:34–38, 2000.

29. Zalman F, Perloff JK, Durant NN, et al: Acute respiratory failure following intravenous verapamil in Duchenne's muscular dystrophy. Am Heart J 105:510–511, 1983.

30. Munoz J, Sanjuan R, Morell JS, et al: Ventricular tachycardia in Duchenne's muscular dystrophy. Int J Cardiol 54:259–262, 1996.

31. Case records of the Massachusetts General Hospital: Weekly clinicopathological exercises: Case 22-1998: A 22-year-old man with a cardiac transplant and creatine kinase elevation. N Engl J Med 339:182–190, 1998.

MYOTONIC MUSCULAR DYSTROPHY

32. Harper PS: Myotonic Dystrophy. London, WB Saunders, 1989.

33. Buxton J, Shelbourne P, Davies J, et al: Detection of an unstable fragment of DNA specific to individuals with myotonic dystrophy. Nature 355:547–548, 1992.

34. Harley HG, Brook JD, Rundle SA, et al: Unstable DNA sequence in myotonic dystrophy. Lancet 339:1125–1128, 1992.

35. Aslanidis C, Jansen G, Amemiya C, et al: Cloning of the essential myotonic dystrophy region and mapping of the putative defect. Nature 355:548–551, 1992.

36. Mahadevan M, Tsilfidis C, Sabourin L, et al: Myotonic dystrophy mutation: An unstable CTG repeat in the 3′ untranslated region of the gene. Science 255:1253–1255, 1992.

37. Redman JB, Fenwick RG Jr, Fu YH, et al: Relationship between parental trinucleotide GCT repeat length and severity of myotonic dystrophy in offspring. JAMA 269:1960–1965, 1993.

38. Tsilfidis C, MacKenzie AE, Mettler G, et al: Correlation between CTG trinucleotide repeat length and frequency of severe congenital myotonic dystrophy. Nat Genet 1:192–195, 1992.

39. Melacini P, Villanova C, Menegazzo E, et al: Correlation between cardiac involvement and CTG trinucleotide repeat length in myotonic dystrophy. J Am Coll Cardiol 25:239–245, 1995.

40. Tokgozoglu LS, Ashizawa T, Pacifico A, et al: Cardiac involvement in a large kindred with myotonic dystrophy: Quantitative assessment and relation to size of CTG repeat expansion. JAMA 274:813–819, 1995.

41. Hayashi Y, Ikeda U, Kojo T, et al: Cardiac abnormalities and cytosine-thymine-guanine trinucleotide repeats in myotonic dystrophy. Am Heart J 134:292–297, 1997.

42. Lazarus A, Varin J, Ounnoughene Z, et al: Relationships among electrophysiological findings and clinical status, heart function, and extent of DNA mutation in myotonic dystrophy. Circulation 99:1041–1046, 1999.

43. Behrens MI, Jalil P, Serani A, et al: Possible role of apamin-sensitive K+ channels in myotonic dystrophy. Muscle Nerve 17:1264–1270, 1994.

44. Timchenko L, Nastainczyk W, Schneider T, et al: Full-length myotonin protein kinase (72 kDa) displays serine kinase activity. Proc Natl Acad Sci U S A 92:5366-5370, 1995.

45. Reddy S, Smith DB, Rich MM, et al: Mice lacking the myotonic dystrophy protein kinase develop a late onset progressive myopathy. Nat Genet 13:325–335, 1996.

46. Jansen G, Groenen PJ, Bachner D, et al: Abnormal myotonic dystrophy protein kinase levels produce only mild myopathy in mice. Nat Genet 13:316–324, 1996.

47. Berul CI, Maguire CT, Aronovitz MJ, et al: DMPK dosage alterations result in atrioventricular conduction abnormalities in a mouse myotonic dystrophy model. J Clin Invest 103:R1–R7, 1999.

48. Brink PA, Ferreira A, Moolman JC, et al: Gene for progressive familial heart block type I maps to chromosome 19q13. Circulation 91:1633–1640, 1995.

49. Annane D, Duboc D, Mazoyer B, et al: Correlation between decreased myocardial glucose phosphorylation and the DNA mutation size in myotonic dystrophy. Circulation 90:2629–2634, 1994.

50. Annane D, Merlet P, Radvanyi H, et al: Blunted coronary reserve in myotonic dystrophy: An early and gene-related phenomenon. Circulation 94:973–977, 1996.

51. Ashizawa T, Dunne CJ, Dubel JR, et al: Anticipation in myotonic dystrophy: I. Statistical verification based on clinical and haplotype findings. Neurology 42:1871–1877, 1992.

52. Motta J, Guilleminault C, Billingham M, et al: Cardiac abnormalities in myotonic dystrophy: Electrophysiologic and histopathologic studies. Am J Med 67:467–473, 1979.

53. Nguyen HH, Wolfe JTD, Holmes DR Jr, et al: Pathology of the cardiac conduction system in myotonic dystrophy: A study of 12 cases. J Am Coll Cardiol 11:662–671, 1988.

54. Child JS, Perloff JK: Myocardial myotonia in myotonic muscular dystrophy. Am Heart J 129:982–990, 1995.

55. Hiromasa S, Ikeda T, Kubota K, et al: Myotonic dystrophy: Ambulatory electrocardiogram, electrophysiologic study, and echocardiographic evaluation. Am Heart J 113:1482–1488, 1987.

56. Phillips MF, Harper PS: Cardiac disease in myotonic dystrophy. Cardiovasc Res 33:13–22, 1997.

57. Fragola PV, Calo L, Antonini G, et al: Signal-averaged electrocardiography in myotonic dystrophy. Int J Cardiol 50:61–68, 1995.

57a. Babuty D, Fauchier L, Tena-Carbi D, et al: Significance of late ventricular potentials in myotonic dystrophy. Am J Cardiol 84:1099–1101, 1999.

58. Moorman JR, Coleman RE, Packer DL, et al: Cardiac involvement in myotonic muscular dystrophy. Medicine (Baltimore) 64:371–387, 1985.

59. Olofsson BO, Forsberg H, Andersson S, et al: Electrocardiographic findings in myotonic dystrophy. Br Heart J 59:47–52, 1988.

60. Florek RC, Triffon DW, Mann DE, et al: Electrocardiographic abnormalities in patients with myotonic dystrophy. West J Med 153:24–27, 1990.

61. Hawley RJ, Milner MR, Gottdiener JS, et al: Myotonic heart disease: A clinical follow-up. Neurology 41:259–262, 1991.

62. Berger RD, Orias D, Kasper EK, et al: Catheter ablation of coexistent bundle branch and interfascicular reentrant ventricular tachycardias. J Cardiovasc Electrophysiol 7:341–347, 1996.

63. Cohen MB, Snow JS, Merkatz KA, et al: Suppression of ventricular tachycardia by sotalol in myotonic dystrophy. Am Heart J 132:446–449, 1996.

64. Tamura K, Tsuji H, Matsui Y, et al: Sustained ventricular tachycardias associated with myotonic dystrophy. Clin Cardiol 19:674–677, 1996.

65. Merino JL, Carmona JR, Fernandez-Lozano I, et al: Mechanisms of sustained ventricular tachycardia in myotonic dystrophy: Implications for catheter ablation. Circulation 98:541–546, 1998.

66. de Die-Smulders CE, Howeler CJ, Thijs C, et al: Age and causes of death in adult-onset myotonic dystrophy. Brain 121:1557–1563, 1998.

67. Mathieu J, Allard P, Potvin L, et al: A 10-year study of mortality in a cohort of patients with myotonic dystrophy. Neurology 52:1658–1662, 1999.

68. Stollberger C, Finsterer J, Keller H, et al: Progression of cardiac involvement in patients with myotonic dystrophy, Becker's muscular dystro-

phy and mitochondrial myopathy during a 2-year follow-up. Cardiology 90:173–179, 1998.

69. Colleran JA, Hawley RJ, Pinnow EE, et al: Value of the electrocardiogram in determining cardiac events and mortality in myotonic dystrophy. Am J Cardiol 80:1494–1497, 1997.

70. Hawley RJ, Gottdiener JS, Gay JA, et al: Families with myotonic dystrophy with and without cardiac involvement. Arch Intern Med 143:2134–2136, 1983.

EMERY-DREIFUSS MUSCULAR DYSTROPHY

71. Emery AE: X-linked muscular dystrophy with early contractures and cardiomyopathy (Emery-Dreifuss type). Clin Genet 32:360–367, 1987.

72. Emery AE: Emery-Dreifuss syndrome. J Med Genet 26:637–641, 1989.

73. Bione S, Maestrini E, Rivella S, et al: Identification of a novel X-linked gene responsible for Emery-Dreifuss muscular dystrophy. Nat Genet 8:323–327, 1994.

74. Nigro V, Bruni P, Ciccodicola A, et al: SSCP detection of novel mutations in patients with Emery-Dreifuss muscular dystrophy: Definition of a small C-terminal region required for emerin function. Hum Mol Genet 4:2003–2004, 1995.

75. Nagano A, Koga R, Ogawa M, et al: Emerin deficiency at the nuclear membrane in patients with Emery-Dreifuss muscular dystrophy. Nat Genet 12:254–259, 1996.

76. Manilal S, Nguyen TM, Sewry CA, et al: The Emery-Dreifuss muscular dystrophy protein, emerin, is a nuclear membrane protein. Hum Mol Genet 5:801–808, 1996.

77. Bonne G, Di Barletta MR, Varnous S, et al: Mutations in the gene encoding lamin A/C cause autosomal dominant Emery-Dreifuss muscular dystrophy. Nat Genet 21:285–288, 1999.

78. Manilal S, Sewry CA, Man N, et al: Diagnosis of X-linked Emery-Dreifuss muscular dystrophy by protein analysis of leucocytes and skin with monoclonal antibodies. Neuromuscul Disord 7:63–66, 1997.

79. Mora M, Cartegni L, Di Blasi C, et al: X-linked Emery-Dreifuss muscular dystrophy can be diagnosed from skin biopsy or blood sample. Ann Neurol 42:249–253, 1997.

79a. Zacharias AS, Wagener ME, Warren ST, et al: Emery-Dreifuss muscular dystrophy. Semin Neurol 19:67–79, 1999.

80. Merlini L, Granata C, Dominici P, et al: Emery-Dreifuss muscular dystrophy: Report of five cases in a family and review of the literature. Muscle Nerve 9:481–485, 1986.

81. Rakovec P, Zidar J, Sinkovec M, et al: Cardiac involvement in Emery-Dreifuss muscular dystrophy: Role of a diagnostic pacemaker. Pacing Clin Electrophysiol 18:1721–1724, 1995.

82. Fishbein MC, Siegel RJ, Thompson CE, et al: Sudden death of a carrier of X-linked Emery-Dreifuss muscular dystrophy. Ann Intern Med 119:900–905, 1993.

83. Cartegni L, di Barletta MR, Barresi R, et al: Heart-specific localization of emerin: New insights into Emery-Dreifuss muscular dystrophy. Hum Mol Genet 6:2257–2264, 1997.

84. Manilal S, Sewry CA, Pereboev A, et al: Distribution of emerin and lamins in the heart and implications for Emery-Dreifuss muscular dystrophy. Hum Mol Genet 8:353–359, 1999.

85. Bialer MG, McDaniel NL, Kelly TE: Progression of cardiac disease in Emery-Dreifuss muscular dystrophy. Clin Cardiol 14:411–416, 1991.

86. Yoshioka M, Saida K, Itagaki Y, et al: Follow up study of cardiac involvement in Emery-Dreifuss muscular dystrophy. Arch Dis Child 64:713–715, 1989.

87. Jensen V: The anaesthetic management of a patient with Emery-Dreifuss muscular dystrophy. Can J Anaesth 43:968–971, 1996.

LIMB GIRDLE MUSCULAR DYSTROPHY

88. Panegyres PK, Mastaglia FL, Kakulas BA: Limb girdle syndromes: Clinical, morphological and electrophysiological studies. J Neurol Sci 95:201–218, 1990.

89. Beckmann JS, Fardeau M: Limb-girdle muscular dystrophies. In Emery AE (ed): Neuromuscular Disorders: Clinical and Molecular Genetics. Chichester, John Wiley & Sons, 1998, p 127.

90. Piccolo F, Roberds SL, Jeanpierre M, et al: Primary adhalinopathy: A common cause of autosomal recessive muscular dystrophy of variable severity. Nat Genet 10:243–245, 1995.

91. Fadic R, Sunada Y, Waclawik AJ, et al: Brief report: Deficiency of a dystrophin-associated glycoprotein (adhalin) in a patient with muscular dystrophy and cardiomyopathy. N Engl J Med 334:362–366, 1996.

92. van der Kooi AJ, de Voogt WG, Barth PG, et al: The heart in limb girdle muscular dystrophy. Heart 79:73–77, 1998.

93. Stubgen JP: Limb girdle muscular dystrophy: A non-invasive cardiac evaluation. Cardiology 83:324–330, 1993.

94. van der Kooi AJ, van Meegen M, Ledderhof TM, et al: Genetic localization of a newly recognized autosomal dominant limb-girdle muscular dystrophy with cardiac involvement (LGMD1B) to chromosome 1q11-21. Am J Hum Genet 60:891–895, 1997.

95. Fang W, Huang CC, Chu NS, et al: Childhood-onset autosomal-dominant limb-girdle muscular dystrophy with cardiac conduction block. Muscle Nerve 20:286–292, 1997.

96. Ng W, Lau CP: Cardiac arrhythmias as presenting symptoms in patients with limb-girdle muscular dystrophy. Int J Cardiol 59:157–160, 1997.

FACIOSCAPULOHUMERAL MUSCULAR DYSTROPHY

97. Wijmenga C, Sandkuijl LA, Moerer P, et al: Genetic linkage map of facioscapulohumeral muscular dystrophy and five polymorphic loci on chromosome 4q35-qter. Am J Hum Genet 51:411–415, 1992.

98. Gilbert JR, Stajich JM, Wall S, et al: Evidence for heterogeneity in facioscapulohumeral muscular dystrophy (FSHD). Am J Hum Genet 53:401–408, 1993.

99. Fisher J, Upadhyaya M: Molecular genetics of facioscapulohumeral muscular dystrophy (FSHD). Neuromuscul Disord 7:55–62, 1997.

100. A prospective, quantitative study of the natural history of facioscapulohumeral muscular dystrophy (FSHD): Implications for therapeutic trials. The FSH-DY Group. Neurology 48:38–46, 1997.

101. de Visser M, de Voogt WG, la Riviere GV: The heart in Becker muscular dystrophy, facioscapulohumeral dystrophy, and Bethlem myopathy. Muscle Nerve 15:591–596, 1992.

102. Stevenson WG, Perloff JK, Weiss JN, et al: Facioscapulohumeral muscular dystrophy: Evidence for selective, genetic electrophysiologic cardiac involvement. J Am Coll Cardiol 15:292–299, 1990.

103. Laforet P, de Toma C, Eymard B, et al: Cardiac involvement in genetically confirmed facioscapulohumeral muscular dystrophy. Neurology 51:1454–1456, 1998.

FRIEDREICH ATAXIA

104. Chamberlain S, Shaw J, Rowland A, et al: Mapping of mutation causing Friedreich's ataxia to human chromosome 9. Nature 334:248–250, 1988.

105. Campuzano V, Montermini L, Molto MD, et al: Friedreich's ataxia: Autosomal recessive disease caused by an intronic GAA triplet repeat expansion. Science 271:1423–1427, 1996.

106. Babcock M, de Silva D, Oaks R, et al: Regulation of mitochondrial iron accumulation by Yfh1p, a putative homolog of frataxin. Science 276:1709–1712, 1997.

107. Wilson RB, Roof DM: Respiratory deficiency due to loss of mitochondrial DNA in yeast lacking the frataxin homologue. Nat Genet 16:352–357, 1997.

108. Branda SS, Yang ZY, Chew A, et al: Mitochondrial intermediate peptidase and the yeast frataxin homolog together maintain mitochondrial iron homeostasis in Saccharomyces cerevisiae. Hum Mol Genet 8:1099–1110, 1999.

109. Wong A, Yang J, Cavadini P, et al: The Friedreich's ataxia mutation confers cellular sensitivity to oxidant stress which is rescued by chelators of iron and calcium and inhibitors of apoptosis. Hum Mol Genet 8:425–430, 1999.

110. Durr A, Cossee M, Agid Y, et al: Clinical and genetic abnormalities in patients with Friedreich's ataxia. N Engl J Med 335:1169–1175, 1996.

111. Filla A, De Michele G, Cavalcanti F, et al: The relationship between trinucleotide (GAA) repeat length and clinical features in Friedreich ataxia. Am J Hum Genet 59:554–560, 1996.

112. Isnard R, Kalotka H, Durr A, et al: Correlation between left ventricular hypertrophy and GAA trinucleotide repeat length in Friedreich's ataxia. Circulation 95:2247–2249, 1997.

113. Casazza F, Morpurgo M: The varying evolution of Friedreich's ataxia cardiomyopathy. Am J Cardiol 77:895–898, 1996.

114. Maione S, Giunta A, Filla A, et al: May age onset be relevant in the occurrence of left ventricular hypertrophy in Friedreich's ataxia? Clin Cardiol 20:141–145, 1997.

114a. Dutka DP, Donnelly JE, Nihoyannopoulos P, et al: Marked variation in the cardiomyopathy associated with Friedreich's ataxia. Heart 81:141–147, 1999.

115. James TN, Cobbs BW, Coghlan HC, et al: Coronary disease, cardioneuropathy, and conduction system abnormalities in the cardiomyopathy of Friedreich's ataxia. Br Heart J 57:446–457, 1987.

116. Zimmermann M, Gabathuler J, Adamec R, et al: Unusual manifestations of heart involvement in Friedreich's ataxia. Am Heart J 111:184–187, 1986.

117. Unverferth DV, Schmidt WR, Baker PB, et al: Morphologic and functional characteristics of the heart in Friedreich's ataxia. Am J Med 82:5–10, 1987.

PERIODIC PARALYSIS

118. Bulman DE: Phenotype variation and newcomers in ion channel disorders. Hum Mol Genet 6:1679–1685, 1997.

119. Fontaine B, Vale-Santos J, Jurkat-Rott K, et al: Mapping of the hypokalaemic periodic paralysis (HypoPP) locus to chromosome 1q31-32 in three European families. Nat Genet 6:267–272, 1994.

120. Ptacek LJ, Tawil R, Griggs RC, et al: Dihydropyridine receptor mutations cause hypokalemic periodic paralysis. Cell 77:863–868, 1994.

121. Ptacek LJ: Channelopathies: Ion channel disorders of muscle as a paradigm for paroxysmal disorders of the nervous system. Neuromuscul Disord 7:250–255, 1997.

122. Cannon SC, Brown RH Jr, Corey DP: A sodium channel defect in hyperkalemic periodic paralysis: Potassium-induced failure of inactivation. Neuron 6:619–626, 1991.

123. Sansone V, Griggs RC, Meola G, et al: Andersen's syndrome: A distinct periodic paralysis. Ann Neurol 42:305–312, 1997.

124. Brown RH Jr: Ion channel mutations in periodic paralysis and related myotonic diseases. Ann NY Acad Sci 707:305–316, 1993.

125. Gould RJ, Steeg CN, Eastwood AB, et al: Potentially fatal cardiac dysrhythmia and hyperkalemic periodic paralysis. Neurology 35:1208–1212, 1985.

MITOCHONDRIAL ENCEPHALOMYOPATHIES

126. Simon DK, Johns DR: Mitochondrial disorders: Clinical and genetic features. Annu Rev Med 50:111–127, 1999.
127. Santorelli FM, Mak SC, Vazquez-Acevedo M, et al: A novel mitochondrial DNA point mutation associated with mitochondrial encephalocardiomyopathy. Biochem Biophys Res Commun 216:835–840, 1995.
128. Berenberg RA, Pellock JM, DiMauro S, et al: Lumping or splitting? "Ophthalmoplegia-plus" or Kearns-Sayre syndrome? Ann Neurol 1:37–54, 1977.
129. Anan R, Nakagawa M, Miyata M, et al: Cardiac involvement in mitochondrial diseases: A study on 17 patients with documented mitochondrial DNA defects. Circulation 91:955–961, 1995.
130. Akaike M, Kawai H, Yokoi K, et al: Cardiac dysfunction in patients with chronic progressive external ophthalmoplegia. Clin Cardiol 20:239–243, 1997.
131. Roberts NK, Perloff JK, Kark RA: Cardiac conduction in the Kearns-Sayre syndrome: Report of 2 cases and review of 17 published cases. Am J Cardiol 44:1396–1400, 1979.
132. Nikoskelainen E, Vilkki J, Huoponen K, et al: Recent advances in Leber's hereditary optic neuroretinopathy. Eye 5:291–293, 1991.
133. Ito T, Hattori K, Tanaka M, et al: Mitochondrial cytopathy. Jpn Circ J 54:1214–1220, 1990.
134. Kobayashi M, Morishita H, Sugiyama N, et al: Two cases of NADH-coenzyme Q reductase deficiency: Relationship to MELAS syndrome. J Pediatr 110:223–227, 1987.

SPINAL MUSCULAR ATROPHY

135. Melki J: Spinal muscular atrophy. In Emery AE (ed): Neuromuscular Disorders: Clinical and Molecular Genetics. Chichester, John Wiley & Sons, 1998, pp 421–422.
136. Melki J, Lefebvre S, Burglen L, et al: De novo and inherited deletions of the 5q13 region in spinal muscular atrophies. Science 264:1474–1477, 1994.
137. Lefebvre S, Burglen L, Reboullet S, et al: Identification and characterization of a spinal muscular atrophy-determining gene. Cell 80:155–165, 1995.
138. Lefebvre S, Burlet P, Liu Q, et al: Correlation between severity and SMN protein level in spinal muscular atrophy. Nat Genet 16:265–269, 1997.
139. Munsat TL, Davies KE: International SMA consortium meeting. Neuromuscul Disord 2:423–428, 1992.
140. Burglen L, Spiegel R, Ignatius J, et al: SMN gene deletion in variant of infantile spinal muscular atrophy. Lancet 346:316–317, 1995.
141. Elkohen M, Vaksmann G, Elkohen MR, et al: Cardiac involvement in Kugelberg-Welander disease: A prospective study of 8 cases. Arch Mal Coeur Vaiss 89:611–617, 1996.

GUILLAIN-BARRÉ SYNDROME

142. Lange DJ, Latov N, Trojaborg W: Acquired neuropathies. In Rowland LP (ed): Merritt's Textbook of Neurology. Baltimore, Williams & Wilkins, 1995, pp 657–676.
143. Winer JB, Hughes RA: Identification of patients at risk of arrhythmia in the Guillain-Barré syndrome. Q J Med 68:735–739, 1988.
144. Minahan RE Jr, Bhardwaj A, Traill TA, et al: Stimulus-evoked sinus arrest in severe Guillain-Barré syndrome: A case report. Neurology 47:1239–1242, 1996.

145. Fagius J, Wallin BG: Microneurographic evidence of excessive sympathetic outflow in the Guillain-Barré syndrome. Brain 106:589–600, 1983.

MYASTHENIA GRAVIS

146. Penn AS, Rowland LP: Disorders of the neuromuscular junction. In Rowland LP (ed): Merritt's Textbook of Neurology. Baltimore, Williams & Wilkins, 1995.
147. Hofstad H, Ohm OJ, Mork SJ, et al: Heart disease in myasthenia gravis. Acta Neurol Scand 70:176–184, 1984.
148. Mygland A, Aarli JA, Hofstad H, et al: Heart muscle antibodies in myasthenia gravis. Autoimmunity 10:263–267, 1991.
149. Arsura EL, Brunner NG, Namba T, et al: Adverse cardiovascular effects of anticholinesterase medications. Am J Med Sci 293:18–23, 1987.
150. Genkins G, Kornfeld P, Papatestas AE, et al: Clinical experience in more than 2000 patients with myasthenia gravis. Ann NY Acad Sci 505:500–513, 1987.

ACUTE CEREBROVASCULAR DISEASE

151. Davis TP, Alexander J, Lesch M: Electrocardiographic changes associated with acute cerebrovascular disease: A clinical review. Prog Cardiovasc Dis 36:245–260, 1993.
152. Rudehill A, Olsson GL, Sundqvist K, et al: ECG abnormalities in patients with subarachnoid haemorrhage and intracranial tumours. J Neurol Neurosurg Psychiatry 50:1375–1381, 1987.
153. Zaroff JG, Rordorf GA, Newell JB, et al: Cardiac outcome in patients with subarachnoid hemorrhage and electrocardiographic abnormalities. Neurosurgery 44:34–39; discussion 39–40, 1997.
154. Andreoli A, di Pasquale G, Pinelli G, et al: Subarachnoid hemorrhage: Frequency and severity of cardiac arrhythmias: A survey of 70 cases studied in the acute phase. Stroke 18:558–564, 1987.
155. Chen HI: Hemodynamic mechanisms of neurogenic pulmonary edema. Biol Signals 4:186–192, 1995.
156. Simon RP: Neurogenic pulmonary edema. Neurol Clin 11:309–323, 1993.
157. Asplin BR, White RD: Subarachnoid hemorrhage: Atypical presentation associated with rapidly changing cardiac arrhythmias. Am J Emerg Med 12:370–373, 1994.
158. Marion DW, Segal R, Thompson ME: Subarachnoid hemorrhage and the heart. Neurosurgery 18:101–106, 1986.
159. Grossman MA: Cardiac arrhythmias in acute central nervous system disease: Successful management with stellate ganglion block. Arch Intern Med 136:203–207, 1976.
160. Brouwers PJ, Wijdicks EF, Hasan D, et al: Serial electrocardiographic recording in aneurysmal subarachnoid hemorrhage. Stroke 20:1162–1167, 1989.
160a. Zaroff JG, Rordorf GA, Newell JB, et al: Cardiac outcome in patients with subarachnoid hemorrhage and electrocardiographic abnormalities. Neurosurgery 44:34–39, 1999.
161. Galinanes M, Hearse DJ: Brain death–induced impairment of cardiac contractile performance can be reversed by explantation and may not preclude the use of hearts for transplantation. Circ Res 71:1213–1219, 1992.
162. Bittner HB, Kendall SW, Chen EP, et al: Myocardial performance after graft preservation and subsequent cardiac transplantation from brain-dead donors. Ann Thorac Surg 60:47–54, 1995.
163. Szabo G, Sebening C, Hackert T, et al: Effects of brain death on myocardial function and ischemic tolerance of potential donor hearts. J Heart Lung Transplant 17:921–930, 1998.

Chapter 72

Renal Disorders and Cardiovascular Disease

HARISIOS BOUDOULAS · CARL V. LEIER

The kidneys can be viewed as components of the circulatory system. Within this integrated system, the function, regulation, and adjustments of the heart and vasculature are closely linked to those of the kidneys. Renal dysfunction and failure adversely affect cardiovascular function, frequently leading to a cardiovascular disorder or failure and, consequently, further impairment of renal performance. Cardiovascular disease, dysfunction, and failure, in turn, can disturb renal function, occasionally to the point of evoking acute or chronic renal failure (CRF), which then causes further deterioration of the cardiovascular condition.

Clinicians have for years appreciated the fact that failure of one component of the cardiorenal system (e.g., renal failure) greatly amplifies the difficulty in clinical management of the failure of another component (e.g., heart failure).

The effects of heart failure and cardiogenic shock on renal function are described in Chapters 16 and 35, respectively. This chapter discusses other cardiovascular disorders that commonly affect renal performance and the primary renal conditions responsible for altering cardiovascular structure and function.

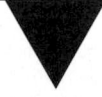

Cardiovascular Conditions That Affect Renal Function

INFECTIVE ENDOCARDITIS
(See also Chap. 47)

In the preantibiotic era, 10 to 15 percent of deaths due to infective endocarditis were attributable to renal failure. Early recognition, precise identification of the infecting organism, and prompt, aggressive antibiotic therapy specifically directed at the offending organism have greatly reduced the renal complications of infective endocarditis, particularly renal failure. Nevertheless, more than 60 percent of patients with documented infective endocarditis have clinical, laboratory, or biopsy evidence of renal involvement.[1-4] The manifestations of endocarditic renal disease range from none to hematuria, pyuria, proteinuria, and occasional renal failure. As many as one-third of patients with infective endocarditis present with serum creatinine values of 2.0 mg/dl or higher.[4]

The deposition of immune complex material in glomeruli represents the most common mechanistic link between infective endocarditis and its renal consequences. Circulating immune complexes and their subsequent deposition in kidneys (and elsewhere) account for the common laboratory finding of reduced serum levels of certain complements (e.g., C3, C4, C1q) in affected individuals. The resultant glomerular lesions are generally proliferative in histological type, with demonstrable immune deposits of IgG, IgM, and C3 along the basement membrane and in the mesangium. The distribution of the glomerular lesions ranges from focal/segmental to diffuse, and their clinical behavior from subclinical to rapidly progressive.

FOCAL/SEGMENTAL PROLIFERATIVE GLOMERULONEPHRITIS. This is the most commonly encountered glomerulopathy in infective endocarditis and represents a wide spectrum of involvement, including focal inflammation of single tufts of glomeruli, sporadic glomerular inflammation and fibrosis, and inflammation and fibrosis of most glomeruli within a renal segment(s) in the midst of normal-appearing kidney.[1-3] The demonstration of immune complex components in the involved glomeruli and the observation that similar glomerular lesions can occur in isolated right-sided heart endocarditis, nonendocarditic infections, and noninfectious inflammatory conditions implicate immunological mechanisms as the cause of the focal/segmental glomerulonephritis of infective endocarditis. The focal/segmental glomerulonephritis can be widespread, such that occasionally it is indistinguishable from diffuse proliferative glomerulonephritis. Although the urine of patients with focal/segmental glomerulonephritis may not be unusual. It customarily shows microscopic hematuria, sterile pyuria, or mild proteinuria.

DIFFUSE PROLIFERATIVE GLOMERULONEPHRITIS. This lesion, viewed by many simply to represent a more severe and extensive form of focal/segmental glomerulonephritis, attacks most glomeruli with a very proliferative cellular process, usually involving the entire glomerulus. The clinical consequences of systemic hypertension, nephritic proteinuria, and CRF are considerably more prevalent with the diffuse forms of proliferative glomerulonephritis. Hematuria, sterile pyuria, proteinuria, and heme or red blood cell casts are common features on urinalysis.

Renal biopsy reveals considerable proliferation and swelling of endothelial, epithelial, and mesangial cells, giving the typically involved glomerulus a packed cellular, even avascular, appearance. Rapidly progressive glomerulonephritis with widespread glomerular crescent formation can occasionally occur in infective endocarditis and is often the explanation for rapid loss of renal function.

MANAGEMENT. Prompt identification and aggressive antibiotic treatment of the infecting organism are the principal means of preventing endocarditic renal disease. Antibiotic therapy has lowered the incidence of diffuse proliferative glomerulonephritis during infective endocarditis from 55 to 80 percent to less than 15 percent.[1-3, 5, 6] Pharmacological control of systemic hypertension and dialysis for renal failure occasionally are necessary supportive measures.

RENAL EMBOLIZATION. Although evidence of renal embolization is found at necropsy in 60 to 70 percent of patients who die of infective endocarditis, less than 25 percent have clinically recognizable renal emboli[1-3, 7] Hematuria is the most common sign of renal emboli. Back or flank pain and renal hemorrhage, rarely fatal, can occur with a large embolus and sizable renal infarction. Larger emboli most often originate from prosthetic valves or from valvular infections caused by *Staphylococcus aureus*, *Neisseria gonococcus*, *Streptococcus pneumoniae*, or fungi. On rare occasions, an infected embolus can evolve into a renal abscess. Currently available imaging methods (e.g., echocardiography) do not yet provide the information needed to reliably identify those at risk for systemic or renal embolization.[8-10]

THROMBOEMBOLIC DISEASE

CAUSES. Table 72-1 presents the major cardiovascular conditions responsible for renal embolization. Because 14 to 20 percent of cardiac output passes through the kidneys and because of their direct proximity to the commonly diseased aorta, the kidneys represent favorite targets for arterial embolization.[11-19] The atherosclerotic aorta is a common source of fibrin, plaque, and cholesterol emboli (see Chap. 40). Suprarenal aneurysms, aortic surgery, intraaortic balloon counterpulsation, cardiac or aortic catheterization, anticoagulation, and thrombolytic therapy increase the risk

▼ **TABLE 72-1. MAJOR CARDIOVASCULAR SOURCES, CAUSES, AND PREDISPOSING FACTORS FOR EMBOLIZATION TO KIDNEYS**

AORTA
Atherosclerotic disease
Extensive atherosclerotic plaque formation; rupture, thrombus and cholesterol embolization
Suprarenal aortic aneurysm
Cardiac and aortic catheterization
Intraaortic balloon counterpulsation therapy
Anticoagulation
Thrombolytic therapy
Aortic surgery

ATRIA
Atrial fibrillation
Atrial enlargement
Cardiomyopathy
Atrial septal aneurysms
Paradoxical embolization
Myxoma (less commonly located in ventricles and on valves)
States of hypercoagulation (e.g., neoplastic diseases; protein C, protein S, or antithrombin III deficiency)

VENTRICLES
Mural thrombus
  Myocardial infarction
  Cardiomyopathy
Cardiac tumors
States of hypercoagulation (see Atria, above)

VALVES
Mitral stenosis (via atrial or valvular thrombus calcification)
Prosthetic valves
Endocarditis
  Infective
  Marantic (noninfective thrombotic)
Mitral annular calcification

of renal embolization from the atherosclerotic aorta. Massive embolization to skeletal muscle can exacerbate or cause renal dysfunction and failure via myoglobinemia-myoglobinuria. The more common cardiac conditions serving as embolic sources are atrial fibrillation, mural thrombi of the left ventricle, mitral stenosis, and prosthetic heart valves (see Table 72-1).

Renal pathology ranges from isolated occlusion of an arteriole with minimal histological change, to segmental infarction ("white infarcts" and scarring), to complete occlusion of a renal artery with unilateral loss of renal function and mass. Cholesterol clefts and calcified debris are histological features of atherosclerotic emboli. Capsular rupture and retroperitoneal hemorrhage can complicate a large infarction.

Similar to embolization elsewhere, the majority are not likely to be detected clinically. Clinical manifestations include various degrees of hematuria, proteinuria, back or flank pain, systemic hypertension (secondary to elevated plasma renin), and renal dysfunction. Extensive embolization to both kidneys or a large embolus of a sole functioning kidney can result in anuria. Eosinophilia, depressed serum levels of C3 and C4, and rarely, lipid droplets floating in a urine sample can be noted with cholesterol emboli. The renal manifestations of atherosclerotic or cholesterol emboli are commonly part of an embolic multisystem "polyarteritis" presentation. Clinical suspicion of renal emboli is raised in patients with an obvious predisposition (e.g., prosthetic heart valve, atherosclerotic aorta, aortic surgery, recent cardiovascular catheterization). Perfusion defects secondary to large emboli are detectable with renal radionuclide scanning. Renal arteriography generally shows a cutoff sign at the point of occlusion, with few vascular markings distal to the occlusion. The rim sign (subcapsular contrast overlying regions of noncontrast) may be seen with extensive or large embolization.

MANAGEMENT. This is generally directed at correcting the source of embolization with supportive therapy for accompanying systemic hypertension or renal failure. For large renal emboli, local thrombolytic therapy, angioplasty, retrieval via catheter, and surgical embolectomy are the principal interventional options.[18, 19] The approach to atherosclerotic-cholesterol emboli is somewhat limited; an obvious source (e.g., suprarenal atherosclerotic aortic disease or aneurysm) should be considered for resection, with the understanding that the aorta is usually diffusely involved with atherosclerosis and that further embolization may occur during and after surgery. Options to be considered in long-term medical management include lipid-lowering agents (particularly the statins), anticoagulation, and perhaps antiplatelet agents, although the effectiveness of these therapeutic modalities remains to be proved in this setting.[14, 17]

Other Cardiovascular Conditions

Aortic Aneurysm and Dissection (See also Chap. 40)
Atherosclerotic aneurysms can threaten renal function in a number of ways, including thromboembolism from a suprarenal location (see Thromboembolic disease, earlier), reduction of renal blood flow by local involvement or encroachment, rupture with hypovolemic shock, aortorenal vein fistula, ureteral obstruction, and the consequences of its surgical repair.[11, 20-22] Ten to 20 percent of atherosclerotic aortic aneurysms are complicated by renal artery stenosis. Clinical suspicion of renal involvement by an atherosclerotic aneurysm is prompted by recent onset or acceleration of systemic hypertension, location near the renal arteries, hematuria, proteinuria, occasional eosinophilia (in cases of atheroemboli), and renal dysfunction and failure. Aneurysmectomy with renal revascularization (when renal arteries are involved) is generally the treatment of choice.

Renal involvement by aortic dissection takes the form of renal artery occlusion or renal dysfunction secondary to compromised hemodynamics from hemorrhagic-hypovolemic shock, cardiac tamponade, or acute heart failure caused by acute aortic valvular insufficiency or acute myocardial infarction.[23, 24] Partial or total renal artery occlusion can occur via an ostial flap or displacement of the intima-media into the lumen as the dissecting hematoma moves into the renal artery. Renal manifestations can include proteinuria, hematuria, systemic hypertension (high plasma renin), renal infarction, azotemia, and renal failure. Anuria should bring bilateral renal artery occlusion (unilateral for a sole functioning kidney) into consideration. Operative correction of the dissection with renal revascularization remains the intervention of choice in most instances.[25, 26]

Congenital Heart Disease

CYANOTIC CONGENITAL DISEASE. The clinical course of cyanotic congenital heart disease is often accompanied by the development of renal dysfunction.[27–29] Although the mechanism for the renal dysfunction is not known, its severity appears to be related to the level and duration of arterial desaturation, the degree of polycythemia, age, severity of right-sided heart failure, and elevation of systemic venous pressure. Histologically, the glomeruli enlarge ("glomerulomegaly") with mesangial hypercellularity, capillary congestion, focal glomerulosclerosis, and localized thickening of the basement membrane. Functionally, the disorder behaves as a glomerulopathy, with proteinuria occurring in 30 percent and microscopic hematuria in 15 to 20 percent of patients.[27, 29] Five to 10 percent develop considerable proteinuria and occasionally the nephrotic syndrome, usually after the

age of 21 years.[27, 28] Tubular dysfunction can occur. Because of increased uric acid production during polycythemia and the tubular dysfunction, hyperuricemia is a common metabolic complication of cyanotic heart disease. A reduction in renal blood flow, glomerular filtration rate (GFR) and urea clearance also occurs over time. Most of the glomerular lesions, renal dysfunction, and urinary findings are reversible and usually return toward normal after successful surgical correction of the cardiac defect and subsequent improvement in hemodynamics, oxygen delivery, and hematocrit.

COARCTATION OF THE AORTA. This malformation has a significant impact on renal physiology and function.[30–33] The lower renal perfusion pressure (distal to the coarctation) evokes sustained release of renin, which contributes to the characteristic hypertension present in the vascular system located above the coarctation. Depending somewhat on the age of the patient and duration of the condition, surgical or angioplasty correction usually does not immediately lower systemic blood pressure (in fact, it may initially increase), and systemic hypertension can persist long term after correction in up to one-third of the patients.[30, 32, 33] Congestive heart failure (CHF), infective endocarditis, and aortic dissection are other complications of coarctation, which, in addition to postrepair systemic hypertension, can adversely affect renal function. Fibromuscular dysplasia and developmental hypoplasia of the renal arteries have been reported in association with coarctation or hypoplasia of the abdominal aorta.[34, 35]

Effects of Renal Failure on the Cardiovascular System

CARDIAC FAILURE CAUSED BY RENAL FAILURE

Left ventricular (LV) dysfunction and CHF are common complications of CRF.[1, 36–44a] Factors that contribute to myocardial damage and dysfunction in patients with this condition are depicted in Figure 72–1. Because it is usually difficult to attribute a predominant causative role to any one of these factors or events, the term *uremic cardiomyopathy* is often used to identify the cardiac disorder resulting from the integration of the various disruptive factors of CRF.

Factors Contributing to the Development of Congestive Heart Failure

The conditions contributing to the development of CHF in patients with CRF are presented in Figure 72–2.

VOLUME OVERLOAD. Loss of renal function allows salt and fluid retention and the development of volume overload. Other factors that contribute to volume overload are chronic anemia and the arteriovenous (AV) access fistula. Normochromic, normocytic anemia is common in CRF, with nontreated hematocrit values ranging from 20 to 30 percent and hemoglobin from 7 to 9 gm/dl; the introduction of erythropoietin therapy in CRF has reduced the degree and consequences of anemia. In general, the overall hemodynamic effect of the typical upper-extremity AV access fistula is small; however, the fistula may contribute to the development of CHF in patients with LV dysfunction.

The contribution of volume overload to the development of CHF in CRF is related to the magnitude and time course of volume expansion and to the concomitant status of cardiac function. A sudden rise in plasma volume can increase LV end-diastolic pressure to levels that produce pulmonary edema, even in the presence of normal resting LV systolic function. In contrast, a gradual increase in plasma volume can allow compensatory ventricular dilatation and hypertrophy with less immediate elevations in LV diastolic pressure.

PRESSURE OVERLOAD. Systemic hypertension, a common finding in patients with CRF, contributes considerably to the generation of acute and chronic CHF by placing an excessive afterload burden on the dysfunctional heart. Increased afterload in CRF is also a result of reduced compli-

FIGURE 72–1. Factors contributing to myocardial damage in patients with chronic renal failure. ATPase = adenosine triphosphatase. (Modified from Leier CV, Boudoulas H: Cardiorenal Disorders and Diseases. Armonk, NY, Futura, 1992.)

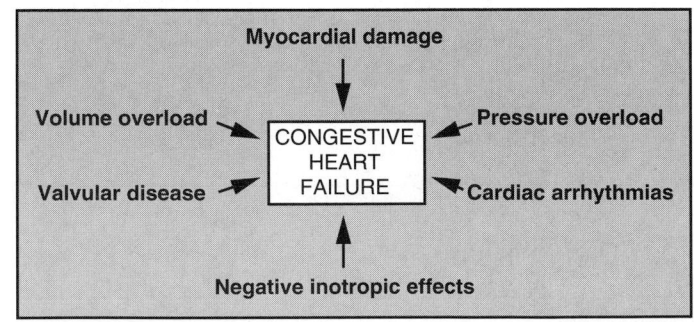

FIGURE 72–2. Factors contributing to the development of congestive heart failure in patients with chronic renal failure. (Modified from Leier CV, Boudoulas H: Cardiorenal Disorders and Diseases. Armonk, NY, Futura, 1992.)

ance of the aorta and large arteries.[45] Renal artery stenosis with secondary or concomitant CRF can cause episodic, marked systemic hypertension and consequently evoke intermittent acute heart failure and pulmonary edema.[46]

NEGATIVE INOTROPIC EFFECTS. Several factors in CRF may decrease myocardial contractility. These include hypoxemia (may occur during hemodialysis), subendocardial ischemia, certain buffers (e.g., acetate) added to the hemodialysis fluid, elevated parathormone levels, various metabolic and electrolyte abnormalities, and "uremic toxins."

EFFECTS OF DIALYSIS AND RENAL TRANSPLANTATION ON THE HEART

DIALYSIS. During dialysis, changes in preload, afterload, arterial PO_2, adrenergic activity, concentrations of electrolytes, ionized calcium, "uremic toxins," and other metabolites and the composition of the dialysis solution affect cardiac-ventricular performance (Fig. 72–3).[1, 28–40b] The baseline status of LV function before the initiation of dialysis therapy is a major determinant of LV performance during dialysis. In general, patients with normal LV function experience little change or a modest decrease in LV performance during dialysis, whereas LV performance in those with baseline systolic dysfunction often improves during the procedure. These observations are due in part to the fact that the preload reduction of dialysis has less effect on LV systolic performance in the dysfunctional (systolic) LV compared with the normal LV, whereas the opposite responses occur during shifts in afterload. Preload reduction during dialysis can adversely affect LV systolic performance and overall hemodynamics in patients with predominant LV diastolic dysfunction.

Changes in preload and afterload during peritoneal dialysis are more gradual and less in magnitude, and thus the effects of peritoneal dialysis on LV performance are not as marked as those of hemodialysis. However, large amounts of intraperitoneal fluid can impair LV systolic performance by reducing venous return and raising afterload.[1, 40]

RENAL TRANSPLANTATION. LV systolic and diastolic volumes and ventricular mass decrease and ejection fraction generally increases over 3 to 4 months after renal transplantation. These changes are likely related to favorable alterations of LV preload and afterload, an increase in hematocrit value, and correction of the various metabolic/endocrinological abnormalities already discussed.[1, 43] Because commonly used immunosuppressive agents (e.g., cyclosporine) can evoke systemic hypertension, blood pressure should be checked regularly and treated appropriately in posttransplant patients.

Management of Heart Failure in Patients with Renal Failure

The clinical presentation and evaluation of CHF in patients with CRF are similar to those of patients without this condition (see Chap. 17). As in patients without CRF, the principles of CHF management in CRF include correcting remedially reversible lesions (e.g., operable occlusive coronary disease), improving contributory conditions (e.g., severe anemia), and optimizing preload, afterload, and cardiac rhythm. Restriction of dietary sodium to 2 gm/day or less is recommended. Angiotensin-converting enzyme inhibitors, digitalis, and vasodilators are often useful in this setting.[1] The duration of dialysis may be lengthened to increase fluid removal or to remove the usual amount of fluid volume more gradually and thus avoid hypotension. Peritoneal dialysis should be considered if problematic hypotension occurs during hemodialysis in patients with both CRF and CHF. Erythropoietin is an effective and safe means of increasing the hematocrit of CRF anemia, and an oversized AV access shunt may have to be modified. Long-term administration of 1α-hydrocholecalciferol may improve LV performance by reducing circulating parathormone and improving cellular calcium, phosphorus, and magnesium metabolism. Renal transplantation usually improves LV performance, hemodynamics, and CHF symptoms. In select patients with end-stage myocardial and kidney disease, combined cardiac and renal transplantation, preferably from the same donor, should be considered.[43, 47]

HYPERTROPHIC CARDIOMYOPATHY
(See also Chap. 48)

For yet undetermined reasons, hypertrophic cardiomyopathy and asymmetrical septal hypertrophy are not uncommon complications of CRF.[1] Patients with CRF with hypertrophic cardiomyopathy also invariably have LV diastolic dysfunction, which, when combined with a LV outflow tract gradient, makes them particularly vulnerable to the occurrence of systemic hypotension during hemodialysis. Special care must be taken to avoid volume depletion during hemodialysis in these patients, with consideration for peritoneal dialysis in those who experience problematic hypotension. If symptoms or complications during dialysis appear to be exacerbated by high adrenergic tone, beta-adrenergic blockade is a reasonable option.

ACCELERATED CORONARY ATHEROSCLEROSIS
(See also Chap. 31)

Atherogenic Factors in Chronic Renal Failure

CHRONIC RENAL FAILURE AND DIALYSIS. Cardiovascular mortality remains high in these patients. This is in large part related to aging of the affected population and to the increased number of diabetic patients undergoing long-term dialysis. Thirty to 35 percent of patients on long-term dialysis management have overt diabetes mellitus. Women with CRF develop coronary artery disease (CAD) as frequently and severely as age-matched men with CRF, perhaps because of earlier menopause and alterations in the pituitary-gonadal axis in these women.[1, 36, 44] For yet unknown rea-

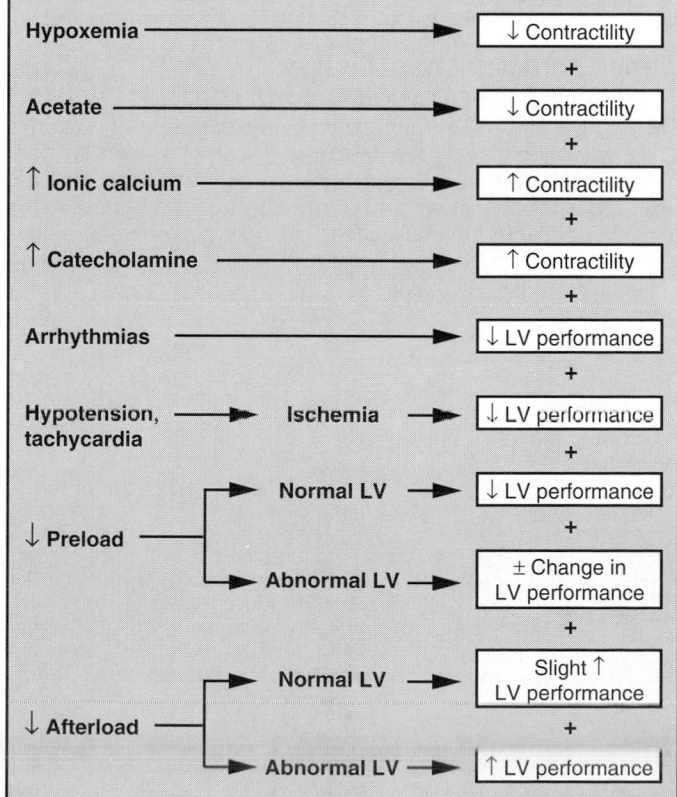

FIGURE 72–3. Effects of multiple factors and events during dialysis on left ventricular (LV) performance. (Modified from Leier CV, Boudoulas H: Cardiorenal Disorders and Diseases. Armonk, NY, Futura, 1992.)

sons, patients with chronic pyelonephritis or interstitial renal disease develop CAD more frequently than patients with other forms of CRF.

The principal atherogenic factors of CRF are shown in Figure 72–4. Carbohydrate and lipid abnormalities, including lipoprotein (a), occur early in chronic renal insufficiency (serum creatine levels >3 mg/dl) and persist as the patient's condition advances into end-stage renal failure and necessitates long-term dialysis. Glucose intolerance and insulin resistance have been demonstrated in a large proportion of patients who have CRF and who are not overtly diabetic, and patients undergoing long-term dialysis develop carbohydrate and lipid disturbances similar to those of diabetes mellitus (insulin resistance, glucose intolerance, increased triglycerides). Although the total cholesterol concentration in serum of patients with CRF on maintenance dialysis can be normal, the level of the high-density lipoproteins is usually depressed. Caucasian men with CRF have lower levels of high-density lipoproteins than African American men so affected, which may account for the higher incidence of CAD in the former group.[1, 48-52] Other abnormalities that likely augment the atherosclerotic process include carnitine deficiency (adversely affects lipoprotein metabolism), secondary hyperparathyroidism, vascular calcification, increased homocystine, various states of hypercoagulation, and enhanced fibrin and platelet deposition.[53-55] Depressed nitric oxide and elevated local and circulating levels of endothelin in patients with CRF may also have a role.[56, 57]

NEPHROTIC SYNDROME. Elevation of serum lipid values is a major feature of the nephrotic syndrome. Total cholesterol and low-density lipoprotein cholesterol concentrations are generally elevated, and high-density lipoprotein cholesterol level is normal or low.[1, 58] These lipid derangements can persist for some time after remission of the nephrotic syndrome, particularly in children. Chronic hypertension and corticosteroid therapy further accelerate atherosclerosis in this subgroup of patients.

RENAL TRANSPLANTATION. Cardiovascular disease contributes heavily to mortality after kidney transplantation. Many patients with CRF have generalized arteriosclerosis-atherosclerosis at the time of transplantation, and thus their pretransplant and posttransplant cardiovascular disease represents a continuum, perpetuated by the persistence, worsening, and accumulation of atherogenic risk factors (e.g., age, hypertension, diabetes, hyperlipidemia, immunosuppressive drugs)[1, 59, 60] (see Fig. 72–4). The number of acute rejection episodes is also linked as an independent risk factor to the development of cardiovascular disease.[1] Significant proteinuria occurs in 10 to 15 percent of transplant recipients and usually indicates various degrees of graft rejection or failure; urinary protein excretion exceeding 0.5 gm daily in posttransplant patients is associated with a significant rise in low-density and very low-density lipoprotein cholesterol and in total triglyceride values. Immunosuppressive therapy with corticosteroids evokes insulin resistance and hyperlipoproteinemia. Cyclosporine increases total cholesterol by elevating the level of low-density lipoprotein cholesterol.[59, 60] Therefore, the cumulative atherogenic risk factors—long-term dialysis, renal transplantation, and periodic graft rejection—account for the high prevalence of morbid cardiovascular disease in renal transplant recipients.

FACTORS AFFECTING MYOCARDIAL OXYGEN SUPPLY AND DEMAND IN CHRONIC RENAL FAILURE

Although the general determinants of myocardial oxygen supply and demand in these patients are similar to those of patients without renal failure, CRF adds several conditions that can evoke myocardial ischemia, even without occlusive CAD. CRF adversely affects coronary perfusion pressure, diastolic perfusion time, and oxygen-carrying capacity of blood (Fig. 72–5). Volume and pressure overload increase ventricular diastolic pressure and thus can decrease coronary perfusion pressure (coronary perfusion pressure during diastole equals coronary artery pressure minus LV diastolic pressure). In the presence of occlusive CAD, coronary artery pressure distal to a high-grade obstruction is not only low but is also not significantly affected by the usual changes in aortic diastolic pressure. Therefore, distal to an obstruction, only changes in LV diastolic pressure can significantly alter coronary perfusion pressure in that region of the heart.[61] An increase in heart rate (as occurs with dialysis, AV shunt, or anemia) reduces myocardial blood flow simply by decreasing diastolic perfusion time.

Because the majority of coronary blood flow occurs in diastole and the duration of diastole (diastolic perfusion time) has a nonlinear inverse relationship with heart rate, even small increases in heart rate can substantially reduce diastolic perfusion time.[62] Anemia, a common feature of CRF, reduces the oxygen-carrying capacity of blood. Hemodialysis with accompanying hypotension, tachycardia, and leftward shift in the arterial hemoglobin-oxygen dissociation curve can be especially threatening to myocardial oxygenation. Coronary blood flow has been shown to decrease in some patients during hemodialysis.[63]

Chronic Coronary Artery Disease

CLINICAL PRESENTATION AND DIAGNOSTIC EVALUATION. CRF modifies the clinical presentation of chronic CAD with a greater prevalence of painless ischemia, partially attributable to a large proportion of patients with CRF with diabetes mellitus, and with chest pain secondary to various nonischemic causes (e.g., uremic pericarditis, neuri-

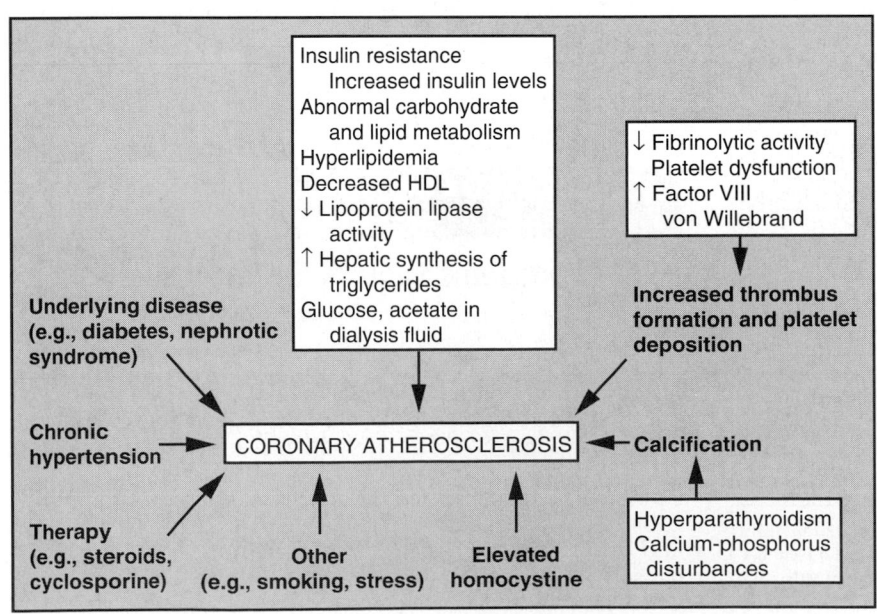

FIGURE 72–4. Factors contributing to the development and acceleration of coronary atherosclerosis in patients with chronic renal failure. HDL = high-density lipoproteins. (Modified from Leier CV, Boudoulas H: Cardiorenal Disorders and Diseases. Armonk, NY, Futura, 1992.)

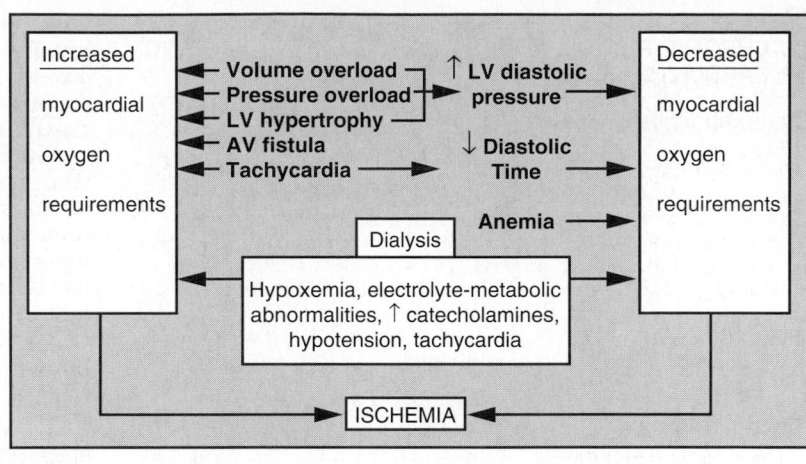

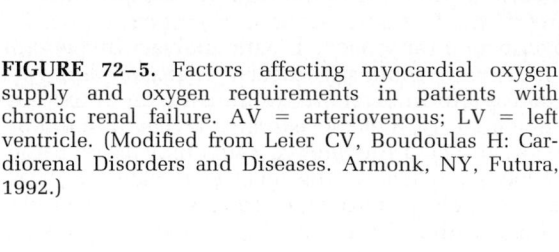
FIGURE 72-5. Factors affecting myocardial oxygen supply and oxygen requirements in patients with chronic renal failure. AV = arteriovenous; LV = left ventricle. (Modified from Leier CV, Boudoulas H: Cardiorenal Disorders and Diseases. Armonk, NY, Futura, 1992.)

tis).[1] Electrocardiographic findings similar to those of myocardial ischemia (e.g., ST segment depression, T wave inversion) are present in many patients with CRF without significant CAD (especially during and after dialysis), thereby limiting the specificity of this diagnostic method. The sensitivity of radionuclide exercise testing for detecting obstructive CAD in CRF is low, perhaps because of generally poor exercise capacity,[1, 64] and data defining the sensitivity and specificity of radionuclide-perfusion imaging after dipyridamole administration are insufficient. Dobutamine-stress echocardiography has been shown to be a promising means of detecting significant CAD in CRF.[36, 65] Coronary arteriography is often required in patients with suspected or problematic CAD to define their coronary artery anatomy and pathology and to develop the most appropriate management plan.

USE OF CONTRAST RADIOGRAPHY. To minimize the renal complications of radiocontrast angiography in patients who have serum creatinine concentrations greater than 2 mg/dl and who are not yet undergoing long-term dialysis, preprocedural hydration and postprocedural volume replacement (saline solution for urine volume) are the most effective interventions.[66, 67] Routine administration of 20 percent mannitol solution is no longer advocated in this clinical setting. The smallest possible amount of radiocontrast agent should be used, because the degree of nephrotoxicity is closely related to the quantity injected. Acute renal failure requiring dialysis is extremely unusual in patients who receive less than 100 ml of contrast agent. Patients with renal artery stenosis are especially susceptible to contrast-induced nephropathy. The osmotic and volume load of radiocontrast material can also provoke acute pulmonary edema in patients with CRF and underlying volume overload or LV dysfunction. Nonionic contrast material evokes less intravascular volume expansion and should generally be used in CRF. To further reduce the amount and risk of administered radiocontrast agent, information about ventricular size and function should be obtained via two-dimensional echocardiography or radionuclide angiography. Avoidance of other nephrotoxic drugs, such as nonsteroidal antiinflammatory agents, is prudent. When renal failure requiring dialysis occurs in the days after the procedure, it is associated with a high in-hospital mortality and poor long-term survival.

MANAGEMENT. The general management approach to CAD in CRF is similar to that for patients without this condition (see Chap. 37), but certain aspects of management are unique to CRF.[1, 68-79] A diet weighted with polyunsaturated fats and a carbohydrate content of approximately 20 percent of total caloric intake is generally recommended. Lipid-lowering agents are usually effective in this clinical setting, and HMG-CoA reductase inhibitors are generally better tolerated in CRF than most other agents. Because of

an increased risk of developing skeletal myopathy and rhabdomyolysis, the HMG-CoA reductase inhibitors must be used with caution in patients receiving cyclosporine. Disturbed calcium-phosphorus metabolism and resultant peripheral and coronary vascular calcification are approached with long-term oral administration of phosphate-binding agents (e.g., calcium carbonate, calcium acetate). For problematic CAD, it is often necessary to administer erythropoietin to keep hemoglobin values at 10 gm/dl or greater. Inadequate hemodialysis is associated with a suboptimal response to erythropoietin therapy. Increasing the intensity of dialysis in patients who have anemia and who are receiving inadequate dialysis results in a significant increase in the hematocrit value.

Oxygen administration at a flow rate of 2 to 3 liters/min may be useful in reducing hypoxemia and ischemic events during hemodialysis. When possible, sodium bicarbonate instead of sodium acetate should be used as the dialysis buffer. This maneuver improves arterial oxygenation, evokes less hypotension, and reduces the tendency of this procedure to precipitate myocardial ischemia. Certain patients with severe CAD and ventricular dysfunction cannot tolerate hemodialysis because of problematic dialysis-induced reduction in cardiac output or blood pressure; some of these patients require cardioactive drug support (e.g., dopamine, dobutamine) during hemodialysis, and others are best treated with peritoneal dialysis.

Percutaneous coronary intervention can be performed in these patients; however, the restenosis rate is rather high. The high rate of angiographic restenosis in patients with end-stage renal disease seems to be related to the size of the vessel dilated and to an increased prothrombotic risk, as indicated by higher fibrinogen concentrations.[69, 72]

Coronary artery bypass graft surgery (CABG) can be performed with increased but acceptable morbidity and mortality in patients undergoing long-term dialysis. Further, mild renal insufficiency, even in the absence of dialysis, increases the risk of blood transfusion, low-output syndrome, and prolongs the length of intensive care unit and postoperative stay. CABG surgery results in considerable improvement in symptoms and functional status in this group of patients; long-term survival, however, is considerably less than in patients without CRF.[68, 71, 74]

PERIOPERATIVE MANAGEMENT

Table 72-2 lists the major recommendations for perioperative treatment of patients who have CRF and are undergoing cardiac surgery. Intravascular volume, serum potassium level, hematocrit value, and drug administration must be carefully monitored during the perioperative period.[1, 68] Preoperatively, daily dialysis (usually of shorter duration) against a low-potassium bath should be considered to control serum and whole-body potassium content. Hemoglobin and hematocrit values should be raised to 10 gm/dl or greater and 30 percent or greater, respectively, with erythropoietin administration or via red blood cell transfusion during dialysis in more urgent situations.[79, 82]

▼ **TABLE 72–2. PERIOPERATIVE MANAGEMENT OF CHRONIC RENAL FAILURE IN PATIENTS UNDERGOING CARDIAC SURGERY**

PREOPERATIVE
Dental evaluation and correction (in valvular disease)
Decrease intake of sodium, potassium, and fluid volume
Short dialysis daily (low potassium bath)
Beta-blockade therapy throughout perioperative period
Antibiotic prophylaxis (start immediately before surgery and continue for 2 d after surgery)
Raise hemoglobin/hematocrit above 10 gm/dl/30 percent

INTRAOPERATIVE
Keep fluid administration to minimum
Do not administer potassium
Special effort to preserve arm vessels and arteriovenous access fistula
Hemodynamic monitoring (during and after surgery) as needed

POSTOPERATIVE
Determine serum potassium levels and arterial blood gases every 4 hr during first 24 hr
Perform dialysis as indicated
Use regional anticoagulation during dialysis over first 5 to 10 postoperative days

Patients should go to surgery at near "dry weight." Intravenously administered fluids are kept to a minimum, with little or no potassium administration. To prevent excessive hemodilution during cardiopulmonary bypass, both blood and lactated Ringer's solution are used to prime the extracorporeal pump. Beta-adrenergic blockade should be continued throughout the perioperative period to avert the myocardial and dysrhythmic complications of the hyperadrenergic state of cardiac surgery. Intraoperative hemofiltration can be used to treat any excessive intravascular volume accumulated during cardiopulmonary bypass.

Postoperatively, dialysis is used to reverse hyperkalemia, significant azotemia, or volume overload. Regional heparinization or citration should be considered during the first 5 to 10 postoperative days as a means of controlling bleeding complications during hemodialysis. The perioperative management used for patients with CRF on regular dialysis also applies to nondialyzed patients with CRF undergoing cardiac surgery; renal function in the latter patients may have to be supported with dialysis over several postoperative days.[71, 73, 74, 77, 78] Patients with a functioning transplanted kidney can be managed in a near-routine (non-CRF) manner, with special attention directed at providing adequate corticosteroid support, avoiding nephrotoxic drugs, and maintaining adequate urine output.

Pericarditis is a common complication of CRF; total pericardiectomy should be considered as a reasonable elective addition to the cardiac surgical procedure in patients with CRF.

Acute Myocardial Ischemic Syndromes

The clinical presentation, diagnostic steps, and therapeutic measures for patients with CRF and acute ischemic syndromes are generally similar to those directed at patients without CRF. Renal artery stent implantation may improve symptoms in patients with significant renal artery stenosis presenting with acute ischemic syndromes, congestive heart failure, or both; these benefits most likely are related to neurohumoral and hemodynamic improvements. Unfortunately, patients with CRF also frequently exhibit abnormal electrocardiographic ST segment and T wave abnormalities and elevated serum cardiac enzyme values in the absence of myocardial ischemia-necrosis. Because of impaired renal clearance, total creatine phosphokinase (CK) and lactate dehydrogenase levels are often elevated. However, the total CK usually comprises brain band CK (CK-BB, increased in about 30 percent of patients with CRF) or skeletal muscle band (CK-MM). Therefore, when myocardial ischemia and infarction is suspected, careful monitoring of the myocardial band (CK-MB) over the ensuing 24 to 48 hours becomes important; new or transient elevation of the CK-MB fraction can usually be regarded as an indication of acute myocardial necrosis. Troponins are more likely to be elevated in dialyzed patients than in other patients with renal

failure who are not on dialysis. The ability of cardiac troponin T and cardiac troponin I to predict risk for subsequent adverse outcomes in patients presenting with suspected acute coronary syndromes is reduced in the presence of renal disease.[36, 75, 79, 83]

Fluid overload is approached with dialysis in patients who have CRF with acute myocardial infarction and who are nonresponsive to intravenous administration of loop diuretics in moderate to high doses. Hemodynamic monitoring with a flow-directed indwelling pulmonary artery catheter is appropriate when a low perfusion state or heart failure develops. Electrolyte and metabolic abnormalities are controlled with dietary measures and dialysis as needed.

CARDIOVASCULAR CALCIFICATION

Dystrophic (metastatic) calcification commonly occurs in patients who have CRF and who are receiving maintenance dialysis; it can involve all tissues, including heart, vasculature, and kidneys. Hyperphosphatemia with elevation of the calcium–phosphorus product, shifts in plasma and tissue pH during and after dialysis, and secondary hyperparathyroidism are regarded as the most important factors responsible for tissue calcification in CRF (Table 72–3).[37, 39, 40, 84] The calcification is exacerbated by excessive intake of milk, use of certain antacids, and calcium extraction from calcium polystyrene materials and surfaces (e.g., certain dialysis units).

The mitral annulus and valve and aortic valve are the cardiac sites predisposed to dystrophic calcification in CRF (see Table 72–3). Consequently, hemodynamically significant valvular stenosis and/or regurgitation, usually manifested clinically as murmurs and occasionally as symptoms and signs of heart failure, are common complications of cardiac calcification in CRF. Myocardial calcification can cause conduction abnormalities (most commonly atrioventricular or bundle branch block), various arrhythmias, ventricular dysfunction, and CHF. Significant annular, valvular, and coronary artery calcification and regions of dense calcification elsewhere in the heart are usually detectable by image-amplified fluoroscopy, echocardiography, or magnetic resonance imaging. Technetium pyrophosphate scintigraphy may demonstrate uptake in areas of myocardial calcification. Pericardial calcification, usually microscopic in degree, contributes to the pathological process of uremic

▼ **TABLE 72–3. METASTATIC CALCIFICATION OF CHRONIC RENAL FAILURE: CONTRIBUTING FACTORS AND COMMON CARDIOVASCULAR SITES OF INVOLVEMENT**

POSSIBLE CONTRIBUTING FACTORS	CARDIOVASCULAR SITES
Hyperphosphatemia	Mitral annulus and valve
Increased ionized calcium	Aortic valve
Increased calcium-phosphorus product	Atrioventricular node-conduction system
Increased parathormone levels	Myocardium
Acute changes in blood pH	Interventricular septum
Increased calcium ingestion	Coronary arteries
Certain antacids	Pericardium
Extraction from calcium-containing polymers and materials	
Vitamin D preparations	

Modified from Leier CV, Boudoulas H: Cardiorenal Disorders and Diseases. Armonk, NY, Futura, 1992.

pericarditis. Dense pericardial calcification is not a feature of CRF and implicates another disease process.

Prevention of cardiovascular calcification is an important component of the management of CRF. Phosphate-binding agents and dietary measures (restriction of phosphate and avoidance of excessive calcium intake) are used for this purpose. Regression of calcification has been achieved by lowering serum phosphorus levels with oral phosphate-binding agents, parathyroidectomy, and renal transplantation; cardiovascular calcification, however, does not appear to be as readily reversible. Management of the CHF, AV block, and cardiac arrhythmias caused by cardiac calcification is directed at controlling symptoms.

HEART MURMURS AND VALVULAR HEART DISEASE

Heart murmurs and acquired valvular abnormalities are common in CRF. Dystrophic calcification (discussed earlier), infectious and noninfectious endocarditis, and certain renal diseases (e.g., polycystic kidney disease) are associated with structural abnormalities of heart valves.[1, 85, 86] However, heart murmurs are frequently noted in CRF without obvious underlying valvular abnormalities and are probably evoked by anemia, the AV access fistula, hyperadrenergic tone, and volume and pressure overload. Early diastolic murmurs of functional aortic or pulmonic regurgitation, generally related to pressure and volume overload, can appear during advanced stages of renal failure and often disappear after hemodialysis. An occasional murmur audible over the anterior aspect of the chest may be transmitted from an AV access fistula located in the upper limb. In patients with forearm shunt access, bruits can be heard in the ipsilateral axillary, clavicular, and cervical regions. Cervical venous hums are also common in these patients. Thus, murmurs in CRF can represent valvular disease, functional pulmonic or aortic valvular flow or regurgitation, transmission from an AV fistula, or a venous hum.

As in other conditions, each murmur requires clinical assessment to define the underlying cause and, if associated with valvular or congenital heart disease, evaluation of the severity of the lesion. A precordial systolic murmur secondary to high flow or transmission from the AV fistula can be easily distinguished from other murmurs by observing the response of the murmur to transient obstruction of the fistula. Functional murmurs secondary to pressure or volume overload decrease considerably with control of hypertension, reduction of fluid overload, correction of anemia, and so forth. Venous hums are usually audible throughout the cardiac cycle; are loudest at the base of the neck, in the upright position and during inspiration; and are abolished by compression of the neck veins or by the Valsalva maneuver.

Laboratory evaluation and overall management of valvular heart disease in patients with CRF is similar to that recommended for patients without CRF (see Chap. 46). Cardiac valve replacement can be done with acceptable operative mortality and reasonably good cardiac rehabilitation in patients undergoing prolonged hemodialysis. Long-term survival for most of these patients is still limited by the clinical course and complications of CRF, but quality of life is generally improved after valve replacement.

Preoperative dental evaluation is mandatory, and dental treatment should be completed several weeks before cardiac surgery. Preparation otherwise is similar to that described for CABG (see Table 72–2). Patients who have CRF and who are undergoing open-heart surgery—especially placement of prosthetic heart valves—are at high risk for infective endocarditis. In the perioperative period, S. aureus, coagulase-negative staphylococci, and diphtheroids are the most common infecting organisms. No single antibiotic agent is effective against all of these organisms, and prolonged use of broad-spectrum antibiotics predisposes patients to superinfection with unusual or resistant organisms. Thus, antibiotic prophylaxis at the time of valvular surgery is primarily directed against staphylococci and should be started immediately before the operative procedure and continued postoperatively for approximately 2 days. The choice of mechanical versus bioprosthetic valve for replacement in CRF remains controversial.[1, 86, 87] When technically feasible, reconstructive valvular repair should be considered for problematic mitral regurgitation.[85, 86]

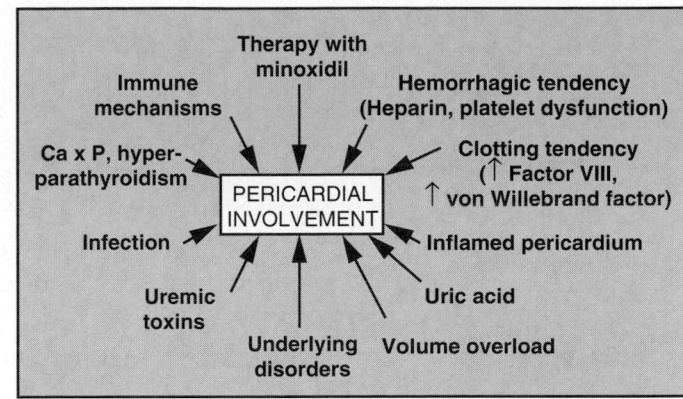

FIGURE 72–6. Factors contributing to the development of pericardial disease in patients with chronic renal failure. Ca = calcium; P = phosphorus. (Modified from Leier CV, Boudoulas H: Cardiorenal Disorders and Diseases. Armonk, NY, Futura, 1992.)

PERICARDIAL DISEASE

Pericardial disease remains a relatively common complication in these patients. The contributory factors are depicted in Figure 72–6, and the evaluation and management of pericardial disorders are presented in Chapter 50 (see also Chap. 72).

SYSTEMIC HYPERTENSION

HYPERTENSION-ASSOCIATED WITH CHRONIC RENAL FAILURE (see also Chap. 28). Systemic hypertension occurs in more than 80 percent of CRF patients before initiation of dialysis. Patients who have CRF and who remain normotensive most often have tubular and interstitial disease or obstructive uropathy as the underlying pathological process. In contrast, arterionephrosclerosis and glomerulopathies are usually associated with hypertension, often marked. The various factors that contribute to the development of systemic hypertension in CRF are presented in Figure 72–7.[88–91, 91a]

HYPERTENSION ASSOCIATED WITH RENAL TRANSPLANTATION. The incidence of systemic hypertension after renal transplantation varies widely (25 to 80 percent) and is highest during the early months after transplantation. The incidence 5 years after transplantation is about 40 to 50 percent. Renal graft failure is increased considerably in the setting of poorly controlled systemic hypertension.[92] Renal artery stenosis (of the transplanted kidney or native kidneys), chronic rejection, native kidney disease, therapy with corticosteroids or cyclosporine, and essential hypertension before transplantation are the leading causes of systemic hypertension in posttransplant patient. Recipients of cadaveric kidneys from donors with a family history of essential hypertension are also more likely to experience posttransplant hypertension. On the other hand, essential hypertension can undergo remission for up to 8 to 10 years after successful transplantation of a kidney from a normotensive donor.

MANAGEMENT. Diagnostic studies should be undertaken in patients with renal failure and hypertension to preclude a reversible renovascular cause (see Chap. 28) and determine the nature of the underlying renal disease. Distinguishing hypertension secondary to renal parenchymal disease from essential hypertension with resultant hypertensive renal disease is often difficult at this stage. The medical history may identify patients who have had long-standing essential hypertension and a familial tendency for

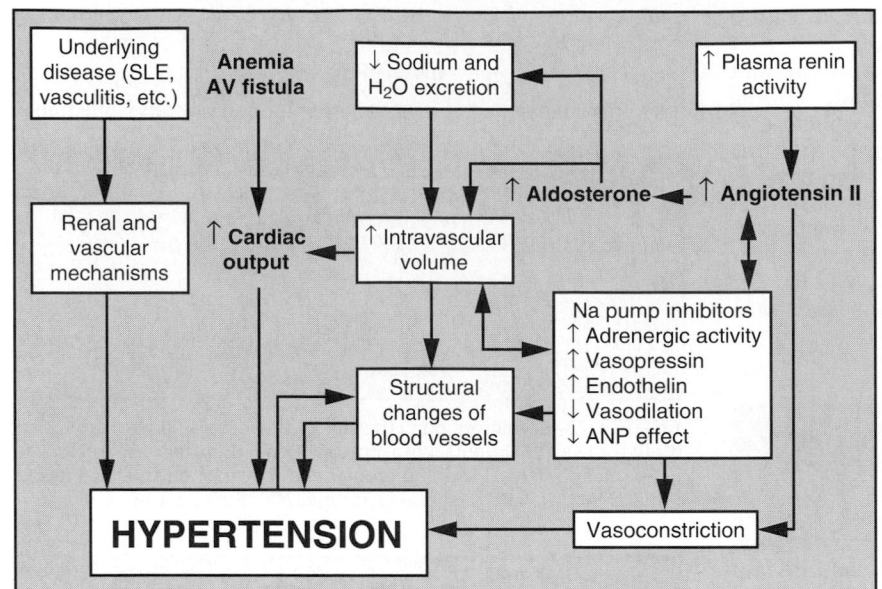

FIGURE 72–7. Pathophysiological mechanisms contributing to the development of systemic hypertension in patients with parenchymal renal disease and failure. ANP = atrial natriuretic peptide; SLE = systemic lupus erythematosus. (Modified from Leier CV, Boudoulas H: Cardiorenal Disorders and Diseases. Armonk, NY, Futura, 1992.)

such, diabetes mellitus, or an episode of glomerulonephritis before developing renal failure.

The treatment of systemic hypertension in patients with active glomerulonephritis and/or CRF is similar to that of essential hypertension (see Chap. 29). However, in patients with CRF, the dosage schedule of drugs cleared by the kidneys has to be modified to match renal function to avoid the deleterious effects of accumulated drug or metabolite. Dialysis should be considered for patients with a substantial reduction of renal function and hypertension refractory to medical management (Fig. 72–8).[1, 93] Early initiation of dialysis decreases the consequences of uremia, allows easier control of hypertension, and reduces the complications of chronic hypertension.

Bilateral nephrectomy is reserved for severely hypertensive CRF patients whose hypertension is refractory to aggressive hemodialysis and optimal drug therapy. The results of nephrectomy are best in patients with markedly elevated plasma renin activity. The major but correctable disadvantages of nephrectomy are a further drop in the hemoglobin and hematocrit values (reduced erythropoietin) and ex-

acerbation of renal osteodystrophy (depressed generation of certain forms of vitamin D). The availability of potent oral antihypertensive agents, such as central sympatholytic drugs (e.g., clonidine), high-dose angiotensin-converting enzyme inhibitors, and minoxidil, has now made bilateral nephrectomy an uncommon procedure in CRF.

The management of systemic hypertension is often complicated by drug therapy needed for the management of the renal disease. This is particularly relevant to posttransplant patients.[1, 94] Corticosteroids adversely affect hypertension control by increasing blood volume and insulin resistance and blunting responsiveness to antihypertensive drugs. Cyclosporine commonly provokes or exacerbates systemic hypertension, occasionally to extremely high levels of blood pressure; calcium channel blocking drugs are usually effective in controlling cyclosporine-induced hypertension. A marked and often refractory increase in systemic blood pressure and occasionally renal interstitial disease can follow administration of nonsteroidal antiinflammatory agents.

Because spontaneous improvement of systemic hypertension in posttransplant patients with obstructing renal artery lesions (usually at the site of vascular anastomosis) is not uncommon, conservative management is generally recommended for transplant recipients who have stable, adequate renal function and whose hypertension is amenable to medications. When stenosis-induced hypertension becomes difficult to control or renal function falls, percutaneous transluminal angioplasty of the arterial lesion becomes a therapeutic option. Surgical intervention may become necessary if angioplasty is not feasible or is unsuccessful. Effective treatment of posttransplant hypertension is very important for the long-term health and survival of both graft and patient.[88, 92]

CARDIAC ARRHYTHMIAS

Cardiac arrhythmias constitute a major clinical problem in CRF because of their increased prevalence and potentially serious complications; their episodic nature also makes identification and characterization difficult. A multicenter study of longstanding hemodialyzed patients showed that ventricular arrhythmias, as assessed by 48-hour ambulatory monitoring, were present in 76 percent of patients[95]; 39 percent had two or more events of two or more sequential ventricular ectopic beats (i.e., couplets or nonsustained ventricular tachycardia) per hour. The frequency of ventricular arrhythmias rose significantly after the second hour of hemodialysis and lasted up to 5 hours following dialysis. The independent risk factors for the presence of ventricular arrhythmias were age over 55 years and LV dysfunction. The frequency of ventricular ectopic beats also appeared to vary directly with resting heart rate. Sixty-nine percent of the patients who had CRF and who were undergoing long-term dialysis had supraventricular arrhythmias, mostly nonsustained. Table 72–4 lists the major factors in CRF

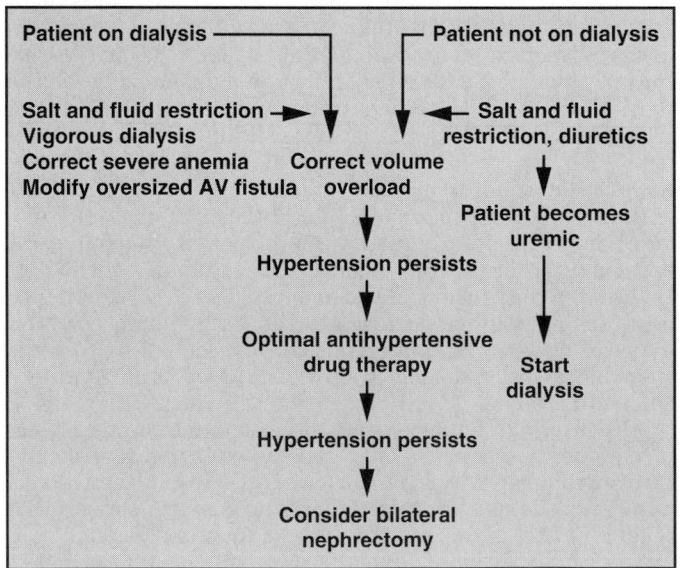

FIGURE 72–8. General management of arterial hypertension caused by renal parenchymal disease. AV = arteriovenous. (Modified from Leier CV, Boudoulas H: Cardiorenal Disorders and Diseases. Armonk, NY, Futura, 1992.)

▼ TABLE 72–4. FACTORS CONTRIBUTING TO DEVELOPMENT OF CARDIAC ARRHYTHMIAS IN PATIENTS WITH CHRONIC RENAL FAILURE

Underlying Cardiac Disease
Myocardial disease (left ventricular hypertrophy, left ventricular dysfunction)
Coronary artery disease—myocardial ischemia
Pericardial disease—myocardial inflammation
Cardiac calcification

Hemodialysis
Rapid changes in serum electrolytes
Rapid changes in blood pH
Hypoxemia

Autonomic Dysfunction

High Calcium-Phosphorus Product

High Parathormone Levels(?)

From Leier CV, Boudoulas H: Cardiovascular Disorders and Diseases. Armonk, NY, Futura, 1992.

likely to contribute to the development of cardiac arrhythmias.[96–98]

MANAGEMENT. As in other patients, the initial approach is directed at treating remediable cardiac disease and at reversing contributory factors (see Table 72–4). Caffeine and other cardiac stimulants should be avoided by patients with CRF and tachyarrhythmias. If arrhythmias are related to hemodialysis, attention should be directed to the potassium concentration of the dialysis bath. A low potassium concentration of the dialysate can lead to hypokalemia and serious rhythm disturbances, particularly in patients who are receiving digitalis or are afflicted with CAD, LV hypertrophy, or LV dysfunction. A dialysate potassium concentration of 3.5 mEq/liter usually abolishes dialysis-related ventricular arrhythmias. If the dialysate potassium concentration exceeds 3.5 mEq/liter, dietary potassium restriction is usually necessary between hemodialysis runs to prevent life-threatening hyperkalemia. Arrhythmias secondary to pericarditis tend to respond to treatment of the inflammatory component, when present. Increased sympathetic activity contributes to cardiac arrhythmias in patients with chronic renal disease. Physical training in patients undergoing hemodialysis augments cardiac vagal activity and may decrease vulnerability to arrhythmia. Angiotensin-converting enzyme inhibition also decreases sympathetic hyperactivity.[96–98]

PREDISPOSITION FOR CARDIOVASCULAR INFECTIONS

Infections are common in patients with end-stage renal disease. Because these patients undergo dialysis 100 to 180 times a year, it is not surprising that infections often involve the AV access site or the abdominal catheter in patients receiving peritoneal dialysis. It is estimated that up to 6 percent of hemodialyzed patients will develop infective endocarditis sometime during the course of their disease; the most common culprit organism is *S. aureus*, followed by *Streptococcus viridans* and enterococci; the aortic valve is the usual target, followed by the mitral valve.[1]

Proper sterile technique during the entire dialysis procedure is mandatory to prevent infectious disease in this very susceptible patient population. Patients should maintain good oral health and personal hygiene to reduce other potential sources for bacteremia and infective endocarditis. Skin flora of dialyzed patients and the dialysis staff should be controlled with bactericidal soap. The staff (via nasal discharge, skin, and other sites) is not an uncommon source for culprit organisms.[99, 100] Patients who are undergoing long-term hemodialysis and who have prosthetic valves and those who have had renal transplantation should receive antibiotics prophylactically.

Recurrent or prolonged bacteremia and septicemia in patients who have CRF and are receiving dialysis implicates persistent infection of the access shunt or catheter or infective endocarditis. Appropriate antibiotic therapy, based on blood culture and antibiotic sensitivity data, should be initiated as soon as possible in these patients. Surgical consultation is indicated when access shunts show abscess or aneurysm formation, thrombosis, or bleeding. Clinical recognition of infective endocarditis in the setting of CRF is often difficult, because many features (e.g., recurrent bacteremia, anemia, and encephalopathy) can occur in patients with end-stage renal failure without infective endocarditis. It is prudent to suspect infective endocarditis in any such patient with fever, leukocytosis, or bacteremia, particularly if associated with an infected access site. The appearance of new murmurs or changes in murmurs increases the likelihood of infective endocarditis. Demonstration of valvular vegetations by echocardiog-

raphy is most informative and can be diagnostic in the presence of other clinical manifestations of infective endocarditis.

AUTONOMIC DYSFUNCTION

Derangements of the autonomic nervous system in CRF most commonly manifested as postural or dialysis-induced hypotension, abnormal hemodynamic responses to Valsalva and other maneuvers, decreased heart rate variability,[96, 97] impairment of perspiration, and alterations in gastric motility, can evoke major symptoms and disability. The cause of autonomic dysfunction in these patients is multifactorial and attributable in some cases to the underlying cause of CRF (e.g., diabetes mellitus, amyloidosis), antihypertensive drugs (e.g., sympatholytic agents), aluminum intoxication from certain antacids, and the uremic syndrome itself.[101–103] Determination of the specific type of autonomic dysfunction can be difficult and may require additional diagnostic testing (e.g., nerve conduction, bladder and sphincter function, tilt studies). Informative yet simple and inexpensive clinical maneuvers include blood pressure and heart rate responses to upright posture or the Valsalva maneuver, heart rate response to normal and deep inspiration, and determination of heart rate variability.[96, 97] In general, specific therapy for the autonomic dysfunction of renal disease is rather limited, and symptomatic therapy is used in most instances.

CARDIOVASCULAR DRUG THERAPY IN PATIENTS WITH RENAL DISEASE

Patients with acute or chronic renal failure are often treated with drugs primarily cleared or metabolized by the kidneys. In comparison with patients with normal renal function, any dose or dosage schedule of such agents in patients with renal failure usually produces higher plasma concentrations for longer duration. In addition, patients with renal failure can react unpredictably and atypically to pharmacological agents; thus, the adverse effects of a drug in this clinical setting are often related to factors other than plasma drug concentration. For example, nausea and vomiting after ingestion of certain agents (e.g., analgesics, potassium elixirs) occur more frequently in patients with CRF because of preexisting chronic inflammation of the gastrointestinal mucosa, and the adverse effects of digitalis and antiarrhythmic agents are exacerbated by abnormalities in serum potassium, magnesium, and calcium levels; hypoxemia; and the hyperadrenergic state of renal disease and dialysis. Side effects of a drug must always be considered when a patient with CRF experiences unexpected or unusual symptoms.

Renal failure often modifies the pharmacokinetics and pharmacodynamics of a drug[1, 93, 104–107a]; many of these variations, however, are not directly linked to the simple reduction in renal function and GFR. The pharmacokinetic pharmacodynamic modifications of CRF are also related to greater variability in drug absorption, protein binding, metabolism, and receptor affinity, sensitivity, and responsiveness. Lower protein binding for many agents is related to hypoproteinemia or hypoalbuminemia, an alteration of the protein molecule, or competition for protein-binding sites by endogenous substances and other types of CRF therapy. Nonesterified fatty acids, increased in CRF and with heparin administration, can displace certain drugs from their binding sites. Anemia with reduced red blood cell binding increases the plasma concentration of certain drugs. Patients with renal failure are commonly treated with several agents; drug-drug interactions can affect gastrointestinal absorption, protein binding, tissue distribution, drug metabolism and clearance, and pharmacodynamic properties.

For drugs cleared by the kidneys, dosing is adjusted for renal function. Three dosing modifications can be used: the dosing interval can be lengthened without altering the dose amount, the dose amount can be lowered without changing the dosing schedule, or a combination of both. The second approach is preferable in most patients because it averts wide swings in plasma drug concentration. Precise adjustment of dosing is usually not necessary for drugs with few

Text continued on page 2295

▶ TABLE 72–5. CARDIOVASCULAR DRUG THERAPY IN RENAL FAILURE

DRUG	THERAPEUTIC RANGE/ml (PLASMA LEVELS)	ELIMINATION AND METABOLISM	HALF-LIFE—hr Normal	HALF-LIFE—hr Renal Failure	PROTEIN BINDING % Normal	PROTEIN BINDING % Renal Failure	ADJUSTMENT FOR RENAL FAILURE	REMOVAL BY DIALYSIS	COMMENTS
CARDIAC GLYCOSIDES									
Digoxin	0.8–2.0 ng	75% renal	45	72–96	25	18	Yes	No	Radioimmunoassay may overestimate serum levels in renal failure
Digitoxin	20–35 ng	95% hepatic	145	Unchanged	90–97	86–97	Decrease dose when creatinine clearance <10 ml/min	No	8% converted to digoxin; protein binding decreases slightly by dialysis
Quabain		40–50% excreted unchanged	21	60–70	40	Unknown	↓ dose	No	
ANTIARRHYTHMIC AGENTS									
Procainamide	4.0–10.0 µg	50% renal 50% hepatic	3–4	11–20	15–20	Unchanged	Yes	Yes, hemodialysis	Some patients require higher plasma concentrations (10–25 µg/ml)
N-Acetylprocainamide	10–20 µg	Renal	6–8	35–70	10	Unchanged	Yes	Yes, hemodialysis	Active metabolite of procainamide
Quinidine	2.0–5.0 µg	85% hepatic 15% renal	6	5–14	80–85	↑	No	Yes, hemodialysis	May increase serum digoxin levels
Disopyramide	0.5–2.0 µg	60% renal 40% hepatic	5–7	10–18	40–90	—	Yes	Yes, hemodialysis	Protein binding concentration dependent
Lidocaine	1.5–5.0 µg	90% hepatic	1.2–2.2	1.3–3	60–66	Unchanged	No	No	Protein binding may be concentration dependent
Tocainide	4–10 µg	40% renal	15	—	10	—	Yes	—	—
Mexiletine	2–7 µg	Hepatic Renal	7–11	↑	57–69	—	Yes	—	—
Phenytoin	10.0–18.0 µg	Hepatic	24	May be shorter	90–95	70–85	No	No	Protein binding in renal failure decreased
Encainide	250 µg	Hepatic (93% population)	2.3	—	60–80	—	No	—	
		Hepatic-renal (7% population)	11.3	—	70–80	—	Yes	—	
a. O-desmethylencainide	30 µg	Hepatic Renal	3.5	—	—	—	Yes	—	
b. 3-Methoxy-O-desemethylencainide	100 ng	Hepatic Renal	6.4	—	—	—	Yes	—	
Flecainide	0.4–0.8 µg	Hepatic Renal (40%)	8–14	↑	50–70	—	Yes	—	
Propafenone	—	Hepatic	2–10	—	85–87	—	—	—	
Moricizine	—	Hepatic	—	—	85	—	Yes	—	
Amiodarone	0.5–3.0 µg	Hepatic	53 days	—	>95	—	—	—	
Brethlium	—	80% renal 20% nonrenal	6.0	13.6	—	—	Yes	—	Avoid when creatinine clearance <10 ml/min
Adenocine	—	<5% excreted unchanged	<10	Unchanged	40	Unknown	No	No	
Cibenzoline	—	50–60% excreted unchanged	7	22	50	Unknown	↓ dose if GFR <10 ml/min	No	
BETA-ADRENERGIC BLOCKERS									
Acebutolol	—	Hepatic	8	22	15–20	—	No	Yes, hemodialysis	Accumulation of active metabolite diacetolol
Alprenolol	—	Hepatic	1–3	2–3	85	—	No	—	

Drug		Elimination	Half-life (normal)	Half-life (renal failure)	Protein binding (%)		Dose adjustment	Dialysis	Comments
Atenolol	—	Renal	6–9	15–35	<5	—	Yes	Yes, hemodialysis	Significant accumulation in renal failure
Metoprolol	—	Hepatic	2.5	4.5	12	—	No	Yes, hemodialysis	Significant accumulation in renal failure
Nadolol	—	Renal	14–24	45	25–30	—	Yes	Yes, hemodialysis	
Oxprenolol	—	Hepatic	2–3	2–3	80	—	No	—	
Pindolol	—	Hepatic	3–4	3–4	40–55	—	No	—	
Propranolol	—	Hepatic	2–4	2–4	90–95	—	No	Yes, hemodialysis	Active metabolites may accumulate
Sotalol	—	Renal (60%)	8	15–50	50	—	Yes	Yes, hemodialysis	
Timolol	—	Hepatic	4–6	4–6	10	—	No	Yes, hemodialysis	
Esmolol	—	Hepatic	.06–2	—	55	—	No	No	For IV use only
Labetolol	—	Mostly hepatic	6–8	—	50	—	—	—	
Carteolol	—	60–70% renal	6	23–30	23–30	—	Yes	No	
Penbutolol	—	Hepatic	5	5	80–98	—	—	—	
Betaxolol	—	Primarily hepatic, renal	14–22	30–40	50	—	Yes	Small amount	
Bisoprolol		50% excreted unchanged	9–13	8–24	30–35	Unknown	↓ dose if GFR <50 ml/min	Unknown	
Bopindolol		<10% excreted unchanged	4–10	Unchanged	Unknown	Unknown	No	No	
Carvedilol		<2% excreted unchanged	5–8	Unchanged	95	Unknown	No	No	
Celiprolol		<10% excreted unchanged	4–5	5	Unknown	Unknown	↓ dose if GFR <10 ml/min	Hemo—unknown CAPD—no	
Dievalol		<5% excreted unchanged	8–12	19–30	75	Unknown	No	No	
Amlodipine		<10% excreted unchanged	30–50	50	>95	Unknown	No	No	
Nisoldipine		<10% excreted unchanged	6.6–7.9	6.8–9.7	99	Unknown	No	No	
CALCIUM CHANNEL BLOCKERS									
Verapamil	—	Hepatic	3	??	90	≈90	No	Yes	
Diltiazem	—	Hepatic	2	?8	83	—	No	—	
Nifedipine	—	Hepatic	4	?5.5	95	—	No	—	
Nicardipine	—	Hepatic	1–1.6	—	89–99	—	No	—	
Nimodipine	—	Hepatic	8–9	—	95; binding concentration dependent	—	No	—	
Bepridil hydrochloride	—	Liver 70%; urine excretion of metabolites	—	—	99	—	—	—	Type 1A antiarrhythmic properties
Isradipine	—	Hepatic	Early 1.5–2 Terminal 8	—	95	—	—	—	
Felodipine	—	Hepatic	11–16	—	>99	—	No	—	
ANTIHYPERTENSIVES									
Methyldopa	—	Mostly renal	5–8	7–16	<15	—	May be necessary when creatinine clearance <50 ml/min	Yes, peritoneal and hemodialysis	Retention of active metabolites in renal failure
Clonidine	—	Renal	6–23	39–42	20–40	—	Yes, when creatinine clearance <10 ml/min	No	Rebound hypertension can occur if drug stopped abruptly
Guanfacine	—	Hepatic, renal	12–24	—	—	—	—	—	Withdrawal syndrome may appear

Table continued on following page

▼ **TABLE 72–5. CARDIOVASCULAR DRUG THERAPY IN RENAL FAILURE** *Continued*

DRUG	THERAPEUTIC RANGE/ml (PLASMA LEVELS)	ELIMINATION AND METABOLISM	HALF-LIFE—hr Normal	HALF-LIFE—hr Renal Failure	PROTEIN BINDING % Normal	PROTEIN BINDING % Renal Failure	ADJUSTMENT FOR RENAL FAILURE	REMOVAL BY DIALYSIS	COMMENTS
Guanabenz	—	Hepatic	4–6	—	—	—	—	—	
Trimethaphan	—	—	—	—	—	—	—	—	Ganglionic blocking drug for IV use with short duration of action
Mecamylamine	—	Renal	—	—	—	—	Contraindicated in uremic patients	—	
Guanethidine	—	Mostly renal, less nonrenal	48–72	96–196	0	—	Yes	—	Orthostatic hypotension common side effect
Reserpine	—	Hepatic, nonrenal	50–170	87–320	40	—	Avoid when creatinine clearance <10 ml/min	No	Long biological half-life
Minoxidil	—	Hepatic	2.8–4.2	—	0	—	No	Yes, hemodialysis	May induce pericardial effusion and pericarditis
Hydralazine	—	Hepatic, nonrenal	2.5–5	7–16	87	—	May be necessary when creatinine clearance <50 ml/min	No	—
Diazoxide	—	Mostly renal	17–31	>30	>90	Decreased	No	Yes, peritoneal dialysis, hemodialysis	May produce sodium and water retention and hyperglycemia; protein binding decrease in renal failure
Guanadril	—	30–40% excreted unchanged	4–10	19	20	No data	↓ dose if GFR <50 ml/min	Unknown	
Ketanserin	—	<2% excreted unchanged	14–19	25–35	95	↓ In uremia	No	No	
Prazosin	—	Mostly hepatic, some renal	2–3	—	97	—	No	No	
Doxazosin	—	Liver	22	—	98	—	—	Yes	
Terazosin	—	10% urine	12	—	90–94	—	—	—	
Nitroglycerin (sublingual)	—	Hepatic	2–4 (min)	2–4 (min)	—	—	No	—	
Isosorbide-2-mononitrate	—	Hepatic	1.5–2.4	—	—	—	Yes	—	
Isosorbide-5-mononitrate	—	Hepatic	4.0–5.0	—	—	—	—	—	
Nitroprusside	—	Nonrenal	<10 min	<10 min	—	—	No	Hemodialysis	Thiocyanate and cyanide may accumulate
CONVERTING ENZYME INHIBITORS									
Captopril	—	Mostly renal, some hepatic	1.9	Prolonged	25–30	—	May be necessary when creatinine clearance <10 ml/min	Yes, hemodialysis	Deterioration of renal function in patients with bilateral renal artery stenosis
Enalapril	—	Mostly renal	11	—	—	—	When creatinine clearance <30 ml/min	—	Deterioration of renal function in patients with bilateral renal artery stenosis
Lisinopril	—	Renal	12	—	—	—	When creatinine clearance <30 ml/min	—	
Enalaprilat	—	Renal	11	—	—	—	When creatinine clearance <30 ml/min	Yes	For IV injection

Benazepril	—	—	10–11	—	96.7	—	—	—	—
Fosinopril sodium	—	50% Urine	12	—	≥95	—	When plasma creatinine >3 mg/dl	—	—
Ramipril	—	60% Urine	13–17	—	—	—	No	—	—
Cilarapril	—	80–90% excreted unchanged	40–50	>50	No data	Unknown	When plasma creatinine >2.5 mg/dl	No	The active moiety is formed in liver
Pentopril	—	80–90% excreted unchanged	2–3	10–40	60	Unknown	↓ Dose	Unknown	—
Perintopril	—	<10% excreted unchanged	5	27	20	Unknown	↓ Dose if GFR <50 ml/min	Hemo—yes CAPD—unknown	—
Quinapril	—	30% excreted unchanged	1–2	6–15	97	Unknown	↓ Dose if GFR <50 ml/min	Hemo—yes CAPD—unknown	—
ANGIOTENSIN RECEPTOR BLOCKERS									
Losartan	—	10–15% excreted unchanged	3–10	4–6	30	Unknown	No	Unknown	—
DIURETICS									
Thiazides	—	Renal	1–2	4–6	70	—	Yes	—	May be ineffective when creatinine clearance <30 ml/min
Metolazone	—	—	—	—	—	—	—	—	Can produce marked diuresis
Furosemide	—	Mostly renal	1	3	95	—	—	Yes, hemodialysis	Large doses necessary in renal failure
Ethacrynic acid	—	Renal, hepatic	3	—	90	—	Yes	Yes, hemodialysis	Large doses necessary in renal failure
Bumetanide	—	Renal, hepatic	1	—	90	—	No	—	Can be effective in patients with renal failure
Acetazolamide	—	Renal	8	Prolonged	80	—	Yes	—	Ineffective when GFR <10 ml/min
Amiloride	—	Renal	7.5	Prolonged	Low	—	Yes	—	May cause hyperkalemia
Triamterene	—	Hepatic, renal	2–12	10	60	Decreased	Yes, avoid when creatinine clearance <30 ml/min	—	Active metabolites have long half-life; may cause hyperkalemia
Spironolactone	—	Hepatic	10–35	98	98	—	Yes, avoid when creatinine clearance <30 ml/min	—	May cause hyperkalemia
Indapamide	—	Mostly renal, some hepatic	14	—	71–79	—	—	—	Oral antihypertensive-diuretic; has little or no diuretic effect in renal failure
Chlorthalidone	—	50% excreted unchanged	44–80	Unknown	76–94	Unknown	Avoid if GFR <10 ml/min	Not applicable	Ineffective with low GFR
Piretanide	—	30–40% excreted unchanged	1.4	1.6–3.4	94	Unknown	No	None	High doses effective in ESRD, ototoxicity
Torasemide	—	25% excreted unchanged	2–4	4–5	97–99	Unknown	No	None	High doses effective in ESRD, ototoxicity

Table continued on following page

▶ TABLE 72–5. CARDIOVASCULAR DRUG THERAPY IN RENAL FAILURE *Continued*

DRUG	THERAPEUTIC RANGE/ml (PLASMA LEVELS)	ELIMINATION AND METABOLISM	HALF-LIFE—hr		PROTEIN BINDING %		ADJUSTMENT FOR RENAL FAILURE	REMOVAL BY DIALYSIS	COMMENTS
			Normal	Renal Failure	Normal	Renal Failure			
ANTICOAGULANTS									
Heparin	—	Nonrenal	0.3–2.0	0.5–3.0	>90	—	No	Yes, hemodialysis and peritoneal dialysis	May potentiate uremic bleeding
Warfarin	—	Hepatic	40	40	99	Decreased	No	—	May decrease protein binding of other drugs; may potentiate uremic bleeding
THROMBOLYTICS									
Streptokinase	—	—	0.38	—	—	—	No	—	May potentiate uremic bleeding
Anistreplase	—	—	1–2	—	—	—	—	—	May potentiate uremic bleeding
Urokinase	—	Hepatic	0.33	—	—	—	—	—	May potentiate uremic bleeding
Tissue plasminogen activators (t-PA)	—	Hepatic	0.05	—	—	—	—	—	May potentiate uremic bleeding
Alteplase	—	Unknown	0.5	Unknown	Unknown	Unknown	No	Unknown	Tissue-type plasminogen activator
LIPID-LOWERING AGENTS									
Cholestyramine	—	Not absorbed	—	—	—	—	No	—	May cause hyperchloremic acidosis
Colestipol	—	Not absorbed	—	—	—	—	No	—	May cause hyperchloremic acidosis
Clofibrate	—	Renal (40–60%), hepatic	17	46–110	96	96	Yes	Hemodialysis	Restricted use because of high profile of adverse effects
Gemfibrozil	—	Renal, fecal	1.5	—	Low	—	Yes	—	Frequent adverse effects in patients with renal failure; aspirin may reduce flushing
Nicotinic acid	—	Hepatic, renal	0.5–1.0	—	—	—	Yes	—	—
Lovastatin	—	Hepatic, renal	—	—	95	—	No	—	—
Fluvastatin	—	<1% excreted unchanged	0.5–1.0	Unknown	98	Unknown	No	Unknown	—
Pravastatin	—	<10% excreted unchanged	0.8–3.2	Unchanged	40–60	Unknown	No	Unknown	—
Simvastatin	—	<0.5% excreted unchanged	2.0	Unknown	>95	Unknown	No	Unknown	—
Probucol	—	Hepatic	—	—	—	—	—	—	—
MISCELLANEOUS									
Dobutamine	—	<10% excreted unchanged	2–3 min	Unknown	Unknown	Unknown	No	Unknown	—
Amrinone	—	10–40% excreted unchanged	2.6–8.3	Unknown	20–40	Unknown	↓ Dose if GFR <10 ml/min	Unknown	Thrombocytopenia; nausea, vomiting in ESRD
Milrinone	—	80–85% excreted unchanged	1–2	1.5–3	Unknown	Unknown	↓ Dose if GFR <10 ml/min	Unknown	—
Midodrine	—	75–80% excreted unchanged	0.5	Unknown	Unknown	Unknown	Unknown	Hemo—yes CAPD—unknown	—

CAPD = continuous ambulatory peritoneal dialysis; ESRD = end-stage renal disease; GFR = glomerular filtration rate.
Modified from Leier CV, Boudoulas H: Cardiovascular Disorders and Diseases. Armonk, NY, Futura, 1992.

adverse effects and a large therapeutic index (safety margin). Pharmacokinetic and dose-adjustment information about the more commonly used cardiovascular drugs in renal disease is presented in Table 72–5.[1, 93] In most instances, the application and monitoring of drug therapy in CRF are based on pharmacodynamic and clinical responses, occasionally supplemented by determination of the drug's plasma concentration (e.g., digitalis) or another laboratory endpoint (e.g., prothrombin time for warfarin).

The therapeutic objectives are fairly well defined for most cardiovascular drugs. For example, for drugs used to control systemic hypertension or edema, the therapeutic endpoints are clear (decrease arterial pressure, reduce edema) and are best followed by clinical observations (blood pressure, physical examination, body weight) for proper drug and dose selection. Angiotensin-converting enzyme inhibitors, most vasodilators, and calcium channel blockers have reasonably well-defined clinical endpoints (e.g., decrease arterial pressure, improve symptoms of heart failure, control angina pectoris). The therapeutic objectives of beta-adrenergic blocking drugs can be followed clinically in most patients (e.g., reduce arterial pressure, myocardial ischemia, and angina; control cardiac rhythms). For digitalis and antiarrhythmic drugs, the clinical endpoints are more elusive and are threatened by potentially serious adverse effects; determination of plasma drug concentrations for such agents often becomes an important component of optimally effective, safe dosing.

CARDIOVASCULAR COMPLICATIONS DURING DIALYSIS

SYSTEMIC HYPOTENSION. Removal of fluid volume, redistribution of plasma volume, baroreceptor disturbances, dysfunction of the autonomic nervous system, depressed responsiveness to alpha-adrenergic receptor stimulation, concomitant drug therapy (e.g., antihypertensive agents), and LV diastolic dysfunction contribute to the propensity of patients with CRF to develop hypotension during hemodialysis. Interestingly, some patients who have renal disease with dialysis-induced hypotension have higher plasma concentrations of atrial natriuretic peptide and lower norepinephrine levels compared with patients with CRF without hypotension.[37, 39, 108]

Symptomatic depletion of fluid volume during dialysis can be averted by allowing a modest amount of weight gain between dialysis treatments. When feasible, antihypertensive therapy and other potential hypotension-inducing drugs (e.g., nitrates) can be withheld 4 to 6 hours before dialysis to minimize their contribution to the problem. Of the antihypertensive agents, minoxidil is least likely to cause unpredictable changes in blood pressure during hemodialysis; however, drug-induced hirsutism and occasional pericarditis make this drug unacceptable to some patients, particularly women. Small doses of noncardioselective beta-adrenergic blocking drugs can be effective in maintaining acceptable arterial pressure; the beta$_1$- and beta$_2$-receptor blockade allows circulating norepinephrine to evoke unopposed alpha-adrenergic receptor stimulation and vasoconstriction. Either peritoneal dialysis or renal transplantation is the best option for patients who have CRF and who poorly tolerate hemodialysis because of hypotension.

HYPOXEMIA. The mechanisms for hemodialysis-induced hypoxemia have not been definitively established; leading explanations include nonbicarbonate buffers (e.g., acetate) used in the dialysis bath, Cupraphane membranes, and pulmonic ventilation-perfusion mismatch elicited by systemic hypotension. Acetate buffer evokes a significant leftward shift in the hemoglobin-oxygen dissociation curve and can disturb ventilation-perfusion of the lungs through its vasodilatory properties. Activation of complement along Cupraphane exchange membranes can result in sequestration of leukocytes within pulmonary vessels, ventilation and perfusion abnormalities, and hypoxemia; this complication has been reduced considerably with the use of biocompatible dialyzers.[1]

ELECTROLYTE AND OTHER METABOLIC ABNORMALITIES. Electrolyte disturbances, metabolic acidosis, and other metabolic abnormalities likely contribute to the development of various cardiovascular derangements in CRF (e.g., cardiac arrhythmias, depression of myocardial contractility). The rate of change in pH, electrolyte concentrations, and other metabolic factors during dialysis is probably as important as the actual degree of change with respect to the clinical consequences of these disturbances. The most common and crucial electrolyte disturbances in patients undergoing hemodialysis involve potassium. Hyperkalemia is a common problem in these patients, and plasma and whole-body potassium levels can be dramatically altered by hemodialysis. The dialysis buffer, acetate, transiently decreases serum bicarbonate level, and with repeated dialysis patients with CRF can become depleted of bicarbonate; bicarbonate has now largely replaced acetate as the dialysis buffer at most modern facilities.[1, 37, 39]

COMPLICATIONS OF THE ARTERIOVENOUS ACCESS FISTULA DURING HEMODIALYSIS. The external access vascular shunt is used when a patient is expected to require only short-term dialysis (days to a few weeks). Because of fewer complications (e.g., lower infection rate and less thrombogenic) over time, the surgically constructed subcutaneous AV fistula is used for long-term dialysis management. In certain patients, particularly the elderly and those with peripheral vascular disease or diabetes mellitus, reduction of blood flow distal to the fistula can lead to local ischemia and infarction, occasionally requiring amputation of a digit or distal extremity.[1, 37, 39] An infrequent complication during hemodialysis involves a "steal syndrome," which may occur when the radial artery distal to a forearm fistula has not been ligated; this vascular arrangement can allow blood to flow from the ulnar artery through the palmar arch (as nonnutritive flow), retrograde into the radial artery and access fistula.

OTHER DIALYSIS-INDUCED COMPLICATIONS. Air embolization and hemolysis, although rare, are serious complications. Hemolysis can occur from improper composition or chemical contamination of the dialysate. Severe illness and death have resulted from dialysate contaminated with excessive aluminum, calcium, or fluoride.[1, 37, 39, 109] Other substances, such as polyvinylchloride, have been leached from membranes, dialyzer shells, and tubing to cause systemic and cardiovascular toxicity.[110] With the use of high-flux polyacryonitrile AN 69 exchange membranes, patients who have CRF and are receiving angiotensin-converting enzyme inhibitors appear to be somewhat more susceptible to anaphylactoid reactions during hemodialysis.[1, 37, 39, 110]

REFERENCES

CARDIOVASCULAR CONDITIONS THAT AFFECT RENAL FUNCTION

1. Leier CV, Boudoulas H: Cardiorenal disorders and diseases. Mount Kisco, NY, Futura, 1992.
2. Neugarten J, Baldwin DS: Glomerulonephritis in bacterial endocarditis. Am J Med 77:297, 1984.
3. Feinstein EI, Eknoyan G, Lister BJ, et al: Renal complications of bacterial endocarditis. Am J Nephrol 5:457, 1985.
4. Conlon PJ, Jefferies F, Krigman HR, et al: Predictors of prognosis and risk of acute renal failure in bacterial endocarditis. Clin Nephrol 49:96–101, 1998.
5. Orfila C, Lepert JC, Modesto A, et al: Rapidly progressive glomerulonephritis associated with bacterial endocarditis: Efficacy of antibiotic therapy alone. Am J Nephrol 13:218–222, 1993.
6. Daimon S, Mizuno Y, Fugii S, et al: Infective endocarditis-induced crescentic glomerolonephritis dramatically improved by plasmaphenesis. Am J Kidney Dis 32:309–313, 1998.
7. Millaire A, Leroy O, Gaday V, et al: Incidence and prognosis of embolic events and metastatic infections in infective endocarditis. Eur Heart J 18:677–684, 1997.
8. Steckelberg JM, Murphy JG, Ballard D, et al: Emboli in infective endocarditis: The prognostic value of echocardiography. Ann Intern Med 114:635–640, 1991.
9. Sanfilippo AJ, Picard MH, Newell JB, et al: Echocardiographic assessment of patients with infectious endocarditis: Prediction of risk for complications. J Am Coll Cardiol 18:1191–1199, 1991.
10. Heinle S, Wilderman N, Harrison JK, et al: Value of transthoracic echocardiography in predicting embolic events in active infective endocarditis. Am J Cardiol 74:799–801, 1994.
11. Kronzon I, Tunick PA: Atheromatous disease of the thoracic aorta: Pathologic and clinical implications. Ann Intern Med 126:629–637, 1997.
12. Gupta BK, Spinowitz BS, Charytan C, Wahl SJ: Cholesterol crystal embolization-associated renal failure after therapy with recombinant tissue-type plasminogen activator. Am J Kidney Dis. 21:659, 1993.
13. Hyman BT, Landas SK, Ashman RF, et al: Warfarin-related purple toes syndrome and cholesterol microembolization. Am J Med 82:1233, 1987.
14. Thadhani RI, Camargo CA Jr, Xavier RJ, et al: Atheroembolic renal failure after invasive procedures: Natural history based on 52 histologically proven cases. Medicine (Baltimore) 74:350–358, 1995.
15. Schepens MA, Defauw JJ, Hamerlijnck RP, et al: Surgical treatment of thoracoabdominal aortic aneurysms by simple cross-clamping: Risk factors and late results. J Thorac Cardiovasc Surg 107:134–142, 1994.
16. Hausman DS, Qalam V, Weber MF, et al: Risk of catheter-related infection in patients with atherosclerotic debris in the thoracic aorta. Am Heart J 131:1149–1155, 1996.
17. Ferrari E, Vidal R, Chevallier T, Baudouy M: Atherosclerosis of the thoracic aorta and aortic debris as a marker of poor prognosis: Benefit of oral anticoagulants. J Am Coll Cardiol 33:1317–1322, 1999.
18. Salam TA, Lumsden AB, Martin LG: Local infusion of fibrinolytic agents for renal artery thromboembolism. Ann Vasc Surg 7:21, 1993.

19. Bonttier S, Valverde JP, Lacombe M, et al: Renal artery emboli: The role of surgical treatment. Ann Vasc Surg 2:161, 1988.

20. Spittel JA Jr, Hunt JC: Abdominal aortic aneurysms and the kidney. Med Clin North Am 50:1021, 1966.

21. Moore HD: Abdominal aortic aneurysm. J Cardiovasc Surg 17:47, 1976.

22. Kashyap VS, Cambria RP, Davison JK, L'Italien GJ: Renal failure after thoracoabdominal aortic surgery. J Vasc Surg 26:949–955, 1997.

23. DeSanctis RW, Doroghazi RM, Austen WG, Buckley MJ: Aortic dissection. N Engl J Med 317:1060, 1987.

24. O'Gara PT, DeSanctis RW: Acute aortic dissection and its variants. Circulation 92:1376–1378, 1995.

25. Erbel R, Oelert H, Meyer J, et al: Effect of medical and surgical therapy on aortic dissection evaluated by transesophageal echocardiography. Circulation 87:1604–1615, 1993.

26. Walker PJ, Dake MD, Mitchell RS, Miller DC: The use of endovascular techniques for the treatment of complications of aortic dissection. J Vasc Surg 18:1042–1051, 1993.

27. Flanagan MF, Hourihanm M, Keane JF: Incidence of renal dysfunction in adults with cyanotic congenital heart disease. Am J Cardiol 68:403, 1991.

28. Krull F, Ehrich JH, Wurster U, et al: Renal involvement in patients with congenital cyanotic heart disease. Acta Pediatr Scand 80:1214, 1991.

29. Dittrich S, Haas NA, Buhrer C, et al: Renal impairment in patients with long-standing cyanotic congenital heart disease. Acta Paediatr 87:949–954, 1998.

30. Cohen M, Fuster V, Steele PM, et al: Coarctation of the aorta: Long-term follow-up and prediction of outcome after surgical correction. Circulation 80:840, 1989.

31. Johnson MC, Canter CE, Strauss AW, Spray TL: Repair of coarctation of the aorta in infancy: Comparison of surgical and balloon angioplasty. Am Heart J 125:464–468, 1993.

32. Shaddy RE, Boucek MM, Sturtevant JE, et al: Comparison of angioplasty and surgery for unoperated coarctation of the aorta. Circulation 87:793–799, 1993.

33. Fawzy ME, Sivanandam V, Galal O, et al: One- to ten-year follow-up results of balloon angioplasty of native coarctation of the aorta in adolescents and adults. J Am Coll Cardiol 30:1542–1546, 1997.

34. Hallett JW, Brewster DC, Darling RC, O'Hara PJ: Coarctation of the abdominal aorta. Ann Surg 191:430, 1980.

35. Bergamini TM, Bernard JD, Mavoudis C, et al: Coarctation of the abdominal aorta. Ann Vasc Surg 9:352–356, 1995.

EFFECTS OF RENAL FAILURE ON THE CARDIOVASCULAR SYSTEM

36. Herzog CA: Dialysis patients: A cardiologist's perspective. ACC Curr J Rev November/December 32–35, 1997.

37. Ifudo O: Care of patients undergoing hemodialysis. N Engl J Med 339:1054–1062, 1988.

38. Chakko S, Girgis I, Contreras G, et al: Effects of hemodialysis on left ventricular diastolic filling. Am J Cardiol 106–108, 1997.

39. Pastan S, Bailey J: Dialysis therapy. N Engl J Med 338:1428–1437, 1998.

40. Gokal R, Mallick NP: Peritoneal dialysis. Lancet 353:823–828, 1999.

40a. Mizushige K, Tokudome T, Seki M, et al: Sensitive detection of myocardial contraction abnormality in chronic hemodialysis patients by ultrasonic tissue characterization with integrated backscatter. J Vasc Dis 51:223, 2000.

40b. Miyazaki H, Matsuoka H, Itabe H, et al: Hemodialysis impairs endothelial function via oxidative stress: Effects of vitamin E–coated dialyzer. Circulation 101:1002, 2000.

41. Ma KW, Greene EL, Raij L: Cardiovascular risk factors in chronic renal failure and hemodialysis populations. Am J Kidney Dis 19:505, 1992.

42. Sohn HJ, Stokes GS, Johnston H: An Na, K-ATPase inhibitor from ultrafiltrate obtained by hemodialysis of patients with uremia. J Lab Clin Med 120:264, 1992.

43. Burt RJ, Gupta-Burt S, Suki WN, et al: Reversal of left ventricular dysfunction after renal transplantation. Ann Intern Med 111:635, 1989.

44. Khan IH, Catto GRD, Edward N, et al: Influence of coexisting disease on survival on renal-replacement therapy. Lancet 1:415, 1993.

44a. Dries DL, Exner DV, Domanski MJ, et al: The prognostic implications of renal insufficiency in asymptomatic and symptomatic patients with left ventricular systolic dysfunction. J Am Coll Cardiol 35:681, 2000.

45. Boudoulas H, Toutouzas P, Wooley CF: Functional Abnormalities of the Aorta. Mount Kisco, NY, Futura 1996.

46. Pickering TG, Devereux RB, James GD, et al: Recurrent pulmonary edema in hypertension due to bilateral renal artery stenosis: Treatment by angioplasty or surgical revascularization. Lancet 2:551, 1988.

47. Huting J: Course of left ventricular hypertrophy and function in end-stage renal disease after renal transplantation. Am J Cardiol 70:1481, 1992.

48. Cressman MD, Hoogwerf BJ, Schreiber MJ, Cosentino FA: Lipid abnormalities and end-stage renal disease: Implications for atherosclerotic cardiovascular disease. Miner Electrolyte Metab 19:180, 1993.

49. Joven J, Vilella E, Ahmad S, et al: Lipoprotein heterogeneity in end-stage renal disease. Kidney Int 43:410, 1993.

50. Sechi LA, Zingaro L, De Carli S, et al: Increased serum lipoprotein(a) levels in patients with early renal failure. Ann Intern Med 129:457–461, 1998.

51. Senti M, Romero R, Pedro-Botet, J, et al: Lipoprotein abnormalities in hyperlipidemic and normolipidemic men on hemodialysis with chronic renal failure. Kidney 41:1394, 1992.

52. Burrell DE, Antignani A, Goldwasser P, et al: Lipid abnormalities in black renal patients. N Y State J Med 91:192, 1991.

53. Robinson K, Gupta A, Dennis V, et al: Hyperhomocysteinemia confers an independent increased risk of atherosclerosis in end-stage renal disease and is closely linked to plasma folate and pyridoxine concentrations. Circulation 94:2743–2748, 1996.

54. Bostom AG, Gohh RY, Beaulieu AJ, et al: Treatment of hyperhomocysteinemia in renal transplant recipients: A randomized, placebo-controlled trial. Ann Intern Med 127:1089–1092, 1997.

55. Moustapha A, Naso A, Nahlawi M, et al: Prospective study of hyperhomocysteinemia as an adverse cardiovascular risk factor in end-stage renal disease. Circulation 97:138–141, 1998.

56. Tolins JP: Mechanisms of glucagon-induced renal vasodilation: Role of prostaglandins and endothelium-derived relaxing factor. J Lab Clin Med 120:941, 1992.

57. Moore K, Wendon J, Frazer M, et al: Plasma endothelin immunoreactivity in liver disease and the hepatorenal syndrome. N Engl J Med 327:1774, 1992.

58. Wanner C, Rader D, Bartens W, et al: Elevated plasma lipoprotein(a) concentrations in patients with nephrotic syndrome. Ann Intern Med 119:263, 1993.

59. Webb AT, Reaveley DA, O'Donnell M, et al: Does cyclosporin increase lipoprotein(a) concentrations in renal transplant recipients? Lancet 1:268, 1993.

60. Burke JF Jr, Pirsh JD, Ramos EL, et al: Long-term efficacy and safety of cyclosporine in renal-transplant recipients. N Engl J Med 331:358, 1994.

61. Boudoulas H, Leier CV: Myocardial perfusion in the age of afterload reduction. ACC Curr J Rev March-April 14–18, 1994.

62. Boudoulas H, Rittgers SE, Lewis RP, et al: Changes in diastolic time with various pharmacologic agents: Implications for myocardial perfusion. Circulation 60:164, 1979.

63. Kenny A, Sutters M, Evans DB, Shapiro LM: Effects of hemodialysis on coronary blood flow. Am J Cardiol 74:291, 1994.

64. Holley JL, Fenton RA, Arthur RS: Thallium stress testing does not predict cardiovascular risk in diabetic patients with end-stage renal disease undergoing cadaveric renal transplantation. Am J Med 90:563, 1991.

65. Reis G, Marcovitz PA, Leichtman AB, et al: Usefulness of dobutamine stress echocardiography in detecting coronary artery disease in end-stage renal disease. Am J Cardiol 75:707, 1995.

66. Soleman R, Werner C, Mann D, et al: Effects of saline, mannitol and furosemide on acute decreases in renal function induced by radiocontrast agents. N Engl J Med 331:1416, 1994.

67. McCullough PA, O'Neill WW: Acute renal failure after coronary intervention. ACC Educational Highlights 7–9, 1997.

68. Manske CL, Wang Y, Rector T, et al: Coronary revascularization in insulin-dependent diabetic patients with chronic renal failure. Lancet 340:998, 1994.

69. Reusser LM, Orebon LA, White HJ, et al: Increased morbidity after coronary angioplasty in patients on chronic hemodialysis. Am J Cardiol 73:965, 1994.

70. Thomas ME, Harris KP, Ramaswamy C, et al: Simvastatin therapy for hypercholesterolemic patients with nephrotic syndrome or significant proteinuria. Kidney Int 44:1124, 1993.

71. Jahangiri M, Wright J, Edmondson S, Magee P: Coronary artery bypass graft surgery in dialysis patients. Heart 78:343–345, 1997.

72. Schoebel FC, Gradaus F, Ivens K, et al: Restenosis after elective coronary balloon angioplasty in patients with end-stage renal disease: A case-control study using quantitative coronary angiography. Heart 78:337–342, 1997.

73. Mangano CM, Diamondstone LS, Ramsay JG, et al: Renal dysfunction after myocardial revascularization: Risk factors, adverse outcomes, and hospital resource utilization. Ann Intern Med 128:194–203, 1998.

74. Rao V, Weisel RD, Buth KJ, et al: Coronary artery bypass grafting in patients with non–dialysis-dependent renal insufficiency. Circulation 96 (Suppl II): II-38, 1997.

75. Van Lente F, McErlean ES, DeLuca SA, et al: Ability of troponins to predict adverse outcomes in patients with renal insufficiency and suspected acute coronary syndromes: A case-matched study. J Am Coll Cardiol 33:471, 1999.

76. Marso SP, Gimple LW, Philbrick JT, DiMarco JP: Effectiveness of percutaneous coronary interventions to prevent recurrent coronary events in patients on chronic hemodialysis. Am J Cardiol 82:378, 1998.

77. Chertow GM, Lazarus JM, Christiansen CL, et al: Preoperative renal risk stratification. Circulation 95:878, 1997.

78. Suen WS, Mok CK, Chiu SW, et al: Risk factors for development of acute renal failure (ARF) requiring dialysis in patients undergoing cardiac surgery. Angiology 49:789, 1998.

79. Roppolo LP, Fitzgerald R, Dillow J, et al: A comparison of troponin T and troponin I as predictors of cardiac events in patients undergoing chronic dialysis at a veteran's hospital: A pilot study. J Am Coll Cardiol 34:448, 1999.

80. Adamson JW, Eschbach JW: Erythropoietin for end-stage renal disease. N Engl J Med 339:625, 1998.

81. Ifudo O, Feldman J, Friedman EA: The intensity of hemodialysis and the response to erythropoietin in patients with end-stage renal disease. N Engl J Med 334:420, 1996.

82. Kaufman JS, Reda DJ, Fye CL, et al: Subcutaneous compared with intravenous epoetin in patients receiving hemodialysis. N Engl J Med 339:578, 1998.

83. Adams JE, Abendschein DR, Jaffe AS: Biochemical markers of myocardial injury: Is MB creatinine kinase the choice for the 1990s? Circulation 88:750, 1993.

84. Wade MR, Chen YJ, Soliman M, et al: Myocardial texture and cardiac calcification in uremia. Miner Electrolyte Metab 19:21, 1993.

85. Sim EK, Mestres CA, Lee CN, Adebo O: Mitral valve repair in patients on chronic hemodialysis. Ann Thorac Surg 52:341, 1992.

86. Straumann E, Meyer B, Misteli M, et al: Aortic and mitral valve disease in patients on chronic hemodialysis. Ann Thorac Surg 52:341, 1992.

87. Lucke JC, Samy RN, Atkins Z, et al: Results of valve replacement with mechanical versus biological prosthesis in patients on chronic renal dialysis [abstract]. J Am Coll Cardiol 25:429, 1995.

88. Khosla S, White CJ, Collins TJ, et al: Effects of renal artery stent implantation in patients with renovascular hypertension presenting with unstable angina or congestive heart failure. Am J Cardiol 80:363–366, 1997.

89. Johansson M, Elam M, Rundqvist B, et al: Increased sympathetic nerve activity in renovascular hypertension. Circulation 99:2537–2542, 1999.

90. Argiles A, Mourad G, Mion C: Seasonal changes in blood pressure in patients with end-stage renal disease treated with hemodialysis. N Engl J Med 339:1364–1370, 1998.

91. Klag MJ, Whelton PK, Randall BL, et al: Blood pressure and end-stage renal disease in men. N Engl J Med 334:13–18, 1996.

91a. van Jaarsveld BC, Krijnen P, Pieterman H, et al: The effect of balloon angioplasty on hypertension in atherosclerotic renal-artery stenosis. N Engl J Med 341:1007, 2000.

92. Cosio FG, Dillon JJ, Falkenhain ME, et al: Racial differences in renal allograft survival: The role of systemic hypertension. Kidney Int 47:1136, 1995.

CARDIOVASCULAR DRUG THERAPY IN PATIENTS WITH RENAL DISEASES

93. Aronoff GR, Berns JS, Brier ME, et al: Drug Prescribing in Renal Failure. 4th ed. Philadelphia, American College of Physicians, 1999.

94. Carter PL: Dosing of antihypertensive medications in patients with renal failure. J Clin Pharmacol 35:81, 1995.

95. Gruppo Hemodialisi E Pathologie Cardiovascolari: Multicenter, cross-sectional study of ventricular arrhythmias in chronically hemodialyzed patients. Lancet 2:305, 1988.

96. Steinberg AA, Mars RL, Goldman DS, Percy RF: Effect of end-stage renal disease on decreased heart rate variability. Am J Cardiol 82:1156–1158, 1988.

97. Deligiannis A, Kouidi E, Tourkantonis A: Effects of physical training on heart rate variability in patients on hemodialysis. Am J Cardiol 84:197–202, 1999.

98. Ligtenberg G, Blankestijn PJ, Oey PL, et al: Reduction of sympathetic hyperactivity by enalapril in patients with chronic renal failure. N Engl J Med 340:1321–1328, 1999.

99. Luzar MR, Coles GA, Faller B, et al: *Staphylococcus aureus* nasal carriage and infection in patients on continuous ambulatory peritoneal dialysis. N Engl J Med 322:505, 1990.

100. Marr KA, Sexton DJ, Conlon PJ, et al: Catheter-related bacteremia and outcome of attempted catheter salvage in patients undergoing hemodialysis. Ann Intern Med 127:275–280, 1997.

101. Robertson D, Hollister AS, Biaggioni I, et al: The diagnosis and treatment of baroreflex failure. N Engl J Med 329:1449, 1993.

102. Converse RL Jr, Jacobsen TN, Toto RD, et al: Sympathetic overactivity in patients with chronic renal failure. N Engl J Med 327:1912, 1992.

103. Crum R, Fairchild R, Bronsther O, et al: Neuroendocrinology of chronic renal failure and renal transplantation. Transplantation 52:818, 1991.

104. Hoyer J, Schulte KL, Lentz T: Clinical pharmacokinetics of angiotensin-converting enzyme (ACE) inhibitors in renal failure. Clin Pharmacokinet 24:230, 1993.

105. Ujhelyi MR, Robert S, Cummings DM, et al: Influence of digoxin immune fab therapy and renal dysfunction on the disposition of total and free digoxin. Ann Intern Med 119:273, 1993.

106. Kovarik JM, Mueller EA, Gaber M, et al: Pharmacokinetics of cyclosporine and steady-state aspirin during coadministration. J Clin Pharmacol 33:513, 1993.

107. Talbert RL: Drug dosing in renal insufficiency. J Clin Pharmacol 34:99, 1994.

107a. Pedro AA, Gehr TWB, Brophy DF, et al: The pharmacokinetics and pharmacodynamics of Losartan in continuous ambulatory peritoneal dialysis. J Clin Pharmacol 40:389, 2000.

108. Morrissey EC, Wilner KD, Barager RR, et al: Atrial natriuretic factor in renal failure and posthemodialytic postural hypotension. Am J Kidney Dis 12:510, 1988.

109. Arnow P, Bland LA, Garcia-Houchings S, et al: An outbreak of fatal flouride intoxication in a long-term hemodialysis unit. Ann Intern Med 121:339, 1994.

110. Burhop KE, Johnson RJ, Simpson J, et al: Biocompatibility of hemodialysis membranes: Evaluation in an ovine model. J Lab Clin Med 121:276, 1993.

111. Verresen L, Waer M, Vanrenterghen Y, Michaelson P: Angiotensin converting enzyme inhibitors and anaphylactoid reaction to high-flux membrane dialysis. Lancet 2:136, 1990.

Index

Note: Page numbers in *italics* indicate illustrations; those followed by t indicate tables. **Boldface page numbers** indicate main discussion. **Plate numbers** indicate color plates.